TIETZ TEXTBOOK OF LABORATORY MEDICINE

SEVENTH EDITION

NADER RIFAI, PhD
Professor of Pathology
Harvard Medical School;
The Louis Joseph Gay-Lussac Chair in
Laboratory Medicine
Director of Clinical Chemistry
Boston Children's Hospital
Boston, Massachusetts

ROSSA W.K. CHIU, MBBS, PhD,
FHKAM, FRCPA
Professor of Chemical Pathology
The Chinese University of Hong Kong
Hong Kong SAR

IAN YOUNG, MD, FRCP, FRCPATH
Professor of Medicine
Centre for Public Health
Queen's University Belfast
Belfast, United Kingdom

CAREY-ANN D. BURNHAM, PhD,
D(ABMM), F(IDSA), F(AAM)
Professor of Pathology and Immunology
Washington University School of Medicine;
Medical Director of Clinical Microbiology
Barnes-Jewish Hospital
Saint Louis, Missouri

CARL T. WITTWER, MD, PhD
Professor Emeritus of Pathology
University of Utah
Salt Lake City, Utah

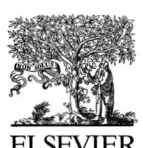

ELSEVIER

Elsevier
3251 Riverport Lane
St. Louis, Missouri 63043

Content Strategist: Heather Bays-Petrovic
Senior Content Development Manager: Luke Held
Senior Content Development Spe«alist: Maria Broeker
Publishing Services Manager: Julie Eddy
Senior Project Manager: Rachel E. McMullen
Design Direction: Maggie Reid

Printed in the United States of America

Last digit is the print number: 9 8 7 6 5 4 3 2 1

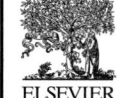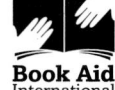

To our families
To the future generation

PREFACE

We are pleased to introduce the seventh edition of the *Tietz Textbook*, now entitled, *Tietz Textbook of Laboratory Medicine*. We have expanded the scope of chapters from the sixth edition to include various specialties throughout laboratory medicine. In addition, we further refined and enriched the *Platform*, a concept we introduced in the sixth edition, of which the Textbook is only a component.

Although the textbook is available in print for selected chapters, the comprehensive product is only available electronically on the Platform. The chapters in the print version of the textbook are meant to give readers a taste of the entire product and to demonstrate its broad scope. Using Elsevier's Expert Consult electronic system, the Platform encompasses:

- A textbook covering all major disciplines of laboratory medicine including clinical chemistry, genetic metabolic disorders, molecular diagnostics, hematology and coagulation, clinical microbiology, transfusion medicine, and clinical immunology. Thirty additional chapters are devoted to analytical techniques and basic practices in laboratory medicine, and an extensive compilation of reference intervals is included. Compared to the previous edition, the number of chapters has increased from 81 to 100
- Electronic search capability and a built-in medical dictionary
- Curriculum-based courses utilizing the concept of adaptive learning provide the users with a personalized education experience (https://rhapsode.com/laboratorymedicine/). Over 100 courses, which span across all disciplines of laboratory medicine, encompass more than 15,000 learning objectives and are authored by world-renowned scientists and physicians; almost 50% of these courses were prepared or reviewed by authors participating in this textbook. Courses are linked to the appropriate chapters
- Multimedia and Educational Resources for an enhanced learning experience that include:
  1. The largest compilation ever assembled of clinical cases in laboratory medicine
  2. Animation films to explain complex mechanisms and concepts
  3. Podcasts
  4. Lecture series
  5. Biochemical calculations
  6. Collections of morphologic images and electrophoretic patterns
  7. Banks of multiple-choice and short-answer questions
  8. Important documents, monographs, and guidebooks

The above-described features are linked to the appropriate chapters for the convenience of the reader. These resources were either previously created by prominent laboratory medicine professionals (e.g., Allan Deacon, Michael J. Murphy, Rajeev Srivastava, Allan Gaw, Bobbi Pritt, Ellen F. Foxman, Julie E. Buring, Pamela Rist, Roy Peake, Morayma Reyes Gil, Matthew Diggle, Vera Paulson, Christina Lockwood, Gifford Batstone, Gary Weaving, Kate Shipman, Tamsyn Cromwell, and John Coakley), prestigious journals (e.g., *Journal of Clinical Microbiology*, *Clinical Chemistry*, *Transfusion*, *American Journal of Hematology* and *Blood*) and leading international scientific societies (e.g., the Association for Clinical Biochemistry and Laboratory Medicine-United Kingdom, Association of Clinical Biochemists-Ireland, Royal Society of Chemistry-London, Imperial College-London, Association of Molecular Pathology, and American Association for Clinical Chemistry), or produced de novo by accomplished scientists and physicians using materials from their own institutions (e.g., Mayo Medical Laboratories, ARUP, HudsonAlpha Institute for Biotechnology, Hôpital Universitaire La Pitié Salpêtrière-Paris, Pathology Queensland-Australia, and Boston Children's Hospital).

- A *living product*, where materials are periodically added and information updated as necessary

Our hope for this Platform is to serve as a resource center where important materials in laboratory medicine are deposited for use by and for the benefit of the community at large. Therefore, we encourage those who have similar materials and wish to have them considered for the Platform to contact one of the editors. The Platform can only be enhanced by further efforts.

Unlike most other textbooks, all chapters in this edition were reviewed by three individuals: a reviewer, an associate editor, and a senior editor. We believe that these efforts have

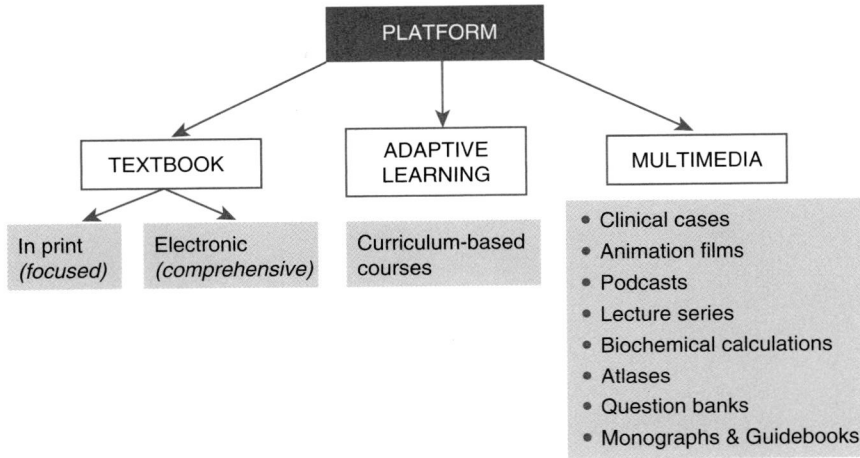

led to a better product. In addition, we made a concerted effort to create an *International* rather than an *American* Platform; about one third of the authors, reviewers, and editors reside outside the United States. We have strongly encouraged authors to include European, Australasian, and other international guidelines in addition to the American ones in order to present different practices and points of view. Furthermore, all measurements are presented both in traditional and SI units.

We aimed to harmonize the presentation of information among chapters while retaining the personality and unique style of each author, hoping for a readable, educational text with enough variety to amuse and occasionally delight.

This ambitious project has been a true group effort and represents the collective intellect, knowledge, and experience of almost 230 leaders in laboratory medicine from 18 countries.

We are in debt not only to the authors, reviewers, and editors of the chapters but also to the contributors of the Multimedia and Educational Resources materials and the Adaptive Learning Courses that greatly enriched the Platform. We are grateful to Elsevier, and particularly to Heather Bays-Petrovic, Maria Broeker, and Rachel McMullen and their team for supporting us throughout this project to realize our vision.

We sincerely hope that this product will be a valuable educational and reference resource for the laboratory medicine community worldwide.

Nader Rifai
Rossa W.K. Chiu
Ian Young
Carey-Ann D. Burnham
Carl T. Wittwer

TEXTBOOK ASSOCIATE EDITORS

Linnea Baudhuin, PhD
Professor of Laboratory Medicine and Pathology
Mayo Clinic
Rochester, Minnesota

Christopher M. Florkowski, MD, MRCP(UK), FRACP, FRCPA, FFSc
Associate Professor of Pathology
University of Otago;
Consultant in Chemical Pathology
Clinical Biochemistry Unit
Canterbury Health Laboratories
Christchurch, New Zealand

Tracy I. George, MD
Professor of Pathology
University of Utah School of Medicine;
President and Chief Medical Officer
ARUP Laboratories
Salt Lake City, Utah

Andy Hoofnagle, MD, PhD
Professor of Laboratory Medicine
University of Washington
Seattle, Washington

Gary Horowitz, MD
Professor of Anatomic and Clinical Pathology
Tufts University School of Medicine;
Chief of Clinical Pathology
Department of Pathology and Laboratory Medicine
Tufts Medical Center
Boston, Massachusetts

Graham Ross Dallas Jones, MBBS, BSc(med), DPhil, FRCPA, FAACB
Conjoint Associate Professor
UNSW;
Senior Staff Specialist
Department of Chemical Pathology
SydPath St Vincent's Hospital
Sydney, New South Wales, Australia

Eric S. Kilpatrick, MD, FRCPath, FRCP Ed
Honorary Professor of Clinical Biochemistry
Hull York Medical School;
Consultant in Chemical Pathology
Department of Clinical Biochemistry
Manchester Royal Infirmary
Manchester University NHS Foundation Trust
Manchester, United Kingdom

Kerry L. O'Brien, MD
Assistant Professor of Pathology
Harvard Medical School;
Medical Director Blood Bank
Beth Israel Deaconess Medical Center
Boston, Massachusetts

Jason Y. Park, MD, PhD
Associate Professor of Pathology
University of Texas Southwestern Medical Center;
Clinical Director of Advanced Diagnostics Laboratory
Department of Pathology
Children's Medical Center of Dallas
Dallas, Texas

Kenneth Andrew Sikaris, BSc(Hons), MBBS, FRCPA, FAACB, FFSc, GAICD
Associate Professor of Pathology
Melbourne University;
Director Clinical Support Systems, Sonic Healthcare
Chemical Pathology
Melbourne Pathology
Victoria, Australia

Arnold von Eckardstein, MD
Professor of Clinical Chemistry
University of Zurich;
Chairman of the Institute of Clinical Chemistry
University Hospital of Zurich
Zurich, Switzerland

Maria Alice Viera Willrich, PhD, DABCC, FAACC
Associate Professor of Laboratory Medicine and Pathology
Mayo Clinic
Rochester, Minnesota

Melanie L. Yarbrough, PhD
Assistant Professor of Pathology and Immunology
Washington University School of Medicine
St. Louis, Missouri

TEXTBOOK REVIEWERS

Jude Abadie, PhD, DABCC, FAACC, DABMGG
Associate Professor of Pathology
Director of Clinical Pathology
Laboratory Director of El Paso Public Health Laboratory
United States Army, Retired
Texas Tech University Health Sciences Center
El Paso, Texas

Archana M. Agarwal, MD
Associate Professor of Pathology
University of Utah
ARUP Laboratories
Salt Lake City, Utah

Joshua Bornhorst, PhD, DABCC
Senior Associate Consultant
Department of Laboratory Medicine and Pathology
Mayo Clinic
Rochester, Minnesota

Niels V. Casteele, PharmD, PhD
Professor of Medicine
UC San Diego
La Jolla, California

Christa Cobbaert, PhD, EurSpLM
Professor of Clinical Chemistry and Laboratory Medicine
Leiden University Medical Centre (LUMC)
Leiden, Netherlands

Marc Roger Couturier, PhD, D(ABMM)
Associate Professor of Pathology
University of Utah
ARUP Laboratories
Salt Lake City, Utah

Julio C. Delgado, MD, MS
Professor of Pathology
University of Utah
Salt Lake City, Utah

Helen Fernandes, PhD
Professor of Pathology
Columbia University Medical Center
New York, New York

Paul Kevin Hamilton, BSc (Hons), MB, BCh, BAO (Hons), MD, FRCP (Edin), FRCPath
Clinical Lecturer
Centre for Medical Education
Queen's University Belfast;
Consultant Chemical Pathologist
Clinical Biochemistry
Belfast Health and Social Care Trust
Belfast, United Kingdom

Mark Kellogg, PhD
Assistant Professor of Pathology
Harvard Medical School;
Director of Quality Programs
Laboratory Medicine
Boston Children's Hospital
Boston, Massachusetts

Attila Kumanovics, MD
Senior Associate Consultant
Department of Laboratory Medicine and Pathology
Mayo Clinic
Rochester, Minnesota

Leslie C.C.L. Lai, MBBS, MSc, MD, FRCPath, FRCP (Edinburgh), FFSc(RCPA), FAMM
Department of Endocrinology
Gleneagles Kuala Lumpur
Kuala Lumpur, Malaysia

Eszter Lázár-Molnár, PhD, D(ABMLI), F(ACHI)
Associate Professor of Pathology
University of Utah School of Medicine
Salt Lake City, Utah

Michael Murphy, MD
Biochemical Medicine
University of Dundee
Dundee, United Kingdom

Robert D. Nerenz, PhD, DABCC
Assistant Professor of Pathology and Laboratory Medicine
The Geisel School of Medicine at Dartmouth
Hanover, New Hampshire;
Assistant Director of Clinical Chemistry
Dartmouth-Hitchcock Health System
Lebanon, New Hampshire

Evangelos Ntrivalas, MD, PhD
Assistant Attending Immunologist
Department of Laboratory Medicine
Memorial Sloan Kettering Cancer Center
New York, New York

Adnan Sharif, MD, FRCP
Department of Nephrology and Transplantation
University Hospitals Birmingham
Birmingham, United Kingdom

TEXTBOOK CONTRIBUTORS

Aasne K. Aarsand, MD, PhD
Consultant Medical Biochemist
Norwegian Porphyria Centre (NAPOS) and Department
    of Medical Biochemistry and Pharmacology
Haukeland University Hospital;
Consultant Medical Biochemist
Norwegian Organization for Quality Improvement
    of Laboratory Examinations
Haraldplass Deaconess Hospital
Bergen, Norway

April N. Abbott, PhD, D(ABMM)
Adjunct Assistant Professor of Microbiology and Immunology
Indiana University School of Medicine;
Director of Microbiology and Molecular Diagnostics
Deaconess Health System
Evansville, Indiana

Roshini S. Abraham, PhD, D(ABMLI), FAAAAI
Professor of Clinical Pathology
Ohio State University College of Medicine;
Director, Diagnostic Immunology Laboratory
Department of Pathology and Laboratory Medicine
Nationwide Children's Hospital
Columbus, Ohio

Khosrow Adeli, PhD, FCACB, FACB, DABCC
Professor of Clinical Biochemistry
Department of Laboratory Medicine and Pathobiology
University of Toronto;
Director of Clinical Biochemistry
Department of Paediatric Laboratory Medicine
The Hospital for Sick Children
Toronto, Ontario, Canada

Mariam Priya Alexander, MD
Associate Professor of Laboratory Medicine and Pathology
Mayo Clinic
Rochester, Minnesota

Catherine Alix-Panabières, PhD
Laboratory of Rare Human Circulating Cells (LCCRH)
Oncobiology
University Medical Center
Montpellier, France

David Alter, MD, MPH
Associate Professor of Pathology
Department of Pathology and Laboratory Medicine;
Director of Clinical Chemistry
Emory University School of Medicine
Atlanta, Georgia

Neil W. Anderson, MD
Associate Professor of Pathology and Immunology
Washington University School of Medicine
Saint Louis, Missouri

Fred S. Apple, PhD
Professor of Laboratory Medicine and Pathology
University of Minnesota;
Principal Investigator Cardiac Biomarkers Trials Laboratory
    (CBTL)
Hennepin Healthcare Research Institute;
Medical Director of Clinical and Forensic Toxicology
    Laboratories
Laboratory Medicine and Pathology
Hennepin County Medical Center
Minneapolis, Minnesota

Ruth M. Ayling, PhD, FRCPath, FRCP
Consultant Chemical Pathologist
Clinical Biochemistry
Barts Health NHS Trust
London, United Kingdom

Daniel Babu, MD
Assistant Professor of Pathology
University of New Mexico Health Sciences Center
Albuquerque, New Mexico

Michael N. Badminton, BSc, MBChB, PhD, FRCPath
Professor
Institute for Medical Education
School of Medicine, Cardiff University;
Professor of Medical Biochemistry
University Hospital of Wales
Cardiff, Wales, United Kingdom

**Tony Badrick, BAppSc, BSc, BA, MLitSt, MBA, PhD,
    FAACB, FAIMS, FRCPA (Hon), FACB, FFScRCPA**
Associate Professor
Faculty of Health Sciences and Medicine
Bond University
Robina, Queensland, Australia;
CEO
RCPA Quality Assurance Programs
Sydney, New South Wales, Australia

Niaz Banaei, MD
Professor of Pathology
Stanford University School of Medicine
Stanford, California

Linnea M. Baudhuin, PhD
Professor of Laboratory Medicine and Pathology
Mayo Clinic
Rochester, Minnesota

Lindsay A.L. Bazydlo, PhD, DABCC, FAACC
Associate Professor of Pathology
University of Virginia
Charlottesville, Virginia

Laura K. Bechtel, PhD, DABCC
Director of Chemistry and Toxicology
Kaiser Permanente—Colorado;
CLIA Laboratory Director
Colorado Antiviral Pharmacology Laboratory (CVAP)
Skaggs School of Pharmacy and Pharmaceutical Sciences
Denver, Colorado

John Benco, PhD
Sr. Director
Research and Development
Siemens Healthcare Diagnostics
Norwood, Massachusetts

Andrew J. Bentall, MBChB, MD
Assistant Professor of Medicine
Division of Nephrology and Hypertension
Mayo Clinic
Rochester, Minnesota

Marc Berg, MD
Clinical Professor of Pediatrics
Stanford University;
Attending Physician of Pediatrics
Lucile Packard Children's Hospital
Palo Alto, California

Roger L. Bertholf, PhD, DABCC, FAACC, MASCP
Professor of Clinical Pathology and Laboratory Medicine
Weill Cornell Medicine
New York, New York;
Medical Director of Clinical Chemistry
Department of Pathology and Genomic Medicine
Houston Methodist Hospital
Houston, Texas

D. Hunter Best, PhD, FACMG
Associate Professor of Pathology
University of Utah School of Medicine;
Medical and Scientific Director of Genomics
ARUP Laboratories
Salt Lake City, Utah

Vanja Radisic Biljak, PhD
Specialist in Laboratory Medicine
Department of Medical Laboratory Diagnostics
University Hospital Sveti Duh
Zagreb, Croatia

Darci R. Block, PhD, DABCC, FAACC
Assistant Professor of Laboratory Medicine and Pathology
Mayo Clinic
Rochester, Minnesota

Lee M. Blum, PhD, FABFT
Assistant Laboratory Director/Toxicologist
NMS Labs
Horsham, Pennsylvania

Olaf A. Bodamer, MD, PhD
Associate Professor of Pediatrics
Harvard Medical School;
Park Gerald Chair in Genetics and Genomics
Division of Genetics and Genomics
Boston Children's Hospital
Boston, Massachusetts

Benjamin Boh, DO, MS
Assistant Professor of Medicine
Geisel School of Medicine at Dartmouth
Hanover, New Hampshire;
Faculty
Department of Medicine, Section of Endocrinology
Dartmouth-Hitchcock Medical Center
Lebanon, New Hampshire

Mary Kathryn Bohn, BSc
PhD Student, Department of Laboratory Medicine and Pathobiology
University of Toronto;
Department of Paediatric Laboratory Medicine
The Hospital for Sick Children
Toronto, Ontario, Canada

Patrick M.M. Bossuyt, PhD
Clinical Epidemiology, Biostatistics and Bioinformatics
Amsterdam University Medical Centers
Amsterdam, Netherlands

Xavier Bossuyt, MD, PhD
Professor of Microbiology, Immunology and Transplantation
Katholieke Universiteit Leuven;
Head of Clinic
Laboratory Medicine
University Hospital Leuven
Leuven, Belgium

James Clark Boyd, MD
Associate Professor Emeritus of Pathology
University of Virginia Health System
Charlottesville, Virginia

Julie A. Braga, MD
Assistant Professor of Obstetrics and Gynecology
Dartmouth Hitchcock Medical Center
Lebanon, New Hampshire

Blake W. Buchan, PhD, DABMM
Associate Professor of Pathology
The Medical College of Wisconsin;
Associate Director of Microbiology and
　Molecular Diagnostics
Wisconsin Diagnostic Laboratories
Milwaukee, Wisconsin

David Buchbinder, MD, MSHS
Associate Professor of Pediatrics
UC Irvine;
Staff Physician in Hematology
CHOC Children's Hospital
Orange, California

Leslie Burnett, MBBS, PhD, FRCPA, FHGSA
Honorary Professor in Pathology and Genomic Medicine
Northern Clinical School
University of Sydney
St Leonards, New South Wales, Australia;
Conjoint Professor
St Vincent's Clinical School
University of NSW Sydney
Sydney, New South Wales, Australia;
Genetic Pathologist
Garvan Institute of Medical Research
Darlinghurst, New South Wales, Australia

Carey-Ann D. Burnham, PhD, DABMM,
　FIDSA, FAAM
Professor of Pathology and Immunology
Washington University School of Medicine;
Medical Director of Clinical Microbiology
Barnes-Jewish Hospital
Saint Louis, Missouri

Theresa Ambrose Bush, PhD, DABCC, RAC
Principal Global Regulatory Director—Medical Devices
Pharma Development Regulatory—Personalized Health
　Care
Genentech, Inc., a Member of the Roche Group
South San Francisco, California

Cory Bystrom, BS, MS, PhD
Laboratory Director
Precision Biomarkers Laboratory
Cedars Sinai
Los Angeles, California

Marco Cattaneo, MD
Professor
Dipartimento di Scienze della Salute
Università degli Studi di Milano
Milano, Italy

Adam J. Caulfield, PhD, DABMM
Director of Clinical Microbiology
Microbiology Department
Spectrum Health
Grand Rapids, Michigan

Mark A. Cervinski, PhD
Associate Professor of Pathology and Laboratory Medicine
The Geisel School of Medicine at Dartmouth
Hanover, New Hampshire;
Director of Clinical Chemistry
Pathology and Laboratory Medicine
Dartmouth-Hitchcock Medical Center
Lebanon, New Hampshire

Devon S. Chabot-Richards, MD
Associate Professor of Pathology
University of New Mexico;
Director of Molecular Diagnostics and Oncology
Tricore Laboratories
Albuquerque, New Mexico

Shanmuganathan Chandrakasan, MD
Associate Professor
Bone Marrow Transplantation Program
Aflac Cancer and Blood Disorders Center
Children's Healthcare of Atlanta
Emory University School of Medicine
Atlanta, Georgia

Derrick J. Chen, MD
Director of Clinical Microbiology
Pathology and Laboratory Medicine
University of Wisconsin-Health
Madison, Wisconsin

Dong Chen, MD, PhD
Professor of Laboratory Medicine and Pathology
Division of Hematopathology
Mayo Clinic
Rochester, Minnesota

Rossa W.K. Chiu, MBBS, PhD, FHKAM, FRCPA
Professor of Chemical Pathology
The Chinese University of Hong Kong
Hong Kong SAR

Nigel J. Clarke, BSc (Hons), PhD
Vice President
R&D
Quest Diagnostics Nichols Institute
San Juan Capistrano, California

Timothy J. Cole, BSc(Hons), PhD
Associate Professor of Biochemistry and Molecular Biology
Monash University
Melbourne, Victoria, Australia

Mark Cooper, BMBCh, PhD, FRCP, FRACP
Professor of Medicine
University of Sydney;
Department of Endocrinology
Concord Repatriation General Hospital
Sydney, New South Wales, Australia

Martin Crook, BSc, MBBS, MA, PhD, FHEA, FRCP, FRCPath
Professor in Biochemical Medicine
Clinical Biochemistry
Guys Hospital
London, United Kingdom

Maite de la Morena, MD
Professor of Pediatrics
University of Washington;
Medical Director, Division of Immunology
Seattle Children's Hospital
Seattle, Washington

Michael P. Delaney, BSc, MD, FRCP, LLM
Renal Medicine
East Kent Hospitals University NHS Foundation Trust
Canterbury, Kent, United Kingdom

Julio C. Delgado, MD, MS
Professor of Pathology
University of Utah School of Medicine
Salt Lake City, Utah

Stanley C. Deresinski, MD
Clinical Professor of Medicine
Division of Infectious Diseases and Geographic Medicine
Stanford University School of Medicine
Stanford, California

Dennis J. Dietzen, PhD, DABCC, FAACC
Professor of Pathology and Immunology
Washington University School of Medicine;
Medical Director of Laboratory Services
St. Louis Children's Hospital
St. Louis, Missouri

Anh P. Dinh, MD
Assistant Professor of Pathology and Laboratory Medicine
Perelman School of Medicine, University of Pennsylvania;
Assistant Director of the Immunogenetics Laboratory
Pathology and Laboratory Medicine
The Children's Hospital of Philadelphia
Philadelphia, Pennsylvania

Christopher D. Doern, PhD
Director of Microbiology
Department of Pathology
Virginia Commonwealth University Health System
Richmond, Virginia

Lora Dukić, PhD
Assistant Professor and Specialist in Laboratory Medicine
Head of the Immunology Laboratory
Department of Medical Laboratory Diagnostics
University Hospital Sveti Duh
Zagreb, Croatia

Graeme Eisenhofer, PhD
Professor and Chief, Division of Clinical Neurochemistry
Institute of Clinical Chemistry and Laboratory Medicine
    and Department of Medicine III
Faculty of Medicine Technische Universität Dresden
Dresden, Germany

Joe M. El-Khoury, PhD, DABCC, FAACC
Associate Professor of Laboratory Medicine
Yale School of Medicine;
Director of Clinical Chemistry
Yale-New Haven Health
New Haven, Connecticut

Christina Ellervik, MD, PhD, DMSci
Associate Professor of Department of Clinical Medicine
Faculty of Health and Medical Sciences
University of Copenhagen
Copenhagen, Denmark;
Assistant Professor
Department of Pathology
Harvard Medical School;
Associate Medical Director
Department of Laboratory Medicine
Boston Children's Hospital
Boston, Massachusetts

Christopher M. Florkowski, MD, MRCP(UK), FRACP, FRCPA, FFSc
Associate Professor of Pathology
University of Otago;
Consultant in Chemical Pathology
Clinical Biochemistry Unit
Canterbury Health Laboratories
Christchurch, New Zealand

William Duncan Fraser, BSc (Hons), MB ChB, MD (Hons), FRCP, FRCPath, Eur Clin Chem
Professor of Medicine
University of East Anglia, Norwich;
Honorary Consultant of Clinical Biochemistry
Norfolk and Norwich University Hospital, Norfolk
Norfolk, United Kingdom

Manish J. Gandhi, MD
Professor of Laboratory Medicine and Pathology
Mayo Clinic School of Medicine;
Director of Histocompatibility Laboratory
Division of Transfusion Medicine
Mayo Clinic
Rochester, Minnesota

Jonathan R. Genzen, MD, PhD
Associate Professor of Pathology
University of Utah;
Chief Operations Officer
ARUP Laboratories
Salt Lake City, Utah

Tracy I. George, MD
Professor of Pathology
University of Utah School of Medicine;
President and Chief Medical Officer
ARUP Laboratories
Salt Lake City, Utah

Paul Glasziou, MD, PhD, FRACGP
Faculty of Health Sciences and Medicine
Bond University
Robina, Queensland, Australia

Russell P. Grant, PhD
VP Research and Development
Laboratory Corporation of America
Burlington, North Carolina

Ralph Green, MD, PhD
Distinguished Professor of Pathology and Laboratory Medicine
University of California Davis;
Distinguished Professor of Internal Medicine
University of California Davis
Sacramento, California

David S. Hage, PhD
Hewett University Professor
Chemistry Department
University of Nebraska
Lincoln, Nebraska

David John Halsall, PhD
Blood Sciences
Cambridge University Hospitals NHS Trust
Cambridge, United Kingdom

Charles D. Hawker, PhD, MBA, FACSc, FAACC
Adjunct Professor of Pathology (retired)
University of Utah;
Scientific Director, Automation and Special Projects (retired)
ARUP Laboratories
Salt Lake City, Utah

Shannon Haymond, PhD
Associate Professor of Pathology
Northwestern University Feinberg School of Medicine;
Vice Chair for Computational Pathology
Ann & Robert H. Lurie Children's Hospital of Chicago
Chicago, Illinois

Phillip Heaton, PhD, DABMM
Medical Laboratory Scientific Director: Microbiology
Department of Pathology and Laboratory Medicine
HealthPartners
Bloomington, Minnesota

Russell A. Higgins, MD
Professor of Clinical Pathology and Laboratory Medicine
University of Texas Health Science Center at San Antonio
San Antonio, Texas

Victoria Higgins, PhD
Clinical Lecturer of Laboratory Medicine and Pathology
University of Alberta;
Clinical Chemist
DynaLIFE Medical Labs
Edmonton, Alberta, Canada

Ingibjörg Hilmarsdóttir, MD
Assistant Professor
Faculty of Medicine
University of Iceland;
Consultant Microbiologist
Department of Microbiology
Landspítali—The University Hospital of Iceland
Reykjavík, Iceland

Matthew M. Hitchcock, MD, MPH
Assistant Professor of Infectious Diseases
Virginia Commonwealth University School of Medicine;
Staff Physician in Infectious Diseases
Division of Infectious Diseases
Central Virginia VA Health Care System
Richmond, Virginia

Catherine A. Hogan, MDCM, MSc
Clinical Assistant Professor
University of British Columbia;
Medical Microbiologist
British Columbia Centre for Disease Control
Vancouver, British Columbia, Canada

Daniel Thomas Holmes, BSc, MD, FRCPC
Clinical Professor of Pathology and Laboratory Medicine
University of British Columbia;
Department Head and Medical Director
Department of Pathology and Laboratory Medicine
St. Paul's Hospital
Vancouver, British Columbia, Canada

Christopher P. Holstege, MD
Professor of Emergency Medicine and Pediatrics
University of Virginia School of Medicine;
Chief of Division of Medical Toxicology
University of Virginia School of Medicine;
Director of Blue Ridge Poison Center
University of Virginia Health
Charlottesville, Virginia

Andrew N. Hoofnagle, MD, PhD
Professor of Laboratory Medicine
University of Washington
Seattle, Washington

Gary Horowitz, MD
Professor of Anatomic and Clinical Pathology
Tufts University School of Medicine;
Chief of Clinical Pathology
Department of Pathology and Laboratory Medicine
Tufts Medical Center
Boston, Massachusetts

Andrea R. Horvath, MD, PhD, FRCPath, FRCPA
Department of Chemical Pathology
New South Wales Health Pathology
Sydney, New South Wales, Australia

John Greg Howe, PhD, FABMG, DABCC
Professor of Laboratory Medicine
Yale University School of Medicine
New Haven, Connecticut

Romney M. Humphries, PhD, DABMM
Professor of Pathology, Microbiology and Immunology;
Director of Clinical Microbiology
Vanderbilt University Medical Center
Nashville, Tennessee

Ilenia Infusino, BSc
Research Centre for Metrological Traceability in Laboratory
    Medicine (CIRME)
University of Milan, Milano
Milano, Italy

Allan Stanley Jaffe, MD
Professor of Medicine/Cardiology,
Professor of Laboratory Medicine and Pathology
Mayo Clinic
Rochester, Minnesota

**Graham Ross Dallas Jones, MBBS, BSc(med), DPhil,
    FRCPA, FAACB**
Conjoint Associate Professor
University of New South Wales;
Senior Staff Specialist
Department of Chemical Pathology
SydPath St Vincent's Hospital
Sydney, New South Wales, Australia

Patricia M. Jones, PhD, DABCC, FAACC
Professor of Pathology
University of Texas Southwestern Medical Center;
Clinical Director, Chemistry
Children's Medical Center
Dallas, Texas

Randall K. Julian, Jr., PhD
Adjunct Professor of Chemistry
Purdue University
West Lafayette, Indiana;
CEO, Indigo BioAutomation
Carmel, Indiana

Peter A. Kavsak, PhD
Professor of Pathology and Molecular Medicine
McMaster University;
Clinical Chemist
Department of Laboratory Medicine
Hamilton Health Sciences
Hamilton, Ontario, Canada

Mark Kellogg, PhD
Assistant Professor of Pathology
Harvard Medical School;
Director of Quality Programs
Department of Laboratory Medicine
Boston Children's Hospital
Boston, Massachusetts

Aaruni Khanolkar, MBBS, PhD, DABMLI
Assistant Professor of Pathology
Northwestern University;
Director, Diagnostic Immunology and Flow Cytometry
    Laboratory
Ann and Robert H. Lurie Children's Hospital of Chicago
Chicago, Illinois

Sarah E. Kidd, BMedSc (Hons), PhD, FASM
Head, National Mycology Reference Centre
Microbiology and Infectious Diseases
SA Pathology
Adelaide, South Australia, Australia

Steve Kitchen, PhD
Department of Coagulation
Sheffield Teaching Hospitals
Sheffield, United Kingdom

Justin D. Kreuter, MD
Assistant Professor of Laboratory Medicine and Pathology
Mayo Clinic
Rochester, Minnesota

Mark M. Kushnir, PhD
Adjunct Associate Professor of Pathology
University of Utah;
Scientific Director, Mass Spectrometry R&D
ARUP Institute for Clinical and Experimental Pathology
ARUP Laboratories
Salt Lake City, Utah

William D. Lainhart, PhD, DABMM
Assistant Professor of Pathology and Medicine
University of Arizona College of Medicine;
System Clinical Director
Infectious Diseases Division
Banner Health/Sonora Quest Laboratories
Tucson, Arizona

Edmund J. Lamb, BSc, MSc, PhD, FRCPath
Clinical Director of Pathology and Consultant Clinical
  Scientist
Department of Pathology
East Kent Hospitals University NHS Foundation Trust
Canterbury, Kent, United Kingdom

James P. Landers, BS, PhD
Professor of Chemistry
University of Virginia
Charlottesville, Virginia

Loralie J. Langman, PhD
Professor of Laboratory Medicine and Pathology
Mayo Clinic College of Medicine
Rochester, Minnesota

Omar Fernando Laterza, PhD, DABCC
Executive Director
Translational Molecular Biomarkers
Merck & Co., Inc.
Kenilworth, New Jersey

Anna F. Lau, PhD, DABMM
Chief of Sterility Testing Service
Department of Laboratory Medicine
National Institutes of Health
Bethesda, Maryland

Eszter Lázár-Molnár, PhD, DABMLI, FACHI
Associate Professor of Pathology
University of Utah School of Medicine
Salt Lake City, Utah

Rachael M. Liesman, PhD, DABMM
Director of Clinical Microbiology
Department of Pathology and Laboratory Medicine
University of Kansas Health System
Kansas City, Kansas

Kristian Linnet, MD, DMSc
Professor of Forensic Chemistry
University of Copenhagen
Copenhagen, Denmark

Stanley F. Lo, PhD
Professor of Pathology
Medical College of Wisconsin;
Associate Director of Clinical Laboratories
Department of Pathology and Laboratory Medicine
Children's Wisconsin Hospital
Milwaukee, Wisconsin

Yuk Ming Dennis Lo, DM, DPhil
Li Ka Shing Professor of Medicine
Department of Chemical Pathology
The Chinese University of Hong Kong
Shatin, New Territories, Hong Kong

Nicola Longo, MD, PhD
Professor and Chief of Pediatrics (Medical Genetics),
Adjunct Professor of Pathology
University of Utah;
Co-Director
Biochemical Genetics and Newborn Screening
ARUP Laboratories
Salt Lake City, Utah

Elaine Lyon, PhD
Director of Clinical Services Lab
HudsonAlpha Institute for Biotechnology
Huntsville, Alabama

**Edmond S.K. Ma, MD(HK), FRCP, FRCPath, FRCPA,
  FHKCPath, FHKAM(Pathology)**
Honorary Clinical Associate Professor of Pathology
The University of Hong Kong;
Clinical Associate Professor (Honorary)
Anatomical and Cellular Pathology
The Chinese University of Hong Kong;
Director of Clinical and Molecular Pathology
Hong Kong Sanatorium and Hospital, Happy Valley;
Chairman of Children's Thalassaemia Foundation
Hong Kong

Mark Mackay, MSc (Hons)
Honorary Consultant
Key Incident Management and Monitoring System
RCPA Quality Assurance Programs Pty Ltd
St Leonards, New South Wales, Australia

Manisha Madkaikar, MBBS, MD
Director, Scientist G
Pediatric Immunology and Leukocyte Biology
ICMR-National Institute of Immunohaematology
Mumbai, India

John P. Manis, MD
Associate Professor of Pathology
Harvard Medical School;
Department of Laboratory Medicine
Boston Children's Hospital
Boston, Massachusetts

Elaine R. Mardis, PhD
Professor of Pediatrics
The Ohio State University College of Medicine;
Co-executive Director
Rasmussen Institute for Genomic Medicine
Nationwide Children's Hospital
Columbus, Ohio

Stephen R. Master, MD, PhD
Associate Professor of Pathology and Laboratory Medicine
Perelman School of Medicine, University of Pennsylvania;
Chief, Division of Laboratory Medicine
Department of Pathology and Laboratory Medicine
Children's Hospital of Philadelphia
Philadelphia, Pennsylvania

Blaine A. Mathison, BS, MASCP
Scientist
Institute for Clinical and Experimental Pathology
ARUP Laboratories
Salt Lake City, Utah

Erin McElvania, PhD
Clinical Assistant Professor of Pathology
University of Chicago
Chicago, Illinois;
Director of Clinical Microbiology
Pathology
NorthShore University HealthSystem
Evanston, Illinois

Gwendolyn Appell McMillin, PhD, DABCC
Professor of Pathology
University of Utah;
Medical Director of Clinical Toxicology and
    Pharmacogenomics
ARUP Laboratories
Salt Lake City, Utah

Jeffrey W. Meeusen, PhD
Co-Director of Cardiovascular Laboratory Medicine
Department of Laboratory Medicine and Pathology
Mayo Clinic
Rochester, Minnesota

Thomas F. Michniacki, MD
Clinical Assistant Professor of Pediatric Hematology/
    Oncology and Bone Marrow Transplantation
University of Michigan
Ann Arbor, Michigan

Melissa B. Miller, PhD, DABMM, FAAM
Professor of Pathology and Laboratory Medicine
UNC School of Medicine;
Director of Clinical Microbiology and Molecular
    Microbiology Laboratories
University of North Carolina Medical Center
Chapel Hill, North Carolina

W. Greg Miller, PhD
Professor of Pathology
Virginia Commonwealth University;
Co-Director of Clinical Chemistry
Director of Pathology Information Systems
Virginia Commonwealth University Medical Center
Richmond, Virginia

Michael C. Milone, MD, PhD
Associate Professor of Pathology and Laboratory Medicine;
Associate Director, Toxicology Laboratory
Hospital of the University of Pennsylvania
Philadelphia, Pennsylvania

Brian Mochon, PhD, DABMM
System Medical Director
Infectious Diseases Division
Banner Health/Sonora Quest Laboratories
Phoenix, Arizona

Karel G.M. Moons, PhD
Professor, Julius Centre for Health Sciences
    and Primary Care
University Medical Center Utrecht, Utrecht University
Utrecht, Netherlands

Heba H. Mostafa, MD, PhD, DABMM
Assistant Professor of Pathology
Director of Molecular Virology
Johns Hopkins School of Medicine
Baltimore, Maryland

Robert D. Nerenz, PhD, DABCC
Assistant Professor of Pathology and Laboratory Medicine
The Geisel School of Medicine at Dartmouth
Hanover, New Hampshire;
Assistant Director of Clinical Chemistry
Dartmouth-Hitchcock Medical Center
Lebanon, New Hampshire

Børge G. Nordestgaard, MD, DMSc
Professor of Genetic Epidemiology
Clinical Medicine, Faculty of Health and Medical Sciences
University of Copenhagen
Copenhagen, Denmark;
Chief Physician of Clinical Biochemistry
Herlev Gentofte Hospital, Copenhagen University Hospital
Herlev, Denmark

Birte Nygaard, MD, PhD
Associate Professor
Herlev Gentofte Hospital
Department of Internal Medicine
University of Copenhagen
Herlev, Denmark

Maurice O'Kane, MD, FRCPath, FRCPEdin
Consultant Chemical Pathologist
Clinical Chemistry Laboratory
Altnagelvin Hospital, Western Health and Social Care Trust
Londonderry, Northern Ireland, United Kingdom

Monica B. Pagano, MD
Associate Professor of Laboratory Medicine and Pathology;
Adjunct Associate Professor of Medicine
University of Washington
Seattle, Washington

Prasad V.A. Pamidi, PhD
Senior Director of Sensor Development
Acute Care Diagnostics R&D
Instrumentation Laboratory
Bedford, Massachusetts

Mauro Panteghini, MD
Professor of Clinical Biochemistry and Clinical Molecular
    Biology
Department of Biomechanical and Clinical Sciences
"Luigi Sacco"
University of Milan;
Director Clinical Pathology Laboratory
ASST Fatebenefratelli-Sacco
Milan, Italy

Klaus Pantel, MD, PhD
Professor of Tumor Biology
UKE
Hamburg, Germany

Jason Y. Park, MD, PhD
Associate Professor of Pathology
University of Texas Southwestern Medical Center;
Clinical Director of Advanced Diagnostics Laboratory
Department of Pathology
Children's Medical Center of Dallas
Dallas, Texas

Marzia Pasquali, PhD, FACMG
Professor of Pathology
University of Utah
ARUP Laboratories
Salt Lake City, Utah

Jay L. Patel, MD, MBA
Associate Professor of Pathology
University of Utah;
Medical Director of Hematopathology and Molecular
    Oncology
ARUP Laboratories
Salt Lake City, Utah

Khushbu Patel, PhD, DABCC
Assistant Professor of Pathology and Laboratory Medicine
University of Pennsylvania;
Director, Clinical Chemistry and Point-of-Care
Department of Pathology and Laboratory Medicine
Children's Hospital of Philadelphia
Philadelphia, Pennsylvania

Robin Patel, MD
Elizabeth P. and Robert E. Allen Professor of Individualized
    Medicine, Professor of Medicine, Professor of
    Microbiology
Division of Clinical Microbiology
Mayo Clinic
Rochester, Minnesota

Roy W.A. Peake, PhD
Instructor of Pathology
Harvard Medical School;
Associate Director of Clinical Chemistry
Department of Laboratory Medicine
Boston Children's Hospital
Boston, Massachusetts

Morgan A. Pence, PhD, DABMM
Director, Clinical and Molecular Microbiology
Cook Children's Medical Center
Fort Worth, Texas

Peter L. Perrotta, MD
Professor and Chair of Pathology, Anatomy and Laboratory
    Medicine
West Virginia University
Morgantown, West Virginia

Tahir S. Pillay, MBChB, PhD (Cantab), FRCPath (Lon)
Professor and Chair of Chemical Pathology,
University of Pretoria;
Chief Specialist
National Health Laboratory Service
Pretoria, Gauteng, South Africa

Jacqueline N. Poston, MD
Assistant Professor of Medicine and Pathology
Larner College of Medicine at the University of Vermont
Burlington, Vermont

Victoria M. Pratt, PhD, FACMG
Professor of Medical and Molecular Genetics
Indiana University School of Medicine;
Director of Pharmacogenomics and Molecular Genetics
    Laboratories
Indianapolis, Indiana

Bobbi S. Pritt, MD, MSc, DTMH
Professor of Laboratory Medicine and Pathology
Mayo Clinic
Rochester, Minnesota

Gary W. Procop, MD, MS
Medical Director and Professor of Pathology
Pathology and Laboratory Medicine Institute
Cleveland Clinic
Cleveland, Ohio

Minke A.E. Rab, MD, PhD
Fellow Hematology/Assistant Professor
Central Diagnostic Laboratory
University Medical Center Utrecht
Utrecht, Netherlands

Lokinendi V. Rao, PhD, HCLD, FAACC
Professor of Pathology
University of Massachusetts
Chan Medical School
Worcester, Massachusetts;
Executive Scientific Director
Quest Diagnostics, North
Marlborough, Massachusetts

Brian A. Rappold, BS
Director of Mass Spectrometry and Integrated Genetics
Laboratory Corporation of America
Research Triangle Park, North Carolina

Hooman H. Rashidi, MD
Professor of Pathology and Laboratory Medicine
University of California Davis School of Medicine
Sacramento, California

Alan T. Remaley, MD, PhD
Senior Scientist
National Institutes of Health
NHLBI
Bethesda, Maryland

Nader Rifai, PhD
Professor of Pathology
Harvard Medical School;
The Louis Joseph Gay-Lussac Chair in Laboratory Medicine
Director of Clinical Chemistry
Boston Children's Hospital
Boston, Massachusetts

Alan L. Rockwood, PhD, DABCC
Professor (Clinical) Emeritus of Pathology
University of Utah School of Medicine;
President of Rockwood Scientific Consulting
Salt Lake City, Utah

Thomas Røraas, PhD†
Mathematician
Haraldsplass Deaconess Hospital
Noklus
Bergen, Vestland, Norway

William Malcolm Charles Rosenberg, MA, MB, BS, DPhil, FRCP
Peter Scheuer Chair of Liver Diseases
Institute for Liver and Digestive Health, Division of Medicine
University College London
London, United Kingdom

David B. Sacks, MB, ChB, FRCPath
Adjunct Professor of Medicine
Georgetown University;
Clinical Professor of Pathology
George Washington University
Washington, DC, District of Columbia;
Senior Investigator
Laboratory Medicine
National Institutes of Health
Bethesda, Maryland;
Honorary Professor
Clinical Laboratory Sciences
University of Cape Town
Cape Town, South Africa

Sverre Sandberg, MD, PhD
Professor of the Institute of Public Health and Primary Health Care
University of Bergen;
Director of the Norwegian Organisation for Quality Improvement of Laboratory Examinations, Noklus
Haraldsplass Deaconess Hospital;
Director of the Norwegian Porphyria Centre
Haukeland University Hospital
Bergen, Norway

Ronald Schifman, MD
Emeritus Professor of Pathology
University of Arizona College of Medicine
Tucson, Arizona

Caroline Schmitt, PharmD, PhD
Associate Professor of Biochemistry and Molecular Biology
Université de Paris
Paris, France

Amar Akhtar Sethi, MD, PhD
Associate Vice President
Clinical Development at Omeros Corporation
Seattle, Washington

Howard M. Shapiro, MD†
President
One World Cytometry, Inc.
West Newton, Massachusetts

Leslie Michael Shaw, PhD
Professor of Pathology and Laboratory Medicine;
Director Toxicology Laboratory;
Director, Biomarker Research Laboratory
Perelman School of Medicine
University of Pennsylvania
Philadelphia, Pennsylvania

†Deceased.

Roy Alan Sherwood, BSc, MSc, DPhil
Professor of Clinical Biochemistry
King's College London
London, United Kingdom

Ana-Maria Simundic, PhD
Professor of Medical Biochemistry and Hematology
Faculty of Pharmacy and Biochemistry
University of Zagreb;
Specialist in Laboratory Medicine
Head of Department of Medical Laboratory Diagnostics
University Hospital Sveti Duh
Zagreb, Croatia

Melissa R. Snyder, PhD
Associate Professor of Laboratory Medicine and Pathology
Mayo Clinic
Rochester, Minnesota

**Jason C.C. So, BSc, MBBS, FRCPath, FHKCPath,
    FHKAM(Pathology)**
Chief of Service and Consultant Hematopathologist
Department of Pathology
Hong Kong Children's Hospital
Hong Kong, China

Ravinder Sodi, PhD, CSci, EuSpLM, FRCPath
Consultant Clinical Biochemist
Department of Blood Sciences
University Hospitals Dorset
Poole, Dorset, United Kingdom;
Visiting Fellow
Faculty of Health and Social Sciences
Bournemouth University
Bournemouth, United Kingdom

Frederick G. Strathmann, PhD, MBA, DABCC (CC, TC)
Assistant Laboratory Director,
Senior Vice President of Operations
NMS Labs
Horsham, Pennsylvania

Catharine Sturgeon, BSc, PhD, FRCPath
Department of Laboratory Medicine
Royal Infirmary of Edinburgh
Edinburgh, United Kingdom

Dorine W. Swinkels, MD, PhD
Professor of Laboratory Medicine
Translational Metabolic Laboratory
Radboudumc
Nijmegen, Netherlands

Valérie Taly, PhD
Centre de Recherche des Cordeliers
INSERM, Sorbonne Université, Université de Paris, CNRS,
    Equipe labellisée Ligue Nationale contre le cancer
Paris, France

Sudeep Tanwar, PhD, MBBS, MRCP
Department of Gastroenterology
Barts Health NHS Trust
London, United Kingdom

Anne E. Tebo, PhD
Senior Associate Consultant
Department of Laboratory Medicine and Pathology
Mayo Clinic
Rochester, Minnesota

Michael TeKippe, MD, PhD
Attending Physician
Pediatric Infectious Diseases
Advocate Children's Hospital
Oak Lawn, Illinois

Stephanie A. Thatcher, BS, MS
Vice President
Molecular Systems
BioFire Diagnostics/bioMerieux
Salt Lake City, Utah

Nam K. Tran, PhD, MS, MAS
Professor and Senior Director of Clinical Pathology
University of California, Davis Health
Sacramento, California

Gregory J. Tsongalis, PhD, HCLD, CC
Professor and Vice Chair for Research,
Director, Laboratory for Clinical Genomics and Advanced
    Technology (CGAT)
Department of Pathology and Laboratory Medicine
Dartmouth Hitchcock Health System and The Audrey and
    Theodor Geisel School of Medicine at Dartmouth
Lebanon, New Hampshire

Masako Ueda, MD
Medical Geneticist
Department of Medicine
University of Pennsylvania
Philadelphia, Pennsylvania

Richard van Wijk, PhD
Associate Professor
Central Diagnostic Laboratory
University Medical Center Utrecht
Utrecht, Netherlands

Jim B. Vaught, PhD
Editor-in-Chief
Biopreservation and Biobanking
Kensington, Maryland

Cindy L. Vnencak-Jones, PhD, FACMG
Professor of Pathology, Microbiology and Immunology;
  Professor of Pediatrics;
Medical Director, Molecular Diagnostics Laboratory
  Medicine Division
Vanderbilt University Medical Center
Nashville, Tennessee

Mia Wadelius, MD, PhD
Professor of Medical Sciences
Clinical Pharmacogenomics
Uppsala University;
Senior Physician
Clinical Pharmacology
Uppsala University Hospital
Uppsala, Sweden

Kelly Walkovich, MD
Associate Professor of Pediatric Hematology/Oncology
University of Michigan Medical School
Ann Arbor, Michigan

Natalie E. Walsham, MBiochem, MSc, DipRCPath
Consultant, Clinical Scientist
Biochemistry, North Kent Pathology Services
Dartford and Gravesham NHS Trust
Kent, United Kingdom

Ping Wang, PhD
Professor of Pathology and Laboratory Medicine
University of Pennsylvania;
Director of Clinical Chemistry and Core Laboratory
Hospital of the University of Pennsylvania
Philadelphia, Pennsylvania

David A. Wells, PhD
Founder and Principal Scientist
Bioanalysis, Metabolism and Automation
Wells Medical Research Services
Laguna Hills, California

Nancy L. Wengenack, PhD
Professor of Laboratory Medicine and Pathology
Mayo Clinic
Rochester, Minnesota

Sharon D. Whatley, BSc, MSc, PhD, FRCPath
Institute of Medical Genetics
University Hospital of Wales
Cardiff, United Kingdom

Maria Alice Vieira Willrich, PhD, DABCC, FAACC
Associate Professor of Laboratory Medicine and
  Pathology
Mayo Clinic
Rochester, Minnesota

William E. Winter, MD
Professor of Pathology, Immunology and Laboratory
  Medicine, Pediatrics, and Molecular Genetics and
  Microbiology
University of Florida
Gainesville, Florida

Carl T. Wittwer, MD, PhD
Professor Emeritus of Pathology
University of Utah
Salt Lake City, Utah

Timothy Wood, PhD
Assistant Professor
University of Colorado Anschutz Medical Campus
Director of Biochemical Genetics Laboratory
Children's Hospital Colorado
Aurora, Colorado

Edward J. Yoon, MD
Assistant Professor of Pathology
Lewis Katz School of Medicine, Temple University;
Associate Director, Transfusion Medicine
Department of Pathology and Laboratory Medicine
Temple University Hospital
Philadelphia, Pennsylvania

Ian Young, MD, FRCP, FRCPath
Professor of Medicine
Centre for Public Health
Queen's University Belfast
Belfast, United Kingdom

Qian-Yun Zhang, MD, PhD
Professor of Pathology
University of New Mexico
Albuquerque, New Mexico

Stefan Zimmermann, MD
Head of Division Bacteriology
Department of Infectious Diseases
University Hospital Heidelberg
Heidelberg, Germany

TEXTBOOK CONTENTS

---

*Full versions of these chapters are available electronically on ExpertConsult.com.

*Full versions of these chapters are available electronically on ExpertConsult.com.

---

*Full versions of these chapters are available electronically on ExpertConsult.com.

MULTIMEDIA & EDUCATIONAL RESOURCES ASSOCIATE EDITORS

Roy W.A. Peake, PhD
Instructor of Pathology
Harvard Medical School;
Associate Director of Clinical Chemistry
Department of Laboratory Medicine
Boston Children's Hospital
Boston, Massachusetts

Shannon Haymond, PhD
Associate Professor of Pathology
Northwestern University Feinberg School of Medicine;
Vice Chair for Computational Pathology
Ann & Robert H. Lurie Children's Hospital of Chicago
Chicago, Illinois

MULTIMEDIA & EDUCATIONAL RESOURCES CONTRIBUTORS

Gifford F. Batstone, MBBS, BSc (Biochemistry), MSc (Medical Education), FRCPath
Consultant Chemical Pathology and Metabolic Medicine (Retired)
Winchester, United Kingdom

David Bick, MD, FACMG
Associate Director
HudsonAlpha Clinical Services Lab, LLC
Huntsville, Alabama

Julie E. Buring, ScD
Professor of Medicine
Harvard Medical School;
Senior Epidemiologist
Brigham and Women's Hospital
Boston, Massachusetts

Sheldon Campbell, MD, PhD
Professor of Laboratory Medicine
Yale School of Medicine;
Associate Chief for Laboratory Medicine
VA Connecticut Health Care
New Haven, Connecticut

Nagarjuna R. Cheemarla, PhD
Postdoctoral Associate of Laboratory Medicine
Yale School of Medicine
New Haven, Connecticut

Pak Leng Cheong, MB ChB, DPhil, FRCPA
Clinical Senior Lecturer
University of Sydney;
Genetic Pathologist
Department of Medical Genomics
Royal Prince Alfred Hospital
Sydney, Australia

John C. Coakley, MD, FRACP, FRCPA, MAACB
Head of Biochemistry (Retired)
The Children's Hospital at Westmead
Sydney, Australia

Meagan Cochran, MS, CGC
Genetic Counselor
HudsonAlpha Clinical Services Lab, LLC
Huntsville, Alabama

Tamsyn Cromwell, BSc, MSc, PhD, FRCPath
Clinical Scientist
University Hospitals Sussex
Brighton, United Kingdom

Allan Deacon, PhD, DipCB, FRCPath,
Consultant Clinical Scientist (Retired)
Bushmead, Luton, United Kingdom

Julio C. Delgado, MD, MS
Professor of Pathology
University of Utah;
Chief Medical Officer
ARUP Laboratories
Salt Lake City, Utah

Mathew A. Diggle, PhD, FRCPath
Associate Professor of Laboratory Medicine & Pathology
University of Alberta;
Clinical Microbiologist
University of Alberta Hospital, Provincial Laboratories
Edmonton, Alberta, Canada

Ellen F. Foxman, MD, PhD
Assistant Professor of Laboratory Medicine and Immunobiology
Yale School of Medicine;
Assistant Director of Clinical Virology and Clinical Immunology
Yale-New Haven Hospital
New Haven, Connecticut

Allan Gaw, MD, PhD, FRCPath
Associate Director for Educational Quality Standards (Retired)
NIHR, University of Leeds
Leeds, United Kingdom

Jonathan R. Genzen, MD, PhD
Associate Professor of Pathology
University of Utah;
Chief Operations Officer
ARUP Laboratories
Salt Lake City, Utah

Morayma Reyes Gil, MD, PhD
Director of Thrombosis and Hemostasis Laboratories
Department of Laboratory Medicine;
Robert J. Tomsich Pathology & Laboratory Medicine Institute
Cleveland Clinic
Cleveland, Ohio

Veronica Greve, MS, CGC
Genetic Counselor
HudsonAlpha Clinical Services Lab, LLC
Huntsville, Alabama

Robert B. Hamilton, MD
Resident in Pathology
Dartmouth-Hitchcock Medical Center
Lebanon, New Hampshire

Lisa M. Johnson, PhD
Assistant Professor of Pathology
University of Utah School of Medicine;
Medical Director of Clinical Chemistry
ARUP Laboratories
Salt Lake City, Utah

Christina M. Lockwood, PhD
Associate Professor of Laboratory Medicine and Pathology
University of Washington;
Director of Laboratory Genomics
University of Washington Medical Center
Seattle, Washington

Stephen P. Miller, BSc (Biomedical Science)
Senior Scientist Haematology
Pathology Queensland Central Laboratories
Royal Brisbane and Women's Hospital Campus
Herston, Queensland, Australia

David L. Murray, MD, PhD
Assistant Professor of Laboratory Medicine and Pathology
Mayo Clinic
Rochester, Minnesota

Michael Murphy, MD
Biochemical Medicine
University of Dundee
Dundee, United Kingdom

Ghunwa Nakouzi, PhD, FACMG
Associate Director
HudsonAlpha Clinical Services Lab, LLC
Huntsville, Alabama

Vijayalakshmi (Viji) Nandakumar, PhD, DABCC
Assistant Professor of Pathology
University of Utah;
Medical Director, Clinical Immunology
ARUP Laboratories
Salt Lake City, Utah

Vera A. Paulson, MD, PhD
Assistant Professor of Laboratory Medicine and Pathology
University of Washington;
Associate Director of UW Medicine's Genetics and Solid
Tumor Lab;
Associate Director of Genetics Preanalytical Services
University of Washington Medical Center
Seattle Cancer Alliance
Harborview Medical Center
Seattle Children's Hospital
Seattle, Washington

Roy W.A. Peake, PhD
Instructor of Pathology
Harvard Medical School;
Associate Director of Clinical Chemistry
Department of Laboratory Medicine
Boston Children's Hospital
Boston, Massachusetts

Lisa K. Peterson, PhD, DABMLI
Assistant Professor of Pathology (Clinical)
University of Utah;
Medical Director of Immunology
ARUP Laboratories
Salt Lake City, Utah

Victoria M. Pratt, PhD, FACMG
Professor and Director of Pharmacogenomics and Molecular
Genetics Laboratories
Medical and Molecular Genetics
Indiana University School of Medicine
Indianapolis, Indiana

Bobbi S. Pritt, MD, MSc, DTMH
Professor of Laboratory Medicine and Pathology
Mayo Clinic
Rochester, Minnesota

Pamela M. Rist, ScD
Assistant Professor of Medicine
Harvard Medical School;
Assistant Professor of Epidemiology
Harvard T.H. Chan School of Public Health;
Associate Epidemiologist
Brigham and Women's Hospital
Boston, Massachusetts

Kate E. Shipman, BMBCh, MA (Hons Oxon), MRCP, FRCPath
Honorary Clinical Lecturer
Brighton and Sussex Medical School;
Consultant Chemical Pathologist
University Hospitals Sussex
Worthing, Western Sussex, United Kingdom

Melissa R. Snyder, PhD
Associate Professor of Laboratory Medicine and Pathology
Mayo Clinic
Rochester, Minnesota

Rajeev Srivastava MS, FRCS, FRCPath
Consultant Chemical Pathologist
Queen Elizabeth University Hospital
Glasgow, United Kingdom

Jillian R. Tate, MSc, FFSc (RCPA)†
Senior Scientist, Chemical Pathology
Royal Brisbane and Women's Hospital
Brisbane, Australia

Gary Weaving, DPhil
Clinical Scientist
University Hospitals Sussex
Brighton, East Sussex, England

Liying Zhang, MD, PhD
Professor of Pathology and Laboratory Medicine
University of California, Los Angeles (UCLA);
Director of Advanced Molecular Diagnostics Service
Los Angeles, California

---

†Deceased.

MULTIMEDIA & EDUCATIONAL RESOURCES CONTENTS

ADAPTIVE LEARNING EDITORS

EDITORS-IN-CHIEF

Nader Rifai
Christina Ellervik

EDITORS

- *Basics in Laboratory Medicine, Analytical techniques, Clinical Chemistry and Genetic Metabolic Disorders*
  Christina Ellervik, Danyel Tacker, Li Zha
- *Laboratory Genomics*
  Linnea M. Baudhuin, Christina Lockwood, Heather Mason-Suares
- *Hematology & Coagulation*
  Kristian T. Schafernak, Rachel Mariani
- *Transfusion Medicine*
  Kerry O'Brien
- *Clinical Microbiology*
  Blake W. Buchan, Ingibjörg Hilmarsdóttir, Derrick Chen
- *Clinical Immunology*
  Melissa R. Snyder, Lusia Sepiashvili

https://rhapsode.com/laboratorymedicine/

ADAPTIVE LEARNING COURSES CONTENTS

[a]Courses will be released in 2022.

Basics of Laboratory Medicine

Exam questions, case studies, and additional resources are available on ExpertConsult.com.
*Full versions of these chapters are available electronically on www.ExpertConsult.com.

1

Laboratory Medicine

Nader Rifai, Rossa W.K. Chiu, Ian Young, Carey-Ann D. Burnham, and Carl T. Wittwer[a]

ABSTRACT

Background

Laboratory medicine is a complex field that measures biomarkers and microorganisms in bodily specimens or tissues to diagnose and manage diseases. It encompasses multiple disciplines including clinical chemistry, hematology and coagulation, clinical microbiology, clinical immunology, molecular diagnostics, and transfusion medicine. Laboratory medicine is driven by technology that helps define the boundaries among its disciplines. Although laboratory medicine specialists are diverse in terms of their education, training, and career paths, their practice of the profession and their adherence to its guiding principles are similar. The goal is to generate relevant chemical, cellular, and molecular data that can be integrated with clinical and other information and interpreted to aid clinical decision making.

Content

This chapter describes the evolution of laboratory medicine and examines the international practice of the profession, the disciplines it encompasses, academic and postgraduate training, certification, career opportunities, and the skills and roles of laboratory medicine specialists in both clinical laboratory and industry settings. This chapter also discusses the guiding principles of practicing the profession, which include maintaining confidentiality of medical information, using available resources appropriately, abiding by codes of conduct, avoiding conflict of interest, and following ethical publishing rules.

INTRODUCTION

Laboratory medicine is a broad and heterogeneous field that deals with the measurement of chemical, biochemical, cellular, and genetic biomarkers; it encompasses multiple disciplines including clinical chemistry, hematology and coagulation, clinical microbiology (including serology and virology), clinical immunology, molecular diagnostics, and, in certain countries, transfusion medicine. Tissue pathology and cytology, although part of the broad definition of laboratory medicine that includes all testing of human tissue, are not included in this textbook. Although the various fields of laboratory medicine overlap in a continuous dynamic evolution (Fig. 1.1), specific disciplines elicit different images. For clinical chemistry, one thinks of pH measurements or large chemistry analyzers; for hematology or microbiology, microscopic examination is what first comes to mind; and molecular diagnostics conjures up the human genome project, companion diagnostics, and personalized and precision medicine. Whereas clinical chemistry and molecular diagnostics are heavily dependent on technological developments, where the former excels in random access testing and the latter has evolved massively parallel methods, the practice of transfusion medicine and hematology is decidedly clinical. Furthermore, certain disciplines like transfusion medicine are well

defined and consistently practiced internationally, while others such as clinical chemistry and clinical microbiology may vary in content depending on the country in which they are practiced. According to the definition of the International Federation of Clinical Chemistry and Laboratory Medicine (IFCC), "Clinical Chemistry is the largest subdiscipline of Laboratory Medicine which is a multidisciplinary medical and scientific specialty with several interacting subdisciplines, such as hematology, immunology, clinical biochemistry, and others. Through these activities clinical chemists influence the practice of medicine for the benefit of the public."[1]

Hospital-based laboratory medicine departments and commercial clinical laboratories provide in vitro testing of a variety of biomarkers in various fluids or tissues of the human body to screen for a disease, confirm or exclude a diagnosis, help to select or monitor a treatment, or assess prognosis. The popular claim that 60 to 70% of clinical decisions are based on laboratory tests cannot be easily justified by objectively measured data.[2,3] Nevertheless, laboratory testing impacts healthcare delivery to virtually every patient.

LOOKING BACK

The examination of body fluids for the diagnosis of disease is certainly not a modern concept. The Greeks noticed before 400 BC that ants are attracted to "sweet urine." Laboratory testing, however, was not always appreciated by clinicians; the famous Dublin physician Robert James Graves (1796–1853) once remarked, "Few and scanty, indeed, are the rays of light

[a]The authors gratefully acknowledge the contributions by David E. Bruns, Edward R. Ashwood, Carl A. Burtis, and A. Rita Horvath on which portions of this chapter are based.

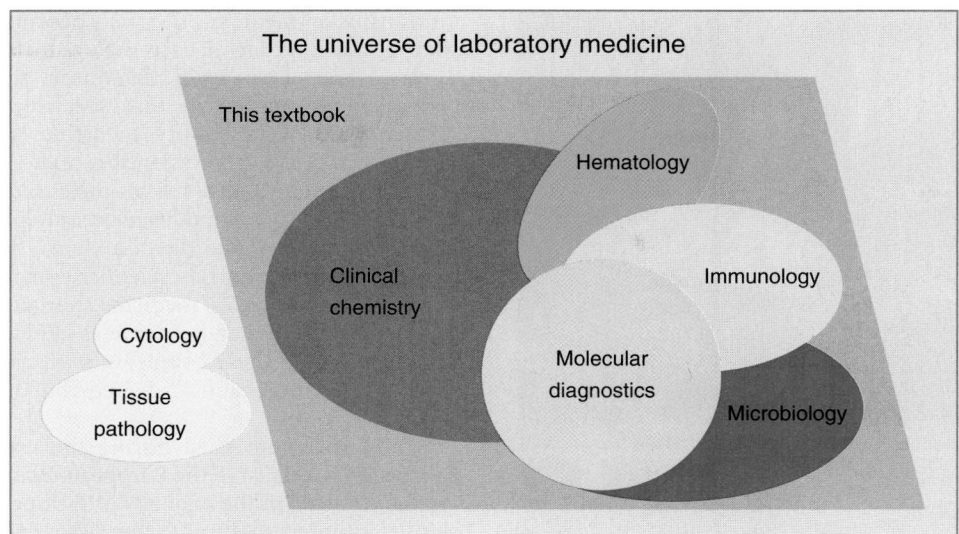

FIGURE 1.1 The interacting disciplines of laboratory medicine. Laboratory medicine encompasses testing and associated activities for the assessment, diagnosis, treatment, management, and prevention of human disease. Although in certain countries tissue pathology and cytology are part of laboratory medicine, their focus on morphology and image analysis sets them apart from other areas of laboratory medicine and they are not considered in this textbook. The largest divisions of laboratory medicine considered within include clinical chemistry, clinical microbiology, clinical immunology, hematology, and molecular diagnostics. These disciplines overlap and evolve over time. *The sizes of the circles are not meant to reflect those of the disciplines.*

which chemistry has flung on the vital mysteries," and the pioneer Max Josef von Pettenkofer (1818–1901) stated that clinicians use their chemistry laboratory services only when needed for "luxurious embellishment for a clinical lecture."[4] Such views have changed throughout the years, and laboratory testing has proven to be a useful tool to clinicians who have grown to depend and rely on the clinical laboratory in the routine management of their patients.

Although it may be difficult to pinpoint the exact date at which the concept of the clinical laboratory was born, a relevant article titled "Hospital Construction" by Francis H. Brown that was published in the *Boston Medical and Surgical Journal*, the precursor of the *New England Journal of Medicine*, in 1861. Dr. Brown stated: "[Every hospital should have] a small room at the end of the ward to serve as a general laboratory … necessary small cooking might be accomplished here; dishes and other articles washed etc.; and it would serve as a general store-room for brooms, pails, and other articles." Although Baron Justus von Liebig (1803–1873) once boasted that his clinical laboratory performed more than 400 tests per annum, the average mid- to large-sized laboratory today performs several million tests yearly; the images presented in Fig. 1.2 depict this striking contrast between the legendary Otto Folin in his biochemistry laboratory at McLean Hospital in Boston in 1905 and the University of Utah Clinical Laboratory/ARUP Laboratories more than a century later.

One of the first laboratories attached to a hospital was established in 1886 in Munich, Germany, by Hugo Wilhelm von Ziemssen.[5] In the United States, the first clinical laboratory recorded was The William Pepper Laboratory of Clinical Medicine, established in 1895 at the University of Pennsylvania in Philadelphia.[6] While there may be some uncertainty about the first hospital laboratory, the concept had become sufficiently well established by the late 1880s to enter popular

culture. Arthur Conan Doyle, writing in 1887, set the first meeting of Sherlock Holmes and Dr. Watson in 1881 in the chemical laboratory in St. Bartholomew's Hospital, London, where Holmes had just discovered a reagent that "is precipitated by haemoglobin, and by nothing else" (A Study in Scarlet). Hopefully, the excitement experienced by Holmes at this discovery is still felt by laboratory specialists today.

Basic research usually precedes clinical application. Hematology began with the microscopic observation of red blood cells by Anthony van Leeuwenhoek (1632–1723). The father of microbiology is considered to be Louis Pasteur (1822–1895), who confirmed the germ theory of disease by experimentation. Immunology arose as a combination of the "cellularists," observing phagocytosis, and the "humoralists," who observed that immunity could be transferred as a soluble substance (antibodies and/or complement) in the late nineteenth century.

Molecular diagnostics has more recent origins than the other disciplines of laboratory medicine. "Molecular Diagnosis" was first mentioned in 1968 as the title of a *New England Journal of Medicine* editorial, commenting on a new inborn error of metabolism that overproduced oxalic acid, resulting in kidney stones.[7] "Molecular" referred to an enzymatic pathway and the substrates, not nucleic acid variants. Twenty years later, additional articles describing "molecular diagnostics" began to appear. In 1986, molecular diagnostics was defined as, "…the detection and quantification of specific genes by nucleic acid hybridization procedures," exemplified by speciation of plant nematodes.[8] In 1987, molecular diagnostics was used to describe mapping of antigenic substances by affinity chromatography using immobilized antibodies.[9] In 1988, the term was used to describe methods for detecting gene amplification and rearrangement using Southern blotting.[10] With the advent of polymerase chain reaction (PCR),

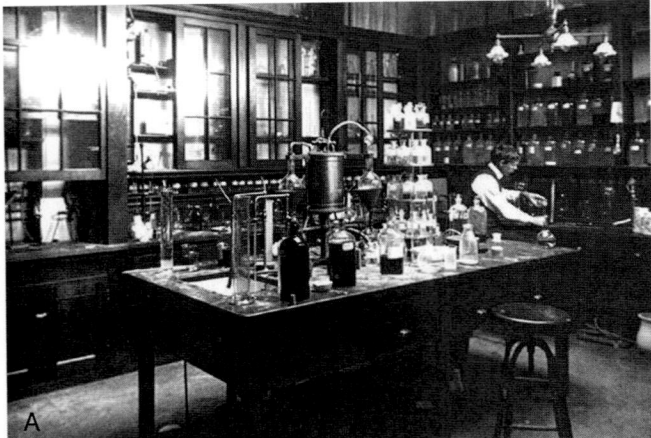

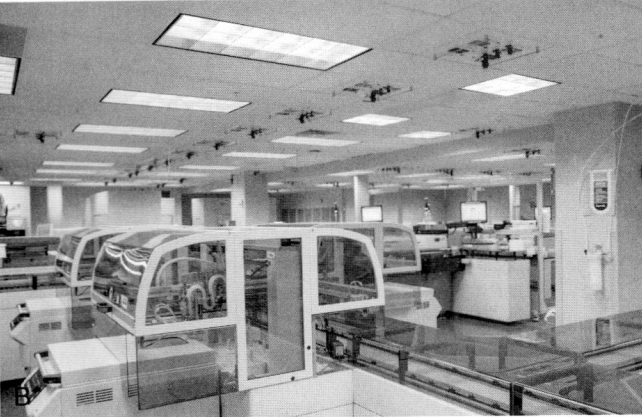

FIGURE 1.2 Early and modern clinical laboratories. The legendary Otto Folin in his biochemistry laboratory at McLean Hospital in Boston in 1905 and the University of Utah Clinical Laboratory/ARUP Laboratories, Salt Lake City, UT, more than a century later. (Image 1 from http://en.wikipedia.org/wiki/File:1905_Otto_Folin_in_biochemistry_lab_at_McLean_Hospital_byAHFolsom_Harvard.png; Image 2 courtesy ARUP Laboratories.)

the term "molecular diagnostics" became more common, its use doubling in the medical literature every 6 to 7 years.[11] By 1997, commercial real-time PCR instruments solidified "molecular diagnostics" as a branch of laboratory medicine.

TRAINING IN LABORATORY MEDICINE

Clinical laboratory professionals are individuals with a medical or a doctoral degree (pharmacy, chemistry, biology, biochemistry, microbiology) who are focused on clinical service. In North America, Australia, and Europe, a minimum of 9 years of academic education (a medical or a doctoral degree) and postgraduate professional training (residency and postdoctoral) is required before an individual becomes an independently practicing specialist (Fig. 1.3).[12] The requirements and training in laboratory medicine to become a specialist differ around the world. For example, in the United States, either those with a medical or a doctoral degree can direct a clinical laboratory after obtaining the appropriate board certification. Those with a medical degree usually do a residency in clinical or clinical/anatomical pathology to direct a general clinical laboratory. However, if they chose to direct a discipline-specific laboratory such as clinical chemistry, microbiology,

or transfusion medicine, they may need to complete a fellowship in that specialty. Those with a doctoral degree tend to direct a discipline-specific laboratory and must complete postdoctoral training in that specialty. In the European Union, 40% of laboratory medicine specialists are from medical, 30% are from scientific, and 30% are from pharmacy backgrounds. In some countries such as Austria, Lithuania, Estonia, Malta, and Sweden, only physicians can practice the profession and direct a clinical laboratory. In most other European countries, scientists, pharmacists, and physicians can be laboratory medicine specialists, yet those with a pharmacy degree may not serve as clinical laboratory directors in some of these countries, such as Italy. A pharmacy degree is a "professional" degree (but not equivalent to a PhD) in France.

The curriculum used during the training of a clinical laboratory specialist in the European Union varies depending on the country. In the majority of European countries, trainees get exposed to clinical chemistry (45% of the curriculum), hematology (30%), microbiology (15%), and genetics (10%).[1,12] Molecular diagnostics (nucleic acid testing) is considered a technique and is included in all fields. In contrast, in the United Kingdom and Ireland, chemical pathology training is restricted to the traditional subdiscipline of clinical chemistry. This diversity of subspecialties is reflected in the heterogeneity of postgraduate training across countries.[13]

Postgraduate professional training and certification examinations at the end of the training are not mandated in all countries (see Fig. 1.3). The EFLM Register of Specialists in Laboratory Medicine (EuSpLM) (https://www.eflm.eu/site/page/a/1305) is attempting to standardize the minimum requirements for education and training for laboratory medicine specialists to facilitate the comparability of their professional training within the European Union.[1,12,13] These issues add to the complexity of defining the qualifications of clinical laboratory directors.

EXPANDING BOUNDARIES DEFINED BY TECHNOLOGY

The diversity of background, training, and subspecialization has led to heterogeneity in what the profession is called throughout the world. Name designations include clinical chemistry, clinical biochemistry, chemical pathology, hematology, clinical microbiology, transfusion medicine, clinical pathology, laboratory diagnostics, clinical or medical biology, clinical laboratory, laboratory medicine, clinical analysis, and so on. The EC4 Register (now the EuSpLM) adopted the name "specialist in laboratory medicine" to represent clinical laboratorians in Europe.

Everyone, including lay people, knows what a cardiologist is and does; the same is true for an infectious diseases specialist and a surgeon. Within laboratory medicine, the function of certain specialists, such as clinical microbiologists, hematologists, or blood bankers, is also clear. It is more difficult, however, to characterize a clinical chemist. Perhaps, unlike other specialties in laboratory medicine, clinical chemistry is very much influenced and shaped by technology. No discipline in laboratory medicine uses more technologies than clinical chemistry. Technologies that evolved over time not only changed practice but remodeled the boundaries of the traditional clinical chemistry laboratory. For example, with

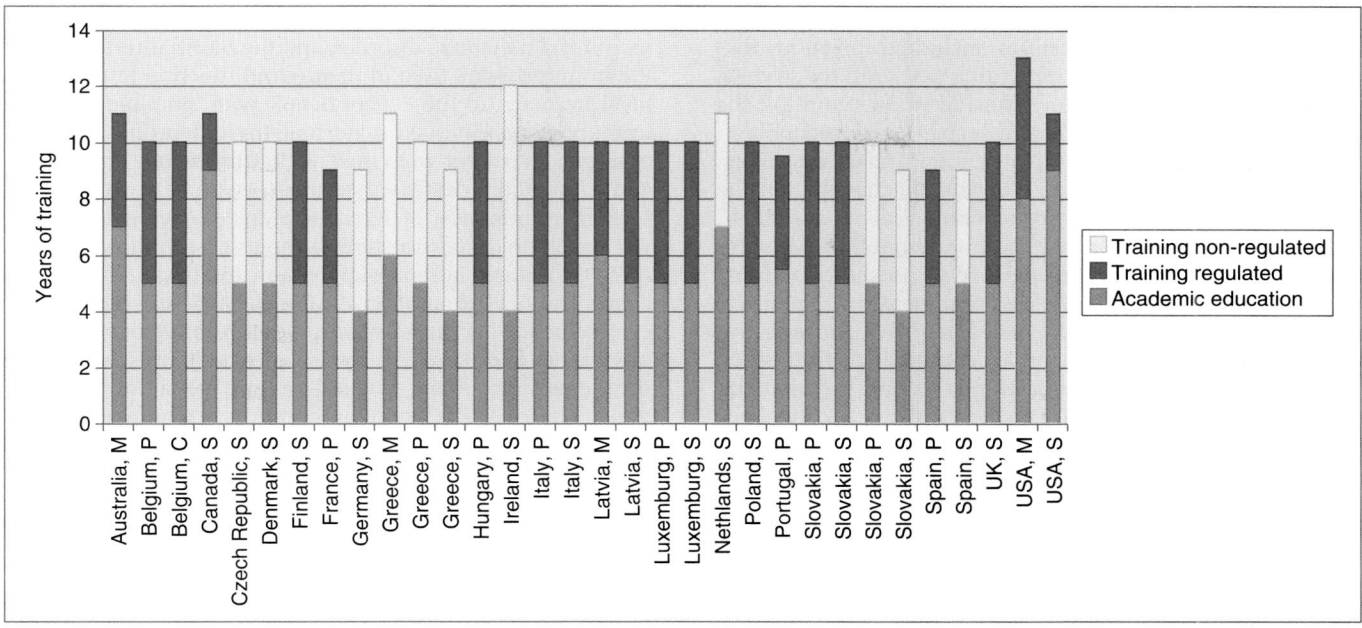

FIGURE 1.3 The number of years of education and training required to practice as clinical laboratory specialist in different countries varies from 9 to 13 years. Different training routes include medical *(M)*, pharmacy *(P)*, chemistry *(C)*, and scientific *(S)*. Both academic education *(light red bars)* and postgraduate training are required. Postgraduate training may be regulated *(dark red bars)* or nonregulated *(pink bars)* in different countries and even within the same country. (Modified from EU Directive 2013/55/EU. The recognition of professional qualifications. Proposing a common training framework for specialists in laboratory medicine across the European Union 2013. http://www.ukipg.org.uk/meetings/international_and_european_forum/ctf_e4_bid.)

the emergence of immunochemical techniques in the 1970s, the US Food and Drug Administration approved many tests for the measurement of proteins, small molecule hormones, and drugs, a development that profoundly changed clinical chemistry and its armamentarium of testing at the time. Integrated automated platforms later enabled the measurement of hormones and therapeutic drugs by immunoassays simultaneously with electrolytes, glucose, and other general chemistry tests, thus subsuming the "endocrine lab" and the "drug lab."

Serologic tests for hepatitis and HIV and assays for the evaluation of autoimmune diseases also moved from their traditional home in microbiology and immunology to chemistry analyzers. Immunoglobulin analysis followed a similar path. In certain countries, coagulation is considered part of clinical chemistry because the measurement of coagulation proteins uses similar instruments to those used in the clinical chemistry laboratory. As a result, the typical clinical chemistry laboratory includes testing for general chemistries, specific proteins and immunoglobulins, therapeutic and abused drugs, blood gases, hormones, biogenic amines, porphyrins, vitamins, and trace elements. Testing for inborn errors of metabolism (such as the measurements of amino acids and organic acids), measurements of coagulation factors, general hematologic testing, and serologic assays can belong either to the clinical chemistry laboratory or to another subspecialty, depending on the institution and country. If amino acids and organic acids are measured in the clinical chemistry laboratory, that does not preclude a biochemical geneticist from providing the clinical interpretation. Similar arguments can be made for coagulation, hematology, and serology testing.

Clinical laboratory professionals have embraced technology over the years and used it effectively to derive answers to clinical questions. In modern clinical laboratories, technologies include spectrophotometry, atomic absorption, cytometry, flame emission photometry, nephelometry, electrochemical, and optical sensor technologies, electrophoresis, and chromatography. The influence of automation, information technology, and miniaturization is evident in today's clinical laboratory. Mass spectrometry, once thought of as a research tool, is playing an ever-growing role in clinical chemistry for the measurement of both small molecules and peptides and more recently proteins. In fact, matrix-assisted laser desorption ionization time-of-flight (MALDI-TOF) mass spectrometry is now routinely used in the identification of microorganisms (including bacteria, mycobacteria and fungi), so it is likely that the evolution in this technology will also bring the clinical chemistry and microbiology laboratories closer. In addition, clinical microbiology laboratories are becoming increasingly automated, with total laboratory automation systems, including fluidic handling and high-resolution digital imaging systems, being adopted with increasing frequency.[14] Molecular diagnostics has forever changed virology and microbiology, introducing faster and more sensitive methods based on nucleic acid detection rather than microbial replication. Nanotechnology, microfluidics, electrical impedance, reflectance spectroscopy, and time-resolved fluorescence are only a few of the technologies used in point-of-care testing for proteins, drugs, DNA, and analysis of metabolites in small samples of whole blood. Point-of-care testing is a disruptive innovation that decentralizes laboratory testing and presents the clinical laboratory specialist with many challenges and opportunities. Molecular diagnostics in particular impacts diverse specialties, including infectious disease, genetics, and oncology, providing new tools for study at a molecular detail never before considered. In summary, the boundaries of laboratory medicine expand with technology, making the profession vibrant, interesting, and ever evolving.

The scope of the profession is constantly changing for the very same reasons. Scientific and technological developments, medical needs, patient demands, and economic pressures bring various disciplines of medicine closer together, and further integration of diagnostic and therapeutic disciplines is envisaged in the pursuit of more integrated and effective healthcare delivery. For example, companion diagnostics, which help predict therapeutic responses and individualize patient treatment options, bring together pharmacy and medical laboratories. Point-of-care testing and use of biomarker measurements in real time with medical interventions break the walls of laboratories and bring the profession closer to clinicians and patients. Integrated diagnostics (a term coined by the medical device industry), whereby in vitro laboratory technology is combined with in vivo imaging technology, intends to provide fully coordinated, interpreted, action-oriented results for managing patient conditions, *and* it places laboratory testing into an integrated patient care pathway (see an example at http://www.healthcare.siemens.com.au/clinical-specialities/reproductive-endocrinology/integrated-diagnostics). New disruptive technologies (e.g., "lab on a chip," nanotechnology, home monitoring) and movement toward patient empowerment and direct-to-consumer testing bring laboratory testing closer to patients. All of these developments present special challenges to the future generations of clinical laboratory specialists both in terms of how they should be trained and how they will have to practice.

Technology alone is not the answer to more effective clinical practice. There must be meaningful, clinically actionable results as a consequence of the data obtained. The generation of more data does not necessarily lead to better patient management. Some technology platforms are useful discovery tools, but seldom provide cost-effective diagnostic or prognostic information that changes patient care. In the 1960s and 1970s, with the advent of automated clinical analyzers, pathologists reported (and charged for) chemistry panels of 10 to 20 results. Many were later sued for excessive production of data that increased their income without commensurate value to patient care. More recently, dense data from expression arrays, genome-wide association studies, epigenomics, and microRNA analyses excel in discovery research, but translation to clinical practice has been slower than anticipated. The promise of greater clinical significance with larger data sets seems intuitive, but history suggests caution.

Clinical laboratorians in this world of "big data" translate high-quality measurement *data* into clinically relevant *information*. This information—when integrated with clinical history and presentation, clinical signs, and an understanding of pathophysiology—becomes *knowledge*. Knowledge, in the context of the experience and judgment of the clinician, is converted to *wisdom* that translates to clinical action for improved patient outcomes. For example, a 2-week-old boy with a suspected inborn error of metabolism had a suppressed thyroid stimulating hormone and increased free T_4 concentrations. Acting on the basis of the data alone would have suggested treatment with methimazole for thyrotoxicosis.

However, the patient was receiving biotin as part of his treatment for a metabolic disorder, and the biotin interfered with the immunoassays used in the thyroid function tests. Repeat measurement of these parameters with non–biotin-based immunoassays revealed a normal thyroid profile. Another example: A patient presented with Cushingoid appearance and a markedly decreased serum cortisol concentration. A further examination of his clinical history revealed that he was using topical corticosteroids for a skin condition, a treatment that caused adrenal suppression and thus a low cortisol concentration. Yet another example: A 55-year-old woman complained to her primary care physician about long-standing bony aches and pains. All results to exclude musculoskeletal problems came back normal except for a low alkaline phosphatase (ALP) enzyme activity. After excluding potential preanalytical errors [e.g., contamination of sample by K-EDTA (potassium ethylenediaminetetraacetic acid) anticoagulant], the laboratory proposed the diagnosis of hypophosphatasia, and testing for mutations of the tissue nonspecific ALP gene confirmed the diagnosis both in the patient and in her daughter. The world of laboratory medicine is full of such examples that demonstrate the value of acting on information beyond the generated numbers. Knowledge is what we must provide to clinicians to support informed clinical decision making and for achieving improved patient outcomes.

HOW IS LABORATORY MEDICINE PRACTICED?

Both the training of laboratory medicine professionals and their career paths are heterogeneous. Although the majority of our colleagues choose a career in a clinical laboratory environment, many work in the in vitro diagnostics (IVD) and pharmaceutical industries. Clinical laboratorians, by virtue of their training, are translational researchers who are equipped for and capable of developing, evaluating, and validating biochemical, cellular, and genetic assays for clinical use; they develop skills that are essential for new biomarker assays, reagent kits, and companion diagnostics. Laboratory medicine professionals also provide interfaces between researchers, clinicians, the clinical laboratory, and the IVD industry and help to translate biomarker research into clinically meaningful decisions and actions.

The functions of a clinical laboratorian include:
- Develop and validate de novo laboratory tests to meet clinical needs.
- Evaluate and characterize the analytical and clinical performance of laboratory tests.
- Present laboratory results to clinicians in an effective manner.
- Provide education and advice on the selection and interpretation of laboratory tests as part of the clinical team.
- Determine the cost-effectiveness and intrinsic value of laboratory tests.
- Participate in the development of clinical testing algorithms and clinical practice guidelines.
- Assure compliance with regulatory requirements.
- Participate in quality assurance and improvement of the laboratory service.
- Teach and train future generations of laboratory specialists.
- Participate in basic or clinical research.

Laboratory medicine specialists practicing in the IVD or the pharmaceutical industry may not need to routinely interact with clinicians or interpret laboratory results, but they understand and appreciate the clinical utility and relevance of the assays and companion diagnostics they are developing and thus contribute more effectively to the development of diagnostics that improve health. The daily practice of the profession has changed over time. In the 1960s and 1970s, clinical chemists, for example, developed laboratory tests. However, as the profession matured and the instrumentation changed from open systems to "black boxes" that relied on manufacturers for assays, the traditional analytical focus of the profession has significantly diminished. At present, de novo assay development is still active only in certain areas such as chromatography, mass spectrometry, and molecular diagnostics.

Laboratory medicine specialists are now more active in the preanalytical and postanalytical phases of testing and in establishing processes such as how best to select the right test for the right patient and to communicate test results to clinicians in a medically meaningful way, how to build laboratory processes that reduce error, and how to continuously improve the quality of laboratory practice. In today's healthcare environment, there is increasing emphasis on clinical impact and cost-effectiveness. Laboratories are expected to demonstrate evidence of improved measurable clinical outcomes and the usefulness and added value of tests to clinical decision making. Proving the fact that laboratory testing contributes to improved patient outcomes is challenging because the relationship between testing and clinical outcomes is mostly indirect. Nevertheless, laboratory medicine specialists should move away from being just providers of high-quality data. Transforming laboratory data to information and knowledge requires more skills in information and information management technology, evidence-based medicine, epidemiology, data mining, and translational research. It also requires a shift of thinking from essentialism to consequentialism and from technology-driven to customer-focused and patient-centered laboratory medicine.[15,16]

To summarize, today's clinical laboratorians are professionals who are trained in pathophysiology and technology. The execution of their daily duties, which are more clinically or technology oriented, is influenced by their training (such as MD vs. PhD), interests, institutional needs, and the country where they practice. Clearly the practice of our profession has evolved over the past half a century, and there are even more challenges on the horizon that will expand and change its scope and role and enhance its diversity.

GUIDING PRINCIPLES OF PRACTICING THE PROFESSION

As in all branches of medicine, practitioners in the clinical laboratory are faced with ethical issues, often on a daily basis; examples are listed in Box 1.1.

BOX 1.1 Ethical Issues in Laboratory Medicine

- Confidentiality of patient medical information
- Allocation of resources
- Codes of conduct
- Publishing issues
- Conflicts of interest

Confidentiality of Patient Information

Safeguarding the confidentiality of a patient's personal and medical information is one of the fundamental ethical principles of the practice of medicine. Upholding of these principles prescribes how some laboratory activities are practiced. The laboratory holds vast amounts of data covering a patient's identifiers and demographics, as well as health and disease status. The patient's morbid state and future risks for illnesses and death are conferred by such information. While laboratory information systems are built to facilitate timely access to the data, the data must be stored in a secure format with measures in place to prevent unwarranted access.

On the other hand, development of new tests requires the use of patient samples and access to patient medical information by the laboratory.[17] Ethical judgments are required regarding the type of informed consent that is needed from patients for use of their samples and clinical information. Clinical laboratory physicians and scientists often serve on institutional review boards that examine proposed research on human subjects. In these discussions, ethical concepts such as clinical equipoise (the genuine uncertainty in the expert medical community over whether a particular treatment or test will be beneficial) and preservation of confidentiality of medical information are central to these decisions.

Broad coverage genetic testing is becoming more of a routine affair. Prominent in the news in the first and second decades of this millennium has been the issue of confidentiality of genetic information. Legislation was considered necessary to prevent denial of health insurance or employment to people found by DNA testing to be at risk of disease. The power of DNA information lies in its heritability. Predictions can be made on the phenotypes and traits of a person's parents, relatives, and offspring based on an individual's DNA profile. In the event of having identified a clinically significant incidental finding, the right to personal confidentiality against the potential duty to disclose the information to at-risk family members is a current subject of debate among stakeholders. Clinical laboratory professionals are actively participating in the development of such disclosure and clinical management guidelines that will need to adapt to the changing standards of information disclosure or nondisclosure.

Allocation of Resources

Because resources are finite, clinical laboratory professionals must make ethically responsible decisions about allocation of resources. There is often a trade-off between cost and quality and/or speed (turnaround time). What is best for patients generally? How can the most good be done with the available resources?

Codes of Conduct

Most professional organizations publish a code of conduct that requires adherence by their members. For example, the American Association for Clinical Chemistry (AACC) has published ethical guidelines that require AACC members to endorse principles of ethical conduct in their professional activities, including (1) selection and performance of clinical procedures, (2) research and development, (3) teaching, (4) management, (5) administration, and (6) other forms of professional service. A similar code of conduct has been developed and approved by the EC4 Register Commission and the European Federation of Clinical Chemistry and Laboratory Medicine.[18]

Publishing Issues

Publication of documents having high scientific integrity depends on editors, authors, and reviewers all working in concert in an environment governed by high ethical standards.[19]

Editors are responsible for the overall process, including identifying reviewers, evaluating the reviews and the authors' response to them, and making the final decision of whether to accept or reject a manuscript. Editors are also responsible for establishing policies and procedures to assure consistency in the editorial process. Finally, the editor-in-chief is responsible for developing a conflict of interest policy and monitoring it among his or her editors. Publishers, being commercial or scientific societies, should monitor any conflicts of interest of the editor-in-chief.

Authors are responsible for honest and complete reporting of original data produced in ethically conducted research studies. Practices such as fraud, plagiarism (verbatim, mosaic), and falsification or fabrication of data (including image manipulation) are unacceptable. The International Committee of Medical Journal Editors (ICMJE)[20] and the Committee on Publication Ethics (COPE)[21] have published policies that address such behavior. Other practices to be avoided include duplicate publication, redundant publication, and inappropriate authorship credit. In addition, ethical policies require that factors potentially influencing the interpretation of study findings must be revealed, such as (1) the role of the commercial sponsor in the design and conduct of the study, (2) interpretation of results, and (3) preparation of the manuscript. Additional undesirable and harmful practices are publication bias and selective reporting in which only studies with positive findings are reported and authors use "data dredging" and meaningless subanalyses to find positive association rather than reporting the original hypothesis that was negative.[19] These practices inflate the actual value of observations or utility of markers and diminish the quality of meta-analyses. As a result, a comprehensive registry of diagnostic and prognostic studies, similar to the registry of clinical trials, has been advocated.[19,22,23]

To avoid publication of biased study results, reporting guidelines have been published for the main study types on the website of the EQUATOR Network (http://www.equator-network.org). For the laboratory profession, the STARD and TRIPOD statements for diagnostic and prognostic studies are probably the most important,[24,25] but reporting guidelines for randomized controlled trials (CONSORT), observational studies (STROBE), systematic reviews (PRISMA), quality improvement studies (SQUIRE), and economic evaluations (CHEERS) are also relevant for the work of laboratory scientists active in research and publication.

Reviewers must provide a timely, fair, and impartial assessment of manuscripts. They must maintain confidentiality and never contact the authors until after the publication of the report. Finally, reviewers must excuse themselves from the review process if they perceive a conflict of interest.

Most journals now require authors to complete conflict of interest forms and delineate each author's contribution. Some journals, including *Clinical Chemistry,* publish this information along with the article for enhanced transparency.

Conflicts of Interest

The interrelationships between practitioners in the medical field and commercial suppliers of drugs, devices, and equipment can be positive or negative.[26] Concerns led the National Institutes of Health in 1995 to require official institutional review of financial disclosure by researchers and management in situations when disclosure indicates potential or actual conflicts of interest. In 2009, the Institute of Medicine issued a report[27] that questioned inappropriate relationships between pharmaceutical device companies and physicians and other healthcare professionals.[26] Similarly, the relationship between clinical laboratory professionals and manufacturers and providers of diagnostic equipment and supplies has been scrutinized.

As a consequence of these concerns and as a result of the enactment of various laws designed to prevent fraud, abuse, and waste in Medicare, Medicaid, and other federal programs, professional organizations that represent manufacturers of IVD and other device and healthcare companies have published codes of ethics. For example, the Advanced Medical Technology Association (AdvaMed) has published a revised code of ethics that became effective on January 1, 2020.[28] Topics discussed in this revised code include gifts and entertainment, consulting arrangements and royalties, reimbursement for testing, and education. Similarly, MedTech Europe has recently published a code of ethics.[29] In this document, topics include member-sponsored product training and education, support for third-party educational conferences, sales and promotional meetings, arrangements and consultants, gifts, provision of reimbursements and other economic information, and donations for charitable and philanthropic purposes. Both the AdvaMed and the MedTech Europe documents address demands from regulators while nurturing the unique role that clinical chemists and other healthcare professionals play in developing and refining new technology.[26]

WHAT IS IN THIS TEXTBOOK?

In this textbook, we have assembled what is essential to effectively practice laboratory medicine. We begin with introductory chapters that describe the basics of laboratory medicine, including statistics, sample handling, preanalytical processes, reference intervals, quality management, quality control, standardization and harmonization, evidence-based laboratory medicine, biobanking, and biomarker and laboratory support for the pharmaceutical and IVD industries, machine learning, test utilization, and laboratory safety. This is followed by a section on analytical techniques and applications, including mass spectrometry and the specialized topics of microfabrication and microfluidics, cytometry, and point-of-care testing. Next, all the major analytes in clinical chemistry, including enzymes, tumor markers, therapeutic drugs, and many others are discussed. Pathophysiology, covering disease states and malfunction of different organ systems that correlate with abnormal laboratory findings follows. A section on genetic metabolic testing discussing newborn screening and inborn error of metabolism is next. This is followed by a section dedicated to molecular diagnostics, perhaps the fastest growing field in laboratory medicine. Then, there is a section discussing automated hematology and white and red blood cell morphologies, as well as hemostasis and coagulation. Following this is coverage of clinical microbiology including antimicrobial stewardship and infection prevention, infectious disease, antimicrobial susceptibility, bacteriology, virology, mycobacteriology, mycology, and parasitology. A transfusion medicine section then presents blood groups, blood components, indications for blood transfusion, and transfusion reactions. Finally, our last section focuses on clinical immunology including systemic autoimmune disease, transplantations, immunogenetics, allergy testing, immunogenicity of biologics, and primary and secondary immunodeficiencies. An appendix tabulates reference intervals for the clinical laboratory. The online version includes all of the above topics, whereas the print version is more selective to keep the tome manageable.

In addition to the above-mentioned chapters, the online version contains a wealth of other information including biochemical calculations, animation films to illustrate complex mechanisms, clinical cases, numerous atlases, podcasts, important documents, lecture series, adn adaptive learning courses.

This is an exciting time to be a laboratory medicine professional. Our aim in this book is to provide current scientific and practical knowledge to support laboratory professionals as a knowledge resource and an interface between science and technology on the one hand and the clinician and the patient on the other.

POINTS TO REMEMBER

- Laboratory medicine is a heterogeneous field with multiple disciplines including clinical chemistry, hematology and coagulation, clinical microbiology, molecular diagnostics, clinical immunology, and transfusion medicine.
- Laboratory medicine is a profession that has been shaped and defined by technology.
- Training of laboratory medicine specialists is heterogeneous and includes physicians and doctoral scientists in chemistry, pharmacy, biology, biochemistry, and microbiology.
- The role of clinical laboratory specialists evolved over time from analytically and technology focused to customer and patient centered.
- Clinical laboratory specialists are translational researchers who convert laboratory data to clinical knowledge.
- Career paths of clinical laboratory specialists are heterogeneous and include work in clinical laboratories and IVD and pharmaceutical industries.
- Clinical laboratory specialists must adhere to guiding principles of practicing the profession, which include maintaining confidentiality of medical information, using resources appropriately, abiding by codes of conduct, following ethical publishing rules, and managing and disclosing conflict of interest.

SELECTED REFERENCES

1. McMurray J, Zerah S, Hallworth M, et al. The European Register of Specialists in Clinical Chemistry and Laboratory Medicine: guide to the Register, version 3-2010. Clin Chem Lab Med 2010;48:999–1008.

3. Hallworth MJ. The "70% claim": what is the evidence base? Ann Clin Biochem 2011;48:487–8.

6. Young DS, Berwick MC, Jarett L. Evolution of the William Pepper Laboratory. Clin Chem 1997;43:174–9.

12. EU Directive 2013/55/EU. The recognition of professional qualifications. Proposing a common training framework for specialists in laboratory medicine across the European Union 2013. <http://www.ukipg.org.uk/meetings/international_and_european_forum/ctf_e4_bid>; 2013.

13. Jassam N, Lake J, Dabrowska M, Queralto J, Rizos D, Lichtinghagen R, et al. The European Federation of Clinical Chemistry and Laboratory Medicine syllabus for post graduate education and training for specialists in laboratory medicine: version 5-2018. Clin Chem Lab Med 2018;56:1846-63.

14. Bailey AL, Ledeboer N, Burnham CAD. Clinical microbiology is growing up: the total laboratory automation revolution. Clin Chem 2019;65:634-43.

15. Hallworth MJ, Epner PL, Ebert C, et al. Current evidence and future perspectives on the effective practice of patient-centered laboratory medicine. Clin Chem 2015;61(4):589–99.

17. Council of Europe. Additional protocol to the convention for the protection of human rights and dignity of the human being with regard to the application of biology and medicine on biomedical research. Law Hum Genome Rev 2004;21:201–14.

18. McMurray J, Zerah S, Hallworth M, et al. The European Register of Specialists in Clinical Chemistry and Laboratory Medicine: code of conduct, version 2—2008. Clin Chem 2009;47:372–5.

19. Annesley TM, Boyd JC, Rifai N, et al. Publication ethics: clinical chemistry editorial standards. Clin Chem 2009;55:1–4.

20. International Committee of Medical Journal Editors. Uniform requirements for manuscripts submitted to biomedical journals: writing and editing for biomedical publication. <http://www.icmje.org/recommendations/browse/manuscript-preparation/>.

21. Graf CWE, Bowman A, Fiack S, et al. Best practice guidelines on publication ethics: a publisher's perspective. Int J Clin Pract Suppl 2007;61:1–26.

22. Rifai N, Bossuyt PM, Ioannidis JP, et al. Registering diagnostic and prognostic trials of tests: is it the right thing to do? Clin Chem 2014;60:1146–52.

24. Bossuyt PM, Reitsma JB, Bruns DE, et al. The STARD statement for reporting studies of diagnostic accuracy: explanation and elaboration. Clin Chem 2003;49:7–18.

27. Institute of Medicine. Conflict of interest in medical research, education and practice. <http://www.nationalacademies.org/hmd/Reports/2009/Conflict-of-Interest-in-Medical-Research-Education-and-Practice.aspx>.

28. Advanced Medical Technology Association. Code of Ethics on interactions with health care professionals. https://www.advamed.org/sites/default/files/resource/advamed-code-of-ethics-2020.pdf.

29. European Diagnostics Manufacturers Association. Part A: interaction with health care professionals. https://www.medtecheurope.org/resource-library/medtech-europe-code-of-ethical-business-practice/.2019.

2

Statistical Methodologies in Laboratory Medicine
Analytical and Clinical Evaluation of Laboratory Tests

Kristian Linnet, Karel G.M. Moons, and James Clark Boyd

ABSTRACT

Background

The careful selection and evaluation of laboratory tests are key steps in the process of implementing new measurement procedures in the laboratory for clinical use. Method evaluation in the clinical laboratory is complex and in most countries is a regulated process guided by various professional recommendations and quality standards on best laboratory practice.

Content

This chapter deals with the statistical aspects of both analytical and clinical evaluations of laboratory assays, tests, or markers. After a short overview on basic statistics, aspects such as accuracy, precision, trueness, limit of detection, and selectivity are considered in the first part. After dealing with comparison of assays in detail, including using difference plots and regression analysis, the focus is on quantification of the (added) diagnostic value of laboratory assays or tests. First, the evaluation of tests in isolation is outlined, which corresponds to simple diagnostic scenarios, when only a single test result is decisive (e.g., in the screening context). Subsequently, the chapter addresses the more common clinical situation in which a laboratory assay or test is considered as part of a diagnostic workup and thus a test's added value is at issue. This involves use of receiver operating characteristic (ROC) areas, reclassification measures, predictiveness curves, and decision curve analysis. Finally, principles for considering the clinical impact of diagnostic tests on actual decision making and patient outcomes are discussed.

ASSAY SELECTION OVERVIEW

The introduction of new or revised laboratory tests, markers, or assays is a common occurrence in the clinical laboratory. Test selection and evaluation are key steps in the process of implementing new measurement procedures (Fig. 2.1). A new or revised test must be selected carefully and its analytical and clinical performance evaluated thoroughly before it is adopted for routine use in patient care (see later in this chapter and Chapter 10). Establishment of a new or revised laboratory test may also involve evaluation of the features of the automated analyzer on which the test will be implemented. When a new test is to be introduced to the routine clinical laboratory, a series of technical or analytical evaluations is commonly conducted. Assay imprecision is estimated, and comparison of the new assay versus an existing one is commonly undertaken. The allowable measurement range is assessed with estimation of the lower and upper limits of quantification. Interferences and carryover are evaluated when relevant. Depending on the situation, a limited verification of manufacturer claims may be all that is necessary, or, in the case of a newly developed test or assay, a full validation may be carried out. Subsequent subsections provide details for all these test evaluations. With regard to evaluation of reference intervals or medical decision limits, readers are referred to Chapter 9.

Evaluation of tests, markers, or assays in the clinical laboratory is influenced strongly by guidelines and accreditation or other regulatory standards.[1–3] The Clinical and Laboratory Standards Institute (CLSI, formerly the National Committee for Clinical Laboratory Standards [NCCLS]) has published a series of consensus protocols (Clinical Laboratory Improvement Amendments [CLIAs]) for clinical chemistry laboratories and manufacturers to follow when evaluating methods (see the CLSI website at http://www.clsi.org). The International Organization for Standardization (ISO) has also developed several documents related to method evaluation (ISOs). In addition, meeting laboratory accreditation requirements has become an important aspect in the evaluation process with accrediting agencies placing increased focus on the importance of total quality management and assessment of trueness and precision of laboratory measurements. An accompanying trend has been the emergence of an international nomenclature to standardize the terminology used for characterizing laboratory test or assay performance.

This chapter presents an overview of considerations in and methods for the evaluation of laboratory tests. This includes explanation of graphical and statistical methods that are used to aid in the test evaluation process; examples of the application of these methods are provided, and current terminology within the area is summarized. Key terms and abbreviations are listed in Box 2.1.

Medical Need and Quality Goals

The selection of the appropriate clinical laboratory assays is a vital part of rendering optimal patient care. Advances

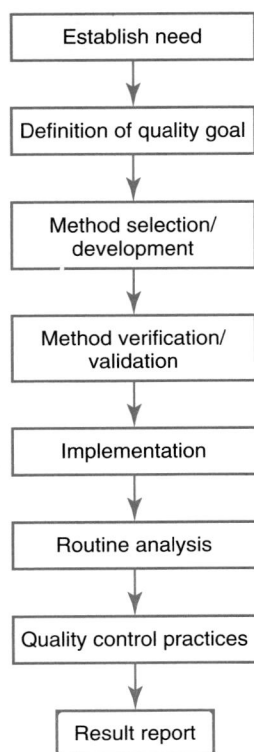

FIGURE 2.1 A flow diagram that illustrates the process of introducing a new assay into routine use.

in patient care are frequently based on the use of new or improved laboratory tests or measurements. Ascertainment of what is necessary clinically from a new or revised laboratory test is the first step in selecting the appropriate candidate test. Key parameters, such as desired turnaround time and necessary clinical utility for an assay, are often derived by discussions between laboratorians and clinicians. When new diagnostic assays are introduced, for example, reliable estimates of its diagnostic performance (e.g., predictive values, sensitivity and specificity) must be considered. With established analytes, a common scenario is the replacement of an older, labor-intensive test with a new, automated assay that is more economical in daily use. In these situations, consideration must be given to whether the candidate assay has sufficient precision, accuracy, analytical measurement range, and freedom from interference to provide clinically useful results (see Fig. 2.1).

Analytical Performance Criteria

In evaluation of a laboratory test, (1) trueness (formerly termed accuracy), (2) precision, (3) analytical range, (4) detection limit, and (5) analytical specificity are of prime importance. The sections in this chapter on laboratory test evaluation and comparison contain detailed outlines of these concepts. Estimated test performance parameters should be related to analytical performance specifications that ensure acceptable clinical use of the test and its results. For more details related to the recommended models for setting analytical performance specifications, readers are referred to Chapters 6 and 8. From a practical point of view, the "ruggedness" of the test in routine use is of importance and reliable performance, when used by different operators and with different batches of reagents over long time periods, is essential.

When a new laboratory analyzer is at issue, various instrumental parameters require evaluation, including (1) pipetting, (2) specimen-to-specimen carryover, (3) reagent lot-to-lot variation, (4) detector imprecision, (5) time to first reportable result, (6) onboard reagent stability, (7) overall throughput, (8) mean time between instrument failures, and (9) mean time to repair. Information on most of these parameters should be available from the instrument manufacturer; the manufacturer should also be able to furnish information on what studies should be conducted in estimating these parameters for an individual analyzer. Assessment of reagent lot-to-lot variation is especially difficult for a user, and the manufacturer should provide this information.

Other Criteria

Various categories of laboratory tests may be considered. New tests may require "in-house" development. (Note: Such a test is also referred to as a laboratory-developed test [LDT].) Commercial kit assays, on the other hand, are ready for implementation in the laboratory, often in a "closed" analytical system on a dedicated instrument. When prospective assays are reviewed, attention should be given to the following:

1. Principle of the test or assay, with original references
2. Detailed protocol for performing the test
3. Composition of reagents and reference materials, the quantities provided, and their storage requirements (e.g., space, temperature, light, humidity restrictions) applicable both before and after the original containers are opened
4. Stability of reagents and reference materials (e.g., their shelf lives)
5. Technologist time and required skills
6. Possible hazards and appropriate safety precautions according to relevant guidelines and legislation
7. Type, quantity, and disposal of waste generated
8. Specimen requirements (e.g., conditions for collection and transportation, specimen volume requirements, the necessity for anticoagulants and preservatives, necessary storage conditions)
9. Reference interval of the test and its results, including information on how such interval was derived, typical values obtained in both healthy and diseased individuals, and the necessity of determining a reference interval for one's own institution (see Chapter 9 for details on how to generate a reference interval of a laboratory test.)
10. Instrumental requirements and limitations
11. Cost-effectiveness
12. Computer platforms and interfacing with the laboratory information system
13. Availability of technical support, supplies, and service

Other questions concerning placement of the new or revised test in the laboratory should be taken into account. They include:

1. Does the laboratory possess the necessary measuring equipment? If not, is there sufficient space for a new instrument?
2. Does the projected workload match the capacity of a new instrument?
3. Is the test repertoire of a new instrument sufficient?
4. What is the method and frequency of (re)calibration?
5. Is staffing of the laboratory sufficient for the new technology?
6. If training the entire staff in a new technique is required, is such training worth the possible benefits?

BOX 2.1 **Abbreviations and Vocabulary Concerning Technical Validation of Assays**

Abbreviations

CI	Confidence interval
CV	Coefficient of variation (=SD/x, where x is the concentration)
CV%	= CV × 00%
CV_A	Analytical coefficient of variation
CV_G	Between-subject biological variation
CV_I	Within-subject biological variation
CV_{RB}	Sample-related random bias coefficient of variation
DoD	Distribution of differences (plot)
ISO	International Organization for Standardization
IUPAC	International Union of Pure and Applied Chemistry
OLR	Ordinary least-squares regression analysis
SD	Standard deviation
SEM	Standard error of the mean ($5SD/\sqrt{N}$)
SD_A	Analytical standard deviation
SD_{RB}	Sample-related random bias standard deviation
x_m	Mean
x_{mv}	Weighted mean
WLR	Weighted least-squares regression analysis

Vocabulary[a]

Analyte Compound that is measured.

Bias Difference between the average (strictly the expectation) of the test results and an accepted reference value (ISO 3534-1). Bias is a measure of trueness.[11]

Certified reference material (CRM) is a reference material, one or more of whose property values are certified by a technically valid procedure, accompanied by or traceable to a certificate or other documentation that is issued by a certifying body.

Commutability Ability of a material to yield the same results of measurement by a given set of measurement procedures.

Limit of detection The lowest amount of analyte in a sample that can be detected but not quantified as an exact value. Also called lower limit of detection or minimum detectable concentration (or dose or value).[23]

Lower limit of quantification (LLOQ) The lowest concentration at which the measurement procedure fulfills specifications for imprecision and bias (corresponds to the *lower limit of determination* mentioned under *Measuring interval*).

Matrix All components of a material system except the analyte.

Measurand The "quantity" that is actually measured (e.g., the concentration of the analyte). For example, if the analyte is glucose, the measurand is the concentration of glucose. For

an enzyme, the measurand may be the enzyme *activity* or the *mass concentration* of enzyme.

Measuring interval Closed interval of possible values allowed by a measurement procedure and delimited by the *lower limit of determination* and the *higher limit of determination*. For this interval, the total error of the measurements is within specified limits for the method. Also called the *analytical measurement range*.

Primary measurement standard Standard that is designated or widely acknowledged as having the highest metrologic qualities and whose value is accepted without reference to other standards of the same quantity.[73]

Quantity The amount of substance (e.g., the concentration of substance).

Random error Arises from unpredictable variations in influence quantities. These random effects give rise to variations in repeated observations of the measurand.

Reference material (RM) A material or substance, one or more properties of which are sufficiently well established to be used for the calibration of a method or for assigning values to materials.

Reference measurement procedure Thoroughly investigated measurement procedure shown to yield values having an uncertainty of measurement commensurate with its intended use, especially in assessing the trueness of other measurement procedures for the same quantity and in characterizing reference materials.

Selectivity or specificity Degree to which a method responds uniquely to the required analyte.

Systematic error A component of error that, in the course of a number of analyses of the same measurand, remains constant or varies in a predictable way.

Traceability "The property of the result of a measurement or the value of a standard whereby it can be related to stated references, usually national or international standards, through an unbroken chain of comparisons all having stated uncertainties."[43] This is achieved by establishing a chain of calibrations leading to primary national or international standards, ideally (for long-term consistency) the Système International (SI) units of measurement.

Uncertainty A parameter associated with the result of a measurement that characterizes the dispersion of values that could reasonably be attributed to the measurand. More briefly, *uncertainty* is a parameter characterizing the range of values within which the value of the quantity being measured is expected to lie.

Upper limit of quantification (ULOQ) The highest concentration at which the measurement procedure fulfills specifications for imprecision and bias (corresponds to the *upper limit of determination* mentioned under *Measuring interval*).

[a]A listing of terms of relevance in relation to analytical methods is displayed. Many of the definitions originate from Dybkær[12] with statement of original source where relevant (e.g., International Organization for Standardization document number). Others are derived from the Eurachem/Citac guideline on uncertainty.[79] In some cases, slight modifications have been performed for the sake of simplicity.

---

7. How frequently will quality control (QC) samples be run?
8. What materials will be used to ensure QC?
9. What approach will be used for proficiency testing?
10. What is the estimated cost of performing an assay using the proposed method, including the costs of calibrators, QC specimens, and technologists' time? Questions applicable to implementation of new instrumentation in a particular laboratory may also be relevant. Does the instrument satisfy local electrical safety guidelines? What are the power, water, drainage, and air conditioning requirements of the instrument? If the instrument is large, does the floor have sufficient load-bearing capacity?

A qualitative assessment of all these factors is often completed, but it is possible to use a value scale to assign points to the various features weighted according to their relative importance; the latter approach allows a more quantitative test evaluation process. Decisions are then made regarding the assays that best fit the laboratory's requirements and that have the potential for achieving the necessary analytical quality for clinical use.

BASIC STATISTICS

In this section, fundamental statistical concepts and techniques are introduced in the context of typical analytical investigations. The basic concepts of (1) populations, (2) samples, (3) parameters, (4) statistics, and (5) probability distributions are defined and illustrated. Two important probability distributions—Gaussian and Student *t*—are introduced and discussed.

Frequency Distribution

A graphical device for displaying a large set of laboratory test results is the *frequency distribution,* also called a *histogram.* Fig. 2.2 shows a frequency distribution displaying the results of serum gamma-glutamyltransferase (GGT) measurements of 100 apparently healthy 20- to 29-year-old men. The frequency distribution is constructed by dividing the measurement scale into cells of equal width; counting the number, n_i, of values that fall within each cell; and drawing a rectangle above each cell whose area (and height because the cell widths are all equal) is proportional to n_i. In this example, the selected cells were 5 to 9, 10 to 14, 15 to 19, 20 to 24, 25 to 29, and so on, with 60 to 64 being the last cell (range of values, 5 to 64 U/L). The ordinate axis of the frequency distribution gives the number of values falling within each cell. When this number is divided by the total number of values in the data set, the relative frequency in each cell is obtained.

Often, the position of the value for an individual within a distribution of values is useful medically. The *nonparametric* approach can be used to directly determine the *percentile* of a given subject. Having ranked N subjects according to their values, the *n*-percentile, $Perc_n$, may be estimated as the value of the $[N(n/100) + 0.5]$ ordered observation.[4] In the case of a noninteger value, interpolation is carried out between neighbor values. The 50th percentile is the median of the distribution.

Population and Sample

It is useful to obtain information and draw conclusions about the characteristics of the test results for one or more target populations. In the GGT example, interest is focused on the location and spread of the population of GGT values for 20- to 29-year-old healthy men. Thus a working definition of a *population* is the complete set of all observations that might occur as a result of performing a particular procedure according to specified conditions.

Most target populations of interest in clinical chemistry are in principle very large (millions of individuals) and so are impossible to study in their entirety. Usually a subgroup of observations is taken from the population as a basis for forming conclusions about population characteristics. The group of observations that has actually been selected from the population is called a *sample.* For example, the 100 GGT

values make up a sample from a respective target population. However, a sample is used to study the characteristics of a population only if it has been properly selected. For instance, if the analyst is interested in the population of GGT values over various lots of materials and some time period, the sample must be selected to be representative of these factors, as well as of age, sex, and health factors of the individuals in the targeted population. Consequently, exact specification of the target population(s) is necessary before a plan for obtaining the sample(s) can be designed. In this chapter, a sample is also used as a specimen, depending on the context.

Probability and Probability Distributions

Consider again the frequency distribution in Fig. 2.2. In addition to the general location and spread of the GGT determinations, other useful information can be easily extracted from this frequency distribution. For instance, 96% (96 of 100) of the determinations are less than 55 U/L, and 91% (91 of 100) are greater than or equal to 10 but less than 50 U/L. Because the cell interval is 5 U/L in this example, statements such as these can be made only to the nearest 5 U/L. A larger sample would allow a smaller cell interval and more refined statements. For a sufficiently large sample, the cell interval can be made so small that the frequency distribution can be approximated by a continuous, smooth curve, similar to that shown in Fig. 2.3. In fact, if the sample is large enough, we can consider this a close representation of the "true" target *population frequency distribution.* In general, the functional form of the population frequency distribution curve of a variable x is denoted by $f(x)$.

The population frequency distribution allows us to make probability statements about the GGT of a randomly selected member of the population of healthy 20- to 29-year-old men. For example, the probability $Pr(x > x_a)$ that the GGT value x of a randomly selected 20- to 29-year-old healthy man is greater than some particular value x_a is equal to the area under the population frequency distribution to the right of x_a. If $x_a = 58$, then from Fig. 2.3, $Pr(x > 58) = 0.05$. Similarly, the probability $Pr(x_a < x < x_b)$ that x is greater than x_a but less than x_b is equal to the area under the population frequency distribution between x_a and x_b. For example, if $x_a = 9$ and $x_b = 58$, then from Fig. 2.3, $Pr(9 < x < 58) = 0.90$. Because the population frequency distribution provides all information related to probabilities of a randomly selected member of the population, it is called the probability distribution of the population. Although the true probability distribution is never exactly known in practice, it can be approximated with a large sample of observations, that is, test results.

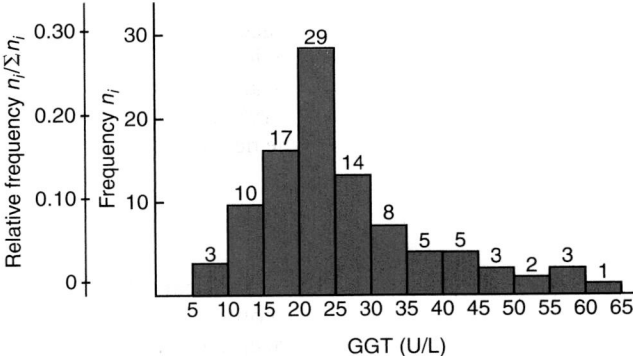

FIGURE 2.2 Frequency distribution of 100 gamma-glutamyltransferase *(GGT)* values.

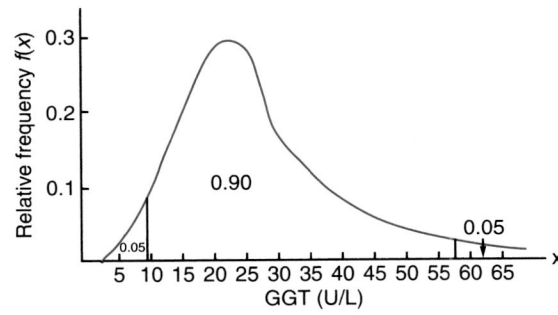

FIGURE 2.3 Population frequency distribution of gamma-glutamyltransferase *(GGT)* values.

Parameters: Descriptive Measures of a Population

Any population of values can be described by measures of its characteristics. A *parameter* is a constant that describes some particular characteristic of a population. Although most populations of interest in analytical work are infinite in size, for the following definitions, we shall consider the population to be of finite size N, where N is very large.

One important characteristic of a population is its *central location*. The parameter most commonly used to describe the central location of a population of N values is the *population mean* (μ):

$$\mu = \frac{\sum x_i}{N}$$

An alternative parameter that indicates the central tendency of a population is the *median*, which is defined as the 50th percentile, $Perc_{50}$.

Another important characteristic is the *dispersion* of values about the population mean. A parameter very useful in describing this dispersion of a population of N values is the *population variance* σ^2 (sigma squared):

$$\sigma^2 = \frac{\sum (x_i - \mu)^2}{N}$$

The *population standard deviation (SD)* σ, the positive square root of the population variance, is a parameter frequently used to describe the population dispersion in the same units (e.g., mg/dL) as the population values. For a Gaussian distribution, 95% of the population of values are located within the mean $\pm 1.96\ \sigma$. If a distribution is non-Gaussian (e.g., asymmetric), an alternative measure of dispersion based on the percentiles may be more appropriate, such as the distance between the 25th and 75th percentiles (the interquartile interval).

Statistics: Descriptive Measures of the Sample

As noted earlier, clinical chemists usually have at hand only a sample of observations (i.e., test results) from the overarching targeted population. A *statistic* is a value calculated from the observations in a sample to estimate a particular characteristic of the target population. As introduced earlier, the sample mean x_m is the arithmetical average of a sample, which is an estimate of μ. Likewise, the sample SD is an estimate of σ, and the coefficient of variation (CV) is the ratio of the SD to the mean multiplied by 100%. The equations used to calculate x_m, SD, and CV, respectively, are as follows:

$$x_m = \frac{\sum x_i}{N}$$

$$SD = \sqrt{\frac{\sum (x_i - x_m)^2}{N-1}} = \sqrt{\frac{\sum x_i^2 - \frac{\left(\sum x_i\right)^2}{N}}{N-1}}$$

$$CV = \frac{SD}{x_m} \times 100\%$$

where x_i is an individual measurement and N is the number of sample measurements.

The SD is an estimate of the dispersion of the distribution. Additionally, from the SD, we can derive an estimate of the uncertainty of x_m as an estimate of μ (see later discussion).

Random Sampling

A random sample of individuals from a target population is one in which each member of the population has an equal chance of being selected. A *random sample* is one in which each member of the sample can be considered to be a random selection from the target population. Although much of statistical analysis and interpretation depends on the assumption of a random sample from some population, actual data collection often does not satisfy this assumption. In particular, for sequentially generated data, it is often true that observations adjacent to each other tend to be more alike than observations separated in time.

The Gaussian Probability Distribution

The *Gaussian* probability distribution, illustrated in Fig. 2.4, is of fundamental importance in statistics for several reasons. As mentioned earlier, a particular test result x will not usually be equal to the true value μ of the specimen being measured. Rather, associated with this particular test result x will be a particular measurement error $\varepsilon = x - \mu$, which is the result of many contributing sources of error. Pure measurement errors tend to follow a probability distribution similar to that shown in Fig. 2.4, where the errors are symmetrically distributed, with smaller errors occurring more frequently than larger ones, and with an expected value of 0. This important fact is known as the central limit effect for distribution of errors: if a measurement error ε is the sum of many independent sources of error, such as $\varepsilon_1, \varepsilon_2, \ldots, \varepsilon_k$, several of which are major contributors, the probability distribution of the measurement error ε will tend to be Gaussian as the number of sources of error becomes large.

Another reason for the importance of the Gaussian probability distribution is that many statistical procedures are based on the assumption of a Gaussian distribution of values; this approach is commonly referred to as *parametric*. Furthermore, these procedures usually are not seriously invalidated by departures from this assumption. Finally, the magnitude of the uncertainty associated with sample statistics can be ascertained based on the fact that many sample statistics computed from large samples have a Gaussian probability distribution.

The Gaussian probability distribution is completely characterized by its mean μ and its variance σ^2. The notation

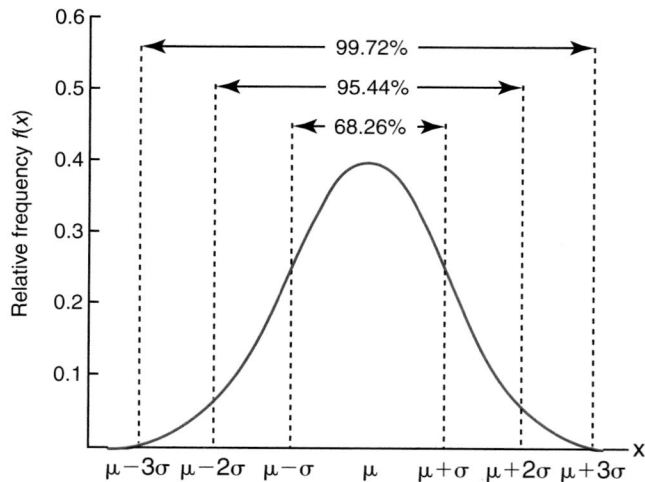

FIGURE 2.4 The Gaussian probability distribution.

$N(\mu, \sigma^2)$ is often used for the distribution of a variable that is Gaussian with mean μ and variance σ^2. Probability statements about a variable x that follows an $N(\mu, \sigma^2)$ distribution are usually made by considering the variable z,

$$z = \frac{x - \mu}{\sigma}$$

which is called the *standard Gaussian variable*. The variable z has a Gaussian probability distribution with $\mu = 0$ and $\sigma^2 = 1$, that is, z is $N(0, 1)$. The probably that x is within 2 σ of μ [i.e., $Pr(|x - \mu| < 2 \sigma) =$] is 0.9544. Most computer spreadsheet programs can calculate probabilities for all values of z.

Student *t* Probability Distribution

To determine probabilities associated with a Gaussian distribution, it is necessary to know the population SD σ. In actual practice, σ is often unknown, so we cannot calculate z. However, if a random sample can be taken from the Gaussian population, we can calculate the sample SD, substitute SD for σ, and compute the value t:

$$t = \frac{x - \mu}{SD}$$

Under these conditions, the variable t has a probability distribution called the *Student* t *distribution*. The t distribution is really a family of distributions depending on the degrees of freedom (df) ν ($= N - 1$) for the sample SD. Several t distributions from this family are shown in Fig. 2.5. When the size of the sample and the df for SD are infinite, there is no uncertainty in SD, so the t distribution is identical to the standard Gaussian distribution. However, when the sample size is small, the uncertainty in SD causes the t distribution to have greater dispersion and heavier tails than the standard Gaussian distribution, as illustrated in Fig. 2.5. At sample sizes above 30, the difference between the t-distribution and the Gaussian distribution becomes relatively small and can usually be neglected. Most computer spreadsheet programs can calculate probabilities for all values of t, given the df for SD.

The Student t distribution is commonly used in significance tests, such as comparison of sample means, or in testing conducted if a regression slope differs significantly from 1. Descriptions of these tests can be found in statistics textbooks.[5] Another important application is the estimation of confidence intervals (CIs). CIs are intervals that indicate the uncertainty of a given sample estimate. For example, it can be

proved that $X_m \pm t_{alpha}$ $(SD/N^{0.5})$ provides an approximate $2alpha$-CI for the mean. A common value for *alpha* is 0.025 or 2.5%, which thus results in a 0.95% or 95% CI. Given sample sizes of 30 or higher, t_{alpha} is ca. 2. $(SD/N^{0.5})$ is called the standard error (SE) of the mean. A CI should be interpreted as follows. Suppose a sampling experiment of drawing 30 observations from a Gaussian population of values is repeated 100 times, and in each case, the 95% CI of the mean is calculated as described. Then, in 95% of the drawings, the true mean μ is included in the 95% CI. The popular interpretation is that for an estimated 95% CI, there is 95% chance that the true mean is within the interval. According to the central limit theorem, distributions of mean values converge toward the Gaussian distribution irrespective of the primary type of distribution of x. This means that the 95% CI is a robust estimate only minimally influenced by deviations from the Gaussian distribution. In the same way, the t-test is robust toward deviations from normality.

Nonparametric Statistics

Distribution-free statistics, often called nonparametric statistics, provides an alternative to parametric statistical procedures that assume data to have Gaussian distributions. For example, distributions of reference values are often skewed and so do not conform to the Gaussian distribution (see Chapter 9 on reference intervals). Formally, one can carry out a goodness of fit test to judge whether a distribution is Gaussian or not.[5] A commonly used test is the Kolmogorov-Smirnov test, in which the shape of the sample distribution is compared with the shape presumed for a Gaussian distribution. If the difference exceeds a given critical value, the hypothesis of a Gaussian distribution is rejected, and it is then appropriate to apply nonparametric statistics. A special problem is the occurrence of outliers (i.e., single measurements highly deviating from the remaining measurements). Outliers may rely on biological factors and so be of real significance (e.g., in the context of estimating reference intervals or be related to clerical errors). Special tests exist for handling outliers.[5]

Given that a distribution is non-Gaussian, it is appropriate to apply nonparametric descriptive statistics based on the percentile or quantile concept. As stated under the earlier section Frequency Distribution, the n-percentile, $Perc_n$, of a sample of N values may be estimated as the value of the $[N(n/100) + 0.5]$ ordered observation.[4] In the case of a non-integer value, interpolation is carried out between neighbor values. The median is the 50th percentile, which is used as a measure of the center of the distribution. For the GGT example mentioned previously, we would order the $N = 100$ values according to size. The median or 50th percentile is then the value of the $[100(50/100) + 0.5 = 50.5]$ ordered observation (the interpolated value between the 50th and 51st ordered values). The 2.5th and 97.5th percentiles are values of the $[100(2.5/100) + 0.5 = 3]$ and $[100(97.5/100) + 0.5 = 98]$ ordered observations, respectively. When a 95% reference interval is estimated, a nonparametric approach is often preferable because many distributions of reference values are asymmetric. Generally, distributions based on the many biological sources of variation are often non-Gaussian compared with distributions of pure measurement errors that usually are Gaussian.

The nonparametric counterpart to the t-test is the Mann-Whitney test, which provides a significance test for the difference

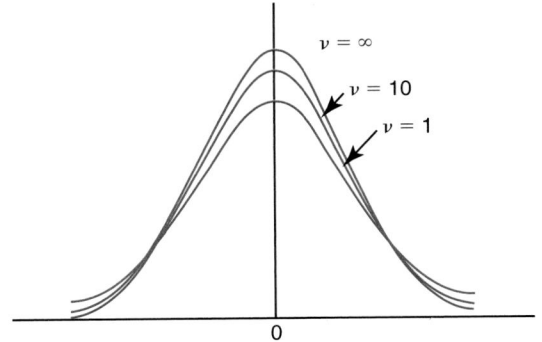

FIGURE 2.5 The t distribution for $\nu = 1$, 10, and ∞.

between median values of the two groups to be compared.[5] When there are more than two groups, the Kruskal-Wallis test can be applied.[5]

Categorical Variables

Hitherto focus has been on quantitative variables. When dealing with qualitative tests and in the context of evaluating diagnostic testing, categorical variables that only take the value positive or negative come into play. The performance is here given as proportions or percentages, which are proportions multiplied by 100. For example, the diagnostic sensitivity of a test is the proportion of diseased subjects who have a positive result. Having tested, for example, 100 patients, 80 might have had a positive test result. The sensitivity then is 0.8 or 80%. We are then interested in judging how precise this estimate is. Exact estimates of the uncertainty can be derived from the so-called binomial distribution, but for practical purposes, an approximate expression for the 95% CI is usually applied as the estimated proportion $P \pm 2SE$, where the SE in this context is derived as:

$$SE = [P(1 - P)/N]^{0.5}$$

where P is here a proportion and not a percentage.[5] In the example, the SE equals 0.0016 and so the 95% CI is 0.77 to 0.83 or 77 to 83%. The applied approximate formula for the SE is regarded as reasonably valid when NP and $N(1 - P)$ both are equal to or higher than 5.

POINTS TO REMEMBER

- Statistics as means, SDs, percentiles, proportions, and so on are computed from a sample of values drawn from a population and provide *estimates* of the unknown population characteristics.
- Whereas parametric statistics rely on the assumption of a Gaussian population of values, which typically applies for measurement errors, nonparametric statistics is a distribution-free approach that apply to, for example, asymmetric distributions often observed for biologic variables.
- The Gaussian distribution is characterized by the mean and the SD, and other types of distributions are described by the median and the percentile (quantile) values.
- Distributions of categorical variables are characterized by proportions or percentages and their SEs.

TECHNICAL VALIDITY OF ANALYTICAL ASSAYS

This section defines the basic concepts used in this chapter: (1) calibration, (2) trueness and accuracy, (3) precision, (4) linearity, (5) limit of detection (LOD), (6) limit of quantification, (7) specificity, and (8) others (see Box 2.1 for definitions).

Calibration

The calibration function is the relation between instrument signal (y) and concentration of analyte (x), that is,

$$y = f(x)$$

The inverse of this function, also called the measuring function, yields the concentration from response:

$$x = f^{-1}(y)$$

This relationship is established by measurement of samples with known quantities of analyte[6] (calibrators). One may distinguish between solutions of pure chemical standards and samples with known quantities of analyte present in the typical matrix that is to be measured (e.g., human serum). The first situation applies typically to a reference measurement procedure that is not influenced by matrix effects; the second case corresponds typically to a routine method that often is influenced by matrix components and so preferably is calibrated using the relevant matrix.[7] Calibration functions may be linear or curved and, in the case of immunoassays, may often take a special form (e.g., modeled by the four-parameter logistic curve).[8] This model (logistic in log x) has been used for immunoassay techniques and is written in several forms (Table 2.1). An alternative, model-free approach is to estimate a smoothed spline curve, which often is performed for immunoassays; however, a disadvantage of the spline curve approach is that it is insensitive to aberrant calibration values, fitting these just as well as the correct values. If the assumed calibration function does not correctly reflect the true relationship between instrument response and analyte concentration, a systematic error or bias is likely to be associated with the analytical method. A common problem with some immunoassays is the "hook effect," which is a deviation from the expected calibration algorithm in the high-concentration range. (The hook effect is discussed in more detail in Chapter 26.)

The precision of the analytical method depends on the stability of the instrument response for a given quantity of analyte. In principle, a random dispersion of instrument signal (vertical direction) at a given true concentration transforms into dispersion on the measurement scale (horizontal direction), as is shown schematically (Fig. 2.6). The detailed statistical aspects of calibration are complex,[5,9] but in the following sections, some approximate relations are outlined. If the calibration function is linear and the imprecision of the signal response is the same over the analytical measurement range, the analytical SD (SD_A) of the method tends to be constant over the analytical measurement range (see Fig. 2.6). If the imprecision increases proportionally to the signal response, the analytical SD of the method tends to increase proportionally to the concentration (x), which means that the *relative* imprecision ($CV = SD/x$) may be constant over the analytical measurement range if it is assumed that the intercept of the calibration line is zero.

With modern, automated clinical chemistry instruments, the relation between analyte concentration and signal can in some cases be very stable, and where this is the case, calibration is necessary relatively infrequently[10] (e.g., at intervals of

---

TABLE 2.1 The Four-Parameter Logistic Model Expressed in Three Different Forms

Algebraic Form	Variables[a]	Parameters[b]
$y = (a - d)/[1 + (x/c)^b] + d$	(x, y)	a, b, c, d
$R = R_0 +$ $K_c/[1 + \exp(-\{a + b \log[C]\})]$	(C, R)	R_0, K_c, a, b
$y = y_0 + (y_* - y_0)(x^d)/(b + x^d)$	(x, y)	y_0, y_*, b, d

[a]Concentration and instrument response variables shown in parentheses.

[b]Equivalent letters do not necessarily denote equivalent parameters.

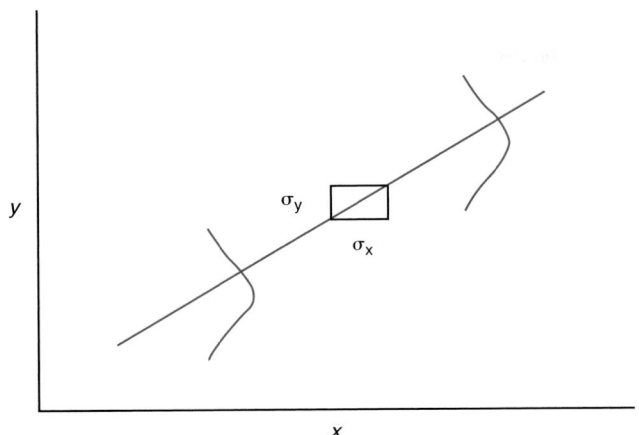

FIGURE 2.6 Relation between concentration *(x)* and signal response *(y)* for a linear calibration function. The dispersion in signal response (σ_y) is projected onto the *x*-axis and is called assay imprecision $[\sigma_x\,(=\sigma_A)]$.

TABLE 2.2 An Overview of Qualitative Terms and Quantitative Measures Related to Method Performance	
Qualitative Concept	**Quantitative Measure**
Trueness	Bias
Closeness of agreement of mean value with "true value"	A measure of the systematic error
Precision	Imprecision (SD)
Repeatability (within run)	A measure of the
Intermediate precision (long term)	dispersion of random
Reproducibility (inter-laboratory)	errors
Accuracy	*Error of measurement*
Closeness of agreement of a single measurement with "true value"	Comprises both random and systematic influences

SD, Standard deviation.

several months). Built-in process control mechanisms may help ensure that the relationship remains stable and may indicate when recalibration is necessary. In traditional chromatographic analysis (e.g., high-performance liquid chromatography [HPLC]), on the other hand, it is customary to calibrate each analytical series (run), which means that calibration is carried out daily.

Trueness and Accuracy

Trueness of measurements is defined as closeness of agreement between the average value obtained from a large series of results of measurements and the true value.[11]

The difference between the average value (strictly, the mathematical expectation) and the true value is the *bias,* which is expressed numerically and so is inversely related to the trueness. *Trueness* in itself is a qualitative term that can be expressed, for example, as low, medium, or high. From a theoretical point of view, the exact true value for a clinical sample is not available; instead, an "accepted reference value" is used, which is the "true" value that can be determined in practice.[12] Trueness can be evaluated by comparison of measurements by the new test and by some preselected reference measurement procedure, both on the same sample or individuals.

The ISO has introduced the trueness expression as a replacement for the term *accuracy,* which now has gained a slightly different meaning. *Accuracy* is the closeness of agreement between the result of a measurement and a true concentration of the analyte.[11] Accuracy thus is influenced by both bias and imprecision and in this way reflects the total error. Accuracy, which in itself is a qualitative term, is inversely related to the "uncertainty" of measurement, which can be quantified as described later (Table 2.2).

In relation to trueness, the concepts *recovery, drift,* and *carryover* may also be considered. *Recovery* is the fraction or percentage increase in concentration that is measured in relation to the amount added. Recovery experiments are typically carried out in the field of drug analysis. One may distinguish between *extraction recovery,* which often is interpreted as the fraction of compound that is carried through an extraction process, and the recovery measured by the entire analytical procedure, in which the addition of an internal standard compensates for losses in the extraction procedure. A recovery close to 100% is a prerequisite for a high degree of trueness, but it does not ensure unbiased results because possible nonspecificity against matrix components (e.g., an interfering substance) is not detected in a recovery experiment. *Drift* is caused by instrument or reagent instability over time, so that calibration becomes gradually biased. Assay *carryover* also must be close to zero to ensure unbiased results. Carryover can be assessed by placing a sample with a known, low value after a pathological sample with a high value, and an observed increase can be stated as a percentage of the high value.[13] Drift or carryover or both may be conveniently estimated by multifactorial evaluation protocols (EPs).[14,15]

Precision

Precision has been defined as the closeness of agreement between independent replicate measurements obtained under stipulated conditions.[12] The degree of precision is usually expressed on the basis of statistical measures of imprecision, such as SD or CV (CV = SD/*x*, where *x* is the measurement concentration), which is inversely related to precision. Imprecision of measurements is solely related to the random error of measurements and has no relation to the trueness of measurements.

Precision is specified as follows[11,12]:

Repeatability: closeness of agreement between results of successive measurements carried out under the same conditions (i.e., corresponding to within-run precision)

Reproducibility: closeness of agreement between results of measurements performed under changed conditions of measurements (e.g., time, operators, calibrators, reagent lots). Two specifications of reproducibility are often used: total or between-run precision in the laboratory, often termed *intermediate precision,* and interlaboratory precision (e.g., as observed in external quality assessment schemes [EQAS]) (see Table 2.2).

The total SD (σ_T) may be divided into within-run and between-run components using the principle of analysis of variance of components[5] (variance is the squared SD):

$$\sigma^2 T = \sigma^2{}_{Within-run} + \sigma^2{}_{Between-run}$$

It is not always clear in clinical chemistry publications what is meant by "between-run" variation. Some authors use the term to refer to the total variation of an assay, but others apply the term *between-run variance component* as defined earlier. The distinction between these definitions is important but is not always explicitly stated.

In laboratory studies of analytical variation, estimates of imprecision are obtained. The more observations, the more certain are the estimates. It is important to have an adequate number so that that analytical variation is not underestimated. Commonly, the number 20 is given as a reasonable number of observations (e.g., suggested in the CLSI guideline for manufacturers).[16] To verify method precision by users, it has been recommended to run internal QC samples for five consecutive days in five replicates.[17] If too few replications are applied, it is likely that the analytical variation will be underestimated.

To estimate both the within-run imprecision and the total imprecision, a common approach is to measure duplicate control samples in a series of runs. Suppose, for example, that a control is measured in duplicate for 20 runs, in which case 20 observations are present with respect to both components. The dispersion of the means (x_m) of the duplicates is given as follows:

$$\sigma_{x_m}^2 = \sigma_{\text{Within-run}}^2 / 2 + \sigma_{\text{Between-run}}^2$$

From the 20 sets of duplicates, we may derive the within-run SD using the following formula:

$$\text{SD}_{\text{Within-run}} = \left[\sum d_i^2 \Big/ (2 \times 20) \right]^{0.5}$$

where d_i refers to the difference between the *i*th set of duplicates. When SDs are estimated, the concept df is used. In a simple situation, the number of df equals $N - 1$. For N duplicates, the number of df is $N(2 - 1) = N$. Thus both variance components are derived in this way. The advantage of this approach is that the within-run estimate is based on several runs, so that an average estimate is obtained rather than only an estimate for one particular run if all 20 observations had been obtained in the same run. The described approach is a simple example of a *variance component analysis*. The principle can be extended to more components of variation. For example, in the CLSI EP05-A3 guideline,[16] a procedure is outlined that is based on the assumption of two analytical runs per day, in which case within-run, between-run, and between-day components of variance are estimated by a *nested* component of variance analysis approach.

Nothing definitive can be stated about the selected number of 20. Generally, the estimate of the imprecision improves as more observations become available. Exact confidence limits for the SD can be derived from the χ^2 distribution. Estimates of the variance, SD^2, are distributed according to the χ^2 distribution (tabulated in most statistics textbooks) as follows: $(N-1)\,\text{SD}^2/\sigma^2 \approx \chi^2_{(N-1)}$, where $(N-1)$ is the df.[5] Then the two-sided 95% CI is derived from the following relation:

$$\Pr\left[\chi^2_{97.5\%(N-1)} < (N-1)\text{SD}^2/\sigma^2 < \chi^2_{2.5\%(N-1)} \right] = 0.95$$

which yields this 95% CI expression:

$$\text{SD} \times \left[(N-1)\Big/ \chi^2_{2.5\%(N-1)} \right]^{0.5} < \sigma < \text{SD} \times \left[(N-1)\Big/ \chi^2_{97.5\%(N-1)} \right]^{0.5}$$

Example

Suppose we have estimated the imprecision as an SD of 5.0 on the basis of $N = 20$ observations. From a table of

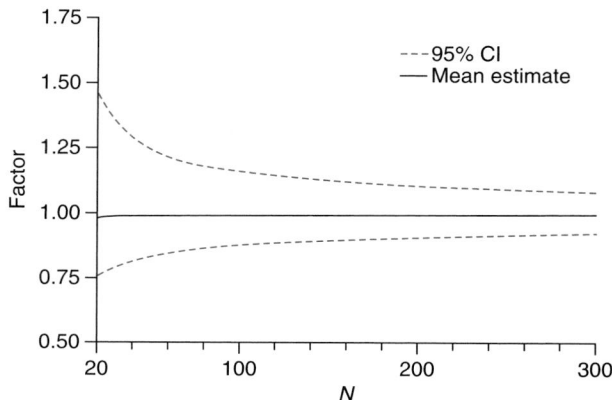

FIGURE 2.7 Relation between factors indicating the 95% confidence intervals *(CIs)* of standard deviations (SDs) and the sample size. The true SD is 1, and the solid line indicates the mean estimate, which is slightly downward biased at small sample sizes.

the χ^2 distribution, we obtain the following 2.5 and 97.5 percentiles:

$$\chi^2_{2.5\%(19)} = 32.9 \text{ and } \chi^2_{97.5\%(19)} = 8.91$$

where 19 within the parentheses refers to the number of df. Substituting in the equation, we get

$$5.0 \times (19/32.9)^{0.5} < \sigma < 5.0 \times (19/8.91)^{0.5}$$

or

$$3.8 < \sigma < 7.3$$

A graphical display of 95% CIs at various sample sizes is shown in Fig. 2.7. For individual variance components, the relations are more complicated.

Precision Profile

Precision often depends on the concentration of analyte being considered. A presentation of precision as a function of analyte concentration is the precision profile, which usually is plotted in terms of the SD or the CV as a function of analyte concentration (Fig. 2.8). Some typical examples may be considered. First, the SD may be constant (i.e., independent of the concentration), as it often is for analytes with a limited range of values (e.g., electrolytes). When the SD is constant, the CV varies inversely with the concentration (i.e., it is high in the lower part of the range and low in the high range). For analytes with extended ranges (e.g., hormones), the SD frequently increases as the analyte concentration increases. If a proportional relationship exists, the CV is constant. This may often apply approximately over a large part of the analytical measurement range. Actually, this relationship is anticipated for measurement error that arises because of imprecise volume dispensing. Often a more complex relationship exists. Not infrequently, the SD is relatively constant in the low range, so that the CV increases in the area approaching the lower limit of quantification (LLOQ). At intermediate concentrations, the CV may be relatively constant and perhaps may decline somewhat at increasing concentrations. A square root relationship can be used to model the relationship in some situations as an intermediate form of relation between the constant and the proportional case. The relationship between the SD and the concentration is of importance (1) when method specifications over the analytical measurement

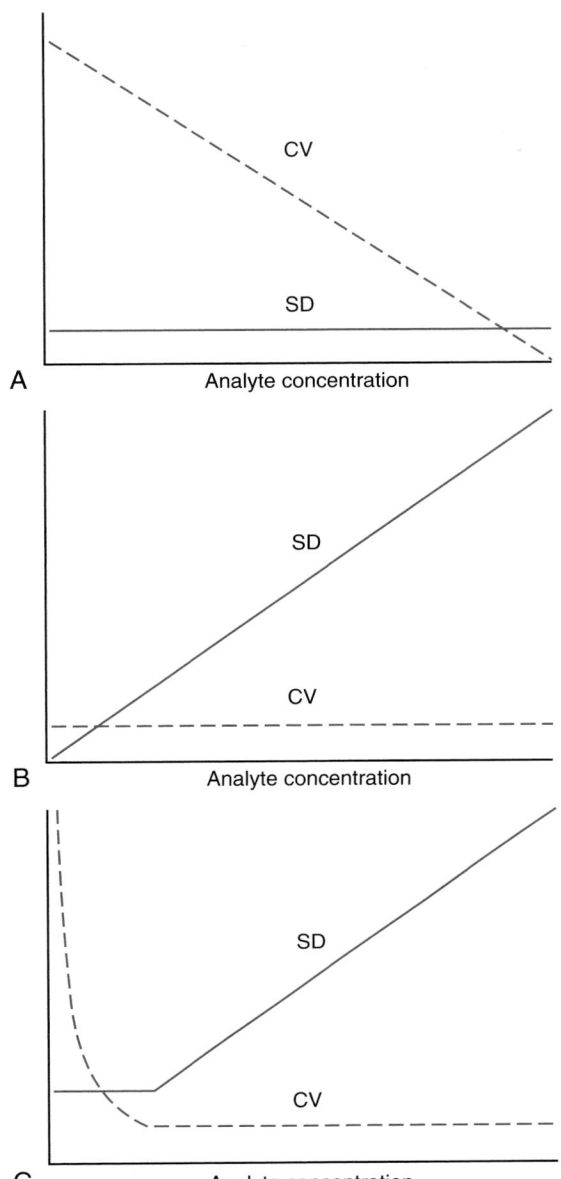

FIGURE 2.8 Relations between analyte concentration and standard deviation *(SD)*/coefficient of variation *(CV)*. **A,** The SD is constant, so that the CV varies inversely with the analyte concentration. **B,** The CV is constant because of a proportional relationship between concentration and SD. **C,** A mixed situation with constant SD in the low range and a proportional relationship in the rest of the analytical measurement range.

range are considered, (2) when limits of quantification are determined, and (3) in the context of selecting appropriate statistical methods for method comparison (e.g., whether a difference or a relative difference plot should be applied, whether a simple or a weighted regression analysis procedure should be used) (see the "Relative Distribution of Differences Plot" and "Regression Analysis" sections later).

Linearity

Linearity refers to the relationship between measured and expected values over the analytical measurement range. Linearity may be considered in relation to actual or relative analyte concentrations. In the latter case, a dilution series of a sample may be examined. This dilution series examines whether the measured concentration changes as expected according to the proportional relationship between samples introduced by the dilution factor. Dilution is usually carried out with an appropriate sample matrix (e.g., human serum [individual or pooled serum] or a verified sample diluent).

Evaluation of linearity may be conducted in various ways. A simple, but subjective, approach is to visually assess whether the relationship between measured and expected concentrations is linear. A more formal evaluation may be carried out on the basis of statistical tests. Various principles may be applied here. When repeated measurements are available at each concentration, the random variation between measurements and the variation around an estimated regression line may be evaluated statistically[18] (by an *F*-test). This approach has been criticized because it relates only the magnitudes of random and systematic error without taking the absolute deviations from linearity into account. For example, if the random variation among measurements is large, a given deviation from linearity may not be declared statistically significant. On the other hand, if the random measurement variation is small, even a very small deviation from linearity that may be clinically unimportant is declared significant. When significant nonlinearity is found, it may be useful to explore nonlinear alternatives to the linear regression line (i.e., polynomials of higher degrees).[19]

Another commonly applied approach for detecting nonlinearity is to assess the residuals of an estimated regression line and test whether positive and negative deviations are randomly distributed. This can be carried out by a runs test (see "Regression Analysis" section).[20] An additional consideration for evaluating proportional concentration relationships is whether an estimated regression line passes through zero or not. The presence of linearity is a prerequisite for a high degree of trueness. A CLSI guideline suggests procedure(s) for assessment of linearity.[21]

Analytical Measurement Range and Limits of Quantification

The analytical measurement range (measuring interval, reportable range) is the analyte concentration range over which measurements are within the declared tolerances for imprecision and bias of the method.[12] Taking drug assays as an example, there exist (arbitrary) requirements of a CV% of less than 15% and a bias of less than 15%.[22] The measurement range then extends from the lowest concentration (LLOQ) to the highest concentration (upper limit of quantification [ULOQ]) for which these performance specifications are fulfilled.

The LLOQ is medically important for many analytes. Thyroid-stimulating hormone (TSH) is a good example. As assay methods improved, lowering the LLOQ, low TSH results could be increasingly distinguished from the lower limit of the reference interval, making the test increasingly useful for the diagnosis of hyperthyroidism.

The LOD is another characteristic of an assay. The LOD may be defined as the lowest value that confidently exceeds the measurements of a blank sample. Thus the limit has been estimated on the basis of repeated measurements of a blank sample and has been *reported* as the mean plus 2 or 3 SDs of the blank measurements. In the interval from LOD up to LLOQ, one should report a result as "detected" but not provide a quantitative result. More complicated approaches for estimation of the LOD have been suggested.[23]

Analytical Sensitivity

The LLOQ of an assay should not be confused with analytical sensitivity. That is defined as ability of an analytical method to assess small differences in the concentration of analyte.[6] The smaller the random variation of the instrument response and the steeper the slope of the calibration function at a given point, the better is the ability to distinguish small differences in analyte concentrations. In reality, analytical sensitivity depends on the precision of the method. The smallest difference that will be statistically significant equals $2\sqrt{2}$ SD_A at a 5% significance level. Historically, the meaning of the term *analytical sensitivity* has been the subject of much discussion.

Analytical Specificity and Interference

Analytical specificity is the ability of an assay procedure to determine the concentration of the target analyte without influence from potentially interfering substances or factors in the sample matrix (e.g., hyperlipemia, hemolysis, bilirubin, antibodies, other metabolic molecules, degradation products of the analyte, exogenous substances, anticoagulants). Interferences from hyperlipemia, hemolysis, and bilirubin are generally concentration dependent and can be quantified as a function of the concentration of the interfering compound.[24] In the context of a drug assay, specificity in relation to drug metabolites is relevant, and in some cases, it is desirable to measure the parent drug, as well as metabolites. A detailed protocol for evaluation of interference has been published by the CLSI.[25]

POINTS TO REMEMBER

- Technical validation of analytical methods focuses on (1) calibration, (2) trueness and accuracy, (3) precision, (4) linearity, (5) LOD, (6) limit of quantification, (7) specificity, and (8) others.
- The difference between the average measured value and the true value is the *bias*, which can be evaluated by comparison of measurements by the new test and by some preselected reference measurement procedure, both on the same sample or individuals.
- The degree of precision is usually expressed on the basis of statistical measures of imprecision, such as SD or CV ($CV = SD/x$, where x is the measurement concentration).
- The measurement range extends from the lowest concentration (LLOQ) to the highest concentration (ULOQ) for which the analytical performance specifications are fulfilled (imprecision, bias).
- Analytical specificity is the ability of an assay procedure to determine the concentration of the target analyte without influence from potentially interfering substances or factors in the sample matrix.

QUALITATIVE METHODS

Qualitative methods, which currently are gaining increased use in the form of point-of-care testing (POCT), are designed to distinguish between results below and above a predefined cutoff value. Note that the cutoff point should not be confused

with the detection limit. These tests are assessed primarily on the basis of their ability to correctly classify results in relation to the cutoff value.

Diagnostic Accuracy Measures

The probability of classifying a result as positive (exceeding the cutoff) when the true value indeed exceeds the cutoff is called *sensitivity*. The probability of classifying a result as negative (below the cutoff) when the true value indeed is below the cutoff is termed *specificity*. Determination of sensitivity and specificity is based on comparison of test results with a gold standard. The gold standard may be an independent test that measures the same analyte, but it may also be a clinical diagnosis determined by definitive clinical methods (e.g., radiographic testing, follow-up, outcomes analysis). Determination of these performance measures is covered later on in the diagnostic testing part. Sensitivity and specificity may be given as a fraction or as a percentage after multiplication by 100. SEs of estimates are derived as described for categorical variables. The performance of two qualitative tests applied in the same groups of nondiseased and diseased subjects can be compared using the McNemar's test, which is based on a comparison of paired values of true and false-positive (FP) or false-negative (FN) results.[26]

One approach for determining the recorded performance of a test in terms of sensitivity and specificity is to determine the true concentration of analyte using an independent reference method. The closer the concentration is to the cutoff point, the larger the error frequencies are expected to be. Actually, the cutoff point is defined in such a way that for samples having a true concentration exactly equal to the cutoff point, 50% of results will be positive, and 50% will be negative.[27] Concentrations above and below the cutoff point at which repeated results are 95% positive or 95% negative, respectively, have been called the "95% interval" for the cutoff point for that method, which indicates a grey zone where the test does not provide reliable results (Fig. 2.9).[27,28]

Agreement Between Qualitative Tests

As outlined previously, if the outcome of a qualitative test can be related to a true analyte concentration or a definitive

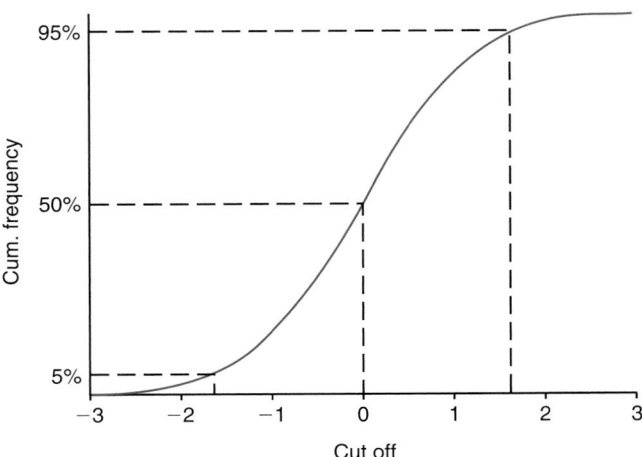

FIGURE 2.9 Cumulative frequency distribution of positive results. The *x*-axis indicates concentrations standardized to zero at the cutoff point (50% positive results) with unit standard deviation.

TABLE 2.3	**2 × 2 Table for Assessing Agreement Between Two Qualitative Tests**		
		TEST 1	
		+	−
Test 2	+	a	b
	−	c	d
Total		a + c	b + d

TABLE 2.4	**2 × 2 Table With Example of Agreement of Data for Two Qualitative Tests**			
		TEST 1		
		+	−	**Total**
Test 2	+	60	20	80
	−	15	40	55
Total		75	60	135

clinical diagnosis, it is relatively straightforward to express the performance in terms of clinical specificity and sensitivity. In the absence of a definitive reference or "gold standard," one should be cautious with regard to judgments on performance. In this situation, it is primarily *agreement* with another test that can be assessed. When replacement of an old or expensive routine assay with a new or less expensive assay is considered, it is of interest to know whether similar test results are likely to be obtained. If both assays are imperfect, however, it is not possible to judge which test has the better performance unless additional testing by a reference procedure is carried out.

In a comparison study, the same individuals are tested by both methods to prevent bias associated with selection of patients. Basically, the outcome of the comparison study should be presented in the form of a 2 × 2 table, from which various measures of agreement may be derived (Table 2.3). An obvious measure of agreement is the overall fraction or percentage of subjects tested who have the same test result (i.e., both results negative or positive):

$$\text{Overall percent agreement} = (a + d)/(a + b + c + d) \times 100\%$$

If agreement differs with respect to diseased and healthy individuals, the overall percent agreement measure becomes dependent on disease prevalence in the studied group of subjects. This is a common situation; accordingly, it may be desirable to separate this overall agreement measure into agreement concerning negative and positive results:

$$\text{Percent agreement given test 1 positive: } a/(a + c)$$

$$\text{Percent agreement given test 1 negative: } b/(b + d)$$

For example, if there is a close agreement with regard to positive results, overall agreement will be high when the fraction of diseased subjects is high; however, in a screening situation with very low disease prevalence, overall agreement will mainly depend on agreement with regard to negative results.

A problem with the simple agreement measures is that they do not take agreement by chance into account. Given independence, expected proportions observed in fields of the 2 × 2 table are obtained by multiplication of the fraction's negative and positive results for each test. Concerning agreement, it is excess agreement beyond chance that is of interest. More sophisticated measures have been introduced to account for this aspect. The most well-known measure is kappa, which is defined generally as the ratio of observed excess agreement beyond chance to maximum possible excess agreement beyond chance.[29] We have the following:

$$\text{Kappa} = (I_o - I_e)/(1 - I_e)$$

where I_o is the observed index of agreement and I_e is the expected agreement from chance. Given complete agreement, kappa equals +1. If observed agreement is greater than or equal to chance agreement, kappa is larger than or equal to zero. Observed agreement less than chance yields a negative kappa value.

Example

Table 2.4 shows a hypothetical example of observed numbers in a 2 × 2 table. The proportion of positive results for test 1 is 75/(75 + 60) = 0.555, and for test 2, it is 80/(80 + 55) = 0.593. Thus by chance, we expect the + + pattern in 0.555 × 0.593 × 135 = 44.44 cases. Analogously, the −−pattern is expected in (1 − 0.555) × (1 − 0.593) × 135 = 24.45 cases. The expected overall agreement percent by chance I_e is (44.44 + 24.45)/135 = 0.51. The observed overall percent agreement is I_o = (60 + 40)/135 = 0.74. Thus we have

$$\text{Kappa} = (0.74 - 0.51)/(1 - 0.51) = 0.47$$

Generally, kappa values greater than 0.75 are taken to indicate excellent agreement beyond chance, values from 0.40 to 0.75 are regarded as showing fair to good agreement beyond chance, and values below 0.40 indicate poor agreement beyond chance. An SE for the kappa estimate can be computed.[29] Kappa is related to the intraclass correlation coefficient, which is a widely used measure of interrater reliability for quantitative measurements.[29] The considered agreement measures, percent agreement, and kappa can also be applied to assess the reproducibility of a qualitative test when the test is applied twice in a given context.

Various methodological problems are encountered in studies on qualitative tests. An obvious mistake is to let the result of the test being evaluated contribute to the diagnostic classification of subjects being tested (circular argument). This is also termed *incorporation bias*.[30,31] Another problem is partial as opposed to complete verification. When a new test is compared with an existing, imperfect test, a partial verification is sometimes undertaken, in which only discrepant results are subjected to further testing by a perfect test procedure. On this basis, sensitivity and specificity are reported for the new test. This procedure (called *discrepant resolution*) leads to biased estimates and should not be accepted.[30–33] The problem is that for cases with agreement, both the existing (imperfect) test and the new test may be wrong. Thus only a measure of agreement should be reported, not specificity and sensitivity values. In the biostatistical literature, various procedures have been suggested to correct for bias caused by imperfect reference tests, but unrealistic assumptions concerning the independence of test results are usually put forward.

ASSAY COMPARISON

Comparison of measurements by two assays is a frequent task in the laboratory. Preferably, parallel measurements of a set of patient samples should be undertaken. To prevent artificial matrix-induced differences, fresh patient samples are the optimal material. A nearly even distribution of values over the analytical measurement range is also preferable. In an ordinary laboratory, comparison of two routine assays is the most frequently occurring situation. Less commonly, comparison of a routine assay with a reference measurement procedure is undertaken. When two routine assays are compared, the focus is on observed differences. In this situation, it is not possible to establish that one set of measurements is the correct one and thereby know by how much measurements deviate from the presumed correct concentrations. Rather, the question is whether the new assay can replace the existing one without a systematic change in result values. To address this question, the dispersion of observed differences between paired measurements may be evaluated by these assays. To carry out a formal, objective analysis of the data, a statistical procedure with graphics display should be applied. Various approaches may be used: (1) a frequency plot or histogram of the distribution of differences (DoD) with measures of central tendency and dispersion (DoD plot), (2) a difference (bias) plot, which shows differences as a function of the average concentration of measurements (Bland-Altman plot), or (3) a regression analysis. In the following, a general error model is presented, and some typical measurement relationships are considered. Each of the statistical approaches mentioned is presented in detail along with a discussion of their advantages and disadvantages.

Basic Error Model

The occurrence of measurement errors is related to the performance characteristics of the assay. It is important to distinguish between pure, random measurement errors, which are present in all measurement procedures, and errors related to incorrect calibration and nonspecificity of the assay. Whereas a reference measurement procedure is associated only with pure, random error, a routine method, additionally, is likely to have some bias related to errors in calibration and limitations with regard to specificity. Whereas an erroneous calibration function gives rise to a systematic error, nonspecificity gives an error that typically varies from sample to sample. The error related to nonspecificity thus has a random character, but in contrast to the pure measurement error, it cannot be reduced by repeated measurements of a sample. Although errors related to nonspecificity for a group of samples look like random errors, for the individual sample, this type of error is a bias. Because this bias varies from sample to sample, it has been called a *sample-related random bias*.[34–36] In the following section, the various error components are incorporated into a formal error model.

Measured Value, Target Value, Modified Target Value, and True Value

Upon taking into account that an analytical method measures analyte concentrations with some random measurement error, one has to distinguish between the actual, measured value and the average result we would obtain if the given sample was measured an infinite number of times. If the assay is a reference assay without bias and nonspecificity, we have the following, simple relationship:

$$x_i = X_{\text{True}i} + \varepsilon_i$$

where x_i represents the measured value, $X_{\text{True}i}$ is the average value for an infinite number of measurements, and ε_i is the deviation of the measured value from the average value. If we were to undertake repeated measurements, the average of ε_i would be zero and the SD would equal the analytical SD (σ_A) of the reference measurement procedure. Pure, random, measurement error will usually be Gaussian distributed.

In the case of a routine assay, the relationship between the measured value for a sample and the true value becomes more complicated:

$$x_i = X_{\text{True}i} + \text{Cal-Bias} + \text{Random-Bias}_i + \varepsilon_i$$

The *cal-bias* term (calibration bias) is a systematic error related to the calibration of the method. This systematic error may be a constant for all measurements corresponding to an offset error, or it may be a function of the analyte concentration (e.g., corresponding to a slope deviation in the case of a linear calibration function). The *random-bias*$_i$ term is a bias that is specific for a given sample related to nonspecificity of the method. It may arise because of codetermination of substances that vary in concentration from sample to sample. For example, a chromogenic creatinine method codetermines some other components with creatinine in serum.[37] Finally, we have the random measurement error term ε_i.

If we performed an infinite number of measurements of a specific sample by the routine method, the random measurement error term ε_i would be zero. The cal-bias and the random-bias$_i$, however, would be unchanged. Thus the average value of an infinite number of measurements would equal the sum of the true value and these bias terms. This average value may be regarded as the target value ($X_{\text{Target}i}$) of the given sample for the routine method. We have:

$$X_{\text{Target}i} = X_{\text{True}i} + \text{Cal-Bias} + \text{Random-Bias}_i$$

As mentioned, the calibration bias represents a systematic error component in relation to the true values measured by a reference measurement procedure. In the context of regression analysis, this systematic error corresponds to the intercept and the slope deviation from unity when a routine method is compared with a reference measurement procedure (outlined in detail later). It is convenient to introduce a modified target value expression ($X'_{\text{Target}i}$) for the routine method to delineate this systematic calibration bias, so that:

$$X'_{\text{Target}i} = X_{\text{True}i} + \text{Cal-Bias}$$

Thus for a set of samples measured by a routine method, the $X_{\text{Target}i}$ values are distributed around the respective $X'_{\text{Target}i}$ values with an SD, which is called σ_{RB}.

If the assay is a reference method without bias and nonspecificity, the target value and the modified target value equal the true value, that is,

$$X_{\text{Target}i} = X'_{\text{Target}i} = X_{\text{True}i}$$

The error model is outlined in Fig. 2.10.

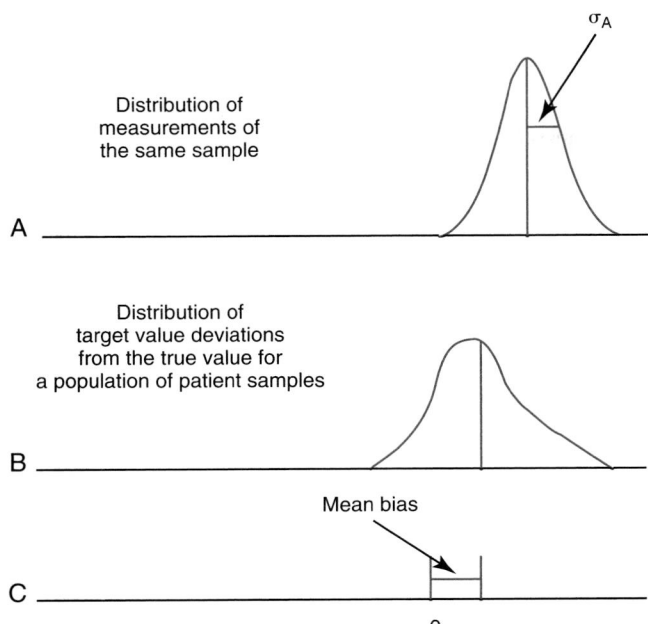

FIGURE 2.10 Outline of basic error model for measurements by a routine assay. **A,** The distribution of repeated measurements of the *same* sample, representing a normal distribution around the target value ($X_{\text{Target}i}$) *(vertical line)* of the sample with a dispersion corresponding to the analytical standard deviation, σ_A. **B,** Schematic outline of the dispersion of target value deviations from the respective true values for a population of patient samples. A distribution of an arbitrary form is displayed. The standard deviation equals σ_{RB}. The vertical line indicates the mean of the distribution. **C,** The distance from zero to the mean of the target value deviations from the true values represents the calibration bias (mean bias = cal-bias) of the assay.

Calibration Bias and Random Bias

For an individual measurement, the total error is the deviation of x_i from the true value, that is,

$$\text{Total error of } x_i = \text{Cal-Bias} + \text{Random-Bias}_i + \varepsilon_i$$

Estimation of the bias terms requires parallel measurements between the method in question and a reference method as outlined in detail later. With regard to calibration bias, one should be aware of the possibility of lot-to-lot variation in analytical kit sets. The manufacturer should provide documentation on this lot-to-lot variation because often it is not possible for the individual laboratory to investigate a sufficient number of lots to assess this variation. Lot-to-lot variation shows up as a calibration bias that changes from lot to lot.

The previous exposition defines the total error in somewhat broader terms than is often seen. A traditional total error expression is[38]:

$$\text{Total error} = \text{Bias} + 2\,\text{SD}_A$$

which often is interpreted as the calibration bias plus $2\,\text{SD}_A$. If a one-sided statistical perspective is taken, the expression is modified to Bias + $1.65\,\text{SD}_A$, indicating that 5% of results are located outside the limit. If a lower percentage is desired, the multiplication factor is increased accordingly, supposing a normal distribution. Interpreting the bias as identical with the calibration bias may lead to an underestimation of the total error.

Random bias related to sample-specific interferences may take several forms. It may be a regularly occurring additional random error component, perhaps of the same order of magnitude as the analytical error. In this context, it is natural to quantify the error in the form of an SD or CV. The most straightforward procedure is to carry out a method comparison study based on a set of patient samples in which one of the methods is a reference method, as outlined later. Krouwer[34] formally quantified sample-related random interferences in a comparison experiment of two cholesterol methods and found that the CV of the sample-related random interference component exceeded the analytical CV. Another form of sample-related random interference is more rarely occurring gross errors, which typically are seen in the context of immunoassays and are related to unexpected antibody interactions. Such an error usually shows up as an outlier in method comparison studies. A well-known source is the occurrence of heterophilic antibodies. Outliers should not just be discarded from the data analysis procedure. Rather, outliers must be investigated to identify their cause, which may be an important limitation in using a given assay. Supplementary studies may help clarify such random sample-related interferences and may provide specifications for the assay that limit its application in certain contexts (e.g., with regard to samples from certain patient categories).

Assay Comparison Data Model

Here we consider the error model described earlier in relation to the method comparison situation. For a given sample measured by two analytical methods, 1 and 2, we have

$$x1_i = X1_{\text{Target}i} + \varepsilon1_i = X_{\text{True}i} + \text{Cal-Bias1} + \text{Random-Bias1}_i + \varepsilon1_i$$
$$x2_i = X2_{\text{Target}i} + \varepsilon2_i = X_{\text{True}i} + \text{Cal-Bias2} + \text{Random-Bias2}_i + \varepsilon2_i$$

From this general model, we may study some typical situations. First, comparison of a routine assay with a reference measurement procedure will be treated. Second, comparison of two routine assays is considered.

Comparison of a Routine Assay With a Reference Measurement Procedure

Assuming that method 1 is a reference method, the bias components disappear by definition, and we have the following situation:

$$x1_i = X1_{\text{Target}i} + \varepsilon1_i = X_{\text{True}i} + \varepsilon1_i$$
$$x2_i = X2_{\text{Target}i} + \varepsilon2_i = X_{\text{True}i} + \text{Cal-Bias2} + \text{Random-Bias2}_i + \varepsilon2_i$$

The paired differences become

$$(x2_i - x1_i) = \text{Cal-Bias2} + \text{Random-Bias2}_i + (\varepsilon2_i - \varepsilon1_i)$$

We thus have an expression consisting of a systematic error term (calibration bias of method 2) and two random terms. The random-bias2 term is distributed around cal-bias2 according to an undefined distribution. $(\varepsilon2_i - \varepsilon1_i)$ is a difference between two random measurement errors that are independent and, commonly, Gaussian distributed. However, we remind readers that the SD for analytical methods often depends on the concentration, as mentioned earlier. For analytes with a wide analytical measurement range (e.g., some hormones), both sample-related random interferences and analytical SDs are likely to depend on the measurement concentration, often in a roughly proportional manner. It may then be more useful to evaluate the *relative* differences—$(x2_i - x1_i)/[(x2_i + x1_i)/2]$—and accordingly express mean and random bias and analytical error as proportions. An alternative is to partition the total analytical measurement range into segments (e.g., three parts) and consider calibration bias, random bias, and analytical error separately for each of these segments. The segments may be divided preferably in relation to important decision concentrations (e.g., in relation to reference interval limits, treatment decision concentrations, or both).

Comparison of Two Routine Assays
In the comparison of two routine methods, the paired differences become

$$(x2_i - x1_i) = (\text{Cal-Bias2} - \text{Cal-Bias1}) + (\text{Random-Bias2}_i - \text{Random-Bias1}_i) + (\varepsilon2_i - \varepsilon1_i)$$

The expression again consists of a constant term, the difference between the two calibration biases, and two random terms. The first random term is a difference between two random-bias components that may or may not be independent. If the two field methods are based on the same measurement principle, the random bias terms are likely to be correlated. For example, two chromogenic methods for creatinine are likely to be subject to interference from the same chromogenic compounds present in a given serum sample. On the other hand, a chromogenic method and an enzymatic creatinine method are subject to different types of interfering compounds, and the random bias terms may be relatively independent. In the $\varepsilon2_i - \varepsilon1_i$ term, the same relationships as described previously are likely to apply. One may note that the general form of the expressed differences is the same in the two situations. Thus the same general statistical principles actually apply. In the following sections, we will consider the DoD under various circumstances, as well as the measurement relations between methods 1 and 2 on the basis of regression analysis.

Preliminary Practical Work in Relation to a Method Comparison Study
When a method comparison study is to be conducted, the analytical methods to be examined first should be established in the laboratory according to written protocols and should be stable in routine performance. Reagents are commonly supplied as ready-made analytical kits, perhaps implemented on a dedicated analytical instrument (open or closed system). Technologists performing the study should be trained in the procedures and associated instrumentation. Furthermore, it is important that a QC system is in place to ensure that the methods being compared are running in an in-control state.

Planning a Method Comparison Study
In the planning phase of a method comparison study, several points require attention, including the (1) number of samples necessary, (2) distribution of analyte concentrations (preferably uniform over the analytical measurement range), and (3) representativeness of the samples. To address the latter point, samples from relevant patient categories should be included, so that possible interference phenomena can be discovered. For example, it may, in a given context, be relevant to include samples from patients with diabetes to

exclude the possibility that aberrations in glucose metabolism may influence test results. Practical aspects related to storage and treatment of samples (e.g., container) and possible artifacts induced by storage (e.g., freezing of samples) and addition of anticoagulants should be considered. Comparison of measurements should preferably be undertaken over several days (e.g., at least 5 days) so that the comparison of methods does not become dependent on the performance of the methods in one particular analytical run. Finally, ethical aspects (e.g., informed consent from patients whose samples will be used) should be considered in relation to existing legislation.

When the comparison protocol is considered, various guidelines may be consulted. The CLSI EP guidelines give advice on various aspects. For example, the CLSI guideline EP-09-A3, "Method Comparison and Bias Estimation Using Patient Samples," suggests measurement of 40 samples in duplicate by each method when a new method is introduced in the laboratory as a substitute for an established one.[39] In addition, it is proposed that a vendor of an analytical test system should have made a comparison study based on at least 100 samples measured in duplicate by each method. The principle of a more demanding requirement for vendors appears reasonable. This initial validation should be comprehensive to disclose the performance of the assay system in detail. Then the requirement for the ordinary user may be more modest. The EP15 guideline "User Verification of Manufacturer's Claims" suggests a more condensed approach based on a bias or difference plot, which does not involve regression analysis and can be carried out using 20 samples.[17] Although these general guidelines on sample size are useful, additional aspects are important. The probability of detecting rarely occurring interferences showing up as outliers should be taken into account when the necessary sample size is considered. Finally, in relation to evaluation of automated methods, special consideration should be given to the sample sequence to evaluate drift, carryover, and nonlinearity (e.g., by a multifactorial design).[14]

Distribution of Differences Plot
From the end-user viewpoint, it is the differences per se that matter. Thus with regard to the outcome of replacing an established routine method with a new one that perhaps is less expensive or more practical, it is important to focus on the DoD between paired measurements by the old and the new method. A graphic display with assessment of the central tendency and dispersion of differences in the form of an ordinary histogram or frequency polygon plot is useful. The differences may or may not be Gaussian distributed. Because both analytical error components and sample-related random interferences may contribute to the differences, the distribution may be irregular, and outliers may occur. Furthermore, the random dispersion elements may be dependent on analyte concentration. This is also termed the *heteroscedasticity* of the measurement. Therefore a nonparametric approach for interpreting the DoD may generally be preferable as a starting point.

Nonparametric Approach
Both the central tendency (median) and extreme percentiles are of interest when the nonparametric approach to the DoD is used. With a traditional 95% level, the 2.5 and 97.5 percentiles

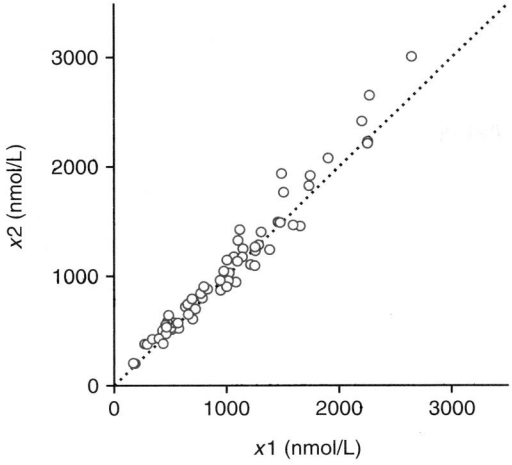

FIGURE 2.11 A scatter plot of $n = 65$ ($x1$, $x2$) data points for comparison of two drug assays. The *dashed line* is the line of identity.

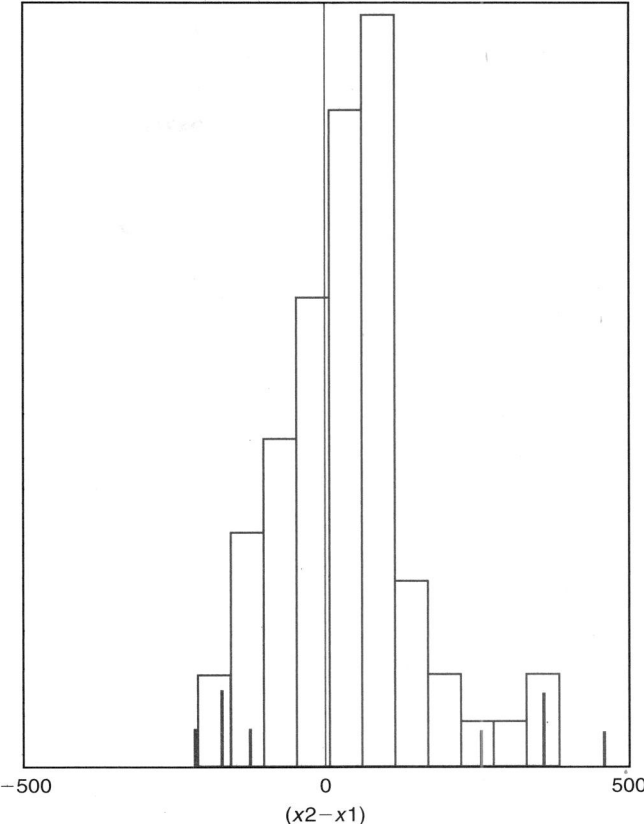

FIGURE 2.12 Distribution of differences plot for comparison of two drug assays: nonparametric analysis. A histogram shows the relative frequency of $n = 65$ differences with demarcated 2.5 and 97.5 percentiles determined nonparametrically. The 90% confidence intervals of the percentiles are shown. These were derived by the bootstrap technique.

are considered. A 99% or higher extreme level may be selected, and the related percentiles (0.5 and 99.5 percentiles, or more extreme ones) may then be applied for a description of method differences. Nonparametric estimation of the 2.5 and 97.5 percentiles requires 2.5 times as many observations as the parametric approach to obtain the same uncertainty, which implies that sample sizes cannot be too small.[40] Estimating confidence limits of the percentiles can give an indication of their imprecision. The CIs can be estimated from the ordered observations as described in Chapter 9 in the section on nonparametric estimation of the 95% reference interval. Alternatively, a bootstrap procedure can be applied as described.[40] The advantage of the bootstrap procedure is that SEs can be derived using smaller sample sizes than are used with the simple nonparametric approach.[41]

A method comparison example from the laboratory of one of the authors (K.L.) is considered. Two drug assays developed in house for serum concentrations of the antipsychotic drug clozapine are compared. The established assay (method 1) is an HPLC method based on manual liquid–liquid extraction. The new method (method 2) is an HPLC method with an automated on-column extraction step. An initial impression of the relation between $x1$ and $x2$ measurements can be obtained from a scatter plot of the 65 measurement sets ($x1$, $x2$) with the identity line outlined (Fig. 2.11). The $x1$ measurements range from 177 to 2650 nmol/L, and the range of $x2$ values is from 200 to 3004 nmol/L (i.e., we have a relatively wide analytical measurement range in the present example). A histogram of the difference ($x2 - x1$) is shown in Fig. 2.12. Applying a nonparametric data description, we order the observed differences according to size and derive the median difference as the value of the $(0.5N + 0.5)$ th ordered observation, here 26 nmol/L. In case the order is a noninteger, interpolation between neighbor-ordered values is carried out. A paired nonparametric test, the Wilcoxon test,[5] shows that the median difference was significantly different from zero ($P < .02$). The 2.5 and 97.5 percentiles correspond to the values of the $(0.025N + 0.5)$th and $(0.975N + 0.5)$th ordered observations, respectively, as displayed in Table 2.5.[4,40] For a sample size smaller than 120, it is not possible to derive CIs for the percentiles by the simple nonparametric procedure.

Therefore we also applied the bootstrap procedure to estimate nonparametric percentiles with 90% CIs (see Table 2.5).[40,42] The bootstrap procedure, which is based on computerized random resampling of the observations, provides slightly different percentile estimates, as shown in Table 2.5. In this way, we obtain an estimation of the size of negative and positive differences with uncertainties. The present example shows a considerable range of differences, with the 2.5 percentile being -169 nmol/L (90%-CI: -214 to -123) and the 97.5 percentile being 356 nmol/L (90% CI: 255 to 457). These relatively large differences should be related to the considerable analytical measurement range for the analyte, and an evaluation of *relative* differences may be more relevant for the present example (see later in this chapter).

In the presented examples, no evident outliers were present. However, outliers deserve special attention.[4] Unless they are related to obvious method or apparatus malfunction, discarding of outliers should be considered with caution. Outliers may indicate the presence of large sample-related random interferences, which may be of major clinical importance (e.g., interference by antibodies or degradation products that occur only rarely). Thus a special investigation of outlying results with reanalysis and exploration of the reasons for the outlying observations should be considered.

TABLE 2.5 **Analysis of Distribution of Differences for the Comparison of Drug Assays Example[a]**

Total range of x1 measurements	177 to 2650		
Total range of x2 measurements	200 to 3004		
Total range of differences (x2 − x1)	−210.00 to 437.00		
Test for normality of differences (Anderson-Darling test)	P < .01		

Statistical Analysis of Differences	Simple Nonparametric	Bootstrap	Parametric
Median	26.00 (P < .02)		
Mean			42.00 (P < .01)
SD			124.42
Coefficient of skewness			+0.83
Coefficient of kurtosis			+1.27
Outlier test (4 SD)			NS
2.5-percentile	−166.00	−169.11	−201.86
97.5 percentile	372.38	355.90	285.86
90% CI for 2.5 percentile		−214.73 to −123.50	−245.24 to −158.47
90% CI for 97.5 percentile		255.03 to 456.77	242.47 to 329.24

[a]$n = 65$ single (x1, x2 measurements). The units are nmol/L.
CI, Confidence interval; NS, not significant; SD, standard deviation.

Parametric Approach

If application of a goodness-of-fit test does not disprove that the DoD is Gaussian distributed, a parametric statistical approach may be undertaken. In the example presented, a significant deviation from normality was present, as assessed by the Anderson-Darling test[43] ($P < .01$); therefore a parametric analysis in principle should not be carried out. However, to demonstrate the procedure, the parametric approach is also carried out (Fig. 2.13 and Table 2.5). The mean and SD (SD$_{Dif}$) of the paired differences (x2 − x1) are estimated according to standard procedures. A paired t-test is used to determine whether the mean difference is significantly different from zero ($P < .01$ in this case). The 2.5 and 97.5 percentiles for the differences are estimated as the mean $\pm t_{0.025(N-1)}$ SD$_{Dif}$. An SE for the percentiles (SE$_{perc}$) may be computed, and the 90% CI limits are then derived as ± 1.65 SE$_{perc}$ around the percentiles (see Fig. 2.13 and Table 2.5). The parametrically derived 2.5 and 97.5 percentiles (−202 and 286 nmol/L) differ somewhat from the nonparametrically derived percentiles, which in the present context with proven non-normality may be regarded as the most reliable estimates.

Relative Distribution of Differences Plot

In some cases in which a wide analytical measurement range (i.e., corresponding to 1 or several decades) is used, the random error components depend on the concentration, as previously mentioned. Analytical SDs may be approximately proportional to the concentration over the major part of the analytical measurement range. In the present example, the initial scatter plot of (x1, x2) values suggests that the random error of the differences increases with the concentration (see Fig. 2.11). A formal test for this possible relation is to compute the correlation coefficient between the average concentration and the *absolute* value of the differences. This correlation coefficient, r, is +0.57, which is significantly different from zero ($P < .001$), and it confirms the relationship of scatter increasing with concentration, which also can be visualized in a scatter plot of the absolute differences against the average concentration (Fig. 2.14). A natural next step is to

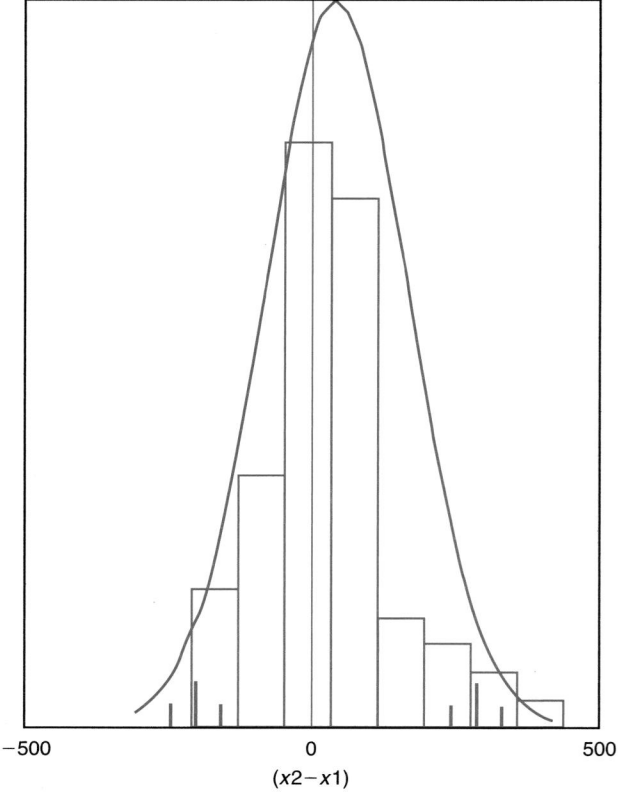

FIGURE 2.13 Distribution of differences plot for comparison of two drug assays: parametric analysis. A histogram shows the relative frequency of $n = 65$ differences with the estimated Gaussian density distribution. Parametrically estimated 2.5 and 97.5 percentiles are shown with 90% confidence intervals.

assess the *relative* differences in relation to the average concentration. The correlation coefficient between the absolute values of the relative differences $[|x2 − x1|/(\{x1 + x2\}/2)]$ and the average concentration $[(x1 + x2)/2]$ was not significantly different ($P > .05$) from zero ($r = −0.15$); a scatter plot also

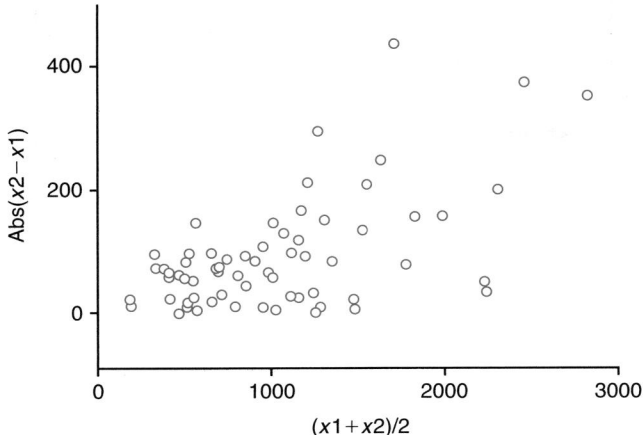

FIGURE 2.14 Plot of absolute differences (ordinate) against average concentration (abscissa) for the comparison of drug assays example. The scatter increases with the average concentration ($r = +0.57$).

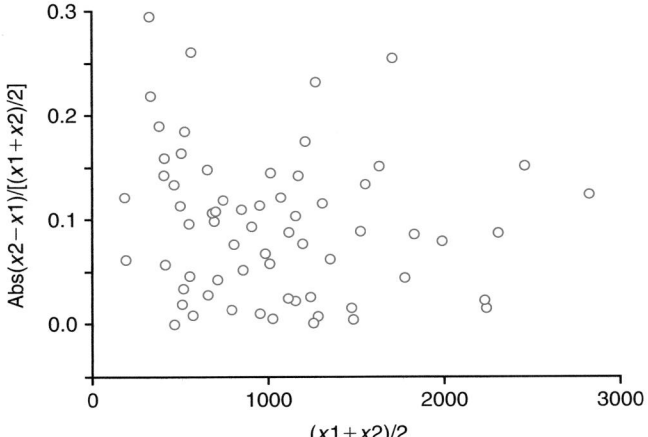

FIGURE 2.15 Plot of absolute *relative* differences (ordinate) against average concentration (abscissa) for the comparison of drug assays example. The scatter is not significantly correlated with the average concentration ($r = -0.15$, not significant).

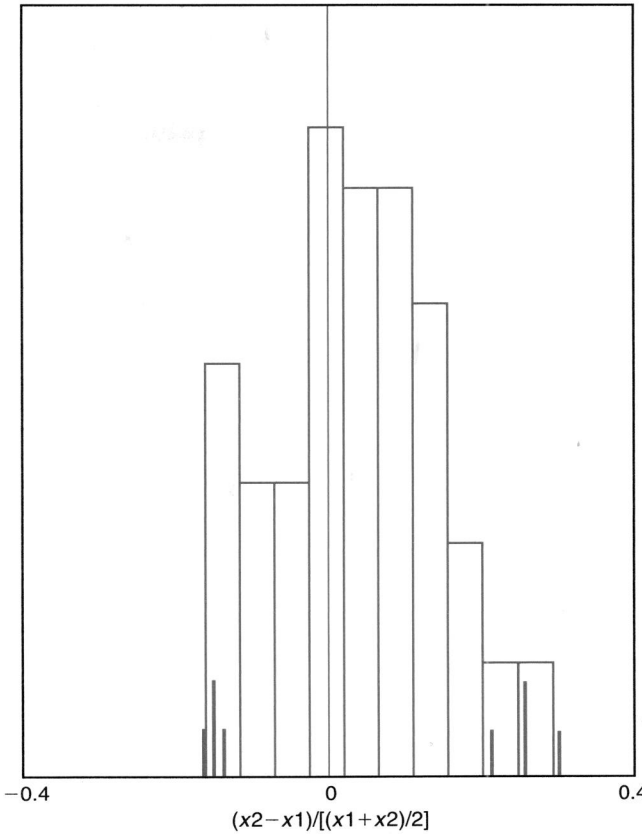

FIGURE 2.16 Relative distribution of differences plot for comparison of two drug assays: nonparametric analysis. A histogram shows the relative frequency of relative differences with demarcated 2.5 and 97.5 percentiles determined nonparametrically. The 90% confidence intervals (bootstrap) of the percentiles are shown.

suggests a more homogeneous dispersion (Fig. 2.15). In this situation, it is more reasonable to deal with *relative* differences or percentage differences $[(\{x2 - x1\}/\{x1 + x2\}/2) \times 100\%]$. The same nonparametric descriptive measures as used earlier may be applied for the central tendency and the dispersion (Fig. 2.16). The median relative difference amounts to 0.042, or 4.2%, which is significantly higher than zero ($P < .01$; Wilcoxon test; Table 2.6). The 2.5 and 97.5 percentiles are -0.15 and 0.26, respectively. The 90% CIs derived by the bootstrap procedure were -0.16 to -0.14 and 0.21 to 0.30, respectively. Thus from this analysis, we may conclude that the 95% interval for percentage differences ranges from about -15 to $+26\%$.

Finally, we may consider a parametric analysis of the relative differences (Fig. 2.17 and Table 2.6). A goodness-of-fit test (Anderson-Darling test; $P > .05$) showed that the relative differences did not depart significantly from a normal distribution, which in this case supports the parametric approach (Fig. 2.18). The parametric 2.5 and 97.5 percentiles were -0.18 and 0.26, respectively. The mean was 0.042, and the SD

of the relative differences was 0.11. Thus we may conclude that there is an average bias of about 4%, which might rely on a calibration difference (an estimate of [cal-bias2 $-$ cal-bias1]), and a random error corresponding to a CV of 11%. The random error CV of 11% is an estimate of the combined dispersion of $[(\text{Random-Bias2}_i - \text{Random-Bias1}_i) + (\varepsilon 2_i - \varepsilon 1_i)]$. If we ascribe the random variation equally to the two assays, it corresponds to a random error level of $11\%/\sqrt{2} = 7.8\%$ for each assay. In the present example, the average bias of 4% and the estimated random variation of differences between the two assays were considered acceptable in relation to the clinical use of the assay, and it was decided to replace the manual assay with the new, automated assay.

Verification of Distribution of Differences in Relation to Specified Limits

In situations in which a field method is being considered for implementation, it may be desired primarily to *verify* whether the differences in relation to the existing method are located within given specified limits rather than *estimating* the DoD. For example, one may set limits corresponding to $\pm 15\%$ as clinically acceptable and may desire that a majority (e.g., 95% of differences) are located within this interval.

By counting, it may be determined whether the expected proportion of results is within the limits (i.e., 95%). One may accept percentages that do not deviate significantly from the

TABLE 2.6   Analysis of Distribution of *Relative* Differences for the Comparison of Drug Assays Example; *n* = 65

Total range of relative differences	−0.1598 to 0.2953		
Test for normality (Anderson-Darling test)	NS		
Statistical Analysis	**Simple Nonparametric**	**Bootstrap**	**Parametric**
Median	0.0467 (*P* < .01)		
Mean			0.0418 (*P* < .01)
SD			0.1109
Coefficient of skewness			+0.05
Coefficient of kurtosis			−0.60
Outlier test			NS
2.5 percentile	−0.1487	−0.1492	−0.1754
97.5 percentile	0.2607	0.2570	0.2591
90% CI for 2.5 percentile		−0.1627 to −0.1357	−0.2141 to −0.1368
90% CI for 97.5 percentile		0.2135–0.3005	0.2204 to 0.2978

CI, Confidence interval; *NS,* not significant; *SD,* standard deviation.

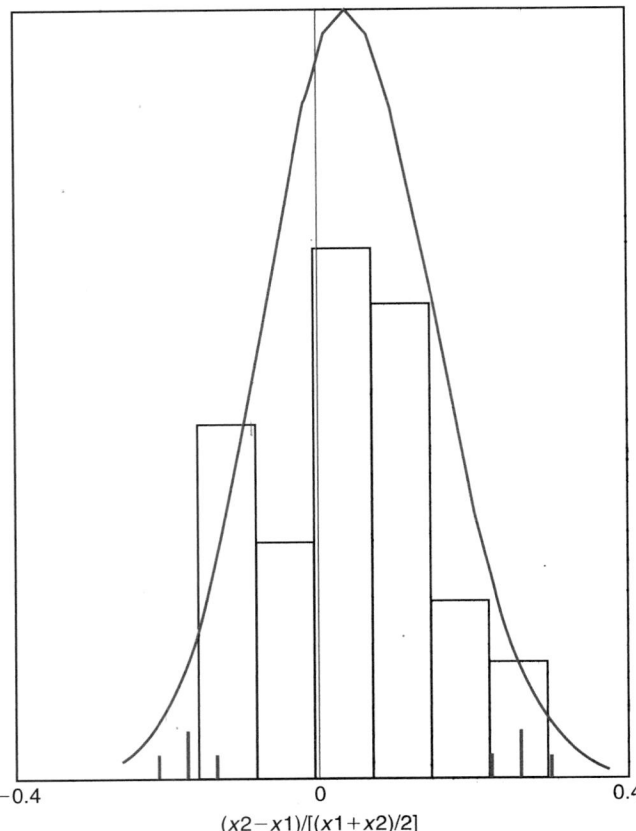
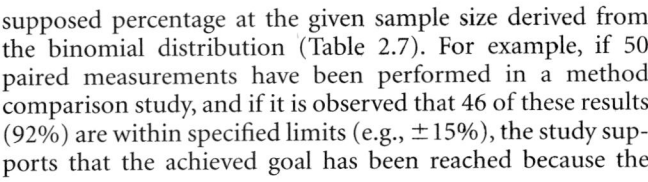

FIGURE 2.17 Distribution of *relative* differences plot for comparison of two drug assays: parametric analysis. A histogram shows the relative frequency of relative differences with the estimated Gaussian density distribution. Parametrically estimated 2.5 and 97.5 percentiles are shown with 90% confidence intervals.

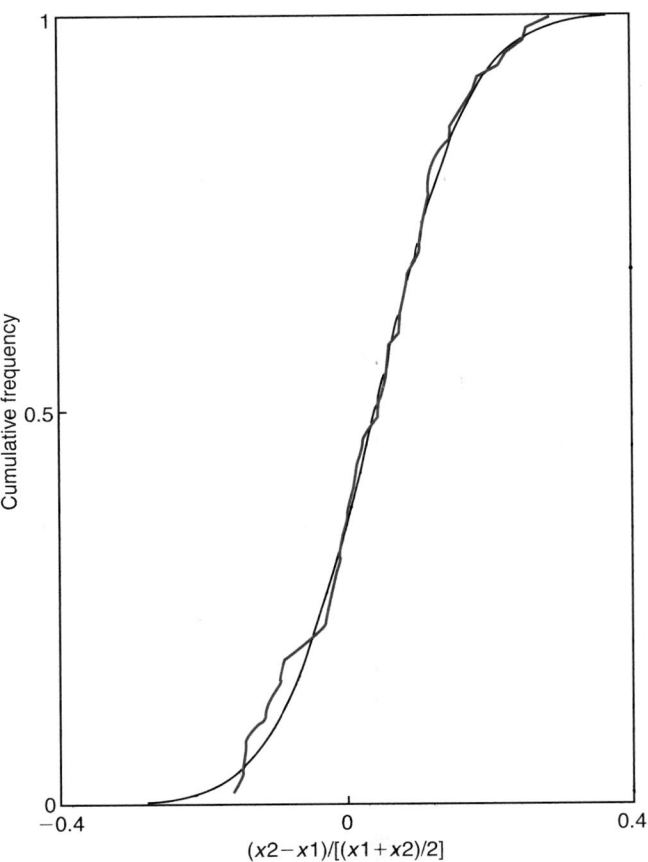

FIGURE 2.18 Cumulative frequency distribution of relative differences for the comparison of drug assays example. The black curve indicates the Gaussian cumulative frequency distribution curve. In accordance with the test for normality, good agreement is observed.

supposed percentage at the given sample size derived from the binomial distribution (Table 2.7). For example, if 50 paired measurements have been performed in a method comparison study, and if it is observed that 46 of these results (92%) are within specified limits (e.g., ±15%), the study supports that the achieved goal has been reached because the lower boundary for acceptance is 90%. It is clear that a reasonable number of observations should be obtained for the assessment to have acceptable power. If very few observations are available, the risk is high of falsely concluding that at least 95% of the observations are within specified limits in case it is not true (i.e., committing a type II error).

TABLE 2.7 Lower Bounds (One-Sided 95% Confidence Interval) of Observed Proportions (%) of Results Being Located Within Specified Limits for Paired Differences That Are in Accordance With the Hypothesis of at Least 95% of Differences Being Within the Limits	
n	**Observed Proportions**
20	85
30	87
40	90
50	90
60	90
70	90
80	91
90	91
100	91
150	92
200	93
250	93
300	93
400	93
500	93
1000	94

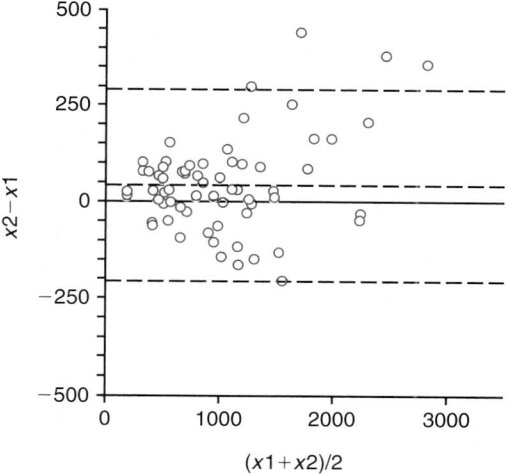

FIGURE 2.19 Bland-Altman plot of differences for the drug comparison example. The differences are plotted against the average concentration. The mean difference (42 nmol/L) with ±2 standard deviation of differences is shown *(dashed lines)*.

Difference (Bland-Altman) Plot

The difference plot suggested by Bland and Altman is widely used for evaluating method comparison data.[44,45] The procedure was originally introduced for comparison of measurements in clinical medicine, but it has also been adopted in clinical chemistry.[46-48] The Bland-Altman plot is usually understood as a plot of the differences against the average results of the methods. Thus the difference plot in this version provides information on the relation between differences and concentration, which is useful in evaluating whether problems exist at certain ranges (e.g., in the high range) caused by nonlinearity of one of the methods. It may also be of interest to observe whether differences tend to increase proportionally with the concentration or whether they are independent of concentration. In some situations, particular interest may be directed toward the low-concentration region. Information on the relation between differences and concentration is useful in the context of how to adjust for an irregularity (e.g., by changing the method to correct for nonlinearity, by restricting the analytical measurement range).

The basic version of the difference plot requires plotting of the differences against the average of the measurements. Fig. 2.19 shows the plot for the drug assay comparison data. The interval ±2 SD of the differences is often delineated around the mean difference (i.e., corresponding to the mean and the 2.5 and 97.5 percentiles considered in the parametric distribution of differences plot [DoD plot][45]). To assess whether the bias is significantly different from zero, the SE of the mean difference is estimated as the SD divided by the square root of the number of paired measurements (SE = $SD/N^{0.5}$) and tested against zero by a *t*-test ($t = [Mean - 0]/SE$).

Nonparametric limits may also be considered. The distribution of the differences as measured on the *y*-axis of the

coordinate system corresponds to the relations outlined for the DoD plot, which represents a projection of the differences on the *y*-axis. A constant bias over the analytical measurement range changes the average concentration away from zero. The presence of sample-related random interferences increases the width of the distribution. If the calibration bias depends on the concentration, if the dispersion varies with the concentration, or if both occur, the relations become more complex, and the interval mean ±2 SD of the differences may not fit very well as a 95% interval throughout the analytical measurement range.

The displayed Bland-Altman plot for the drug assay comparison data (see Fig. 2.19) shows a tendency toward increasing scatter with increasing concentration, which is a reflection of increasing random error with concentration, as considered in detail in previous paragraphs. Thus a plot of the relative differences against the average concentration is of relevance (Fig. 2.20). This plot has a more homogeneous dispersion of values, agreeing with the estimated limits for the dispersion, that is, the relative mean difference ± $t_{0.025(N-1)}$ SD_{RelDif} equal to 0.042 ± 1.998 × 0.11 corresponding to −0.18 and 0.26, analogous to the situation with the relative DoD plot considered earlier.

Use of *relative* differences in situations with a proportional random error relationship prevents very large differences in the high-concentration range from dominating the analysis and making a balanced interpretation difficult. In the low range, the proportional relationship may not necessarily hold true, and sometimes the relative difference plot overcompensates for lack of proportionality in this region. It is then possible to truncate the proportional relationship at some lower limit and assume a constant SD for differences below this limit[49] (i.e., corresponding to the relationship in Fig. 2.3C). In the actual drug example (see Fig. 2.20) with a slightly negative correlation coefficient between relative differences and average concentration, a tendency toward this pattern is seen. An alternative to the relative difference plot is to plot the logarithm of the differences against the average concentration, but this type of plot is more difficult to interpret, because the scale is changed.

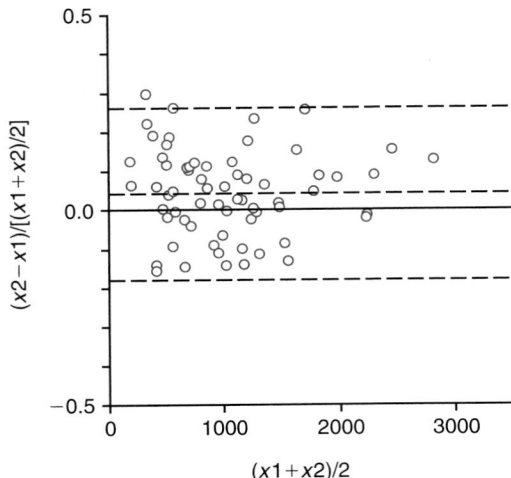

FIGURE 2.20 Bland-Altman plot of *relative* differences for the drug comparison example. The differences are plotted against the average concentration. The mean relative difference (0.042) with ±2 standard deviation of relative differences is shown *(dashed lines)*.

Although it is customary to display the *estimated* limits for the differences (often, mean ± 2 SD_{dif}), one may, as an alternative, display specification limits considered reasonable, as mentioned for the DoD plot.[47] It may then be assessed whether the observed differences conform to these limits, as discussed earlier (see Table 2.7). Application of the difference plot in various specific contexts has been considered.[50,51] It has also been suggested to estimate a regression line for the differences as a function of the average measurement concentration.[52]

A Caution Against Incorrect Interpretation of Paired *t*-Tests in Method Comparison Studies

In association with the difference plot, the paired *t*-test is usually applied as described earlier,[44] but one should be careful with regard to the interpretation. For example, consider the case shown below, in which method 2 (*x2*) measurements tend to exceed method 1 (*x1*) measurements in the low range and vice versa at high concentrations (Fig. 2.21A). This corresponds to a positive calibration bias in the low range, changing to a negative calibration bias in the high range. In this situation, the overall averages of both sets of measurements are nearly equal, and the paired *t*-test yields a nonsignificant result because the average paired difference (i.e., the overall bias) is close to zero (Table 2.8). This does not mean that the measurements are equivalent. Subjecting the data to Deming regression analysis (see the next section) clearly discloses the relation (Fig. 2.21B).[53] Results of the regression analysis confirm the existence of both a systematic constant error (intercept different from zero) and a systematic proportional error (slope different from 1). Therefore as pointed out previously, the statistical significance revealed by the paired *t*-test cannot be used to indicate whether measurements are equivalent. The paired *t*-test is just a test for the average bias; it does not say anything about the equivalency of measurements throughout the analytical measurement range.

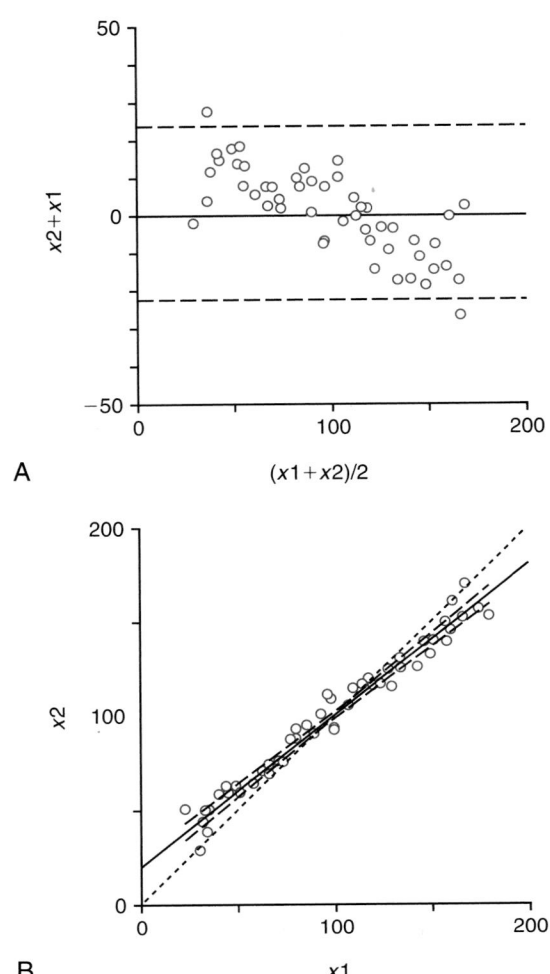

A

B

FIGURE 2.21 Simulated example with positive and negative differences in the low and high ranges, respectively. **A,** Bland-Altman plot. **B,** *x-y* Plot with diagonal *(dotted straight line)* and estimated Deming regression line *(solid line)* with 95% confidence curves *(dashed lines)*.

TABLE 2.8 Comparison of Paired *t*-Test Results and Deming Regression Results for a Simulated Method Comparison Example With Positive Intercept ($a_0 = 20$) and Slope Below Unity ($b = 0.80$), $n = 50$ ($x1$, $x2$) Measurements

	Paired *t*-Test	Regression Analysis (Deming)
Mean difference (SEM)	0.78 (1.63)	
t = mean difference/ SEM	0.78/1.63 = 0.48 (NS)	
Slope *(b)* [SE*(b)*]		0.80 (0.027)
$t = (b - 1)/SE(b)$		−7.4 ($P < .001$)
Intercept (a_0) [SE(a_0)]		20.3 (2.82)
$t = (a_0 - 0)/SE(a_0)$		7.2 ($P < .001$)

NS, Not significant; *SEM,* standard error of the mean.

Regression Analysis

Regression analysis is commonly applied in comparing the results of analytical method comparisons. Typically, an experiment is carried out in which a series of paired values is collected when a new method is compared with an established method. This series of paired observations $(x1_i, x2_i)$ is then used to establish the nature and strength of the relationship between the tests. This discussion outlines various regression models that may be used, gives criteria for when each should be used, and provides guidelines for interpreting the results.

Regression analysis has the advantage that it allows the relation between the target values for the two compared methods to be studied over the full analytical measurement range. If the systematic difference between target values (i.e., the calibration bias between the two methods, or the systematic error) is related to the analyte concentration, such a relationship may not be clearly shown when the previously mentioned types of difference plots are used. Although nonlinear regression analysis may be applied, the focus is usually on linear regression analysis. In linear regression analysis, it is assumed that the systematic difference between target values can be modeled as a constant systematic difference (intercept deviation from zero) combined with a proportional systematic difference (slope deviation from unity), usually related to a discrepancy with regard to calibration of the methods. In situations when random errors have a constant SD, unweighted regression procedures are used (e.g., Deming regression analysis). For cases with SDs that are proportional to the concentration, the weighted Deming regression procedure is preferred.

Error Models in Regression Analysis

As outlined previously, we distinguish between the measured value (x_i) and the target value $(X_{Targeti})$ of a sample subjected to analysis by a given method. In linear regression analysis, we assume a linear relationship between values devoid of random error of any kind.[54,55] Thus to operate with a linear relationship between values without random measurement error and sample-related random bias, we have to introduce modified target values:'

$$X1_{Targeti} = X1'_{Targeti} + \text{Random-Bias}1_i$$
$$X2_{Targeti} = X2'_{Targeti} + \text{Random-Bias}2_i$$

where we now assume a linear relationship between these modified target values:

$$X2'_{Targeti} = \alpha_0 + \beta X1'_{Targeti}$$

In this model, α_0 corresponds to a constant difference with regard to calibration, and $(\beta - 1)$ is a proportional deviation. Thus the systematic error or calibration difference between the measurements corresponds to

$$X2'_{Targeti} - X1'_{Targeti} = \alpha_0 + (\beta - 1)X1'_{Targeti}$$

Because of sample-related random interferences and measurement imprecision (of the type that can be described by a Gaussian distribution, e.g., caused by pipetting variability, signal variability), individually measured pairs of values $(x1_i, x2_i)$ will be scattered around the line expressing the relationship between $X1'_{Targeti}$ and $X2'_{Targeti}$. Fig. 2.22 outlines schematically

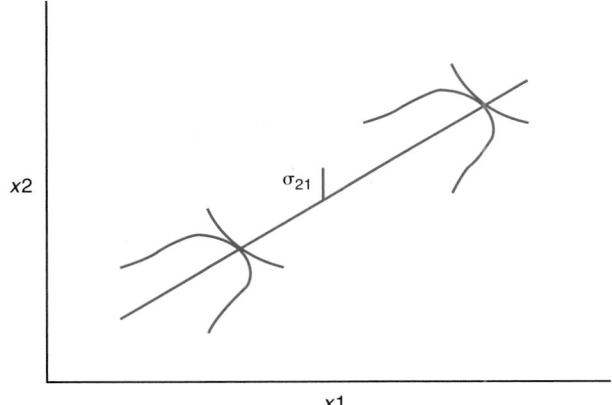

FIGURE 2.22 Outline of the relation between $x1$ and $x2$ values measured by two assays subject to random errors with constant standard deviations over the analytical measurement range. A linear relationship between the modified target values $(X1'_{Targeti}, X2'_{Targeti})$ is presumed. The $x1_i$ and $x2_i$ values are Gaussian distributed around $X1'_{Targeti}$ and $X2'_{Targeti}$, respectively, as schematically shown. σ_{21} (σ_{yx}) is demarcated.

how the random distribution of $x1$ and $x2$ values occurs around the regression line. We have

$$x1_i = X1_{Targeti} + \varepsilon 1_i = X1'_{Targeti} + \text{Random-Bias}1_i + \varepsilon 1_i$$
$$x2_i = X2_{Targeti} + \varepsilon 2_i = X2'_{Targeti} + \text{Random-Bias}2_i + \varepsilon 2_i$$

The random error components may be expressed as SDs, and generally we can assume that sample-related random bias (SD σ_{RB}) and analytical imprecision (SD σ_A) are independent for each analyte, yielding the relations

$$\sigma_{ex1}^2 = \sigma_{RB1}^2 = \sigma_{A1}^2$$
$$\sigma_{ex2}^2 = \sigma_{RB2}^2 = \sigma_{A2}^2$$

σ_{ex1} and σ_{ex2} are the total SDs of the distributions of $x1_i$ and $x2_i$ around their respective modified target values, $X1'_{Targeti}$ and $X2'_{Targeti}$. The sample-related random bias components for methods 1 and 2 may not necessarily be independent. They also may not be Gaussian distributed, contrary to the analytical components. Thus when a regression procedure is applied, the explicit assumptions to take into account should be considered. In situations without random bias components of any significance, the relationships simplify to

$$\sigma_{ex1}^2 = \sigma_{A1}^2$$
$$\sigma_{ex2}^2 = \sigma_{A2}^2$$

In this situation, it usually can be assumed that the error distributions are Gaussian, and estimates of the analytical SDs may be available from QC data.

Another methodologic problem concerns the question of whether the dispersion of sample-related random bias and the analytical imprecision are constant or change with the analyte concentration, as considered previously in the difference plot sections. In cases with a considerable range (i.e., a decade or longer), this phenomenon should also be taken into account when a regression analysis is applied. Fig. 2.23 schematically shows how dispersions may increase proportionally with concentration.

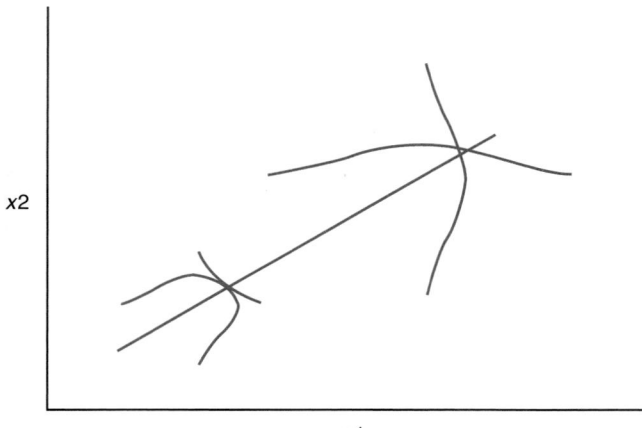

FIGURE 2.23 Outline of the relation between $x1$ and $x2$ values measured by two assays subject to proportional random errors. A linear relationship between the modified target values is assumed. The $x1_i$ and $x2_i$ values are Gaussian distributed around $X1'_{Target i}$ and $X2'_{Target i}$, respectively, with increasing scatter at higher concentrations, as is shown schematically.

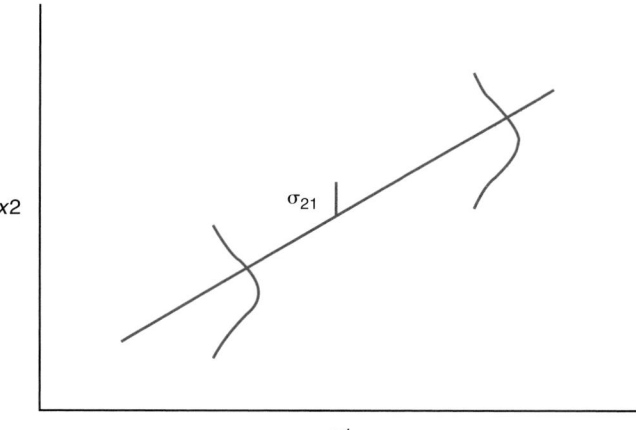

FIGURE 2.24 The model assumed in ordinary least-squares regression. The $x2$ values are Gaussian distributed around the line with constant standard deviation over the analytical measurement range. The $x1$ values are assumed to be without random error. σ_{21} (σ_{yx}) is shown.

Deming Regression Analysis and Ordinary Least-Squares Regression Analysis (Constant Standard Deviations)

To reliably estimate the relationship between modified target values (i.e., a_0 for α_0 and b for β), a regression procedure taking into account errors in both $x1$ and $x2$ is preferable[6] (i.e., Deming approach; see Fig. 2.22). Although the ordinary least-squares (OLR) procedure is commonly used in method comparison studies, it does not take errors in $x1$ into account but is based on the assumption that only the $x2$ measurements are subject to random errors (Fig. 2.24). In the Deming procedure, the sum of squared distances from measured sets of values ($x1_i$, $x2_i$) to the regression line is minimized at an angle determined by the ratio between SDs for the random variations of $x1$ and $x2$. It can be proven theoretically that, given Gaussian *error* distributions, this estimation procedure is optimal. It should here be noted that it is the *error* distributions that should be Gaussian, not the dispersion of values over the measurement range. This is often misunderstood. In Fig. 2.25, the symmetric case is illustrated with a regression slope of 1 and equal SDs for the random variations of $x1$ and $x2$, in which case the sum of squared distances is minimized orthogonally in relation to the line.

OLR regression is not recommended except in special situations. In OLR, the sum of squared distances is minimized in the vertical direction to the line (see Fig. 2.25). It can be proven theoretically that neglect of the random error in $x1$ induces a downward biased slope estimate

$$\beta' = \beta\left[\sigma^2_{X1'_{target}}\Big/\left(\sigma^2_{X1'_{target}} + \sigma^2_{ex1}\right)\right] = \beta\Big/\left[1 + \left(\sigma_{ex1}\Big/\sigma_{X1'_{target}}\right)^2\right]$$

where $\sigma_{X1'target}$ is the SD of $X1'$ target values.[5] The magnitude of the bias depends on the ratio between the SD for the random error in $x1$ and the SD of the $X1'$ target values. Fig. 2.26 shows the bias as a function of the ratio of the random error SD to the SD of the $X1'$ target value dispersion. For a ratio up to 0.1, the bias is less than 1%. At a ratio of 0.33, the bias amounts to 10%; it increases further for increasing ratios. In a given case, one can take the analytical SD (e.g., from QC data)

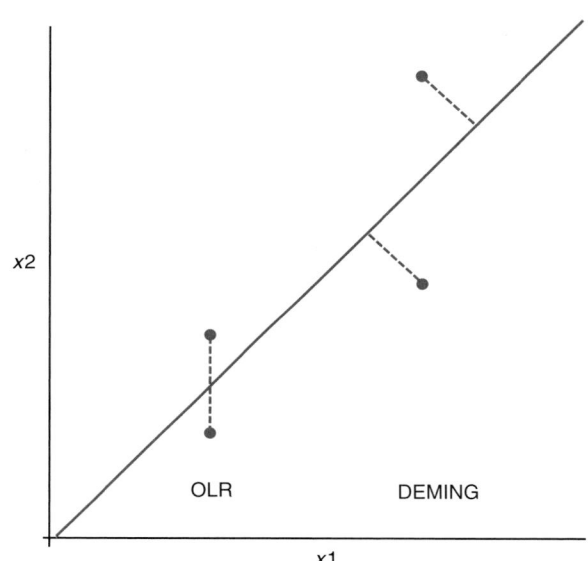

FIGURE 2.25 In ordinary least-squares regression *(OLR)*, the sum of squared deviations from the line is minimized in the vertical direction. In Deming regression analysis, the sum of squared deviations is minimized at an angle to the line, depending on the random error ratio. Here the symmetric case is displayed with orthogonal deviations. (From Linnet K. The performance of Deming regression analysis in case of a misspecified analytical error ratio. *Clin Chem* 1998;**44**:1024–31.)

and divide by the SD of the measured $x1$ values, which approximately equals the SD of $X1'$ target values. As an example, a typical comparison study for two serum sodium methods may be associated with a downward directed slope bias of about 10% (Fig. 2.27).

In the example presented previously, the ratio of the analytical SD to the SD of the target value distribution is large because of the tight physiologic regulation of electrolyte concentrations, which means that the biological variation is limited. Most other types of analytes exhibit wider distributions, and the ratio of error to target value distribution is

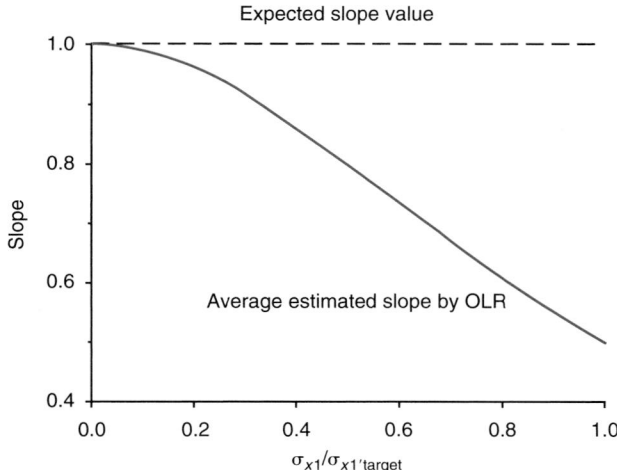

FIGURE 2.26 Relations between the true (expected) slope value and the average estimated slope by ordinary least-squares regression *(OLR)*. The bias of the OLR slope estimate increases negatively for increasing ratios of the standard deviation (SD) random error in *x*1 to the SD of the *X*1 target value distribution.

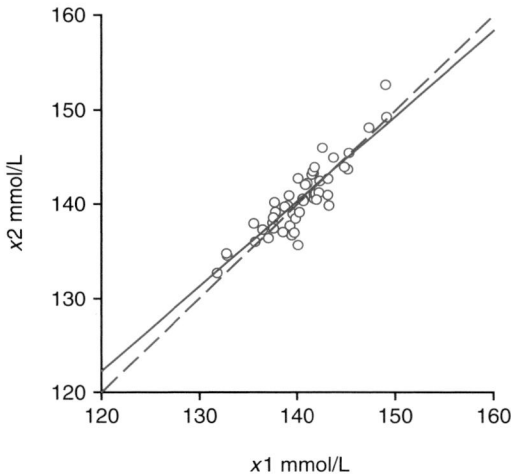

FIGURE 2.27 Simulated comparison of two sodium methods. The *solid line* indicates the average estimated ordinary least-squares regression (OLR) line, and the *dotted line* is the identity line. Even though no systematic difference is evident between the two methods, the average OLR line deviates from the identity line corresponding to a downward slope bias of about 10%.

smaller. For example, for analytes with a distribution of longer than 1 decade and an analytical error corresponding to a CV of 5% at the middle of the analytical measurement range, the OLR slope bias amounts to about -1%.

Computation Procedures for Ordinary Least-Squares Regression and Deming Regression

Assuming no errors in *x*1 and a Gaussian error distribution of *x*2 with constant SD throughout the analytical measurement range, OLR is the optimal estimation procedure, as proved by Gauss in the eighteenth century. Given errors in both *x*1 and *x*2, the Deming approach is the method of choice.[56] It should be noted for these parametric procedures that only the *error* distributions must be Gaussian or normal. The least-squares principle does not require normality to be

applied, but it is optimal under normality conditions, and the nominal type I errors for associated statistical tests for slope and intercept hold true under this assumption. The procedures are generally robust toward deviations from normality, but they are sensitive to outliers because of the squaring principle. Finally, the distribution of the *x*1 and *x*2 values over the measurement range does not have to be normal. A uniform distribution over the analytical measurement range is generally of advantage, but the distribution in principle may take any form. For both procedures, we may evaluate the SD of the dispersion in the *vertical* direction around the line (commonly denoted $SD_{y \cdot x}$ and here given as SD_{21}). We have

$$SD_{21} = \left[\sum \left(x2_i - X2'_{Targetesti} \right) 2 / (N = 1) \right]^{0.5}$$

Further discussion regarding the interpretation of SD_{21} will be given later.

To compute the slope in Deming regression analysis, the ratio between the SDs of the random errors of *x*1 and *x*2 is necessary, that is,

$$\lambda = \left(\sigma^2_{RB1} + \sigma^2_{A1} \right) / \left(\sigma^2_{RB2} + \sigma^2_{A2} \right)$$

SD_As can be estimated from duplicate sets of measurements as

$$SD^2_{A1} = (1/2N) \left[\sum \left(x1_{2i} - x1_{1i} \right)^2 \right]$$
$$SD^2_{A2} = (1/2N) \left[\sum \left(x2_{2i} - x2_{1i} \right)^2 \right]$$

or they may be available from QC data. The latter is a practical approach that avoids the need for duplicate measurements by each measurement procedure.

If a specific value for λ is not available and the two routine methods that are compared are likely to be associated with random errors of the same order of magnitude, λ can be set to 1. The Deming procedure is generally relatively insensitive to a misspecification of the λ value.[57]

Formulas for computing slope (β), intercept (α_0), and their SEs are available from other sources[5,49,56] and are not provided here.

Evaluation of the Random Error Around an Estimated Regression Line

The estimated slope and intercept provide an estimate of the systematic difference or calibration bias between two methods over the analytical measurement range. Additionally, an estimate of the random error is important. It is common to consider the dispersion around the line in the vertical direction, which is quantified as $SD_{y \cdot x}$ (here denoted SD_{21}). SD_{21} was originally introduced in the context of OLR, but it also can be considered in relation to Deming regression analysis.

Interpreting $SD_{y \cdot x}$ (SD_{21}) With Random Errors in Both x1 and x2

With regard to σ_{21}, we have here without sample-related random interferences

$$\sigma^2_{21} = \beta^2 \sigma^2_{A1} + \sigma^2_{A2}$$

Thus σ_{21} reflects the random error both in *x*1 (with a rescaling) and in *x*2. Often β is close to unity, and in this case, σ^2_{21} becomes approximately the sum of the individual squared SDs. This relation holds true for both Deming and OLR analyses. Frequently, OLR is applied in situations associated with random measurement error in both $x1$ and $x2$, and in these situations, σ_{21} reflects the errors in both.

The presence of sample-related random interferences in both $x1$ and $x2$ gives the following expression:

$$\sigma_{21}^2 = \left(\beta^2 \sigma_{A1}^2 + \sigma_{A2}^2\right) + \left(\beta^2 \sigma_{RB1}^2 + \sigma_{RB2}^2\right)$$

Thus the σ_{21} value is influenced by the slope value and the analytical error components σ_{A1} and σ_{A2} (grouped in the first bracket) and σ_{RB1} and σ_{RB2} (grouped in the second bracket). In many cases, the slope is close to unity, in which case we have simple addition of the components. As mentioned earlier, the sample-related random interferences may not be independent. In this case, simple addition of the components is not correct because a covariance term should be included. However, in a real case, we can estimate the combined effect corresponding to the bracket term. Information on the analytical components is usually available from duplicate sets of measurements or from QC data. On this basis, the combined random bias term in the second bracket can be derived by subtracting the analytical components from σ_{21}. Overall, it can be judged whether the total random error is acceptable or not. The systematic difference can be adjusted for relatively easily by rescaling one of the sets of measurements. However, if the random error term is very large, such a rescaling does not ensure equivalency of measurements with regard to individual samples. Thus it is important to assess both the systematic difference and the random error when deciding whether a new routine method can replace an existing one.

Assessment of Outliers

The principle of minimizing the sum of squared distances from the line makes the described regression procedures sensitive to outliers, and an assessment of the occurrence of outliers should be carried out routinely. The distance from a suspected outlier to the line is recorded in SD units, and the outlier is rejected if the distance exceeds a predetermined limit (e.g., 3 or 4 SD units). In the case of OLR, the SD unit equals SD_{21}, and the vertical distance is considered. For Deming regression analysis, the unit is the SD of the deviation of the points from the line at an angle determined by the error variance ratio λ. A plot of these deviations, a so-called residuals plot, conveniently illustrates the occurrence of outliers.[54] Fig. 2.28 A illustrates an example of Deming regression analysis with occurrence of an outlier and the associated residuals plot (B), which clearly shows the outlier pattern. In this example, the residuals plot was standardized to unit SD. Use of an outlier limit of 4 SD units in this example led to rejection of the outlier, and a reanalysis was undertaken. In this example, rejection of the outlier changed the slope from 1.14 to 1.03. With regard to outliers, these measurements should not be rejected automatically; the reason for their presence should be investigated as a method limitation (e.g., possibly a nonspecificity for the analyte).

The Correlation Coefficient

Now that the random error components related to regression analysis have been outlined, some comments on the correlation coefficient may be appropriate. The ordinary correlation coefficient, ρ, also called the Pearson product moment

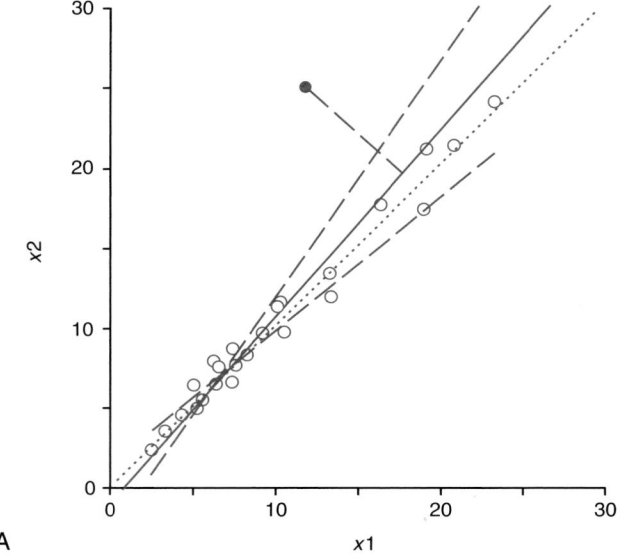

A

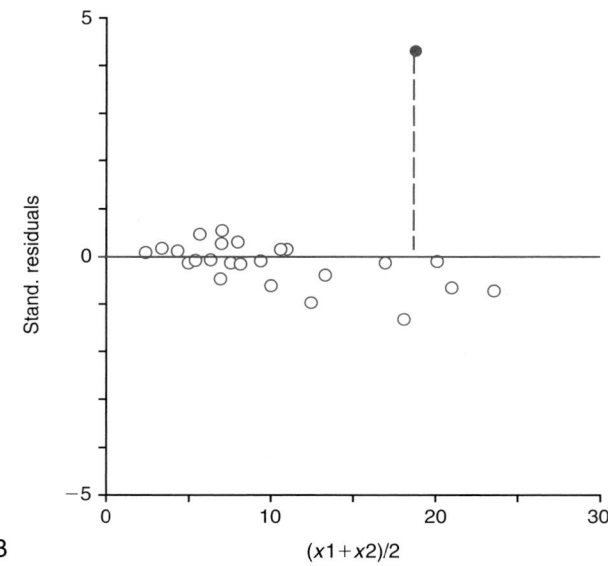

B

FIGURE 2.28 **A,** A scatter plot with the Deming regression line *(solid line)* with an outlier *(filled point)*. The *dotted straight line* is the diagonal, and the *curved dashed lines* demarcate the 95% confidence region. **B,** Standardized residuals plot with indication of the outlier.

correlation coefficient, is estimated as r from sums of squared deviations for $x1$ and $x2$ values as follows:

$$r = p/(uq)^{0.5}$$

where

$$P = \sum \left(x1_i - x1_m\right)\left(x2_i - x2_m\right)$$

$$u = \sum \left(x1_i - x1_m\right)^2 \quad \text{and} \quad q = \sum \left(x2_i - x2_m\right)^2$$

and

$$x1_m = \sum x1_i / N \quad \text{and} \quad x2_m = \sum x2_i / N$$

A look at the theoretical model reveals that ρ is related to the ratio between the SDs of the distributions of target values

($\sigma_{X1'target}$ and $\sigma_{X2'target}$) and the associated independent total random error components[58] (σ_{ex1} and σ_{ex2}):

$$\rho = \sigma_{X1_{target}} \sigma_{X2_{target}} \Big/ \left[\left(\sigma^2_{X1_{target}} + \sigma^2_{ex1} \right) \left(\sigma^2_{X2_{target}} + \sigma^2_{ex2} \right) \right]^{0.5}$$

The total random error components comprise both imprecision error and sample-related random interferences (i.e., $\sigma^2_{ex1} = \sigma^2_{A1} + \sigma^2_{RB1}$ and $\sigma^2_{ex2} = \sigma^2_{A2} + \sigma^2_{RB2}$). Thus ρ is a relative indicator of the amount of dispersion around the regression line. If the numeric interval of values is short, ρ tends to be low and vice versa for a long range of values. For example, consider simulated examples, where the random errors of $x1$ and $x2$ are the same but the width of the distributions of measured values differs (Fig. 2.29A and B). In A, the target values are uniformly distributed over the range 1 to 3, and in B, the range is 1 to 6. The random error SD is presumed constant, and it is set to 0.15 for both $x1$ and $x2$, corresponding to a CV of 5% at the value 3. Given sets of 50 paired measurements, the correlation coefficient is 0.93 in case A and 0.99 in case B. Furthermore, a single point located outside the range of the rest of the observations exerts a strong influence (Fig. 2.29C). In C, 49 of the observations are distributed within the range 1 to 3, with a single point located apart from the others around the value 6, other factors being equal. The correlation coefficient here takes an intermediate value, 0.97. Thus a single point located away from the rest has a strong influence (a so-called influential point). Note that it is not an outlying point, just an aberrant point with regard to the range.

Although σ_{21} is the relevant measure for random error in method comparison studies, ρ is still incorrectly used as a supposed measure of agreement between two methods. It should be noted that a systematic difference due to a difference with regard to calibration is not expressed through ρ but solely in the form of an intercept (α_0) deviation from zero or a slope (β) deviation from unity. Thus even though the correlation coefficient is very high, a considerable calibration bias may be noted between the measurements of two methods.

Regression Analysis in Cases of Proportional Random Error

As discussed in relation to the precision profile, for analytes with extended ranges (e.g., 1 or several decades), the SD_A is seldom constant. Rather, a proportional relationship may apply. This may also be true for the random bias components. In this situation, the regression procedures described previously may still be used, but they are not optimal because the SEs of slope and intercept become larger than is the case when a weighted form of regression analysis is applied. The optimal approaches are weighted forms of regression analysis that take into account the relationship between random error and analyte concentration.[49,54] Given a proportional relationship, a weighted procedure assigns larger weights to observations in the low range; low-range observations are more precise than measurements at higher concentrations that are subject to larger random errors. More specifically, weights are applied in the computations that are inversely proportional to the squared SDs (variances) that express the random error. In the weighted modification of the Deming procedure, distances from ($x1_i$, $x2_i$) to the line are inversely weighted according to the squared SDs at a given concentration

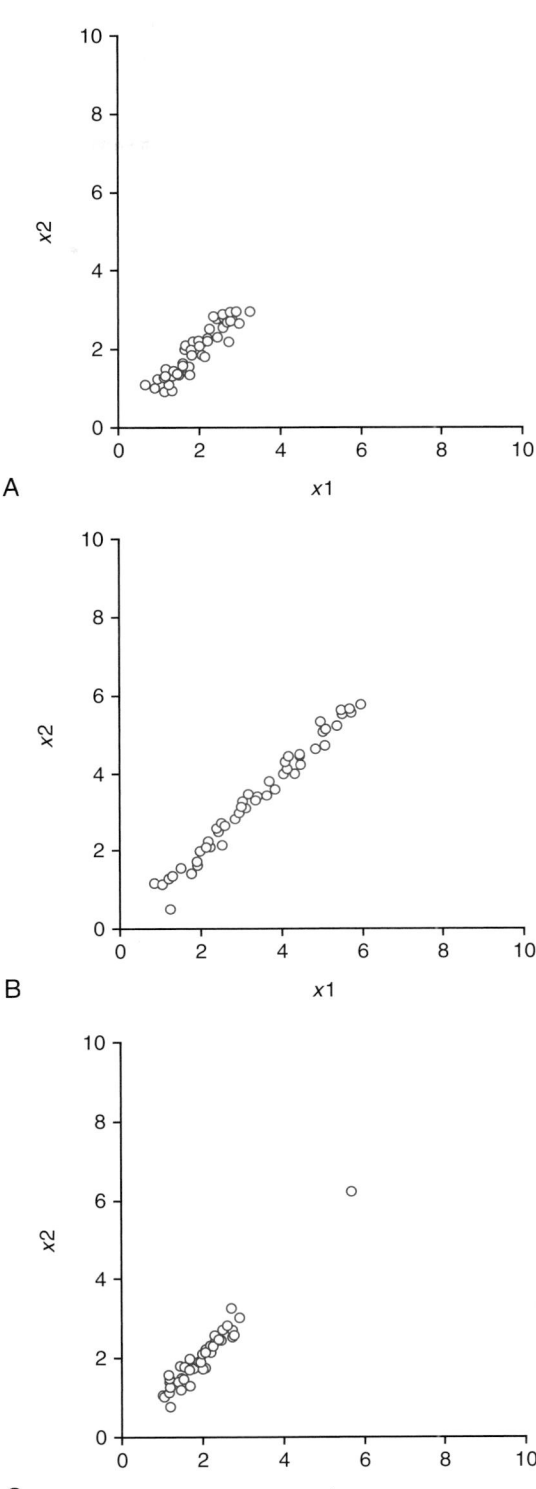

FIGURE 2.29 Scatter plots illustrating the effect of the range on the value of the correlation coefficient ρ. **A,** Target values are uniformly distributed over the range 1 to 3 with random errors of both $x1$ and $x2$ corresponding to a standard deviation (SD) of 5% of the target value at 3 (constant error SDs). **B,** The range is extended to 1 to 6 with the same random error levels. The correlation coefficient equals 0.93 in A and 0.99 in B. **C,** The effect of a single aberrant point is shown. Forty-nine of the target values are distributed over the range 1 to 3, with a single point at 6. The correlation coefficient is 0.97.

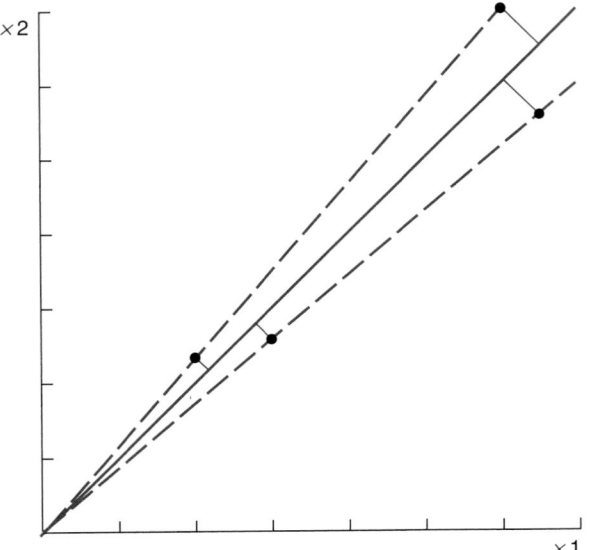

FIGURE 2.30 Distances from data points to the line in weighted Deming regression assuming proportional random errors in $x1$ and $x2$. The symmetric case is illustrated with equal random errors and a slope of unity yielding orthogonal projections onto the line. (Modified from Linnet K. Necessary sample size for method comparison studies based on regression analysis. *Clin Chem* 1999;45:882–94. Used with permission.)

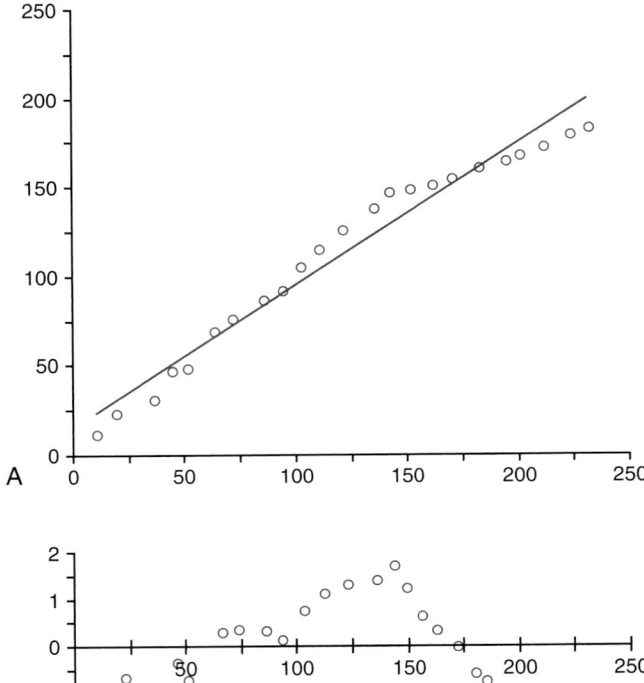

FIGURE 2.31 A, Scatter plot showing an example of nonlinearity in the form of downward-deviating $x2$ values at the upper part of the range. **B,** Plot of residuals showing the effects of nonlinearity. At the upper end of the analytical measurement range, a sequence (run) of negative residuals is present.

(Fig. 2.30). The regression procedures are most conveniently performed using dedicated software.

Testing for Linearity

Splitting of the systematic error into a constant and a proportional component depends on the assumption of linearity, which should be tested. A convenient test is a runs test, which in principle assesses whether negative and positive deviations from the points to the line are randomly distributed over the analytical measurement range. The term *run* here relates to a sequence of deviations with the same sign. Consider, for example, the situation with a downward trend of $x2$ values at the upper end of the analytical measurement range (Fig. 2.31A). The SDs from the line (i.e., the residuals) will tend to be negative in this area instead of being randomly distributed above and below the line (Fig. 2.31B).[20] Given a sufficient number of points, such a sequence will turn out to be statistically significant in a runs test.

Nonparametric Regression Analysis (Passing-Bablok Procedure)

The slope and the intercept may be estimated by a nonparametric procedure, which is robust to outliers and requires no assumptions of Gaussian error distributions.[59,60] The method takes measurement errors for both $x1$ and $x2$ into account, but it presumes that the ratio between random errors is related to the slope in a fixed manner:

$$\lambda = \left(SD_{RB1}^2 + SD_{A1}^2\right) / \left(SD_{RB2}^2 + SD_{A2}^2\right) = 1/\beta^2$$

Otherwise, a biased slope estimate is obtained.[49,60] The procedure may be applied both in situations with random errors with constant SDs and in cases with proportional SDs. The

method is not as efficient as the corresponding parametric procedures[49] (i.e., Deming and weighted Deming procedures). Slope and intercept with CIs are provided, together with Spearman's rank correlation coefficient. A software program is required for the procedure.

Interpretation of Systematic Differences Between Methods Obtained on the Basis of Regression Analysis

A systematic difference between two methods is identified if the estimated intercept differs significantly from zero or if the slope deviates significantly from 1. This is decided on the basis of *t*-tests:

$$t = (a_0 - 0)/SE(a_0)$$

$$t = (b - 1)/SE(b)$$

The *t*-tests can be supplemented with 95% CIs.

SE(a_0) and SE(b) are the SEs of the estimated intercept a_0 and the slope b, respectively. SEs can be derived by a computerized resampling principle called *the jackknife procedure*, which in practice can be carried out using appropriate software.[61] Having estimated a_0 and b, we have the estimate of the systematic difference between the methods, D_c, at a selected concentration, $X1'_{Targetc}$:

$$D_c = X2'_{Targetestc} - X1'_{Targetc} = a_0 + (b - 1) X1'_{Targetc}$$

$X2'_{Targetestc}$ is the estimated $X2'$ target value at $X1'_c$. Note that D_c refers to the *systematic* difference (i.e., the difference between modified target values corresponding to a calibration difference). The SE of D_c can be derived by the jackknife procedure using a software program. By evaluating the SE throughout the analytical measurement range, a confidence region for the estimated line can be displayed. If method comparison is performed to assess the calibration to a reference measurement procedure, correction of a significant systematic difference $Delta_c$ will often be performed by recalibration [$x2_{rec} = (x1 - a_0)/b$]. The associated standard uncertainty is the SE of $Delta_c$. Even though the intercept and the slope are not significantly different from zero and 1, respectively, the combined expression $Delta_c$ may be significantly different from zero.

Example of Application of Regression Analysis (Weighted Deming Analysis)

Application of weighted Deming regression analysis may be illustrated by the comparison of drug assays example [$N = 65$ ($x1$, $x2$) single measurements]. As outlined in the section on the Bland-Altman plot (see Fig. 2.15), in this example the random error of the differences increases with the concentration, suggesting that the weighted form of Deming regression analysis is appropriate. Fig. 2.32 shows (A) the estimated regression line with 95% confidence bands and (B) a plot of normalized residuals. The nearly homogeneous scatter in the residuals plot supports the assumed proportional random error model and the assumption of linearity. The slope estimate (1.014) is not significantly different from 1 (95% CI: 0.97 to 1.06), and the intercept is not significantly different from zero (95% CI: −6.7 to 47.4) (Table 2.9). A runs test for linearity does not contradict the assumption of linearity. The amount of random error is quantified in the form of the SD_{21} proportionality factor equal to 0.11, or 11%. In the present example, with a slope close to unity and two routine methods with assumed random errors of about the same magnitude, we divide the random error by the square root of 2 and get $CV_{x1} = CV_{x2} = 7.8\%$. QC data in the laboratory have provided CV_As of 6.1% and 7.2% for methods 1 and 2, respectively. Thus in this example, the random error may be attributed largely to analytical error. The assay principle for both methods is HPLC, which generally is a rather specific measurement principle; considerable random bias effects are not expected in this case.

In Table 2.9, estimated systematic differences at the limits of the therapeutic interval (300 and 2000 nmol/L) are displayed (24.6 and 48.9 nmol/L, respectively). This corresponds to percentage values of 8.2% and 2.4%, respectively. Estimated SEs by the jackknife procedure yield the 95% CIs, as shown in the table. At the low concentration, the difference is significant (95% CI: 5.7 to 44 nmol/L; does not include zero), which is not the case at the high level (95% CI: −19 to 117 nmol/L). Even though the intercept and slope estimates separately are not significantly different from the null hypothesis values of 0 and 1, respectively, the combined difference $Delta_c$ is significant at low concentrations in this example. If the difference is considered of medical importance and both methods are to be used simultaneously in the laboratory, recalibration of one of the methods might be considered.

Discussion of Application of Regression Analysis

Generally, it is recommended that Deming or weighted Deming regression analysis should be used to operate with a type of regression analysis that is based on a correct error model.

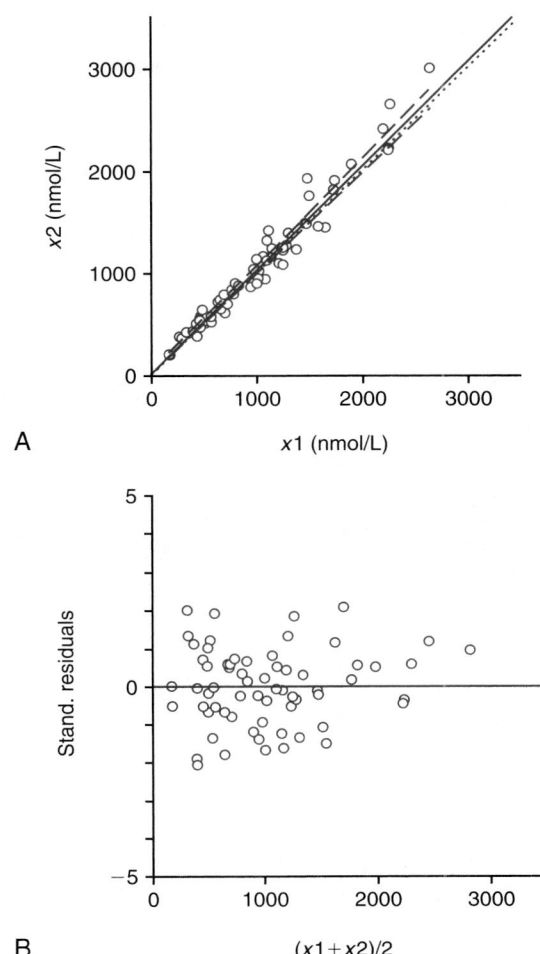

FIGURE 2.32 An example of weighted Deming regression analysis for the comparison of drug assays. **A,** The *solid line* is the estimated weighted Deming regression line, the *dashed curves* indicate the 95%-confidence region, and the *dotted line* is the line of identity. **B,** A plot of residuals standardized to unit standard deviation. The homogeneous scatter supports the assumed proportional error model and the assumption of linearity.

TABLE 2.9 Results of Weighted Deming Regression Analysis for the Comparison of Drug Assays Example, $n = 65$ Single ($x1$, $x2$) Measurements

	Estimate	SE	95% CI
Slope (b)	1.014	0.022	0.97 to 1.06
Intercept (a_0)	20.3	13.5	−6.7 to 47.4
Weighted correlation coefficient	0.98		
SD_{21} proportionality factor	0.11		
Runs test for linearity	NS		
$Delta_c = X_2 - X_1$ at X_c = 300	24.6	9.5	5.72 to 43.6
$Delta_c = X_2 - X_1$ at X_c = 2000	48.9	34.2	−19.3 to 117

CI, Confidence interval; *NS,* not significant; *SD,* standard deviation; *SE,* standard error.

Most published method evaluations are based on unweighted regression analysis; here the use of unweighted analysis is considered in the setting of proportional random errors.

Basically, the Deming procedure provides unbiased estimates of slope and intercept when the SDs vary, provided that their ratio is constant throughout the analytical measurement range. This aspect is important and means that generally the estimates of slope and intercept are reliable in this frequently encountered situation. However, application of the unweighted Deming analysis in cases of proportional SD_As is less efficient than applying the weighted approach. For uniform distributions of values with range ratios from 2 to 100, 1.2 to 3.7 times as many samples are necessary to obtain the same uncertainty of the slope estimated by the unweighted compared with the weighted approach.[61] Thus the larger the range ratio, the more inefficient is the unweighted method.

POINTS TO REMEMBER

- Comparison of two analytical methods is usually based on parallel measurement of a suitable number of patient samples (e.g., 40 in a laboratory and 100 for a vendor of analytical kit methods).
- Data analysis can be based on either a difference plot or regression analysis, the latter providing more details.
- Differences between measurement results may rely on calibration differences, random measurement errors, and biologically based bias sources.
- The optimal regression technique takes measurement errors by both methods into account (e.g., the parametric Deming approach or the nonparametric Passing-Bablok procedure).

MONITORING SERIAL RESULTS

An important aspect of clinical chemistry is monitoring of disease or treatment (e.g., tumor markers in cases of cancer, drug concentrations in cases of therapeutic drug monitoring). To assess changes in a rational way, various imprecision components have to be taken into account. Biologic within-subject variation (SD_I) and preanalytical (SD_{PA}) and analytical variation (SD_A) all have to be recognized.[62] We assume in the following discussion that preanalytical variation is already included in the estimated within-subject variation SD, which often is the case. On this basis, using the principle of adding squared SDs (variances), a total SD (SD_T) can be estimated as follows:

$$SD_T^2 = SD_{Within\ B}^2 + SD_A^2$$

The limit for statistically significant changes then is $k\sqrt{2}\ SD_T$, where k depends on the desired probability level. Considering a two-sided 5% level, k is 1.96. The corresponding one-sided factor is 1.65. If a higher probability level is desired, k should be increased.

Limits for statistically significant changes ($Delta_{stat}$) may be related to changes that are considered of medical importance by clinicians[63] (i.e., action limits [$Delta_{med}$]). Here we will consider a one-sided situation in which an increase is of importance and a 5% significance level is selected (i.e., $Delta_{stat} = 1.65\sqrt{2}\ SD_T = 1.65\ SD_{Delta}$). Suppose as a starting point that the true change ($Delta_{true}$) for a patient is zero (Fig. 2.33A). If $Delta_{stat}$ is less than $Delta_{med}$, the frequency of FP alarms will be

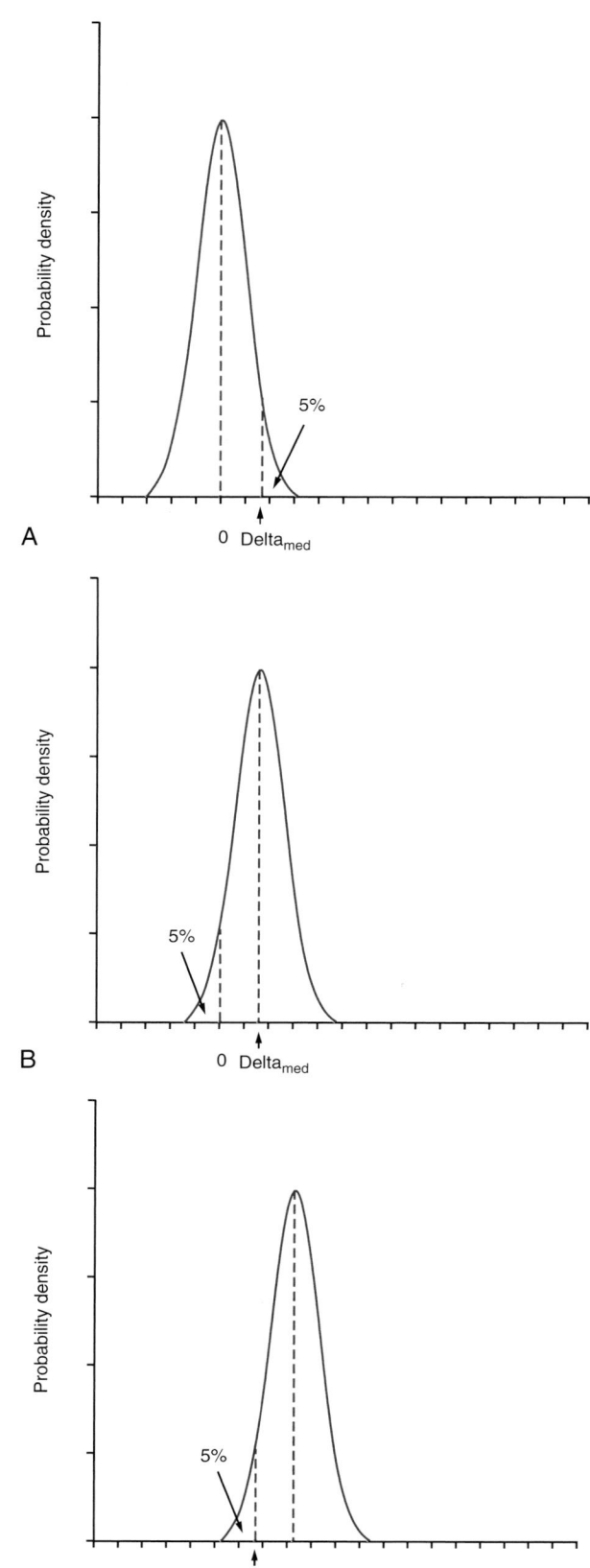

FIGURE 2.33 The monitoring situation. **A,** Distribution of observed changes given a true change of zero. **B,** A true change equal to $Delta_{med}$. **C,** A true change of ($Delta_{med}$ + 1.65 SD_{delta}). $Delta_{stat}$ (=1.65 SD_{delta}) equals $Delta_{med}$ in these examples.

less than 5%. If, on the other hand, Delta$_{stat}$ exceeds Delta$_{med}$, the frequency of FP alarms will exceed 5% (i.e., medical action will be taken too frequently). Fig. 2.33A illustrates the situation with Delta$_{stat}$ equal to Delta$_{med}$. We now consider the situation with a true change equal to the medically important change (i.e., Delta$_{true}$ = Delta$_{med}$) (see Fig. 2.33B), where exactly 50% of observed changes exceed the medically important limit. If Delta$_{stat}$ is less than or equal to Delta$_{med}$, fewer than 5% of patients will exhibit an observed delta value in the opposite direction of the true change (an obviously misleading trend). If the condition is not met, more than 5% will have a misleading change. Finally, when the true change equals the sum of Delta$_{med}$ and Delta$_{stat}$ (see Fig. 2.33C), more than 95% of observed changes exceed the medically important change, and appropriate action will be taken for most patients.

The outline presented previously illustrates that in the monitoring situation, not only the requirement for statistical significance (i.e., the type I error problem concerning false alarms) but also the type II error problem or the risk of overlooking changes should be addressed; the latter is an aspect that often is overlooked.[64] Provided that Delta$_{stat}$ is small relative to Delta$_{med}$, both type I and type II errors can be kept small. On the other hand, if Delta$_{stat}$ equals or exceeds Delta$_{med}$, the relative importance of type I and type II errors may be weighed against each other. If the consequences of overlooking a medically important change are serious, one should keep the type II error small and accept a relatively large type I error (i.e., accept the occurrence of false alarms). On the contrary, if overlooking changes only gives rise to minor or transient problems, the priority may be to keep the type I error small. In addition to simple evaluation of a shift between two measurements, as considered here, sequential results may be analyzed using more refined time-series models.[65]

TRACEABILITY AND MEASUREMENT UNCERTAINTY

As outlined previously in the error model sections, laboratory results are likely to be influenced by systematic and random errors of various types. Obtaining agreement of measurements between laboratories or agreement over time in a given laboratory often can be problematic.

Traceability

To ensure reasonable agreement between measurements of routine methods, the concept of traceability comes into focus. (See also the "Calibration Traceability to a Reference System and Commutability Considerations" section in Chapter 7.) Traceability is based on an unbroken chain of comparisons of measurements leading to a known reference value (Fig. 2.34). A hierarchical approach for tracing the values of routine clinical chemistry measurements to reference measurement procedures was proposed by Tietz[66] and has been adapted by the ISO. For well-established analytes, a hierarchy of methods exists with *a reference measurement procedure* at the top, *selected measurement procedures* at an intermediate level, and finally *routine measurement procedures* at the bottom.[66–68] A reference measurement procedure is a fully understood procedure of highest analytical quality containing a complete uncertainty budget given in Système Internationale (SI) units.[12,69] Reference procedures are used to measure the analyte concentration in *secondary reference*

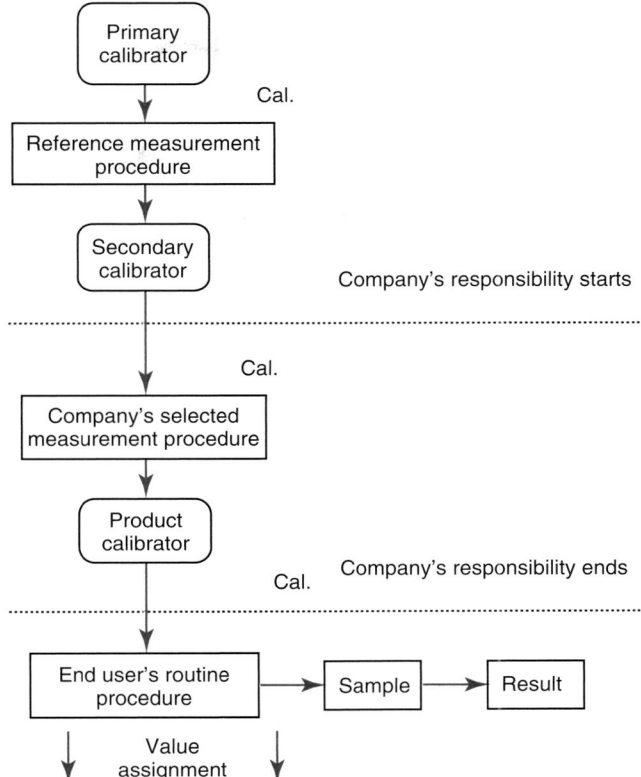

FIGURE 2.34 The calibration hierarchy from a reference measurement procedure to a routine assay. The uncertainty increases from top to bottom. *Cal., Calibration.*

materials, which typically have the same matrix as samples that are to be measured by routine procedures (e.g., human serum). Secondary reference materials are usually of high analytical quality, and certified secondary reference materials must be validated for commutability with clinical samples if they are intended for use as trueness controls for routine methods.[70,71] Otherwise, their use is restricted to selected measurement procedures for which they are intended. The certificate of analysis should state the methods for which the secondary reference materials have been validated to be commutable with clinical samples. When no information is given for commutability, it must be assumed that the reference material is not commutable with clinical samples, and the user has the responsibility to validate commutability for the methods of interest.[72] Uncertainty of the measurement procedure results in increases from the top level to the bottom. ISO guidelines (15193 and 15194) address requirements for reference methods and reference materials.[69,73]

The measurement uncertainty down the traceability chain can end up being too high. By repetition of independent measurements at each step, it may be possible to reduce the overall uncertainty so that it becomes acceptable in relation to analytical performance specification (e.g., those based on biological variation).[74] For more detailed information on analytical performance specifications see "Performance of a Measurement Procedure for Its Intended Medical Use" section of Chapter 7 and the "Analytical Performance Specifications Based on Biological Variation" section of Chapter 8.

Using cortisol as an example, the primary reference material is crystalline cortisol with a chemical analysis for impurities[71]

(National Institute of Standards and Technology [NIST] standard reference material 921, cortisol [hydrocortisone]). A primary calibrator is then a cortisol preparation with a stated mass fraction (purity) (e.g., 0.998 and a 95% CI of ±0.001). The reference measurement procedure is an isotope-dilution gas chromatography–mass spectrometry method that is calibrated with the primary calibrator. A panel of individual frozen serum samples that have values assigned by the primary reference measurement procedure is available from the Institute for Reference Materials and Measurements (IRMM) as secondary reference materials (European Reference Material [ERM]-DA451/International Federation of Clinical Chemistry and Laboratory Medicine [IFCC]). A manufacturer's *selected measurement* procedure is calibrated with the secondary reference materials and is used for measurement of the quantity in the manufacturer's *product calibrator,* which is the calibrator used for the routine method in clinical laboratories.

At the time of writing, the Joint Committee for Traceability in Laboratory Medicine (JCTLM) Database (http://www.bipm.org/jctlm) lists reference materials, either pure or matrix matched, for more than 95 measurands, of which over 50 are traceable to the SI (list I). SI traceable measurands include electrolytes, some metabolites (e.g., glucose, creatinine, urea, uric acid), drugs, metals, steroids, and thyroid and other hormones. Analytes listed in the database that are not traceable to the SI (list II) include 13 plasma proteins (e.g., albumin, α1 acid glycoprotein, α1 antitrypsin, transferrin, transerythretin), using the ERM-DA470k/IFCC. The database also lists reference measurement procedures that define the top of the traceability chain for eight serum enzymes. There are also analytes traceable to higher-order international reference preparations not listed in the JCTLM database, which have been produced by National Measurement Institutes (e.g., pH, PCO_2, PO_2, and ammonia) or by the World Health Organization (http://www.who.int/bloodproducts/catalogue/en) (e.g., for allergens, various proteins and antigens, coagulation factors, and various hormones); however, these are not traceable to the SI. With protein hormones, the existence of heterogeneity or microheterogeneity complicates the problem of traceability.[75,76]

In case a reference measurement procedure exists for an analyte (measurand), comparable results among measurement procedures can be achieved as described earlier, so-called standardization. When reference measurement procedures are not available, so-called harmonization refers to the process of establishing comparable results among measurement procedures for the given analyte.[77] Harmonization is typically based on distribution among laboratories of commutable secondary reference materials with arbitrarily set target values. For more information on harmonization, readers are referred to the "Calibration Traceability to a Reference System and Commutability Considerations" section of Chapter 7.

Harmonization and standardization are especially important when disease is defined by clinical biochemistry results. This pertains to, for example, the diagnosis of diabetes based on plasma glucose determinations. The analytical quality in this instance becomes very critical for a correct evaluation. An analytical bias results in misclassification of subjects into diseased and nondiseased groups. With regard to imprecision, repeat testing may partly circumvent classification errors.[78]

The Uncertainty Concept

To assess in a systematic way errors associated with laboratory results, the *uncertainty* concept has been introduced into laboratory medicine.[79,80] According to the ISO's "Guide to the Expression of Uncertainty in Measurement" (GUM), *uncertainty* is formally defined as "a parameter associated with the result of a measurement that characterizes the dispersion of the values that could reasonably be attributed to the measurand." In practice, this means that the uncertainty is given as an interval around a reported laboratory result that specifies the location of the true value with a given probability (e.g., 95%). In general, the uncertainty of a result, which is traceable to a particular reference, is the uncertainty of that reference together with the overall uncertainty of the traceability chain.[79] Updated information on traceability aspects is available on the website of the Joint Committee on Traceability in Laboratory Medicine (www.bipm.org/jctlm/).

The Standard Uncertainty (u_{st})

The uncertainty concept is directed toward the end user (clinician) of the result, who is concerned about the total error possible and who is not particularly interested in the question of whether the errors are systematic or random. In the outline of the uncertainty concept, it is assumed that any known systematic error components of a measurement method have been corrected, and the specified uncertainty includes uncertainty associated with correction of the systematic error(s).[80] Although this appears logical, one problem may be that some routine methods have systematic errors dependent on the patient category from which the sample originates. For example, kinetic Jaffe methods for creatinine are subject to positive interference by 2-OXO compounds and to negative interference by bilirubin and its metabolites, which means that the direction of systematic error will be patient dependent and not generally predictable.

In the theory on uncertainty, a distinction between type A and B uncertainties is made. Type A uncertainties are frequency-based estimates of SDs (e.g., an SD of the imprecision). Type B uncertainties are uncertainty components for which frequency-based SDs are not available. Instead, uncertainty is estimated by other approaches or by the opinion of experts. Finally, the total uncertainty is derived from a combination of all sources of uncertainty. In this context, it is practical to operate with *standard uncertainties* (u_{st}), which are equivalent to SDs. By multiplication of a standard uncertainty with a *coverage factor (k)*, the uncertainty corresponding to a specified probability level is derived. For example, multiplication with a coverage factor of two yields a probability level of approximately 95%, given a Gaussian distribution. When the total uncertainty of an analytical result obtained by a routine method is considered (u_{st}), preanalytical variation (u_{PAst}), method imprecision (u_{Ast}), sample-related random interferences (u_{RBst}), and uncertainty related to calibration and bias corrections (traceability) (u_{Tracst}) should be taken into account. In expressing the uncertainty components as standard uncertainties, we have the following general relation:

$$u_{st} = \left[u_{PAst}^2 = u_{Ast}^2 = u_{RBst}^2 = u_{Tracst}^2 \right]^{0.5}$$

Uncertainty can be assessed in various ways; often a combination of procedures is necessary. In principle, uncertainty can be judged *directly* from measurement comparisons ("top down")[81,82] or *indirectly* from an analysis of individual error sources according to the law of error propagation ("error budget," bottom up").[80] Measurement comparison may consist of a method comparison study with a reference method based on patient samples according to the principles outlined previously or by measurement of commutable certified matrix reference materials (CRMs). This approach demonstrates the actual uncertainty, which is an advantage. The indirect procedure, on the other hand, builds on an assumed error model, which may or may not be correct and so the uncertainty estimate. It may depend on the circumstances which procedure is feasible. Below, examples of the two types of approaches are outlined.

Example of Direct Assessment of Uncertainty on the Basis of Measurements of a Commutable Certified Reference Material

Suppose a CRM is available that was validated to be *commutable* with patient samples for a given routine method with a specified value 10.0 mmol/L and a standard uncertainty of 0.2 mmol/L. Ten repeated measurements in independent runs give a mean value of 10.3 mmol/L with SD 0.5 mmol/L. The SE of the mean is then $0.5/\sqrt{10} = 0.16$ mmol/L. The mean is not significantly different from the assigned value $[t = (10.3 - 10.0)/(0.2^2 + 0.16^2)^{0.5} = 1.17]$. The total standard uncertainty with regard to traceability is then $u_{\text{Trac st}} = (0.16^2 + 0.2^2)^{0.5} = 0.26$ mmol/L. If the bias had been significant, one might have considered making a correction to the method, and the standard uncertainty would then be the same at the given concentration. Thus measurements of the CRM provide an estimate of the uncertainty related to traceability, *given the assumption of commutability with patient samples*. The other components have to be estimated separately. Concerning method imprecision, long-term imprecision (e.g., observed from QC measurements) should be used rather than the short-term SD observed for CRM material. Here we suppose that the long-term SD_A is 0.8 mmol/L. Data on preanalytical variation can be obtained by sampling in duplicates from a series of patients or can be a matter of judgment (type B uncertainty) based on literature data or data on similar analytes. We here suppose that SD_{PA} equals half the analytical SD (i.e., 0.4 mmol/L). Finally, we lack data on a possible sample-related random bias component, which we may choose to ignore in the present example. The standard uncertainty of the results then becomes

$$u_{st} = \left[u_{PAst}^2 + u_{Ast}^2 + u_{RBst}^2 + u_{Tracst}^2 \right]^{0.5}$$
$$= \left(0.4^2 + 0.8^2 + 0.26^2 \right)^{0.5}$$
$$= 0.93 \, (\text{mmol/L})$$

In this case, the major uncertainty component is the long-term imprecision in the laboratory. To attain a reasonably precise uncertainty estimate, estimated SDs should be based on an appropriate number of repetitions. In the subsection on method precision, it can be seen that $N = 30$ repetitions provides SD estimates with 95% CIs extending from about 20% below to 35% above an estimated value (see Fig. 2.7), which may be regarded as reasonable.

Example of Direct Assessment of Uncertainty on the Basis of a Method Comparison Study With a Reference Measurement Procedure Using Patient Samples

Suppose a set of patient samples has been measured by a routine method ($X2$) in parallel with a reference measurement procedure ($X1$) and that a linear relationship exists between measurements. We want to assess a possible calibration bias and evaluate the standard uncertainty of results of the routine method on the basis of regression analysis results and information on standard uncertainty related to the traceability of reference method results. The imprecision of the reference method is 2.5% or, as a fraction (used in the following), 0.025 ($=CV_{A1}$), and the component related to the uncertainty of the traceability chain for the reference method is 0.020 ($=u_{\text{trac st}}$). Proportional measurement errors are assumed for both methods, and a weighted form of Deming regression analysis is applied. The error variance ratio λ is not known exactly, but the reference method is devoid of sample-related random bias, so it is assumed that the random error is about half that of the routine method (i.e., λ is set to $\frac{1}{2}^2 = \frac{1}{4}$). At a decision point ($X1'_{\text{Targetc}}$) (e.g., corresponding to the upper limit of the 95% reference interval), the systematic difference between methods ($D_c = a_0 + [b - 1] X1'_{\text{Targetc}}$) is estimated with SE (see section on regression):

$$D_c = X2'_{\text{Targetc}} - X1'_{\text{Targetc}} = 20 \, \text{mg/L with SE} \left(D_c \right) = 1.0 \, \text{mg/L}$$

corresponding to a relative $SE(D_c)$ of 0.050 ($=[1.0 \, \text{mg/L}]/[20 \, \text{mg/L}]$). For the Deming procedures, the SE can be conveniently computed by the jackknife procedure. We observe that the difference is highly significant and decide to recalibrate the routine method in relation to the reference method using the estimated slope and intercept (i.e., the recalibrated $x2$ values equals $[x2 - a_0]/b$). Having done this, the routine method is assumed to have no systematic error in relation to the reference method, but when the uncertainty of the results is considered, we have to add the standard uncertainty of the bias correction. The uncertainty related to traceability for the routine method is now obtained as the uncertainty inherent to the reference method and the comparison step, that is,

$$u_{\text{Tracst}} = (0.020^2 + 0.050^2)^{0.5} = 0.054$$

We are now further interested in deriving estimates of random error components for the routine method from regression analysis results. Both analytical error (e.g., estimated from QC data) and sample-related random bias should be assessed, and it should be recognized that the observed total random error is the result of contributions from both measurement methods. Suppose that CV_{21} of the regression analysis has been calculated to be 0.10 (CV_{21} is analogous to SD_{21} or SD_{yx}), given constant measurement errors over the analytical measurement range (i.e., an expression for the random error in the vertical direction in the x-y plot). From the regression section, we have

$$CV_{21}^2 = \left[CV_{A1}^2 + CV_{A2}^2 \right] + \left[CV_{RB1}^2 + CV_{RB2}^2 \right]$$

By substituting $CV_{A1} = 0.025$, $CV_{RB1} = 0$, and $CV_{21} = 0.10$, we derive

$$CV_{RB2}^2 + CV_{A2}^2 = 0.009375$$

and get

$$\left[CV_{RB2}^2 + CV_{A2}^2\right] = 0.0968$$

Thus the total random error of the routine method corresponds to a CV of 0.097. If we had measured samples in duplicate in the method comparison experiment or had available QC data, we could split the total random error into its components. CV_{A2} was here determined to be 0.035 from QC data, which gives 0.090 corresponding to CV_{RB2}. We may here note that the assumed error ratio λ of $(\frac{1}{2})^2$ is not quite correct. According to our results, λ should be $(0.025/0.0968).^2$ Although the Deming regression principle is rather robust toward misspecified λ values, we could choose to carry out a reanalysis with the more correct λ value—a process that could be iterated. Finally, assuming a value of 0.03 for the preanalytical CV, we derive a total standard uncertainty estimate of

$$u_{st} = \left[u_{PAst}^2 + u_{Ast}^2 + u_{RBst}^2 + u_{Tracst}^2\right]^{0.5}$$
$$\left(0.03^2 + 0.0968^2 + 0.054^2\right)^{0.5} = 0.115$$

At the given decision level of 20 mg/L and with a coverage factor of 2, we obtain the 95% uncertainty interval of a single routine measurement as

20 mg/L $\pm$ (2 $\times$ 0.115 $\times$ 20) mg/L =15.4 − 24.6 mg/L

Having estimated the uncertainty as outlined, additional uncertainty sources should be considered. If the comparison was undertaken within a short time period, one might consider adding an additional long-term imprecision component as a variance component to the standard uncertainty expression.

When the two approaches briefly outlined are compared, the latter is the more informative. Using a series of patient samples instead of a pooled sample, individual random bias components are included in the uncertainty estimation, assuming that the patient samples are representative. Also, natural patient samples are preferable to a stabilized pool that perhaps is distributed in freeze-dried form, which may introduce artefactual errors into some analytical systems. Using a commutable CRM, on the other hand, is more practical and in many situations is the only realistic alternative.

Care is necessary in estimating the uncertainty when it is derived from a comparison study of patient samples. First, it is important to correctly estimate the SE of the difference at selected decision points or at points covering the analytical measurement range (i.e., at the lower limit, in the middle part, and at the upper limit). From the expression of the estimated difference $[D_c = a_0 + (b - 1) X1'_{Targetc}]$, initially, one might estimate the SE (standard uncertainty) by adding (squared) the SEs of the intercept and the slope. However, simple squared addition of SEs is correct only when the independence of estimates is given (see later). Estimates of intercept and slope in regression analysis are negatively correlated, which implies that simple squared addition of SEs leads to an overestimation of the total standard uncertainty.[83] Rather, a direct estimation procedure for the SE should be applied, as mentioned earlier.

As mentioned earlier a method comparison study based on genuine patient samples represents a real assessment of traceability. In Fig. 2.34, the focus is on the calibration aspect

intended to *mediate* traceability. One should recognize that the matrix of product calibrators for practical reasons often is artificial (e.g., the matrix of a calibrator may be bovine albumin instead of human serum). Many routine methods are matrix sensitive, which implies that calibrators and patient samples are not commutable. To ensure traceability in this situation, the assigned concentration of a calibrator has to be different from the real concentration.

Indirect Evaluation of Uncertainty by Quantification of Individual Error Source Components

On the basis of a detailed quantitative model of the analytical procedure, the standard approach is to assess the standard uncertainties associated with individual input parameters and combine them according to the law of propagation of uncertainties.[79,84] The relationship between the combined standard uncertainty $u_c(y)$ of a value y and the uncertainty of the *independent* parameters $x_1, x_2, \ldots x_n$, on which it depends, is

$$u_c\left[y(x_1, x_2, \cdots)\right] = \left[\sum c_i^2 u(x_1)^2\right]^{0.5}$$

where c_i is a sensitivity coefficient (the partial differential of y with respect to x_i). These sensitivity coefficients indicate how the value of y varies with changes in the input parameter x_i. If the variables are not independent, the relationship becomes

$$u_c\left[y(x_1, x_2, \cdots)\right] = \left[\sum c_i^2 u(x_1)^2 + \sum c_i c_k u(x_1, x_k)^2\right]^{0.5}$$

where $u(x_i, x_k)$ is the covariance between x_i and x_k, and c_i and c_k are the sensitivity coefficients. The covariance is related to the correlation coefficient ρ_{ik} by

$$u(x_i, x_k) = u(x_i)u(x_k)\rho_{ik}$$

This is a complex relationship that usually will be difficult to evaluate in practice. In many situations, however, the contributing factors are independent, thus simplifying the picture. Below, some simple examples of combined expressions are shown.[84] The rules are presented in the form of combining SDs or CVs given *independent* input components.

$q = x + y$	$SD(q) = [SD(x)^2 + SD(y)^2]^{0.5}$
$q = x - y$	$SD(q) = [SD(x)^2 + SD(y)^2]^{0.5}$
$q = ax$	$SD(q) = a\, SD(x)$ and $CV(q) = CV(x)$
$q = x^p$	$CV(q) = pCV(x)$
$q = xy$	$CV(q) = [CV(x)^2 + CV(y)^2]^{0.5}$
$q = x/y$	$CV(q) = [CV(x)^2 + CV(y)^2]^{0.5}$

The formulas shown may be used, for example, to calculate the combined uncertainty of a calibrator solution from the uncertainties of the reference compound, the weighting, and dilution steps (see later).

The SD for certain non-Gaussian distributions may also be of relevance for uncertainty calculations (type B uncertainties) (Table 2.10). For example, if the uncertainty of a CRM value is given with some percentage, it may be understood as referring to a rectangular probability distribution. In relation to calibration of flasks, the triangular distribution is often assumed.

TABLE 2.10	Relations Between Standard Deviation and Range for Various Types of Distributions		
Normal Distribution		**Rectangular Distribution**	**Triangular Distribution**
SD = Half width of 95% interval/$t_{0.975}(\nu)$ ≈ Half width of 95% interval/2		SD = Half width $\sqrt{3}$	SD = Half width $\sqrt{6}$

SD, Standard deviation.

It has been suggested to apply the standard uncertainty estimate as the smallest analyte reporting interval.[85] Using a coverage factor of two, the uncertainty of a result becomes twice the smallest reporting interval, and the reference change value (RCV) becomes approximately three times (2sqrt[2]) the smallest reporting interval.

Example. Briefly, computation of the standard uncertainty of a calibrator solution will be outlined. The concentration C equals the mass M divided by the volume $V (C = M/V)$. We will here express the standard uncertainties as relative values and will derive the approximate total standard uncertainty by squared addition of the individual contributions. Starting with the mass, the purity is stated on the certificate as 99.4 ± 0.4%. Assuming a rectangular distribution, the relative SD becomes $0.004/\sqrt{3} = 0.0023$. The uncertainty of the weighing process is known in the laboratory to have a CV of 0.1%, or 0.0010. Thus the relative standard uncertainty of the mass becomes

$$u_{Mst} = (0.0023^2 + 0.0010^2)^{0.5} = 0.0025$$

The certificate of the flask (50 mL at 20 °C) indicates ±0.1 mL as uncertainty. Assuming here a triangular distribution, we derive the standard uncertainty as 0.10 mL/$\sqrt{6}$ = 0.0408 mL, which is converted to a relative value of 0.000816. The temperature expansion coefficient is given as 0.020 mL per degree change of temperature. Assuming a variability of 20 ± 4 °C, this contribution amounts to ±0.080 mL. Assuming here a rectangular distribution, we get an SD of 0.080/$\sqrt{3}$ mL, or 0.00092 as a relative SD. The repeatability of the volume dispensing process in the laboratory has been assessed to 0.020 mL expressed as an SD, which corresponds to a relative value of 0.00040. The total standard uncertainty of the volume dispensing process becomes

$$u_{Vst} = (0.000816^2 + 0.00092^2 + 0.00040^2)^{0.5} = 0.0013$$

The total standard uncertainty of the calibrator solution is

$$u_{Cal\,st} = \left(u_{M\,st}^2 + u_{v\,st}^2\right)^{0.5}$$
$$= (0.0025^2 + 0.0013^2)^{0.5}$$
$$= 0.0028, \text{ or } 0.28\%$$

Generally, when squared CVs are added, minor contributions in practice can be ignored (e.g., CVs less than a third or a quarter of the other components).[79]

The indirect procedure is mainly of relevance for relatively simple procedures. For closed, automated clinical chemistry procedures, it is often not possible to discern the individual error elements. Furthermore, the correlation aspect is difficult to take into account in practice. In these cases, the direct procedure of measurement comparison is preferable. However, the indirect procedure has been applied in clinical chemistry.[86,87]

In some situations, a simulation model of a complex analytical method may be established to estimate the combined uncertainty of the method on the basis of input uncertainties.[88,89] Farrance and Frenkel[89] investigated Monte Carlo simulations using Microsoft Excel for the calculation of uncertainties building on functional relationships and taking into account uncertainties in empirically derived constants. In this way, complex relationships can be evaluated relatively easily and a resulting standard uncertainty estimate of an analytical result estimated. This procedure is useful for generating standard uncertainties of derived expressions, such as the estimated glomerular filtration rate or the expression for the anion gap.

Uncertainty in Relation to Traditional Systematic and Random Error Classifications

As mentioned previously, systematic errors are not included in the uncertainty expression because it is assumed that they have been corrected. Therefore the uncertainty of the correction procedure should be taken into account. Otherwise, systematic errors have been added linearly or squared in error propagation models.[90,91] One may further consider that the distinction between systematic effects and random effects may be a matter of the reference frame. For example, a systematic error over time may turn into a random error because a bias may change over time. Lot-to-lot reagent effects may be interpreted as systematic or random errors. When a laboratory changes from an old to a new lot, a shift in measurement values may occur. Initially, this will be considered a systematic change. However, over a long time period involving several lots of reagents, the recorded shifts typically will be up and down and will be regarded as a long-term random error component. Additionally, a bias in a particular laboratory may be viewed as a random error component when dealing with a whole group of laboratories because individual laboratory biases appear randomly distributed and are quantified as the interlaboratory SD. Thus there are arguments for using the uncertainty concept as outlined earlier to end up with one overall uncertainty expression directed toward the end user of the laboratory result. Still, as mentioned previously, systematic errors linked to samples from specific patient subcategories may constitute a problem because a general correction is not possible. A way to quantify this error contribution is to include samples from all patient subgroups in a balanced way in a method comparison study so that this error type is incorporated into the uncertainty component related to traceability. Another problem with systematic errors is that they often depend on the analyte concentration. Thus if a commutable CRM is measured at a particular concentration, one should consider whether a bias correction is valid only at the given concentration or generally over the analytical measurement range. Furthermore, the occurrence of outliers caused by rarely occurring interference (e.g., heterophilic antibodies in relation to immunoassays) constitutes a problem.[92] If the uncertainty estimation is based on parametric statistics (standard uncertainty expanded by a coverage factor), inclusion of gross outliers may increase the standard uncertainty considerably and make the uncertainty specification useless. A solution here might be to omit the outliers in the first hand, compute the 95% uncertainty interval, and then finally add a special note with regard to the probability of occurrence of outliers in the uncertainty specification.

Although it may appear complicated to specify the uncertainty in a detailed manner, a rough estimate may be obtained by adding the squares of CVs corresponding to essential uncertainty elements (e.g., grouped as factors outside the laboratory) (derived from the traceability chain), the analytical factors inside the laboratory (intermediate precision), and the preanalytical elements.[93] In estimating uncertainty, it is important to include relevant elements, but one must be careful to avoid counting the same elements twice. Application of the uncertainty concept and the pros and cons of "top-down" versus "bottom-up" approaches in the field of clinical chemistry are subject to some discussion.[81,92,94] Further reading and case studies with worked example calculations can be found in freely downloadable resources.[81,82]

POINTS TO REMEMBER

- For well-established analytes, a hierarchy of methods exists with *a reference measurement procedure* at the top, *selected measurement procedures* at an intermediate level, and finally *routine measurement procedures* at the bottom.
- The uncertainty is given as an interval around a reported laboratory result that specifies the location of the true value with a given probability (e.g., 95%).
- The uncertainty of a result, which is traceable to a particular reference, is the uncertainty of that reference together with the overall uncertainty of the traceability chain.
- The uncertainty can be judged *directly* from measurement comparisons ("top down") or *indirectly* from an analysis of individual error sources according to the law of error propagation ("error budget," bottom up).

DIAGNOSTIC ACCURACY OF LABORATORY TESTS[a]

Application of diagnostic assays or tests represents a form of medical intervention and therefore requires systematic evaluation before the tests are put into clinical use. We here consider the basic steps for evaluation of the clinical accuracy of laboratory tests, although it applies to any type of diagnostic test, including imaging or electrophysiologic tests. In diagnostic accuracy studies, the measurements or results of one (or more) laboratory test under evaluation (i.e., the so-called index test) are compared with the results of a reference standard or method. This reference is the best prevailing test or strategy that is used to establish the presence or absence of the disease of interest (i.e., the so-called target disease that is to be detected or excluded by the index tests). This reference standard is conducted and its results interpreted as blindly for and independently from the index test(s) results as possible. Test accuracy studies show the concordance in results of the index test(s) with the presence or absence of disease as

defined by the reference standard results.[98–100] These studies provide information regarding the frequency of types of errors (i.e., FP and FN test results) by the index test in relation to the reference standard.

Diagnostic Accuracy of a Test in Isolation
Diagnostic Accuracy, Sensitivity, and Specificity

A systematic and unbiased evaluation and comparison of tests is important.[101–103] The basic approach for any diagnostic accuracy study is one in which the results of the index test are compared with those of a reference test in the same individuals, all of whom are suspected to have the target disease. The simplest situation is a comparison of a single index test, with only two result categories (i.e., a dichotomous or binary index test) to a reference standard (i.e., a single-test accuracy study). The ideal dichotomous index test correctly identifies all individuals as diseased or nondiseased with an error rate of zero. A zero error rate is only possible when there is no overlap between index test results in the diseased and nondiseased individuals. However, when there is overlap in index test results, some individuals are classified wrongly as shown below in an example concerning the diagnosis of deep venous thrombosis (DVT) using a D-dimer index test. When using a quantitative (continuous) index test to classify individuals as diseased or nondiseased, a cutoff value needs to be chosen to estimate these error rates. This results in a so-called dichotomized index test.

Values of the dichotomous or dichotomized index test that exceed the cutoff in individuals having the target disease are classified as true positives (TP) (Fig. 2.35). Similarly, index test results lower than the cutoff in nondiseased individuals are true negatives (TN). Accordingly, index test results below the cutoff in truly diseased subjects are FN, and correspondingly, index test results exceeding the cutoff in truly nondiseased subjects are FP. Based on the frequencies of FN and FP results, an overall error rate or nonerror rate can be derived. The overall diagnostic accuracy of an index test is then defined as the fraction of true classifications out of all classifications:

$$\text{Diagnostic accuracy} = (TB + TP)/(TN + TP + FP + FN)$$

This is an overall nonerror rate that can be subdivided into the nonerror rate of the nondiseased individuals, which is the specificity of the test, and the nonerror rate of diseased individuals, which is the sensitivity of the test

$$\text{Specificity} = TN/(TN + FP)$$
$$\text{Specificity} = TP/(TP + FN)$$

Whereas a very specific test provides negative results for all or almost all subjects who are free of the target disease, a very sensitive test detects all or almost all diseased subjects.

Test result	Disease status	
	Diseased	Nondiseased
Positive	TP	FP
Negative	FN	TN

FIGURE 2.35 The basic 2 × 2 table for estimating the diagnostic accuracy of a dichotomized quantitative test result. Positive test results are divided into true positives *(TPs)* and false positives *(FPs)* and negative results into true negatives *(TNs)* and false negatives *(FNs)*. (From Linnet K, Bossuyt PM, Moons KG, Reitsma JB. Quantifying the accuracy of a diagnostic test or marker. *Clin Chem* 2012;**58**:1292–301.)

[a]This section relies on three published papers.[95–97]

TABLE 2.11 Relationship Between Sample Size and 95% Confidence Intervals of a Proportion (e.g., a Sensitivity or Specificity): Selected Examples of Proportions of 0.05 and 0.8

Sample Size	95% CI of a Proportion of 0.05	95% CI of a Proportion of 0.80
20	0.00–0.25	0.56–0.94
60	0.01–0.14	0.68–0.90
100	0.02–0.11	0.71–0.87
500	0.03–0.07	0.76–0.83
1000	0.04–0.07	0.77–0.82

CI, Confidence interval.

Confidence Intervals of Diagnostic Accuracy, Sensitivity, and Specificity

To assess the (im)precision of these estimates, CIs for either the estimates or the SEs should be specified. If the cutoff value of a quantitative index test is fixed and has not been estimated from the results obtained in the study, the binomial distribution can be applied. Given random sampling, the 95% CI of a proportion can be derived from tables or by applying simple computer programs. An approximation of the binomial to the normal distribution is often used for estimation of the 95% CI of proportions such as a sensitivity and specificity, that is, ± 2 SE(P), where SE(P) = $[P(1 - P)/N]^{0.5}$ (P, proportion; N, sample size).

The normal approximation does not work well with small sample sizes or proportions close to 0 or 1. Both situations occur frequently in diagnostic accuracy research. The method of Wilson is an alternative.[104] Table 2.11 displays the widths of the 95% CIs at various sample sizes of 20 to 1000 for two selected proportions, corresponding to either a sensitivity or a specificity (for that threshold) of an index test. For example, at a sample size of 20, the 95% CI extends from 0.56 to 0.94 for a proportion of 0.80. Thus rather wide estimates of specificity or sensitivity are obtained for small samples. Bachmann and colleagues[105] reported that for 43 nonscreening studies on diagnostic accuracy of tests, the median sample size was 118 (interquartile range, 71 to 350). For the diseased group, the median sample size was only 49 (interquartile range, 28 to 91), but for the nondiseased group, it was 76 (interquartile range, 27 to 209). The specificity and sensitivity of two tests applied in the same study subjects can be statistically compared using the McNemar's test, which is based on a comparison of paired values of true and FP or FN results.[26]

Clinical Example: Accuracy of D-Dimer Test in Diagnosis of Deep Venous Thrombosis

We illustrate the concepts using some of the empirical data of a previously published study in primary care patients suspected of having DVT, the target disease (Fig. 2.36).[106,107] The data given here are used for illustration purposes only and not to quantify the true diagnostic accuracy of the index test for this clinical situation.

The study consisted of 2086 patients suspected of DVT, where DVT was defined as present in patients manifesting at least one of the following symptoms or signs: presence of swelling, redness, or pain in the leg. All patients were given a

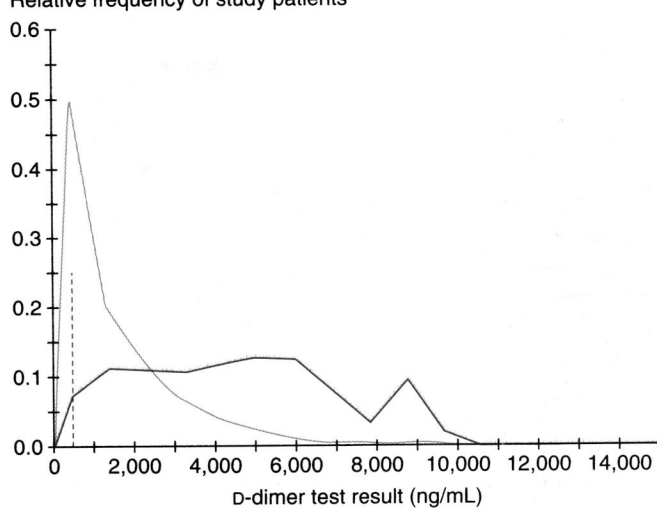

Relative frequency of study patients

FIGURE 2.36 Distribution of the quantitative D-dimer values for deep venous thrombosis (DVT) and non-DVT subjects in the example study. *Light red line,* non-DVT; *red line,* DVT. The *dashed line* indicates the commonly used cutoff value of 500 μg/L. (From Linnet K, Bossuyt PM, Moons KG, Reitsma JB. Quantifying the accuracy of a diagnostic test or marker. *Clin Chem* 2012;58: 1292–301.)

standardized diagnostic workup, including medical history; clinical examination; and testing for D-dimer, the (quantitative) index test. The reference procedure consisted of repeated compression ultrasonography tests and was performed in all patients, blinded to and independent of the index test results. A total of 416 (20%) of the 2086 included patients had DVT. It should be noted that although the reference test is applied currently, it may not be infallible. The potential consequences of applying imperfect reference tests and how to cope with this problem are very important, but these aspects are beyond the scope of this chapter, and for this, we refer to the literature.[108–113]

Applying a commonly used cutoff of 500 μg/L or greater for the (originally) quantitative D-dimer assay (dashed line in Fig. 2.36), the sensitivity was 0.97 (i.e., 3% of the subjects with DVT had a value <500 μg/L). The specificity was only 0.37. The resulting overall diagnostic accuracy was 0.50. Whereas the test displayed good sensitivity at this threshold, detecting all but 3% of those having DVT, its specificity at this test threshold was relatively low, resulting in many FP results. The sample size was high enough to provide precise estimates of specificity and sensitivity. The SEs were 0.012 for the specificity and 0.008 for the sensitivity, resulting in CIs of 0.356 to 0.402 and 0.955 to 0.987, respectively.

Receiver Operating Characteristic Curves

As said, for a quantitative index test, the specificity and sensitivity depend on the selected cutoff point. A plot of the sensitivity and specificity pairs for all possible cutoff values over the measurement range provides the so-called ROC curve, which is shown in Fig. 2.37 for the D-dimer example.[114–117] Usually, sensitivity *(y)* is plotted against (1 − specificity) *(x)* at each possible cutoff value. The better the performance of the test, the higher the ROC curve is located in the left, upper region of the plot. With use of the ROC curve, an appropriate combination of specificity and sensitivity, or rather for an

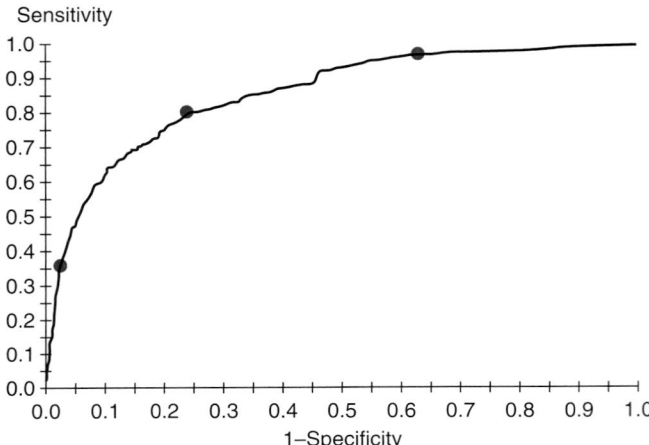

FIGURE 2.37 Receiver operating characteristic curve of the D-dimer assay result for diagnosis of deep venous thrombosis in our example study. The *red markers* correspond to various cutoff choices (from left to right, 5435, 2133, and 500 μg/L). (From Linnet K, Bossuyt PM, Moons KG, Reitsma JB. Quantifying the accuracy of a diagnostic test or marker. *Clin Chem* 2012;**58**: 1292–301.)

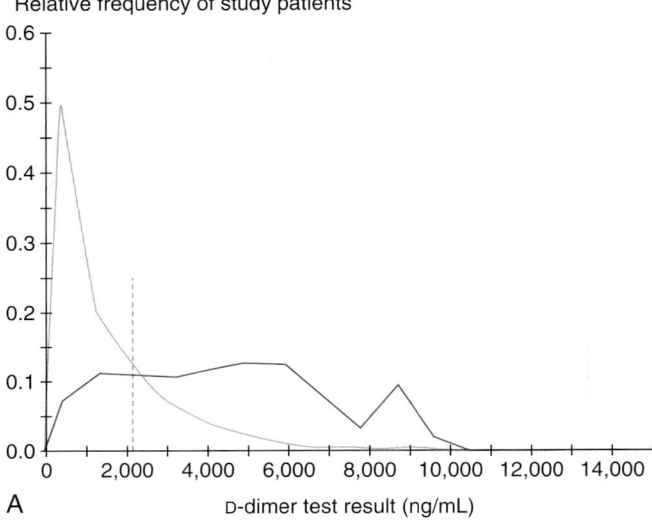

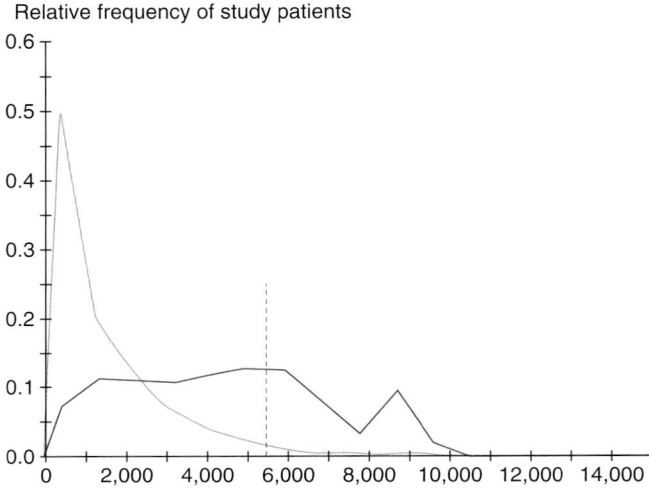

FIGURE 2.38 Alternative cutoffs to 500 μg/L in the D-dimer example. **A,** Cutoff (2133 μg/L) giving maximum value of the sum of the specificity and sensitivity. **B,** Cutoff (5435 μg/L) providing a high specificity (0.975). *Light red line,* non–deep venous thrombosis (DVT); *red line,* DVT. The *dashed line* indicates the cutoff value. (From Linnet K, Bossuyt PM, Moons KG, Reitsma JB. Quantifying the accuracy of a diagnostic test or marker. *Clin Chem* 2012;**58**:1292–301.)

acceptable FN and FP proportion, may be chosen, and the corresponding cutoff then selected. For the D-dimer test, in the example given, the commonly used cutoff of 500 μg/L corresponds to a sensitivity of 0.97 and (1 − specificity) of 0.63.

An area under the ROC curve (i.e., the ROC area or so-called concordance or c-index) can be assessed statistically. The approach used for assessment should emulate the approach used to estimate the ROC curve, either parametric or nonparametric, of which the latter approach generally is preferable. Standard computer programs to perform these calculations are widely available. Given an SE of the ROC area or c-index, it is possible to test whether the area significantly exceeds 0.5, which would demonstrate that the index test performs better than chance. A worthless test has an area of 0.5. Furthermore, using the SE also a 95% CI can be derived for the ROC area or c-index. For the D-dimer test in the earlier example, the area under the ROC curve was 0.86 (SE, 0.011), with a 95% CI of 0.84 to 0.88.

The ROC area provides an overall measure of an index test's diagnostic ability. It can be shown that the area under the ROC curve indicates, for all possible pairings of individuals, one with and one without the target disease, the proportion of pairs in which diseased individuals have a higher (more severe) index test result than individuals without the disease.[114–117] Although ROC curve evaluation has various advantages, it also has some drawbacks.[117–119] The ROC curve does not reflect directly the index test performance for a given cutoff value but can be used for this purpose depending on the desired sensitivity and specificity, or rather the acceptable FN and FP proportions; Fig. 2.37 also displays the sensitivity and specificity at various D-dimer cutoff points (including 500 μg/L, as well as the cutoff values used in Fig. 2.38 below).

Selection of Cutoff Value in Case of Quantitative Index Tests
The specificity and sensitivity determined for an index test usually vary inversely over the range of possible cutoffs. One may select the cutoff point that provides the maximum of the

sum of the specificity and sensitivity. In the D-dimer example, this cutoff would be close to 2000 μg/L, yielding a specificity of 0.76 and a sensitivity of 0.80 (see Fig. 2.38A). However, this method of cutoff selection is commonly not recommended. The selection should rather be based on the intended purpose of the index test. If an index test is applied primarily to rule out the presence of disease (e.g., in the case of the D-dimer assay for exclusion of DVT), the cutoff point should be at the lower end of the distribution of values of diseased individuals (see Fig. 2.36) (e.g., a cutoff of 500 μg/L). At this cutoff, the sensitivity approaches 1.0. But attaining such a high sensitivity is at the cost of a loss of specificity. How low the specificity becomes depends on the extent of overlap of test values in the diseased and nondiseased individuals.

Conversely, when FP results are judged unacceptable, the cutoff should be toward the upper limit of the distribution of values for the nondiseased group. For the D-dimer test example, a cutoff value corresponding to the 97.5 percentile of the distribution of values for those not having DVT (5435 μg/L) resulted in a specificity of 0.975, but now the sensitivity was only 0.36 (i.e., nearly the opposite of the situation with a cutoff of 500 μg/L) (see Fig. 2.38B).

The estimation of an optimal cutoff point can be biased when the cutoff value is selected in the same study in which sensitivity and specificity of the index test have been estimated.[26,120] A good rule is to use independent samples for estimation of the optimal diagnostic cutoff value of the index test and for estimating the diagnostic accuracy measures. Evaluation of the index test in an independent sample also gives an indication of the robustness of the index test.

Posterior Probabilities (Predictive Values)

A straightforward question arising after the application of a diagnostic index test is what is the probability that the target disease is present given the index test value ($P[D|Tpos]$)? The sensitivity and specificity of a test do not directly relate to this question. The probability of presence of target disease given the index test result is an example of a so-called posterior disease probability, where the prior probability corresponds to the prevalence of the disease in the given situation. The prevalence of disease (P[D]) in the study sample is the a priori (pretest) probability of disease.

Given a positive test result (Tpos), the posterior disease probability is estimated as the fraction of TP out of all test result positives:

$$P(D|Tpos) = TP/(TP + FP)$$

Analogously for a negative result (Tneg), the probability that the given disease is absent is

$$P(Non\text{-}D|Tneg) = TN/(TN + FN)$$

Just as with sensitivity and specificity values, these posterior disease probabilities depend on the selected cutoff point for a quantitative test. In case of a dichotomous or dichotomized index test, these posterior probabilities are also called predictive values.[121] They are highly dependent on the disease prevalence. From the Bayes rule, the following relations exist:

$$P(D|Tpos) = [Sensitivity \times P(D)]/[Sensitivity \times P(D)] + (1 - Specificity)(1 - P(D))]$$

$$P(Non\text{-}D|Tneg) = [Sensitivity \times (1 - P(D))]/ [Sensitivity \times (1 - P(D))] + P(D) \times (1 - Specificity)]$$

Likelihood Ratios and Odds Ratios

Besides the above parameters, one may also estimate the so-called diagnostic likelihood ratio (LR) for index test results. From relative frequency distributions for results of the index test in the nondiseased and diseased groups, one may calculate the LR of an index test result (X) as the ratio between the heights of the relative frequency (f) distributions at that specific test value.[122] We get:

$$LR(X) = f_D(X)/f_{Non\text{-}D}(X)$$

In case the relative frequency of the distribution of diseased individuals is higher than that of the nondiseased individuals, the ratio exceeds 1. This indicates that disease is more likely than nondisease given this particular index test result. More formally, the ratio can be used to calculate posterior disease probabilities given specific values of the index test (X) and the disease prevalence (D):

$$P(D|X) = P(D) \times LR(X)/[P(D) \times LR(X) + (1 - P(D))]$$

or a simpler calculation can be carried out using odds instead of probabilities:

$$Odds(D|X) = Odds(D) \times LR(X)$$

based on the relation

$$Odds = P(1 - P)$$

Odds is an alternative way of expressing probabilities commonly used in betting games in Anglo-Saxon countries. For example, a probability of 0.80, or 80%, corresponds to an odds value of 4 according to the formula above. The higher the odds, the closer a probability is to one. From the equation, the posterior odds are equal to the prior odds multiplied by the diagnostic LR for the result X.

For a dichotomous or dichotomized index test, the following relationships apply:

$$LR(pos) = Sensitivity/(1 - Specificity)$$

$$LR(neg) = (1 - Sensitivity)/Specificity$$

Although the LR approach has been tried in various situations, generally the application of diagnostic LRs has been limited in clinical chemistry. Specific conditions are required for the concept to be applied in a practical and reliable way. A simple way of achieving the posttest probability of disease from the prevalence (pretest probability of disease) and the diagnostic LR is to use the Fagan nomogram.[123] A recent example is the estimation of the probability of DVT from testing for D-dimer.[124] Finally, it can be noted that the diagnostic LR of a result X equals the slope of the ROC curve at that index test value.

Comparison of Diagnostic Accuracy of Two Tests in Isolation

The diagnostic accuracy—that is, the ability to detect or exclude the target disease as determined by the reference method—of a new diagnostic index test is usually compared with another, established, index test. We here focus on the pure performances of the tests without consideration of other tests (i.e., we consider each test in isolation). When comparing the accuracy of two or more diagnostic index tests, a paired design is generally preferable for reasons of both validity and efficiency. In the target disease-suspected patients, the two index tests under comparison and the reference standard are performed on all subjects, again independently and blinded with regard to each other's test results. Because both index tests are applied to the same nondiseased and diseased individuals (as classified by the same reference standard), any bias effects caused by differences in disease spectrum or comorbidity are automatically balanced.

A paired comparison of, for example, the sensitivities or specificities for two dichotomous or dichotomized index tests can be evaluated using the McNemar's test.[26,125] The principle of this statistical procedure is that the number of preferences for index test A (cases detected by index test A but not by index test B) is compared with the number of preferences for index test B, and if the difference exceeds some critical value, one index test is found to be superior to the other.

Receiving operating characteristic curve areas may also be compared. Here, a paired comparison should also be undertaken when the index tests have been applied in the same groups of individuals. An example of a paired comparison is displayed in Fig. 2.39. Parametric and nonparametric statistical procedures exist that usually are performed by computer programs.[116,126] Overall, the index test having the largest area under the ROC curve represents the best test, although this assessment becomes more difficult if the ROC curves of tests cross each other.[119] Preferably, CIs of areas and differences of areas should be provided.

Shortcomings of Diagnostic Accuracy Studies of Tests in Isolation

The accuracy of a diagnostic test highly depends on the context. The estimated diagnostic accuracy measures of an index test (posterior probabilities, sensitivity, specificity, LR, or ROC area) preferably obtained from data of a cohort of target disease–suspected patients are not constant; they vary across other index test results, patient characteristics, disease prevalence, or disease severities.[127–129] We illustrate this for our D-dimer example in Table 2.12. The overall sensitivity and specificity for the 500 µg/L threshold were 0.97 and 0.37, respectively (upper row). However, when estimating these measures for patient subgroups within the study sample defined by other test results from patient history and physical

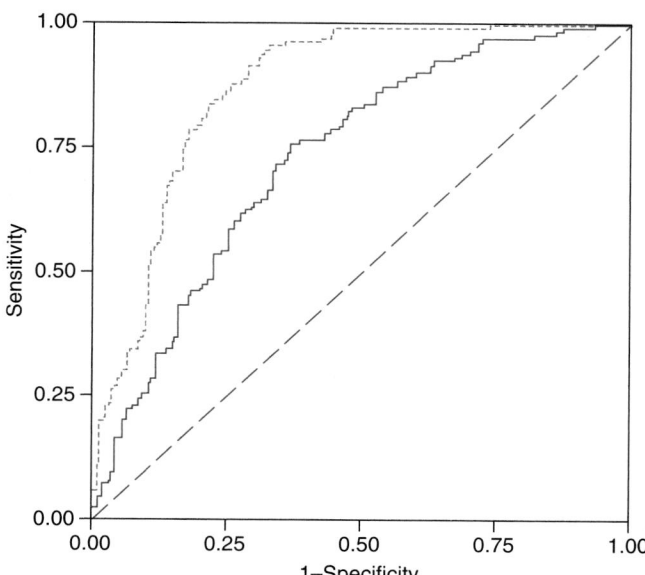

FIGURE 2.39 Comparison of the receiver operating characteristic curves of two hypothetical index tests for the same target disease undertaken in the same individuals. The *dotted, red curve* represents a superior diagnostic test, both with regard to sensitivity and specificity over all possible cutoff points. The *dashed diagonal* represents a worthless test, with equal probability of a false-positive (1−Specificity) and false-negative (1−Sensitivity) result across all cutoff values (i.e., flipping a coin test). (From Linnet K, Bossuyt PM, Moons KG, Reitsma JB. Quantifying the accuracy of a diagnostic test or marker. *Clin Chem* 2012;**58**:1292–301.)

TABLE 2.12 Variations in the Sensitivity and Specificity (at Cutoff Values 500 ng/mL and 1000 ng/mL) and the Receiver Operating Characteristic Area of the D-Dimer Test According to Various Other Test Results or Patient Characteristics.

	D-DIMER > 500 ng/mL		D-DIMER > 1000 ng/mL		D-Dimer (Continuous)
	Sensitivity	Specificity	Sensitivity	Specificity	AUC (CI)
Overall	0.97	0.37	0.89	0.55	0.86 (0.84;0.88)
Previous lung embolism					
Yes (*n* = 173)	1.00	0.37	0.84	0.53	0.82 (0.75;0.90)
No (*n* = 1913)	0.97	0.37	0.89	0.55	0.86 (0.84;0.88)
Malignancy					
Yes (*n* = 115)	0.95	0.25	0.95	0.44	0.86 (0.79;0.93)
No (*n* = 1971)	0.97	0.38	0.89	0.55	0.84 (0.83;0.87)
Recent surgery					
Yes (*n* = 278)	0.96	0.22	0.90	0.38	0.84 (0.78;0.90)
No (*n* = 1808)	0.97	0.39	0.89	0.57	0.86 (0.84;0.88)
Leg trauma					
Yes (*n* = 344)	0.96	0.32	0.85	0.48	0.79 (0.72;0.87)
No (*n* =1742)	0.97	0.38	0.89	0.56	0.86 (0.84;0.89)
Pitting edema					
Yes (*n* = 1301)	0.97	0.32	0.88	0.50	0.84 (0.82;0.87)
No (*n* = 785)	0.97	0.46	0.90	0.62	0.87 (0.84;0.91)
Pregnancy					
Yes (*n* = 45)	1.00	0.28	1.00	0.55	0.98 (0.00;1.00)
No (*n* = 2041)	0.97	0.37	0.89	0.55	0.85 (0.83;0.88)

AUC, Area under the receiver operating characteristic curve; *CI,* 95% confidence interval.

examination, substantial differences appear with regard to specificity, especially for the malignancy, recent surgery, and pitting-edema subgroups. At a higher threshold (1000 µg/L) variations in sensitivity also occur, for example, in the pregnancy and previous embolism subgroups. The last column of Table 2.12 reveals that this variation in single-test accuracy measures also holds true for non–threshold-dependent measures such as the ROC area. The ROC area was from 0.79 to 0.98, with 0.86 for the total study group. Although all these differences should not be overinterpreted, one must always be careful when judging a single test's diagnostic accuracy measures. A diagnostic laboratory test should always be considered in relation to a specific clinical situation and its results judged within the diagnostic pathway (i.e., in view of the results of other usually applied tests) in which the test under study is to be applied.[128–130] How to do so is covered in the next section.

The Standards for Reporting of Diagnostic Accuracy Studies (STARD) initiative, originally launched in 2003[101] and updated in 2015,[102] aims to improve the quality and reporting of diagnostic accuracy studies. A checklist guides investigators regarding what information to report on patient selection, the order of test application, and the number of individuals undergoing the test under evaluation, the reference test, or both, and other characteristics important for unbiased study design (Box 2.2).[102] Similarly, the so-called Quality Assessment Tool for Diagnostic Accuracy Studies (QUADAS-2) tool to critically appraise and assess risk of bias in primary diagnostic accuracy studies has been developed to assist systematic reviews of diagnostic accuracy studies (http://www.quadas.org).[131] For more information on STARD and QUADAS and the Diagnostic Test Accuracy Review Group of the Cochrane Collaboration, see Chapter 10 on evidence-based laboratory medicine.

POINTS TO REMEMBER

- The diagnostic accuracy of a test indicates the frequency and type of errors that a test will produce when differentiating between patients with and without the target disease.
- The cohort design based on patients suspected of the diseases targeted by the index test is generally preferable for evaluating diagnostic accuracy.
- It is not meaningful to regard estimates of diagnostic performance as properties of the test itself but rather to interpret them as depending on the setting in which the index test was applied and dependent on other tests that are commonly used in that setting.

Diagnostic Accuracy of a Test in the Clinical Context

The diagnostic process in practice begins with a patient having particular symptoms or signs. These symptoms and signs may direct the suspicion toward several possible diseases (the differential diagnosis). The diagnostic workup is often primarily targeted to include or exclude a particular disease or disorder, the so-called target disease, among several possible differential diagnoses.[99,101,132–135] For example, a woman showing up with a red, swollen leg may be suspected of having DVT; a man with blood in his stool may be suspected of having colon carcinoma; and a child with convulsions may be suspected of having

bacterial meningitis. The target disorder in question can be the most severe disorder of the differential diagnoses ("the one not to miss") but also the most probable one.

The diagnostic process commonly consists of a series of sequential steps in which much diagnostic information (i.e., diagnostic test results) is acquired. After each step, the physician intuitively judges the probability of the target disease being present. The initial step always consists of patient history and physical signs. If uncertainty about the presence and type of disease remains, subsequent tests are performed, often in another stepwise fashion. These supplementary tests may consist of simple blood or urine tests or be imaging, electrophysiology, or genetic tests or even later in the process more invasive testing such as biopsy, angiography, or arthroscopy. The supplementary information of each subsequent test is implicitly added to the yet collected diagnostic information, and the target disease probability is constantly updated. This process continues until the target disease can be included or excluded with sufficient certainty and some therapeutic management can be started, including the decision to refrain from treatment.

Hardly any diagnosis is based on a single test; for example, information from the history and the physical examination are almost always collected before any laboratory test is applied. Rather, the diagnostic context involves a multivariable (multiple-test) and phased process in which physicians decide whether the next test will add information to what is already established.[129,136,137]

Investigations of diagnostic laboratory tests should incorporate this multivariable clinical context in their studies. Laboratory tests should not be evaluated in isolation; rather, their studies should reflect the steps in the diagnostic process so that the added value of such tests in excess of the information that is already present can be assessed. Depending on the situation, studies may reveal that the diagnostic information of any subsequent test is already supplied by the simpler previous test results. When regarded in isolation such subsequent test or marker may indeed show diagnostic accuracy or value, but when assessed in the overall diagnostic workup, it does not. Such a case can arise because different tests may gauge the same underlying pathologic processes to varying degrees and thus provide related diagnostic information. From a statistical point of view, the various test values, whether obtained from patient history, physical signs, or subsequent testing, are to varying degrees mutually correlated.[127,128,130] The main point in diagnostic accuracy assessment, therefore is not what the diagnostic accuracy of a particular (laboratory) test is, as covered in the previous section, but rather whether it is going to improve the diagnostic accuracy of the existing setup beyond what is present from the already acquired diagnostic information.

In the following, we focus on the extent to which a certain laboratory test adds information to test results that have already been obtained. How much the new test adds in terms of improved discrimination between the presence or absence of the target disease in relation to a reference standard is of interest in this section.

Clinical Example: Added Value of D-Dimer Testing in the Diagnosis of Suspected Deep Venous Thrombosis

The concept of assessing the added value of a subsequent diagnostic test will be illustrated by the same DVT case study

BOX 2.2 STARD 2015

An Updated List of Essential Items for Reporting Diagnostic Accuracy Studies

Title or Abstract

1. Identification as a study of diagnostic accuracy using at least one measure of accuracy (e.g., sensitivity, specificity, predictive values, AUC)

Abstract

2. Structured summary of study design, methods, results, and conclusions (for specific guidance, see STARD for Abstracts)

Introduction

3. Scientific and clinical background, including the intended use and clinical role of the index test
4. Study objectives and hypotheses

Methods

Study Design

5. Whether data collection was planned before the index test and reference standard were performed (prospective study) or after (retrospective study)

Participants

6. Eligibility criteria
7. On what basis potentially eligible participants were identified (e.g., symptoms, results from previous tests, inclusion in registry)
8. Where and when potentially eligible participants were identified (setting, location, and dates)
9. Whether participants formed a consecutive, random, or convenience series

Test Methods

10a. Index test, in sufficient detail to allow replication
10b. Reference standard, in sufficient detail to allow replication
11. Rationale for choosing the reference standard (if alternatives exist)
12a. Definition of and rationale for test positivity cutoffs or result categories of the index test, distinguishing prespecified from exploratory
12b. Definition of and rationale for test positivity cutoffs or result categories of the reference standard, distinguishing prespecified from exploratory
13a. Whether clinical information and reference standard results were available to the performers or readers of the index test

13b. Whether clinical information and index test results were available to the assessors of the reference standard

Analysis

14. Methods for estimating or comparing measures of diagnostic accuracy
15. How indeterminate index test or reference standard results were handled
16. How missing data on the index test and reference standard were handled
17. Any analyses of variability in diagnostic accuracy, distinguishing prespecified from exploratory
18. Intended sample size and how it was determined

Results

Participants

19. Flow of participants, using a diagram
20. Baseline demographic and clinical characteristics of participants
21a. Distribution of severity of disease in those with the target condition
21b. Distribution of alternative diagnoses in those without the target condition
22. Time interval and any clinical interventions between index test and reference standard

Test Results

23. Cross-tabulation of the index test results (or their distribution) by the results of the reference standard
24. Estimates of diagnostic accuracy and their precision (e.g., 95% CIs)
25. Any adverse events from performing the index test or the reference standard

Discussion

26. Study limitations, including sources of potential bias, statistical uncertainty, and generalizability
27. Implications for practice, including the intended use and clinical role of the index test

Other Information

28. Registration number and name of registry
29. Where the full study protocol can be accessed
30. Sources of funding and other support; role of funders

AUC, Area under the curve; *CI,* confidence interval; *STARD,* Standards for Reporting of Diagnostic Accuracy Studies.
From Bossuyt PM, Reitsma JB, Bruns DE, Gatsonis CA, Glasziou PP, Irwig L, et al. STARD Group. STARD 2015: an updated list of essential items for reporting diagnostic accuracy studies. Clin Chem 2015;61(12):1446–52.

described earlier.[106,107] In short, 2086 patients were suspected of DVT, having at least one of the following symptoms: swelling, redness, or pain in the leg. All patients had a standardized diagnostic workup consisting of index tests from medical history taking, physical examination, and quantitative D-dimer testing. The reference standard was repeated compression ultrasonography, according to current clinical practice. This reference test was carried out in all patients independent of the results of the index tests and blinded with regard to all preceding collected index test results. In total, 416 of the 2086

included patients (20%) had DVT confirmed by ultrasonography. In this section, we focus on estimating the added value of D-dimer testing to the information provided by history taking and physical examination (Table 2.13).

Table 2.13 displays the relationship between each diagnostic test result and the presence or absence of DVT. The values in fact correspond to single-test accuracy values, as discussed in the preceding section. It would be difficult, if not impossible, to select the most promising index tests from these single-test accuracy values. None of the history and physical

TABLE 2.13 Distribution and Accuracy of Each Diagnostic Variable Compared With the Reference Standard Outcome (Deep Venous Thrombosis Present or Absent Based on Repeated Compression Ultrasonography)

| | DEEP VENOUS THROMBOSIS | | | | | | |
| | Yes (n = 416) | | | No (n = 1670) | | | |
	n	Sens (%) (95% CI)	PPV (%) (95% CI)	n	Spec (%) (95% CI)	NPV(%) (95% CI)	ROC Area[a] (95% CI)
Male gender	194	47 (42–51)	25 (22–29)	569	66 (64–68)	83 (81–85)	—
Mean age in years (SD)	62 (17)	—	—	59 (18)	—	—	0.53 (0.50–0.56)
Presence of malignancy	40	10 (7–13)	35 (27–44)	75	96 (94–96)	81 (79–83)	—
Recent surgery	76	18 (15–22)	27 (22–33)	202	88 (86–89)	81 (79–83)	—
Absence of recent leg trauma	47	89 (85–91)	21 (19–23)	297	18 (16–20)	86 (82–90)	—
Vein distension	115	28 (24–32)	28 (24–32)	302	82 (80–84)	82 (80–84)	—
Pain on walking	344	83 (79–86)	21 (19–23)	1325	21 (19–23)	83 (79–86)	—
Swelling whole leg	247	59 (55–64)	26 (23–29)	699	58 (56–60)	85 (83–87)	—
Mean difference in calf circumference in cm (SD)	3 (2)	—	—	2 (2)	—	—	0.69 (0.67–0.72)
Mean D-dimer in ng/mL (SD)	4549 (2665)	—	—	1424 (1791)	—	—	0.86 (0.84–0.88)

[a]A receiving operator characteristic (ROC) area lower than 0.5 means that overall this test result was better for excluding than including deep venous thrombosis (DVT) presence.

NPV, Negative predictive value, the proportion of subjects labeled no DVT by the diagnostic test with true absence of DVT; *PPV,* positive predictive value, the proportion of subjects labeled DVT by the diagnostic test with true DVT; *Sens,* sensitivity, the proportion of subjects with true DVT who are labeled as DVT by the diagnostic test; *Spec,* specificity, the proportion of subjects with true absence of DVT who are labeled as no DVT by the diagnostic test.

examination tests was pathognomonic for DVT. Some tests or investigations had a high sensitivity but a low specificity (e.g., absence of leg trauma and pain on walking), but other tests exhibited a high specificity and low sensitivity (e.g., presence of malignancy or recent surgery). Some tests would serve better for exclusion, others for inclusion. The ROC areas for the continuous tests, age and difference in calf circumference (but also for the D-dimer test), were all below 1 and above 0.5. One questions whether combinations of history and physical examination test results have better accuracy compared with their individual accuracy values and whether the D-dimer biomarker has incremental accuracy.

A multivariable statistical approach is needed to assess the diagnostic accuracy of combined index test results. Given a dichotomous outcome (DVT present or not), multivariable logistic regression modeling is the most appropriate approach. Logistic regression models express the probability of DVT (on the logit scale) as a linear function of the included index test results. Note that index test results may be included as binary, categorical, or even continuous results. The latter two do by no means need to be dichotomized first. Indeed, this is even contraindicated because it may often lose diagnostic value to the index test. Table 2.14 (model 1) shows the results from history and physical examination test results that were significantly related to DVT in the multivariable analysis, here defined as a multivariable odds ratio significantly ($P < .05$) different from 1 (no association).

To quantify whether the quantitative D-dimer assay value has added diagnostic value beyond the history and physical examination results combined, the basic model 1 was simply extended by including the index test D-dimer value, resulting in model 2 (see Table 2.14). After the inclusion of the D-dimer assay result, the regression coefficients of most history and physical tests in model 2 are found to be different from those in model 1: They now express the contribution of the corresponding test results, given a specific D-dimer result. This change reveals that the history and physical and the D-dimer results are indeed correlated and partly provide the same diagnostic information regarding whether DVT is present or not. The trend of lower regression coefficients of most findings can be interpreted as follows: A portion of the information supplied by the history and physical items is now replaced by the D-dimer assay result. Notice that the influence of the variable, recent surgery, has completely disappeared after the addition of the D-dimer biomarker.

Diagnostic Accuracy of Combinations of Diagnostic Tests: Receiver Operating Characteristic Area

The multivariable diagnostic model, which is based on a combination of diagnostic index tests, as exemplified in models 1 and 2 in Table 2.14, can actually be considered as a single (overall or combined) quantitative index test, consisting of a composite of individual index tests. The test result of this "combined index test model" for each study patient is simply the calculated posterior probability of DVT presence given the observed pattern of the individual index test results in that patient. (See the footnote to Table 2.14 on how to calculate this probability of disease presence.) Note that this posterior probability is now the probability of DVT based on combination of multiple index test results rather than of a single index test result.

As for single continuous index tests described earlier, also for "test combinations" combined into a single multivariable model, one can calculate the ROC area (*c*-statistic) to indicate

TABLE 2.14 **The Basic and Extended Multivariable Diagnostic Model to Discriminate Between Deep Venous Thrombosis Presence versus Absence[a]**

	MODEL 1 (BASIC MODEL)			MODEL 2 (BASIC MODEL + D-DIMER)		
	Regression Coefficient (SE)	OR (95% CI)	*P*	Regression Coefficient (SE)	OR (95% CI)	*P*
(Intercept)	−3.70 (0.26)	—	<.01	−4.94 (0.32)	—	<.01
Presence of malignancy	0.62 (0.22)	1.9 (1.2–2.9)	<.01	0.22 (0.26)	1.2 (0.7–2.1)	.41
Recent surgery	0.44 (0.16)	1.6 (1.1–2.1)	<.01	0.003 (0.19)	1.0 (0.7–1.5)	.99
Absence of leg trauma	0.75 (0.18)	2.1 (1.5–3.0)	<.01	0.67 (0.20)	2.0 (1.3–2.9)	<.01
Vein distension	0.48 (0.13)	1.6 (1.1–2.1)	<.01	0.25 (0.16)	1.3 (0.9–1.8)	.12
Pain on walking	0.41 (0.15)	1.5 (1.1–2.0)	<.01	0.46 (0.18)	1.6 (1.1–2.3)	.01
Swelling whole leg	0.36 (0.12)	1.4 (1.1–1.8)	<.01	0.47 (0.14)	1.6 (1.2–2.1)	<.01
Difference in calf circumference (per cm)	0.36 (0.04)	1.4 (1.3–1.5)	<.01	0.29 (0.04)	1.3 (1.2–1.4)	<.01
D-Dimer (per 500 ng/mL)	NA	NA	NA	0.29 (0.02)	1.3 (1.3–1.4)	<.01

[a]Exp(regression coefficient) is the odds ratio (OR) of a diagnostic test result. For example, an odds ratio of 2 for absence leg trauma (model 2) means that a suspected patient without a recent leg trauma has a two times higher chance of having deep venous thrombosis (DVT) than a patient with a recent leg trauma (because in the latter the leg trauma would more likely be the cause of the presenting symptoms and signs). Similarly, an odds ratio of 1.3 for calf difference in cm (model 2) means that for every centimeter increase in calf circumference difference, a patient has a 1.3 times (or 30%) higher chance of having DVT.
A diagnostic model can be considered as a single overall or combined test consisting of different test results, with the probability of DVT presence as its test result. For example, for a male subject without malignancy, recent surgery, or leg trauma but with vein distension and a painful not swollen leg when walking with a calf difference of 6 cm the formula is (model1):
$Z = -3.70 + 0.62*0 + 0.44*0 + 0.75*0 + 0.48*1 + 0.41*1 + 0.36*0 + 0.36*6 = -0.65$.
The probability for this patient of the presence of DVT based on the basic model then is exp(−0.65)/[1 + exp(−0.65)] = 34%.

the ability of this "test combination" to discriminate between the presence versus absence of the target disease (here DVT).[115,138] Here the ROC area expresses the proportion out of all possible pairs of patients with and without DVT for which the patient with DVT has a higher estimated probability by the model than the patient without DVT. Fig. 2.40 shows the ROC curves and areas for models 1 and 2, which is not much different from the comparison of two continuous index tests in isolation described earlier except that in this section, all tests are not considered in isolation but in combination or within the diagnostic pathway.

Fig. 2.40 displays how adding the quantitative D-dimer assay to model 1 mediated an increase in the ROC area from 0.72 to 0.87, a considerable and statistically significant gain (*P* < .01),[115,116] which can be estimated using the same method described earlier for comparing two quantitative index tests in isolation. This implies that the overall diagnostic accuracy of the information from patient history and physical examination can be improved substantially by addition of the D-dimer test.

The use of the difference in ROC area to express the added value of a new test or biomarker has been subject to criticism.[139–141] First, the area under the receiver operating characteristic curve (AUC) is a summary measure of discrimination and has no direct clinical implication in terms of correct or incorrect diagnostic classifications or absolute patient numbers. Various investigators have noticed that the increase in AUC commonly may be relatively small by adding new but still relevant biomarkers, particularly when the AUC of the baseline model already is large.[140–143] Several alternative measures have been suggested to quantify the added value of a novel test or biomarker to circumvent these limitations.

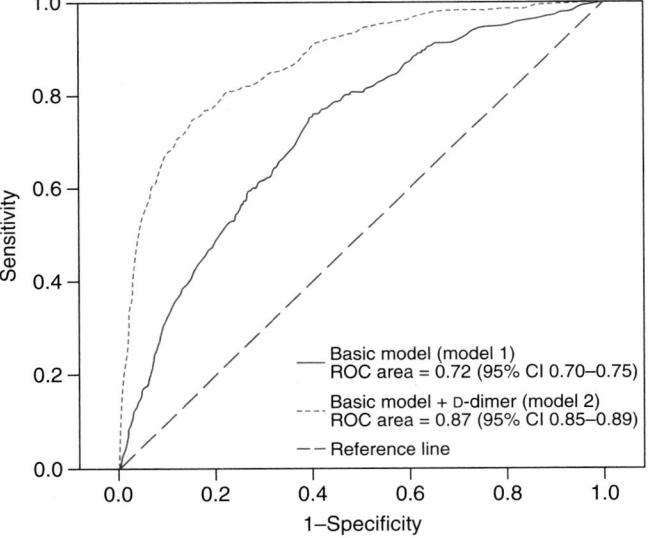

FIGURE 2.40 Receiver operating characteristic *(ROC)* curves for the combination of history and physical examination tests before and after addition of the D-dimer assay result. *CI,* Confidence interval. (From Moons KG, de Groot JA, Linnet K, Reitsma JB, Bossuyt PMM. Quantifying the added value of a diagnostic test or marker. *Clin Chem* 2012;**58**:1408–17.)

Reclassification Measures

To handle the problems associated with the difference in ROC areas, reclassification analysis has been proposed.[144] The reclassification table displays how many patients actually are regrouped by adding a new test to (a combination of) existing tests after defining a threshold for a given posterior probability for presence of disease. The reclassification table with

TABLE 2.15   Reclassification Table From The Basic and Extended (With D-Dimer) Model at an Arbitrary Deep Venous Thrombosis Probability Threshold of 25%[a]

DVT Yes (n = 416)

		Model 2 with D-Dimer		
DVT probability threshold		≤25%	>25%	Total
Model 1 without D-dimer	≤25%	92	123	215
	>25%	26	175	201
	Total	118	298	416

DVT No (n = 1670)

		Model 2 with D-Dimer		
DVT probability threshold		≤25%	>25%	Total
Model 1 without D-dimer	≤25%	1223	116	1339
	>25%	227	104	331
	Total	1450	220	1670

[a]A patient with a model's probability of greater than 25% is considered high probability of having deep venous thrombosis (DVT) and is further worked up or managed for DVT.

a threshold at 25% is shown in Table 2.15. This means, in this theoretical example, that patients with a calculated posterior probability of 25% or higher are considered to be at high risk of having DVT and need to be referred for reference testing, but those of less than 25% receive no reference testing.

Table 2.15 displays the reclassification of patients according to model 2 instead of model 1 at a DVT probability threshold of 25%. For example, in patients with DVT, 36% (123/416 + 26/416) were reclassified by model 2 compared with model 1. For patients without DVT, this percentage was 21% (227/1670 + 116/1670).

The simple change in classification of individuals to different posterior probability categories of DVT presence, however, is not satisfactory for assessing improvement in diagnostic accuracy by a new test or biomarker; the changes should also be in the right direction. Otherwise, an increase in posterior probability categories for subjects with DVT implies improved diagnostic classification, and any movement in the other direction implies worse diagnostic categorization. The picture is opposite for individuals without DVT present.[145]

The overall improvement in diagnostic reclassification can be expressed in various ways depending on the selected denominators, but commonly it is quantified as the difference between two differences. This is done by first calculating the difference between the proportions of individuals moving up and the proportion of subjects moving down for those with DVT, computing the corresponding difference in proportions for those without DVT, and then taking the difference of these two differences. This measure has been proposed as the net reclassification improvement (NRI).[146] The NRI is thus estimated as follows:

$$\text{NRI} = [P(\text{up}|D=1) - P(\text{down}|D=1)] \\ - [P(\text{up}|D=0) - P(\text{down}|D=0)]$$

where P is the proportion of patients, upward movement (up) is defined as a change into a higher probability of disease presence category based on model 2, and downward movement (down) is defined as a change in the opposite direction. D denotes the disease classification (in this case, DVT), present (1) or absent (0).

The NRI results for addition of D-dimer assay to the combination of history and physical examination using the numbers displayed in Table 2.15 were $(0.30 - 0.06) - (0.07 - 0.14) = 0.31$ (95% CI, 0.24 to 0.36). For 123 of 416 (i.e., 0.30) of patients who experienced DVT events, classification improved with the model with D-dimer, and for 26 of 416 (0.06) people, it became worse, resulting in a net gain in reclassification proportion of 0.24. In subjects who did not have DVT, 116 of 1670 (0.07) individuals were reclassified worse by the model with the D-dimer, and 227 of 1670 (0.14) were reclassified better, resulting in a net gain in reclassification proportion of 0.07. The overall net gain in reclassification proportion therefore was $0.24 + 0.07 = 0.31$. This estimate was significantly different from 0 ($P < .001$). The 95% CI around the NRI estimate was computed as suggested by Pencina and colleagues.[146]

Most investigators use three or four categories. But the NRI is clearly highly dependent on what probability threshold(s) are selected. Different thresholds may result in very different NRIs for the same added test result. To circumvent this problem of arbitrary cutoff choices, another possibility is to compute the so-called integrated discrimination improvement (IDI), which determines the magnitude of the reclassification probability improvements or deteriorations by a new test or biomarker over all possible categorizations or probability thresholds.[145–147]

The IDI is calculated as follows:

$$\text{IDI} = [(P_{\text{extended}}|D=1) - (P_{\text{basic}}|D=1)] \\ - [(P_{\text{extended}}|D=0) - (P_{\text{basic}}|D=0)]$$

In this equation, $P_{\text{extended}}|D=1$ and $P_{\text{extended}}|D=0$ are the means of the predicted DVT probability by the extended model 2 (see Table 2.14) for, respectively, the patients with DVT and the patients without DVT, and $P_{\text{basic}}|D=1$ and $P_{\text{basic}}|D=0$ are the means of the predicted DVT probability by model 1 see (Table 2.14) for, respectively, the patients with DVT and the patients without DVT. The 95% CI around the NRI estimate again was calculated as outlined by Pencina and colleagues.[146]

The IDI for the DVT example was $(0.49 - 0.13) - (0.28 - 0.18) = 0.26$ (95% CI, 0.23 to 0.28).

This implies that adding D-dimer to history and physical examination increased the difference in mean predicted probability between patients with DVT and patients without DVT by 0.26. This can also be interpreted as corresponding to the increase in mean sensitivity given an unchanged specificity.[146]

Although very popular and increasingly requested in reports on added value estimations, the NRI and IDI are only measures of discrimination between disease and nondiseased, as is also the case for ROC area. They give no information about whether the diagnostic probabilities calculated with a diagnostic model are in agreement with the observed disease prevalence (i.e., whether the models' DVT probabilities are over- or underestimated compared with the observed DVT prevalence), nor do they account in any way for the consequences of diagnostic misclassifications when a diagnostic biomarker or test is added.[148,149] The following methods better address these issues.

Predictiveness Curve

The predictiveness curve[147,150] is a graphic outline of the distribution of the predictive disease probabilities. Accordingly, the predictive probabilities of model 1 (without D-dimer) are ordered from lowest to highest and then plotted (Fig. 2.41).

The x-axis delineates the cumulative percentage over all individuals in the study; the y-axis shows the probabilities according to model 1. Looking first at the results only for model 1, we observe for the DVT example that if individuals who have a posterior risk (after history and physical examination) of more than 25% are selected for further investigation (regarded as positive), then 74% of patients will actually be negative and 26% will be positive (vertical dividing line in Fig. 2.41).

The four areas defined by the vertical dividing line represent, respectively, the TNs (64%), FPs (16%), FNs (10%), and TPs (10%).

In this example (threshold of >25%), the sensitivity becomes TP/Prevalence × 100 = 0.10/0.2 × 100 = 50%.

The specificity becomes

TN/(1 − Prevalence) × 100 = 0.64/0.8 × 100 = 80%

The graph thus displays the estimated probabilities associated with the history and physical examination mode when applied to the source population from which the study patients theoretically originated.[151]

The graph may also be used to assess the two different diagnostic models and, accordingly, the added value of the D-dimer test for correct estimation of the probability of DVT

presence. The predictiveness curve for model 1 is substantially inferior to that of the more comprehensive model including the D-dimer results (Fig. 2.42). For example, if we set less than 0.1 as a cutoff for low risk and greater than 0.4 as a threshold for high risk (on the y-axis), we observe that 90 − 20 = 70% of the predictions of model 1 are in the equivocal zone between these thresholds, but only 85 − 50 = 35% fall between these thresholds for the predictions of model 2. Thus model 2 performs much better with regard to classifying patients into low (<0.1) versus high (>0.4) risk, as can be directly seen from the difference in steepness or slope of the predictiveness curve of the model with D-dimer (steeper) as opposed to the model without.[151]

Decision Curve Analysis

Decision curve analysis, according to Vickers and Elkin,[152] is a procedure that focuses on the explicit quantification of the clinical usefulness of a new index test when added to established ones in the intended clinical context. As opposed to the NRI, which is based on a single predefined probability threshold, this approach allows each professional (or even patient) to select his or her individual threshold to determine whether to take further steps such as referral for supplemental diagnostic investigations or for treatment initiation in the context of the intended use of the index test or index model. Accordingly, the corresponding net benefits can be considered without explicitly assigning weights or utilities to the wrong diagnostic classifications.

As displayed in Fig. 2.43, a posterior probability threshold of 50% would indicate that an incorrect referral (FP) is equivalent in consequences to a missed thrombosis (FN). To reduce the risk, the physician or patient might prefer reference testing or further management at a lower posterior probability threshold. This would be of particular relevance

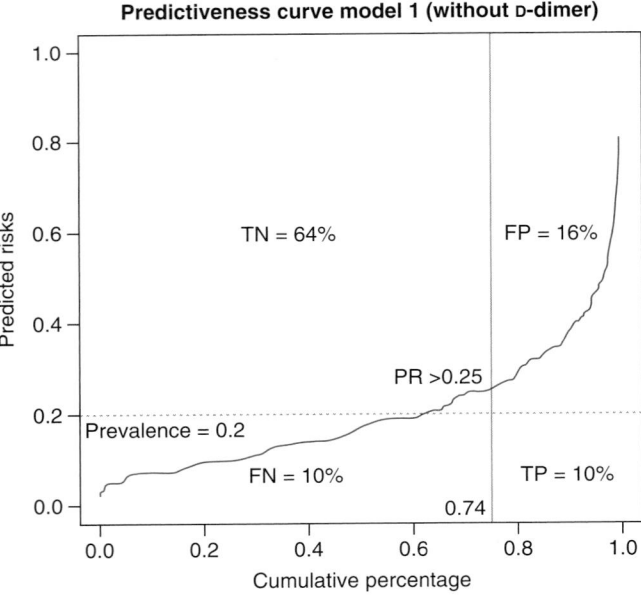

FIGURE 2.41 Predictiveness curve for model 1 (without D-dimer) showing the distribution of positive and negative patients at a posterior risk *(PR)* cutoff of 0.25. *FN,* False-negative; *FP,* false-positive; *TN,* true negatives; *TP,* true positives. (From Moons KG, de Groot JA, Linnet K, Reitsma JB, Bossuyt PMM. Quantifying the added value of a diagnostic test or marker. *Clin Chem* 2012;**58**:1408–17.)

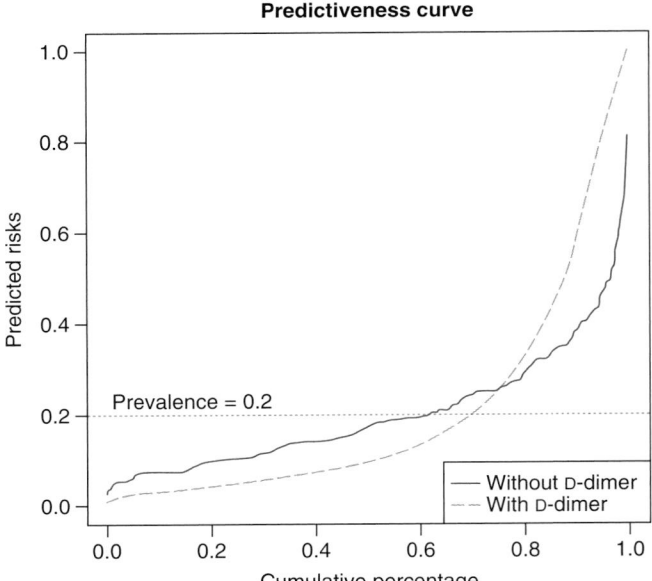

FIGURE 2.42 Comparison of predictiveness curves for the two models of Table 2.16 with and without D-dimer. (From Moons KG, de Groot JA, Linnet K, Reitsma JB, Bossuyt PMM. Quantifying the added value of a diagnostic test or marker. *Clin Chem* 2012;**58**:1408–17.)

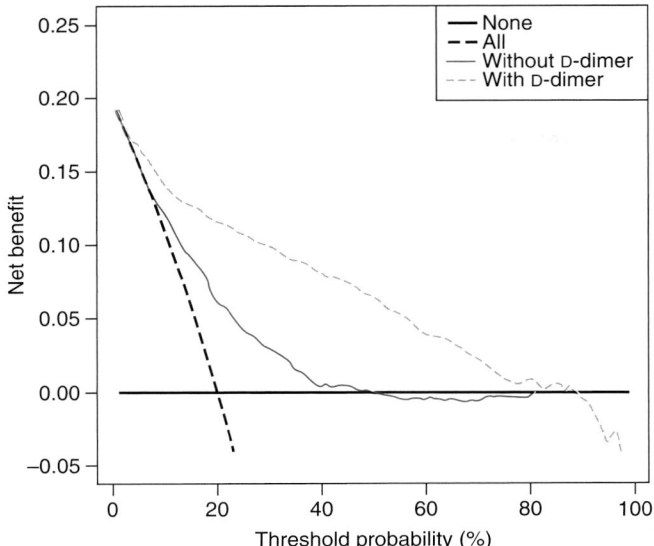

FIGURE 2.43 Decision curve analysis showing the net benefit of referring none of the patients for reference testing, referring all patients for reference testing, the basic prediction model, and the extended prediction model, in relation to the selected probability threshold for referral. (From Moons KG, de Groot JA, Linnet K, Reitsma JB, Bossuyt PMM. Quantifying the added value of a diagnostic test or marker. *Clin Chem* 2012;**58**:1408–17.)

TABLE 2.16 **The Relationship Between True Deep Venous Thrombosis Status and the Result of the Basic and Extended Prediction Model With Thresholds of 20% and 70% Predicted Probability**

		DVT (n = 2086)	
		Present	Absent
Basic model (model 1):	Yes	263	528
probability of DVT ≥20%	No	153	1142
Extended model (model 2):	Yes	319	301
probability of DVT ≥20%	No	97	1369
Basic model (model 1):	Yes	3	6
probability of DVT ≥70%	No	413	1664
Extended model (model 2):	Yes	123	31
probability of DVT ≥70%	No	293	1639

DVT, Deep venous thrombosis.

if the further testing were simple, noninvasive, or inexpensive or if the given treatment had relatively low risk of adverse reactions. In such a situation, the risk of DVT could be, for example, 20%. Such a lower cutoff for referral would lead to acceptance of a larger percentage of incorrect referrals (FPs) rather than missing a diseased DVT subject (FN) (i.e., implicitly a higher weight is assigned to FN cases than to FP cases). On the contrary, another one might pay more attention to the costs or burden of further testing or initiation of treatment. This might be the case if the subsequent test was very invasive or complicated or therapy implied a heavy risk of adverse reactions. In this situation, a higher probability threshold of, for example, 70% might be relevant, implying a higher weight to incorrect referral of patients without the disease (FPs) and less weight to missed cases (FNs) with disease (DVT).

The graph displays the whole range of probability thresholds for further management on the x-axis and the net benefit of the diagnostic strategies or models on the y-axis.[153] To compute the net benefit, the proportion of all patients who are FP is subtracted from the proportion of all patients who are TP, weighting by the relative cost of an FP and an FN classification.[152] A numerical example shows the relations.

Table 2.16, presenting results for this empirical study on DVT, shows for the above-mentioned threshold of 20% that the TP count for model 1 was 263, and the FP count was 528. The total number of patients *(n)* was 2086. The net benefit for model 1 at the threshold of 20% was $(263/2086) - (528/2086) \times (0.2/0.8) = 0.06$. The net benefit ratio 0.2/0.8 explicitly reveals that less weight is now assigned to the FPs compared with the FNs, as considered earlier. For model 2, the net benefit at the cutoff of 20% was $(319/2086) - (301/2086) \times (0.2/0.8) = 0.12$, two times larger. Although model 2 outperforms model 1, it should be noted that when the extended model is used at this threshold, 97 of 416 known

cases would be missed and thus not treated or referred for additional testing. This implies that the overall diagnostic performance of our shown model 2 is relatively poor for this theoretically selected threshold.

At the threshold of 70%, the net benefit of model 1 was $(3/2086) - (6/2086) \times (0.7/0.3) = -0.01$, and for model 2, it was $(123/2086) - (31/2086) \times (0.7/0.3) = 0.02$.

The net benefit of model 1 of 0.06 for a threshold of 20% can be expressed as: "Compared with the case of no referrals, referral by model 1 is the equivalent of a strategy that correctly refers 6 patients with DVT of 100 suspected patients without having any unnecessary (i.e., FP) referrals."

The important point of the decision curve (see Fig. 2.43) is to observe which diagnostic strategy provides the best net benefit given the doctor's or patient's individual choice for a probability cutoff. The horizontal black line along the x-axis in Fig. 2.43 presupposes that no patients will be referred to reference testing. Because this strategy refers 0 patients, the net benefit of this strategy becomes 0 (i.e., corresponding to incorrect handling of all patients with DVT). The grey steep declining line in Fig. 2.43 shows the net benefit of the strategy of simply subjecting all individuals to reference testing. This line intersects the x-axis at the threshold probability of 20% (i.e., the prevalence in the study). Accordingly, model 2 has the greatest net benefit (i.e., it is the highest line) for all threshold probabilities. Thus we can conclude that, irrespective of the applied probability thresholds, the extended model with D-dimer added is better than the basic model.

POINTS TO REMEMBER

- Focus has been on approaches and measures for quantification of the diagnostic accuracy of combinations of index tests and of the added value of a new diagnostic test beyond existing diagnostic tests.
- Reporting on the increase in discrimination and in (re)classification is important to gain insight into the full clinical value of a biomarker.
- Decision-curve analysis implicitly accounts for the consequences of the FP and FN classifications, complementing the information from the other measures.

Test Evaluation Beyond Diagnostic Accuracy

Despite the methods we have presented in this chapter for the evaluation of the analytical performance and diagnostic accuracy of laboratory tests, increasingly more information is demanded about the actual impact laboratory tests and test results have on medical decision making and indeed on patient outcomes.[97,137,154-161] For instance, government health policymakers and private insurers in the United States now want to see empirical evidence that testing quantifiably improves actual patient outcomes in relevant patient populations or that it enhances healthcare quality, efficiency, and cost-effectiveness before recommending diagnostic tests and markers for clinical use and before deciding on their reimbursement.[162] In Europe, a visionary document was recently issued stressing the importance of evaluating medical technology, including diagnostic devices, on their ability to actually improve medical care and patient outcomes.[163] When making decisions and considering recommendations about diagnostic tests, clinicians and other decision makers have to consider the (cost-)effectiveness of the test use.

Restricting ourselves to the above explained traditional diagnostic accuracy study designs and statistical measures (e.g., sensitivity, specificity, predictive values, ROC curves), we cannot easily infer on a test's actual impact on patient health or healthcare. Addressing these challenges ideally requires comparative studies, wherein the use of a certain (new) test is examined in the clinical context compared with the current best alternatives of care, such as other form(s) of testing or no testing at all. Downstream effects of testing on clinical decision making and patient care and patients' health outcomes can be compared between both strategies. Furthermore, such studies allow for in-depth examination whether the diagnostic test improves patient outcomes and healthcare quality, efficiency, and cost-effectiveness at large.[97,137,154-159,161] The terms *clinical utility* or *clinical effectiveness* and *impact* of a diagnostic test are often used to express the extent to which diagnostic testing or diagnostic test results improve decision making, patient outcomes, or (cost-)effectiveness of healthcare. A more detailed discussion of clinical effectiveness and the overall impact of diagnostic tests is provided in Chapter 10 on evidence-based laboratory medicine.

How Does Testing Yield Health(care) Benefits?

Tests, including laboratory tests that are diagnostic, prognostic, monitoring, or screening tests, do not by themselves alleviate diseases, symptoms, or signs directly but rather *indirectly*.[99,154,155,158,159,163] A test provides information to a user (e.g., healthcare professional or patient), which in turn indicates subsequent actions or interventions, such as therapies or lifestyle changes. For example, a test provides information (test results) that can be used to better identify patients who will and who will not benefit from helpful downstream management actions, such as administration of effective interventions or actions in individuals with certain (positive) test results and alternative or no treatment for those with other (negative) results. These interventions or actions, if beneficial, yield benefits in terms of improved health outcomes of individuals or patients. Diagnostic tests may affect patient outcomes and healthcare cost-effectiveness by improving the selection of the most effective treatment modalities or methods; examples include companion diagnostics, molecular imaging devices, and imaging devices to

guide surgery. Moreover, a certain (new) diagnostic test may be beneficial because it allows for less invasive or less costly detection of disorders. A new screening or monitoring test that leads to early detection makes it possible to administer the appropriate treatment at an early stage. Also, knowing certain diagnostic test results may affect the cognition, behavior, and lifestyle of individuals, which in turn may affect their health outcomes. Finally, besides intended effects (benefits) of testing, some tests may also lead to unintended (side) effects.

The Working Pathway

When thinking about approaches to evaluate the impact of diagnostic tests on medical decision making, patient outcomes, and healthcare at large, it is useful to describe the pathways through which benefits (and risks) of using the test are likely to occur. This so-called *working pathway* provides a framework (Fig. 2.44) to explain how a given test leads to benefits or risks for patients' health or healthcare. Such working pathways include:

1. The anticipated technical or analytical capabilities of the test
2. The unintended and intended results and effects of the test when applied in the targeted context
3. In whom these effects are likely to occur (e.g., in the targeted patients or in the care providers)
4. The anticipated mechanisms through which these potential effects will occur
5. Existing care in the targeted context and individuals
6. The expected time frame in which potential risks and benefits might occur

A clear description of the working pathway of a new test can determine the current benefits (and risks) of prevailing care in the intended medical context. It also helps determine what added value or benefits the new test must provide to improve existing care and what evidence is necessary to quantify whether these (added) benefits are indeed achieved at what risks or costs.

Having a detailed description of the working pathway at an early stage is particularly useful for invasive and costly (new) tests. A detailed description of the working pathway can also be used when evidence is interpreted from different studies (e.g., technical, safety, and clinical studies). For instance, if analytical performance studies fail to provide evidence for the intended technical capabilities of a test, further studies are unnecessary. If safety and analytical performance studies of a new version (modification) of an existing test show that its safety and analytical performance is similar to the preceding version but that it is less burdensome or cheaper to use, then subsequent studies may not be needed.

Comparative Tests: Treatment Studies to Quantify the Impact of Tests

One could design a longitudinal study to validly quantify whether a certain (new) test has impact on patient's health or healthcare beyond what is achieved by current practice.[156,157,161,163-168] This is in fact a similar approach used to evaluate the *effectiveness* (not the efficacy) of medical drugs: so-called comparative or pragmatic randomized trial. The study should:

- Investigate the (new) test in the same targeted individuals (e.g., professionals and patients) as it is intended to be used in practice.

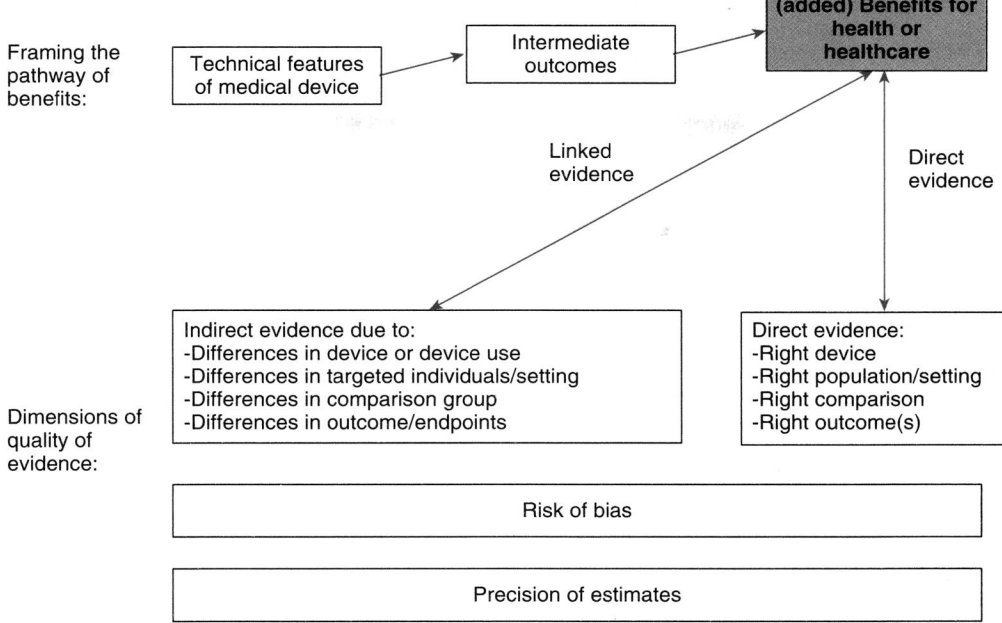

FIGURE 2.44 Relationship between the pathway through which devices may lead to benefits or added benefits for health or healthcare and the three dimensions of quality for evidence (indirectness of evidence, risk of bias, precision of estimates). (From KNAW. Evaluation of new technology in health care. In need of guidance for relevant evidence. Amsterdam: KNAW, 2014.)

- Investigate the test in the clinical pathway in which it is intended to be used in practice.
- Study the use of the test in combination with any subsequent management (e.g., therapeutic) actions indicated by the test or its results.
- Compare the test and subsequent management actions to the best prevailing care. Ideally, this would be a randomized comparison: Individuals are allocated randomly to either the new test use or to the comparative strategy.
- Measure all outcomes or endpoints relevant for the targeted individuals, professionals, and ideally for society at large, including unintended outcomes, intended health outcomes (for patient and users), burden and ease of test use, speed of administering subsequent management, and even costs of test use.
- Be sufficiently long to investigate the long-term healthcare effects.
- Be sufficiently large to obtain precise estimates of the safety and health benefits of the test use.

The two comparison groups are thus created randomly. In the index group, the new test is used in combination with subsequent management or therapeutic actions, with the prevailing tests and management being applied in the comparison (control) group. Provided the two groups are large enough, any observed differences between the two groups in terms of benefits (and risks) can then be ascribed to the difference in tests plus subsequent management. Such randomized studies compare the use of the index test or tests combined with subsequent actions, directly with the best alternative strategy in the right population, measuring all relevant outcomes (for patients, users, and healthcare) in the short and long terms. Such studies thus generate the most *direct* and *valid evidence* as to whether the test use will indeed produce the intended relevant benefits at an acceptable level of risks and costs compared with prevailing care.

This randomized comparative study approach is not always feasible or possible.[156,157,161,168] Numerous alternative comparative study approaches may also produce (direct) evidence of the (added) benefits of test use for the relevant health outcomes in the intended medical context. These approaches may include alternative randomized designs as described.[169,170] Furthermore, there are also many nonrandomized comparative study approaches, ranging from quasi-randomized studies to controlled before-and-after studies and comparative cohort or even case-control studies.[133,171,172] These nonrandomized comparative studies are more prone to bias because of differences in demographic and clinical characteristics between the two groups being compared. Fortunately, there are various approaches to controlling or adjusting for such biases, for which we refer to the literature.[133,171,172]

Linked-Evidence Approaches to Quantify the Impact of Tests

Besides technical performance and cross-sectional diagnostic test accuracy studies described earlier, many clinical studies of (new) laboratory tests focus on measuring intermediate effects or outcomes along the working pathway for a given test. Each of these studies by themselves often do not allow for inferring on the desired longer-term (added) benefits and risks of the test use. However, it is possible to use the so-called quantitative linked-evidence approach in which the evidence of these different types of diagnostic test studies are quantitatively combined to estimate a test's effect on relevant health or healthcare outcomes.[158,159,173–177]

An example is the assessment of the analytical performance requirements for glucose monitoring devices to achieve clinically useful glucose control. Rather than conducting large-scale longitudinal comparative, expensive randomized studies using many different measuring devices as comparators, computers using a variety of underlying modeling schemes have been used to generate simulated glucose results from glucose measurement devices having varying amounts of bias and imprecision. The patient data used in these studies were derived from physiologic models of glucose metabolism or hospitalized patients.[178] The results of such linked-evidence modeling approaches can be used to evaluate the effects of measurement bias and imprecision on quantifiable intermediate results such as the percentage of the time glucose falls within the desired therapeutic range, the frequency and duration of hypoglycemic episodes, and the within-patient variability of glucose. Such intermediate results are known to have direct relationships with the rates of clinical complications in individuals with poor glucose control. For the evaluation of the impact or utility of (new) laboratory tests on patient and healthcare outcomes in the intended medical context, linked-evidence approaches offer an attractive alternative when direct evaluation of a test's benefits on long-term, patient-relevant outcomes is difficult or impossible. For the glucose example, it would be difficult to gain ethical approval for a randomized trial in which yet imprecise glucose analyzers were evaluated for their effects when used for patient glucose monitoring. The validity of a linked-evidence approach is dependent on how predictive the existing study results and evidence are and the relation of these intermediate outcomes with the long-term, relevant health or healthcare outcomes.

Linked-evidence studies can be particularly useful for laboratory test studies when there is evidence from cross-sectional studies on the diagnostic accuracy of a test and results of therapeutic studies provide a link to health outcomes. Simple modeling approaches might be used to link both types of evidence and to actually quantify the benefits (and risks) of the test use on these health outcomes. Such linked-evidence models might include various sensitivity analyses, for example, to account for the risks of using various types of evidence taken from different sources.[158,159,173–176] For example, a so-called Markov model was used to combine evidence from analytical performance studies, cross-sectional diagnostic accuracy studies, and long-term management studies to quantify the long-term cost-effectiveness of point-of-care D-dimer tests compared with the use of central laboratory D-dimer tests to rule out DVT in primary care.[179]

POINTS TO REMEMBER

- It is important to assess information concerning the actual impact or utility of the use of a diagnostic test on patient outcomes or healthcare at large.
- The impact of diagnostic tests on medical decision making and patient outcomes can be considered by describing the pathways through which benefits (and risks) of using the test are likely to occur (the so-called *working pathway*).
- *Direct and valid evidence* as to whether the new test will indeed produce the intended relevant benefits can be assessed by randomized studies comparing the outcome of use of the new test with that of the index test.
- A supplementary approach is the so-called quantitative linked-evidence procedure in which the evidence of different types of diagnostic test studies are quantitatively combined to estimate a test's effect on relevant health or healthcare outcomes.

SELECTED REFERENCES

5. Snedecor GW, Cochran WG. Statistical methods. 8th ed. Ames, Iowa: Iowa State University Press; 1989. p. 75, 121, 140–2, 170–4, 177, 237–8, 279.

12. Dybkær R. Vocabulary for use in measurement procedures and description of reference materials in laboratory medicine. Eur J Clin Chem Clin Biochem 1997;35:141–73.

35. Krouwer JS. Setting performance goals and evaluating total analytical error for diagnostic assays. Clin Chem 2002; 48:919–27.

40. Linnet K. Nonparametric estimation of reference intervals by simple and bootstrap-based procedures. Clin Chem 2000;46: 867–9.

44. Bland JM, Altman DG. Statistical methods for assessing agreement between two methods of clinical measurement. Lancet 1986;i:307–10.

49. Linnet K. Evaluation of regression procedures for methods comparison studies. Clin Chem 1993;39:424–32.

53. Linnet K. Limitations of the paired t-test for evaluation of method comparison data. Clin Chem 1999;45:314–15.

54. Linnet K. Estimation of the linear relationship between the measurements of two methods with proportional errors. Stat Med 1990;9:1463–73.

60. Passing H, Bablok W. Comparison of several regression procedures for method comparison studies and determination of sample sizes. J Clin Chem Clin Biochem 1984;22:431–45.

71. Vesper HW, Thienpont LM. Traceability in laboratory medicine. Clin Chem 2009;55:1067–75.

95. Linnet K, Bossuyt PM, Moons KG, et al. Quantifying the accuracy of a diagnostic test or marker. Clin Chem 2012;58:1292–301.

96. Moons KG, de Groot JA, Linnet K, et al. Quantifying the added value of a diagnostic test or marker. Clin Chem 2012;58:1408–17.

97. Bossuyt PMM, Reitsma JB, Linnet K, et al. Beyond diagnostic accuracy: the clinical utility of diagnostic tests. Clin Chem 2012;58:1636–43.

102. Bossuyt PM, Reitsma JB, Bruns DE, et al. An updated list of essential items for reporting diagnostic accuracy studies. Clin Chem 2015;in press.

106. Oudega R, Moons KG, Hoes AW. Ruling out deep venous thrombosis in primary care. A simple diagnostic algorithm including D-dimer testing. Thromb Haemost 2005;94:200–5.

118. Obuchowski NA, Lieber ML, Wians FH Jr. ROC curves in clinical chemistry: uses, misuses, and possible solutions. Clin Chem 2004;50:1118–25.

137. Moons KG. Criteria for scientific evaluation of novel markers: a perspective. Clin Chem 2010;56:537–41.

143. Pencina MJ, D'Agostino RB, Vasan RS. Statistical methods for assessment of added usefulness of new biomarkers. Clin Chem Lab Med 2010;48:1703–11.

177. Horvath AR, Lord SJ, StJohn A, et al. From biomarkers to medical tests: the changing landscape of test evaluation. Clin Chim Acta 2014;427:49–57.

179. Hendriksen JMT, Geersing GJ, van Voorthuizen SC, et al. The cost–effectiveness of point-of-care D-dimer tests compared with a laboratory test to rule out deep venous thrombosis in primary care. Expert Rev Mol Diagn 2015;15:125–36.

Governance, Risk, and Quality Management in the Medical Laboratory*

Leslie Burnett, Mark Mackay, and Tony Badrick

ABSTRACT

The aspirational goal of diagnostic pathology laboratories is to always provide the right result for the right test on the right patient at the right time and with the right support. To deliver this outcome systematically, reliably, and safely for the patient, has required the long-term development of an organizational culture and framework by the international laboratory medicine community.

Background

Quality management (QM) is a set of principles for coordinating management and improvement activities to ensure that an organization continuously meets the requirements of its customers (users), even as those needs change. There are many approaches to and tools for deploying these principles, some tools focusing only on selected principles. It is widely regarded as best management practice when these principles are fully adopted as an organizational framework.

Quality management systems (QMS) are consensus-driven structured frameworks for ensuring consistency in the quality of products and services to meet customer needs. Both QM and QMS evolved from technical quality, namely, quality control (QC) and external quality assessment/proficiency testing (EQA/PT) activities, and these elements still play important roles. The International Organization for Standardization (ISO) has developed ISO 15189 as an internationally accepted QMS standard suitable for accreditation of medical laboratories. In some countries, alternative or additional standards or accreditation requirements may apply.

Further evolution and development of this framework is continuing. Laboratory medicine is different to many other industries because it includes the patient, and thus carries additional ethical and legal responsibilities for maintaining patient safety and optimizing and improving patient care—this is addressed under the banner of clinical governance. There is also increasing recognition of the need to prioritize and focus efforts on those organizational activities most vulnerable to failure or with the greatest consequences—this is addressed through risk management. And layered on top of these frameworks and standards is the recognition that leadership and accountability are required to drive and maintain quality improvement.

Content

The most widely adopted QMS used internationally (ISO 15189) is described in some detail and is compared with an alternative or supplementary framework (Clinical and Laboratory Standards Institute [CLSI] QMS01). The role of standards and guidelines in self-assessment and in the accreditation and regulation of medical laboratories, and the differences between accreditation and certification are explained. The principles of clinical governance and risk management are described and their links to QMS are explored. Finally, the philosophy and principles of QM are described, and within this, the rationale is explained for a QMS as a means of maintaining and controlling existing operations, as well as systematically improving the quality of test results and organizational services. Various pathways taken by laboratories to implementing QM are considered, and various structured quality improvement tools and management approaches are described.

*The full version of this chapter is available electronically on ExpertConsult.com.

Specimen Collection and Processing

Khushbu Patel and Patricia M. Jones

ABSTRACT

Background
Proper specimen collection and processing are critical to avoiding common preanalytical errors and ensuring accurate test results. Specific steps, recommendations, and procedures are designed to protect both the patient and the individual collecting the specimen.

Content
This chapter addresses in detail the issues related to specimen collection. The most common types of specimens collected are discussed with the collection method(s) outlined, and some caveats for special populations, such as pediatric patients, are included. Details on collection devices and preservatives, and their appropriate use for individual test requests are outlined with attention to how to recognize when an incorrect sample is submitted for testing. The chapter concludes with the equally important details on proper specimen processing, handling, and transport to the testing facility. It is stressed that specimen collection and handling must be done in a manner that is validated for the tests that will be performed. The information provided is designed to assist laboratorians in mitigating preanalytical errors associated with specimen collection and ensure accurate and quality results.

INTRODUCTION

Proper collection, processing, storage, and transport of common sample types associated with requests for diagnostic testing are critical to the provision of quality test results. Each of the steps involved, as well as factors associated with the patient from whom the sample is being collected, can be the source of errors that cause inaccurate results. Minimizing these errors through careful adherence to the concepts discussed here and to individual institutional policies will result in more reliable information for use by healthcare professionals in providing quality patient care.

This chapter provides a review of the most common specimen types and discusses how they are (1) collected, (2) identified, (3) processed, (4) stored, and (5) transported. Body fluids other than blood and urine are covered in detail elsewhere (see Chapter 45) as are additional preanalytical factors (see Chapter 5). Attention to the differences between adult and pediatric collection are also discussed.

PATIENT IDENTIFICATION

Before any specimen is collected, the phlebotomist must confirm the identity of the patient. Two or three items of identification should be used (e.g., full name, medical record number, date of birth, telephone number, or other person-specific identifier). The Joint Commission, a US hospital accreditation body, requires at least two of these unique identifiers be used to properly identify the patient.[1] In specialized situations, such as paternity testing or other tests of medicolegal importance, establishment of a chain of custody for the specimen may require that additional patient identification, such as a photograph, be provided as part of the identification process or taken to confirm the identity of the patient.

Identification must be an active process. When possible, the patient should state his or her full name and date of birth or other identifier, and the phlebotomist should verify information on the patient's wrist band if the patient is hospitalized. If the patient is an outpatient, the phlebotomist should ask the patient to state his or her full name and date of birth and should confirm the information on the test requisition form with identifying information provided by the patient. In the case of pediatric patients, the parent or guardian should be present and should provide active identification of the child such as: "Please tell me the name of your child." Parents with young children are often distracted or worried about the upcoming procedure and may answer without paying attention to the question, so the question should always be posed in a manner to prevent a yes or no answer. Strict adherence to institutional policies is required.

TYPES OF SPECIMENS

Types of biologic specimens that are analyzed in clinical laboratories include (1) whole blood; (2) serum; (3) plasma; (4) urine; (5) stool; (6) saliva; (7) other body fluids such as spinal, synovial, amniotic, pleural, pericardial, and ascitic fluids; and (8) cells and various types of solid tissue. The

TABLE 4.1 Clinical and Laboratory Standards Institute Documents Related to Specimen Collection, Processing, and Transport

Document Name	Document Number
Accuracy in patient and sample identification, 2nd ed.	GP33
Blood collection on filter paper for newborn screening programs: approved standard, 6th ed.	NBS01-A6
Body fluid analysis for cellular composition: approved guideline, 1st ed.	H56-A
Collection, transport, and processing of blood specimens for testing plasma-based coagulation assays and molecular hemostasis assay: approved guideline, 5th ed.	H21-A5
Collection, transport, preparation, and storage of specimens for molecular methods: approved guideline, 1st ed.	MM13-A
Ionized calcium determinations: precollection variables, specimen choice, collection, and handling: approved guideline, 2nd ed.	C31-A2
Procedures and devices for the collection of diagnostic capillary blood specimens: approved standard, 6th ed.	GP42-A6
Collection of diagnostic venous blood specimens	GP41
Tubes and additives for venous and capillary blood specimen collection: approved standard, 6th ed.	GP39-A6
Procedures for the handling and processing of blood specimens for common laboratory tests: approved guideline, 4th ed.	GP44-A4
Protection of laboratory workers from occupationally acquired infections: approved standard, 4th ed.	M29-A4
Quality management system: qualifying, selecting and evaluating a referral laboratory: approved guideline, 2nd ed.	QMS05-A2
Sweat testing: sample collection and quantitative chloride analysis, 4th ed	C34-A4

World Health Organization[2] and the Clinical and Laboratory Standards Institute (CLSI) have published several guidelines for collecting many of these specimens under standardized conditions (Table 4.1). In addition, the CLSI has published documents related to sample collection and analysis for specialized tests such as sweat chloride collection and testing (CLSI C34-A4, see Table 4.1).

Blood

Blood for analysis may be obtained from veins, arteries, or capillaries. Venous blood is usually the specimen of choice, and venipuncture is the method for obtaining this specimen. Arterial puncture is used mainly for blood gas analyses. In young children and for many point-of-care tests, skin puncture is frequently used to obtain capillary blood. The process of collecting blood is known as phlebotomy (from *phleb*, which means vein, and *tome*, to cut or incise) and should always be performed by a trained phlebotomist.

Venipuncture

In the clinical laboratory, venipuncture is defined as all of the steps involved in obtaining an appropriate and identified blood specimen from a patient's vein (CLSI GP41, see Table 4.1).

Preliminary steps. Before venipuncture is started the patient should be asked about latex allergies. If latex allergy is present and if latex gloves or a latex tourniquet may be used, the phlebotomist should secure an alternative tourniquet and put on gloves that are latex free. Finally, for some specialized tests such as testing for genetic diseases, the performing laboratory may request the use of a special requisition. When these are required, in general they should be provided by the requesting physician and be brought by the patient to the collection.

Before collection of a specimen, the phlebotomist should dress in personal protective equipment (PPE), such as an impervious gown and gloves applied immediately before approaching the patient, and adhere to standard precautions against potentially infectious material; the goal is to limit the spread of infectious disease from one patient to another and to promote the safety of the patient and phlebotomist. Because small children are often frightened of anyone in a white coat or gown, pediatric phlebotomists often dress in bright, cheerful colors, including colored PPE rather than standard white. Pediatric drawing stations are also often brightly colored with lots of distracters for the patient. If the phlebotomist must collect a specimen from a patient in isolation in a hospital, the phlebotomist must put on a clean gown and gloves and a face mask and goggles before entering the patient's room. The face mask limits the spread of potentially infectious droplets, and the goggles limit the possible entry of infectious material into the eye. The extent of the precautions required varies with the nature of the patient's illness and the institution's policies and bloodborne pathogen plan to which a phlebotomist must adhere. For example, if airborne precautions are indicated, the phlebotomist must wear an N95 tuberculosis respirator in the United States.

If required, the phlebotomist should verify that the patient has fasted, identify what medications are being taken or have been discontinued as required, and determine any other relevant information required. Chapter 5 describes in more detail the effects of diet and fluid intake and the recommended steps for patient preparation, including fasting, before phlebotomy. The patient should be comfortable, seated or supine (if sitting is not feasible), and should have been in this position for as long as possible before the specimen is drawn. The correct interpretation of certain tests (e.g., aldosterone, renin, plasma metanephrines) requires that the patient be in a supine position for at least 30 minutes before venipuncture. (For details on the effects of position, refer to Chapters 5 and 53.) For an outpatient, it is generally recommended that patients be seated before completion of the identification process to maximize their relaxation. At no time should venipuncture be performed on a standing patient.

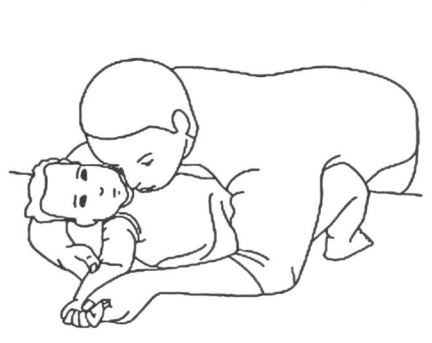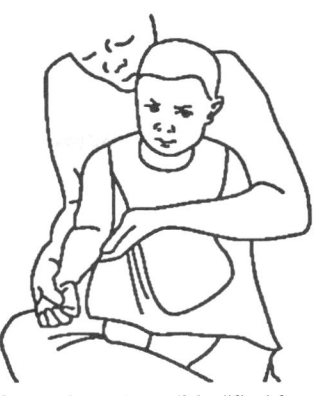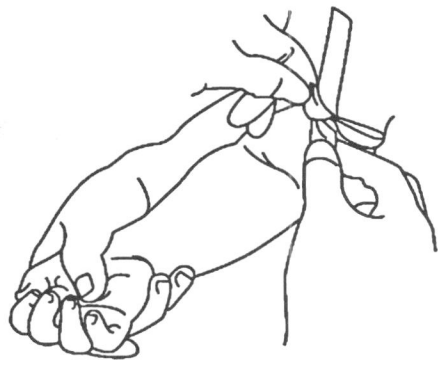

FIGURE 4.1 Holding a child for venipuncture. (Modified from World Health Organization. *WHO guidelines on drawing blood: best practices in phlebotomy. Pediatric and neonatal blood sampling.* Geneva: World Health Organization; 2010. http://www.ncbi.nlm.nih.gov/books/NBK138647.)

Infants and young children may need to be held in order to restrain them and prevent movement. Young children may be held sitting upright in a parent's lap with the parent helping to support and hold the patient and arm still (Fig. 4.1).[2] Infants' blood is often drawn with the infant in a supine position, and the infant may be swaddled in a blanket, or a papoose board may be used to restrain movement. Occasionally, the parents will be more anxious than the child or will wish not to be associated with a procedure which causes the child pain, and the phlebotomist will need to make the decision to request help from a colleague phlebotomist to properly and safely perform the collection.[3,4]

Either of the patient's arms should be extended in a straight line from the shoulder to the wrist. An arm with an inserted intravenous (IV) line should be avoided, as should an arm with extensive scarring or a hematoma at the intended collection site. If a woman has had a mastectomy, arm veins on that side of the body should not be used because the surgery may have caused lymphostasis (blockade of normal lymph node drainage), affecting the blood composition. If a woman has had a double mastectomy, blood should be drawn from the arm of the side on which the first procedure was performed. If the surgery was done within 6 months on both sides, a vein on the back of the hand or at the ankle should be used.

Before performing a venipuncture, the phlebotomist should estimate the volume of blood to be drawn and should select the appropriate number and types of tubes for the blood, plasma, or serum tests requested. In many settings, this is facilitated by computer-generated collection recommendations and should be designed to collect the minimum amount necessary for testing. Estimating volume of blood to be drawn is especially critical in a pediatric setting. An average-weight newborn infant has a total blood volume of approximately 350 mL. Collecting too much blood from an infant in a hospital setting will eventually result in the need to give the infant blood back in the form of a transfusion, risking exposure to bloodborne pathogens. Blood collection in the pediatric population should not exceed recommended volumes for the pediatric patient's weight.[5] The later sections on "Order of Draw for Multiple Collections" and "Collection with Evacuated Blood Tubes" discuss in greater detail the recommended order in which to draw multiple specimens and the types of tubes to be used. Careful consideration

should also be taken in the case of an adult patient, as one study showed that on average, every 100 mL of phlebotomy was associated with a decrease in hemoglobin of 7.0 g/L and hematocrit of 1.9%.[6] Such iatrogenic blood loss can lead to the same possible unnecessary required blood transfusion and an increased risk of exposure to bloodborne pathogens in adults as in children.

In addition to tubes, an appropriate needle must be selected. The most commonly used sizes for adults are 19 to 22 gauge (the larger the gauge number, the smaller the bore). The usual choice for an adult with normal veins is 20 gauge; if veins tend to collapse easily, a size 21 is preferred. For volumes of blood from 30 to 50 mL, an 18-gauge needle may be required to ensure adequate blood flow. In pediatric patients, 23- to 25-gauge needles are most commonly used, with 23-gauge being the preferred size. Venipuncture on infants and children younger than 2 years old is often performed on dorsal hand veins rather than arm veins, and the veins in either place are very small in this age group. Even for larger volumes of blood, rarely will a needle larger than a 21 gauge be used because it will not fit into the vein easily. A needle is typically 1.5 inches (3.7 cm) long, but 1-inch (2.5-cm) needles, usually attached to a winged or butterfly collection set, are also used and are common in pediatrics. All needles must be sterile and sharp and without barbs. If blood is drawn for trace element measurements, the needle should be stainless steel and should be known to be free from contamination.

Finally, the phlebotomist should ensure that all postdraw safety devices are in place. These include (for the person drawing) quick, convenient, and safe access to proper disposal devices for all (now) contaminated needles and associated devices and (for the patient) the appropriate post–blood draw supplies (gauze and bandage) are in place to ensure no adverse events might affect the patient.

Timing. The time at which a specimen is obtained is important for blood constituents that undergo marked diurnal variation (e.g., corticosteroids, iron), for those for which a fasting sample has been requested, and for those used to monitor drug therapy. In each case, the timing should match the conditions under which reference intervals or clinical decision points were determined (see Chapter 9). Furthermore, timing is important in relation to specimens for alcohol or drug measurements in association with medicolegal considerations.

Location. The median cubital vein in the antecubital fossa, or crook of the elbow, is the preferred site for collecting venous blood in adults because the vein is large and is close to the surface of the skin (CLSI GP41, see Table 4.1). Veins on the back of the hand or at the ankle may be used, although these are less desirable and should be avoided in people with diabetes and other individuals with poor circulation. However, in infants and children younger than 2 years old, collection from superficial veins is recommended, and these sites may be preferred over the median cubital vein. In the inpatient setting, it is appropriate to collect blood through a cannula that is inserted for long-term fluid infusions at the time of first insertion to avoid the need for a second stick. This method of collection may increase the chances of a hemolyzed sample and contamination of the collected sample with fluids being infused. Careful adherence to withdrawal of a discard volume and discussions with the clinical team on alternative site for phlebotomy can greatly reduce these preanalytical variables. For severely ill individuals and those requiring many IV injections, an alternative blood-drawing site should be chosen. Selection of a vein for puncture is facilitated by palpation. An arm containing a cannula or an arteriovenous fistula should not be used without consent of the patient's physician. If fluid is being infused intravenously into a limb, the fluid should be shut off for at least 3 minutes (with clinician consent) before a specimen is obtained and a suitable note made in the patient's chart and on the result report form and the recommencement of the infusion must be ensured. Specimens obtained from the opposite arm are preferred. Specimens below the infusion site in the same arm may be satisfactory for most tests, except for analytes that are contained in the infused solution (e.g., glucose, electrolytes).

Preparation of the site. The area around the intended puncture site should be cleaned with whatever cleanser is approved for use by the institution. Three commonly used materials are a prepackaged alcohol swab, a gauze pad saturated with 70% isopropanol, and a benzalkonium chloride solution (e.g., Zephiran chloride solution, 1:750). Cleaning of the puncture site should be done with a circular motion from the site outward. The skin should be allowed to dry in the air. No alcohol or cleanser should remain on the skin because traces may cause hemolysis and invalidate test results. After the skin has been cleaned, it should not be touched until after the venipuncture has been completed.

Venous occlusion. After the skin is cleaned, a blood pressure cuff or a tourniquet is applied 4 to 6 inches (10 to 15 cm) above the intended puncture site (distance for adults). This obstructs the return of venous blood to the heart and distends the veins (venous occlusion). When a blood pressure cuff is used as a tourniquet, it is usually inflated to approximately 60 mm Hg (8.0 kPa). Tourniquets typically are made from precut soft rubber strips or from Velcro. If a dorsal hand vein is being accessed in infants and young children, no tourniquet is used. The phlebotomist applies enough pressure with the hand holding the patient's wrist and hand to occlude and distend the vein.

It is rarely necessary to leave a tourniquet in place for longer than 1 minute after venous access is secured and the tourniquet is removed, but even within this short time, the composition of blood changes, and adherence to institutional policies must be followed. Although the changes that occur in 1 minute are slight, marked changes have been observed after 3 minutes for some chemistry analytes. The composition of blood drawn first—that is, the blood closest to the tourniquet—is most representative of the composition of circulating blood and the least affected by fluid shifts where protein bound components and other large molecules will be concentrated; water-soluble smaller molecules such as electrolytes may be less affected. The first-drawn specimen should therefore be used for analytes such as calcium and other analytes that are both protein bound and pertinent to critical medical decisions and that may be affected by the collection process.[7,8] A uniform procedure for the order of draw for tests should therefore be established (see later discussion). If it is only possible to collect a small volume of blood, the priority of which tests to perform should be established.

Two special notes on the collection process: Pumping of the fist before venipuncture should be avoided because it causes an increase in plasma potassium, phosphate, and lactate concentrations. The lowering of blood pH by accumulation of lactate also causes the plasma ionized calcium concentration to increase.[7] The ionized calcium concentration reverts to normal 10 minutes after the tourniquet is released.[8] Importantly, the stress associated with blood collection and/or hospitalization can have effects on patients at any age. As a consequence, plasma concentrations of analytes affected by stress, such as cortisol, thyroid-stimulating hormone, and growth hormone, may increase. Stress occurs particularly in young children who are frightened, struggling, and held in physical restraint. Collection under these conditions may cause adrenal stimulation, leading to an increased plasma glucose concentration, or may create increases in the serum activities of enzymes that originate in skeletal muscle.

Order of draw for multiple blood specimens. In a few patients, backflow from blood tubes into veins occurs owing to a decrease in venous pressure. The dangerous consequences of this occurrence are prevented by using only sterile tubes for collection of blood. Backflow is minimized if the arm is held downward and blood is kept from contact with the stopper during the collection procedure. When collecting multiple specimens with an evacuated tube system, one of the primary concerns is to prevent cross-contamination between tubes. For example, potassium ethylenediaminetetraacetic acid (EDTA) contamination can cause an erroneously reported hyperkalemia or hypocalcemia when an inappropriate tube type is used.[9] To minimize problems if backflow occurs and to optimize the quality of specimens by preventing cross-contamination with anticoagulants, blood should be collected into tubes in the order outlined in Table 4.2, which generally follows a process of no anticoagulant to mild anticoagulant to strong anticoagulant. This table also provides the recommended number of inversions for each tube type because it is critical that complete mixing of any additive with the blood collected be accomplished as quickly as possible. In addition, completing a blood collection within 2 minutes of starting, and getting the tubes mixed correctly as soon as possible, helps to prevent clotting in anticoagulated tubes. The order of collection when multiple tubes are drawn from a skin puncture is different than when an evacuated tube system is used (see the later section on skin puncture).

Collection with evacuated blood tubes. Evacuated blood tubes are usually considered to be safer, less expensive, more convenient, and easier to use than syringes and thus are the

TABLE 4.2 Recommended Order of Draw for Multiple Blood Specimen Collection

Stopper Color	Contents	Inversions
Yellow	Sterile media for blood culture	8
Royal blue	No additive	0
Clear	Nonadditive; this is a discard tube if no royal blue is collected, used to fill collection set spaces prior to collecting coagulation (sodium citrate) tube	0
Light blue	Sodium citrate	3–4
Gold/red	Serum separator tube	5
Red/red, orange/yellow, royal blue	Serum tube, with or without clot activator, with or without gel	5
Green	Heparin tube with or without gel	8
Tan (glass)	Sodium heparin	8
Royal blue	Sodium heparin, sodium EDTA (trace metal free)	8
Lavender, pearl white, pink/pink, tan (plastic)	EDTA tubes, with or without gel	8
Gray	Glycolytic inhibitor	8
Yellow (glass)	ACD for molecular studies and cell culture	8

ACD, Acid citrate dextrose; *EDTA,* ethylenediaminetetraacetic acid.
Modified from information in Clinical and Laboratory Standards Institute. *Tubes and additives for venous blood specimen collection: CLSI-approved standard GP39-A6.* 6th ed. Wayne, PA: Clinical and Laboratory Standards Institute; 2010; and Garza D, Becan-McBride K. Venipuncture procedures. In: Garza D, Becan-McBride K, editors. *Phlebotomy handbook: blood specimen collection from basic to advanced.* 10th ed. Upper Saddle River, NJ: Pearson Prentice Hall; 2019. p. 308–70.

collection device of choice in many institutions. Evacuated blood tubes may be made of soda-lime or borosilicate glass or plastic (polyethylene terephthalate). Because of the decreased likelihood of breakage and subsequent exposure to infectious materials, many, if not most, laboratories have converted from glass to plastic tubes. Several types of evacuated tubes may be used for venipuncture collection. They vary by the type of additive added and the volume of the tube. The different types of additives are identified by the color of the stopper used. Color coding of specimen collection tubes is not yet harmonized and may vary according to manufacturers. Table 4.3 presents the most common forms of color codes of various tube types. Serum or plasma separator tubes are available that contain an inert, polymer gel material with a specific gravity of approximately 1.04. Aspiration of blood into the tube and subsequent centrifugation displaces the gel, which settles like a disk between cells and supernatant when the tube is centrifuged. A minimum relative centrifugal force (RCF) of 1100 × g is required for gel release and barrier formation in most tubes. Release of intracellular components into the supernatant is prevented by the barrier for several hours or, in many cases, for 7 days or more, allowing for additional testing ("add-ons") from samples collected at a specific time in the patient's care. However, all laboratories need to review the specific manufacturers' recommendations of what may be allowed based on provided data or perform their own validation studies. Most importantly, these separator tubes may be used as primary containers from which serum or plasma can be directly aspirated by a number of analytical instruments, avoiding aspiration of red blood cells (RBCs) or possible errors of patient or sample identification during aliquoting. Additional tubes, not listed, are sold for special applications, such as RNA isolation. As with all specimen collection containers, these less common tubes must be validated by each laboratory before use if not approved by the manufacturer for the specific analysis to be conducted.

Stoppers may contain zinc, invalidating the use of evacuated blood tubes for zinc measurement, and tris(2-butoxyethyl) phosphate (TBEP), also a constituent of the stopper, which may interfere with the measurement of certain drugs. With time, the vacuum in evacuated tubes is lost and their effective draw diminishes. The silicone coating also decays with age. Therefore the stock of these tubes should be rotated and careful attention paid to the expiration date. Blood collected into a tube containing one additive should never be transferred into other tubes because the first additive may interfere with tests for which a different additive is specified. Additionally, cross-contamination of additives from one tube to another during multiple tube draws should be minimized (or adverse effects reduced) through strict adherence to recommendations for order of tube use (see Table 4.2).

Typical systems for collecting blood[10] are shown in Fig. 4.2. Single-use devices incorporate a cover that is designed to be placed over the needle when collection of the blood is complete, thereby reducing the risk of puncture of the phlebotomist by the now contaminated needle. A needle or winged (butterfly) set is screwed into the collection tube holder, and the tube is then gently inserted into this holder. The tube should be gently tapped to dislodge any additive from the stopper before the needle is inserted into a vein; this prevents aspiration of the additive into the patient's vein.

After the skin has been cleaned, the needle should be guided gently into the patient's vein; when the needle is in place, the tube should be pressed forward into the holder to puncture the stopper and release the vacuum. As soon as blood begins to flow into the tube, the tourniquet should be released without moving the needle (see earlier discussion on venous occlusion). The tube is filled until the vacuum is exhausted. It is critically important that the evacuated tube be filled completely. Many additives, particularly for coagulation testing, are provided at concentrations in the tube based on a specified volume requirement; both short and too-full draws can be a source of preanalytical error because they can significantly affect the established testing parameters that are based on a properly collected sample. Therefore a vacuum tube should always be filled using the vacuum that is designed

TABLE 4.3 Coding of Stopper Color to Indicate Additive in Evacuated Blood Tube

Tube Type	Additive	Stopper Color	Alternative
Gel separation tubes	Polymer gel/silica activator	Red/black	Gold
	Polymer gel/silica activator/lithium heparin	Green/gray	Light gray
Serum tubes (nonadditive)	Silicone-coated interior	Red	None
	Uncoated interior	Red	Pink
Serum tubes (with additives)	Thrombin (dry additive)	Gray/yellow	Orange
	Particulate clot activator	Yellow/red	Red
	Thrombin (dry additive)	Light blue	Light blue
Whole blood/plasma tubes	K_2 EDTA (dry additive)	Lavender	Lavender
	K_3 EDTA (liquid additive)	Lavender	Lavender
	Na_2 EDTA (dry additive)	Lavender	Lavender
	Citrate, trisodium (coagulation)	Light blue	Light blue
	Citrate, trisodium (erythrocyte sedimentation rate)	Black	Black
	Sodium fluoride (antiglycolic agent)	Gray	Light/gray
	Heparin, lithium (dry or liquid additive)	Green	Green
	Potassium oxalate/sodium fluoride	Light gray	Light gray
	Lithium heparin/iodoacetate	Light gray	Light gray
Specialty Tubes (Microbiology)			
Blood culture	Sodium polyanethol sulfonate (SPS)	Light yellow	Light yellow
Specialty Tubes (Chemistry)			
Lead	Heparin, potassium (liquid additive)	Tan	Tan
	Heparin, sodium (dry additive)	Royal blue	Royal blue
Trace elements	Silicone-coated interior (serum tube)	Royal blue	Royal blue
Stat chemistry	Thrombin	Gray/yellow	Orange
Specialty Tubes (Molecular Diagnostics)			
Plasma	K_2 EDTA (dry additive)/polymer gel/silica activator	Opalescent white	Opalescent white
	ACD solution A (Na_3 citrate, 22.0 g/L; citric acid, 8.0 g/L; dextrose, 24.5 g/L)	Bright yellow	Bright yellow
	ACD solution B (Na_3 citrate, 13.2 g/L; citric acid, 4.8 g/L; dextrose, 14.7 g/L)	Bright yellow	Bright yellow
Mononuclear cell preparation tube	Sodium citrate with density gradient polymer fluid	Blue/black	Blue/black
	Sodium heparin with density gradient polymer fluid	Green/red	Green/red

ACD, Acid citrate dextrose; *EDTA,* ethylenediaminetetraacetic acid.
Modified from information in Clinical and Laboratory Standards Institute. *Tubes and additives for venous blood specimen collection: CLSI-approved standard GP39-A6*. 6th ed. Wayne, PA: Clinical and Laboratory Standards Institute; 2010; and Becton Dickinson. http://www.bd.com.

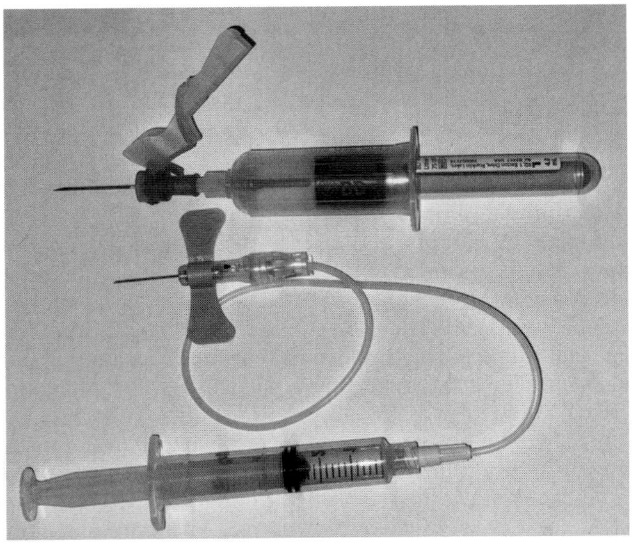

FIGURE 4.2 Assorted venipuncture collection devices.

to fill it correctly. These tubes should never be opened and filled from a syringe or other source. After the tube is filled completely, it should be withdrawn from the holder, mixed gently by inversion, and replaced by another tube if necessary. Other tubes may be filled using the same technique with the holder in place.

Blood collection with a syringe. Syringes are customarily used for patients with difficult veins, including very small veins, and for blood gas analysis. If a syringe is used, the needle is placed firmly over the nozzle of the syringe, and the cover of the needle is removed. If the syringe has an eccentric nozzle, the needle should be arranged with the nozzle downward but the bevel of the needle upward. The syringe and the needle should be aligned with the vein to be entered and the needle pushed into the vein at an angle to the skin of approximately 15 degrees. When the initial resistance of the vein wall is overcome as it is pierced, forward pressure on the syringe is eased, and the blood is withdrawn by very gently pulling back the plunger of the syringe. If a second syringe is necessary, a gauze pad may be placed under the hub of the needle to absorb the spill; the first syringe is then quickly disconnected, and the second is put in place to continue the blood draw.

After filling the syringe and completing the collection, if the sample needs to be transferred to an evacuated tube, a transfer device should be used to puncture the cap of the tube. Use of transfer devices prevents having to puncture an evacuated tube with a needle and risking a needle-stick injury. The tube should be allowed to fill passively using its vacuum; uncapping the evacuated tube is not recommended for the reasons stated earlier. Vigorous withdrawal of blood into a syringe during collection or forceful transfer from the syringe to the receiving vessel may cause hemolysis of blood and will likely make the sample not valid for testing. Communication of this common preanalytical error to those not trained in routine sample collection is the responsibility of all laboratory directors and the experts, the phlebotomy team. Although safe use and disposal of sharps is important with any collection device, this is particularly important with the use of a needle and syringe. The phlebotomist must ensure an appropriate sharps disposal bin is available at the point of collection, that the location is free of interference or distractions that may increase the risk of a needle-stick injury, and that he or she has been trained in all procedures.

Completion of collection. When blood collection is complete and the needle withdrawn, the patient should be instructed to hold a dry gauze pad tightly over the puncture site with the arm raised to stop residual bleeding and promote the clotting process. The pad should then be held in place firmly by a bandage or by a nonadhesive strap (which avoids pulling hairs on the arm when it is removed); these may be removed after 15 minutes. With a collection device, such as that shown in Fig. 4.2, the needle is covered, and the needle and the tube holder are immediately discarded into a sharps container that should be conveniently and safely positioned. In the event that a winged (butterfly) set is used, the wings are pushed forward to cover the needle, or with newer available equipment, a button is pressed, releasing a spring that retracts the needle. If a syringe was used, the needle should not be removed because of the danger of a needlestick on the part of the phlebotomist. All used supplies should be discarded in a hazardous waste receptacle.

All tubes should then be labeled per institutional policy. Most institutions have a written procedure prohibiting the advance labeling of tubes because this is seen as providing the potential for mislabeling, one of the most common sources of preanalytical error. Collectors should ensure that the correct labels are applied. Incorrect labels which have been mistakenly filed in patient notes, files, or are in the room of a hospitalized patient, are a major source of mislabeling and preanalytical error. Many US institutions recommend showing the labeled tube to the patient to further confirm correct identification. At the conclusion of this process, gloves should be discarded in a hazardous waste receptacle if visibly contaminated or in uncontaminated trash if not visibly contaminated. Before applying new gloves and proceeding to the next patient, and depending on institutional policy, all caregivers including phlebotomists should use an alcohol-based cleanser or soap and water to wash their hands.

Venipuncture in children. The techniques for venipuncture in children and adults are similar. However, children are likely to make unexpected movements, and assistance in holding them still is often desirable. Although a syringe or an evacuated blood tube system may be used to collect specimens, a syringe with a winged butterfly collection set is more commonly used in younger children. The pressure on a syringe can be more easily controlled by the phlebotomist than the vacuum pressure in an evacuated tube, thus preventing the pressure from pulling small veins closed instead of drawing blood from them. A syringe should be the tuberculin type or should have a 3-mL capacity, except when a large volume of blood is required for analysis. A 21- to 23-gauge needle or a 20- to 23-gauge butterfly needle with attached tubing is appropriate to collect specimens. In the pediatric population, alternative collection through skin puncture is often used.

Skin Puncture

Skin puncture is an open collection technique in which the skin is punctured by a lancet and a small volume of blood is collected into a micro device. In practice, skin puncture is used in situations in which (1) sample volume is limited (e.g., pediatric applications), (2) repeated venipunctures have resulted in severe vein damage, or (3) patients have been burned or bandaged and veins therefore are unavailable for venipuncture. This technique is also commonly used when the sample is to be applied directly to a testing device in a point-of-care testing situation or to filter paper. It is most often performed on the tip of the finger or the heels of infants. For example, in an infant younger than 6 months, the lateral or medial plantar surface of the foot should be used for skin puncture; suitable areas are illustrated in Fig. 4.3. These areas are the fleshiest part of the foot in an infant, with the most distance between the skin surface and the underlying bone. Risk of inadvertently hitting bone and causing a bone infection is the lowest when these areas are used for a heel stick. For this reason, the back of the heel and the toes should not be used.[11] Blood collection from anywhere on the foot should be avoided on ambulatory patients; thus when an infant starts walking, a heel stick should no longer be performed. In addition, devices are made specifically for a heel stick or a finger stick, and they should not be used interchangeably. These devices have different tip lengths and thus make a shallower or a deeper puncture (Table 4.4). The finger-stick procedure should not be performed on infants younger than 6 months old because no commercially available device punctures shallow enough to avoid bones. The complete procedure for collecting blood from infants using skin puncture is described in a CLSI document (CLSI GP42-A6, see Table 4.1).

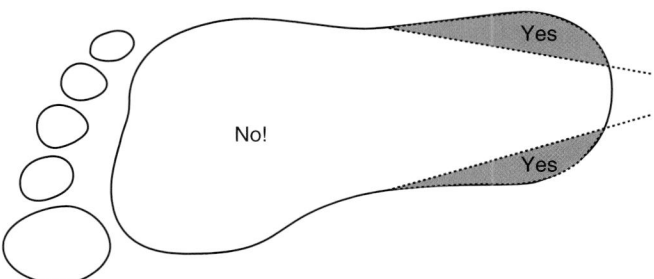

FIGURE 4.3 Acceptable sites for skin puncture to collect blood from an infant's foot. (Modified from Blumenfeld TA, Turi GK, Blanc WA. Recommended site and depth of newborn heel punctures based on anatomical measurements and histopathology. *Lancet* 1979;**1**:230–33. Reprinted with permission from Elsevier.)

TABLE 4.4 Tip Lengths in Finger- and Heel-Stick Devices

Collection Type and Age of Use	Tip Length (mm)
Heel stick: premature infants	0.85
Heel stick: term infants to 6 months old	1.0
Heel stick: 6 months to 1 year	1.25
Finger stick: walking to 8 years	1.5
Finger stick: >8 years	1.75–2.0

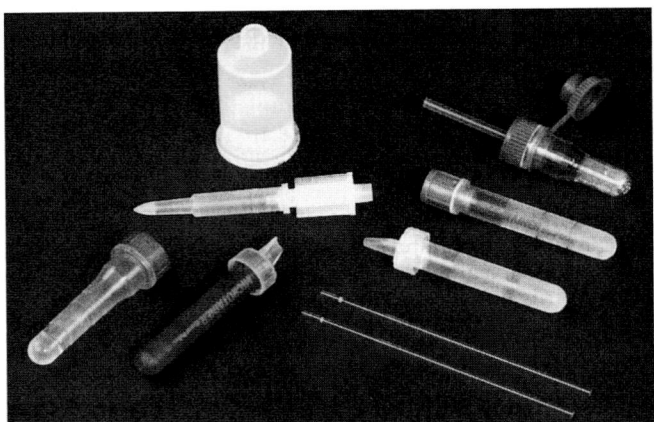

FIGURE 4.4 Microcollection tubes. (From Flynn JC. *Procedures in phlebotomy.* 3rd ed. St. Louis, MO: Saunders; 2005.)

To collect a blood specimen by skin puncture, the phlebotomist first thoroughly cleans the skin with a gauze pad saturated with an approved cleaning solution, as outlined earlier for venipuncture. If an alcohol swab is used, the alcohol must be allowed to evaporate from the skin so that hemolysis does not occur. When the skin is dry, it is quickly punctured by a sharp stab with a lancet. The depth of the incision should be less than 2.0 mm to prevent contact with bone. To minimize the possibility of infection, a different site should be selected for each puncture. The finger should be held in such a way that gravity assists collection of blood at the fingertip and the lancet held to make the incision as close to perpendicular to the fingernail as possible.[11] Massaging of the finger to stimulate blood flow should be avoided because it causes the outflow of debris and tissue fluid, which does not have the same composition as plasma. To improve circulation of the blood, the finger (or the heel in the case of a heel stick) may be warmed by application of a warm, wet washcloth or a specialized device, such as a heel warmer, for 3 minutes before the lancet is applied. Warming the heel or finger properly will not only cause the capillary blood to be free flowing and improve the ability to collect the sample, but the analytes in the sample will also approach arterial blood values in a properly warmed heel stick. In a cold heel, the values more approximate venous blood. Warming thus may be especially important for capillary blood gas collections. The first drop of blood is wiped off, and subsequent drops are transferred to the appropriate collection tube by gentle contact. Filling should be done rapidly to prevent clotting, and introduction of air bubbles should be prevented.

As the name suggests, blood is collected into capillary blood tubes by capillary action. A variety of collection tubes are commercially available (Fig. 4.4). Containers are available that contain different anticoagulants, such as sodium and lithium heparin, and some are available in brown glass for collection of light-sensitive analytes, such as bilirubin (see later section on anticoagulants). As with evacuated blood tubes and to prevent the possibility of breakage and the spread of infection, capillary devices frequently are plastic or coated with plastic. A disadvantage of some of the collection devices shown in Fig. 4.4 is that blood tends to pool in the mouth of the tube and must be flicked down the tube, creating a risk of hemolysis. Drop-by-drop collection and scooping along the skin with the edge of the tube to collect the blood should be avoided because both practices increase hemolysis. The correct order of filling of these devices is different than evacuated blood tubes because the concerns are different.[11,12] These samples are collected by dripping or capillary action from the puncture site into the small tubes that hold less than 1 mL each. There is less chance of cross-contamination with anticoagulant between tubes; however, the flow of blood also clots quickly in a heel or finger stick, and platelet levels drop quickly as the clots form. Thus the anticoagulant tubes, especially the EDTA tube for the complete blood count (CBC), are drawn first rather than last. The serum tubes are drawn last (Table 4.5) because it does not matter if clots are formed in the sample.[13,14]

For collection of blood specimens on filter paper for molecular genetic testing and neonatal screening, the skin is cleaned and punctured as described previously. The first drop of blood should be wiped away. Then the filter paper is gently touched against a large drop of blood that is allowed to soak into the paper to fill the marked circle. Only a single application per circle should be made to prevent nonuniform analyte concentration. The paper is examined to verify that there has been complete penetration of the paper. The procedure is repeated to fill all the circles. As with all skin puncture collections, avoid milking or squeezing the finger or foot because this procedure contributes tissue fluids to the sample. The filter papers should be air dried (generally for 2 to 3 hours and horizontally placed to prevent mold or bacterial overgrowth and possible separation of blood components, respectively) before storage in a properly labeled envelope. Blood should never be transferred onto filter paper after it has been collected in non-anticoagulated capillary tubes because partial clotting may have occurred, compromising the quality of the specimen. However, blood collected into any type of tube containing an anticoagulant may be applied directly to the filter paper. Dried blood spots

TABLE 4.5 Order of Draw for Skin Puncture: Capillary Blood

Usage or Additive	Tube Top Color
Blood gases (heparin)	Microhematocrit tubes
EDTA	Lavender
Heparin	Green
Other additives	Light blue, gray
Nonadditives	Red, tiger, yellow

EDTA, Ethylenediaminetetraacetic acid.

on filter paper are a convenient way to store a sample for possible future molecular testing (with patient consent). These blood spots are handled in the same manner as neonatal screening specimens, with air drying and storage in a dry protected environment.

Arterial Puncture

Arterial puncture requires considerable skill and is usually performed only by physicians or specially trained technicians or nurses. Preferred sites of arterial puncture are, in order, the (1) radial artery at the wrist, (2) brachial artery in the elbow, and (3) femoral artery in the groin. Because leakage of blood from the femoral artery tends to be greater, especially in older adults, sites in the arm are used most often. The proper technique for arterial puncture has been described.[15,16]

In neonates, an indwelling catheter in the umbilical artery is best to obtain specimens for blood gas analysis. In older children and adults in whom it is impossible to perform an arterial puncture, a capillary puncture may be performed to obtain arterialized capillary blood. Such a specimen yields acceptable values for pH and PCO_2 but not always for PO_2 unless the site is properly warmed. In children and adults, the preferred puncture site for arterialized capillary blood is the finger; in infants, it is the heel. Capillary blood specimens are particularly inappropriate when blood circulation is poor and thus should be avoided when a patient has reduced cardiac output, hypotension, or vasoconstriction or has a condition of fluid overload. For each capillary puncture, the skin should be warmed first with a hot, moist towel to improve the circulation. The puncture itself should be performed as described previously; a free flow of blood is essential. Heparinized capillary tubes containing a small metal bar can be used to collect the blood. Tubes should be sealed quickly and the contents mixed well by using a magnet to move the metal bar up and down in the tube so that a uniform specimen is available for analysis.

Anticoagulants and Preservatives for Blood

Serum is defined as that portion of blood that remains after coagulation has occurred and the cells have been removed. Serum is the specimen of choice for many analyses, including viral and antibody screening and protein electrophoresis. Samples are collected into tubes with no additive or with a clot activator and must be allowed to complete the coagulation process before further processing. Plasma is defined as the noncellular component of anticoagulated whole blood after the cellular components have been removed. There are multiple ways to produce a plasma sample as detailed later. Heparinized plasma is increasingly being used for routine chemistry testing to decrease turnaround time, because it is not necessary to wait for the blood to clot. Sometimes considerable differences may be observed between the concentrations of analytes in serum and in plasma, as shown in Table 4.6. For molecular diagnostics, anticoagulated whole blood or plasma is more likely to be the specimen of choice for either genomic DNA isolation from the white blood cells (WBCs) still intact from a whole blood collection or from plasma that will yield viral identification and quantification. A number of anticoagulants are available, including heparin, EDTA, sodium fluoride (NaF), citrate, acid citrate dextrose (ACD), oxalate, and iodoacetate, which are covered in detail later.

TABLE 4.6   Differences in Composition Between Heparin Plasma and Serum[a,b]

Plasma Value > Serum Value (%)		No Difference Between Serum and Plasma Values	Plasma Value < Serum Value (%)	
Lactate dehydrogenase	2.7	Bilirubin	Glucose	5.1
Total protein	4.0	Cholesterol	Phosphorus	7.0
		Creatinine	Potassium	8.4

[a]To estimate the probable effect of a factor on results, relate the percent increase or decrease shown in the table to analytical variation (±% coefficient of variation) routinely found for analytes.
[b]This list includes only differences that are of clinical significance and may need to be annotated with a comment on patient results that general (plasma) reference intervals may not apply.
Modified from Ladenson JH, Tsai L-MB, Michael JM, Kessler G, Joist JH. Serum versus heparinized plasma for eighteen common chemistry tests. *Am J Clin Pathol* 1974;**62**:545–52. Copyright 1974 by the American Society of Clinical Pathologists. Reprinted with permission.

For any assay provided for clinical use, manufacturers specify the appropriate sample type(s) for which they have validated the assay. Use of different sample types is acceptable only if the laboratory has validated the alternate type(s). For example, care should be taken with gel tubes because they may vary among tube manufacturers. Acceptability of a wide range of sample types can be advantageous because it can reduce the need for recollections if the preferred tube is not provided.

Heparin. Heparin is the most widely used anticoagulant for chemistry testing. It is a mucoitin polysulfuric acid and is available as sodium, potassium, lithium, and ammonium salts, all of which can adequately prevent coagulation. This anticoagulant accelerates the action of antithrombin III, which neutralizes thrombin and thus prevents the formation of fibrin from fibrinogen. Most blood tubes are prepared with approximately 0.2 mg of heparin for each milliliter of blood (18 units/mL) to be collected. The heparin is usually present as a dry powder that is hygroscopic and dissolves rapidly assuming that the tube of blood is correctly mixed (see Table 4.2). Heparin is a naturally occurring anticoagulant and has the disadvantages of high cost and a more temporary action of anticoagulation than is attained by the chemicals discussed later. It produces a blue background in blood smears that are stained with Wright's stain. In addition, heparin can interfere with the binding of calcium to EDTA in analytical methods for calcium involving complexing with EDTA. Heparin, which is negatively charged, binds calcium and can reduce results for ionized calcium measurements. Thus either serum tubes are required or blood gas syringes with either low heparin concentrations or so-called "balanced heparin" with added calcium to block the binding of further calcium are used. Of course, the use of lithium or ammonium heparin is unacceptable for lithium and ammonia measurements, respectively, because the tube contains an amount similar to that found in treated patients (lithium) or can elevate the clinically actionable value (ammonia). Heparin tubes are also unsuitable for protein electrophoresis as the fibrinogen in the unclotted sample causes an interfering band. This fibrinogen is also the cause of a higher total protein in heparin tubes than in serum tubes.

It should be noted that heparin is unacceptable for most tests performed using polymerase chain reaction (PCR) because of inhibition of the polymerase enzyme by this large molecule. In some special circumstances, a heparin tube can be shared with a molecular diagnostic laboratory if a non-heparinized tube is not available. DNA can be extracted from heparinized samples, but amplification may be reduced, and the effect of heparin on any molecular diagnostic assay should be assessed as part of a method validation study.

Ethylenediaminetetraacetic acid. EDTA is a chelating agent of divalent cations such as Ca^{2+} and Mg^{2+} that is particularly useful for (1) hematologic examinations including transfusion medicine applications, (2) measurement of intracellular drugs such as cyclosporine or tacrolimus, (3) HbA_{1c} analysis, (4) isolation of genomic DNA, and (5) qualitative and quantitative virus determinations by molecular techniques because it preserves the cellular components of blood. It is used as the disodium, dipotassium, or tripotassium salt, the last two being more soluble with the tripotassium salt commonly provided as a liquid in the collection tube. It is effective at a final concentration of 1 to 2 g/L of blood. Higher concentrations hypertonically shrink the RBCs. EDTA prevents coagulation by binding calcium, which is essential for the clotting mechanism. EDTA tubes are also available with a gel barrier to separate plasma from cells when EDTA plasma is required (white tubes; see Table 4.3). In blue/black tubes, incorporation of a density gradient allows recovery of nucleated cells after centrifugation, thus increasing the yield of DNA.

Because it chelates calcium, magnesium, and iron, EDTA is unsuitable for specimens for these analyses using the most common photometric or titrimetric techniques. For many laboratories, an undetectable calcium value or a critical potassium value in an otherwise stable patient is often used as a flag that an inappropriate specimen type has been submitted for just this reason. Additionally, EDTA, probably by chelation of required metallic cofactors, inhibits alkaline phosphatase and creatine kinase activities. As an anticoagulant, it has little effect on other clinical tests, although the concentration of cholesterol has been reported to be decreased by 3% to 5%.

Sodium fluoride. NaF is a weak anticoagulant that is often added as a preservative for blood glucose and lactate.[17,18] As a preservative, together with another anticoagulant such as potassium oxalate, it is effective at a concentration of approximately 2 g/L blood. It exerts its preservative action by inhibiting enolase, a downstream enzyme in the glycolysis pathway. Therefore the inhibition is not immediate,[17] and a certain amount of degradation occurs during the first 1 to 2 hours after collection. Most specimens are then stable at 25 °C for at least 24 hours or at 4 °C for 48 hours. Without an antiglycolytic agent, the blood glucose concentration decreases approximately 10 mg/dL (0.56 mmol/L) per hour at 25 °C. The rate of decrease is faster in newborns because of the increased metabolic activity of their erythrocytes and in leukemic patients because of the high metabolic activity of the WBCs. NaF is poorly soluble, and blood must be well mixed for NaF to be effective (see Table 4.2). Because of the delay in onset of action, recent protocols recommend placing the tube on ice until the sample can be separated to ensure

accurate glucose measurements. Newer NaF combination tubes include tubes containing NaF–citrate buffer–Na_2EDTA, NaF–Na-heparin, NaF–K_2oxalate, NaF–citrate, and NaF–Na_2EDTA. Acidification of specimens by citrate and addition of EDTA to a fluoride tube immediately inhibit glycolysis and preserve glucose in the specimen for at least 24 hours. These various tubes have all been found to be suitable for glucose preservation,[18] but care must be taken to ensure use according to manufacturers' guidelines when using different tube types.[19]

If NaF is used alone for anticoagulation, three to five times greater concentrations than the usual 2 g/L are required. This high concentration and inhibition of the glycolytic cycle are likely to cause fluid shifts and a change in the concentration of some analytes. Fluoride is also a potent inhibitor of many serum enzymes and in high concentrations also affects urease, which is used to measure urea nitrogen in many analytical systems.

Citrate. Sodium citrate solution, at a concentration of 34 to 38 g/L in a ratio of 1 part to 9 parts of blood, is widely used for coagulation studies. The correct ratio of blood to anticoagulant is critical (refer to the earlier discussion concerning proper filling of vacuum blood tubes) to achieve proper coagulation measurements because the anticoagulant effect is reversed by addition of standard amounts of Ca^{2+} that are based on a proper collection volume. Because citrate chelates calcium, it is unsuitable as an anticoagulant for specimens for measurement of this element. It also inhibits aminotransferases and alkaline phosphatase but stimulates acid phosphatase when phenylphosphate is used as a substrate. Because citrate complexes molybdate, it decreases the color yield in phosphate measurements that involve molybdate ions and produces low results.

Acid citrate dextrose. As indicated previously, the collection of specimens into EDTA is often used for isolation of genomic DNA from the patient. However, additional and complementary diagnostic tests, such as cytogenetic testing, may be requested at the same time. For this reason, samples for molecular diagnostics with an accompanying cytogenetic request are often collected into ACD anticoagulant so as to preserve both the form and the function of the cellular components. There are two ACD tube designations: ACD A and ACD B. These differ only by the concentrations of the additives (see Table 4.3). Both enhance the vitality and recovery of WBCs for several days after collection of the specimen; thus they are suitable for both molecular diagnostic testing and cytogenetic testing.

Whereas solution A is used for an 8.5-mL blood draw (10 mL total volume), solution B is used for a 3- or a 6-mL blood draw (7 mL total volume). The specific test(s) requested will determine the size of tube necessary for specimen collection.

Oxalates. Sodium, potassium, ammonium, and lithium oxalates inhibit blood coagulation by forming rather insoluble complexes with calcium ions. Potassium oxalate ($K_2C_2O_4 \cdot H_2O$), at a concentration of approximately 1 to 2 g/L of blood, is the most widely used oxalate. At concentrations of greater than 3 g oxalate per liter, hemolysis is likely to occur.

Combined ammonium and/or potassium oxalate does not cause shrinkage of erythrocytes. However, other oxalates have been known to cause shrinkage by drawing water into the plasma. Reduction in hematocrit may be as much as

10%, causing a reduction in the concentration of plasma constituents of 5%. As fluid is lost from the cells, an exchange of electrolytes and other constituents across the cell membrane occurs. Oxalate inhibits several enzymes, including acid and alkaline phosphatases, amylase, and lactate dehydrogenase (LDH), and may cause precipitation of calcium as the oxalate salt.

Iodoacetate. Sodium iodoacetate at a concentration of 2 g/L is an effective antiglycolytic agent (with the caveats mentioned earlier) and a substitute for NaF. Because it has no effect on urease, it can be used when glucose and urea tests are performed on a single specimen. It inhibits creatine kinase but appears to have no notable effects on other clinical tests.

Influence of Site of Collection on Blood Composition

Blood obtained from different sites differs in composition. In general, skin puncture blood is more similar to arterial blood than venous blood, depending on the collection condition as described earlier. Thus there are no clinically significant differences between freely flowing capillary blood and arterial blood in pH, PCO_2, PO_2, and oxygen saturation. The PCO_2 of venous blood is up to 6 to 7 mm Hg (0.8 to 0.9 kPa) higher. Venous blood glucose is as much as 7 mg/dL (0.39 mmol/L) less than capillary blood glucose.

Blood obtained by skin puncture is contaminated to some extent with interstitial and intracellular fluids. The major differences between venous serum and capillary serum are illustrated in Table 4.7.

Collection of Blood From Intravenous or Arterial Lines

When blood is collected from a central or peripheral venous catheter or arterial line, it is necessary to ensure that the composition of the specimen is not affected by the fluid that is infused into the patient. With clinical approval, fluid may be shut off using the stopcock on the catheter, and 10 mL of blood is aspirated through the stopcock and discarded before the specimen for analysis is withdrawn. In pediatric patients, 10 mL of blood going to waste is often not feasible, so lesser volumes are aspirated, although the goal is still to aspirate roughly three times the dead space of the line before collecting the sample for testing. Any infused fluid contamination may affect basic biochemical tests such as electrolytes, lactate, or glucose. Aspirating this blood and clearing the lines is

TABLE 4.7 Difference in Composition of Capillary and Venous Serum[a]

Capillary Value > Venous Value (%)		No Difference Between Capillary and Venous Values	Capillary Value < Venous Value (%)	
Glucose	1.4	Phosphate	Bilirubin	5.0
Potassium	0.9	Urea	Calcium	4.6
			Chloride	1.8
			Sodium	2.3
			Total protein	3.3

[a]To estimate the probable effect of a factor on results, relate the percent increase or decrease shown in the table to analytical variation (± % coefficient of variation) routinely found for analytes. From Kupke IR, Kather B, Zeugner S. On the composition of capillary and venous blood serum. *Clin Chim Acta* 1981;**112**:177–85.

equally important for molecular diagnostics and coagulation testing because the stopcock is often heavily saturated with heparin to prevent clotting. Collection of samples for therapeutic drug monitoring should not be done from the line used for the infusion irrespective of the time since infusion or amount of blood aspirated because the drug may adhere to the line and leak into the collected sample, causing false elevations. Additionally, blood collected from a heparinized catheter line cannot be used for coagulation testing as it will significantly affect results.[20]

In theory, blood may be collected from the veins of an arm below an IV line without interference from the fluid being infused because retrograde blood flow does not occur in the veins and the fluid that is infused must first circulate through the heart and return to the tissue before it reaches the sampling site. However, as stated previously, collection from the arm without the IV line is strongly recommended.

Hemolysis

Hemolysis is defined as the disruption of the RBC membrane, resulting in the release of hemoglobin, and may be the consequence of intravascular events (in vivo hemolysis) or may occur subsequent to or during blood collection (in vitro hemolysis). In vitro hemolysis is perhaps the single biggest preanalytical factor affecting test results and has many causes. Mechanical disruption of the cells may occur from improper mixing of sample and anticoagulant after collection. Improper collection may occur, including applying high shear forces on the sample from too rapid collection of the sample into the collection device or performing the collection through an inadequately cleared IV line. Higher rates of hemolysis are commonly seen when collection is done through IV lines and in samples collected in the emergency department. This may be due to a combination of rapid collection in a high-stress environment, poor collection technique causing contamination between tubes, and improper mixing. Low-volume evacuated tubes are available which have reduced vacuum and cause lower shear force on the RBCs. These tubes also collect less blood, but can be used to help reduce the percentage of hemolyzed samples being collected. In pediatrics and especially with neonates, in vitro hemolysis is a considerable and constant problem. The shear forces generated on the cells when collecting a blood sample are exacerbated by the small-bore needles necessary to get into tiny veins. Additionally, most samples from neonates are collected via heel-stick skin puncture, and this collection technique commonly results in hemolyzed samples. Finally, neonates have larger, more fragile RBCs with a shorter half-life that are prone to hemolyze. Again, low-volume evacuated tubes can help reduce hemolysis rates, as can continuous education on proper collection techniques for heel sticks and careful handling of the collected samples.

Serum and plasma show visual evidence of hemolysis when the hemoglobin concentration exceeds 50 mg/dL (7.7 μmol/L). When the level exceeds 150 to 200 mg/dL (23 to 31 μmol/L), the plasma will appear bright red to most observers. Slight hemolysis has little effect on most but not all test values. A clinically significant interpretation of results at this lower concentration may be observed on those constituents that are present at a higher concentration in erythrocytes than in plasma. Thus plasma activities or concentrations of LDH, aspartate transaminase (AST), potassium, magnesium, and phosphate are particularly increased by even a slight degree of hemolysis and may need to be explained to the care team to determine whether or not the result(s) represent in vivo or in vitro hemolysis and determine the implication(s) of the test result. Most manufacturers provide data on the effects of hemolysis on the analytical performance of individual tests, and this should be evaluated in the selection of individual methods. Each laboratory must define at what level of hemolysis results should be held and not reported to prevent poor clinical action on such unreliable test results.

Although the amount of free hemoglobin could be measured and a calculation made to correct test values affected by hemoglobin, this practice is undesirable because factors other than hemoglobin could contribute to the altered test values, and it would be impossible to assess their impact. Hemolysis may affect many un-blanked or inadequately blanked analytical methods.[21] Currently, most large chemistry analyzers have the capability of measuring the amount of hemolysis, icterus, and lipemia (the HIL indices) in samples placed on the instrument. These are the three main interferents present in patient samples, and the instrument can be programmed to prevent release of results affected by a specific level of each of these. For some analytes, the effect of hemolysis is time dependent (e.g., the degradation of insulin by released intracellular enzymes), and any hemolysis may give falsely low results. For more details about HIL indices and their assessment and management in the laboratory, refer to Chapter 5.

In molecular diagnostic testing, hemoglobin may interfere with the amplification reaction, particularly when reverse transcriptase (RT)-PCR is the first step in the analysis of RNA. In some situations, the isolation of nucleic acid is sufficiently selective that free hemoglobin from the ruptured cells is removed and will not cause a problem. However, with hemolyzed blood, alternative or additional extraction methods are usually needed to ensure that RNA is fully and accurately transcribed and that the greatest amplification of DNA is achieved.

Urine

The type of urine specimen to be collected is dictated by the tests to be performed. Untimed or random specimens are suitable for only a few chemical tests; usually, urine specimens must be collected over a predetermined interval of time, such as 4, 12, or 24 hours. A clean, early morning, fasting specimen is usually the most concentrated specimen and thus is preferred for microscopic examinations and for detection of constituents, such as proteins, especially albumin, or human chorionic gonadotropin. The clean timed specimen is one obtained at specific times of the day or during certain phases of the act of micturition. Whereas bacterial examination of the first 10 mL of urine voided is most appropriate to detect urethritis, the midstream specimen is best for investigating bladder disorders. The double-voided specimen is the urine excreted during a timed period after complete emptying of the bladder; it is used, for example, to assess glucose excretion during a glucose tolerance test. Its collection must be timed in relation to the ingestion of glucose. Similarly, in some metabolic disorders, urine must be collected during or immediately after symptoms of the disease appear (see Chapters 41 and 61).

When used for testing alcohol and drugs of abuse content, urine specimens are collected under rigorous conditions.

Such collections may begin with a requirement for formal identification such as a driver's license or other picture identification as discussed earlier. Patients are asked to leave all personal belongings outside of the restroom facility to prevent substitution of the patient's urine with urine brought from outside. Many locations that routinely perform these collections have the capacity to turn running water off to prevent dilution or put a coloring agent in the toilet water so such dilution attempts are easily identified; the temperature of the urine is often recorded as well to detect such attempts. Finally, patients are often asked to put their initials on the urine cup and sign the paperwork, accepting the sample as theirs. This chain of custody documentation is then sealed in a transport bag with the sample (also sealed) and transported to the testing laboratory directly, where the chain of custody documentation will be continued throughout the testing process. It is necessary for laboratories to be aware of the relevant legal requirements for this type of testing and plan in advance how these samples and the supporting paperwork will be collected and handled. Institutional policies should be in place and adhered to in all cases.

Catheter specimens are used for microbiologic examination in critically ill patients and in those with urinary tract obstruction but should not normally be obtained just for examination of chemical constituents. The suprapubic tap specimen is a useful alternative because the tap is unlikely to cause infection. After appropriate cleaning of the skin over the full bladder, a 22-gauge spinal needle is passed through a small wheal made by a local anesthetic. The bladder is penetrated and the urine withdrawn into the syringe.

Even though tests in the clinical laboratory are not usually affected by lack of sterile collection procedures, the patient's genitalia should be cleaned before each voiding to minimize the transfer of surface bacteria to the urine. Cleansing is essential if the true concentration of WBCs is to be obtained.

Currently, urine is an uncommon specimen type in the molecular diagnostic laboratory for genomic testing, although some laboratories use urine samples for bladder cancer screening and monitoring of therapy for bladder cancer. However, urine is frequently used for molecular testing for infectious agents, such as *Chlamydia*, a common sexually transmitted organism, or BK virus (also known as polyomavirus hominis 1), associated with potential rejection or failure of transplanted kidneys. Because most requests involve a specific organism, an untimed or random urine specimen collected into a sterile container with no preservative is usually acceptable.

Timed Urine Specimens

The collection period for timed specimens should be long enough to minimize the influence of short-term biologic variations. When specimens are to be collected over a specified period of time, the patient's close adherence to instructions is critically important, and a common source of a preanalytical variable. The bladder must be emptied at the time the collection is to begin and this urine discarded. Thereafter, all urine must be collected until the end of the scheduled time, including emptying of the bladder at the end of the collection period. If a patient has a bowel movement during the collection period, precautions should be taken to prevent fecal contamination of the urine. If the collection has to be made over several hours, urine should be passed into a separate container at each voiding and then emptied into a larger container for the complete specimen. This two-step procedure prevents the danger of patients splashing themselves with a preservative, such as acid that may be included in the timed collection device. The large container generally should be stored at 4 °C during the entire collection period.

Before beginning a timed collection, a patient should be given written instructions with regard to diet or drug ingestion, if appropriate, to avoid interference of ingested compounds with analytical procedures. For example, instructions for collection of specimens for 5-hydroxyindoleacetic acid measurements should specify avoidance of avocados, bananas, plums, walnuts, pineapples, eggplant, acetaminophen, and cough syrups containing glyceryl guaiacolate (guaifenesin). These dietary components are sources of 5-hydroxytryptamine and should be avoided for this reason; the other compounds interfere with certain analytical procedures but may not interfere with highly specific analytical methods. Each laboratory should determine its own requirements. See also specimen information for specific analytes in the respective chapters.

For 2-hour specimens, a prelabeled 1-L bottle is generally adequate. For a 12-hour collection, a 2-L bottle usually suffices; for a 24-hour collection, a 3- or 4-L bottle is appropriate for most patients. A single bottle allows adequate mixing of the specimen and prevents possible loss of some of the specimen if a second container does not reach the laboratory. Urine should not be collected at the same time for two or more tests requiring different preservatives. Aliquots for an analysis such as a microscopic examination should not be removed while a 24-hour collection is in process. Removal of aliquots during collection is not permissible even when the volume removed is measured and corrected because excretion of most compounds varies throughout the day, and test results will be affected. Appropriate information regarding the collection, including warnings with respect to handling of the specimen, should appear on the bottle label.

When a timed collection is complete, the specimen should be delivered without delay to the clinical laboratory, where the volume should be measured. This may be done by using graduated cylinders or by weighing the container and the urine when preweighed or uniform containers are used. The mass in grams may be reported as if it were the volume in milliliters. There is rarely a need to measure the specific gravity of a weighed specimen because errors in analysis usually exceed the error arising from failure to correct the volume of urine for its mass.

Before a specimen is transferred into small containers for each of the ordered tests, it must be thoroughly mixed to ensure homogeneity because the specific gravity, volume, and composition of the urine all may vary throughout the collection period. The small container into which an aliquot is transferred should not be a plastic bottle if toluene or another organic compound has been used as a preservative; metal-free containers must be used for trace metal analyses. See the later discussion on appropriate labeling of such secondary containers.

Collection of Urine From Children

Collection of any type of urine specimen from an infant is difficult, with timed collections being the most problematic. Fortunately, timed collections are rarely required in neonates. The approved method for collecting a random urine

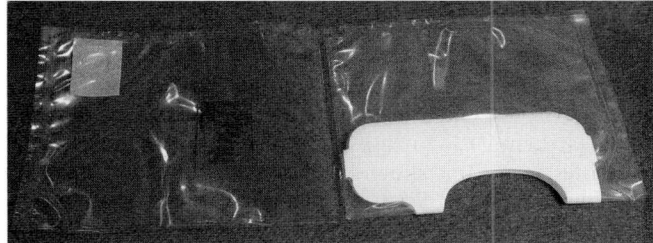

FIGURE 4.5 Urine collection device used in children.

specimen from an infant involves a process known as bagging. The scrotal or perineal area is cleaned and dried first, and any natural or applied skin oils are removed. Then a plastic bag (e.g., U-Bag, Hollister, Chicago, IL, or Tink-Col, C.R. Bard, Murray Hill, NJ) is placed around the infant's genitalia and held in place by a mild adhesive (Fig. 4.5). The baby's diaper is reapplied to help hold the bag in place. As soon as voiding has occurred, the bag containing the urine sample is removed and emptied into a regular urine collection cup. The mild adhesive on the bag will often fail when it becomes wet with urine, so the infant should be monitored and the bag removed as soon as the urine sample is collected. Even a random or spot urine collection for something as simple as a urinalysis may require either catheterization or a suprapubic tap collection in an infant, especially if there is difficulty getting the infant to urinate or in collecting the sample when the infant does urinate. In infants and very young children requiring a rare 24-hour urine collection, hospitalization and catheterization are often required to obtain a complete collection.

Urine Preservatives

The most common preservatives and the tests for which preservatives are required are listed in Table 4.8. Preservatives have different roles but usually are added to reduce bacterial action or chemical decomposition or to solubilize constituents that otherwise might precipitate out of solution. Another application is to decrease atmospheric oxidation of unstable compounds. Some specimens should not have *any* preservatives added because of the possibility of interference with analytical methods.

One of the most acceptable forms of preservation of urine specimens is refrigeration immediately after collection; it is even more successful when combined with chemical preservation. Urinary preservative tablets that contain a mixture of chemicals, such as potassium acid phosphate, sodium benzoate, benzoic acid, hexamethylene tetramine, and sodium bicarbonate have been used for chemical and microscopic examination. Because these tablets contain sodium and potassium salts, among others, they should not be used for analysis of these analytes. The preservative tablets act mainly by lowering the pH of the urine and by releasing formaldehyde. Formalin has also been used for preserving specimens, but in large amounts it precipitates urea and inhibits certain reactions (e.g., the dipstick esterase test for leukocytes). Acidification to below a pH of 3 is widely used to preserve 24-hour specimens and is particularly useful for specimens for determination of calcium, steroids, adrenaline, noradrenaline, and vanillylmandelic acid. However, precipitation of

TABLE 4.8 Commonly Used Urine Preservatives

Preservative	Concentrations or Volumes	Common Usage (Analytes)
HCl	6 mol/L; 30 mL per 24-h collection	Acidification/common preservative for 24-h urine collections
Acetic acid	50%; 25 mL per 24-h collection	Acidification/preservative for 24-h urine collections (Aldosterone, Catecholamines, Serotonin, 5-hydroxyindoleacetic acid [5-HIAA], homovanillic acid/vanillylmandelic acid [HVA/VMA])
Na_2CO_3	5 g per 24-h collection	Alkalinization/ preservative for 24-h urine collections (porphyrins, urobilinogen, uric acid)
HNO_3	6 mol/L; 15 mL 24-h hour collection	Acidification/preservative for 24-h urine collections (used sometimes for trace metal analysis)
Boric acid	10 g per 24-h collection	Acidification/preservative for 24-h urine collections (Urea, glucose, cortisol, aldosterone, other corticosteroids)
Toluene	30 mL per 24-h collection	Bacteriostatic agent/preservative for 24-h urine collections (oxalate, cystine, lysine, ornithine, arginine)
Thymol	10% in isopropanol; 10 mL per 24-h collection	Microscopy (not commonly used)

Modified from information provided in Clinical and Laboratory Standards Institute. *Routine urinalysis and collection, transportation, and preservation of urine specimens: CLSI-approved guideline GP16-A3.* Wayne, PA: Clinical and Laboratory Standards Institute; 2009.

urates will occur, thereby rendering a specimen unsuitable for measurement of uric acid.

Sulfamic acid (10 g/L urine) has also been used to reduce pH. Boric acid (5 mg/30 mL) has been used, but it also causes precipitation of urates. Thymol and chloroform were widely used in the past to preserve specimens for chemical and microscopic urinalysis, and thymol is still used in some cases. For many analytes, it is now recognized that specimens should be analyzed immediately and that the addition of preservatives is both largely ineffective and a source of interference with several analytical methods. Toluene is the only organic solvent that is still regularly used as a preservative. When present in a large enough amount, it acts as a barrier between the air and the surface of the specimen. Toluene, however, does not prevent the growth of anaerobic microorganisms and, because of its flammable nature, is a safety hazard. A mild base, such as sodium bicarbonate or a small amount of sodium hydroxide, is used to preserve porphyrins, urobilinogen, and uric acid. A sufficient quantity should be added to adjust the pH to between 8 and 9.

Stool

Small aliquots of stool are frequently analyzed to detect the presence of "hidden" blood, so-called occult blood. Occult blood screening is included as part of many periodic health examinations. Guaiac-based occult blood tests are subject to many interferences (aspirin, vitamin C, steroids, various drugs, red meat, alcohol), causing both false-positive and false-negative results, and should be interpreted cautiously unless the intent is to identify current bleeding in any portion of the gastrointestinal (GI) tract in an emergent patient. Newer immunochemical-based tests, immunochemical fecal occult blood (iFOB) tests, have decreased the interfering effects of food intake greatly for the purpose of identifying a lower GI tract bleed that may indicate the presence or possibility of malignant growth. In either case, tests for occult blood should be done on aliquots of excreted stools rather

than on material obtained on the glove of a physician doing a rectal examination because this procedure may cause enough bleeding to produce a positive result. Conversely, the small amount of stool present on the glove may not be representative of the whole, so bleeding may not be recognized.

In newborns, the first specimen from the bowel (meconium) may be used for detection of maternal drug use during the gestational period, which requires specific attention to the details of collection and identification similar to the chain of custody procedure for urine collection discussed earlier. Stool from infants and children may be screened for tryptic activity or for increased fecal fat concentrations, both of which can be indicators of cystic fibrosis. Fecal material is also commonly collected in childhood for the detection of parasites (ova and parasites [O & P]), enteric disease organisms such as *Salmonella* and *Shigella*, and viruses, all of which are useful in sorting out the differential diagnosis of diarrhea. Fecal testing is also used for helping to determine causes of malabsorption. In infants, fecal material for these tests is usually recovered from the diaper.

In adults and children, measurement of fecal nitrogen and fat in 72-hour specimens is used to assess the severity of malabsorption; measurement of fecal porphyrins is occasionally required to characterize the type of porphyria. Usually, no preservative is added to the stool, but the container should be kept refrigerated throughout the collection period, and care should be taken to prevent contamination from urine. When the collection is complete, the container and stool are weighed, and the mass of excreted stool is calculated. The specimen is homogenized and aliquoted so that the amount of fat or nitrogen excreted per day and the proportion of dietary intake excreted can be calculated.

For metabolic balance studies, collections of stool are usually made over a 72-hour period. Many balance studies are carried out in conjunction with research on the metabolism of such elements as calcium. It is important for such studies that a patient be on a controlled diet for a sufficiently long time before commencement of the study, so that a steady state has been attained.

DNA isolated from fecal samples is representative of the genetic composition of the colonic mucosa at the time of stool collection. The analysis of stool DNA is recommended by the American Cancer Society as a sensitive and specific biomarker useful for the detection of colorectal cancer.[22]

Other Body Fluids

Specimens may be collected for analysis from a range of different body fluids. These include cerebrospinal fluid (CSF), pleural fluid, ascitic fluid, pericardial fluid, amniotic fluid, synovial fluid, and others.[23–25] Readers are referred to Chapter 45 for a complete discussion of collection, analysis, and interpretation for these specimens.

Bronchoalveolar Lavage

Bronchoalveolar lavage (BAL) samples are another type of fluid sample that may be received in a laboratory. BAL is performed by a skilled clinician and involves passing a bronchoscope into a part of the lung, squirting a small amount of saline into that section, and then aspirating it back for examination. BAL is the most common method of sampling the internal lung milieu in the lower respiratory tract and is especially useful in patients with cystic fibrosis; immunocompromised patients; patients with pneumonia on ventilators; and patients with lung diseases, including cancers. Tests that are commonly ordered on BAL samples include cell count and WBC differential; cytospin and various histology slides for staining; and aerobic and anaerobic bacterial, mycobacterial, fungal, and viral cultures. Respiratory viral panels by PCR are also commonly ordered on BAL samples, as are acid-fast bacilli culture and stain and *Mycobacterium tuberculosis*–specific PCR testing.

Chorionic Villus Sampling

Chorionic villus sampling (CVS) testing can be performed at a gestation period of 10 to 12 weeks, but with amniotic fluid, testing generally is not performed until week 15 to 20 of gestation. CVS is the technique of inserting a catheter or needle into the placenta and removing some of the chorionic villi, or vascular projections, from the chorion. This tissue mostly has the same chromosomal and genetic makeup as the fetus and can be used to test for disorders that may be present in the fetus. When chorionic villus is sampled, ultrasonography is performed to assess the placenta and determine its position. The sample of the placenta is obtained through the vagina or through the abdomen, depending on the location of the placenta

Maternal cell contamination testing is used to definitively identify the source of isolated cells in an amniotic fluid sample and in CVS. Such confirmation of the source of the sample is strongly recommended for any prenatal diagnostic testing and may be required as a quality monitor in some laboratories. Of note, measurement of circulating nucleic acids in maternal plasma has become the method of choice and has led to a worldwide reduction of such invasive procedures for prenatal diagnosis of genetic and chromosomal abnormalities (see Chapter 72).

Buccal Cells

Collection of buccal cells (cells of the oral cavity of epithelial origin) has been identified as providing an excellent source of genomic DNA. Collection of buccal cells is often viewed as less invasive than collection of blood. It is particularly useful for collecting cells with the patient's genomic DNA when the patient has had blood transfusions and thus has blood with another person's (or persons') DNA. Similarly, it is useful after bone marrow transplantation when the circulating blood cells are derived wholly or partially from the donor of the bone marrow. Two methods are used commonly to collect buccal cells: rinsing with mouthwash and using swabs or cytobrushes.

Rinsing of the oral cavity generally provides a higher yield of cells than can be obtained by using swabs. For these collections, the patient is provided with a small amount of mouthwash and is instructed to rinse well for a minimum of 60 seconds; then the patient returns the mouthwash to a collection tube. There is no harm in doing this longer than 60 seconds, but shortening the time may decrease the yield of buccal cells. Mouthwash solutions high in phenol and ethanol are destructive to recovered cells and should be avoided. It is necessary for each laboratory to validate a list of acceptable solutions.

Swabs or cytobrushes have also been used to collect buccal cells for molecular genetics testing. For swabs, a sterile Dacron or rayon swab with a plastic shaft is preferred because calcium alginate swabs or swabs with wooden sticks may contain substances that inhibit PCR-based testing. After collection, the swab or cytobrush should be stored in an air-tight plastic container or immersed in liquid, such as phosphate-buffered saline or viral transport medium. In general, the yield of cells and nucleic acid is lower with physical scraping using swabs or cytobrushes than with rinsing.

Although collection of buccal cells from children is rare except in the situation of identification of paternity or maternity, the same process is followed.

Solid Tissue

Traditionally, the solid tissue most often analyzed in the clinical laboratory was malignant tissue from the breast for estrogen and progesterone receptors. During surgery, at least 0.5 to 1 g of tissue is removed and trimmed of fat and nontumor material. This tissue is quickly frozen, within 20 minutes, preferably snap frozen in liquid nitrogen or in a mixture of dry ice and alcohol. A histologic section should always be examined at the time of analysis of the specimen to confirm that the specimen is indeed malignant tissue. Another traditional use of solid tissue analysis is measurement of liver iron or copper to assist with the diagnosis of hemochromatosis or Wilson's disease, respectively.

The same procedure may be used to obtain and prepare solid tissue for elemental or toxicologic analysis; however, when trace element determinations are to be made, all materials used in the collection or handling of the tissue should be made of plastic or materials known to be free of contaminating trace elements.

Somatic gene analysis such as T and B cell clonality and the identification of possible clinically actionable mutations in malignant tissue (*KRAS* mutations, *MGMT/MLH* methylation status) are now proving to be of increasing importance for clinicians in both diagnosis and direction of appropriate therapeutic options for the patient. For these studies, the molecular diagnostic laboratory often receives tissue that has been formalin-fixed and paraffin-embedded (FFPE) rather than fresh tissue because the request for further testing is generally made after the pathologist's diagnosis of the particular malignancy. In general, neutral buffered formalin, containing no heavy metals, will not interfere with amplification reactions. However, recovery of nucleic acids is greatly decreased if the tissue has been over-fixed or if a decalcification process has been applied to, for example, bone marrow samples. DNA can still be extracted from tissue embedded in paraffin, but the DNA will be degraded to low-molecular-weight fragments. In most cases, segments of DNA will amplify in a PCR reaction, but Southern blot methods are problematic because most require high-molecular-weight DNA.

Tissue structure and better recovery of DNA can be retained without permanent fixation by freezing specimens in an optimal cutting temperature compound (OCT). OCT is a mixture of polyvinyl alcohol and polyethylene glycol that surrounds but does not infiltrate the tissue. The sample is then frozen at about $-80\ °C$, and sections are prepared for review by a pathologist. OCT is fully water soluble and should be completely removed from a tissue specimen before it is used as a source of DNA. In general, DNA of higher molecular weight can be extracted from OCT-fixed tissues compared with that extracted from FFPE samples.

Hair and Nails

Hair and fingernails or toenails have been used for trace metal and drug analyses with the potential advantage of timing of exposure if separate segments of longer hair are analyzed, although no current standards for such testing currently exist. For the latter examinations, clear labeling of the follicular end of the sample is required. However, collection procedures have been poorly standardized, and quantitative measurements are better obtained from blood or urine. Use of such samples requires each laboratory to validate the processes because, again, there are no published standards for this unusual specimen type. Currently, the use of hair or nails in molecular diagnostics is limited to forensic analysis (genomic DNA identification).

HANDLING OF SPECIMENS FOR ANALYSIS

Steps that are important for obtaining a valid specimen for analysis include (1) identification, (2) preservation, (3) separation and storage, and (4) transport.

Maintenance of Specimen Identification

Although the collection of an acceptable specimen is a key aspect of excellent testing, proper identification of the specimen must be maintained at each step of the testing process to ensure that the correct result is reported for the correct patient at all times. The minimum information on any label associated with a specific specimen should include the patient's name, location, and identifying number, as well as the date and time of collection. Many institutions also require the collecting person's initials or some means of identifying the person who collected the sample be included on the label. All labels should conform to the laboratory's stated requirements to facilitate proper processing of specimens. In the United States, no specific labeling should be attached to specimens from patients with infectious diseases that are submitted to the routine laboratory to suggest that these specimens should be handled with special care. Universal precautions

should always be used, meaning that all specimens should be treated as if they are potentially infectious with the following caveat. The exception will be samples from patients suspected to have known, high-risk pathogens (e.g., hemorrhagic viruses such as Ebola) that must have separate, pre-prepared sample handling protocols that may or may not involve the routine laboratory. Proactive procedures must be in place including by whom and where such samples might be analyzed unless the sample can be rendered safe (e.g., by heat treatment), in which case again standard universal precautions should be used.

In practice, every specimen container must be adequately labeled even if the specimen must be placed in ice or if the container is so small that a label cannot be placed along the tube, as might happen with a capillary blood tube. Direct labeling of a capillary blood tube by folding the label like a flag around the tube is preferred or recommended by most laboratories. For small volumes of urine submitted in screw-cap urine cups and any specimen submitted in a screw-cap test tube or cup, the label should be placed on the cup or tube directly, not just on the cap.

It is critical that samples be positively identified through all steps of processing and analysis, and this is especially important in pediatrics because the samples are often collected in small tubes that cannot be sampled from directly by an automated instrument. Aliquoting a sample from the primary collection container to one or more other containers configured for the instrumentation requires close attention to proper labeling and tracking of the sample identifiers to ensure samples are not switched. Good work practice includes "piece work" in which only a single patient's samples are in the work area at one time, the area is clean with no old labels present, and the worker is not disturbed. Although this may not be possible in a large laboratory facility, training that emphasizes the criticality of this function to achieve best patient care and adherence to all policies can be equally effective. Because the majority of samples received from pediatric patients are in microtubes, many samples need to be aliquoted; poured into a microsampling device; or hand entered into instruments that use whole blood, such as hematology instruments, because these systems are not made to deal with such small tubes. Additionally, many times bar codes do not fit these tubes. Bar code readers in instruments cannot be used unless the sample is aliquoted into a larger tube. This extra handling of the specimens offers more opportunities for error and thus requires stricter attention to detail and analysis of the possible risks during design of the process. Special attention should be placed on molecular diagnostics, forensic specimens, and transfusion medicine specimens as applicable.

Preservation of Specimens

The practitioner must ensure that specimens are collected into the correct container and are properly labeled; in addition, specimens must be properly treated both during transport to the laboratory and from the time the serum, plasma, or cells have been separated until analysis. For some tests, it is crucial that the sample be analyzed immediately from the time the blood is drawn to minimize metabolism and degradation of sample components. Examples are specimens for ammonia and blood gas determinations, such as PCO_2, PO_2, and blood pH, which should be analyzed within 30 minutes after collection. Specimens for lactate, pyruvate, and certain hormone tests (e.g., adrenocorticotropic hormone [ACTH], gastrin and renin activity) are also time sensitive and may require transport of the specimen on ice after collection. A notable decrease in pyruvate and increase in lactate concentration occurs within a few minutes at ambient temperature. Information on sample stability is generally provided by kit manufacturers, however this often does not cover all circumstances, for example, stability in whole blood prior to centrifugation, and the manufacturer may not have provided information for the required time period. Laboratories should gain extra information from the literature or conduct local studies as needed.

For all test constituents that are thermally labile, serum and plasma should be separated from cells in a refrigerated centrifuge. Specimens for bilirubin or carotene and for some drugs, such as methotrexate, may need to be protected from both daylight and fluorescent light to prevent photodegradation, although the use of plastic rather than glass tubes has decreased this preanalytical variable.

For molecular diagnostic laboratories, a substantial challenge is the recovery of RNA from transported specimens. Depending on the tissue source, RNA yields vary, primarily because of the amount of RNA present at the time of collection. Specimens from the liver, spleen, and heart have larger amounts of RNA than specimens from skin, muscle, and bone. Increasingly, creative solutions to this issue continue to be produced with collection kits that contain stabilizers and even the first reagents required for extraction, all of which have the effect of maximizing the recoverable nucleic acid. Tissue samples should be frozen immediately. Alternatively, a blood specimen should never be frozen before separation of the cellular elements because of hemolysis and released hemoglobin that may interfere with subsequent amplification processes. For tissue samples, it is critical to choose the disruption method best suited for the specific type of tissue. Thorough cellular disruption is critical for high RNA quality and yield. RNA that is trapped in intact cells is often removed with cellular debris by centrifugation.[26]

For specimens that are collected in a remote facility with infrequent transportation by courier to a central laboratory, proper specimen processing must be done in the remote facility so that appropriately separated and preserved plasma or serum is delivered to the laboratory. This necessitates that the remote facility has ready access to appropriately calibrated centrifuges, all commonly used preservatives, and wet ice.

Add-on Requests

In the interest of preventing additional phlebotomies and to assess a clinical situation from a specimen collected at a specific time, many physicians request an "add-on" test, that is, for the laboratory to perform a test on a sample already in the laboratory and processed. This is especially true in specimens collected from pediatric patients, in whom more blood may not be able to be collected promptly, and for patients from an emergency department, where additional testing from the time of presentation with specific symptoms may be needed after a clinical diagnosis has been made or narrowed by the clinician. Each laboratory must establish its own guidelines for what will be allowed in what time frame. For example, evaporation of small or even routine samples with requests for volatile compounds such as ethanol or methanol can

make them unsuitable for additional testing, so storage conditions and time in the laboratory are important considerations. Also, most samples are stored at refrigerated temperatures after initial analysis; this makes them unacceptable for LDH analysis later but does not affect, for example, alkaline phosphatase or electrolyte analysis, provided that evaporation and air exposure has been kept to a minimum.

Separation and Storage of Specimens

Plasma or serum should be separated from cells as soon as possible and certainly within 2 hours[27] for some but not all analytes. Premature separation of serum, however, may permit continued formation of fibrin, which can clog sampling devices in testing equipment. If it is impossible to centrifuge a blood specimen within 2 hours, the specimen should be held at room temperature rather than at 4 °C to decrease any effect on potassium measurement caused by leakage from the RBCs by inhibition of the Na/K ATPase pump. For most plasma samples used for molecular diagnostics, the plasma should be removed from the primary tube promptly after centrifugation and held at −20 °C in a freezer capable of maintaining this temperature. In all instances of freezing a sample, frost-free freezers should be avoided because they have a wide temperature swing during the freeze–thaw cycle. Although changes in concentration of test constituents have been observed when serum or plasma is stored in a gel separator tube in a refrigerator for 24 hours, these changes do not appear to be large enough to be of clinical significance.

Primary specimen tubes should always be centrifuged with the original cap in place. Such containment reduces evaporation, which occurs rapidly in a warm centrifuge with the air currents set up by centrifugation. Caps on the original tube also prevent aerosolization of infectious particles and thus provide a further safeguard for laboratorians. Specimen tubes with requested test for volatiles, such as ethanol, *must* have the initial cap in place while they are spun to prevent release of the volatile compound and result in an artificially reduced measurement of ethanol, methanol, or such compounds. Centrifuging specimens with the cap in place also maintains anaerobic conditions, which are important in the measurement of carbon dioxide and ionized calcium. Removal of the stopper before centrifugation allows loss of carbon dioxide and an increase in blood pH. Control of pH is especially important for the accurate measurement of ionized calcium.

Cryopreservation of WBC and DNA is one method to store and maintain samples for extended periods of time. Whole blood specimens can be centrifuged and WBCs removed and cryopreserved at −20 °C in a temperature-controlled freezer until these cells are required for DNA extraction. For even longer periods of storage, isolated DNA can be stored at −70 °C, although 4 °C may be adequate for most purposes. The extracted DNA should not be exposed to repetitive cycles of freezing and thawing because this can lead to shearing of the DNA. After these extracted DNA samples have completely thawed, it is important to fully mix the sample to ensure a homogeneous specimen.

Transport of Specimens

Hemolysis may occur in pneumatic tube systems unless the tubes are completely filled and movement of the blood tubes inside the specimen carrier is prevented.[28] The pneumatic tube system should be designed to eliminate sharp curves and sudden stops of specimen carriers because these factors are responsible for much of any in vitro hemolysis that may occur. With many systems, however, the plasma hemoglobin concentration may be increased, and the serum activity of RBC enzymes, such as LDH and AST, may also be increased (see the earlier discussion on the effect of hemolysis). Nonetheless, the amount of hemolysis from transport issues is usually so small that it can be ignored. In special cases, such as a patient undergoing chemotherapy whose cells are fragile or leukemia patients with fragile leukocytes, samples should be centrifuged before they are placed in the pneumatic tube system or identified as "messenger delivery only" and delivered rapidly to the laboratory. There are also occasional tests that cannot be transported to the laboratory via a pneumatic tube system because of the effect the transport has on the test results. For example, sending blood gas samples through the tube system has been shown to adversely affect PO_2 results,[29] and samples for thromboelastography and rotational thromboelastometry or platelet function testing may also require hand delivery to the laboratory.

Although the remaining discussion uses the specific example of referral laboratory testing by another laboratory, many of the issues discussed, such as regulations related to shipping, are also relevant to a laboratory that receives specimens from outlying clinics via a courier service, which may be laboratory owned or operated. This may involve validating specific transport or storage conditions that are not specified in or in conflict with existing CLSI recommendations.[30] For example, a laboratory may have a clinic that provides sweat chloride collection and sends the sweat samples to the main laboratory for chloride analysis through a courier service. In all cases, the appropriate transport parameters for these samples must be validated.

Before a referral laboratory is used for any tests, the quality of its work should be verified by the referring laboratory. Guidelines for selection and evaluation of a referral laboratory have been published (QMS05-A2, see Table 4.1). For laboratories accredited by the College of American Pathologists (CAP), it is a requirement that the referring laboratory validate that the referral laboratory is CLIA'88 certified by obtaining a copy of the Clinical Laboratory Improvement Act (CLIA) certificate before specimens are shipped. For molecular diagnostic testing, this is of particular importance because often the latest genetic test being requested by a physician has not yet been moved from research interest status to patient care status and may not be available in a CLIA-certified laboratory.

Specimen type and quantity and specimen handling requirements of the referral laboratory must be observed, and in laboratories operating under CLIA'88 regulations, test results reported by a referral laboratory must be identified as such when they are filed in a patient's medical record. The director of a referring laboratory has the responsibility to ensure that specimens will be adequately transported to the referral laboratory. Also, the director should determine the benefits of different services and should keep in mind that the fastest service may be the most expensive. The director should also know that specimens should not be sent to a referral laboratory at the end of the week or in a holiday period because more delays in transit occur during these times than during the working week, and deterioration of specimens is more likely.

It should be assumed that transport from a referring laboratory to a referral laboratory may take as long as 72 hours.

Under optimal conditions, a referring laboratory should retain enough of the original specimen for retesting in case an unanticipated problem arises during shipment, although this essentially never happens in pediatric laboratories where sample volume is at a minimum. Most reference laboratories have lower minimum volume requirements for pediatric specimens than for adult specimens, but these lower minimums generally preclude being able to retest the sample if there is a problem with the initial analysis. The tube and transport condition for the specimen should be constructed such that the contents do not escape if the container is exposed to extremes of heat, cold, or sunlight. Reduced pressure of 0.50 atmosphere (50 kPa) may be encountered during air transport, together with vibration, and specimens should be protected from these adverse conditions by a suitable container. Variability in temperature is a significant factor causing instability of test constituents.

Polypropylene and polyethylene containers are usually suitable for specimen transport. Glass should be avoided. Polystyrene is unsuitable because it may crack when frozen. Containers must be leak-proof and should have a Teflon-lined screw cap that does not loosen under the variety of temperatures to which the container may be exposed. The materials of both stopper and container must be inert and must not have any effect on the concentration of the analyte.

In situations in which sample delivery for molecular analysis will be delayed, extracted nucleic acid, usually DNA only, can be transported in a buffer solution or water, or it can be dried down and shipped as a loose powder. With either method, DNA should be transported at ambient temperatures and should not be exposed to extremely high temperatures for an extended period of time because it will begin to degrade and testing may be compromised. Because dried blood spot samples are so easy to store and transport, and with an increasing number of DNA tests being developed using dried blood spots (e.g., PCR testing for cystic fibrosis and severe combined immunodeficiency), such samples may become one of the best ways to collect, store, and ship samples for DNA testing.

The shipping or secondary container used to hold one or more specimen tubes or bottles must be constructed to prevent the tubes from contact with another specimen. Corrugated, fiberboard, or Styrofoam boxes designed to fit around a single specimen tube are commonly used. A padded shipping envelope provides adequate protection for shipping single specimens. When specimens are shipped as drops of blood on filter paper (e.g., for neonatal screening), the paper should be enclosed in a paper envelope to ensure that the sample remains dry. The initial paper envelope can be placed in a shipping envelope and transported to the testing facility; rapid shipping is rarely required for dried blood on paper.

For transport of frozen or refrigerated specimens, a Styrofoam container should be used. The container walls should be 1 inch (2.5 cm) thick to provide effective insulation. The container should be vented to prevent buildup of carbon dioxide under pressure and a possible explosion. Solid carbon dioxide (dry ice) is the most convenient refrigerant material for keeping specimens frozen, and temperatures as low as −70 °C can be achieved. The amount of dry ice required in a container depends on the size of the container, the efficiency of its insulation, and the length of time for which the specimens must be kept frozen. One piece of solid dry ice (about 3 inches × 4 inches × 1 inch) in a container with 1-inch Styrofoam walls and a volume of 125 cubic inches (2000 cm³) will maintain a single specimen frozen for 48 hours. More commonly, smaller pieces of the solid will be used and it is critical that the specimen be buried rather than sitting on top of this refrigerant.

Various laws and regulations apply to the shipment of biologic specimens. Although such regulations theoretically apply only to etiologic agents (known infectious agents), all specimens should be transported as if the same regulations apply. In many countries, airlines have rigid regulations covering the transport of specimens. Airlines deem dry ice a hazardous material; therefore the transport of most clinical laboratory specimens is affected by the regulations and those who package the specimens should be trained in the appropriate regulations, such as those put forth by the US International Air Transport Association.

The various modes of transport of specimens influence the shipping time and cost, and each laboratory needs to make its own assessment as to adequate service. The objective is to ensure that the properly collected, processed, and identified specimen arrives at the testing facility in time and under the correct storage conditions so that the analytical phase can then proceed.

CONCLUSION

Accurate test results (i.e., the right result for the right patient) begin and end with the integrity of the sample being tested. Integrity can only be assured by proper preparation of the patient; choice of sample container; collection of the sample; and finally transport, processing, and storage of the collected sample with each step maintaining proper identification. Every step of the process affects the quality of the end result. For these reasons, best laboratory practice demands attention to detail and following appropriate protocols. It is incumbent on laboratories and laboratory professionals to fully delineate their processes in complete policies and procedures that not only cover the routine and correct procedures but also cover the unusual. These should include how to handle the process when the system breaks down and steps are not properly performed and may need to be addressed case-by-case by the laboratory director. Finally, laboratories should fully validate protocols that may not be covered under normal procedures or that may deviate from local regulatory guidelines (e.g., the US Food and Drug Administration or CLIA). Preanalytical variables can be lessened or even avoided if these steps are followed.

POINTS TO REMEMBER

- Proper identification of the patient is essential, and the sample should be properly labeled at all steps, including when separated from the primary collection container.
- Policies designed to ensure the safety of both the patient and the person collecting any sample should always be followed.
- Collection of all samples must be in the correct primary container, and those collecting specimens should understand the biochemical or chemical actions of any additive and possible implications on the test result.

- Attention to the details related to processing of the collected sample (time, temperature, special handling) should always follow validated local policies.
- The accurate result for any patient's sample that will be acted on by the clinician depends on adherence to all policies and procedures, and personnel collecting specimens bear a tremendous responsibility to ensure that they do not contribute to errors that may impact patient care.

SELECTED REFERENCES

1. The Joint Commission. National Patient Safety Goals. https://www.jointcommission.org/en/standards/national-patient-safety-goals/hospital-2020-national-patient-safety-goals/ [accessed 2/10/2020].
2. WHO Guidelines on Drawing Blood: Best practices in phlebotomy. Pediatric and neonatal blood sampling. World Health Organization; 2010 [Chapter 6] <http://www.ncbi.nlm.nih.gov/books/NBK138647/>; [accessed 2/10/2020].
7. Renoe BW, McDonald JM, Ladenson JH. The effects of stasis with and without exercise on free calcium, various cations, and related parameters. Clin Chim Acta 1980;103:91–100.
8. McNair P, Nielsen SL, Christiansen C, et al. Gross errors made by routine blood sampling from two sites using a tourniquet applied at different positions. Clin Chim Acta 1979;98:113–18.
9. Cornes MP, Ford C, Gama R. Spurious hyperkalemia due to EDTA contamination: common and not always easy to identify. Ann Clin Biochem 2008;45:601–3.
7. Mikesh LM, Bruns DE. Stabilization of glucose in blood specimens: mechanism of delay in fluoride inhibition of glycolysis. Clin Chem 2008;54:930–2.
18. Fokker M. Stability of glucose in plasma with different anticoagulants. Clin Chem Lab Med 2014;52:1057–60.
27. Laessig RH, Indriksons AA, Hassemer DJ, et al. Changes in serum chemical values as a result of prolonged contact with the clot. Am J Clin Pathol 1976;66:598–604.
28. Farnsworth CW, Webber D, Budelier M, Bartlett N, Gronowski AM. Parameters for validating a hospital pneumatic tube system. Clinical Chemistry. 2019;65(5):694-702.
29. Victor PJ, Patole S, Fleming JJ, et al. Agreement between paired blood gas values in samples transported either by a pneumatic tube system or by human courier. Clin Chem Lab Med 2011;49:1303–9.
30. Haverstick DM, Brill LB, Scott MG, et al. Preanalytical variables in measurement of free (ionized) calcium in lithium heparin-containing blood collection tubes. Clin Chim Acta 2009;403:102–4.

5

Preanalytical Variation and Pre-Examination Processes

Ana-Maria Simundic, Lora Dukić, and Vanja Radisic Biljak

ABSTRACT

Background

The preanalytical phase has long been recognized as a source of substantial variability in laboratory medicine. Laboratory errors, mostly due to some defect in the preanalytical phase, may lead to diagnostic errors. Understanding preanalytical variation and reducing errors in the pre-examination phase of the testing process are therefore important for improved safety and quality of laboratory services delivered to patients.

Content

There are numerous preanalytical factors that may affect the concentration of the analyte, the measurement procedure, or the test result. These factors may be divided into two major groups: influencing and interference factors. Influencing factors are effects on laboratory results of biological origin that most commonly occur in vivo but can also be derived from the sample in vitro during transport and storage. Biological influence factors lead to changes in the quantity of the analyte in a method-independent way. Interference factors (interferences) are defined as mechanisms and factors that lead to falsely increased or decreased results of laboratory tests of a defined analyte. Interference factors and their mechanisms differ with respect to the intended analyte and analytical method. Interference factors do not affect the concentration of the analyte. On the contrary, they alter the test result for a specific analyte after the sample has been collected. They are different from the measured analyte and interfere with the analytical procedure. Therefore their effect is method dependent and may thus be reduced or eliminated by selecting a more specific method. This chapter describes the most common preanalytical sources of variability (influences and interferences) and provides recommendations on how to deal with them in everyday practice.

INTRODUCTION

The incidence of premature patient deaths associated with some kind of preventable medical error has been estimated to be 98,000 per year.[1] More recent data indicate that the actual mortality caused by preventable medical errors is fourfold higher.[2] According to the European Commission (EC) and World Health Organization (WHO), 1 in 10 patients is being harmed while receiving hospital care in developed countries.[3,4] Errors in laboratory medicine can lead to increased health care expenditure, cause patient harm to various degrees, and lead to different diagnostic errors (i.e., missed diagnosis, misdiagnosis, and delayed diagnosis).[5]

It has been suggested that laboratory test results affect approximately 70% of medical decisions, and this clearly explains why laboratory errors have a large contribution to the overall error frequency in health care.[6,7] Almost 40% of diagnostic errors are attributed to some error that has occurred within the area of radiology or laboratory medicine, and the majority of those laboratory errors are due to some defect in the preanalytical phase of the total testing process (TTP).[8]

Historical Perspective

The preanalytical or, according to ISO 15189 terminology, *pre-examination* phase of the laboratory testing process has been recognized since the early 1970s as an important source of variability, and it still represents one of the greatest challenges for specialists in laboratory medicine.[9,10]

In the second half of the 20th century, when quality assurance programs were introduced for the analytical processes, laboratories became aware that some factors outside the analytical phase also significantly impacted laboratory results.[11] Results that did not correspond with the patient's clinical condition have often been called "laboratory errors." It also became clear that these variables could not be standardized or controlled by analytical quality assurance programs. In the late 1970s, Statland and Winkel defined the phase prior to analysis as the "preinstrumental phase,"[12] which was later changed to the "preanalytical phase."[13]

Even before the preanalytical phase was recognized as an important issue in laboratory medicine, some experts from different areas of laboratory medicine defined these variables as *influencing* and *interference* factors,[14,15] which were not immediately recognized as important sources of "laboratory errors." It took some time for laboratory medicine professionals to gather knowledge about their causes and mechanisms and acknowledge their importance.

After years of discussion within several national and international expert groups in the 1960s and 1970s,[12–16] the term *biological influence factor* was introduced and distinguished from interference factors. This led to the definitions established in the 1980s,[17,18] which are still valid today.[19]

The Preanalytical Phase Today

The preanalytical phase is recognized as the most vulnerable part of the TTP, and it accounts for two-thirds of all laboratory errors.[20] Preanalytical errors can occur at any step of the preanalytical phase—for example, during test requesting, patient preparation, sample collection, sample transport, handling, and storage.[21] This high frequency of preanalytical errors may be attributed to various reasons. Many preanalytical steps are performed outside the laboratory and are not under the direct supervision of laboratory staff. Furthermore, many individuals are involved in various preanalytical steps, and those individuals have different levels of education and professional background. Finally, safe practice standards for many activities and procedures are either not available, or are available but not evidence-based, or the level of compliance with those standards is low.

The ISO 15189 accreditation standard clearly defines that medical laboratories are responsible for the management and quality of the pre-examination phase.[21] It is the role of the laboratorian that the right sample be taken from the right patient at the right time, and that correct test results are provided to the requesting physician in a timely manner. If the quality of the specimen is compromised to a degree where the expected effect is larger than the allowable error, thus causing clinically significant bias, the sample should be rejected for analysis. Our guiding principle should be "No result is always better than a wrong result." Patient benefit should always be the top priority.

Influencing and Interference Factors

Influencing Factors

Influencing factors are the effects on laboratory results of biological origin that most commonly occur in vivo but can also be derived from the sample in vitro during transport and storage. Biological influence factors lead to changes in the quantity of the analyte to be measured in a defined matrix. They modify the concentration of the measured (affected) analyte in a method-independent way.

These factors are either present in the healthy individual, like circadian rhythms, or they appear as side effects of a disease and its treatment. Influencing factors may be modifiable, such as diet, time of the day, or time of the year (season), or unmodifiable, such as gender, race, ethnicity, genetic background, and so on. Some modifiable biological influence factors can be controlled by patient action—for example, diet—whereas others—for example, age—are not controllable. Particular care should be taken with the influencing factors whose effects may be reduced through standardization of preanalytical conditions.

As already mentioned, modification of the concentration of certain analytes can also occur in vitro. For example, glucose concentration will decrease during prolonged storage of unseparated blood due to cell metabolism, whereas potassium concentration will increase if blood is kept at lower temperatures or refrigerated ($+4\,°C$). Such increase in potassium will occur even without visible hemolysis.

Interference Factors

Interferences are defined as mechanisms and factors that lead to falsely increased or decreased laboratory test results for a defined analyte. Interferences may be endogenous (i.e., biological constituents of the sample) or exogenous. Exogenous interferences occur in the preanalytical phase due to the action of some external factors or conditions that are not normally present in properly collected, transported, handled, and stored specimens.[22] Interference factors and their mechanisms differ with respect to the intended analyte and analytical method, and they alter the result of a sample constituent after the specimen has been collected. They are different from the measured analyte and interfere with the analytical procedure. Therefore their effect is method dependent and may thus be reduced or eliminated by selecting a more specific method.[14]

Possible interferents include the following:
1. Biological constituents of the sample (e.g., free hemoglobin, lipids, bilirubin, paraproteins, fibrin, fibrin clots, etc.)
2. Exogenous molecules present in the sample (e.g., drugs, herbal supplements, contrast media)
3. Exogenous molecules added to the sample during sampling or after the sampling procedure (e.g., anticoagulants, tube additives, intravenous infusions, etc.)

Because interference factors are analyte and method specific, they may be eliminated or at least reduced by changing the measurement method.

Although exogenous preanalytical interferences are not rare, they are often neglected and overlooked in everyday routine work. If they go undetected, preanalytical interferences may cause unnecessary harm to the patient and increase health care–related costs. Some examples of harmful results due to erroneous immunoassay findings are listed in Table 5.1.

It is very important that laboratory staff has a thorough knowledge and understanding of the assays and instruments in use in their laboratory and potential interferents which may affect laboratory measurements. This chapter provides an overview of the most common preanalytical sources of variability (influences and interferences) and provides recommendations on how to deal with them in practice.

POINTS TO REMEMBER

Influencing and Interference Factors
- Influencing factors lead to changes in the quantity of the analyte in a method-independent way.
- Influencing factors may be changeable (e.g., diet, time of sample collection during the day) or unchangeable (e.g., gender, race, ethnicity, genetic background).
- The effect of influencing factors may be reduced through standardization of preanalytical conditions.
- Interferences are mechanisms and factors that lead to falsely increased or decreased results of laboratory tests.
- Interference factors and their mechanisms differ with respect to the intended analyte and analytical method and may be reduced or eliminated by selecting a more specific method.

INFLUENCING FACTORS

The effect of most modifiable influencing factors can be either minimized or even entirely eliminated by standardization of preanalytical processes. Several local and international guidelines provide recommendations for efficient standardization of patient preparation and sample collection.[24,25] These documents provide guidance on timing of

TABLE 5.1 Effects of Laboratory Errors on Patient Outcome	
Wrong Result	**Consequence**
Falsely Increased Concentration	
High human chorionic gonadotrophin indicating gonadal tumor	Unnecessary surgery, chemotherapy
High calcitonin indicating medullary thyroid cancer	Unnecessary fine-needle aspiration
High prolactin	Misdiagnosis of prolactinoma
High urine free cortisol	Unnecessary diagnostic follow-up
High testosterone in women	Unnecessary diagnostic follow-up
High luteinizing hormone and follicle-stimulating hormone	Unnecessary diagnostic follow-up
Falsely Decreased Concentration	
Low 25-hydroxyvitamin D result despite replacement therapy	Incorrect diagnosis of hypovitaminosis D
Negative human chorionic gonadotropin result	Missed diagnosis of choriocarcinoma
Low digoxin	Wrong treatment (overdosing with digoxin, risk of digoxin toxicity)
Low insulin	Missed diagnosis of insulinoma
Negative troponin result	Missed diagnosis of myocardial infarction

Modified from Jones, A.M. & Honour, J.W. Unusual results from immunoassays and the role of the clinical endocrinologist. *Clin Endocrinol (Oxf)* 2006;64:234–44.

sampling, diet and activities before sampling, body position and disinfection during sampling, and regulations regarding documentation of these variables for diagnostic and/or therapeutic purposes.

On the other hand, since the effects of unmodifiable factors cannot be eliminated by standardization, they are addressed by assigning appropriate reference intervals (e.g., gender-specific, age-specific, etc.).

Controllable Variables

Time of Sampling

Time of sampling matters for all analytes which are subject to substantial biological variation. Changes of the concentration of an analyte due to biological variation may significantly affect the given result of a particular laboratory test and their nature can be either linear or cyclic. Linear changes occur in a chronological order, while cyclic changes are of repetitive nature, such as seasonal changes, or changes due to the menstrual cycle. Knowledge about the time of the sample collection is therefore necessary for correct test result interpretation and as such is an important preanalytical factor which should be carefully considered.

Several analytes tend to fluctuate in terms of their plasma concentration over the course of a day, and for this reason reference intervals are preferentially defined for sampling between 7 and 9 am.[26] For example, the concentration of potassium is lower in the afternoon than in the morning, whereas that of cortisol decreases during the day and increases at night (Fig. 5.1).[29] Furthermore, the cortisol circadian rhythm may well be responsible for the poor results obtained from oral glucose tolerance testing in the afternoon.

For many years, it was believed that iron has a substantial circadian variation, with an early morning peak and a decrease in the afternoon; that was the main reason most of the blood collections for iron were done in the morning. It was only recently demonstrated that iron concentration is quite sustainable throughout the day, up until 3 pm, when it starts to decrease, whereas the lowest iron concentrations were observed with collection times past 4 pm.[27]

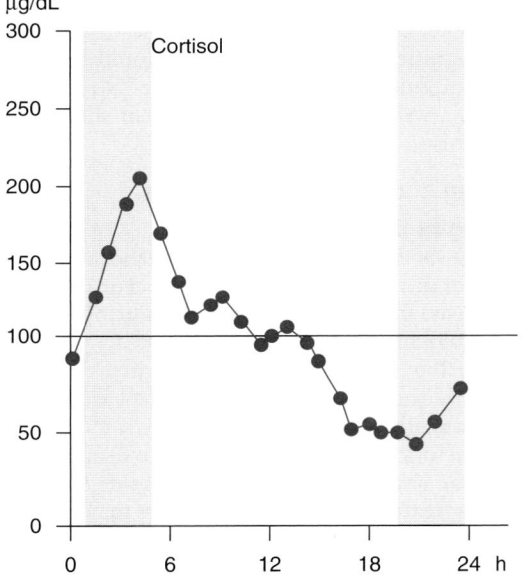

FIGURE 5.1 Daily variation of plasma concentrations of cortisol (shaded area = sleep period). (Modified from: Evans K, Laker MF. Intraindividual factors affecting lipid, lipoprotein and apolipoprotein measurement: a review. *Ann Clin Biochem* 1995;32:261–80.)

In some cases, seasonal influences also have to be considered. For example, total triiodothyronine (T3) is 20% lower in the summer than in the winter,[28] whereas 25 OH-cholecalciferol exhibits higher serum concentrations in the summer than in the winter.[29]

Some analytes can exhibit significant changes due to the hormone biological variations that occur during menstruation cycle. For example, aldosterone concentration in plasma is twice as high before ovulation than in the follicular phase, concentration of renin is increased preovulatory, cholesterol exhibits a significant decrease during ovulation, while the concentration of phosphate and iron decreases during menstruation.[28]

Influence of Diagnostic and Therapeutic Procedures

Time of sampling is not only important to eliminate confounding effects of biological variation, but is also extremely important for patients receiving some diagnostic and/or therapeutic procedures which may cause some in vivo (influencing effect, very frequent) or in vitro (interference effect, much less common) effects on laboratory tests.[30,31] Some examples of these diagnostic and/or therapeutic procedures are listed below:

- Surgical operations
- Infusions and transfusions
- Punctures, injections, biopsies, palpations, whole-body massage
- Endoscopy
- Dialysis
- Physical stress (e.g., ergometry, exercise, ECG)
- Function tests (e.g., oral glucose tolerance test)
- Immunoscintigraphy
- Contrast media
- Drugs, herbal supplements and over-the-counter medicines
- Mental stress
- Ionizing radiation

Plateletpheresis procedure is used in Transfusion Medicine to obtain platelets needed for treatment of thrombocytopenia. Citrate used in this procedure has chelating effect on ionized calcium and magnesium and along with decreases in some hematology parameters, can also lead to acute ionized hypocalcemia and hypomagnesemia.[32,33] Citrate chelation can also lead to decreased ionized calcium concentration in critically ill patients with high risk of bleeding and acute renal failure who are subjected to citrate-anticoagulated continuous venovenous hemofiltration. In this situation, hypocalcemia reflects citrate overdose. Due to citrate effect, lower concentrations of ionized calcium and magnesium have also been observed in patients receiving high volumes of transfused blood.

Administration of hypertonic saline in patients having severe head trauma with therapeutic target sodium concentration of 155 mmol/L (or mEq/L) and should not be misinterpreted as contamination with saline intravenous fluid.[34]

Iodinated contrast media used in computed tomography (CT) have high osmolality and high iodine content.[35] Application of these iodinated contrast media for imaging purposes in the pediatric population exceeds normal daily intake of iodine, carries a risk of thyroid dysfunction, and prompts close monitoring of pediatric patients after exposure.[36]

Contrast media may also affect some coagulation and inflammatory parameters. For example, ioxaglate and iodixanol, radiographic contrast media used in diagnostic and therapeutic angiography, may inhibit generation of thrombin in studies performed on platelet-poor and platelet-rich plasma (PRP).[37] The effect of contrast media during coronary angiographic procedure on the inflammatory markers interleukin-6 (IL-6) and soluble (s) receptors (R) for tumor necrosis factor alpha (TNFα) sTNFRα1 and sTNFRα2 has also been reported. Ioxaglate causes the increase in inflammatory markers after contrast media administration, and this effect is more pronounced after the administration of ionic (ioxaglate) compared to nonionic (iohexol and iodixanol) contrast media.[38]

Many drugs, herbal supplements, and over-the-counter medicines may cause various in vivo changes of the composition of the blood and subsequently influence the measurement of many laboratory parameters. For example, long-term treatment with proton pump inhibitors leads to the increase in the concentration of the neuroendocrine tumor marker chromogranin A by stimulating enterochromaffine-like cells. In order to avoid unnecessary diagnostic procedures, it is therefore advised to cease proton pump inhibitors at least 2 weeks before chromogranin A testing.[39]

Another example of the drug which exerts in vivo influencing effect is azithromycin. In patients on azithromycin, there is a risk of the occurrence of drug-induced immune thrombocytopenia.[40] Alemtuzumab infusion to patients with active relapsing-remitting multiple sclerosis has remarkable effect on several hematology and biochemistry tests.[41] Cross-sectional data analysis of the Rotterdam study on 9820 participants has demonstrated the significant association of thiazide diuretics use with the increased risk of hypomagnesemia.[42] Trimethoprim, a drug commonly prescribed together with other antibiotics for urinary tract infection treatment, may cause reversible increase in serum creatinine concentration; this increase affects calculation of estimated glomerular filtration rate. Lack of information about this in vivo effect of trimethoprim can cause misinterpretation and erroneous clinical decision.[43]

The influencing effect of herbal supplements is exerted through toxicity or enzyme induction. Since herbal supplements are categorized as dietary supplements, they are not subject to strict regulations like drugs. Such permissive regulation carries a significant risk due to the uncontrolled use of herbal supplements alone or in combination with other supplements or drugs.[44-46] Obviously, there is a need to increase the level of awareness about potential risks associated with the use of herbal supplements.[47]

Kava is a traditional medicinal substance used in the Pacific region. It has relaxing effect and is consumed to treat anxiety, as an aqueous nonalcoholic drink made of kava rhizome. Cases of heavy kava consumption are associated with the 70- and 60-fold increase of alanine aminotransferase (ALT) and aspartate aminotransferase (AST) activity, as well as largely increased alkaline phosphatase (ALK), γ-glutamyltransferase (GGT), lactate dehydrogenase (LD), and total and conjugated bilirubin concentration and in extreme cases even with fulminant hepatic failure.[48]

The most probable underlying mechanism of hepatotoxicity is related to metabolic interaction of alcohol with kava, although multiple factors, involving genetic defects in hepatic metabolism, contribute to development of extreme reactions.[49] Some other dietary supplements such as LipoKinetix and Centella asiatica which are largely used for weight loss, may also cause hepatotoxicity and even lead to fulminant hepatic failure associated with extreme increase of liver enzymes, which can be resolved after discontinuation of consumption.[50,51]

Kelp, a kind of seaweed used in Asia as a selenium supplement, is rich in iodine. Patients taking kelp commonly have high serum and urine iodine concentration even if on low-iodine diet, which is mandatory for radioiodine therapy.[52,53]

To prevent the confounding effect of these factors, samples should always be collected before any diagnostic or therapeutic procedure with potential influencing or interfering effects. Likewise, drugs exerting influencing or interfering effects should be administered exclusively after collecting a blood sample, if not advised differently by the requesting physician (Note: time of sampling for therapeutic drug monitoring is discussed in Chapter 42).

For all the above-mentioned reasons, and given the fact that in some circumstances a sample taken at the wrong time might be worse than taking no sample, exact time of sample collection always needs to be provided to the laboratory.

For effective standardization of the time of sampling, laboratories should ensure that:
- the best time of sampling for each analyte is known (taking into account how the concentration of the particular analyte changes over time),
- blood is always taken at the recommended time,
- the exact time of sampling is known for each sample and is recorded into the laboratory information system (LIS) by the health care staff,
- patients and the health care staff are educated about when blood samples should be collected for laboratory testing, as well as about the importance of the time of blood sampling and its effect on laboratory test results.

Diet

Prior to blood sampling, the confounding influences of food and fluid intake should be excluded. Diet and fluid intake substantially affect the composition of plasma. Differences in serum composition may occur respective to the source of nutrients, number of meals, and proportion of nutrients in a diet. Moreover, malnutrition or obesity, prolonged fasting, starvation, and vegetarianism may also influence plasma composition. The effects from diet can be divided into long-term and acute effects.

Long-term effects of diet. It is well known that changes in protein intake that occur over a couple of days may affect the composition of nitrogenous components of plasma and the excretion of end products of protein metabolism. Creatinine is an important example of the effect of diet on the composition of plasma. It has been shown that an increase of up to 20% of plasma creatinine concentration (measured by kinetic Jaffe method) is observed after ingesting cooked meat.[54] Protein-rich food affects not only the concentration of serum creatinine but also the concentration of urea and urate in serum.

A diet rich in fat leads to increased serum triglyceride concentration, reduced serum urate, and a depletion of the body's nitrogen pool. The nitrogen pool is affected because excretion of ammonium ions is required to maintain acid-base homeostasis.[55,56] The relative ratio in which various dietary fats are consumed closely relates to serum lipid concentrations. A diet rich in monounsaturated and polyunsaturated fats causes a reduction of low-density lipoprotein (LDL) and high-density lipoprotein (HDL) cholesterol concentrations,[57] although in some situations HDL cholesterol may be increased.

A diet rich in carbohydrates decreases serum protein and lipid concentrations (triglycerides, and total and LDL cholesterol).[58] It should be emphasized that not only the proportion but also the source of nutrients in the diet affect the composition of serum. For example, some early studies have shown that serum ALP and LD activities are higher, whereas AST and ALT activities are lower in individuals who consume carbohydrates rich in sucrose or starch rather than other sugar types.[59] Moreover, total, LDL, and HDL cholesterol concentrations tend to be much lower in those who consume

the same amount of food in many small meals throughout the day than in individuals who eat three meals per day.[55]

Compared to omnivorous subjects, vegetarians tend to have lower concentrations of plasma cholesterol, triglycerides, and creatinine, with reduced urinary excretion of creatinine and a higher urinary pH as a result of reduced intake of precursors of acid metabolites.[55] In malnourished individuals, the activity of most of the commonly measured proteins and enzymes is reduced.[60,61] Most of the above-described changes normalize following the restoration of good nutrition.

Acute effects of diet and other influencing factors. While it is clear that many analytes are affected by acute ingestion of food, the direction and magnitude of the change still remain largely unclear, mainly due to substantial differences in the design of the original studies published so far. Some of the methodological aspects of these studies which might be responsible for the observed differences are: time of blood collection (morning, afternoon, etc.), time intervals at which blood collection was done (i.e., length of time after the meal), sample type (serum, plasma), assay (method principle, manufacturer), measurement equipment, baseline concentration of the analyte, measurement unit (i.e., mmol/L, mg/dL), type of the meal, food composition, and other patient-related characteristics (e.g., health status, age, gender, ethnicity, physical activity, smoking status, and consumption of alcohol and coffee).[62,63] Moreover, while some postprandial effects are a result of the in vivo physiologic changes, some effects occur due to the interfering effect of sample turbidity caused by the increase of triglyceride (chylomicrons) concentration, and as such are method- and instrument-dependent. Table 5.2 shows the maximal postprandial effects observed anywhere within 1 to 4 hours after a meal on some most common chemistry analytes and hormones.

Certainly, not all changes are clinically significant, but for those analytes for which postprandial changes are clinically significant, fasting prior to blood collection is recommended to overcome this problem. The most pronounced change after a recent meal among chemistry tests is observed in triglycerides. Triglyceride concentrations in serum increase almost twofold during the absorptive phase, within 1 to 2 hours after the meal, and the magnitude of the increase obviously depends on the type of meal and time of sample collection after the meal.

Whereas the nature of the change for most analytes is mostly unidirectional, some analytes, like phosphate, exhibit a characteristic bi-phase change. Concentration of phosphor initially drops for -2.7 to -8% within 1 hour after the meal and is followed by an increase of up to 12.6% 4 hours after the meal.[65,67]

It is noteworthy to point out that not only chemistry tests but also some hormones (e.g., thyroid stimulating hormone [TSH], free thyroxine [fT4], cortisol, insulin) are significantly affected by acute food ingestion.

Acute food ingestion also affects hematology and coagulation parameters. Tables 5.3 and 5.4 show the maximal postprandial effects observed anywhere within 1 to 8 hours after a meal on complete blood count (CBC) and coagulation parameters.

There is an evident postprandial increase in neutrophil count, along with a decrease in red blood cell (RBC) count, as well as some RBC indices. Variations in RBC count and

TABLE 5.2 Results of Four Original Studies Demonstrating the Postprandial Effects (% Change) on the Concentration of Some Most Common Chemistry Analytes and Hormones

	Guder, 2009[64]	Lima-Oliveira, 2012[65]	Kackov, 2013[66]	Bajana, 2019[67]
Type of meal	Standard meal	Light meal, containing standardized amounts of carbohydrates, protein, and lipids.	Standardized High-calorie meal (823 kcal)	Andean breakfast, containing standardized amounts of carbohydrates, protein, and lipids.
Blood collection time points	Baseline and 2 h after the meal	Baseline and 1 h, 2 h, 4 h after the meal	Baseline and 3 h after the meal	Baseline and 1 h, 2 h, 4 h after the meal
Analyte				
Triglycerides	78%	28%	71.4%	85%
CRP	NA	25%	−5%	6%
Urea	0% (no change)	−4%	NA	26%
Creatinine	NA	−2.2%	NA	33%
AST	25%	14%	NA	5%
ALT	5.5%	18%	NA	4.3%
Albumin	1.8%	3.4%	NA	4.4%
Bilirubin (total)	16%	−16%	NA	−29%
Bilirubin (direct)	NA	−24%	NA	−29%
Calcium	1,6%	3,5%	NA	4%
Magnesium	NA	3,4%	NA	9%
Iron	NA	10%	NA	−35%
Potassium	5.2%	5.8%	NA	3%
Uric acid	NA	−5%	NA	−3.6%
TSH	NA	NA	NA	27%
fT4	NA	NA	NA	6.6%
Cortisol	NA	NA	NA	−29%

Note: Presented are maximal deviations (% change) that occur anywhere within the observed period of time. *Red fields* show parameters with an increase, *light red fields* show parameters with a decrease.
ALT, Alanine aminotransferase; *AST*, aspartate aminotransferase; *CRP*, C-reactive protein; *fT4*, free thyroxine; *TSH*, thyroid stimulating hormone.

TABLE 5.3 Results of the Four Original Studies Demonstrating the Postprandial Effects (% Change) on Complete Blood Count Parameters

	van Oostrom, 2003[68]	Lippi, 2010[69]	Kościelniak, 2017[70]	Arredondo, 2019[71]
Type of meal	Standardized oral-fat loading test.	Light meal, containing standardized amounts of carbohydrates, protein, and lipids.	Light meal, containing standardized amounts of carbohydrates, protein, and lipids (300–700 kcal).	Chilean breakfast, containing standardized amounts of carbohydrates, protein, and lipids.
Blood collection time points	Baseline and 2 h, 4 h, 6 h, 8 h after the meal	Baseline and 1 h, 2 h, 4 h after the meal	Baseline and 1 h, 2 h after the meal	Baseline and 1 h, 2 h, 4 h after the meal
Analyte				
WBC	NA	NA	16%	16.9%
Neutrophils	42%	7.6%	37%	27.4%
Lymphocytes	42%	−18.7%	−12%	15.9%
Monocytes	No change	−6.9%	No change	25.0%
Eosinophils	NA	−23.2%	No change	No change
RBC	No change	−3.3%	−7%	−3.4%
Hgb	NA	No change	−8%	−2.7%
Hct	NA	−3.9%	−6%	−4.4%
MCV	NA	No change	No change	−2.1%
MCH	NA	1.6%	No change	No change
Plt	NA	No change	−6%	6.9%
MPV	NA	−2.3%	No change	−8.5%

Note: Presented are maximal deviations (% change) that occur anywhere within the observed period of time. *Red fields* show parameters with an increase, *light red fields* show parameters with a decrease.
Hct, Hematocrit; *Hgb*, hemoglobin; *MCH*, mean cell hemoglobin; *MCV*, mean corpuscular volume; *MPV*, mean platelet volume; *Plt*, platelets; *RBC*, red blood cells; *WBC*, white blood cells.

TABLE 5.4   Results of the Two Original Studies Demonstrating the Postprandial Effects (% Change) on Coagulation Parameters

Analyte	Lima-Oliveira, 2014[72]	Arredondo, 2019[10]
Activated partial thromboplastin time (aPTT)	−6.2	−4.5
Fibrinogen	No change	−3.1
Antithrombin III	3.7	1.8
Type of meal	Light meal, containing standardized amounts of carbohydrates, protein, and lipids (563 kcal).	Chilean breakfast, containing standardized amounts of carbohydrates, protein, and lipids.
Blood collection time points	Baseline and 1 h, 2 h after the meal	Baseline and 1 h, 2 h, 4 h after the meal

Note: Presented are maximal deviations (% change) that occur anywhere within the observed period of time. *Red fields* show parameters with an increase, *light red fields* show parameters with a decrease.

indices are most likely attributable to hemodilution caused by the ingestion of food and fluids. Postprandial neutrophil increase is suggested to play a role in the pathogenesis of atherosclerosis.[68] The effect of acute ingestion of food and fluid on lymphocyte and platelet count is less clear and is most likely instrument-dependent.

Postprandial triglyceridemia causes a transient increase of the plasma levels of the activated factor VII (FVIIa) and plasminogen activator inhibitor (PAI-1); mechanism of this phenomenon is still not completely understood.[73,74] As FVIIa is the first enzyme of the blood coagulation system, postprandial phase fluctuations can trigger the coagulation cascade and significantly change some of the plasma coagulation parameters.[75] It should be emphasized that activated partial thromboplastin time (aPTT) is shortened in the postprandial state and this is why monitoring of unfractionated heparin could be jeopardized if samples are taken in a nonfasting state. Considering the above, a period of fasting is required before hemostasis testing.

Finally, the human body experiences a mild postprandial metabolic alkalosis in response to a meal. This alkalosis occurs due to the secretion of the hydrochloric acid in the parietal cells of the stomach, which is followed by extraction of chloride from the plasma and the release of bicarbonate into the plasma in order to maintain electrical neutrality. Thus venous blood leaving the stomach is enriched with bicarbonates, and this phenomenon is responsible for postprandial metabolic alkalosis (i.e., the alkaline tide) with concomitant increase of pCO_2 and a subsequent reduction of ionized calcium by 0.2 mg/dL (0.05 mmol/L).[55]

To avoid any misinterpretation due to the above-described effects, blood collection should preferably be done after an overnight (12 hours) fast (discussed in more details later in the section entitled Preparing for Blood Sampling).

Effects of Fluid Intake Before Sampling

Whereas drinking coffee or small amounts of alcohol is largely seen as part of normal life and therefore not worth reporting to the physician, one should be aware of the influence of the intake of various fluids on the concentration of different analytes. Ingestion of various fluids may also exert acute and chronic effects.

Caffeinated beverages. Many beverages, such as tea, coffee, and cola drinks, contain caffeine. Caffeine stimulates the adrenal cortex and medulla, leading to the subsequent increase of the concentration of catecholamines and their

metabolites, as well as free cortisol, 11-hydroxycorticoids, and 5-hydroxyindoleacetic acid (5-HIAA) in serum. These hormonal changes are followed by the increase in plasma glucose concentration. Plasma renin activity may also be increased following caffeine ingestion.[55,76] Caffeine induces diuresis and inhibits the reabsorption of electrolytes, thus leading to a transient increase in their excretion and this effect is dose-dependent. Total urine output of water and electrolytes (calcium, magnesium, sodium, chloride, potassium) increases within 2 hours following caffeine ingestion, and caffeine-induced urinary loss of calcium and magnesium is therefore largely attributable to a reduction of the renal reabsorption of calcium and magnesium.[77] Caffeine also has a marked effect on lipid metabolism. Ingestion of coffee increases the rate of lipid catabolism, thus leading to an increase of plasma free fatty acids, glycerol, and lipoproteins.[78,79] Finally, caffeine is a strong stimulant of gastrin release and gastric acid secretion and also induces the secretion of pepsin.[80]

Alcohol. Alcohol consumption, depending on its duration and extent, may affect a number of analytes. Among alcohol-related changes, acute and chronic effects should be considered separately. The decrease of plasma glucose and increase of lactate are the acute effects that occur within 2 to 4 hours of ethanol consumption. Ethanol is metabolized to acetaldehyde and then to acetate. This increases hepatic formation of uric acid[81] and inhibits renal urea excretion, thus causing an increase of uric acid in plasma.[82] Together with lactate, acetate decreases plasma bicarbonate, resulting in mild to severe metabolic acidosis, depending on the amount of ingested alcohol.

Acute alcohol ingestion increases the activity of serum GGT and some other enzymes (e.g., isocitrate dehydrogenase, ornithine carbamoyltransferase).[83] Chronic effects of ethanol ingestion include the increase in serum triglyceride concentration due to decreased plasma triglyceride breakdown and an increase in the serum activity of many enzymes (GGT, AST, and ALT).

Moreover, chronic alcohol consumption affects pituitary and adrenal function and is associated with numerous biochemical abnormalities.[84,85] It affects lipid metabolism and inhibits the sialylation of transferrin that leads to increased serum concentration of carbohydrate-deficient forms of transferrins (CDT).[86] Increased mean corpuscular volume (MCV) is related to the direct toxic effect of alcohol on erythropoietic cells or a deficiency of folate.[87] Increased urine ethanol excretion leads to a decreased formation of vasopressin with increasing diuresis. Enhanced diuresis is followed by increased secretion of renin and aldosterone.[88]

To assess the effect of alcoholic drinks on test results and to avoid misinterpretation of laboratory results, it is recommended that the history of alcohol intake (i.e., the ingested amount and frequency/time of ingestion) be documented in clinical records.

Smoking Tobacco

Smoking tobacco leads to a number of acute and chronic changes in analyte concentrations, with the chronic changes being rather modest. Smoking increases the serum concentrations of fatty acids, epinephrine, free glycerol, aldosterone, and cortisol.[26] These changes occur within 1 hour of smoking a cigarette. Through adrenal gland stimulation, nicotine causes the increase of the concentration of epinephrine in the plasma and the urinary excretion of catecholamines and their metabolites.[89] Smoking leads to the acute increase in serum triglyceride, and total and LDL cholesterol concentrations.[90] Glucose metabolism is also dramatically affected by nicotine. Within only 10 minutes of smoking a single cigarette, glucose concentration increases by up to 10 mg/dL (0.56 mmol/L). This increase may persist for 1 hour.

Alterations in analytes induced by chronic smoking affect numerous blood components such as CBC, some enzymes, lipoproteins, carboxyhemoglobin, hormones, vitamins, tumor markers, and heavy metals (Fig. 5.2). These changes are induced by nicotine and its metabolites and reflect pathophysiologic responses to toxic effects. To avoid a risk of misinterpretation of laboratory test results, smoking habits should be documented in clinical records.

In heavy smokers blood leukocyte count may be increased by as much as 30%, with a proportional increase of

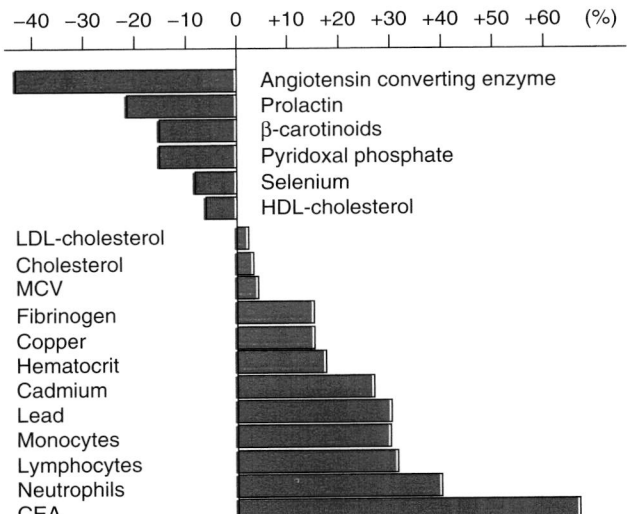

FIGURE 5.2 Chronic effects of smoking. Deviation (%) of blood analyte concentrations between current smokers and nonsmokers. *CEA,* Carcinoembryonic antigen; *HDL-cholesterol,* high density cholesterol; *LDL-cholesterol,* low density cholesterol; *MCV,* mean corpuscular volume. (Reproduced from Guder WG, Narayanan S, Wisser H, & Zawta B. *Diagnostic Samples: From the Patient to the Laboratory.* 4th updated ed. Weinheim: Wiley-Blackwell; 2009, with permission by Wiley-VCH-Verlag, Weinheim, Germany.)

the lymphocyte count.[55] For carcinoembryonic antigen (CEA), different reference limits should be applied for smokers and nonsmokers due to the large differences between the two groups. The higher concentration found in smokers is caused by an increased synthesis and secretion of CEA in the colon. Tobacco smokers have higher carboxyhemoglobin concentration. To compensate for the impaired capacity for oxygen transport in heavy smokers, there is also an increase in RBC count. Partial pressure of oxygen (pO_2) is lower in tobacco smokers than in nonsmoking individuals by about 5 mm Hg (0.7 kPa).[55] Like caffeine, nicotine is also a very potent stimulant of the secretion of gastric juice and an inhibitor of duodenal bicarbonate secretion.[91] These effects may be observed within 1 hour of smoking several cigarettes. Smoking also affects the body's immune response and male fertility by affecting the sperm count, morphology, and motility.[55,92] The effect of smoking may persist even after smoking cessation. It usually takes 5 years, or even longer, for most parameters to normalize (e.g., C-reactive protein [CRP] and fibrinogen concentrations, hematocrit). Interestingly, for some parameters (e.g., white blood cell [WBC] count), it may take up to 20 years to return to baseline value.[93]

Body Position and Tourniquet

Body posture influences blood constituent concentrations. This is caused by the net capillary filtration (i.e., the net result of the differences in the membrane permeability, hydrostatic pressure, colloid osmotic pressure of plasma, and interstitial fluid). Capillary filtration is especially increased in the lower extremities when changing from the supine to the upright position. The change in body posture from the supine to sitting and from sitting to the upright position leads to a significant decrease in plasma volume with a subsequent increase in the concentration of all constituents that usually do not pass the capillary filtration barrier (e.g., blood cells, large molecular weight molecules). Although this effect is observed in healthy and diseased individuals, the degree of the change is usually greater in some disease states—for example, in cardiac insufficiency.

Variations in the plasma volume subsequent to the change of the body position alter blood cell count (RBC, WBC, and platelets), concentrations of hemoglobin, and hematocrit; a short period of 10 minutes is usually enough for the vascular volumes to re-equilibrate and to adapt to the new posture.[94–96] It was also demonstrated that patient posture might have a significant impact on results of routine hemostasis testing, decreasing the prothrombin time (PT) values, and increasing the fibrinogen concentration when patient position is changed from supine to sitting.[97] Finally, net capillary filtration effect due to the change in body posture also affects small molecular weight molecules which are transported in blood bound to proteins. For example, while the concentration of free calcium is not affected, total calcium concentration increases by 5 to 10%[98] when changing from the supine to the upright position. To minimize the effect of this preanalytical source of potential bias, reference intervals should ideally be obtained under identical conditions with regard to body posture. Blood sampling should be performed after at least 15 minutes of rest in a supine or sitting position.[25]

A similar mechanism occurs when a tourniquet is applied to facilitate finding appropriate veins for venipuncture. The higher pressure obtained in veins leads to the loss of water and low molecular weight substances, increasing the concentration of proteins and analytes bound to them, cells, hemoglobin concentration, and hematocrit.[99,100] This becomes clinically significant after 1 to 2 minutes of tourniquet application.[55] Prolonged venous stasis can also cause a significant increase of fibrinogen and a shortening of aPTT and PT.[101] Therefore the tourniquet should be released 1 minute after it has been applied.

Muscular Activity

Physical activity of varying duration and intensity may lead to substantial changes in the plasma composition, and the extent of this change depends on several factors, such as training status, intake of fluid, electrolytes and carbohydrates, and even the ambient temperature.[102,103] For example, even a mild physical effort, like clenching the fist during venous blood sampling, can increase the concentration of potassium and should therefore be avoided.[104] This occurs due to the release of potassium from skeletal muscles and even without a tourniquet.

Intensive exercise is associated with transient increases in cardiac biomarkers, markers of muscle damage, platelet aggregation, tissue-plasminogen activator, activation of the fibrinolytic system, and a decrease in the ability of the blood to clot and generate thrombin, as well as with leukocytosis.[105–108] Cardiac troponin (cTn) rises after a maximal bicycle stress test.[109] The majority of changes are of transient nature and most of the parameters return to baseline within 3 hours after the exercise, although it was observed that some hematologic indices, such as red cell distribution width (RDW), continue to increase after the half-marathon run, reaching a peak 20 hours after the run.[110] Furthermore, it has been demonstrated that in individuals who are physically active more than 12 hours per week, concentrations of creatine kinase (CK), Creatine kinase MB (CK-MB), ALT, and LD are increased for a prolonged period of time.[111]

Due to such substantial changes in plasma composition, in professional athletes (e.g., marathon runners), a large proportion of laboratory results may fall outside the usual reference intervals.[112]

Intensive physical activity (within 12 hours before blood sampling) may also affect homeostasis for numerous hormones including catecholamines and their derivatives, epinephrine, norepinephrine, dopamine, corticotropin (ACTH) and vasopressin, gastrin, TSH, prolactin, growth hormone, aldosterone, cortisol, testosterone, human chorionic gonadotropin (hCG), insulin, glucagon, and β-endorphin.[113–116]

Preparing for Blood Sampling

Because food, fasting time, circadian rhythm, muscular activity, smoking, drugs, and ethanol consumption can affect the concentration of numerous analytes, standardization of all those controllable variables is highly recommended. Proper standardization of controllable variables leads to significant reduction of preanalytical variability. In the past, there has been a great heterogeneity in the definition of *fasting state* used for different analytes by different health care facilities and in the literature. To facilitate the agreement on the definition of *fasting state* and encourage uniform and consistent compliance the European Federation for Clinical Chemistry and Laboratory Medicine (EFLM) Working Group for Preanalytical Phase WG-PRE has published a recommendation for the definition

of fasting requirements as a guiding framework for harmonization of this important preanalytical aspect.[117]

According to these recommendations, the following general requirements should be applied to all blood tests:

1. Blood should be drawn preferably in the morning between 7 am and 9 am
2. Fasting should last for 12 hours, during which only water consumption is permitted.
3. Alcohol should be avoided for 24 hours before blood sampling.
4. In the morning before blood sampling, patients should refrain from cigarette smoking and caffeine-containing drinks (tea, coffee, etc.).

Professional associations and laboratories worldwide are encouraged to adopt, implement, and disseminate the EFLM WG-PRE recommendation for the definition of *fasting*. Moreover, laboratories worldwide should have policies for sample acceptance criteria related to fasting samples. Blood samples for routine testing should not be taken if a patient has not been appropriately prepared for sample collection.

Noncontrollable Variables

Various unavoidable biological factors can lead to changes in analyte concentration and can therefore only be considered during interpretation with the respective knowledge. Table 5.5 summarizes some of these factors and their respective effects. These factors should be considered when interpreting laboratory results because their influence cannot be prevented by preanalytical standardization.

Age and Gender

Due to dramatic physiologic changes associated with growth and development, the reference intervals for many analytes differ substantially with respect to an individual's age and gender (see Chapter 9 and the Appendix). In newborn subjects, the body fluids reflect the trauma of birth and early postnatal events related to the adaptation of the baby to new extrauterine life. Immediately after birth, infants usually experience a mild metabolic acidosis of transient nature, due to the accumulation of lactates. This acid-base disturbance is usually normalized within the first day after birth.[55] The CALIPER study is an excellent source of reference intervals in childhood (see the Appendix).[126] In the early hours of extrauterine life, the concentration of some biochemical markers (AST, direct bilirubin, total bilirubin, creatinine, CRP, GGT, immunoglobulin G [IgG], LD, magnesium, phosphate, rheumatoid factor, uric acid) is increased, thus reflecting the maternal concentrations, but it then declines within the first 2 weeks of life.[127] Concentrations of other markers (e.g., amylase, transferrin, antistreptolysin O [ASO], cholesterol, IgA, IgM) are very low in the neonatal period and gradually increase within the first 2 weeks of extrauterine life. This upward trend in analyte concentrations continues over time from birth to 18 years. Most of the biochemistry parameters (albumin, ALP, AST, total bilirubin, creatinine, IgM, iron, lipase, transferrin, HDL cholesterol, and uric acid) exert differences between genders during the early childhood years. However, these changes are most significant during puberty (age 14 to 18 years), due to the strong influence of sexual development and growth.[127]

Hemoglobin concentration, hematocrit, and the other RBC indices follow a similar pattern, showing the gradual

TABLE 5.5 Unavoidable Influences on Laboratory Results

Influence (Reference)	Examples of Analyte Concentrations Changed	Remarks
Age[118-120]	ALP, LDL cholesterol, hormones, creatinine, total WBC count, WBC subpopulations, RBC, hemoglobin, hematocrit, RBC indices, VWF, AT, PC, PS, plasminogen.	Provide age-dependent reference intervals
Race[119-123]	CK higher in black than in white males. Creatinine higher in black than in white males. Granulocytes higher in white than in black males. Hematocrit, hemoglobin, and MCV lower in African Americans than Caucasians. Hematocrit, hemoglobin, MCH, MCHC, and MPV lower in Asians than Caucasians.	Provide race-specific reference intervals
Gender[118,124,120]	ALT, γ-GT, creatinine, hemoglobin, hematocrit, RBC, WBC, PLT	Provide gender-specific reference intervals
Pregnancy[26,64,125]	Triglycerides ↑, homocysteine ↓, WBC ↑, d-dimers ↑, PT ↑, fibrinogen ↑	Document months of pregnancy with laboratory results
Altitude[64,120]	CRP, hemoglobin ↑, hematocrit ↑, RBC ↑, transferrin↓	Consider weeks of adaptation, when coming from or going to high altitude

ALP, Alkaline phosphatase; *ALT*, alanine aminotransferase; *AT*, antithrombin; *CK*, creatine kinase; *CRP*, C-reactive protein; γ-*GT*, gamma-glutamyltransferase; *LDL*, low density lipoprotein; *MCH*, mean corpuscular hemoglobin; *MCHC*, mean corpuscular hemoglobin concentration; *MCV*, mean corpuscular volume; *MPV*, mean platelet volume; *PC*, protein C; *PLT*, platelets; *PS*, protein S; *PT*, prothrombin time; *RBC*, red blood cell; *VWF*, von Willebrand Factor; *WBC*, white blood cell.

increase during the first 10 years of life. First gender differences are observed at the age of 10 years, when values in boys show a sharp increase during puberty and adolescence. Concentrations in females are much lower, but they also slowly increase throughout puberty. Such gender differences are related to the lower metabolic demand, decreased muscle mass, and lower iron stores in females.[128]

Concentration of thrombopoietin peaks shortly after birth and then slowly decreases. Subsequent to the change of thrombopoietin concentration, immediately after birth there is a peak in platelet count, followed by a decline during childhood and into adulthood. The WBC count is also higher in the early extrauterine days and throughout the first couple of years of childhood; values decline in older children. Females have slightly higher platelet count than males during adolescence and adulthood.[128]

POINTS TO REMEMBER

Influencing Factors
- Samples should be taken before any therapeutic and diagnostic procedures that have a potential influencing effect.
- Tobacco smoking leads to several acute and chronic changes in the concentrations of numerous analytes.
- Even within only 1 hour of smoking one to five cigarettes, there is an increase in serum concentration of fatty acids, epinephrine, free glycerol, aldosterone, and cortisol.
- Diet substantially affects the composition of plasma. The effects of diet can be long term and acute.
- Physical activity of varying duration and intensity leads to changes in the plasma composition of many analytes. The extent of this change depends on training status, intake of liquid, electrolytes and carbohydrates, and even the ambient temperature.
- Most of the reference interval data for children are obtained from the CALIPER study.

Although bone marrow cellularity decreases with age, in the absence of disease WBC, hemoglobin, platelets, and differential are maintained within adult reference intervals in individuals older than 65 years.[120,129-131]

Hemostasis develops during fetal development and changes with gestational age. In neonates, the concentrations of the proteins of the prothrombin and contact factor groups are lower than in adults, due to liver immaturity, and reach adult values only after 6 months of age.[120]

INTERFERENCE FACTORS

As mentioned earlier, interference factors have the ability to interfere with the analytical procedure and alter the test results. The effect of interference factors depends on the method—that is, the same interferent may not necessarily affect two different methods used to measure the same analyte. Common interference factors are hemolysis, lipemia, icterus, drugs, paraproteins, and various sample contaminants such as gels, tube additives, and fibrin clots.

Interfering factors are considered clinically relevant when the bias caused by their interference is greater than the maximum allowable deviation of a measurement procedure. How this "maximum allowable deviation" should be established is still debated. The Clinical Laboratory Standards Institute (CLSI) EP7-A2 guideline, for example, sets this criterion at ±10% as a rule of thumb. Others would argue that the degree of allowable deviation caused by interfering factors should be derived (I) from data on the biological variation of the analyte, (II) by simulation modeling based on the effect of preanalytical and analytical performance on clinical decisions or patient outcomes, or (III) from information on the state-of-the-art.[132] The choice of the method for determining the maximum allowable deviation for a certain analyte not only depends on the medical use of the test but also on the national and international regulations in use.

Interferences can be endogenous and exogenous. Endogenous interferences originate from the substances present in the patient sample, whereas exogenous interferences relate to the effect of various substances added to the patient sample, such as separator gels, anticoagulants, surfactants, and so on, all of which may cause significant interference.[133,134]

Hemolysis

Definition and Background

Hemolysis is defined as a process of membrane disruption of erythrocytes and other blood cells, accompanied by the subsequent release of cell components into the plasma and red coloration of the serum (or plasma) to various degrees after centrifugation.[135,136] Though hemoglobin is the most abundant protein in RBC, hemolysis is not necessarily always associated with the release of hemoglobin into the surrounding extracellular fluid. For example, if the blood sample is stored at a low temperature, low molecular intracellular components like electrolytes diffuse from the cells, but hemoglobin will not. Furthermore, efflux of cell components due to cell lysis affects all blood cells (i.e., platelets and WBC) and not only erythrocytes. Therefore it is important to remember that red coloration of the serum or plasma can never accurately predict the concentration of blood cell components.

Hemolysis is the most common preanalytical error and the most common cause of sample rejection. It occurs with a frequency of up to 30%[137,138] and accounts for almost 60% of unsuitable specimens.[139] The frequency of hemolysis largely depends on the collection facility, characteristics of the patient population, and the type of professional who is doing the phlebotomy. The highest frequency of hemolysis has been observed in samples from emergency departments, pediatric departments, and intensive care units, whereas hemolysis has proven to be the least frequent in outpatient phlebotomy centers, where blood sampling is done by specialized laboratory staff.[140,141] These differences are due to the level of knowledge and skills of the staff who perform the blood collection.[24] One large study in Australia of five hospitals from October 2009 to September 2013 found that the hemolysis rate is much higher in emergency departments (up to 8.73%, depending on the triage category) than in other inpatient settings (<4%). Interestingly, the hemolysis rate was highest in patients who were triaged in the most urgent category. Also, the hemolysis rate was higher if the phlebotomy was done by the clinical staff than by laboratory phlebotomists.[142]

The two major sources of hemolysis are in vivo hemolysis and in vitro hemolysis. In vivo hemolysis is a result of a pathologic condition and occurs within the body before the blood has been drawn. It may occur as a result of numerous biochemical (enzyme deficiencies, erythrocyte membrane defects, hemoglobinopathies), physical (prolonged marching, drumming, prosthetic heart valves), chemical (ethanol, drug overdose, toxins, snake venom), or immunologic (autoantibodies) mechanisms, and infections (babesiosis, malaria). In vivo hemolysis can further be categorized as intravascular and extravascular, depending on the site of the destruction of RBC. Intravascular hemolysis occurs as a direct and immediate disruption of RBC due to the cell injury within the vasculature, whereas in extravascular hemolysis, RBC membranes are damaged by the reticuloendothelial system, primarily in the spleen.[143] The most common causes of in vivo hemolysis are reaction to incompatible transfusion and autoimmune hemolytic anemia.

In vivo hemolysis is not very common and accounts for only 3% of all hemolyzed samples.[144] Nevertheless, in vivo hemolysis is of great clinical importance because it reflects an underlying pathologic process in a patient. Laboratories should therefore have a procedure in place for distinguishing in vivo and in vitro hemolysis. In vivo hemolysis should always be suspected when patient blood is hemolyzed over a longer period after different types of samples (e.g., citrate, serum, and heparinized tube) are hemolyzed or repeated blood sampling, even after special care has been taken to avoid hemolysis.

Common findings associated with in vivo hemolysis which may help in distinguishing in vivo from in vitro hemolysis:
- dark brown serum/plasma and urine,
- ↓↓↓ serum/plasma haptoglobin,
- hemoglobinuria (free hemoglobin in urine) and methemoglobinuria,
- ↑ indirect bilirubin concentration in serum/plasma,
- ↑ reticulocyte count (compensatory bone marrow response),
- normal potassium concentration in serum/plasma,
- ↑↑ LDH in serum/plasma,

Decreased concentrations of haptoglobin in serum and free hemoglobin in urine are the most pronounced and specific laboratory signs of in vivo hemolysis. Haptoglobin is a protein that binds free hemoglobin in the circulation to prevent oxidative damage induced by hemoglobin.[145] Once released from the erythrocyte into the plasma, hemoglobin forms complexes with haptoglobin, and those complexes are removed from the circulation by macrophages. In more pronounced cases of in vivo hemolysis, haptoglobin in serum can be undetectable (i.e., below the detection range), whereas its concentration in cases of in vitro hemolysis remains unchanged.[146,147] When in vivo hemolysis is confirmed, the laboratory should not reject hemolyzed samples for analysis, because parameters in hemolyzed samples reflect the actual patient condition and are extremely relevant for adequate patient care (diagnosis, therapy management, monitoring).

In vitro hemolysis occurs outside the patient at many steps of the preanalytical phase: blood sampling, sample handling and delivery to the laboratory, and sample storage. Causes of in vitro hemolysis are described in Chapter 4.

Mechanisms of Hemolysis Interference

Hemolysis is an endogenous interference that causes clinically relevant bias of patient results through the several distinct mechanisms described in the following.

Spectrophotometric interference. Spectrophotometric interference of hemolysis occurs due to the ability of hemoglobin to absorb light at 415-, 540-, and 570-nm wavelengths.[148] This characteristic of hemoglobin causes optical interference that can lead to either falsely increased or decreased concentrations of the measured parameters. The direction and degree of the interference largely depend on the analyte and the method.

Release of the cell components into the sample. Some components are present in blood cells in concentrations that are several times higher than those in the extracellular space (i.e., plasma or serum). Table 5.6 shows some of the most pronounced differences between intracellular and extracellular concentration in RBC.[149–152]

From this it follows that there is a dramatic increase in the concentration of the listed analytes measured in hemolyzed

TABLE 5.6 Ratio Between Intracellular and Extracellular Concentration of Various Analytes in Red Blood Cells	
Analyte	**Intracellular Concentration (Compared to Extracellular)**
Lactate dehydrogenase	↑ 160×
Inorganic phosphate	↑ 100×
Potassium	↑ 40×
Aspartate aminotransferase	↑ 40×
Folic acid	↑ 30×
Alanine aminotransferase	↑ 7×
Magnesium	↑ 3×

TABLE 5.7 Chemical Mechanisms of Hemolysis Interference	
Direct mechanism	**Indirect mechanism**
• Competition for a substrate or any other component of the assay reaction mixture (e.g., creatine kinase assay) • Inhibition of the assay (e.g., pseudo-peroxidase activity of free hemoglobin)	• Complexation • Proteolysis (cathepsin E) • Precipitation of the analyte or any other component of the assay reaction mixture

plasma (or serum) due to the efflux of those substances from erythrocytes into the sample. The most pronounced effect of hemolysis is seen for LD. LD activity may be increased by over 20% in mildly hemolyzed samples (at a concentration of only 0.27 g/L of free hemoglobin), by over 60% at 0.75 g/L of free hemoglobin, and up to over 350% in grossly hemolyzed samples with 3.34 g/L of free hemoglobin.[153]

Because intracellular components may also escape from platelets during clotting, there is a marked difference in the potassium concentration between serum and plasma. The mean estimated difference in the concentration of potassium in serum and plasma is 0.36 ± 0.18 mmol/L, and this difference is positively associated with the platelet count.[154] Plasma is therefore the recommended sample type for the accurate measurement of potassium.

Sample dilution. Some analytes are present in much higher concentrations in plasma than in blood cells like albumin, bilirubin, glucose, sodium, and a few others.[150] For those parameters, hemolysis will cause a dilution effect, and their concentrations will be lower in hemolyzed samples. The effect of sample dilution causes clinically significant bias only at higher degrees of hemolysis. For example, glucose is negatively affected by severe hemolysis (−8.3%) only at the concentration of 3.34 g/L of free hemoglobin if measured by the Beckman Coulter chemistry analyzer and reagents (Olympus AU2700, Beckman Coulter, O'Callaghan's Mills, County Clare, Ireland).[153]

Chemical interference. Various blood cell components may affect the analyte measurement procedure by directly or indirectly modifying the analyte (Table 5.7).

An example of the direct interference through competition is the effect caused by the enzyme adenylate kinase, which is present in both erythrocytes and platelets.[155] Adenylate kinase (EC 2.7.4.3) is an enzyme that catalyzes the reversible conversion of ATP and AMP to two ADP molecules and maintains the adenine nucleotide cell content.[156] When released from the cells during hemolysis, adenylate kinase may compete for ADP with CK in a CK assay if inhibitors are not supplied in the reaction mixture.[157]

Hemoglobin released from erythrocytes during hemolysis may interfere with various assays through its pseudo-peroxidase activity. Pseudo-peroxidase activity of free hemoglobin released from erythrocytes interferes in the assay for measurement of bilirubin concentration through the inhibition of the formation of diazonium salt.[158]

Hemolysis may cause a clinically significant interference on a wide range of analytes in immunochemistry assays. This interference is caused by modifying the reaction analytes (antigens and antibodies) by the proteolytic action of cathepsin E, the major proteolytic enzyme in mature erythrocytes. Proteolytic enzymes released from erythrocytes may mask or potentially enhance epitope recognition in various immunoassays. Interference caused by proteolytic activity may cause measurement bias of various degrees and various directions, depending on the assay. For example, current cTn assays have variable susceptibility to hemolysis interference.

Hemolysis has been shown to cause negative interference with concentrations of cTnT, insulin, cortisol, testosterone, and vitamin B12, and false-positive increases for prostate-specific antigen (PSA) and cTnI in a concentration-dependent manner.[159-161] However, the degree and direction of bias are analyte and method dependent. For example, hemolysis causes falsely decreased concentrations of cTnT assayed with the Roche hs cTnT assay on the Elecsys E170 immunochemistry analyzer, whereas concentrations of cTnI measured using the Ortho Clinical Diagnostics TnI ES assay on the Vitros 5600 Integrated System (Ortho Clinical Diagnostics, Rochester, NY) are falsely increased in hemolyzed samples.[162] Abbott Architect TnI assay appears to be more robust against interference from hemolysis.[163] The microparticle enzyme immunoassay for cTnI (Abbott Laboratories, Abbott Park, IL) is not affected by moderate hemolysis and exerts clinically relevant bias only for grossly hemolyzed samples.[164]

Lipemia

Lipemia is defined as a turbidity of the sample visible to the naked eye. Turbidity of the sample is caused by the light scattering due to the presence of large lipoprotein particles (chylomicrons). The increase in concentration of lipoproteins in blood most commonly occurs due to postprandial triglyceride increase, parenteral lipid infusions, or some lipid disorders. Not all lipoproteins have equal contribution to the sample turbidity. The effect of lipoprotein particles on the sample turbidity depends on the size of the particles. Chylomicrons and very low-density lipoproteins (VLDL), the largest lipoprotein particles in the circulation, have the greatest contribution to the sample turbidity. To avoid postprandial lipemia, patients are therefore requested to fast for 12 hours before the blood sampling.[117]

Mechanisms of Interference Caused by Lipemia

Lipemia is an important endogenous interference that may cause clinically relevant bias of patient results through the several mechanisms described below.

Spectrophotometric interference. Lipemia causes interference by light absorbance and light scattering. The lipemic sample absorbs light, causing a decrease in the intensity of the light passing through the sample. The ability of lipoprotein particles to absorb light is manifested in the range of wavelengths (300 to 700 nm). Sample absorbance rises with the decreasing wavelengths and is maximal in the ultraviolet range. That is why many enzymatic methods in which the end product is measured at 340 nm (NAD[P] or NADP[H]) are strongly affected by lipemia.

Lipemic samples also cause light scattering. Light scattering occurs in all directions, and its intensity depends on the number and size of lipoprotein particles and the wavelength of measurement.[165] For this reason, light scattering of lipoprotein particles causes significant interference with turbidimetry and nephelometry. In methods where the transmittance of light is inversely proportional to the concentration of the analyte, in the absence of the sample blank, sample turbidity causes positive bias. However, in some competitive assays where the transmittance of light is directly proportional to the concentration of the analyte, sample turbidity will cause negative bias.

Interference caused by the volume depletion effect. Plasma in healthy individuals in the fasting state consists of only minor portion of lipids (<10% of the total plasma volume). The rest of the plasma is water. The increase in the concentration of lipoprotein particles leads to an increase in the plasma volume occupied by lipids. Particles that are not lipid soluble are displaced by the lipids to the water part of the plasma. Therefore lipemia leads to a false decrease in the concentration of the measured analyte in all methods in which the concentration of respective analyte is measured in the total plasma volume.

One example of interference caused by the volume depletion effect is the bias in electrolyte measurement, leading to so-called pseudo-hyponatremia. This type of interference affects electrolytes only if measured by flame photometry and by indirect measurement using ion-selective electrodes (ISEs) but not in direct potentiometry (for more details, see Chapters 17 and 37). However, it must be noted that the volume displacement effect of the lipemic sample will affect the electrolyte measurement only in grossly lipemic samples with concentrations of triglycerides greater than 17 mmol/L (1504 mg/dL).[166]

Interference caused by partitioning of the sample. Upon centrifugation of a lipemic sample, lipoproteins are not homogeneously distributed in the serum or plasma due to the lipid gradient (Fig. 5.3). Water-soluble analytes are more concentrated in the lower layer of the plasma or serum, whereas lipids and lipid-soluble analytes, such as drugs and some lipid-soluble hormones, are more concentrated in the top lipid-rich layer. This is especially important in automated chemistry analyzers with fixed path lengths of the sample probe. Test results may differ for those analytes that are not evenly distributed between the lipid and water portion of the sample, depending on the part of the sample from which the sample probe is taking the sample for analysis.

Interference caused by physicochemical mechanisms. An excess of lipoproteins in the blood may interfere in electrophoretic and chromatographic methods by causing abnormal peaks. Increased concentrations of triglycerides and lipoprotein particles may disturb the electrophoretic pattern and morphology, as well as falsely increase the relative percentage of the prealbumin, albumin, and α1- and α2-globulin regions.[167,168] Moreover, lipemia may even affect some immunochemistry assays by masking the binding sites on antigens and antibodies and thus physically interfering with antigen–antibody binding.[169]

One additional complication of excessive lipemia is the increased sample susceptibility to hemolysis leading to the specific turbid and reddish appearance of the sample (the so-called "strawberry milk" appearance). This effect is most probably caused by the increased fragility of the erythrocyte membranes due to the alterations in the content of the phospholipid membrane layer and is more pronounced with the increase in lipid (particularly triglycerides) concentrations.[170]

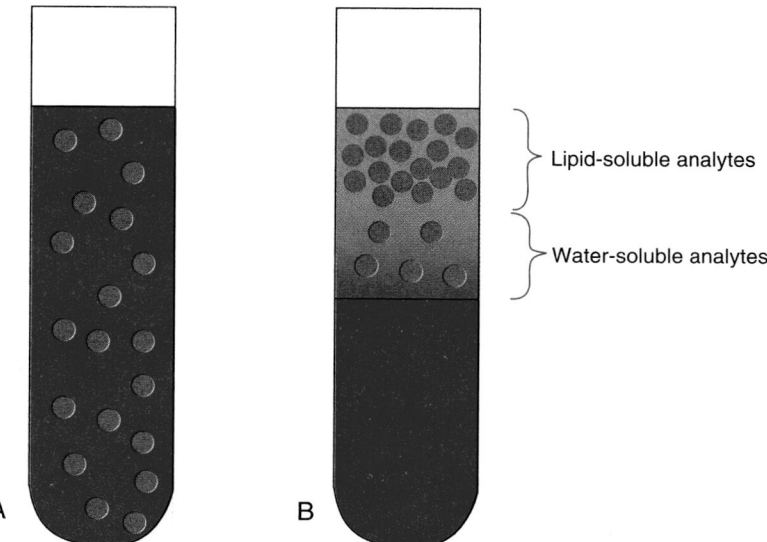

FIGURE 5.3 (A) Lipids are distributed evenly in whole blood prior to centrifugation. (B) Lipid gradient in centrifuged sample. Top lipid-rich layer contains lipid-soluble analytes. Lower plasma layer contains water-soluble analytes.

Removal of Lipids From the Sample

In the hospital environment, lipemic samples are not infrequent. They most often originate from emergency departments, intensive care units, and endocrinology and gastrointestinal clinics from patients suffering from conditions that include acute pancreatitis, acute or chronic kidney failure, thyroid or lipid disorders, and diabetes mellitus. Lipemic samples quite commonly require immediate results. Unlike hemolysis, the interference caused by lipemia can be fully eliminated, or at least reduced, by removing the excess of lipids from the sample. Still, even if lipids have been successfully removed from the sample, any visible turbidity of a sample should be documented and reported with the test results because it offers clinically useful information about the patient.[166] Moreover, lipid testing and testing for lipid-soluble drugs (e.g., benzodiazepines) and hormones (e.g., thyroid hormones) should always be done on the native sample, before delipidation. Methods for lipid removal include ultracentrifugation, high-speed centrifugation, and some lipid-clearing agents.

Lipid removal by ultracentrifugation and high-speed centrifugation. According to the CLSI C56-A standard for Hemolysis, Icterus, and Lipemia/Turbidity Indices as Indicators of Interference in Clinical Laboratory Analysis, ultracentrifugation is the recommended method for the removal of the excess of lipids in the sample.[171] Ultracentrifuges use the centrifugation force of almost 200,000 g and are very effective in clearing lipemic sera by separating lipids, especially chylomicrons (top layer) from the aqueous part (lower layer) of the sample. After centrifugation, the infranatant (lower part of the sample) can be transferred into the clean tube and analyzed. It should be kept in mind that by removing the upper lipid layer, one also removes lipid-soluble analytes like drugs and hormones. Results reported from ultracentrifuged samples or samples from which lipids have been removed in any other way should be appropriately annotated to ensure clinicians are aware that the sample has been manipulated to obtain the reported results.

Though considered a gold standard, ultracentrifugation is not widely available in many laboratories. High-speed centrifugation using the microcentrifuge with a maximum centrifugation speed of up to 20,000 g may therefore serve as an acceptable alternative and is the method of choice for most laboratories.[172] The effectiveness of high-speed centrifugation depends on the concentration of lipids in the lipemic sample. However, it must be emphasized that ultracentrifugation is superior to high-speed centrifugation for grossly lipemic samples. By using the ultracentrifuge, triglyceride concentration may be reduced 7-fold (from 59.2 to 8.1 mmol/L; or 5239 to 717 mg/dL), whereas the high-speed centrifuge may achieve only 3.4-fold reduction.[173]

Lipid removal by lipid-clearing agents. Lipid-clearing agents are widely used in many laboratories due to their low cost, convenience, and ease of use. Those agents (cyclodextrin, polyethylene glycol, dextran sulphate, hexane, and others) may vary in their ability to extract lipids from a lipemic sample and may also lead to reduction of a significant amount of protein from the sample.[174] It is therefore extremely important for laboratories to verify the performance of such reagents before their routine use because they may not be appropriate for a wide range of analytes due to their low recovery. For example, LipoClear spin columns (Iris International Inc., Westwood, MA) may lead to serious underestimation of CRP (−92%), CK-MB (−25%), and GGT (−30%) and overestimation of cTnT (+20%) and phosphates (+7%) (Fig. 5.4).[175]

Lipid removal takes time and may cause delays in reporting the results. It is up to each individual laboratory to establish its own procedure for managing lipemic samples, bearing in mind to ensure the highest possible accuracy of results and

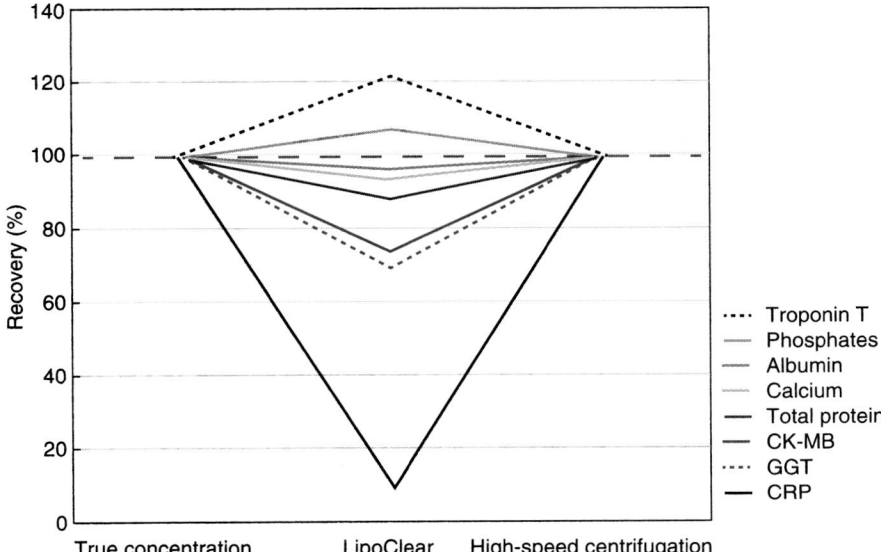

FIGURE 5.4 Recoveries for several chemistry assays after lipid removal from a lipemic sample with a lipid clearing agent (LipoClear, Iris International Inc., Westwood, MA) and high-speed centrifugation in Eppendorf Mini Spin centrifuge (Eppendorf, Hamburg, Germany) at 12,100 g for 5 minutes. *CK-MB,* Creatine kinase MB; *CRP,* C-reactive protein; *GGT,* gamma-glutamyl transferase. (Data from Saracevic A, Nikolac N, Simundic AM. The evaluation and comparison of consecutive high-speed centrifugation and LipoClear reagent for lipemia removal. *Clin Biochem* 2014;47:309–14.)

speed. To minimize the prolongation of the turnaround time and subsequent delays in reporting the results for grossly lipemic samples, laboratories may consider analyzing electrolytes using the blood gas analyzers (direct ion selective electrode methodology) while manipulating the rest of the sample to remove the lipids.

Intravenous Lipid Emulsion Therapy as an Antidote to Drug Overdose

Lipid emulsions were introduced in 2006 as a remedy for systemic toxic effects caused by local anesthetic and are used increasingly today in emergency settings to treat patients who have overdosed on antiepileptic, cardiovascular, or psychotropic drugs.[176,177] Their use is recommended in patients suffering from severe systemic cardiovascular toxic effects who have not otherwise responded to conventional resuscitation protocol and antidotal therapies.[176] The American College of Medical Toxicology recommends it as a reasonable therapeutic option in circumstances where there is serious hemodynamic or other instability from a lipid-soluble drug, even if the patient is not in cardiac arrest.[178] The exact mechanism of action of lipid emulsions is not known. In patients treated with large doses of lipid emulsions, possible side effects include severe hypertriglyceridemia, pancreatitis, lipemia, and numerous interferences in laboratory assays.[179] To avoid compromising patient outcome caused by reporting of incorrect results and delays in reporting of critical results, it is important that blood samples in such cases are collected prior to initiating the intravenous lipid emulsion therapy whenever possible.[180] If intravenous lipid emulsion therapy has already been initiated before the blood sampling, the laboratory should make an effort to remove the lipids and ensure acceptable accuracy of results and turnaround time. Good communication between the laboratory and the clinical staff in such cases of life-threatening toxicity from lipophilic drugs is of paramount importance.

Icterus

The normal concentration of bilirubin in human plasma (or serum) is up to 20 μmol/L (1.2 mg/dL). Change in the color of the serum (or plasma) becomes detectable when bilirubin concentration exceeds 34 μmol/L (2 mg/dL). Bilirubin concentrations above 100 μmol/L (5.9 mg/dL) are clinically defined as *icterus*. Icteric plasma is commonly seen in patients from intensive care units, gastroenterology centers, and pediatric clinics. Bilirubin interferes with numerous chemistry tests such as enzymes (ALT, ALK, CK, lipase), electrolytes, metabolites (urea, creatinine, glucose), lipids (cholesterol, triglycerides), proteins (albumin, total proteins, IgG), hormones (estradiol, beta-HCG, free triiodothyronine [FT3]), and even some drugs (gentamicin, phenobarbital, theophylline, tobramycin).[181–183]

Just as with hemolysis and lipemia, interference caused by bilirubin differs among instruments and assays. For example, bilirubin exerts interference of different magnitudes (strong, moderate, or negligible) and directions (positive and negative interferences), both with Jaffe and enzymatic methods for the measurement of serum creatinine from different manufacturers. While some methods are not affected by bilirubin at all, others may exhibit strong interference by bilirubin, causing clinically significant bias for creatinine measurement and compromising the adequate management of patients with

kidney disease.[184,185] It has been demonstrated that even if two methods have identical reagents, differences in their susceptibility to interference by bilirubin may still occur. These differences may be due to the different incubation times and temperatures and some other parameters related to the assay setup.[186] Interestingly, although enzymatic methods are often considered the method of choice due to being less susceptible to various interferences, bilirubin has been reported to cause greater interference in some enzymatic creatinine assays than in Jaffe methods.[187]

Bilirubin is present in the blood in several distinct forms: as unconjugated and conjugated (mono- and diglucuronide conjugates). Unconjugated bilirubin is not soluble in water and is therefore transported in blood bound to albumin. Bilirubin conjugates are soluble in water. Additionally, bilirubin photoisomers may be found in the blood of neonates.[188] All these different molecular forms of bilirubin have different physical and chemical properties and behave differently in different chemistry assays. The total amount of measured bilirubin in the patient is a mixture of these different forms. Different forms of bilirubin cause interference to various degrees with different laboratory methods, and the same forms of bilirubin can act differently with the same assays on different instruments.

Most interference studies performed by manufacturers and most original studies published by different authors were done on commercially available forms of unconjugated bilirubin that may not correspond to what is found in the blood. This is why sometimes data obtained by interference studies does not mimic real scenarios in human blood and cannot be extrapolated to define rules for adequate detection and management of icteric samples.

Unfortunately, laboratories cannot do much about removing or minimizing the effect of icteric interference. Bilirubin oxidase and blanking procedures have been recommended.[19] Possible options are dilution of the sample (possible only for analytes present at high enough concentrations in the blood) and testing the requested analytes with a different method or on a different instrument for which icterus does not cause clinically significant interference. For maximal patient benefit, laboratories may consider having special protocols (dilutions or different methods) for some critical analytes in icteric samples to avoid unnecessary sample rejections.

Mechanisms of Interference Caused by Icterus

Icterus interferes through two mechanisms: spectrophotometric interference and by interfering with chemical reaction. It is important to recognize that both mechanisms may occur simultaneously in one sample.

Spectrophotometric interference of bilirubin. Bilirubin causes spectrophotometric interference due to its ability to absorb light in the wide range of wavelengths between 400 and 540 nm.

Chemical interference of bilirubin. Bilirubin produces negative bias on assays that involve H_2O_2 as an intermediate reaction (e.g., cholesterol, glucose, uric acid, triglycerides).

Detection of Hemolytic, Icteric, and Lipemic Samples

Hemolysis becomes visible at the concentration of 0.3 to 0.5 g/L of free hemoglobin, and the intensity of the red color of the serum or plasma further increases with the increase in

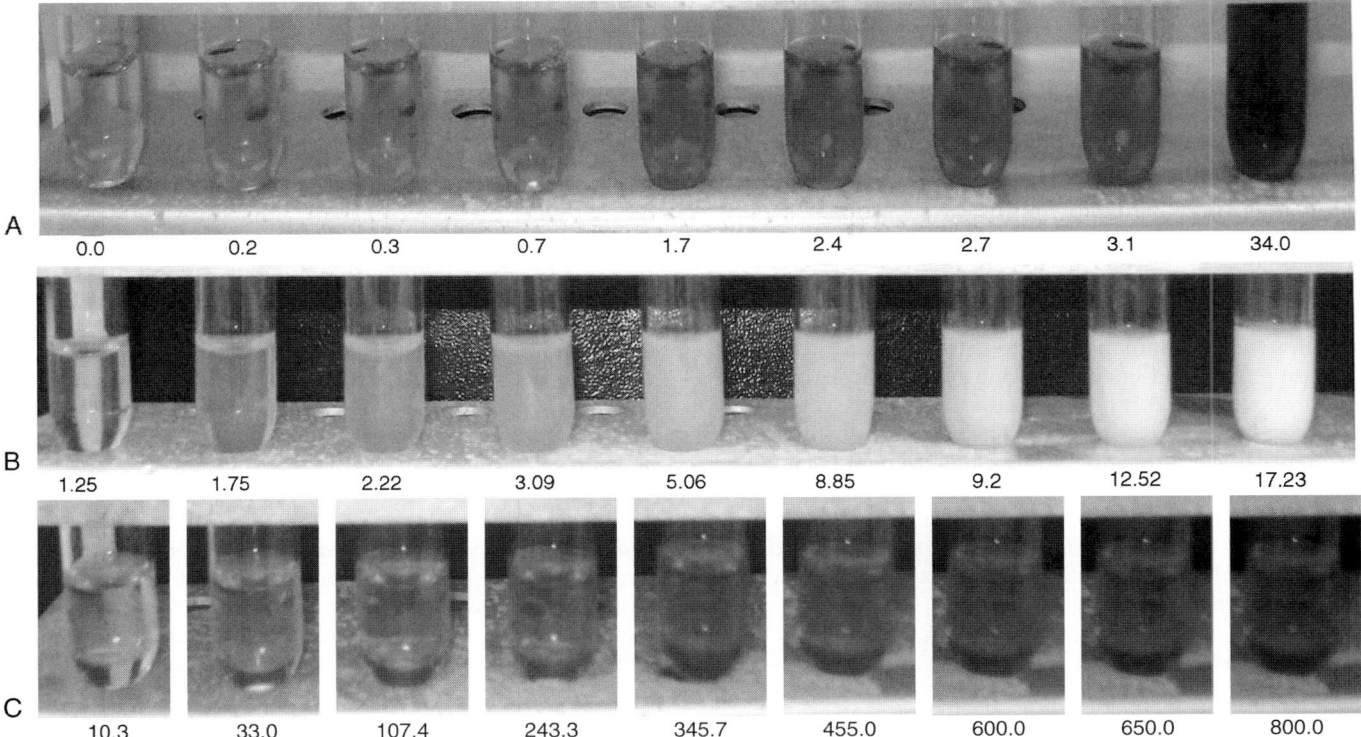

FIGURE 5.5 (A) Hemolysis: the intensity of the red color of the serum and corresponding concentrations of free serum hemoglobin (in g/L). (B) Lipemia: the degree of turbidity and corresponding concentrations (in mmol/L) of triglycerides. (C) Icterus: the intensity of the yellow color of the serum and corresponding concentrations of bilirubin (in μmol/L). (Color standard scales provided by Clinical Institute of Chemistry, University Hospital Center "Sestre milosrdnice," Zagreb, Croatia. Please see the online version of this figure for full color.)

concentration of free serum hemoglobin (Fig. 5.5A). Lipemia causes sample turbidity, which approximately corresponds to the concentration of serum triglycerides (Fig. 5.5B). Increased concentrations of serum bilirubin lead to yellow to orange coloration of the serum, and the change of the color correlates to the increasing concentration of the bilirubin in the serum (Fig. 5.5C).

Free hemoglobin, triglycerides, and bilirubin have characteristic absorption peaks in a wide wavelength range of 300 to 600 nm. This is also the range where sample absorbance is measured in spectrophotometric methods, and that is why hemolysis, icterus, and lipemia cause spectral interferences. Fig. 5.6 presents the characteristic absorption curves of oxyhemoglobin, triglycerides, and bilirubin. Serum indices may be detected by visual inspection and by the use of automated detection systems.

Visual Detection of Serum Indices

Although detection of the degree of hemolysis, icterus, or lipemia has historically been done by visual inspection, such an approach is highly unreliable.[189] Laboratory personnel are not able to accurately assess the degree of hemolysis, icterus, or lipemia in serum, even if well trained and when using a color standard for comparison.[190] Moreover, there is a poor interrater agreement (reproducibility) in estimating the degree of serum indices between different members of laboratory staff,

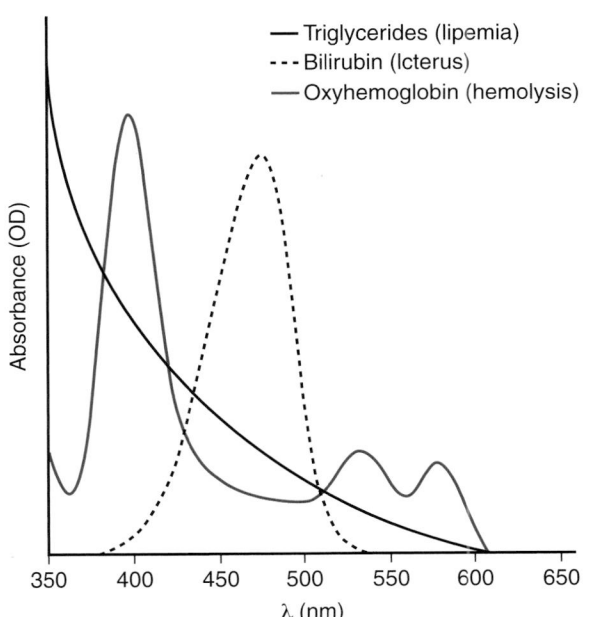

FIGURE 5.6 Absorption curves of oxyhemoglobin in serum with characteristic peaks at 415, 540, and 570 nm *(red line)*; triglycerides absorption curve covers wide range of wavelengths, with a maximum in the lower part of the spectrum *(dotted black line)*; bilirubin has one distinct peak at 460 nm *(black line)*.

reflecting the substantial interindividual differences in visual sensitivity to different colors.[191] For example, it has been demonstrated that visual inspection of the degree of hemolysis is influenced by the sample type (serum or plasma) and the test requested, thus leading to either over- or underestimation of the actual degree of hemolysis, depending on the expected effect of hemolysis on the measured analyte.[192] The ability to detect hemolysis by visual inspection is further impaired in samples that are both hemolyzed and icteric.[193] This is especially important in neonatal samples, where increased bilirubin concentrations are quite common.

Other substances, such as medical contrast media, may also influence the human ability to detect not only hemolysis but also icterus and lipemia.[194] One such example is Patent Blue dye, which is commonly used for sentinel lymph node biopsy in breast cancer patients. The presence of this dye in serum negatively affects the ability of laboratory personnel to reliably detect hemolysis, as well as icterus and lipemia. For the above-mentioned reasons, visual detection of the degrees of hemolysis, lipemia, and icterus is not recommended and should be replaced with automated detection systems whenever and wherever possible.

Automated Serum Indices

Today, most mainstream chemistry analyzers can detect serum indices by the use of semiquantitative, spectrophotometric measurement and grading the interfering substances into categories. The serum index is automatically reported for every sample and can be used to determine the degree of interference and its effect on the requested parameters. Where an automated detection system for serum indices is not available, grading of interference factors by visual inspection is still a practical alternative used by many laboratories.[195–197]

Automated serum index detection systems have numerous advantages over visual detection (Table 5.8).

Such systems are highly reproducible and provide an objective and standardized way to screen for common interferences and manage specimen rejection via built-in rules. Moreover, their implementation improves laboratory turnaround time, leads to an increase in laboratory efficiency, and minimizes waste by reducing the number of rejected samples.[198] However, there are still some problems and challenges

associated with the automated detection of serum indices on various analytical platforms, which are detailed below.

Variability between different analytical platforms. There is a large variability across different chemistry analyzers in analytical characteristics of their serum index measurement. Different analyzers have different sensitivities, measurement ranges of, and decision thresholds for hemolysis, icterus, and lipemia. Moreover, they differ in the sample volume necessary for the estimation of serum indices and the type of solution used (saline, sample diluent, etc.). Different analyzers measure sample absorbance at various wavelengths and use different algorithms for determining the degree of serum indices. Finally, different manufacturers have employed different reporting systems to report the results of serum indices. Some are reporting qualitative results using the ordinal scale, whereas others are reporting semiquantitative results using actual concentrations of the interferent.[199,200]

Necessity to verify manufacturers' claims. It is the responsibility of the manufacturers of in vitro diagnostic systems and reagents to validate the analytical performance characteristics of their reagents and provide this information to the customer. The instructions for use must particularly contain the information about the effect of all known relevant interferences (e.g., serum indices) on laboratory assays. The CLSI EP7-A2 standard for interference testing in clinical chemistry[201] recommends that validation of the effect of an interferent on clinical chemistry assay be done at two concentrations of an analyte and at five concentrations of an interferent. The maximum concentration of an interferent must reflect the maximum expected concentration of that interferent in the clinical laboratory on patient samples. Moreover, the acceptance limits for allowable interference should be derived whenever possible from biological variability or clinically established thresholds. Due to financial constraints and the lack of time and staff, laboratories often rely on the information provided by the manufacturers, and only a minority of laboratories verifies manufacturer declarations.[195] However, manufacturers do not always comply with the recommended procedure for testing interferences, and their claims are often not accurate, reproducible, or reliable.[202,203] It is therefore a good practice for a laboratory to perform its own verification of serum indices. Alternatively, laboratories may rely on the evidence from the literature if it exists and only if the evidence is of adequate quality.

Necessity to implement a systematic approach to internal and external quality control of serum indices. Like all other laboratory methods, analytical quality of the method for detection of serum indices should be continuously monitored by using appropriate internal quality control (IQC) and through participation in an external quality assessment program (EQA). The ISO 15189:2012 International Standard for medical laboratories states, "EQA programs should, as far as possible, provide clinically relevant challenges that mimic patient samples and have the effect of checking the entire examination process, including pre- and postexamination procedures."[21] EQA for serum indices may be conducted by sending samples with varying degrees of lipemia, hemolysis, and icterus to laboratories, and then participants provide their serum indices value and report results as they would for a patient sample.[204,205] Unfortunately, IQC and EQA are not widely available for serum indices. EQA for serum indices is currently available only from few providers (WEQAS and

TABLE 5.8   Advantages and Disadvantages of Visual and Automated Detection of Serum Indices

Visual detection	Automated serum indices
• Subjective	• Objective
• Time-consuming	• Reduces turn-around time (compared to visual detection)
• Requires available staff	• Reproducible
• Low reproducibility	• Reliable
• Unreliable	• Potential problems:
	• Presence of paraproteins
	• Cross-reactivity of serum indices
	• Interference caused by drugs, contrast media, and other interferents

RCPA-QAP), and IQC material for serum indices has been recently made commercially available by a single manufacturer.[206] To overcome this problem, laboratories are encouraged to produce their own in-house prepared IQC materials and manage them in the same way as all other conventional laboratory IQC procedures.[207] For additional discussion on IQC and EQC, refer to Chapter 6.

Potential sources of interferences affecting serum indices. Some medical contrast media are known to interfere with serum indices and impair the accurate determination of hemoglobin, bilirubin, and sample turbidity. It is important that laboratory staff be aware of this issue and that each sample be visually checked whenever serum index measurements raise suspicion or do not match the sample appearance or clinical condition of the patient. Patent Blue dye, which negatively affects the ability to detect changes in the sample's color, has also been found to interfere with serum indices measurement on the Roche Modular Pre-Analytics system and the Abbott Architect chemistry analyzer.[208,209] Patent Blue exerts positive interference on the lipemia index and a negative interference on hemolytic and icteric indices in a linear, dose-responsive fashion.

Rose Bengal has a peak absorbance at 562 nm and is a component of a drug that is used for intralesional therapy in patients with refractory cutaneous or subcutaneous metastatic melanoma.[210] Used in a treatment trial for severe melanoma lesions, it was found to cause false-positive interference on the hemolysis index on Roche Modular D in a sample with a red/pink tinge collected 20 minutes after the injection of a drug.[211]

Monoclonal proteins may also give an abnormal reading of serum lipemic index in apparently clear serum.[212] Markedly increased serum lipemia indices in clear sera were also quite frequently observed in patients with high concentrations of polyclonal immunoglobulins.[213] Nevertheless, unusually high lipemia indices in otherwise clear sera do not occur in all patients with monoclonal or biclonal peaks.

One serum index may also adversely affect the other when two or three HIL indices are abnormal in the same sample (e.g., serum hemolyzed and icteric, hemolyzed and lipemic). In these cases, the magnitude and direction of the bias of one index on the measurement of the other will vary greatly among different instruments and will depend on the respective wavelengths used.[171]

Management of Hemolytic, Icteric, and Lipemic Samples

Laboratories should be aware of the effect of preanalytical interferences on their assays. When there is a significant deviation from the true value of the analyte caused by the presence of cell compounds released by sample hemolysis, bilirubin, or increased concentration of serum lipids, such a result is a threat to patient safety. Biased and inaccurate results may cause diagnostic errors and affect patient management. To ensure the accuracy of their results, laboratories should have procedures in place to systematically detect the presence of potential interferences and how to address them. Unfortunately, there is a large discrepancy among the ways results are reported from samples with interferences, among different countries, institutions, and even individuals (e.g., analyze and report all components, reject the sample and not analyze anything, or analyze only selected components that

are not affected by the interferent).[142,171,196,197] There is room for improvement and harmonization in this respect.

When interferences from hemolysis, icterus, and lipemia are causing unacceptable bias and results are clinically inaccurate, such results should not be reported and sample redraw should be requested.[214,215] Such a test report should always be accompanied with comments informing the clinical staff about the reasons for not reporting the originally requested test results. It is also important that a laboratory notifies the medical staff when sample appearance (color, turbidity) deviates from a normal state by including a comment on a test report (e.g., sample hemolyzed, icteric, lipemic, or turbid), even if the tests are not affected by this change in appearance. Such comments provide useful information to the clinicians. Comments should also indicate if the sample has been treated in any way to minimize the effect of interfering substances (e.g., delipidation).

Unfortunately, each time a redraw is requested, there is a delay in providing the requested test results, and this leads to delays in patient management. In a previously mentioned study by Vecellio and colleagues, the length of stay (LOS) in emergency departments of five large Australian hospitals was on average 18 minutes longer if one or more samples for a particular patient were hemolyzed.[142] To avoid such delays, a laboratory should make a thorough investigation of the causes of the unsuitable specimens and be actively engaged in process improvement to reduce the frequency of errors that affect the quality of the sample.

POINTS TO REMEMBER

Hemolysis, Lipemia, and Icterus
- Visual assessment of the degree of hemolysis, lipemia, and icterus is not reliable and leads to errors.
- Hemolysis is the most common preanalytical error and most common cause of sample rejection.
- Hemolysis may cause clinically relevant bias through spectrophotometric and chemical interference, sample dilution, and release of the cell components into the sample.
- Lipemia causes interference by spectrophotometric interference (light absorption and light scattering), the volume depletion effect, partitioning of the sample, and physicochemical mechanisms (e.g., disturbance of the electrophoretic pattern).
- Laboratories should verify the performance of lipid removal reagents before their routine use because they may not be appropriate for a wide range of analytes due to their low recovery.
- Different forms of bilirubin cause varying degrees of interference with different laboratory methods, and the same forms of bilirubin act differently with the same assays on different instruments.

Interferences Caused by Paraproteins

Paraprotein interferences are not uncommon. The frequency of paraprotein interference has been estimated to be as high as 3 or 4% in hospitals,[216] and it has been reported to affect numerous laboratory assays (Table 5.9). Laboratory staff should carefully review every case in which a measured concentration of an analyte does not correlate with the clinical condition of the patient after all potential sources of errors have been investigated.

TABLE 5.9 Paraprotein Interference With Different Assays

Group of Analytes	Molecule
Enzymes	Alkaline phosphatase[217]
	Gamma-glutamyl transferase[218]
	Lactate dehydrogenase[217]
Electrolytes, minerals, and microelements	Calcium[219]
	Inorganic phosphorus[220–224]
	Iron[225]
Metabolites	Bilirubin[226–229]
	Cholesterol[226,230,231]
	Creatinine[230]
	Glucose[218]
	Urea[232]
	Uric acid[217]
Proteins	C-reactive protein[230,233,234]
	IgA, IgG[235]
Hormones	Thyroid-stimulating hormone[236,237]
	Human chorionic gonadotropin[236]
Drugs	Gentamicin[238]
	Vancomycin[238–241]
	Valproic acid[238]
	Phenytoin[242]
Cardiac markers	Troponin I[236]
Tumor markers	α-Fetoprotein[236]
	CA-125[236]

Paraprotein interferences have been observed on different analytical instruments, and they appear to be methodology and concentration dependent. They affect not only measurements by turbidimetry and nephelometry but also some common chemistry assays with spectrophotometric detection. The likelihood of paraprotein-caused interferences increases with an increasing paraprotein concentration.[229]

Mechanisms of Paraprotein Interference

Paraprotein interference may affect chemistry assays through several distinct mechanisms, including precipitation, volume displacement, and change of sample viscosity.

Precipitation of the paraprotein. A case of paraprotein interference has been reported in a 93-year-old female with severe dementia who presented with cellulitis on the leg and sepsis. Gentamicin was not measurable due to the paraprotein interference caused by the IgM monoclonal protein.[238] The IgM concentration was 18.9 g/L (reference interval: 0.4 to 2.3 g/L). Paraprotein interference was observed on a Beckman DxC600 general chemistry analyzer with a particle-enhanced turbidimetric inhibition immunoassay method (Beckman Coulter, Brea, CA), and it was a result of the persistent high blank absorbance readings. Gentamicin concentration for that patient was successfully measured (3.3 mg/L) on a Roche Cobas system (Roche Diagnostics, Mannheim, Germany) where interference was not present.

Paraprotein interference can be detected by reviewing the reaction curve on the instrument for that specific patient. The reaction curve for the sample without interference shows that precipitation of the gentamicin occurs when precipitating reagent is added to the reaction mixture. The reaction curve for the affected sample shows that IgM precipitation

has occurred in the blanking phase, even before precipitating reagent is added to the reaction mixture. This phenomenon was also observed in a sample that was diluted with a normal saline at a ratio of 1:20 (Fig. 5.7A–C). The manufacturer's instructions for the gentamicin assay states that there is no interference by IgM up to 5 g/L; IgM concentration in this patient was fourfold higher.

Precipitation depends on various assay parameters, such as reaction components, presence of assay additives such as preservatives and surfactants, ionic strength, pH (protein precipitation can occur at both very low and very high pH), and the physicochemical characteristics of the paraprotein. This explains why some assays are affected and others are not by the same paraprotein on the same instrument.

Monoclonal proteins have been reported to appear in serum with a concentration of up to 104.1 g/L.[228] Manufacturers should improve the way in which they test and report data from interference studies. Paraprotein interference should be studied in the whole range of expected concentrations of paraproteins. Laboratories must carefully read the declarations provided by manufacturers and perform their own interference studies to verify the absence or presence of paraprotein interference.

Paraprotein interference may vary according to the type of specimen or the choice of anticoagulant used in sample collection. For example, IgM interfered with a hexokinase method for glucose and a Szasz method for GGT using the Hitachi Modular D and P systems (Roche Diagnostics GmbH).[218] Glucose in lithium heparinized plasma was extremely low in that patient, but the interference was not present in the actual collection tube. Moreover, the interference was absent when glucose and GGT were tested with dry chemistry on a Vitros 950 analyzer (Ortho Clinical Diagnostics). Precipitation of a paraprotein has occurred due to fibrinogen precipitation resulting from the action of heparin. In this case, the best solution is to request a serum sample for that patient or to run the tests affected by the interference using a different method.

Precipitation of paraprotein may occur due to the reaction of paraprotein and the solubilizing agent in the reagent used for the measurement of the concentration for total bilirubin. This mechanism of paraprotein interference has been reported to affect bilirubin measurement by Hitachi Modular P random access autoanalyzer using Roche test kits (Roche Diagnostics GmbH). Such interference leads to a false increase of bilirubin concentration in serum with otherwise normal (anicteric) appearance and in the absence of hemolysis or lipemia.[228,243]

Binding of paraprotein to assay components. Paraproteins may bind to the analyte or any other component of the reaction mixture. The effect of such interference depends on the component to which the paraprotein is bound. Binding of an IgM paraprotein to latex particles resulted in high CRP and ASO values in a young Japanese female myeloma patient.[234] The IgM concentration was grossly increased at 70.0 g/L (reference interval: 1.31 to 2.83 g/L). Concentrations of CRP, ASO, IgG, IgA, and IgM were measured by a Behring nephelometer II automated analyzer (Behringwerke AG, Marburg, Germany) that used latex particles coated with anti-CRP rabbit antibody, streptolysin-O antigen, and anti-human IgG, IgA, and IgM rabbit antibody (Behringwerke AG), respectively. When measured with another method, CRP and ASO concentrations were within the reference interval.

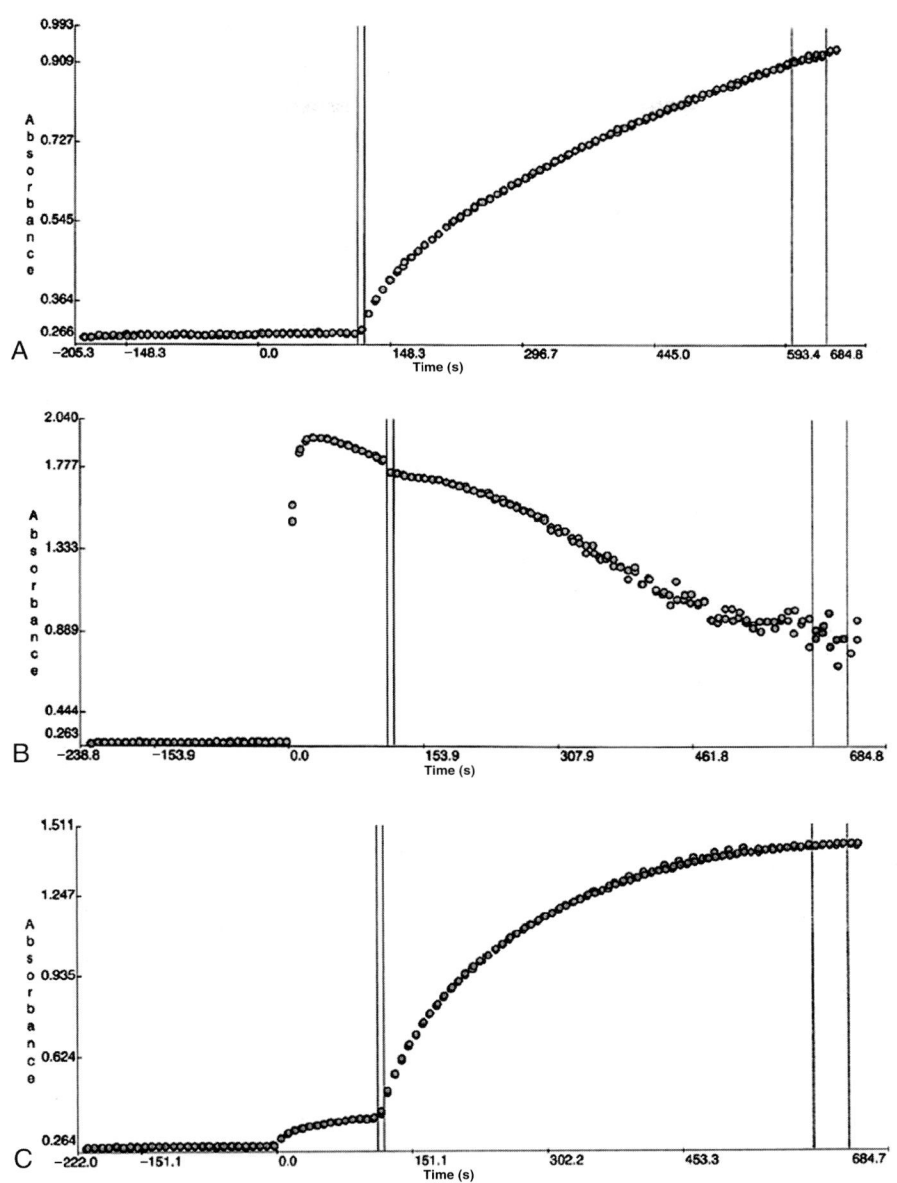

FIGURE 5.7 Reaction curve for the gentamicin particle–enhanced turbidimetric inhibition immunoassay method on the Beckman DxC600 general chemistry analyzer in a patient in whom gentamicin was not measurable due to the paraprotein interference caused by the IgM monoclonal protein. (A) Precipitation of the analyte occurs when precipitating reagent is added to the reaction mixture. The reaction curve for the sample is affected by the paraprotein interference (IgM). (B) Precipitation of the analyte occurs in the blanking phase (unexpectedly high blank absorbance readings), even before the precipitating reagent is added to the reaction mixture. (C) The change in the reaction curve is visible even in a sample that has been diluted with a normal saline in a ratio of 1:20. (From Dimeski G, Bassett K, Brown N. Paraprotein interference with turbidimetric gentamicin assay. *Biochem Med* 2015;25:117–24, with permission by the Croatian Society of Medical Biochemistry and Laboratory Medicine.)

This kind of interference does not cause sample turbidity. Reaction kinetics for the unaffected sample and a sample with an interfering paraprotein are very similar, and therefore this type of interference cannot be detected by reviewing the reaction curve on the instrument (Fig. 5.8).[244]

Paraprotein interference due to volume displacement. Paraproteins affect chemistry assays by the same mechanism as lipemia—that is, due to the volume displacement effect. Most pronounced are changes in serum electrolytes and especially in serum sodium measurement by indirect ISE technology (ISE). A high concentration of paraproteins leads to false hyponatremia if sodium is measured by indirect ISE. As a general rule, in samples with total protein concentration greater than 100 g/L or less than 40 g/L, electrolytes (and

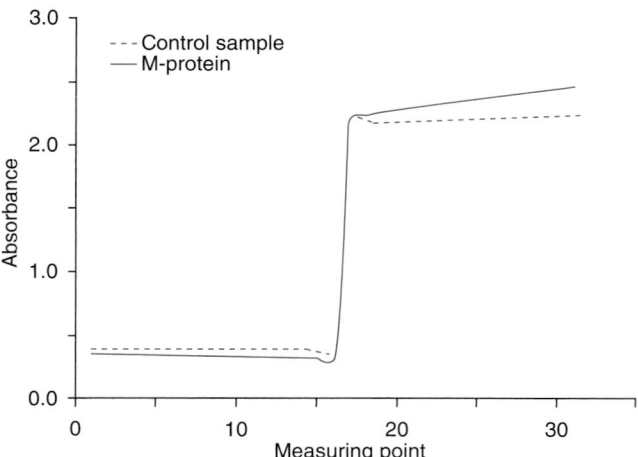

FIGURE 5.8 An example of IgM (7.45 g/L) paraprotein interference with measurement of ferritin concentration on the Roche/Hitachi 911 analyzer, caused by binding of the paraprotein to the components of the reaction mixture. The ferritin concentration was 492 mg/L on the Roche/Hitachi 911 analyzer and six times lower (80 mg/L) when measured with a different assay on another instrument. (From Bakker AJ, Mücke M. Gammopathy interference in clinical chemistry assays: Mechanisms, detection and prevention. *Clin Chem Lab Med* 2007;45:1240–43, with permission by Walter de Gruyter.)

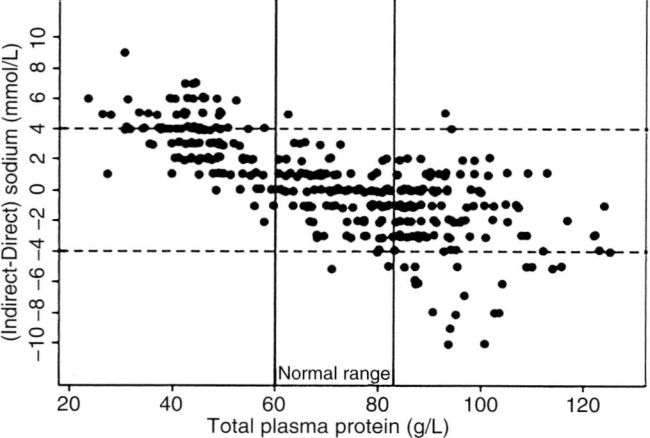

FIGURE 5.9 The association of the difference between direct and indirect ion-selective electrode measurement of plasma sodium relative to plasma protein concentration. Vertical lines demonstrate the reference interval for total plasma protein. Dashed line shows disagreement of 4 mmol/L or greater in sodium measurements. (From Dimeski G, Morgan TJ, Presneill JJ, Venkatesh B. Disagreement between ion selective electrode direct and indirect sodium measurements: Estimation of the problem in a tertiary referral hospital. *J Crit Care* 2012;27:326.e9–16, with permission from Elsevier.)

especially sodium) should be measured by direct ISE technology.[245,246] Otherwise, clinically significant bias is possible and may lead to adverse patient outcomes.

The concentration of plasma sodium, measured by indirect ISE methods, is inversely proportional to the concentration of plasma proteins. The greater the concentration of plasma proteins, the lower the concentration of plasma sodium (Fig. 5.9).

Paraprotein interference due to change in sample viscosity. Paraproteins may exert their interference simply by affecting the viscosity of the sample. Viscosity is much higher in samples with very high paraprotein concentration or in refrigerated samples in which a gel has been formed (e.g., in the case of cryoglobulinemia). Sample viscosity affects the volume of the sample pipetted in the reaction mixture. Many instruments are able to detect such changes in sample viscosity and trigger an alarm if viscosity is not within predefined limits. In such cases, a rerun in a dilution mode is the recommended corrective action, provided the analyte can be accurately measured in the diluted specimen. In instruments where this feature is not available, increased sample viscosity may lead to incorrect sample volume and cause falsely increased or decreased results, depending on the assay format.

How to Detect and Deal With Paraprotein Interference.

Laboratories can put safeguards in place to automatically detect interference caused by paraproteins:

- Have the instrument sound an alarm if the difference in absorbance between selected points is unexpectedly greater than some predetermined value
- In cases of interference of paraproteins on bilirubin concentration, have the instrument flag the results for confirmation when the bilirubin concentration in a sample is higher than some predetermined value and the icterus index is normal
- Have the instrument flag and block all test results that are preceded by a minus sign
- Have the instrument block all test results for patients who have erroneous results, such as higher direct bilirubin than total bilirubin or higher albumin than total proteins

Hopefully, future chemistry analyzers will be able to monitor analytical reactions in real time and automatically screen for potential interferences similarly to the detection of serum indices.

Laboratories may also apply various approaches to eliminate paraprotein interference[173]:

- Samples can be analyzed on an alternative instrument with a different method
- Proteins in the sample can be precipitated by a blocking agent, ethanol, ammonium sulphate, or polyethylene-glycol, while the analyte of interest remains in the supernatant
- Serial dilutions of the sample may be performed
- The sample can be filtered to remove the proteins

Exogenous Interferences

Exogenous interferent is defined as a substance originating outside of the body (e.g., a drug or its metabolites, a specimen preservative, or a sample contaminant) that causes interference with the analysis of another substance in the specimen.[247] Exogenous interferences are quite complex and difficult to identify and deal with.[173,201] Interferences can be introduced into the sample via several different sources:

- prescribed medication used for patient treatment
- supportive medical therapy, including parenteral emulsions, contrast media agents, and infusion solutions
- natural preparations (herbal and animal remedies) and dietary supplements
- accidental exposures and poisonings
- contamination during sample handling (from rubber tube stoppers, lubricants, anticoagulants, or surfactants) or sample analysis (antibiotics used for reagent and buffer stability)

Mechanisms of Interference

Drugs interfere in laboratory testing in two ways: in vivo, through pharmacologic effect of the drug on a specific analyte, and in vitro during the actual analysis. The comprehensive database of the physiologic (in vivo) and analytical (in vitro) drug effects is available as an on-line resource.[248]

Analytical (chemical) in vitro interference is caused when the presence of the drug directly or indirectly leads to falsely increased or decreased concentration of a measured analyte.

There are different mechanisms of drug in vitro interference:

- the parent drug or its metabolite cross-reacts with the substrate, due to the structural similarity with the tested analyte
- the parent drug or its metabolite interferes with the chemical reaction by accelerating or inhibiting it
- the parent drug or its metabolite affects sample turbidity or absorbance and causes overlap of drug and chromogen absorption peaks[249,250]
- some drugs can interfere with the integrity of the sample by changing sample density (viscosity) and cause obstruction problems on analytical systems (e.g., iodine-based contrast media)

Chemical mechanisms of interference are discussed in more detail later in this chapter.

Manufacturer Claims Regarding Drug Interferences

The impact of exogenous interferent on patient condition could range from harmless to fatal. Manufacturers of laboratory reagents are responsible to conduct extensive interference testing and provide all relevant information about any possible interference susceptibility of their assays to their end-users. According to the CLSI EP07-ED3:2018 standard, interference testing is composed of the following steps:

- selection of appropriate analyte concentrations for interference testing (concentrations at medical decision points)
- selection of substances which could interfere with assay
- selection of appropriate tested interferent concentrations
- assurance of reliability of testing procedures during interference evaluation
- paired testing of sample without and with added interferent drug in concentration three times the highest recorded concentration during therapeutic drug monitoring
- if difference in concentration of tested analyte does not exceed defined acceptance criteria, there is no need for additional interference testing
- if acceptance criteria have been exceeded, dose-response experiment has to be performed
- when dose-response experiment is completed, interference should be reported.[247]

Laboratory professionals are responsible for verifying manufacturer interference claims, investigating any discrepant result that might be caused by an interfering substance, and providing feedback to the manufacturers.[201] End-users are also responsible for reporting any inconsistencies in the use of diagnostic products which could impact patient safety to the local agencies responsible for postmarket surveillance. Moreover, it is important that laboratory professionals have safe procedures in place for effective detection of new potential sources of exogenous interferences and the knowledge about the type and quantity of potential exogenous interferents used in patient management in order to prevent possible negative outcome.

Exogenous interferences are not easy to detect and it is quite unlikely that a laboratory will have an error-proof system, consistent policy, and procedures in place to safeguard from exogenous interferences. Most commonly, a suspicion is raised when test results do not match the clinical condition of the patient or when there is a sudden change in patient test results. Different strategies are suggested for investigation of suspected exogenous interference. Table 5.10 provides a list of some most common exogenous interferents and measures which should be undertaken in case of their occurrence.

Whenever there is a clinical suspicion, due to the sudden change in laboratory test results, that some other tube components might have caused some interference, it is recommended to recollect the sample using different tube type and/or to perform the analysis on a different analytical platform and/or method.

Besides interferences of endogenous components that are listed in manufacturers' claims (lipids, hemoglobin, bilirubin, proteins), manufacturers usually include the results of interference testing for drugs that could potentially affect the measurement. The drug list is adjusted for any specific analyte. Drugs and metabolites that are likely to interfere on the basis of their chemical and physical properties and those most often prescribed in the patient population for which the test is ordered should be tested.[201] Tested drug concentrations should cover the entire range of the expected blood drug concentrations. To minimize the risk of unrecognized drug effect due to the low tested concentration, the highest expected drug concentration should be tested at least three times. A list of proposed tested drug concentrations is provided in CLSI document EP7-A2, *Interference Testing in Clinical Chemistry*.[201] Table 5.11 presents an example of drug interferences listed in the reagent insert sheet provided with the Abbott Hemoglobin A1c enzymatic assay (Abbott Laboratories, Lake Bluff, IL).

Unfortunately, information about patient medication is often not available to laboratory staff. Hospital electronic medical records can help identify whether any potentially interfering drug is prescribed to the patient. However, in most cases there is no way of knowing if the drug concentration in patient blood exceeds the allowable threshold. For most of the drugs listed in Table 5.11, concentration can be measured only in specialized laboratories. Therefore many drug interferences remain undetected and only a clear discrepancy between the test result and clinical information prompts the laboratory staff to suspect drug interference and proceed to further investigation, as already described above.[251]

Drug interference in laboratory tests is a major cause of concern. Lack of information on influence and interference of specific drugs carries risk of reporting of erroneous results that could lead to faulty patient management. Unfortunately, these interactions are still largely unrecognized and only a minority of drug labels contain information on drug-laboratory test interaction. The way forward to solve this problem would be to establish an on-line database, continuously updated, with information on possible impacts of drugs and other exogenous interferents on laboratory measurements.[252,253]

Prescribed Medication

Prescribed medication can often interfere with the measurement and cause erroneous laboratory results. There are numerous reports describing the interference of prescribed

TABLE 5.10   A Summary of Common Exogenous Interferences and How to Identify and Investigate Them

Contaminant	Common Potentially Affected Analytes (Not an Exhaustive List)	When to Suspect	Point of Occurrence of the Interference	Initial Investigations
Drugs/herbal remedies	All analytes could be affected	Sudden change in value Clinical suspicion	Patient	Literature search Recollect the sample after removal of medication
Skin disinfectants	Electrolytes, LD, AST, bilirubin, phosphate, folate, urate	Hemolysis Sudden change in value Clinical suspicion	Phlebotomy	Recollect the sample Check indices values
EDTA	Potassium, calcium, zinc, magnesium, iron, ALP	Sudden change in value Clinical suspicion Potassium very high	Phlebotomy	Check divalent cations Measure EDTA Recollect the sample
Sodium citrate	Sodium	Sudden change in value Clinical suspicion Sodium very high	Phlebotomy	Check chloride Check osmolar gap Recollect the sample
Heparin	Sodium, analytes measured by immunoassays, thyroid Function tests	Sudden change in value Clinical suspicion	Patient or phlebotomy	Recollect the sample once source of heparin has been removed
Fluoride oxalate	Hematocrit, electrolytes	Sudden change in value Clinical suspicion	Phlebotomy	Recollect the sample
Gel separators	Hydrophobic drugs, drugs and hormones measured by mass Spectrometry, e.g. testosterone	Sudden change in value Clinical suspicion Interfering peaks	Phlebotomy	Recollect the sample using different tube type
Contrast media	Sample potentially unsuitable for all analytes measured by spectrophotometric assays Divalent cations Indices value	Sudden change in value Clinical suspicion Gel barrier incorrectly positions after centrifugation Instrument flags	Patient	Recollect the sample when source has been removed
Antibody therapies	Analytes measured by immunoassays	Sudden change in value Clinical suspicion Instrument flags	Patient	Try different analytical method/platform Remove treatment
IV infusion	Potassium, sodium, glucose Dilution of analytes not being infused	Sudden change in value Clinical suspicion Reagent lots of low analyte concentrations (with normal sodium if saline)	Patient	Recollect the sample from other arm, or when infusion is finished
Analyzer problems or Contamination	All analytes could be affected	Sudden change in value across multiple patients Clinical suspicion	Laboratory	Run samples on another analyzer Recalibrate analyzer Maintain analyzer

ALP, Alkaline phosphatase; *AST*, aspartate aminotransferase; *LD*, lactate dehydrogenase.
Modified from Cornes MP. Exogenous sample contamination. Sources and interference. *Clin Biochem* 2016;49:1340–5.

medication in the measurement of various analytes in different matrices, such as whole blood, serum, plasma, and urine samples. The type and magnitude of the interference is dependent on a number of factors such as drug dose, timing, route of administration, duration of drug application, concomitant use of other drugs and herbal supplements, method of analyte determination, reagent composition, analyzer used, age of detecting components, sample type, etc.

Although all laboratory methods can potentially be affected by drug interferences, specific enzymatic chemistry methods are usually not as susceptible as colorimetric tests. Creatinine is one of the most commonly measured parameters in a clinical chemistry laboratory. Laboratories worldwide use either the Jaffe colorimetric assay with alkaline

picrate or an enzymatic assay for creatinine measurement (Fig. 5.10).

Some commonly prescribed antibiotics and analgesic drugs can interfere with creatinine measurement. For example, cephalosporin antibiotics cause falsely increased creatinine concentrations (measured by the Jaffe method) in sera drawn shortly after intravenous administration of cefpirome.[254,255] Falsely increased creatinine concentration measured by the Jaffe method has also been observed after adding subtherapeutic, therapeutic, and toxic concentrations of acetaminophen, acetylsalicylic acid, or metamizole to the serum. Although the Jaffe method has always been considered to be more susceptible to interference compared to the enzymatic assay, it is now known that even the enzymatic assay is not free from the interfering

TABLE 5.11   List of Interfering Drugs Tested for Potential Interference With HbA$_{1c}$ Enzymatic Assay

| Interfering Substance | HIGH TEST LEVEL | | % INTERFERENCE | |
	Conventional Units	SI Units	6.0–7.0% HbA$_{1c}$ Value	≥8.0% HbA$_{1c}$ Value
Acarbose	50 mg/dL	0.77 mmol/L	0.0	0.0
Acetaminophen	200 µg/mL	1324 µmol/L	−1.5	−1.1
Acetylsalicylate	50.8 mg/dL	2.82 mmol/L	0.0	0.0
Atorvastatin	600 µg Eq/L	600 µg Eq/L	0.0	0.0
Captopril	0.5 mg/dL	23 µmol/L	−1.5	−1.1
Chlorpropamide	74.7 mg/dL	2.7 mmol/L	0.0	0.0
Cyanate	50 mg/dL	6.16 mmol/L	0.0	1.1
Furosemide	6.0 mg/dL	181 µmol/L	0.0	0.0
Gemfibrozil	7.5 mg/dL	300 µmol/L	0.0	0.0
Ibuprofen	0.5 mg/mL	2524 µmol/L	0.0	0.0
Insulin	450 µU/mL	450 µU/mL	0.0	0.0
Losartan	5 mg/dL	0.11 mmol/L	0.0	0.0
Metformin	5.1 mg/dL	310 µmol/L	0.0	0.0
Nicotinic acid	61 mg/dL	4.95 mmol/L	0.0	0.0
Propranolol	0.2 mg/dL	7.71 µmol/L	0.0	0.0
Repaglinide	60 ng/mL	132.57 nmol/L	0.0	0.0

Interference effects were assayed by comparing test samples containing potential drug interferents to the reference samples. According to the CLSI EP7-A2 protocol for interference testing in clinical chemistry, two clinically relevant analyte concentrations were used (6.0 to 7.0% and ≥8.0% HbA$_{1c}$). Various potential interfering drugs are added into the samples (listed in column 1). Concentrations of the analyte (HbA$_{1c}$) were measured in the sample with added interferent (test result) and in the reference sample without interferent (control result). Interference effect was calculated as bias according to the formula: Interference = (Test result − Control result)/Control result × 100%.
However, calculated bias values are representative of potential drug interferences only up to the tested concentrations listed in columns 2 and 3. Some of these drugs might have a stronger impact on HbA$_{1c}$ concentration measurements when they are present in higher concentrations.

From reagent insert sheet provided with the Abbott HbA$_{1c}$ reagent (REF 4P52-21). From Abbott Laboratories, Lake Bluff, IL.

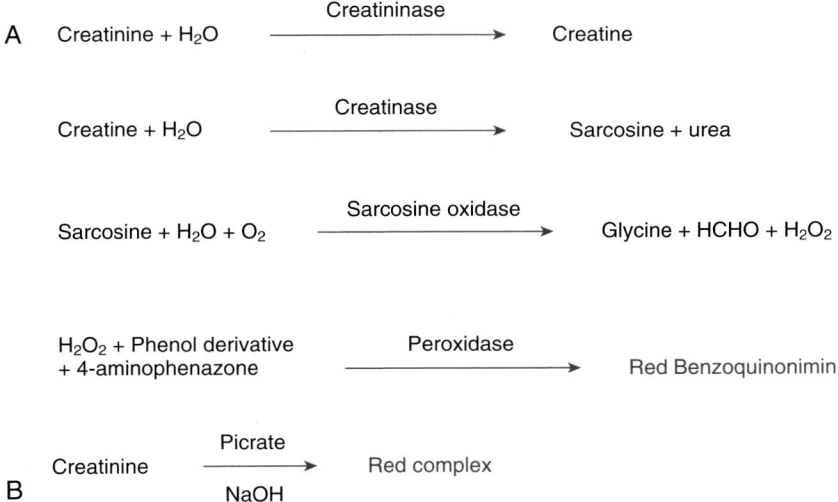

FIGURE 5.10 Methods for the measurement of creatinine. (A) Enzymatic assay: the absorption at 546 nm of the red-colored product of the indicator reaction is proportional to creatinine concentration. (B) Jaffe colorimetric assay: creatinine reacts with picrate in alkaline media and forms a red complex. Change in absorption at 509 nm is proportional to creatinine concentration.

effects of various drugs. An in vitro study has demonstrated that the addition of toxic concentrations of metamizole to serum pool causes falsely decreased creatinine concentrations measured by the enzymatic method (Fig. 5.11).[256] It has also been demonstrated that metamizole causes significant negative interference with several isotopic dilution mass spectrometric traceable enzymatic creatinine methods and some other routine biochemistry analytes.[257,258] To avoid the interference of metamizole, it has been suggested that creatinine measurements are done at least 3 hours after drug injection.[257]

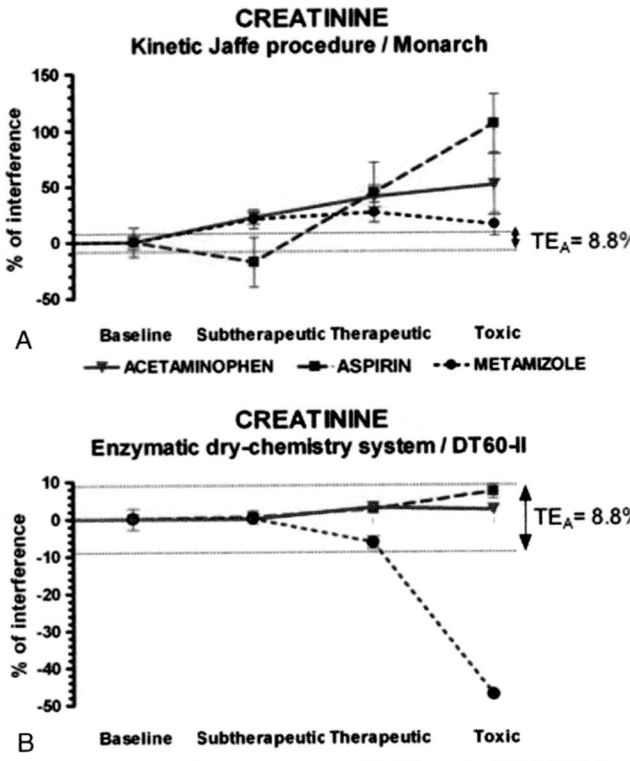

CREATININE
Kinetic Jaffe procedure / Monarch

A

Baseline Subtherapeutic Therapeutic Toxic
ACETAMINOPHEN ASPIRIN METAMIZOLE

CREATININE
Enzymatic dry-chemistry system / DT60-II

B

Baseline Subtherapeutic Therapeutic Toxic
ACETAMINOPHEN ASPIRIN METAMIZOLE

FIGURE 5.11 Analgesic drug interference with creatinine measurement. (A) Interference of acetaminophen, acetylsalicylic acid (aspirin), and metamizole on creatinine measurement by Jaffe method. All tested drugs cause interference error over acceptance criteria based on biological variations (dashed line; total error = 8.8%). (B) Interference of acetaminophen, acetylsalicylic acid (aspirin), and metamizole on creatinine measurement by enzymatic method. Only toxic concentrations of metamizole cause a falsely decreased concentration of creatinine. (Reproduced from Luna-Záizar H, Virgen-Montelongo M, Cortez-Álvarez CR, et al. In vitro interference by acetaminophen, aspirin, and metamizole in serum measurements of glucose, urea, and creatinine. *Clin Biochem* 2015;48:538–44, with permission by Elsevier.)

Ethamsylate is a hemostatic drug indicated in cases of capillary bleeding.[259] This drug causes a significant decrease in creatinine concentration (approximately 50%) measured by enzymatic assay. Interestingly, the Jaffe method is not influenced by ethamsylate. The interference is probably caused by the presence of a hydrochinone structure in the ethamsylate molecule. Hydrochinone interferes in the last reaction of creatinine quantification (see Fig. 5.10A). Therefore the other methods that are using the same indicator reaction are also affected by the administration of this drug. There is evidence that ethamsylate also causes significant false decrease in the concentrations of cholesterol (9.2%), triglycerides (15.6%), and uric acid (15.4%).[260,261] A similar problem with the enzymatic creatinine assay was found in the presence of high concentrations of therapeutically administered catecholamines. Dopamine, dobutamine, epinephrine, and norepinephrine cause strong negative interference with the Creatinine Plus enzymatic (Roche Diagnostics GmbH, Penzberg, Germany) assay. The Vitros (Ortho Clinical Diagnostics) enzymatic creatinine assay demonstrates slight negative interference, while

the i-STAT enzymatic (Abbott) and Jaffe methods (Roche Diagnostics and Siemens [Siemens Healthcare Diagnostics, Munich, Germany]) are unaffected by the presence of therapeutically administered catecholamines.[262]

Due to its hepatotoxicity, eltrombopag, a thrombopoietin receptor agonist used for treatment of immune thrombocytopenia, requires careful monitoring of liver function tests.[263] It has been shown that eltrombopag is a colored drug and as such has the potential to interfere with many routine chemistry spectrophotometric assays. The color of eltrombopag is pH dependent. In alkaline pH, the color of eltrombopag is reddish brown, while it is yellow in acidic pH. Therefore this drug may cause interference with varying degree on different instruments, depending on the assay design and pH of the reaction solution. For example, the pH-dependent color change interferes with the total bilirubin assay and some other routine chemistry tests with varying degree on several chemistry instruments (Beckman Coulter DxC, Roche Cobas, Siemens Advia and Abbott Architect), whereas total bilirubin assay on Beckman Coulter AU analyzer is resistant to this interference due to the existence of separate total and blank channels with identical pH reagents.[263]

Ionized calcium is the best indicator of calcium homeostasis in patients with suspected or known derangements of calcium metabolism.[264] Direct potentiometric determination of ionized calcium is known to be susceptible to the interference caused by several drugs. Degree of positive or negative drug interference is dependent on half-life of drug, specific manufacturer design, and age of the electrode. One such example is the active metabolite of leflunomide (teriflunomide), a synthetic isoxazole-derivative drug with immunosuppressive and antiviral properties, which exerts interference with ionized calcium. In kidney transplant patients treated with leflunomide, low ionized calcium concentrations are sometimes observed without any clinical signs of hypocalcemia. This interference is caused by an active metabolite of leflunomide. Shortly after oral administration, leflunomide is rapidly converted into its active metabolite teriflunomide, which is responsible for this falsely decreased ionized calcium concentration. The interference is dependent on the type of the blood gas analyzer used for the measurement of ionized calcium; it was found to affect the Rapidlab-1265 (Siemens Diagnostics) and i-Stat point-of-care analyzer (Abbott), but not the ABL800-FLEX blood gas analyzer (Radiometer, Copenhagen, Denmark).[265] Because this drug is widely used not only in kidney transplant patients but also in patients with rheumatoid arthritis, every hypocalcemia in laboratories using RAPIDlab or i-Stat point-of-care analyzers should be interpreted with caution and compared with the patient's clinical condition. Unfortunately, this is not the only reported interference for ionized calcium measurement. Sodium perchlorate, which is used as an oral drug to treat hyperthyroidism, causes a significant false decrease in calcium results when using Radiometer and Siemens RAPIDlab POCT instruments for measuring ionized calcium.[266]

Another example of interference with indirect potentiometry is related to electrolyte measurement. Measurement of chloride concentration is important in the management of critically ill patients, where acid-base balance is compromised and information on anion gap is essential for correct patient management. It has been demonstrated that bicarbonates interfere with chloride measured by ISE on Roche cobas 6000 c501 analyzer; the chloride concentration increase is proportional to the bicarbonate concentration.[267]

Thiopental is a barbiturate used for the treatment of increased intracranial pressure. The central laboratory analyzer Dimension Vista (Siemens), which uses the V-LYTE Integrated Multisensor Technology system for electrolyte measurement, produces falsely increased sodium concentrations in the presence of thiopental. However, when the sodium is measured on a point-of-care analyzer using direct potentiometry (RAPIDlab 1200, Siemens), there is no evidence of thiopental interference.[268]

Drug interferences are also observed in coagulation testing. Dabigatran etexilate, a new oral direct thrombin inhibitor, is used as an anticoagulant drug. Application of this drug causes significant bias in many coagulation tests. Dabigatran causes dose-dependent prolongation of PT and aPTT, and thus significantly changes the results of various other coagulation tests, including antithrombin III and coagulation factors II, V, VII, VIII, IX, X, XI, XII, and XIII. Falsely decreased factor activities and falsely positive misdiagnosis of lupus anticoagulant are observed in the presence of dabigatran.[269]

Another example of the interference in coagulation testing is telavancin, an antibiotic used for the treatment of methicillin-resistant *Staphylococcus aureus* (MRSA). Telavancin was found to interact with the artificial phospholipid reagent Dade Behring Innovin for PT measurement, causing falsely decreased values.[270]

Carbohydrate-deficient transferrin (CDT) is a biomarker for long-term alcohol consumption. The evidence shows that the sensitivity of the test for its measurement can be affected by the use of several dugs like amlodipine (calcium channel blocker), perindopril (ACE inhibitor), atorvastatin (statin), isosorbide mononitrate (nitrate), carvedilol (beta blocker), ticlopidine (inhibitor of platelet aggregation), and pantoprazole (gastric acid pump inhibitor).[271] It is still unclear whether the false-negative measurement is a result of polytherapy where unexpected metabolic pathways can be activated. Even if some or all of the drugs are listed as potential interfering substances, manufacturers usually do not declare what effects can occur in vivo when multiple drugs are combined.

The most common drug interferences are reported for urine matrix and most common among them are interferences related to screening for drugs of abuse and dipstick tests. This is why urine drugs of abuse screening for employment or employee control demands confirmatory testing with more reliable methods.[272] Regular use of substances like bupropion, an antidepressant and an aid for smoking cessation, could have an impact on urine drug testing. Bupropion metabolite at concentrations higher than 500 ng/mL cross-reacts with two enzyme-linked immunosorbent assays for urine amphetamine, giving false positive results.[273] Hydrochloroquine, a drug used for rheumatoid arthritis treatment, was also shown to interfere with drugs of abuse urine tests.[274] Long-term, high-dose morphine therapy in hospice patients could cause an appearance of low concentration of hydromorphone in urine, rather as morphine metabolite, than as an indicator of opioid abuse.[275] Quinolone antibiotics and drugs derived from quinine interfere with urine test strip Multistix 10 SG protein detection and with quantitative urine protein test method using pyrogallol red-molibdate.[276] Ciprofloxacin, quinine, and chloroquine in supratherapeutic concentrations and chloroquine in therapeutic concentration

give spurious proteinuria results when using Multistix 10 SG urine tests strips.[277]

Even highly specific and sensitive methods employed for measurement specific analytes in 24-hour urine sample, like high-performance liquid chromatography with electrochemical detection (HPLC/ECD) and liquid chromatography with tandem mass spectrometry (LC-MS/MS), are susceptible to drug interference. Sulfasalazine interference caused falsely high normetanephrine concentration in 24-hour urine sample.[278] Determination of free cortisol concentration in 24-hour urine by liquid chromatography coupled to atmospheric pressure ionization tandem mass spectrometry (LC-ESI-MS/MS) was shown to be affected by the antibiotic piperacillin; one way to circumvent this problem is to adjust urine sampling according to the kinetics of the interfering drug.[279]

Electrophoresis-based methods are also susceptible to this interference and may give false-positive findings, if unrecognized.[280] False positive electrophoresis and serum immunofixation electrophoresis results showing monoclonal IgG-kappa were reported in patients taking ofatumumab, a monoclonal antibody used in the treatment of patients with Waldenstrom macroglobulinemia.[281] Another example is siltuximab, a monoclonal antibody directed to IL-6, intended for treatment of malignancies in clinical trials, which is known to interfere with serum protein electrophoresis. Interference was observed in patients with IgDκ multiple myeloma, who had spurious finding of IgG heavy chain immunoglobulin.[282]

Last, but not the least, interference of monoclonal antibodies used for therapeutic purposes are now receiving increasing attention due to the fast-growing production of antigen-directed monoclonal antibodies which enable targeted, effective, personalized patient treatment. Monoclonal antibodies are used for the treatment of malignancies, autoimmune diseases, transplant-related conditions, and inflammatory diseases. They have a significant impact on different laboratory tests that may lead to diagnostic errors. Most compromised are those methods which utilize monoclonal antibodies such as immunoassays, cytometric analysis, immunohistochemistry assays, etc. One such example is alemtuzumab, therapeutic immunoglobulin which interferes with flow cytometry, giving false positive finding of light chain clonality, thus raising the risk of misdiagnosis of B-cell neoplasms.[283] Another example is a monoclonal anti-CD47 which has been recognized as a promising treatment option for hematologic and solid malignancies. It was observed that it interferes in pretransfusion erythrocyte and platelet compatibility testing.[284] There are also studies reporting the interference of daratumumab, a monoclonal antibody used for the treatment of multiple myeloma, in electrophoretic and immunofixation testing[285-287] and in immunohematologic assays.[288] Other therapeutic monoclonal antibodies have also been known to interfere with serum protein electrophoresis and several strategies for resolving this type of interference have been suggested.[289-291]

It should be pointed out again that this interference depends on the assay and instrument. This has been nicely demonstrated by the College of American Pathologists (CAP) survey aimed to explore the impact of the therapeutic monoclonal antibody omalizumab, intended for treatment of asthma patients, on IgE immunoassay performance. Plasma specimens of atopic patients incubated with omalizumab were sent to 159 laboratories—participants of Allergy Proficiency CAP Survey—and the results have shown that all manufacturers except Pharmacia ImmunoCAP total and specific IgE assays are susceptible to interference by omalizumab.[292]

Potential drug interferences are numerous, and not all of them can be recognized or predicted. The largest available online source for analytical interferences is the *Effects on Clinical Laboratory Tests* series, edited by Young and colleagues.[293,294] This database has compiled the largest body of evidence from the published literature and is the most extensive source of analytical interferences. For example, the database lists 307 results of potential drug interferences for creatinine.

Supportive Medical Therapy

Medical contrast media are used during medical imaging procedures to enhance the contrast of organs and fluids. Iodine-based compounds (iohexol, iodixanol, and ioversol) are mostly used for the x-ray methods, while gadolinium contrast agents (ionic, neutral, albumin-bound, or polymeric) are typically used in magnetic resonance imaging.[194] Due to their specific chemical characteristics, effects of contrast media on laboratory tests cover a broad spectrum, some of which are listed below:

- gel displacement in blood collection tubes
- abnormal peak in electrophoresis
- chemical interference (contrast media interfere with the chemical reaction in various ways)
- chelating effect.

The type and magnitude of interference of the medical contrast media on laboratory tests depend on the agent, its concentration and half-life, mode of application, assay used, and instrument on which specific analyte is measured.

Blood collection from a patient who has recently received iodinated contrast media such as iohexol or iodixanol may cause some serious problems in sample processing, such as needle blockage, if serum/plasma gel separator tubes are used; iodine molecules have high density and can prevent proper formation of the barrier in the serum gel separator tubes. Upon centrifugation, instead of positioning between cell and serum/plasma layer, gel remains on the top and blocks the access of the needle to the serum/plasma.[295–297] This problem may cause considerable disruption in workflow and damage in highly automated laboratories, where visual inspection of the sample, after centrifugation, is not done.

Also, some specific interferences of the medical contrast media with chemistry tests have been observed. Iopromide is used as a contrast media agent in coronary angiography. A false increase in cTnI concentration measured by Opus Magnum reagent (Opus cTnI immunoassay system; Behring Diagnostics, Siemens) is detected if the sample is taken immediately after the procedure. This interference was deemed to be reagent-specific since no similar finding was observed when using cTn assay by a different manufacturer (ACCESS cTnI immunoassay; Beckman Coulter, Tokyo, Japan).[298]

Gadolinium (Gd) contrast agents act as chelators, and that seems to be the main mechanism of their interference with clinical laboratory assays. Gd contrast agents interfere with many clinical chemistry assays such as angiotensin-converting enzyme, total iron-binding capacity, zinc, magnesium, bilirubin, and creatinine.[299–301] Interestingly, calcium measurement is one of the parameters, which is most affected by the presence of Gd-based compounds. Colorimetric calcium assays (o-cresol-phthalein complexone or methylthymol blue) are affected by the presence of gadodiamide, while ion selective electrode and inductively coupled plasma-atomic emission spectroscopy assays can reliably determine calcium concentration.[302–304]

Inductively coupled mass spectrometry (ICP-MS) is often used for the measurement of trace elements (see Chapter 44). There is ample evidence that Gd interferes with ICP-MS measurement of selenium (Se) and causes false increases in patients undergoing magnetic resonance imaging. Ryan and colleagues published a case report of a 30-year-old man with no history of Se exposure or toxicity symptoms who had lethal concentrations of plasma Se measured by ICP-MS.[305] This patient had undergone magnetic resonance imaging with a Gd contrast agent prior to measurement of Se concentration. It was postulated that the Gd^{2+} isotope was causing interference with $^{78}Se^{+}$, the isotope used for the Se measurement, by having an identical mass-to-charge ratio. If this interference is not recognized, potential Se exposure can be suspected for these patients, and the patient could be misdiagnosed and mistreated. To avoid this interference, another Se isotope (^{82}Se) that has a different mass-to-charge ratio, and thus is not affected by Gd, should be measured, or pure hydrogen should be used in the collision cell.[306,307]

Any chemical substance that absorbs light at the same wavelength as the peptide bond (200 nm) has the potential to interfere with protein detection in capillary electrophoresis (CE). Iodinated contrast media may mimic abnormal peaks in α2- or β-globulin fraction on CE, because their absorbance (200 to 275 nm) overlaps with that of protein absorbance (200 nm).[308] The magnitude of the interfering effect largely depends on the compound, its half-life, concentration, time of sampling, and patient kidney function. Due to their short plasma half-life, most contrast media are rapidly eliminated by the kidney in individuals with normal glomerular filtration rate. Therefore in most patients with normal kidney function, interference caused by iodinated contrast media is usually cleared from the serum/plasma 24 hours after the contrast infusion.[309]

To avoid possible interferences caused by contrast media, it is recommended to perform blood/urine sampling before administration of contrast media. If blood collection has to be done after the imaging, care should be taken to allow that sufficient time has elapsed from the application of the contrast media, taking into account the half-life of contrast used and patient renal function. Also, as a precautionary measure, whenever an additional narrow peak on the CE is detected, especially in a patient with impaired kidney function, care should be taken to exclude contrast media as a potential interfering cause. Another electrophoretic evaluation may be done after 24 hours to exclude or confirm this interference.[310]

Natural Preparations

Today, it is becoming more common to use natural preparations for self-medication or supportive therapy. Patients consume herbal and other dietary products, but they fail to report the usage to their doctors or to the laboratory staff during phlebotomy.[311] The influence of these products on laboratory tests is not fully appreciated. Herbal medicines can cause direct interference with immunoassays due to cross-reactivity. Due to their structural similarity to the tested analyte, active compounds that are present in herbal products can react with the antibody in the assay and, based on the structure and design of the immunoassay, result in both falsely increased or decreased analyte concentration. The concept of cross-reactivity in immunoassays is described in more detail in Chapter 26.

Another potential problem is the unexpected reactions since the exact content of these preparations is not always known.[312] Preparations used in Chinese medicine, like Chan Su, can contain some physiologically highly active molecules, like bufadienolides (bufalin, cinobufagin, and resibufogenin) that are extracted from the glands of Chinese toads. This preparation is used for the treatment of a variety of conditions, such as tonsillitis, sore throat, furuncle, and heart palpitations.[313] The structural similarity of bufadienolides and digoxin is responsible for both cardiotoxicity and interference with immunoassays. Ingestion of this medicine can cause both false-positive and false-negative results for digoxin, depending on the assay format. The most affected assays are those using polyclonal antibodies, like fluorescence polarization immunoassay or microparticle enzyme immunoassay; the assays using monoclonal antibodies are also susceptible to interference by bufadienolides.[314,315] Herbal supplements that are used widely throughout the world, like ginseng, can also interfere with digoxin measurement, even though some more recently introduced chemiluminescent microparticle assays seem to be free of such interference.[316,317] Labeling of herbal products may not accurately reflect their content, and adverse events or interactions attributed to a specific herb may be due to misidentification of plants, contamination of plants with pharmaceuticals or heavy metals, or quality control problems. For example, it has been recognized that some Chinese herbal remedies may contain steroids, with the potential of interfering with some assays and causing suppression of the hypothalamic-pituitary-adrenal axis.[318] Similarly, it is also well documented that some Ayurvedic herbal medicine products may be contaminated with lead, with the potential to cause toxicity.[319]

Besides being used for therapeutic purposes in patients with multiple sclerosis and metabolic disorders, biotin is increasingly being used as an over-the-counter dietary supplement to treat hair loss and problems with nails and skin.[320] Supplements are available in doses which are much higher than the recommended daily intake. This increasing trend in high-dose biotin supplementation poses a significant risk for interference in immunoassays. The body of evidence related to this interference is growing and numerous case reports and in vivo and in vitro studies are now available in the literature.[321] The mechanism of biotin interference depends on the format of the immunoassay. In sandwich immunoassays, biotin causes false negative results, whereas in competitive immunoassays it causes false positive results.[322]

Upon ingestion, biotin absorption is rather fast and plasma concentrations peak within 1 to 2 hours. Low-dose elimination half-life is 2 hours and biotin is cleared almost completely from the circulation of healthy individuals within 8 hours. Regular daily biotin supplementation leads to the accumulation of biotin in the body and steady state is usually achieved on the third day. In patients on high doses of biotin supplementation, half-life may be as long as 18 to 19 hours.[323]

In order to prevent unfavorable outcomes, in vitro diagnostics manufacturers were encouraged to conduct additional interference studies and update their instructions for use with warnings about potential biotin interference and biotin threshold for interference, while reformulation of the assays was suggested as a long-term solution of the problem.[324]

Several approaches have been suggested when biotin interference is suspected[323,325]:

- to re-analyze the sample using a different, biotin-free immunoassay
- to dilute the sample, with the dedicated assay diluent
- to remove the excess of biotin by the use of streptavidin-coated beads
- to measure the concentration of biotin in the sample (if such method is available)
- to repeat the analysis after the wash-out period (minimum of 8 hours in patients taking 5 to 10 mg biotin daily, and $\geq$ 72 hours in patients who are prescribed a high-dose biotin therapy, i.e., $\geq$ 100 mg/day). Patients with impaired kidney function would need a longer wash-out period.

Accidental Exposures and Poisonings

In the case of accidental poisonings with herbs, household cleaning products, or any other exogenous compounds, interferences with laboratory test results can potentially delay the diagnostic procedures in acute patient care and cause harm to the patient. Due to their structural similarity to the digoxin molecule, cardiotonic glycosides can interfere with the digoxin measurement. Numerous cases of poisonings by cardiac glycoside–containing plants like lily of the valley (*Convallaria majalis*) or oleander (*Nerium oleander*) are reported. Ingestion of oleander is potentially fatal due to the cardiotoxicity of its active component, oleandrin. Positive and negative interferences of oleandrin and oleander extract on a Loci digoxin assay using the Vista 1500 analyzer have been reported.[326] Convallatoxin is a glycoside extracted from *Convallaria majalis*. Due to the significant cross-reactivity between convallatoxin and digoxin, the digoxin assay was suggested to be used as a screening tool for the detection of convallatoxin ingestion.[327]

Accidental intoxications often occur as a result of children ingesting cleaning products commonly found in the home. Miniature racing cars run on nitromethane, which has been shown to interfere with creatinine measurement, producing a falsely increased concentration.[328–330] Nitromethane is also used in racing cars to enhance combustion. Extreme creatinine concentration (8270 μmol/L; 93.6 mg/dL) without evident renal failure has been observed in a suicide attempt in which Blue Thunder fuel containing nitromethane was ingested.[331] In a Jaffe method, nitromethane also reacts with alkaline picrate and forms a red chromophore with absorbance similar to the creatinine picrate chromophore. This reaction causes falsely increased creatinine concentration. When an enzymatic assay is used (as opposed to Jaffe), creatinine can be accurately measured in the presence of nitromethane.[332,333]

Laboratory professionals should be alerted by any unexpected result and discuss it with the clinical staff. If the source of suspected interference cannot be determined, laboratories should try to involve manufacturers of the reagents to identify the potential interfering substance and quantify its effect.

Sample Contaminants

Blood samples can be contaminated by several different exogenous substances during phlebotomy, sample handling, or even test measurement. Several components of the blood collection systems (i.e., blood tube, needle, holder) can interfere with the measurement and influence laboratory results, including lubricants, needles, surfactants, separator gels, clot activators, and anticoagulants.[133]

Tube additives. Needles are made of stainless steel, which contains a minimum of 11% of chromium, to prevent oxidative needle corrosion. Due to the leaching of chromium into the sample, falsely increased chromium concentrations may be observed.[334] Lubricants like silicone oils and glycerol facilitate insertion and removal of the stoppers. Glycerol should not be used for the lubrication of stoppers in tubes that will be used for triglyceride measurement because glycerol interferes with most triglyceride assays.[335] Silicone-based lubricants are less likely to interfere with assays, although silicone can falsely increase ionized magnesium and T3 concentrations.[336] Additional peaks in mass spectrometry in the presence of silicone-based lubricants can interfere with interpretation of results.[337] Plastic tubes require clot activators to ensure rapid clot formation. Some clot activators based on silica particles affect the measurement of some analytes like lithium[338] and testosterone.[339] Bovine thrombin in some serum tubes causes falsely decreased parathyroid hormone concentration.[340] Silicone surfactants used to decrease nonspecific adsorption of components on tube walls may interfere with measurement of vitamin B12 and cancer antigen 15-3.[336]

Separator gels. Separator gels are used to ensure rapid and prolonged separation of serum and plasma from clotted blood and cells, respectively. Sample separation is enabled by the specific gravity of the gel (1.03–1.06 kg/L), its ability to undergo a temporary change in viscosity during centrifugation, and its ability to lodge between the packed cells and the top serum/plasma layer.[134]

Hydrophobic compounds may bind to the gel, which is why tubes containing separator gels are not appropriate for some hydrophobic drugs and hormones such as the following[341–344]:
1. Drugs: phenytoin, phenobarbital, carbamazepine, tricyclic antidepressants, quinidine, lidocaine
2. Hormones: testosterone, estradiol, cortisol, fT4, fT3.

Due to differences in the gel composition among different manufacturers, it is quite possible that one manufacturer's gel tube may be used for a particular analyte but not another.

Moreover, if kept under improper storage conditions (time and temperature), the gel may degrade and release small particles or globules into the supernatant. These particles may affect instrument performance by interfering with the sample probe, coating the inner surface of the reaction cuvettes, and causing interference in immunoassays.[133] It is therefore important to strictly follow recommendations provided by the tube manufacturers on the appropriate storage and handling of gel tubes.

Anticoagulants. Although serum is still the predominant sample type in clinical chemistry testing worldwide, more laboratories are transitioning from the use of serum to plasma because of the shorter plasma separation time, greater plasma yield, and the ability to eliminate the problem of fibrin clots formation.[345] Particularly for urgent or stat testing, such as for cardiac markers, plasma has always been the preferred specimen.[346] Nevertheless, due to the interfering effect of some plasma additives (EDTA, heparin, sodium citrate) with some cardiac markers assays, serum is an acceptable alternative.

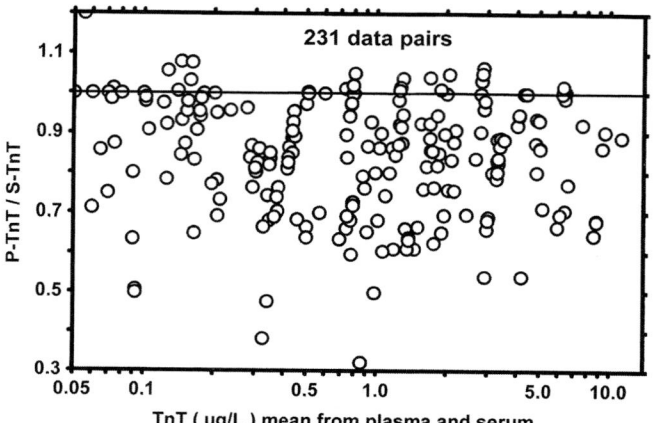

FIGURE 5.12 Differences (ratio) in the concentration of cardiac troponin T (cTnT) in plasma versus serum (P-TnT/S-TnT) relative to the average troponin concentrations in plasma and serum (log transformed and presented as natural logarithm). (From Gerhardt W, Nordin G, Herbert AK, Burzell BL, Isaksson A, Gustavsson E, et al. Troponin T and I assays show decreased concentrations in heparin plasma compared with serum: Lower recoveries in early than in late phase of myocardial injury. *Clin Chem* 2000;46:817–21, with permission by American Association for Clinical Chemistry.)

Heparin interferes with numerous immunoassays by affecting the binding of antibody and antigen and thus affecting the rate of reaction.[133] Heparinized plasma has been documented to cause significant negative bias (up to 30%) in cTn results with some earlier-generation cTn assays from different manufacturers.[347,348] The observed bias did not correlate with the concentration of cTn (Fig. 5.12). Heparin interference occurs due to its negative charge and its binding to positively charged cTn. Binding of heparin and cTn leads to the conformational change of cTn and affects the antibody-antigen interaction. This interference was neutralized in the fourth-generation cTnT assay by adding cationic heparin blocking agent to the assay's mixture, although in certain cases there is still poor comparability between serum and plasma values.[349] For this reason, it is essential that the sample type for cTn testing remain consistent within a given patient.[350]

EDTA is a commonly used additive, especially in hematology and in some countries in endocrinology, because it offers increased stability of cells and analytes.[351] Most hormones (except adrenocorticotropic hormone or ACTH) are stable for up to 5 days in EDTA plasma if they are kept refrigerated at 4 °C.[352] The main action of EDTA is chelation of cations (e.g., calcium, magnesium, and zinc). If EDTA is present in higher concentrations in the sample (when tubes are underfilled), its chelating activity is enhanced. This may lead to interferences in some chemiluminescence immunoassays that use conjugated ALP as a secondary enzyme in their reactions. For example, it has been shown that underfilling the EDTA tubes by half or more causes clinically significant bias (the reported concentration was <75% of the true value) in the measurement of intact parathyroid hormone with the DPC IMMULITE assay.[353]

Potassium oxalate also acts as calcium chelating anticoagulant and is often combined with antiglycolytic agents (sodium fluoride and sodium iodoacetate). As with EDTA, oxalate can also inhibit some enzymes (e.g., amylase, LD, ALP) by chelating bivalent cations that are necessary for their activity.[134]

Intravenous fluids. Contamination of blood sample with intravenous fluids is often caused by inadequate volume of discarded blood prior to sampling from a catheter or canula. This could cause a considerable effect on results of hematology, biochemistry, and coagulation tests, depending on the type of administered intravenous fluid. One example is a trisodium citrate solution (Citra-Lock solution), commonly used in dialysis catheters to prevent infection and thrombosis between dialysis sessions, which contains 35 times higher sodium concentration than serum. Sample contamination with a trisodium citrate solution may lead to gross hypernatremia with sodium results up to five times higher than the upper reference interval. To avoid the risk of contamination, first draw should be discarded when collecting a sample from a vascular access device (VAD).[354]

Other Mechanisms of Interference
Formation of Fibrin Clots
Under optimal clotting conditions, serum is considered to be free of fibrin, fibrinogen, and cells, and it is a preferred matrix for most immunoassays. To allow complete clot formation, serum tubes should be allowed to stand for a minimum of 30 minutes. This delay, which is due to clotting time, is a major shortcoming for serum use, especially in emergency settings. However, with new tube types containing clot activators (thrombin-based clotting agent), serum clotting time is substantially reduced (on average <2.5 minutes) without compromising the sample quality and stability for most chemistry analytes.[355,356]

Blood from patients who are receiving heparin therapy may require a longer time to completely clot, and there is a greater likelihood for latent post-centrifugation clot formation. Insoluble fibrin has been found in both serum and plasma.[357–360] Insoluble fibrin, fibrin strands, and microclots formed as a result of delayed and latent clotting may affect instrument performance and cause interferences. Some analyzers have the ability to detect clots and flag such samples for rerun, but if this feature is not available on the instrument being used, clots may interfere with assays and cause erroneous results and unnecessary delays.

If fibrin is aspirated for analysis and goes undetected, there is a high likelihood of getting false-positive results for that sample.[357] This is manifested by duplicate measurement errors (i.e., unacceptable deviations in two measurements on the same sample). The false-positive result is caused by the nonspecific binding of insoluble fibrin strands present in the sample. Duplicate errors due to latent clotting or incomplete fibrin removal during centrifugation have been repeatedly reported for cTn measurements (Fig. 5.13), and laboratories have been implementing different strategies to minimize the risk of reporting erroneous cTn results due to fibrin clots.[361,362] A possible approach is to recentrifuge all positive cTn samples (e.g., cTnI concentration >0.1 mg/L, measured on DxI 800 analyzer, Beckman Coulter) at a high speed (6700 g for 5 min) and then repeat the analysis.[363] This approach, however, has been questioned by some authors and is not widely implemented.[364] Another approach employs a reflex rule to analyze samples in duplicate whenever the result is below or above some predefined value (e.g., cTnI concentration <0.04 or >5.00 µg/L). If a reflex measurement exceeds the limits of acceptance (>20%), an aliquot is recentrifuged and the sample is reanalyzed.[357]

Unfortunately, many instruments cannot consistently detect and appropriately respond to samples of questionable quality due to residual and latent fibrin strands. Until the quality of blood collection systems and instrument performance is improved, laboratory professionals must stringently monitor reported results and implement corrective strategies to minimize the risk of such preanalytical errors.

Interference Caused by Sample Carryover
Sample carryover in automated analyzers occurs as a result of inefficient probe and cuvette washing and the subsequent inability of an instrument to successfully remove any remnants of the sample or reagent. Due to improper washing, a certain amount of reagent or analyte can be transferred (carried) by the measuring system from one assay reaction to a subsequent reaction, thereby erroneously affecting test results. Those instruments that do not use disposable probes are more susceptible to carryover problems with some highly sensitive assays. Carryover is, of course, not unique to immunoassays and may occur in all assay types. Nevertheless, the effect of carryover is more pronounced in sensitive assays, such as highly sensitive immunoassays and in assays measuring analytes with a very wide range of concentrations.

Sample carryover has been reported for the Enzymun-Test CEA assay on the ES-300 automated immunochemistry instrument (Boehringer-Mannheim, Germany).[365] Carryover was observed in samples being tested subsequent to those with extremely high CEA concentrations.

Though not confirmed by all participating laboratories in the study,[366] sample carryover as a cause of faulty results was also reported for cTnI on Beckman Access 2, UniCel DxI600, and UniCel DxI800 immunochemistry analyzers (Beckman Coulter, Inc.). Specimens with extremely high cTn concentrations have been causing false increases that resulted in clinically significant changes in subsequent patients tested for cTnI.[367,368] To mitigate this problem, a reflex rule may be implemented to reanalyze cTnI in two subsequent specimens. Also, additional probe and cuvette washing may be performed after extremely high results that are associated with an increased risk of carryover.

Finally, it is highly recommended that laboratories perform testing for interferences due to sample carryover where evidence for the absence of an analyte is of clinical importance (i.e., at the limit of quantification), such as cardiac markers, tumor markers, and infectious disease (e.g., hepatitis) markers.

According to International Union of Pure and Applied Chemistry (IUPAC), sample carryover testing is performed by running one sample with high concentration of an analyte at least two times, followed by at least three runs of a sample with low concentration of that analyte.[369] If the instrument probe washing procedure is not done correctly, the results in the sample with low analyte concentration will be higher, and subsequent results will show a gradually decreasing pattern. The performance of the cuvette washing procedure is somewhat more difficult to assess because it may require multiple runs of a sample with high and low analyte concentrations (the exact number of runs depends on the number of cuvettes).[173]

According to CLSI, carryover testing for immunoassays is done by running four consecutive analyses of two samples at different concentrations (samples with extremely high analyte concentrations (A), followed by samples with very low

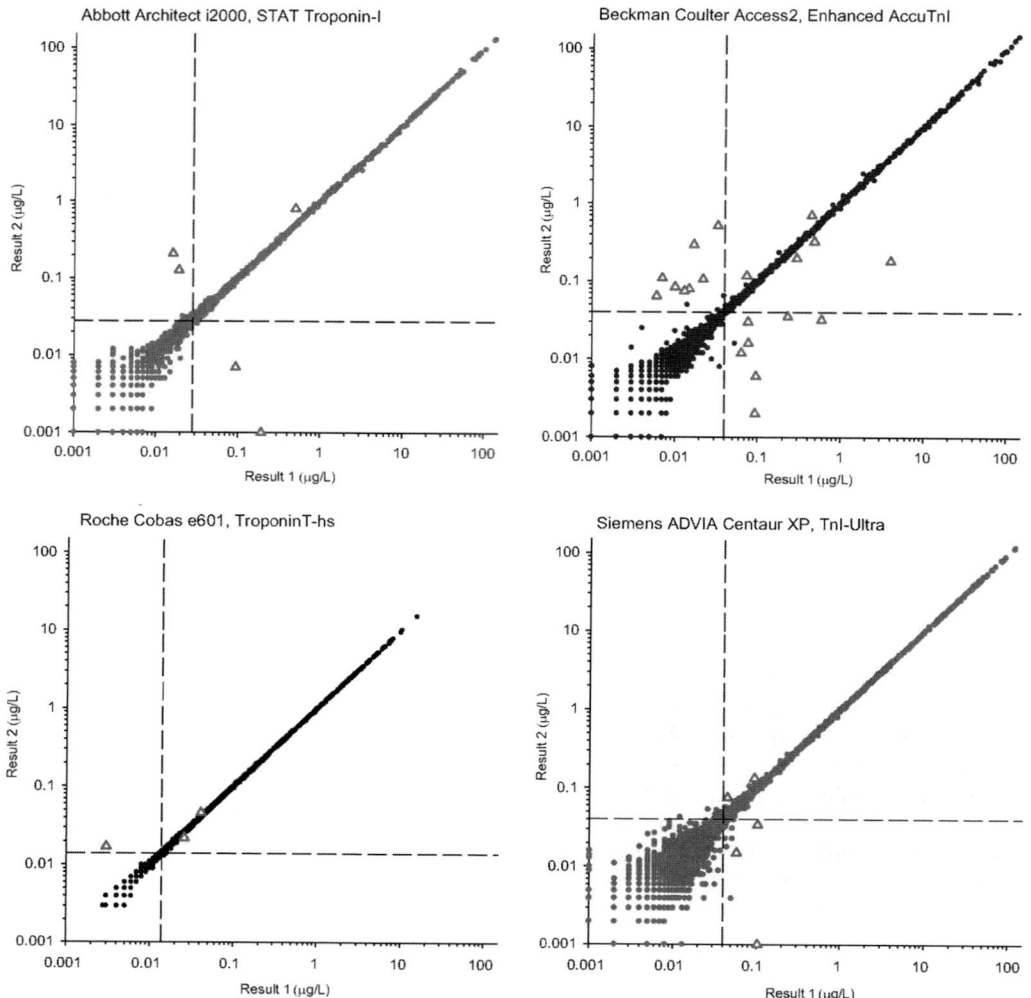

FIGURE 5.13 Distribution of duplicate results for cardiac troponin measurement on four analyzers for a series of duplicate measurements in 2391 patient sera. Samples were analyzed with (1) Abbott Architect i2000SR analytical system with STAT Troponin-I reagent (Abbott Diagnostics); (2) Beckman Coulter Access2 analyzer with Enhanced AccuTnI reagent; (3) Roche Cobas e601 with TroponinT hs reagent (Roche Diagnostics); and (4) Siemens ADVIA Centaur XP with TnI-Ultra reagent (Siemens Healthcare Diagnostics). Dashed line marks the 99th percentile, as declared by the manufacturer. Red triangles represent outliers. (From Pretorius CJ, Dimeski G, O'Rourke PK, Marquart L, Tyack SA, Wilgen U, Ungerer JP. Outliers as a cause of false cardiac troponin results: Investigating the robustness of four contemporary assays. *Clin Chem* 2011;57:710–8, with permission by American Association for Clinical Chemistry.)

(B) concentrations for the same analyte).[370] The order of samples may be as follows:

$$A1, A2, A3, A4, B1, B2, B3, B4$$

According to the IUPAC protocol, carryover is expressed as the amount of analyte transferred from sample A2 to sample B1 (Fig. 5.14),

$$\text{Carryover, }\% = 100 \times (B1 - B3)/(A2 - B3)$$

Interference Caused by Antibiotics

Antibiotics are commonly added into reagents and buffer solutions to prevent microbial growth. Carryover from reagents containing gentamicin may cause spuriously high gentamicin results. Gentamicin is present in some diagnostic reagents

(glucose, urate, direct bilirubin, CK, ALT, AST, betahydroxybutyrate) as an antibacterial additive and is known to cause spuriously high gentamicin results on the Beckman Coulter AU480 analyzer (Beckman Coulter, Inc.) due to reagent carryover.[371,372] Therefore gentamicin measurement should be processed in a separate batch (i.e., before or after the measurement of any of the listed parameters) to prevent carryover.

SPECIFIC CONSIDERATIONS

Besides the general features of preanalytical quality (i.e., patient and sample identification, controllable and noncontrollable variables), some specific aspects related to urine, saliva, and blood gas testing are of particular relevance to laboratory medicine. The following sections examine the preanalytical

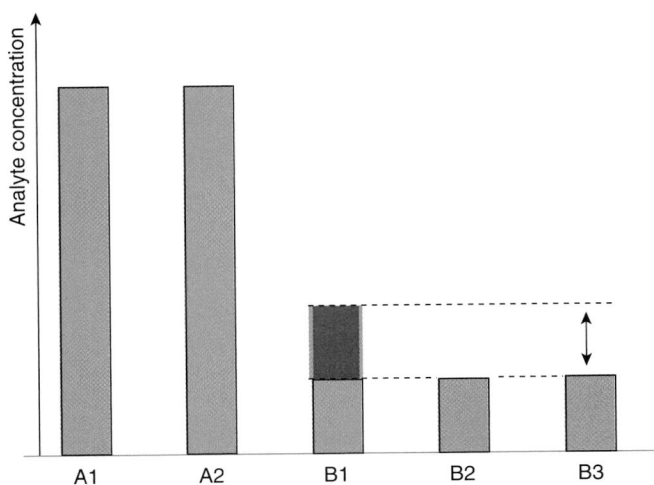

FIGURE 5.14 Carryover analysis. Samples A1 and A2 Have a high concentration of an analyte. Samples B1, B2, and B3 have a low concentration of the same analyte. The red rectangle depicts the amount of an analyte transferred from sample A2 to sample B1.

TABLE 5.12 Urine Specimens and Their Diagnostic Use	
Urine Type	**Use**
First morning urine	Qualitative urinalysis
Second morning urine	Proteins measurement, urinalysis
Timed urine (6–24 h)	Hormones and drugs measurement and detection
First void urine	Chlamydia
Midstream urine	Urinalysis, microbiological examination
Urine obtained through a catheter or sterile suprapubic aspiration	Exclusion and confirmation of urinary tract infection

aspects of sample types other than serum and plasma, and other types of testing that deserve special preanalytical considerations. For additional discussion on body fluids, refer to Chapter 45.

Urine

Urine composition is usually more variable and exhibits a broader reference interval compared to plasma.[373] Fluid intake, feeding, starvation, and muscular activity all influence the excreted amounts of urine constituents. Immobilization has also been shown to affect calcium excretion.[374] Calcium excretion increased 2.5-fold over 6 weeks of immobilization, reflecting bone degradation, and returned to normal when the patient was remobilized.[29]

Some of the most important preanalytical issues in the analysis of urine relate to patient preparation, choice of urine type, type of collection vessel, sample stability during transport and storage, sample homogeneity, and sample contamination.[375,376] These aspects are covered below.

Types of Urine

Not every urine sample is suitable for every type of laboratory testing. Whereas some samples are well suited for hormone or drug testing, other types are appropriate for microbiological examinations. The possible types of urine samples and their intended uses are described in Table 5.12.

When collecting urine specimens and to prevent contamination with bacteria that normally reside on the skin, hygiene of the hands and genitalia is essential. Hands should be washed with soap, thoroughly rinsed with water, and dried. The positive predictive value of urinalysis for urinary tract infection is significantly higher and the contamination rate is much lower in urine specimens collected after proper hand and genital hygiene.[377] Thorough rinsing is also extremely important because baby soaps, for example, are known to cause significant interference with tetrahydrocannabinol (THC) immunoassays.[378] To prevent sample contamination by skin microorganisms, it is very important not to touch the inner surface of the cap and the container during collection.

Urine should be collected while holding the skin folds (labia) apart (females) or retracting the foreskin (uncircumcised men) during voiding.

First morning urine (also called "overnight" or "early morning" specimen) is collected immediately after arising from bed. In the cases of patients who suffer from insomnia or work the night shift, another 8-hour period can be used for first morning urine collection. It is important that the patient's bladder is emptied immediately before going to sleep and that any amount of urine voided during the night is also collected and added to the first morning voided specimen.[379]

Timed urine specimens are collected at a specified time or in relation to some activity (before a meal, after a meal, before therapy, after exercise, etc.) during the 24-hour period. The exact time of the collection should always be indicated in the test report.

First void urine comprises the first portion of the urine (usually the first 15 to 50 mL) voided at any time of the day. It is collected after a patient has not urinated for at least 1 to 2 hours. The exact time depends on the sensitivity of the actual test method and is usually designated on the method insert sheet.

Midstream urine (also called a "clean catch specimen") is a urine specimen collected during the middle of a urine flow after the urinary opening has been carefully cleaned. The first few drops of urine should go into the toilet. This prevents contamination with skin, vaginal, or urethral cells and bacteria. The midstream of the urine is collected, and once the container is filled, the rest of urine is voided into the toilet until the bladder is emptied.

Suprapubic aspiration and catheterization are procedures that are usually used in bacteriologic studies to obtain uncontaminated bladder urine. A catheter specimen is collected after inserting a catheter into the bladder through the urethra. A suprapubic specimen is collected by aspirating urine from the distended bladder through the abdominal wall. Both collection methods use sterile techniques and serve as an alternative to traditional methods of obtaining urine due to their high sensitivity and low risk of contamination.

Patient Preparation and Sampling

European Urinalysis Guidelines provide recommendations on the proper patient preparation and sampling techniques to ensure the most accurate and reliable test results.[373] It is the responsibility of the laboratory to explain to a patient why a urine specimen needs to be collected and provide correct information regarding optimal preparation and sampling procedure. Proper interpretation of laboratory reports is possible only if these conditions are fulfilled. Patients should be informed of all practical aspects of urine sampling and the possible effects of diet and fluid intake, diuresis, exercise, and other interferents.

The ideal container for any urine specimen is a wide-mouthed bottle of appropriate size. Containers should be clean, inert, leakproof, particle-free, and preferably made of a clear, disposable material that is inert with regard to urinary constituents.[379] The use of various "re-used" home items are discouraged, as they may lead to erroneous results due to the interaction of bottle material, detergent, or remnant bottle content with the urinary constituents.[373] If the urine is to be transported, the container should have a secure lid that will not leak during transport. If the urine is to be analyzed bacteriologically, the container must be sterile.

Nonspecific adsorption of various compounds (hormones, drugs, and proteins) to container surfaces in which the samples are collected, stored, or processed can cause analyte losses and affect the accuracy of quantification methods.[380,381] This is especially significant for protein analytes present in urine in low concentrations. For example, at low albumin concentrations, the adsorption of albumin to the surface of the urine container can cause a significant relative loss.[382] Analyte absorption to the vessel wall is avoided, or at least minimized, by the addition of some agents that either increase analyte solubility or minimize the interaction of analytes with the surface of a urine container.[383]

For pediatric and newborn patients, urine specimen collection bags with hypoallergenic skin adhesive should be used. First, the pubic and perineal areas should be cleaned with soap and water. Then the adhesive strip should be pressed all around the vagina or the bag fixed over the penis and the flaps pressed to the perineum.

Transport and Storage of the Sample

Because some urine parameters have limited stability in unpreserved urine, temperature and time conditions during transport and storage of urine are of utmost importance for adequate sample quality. The stability of different particles in urine (Table 5.13) and test strip parameters (Table 5.14) is limited and decreases during prolonged storage and at higher temperatures.

Urine samples may be stored for up to 1 hour at room temperature and up to 4 hours if refrigerated without significant variation in the results of the physical, chemical, and morphologic analyses of particles.[373,384] With prolonged storage, urine particles lyse and bacteria grow. Bacterial growth causes the increase of urine pH. The stability of urine particles is lower in urine with alkaline pH (vegetarian diet), low relative density, and low osmolality (polyuria). Also, some preservatives (e.g., ethanol, polyethylene glycol, sodium fluoride, mercuric chloride, boric acid, formaldehyde- and formate-based solutions, etc.) may enhance the stability of urine particles.

As a general rule, if test strip analysis is performed within 2 to 4 hours from urine collection and urine has been kept at room temperature, preservatives for chemical constituents examined with test strips are not necessary. In unrefrigerated urine, bacterial growth may occur, leading to false-positive test strip results.

The addition of stabilizers inhibits the bacterial growth, metabolic processes, and degradation of urine analytes and

TABLE 5.13 Stability of Urine Particles at Different Storage Conditions (Temperatures)

Particle	−20 °C	4–8 °C	20–25 °C
Red blood cell	NA	1–4 h	1–24 h (>300 mOsmol/kg)
White blood cell	NA	1–4 h	1 h (pH >7.5) to 24 h (pH <6.5)
Acanthocytes	NA	2 days	1 day (>300 mOsmol/kg)
Casts	Not allowed	NA	2 days
Bacteria	NA	24 h	1–2 h
Epithelial cells	NA	NA	3 h

NA, Data not available.
From Delanghe J, Speeckaert M. Preanalytical requirements of urinalysis. *Biochem Med* 2014;24:89–104, with permission by Croatian Society of Medical Biochemistry and Laboratory Medicine.

TABLE 5.14 Effect of Urine Storage Temperature on Chemical Constituents Examined by Urine Test Strips

Analyte	4–8 °C	20–25 °C
Red blood cells	1–3 h	4–8 h
White blood cells	1 day	1 day
Proteins	NA	>2 h (unstable at pH >7.5)
Glucose	2 h	<2 h
Nitrites	8 h	4 days

NA, Data not available.
From Delanghe J, Speeckaert M. Preanalytical requirements of urinalysis. *Biochem Med* 2014;24:89–104, with permission by Croatian Society of Medical Biochemistry and Laboratory Medicine.

TABLE 5.15 Stability of Urine Particles in the Most Commonly Used Urinary Preservatives

Particle	Borate + Formate + Sorbitol	10 mL/L Formaline 0.15 mol/L NaCl	80 mL/L Ethanol + 20 g/L PEG
Red blood cell	Good	Not good	Not good
White blood cell	Very good	Very good	Very good
Casts	Good	Not good	Not good
Epithelial cells	Very good	Good	Not good
Bacteria	Very good	Very good	Good

From Delanghe J, Speeckaert M. Preanalytical requirements of urinalysis. *Biochem Med* 2014;24:89–104, with permission by Croatian Society of Medical Biochemistry and Laboratory Medicine.

particles. While the addition of some preservatives and the use of commercially available preservative tubes may be beneficial if sample transport time is more than 2 hours, it must be kept in mind that these preservatives can affect some chemical properties of the urine and particle integrity.[385] It is therefore important to select appropriate preservatives, taking into account potential effects on the analyte of interest. Table 5.15 provides data on the influence of the most

TABLE 5.16 The Influence of Preservatives on the Stability of Some Chemical Constituents Examined by Urine Test Strips

Analyte	Boric Acid	Formaldehyde	Hg Salts	Chloral Hexidine
Red blood cells	Stabilization	No stabilization	Stabilization	Limited stabilization
White blood cells	No stabilization	No stabilization	Limited stabilization	Limited stabilization
Proteins	No stabilization	Stabilization	Stabilization	Stabilization
Glucose	No stabilization	No stabilization	No stabilization	No stabilization
pH	No stabilization	No stabilization	No stabilization	No stabilization
Bacteria	Stabilization	Stabilization	Stabilization	Stabilization

From Delanghe J, Speeckaert, M. Preanalytical requirements of urinalysis. *Biochem Med* 2014;24:89–104 with permission by Croatian Society of Medical Biochemistry and Laboratory Medicine.

common preservatives on the stability of urine particles. Data about the influence of preservatives on the stability of some chemical constituents examined by urine test strips are provided in Table 5.16.

POINTS TO REMEMBER

Urine
- The contamination rate is much lower in urine specimens collected after proper hand and genital hygiene.
- Laboratories should provide instructions to patients about reasons for urine collection, how to prepare for urine sampling (e.g., effects of diet and fluid intake, diuresis, exercise, and other interferents), and how to properly collect urine.
- The stability of different analytes in urine is limited and decreases during prolonged storage and at higher temperatures.
- Preservatives like ethanol, polyethylene glycol, sodium fluoride, mercuric chloride, boric acid, and formaldehyde- and formate-based solutions may enhance the stability of urine particles.
- The addition of urine stabilizers inhibits the bacterial growth, metabolic processes, and degradation of urine analytes and particles.

Saliva

Saliva is produced by the major salivary glands (parotid, submandibular, and sublingual glands) and by oral secretion of the mucus by hundreds of minor salivary glands. The major function of saliva is to provide oral protection by lubrication, digestion, and immune response.[386] Saliva is an attractive alternative to blood because it is collected noninvasively. As a diagnostic sample, saliva offers many advantages and some challenges (Box 5.1).

Today, saliva is increasingly used for assessing the genetic susceptibility to various conditions and for testing numerous analytes, as shown in Table 5.17.[387,388]

Types of Saliva Samples

The easiest way to collect saliva is to collect whole oral fluid (whole saliva). Whole saliva is representative of the oral milieu. However, depending on the intended aim of the sample collection and analyte to be tested, some other sample types are also possible. Various sampling techniques and devices

BOX 5.1 Advantages and Challenges of Using Saliva as a Diagnostic Specimen

Advantages
- Rapid and easy collection by minimally trained individuals
- Sampling can be done by patients, at home, or outside hospital
- Multiple sample collection is possible
- Procedure is safe and painless for the patient
- Convenient in children, psychiatric patients, and stress research
- Availability
- Low cost associated with sampling (skilled staff not required)
- Convenient method for population screening programs
- Low risk of infections associated with sampling

Challenges
- Low analyte concentration
- Some analytes may be affected by circadian cycle
- Questionable recovery for some analytes
- Risk of contamination during collection
- Difficult sampling and low patient compliance (in small children).

are available. Whereas collection of whole oral fluid is an easy procedure, other sampling methods are more complicated, require trained staff, and are not commonly used.[389] See Chapter 4.

Whole saliva may be collected as both unstimulated and stimulated samples. Stimulation of saliva is obtained by oral movements (yawning, chewing gum) or by the use of a cotton ball soaked with citric acid. It must be noted that stimulated and unstimulated saliva are of different origins (produced by different salivary glands) and compositions (concentration of some analytes may vary) and are thus not equally suitable for all assays.[390] Unstimulated saliva is mostly produced by the submandibular glands, while stimulated saliva predominantly originates from the parotid glands.[391] Moreover, saliva stimulated by citric acid has a much lower pH (~3.0), and this may affect antigen antibody binding and interfere with immunoassays.[392]

Several commercially available devices may be used for the collection of saliva. Unstimulated whole saliva can be collected by passive drooling into a plastic vial or spitting into a collector vial. Passive drooling is considered by many to be the gold standard collection method for many analytes because it enables collection of a representative portion of saliva

TABLE 5.17 Suitability of Different Specimen Types for Downstream Analyses

	Whole Blood	Plasma	Serum	Buffy Coat	ACP	DBS	Urine	Saliva
Chemistry		✓	✓			✓	✓	✓
Hematology	✓					✓	✓	
Coagulation		✓						
Glucose	✓	✓				✓	✓	✓
Hemoglobin A$_{1c}$	✓					✓		
Hormones		✓	✓			✓	✓	✓
Inflammation		✓	✓			✓	✓	✓
Cytokines			✓			✓	✓	✓
Vitamins			✓			✓		
Live cells				✓				
Proteomics		✓	✓			✓	✓	✓
Metabolomics		✓	✓			✓	✓	✓
Genomics/germline DNA	✓			✓	✓	✓	✓	✓
ccfDNA		✓					✓	✓
Transcriptomics/mRNA	✓			✓		✓	✓	✓
miRNA (circulating)		✓	✓				✓	✓

ACP, All-cell pellet; *ccfDNA,* circulating cell-free DNA; *DBS,* dried blood spot; *miRNA,* microRNA.
From Ellervik C, Vaught J. Preanalytical variables affecting the integrity of human biospecimens in biobanking. *Clin Chem* 2015;61:914–34, with permission by American Association for Clinical Chemistry.

in the oral cavity.[393] Moreover, passive drooling is preferred over spitting because saliva collected by spitting is more likely to be contaminated with bacteria.[394]

Stimulated saliva can be obtained by adsorbing saliva with cotton balls, cotton swabs, or filter paper. Cotton is not an ideal collection material because of its unpleasant texture and because it may induce some variations in salivary immunoassays (some analytes are difficult to elute from cotton). To address this problem, some synthetic materials were made available, like inert polymers, polystyrene, rayon, and polyester.[389] Saliva is collected by placing the cotton ball in the patient's mouth. Placement of the ball or swab may vary depending on the analyte of interest. The ball is gently chewed for a couple of minutes and then placed in the vial. Saliva is obtained from the ball by centrifugation or expressed by a syringe. It must be emphasized that the composition of saliva collected by the use of various adsorbent devices may differ from the whole saliva because adsorbent devices mostly collect localized saliva. It is therefore important to be well aware of the collection method, its characteristics, and its performance.

Saliva collection in the elderly may be challenging, mostly due to xerostomia (dry mouth), which is quite common in the geriatric population, and low compliance. Challenges characteristic to infants and small children include the following[392]:
- Irregular cycles of sleep and periods of being awake
- Frequent napping (small babies often fall asleep, even during collection)
- Residue from liquids (e.g., milk in babies, juices in children) in the patient's mouth
- Food residue in an infant's mouth
- Anxiety about strangers (in children)
- Low compliance

Patient Preparation for Saliva Sampling

The laboratory is responsible for providing information to the patient about the purpose of saliva collection, as well as how to prepare for collection and how to collect saliva. Gloves should be worn during saliva collection to avoid sample contamination. Here are some important measures to minimize errors and ensure a high-quality saliva sample:
- If not otherwise decided by the requesting physician, saliva should be collected in the morning, preferably in the fasting state (the exact time of collection is important because some analytes may have diurnal variations).
- The patient should wash his or her face with water and soap and rinse it thoroughly to avoid contamination with facial creams and lotions.
- The patient should not consume alcohol 12 hours before the collection.
- The patient should not brush or floss his or her teeth at least 30 minutes before the collection.
- The patient should not have any dental work done 2 days before the collection (dental bleeding may affect test results).
- The patient should not ingest any food or drink (except water) within 30 minutes before the collection.
- The patient should not chew gum for at least 30 minutes before collection.
- Before the collection, the patient should rinse his or her mouth with water to remove any food particles. To avoid sample dilution with water, the sample should be collected 10 to 15 minutes after rinsing the mouth.

Any sample that is visibly contaminated with blood or food remnants should be rejected for analysis, and sample recollection should be requested.

Storage of Saliva

After taking the sample, the saliva should be properly stored to prevent bacterial growth and protein degradation and to maintain sample integrity. Storage recommendation depends on the intended use of the saliva and duration of storage (Table 5.18). Some additives may also be used to inhibit the protease activity and retard bacterial growth (sodium azide).[387]

TABLE 5.18 Recommendations for Different Storage Conditions for Saliva Specimens

Storage Condition	Storage Time
Room temperature	30–90 min
+4 °C	3–6 h
−80 °C	Several months

From Chiappin S, Antonelli G, Gatti R, et al. Saliva specimen: a new laboratory tool for diagnostic and basic investigation. *Clin Chim Acta* 2007;383:30–40.

POINTS TO REMEMBER

Saliva

- Saliva is increasingly used for assessing the genetic susceptibility to various conditions and for testing numerous analytes.
- The advantages of saliva as a diagnostic specimen are that it is inexpensive, convenient, rapid, easy, safe, and painless.
- The easiest way to collect saliva is to collect whole oral fluid (whole saliva), which is representative of the oral milieu.
- Whole saliva may be collected as either an unstimulated or a stimulated sample.
- Stimulation of saliva is obtained by oral movements (yawning, chewing gum) or by using a cotton ball soaked with citric acid.
- Stimulated and unstimulated saliva are of different origin and composition.

Arterial Blood Gas Testing

Arterial blood gas testing requires attention for several reasons[395]:

- Blood gas testing is commonly requested in patients with a critical, life-threatening condition or who are experiencing some unexpected deterioration. Such patients may have a serious metabolic (acute complications of diabetes mellitus, drug intoxication) or respiratory disorder (respiratory failure, sepsis, or multiorgan failure) and need immediate medical intervention.
- Arterial blood sampling is an invasive procedure associated with a risk of complications such as bruising, bleeding, infections, and arterial thrombosis.
- Arterial blood samples have very limited stability. Due to the low biological variability of many blood gas parameters, allowable total error is quite low, and even small differences in serial measurements can be clinically meaningful.

International standards are available and may serve as a good resource for standardization of preanalytical steps respective to laboratory testing for blood gases, pH analysis, and ionized calcium.[396–398] See Chapters 37 and 50 for further discussion.

Patient Condition

To ensure that test results reflect the actual condition of the patient, blood sampling should be done when a patient is in a stable, resting state. Furthermore, the exact time of the blood collection should always be recorded and reported with a test result. Any deviation from the steady state should be noted as a comment and accompany the test result in order to allow proper interpretation of the results and patient management.

Relevant patient condition determinants (at the time of blood collection) include the following:

- Patient status (resting, exercising, crying (children), anxious)
- Ventilatory setting (spontaneous breathing or assisted mechanical ventilation)
- Mode of oxygen delivery (fraction of inspired oxygen (FiO_2) through nasal cannula or Venturi mask)
- Respiratory rate (hyperventilation, hypoventilation)
- Body temperature

If the patient's condition is changing, a sufficient time should be allowed for the patient to stabilize.[399,400] For example, crying leads to a rapid decrease of oxygen saturation.[401] It has been shown that even a short walk or mild exercise may lead to a significant decrease in oxygen saturation in patients who are suffering from chronic obstructive pulmonary disease.[402] Hypoventilation and increasing body temperature are associated with an increase in ionized calcium and pCO_2 and a decrease in pH.[403] Thus if patient temperature deviates from normal body temperature, information about that should accompany the test report to allow proper interpretation of results. Although blood gas instruments offer temperature-corrected values, their use is not recommended because currently data are not available to quantify the balance between oxygen delivery and oxygen demand at temperatures other than 37 °C.[404] If the temperature-adjusted results are reported anyway, it is absolutely mandatory that the report be clearly labeled as such and that the uncorrected values (at 37 °C) are also made available on the test report.[405]

If there has been any change in the ventilatory setting or mode of oxygen delivery, the patient should be left in a resting state to stabilize. For patients without pulmonary disease, a period of 3 to 5 minutes is usually enough to stabilize. However, in patients with pulmonary disease, this period is significantly longer. According to the CLSI C46-A2 standard for blood gas and pH analysis and related measurements, adequate time for most patients to reach a stable state following ventilatory changes is 20 to 30 minutes.[397]

Sample Type

In healthy individuals, oxygen content in arterial blood is higher than in venous blood. The composition of arterial blood is constant throughout the body, whereas the composition of venous blood largely depends on the time of blood sampling, local and global circulatory conditions, and metabolic activity of the organ or tissue from which it carries blood to the heart. The major difference between arterial and venous blood is in their oxygen content. However, other parameters (pCO_2, pH) may also vary. The differences are more pronounced in conditions associated with compromised local or global circulation. Although venous blood is the specimen of choice for most routine laboratory tests, it is not the appropriate sample choice for the assessment of oxygen content in the blood. Arterial blood collected under anaerobic conditions is therefore the only acceptable sample type for an accurate evaluation of the gas exchange function of the lungs (pO_2 and pCO_2).[405]

If arterial blood is not available (e.g., neonates, small children, patients with burns) and during medical transport and prehospital critical care, a capillary sample is an acceptable alternative. Capillary blood is obtained by puncturing the dermis layer of the skin and collecting it from the capillary beds running through the subcutaneous layer of the skin. Capillary blood is therefore a mixture of unknown proportions of the blood from the smallest veins (venules) and arteries (arterioles), the capillaries, and surrounding interstitial and intracellular fluids. Due to large differences in oxygen content between arterial and capillary blood, the results obtained from a capillary sample should be interpreted with extra caution.

Whereas capillary blood, if sampled properly, may accurately reflect arterial pCO_2 and pH over a wide range of values, unfortunately, it may never serve as an adequate substitute for arterial blood for accurate pO_2 measurement.[406,407] The difference in oxygen content between arterial and capillary blood is even more pronounced in hypotensive patients and in patients with an increase of arterial pO_2.[408,409] Moreover, capillary blood sampling is not recommended in patients with circulatory shock or with poorly perfused (cyanotic), infected, inflamed, swollen, or edematous tissues. Capillary blood should be collected using an arterialization technique by warming the skin to 40 to 45 °C with a warm towel or by using a vasodilating cream containing, for example, methyl nicotinate or capsaicin. Arterialization increases the blood flow through the capillary beds and thus the proportion of arterial blood relative to venous blood in the capillary sample. An earlobe is a better sampling site than a fingertip because the blood sampled from an arterialized earlobe better reflects arterial blood values. Arterialized earlobe capillary blood gas sampling is widely used across primary and secondary health care settings, especially in patients requiring frequent monitoring of blood gas parameters.[410] To circumvent difficulties in capillary blood collection from an earlobe and minimize room air contamination, some special devices have been designed and are currently being evaluated.[411] These devices have been primarily designed to improve medical emergency management of patients in some extreme environments (e.g., space, high altitudes), but they could also become routinely used in the near future.

Anticoagulants

The recommended anticoagulant for arterial blood gas and ionized calcium testing is lyophilized balanced Li-heparin. According to the CLSI C46-A2 standard on blood gas and pH analysis and related measurements, the final heparin concentration in the sample should be 20 IU/mL blood. Because the pH of heparin is 7.0 (slightly acidic) and its pO_2 and pCO_2 values are near room air values, the excess of heparin in the sample can alter sample pH, pO_2, and pCO_2.[412]

Why use balanced heparin? Heparin is traditionally used to prevent blood sample coagulation. However, heparin is negatively charged and binds various cations (e.g., Ca^{++}, Na^+, K^+) in a dose-dependent manner. This may cause underestimation of electrolyte concentration. To prevent such direct binding of heparin and cations from the sample, balanced heparin was introduced. The binding sites of balanced heparin are presaturated with calcium.

Why use lyophilized heparin? Most commercially available dedicated syringes for arterial blood sampling contain spray-dried balanced heparin as an anticoagulant. Syringes with liquid heparin are also available. Whereas liquid heparin

enables better sample mixing, it may introduce sample dilution in cases of incomplete draw. Using ordinary syringes (without heparin) and flushing them before use are strongly discouraged. Flushing the syringe with liquid heparin causes sample contamination with heparin and sample dilution, resulting in significant differences among blood gas parameters (Fig. 5.15).[413]

Sample Contamination

Sample contamination may substantially affect blood sample quality and cause significant bias. Arterial blood gas samples are most commonly contaminated with liquid heparin (discussed above), venous blood, or air bubbles. Contamination of an arterial sample with venous blood occurs if a vein is accidentally punctured. This may happen if the needle is not correctly positioned during arterial blood sampling. In an arterial blood sample contaminated with venous blood, pO_2 and sO_2 may be falsely decreased, while pCO_2 may be falsely increased.

When making an arterial puncture, the needle should be inserted at a 30 to 45-degree angle. Moreover, it is also recommended that short-beveled needles be used because they are much easier to position inside the artery. Self-filling dedicated syringes are also highly recommended. These syringes fill more quickly and easily when a needle is puncturing an artery instead of a vein as a result of the difference in blood pressure between the vein and the artery.[414]

The aspiration of air during arterial blood sampling or bubble formation can result in significant changes in the concentration of some blood gas parameters ($\uparrow$pH, $\uparrow pO_2$, $\uparrow sO_2$, $\downarrow pCO_2$). The exchange between the air bubble and the arterial blood sample is rapid. It starts immediately and becomes significant after only 1 to 2 minutes. The exchange rate does not depend on the size of the bubble.[415] The longer the delay between blood sampling and sample analysis, the greater the effect of the contamination with atmospheric air and deviation from the true patient values. It should be noted that even a bubble as small as 1% of the total sample volume may cause significant changes in the oxygen content of the specimen.

Contamination with air bubbles can be prevented by visual inspection of the specimen immediately after blood sampling. If air bubbles are present in the sample, they should be expelled as soon as possible and certainly prior to the sample mixing. If there is a visible froth in the sample, such samples should not be analyzed because froth may contain a significant amount of atmospheric air.

The degree of contamination also depends on sample agitation during transport. The increment in pO_2 in the presence of air bubbles in the sample is even more pronounced if the samples are transported by pneumatic tubes due to the exaggerated oxygen movement between the blood sample and ambient air caused by sample turbulences in the pneumatic tube.[416–418] Pneumatic tubes are thus not recommended for the transport of arterial blood samples.

The use of blood gas syringes with a vented mechanism is also recommended to avoid sample contamination with air. Once such a syringe has been filled up to the dedicated volume, the vent allows the air to be pushed out from the syringe. After the air has been pushed out, the vent is closed, preventing the subsequent contamination of the sample with atmospheric air.

Hemolysis

Sample hemolysis is another big concern related to blood gas testing. Although sample hemolysis is difficult (or almost impossible) to assess in arterial blood samples, it has been demonstrated that a significant proportion (up to 4%) of arterial blood samples are hemolyzed.[419,420] Hemolysis leads to a significant decrease in pO_2 and an increase in pCO_2.[421] Electrolyte concentrations (potassium, calcium) are also dramatically affected by hemolysis. Hemolysis can occur during sampling and due to inadequate transport and storage conditions.

Because sample hemolysis cannot be detected in arterial blood gas samples, all necessary precautions should be taken to minimize the risk of sample hemolysis. The following conditions should be avoided to minimize the risk of hemolysis:

• Vigorous mixing. Sample mixing should be done gently.
• Any source of sample turbulence
• Pneumatic tube systems
• High force during sample aspiration
• Cooling the sample directly on ice cubes. If the sample needs to be cooled, an ice slurry should be used instead.

If capillary blood is collected, excessive pressure ("milking") should be avoided. Sample milking leads to significant hemolysis and contamination of the sample with surrounding tissue fluid (see Chapter 4). If milking is applied, many parameters in the sample will substantially deviate from the

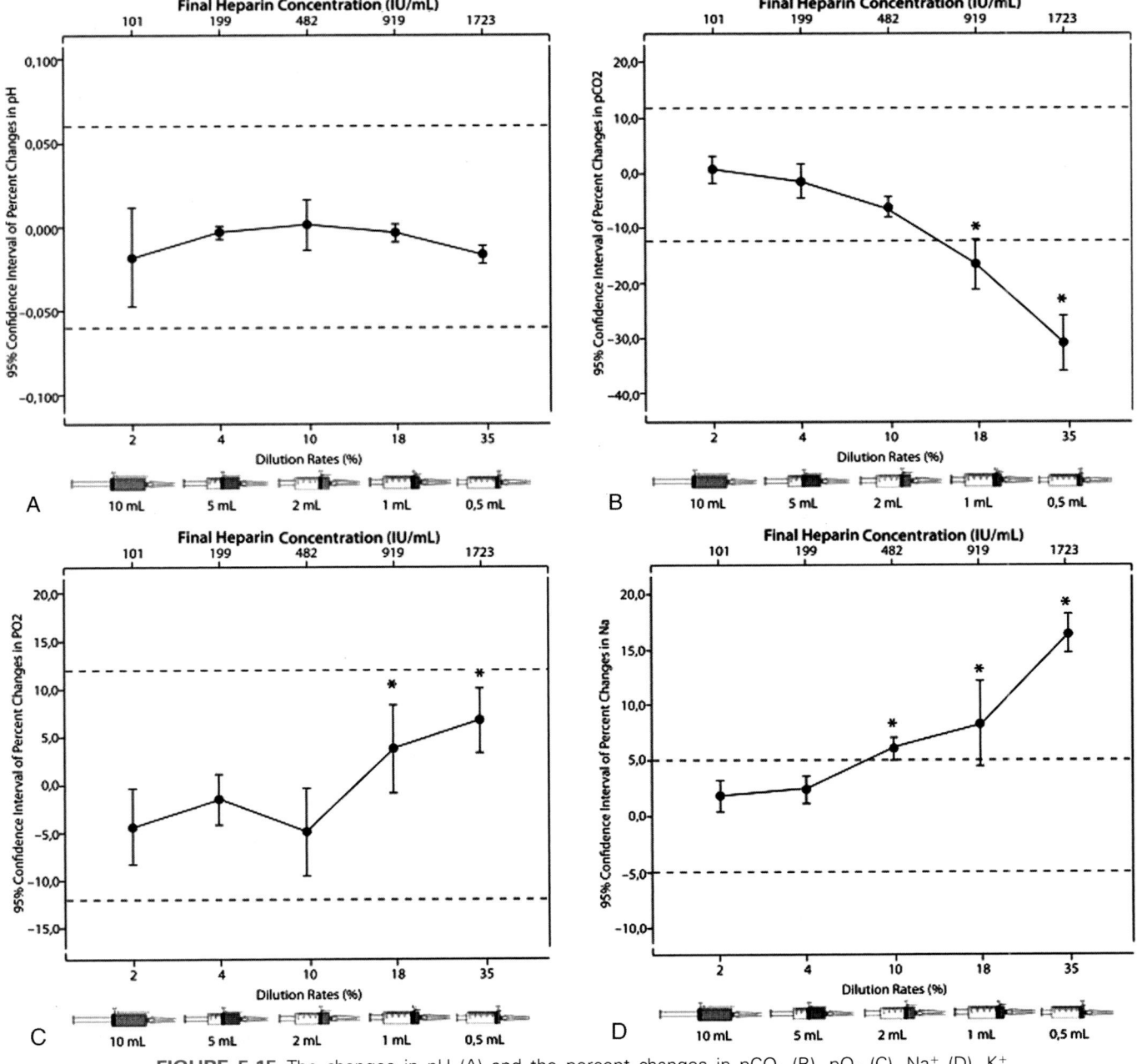

FIGURE 5.15 The changes in pH (A) and the percent changes in pCO_2 (B), pO_2 (C), Na^+ (D), K^+

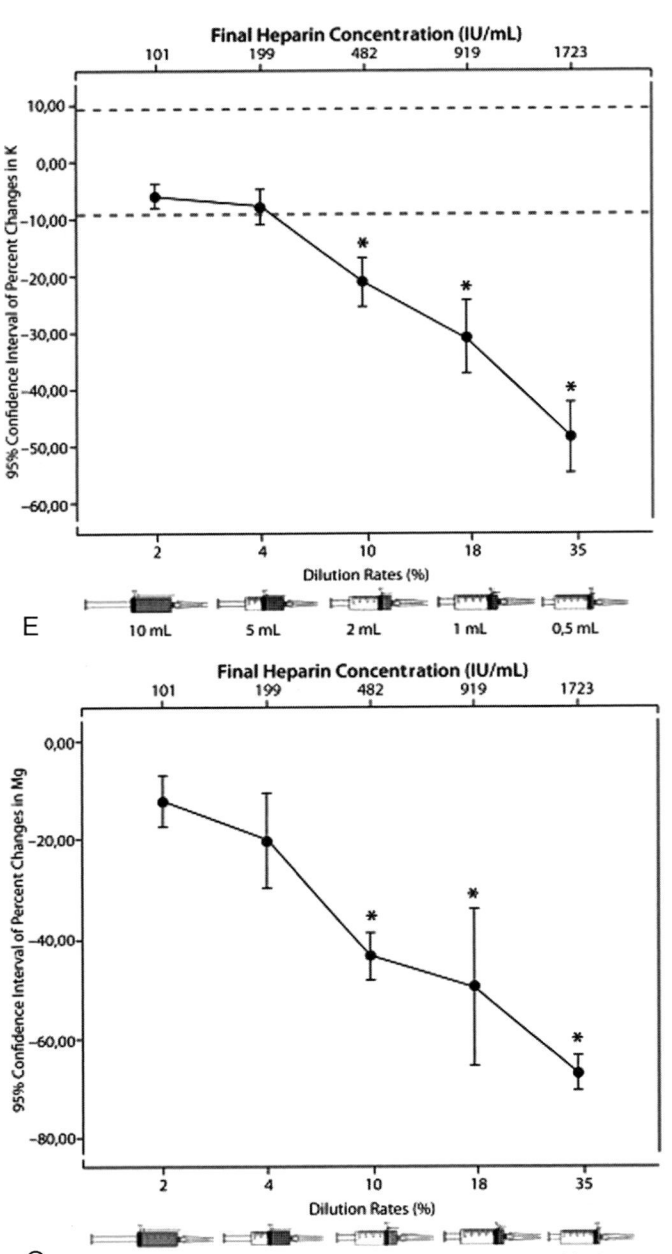

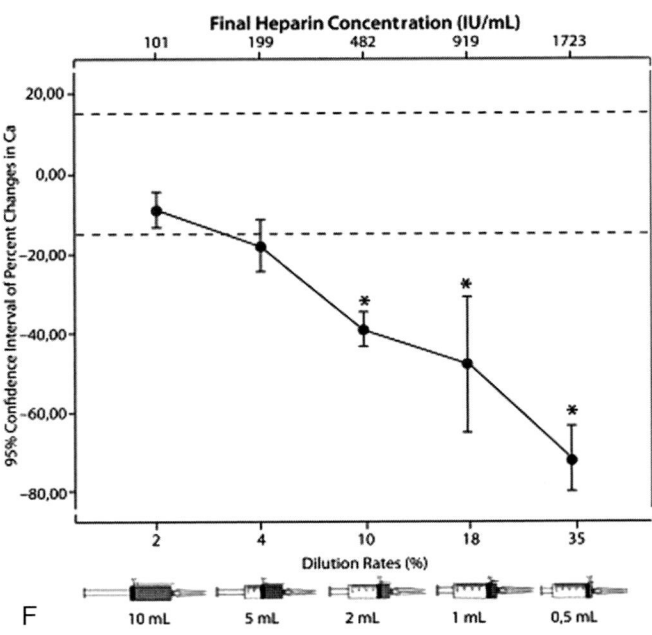

FIGURE 5.15 cont'd (E), iCa+2 (F), and iMg+2 (G) at different dilutions and final heparin concentrations. The horizontal dotted line indicates the acceptable total analytical error (TEa) limits according to RiliBAK. *$P < .05$ for differences from the true values (full sampling done to the full volume without dilution). (From Kume T, Sisman AR, Solak A, Tuglu B, Çinkoglu B, Çoker C. The effects of different syringe volume, needle size and sample volume on blood gas analysis in syringes washed with heparin. *Biochem Med* 2012;22:189–201, with permission from Croatian Society of Medical Biochemistry and Laboratory Medicine.)

true values (Fig. 5.16). Possible difficulties during capillary blood sampling should always be recorded and reported with the test results to enable proper interpretation of test results by the clinician.

Sample Mixing

Blood samples must be properly mixed to prevent clot formation, promote heparin dissolution, and ensure that blood cells are uniformly suspended in the sample. Blood samples should be mixed immediately after the sampling but only after visible air bubbles have been expelled. Mixing should be done gently to avoid hemolysis. Samples can be mixed manually and automatically. Manual sample mixing is done by gently inverting the syringe several times and rolling it between the palms (Fig. 5.17). If manual mixing

is not performed properly, the sample is unsuitable for analysis. The automatic arterial sample mixing is done with the use of a small metal ball located in the syringe barrel. The ball in the sample is moved through the sample by the force of an external magnet.

A clotted sample will cause analyzer malfunction. Moreover, if a clotted sample is analyzed, potassium concentration will be increased due to the efflux of the potassium from the platelets during blood clotting.

If the analysis is not done immediately and the sample needs to be transported to another location, the sample must be mixed again immediately prior to analysis. This is necessary to obtain a homogeneous sample and to ensure accurate test results. Mixing time depends on the time span between the sample collection and analysis. A shorter mixing time

ELECTROLYTES	Without milking	ELECTROLYTES	Milking applied
Na$^+$	140.1	Na$^+$	137.1
K$^+$	3.76	K$^+$	4.12
Ca^{++}	0.97 ↓	Ca^{++}	0.70 ↓
Ca^{++} (7.4)	0.99	Ca^{++} (7.4)	0.71
Cl$^-$	104	Cl$^-$	101

FIGURE 5.16 Example of the effect of excessive repetitive pressure (the so-called sample "milking") on sample hemolysis and sample contamination with tissue fluid. These two samples were obtained from the same patient in the resting state within 2 minutes. Sample without milking was obtained after an arterialization with a warm towel, while the other sample was obtained by the use of excessive finger pressure. (Laboratory data from the Clinical Institute of Chemistry, Clinical Hospital Center "Sestre milosrdnice," Zagreb, Croatia. Data used with patient consent.)

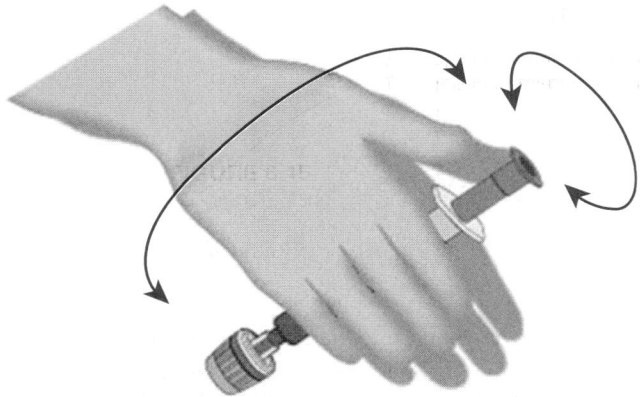

FIGURE 5.17 Manual sample mixing is done by gently inverting the syringe several times and rolling it between the palms. If manual sample mixing is not done properly, the sample is unsuitable for analysis.

(<1 minute) is acceptable if the time span from sampling to analysis is no longer than a couple of minutes. If longer delays occur between sampling and analysis, longer mixing intervals are required. The longer the time span, the longer the mixing time required. In samples that have been left to stand for 20 to 30 minutes, the homogeneity of the samples can be achieved by continuous mixing for at least 2 minutes.[422]

Sample Transport

Arterial blood samples should be transported by hand and at room temperature. As already mentioned, vigorous movement during sample transport should be avoided. Time is a critical variable in blood gas testing. It is important to avoid delays and to analyze the sample as soon as possible. Prolonged storage prior to analysis introduces significant bias due to cell metabolism and oxygen exchange between the sample and the atmosphere. Moreover, prolonged storage may also cause spurious results due to blood sedimentation. To avoid that, samples should be visually inspected and properly mixed to homogenize the blood inside the syringe.

As a general rule, samples drawn in plastic syringes should be analyzed immediately. If analysis is delayed, the samples should be stored in glass syringes.[423] Plastic syringes should not be cooled because plastic molecules contract when cooled to 0 to 4 °C. Contraction of plastic molecules creates pores in the syringe wall through which oxygen easily diffuses. Because carbon dioxide is a much larger molecule than oxygen, it cannot diffuse through the syringe wall (Fig. 5.18). The deviation in an inappropriately cooled plastic syringe is therefore greatest for oxygen and oxygen-related parameters.

According to the CLSI C46-A2 standard (blood gas and pH analysis and related measurements), samples should be transported by hand in a plastic syringe at room temperature and analyzed within 30 minutes of collection. In cases when expected delivery time is longer than 30 minutes, glass syringes should be used and the sample should be transported on ice to reduce the rate of metabolism and exchange of gases between the sample and the ambient air.[397] For more information on blood gas measurement and interpretation of results, refer to Chapter 37.

Hemostasis Testing

Many preanalytical variables may affect the results of routine coagulation testing, including general requirements regarding adequate test selection and ordering, patient preparation, patient identification, as well as all of the well-known potential sources of variation regarding sampling technique (fasting state, length of the venous stasis, order of draw, sampling from a catheter, sample handling (centrifugation), transport, and storage prior to analysis).[424–431] Some specific considerations related to hemostasis testing are explained further in the text.

One of the major preanalytical issues in hemostasis testing is clotted samples. Samples that contain visible clots should not be accepted for analysis and must be rejected. To prevent clot formation, some precautionary measures should be taken during blood sampling, handling, and transport; the following errors should be avoided:

- Inappropriate anticoagulant
- Too slow blood flow (during blood sampling)
- Transferring to citrated tube after sample collection with a syringe
- Underfilled tubes
- Prolonged use of a tourniquet
- Considerable manipulation of the vein by the needle
- Incomplete mixing

Clot formation induces the activation of platelets and clotting factors and allows the release of granules from the platelets; these factors may lead to false results in coagulation assays. It is very important to keep in mind that even small clots that are invisible to the human eye may significantly impact coagulation assays. Longer venous stasis should be avoided because it results in hemoconcentration, activation of fibrinolysis, and other changes, such as an increase in fibrinogen and factors VII, VIII, and XII.[432] Clotted samples must be rejected.

Choice of Anticoagulant

Historically, tubes made of glass have been used to collect blood samples. Since the coagulation cascade can be activated by contact with glass surface, these tubes must be siliconized to prevent glass-induced coagulation activation.[433] In the past

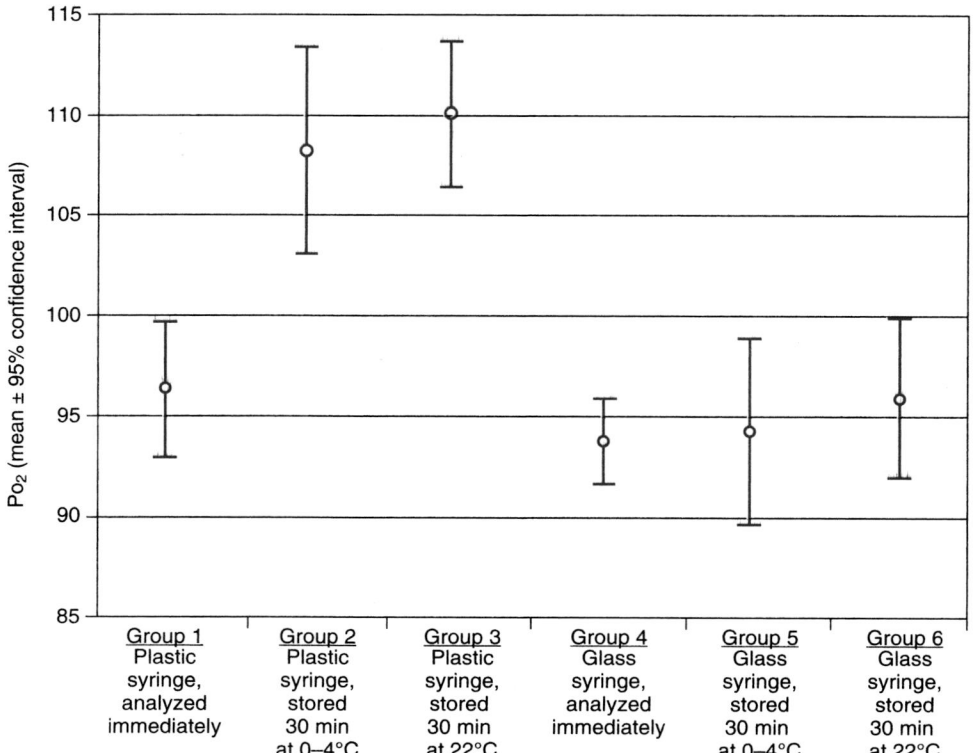

FIGURE 5.18 Plastic syringes should not be cooled because plastic molecules contract when cooled to 0 to 4 °C. Contraction of plastic molecules creates pores in the syringe wall, through which oxygen easily diffuses. If samples must be cooled, glass syringes should be used to avoid the exchange of oxygen through the syringe wall. This graph shows the differences in pO$_2$ values in arterial blood samples stored at different temperatures for different periods of time. (From Knowles TP, Mullin RA, Hunter JA, Douce FH. Effects of syringe material, sample storage time, and temperature on blood gases and oxygen saturation in arterialized human blood samples. *Respir Care* 2006;51:732–36, with permission by Dallas, Texas: Daedalus Enterprises for the American Association for Respiratory Therapy.)

decade blood collection tubes made of a variety of plastic materials have started to replace glass tubes, thus providing improved safety due to their increased shock resistance and tolerance to higher centrifugation speed; evidence showed equality in performance between the two types of tubes.[434] However, such plastic tubes should contain polypropylene as a nonactivating material.[435,436] Samples for hemostasis testing should be anticoagulated with 3.2% sodium citrate, although 3.8% may also be acceptable. It is important that the same concentration of sodium citrate be used within the laboratory because clotting times may be longer in 3.8% than in 3.2% sodium citrate.[435] As 3.8% sodium citrate binds more assay-added calcium than 3.2%, it has been reported that PT and aPTT may be overestimated in 3.8% sodium citrate, whereas fibrinogen is underestimated compared to values obtained in 3.2% citrated samples.[437,438] Additionally, it is important to emphasize that only 3.2% trisodium citrate is used for thromboplastin international sensitivity index (ISI) assignment that is also recommended by Scientific and Standardization Committee (SSC) of the International Society on Thrombosis and Hemostasis, so the anticoagulant of choice should preferably be 3.2% sodium citrate.

Other anticoagulants (e.g., EDTA or heparin) are not acceptable for hemostasis testing because they can lead to erroneous results and can cause clinically significant errors. For some analyses, especially platelet function assays, buffered citrate solution or other anticoagulants, such as lepirudin or synthetic inhibitors of thrombin and factor Xa, are used.[439–441]

Blood/Anticoagulant Ratio
The required blood to anticoagulant ratio is 9:1; it is therefore very important that tubes for coagulation assays be filled to the mark noted on the tube.[435] As filling volume decreases, clotting time in seconds tend to increase. This effect is more pronounced in tubes with 3.8% sodium citrate, compared to 3.2%. Acceptable deviation is maximum 10% of the total volume; filling the tube over 10% (overfilling) or less than 10% (underfilling) of the designated volume is strictly discouraged because this can introduce bias into test results. Although there is a great deal of evidence in the literature that demonstrates that unbiased results can be observed in 3.2% citrate tubes filled as low as 60%, especially in samples with low hematocrit value,[442–444] the general rule of thumb is to reject citrate anticoagulant tube filled below 90%.[435,445] Laboratories should have preanalytical procedures in place for the rejection of over- or underfilled tubes.

Order of Draw
In the past, a discard tube was recommended whenever the coagulation tube was the first tube.[446] However, more recent

evidence suggests that a "discard" tube may not be necessary[447-451]; CLSI stopped that recommendation, except in selected circumstances.

When the coagulation tube is collected as the first or the only tube:

- and a straight needle is used for blood collection, no discard tube is needed
- and a winged blood collection set (butterfly devices) is used, a discard tube must be collected to prevent underfilling[435,452]

If a safe venipuncture is not possible, blood specimens have to be obtained through a VAD. If intravenous catheter systems are used for blood sampling, it is recommended to flush the central catheter with saline and to discard the first 5 mL of blood or the catheter dead space volume corresponding to six times the line volume prior to tube collection for coagulation testing.[435,436] If blood is obtained from a normal saline lock, two dead space volumes of the catheter and extension set should be discarded.[435] If the catheter might be contaminated with heparin due to heparin infusion or flushing with heparin-containing fluid, the option of heparin neutralization of the sample should be considered.[435]

The order of draw should be followed without exceptions during every blood collection.

Mixing

Mixing of samples is extremely important for adequate coagulation testing. Samples must be promptly mixed to avoid in vitro clot formation. Tubes should be mixed by gently inverting the tubes (at 180 degrees) several times. For proper mixing, instructions from the tube manufacturer should be followed. Vigorous mixing and shaking of the tubes are discouraged because this may lead to sample hemolysis; the activation of platelets and coagulation factors, resulting in false shortening of clotting times; and even possibly a false increase in clotting factor activity.[425,427,430]

Transport

Following collection, citrated samples should ideally be transported to the laboratory immediately and at room temperature but no later than within 1 hour from blood draw.[424] Transport of samples by pneumatic tubes is still under debate. While some claim that pneumatic tube transport is acceptable for the transport of samples for routine hematology and coagulation parameters,[428,453] others argue that samples transported by pneumatic tube are not suitable for platelet aggregation assays.[454] It is therefore recommended that each institution verifies the acceptability of its tube transport systems by conducting a comparison study.

Centrifugation

Whole blood coagulation assays should be performed within 4 hours after blood sampling. For platelet function assays, samples should rest (at room temperature) for 30 minutes before analysis. Centrifugation is normally performed at 1500 g at room temperature for 10 to 15 minutes to obtain platelet-poor plasma.[435] Although there are many studies that aim to optimize centrifugation of coagulation samples at higher speeds with shorter centrifugation times,[455-457] these shortened protocols are not recommended because they may induce hemolysis and activation of platelets. Moreover, centrifuge breaks should also be avoided to prevent remixing of samples.[427,458]

The preparation of PRP for platelet function assays requires special care, and centrifugation speeds and duration need to be carefully optimized to ensure optimal results. Generally, centrifugation is performed at 200 to 250 g for 10 minutes without application of a rotor brake.[459,460]

Stability and Storage

Blood samples for coagulation testing must be kept at room temperature (20 to 25 °C) until analysis. Storage at lower temperatures or on ice is discouraged because cold temperature activates some coagulation factors. For example, in citrated whole blood stored in an ice bath or refrigerated (2 to 8 °C), the activation of platelets, activation of factor VII, and significant time-dependent loss of both FVIII and von Willebrand factor (VWF) will occur.[424] PT and aPTT should generally be performed using fresh plasma within 4 hours after blood sampling and stored at room temperature.[461] If the centrifuged plasma is left to sit on the blood cells, this may result in shortening of PT and prolongation of aPTT.[462] Stability data for screening coagulation test according to CLSI *Collection, Transport, and Processing of Blood Specimens for Testing Plasma-Based Coagulation Assays and Molecular Hemostasis Assays* H21-A5,[435] and CLSI *Quantitative d-dimer for the Exclusion of Venous Thromboembolic Disease* H59-A[463] guidelines are listed in Table 5.19.

Stability data for all coagulation factors can be found in the literature.[435,464] Although sample stability for coagulation assays has been extensively investigated by ample studies, and results are discrepant from aforementioned guidelines,[465-468] the samples should be routinely processed according to current CLSI H21-A5 guidelines.[435] If possible, all coagulation analyses should be performed using fresh material; freezing of samples should be an exception.[469] Previously frozen samples should be rapidly thawed in a 37 °C water bath for 5 to 10 minutes or until completely thawed. The samples should not be allowed to sit in the water bath for an extended period of time due to some thermolabile factors (FVIII, FV). Once thawed, samples should be thoroughly and adequately mixed prior to testing.[470,471]

For more information on coagulation and platelet function tests and interpretation of results, refer to Chapters 80 and 81.

Hematology

CBC is the most prevalent laboratory test, even across different continents, and regardless of the country's income.[472] However, even with the high prevalence of CBC determinations, reported frequency of preanalytical errors in the hematology laboratory is low, a mere ~1%.[137,473-477] Errors in patient identification and specimen labelling are pan-disciplinary and not related specifically to hematology testing.[478] Of the preanalytical errors related to samples for hematology testing, some of the most commonly reported problems are related to the clotting of samples and samples with an inappropriate blood-to-anticoagulant ratio (Table 5.20).

Some of the most common variables leading to an unsatisfactory sample for hematology testing are listed further in the text.

Choice of Anticoagulant

Being efficacious for preserving cellular morphology, EDTA is the anticoagulant of choice for hematology testing. EDTA

TABLE 5.19   Stability data for screening coagulation tests and D-dimer[435,463]

	STORED AS WHOLE BLOOD			PROCESSED AND PLASMA ALIQUOTED			
Assay	Room Temp	Refrigerated	Frozen	Room Temp	Refrigerated	Frozen −20 °C	Frozen ≥−70 °C
PT	24 h	Unacceptable	Unacceptable	24 h	Unacceptable	2 weeks	12 months
aPTT	4 h	Unknown	Unknown	4 h	4 h	2 weeks	12 months
D-dimer	NA	NA	NA	24 h	24 h	24 months	24 months

aPTT, Activated partial thromboplastin time; *PT*, prothrombin time.
Adapted from Clinical and Laboratory Standards Institute (CLSI). Collection, Transport, and Processing of Blood Specimens for Testing Plasma-Based Coagulation Assays and Molecular Hemostasis Assays; Approved Guideline—Fifth Edition. CLSI document H21-A5. Clinical and Laboratory Standards Institute, Wayne, Pennsylvania, USA, 2008; Clinical and Laboratory Standards Institute (CLSI). Quantitative D-dimer for the Exclusion of Venous Thromboembolic Disease; Approved Guideline. CLSI document H59-A. WaYNE, PA: Clinical and Laboratory Standards Institute; 2011.

TABLE 5.20   Comparison of Prevalence of Reported Preanalytical Errors in Hematology Laboratory

	Lippi, 2007[473]	Simundic, 2010[137]	Upreti, 2013[474]	Narang, 2016[475]	Arul, 2018[476]	Narula, 2019[477]
Wrong/missing identification	3.0%	27.1%	36.0%	2.6%	4.5%	23.4%
Inappropriate container	9.4%	0.4%	16.5%	5.3%	11.7%	2.3%
Inappropriate volume	7.0%	14.2%	19.7%	18.2%	45.8%	67.4%
Clotted samples	76.8%	31.5%	13.4%	73.9%	27.1%	2.3%
Contamination	3.8%	NA	4.3%	NA	4.5%	NA
Hemolysis	NA	23.7%	10.1%	NA	6.4%	NA
Samples lost/not found	NA	7.8%	NA	NA	NA	2.3%
Samples damaged in transport	NA	3.8%	NA	NA	NA	2.3%

Percentages are calculated as number of observed samples within category/total number of unsuitable samples.
Highest observed prevalence among preanalytical errors in hematology laboratory is marked in *light red*.

was chosen for hematologic tests when aniline-derived dyes were proposed for preparing blood smear from peripheral venous blood.[479] Anticoagulant function of EDTA is exerted through its potential to chelate calcium. Because EDTA as a free acid is not water soluble, it comes as disodium, dipotassium, and tripotassium salt. Potassium EDTA salts are more soluble than sodium salts. EDTA salts cause osmotically induced cell shrinkage and swelling to a different degree. Also, pH of EDTA increases with the number of ions bound to EDTA. Whereas the pH of EDTA in a free acid form is 2.5, tripotassium EDTA (K_3EDTA) has a pH of 7.5. In dipotassium and disodium EDTA, cell swelling is counteracted by cell shrinkage (due to the lower pH in dipotassium salts). Because cell shrinkage is less apparent, dipotassium EDTA (K_2EDTA) salts are superior to K_3EDTA. Also, mean cell corpuscular volume (MCV) based on the minihematocrit values in disodium and K_2EDTA samples provide acceptable results, as opposed to K_3EDTA samples.[480] Additionally, EDTA allows optimal dying with May-Grünwald Giemsa stain and optimal extended stabilization of blood cells and particles.[479] For these reasons, due to its higher solubility, lower osmotic effect, and best overall performance, the International Council for Standardization in Haematology (ICSH) recommends K_2EDTA salt as the anticoagulant of choice for hematology testing.[481] However, it is important to emphasize that these recommendations were based exclusively on the liquid form of K_3EDTA, and the conclusions drawn based on those type of tubes. Since the release of the recommendations, various studies have been published comparing K_2 and K_3EDTA in

the automated CBC analysis, using glass and plastic tubes, and the results only partially agree with the recommendation.[482] Van Cott and colleagues concluded that the differences between results obtained with K_3EDTA glass tubes versus K_2EDTA plastic tubes are minimal and unlikely to be of any clinical significance.[483] With the release of spray-dried K_3EDTA tubes, some authors demonstrated the equivalence of spray-dried K_2EDTA, spray-dried K_3EDTA, and liquid K_3EDTA blood collection tubes for routine donor center or transfusion service testing.[484] It was confirmed that new K_3EDTA spray-dried tubes do not represent a clinically relevant new source of error in the clinical laboratory for several routine hematologic laboratory parameters.[485] Even the manufacturers themselves (Greiner Bio-One) have challenged the ICSH recommendation and demonstrated substantially equivalent performance of spray-dried K_3EDTA tubes to spray-dried K_2EDTA tubes.[486] Nevertheless, up to now, the recommended anticoagulant for hematology testing remains K_2EDTA. However, laboratory managers should be aware that the use of K_2EDTA vacuum tubes from different manufacturers may represent a clinically relevant source of variation for some CBC parameters.[487]

Blood-to-Anticoagulant Ratio

According to CLSI GP39-A6 standard, EDTA tubes have a fixed fill volume that gives the optimum concentration of anticoagulant and should be filled to ±10% of the stated draw volume.[488] In underfilled EDTA tubes, cell count and hematocrit might be falsely decreased due to the excess

EDTA, which leads to cell shrinkage. On the other side, tube overfilling may lead to clot formation and platelet clumping, because sample mixing becomes difficult due to the small head space.

These recommendations are based on some outdated studies, some of which are based on collection tubes with liquid anticoagulant.[489–491] Today, the predominant tubes for hematologic testing are spray-dried tubes, and evidence is emerging that shows that even underfilled spray-dried EDTA tubes might be acceptable for automated CBC counting.[492–494] Nevertheless, until some new studies prove differently tube overfilling is strongly discouraged.

Contamination

Contamination with infusion fluids may be a cause of spurious anemia.[478] An unexplained decrease in CBC parameters may be due to IV contamination. A sudden shift of 4 to 5 fL in MCV, a parameter which should not fluctuate more than 1 to 2 fL within an individual, in the absence of a recent transfusion, is another reliable indicator of intravenous (IV) fluid contamination.[495] The fluid inside the RBC is hypertonic compared to the IV fluid which causes a shift of fluid into the cells, thus increasing their volume. Delta checks, the process of flagging differences in specific analytes between consecutive analyses, are one way to detect such problems. Delta checks are most efficient when done on parameters with low short-term biologic variability (e.g., within 24 hours), such as MCV and mean cell hemoglobin concentration (MCHC).[496]

Whenever possible, specimens should be collected from the arm opposite the line to avoid contamination. Specimens should not be collected distal to a catheter because fluids tend to pool in the periphery of the limb. Collection of samples proximal to a catheter will be diluted by the infusion fluid. When vascular access is limited, a specimen may need to be collected from the line. This decision should only be made after weighing the risk of specimen contamination versus the risk of phlebotomy from another site. Before drawing a specimen from the line, the infusion fluid should be completely stopped for several minutes and an amount of blood equal to three or more times the dead space of the catheter should be discarded.

Tube Mixing

Blood should be mixed immediately after the specimen is drawn to allow proper mixing of the additive with blood and to prevent sample clotting. Poor sample mixing may lead to sample clotting. Clotted specimens are among the most common reasons for sample rejection in automated cell counting and coagulation.[475,478,497] While some authors have argued that mixing may be avoided, because blood is mixed with anticoagulant spontaneously, during the blood draw,[498] tube mixing is still recommended as an essential step which ensures the quality of hematology samples.

Tubes should also be mixed immediately before the analysis to achieve sample homogeneity.

Adequate mixing is achieved by gently inverting the tube at 180° and back to the upright position. For optimal results, the number of full rotations should correspond to manufacturers' instructions.[499] Although it has been suggested that vigorous mixing does not promote laboratory variability,[500] general advice is that vigorous mixing should be avoided.

Sample Stability

Sample stability is a crucial aspect for the quality of results in the hematology laboratory. Although the official recommendations of the ICSH evolved with time,[501,502] as a general rule, the EDTA anticoagulated blood should be stored at room temperature and analyzed within 3 hours of collection. It should be noted that analyte stability may differ depending on the parameters that are being measured, instrument type, and transport and storage conditions.[503–506] Therefore on some occasions, a shorter storage time is necessary to ensure accurate and reliable results, whereas some parameters show excellent stability even over much longer time intervals. Some parameters are very stable (hemoglobin and RBC), while others appear less stable (reticulocytes, MCV, and hematocrit). The stability of hematologic parameters is improved if samples are kept at 4 °C. Medium to long-term storage of whole blood samples at high temperatures (37 °C) should absolutely be avoided, both during transportation and within the laboratory.[504] Special attention should be paid to sample stability for preparation of peripheral blood smears. Morphologic changes in anticoagulated blood begin within 30 minutes in neutrophils and other granulocytes and consist of swelling, nuclear lobe structure, loss of cytoplasmic granulation, and vacuolization in anticoagulated blood.[501] These changes are attenuated with the time and conditions of blood storage. Some most relevant changes observed for WBC after prolonged storage at room temperature are abnormal chromatin clumping, abnormal band forms (so called "pseudo-bands"), loss of cytoplasmic margin definition, neutrophil and/or basophil degranulation, smudge cells, and so on.[507]

Although some of the changes are delayed in samples stored at 4°C, they are not eliminated, and for this reason, it is important to make smears as soon as possible.[502]

The ICSH data on the stability of some hematology parameters are summarized in Table 5.21.

TABLE 5.21 International Council for Standardization in Haematology Data on the Stability of Some Hematology Parameters[502]

Parameter	Storage Conditions	
	Room Temperature (18–25 °C)	4 °C
Hemoglobin	NA	72 h
RBC count	NA	72 h
MCV (Hct)	1–4 h	6–12 h
Reticulocyte count	NA	24–72 h
Platelets	NA	24–72 h
WBC count	6 h	24–72 h
Automated differential count	6 h	24–72 h
Peripheral blood smear	<3 h	8 h

Hct, Hematocrit; *MCV,* mean corpuscular volume; *RBC,* red blood cell; *WBC,* white blood cell.
Adapted from Zini G. International Council for Standardization in Haematology (ICSH): stability of complete blood count parameters with storage: toward defined specifications for different diagnostic applications. *Int J Lab Hematol* 2014;36:111–3.

As already emphasized above, the stability may vary depending on the instrument used. It is therefore the responsibility of the individual laboratory to verify the stability of the hematologic parameters on their instruments.

Antibodies

Antibodies may affect the cell count of erythrocytes, leukocytes, and platelets. The following antibodies are known to interfere with hematologic analytes:

- EDTA-dependent antibodies with thrombocyte and leukocyte specificity
- Cold agglutinins (erythrocyte specific)
- Cryoglobulins

EDTA pseudothrombocytopenia. EDTA may in some individuals cause pseudothrombocytopenia—that is, platelet clumping or platelet satellitism (platelets adhering to neutrophils) and subsequently inaccurate platelet results.[508,509] Although EDTA-dependent pseudothrombocytopenia is a rare phenomenon (around 0.1% in the general population),[510,511] the reliable and timely identification is essential since it can lead to inappropriate clinical decisions.[512] The phenomenon was described more than 50 years ago and has been observed in healthy and diseased individuals, unrelated to gender, age, age of onset, disease, hemostasis alterations, or ingestion of specific drugs.[513,514] The hypothesized mechanism in pseudothrombocytopenia involves IgM autoantibodies directed against platelet IIb/IIIa fibrinogen receptors. EDTA induces steric conformation on negatively charged phospholipids and membrane receptors which then react with autoantibodies that triggers platelet activation through enhanced expression of GMP140, Gp55, and thrombospondin, activation of the tyrosine kinase pathway, and finally platelet agglutination and clumping in vitro (Fig. 5.19).[512]

This is further supported by the fact that platelets from patients with Glanzmann thrombasthenia (in which platelets have either defective or low concentrations of glycoprotein IIb/IIIa) do not react to autoantibodies from pseudothrombocytopenic patients.[515] Transplacental transmission from mother to child during pregnancy has also been described.[516,517] Major criteria for establishing a diagnosis of EDTA-dependent pseudothrombocytopenia are as follows[512]:

1. Platelet count typically $<100 \times 10^9$/L
2. Onset in only EDTA-anticoagulated sample kept at room temperature
3. Time-dependent fall of the platelet count in EDTA specimens
4. Presence of platelet aggregates and clumps in EDTA-anticoagulated samples
5. Lack of clinical signs or symptoms of platelet disorder

Because most cell counters are not able to identify this preanalytical problem, platelets are thus counted as WBC, resulting in spurious leukocytosis and false thrombocytopenia.[518] Although there were some efforts in screening for EDTA-dependent deviations in platelet counts by exploring platelet distribution histograms on hematology analyzers,[519] visual evaluation of blood smears is regarded as the gold standard for detection of EDTA-pseudothrombocytopenia, showing a typical pattern of platelet aggregates (Fig. 5.20).[520,521]

Although promising in many aspects of morphologic assessment of the blood smear, digital morphology analyzers have shown insufficient sensitivity for platelet clump detection; a manual microscopic review is recommended.[522]

Several approaches have been described to resolve this in vitro phenomenon. Platelet aggregation was not observed in samples anticoagulated with mixtures of EDTA and aminoglycosides.[523] Magnesium sulfate, previously used as anticoagulant for estimating manual platelet count, has also been proven promising as an alternative anticoagulant for platelet counts estimation in EDTA-pseudothrombocytopenia,[524] and some novel methods to dissociate platelet clumps based on the pathophysiologic mechanism were described.[525] Nevertheless, the most suitable and practical approach for most

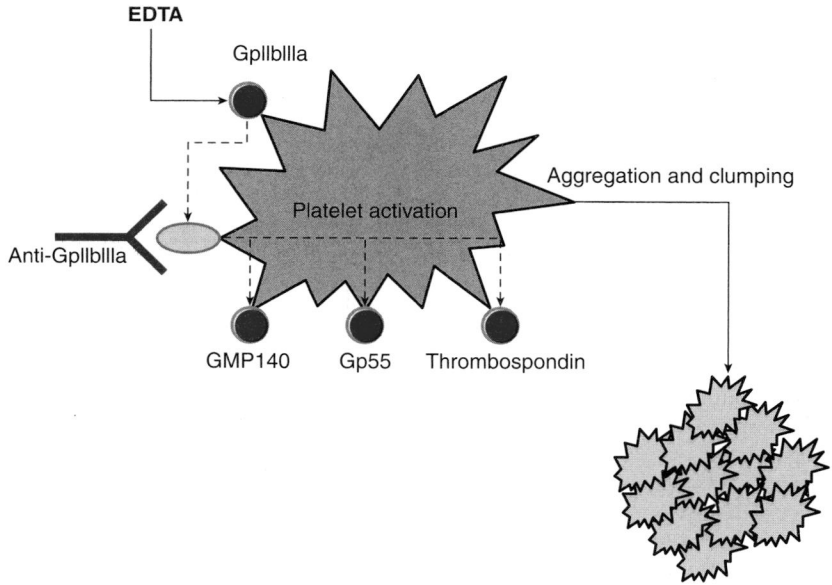

FIGURE 5.19 Pathogenesis of EDTA-dependent pseudothrombocytopenia.[512] EDTA from the anticoagulant enables IgM autoantibodies binding against platelet IIb/IIIa fibrinogen receptors. This triggers platelet activation and, finally, platelet agglutination and clumping in vitro.

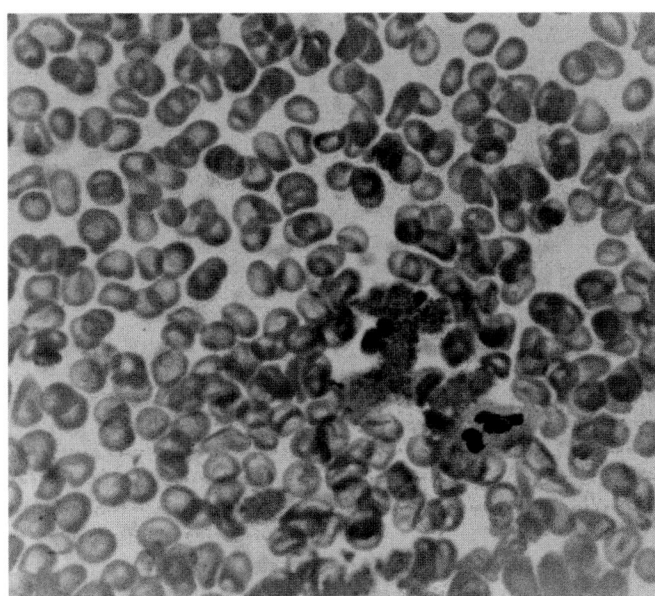

FIGURE 5.20 EDTA induced platelet aggregates in the peripheral blood smear. (Figure provided by the Department of Medical Laboratory Diagnostics, Clinical Hospital Sveti Duh, Zagreb, Croatia. Photo taken by Vanja Radisic Biljak.)

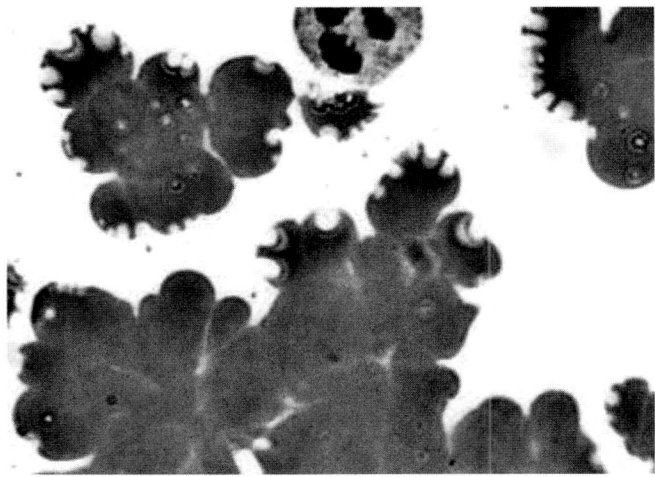

FIGURE 5.21 Cold agglutinins in peripheral blood smear with typical clusters of erythrocytes, May-Grünwald—Giemsa stain, 1000x. Cold agglutinins bind to the erythrocyte surface antigen at a temperature optimum of 0 to 4 °C, which causes agglutination of erythrocytes. Red blood cells cluster together in an irregular mass giving the "bunch of grapes" appearance, unlike rouleaux formation which resembles a "stack of coins" agglutinates.[531]

clinical laboratories will be recollection of specimens using tubes with other anticoagulant (sodium citrate, CPT, $CaCl_2$/heparin), and immediate processing of those blood samples.

Cold agglutinins. Cold agglutinins are antibodies that are specific for erythrocyte surface carbohydrate antigens, which bind to the erythrocyte surface at temperatures of 0 to 4 °C. Binding of agglutinins causes agglutination of erythrocytes, induces complement activation and hemolysis, and impairs peripheral circulation.[526] Cold agglutinins may be monoclonal or polyclonal. Monoclonal agglutinins are found in patients with idiopathic forms of cold agglutinin disease or lymphoproliferative disorders, whereas polyclonal antibodies are often found in patients recovering from some infectious diseases.[527] Some rare cases of cold agglutinins toward platelets have also been described, causing pseudothrombocytopenia independent of EDTA.[528]

Cold agglutinins, if undetected, may cause diagnostic confusion and lead to subsequent extensive diagnostic workup and incorrect and unnecessary therapy, risking patient safety and increasing health care costs. It is therefore very important to recognize cold agglutinins promptly. Cold agglutinins should be suspected if the following anomalies are observed[529,530]:

- RBC counts too low, even at normal hemoglobin concentration, with a false decrease in hematocrit
- Falsely increased Red Cell Distribution Width (RDW) values
- Grossly enhanced MCV values due to measurements of erythrocyte clumps
- Falsely increased MCH and MCHC values without any obvious explanation.

Since hemoglobin is measured after RBC are lysed, it is generally not affected. The blood smear will show agglutination of erythrocytes (Fig. 5.21).[531]

For adequate analysis of samples in which cold agglutinins are suspected, it is essential to warm up the EDTA blood sample at 37 °C and analyze immediately afterward.[529,530,532] This anomaly will appear again if a sample is kept at 4 °C and analyzed while it is cold. Samples in which cold agglutination is suspected should be examined by microscopic observation of a blood smear. In such cases, both the sample and the glass slide should be prewarmed to avoid agglutination.[533] A schematic overview of a proposed laboratory procedure to prevent preanalytical errors caused by cold agglutinins is presented in Fig. 5.22.[534]

Cryoglobulins. Cryoglobulins are immunoglobulins that precipitate in vitro at cold temperature and dissolve at 37 °C.[535] Cryoglobulins are often associated with infections, autoimmune disorders, and malignancies, and they can cause organ damage through immune-mediated mechanisms and vascular damage due to increased viscosity of the blood.[536] Precipitation of cryoglobulins depends on the immunoglobulin class to which they belong. Also, precipitation is absent at pH less than 5.0 or greater than 8.0.

In samples kept at room temperature, cryoglobulins tend to form globular or cylindric precipitates that are then counted by automated hematologic analyzers as cells, thus affecting hematologic laboratory tests and leading to false leukocytosis (pseudoleukocytosis) or false thrombocytosis (pseudothrombocytosis), while RBC values are generally unaffected in cryoglobulinemias. The degree of pseudoleukocytosis and pseudothrombocytosis depends on the time of exposure, temperature, cryoglobulin concentration, and the interaction of cryoglobulins with other plasma proteins.[537] Recognition of the hematologic abnormalities may be the first clue leading to the diagnosis of cryoglobulinemia.[538,539] The following indices may point to the presence of cryoglobulins[538]:

1. Abnormalities in automated WBC and/or platelet counts
2. Visualization of the cryoglobulins as blue sediments in differential count samples
3. In a sample warmed up to 37 °C, significantly lower cell counts

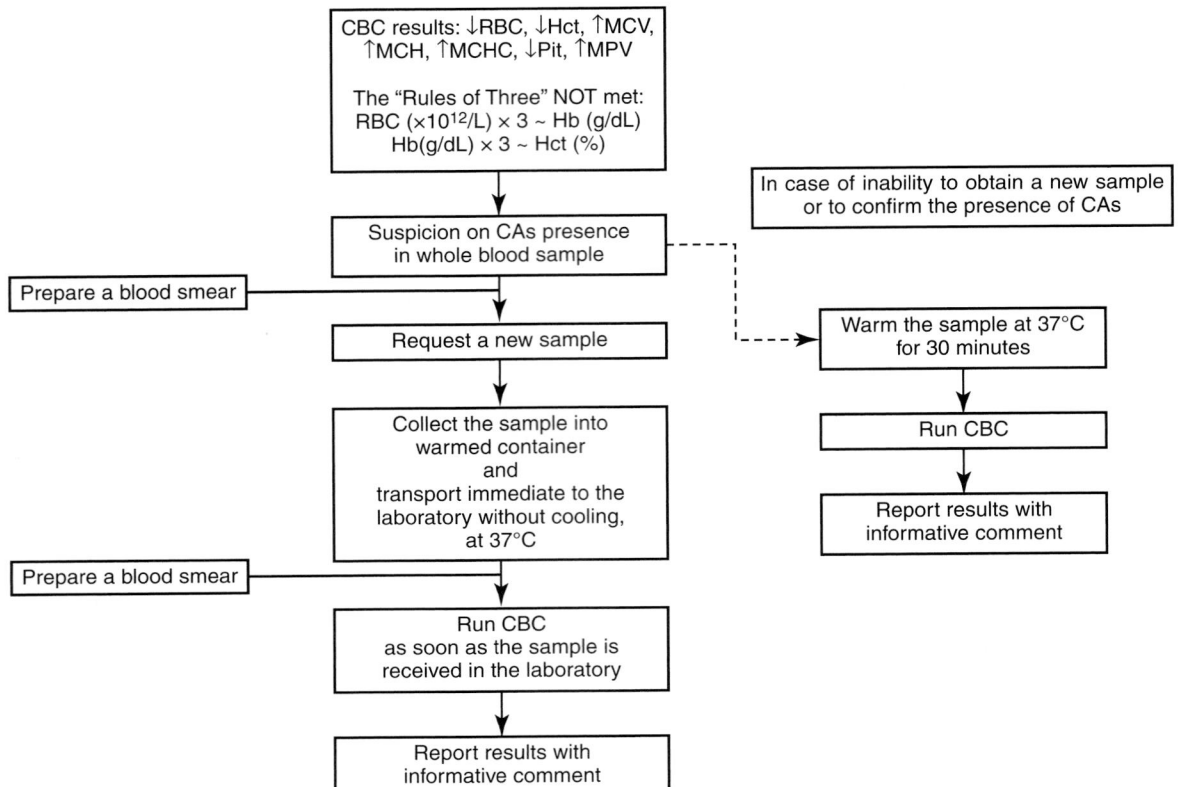

FIGURE 5.22 Laboratory algorithm for investigating suspected cold agglutinins in whole blood samples. *CAs,* Cold agglutinins; *CBC,* complete blood count; *Hct,* hematocrit; *MCH,* mean corpuscular hemoglobin; *MCV,* mean corpuscular volume; *MCHC,* mean corpuscular hemoglobin concentration; *MPV,* mean platelet volume; *Plt,* platelet; *RDW,* red cell distribution width; *WBC,* white blood cell count (From Topic A, Milevoj Kopcinovic L, Bronic A, et al. Effect of cold agglutinins on red blood cell parameters in a trauma patient: a case report. *Biochem Med* 2018;28:031001, with permission by Croatian Society of Medical Biochemistry and Laboratory Medicine.)

Diagnosis of cryoglobulinemia is further confirmed by biochemical analysis of the serum, followed by isolation, purification, and immunochemical analysis of cryoglobulins. As in the case of cold agglutinins, for adequate analysis of samples in which cryoglobulins are suspected, preincubation of blood samples at 37 °C for 10 to 15 minutes often yields reliable CBC results, especially if analyzed immediately afterward.[540]

MANAGEMENT OF THE QUALITY OF THE PREANALYTICAL PHASE

The ultimate goal of preanalytical quality management is not to improve the quality of the sample per se but to improve patient outcome.[205] Preanalytical quality management achieves its primary goal only if (1) the importance of preanalytical processes in the TTP is fully understood; (2) all sources of preanalytical variability and their effects are known; (3) patient-centered and evidence-based guidelines are available; (4) compliance with guidelines can be ensured; and (5) quality is continuously monitored and improved.[205]

Unfortunately, the preanalytical part of the TTP is not fully understood by all involved (laboratory staff, nurses, clinicians, and patients). Patients are usually not aware of the importance of proper preanalytical procedures and how improper sample collection could affect the results of requested tests.[541,542] Education is the key to the improvement of the

level of understanding of the importance of the preanalytical phase.[543–545] However, the effects of educational interventions are usually short-lived, and education should therefore be a continuous quality improvement activity.

Outcome-based Preanalytical Studies

Although many potential sources of variability and how they affect the quality of samples and test results are well recognized, there is little evidence demonstrating the effect of preanalytical variation on patient outcomes and how particular errors may affect health care organization and expenditure. Most studies so far have been descriptive and reported failures of processes without linking those to patient harm. Quality improvement should focus on reducing patient harm rather than just eliminating process defects and waste.[546] Original studies need to focus more on patient-relevant outcomes—for example, how some preanalytical errors, such as improper sampling, delayed transport, or hemolyzed or clotted samples, may lead to patient discomfort, additional diagnostic workup, increased LOS in the hospital, increased costs, disease prevalence, and so on.[547–550] Error reduction strategies should focus on those most critical errors that have the greatest potential to impact patient outcomes.

Quality Indicators

Preanalytical quality should continuously be monitored and improved. To measure the degree of improvement, quality indicators (QI) should be used (see Chapter 3). QI are measurable, objective, quantitative measures of key system elements that show to what extent a laboratory meets the needs and expectations of the customers.[551] To allow consistent and comparable use across settings over time, a unique definition is needed for QIs.[552–554] While different professional groups have proposed some interesting programs on the use of QI in the TTP, until very recently there was no consensus on the definition, measurement methodology, and reporting practices for QI. Recently, a harmonized model of QI has been established by an expert panel during a consensus conference in Padua in October 2013.[555] The proposed QI model is based on a patient-centered approach, and the essential prerequisites taken into account were the following:

1. Importance and applicability to a wide range of clinical laboratories worldwide

2. Scientific soundness (focused on some most important areas in laboratory medicine)
3. Definition of evidence-based thresholds for acceptable performance
4. Timeliness and possible utilization as a measure of laboratory improvement

The model proposes 22 high-priority and 6 lower-priority preanalytical QIs (Table 5.22).

QIs enable the measurement of the quality of care and services, with the aim of assisting in quality improvement efforts. Collecting data on QI per se does not automatically mean quality improvement. Laboratories should strive for a system of continuous preanalytical quality improvement based on the "plan-do-check-act" cycle and using corrective and preventive actions with subsequent system redesign. Only then can patient outcomes be improved, preanalytical errors be reduced, and waste be eliminated.

TABLE 5.22 Proposed Preanalytical (Priority 1) Quality Indicators Based on a Harmonized Consensus Model

Quality Indicator	Reporting Systems
Misidentification errors	Samples suspected to be from wrong patients
	Percentage of "Number of misidentified requests/Total number of requests"
	Percentage of "Number of misidentified samples/Total number of samples"
	Percentage of "Number of samples with fewer than two identifiers initially supplied/Total number of samples"
	Percentage of "Number of unlabeled samples/Total number of samples"
Test transcription errors	Percentage of "Number of outpatient requests with erroneous data entry (test name)/Total number of outpatient requests"
	Percentage of "Number of outpatient requests with erroneous data entry (missed test)/Total number of outpatient requests"
	Percentage of "Number of outpatient requests with erroneous data entry (added test)/Total number of outpatient requests"
	Percentage of "Number of inpatient requests with erroneous data entry (test name)/Total number of inpatient requests"
	Percentage of "Number of inpatient requests with erroneous data entry (missed test)/Total number of inpatient requests"
	Percentage of "Number of inpatient requests with erroneous data entry (added test)/Total number of inpatient requests"
Incorrect sample type	Percentage of "Number of samples with wrong or inappropriate type (i.e., whole blood instead of plasma)/Total number of samples"
	Percentage of "Number of samples collected in wrong containers/Total number of samples"
Incorrect fill level	Percentage of "Number of samples with insufficient sample volume/Total number of samples"
	Percentage of "Number of samples with inappropriate sample-anticoagulant volume ratio/Total number of samples with anticoagulant"
Unsuitable samples for transportation and storage problems	Percentage of "Number of samples not received/Total number of samples"
	Percentage of "Number of samples not properly stored before analysis/Total number of samples"
	Percentage of "Number of samples damaged during transportation/Total number of samples"
	Percentage of "Number of samples transported at inappropriate temperature/Total number of samples"
	Percentage of "Number of samples with excessive transportation time/Total number of samples"
Contaminated samples	Percentage of "Number of contaminated samples rejected/Total number of samples"
Samples hemolyzed	Percentage of "Number of samples with free hemoglobin >0.5 g/L/Total number of samples (clinical chemistry)"[a]
Samples clotted	Percentage of "Number of samples clotted/Total number of samples with an anticoagulant"

[a]Clinical chemistry: all samples that are analyzed on the chemistry analyzer that is used for detection of HIL indices. If laboratories are detecting hemolysis visually, they count all samples with visible hemolysis (clinical chemistry). A color chart should be provided for this purpose.
From Plebani M, Astion ML, Barth JH, Chen W, de Oliveira Galoro CA, Escuer MI, et al. Harmonization of quality indicators in laboratory medicine: a preliminary consensus. *Clin Chem Lab Med* 2014;52:951–8, with permission by Walter de Gruyter.

POINTS TO REMEMBER

Management of the Quality of the Preanalytical Phase
- Quality improvement should focus on how to improve patient outcomes and reduce patient harm rather than to eliminate process defects and waste.
- Original studies need to focus more on outcomes and provide evidence for the effect of preanalytical errors (e.g., improper sampling, delayed transport, hemolyzed or clotted sample) on patient discomfort or harm, additional diagnostic workup, increased length of stay, increased costs, disease prevalence, and so on.
- Knowing the errors with the greatest potential to impact patient outcomes helps to prioritize error-reduction strategies and focus on the most critical errors.

SUGGESTED READING

9. Guder WG. History of the preanalytical phase: a personal view. Biochem Med 2014;24:25–30.
24. Simundic AM, Cornes M, Grankvist K, et al. Survey of national guidelines, education and training on phlebotomy in 28 European countries: an original report by the European Federation of Clinical Chemistry and Laboratory Medicine (EFLM) working group on the preanalytical phase (WG-PA). Clin Chem Lab Med 2013;51:1585–93.
25. Simundic AM, Bölenius K, Cadamuro J, et al. Joint EFLM-COLABIOCLI recommendation for venous blood sampling. Clin Chem Lab Med 2018;56(12):2015–38. doi:10.1515/cclm-2018-0602.
103. Sanchis-Gomar F, Lippi G. Physical activity—an important preanalytical variable. Biochem Med 2014;24:68–79.
117. Simundic AM, Cornes M, Grankvist K, et al. Standardization of collection requirements for fasting samples: for the Working Group on Preanalytical Phase (WG-PA) of the European Federation of Clinical Chemistry and Laboratory Medicine (EFLM). Clin Chim Acta 2014;432:33–7.
133. Bowen RA, Remaley AT. Interferences from blood collection tube components on clinical chemistry assays. Biochem Med 2014;24:31–44.
135. Simundic AM, Baird G, Cadamuro J, Costelloe SJ, Lippi G. Managing hemolyzed samples in clinical laboratories. Crit Rev Clin Lab Sci 2020;57(1):1–21. doi:10.1080/10408363.2019.1664391.
142. Vecellio E, Li L, Mackay M, et al. A benchmark study of the frequency and variability of haemolysis reporting across pathology laboratories—The implications for quality use of pathology and safe and effective patient care. Report to Royal College of Pathologists Australasia. Australian Institute of Health Innovation, Macquarie University, Sydney; July 2015.
166. Nikolac N. Lipemia: causes, interference mechanisms, detection and management. Biochem Med 2014;24:57–67.
169. Tate J, Ward G. Interferences in immunoassay. Clin Biochem Rev 2004;25:105–20.
173. Dimeski G. Interference testing. Clin Biochem Rev 2008;29(Suppl 1):S43–8.
203. Nikolac N, Simundic AM, Miksa M, et al. Heterogeneity of manufacturers' declarations for lipemia interference—An urgent call for standardization. Clin Chim Acta 2013;426:33–40.
323. Li D, Ferguson A, Cervinski MA, et al. AACC guidance document on biotin interference in laboratory tests. J Appl Lab Med 2020;5(3):575–87.
375. Delanghe J, Speeckaert M. Preanalytical requirements of urinalysis. Biochem Med (Zagreb) 2014;24:89–104.
388. Ellervik C, Vaught J. Preanalytical variables affecting the integrity of human biospecimens in biobanking. Clin Chem 2015;61:914–34.
395. Baird G. Preanalytical considerations in blood gas analysis. Biochem Med 2013;23:19–27.
424. Bonar R, Favaloro EJ, Adcock DM. Quality in coagulation and haemostasis testing. Biochem Med 2010;20:184–99.
431. Gosselin RC, Marlar RA. Preanalytical variables in coagulation testing: Setting the stage for accurate results. Semin Thromb Hemost 2019;45:433–48.
551. Simundic AM, Topic E. Quality indicators. Biochem Med 2008;18:311–19.
554. Plebani M, Sciacovelli L, Aita A, et al. Harmonization of pre-analytical quality indicators. Biochem Med 2014;24:105–13.

6

Quality Control of the Analytical Examination Process

W. Greg Miller and Sverre Sandberg[a]

ABSTRACT

Quality control (QC), also called internal QC, monitors a measurement procedure to verify that results for patient samples meet performance specifications appropriate for patient care or that an error condition exists that must be corrected. QC samples are measured at intervals along with patient samples. Recovery of the expected target values for the QC samples allows the laboratory to verify that a measurement procedure is working correctly and the results for patient samples can be reported. The QC plan specifies the number of controls, the frequency they are to be measured, and the rules to determine if the QC results are consistent with expected measurement procedure performance. External QC, also called external quality assessment (EQA) or proficiency testing (PT), is an assessment process in which control samples are received from an independent external organization and the expected values are not known by the laboratory. The results for the EQA/PT samples are compared with target values assigned to the samples to verify that a laboratory's measurement procedures conform to expected performance. EQA/PT schemes that use commutable samples assess trueness of patient sample results when a reference measurement procedure is used for target value assignment, or harmonization among results when no reference measurement value is available.

patient to assist with diagnosis, to guide or monitor therapy, or to assess risk for developing a disease or for progression of a disease. QC, also called internal QC, monitors a measurement procedure to verify that it meets performance specifications appropriate for patient care or that an error condition exists that must be corrected.

Content
Internal QC ensures that measurement procedures meet specifications at the time patient testing occurs. QC samples are measured at intervals along with patient samples. Recovery of the expected target values for the QC samples allows the laboratory to verify that a measurement procedure is working correctly and the results for patient samples can be reported. The QC plan specifies the number of controls, the frequency they are to be measured, and the rules to determine if the QC results are consistent with expected measurement procedure performance. External QC, also called *external quality assessment (EQA)* or *proficiency testing (PT)*, is an assessment process in which control samples are received from an independent external organization and the expected values are not known by the laboratory. The results for the EQA/PT samples are compared with target values assigned to the samples to verify that a laboratory's measurement procedures conform to expected performance. In addition to internal and external QC, the results from patient sample testing (e.g., medians of patient results) can be used to assess and monitor the performance of measurement procedures.

Background
The purpose of a clinical laboratory test is to provide information on the pathophysiologic condition of an individual

INTRODUCTION

The purpose of a clinical laboratory test is to provide information on the pathophysiologic condition of an individual patient to assist with diagnosis, to guide or monitor therapy, or to assess risk for developing a disease or for progression of a disease. Quality control (QC) monitors a measurement procedure to verify that it meets performance specifications

appropriate for patient care or that an error condition exists that must be corrected. QC includes both internal and external components.

Internal QC includes control procedures applied within a laboratory to assess the performance of an analytical examination procedure. The most common approach is to substitute surrogate QC samples that are intended to simulate clinical samples from patients. The QC samples are measured at intervals along with patient samples. Recovery of the expected target values for the QC samples allows the laboratory to verify that a measurement procedure is working correctly and the results for patient samples are reliable enough to be

[a]Some of this material was previously published in McPherson RA and Pincus MR, editors. *Henry's clinical diagnosis and management by laboratory methods.* 24th ed. St. Louis: Elsevier; 2020.

reported. Note the term internal QC is distinct from control processes and fluids that are "built-in" to a measurement technology or to the reagent cartridges or strips used by a measurement procedure. The performance of a measurement procedure can, for some measurands, also be monitored using the consistency of results from patient samples as part of the internal or external QC process.

External QC, also called external quality assessment (EQA) or proficiency testing (PT), is a monitoring process in which surrogate samples are received from an independent external organization and the expected values are not known by the laboratory. The results for the EQA/PT samples are sent to the provider and compared with results from other laboratories to examine if a laboratory's measurement procedures conform to expected performance. When commutable EQA samples are used (see later section on EQA) the performance can be assessed for agreement with a true value assigned by a reference procedure. Some EQA providers also provide follow up of erroneous results with advice and site visits to individual participants. In these organizations, the acronym EQA stands for external quality *assurance*.

As illustrated in Fig. 6.1, internal QC evaluates a measurement procedure by periodically measuring a QC sample for which the expected result is known in advance. If the result

for a QC material is within acceptable limits of the expected value (see Fig. 6.1A), the measurement procedure is verified to be stable, which means that it is performing as expected, and results for patient samples can be reported with high probability that they are suitable for clinical use. If a QC result is not within acceptable limits (see Fig. 6.1B), the measurement procedure is not performing correctly, there is a high probability that results for patient samples are not suitable for clinical use, and corrective action is necessary. Note that QC acceptance criteria may be designed to provide a warning of, for example, calibration drift that can be corrected before the error becomes large enough to adversely affect patient results. If corrective action is indicated, patient sample measurements will need to be repeated when the measurement procedure has been restored to its stable performance condition. If erroneous results have already been reported before an error condition is identified, a corrected report must be issued.

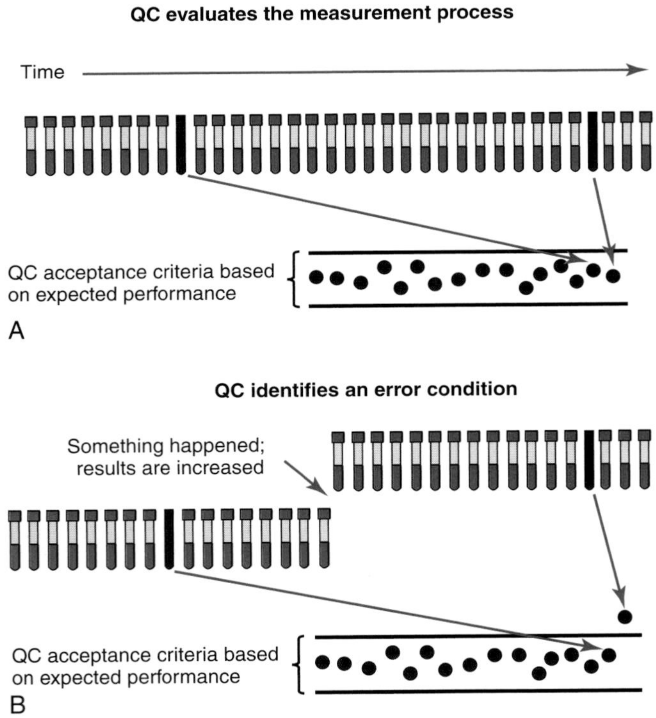

Measurement procedures fall into one of two general categories from a QC plan perspective. One type of procedure is a "batch" measurement process in which the results for patient samples and QC samples are completed before the results are reported. For batch measurement procedures, results are not reported if an error condition is identified by the QC sample measurements. The other type of procedure, which is becoming more common, is a "continuous" measurement process in which patient sample results are reported during the interval between QC sample measurements and continue to be reported after a QC measurement event with no intervention made to the measuring system. For continuous measurement procedures, there is a possibility that erroneous results have already been reported if an error condition is identified by the next QC sample measurement(s). In either category, a random measurement error that affects only one or a few patient results, called a nonpersistent error, may not be identified by the results for the QC samples. QC procedures only identify persistent error conditions at the point in time when a QC sample is actually measured. Consequently, the choice of criteria to evaluate QC results and the frequency that QC results are measured become important QC plan design considerations.

The design of a QC plan must consider the analytical performance capability of a measurement procedure and the risk of harm to a patient that might occur if an erroneous laboratory test result is used for a clinical care decision. An erroneous laboratory test result is a hazardous condition that may or may not cause harm to a patient depending on how the laboratory test is used for patient monitoring and treatment, the magnitude of error, and what action or inaction is taken by a clinical care provider based on the erroneous result. The following sections in this chapter explain how to establish a QC plan for monitoring a measurement procedure based on information about a measurement procedure's analytical performance, the analytical performance required to meet medical care requirements, and the risk of harm from an erroneous result. However, establishing the analytical performance specifications to meet medical requirements and evaluating the probability of harm from an erroneous result are challenging because the link between analytical performance and the outcome for the patient can be difficult to establish.[1]

QC evaluates the measurement process

Time

QC acceptance criteria based on expected performance

A

QC identifies an error condition

Something happened; results are increased

QC acceptance criteria based on expected performance

B

FIGURE 6.1 Quality control *(QC)* process for a measurement procedure. **(A)** QC samples *(black)* are periodically measured in place of patient samples *(red/grey)* to determine if the results for QC samples are within expected performance limits for a measurement procedure. **(B)** If an error occurs in the measuring system, such as a shift to higher results, a QC result can identify that a measurement error condition occurred at some point in time since the last acceptable QC result was measured.

MEASUREMENT PROCEDURE PERFORMANCE AS A PREREQUISITE FOR A QUALITY CONTROL PLAN

Calibration Traceability to a Reference System

Chapter 7 describes that calibration of clinical laboratory measurement procedures should, whenever possible, be traceable to a higher order reference measurement procedure (RMP) or certified reference material.[2–4] Such calibration ensures that results for patient samples are equivalent within medically acceptable limits irrespective of the measurement procedure or laboratory making the measurements. Calibration is provided by the in vitro diagnostic (IVD) manufacturer for commercially available measurement procedures. In the case of a laboratory developed test, the clinical laboratory produces the measurement procedure and is responsible for its calibration hierarchy including traceability to a reference system when available.

Internal QC is not intended to verify that a measurement procedure is calibrated to a higher order reference system. Rather, QC is intended to verify that the performance, for example, the bias and imprecision, of a measurement procedure remains within acceptable limits during use. A clinical laboratory may wish to verify that a measurement procedure's calibration conforms to an IVD manufacturer's claim for traceability to the reference system used for a given measurand. Some measurement procedure manufacturers provide materials specifically intended for this purpose. Such materials may be provided as measurement procedure-specific QC materials that typically have matrix characteristics and target values that are intended only for use with the specific measurement procedures claimed in the instructions for use and cannot be used with any other manufacturer's measurement procedure.

A clinical laboratory has limited resources to verify the calibration traceability of a commercially available or laboratory developed measurement procedure. National and international certified reference materials are available for some measurands. As described in Chapter 7, certified reference materials can be used to verify calibration when those certified reference materials are commutable with clinical samples for use with a specific measurement procedure. The certificate or published validation of a certified reference material should be reviewed for commutability documentation. A laboratory can split clinical samples with a laboratory that offers an RMP to verify calibration. In most cases, a clinical laboratory is dependent on the IVD manufacturer for metrologic traceability of calibration of measurement procedures.

Third-party QC materials intended for statistical process control (i.e., those provided by a manufacturer other than the routine measurement procedure's manufacturer) are not suitable to verify calibration traceability. These materials are not validated for commutability with clinical samples for different routine measurement procedures, and they do not have target values that are traceable to higher-order RMPs. Such QC materials are designed to be used as QC samples, with target values and standard deviation (SD) values assigned as described later in this chapter. When third-party QC materials are used in an interlaboratory comparison program with measurement procedure-specific peer group mean values, these values can be used to confirm that a laboratory is using a specific measurement procedure in conformance with other users of the same measurement procedure when the results are not influenced by different reagent lots (see External Quality Assessment or Proficiency Testing section).

Analytical Bias and Imprecision

Fig. 6.2 illustrates the meaning of bias and imprecision that must be known to develop a QC plan for a measurement procedure. In Fig. 6.2A, the horizontal axis represents the numeric value for an individual result, and the vertical axis represents the number of repeated measurements with the same value made on aliquots of a QC material. The *red line* shows the dispersion of results for repeated measurements

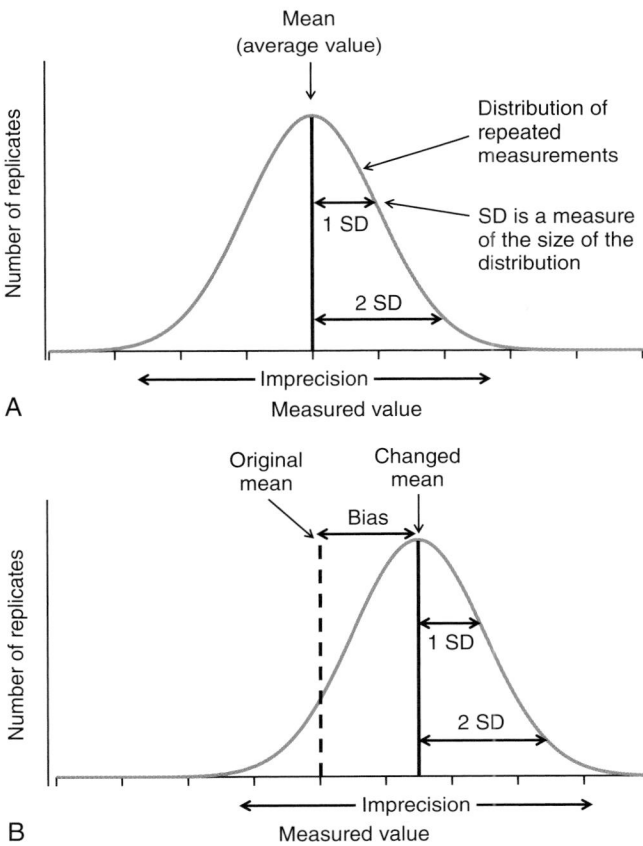

FIGURE 6.2 (A) Distribution of results showing the mean value and distribution of results (standard deviation, *SD*) for repeated measurements of a quality control sample. (B) Bias when a change in calibration has occurred. (From Miller WG. Quality control. In: McPherson RA, Pincus MR. *Henry's clinical diagnosis and management by laboratory methods.* 24th ed. Philadelphia: Elsevier; 2020.)

of aliquots of the same QC material, which is the random imprecision of the measurement. Assuming that the dispersion of results follows a Gaussian (normal) distribution, it is described by the SD. The SD is a measure of expected imprecision in a measurement procedure when it is performing within specifications. Note that results near the mean (average value) occur more frequently than results farther away from the mean. An interval of ±1 SD includes 68% of the measured values, ±2 SDs includes 95% of the values. A result that is more than 2 SDs from the mean is expected to occur 5% of the time (100%–95%) with 2.5% of results in a positive and 2.5% of results in a negative direction from the mean value. Correct calibration of a measurement procedure eliminates systematic bias (within uncertainty limits), so the mean of repeated measurements of a QC sample becomes the expected or target value for that QC sample when the measurement procedure is performing within specifications.

Fig. 6.2B, illustrates that if the calibration changes for any reason, a systematic bias is introduced into the results. The bias is the difference between the observed mean and the expected value for a QC material (for more discussion on bias, refer to Chapter 2). Note that the imprecision is the same as before the bias occurred because it is unlikely, although not impossible, that a change in imprecision would occur at the same time as a bias shift. The primary purpose of measuring QC samples is to statistically evaluate the measurement procedure performance to verify that it continues to perform within the specifications consistent with its acceptable expected stable condition or to identify that a change in performance occurred that needs to be corrected. Acceptance criteria for QC results, discussed in a later section, are based on the probability for an individual QC result to be different from the variability in results expected when the measurement procedure is performing within specifications.

The term *accuracy* is used for closeness of agreement of an individual result and a true value and is the combination of bias and imprecision that occurred for that specific measurement

(refer to Chapter 2 for more discussion on accuracy). The bias for an individual patient sample includes any systematic bias in the measurement procedure and the influence of any interfering substances that could be present in that sample. An individual QC sample is only influenced by systematic bias and imprecision of the measurement procedure. Statistical QC does not evaluate possible interfering substances that may affect results for an individual patient sample. The influence of interfering substances needs to be examined during the evaluation that a measurement procedure is suitable for use (refer to Chapter 5 for additional discussion on interference). However, the imprecision observed for QC results provides a measure of the variability expected for an individual patient result caused by the inherent imprecision of a measurement procedure and is usually independent of interfering substances that typically affect the bias for an individual patient result.

The term *trueness* is inversely related to a bias that may be present in a measurement procedure. Trueness is an attribute of a measurement procedure that reflects how correctly its calibration is traceable to a reference system.

Fig. 6.3 shows a Levey-Jennings[5] plot that was an adaptation for clinical laboratory measurements of the Shewhart[6] plot developed for statistical process control in manufacturing. The Levey-Jennings plot is the most common presentation for evaluating QC results. This format shows each QC result sequentially over time and allows a quick visual assessment of performance. Assuming the measurement procedure is performing in a stable condition consistent with its specifications, the mean value represents the target (or expected) value for the QC result, and the SD lines represent the expected imprecision. Assuming a Gaussian (normal) distribution of imprecision, the results should be distributed uniformly around the mean with results observed more frequently closer to the mean than near the extremes of the distribution. Note that a few results in Fig. 6.3 are greater than 2 SDs, and two results slightly exceed 3 SDs, which is expected for a Gaussian distribution of imprecision. For a

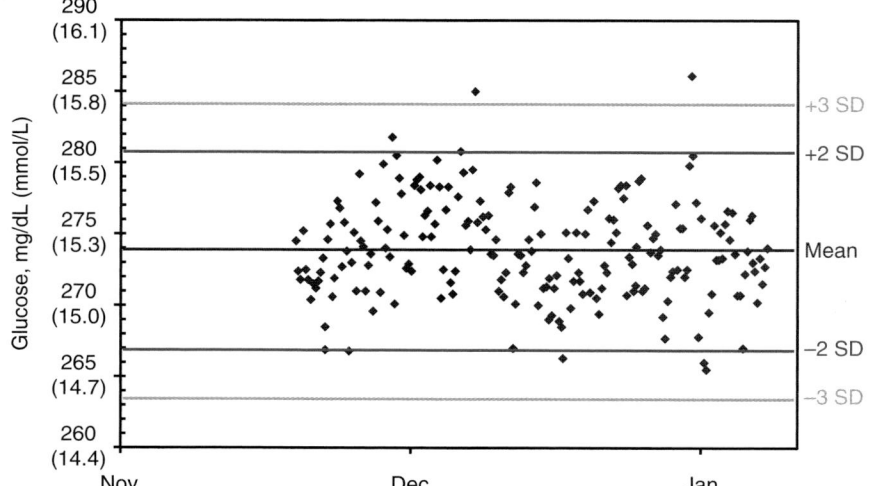

FIGURE 6.3 Levey-Jennings plot of quality control (QC) results (*n* = 199) for a single lot of QC material used for a 49-day period. *SD,* Standard deviation. (From Miller WG. Quality control. In: McPherson RA, Pincus MR. *Henry's clinical diagnosis and management by laboratory methods.* 24th ed. Philadelphia: Elsevier; 2020.)

large number of repeated measurements, the number of results expected within the SD intervals is as follows:
- ± 1 SD $= 68.3\%$ of observations
- ± 2 SD $= 95.4\%$ of observations
- ± 3 SD $= 99.7\%$ of observations

Interpretation of an individual QC result is based on its probability to be part of the expected distribution of results for the measurement procedure when the procedure is performing correctly. A later section provides details regarding interpretive rules for evaluation of QC results. Note that evaluation of individual QC results may be performed by computer algorithms without visual examination of a Levey-Jennings chart. However, the underlying logic of such algorithms is illustrated by the Levey-Jennings chart example.

Performance of a Measurement Procedure for Its Intended Medical Use

It is necessary to determine how the performance of a measurement procedure relates to the intended medical use for interpreting results in order to determine the frequency to measure QC samples and the criteria to use to evaluate the QC results. The sigma metric is commonly used to assess how well a measurement procedure performs relative to the analytical performance specifications that ideally should be based on the intended medical use of the results. Sigma is the Greek letter used to denote SD. The sigma scale expresses the variability of a measurement process in SDs in relation to the variability that is acceptable because it will not cause an error in diagnosis or treatment of a patient.

For laboratory measurements, the sigma metric is calculated as:

$$\text{Sigma} = \frac{(\text{TE}_a - \text{bias})}{\text{SD}}$$

where TE_a is the total error allowed based on analytical performance specifications that ideally should be related to the intended medical use for interpreting results, and bias and SD refer to performance characteristics of the measurement procedure. The SD is estimated from the QC data as previously described. It is critically important that the estimate of SD be made using QC data that represent all or most components of variability that occur over an extended time period (see the section called Establishing the Quality Control Target Value and Standard Deviation That Represent a Stable Measurement Operating Condition). The bias is difficult for a laboratory to estimate because it is difficult to evaluate if a particular measurement procedure has a bias compared with a reliable estimate of a true value such as based on an RMP. For internal QC, a laboratory is usually interested to determine if a bias has occurred compared with the condition established by calibration of a measurement procedure. Such a bias represents a QC result that is sufficiently different from its target value that corrective action is needed. Consequently, the bias is usually assumed to be zero for calculating sigma.

However, a bias term may be needed in situations when there are two or more different measurement procedures used for the same measurand and those different measurement procedures have a bias between them that cannot be removed, or when changes in lots of reagents or calibrators introduce shifts in bias that cannot otherwise be corrected. Note that it is preferable to adjust the calibration of different measurement procedures or different lots of reagents or

calibrators to provide equivalent results, but this solution may not be applicable for some technologies. In such cases, this relative bias can be estimated based on comparison of results for patient samples following a procedure such as described in Clinical and Laboratory Standards Institute (CLSI) document EP9[7]. That bias should be considered in determining the sigma metric and in establishing a QC plan for such measurement procedures.

TE_a represents the measurement procedure performance required to enable suitable medical decisions based on a test result. A test result may be used for different medical decisions in different disease conditions. In a main lab setting where samples from different medical practices are measured, the most stringent decision parameter should be used as the basis for the TE_a. In a setting where the samples are used for one specific clinical situation, for example, in a point-of-care (POC) setting, the medical requirements of the setting can be used as the basis for the TE_a. TE_a can be estimated using three models.[8] The preferred model (model 1) to set a performance specification is to base it on an outcome study (i.e., investigating the impact of analytical performance of the measurement procedure on the clinical outcome). Outcome studies can be direct assessment of clinical outcome for a group of patients or "indirect" outcome when the consequences of analytical performance on, for example, clinical classifications or decisions and thereby on the probability of patient outcomes can be investigated. These probabilities can be discussed with clinical experts who then can recommend a performance specification.[8]

Indirect outcome studies are often used to set TE_a in laboratory practice guidelines. For example, the National Cholesterol Education Program recommends that total cholesterol be measured with a TE_a of 9% or less,[9] and the National Kidney Disease Education Program recommends that creatinine be measured with a TE_a of less than 7 to 10% in the concentration interval 1 to 1.5 mg/dL (76.3 to 114.4 mmol/L).[10] The limitation of this model is that it is only useful when the links between the measurand, clinical decision-making, and clinical outcomes are strong, which is the case for a minority of measurands.

Another model (model 2) tries to minimize the ratio of the "analytical" noise to the "biologic signal" with an assumption that a small ratio will identify measurement procedure performance that relates to the medical requirements. The biological variation is composed of within and between subject variation. Performance specifications for imprecision, bias, and TE_a are based on a fraction of the within and between individual biologic variations of the measurand.[11,12] Tables of optimal, desirable, and minimal TE_a based on biologic variation are available and may provide useful information.[13,14] However, biologic variation–based estimates of TE_a should be used with caution because the estimates of biologic variation in many cases are based on limited data, and the experimental designs of the estimates and the process to select the estimates to list in the tables have been challenged.[15–17] Estimates of biologic variation typically vary among different investigations.[18–20] The newly established EFLM database on biological variation[14] evaluates published reports on biological variation using a critical appraisal checklist[21] and calculates point estimates with confidence intervals for each measurand after a meta-analysis of eligible reports. In addition, the way the TE_a is calculated is flawed because the calculation combines maximum allowable imprecision with maximum allowable bias (both based on a fraction of biologic variation) that has no theoretical basis and leads to overestimation of the TE_a.[15] Another limitation is that the biologic variability has typically been derived from data for nondiseased individuals and may be different for pathologic conditions. Additional examples and discussion of biologic variation are provided in Chapter 8.

Model 3 bases the performance specifications on the "state of the art." The advantage of this model is that data are readily available from QC and EQA/PT information. The disadvantage is that there may be no relationship between what is technically achievable and what is needed to make a medical decision for diagnosis or treatment of a patient. It is generally agreed that preference should be given to model 1 whenever such information is available or to model 2 as a starting point to estimate TE_a.[8,22] A laboratory director should consult with clinical care providers to agree on an appropriate TE_a for the patient population served. An extended presentation of analytical performance specifications is given in Chapter 8.

Because sigma assumes a Gaussian or normal distribution for repeated measurements, the probability of a defect (i.e., an erroneous laboratory result) can be predicted as shown in Table 6.1. The sigma metric represents the probability that a given number of erroneous results that could cause risk of harm to a patient are expected to occur when the test measurement procedure is performing to its specifications. The phrase "six sigma" refers to a condition when the variability in the measurement process is sufficiently smaller than the medical requirement that erroneous results are very uncommon. A "four-sigma" measurement procedure would be less robust and have a higher probability that erroneous results could be produced but still at a fairly low frequency. A "two-sigma" measurement procedure would produce enough erroneous results even though it met its performance specifications that it would not be very reliable for patient care.

Fig. 6.4 shows how the sigma metric describes the performance of a laboratory test relative to the TE_a. Parts *A* and *B* show that a measurement procedure with the same analytical performance characteristics can have different sigma metrics depending on how the imprecision relates to the TE_a. Fig. 6.4A shows a "six-sigma" measurement procedure that has the TE_a limits 6 SDs away from the center point of the distribution of variability in measurements when the measurement procedure is performing to its analytical specifications. In the "six-sigma" situation, a small amount of bias or increased imprecision will have little influence on the number of erroneous results produced, and less stringent QC will be appropriate because the risk of producing an erroneous result even with some loss of performance is very low.

Fig. 6.4B shows a "three-sigma" measurement procedure that has the TE_a limits 3 SDs away from the center point of the expected distribution of variability in measurements when the measurement procedure is performing to its analytical specifications. In the "three-sigma" situation, a small amount of bias or increased imprecision will cause the number of erroneous results to increase substantially, and more stringent QC is needed to identify when such an error condition occurs so that corrective action can be initiated. Note that no amount of QC will improve the performance of a marginal measurement procedure. However, more frequent QC and more stringent acceptance criteria will allow the

TABLE 6.1   Probability of Acceptable or Erroneous Results Based on the Sigma Scale[a]

Sigma Value	Percent of Results Within Specification	Percent of Results With an Error (Defect)	Errors (Defects) per Million Opportunities
1	68	32	317,311
2	95.5	4.5	45,500
3	99.7	0.3	2700
4	99.994	0.006	63
5	99.99994	0.00006	0.6
6	99.9999998	0.0000002	0.002

[a]The values in this table are based on a Gaussian statistical distribution and do not include the "1.5 sigma shift" frequently introduced to recognize that many manufacturing processes have been observed to have a long-term drift approximately ±1.5 SD when operating in a stable condition. The 1.5 sigma shift is not used for QC rules design.
From Miller WG. Quality control. In: McPherson RA, Pincus MR. *Henry's clinical diagnosis and management by laboratory methods.* 24th ed. Philadelphia: Elsevier; 2020.

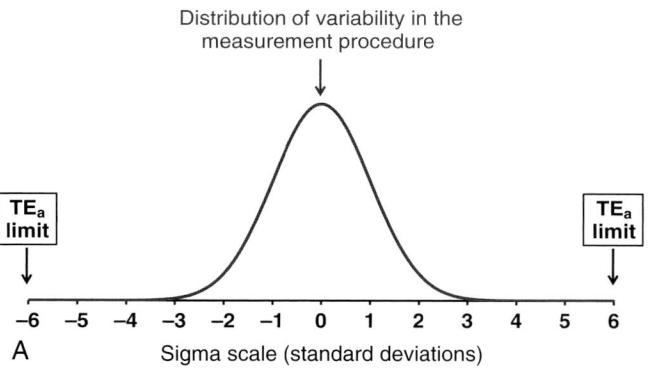

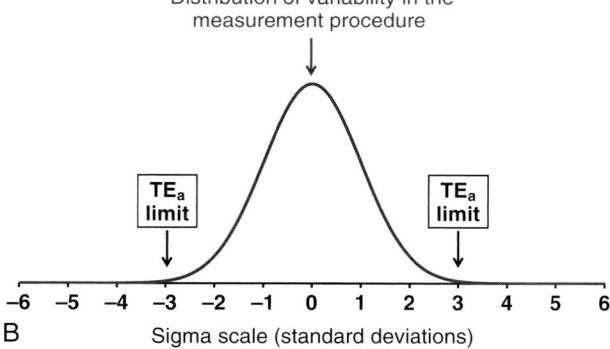

FIGURE 6.4 Measurement procedure performance relative to the sigma scale to describe how well performance meets medical requirements expressed as the allowable total error *(TE_a)*. **(A)** A "six-sigma" measurement procedure. **(B)** A "three-sigma" measurement procedure. (From McPherson RA, Pincus MR. *Henry's clinical diagnosis and management by laboratory methods.* 24th ed. Philadelphia: Elsevier; 2020.)

laboratory to more quickly identify when small changes in performance occur so they can be corrected to minimize the risk of harm to a patient from erroneous results being acted on to make medical care decisions. It is important to emphasize that the sigma calculations are dependent on what TE_a is chosen. As discussed earlier, an "objective" TE_a is often difficult to establish, and good data to set a TE_a are often lacking.

POINTS TO REMEMBER

Measurement Procedure Performance as a Prerequisite for a Quality Control Plan
- The performance characteristics of a measurement procedure when it is performing in a stable in-control condition must be understood.
- The allowable total error for a measurement procedure must be established based on analytical performance specifications that ideally should be based on the intended medical use of a laboratory result in patient care decisions.
- The sigma metric represents the probability that a given number of erroneous results that could cause risk of harm to a patient are expected to occur when the test measurement procedure is performing to its specifications.

DEVELOPING A QUALITY CONTROL PLAN AND IMPLEMENTING QUALITY CONTROL PROCEDURES

Selection of Quality Control Materials

Generally, two different concentrations are necessary for adequate statistical QC. For quantitative measurement procedures, QC materials should be selected to provide measurand concentrations that monitor the analytical measuring interval of the measurement procedure. In practice, laboratories are frequently limited by concentrations available in commercial QC products. When possible, it is important to confirm that measurement procedure performance is stable near the limits of its analytical measuring interval because defects may affect these concentrations before others. Many quantitative measurement procedures have a linear response over the analytical measuring interval, and it is reasonable to assume that their performance over the interval is acceptable if the results near the interval limits are acceptable. In the case of nonlinear analytical response, it may be necessary to use additional controls at intermediate concentrations. Concentrations of control materials close to clinical decision values (e.g., glucose, therapeutic drugs, thyroid-stimulating hormone, prostate-specific antigen, hemoglobin A_{1c} [HbA_{1c}], troponin) may also be appropriate for additional QC monitoring. In many cases, the imprecision near the limit of quantitation may be relatively large, in which case the concentration should be chosen to provide adequate SD for practical evaluation of QC results. For procedures with extraction or other pretreatment steps, controls must be used that are subject to the same pretreatment steps.

This chapter primarily focuses on QC procedures for quantitative measurement procedures. However, the principles can be adapted to most qualitative procedures with allowances for the lack of numeric results. For measurement

procedures based on qualitative interpretation of quantitative measurements (e.g., drugs of abuse, human chorionic gonadotropin, hepatitis markers), the same principles of QC assessment can be applied to the numeric results even if they are only expressed as instrument signal values. For qualitative results, the negative and positive controls should be selected to have concentrations relatively near the clinical decision threshold to adequately control for discrimination between negative and positive. For qualitative procedures with graded responses (e.g., dipstick urinalysis), negative, positive, and graded response controls are required. For qualitative tests based on other properties (e.g., electrophoretic procedures, stain adequacy, immunofluorescence, organism identification), it is necessary to ensure that the QC procedure will appropriately evaluate that the measurement procedure correctly discriminates normal from pathologic conditions.

The QC samples selected must be manufactured to provide stable materials that can be used for an extended time period, preferably 1 or more years for stable measurands. Use of a single lot for an extended period allows reliable interpretive criteria to be established that will permit efficient identification of a measurement procedure problem, avoid false alerts caused by poorly defined expected ranges for the QC results, and minimize limitations in interpreting values after reagent and calibrator lot changes.

Limitations of Quality Control Materials

Limitations are inherent in most commercially available QC materials. One limitation is that the QC material is frequently noncommutable with patient samples. Commutability is a property of a reference or control material that refers to how well that material mimics patient samples in measurement procedures. A commutable QC material is one that reacts in a measurement procedure to give a result that would closely agree with that expected for a patient sample containing the same amount of measurand. Fig. 6.5A shows that results from patient samples and from commutable QC (or EQA/PT) samples have the same relationship between two measurement procedures or between two reagent lots used with the same measurement procedure. Fig. 6.5B shows that noncommutable samples have a different relationship than observed for patient samples.

QC, as well as EQA/PT materials, are typically noncommutable with patient samples because the serum or other biologic fluid matrix is usually altered from that of a patient sample.[23-27] The matrix alteration is due to processing of the biologic fluid during product manufacturing; use of partially purified human and nonhuman additives to achieve desired concentrations of the measurands; and various stabilization processes that alter proteins, cells, and other components. The impact of the matrix alteration on measurement of a measurand is not predictable and is frequently different for different lots of QC material, for different lots of reagent within a given measurement procedure, and for different measurement procedures.[28,29] Because of the noncommutability limitation, special procedures are required (discussed in later sections) when changing lots of reagent or comparing QC results among two or more measurement procedures.

A second limitation of QC materials is deterioration of the measurand during storage. Measurand stability during unopened storage is generally excellent, but slow deterioration eventually limits the shelf life of a product and can introduce

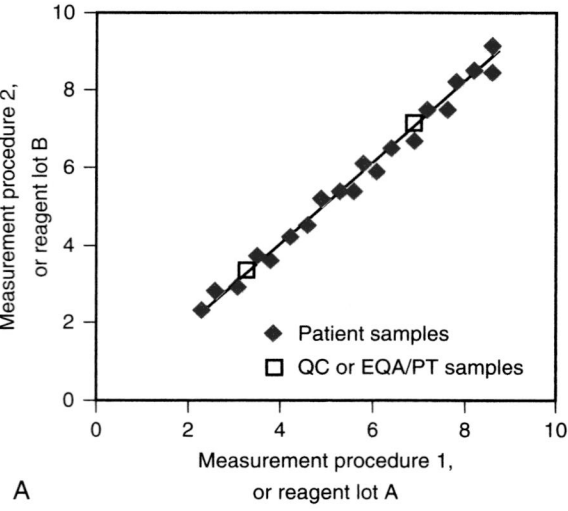
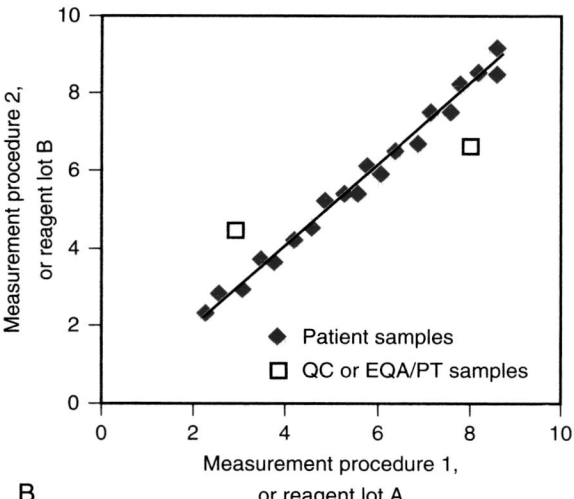

FIGURE 6.5 Illustration of commutable and noncommutable samples. **(A)** Quality control *(QC)* or external quality assessment/proficiency testing *(EQA/PT)* samples *(open white squares)* are commutable when they have the same relationship between two measurement procedures, or two reagent lots, as observed for patient samples *(red diamonds)*. **(B)** Noncommutable QC or EQA/PT samples have a different relationship than observed for patient samples.

a gradual drift into QC data that may require correction over the life of a lot of QC material. Measurand stability after reconstitution, thawing, or vial opening can be an important source of variability in QC results and can vary substantially among measurands in the same vial. Variables to be controlled are the time spent at room temperature and the time spent uncapped with the potential for evaporation. An expiration time after opening is provided by the QC material manufacturer but may need to be established by a laboratory for each QC material under the conditions of use in that laboratory and may be different for different measurands in the same QC product. For QC materials reconstituted by adding a diluent, vial-to-vial variability can be minimized by standardizing the pipetting procedure (e.g., using the same pipet or filling device, preferably an automated device, and having the same person prepare the controls) whenever practical.

Another limitation of QC materials is that measurand concentrations in multiconstituent control materials may not be at levels optimal for all measurement procedures. This limitation may be caused by solubility considerations or potential interactions between different constituents, particularly at higher concentrations. It may be necessary to use supplementary QC materials to adequately monitor the measuring interval and clinically important decision concentrations.

Frequency to Measure Quality Control Samples

Determining the frequency to measure QC samples should use a risk assessment approach. The frequency to measure QC samples is a function of several parameters:
- Analytical stability of the measurement procedure
- Risk of harm to a patient from clinical action being taken before a significant error is detected at the next scheduled QC event
- Number of patient results produced in a period of time when an error condition could exist but is not yet detected
- Scheduled events such as recalibration or maintenance that may alter the current performance condition of the measurement procedure

- Training and competency of the test operator, particularly for manual or semiautomated measurement procedures

Analytical Stability of the Measurement Procedure

The stability of the measurement procedure is a fundamental determinant of how frequently a QC sample needs to be measured. The more stable the measurement procedure, the less frequently a QC evaluation needs to be performed. Note, however, that all of the considerations in the preceding list must be evaluated together to determine a suitable frequency to perform QC. Some measurement procedures have been designed with sophisticated built-in control procedures to mitigate the risk that an erroneous result may be produced. Built-in control procedures may include calibrators and QC materials integrated with reagent packaging, and sensors that monitor electronic components and the measurement process with algorithms that prevent a result from being produced if any monitored conditions fail to meet criteria. Examples of built-in controls are frequently found in POC instruments. These measurement systems may be sufficiently stable and self-monitored to justify reduced frequency of traditional surrogate QC sample testing. However, there is little information in the literature that has examined the optimal frequency or control rules to be used in these cases.

Risk of Harm to a Patient and Number of Patients Who May Be at Risk

The risk of clinical action being taken before a significant measurement error is detected is an important consideration for more frequent QC measurements than one based strictly on analytical stability of the measurement procedure or on regulatory minimum requirements. More frequent QC measurements are appropriate to avoid the situation of discovering a measurement procedure defect many hours after a physician has made a clinical treatment or nontreatment decision based on an erroneous result. For example, QC sampling performed on a 24-hour cycle might be performed at 9 A.M. If the next QC results indicate a measurement procedure problem, the erroneous condition could have started at any time during the previous 24 hours. If the problem had occurred at 3 P.M. the previous day, erroneous results could have been reported for 18 hours, likely putting a large number of patients at risk of an inappropriate medical decision. Parvin[30] reported an assessment of the frequency of QC testing and the number of potentially incorrect patient results that could be reported before errors of different magnitudes were detected.

The medical risk of harm to a patient from erroneous results must be considered and the frequency of QC testing established to reduce the risk to an acceptable level. From a practical perspective, the cost of a medical error, or simply the cost of repeating questionable patient samples since the last acceptable QC results, could be more expensive than a more frequent QC measurement schedule that would detect an error condition in a more timely manner.

The CLSI has published guideline EP23 addressing risk-based QC procedures.[31] The document provides guidance to clinical laboratories on how to develop a QC plan based on evaluation of risk of harm to a patient and assessment of the effectiveness of risk mitigation procedures, including QC, used with a measurement procedure. Information about measurement procedure performance is obtained from the manufacturer, from laboratory validation and QC data, and from other literature sources that is combined with the clinical requirements of the local health care setting. In general terms, the laboratory director is responsible for ensuring that a result has a high probability of being correct at the time it is reported for clinical use. To make this judgment, the laboratory director needs to understand the risks that can cause a measurement technology to perform incorrectly, needs to evaluate the effectiveness of built-in control processes to mitigate those risks, and needs to ensure that adequate control procedures are in place to confirm that a result is correct at the time it is reported. A combination of built-in and QC samples-based monitoring procedures can be used to ensure that all risks have been appropriately mitigated or monitored at a frequency commensurate with the risk of malfunction and the risk of harm to a patient if an incorrect result was reported.

Measurement of Quality Control Samples Based on Scheduled Events

Laboratory operations typically implement two types of testing schedules. Batch processes measure a group of clinical samples as a batch and testing for all samples is completed before reporting the results. For batch processes, QC samples can be measured concurrent with the patient samples, for example, multiple well reaction plates, or at the beginning and end of a sequential series of measurements to ensure all results have a high probability of being correct before reporting.

Continuous measurement processes are common in higher-volume settings, for example, automated chemistry or hematology, when patient samples are measured and results reported continuously as they are received in the laboratory with QC sample measurements made periodically during the course of the process. When using a continuous measurement system, scheduled events such as recalibration or maintenance are performed to ensure the measurement conditions continue to meet specifications and to correct for any calibration drift or component deterioration that may have

occurred. Measuring QC samples before such scheduled events allows the laboratory to verify that no significant errors in results have occurred since the last time QC samples were measured.[32] If QC samples are not measured before such scheduled events, a laboratory will not know if erroneous results for patient samples were reported since the time of measuring the last QC samples and initiation of the scheduled event.

The laboratory director uses a risk assessment approach to determine when QC samples should be measured before a scheduled event. For example, daily cleaning procedures are intended to maintain the measuring system in good working condition and may not require QC assessment before the event. Whereas, a maintenance event that replaces components will produce an altered measuring system and QC assessment before the event is the only way to determine that no erroneous results were reported since the last acceptable QC results before the event. QC samples should be measured after scheduled events to verify that the operations were performed correctly, and that measurement procedure performance meets specifications before restarting to measure patient samples.

If a malfunction occurs during a continuous measurement process such that the measuring system becomes nonoperable, that condition must be treated as a QC failure with follow up to repeat and confirm the acceptability of already reported patient sample results. This follow up action is required because the malfunction prevents measuring QC samples to determine if erroneous results were reported since the time of the last acceptable QC assessment.

Establishing the Quality Control Target Value and Standard Deviation That Represent a Stable Measurement Operating Condition

QC target values and acceptable performance limits are established to optimize the probability of detecting a measurement defect that is large enough to have an impact on clinical care decisions while minimizing the frequency of "false alerts" caused by statistical limitations of the criteria used to evaluate QC results. The measurement system must be correctly calibrated and operating within acceptable performance specifications before the statistical parameters to establish QC interpretive rules can be established. Some sources of measurement variability that are expected to occur during typical operation of a measurement procedure are listed in Table 6.2. Measurement variability includes sources with short time interval frequencies, many of which can be described by Gaussian error distributions, and intermittent and longer time interval sources, which can cause cyclic fluctuations over several days or weeks, gradual drift over weeks or months, and intermittent abrupt small shifts in results. The SD used in QC interpretive rules needs to adequately represent all sources of variability in results that are expected to occur over time when the measurement procedure is performing to specifications.

Quality Control Material Target Value

A QC material must have a reliable target value that represents the condition when systematic bias is as small as possible. This condition requires the measurement procedure to be calibrated correctly. For practical reasons, the sources of

TABLE 6.2   Common Sources of Measurement Variability

Source	Time Interval for Fluctuation	Likely Statistical Distribution
Pipet volume	Short	Gaussian
Pipet seal deterioration	Long	Drift
Instrument temperature control	Short or long	Gaussian or other
Electronic noise in the measuring system	Short	Gaussian
Calibration cycles	Short to long	Gaussian or periodic drift/shift
Reagent deterioration in storage	Long	Drift
Reagent deterioration after opening	Intermediate	Cyclic, periodic drift or shift
Calibrator deterioration in storage	Long	Drift
Calibrator deterioration after opening	Intermediate	Cyclic, periodic drift or shift
Control material deterioration in storage	Long	Drift
Control material deterioration after opening	Intermediate	Cyclic, periodic drift or shift
Environmental temperature and humidity	Variable	Variable
Reagent lot changes[a]	Long	Periodic shift
Calibrator lot changes	Long	Periodic shift
Instrument maintenance	Variable	Cyclic or periodic shift
Deterioration of instrument components	Variable	Cyclic, periodic drift or shift

[a]Note that reagent lot changes can have an artifactual influence on quality control values and require special handling as discussed in the section Verifying Quality Control Evaluation Parameters After a Reagent Lot Change.
From Miller WG. Quality control. In: McPherson RA, Pincus MR. *Henry's clinical diagnosis and management by laboratory methods.* 24th ed. Philadelphia: Elsevier; 2020.

variability in Table 6.2 are not represented in the time available to establish a target value. Consequently, the target value has uncertainty and needs to be refined over time to reflect the expected variability in measurement conditions within the performance specifications for a measurement procedure.

The generally accepted minimum protocol for target value assignment is to use the mean value from at least 10 measurements of the QC material on 10 different days.[32] The 10 or more measurements can be performed over a longer time interval to include other important sources of variability in the estimate of target value. When applicable, more than one calibration should be represented in the 10 measured values to include this source of variability in the target value. If a QC material will be used for longer than 1 day, a single vial should be stored correctly and measured on as many days as the material is planned to be used to allow variability caused by opened storage to be represented in the target value. If a 10-day protocol is not possible (e.g., if an emergency replacement of a lot of QC material is necessary), a provisional target value can be established with fewer data but should be updated when additional replicate results are available.

Because all sources of variability cannot be captured in 10 measurements, it is recommended to update the target value after more data have been acquired during use of the QC material. Target values may also need to be updated after reagent lot changes or other alterations in measurement conditions as described in a later section called Verifying Quality Control Evaluation Parameters After a Reagent Lot Change.

Quality Control Material Standard Deviation

SD is the conventional way to express measurement procedure variability and assumes the QC data can be described by a Gaussian (normal) distribution even though non-Gaussian components of variability influence the QC results. The statistical QC packages in instrument and laboratory computer systems are designed with the assumption that the SD for

a Gaussian distribution is used for the QC rules criteria. Because there are non-Gaussian components to measurement variability over time, it is very important that they be represented in the data used to estimate an SD used to make conclusions regarding the acceptability of an individual QC value. The SD must be as realistic as possible to represent the variability expected for a measurement procedure when its performance meets its specifications.

When a measurement procedure has been established in a laboratory and a new lot of QC material is being introduced, the target value for the new lot of QC material is used along with the well-established long-term SD from the previous lot. This practice is appropriate because in most cases, measurement imprecision is a property of the measurement procedure and equipment used and is unlikely to change with a different lot of QC material.[32] **The SD from a small number of replicate measurements made on a new lot of QC material should not be used because it will not include most sources of variability, will underestimate the SD, and thus cause meaningless false positive QC rule failures.** When a new QC material from a different manufacturer is introduced, it is possible for the observed SD to be different than the historic value because of matrix differences, and the SD should be monitored and adjusted as experience with the new material is accumulated. If target values for the old and new lots are substantially different, a different SD may be needed. Assuming the coefficient of variation (CV) is approximately constant over the difference in concentration between target values for the old and new QC lots, the SD can be calculated by applying the existing CV to the new target value and then converting to the corresponding SD value. Because it is possible for the SD to be influenced by a lot of QC material, adjustment to the SD may be necessary as additional experience with the new lot is accumulated.

If a new measurement procedure is introduced for which no historical performance information is available, the SD for stable performance can be established using QC data obtained during the measurement procedure validation. A minimum of 20 results on different days is recommended for the initial estimation of the SD.[32] Not all of the sources of variability in Table 6.2 will be included in the initial estimate of SD and this SD will likely be smaller than an estimate based on longer-term data that includes most sources of variability. It is desirable to have some of the events that contribute to measurement variability, in particular calibration and maintenance, included during the time interval over which the SD is estimated. Note that reagent lot changes should not be included in the estimate of SD because QC results are frequently artifactually influenced by different reagent lots (see the section Verifying Quality Control Evaluation Parameters After a Reagent Lot Change). The CLSI document EP05 provides guidance on establishing the SD for a measurement procedure.[33] Note that EP05 does not include longer-term sources of variability, so the long-term SD is underestimated by this protocol.

When a new measurement procedure replaces an existing procedure, the SD for the existing procedure can in many cases be used to inform the initial estimate of the SD for the new measurement procedure. With the assumption that the SD for the existing measurement procedure was appropriate to ensure the results were suitable for use in medical decisions, that SD can be used as the basis for QC decisions for the new measurement procedure. This approach is suitable when the initial estimates of SD for the new procedure are smaller than the SD in use for the old procedure. This approach may allow an initial estimate of SD that is consistent with the intended use of the results for medical decisions until sufficient QC results have been obtained for the new measurement procedure to estimate a new SD that includes sources of variability that are not possible to include in the initial estimate of SD determined during validation of the new measurement procedure.

The initial estimate of SD will likely not include contributions from all expected sources of variability and will need to be updated when additional QC data are available. An estimate of SD can vary with measurement conditions over different time intervals with more robust values obtained for longer time intervals that include most sources of variability.[34] An SD that represents stable measurement performance can usually be estimated from the cumulative SD over a 6- to 12-month period, ideally for a single lot of QC material and reagent. Fig. 6.6 illustrates the fluctuation in SD that occurred when calculated for monthly intervals compared with the relatively stable value observed for the cumulative SD after a period of 6 months. Note that the cumulative SD is not the average of the monthly values but is the SD determined from all individual results obtained over a time interval since the lot of QC material was first used. Different sources of long-term variability occur at different times during the use of a measurement procedure. The monthly SD does not adequately reflect the longer-term components of variability. Consequently, the cumulative SD is typically larger than the monthly values because it includes more sources of variability (see Table 6.2) and better represents the actual variability of the measurement procedure. If the SD expected during normal stable operation is underestimated, the acceptable range for QC results will be too small, and the false-alert rate will be unacceptably high. If SD for the stable condition is overestimated, the acceptable range will be too large, and a significant measurement error might go undetected.

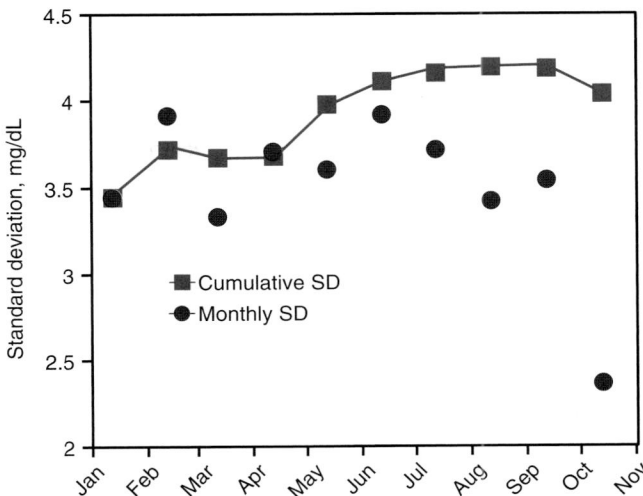

FIGURE 6.6 Cumulative standard deviation *(SD)* versus single monthly values calculated from the data in Fig. 6.9. (From Miller WG. Quality control. In: McPherson RA, Pincus MR. *Henry's clinical diagnosis and management by laboratory methods.* 24th ed. Philadelphia: Elsevier; 2020.)

Data can be combined from more than one lot of QC material or for more than one lot of reagent using a statistical pooling approach to obtain a long-term estimate of SD that represents most sources of variability in a measurement procedure. For example, this approach may be needed when the stability of a QC product is limited, and a single lot is not available for an extended time interval or when reagent stability is limited, and a new reagent lot must be used frequently. See the later section called Verifying Quality Control Evaluation Parameters After a Reagent Lot Change that explains why QC results can be artifactually influenced by reagent lot changes. Pooling of data to obtain an SD requires the SD for each stable interval of use to be determined separately; then the SD for each stable interval can be combined using the following formula where n is the number of QC results in a given time interval from 1 to i.

$$SD_{pooled} = \frac{\sqrt{(n_1-1)\times SD_1^2 + (n_2-1)\times SD_2^2 + \cdots + (n_i-1)\times SD_i^2}}{n_1 + n_2 + \cdots + n_i - i}$$

It is important to include all valid QC results in the calculation of SD to ensure that the SD correctly represents expected measurement procedure variability. A valid QC result is one that was, or would have been in the case of preliminary value assignment, used to verify acceptable measurement procedure performance and supported reporting patient results. Only QC results that were, or would have been, responsible for not reporting patient results should be excluded from summary calculations.

Quality Control Materials With Preassigned Values

Some QC materials are provided by the measurement procedure manufacturer with preassigned target values and acceptable ranges intended to confirm that the measurement procedure meets the manufacturer's specifications. Such assigned values may be used to verify the manufacturer's specifications. However, it is recommended that both the target value and the SD should be reevaluated and assigned by the laboratory after adequate replicate results have been obtained because the QC interpretive rules used in a single laboratory should reflect performance for the measurement procedure in that laboratory. The acceptability limits (product insert ranges) suggested by a manufacturer typically account for sources of variability, such as among instruments, among reagent lots, and among calibrator lots, that will be greater than the variability expected in an individual laboratory. Use of product insert ranges that are too large will reduce a laboratory's ability to detect an erroneous measurement condition. It is often a problem for POC devices that the manufacturer's preset limits must be used that can reduce the possibilities to detect errors. A laboratory can institute additional QC testing, but such options may be limited for some technologies.

QC materials with assigned target values and SDs are also available from third-party manufacturers (i.e., manufacturers not affiliated with the measurement procedure manufacturer) and typically have values that are applicable to specifically stated measurement procedures to accommodate the influence of noncommutability. Caution should be used with target values and SDs assigned by third-party QC material providers because the target values may have been assigned by a small number of measurements and using reagent and calibrator lots that are no longer available. The SD values will not be suitable for use in QC acceptance rules because they do not reflect the measurement conditions in an individual laboratory. Of particular concern is, for example, when a QC material manufacturer assigned SD is larger than that observed in an individual laboratory, the acceptable limits for QC results will be too large, and an erroneous measurement condition may not be identified appropriately.

Some QC material providers offer an interlaboratory comparison program to which participants send QC results for aggregation with those of other laboratories. Such interlaboratory summary data are similar to those from EQA/PT programs and can be useful to laboratories to compare their target values to those from a group of laboratories using the same measurement procedure and lot of QC material (see the section called External Quality Assessment or Proficiency Testing). The within group SD values from aggregated QC data are not suitable for use in an individual laboratory because the values do not reflect the measurement conditions in an individual laboratory. The SD from aggregated QC data is likely to be larger than the SD in an individual laboratory causing the acceptable limits for QC results to be too large, and an erroneous measurement condition to not be identified appropriately.

Establishing Rules to Evaluate Quality Control Results

The acceptable range and rules for interpretation of QC results are based on the probability of detecting a significant analytical error condition with an acceptably small false-alert rate. The desired process control performance characteristics must be established for each measurand before the appropriate QC rules can be selected.

The conventional way to express QC interpretive rules is by using an abbreviation nomenclature popularized among clinical laboratories by Westgard[35] and summarized in Table 6.3. Note that fractional standard deviation intervals (SDIs) can be used as in the $2_{2.5S}$ and $8_{1.5S}$ examples and that combinations of numbers of controls and limits can be used as appropriate for QC interpretive rules. Statistical procedures, such as cumulative sum (CUSUM), moving average, or exponentially weighted moving average (EWMA), are preferred to

---

TABLE 6.3 Abbreviation Nomenclature for Quality Control Evaluation Rules

Rule	Meaning	Detects
1_{2S}	One observation exceeds 2 SDs from the target value. The 1_{2S} rule has a large false-alert rate and is not recommended except for low sigma measurement procedures.	Bias or imprecision (use with caution)
1_{3S}	One observation exceeds 3 SDs from the target value.	Bias or large imprecision
2_{2S} $(2_{2.5S})$	Two sequential observations, or observations for two QC samples measured at approximately the same time, exceed 2 SDs (or 2.5 SDs) from the target value in the same direction.	Bias
$2of3_{2S}$	Two observations for three QC samples measured at approximately the same time exceed 2 SDs from the target value in the same direction. Note that this type of rule is used when three QC materials are used for a measurement procedure.	Bias
R_{4S}	Range between observations for two QC samples measured at approximately the same time, or for two sequential observations of the same QC sample, exceeds 4 SDs.	Imprecision
10_x or 10_m	Ten sequential observations for the same QC sample are on the same side of the target value (x or mean). The 10_x rule is not recommended because it has a large false-alert rate.	Bias trend (not recommended)
8_{1S} $(8_{1.5S})$	Eight sequential observations for the same QC sample exceed 1 SD (or 1.5 SD) in the same direction from the target value.	Bias trend
CUSUM	Cumulative sum of SDI for a specified number of previous results.	Bias trend
MA	Moving average for a specified number of previous results.	Bias trend
EWMA	Exponentially weighted moving average with newer results having more influence (weight).	Bias trend

CUSUM, cumulative sum; *EWMA*, exponentially weighted moving average; *MA*, moving average; *QC*, quality control; *SD*, standard deviation; *SDI*, standard deviation interval.

Modified from Miller WG. Quality control. In: McPherson RA, Pincus MR. *Henry's clinical diagnosis and management by laboratory methods.* 24th ed. Philadelphia: Elsevier; 2020.

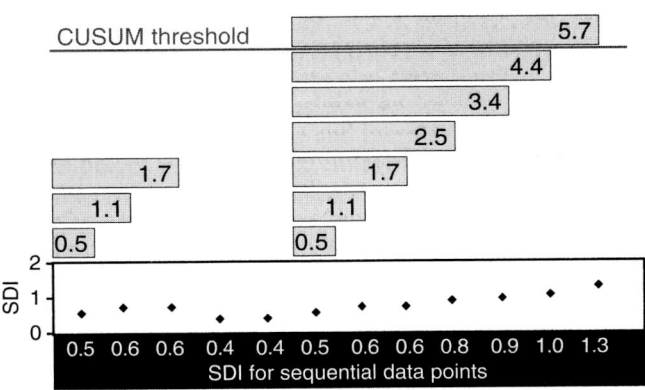

FIGURE 6.7 Cumulative sum *(CUSUM)* process to identify trends in sequential results. The standard deviation interval (*SDI* for a result vs. its target value) to initiate a CUSUM is 0.45, and the threshold for an alert is 5.0.

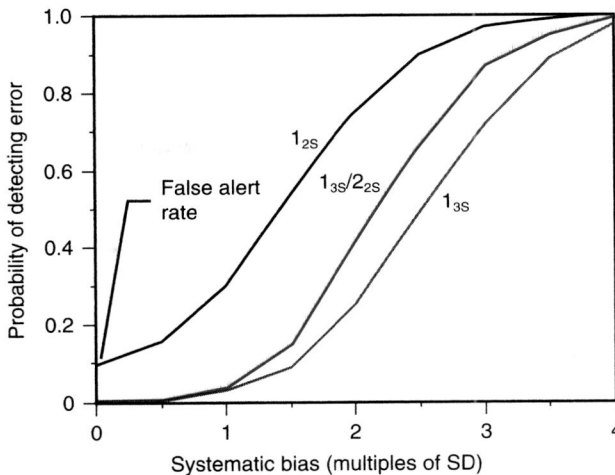

FIGURE 6.8 Power function graphs for the ability of different quality control interpretive rules to detect systematic error using two controls. Systematic error is expressed as number of standard deviations *(SDs)* from the target value. (Modified with permission from Westgard JO, Groth T. Power functions for statistical control rules. *Clin Chem* 1979;25:863–9.)

monitor for bias trends.[36] One of these more advanced trend detection procedures is recommended if supported by an available computer system because they are more powerful for detecting trends than approaches based on a number of sequential observations exceeding a specified SD interval from the target value.

CUSUM expresses the difference between a QC result and its target value as an SDI, or z-score. For example, if the target value is 25.3 and the SD is 1.4, a QC result of 27.5 would have an SDI of $(27.5 - 25.3)/1.4 = 1.6$. Fig. 6.7 illustrates the CUSUM of SDI values for the most recent QC result and previous results for the same QC material since the last CUSUM reset. A minimum value for the SDI is used to initiate the cumulative summation to prevent relatively small increments from giving false alerts. If a QC value does not exceed the minimum SDI, the CUSUM is reset to zero. When the CUSUM exceeds a threshold value, an alert is given. The CUSUM alert may occur before a trend in bias causes the result for an individual QC value to be recognized as exceeding its QC evaluation rules. The threshold value for the CUSUM and the minimum value for the SDI to initiate the summation are set to provide a high probability to identify a trend in bias that may represent a defect in the measurement procedure that needs to be investigated. The threshold can be set to provide a warning that may not require immediate corrective action but rather an alert to a potential problem.

Moving average or EWMA operates similarly to CUSUM by taking the average of the most recent QC result and a specified number of previous results. For EWMA, a function in the calculation decreases the "weights" of each result in an exponential manner such that recent results contribute a greater proportion, and older results contribute a smaller proportion to the "average" value. The moving average or EWMA value represents a bias trend in the QC results, and a threshold is set that represents a defect in the measurement procedure that needs to be investigated. As for CUSUM, the threshold can be set to provide a warning that may not require immediate corrective action but rather an alert to a potential problem.

Power function graphs have been used to express the probability that a QC interpretive rule will detect an analytical error of a given magnitude.[37] Software to calculate power function graphs assumes Gaussian (normal) error distributions. Consequently, because there are influences on QC

results that are non-Gaussian, the conclusions about QC rule performance from power function graphs are most useful as general guidance for selecting rules to interpret QC data. Other literature reports have addressed rule selection criteria using various statistical models and assumptions regarding distribution of errors.[38–41]

Power function graphs are useful to indicate relationships and relative effectiveness among different QC rules. Fig. 6.8 shows an example power function graph that plots the probability to detect a measurement error (*y*-axis), which is the probability that a result will exceed a particular interpretive rule, versus a systematic bias of known magnitude in a result (*x*-axis) with a fixed random imprecision of 1 SD when there are two QC samples being measured. The three lines in Fig. 6.8 represent the probabilities of different interpretive rules to detect biases of various magnitudes. For example, for the 1_{2S} rule, a result with a bias of 1 SD (*x*-axis) has a 0.35 (35%) probability (*y*-axis) of violating the rule (i.e., of having a result >2 SDs from the target value). Note that this figure shows only bias as SD on the *x*-axis, and a result with 1 SD bias will also have an imprecision component that may cause the 1_{2S} rule to be exceeded. A 1_{2S} interpretive rule has approximately 35% probability to detect a systematic error that is 1 SD in magnitude and approximately 80% probability to detect a systematic error that is 2 SD in magnitude. Similar graphs can be created for other interpretive rules for both bias and imprecision error conditions.

Note in Fig. 6.8 that none of these interpretive rules has a 100% probability to detect a systematic bias until the error becomes relatively large. The 1_{2S} rule has a good probability of detecting errors (e.g., almost 90% probability of detecting a 2.5-SD bias) but has a high false-alert rate as indicated by the *y*-intercept that indicates that because of imprecision, the probability of indicating an error condition for zero bias is approximately 10%. Because of this high false-alert rate, it is generally not recommended to use a 1_{2S} rule unless the measurement procedure has marginal performance (i.e., is a "low sigma" measurement procedure) and the laboratory desires to identify small biases that could cause inappropriate risk for a patient care decision. The 1_{3S} rule has a low false-alert rate but a lower probability to detect an error (e.g., a 50% probability to detect a 2.5-SD bias).

Combining two or more rules and applying them simultaneously as multi-rule criteria is recommended to improve the efficiency of QC interpretive rules. For example in Fig. 6.8, the $1_{3S}/2_{2S}$ multi-rule identifies an error condition if one control exceeds ± 3 SD from the target value or if two controls exceed ± 2 SDs in the same direction from the target value. The $1_{3S}/2_{2S}$ multi-rule has a low false-alert rate similar to the 1_{3S} rule but improved probability to detect an error (e.g., a 65% probability to detect a 2.5-SD bias and a 90% probability to detect a 3.2-SD bias). In this multi-rule example, the 1_{3S} component is sensitive to imprecision or large bias, the 2_{2S} component is sensitive to bias.

A challenge in selecting interpretive rules for evaluating QC results is that the different longer-term sources of variation listed in Table 6.2 occur at different times when using a measurement procedure. These types of variability are not adequately described by Gaussian models for rules selection. At certain periods of time, the short-term SD will be noticeably smaller than the long-term cumulative value (see Fig. 6.6). One must avoid concluding, based on a short-term estimate of SD, that the SD used for evaluation is too large because, over time, the cumulative value will be more consistent with measurement procedure performance as periodic sources of variability are encountered. Using an estimate of SD that is inappropriately small will lead to increased frequency of false alerts.

Fig. 6.9 shows how non-Gaussian error sources influenced results for a single lot of QC material used over a 10-month period for an automated glucose measurement procedure. The stability and performance over the 10 months were considered acceptable for clinical use. Data for the first 49 days are the same as in Fig. 6.3 and represent the initial experience with this lot of QC material. Examination of these data shows several fluctuations that cannot be described by a Gaussian statistical model. The first reagent lot change caused a step shift to higher values that was too small to initiate a change in target value. The second reagent lot change had no effect on QC results. Between March and April, a transition to lower values occurred that did not correspond to any maintenance, reagent lot change, or calibration events. Throughout the 10-month period, intervals of several weeks in duration occurred when the imprecision was better or worse than at other time periods (also see Fig. 6.6 calculated from the same data).

In practice, empirical judgment is frequently used to establish acceptance criteria (rules) to evaluate QC results based on data acquired over a long enough time to adequately estimate the expected variability when a measurement procedure is working correctly. QC rules should not be selected based only on Gaussian models of imprecision because the rules will not correctly accommodate all the types of variability observed for many analytical measuring systems.

Table 6.4 gives an example of an empirically developed multi-rule based on the data in Fig. 6.9. An empirical approach can be used by obtaining a set of QC data that represents a time interval expected to include most sources of variability. Using those QC data, the false-alert rate for a rule can be determined, and bias errors of different magnitudes can be added to estimate the ability of a rule, or a combination of rules, to identify that error. This multi-rule had 0.6% false alerts when applied to the data in Fig. 6.9 using the mean from the November to January (see Fig. 6.3) period as the target value and the cumulative SD for the 10-month period to represent overall imprecision. If a 2_{2S} rule was used instead of a $2_{2.5S}$ rule, the false-alert rate would increase by 1.2%, but the rule would detect slightly smaller biases. An $8_{1.5S}$ rule was used to provide detection of bias

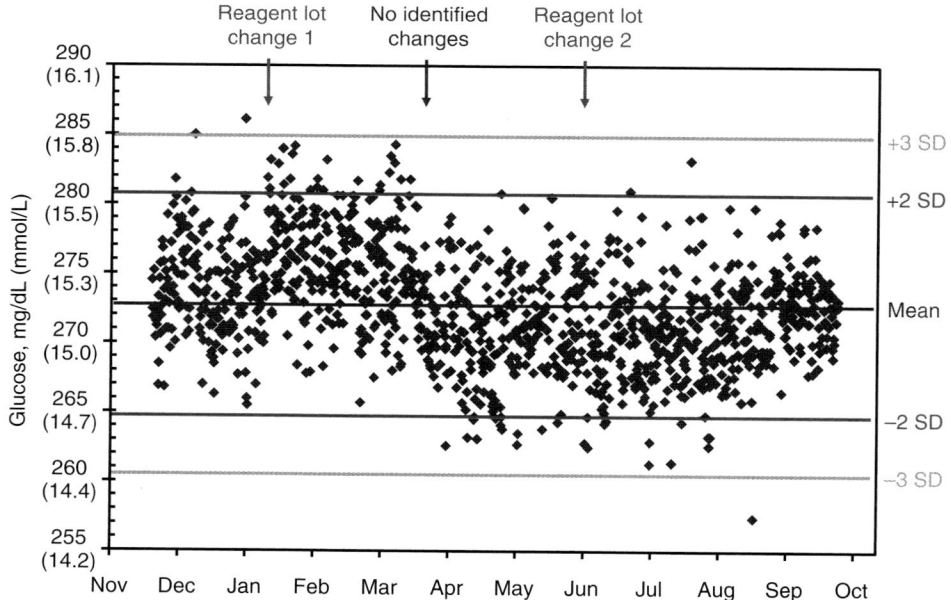

FIGURE 6.9 Levey-Jennings plot of quality control *(QC)* results ($n = 1232$) for a single lot of QC material used over a 10-month period. *SD,* Standard deviation. (Adapted with permission from Miller WG, Nichols JH. Quality control. In: Clarke WA, editor. *Contemporary practice in clinical chemistry.* 2nd ed. Washington, DC: AACC Press; 2010.)

TABLE 6.4 Empirical Multi-Rule for the Quality Control Data Presented in Fig. 6.11

Multi-Rule Components	Type of Variability Detected
1_{3S}	Imprecision or bias
$2_{2.5S}$	Bias
R_{4S}	Imprecision
$8_{1.5S}$	Bias trend

QC, Quality control.
From Miller WG. Quality control. In: McPherson RA, Pincus MR. *Henry's clinical diagnosis and management by laboratory methods.* 24th ed. Philadelphia: Elsevier; 2020.

trends because it had a 0% false-alert rate (compared with 0.5% for an 8_{1S} rule) and was adequate to detect a developing trend before it became clinically important because the CV was small, 1.5%, at the concentration of the QC material. If a 10% TE$_a$ is considered acceptable for glucose at this concentration, then the sigma metric for this measurement procedure is 6.7, suggesting that it has a very low error rate, and these QC rules with a low false-alert rate will be suitable to alert the laboratory to an error condition large enough to affect patient care decisions. Such control rules should allow the laboratory to detect errors before they are of a magnitude that will affect clinical actions. At other clinical concentration ranges or for other analytes, a different set of QC evaluations rules may be more appropriate. A 10_x rule was not used because it would have increased the false-alert rate by 10.6%. A 10_x rule or other rule that counts the number of sequential QC results on one side of the target value is not recommended because this condition does not indicate a problem with clinical interpretation of patient results when the magnitude of the difference from the target value is small. Counting the number of sequential results that exceed a larger SD from the target value, such as $8_{1.5S}$ in this example, is more likely to represent a measurement condition that might need investigation.

The balance between false alerts and the probability of detecting an error is improved when multiple rules are used in combination. When establishing rules to interpret QC results, it is important to remember that statistical process control can only verify at a point in time that a measurement procedure is producing results that conform to the expected variability when the procedure is performing in a stable operating condition. It is important to remember that periodic measurement of QC samples does not identify random events (e.g., a temporary clot in a sample pipet, a random reagent pipetting error) that do not persist until the next QC sample is measured. QC rules are chosen to detect changes in calibration and changes in imprecision that persist until the next QC measurement and are significant enough to require correction before patient results are reported.

Poorly Performing Measurement Procedures

In the process of reviewing statistical parameters for QC data, a measurement procedure's performance may be identified as marginal or inadequate to meet medical requirements. Determining the sigma metric is helpful to make this assessment because the sigma value gives a prediction of the number of erroneous results expected. If the measurement procedure performance cannot be improved and a better measurement procedure is not available, the laboratory can either discontinue

the test if the performance is inadequate or apply more stringent QC practices to identify small deviations from the expected performance. More stringent QC practices include selecting rules that will give an alert at smaller error conditions, using additional rules in a multi-rule set, measuring QC more frequently, using more than two QC samples, and not releasing patient results until QC assessment is complete for the time interval during which patient samples were measured. Lower sigma measurement procedures usually require more frequent measurement of QC samples, more stringent criteria for accepting QC results, as well as applying patient-based QC monitoring when possible.

More stringent QC rules will not improve measurement procedure performance but will identify smaller changes in measurement procedure performance that could affect patient care decisions based on the results. More stringent QC rules will have more false alerts, but this is an unavoidable cost when lower sigma measurement procedures are used. Because the analytical requirements are not easy to establish and are themselves somewhat uncertain, one should regularly reassess the requirements to see if they remain appropriate or should be updated, and should reconsider that the QC rules are appropriate to identify an error condition. In addition, the measurement procedure limitations should be communicated to patient care providers.

Specifying the Quality Control Plan

The preceding subsections describe the considerations for each component in a QC plan. The laboratory director is responsible for considering the components, making judgments regarding the considerations, and approving the final plan for each analyte measured in a laboratory. A plan for internal QC using surrogate samples specifies the following components:
- The number of controls to be measured and the approximate concentrations of analytes in those controls
- The target values for each control
- The SD to be used in the QC rules
- The rules for evaluating the QC results
- The frequency to test the QC samples

Overall, the choice of the parameters in the QC plan depends on the performance characteristics of the measurement procedure, the number of potentially erroneous patient results that could occur before the error condition is identified, and the risk of harm to a patient if potentially erroneous results were used in medical care decisions. Yundt-Pacheco and Parvin described a methodology using a Gaussian statistical model to compute the expected number of unreliable patient results produced based on an out-of-control condition and the performance characteristics of a measurement procedure.[41]

Considerations for Point-of-Care Testing

Internal QC of POC instruments offers extra challenges compared with those addressed at the central laboratory. The main reasons for this are that POC instruments are often operated by persons without laboratory training; they often use methodologic principles that are different from those in the central laboratory; they often have "built-in" controls; and the number of measurements is rather small, making the use of QC samples in the traditional way expensive. Because the instruments are used by nonlaboratory personnel who also should run the QC program, these people have to be convinced that measuring QC samples is useful and will detect errors important for patient safety. Unfortunately, the evidence for measuring QC samples is scarce, probably because there is little agreement on how to implement QC for POC instruments and how to handle the QC alerts. The ISO 22870 document[42] states that if an institution wants to be accredited to this standard, internal and external QC of POC instruments should be done, but it is not stated how this should be done. Recommendations from different countries generally state that it is "mandatory" to measure QC samples, but they are usually vague concerning how it should be done, from analyzing two levels of QC materials a day to one level of QC material every sixth month or as "recommended by the manufacturer" or "recommended to use control material independent from the manufacturer" and use specifications as defined by the local laboratory.[43–45]

It is not surprising that there are no uniform or concrete recommendations because POC instruments use different methodologies and technologies, and they are used at different locations, from wards at a hospital to remote areas. Before establishing an internal QC program for POC instruments, at least three issues should be taken into consideration: (1) the type of POC instrument and what "built-in" control processes it has, (2) the location of the instrument, and (3) the operator of the instrument. Broadly, the current instruments have been divided into three categories: (1) instruments that are similar to the wet chemistry instruments used in the central laboratory, (2) cartridge-based instruments, and (3) strip-based instruments,[46] although there is a significant "overlap" between the two last categories. The instruments using wet chemistry and similar technologies to those used in the central laboratory should follow the principles for internal QC as outlined in this chapter albeit taking into consideration the number of measurements per day. In cartridge-based and some strip-based instruments, the manufacturer often has placed the technology in the cartridge or strip together with QC materials, and in some cases, QC rules are built in so that patient results cannot be reported unless the QC is "satisfactory."[47] The instrument is then merely an electronic reader that often has incorporated an "electronic quality control" where the electronics of the measurement procedure are verified. The electronic instrument checks do not verify the reagents in the cartridges or strips, and unless each cartridge has internal QC materials, the reagent cartridges or strips should be checked at delivery and then at intervals (e.g., with the arrival of a new shipment or lot or at a suitable interval such as monthly or based on the number of patient measurements in a time interval).

Not all POC instruments include enhanced QC features. In these cases, one must rely on daily liquid surrogate QC performed by the operator.[48] The limitation of using the liquid QC sample in this situation is that it only checks if one disposable cartridge or strip meets the performance specifications. This limitation requires an assumption that all devices in a lot were manufactured uniformly and will perform equivalently. Some tests, such as dipstick urinalysis, require liquid QC because there are no built-in control mechanisms. Others, such as urine pregnancy tests, have a built-in positive control band to ensure that the device is functioning properly, but this may not be an adequate substitute for a traditional QC sample that can assess suitable recovery of concentrations. Some POC protocols run patients' samples on a POC instrument and send the same samples to a central laboratory

as a form of internal QC. It has been shown for international normalized ratio that this periodic split patients' samples procedure cannot be recommended because it had a lower probability of error detection and a higher rate of false alarms compared with using commercial lyophilized QC material.[48] The operator of the instrument is also important. In patient self-testing, it is difficult to implement internal QC procedures other than what is built into the instruments or strips or cartridges.

How internal QC should be performed and supervised also depends on the location of the POC instruments. In a hospital, it is now possible with real-time bidirectional connectivity between the POC devices and the central laboratory to transfer both patient and QC results and to set lockout parameters for conformance to a QC protocol. As technology advances, the general trend is for more sophisticated POC devices with built-in control systems to be incorporated to minimize or prevent the possibility for an incorrect result.[49]

Corrective Action When a Quality Control Result Indicates a Measurement Problem

A QC alert occurs when a QC result fails an evaluation rule, which indicates that an analytical problem may exist. A QC alert means there is a high probability that the measurement procedure is producing results that have the potential to be unreliable for patient care. Some types of QC rules, for example, trend rules, can be established as warnings intended to initiate an investigation but not require immediate discontinuing reporting of results. Other types of QC rules are intended to indicate error conditions for which discontinuing reporting patients' results is indicated. Fig. 6.10 presents a generalized troubleshooting sequence. Remeasuring the same QC sample is not recommended because, with properly designed control rules, it is more likely that a measurement procedure problem exists than the QC result was a statistical outlier or gave a false alert. However, QC materials can deteriorate after opening because of improper handling and storage or because of unstable measurands. Thus repeating the measurement on a new vial of the QC material is a useful step to determine if the alert was caused by deteriorated QC material rather than by a measurement procedure problem. In this situation, if the result for the new QC sample is acceptable, testing of patient samples can resume. One caution when the repeat QC result is near acceptability limits is to consider

1. Stop reporting results
2. Measure a new container of control

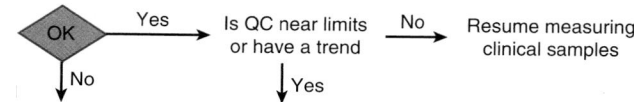

3. Identify and correct the measurement defect
4. Repeat controls

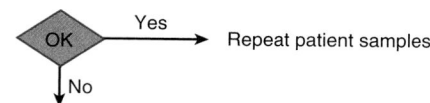

5. Further technical investigation

FIGURE 6.10 Generalized troubleshooting sequence showing the initial steps after an unacceptable quality control *(QC)* result. The details of troubleshooting the defect may be different for different rules violations or if more than one unacceptable QC result was obtained.

whether the repeat and original results are essentially the same. In this situation, the probability is fairly high that a measurement problem exists, and this possibility should be investigated. In addition, current and preceding QC results should be examined for a trend in bias that indicates a measurement issue that needs to be corrected. These precautions in evaluating repeat results for a new QC sample can be challenging or impossible for automated evaluation by computer systems, thus requiring the laboratory technologist to be vigilant in reviewing results.

When repeat testing of a new QC sample does not resolve the alert situation, the instrument and reagents should be inspected for component deterioration, empty reagent containers, mechanical problems, and so on. In many cases, recalibration is indicated.

When the problem is identified and corrected, QC samples should be measured to verify the correction, and all patient samples since the time of the last acceptable QC results, or the time when the error condition occurred, should be measured again. It may be difficult to establish the time when an error condition occurred but repeating selected patient results may be considered. For example, every few samples can be repeated back to the time of the last acceptable QC results. The repeated results are then compared with acceptable criteria for repeated results agreement (see next paragraph) to identify a point in time when the error condition occurred. When selecting the samples to repeat, it is important to ensure that a substantial representation of the potentially erroneous samples is repeated and that samples at a concentration consistent with that of the unacceptable QC are represented. Alternatively, groups of 10 patient samples can be repeated, again ensuring that samples at a concentration consistent with that of the unacceptable QC are represented, until all repeat results in at least two sequential groups are within acceptable criteria for repeated results. When the point at which the error condition was likely to have occurred is identified, all patient samples must be repeated from that point until the unacceptable QC result was obtained. Any assessment of the point at which an error condition occurred by repeating selected patient samples has a risk to incorrectly identify that point and laboratories must repeat enough patient samples to have confidence in the assessment.

The laboratory director must establish acceptable criteria to determine if the repeat results agree adequately to permit reporting of original results without issuing a corrected report. Otherwise, corrected results must be reported. As an example, Table 6.5 lists empirical criteria used in one author's laboratory for this purpose. The criteria for acceptability of repeated tests are based on measurement procedure performance characteristics and the intended medical use of the results. The considerations for determining the TE_a described in the section Performance of a Measurement Procedure for its Intended Medical Use and in Chapter 8 related to the reference change value may be helpful to set acceptance criteria for repeated patient sample results.

In some cases, residual sample volume may not be adequate for repeat testing (quantity not sufficient [QNS]). In these situations, no results can be reported unless it is documented that the impact of the measurement procedure defect on the original results was small enough to have minimal effect on clinical interpretation. A protocol to evaluate the clinical impact of the measurement defect involves repeating

TABLE 6.5 Example for Selected Chemistry Analytes of Empirical Criteria for Patient Test Result Agreement Between Repeated Assays and for Agreement Among Results for a Single Patient Sample Measured on Multiple Instruments

Analyte	Acceptance Criteria (Difference Between Results)
Albumin	0.4 g/dL (4.0 g/L)
ALP	10 U/L or 10%[a]
ALT	10 U/L or 10%[a]
Amylase	15 U/L or 10%[a]
AST	10 U/L or 10%[a]
Bilirubin, total	0.3 mg/dL (5 μmol/L) or 10%[a]
Calcium, total	0.5 mg/dL (0.125 mmol/L)
Chloride	4 mmol/L
Cholesterol	5%
CK	10 U/L or 10%[a]
CO_2	4 mmol/L
Creatinine	0.2 mg/dL (18 μmol/L) or 10%[a]
GGT	10 U/L or 10%[a]
Glucose	6 mg/dL (0.33 mmol/L) or 5%[a]
Iron	10 μg/dL (1.8 μmol/L) or 10%[a]
Lactate	0.32 mmol/L
LDH	10 U/L or 10%[a]
Lipase	10 U/L or 10%[a]
Magnesium	0.3 mg/dL (0.1 mmol/L)
Phosphorus	0.4 mg/dL (0.13 mmol/L)
Potassium	0.3 mmol/L
Protein, total	0.4 g/dL (4.0 g/L)
Sodium	4 mmol/L
Triglycerides	10%
Urea nitrogen (BUN)	3 mg/dL (1.1 mmol/L urea) or 10%[a]
Uric acid	0.4 mg/dL (24 μmol/L)

[a]Whichever is greater.
ALP, Alkaline phosphatase; *ALT*, alanine aminotransferase; *AST*, aspartate aminotransferase; *BUN*, blood urea nitrogen; *CK*, creatine kinase; CO_2, carbon dioxide; *GGT*, γ-glutamyl transferase; *LDH*, lactate dehydrogenase.
From Miller WG. Quality control. In: McPherson RA, Pincus MR. *Henry's clinical diagnosis and management by laboratory methods.* 24th ed. Philadelphia: Elsevier; 2020.

those samples that have adequate volume. The repeated samples must represent the concentration range of the QNS samples and the time span since the previous acceptable QC results and should include a substantial proportion of the total samples originally assayed while the measurement procedure was in the unacceptable condition. If the repeat results for this subgroup are within established "acceptable" criteria for repeat testing of patient samples, the original results for the QNS samples can be reported. Otherwise, the original results for the QNS samples are considered erroneous; no results can be reported, and any original results already reported need to be corrected to a "no result" condition.

Alternatively, for QNS samples, when there was not an outright malfunction but rather a drift or shift in calibration, it may be possible to estimate the magnitude of a bias error from the results for other patient samples that were repeated, apply that bias as a correction to the QNS samples, and report the corrected result with a comment regarding the increased uncertainty in the values. When there are inadequate data to estimate a correction factor from repeated results for other patients, the laboratory may consider reporting the original result for a QNS sample with a comment regarding its uncertainty. This approach can be useful especially in cases when it might be difficult or take a long time to obtain a new sample, or in cases when the clinical question can be answered by whether the result is very high or very low (e.g., hypo- or hyperthyroidism). The laboratory director should be consulted for guidance in reporting results for QNS samples that may have greater uncertainty than the usual quality performance for a laboratory.

Verifying Quality Control Evaluation Parameters After a Reagent Lot Change

Changing reagent lots can have an unexpected impact on QC results. Careful reagent lot crossover evaluation of QC target values is necessary. Because the matrix-related interaction between a QC material and a reagent can change with a different reagent lot, QC results may not be a reliable indicator of a measurement procedure's performance for patient samples after a reagent lot change. In a large study of 661 reagent lot changes for eight QC materials measured for 82 analytes using seven different instrument platforms, 41% of 1483 QC material–reagent lot combinations had significant differences in QC values between the reagent lots that were not observed for patient samples.[28] In the example in Fig. 6.11, QC values for the high-concentration control shifted after the change to a new lot of reagents, but there was no change in results for the low control. A comparison of results for a panel of patient samples measured using the new and old reagent lots, as shown in Fig. 6.12, verified that patient results were the same when either lot of reagents was used. Patient results spanning the measuring interval had nearly identical values, as indicated by the slope of 1.00 and the small intercept of −3 mg/dL (0.17 mmol/L). Consequently, the change in values for the high-concentration QC material was due to a difference in matrix-related bias between the QC material and each of the reagent lots.

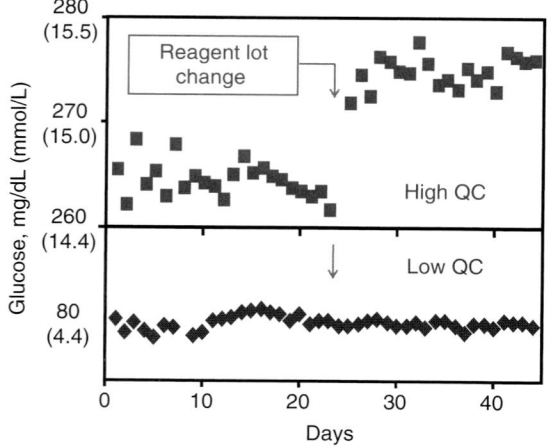

FIGURE 6.11 Levey-Jennings plot showing impact of a reagent lot change on matrix bias with quality control *(QC)* samples. (Modified with permission from Miller WG, Nichols JH. Quality control. In: Clarke WA, editor. *Contemporary practice in clinical chemistry.* 2nd ed. Washington, DC: AACC Press; 2010.)

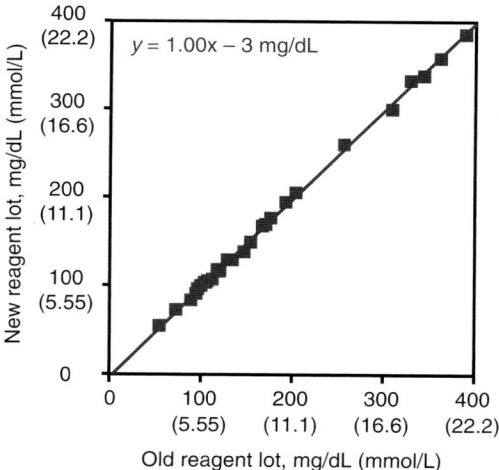

FIGURE 6.12 Deming regression analysis of results from a patient sample comparison between the same old and new lots of reagent shown in Fig. 6.11 for quality control samples. (From Miller WG. Quality control. In: McPherson RA, Pincus MR. *Henry's Clinical diagnosis and management by laboratory methods.* 24th ed. Philadelphia: Elsevier; 2020.)

Clinical patient samples must be used to verify the consistency of results between old and new lots of reagents because of the unpredictability of a matrix-related bias being present for QC materials. Fig. 6.13 presents a protocol to verify or adjust QC material target values after a reagent lot change. A group of patient samples and the QC samples are measured using both the current (old) and new reagent lots. The first step is to verify that results for a group of patient samples measured with the new reagent lot are consistent with results from the current (old) lot. The patient sample results, not the QC results, provide the basis for verifying that the new reagent lot is acceptable for use. If a problem is identified, the calibration of the new reagent lot must be investigated and corrected, or the new reagent lot may be defective and should not be used. When evaluating the patient results, keep in mind that the calibration of the old reagent lot may have drifted and should be verified before concluding that the new reagent lot is not giving acceptable results for the patient samples.

The number of patient samples to use for verifying the performance of a new reagent lot will depend on the measuring interval, the imprecision of a measurement procedure, and the concentrations at which clinical decisions are made. CLSI document EP26[50] recommends a minimum of three patient samples and more patient samples depending on the number of important clinical decision concentrations and the imprecision of a measurement procedure. This CLSI guideline includes a statistical analysis to determine if a difference in patient results is less than a critical difference that would represent risk for an inappropriate patient care decision based on a particular laboratory test result. An alternate approach is to select 10 or more patient samples that span the measuring interval and use orthogonal regression analysis or a difference plot to evaluate average performance over the interval of concentrations represented by the patient samples.

There are no well-established clinical acceptance criteria for agreement between results; consequently, the laboratory must establish acceptance criteria consistent with the

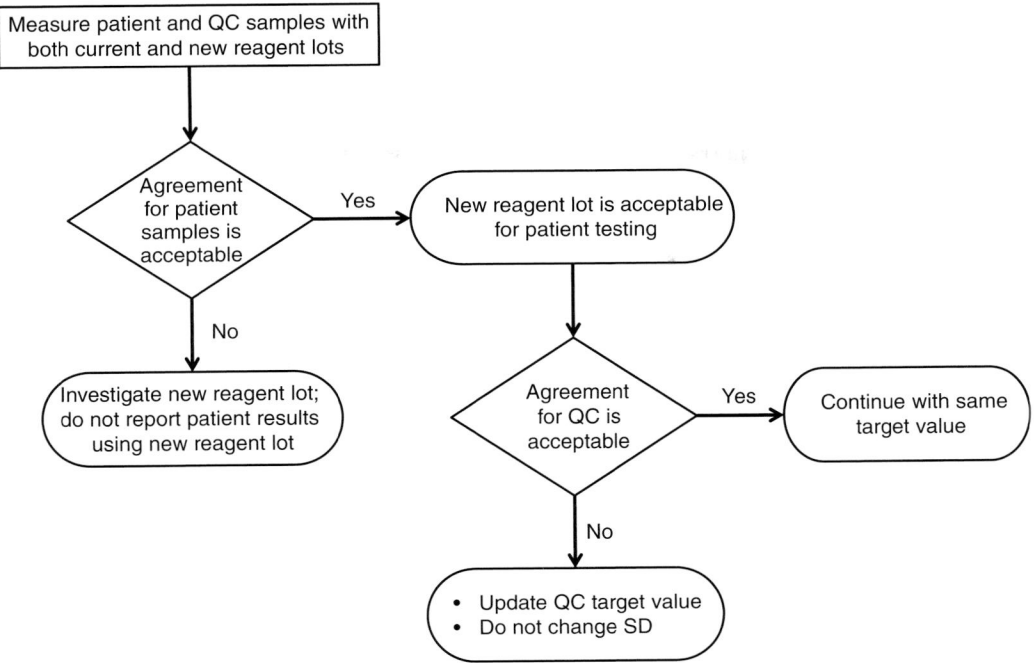

FIGURE 6.13 Process for assessment of potential matrix impact on quality control *(QC)* samples after a reagent lot change. *SD,* Standard deviation. (From Miller WG. Quality control. In: McPherson RA, Pincus MR. *Henry's clinical diagnosis and management by laboratory methods.* 24th ed. Philadelphia: Elsevier; 2020.)

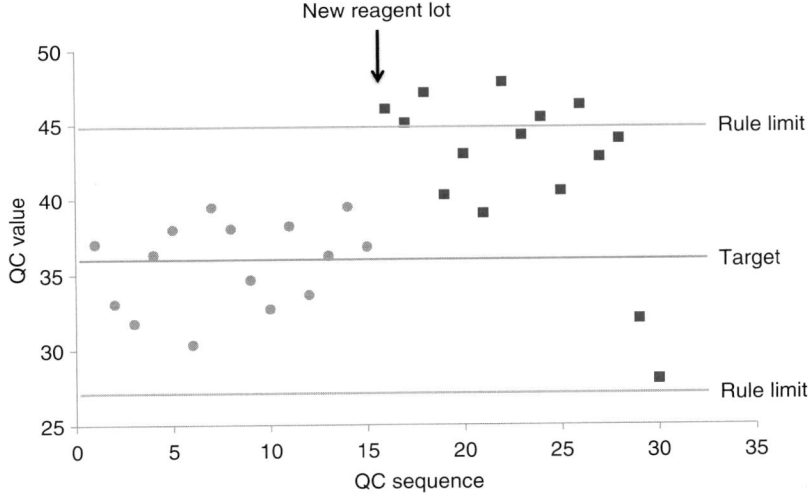

FIGURE 6.14 Illustration of the influence on the failure rate for a quality control *(QC)* rule when failing to adjust the target value for a matrix-related shift. QC results before a new reagent lot are shown as *gray circles* and after the new reagent lot as *red squares. SD,* Standard deviation. (From Miller WG. Quality control. In: McPherson RA, Pincus MR. *Henry's clinical diagnosis and management by labora-tory methods.* 24th ed. Philadelphia: Elsevier; 2020.)

relatively small number of samples used, the analytical performance characteristics of a measurement procedure, and the intended medical use for interpreting results. As an example, empirical acceptance criteria used in one author's laboratory for assessment of individual results are provided in Table 6.5.

When the results for patients' samples are acceptable, the second step in Fig. 6.13 evaluates results for each QC material to determine if its target value is correct for use with the new

lot of reagent(s). If the target value has changed, it must be adjusted to correct for the change in matrix-related bias between old and new lots of reagent(s). This adjustment keeps the expected variability centered around the QC target value so that QC interpretive rules will remain valid. Failure to make a target value adjustment will introduce an artifactual bias in subsequent QC results, causing both an increased false-alert rate and a decreased ability to detect some error conditions. These effects are illustrated in Fig. 6.14 where the shift in target value would cause some of the results shown by *red squares* to exceed the old upper QC rule limit when in reality there is no defect in patient results because the QC results are artifactually increased because of the matrix-related bias with the new reagent lot. Similarly, the increased magnitude of the gap to the old lower QC rule limit will permit a low bias condition, as shown by the square red points at sequence number 29 and 30, to be undetected until the low bias becomes larger than the QC rule is intended to detect.

The SD used to evaluate QC results will not typically change when a new lot of reagent(s) is put into use. The SD represents expected variability when the measurement procedure is stable and is performing according to specifications. In most cases, the variability of a measurement procedure will be the same with any lot of reagent(s). However, occasional exceptions may occur; for example, if the new reagent lot is a reformulation, it may be necessary to adjust the SD after additional numbers of QC results are accumulated with the new reagent lot. A reagent lot verification is typically performed on a single day and will likely provide only a few QC results from which to evaluate if the target value has changed. Consequently, it is necessary to carefully monitor QC results as more data are acquired using the new reagent lot and, if needed, to further refine the new target value.

Note that a reagent lot induced matrix-related change in the numeric values for the QC results will cause an artifactual increase in the cumulative SD, thus making it larger than the inherent measurement variability and not suitable for use in QC rules. For this reason, it is recommended to use the cumulative SD from a single reagent lot or the pooled SD from more than one reagent lot (see subsection called Quality Control Material Standard Deviation) when determining the SD to use for interpreting QC rules.

Experience in clinical laboratories has shown that there are changes, other than reagent lot changes, in measurement procedures that can also affect the QC values but not the results for patient samples. Such changes could be caused by instrument component replacement or other causes. In theory, there should be an assignable cause for such effects, but such a cause is not always identifiable. In practice, any condition that affects QC results but does not affect patient results is treated in the same manner as described for reagent lot changes.[32] The important QC principle is that if the results for patient samples are consistent between the two conditions, then the target value for the QC sample should be adjusted, if necessary, to reflect its value under the new condition. Failure to adjust the QC target value will cause inappropriate acceptability criteria to be used for evaluating the QC results and incorrect QC rules evaluation with increased false alerts and some potential error conditions missed (see Fig. 6.14).

Verifying Measurement Procedure Performance After Use of a New Lot of Calibrator

When a new lot of calibrator is used, with no change in reagents, there is no change in matrix interaction between the QC material and the reagents. In this situation, QC results provide a reliable indication of calibration status with the new lot of calibrator. If the QC results indicate a bias after use of a new lot of calibrator, the calibration has changed and needs to be corrected to ensure consistent results for patient samples.

Some measurement procedures are packaged as kits that include reagents, calibrators, and QC materials. In this case, QC results could fail to identify a calibration shift when a new kit lot is used, and it is necessary to measure patient samples with the old and new kit lots to verify consistency of patient results. When possible, it is recommended to use QC materials that are independent of the kit lot and to avoid changing lots of QC material at the same time as changing lots of reagent or calibrators. Measuring patient samples always provides a reliable approach to verify the consistency of results after changes in lots of reagents or calibrators and changes in other measurement conditions.

Review of Quality Control Data and the Effectiveness of the Quality Control Plan

The immediate use of QC data is to determine if the results for patient samples can be reported for use in clinical care decisions as described in the preceding sections. In addition, QC data must be reviewed by laboratory management on a regular schedule. Typical review schedules are weekly by senior technologists or supervisors and at least monthly by the laboratory director. However, the laboratory director should promptly review items such as reagent or calibrator lot change validations, changes in QC target values associated with reagent lot or other changes, EQA/PT results review, and other occurrences that may affect quality of the laboratory results.

The weekly review process should determine that correct follow up of any QC alerts was conducted, that all patient samples that may have had erroneous results were repeated, that any corrected reports were issued, and that the process was properly documented in QC records. The monthly review should include any issues identified by the weekly review process and examination of the Levey-Jennings chart or other tool to identify trends or changes in assay performance that may need to be addressed before they have effects on clinical care decisions. Note that automated systems to assist in the review of QC data are acceptable, and individual Levey-Jennings charts do not need to be examined every month. A report that compares the mean and SD for QC results over a defined time interval, such as 1 month, to the expected values consistent with stable performance can be useful to focus the review on measurement procedures that may need attention. For example, the report might identify a QC mean value that is more than a specified amount, such as 1 SD, from its target value, an SD that exceeds its expected value, or the number of individual results that exceed 2 or 3 SDs from the target value. QC values that are identified as needing further examination can then be followed up with review of a Levey-Jennings chart or other records of measurement procedure performance such as maintenance, calibration, and reagent change. The monthly review should also include any patient data–based QC procedures described in the following sections, as well as notation of any adjustments made to QC parameters during the month.

The QC review process serves three major functions, which are to (1) verify that the measurement procedures are stable and meeting their performance specifications, (2) identify measurement procedures that may need intervention to address performance issues, and (3) make adjustments as needed to the QC plan based on review of relevant quality indicators. Quality indicators and implementation of

TABLE 6.6 Examples of Quality Indicators for the Examination Process

Quality Indicator	Interpretation
Frequency of QC alerts	Compare with the frequency expected for the measurement procedure sigma metric and QC rules used. A higher frequency may indicate an issue with the measurement procedure or inappropriate QC rules. A lower frequency may indicate inappropriate QC rules.
Frequency of recalibration based on QC alerts	May indicate that recalibration should be performed more frequently.
Number of reagent changes due to QC alerts	May indicate that reagents are not stable and smaller quantities should be used or perhaps more frequent recalibration should be performed to compensate for reagent changes.
Number of times controls were repeated without confirming a measurement error	May indicate that the QC rules allow too high frequency of false alerts or the QC material is not stable after opening, is stored incorrectly, or other QC handling issue.
Frequency of unscheduled maintenance due to QC alerts	May indicate that maintenance is needed on a more frequent schedule.
Number of patient samples repeated based on QC alerts	May indicate that QC should be performed more frequently to minimize the risk of an erroneous result causing harm to a patient.
Frequency that patient samples are repeated based on QC alerts	May indicate inadequate calibration or maintenance schedules, that QC rules are inappropriate, or the QC sample target value or SD is not a correct reflection of measurement procedure performance.
Number of patient results corrected	May indicate an unstable measurement procedure and that QC should be performed more frequently to minimize the risk of an erroneous result causing harm to a patient.
Number of EQA/PT unacceptable results	May indicate that a measurement procedure is not calibrated correctly or some part of the measurement is not being performed correctly.

EQA, External quality assessment; *PT*, proficiency testing; *QC*, quality control; *SD*, standard deviation.

the laboratory quality management program are described in Chapter 3. Table 6.6 lists some useful quality indicators related to the examination process and its QC plan. The quality indicators should be reviewed at regular intervals as part of the overall quality management program and can also be reviewed at suitable intervals during regularly scheduled QC review meetings to determine if changes in the QC plan may be needed.

POINTS TO REMEMBER

Internal Quality Control/Statistical Process Control
- QC samples are measured along with patient samples.
- The target value and SD expected for a QC sample are established by the laboratory.
- Results from QC samples are evaluated using interpretive rules that are established after considering the probability of detecting errors that represent a risk of harm to a patient and the probability of false alerts.
- The QC plan is designed to confirm acceptable performance of a measurement procedure and to identify error conditions that may cause risk of harm to a patient.

USING PATIENT DATA IN QUALITY CONTROL PROCEDURES

In addition to using patient samples to verify consistency of patient results when changing lots of reagent or calibrators for a measurement procedure discussed previously, patient data are used in other QC applications. A delta check process compares current with previous results for a patient to identify inconsistencies that may represent a pre-examination or measurement error. Comparison of patient results among different measurement procedures used in a healthcare system for the same measurand is used to ensure that calibration of the different measurement procedures produces consistent results. There is increasing interest in using patient results to monitor the performance of a measurement procedure in real time as a supplement to the surrogate QC sample approach. Each of these patient data-based techniques is described in more detail in the next sections.

Delta Check With a Previous Result for a Patient

Some types of laboratory errors can be identified by comparing a patient's current test result against a previous result for the same measurand. This comparison is called a "delta check." If there is a difference between the two results exceeding the delta check value, this difference can be caused either by a pre-examination error, a laboratory error, or a change in the patient's physiologic condition. Delta check values can be developed in three ways. The first approach is to set delta check values based empirically on experience and then adjust them with time so as not to generate too many false delta check failures. The second involves collecting large numbers of consecutive pairs of patient results for the same measurand from a population that is representative of the patient population to which the delta check values will be applied. The population of delta values, which are actually empirically obtained reference change values (see Chapter 8), are plotted in a frequency distribution histogram. Delta check values are then identified to flag a certain percentage, for example, 5% or 1%, of the population of observed delta values. The third approach is to calculate the reference change value based on analytical and within-subject biologic variation. Reference change values can then be used to flag reports to alert users to those serial results in an individual where, for example, there is less than 1% probability that the change can be explained by the combined

TABLE 6.7   Example Delta Check Criteria Intended to Identify Samples That Are Potentially Mislabeled or Contaminated With Intravenous Fluids Because of Incorrect Collection

Test	Delta Criteria
Sodium	5% change within previous 48 h
Urea nitrogen	60% change within previous 48 h
Creatinine	50% change within previous 48 h
Calcium	25% change within previous 48 h
Osmolality	5% change within previous 48 h

From Miller WG. Quality control. In: McPherson RA, Pincus MR. *Henry's clinical diagnosis and management by laboratory methods.* 24th ed. Philadelphia: Elsevier; 2020.

influence of pre-examination error, examination (or analytical) error, and biologic variation.

The most common use of delta checks is to identify mislabeled samples and samples altered by dilution with intravenous fluid. The difference between results that causes a delta check alert must be sufficiently large to avoid excessive numbers of false alerts yet adequate to allow identification of samples that may be compromised and require follow-up investigation. Table 6.7 shows, as an example, the delta check parameters for automated chemistry used in one author's laboratory designed to identify compromised patient samples. A relatively small number of measurands are sufficient to identify potentially compromised specimens. The delta criteria were based on assessment of the delta values for consecutive pairs of results from the same patient that had differences larger than the 99 percentile of all the differences found, that is, an alert rate less than 1%.

Delta checks can detect analytical measurement errors; however, the threshold values necessary to identify analytical errors are usually fairly small compared with physiologic changes and may cause a large number of false alerts that reduce the efficiency of laboratory workflow. A well-designed statistical QC plan is more effective to detect analytical errors. However, delta checks might be useful to identify an interfering substance (e.g., from a drug) that may appear in a patient's sample. Kazmierczak[51] has reviewed and presented recommendations for using delta check and other patient data–based QC procedures. CLSI has published guideline EP33 for using delta checks in the clinical laboratory.[52]

Verify Consistency of Results Between More Than One Instrument or Measurement Procedure

Another common use of patient results as part of the QC process is to verify the consistency of patient results when a measurand is measured using more than one instrument or measurement procedure within the same health delivery system. Verification of consistent results is necessary even when identical measurement procedures from the same manufacturer are used. Good laboratory practice requires that multiple instruments or measurement procedures for the same measurand be calibrated to produce the same results for patient samples whenever possible. It may be necessary to modify the calibration settings of one measurement procedure so that results for patient samples will be equivalent to

those for another measurement procedure. This strategy allows a common reference interval to be used, provides continuity in results among different laboratory testing locations, and avoids clinical confusion regarding interpretation of laboratory results.

As illustrated in Fig. 6.15, consistency of patient results is verified by measuring aliquots of patient samples using each of two or more measurement procedures to evaluate and, if necessary, adjust the calibration or use a postmeasurement correction function as needed to achieve agreement in results for patient samples. Such an analysis design is called a "round robin." One procedure may be chosen to represent the primary measurement procedure (or designated comparison measurement procedure) to which others will be adjusted to achieve equivalent results. The primary measurement procedure should be chosen based on quality and reliability of results with consideration of its calibration traceability to a national or international reference system, its performance stability, its analytical selectivity for the analyte, and its susceptibility to interfering substances. An alternate approach is to evaluate each measurement procedure for agreement with the mean of all measurement procedures and to adjust the calibration of any measurement procedures as necessary to produce equivalent results among the group.

There are no well-established guidelines regarding the number of samples to use for a round-robin exchange. The laboratory needs to establish the frequency of evaluation and the number of samples based on the stability of the measurement procedures, the frequency of reagent and calibrator lot changes, and the intended medical use of results in the health delivery system. Common practices include a round-robin exchange of one or more individual patient samples or a pool prepared from several samples on a weekly basis for high-volume measurement procedures or on a monthly or quarterly basis for lower-volume or very stable measurement procedures. For frequent comparisons with one or two samples, concentrations should be chosen to evaluate the measuring interval over a period of several examinations. For less frequent comparisons, a larger number of patient samples is recommended to cover the measuring interval. When establishing interpretation criteria, the laboratory needs to consider the limited statistical power for the number of results available. CLSI document EP31 provides a statistical approach suitable for using one to five samples in a comparison.[53]

Table 6.5 provides, as an example, empirical criteria used in one author's laboratory for evaluation of agreement among results for a single patient sample assayed weekly among multiple analyzers. These criteria were established based on the expected imprecision of the measurement procedures used and the influence of discrepant results on medical decisions. To allow for the limitations of a single measurement of a single sample in a comparison, a result outside a criterion is typically not acted on unless the magnitude of a difference is much larger than the criterion or the situation persists for 2 or more weeks.

Patient samples are recommended to verify agreement between multiple measurement procedures or instruments of the same type even when from the same manufacturer. Results for QC materials should not be used for the purpose of verifying consistency of results for patient samples measured using different measurement procedures or instruments. As discussed in an earlier section, QC materials are not validated

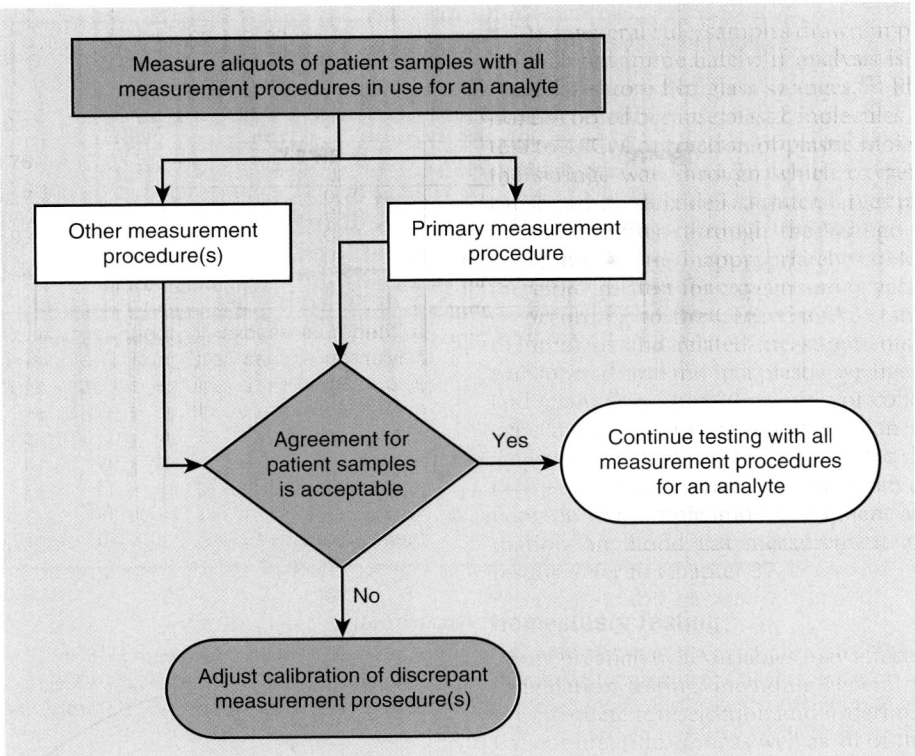

FIGURE 6.15 Process used to evaluate agreement between measurement procedures and to adjust calibration, if necessary, to achieve equivalent results from different measurement procedures. (From Miller WG. Quality control. In: McPherson RA, Pincus MR. *Henry's clinical diagnosis and management by laboratory methods.* 24th ed. Philadelphia: Elsevier; 2020.)

to be commutable with patient samples between different measurement procedures. Even when more than one measurement procedure from the same manufacturer is used, differences may be seen in the measured values for QC materials between different reagent lots and different instruments.[34] In principle, if more than one of the same model of an instrument with the same reagent lots is used, all should have the same results for the same lot of QC material. In practice, differences in measurement details or maintenance condition between different instruments frequently cause small differences in QC results. The acceptance criteria for a QC result can be set to allow for such differences. However, more reliable conclusions will be drawn when patient samples are used to evaluate agreement among different instruments.

Using Patient Data for Statistical Quality Control

Patient results can be used in a statistical QC process to monitor measurement procedure performance. For a sufficiently large number of results, the mean (or preferably, median) value may be sufficiently stable to be used as an indicator of measurement procedure consistency over time. This approach can be used on a periodic basis by extracting data for a specified time period (e.g., 1 day, week, month depending on the number of results available), calculating the mean and SD for the distribution of results, and comparing one time period versus another to determine whether any changes have occurred. This type of periodic evaluation can identify changes in calibration stability or in overall imprecision for a measurement procedure. The mean and SD can also be compared for consistency among two or more measurement procedures for the same measurand.

An important limitation for using patient data to evaluate consistency within a single measurement procedure or between different measurement procedures for the same measurand is the physiologic homogeneity of results. Fig. 6.16 shows an example of the potential impact of a non-homogeneous sample of patients on distribution of serum albumin results for hospital general medicine inpatients compared with a student health outpatient clinic. The histograms are very different because the two patient groups differ in severity of disease and in recumbent versus supine position for blood collection, which influences vascular water volume and the concentration of albumin. Using patient data for process control for albumin measurement, similar to other measurands, requires partitioning of the patient population into a homogeneous subgroup.

Automated approaches to use the mean (or median) for groups of sequential patient results as a continuous process control parameter have been described.[51,54–60] These approaches are called "average of normals" (a misnomer because not all results are from normal individuals) or "moving average" techniques and are suitable for use in higher-volume measurement procedures in chemistry and hematology. In general, these approaches evaluate sequential patient results over time intervals from minutes to hours or days. The time interval that can be confidently used depends on the number of results in the time interval and the relative homogeneity of

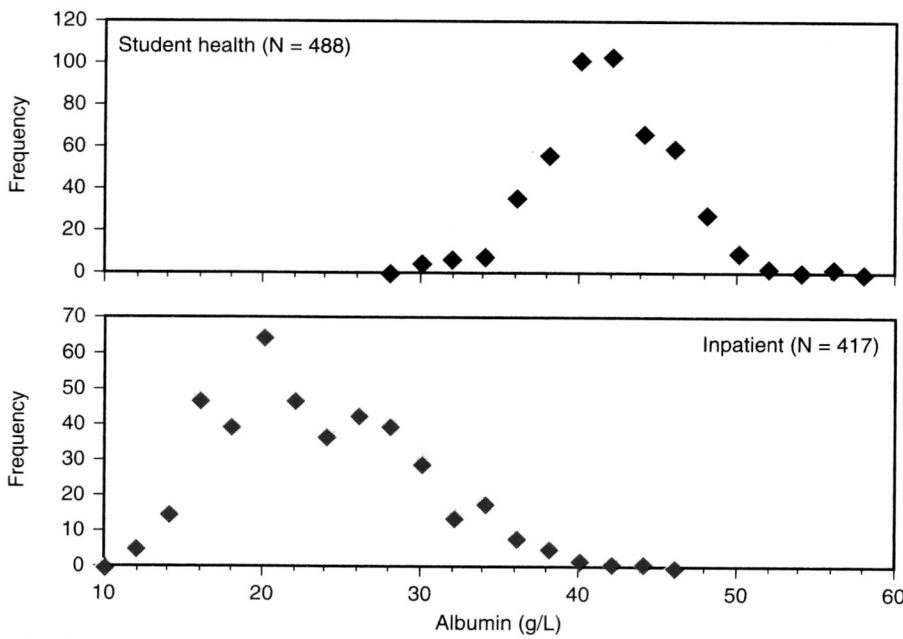

FIGURE 6.16 Histograms for distribution of sequential patient results for albumin from a student health outpatient clinic and a hospital general medicine inpatient unit. (From Miller WG. Quality control. In: McPherson RA, Pincus MR. *Henry's clinical diagnosis and management by laboratory methods.* 24th ed. Philadelphia: Elsevier; 2020.)

the clinical conditions represented in the patients' results. For some measurands, patients may need to be partitioned to obtain subgroups whose results are expected to be homogeneous. Considerations for partitioning include age, gender, ethnicity, and disease conditions. It is easier to obtain homogenous groups when monitoring one laboratory than when comparing several laboratories. Some approaches have arbitrarily ignored abnormal results in an attempt to restrict results to more normal health conditions. Removing abnormal results must be used with caution because excessive deletion will create an artificial subset of results that may not reflect a measurement procedure's calibration condition. The median of a group of patient results is sensitive to the overall distribution of results but is minimally influenced by extreme values and is recommended as the most robust estimate for tracking measurement procedure stability over time.

There is no consensus regarding the number of sequential patient results to include in a group for which the mean or median is calculated. An empirical approach based on extracting patient data from the laboratory computer system and simulating different group sizes in a spreadsheet can identify group sizes that have sufficiently small variation over time to provide useful information for tracking consistency of a measurement procedure. The same data can be used to assess the influence of partitioning considerations and to determine the statistical parameters to use for interpreting the data described in the next paragraph.

The mean or median for groups of patient results is tracked over sequential time intervals to monitor measurement procedure performance. The mean or median for groups of patient results can be treated as a QC sample value. A target value for the average mean or median and an SD for the distribution of mean or median values is determined, and these parameters are used to establish acceptance rules

similar to those used to interpret an individual surrogate QC sample result. Process control using patient data is primarily useful to identify bias and is less useful to identify changes in precision because of the inherent differences in measurand values among a group of patient results. Statistical procedures such as moving average, EWMA, or CUSUM are used to monitor trends in calibration status based on patient data.

Moving averages are frequently applied in hematology blood count measurement procedures based originally on the Bull's Algorithm approach.[61] Other than this application, patient results-based QC monitoring procedures have not been widely adopted because of lack of consensus guidelines for their use and lack of computer support from instrument and laboratory information system (LIS) suppliers. When computer support is available, patient data-based statistical monitoring is a useful addition to conventional QC measurements especially for analytes such as calcium, sodium, and others with low sigma metric performance capability. The advantage is that aggregated patient results give information in real time, the results are free from any matrix effects (i.e., the patients' samples are by definition "commutable"), and the results also include the pre-examination (preanalytical) variation. The disadvantage is that to obtain reliable results, the patient populations need to be stable[59,60] or be partitioned into stable subgroups as shown in the albumin example.

EXTERNAL QUALITY ASSESSMENT OR PROFICIENCY TESTING

EQA/PT is a program used to evaluate measurement procedure performance by comparing a laboratory's results with those of other laboratories for the same set of samples.[62] EQA/PT providers circulate a set of samples among a group

TABLE 6.8 Evaluation Capabilities of External Quality Assessment or Proficiency Testing Related to Scheme Design

	SAMPLE CHARACTERISTICS			EVALUATION CAPABILITY						
				Accuracy					Standardization or Harmonization[a]	
				Individual Laboratory					Measurement Procedure Calibration Traceability	
				Relative to Participant Results			Reproducibility			
Category	Commutable	Value Assigned With RMP or CRM	Replicate Samples in Survey	Absolute vs. RMP or CRM	Overall	Peer Group	Individual Laboratory Intralaboratory CV	Measurement Procedure Interlaboratory CV	Absolute vs. RMP or CRM	Relative to Participant Results
1	Yes	Yes	Yes	X	X	X	X	X	X	X
2	Yes	Yes	No	X	X	X		X	X	X
3	Yes	No	Yes		X	X	X	X		X
4	Yes	No	No		X	X		X		X
5	No	No	Yes			X	X	X		
6	No	No	No			X		X		

[a]Standardization when patient results are equivalent between measurement procedures and calibration is traceable to the Système Internationale using a reference measurement procedure, harmonization when patient results are equivalent between measurement procedures, and calibration traceability is not based on a reference measurement procedure.

CRM, Certified reference material; *CV*, coefficient of variation; *RMP*, reference measurement procedure.

Reproduced with permission from Miller WG, Jones GRD, Horowitz GL, Weykamp C. Proficiency testing/external quality assessment: current challenges and future directions. *Clin Chem* 2011;**57**:1670–80.

of laboratories. Each laboratory measures the EQA/PT samples as if they were patient samples and reports the results to the EQA/PT provider for evaluation. The EQA/PT provider assigns a target value for the EQA/PT samples and determines if the results for an individual laboratory are in close enough agreement with the target value to be consistent with acceptable measurement procedure performance.

Ideally, an EQA/PT program should circulate commutable materials that are measured in replicates by the participating laboratories to provide participants with results that inform them if their measurement procedure has a bias from a true value assigned using an RMP or RM, or with results from all other measurement procedures. Unfortunately, commutable materials are often not used, and in some cases, circulation of unsuitable EQA/PT materials can cause harm by misclassifying measurement procedure performance.

EQA/PT is not available for some measurands because a particular measurement procedure may be new to the clinical laboratory, is not commonly performed, or because measurand stability makes it difficult to include in an EQA/PT material. In these situations, the laboratory should use an alternate approach to periodically verify acceptable performance of the measurement procedure. CLSI guideline QMS24 provides approaches for verifying measurement procedure performance when formal EQA/PT is not available.[63]

Before enrolling in an EQA/PT program, the laboratory should consider the quality of the program. The following questions have to be addressed: (1) Is the EQA/PT material commutable with patient samples? (2) How many replicates are measured? (3) How is the target value established? (4) What is the number of participants in the scheme and in a particular method group? (5) How is the measurement method group established? And (6) How are the performance specifications set? This information is necessary to be able to interpret the feedback report from the organizer in a sensible way. Types of EQA/PT schemes are summarized in Table 6.8, with the most desirable type of program listed first and schemes that provide less information at the bottom.

External Quality Assessment or Proficiency Testing Programs That Use Commutable Samples

EQA/PT programs that use commutable samples are preferred whenever available.[62] Refer to Fig. 6.5 for an explanation of commutability. Commutable samples are typically prepared by using an individual donor's specimen or by pooling patient samples with minimal processing or additives to avoid any alteration of the sample matrix. To achieve samples with abnormal values for measurands, donors can be identified with known pathologic conditions, or blood, plasma, serum, or urine units from a general donor population can be prescreened for a selected measurand. Supplementing donor samples or pools with purified analytes may be acceptable in some cases, but assessment of commutability should be performed to confirm that supplementation did not inappropriately alter the matrix.[64]

When commutable EQA/PT samples can be prepared, the results reflect what would be expected if individual patient samples were sent to each of the different laboratories. Thus agreement among different laboratories and measurement procedures (harmonization) can be correctly evaluated. The agreement between an individual laboratory result measured in singlicate and a reference measurement result gives an assessment of accuracy, the agreement between an individual laboratory result measured in replicate and a reference measurement result gives an assessment of trueness, and the agreement between a measurement procedure group mean value and the reference measurement result gives an assessment of trueness and calibration traceability for the measurement procedure group. The latter information is of particular interest to the producers of measurement procedures and can be used as part of a surveillance program for the metrologic traceability scheme.[65]

For example, EQA/PT programs for HbA_{1c} in many countries use pooled, freshly collected whole blood from both normal and diabetic donors. The target values for the pooled blood are assigned by RMPs for HbA_{1c}. In these surveys, the accuracy of individual laboratory results and the trueness of measurement procedure group means versus the RMP values can be evaluated because the EQA/PT samples are commutable with clinical patient samples. In these cases, the performance of different measurement procedures has been used to monitor and improve the calibration traceability processes used by the measurement procedure manufacturers for the benefit of improved patient care decisions regarding diabetes.[66,67]

Sufficient volumes of commutable materials have been challenging to prepare for use in large EQA/PT programs. An alternative is to combine commutable and noncommutable samples in the same EQA/PT event. An example from such a survey is shown in Fig. 6.17. The measurement procedure bias was evaluated based on results from a smaller group of the participating laboratories that measured the commutable samples, and individual participant's performance was evaluated based on agreement within a measurement procedure peer group using the noncommutable materials.[68] Use of commutable materials adds substantial value to the information obtained from EQA/PT survey results and is recommended whenever possible.[62] Refer to Chapter 7 for information on procedures to validate the commutability of QC, EQA/PT, and reference materials.[64,69–73]

External Quality Assessment or Proficiency Testing Programs That Use Noncommutable Samples

Table 6.8 includes EQA/PT programs that use noncommutable samples. The materials commonly used for EQA/PT samples are derived from blood, urine, or other body fluids but are altered in the process to manufacture EQA/PT samples such that the matrix is modified and the samples frequently do not have the same measurement characteristics as observed for unaltered clinical patient samples.[24–27,62,73] In addition, some EQA/PT samples (e.g., cerebrospinal fluid or blood gas) are prepared as synthetic materials that are not derived from patient fluids. Consequently, many EQA/PT samples, as for QC samples, are noncommutable with authentic patient samples. The results for a noncommutable EQA/PT sample will have a different relationship in their numeric values between different measurement procedures and sometimes for different reagent lots within a measurement procedure than would be observed for patient samples.

Because EQA/PT samples are frequently noncommutable with patient samples, it is a common practice for EQA/PT providers to organize results into "peer groups" of measurement procedures that represent similar technology expected to have the same result for a noncommutable EQA/PT sample. The mean or median value of the peer group results is the target value. Because the peer group mean value may be influenced by a matrix-related bias, that value can only be used to evaluate laboratories using the same or very similar

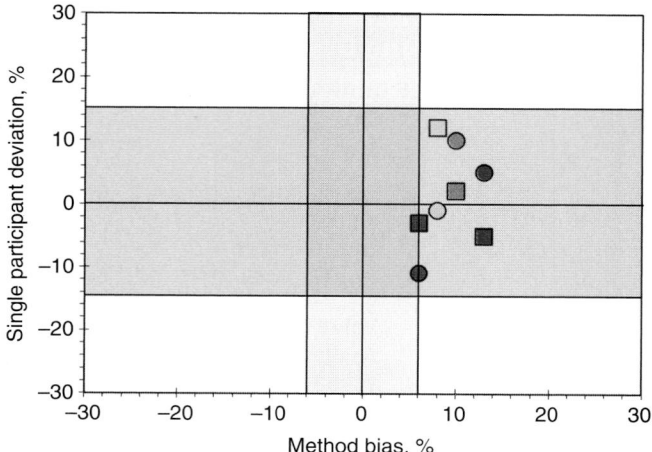

FIGURE 6.17 Example of part of an international normalized ratio external quality control report from the Norwegian Organisation for Quality Improvement of Laboratory Examinations (Noklus). The bias of each measurement procedure from the conventional true value was obtained using patient samples for each measurement procedure (*x*-axis). A single participant was evaluated against the peer group target value for a given measurement procedure (*y*-axis). *Vertical lines* represent acceptable bias for measurement procedure performance, and *horizontal lines* represent acceptable deviation from a peer group target value. The *circle* and *square* represent two samples in one survey with each color representing a different survey (four surveys). The results show that, whereas the measurement procedures had a bias of about 10%, the participant's deviations from the peer group target value were within the performance specifications. This graph indicates that the participants perform the measurement procedures correctly, but the measurement procedures had an unacceptable positive bias. (Modified with permission from Stavelin A, Petersen PH, Sølvik UØ, Sandberg S. External quality assessment of point-of-care methods: model for combined assessment of method bias and single-participant performance by the use of native patient samples and noncommutable control materials. *Clin Chem* 2013;59:363–71.)

measurement procedures and cannot be used to evaluate if results from different measurement procedures agree with each other. Peer groups may be formed arbitrarily based on the apparent agreement among results for different measurement procedures, but there is no scientific basis for this practice, and unexpected changes may occur, such as when new reagent lots or formulations are introduced by a manufacturer. The measurement procedures included in an arbitrarily formed peer group may not be similar. In this situation, one of the measurement procedures in the "peer group" may dominate the number of results and inappropriately influence the target value if set as the mean/median of all results. An alternative is to set the target value not as the mean/median of all results, but as a mean/median of the means/medians determined for each different measurement procedure in the peer group.

However, even within a peer group using the same measurement procedure, differences can occur because of different reagent lots used in different laboratories because the matrix of the EQA/PT material can influence the results from different reagent lots even if the patient samples give similar results.[29] Therefore in some cases, reagent lots should be registered, and even reagent lot–specific target values may need

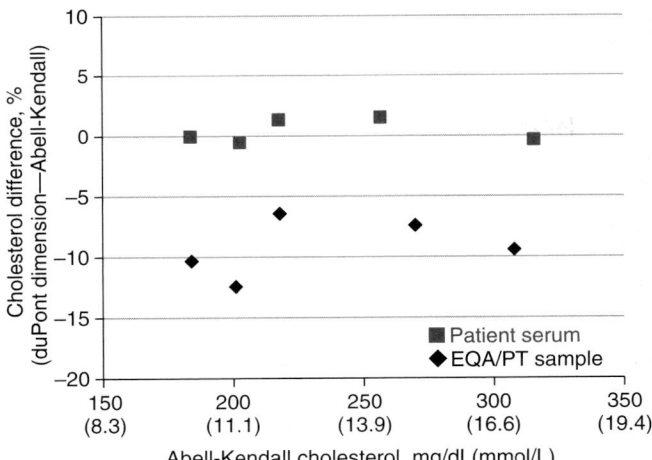

FIGURE 6.18 Example of noncommutable results between proficiency testing samples and pooled patient serum samples for a specific measurement procedure. *EQA*, External quality assessment; *PT*, proficiency testing. (Data replotted from Naito HK, Kwak YS, Hartfiel JL, Park JK, Travers EM, Myers GL, et al. Matrix effects on proficiency testing materials: impact on accuracy of cholesterol measurement in laboratories in the nation's largest hospital system. *Arch Pathol Lab Med* 1993;117:345–51.)

to be assigned.[74,75] When target values are set for noncommutable materials, it is important how the target values are calculated, how outlier results are treated, and what uncertainty is associated with the target value. When target values are assigned from relatively small numbers of results in a peer group, the target value should be given with an uncertainty and the criteria for acceptable performance should be "extended" to high and low values that include the uncertainty.

Fig. 6.18 illustrates the effects of noncommutable materials on interpretation of EQA/PT results and demonstrates why "peer group" evaluation is used. In this older but still valid example, pooled patient sera and EQA/PT samples were measured by the DuPont Dimension Analyzer and by the Abell-Kendall RMP for cholesterol.[76] The Abell-Kendall measurement procedure was shown to be unaffected by matrix-induced changes in EQA/PT samples.[77] The patient samples showed excellent agreement between the two measurement procedures (average bias, 0.2%). However, the EQA/PT samples had a large negative bias (average −9.5%) between measurement procedures, caused by a matrix-related bias with the DuPont measurement procedure that was not present with the RMP.[78]

In this example, the routine measurement procedure was correctly calibrated and produced results for patient samples that were traceable to the RMP. However, EQA/PT results gave an incorrect impression of the measurement procedure's calibration relationship to the RMP. If the routine measurement procedure's calibration had been erroneously adjusted on the basis of EQA/PT results, the results for patient samples would then be incorrect. EQA/PT results were useful for evaluating the performance of all laboratories using the DuPont measurement procedure because the matrix-related bias was uniform within this peer group. Consequently, if an individual laboratory's results agreed with those of the peer group, the individual laboratory could conclude that the measurement procedure was performing in conformance

with the manufacturer's specifications. In general, an individual laboratory depends on the manufacturer to correctly calibrate a clinical laboratory measurement procedure to be traceable to the reference system for a measurand.

QC material manufacturers may provide a data analysis service that compares results from different laboratories using the same lot of QC material by calculating group statistics for performance evaluation. This type of interlaboratory QC data analysis provides similar information to that from EQA/PT programs that use noncommutable samples. Interlaboratory QC data comparison allows a laboratory to verify that it is producing QC results that are consistent with those of other laboratories using the same measurement procedure and lot of QC material. This information can be helpful for troubleshooting measurement procedure issues and for assessing performance of a new measurement procedure being introduced to a laboratory.

External Quality Assessment or Proficiency Testing Programs for Measurements on a Nominal or Ordinal Scale

Many constituents in laboratory medicine can be measured on a nominal scale (all types of classification without any quantitative value, e.g., identity of a bacteria as *Escherichia coli*, Group A Strep, or Klebsiella; a virus as SARS-COV-2 or different mutations) or an ordinal scale (all types of graded response, e.g., urine strips with values 0, 1, 2, 3, 4 for increasing amounts of analyte present). Often, measurements performed on an ordinal scale are measurements that can also be performed on a ratio or interval (numeric) scale. The quantities are often measured on an ordinal scale because a more rapid result can be obtained and because such tests can be performed by nonprofessional users (e.g., in a physician's office or by lay people using a POC device). When setting up an EQA/PT program for such measurement procedures, it is important to note that all aspects regarding commutability of the QC samples and thereby establishing target values will be the same as for measurement procedures on the interval or ratio scale (quantitative measurements).

EQA/PT programs addressing identifications of species or mutations often circulate multiple samples where different mutations of species should be identified and the participants are classified according to the percentage of correct identifications.[79,80] Results from measurement procedures using the ordinal scale can be dichotomous (often called qualitative tests) or multinary with more steps (often called semiquantitative tests) in which each category can be considered as a dichotomous test. It is possible to evaluate the results from these tests using a rankit ordinal model.[81,82] The performance characteristics of the measurement procedure should be described from the manufacturer giving a detection limit for dichotomous tests and, for example, the concentrations below which 5% of the samples should be negative, the concentration at which 50% of the samples should be positive, and the concentration above which 95% of the samples should be positive (C_5, C_{50}, C_{95}, respectively) when related to a ratio scale. Performance specifications for such measurement procedures should use the same models as described earlier[8] and can, for example, relate to the percentage of results that should be positive or negative above or below a certain concentration.[82] These performance specifications are, however, easier to apply for method evaluation than for single participant evaluation in an EQA/PT scheme because numerous samples with different concentrations are necessary.

In an EQA/PT assessment, it is useful to circulate samples with concentrations that are expected to give "positive" or "negative" results and samples with an intermediate concentration that can have both positive and negative results. In the feedback report, participants will typically be evaluated with respect to the positive or negative samples because failure to obtain the expected results will be evaluated as "poor" performance. Samples with intermediate concentrations may be included to assess the robustness of threshold values by reporting to the participants how many obtained positive results and how many obtained negative results. However, intermediate concentrations are typically not graded because the results are expected to be mixed between "positive" and "negative." Such information is useful to assess and to monitor the performance of the measurement procedure. For example, a study using EQA/PT results showed that six of eight POC measurement procedures for human chorionic gonadotropin gave 3 to 11% false-positive results.[82] Using a commutable EQA/PT material, different measurement procedures can be compared and monitored over time, and it is possible to identify opportunities when the threshold discrimination needs to be improved among different measurement procedures.[83,84]

Some EQA/PT programs, often for rare diseases, are examining the whole testing procedure (e.g., the correct measurands to request for a certain diagnostic problem, the appropriate sample collection and transportation, the performance of the analytical measurement procedures, the adequacy of the diagnosis, and the report provided to the clinicians).[79,85,86] These programs are often run on an international level.

Reporting External Quality Assessment or Proficiency Testing Results When One Measurement Procedure Is Adjusted to Agree With Another Measurement Procedure

It is good laboratory practice to adjust the calibration of different measurement procedures for the same measurand used within a large hospital system that can have several satellite laboratories or a collection of several hospitals with the same management structure so that the results for patient samples are consistent, irrespective of which measurement procedure is used. Such harmonization of results is important for uniform use of reference intervals and decision thresholds within a hospital or clinic system.

It is important to report EQA/PT results such that they can be properly evaluated against a true target value or the peer group target value that reflects the calibration established by the measurement procedure manufacturer. When a laboratory has applied a calibration correction, it is important to inform the EQA provider what result is provided. Usually the individual EQA/PT result should be reported to the EQA/PT provider after removing any calibration adjustments so that the reported result is consistent with the manufacturer's nonadjusted calibration. The most convenient way to remove a calibration adjustment is to first measure the EQA/PT samples with the calibration adjustment applied to

the measurement procedure, as would be the usual measurement process for patient samples. After the measurement, the EQA/PT results should be adjusted "in reverse" by mathematically removing the calibration adjustment factors, and the results should be reported to the EQA/PT provider with any adjustment factors removed. One should not recalibrate the instrument with a new set of calibrators for the purpose of measuring the EQA/PT samples because this practice would violate regulations requiring the EQA/PT material to be measured in the same manner as patient samples.

For example, a laboratory has performed a patient sample comparison between measurement procedure A used in the main laboratory and measurement procedure B used in a satellite laboratory. Measurement procedure B consistently gave 10% higher results (i.e., a slope of 1.10 and a negligible intercept were observed for a regression analysis). Measurement procedure B was adjusted to agree with measurement procedure A by putting the adjustment factor $1/1.10 = 0.9091$ in the measurement procedure B instrument to automatically multiply each measured result by 0.9091 to lower the reported result to be equivalent to a value that would have been reported by method A. When EQA/PT results from measurement procedure B are reported, it is necessary to remove the 0.9091 factor to allow the reported result to be compared with the peer group mean of results from all laboratories using measurement procedure B. Removing the 0.9091 factor is accomplished by multiplying the reported EQA/PT result from measurement procedure B by the factor $1/0.9091 = 1.100$ to increase its numeric value by 10% to the nonadjusted value that was actually measured according to the manufacturer's defined calibration procedure for measurement procedure B. This process allows the EQA/PT result measured by measurement procedure B to be appropriately evaluated in comparison with its peer group mean, which will reflect the manufacturer's established calibration. This process permits the EQA/PT sample to be measured in the same manner as patient samples and the numeric result reported to the EQA/PT provider to reflect the actual measured result using the manufacturer's calibration settings.

Interpretation of External Quality Assessment or Proficiency Testing Results

Many countries have regulations requiring EQA/PT and specifying the evaluation criteria for acceptable performance. When criteria are set by regulations, an EQA/PT provider is required to use them. When criteria are not set by regulations, the EQA/PT provider sets evaluation criteria on the basis of clinically acceptable performance, biologic variation, or the analytical capability of the measurement procedures in use. EQA/PT evaluation criteria are usually designed to evaluate the accuracy of a single measurement. In some cases, measurements are made several times, and it is possible to separately assess the bias and the imprecision. The acceptability limits for EQA/PT include bias and imprecision components considered acceptable for a measurand plus other error components that are unique to EQA/PT samples such as between-laboratory variation in calibration; variable matrix-related bias with different lots of reagent within a peer group; uncertainty in the target value; stability variability in the EQA/PT material, both in storage and shipping, and after reconstitution or opening in the laboratory; and homogeneity of the EQA/PT material vials. Consequently, the acceptability limits for EQA/PT samples are frequently larger than what might be expected for clinically acceptable total error with patient samples.

The acceptability limits are partly dependent on the quality of the EQA/PT material (e.g., its commutability, stability, homogeneity, and methods of reconstitution). A commutable EQA/PT material often has a target value assigned by an RMP or by value transfer from suitable measurement procedures calibrated using commutable certified reference materials. A commutable EQA/PT material should in principle have the same results for all measurement procedures and lots of reagent and measurement procedure calibrator. In this case, the variation in the results will reflect the different measurement procedures, reagent lots, and calibrator lots in use from all of the manufacturers represented in the survey. For example, a multi-country European EQA/PT program that used commutable samples documented the performance of 17 measurands among six commercially available measurement procedures.[87]

With a noncommutable EQA/PT material, the target value is set by the mean or median of the peer group that should include only very similar measurement procedures, and the acceptance criteria could be stricter because the variability only includes variation within the same measurement procedure. However, in some cases, a noncommutable EQA/PT material is not even commutable among reagent lots for the same measurement procedure, and in theory, each reagent lot could have its own target value with even stricter acceptability limits.[28,29,74,75]

Fig. 6.19 is an example of a typical evaluation report sent to a participating laboratory when noncommutable samples were used. Each reported result is compared with the mean result for the peer group using the same measurement procedure. The report also includes the SD for the distribution of results in the peer group, the number of laboratories in the peer group, and the SDI, which expresses the reported result as the number of SDs it is from the mean value (SDI = [Result − Mean]/SD). The limits of acceptability are shown. Acceptability

A External Quality Assessment (Proficiency Testing) Participant Report
Shipment date: 1 May 2015
Evaluation date: 12 June 2015

Analyte Units Method	Specimen	Reported Result	Mean	SD	Labs (*n*)	SDI	Limits of Acceptability Lower	Limits of Acceptability Upper
Calcium	1	9.6	9.92	0.23	587	−1.4	8.9	11.0
mg/dL	2	8.8	8.86	0.26	592	−0.2	7.8	9.9
Arsenazo dye	3	7.5	7.65	0.23	587	−0.7	6.6	8.7
Manufacturer A	4	8.2	8.43	0.23	590	−1.0	7.4	9.5
	5	10.8	10.87	0.25	589	−0.3	9.8	11.9
Iron	1	190	192.5	7.0	397	−0.4	154	232
μg/dL	2	65	65.0	3.4	394	0.0	51	78
Pyridylazo dye	3	74	69.2	3.2	395	+1.5	55	83
Manufacturer A	4	124	107.9	4.6	395	+3.5	86	130
	5	277	260.9	8.8	396	+1.8	208	314

B External Quality Assessment (Proficiency Testing) Participant Report
Shipment date: 1 May 2015
Evaluation date: 12 June 2015

Analyte Units Method	Specimen	Reported Result	Mean	SD	Labs (*n*)	SDI	Limits of Acceptability Lower	Limits of Acceptability Upper
Calcium	1	2.40	2.48	0.06	587	−1.4	2.22	2.74
mmol/L	2	2.20	2.21	0.06	592	−0.2	1.95	2.47
Arsenazo dye	3	1.87	1.91	0.06	587	−0.7	1.65	2.17
Manufacturer A	4	2.05	2.10	0.06	590	−1.0	1.85	2.37
	5	2.69	2.71	0.06	589	−0.3	2.45	2.97
Iron	1	34.0	34.5	1.3	397	−0.4	27.6	41.5
μmol/L	2	11.6	11.6	0.6	394	0.0	9.1	14.0
Pyridylazo dye	3	13.3	12.4	0.6	395	+1.5	9.8	14.9
Manufacturer A	4	22.2	19.3	0.8	395	+3.5	15.4	23.3
	5	49.6	46.7	1.6	396	+1.8	37.2	56.2

FIGURE 6.19 Example of an external proficiency testing evaluation report sent to a participating laboratory. **(A)** conventional units; **(B)** SI units. The *red* value represents a large SDI. *SD,* Standard deviation; *SDI,* standard deviation interval. (A, from Miller WG. Quality control. In: McPherson RA, Pincus MR. *Henry's clinical diagnosis and management by laboratory methods.* 24th ed. Philadelphia: Elsevier; 2020.)

criteria may be a number of SDs from the mean value, a fixed percent from the mean value, or a fixed concentration from the mean value. For example, in Fig. 6.19, calcium acceptability criteria are ±1 mg/dL (0.25 mmol/L) from the mean value, and iron criteria are ±20% from the mean value.

Peer group evaluation allows a laboratory to verify that its EQA/PT results are consistent with those of other laboratories using the same measurement procedure and by extension that its results for patient results are in agreement with those of other laboratories in the peer group. Consequently, the laboratory can conclude that it is using a commercially available measurement procedure according to the manufacturer's specifications.[62] In Fig. 6.19, the calcium results are in close agreement with the peer group mean (SDI ranges from −0.2 to −1.4). However, the iron results show greater variability, with one result +3.5 SDI. Although this iron result is within the acceptability criteria, it is recommended to investigate the measurement procedure because a +3.5 SDI is more likely to be different from, than to be in agreement with, the peer group.

Fig. 6.20 shows a typical evaluation report sent to a primary care office for POC measurement of HbA_{1c} for one of two EQA/PT samples. In this situation, the EQA/PT provider is communicating directly with the user of the measurement procedure, the clinician or the coworker in the general practice office, and the feedback must be easy to understand for nonlaboratory professionals. The EQA/PT result is evaluated

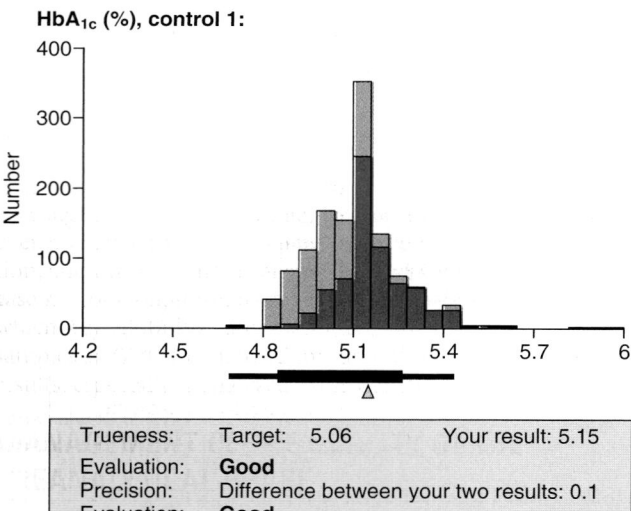

FIGURE 6.20 Example of part of a feedback report to hemoglobin A_{1c} (HbA_{1c}) point-of-care (POC) users in a survey for general practitioners' offices and nursing homes. Commutable EQA/PT material was measured in duplicate. The participant is informed about the bias (mean of the two results) compared with a reference measurement procedure target (x-axis) and "precision" as the difference between the two results. The histogram represents the distribution of results among all participants *(pink)* and for the participant's method group *(red)*. The *thick black line* represents the interval for "good" results, and the *thin black line* represents the interval for "acceptable" results. Results outside these limits are characterized as "poor." The *triangle* points to the result of the participant. (Modified with permission from the Norwegian Organisation for Quality Improvement of Laboratory Examinations (Noklus), the external quality assessment provider in Norway.)

as "good," "acceptable," or "poor." The lot numbers of the reagent are always registered so that the participant, in case of an aberrant result, can get information if the result was due to the measurement procedure used, the reagent lot used, or the performance of the user. In this case, commutable samples were used and in addition to participant reports, the manufacturers were informed of aberrant reagent lots. In cases when noncommutable samples are used, comments to results for aberrant reagent lots typically include a sentence that the EQA/PT result may not necessarily reflect results for patient samples. In all cases, the participants are encouraged to contact the organizers to sort out problems.

Fig. 6.21 shows a similar report from the same HbA_{1c} survey provided to hospital laboratories. In addition to the figures about the distribution of results, information is provided on how different measurement procedures performed and a historical overview of performance on consecutive EQA/PT samples and performance related to the concentration of the sample. The EQA/PT material used for the HbA_{1c} is pooled fresh patient blood (commutable), and the target value was set by an RMP and is therefore the same for all measurement procedures. Each sample was measured in duplicate (as requested by the EQA/PT provider), and the mean of the duplicates was used to estimate bias versus the RMP. In the present example, the performance was within the acceptability limits but with a generally high bias during the whole period. Because this observation was true for all the participants using this measurement procedure, the EQA/PT organizer discussed the results with the manufacturer to solve the problem. Until the problem was solved (the manufacturer had to make a new calibrator), the participants were advised by the EQA/PT provider to use a correction factor when reporting their results for patient samples.[88]

If an unacceptable EQA/PT result is identified, the measurement procedure must be investigated for possible causes and the necessary corrective action taken. Even when an EQA/PT result is within acceptability criteria, it is a good laboratory practice to investigate results that are more than approximately 2.5 SDI from the peer group mean. When the SDI is 2.5, there is only a 0.6% probability that the result will be within the expected distribution for the peer group; consequently, the probability is reasonable that a measurement procedure problem may need to be corrected. In addition, EQA/PT results that have been near the failure limit for more than one EQA/PT event, even if the results have met the EQA/PT acceptance criteria, should initiate a review for systematic problems with the measurement procedure. These practices support identification of potential problems before they progress to more serious situations. When results are investigated, a limitation of SD-based grading criteria should be considered. A peer group with very precise measurement procedures may have a very small SD, and even if a result is outside an SD limit, the finding may be inconsequential regarding the intended use of results for medical decisions.

Common causes for EQA/PT failure are listed in Box 6.1. Incorrect handling and reporting are unique to EQA/PT events and may not reflect the process used in the laboratory for patient samples. Nonetheless, these situations reflect the attention to detail, which is a necessary attribute for quality laboratory testing. Occasionally, the EQA/PT material may have a defect that causes it to perform inappropriately for all or a subgroup of measurement procedures or reagent lots. In

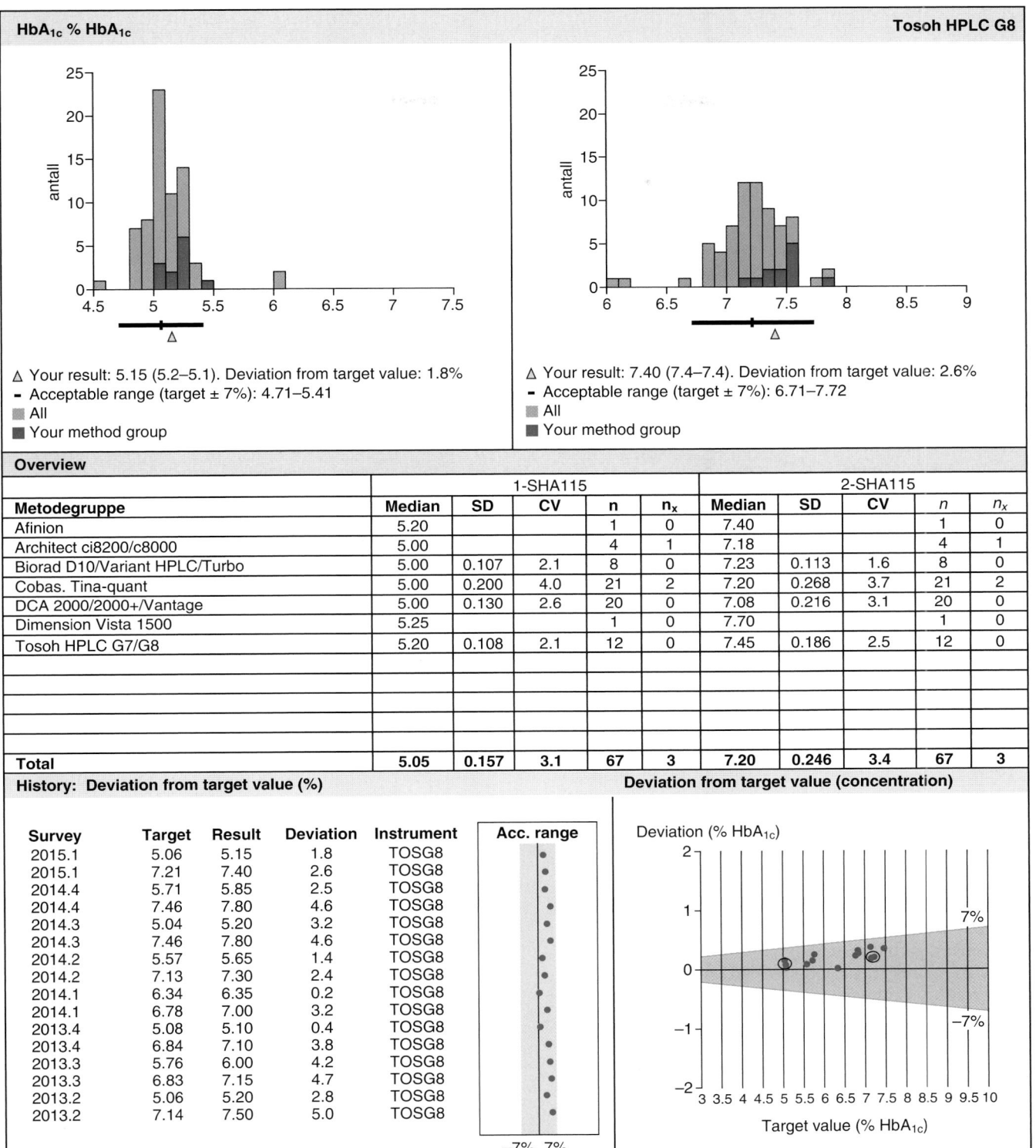

FIGURE 6.21 Example of a part of a feedback report to hemoglobin A$_{1c}$ (HbA$_{1c}$) users in hospital laboratories. Same survey and same materials as presented in Fig. 6.20. The histogram represents the distribution of results among all participants *(pink)* and for the participant's method group *(red)*. Only limits for "acceptable" results are given *(black lines* in figures). Information about performance of measurement procedures is given in addition to a historical overview of percentage deviation from target values dependent on time and concentration of HbA$_{1c}$. Shaded area represents the limits of acceptable performance. *CV,* Coefficient of variation; *HPLC,* high pressure liquid chromatography; *SD,* standard deviation. (Modified with permission from the Norwegian Organization for Quality Improvement of Laboratory Examinations (Noklus), the external quality assessment provider in Norway.)

BOX 6.1   Classification of Potential Problems Identified When Investigating Unacceptable External Quality Assessment or Proficiency Testing Results[a]

1. Clerical errors
    Incorrectly transcribed EQA/PT result from the instrument read-out to the report form
    The EQA/PT sample was mislabeled in the laboratory
    Incorrect instrument or measurement procedure was reported on the results submission form
    Incorrect units were reported
    Decimal point was misplaced
2. Measurement procedure problems
    Inadequate standard operating procedure (SOP)
    Problem with manufacture or preparation of reagents or calibrators (e.g., unstable)
    Lot-to-lot variation in reagents or calibrators
    Incorrect value assignment of calibrators
    Measurement procedure lacks adequate specificity for the measurand
    Measurement procedure lacks adequate sensitivity to measure the concentration
    Carry-over from a previous sample
    Inadequate QC procedures used
3. Equipment problems
    Obstruction of instrument tubing or orifice by clot
    Misalignment of instrument probes
    Incorrect instrument data processing functions
    Incorrect instrument setting
    Automatic pipetter not calibrated to acceptable precision and accuracy

    Equipment component malfunction (e.g., light source, membrane, fluidics, detector)
    Incorrect instrument conditions (e.g., water quality, surrounding temperature)
    Instrument maintenance not performed appropriately
4. Technical problems caused by personnel errors
    Did not operate equipment correctly or did not conform to measurement procedure SOP
    Incorrect storage, preparation, or handling of reagents or calibrators
    Delay causing evaporation or deterioration of the EQA/PT sample
    Failure to follow recommended instrument function checks or maintenance
    Pipetting or dilution error
    Calculation error
    Misinterpretation of test result
5. A problem with the EQA/PT material such as:
    Incorrect storage, preparation, or handling of EQA/PT materials
    Differences between EQA/PT samples and patient samples (e.g., matrix, additives, stabilizers)
    Sample deteriorated in transit or during laboratory storage
    Sample had weak or borderline reaction
    Sample contained interfering factors (which may be measurement procedure specific)
    Sample was not homogeneous among vials

[a]This classification scheme assists in developing an appropriate corrective action plan.
EQA, External quality assessment; *PT,* proficiency testing; *QC,* quality control.
From Miller WG, Jones GRD, Horowitz GL, Weykamp C. Proficiency testing/external quality assessment: current challenges and future directions. *Clin Chem* 2011;**57**:1670–80.

---

this case, the EQA/PT provider should recognize the problem and not grade participants for that sample. Because the influence of reagent lots on noncommutability related bias is well documented,[28,29,74,75] EQA/PT programs are recommended to register reagent lots as part of the reporting process so this limitation can be more appropriately addressed in the scoring and investigating schemes.[74,75]

EQA/PT results are usually received several weeks after the date of testing. Consequently, investigation of unacceptable results requiring review of QC, reagent lots, calibration frequency and lots, and maintenance records for the date of the test and the preceding several weeks or months is necessary. It is common practice to save any remaining EQA/PT samples for use to investigate an unacceptable result. Care must be taken to store the residual EQA/PT samples to preserve the stability of the measurands. In some cases, the measurand will not be stable during storage. In addition, degradation that could affect any remeasured value may have occurred during storage, for example freeze-thaw, or possibly before storage while the materials were still being tested in the laboratory for the EQA/PT event. It may be possible to obtain additional vials from the EQA/PT provider. If a review of records suggests a stable operating condition, and a review of the EQA/PT material handling and documentation does not identify a cause for the erroneous EQA/PT result, one can

conclude that the EQA/PT failure was a random event. Investigative steps, data reviews, conclusions, and all corrective actions must be documented in a written report to address the unacceptable EQA/PT results and reviewed by the laboratory director. Some EQA/PT programs provide the participants with flow charts or checklists to be used to identify the reason for the EQA/PT failure.

Interpreting External Quality Assessment or Proficiency Testing Summary Reports

EQA/PT providers typically provide a summary report, which includes the mean and SD for all peer groups represented by the participants' results (see Figs. 6.19 to 6.21). When commutable materials were used in the surveys, the trueness compared with an RMP or the harmonization among different measurement procedures can be assessed.

When summary reports are for surveys with noncommutable materials, assessment of mean results among different peer groups or to an RMP is not possible. The EQA/PT results from noncommutable samples are not reliable to infer agreement or lack of agreement for patient results among different measurement procedures for the same measurand. In this case, the peer group mean and SD are useful for evaluating the uniformity of results among laboratories using the same measurement procedure, and to evaluate the consistency of an individual measurement procedure's performance over time intervals from one EQA/PT event to the next (trend monitoring). A limitation using EQA/PT results for trend monitoring is that differences in matrix-related bias in different sample materials can be different within the same peer group over time.

Summary information also allows evaluation of the imprecision of various measurement procedure groups, within the limitations of EQA/PT material and reagent lot matrix-bias differences. The number of users in each measurement procedure group reveals which measurement procedures are commonly used.

Using Patient Medians for External Quality Assessment

One of the main objectives of EQA/PT is to compare results between different measurement procedures and, if possible, to compare them with a true value obtained by an RMP or reference material. This information is important both for the laboratory and also for the IVD manufacturers. However, a comparison between measurement procedures is only possible by using commutable samples. Commutable samples can be difficult to prepare for numerous measurands since they are often more expensive, unstable, and not possible to obtain for many measurands.

Comparison of results between measurement procedures can be done by comparing medians of patient results between measurement procedures performed in different laboratories. It is then possible in real time to monitor the effect of harmonization and standardization efforts. One prerequisite for using patient medians for this purpose is that the patient medians originate from similar patient populations. Patient medians also include pre-examination (preanalytical) factors in addition to measurement biases. Commutable EQA/PT samples can be circulated to the same laboratories to validate that differences in patient medians between measurement procedures reflect "real" measurement procedure differences if these differences can be reproduced with the commutable samples.

An example of such a comparison is shown in Fig. 6.22 where results of patient medians reflect the same differences as observed for fresh frozen patient samples.[89] When this relationship is established, daily or weekly monitoring of the measurement procedures can be performed using the patient medians. A laboratory can then monitor in a "continuous" manner its own measurement procedure in comparison with others to determine: (i) results comparability, (ii) measurement procedure stability including lot-to-lot reagent and calibrator changes, and (iii) individual laboratory bias, for example, caused by changes in preanalytical conditions. This

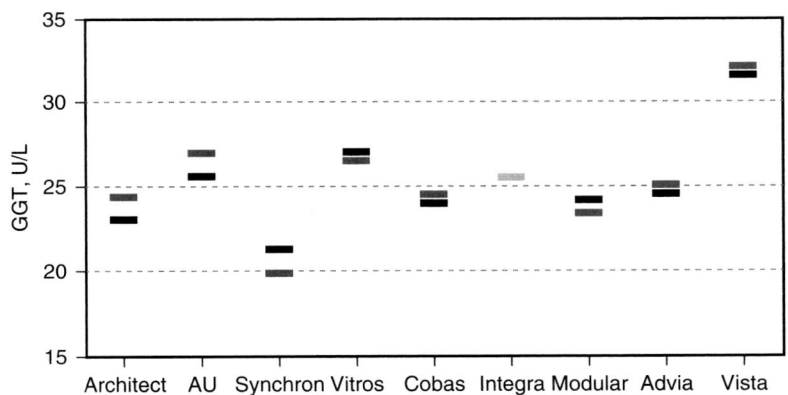

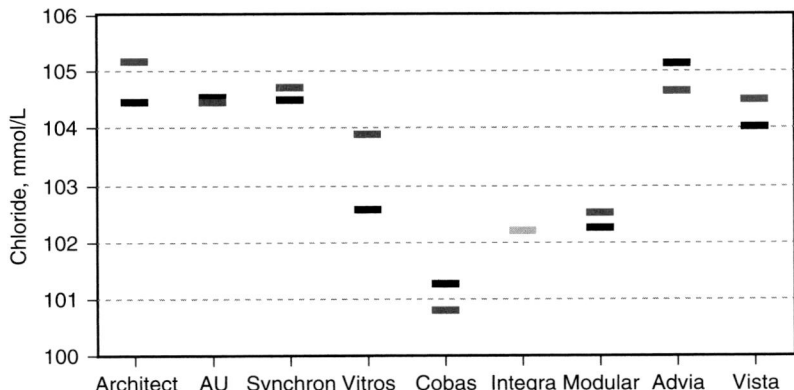

FIGURE 6.22 Comparison of medians of patient results *(black bars)* from 100 laboratories with a total of 182 devices with the results from peer group medians *(red bars)* of 20 fresh frozen serum samples analyzed by 20 laboratories per peer group for chloride and gamma-glutamyl transferase (GGT). (From De Grande LAC, Goossens K, Van Uytfanghe K, Stöckl D, Thienpont LM The empower project—a new way of assessing and monitoring test comparability and stability. *Clin Chem Lab Med* 2015;**53**:1197–204.)

near-continuous monitoring allows remediation shortly after an event takes place.

It is also possible to calculate the percentage of patient results that is outside a reference interval or a specific clinical cut-off interval. Thus the consequences for patients of any changes in measurement performance can be easily shown. For example, Fig. 6.23 shows moving daily patient medians for the previous 16 days for serum calcium and the percent of median results that are above or below the reference interval limits. The moving median could be determined from other time periods, for example, 5 days or 8 days as appropriate for a given measurand. The laboratory can, in addition to being compared with all laboratories, choose to be compared with their own instrument group.

Development of more sophisticated information management systems makes it easier for laboratories to obtain

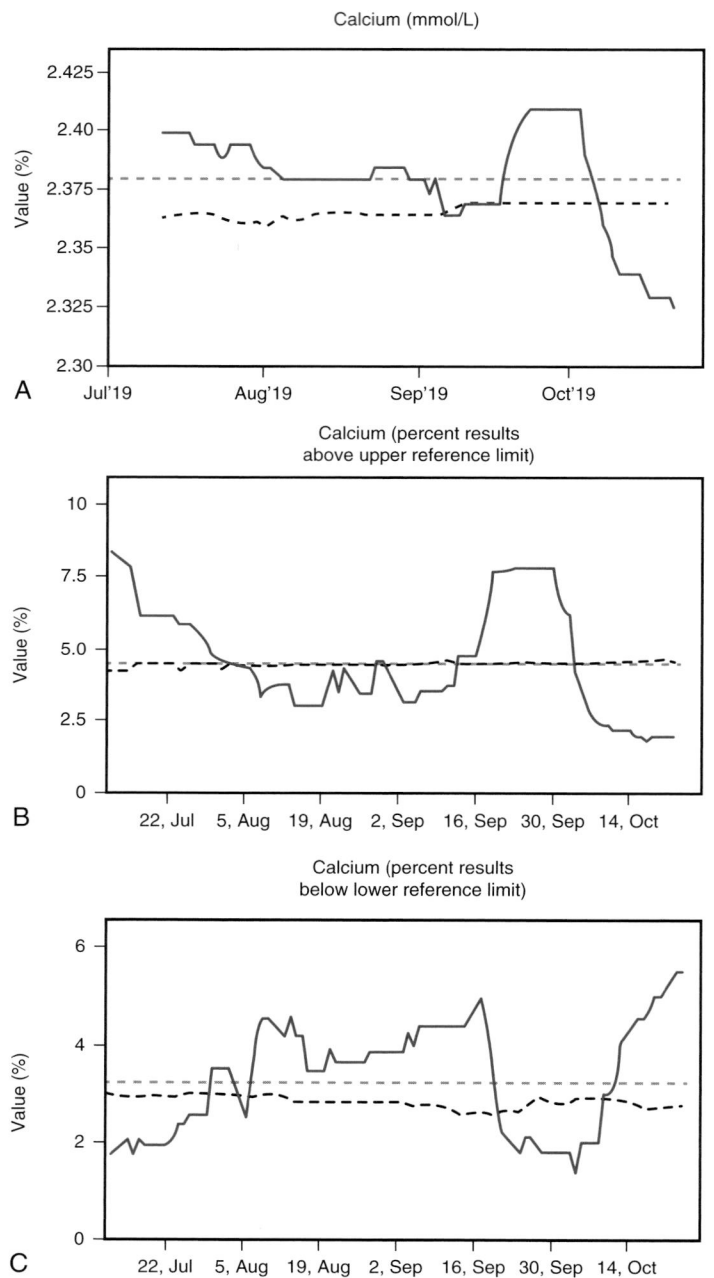

FIGURE 6.23 Moving daily patient median (average medians of the last 16 days) of (**A**) the concentration of calcium (mmol/L); (**B**) the percentage of calcium results outside the upper reference limit; and (**C**) the percentage of results below the lower reference limit. The *red* line represents the results from one laboratory, the grey broken line represents the long-term median of the laboratory, and the black broken line represents the results from the moving median (16 days) from all the laboratories participating in the program (≈150 laboratories). (Reprinted with permission from the Norwegian Organization for Quality Improvement of Laboratory Examinations (Noklus), the external quality assessment provider in Norway.)

patient medians and percentage of results outside defined cut-offs, and to aggregate the data as an EQA process. Preferably, the calculations are done in the laboratory by an automatic function either in the LIS or via a middleware or homemade solution and then transferred, preferably on a daily basis, or batch-wise (frequency as convenient). Some LIS providers and IVD manufacturers offer their customers a solution for these patient data-based transfers.[90]

It is likely that such systems based on patient data will be a valuable supplement to traditional EQA programs.

Responsibility of the External Quality Assessment or Proficiency Testing Provider

The EQA/PT provider is responsible for producing programs that fulfill the goal of evaluating a measurement procedure's performance in a single laboratory to that of other laboratories, or to a true value when possible.[91] EQA/PT providers should strive to use commutable materials whenever possible.[62] The frequency of distribution and the number of EQA/PT samples must address the need of the laboratory and conform to applicable regulatory requirements.

The EQA/PT provider should have the knowledge to advise the participants when they have questions regarding their EQA/PT results. Some EQA/PT providers organize "user meetings" to address and evaluate the results of the different schemes, facilitate discussions on topics of common interest, provide a "national overview" of the performance of measurement procedures and laboratories, and develop national "expert" groups within different topics.[92,93]

The EQA/PT providers should communicate directly with manufacturers concerning findings related to their measurement procedures. Furthermore, they should, especially when commutable samples are used, perform postmarketing surveillance and report any deficiency that could affect patient safety to the appropriate regulatory body.[94]

POINTS TO REMEMBER

External Quality Assessment or Proficiency Testing
- An independent external organization circulates samples with unknown target values.
- The quality of the EQA/PT sample is critical for interpretation of the results.
- When commutable, "patient-like," samples are used, a laboratory can compare its own results with results from all other measurement procedures and often with a true value from an RMP.
- When noncommutable samples are used, a laboratory can only compare its own results with results from participants using a similar measurement procedure.

SELECTED REFERENCES

1. Horvath AR, Bossuyt PMM, Sandberg S, et al. Setting analytical performance specifications based on outcome studies—is it possible? Clin Chem Lab Med 2015;53:841–8.
8. Sandberg S, Fraser CG, Horvath AR, et al. Defining analytical performance specifications: consensus statement from the 1st Strategic Conference of the European Federation of Clinical Chemistry and Laboratory Medicine. Clin Chem Lab Med 2015;53:833–5.
14. European Federation of Clinical Chemistry and Laboratory Medicine on-line biological variation database. <https://biologicalvariation.eu> [accessed 2020.07.04].
16. Roraas T, Petersen PH, Sandberg S. Confidence intervals and power calculations for within-person biological variation: effect of analytical imprecision, number of replicates, number of samples, and number of individuals. Clin Chem 2012;58:1306–13.
17. Aarsand AK, Røraas T, Sandberg S. Biological variation—reliable data is essential. Clin Chem Lab Med 2015;53:153–4.
21. Aarsand AK, Roraas TR, Fernandez-Calle P, et al. The Biological Variation Data Critical Appraisal Checklist: A Standard for Evaluating Studies on Biological Variation. Clin Chem 2018:64,501–14.
22. Panteghini M, Sandberg S. Defining analytical performance specifications 15 years after the Stockholm conference. Clin Chem Lab Med 2015;53:829–32.
28. Miller WG, Erek A, Cunningham TD, et al. Commutability limitations influence quality control results with different reagent lots. Clin Chem 2011;57:76–83.
30. Parvin CA. Assessing the impact of the frequency of quality control testing on the quality of reported patient results. Clin Chem 2008;54:2049–54.
31. CLSI. Laboratory quality control based on risk management; approved guideline EP23-A. Wayne, PA: Clinical and Laboratory Standards Institute; 2011.
32. CLSI. Statistical quality control for quantitative measurement procedures: principles and definitions; approved guideline C24-A4. Wayne, PA: Clinical and Laboratory Standards Institute; 2016.
50. CLSI. User evaluation of between-reagent lot variation; approved guideline EP26-A. Wayne, PA: Clinical and Laboratory Standards Institute; 2013 (under revision at the time of publication).
53. CLSI. Verification of comparability of patient results within one healthcare system; approved guideline EP31-A-IR. Wayne, PA: Clinical and Laboratory Standards Institute; 2012.
58. Ng D, Poliyo FA, Cervinski MA. Optimization of a Moving Averages Program Using a Simulated Annealing Algorithm: The Goal is to Monitor the Process Not the Patients. Clin Chem 2016;62:1361-71.
59. Bennett ST. Continuous Improvement in Continuous Quality Control. Clin Chem 2016;62:1299-1301.
60. Badrick T, Bietenbeck A, Cervinski MA, et al. Patient-Based Real-Time Quality Control: Review and Recommendations. Clin Chem 2019;65:962-71.
62. Miller WG, Jones GRD, Horowitz GL, et al. Proficiency testing/external quality assessment: current challenges and future directions. Clin Chem 2011;57:1670–80.
74. Stavelin A, Riksheim BO, Christensen NG, et al. The Importance of reagent lot registration in external quality assurance/proficiency testing schemes. Clin Chem 2016;62:708–15.
75. Miller WG. Time to pay attention to reagent and calibrator lots for proficiency testing. Clin Chem 2016;62:666–7.
89. De Grande LAC, Goossens K, Van Uytfanghe K, et.al. The Empower project - a new way of assessing and monitoring test comparability and stability. Clin Chem Lab Med 2015;53:1197–204.

Standardization and Harmonization of Analytical Examination Results*

W. Greg Miller

ABSTRACT

Background

The purpose of a clinical laboratory test is to provide information on the pathophysiologic condition of an individual patient to assist with diagnosis, to guide or monitor therapy, or to assess risk for a disease. Results for the same measurand must be equivalent when measured using different measurement procedures (MPs) to avoid medical errors when using clinical decision values to interpret those results. Standardization or harmonization of results is accomplished by metrological traceability of calibration to the same reference system and by MPs having adequate selectivity for the measurand being measured.

Content

The purpose of a clinical laboratory test is to provide information on the pathophysiologic condition of an individual patient to assist with diagnosis, to guide or monitor therapy, or to assess risk for a disease. Results for the same measurand must be equivalent when measured using different MPs to avoid medical errors when using clinical decision values to interpret those results. Standardization or harmonization of results is accomplished by metrological traceability of calibration to the same reference system and by MPs having adequate selectivity for the measurand being measured.

The International Organization for Standardization (ISO) has published a series of standards that describe requirements for metrological traceability of results for patients' samples to higher-order references, including a harmonization protocol, for reference materials (RMs) and reference MPs used in metrological traceability, and for calibration laboratories that offer reference measurement services. The Joint Committee for Traceability in Laboratory Medicine reviews and approves RMs and reference MPs that conform to the ISO standards.

In vitro diagnostic manufacturers of end-user MPs used in clinical laboratories, including clinical laboratories that develop test procedures, establish metrological traceability to the available higher-order reference system for a measurand. When metrological traceability is successful, results for patients' samples agree among different MPs. Important limitations in achieving harmonized results are that higher-order references are available for only a little over 100 measurands and some matrix-based RMs in use are not commutable with patients' samples, which causes disagreement among results from different MPs. External quality assessment or proficiency testing using commutable samples is an important procedure to monitor the success of harmonization and provide feedback to identify measurands that need better harmonization of results.

---

*The full version of this chapter is available electronically on ExpertConsult.com.

Biological Variation and Analytical Performance Specifications*

Sverre Sandberg, Thomas Røraas, and Aasne K. Aarsand

ABSTRACT

Background

There are many sources of variation in numerical results generated by examinations performed in laboratory medicine. Some measurands have biological variations over the span of life and others have predictable cyclical or seasonal variations. Most measurands in an individual display random variation around homeostatic set points and this is termed within-subject biological variation. The homeostatic set points vary between individuals and the variation between the set points of different individuals is termed between-subject biological variation. An understanding of these sources of variation is required to enable appropriate application of clinical laboratory measurements.

Content

In this chapter, we explain that numerical estimates of analytical, within-subject, and between-subject biological variation are usually generated by prospective studies; series of specimens from a cohort of individuals are examined, followed by statistical analysis to identify and quantify the different types of variation. Furthermore, sources of evidence-based data on biological variation and tools for the appraisal of the quality of biological variation studies are presented. The chapter also provides an overview of what applications biological variation data have in laboratory medicine such as the "index of individuality" and "reference change value" where the latter is used to determine whether changes in serial results from an individual can be explained by analytical and within-subject biological variation only. Additionally, models for setting analytical performance specifications, for imprecision, bias, total error, and measurement uncertainty, which can be created using estimates of within-subject and between-subject variation, are presented.

---

*The full version of this chapter is available electronically on ExpertConsult.com.

Establishment and Use of Reference Intervals

Gary Horowitz and Graham Ross Dallas Jones

ABSTRACT

Background

One of the most important elements of a laboratory test result is the reference interval, a set of values against which physicians compare their patients' test results, facilitating interpretation. It is extremely important, therefore that the laboratory community devotes sufficient resources to ensure the reference limits they provide are well-founded. Most frequently, these reference limits represent values for healthy, adult patients, but other sets of values can be provided (such as values for pregnancy or for children). Sometimes, clinical decision limits are provided in place of conventional reference limits (such as for treating patients with diabetes or for diagnosing acute coronary syndromes).

Content

In this chapter, we describe the techniques for properly establishing reference intervals, including selection of appropriate reference individuals, implementation of preanalytical standardization, considerations for eliminating outliers, partitioning the reference group, and performance of statistical methods to calculate reference limits and their confidence intervals. In addition, since formal establishment of reference intervals may be beyond the capacity of many laboratories, we discuss alternative sources for reference limits (including manufacturers' package inserts, peer-reviewed literature, multicenter trials, historical laboratory data), along with techniques to verify the transferability of these data and common reference intervals. Consideration will be given to issues related to enhancing the display of patient test results with the appropriate reference limits. Even though most of the chapter is devoted to single tests (univariate) and population-based reference limits, we will also briefly describe the concept of subject-based and multivariate reference intervals. Lastly, we discuss techniques for ongoing verification of reference limits.

CONCEPT OF REFERENCE LIMITS

Interpretation by Comparison

Laboratory test results play a vital role in clinical medicine. Physicians use these results when screening for diseases in apparently healthy people, for confirming, excluding, or changing the probability of the diagnosis of specific diseases in patients with certain symptoms and signs, and for monitoring changes in a patient over time. To achieve these goals, interpretation is made by comparison with population reference limits, clinical decision limits, or previous results from the same patient. Population reference limits are generally derived from subjects without diseases, whereas clinical decision limits are generally based on clinical categories or outcomes of patients which can be separated on the basis of laboratory results. To facilitate these comparisons it is critical that laboratories provide not only the patient's test result but appropriate *reference limits* with which the patient's results can be compared. Ideally, for comparison with population limits, such reference limits should be available not only from healthy individuals but also from patients with relevant diseases, to assess whether a result is within the expected range for a clinical condition under consideration. Usually only health-associated reference limits are available in pathology reports with expected values in diseases often estimated by doctors based on training and experience. Reference limits have been described as the most common decision support tool in laboratory medicine, and their inclusion on a pathology report is endorsed by the international clinical laboratory standard ISO 15189[1] and required by the College of American Pathologists (CAP).[2] A detailed history and commentary on the development of reference intervals is available.[3]

Normal Values/Normal Ranges: Obsolete Terms

Historically, the term *normal values* was used to describe the laboratory data provided for purposes of comparison, and *normal ranges* as the expression of these on pathology reports. However, use of these terms often leads to confusion because the word "normal" has several different connotations.[4] For example, three medically important but very different meanings of "normal" are:

1. *Statistical sense:* Values can be described as "normal" if their observed distribution seems to follow closely the theoretical *normal distribution* of statistics—the Gaussian probability distribution. This use of "normal" has sometimes misled people to believe that the distribution of biological data is always symmetric and bell shaped, like the Gaussian distribution. However, on closer examination,

this usually is not correct. To exorcise the "ghost of Gauss," Elveback and colleagues recommend not using the term *normal limits*.[5] For a similar reason, the term *normal distribution* should be avoided and replaced by the term *Gaussian distribution*.

2. *Epidemiologic sense:* Another meaning of "normal" is illustrated by the following statement: It is "normal" to find that the activity of gamma-glutamyltransferase (GGT) in serum is between 7 and 47 IU/L, whereas it is considered "abnormal" to have a serum GGT value outside these limits. Here a more exact statement would read as follows: Approximately 95% of the values obtained, when the activity of GGT in sera collected from individuals considered to be healthy is measured, are included in the interval 7 to 47 IU/L. The obsolete concept of *normal values* in part carried this meaning. Alternative terms for "normal" in this sense are *common, frequent, habitual, usual,* and *typical*.

3. *Clinical sense:* The term "normal" also is often used to indicate that values show the absence of certain diseases or the absence of risks for the development of diseases. In this sense, a *normal value* is considered a sign of health. Better descriptive terms for such values are *healthy, nonpathologic,* and *harmless*. As a corollary, when results are discussed with patients, it may be unhelpful to describe results outside reference limits as "abnormal" because this may be taken to indicate the presence of disease or ill health and therefore create unnecessary anxiety or concern.

Because of confusion resulting from the different meanings of normal, the terms *normal values* and *normal ranges* are obsolete and should not be used.

To prevent the ambiguities inherent in the term *normal values,* the concept of *reference values,* from which the terms *reference intervals* and *reference limits* are derived, was introduced and implemented in the 1980s.[6,7] The term *reference* is appropriate because these values provide something to refer to when interpreting a result. This was an important event in establishing a scientific basis for clinical interpretation of laboratory data.[8] The term *reference range* is sometimes used in place of the term *reference interval* recommended by the International Federation of Clinical Chemistry and Laboratory Medicine (IFCC). This use is incorrect because the statistical term *range* denotes the difference (a single value!) between maximum and minimum values in a distribution.[9]

Terminology

The IFCC recommends use of the term *reference individuals* and related terms such as *reference value, reference limit, reference interval,* and *observed values*.[7,10–15] The definitions and the presentation in the following sections of this chapter are in accordance with IFCC recommendations,[10–15] which have been adopted by the Clinical Laboratory Standards Institute (CLSI).[16]

Reference individual: An individual selected for comparison using defined criteria.

As mentioned previously, for the interpretation of values obtained from an individual under clinical investigation, appropriate comparison values are needed. To provide such values, suitable individuals must be selected. The characteristics of the individuals in each group chosen for comparison should be clearly defined. Their age and sex must be specified and whether they should be healthy or have a certain disease. The definition of a reference individual also covers cases in

which the individual under clinical investigation is his or her own reference, as discussed in a later section on subject-based reference values.

Reference population: The entire set of reference individuals.

Reference value: A value obtained by observation or measurement of a particular type of quantity on a reference individual.

If, for example, the activity of GGT is measured in sera collected from a group of reference individuals selected for comparison according to a sufficiently exact set of criteria, the GGT results are considered reference values.

Reference distribution: The distribution of the reference values.

Reference limits: The upper and lower bounds of the specified fraction of the reference distribution, typically the central 95% of the distribution.

Reference interval: The spread of values defined by the upper and lower reference limits.

Observed value: A value of a particular type of quantity obtained by observation or measurement and produced to make a medical decision. Observed values can be compared with reference values, reference distributions, reference limits, or reference intervals.

Or, rephrased: An observed value is the result obtained by analysis of a specimen collected from *an individual under clinical investigation*. The equivalent term used in the International Vocabulary of Metrology (VIM) is *measurement result*.[17]

The IFCC also defines other terms related to the concept of *reference values:* reference sample group, reference distribution, reference limit, and reference interval.[10–15] Some of these terms are introduced in later sections of this chapter.

Clinical Decision Limits

The terms *reference limits* and *clinical decision limits* should not be confused.[8,18] *Reference limits* are descriptive of the distribution of results in the selected subset of reference individuals; they tell us something about the expected variation of values in the reference population. Comparison of new values with these limits conveys information about similarity to the given reference values. In contrast, *clinical decision limits* provide separation based on clinical categories or outcomes. The latter limits may be based on analysis of reference values from several groups of individuals (healthy persons and patients with relevant diseases) and are used for the purpose of differential diagnosis.[18–20] Alternatively, such values are established on the basis of outcome studies and are used as clinical guidelines for treatment. Examples of current decision limits include recommended concentrations for therapeutic drug levels (see Chapter 42), the National Cholesterol Education Program guidelines related to cholesterol,[21] the American Diabetes Association recommendations for diagnosis of diabetes with HbA_{1c} or plasma glucose,[22] and the American Academy of Pediatrics guidelines on neonatal bilirubin.[23] A key factor with clinical decision limits is that each assumes that measurements of the involved analytes are accurate, with the metrological traceability similar to the method used in the clinical studies on which the clinical decision points were established (see Chapter 7).

In this context, it is critical to point out another difference between reference limits and clinical decision limits. For most analytes, a laboratory should establish (or verify) its own reference limits. The processes to do this are described later in this chapter. But for analytes interpreted using clinical decision limits such as national or international laboratory guidelines, efforts that once would have been dedicated to establishing or verifying reference intervals should be redirected toward establishing accuracy (trueness). In the 2010 CLSI guidelines,[16] this point is given much-deserved emphasis. It does little good to establish one's own reference limits if physicians will (and should) use national guidelines or if the laboratory gives results which are biased compared with the results used to determine the clinical decision points. Methods to establish the accuracy of one's method are discussed in Chapter 7. It is also important for laboratories to communicate to clinicians the nature of reference limits provided with results, specifying whether these are population reference intervals or clinical decision limits, as well as any additional information required for appropriate use. In particular, information on populations with and without specified diseases allows for determination of important characteristics of diagnostic tests, including their sensitivity, specificity, predictive values, and likelihood ratios, all of which are discussed in detail in Chapter 2.

Types of Reference Limits

In practice it is often necessary or convenient to give a short description associated with the term *reference limits,* such as *health-associated reference limits* (close to what was understood by the obsolete term *normal values*). With conditions such as obesity, which are prevalent in many populations and associated with poorer health outcomes, the definition of health-associated reference limits becomes more difficult, both to define (this is discussed in subsequent text with exclusions from the reference population) and to communicate to the end-user. Other examples of such qualifying words could be *hospital inpatient, pregnancy,* and *patients with well-controlled diabetes.* These short descriptions prevent the common misunderstanding that reference values are associated only with health.

Subject-Based and Population-based Reference Values

Subject-based reference values are previous values from the same individual, obtained when he or she was in a known state of health. *Population-based* reference limits are those obtained from a group of well-defined reference individuals and are usually the types of values referred to when the term *reference limits* is used with no qualifying words. This chapter deals primarily with population-based values. It should be noted, however, that for some tests, intraindividual variation may be small relative to interindividual differences. The relationship of within- to between-individual variation is known as the index of individuality (see Chapter 8), and in cases in which this is low (e.g., creatinine,[24] immunoglobulins[25]), the use of population-based reference intervals may distract from clinically significant intraindividual changes, as noted later in this chapter. In this setting the concept of "reference change value" (RCV) can be seen as analogous to a population reference limit, as the RCV is defined using data from reference subjects from a reference population, and a statistical analysis used to determine significant changes.

It is also important to note that this chapter focuses on population-based *univariate reference limits* and quantities derived from them. For example, if separate reference limits

for calcium and parathyroid hormone (PTH) in plasma are used, two sets of univariate reference limits are produced. The term *multivariate reference limits* denotes that results of two or more analytes obtained from the same set of reference individuals are treated in combination. Plasma calcium and PTH values may be used, for example, to define a bivariate reference region, which would reflect the fact that, as calcium concentrations decrease, even within healthy reference limits, PTH levels rise. Thus a PTH level that is within health-associated univariate reference limits might not be within the health-associated bivariate reference limits. This subject is addressed briefly in a later section.

Requirements for Valid Use of a Reference Interval

Certain conditions apply for a valid comparison between a patient's laboratory results and reference values[26]:
1. The reference individuals for each test should be clearly defined.
2. The patient examined should sufficiently resemble the reference individuals in all respects other than those under investigation.
3. The conditions under which the reference specimens were obtained and processed for analysis should be known and these conditions should be the same as for the patient specimen.
4. The measurand under examination in the patient and the reference individuals should be the same.
5. All laboratory results should be produced using adequately standardized methods under sufficient analytical quality control (see Chapters 6 and 7). The standardization should be sufficient that any bias or difference in precision or analytical specificity between the analytical system used for the patient sample and that used for the reference samples does not affect the interpretation.

To these general requirements one may add others that become necessary when more detailed and sophisticated approaches to decision making are applied.[8]
6. Stages in the pathogenesis of diseases that are the objectives for diagnosis should be demarcated beyond the separation between presence and absence of the disease. For example, although some overlap occurs, the clinical grades of congestive heart failure (CHF) are distinguished by progressive increases in levels of N-terminal pro-brain natriuretic peptide (NTproBNP).[27]
7. Clinical diagnostic sensitivity and specificity, prevalence, and clinical costs of misclassification should be known for all laboratory tests used. For example, in some instances, one might want to know whether a given NTproBNP value is "healthy," in which case one would want to use reference limits for age- and sex-matched individuals with no evidence of CHF. In contrast, when faced with a patient complaining of shortness of breath in the emergency room, one might want instead to know, not so much whether any degree of CHF is present, but whether the patient's CHF is sufficiently advanced to be the cause of the shortness of breath.[28,29]

SELECTION OF REFERENCE INDIVIDUALS

A set of *selection criteria* determines which individuals should be included in the group of reference individuals.[7,10–15] Such selection criteria include statements describing the source population and specifications of criteria for health or for the disease of interest.

Often, separate reference values for each sex and for different age groups,[30] as well as other criteria, are necessary. The overall group of reference individuals therefore may have to be divided into more homogeneous subgroups. For this purpose, specific rules for the division, called *stratification* or *partitioning criteria,* are needed.

It is important to distinguish between selection and partitioning criteria. First, selection criteria are applied to obtain a group of reference individuals. Thereafter, this group is divided into subgroups using partitioning criteria. Whether a specific criterion (e.g., sex) is a selection or a partitioning criterion depends on the purpose of the actual project. For example, sex is a selection criterion if reference values only from female subjects are necessary. Sex can also be a selection criteria where the data will be partitioned using this criterion to ensure sufficient numbers of each sex are collected.

Concept of Health in Relation to Reference Values

There is an obvious requirement for health-associated reference values for quantities measured in the clinical laboratory. But the concept of health is problematic; as Grasbeck stated "Health is characterized by a minimum of subjective feelings and objective signs of disease, assessed in relation to the social situation of the subject and the purpose of the medical activity, and it is in the absolute sense an unattainable ideal state."[31] Much confusion may arise if the selection criteria for health are not clearly stated for a specific project.

When reference values are produced, the following questions are asked: (1) Why are these values needed? (2) How are they going to be used? (3) To what extent does the intended purpose of the project determine how health is identified? For example when setting reference limits for cardiac-specific troponins, a "cardio-healthy" population is required that is in other ways similar to the patients who are likely to present with possible acute coronary syndrome (i.e., they should be of similar age and gender, and they may have hypertension or hyperlipidemia).[32,33]

Strategies for Selection of Reference Individuals

Several methods have been suggested for the selection of reference individuals. Table 9.1 shows a variety of concepts that may be used to describe a sampling scheme. The concepts can be considered as pairs, each of which is mutually exclusive. For example, the sampling may be direct or indirect, and direct sampling may be a priori or a posteriori.

The merits and disadvantages of these strategies are described in the following sections. It is not possible to recommend one sampling scheme that is superior in all respects and applicable to all situations. One must choose the optimal approach for a given project and state clearly what has been done.

Direct or Indirect Sampling?

Selection of reference intervals by *direct* sampling involves collection of specimens from selected members of the reference population for the purpose of establishing reference limits. *Indirect* sampling involves deriving reference limits from using results of samples collected for other purposes. Direct selection of reference individuals (see Table 9.1) concurs with the concept of reference values as recommended by

TABLE 9.1	Strategies for Selection of Reference Individuals
Direct Versus Indirect	
Direct	Individuals are selected from a parent population using defined criteria
Indirect	Individuals are not considered, but certain statistical methods are applied to analytical values in a laboratory database
A Priori Versus A Posteriori	
A Priori	Individuals are selected for specimen collection and analysis if they fulfill defined inclusion criteria
A Posteriori	Use of an already existing database containing both relevant clinical information and analytical results. Values of individuals meeting defined inclusion criteria are selected.
Random Versus Nonrandom	
Random	Process of selection giving each item (individual or test result) in the parent population an equal chance of being chosen
Nonrandom	Process of selection that does not ensure that each item in the parent population has an equal chance of being chosen

the IFCC,[10–15] and it is the basis for the presentation in this chapter. Its major disadvantages are the problems and costs of obtaining a representative group of reference individuals.

These practical problems have led to the search for simpler and less expensive approaches such as *indirect* methods.[6,34] Historically the indirect approach has been taken using results in a routine pathology database, often from laboratories serving a largely inpatient population. While these may be the only data available for some laboratories, the indirect approach may be applied to other data sources, such as samples collected for research, epidemiology, or "wellness testing," where the expected prevalence of disease may be low. A key starting point with any indirect method is an understanding of the population from which the samples have been drawn, even if specific criteria have not been applied at the time of collection.

The indirect approach is based on the observation that many analysis results produced in the clinical laboratory seem to be "normal," or at least unaffected by the reason for the sample collection. Two main concepts have been used to extract information about reference distributions from this type of data. The first is the use of statistical methods which allow identification of a distribution within the database which is then taken to represent the reference population. Note that for this approach no attempt is made to classify individual results as representing the reference population. The alternate method is to use additional clinical information to classify individual results and exclude those which are more likely to be from individuals with relevant disease or other factors which may affect the results. Typically both methods are applied in the development of reference intervals using the indirect approach.

An example of the results from a pathology database is shown in Fig. 9.1. As seen, the values of serum sodium

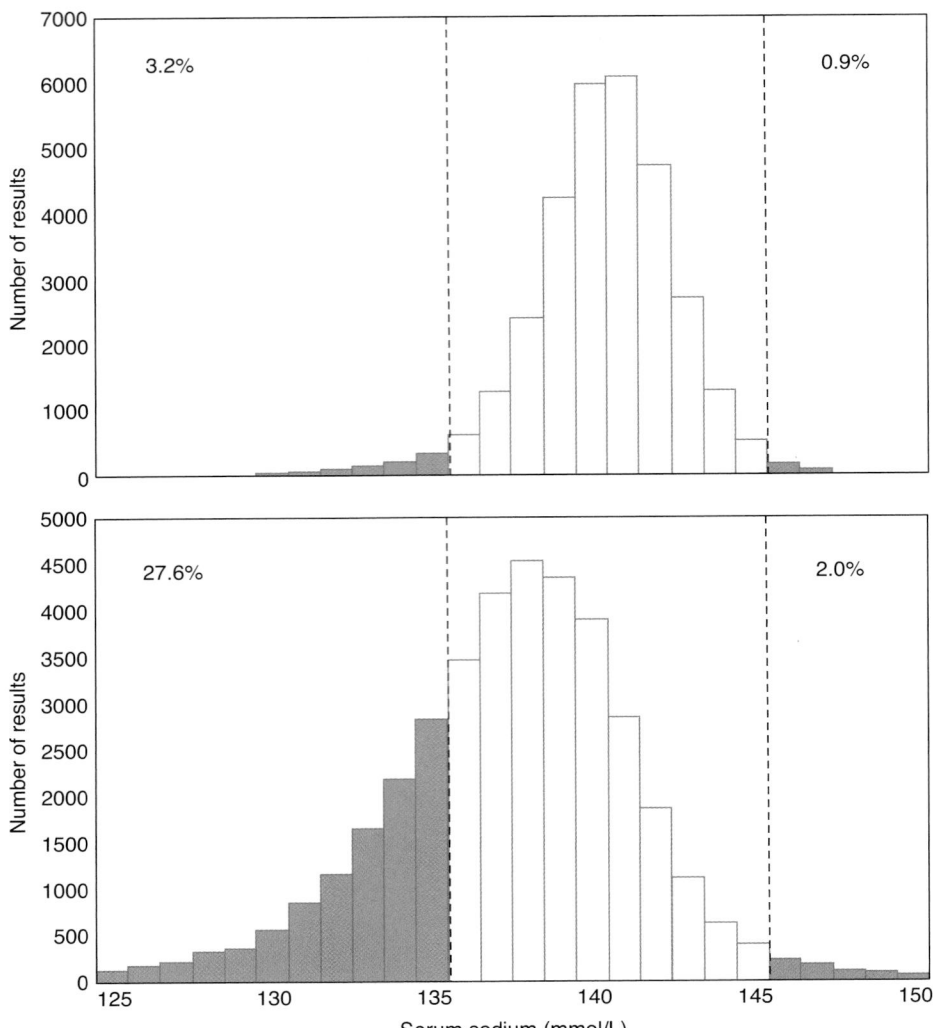

FIGURE 9.1 Distribution of serum sodium concentrations obtained in a routine laboratory over 1 year. The top histogram **(A)** shows 31,183 sequential results from general practice sites and the lower histogram **(B)** shows 38,751 from hospital wards. The dark shaded areas and attached percentages show the fractions of the two populations outside the reference interval derived by direct methods in the same population (represented by the dashed vertical lines, 136 to 145 mmol/L) (From Koerbin G, Cavanaugh JA, Potter JM, Abhayaratna WP, West NP, Glasgow N, et al. "Aussie normals": an a priori study to develop clinical chemistry reference intervals in a healthy Australian population. *Pathology*. 2015;47:138–44).

concentrations from outpatients have a distribution with a preponderant central peak and a shape similar to a Gaussian distribution. The underlying assumption of the indirect method is that this peak is composed mainly of *normal values* or, more precisely, is derived from patients without the condition of interest or diseases that may affect the analyte under consideration. Advocates of the method therefore claim that it is possible to estimate a *reference interval* if the distribution of unaffected values from this distribution is extracted. Fig. 9.1 also shows serum sodium results from hospital inpatients showing both lower results on average, as well as an increased proportion of lower results (the data set is left skewed). This may be due to the presence of a significant proportion of the samples being derived from patients with a condition affecting the results, for example, in the case of

serum sodium, diuretic use, dehydration, and other fluid imbalances. It may also be due to systematic preanalytical differences, such as recumbence in inpatients compared with ambulatory outpatients. This shows the importance of selection of the data set to use for indirect analysis. Several mathematical methods have been used to extract a distribution for the derivation of reference limits from routine laboratory data.[35–38]

In short, the indirect method has at least two potential major deficiencies:
1. Estimates of the reference limits can depend heavily on the particular mathematical method used and on its underlying assumptions.
2. Estimates of the reference limits can be affected by the prevalence, nature, and severity of disease included in the laboratory database. This may be a particular problem

with databases containing only hospital inpatients. The use of ambulatory outpatients and general practice patients can reduce this variability considerably.

However, if appropriate exclusion criteria are applied, data derived by indirect sampling from pathology databases may be used for the establishment of reference values in a way that is fully concordant with IFCC recommendations.[35–37,39,40] The requirement for this approach is that laboratory results should be *combined with other information* (i.e., to combine an a posteriori strategy with the indirect method). Laboratory results are to be used as reference values only if stated clinical criteria are fulfilled. The types of data which can be used include demographic information such as age, sex, source (e.g., inpatient, outpatient, specific clinics); patient sampling related information (e.g., by excluding multiple results from the same patient or limiting samples to those where only a single request for that test has been made in a specified time); information from other pathology results (e.g., using HbA_{1c} or fasting glucose results to reduce the likelihood of overweight or obesity related effects); or from other clinical information available by linking with clinical databases. In practice the factors applied are analyte-specific and depend on what is available, and detailed understanding of the pathophysiology of the analyte being examined is required. For example results from inpatients should be excluded for analytes affected by recumbency (e.g., serum albumin or sodium) or intercurrent disease (e.g., C-reactive protein [CRP], other acute phase reactants). For tests used for both diagnosis and monitoring (e.g., serum creatinine, tumor markers), restricting analysis to patients with a single result may be preferred. This can also be seen as an acceptance by the treating doctor that further investigation was not warranted based on the results.

Reference values produced by indirect sampling techniques have a number of significant potential advantages over those based on direct sampling. With any indirect method, the preanalytical and analytical factors are exactly the same for the patient sample and the reference setting process, and also the reference population matches that of the patient. This can provide a more appropriate comparison group, as the role of clinical decision-making is to separate patients with the same clinical presentation on the basis of disease, rather than separating sick from healthy. For example, the need, in patients with chest pain, is to distinguish those having a myocardial infarction from those who are not.

The indirect approach can also be used in settings where collection of samples for reference interval studies may be particularly problematic such as extremes of age or during pregnancy. Additionally the numbers of samples which may be available for indirect techniques can be vastly greater than direct techniques, in the many tens or even hundreds of thousands and the costs are a fraction of those of direct studies. If direct studies are available for comparison, indirect studies will enable an assessment of whether there are differences in the local population, specimen collection techniques, or analytical methods. It is however important to note that the indirect approach is continuing to evolve and that if poorly performed, an indirect study can give misleading results.

A Priori or A Posteriori Sampling?

When carefully performed, both *a priori* (before) and *a posteriori* (after) sampling (see Table 9.1) may result in reliable reference values. The use of the *a priori* approach is limited to direct reference interval studies, but as discussed above, the *a posteriori* approach can be applied to direct and indirect studies. The choice is often a question of practicality. Both require the same set of successive steps, but the order of some of these operations differs depending on the mode of selection: a priori or a posteriori.[6]

The first step in the process of producing reference values for a laboratory test should always be the collection of quantitative information about sources of biological, preanalytical, and analytical variation for the analyte studied. In this setting, biological variation includes expected variation with time of day, with meals, with seasons, and with life stages. A search through relevant literature may yield the required information.[41,42] If relevant information cannot be found in the literature, pilot studies may be necessary before the selection of reference individuals is planned in detail. Serum sodium is an example of a biological analyte that is affected by only a few sources of biological variation. However, the list of factors may be rather long for other analytes, such as serum enzymes, proteins, and hormones.

It is important to distinguish between controllable and noncontrollable sources of biological variation. Some factors may be controlled by standardization of the procedure for preparation of reference individuals and specimen collection such as fasting status and time of day (see a later section of this chapter). Other factors, such as age and gender, may be relevant partitioning criteria. Remaining sources of variation should be considered when criteria for the selection of reference individuals are defined.

The *a priori* strategy is best suited for smaller studies and for analytes for which there are very specific confounding factors or for which the analytical process is very difficult or expensive. One such example is male sex hormone–related reference intervals.[43] Potential reference individuals from the parent population should be interviewed and examined clinically and by selected laboratory methods to decide whether they fulfill the defined inclusion criteria. If they do, specimens for analysis are collected by a standardized procedure (including the necessary preparation of individuals before the collection).

The *a posteriori* method is based on the availability of a large collection of data on medically examined individuals and measured quantities. Studies thoroughly planned by centers for health screening or preventive medicine may provide such data. It is important that data be collected by a strictly standardized and comprehensive protocol concerning (1) sampling from the parent population, (2) registration of demographic and clinical data on participating individuals, (3) preparation for and execution of specimen collection, and (4) handling and analysis of the specimens. If these requirements are met, values may be selected after application of the defined inclusion criteria to individuals found in the database. The selection of individuals from large pathology databases (see earlier discussion) is another example of the application of an a posteriori method. In this case, however, the quality of data may be lower than that in well-planned population studies.

A study performed in Kristianstad, Sweden,[44] highlights a practical problem often met when reference individuals are selected: the number of subjects fulfilling the inclusion criteria may be too small. In this study, only 17% of participants were accepted into the study, according to the criteria used, leaving an insufficiently sized reference sample group and a risk of selection bias. The frequency of exclusion was higher among women and in older age groups, exacerbating the issues in these groups.

This problem has two possible solutions:

1. The exclusion criteria may be relaxed. As already discussed, the set of relevant sources of biological variation differs among different analytes. One may define a minimum set of exclusion criteria for a given laboratory test. In the Kristianstad study, the complete group of individuals could probably be used for establishment of reference values for serum sodium, and most of the individuals would be acceptable for the determination of reference values for several other analytes.[44]

2. Another design of the sampling procedure could reduce the practical problems and costs of obtaining a sufficiently large group of reference individuals. The Kristianstad study showed that 75% of excluded subjects could have been identified using only a simple questionnaire.[44] In the upper age group, this percentage was even higher. Therefore preliminary screening of a large number of individuals from the parent population, using a carefully designed questionnaire (i.e., of or related to the current or previous medical history of a patient), would result in a much smaller sample of individuals for examination clinically and by laboratory methods. If 3000 individuals had been prescreened in Kristianstad, and if only the individuals remaining in the reduced sample were subjected to a closer examination, a group of 240 reference individuals would have been obtained.

The two modifications of the protocol may also be combined.

Random or Nonrandom Sampling?

Ideally, the group of reference individuals should be a random sample of all individuals fulfilling the inclusion criteria defined in the parent population. Statistical estimation of distribution parameters (and their confidence intervals) and statistical hypothesis testing require this assumption.

For several reasons, most collections of reference values are, in fact, obtained by a nonrandom process.[45] This means that all possible reference individuals in the entire population under study do not have an equal chance of being chosen for inclusion in the usually much smaller sample of individuals studied. A strictly random sampling scheme in most cases is impossible for practical reasons. It would imply the examination of and application of inclusion criteria to the entire population (thousands or millions of persons), and then the random selection of a subset of individuals from among those accepted. This approach has been used in selecting individuals at random to provide a cohort that is representative of the full population by several national organizations, such as the National Health and Nutrition Examination Survey (NHANES)[46] in the United States, the Canadian Health Measures Survey in Canada,[47] and the Australian Bureau of Statistics.[48]

Usually the situation is less satisfactory. The sampling process is highly affected by convenience and cost. For example, samples of reference individuals are commonly obtained by selecting (1) from blood donors, (2) from persons working in a nearby factory, (3) from hospital staff, or (4) from hospital databases, none of which represent a random sampling of possible reference individuals in the general population.

The conclusions are obvious: (1) the best reference sample obtainable should be used with a balance between practical considerations and consideration of possible biases that may be introduced by the selection process, and (2) the data should be used and interpreted with due caution, with awareness of the possible bias introduced by the nonrandomness of the sample selection process. For example, lower iron stores may be expected in a sample of regular blood donors, and higher vitamin D concentrations may be expected in a sample drawn from outdoor workers. An additional effect of nonrandomness is an increased chance that results of different reference studies may produce different results even when the defined reference population is intended to be the same.

Selection Criteria and Evaluation of Subjects

The selection of reference individuals consists essentially of applying defined criteria to a group of examined candidate persons.[10–15] The required characteristics of the reference values determine which criteria should be used in the selection process. Table 9.2 lists some important criteria to consider when production of health-associated reference values is the aim.

In practice, consideration of which *diseases* and *risk factors* to exclude is difficult (see the discussion on the concept of health earlier in this chapter). The answer lies in part in the intended purpose of establishing reference values; the project must be goal oriented.

Once a factor has been selected as an exclusion factor, a relevant and practical definition is required. For example, obesity is a common condition that is associated with a

TABLE 9.2 Examples of Exclusion and Partitioning Criteria[a]	
Exclusion	**Partitioning**
Age	Age
Alcohol intake	Blood group
Blood donation (recent)	Circadian variation
Drug abuse	Ethnicity
Exercise intensity (recent)	Exercise intensity (recent)
Fasting vs. nonfasting	Fasting vs. nonfasting
Sex	Sex
Hospitalization (recent)	Menstrual cycle (by stage)
Hypertension	
Illness (recent)	
Lactation	
Obesity	Obesity
Occupation	Posture (when sampled)
Oral contraceptives	
Pregnancy	Pregnancy (by stage)
Prescription drugs	Prescription drugs
Recent transfusion	

[a]As indicated by the *shaded boxes*, some criteria may be considered as either exclusion criteria or partitioning criteria.

number of diseases; however, the definition of *obesity* is problematic. A definition might be based on a known assumed contribution to the risk of a development of specified disease. However, scientific data of this type are seldom available for the studied population. Another possibility for establishing obesity is to use upper limits based on weight measurements in different age, gender, and height groups of the general population (e.g., more than 20% above the national age-, sex-, and height-specific mean weight). For obesity, a common approach is to use definitions based on the body mass index (BMI),[49] although limiting subjects to the healthy range will exclude over 50% of some populations. Tables of optimum or ideal weights have been published by life insurance companies; they may be more appropriate for delineation of obesity. Similar problems relate to the definition of hypertension. And what if a potential reference individual is no longer obese as a result of bariatric surgery or is currently normotensive on drug therapy?

In addition, is it permissible to use exclusion criteria based on *laboratory measurements*? It has been argued that a circular process might happen when laboratory tests are used to assess the health of subjects who are subsequently used as healthy control subjects for laboratory tests. But actually there is no difference, in this context, between measuring height, weight, and blood pressure and performing selected laboratory tests, provided that these laboratory tests are neither those for which reference values are produced nor tests that are significantly correlated with them.[31]

The removal of reference results based on other laboratory results has been used in a process termed latent abnormal values exclusion (LAVE). In a multinational study it was shown that this process, using a standard group of exclusion tests and criteria, affected some analytes but had little effect on others.[50] As stated above, care should be taken that tests with correlated results are not used for this purpose. It is particularly difficult to define selection criteria when establishing reference values for older patients.[51] In older age groups, it is "normal" (i.e., common) to have minor or major diseases and to take therapeutic drugs. One solution is to collect values at one time and to use the values of survivors after a defined number of years.[31,52]

Usually the clinical evaluation of candidate individuals is based on (1) a detailed interview or questionnaire (i.e., the complete history recalled and recounted by a patient), (2) a physical examination, and (3) supplementary investigations. Questionnaires and examination forms tailored to the requirements of the actual project facilitate the evaluation and document the decisions made.

Partitioning of the Reference Group

It may also be necessary to define *partitioning criteria* for the subclassification of the set of selected reference individuals into more homogeneous groups (see Table 9.2).[10–15] (The question of determining when stratification of the reference sample group is necessary and justified is discussed in later sections.) In practice, the number of partitioning criteria should usually be kept as small as possible to ensure sufficient sample sizes to derive valid estimates.

Age and *sex* are the most frequently used criteria for subgrouping, because several analytes vary notably among different age and sex groups.[41,51,53] Age may be categorized by equal intervals (e.g., by decades) or by intervals that are narrower in the periods of life when greater variation is observed. In some cases, more appropriate intervals can be obtained from qualitative age groups, such as (1) postnatal, (2) infancy, (3) childhood, (4) prepubertal, (5) pubertal, (6) adult, (7) premenopausal, (8) menopausal, and (9) geriatric. Further subdivision may also be needed based on Tanner stage of puberty or based on phase of the menstrual cycle. Height and weight also have been used as criteria for categorizing children. The use of age and sex for partitioning has the advantage that reference limits derived from subpopulations on these criteria can be easily applied on pathology reports where these factors are usually known about the patient. In contrast, the application of limits based on other criteria requires knowledge not usually available to the laboratory.

SPECIMEN COLLECTION

Several preanalytical factors can influence the values of measured biological quantities, such as the concentrations of components in a blood sample or the amount excreted in feces, urine, or sweat.[54,55] This topic is covered elsewhere (see Chapters 4 and 5). In this discussion, only aspects of special relevance to the generation of reliable reference values are highlighted.[10–15,54]

Standardization of the (1) preparation of individuals before specimen collection, (2) procedure of specimen collection itself, and (3) handling of the specimen before analysis may eliminate or minimize bias or variation from these factors. This reduces the "noise" that might otherwise conceal important biological "signals" of disease, risk, or treatment effect.

Preanalytical Standardization

Preanalytical procedures used before routine analysis of patient specimens and when reference values are established should be as similar as possible. In general, it is much easier to standardize routines for studies of reference values than those used in the daily clinical setting, especially when specimens are collected in emergency or other unplanned situations. Thus two general approaches have been suggested:
1. Only such factors that may be relatively easily controlled in the clinical setting should be part of the standardization when reference values are produced.
2. The rules for preanalytical standardization when reference values are produced should also be used for the clinical situation. Such rules include food and beverage restrictions, exercise restrictions, time sitting (or lying down) prior to phlebotomy, and tourniquet time. It has been shown that it is possible to apply these rules rather closely in the clinical setting for both hospitalized and ambulatory patients.[7] The same philosophy forms the basis for recommendations concerning sample preparation preceding analysis.

However, either philosophy is concordant with the concept of reference values, provided that the conditions under which reference values are produced are clearly stated.

Analyte-Specific Considerations

The types and magnitudes of preanalytical sources of variation clearly are not equal for different analytes (see Chapter 5).[42] In fact, some believe that only those factors that cause unwanted variation in the biological quantities for which reference values are being generated should be considered. For example, body posture during specimen collection is highly relevant for the establishment of reference values for analytes that do not diffuse across blood vessel walls, such as albumin in serum or red cell count in blood, but posture is irrelevant for establishment of serum sodium values.[42,55]

Alternatively, several constituents are analyzed routinely in the same clinical specimen and therefore it would be impractical to devise special procedures for every single type of quantity.[7] Consequently, three standardized procedures for blood specimen collection by venipuncture have been recommended[6,54]: (1) collection in the morning from hospitalized patients, (2) collection in the morning from ambulatory patients, and (3) collection in the afternoon from ambulatory patients. Such schemes have to be modified depending on local conditions and necessities and on the intended use of the reference values produced. Published checklists[7,10–15] may be helpful in the design of a scheme.

A special problem is caused by drugs taken by individuals before specimen collection,[56,57] and it may be necessary to distinguish between indispensable and dispensable medications. If possible, dispensable medication should be avoided for at least 48 hours. The use of indispensable drugs, such as contraceptive pills or essential medication, may be a criterion for exclusion or partitioning if these affect the analyte of interest.

In emergency or other unplanned clinical situations, even a partial application of the standardized procedure for collection has been shown to be of great value.[6] When collections have been made under conditions other than those specified for a specific analyte, interpretation of results against reference limits requires awareness of the type and magnitude of variation that may be expected under those circumstances. For example, a serum cortisol collected in the evening cannot usually be compared with reference limits established for morning collections, the exception being that a high result is still of great clinical relevance because the upper limit for evening values is typically much lower than the upper limit for morning values.

Necessity for Additional Information

The clinical situation is often different from a controlled research situation; for example, specimens have to be taken (1) during operations, (2) in emergency situations, and (3) when patients are unwilling or unable to follow instructions. Therefore the clinician may need additional information for interpretation of a patient's values in relation to reference values obtained under fairly standardized conditions.

An *empirical approach*[7] is to produce other sets of reference values, such as postprandial values, postexercise values, or postpartum values.[6] Such a method, however, is very expensive and does not cover all situations that could possibly arise. This approach is also limited by the variability in these events (i.e., for postprandial samples, the size of the meal, the types of food consumed, and the number of hours since the meal).

Another, more general solution to the problem is called the *predictive approach*.[7] Starting from a set of ordinary reference values and using quantitative information on the effects of various factors (e.g., intake of food, alcohol, and drugs; exercise; stress; posture; or time of day), expected reference

values that fit the actual clinical setting could be estimated.[41,42] An interesting example is provided by thyroid-stimulating hormone (TSH), where the effect of diurnal variation needs to be considered.[58]

More studies of such effects are needed, especially for the combined effect of two or more sources of variation. For example, is the combined effect of alcohol and contraceptive drugs on GGT activity in serum less than, equal to, or greater than the sum of their individual effects?

ANALYTICAL PROCEDURES AND QUALITY CONTROL

Essential components of the required definition of a set of reference values are specifications concerning (1) the analysis method (including information on metrological traceability, equipment, reagents, calibrators, type of raw data, and calculation method; see Chapter 7), (2) quality control (see Chapter 6), and (3) reliability criteria.[6,10–15]

Specifications should be so carefully described that another investigator will be able to reproduce the study and that a user of reference values will be able to evaluate their comparability with values obtained by methods used for producing the patients' values in a routine laboratory. To ensure comparability between reference values and observed values a method with the same performance characteristics of traceability, reproducibility, and analytical specificity should be used.

It is often claimed that analytical quality should be better when reference values rather than routine values are produced. This is certainly correct for trueness; all measures should be taken to select an appropriate reference standard (materials or methods) for traceability base and minimizing bias from that standard. The use of methods traceable to the Joint Committee for Traceability in Laboratory Medicine (JCTLM)-listed reference materials, methods, and services[59] (if available) increases the likelihood that reference limits are transferable among different laboratories. The question of imprecision is more difficult because it depends in part on the intended use of the reference values. Increases in analytical random variation result in widening of the reference interval.[6,a] For some special uses of reference values, the narrower reference interval obtained by a more precise analytical method may be appropriate. However, this usually is not true for routine clinical use of reference values. Interpretation is simplest if a patient's values and reference values are comparable with regard to analytical imprecision. For the same reason, it is advisable to analyze specimens from reference individuals in several runs to include between-run components of variation. A safe way to obtain comparability is to include these specimens in routine runs together with real patient specimens. Particular care must be taken with

---

[a]The width of a reference interval is a combination of the within-subject biological variation (coefficient of variation [CV_I]), the between-subject biological variation (CV_G), the preanalytical variation (CV_{PA}), and the analytical variation (CV_A). Assuming for demonstration that these factors are all distributed in a Gaussian manner, the CV of the results produced in a reference interval study (CV_{RI}) is $\sqrt{CV_i^2 + CV_g^2 + CVpa^2 + CVa^2}$. Thus a greater analytical imprecision leads to a wider reference interval.

analytical quality if multisite studies are performed with measurements performed at different locations. There is likely to be increased analytical variation due to between-instrument and between-laboratory factors, which must be kept small enough so that it does not adversely affect the results.

STATISTICAL TREATMENT OF REFERENCE VALUES

This section deals with two main topics: the partitioning of reference values into more homogeneous classes, and the determination of reference limits and intervals.[60] The subject matter is presented in the order in which data are often treated. Fig. 9.2 gives an outline and refers to corresponding sections in the text. Before the presentation of methods, some statistical concepts used are briefly discussed (see also Chapter 2). A textbook by Harris and Boyd gives an excellent summary of the statistical bases of reference values in laboratory medicine.[61]

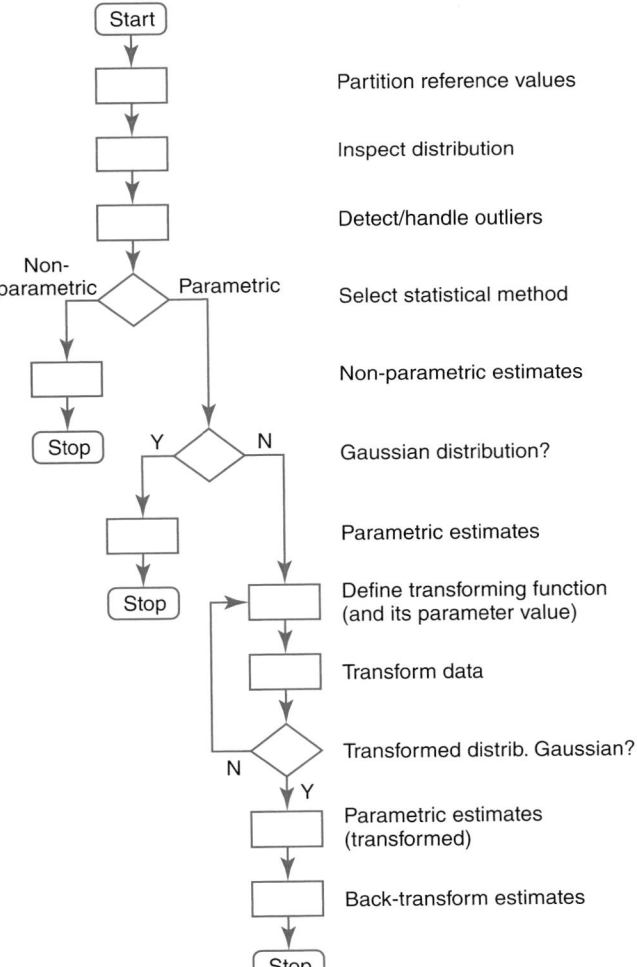

FIGURE 9.2 The statistical treatment of reference values. The *boxes* in the flow chart refer to sections in the text. The order of the first three actions (partitioning, inspection, and detection and/ or handling of outliers) may vary, depending on the distribution and the statistical methods applied. *N*, No; *Y*, yes.

Basic Statistical Concepts

Sample

The first step in the establishment of reference values is the selection of a group of reference individuals. In practice, it is not feasible to gather observations on all possible reference individuals of a certain category of the general population. Therefore a smaller group (sometimes called the reference *sample* group) is examined. This *subset* is chosen so that it is expected to give the desired information about the characteristics of the complete *set* of individuals (the reference *population*).[10–15]

The reference *population* is often considered to be *hypothetical* because its characteristics are not observed directly; neither the number (the set size) nor the properties of all of its individuals are known. An obvious requirement is that individuals in the subset are typical of those in the complete set. Statistical theory usually assumes that items in the subset are selected at *random* from among those in the set; otherwise, the subset may be biased. If items are not randomly selected, statistical techniques are still used, but only with due caution and with awareness of the possible bias introduced.

Two main types of inference may be made from values obtained from the subset (sample group) to the set (total reference population): estimating properties of the reference population (e.g., midpoint estimate and reference limits) and testing hypotheses related to the reference population (e.g., whether the distribution is Gaussian).

Estimating Properties

In practice, properties of the set are estimated. A *reference limit* (a percentile) of a biological quantity, such as the activity of serum GGT, based on subset reference values, is an example of a *point estimate* (a single value). It is considered representative of the property that might have been found if all possible values in the set had been observed. If many randomly selected subsets from the same set are examined, several estimates with some variation around the "true" value of the set are obtained. Also, it is possible to produce an *interval estimate* bounded by limits within which the "true" value is located with a specified confidence: the *confidence interval*. The parameter is expressed as a percentage between 0 and 100%, indicating the degree on the scale between "never" and "always" that the point estimate lies within the interval estimate. A reference limit for serum GGT can thus be associated with a confidence interval showing its region of uncertainty (e.g., the 97.5th percentile for serum GGT is 47 IU/L, with 90% confidence limits of 39 to 50 IU/L).

Testing Hypotheses

Hypotheses about the population distribution can be also tested. For example, one can state the *null hypothesis* that the distribution of values for serum GGT activities is Gaussian. If true, this will enable determination of the reference limits with relatively few points. If deviations of subset values from the Gaussian distribution are small, they can be ascribed to variation caused by chance alone. In that case, it is reasonable to use statistical methods based on the Gaussian distribution. However, the hypothesis must be rejected if it is unlikely that observed deviations from the Gaussian distribution are caused by chance alone. *Statistical tests* provide quantitative approaches to these types of decisions; the null hypothesis is rejected if the statistical test shows that the probability of the hypothesis being true is less than a stated *significance level.* The *probability (P)* is a number in the interval of 0 to 1, with higher values indicating a greater certainty. If a significance level of 0.05 is stated, the Gaussian hypothesis is tested for the distribution of serum GGT activities; it should be rejected if the probability obtained by the test is below this value (e.g., if *P* = .01, there is only a 1% chance that the distribution is Gaussian). Then the alternative hypothesis that the distribution is non-Gaussian is accepted. The *power* of a statistical test is the probability of rejection when the null hypothesis is false.

Describing the Distribution

In the following sections, the term *reference distribution*[10–15] is used for the distribution of reference values *(x)*. For Gaussian distributions the two statistics *arithmetic mean* $(\bar{x})$ and *standard deviation (SD)* (s_x) are measures of the location (based on a measure of the center of the distribution) and the dispersion of values in it, respectively. They are defined as follows:

$$\bar{x} = \frac{\sum x}{n}$$

$$S_x = \sqrt{\frac{\sum (x - \bar{x})^2}{n-1}} = \sqrt{\frac{\sum x^2 - \frac{(\sum x)^2}{n}}{n-1}}$$

where *x* represents each of the *n* reference values in the subset (or a subclass of it). The equations can be described in words to facilitate understanding. The arithmetic mean is the sum of all the values divided by the number of values. The SD is the square root of the result of the following calculation: the sum of the squares of all the differences of each value from the arithmetic mean divided by the number of samples minus one.

An observed distribution should be presented as a table or, preferably, as a graph (histogram) showing the number of observations in small intervals (Fig. 9.3). The number of observations in an interval divided by the total number of observations in the distribution (its size) is an estimator of the probability of finding a value in the corresponding interval of the hypothetical *probability distribution* of the population (assuming random sampling). By consecutive summing of all

these ratios, starting with the leftmost interval of the observed distribution, an estimate is obtained of the hypothetical *cumulative probability distribution,* shown as a normal probability plot in Fig. 9.4B.

Reference Limits: Interpercentile Interval

As mentioned previously, reference values provide a basis for interpretation of laboratory data. In clinical practice, one

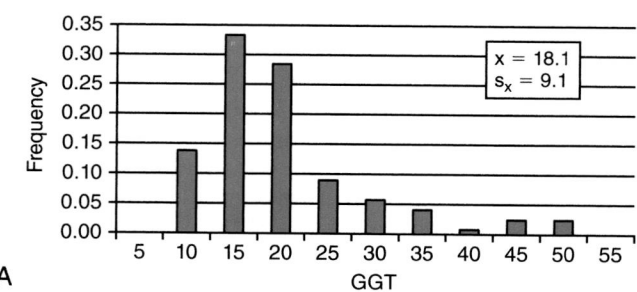

A

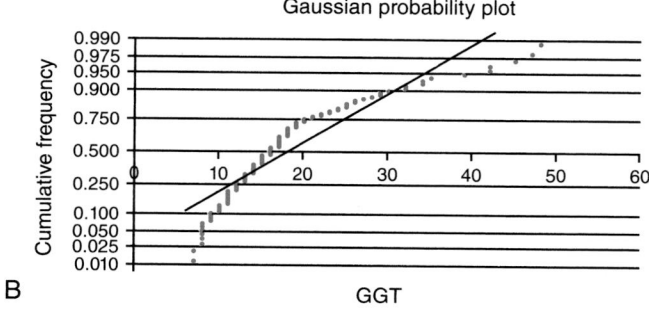

Gaussian probability plot

B

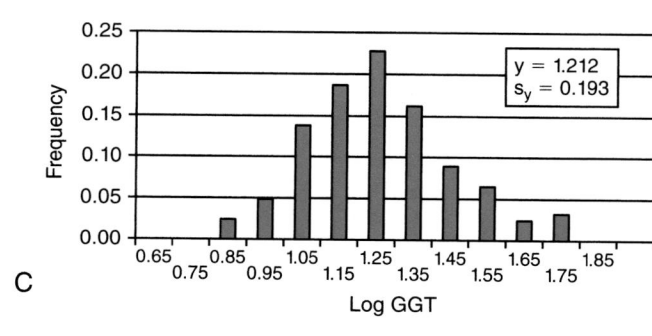

C

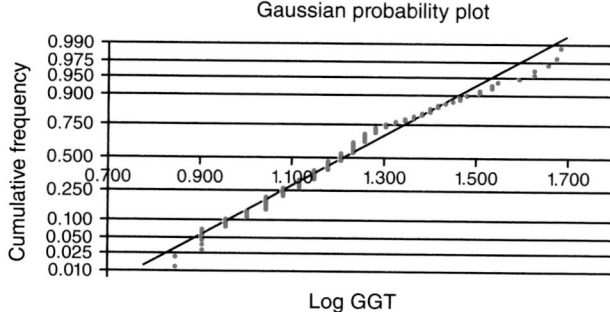

Gaussian probability plot

D

FIGURE 9.4 Distribution of 123 remaining gamma-glutamyl-transferase *(GGT)* values from reference subjects **(A)** is a histogram of the original, untransformed data, **(B)** shows the cumulative frequency of the data from (A) plotted on Gaussian probability paper, **(C)** is a histogram of the logarithmic transformed data, **(D)** shows the cumulative frequency of the data from (C) using a "normal probability plot."

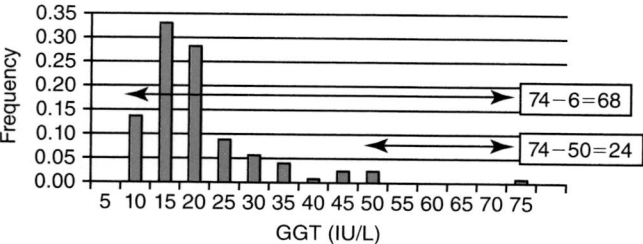

FIGURE 9.3 Observed distribution of 124 gamma-glutamyltransferase *(GGT)* values in serum (IU/L). The *upper arrow* indicates the range of the observed values (highest − lowest, or 74 − 6 = 68); the *lower arrow* indicates the difference between the highest value and the next highest value (74 − 50 = 24). Since the quotient (24/68 = 0.35) exceeds 0.33, Dixon's range test indicates that the highest value is an outlier and is therefore omitted from all further analyses.

usually compares a patient's result with the corresponding *reference interval*, which is bounded by a pair of *reference limits*.[10–15] This interval, which may be defined in different ways, is a useful condensation of the information carried by the total set of reference values.

This discussion will be confined to the *interpercentile interval*, which is (1) simple to estimate, (2) commonly used, and (3) recommended by the IFCC[10–15] and CLSI.[16] It is defined as an interval bounded by two percentiles of the reference distribution. A *percentile* denotes a value that divides the reference distribution such that specified percentages of its values have magnitudes less than or equal to the limiting value. For example, if 47 IU/L is the 97.5th percentile of serum GGT values, then 97.5% of the values are equal to or below this value.

It is an arbitrary but common convention to define the reference interval as the *central 95%-interval* bounded by the 2.5th and 97.5th percentiles.[10–15] Another size or an asymmetric location of the reference interval may be more appropriate in particular cases. For example, the 99th percentile has been recommended for cardiac troponins,[62] and the 80th percentile for lipoprotein(a).[63] To prevent ambiguity, the definition of the interval should always be stated. The estimation of percentiles presented in the following sections is based on the conventional central 95% interval, but the techniques are easily adapted to other locations of the limits.

The percentiles are point estimates of population parameters. Accordingly, they are unbiased estimates only if the subset of values was selected randomly from the population. But, as was discussed earlier, random sampling is often difficult to achieve. An interpercentile interval may always be used, however, as a summary or description of the *subset* reference distribution.

The precision of a percentile as an estimate of a population value depends on the size of the subset and the scatter of results around the percentile; it is less precise when few observations are reported or when data points are more widely scattered. If the assumption of random sampling is fulfilled, the *confidence interval* of the percentile (i.e., the limits within which the true percentile is located with a specified degree of confidence) can be determined. The 90% confidence interval of the 2.5th percentile (lower reference limit) for serum GGT values may, for example, be 6 to 8 IU/L, whereas the 90% confidence interval of the 97.5th percentile could be 39 to 50 IU/L. The upper limit confidence interval is wider because of a skewed distribution leading to more scattered data points.

Methods Used to Determine Interpercentile Intervals

The interpercentile interval is typically determined based on one of two major method principles: parametric or nonparametric (Table 9.3).[10–16]

The *parametric method* has as its major advantage the need for fewer reference values to determine percentiles and their confidence intervals. It can be applied when the distribution can be described completely by a small number of population parameters. For example, in a Gaussian distribution, determination of the mean and SD allow for calculation of the 2.5th and 97.5th reference limits as the values located roughly two SDs below and above the mean. In fact, most of the parametric methods are based on the Gaussian distribution. If the reference distribution does not appear to be Gaussian, mathematical functions may be used to transform

TABLE 9.3	Notable Differences Between Analysis Methods	
	Nonparametric	**Parametric**
Sample size (minimum number of reference individuals per partition)	120	40
Reference value distribution	No requirements Any distribution is acceptable	Gaussian distribution required
Ease of analysis	Straightforward No expertise required	Can be complicated Proof that distribution is Gaussian required Transformation of data may be required
Endorsements	IFCC, CLSI	

CLSI, Clinical Laboratory Standards Institute; *IFCC,* International Federation of Clinical Chemistry and Laboratory Medicine.

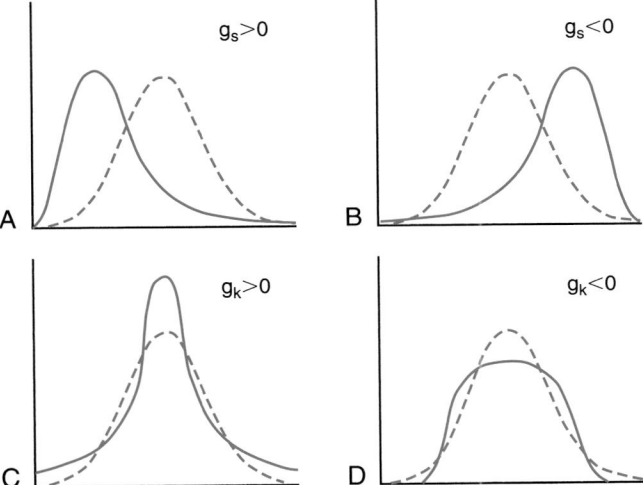

FIGURE 9.5 Skewness and kurtosis. The two *upper figures* show asymmetric distributions (**A**, positive skewness; **B**, negative skewness). The two *lower figures* show distributions with non-Gaussian peakedness (**C**, positive kurtosis; **D**, negative kurtosis). The Gaussian distribution *(dashed curve)* is shown in all graphs for comparison. The values of the coefficients of skewness *(g_s)* and kurtosis *(g_k)* are also shown.

data to a distribution that approximates a Gaussian shape. Some positively skewed distributions (Fig. 9.5A) may, for example, be made symmetric by using logarithmic, Box-Cox, or other transformations of the data values.

In contrast, the *nonparametric method* has as its major advantage that it makes no assumptions concerning the type of distribution and does not use estimates of distribution parameters. Percentiles are determined simply by eliminating the required percentage of values in each tail of the subset reference distribution (typically 2.5%).

The simple nonparametric method for determination of percentiles is recommended by IFCC[10–15] and CLSI.[16] The parametric method, which can be fairly complex, is seldom necessary, but it will be presented here because of its popularity and frequent misapplication.

Two other methods will be mentioned later in this chapter, but they are more complex and require the use of computer techniques (though these techniques are widely available in commercial software). It is worth emphasizing that, when results obtained using proper application of any of these methods are compared, it is usually found that estimates of the percentiles are very similar. Indeed if dissimilar results are obtained, investigation should be undertaken to consider possible causes. Detailed descriptions of nonparametric and parametric methods are given later in this chapter.

Sample Size

For the parametric method, the theoretical lower limit of the sample size required for estimation of the $100p$ and $100(1 - p)$ percentiles is equal to $1/p$. Thus estimation of the 2.5th percentile requires at least $1/0.025 = 40$ observations (per partition).

In contrast, for the nonparametric approach, a sample size of at least 120 reference values (per partition) has been recommended (the actual minimum is 119; however, this is commonly rounded up to 120); otherwise, one cannot determine confidence intervals for the reference limits.[10–16] It is important to note that 120 reference values allows for calculation of statistically valid 90% confidence limits; it does not necessarily provide the user with reference limits that would be considered clinically adequate. It is up to the scientists managing the study to determine whether the uncertainty of the estimates of the reference intervals meets the clinical need.

It should be noted that for any method (parametric or nonparametric), the precision of the percentile estimates improves as the number of observations increases. Additionally, different numbers of samples are required for different percentiles. For example, it requires 299 samples to determine the 90% confidence limit for the 99th percentile (vs. 120 for the 97.5th percentile). Also, the more highly skewed a distribution is, the larger is the number of reference values needed to obtain clinically reasonable confidence intervals at the tail end of the distribution.[64] The Nordic Reference Interval Project (NORIP)[65] provides a particularly good example of this phenomenon. The value for the 97.5th percentile for serum alanine aminotransferase (ALT) in males was 68, with 90% confidence limits of 63.4 to 73.6. Even though the study was based on 1080 subjects, the confidence interval represented more than 15% of the reference interval.

Partitioning of Reference Values

The best order of the first three actions outlined in Fig. 9.2 (1—partitioning of reference values, 2—inspection of the distribution, and 3—detection/handling of outliers) may in some cases be different from that shown in the figure. For example, it might be more appropriate to detect outliers before testing for partitioning. No strict rules for the order of these actions can be given because it depends on data and the statistical methods applied. In addition, it can be argued that inspection of the data is important at each of the processes in the figure. With these cautions in mind, the presentation in this chapter follows Fig. 9.2.

The subset of reference individuals and corresponding reference values may be partitioned according to sex, age, and other characteristics (see Table 9.2). The process of partitioning is also referred to as stratification, categorization, or subgrouping, and its results have been called partitions, strata, categories, classes, or subgroups. In this chapter, the terms *partitioning* (for the process) and *(sub)classes* (for its result) are used.

The aim of partitioning is to create more homogeneous subsets of data so as to provide a better basis for comparison of clinical laboratory results: *class-specific* reference intervals (e.g., age- and sex-specific reference intervals). An initial step is to graph the data against the relevant parameter. For example, plotting reference values against age will allow assessment as to whether partitioning is likely to be needed and, if so, which ages should be included in each class.

Various statistical criteria for partitioning have been suggested.[61,66] For example, an intuitive criterion states that partitioning is necessary if differences between classes are statistically significant (rejection of the "null" hypothesis of equal distributions). The distribution of reference values in the classes may show different locations (the mean values vary) or different intraclass variations (the SDs vary). These differences may be tested by statistical methods, which are not described here. The reader is referred to Chapter 2 and to standard textbooks of parametric[67,68] and nonparametric statistics.[69]

Differences in location or variation, however, may be statistically significant and still may be too small to justify replacing a single total reference interval with several class-specific intervals. In practice it is common to use a clinical assessment as to whether the proposed differences are likely to be important for patient care. For example, a difference within the analytical variation of the assay may be deemed sufficiently small to ignore. Alternatively, statistically nonsignificant differences can lead to situations in which the proportions of each subclass above the upper or below the lower reference limits (without partitioning) are much different from the desired 2.5% on each side. Harris and Boyd[61] therefore suggested criteria based on the ratio between subclass SDs, a normal deviate test of means, and calculation of critical decision values dependent on the sample size. Lahti and coworkers[66,70] suggested focusing directly on the proportions of each subgroup falling outside the combined population reference limits in order to determine whether partitioning is indicated. According to their approach, subgroup-specific reference limits are needed when more than 4.1% or less than 0.9% of any subgroup falls outside the combined reference limits. Advantages of their method are that it can be used with non-Gaussian and Gaussian distributions and that it takes into account differences in subgroup prevalences.

Partitioning requires large samples of reference values. If these are not used, subclass sizes may be too small for reliable estimates of reference intervals and there may be limited statistical power to identify true differences between classes.

To solve the subclass size problem, it has been suggested to estimate regression-based reference intervals. Instead of dividing, for example, the total material into several age classes, one may construct continuous age-dependent reference limits and their confidence regions. Simulation studies have shown that this method produces reliable estimates with smaller sample sizes.[71,72] When the intended purpose of the reference interval is to detect individual changes in biochemical status, subject-based reference values may be more appropriate than class-specific reference intervals for interpretation.[61,73,74]

In the following sections, a homogeneous reference distribution and either the complete distribution (if partitioning has been shown to be unnecessary) or a subclass distribution (after partitioning) are assumed.

Inspection of the Distribution

It is always advisable to display the reference distribution graphically and to inspect it. A *histogram,* as shown in Fig. 9.3, is easily prepared and is the type of data display best suited for visual inspection. Examination of the histogram serves as a safeguard against misapplication or misinterpretation of statistical methods, and it may reveal valuable information about the data. Data should be evaluated for the following characteristics of the distribution:

1. Highly deviating values *(outliers)* may represent erroneous values.
2. *Bimodal* or *polymodal* distributions have more than one peak and may indicate that the distribution is nonhomogeneous because of mixing of two or more distributions. If so, the criteria used to select reference individuals should be reevaluated, or partitioning of the values according to age, sex, or other relevant factors should be attempted.
3. The shape of the distribution should be noticed. It may be asymmetrical, or it may be more or less peaked than the symmetrical and bell-shaped Gaussian distribution (see Fig. 9.5). The asymmetry most frequently observed with clinical chemistry data is positive *skewness* (see Fig. 9.5A). A symmetric distribution with positive *kurtosis* has a high and slim peak and a greater number of values in both tails than the Gaussian type of distribution (see Fig. 9.5C). Conversely, negative kurtosis indicates that the distribution has a broad and flat top with relatively few observations in the tails (see Fig. 9.5D). Asymmetry and non-Gaussian peakedness may be combined.

The visual inspection may also provide initial estimates of the location of reference limits that are useful as checks on the validity of computations. Assessment of the shape of the distribution can lead to a number of actions. It can guide the choice of approach (i.e., parametric or nonparametric) or the necessity for transformation before using a parametric approach. As noted earlier, a skewed distribution may be a true reflection of the population, but it, or a secondary population, may also raise a question about possible causes: for example, the effect of a covariate (e.g., age affecting part of the population), an analytical problem (e.g., bias during one analytical run), or a preanalytical problem (e.g., samples from one site handled differently from other sites). Visual inspection can also be a valuable tool to assess for data quality and a possible need for partitioning. Viewing the data with age, sex, or time of collection/analysis on the *x*-axis may highlight important changes with these parameters.

Identification and Handling of Erroneous Values

An *erroneous value* may occur due to a gross deviation from the prescribed procedure for establishment of reference values.[45] Such values may deviate significantly from proper reference values *(outliers)* or may be hidden in the reference distribution. Only a strict experimental protocol, with adequate controls at each step, can eliminate the latter type of erroneous values.

An outlier has been defined as "the observation in a sample, so far separated in value from the remainder as to suggest that it may be from a different population, or the result of an error in measurement."[75] This definition has some particular utility because it focuses on the possible nature of the expected distribution as outlined in the subsequent text.

As stated previously, *visual inspection* of a histogram is useful in screening for identification of possible outliers. It is important to keep in mind, however, that values far out in the long tail of a skewed distribution may easily be misinterpreted as outliers. If the distribution is positively skewed, inspection of a histogram after logarithmic or some other transformation of the values may aid in the visual identification of outliers. In the end, though, statistical tests must be used to make a final determination.

Some outliers may be identified by statistical tests independent of visual inspection, but no single method is capable of detecting outliers in every situation that may occur. The number of techniques suggested or recommended is, for this reason, very large.[61,76,77] The two main problems encountered can be described as follows:

1. Many tests assume that the type of the true distribution is known before the test is used. Some of these specifically require that the distribution be Gaussian. However, biological distributions often are non-Gaussian, and their types are seldom known in advance. Furthermore, statistical tests of types of distribution are unreliable in the presence of outliers. This unreliability poses a difficult dilemma; some tests for outliers assume that the type of distribution is known, but tests for determining the type of distribution require that outliers be absent! As a consequence, it may be difficult to transform the distribution to Gaussian form before outliers are identified by statistical tests. Some tests are relatively insensitive to departures from a Gaussian distribution. This is the case with Dixon's *range test*, in which a value is identified as an extreme outlier if the difference between the two highest (or lowest) values in the distribution exceeds one third of the range of all values (see Fig. 9.3).[10–15,61,78]
2. Several tests for outliers assume that a data set contains only a single outlier. The limitation of these tests is obvious. Some tests may detect a specified number of outliers, or they may be run several times, discarding one outlier in each pass of data. The range test, however, usually fails in the presence of several outliers. It is possible to estimate the SD using data remaining after *trimming* of both tails of the distribution by a specified percentage of observations.[61,79] Outliers could be identified by this method as the values lying 3 or 4 SDs from the arithmetic mean. This method assumes, however, that the true distribution is Gaussian.

Horn and coworkers[80] published a novel method in two stages for outlier detection that seems to provide a promising solution to both of the problems just mentioned. With this method, one executes the following:

1. Mathematically transform the data to approximate a Gaussian distribution. Horn used the Box-Cox transformation,[81] but other transformations that correct for skewness (see later) probably would also work. As mentioned earlier, it is impossible to achieve exact symmetry by transformation in the presence of outliers, but this does not seem to be critical with Horn's method.
2. Identify (or eliminate) outliers using a criterion based on the central 50% of the distribution, thus reducing the

masking effect of several outliers. Compute the interquartile range (IQR) between the lower and upper quartiles of the distribution (Q_1 and Q_3, respectively): $IQR = Q_3 - Q_1$. Then identify as outliers data lying outside the two fences

$$Q_1 - 1.5 \times IQR \text{ and } Q_3 + 1.5 \times IQR$$

Deviating values identified as possible outliers cannot always be discarded automatically. Values should be included or excluded on a rational basis. For example, records of the dubious values should be checked and errors corrected. In some cases, deviating values should be rejected because noncorrectable causes have been found, such as in previously unrecognized conditions that qualify individuals for exclusion from the group of reference individuals or analytical errors.

Methods for Determining Reference Limits—Suitable for Direct Sampling

More details regarding four different approaches to determining reference limits are discussed in this section. In addition to the nonparametric and parametric methods described in general terms earlier, overviews of the bootstrap and robust methods are provided. In all four cases, it is important to remember that, at this stage, a homogeneous reference distribution, with outliers removed, is assumed.

Nonparametric Method

The nonparametric method is notable for at least three reasons: it is simple to perform, it does not require that the distribution is Gaussian, and it is recommended by both IFCC[10–15] and CLSI.[16] On the other hand, for estimates of the central 95 percentiles, it does require a minimum of 120 values (per partition). It consists essentially of eliminating a specified percentage of the values from each tail of the reference distribution. Very simple and reliable methods are based on *rank numbers*.[10–15,78,82] These methods also allow nonparametric estimation of the confidence intervals of the percentiles[78] and can easily be applied manually or with a spreadsheet program.

The rank-based method as recommended by the IFCC[10–15] and CLSI[16] requires the following steps:
1. First, the *n* reference values are sorted in ascending order of magnitude.
2. Next, the individual values are ranked. For example, the minimum value has rank number 1, the next value has rank number 2, and so on, until the maximum value, which has rank number *n*. Consecutive rank numbers should be given to two or more values that are equal ("ties").
3. The rank numbers of the $100p$ and $100(1 - p)$ percentiles are computed as $p(n + 1)$ and $(1 - p)(n + 1)$, respectively. Thus the limits of the conventional 95% reference interval have rank numbers equal to $0.025(n + 1)$ and $0.975(n + 1)$; in a data set of 120, these are the 3rd and 118th ranked results.
4. The percentiles are determined by finding the original reference values that correspond to the computed rank numbers, provided that the rank numbers are integers. Otherwise, one should interpolate between the two limiting values. Note that the final values selected should have the same number of significant figures as will be used to report clinical results.
5. Finally, the confidence interval of each percentile is determined by using the binomial distribution.[78] Table 9.4

TABLE 9.4 Nonparametric Confidence Intervals of Reference Limits

	RANK NUMBERS		
Sample Size	Lower 0.90 CI Limit	2.5th Percentile	Upper 0.90 CI Limit
119–132	1	4	7
133–160	1	4	8
161–187	1	5	9
188–189	2	5	9
190–200	2	5	10
201–219	2	6	10
219–240	2	7	10
240–248	2	7	11
249–249	2	7	12
250–279	3	7	12
280–307	3	8	13
308–309	4	8	13
310–320	4	8	14
321–340	4	9	14
341–360	4	9	15
361–363	4	10	15
364–372	5	10	15
373–400	5	9	16
401–403	5	11	16
404–417	5	11	17
418–435	6	11	17
436–440	6	11	18
441–468	6	12	18
469–470	6	12	19
471–481	6	13	19
471–500	7	13	19

The table shows the rank numbers of the 2.5th percentile together with the lower and upper limits of the 0.90 confidence interval for samples with 119 to 500 values. To obtain the corresponding rank numbers of the 97.5th percentile, subtract the rank numbers in the table from ($n + 1$), where n is the sample size. Note that the 2.5th percentile values are the nearest number from the data set and may differ from results derived from statistical software packages that commonly derive the percentile values by interpolation between results from the data set when the rank value does not correspond to the exact percentile.
CI, Confidence interval.

provides data for the 0.90 confidence interval of the 2.5th and 97.5th percentiles. For the relevant sample size *n*, rank numbers for the lower and upper limits should be found for the 2.5th percentile; those same values are subtracted from ($n + 1$) to find the rank numbers for the 97.5th percentile. Several software packages are available to determine the percentiles and their uncertainties.[83–85]

Table 9.5 provides a detailed example of the nonparametric determination of 95% reference limits using the serum GGT reference values first shown in Fig. 9.3.

It is claimed that the nonparametric process is less affected by outliers than parametric methods, a statement that has some truth. For example, a single extreme outlier in a set of 120 results will affect the calculated mean and SD, but it will not affect the 2.5th and 97.5th percentiles. It will, however, affect the 90% confidence interval of the nonparametric method, as the extreme result is the boundary of the confidence

TABLE 9.5 Nonparametric Determination of Reference Interval

				GGT Value	Frequency	Rank Order
Calculation of Rank Numbers of Percentiles				6	1	1
Lower:		0.025 (123 + 1) = 3.1 (i.e., Rank #3)		7	2	2, 3
Upper:		0.975 (123 + 1) = 120.9 (i.e., Rank #121)		8	6	4–9
				9	4	10–13
				10	4	14–17
				11	9	18–26
				12	7	27–33
Original Values Corresponding to These Rank Numbers				13	7	34–40
Lower limit (2.5th percentile):		7 IU/L		14	9	41–49
Upper limit (97.5th percentile):		47 IU/L		15	9	50–58
				16	8	59–66
				17	11	67–77
				18	8	78–85
				19	5	86–90
Rank Numbers and Values of the 0.90-Confidence Limits				20	3	91–93
Lower Reference Limits				21	2	94, 95
Rank numbers (see Table 8.4):		#1 and #7		22	2	96, 97
Values:		6 and 8 IU/L		23	2	98, 99
Upper Reference Limits				24	2	100, 101
Rank numbers (see Table 8.4):		(123 + 1) − 7 = #117 and (123 + 1) − 1 = #123		25	3	101–104
Values:		39 and 50 IU/L		26	2	105, 106
				27	1	107
				28	1	108
				29	2	109, 110
				30	1	111
				32	2	112, 113
				34	2	114, 115
				35	1	116
				39	1	117
Summary				42	2	118, 119
Lower reference limit:		7 (6 to 8) IU/L		45	1	120
Upper reference limit:		47 (39 to 50) IU/L		47	1	121
				48	1	122
				50	1	123

This table shows an example using the 123 serum gamma-glutamyltransferase (GGT) values displayed in Fig. 9.4A. See text for a description of the nonparametric method.

limit with these numbers. It can be easily seen, however, that a larger number of outliers will influence the percentile limits as well.

It should be emphasized that Table 9.4 is specific for the 2.5th and 97.5th percentiles and 90% confidence limits. It can be seen from the table that 0.90 CI are not available for fewer than 119 samples. For this reason, when fewer than 120 samples are included in reference interval studies provided by manufacturers, a narrower reference interval is sometimes provided [e.g., the central 90% (5th through 95th percentiles)]. As noted previously, a larger number of samples is required to generate 0.90 CI for wider reference intervals (e.g., the central 98%, or 1st through 99th percentiles); a smaller number is required for narrower reference limits (e.g., the central 90%, or 5th through 95th percentiles).

Parametric Method

Although it can be more complicated, usually involving statistical software, the parametric method is advantageous (in comparison to the nonparametric method) in requiring fewer reference values to determine reference limits. The method is presented here under separate headings for testing the type of distribution, for transforming the data, and for estimating percentiles and their confidence intervals.

It should be noted that commonly used statistical computer program packages aid in the estimation of reference limits, but these packages may lack some of the techniques described in this chapter. Several programs have been designed with clinical laboratories in mind and have specific functions to perform many of these processes, including CB-stat,[83] MedCalc,[84] and Analyse-it.[85] The availability of these and other specialized programs will change over time, but it can be most useful to select a program that meets the needs of the laboratory, gain skills in its correct use, and maintain use of the same program over time. Basic statistical analysis can also be performed in common spreadsheet programs (e.g., Microsoft Excel), but the more sophisticated features like confidence limits may require writing special functions into the spreadsheet.

Testing fit to Gaussian distribution. The parametric method for estimating percentiles assumes that the true distribution is Gaussian. This fact was frequently ignored in the past and caused Elveback[5] to warn against "the ghost of Gauss." This assumption may result in seriously biased estimates of reference limits.[86] Simple signs that a distribution is highly unlikely to be Gaussian are skewed distribution on visual inspection of the distribution, a mean and median that are markedly different, and S_x above approximately 30% of the mean value. In any of these cases, formal assessment for Gaussian distribution is unnecessary. After elimination of the outlier from the GGT reference values in Fig. 9.3, the mean and SD of the remaining 123 serum GGT reference values are 18.1 and 9.1 (see Fig. 9.4A), from which the reference interval is calculated as $\bar{x} \pm 1.96 \times S_x$, or 0 to 36 IU/L (vs. the nonparametric values of 7 and 47 IU/L; Table 9.6). More highly positively skewed distributions may even result in negative values for the lower reference limit.

TABLE 9.6 Summary of Gamma-Glutamyltransferase Reference Interval Determination by Three Methods

Method	Midpoint	Lower Limit (CI)	Upper Limit (CI)	Values Below Lower Limit	Values Above Upper Limit
Nonparametric	16	7 (6 to 8)	47 (39–50)	1	2
Parametric—untransformed data	18	0 (−2 to 2)	36 (34–38)	0	7
Parametric—transformed data	16	7 (6 to 8)	40 (35–44)	1	6

The table summarizes the midpoint, central 95% and associated 90% confidence limits of the reference intervals generated by each of three methods for the same data set. The numbers of observed values deemed lower and higher than the corresponding interval for each method are given in the last two columns. Because the original data are positively skewed, note that the parametric techniques generate intervals that are biased low. Note, also that the parametric technique on untransformed data has a lower confidence interval, which is actually less than 0. *CI*, Confidence interval.

Therefore a critical phase in the parametric method is testing the goodness-of-fit of the reference distribution to a hypothetical Gaussian distribution. If the Gaussian hypothesis must be rejected at a specified significance level, one is left with two alternatives (see Fig. 9.2): either the nonparametric method can be used, or a mathematical transformation of data can be applied to approximate the Gaussian distribution. Only when the Gaussian hypothesis is not rejected by the test can one pass directly to parametric estimation of percentiles and their confidence intervals (see Fig. 9.2).

Formal goodness-of-fit tests have been reviewed by Mardia.[87] These tests can be broadly classified as (1) graphical procedures, (2) coefficient-based tests, and (3) tests that are based on shape differences between observed and theoretical distributions.

1. *The graphical procedure* consists of plotting the cumulative distribution on probability paper, which has a nonlinear vertical axis based on the Gaussian distribution (see Fig. 9.4B and D). The plot should be close to a straight line if the distribution is Gaussian.
2. *Coefficient-based tests* use statistical measures of skewness and kurtosis (see Fig. 9.5). Formulas for calculating these parameters are available elsewhere,[10–15] or they may be produced by statistical or reference interval software.[83–85] For Gaussian (and other symmetric distributions), the *coefficient of skewness* is zero; the sign of a nonzero coefficient indicates the type of skewness present in the data (see Fig. 9.5A and B). The *coefficient of kurtosis* is approximately zero for the Gaussian distribution. The sign of a nonzero coefficient indicates the type of kurtosis present in the data (see Fig. 9.5C and D). The statistical significance of these two coefficients may be found by referring to tables for testing skewness and kurtosis.[68]
3. Tests of *shape differences* that have been used to evaluate goodness-of-fit include the (1) Kolmogorov-Smirnov, (2) Cramer-von Mises, and (3) Anderson-Darling tests.[10–15,88] The Anderson-Darling test is recommended by the IFCC.[10–15]

Transformation of data. In the previous section, it was shown that $\bar{x} \pm 1.96 \times S_x$ of the serum GGT data in Fig. 9.4A resulted in biased reference limits (too low values), as was to be expected with this positively skewed distribution. However, it is often possible to transform data mathematically to obtain a distribution of transformed values that approximates a Gaussian distribution. With these new values, the 2.5th and 97.5th percentiles are again localized at 1.96 SDs on both sides of the mean. The estimates may then be transformed back to the original measurement scale by using the inverse mathematical function.

It is frequently observed that *logarithmically transformed* values, $y = log(x)$, of a positively skewed distribution fit the Gaussian distribution rather closely. In other cases, *square roots* of the values, $y = \sqrt{x}$, result in a better approximation to the Gaussian distribution. In theory, any mathematical transformation of the data can be used. From a practical perspective, the family of Box-Cox transformations provides solutions in the vast majority of situations where the transformation parameter (λ) can be selected to transform right-skewed distributions which may be more or less skewed than a logarithmic distribution.[86]

The following example uses the logarithmic transformation for convenience, but any other transformation can be used in the same way. The procedure is as follows:

1. Test the fit of the distribution of original data to the Gaussian distribution. If the distribution has approximately a Gaussian shape, the 2.5th and 97.5th percentiles are calculated directly as $\bar{x} \pm 1.96 \times S_x$. Otherwise, continue with the following steps.
2. Transform data by the logarithmic function $y = log(x)$ (or by another selected function), then test the fit to the Gaussian distribution. If the transformed distribution is significantly different from Gaussian shape, try another transformation or estimate the percentiles by the nonparametric method (see earlier in this chapter). Continue with the next step if the transformation resulted in a Gaussian distribution.
3. Compute the mean $\bar{y}$ and the SD s_y of transformed data. Then estimate the 2.5th and 97.5th percentiles in the transformed data scale as $\bar{y} \pm 1.96 \times S_y$.
4. The final step is reconversion of these percentiles to the original data scale. The inverse function for the logarithmic transformation $y = log\,x$ is $x = 10^y$.
5. It is now possible to use the properties of the Gaussian distribution to estimate the reference limits and their confidence intervals. This method is presented in a later section.

Example: As noted earlier, the original GGT data reference distribution is not Gaussian but is, as with many biological distributions, skewed to the right (see Fig. 9.4A). However, by using the logarithm of the serum GGT values, a distribution very close to Gaussian shape (see Fig. 9.4C) is obtained. This observation is confirmed in Fig. 9.4B and D where the cumulative probabilities are shown graphed on Gaussian probability paper; the original data are not linear, but the transformed data form a reasonably good line.

Parametric estimates of percentiles and their confidence intervals. Once the distribution of reference data (original or transformed) is shown to be Gaussian, calculations of the $100p$ and $100(1 - p)$ percentiles and their 0.90 confidence intervals are straightforward:

As noted earlier, the $100p$ and $100(1 - p)$ *percentiles* are calculated as follows:

$$\text{mean} \pm c \times (\text{standard deviation})$$

where c is the $(1 - p)$ standard Gaussian deviate, as can be found in statistical tables. For the 2.5th and 97.5th percentiles, the $(1 - 0.025) = 0.975$ standard Gaussian deviate, c, has a value of 1.960.

The 0.9-*confidence intervals* of these percentiles are then determined as follows[7,10–15]:

$$\text{percentile} = \pm 2.81 \frac{s_y}{\sqrt{n}}$$

where s_y is the SD of the reference values (original or transformed) and n is the number of values.[b]

Example: The mean and SD of the transformed data in Fig. 9.4 are $\bar{y} = 1.212$ and $s_y = 0.193$, respectively; that is, the mean value is 1.212 (corresponding to $10^{1.212}$, or 16 in the original scale). The transformed 2.5th percentile is then $1.212 - (1.960 \times 0.193) = 0.835$. On reconversion to the original data scale, a value of $10^{0.835} = 6.84$ is obtained. The lower reference limit of serum GGT is thus 7 IU/L. Similarly, it is found that the upper reference limit is 39 IU/L. These values are in closer agreement with those found by the nonparametric method: 7 and 47 IU/L (see Tables 9.5 and 9.6).

The 0.90 confidence limits of the lower percentile are then

$$0.835 - 2.81* \left(0.193/\sqrt{123}\right) = 0.786 \quad 10^{0.786} = 6.1$$

$$0.835 + 2.81* \left(0.193/\sqrt{123}\right) = 0.884 \quad 10^{0.884} = 7.7$$

Thus the complete estimate of the 2.5th percentile (and its 0.90 confidence interval) is 7 (6 to 8) IU/L. The 97.5th percentile is, by the same method, found to be 39 (35 to 43) IU/L.

Table 9.6 summarizes data from the three methods used to determine reference intervals from GGT data. It can be seen that the application of parametric statistics to transformed data yields similar reference limits to those obtained by nonparametric methods. While nonparametric methods have the advantage of simpler mathematical processes and determining reference limits without assumptions on the underlying distribution, there can be some advantages to using parametric methods. If an underlying distribution can be defined, it can assist in assessing the likelihood of a result being a member of the reference population based on the parameters defining the population.

Other Methods

As a brief introduction to the bootstrap and robust methods for determining reference limits, it is worth noting that they share two characteristics. First, neither of these methods makes assumptions about the underlying distribution; it need not be Gaussian. Second, both require the use of computer software because they involve numerous iterations and somewhat complicated calculations. These methods are appropriate for use in direct reference interval studies or indirect studies provided the likelihood of nonhealthy subjects can be made sufficiently small.

Bootstrap method. There are a number of variations on the "bootstrap" method, all of which can be used to generate reliable reference limits.[61,82,89] In principle, the technique is simple, but it involves many iterations (100 to 1000) and thus requires computers. As is the case with the nonparametric method, there is no requirement that the distribution be Gaussian. For reliable estimates of confidence intervals for the reference limits, it is recommended that there be a minimum of 100 reference values (per partition).[82] The following steps are involved in a typical bootstrap procedure:

1. First, random samples, each of size *m,* are selected, with replacement, from the original set of *n* reference values. One selects "with replacement" if each value randomly selected from the original set remains available, so that it may be selected again in the random selection of the next value. In other words, even if there is only one occurrence of a specific value in the original set of *n* values, it may appear more than once in one, or more, random samples of size *m.* The number of resamples should be high (500 is a reasonable number of iterations).
2. For each resample, the upper and lower reference limits (percentiles) are next estimated by the rank-based nonparametric procedure described previously. These estimates from each iteration are saved.
3. Upon completion of all iterations, the final lower reference limit is calculated as the mean of the estimates of the lower reference limit; similarly, the final upper reference limit is calculated as the mean of the estimates of the upper reference limit.
4. Finally, the 0.90 confidence interval of each reference limit is calculated from the distribution of the percentile estimates, that is, with 500 iterations, the confidence interval for the 2.5th percentile (the mean of ranks 13) would be the means of ranks 7 and of ranks 19.

The reader should note that the bootstrap version described here uses rank-based nonparametric percentile estimates. However, the bootstrap principle may be employed with any kind of estimation, parametric or nonparametric.

Robust method. The robust method has the form of the parametric method described earlier, but instead of using the mean and the SD of the sample, it uses robust measures of location and spread. For example, instead of using the mean, it uses the median: in a series of 10 values, if the highest value is doubled, the mean changes appreciably, but the median does not change at all. The process involves weighting the data to place more value on results near the middle of the distribution and less weight on more distant results. The rationale is that the scattered data are more likely to reflect results that are not members of the desired distribution. This resistance to the effect of outliers is the basis for the term *Robust Method.* This method has particular value with small sample sizes.

[b]This formula is a special case of a general formula that can be used for confidence intervals of other sizes or for other percentiles derived from Gaussian distributions. CI for percentiles are calculated as follows: mean $\pm z_1 \times s_y \pm z_2 \times [s_y^2/n + (z_1^2 \times s_y^2)/(2 \times n)]^{0.5}$ where mean is the population mean, s_y is the population SD, n is the sample size, z_1 is the probit value related to the selected percentile ($=1.96$ for 97.5th percentile), and z_2 is the covering factor for the CI ($=1.64$ for 90%). (http://www.statsdirect.com/help/Default.htm#parametric_methods/reference_range.htm.)

Briefly, the steps involved are as follows:

1. Symmetry of the data is ensured, using transformations if necessary (e.g., Box-Cox transformation[81]).
2. Initial robust measures of location (median) and spread (median absolute deviation) are found.
3. Using a *biweight estimation* technique, in which more weight is given to observations closer to the center and progressively less to values farther from the center, new estimates of location and spread are found until successive results are satisfactorily close.
4. With final robust values of location and spread, the upper and lower limits are calculated, in a manner analogous to that described for the parametric technique.
5. Confidence intervals are then estimated using the bootstrapping technique described in the previous section.

Similar to the bootstrap method, this method does not require a Gaussian distribution. It is resistant to outliers and may be applied to very small numbers of observations. Details on the method are available.[90]

Methods for Determining Reference Limits—Suitable for Indirect Sampling

The methods above are recommended for direct reference interval studies, but they are not suitable for indirect studies when appreciable numbers of results from diseased subjects is likely. To address this issue, a number of statistical approaches have been developed to minimize the effect of the presence of results not representing the reference population.[37]

Graphical-Based Methods

In the precomputer era, a number of alternate methods for computing reference intervals were developed based on analysis of graphical display of reference values. The best known of these are the Hoffmann[35] and Bhattacharya[36] methods. Many reference interval studies have been performed using these tools. Both methods can be performed using basic computer spreadsheets or with third-party software. The methods are based on finding a Gaussian distribution in the midst of other data. With care and the right data set, both methods can provide useful results. Each method has some user-defined steps which can affect the accuracy, and therefore care and understanding of the processes is required to ensure accurate results are produced. The methods are more robust with larger numbers of values; while no minimum has been determined, inclusion of several thousand results is likely to lead to more accurate reference intervals. Approaches to minimize risk of such errors include the use of more than one statistical method to estimate the reference limits and, as mentioned previously, the visual inspection of the original data with the derived reference intervals. For both the Hoffmann and Bhattacharya techniques, a key factor is the use of transformations such as logarithms or one of the Box-Cox family. For analytes with a narrow, symmetrical between-person variation (e.g., serum sodium, calcium, albumin, and other analytes with a group coefficient of variation (CV_G) less than about 15%) a good Gaussian fit is often possible on untransformed data. For analytes with a wider, skewed distribution, transformation is required. One approach may be to use a transformation (e.g., a value for lambda in a Box-Cox distribution) which has been shown to describe a healthy distribution from a direct study.[50] Applying a transformation to give the best fit on the data may "normalize" pathology by bringing it into the central data peak. An example may be liver transaminases under the effect of fatty liver, where the "best fit" transformation may wrongly include subjects with this condition being included within the reference limits.[50] An important limitation of these methods is the lack of a confidence interval for the reference limits.

Hoffmann Method. The Hoffmann technique was developed in 1963 and is based on a display of the data as a cumulative distribution using normal probability paper (or electronic equivalent) and identifying the linear section which indicates a Gaussian distribution.[35] The assumption of this technique is that the majority of the data in the central region has a Gaussian distribution, and one of its key advantages is that distant outliers have no effect on the outcome. Key risks with the use of this procedure are closely overlapping distributions which may not be separated or the presence of a secondary population of significant size.[91] The decisions that must be made are whether any transformation of the original data is indicated and how much of the final data set to include as reflecting a Gaussian distribution. A revised version described as "computerized Hoffmann method" has been developed[92,93] although this does not use the normal probability data analysis and should be considered a separate method[94] with less satisfactory performance.[95]

Bhattacharya Method. The Bhattacharya method, like Hoffmann, is also a graphical method for identifying a Gaussian distribution in the midst of other data.[36] The procedure is able to separate overlapping distributions after graphical display.[36,91] Computer-based versions have been developed in Microsoft Excel and R programming language. The Bhattacharya method has been shown to be less influenced by data not included in the Gaussian distribution than is Hoffmann.[91] This method has been subject to review[34,96,97] and has been used in a number of published papers.[98,99] The variables that must be selected are the bin size and bin location to use in analyzing the data and, as with the Hoffmann technique, whether any transformation of the original data is indicated and how much of the final data set to include as reflecting a Gaussian distribution. An additional factor after transformation is variation in bin sizes of the data which can produce results which are difficult to model. The use of extra significant figures in the raw data can minimize this effect.

Special Computerized Approaches

The key limitations to the graphical methods above are the quality of the separation of a deemed healthy subpopulation from other subpopulations that may be affected by disease, and the handling of data transformation. Computer-based solutions that address both of these issues have been developed.

DGKL Reference Limit Estimator. Developed by the German scientific society for Clinical Chemistry and Laboratory Medicine (DGKL) working group on reference intervals, a description and software is available on the DGKL website.[100] In this process a Gaussian distribution is automatically fitted to the majority of the data with an optimal transformation, and this fit is used to define the reference limits with the distribution of pathologic results also determined.[38] Additionally the software calculates possible clinical decision limits as the intersection point of the nonpathologic and pathologic density curves (bimodal reference limit with the highest diagnostic efficiency) and checks for possible analytical trend during the time of data collection and considers automatic stratification according to sex and age.

Mixed Likelihood Techniques An alternate method is based on mixed likelihood techniques used in other fields.[95,101] This method separates likely healthy and diseased subpopulations, each of which may have Gaussian or skewed distributions and may overlap to varying degrees. There are a number of statistical tools available for this approach and superiority over Hoffmann and Bhattacharya has been claimed.[95]

TRANSFERABILITY OF REFERENCE LIMITS FROM OTHER SOURCES

Determination of reliable reference values for each test in the laboratory's repertoire is a major task that is often far beyond the capabilities of the individual laboratory. This is especially important when ethical or practical considerations limit the number of available individuals (e.g., when establishing pediatric or cerebrospinal fluid [CSF] reference values). However, even in the absence of such considerations, most of the methods discussed in the previous sections require qualification of, and analysis of samples from, relatively large numbers of reference individuals.

Two issues are critical in considering adopting reference intervals derived from the other sources discussed in the following sections. First, the populations under consideration must be comparable (i.e., no major ethnic, social, or environmental differences should be noted between them that may be relevant to the analyte in question). If they are not, a separate reference interval study may well need to be done. Second, even if the populations are comparable, the analytical methods under consideration must be comparable. The optimal, but often unrealistic, situation assumes that analytical methods, including their calibration and quality assurance, are identical in the laboratories. The provision of methods from different manufacturers that are all traceable to equivalent higher-order reference materials and methods, such as are listed on the JCTLM database, facilitates the sharing of reference intervals.[102] In the absence of verified traceable methods, a pragmatic approach involves (1) standardization of analytical protocols, (2) common calibration, (3) design of a sufficiently efficient external quality control scheme, and (4) the use of mathematical transfer functions if results still are not directly comparable.[103] The parameters of transfer functions may be estimated from results obtained by analysis of a sufficient number of patient specimens spanning the relevant range of concentrations in all participating laboratories.[16] Provided both assays are linear, functions of the form $y = \alpha \times x + \beta$ are generally appropriate, where the constant term β compensates for systematic shifts among methods, whereas the coefficient term α adjusts for proportional differences. Care should be taken to ensure that errors do not occur due to the use of inappropriate statistical techniques. For example, simple linear regression can be affected by outlier values, variation in data dispersion at different analyte concentrations (heteroscedasticity), and a limited range of analyte concentrations. The use of Passing and Bablok[104] (or

weighted linear regression) provides a more robust estimate of the linear function (see Chapter 2). It should be noted that the mentioned transfer functions account only for analytical bias; however, adjustments for differences in imprecision may also be designed.

Other Sources for Reference Limits

The reference limits used by clinical laboratories are often those provided by the manufacturers of diagnostic equipment. At the outset, it is important to note that, in some cases, manufacturers do not actually perform reference limit studies with their methods but instead cite other literature as the source for their reference limits (including earlier versions of this textbook). As stated earlier, some manufacturers' limits are central 90% rather than the usual central 95%. If, however, the manufacturer has indeed performed a good reference limit study using its method, and the laboratory uses the method exactly as prescribed by the manufacturer, it is reasonable to infer that the issue of method comparability has been addressed. Even after method comparability has been assured, though, it remains to be shown that the package insert data addresses the population comparability. Because supporting information is commonly not supplied in the manufacturers' Instructions for Use, it may be necessary to contact the manufacturer. The information required should include the age and sex distribution of the reference population, exclusion criteria, confidence intervals of the reference limits, and the statistical processes used. If relevant, additional information (e.g., ethnicity; lifestyle factors; body composition data, such as BMI or waist circumference) may be helpful. For example, the creatine kinase (CK) upper reference limits cited in a package insert based on a Caucasian population underestimated, by several-fold, the upper reference limits for blacks and Asians.[105]

A second source for reference limits is peer-reviewed publications. In this case, both method comparability and population comparability are at issue. Laboratories seeking to adopt these limits must proceed carefully, but it may well be considerably easier to address these issues than it would be to repeat the studies themselves. To return to the CK example just cited,[105] laboratories using the same method that was used in that publication, or other methods with demonstrated traceability to the same reference method (which is stated in the paper), could presumably adopt the reference limits determined in the study, whereas laboratories using other methods without this traceability would be aware of a potential problem but could not simply adopt those same reference limits for those ethnic groups. Another excellent example is the CALIPER initiative,[53] which established, using the methods described earlier, pediatric reference intervals, partitioned by age, sex, and ethnicity, for 40 different assays. As the authors emphasized, the published reference limits were specific to the methods they used. (In later publications[106] the authors provide reference limits for additional analytical methods based on transference studies alluded to in the previous section.) A third example, involving adult reference intervals, was structured along the same lines as the original CALIPER studies.[107]

A recent enhancement of this technique is reflected in the HAPPI Kids study in Australia, where a single set of collected specimens was analyzed by multiple methods to generate reference intervals, thereby allowing adoption in a larger number of laboratories sooner.[108]

A third source for reference limits is multicenter trials. In contrast to the CALIPER initiative, in which all the analyses were done in a single laboratory, these studies seek to pool data from many laboratories spread over large regions and potentially among different countries. Although this decreases the number of reference individuals needed to be recruited from each laboratory, it also typically increases the number of analytical methods involved for each assay. Despite global efforts at harmonization and standardization, these multicenter trials have repeatedly shown that current methods do not always produce interchangeable results, and therefore methods to ensure method comparability are still needed. Nonetheless, once these issues have been addressed, multicenter trials are proving to be an excellent way to generate data for establishing reference limits.[65,109]

Another potential source of data to generate reference limits is a laboratory's own historical data. A laboratory's database is attractive on several counts: it encompasses the laboratory's own populations; it is generated with the laboratory's own methods and own preanalytical conditions; and it may include large quantities of data. The major limitation associated with this data is that it almost certainly includes data from unhealthy subjects and healthy subjects. However, as described previously, careful application of any of several indirect techniques has been used with data of this type to generate reliable reference limits.[98,110]

In summary, there are multiple different sources of information on reference intervals, including local formal reference interval studies, manufacturers' data, peer-reviewed publications, data mining techniques, and textbooks, including a compilation of reference interval data in various chapters and at the end of this textbook. Such information can be used as yet another source of data, with the same caveats noted at the beginning of this section and in the following section on verification. As is the case with any scientific process, it is good practice, when setting reference intervals, to access all available sources of information. This process allows for identification of discordant data sources and unexpected causes of variation, as well as for confirmation when different data sources provide the same information.

POINTS TO REMEMBER

Sources for Reference Limits (Other Than Establishing One's Own)

- Manufacturers' package inserts[c]
- Peer-reviewed literature[c]
- Multicenter trials[c]
- Analysis of laboratory's own historical data ("data mining")[a]

[a]Verification of the transferability of these values is *required*.

Verification of Transferability

Whether a laboratory adopts reference values from (1) a manufacturer's package insert, (2) a peer-reviewed publication or textbooks, (3) a multicenter trial, or (4) a data mining exercise, it is important that the laboratory verifies the appropriateness of those values for its own use.[61] This verification is the final check that the laboratory has implemented the analytical method correctly, and that the laboratory's own population is comparable with that used for the original reference value study.

Comparison of a locally produced, small subset of values with the large set produced elsewhere using traditional statistical tests often is not appropriate because the underlying statistical assumptions are not fulfilled and the sample sizes are unbalanced. Relatively sophisticated methods using nonparametric tests[111] or Monte Carlo sampling[100,112] have been described. In addition to providing its own recommendations for relatively sophisticated tests for verification, CLSI suggests a reasonably practical alternative that most laboratories should be able to adopt: with a sample size of 20 reference values, one verifies the appropriateness of a proposed reference interval so long as no more than two values are outside the proposed limits.[16] One obvious deficiency of this test is that it does not detect the situation in which the reference interval of the local group is narrower than that of the study group. Nonetheless, it does provide reasonable assurance that a proposed reference interval can be used. The use of a larger number of local samples can give greater assurance that the intervals are satisfactory and more chance to detect inappropriate intervals. If the data exists, local data mining techniques can also be used to verify, or at least assess, transferred reference intervals.[113] For example, the median or mode of an outpatient population should be close to the central point of the transferred reference interval, and the effect of the transferred interval on flagging rates, high and low, can be assessed.

PROCESS OF SELECTING REFERENCE INTERVALS

Laboratories are responsible for, and usually take the lead in, providing reference limits for their test results. However, as indicated in the previous sections of this chapter, there are a large number of potentially complicated decisions involved in the process, and the final selection of reference limits will influence the decisions of many physicians about their patients. As a result, it is important for organizations to include individuals from outside the laboratory in the process of selecting reference limits for use. A multidisciplinary group should be involved in making decisions, such as whether to perform a reference interval study or to transfer intervals from another source; if the decision is made to do a local study, whether partitioning will be necessary (which will affect the number of subjects), and which preanalytical variables are relevant; and if limits will be transferred from another source, whether the methods and populations from that source are comparable. Some issues are more subjective: whether to set exclusion criteria in an effort to change sensitivity (e.g., exclude individuals who are obese or drink alcohol in order to increase sensitivity to detect the effects of these conditions); whether statistically significant differences in partitions are clinically significant; consideration of "rounding" the reference limits for ease of memory and to avoid an unwarranted impression of precision (e.g., whether the GGT upper limit calculated earlier could be rounded from 47 to 50 IU/L). As suggested earlier, even if a local reference limit study is performed, it is appropriate to review all available data from the literature and from local data mining. When all data sources are concordant, there can be greater confidence in the limits. In contrast, when there is variability among the sources, it serves as a flag to assess possible reasons for the differences. There should be a written record of the people, decisions, and data used in selecting reference intervals, which will facilitate review and understanding in the future.

Common Reference Intervals

As stated in the previous sections, there is a considerable amount of work involved in setting a reference interval. The usual concept of individual laboratories performing this work for all their tests is potentially overwhelming, even for large well-resourced laboratories. Additionally, when laboratories do determine their own, there are often variations in the final reference intervals that are not supported by analytical or population differences.[114,115] There is also an increasing need to reduce unnecessary variation among laboratories as patients move between health locations, data is combined in common databases, and patients view their results directly and wonder about small differences and the changes in classification that these may cause. One approach that is gaining in acceptance is to recommend common reference intervals for a country, region, or other grouping of laboratories. The aim is to gather an appropriately experienced group to assess all available data (as described in the previous section), including analytical and possibly population differences, and then to select reference intervals for participating laboratories. As well as the advantages of sharing the workload, better decisions may be made by involving a wider range of parties in the decisions. It is important to realize that common reference intervals are likely to be a little wider than single-site reference intervals, at least in part because of the greater analytical variation expected from a group of laboratories versus a single laboratory. For this reason, a single laboratory may observe that fewer than 5% of its patients are outside the traditional 95% limits. Approaches that have been used vary between sites, but work of this type has begun in Australia, Canada, and the Netherlands.[102,110,116,117]

PRESENTATION OF AN OBSERVED VALUE IN RELATION TO REFERENCE VALUES

The purpose of reference limits is to allow a point of comparison for an observed value (patient's value). This comparison is similar to hypothesis testing, but it is seldom statistical testing in the strict sense. Ideally, the patient and the reference individuals should match (i.e., the hypothesis is stated that they were all picked from the same set [population]) in all aspects other than the presence of the medical condition for which the test has been requested. Often, however, this is not the case. Thus it is advisable to consider the reference values as the yardstick for a less formal assessment than hypothesis testing. It is this less formal assessment that typically directs the attention of the interpreting doctor to those results most likely to represent pathology. Indeed the results flagged as outside the reference intervals are commonly used as the starting point to begin interpretation of a report and to assess for possible major or urgent pathology.

The convenient presentation of an observed value in relation to reference values and clear flagging of results outside the intervals may be of great help for the busy clinician.[6,10–15,26,118] The most common presentation format for reference limits is the provision of the upper and lower reference limits on the same line of a report as the test name, test result (observed value), and units used for the result. Typically, when the result is outside the reference limits, the test result is accompanied by a "flag," which may be an asterisk, the letter H for "High" (i.e., above the upper reference limit), the letter L for "Low" (i.e., below the lower reference limit), or some other combinations of symbols. This format for reference limits has some significant strengths and weaknesses. The key strengths are the close proximity of the limits to the results, the ability to highlight values outside the reference limits, and the potential to tailor the displayed limits based on patient demographics typically available to the laboratory (such as age, sex, and fasting status). To the extent that additional factors about the patient are available (e.g., time since last drug dose or stage of pregnancy), even more specific limits can be supplied with the result. Limitations to this process include situations in which relevant factors are not available (e.g., stage of puberty or phase of the menstrual cycle). In these cases, a list of reference limits covering those factors can be included in the report, and the ordering clinician with knowledge of the patient can make the correct interpretation.

The preceding comments relate to reports in paper format and rendered electronic formats (e.g., portable document format [PDF]), situations in which the laboratory controls the way the data are presented. Recognizing that ease of reading pathology reports is a patient safety issue (a misread report can lead to a wrong medical decision; a report that is difficult to read will waste important clinical time), an Australian group has recommended strict formatting requirements for reports, including the placement and formatting of reference limits and flagging (e.g., columns of numerical results right-aligned, flagged with L or H to the right of results following a clear space, reference intervals in brackets to the right of results, and units of measure further to the right).[119]

A more difficult, and often under-appreciated, issue is the need to transfer reference limits along with patient results when they are communicated in other ways. For example, when individual patient values are transferred into third-party systems or common pathology databases, it is important to ensure that the laboratory-specific reference limits be as easily accessible as the patient values themselves. This issue is one driver toward developing common reference intervals.[120]

In addition, a very informative presentation of the observed value involves showing its location graphically relative to the reference limits. In the era of information overload, and review of pathology reports by patients and other non-medical personnel, a number of graphical tools are being developed to convey the information contained in a result and its relationship to reference limits.[121]

As stated earlier, results outside the reference limits may be flagged. A more detailed division of these results has been advocated to indicate how unusual the observed value is. For example, some laboratories highlight critical or extreme values with different flags such as C for critical, HH and LL for extremely high or low results respectively. In such cases, it is important for laboratories to educate their clinicians about these flags because their use and meaning may vary considerably between laboratories and among tests. Similarly, subdivisions within the reference interval may also have clinical meaning and require communication to clinicians. For example, high-sensitivity C-reactive protein (hsCRP) results may be used not only for cardiovascular risk prediction but also as an indicator of acute inflammation.

Another method that can be used to express the observed value is by a *statistical distance measure*. All such distances are ratios of the following type:

$$\frac{\text{observed value} - \text{measure of location}}{\text{measure of dispersion}}$$

The *SD unit*, or normal equivalent deviate, is such a measure. It is calculated as the difference between the observed value and the mean of the reference values divided by their SD.[122] Several similar ratios under different names have been suggested and discussed.[51,123-125] This approach can be used to produce a graphical report for multiple analytes where the reference limits for different tests are aligned, and the observed values plotted as an SD unit against the reference limits. This allows a rapid assessment as to which results on a report are the "most abnormal." One issue with these protocols is the need to develop methods for non-Gaussian distributions. Such methods include using transformed data[126] or using split data with different SDs for the upper and lower half of the reference population.[127]

A related concept is the use of *multiples of the median* (MoM), where observed values are expressed as a multiple of the median reference value. This is most commonly used in antenatal testing. By maintaining a current database comprising a large number of subjects unaffected by disease, this process seeks to reduce the effect of analytical bias by normalizing current reported values against current assay performance; the extent to which this is achieved has been questioned.[128]

Reporting the observed value as a *percentile* of the reference distribution provides a very accurate measure of the relation for results within the interval.[26,129] An observed serum GGT value of 48 IU/L may, for example, be reported as 48 IU/L (99th percentile). Results outside the reference interval will have very high or low percentiles and the accuracy of the assignment is likely to be limited. Alternatively, the probability of finding a value closer to the mean than the observed value, the *index of atypicality*, can be estimated.[118,130]

No matter how a reference interval is displayed, the clinician should always have access to as much information about the reference values as needed to use them appropriately. Reference values for all laboratory tests may be presented to clinicians in a booklet, web page, or other medium, together with information about (1) analytical methods, (2) their imprecision, and (3) descriptions of the reference values (e.g., whether they represent the central 90% rather than 95% of values) and any relevant limitations necessary for basic interpretation (e.g., diurnal variation). Graphical representations of the reference distributions can be informative (e.g., the use of a histogram [see Fig. 9.4A and C]), or a plot of the cumulative distribution [see Fig. 9.4B and D]), particularly with skewed distributions and tests with which the clinician is less familiar. If a reference limit is a clinical decision limit, it is important to make this distinction and to provide supporting documentation. The goal is to provide sufficient information to clinicians for them to make rational clinical judgments.

ADDITIONAL TOPICS

Multivariate, Population-Based Reference Regions

The topic of previous sections of this chapter has been univariate population-based reference values and quantities derived from them. However, such values do not fit the common clinical situation in which observed values of several different laboratory tests are available for interpretation and decision making. For example, the average number of individual clinical chemistry tests requested on each specimen received in the authors' laboratories is roughly 10; in many laboratories, this number is even larger. Two models are used for interpretation by comparison in this situation. Each observed value can be compared with the corresponding reference values or interval (i.e., a *multiple, univariate comparison is performed*), or the set of observed values can be considered as a single multivariate observation and can be interpreted as such by a *multivariate comparison*. In this section, the relative merits of these two approaches are discussed, and methods for the latter type of comparison are presented.

Multivariate Concept

A univariate observation, such as a single laboratory result, may be represented graphically as a point on a line—the axis. Results obtained by two different laboratory tests performed on the same specimen (a bivariate observation) are then displayed as a point in a plane defined by two perpendicular axes. With three results, a trivariate observation and a point in a space are defined by three perpendicular axes, and so forth. The possibility of visualization of a multivariate observation is lost when there are more than three dimensions. Still, one can consider the multivariate observation as a point in a multidimensional hyperspace with as many mutually perpendicular axes as there are results of different tests. The prefix *hyper-* signifies, in this context, "more than three dimensions." Such multivariate observations are also called *patterns* or *profiles*. A multivariate distribution thus is represented by a cluster of points on a plane, in a space, or in a hyperspace, depending on the dimensionality of the observation.[76,126,131,132] Several statistical methods are based on multivariate methods, some of which are straightforward extensions of well-known univariate methods.[133]

Multiple, Univariate Reference Region

The univariate reference interval is bounded by two reference limits (lower and upper) on the result axis. Fig. 9.6 shows the univariate reference intervals for two laboratory tests: one depicted on the *x*-axis and the other on the *y*-axis. Together, they describe a square in the plane of the two axes. Similarly, three or more univariate reference intervals define boxes or hyperboxes in the (hyper)space. By multiple, univariate comparison, it can be decided whether a multivariate observation point lies inside or outside this square, box, or hyperbox. However, this method has two very serious deficiencies[134]: an observation may lie outside the limits of the region without being unusual (see Fig. 9.6, point *a*), or it may be found on the inside and still be an atypical observation (see Fig. 9.6, point *b*). If the central 95% interval is used, 5% of the values by definition are expected to be located in the two tails of the univariate reference distribution. However, more than 5% of the values would be located outside the square or (hyper)box created by several 95% intervals. To be exact, $100(1 - 0.95^m)$

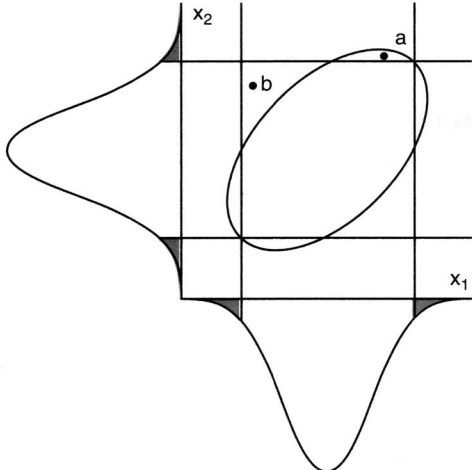

FIGURE 9.6 Bivariate reference region *(ellipse)* compared with the region defined by the two univariate reference intervals *(box).*

percent of multivariate reference values would be excluded by the method of multiple, univariate comparison (*m* being the number of different tests, or the dimensionality). For example, provided the results are independent of each other, one would expect to find $100(1 - 0.95^{10}) = 40\%$ of healthy subjects (members of the reference population) to have at least one result flagged as "abnormal" (i.e., 40% of healthy subjects will have false-positive results when 10 laboratory tests are performed). While this description is based on a multidimensional analysis, it is a model of standard laboratory practice. Additionally, an unusual combination (e.g., a low serum urea and high serum creatinine, each within its reference interval) would not be detected as abnormal, reflecting a limited sensitivity for abnormal patterns of results. This discouraging result has been verified in several multiphasic screening programs. Therefore a better method is needed.

Multivariate Reference Region

It is possible to define a common multivariate reference region[61,130–132,134,135] on the basis of joint distribution of reference values for two or more laboratory tests. This multivariate region is not a right-angled area, or hyperbox, but is more like an ellipse in the plane (see Fig. 9.6) or an ellipsoid hyperbody in hyperspace. This region may be a straightforward extension of the univariate 95% interval to the multivariate situation; it may be set to enclose 95% of central multivariate reference data points. In this case, one would expect to find only 5% false positives.

The use of multivariate reference regions usually requires the assistance of a computer program, which takes a set of results obtained by several laboratory tests on the same clinical specimen and calculates an index. Interpretation of a multivariate observation in relation to reference values is then the task of comparing the index with a threshold value estimated from the reference values. Obviously, this is much simpler than comparing each result with its proper reference interval.

This index is essentially a distance measure and is known as *Mahalanobis' squared distance* (D^2). It is analogous to the square of the SD for single reference values. It expresses the multivariate distance between the observation point and the common mean of the reference values, taking into account the dispersion and the correlation of the variables.[61,130–132,134,135] More interpretational guidance may be obtained from this distance by expressing it as a percentile analogous to the percentile presentation of univariate observed values.[135] Also, the index of atypicality has a multivariate counterpart.[130,131]

Although the theory of multivariate reference regions has been known for a while, surprisingly few applications of it have been reported in the literature. Some recent examples are two- and three-dimensional regions for thyroid function tests[136] and an outcome study in intensive care showing improved prediction with result pairs than with individual results.[137] An important report reviews the topic and presents the results of a very careful study on the multivariate 95% region for a 20-test chemistry profile.[135] Some of the most important findings can be summarized as follows:

1. Sixty-eight percent of subjects had at least one test result outside univariate reference intervals, which was close to what was theoretically expected: $100(1 - 0.95^{20}) = 64\%$.
2. By contrast, only 5% of patterns were outside the multivariate reference region (as expected).
3. Transformation to approximately Gaussian shape of the univariate distributions was necessary.
4. A test profile may be distinctly unusual in the multivariate sense even though each individual result is within its proper reference interval (e.g., see point *b* in Fig. 9.6).
5. The multivariate reference region could detect minor deviations of multiple analytes.
6. Conversely, it could also be insensitive to highly deviating results for a single analyte.
7. Sensitivity could be increased by defining multivariate reference regions for subsets of physiologically related tests.

Subject-Based Reference Values

Fig. 9.7 depicts the inherent problem associated with population-based reference values. It shows two hypothetical reference distributions. One represents the common reference distribution based on single specimens obtained from a group of

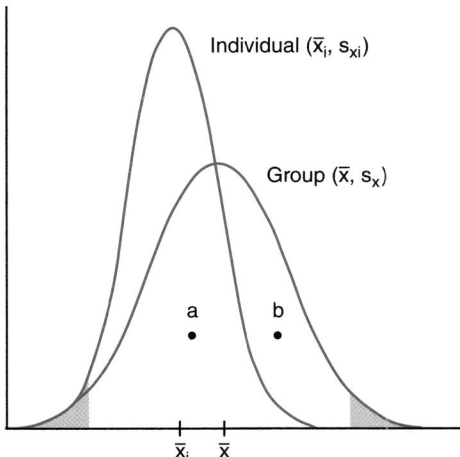

FIGURE 9.7 Relationship between population- and subject-based reference distributions and reference intervals. The example is hypothetical, and the two distributions are, for simplicity, Gaussian. Note that both points *a* and *b* are within the population-based reference interval, but only point *a* would be "normal" for this particular subject. (Modified from Harris EK. Effects of intraindividual and interindividual variation on the appropriate use of normal ranges. *Clin Chem* 1974;20:1536.)

different reference individuals. It has a true (hypothetical) mean $\bar{x}$ and a SD s_x. The other distribution is based on several specimens collected over time in a single individual, the ith individual. Its hypothetical mean is $\bar{x}_i$ and its SD s_{xi}.

If an observed value is located outside the subject's 2.5th and 97.5th percentiles, the personal or *subject-based reference interval*, the cause may be a change in biochemical status, suggesting the presence of disease. Fig. 9.7 shows that such an observed value may still be within the population-based reference interval. The sensitivity of the latter interval to changes in a subject's biochemical status depends accordingly on the location of the individual's mean x_i relative to the common mean x and to the relative magnitudes of the corresponding SDs s_{xi} and s_x. A mean s_{xi} close to s_x and a small s_{xi} relative to s_x may conceal the individual's changes entirely within the population-based reference interval.

Harris[73,74] analyzed this topic and found that the ratio R of intraindividual (personal) variation over interindividual (among subjects) variation provides a criterion for the usefulness of the population-based reference interval. This is now known as the Index of Individuality (II). The population-based reference interval has less than the desired sensitivity to changes in biochemical status if II is ≤ 0.6. The interval is a more trustworthy reference if II is greater than 1.4, at least for the individual whose SD σ_i is close to the average value. Published data[73,138] usually show that homeostatically tightly controlled quantities, such as serum electrolytes, have high ratio values. Population-based reference intervals of such analytes suffice for clinical use. In contrast, serum proteins and enzymes have very low ratios because they are not under the same degree of metabolic control. Here, subject-based reference intervals seem more appropriate, although limitations to the meaning of a low value for the II have been raised.[139]

Two specific examples mentioned earlier may help to clarify this concept further. Fig. 9.8 depicts immunoglobulin (Ig)M values from several healthy individuals over the course

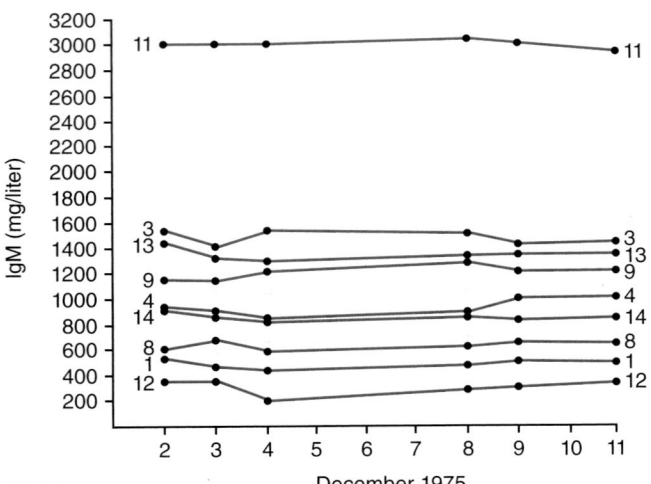

FIGURE 9.8 Serial immunoglobulin (Ig)M values over several days from reference individuals. Note that the intraindividual variability is very small compared to the interindividual variability. (From Statland BE, Winkel P, Killingsworth LM. Factors contributing to intra-individual variation of serum constituents: physiological day-to-day variation in concentrations of 10 specific proteins in sera. *Clin Chem* 1976;22:1635–8.)

of several days. As illustrated, the intraindividual differences are small compared with interindividual differences. Even though the population-based reference interval might extend from 200 to 1600 mg/dL, it would be most unusual (abnormal) for any patient's IgM value to change by more than 200 mg/dL, even if the value remained within the population-based reference interval. Similarly, it is well known that any given patient's serum creatinine value is reasonably constant,[24] which is related both to glomerular filtration rate (GFR) and to lean muscle mass. If the latter is constant, then changes in GFR are inversely proportional to the serum creatinine (see Chapter 34). That is, even though a typical (population-based) reference interval for serum creatinine might extend from 62 to 106 μmol/L (0.7 to 1.2 mg/dL), a change from 65 to 105 μmol/L in a given patient would be distinctly abnormal, representing the loss of almost half of the GFR, a finding of great clinical importance.

Two solutions can be proposed to the problem of the clinical insensitivity of population-based reference intervals:
1. One can try to reduce variation in reference values by *partitioning* into more homogeneous subclasses, as was discussed in a previous section. However, increasing the index of individuality (II), for example, from 0.6 to 1.4 by partitioning requires that one can obtain the rather dramatic reduction of 37% in SD.[74] This is often difficult to attain in practice.
2. The other possibility is to use the patient's previous values, obtained when the patient was in a defined state of health, as the reference for any future value. Application of *subject-based reference values* becomes more feasible as health screening by laboratory tests and computer storage of results become available to large segments of the general population.

The current approach to adopting the second solution above is to use one or more previous results as the best estimate of the patient's previous state, and then assess whether a subsequent result is likely to be different from that baseline. There are many similarities in this approach with the descriptions of population reference intervals previously described in this chapter. The amount of change in analyte concentration which is considered significant, known as the RCV, although previously referred to as the *critical difference*, is commonly set at a 5% probability of the change being due to random effects. Just as this mirrors the 5% probability of a member of the reference population being outside standard reference limits, it is possible to set RCVs based on different probabilities. The RCV is a combination of the analytical variation, the within-subject biological variation (CV_I), and the desired probability. For population reference intervals these also include the between-subject variation. It is recommended that values for CV_I are determined in formal studies with reference individuals under controlled conditions,[140] but methods have been developed to determine values for CV_I from laboratory databases,[141] these two approaches mirroring the direct and indirect approaches of population reference intervals. More information on biological variation, RCVs, and the relationship with population reference intervals is found in Chapter 8.

When "Normal" May Appear to Be "Abnormal" and Vice Versa

Some, if not many, clinical laboratory test results are related to other clinical laboratory test results in a way that affects their interpretation. For example, consider the relatively common situation of a patient with a low serum albumin. Because of the physiologic relationship between total calcium and albumin in serum (see Chapter 54), a total serum calcium concentration in the healthy reference interval might actually be pathologically high in this patient, and a total serum calcium concentration below the lower reference limit might be healthy. (For this reason, clinicians may choose to calculate an "adjusted calcium concentration" or to measure the "free calcium" concentration in these patients.) In these types of situations, it is important not to consider the normal (or abnormal) test results out of context. In most cases, laboratory reports, including reference intervals, do not take these situations into account.

As another example, consider a pregnant woman with typically high concentrations of serum binding proteins, including thyroxine binding globulin. She might well have what appears to be an "abnormally" high concentration of serum total thyroxine when compared with conventional reference limits (see Chapter 57), when in fact this is typical of a healthy pregnant state. Similarly, high concentrations of ceruloplasmin in pregnancy and other high estrogen states such as the oral contraceptive pill can produce high concentrations of serum copper, which does not indicate any change in copper metabolism. Other such examples in clinical medicine abound. Consider the prostate specific antigen (PSA) level in a postprostatectomy patient or the thyroglobulin level in a post-thyroidectomy patient. In these cases, it would be "healthy" to have abnormally low (undetectable) concentrations of these measurands, and it would be distinctly "unhealthy" to have levels in the healthy reference interval. Another scenario is urine sodium in investigation of acute kidney injury. If the kidney is "healthy" (i.e., with prerenal causes of acute kidney injury [AKI]), the urine sodium will be lower than the population reference interval, and a "healthy" result is consistent with intrinsic damage to the kidney. In all of these cases, the problem is that the traditional reference population (nonpregnant, healthy individuals) is not appropriate for the specific clinical setting.

Indeed, interpretations in much of the field of endocrinology are based not so much on "healthy" concentrations but rather on "appropriate" concentrations. For example, in a patient with a very high free T4 concentration, a thyroid stimulating hormone (TSH) within the traditional reference limits is used for differential diagnosis rather than likelihood of health. It should be undetectable in primary hyperthyroidism; otherwise, it may well represent secondary or tertiary hyperthyroidism (see Chapter 57). Similarly, in a patient with hypercalcemia, a PTH within the traditional healthy reference limits is distinctly abnormal.

In other words, even when reference limit studies are done well, one needs to remember there are dependencies that can render those reference limits misleading.

Special Populations

As noted in the previous section, there are groups of patients for whom the typical populations used in establishing reference limits may not be appropriate. Such groups include, but are not limited to, children, pregnant women, and the elderly. Even within these groups there may be important subgroups (partitions): for example, children may need to be further divided by age, sex, ethnicity, and/or Tanner stage; pregnant women, by trimester or week; elderly, by age, sex, and ethnicity. Over the past decade a number of studies have been conducted to establish reference intervals for these populations.

As noted earlier, the CALIPER initiative, a multicenter trial, recruited several thousand healthy pediatric subjects from across Canada and established reference limits, partitioned by age, sex, and ethnicity, for 40 measurands using one analytical system.[53] Its database was later extended by transference to several additional analytical systems and to an additional 29 measurands.[106] A recent study from Denmark established reference limits for 36 measurands based on 801 normal pregnancies in Caucasian women.[142] These limits might be extended to other analytical systems by transference, but additional pregnancies in non-Caucasian women will be required to determine whether the limits can be extended to other ethnic groups. Another study from Denmark established reference limits for 27 measurands based on 1016 70-year-old Caucasians.[143] Again, this involved a single set of analytical systems and a single ethnic group, so the authors were careful to point out that additional work will be required to determine to what extent their reference limits can be adopted by others.

In each of these cases, important differences from the traditional reference intervals were uncovered.

Special Cases of Laboratory Test Result Interpretation

In the search for improved diagnostic performance, several individual test results may be combined to form an index or score with the aim of combining the discriminating power of the individual results. Examples include the "triple" and "quad" screens used to calculate risk for Down syndrome and trisomy 18 in early pregnancy (see Chapter 59), a variety of proprietary "liver fibrosis" screens[144] to estimate the likelihood of cirrhosis (see Chapter 51), and the prostate health index from Beckman Coulter.[145] Although a discussion of these methods is beyond the scope of this chapter, the basic concepts of reference populations, sampling, outlier exclusion, and so on remain vital to the process. Typically, the reference limit is a clinical decision point rather than a population reference interval limit. In these cases, the goal is not so much to determine whether the patient is healthy but to determine whether the likelihood of abnormality is high enough that additional testing is warranted (triple and quad screens) or to determine whether certain therapies are likely to be helpful without resorting to an invasive liver[144] or prostate biopsy.[145] More common examples are calculated tests such as the anion gap, osmolar gap, serum globulins, and calculated free testosterone. In each case there is a tendency for reference intervals to be derived from textbooks without taking the test methodology into account. Laboratories need to consider and promote accurate reference intervals for these tests with the same care as for individual tests.

Ongoing Verification of Reference Limits

Whether a laboratory establishes values with its own reference limit studies or adopts reference limits after verification from another source, it is rare for any laboratory to assess those reference limits on a regular basis. Typically, the reference limits are not reevaluated until the laboratory implements new instrumentation, at which point it may be necessary to make changes. Even with changes in methods, though, there is no guarantee that a reassessment will occur. In an interesting report from Australia,[102] studies showed that reference limits for common measurands differed significantly among laboratories, even when they used the same analytical systems; additional studies indicated that common reference intervals for these measurements could, and should, be implemented across all these laboratories.

Laboratories can, however, use "data mining" techniques discussed earlier to perform ongoing audits of reference limits and to investigate specific concerns when they arise. For example, with these techniques, a laboratory could determine the median of the distribution of bicarbonate values from its healthy outpatients, which should be extremely stable.[113,146] Similarly, it could determine what percentage of these values fall outside the reference limits. Assuming those limits were set to include the central 95% of healthy outpatient values, no more than 2.5% of the values should be below the lower limit or above the upper limit. If a change in median occurs, or if too many samples fall outside the limits, there may well be a problem. The laboratory could then investigate further by using the technique to see when the problem started, by reviewing whether any changes in methods were made, by investigating performance on proficiency testing, and even by repeating a short reference interval verification study with 20 individuals as described earlier. These data mining studies are relatively inexpensive, involving only retrieval and manipulation of data that already exists, but they provide great reassurance to the laboratory and its users of the accuracy of its test results and reference limits.

CONCLUSION

In this chapter, we have emphasized the importance of reference limits, which provide physicians with values with which they can compare their patients' results, thereby facilitating interpretation. In most, but not all, cases, reference limits reflect values seen in healthy individuals.

When generating, verifying, or reporting reference limits, it is critical that the populations be well-defined and that the patients for whom the limits are used be comparable in terms of gender, age, and ethnicity where relevant, and any other measurable characteristics determined to be of importance. We have described in detail ways to ensure collection of high-quality data, methods to eliminate outliers when appropriate, and techniques to analyze the data (including nonparametric [preferred], parametric, graphical, computerized).

Recognizing that many laboratories do not have the resources to generate their own reference limits, we have described alternative sources (including manufacturers' package inserts, peer-reviewed literature, multicenter trials, historical laboratory data) and techniques to verify the transferability of such data.

We have recommended a multidisciplinary approach to selecting and implementing reference limits, as well as support for the concept of common reference intervals amongst groups of laboratories in a region or country, and we have discussed a number of considerations related to the display of reference limits along with patient results.

We have also included discussion of several special topics, including multivariate reference limits, subject-based reference limits, reference limits for special populations, and ongoing verification of reference limits.

It is quite clear that laboratories face many issues and a great deal of effort in ensuring that their reference limits are valid, but we would argue that, in the absence of this effort, much of the data we generate would not be interpretable. The validity of our reference limits is at least as important as the accuracy and precision of our analytical techniques and should therefore warrant at least as much attention.

SELECTED REFERENCES

3. Siest G, Henny J, Grasbeck R, et al. The theory of reference values: an unfinished symphony. Clin Chem Lab Med 2013;51:47-64.
10. Solberg HE. IFCC approved recommendation on the theory of reference values. Part 1. The concept of reference values. J Clin Chem Clin Biochem 1987;25:337-42.
16. Clinical And Laboratory Standards Institute: Defining, establishing, and verifying reference intervals in the clinical laboratory (EP28-A3c). Wayne, PA: Clinical and Laboratory Standards Institute; 2010.
20. Ozarda Y, Sikaris K, Streichert T, Macri J. Distinguishing reference intervals and clinical decision limits - A review by the IFCC Committee on Reference Intervals and Decision Limits. Critical reviews in clinical laboratory sciences 2018;55:420-31.
37. Jones GRD, Haeckel R, Loh TP, et al. Indirect methods for reference interval determination - review and recommendations. Clin Chem Lab Med 2018;57:20-9.
50. Ichihara K, Ozarda Y, Barth JH, et al. A global multicenter study on reference values: 1. Assessment of methods for derivation and comparison of reference intervals. Clin Chim Acta 2017;467:70-82.
53. Colantonio DA, Kyriakopoulou L, Chan MK, et al. Closing the gaps in pediatric laboratory reference intervals: a CALIPER database of 40 biochemical markers in a healthy and multiethnic population of children. Clin Chem 2012;58:854-68.
60. Ichihara K, Boyd JC. An appraisal of statistical procedures used in derivation of reference intervals. Clin Chem Lab Med 2010;48:1537-51.
61. Harris EK, Boyd JC. Statistical bases of reference values in laboratory medicine. New York: Marcel Dekker; 1995.
65. Rustad P, Felding P, Franzson L, et al. The Nordic Reference Interval Project 2000: recommended reference intervals for 25 common biochemical properties. Scand J Clin Lab Invest 2004;64:271-84.
86. Pavlov IY, Wilson AR, Delgado JC. Reference interval computation: which method (not) to choose? Clin Chim Acta 2012;413:1107-14.
90. Horn PS, Pesce AJ. Reference intervals: a user's guide. Washington, DC: AACC Press; 2005.
92. Katayev A, Fleming JK, Luo D, Fisher AH, Sharp TM. Reference intervals data mining: no longer a probability paper method. Am J Clin Pathol 2015;143:134-42.
95. Holmes DT, Buhr KA. Widespread Incorrect Implementation of the Hoffmann Method, the Correct Approach, and Modern Alternatives. Am J Clin Pathol 2019;151:328-36.
102. Tate JR, Sikaris KA, Jones GR, et al. Harmonising adult and paediatric reference intervals in australia and new zealand: an evidence-based approach for establishing a first panel of chemistry analytes. Clin Biochem Rev 2014;35:213-35.
106. Karbasy K, Ariadne P, Gaglione S, Nieuwesteeg M, Adeli K. Advances in Pediatric Reference Intervals for Biochemical Markers: Establishment of the Caliper Database in Healthy Children and Adolescents. J Med Biochem 2015;34:23-30.
113. Jones GR. Validating common reference intervals in routine laboratories. Clin Chim Acta 2014;432:119-21.
117. Koerbin G, Sikaris K, Jones GRD, Flatman R, Tate JR. An update report on the harmonization of adult reference intervals in Australasia. Clin Chem Lab Med 2018;57:38-41.
119. Flatman R, Legg M, Jones GR, Graham P, Moore D, Tate J. Recommendations for reporting and flagging of reference limits on pathology reports. Clin Biochem Rev 2014;35:199-202.
121. O'Connor JD. Reducing post analytical error: perspectives on new formats for the blood sciences pathology report. Clin Biochem Rev 2015;36:7-20.

Evidence-Based Laboratory Medicine*

Patrick M.M. Bossuyt, Paul Glasziou, and Andrea R. Horvath

ABSTRACT

Background
Evidence-based laboratory medicine (EBLM) is an approach to medical practice that integrates the best available research evidence about laboratory investigations with the clinical expertise of clinicians, to improve the health and health care outcomes of individual patients. Practicing EBLM enables laboratory professionals to translate test results to clinically relevant information that helps clinicians in delivering effective and cost-effective patient care.

Content
This chapter provides an overview on how evidence about laboratory tests is generated, how it is synthesized, and how it can be applied to questions about diagnosis, screening, prognosis, or monitoring. The topics covered here introduce the reader to the methodological and practical aspects of EBLM. They include (1) the process and methods of practicing EBLM, (2) the key components and types of evidence used in the evaluation of biomarkers, (3) tools for the assessment of the validity and applicability of the evidence, (4) key aspects of synthesizing the evidence in systematic reviews and meta-analyses, (5) basic principles of how EBLM is applied to other purposes of testing than diagnosis, (6) the challenges and tools of implementing the evidence for achieving best laboratory practice, and (7) the history and future challenges of EBLM.

---

*The full version of this chapter is available electronically on ExpertConsult.com.

Biobanking*

Christina Ellervik and Jim B. Vaught

ABSTRACT

Background
Biobanks may be established for nonresearch purposes, such as diagnostic, therapeutic, treatment, forensic, transplantation, and transfusion, or for research purposes as part of epidemiologic studies and clinical trials. Biobank planning is essential for biospecimen integrity in support of such research, but also for the establishment, governance, management, operation, access, use, sustainability, and discontinuation of biobanks.

Content
We focus on best practices procedures for collection, processing, storage, and retrieval of biospecimens with regard to

downstream analyses for blood, urine, and saliva. Security measures, disaster planning, quality management, accreditation and certification, staff education, chain-of-custody, annotation of data, cost, and sustainability issues are reviewed. Adoption of various internal and external standards is discussed. Ethical, legal, and social issues, as well as administrative issues regarding governance, ownership, stewardship, and access criteria are discussed.

*The full version of this chapter is available electronically on ExpertConsult.com.

Laboratory Support of Pharmaceutical, In Vitro Diagnostics, and Epidemiologic Studies*

Omar Fernando Laterza, Amar Akhtar Sethi, Theresa Ambrose Bush, and Nader Rifai[a]

ABSTRACT

Background

Biomarkers are used in the clinical laboratory for routine patient care, and in the pharmaceutical industry during drug development, and in establishing safety and efficacy of a candidate drug. Biomarkers are also used in clinical and epidemiologic research to gain a better insight into pathophysiology, to identify predictors of disease, and to refine treatment strategies. The in vitro diagnostic (IVD) industry develops most of the biomarker assays and makes them commercially available. The pharmaceutical and IVD industries, as well as epidemiologic researchers, often seek the help of clinical laboratories in their biomarker studies, thus providing a mutually beneficial and rewarding relationship.

Content

This chapter describes, in detail, the various areas in which the pharmaceutical and IVD industries and epidemiologic and clinical researchers use biomarkers and illustrates the ways in which the clinical laboratory can be involved in providing such services, which can be both financially and intellectually rewarding. However, these opportunities have their own challenges, including the need for strict regulatory rules, extensive documentation requirements, and particular data access and storage specifications. The regulatory requirements for performing biomarker testing are described in this chapter; results may be used in premarket submissions to governmental agencies, for both drugs and assay kits. The relevant documents for analytical and clinical evaluations of biomarkers are identified and discussed. Due to the daunting task of summarizing worldwide regulations, the regulatory requirements in the United States are primarily referred to as examples. The reader should refer to their local agencies when assessing the exact needs applicable to their situation. Overall, the goal of this chapter is to provide a general overview to those in the clinical laboratory who are interested in biomarker research collaborations.

*The full version of this chapter is available electronically on ExpertConsult.com.

[a]The authors acknowledge the contributions of Mark J. Sarno to the earlier version of the chapter in the 6th edition. The authors also acknowledge that a small portion of this chapter was based on Cole TG, Warnick GR, Rifai N. Providing laboratory support for clinical trials, epidemiologic studies, and in vitro diagnostic evaluations. In: Rifai N, Warnick GR, Dominiczak MH, editors. *Handbook of Lipoprotein Testing*. AACC Press, with permission.

Machine Learning and Big Data in Laboratory Medicine*

Stephen R. Master, Randall K. Julian, Jr., and Shannon Haymond

ABSTRACT

Background

The large number of test results generated by clinical laboratories has led to challenges in data management and analytics. Because of the potential diagnostic value of examining these results in aggregate, it is important to utilize emerging tools for the analysis of high-dimensional data. Machine learning uses a variety of computational algorithms to analyze complex datasets and make robust predictions.

Content

This chapter discusses the varied definitions of *big data* and their application to laboratory medicine. It also presents workflows, concepts, common algorithms, infrastructure, and applications related to the use of machine learning in the clinical laboratory. The chapter is a more technical and extensive version of one previously authored on these topics.[1]

Because each biomarker measured in a patient can be plotted as a single number, the collection of biomarkers measured in this patient can be represented in a high-dimensional space. Unsupervised learning methods are used to find patterns in this high-dimensional space, and supervised learning methods use known outcomes from a set of subjects to develop a model to predict the outcome in a new, unknown subject. A variety of different algorithms, each with different advantages and disadvantages, has been used for these machine learning tasks. Implementing machine learning in the laboratory requires not only understanding the basic algorithmic concepts, but also deploying an appropriate computational infrastructure. Machine learning has been successfully deployed in laboratory medicine settings using a variety of underlying datasets, including traditional laboratory values, next-generation sequencing data, and images.

---

*The full version of this chapter is available electronically on ExpertConsult.com.

14

Laboratory Stewardship and Test Utilization*

Gary W. Procop, Ronald B. Schifman, and Peter L. Perrotta

ABSTRACT

Laboratory tests substantially impact clinical care, but their overuse, misuse, or underuse can cause patient harm and dissatisfaction, suboptimal patient care, and increased costs. Traditionally, the first consideration of pathology and laboratory medicine has been centered on optimizing the analytic phase of testing, which, of course, is critical for producing reliable and meaningful test results. Subsequently, it has become clear that specimen acquisition, transport and processing (preanalytics) and the accurate and timely reporting of results (postanalytics) substantially affect the reliability of test results. Finally, proper test selection (pre-preanalytics), and accurate interpretation of results (post-postanalytics) are the other important components of laboratory testing that impact value and outcomes. All of these functions are within the scope of practice for pathologists and clinical laboratorians,

who are responsible for the overall quality of laboratory testing. This chapter outlines the reasons for suboptimal test use, lists potential outcomes of improper test use, describes how to create and maintain a test utilization or laboratory stewardship program, provides insights on the management of test utilization projects, and provides examples of specific interventions that can improve test utilization patterns. Finally, this chapter will underscore the importance of collaborative engagement of pathologists and clinical laboratorians with stakeholders to promote the optimal use and performance of laboratory testing from the moment testing is considered through to the clinical response to the results. In addition, because the area of Laboratory Stewardship is a relatively new and evolving field, the authors include examples of implementation of these practices.

*The full version of this chapter is available electronically on ExpertConsult.com.

Principles of Basic Techniques and Laboratory Safety*

Tahir S. Pillay and Stanley F. Lo[a]

ABSTRACT

Background

To appropriately interpret clinical laboratory test results and adequately validate assays, the basic principles and techniques of analytical chemistry need to be understood. These techniques should be used by laboratory professionals in a safe testing environment.

Content

Factors that affect the analytical process and operation of the clinical laboratory are described in this chapter. The concepts of solute and solution, and the international system of units used to standardize their expression and reporting are described. These solutions are composed of various types of chemicals used in the development of clinical laboratory assays. The importance of water purity, appropriate reagent preparation, and the different types of reference materials are addressed. The principles of basic techniques in the clinical laboratory, including pipetting, centrifugation, radioactivity, gravimetry, and thermometry, are also discussed. These techniques are used in a variety of laboratory tasks such as making buffers, performing dilutions, evaporation, lyophilization, and filtration. Safety is a constant and crucial concern for laboratory personnel. Each laboratory must create a comprehensive safety program. Plans for the handling of chemicals, exposure to blood-borne pathogens, tuberculosis, and other highly infectious agents are necessary components of a safety plan. The training of laboratory personnel to identify various types of biological, chemical, and electrical hazards and to react appropriately to fire must be addressed in such a plan.

*The full version of this chapter is available electronically on ExpertConsult.com.
[a]The author gratefully acknowledges the original contributions of Drs. Edward W. Bermes, Stephen E. Kahn, Donald S. Young, Edward R. Powsner, and John C. Widman, on which portions of this chapter are based.

199

Analytical Techniques

Exam questions, case studies, and additional resources are available on ExpertConsult.com.
*Full versions of these chapters are available electronically on www.ExpertConsult.com.

Optical Techniques

Khushbu Patel and Jason Y. Park[a]

ABSTRACT

Background

Measurement of radiant energy (light) is used throughout the clinical laboratory to measure analytes, including proteins, metals, enzymes, antigens, and antibodies.

Content

This chapter describes the range of optical techniques used in clinical laboratory analysis. The techniques and instrumentation used for these measurements range from simple visualization by the naked eye to complex analysis with semiconductor-based lasers matched to solid-state, charge-coupled detectors (CCDs). With the naked eye, white light is the radiant energy that is used to observe the presence or absence of turbidity or a chromogen (e.g., latex agglutination or lateral-flow point-of-care test). In sophisticated instrumentation, the radiant energy may take the form of white light (e.g., halogen light bulb), but the radiant energy may also be selectively chosen for a specific wavelength or range of wavelengths (e.g., laser excitation of a fluorophore). The radiant energy in an instrument may be used to energize or be scattered by molecules of interest. The basic components of all optical analytical systems include a source for radiant energy, a device for selecting wavelength(s) of light, and a detector.

Although the optical components of a test system may be hidden away in the deep recesses of high-throughput instrumentation, electromagnetic radiation is a critical component of modern clinical chemistry methods (e.g., spectrophotometry, fluorometry, nephelometry, turbidimetry).

Many determinations made in the clinical laboratory are based on measurements of radiant energy emitted, transmitted, absorbed, scattered, or reflected under controlled conditions. The principles involved in such measurements are considered in this chapter.

NATURE OF LIGHT

Electromagnetic radiation includes radiant energy that extends from cosmic rays with wavelengths as short as 10 nm up to radio waves longer than 1000 km. However, in this chapter, the term *light* is used to describe radiant energy from the ultraviolet (UV) and visible portions of the spectrum (380 to 750 nm).

The wavelength of light is defined as the distance between two peaks as the light travels in a wavelike manner. This distance is expressed in nanometers (nm) for wavelengths commonly used in photometry. Other units include:

1 nm = 1 millimicron (mμ) = 10 Angstroms (A) 10^{-9} m

In addition to possessing wavelength characteristics, light has properties that indicate that it is composed of discrete energy packets called *photons*. The relationship between the energy of photons and their frequency is given by Planck's equation:

$$E = h\nu \qquad (16.1)$$

where E = energy in joules, v = frequency of light in cycles per second, and h = Planck's constant (6.626×10^{-34} joule seconds). The v is related to the wavelength by an equation:

$$\nu = \frac{c}{\lambda} \qquad (16.2)$$

where c = speed of light in a vacuum (3×10^{10} cm/s), and λ = wavelength in centimeters. Combining Eqs. (16.1) and (16.2) results in:

$$E = \frac{hc}{\lambda} \qquad (16.3)$$

This equation shows that the energy of light is inversely proportional to the wavelength. For example, UV radiation at 200 nm possesses greater energy than infrared (IR) radiation at 750 nm.

The human eye detects radiant energy with wavelengths between approximately 380 and 750 nm, but modern instrumentation permits measurements at both shorter wavelength (UV) and longer wavelength (IR) portions of the spectrum. Sunlight, or light emitted from a tungsten filament, is a mixture of wavelengths or a spectrum of radiant energy of different wavelengths that the eye recognizes as "white." Table 16.1 shows approximate relationships between wavelengths and color characteristics for the UV, visible, and short IR portions of the spectrum. Thus a solution will appear green when

[a]The authors gratefully acknowledge the original contributions by Drs. Merle A. Evenson, Thomas O. Tiffany, and Larry Kricka upon which portions of this chapter are based.

TABLE 16.1   Ultraviolet, Visible, and Short Infrared Spectrum Characteristics

Wavelength (nm)	Region Name	Color Observed[a]
<380	UV[b]	Invisible
380–440	Visible	Violet
440–500	Visible	Blue
500–580	Visible	Green
580–600	Visible	Yellow
600–620	Visible	Orange
620–750	Visible	Red
800–2,500	Near infrared	Not visible
2,500–15,000	Mid infrared	Not visible
15,000–1,000,000	Far infrared	Not visible

[a]Because of the subjective nature of color, the wavelength intervals shown are only approximations.
[b]The ultraviolet (UV) portion of the spectrum is sometimes further divided into "near" UV (200–380 nm) and "far" UV (<220 nm). This arbitrary distinction has a practical basis because silica used to make cuvets transmits light effectively at wavelengths ≥220 nm.

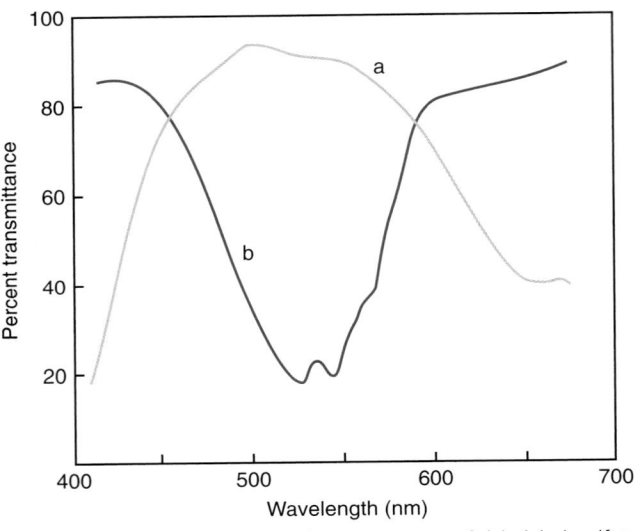

FIGURE 16.1 Spectral transmittance curves of *(a)* nickel sulfate and *(b)* potassium permanganate. Arbitrary concentrations read versus water as a blank (Beckman DB-G spectrophotometer).

viewed against white light if it transmits light maximally between 500 and 580 nm but absorbs light at other wavelengths. Similarly, a solid object appears green if it reflects light in this region (500 to 580 nm) but absorbs light at other portions of the spectrum. In general, if the intensity of light transmitted by a colored solution is compared with that of a reference solution over the entire spectrum, a typical spectral transmittance curve characteristic for that spectrum is obtained. Such curves are shown in Fig. 16.1 for solutions of *(a)* nickel sulfate and *(b)* potassium permanganate. Inspection of the curves should lead to the prediction that the color of the solution *(a)* is green because light is transmitted maximally near the green portion of the spectrum. In contrast, curve *(b)* illustrates a $KMnO_4$ solution that absorbs in the green-yellow region (550 nm) and transmits light maximally in the blue, violet, and red portions of the spectrum. The eye recognizes this mixture of colors as purple.

POINTS TO REMEMBER

Radiant Energy
- Wavelength size has a wide distribution, ranging from as small as 10 nm to greater than 1000 km.
- The visible portion of the spectrum ranges from approximately 380 to approximately 750 nm.
- The energy of light is inversely proportional to the wavelength; shorter wavelengths have greater energy.
- Light possesses both wavelength and energy packet characteristics; the packets are described as photons.

SPECTROPHOTOMETRY

Photometry is defined as the measurement of light; spectrophotometry is defined as the measurement of the intensity of light at selected wavelengths. Spectrophotometric analysis is a widely used method of quantitative and qualitative analysis in the chemical and biological sciences. The method depends on the light-absorbing properties of the substance or a derivative of the substance being analyzed. The intensity of transmitted light passing through a solution containing an absorbing substance (chromogen) is decreased by the absorbed fraction. This fraction is detected, measured, and used to relate the light transmitted or absorbed to the concentration of the analyte in question.

Basic Concepts

Consider an incident light beam with intensity I_0 passing through a square cell containing a solution of a compound that absorbs light of a certain wavelength, λ. Because the intensity of the transmitted light beam is I_S, then transmittance (T) of light is defined as:

$$T = \frac{I_S}{I_0} \qquad (16.4)$$

However, a portion of the incident light may be reflected by the surface of the cell or may be absorbed by the cell wall or solvent. To focus attention on the compound of interest, elimination of these factors is necessary. This is achieved using a reference cell identical to the sample cell, except that the compound of interest is omitted from the solvent in the reference cell (i.e., reference blank). The transmittance (T) through this reference cell is I_R divided by I_0; the transmittance for the compound in solution is then defined as I_S divided by I_R. In practice, the light beam is blocked, the detector signal is set to zero transmittance, then a reference cell is inserted, and the detector signal is adjusted to an arbitrary scale reading of 100 (corresponding to 100% transmittance), followed by the cell containing the sample to be measured, and the percent transmittance reading is made on the sample. As the concentration of the compound in solution is increased, the transmittance varies inversely and logarithmically with the concentration (Fig. 16.2). Consequently, it is more convenient to define a new term, absorbance (A), which will be directly proportional to the concentration. Thus the amount of light absorbed (A) as the incident light passes through the sample is equivalent to:

$$A = -\log\frac{I_S}{I_R} = -\log T \qquad (16.5)$$

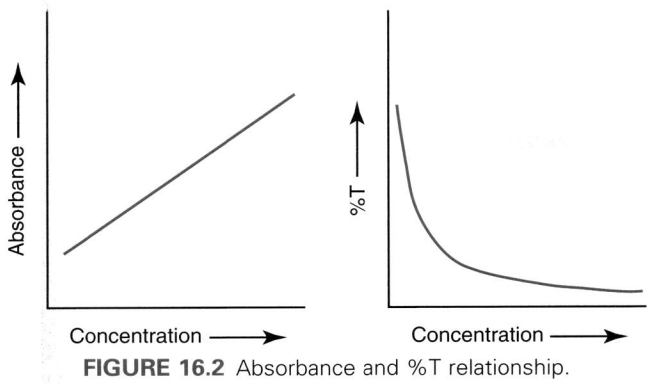

FIGURE 16.2 Absorbance and %T relationship.

TABLE 16.2	Spectrophotometry Nomenclature	
Name	**Symbol**	**Definition**
Absorbance	A	$-\log T$ or $\log I_0/I$
Absorptivity	a	A/bc (c in g/L)
Molar absorptivity	ε	A/bc (c in mol/L)
Path length	b	Internal cell or sample length, in cm
Transmittance	T	I_s/I_0[a]
Wavelength unit	nm	10^{-9} m
Absorption maximum	λmax	Wavelength at which maximum absorption occurs

[a]I_s/I_0 is the ratio of the intensity of transmitted light to incident light.

Analytically, the amount of light absorbed or transmitted is related mathematically to the concentration of the analyte in question by Beer's law.

Beer's Law: Relationship Among Transmittance, Absorbance, and Concentration

Beer's law (also known as the Beer-Lambert law) states that the concentration of a substance is directly proportional to the amount of light absorbed or inversely proportional to the logarithm of the transmitted light (see Fig. 16.2). Mathematically, Beer's law is expressed as:

$$A = abc \qquad (16.6)$$

where A = absorbance; a = proportionality constant defined as absorptivity; b = light path (in centimeters); and c = concentration of the absorbing compound (usually expressed in moles per liter).

This equation forms the basis of quantitative analysis by absorption photometry. When b is 1 cm and c is expressed in moles per liter, the constant a is called the molar absorptivity. The value for a is a constant for a given compound at a given wavelength under prescribed conditions of solvent, temperature, pH, and so forth. The nomenclature of spectrophotometry is summarized in Table 16.2. Values for a are useful for characterizing compounds, establishing their purity, and comparing the sensitivity of measurements obtained on derivatives. Pure bilirubin, for example, when dissolved in chloroform at 25 °C, has a molar absorptivity of 60,700 ± 1600 $cm^{-1}M^{-1}$ at 453 nm. The molecular weight of bilirubin is 584. Hence, a solution containing 5 mg/L (0.005 g/L) should have a concentration c of 0.005 g/L × (584 g/mole)$^{-1}$ which is 0.005/584 moles/L (M). This results in:

$$A = abc = \left(\frac{60,700}{cm \cdot M}\right) \times \left(1\,cm\right) \times \left(\frac{0.005}{584}\right) = 0.520 \quad (16.7)$$

The molar absorptivity of the complex between ferrous iron and s-tripyridyltriazine is 22,600, whereas that with 1,10-phenanthroline is 11,000. Thus for a given concentration of iron, s-tripyridyltriazine produces a complex with an absorbance approximately twice that of the complex with 1,10-phenanthroline. Consequently, s-tripyridyltriazine is a more sensitive reagent to use in the measurement of iron.

Application of Beer's Law

In practice, a calibration relationship between absorbance and concentration is established experimentally for a given instrument under specified conditions using a series of reference solutions that contain increasing concentrations of analyte. Frequently, a linear relationship exists up to a certain concentration or absorbance. When this linear relationship exists, the solution is said to obey Beer's law up to this point. Within this limitation, a calibration constant may be derived and used to calculate the concentration of an unknown solution by comparison with a calibrating solution.

Certain precautions must be observed with the use of such calibration constants. For example, under no circumstances should the calibration constants be used when the calibrator or unknown readings exceed the linear portion of the calibration relationship. In other words, calibration constants are used only when the curve obeys Beer's law. At least two and preferably more calibrators should be included in each series of determinations to permit direct comparison of unknown readings with calibrators or to calculate the calibration constant. These multiple calibrators are necessary because variations in reagents, working conditions, and cell diameters, and deterioration or changes in instruments may result in day-to-day changes in the absorbance value for the calibrator. A nonlinear calibration curve may be used if a sufficient number of calibrators of varying concentrations are included to cover the entire range encountered for readings of unknowns.

In some cases, a pure reference material may not be readily available, and constants may be provided that were obtained on pure materials and reported in the literature. In general, published constants should only be used if the method is followed in detail and readings are made on a spectrophotometer capable of providing light of high spectral purity at a verified wavelength. Use of broader band light sources usually leads to some decrease in absorbance. For example, the absorbance of nicotinamide adenine dinucleotide at 340 nm is frequently used as a reference for determination of enzyme activity, based on a molar absorptivity of 6220 $cm^{-1}M^{-1}$ (see Chapter 25). This value is acceptable only under the carefully controlled conditions previously described and should not be used unless these conditions are met. Published values for molar absorptivities and absorption coefficients should be used only as guidelines until they are verified by readings on pure reference materials for a given instrument. In addition, Beer's law is followed only if the following conditions are met:
- Incident radiation on the substance of interest is monochromatic.
- The solvent absorption is insignificant compared with the solute absorbance.

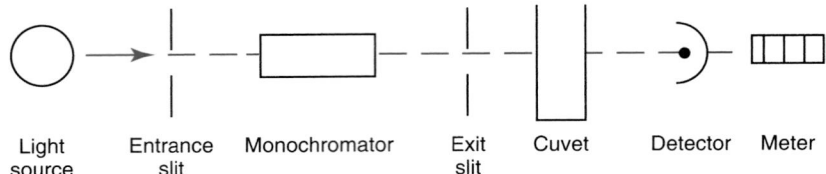

Light source — Entrance slit — Monochromator — Exit slit — Cuvet — Detector — Meter

FIGURE 16.3 Major components of a single-beam spectrophotometer.

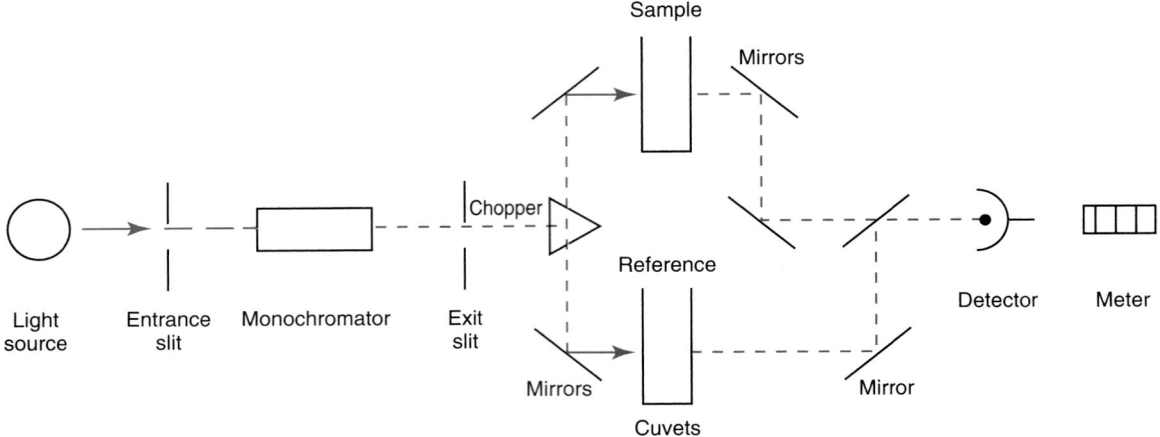

FIGURE 16.4 Major components of a double-beam spectrophotometer.

- The solute concentration is within given limits.
- An optical interferent is not present.
- A chemical reaction does not occur between the molecule of interest and another solute or solvent molecule.

Instrumentation

Modern instruments isolate a narrow wavelength range of the spectrum for measurements. Those that use filters for this purpose are referred to as filter photometers; those that use prisms or gratings are called spectrophotometers. Spectrophotometers are classified as single or double beam.

The major components of a single-beam spectrophotometer are shown in Fig. 16.3. In such an instrument, a beam of light is passed through a monochromator that isolates the desired region of the spectrum to be used for measurements. The light next passes through an absorption cell (cuvet), where a portion of the radiant energy is absorbed, depending on the nature and concentration of the substance in the solution. Any light not absorbed is transmitted to a detector, which converts light energy to electrical energy that is registered on a meter or recorder, or digitally displayed.

In operation, an opaque block is substituted for the cuvet, so that no light reaches the photocell, and the meter is adjusted to read 0% *T*. Next, a cuvet containing a reagent blank is inserted, and the meter is adjusted to read 100% *T* (zero absorbance). The composition of the reagent blank should be identical to that of the calibrating or unknown solutions except for the substance to be measured. Calibrating solutions containing various known concentrations of the substance are inserted, and readings are recorded. Finally, a reading is made of the unknown solution, and its concentration is determined by comparison with readings obtained on the calibrators. In most spectrophotometers, digital hardware

and software are integral components and perform these functions automatically.

Fig. 16.4 illustrates a typical double-beam instrument that uses a light-beam chopper (a rotating wheel with alternate silvered sections and cutout sections) inserted after the exit slit. A system of mirrors passes portions of the light reflected off the chopper alternately through the sample and a reference cuvet onto a common detector. The chopped-beam approach, using one detector, compensates for light source variation and for sensitivity changes in the detector.

Components

The basic components of a spectrophotometer include (1) a light source, (2) a device to isolate light of a desired wavelength, (3) a cuvet, (4) a photodetector, (5) a readout device, and (6) a data system.

Light sources. Types of light sources used in spectrophotometers include incandescent lamps, xenon discharge lamps, lasers, and light-emitting diodes (LEDs).

Incandescent, arc, and cathode lamps. The light source for measurements in the visible portion of the spectrum is usually a tungsten light bulb. The lifetime of a tungsten filament is greatly increased by the presence of a low pressure of iodine or bromine vapor within the lamp. An example is the quartz-halogen lamp, which has a fused-silica envelope and provides high-intensity light over a wide spectrum for extended operating periods (2000 to 5000 hours) before replacement is necessary.

However, a tungsten light source does not supply sufficient radiant energy for measurements in the UV region (<320 nm). In the UV region of the spectrum, hydrogen and deuterium lamps, as well as high-pressure mercury and xenon arc lamps, are sources of continuous spectra in the

UV region with sharp emission lines. These sources are more commonly used in UV absorption measurements. Low-pressure mercury vapor lamps also provide spectra in the UV region and are useful for calibration purposes, but because of their limited wavelengths, they are not practical for absorbance measurements.

Mercury arc lamps emit an intense 254-nm resonance line and are widely used as detectors in high-pressure liquid chromatography (HPLC) (see Chapter 19). Alternatively, some HPLCs use a miniature hollow cathode lamp as a very narrow wavelength intense source. For example, a zinc hollow cathode lamp emits a line at 214 nm that is close to the maximum wavelength of peptide bond absorption (206 nm); this emission property permits the usage of such lamps to measure peptides and proteins. Details on the hollow cathode lamp are found in the section on Atomic Absorption Spectrophotometry. The hollow cathode lamp also has a long, useful lifetime if a lower current, nonpulsed power supply is used.

Laser sources. A laser (light amplification by stimulated emission of radiation) is a device that controls the way that energized atoms release photons; lasers are used as light sources in spectrophotometers because they provide intense light of a narrow wavelength. Through selection of different materials, different wavelength(s) of light are emitted by different types of lasers (Table 16.3).

Three properties of laser sources distinguish them from "conventional" sources: (1) spatial coherence is a property of lasers that allows beam diameters in the range of several micrometers; (2) lasers produce monochromatic light; and (3) lasers have pulse widths that vary from microseconds (flash lamp–pulsed lasers) to nanoseconds (nitrogen lasers) to picoseconds or less (mode-locked lasers) in duration. Air-cooled argon ion lasers produce approximately 25 mW of energy output at 488 nm and have plasma tube lifetimes of 6000 hours or longer. Continuous-wave dye lasers typically use an argon ion laser with an output of 1 W or less as an energy pump and use different fluorescent dyes to achieve excitation wavelength ranges of 400 to 800 nm. Helium-neon and helium-cadmium lasers are useful because of their low cost and ease of operation, and because they emit a number of excitation wavelengths; however, the power output of helium-neon lasers has been limited to approximately 2 mW at 594 nm.

Diode lasers are used in compact disc players and laser printers, and in bar code readers (see Chapter 29). They are solid-state devices, typically constructed of gallium arsenide, and energy is pumped into them at a low potential of −1.5 V. Depending on its construction, the wavelength output of the laser ranges from 350 to 29,000 nm. Development of inexpensive near-IR lasers has led to interest in using reflective techniques in the near-IR region of the spectrum (0.8- to 2.5-μm wavelength). Reflectance spectrophotometry is now used clinically for the transcutaneous measurement of bilirubin in neonates (see Chapter 51).[1] Another application of reflectance spectrophotometry is measurement of blood oxygen saturation in near-IR and IR regions.

Spectral isolation. Radiant energy of a desired wavelength can be isolated and that of other wavelengths excluded in various ways, including the use of (1) filters (interference or dichroic filters), (2) prisms, and (3) diffraction gratings. Combinations of lenses and slits may be inserted before or after the monochromatic device to render light rays parallel or to isolate narrow portions of the light beam. Variable slits may be used to permit adjustments in total radiant energy to reach the photocell.

Filters. The simplest type of filter is a thin layer of colored glass. Certain metal complexes or salts, dissolved or suspended in glass, produce colors corresponding to the predominant wavelengths transmitted. The spectral purity of a filter or other monochromator is usually described in terms of its spectral bandwidth. This is defined as the width, in nanometers, of the spectral transmittance curve at a point equal to one half the peak transmittance. Glass filters have spectral bandwidths of approximately 50 nm, and are referred to as wide bandpass filters.

Other glass filters include narrow bandpass and sharp cutoff types. Operationally, a cutoff filter typically shows a sharp rise in transmittance over a narrow portion of the spectrum and is used to eliminate light below a given wavelength. Historically, narrow bandpass filters were constructed by combining two or more sharp cutoff filters or regular filters. Currently, however, the availability of high-intensity light sources now favors the use of narrow bandpass interference filters.

A narrow bandpass interference or dichroic filter uses a dielectric material of controlled thickness sandwiched between two thinly silvered pieces of glass. The thickness of the layer determines the wavelength of energy transmitted after constructive and destructive wavelength interference caused by reflections between the glass surfaces separated by the dielectric spacing. These filters have narrow spectral bandwidths, usually from 5 to 15 nm. Because they also transmit harmonics, or multiples, of the desired wavelength, accessory glass filters are required to eliminate undesired wavelengths. For example, an interference filter designed for 620 nm will also transmit some radiation at 310 and 1240 nm unless accessory cutoff filters are provided to absorb this undesired stray light.

TABLE 16.3 Various Types of Lasers and the Wavelengths at Which They Operate

Laser	Wavelengths (nm)
Argon fluoride	193
Krypton fluoride	248
Helium-cadmium	325 or 442
Nitrogen	337
Argon (blue)	488
Argon (green)	514
Helium-neon (green)	543
Light-emitting diode (GaP)	550 or 700
Rhodamine 6G dye (tunable)	570–650
Laser diode (AlGaInP, AlGaAs)	633–1660
Helium-neon (red)	633
Ruby (CrAlO₃) (red)	694
Light-emitting diode (GaAs)	880
Light-emitting diode (Si)	1100
Neodymium-YAG (yttrium aluminum garnet)	1064
Carbon dioxide	9300, 9600, 10,300, or 10,600

AlGaInP, Aluminum gallium indium phosphide; *AlGaAs,* aluminum gallium arsenide; *GaAs,* gallium arsenide; *GaP,* gallium phosphide; *Si,* silicon.

Prisms and gratings. Prisms and diffraction gratings are widely used as monochromators. A prism separates white light into a continuous spectrum because shorter wavelengths are bent, or refracted, more than longer wavelengths as they pass through the prism. A diffraction grating is prepared by depositing a thin layer of aluminum-copper alloy on the surface of a flat glass plate, and then fabricating many small parallel grooves into the metal coating. Better gratings contain 1000 to 2000 lines/mm and must be made with great care. These are then used as molds to prepare less expensive replicas for general use in instruments.

Modern holographic gratings are made using a laser in a "high-precision machining" mode. The focused beam of the laser is accurately scanned over a photosensitive material termed a photoresist. After multiple lines have been scribed on the photoresist, chemicals are used to dissolve and elute the exposed photoresist to create channels that become the lines of the grating. A layer of a highly reflective material is then deposited onto the surface of the laser-etched channels, and the grating is then ready for use. A flat photoresistive surface or a concave surface can be used to make this type of grating. These types of gratings are extremely accurate, have low light scatter, and are widely used in the spectrophotometers found in clinical chemistry instruments. For example, most UV-visible spectrophotometers and virtually all IR spectrophotometers use reflective gratings. In addition, HPLC detectors frequently use a concave holographic reflective grating in their optical system.

Each line ruled on the grating, when illuminated, reflects light and gives rise to a tiny spectrum. An array of parallel wavefronts is formed that reinforce those wavelengths in phase and cancel those wavelengths not in phase. The net result is a uniform linear spectrum. Instruments contain diffraction gratings that produce spectral bandwidths in the range of 0.5 to 20 nm.

The flat surface grating discussed previously is called a plane transmission grating. Lines are engraved on the surface of a mirror, which may be a polished metal slab or a glass plate on which a thin, metallic film has been deposited. A grating may also be ruled at a specified angle, so that a maximum fraction of the radiant energy is directed into wavelengths diffracted at a selected angle. This type of grating is called an echelette and is said to have been given a blaze at a particular angle or to have been blazed at a certain wavelength (e.g., 250 nm).

Selection of a wavelength isolation device. The type of monochromator chosen depends on the analytical purpose for which it is to be used. For example, narrow spectral bandwidths are required in spectrophotometers for resolving and identifying sharp absorption peaks that are closely adjacent. Lack of agreement with Beer's law will occur when a part of the spectral energy transmitted by the monochromator is not absorbed by the substance being measured. This is more commonly observed with wide bandpass instruments. In practice, an increase in absorbance and improved linearity with concentration are usually observed with instruments that operate at narrower bandwidths of light. This is especially true for substances that exhibit a sharp peak of absorption.

The natural bandwidth of an absorbing substance is the bandwidth of the spectral absorbance at half the maximum absorbance. As a general rule, the spectral bandwidth should not exceed 10% of the natural bandwidth for peak absorbance readings to be within 99.5% of true values. For example, many chemistry procedures used in the clinical laboratory produce an absorbing species for which the natural bandwidth ranges from 40 to more than 200 nm. The natural bandwidth of nicotinamide adenine dinucleotide is 58 nm (λmax = 339 nm). Therefore for accurate measurements of this compound, a spectral bandwidth of 6 nm or less should be used.

In practice, the wavelength selected is usually at the peak of maximum absorbance to attain the maximum measurement; however, it may be desirable to choose another wavelength to minimize interfering substances. For example, turbidity readings on a spectrophotometer are greater in the blue region than in the red region of the spectrum, but the latter region is chosen for turbidity measurements to avoid absorption of light by bilirubin (460 nm) or hemoglobin (417 and 575 nm). The absorbing species developed in the alkaline picrate procedure for creatinine produces a relatively flat peak in the visible region of the spectrum at approximately 480 nm, but the reagent blank itself absorbs light strongly at less than 500 nm. A compromise is made by selecting a wavelength at 520 nm to minimize the contribution of the blank. Blank readings should be kept to a minimum. A small difference between two large numbers is subject to greater uncertainty; hence, minimizing absorbance of the blank improves precision and accuracy. The linear working range of a method can be expanded by not measuring at the peak absorbance. However, measurements should not be taken on the steep slope of an absorption curve, because a slight error in wavelength adjustment will introduce a significant error in absorbance readings.

Cuvets. A cuvet (also often termed a cuvette) is a small vessel used to hold a liquid sample to be analyzed in the light path of a spectrometer. Cuvets may be round, square, or rectangular, and are constructed from glass, silica (quartz), or plastic. Square or rectangular cuvets have plane-parallel optical surfaces and a constant light path. The most popular cuvets have a 1.0-cm light path, held to close tolerances. Ordinary borosilicate glass or plastic cuvets are suitable for measurements in the visible portion of the spectrum. However, quartz cells are usually required for readings at less than 340 nm. Some plastic cells have good clarity in both the visible and UV range, but they can present problems related to tolerances, cleaning, etching by solvents, and temperature deformations. Many plastic cuvets are designed for disposable, single-use applications. However, in many clinical analyzers, cuvets are cleaned and reused many times before optical degradation requires them to be replaced.

Cuvets must be clean and optically clear, because etching or deposits on the surface affect absorbance values. Cuvets used in the visible range are cleaned by copious rinsing with tap water and distilled water. Alkaline solutions should not be left standing in cuvets for prolonged periods, because alkali slowly dissolves glass and produces etching. Cuvets may be cleaned in mild detergent or soaked in a mixture of concentrated hydrogen chloride to water to ethanol (1:3:4). Cuvets should never be soaked in dichromate cleaning solution because the solution is hazardous and tends to adsorb onto and discolor the glass.

Cuvets used for measurements in the UV region should be handled with special care. Invisible scratches, fingerprints, or residual traces of previously measured substances may be present and may absorb significantly. A good practice is to fill all such cuvets with distilled water and measure the absorbance for each against a reference blank over the wavelengths to be used. This value should be essentially zero.

Photodetectors. A photodetector is a device that converts light into an electric signal that is proportional to the number of photons striking its photosensitive surface. The photomultiplier tube (PMT) is a commonly used photodetector for measuring light intensity in the UV and visible regions of the spectrum. Alternatively, photodiodes are solid-state devices that are also used in modern instruments. In older instruments, barrier layer cells (also known as photovoltaic cells) were used as photodetectors, because they were more durable and less expensive.

Photomultiplier tubes. A PMT contains (1) a cathode, (2) a light-sensitive metal, and (3) a series of dynodes, all of which are enclosed in an evacuated glass enclosure. As many as 10 to 15 stages or dynodes are present in common photomultipliers. Photons that strike the photoemissive cathode emit electrons that are accelerated toward the dynodes. Additional electrons are generated at each dynode. Depending on the number of dynodes and the accelerating voltage, the cascading effect creates 10^5 to 10^7 electrons for each photon hitting the first cathode. This amplified signal is finally collected at the anode, where it can be measured.

When such a tube is operated, voltage is applied between the photocathode and each successive stage. The normal incremental increase in voltage at each photomultiplier stage is from 50 to 100 V greater than that of the previous stage (Fig. 16.5). Typically, a conventional PMT tube has approximately 1500 V applied to it.

PMTs have (1) extremely rapid response times, (2) are very sensitive, and (3) are slow to fatigue. Because these tubes are very sensitive and have a rapid response, they must be carefully shielded from all stray light. A PMT with the voltage applied should never be exposed to room light because it will burn out. The rapid response times of PMTs are needed when a spectrophotometer is being used to determine an absorption spectrum of a compound. Also, PMTs are sensitive over a wide range of wavelengths.

When voltage is applied to a PMT in the absence of any incident light, some current is usually produced. This current is called dark current. It is desirable to have the dark current of a PMT at its lowest level because this current appears as background noise.

Photodiodes. Photodiodes are solid-state photodetectors that are fabricated from photosensitive semiconductor materials such as (1) silicon, (2) gallium arsenide, (3) indium antimonide, (4) indium arsenide, (5) lead selenide, and (6) lead sulfide. These materials absorb light over a characteristic wavelength range (e.g., 250 to 1100 nm for silicon). Their development and use as detectors in spectrophotometers have resulted in instruments capable of measuring light at a multitude of wavelengths. When a photodetector consists of two-dimensional arrays of diodes, it is known as a photodiode array. Each photodetector within the array responds to a specific wavelength. For example, photodiode arrays have been designed to have a 2-nm resolution per diode from 200 to 340 nm, and a 1-nm resolution per diode from 340 to 800 nm.

In practice, all diodes are initially charged to 5 V, and they discharge when they are struck by light. Each diode then is

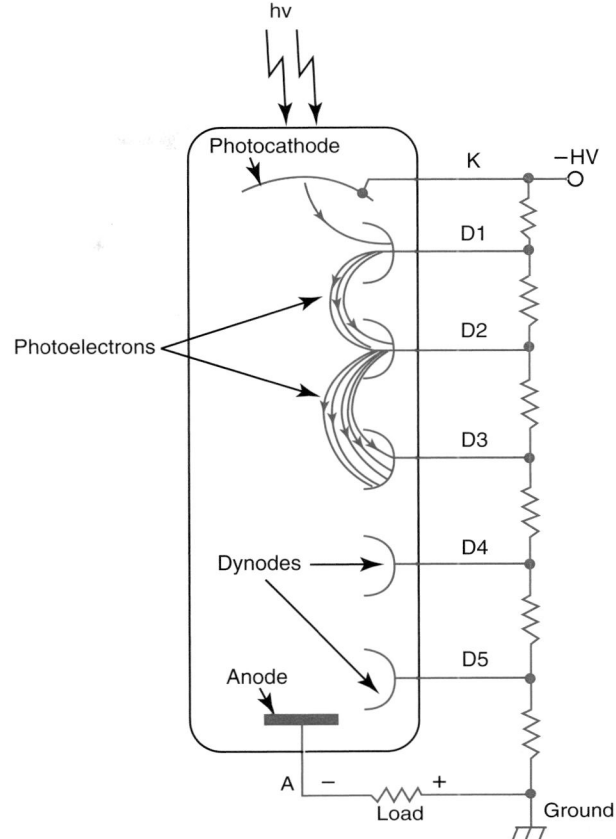

Figure 16.5 Schematic diagrams of a glass photomultiplier tube. Energy from photons of light (hv) are converted into electrons at the photocathode. Electrons from the photocathode travel to the chain of dynodes *(D1, D2, D3, D4, D5)* (HV, high voltage). At each dynode, additional electrons are generated, leading to a multiplying effect. The photoelectrons terminate at the anode.

sequentially scanned and recharged to 5 V. The amount of energy required for recharging is proportional to the quantity of light striking that diode. Because scan time for all diodes is in the millisecond range, many scans are typically taken. The resultant data are processed using a variety of algorithms, including signal averaging, background subtraction, and correction for scattered light. Consequently, an optical spectrum of an ongoing chemical reaction can be monitored as a function of time with a high degree of resolution and accuracy.

Readout devices. Electrical energy from a detector is displayed on some type of meter or readout system. In the past, analog devices were widely used as readout devices in spectrophotometers. However, they have been replaced by digital readout devices that provide a visual numeric display of absorbance or converted values of concentrations. Spectrophotometers may be equipped with recorders in addition to or instead of a digital display. These are synchronized to provide line traces of transmittance or absorbance as a function of time or wavelength. When a continuous tracing of absorbance versus wavelength is recorded, the resultant display is called an absorption spectrum. If a substance absorbs light, distinct peaks of absorbance will be observed (see Fig. 16.1). Measuring the absorption spectra of an unknown sample and comparing them with spectra from known compounds is useful for qualitative purposes. For example, this type of procedure is especially useful for identification of drugs that absorb in the UV region.

Performance Parameters

In most spectrophotometric analytical procedures, the absorbance of an unknown is compared directly with that of a calibrator or a series of calibrators. Under these circumstances, minor errors in wavelength calibration, variation in spectral bandwidths, and the presence of stray light are compensated for and usually do not contribute serious errors. Use of a series of calibrators covering a wide range of concentrations also provides a measure of linearity (i.e., agreement with Beer's law for a given procedure and instrument). However, when calculations are based on published or previously determined values for molar absorptivities or absorption coefficients, the spectrophotometer must be checked more rigorously. Performance verification of spectrophotometers on a periodic basis also improves reliability of routine comparative analyses.

To verify that a spectrophotometer is performing satisfactorily, the following parameters should be tested: (1) wavelength accuracy, (2) spectral bandwidth, (3) stray light, (4) linearity, and (5) photometric accuracy.

The National Institute of Standards and Technology (NIST) provides several standard reference materials (SRMs) for spectrophotometry that are useful in the calibration or verification of the performance of photometers or spectrophotometers (e.g., SRM 930e is for the verification and calibration of the transmittance and absorbance scales of visible absorption spectrometers) (http://www.nist.gov/srm).

The Institute for Reference Materials and Measurements (IRMM) belongs to the European Commission and provides reference materials for verification of the performance of photometers or spectrophotometers. These materials are listed in the Joint Research Centre's Reference Materials Catalogue (https://ec.europa.eu/jrc/en/reference-materials).

Wavelength calibration. With narrow spectral bandwidth instruments, a holmium oxide glass may be scanned over the range of 280 to 650 nm. This material shows sharp absorbance peaks at defined wavelengths, and the operator may compare the wavelength scale readings that produce maximum absorbance with established values. If compared values do not coincide, a calibration correction table can be constructed to relate scale readings to true wavelengths. A typical spectral transmittance curve for holmium oxide glass is shown in Fig. 16.6. Selected absorption peaks for this filter, which are suitable for calibration purposes, occur at the following wavelengths: 360, 418, 445, 453, 460, 536, and 637 nm. Solutions of holmium oxide in dilute perchloric acid have also been recommended and may be used with any spectrophotometer.

With broader bandpass instruments, a didymium filter may be used to verify wavelength settings. These filters should show a minimum percent transmittance at 530 nm against an air blank (Fig. 16.7). Because didymium has several absorption peaks, the setting should be verified grossly by visual examination of transmitted light. This light should appear green at 530 nm.

Spectral bandwidth. The apparent width of an emission band at half-peak height is taken to be the spectral bandwidth

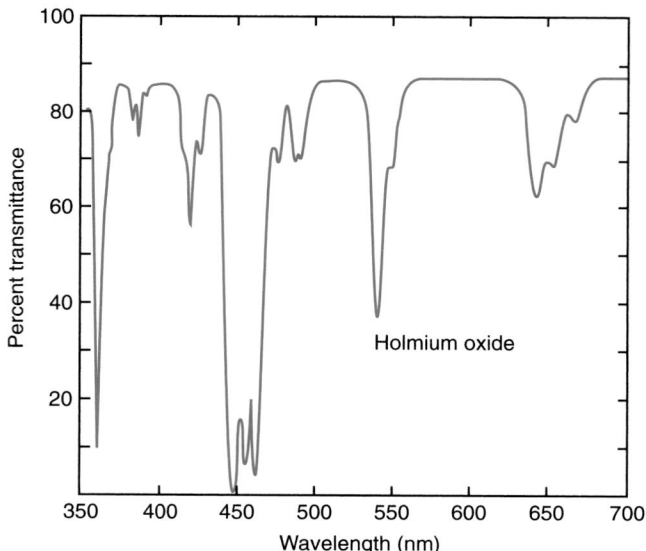

FIGURE 16.6 Spectral transmittance curve of holmium oxide filter.

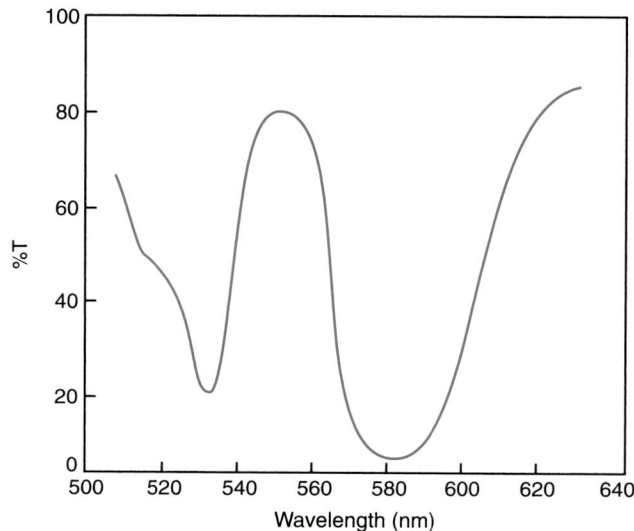

FIGURE 16.7 Spectral transmittance curve of a didymium filter (Perkin-Elmer Model 35 spectrophotometer, 8-nm nominal spectral bandwidth).

of the instrument. The spectral bandwidth may also be calculated from the manufacturer's specifications. Interference filters with spectral bandwidths of 1 to 2 nm are available and may be used to check those instruments with a nominal spectral bandwidth of 8 nm or more.

Stray light. Stray light, in general terms, is radiation of wavelengths outside the narrow band nominally transmitted by the monochromator that hits the detector. A perfect monochromator would transmit light only within its bandpass. In practice, scattering and diffraction inside the monochromator generate light of other wavelengths into the exit beam. This light is further modified by other components of the spectrophotometer and by the sample itself. Stray light is usually defined as a ratio or percent to the total detected light.

Other sources of unwanted light include light leaks and fluorescence of the sample. Light leaks should be excluded by covering the cell compartments. Light arising from fluorescence can increase the signal to the detector and cause an apparent decrease in absorbance. These sources of light are not included in the usual definition of stray light.

The major effect of stray light on the performance of a spectrophotometer is an absorbance error, especially in the upper end of the absorbance range of the instrument. Most spectrophotometers are equipped with one or more stray-light filters. Thus a blue filter is used with a tungsten lamp for wavelength settings below approximately 400 nm. For example, when the spectrophotometer is set to 350 nm, most of the stray light is of wavelengths in the visible range. The blue filter absorbs most of the visible light but transmits well in the UV portion of the spectrum. Similarly, a red filter is used for wavelengths in the range of 650 to 800 nm.

Cutoff filters are satisfactory for the detection of stray light. These may be of glass, similar to the stray-light filters discussed previously, and produce a sharp cut in the spectrum, with almost complete absorption on one side and high transmittance on the other. Liquid cutoff filters are satisfactory and convenient in the UV range, where stray light is usually more of a problem. A 50 g/L aqueous solution of sodium nitrite should show essentially 0% T when read against water over the range of 300 to 385 nm. Acetone, read against water, should show 0% T over the range of 250 to 320 nm.

Photometric accuracy. Neutral density filters (e.g., SRM 1930; NIST) are used to check an instrument's photometric accuracy. In addition, solutions of potassium dichromate ($K_2Cr_2O_7$) may be used for overall checks on photometric accuracy. In practice, analytical reagent grade $K_2Cr_2O_7$ is dried at 110 °C for 1 hour, and then the following solutions in 0.005 mol/L sulfuric acid are prepared: (1) solution A: 0.0500 g/L for the absorbance range from 0.2 to 0.7; and (2) solution B: 0.1000 g/L for the absorbance range from 0.4 to 1.4.

Measurements are made in 10-mm cells with the temperature controlled in the range of 15 to 25 °C, using 0.005 mol/L sulfuric acid as the reference. Table 16.4 gives the expected values for the two absorbance maxima and minima of the solutions based on literature values. Because the natural bandwidth of solution A at 350 nm is approximately 63 nm, the values shown are applied strictly to spectrophotometers with a spectral bandwidth of 6 nm or less.

Multiple-wavelength readings. Background interference due to interfering chromogens can often be eliminated or minimized by inclusion of blanks or by reading absorbance at two or three wavelengths. In one approach, termed bichromatic,

absorbance is measured at two wavelengths—one corresponding to peak absorbance and another at a point near the base of the peak that serves as a baseline. The difference in absorbance at the two wavelengths is related to concentration.

Before the correction is used, knowledge of the shape of the absorption curve for the substance of interest and of the interference is required. The linearity of the baseline shift should be verified by measuring the absorption spectrum of commonly encountered interferences. Care should be exercised in the use of the correction because if it is not properly used, it may introduce larger errors than would be observed without correction. For example, such a situation may occur if the background reading is not linear over the region measured.

REFLECTANCE PHOTOMETRY

In reflectance photometry, diffuse reflected light is measured. The reaction mixture in a carrier is illuminated with diffused light, and the intensity of the reflected light from the chromogen is compared with the intensity of light reflected from a reference surface. Because the intensity of reflected light is nonlinear in relation to the concentration of the analyte, the Kubelka-Munk equation or the Clapper-Williams transformation is commonly used to convert the data into a linear format. The electro-optical components used in reflectance photometry are essentially the same as those required for absorbance photometry, except that the geometry of the system is modified so that the light source and the detector are located next to each other on one side of the sample, as opposed to on opposite sides of the sample cuvet, as in absorption photometry. Reflectance photometry is used as the measurement method with dry-film chemistry systems.

FLAME EMISSION, INDUCTIVELY COUPLED PLASMA SPECTROPHOTOMETRY, AND ATOMIC ABSORPTION SPECTROSCOPY

Flame emission spectrophotometry is based on the characteristic emission of light by atoms of many metallic elements when given sufficient energy, such as that supplied by a hot flame. The wavelength to be used for the measurement of an element depends on the selection of a line of sufficient intensity to provide adequate sensitivity and freedom from other interfering lines at or near the selected wavelength. For example, lithium produces a red, sodium a yellow, potassium a violet, rubidium a red, and magnesium a blue color in a flame. These colors are characteristic of the metal atoms that are present as cations in solution. Under constant and controlled conditions, the light intensity of the characteristic wavelength produced by each of the atoms is directly proportional to the number of atoms that are emitting energy, which in turn is directly proportional to the concentration of the substance of interest in the sample. Although this technique once was used widely for analysis of sodium, potassium, and lithium in body fluids, it now has been replaced largely by electrochemical techniques.

Inductively coupled plasma (ICP) atomic emission spectroscopy is a technique for elemental analysis (e.g., trace metals) that uses an ICP to produce excited species that emit light at wavelengths characteristic of a particular element present in the sample. An ICP spectrometer consists of an optical

Wavelength (nm)	ABSORBANCE	
	Solution A	Solution B
235 (min)	0.626 ± 0.009	1.251 ± 0.019
257 (max)	0.727 ± 0.007	1.454 ± 0.015
313 (min)	0.244 ± 0.004	0.488 ± 0.007
350 (max)	0.536 ± 0.005	1.071 ± 0.011

TABLE 16.4 Absorbance Values for Acidic Potassium Dichromate Solutions on a Calibrated Spectrophotometer

spectrometer and an ICP torch. The torch produces argon gas plasma (10,000 K) using a radiofrequency induction coil and an electric spark. A nebulized sample is injected into the argon gas plasma; elements in the sample become excited, and the electrons emit energy at a characteristic wavelength as they return to ground state. The emitted light is then measured by optical spectrometry.

Atomic absorption (AA) spectroscopy is used in clinical laboratories to measure elements such as aluminum, calcium, copper, lead, lithium, magnesium, zinc, and other metals. A method for metal analysis that has begun to replace AA is inductively coupled plasma mass spectrometry (ICP-MS). AA retains advantages over ICP-MS in terms of overall cost and ease of use. However, a single ICP-MS instrument has greater flexibility in measuring multiple metals simultaneously and with greater sensitivity (see Chapters 39 and 44).

Basic Concepts

AA is an absorption spectrophotometric technique in which a metallic atom in the sample absorbs light of a specific wavelength. However, the element is not appreciably excited in the flame, but is merely dissociated from its chemical bonds (atomized) and placed in an unexcited or ground state (neutral atom). Thus the ground state atom absorbs radiation at a very narrow bandwidth corresponding to its own line spectrum. A hollow cathode lamp with the cathode made of the material to be analyzed is used to produce a wavelength of light specific for the atom. Thus if the cathode were made of sodium, sodium light at predominantly 589 nm would be emitted by the lamp. When the light from the hollow cathode lamp enters the flame, some of it is absorbed by the ground-state atoms in the flame, resulting in a net decrease in the intensity of the beam from the lamp. This process is referred to as atomic absorption.

A specific hollow cathode lamp serves as the light source, and the sample heated in the flame is the sample in the cuvet. The path length of the flame is the light path through the cuvet. Hence, most of the atoms are in the ground state and are able to absorb light emitted by the cathode lamp. In general, AA methods are approximately 100 times more sensitive than flame emission methods. In addition, because of the unique specificity of the wavelength from the hollow cathode lamp, these methods are highly specific for the element being measured.

Instrumentation

Fig. 16.8 shows the basic components of an AA spectrophotometer. The hollow cathode lamp is made of the metal of the substance to be analyzed and is different for each metal analysis. In some cases, an alloy is used to make the cathode, resulting in a multielement lamp. The hollow cathode lamp usually contains argon or neon gas at a pressure of a few

millimeters of mercury. An argon-filled lamp produces a blue-to-purple glow during operation, and the neon produces a reddish-orange glow inside the hollow cathode lamp. Quartz, or a special glass that allows transmission of the proper wavelength, is used as a window. A current is applied between the two electrodes inside the hollow cathode lamp, and metal is deposited from the cathode into the gases inside the glass envelope. When the metal atoms collide with the neon or argon gases, they lose energy and emit their characteristic radiation. Calcium has a sharp, intense, analytical emission line at 422.7 nm, which is used most frequently for calcium analysis. In an ideal interference-free system, only calcium atoms absorb the calcium light from the hollow cathode as it passes through the flame.

A pulsed hollow cathode lamp and a tuned amplifier are incorporated into most AA instruments. Operationally, the power to the hollow cathode lamp is pulsed, so that light is emitted by the lamp at a certain number of pulses per second. In contrast, all of the light originating from the flame is continuous. When light leaves the flame, it is composed of pulsed, unabsorbed light from the lamp and a small amount of nonpulsed flame spectrum and sample emission light. The detector senses all light, but the amplifier is electrically tuned to the pulsed signals and can subtract the background light measured when the lamp is off and the total light that includes both the lamp and flame background light. In this way, the electronics, in conjunction with the monochromator, discriminates between the flame background emission and the sample AA.

Fig. 16.9 shows a laminar flow premix burner and illustrates how the sample is aspirated, volatilized, and burned to form atoms of the metal in the gas phase. Note that the gases are mixed and the sample is atomized before it is burned. An advantage of this system is that the larger droplets go to waste while the fine mist enters the flame, thus producing a less noisy signal.

In flameless AA techniques (carbon rod or "graphite furnace"), the sample is placed in a depression on a carbon rod in an enclosed chamber. Strips of tantalum or platinum metal may also be used as sample cups. In successive steps, the temperature of the rod is raised to dry, char, and, finally, atomize the sample into the gas phase in the chamber. The atomized element then absorbs energy from the corresponding hollow cathode lamp. This approach is more sensitive than conventional flame methods and permits determination of trace metals in small samples of blood or tissue.

With flameless AA, a novel approach used to correct for background absorption is called the Zeeman correction.[2] In Zeeman background correction, the light source or the atomizer is placed in a strong magnetic field. In practice, because Zeeman correction requires special lamps, the analyte is placed in the magnetic field. The intense magnetic field splits

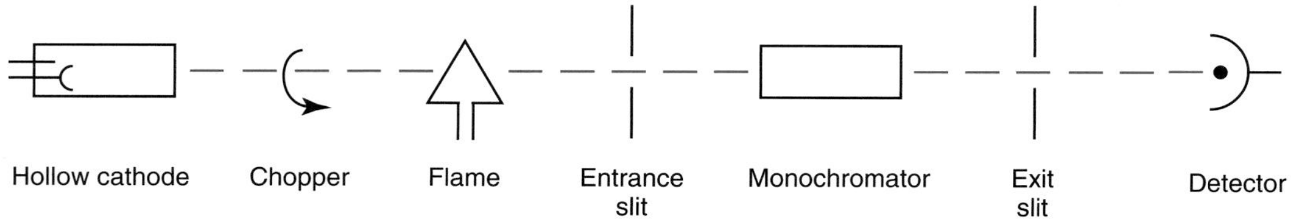

FIGURE 16.8 Basic components of an atomic absorption spectrophotometer.

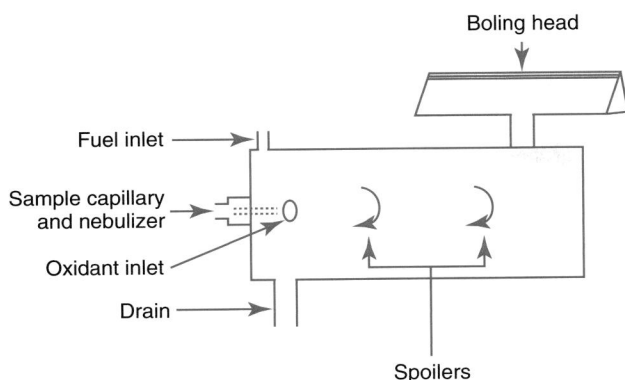

FIGURE 16.9 Laminar flow pre-mix burner.

the degenerate (i.e., of equal energy) atomic energy levels into two components that are polarized parallel and perpendicular to the magnetic field, respectively. The parallel component is at the resonance line of the source, whereas the two perpendicular components are shifted to different wavelengths. The two components interact differently with polarized light. A polarizer is placed between the source and the atomizer, and two absorption measurements are taken at different polarizer settings. One measures both analyte and background absorptions, A_t, the other only the background absorption, A_{bc}. The difference between the two absorption readings is the corrected absorbance.

The major advantage of the Zeeman correction method is that the same light source at the same wavelength is used to measure the total and the background absorption. The implementation is complex and expensive, and the strength of the magnetic field needs to be optimized for every element, but the method gives more accurate results at higher background levels than those attained with the other correction techniques.

Interferences in Atomic Absorption Spectrophotometry

Interferences in AA spectroscopy are divided into spectral and nonspectral interferences.

Spectral Interferences

Spectral interferences include absorption by other closely absorbing atomic species, absorption by molecular species, scattering by nonvolatile salt particles or oxides, and background emission (which can be electronically filtered). Absorption by other atomic species usually is not a problem because of the extremely narrow bandwidth (0.01 nm) used in the absorption measurements. Absorption and scattering by molecular species are particularly problematic in lower atomizing temperatures.

Nonspectral Interferences

Nonspectral interferences may be nonspecific or specific. Nonspecific interferences affect nebulization by altering the viscosity, surface tension, or density of the analyte solution, and consequently, the sample flow rate. Certain contaminants also decrease desolvation and atomization efficiency by lowering the atomizer temperature. Specific interferences are also called chemical interferences because they are more analyte dependent. Solute volatilization interference refers to the situation in which the contaminant forms nonvolatile species

with the analyte. An example is phosphate interference in the determination of calcium that is caused by the formation of calcium–phosphate complexes. The phosphate interference is overcome by adding a cation, usually lanthanum or strontium; the cation competes with the calcium for the phosphate. Enhancement effects are also observed, in which the addition of contaminants increases the volatilization efficiency. Such is the case with aluminum, which normally forms nonvolatile oxides, but in the presence of hydrofluoric acid forms more volatile aluminum fluoride. Dissociation interferences affect the degree of dissociation of the analyte. Analytes that form oxides or hydroxides are especially susceptible to dissociation interferences. Ionization interference occurs when the presence of an easily ionized element, such as potassium, affects the degree of ionization of the analyte, which leads to changes in the analyte signal. Ionization interference is controlled by adding a relatively high concentration of an element that is easily ionized to maintain a more consistent concentration of ions in the flame and to suppress ionization of the analyte. In the case of excitation interference, the analyte atoms are excited in the atomizer, with subsequent emission at the absorption wavelength. This type of interference is more pronounced at higher temperatures.

FLUOROMETRY

Fluorescence refers to the condition where a molecule absorbs light at one wavelength and reemits light at a longer wavelength. An atom or molecule that fluoresces is termed a fluorophore. Fluorometry is defined as the measurement of emitted fluorescent light. Fluorometric analysis is widely used for quantitative measurement in the chemical and biological sciences due to its high accuracy and sensitivity.

Basic Concepts

Fig. 16.10 illustrates the relationship among absorption, fluorescence, and phosphorescence. As indicated, each molecule contains a series of closely spaced energy levels. Absorption

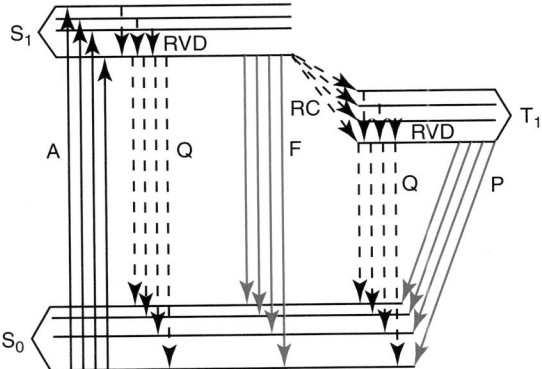

FIGURE 16.10 Luminescence energy-level diagram of typical organic molecule. *A*, Absorption process; *F*, fluorescence process from the first excited singlet state; *P*, phosphorescence process from the first excited triplet state; *Q*, quenching of the excited singlet or triplet state; *RC*, radiation-less crossover from the first excited singlet state to the first excited triplet state; *RVD*, radiation-less vibrational deactivation; *S₀*, ground-level singlet state; *S₁*, first excited singlet state; *T₁*, first excited triplet state.

of a quantum of light energy by a molecule causes the transition of an electron from the singlet ground state to one of a number of possible vibrational levels of its first singlet state. The actual number of molecules in the excited state under typical reaction conditions and excited with a typical 150-W light source is very small and is estimated to be approximately 10^{-13} mol/mol of fluorophore. Once the molecule is in an excited state, it returns to its original energy state in several ways. These include (1) radiation-less vibrational equilibration, (2) the fluorescence process from the excited singlet state, (3) quenching of the excited singlet state, (4) radiation-less crossover to a triplet state, (5) quenching of the first triplet state, and (6) the phosphorescence process of light emission from the triplet state.

As shown in Fig. 16.10, vibrational equilibration before fluorescence results in some loss of the excitation energy. The emitted fluorescence is therefore of less energy or has a longer wavelength than the excitation light. The difference between the maximum wavelength of the excitation light and the maximum wavelength of the emitted fluorescence is a constant referred to as the Stokes shift. This constant is a measure of energy lost during the lifetime of the excited state (radiation-less vibrational deactivation) before returning to the ground singlet level (fluorescence emission).

Time Relationships of Fluorescence Emission

The time required for a molecule to absorb radiant energy and to be promoted to an excited state is approximately 10^{-15} s. The length of time for vibrational equilibration to occur to the lowest excited state is 10^{-14} to 10^{-12} s. The length of time required for fluorescence emission to occur is 10^{-8} to 10^{-7} s. Relatively speaking, there is a considerable time delay among the (1) absorption of light energy, (2) return to the lowest excited state, and (3) emission of light energy. This time relationship is shown in Fig. 16.11. In this figure, phase I represents the time period between the absorbance of light energy and the radiation-less loss of energy during vibrational rearrangement to the lowest excited energy state. This time period is represented by the up and down arrows in the diagram. Phase II shows the emission and decay of a (b) short- and (a) a long-lived fluorophore. If the fluorescence

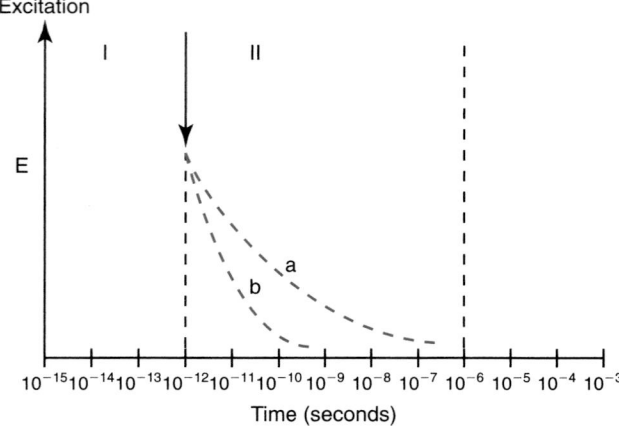

FIGURE 16.11 Fluorescence decay process. *a*, Long fluorescence decay time; *b*, short fluorescence decay time; *E*, absorption of energy; *I*, vibrational deactivation time phase; *II*, fluorescence emission time phase.

emission is measured over time following a pulse of light from an excitation source, such as a xenon lamp or laser, the intensity of the emitted light decays as a first-order process similar to radioactive decay (i.e., phase II of Fig. 16.11). The time required for the emitted light to reach $1/e$ of its initial intensity, where e is the Naperian base 2.718, is called the average lifetime of the excited state of the molecule, or the fluorescence decay time.

The time delay between absorption of quanta of energy and fluorescence is used in fluorescence instrumentation called time-resolved fluorometers. Advantages of a time-resolved fluorometer include the elimination of background light scattering due to Rayleigh and Raman signals and a short-lived fluorescence background with a consequent dramatic increase in signal-to-noise and detection sensitivity.

Time-resolved fluorometry[3] falls into one of two categories, depending on how the fluorescence emission response is measured: (1) pulse fluorometry, in which the sample is illuminated with an intense brief pulse of light and the intensity of the resulting fluorescence emission is measured as a function of time with a fast detector system; or (2) phase fluorometry, in which a continuous-wave laser illuminates the sample, and the fluorescence emission response is monitored for impulse and frequency response.

Relationship of Concentration and Fluorescence Intensity

The relationship of concentration to the intensity of fluorescence emission is derived from the Beer-Lambert law. By expansion through a Taylor series, rearrangement, logarithm base conversion, and basic assumptions about dilute solutions, the following equation is obtained:

$$F = \varphi[I_0(2.3 - abc)] \tag{16.8}$$

where F = relative fluorescence intensity; φ = fluorescence efficiency (i.e., the ratio between quanta of light emitted and quanta of light absorbed); I_0 = initial excitation intensity; a = molar absorptivity; b = volume element defined by geometry of the excitation and emission slits; and c = the concentration in moles per liter.

Eq. (16.8) indicates that fluorescence intensity is directly proportional to the concentration of the fluorophore and the excitation intensity. This relationship holds only for dilute solutions, in which absorbance is less than 2% of the exciting radiation; the fluorescence intensity becomes nonlinear as the absorbance of the solution increases to greater than 2% of the exciting radiation. This phenomenon, called the inner filter effect, is discussed in more detail in a later section. Other factors influencing the measurement of fluorescence intensity include the sensitivity of the detector and the degree of background light scatter seen by the detector.

Fluorescence intensity measurements are more sensitive than absorbance measurements. The magnitude of absorbance of a chromophore in solution is determined by its concentration and the path length of the cuvet. The magnitude of fluorescence intensity of a fluorophore is determined by its concentration, the path length, and the intensity of the light source. The sensitivity of fluorescence measurements can be 100 to 1000 times greater than the sensitivity of absorbance measurements using more intense light sources, digital signal filtering techniques, and sensitive emission photometers. All of these are incorporated into conventional spectrofluorometric instrumentation, described later in this chapter.

Frequently, fluorescence measurements are expressed in units of relative intensity (relative fluorescence unit [RFU]). The word *relative* is used because the intensity measured is not an absolute quantity. It is a small part of the total fluorescence emission, and its magnitude is defined by the instrument slit width, detector sensitivity, monochromator efficiency, and excitation intensity. Because these are instrument-related variables, establishing an absolute intensity unit for a given concentration of a fluorophore that is valid from instrument to instrument is difficult, if not impossible.

Fluorescence Polarization

Light is composed of electrical and magnetic waves at right angles to each other. Light waves produced by standard excitation sources have their electrical vectors oriented randomly. Light waves, passed through certain crystalline materials (polarizers), have their electrical vectors oriented in a single plane and are said to be plane-polarized. Fluorophores absorb light most efficiently in the plane of their electronic energy levels. If their rotational relaxation (Brownian movement) is slower than their fluorescence decay time, as is the case for large, fluorescent-labeled molecules, the emitted fluorescence light will remain polarized. Because small molecules have rotational relaxation times that are much shorter than their fluorescence decay time, their emitted fluorescence light is depolarized. However, if the small fluorescent molecule is attached to a macromolecule, or if it is placed in a viscous solution, the small molecule will emit polarized light. Fluorescence polarization, P, is defined by the following equation:

$$P = \frac{(I_v - I_h)}{(I_v + I_h)} \qquad (16.9)$$

where I_v = intensity of the emitted fluorescence light in the vertical plane, and I_h = intensity of the emitted fluorescence light in the horizontal plane.

As indicated, P is the difference between the two observed intensities divided by their sum. Fluorescence polarization is measured by placing a mechanically or electrically driven polarizer between the sample cuvet and the detector. A diagram of a fluorescence polarization measurement system is shown in Fig. 16.12. In the normal instrumentation mode, the sample is excited with polarized light to obtain maximum sensitivity. First, the polarization analyzer is positioned to measure the intensity of the emitted fluorescence light in the vertical plane (I_v), then the polarization analyzer is rotated 90° to measure the emitted fluorescence light intensity in the horizontal plane (I_h). P is then calculated manually or automatically by using Eq. (16.9).

Fluorescence polarization is used to quantitate analytes by using the change in fluorescence depolarization following immunologic reactions (see Chapter 26). Quantitation is accomplished by adding a known quantity of fluorescent-labeled analyte molecules to a reaction solution containing an antibody specific to the analyte. The labeled analyte binds to the antibody, and the slowed rotation and longer relaxation time results in an increased degree of fluorescence polarization. The addition of a nonlabeled analyte, such as an unknown quantity of a therapeutic drug in a serum specimen, will result in competition for binding to the antibody with the fluorescent-labeled analyte. This change in binding of the fluorophore-labeled analyte causes a change in

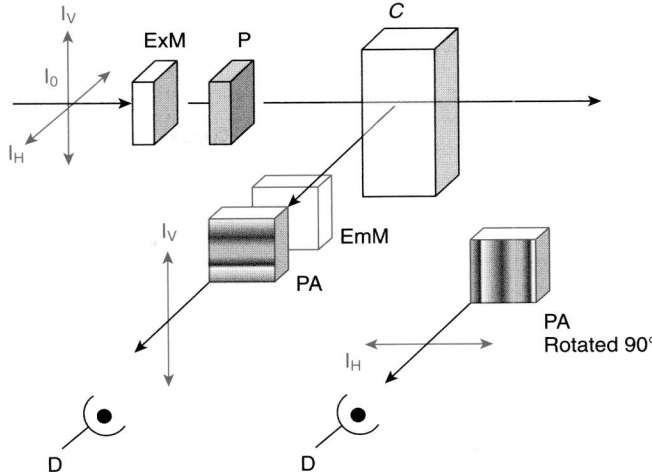

FIGURE 16.12 Schematic diagram of a fluorescence polarization analyzer. The nonpolarized excitation light *(I₀)* has both vertical *(Iᵥ)* and horizontal *(Iₕ)* components *(left)*. The light travels through excitation monochromator and polarizer to energize the sample in the cuvet. The light from the sample travels through the emission monochromator and polarizer analyzer as light in the vertical plane *Iᵥ*, which is measured by the detector. In contrast, when the polarizer analyzer has been rotated 90 degrees the light in the horizontal plane *Iₕ* is measured by the detector *(right)*. *C*, Reaction cell or cuvet; *D*, detector; *EmM*, emission monochromator; *ExM*, excitation monochromator; *P*, polarizer used to provide polarized excitation light; *PA*, polarizer analyzer, which is rotated to provide measurements of parallel and perpendicular polarized fluorescence emission intensity.

fluorescence polarization that is inversely proportional to the amount of analyte contained in a given sample. Because the change in fluorescence polarization is a direct response to the reaction mixture, the bound fluorophore need not be separated from free fluorophore. Thus fluorescence polarization is applicable to homogeneous assays of low-molecular-weight analytes, such as therapeutic drugs.[4]

Instrumentation

Fluorometers and spectrofluorometers are used to measure fluorescence and operationally may have similar components with absorption spectrophotometers.

Components

Basic components of fluorometers and spectrofluorometers include (1) an excitation source, (2) an excitation monochromator, (3) a cuvet, (4) an emission monochromator (EmM), and (5) a detector.

Excitation source. The absorption spectra of most fluorescent compounds of interest are in the spectral region of 300 to 700 nm. The fluorescence emission intensity is proportional to the initial excitation intensity and to the concentration and size of the volume element being measured in the sample cell. Therefore an intense lamp capable of emitting radiant energy over a large spectral region is desirable. Excitation sources used in fluorometers and spectrophotometers include xenon, quartz halogen, and mercury arc lamps and lasers. Some provide high-intensity spectra at one or more wavelengths; others provide a continuum over the spectral range of interest.

Xenon lamp. The xenon lamp is a popular excitation source because it provides a continuum of relatively high-intensity radiant energy over the spectral region of 250 to 800 nm. It is widely used for certain fluorescence applications because of its high energy output, stability of lamp flashes, and higher UV and visible spectral output. These flash lamps can be pulsed at rates up to 2500 pulses/s. Light output is typically in the 0.01- to 0.1-J interval, with a spectral distribution ranging from 250 to 800 nm. The life of flash lamps varies from 10^6 to 10^9 flashes, with spectral stability maintained throughout the life of the flash lamp. A limitation of xenon lamps for analytical use is arc wandering or flicker. However, the use of current-stabilized power supplies has minimized this problem and improved the performance of fluorescence instrumentation using xenon lamps.

Lasers. Laser sources (discussed earlier in the Spectrophotometry section) are widely used in fluorescence applications in which highly intense, well-focused, and essentially monochromatic light is required. Examples of these applications include time-resolved fluorometry, flow cytometry, pulsed laser confocal microscopy, laser-induced fluorometry, and light scattering measurements for particle size and shape. Several different types of lasers are available as an excitation source for fluorescence measurements (see Table 16.3).

Light-emitting diode. LEDs are similar to laser diodes in that they are both solid-state devices, which produce monochromatic light. However, LEDs are fabricated from different semiconductor materials and produce incoherent light, compared with the coherent, narrow wavelength of light from laser diodes.[5] Laser diodes are used for spectrophotometry and fluorometry applications where coherent, narrow wavelength light are preferred. Coherent light has not only the same wavelength (monochromatic) but also the same frequency (in phase). Incoherent light may have the same wavelength, but the photons are not at the same frequency (out of phase). LED light sources with incoherent light can be used instead of conventional light sources (mercury vapor lamp) in fluorescence microscopy.

Excitation and emission monochromators. Monochromators used in fluorescence instrumentation include interference filters, colored glass filters, gratings, and prisms. Most modern analytical instruments using interference filters use the all-dielectric multicavity filter or a hybrid Fabry-Perot–coupled dielectric layer filter (a filter with metal reflective layers). Either type of filter is combined with appropriate sharp cutoff glass filters to form a single filter package, which removes undesired transmission of higher orders and provides narrow bandwidth, higher peak wavelength transmission, and increased band slope. The increased slope of the spectral band makes the transition from peak transmission to nontransmission more abrupt, which is very important for the spectral separation of excitation and emission bands with a small Stokes shift.

Colored glass filters selectively absorb certain wavelengths of light. These filters have been used for both excitation and emission wavelength selection, but they are more susceptible to transmitting stray light and unwanted fluorescence.

Grating monochromators are devices that isolate regions of the spectrum. The spectral resolution of the light at the slit is a function of slit width and resolution of the grating. Spectrofluorometers generally use larger slit widths than absorbance spectrophotometers to obtain higher excitation

intensities. An advantage of the grating monochromator is that it provides selectivity of the excitation and emission wavelengths required when working with new fluorophores with absorbance and emission maxima for which specially fabricated interference filters may not exist. The rotation of the grating is digitally controlled when spectral scans of fluorescence excitation and emission are automated. In the conventional operation of a spectrofluorometer, the excitation wavelength or the emission wavelength is held constant, and the other is scanned. With more automated instrumentation, both excitation and EmMs are synchronized and scanned together at programmed rates. This provides a change in emission intensity as a function of change in excitation and emission wavelength and gives an additional dimension of specificity to fluorescence measurements. Because of their high degree of monochromaticity, lasers are used as both the excitation light source and the monochromator. When a laser is used as a combination excitation source and monochromator, a narrowband interference filter is usually placed before the detector to eliminate additional orders of emission.

Cuvet. As with spectrophotometers, cuvets are used in fluorometers and spectrofluorometers to hold the liquid sample to be analyzed. For fluorescence instruments, the cuvets used are typically square or rectangular, and are constructed from a material that allows the excitation and the emitting light to pass (glass or plastic for visible light; quartz for UV light). However, some plastic cuvets contain UV absorbers that fluoresce, causing unwanted background signal and loss of sensitivity.

With fluorometers and spectrofluorometers, placement of the cuvet and excitation beam relative to the photodetector is critical in establishing the optical geometry for fluorescence measurements. Because fluorescence is emitted in all directions from a molecule, several excitation and/or emission geometries are used to measure fluorescence (Fig. 16.13). Although the end-on approach allows the adaptation of a fluorescence detector to existing 180-degree absorption instruments, it is not widely used because its sensitivity is limited by the quality of the excitation and/or emission interference filter pair, the excitation and/or emission spectral band overlap, and the inner filter effect. In practice, most commercial spectrofluorometers and fluorometers use the right angle–detector approach because it minimizes the background signal that limits analytical sensitivity. The front surface approach provides the greatest linearity over a broad range of concentration because it minimizes the inner filter effect. The front surface approach shows similar sensitivity to the right-angle detectors but is more susceptible to background light scatter (see section on Inner Filter Effects). Front surface fluorometry has been widely applied to heterogeneous solid-phase fluorescence immunoassay systems.

To accommodate these different geometries, the sample cell is oriented at different angles in relation to the excitation source and the detector. Major concerns related to the geometry of the sample cell include light scattering, the inner filter effect, and the sample volume element seen by the detector. Fig. 16.14A shows the sample cell and slit arrangement for a conventional fluorescence spectrophotometer, with the excitation and emission slits oriented at a right angle. $Slit_1$ and $Slit_2$ designate the excitation and emission slits, respectively. The position of the emission slit and the width of the slit are important. If the emission slit is located near the front edge

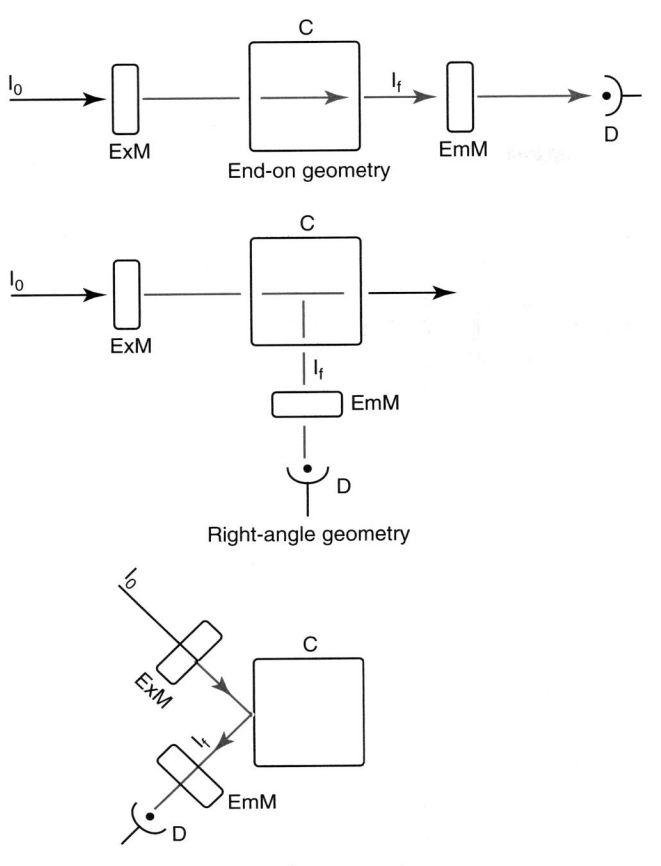

FIGURE 16.13 Fluorescence excitation/emission geometries. *C*, Sample cuvet; *D*, detector; *EmM*, emission monochromator; *ExM*, excitation monochromator; *I₀*, initial excitation energy; *Iᵢ*, fluorescence intensity.

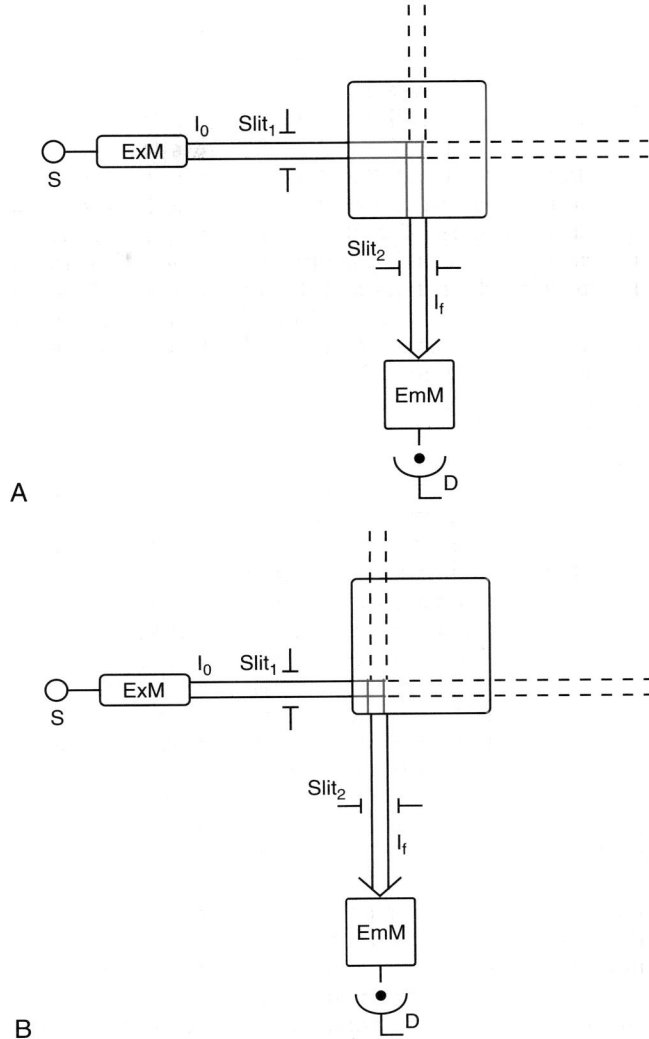

FIGURE 16.14 Two right-angle fluorescence sample cuvet positions. **A**, The standard 90-degree configuration. **B**, The offset positioning of the cuvet to minimize the inner filter effect. *D*, Detector; *ExM*, excitation monochromator; *EmM*, emission monochromator; *I₀*, Initial excitation energy; *Iᵢ*, fluorescence intensity; *S*, excitation source; *Slit₁*, excitation slit; *Slit₂*, emission slit.

of the sample cell, as shown in Fig. 16.14B, the inner filter effect is minimized. If the emission slit width is increased, sensitivity will increase, but specificity may decrease.

Photodetectors. As with spectrophotometric instruments, a number of devices are used as photodetectors in fluorometric instruments, including the PMT and the CCD. In addition, visual observation is used for some applications.

Visual observation. Because the human eye is a sensitive detector with a wide range of spectral recognition, qualitative fluorescent thin-layer chromatographic (TLC) methods in the clinical laboratory use short- and long-wavelength UV lamp sources coupled with visual observation. TLC is used as a routine screening method in analytical toxicology laboratories and in testing for counterfeit drugs in resource poor settings (Global Pharma Health Fund–Minilab).[6]

Photomultiplier tube. For quantitative assays, the most commonly used detector in fluorometers and spectrofluorometers is the PMT. Important features of the PMT for fluorescence measurements consist of (1) a wide choice of spectral responses, (2) nanosecond photon response time, and (3) sensitivity. Sensitivity is due to the possible gain of 10^6 electrons at the anode of the PMT for each incident photon hitting the photo cathode.

Depending on the light level (photon flux) striking the PMT cathode and the desired sensitivity, measurement of electron flow at the PMT anode is accomplished in different ways. At high light intensities, analog techniques for measurement of PMT current are used. The analog signal is converted to a digital signal for computer use or for panel digital display. At low light levels, spikes or pulses generated at the cathode of the PMT are counted. The number of pulses that occur per unit of time is directly proportional to the intensity of emitted fluorescence light striking the PMT. This method is called photon counting. The use of photon counting increases the signal-to-noise ratio and decreases the lower limit of detection of the measurement of fluorophores at low concentrations.

Charge-coupled detector. CCDs are multichannel devices with a dynamic range and a signal-to-noise ratio that is superior to those of PMTs; this enhanced sensitivity of CCDs has resulted in its implementation into diverse fields including astronomy.[7] These solid-state devices are composed of a large number of photo-detecting shift registers that are read horizontally and vertically. CCDs were first used for astronomy applications and in ground-based optical telescopes, in which sensitive low-light measurements are required. Because of their ability to detect low levels of light, they have been used for molecular fluorescence measurement of low concentrations of fluorescent molecules and as quantitative electronic imagers for quantitative confocal microscopy.[8] A data-reading technique called *binning* has been developed that allows multielement devices to have functional elements linked together, much like rectangular slit widths. A related solid-state device, the avalanche photodiode, is also finding use for low-level light detection as a detector in confocal microscopy.[8]

Performance Verification

As with spectrophotometers, NIST provides a number of SRMs for use in calibration or verification of the performance of fluorometers or fluorospectrophotometers. These include SRM 936a (quinine sulfate dihydrate) for calibrating such instruments and SRM 1932 (fluorescein) for establishing a reference scale for fluorescence measurements (http://www.nist.gov/srm).

Types of Fluorometers and Spectrofluorometers

Fluorometers and fluorescence spectrophotometers that offer a variety of features are available. These features include ratio referencing, microprocessor-controlled excitation and EmMs, pulsed xenon light sources, photon counting, rhodamine cells for corrected spectra, polarizers, flow cells, front-surface viewing adapters, multiple cell holders, and microprocessor-based data reduction systems.

In addition to the basic spectrofluorometer discussed earlier, other types of fluorometric instruments include a ratio-referencing spectrofluorometer, a time-resolved fluorometer, a flow cytometer, and a hematofluorometer.

Ratio-referencing spectrofluorometer. The xenon lamp energy source in single-beam spectrofluorometers is unstable (i.e., arc flicker and lamp decay). This is a source of laboratory error and requires frequent calibration. The unstable energy source in single-beam spectrofluorometry can be addressed by ratio-referencing spectrofluorometry. The ratio-referencing spectrofluorometer splits the energy from the light source to energize both a sample PMT and a reference PMT. Thus any instability of the energy source will affect both the reference and sample PMT and reduce the possibility of measurement error.

A typical ratio-referencing spectrofluorometer is illustrated in Fig. 16.15. Basically, this is a right-angle instrument that uses two monochromators (exciter monochromator [ExM] and EmM), two PMT detectors (D1 and D2, the reference, and sample PMTs), and a xenon lamp source. The light from the ExM is split, and a small portion (10%) is directed to the reference PMT (D1) for ratio-referencing purposes. The remaining excitation light is focused into the sample compartment. Emission optics are positioned at a right angle to the excitation optics. An EmM is used to select or scan the desired portion of the emission spectra, which is directed to the sample PMT (D2) for measurement of emission intensity. Output signals from the reference and sample PMTs are amplified, and the ratio of the sample to the reference signal is provided by a digital display or a chart recorder. The operational mode of a ratio fluorometer is similar to that of a spectrofluorometer; however, only discrete excitation and emission wavelengths are available, and use of this type of instrument is precluded from scanning fluorophores to obtain emission and excitation spectra. The ratio filter

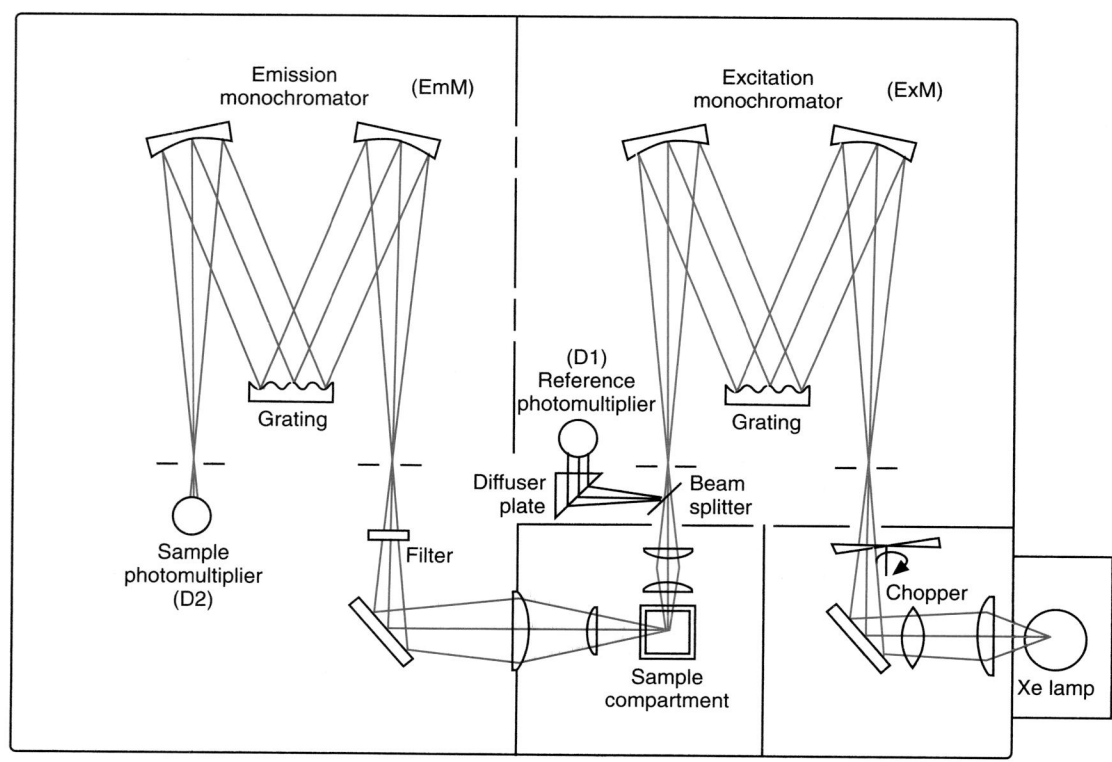

FIGURE 16.15 Diagram of a typical ratio-referencing spectrofluorometer. *Xe,* Xenon.

fluorometer is most useful for obtaining concentration measurements at defined excitation and emission wavelengths.

The ratio-referencing spectrofluorometer is operated at fixed excitation and emission wavelength settings for concentration measurements; alternatively, it is used to measure the excitation or emission spectrum of a given compound. Measurement of the concentration of a specimen is accomplished in a similar manner as with a single-beam fluorometer. A blank and a calibrating solution are measured first; then the unknown specimens are measured (see Fig. 16.15).

Time-resolved fluorometer. The time-resolved fluorometer[9] is similar to the ratio-referencing fluorometer, with the exceptions that the light source is pulsed, and the detector monitors the exponential decay of the fluorescence signal after excitation in a fast photon-counting mode. Time-resolved fluorometry requires the use of long-lived fluorophores, such as the lanthanide (rare earth) metal ions europium (Eu^{3+}) and samarium (Sm^{3+}). Although most fluorescence compounds have decay times of 5 to 100 ns, Eu^{3+} chelates decay in 0.6 to 100 s. Thus time-resolved fluorescence assays take advantage of the difference in lifetimes of fluorophore and background fluorescence by measuring the decaying fluorescence signal. This eliminates background interferences and at the same time averages the signal to improve the precision of measurement. Detection limits of approximately 10^{-13} mol/L can be achieved with time-resolved fluorometry; this is an improvement of approximately four orders of magnitude compared with conventional fluorometric measurements.

Flow cytometer. Cytometry refers to the measurement of physical and/or chemical characteristics of cells, or by extension, of other biological particles (for additional information on cytometry, refer to Chapter 28). Flow cytometry is a process in which such measurements are made while cells or particles pass, preferably in single file, through the measuring apparatus in a fluid stream. Flow sorting extends flow cytometry by using electrical or mechanical means to divert and collect cells with one or more measured characteristics that fall within a range or ranges of values set by the user.[10]

Operationally, flow cytometry combines laser-induced fluorometry with particle light scattering analysis that allows different populations of molecules, cells, or particles to be differentiated by size and shape using low-light and right-angle light scattering. The use of a laser is ideally suited for low-angle light scattering. These cells, molecules, or particles are labeled with specific fluorescent labels, such as β-phycoerythrin, fluorescein isothiocyanate, rhodamine-6G, and other dye-labeled antibodies. As they move in a fluid stream through the flow cell, simultaneous fluorescence and light scattering measurements are automatically performed by the flow cytometer. Most flow cytometers incorporate two or more fluorescence emission detection systems, so that multiple fluorescent labels can be used. In this manner, molecules, cells, or particles can be classified by size, shape, and type according to their light scattering and fluorescent properties. A schematic diagram of a flow cytometer is shown in Fig. 16.16. An optical stop is placed in the 180° beam after the flow capillary to block the main laser beam and permit low-angle forward light scattering measurements. The 90° emission signal is split and directed to two PMTs to determine right-angle light scattering and detect at least two separate fluorescence emission signals. Two narrow bandpass interference filters (530 and 596 nm) are placed in front of the two 90° fluorescence emission PMTs. A computer with substantial resident software is used to reduce the acquired data to appropriate histograms for final result reporting. Cell-sorting electrodes are shown in the schematic drawing. Most commercial flow cytometers use one or more laser light sources. For example, the LSR II (BD Biosciences, Rockville, Maryland) can be equipped with seven lasers (355 nm [UV], 405 nm [violet], 488 nm [blue], 532 nm [green], 594 nm [yellow], 638 nm [red], and 785 nm [IR]), which are used to simultaneously measure 18 emission spectra.

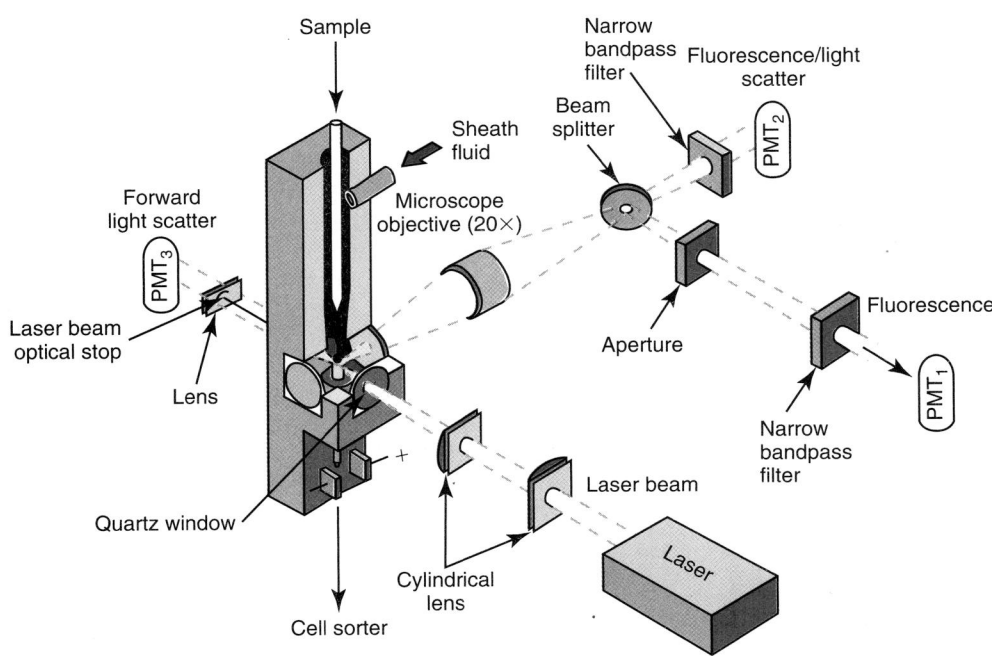

FIGURE 16.16 Schematic diagram of a flow cytometer. *PMT,* Photomultiplier tube.

Flow cytometers are able to measure multiple parameters, including cell size (forward scatter), granularity (90°; side scatter), DNA content, RNA content, DNA (A + T)/(G + C) nucleotide ratios, chromatin structure, antigens, total protein content, cell receptors, membrane potential, and calcium ion concentration as a function of pH. These parameters are used in hematology, immunology (e.g., in T-cell subsets, tissue typing, lymphocyte stimulation, and antigen antibody reactions), oncology (e.g., in diagnosis, prognosis, and treatment monitoring), microbiology (e.g., in bacterial identification and antibiotic sensitivity), virology (e.g., viral particles), and genetics (e.g., in karyotyping and carrier state detection) (additional information can be found in Chapter 28). Flow cytometry also has potential applications for the development of sensitive laser-induced fluoroimmunoassays. Phycoerythrin is a large phycobiliprotein molecule (molecular weight = 250,000 Da) with the fluorescence emission equivalent of 25 rhodamine-6G molecules, a quantum yield of 0.98, a broad emission spectrum of 530 to 630 nm, and low photodecomposition. It is an excellent label for cells and possibly for use in new fluoroimmunoassays.

The development and use of particle-based flow cytometric assays should be noted. With this technology, a flow cytometer is combined with microspheres that are used as the solid support for conventional immunoassay, affinity assay, or DNA hybridization assay.[11] The microspheres are comprised of different proportions of two fluorescent dyes to generate 100 different signatures. Each of these signatures can be assigned to a specific analyte to multiplex 100 analytes in the same sample. The resultant system is flexible, and its use has led to the development of small volume assays that simultaneously assess a wide variety of analytes in the same sample (see additional discussion on Luminex multiplex technology in Chapter 26).

Hematofluorometer. The hematofluorometer is a single-channel, front-surface photofluorometer dedicated to the analysis of zinc protoporphyrin in whole blood (see Chapter 41). A typical hematofluorometer uses a quartz-tungsten lamp, a narrow bandpass excitation filter (420 nm), front-surface optics, a narrow bandpass filter (594 nm), and a PMT. A drop of whole blood is placed on a small rectangular glass slide that serves as a cuvet. Zinc protoporphyrin (ZPP) analysis by a hematofluorometer may be used for lead screening in adults. Historically ZPP was used for lead screening in asymptomatic children, however, it has poor sensitivity and specificity which limits its utility. ZPP has been proposed for iron deficiency screening in pediatric populations.[12]

Limitations of Fluorescence Measurements

Factors that influence fluorescence measurements include concentration effects (e.g., inner filter effects, concentration quenching), background effects (due to Rayleigh and Raman scattering), solvent effects (e.g., interfering nonspecific fluorescence, quenching from the solvent), sample effects (e.g., light scattering, interfering fluorescence, sample adsorption), temperature effects, and photodecomposition (bleaching) of the sample.

Inner Filter Effects

The linear relationship between concentration and fluorescence emission (Eq. 16.8) is valid when solutions that absorb less than 2% of the exciting light are used. As the absorbance of the solution increases above this amount, the relationship becomes nonlinear, a phenomenon known as the inner filter effect. It is caused by loss of excitation intensity across the cuvet path length as excitation light is absorbed by the fluorophore. Thus as the fluorophore becomes more concentrated, absorbance of the excitation intensity increases, and loss of the excitation light as it travels through the cuvet increases. This effect is most often encountered with a right-angle fluorescence instrument, in which the emission slits are set to monitor the center of the sample cell, where absorbance of excitation light is greater than that at the front surface of the cuvet. Therefore it is less problematic if a front-surface fluorescence instrument is used. However, most fluorescence measurements are made on dilute solutions, and therefore the inner filter effect is not a problem.

Concentration Quenching

Another related phenomenon that results in a lower quantum yield than expected is called concentration quenching. This can occur when a macromolecule, such as an antibody, is heavily labeled with a fluorophore, such as fluorescein isothiocyanate. When this compound is excited, the fluorescence labels are in such close proximity that radiation-less energy transfer occurs. Thus the resulting fluorescence is much lower than expected for the concentration of the label. This is a common problem in flow cytometry and laser-induced fluorescence when attempts are made to enhance detection sensitivity by increasing the density of the fluorescing label.

Light Scattering

Light scattering—Rayleigh and Raman—limits the use of fluorescence measurements. Rayleigh scattering occurs with no change in wavelength. For fluorophores with small Stokes shifts, the excitation and emission spectra overlap and are particularly susceptible to loss of sensitivity because of background light scatter. Rayleigh-type light scatter is controlled by using well-defined emission and excitation interference filters or by appropriate monochromator settings and the use of polarizers.

Raman scattering occurs with lengthening of a wavelength. This type of light scattering is independent of excitation wavelength and is a property of the solvent. Because Raman light scattering appears at longer wavelengths than the exciting radiation, it is a difficult interference to eliminate when working at very low fluorophore concentrations. As an example, the wavelength shift in water is approximately 50 nm at an excitation wavelength of 365 nm and approximately 75 nm at an excitation wavelength of 436 nm. This shift will represent a problem if the excitation maximum of a fluorophore is 365 nm, and the emission maximum is 415 nm. Raman light scattering is controlled by setting the excitation and emission wavelengths far enough apart. It is also controlled by narrowing the slit width on the excitation monochromator. However, both options tend to decrease sensitivity.

Cuvet Material and Solvent Effects

Certain quartz glass and plastic materials that contain UV absorbers will fluoresce. Some solvents, such as ethanol, are also known to cause appreciable fluorescence. It is therefore important when developing a fluorescence assay to assess the background fluorescence of all components of the reaction mixture. Solvents and cuvets with minimal fluorescence emissions are commercially available; these reagents minimize background fluorescence problems.

Quenching by the solvent can be a problem and should be investigated when a new fluorometric method is established. Quenching is related to the interaction of the fluorophore with the solvent or with a solute dissolved in the solvent. Such interaction results in loss of fluorescence because of energy transfer or other mechanisms, but no effect on the absorbance spectrum of the fluorophore has been noted. Although unintended fluorescence quenching can be detrimental in fluorometric assays, fluorescence quenching has been used in assays for analytical measurements. In TaqMan DNA probes (Thermo Fisher Scientific Inc., Waltham, Massachusetts), a reporter fluorescent dye is linked to a nearby quencher fluorescent dye. In the presence of target DNA sequence, the exonuclease activity of Taq polymerase separates the quencher from the reporter, allowing the reporter fluorescent dye to be detected (see Chapter 64). Quenching can be a useful tool for studying molecular structure because fluorescence emission is sensitive to and specific for changes in atomic and molecular structure.

Sample Matrix Effects

A serum or urine sample contains many compounds that fluoresce. Thus the sample matrix is a potential source of unwanted background fluorescence and must be examined when new methods are developed. The most serious contributors to unwanted fluorescence are proteins and bilirubin. However, because protein excitation maxima are in the spectral region of 260 to 290 nm, their contribution to overall background fluorescence is minor when excitation at more than 300 nm occurs.

Light scattering of proteins and other macromolecules in the sample matrix has been known to cause unwanted background signal. For example, lipemic samples are noted for their intense light scattering, and the relative contributions of lipids to the background signal of a fluorescence measurement should be investigated when setting up a new method.

In addition to background interferences, dilute solutions of some fluorophores in the concentration range of 10^{-9} mol/L or less will adsorb to the walls of glass cuvets and other reaction vessels. Also, dilute solutions of fluorophores, when excited over long periods of time, are susceptible to photodecomposition by intense excitation light. Operationally, these problems are avoided by selecting proper reaction vessels, adding wetting agents, and minimizing the length of time a sample is exposed to the excitation light.

Temperature Effects

The fluorescence quantum efficiency of many compounds is sensitive to temperature fluctuations. Therefore the temperature of the reaction must be regulated to within ±0.1 °C. In general, fluorescence intensity decreases with increasing temperature by approximately 1% to 5% per degree Celsius. Increased temperatures result in more frequent molecular collisions and quenching. Collisional quenching can be decreased by lowering the temperature or by increasing the viscosity.

Photodecomposition

In conventional fluorometry, excitation of weakly fluorescing or dilute solutions with intense light sources will cause photochemical decomposition of the analyte (photobleaching).

The following steps help to minimize photodecomposition effects:
1. Always use the longest feasible wavelength for excitation that does not introduce light scattering effects.
2. Decrease the duration of excitation of the sample by measuring the fluorescence intensity immediately after excitation.
3. Protect unstable solutions from ambient light by storing them in dark bottles.
4. Remove dissolved oxygen from the solution.

In addition, fluorescence-based assays for analytes at ultralow concentrations require optimization of laser intensity and use of a sensitive detector. Highly intense laser light sources with an energy output greater than 5 to 10 mW have higher sensitivity and are used in applications that have low concentrations of analyte, such as flow cytometry, fluorescence microscopy, and laser-induced fluorescence measurements. However, these intense light sources rapidly photodecompose some fluorescence analytes. This decomposition introduces nonlinear response curves and loss of most of the sample fluorescence. Thus optimization of laser intensity balances higher sensitivity with increased photodecomposition.

PHOSPHORESCENCE

Phosphorescence is the luminescence produced by certain substances (e.g., zinc sulfide) after radiant energy or other types of energy are absorbed. Phosphorescence is distinguished from fluorescence in that phosphorescence results from the relaxation of molecules in an excited triplet electronic state, as opposed to the excited singlet electronic state observed in fluorescence emission. The decay time of emission of phosphorescence is usually longer (10^{-4} to 10^2 s) than the decay time of fluorescence emission because of the longer lifetime of molecules in an excited triplet state. Phosphorescence shows a larger shift in emitted light wavelength than that seen with fluorescence. There have been many proposed assay formats based on phosphorescence, but few of them are currently commercialized (see Chapters 17 and 26).

CHEMILUMINESCENCE, BIOLUMINESCENCE, AND ELECTROCHEMILUMINESCENCE

Chemiluminescence, bioluminescence, and electrochemiluminescence are types of luminescence in which the excitation event is caused by a chemical,[13] biochemical, or an electrochemical reaction, and not by photoillumination.

Basic Concepts

The physical event of light emission in chemiluminescence, bioluminescence, and electrochemiluminescence is similar to fluorescence in that it occurs from an excited singlet state, and light is emitted when the electron returns to the ground state.

Chemiluminescence and Bioluminescence

Chemiluminescence is the emission of light when an electron returns from an excited or higher energy level to a lower energy level. The excitation event is caused by a chemical reaction and involves the oxidation of an organic compound, such as luminol, isoluminol, acridinium esters, or luciferin, by an oxidant (e.g., hydrogen peroxide, hypochlorite, oxygen);

light is emitted from the excited product formed in the oxidation reaction. These reactions occur in the presence of catalysts, such as enzymes (e.g., alkaline phosphatase, horseradish peroxidase), metal ions, or metal complexes (e.g., hemin).

Bioluminescence is a special form of chemiluminescence found in biological systems. In bioluminescence, an enzyme or a photoprotein increases the efficiency of the luminescence reaction. Luciferase and aequorin are two examples of these biological catalysts. The quantum yield (e.g., total photons emitted per total molecules reacting) is approximately 0.1 to 10% for chemiluminescence, and typically 10 to 30% for bioluminescence.

Chemiluminescence assays are ultrasensitive (attomole to zeptomole detection limits) and have wide dynamic ranges. They are now widely used in automated immunoassay and DNA probe assay systems (e.g., acridinium ester and acridinium sulfonamide labels, 1,2-dioxetane substrates for alkaline phosphatase labels, enhanced luminol reaction for horseradish peroxidase labels [see Chapter 26]).

Electrochemiluminescence

Electrochemiluminescence differs from chemiluminescence in that the reactive species that produce the chemiluminescent reaction are electrochemically generated from stable precursors at the surface of an electrode.[14] A ruthenium, tris(bipyridyl) chelate is the most commonly used electrochemiluminescent label, and electrochemiluminescence is generated at an electrode via an oxidation reduction–type reaction with tripropylamine. This chelate is stable and relatively small, and has been used to label haptens or large molecules (e.g., proteins, oligonucleotides). The electrochemiluminescence process has been used in both immunoassays and nucleic acid assays. Advantages of this process include (1) improved reagent stability, (2) simple reagent preparation, and (3) enhanced sensitivity. With its use, detection limits of 200 fmol/L and a dynamic range extending over six orders of magnitude can be obtained.

Instrumentation

Luminometers are instruments used to measure chemiluminescence and electrochemiluminescence. Basic components are (1) the sample cell housed in a light-tight chamber, (2) the injection system used to add reagents to the sample cell, and (3) the detector. The detector is usually a PMT. However, CCD, x-ray film, or photographic film has been used to image chemiluminescent reactions on a membrane or in the wells of a microplate. For electrochemiluminescence, the reaction vessel incorporates an electrode, at which electrochemiluminescence is generated.

Limitations of Chemiluminescence and Electrochemiluminescence Measurements

Light leaks, light piping, and high background luminescence from assay reagents and reaction vessels (e.g., plastic tubes exposed to light) are common factors that degrade analytical performance. The extreme sensitivity of chemiluminescent assays requires stringent controls on the purity of reagents and the solvents (e.g., water) used to prepare reagent solutions. Efficient capture of light emission from reactions that produce a flash of light requires an efficient injector that provides adequate mixing when the triggering reagent is added to the reaction vessel. Chemiluminescent and electrochemiluminescent assays have a wide linear range

that are usually several orders of magnitude, but high-intensity light emission can lead to pulse pile-up in PMTs, and this can lead to a serious underestimation of true light emission intensity.

NEPHELOMETRY AND TURBIDIMETRY

Light scattering is a physical phenomenon that results from the interaction of light with particles in solution. Nephelometry and turbidimetry are analytical techniques used to measure scattered light. Light scattering measurements have been applied to immunoassays of specific proteins and haptens (for additional information, refer to Chapter 26).

Basic Concepts

Light scattering occurs when radiant energy passing through a solution encounters a molecule in an elastic collision, which results in scattering of the light in all directions. Unlike fluorescence emission, the scattered light is of the same frequency as the incident light.

Factors that influence light scattering include particle size, wavelength dependence, distance of observation, polarization of incident light, concentration of the particles, and molecular weight of the particles.

Particle Size

The Rayleigh scattering equation (see next section) applies to the scattering of light from small particles with much smaller dimensions than the wavelength of incident light (e.g., particle size less than $\lambda/10$). When the dimensions of the particles are much smaller than the wavelength of the incident light, each particle is subjected to the same electric field strength at the same time. Reradiated or scattered light waves from the small particle are in phase and reinforce each other. As the particles become larger than the incident light wave, radiated light waves are no longer all in phase. Reinforcement of radiation occurs in some directions, and destructive interference occurs in others. Scattering patterns from these large particles are characteristic of the size and shape of the particle.

Wavelength Dependence of Light Scattering

The Rayleigh scattering equation demonstrates the relationship of the intensity (I_S) of scattered light to the intensity (I_0) of incident light:

$$\frac{I_S}{I_0} = \frac{16\pi^2 a \sin^2 \Phi}{\lambda^4 r^2} \tag{16.10}$$

where I_s = intensity of scattered light; I_0 = intensity of the excitation light; a = polarizability of the small particle; Φ = angle of observation with the z-axis; λ = wavelength of incident light; *and* r = distance from light scattering to the detector.

As indicated, the intensity of light scattering is inversely proportional to the wavelength of the incident light. Another useful observation is that scattered light intensity is also inversely proportional to the distance r from the light scattering to the detector. Thus the detector should be located close to the analytical cell by the juxtaposition of the cell to the detector or by the use of good collection optics. Eq. (16.10) expresses light scattering from small particles if excited by polarized light.

With polarized light, there is less scattering compared with nonpolarized light. Therefore if a polarizer is used in front of the emission detector, there is a reduction in background signal due to light scattering. An additional feature of light scattering is that it is directly proportional to both the concentration of particles and the molecular weight of particles.

Angular Dependence of Light Scattering

The angular dependence of light scattering from small particles (i.e., less than $\lambda/10$) shows that the intensity of forward scatter and back scatter (I_0 at 0 degree and 180 degrees) from small particles excited by nonpolarized light is equal. However, light scatter intensity at 90 degrees is much less than forward and back scatter. As particles become larger (i.e., greater than $\lambda/10$), the light scattering intensities at forward and back angles are not equal; forward scatter intensity is much larger. Also, light scattering intensity at 90 degrees is much less than the intensity at the forward (0 degree) angle. As particles become even larger, this dissymmetry between forward and back scatter intensities increases even further. This dissymmetry and the change in angular dependence of light scattering with change in the size of particles are very useful for characterization and differentiation of various classes of macromolecules and cells. As was previously mentioned, this property of light scattering is being used in the design of flow cytometers. These instruments measure near-forward light scattering and right-angle light scattering from cellular particles flowing through an optical cell and excited by a high-intensity laser. The ratio of near-forward light scattering intensity to right-angle light intensity is used in these instruments to distinguish among cell sizes.

Light Scattering and Plasma Proteins

The expression for light scattering given in Eq. (16.10) holds true in dilute solution for small particles if the largest dimension is less than one-tenth the wavelength of the incident light. Thus the upper limit on the size of particles exhibiting Rayleigh scattering is approximately 40 nm when visible light is used at 400 nm. Many of the plasma proteins—such as immunoglobulins, β-lipoproteins, and albumin—are below this limit. For larger particles (approximately 40 to 400 nm), the angular dependence of the scattered light loses symmetry around the 90-degree axis and shows an increase in forward scattering. Some plasma proteins of the immunoglobulin-M class, chylomicrons, and aggregating immunoglobulin–antigen complexes fall into the size range described by Rayleigh-Debye scattering. Particles such as red blood cells and bacteria are even larger (i.e., 7000 to 40,000 nm). These particles show a complex angular dependence of light scattering, and this type of scattering from large particles is called Mie scattering. These large particles produce a predominance of scattered light in a narrow angular region in the forward direction.

Measurement of Scattered Light

Turbidimetry and nephelometry are methods used to measure scattered light. Such measurement has proven useful for the quantitation of serum proteins (see Chapter 31). The choice between turbidimetry and nephelometry depends on the application and the available instrumentation.

Turbidimetry

Because of the light scattering that occurs with turbidity, the intensity of light reaching the detector at 180 degrees is reduced. Measurement of this decrease in intensity is called turbidimetry. Analogous to absorption spectroscopy, turbidity is defined as follows:

$$I = I_0 e^{-bt} \qquad (16.11)$$

or

$$t = \frac{1}{b} \ln \frac{I_0}{I} \qquad (16.12)$$

where t = turbidity; b = path length of incident light through the solution of light scattering particles; I = intensity of transmitted light; and I_0 = intensity of incident light.

Turbidity is measured at 180 degrees from the incident beam, or more simply, in the same manner as absorbance measurements are made in a spectrophotometer. Turbidity can be measured on most spectrophotometers and automated clinical chemistry analyzers. The stability and resolution of modern microprocessor-driven spectrophotometers and photometers have greatly improved their ability to measure turbidity with accuracy and precision.

Turbidimetric measurements are performed on photometers or spectrophotometers and require little optimization. The principal concern of turbidimetric measurements is signal-to-noise ratio. Photometric systems with electro-optical noise in the range of ± 0.0002 absorbance unit or less are useful for turbidity measurements.

Nephelometry

Nephelometry is defined as the detection of light energy scattered or reflected toward a detector that is not in the direct path of the transmitted light. Common nephelometers measure scattered light at right angles to the incident light. The ideal nephelometric instrument would be free of stray light, and neither light scatter nor any other signal would be seen by the detector when the solution in front of the detector is free from particles. However, because of stray light-generating components in the optical system and in the sample cuvet or the sample itself, a truly dark field situation is difficult to obtain when making nephelometric measurements. Some nephelometers are designed to measure scattered light at an angle other than 90 degrees to take advantage of the increased forward scatter intensity caused by light scattering from larger particles (e.g., immune complexes).

Although light scattering can be measured with standard analytical fluorometers or photometers, the angular dependence of light scattering intensity has resulted in the design of special nephelometers. These devices place the PMT detector at appropriate angles to the excitation light beam. The design principle of a nephelometer is similar to the design principle applied in fluorescence measurement. The major operational difference between the fluorometer and the nephelometer is that the excitation and detection wavelengths will be set to the same value when operating a nephelometer. The principal concerns of light scatter instrumentation include excitation intensity, wavelength, distance of the detector from the sample cuvet, and minimization of external stray light. As shown in Fig. 16.17, the basic components of a nephelometer include (1) a light source, (2) collimating optics, (3) a sample cell, and (4) collection optics, which include light scattering optics, a detector optical filter, and a detector. The schematic diagram also shows the different angles from the incident light beam where the detector, filter, and optics are placed to measure light scattering. Fig. 16.17a shows the straight-through arrangement for turbidimetry, whereas Fig. 16.17b and c show arrangements frequently found in nephelometers. The detector arrangement shown in Fig. 16.17b is used for measurement of forward scatter at 30 degrees, which is the optical arrangement used with some commercial nephelometers.

Operationally, the optical components used in turbidimeters and nephelometers are similar to those used in fluorometers and photometers. For example, the light sources commonly used are quartz-halogen lamps, xenon lamps, and lasers. Helium-neon lasers, which operate at 633 nm, typically have been used for light scattering applications, such as nephelometric immunoassays, and particle size and shape determinations. The laser beam is used specifically in some nephelometers because of its high intensity; in addition, the coherent nature of laser light makes it ideally suited for nephelometric applications. In addition, ratio-referencing fluorometers are well suited for nephelometric measurements.

Limitations of Light Scattering Measurements

Antigen excess and matrix effects are limitations encountered in the use of turbidimeters and nephelometers for measurement of analytes of clinical interest in some situations.

Antigen Excess

Antigen–antibody reactions are complex and appear to result in a mixture of aggregate sizes. As turbidity increases during addition of antigen to antibodies, the signal increases to a maximum value and then decreases. The point at which the decrease begins marks the beginning of the phase of antigen excess; this phenomenon is explained in Chapter 26. Consequently, light scattering methods for quantitation of antigen–antibody reactions must provide a method for detecting antigen excess. The kinetics of immune complex formation measured by nephelometry or turbidimetry is sufficiently different in each of the three phases—antibody excess, equivalence, and antigen excess—that computer algorithms that detect antigen excess need to be included in a test system.[15,16]

Matrix Effects

Particles, solvent, and all serum macromolecules scatter light. Lipoproteins and chylomicrons in lipemic serum provide the highest background turbidity or nephelometric intensity.

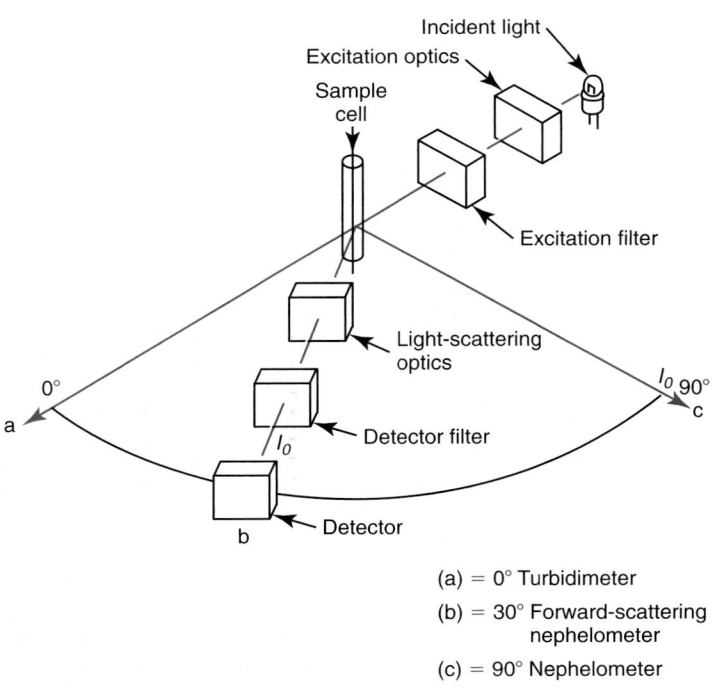

FIGURE 16.17 Schematic diagram of light scattering instrumentation showing *(a)* the optics position for a turbidimeter, *(b)* the optics position for a forward scattering nephelometer, and *(c)* the optics position for a right-angle nephelometer.

With appropriate dilutions, the relative intensity of light scattering from a lipemic sample is less than that of the antiserum blank. However, as the concentration of the antigen in serum decreases and correspondingly less dilute samples are used, background interference from lipemic samples becomes greater. An effective method for minimizing this background interference is the use of rate measurements, in which the initial sample blank is eliminated. Large particles, such as suspended dust, also cause significant background interference. This background interference is controlled by filtering all buffers and diluted antisera before analysis is attempted.

POINTS TO REMEMBER

Light Scattering Assays
- Turbidity assays measure light scattering to determine the formation of antigen–antibody complexes.
- Interferences in light scattering include:
  - an excess of antigen decreases the turbidity
  - macromolecules, such as lipoproteins, chylomicrons, and dust in the sample matrix, which will increase the background turbidity
- Macromolecule interference in light scattering can be decreased by using rate measurements rather than directly assessing light scattering.

REFERENCES

1. Nagar G, Vandermeer B, Campbell S, Kumar M. Reliability of transcutaneous bilirubin devices in preterm infants: a systematic review. Pediatrics 2013;132:871–81.
2. Gleisner H, Eichardt K, Welz B. Optimization of analytical performance of a graphite furnace atomic absorption spectrometer with Zeeman-effect background correction using variable magnetic field strength. Spectrochimica Acta Part B: Atomic Spectroscopy 2003;58:1663–1678.
3. Valeur B. Pulse and phase fluorometries: An objective comparison. In: Hof M, Hutterer R, Fidler V, eds. Fluorescence Spectroscopy in Biology, vol. 3. Berlin, Heidelberg: Springer 2005. p. 30–31.
4. Yamanishi CD, Chiu JH, Takayama S. Systems for multiplexing homogeneous immunoassays. Bioanalysis 2015;7:1545–56.
5. Bergh AA. Blue laser diode (LD) and light emitting diode (LED) applications. Physica Status Solidi (a) 2004;201:2740–54.
6. Visser BJ, Meerveld-Gerrits J, Kroo D, et al. Assessing the quality of anti-malarial drugs from Gabonese pharmacies using the MiniLab: a field study. Malar J 2015;14:273.
7. Nather RE, Mukadam AJ. A CCD time-series photometer. ApJ 2004;605:846.
8. Michalet X, Colyer RA, Scalia G, et al. Development of new photon-counting detectors for single-molecule fluorescence microscopy. Phil Trans R Soc B 2013;368.
9. Ankelo M, Westerlund A, Blomberg K, et al. Time-resolved immunofluorometric dual-label assay for simultaneous detection of autoantibodies to GAD65 and IA-2 in Children with Type 1 diabetes. Clin Chem 2007;53:472–9.
10. Cossarizza A, Chang HD, Radbruch A, et al. Guidelines for the use of flow cytometry and cell sorting in immunological studies. Eur J Immunol 2017;47:1584–1797.
11. Nolan JP, Mandy F. Multiplexed and microparticle-based analyses: Quantitative tools for the large-scale analysis of biological systems. Cytometry A 2006;69:318–25.
12. Magge H, Sprinz P, Adams WG, et al. Zinc protoporphyrin and iron deficiency screening. JAMA Pediatr 2013;167:361–7.
13. Rodríguez-Orozco AR, Ruiz-Reyes H, Medina-Serriteño N. Recent applications of chemiluminescence assays in clinical immunology. Mini Rev Med Chem 2010;10:1393–400.
14. Gross EM, Maddipati SS, Snyder SM. A review of electrogenerated chemiluminescent biosensors for assays in biological matrices. Bioanalysis 2016;8:2071–89.
15. Urdal P, Amundsen EK, Toska K, Klingenberg O. Automated alarm to detect antigen excess in serum free immunoglobulin light chain kappa and lambda assays. Scand J Clin Lab Invest 2014;74:575–81.
16. Zaydman MA. Kinetic Approach Extends the Analytical Measurement Range and Corrects Antigen Excess in Homogeneous Turbidimetric Immunoassays. J Appl Lab Med 2019 Sep;4(2):214–223.

17

Electrochemistry and Chemical Sensors*

Prasad V.A. Pamidi[a]

ABSTRACT

Background

Chemical sensors utilizing electrochemical and optical detection methods have become routine analytical tools in clinical chemistry applications, especially for measurement of critical care analytes (blood gases, electrolytes, metabolites) directly in whole blood at point of care or near patient testing. Coupling electrochemical or optical transducers together with chemical or biological recognition elements has expanded the role of chemical sensors for measurement of analytes without direct electrochemical or optical activity.

Content

This chapter reviews fundamental aspects of electrochemical and optical measurements and their applications in routine clinical practice for measurements of blood gases (pH, partial pressure of oxygen [PO_2], partial pressure of carbon dioxide [PCO_2]), electrolytes (sodium [Na^+], potassium [K^+], calcium [Ca^{2+}], chloride [Cl^-], magnesium [Mg^{2+}], lithium [Li^+]), hematocrit [HCT], and toxic metals (lead [pb^{2+}]) directly in whole blood. The base principles of these electrochemical and optical sensors are applied as building blocks for enzyme-based biosensors for measurement of important metabolites directly in whole blood (glucose, lactate, urea,

creatinine). Recent advances in miniaturization of enabling technologies and the demand for direct whole blood measurements have transformed these sensors as ideal measurement technologies for point-of-care testing, near patient testing, or at-home monitoring. Affinity sensors utilizing antibodies, nucleic acids, and aptamers are expanding the role of biological recognition elements in biosensors. These molecules, when coupled to electrochemical, optical, and other transducers, produce biosensors for sensitive detection of biomarkers for cancer, cardiac disease, and genetic testing. Although there are several commercial applications of affinity sensors in clinical use, continued growth in research publications and patents points to future possibilities for expanding applications to other clinical markers. This chapter discusses nanotechnology to further enhance sensitivity of biosensors. The sensor technologies routinely applied for in vitro measurements of critical care analytes (blood gases, glucose) are being adapted for in vivo and minimally invasive or noninvasive wearable applications, through developing solutions to address problems such as biocompatibility and calibration stability. Commercial products for continuous glucose monitoring (CGM) and health vital sign monitoring are a few examples of wearable sensors that are increasingly available.

---

*The full version of this chapter is available electronically on ExpertConsult.com.
[a]The author gratefully acknowledges the contributions of Drs. Paul D'Orazio, Richard A. Durst, Ole Siggard-Andersen, and Mark E. Meyerhoff for earlier versions of this chapter.

18

Electrophoresis

Lindsay A.L. Bazydlo and James P. Landers[a]

ABSTRACT

Background

Developments in DNA testing, improvements in ease of performance through automation, and advantages of speed and miniaturization afforded by the technique of *capillary electrophoresis (CE)* have led to a renaissance and growth of *electrophoresis* as an analytical tool that is widely used in clinical laboratories. These developments and improvements have enabled clinical laboratories to keep pace with higher volumes of testing and to introduce more sophisticated technology to meet the demands of modern clinical practice.

Content

This chapter will review the principles and practice of the technique and will separately discuss conventional, capillary, and microchip electrophoresis. Traditional electrophoresis has been performed in the slab gel format, and many laboratories nowadays still use that approach. Based on the same inherent principles, CE has recently been gaining popularity in clinical laboratory use. Capillary zone electrophoresis (CZE) allows for higher voltages to be applied to facilitate the separation, which can translate to faster separation times. Taking faster separations one step further, electrophoresis also can be performed in the microfluidic format. This allows for even faster separations, and recent years have seen an increase in the commercialization of this approach. Clinical applications are mentioned throughout the chapter to illustrate the utility of this technique and the analysis of relevant biological analytes.

BASIC CONCEPTS AND DEFINITIONS

Electrophoresis is a comprehensive term that refers to the migration of charged solutes or particles of any size in a liquid medium under the influence of an electrical field. *Iontophoresis* and *isotachophoresis* (ITP) are similar terms but refer specifically to the migration of small ions. The first electrophoresis method used to study proteins was the free solution or moving boundary method devised by Tiselius in 1937. This technique was used in research to measure electrophoretic mobility and study protein-protein interaction. It was able to resolve the serum proteins into only four component mixtures, with the α_1 fraction incompletely separated from albumin.

Zone electrophoresis refers to the migration of charged molecules of proteins, usually in a porous supporting medium such as agarose gel film, so that each protein zone is sharply separated from neighboring zones by a protein-free area. Zones are visualized by staining with a protein-specific stain to produce an *electropherogram* that is then scanned and quantified using a densitometer. The support medium also can be handled after drying and kept as a permanent record. This is the most commonly applied technique in clinical chemistry and is used to separate proteins in serum, urine, cerebrospinal fluid (CSF), other physiologic fluids, erythrocytes and tissue, and nucleic acids in various tissue cells.

Although electrophoretic separation of biologically relevant macromolecules in gels (or paper) has been the workhorse of modern biomedical research, the advent of *capillary electrophoresis* (CE) has revolutionized separations. Intense interest in carrying out electrophoretic separation in capillaries with inner diameters ranging from 20 to 75 μm has resulted from its unprecedented resolving power, separation speed, and small sample analysis capabilities. However, the true significance of CE to the separations community can be seen in its ability to apply these separation principles in a multimodal approach to a variety of analytes that obviously included proteins and polynucleic acids, but also peptides, small drug-like molecules, and even ions.

THEORY OF ELECTROPHORESIS

Depending on the charge they carry, ionized solutes move toward either the cathode (negative electrode) or the anode (positive electrode) in an electrophoresis system. For example, positive ions (cations) migrate to the cathode and negative ions (anions) to the anode. An ampholyte (a molecule that is either positively or negatively charged, formerly called a *zwitterion*) becomes positively charged in a solution that is more acidic than its isoelectric point (pI)[b] and migrates toward the cathode. In a more alkaline solution, the ampholyte becomes negatively charged and migrates toward the anode.

---

[a]The authors gratefully acknowledge the original contributions of Drs. Emmanuel Epstein, Raymond Karcher, and Kern L. Nuttall, on which portions of this chapter are based.

[b]The isoelectric point of a molecule is the pH at which it has no net charge and will not move in an electrical field.

Because proteins contain many ionizable amino ($-NH_2$) and carboxyl ($-COOH$) groups and because the bases in nucleic acids also may be positively or negatively charged, they both behave as ampholytes in solution.

The rate of migration of ions in an electrical field depends on the factors listed in Box 18.1. The equation expressing the driving force in such a system is given by the following:

$$F = (X)(Q) = \frac{(EMF)(Q)}{d}$$

where

F = the force exerted on an ion
X = the current field strength (V/cm) (i.e., voltage drop per unit length of medium)
Q = the net charge on the ion
EMF = the electromotive force [voltage (V) applied]
d = the length of the electrophoretic medium (cm)

Steady acceleration of the migrating ion is counteracted by a resisting force characteristic of the solution in which migration occurs. This force, expressed by Stokes law, is

$$F' = 6\pi r \eta v$$

where

F' = the counter force
π = 3.1416
r = the ionic radius of the solute
η = the viscosity of the buffer solution in which migration is occurring
v = the rate of migration of the solute = velocity, length *(l)* traveled per unit of time (cm/s)

The force F' counteracts the acceleration that would be produced by F if no counter force were present, and the result of the two forces is a constant velocity. Therefore when

$$F = F'$$

then

$$6\pi r \eta v = (X)(Q)$$

or

$$\frac{v}{X} = \frac{1 \times d}{t \times E} = \frac{Q}{6\pi r \eta} = \mu$$

where v/X is the rate of migration (cm/s) per unit field strength (E/cm), defined as the electrophoretic mobility and expressed by the symbol μ.

Electrophoretic mobility is directly proportional to the net charge and inversely proportional to the size of the molecule and the viscosity of the electrophoresis medium. Mobility may be positive or negative, depending on whether a protein migrates in the same or the opposite direction as the electrophoretic field (defined as extending from the anode to the cathode).

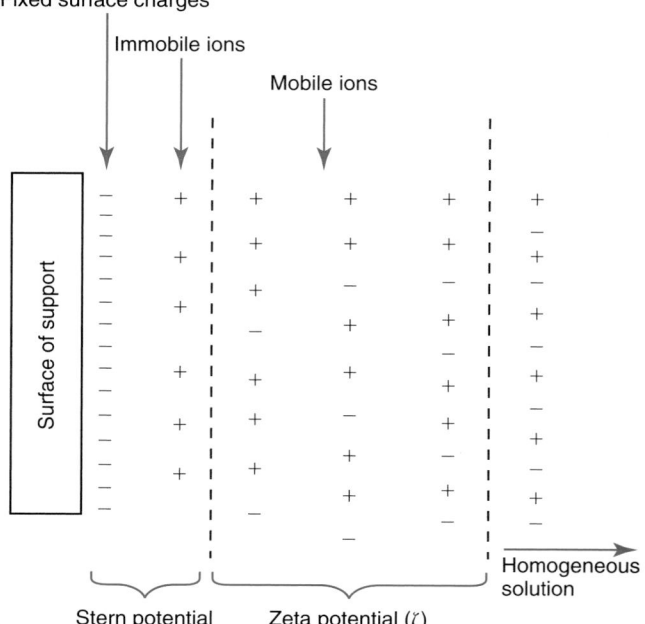

FIGURE 18.1 Distribution of + and − ions around the surface of an electrophoretic support. Fixed on the surface of the solid is a layer of − ions. (These may be + ions under suitable conditions). A second layer of + ions is attracted to the surface. These two layers compose the Stern potential. The large, diffuse layer containing mostly + ions is the electrokinetic or zeta potential. Extending farther from the surface of the solid is homogeneous solution. The Stern potential plus the zeta potential equals the electrochemical potential, or epsilon potential.

In addition to the factors listed in Box 18.1, other factors that affect electrophoretic mobility include electroendosmosis and wick flow. Electroendosmosis, also known as electroosmotic flow (EOF), affects mobility by causing uneven movement of water through the support medium. An electrophoretic support medium, such as a gel in contact with water, takes on a negative charge caused by adsorption of hydroxyl ions. These ions are fixed to the surface and are immobile. Positive ions in solution cluster about the fixed negative charge sites, forming an ionic cloud of mostly positive ions. The number of negative ions in the solution increases with increasing distance from the fixed negative charge sites until eventually positive and negative ions are present in equal concentrations (Fig. 18.1).

When current is applied to such a system, charges attached to the immobile support remain fixed but the cloud of ions in solution moves to the electrode of opposite polarity. Because ions in solution are highly hydrated, this results in movement of the solvent as well. Movement of solvent and its solutes relative to the fixed support is EOF and causes preferential movement of water in one direction. Macromolecules in solution that move in the direction opposite this flow may remain immobile or even may be swept back toward the opposite pole if they are insufficiently charged. In media in which EOF is strong, such as conventional cellulose acetate and unpurified agarose gel, γ-globulins are swept back from the application point. Because the inner surface of a glass capillary contains many such charged groups, EOF is very strong and is actually the primary driving force for migration in CE systems.

However, the conditions in CE can be manipulated to modify the magnitude of the EOF effect. In electrophoretic media in which surface charges are minimal (starch gel, purified agarose gel, or polyacrylamide gel), EOF is minimal.

Wick flow results from the movement of buffer into the support medium. During electrophoresis, heat that evolves because of the passage of current through a resistive medium can cause evaporation of solvent from the electrophoretic support. This drying effect draws buffer into the support, and, if significant, the flow of buffer can affect protein migration and hence the calculated mobility.

POINTS TO REMEMBER

Electrophoresis
- Refers to the migration of ions in an electrical field
- Separation occurs based on the inherent electrophoretic mobility of an analyte
- Electrophoretic mobility is directly proportional to the net charge and inversely proportional to the size of the molecule and the viscosity of the electrophoresis medium

---

CLINICAL ELECTROPHORESIS

In this section, focus will be on the electrophoresis methodology that is frequently used in clinical laboratories. Refer to Chapter 31 for a thorough discussion on the various electrophoretic fractions present in clinical protein electrophoresis.

Slab Gel Electrophoresis

Traditional methods, using a rectangular gel, are referred to collectively by the term *slab gel electrophoresis*. Its main advantage is its ability to simultaneously separate several samples in one run. Starch, agarose, and polyacrylamide media have been used in this format. It is the primary method used in clinical chemistry laboratories for separation of various classes of serum or CSF proteins and DNA and RNA fragments. Gels (usually agarose) may be cast on a sheet of plastic backing or completely encased within a plastic-walled cell, which allows horizontal or vertical electrophoresis and submersion for cooling, if necessary.

General Operations

General operations performed in conventional electrophoresis include separation, detection, and quantification, and "blotting" techniques.

Electrophoretic separation. When electrophoresis is performed on precast microzone agarose gels, the following steps are typical: (1) excess buffer is removed from the support surface by blotting, taking care that bubbles are not present; (2) 5 to 7 μL of sample is applied using a comb or a plastic template and is allowed to diffuse into the gel; it is then blotted to remove the excess; (3) the gel is placed into the electrode chamber; (4) electrophoresis is performed at specified current, voltage, or power; (5) the gel is fixed, rinsed, and then dried; (6) the gel is stained and redried; and (7) the gel is scanned in a densitometer. If isoenzymes are to be determined, substrate dye solution is incubated on the gel to stain zones before fixing and drying. Alternative procedures would be required if the more sophisticated methods described later are used.

TABLE 18.1   Suggested Wavelengths for Quantitation of Protein Zones by Direct Densitometry

Separation Type	Stain	Nominal Wavelength (nm)
Serum proteins in general	Amido Black (Naphthol Blue Black)	640
	Coomassie Brilliant Blue G–250 (Brilliant Blue G)	595
	Coomassie Brilliant Blue R–250 (Brilliant Blue R)	560
	Ponceau S	520
Isoenzymes	Nitrotetrazolium Blue	570
Lipoprotein zones	Fat Red 7B (Sudan Red 7B)	540
	Oil Red O	520
	Sudan Black B	600
DNA fragments	Ethidium bromide (fluorescent)	254 (Ex) 590 (Em)
CSF proteins	Silver nitrate	—

CSF, Cerebrospinal fluid; *Em*, emission; *Ex*, excitation.

Detection and quantification. Once separated, proteins may be detected by staining followed by quantification using a densitometer or by direct measurement using an optical detection system set at 210 nm.

Staining. If staining is used to visualize separated proteins, the proteins usually are fixed first by precipitating them in the gel with a chemical agent such as acetic acid or methanol. This prevents diffusion of proteins out of the gel when submersed in the stain solution. The amount of dye taken up by the sample is affected by many factors, such as the type of protein and the degree of denaturation of the proteins by fixing agents.

Table 18.1 lists dyes commonly used in electrophoresis, along with suggested wavelengths for quantification by densitometry. Most commercial methods for serum protein electrophoresis use Amido Black B or members of the Coomassie Brilliant Blue series of dyes for staining. Isoenzymes are typically visualized by incubating the gel in contact with a solution of substrate, which is linked structurally or chemically to a dye before fixing. Silver nitrate and silver diamine stain proteins and polypeptides with sensitivity 10- to 100-fold greater than that of conventional dyes.[1] Selective fixing and staining of protein subclasses also can be achieved by combining a stain molecule with an antiglobulin, as is done in immunofixation electrophoresis (IFE).

Improvements in conducting sensitive measurements have been achieved by linking an enzyme such as alkaline phosphatase or peroxidase to a single or double antibody specific for particular proteins such as oligoclonal immunoglobulin (Ig)[2] or by spraying separated proteins with luminal and peroxide to develop chemiluminescence, which, in turn, exposes x-ray film to form a permanent image.[3] Chemiluminescence has been used in this way to quantify IgE (Lumi-Phos 530, Lumigen, Southfield, Mich),[4] and DNA fragments have been detected by linking with a fluorescent dye label.[5]

In practice, a typical stain solution may be used several times before it is replaced. A good rule of thumb is that a stain solution of 100 mL may be used for a combined total of 387 cm^2 (60 in^2) of agarose film. The stain solution may be considered faulty if leaching of stained protein zones occurs in the 5% acetic acid wash solution. Whenever protein zones appear too lightly stained, the stain or substrate reagent—in the case of isoenzymes—always should be suspected. Stain solution must be stored tightly covered to prevent evaporation.

Quantification. A *densitometer* is used to quantify stained zones. This instrument measures the absorbance of each fraction as the gel (or other medium) is moved past a photometric optical system and displays an *electropherogram* on a computer display. The software is able to automatically integrate the area under each peak and report each as a percentage of total or as absolute concentration or activity computed from the total protein or activity of enzyme in the sample.

Reliable densitometric quantitation requires (1) light of an appropriate wavelength, (2) linear response from the instrument, and (3) a transparent background in the medium being scanned. Linearity may be tested with a neutral density filter designed with separated or adjacent areas of linearly increasing density. The densities are permanent and have expected absorbance values. The very small sample sizes used and the transparency of agarose gels satisfy the requirement for a clear background. Nevertheless, problems can occur with densitometry because of differences in the quantity of stain taken up by individual proteins and differences in protein zone sizes. In addition, comigrating proteins cannot be distinguished by densitometry and can falsely increase the concentration of a specific protein.

Essential features of a densitometer include (1) the ability to scan gels 25 to 100 mm in length; (2) electronic adjustment of the most intense peak to full scale; (3) automatic background zeroing (peaks are not lost or "cut off"); (4) variable wavelength control over the range of 400 to 700 nm; (5) variable slits to allow adjustment of the beam size; (6) an integrating device with both automatic and manual selection of cut points between peaks; and (7) automatic indexing, a feature that advances the electrophoresis strip from one sample channel to the next.

Desirable features of a densitometer include computerized integration and printout, built-in diagnostics for instrument troubleshooting, choice of one of several scanning speeds, and ability to measure in the reflectance mode. Models with a separate computer for data processing permit storage and reformatting of data, if desired, and reprinting or delayed transmission to a host computer.

DNA analysis requires the ability to scan larger gels, which may contain several dozen bands of DNA fragments of different length. Modern automated electrophoresis systems also use larger gels containing 30 or more samples, which are scanned on a new generation of densitometers referred to as *flatbed scanners* or *digital image analyzers*. These instruments are capable of scanning and storing digitized light intensity readings from large areas and use ultrasensitive charge-coupled device detectors having a resolution of up to 1200 dots per inch (21 μm). Sophisticated data processing software permits manipulation of stored image information to produce conventional scans and computations or more complex outputs, such as overlaying and subtraction of patterns from two different samples.

Blotting techniques. In 1975, Edward Southern developed a technique that is widely used to detect fragments of DNA.

This technique, known as *Southern blotting*,[6] first requires electrophoretic separation of DNA or DNA fragments by agarose gel electrophoresis (AGE). Next, a strip of nitrocellulose or a nylon membrane is laid over the agarose gel, and the DNA or DNA fragments are transferred or "blotted" onto it by capillary blotting, electro-blotting, or vacuum blotting. They are then detected and identified by hybridization with a labeled, complementary nucleic acid probe. This technique is widely used in molecular biology for identifying a particular DNA sequence; determining the presence, position, and number of copies of a gene in a genome; and typing DNA.

Northern and *Western* blotting techniques,[6] named by analogy to Southern blotting, were subsequently developed to separate and detect RNAs and proteins, respectively. Northern blotting is carried out identically to Southern blotting except that a labeled RNA probe is used for hybridization. Western blotting is used to separate, detect, and identify one or more proteins in a complex mixture. It involves first separating the individual proteins by polyacrylamide gel and then transferring or blotting onto an overlying strip of nitrocellulose or a nylon membrane by electro-blotting. The strip or membrane is then reacted with a reagent that contains an antibody raised against the protein of interest.

Instrumentation

Although modern electrophoresis equipment and systems vary considerably in form and degree of automation, the essential components common to all systems (Fig. 18.2) include two reservoirs (1), which contain the buffer used in the process, a means of delivering current from a power supply via platinum or carbon electrodes (2), which contact the buffer, and a support medium (3) in which separation takes place connecting the two reservoirs. In some systems, wicks (4) may connect the medium to the buffer solution or directly to the electrodes. The entire apparatus is enclosed (5) to minimize evaporation and protect both the system and the operator. The direct current power supply sets the polarity of the electrodes and delivers current to the medium.

Power supplies. The power supply drives the movement of ionic species in the medium and allows adjustment and control of the current or the voltage. With more sophisticated units, the power may be controlled as well, and conditions may be programmed to change during electrophoresis. Capillary systems use power supplies capable of providing voltages in the kilovolt range.

Current flowing through a medium that has resistance produces heat:

$$\text{Heat} = (E)(I)(t)$$

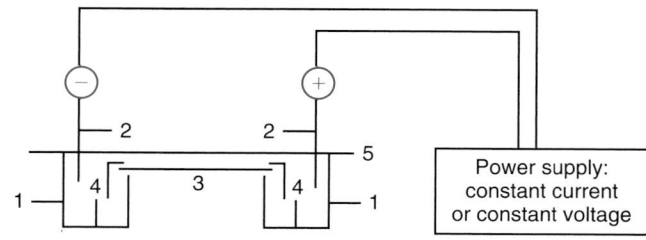

FIGURE 18.2 A schematic diagram of a typical electrophoresis apparatus showing two buffer boxes with baffle plates *(1)*, electrodes *(2)*, electrophoretic support *(3)*, wicks *(4)*, cover *(5)*, and power supply.

where

E = electromotive force (EMF) in volts (V)

I = current in amperes (A)

T = time in seconds (s)

This heat is released into the medium and increases the thermal agitation of all dissolved ions and therefore the conductance of the system (decreases resistance). With constant-voltage power supplies, the resultant rise in current increases both protein migration and evaporation of water from the medium. Any water loss increases the ion concentration and further decreases the resistance (R). Under these circumstances, the current and therefore the migration rate will progressively increase. To minimize these effects, it is best to use a constant-current power supply. According to Ohms law,

$$E = (I)(t)$$

Therefore if R decreases, the applied EMF also decreases, keeping the current constant. This in turn decreases the heat effect and stabilizes the migration rate.

Buffers. Buffer ions have a twofold purpose in electrophoresis: they carry the applied current, and they fix the pH at which electrophoresis is carried out. Thus they determine (1) the type of electrical charge on the solute; (2) the extent of ionization of the solute, and therefore (3) the electrode toward which the solute will migrate. The buffer's ionic strength determines the thickness of the ionic cloud (buffer and nonbuffer ions) surrounding a charged molecule, the rate of its migration, and the sharpness of the electrophoretic zones. With increasing concentration of ions, the ionic cloud increases in size and the molecule becomes more hindered in its movement.

According to Joule law, power produced when current flows through a resistive medium is dissipated as heat. This heat increases in direct proportion to the resistance but also in proportion to the square of the current. The reduction in resistance caused by a high-ionic-strength buffer therefore leads to increased current and excessive heat. These buffers yield sharper band separations, but the benefits of sharper resolution are diminished by the Joule (heat) effect that leads to denaturation of heat-labile proteins or degradation of other components.

Ionic strength (also denoted by the symbol μ) is computed according to the following:

$$\mu = 0.5 \sum c_i z_i^2$$

where

c_i = ion concentration in mol/L

z_i = the charge on the ion

The ionic strength μ of an electrolyte (buffer) composed of monovalent ions is equal to its molarity (mol/L). The ionic strength of a 1-mol/L electrolyte solution with one monovalent and one divalent ion is 3 mol/L, and for a doubly divalent electrolyte it is 4 mol/L.

A buffer of relatively high ionic strength used in *high-resolution electrophoresis* improves the separation of serum proteins into as many as 13 bands (compared with 6 bands on traditional protein electrophoresis), with 2 or more bands in the α_1-, α_2-, and β-globulin regions and 1 or more additional bands seen in various pathologic conditions. Because of higher conductivity and the associated heat produced, it is necessary to reduce the temperature of the system to between 10 to 14 °C. "Submarine" techniques, in which gels are submersed in circulating buffer cooled by an external cooling device or are supported on an electrophoresis chamber cooled by circulating water or an integral Peltier plate, provide exact temperature control. Effective cooling with less-precise temperature control also may be achieved using chambers designed with a sealed compartment of cooled ethylene glycol, which is in contact with the gel during running.

Because buffers used in electrophoresis are good culture media for the growth of microorganisms, they should be refrigerated when not in use. Moreover, a cold buffer is preferred in an electrophoretic run because it improves resolution and decreases evaporation from the electrophoretic support. Buffer used in a small-volume apparatus should be discarded after each run because of pH changes resulting from the electrolysis of water that accompany electrophoresis.

Support media. The support medium provides the matrix in which protein separation takes place. Various types of support media have been used in electrophoresis and range from pure buffer solutions in a capillary to insoluble gels (e.g., sheets, slabs, or columns of starch, agarose, or polyacrylamide) or membranes of cellulose acetate. Gels are cast in a solution of the same buffer to be used in the procedure and may be used in a horizontal or vertical direction. In either case, maximum resolution is achieved if the sample is applied in a very fine starting zone. Separation is based on differences in charge-to-mass ratio of the proteins and, depending on the pore size of the medium, possibly molecular size.

Cellulose acetate. Cellulose acetate, a thermoplastic resin made by treating cellulose with acetic anhydride to acetylate the hydroxyl groups, also is primarily of historical interest. When dry, the membranes contain approximately 80% air space within the interlocking cellulose acetate fibers and are opaque, brittle films. As the film is soaked in buffer, the air spaces fill with liquid and it becomes pliable. Samples are applied with a twin-wire applicator or the edge of a glass slide. Because of their opacity, stained membranes need to be made transparent (cleared) for densitometry by soaking in 95:5 methanol to glacial acetic acid. Cleared membranes are strong and could be stored as a permanent record, but because of the necessity for presoaking and clearing, cellulose acetate has largely been replaced by agarose gel in most clinical applications.

Agarose. Agarose is a linear polymer containing alternating D-galactose and 3,6-anhydro-L-galactose monomers. It is the purified, essentially neutral fraction of agar obtained by separating agarose from agaropectin, a more highly charged fraction containing acidic sulfate and carboxylic side groups. Because the pore size in agarose gel is large enough for all proteins to pass through unimpeded, separation is based only on the charge-to-mass ratio of the protein. Advantages of agarose gel include its lower affinity for proteins and its native clarity after drying, which permits excellent densitometry.

Most routine procedures for AGE are now performed using commercially produced, prepackaged microzone gels, and the sample is applied by means of a comb or a thin plastic template, with small slots corresponding to sample application points. The template is placed on the agarose surface, and 5- to 7-μL samples are placed on each slot. The serum sample is allowed to diffuse into the agarose for 5 minutes, excess sample is removed by blotting, and the template is removed. AGE separation for most routine serum applications requires an electrophoresis time of 20 to 30 minutes.

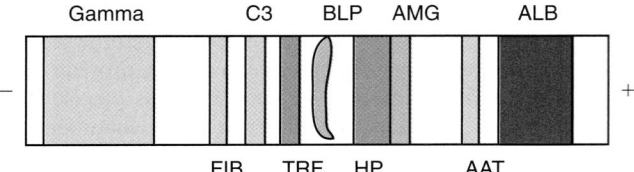

FIGURE 18.3 A simplified schematic drawing of a protein pattern from the serum of a subject with haptoglobin type 2-1 (separation by polyacrylamide gel electrophoresis [PAGE]). Some zones contain more than the one protein shown, as demonstrated by immunologic techniques. *AAT*, α₁-Antitrypsin; *ALB*, albumin; *AMG*, α₂-macroglobulin; *BLP*, β-lipoprotein; *C3*, complement 3; *FIB*, fibrinogen; *gamma*, γ-globulin; *HP*, haptoglobin; *TRF*, transferrin.

Polyacrylamide gel. Polyacrylamide is a polymeric matrix consisting of linear chains of acrylamide cross-linked with bisacrylamide. It is thermostable, transparent, strong, and relatively chemically inert and—depending on concentration—can be made in a wide range of pore sizes. Its average pore size in a typical 7.5% gel is approximately 5 nm (50 Å)—large enough to allow most serum proteins to migrate unimpeded. However, proteins with a molecular radius and/or length that exceeds critical limits will be impeded in their migration. Some of these proteins are fibrinogen, β-lipoprotein, α₂-macroglobulin, and γ-globulins; a schematic representation of serum protein electrophoresis by polyacrylamide gel electrophoresis (PAGE) is shown in Fig. 18.3. The separation is based on both charge-to-mass ratio and molecular size (a phenomenon referred to as *molecular sieving*), and serum proteins can be resolved into more individual fractions than with agarose gel. Furthermore, these gels are uncharged, thus eliminating EOF. Precast minigels are available in a variety of concentrations and ratios of acrylamide to bisacrylamide suitable for most protein or nucleic acid separations. Because of the known neurotoxicity of acrylamide, however, appropriate caution must be exercised when handling this material if gels are prepared by hand.

Attempts to improve the hydrophilic nature of polyacrylamide have led to the development of monosubstituted and disubstituted monomers, one of which is *N*-acryloyl-tris(hydroxymethyl)aminomethane, or poly(NAT) (Elchrom Scientific, Cham, Switzerland).[7] This material is more hydrophilic than polyacrylamide and its matrix has larger pores, thereby presenting less resistance to the passage of large molecules. It is ideally suited to the separation of DNA fragments up to 20 kilobases (kb) using a homogeneous (nonpulsed) electric field. Fragments that differ in size by as little as 2% can be resolved. Gels are submersed in buffer during use, allowing temperatures to be tightly controlled at values between 50 and 60 °C. Use of increased temperatures results in shorter run times and more reproducible band migration.

Automated systems. Because of increased volume of testing, primarily for serum proteins, many laboratories are converting to automated systems for electrophoresis. Such a system is the Helena SPIFE 4000 (Helena Laboratories, Beaumont, TX), an automated electrophoresis system providing automated reagent application and a variety of gel sizes that permit analysis of 10 to 100 samples simultaneously. It also features inline sample application, automated electrophoretic separation and staining of analytes, multiple stain ports, and

positive sample identification. The Interlab Microgel system (Interlab Srl, Rome, Italy) also fully automates the process and integrates sample application, temperature-controlled electrophoresis, staining, and densitometry into a single unit with the capability of managing four gels simultaneously. Other systems that have partially automated the procedure or incorporated the ability to sequentially process multiple gels of different compositions include the Phast System (Pharmacia LKB, Gaithersburg, MD), the HITE Fractoscan (Olympus, Invicon, München, Germany), the Hydragel-Hydrasys (Sebia, Durham, NC), and the High-Performance Gel Electrophoresis (HPGE)-1000 system (LabIntelligence, Belmont, CA). Most CE systems (see section on Capillary Electrophoresis) have autosampling capability for sequentially processing specimens, but the Sebia Capillarys permits simultaneous processing of seven samples by using multiple capillaries. Newer microchip-based analyzers such as the Agilent 2100 Bioanalyzer (Agilent Technologies, Santa Clara, CA) significantly miniaturize and increase the speed of the process for separating proteins, nucleic acids, or even entire cells. These advances substantially reduce the labor component associated with this technique.

Capillary Electrophoresis

With CE, the classic techniques of zone electrophoresis, ITP, isoelectric focusing (IEF), and gel electrophoresis are carried out in a small-bore (10- to 100-μm internal diameter) fused silica capillary tube, 20 to 200 cm in length.[8]

Two distinct advantages of the capillary format include the ability to apply much higher voltages than in traditional electrophoresis and the ease of automation. Applications are also more extensive and include separation of low-molecular-weight ions, in addition to proteins and other macromolecules. Even uncharged molecules can be separated using CE in the micellar electrokinetic chromatography (MEKC) mode, discussed later. CE has also proven useful for separation of inorganic ions, amino acids, organic acids, drugs, vitamins, porphyrins, carbohydrates, oligonucleotides, proteins, and DNA fragments.[9–12]

General Operations

A schematic diagram of a typical instrumental configuration for CE is shown in Fig. 18.4. As indicated, the capillary serves as an electrophoretic chamber, analogous to a lane on a gel,

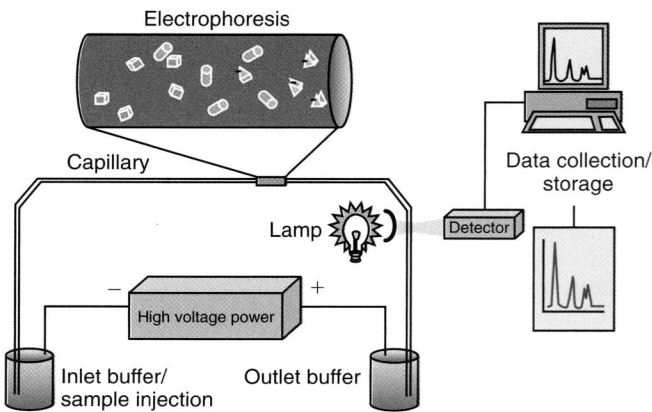

FIGURE 18.4 A schematic for capillary electrophoresis instrumentation.

which is connected to buffer reservoirs at both ends, which, in turn, are connected to a high-voltage power supply. It is important to note that at some point along the length of the capillary (typically close to the end), a detector is interfaced for online detection. Improved heat dissipation from the capillary (as opposed to a slab gel) permits the application of voltages in the range of 10 to 30 kV, which enhances separation efficiency and reduces separation time, in some cases to less than 1 minute. Only a few microliters of the sample are required, with injected volumes in the nanoliter range. The small sample plug volume minimizes distortions in the applied field caused by the presence of analytes or other sample species.

In contrast to the cumbersome and time-consuming tasks of conventional electrophoresis, CE is easily automated. Analogous to high-performance liquid chromatography (HPLC) technology, samples typically are stored in a temperature-controlled environment and are automatically injected into the capillary, with a variety of detector types available; the resulting electropherograms are analyzed and manipulated in much the same manner as chromatograms.

The capillaries used as separation columns in CE are most commonly made from fused silica (i.e., pure glass) coated with a thin exterior covering of polyimide to provide strength and flexibility. Although capillaries can be made from other materials, such as polyethylene or Teflon, such capillaries have seen limited use. The polyimide coating is usually removed from a small portion of the capillary close to the terminal end, creating a window for online optical detection. The outer diameter of the capillary tubing typically varies from 180 to 375 μm, the inner diameter from 20 to 180 μm, and the total length from 20 cm up to several meters. Noncylindrical capillary tubing suitable for CE is available from some commercial providers. For example, rectangular capillaries (Polymicro Technologies, Phoenix, AZ) provide a flat surface that is more amenable to optical detection than their curved counterparts.

Sample injection. In CE, sample volumes of 1 to 50 nL are loaded into the capillary by *hydrodynamic injection* or *electrokinetic (EK) injection.* With hydrodynamic injection, an aliquot of a sample is introduced by applying positive pressure at the inlet vial or vacuum at the outlet vial. The volume of sample loaded is governed by a number of parameters, including (but not restricted to) (1) the inner diameter of the capillary, (2) buffer viscosity, (3) applied pressure, (4) temperature, and (5) time. With some earlier commercial or homemade systems, gravity was used as the source of pressure by raising the inlet vial (or lowering the outlet vial), thus allowing "siphoning" to occur for a timed interval. With EK injection, an aliquot of a sample is introduced by applying a voltage for a timed interval. The magnitude of the voltage depends on the analyte and buffer system used but typically involves a field strength three to five times lower than that used for separation. It is important to note that although hydrodynamic methods introduce a sample representative of the bulk specimen, EK injection favors the preferential movement of more electrokinetically mobile analytes into the capillary.

In practice, to maintain high separation efficiency, the sample plug length is usually less than 2% of the total capillary length.

Direct detection. With CE, separated analytes are detected and measured as they migrate past a point on the capillary that is optically interrogated. Optical detection is based on classic methods, such as photometric absorbance, refractive index, and fluorescence (see Chapter 16). As with HPLC, ultraviolet (UV)-visible photometers are widely used as detectors to monitor CE separations.[13] To interface such online detectors with the capillary, a *detection window* is created toward the outlet end of the capillary. This "window," which serves as an inline cuvet, typically is formed by burning off the polyimide with a small flame and cleaning the window with ethanol. Although this configuration allows high-efficiency separation, the inner diameter of the capillary tube defines the optical path length (OPL) of the inline cuvet. Because absorbance is directly proportional to the length of the cuvet used in an optical system, the 20- to 100-μm inner diameter of the capillary limits UV-visible absorbance detection limits to concentrations of 10^{-8} to 10^{-6} molar.

More sensitive optical techniques that have been used with CE include (1) fluorescence, (2) refractive index, (3) chemiluminescence, (4) Raman spectrophotometry, and (5) circular dichroism.[11] The most sensitive optical detection method used in CE is laser-induced fluorescence (LIF), which is capable of detection limits in the 10^{-9} to 10^{-12} molar (or better) range. This detection mode is easily accomplished with analytes that may be labeled with a fluorescent substrate (e.g., intercalators for double-stranded [ds]DNA) or may be naturally fluorescent (e.g., proteins or peptides containing tryptophan). CE systems also have been interfaced with mass spectrometers,[14] and electrochemical detection devices[15] have been developed, although such detectors must be isolated electrically from the electrophoretic voltages.

Indirect detection. When strong chromophores are lacking in the analyte of interest, absorbance and fluorescence detection have been used in an indirect mode.[16–18] In this mode, a strongly absorbing ion is added to the running electrolyte and is monitored at a wavelength that gives a constant high background absorbance. As solute ions move into their discrete zones during the electrophoretic process, they displace the indirect detection agent through mutual repulsion, and this produces a decrease in background absorbance as the zone passes through the detector. Reagents with appropriate fluorescence properties have been used in a similar manner. Indirect detection of amino acids by CE has been demonstrated, with the potential for use in diagnosis of aminoacidurias.[19] Investigators have demonstrated the direct extrapolation of this technique to microchip detection when UV detection is difficult, if not impossible.

Types of Electrophores

Capillary zone electrophoresis. CZE, also called *open-tube* or *free-solution* CE, is the simplest form of CE. It includes *capillary ion electrophoresis,* which refers to the analysis of inorganic ions by CZE, often using indirect detection. The power of the CZE mode is its ability to electrophoretically resolve charged species without a sieving matrix; this applies to a broad spectrum of analytes ranging from proteins, peptides, and amino acids to small molecules (e.g., drugs) and ions.

Capillary gel electrophoresis. Capillary gel electrophoresis (CGE) is directly comparable with traditional slab or tube gel electrophoresis because the separation mechanisms are identical. Size separation is achieved with a suitable polymer, which acts as a molecular sieve or sizing mechanism. As charged analytes migrate through the polymer network, they become hindered to a degree that is governed by their size (larger molecules are hindered more than smaller ones). Macromolecules, such as DNA and sodium dodecyl sulfate (SDS)-saturated proteins, cannot be separated without a gel or some other separation mechanism, because they have a mass-to-charge ratio that is size independent. The term *gel* in CGE is a misnomer, primarily because cross-linked "gels," as we know them in slab format, are not routinely used in CE. A more suitable term is a *sieving matrix* or *soluble polymer network,* a linear polymeric structure that is soluble, has reasonably low viscosity, and is capable of self-entangling in a manner that forms pores through which sieving can occur. A variety of polymeric matrices have been defined for DNA (e.g., polyacrylamide, cellulosic materials) and protein analysis (e.g., dextran-base matrices), provided that pores can be formed inherently that have diameters in the range of tens to hundreds of nanometers. One of the requirements that often accompanies this type of analysis is reduction of EOF. This is accomplished by covalently, adsorptively, or dynamically coating the surface. Cross-linked polyacrylamide was the main polymer of choice for this but recently has been supplanted by a host of polymeric matrices that not only provide effective molecular sieving but also adsorptively coat the capillary surface.[20,21]

POINTS TO REMEMBER

Capillary Electrophoresis
- Capillary zone electrophoresis (CZE) uses electro-osmotic flow (EOF) to mobilize the sample plug past the detector.
- Capillary gel electrophoresis (CGE) is best used with macromolecules such as DNA or large proteins and uses a sieving matrix for separation.
- Higher voltages can be applied because of more efficient dissipation of heat—this can translate to faster separations.

Technical Considerations—Gel

In performing electrophoretic separations, a number of technical and practical aspects need to be considered for optimal performance.

Sampling

To achieve a proper balance between sensitive measurements and resolution, the amount of serum protein applied to an electrophoretic support must be optimal. Albumin is approximately 10 times more concentrated in serum than the smallest fraction, the α_1-globulins. Therefore the amount of serum applied should prevent overloading with albumin but still should be adequate to quantify α_1-globulin. For separation of serum proteins using PAGE, 3 μL of serum containing approximately 210 μg of total protein is applied. For alkaline phosphatase isoenzymes, up to 25 μL of serum may be applied if alkaline phosphatase activity is within the reference interval but smaller volumes may be used if enzyme activity is greatly increased. Urine specimens require 50- to 100-fold concentration or extended application time for adequate sensitivity, and CSF may or may not require concentration, depending on the staining approach used.

Discontinuities in Sample Application

Discontinuities in sample application may be caused by (1) dirty applicators, (2) uneven absorption by sample combs, or (3) inclusion of an air bubble if sample is pipetted onto the gel. The pipette tip should be checked for air bubbles before the sample is applied to the agarose gel template.

Unequal Migration Rates

Unequal migration of samples across the width of the gel may be caused by dirty electrodes, which may cause uneven application of the electric field, or by uneven wetting of the gel. If wicks are used to connect the gel to a power supply, uneven wetting of the wicks could cause unequal migration or bowing of sample lanes at the gel edges. Gels must be kept horizontal during storage to avoid sagging and uneven thickness. Finally, gels that may have been stored too close to heat sources (e.g., in a cabinet over a light fixture) could have partially and unevenly dried areas, contributing to similar problems.

Distorted, Unusual, or Atypical Bands

Distorted protein zones may be caused by (1) bent applicators, (2) incorporation of an air bubble during sample application, (3) overapplication, or (4) inadequate blotting of the sample. Excessive drying of the electrophoretic support before or during electrophoresis may also cause distorted zones. Irregularities (other than broken zones) in the sample application probably are due to excessively wet agarose gels. Portions of applied samples may look washed out.

In most cases, unusual bands are artifacts that may be easily recognized. Hemolyzed samples are frequent causes of increased β-globulin (where free hemoglobin migrates) or an unusual band between the α_2- and β-globulins, the result of a hemoglobin-haptoglobin complex. If plasma samples are tested, a fibrinogen band will be observed at the application point of an electropherogram. Because such a band appears similar to those formed by monoclonal Igs, it may be mistakenly reported as an abnormal, monoclonal protein if plasma is submitted for testing in place of serum. The α- and β-lipoproteins may migrate ahead of their normal positions in some samples. Occasionally, a split albumin zone is observed in the rare, benign, genetically related condition of bisalbuminemia. However, a grossly widened albumin zone could be due to albumin-bound medication and not faulty practice of electrophoresis.

Technical Considerations—Capillary

Temperature and surface effects influence the separation capabilities of CE. Artifacts also have been known to arise with CE.

Temperature Effects

In most slab or tube platforms for electrophoresis, moderate electric fields (up to 1000 V) are used, because the Joule heating that accompanies the use of higher field strengths causes nonuniform temperature gradients, local changes in viscosity, and subsequent zone broadening. CE is distinguished from other forms of electrophoresis by the fact that extraordinarily high fields (30,000 V) are used to obtain rapid, high-efficiency separations. The problems encountered with noncapillary platforms are prevented by effective dissipation of Joule heat by forced air convection or liquid cooling of the capillary, both of which are possible because of the narrow bore of the capillary. The Joule heat produced is a function of (1) buffer type, (2) buffer concentration, (3) voltage applied,

(4) capillary inner diameter, and (5) length and can be determined for any given system by generating an *Ohms law plot,* which allows easy determination of the maximum voltage that can be used effectively.[22] Reducing the inner diameter of the capillary, the ionic strength of the running buffer, or the applied voltage will reduce the heat produced by the electrophoretic process. It should be noted that reducing the inner diameter will compromise the detection limit of UV measurements (smaller OPL); reducing the applied field is less desirable in that resolution is directly proportional to the applied field. Consequently, attempts should be made to alter other parameters before reducing inner diameter or the applied field.

Surface Effects

As in electrophoresis in general, the flow of fluid (EOF) in CE is a consequence of surface charge on the solid support. In CE, EOF has been known to play a significant role in the separation process. The charge on the inner surface of a fused silica capillary is determined by the ionization state of the silanol groups that populate it. Interaction of positively charged buffer species with bound surface anions generates a layer of mobile cations that move toward the cathode when voltage is applied. This induces a very strong EOF that mobilizes all analytes in the same direction, regardless of their charge. The desired separation is consequently achieved because of differences in the electrophoretic migration rates of analytes superimposed on this EOF.

Because the driving force of the flow is distributed along the wall of the capillary, the flow profile is nearly flat or pluglike, contrasting with the laminar or parabolic flow generated by a pressure-driven system caused by shear forces at the wall. A flat flow profile is beneficial because it does not contribute to the dispersion of solute zones. The magnitude and direction of the EOF are influenced by several parameters, including (1) type of electrolyte used, (2) pH, (3) ionic strength, (4) use of additives (e.g., surfactants, organic solvents), and (5) polarity and magnitude of the applied electric field.

Although advantageous for dissipation of Joule heat, the large ratio of surface area to volume of the inner capillary space increases the likelihood of analyte adsorption onto the surface of its inner wall. This causes phenomena such as peak tailing and even total and irreversible adsorption of the analyte. Adsorption is typically noted between cationic solutes and the negatively charged inner wall of the capillary, primarily through ionic interactions (with deprotonated silanols), but also involves hydrophobic interactions (with siloxanes). Because of the numerous charges and hydrophobic regions, significant adsorptive effects have been noted, especially for highly cationic proteins. In practice, adsorption of substances, whether from the sample or from the buffer, to the inner surface of the capillary will alter migration times and other separation characteristics; unaddressed, the capillary eventually may become "fouled." Buffer components and/or additives such as surfactants often can render permanent changes to the inner surface of the capillary (through adsorption) and may warrant dedication of specific capillaries for use with particular surfactants.

To minimize these inner wall effects, capillaries are conditioned by chemical treatment, most commonly with base, to remove adsorbates and rejuvenate the surface. A typical wash method includes flushing the chamber with 10 to 20 capillary

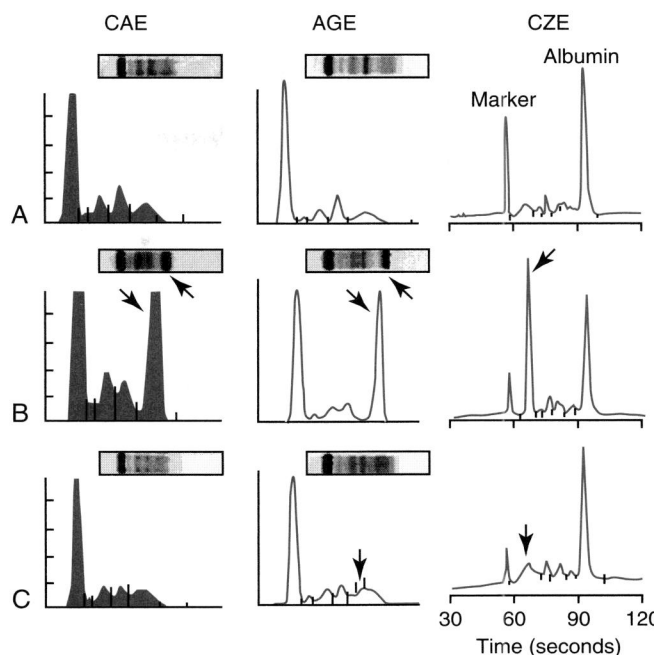

FIGURE 18.5 Rapid protein electrophoresis of serum protein; comparison with scanning densitometry profiles obtained from cellulose acetate *(CAE)* and agarose *(AGE)* electrophoresis. **A,** Normal serum. **B,** Patient serum containing a large M-protein. **C,** Patient serum containing a small monoclonal protein. *Arrows* indicate the position of the monoclonal proteins. *CZE,* Capillary zone electrophoresis.

volumes of 0.1 to 1.0 mol/L NaOH, followed by flushing with "run" buffer. To prevent exposing the capillary surface to drastic fluctuations in pH, conditioning procedures for separations at low pH may be better served by using strong acids (e.g., HNO_3), surfactants (e.g., SDS), or organic solvents, such as acetonitrile or methanol.

Serum Protein Analysis

Compared with AGE and cellulose acetate electrophoresis (CAE), CZE is more advantageous for serum protein analysis.[8,23,24] Fig. 18.5 shows a comparison of the separation of serum proteins by CAE, AGE, and CE. The presence of the classic zones with CE is apparent, albeit in reversed order, as is the identification of serum protein abnormalities in the gamma regions. Retrospective studies have shown CE to be effective for detecting monoclonal proteins, which could then be immunotyped by conventional techniques (immunofixation and IEF).[8] Moreover, one study demonstrated the utility of CE in doing both serum protein electrophoresis and immunotyping for more than 1500 serum samples.[23] These and other studies put forth the same conclusion—that CE is more sensitive than AGE in identifying abnormalities. More recent studies have shown the value of CZE in serum protein analysis. In 2005, Luraschi and associates[25] described the use of CZE coupled with immunosubtraction to detect and characterize low concentrations of free γ heavy chains in serum. In this study, they showed that γ heavy chain disease could be detected by serum protein analysis in CZE in tandem with immunosubtraction. However, although studies have proven the clear utility of CZE for serum protein analysis, Bossuyt and coworkers[26] point to the fact that CZE is not flawless, describing a case in which CZE failed to detect μ heavy chain disease in a 90-year-old woman. This is countered by Maisnar and colleagues,[27] who submit that the laboratory diagnosis of patients with μ heavy chain disease is typically challenging and that detection of the monoclonal protein by standard electrophoretic approaches may fail in up to 75% of cases of μ heavy chain disease. They describe a patient who had multiple malignancies, which included vulvar carcinoma and Hodgkin lymphoma, for whom CZE with immunotyping allowed the detection and characterization of monoclonal μ heavy chains.

Finally, CZE for serum protein analysis is evolving in a high-throughput format that has leveraged the success of multiplexed CE systems developed for DNA analysis. Two commercial systems have evolved: the Beckman Paragon 2000 (Beckman Analytical, Milan, Italy) and Sebia Capillarys. Although several studies have illustrated the potential of these systems for serum paraprotein characterization (essentially supplanting AGE and IFE),[28–30] studies have not yet settled the issue of paraprotein detection sensitivity and specificity for the clinical community.[28,31,32] For example, Yang and associates[33] compared the Capillarys 2 system versus standard serum protein AGE for the detection and identification of monoclonal proteins in patient serum samples. After defining sensitivity for both, they concluded that AGE and CZE had the same specificity for detection of monoclonal proteins but that CZE/immunosubtraction was slightly less sensitive than standard immunofixation in the detection of IgM and free light chains.

Artifacts in Serum Protein Analysis

With CE using online optical detection, artifacts can occur in the form of "system peaks." These often originate from the sample or from the interfaces between the sample and the separation buffer, because any species that absorbs at the detection wavelength will generate a response. This differs from protein slab gel electrophoresis, wherein detection specificity is governed by a protein-specific stain. It is not uncommon, for example, for buffer species present in the sample but not in the separation buffer to generate system peaks.

One problem associated with conventional electrophoresis of serum proteins is its proclivity for point-of-application artifacts. These are bands that result from the fact that electrophoretic mobility (e.g., with AGE) is bidirectional from the point of application. Consequently, the point of application remains part of the scanned area of interest. These bands must be immunotyped to distinguish real monoclonal proteins from artifacts—a process that is costly and time consuming. CE prevents point-of-application artifacts in two ways. First, net mobility in CE results from the vectorial addition of both protein electrophoretic mobility and EOF. As a result of this unidirectional movement (toward the detector), the point of application remains removed from the detector. Second, unlike AGE, in which precipitates cannot exit the loading well and enter the gel (thus appearing as a band in the scanned region of the gel), no gel matrix is present in CZE to impede electrophoretic migration, because analysis occurs in free solution (i.e., CZE). This was demonstrated by Clark and colleagues,[34] who evaluated a small subset of serum samples containing application artifacts resembling monoclonal proteins on agarose gels (and cellulose acetate) but

were eliminated by CZE. These precipitates may be euglobulin or cryoprecipitates and may contain a monoclonal protein; only immunoelectrophoresis or IFE can identify the presence of monoclonal proteins.

Hemoglobin Analysis

CE has been used in the clinical lab for analysis of hemoglobin in two different applications: one is to identify hemoglobinopathies and one for the analysis of hemoglobin A_{1c} (HbA_{1c}). Traditional hemoglobinopathy analysis involves performing acid and/or alkaline gel electrophoresis along with liquid chromatography for this analysis (see Chapter 77 for more details), but more recently, clinical labs have begun to implement CZE. Important benefits of CE include a more automated process and higher throughput of samples. Analytically, hemoglobinopathy detection has displayed favorable comparison with HPLC systems, showing a linear correlation of hemoglobin (Hb)A_2, HbF, and HbS.[35,36]

HbA_{1c} is the fraction of hemoglobin where a glucose has been nonenzymatically attached to the N-terminal valine of the β-chain, which is frequently measured as a means to diagnose and monitor diabetes (see Chapter 47). Historical HbA_{1c} measurement methods in the clinical laboratory have included HPLC, boronate affinity HPLC, and immunoassay. In 1997, CE was evaluated as an analytical tool to measure HbA_{1c} and showed favorable comparison with an HPLC method.[37] Since then, the technology has advanced and commercial systems are available to clinical laboratories. Compared with HPLC systems, CE offers an improved resolution of HbA_{1c}, HbA and HbA_2 peaks, as well as the ability to detect the presence of rare hemoglobins.[38,39]

Improving Limits of Detection

Several approaches have been devised to improve the limit of detection of online CE detectors. These include increasing the length of the OPL and online concentration of the sample.

Increased optical path length. Capillary tubes modified at the detector window with a "bubble" cell (a glass-blown expansion of the internal diameter of the capillary tube) can expand the OPL by almost an order of magnitude, with concomitant lowering of the system's limit of detection. Alternatively, a "Z" geometry has been developed that increases the OPL via detection down the core of the capillary, with possible lengths up to 1 mm.

Online sample concentration. Another technique used in CE systems to increase their limit of detection is preconcentration of the sample. One of the simplest methods for sample preconcentration is to induce a "stacking" effect with the sample components, which is easily accomplished by exploiting the ionic strength differences between the sample matrix and the separation buffer.[40] This results from the fact that sample ions have decreased electrophoretic mobility in a higher conductivity environment. When voltage is applied to the system, sample ions in the sample plug instantaneously accelerate toward the adjacent separation buffer zone. On crossing the boundary, the higher conductivity environment induces a decrease in electrophoretic velocity and subsequent stacking of the sample components into a smaller buffer zone than the original sample plug. Within a short time, the ionic strength gradient dissipates and the charged analyte molecules begin to move from the stacked sample zone toward the cathode. Stacking has been used with hydrostatic or EK injection and typically yields a 10-fold enhancement in sample concentration, resulting in a lower limit of detection.

An alternative approach to stacking is "focusing" that is based on pH differences between the sample plug and the separation buffer. This has been shown to be very useful for analysis of peptides, mainly because of their relative stability over a wide pH range.[41] By increasing the pH of the sample to greater than that of the net pI of the analytes of interest and flanking the sample plug with low-pH separation buffer zones (i.e., an equivalent volume of low-pH separation buffer after introduction of the sample plug), negatively charged peptides are electrophoretically driven toward the anode. On entering the lower pH separation buffer, a pH-induced change in their charge state causes a reversal in their electrophoretic mobility, resulting in "focusing" of the peptides at the interface of the sample (high pH) and low-pH buffer plugs (similar to those in IEF). After the pH gradient dissipates, the peptides, again positively charged, migrate toward the cathode as a sharp zone. This approach has been applied to a variety of analytes but is limited to those able to withstand inherent changes in pH without substantial denaturation and may yield as much as a fivefold enhancement of a system's limit of detection.[42]

Other types of sample concentration enhancement approaches applicable to CE include ITP[43] and those involving concentration of an online solid phase.[44] This latter method shows much promise for both small and large molecules and is discussed in detail in the review by Wettstein and Strausbauch.[45]

SPECIALTY ELECTROPHORESIS TECHNIQUES

With different media in different physical formats and a variety of instrumental configurations, several different types of electrophoretic techniques are used for the separation of a diverse range of analytes.

Starch Gel

Starch gel was the first gel medium to be used for electrophoresis and is only of historical interest. It separated proteins by both charge-to-mass ratio and molecular size, and, because proteins compacted on the surface of the gel before migrating into it, they formed narrow bands with improved resolution.

Disc Electrophoresis

Protein electrophoresis using agarose gel yields only five zones: (1) albumin and (2) α_1-, (3) α_2-, (4) β-, and (5) γ-globulins, although some subfractionation of the α_2- and β-globulins is possible with high-resolution gels. *Disc electrophoresis* was developed by Davis and Ornstein to improve this situation and derived its name from *discontinuities* in the electrophoretic matrix caused by layers of polyacrylamide or starch gel that differ in composition and pore size. These gels may yield 20 or more fractions and were widely used to study individual proteins in serum, especially genetic variants and isoenzymes.

With this technique, samples were separated in a three-gel system prepared in situ. A small-pore *separation gel*, followed by a thin segment of large-pore *spacer gel*, then a thin layer of large-pore monomer solution containing a small amount of serum—approximately 3 µL—was polymerized in open-ended glass tubes. When electrophoresis begins, all protein

ions stack up on the separation gel in a very thin zone. This process improves resolution and concentrated protein components so that preconcentration of specimens with low protein content (e.g., CSF) may not be necessary.

Isoelectric Focusing Electrophoresis

IEF separates amphoteric compounds, such as proteins, with increased resolution in a medium possessing a stable pH gradient. The protein becomes "focused" at a point on the gel as it migrates to a zone where the pH of the gel matches the protein's pI. At this point, the charge of the protein becomes zero and its migration ceases. Fig. 18.6 illustrates the procedure and shows the electrophoretic conditions before and after current is applied. The protein zones are very sharp because the region associated with a given pH is very narrow. Ordinary diffusion is also counteracted by the acquisition of a charge, as a protein varies from its pI position and subsequently migrates back because of electrophoretic forces (Fig. 18.7). Proteins that differ in their pI values by only 0.02 pH unit have been separated by IEF.

The pH gradient is created with *carrier ampholytes,* a group of amphoteric polyaminocarboxylic acids that have slight differences in pKa value and molecular weights of 300 to 1000. Mixtures of 50 to 100 different compounds are added to the medium and create a "natural pH gradient" when individual ampholytes reach their pI values during electrophoresis. They establish narrow buffered zones, with stable but slightly different pH values, through which the slower moving proteins migrate and stop at their individual pIs.

As Fig. 18.6 illustrates, the anode is surrounded by a dilute acid solution and the cathode by a dilute alkaline solution. After focusing, the most negatively charged carrier ampholytes and proteins will be found at the anodal end and the most positively charged near the cathodal end of the electrophoretic matrix. The other carrier ampholytes and proteins

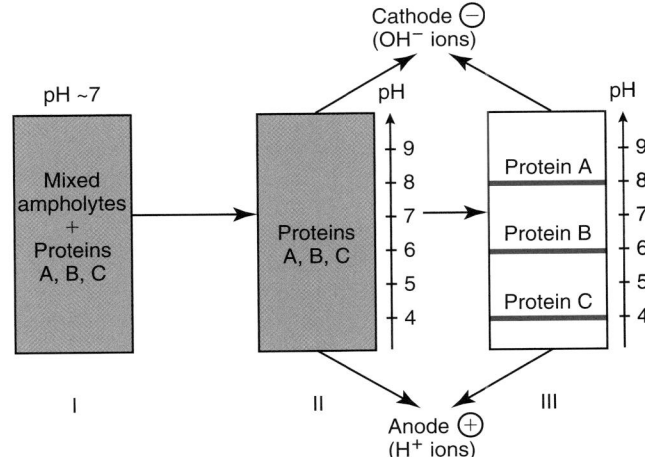

FIGURE 18.6 Schematic of an isoelectric focusing (IEF) procedure. *I,* A homogeneous mixture of carrier ampholytes, pH range 3 to 10, to which proteins A, B, and C, with isoelectric point (pI) of 8, 6, and 4, respectively, were added. *II,* Current is applied and carrier ampholytes rapidly migrate to pH zones where the net charge is zero (the pI value). *III,* Proteins A, B, and C migrate more slowly to their respective pI zones, where migration ceases. The high buffering capacity of the carrier ampholyte creates stable pH zones in which each protein may reach its pI.

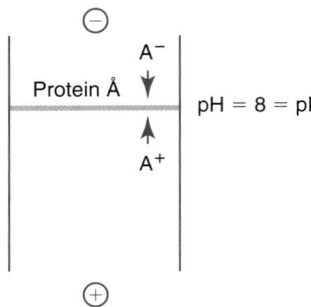

FIGURE 18.7 After the pH where protein A has a net charge of zero (Å) is attained, diffusion toward the cathode bestows a negative charge on A (A⁻), and migration in the electric field forces A⁻ back to Å. Diffusion toward the anode causes A to take on the opposite charge A⁺, and migration is toward the cathode and toward the point where Å exists. Isoelectric focusing processes of this type cause focusing of proteins and formation of sharp zones.

focus at intermediate points according to their pI values. Because carrier ampholytes are generally used in relatively high concentrations, a high-voltage power source (up to 2000 V) is necessary (power is in the vicinity of 2 to 50 W, depending on experimental conditions). As a result, the electrophoretic matrix must be cooled. A modification of this technique (immobilized pH gradient [IPG]-IEF), in which an IPG is produced in the gel before the sample is applied, is reported to improve resolution and reproducibility.[46]

PAGE-IEF is widely used in analytical work, because it is essentially free of EOF. However, the polyacrylamide gel must have a sufficiently large pore size so that protein migration will not be impeded by molecular sieving effects. In actual practice, impeded migration of some proteins, such as IgM, cannot be prevented. AGE-IEF has the advantages that operating conditions are simple and large pore sizes make it unlikely that any proteins will be excluded on the basis of molecular size. IEF has been applied to the separation of alkaline phosphatase isoenzymes and is widely used in neonatal screening programs to test for variant hemoglobins (see Chapter 77). Off-gel techniques carry out the separation in free solution with sample containing ampholytes loaded into each of a linear series of wells separated by semipermeable membranes and in contact with a pH gradient strip. Electrophoresis separates sample proteins into different wells depending on their pI values. Separated fractions can be further resolved in a second similar focusing step or taken directly to further separation by two-dimensional (2D) electrophoresis (see later section) or liquid chromatography tandem mass spectrometry (LC-MS/MS).[47,48] This technique has been useful in the study of the human proteome.

For IEF, a power supply that provides constant power is advisable. During electrophoresis, current drops significantly because of lower conductivity as carrier ampholytes focus at their pI values and because of creation of zones of pure water. If a constant voltage supply is used, frequent voltage adjustments may be necessary. As a result, constant current power supplies are not customarily used in IEF. *Pulsed-power* or *pulsed-field* techniques (see later section) require a power supply that can periodically change the orientation of the applied field relative to the direction of migration.

Isotachophoresis

ITP completely separates smaller ionic substances into adjacent zones that contact one another with no overlap, and all migrate at the same rate. In this technique, background electrolyte (buffer) is not mixed with the sample, so current flow is carried entirely by charged sample ions. An aliquot of a sample is typically placed in a capillary between a leading electrolyte solution that contains faster migrating ions than any in the sample and a trailing solution containing slower migrating ions than any in the sample. Once a faster-moving component separates completely from a slower-moving one, any further separation creates a region of depleted charge and increases the resistance and therefore the local voltage in that region. Increased voltage causes the slower component to migrate faster and close the gap, thereby concentrating it and increasing the conductivity of its zone until it matches that of the faster ion. Ultimately, all ions migrate at the rate of the fastest ion in zones that differ in size depending on their original concentrations. Zone size is determined by measuring UV absorbance, temperature difference, or conductivity as the sample passes a detector. Applications include the separation of small anions and cations, organic and amino acids, and peptides, nucleotides, nucleosides, and proteins.

Pulsed-Field Electrophoresis

In pulsed-field electrophoresis, power is alternately applied to different pairs of electrodes or electrode arrays, so the electrophoretic field is cycled between two directions. The directions can differ spatially by 105 to 180°, and molecules must reorient themselves to the new field direction during each cycle before migration can continue. Because reorientation time depends on molecular size, net migration becomes a function of the frequency of field alteration. This permits separation of very large molecules, such as DNA fragments greater than 50 kb, which cannot be resolved by the relatively small pores in agarose or polyacrylamide gels.[49] Fragments of 50 to 400 kb can be resolved using 10-s pulse times, whereas larger fragments up to 7 Mb in size or intact chromosomes require pulse times of several hours for complete resolution. This technique has been applied to typing various strains of bacterial DNA for research or epidemiologic studies.[50–53]

Two-Dimensional Electrophoresis

In the field of proteomics, *2D electrophoresis* is extensively used to study families of proteins and search for genetic- or disease-based differences or to study the protein content of cells of various types.[54] It also has been applied to the study of human gene mutations[55] and the DNA of various bacteria and tumor cells as a means to establish an earlier diagnosis.[56,57] By combining charge-dependent IEF in the first dimension with molecular weight–dependent electrophoresis in the second, the technique is able to resolve up to 1100 separate protein spots using autoradiographic detection, and up to 400 using Coomassie dyes. The first-dimension separation is carried out in a large-pore medium, such as agarose gel or large-pore polyacrylamide gel. The second dimension is often polyacrylamide in a linear or gradient format.

Conventional 2D electrophoresis uses PAGE-IEF in 130 × 2.5-mm (internal diameter) tubes for the first dimension and covers a pH range of 3 to 10 units. After electrophoresis is complete, the gel is extruded from the tube and placed in contact with a thin, polyacrylamide gradient gel slab that incorporates SDS. At the end of the process, the polypeptides are detected by one of several different methods. SDS is commonly used in the second dimension because it denatures proteins to polypeptides by reducing disulfide bonds and depolymerizing proteins. When native proteins, such as enzymes, are desired for further study, nondenaturing sample preparation and electrophoresis conditions must be used.

Separated proteins are detected with Coomassie dyes, silver staining, radiography (exposure of photographic film to emissions of isotopically labeled polypeptides or chemiluminescence), or fluorographic analysis (x-ray film exposed to tritium-labeled polypeptides in the presence of a scintillator). The latter two methods represent the most sensitive methods and are 100 to 1000 times more sensitive than Coomassie dyes. Difference gel electrophoresis permits two samples to be compared on the same 2D gel by labeling each with a different fluorophore. Although each separated spot contains protein from the two different samples, selective excitation and scanning software allow differences in expression to be qualitatively identified.[58,59]

Newer developments in this area combine analytical techniques to achieve 2D separation by linking, for example, liquid IEF with nonporous silica reverse-phase HPLC (for additional information on chromatography see Chapter 19) and detecting intact proteins by electrospray ionization, time of flight, and mass spectrometry (see Chapter 20).[21,60]

Micellar Electrokinetic Chromatography

MEKC is a hybrid of electrophoresis and chromatography. MEKC, a mode that is separate and distinct from capillary EK chromatography, is an effective electrophoretic technique because it can be used for separation of neutral and charged solutes. The separation of neutral species is accomplished by exploiting micelles formed in the running buffer when the concentration of surfactant exceeds the critical micelle concentration (e.g., 8 to 9 mmol/L for SDS). During electrophoresis, neutral micelles can interact with analytes in a chromatographic manner through hydrophobic interactions in which analytes are micellized based on their degree of hydrophobicity. Under these conditions, partitioning into the micelle is the driving force for separation. With charged micelles (e.g., SDS), analytes also can interact through electrostatic interactions via the charge on the surface of the micelle.[61]

Capillary Isoelectric Focusing Electrophoresis

Capillary isoelectric focusing electrophoresis (cIEF) is comparable with tube IEF and is governed by the same principles and procedures. It differs from conventional IEF in that it can be carried out using a free solution of ampholytes or a precast gel. As expected with a CE mode, and unlike conventional IEF, the focused zones migrate past the online detector during the focusing process or following it. Fig. 18.8 shows an example of this in which separation by cIEF is completed in approximately 15 minutes, circumventing conventional IEF protocols and/or the necessity for other electrophoretic methods (e.g., CAE to detect hemoglobin variants), both of which are much less time efficient.[62]

Capillary Isotachophoresis

Capillary ITP has essentially the same features as ITP in other formats, except that conditions of pure ITP usually are not

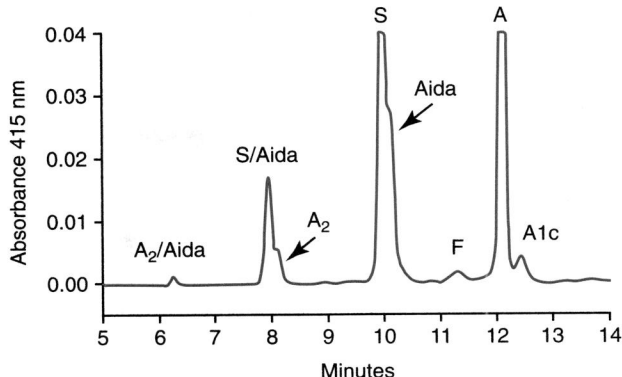

FIGURE 18.8 Capillary electrophoresis (CE)-based identification of uncommon hemoglobin (Hb) variants by capillary isoelectric focusing electrophoresis.[57] Analysis of blood from a patient with HbS/Aida trait detected the presence of seven different normal and abnormal structural Hb variants, some of which are not detectable by conventional electrophoresis because of lack of sensitivity or inadequate resolution. The four abnormal variants include HbS, Aida, S/Aida hybrid, and A_2/Aida. Glycated HbA (HbA$_{1c}$) is also apparent in the electropherogram.

achieved. This is not commonly used as a bona fide CE mode but instead is more typically used for online sample preconcentration (as described earlier). Most of the time, it functions as a preconcentrating step in a mixed mode with CZE, MEKC, or CGE. However, ITP may be undergoing a renaissance. Research being performed by the Santiago Group at Stanford University is beginning to show that rigorous modeling of the process may begin to tease new capabilities and applications out of a technique that has been largely unheralded over the decades since Schoots and Eaverarts first described it as a sample preparation technique for liquid chromatography.[63]

Microchip Electrophoresis

Over the past decade, microchip electrophoresis has undergone substantial development, including integrated microchip designs, advanced detection systems, and new applications.[64–67] In the arena of clinical diagnosis, the main analytes of interest for extrapolation to the microchip platform are proteins and DNA. This section provides a very brief overview; for a more comprehensive discussion, see Chapter 27.

Among the attributes of microchip electrophoresis separation, the most notable is high speed—normally 4-fold to 10-fold faster than conventional CE, and at least an order of magnitude faster than the slab gel format. Other advantages of microchips include simplicity, capability for chip integration of multiple functions, and certainly the potential for automation.

Instrumentation

Although similar in principle, the microchip system differs from its CE counterpart. For example, with the microchip approach, separation channels, sample injection channels, reservoirs, and sample preparation and/or precolumn or postcolumn reactors can be fabricated onto the surface of a microchip, using photolithographic processes defined by the microelectronics industry. Thus creation of a truly multifunctional, "integrated" analytical device embedded in a single monolithic substrate is possible. The classic "cross-T" design of a single-channel microchip involves a short (injection) channel that intersects a longer (separation) channel and includes a reservoir at the end of each of these, as shown in Fig. 18.9. The setup for LIF detection on a single-channel microchip is shown in Fig. 18.10.

When solution volumes required to fill the architecture are compared, it is seen that the volume of the separation channel on a microchip is approximately an order of magnitude smaller (low nanoliters) than conventional capillary systems. With their decreased volume requirements (nanoliter and even picoliter range), pressure injection is more challenging (but not impossible), and for this reason, the EK sample injection mode is primarily used. In practice, an injection voltage of several hundred volts is applied across the sample and sample waste reservoirs to migrate the sample to the injection cross, which typically represents an injection volume of 50 to 100 pL. A separation voltage (1 to 4 kV) is then applied to the separation channel; this induces separation of the analyte zones before they reach the detection window downstream. It is important to note that, although the sample volume injected is approximately 100 to 500 pL, the actual sample volume necessary (for handling) is still approximately 2 to 4 μL, depending on the reservoir size.

Detection with a microchip occurs primarily through LIF, because this is easily implemented with the planar configuration of the microchip (see Fig. 18.10). Limits of detection for fluorescein have been easily demonstrated at 10^{-15} molar.[68] This allows for detection, for example, of polymerase chain reaction (PCR)-amplified DNA fragments at a level that competes with phosphorus-32 autoradiography from Southern blots.[69] Typical microchip separation times are approximately 50 to 200 seconds.

Fabrication of Microchips

Standard cross-T configuration microchips can be obtained commercially from several small vendors, but chips of more complex architecture tend to be fabricated in the laboratories that use them. They can be constructed from substrates such as glass (Pyrex-like or soda lime), silicon (as per microelectronic chips), or a variety of polymeric materials (plastics), or

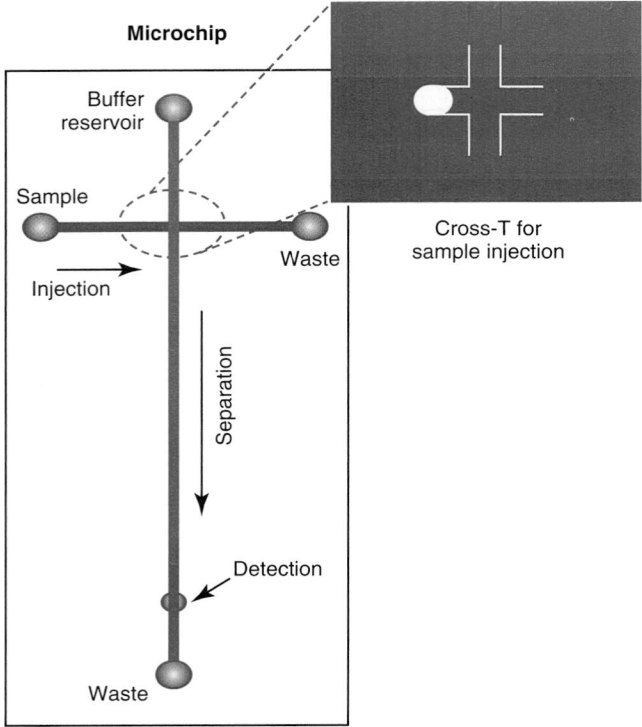

FIGURE 18.9 Simple cross-T microstructure design on chips used for electrophoretic separation.

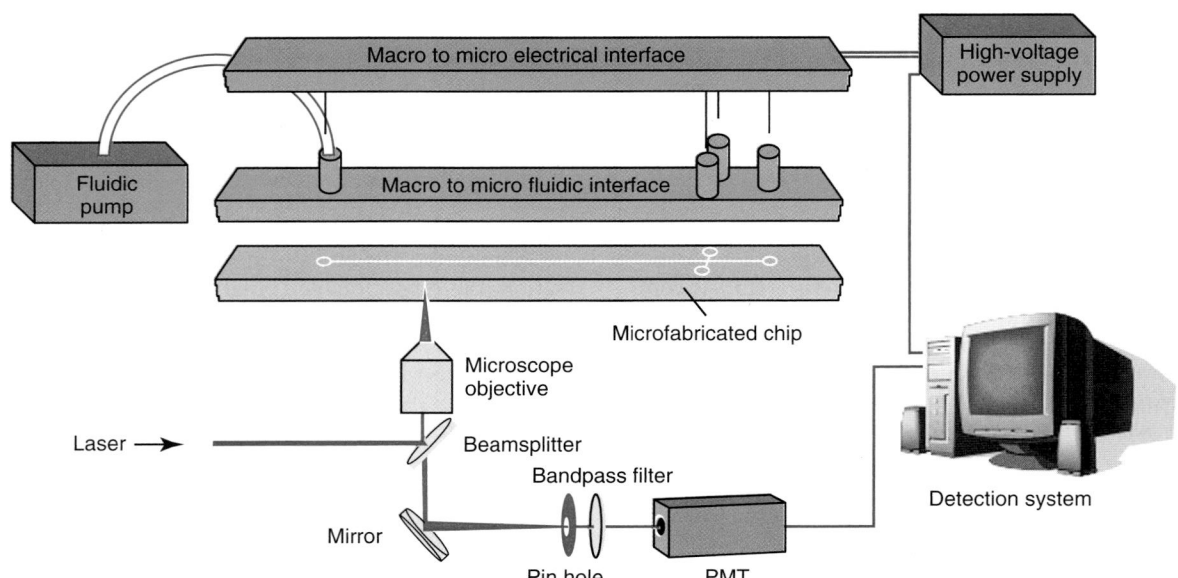

FIGURE 18.10 Detection system for laser-induced fluorescence detection on microchips. Fluidic and electrical interfaces are indirectly fundamental to the detection system. The fluidic interface drives the preparation and flushing of the chip before separation and after separation, and the electrical interface drives the electrophoretic separation and controls the flow of fluid through the chip architecture via electrokinetic valving. *PMT,* Photomultiplier tube.

they may be cast from silicone-like materials (polydimethylsiloxane).[70] Historically, the first two of these types constituted the vast majority of electrophoretic devices described in the literature.

A buffered solution of hydrofluoric acid is used to etch the desired structures into a glass wafer, thereby producing a series of U-shaped troughs (typically 70 µm [w] × 20 µm [d]) that interconnect appropriately. Smooth walls are typically achieved, but channels are U-shaped because of downward and lateral etching by the etch solution. Consequently, features are often designed to be smaller than they have to be to allow for this type of spreading. After successful etching, the etched wafer is bonded to a second piece of glass, into which reservoirs have been drilled, to enclose chambers and channels of the device.

Molecular Diagnostics Using Microchips

As a result of the ease with which dsDNA can be made to fluoresce via high-affinity dsDNA fluorescent intercalators, and the excellent detection sensitivity that results from LIF, DNA separations on microchips have developed more rapidly than protein separations. Consequently, capillary and microchip types of electrophoresis have emerged as alternatives to traditional slab gel electrophoresis for DNA analysis; this is exemplified by sequencing of the human genome by Celera using primarily CE-based separation. A variety of polymers have been defined as *sieving matrices*, effective for molecular sieving and size-based microchip DNA separations, many of which had been used previously in CE.

As described in the CE section, the chemical nature of the microchannel surface is equally important in DNA separation, in which EOF has to be minimized or eliminated. For microchip-based electrophoretic DNA analysis, the chip surface must be passivated to reduce EOF. This can be accomplished through covalent modification with polymers

such as polyacrylamide[71]; however, PCR samples must be desalted to achieve optimal resolution and acceptable longevity.[72,73] More attractive alternatives developed for CE involve polymers that have dual functionality, in that they both coat the microchannel surface and act as effective sieving polymers. Polydimethylacrylamide and the cellulosic polymers hydroxyethyl cellulose and hydroxypropyl cellulose have been shown to be very effective in this respect.[74]

An almost exponential growth of literature has occurred with respect to the application of microchip electrophoresis to the molecular diagnosis of disease based on PCR amplification of DNA.[20] Rudimentary microchip designs have been used to demonstrate the application of this platform in the most simplistic form (i.e., detecting the presence of a PCR product of diagnostic significance). This has been demonstrated with multiple applications, including detection of herpes simplex viral DNA in CSF for diagnosis of encephalitis, detection of gene rearrangements correlative with lymphoproliferative disorders, detection of polymorphisms in the methylenetetrahydrofolate reductase gene, diagnosis of fragile X syndrome, detection of tetranucleotide repeats associated with hypercholesterolemia, and diagnosis of muscular dystrophy (for a recent review, see reference 75). More complicated DNA assays have been accomplished on electrophoretic microchips, including single-stranded conformation polymorphism and heteroduplex analysis for the detection of common mutations in the breast cancer susceptibility genes, *BRCA1* and *BRCA2*.[20]

An example of microchip DNA separation applied to short tandem repeat (STR) analysis is shown in Fig. 18.11.[75,76] Using a separation length of only 4 cm and integrated gold leaf electrodes, this device was capable of separating STR products at a resolution of 2 base pairs in less than 5 minutes. More recent examples are seen in chip-based methods for DNA extraction from sample, PCR amplification of purified

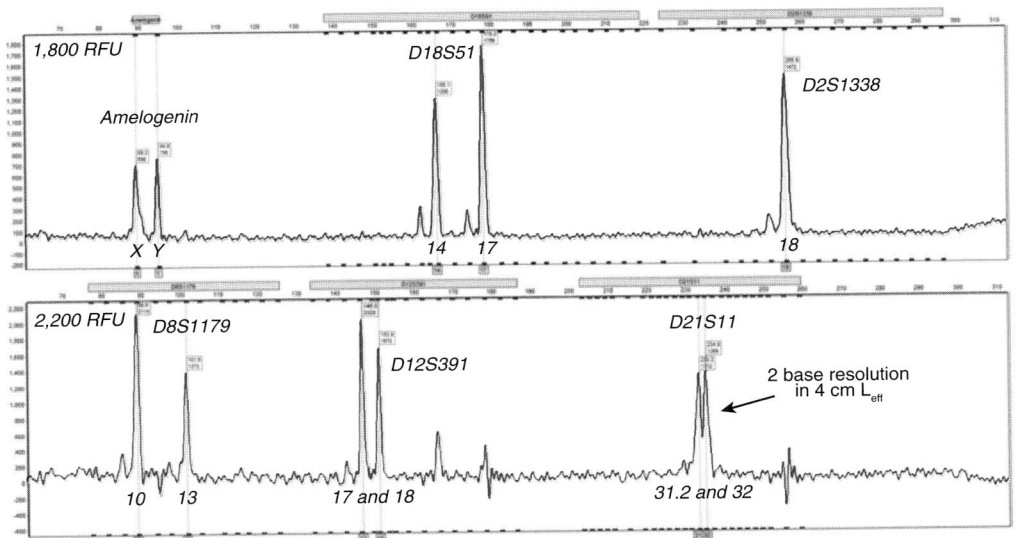

FIGURE 18.11 Electrophoretic detection of short tandem repeat (STR) products. Analysis of six loci was performed on a fully integrated microfluidic device. *Top,* Three of the STR markers labeled with fluorescein. *Bottom,* Three of the STR markers labeled with JOE, achieving two-base resolution. This profile matches the results obtained by the conventional methodology (ABI 310 instrument).

DNA, and a method to inject this material with a DNA ladder for electrophoretic interrogation, with all processes interfaced on a single chip. Using whole blood from a mouse infected with *Bacillus anthracis,* analysis of less than 1 μL of blood allowed the detection of an *anthracis*-specific PCR product in less than 30 minutes, demonstrating the power of integrated microchip-based analysis.[77]

More complicated microchip systems have been developed to address the high-throughput requirements of molecular diagnostics laboratories. For example, high-throughput genetic typing has been performed on a 96-channel radial capillary array electrophoresis microplate with an unprecedented sample throughput of approximately 0.6 samples/s.[67,73] This has been extrapolated to a variety of other applications, including genotyping of the marker gene for diagnosis of hereditary hemochromatosis.[78]

SELECTED REFERENCES

3. Tao Q, Wang Z, Zhao H, et al. Direct chemiluminescent imaging detection of human serum proteins in two-dimensional polyacrylamide gel electrophoresis. Proteomics 2007;7:3481–90.

11. St. Claire RL. Capillary electrophoresis. Anal Chem 1996;68: R569–86.

13. Pentoney SL Jr, Sweedler JV. Optical detection techniques for capillary electrophoresis. In: Landers JP, editor. Handbook of capillary electrophoresis. 2nd ed. Boca Raton, FL: CRC Press; 1997. p. 379–423.

14. Severs JC, Smith RD. Capillary electrophoresis-mass spectrometry. In: Landers JP, editor. Handbook of capillary electrophoresis. 2nd ed. Boca Raton, FL: CRC Press; 1997. p. 791–826.

20. Landers JP. Molecular diagnostics on electrophoretic microchips. Anal Chem 2003;75:2919–27.

26. Marien G, Verhoef G, Bossuyt X. Detection of heavy chain disease by capillary zone electrophoresis. Clin Chem 2005;51:1302–3.

27. Maisnar V, Tichy M, Stulik J, et al. Capillary immunotyping electrophoresis and high resolution two-dimensional electrophoresis for the detection of mu-heavy chain disease. Clin Chim Acta 2008;389:171–3.

31. Lissoir B, Wallemacq P, Maison D. Serum protein electrophoresis: comparison of capillary zone electrophoresis Capillarys (Sebia) and agarose gel electrophoresis hydrasys (Sebia). Ann Biol Clin (Paris) 2003;61:557–62.

33. Yang Z, Harrison K, Park YA, et al. Performance of the Sebia Capillarys 2 for detection and immunotyping of serum monoclonal paraproteins. Am J Clin Pathol 2007;128:293–9.

35. Borbely N, Phelan L, Szydlo R, et al. Capillary zone electrophoresis for haemoglobinopathy diagnosis. J Clin Pathol 2013;66(1):29–39.

36. Agouti I., Merono F., Bonello-Palot N., et al. Analytical evaluation of the Capillarys 2 Flex piercing for routine heamoglobinopathies diagnosis. Int J Lab Hematol 2013;35(2):217–221.

38. Strickland SW, Campbell ST, Little RR, et al. Prevalence of rare hemoglobin variants identified during measurements of Hb A_{1c} by capillary electrophoresis. Clin Chem 2017;63(12):1901–1902.

39. Strickland SW, Campbell ST, Little RR, et al. Recognition of rare hemoglobin variants by hemoglobin A_{1c} measurement procedures. Clin Chim Acta 2018;476:67–74.

42. Shihabi Z. Effects of sample matrix on capillary electrophoretic analysis. In: Landers JP, editor. Handbook of capillary electrophoresis. 2nd ed. Boca Raton, FL: CRC Press; 1997. p. 457–77.

47. Heller M, Michel PE, Morier P, et al. Two-stage off-gel isoelectric focusing: protein followed by peptide fractionation and application to proteome analysis of human plasma. Electrophoresis 2005;26:1174–88.

48. Xiao Z, Conrads TP, Lucas DA, et al. Direct ampholyte-free liquid-phase isoelectric peptide focusing: application to the human serum proteome. Electrophoresis 2004;25:128–33.

53. Sandt CH, Krouse DA, Cook CR, et al. The key role of pulsed-field gel electrophoresis in investigation of a large multiserotype and multistate food-borne outbreak of salmonella infections centered in Pennsylvania. J Clin Microbiol 2006;44:3208–12.

61. Terabe S. Micellar electrokinetic chromatography. In: Landers JP, editor. Handbook of capillary and microchip electrophoresis and associated microtechniques. 3rd ed. Boca Raton, FL: CRC Press; 2008. p. 109–34.

62. Hempe J, Vargas A, Craver R. Clinical analysis of structural hemoglobin variants and Hb A1c by capillary isoelectric focusing. In: Petersen J, Mohammad A, editors. Clinical and forensic applications of capillary electrophoresis. Totowa, NJ: Humana Press; 2001. p. 145–63.

75. Ahrberg CD, Manz A, Chung BG. Polymerase chain reaction in microfluidic devices. Lab Chip 2016;20:3866–3884.

Chromatography

David S. Hage[a]

ABSTRACT

Background

Clinical tests often involve the use of one or more steps to isolate, enrich, or separate a target compound from other chemicals in the sample. Chromatography is one of the most common methods for achieving this type of separation. In this method, the components of a mixture are separated based on their differential interactions with two chemical or physical phases: a mobile phase and a stationary phase that is held in place by a supporting material. There are many forms of chromatography based on the different mobile phases, stationary phases, and supports that can be used in this method, which has led to a wide range of applications for this technique.

Content

This chapter describes the basic principles of chromatography and discusses various forms of this method that are used for chemical analysis or to prepare specimens for analysis by other techniques. The methods of gas chromatography and liquid chromatography are discussed, as well as the techniques of planar chromatography, supercritical fluid chromatography, and multidimensional separations. The mobile phases, stationary phases, and supports that are used in each of these methods are described. The instrumentation and detection schemes that are employed in these methods are also discussed.

Biological fluids are complex mixtures of chemicals. This means that clinical tests for specific components in these fluids often involve the use of one or more separation steps to isolate, enrich, or separate the target compound of interest from other chemicals in the sample. Chromatography is one of the most common methods for achieving this type of separation. This chapter describes the basic principles of chromatography and discusses various forms of this method that are used for chemical analysis or to prepare specimens for analysis by other techniques.

BASIC PRINCIPLES OF CHROMATOGRAPHY

General Terms and Components of Chromatography

Chromatography is a method in which the components of a mixture are separated based on their differential interactions with two chemical or physical phases: a mobile phase and a stationary phase.[1-4] The basic components and operation of a typical chromatographic system are illustrated in Fig. 19.1. The mobile phase travels through the system and carries sample components with it once the sample has been applied or injected. The stationary phase is held within the system by a support and does not move. As a sample's components pass through this system, the components that have the strongest interactions with the stationary phase will be more highly retained by this phase and move through the system more slowly than components that have weaker interactions with the stationary phase and spend more time in the mobile phase. This leads to a difference in the rate of travel for these components and their separation as they move through the chromatographic system.

The type of chromatographic system that is shown in Fig. 19.1 uses a column (or a tube) to contain the stationary phase and support, while also allowing the mobile phase and sample to pass through the system. This approach was first described in 1903 by Mikhail Tswett, who used this method to separate plant pigments into colored bands by using a column that contained calcium carbonate as both the support and stationary phase.[5] Tswett gave the name *chromatography* to this method. This name is derived from Greek words *chroma* and *graphein*, which mean "color" and "to write." This term is still used to describe this technique, even though most modern chromatographic separations do not involve colored sample components.

The type of chromatography that was used by Tswett, in which the stationary phase and support are held within a column, is known as "column chromatography." In chromatography, the stationary phase may be the surface of the support, a coating on this support, or a chemical layer that is cross-linked or bonded to the support.[2,6,7] In column chromatography, the support may be the interior wall of the column or it may be a material that is placed or packed into the column. A column is the most common format for chromatography. However, it is also possible to use a support and stationary phase that are present on a plane or open surface. This second format is known as "planar

[a]The author gratefully acknowledges the contributions of Drs. Glen L. Hortin, Bruce A. Goldberger, M. David Ullman, Carl A. Burtis, and Larry D. Bowers to this chapter in previous editions.

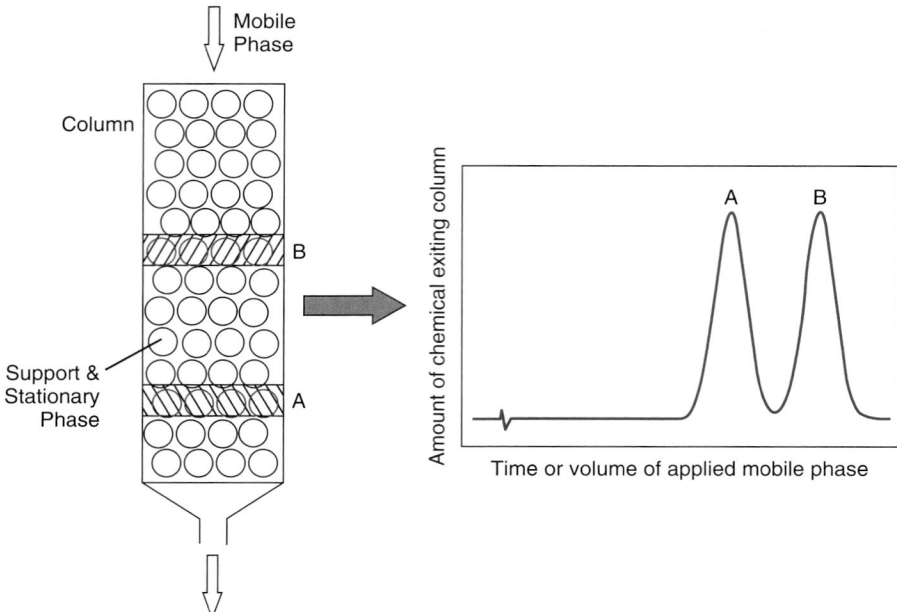

FIGURE 19.1 The general components of a chromatographic system, as illustrated here by using a column to separate two chemicals, *A* and *B*.

chromatography," as will be discussed in more detail later in this chapter.[2,7]

One way of classifying chromatographic methods is based on the type of support that they employ; two examples are the techniques of column chromatography and planar chromatography. Chromatographic methods also can be classified based on the mobile phase that is present. For instance, a chromatographic method that uses a gas mobile phase is called gas chromatography (GC),[8] and a chromatographic method that uses a liquid mobile phase is known as liquid chromatography (LC).[9] It is also possible to divide chromatographic methods according to the type of stationary phase that is present or the way in which this stationary phase is interacting with sample components. Examples of these classifications include the GC methods of gas-solid chromatography (GSC) or gas-liquid chromatography (GLC) and the LC methods of adsorption chromatography, partition chromatography, or ion-exchange chromatography (IEC). Each of these categories, as well as others, will also be discussed later in this chapter.

The instrument that is used to perform a separation in chromatography is known as a chromatograph.[7,10] For instance, in GC the instrument is a gas chromatograph, and in LC the instrument used to carry out this method is a liquid chromatograph. These instruments can provide a response that is related to the amount of a compound that is exiting (or eluting) from the column as a function of the elution time or the volume of mobile phase that has passed through the system. The resulting plot of the response versus time or volume is known as a chromatogram,[7,10] as is illustrated in Figs. 19.1 and 19.2.

The average time or volume that is required for a particular chemical to pass through the column is known as that chemical's retention time (t_R) or retention volume (V_R). These values both increase with the strength and degree to which the chemical is interacting with the stationary phase.

The elution time or volume for a compound that is nonretained or that does not interact with the stationary phase is known as the void time (t_M) or void volume (V_M). If the retention time or retention volume is corrected for the void time or void volume, the resulting measure of retention is known as the adjusted retention time (t_R', where $t_R' = t_R - t_M$) or the adjusted retention volume (V_R', where $V_R' = V_R - V_M$). For two chemicals to be separated by chromatography, it is necessary for these chemicals to have different values for t_R and V_R (or t_R' and V_R').[2,7,10]

Most separations that are used for chemical analysis in column chromatography are carried out by injecting a relatively small volume or amount of sample onto the chromatographic system. This situation results in a chromatogram that consists of a series of peaks that represent the different compounds in the sample as they each elute from the column. The retention time or retention volume of each peak can be used to help identify the eluting compound, whereas the area or height of the peak can be used to measure the amount of the compound that is present.

The width of each peak is also of interest in a chromatogram. The peak width reflects the separating performance or efficiency of the chromatographic system. The width of a peak in a chromatogram is often represented by its baseline width (W_b) or its half-height width (W_h) (Fig. 19.3).[2,7,10] As the widths for the peaks in a chromatogram become sharper, it becomes easier for the chromatographic system to separate two peaks with similar interactions with the system and to separate more peaks in a given amount of time. Sharper peaks are also easier to measure than broader peaks and tend to produce better limits of detection.

Retention and Selectivity

For two chemicals to be separated by chromatography, these chemicals need to have some differences in how they are interacting with the stationary phase versus the mobile phase.

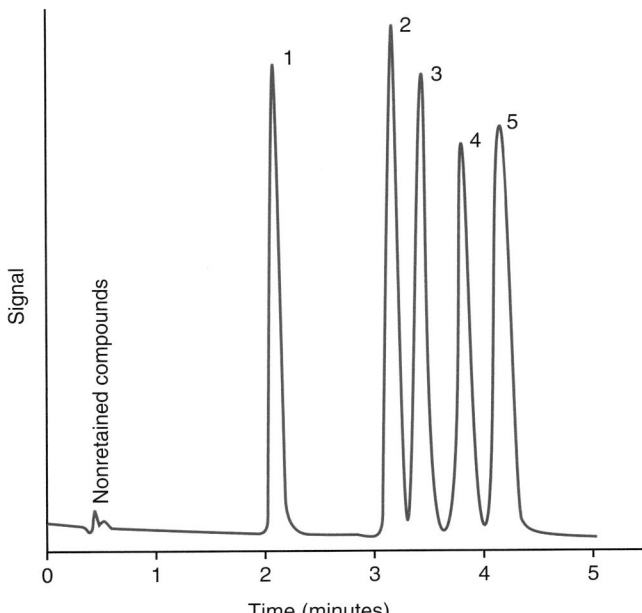

Column: C18, 3 μm, 0.46 ID × 10 cm
Eluent: Isocratic, 0.025 M phosphate
Buffer: pH 3.0 in 25% acetonitrile
Flow rate: 2 mL/min
Detection: 215 nm, 0.1 AUFS

Compounds: 1. Doxepin
            2. Desipramine
            3. Imipramine
            4. Nortriptyline
            5. Amitriptyline

FIGURE 19.2 Chromatogram from a separation of tricyclic antidepressants based on reversed-phase chromatography and high-performance liquid chromatography. Detection was based on the use of an absorbance detector that monitored the column eluent at 215 nm. NOTE: the signal is displayed at 0.1 absorbance units-full scale (AUFS). (Courtesy Hichrom Limited.)

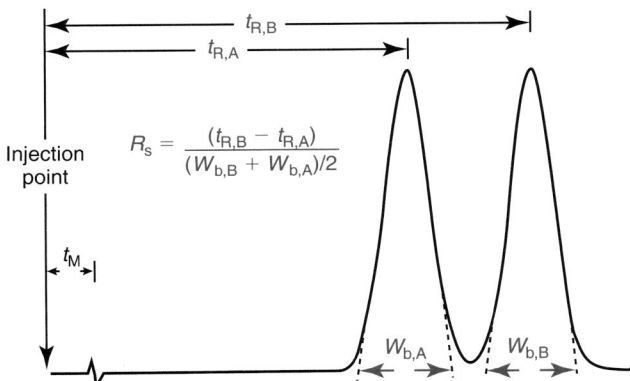

FIGURE 19.3 An example of a general chromatogram that may be obtained when using a column. In this example, compound B is eluted later than compound A. R_s, Resolution; t_M, void time; $t_{R,A}$ and $t_{R,B}$, retention times for solutes A and B; $W_{b,A}$ and $W_{b,B}$, baseline peak widths for compounds A and B.

Besides using the retention time and retention volume (or adjusted retention time and adjusted retention volume) to describe these differences, another way of representing retention in chromatography is by using the retention factor (k). This term is also sometimes represented as k' or called the capacity factor.[7,10] The retention factor is a measure of the average time a chemical resides in the stationary phase versus the time it spends in the mobile phase. This value can be calculated from experimental data by using any of the following equivalent relationships[2,7,10]:

$$k = (t_R - t_M)/t_M = (t_R')/t_M$$

or

$$k = (V_R - V_M)/V_M = (V_R')/V_M$$

As these equations suggest, the retention factor is a unitless number where a value of 0 indicates that no binding or interactions are occurring between a chemical and the stationary phase or that this compound is eluting from the system at the void time. As the chemical undergoes greater interactions with the stationary phase, this will result in longer retention times and an increased value of k. In practice, it is desirable to have a value for k that is between 1 and 10 to provide reasonable separations between compounds without the need for excessive lengths of time for their elution from the column.

The retention factor is useful in describing a compound's retention in chromatography for several reasons. First, the value of k should be independent of the flow rate and column size. Also, k can be directly related to the strength of the interactions that are occurring between a chemical and the stationary phase or mobile phase, as well as the relative amount of stationary phase versus mobile phase that is present in the column. This last feature is illustrated by the following equation for a chromatographic system in which a chemical is separated based on its ability to partition between the mobile phase and stationary phase. Similar relationships can be written for other types of separation mechanisms[2]:

$$k = K_D (V_S/V_M)$$

In this relationship, the value of k is directly related to (1) the distribution equilibrium constant (K_D) for partitioning of the analyte into the stationary phase versus the mobile phase and (2) the relative amount of stationary phase in the column (as represented here by V_S) versus the amount of mobile phase that is present (as represented by V_M, the void volume). The value of k in this situation will increase if there is either an increase in K_D, which reflects the tendency of the chemical to enter the stationary phase over the mobile phase, or the ratio (V_S/V_M), which is a term also known as the *phase ratio*.[2,7]

Any separation in chromatography requires that there be some difference in retention for the chemicals that are to be separated from each other. One way of describing this difference in retention is by using the separation factor or selectivity factor (α).[7,10] The separation factor for two compounds (A and B) is equal to the ratio of their retention factors (k_A and k_B),

$$\alpha = k_B/k_A$$

where the retention factor for the later eluting component is given in the numerator. If two chemicals have the same retention in a chromatographic system, the value of α will equal 1 and no separation will be possible. If the peaks for A and B do have different retention, the value of α will be greater than 1 and will increase as the degree of separation increases.

The values of both the retention factor and selectivity factor are determined by the chemicals that are being separated, as well as the stationary and mobile phases that are present in the chromatographic system. A large difference in retention and a large separation factor are desirable when the goal is to selectively isolate one chemical from others in a sample. However, smaller differences in retention and in separation factors are often used when the chromatographic system is used to separate several chemicals and peaks from the same sample. In this second situation, a value for α of 1.1 or greater represents an adequate separation in many common types of chromatography. However, chromatographic methods that result in broad peaks may need even larger values of α to produce a good separation between two chemicals.

Band-Broadening and Efficiency

Besides needing a difference in retention for a separation to occur, the peaks for two neighboring chemicals must be sufficiently narrow to allow this difference to be observed. The injection of even a sample with a small volume will experience some increase in width, or band-broadening, as this peak travels through the chromatographic system. This broadening of peaks is produced by various processes related to the rate of movement or diffusion of the applied chemicals as they pass around or within the support and within or between the mobile phase and stationary phase. These band-broadening processes, in turn, are affected by factors such as the diameter or type of support within the chromatographic system, the flow rate, the diffusion coefficient of the chemical in the mobile phase and stationary phases, and the degree of retention of the chemical in the column (Box 19.1). Together, these processes and factors determine the overall efficiency or extent of band-broadening obtained.

The efficiency and degree of band-broadening in a chromatographic system are related experimentally to the final observed width of a chemical's peak. This width can be described by measures such as the baseline width (W_b), the half-height width (W_h), or the standard deviation (σ) of the peak. These values, in turn, can be used to find another measure of chromatographic efficiency known as the number of

theoretical plates, or plate number (N). The value of N for any type of chromatographic peak can be calculated by using the following formula,

$$N = (t_R/\sigma)^2$$

where t_R is the retention time for the peak and σ is the standard deviation of the peak in the same units of time as t_R.[7,10] This equation takes on the following two equivalent forms for a Gaussian-shaped peak.[2,7]

$$N = 16(t_R/W_b)^2 \quad \text{or} \quad N = 5.545(t_R/W_h)^2$$

These last two equations make use of the fact that a Gaussian peak has a baseline width, as measured by the intersection of the baseline with tangents along either side of the peak, that is equal to 4 σ, and a half-width width that is equal to 2.355 σ.

The value of N can be thought of as representing the effective number of times that a chemical has been distributed between the mobile phase and stationary phase as this chemical has passed through the chromatographic system. A larger value for N represents many such steps, which makes it easier to distinguish between two chemicals that have only small differences in their retention. Experimentally, a large value of N results in a high chromatographic efficiency and sharp peaks, which are both desirable for either separating chemicals with similar retention or quickly separating many chemicals in the same sample.

There are several other ways in which the efficiency of a chromatographic system can be described. One way is by using the number of theoretical plates (N) per unit length of the chromatographic system (L), as given by the ratio (N/L). This ratio helps in comparing systems with different lengths, because the value of N increases in direct proportion to the length of the column or support bed that is used in a separation for chromatography. Although this means that a longer chromatographic system will always lead to a larger value for N and greater efficiency, the use of a longer system also results in longer separation times.

Another way of describing column efficiency is the height equivalent of a theoretical plate or plate height (HETP, or H).[7,10] The value of H is found by dividing the length of the chromatographic system by the number of theoretical plates for this system.

$$H = L/N$$

The value of H represents the length of the column or chromatographic system that makes up one theoretical plate or one distribution step for a chemical between the mobile phase and stationary phase. Although a large value of N (or N/L) represents a chromatographic system with high efficiency, the same system would be represented by a small value for H (or L/N).

A valuable feature of using H to describe chromatographic efficiency is that this term can be related directly to the parameters and processes that affect band-broadening. A common example of this is the *van Deemter equation*,[11] which shows how the overall value of H is affected by the linear velocity of the mobile phase (u), which is directly related to the flow rate (F) through the relationship $u = (F \times L)/V_M$.[10,12]

$$H = A + B/u + C u$$

BOX 19.1   Factors That Can Affect Chromatographic Efficiency

- Column length (affecting the number of theoretical plates, N, but not the plate height, H)
- Particle size of support (packed bed column) or tube diameter (open tubular column)
- Uniformity in size, shape, and packing of the support
- Flow rate and linear velocity
- Temperature and rate of solute diffusion
- Mobile phase viscosity
- Degree of compound retention
- Initial injection volume
- Volume of connecting tubing, detector, and system components besides the column

The terms A, B, and C in this equation are constants that represent the contributions of several types of band-broadening processes. For instance, the A term represents the contributions of band-broadening processes that are independent of the linear velocity and flow rate, such as eddy diffusion and mobile phase mass transfer. The B term is the contribution to the plate height by longitudinal diffusion, which is a process that becomes more important as the flow rate and linear velocity are decreased. Finally, the C term represents the contributions from processes that lead to an increase in H as the flow rate or linear velocity is increased. The processes that make up the C term are stagnant mobile phase mass transfer and stationary phase mass transfer. The van Deemter equation predicts that the combined effect of these band-broadening processes will be an optimum range of flow rates and linear velocities over which the lowest plate heights, and best efficiencies, will be obtained.[11] In practice, the usual goal in varying the flow rate in chromatography is to identify those conditions that provide the most rapid separation times while still providing adequate resolution of all peaks that are of interest in the samples being separated.

Several factors that affect chromatographic efficiency are listed in Box 19.1. For instance, efficiency can be improved by using longer columns, which increases the value of N but does not alter H. It is also possible to change the flow rate to its optimum value, to use smaller diameter support particles, to use nonporous or pellicular particles instead of fully porous support particles, or to use a relatively narrow-diameter coated capillary instead of a packed bed column. All these latter factors help to lower the value of H, which in turn increases the value of N for a given length of column or chromatographic bed. However, there are practical limits to how much some of these experimental parameters can be changed. As an example, a reduction in the diameter of the support particle will lead to greater efficiency, but it will also result in higher back pressures across the chromatographic system, require the use of lower flow rates, or both.

Resolution and Peak Capacity

The overall extent to which two peaks are separated in chromatography can be described by using a term known as the resolution (R_s), as is illustrated in Fig. 19.3. The resolution between two neighboring peaks can be found by using the following formula[7,10]:

$$R_s = \frac{\left(t_{R,B} - t_{R,A}\right)}{\left(W_{b,B} + W_{b,A}\right)/2}$$

In this equation, $t_{R,A}$ and $t_{R,B}$ are the average retention times for compounds A and B (where B elutes after A), while $W_{b,A}$ and $W_{b,B}$ are the baseline widths for the peaks of these compounds (in time units, in this case). An equivalent equation can be written in terms of the retention volumes of A and B and their baseline widths in volume units. The use of either approach will give a unit-less value for R_s that represents the average number of baseline widths that separate the centers of the two peaks.

Fig. 19.4 shows how the separation of two neighboring peaks changes as the value of R_s increases for these peaks. An R_s value of 0 is obtained when there is no separation between the peaks and they have exactly the same retention times or retention volumes. The degree of peak separation increases as the value of R_s increases. An R_s value of 1.5 or greater is often

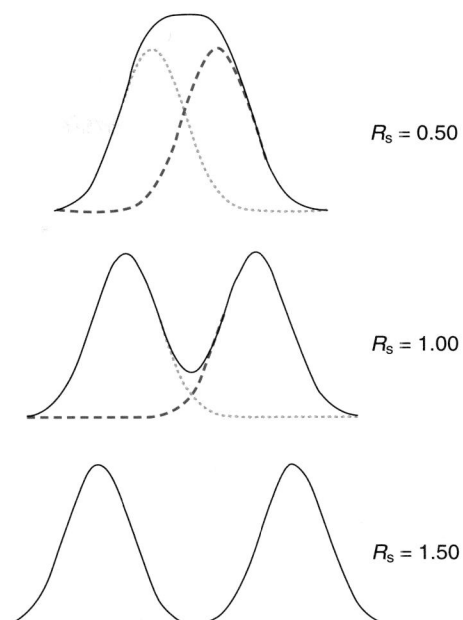

FIGURE 19.4 Degree of separation obtained for two chromatographic peaks that are present in a 1:1 area ratio as the resolution between these peaks (R_s) is varied.

said to represent a complete separation between two equally sized peaks, or baseline resolution. However, for many separations, resolution values between 1.0 or 1.25 and 1.5 also may be adequate, especially if the peaks are about the same size and are to be measured using their peak heights rather than their peak areas.

Several approaches can be used to alter or improve the resolution between two peaks in chromatography (Fig. 19.5). These approaches are indicated by the following expression, which is sometimes known as the resolution equation of chromatography[13]:

$$R_s = [(N^{1/2})/4] \times [(\alpha - 1)/\alpha] \times [k/(1 + k)]$$

In this equation, k is the retention factor for the second of two neighboring peaks, α is the separation factor between the first and second peaks, and N is the number of theoretical plates for the chromatographic system. This relationship indicates that resolution of two peaks in chromatography can be changed in three ways: (1) by altering the efficiency of the system, as represented by N; (2) by changing the overall degree of peak retention, as represented by k; or (3) by changing the selectivity of the column for one compound versus another, as represented by α. An increase in N, such as can be obtained through use of a longer column, will lead to an increase in R_s that is proportional to $N^{1/2}$. An increase in the retention factor (k) or selectivity (α) will also lead to a nonlinear increase in resolution.

Another way of describing a chromatographic separation is in terms of the *peak capacity*. The peak capacity is the maximum number of peaks (or sample components) that can be separated, in theory, during a single chromatographic separation.[14–16] The value of the peak capacity can be found by assuming there is a continuous distribution of peaks that are separated by an average baseline width (or 4 standard deviations). In practice, the number of components that can

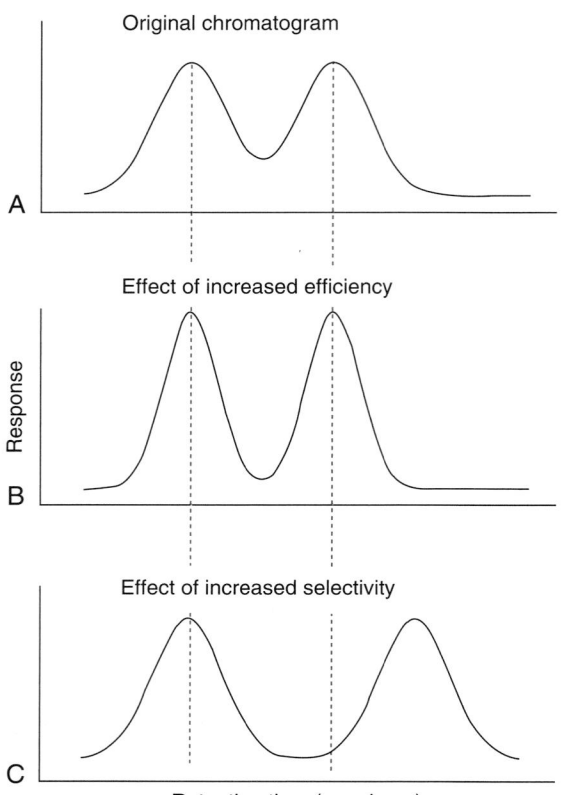

FIGURE 19.5 Effects of selectivity and efficiency on the resolution of peaks in chromatography. These three situations represent cases in which there is (A) poor or moderate resolution between two neighboring peaks, (B) good resolution between the peaks as a result of high column efficiency, or (C) good resolution between the peaks as a result of good column selectivity.

be separated in a single run by a given system will be lower than the theoretical peak capacity because the retention times of their peaks will not be evenly distributed. The peak capacity of a system that is used for high-performance liquid chromatography (HPLC) is usually limited to several hundred peaks, whereas higher values can be obtained in methods such as capillary GC. Factors that can be used to increase the peak capacity include increasing the efficiency of the system (e.g., by using a longer column) and using gradient elution or extended run times. Another approach for increasing the peak capacity is to use a multidimensional separation, as will be discussed later in this chapter.

> ### POINTS TO REMEMBER
>
> **General Ways to Improve Peak Resolution in Chromatography**
> - Increase the efficiency of the system
> - Increase the overall degree of peak retention
> - Increase the selectivity of the column for the peak of one compound versus another

Analyte Identification and Quantification

Chromatography is often used as an analytical tool to qualitatively identify analytes in a sample and to measure the

concentrations of these analytes. For example, the retention time, retention volume, and retention factor for an analyte are all characteristic values that reflect how this chemical is interacting within a particular chromatographic system. These retention values can be compared to those for a known sample of the same compound to help confirm its identity. However, other confirmation also may be needed because other compounds may have similar retention characteristics.

One-way additional confirmation can be obtained is if the unknown compound and reference compound have the same retention under several types of chromatographic conditions, such as on different columns or column/mobile phase combinations. In the case of capillary GC or LC columns, it is possible to simultaneously introduce samples onto two columns that contain different stationary phases and that are connected to separate detectors. If the unknown compound and a reference compound match in their retention properties on the two columns, this greatly enhances the chance for correctly identifying the unknown analyte. An alternative and even more reliable approach for identification is to use a detection method that provides structural information on the analyte, such as mass spectrometry (see Chapters 20 to 23).

The peak area or peak height can be used to produce quantitative information on an analyte that is separated from other sample components by chromatography. Peak areas tend to provide a more precise means for measuring an analyte, whereas peak heights are easier to use if there is not complete resolution between the analyte and its neighboring peaks. Both external and internal calibration techniques can be used in chromatography for such measurements.[2,17] In external calibration, standard solutions containing known quantities of the analytes are processed and separated in the same manner as samples that contain one or more of these analytes (Fig. 19.6). A calibration curve is then constructed by plotting the peak height or peak area (or the spot density, in the case of planar methods) versus the concentration or mass of analyte that was applied in the standard solutions. This curve can then be used with the peak area or peak height that is determined for the same analyte in the samples to find the concentration or amount of this analyte present.

In the method of internal calibration (also called internal standardization), standard solutions of the analyte are again prepared; however, a constant amount of a different compound known as the internal standard is also now added to each standard solution and sample (Fig. 19.7). The internal standard should be a chemical that was not originally present in either the sample or the standard, is similar in its chemical and physical properties to the analyte, and can be measured independently from the analyte. This internal standard is typically added to the samples and standards before they are processed by any pretreatment steps, such as extraction or derivatization. The addition of this agent can help normalize the results for any variations that may occur during the pretreatment steps or during sample/standard injection onto the chromatographic system. This normalization is made by constructing a calibration curve in which the y-axis is based on the ratio of the peak height or peak area for the analyte in a given standard or sample divided by the peak height or peak area for the internal standard in the same standard or sample. This ratio is plotted versus the concentration or amount of analyte in each standard. This calibration plot can then be

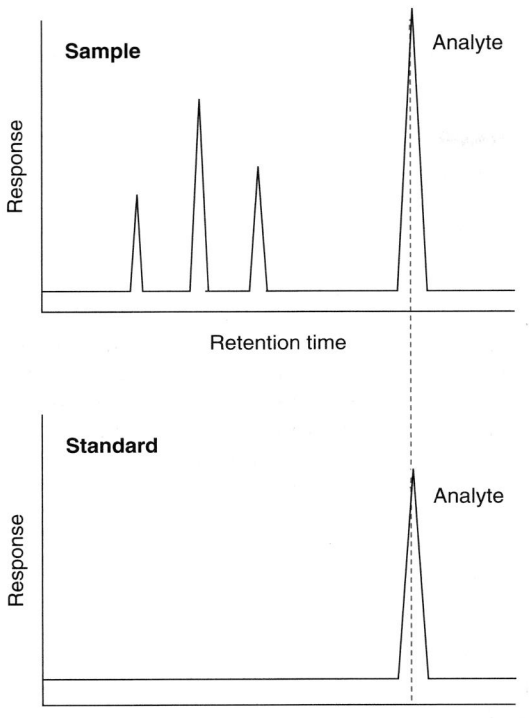

FIGURE 19.6 Use of external calibration and standards to quantify an analyte based on its peak height or area in a chromatogram for an injected sample.

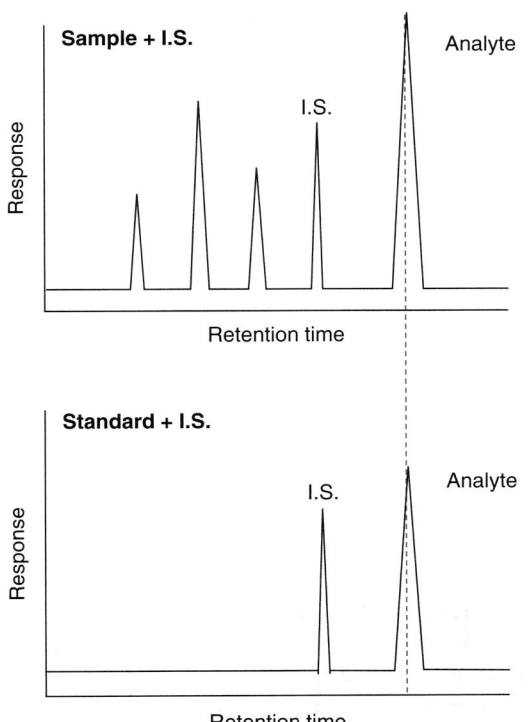

FIGURE 19.7 Use of internal calibration and samples or standards containing an internal standard (I.S.) to quantify an analyte based on its peak height or area in a chromatogram for an injected sample.

used to find the concentration or amount of the analyte that was present in each sample.[2,17]

GAS CHROMATOGRAPHY

GC is a common type of chromatography often used in chemical separations and analysis. GC can be defined as a chromatographic method in which the mobile phase is a gas.[7] The first modern GC system was developed in the mid-1940s by Cremer[18,19] and became popular after work by James and Martin in 1952, who used this method to separate methyl esters of fatty acids.[20]

In GC, a gaseous mobile phase is used to pass a mixture of volatile solutes through a column containing the stationary phase.[7,8] The mobile phase is typically an inert gas such as nitrogen, helium, or argon or a low mass gas such as hydrogen. Because of the low densities of gases under typical GC operating conditions, the compounds injected onto a GC column do not have any appreciable interactions with the gaseous mobile phase. Instead, this gas acts to merely carry samples through the column. As a result, the term carrier gas is commonly used to refer to the mobile phase in GC.[7]

Solute separation in GC is based on differences in the vapor pressures of the injected compounds and in the different interactions of these compounds with the stationary phase. For instance, a more volatile chemical will spend more time in the gaseous mobile phase than a less volatile solute and will tend to elute more quickly from the column. In addition, a chemical that selectively interacts with the stationary phase more strongly than another chemical will tend to stay longer in the column. The overall result is a separation of these chemicals based on their volatility and interactions with the stationary phase.

Types of Gas Chromatography

There are several ways of classifying GC methods based on the type of stationary phase present. These categories include GSC, GLC, and bonded phase GC.

Gas-Solid Chromatography

GSC is a type of GC in which the same material acts as both the stationary phase and the support.[7] In this method, chemicals are retained by their adsorption to the surface of the support. This support is often an inorganic material such as silica or alumina. Other supports that can be used in this method are molecular sieves, which are porous materials that are made from a mixture of silica and alumina, or organic polymers such as porous polystyrene.[2,12,21]

The retention of an analyte on a GSC support will be affected by several factors. These factors include the surface area of the support, the size of the pores in the support, and the types of functional groups that are present on the surface of the support. Using a support with a high surface area will lead to higher retention than a support with a lower surface area. The selection of an appropriate pore size may be important if the analytes are large enough to be able to access the surface within only some of these pores. The functional groups and polarity of the support and its surface will also determine which types of analytes will have the strongest adsorption to this surface. Polar materials such as silica, alumina, and molecular sieves will usually have strong binding to polar compounds and to those that can form hydrogen

TABLE 19.1   Stationary Phases Commonly Used in Gas-Liquid Chromatography and as Bonded Phases in Gas Chromatography

Composition	Polarity	Commercial Examples	Typical Applications
100% Methylpolysiloxane	Nonpolar	OV-1, SE-30	Drugs, amino acid derivatives
5% Phenyl–95% methylpolysiloxane	Nonpolar	OV-23, SE-54	Drugs
50% Phenyl–50% methylpolysiloxane	Intermediate polarity	OV-17	Drugs, steroids, glycols
50% Cyanopropylmethyl–50% phenylmethylpolysiloxane	Intermediate polarity	OV-225	Fatty acid methyl esters, carbohydrate derivatives
Polyethylene glycol	Polar	Carbowax 20M	Acids, alcohols, glycols, ketones

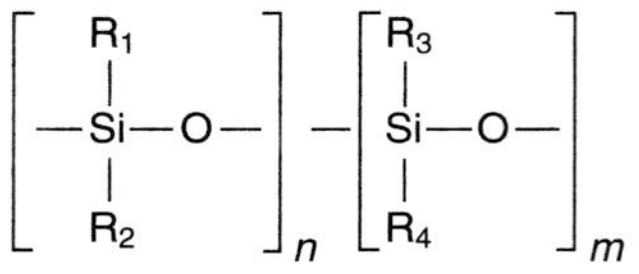

FIGURE 19.8 General structure of a polysiloxane. The side groups are represented by R_1 through R_4, while n and m represent the relative lengths (or amounts) of each type of segment in the overall polymer.

bonds. Polystyrene and other less polar supports will have weaker and less selective interactions with chemicals and tend to give separations that are based more on the volatility of the components in an applied sample.

Gas-Liquid Chromatography and Bonded Phases

In GLC, the stationary phase is a liquid that is placed as a coating or layer on the support.[7] This is the most common type of GC for chemical analysis. Various types of liquids can be used for this purpose (see examples in Table 19.1). All these liquids must have a low volatility to allow them to stay within the column at the high temperatures that are often used in GC separations. Many GLC stationary phases are based on polysiloxanes, which have the basic structure shown in Fig. 18.8.[12] The molar mass of the –Si-O-Si- chain in a polysiloxane can range in size from a few thousand to over a million grams per mole. The side chains that are attached to the silicon atoms in this chain can have structures that range from nonpolar methyl groups to polar cyanopropyl groups. These side chains also can be present in various ratios as mixtures. The overall polarity and types of chemicals that will be retained the most by this type of stationary phase will be determined by the amounts and types of side chains that are present.

One issue in using a liquid as a stationary phase in GC is that some of this liquid will eventually leave the column over time. This loss of the stationary phase is known as column bleed.[12,22] This process is not desirable because it will result in a change in the amount of stationary phase present and a change in the ability of the GC system to retain chemicals. This process also may cause the signal of the GC detector to have a high background or to be noisy as the liquid stationary phase leaves the column and passes through the detector.

Column bleed can be minimized by using a bonded phase instead of a liquid as the stationary phase in the GC column. The resulting method is sometimes known as bonded phase GC. A bonded phase can be produced by reacting functional groups on a stationary phase such as a polysiloxane with silanol groups on the surface of silica. Alternatively, the

stationary phase can be cross-linked to make it less volatile and more stable. Besides providing a stationary phase that is more stable, a bonded phase also can provide a stationary phase that has a thinner and more uniform coating than a stationary phase based on a liquid coating. Although bonded phases are more expensive than liquid stationary phases, bonded phases are often preferred for analytical work because of their better thermal stability and better efficiencies.[12,22]

POINTS TO REMEMBER

Types of Gas Chromatography Based on the Stationary Phase
- Gas-solid chromatography
- Gas-liquid chromatography
- Bonded phase gas chromatography

Gas Chromatography Instrumentation

The typical components of a gas chromatograph are illustrated in Fig. 19.9.[21] The first major component is the source of the gaseous mobile phase, which is used to supply the carrier gas at a controlled pressure and flow rate. Next, there is the injection system, through which samples are placed into the gas chromatograph and converted into a volatile form. This is followed by the column, which contains the support and the stationary phase. This column is held in an oven for temperature control. The fourth part of the GC system is a detector that monitors sample components as they leave the column. Finally, there is a computer or control system that acquires data from the detector and allows control of the GC system.[21]

Carrier Gas Sources and Flow Control

The function of the carrier gas source is to provide the gas that will be used as the mobile phase for the GC separation. The carrier gas is usually supplied by a standard gas cylinder. However, the carrier gas is sometimes provided by using a gas generator that is connected to the GC system. Such a generator can be used to isolate nitrogen from air or produce hydrogen gas through the electrolysis of water.[2]

Good flow control is needed in GC to provide a constant or well-defined flow of the carrier gas. This control makes it possible to maintain good column efficiency and obtain reproducible elution times. Systems that are used to provide constant flow rates may use a simple mechanical device, such as a pressure regulator, or a more sophisticated electronic control device. Methods in GC such as temperature programming, as will be discussed later, require electronic

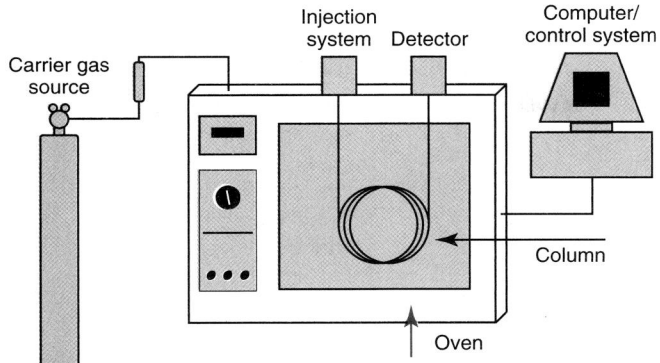

FIGURE 19.9 General design of a gas chromatograph. (Modified from a figure courtesy Restek Corporation, Bellefonte, PA.)

pressure control to regulate the carrier gas flow rate and pressure during a chromatographic run. Such a controller may be operated in a constant-flow or constant-pressure mode. In the constant-flow mode, the pressure required to provide a flow rate that is independent of the carrier gas viscosity is determined and maintained by the system through use of a pressure transducer and pressure regulator.

The magnitude of the carrier gas flow rate will depend on the type of column being used. For example, packed columns require typical flow rates that range from 10 to 60 mL/min (0.17×10^{-3} to 1.0×10^{-3} L/s). Capillary columns use much lower flow rates (e.g., 1 to 2 mL/min, or 1.7×10^{-5} to 3.3×10^{-5} L/s). Because of the greater efficiencies of capillary columns versus packed columns, operating at a consistent flow rate is even more critical for the operation of the capillary columns.

Various gases can be used as the mobile phase in GC. The choice of carrier gas will depend on factors such as the type of column and detector used, as well as the expense, purity, and chemical or physical properties of the gas. Hydrogen and helium are the carrier gases of choice with capillary columns. Only high-purity hydrogen and helium should be used for this purpose. For packed columns, the most frequently used carrier gas is nitrogen.

Carrier gas impurities such as water, oxygen, and hydrocarbons can (1) harm or alter the column, (2) negatively influence the performance of some detectors, and (3) adversely affect the measurement of chemicals. The carrier gas should be as pure as possible to avoid such problems. The carrier gas should be dry, and the tubing used to connect the gas source to the GC system should be free from contamination. Molecular sieve beds and specialized inline traps are often used to remove water, hydrocarbons, oxygen, and particulate matter that may be present in the carrier gas.[23]

Many GC detectors work best with certain types of carrier gases. For instance, work with packed columns often involves the use of nitrogen as the carrier gas when working with a flame ionization detector (FID), electron capture detector (ECD), or thermal conductivity detector (TCD), which are each described in more detail later. Helium is often used with capillary columns and in work with a FID or TCD, whereas nitrogen/argon-methane mixtures are used with an ECD.

Injection Systems and Sample Derivatization
The injection of a sample into a GC system must be done with minimal disruption of gas flow into the column. Most

clinical GC methods make use of liquid-phase samples, for which the sample components are first extracted into or dissolved in a nonaqueous liquid or adsorbed onto a microextraction fiber. This liquid or microextraction fiber is then placed into the chromatographic system by using a precise and rapid online injector (e.g., an autosampler or automated injection system). With packed columns, a glass microsyringe is used to inject a 1- to 10-µL portion of the sample through a septum, which serves as the interface between the injector and the chromatographic system. On the other side of the septum is located a heated injection port. Volatile chemicals in the sample and the solvent are flash-vaporized in this heated port and swept into the column by the carrier gas. To ensure rapid and complete volatilization, the temperature of the heated injection port is usually maintained at a temperature that is at least 30 to 50 °C higher than the column temperature.

Common problems during injection include septum leaks and the adsorption of sample components onto the septum. In addition, because the injection port is heated, thermal decomposition products may be produced here from the sample and enter the column. This process can result in spurious peaks, or "ghost" peaks, in the chromatogram. This type of contamination is most likely to occur at high injection temperatures. A Teflon-coated septum, or low-bleed septum, can be used to minimize this problem. In addition, the inner surface of the septum can be purged with the carrier gas and vented before the purge gas passes into the column. This approach is especially effective in reducing septum-related problems, and most commercial injectors are equipped with continuous-purge capabilities. The septum is a consumable component of the gas chromatograph and should be replaced at least once every 100 injections.

Because of the low sample capacities and slow carrier gas flow rates that are used with capillary columns, split and splitless injection techniques are used to introduce samples into such columns.[2,22] In the method of split injection, only a small portion of the vaporized sample enters the column, with the remainder being passed through a side vent. In splitless injection, most of the sample enters the column.[4] The split flow injection mode is used for samples that contain relatively high concentrations of the target analytes, whereas the splitless mode is used for samples that contain relatively low concentrations of the analytes.

Temperature-programmable injection ports are available and may be used in either the split or splitless injection mode. In this type of port, the sample is injected at a temperature slightly higher than the boiling point of the solvent that contains the sample. Under these conditions, most of the sample components will condense on a glass or fused silica wool insert that is present in the injector, while the solvent is vaporized and removed. The injector is then rapidly heated at rates of up to 100 °C/min. The rapid heating vaporizes the analytes, which then move into the column. This rapid heating is advantageous because any thermally labile compounds that may be present in the sample are exposed to the high temperatures for only a short time. The ability of this approach to provide separate steps for solvent removal and analyte vaporization can allow the injection of sample volumes of up to hundreds of microliters. This ability can improve analyte detection when the amount of sample that is available is not a limiting factor.

Headspace analysis is a sample introduction technique that can be used with aqueous solutions or samples that contain some nonvolatile components.[22] In this method, a portion of the vapor phase (or "headspace") that is above a liquid or solid sample is used for the analysis. This vapor phase contains a portion of some of the more volatile components of the sample and can be directly injected onto a GC system for analysis. Headspace analysis can be carried out using either a static method or a dynamic method. In the static method, the sample is placed in an enclosed container and allowed to reach equilibrium for the distribution of its components between the sample and the vapor phase above the sample. A portion of the vapor phase is then injected onto the GC system for analysis. In the dynamic method, an inert gas is passed through the sample and used to sweep away the volatile components. These components are then captured by a solid adsorbent or a cold trap and later injected onto the GC system for analysis.

Although a fairly large number of low-mass chemicals can be injected directly onto a GC system, many more are not sufficiently volatile or thermally stable for their direct application to a GC system. A common way of making a chemical more volatile and thermally stable is to alter its structure through derivatization.[2,24] This usually involves replacing one or more polar groups on the analyte with less polar groups. This change tends to make the chemical more volatile by reducing dipole-related interactions or hydrogen bonding and often makes the chemical more thermally stable. Various types of reactions can be used for this purpose in GC. A common example is the replacement of an active hydrogen on an alcohol, phenol, amine, or carboxylic acid group with a trimethylsilyl (TMS) group, producing a TMS derivative. Other examples include the use of alkylation (e.g., the formation of a methyl ester through the esterification of a carboxylic acid) or acylation (e.g., the production of an acetate derivative from an alcohol or amine).[24] Along with increasing the volatility and thermal stability of a compound, some of these derivatization reactions also can be used to change the response of the analyte to certain detectors, such as an ECD through the addition of halogen atoms to a compound's structure.

Columns and Supports

Both packed columns and capillary columns are used in GC.[2,7,21,25] Packed GC columns are filled with support particles that are based on either uncoated supports, as used in GSC, or that have liquid coatings or bonded stationary phases, as used in GLC and bonded phase GC. These packed columns vary from 1 to 4 mm in inner diameter and have typical lengths of 1 to 2 m, with the outside of the column being fabricated from tubes of glass or stainless steel. Packed GC columns are useful when it is necessary to apply a relatively large amount of a sample onto the GC system. However, packed columns also tend to have lower efficiencies than capillary columns. This last factor results in packed columns being mainly used for separations in which a relatively small number of compounds are to be separated.

Capillary columns, which are also known as open-tubular columns, consist of a column that has the stationary phase attached to or coated on its interior surface. Capillary columns have typical inner diameters of 0.10 to 0.75 mm and lengths that often range from 10 to 150 m. The capillary columns with narrow bores are more efficient, and the wider bore columns have greater sample capacities. Capillary GC columns are usually made from fused silica capillaries that have a polyimide or aluminum coating on the outside to give the capillary sufficient strength and flexibility for use in a GC system. Although capillary columns have lower sample capacities than packed columns, they also provide better peak resolution and higher efficiencies. These properties make capillary columns the most common type of support used in GC for analytical applications.

There are several types of capillary columns. Three common types are (1) porous-layer open tubular (PLOT) columns, (2) support-coated open tubular (SCOT) columns, and (3) wall-coated open tubular (WCOT) columns.[2,7,21,25] In PLOT columns, a porous layer is placed on the inner wall of the capillary columns. This porous layer is made by either chemical means (e.g., etching) or by depositing a layer of porous particles on the wall from a suspension. The porous layer serves as a support and/or stationary phase for use in GSC. PLOT columns are primarily used for analysis of gases and separation of low-mass hydrocarbons.

SCOT columns have an inner wall with a thin layer of a support onto which a stationary phase is coated or attached. This type of column is used with liquid stationary phases or bonded phases. WCOT columns consist of a capillary tube whose inner wall is coated directly with a liquid stationary phase or a bonded phase. WCOT columns tend to be more efficient than SCOT columns but also have a smaller sample capacity.

In addition to traditional packed columns and capillary columns, research has been carried out in the development of GC columns on microchips.[26] These devices have great potential for use in high-speed GC and miniaturized GC systems.[27]

Temperature Control

All types of GC columns and systems require careful control of temperature. The accurate, precise control of the column and injector temperatures is required to obtain optimal performance and reliable results in a GC system. Control of the column temperature is achieved by using a column oven, in which the column is heated directly by resistive heating.[21,28] The temperatures of the injection system and detectors are also usually controlled by resistive heating. Temperature control of the column is especially important, particularly in applications in which the retention times or volumes of eluting peaks are compared with those of standards for compound identification. For instance, a change of only 1°C in column temperature can lead to a 5% change in retention time.

Depending on the type of GC separation being carried out and the complexity of the sample, the column may be maintained at a constant temperature during the separation (i.e., a method known as isothermal elution) or the temperature may be varied as a function of time (i.e., a technique known as temperature programming).[7] Temperature programming is used for most clinical applications. In temperature programming, the sample components with the lowest boiling points and weakest interactions with the GC column will elute first, followed by chemicals that have higher boiling points and/or stronger interactions with the column. As a result, it is possible with temperature programming to separate a complex mixture of chemicals with a wide range of boiling points and volatilities. Temperature programming also usually provides sharper and more distinct peaks in less time than can be obtained with isothermal elution. The main advantage of isothermal elution is that it can be faster for simple samples that do not contain a wide range of chemicals with different volatilities. Also, it is essential with temperature programming to use computer control to provide a reproducible and well-defined temperature gradient during the analysis.

The thermal stability of the stationary phase is important to consider during the development of a GC method. Because each stationary phase has a specific temperature range over which it is stable, it is necessary to keep the column temperature within this usable range. For nonpolar stationary phases in silica capillary columns, the upper temperature limit is often determined by the stability of the polyimide coating on the capillary. The introduction of aluminum clad columns has broadened this usable temperature range. Oxidation reactions that may occur at high temperatures tend to limit the operating temperature of stationary phases that have an intermediate polarity or that have a higher polarity.

Before any GC column is used for routine analysis, it must be "thermally conditioned" by heating the column at various temperatures and for different lengths of time. This process helps to remove volatile contaminants, including residual monomers from a polymeric stationary phase that may be initially present in the column. Furthermore, the thermal conditioning of used columns can remove nonvolatile contaminants that have accumulated on this column and that can lead to unstable baselines.

To thermally condition a column, the column should be disconnected from the detector and purged for at least 5 minutes with pure carrier gas. The column should then be heated to a temperature that is above 50 °C. The column temperature is then passed through a normal temperature program for three or four cycles. Alternatively, the column can be maintained at the maximum operating temperature for 12 to 24 hours. Thermal conditioning at lower temperatures can prolong the life of the column, but longer conditioning times are required under these conditions to achieve good baseline stability. Preconditioned capillary columns are also available to minimize such problems.

Gas Chromatography Detectors

A variety of detectors can be used in GC systems (Table 19.2). These include universal detectors that can detect a broad range of analytes and more selective devices that may detect only specific groups of analytes. Examples that will be examined in this section include the (1) FID, (2) nitrogen-phosphorus detector, (3) ECD, (4) photoionization detector (PID), (5) TCD, and (6) mass spectrometric detectors.[12,21,22] Many other types of detectors have been used in GC, and it has become common to place two or more detectors in series to enhance the specificity and sensitivity of GC systems.

Flame Ionization Detector. An FID is a common detector used for GC in clinical laboratories.[4,12,21,22] This type of detector is often used during GC analysis of ethanol and other volatiles in blood or other aqueous samples. Typical chromatograms are shown in Fig. 19.10 of volatile compounds that have been examined by using headspace analysis and a GC system equipped with an FID. During the operation of an FID, the carrier gas that is leaving the column is mixed with hydrogen, and the eluting compounds are burned by a flame that is surrounded by air and an oxygen-rich environment. Approximately one organic molecule in 10,000 results in the production of a gas-phase ion. These ions are detected by a

TABLE 19.2 Examples of Detectors Used in Gas Chromatography

Type of Detector	Principle of Operation	Selectivity	Approximate Limit of Detection
Flame ionization detector (FID)	Production of gas phase ions from combustion of organic compounds	General: Organic compounds	10^{-12} g carbon
Nitrogen-phosphorus detector (NPD; thermionic selective detector, TSD)	Heated alkali bead selectively ionizes nitrogen- or phosphorus-containing compounds	Nitrogen- or phosphorus-containing compounds	10^{-14}–10^{-13} g nitrogen or phosphorus
Electron capture detector (ECD)	Capture of electrons by chemicals with electronegative groups	Chemicals with electronegative groups	10^{-15}–10^{-13} g
Mass spectrometry (MS)	Production of gas phase ions, followed by separation/analysis of these ions based on their mass-to-charge ratios	Universal: Full-scan mode Selective: Selected ion monitoring mode (SIM)	10^{-10}–10^{-9} g (full-scan mode) 10^{-12}–10^{-11} g (SIM mode)
Thermal conductivity detector (TCD)	Measurement of change in thermal conductivity of carrier gas as compounds elute from the column	Universal	10^{-9} g
Photoionization detector (PID)	Measurement of gas phase ions that are produced due to chemical ionization with light	General: Organic compounds	10^{-12}–10^{-11} g
Flame photometric detector (FPD)	Phosphorus- and sulfur-containing compounds emit light when burned in a flame; emitted light is detected	Phosphorus and sulfur-containing compounds	10^{-12} g phosphorus 10^{-11} g sulfur
Infrared (IR) spectroscopy	Absorption of IR light	IR-absorbing compounds	10^{-9} g

Portions of this table are based on data from Hage DS, Carr JD. *Analytical chemistry and quantitative analysis*. New York: Pearson; 2011, and references cited therein.

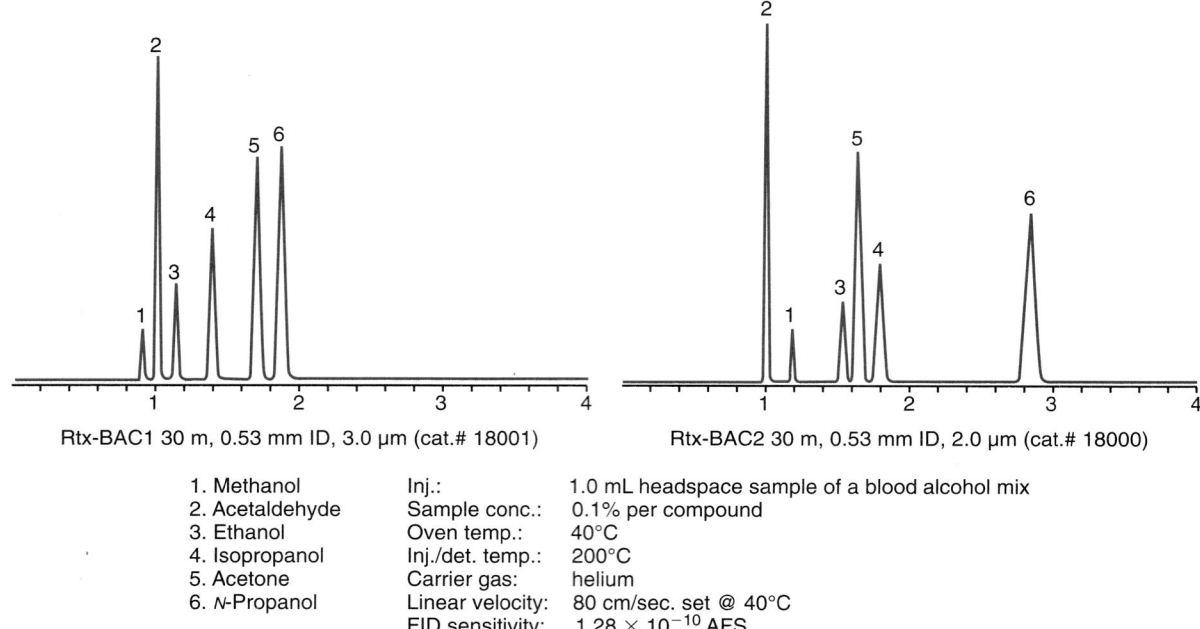

FIGURE 19.10 Chromatograms obtained during the analysis of volatile organic compounds when using headspace analysis and gas chromatography. (Courtesy Restek Corporation, Bellefonte, PA.)

collector electrode that is positioned above the flame. The magnitude of the current that is generated by these ions is related to the mass of carbon that was delivered to the detector. This signal can then be used for both the detection and quantification of organic compounds that are eluting from the column.

The advantages of an FID include its simplicity, reliability, versatility, and ease of operation. Another advantage of using an FID is that this detector gives little or no signal for common carrier gases (e.g., He, Ar, or N_2) or typical contaminants in such gases (e.g., O_2 and H_2O). An FID is easy to use with temperature programming and is a good general detector for the routine clinical analysis of organic compounds. One disadvantage of the FID is its destructive nature, so it cannot be connected directly to other GC detectors. However, an FID still can be used in combination with another detector if part of the carrier gas stream is split between the FID and the other detector.

Nitrogen-Phosphorus Detector. The nitrogen-phosphorus detector (NPD) is also known as a thermionic selective detector (TSD). This detector is similar to an FID but instead of a flame uses an electrically heated alkali bead, which is generally made of rubidium. This heated bead is placed directly above where the mixture of the carrier gas and hydrogen enter the detector.[12,21,22] Ions are generated at or above the surface of the heated alkali bead, which supplies electrons to electronegative compounds that surround the bead and leads to the formation of negatively charged ions. These ions are then collected at an electrode and generate a current that is used to detect and quantify the eluting compounds.

Nitrogen- or phosphorus-containing compounds are especially good at creating ions in an NPD. This feature makes the NPD particularly useful for monitoring low concentrations of analytes that have nitrogen or phosphorus in their structures. The NPD is frequently used in GC for detection of organic bases and acids. This type of detector does not respond to common GC carrier gases or their impurities, and several types of carrier gases can be used with this detector. However, it is necessary to have the alkali bead in this detector changed on a regular basis because this material will slowly degrade over time.

Electron Capture Detector. The ECD is another example of a selective GC detector. The operation of an ECD is based on the capture of secondary electrons by electronegative compounds that are eluting from the column.[12,21,22] High-energy electrons, or beta particles, are provided in an ECD by a radioactive source such as ^{63}Ni or ^{3}H that is housed in the detector. As the beta particles are produced, they collide with the carrier gas and lead to the release of many secondary electrons. When only the carrier gas is passing through this detector, a consistent supply of the secondary electrons is created. These secondary electrons are collected at a positive electrode and measured. When a chemical with electronegative groups elutes from the column, some of these secondary electrons are captured and fewer reach the electrode. The resulting change in current is used to detect and measure the amount of analyte that was eluting from the column.

An ECD can provide both selective and sensitive detection for chemicals that contain electronegative groups. This includes chemicals that contain halogen atoms (I, Br, Cl, and F) or nitro groups ($-NO_2$). It also includes chemicals that are polynuclear aromatic hydrocarbons, anhydrides, or conjugated carbonyl compounds, along with many others. Derivatization with reagents containing polychlorinated or polyfluorinated groups can be used with some chemicals to also allow them to be monitored with an ECD.

Argon and nitrogen are usually employed as the carrier gases for a GC system with an ECD because their relatively large size makes it easy for them to collide with beta particles and produce secondary electrons. Some methane is also usually combined with these carrier gases to produce a steady stream of secondary electrons and provide a stable detector response. It is important that these gases be pure and dry because the presence of oxygen and water can foul this type of detector. Because an ECD uses a radioactive source, this source needs to be replaced on a regular basis by a certified technician.

Mass spectrometry. Mass spectrometers are also used as detectors for GC. This combination is known as gas chromatography/mass spectrometry (GC/MS).[12] GC/MS is a powerful method for identifying analytes and quantifying them as they elute from a GC column. Ionization methods that are often used in GC/MS include electron impact ionization and chemical ionization, which are both discussed in Chapter 20. Some mass analyzers that are commonly used in GC/MS are quadrupole mass analyzers and ion traps (see Chapter 20), although other types of mass analyzers can be used as well.

In the full-scan mode of GC/MS, information is acquired by the MS system on a wide range of ions. This mode is used when the goal is to detect many compounds in a single run or provide data that can be used to identify an unknown compound from its mass spectrum. In this mode, the mass spectrometer acts as a general detector for the GC system. GC/MS also can monitor specific analytes by using selected ion monitoring (SIM). This mode uses the mass spectrometer to monitor only a few ions that are representative of the analytes of interest. SIM is used when selective detection and low detection limits are desired but does require that information be available in advance on the types of ions that will be generated from the analytes.

The response of a GC/MS system can be represented in several ways. For instance, in the full-scan mode a plot can be made of the number of ions measured at each elution time. This type of graph is known as a mass chromatogram, or total ion chromatogram, and can be used to show the overall response of the system to the eluting analytes. It is also possible in the full-scan mode to use all the collected data to show the mass spectrum that is acquired at a given elution time. This plot can be used to help identify a compound that is eluting at that time from the GC/MS system. Finally, a plot can be made of the number of ions that are detected at only specific mass-to-charge ratios as a function of the elution time. This last plot is called a selected ion chromatogram and is used in the SIM mode or the full-scan mode when looking for specific compounds that may be eluting from the GC/MS system.

Other gas chromatography detectors. A variety of other detectors can be part of a GC system. One example is the TCD. A TCD is a general detector that can monitor both inorganic and organic compounds. It detects and measures these compounds based on their ability to change how the carrier gas/analyte mixture will conduct heat away from a hot wire filament (i.e., a property referred to as thermal conductivity).[12,21,22] The carrier gas used with a TCD is often helium or hydrogen, which have the greatest differences in their thermal conductivities from most organic or inorganic compounds. However, nitrogen or other carrier gases also can be used with a TCD.

The primary advantage of a TCD is its ability to detect many types of chemicals, as long as they are present at sufficient quantities to be detected. This detector is nondestructive and can be easily combined with a second detector.

However, a TCD also can respond to contaminants in the carrier gas and can give a change in the background response during temperature programming. In addition, the TCD tends to have much higher detection limits than other common GC detectors.

Another group of GC detectors makes use of the interactions of chemicals with light. One example is the PID.[12,21] The PID is similar in design and operation to an FID in that both use electrodes to detect and measure ions produced from chemicals eluting from the column. However, in the PID these ions are produced through interaction of the eluting chemicals with ultraviolet (UV) radiation rather than through the use of a flame. Another GC detector that makes use of light is a flame photometric detector (FPD).[12] An FPD is a selective detector for phosphorus- or sulfur-containing compounds. Like an FID, an FPD passes the eluting chemicals into a flame, but the FPD measures the release of light from excited-state phosphorus- or sulfur-containing species rather than the production of ions. It is also possible to combine GC with infrared (IR) spectroscopy, giving a method known as gas chromatography/infrared spectroscopy (GC/IR).[12] This combination can be used for both chemical measurement and identification by looking at the absorption of IR radiation by chemicals as they elute from a GC column.

Data Acquisition and System Control

As with most modern analytical instruments, computers are used to both control and automate GC systems, as well as collect and process data from these systems. With regard to system control, the computer can regulate parameters such as (1) the carrier gas composition and flow rate; (2) the column back pressure; (3) the column and detector temperatures, including temperature programming; (4) the sample injection process; (5) detector selection and operation; and (6) the timing steps that are used during system operation and chemical analysis.

In terms of data acquisition and processing, the computer can monitor the signals generated by the GC system's detectors, including the acquisition and storage of data at specified time intervals. From this information, the area or height of each chromatographic peak can be measured, and this information can be used to determine the analyte concentration represented by each peak. Algorithms are available for this process in modern GC systems that allow for the generation of calibration curves or conversion factors based on either internal or external calibration methods. The computer system also can be used to search databases to aid in identification of analytes based on their retention times or response at the detector (e.g., their mass spectra).[21,29] If desired, the data acquisition system can then be used to generate a report on the results for each chromatographic run. Alternatively, these data can be stored for later examination or reprocessing.

Laboratory Safety in Gas Chromatography

Standard safety precautions should be followed when placing and securing the gas cylinder or mobile phase source that is used for GC. If hydrogen is used as the carrier gas, extra precautions should be taken in training laboratory personnel in the handling and use of this flammable and potentially explosive gas. Proper ventilation facilities should be available in the work area to deal with carrier gas that has passed through the GC system. All samples, reagents, and solutions that are used during a GC analysis should also be handled and stored using appropriate laboratory procedures (see Chapter 15).

LIQUID CHROMATOGRAPHY

LC is a type of chromatography in which the mobile phase is a liquid. Separations in LC are based on the distribution of chemicals between a liquid mobile phase and a stationary phase.[9] This was the type of chromatography used by Tswett when he first began to practice column chromatography in 1903. Although LC was mainly a preparative tool until the 1960s, it is now the dominant type of chromatography used for chemical analysis in clinical or biomedical laboratories. A key advantage of this method over GC is the ability of LC to work directly with liquid samples, such as those encountered with clinical or biological specimens.

Before the mid-1960s, the supports used in LC columns were based on large and irregularly shaped particulate supports such as those used in packed columns for GC. These supports were useful in preparative work but were not suitable for many analytical applications because they tended to result in broad peaks and separations with low resolution. In addition, these supports generally had limited mechanical stability and could be used only at relatively low operating pressures.

Developments beginning in the 1960s allowed the production of smaller, more mechanically stable, and more efficient supports for LC, along with the instrumentation that could be used with such materials.[30] This resulted in a method that is now known as HPLC.[10,30–32] The use of these more efficient supports made it possible to obtain narrower peaks, better separations, and lower limits of detection in LC. These reasons, along with the ability of HPLC to be used as an automated method, have made this technique the method of choice for most routine chemical separations and analysis methods in modern laboratories, including those in a clinical setting. Other advantages of HPLC and LC include the wide range of separation mechanisms, stationary phases, solvents, and detectors that can be employed in such methods.

In HPLC, particulate supports with relatively small diameters are often used to hold the stationary phase within the column. Because the pressure drop across a packed bed column is related to the square of a support particle's diameter, relatively high pressures can be required to pump liquids through HPLC columns with even moderate lengths. As a result, this technique has also been referred to as high-pressure liquid chromatography, although HPLC is the preferred name. Most modern HPLC systems can work at pressures up to 5000 to 6000 psi (or 34.5 to 41.4 MPa). Specialized systems that can operate at even higher pressures have recently been developed for a method known as ultra-high-performance liquid chromatography or ultra-high-pressure liquid chromatography.[33–36]

One important difference between LC and GC is that the retention of chemicals in LC can depend on the interactions of these chemicals with both the mobile phase and stationary phase. This means the composition and nature of the mobile phase are important to consider when adjusting the retention of a chemical in an LC system. The term strong mobile phase is used to describe a mobile phase that leads to weak retention for an analyte on a given type of stationary phase. The weakest retention for a chemical will occur when this substance favors staying in the mobile phase instead of the stationary phase. The term weak mobile phase refers to the opposite situation in which a chemical favors the stationary phase versus the mobile phase and has its highest retention within a given column.[2]

POINTS TO REMEMBER

Mobile Phase Strength in Liquid Chromatography
- The mobile phase is a primary determinant of chemical retention.
- A strong mobile phase leads to weak retention for an analyte on a given type of stationary phase and column.
- A weak mobile phase causes a chemical to favor the stationary phase, resulting in high retention within a given column.

Types of Liquid Chromatography

Liquid chromatographic methods are classified according to the chemical or physical mechanisms by which they separate chemicals (Fig. 19.11). The five main types of LC based on the separation mechanism are (1) adsorption chromatography, (2) partition chromatography, (3) IEC, (4) size-exclusion chromatography (SEC), and (5) affinity chromatography.[2,7] Most clinical applications use LC separations that are based on partition chromatography or IEC; however, the other types of LC also have valuable clinical applications.

Adsorption Chromatography

Adsorption chromatography is a type of LC in which chemicals are retained based on their adsorption and desorption at the surface of the support, which also acts as the stationary phase (see Fig. 19.11). This method is also sometimes referred to as liquid-solid chromatography.[10] Retention in this method is based on the competition of the analyte with molecules of the mobile phase as both bind to the surface of the support. The degree of a chemical's retention in adsorption chromatography will depend on (1) the binding strength of this chemical to the support, (2) the surface area of the support, (3) the amount of mobile phase displaced from the support by the chemical, and (4) the binding strength of the mobile phase to the support.[12] Electrostatic interactions, hydrogen bonding, dipole-dipole interactions, and dispersive interactions (i.e., van der Waals forces) all may affect retention in this type of chromatography.[37,38]

The binding strength of the mobile phase with the support in adsorption chromatography is described by the mobile phase's eluotropic strength.[10,12,39] A liquid or solution that has a large eluotropic strength for a given support will act as a strong mobile phase for that material because this mobile phase will tend to bind tightly to the support and cause the analyte to elute more quickly as it spends more time in the mobile phase. As an example, a relatively polar solvent such as methanol will have a higher eluotropic strength for a polar support such as silica than a nonpolar solvent such as carbon tetrachloride. In the same manner, a liquid or solution that has a low eluotropic strength for a support would represent a weak mobile phase for that support in adsorption chromatography (e.g., carbon tetrachloride on silica).

Three types of adsorbents are generally used in adsorption chromatography: (1) polar acidic supports, (2) polar basic supports, and (3) nonpolar supports. The most common polar

Adsorption chromatography
Separation based on adsorption of
chemicals to the surface of a support

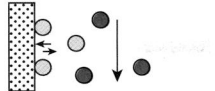

Partition chromatography
Separation based on partitioning of chemicals
into a layer of the stationary phase

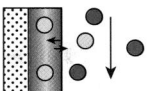

Ion-exchange chromatography
Separation of ions based on their binding to
fixed charges on a support

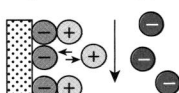

Size-exclusion chromatography
Separation of chemicals based on their size
and ability to enter a porous support

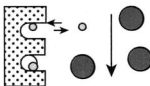

Affinity chromatography
Separation of chemicals based on their interactions
with a biologically related binding agent

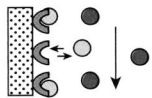

FIGURE 19.11 Main types of liquid chromatography based on their separation mechanisms.

and acidic support used in adsorption chromatography is silica. The surface silanol groups on this support tend to adsorb polar compounds and work particularly well for basic substances. Alumina is the main type of polar and basic adsorbent that is used in adsorption chromatography. Like silica, alumina retains polar compounds, but alumina works especially well for polar acidic substances. Florisil is an alternative polar and basic support that can be used in place of alumina, such as when catalytic decomposition of an analyte is observed with this latter material. Other types of supports that can be used in adsorption chromatography are nonpolar adsorbents such as charcoal and polystyrene.

Partition Chromatography

The second major type of LC based on the separation mechanism is partition chromatography. Partition chromatography is an LC method in which solutes are separated based on their partitioning between a liquid mobile phase and a stationary phase that is coated or bonded onto a solid support (see Fig. 19.11).[40–42] The support in most types of partition chromatography is silica, although other types of supports also can be employed. This method originally involved coatings of liquid stationary phases that were immiscible with the desired mobile phase. However, most current columns used in partition chromatography employ stationary phases that are bonded to the support. These bonded phases are more stable than the coated layers of stationary phases that were initially used in partition chromatography and provide better column efficiencies.

The two main types of partition chromatography based on the polarity of the stationary phase are normal-phase chromatography and reversed-phase chromatography.[7,10,12,39] Normal-phase chromatography is a type of partition chromatography in which a polar stationary phase is used.[7,10,43] This is the first type of partition chromatography that was developed, and it is also known as normal-phase liquid chromatography. The stationary phase in this method typically contains groups that can form hydrogen bonds or undergo

dipole-related interactions. Examples of bonded stationary phases for normal-phase chromatography are those that contain aminopropyl groups, cyano groups, and diol groups. Because this method has a polar stationary phase, it will have its highest retention for polar compounds. A weak mobile phase in this method will be a nonpolar liquid. A strong mobile phase in normal-phase chromatography is a polar liquid, such as methanol or water.

Normal-phase chromatography can be used in many of the same applications as separations in adsorption chromatography that use silica or alumina supports. These applications usually involve the separation or analysis of chemicals that are present in organic solvents and of substances that contain one or more polar functional groups. Examples of chemicals that are of clinical interest and for which normal-phase chromatography has been used include steroids and sugars.[12,31,32,44]

The second major type of partition chromatography is reversed-phase chromatography, which is also known as reversed-phase liquid chromatography. Reversed-phase chromatography is a type of partition chromatography that uses a nonpolar stationary phase.[7,10] It is the most popular type of liquid chromatography and the most common type found in clinical laboratories.[12,31,32,45] One reason for this is that the weak mobile phase in reversed-phase chromatography is a polar solvent, such as water. This property makes this type of LC convenient for the analysis and separation of chemicals in aqueous-based systems, such as serum, urine, and blood.[12,31,32,39] A strong mobile phase in this method is a liquid that is less polar than water, such as acetonitrile or methanol. Because of the presence of a nonpolar stationary phase, nonpolar compounds will have the highest retention in reversed-phase chromatography.

Reversed-phase chromatography has many applications in the areas of clinical chemistry and biomedical research. Examples of chemicals that have been separated or analyzed by this method include drugs, drug metabolites, amino acids, peptides, proteins, carbohydrates, lipids, and bile acids. A separation of antidepressant drugs by reversed-phase chromatography was shown earlier in Fig. 19.2. Compounds representing the greatest challenge for reversed-phase separations are highly polar compounds such as sugars or amino acids, which tend to be weakly retained by reversed-phase columns, and basic compounds, which may exhibit peak tailing as the result of their interactions with silica. Derivatization of some compounds (e.g., amino acids) has been employed to improve their retention on reversed-phase columns.[3] It is also important to consider both the type of analyte and support that are being used in these separations. For instance, large chemicals such as peptides or proteins will require reversed-phase supports with larger pore sizes than those routinely used for the separation of small molecules.[46–48]

A relatively wide range of stationary phases and supports are available for reversed-phase separations.[6,12,49–51] The most common stationary phases used in reversed-phase chromatography are those based on octadecyl (C_{18}), octyl (C_8), phenyl, or butyl (C_4) groups that are attached to a support such as silica. Similar materials are commonly used in solid-phase extraction (see Chapter 20). The retention characteristics of these silica-based columns will depend on (1) the nature of the bonded phase, (2) the amount of the bonded phase (often expressed as the percent of carbon load), (3) the surface area of the support, (4) the pore size of the support, and (5) the quantity of accessible groups on the support (e.g., silanol groups on silica) that can be used to prepare the bonded phase. Alternative reversed-phase materials such as porous graphite, fluorinated hydrocarbons, and hydrophobic stationary phases with embedded polar groups offer different selectivities than C_{18}- or C_8-silica. Silica tends to dissolve slowly at a pH greater than 8.0 or at a pH below 2.0, so separations that make use of silica supports are usually done in this pH range unless the silica has been stabilized by surface treatment.[49] Some of the other supports that are available for reversed-phase chromatography, such as polystyrene or porous graphite, are stable over a broader pH range (e.g., pH 2.0 to 13.0).

During the bonding of a reversed-phase stationary phase to silica, it is usually not possible to cover all the available silanol groups. These remaining silanol groups may interact with some analytes and lead to mixed-mode interactions that produce broad peaks and result in a decrease in peak resolution. For instance, the peak tailing that may occur for some basic compounds on silica is caused by coulombic interactions of these compounds with the conjugate base form of silanol groups. These interactions can be minimized by reacting many of the silanol groups with a small organosilane such as trimethylchlorosilane in a method known as endcapping.[10] In addition, the pH of the mobile phase can be lowered to decrease the amount of silanol groups that are present in their charged form. Additives such as trifluoroacetic acid or triethylamine can be added to the mobile phase to minimize interactions of the silanol groups with analytes.[12,39,44]

The strength of a mobile phase in both normal-phase chromatography and reversed-phase chromatography can be described by using the solvent polarity index. A weak mobile phase for normal-phase chromatography will be a solvent or solvent mixture that has a low value for the solvent polarity index, whereas a strong mobile phase in this method would be one with a high solvent polarity index. The opposite trend occurs in reversed-phase chromatography, in which a weak mobile phase will have a high solvent polarity index, and a strong mobile phase will have a low solvent polarity index. Some large aliphatic stationary phases in reversed-phase chromatography, such as C_{18}-silica, may undergo phase collapse if they are used in only an aqueous mobile phase; this process probably represents the folding of the aliphatic groups down onto the surface to decrease their exposure to water. This effect can be minimized by including a small amount of organic modifier in the mobile phase or by using a bonded phase with a shorter chain length.

Samples are usually applied or injected onto a reversed-phase column in the presence of an aqueous solution or water that contains a low concentration of an organic solvent such as methanol or acetonitrile. The partitioning of chemicals that are weak acids or weak bases can be adjusted in reversed-phase chromatography by changing the pH to minimize the charge of these solutes. Because most acid-base reactions are fast, this situation will usually result in only one observed peak with a retention time that is the weighted average of what would be seen for the acid or base forms of the compound. The same type of effect and shifts in retention can occur for chemicals that undergo other rapid reactions, such as complex formation with mobile phase additives.[12] The mobile phase strength in normal-phase chromatography and reversed-phase chromatography is often changed by using mixtures of solvents or solutions and gradients in which the proportions of solvents or solutions are changed during an analysis (see Fig. 19.12).[52] It is also possible to modify the polarity of aqueous solutions in reversed-phase chromatography by changing the salt concentration of the mobile phase.

This last approach is employed in a variation of reversed-phase chromatography that is known as hydrophobic interaction chromatography (HIC).[12] This method is applied mainly in the separation of large biomolecules such as proteins. HIC

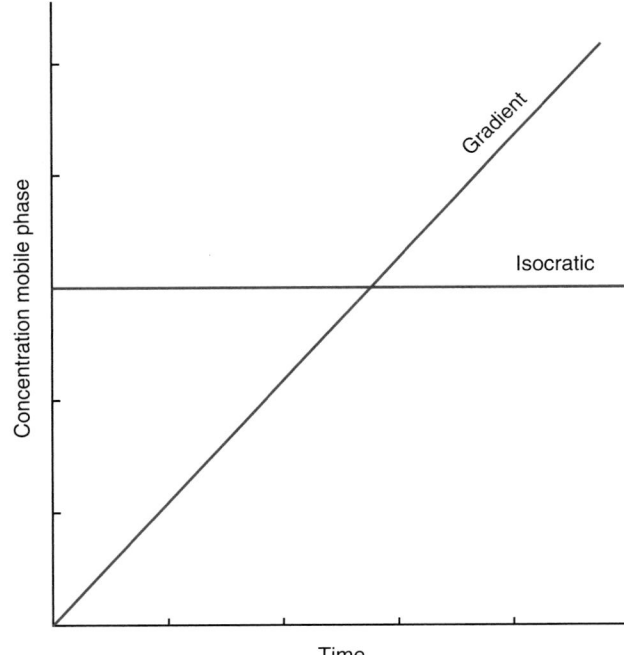

FIGURE 19.12 Examples of isocratic elution (i.e., constant mobile phase composition) or gradient elution based on solvent programming (i.e., varying mobile phase composition).

makes use of a weakly hydrophobic stationary phase that is made up of small nonpolar groups such as phenyl or butyl residues. The weak mobile phase that is used with this type of column, and which promotes the binding of proteins or related biomolecules to the stationary phase, is an aqueous solution that contains a high salt concentration. The retained biomolecules are eluted by using a strong mobile phase that is less polar, which in this case is an aqueous solution that has a lower salt concentration.

Ion-Exchange Chromatography

The third type of liquid chromatography is IEC. IEC is a type of liquid chromatography in which ions are separated by their adsorption onto a support that contains fixed charges on its surface.[7,10] This method relies on the interaction (or exchange) of ions in the sample or mobile phase with fixed ionic groups of the opposite charge that are bound to the support and act as the stationary phase (see Fig. 19.11). Depending on the charge of the groups that make up the stationary phase, the types of ions that bind to the column may be either cations (i.e., positively charged ions) or anions (i.e., negatively charged ions). These two methods are referred to as cation-exchange chromatography and anion-exchange chromatography, respectively.[12]

Supports for cation-exchange chromatography contain negatively charged functional groups. These groups may be the conjugate bases of strong acids, such as sulfonate ions that are formed by the deprotonation of sulfonic acid, or the conjugate bases of weak acids, such as those produced from carboxyl or carboxymethyl groups. The supports used in anion-exchange chromatography are usually the conjugate acids of strongly basic quaternary amines, such as triethylaminoethyl groups, or the conjugate acids of weak bases, such as aminoethyl or diethylaminoethyl groups. Supports that can be modified to contain these charged groups for use in IEC include silica and polystyrene, as well as carbohydrate-based materials such as agarose, dextran, or cellulose.[10,12,44] The carbohydrate-based supports are particularly useful in preparative work with biological agents, which can have strong binding to materials such as underivatized silica or polystyrene. The large pore size of supports such as agarose also makes these materials valuable in separations involving biological macromolecules such as proteins and nucleic acids.[10,12,44]

A strong mobile phase in IEC is usually a mobile phase that contains a high concentration of competing ions. The presence of these competing ions will make it more difficult for a charged analyte to bind to the fixed charges that act as the stationary phase. A weak mobile phase in IEC is one that contains few or no competing ions or that otherwise promotes binding by charged analytes to the column. Changing the competing ion concentration is the most common approach for adjusting the retention of analyte ions in IEC. The retention of ions in this method also may be affected by (1) pH, (2) the type of competing ion used, (3) the type of fixed charges used as the stationary phase, and (4) the density of these fixed charges on the support. Many stationary phases in IEC can exhibit mixed-mode retention through a combination of coulombic interactions and adsorption. As an example, ion-exchange resins that are used for amino acid analysis can separate amino acids with virtually the same charge because of differences in the adsorption of these amino acids onto the stationary phase.

IEC has several clinical applications. Common examples are the use of this method in the separation and analysis of amino acids and hemoglobin variants. IEC is also frequently used as a preparative tool in biomedical research for purifying proteins, peptides, and nucleotides. A modified form of IEC, known as ion chromatography, can be used with a conductivity detector to analyze small inorganic and organic ions.[12] The water purification systems that are used in many laboratories are another important application of IEC. In these purification systems, supports containing a mixture of cation- and anion-exchange groups are used to remove anions and cations from water, in which hydrogen ions are exchanged for other cations and hydroxide ions are exchanged for other anions. Most of these hydrogen ions and hydroxide ions then combine to form deionized water.[2]

Size-Exclusion Chromatography

SEC is an LC technique that separates molecules or other particles based on size (Fig. 19.13, see also Fig. 19.11).[2,12,44] In this method, a porous support is used that has an inert surface and few or no interactions with the injected sample components. This support also should have a range of pore sizes that approach, or are similar to, the sizes of the compounds that are to be separated. As a sample travels through a column that contains this support, small components of the sample can enter all or most of the pores and larger components may enter only a few or none of the pores. The result is a separation based on size or molar mass, in which the larger components elute first from the column.

In SEC, all the injected components will elute in a fairly narrow volume range. This range extends from the volume of mobile phase that is outside of all the pores of the support (also known as the excluded volume, V_E) to the total amount of mobile phase in the column, as represented by the void volume (V_M). The stationary phase in SEC can be thought of as the volume of the mobile phase in the pores of the support that can be entered by a given solute. The extent of retention in this method can be described by using the measured t_R or retention volume V_R for an injected component or by using the ratio K_o, which is calculated by using the following equation[44]:

$$K_o = \frac{(V_R - V_E)}{(V_M - V_E)}$$

The value of K_o represents the fraction of the volume between V_M and V_E in which a given sample component elutes. Small components will have a value for K_o that is equal to or approaches 1, whereas large components will have a K_o value that is equal to or approaches 0. Components with intermediate sizes will have values for K_o between 0 and 1.

Many types of porous supports have been used in SEC. Cross-linked carbohydrate-based supports such as dextran and agarose are often used in this method for work with aqueous-based samples and biological compounds such as proteins or nucleic acids. Polyacrylamide gel and silica or glass beads that have been modified into a diol-bonded form also can be used for aqueous samples and biological compounds. Polystyrene is usually employed as the support when SEC is to be used with synthetic polymers and samples that are present in organic solvents.[12,31,44] For each of these supports, the range of pore sizes that are present will determine the range of sizes for the injected compounds that can be

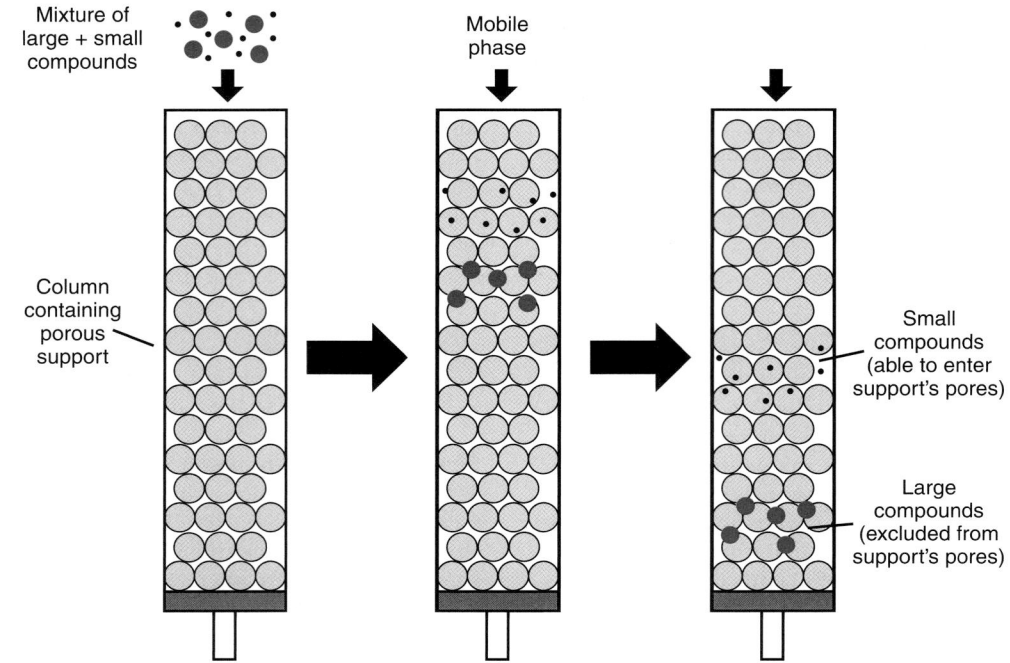

FIGURE 19.13 General principle of size-exclusion chromatography. This method separates compounds based on their size and by using a column that contains a porous support.

separated. In the case of carbohydrate-based supports and polymeric supports, this range will become smaller as the degree of cross-linking of the support is increased.

The mobile phase in SEC can be a polar solvent, such as water, or a nonpolar solvent, which is usually tetrahydrofuran. Because the stationary phase is based on a physical difference in the accessible pore volume for the solutes, rather than on chemical interactions, there is no weak mobile phase or strong mobile phase in this method. The choice of the mobile phase is instead determined by the solubility of the desired analytes and the stability of the support and the column. If water or an aqueous mobile phase is used in SEC (which typically involves a carbohydrate-based support, polyacrylamide or diol-bonded silica or glass), the resulting method is often called gel filtration chromatography. If an organic mobile phase is used (which generally involves the use of polystyrene as the support), the size-exclusion method is referred to as gel permeation chromatography.[10] Other names that are sometimes used for SEC are steric exclusion, molecular exclusion, and molecular sieve chromatography.

SEC in the gel filtration mode allows the separation of molecules under physiologic salt conditions. This feature is useful for identifying intact complexes of agents such as lipoproteins, antibody-antigen complexes, and the binding of proteins with their target compounds. SEC is often used as a rapid preparative technique to exchange buffers or to remove salts from large sample components. In addition, this method can be used to remove small molecules from large biomolecules, such as in the isolation of drugs, fatty acids, and peptides from proteins.

SEC also can be used to estimate the molecular weight of a biomolecule, such as a protein or nucleic acid, or to characterize the distribution of molecular weights for a polymer. This is done by first calibrating the size-exclusion column

with compounds that are similar to the desired analytes in structure but that have known molecular weights.[53] A calibration curve can be made by plotting the logarithm of the molecular weight versus the measured retention time, retention volume, or calculated value of K_0 for each standard compound. This plot is then used to determine the molecular weight of the unknown compounds based on their measured retention on the same column. This approach can be used to provide a good estimate of the molecular weight; however, it is a relatively low-resolution technique that does require substantial differences in molecular weight to create significant shifts in retention. For example, the diameters of globular proteins change in proportion to the cube root of their molecular weights, so roughly an eightfold difference in molecular weight is required to yield a twofold change in diameter.[53] Linear polymers, such as DNA and proteins that have been denatured and treated with sodium dodecyl sulfate or guanidine hydrochloride, have a much larger diameter for the same molecular weight, and their diameter changes approximately in proportion to the square root of molecular weight. This latter effect allows for smaller differences in molecular weight to be observed by SEC for linear molecules compared to globular molecules (e.g., nondenatured globular proteins).

Affinity Chromatography and Chiral Separations
The fifth main type of LC is affinity chromatography. Affinity chromatography is an LC method that makes use of biologically related interactions for the retention and separation of chemicals (see Fig. 19.11).[7,10,54–56] This method uses the selective, reversible interactions found in many biological systems, such as the binding of an antibody with an antigen, the interactions of an enzyme with a substrate or inhibitor, the binding of a hormone with a receptor, and the interactions of a lectin with a carbohydrate. These selective interactions are

used in affinity chromatography by immobilizing one of a pair of interacting compounds onto a support for use as the stationary phase. This immobilized binding agent is called the affinity ligand,[55] and it is used to create a column that can selectively bind and capture the complementary compound from applied samples.

The stationary phase for affinity chromatography is usually prepared by covalently immobilizing the affinity ligand to the support.[55] This is often done through the reaction of amine, sulfhydryl, carboxyl, or carbonyl groups on the affinity ligand with activated sites on the support, although other types of groups can be employed. During this process, the orientation of the affinity ligand and its accessibility to its target compound are both important to consider in providing good activity for the binding agent. Use of a spacer between the surface of the support and the affinity ligand also may be needed with smaller binding agents. Besides covalent immobilization, it is also sometimes possible to adsorb the affinity ligand to the support. This can be done in a general manner, such as through polar or ionic interactions; it also can be done through biospecific adsorption to a secondary binding agent. Examples of this latter approach include the biospecific adsorption of antibodies to an immobilized immunoglobulin-binding protein such as protein A or protein G, and the biospecific adsorption of biotin-labeled agents to immobilized avidin or streptavidin.[55] Another alternative approach for preparing affinity ligands is to form a molecularly imprinted polymer in the presence of the desired target or a target analog.[55,57] In this case, the shape and structure of the binding pockets that remain in the polymer after release of the target template can be used to selectively bind to the same or similar targets from samples.

Affinity chromatography is usually carried out by applying a sample to the column under conditions that allow strong and specific binding of the affinity ligand to its target compound.[55] This is done in the presence of a mobile phase solution, known as the application buffer, which mimics the pH and natural or preferred conditions for binding between the affinity ligand and the target. As the target binds to the column under these conditions, most other sample components are washed away as a result of the selective nature of this interaction. The retained target is then later released from the column by using an elution buffer that either contains a competing agent that will displace the target from the affinity ligand (a method known as biospecific elution) or uses a change in conditions such as pH, ionic strength, or polarity of the mobile phase to decrease the strength of binding between the target and affinity ligand (a technique called nonspecific elution). After the target has been eluted for detection or further use, the application buffer can be passed again through the column and the system is allowed to regenerate before application of the next sample. For systems with weak to moderate binding strengths, it is also possible to use isocratic elution for both sample application and target elution. This second type of elution is usually employed in chiral separations and in a method known as weak affinity chromatography.[55,58]

Various supports can be used in affinity chromatography. For preparative work, it is most common to use carbohydrate-based materials such as cross-linked agarose and various modified forms of cellulose. Silica and glass also have been used as supports for both preparative and analytical applications of affinity chromatography. This first requires that these supports be modified to give them low nonspecific binding for biological molecules and to provide groups that can be used for the immobilization of affinity ligands. In addition, several polymeric materials have been used in this method, ranging from hydroxylated polystyrene to azlactone beads, agarose-acrylamide or dextran-acrylamide copolymers, and derivatives of polyacrylamide or polymethacrylate.[55,59]

The power of affinity chromatography lies in its selectivity and in the wide range of binding agents that can be used in this method. This has led to many applications for this type of LC in work with biological compounds. Bioaffinity chromatography (or biospecific adsorption) is the most common type of affinity chromatography and involves the use of a biological binding agent as the affinity ligand.[55,59] The purification of an enzyme by using an immobilized inhibitor, coenzyme, substrate, or cofactor is an example of this approach.[55,60,61] Another example is the use of affinity ligands that are lectins or nonimmune system proteins that can bind certain types of carbohydrate residues.[55] Lectins such as concanavalin A (Con A, which binds to α-D-mannose and α-D-glucose residues) and wheat germ agglutinin (which binds to D-N-acetylglucosamines) have been popular in recent years for the isolation of carbohydrate-containing compounds, such as glycopeptides, glycoproteins, and glycolipids. This method is sometimes referred to as lectin affinity chromatography.[55] Another set of binding agents that are used in bioaffinity chromatography are immunoglobulin-binding proteins, such as protein A (from *Staphylococcus aureus*) and protein G (from group G streptococci), which have been used for antibody purification and as secondary ligands for the biospecific adsorption of antibodies.[55]

Immunoaffinity chromatography (IAC) is a subset of bioaffinity chromatography that uses an antibody or antibody-related agent as the affinity ligand. The selectivity of this method has made it popular for the isolation of targets that have ranged from antibodies, hormones, and recombinant proteins to receptors, viruses, and cellular components. This method also can be used to detect specific target compounds directly or indirectly in a set of techniques known as chromatographic immunoassays (or flow-injection immunoanalysis).[55,62] Another important application of IAC is as a tool for target isolation and sample pretreatment before analysis by other methods. The use of IAC to isolate a specific target from a sample is known as immunoextraction, which can be combined either off-line or online with other analytical methods.[55,63] A related technique is immunodepletion, which is used to remove certain compounds from a sample before analysis of the remaining sample components. This last approach has been used in proteomics to remove high-abundance proteins from biological samples before the measurement and detection of lower abundance proteins in the same samples.[63] For additional discussion, refer to Chapter 24.

Another group of methods in affinity chromatography are those that use nonbiological binding agents. Dye-ligand affinity chromatography uses an affinity ligand that is a synthetic dye such as Cibacron Blue 3GA, Procion Red HE-3B, or Procion Yellow H-A. This method is commonly used for the large- and small-scale purification of enzymes and proteins, including many protein-based biopharmaceuticals.[55,64] Dye-ligand affinity chromatography is a type of biomimetic affinity chromatography that uses an affinity ligand that is a mimic of a natural compound. Besides synthetic dyes, other binding agents that are used in this method are those generated by combinatorial chemistry and computer modeling or that are derived from peptide libraries, phage display libraries, aptamer libraries, and ribosome display libraries.[55]

Two other types of affinity chromatography that use nonbiological binding agents are immobilized metal-ion affinity chromatography (IMAC) and boronate affinity chromatography. In IMAC, the affinity ligand is a metal ion that is complexed with an immobilized chelating agent, such as Ni^{2+} complexed to a support containing iminodiacetic acid.[55] This technique is frequently used to isolate recombinant histidine-tagged proteins and has been used for the isolation or analysis of phosphorylated proteins in proteomics.[55] Boronate affinity chromatography uses an affinity ligand that is boronic acid or a related derivative. These affinity ligands are able to form covalent bonds with compounds that contain *cis*-diol groups; this feature makes these binding agents useful in the purification and analysis of polysaccharides, glycoproteins, ribonucleic acids, and catecholamines.[55,65] An important clinical application of boronate affinity chromatography is its use in the analysis and isolation of glycosylated hemoglobin in blood samples from diabetic patients.[66,67]

Many biological molecules occur as specific stereoisomers. Examples are amino acids, peptides, and proteins. As a result, it is not unusual for the different chiral forms of a drug to have some variations in their interactions with these biological agents. This, in turn, can lead to differences in the activity and toxicity of these drugs in the body.[68–70] In some cases only a particular stereoisomer of a drug may be active. In the absence of any chiral binding agent, the two mirror-image forms of a drug (or enantiomers) will have identical physical and chemical properties. These forms will not be separated in most types of chromatography, which generally use nonstereoselective (or achiral) stationary phases. However, it may be possible to separate the enantiomers and stereoisomers of a drug or target compound if the stationary phase is also chiral and can interact with these compounds in a stereospecific manner. This type of medium is known as a chiral stationary phase (CSP).[55,68,69]

The use of a CSP can be viewed as a subset of affinity chromatography, in that the resulting separation makes use of a biologically related binding agent or a mimic of such an agent.[55,71–73] For instance, carbohydrates, peptides, and proteins (including some enzymes and serum transport proteins) have all been used as CSPs because they are composed of chiral amino acids and sugars.[55,68] Cyclodextrins, which are cyclic polymers of glucose, are an important set of carbohydrates that have been used for separating many types of chiral compounds in both LC and GC.[68,69] CSPs also can be based on synthetic binding agents or molecularly imprinted polymers.[12,55,68–70] It is further possible in LC to carry out a chiral separation with an achiral column, such as a reversed-phase support, by placing a chiral binding agent such as a cyclodextrin in the mobile phase. In this last case, the separate forms of a chiral drug or compound may have different interactions with this mobile phase additive, which then leads to differences in their observed retention on the column.[68,69]

Hydrophilic Interaction Liquid Chromatography and Mixed-mode Methods

Besides the traditional categories of LC, there are other methods that combine several separation modes. One example is hydrophilic interaction liquid chromatography (HILIC). HILIC is a type of partition chromatography that uses a polar stationary phase and in which chemicals partition between an organic-rich region in the mobile phase and a more polar water-enriched layer that is at or near the surface of a polar support. The surface of the support, which can often undergo hydrogen bonding or dipole-related interactions with the applied solutes, also may have charged groups that can take part in ionic interactions with these compounds while they are in the water-enriched layer.[74–76] These features make HILIC a variation of normal-phase chromatography that is combined with some of the retention characteristics of reversed-phase chromatography and IEC.

Several types of supports can be used in HILIC. The conventional form of HILIC uses a polar but noncharged surface, such as is present on unmodified silica. Other neutral groups that may be present on the supports for HILIC are amide, diol, or cyano groups. One variation of this method is the technique of electrostatic repulsion hydrophilic interaction liquid chromatography (ERLIC, or eHILIC), in which charged groups such as protonated amines or deprotonated carboxylic acids are present on the support and used to repel injected compounds with the same charge. Another form of HILIC is zwitterionic hydrophilic interaction liquid chromatography (ZIC-HILIC), in which zwitterionic groups are present on the support; these groups can interact with analytes that have a positive charge or negative charge or that are also zwitterions.[74–76]

HILIC and related methods have become popular in areas such as proteomics and glycomics. Advantages of these methods include (1) their ability to give better separations for polar compounds than can be obtained by reversed-phase chromatography, (2) the greater ease with which they can be used with aqueous samples and in solubilizing polar compounds compared to normal-phase chromatography, and (3) the ability to couple these methods with mass spectrometry. A possible limitation of HILIC for use in clinical laboratories is that biological fluids are highly polar and include a substantial quantity of salts that also can interact with polar stationary phases. Therefore these specimens may need to be extracted or modified by the addition of a less polar solvent such as acetonitrile to promote compound interactions in HILIC.

Ion-pair chromatography (IPC) is another example of a mixed-mode LC method.[12] This technique combines columns that are used in reversed-phase chromatography with the ability to separate ionic compounds based on their charges, as is done in IEC. This method is carried out by adding an ion-pairing agent to the mobile phase for a reversed-phase column. The ion-pairing agent is usually a surfactant that has a charged group at one end and a nonpolar tail or group at the other end. Examples of ion-pairing agents are sodium dodecyl sulfate and perchlorate, for binding to positively charged ions, and *t*-butyl ammonium, for binding to negatively charged ions.

The purpose of the ion-pairing agent is to combine with ions of the opposite charge in the sample. This may involve the sample ions interacting with the charged end of the ion-pairing agent while the nonpolar tail of the same agent partitions into the nonpolar stationary phase of the reversed-phase column. Alternatively, the sample ion and ion-pairing agent may interact in the mobile phase and form a neutral

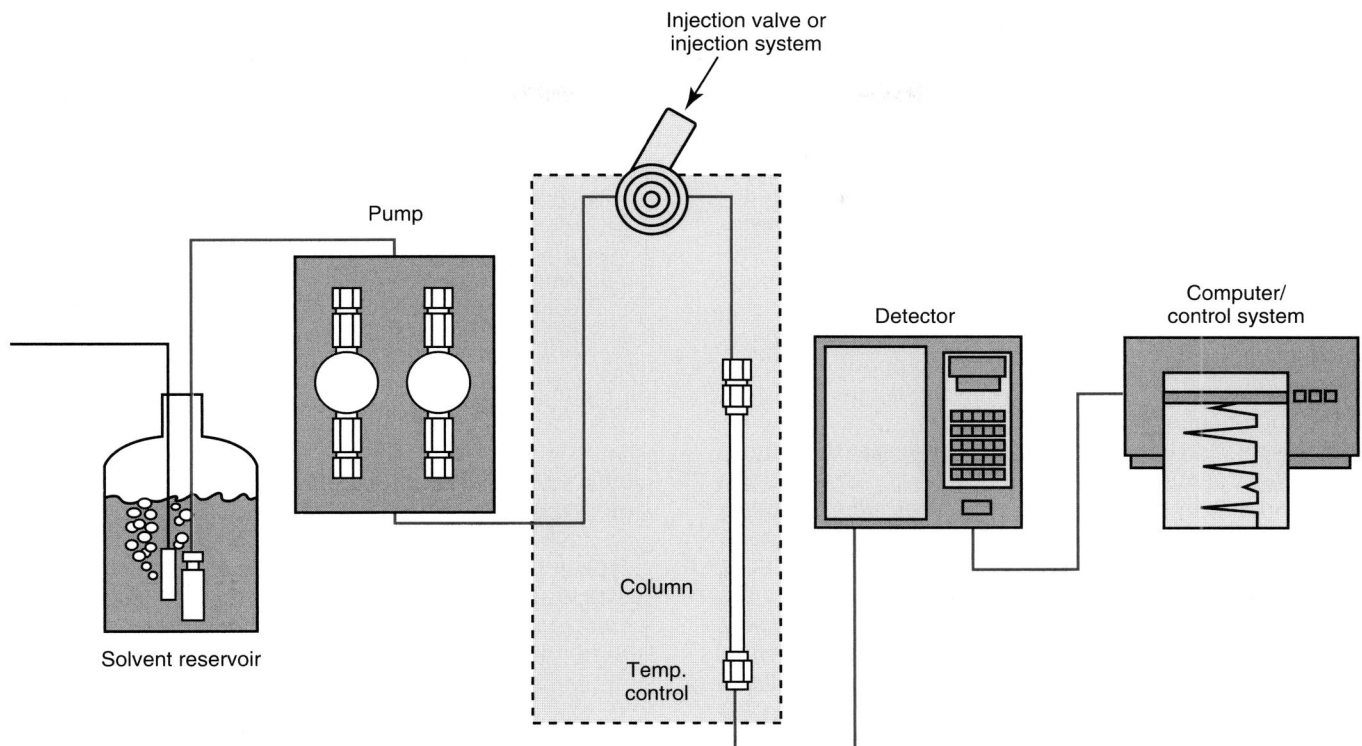

FIGURE 19.14 General design of a liquid chromatograph, as used in high-performance liquid chromatography. (Modified from a figure courtesy Restek Corporation, Bellefonte, PA.)

complex that then interacts with the nonpolar stationary phase. The result in either case is the retention of charged analytes based on their ability to interact with the ion-pairing agent.

IPC is useful in the separation of charged compounds that are poorly resolved by IEC. This method not only combines the better efficiencies that are normally produced by reversed-phase columns, but it also has several parameters that can be varied to control and adjust its separations. These parameters include (1) the strength and type of solvent used in the mobile phase for the reversed-phase column, (2) the concentration and type of ion-pairing agent placed into this mobile phase, and (3) the ion content and pH of the mobile phase. Applications in which IPC has been employed include the separation and analysis of catecholamines, drugs, and nucleic acids.[12]

Restricted access media are a set of supports that combine SEC with another type of LC, which is usually reversed-phase chromatography.[12] This type of material is prepared in a manner so that the exterior of the support is inert or protected by a hydrophilic network with low nonspecific binding for proteins and biological compounds. The interior contains a stationary phase such as a nonpolar bonded phase. If the sizes of the pores or the size-exclusion properties are chosen properly, small solutes such as drugs can pass into the interior and be retained by the stationary phase that is located there. Larger compounds, such as proteins, will not be able to access this inner region and pass nonretained through the column. Columns that contain a restricted access support can be used for the direct injection of biological samples that may contain high concentrations of proteins (i.e., which will elute nonretained) and are being used for measurement of small

analytes. This approach can greatly simplify the process of sample preparation for such analytes.

Liquid Chromatography Instrumentation

The major components of an LC system used in HPLC are shown in Fig. 19.14.[21,77] First, there is a source for the mobile phase, or a solvent reservoir, which supplies a solvent or solution that goes into a pump for delivery to the rest of the LC system. This is followed by an injection valve or injection system, which allows samples to be placed into the mobile phase stream. Next, the mobile phase and sample enter and pass through the column, which contains the support and stationary phase. A control system also may be present to maintain a constant or well-defined temperature within the column. The column is followed by a detector to observe and measure the components of the sample as they exit the system. Modern systems also have a computer or control system to operate the liquid chromatograph and to gather data from the LC detector.

Mobile Phase Reservoirs and Delivery Systems

Solvents and solutions that are used as mobile phases in LC are contained in solvent reservoirs. In their simplest form, these reservoirs are glass bottles or flasks into which feed lines to the pump are inserted. Filters are often placed at the inlets of the feed lines to prevent any particles in the mobile phase from moving on to the rest of the LC system. Most mobile phase reservoirs also have a means of "sparging" the mobile phase by bubbling through a gas such as helium or nitrogen to remove dissolved air or oxygen that may interfere with the response of some detectors. The removal of air and oxygen, or degassing, also can be achieved by applying a vacuum to the reservoir or by placing gas exchange devices or gas filters in the flow path leading from the mobile phase reservoir.[12]

The composition and strength of the mobile phase are factors that can be used to adjust and control a separation in LC. If the same mobile phase is used throughout the separation, this approach is known as isocratic elution.[7,10] If the composition of the mobile phase is varied over time, the method is called solvent programming.[7,12] Solvent programming begins with a weak mobile phase to allow chemicals with weak retention to have their strongest possible interactions with the column. A change is then made over time to a stronger mobile phase to also elute chemicals with moderate or high retention. This change in mobile phase composition can be made in one or more steps and may involve the use of a linear change or a nonlinear change over time.

A variety of techniques have been used to vary the composition of the mobile phase over time.[12,21] For instance, this might be done by using valves that alternate which solvents or solutions are being passed into the LC system at a given time. Solvent gradients may be generated by using the same type of valve linked to two or more solvent reservoirs and that passes these mobile phases into a mixing chamber and onto the inlet of a single pump. This method is known as low-pressure mixing. A second approach, known as high-pressure mixing, uses two or more pumps that are each linked to a different solvent or solution; the flow rates of the mobile phases that are being passed through these pumps are then varied to control the mixing ratio of these solvents or solutions. This combined solution is then passed through a mixing chamber and onto the column. These solvents and solutions can be mixed by using static mixers, which rely on flow-generated turbulence, or dynamic mixers, which use magnetic stirrers. Solvent miscibility and viscosity are two factors to consider when choosing which solvents or solutions are to be used in a solvent program. Both factors can affect the mixing characteristics of the two liquids, where inadequate mixing may result in poor chromatographic performance and inadequate separations.[21]

Several types of pumps have been used in LC.[12,21] Peristaltic and diaphragm-type pumps can be used with columns that can be operated at low pressures, as are encountered in classic and low- to medium-performance LC; however, these pumps are not usually suitable for HPLC. Reciprocating pumps and syringe pumps are instead used to achieve the higher pressures needed to deliver the mobile phase through HPLC columns. Reciprocating pumps are commonly used in HPLC for work at flow rates in the milliliter-per-minute range. In these pumps, a piston moves in and out of the solvent chamber, with check valves being used to keep the flow of the mobile phase moving from the pump inlet to the outlet. The reciprocating action of the piston in this type of pump does generate some pulsation in the pressure and mobile phase flow, which can increase the baseline noise seen with many LC detectors. These pulsations can be minimized by electronic control of the pump and by placing pulse dampers in the flow path. Syringe pumps make use of the continuous application of a syringe to the solvent chamber to deliver the mobile phase to the rest of the system. These pumps can deliver essentially pulse-free flow and can be used at much lower flow rates than reciprocal pumps (e.g., flow rates in the microliter-to-minute range). However, syringe pumps are not as convenient to use as reciprocating pumps

when carrying out solvent programming or during the application of even modest volumes of the mobile phase to a column.[12,21]

Until recently, the upper pressure limit of most HPLC applications has been approximately 6000 psi (41 MPa or 414 bar). In recent years, commercial instrumentation for LC has been developed that can operate up to 15,000 psi (103 MPa or 1034 bar).[33,36,78–80] These higher pressures are needed for work with small-diameter supports, which offer the potential for more efficient separations but also produce higher column back pressures. The use of these smaller support particles and these higher pressures has resulted in a method that is often called ultra-high performance liquid chromatography (UPLC or UHPLC).[33–36] Work at these higher pressures not only requires special pumps that are designed to operate under these conditions, but also requires tubing, connections, and columns that can be used under the same conditions.

Systems for HPLC have pressure sensors to detect any obstruction to flow. These sensors can shut down the entire system once a defined pressure limit has been reached, which is done to prevent damage to the components of the LC system. At very high pressures, some solvents become slightly compressible and a compensation for this solvent compression needs to be made to achieve constant flow rates.[33]

Another extreme condition that may be encountered during the operation of an LC system is when work is to be carried out at quite low flow rates, as might be needed for small-bore microfluidic columns or capillary columns. Work at flow rates below 10 μL/min (1.7×10^{-7} L/s) may require specially designed pumping systems or flow splitting of the output from a standard HPLC pump. The use of low rates in the nanoliter-per-minute range is sometimes called nanoflow chromatography and has been combined with mass spectrometry through the use of nanospray interfaces, which can provide high ionization efficiencies.

Injection Systems and Sample Derivatization

Various approaches can be used to introduce a sample into an LC system.[12,21] The most widely used approach in HPLC is a fixed-loop injector that is switched into or out of the flow path by manual control or through the use of an autoinjector. When this valve is in the inject mode, the sample loop is switched into the flow path and the sample is carried downstream and into the column. The loop continues to be part of this flow path until it is switched back into the load or fill position.

Some important characteristics to consider when selecting an injection system are its (1) reproducibility, (2) the amount of sample carryover from one injection to the next, and (3) the range of volumes that can be injected. Some automated injection systems have the capability of injecting multiple aliquots of the same sample or of mixing a sample and a reagent for derivatization before injection. Some of these systems also are able to control the temperature of the samples before their injection. For instance, the refrigeration of samples before injection may be important during the analysis of specimens or analytes that have limited stability or when large batches of samples are to be analyzed.

Derivatization is sometimes used in LC to improve the response of a given compound or group of compounds to a particular detector (e.g., an absorbance, fluorescence, or electrochemical detector, as will be discussed later). It is also possible to use derivatization in LC to alter the separation of a compound from other chemicals by changing the structure and retention of this compound on the column. The two main ways of carrying out derivatization in LC are (1) precolumn derivatization and (2) postcolumn derivatization. Precolumn derivatization is done before the sample is injected and can be used to alter a compound's retention or to increase its response to a particular type of detector. Postcolumn derivatization is carried out online as compounds elute from a column and is used only to improve the response of one or more of these compounds on the LC detector.[44,81]

Columns and Supports

A wide selection of columns is available for LC. These columns can have various combinations of packing materials and diameters or lengths. Columns for LC, and especially those used in HPLC, often include an inlet filter to remove particulate matter. In the use of LC and HPLC for chemical analysis, a short guard column that contains the same packing material also may be placed before a longer analytical column to protect and extend the usable life of the more expensive analytical column.[12]

The column size in LC will depend on the desired application. For off-line sample pretreatment or the low-performance isolation of compounds, the column size is often determined by the sample capacity that is needed for the separation. Examples of these columns include those used for applications such as desalting, purification of compounds based on IEC, and many types of affinity-based separations for sample pretreatment. Size-exclusion columns, such as small centrifugation columns that are used for desalting, can accommodate specimens with sizes up to about 10% of the column volume. The size of ion-exchange or affinity columns that are used for sample pretreatment and compound isolation will depend on the amount of compound that needs to be separated and the binding capacity of the packing material. This principle also applies to the use of other types of LC for sample pretreatment or compound isolation.

Modern column technology for HPLC has produced columns with various dimensions, with a trend toward smaller internal volumes.[12] These small-volume columns are useful in combining LC with other methods, such as mass spectrometry, to produce hyphenated techniques (see Chapter 20). In the clinical laboratory, most conventional packed HPLC columns consist of tubes that are made of 316 stainless steel; however, polymers that are suitable for work at high liquid pressures also can be employed. These columns have typical internal diameters that range from 4 to 5 mm and lengths ranging from 5 to 30 cm (Table 19.3). Column end fittings, which ideally have a zero dead volume and frits to hold the support particles in the column, are used to connect the column to the injector and to a detector or other postcolumn devices.

In general, better efficiencies and lower detection limits are achieved with HPLC columns that have longer lengths and smaller inner diameters. These smaller inner diameter columns include narrow-bore columns, with approximate inner diameters of 2 to 3 mm, and microbore columns, with approximate inner diameters of 1 to 2 mm. In addition to providing improved efficiencies, these columns with small inner diameters also can require lower flow rates and smaller

TABLE 19.3 Typical Column Sizes Used in Analytical High-Performance Liquid Chromatography

Type of Column	Typical ID and Lengths	Typical Flow Rate Range
Conventional packed column	4–5 mm ID × 5–30 cm	1–3 mL/min (1.7–5.0 × 10⁻⁵ L/s)
Narrow-bore column	2–3 mm ID × 5–15 cm	0.2–0.6 mL/min (0.3–1.0 × 10⁻⁵ L/s)
Microbore column	1–2 mm ID × 10–100 cm	0.05–0.2 mL/min (0.08–0.33 × 10⁻⁵ L/s)
Packed capillary	0.1–0.5 mm ID × 20–200 cm	0.1–20 μL/min (0.17–33 × 10⁻⁸ L/s)
Open tubular column	0.01–0.075 mm ID × 1–100 cm	0.05–2 μL/min (0.083–3.3 × 10⁻⁸ L/s)

ID, Inner diameter.
Portions of the data in this table are based on Poole CF, Poole SK. *Chromatography today.* New York: Elsevier; 1991.

volumes of the mobile phase for their operation than conventional packed columns.

Capillary columns are sometimes used in LC. For instance, packed capillary columns can be used that have inner diameters of 0.1 to 0.5 mm and lengths of 20 to 200 cm. Open tubular capillary columns for LC also can be constructed by placing a thin film or coating of the stationary phase onto the inner wall of a fused silica tube. These open tubular columns have typical inner diameters of 0.01 to 0.075 mm and lengths of 1 to 100 cm. Both types of capillary columns are used with flow rates in the mid-to-low microliter-per-minute range.

Many types of particles and support formats have been developed for LC.[30,82] The most common type of support in LC is a packed bed of small particles.[82] The supports in modern HPLC columns may have particle diameters for porous supports that are in the range of 1.8 to 10 μm, with a typical value of 5 μm. The lower end of this diameter range is representative of the supports that are used in the UPLC.[36] A smaller diameter for these supports provides better efficiency for the chromatographic system, but it also leads to an increase in back pressure across the column. As mentioned previously, the back pressure generated by a packed bed that contains such a support will vary inversely with the square of the particle diameter. Thus a twofold reduction in the particle size will result in approximately a fourfold increase in back pressure. Low-to-medium performance separations, which have much lower operating pressures than HPLC, typically use packing materials such as cross-linked dextran or agarose that have support particles with diameters of 50 to 200 μm.

In the porous support particles that are usually employed in LC, the mobile phase flows around the support but not through the particle. However, this means compounds must travel within the particle by means of diffusion, which is a relatively slow process that can be a major source of band-broadening. The distance that these compounds must diffuse can be reduced by using a nonporous support or a pellicular support, in which the latter has a thin, porous layer or porous shell.[10,30] The use of these supports results in a more efficient separation and less band-broadening because of diffusion-based processes. Another approach for minimizing this band-broadening is to use perfusion particles. This type of support has small pores that contain most of the stationary phase and larger pores that allow the mobile phase to pass both through and around the support particles. The presence of these large flow-through pores decreases the distance compounds must diffuse to reach the stationary phase and helps decrease band-broadening.[10,30]

Another alternative support that can be used to improve efficiency is a monolithic support.[83–85] This type of support consists of a continuous porous bed that is prepared from an inorganic or organic polymer. Monoliths may be made from silica or various polymers. Monolith columns have bimodal pore structures with large pores (approximately a few microns in diameter) that allow the mobile phase to flow through the support and smaller pores (with typical pore sizes of 10 to 20 nm) that provide a large internal surface area to contain the stationary phase. These supports can provide efficient and fast separations, while also providing lower back pressures than particle-based columns at high flow rates. The low back pressure of a monolithic column makes it possible to use this type of column with a flow gradient (e.g., increasing the flow rate at the end of a separation) and allow several such columns to be coupled in series to improve the efficiency and resolution of an LC separation. These columns also can have reasonably high sample capacities. Commercial monolithic rods are encased in inert polytetrafluoroethylene tubing and housed in stainless steel tubes. The inert tubing eliminates voids that may occur at the interface between the stainless steel and the monolith, thus improving the resolution of the column. Capillary monolithic columns also are available. One area of clinical interest in which monolithic columns have been used is in reversed-phase separations of peptides and proteins.[46–48,86]

Temperature Control

The control of column temperature can be an important factor in determining the reproducibility and efficiency of an LC separation.[21] Unlike in GC, in which temperature gradients are often employed, in LC a constant column temperature is usually maintained. Temperature control of an LC column can be achieved by a variety of techniques. These techniques include the use of temperature-controlled (1) column chambers, (2) water jackets, (3) blankets, and (4) heating/cooling blocks. In addition, operation at high flow rates might require a heater/exchanger, which is usually a coil of tubing with good heat exchange properties that is placed before the column inlet.

During the operation of an LC separation, a stable column temperature is required to generate reproducible retention times. In addition, an increase in the column temperature will (1) lower the mobile phase viscosity, (2) increase the rates of mass transfer between mobile phase and stationary phase, and (3) allow the use of higher flow rates, which in turn will lead to a shorter analysis time. The degree to which the temperature can be increased is determined by the boiling point and vapor pressure of the mobile phase, as well as the thermal stability of the analytes in the injected samples. In some instances, the stability of the samples and analytes may require separations to be carried out at reduced temperatures. One common example of this occurs in the use of LC for the isolation and preparation of proteins, which is often performed in cold rooms or in refrigerated cabinets to decrease the rates of protein denaturation and proteolytic degradation. Some systems for temperature control can operate below room temperature through the action of Peltier coolers or other types of refrigeration. Features to consider in selecting a system for temperature control in LC include (1) the usable temperature range of the system, (2) the constancy of the temperatures it can provide, and (3) the number and sizes of columns that the system can accommodate.

Liquid Chromatography Detectors

Many types of detectors can be used in LC (Table 19.4).[12,21] Some common LC detectors are (1) absorbance detectors, (2) fluorescence detectors, (3) electrochemical detectors,

TABLE 19.4   Examples of Detectors Used in Liquid Chromatography

Type of Detector	Principle of Operation	Range of Application	Detection Limit
Absorbance detector	Measures absorbance of light at a given wavelength or set of wavelengths	Compounds with chromophores that can absorb ultraviolet or visible light	10^{-10}–10^{-9} g
Fluorescence detector	Measures ability of chemicals to absorb and reemit light through fluorescence	Compounds with fluorophores	10^{-12}–10^{-9} g
Electrochemical detector	Measures current or charge as a result of chemical oxidation or reduction	Electrochemically active compounds	10^{-11}–10^{-9} g
Conductivity detector	Measures change in conductivity of the mobile phase as ions elute from the column	General for ionic solutes	10^{-9} g
Refractive index detector	Measures change in refractive index of the mobile phase as compounds elute the column	Universal	10^{-7}–10^{-6} g
Mass spectrometry	Production of gas phase ions, followed by separation/analysis of these ions based on their mass-to-charge ratios	Universal: Full-scan mode Selective: Selected ion monitoring mode	10^{-10}–10^{-9} g (full-scan mode) $\leq 10^{-12}$ g (SIM mode)
Evaporative light scattering detector	Light scattering by chemicals after solvent evaporation	Nonvolatile compounds	10^{-9} g
Charged aerosol detector	Measurement of ions produced from chemicals by using a corona discharge	Nonvolatile compounds	$<10^{-9}$ g

Portions of the data in this table are based on Poole CF, Poole SK. *Chromatography today.* New York: Elsevier; 1991.

(4) refractive index detectors, and (5) mass spectrometric detectors. A key component for most of these detectors is the flow cell through which the mobile phase and eluting compounds from the column must pass. As these components travel through the flow cell or into the detector, a signal is generated that can be used to monitor the eluting chemicals and measure the amount of these chemicals that are present. Many LC detectors are nondestructive and can be used individually or linked together in series. In addition, a postcolumn reactor may be present between the column and detector to derivatize some of the eluting compounds and generate products that have a stronger and more specific signal on the detector.

Absorbance detectors. The absorption of UV or visible light is often used to detect compounds as they elute from a liquid chromatographic column.[12,21] Many of the absorbance detectors (also referred to as photometers or spectrophotometers) used in LC can measure the absorption of UV light with wavelengths in the range 190 to 400 nm or of visible light with wavelengths in the range of 400 to 700 nm. Many organic compounds with aromatic groups or double or triple bonds absorb UV light between 250 and 300 nm. Many other organic compounds can absorb in the range of 190 to 220 nm, at which amide bonds, carboxylic acids, and many other groups can have substantial absorption. In addition, some ions, inorganic compounds, and metal complexes can be detected by their absorption of light in the UV or visible range.

There are several types of absorbance detectors that can be used in LC.[2,12,21] Fixed-wavelength absorbance detectors have the simplest design and are used to monitor absorbance at a particular wavelength or wavelength band. For instance, detection is often done with a UV absorbance detector at 254 nm, a wavelength absorbed by many unsaturated organic compounds. This wavelength corresponds to an intense emission line that is produced by a mercury arc lamp. A fixed-wavelength absorbance detector can be extremely sensitive and can operate with detection at 0.005 absorbance units full scale. Fixed-wavelength absorbance detectors that have greater flexibility in their design can be obtained by using other, less intense emission lines of a mercury arc lamp. In addition, a phosphor can be placed between the light source and the flow cell, with the light that is emitted by this agent then passing through the flow cell. This approach is used in dual-wavelength detectors that operate at two fixed wavelengths (e.g., 254 and 280 nm). The intense emission lines at 214 or 229 nm that are produced by a zinc or cadmium arc lamp, respectively, may be used for detection at lower wavelengths, where many organic compounds have strong absorption.

A second type of detector in this category is a variable-wavelength absorbance detector.[2,12,21] This detector operates at a wavelength that is selected from a given wavelength range. The use of a detector that operates at the absorption maximum for a given chemical or set of chemicals can greatly enhance the applicability and selectivity of such a device. Another advantage of this detector is its ability to operate at low-UV wavelengths (e.g., 190 nm), at which a number of clinically important compounds absorb light (e.g., cholesterol). However, at these lower wavelengths many solvents and mobile phases also absorb light. Important exceptions are water, acetonitrile, and methanol, which are frequently used in reversed-phase chromatography.

A photodiode array detector also can be used in LC.[2,12,21] This is an absorbance detector that uses an array of small detector cells to measure the change in absorbance at many wavelengths simultaneously. This array makes it possible to record an entire spectrum for a compound as this chemical elutes from a column, which can be valuable in identifying overlapping peaks.[12,32,44] This type of detector can yield spectral data over a wide wavelength range (e.g., 190 to 600 nm) in approximately 10 ms. During operation, the photodiode array detector passes polychromatic light through the flow cell. The transmitted light is then dispersed by a diffraction grating and directed to a photodiode array, at which the intensity of transmitted light is measured at multiple wavelengths across the spectrum. Such detectors have been helpful in the identification of drugs in samples such as urine and serum.[87]

During the use of an absorbance detector, it is necessary to use solvents, ion-pairing agents, and buffers that have little or no absorption of light at the wavelengths of interest; this is needed to maintain a low background signal. Water, acetonitrile, methanol, isopropanol, and hexane are solvents that allow UV detection down to wavelengths of 200 nm. Phosphate buffers also can be used under these detection conditions. Many other solvents and buffers have substantial UV absorbance, which may limit their use over this wavelength range.

There are several other factors to consider in the use of absorbance detectors. For instance, flow cells with small volumes should be used in absorbance detectors for HPLC to avoid the introduction of significant extracolumn band-broadening. Another issue with the operation of these detectors is the outgassing and bubble formation that can occur as the mobile phase exits the high-pressure region within the column and enters the lower-pressure region in the flow cell. Because these detectors can be quite sensitive, these bubbles can lead to noise in the response and degrade the signal-to-noise ratio. Effective degassing of the mobile phase and the use of some back pressure across the detector can help minimize this bubble formation. However, care must also be taken in this last approach to avoid exceeding the usable pressure range of the detector.

Fluorescence detectors. As discussed in Chapter 16, fluorescence occurs when a chemical absorbs light at one wavelength and reemits light at a different, longer wavelength.[12,21] Fluorescence detectors with flow cells are used in LC to detect fluorescent compounds as they elute from the column. These detectors are generally much more selective and have better limits of detection than absorbance detectors for chemicals that are naturally fluorescent or can be converted into a fluorescent derivative. Both precolumn and postcolumn derivatization have been used to modify chemicals for use with this type of detector.[81] For example, amino acids and other primary amines are often labeled with a dansyl or fluorescamine tag, followed by their HPLC separation and detection through fluorescence. Some fluorescence detectors for LC use fixed wavelengths for both the excitation and emission wavelengths that are employed for monitoring compounds. However, variable-wavelength fluorescence detectors are also available. Deuterium lamps, xenon arc lamps, and lasers have all been used as light sources in such detectors.

Electrochemical and conductivity detectors. Various types of electrochemical detectors can be used in LC. This combination is sometimes known as liquid chromatography/electrochemical detection (LC-EC).[2,12] In an amperometric electrochemical detector (see Chapter 17), an electroactive chemical enters the flow cell, where it may be oxidized or reduced at an electrode that is held at a constant potential; the current needed for or generated by this process is then detected.[2,12,88] The use of multiple electrodes and cyclic changes in the applied voltage can allow the detection of multiple components at different potentials and provides for regular cleaning of the electrode. Electroactive compounds that are of clinical interest and that can be readily examined by HPLC with electrochemical detection include urinary catecholamines (see Chapter 53), ascorbic acid (see Chapter 39), and thiol-containing compounds such as homocysteine (see Chapter 31). In addition, electrochemically active tags (e.g., bromine) can be added to compounds such as unsaturated fatty acids or prostaglandins for use with this type of detector.

Coulometric detectors are also used in LC. This type of detector measures the amount of charge that is required for a given electrochemical reaction. When placed in series, such detectors can be used to detect and measure coeluting compounds that differ in their half-wave potentials (i.e., the potential at half of the maximum signal) by 60 mV or more. These detectors are selective, sensitive, and have reasonably wide linear ranges. Coulometric detectors are used in clinical laboratories during the analysis of metanephrines, vanillylmandelic acid, homovanillic acid, and 5-hydroxyindole acetic acid in human urine (see Chapter 53).

A conductivity detector in LC measures the ability of the mobile phase and its contents to conduct a current when they are placed in an electrical field.[2,12] This type of detector is often used in combination with IEC. For instance, conductivity detectors with relatively low sensitivities have been used to monitor salt gradients during IEC. Conductivity detectors are also used to monitor the elution of charged analytes in ion chromatography.[2,89] The signal resulting from the conductivity of a specific ion will be related to its concentration, charge, and mobility. This means such a detector is best suited for work with small inorganic and organic ions, which have high mobilities. Conductivity detectors have been used to measure compounds such as sulfate in biological fluids.

Refractive index detectors. A refractive index detector in LC measures the change in the refraction of light as chemicals pass with the mobile phase through a flow cell.[12,21] An important advantage for this type of detector is that it can monitor substances such as alcohols, polyethylene glycol, salts, and sugars that do not give a usable response on absorbance or fluorescence detectors.[21,90] An RI detector also can be valuable when the nature or spectroscopic properties of an analyte have not yet been determined. One disadvantage of this type of detector is it does not have limits of detection as low as absorbance or fluorescence detectors, and it has a response that can be sensitive to changes in the mobile phase composition and temperature.

Mass spectrometry. LC can be combined with mass spectrometry, giving a combined technique known as LC-MS.[91–94] This is a sensitive and specific technique that has seen increasing applications in clinical and research laboratories and in fields such as proteomics, metabolomics, and small molecule analysis (see Chapters 20, 23, and 24).[95–99] This method is similar to GC-MS in that the combined use of LC with mass spectrometry makes it possible to both measure chemicals and identify them based on the masses of their molecular

ions or fragment ions. When used in the full-scan mode to look at all or most ions, the mass spectrometer in LC-MS acts as a general detector. If the mass spectrometer is instead used for looking at particular ions, this device then acts as a selective detector.

Several types of ionization methods and mass analyzers can be employed in LC-MS (see Chapter 20). A common combination is the use of electrospray ionization with a quadrupole mass analyzer.[2] Other possible ionization methods that can be used in LC-MS are chemical ionization or photoionization (see Chapter 20). For many applications, the specificity of tandem mass spectrometers allows short HPLC separations to be used because most compounds do not need to be completely separated for them to be detected by the mass spectrometer.

A critical element in linking HPLC to a mass spectrometer is the interface. For example, the interface between a LC and a mass spectrometer has the challenging task of removing solvent from the mobile phase and placing the remaining sample components in a charged form and in the gas phase that can be analyzed by the mass spectrometer. This process requires that the buffers used in LC-MS be sufficiently volatile to avoid overloading and contaminating the interface. For the same reason, a switching valve is often used to divert salts and other nonretained components that elute early in the LC separation to a waste container. The same switching valve can then direct later eluting components to the mass spectrometer for analysis (see Chapter 20 for an extensive discussion of mass spectrometry).

Other liquid chromatography detectors. Several detectors have been developed for LC to detect nonvolatile compounds.[21,90,100] An example is an evaporative light-scattering detector (ELSD).[21] In an ELSD, the solvent is evaporated by nebulizing it with a stream of gas as the mobile phase and its contents exit the column. Nonvolatile chemicals that were present in the mobile phase will remain as particles in the gas phase, and these particles can be detected by measuring their ability to scatter light. The degree of this light scattering will be proportional to the mass of the nonvolatile substances. Potential applications for an ELSD include its use in the analysis of lipids, sugars, and other compounds that are difficult to monitor by absorbance or fluorescence detectors.[21]

Another type of evaporative detector is a charged aerosol detector.[100] This detector ionizes chemicals by using a corona discharge and measures the ion current that is produced. This type of detector has a good response for many compounds. A disadvantage of both the ELSD and the charged aerosol detector is that they are destructive. This means sample components cannot be collected for further analysis after passing through these detectors. Additionally, these detectors cannot be followed directly online by another detector.

A number of other detectors have been used in LC, although many of these have been used primarily for research applications. Dynamic light-scattering detectors measure the scattering of light by chemicals that are eluting from a column, which provides a signal that is related to the size of these chemicals. This type of detector has been useful in characterizing the size of large molecules and complexes.[101] Nuclear magnetic resonance (NMR) spectroscopy has been combined with LC[12] for applications such as lipoprotein analysis (see Chapter 36), metabolomics, and the characterization of drug metabolites.

Data Acquisition and System Control

When using a simple LC system it is possible to perform injections and make pump adjustments manually, with the results being recorded by a computer or comparable data acquisition device. For automated or high-volume applications, there usually is a need to automate both the injection of samples and the chromatographic system. The system controller for an HPLC will often manage (1) sample injections, (2) solvent delivery, (3) system flow rate and temperature, (4) detector operations, and (5) acquisition of data from these detectors. Modern control systems also usually provide an auditable record of the analyst, LC method, calibration conditions, control samples, and specimens that were analyzed.

Data acquisition systems can collect thousands of data points from an individual run. These data can then be used to identify and characterize a set of peaks based on parameters such as the retention times, areas, heights, and widths of these peaks. Comparison of these parameters with those that have been generated by reference materials and standards makes it possible to identify and measure the compounds in these peaks. The hardware and software that are used for data analysis in LC become more critical as the amount of collected data becomes large, as can often occur during the use of photodiode array detectors or LC-MS. Libraries of spectra or other databases can be searched as part of this process to aid in the identification of chemicals (e.g., peptides and nucleic acid sequences) based on the chromatograms and signals that are generated during the separation.

Laboratory Safety in Liquid Chromatography

Standard laboratory procedures for the storage, handling, and disposal of chemicals and solvents should be followed when using LC and HPLC. For instance, many of the organic solvents that are used as mobile phases or solvents in LC are flammable and should be treated with appropriate precautions for such chemicals (see Chapter 15). The waste solvents, samples, and column effluent should be collected in a suitable container and stored appropriately before disposal. The release of pressure in a traditional LC system or HPLC system is not usually a major hazard, because liquids compress only slightly and therefore accumulate little energy; however, work at the higher pressures of UPLC may require some additional precautions.

OTHER CHROMATOGRAPHIC METHODS

In addition to LC and GC, and the use of columns or open tubular supports, there are a variety of other chromatographic methods that can be used for chemical separation and analysis. Some important examples are supercritical fluid chromatography (SFC) and planar chromatography. The use of multidimensional separations based on chromatography is another area of continued interest.

Supercritical Fluid Chromatography

SFC is a type of chromatography in which the mobile phase is a supercritical fluid.[12,102,103] A supercritical fluid is a state of matter that has properties between those of a gas and a liquid and that is formed when the temperature and pressure exceed a particular critical point in a chemical's phase diagram. Carbon dioxide is one chemical that can be easily converted into a supercritical fluid for use in SFC. The formation of supercritical fluid carbon dioxide occurs at or above a temperature of 31.1 °C and at or above a pressure of 73.9 bar (72.9 atm or 7.4 MPa). Under these conditions, carbon dioxide has a density that approaches that of a liquid, so it can interact with and solvate chemicals; this feature allows supercritical fluid carbon dioxide to be used in dissolving many hydrophobic compounds.[104,105] However, a supercritical fluid also has a lower viscosity and a higher diffusion coefficient than a liquid, which allows it to provide efficiencies that are closer to those seen when using a gas as the mobile phase. As a result, SFC has performance characteristics that are between those of LC and GC.[102,103]

SFC can be used with many columns that are available for either LC or GC and can be carried out on systems that are modified versions of LC or GC instruments. It is necessary for these systems to have both pressure and temperature control to keep the mobile phase in the state of a supercritical fluid as it passes through the column. A variety of organic modifiers have been mixed with carbon dioxide to serve as the mobile phase, and solvent programming or temperature programming can be used for elution in this method. It is also common for pressure programming (or density programming) to be used in SFC, as the mobile phase strength of a supercritical fluid will change with its density.[21,102] This technique has been used for the analysis of lipids and other hydrophobic compounds. In addition, SFC has been applied to pharmaceutical research and to the analysis of natural products. However, because of its need for specialized equipment, SFC has found limited use in clinical laboratories.

Planar Chromatography

Another alternative type of chromatographic method is planar chromatography. In planar chromatography, the stationary phase is coated or placed onto a flat surface, or plane.[12] The sample is added as a small spot or band on this surface. This support is then placed into an enclosed container with the bottom edge in contact with the mobile phase and the sample band located above this point of contact (Fig. 19.15). The mobile phase is usually allowed to travel across the plane by means of capillary action. After this movement has occurred for a given period, the support is removed from the mobile phase and dried before the analysis or measurement of the separated sample components.

The planar surface that is used in this method may be a sheet of paper, giving a method known as paper chromatography, or some other type of surface, resulting in a method known as thin-layer chromatography (TLC).[12,106] In paper chromatography, the stationary phase is a layer of water or a polar solvent that is coated onto paper. In TLC, a thin layer of particles (made from a material such as silica, microparticulate cellulose, or alumina) is usually spread uniformly on a glass plate, plastic sheet, or aluminum sheet. When this layer of particles is made up of a material with a small diameter (e.g., silica with diameter of around 4.5 μm), the resulting technique is known as high-performance thin-layer chromatography.[12]

In planar chromatography, retention is described as a function of the distance that compounds have traveled in a given amount of time (Fig. 19.16). This differs from column chromatography or open tubular chromatography, in which retention is instead described by using the time or volume of mobile phase that is needed for compounds to travel a given

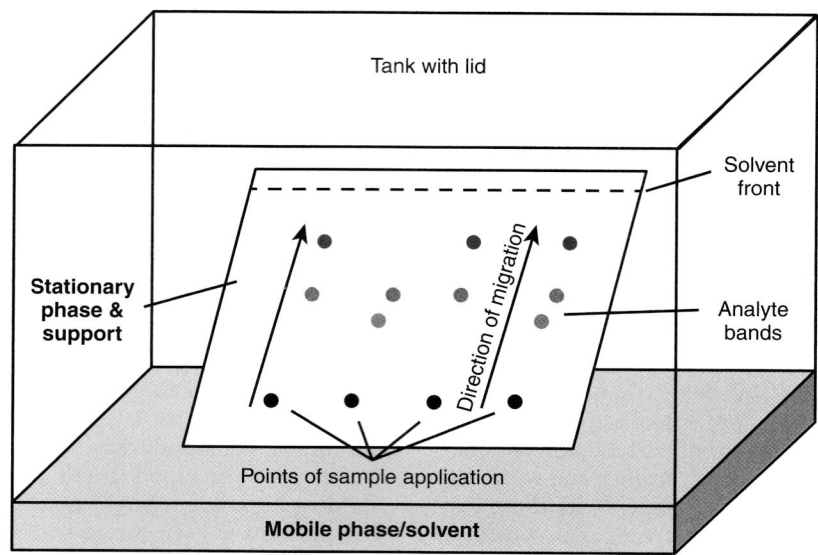

FIGURE 19.15 General operation and system components of thin-layer chromatography. In this example, the mobile phase moves up a glass plate containing a thin layer of adsorbent by means of capillary action.

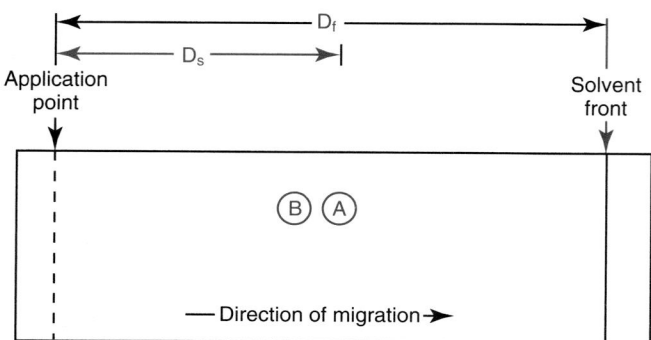

FIGURE 19.16 General example of a separation obtained by planar chromatography. In this example, compound *B* is more strongly retained and migrates a shorter distance than compound *A*. D_f, distance traveled by the mobile phase, or solvent front, from the point of sample application in the same amount of time as allowed for sample migration; D_s, distance traveled by an analyte (*A*, in this example) from the point of sample application.

distance (e.g., the length of the column). The retention of chemicals in methods such as paper chromatography and TLC can be described either in terms of the migration distances that these chemicals have traveled from their point of application in a set amount of time, or by comparing these distances to the distance that has been traveled by the mobile phase in the same amount of time. This second approach can be used to calculate a measure of retention that is known as the retardation factor (R_f), which is defined as follows:

$$R_f = D_s/D_f$$

where D_s is the distance traveled by a chemical from its point of application, and D_f is the distance traveled by the mobile phase, or solvent front, in the same amount of time. The value for R_f will always be between 0 and 1. Chemicals that have high retention with the stationary phase will have low values for R_f, and chemicals that have low retention will have R_f values that approach 1.[7,12]

Chemicals can be identified in planar chromatography based on the position of their bands and by comparing their retention to reference compounds that have been examined on the same plate or surface as the unknown samples. The detection characteristics of the reference compounds also can be compared with the chemicals in the unknown sample. If the R_f value for an unknown substance and the R_f value for a reference compound do not match within the allowed tolerance, the compounds can be said to be different. If the R_f values do match, then confirmation can be made by comparing the detection properties of these compounds (e.g., the color of their bands or their response to a color-forming reagent). Software and databases are also available for compound identification in planar chromatography that allow for searching libraries of both absorption spectra and R_f values. Additional confirmation can be obtained by comparing the unknown compound and the reference compound under a different set of separation conditions.

The separated components in planar chromatography often can be detected by their natural color, by their response to UV light (e.g., through their fluorescence), or through their visualization with chemical reagents that form colored products.[12] In some cases, these chemicals may be allowed to react with labeled antibodies for their detection or they may be detected by using radiolabels and autoradiography. Their bands also may be removed from the planar surface for analysis by a method such as mass spectrometry or NMR spectroscopy.

Paper chromatography and TLC tend to be used primarily for qualitative analysis. In addition, they can be used in multidimensional separations (see next section). Planar chromatography is relatively simple, inexpensive to conduct, and can be used for the simultaneous analysis of multiple samples. However, the application of these methods in clinical laboratories has been decreasing in recent years because of the lack of automation in traditional planar methods and their general lack of ability to perform precise quantitative measurements for chemicals. One application of these techniques in clinical laboratories was the determination of lecithin-to-sphingomyelin ratios in amniotic fluid to evaluate fetal lung maturity. Another application was in the screening of urine for drugs or metabolites such as amino acids that accumulate during hereditary disorders.

Multidimensional Separations

Another topic of growing interest in chromatography is in the area of multidimensional separations. These separations involve the use of two or more separation methods on a sample, in which each of these methods ideally uses a different mechanism for resolving components of the sample. A multidimensional separation can allow a large increase in peak capacity by combining chromatographic methods in which each separation step (or dimension) is performed sequentially.

Multidimensional separations can be carried out in various ways. For instance, this might be done by collecting fractions from one method and then analyzing these fractions by a second method. It is also possible in some cases to couple two chromatographic methods together. This can be done if the second method is faster than the first and if the mobile phase used for elution in the first method is compatible with the conditions needed for sample application in the second method.[14,107]

Planar chromatography is one approach that can be used for two-dimensional separations, but HPLC methods also can be employed. Peak capacities greater than 10,000 have been achieved for two-dimensional HPLC separations; however, this can require prolonged analysis times for the sample and usually means that multiple runs per sample must be conducted in the second dimension.

It is possible to link chromatographic methods with other analytical methods or detectors to create multidimensional methods. One common example is liquid chromatography-tandem mass spectrometry (LC-MS/MS), in which LC is used to separate chemicals based on their interactions with a given mobile phase and stationary phase, while a mass spectrometer is used to separate and analyze the gas phase ions that are generated at any given point in the chromatogram.[91] The addition of another dimension based on mass spectrometry, as occurs in LC-MS/MS to look at fragment ions that are produced from a given parent ion,[92-94,108] can further increase the ability to resolve or detect multiple components without extending the chromatographic component of the analysis time. This combined approach can enable the practical analysis of hundreds or thousands of components in a single specimen, as occurs during the analysis of samples in metabolomics[109] and proteomics.[110]

SELECTED REFERENCES

2. Hage DS, Carr JD. Analytical chemistry and quantitative analysis. New York: Pearson; 2011.
3. Miller JM. Chromatography: concepts and contrasts. 2nd ed. Malden, Mass: Wiley-InterScience; 2009.
8. McNair HM, Miller JM. Basic gas chromatography. 2nd ed. Malden, Mass: Wiley-InterScience; 2009.
9. Snyder LR, Kirkland JJ, Dolan JW. Introduction to modern liquid chromatography. 3rd ed. New York: Wiley; 2009.
21. Ewing GW, editor. Analytical instrumentation handbook. 2nd ed. New York: Marcel Dekker; 1997.
24. Drozd J. Chemical derivatization in gas chromatography. Amsterdam: Elsevier; 1981.
30. Majors RE. A review of HPLC column packing technology. Am Lab 2003;10:46–54.
32. Lough WJ, Wainer IW. High performance liquid chromatography: fundamentals principles and practice. New York: Blackie Academic; 1995.
39. Karger BL, Snyder LR, Horvath C. An introduction to separation science. New York: Wiley; 1973.
44. Ravindranath B. Principles and practice of chromatography. New York: Wiley; 1989.
55. Hage DS, editor. Handbook of affinity chromatography. 2nd ed. Boca Raton: CRC Press; 2005.
64. Janson JC, editor. Protein purification: principles, high resolution methods, and applications. 3rd ed. Hoboken: Wiley; 2011.
68. Allenmark S. Chromatographic enantioseparations: methods and applications. 2nd ed. New York: Ellis Horwood; 1991.
79. Jorgenson JW. Capillary liquid chromatography at ultrahigh pressures. Annu Rev Anal Chem (Palo Alto Calif) 2010;3:129–50.
81. Lunn G, Hellwig GC. Handbook of derivatization reactions for HPLC. New York: Wiley-InterScience; 1998.
85. Svec F, Huber CG. Monolithic materials: promises, challenges, achievements. Anal Chem 2006;78:2100–8.
91. Gross ML, Caprioli RM, Niessen W. The encyclopedia of mass spectrometry, vol. 8. hyphenated methods. Amsterdam: Elsevier; 2006.
92. Shushan B. A review of clinical diagnostic applications of liquid chromatography-tandem mass spectrometry. Mass Spectrom Rev 2010;29:930–44.
103. Taylor LT. Supercritical fluid chromatography. Anal Chem 2008;80:4285–94.
106. Sherma J, Fried B, editors. Planar chromatography. New York: Taylor & Francis; 2003.

20

Mass Spectrometry

Mark M. Kushnir, Alan L. Rockwood, and Nigel J. Clarke[a]

ABSTRACT

Background

Mass spectrometry (MS) is a powerful analytical technique used to identify and quantify analytes using the mass-to-charge ratio *(m/z)* of ions generated from a sample. It is useful for the analysis of a wide range of clinically relevant analytes, including small molecules, proteins, and peptides. When MS is coupled with gas or liquid chromatography (GC or LC), the resultant analyzers have expanded analytical capabilities with widespread clinical applications, including quantitation of analytes in body fluids and tissues. In addition, because of its ability to identify and quantify proteins, MS is widely used in the field of proteomics and emerging health-related "omics" fields, such as metabolomics and lipidomics.

Content

This chapter describes the basic concepts and definitions of MS. Techniques based on MS require an ionization step wherein an ion is produced from neutral atoms or molecules. Electron ionization (EI) and chemical ionization (CI) are often used in GC-MS; in LC-MS, electrospray ionization (ESI) and atmospheric pressure CI are the most commonly used techniques. In microbiology, a desorption/ionization technique termed MALDI (matrix-assisted laser desorption ionization) is used. Once molecules are ionized, resultant ions are analyzed using either beam type analyzers (e.g., quadrupole, or time-of-flight [TOF]) or trapping mass analyzers (e.g., ion trap). Mass analyzers also can be combined to form tandem mass spectrometers, further expanding the capabilities of the technique. Clinical applications of MS are provided to illustrate the role of this technique in the analysis of clinically relevant analytes.

Mass spectrometry (MS) is a powerful qualitative and quantitative analytical technique that is used to identify and quantify a wide range of clinically relevant analytes. When coupled with gas or liquid chromatographs, mass spectrometers allow expansion of analytical capabilities to a variety of clinical applications. In addition, because of its ability to identify and quantify proteins, MS is a key analytical tool in the field of proteomics.

We begin this chapter with a discussion of the basic concepts and definitions of MS, followed by discussions of MS instrumentation and clinical applications, and we end the chapter with a discussion of logistic, operational, and quality issues. In this chapter it is impossible to cover all concepts in a field as vast as MS, even if focus is limited to clinical applications. The Clinical and Laboratory Standards Institute (CLSI) has published recommendations on clinical MS that can serve as a next step to study this topic and a gateway into the extensive literature on this subject.[1,2]

BASIC CONCEPTS AND DEFINITIONS

MS is a branch of analytical chemistry that deals with all aspects of instrumentation and the applications of this technique.[3,4]

Molecular mass (sometimes referred to as *molecular weight*) is measured in *unified atomic mass units* (u), also known as the *dalton* (Da), equal to $\frac{1}{12}$ of the atomic mass of the most abundant isotope of a carbon atom in its lowest energy state.

In MS, the mass-to-charge ratio *(m/z)* is mass of the ion divided by its charge, where *m* is the molecular weight of the ion and *z* is the number of charges present on the molecule. Small molecules (<1000 Da) are typically single charged, and therefore the *m/z* value is the same as the mass of the molecular ion. However, when larger molecules (e.g., proteins, peptides) are ionized, they typically carry multiple charges and therefore the *z* value is an integer greater than 1. In such cases, the *m/z* value will be a fraction of the mass of the ion.

All MS techniques require an initial *ionization* step in which an ion is produced from a neutral atom or molecule. Ions are formed in the ion source of the mass spectrometer. Some ion sources require the targeted analyte to be present in solution in the form of ions, in these cases the ion source function is to transfer the ions from a condensed phase to the gas phase. The development of versatile ionization techniques has allowed MS to become the robust broad-spectrum analytical methodology it is nowadays; this was highlighted in 2002, when John Fenn and Koichi Tanaka shared the Nobel Prize for their development of electrospray[5] and laser desorption[6] ionization techniques, respectively.

[a]The authors gratefully acknowledge the original contributions by Thomas M. Annesley, Nicholas E. Sherman, and Larry D. Bowers on which portions of this chapter are based.

In the most frequently used ion sources of commercially produced MS instruments, ionization in positive ion mode typically results from the addition of one (or more) proton(s) to the basic site(s) on the molecule.[7] This process is referred to as protonation and leads to formation of a positively charged ion. The mass of a single charged protonated ion is greater than the mass of the uncharged neutral molecule by the added mass of one proton, approximately 1 Da. Negatively charged ions (negative ion mode of MS operation) can be generated by the loss of a proton or addition to the molecule of a negatively charged moiety.

Ions may also be produced by removal of one or more electrons from a molecule using EI. Historically, this ionization method was the dominant technique used in MS [most commonly in gas chromatography–mass spectrometry (GC-MS) instruments], and is still used in most of the methods using GC-MS instruments, but other ionization techniques are now more frequently used in clinical MS-based methods.

Ions formed in the ion source are separated according to m/z values in a mass analyzer, and may undergo *fragmentation*, whereby energy is imparted into the ionized analyte, causing internal bonds to break and resulting in the production of multiple fragments of the molecule. Fragmentation may take place within different regions of the mass spectrometer; it may occur due to the deliberate action of the operator, or excessive energy imparted into the parent molecule, as it is being ionized or passes through the vacuum region of the mass analyzer. An unfragmented ion of the intact molecule is referred to as the *molecular ion*, whereas the species that occur on fragmentation of the molecular ion are called the *fragment ions*.

If the ionization of the analyte in the source produces little or no fragmentation, it is referred to as being *soft*, and the most abundant peak in the mass spectrum (the *base* peak) is often the molecular ion. If the ion source produces extensive fragmentation, it is referred to as *hard* ionization, and the base peak in the resulting spectra may be one of the produced fragment ions. By convention, the base peak in a mass spectrum is assigned a relative abundance value of 100%.

Fragment ions that are formed in a dissociation cell (also known as the collision cell) inside a *tandem mass spectrometer* are known as *product ions*, and the technique is called *tandem mass spectrometry (MS/MS)*. Ions that give rise to the product ions are known as *precursor ions*. A tandem mass spectrometer consists of two mass spectrometers operated in sequence (MS/MS in space) or a single mass spectrometer capable of sequential fragmentation and detection of ions within a single region of space but separated by time (MS/MS in time). Most commonly in the MS-based clinical diagnostic methods, precursor ions are dissociated into product ions between the two stages of m/z analysis (MS/MS in space).

A *mass spectrum* is represented by the relative abundance of the detected ions, plotted as a function of m/z (Fig. 20.1). As mentioned earlier, for small molecules, usually the ions are singly charged ($z = 1$); thus the m/z ratio is equal to the mass of the ion, and if ionization occurs by protonation, then the mass of the ion is approximately 1 Da (accurate mass 1.00728 Da) greater than the neutral molecule from which the ion is formed. However, in some cases, the charge may be represented by an integer number greater than 1, in which case the m/z ratio is not equal to the mass of the ion but rather is a fraction of the mass of the ion.

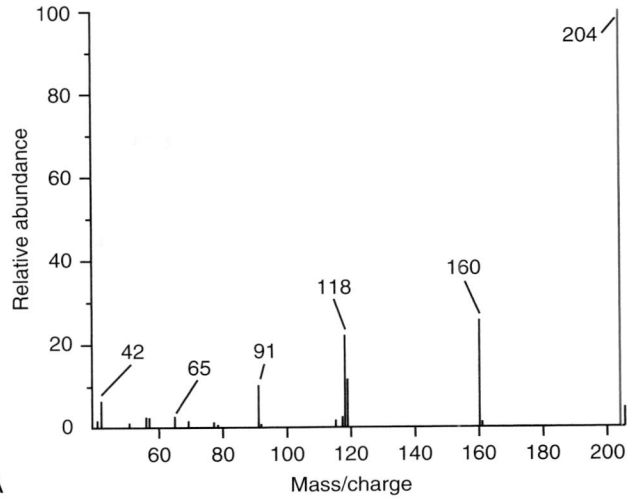

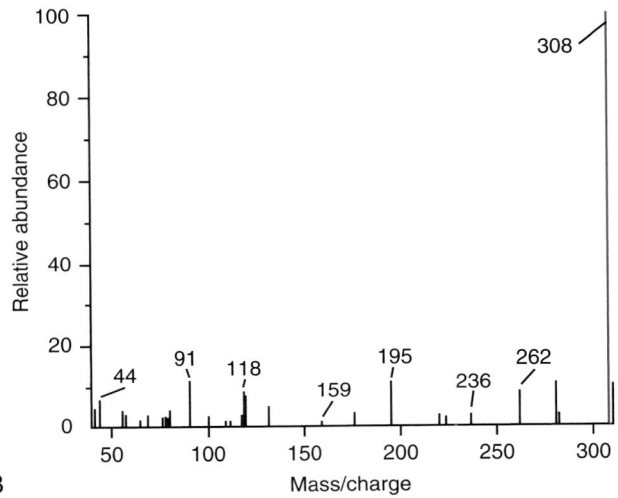

FIGURE 20.1 Mass spectra of pentafluoropropionyl (**A**) and carbethoxyhexafluorobutyryl (**B**), derivatives of D-methamphetamine.

An ion may be positively charged, in which case the number of electrons in the ion is less than the sum of the number of protons in all nuclei of the ion, or negatively charged, in which case the number of electrons is greater than the number of protons. By convention, in MS, z is taken as an absolute value (e.g., $z = 1$ for Na^+ and Cl^-).

Chemical interferences, as well as higher background noise, are more common for analytes with m/z 200 to 500 than for m/z less than 200 and m/z greater than 500. Monitoring ions with higher m/z often results in greater signal-to-noise ratio, because of the lower background noise and lower occurrence of isomers and isobars of the targeted molecules.

A peak in a mass spectrum can be characterized by its *resolution* $[(m/z)/(\Delta m/z)]$, where $\Delta m/z$ is the width of the mass spectral peak. This parameter characterizes the ability of a mass spectrometer to separate nearby masses from each other. Typically, the width of the peak is measured at 50% of the height of the peak and is referred to as the full width at half height (FWHH) or full width half maximum (FWHM) resolution; another frequently encountered definition for resolution is based on the 10% valley ($\Delta m/z$ as the distance

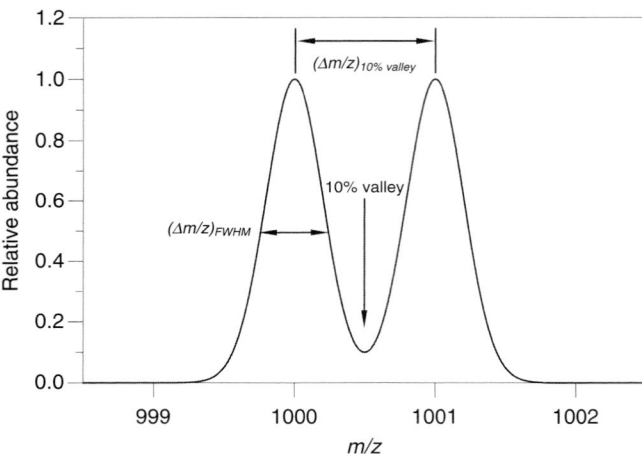

FIGURE 20.2 Parameters used to define resolution in mass spectrometry. *FWHM,* Full width half maximum.

between two peaks of equal intensity with the valley between the peaks of 10% of the peak height) (Fig. 20.2). The 10% valley is a more conservative definition than FWHM because, for a given quoted resolution (e.g., 2000), the peaks are narrower under the 10% valley definition, hence better separated. High resolution is a desirable property in MS because it can help reduce interferences from nearby peaks in the mass spectrum, thereby allowing to achieve a higher specificity.

By setting the relative abundance of the base peak to 100%, relative abundance of the fragment ions can be compared among multiple instruments. Because fragmentation at specific bonds depends on their chemical nature and strength of the bonds, information from the mass spectrum can be used for interpreting molecular structure of the analyte. In some cases, the partial or even complete molecular structure can be deduced (or at least reconciled) with features found in the mass spectrum.

Computer-based libraries of mass spectra are also available to assist with identification of the analyte(s) based on fragmentation pattern. In some applications, the mass spectrum of an analyte may be matched against mass spectra in a database, thereby identifying the analyte by its mass spectral *fingerprint.* In general, an unknown is considered to be identified if the relative abundances of three or four ion fragment ions agree within $\pm20\%$ of those from a reference compound; and the relative abundances of the fragments, monoisotopic and isotopic ions of the molecular ion, are in agreement with the relative abundances of the ions in a reference mass spectrum.

When interfaced to a liquid or gas chromatograph, the mass spectrometer functions as a powerful detector, able to provide structural information on peaks of the analytes. Depending on the operating characteristics of the mass spectrometer and the chromatographic peak width, multiple mass spectral scans can be acquired across the peak. The data also can be displayed as a function of time to yield a *total ion chromatogram (TIC),* where each time point corresponds to the total abundance of all acquired *m/z.*

The mass spectrometer can be considered close to a universal detector, because molecules of many classes (e.g. small molecules, peptides, proteins, lipids) may be ionized and then detected in a mass spectrometer. Furthermore, there are different MS operation modes and different types of fragmentation can be applied to provide different types of data, allowing to obtain complementary information about the measured compound(s). Finally, the instrument data system can analyze and display the collected data in various modes, allowing the operator to selectively process information from the acquired data.

For example, it is possible to display only chromatograms of ions with a preselected *m/z;* the data that come from this preselection is called an *extracted ion* chromatogram (EIC) and is displayed as the intensity of signal on the *y*-axis, plotted against time on the *x*-axis. The height or area of the peaks can be obtained from the data and used for quantitative analysis. Furthermore, the EIC allows selecting data corresponding to the analyte of interest, as identified by its *m/z,* while disregarding data corresponding to the other *m/z* acquired during the analysis. With high-resolution instruments, specificity of analysis can be enhanced by use of narrow *m/z* windows for plotting EIC. Such data processing results in a reduced number of overlapping chromatographic peaks from ions of nearby *m/z* and cleaner baseline, thus improving the quantitative accuracy and the specificity (Fig. 20.3).

Sample preparation is critical for obtaining high-quality MS data, particularly when dealing with highly complex sample matrices, commonly encountered in clinical chemistry. This typically involves one or more of the following steps: (1) protein precipitation followed by centrifugation or filtration, (2) solid-phase extraction, (3) liquid-liquid extraction, (4) affinity enrichment, and (5) *derivatization,* or combination of these techniques (see Chapters 21 and 23).

Derivatization is the process of chemically modifying (addition of a functional group) to the target compound(s), to have more favorable properties for chromatographic separation and/or MS analysis. The goals of derivatization vary, depending on the application, but typically include (1) increased volatility (in the case of GC-MS), (2) greater thermal stability (in the case of GC-MS), (3) modified chromatographic properties (in the case of either GC-MS or LC-MS), (4) greater ionization efficiency (in the case of LC-MS), (5) favorable fragmentation properties (in the case of either GC-MS or LC-MS), or a combination of these.

Analysis by MS can be used to target specific known compounds (*targeted analysis*) or seek to identify one or more unknown compounds in a sample (*screening*). When only one or a few targeted analytes are of interest for quantitative analysis and their mass spectra are known, the mass spectrometer is set to monitor only those ions of interest. This detection technique is known as *selected ion monitoring* (SIM). Because SIM collects data on a limited number of *m/z,* more data points are collected for the selected *m/z,* which results in a greater specificity, improved signal-to-noise ratio for the analyte of interest, and greater sensitivity and enables more accurate quantitation with greater precision. One drawback of SIM is related to specificity of detection. Most biological samples are highly complex, and thus it is not uncommon to have multiple compounds with very close or identical masses to be present in the sample matrix. In those cases, chromatography can aid in separation of these isobars; however, they still can affect a SIM result if a peak of interfering substance is not fully separated from the analyte of interest.

By using a triple-quadrupole mass analyzer, a method known as *selected reaction monitoring* (SRM; or multiple

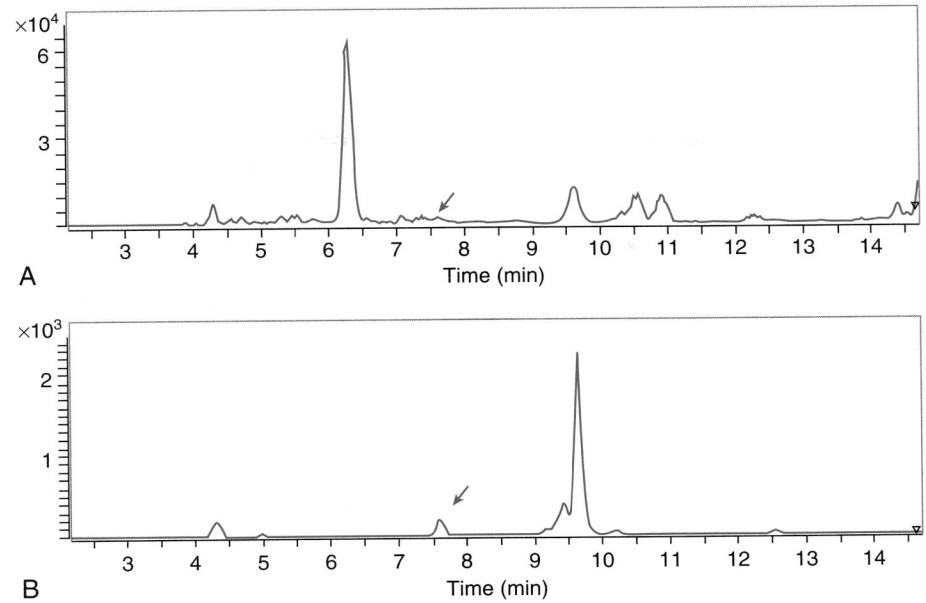

FIGURE 20.3 Extracted ion chromatograms of a peptide (*m/z* 761.3718) using an extraction window of 1 Da (**A**) and 0.0076 Da (**B**). *Arrows* indicate the peak that is completely hidden in the chemical background noise, while resolved from the noise when using a mass extraction window of 0.0076 Da.

reaction monitoring [MRM], if used for the simultaneous detection of number of ions), can be used to help alleviate such potential issues. In a triple-quadrupole mass analyzer, the first quadrupole mass analyzer is set to transmit the *m/z* of the molecular ion, the analyte gets fragmented in the collision cell (the second quadrupole), and the third quadrupole mass analyzer is set to transmit the *m/z* of one or more known fragment ions of the targeted molecule. In this manner, data similar to those gathered by SIM can be acquired but with added specificity from the use of the targeted molecular ion and fragment ions. A more detailed description of MRM mode of data acquisition is given in the section of this chapter describing tandem MS.

Analytical screening methods are used in clinical chemistry laboratories less commonly than the analysis of target compounds. The main task for screening methods is qualitative identification of unknowns in a sample. In most cases, this is performed by matching chromatographic retention time and fragment ion patterns (*m/z* and relative abundance) of either fragment ions generated in the ion source of a single-stage mass spectrometer, or product ions formed in a collision cell in a tandem mass spectrometer.

A chemical element may be composed of a single isotope or multiple isotopes. Isotopes of an element have the same number of protons but different numbers of neutrons. For example, naturally occurring carbon is composed primarily of two isotopes: ^{12}C, whose nuclei contain six protons and six neutrons, and ^{13}C, whose nuclei contain six protons and seven neutrons (abundance of ^{14}C isotope for the purposes of routine MS is negligible, as compared with the other two isotopes). The natural abundance of ^{12}C is approximately 98.9%, and the natural abundance of ^{13}C is approximately 1.1%. Some elements, such as phosphorous and arsenic, have only a single isotope in the naturally occurring state, whereas other elements, such as tin, may have as many as 10 naturally occurring isotopes.

For molecules consisting of multiple atoms, the isotope pattern is a combination of the isotope patterns of the individual atoms.[8,9] As an example, carbon monoxide (CO) has the following combinations of isotopes $^{12}C^{16}O$ (molecular weight 28), $^{13}C^{16}O$ (molecular weight 29), $^{12}C^{17}O$ (molecular weight 29), $^{12}C^{18}O$ (molecular weight 30), and $^{13}C^{18}O$ (molecular weight 31).

Nitrogen (N_2) is isobaric with CO; that is, it has nearly the same mass. However, the accurate masses of the isotope peaks of isobars may differ. For example, the monoisotopic mass of $^{12}C^{16}O^+$ (the isotopic peak composed of the most abundant atomic isotopes) has an accurate mass of 27.9944 Da, whereas N_2^+ has an accurate molecular mass of 28.0056 Da. The accurate mass can be used to infer the chemical formula of a compound or to confirm the identity of a target compound. This technique requires a mass analyzer capable of high mass accuracy (few parts per million), is limited to compounds with molecular weight of a few hundred daltons or less, and is unable to discriminate isomers (compounds that have the same chemical formulas but different molecular structure).

Isotopic information also can be used to infer the chemical formula of an unknown or to confirm chemical identity of a target compound. Using CO^+ and N_2^+ as examples, the monoisotopic and the next two isotopic peaks of CO^+ have a relative abundance of 0.986, 0.011, and 0.002, whereas the monoisotopic and the next two isotopic peaks of N_2^+ have relative abundances of 0.993, 0.007, and 0.000. This technique requires accurate measurement of relative isotopic peak abundances and, if used in conjunction with accurate mass measurements, can be powerful.

A distinct advantage of the mass spectrometer is that it can distinguish between ions of the same chemical formula that have different masses, because of the different isotopic composition. To illustrate with a simple example, $^{12}C^{16}O^+$ has a different mass than $^{12}C^{18}O^+$, and these two forms can be separated and detected in a mass spectrometer. One can take advantage of this fact by using synthetically produced forms of a target analyte. The labeling consists of substitution of one or more monoisotopic atoms with isotopic atoms (e.g., substituting ^{2}H for ^{1}H, ^{13}C for ^{12}C, or ^{15}N for ^{14}N). The stable isotope-labeled analog of the targeted molecule can be chemically synthesized and added to the samples as an internal standard, which behaves nearly identically to the native compounds during sample preparation and chromatographic separation.[1,4] In this respect, ^{13}C or ^{15}N is generally preferred over ^{2}H labeling, because ^{2}H-labeled compounds sometimes exhibit chromatographic shifts compared with unlabeled compounds, whereas ^{13}C- or ^{15}N-labeled compounds generally do not. A quantitative analysis can then be carried out by comparison of the signal from the native compound, relative to the stable isotope labeled version of the compound, added into the samples during the sample preparation.

An internal standard should be selected to have a sufficient number of isotopic atoms so that no naturally occurring isotopes (e.g., ^{2}H or ^{13}C) of the analyte of interest would significantly contribute to the signal of the internal standard.[1] As an example, for the methamphetamine derivatives shown in Fig. 20.4A, an internal standard with at least three ^{2}H or ^{13}C atoms is preferred, because contribution of the natural abundance of these isotopes to the molecular ion [(M + 3)$^+$] would be negligible (<0.1%). The position of the stable isotope atoms within the molecule and the number of isotopic ions within the structure are also important for adequate performance of the methods.[1,10] For example, the m/z 204 ion for methamphetamine represents the aliphatic portion of the molecule (loss of the aromatic ring). If three deuterium atoms were located on the aromatic ring of the pentafluoropropionyl derivative of methamphetamine, the native and the isotope-labeled molecules would both yield the m/z 204 ion. This m/z 204 ion would therefore fail to distinguish the native compound from the isotope-labeled compound and would

therefore not be useful as an internal standard. On the other hand, if ^{2}H labeling were to occur in the aliphatic portion of the molecule, the fragment ion analogous to the m/z 204 would contain three ^{2}H (m/z 207), and the ion could be useful as an internal standard. The same comments apply to the compound illustrated in Fig. 20.4B.

The concepts of internal standard selection are different when applied to tandem MS.[1] For example, it is possible for a native compound and the internal standard to have product ions of the same m/z, because the precursor ion m/z is different for the targeted analyte and the internal standard.

When using deuterium (^{2}H) labeling, the isotopic ions must be located in the positions within the molecule where it will not be exchangeable with hydrogen atoms (in solution or in gas phase). For example, deuterium labeling of an acidic hydrogen position would be useless because the ^{2}H would easily exchange with protons in the matrix, making the original labeling moot. Certain other labeling positions within a molecule, where ^{2}H could exchange with hydrogen (alcohols, amines, amides, and thiols), also must be avoided.

A technique of quantitative analysis of compounds relative to their isotopic analogs added to the samples at known or fixed concentration is called *isotope dilution analysis* or isotope dilution mass spectrometry (IDMS). The IDMS technique is widely used in methods for analysis of clinically relevant biomarkers.

MS is often considered as a highly sensitive technique. *Sensitivity* is a somewhat problematic term because it is used in two different ways. In an official definition it means the slope of a calibration curve (or more generally, a change in signal vs. the change in concentration), but more commonly it is used to signify the ability to detect or quantify an analyte at very low concentration; that is, a more sensitive technique would be able to detect or quantify a lower concentration of the target analyte.

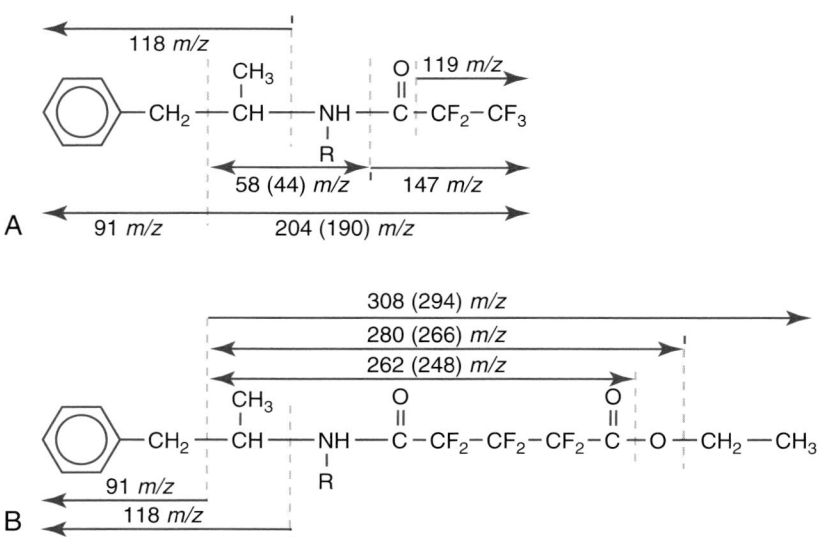

FIGURE 20.4 Fragmentation patterns for pentafluoropropionyl (**A**) and carbethoxyhexafluorobutyryl (**B**), derivatives of methamphetamine (R = CH$_3$) and amphetamine (R = H; *masses in parentheses*). Look at the predicted m/z in the mass spectra shown in Fig. 20.1. Note that for the pentafluoropropionyl derivative, only one ion [204 (190) m/z] is characteristic of the aliphatic portion of the molecule.

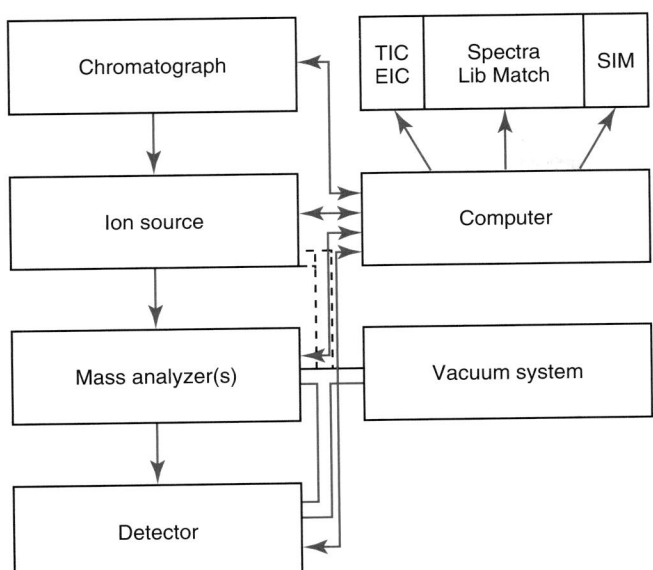

FIGURE 20.5 Block diagram of the components of a chromatograph–mass spectrometer system. The mass analyzer and the detector are always under vacuum. The ion source may be under vacuum or under near-atmospheric pressure conditions, depending on the ionization mode. *EIC*, Extracted ion chromatogram; *SIM*, selected ion monitoring; *TIC*, total ion chromatogram.

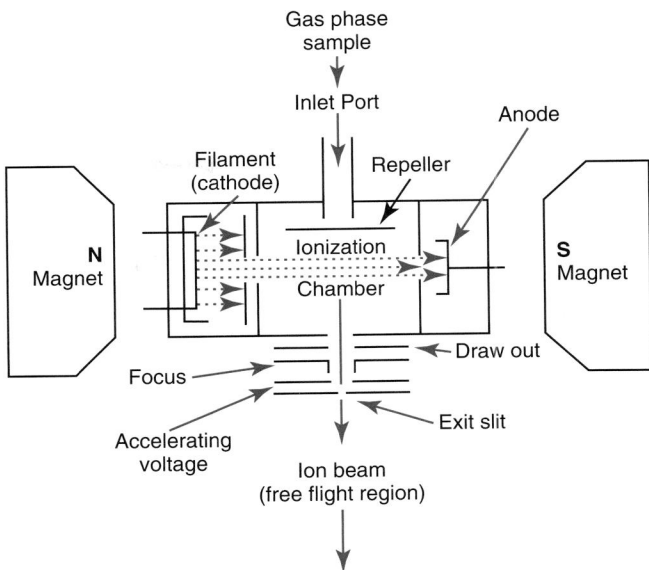

FIGURE 20.6 Electron ionization ion source. The magnets are used to collimate a dense electron beam, which is drawn from a heated filament placed at a negative potential. The electron beam is positioned in front of a repeller, which is at a slightly positive potential (relative to the ion source). The repeller sends positively charged fragment ions toward the opening at the front of the ion source.

INSTRUMENTATION

A mass spectrometer consists of the following components: (1) ion source, (2) vacuum system, (3) mass analyzer, and (4) detector (Fig. 20.5). Most modern mass spectrometers also include a computer for instrument control, data acquisition, and data processing.

Ion Source

Many approaches have been used to form ions in both, high-vacuum and near-atmospheric pressure conditions, but this chapter will limit discussion to ion sources of interest to clinical applications of MS. EI and CI are ionization techniques used when gas-phase molecules are introduced directly into an ion source operated at very low pressure, typically in a gas chromatograph. In high-performance liquid chromatography–mass spectrometry (HPLC-MS), ESI, and *atmospheric pressure chemical ionization* (APCI) ion sources are often used.[11,12] Ionization in these two ion sources takes place at atmospheric pressure. Other commonly used ionization techniques are *inductively coupled plasma* (ICP) and MALDI (see Chapters 22 and 39).[11,13,14] The CLSI documents C50-A and C62-A contain recommendations for matching the capabilities of different types of ion sources to various MS applications.[1,2]

Electron Ionization

In EI, gas-phase molecules are bombarded by electrons emitted from a heated filament, causing extensive fragmentation of the molecules (Fig. 20.6). To make the process robust, prevent filament oxidation, and minimize scattering of the electron beam, the ionization must occur in a vacuum. EI is typically performed using electrons with a kinetic energy of 70 eV; collision of electrons having such energy with most

molecules results in formation of *radical* cations (i.e., a molecular fragment that is both a positively charged ion and a radical).[15] A radical is a molecule or ion containing an unpaired electron. The radical ion then often undergoes intramolecular rearrangement and dissociation to produce a cation and an uncharged radical:

$$AB^{+\bullet} \rightarrow A^+ + B^\bullet$$

Positive ions are drawn out of the ionization chamber by an electrical field and electrostatically focused and introduced into the mass analyzer. EI is primarily used as an ion source in GC-MS. Because the same ion energy (70 eV) is used in all commercial EI-GC-MS instruments and because the fragmentation pattern is only weakly dependent on small deviations from 70 eV, fragmentation patterns observed using an EI source are reproducible and relatively unique for each chemical compound. The fragmentation pattern is therefore often used as a fingerprint to identify compounds by matching mass spectra of unknown compounds to the entries in the mass spectral libraries.[4]

Chemical Ionization

CI is a soft ionization technique in which a proton is transferred (or abstracted from) through a gas phase by reaction with a molecule such as methane, ammonia (NH_3), isobutane, or water vapor. The reagent gas is supplied into a CI ion source at a pressure of approximately 0.1 torr. (*NOTE:* For practical purposes, torr is equivalent to millimeter of mercury and is a unit commonly used in the field of MS). An electron beam produces reactive species through a series of ion-molecule reactions, resulting in formation of reactive intermediates (e.g., methonium [CH_5^+] if methane is the CI reagent gas), leading to ionization of the gas phase molecules,

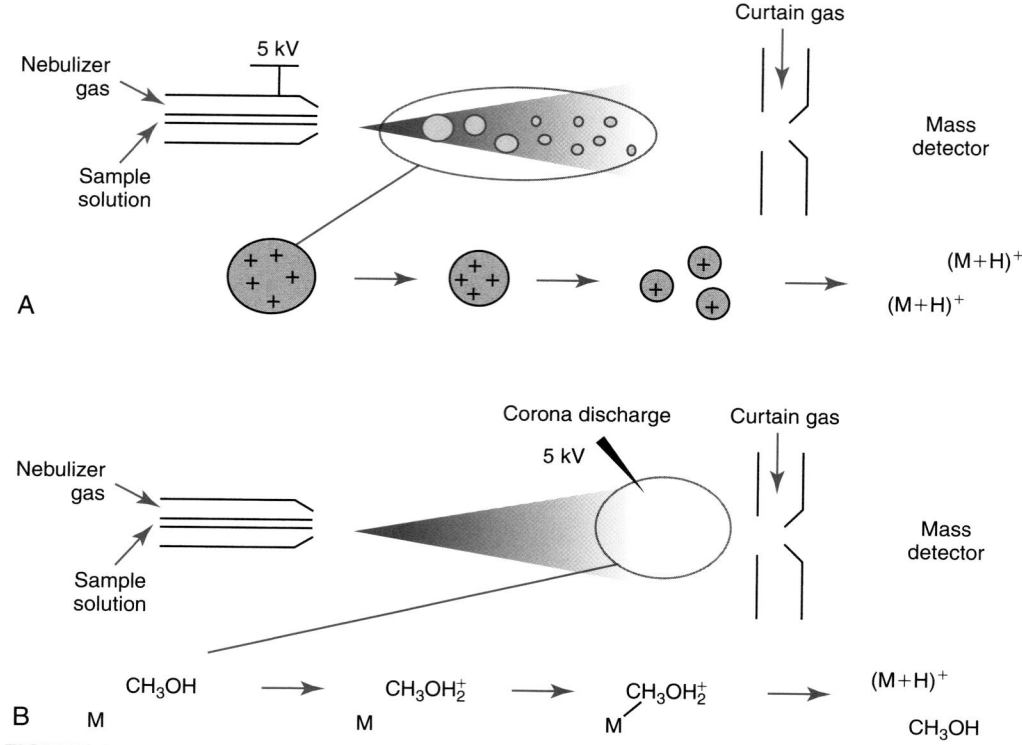

A

B

FIGURE 20.7 Schematics of **(A)** electrospray ionization (ESI) and **(B)** atmospheric pressure chemical ionization (APCI) sources. Note the different points where ionization occurs.

typically via attachment of a proton. In most cases, relatively little fragmentation occurs during this process, and for the majority of the molecules, only molecular ions (in the form of a protonated molecule) are observed in the mass spectra. The lack of fragmentation enhances sensitivity of detection, because the signal is not spread out over a large number of molecular fragments. Although this process enhances sensitivity, it does not allow one to obtain adequate mass spectral information to confirm identity of the analyte.

Negative ion electron capture CI has become popular for quantification of drugs, such as benzodiazepines. Negative ions are formed when thermalized electrons are captured by electronegative functional groups or atoms within the molecule (e.g., chlorine, fluorine). Negative ion CI often enables high sensitivity detection for the molecules, which may efficiently capture an electron.

Electrospray Ionization

ESI, the most frequently used ionization technique in clinical MS, is a soft ionization technique in which a sample is ionized at atmospheric pressure before introduction into the mass analyzer.[12,15] An effluent from a separation device, typically an HPLC, is passed through a narrow metal or fused silica capillary to which a 1- to 5-kV voltage has been applied (Fig. 20.7 *A*). The applied high voltage causes mechanical instability in the liquid, leads to formation of an electrospray cone (also known as Taylor cone), creates aerosol and causes expulsion of charged droplets (Fig. 20.8). In some variations of commercial ESI sources, a nebulizing gas aids in spray formation, and directs and speeds up the evaporative process. As droplets evaporate, while migrating through the atmospheric pressure region, they expel smaller droplets as the

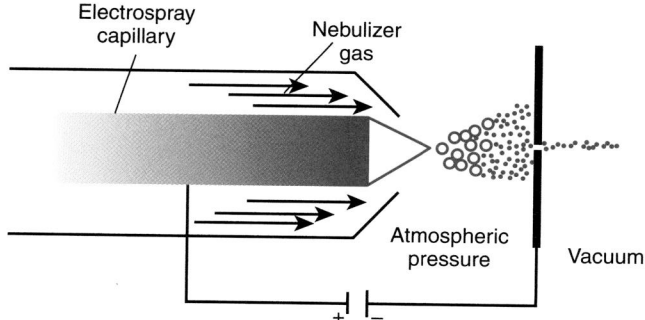

FIGURE 20.8 Simplified conceptual schematic of electrospray ion source showing Taylor cone.

charge-to-volume ratio of the droplets exceeds the Raleigh instability limit, leading to expulsions of ions from the droplets. In most cases, the ionization process produces protonated species as the result of in-solution acid/base chemistry. However, other ionization products are sometimes observed, such as metal ion (Na^+ or K^+) or NH_4^+ adducts, or ions formed by redox processes. Ions then pass through an orifice, sampling cone and one or more extraction cones (skimmers) before entering the high-vacuum region of the mass analyzer.

One feature of ESI is the production of multiple charged ions, particularly from peptides and proteins. It is common to observe approximately one charge for every 10 to 15 amino acid residues in a protein. For example, for a molecule of mass 20,000, 20 charges supplied by the addition of 20 protons, resulting in an ion with m/z of approximately 1000 [or more correctly, m/z 1001 = (20,000 + 20)/20]. The phenomenon of multiple charging results in the formation of a series of peaks in the mass spectrum, with each peak corresponding to a different number of added protons and as a result, extends the accessible mass range of instruments. In addition to proteins and peptides, multiply charged ions are also observed for oligonucleotides in negative ion mode.

It should be noted that Figs. 20.7 and 20.8 represent a simplified illustration of the probe being directed toward the sampling cone of the mass detector. To enhance performance and minimize contamination of the mass analyzer, many modern hardware configurations offset the probe relative to the orifice of the sampling cone; in most of the commercial instruments, the spray is orthogonal to the sampling cone.

ESI tends to be an efficient ion source for polar compounds or for molecules that are present as ions in solution, which includes a majority of biomolecules. ESI and APCI are the most commonly used ion sources in clinical applications of MS.

As already mentioned, ESI is considered a soft ionization source[7]; however, it is possible to generate fragment ions before mass analysis, by applying a higher than typical voltage gradient in the low-pressure region of the electrospray interface, causing collisional heating and fragmentation of the ions.

Atmospheric Pressure Chemical Ionization

In APCI ion sources, as in ESI, the ionization takes place at atmospheric pressure, involves nebulization and desolvation, and uses the same design of the ion extraction cone as ESI. However, in APCI, no high voltage is applied to the inlet capillary. Instead, the mobile phase from the separation device gets evaporated and the vapor passes by a corona discharge needle.[7,12] Somewhat analogously to the processes occurring in a CI source, ions generated by the corona discharge undergo variety of ion-molecule reactions such as the following:

$$CH_3OH + H^+ \rightarrow CH_3OH_2^+$$

$$A(analyte) + CH_3OH_2^+ \rightarrow AH^+ + CH_3OH$$

$$H_2O + H^+ \rightarrow H_3O^+$$

$$A(analyte) + H_3O^+ \rightarrow AH^+ + H_2O$$

Because solvent molecules from the evaporated mobile phase (e.g., water, methanol, acetonitrile) are present in the vapor in excess, relative to the sample constituents, they are predominantly ionized early in the ion molecule cascade of reactions and then act as a reagent gas that reacts secondarily to ionize analyte molecules (see Fig. 20.7B). The products of these secondary reactions may contain clusters of solvent and analyte molecules. A countercurrent flow of heated inert gas, such as nitrogen, is applied in the direction opposite to the direction of the ions entering vacuum region of the mass analyzer, to assist with evaporation of solvent from the sprayed droplets and to minimize number of noncharged molecules entering the vacuum region of the mass analyzer. A decluttering potential is applied at the region where the pressure transitions from atmospheric to the vacuum. This potential causes acceleration of ions entering the vacuum region of the mass analyzer; when the ions acquire enough energy, the adducts break away from the ion, leaving a bare analyte ions.

As with ESI, APCI is a soft ionization technique, resulting in relatively little fragmentation; however, unlike ESI, APCI

typically requires use of higher temperature, which may cause pyrolysis of the thermally labile compounds and may cause issues with quantitative performance of the assays (e.g., deuterium/ hydrogen exchange in deuterium labeled internal standard molecules).

When compared with EI, the mass spectra produced by APCI, ESI, and other soft ionization techniques typically have fewer fragments and are less useful for analyte identification. However, because of the little fragmentation, APCI and other soft ionization sources are well matched to the requirements of tandem MS (discussed later) and are well suited for quantitative analysis. APCI and ESI are the most commonly used ion sources for quantitative analysis in clinical MS. In the case of nonpolar compounds, such as many steroids and some drug molecules, APCI could provide a higher ionization efficiency than ESI.

Inductively Coupled Plasma

ICP, similarly to ESI and APCI, is an atmospheric pressure ionization method.[16] However, unlike most atmospheric pressure ionization methods, which are soft (i.e., produce little fragmentation), ICP is the ultimate in hard ionization, typically leading to complete atomization of the molecules present in a sample during ionization. Consequently, its primary use is for elemental analysis. In the clinical laboratory, ICP-MS is particularly useful for trace element analysis in biological samples. ICP-MS is extremely sensitive (parts per trillion limits of detection) and is capable of a wide dynamic range of measurements.

After sample preparation, which typically includes the addition of an internal standard and in some cases an acid digestion step, the sample is introduced into the ion source, usually via a nebulizer fed by a peristaltic pump. The nebulized sample is transmitted into argon plasma, generated by inductively coupling power into the plasma using a high-powered, radiofrequency (RF) generator (Fig. 20.9). The temperature of the plasma is typically 6000 to 10,000 K (comparable with the temperature on the surface of the Sun). The sample is introduced into the plasma, and the generated ions are transmitted into the mass analyzer. The atmospheric sampling apparatus is conceptually similar to that of other atmospheric pressure ion sources, such as electrospray, except that the device must withstand the extremely high temperatures generated by the plasma.

Compared with MS equipped with other atmospheric pressure ionization sources, ICP-MS is subject to less frequent occurrence of interference. Most interfering species in ICP-MS methods are polyatomic ions formed in the torch via ion-molecule reactions. For example, argon oxide (ArO^+) interferes with iron at m/z 56. One solution to this problem is to use a reaction cell, which consists of a moderate-pressure gas region in front of the mass analyzer, with a reactant gas, such as NH_3, supplied into the reaction cell.[18] The reactant gas reacts with polyatomic interferences and fragments them before introduction into the mass analyzer. A related technique uses a nonreactive collision gas, which removes interferences using collisions, relying on differences in collision cross-sections between polyatomic ions and monoatomic ions. Another approach to removing interferences of the same nominal mass is to use a high-resolution mass spectrometer, which is capable of resolving species with similar nominal

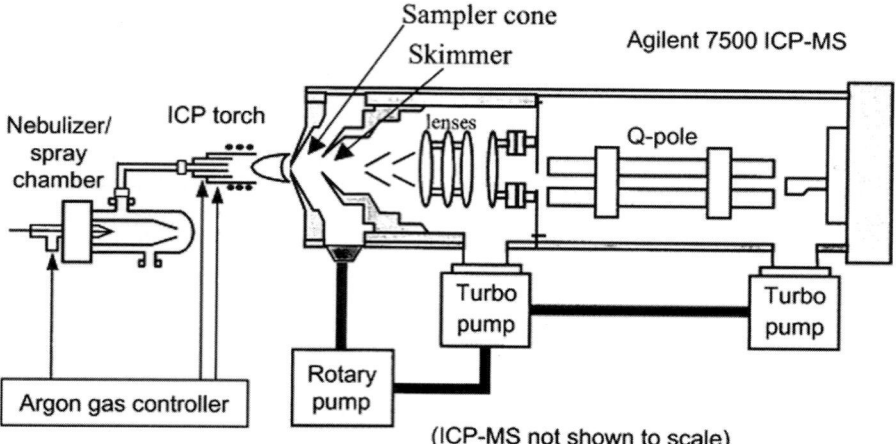

FIGURE 20.9 Simplified conceptual schematic of inductively coupled plasma–mass spectrometer *(ICP-MS). Q-pole,* Quadrupole. (Reprinted with permission from Kannamkumarath SS, Wrobel K, Wrobel K, B'Hymer C, Caruso JA. Capillary electrophoresis-inductively coupled plasma-mass spectrometry: an attractive complementary technique for elemental speciation analysis. *J Chromatogr A* 2002;975[2]:245–66.)

mass.[18] For example, the masses of ArO^+ and $^{56}Fe^+$ differ by 0.022 Da—a difference that may be resolved using a high-resolution mass spectrometer.

Matrix-assisted Laser Desorption Ionization

MALDI is another type of soft ionization technique in which ions are produced through energy transfer from a pulsed laser beam to the sample.[19] Samples for MALDI ionization are prepared as dry spots, consisting of the sample mixed with a matrix (small molecular weight ultraviolet [UV]-absorbing compound), applied on a target and dried. A pulsed laser irradiates the dried spots, triggering ablation and desorption of the sample and matrix material; ions produced in the process are accelerated and enter into the mass analyzer (Fig. 20.10). In other applications, a layer of the solid matrix is deposited on the target and allowed to crystalize, and then the sample is applied on top of the matrix. Application of the liquid sample causes partial solubilization of the matrix followed by recrystallization. With this approach, the sample is maintained in the outer layer of the matrix, in some cases allowing enhancement of the sensitivity and reduction of the background noise.

AMBIENT IONIZATION

Ambient ionization (AI) is a type of ionization in which ions are formed directly from a sample, without, or after minimal sample preparation.[20] Desorption electrospray ionization (DESI) was the first described AI technique. DESI uses an electrospray source to generate charged droplets directed to the tested sample; these charged droplets cause formation of secondary ions, which are introduced into a mass spectrometer. Since the time this technique was introduced, more than 50 other AI-MS approaches have been described. In the described AI methods, ions are formed by one of the following techniques: (a) thermal desorption from a sample, followed by CI; (b) laser ablation, accompanying by ionization; (c) deposition of a drop of solvent on the surface of a sample,

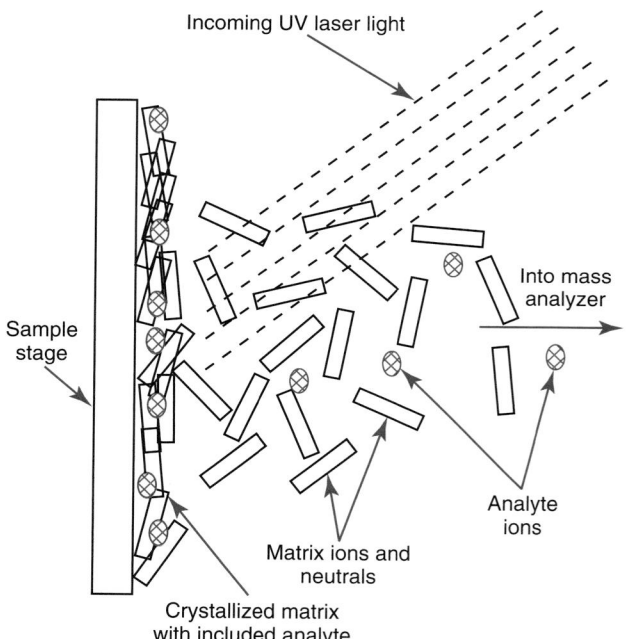

FIGURE 20.10 A generic view of the process of matrix-assisted laser desorption ionization (MALDI). Cocrystallized matrix and analyte molecules are irradiated with an ultraviolet *(UV)* laser. The laser vaporizes the matrix, producing a plume of matrix ions, which ionize neutral molecules. Gas-phase ions are directed into a mass analyzer.

followed by transfer of the droplet into an ion source and subjecting the droplet to ESI; or (d) introduction of a sample in plasma, which results in formation of metastable atoms and reactive ions.

One of the tasks performed by pathologists is microscopic evaluation of tissue cell morphology. AI-MS techniques enable imaging capabilities, which could allow determination of the molecular composition of tissue samples. Such information could be useful for evaluation of surgical margins during cancer surgeries, especially if performed in real time, while the tissue is resected. Several designs of such devices have been developed and evaluated.[21]

Rapid evaporative ionization MS (REIMS or iKnife) was the first described AI-MS technique. Using this device, ions are produced during thermal ablation of the resected tissues and transmitted into a mass spectrometer in real-time during the surgery; the device allowed special resolution of 0.5 to 2 mm.[21] In another design of AI-MS, a drop of water is applied on the tissue during a surgical procedure; after a brief exposure, the droplet is transferred into an ion source of a mass spectrometer, where the sample constituents subjected to ESI. In the evaluated prototype of the device, cycle time from sampling to obtaining the real time mass spectral information was less than 5 seconds.

In the studies performed to date, AI techniques allowed for discrimination between normal and abnormal tissues, with the following classes of molecules serving as biomarkers: (a) fatty acid, (b) lipids, (c) cholesterol metabolites, (d) carbohydrates, and (e) peptides. The ability of the AI-MS to determine marginal regions between pathologic and normal tissue was demonstrated for breast, brain, kidney, prostate, bladder, stomach, and colon cancer tissues.[22] If the technique and the devices will prove to be sufficiently robust and will be commercialized, they could enable surgeons to use real-time information on tumor margins, while performing cancer surgeries, potentially leading to better treatment outcomes.

Vacuum System

With the exception of certain ion trap mass spectrometers, ion separation in mass analyzers requires that the ions do not collide with other molecules during their interaction with magnetic or electric fields. This requires the use of a vacuum, which depending on the type of mass analyzer ranges between 10^{-3} and 10^{-9} torr. Unless collisions play a role in the mass analysis, the length of the ion path in the analyzer must be shorter than the mean free path distance of the ions.

In modern instruments, the most common high-vacuum pumps are turbomolecular (often referred to as "turbo") pumps. In addition to the turbo pumps, the vacuum system of all mass analyzers use mechanical, positive displacement (vacuum) pump (sometimes referred to as a "roughing pump").

A key consideration in the design of the vacuum system of mass analyzers is pumping speed, which is defined as the ability of the pump to maintain vacuum within the mass analyzer by removing gases and solvent vapors entering the system while the instrument is operating or in a standby mode. In general, higher pumping speeds allow for obtaining a higher vacuum, which is associated with lower detection limits and lower noise arising from presence of the background gases inside the mass analyzer.

Mass Analyzers, Tandem Mass Spectrometers, and Ion Detectors

The term *mass spectrometry* is somewhat a misnomer because mass spectrometers do not measure molecular mass, but rather they measure the mass-to-charge ratio. This fact is fundamental to the physical operating principles of mass spectrometers and consequently affects all aspects of instrumentation design, instrument operation, and interpretation of results. The symbol m/z is used to denote mass-to-charge ratio and is expressed in *Dalton* (Da, also known as unified atomic mass units [u]); Da conventionally has been defined as a dimensionless quantity.[23]

Mass Spectrometry: Principles and Instrumentation

Mass spectrometers are broadly classified into two groups: beam-type instruments and trapping-type instruments. In a beam-type instrument, the ions make one pass through the vacuum chamber of the instrument and then strike the detector, where they are destructively detected. The entire process, from the time an ion enters the analyzer until the time it is detected, generally takes microseconds to milliseconds.

In a trapping-type analyzer, ions are held in a spatially confined region through a combination of magnetic and/or electrostatic and/or RF electrical fields. The trapping fields or supplemental fields are applied and manipulated in ways that allow m/z measurements to be performed. Trapping times may range from milliseconds to minutes, although most clinical applications are at the low end of this range.

Examples of trapping-type instruments include quadrupole ion traps (QITs), linear ion traps (which, along with QITs, also depend on RF electric fields), ion cyclotron resonance (ICR) mass spectrometers, electrostatic ion traps, and Orbitraps (which is a type of electrostatic ion trap).

Detection of the ions in a trapping-type instrument may be destructive or nondestructive, depending on the specific type of mass spectrometer used. In this context, *destructive* means that ions are destroyed in the detection process. Additional discussions of mass analyzers, tandem mass spectrometers, and ion detectors can be found in the literature and the CLSI documents C50-A and C62-A, containing recommendations for matching the capabilities of different m/z analyzers to various types of applications.[1,2]

Beam-type designs. The main beam-type mass spectrometer designs are (1) quadrupole, (2) magnetic sector, and (3) TOF. It is convenient to categorize beam-type instruments into two broad categories, those that produce a mass spectrum by scanning a specified m/z range (quadrupole and magnetic sectors) and those that acquire instantaneous snapshots of the mass spectrum (TOF).

Quadrupole. Quadrupole mass analyzers, are currently the most widely used type of mass spectrometers, and the most suitable type of mass spectrometers for quantitative analysis. Quadrupole mass spectrometers offer an attractive and practical set of features that account for their popularity, including (1) ease of use, (2) flexibility, (3) adequate performance for most analytical chemistry applications, (4) relatively low cost, (5) small size, (6) less demanding installation site requirements, and (7) well-developed data collection and data analysis software.

A quadrupole mass analyzer consists of four parallel electrically conductive rods arranged in a square array (Fig. 20.11). The four rods form a channel, through which the ion beam passes. The beam enters near the axis at one end of the array, passes through the array, and exits at the opposite end of the array. The ion beam entering the quadrupole array may contain a mixture of ions of various m/z values. Typically, the instrument is tuned so, at a given point in time, only ions within a narrow m/z range (or a specified m/z) will be transmitted through the device to reach the detector. Ions outside of this specified range are ejected radially. The $\Delta m/z$ range represents a pass band, analogous to the pass band of

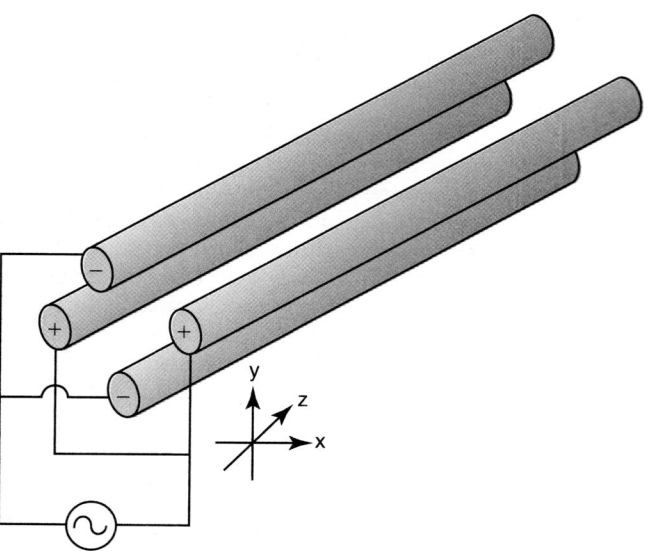

FIGURE 20.11 Diagram of quadrupole mass filter. Radiofrequency voltages applied to quadrupole rod assembly.

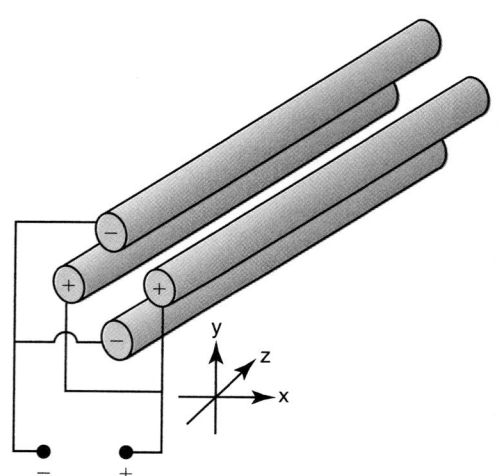

FIGURE 20.12 Diagram of quadrupole mass filter. Direct current voltages applied to quadrupole rod assembly.

an interference filter in optics (see Chapter 16). This is why quadrupole mass spectrometers are often referred to as *mass filters* rather than *mass spectrometers*.

Separation of ions in quadrupole MS is based on a superposition of RF and constant (DC) potentials, applied to the quadrupole rods. The voltages are applied to the electrodes in a quadrupolar pattern. For example, a positive DC potential is applied to electrodes 1 and 3, as indicated in Fig. 20.12, and an equivalent negative DC potential is applied to electrodes 2 and 4. The DC potentials are relatively small, in the order of a few volts. Superimposed on the DC potentials are RF potentials, also applied to the rods in a quadrupolar fashion. RF potentials range up to the kilovolt range, with frequency in the order of 1 MHz. The frequency is typically derived from a fixed-frequency and highly stable crystal-controlled oscillator.

The physical principles underlying the operation of a quadrupole mass spectrometer are described by solutions of the Mathieu equation.[24] When an ion is subjected to a

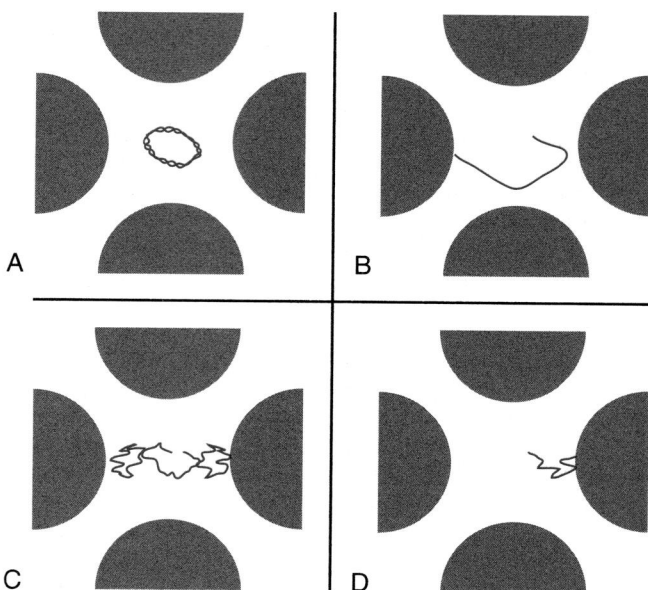

FIGURE 20.13 Ion trajectories showing confinement and ejection of ions in quadrupole mass filters. **A,** Ion confinement by radiofrequency (RF)-only field. **B,** Ion ejection by RF-only field. **C,** Ion confinement with a combination of RF and direct current (DC) fields. **D,** Ion ejection with a combination of RF and DC fields. All trajectories were simulated using Simion software. (Courtesy Scientific Instrument Services, Ringoes, NJ.)

quadrupolar RF field, its trajectory is described qualitatively as a combination of fast and slow oscillatory motions, with the slow component resembling motion of a particle in a fictitious harmonic *pseudopotential*. The frequency of this oscillation is sometimes called the *secular frequency.*

Effective force associated with the pseudopotential is directed inward toward the quadrupolar axis and is proportional to the distance from the axis. It therefore acts as a confining force, preventing ions from being ejected radially from the interquadrupolar space. Fig. 20.13A, shows an example of an ion confined by an RF-only quadrupole. Below a certain *m/z* (which depends on the frequency and amplitude of the RF field), ions are ejected rather than confined. Fig. 20.13B, shows an example of an ion ejected by an RF-only quadrupolar field. This establishes the low mass cutoff for the *m/z* pass band.

The DC part of the quadrupolar potential is independent of *m/z*. Positive ions are attracted toward the negative poles. Negative ions are attracted toward the positive poles. The attraction force increases linearly as the distance from the quadrupolar axis increases. Because a quadrupolar DC potential has both, negative and positive poles, the quadrupolar DC potential always contributes to ejection, regardless of ion polarity. Whether ejection of an ion of a particular *m/z* actually occurs, depends on whether the ejecting force caused by the quadrupolar DC potential overcomes the effective confining force caused by the pseudopotential generated by the RF field. Above a certain *m/z* value, the DC part dominates and ions are ejected radially from the device; this establishes an upper *m/z* limit for ion transmission. Fig. 20.13C and D show examples of ion trajectories under the influence of combined RF-DC fields, one being confined and the other being ejected. Trajectories shown in Fig. 20.13 were calculated using the Simion ion optics computer program.

A rigorous description of low- and high-mass cutoffs is found in so-called stability diagrams. These graphically describe the lower and upper m/z cutoffs of a quadrupole mass spectrometer in terms of parameters related to voltages, frequencies, and m/z. However, a full discussion of the stability diagram is outside of the scope of this chapter.[24]

The combination of lower and upper m/z limits establishes a pass band ($\Delta m/z$) and ultimately a resolution [$(m/z)/(\Delta m/z)$]. With relatively few exceptions, quadrupole instruments are limited to a resolution of a few hundred to several thousand, which is sufficient to achieve isotopic resolution for singly charged ions of m/z as high as several thousand.

A quadrupole MS may be operated in SIM mode or scanning mode. In SIM mode, both DC and RF voltages are fixed; consequently, both the center of the pass band and the width of the pass band are fixed. For example, the mass spectrometer may be set to pass ions of m/z 363 ± 0.5. The desired m/z (or the $\Delta m/z$ range) are selected by the user, and the instrument acquisition software calculates and sets the corresponding DC and RF voltages.

In the scanning mode of operation, the RF and/or DC voltages are continuously varied to scan a range of the specified m/z values within a specified time interval. Usually the scan function is set to maintain a constant $\Delta m/z$ across the full m/z range, thus the mass resolution increases as m/z increases. The value of $\Delta m/z$ is frequently chosen in the range 0.6 to 0.8 (at the half-height of the peak) to resolve isotopic peaks of singly charged ions across the entire m/z range.

Magnetic Sector. Magnetic sector mass spectrometers separate ions in a magnetic field according to the momentum and charge of the ions. Ions are accelerated from the ion source region into the magnetic sector by a 1000 to 10,000 V electric field (significantly greater, as compared with the acceleration field in a quadrupole mass analyzer). As the charged ions pass through the magnetic sector, the magnetic field bends the ion beam in form of an arc. The radius of this arc depends on the m/z of the ions, and the magnetic field strength. These instruments are versatile, reliable, and highly sensitive; and in their "double focusing" design are capable of very high mass resolution and mass accuracy. However, the magnetic sector instruments are significantly larger than modern bench top mass spectrometers, more expensive, and more difficult to operate. Consequently, magnetic sector mass spectrometers are rarely used in clinical laboratories.

Time-of-flight. TOF-MS is a nonscanning technique by which a full mass spectrum is acquired as a snapshot rather than by sweeping through a sequential series of m/z values, while acquiring the data. It is described here as a snapshot because, although ions of different m/z arrive at the detector sequentially (low m/z first), the samples are loaded into the ion source with little or no m/z discrimination with regard to time, and the duration of the acquisition of a single mass spectrum is measured in microseconds. One implication of this is that, if the composition of the sample stream being presented to the mass spectrometer changes with time, there is essentially no distortion of the mass spectrum, whereas with scanning-type mass spectrometers the mass spectrum may be distorted because of the interaction between scan time of the mass spectrometer and the changing concentration in

different segments of a chromatographic peak. This is particularly significant when dealing with fast chromatographic separations (narrow chromatographic peaks) coupled to MS.

As compared with other mass analyzers, TOF mass spectrometers have several advantages, including (1) a nearly unlimited m/z range, (2) high acquisition speed, (3) high mass accuracy, (4) moderate to high resolution, (5) moderate to high sensitivity, and (6) absence of spectral distortions when used in conjunction with fast separations and narrow chromatographic peaks. TOF-MS is also well adapted to pulsed ionization sources, which is an advantage in some applications, particularly with MALDI and related techniques.

A major advantage of modern TOF mass spectrometers is that they are capable of acquiring accurate mass measurements, which is typically accurate to a few parts per million (ppm). This allows for using TOF data for confirmation of the molecular formula of a compound and assisting with identification of unknowns in the mass spectra.

The principle of operation of TOF mass spectrometers is based on the fact that, in vacuum, a lighter ion travels faster than a heavier ion, provided that both have the same kinetic energy.[25] Fig. 20.14 presents a simplified conceptual diagram of a TOF mass spectrometer. It resembles a long tube wherein ions are injected at the source end of the device and then are accelerated by the applied potential of several kilovolts. The ions travel down the flight tube and strike the detector at the far end. The time it takes to traverse the tube is known as the flight time and is related to the mass-to-charge ratio of the ion according to the equation:

$$t = L \left(\frac{m}{2zeVE} \right)^{1/2}$$

$$t = L \left(\frac{m}{z} \right)^{1/2} \left(e\Phi \right)^{-1/2}$$

where L is the distance traveled, e the value of an elementary charge, and Φ is the potential through which the ion was accelerated prior to entering the flight tube. Note that $ze\Phi$ represents the kinetic energy of the ion.

A sample calculation for an ion of molecular weight 200 Da (3.32×10^{-25} kg) and $z = 1$, with a kinetic energy of 10 keV (1.60×10^{-15} J), traveling through a distance of 1 m, yields a flight time of 10.18 μs, and an ion of molecular weight 201 takes just 25 ns longer. To accurately capture such fleeting signals, the data recording system must operate on an approximately 1 ns or shorter timescale. Advances in signal processing electronics allows for such speed of data collection. The TOF analyzers typically have modest cost, and this has been a major factor in the rise in their popularity.

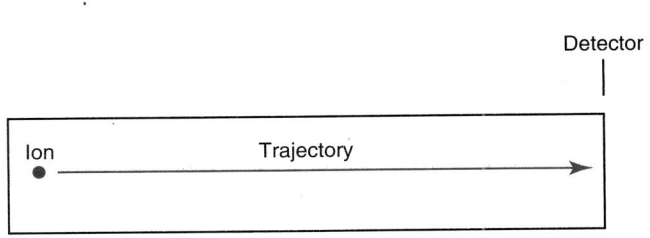

FIGURE 20.14 Simplified diagram of a time-of-flight mass spectrometer.

TOF is inherently a pulsed technique; consequently, it couples readily to pulsed ionization sources, with MALDI being the most common example, although TOF can also be coupled with continuous ion sources such as EI, ESI, and APCI. However, the continuous nature of these non-MALDI sources causes a mismatch between continuous introduction of ions from the ion source and a pulsed detection by TOF-MS. This mismatch is overcome by using a technique known as orthogonal acceleration, in which the ion beam is injected orthogonal to the axis of the TOF-MS. In this technique, during the injection period, the acceleration voltage is turned off. Once the injection region is filled with the ion beam, the acceleration voltage is quickly turned on and the TOF timing cycle starts; the process is cycled repeatedly with high frequency. The overall duty cycle for this method can be more than 10%; this represents a vast improvement over the traditional method of gating the ion beam for TOF analysis. In methods using continuous ion sources and full spectrum data acquisition, orthogonal injection TOF mass spectrometers are considered to have the lowest detection limits, as compared with the other types of mass spectrometers. However, for the monitoring of a single (or a limited number) of m/z rather than a full mass spectrum, the use of SIM mode of quadrupole MS is superior to TOF sensitivity.

In addition to the aforementioned advantages of TOF-MS, orthogonal acceleration minimizes resolution-degrading effects, which would normally accompany the kinetic energy variations of individual ions in the ion beam.

Use of an ion mirror is another technique often used in TOF-MS for improving resolution by compensating for kinetic energy variations. Such a device is known as *reflectron*. To date, TOF-MS has had a limited impact in clinical chemistry with only a few TOF-MS–based assays, such as insulin-like growth factor I and toxicology drug screening, but it could potentially play a greater role in the future. For example, full-spectrum capability, high resolution (up to 40,000), high speed (10 to 100 stored spectra per second), and high mass accuracy of TOF-MS seem well suited to the methods using fast chromatographic separations.

Considering that m/z ranges measured by TOF-MS are nearly unlimited, these analyzers have advantage in analysis of high m/z analytes. MALDI-TOF instruments have gained wide acceptance for identification of microorganisms and pathogens in patient specimens (Chapter 22). The use of TOF-MS is expected to increase in future, as clinical laboratories embrace proteomic-based diagnostic methods.

Trapping mass spectrometers. In contrast to beam-type designs, these mass spectrometers are based on trapping and holding ions for an extended length of time in a small confined space, with the trapping times varying from a fraction of a second to minutes. Compared with beam-type instruments, the division between scanning and nonscanning instruments has less meaning for ion-trapping instruments. The main practical difference between scanning and nonscanning instruments is related to distortions in chromatographic peak shape (or peak skewing). These arise from the finite scan time of a mass spectrometer relative to the timescale relative to the width of a chromatographic peak. The result is that the abundances of the peaks in mass spectra, collected during the rising or falling portions of a chromatographic peak are distorted, relative to the true mass spectrum. As a result, mass spectra collected at the beginning of

a chromatographic peak may have different relative peak intensities compared with those of spectra collected at the end of a chromatographic peak.

Traditionally, ion traps have been classified as (1) QIT, which relies on RF fields to provide ion trapping; (2) linear ion trap, which is closely related to the QIT in its operating principles; (3) ICR-MS, which relies on a combination of magnetic fields and electrostatic fields for trapping; and (4) Orbitrap, a more recent introduction into the field of ion trap MS.

Quadrupole ion trap. QITs are relatively compact, inexpensive, and versatile instruments that are typically used for (1) exploratory studies, (2) structural characterization, and (3) qualitative identification.

Operation of the QIT is based on the same physical principles as the earlier described quadrupole mass spectrometer. Both devices make use of the ability of RF fields to confine ions, while in QIT electric fields trap ions in a confined three-dimensional space, rather than to allow the ions to pass through as in a quadrupole mass analyzer, which confines ions in two dimensions.

Although physical principles of QIT operation are the same as of a quadrupole mass analyzer, the instrument is designed differently. A diagram of an ion trap is shown in Fig. 20.15. By design, QITs consist of a hyperbolic ring electrode and two hyperbolic metal electrodes facing each other. The ions are trapped and manipulated in the space between these three electrodes by oscillating AC and DC voltages. Detection in QIT is performed by ejection of ions from the trap in an m/z-dependent fashion into an externally positioned electron multiplier.

Some advantages of QITs are an ability to perform multiple stages of tandem MS (MS^n), high sensitivity, and decoupling of the mass analysis from scanning. However, ion-ion repulsion effects (caused by the large number of charged ions confined in a small space within the trap) limit the number of ions, which can be simultaneously trapped, causing reduced linear dynamic range and causing m/z miss-assignments at

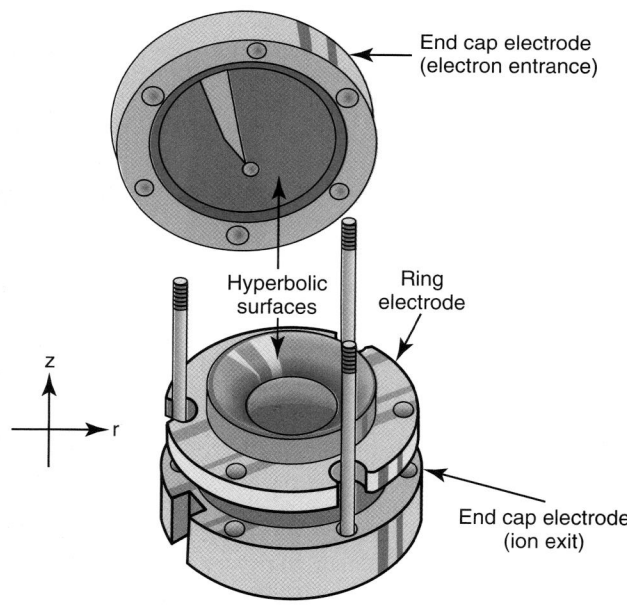

FIGURE 20.15 Diagram of quadrupole ion trap. *r*, Radial direction; *z*, axial direction.

high signal levels. The previously mentioned features make QIT-MS not well suited for quantitative analyses, which are typically required for majority of MS applications in clinical laboratories.

Linear ion trap. The linear trap is an RF ion trap that is based on a modified linear quadrupole mass analyzer. Rather than being a pass-through device, as linear quadrupole mass analyzer, in QIT electrostatic fields are applied at both ends of the quadrupoles, to enable trapping the ions within the quadrupole. When trapped in this manner, ions can be manipulated in a similar way as in a QIT. An advantage of the linear QIT is that the trapping field can be turned off at will and the device may be operated as a traditional quadrupole mass analyzer. Furthermore, the trapping volume available within the quadrupole mass analyzer is much greater than in the traditional QIT, allowing greater capacity of the ions to be trapped before ion-ion repulsion becomes an issue. Thus a single device combines most of the features of a QIT and a quadrupole mass analyzer, making the instrument extremely versatile. Such analyzers, with quadrupole functioning either as a linear trap or as a conventional quadrupole mass spectrometer, are commercially available.

Ion cyclotron resonance. Fourier transform (FT) ICR-MS excels in high-resolution and high mass accuracy measurements. ICR is a trapping technique that shares many of the advantages of RF ion traps (QIT or linear ion traps), including the ability to perform multiple stages of MS/MS (MS[n]) experiments. Measurements at a mass resolution exceeding 1,000,000 are not unusual with the ICR-MS instruments. Furthermore, sampling is decoupled from spectral acquisition, so no peak skewing is seen in chromatographic experiments—a feature that ICR shares with TOF and QIT, while the signal acquisition times are typically longer than for other types of mass analyzers. Because of the aforementioned, ICR detection is not compatible with fast chromatographic separations.

ICR-MS is based on the principle that ions in a high magnetic field, generated using superconducting magnets (3 to 12 tesla), undergo circular (cyclotron) motion, which keeps ions from being lost radially (in the direction perpendicular to the magnetic field). A low (approximately 1 V) potential is applied to the end caps to keep ions from leaving the trap axially. Thus the combination of electric and magnetic fields keeps ions confined within the cell.

Ions circulating in the ICR cell induce an electrical current in two detection electrodes, which are arranged parallel to the magnetic field, and positioned on the opposite sides of the ICR cell. The signal acquired by the detection electrodes is processed using FT mathematical operation, with each cyclotron frequency associated with m/z of the detected ions. Because of the use of FT in ICR, the technique is often referred to as FT-ICR MS.

Although this technique has many advantages (e.g., high mass accuracy, ultra-high resolution, and the ability to perform MS[n]), ICR-MS has several disadvantages, including (1) high instrument costs; (2) very demanding site requirements, in terms of both space and access restrictions; (3) requirement for a high-field superconducting magnet; (4) relatively long signal acquisition time, which limits the number of scans that can be acquired during the elution of a chromatographic peak; (5) safety concerns related to high magnetic fields; (6) demagnetization of magnetically encoded devices (e.g., credit cards);

(7) high costs of operation and maintenance; and (8) requirement for highly skilled staff to operate the instrument. Despite these challenges, one recent pilot study has demonstrated the technical feasibility of using FT-ICR for diagnosis of hemoglobinopaties and thalasemias.[26]

Orbitrap. Orbitrap is the newest type of high-resolution/high-mass-accuracy MS that has been shown to be useful for applications in clinical laboratories.[27] The Orbitrap mass analyzer has resolution and mass accuracy approaching that of an ICR MS; the principles of mass analysis in an Orbitrap are based on trapping ions within electrostatic fields. The actual device is a uniquely shaped spindle-like central electrode, surrounded by a barrel-like outer electrode. When ions are introduced perpendicular to the central electrode and a radial potential is applied between the electrodes, the ions spiral (orbit) around the central electrode and are effectively trapped in a radial direction. Trapping in the axial direction is assisted by the shape of the electrode and the potentials applied to the electrodes. Ion trapping therefore involves both orbital motion around the central electrode and axial oscillations.

The trapping potential in the axial direction is in the form of a harmonic oscillator, and because the frequency of a harmonic oscillator is independent of oscillation amplitude, this frequency is very stable and well behaved. The m/z can be calculated from the frequency of axial oscillation:

$$\omega = 2\pi f = (km/z)^{-1/2}$$

where ω is angular velocity, f is frequency, m/z is the mass-to-charge ratio, and k is a constant determined by the trap geometry, dimensions, and the applied potential.

The image current (current induced by a motion of ions passing near a conductor) made in the outer electrode, induced by the ion motion is acquired in the time domain and can be Fourier-transformed to produce a frequency spectrum that is then converted to m/z using the aforementioned equation.

This instrument is capable of mass resolution greater than 200,000 and up to sub–parts per million mass accuracy; it has four orders of magnitude dynamic range and has sampling decoupled from spectral acquisition (as in the ICR). The mass resolution and mass accuracy of Orbitrap are typically approximately two orders of magnitude greater than for quadrupole mass spectrometers.

With the ability to perform accurate mass measurements, especially when combined with a linear ion trap or quadrupole to form a hybrid tandem mass spectrometer, Orbitrap mass analyzers have excellent capabilities for metabolomics and proteomics type of applications. One recent publication noted anomalous isotope ratios observed under high-resolution operating conditions.[28] The anomaly is compound dependent and generally increases with data acquisition using higher mass resolution. A potential pitfall arising from this issue is that the observed isotope ratios may not be effective in confirming compound identity in cases where the isotopic profile is distorted. A theoretical explanation for these anomalies has been given.[28]

TANDEM MASS SPECTROMETERS

Tandem MS (or MS/MS) has become the dominant MS-based technique used in clinical laboratories for quantitative analysis of routine samples.[29] MS/MS is also a useful technique for structural characterization and compound identification and therefore often used for exploratory work. The most important features of MS/MS are high selectivity, which in turn often conveys an ability to measure very low concentrations of analytes, and ability to multiplex the measurement of multiple analytes in a single method. Susceptibility of MS/MS to interferences is typically very low, especially if it is combined with chromatographic separation. The reason is that a detected compound is separated and characterized by three physical properties: chromatographic retention time, precursor ion m/z, and product ion m/z. Because of its high specificity, low consumable cost, and a potential for high sample throughput, these instruments are widely used for the routine analysis in clinical laboratories.

The physical principle of MS/MS is based on the use of two mass spectrometers (or mass filters) arranged sequentially in tandem, with a collision cell placed between the two mass filters. The first filter is used to select a *precursor ion* of a particular m/z. The precursor ion is directed into the collision cell, where ions collide with background gas molecules and are broken into smaller product ions. The second mass filter acquires the mass spectrum of the product ions or monitors ions of specified m/z.

A variety of scan functions are possible with MS/MS (Fig. 20.16). A product ion scan involves setting the first mass spectrometer (also called MF1, MS1, or Q1) to select a given m/z, and scanning through the full mass spectrum of product ions generated in the collision cell (also called Q2) using the second mass spectrometer or mass filter, MS2 (also called MF2, or Q3). This scan function is often used for structural characterization.

A precursor ion scan reverses this relationship, with the second mass filter, MS2, set to select a specific product ion, and MS1 is scanned through the spectrum of precursor ions.

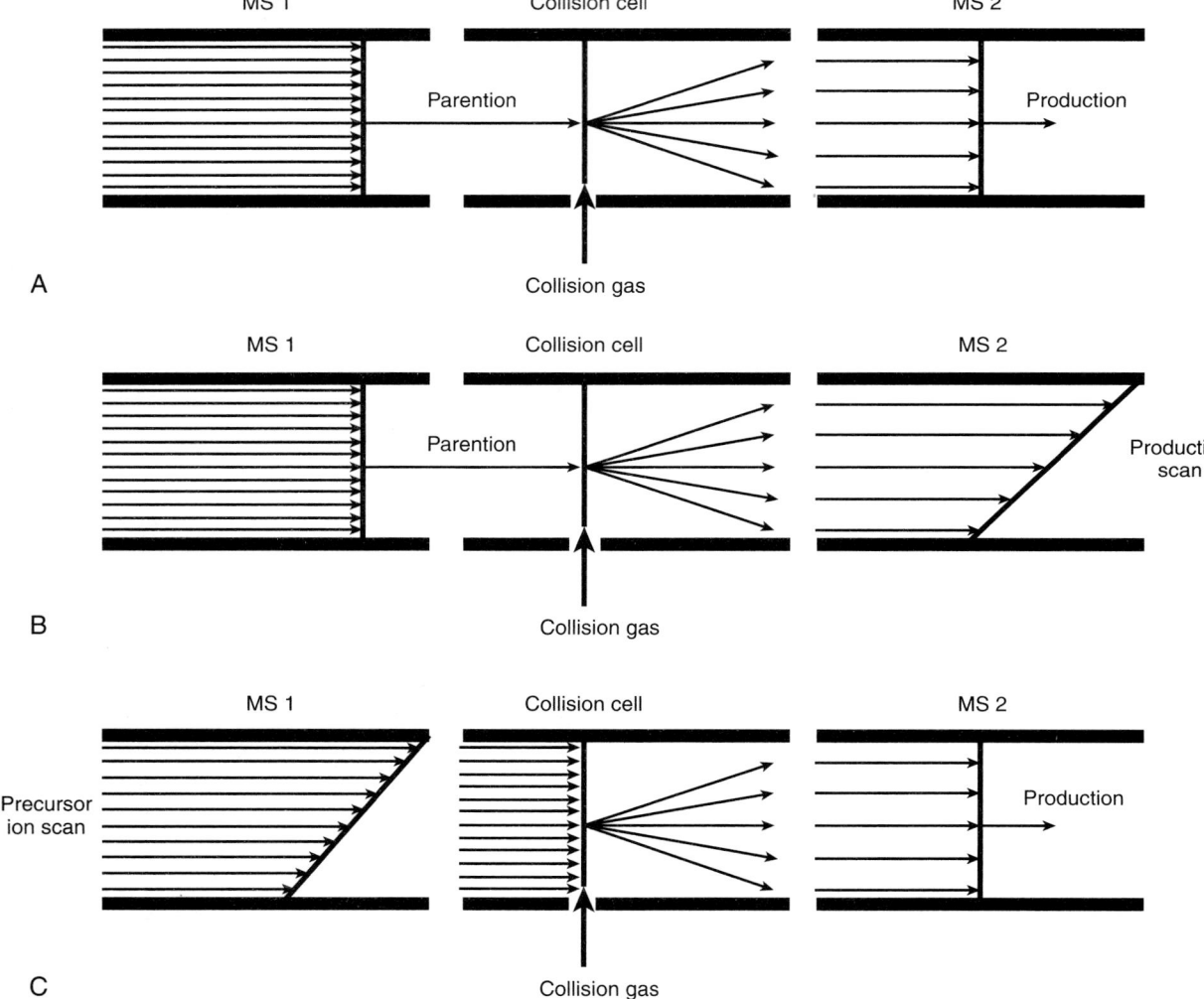

FIGURE 20.16 Scan modes in triple quadrupole mass spectrometry (MS/MS). **A,** Single reaction monitoring (SRM). The first mass analyzer (MS 1) is fixed to monitor a single m/z, and the second mass analyzer (MS 2) is fixed to monitor a single m/z; in cases when multiple mass transitions are monitored in a single experiment, this scan type is named multiple reaction monitoring (MRM). **B,** Product ion scan mode. The first mass analyzer (MS 1) is fixed to monitor a single m/z and the second mass analyzer (MS 2) scans through a range of m/z. **C,** Precursor ion scan mode. The second mass analyzer (MS 2) is fixed to monitor a single m/z, and the first mass filter (MS 1) is scanned through a range of m/z values.

The scan detects precursor ions, which produce a specific product ion; this capability is often used to analyze for specific classes of compounds. For example, acylcarnitines are often analyzed using precursor ion scan mode by acquiring signals from all molecules producing fragment m/z 85. Acylcarnitine analysis based on this principle has found widespread use in newborn screening for metabolic diseases (Chapter 60).[30]

In a neutral loss scan, the two mass filters are scanned synchronously, with a constant m/z offset between the precursor and the product ion. This scan indicates which ions lose a particular neutral fragment. For example, an offset of 176 m/z would select for ions losing a glucuronide moiety in the dissociation process, and a constant neutral loss of 102 targets several amino acids.

The most commonly used type of acquisition in MS/MS is MRM (also referred as SRM). In this type of acquisition, a series of precursor/product ion pairs are monitored, with the mass spectrometer set to step through a list of parent/product ion pairs in a cyclic fashion. MRM acquisition is primarily used for quantitative analysis of target compounds and is an analog to the SIM type of acquisition used in GC-MS.

As with single-stage mass spectrometers, MS/MS are categorized as either beam-type instruments or trapping instruments.[29] The most popular beam-type instrument is the triple quadrupole MS. In this instrument, the first quadrupole (Q1) functions as MF1 and the third quadrupole (Q3) functions as MF2. Between these two quadrupoles is another quadrupole, Q2, which functions as the collision cell. Fragmentation in the collision cell (Q2) is performed by rising pressure to approximately 10^{-3} torr by means of supplying in the collision cell of a nonreactive gas (e.g., nitrogen, argon) to the point that ions traversing Q2 undergo multiple collisions, leading to deposition of energy onto the analyte molecules and subsequent fragmentation of the precursor ion(s) into smaller fragments, followed by separation and detection of the fragment ions in a subsequent stage of mass analysis. The Q2 is operated as an RF-only quadrupole, allowing all ions to pass through, regardless of the m/z. The technique is typically used to fragment molecular ions to obtain analyte-specific fragments, which can be used for elucidating structure of the molecules of interest or in selective analysis of targeted molecules. In cases in which the collision-induced dissociation spectrum contains a large number of ions, the experienced investigator often can deduce the structure of a molecule from the mass spectrum of the product ion.

In hybrid type instruments, two mass spectrometers of different types are used in a tandem arrangement. The combination of a magnetic sector mass spectrometer with a quadrupole mass spectrometer was an early instrument of this type. Widely used hybrid instruments are (1) combination of a quadrupole as the first stage of m/z selection with a TOF as the second m/z analyzer, and (2) ion trap and quadrupole mass analyzers in combination with an Orbitrap. The hybrid type instruments are often used in metabolomics and proteomics research. These instruments cannot perform the true precursor ion scans or constant neutral loss scans, although it is possible to mimic these functions by postprocessing the acquired data, provided the full precursor/product ion scans were generated in the experiments.

QIT, linear ion trap, and ICR mass spectrometers also can be used as MS/MS. Unlike beam-type instruments, which are referred to as "tandem in space," trapping mass spectrometers are "tandem in time," meaning that ions are held in one region of space while the parent ion is selected and dissociated and the product ions are analyzed sequentially in time in the same region of space. The ability to perform MS/MS is inherent in the design of most trapping mass spectrometers. In general, little or no additional hardware is required, and tandem capability is supplied via the software. An exception is the Orbitrap, which is not amenable to MS/MS when used alone, but is capable of such function when incorporated into a hybrid instruments (with linear ion trap or a quadrupole used as the first stage of MS).

Most trap-based instruments are capable of multiple stages of MS. Thus product ions may be further dissociated to produce another generation of product ions (MS/MS/MS, or MS[3]). In principle, any number of dissociation stages may be performed (MS[n]), while additional stages of MS reduce sensitivity of detection. This capability finds its greatest use in structural characterization of unknown molecules and is not useful for quantitative analysis.

Ion Mobility

Although strictly speaking, ion mobility spectrometers (IMSs) are not mass analyzers; they are nevertheless often included as part of the field of MS, either as part of a hyphenated technique (e.g., IMS-MS) or as a substitute for an MS analyzer. Similar to MS, IMSs require the analyte to be in an ionized form, whereas the separation mechanism in IMS is different. Rather than separating ions by their mass-to-charge ratio, ions are separated according to their mobility in an electric field; in this regard, IMS can be viewed as a form of gas phase electrophoresis.[31]

The simplified schematic of a conventional IMS strongly resembles a TOF-MS, but rather than following a collisionless trajectory, ions undergo many collisions as they drift under the influence of an electric field. Other configurations for measuring gas phase mobility are also possible, but these will not be reviewed in detail here.

An IMS may operate at atmospheric pressure or at reduced pressure but not under a high vacuum, because collisions are necessary for its operation. When used in conjunction with a mass spectrometer, it is possible to place the mobility device before the first mass analyzer or following one or more stage of mass analysis.

A technique known as field asymmetric ion mobility spectrometry (FAIMS) is also based on ion mobility, but in this case, ions are not separated strictly according to their mobility. FAIMS, sometimes known as differential mobility spectrometry (DMS), is based on the fact that the mobility of a gas phase ion is not strictly constant; that is, the drift velocity is not simply proportional to the electric field, but rather at high field there is a deviation from the proportional relationship. FAIMS uses a combination of an asymmetric high-voltage RF field and a smaller DC field, allowing separation of ions according to a combination of low-field mobility and high-field mobility.

Detectors

With the exceptions of ICR-MS, Orbitrap, and some ICP-MS instruments, most modern mass spectrometers use electron multipliers for ion detection. The main classes of electron multipliers used as MS detectors include the (1) discrete

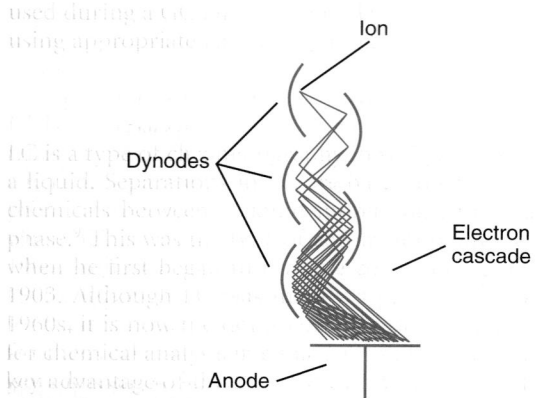

FIGURE 20.17 Discrete dynode electron multiplier showing dynode structure and generation of a cascade of electrons.

dynode multipliers; (2) continuous dynode electron multipliers (CDEMs), also known as channel electron multipliers; and (3) microchannel plate electron multipliers. Although different in design, all three work on the same physical principle. Additional types of detectors used in mass spectrometers are the Faraday cup and image current detection.

Fig. 20.17 presents a conceptual diagram of the operation of a discrete dynode electron multiplier. When an ion strikes the first dynode, it causes ejection of one or more electrons (secondary electrons) from the dynode surface. The electron is accelerated toward the second dynode by a voltage difference of approximately 100 V. On striking the second dynode, each electron causes the ejection of additional electrons. The second group of electrons is then accelerated toward the third dynode, and while striking the third dynode, each electron causes the ejection of additional electrons. This process is repeated through a chain of dynodes (typically 12 to 24). The cascade process typically produces a gain of 10^4 to 10^8, meaning that one ion striking the first electrode produces a pulse of 10^4 to 10^8 electrons at the end of the cascade. The duration of the pulse is very short, typically less than 10 ns. Thus for a brief instant, the output current reaches the microampere range, allowing to detect a single ion, striking the detector.

A CDEM works on the same principle as a discrete dynode electron multiplier but differs in design. The set of dynodes of a discrete dynode electron multiplier is replaced by a single continuous resistive surface that acts both as a (continuous) voltage divider to establish the potential gradient and as the secondary electron-generating surface. A microchannel plate electron multiplier is essentially a monolithic array of miniaturized CDEMs fabricated in a single wafer. Microchannel plates are typically used as detectors in TOF-MS.

The Faraday cup is a charge detector that, when used with an electronic amplifier, measures signal intensity directly, rather than indirectly (as in saturation-prone electron multipliers). The Faraday cup provides an absolute measure of ion current and is useful when the magnitude of the signal is too high for electron multiplier-based detection. Some instruments use both an electron multiplier and Faraday cup–based detection to provide extended dynamic range, which is especially useful for analysis of trace and toxic elements by ICP-MS.

Detection in ICR occurs via image current detection. This type of detection is more similar to the Faraday detection cup in the sense that the ion current is detected directly and is not

multiplied (as in an electron multiplier). One key feature of ICR mass spectrometers is that ions in ICR are not destroyed; thus the signal can be measured as long as necessary. Image current detection is also used in the Orbitrap.

Closely linked to the detection system is the electronic and signal processing system. In instruments that use electron multiplier detection (the vast majority of mass spectrometers), the raw signal from the detector is processed in one of two ways: (1) counting of individual pulses (corresponding to individual ions), as in ion counting systems, or (2) the signal may be converted to a digital representation of the analog signal using an analog-to-digital converter, as in analog detection.

Computer and Software

Because of the high speed of the *m/z* signal acquisition, high mass resolution capabilities, and the enormous amount of the data that need to be processed, modern MS instruments require powerful computers and software. The most important functions of software in MS systems are data collection and processing.

In applications requiring identification of unknown constituents of the samples, an important function of the data system is library-searching capability. Several commercial libraries, including the Wiley Registry of Mass Spectral Data; the NIST Mass Spectral Database; and the Pfleger, Maurer, Weber drug libraries, and PeptideAtlas are available; in addition, many laboratories generate their own mass spectral libraries. The quality and number of available spectra, and the search algorithm, are important factors in spectral matching.

In proteomics and biomarker discovery, complex mass spectra from single proteins, protein mixtures, or protein digests corresponding to complex samples are obtained or generated in silico (in silico means a computer-generated prediction, which can then be compared against an experimentally obtained result. Data systems aid in characterization of spectral data to identify such properties as intact protein mass, amino acid subsequences, and post-translational modifications.

Chromatographic peaks are integrated using data analysis software, and integrated peak intensities or peak areas serve as the basis for quantitative analysis. In methods for quantitative analysis, calibration standards are prepared and analyzed along with the samples; calibration curves are generated during data processing, and quantitative results are determined using the calibration curves. The data systems also allow qualitative confirmation of identity of each substance,[32] evaluation of the quality control (QC), data review, and report generation capabilities.[1,2]

CLINICAL APPLICATIONS

Mass spectrometers coupled with gas or liquid chromatographs (GC-MS or LC-MS) serve as versatile analytical instruments that combine the resolving power of a chromatograph with the specificity of a mass spectrometer.[1,2] Such instruments are powerful analytical tools used by clinical laboratories to identify and quantify biomolecules. The instruments are capable of providing structural and quantitative information on sample constituents. Examples of clinical applications of these instruments can be found in Chapters 21–24, 39, 42–44, 60, and 61.

Gas Chromatography–Mass Spectrometry

GC-MS has been used for the analysis of biological samples for several decades. This technique is used by the US National Institute of Standards and Technology and other agencies for the development of definitive methods to qualify standard reference materials and assign accurate concentration to reference materials of many clinically relevant analytes, including cholesterol, glucose, steroid hormones, creatinine, and urea nitrogen.

One of the most common applications of GC-MS is drug testing for clinical or forensic purposes. Many drugs and drug metabolites have relatively low molecular weight and are relatively nonpolar and volatile, making these compounds suitable for analysis by GC. EI ionization with full scan mass acquisition is a widely used approach for toxicology drug screening, organic acid screening for diagnosing inherited metabolic diseases, screening for pesticides and pollutants, metabolomics studies, etc. In these applications, unknown compounds can be identified by matching mass spectra of the observed peaks with entries of mass spectral libraries. GC triple quadrupole (GC-MS/MS) mass spectrometers expand the capability of GC-MS for use in targeted and untargeted analysis.

One important limitation of GC-MS is the requirement that compounds be sufficiently volatile and thermally stable to allow transfer from the liquid phase to the gas phase (in injection port of an instrument). Although many biological compounds are amenable to chromatographic separation with GC, many molecules of clinical interest are too polar or too large to be analyzed with this technique. In some cases, chemical derivatization can be used to reduce polarity and to make the molecules volatile and suitable to GC separation and MS detection.

Despite some limitations, GC-MS has several useful attributes. This technique allows for achieving high-efficiency chromatographic separation, low limits of quantification, and using commercial mass spectral libraries for identification of sample constituents. For some of the analytes, such as organic acids, GC-MS has an advantage of higher specificity compared with soft ionization techniques used in LC-MS.

GC-based separations often require longer analysis time as compared with LC-based separations, and this can be a disadvantage in high-throughput clinical laboratories.

Liquid Chromatography–Mass Spectrometry

As discussed earlier, several interface techniques have been developed for coupling a liquid chromatograph to a mass spectrometer, notably ESI and APCI, which have allowed LC-MS and LC-MS/MS to be successfully applied to analysis of a wide range of molecules of clinical interest. In theory, as long as a compound can be dissolved in a liquid, it can be introduced into an LC-MS system. Thus in addition to low-molecular-weight polar and nonpolar analytes, large-molecular-weight compounds, such as peptides and proteins, can be analyzed using this technique (see Chapter 24).

The majority of targeted analysis LC-MS/MS methods use MRM acquisition with mass transitions corresponding to the analytes of interest and the internal standards (see Fig. 20.16A). For example, a method can be set up for a subset of the targeted molecules within the chromatographic time window of 1.0 to 2.0 minutes, whereas during the next defined time window, a new set of MRM transitions can be monitored for

another subset of analytes targeted in the assay. A related approach is the use of targeted MRM, in which recognition of a chromatographic peak containing a preselected MRM transition triggers a product ion scan in a process, called *information-dependent acquisition* (or *data-dependent acquisition*). One benefit of this approach is the ability to provide confirmation of the identity of the peaks identified during the analysis.

Coupling of TOF-MS to GC or LC provides enhanced capabilities to the identification of unknowns. Because TOF is capable of achieving high mass resolution and high mass accuracy, an adequate specificity of analysis could be achieved without the additional stage of mass analysis, allowing compound identification based on retention time, accurate mass, and isotope pattern. In addition, the ability to acquire a full mass spectrum with high sensitivity allows for detection and identification of sample constituents without setting the mass spectrometer to acquire specific targets. Thus a data file can be examined after the analysis to identify compounds, which may not have been anticipated to be present in the sample. This is very valuable in a toxicology drug screen, when often the clinician may not know which drugs or toxins might be present in patient's samples.[33]

Since LC-MS/MS was introduced in clinical laboratories, a large number of assays have been developed and implemented in routine diagnostic use. Types of molecules for which LC-MS/MS methods are available in clinical laboratories include (1) drugs and drug metabolites, (2) endogenous small molecule biomarkers (e.g., steroids, small molecule hormones, intermediates and final products of enzymatic reactions), and (3) protein and peptide biomarkers (e.g., therapeutic monoclonal antibodies, protein and peptide hormones, tumor markers).

When quantification of a specific compound is desired, the most effective approach is MRM analysis (see Fig. 20.16B). With MRM acquisition, both mass filters MF1 and MF2 are set in a static mode, whereby only precursor ions specific for the compound of interest are passed through MF1. This preselected precursor ion is then fragmented in the collision cell, and molecule-specific fragment ions derived from the compound of interest are passed by MF2 to the detector. Because only the target-specific ions are transmitted by MF1 and only the target-specific fragment ions are transmitted by MF2, the MRM data acquisition allows for achieving high specificity, as well as lower limits of quantification. Acquisition of the MS/MS transitions for the target compound is multiplexed with MS/MS transitions of an internal standard, allowing accurate quantification of the target.

Another area in which MS/MS is used clinically is screening and confirmation of genetic disorders and inborn errors of metabolism (see Chapters 60 and 61).[34,35] The ability to analyze multiple compounds in a single analytical run makes MS/MS an efficient technique for screening purposes. In this application, MS/MS often is of sufficient selectivity to eliminate the need in LC separation, a simplification that allows high-throughput analysis. Classes of compounds analyzed for detection of inborn errors of metabolism include amino acids, organic acids, acylcarnitines, steroid hormones, and intermediates of the steroid biosynthesis pathway.

One of the difficulties in the methods for analysis of acylcarnitines and amino acids is that these compounds vary widely in their polarity, resulting in uneven ionization efficiency and a wide among-compound difference in sensitivity of detection. To address this issue, methods using a butyl ester derivatization of the carboxyl group have been developed; the approach allowed achieving a more uniform sensitivity among the analytes targeted in the assay.

In screening methods for acylcarnitines, butyl esters of acylcarnitines are often analyzed in a *precursor ion scan* mode of acquisition (see Fig. 20.16*C*). This type of acquisition makes use of the fact that butyl esters of acylcarnitines have a common product ion, produced by collision-induced dissociation (m/z 85, represented by *X* in Fig. 20.16*C*), that is monitored in MF2, while MF1 is set to scan precursors that lose fragment m/z 85, thus detecting and identifying acylcarnitines present in the sample (see Fig. 20.16*C*). By incorporating stable isotope-labeled analogs of the targeted acetylcarnitines in the method, it is possible, in addition to identifying, also determine the concentration of acylcarnitines of interest.

Analysis of amino acids by LC-MS/MS is typically performed using MRM monitoring but also can be performed using a data acquisition mode known as *constant neutral loss* (see Fig. 20.16*D*). Butyl derivatives of α-amino acids share a common neutral product, butylformate, which has mass 102 (represented by *X* in Fig. 20.16*D*). By scanning both product (MF2) and precursor (MF1) ions and by keeping a constant offset between the two mass analyzers (difference of 102), only peaks corresponding to the molecules which may lose a fragment with mass 102 Da will be detected; such detection in combination with an appropriate method of sample preparation would be specific to amino acids.

One advantage of LC-MS/MS, compared with GC-MS, is that in many cases it avoids the need for derivatization; however, at times, derivatization could be beneficial for LC-MS/MS analysis. The most frequent reasons for using derivatization in LC-MS and LC-MS/MS are to achieve improved ionization efficiency and to achieve more favorable fragmentation properties than the underivatized molecules. For example, the dibutyl ester of methylmalonic acid (MMA), when analyzed in positive ion mode ESI, has more favorable MS/MS spectra than the underivatized molecule, analyzed in negative ion mode ESI. In addition, the dibutyl esters of dicarboxylic acids are selectively ionized in positive ion mode ESI, whereas monocarboxylic organic acids are not ionized as efficiently, thus allowing enhancement in the specificity of detection.[36]

Matrix-assisted Laser Desorption Ionization Mass Spectrometry

MALDI (typically coupled to a TOF analyzer) has been used to analyze many different classes of compounds. Notably, it has been widely applied in discovery applications for the detection and identification of proteins and peptides (see Chapter 24). Primary limitations of MALDI include high background noise and a higher coefficient of variation, which is inherent of the MALDI ionization process. In addition, MALDI is essentially a batch-type process that does not interface with online separation processes using chromatographic techniques (e.g., HPLC, capillary electrophoresis).

One clinical application of MALDI-TOF that has proven its great clinical utility is the bacteria species identification (Chapter 22).[13,19] Identification of bacteria is performed by "fingerprinting" proteins and peptides extracted from bacterial culture. The basis of this technique is that different bacteria express unique mixtures of proteins and peptides. When samples are analyzed using MALDI-TOF, the bacteria-specific mass spectra are acquired in the 2- to 20-kDa mass range, followed by database searching and classification based on the lipid and protein mass fingerprint. In this technique, the observed mass spectral fingerprints are compared with a mass spectral library and matched to the library entries, allowing for microbial identification.[37] This technique has proven to be reliable and is widely adopted in routine clinical microbiology laboratories.

MALDI-TOF is often used to determine the identity of proteins through peptide mass fingerprinting. For example, this technique has been used to identify a large number of two-dimensional (2D) gel spots for the bacterial pathogen *Pseudomonas aeruginosa*.[38] The procedure typically involves in-gel tryptic digestion followed by accurate mass measurement of the peptides produced during the digestion. The generated mass list is then compared with the expected theoretical m/z of tryptic peptides of proteins in a database (Fig. 20.18 and Table 20.1). This procedure works best for organisms with annotated genomes; the instrumental analysis is very rapid and allows for identification of a large number of proteins in the samples.

MALDI MS has the reputation of being a nonquantitative technique; however, some progress has been made toward its use in quantitative analysis.[39] If this application becomes routine, it will have major benefits for clinical MS because the time to acquire a mass spectrum by MALDI is only a few seconds per sample; however, to achieve an adequate selectivity, off-line sample preparation will be required.

Laser diode thermal desorption (LDTD) is a related ionization technique that works on the principle of thermal desorption of a dried sample into the gas phase, followed by APCI and MS/MS detection. Methods for quantitative analysis using LDTD-MS/MS have been developed; the technique allows achieving instrumental analysis time of only a few seconds per sample.

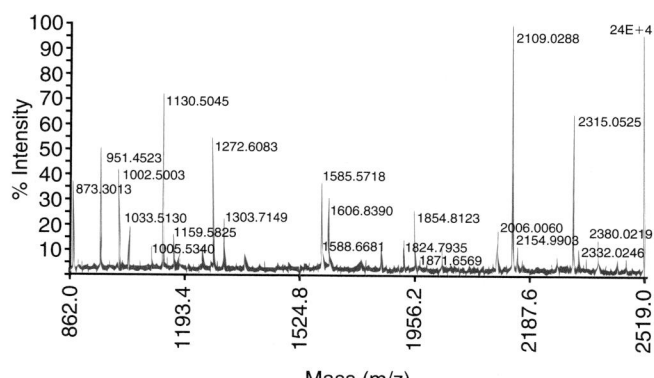

FIGURE 20.18 Example of a matrix-assisted laser desorption ionization–time-of-flight spectrum showing *m/z* of peptides generated in a tryptic digest of a spot cored from a two-dimensional sodium dodecyl sulfate polyacrylamide gel electrophoresis. The 16 most abundant *m/z* values were submitted for search against the nonredundant database. The results for this search are shown in Table 20.1.

TABLE 20.1 Example of a Report of Microbial Identification Through Peptide Mass Fingerprinting Using MALDI-TOF Mass Spectrometry

Rank	Mowse Score	# (%) Masses Matched	Protein MW (Da)/pI	Species	NCBInr.81602 Accession #	Protein Name
1	1.07e+008	14/16 (87%)	101754.9/ 9.15	*Saccharomyces cerevisiae*	6321275	(Z72685) ORF YGL163c

1.14/16 matches (87%). 101,754.9 Da, pI = 9.15. Acc. #6321275. *Saccharomyces cerevisiae*. (Z72685) ORF YGL163c.

m/z Submitted	MH⁺ Matched	Delta ppm	Start	End	Peptide Sequence	Modifications
870.4746	870.4797	−5.8732	598	606	(K) GVGGSQPLR(A)	
873.3981	873.3929	5.9793	774	779	(K) DCFIYR(F)	$C_2H_2O_2$
951.4901	951.4900	0.1050	814	821	(R) LFSSDNLR(Q)	
1002.5385	1002.5373	1.2224	515	522	(K) NFENPILR(G)	
1033.5513	1033.5543	−2.8793	46	55	(K) NTHIPPAAGR(I)	
1130.6349	1130.6322	2.4037	120	128	(R) LSHIQYTLR(R)	
1130.6349	1130.6322	2.4037	514	522	(R) KNFENPILR(G)	
1159.6039	1159.6071	−2.7957	56	67	(R) IATGSDNIVGGR(S)	
1272.6508	1272.6483	1.9865	734	746	(K) AGGCGINLIGANR(L)	$C_2H_2O_2$
1303.7573	1303.7599	−1.9457	270	280	(K) ILRPHQVEGVR(F)	
1585.7190	1585.7215	−1.5602	446	459	(K) NCNVGLMLADEGHR(L)	$C_2H_2O_2$
1606.8861	1606.9029	−10.4650	22	35	(R) LVPRPINVQDSVNR(L)	
2138.0756	2138.0704	2.4250	747	765	(R) LILMDPDWNPAADQQALAR(V)	
2315.1093	2315.0951	6.1321	401	423	(K)SSMGGGNTTVSQAIHAWAQAQGR(N)	
2388.0671	2388.0731	−2.5004	293	313	(K) DYLEAEAFNTSSEDPLKSDEK(A)	

A generated mass list is compared with theoretical tryptic masses of proteins in the database.
MH⁺, Ion formed by attachment of a proton to molecule M; *MOWSE*, MOlecular Weight SEarch method; *MW*, molecular weight; *m/z*, mass-to-charge ratio.

Inductively Coupled Plasma Mass Spectrometry

ICP-MS is used for the determination of trace and toxic elements in biological samples (see Chapters 39 and 44). In clinical laboratories, ICP-MS is used for quantification of trace elements in whole blood, urine, plasma, serum, and tissue biopsy samples. Clinical indications for analyzing biological samples for trace elements include screening and confirmation of suspected heavy metal poisoning and diagnosing/monitoring patients with metabolic disorders (e.g., Wilson disease). In some cases, toxicity depends on the presence of the metal within organic or inorganic molecules and requires determination of the concentration of the element in specific classes of molecules rather than the total concentration of the element in the sample. These applications use sample fractionation with HPLC or capillary electrophoresis to separate various metal-containing molecules before sample introduction in an ICP-MS instrument.

Proteomics and Metabolomics

The term proteomics generally refers to the large-scale studies of proteins and proteomes, but it also refers to the identification and quantification of proteins and their post-translational modifications in a given system. Proteome analysis is a powerful tool for investigating (1) biomarkers of disease, (2) antigens of pathogens, (3) drug target proteins, and (4) post-translational modifications, as well as other investigations. Protein identification and quantitation for clinical diagnostics needs are a challenging task because most of the clinically relevant proteins present in biological fluids at very low concentrations and many proteins present in various isoforms are extensively post-translationally modified (see Chapter 24).[40]

Currently, MS is routinely used to accomplish many tasks in proteomics. The most basic task is protein identification. The typical approach is known as the *bottom-up* method, whereby proteins are separated from the sample matrix and then enzymatically digested. The resulting enzymatic fragments are analyzed and used to identify proteins present in the samples.

Another approach that is used in proteomics, involves sequencing of intact proteins and is known as the *top-down* method. Top-down proteomics involves identification of proteins in complex mixtures without prior digestion of proteins into peptides. Approaches used for protein top-down characterization include extraction of the proteins from samples, sample fractionation, followed by analysis using high-resolution accurate mass MS/MS with CID, higher energy collision dissociation, and electron-transfer dissociation fragmentation. Main benefits of the top-down analysis are in the ability to detect protein isoforms, sequence variants, and proteins containing various post-translational modifications.

The term *proteomics* includes application of MS for the analysis of known protein and peptide biomarkers.[41] Some examples of mass spectrometric methods for quantitative analysis of proteins are LC-MS methods for quantitative analysis of carbohydrate-deficient transferrin, biomarker of congenital disorders of glycosylation, and marker of alcohol abuse; thyroglobulin, a marker of the recurrence of differentiated thyroid cancer,[42–45] IGF-1, marker of growth hormone status[46]; PTH, marker of hypoparathyroidism and hyperparathyroidism[47]; PTHrP, marker of hypercalcemia of malignancy[48]; monoclonal proteins, markers of monoclonal gammopathy[49]; therapeutic antibodies, for monitoring patients undergoing treatment with these biologics[50]; hepcidin, a regulator of iron status; and other protein biomarkers.

Some examples of mass spectrometric methods for qualitative analysis of proteins of clinical significance are methods for characterization of hemoglobinopathies[26]; disorders causing abnormal production or structure of the hemoglobin molecules; amyloidosis subtyping[51] for conditions characterized by extracellular deposition of misfolded proteins resulting in life-threatening organ damage; and insulin analogs, in forensic applications and doping control.

Another area in which MS plays a significant role is *metabolomics*. This scientific area involves the investigation and characterization of small molecules, including intermediates and products of metabolism, present in biological fluids under different conditions that include (1) normal homeostasis, (2) disease states, (3) stress, (4) dietary modification, (5) treatment protocols, and (6) aging. In a fashion similar to a mass spectrum, providing a fingerprint signature for a specific molecule, it has been speculated that panels of compounds identified in metabolomic studies may provide a fingerprint signature for different physiologic states.

In metabolomics studies, the detected peaks are identified by comparison with (1) known reference materials, (2) commercial or in-house developed mass spectral libraries or metabolite databases, (3) interpretation of mass spectra, or (4) ancillary techniques (e.g., nuclear magnetic resonance). As with other applications of MS, both GC-MS and LC-MS have a place in such studies.

Advantages of LC-MS in metabolomics research include the ability to detect molecular ions of substances present in the samples and the ability to analyze a wide range of polar and nonvolatile compounds. Compared with proteomic research, metabolomics faces the added difficulties in that the MS/MS spectra are more difficult to interpret and limited information is available in the existing MS/MS libraries.

Mass spectral imaging of tissue sections is another technology that has potential for clinical applications and holds great promise.[52] The most common approach is to use MALDI MS to image tissue sections. A mass spectrum is acquired at each spot on a regularly spaced array across the sample. From these data, an image is constructed for the *m/z* of interest. Such images provide a spatial map of chemical composition (e.g., peptides, lipids, small molecules) present in the sample. This technique was extended to immunohistochemical imaging by using metal-labeled antibodies and instrumental analysis performed on CyTOF instrument, an MS technique based on ICP MS and TOF-MS detection. In such methods, rare earth metal tags, conjugated to antibodies are used, allowing simultaneous multiplexed imaging of large number of targets in tissue samples.[53] However, it should be noted that, currently, mass spectral imaging is a time-consuming process because the laser beam has to raster across the tissue thousands of times and very large amounts of data need to be processed for the data analysis. At this time, this is mainly a research technique that is not used in routine diagnostic laboratories, although if technical and practical difficulties can be overcome, it has great potential in cancer diagnostics, histology, and cytology.

Practical Aspects of Mass Spectrometry: Logistics, Operations, and Quality

In many respects, the logistics, operations, quality control, and quality assurance processes for clinical MS laboratories follow well-established clinical laboratory standards and guidelines.[1,2,54] However, mass spectrometers are complex instruments and consequently, the adoption of LC-MS/MS places added demands on training, competency, and manufacturers' support beyond other well-established technologies used in clinical laboratories.

In contrast to techniques such as optical spectrophotometry, mass spectrometers tend to require more frequent troubleshooting, tuning, calibration, optimization, and daily performance verification.[4]

The term *calibration* in relation to MS is used in two distinct ways.[1,2] The first is calibration of the *m/z* scale of the instrument, usually referred to as *mass calibration*; the other is a quantitative calibration. Schedules for mass calibration vary among laboratories, types of instruments, instruments of different vendors and types of assays for which an instrument is used. In assays using high-mass-resolution/high-mass-accuracy instruments (e.g., Orbitrap, TOF-MS), frequent mass calibration and real-time mass correction are required. For applications which are less dependent on mass accuracy (quantitative analysis using quadruple mass analyzers), mass calibration is performed less frequently (e.g., monthly mass calibration, with daily verification of the calibration).

Similarly, schedules for quantitative calibration in methods for quantitative analysis may vary. For example, in some laboratories quantitative calibration is performed daily, with multiple batches of samples analyzed per day, whereas in other laboratories the calibration is performed with every batch of samples.

One advantage of MS is that the technique does not require use of highly specialized reagents (e.g., commercial kits of reagents and antibodies). Consumables are mostly generic items (e.g., solvents, common laboratory reagents, chromatographic columns, 96-well plates). This tends to buffer the laboratories from supply disruptions of specialized reagents and, in some cases, can decrease consumable costs as well. However, reagents and consumables used in the assays must be carefully selected and monitored for quality because impurities introduced from reagents and supplies may negatively affect performance of the methods. Solvent quality is of particular concern. For example, multiple studies have documented that variation in the purity of solvents from different suppliers results in a difference in ionization efficiency and cause interferences in the analysis.

Whenever possible, a quantitative method should use isotopically labeled internal standards, which typically differ from the analyte of interest by substitution of monoisotopic ions with isotope labels analogs (typically deuterium, ^{13}C or ^{15}N). However, it is not always possible to obtain isotopically labeled analogs of each target analyte, in which case a closely related chemical analog should be selected as an internal standard. One example of the use of chemical analog of the targeted compound as the internal standard is the use of 32-desmethoxyrapamycin as an internal standard in methods for quantitative analysis of the immunosuppressant drug sirolimus.[55]

MS provides several opportunities for enhancing analytical quality and therefore improving patient care. The high degree of selectivity of MS, particularly when used as a part of hyphenated techniques (GC-MS, LC-MS, LC-MS/MS, etc.), reduces the likelihood of interference compared with immunoassays or separation-based techniques (GC or LC) using nonspecific detection.

In addition to a high degree of selectivity, MS provides a means to detect the presence of interferences when they occur. In methods relying on fragmentation of the targeted analytes (either in the ion source, as in EI, or in a collision cell, as in MS/MS), the fragment ions have reproducible relative intensity. By monitoring one or more ratios of the ion fragments (or ratios of mass transitions, as in MS/MS), and by comparing these ratios to the ratios observed from authentic reference materials measured within the same run, it is possible to detect the presence of interfering compounds on a sample-by-sample basis.[32]

Accurate mass measurements are also useful for detection of interferences if one is using an instrument capable of such measurements (e.g., TOF, Orbitrap MS). To illustrate, the accurate mass of protonated cortisol ($C_{12}H_{31}O_5^+$) is 363.2166 Da, whereas the accurate mass of one of the isotope peaks of protonated molecule of the drug fenofibrate ($C_{20}H_{22}ClO_4^+$) is 363.1180 Da—a difference of 271 ppm.[56] Therefore an interference of fenofibrate (a drug used for treating patients with increased triglycerides) in a cortisol analysis would be detectable on an instrument capable of high mass resolution and high mass accuracy.

Obviously, detection of interferences by accurate mass measurement alone becomes more difficult as the mass of the interfering compound approaches that of the target compound. However, given the ability to detect interferences at a peak intensity of approximately 20% relative to the peak intensity of the targeted analyte, and assuming that a mass spectrometer is able to provide approximately 3-ppm mass accuracy, a reasonable estimate is that interferences could be detected for the compounds with $|\Delta m/z|$ greater than 30 ppm, relative to the compound of interest.

OPTIMIZATION OF INSTRUMENT CONDITIONS

When developing an MS-based method, there are many parameters, which should be optimized. This applies to both the MS and the separation method.

Selection of Mass Transitions and Operating Conditions

MRM is the most commonly used mode of data acquisition in LC-MS/MS methods for targeted analysis. MRM-based methods allow for sensitive and specific quantitation of analytes in samples with complex matrices. Typical MRM chromatograms contain one or a few peaks, which are easy to integrate, particularly if the sample preparation and the instrumental analysis have been well designed.

When developing MRM methods, it is useful to start with the identification of all analyte-specific mass transitions. The typical approach for selection and optimization of mass transitions is through infusion of solution of pure standard of the targeted compound using a syringe pump. During the infusion, the signal can be optimized by adjusting the ion source conditions, declustering potential, the ion transmission conditions, and collisional fragmentation. When ions are transported from atmospheric pressure to the vacuum region, they typically exist in the form of clusters. Application of the declustering potential during the ion focusing causes low-energy collisions, which lead to declustering of the ions.

Methods using MRM data acquisition are set up by specifying *m/z* of the precursor ion (typically the molecular ion) of the targeted molecule and the *m/z* of the molecule-specific fragments, produced by fragmentation in the collision cell. While developing a method, it is important to carefully select the analyte-specific mass transitions to be used in the method. The best sensitivity and specificity are typically achieved using high-intensity unique fragment ions, which have minimal background noise and no peaks coeluting with the analyte of interest. Use of fragment ions corresponding to the loss of water, ammonia, carbonyl (CO), and CO_2 groups (often referred to as *trivial losses*) generally should be avoided because they result in relatively nonspecific mass transitions.

The optimal values of the voltages needed for declustering the molecular ion and the ion transmission are established by scanning the voltages and finding the apex values that correspond to the maximum signal intensity. Optimization of the collision energy (CE) is accomplished by scanning the CE used for fragmentation of the molecular ion and plotting the abundances as a function of CE, a profile, called a *breakdown curve* (Fig. 20.19).

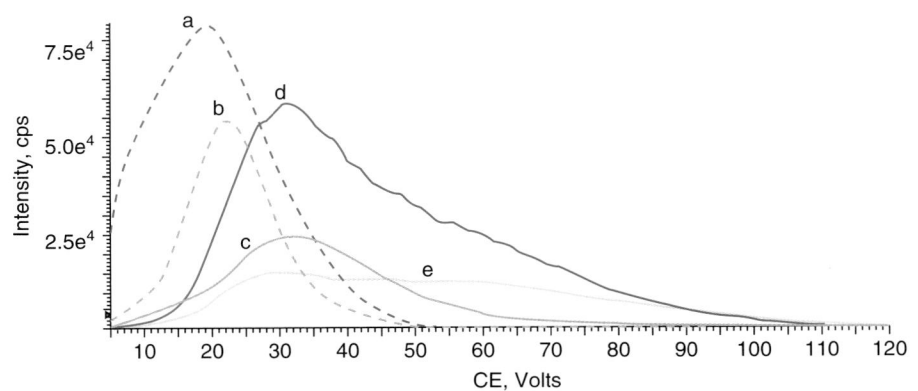

FIGURE 20.19 Breakdown curves for collision energy scans of cortisol. Curves correspond to mass transitions: *a*—*m/z* 363 → 345; *b*—*m/z* 363 → 327; *c*—*m/z* 363 → 171; *d*—*m/z* 363 → 121; *e*—*m/z* 363 → 97. *CE*, Collision energy; *cps*, counts per second.

In the majority of cases, the voltage corresponding to the apex of the breakdown curve is selected for use in the method, and this value provides the maximum signal intensity. A second advantage of operating at the apex is that slight fluctuations in the instrument conditions do not result in large changes in the signal intensity, so the instrument performance is more stable. However, on some occasions, when unresolved chromatographic peaks could interfere with the analysis, it is beneficial to select CE on the leading slope or the trailing slope of the breakdown curve (more commonly on the leading slope) to improve specificity of analysis by avoiding fragmentation of the substance which may potentially interfere with the analyte of interest. This can be useful in cases in which the breakdown curve of an MS/MS transition of a potentially interfering compound partially overlaps that of the target compound. In such cases, by operating on the slope of the breakdown curve of the selected MS/MS transition of the target compound, it could be possible to achieve a greater discrimination of the interfering substances.

In addition to evaluating breakdown curves, CE should be selected with the following principles in mind. If the CE is too low, ion fragmentation will be inefficient, and the signal intensity will be low; if the CE is too high, fragmentation can become too extensive, and the possibility of interfering peaks originating from coeluting isobaric substances may increase.

Depending on the type of ionization source used, ionizability of molecules is influenced by their volatility, solution-phase acidity (pKa), proton affinity, electronegativity, hydrophilicity/hydrophobicity, surfactant properties, solution pH, ionization energy, electron collision cross-section, and other physical and chemical properties. Of the ionization methods most commonly used in the MS applications in clinical laboratories, ESI is typically used for analysis of polar and ionizable molecules and APCI is used for nonpolar molecules. When a new method is being developed, available ionization techniques and polarity modes should be evaluated to assess effect of the conditions on the signal response and specificity of the detection.

The electrospray voltage and ion source conditions have a great effect on the ionization efficiency; the optimal voltage depends on the molecular structure, mobile phase composition, and flow rate. At higher electrospray voltages, greater fluctuation in the ionization efficiency can be observed and a larger number of impurities present in the sample may get ionized, potentially causing the loss of specificity and poor reproducibility. Therefore the lowest voltage resulting in an adequate sensitivity for the analyte is typically preferred. In general, there is a threshold voltage below which ionization is very inefficient; in cases when the ESI voltage is too high, corona discharge, leading to a greater interference potential or other undesirable effects, may occur.

Online Two-dimensional Separations

Two-dimensional chromatographic separation is a technique in which separation is performed using two HPLC columns with stationary phases having different selectivity.[44,48] In one of the configurations, the chromatographic columns are connected to a switching valve, the sample is injected in the first column, and effluent from the column is directed to waste. At the time when the targeted peak is eluted from the first column, the effluent is redirected into the second column by changing position of the switching valve, then during the column reconditioning and equilibration the switching valve

is turned back to the original position. Using this approach, chromatographic columns with complementary (orthogonal or partially orthogonal) selectivity are typically used, so that peaks that are poorly resolved or unresolved from the potential interfering substances by the first column, would be separated on the second column.

In addition to the use of different stationary phases with complementary retention mechanisms, the selectivity may be modified by selecting the optimal mobile phases and temperature for each of the separations. Some advantages of well-designed 2D separations may include greater resolving power, faster analysis time (while the separation takes place on one column, the other column could be conditioned and re-equilibrated), reduced contamination of the mass analyzer (major fraction of the effluent from the first column is directed to waste and not transferred into the second column), and ability to use for the second separation a mobile phase that is favorable for the optimal ionization efficiency. Various coupling strategies for the chromatographic columns have been described; the choice of the specific strategy is method dependent and would affect the robustness of the assay. Two-dimensional separations are more difficult to develop and troubleshoot, but in many cases the observed superior methods' performance outweigh the drawbacks.

Conventional versus Microflow Separations

As more LC-MS methods are developed, greater sensitivity and reduced sample volume are often required. This is especially true for analysis of biomarkers present in samples at very low concentrations or when there is a limited sample volume available for analysis. Other trends in modern analytical laboratories are aimed at reducing the volume of solvents used, the cost of the used mobile phase disposal, and the costs of labor.

The benefits of microflow separations in LC-MS analysis have been widely reported; they include a higher sensitivity, greater efficiency of ion sampling, reduced solvent consumption and waste, and reduced contamination of the ion source. Despite these advantages, there are relatively few microflow-based LC-MS methods used in routine laboratories. The main reasons are related to the fact that these separations historically were insufficiently robust, require greater technical expertise of the staff, and frequently cause interruptions in the workflow of a laboratory. However, recent publications on the comparison of microflow and high-flowrate traditional LC-MS/MS methods have demonstrated the robust method's performance, with up to 10-fold gain in the signal-to-noise ratios and up to 20-fold reduction in the use of solvents, as compared to the methods using traditional HPLC separations.[57] In one recent example, the analysis of thyroglobulin by microflow LC-MS/MS was shown to be more sensitive than methods using traditional HPLC separation and high-sensitivity immunoassays.[45]

ION SUPPRESSION

Ion suppression is another quality issue that should be evaluated during method development and validation.[58,59] Ion suppression is a matrix effect caused by peaks of interfering substances coeluting with the peaks of analytes targeted in an assay, which leads to reduced ionization efficiency. Substances causing ion suppression could be molecules containing highly ionizable functional groups, (ion-pairing agents, salts, lipids, surfactants, etc.), which compete with molecules of the targeted analyte for access to the surface of the droplets and/or transfer of ions of the targeted analyte to the gas phase. Phospholipids present in biological samples and impurities introduced during the sample preparation and analysis are a particular challenge because they are often present in biological samples and have been demonstrated to be major contributors to *ion suppression.*

Ion suppression may have an adverse effect on the accuracy, precision, and sensitivity of the assays, particularly if the internal standard does not perfectly coelute with the peak of the targeted analyte, in which case the internal standard and the analyte may undergo different extent of ion suppression and thus compromise accuracy and sensitivity of the quantitative measurements. This is most likely to happen in methods that use highly deuterated internal standards. Of the different types of ionization techniques used in LC-MS methods, ESI tends to be most susceptible to ion suppression. Methods using APCI are typically less prone to the effects of ion suppression, but the possibility of ion suppression in APCI should not be dismissed without verification.[58,60]

Considering that biological samples contain a large number of endogenous and exogenous compounds, with concentrations ranging over a very wide dynamic range, ion suppression should be evaluated for all new or modified methods and should be performed using a large number of neat patient samples, so as to capture the variability that may occur in the patient population. The presence of ion suppression or other deleterious matrix effects can be evaluated via several experimental protocols.

A preferred protocol for assessment of ion suppression involves postcolumn continuous infusion of a solution containing the targeted analyte into the MS detector, while analyzing samples in a native matrix prepared according to the protocol of the evaluated method. The instrumental setup includes a syringe pump connected via a tee to the column effluent (Fig. 20.20), in front of the ion source of the MS. Because the compound being tested is introduced into the ion source at a constant rate, a constant instrument response should be observed, if no ionization suppression or enhancement occurs, while analyzing biological specimens (Fig. 20.21*A*). Typically, there is suppression of the signal in the portion of the analysis that corresponds to the void volume of the HPLC column (see Fig. 20.21*B*). The void volume is that portion of a chromatographic run corresponding to the time of elution

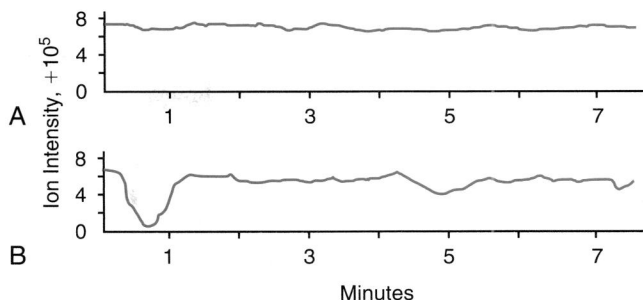

FIGURE 20.21 Chromatograms with data of an experiment on evaluation of ion suppression. **A,** Ion suppression profile corresponding to injection of a solvent. **B,** Ion suppression profile corresponding to injection of extracted plasma sample. Dips in the baseline correspond to the areas of ion suppression.

of the samples' constituents that are not retained by the stationary phase of HPLC column; typically, this is the time it takes for the mobile phase to flow through the column.

Another less commonly used approach for assessment of ion suppression involves comparison of the instrument response for injection of the targeted analyte dissolved in a solvent, and the same amount of the targeted analyte spiked into pre-extracted samples. Data corresponding to the injection of the standard in the solvent provide a relative 100% response value; data corresponding to injection of the same amount of the analyte spiked into pre-extracted samples show the effect of sample matrix (ion suppression) on MS response.

The degree of ion suppression and the recovery time to full response may vary among individual samples, and can be dependent on the sample preparation method, chromatographic column used, and LC separation conditions. Because endogenous and exogenous compounds from the specimen matrix may elute at any time during the chromatographic run, ion suppression is not limited to the column void and is not limited to the analysis time of the evaluated sample. In the case of strongly retained compounds, substances causing ion suppression may elute in subsequent injections. The observed degree of ion suppression also can be dependent on the sample volume aliquotted for the analysis, the injection volume, and the concentrations of the targeted analyte measured in the assay.

To control for ion suppression, it is highly desirable to use matrix-matched calibration standards and controls. It is important to evaluate ion suppression for all types of sample matrices (serum, plasma, urine, etc.) and sample collection tubes intended for the assay; in addition, considering the complexity of biological samples and the between-subject differences, there may be substantial fluctuations in the concentrations of the ion-suppressing species among the individual samples.

As a rule of thumb, the extent of ion suppression decreases as the sample injection volume is reduced or when the final sample injected in the instrument is diluted. This in turn favors the use of high-sensitivity mass spectrometers, which allow for lower injection volumes and the use of higher sample dilutions.

In cases when the peak of the isotope-labeled internal standard does not fully coelute with the peak of the analyte of interest (as with highly deuterated analogs of the targeted in

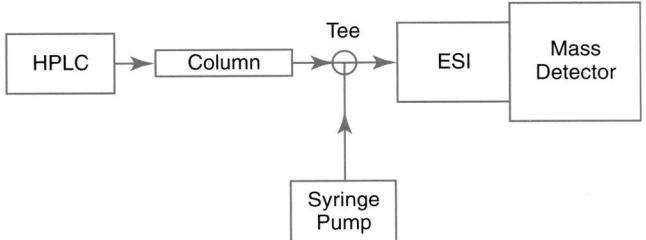

FIGURE 20.20 Diagram of postcolumn infusion for evaluation of ion suppression. Specimen extracts are injected into the high-performance liquid chromatography *(HPLC)* system. Standard of the targeted in the assay analyte is continuously infused post column, mixed with the column effluent in a tee before entering the electrospray ion source (ESI).

the analysis compound), ion suppression cannot be completely compensated by the internal standard, and this may cause significant quantitative errors in the analysis. The ^{13}C- or ^{15}N-labeled compounds are chromatographically retained identically to the unlabeled analogs and are not susceptible to this problem.

Ion suppression is not limited to HPLC-MS or ESI/APCI ion sources. For MALDI analysis, arginine-containing peptides have been reported to dominate the signal as compared to other peptides in protein digests. The presence of ionic detergents, such as Triton X-100 and Tween 20, has also been shown to cause signal suppression in MALDI experiments.

Noise Reduction Techniques

Background noise refers to the sum of electronic and chemical noise in the collected analytical data, which is independent of the analytical data signal. The presence of background noise interferes with the measurements and affects accuracy and specificity of analysis.

Reduction of chemical noise has been one of the aims for improvement since the introduction of MS as an analytical technique. This problem has long been known, and it affects virtually all ionization methods. It should be noted that "chemical noise" is caused by presence of interfering compounds which has different statistical properties than "random noise." For example, random noise can be reduced via signal averaging methods, whereas signal averaging typically does not reduce chemical noise.

Chemical noise is often dominant over electronic noise in MS. Background ions are inherent of atmospheric pressure ionization and are related to the presence of impurities in the samples and in the mobile phases, residues accumulating on the surfaces of the ion source, and in part the high efficiency of atmospheric pressure ionization. Approaches used for noise reduction include optimization of the sample preparation, enhancement of the selectivity of ionization, optimization of the declustering conditions and ion transmission, maintaining cleanliness of the ion sources and the flow path of the separation device, and use of high purity solvents and reagents used during the sample preparation and for preparing the mobile phases.

One effective way for reduction of the effect of background noise on the methods' performance is the use of MS/MS acquisition (MRM, neutral loss scan, product ion scan, and precursor ion scan), which allows substantial improvement of the detection specificity and reduction of the effects of chemical noise. Other approaches for reduction of background noise include the use of mass analyzers with high resolving power (see Fig. 20.3); use of multidimensional separations along with MS, such as ion mobility separations, FAIMS, multidimensional chromatographic separations, and use of additional stages of fragmentation (MS/MS/MS). Software-based approaches (e.g., dynamic background subtraction, active background noise reduction) also have been applied as noise reduction techniques. The software-based techniques allow for a reduction in the interference from the chemical background noise but do not affect its cause. The best approach to the reduction of chemical background noise is the use of more extensive and efficient sample cleanup, as a way of removal of potentially interfering substances prior to the instrumental analysis.

With regard to reducing background noise by using mass analyzers with high resolving power, it is important to understand the relationships among resolution, background noise (primarily chemical noise), electronic noise, and total signal level. A complete discussion of the subject is beyond the scope of this chapter, but a few general concepts can be useful to the clinical chemist without necessarily delving into all of the subtleties.

For example, TOF-MS acquires the full mass spectrum and allows for extracting from the data signal, corresponding to very narrow m/z range (Fig. 20.3). If the m/z window is significantly wider than the mass spectral peak width, the portion of the integrated signal arising from the targeted peak is independent of the peak width; however, the signal arising from chemical noise generally increases with increasing width of the data extraction m/z window. Considering the aforementioned, one would expect the chemical noise to decrease as the width of the data extraction m/z window decreases. In cases when the data extraction m/z window is much narrower than the mass spectrometric peak width, narrowing the integration window reduces chemical noise and target analyte signal nearly equally, so there is very little to be gained in terms of improving the signal-to-noise ratio by making the integration window narrower. Thus in many cases, there is an optimum operating condition wherein the optimal integration window is approximately equal to the peak width of the mass spectrometer. Fig. 20.3 illustrates use of a narrow window m/z for improving selectivity of analysis, and, as one can infer from the earlier discussion, this technique works best when using a high-resolution mass spectrometer.

POINTS TO REMEMBER

- Mass spectrometry (MS) is a highly sensitive and selective technique for analyzing a wide variety of clinically relevant analytes.
- MS relies on ionizing analytes in a sample, followed by separation of the ions according to their mass to charge ratios.
- When coupled with a separation device, such as a gas chromatograph or liquid chromatograph, the hybrid technique is well suited for the quantitative analysis of clinically relevant molecules from bodily fluids and tissues.
- The use of MS for clinical applications has led to the development of highly specific assays that can overcome many of the issues faced when using immunoassays (e.g., cross-reactivity).
- Although highly selective, MS is not immune to interferences; molecules with the same m/z (isomers and isobars) and similar fragmentation pattern may interfere with the analysis.

SELECTED REFERENCES

1. CLSI C62-A Liquid Chromatography-Mass Spectrometry Methods; Approved Guideline, C62AE. Wayne, Pennsylvania Clinical and Laboratory Standards Institute; 2014.
4. Fundamentals of Mass Spectrometry. Hiraoka K, editor. New York: Springer; 2013.
5. Fenn JB. Electrospray wings for molecular elephants (Nobel lecture). Angew Chem Int Ed Engl. 2003;42(33):3871–94.
6. Tanaka K. The origin of macromolecule ionization by laser irradiation (Nobel lecture). Angew Chem Int Ed Engl. 2003; 42(33):3860–70.
8. Rockwood AL, Palmblad M. Isotopic distributions. Methods in Molecular Biology. 2013;1007:65–99.
12. Covey TR, Thomson BA, Schneider BB. Atmospheric pressure ion sources. Mass Spectrometry Reviews. 2009;28(6):870–97.
13. Sandalakis V, Goniotakis I, Vranakis I, Chochlakis D, Psaroulaki A. Use of MALDI-TOF mass spectrometry in the battle against bacterial infectious diseases: recent achievements and future perspectives. Expert Rev Proteomics. 2017;14(3):253–67.
16. Mbughuni MM, Jannetto PJ, Langman LJ. Mass Spectrometry Applications for Toxicology. EJIFCC. 2016;27(4):272–87.
21. Feider CL, Krieger A, DeHoog RJ, Eberlin LS. Ambient Ionization Mass Spectrometry: Recent Developments and Applications. Anal Chem. 2019;91(7):4266–90.
28. Yost RA, Boyd RK. Tandem mass spectrometry: quadrupole and hybrid instruments. Methods Enzymol. 1990;193:154–200.
31. Kushnir MM, Rockwood AL, Nelson GJ, Yue B, Urry FM. Assessing analytical specificity in quantitative analysis using tandem mass spectrometry. Clinical Biochemistry. 2005;38(4):319–27.
32. Wu AH, Gerona R, Armenian P, French D, Petrie M, Lynch KL. Role of liquid chromatography-high-resolution mass spectrometry (LC-HR/MS) in clinical toxicology. Clinical Toxicology (Phila). 2012;50(8):733–42.
33. Chace DH. Mass spectrometry in newborn and metabolic screening: historical perspective and future directions. Journal of Mass Spectrometry. 2009;44(2):163–70.
36. Sandrin TR, Demirev PA. Characterization of microbial mixtures by mass spectrometry. Mass Spectrometry Reviews. 2018;37(3):321–49.
40. Hoofnagle AN, Wener MH. The fundamental flaws of immunoassays and potential solutions using tandem mass spectrometry. J Immunol Methods. 2009;347(1–2):3–11.
41. Hoofnagle AN, Becker JO, Wener MH, Heinecke JW. Quantification of thyroglobulin, a low-abundance serum protein, by immunoaffinity peptide enrichment and tandem mass spectrometry. Clinical Chemistry. 2008;54(11):1796–804.
42. Clarke NJ, Zhang Y, Reitz RE. A novel mass spectrometry-based assay for the accurate measurement of thyroglobulin from patient samples containing antithyroglobulin autoantibodies. J Investig Med. 2012;60(8):1157–63.
43. Kushnir MM, Rockwood AL, Roberts WL, Abraham D, Hoofnagle AN, Meikle AW. Measurement of thyroglobulin by liquid chromatography-tandem mass spectrometry in serum and plasma in the presence of antithyroglobulin autoantibodies. Clinical Chemistry. 2013;59(6):982–90.
45. Bystrom CE, Sheng S, Clarke NJ. Narrow mass extraction of time-of-flight data for quantitative analysis of proteins: determination of insulin-like growth factor-1. Analytical Chemistry. 2011;83(23):9005–10.
57. Matuszewski BK, Constanzer ML, Chavez-Eng CM. Strategies for the assessment of matrix effect in quantitative bioanalytical methods based on HPLC-MS/MS. Anal Chem. 2003;75(13):3019–30.

Sample Preparation for Mass Spectrometry*

David A. Wells

ABSTRACT

Background

Biological samples such as blood, plasma, serum, and urine contain contaminants that are not suitable for direct analysis and must be removed before chromatographic separation and detection by mass spectrometry. This chapter discusses the classic sample preparation techniques performed in drug analysis laboratories in clinical and research settings and introduces high-throughput applications for improved efficiency.

Content

The general techniques discussed are dilution, centrifugation, sonication, and homogenization. Separation techniques discussed are filtration and ultrafiltration, dialysis and microdialysis, desalting, buffer exchange, enzymatic hydrolysis, and acid-base digestion. Protein precipitation is the precipitation technique discussed. Enrichment techniques described consist of evaporation, solvent exchange, and derivatization. Extraction techniques reviewed are liquid-liquid extraction, solid-supported liquid-liquid extraction, salt-assisted liquid-liquid extraction, and solid-phase extraction (offline and online sample processing). The chromatographic techniques discussed include column-switching (single and dual column modes) for turbulent flow chromatography, restricted access media, monolithic columns, and immunoaffinity extraction. The evolving techniques described are dried blood spots, capillary microsampling, and tissue imaging.

---

*The full version of this chapter is available electronically on ExpertConsult.com.

MALDI-TOF Mass Spectrometry Applications in Infectious Diseases*

Phillip Heaton and Robin Patel[a]

ABSTRACT

Background

Matrix-assisted laser desorption/ionization time-of-flight mass spectrometry (MALDI-TOF MS) is a powerful tool in the clinical microbiology laboratory, enabling accurate identification of bacteria, fungi, and mycobacteria grown in culture. First adopted in some European microbiology laboratories, its ease of use, accuracy, rapid turnaround time, and low cost have led to it becoming standard of care in clinical microbiology laboratories around the world.

Content

This chapter briefly discusses the history of MALDI-TOF MS leading to its commercialization and adoption in clinical microbiology laboratories. Identification of aerobic and anaerobic organisms, as well as mycobacteria and fungi, with a focus on the US Food and Drug administration (FDA)-approved/cleared platforms, is discussed. Additional applications, such as direct identification from blood cultures are reviewed as is implementation of MALDI-TOF MS into routine laboratory workflow.

---

*The full version of this chapter is available electronically on ExpertConsult.com.
[a]This chapter expands upon the previous review: Patel R. *Clin Chem* 2015;61:100–111, with permission.

Development and Validation of Small Molecule Analytes by Liquid Chromatography-Tandem Mass Spectrometry*

Russell P. Grant and Brian A. Rappold

ABSTRACT

Background

The application of liquid chromatography coupled to tandem mass spectrometry (LC-MS/MS) represents one of the most compelling opportunities for advancements in human health through the combination of reference measurement procedure capabilities, broad chemical coverage, and a rich history in support of drug development from the 1990s onward. Clinical application of these technologies has begun to gather pace in many laboratories, with diverse applications ranging from expanded newborn screening to identification of emerging toxicants. The promise of these technologies is vast and the need is palpable; however, the journey can be exacting. Perhaps somewhat unique among analytical techniques, LC-MS/MS assay development and validation requires significant knowledge of a number of specialties: a mastery of chemistry (sample preparation, chromatography, ionization), physics (ion manipulation), engineering principles (automation, order of experiments, programming), and mathematics (data reduction and interpretation) applied to questions of a biological origin (normal, disease, metabolism).

Content

This chapter provides a stepwise roadmap for systematically developing and validating an LC-MS/MS assay for small molecule analytes. Starting from first principles (i.e., salt correction in gravimetric weighing), each component of the LC-MS/MS assay (mass spectrometer tuning, ionization enhancements, chromatography, extraction) is detailed with best-practice experiments for development and data reduction techniques to fulfill performance goals. After refinement of each component of the assay, prevalidation experiments are described to enable efficient execution of validation. Finally, an array of validation guidance documents is reduced to a coherent process for burden of proof.

---

*The full version of this chapter is available electronically on ExpertConsult.com.

Proteomics*

Andrew N. Hoofnagle and Cory Bystrom

ABSTRACT

Background
Clinical proteomics has traditionally referred to experiments that attempt to discover novel biomarkers for disease diagnosis, prognosis, or therapeutic management by using tools that measure the abundance of hundreds or thousands of proteins in a single sample. These discovery experiments began with protein electrophoresis, particularly two-dimensional (2D) gel electrophoresis, and have evolved into workflows that rely very heavily on mass spectrometry (MS). Using the workflows developed for discovery proteomics, clinical laboratories have developed quantitative assays for proteins in human samples that solve many of the issues associated with the measurement of proteins by immunoassay. This technology is changing clinical research and is poised to significantly transform protein measurements used in patient care.

Content
This chapter begins with the history of clinical proteomics, with a special emphasis on 2D gel electrophoresis of serum and plasma proteins. It then describes discovery techniques that use MS, including data-dependent acquisition and data-independent acquisition. It finishes with a discussion of targeted quantitative proteomic methods, both bottom-up (proteolysis-assisted) and top-down (intact) as replacement methodologies for immunoassays and Western blotting. Special attention is paid to peptide selection, denaturation and digestion, peptide and protein enrichment, internal standards, and calibration.

---

*The full version of this chapter is available electronically on ExpertConsult.com.

Enzyme and Rate Analysis*

Mauro Panteghini and Ilenia Infusino[a]

ABSTRACT

Background

Enzymes are biological catalysts that can be used in the diagnosis and monitoring of disease and their remarkable properties make them sensitive indicators of pathologic change.

Metabolism can be regarded as an integrated series of enzymatic reactions and some diseases as a derangement of the physiologic pattern of metabolism. Many enzymes exist in multiple forms, and differences in their properties help in differentiating them and understanding organ-specific pathophysiology. Genetically determined variations in enzyme structure among individuals are used to account for such characteristics as differences in sensitivity to drugs and differences in metabolism that manifest as hereditary metabolic diseases.

Content

The properties and mechanism of action of enzymes that influence the specificity and sensitivity of these proteins and enables them to be used in disease management are described. In addition, the existence of multiple forms of some enzymes provides opportunities to increase the diagnostic specificity and sensitivity of enzyme assays in body fluids. The principles of enzyme kinetics are described, as well as how these properties are affected by activators and inhibitors. Kinetic properties are used to develop optimal conditions for measuring catalytic concentrations of enzymes and standardization approaches in order to achieve comparable results in clinical samples have been proposed. Finally, the use of enzymes as biological reagents in the measurement of metabolites and as indicator reactions in many immunoassays is mentioned.

*The full version of this chapter is available electronically on ExpertConsult.com.
[a]The authors gratefully acknowledge the original contributions of R. Bais on which portions of this chapter are based.

Immunochemical Techniques

Jason Y. Park and Khushbu Patel[a]

ABSTRACT

Background
Immunoassay is a powerful qualitative and quantitative analytical technique used to detect and measure a wide range of clinically important analytes. The extreme sensitivity and specificity of immunoassays have allowed detection and quantitation of analytes present at very low concentrations not easily measured by other analytical techniques.

Content
This chapter describes the scope of immunologic assays, including the basics of antigen-antibody binding, antibody production, and nonantibody binding agents (e.g., aptamers, molecularly imprinted polymers, boronates). Qualitative methods described include the precipitin reaction, the agglutination reaction, passive gel diffusion, immunoelectrophoresis (IEP; crossed and counterimmunoelectrophoresis [CIE]), immunofixation, blotting (Western and dot blotting), and cell- and tissue-based immunochemical techniques. Quantitative methods include radial immunodiffusion (RID), electroimmunoassay, turbidimetric and nephelometric assays, surface plasmon resonance–based immunoassay, and labeled immunochemical assays. Important aspects of the latter assay category are considered, including methodologic principles (competitive versus noncompetitive and heterogeneous versus homogeneous immunochemical assays), and analytical and functional sensitivity. Important types of labeled immunoassays are outlined, including radioimmunoassay, enzyme immunoassay (e.g., enzyme-linked immunosorbent assay, enzyme multiplied immunoassay technique, cloned enzyme donor immunoassay, fluoroimmunoassay [e.g., fluorescence resonance energy transfer]), phosphor immunoassay, chemiluminescence and bioluminescence immunoassay, electrochemiluminescence immunoassay, magnetic particle immunoassay, immuno–polymerase chain reaction, bio-barcode immunoassay, and digital immunoassay. Multiplexed immunoassays based on distinguishable labels and location of a solid support (e.g., protein microarray) are illustrated, as well as simplified immunoassays designed for point-of-care applications.

Immunologic assays are prone to interferences, and the scope of these interferences is described and exemplified (e.g., hook effect, false-negative or false-positive results caused by anti–animal immunoglobulin antibodies).

Immunochemical reactions form the basis of a diverse range of sensitive and specific clinical assays. In a typical immunochemical analysis, an antibody is used as a reagent to detect an antigen of interest. The exquisite specificity and high affinity of antibodies for their antigens, coupled with the ability of antibodies to cross-link antigens, allow the identification and quantitation of specific substances by a variety of methods. The principles of the methods most commonly used in the clinical laboratory are discussed in this chapter. This introduction is intended to acquaint the reader with the structure and function of antibodies (immunoglobulins) in relation to their use as reagents in immunoanalysis.

BASIC CONCEPTS

The binding of antibodies and their complementary antigens forms the basis of all immunochemical techniques.

Antibodies

Antibodies are immunoglobulins capable of binding specifically to a wide array of natural and synthetic antigens, including proteins, carbohydrates, nucleic acids, lipids, and other molecules. Immunoglobulins consist of five general classes designated as immunoglobulin (Ig)G, IgA, IgM, IgD, and IgE. IgG is used most commonly in immunochemical reagents. A schematic diagram of the IgG molecule is shown in Fig. 26.1. IgG is a glycoprotein (molecular weight [MW], 158,000 Da) composed of two heavy (γ) and two light (κ or γ) chains joined by disulfide bonds. Each chain (H or L) is the product of three (L) or four (H) distinct gene segments. These are the constant (C), joining (J), diversity (D), and variable (V) genes that undergo combinatorial joining during B cell development. Several hundred germline V genes, 5 to 10 J genes, 15 D genes (H chain only), and a single C gene have been identified for each heavy or light chain class. During B cell development, the V, D, and J (H chain) or V and J (L chain) undergo random rearrangement and splicing, and this recombined product is then spliced to the constant region gene. This combinatorial diversity, along with somatic mutations that occur at the splicing sites, generates a tremendous

[a]The authors gratefully acknowledge the contributions by Drs. Gregory Buffone and Larry Kricka, on which portions of this chapter are based.

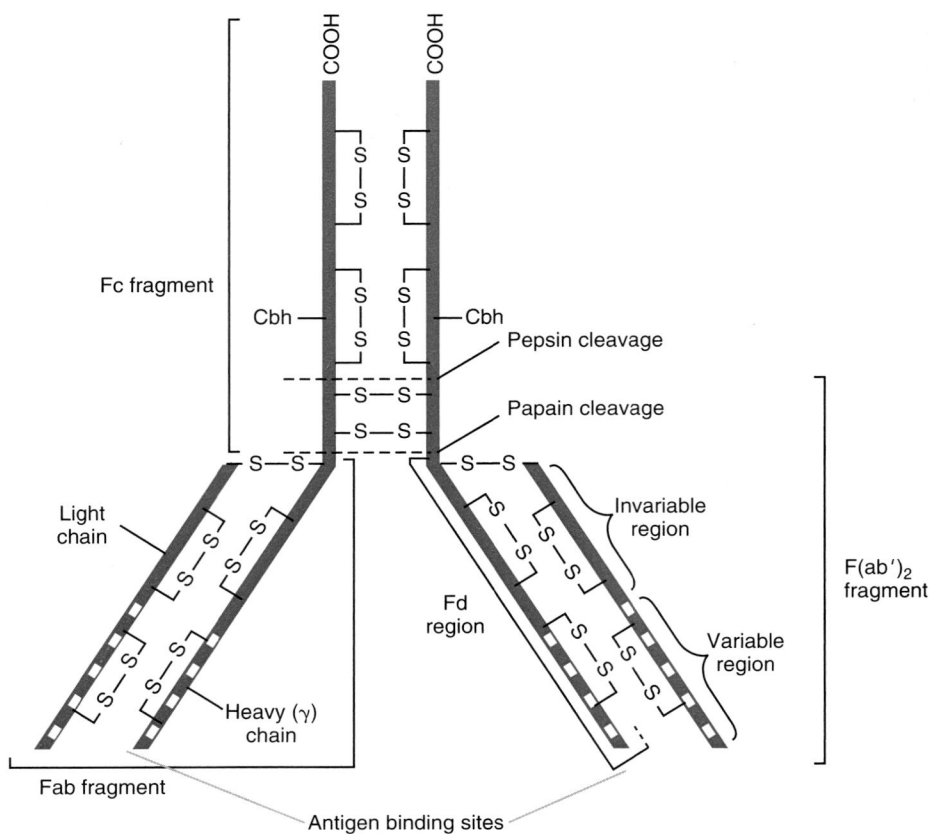

FIGURE 26.1 Schematic diagram of immunoglobulin (Ig)G antibody molecule showing carbohydrate (Cbh), disulfide bonds (—S—S—), and major fragments produced by proteolytic enzyme treatment (F[ab′]₂, Fc, Fab, Fd).

diversity of antibody specificities. When a B-cell clone expressing a particular antibody specificity on its surface is selected by an antigen, it expands and differentiates into a plasma cell that secretes the specific antibody.

The variable amino acid sequence at the amino terminal end (~105 amino acids) of each chain determines the antigenic specificity of the particular antibody. Each unique variable region is a product of a single plasma cell line or clone. A complex antigen is capable of eliciting a multiplicity of antibodies with different specificities that are derived from different cell lines. Antibodies derived in this manner are termed *polyclonal* and exhibit diverse specificities in their reactivity with the immunogen. Each unique region of the antigen molecule that will bind a complementary antibody is termed an *epitope* (antigenic determinant). See Chapter 31 for additional information.

Immunogens

An immunogen is a protein or a substance coupled to a carrier that, when introduced into a foreign host, is capable of inducing the formation of an antibody in the host. The antibody produced may be circulating (humoral) or tissue bound (cellular).

A hapten is a small, chemically defined determinant that, when conjugated to an immunogenic carrier, stimulates the synthesis of antibody specific for the hapten. It is capable of binding an antibody but cannot by itself stimulate an immune response.

Continued stimulation by an immunogen results in increased production of immunoglobulins of different types and of high-affinity binding characteristics for antigens. After the first exposure to an immunogen, a latent period (induction) occurs during which no antibody is present in serum; this period may last from 5 to 10 days.

The strength or energy of interaction between the antibody and the antigen is described by two terms. Affinity refers to the thermodynamic quantity defining the energy of interaction of a single antibody-combining site and its corresponding epitope on the antigen. The affinity can be influenced by thermodynamic factors such as pH and temperature. Avidity refers to the overall strength of binding of an antibody and its antigen and includes the sum of all the individual binding affinities of all the combining sites on the antibody. The avidity is also dependent on the valency and structural arrangement of the antibody and antigen. For example, IgG has two antigen-binding sites, whereas IgM has 10 antigen-binding sites per antibody molecule. For polyclonal antibodies, affinity and avidity are difficult to determine primarily because of the diversity of the antibody population.

Polyclonal antiserum is raised in an animal host in response to immunogen administration. In contrast, monoclonal antibodies are produced in a very different manner and represent the product of a single clone or plasma cell line, rather than a heterogeneous mixture of antibodies produced by many plasma cell clones in response to immunization. Monoclonal antibodies are currently widely used as reagents in immunoassay techniques.[1] The usual method of production of monoclonal antibodies involves fusing antibody-producing plasma cells from the spleens or lymph nodes of immunized mice with a murine myeloma cell line from tissue culture.

Because of the unique ability of a monoclonal antibody to react with a single epitope on a multivalent antigen, the majority of monoclonal antibodies will not cross-link and precipitate macromolecular antigens. Consequently, monoclonal antibodies have not found broad applicability in traditional precipitin methods. A practical advantage of using monoclonal antibodies is that two different antibody specificities can be combined in a single incubation step. A solid-phase antibody specific for a unique epitope and another labeled antibody specific for a different epitope can react with an antigen in a single step. This eliminates the incubating and washing steps that usually would be required for polyclonal antibodies.

Phage display technology provides an in vitro approach for producing antibodies (single-chain Fv fragments, Fab fragments, and whole antibody molecules) that mimic the immune system but do not require B-cell immortalization. V genes coding for the heavy- and light-chain variable domains of immunoglobulin isolated from lymphocytes are amplified by the polymerase chain reaction (PCR) and ligated into a filamentous bacteriophage vector to form combinatorial libraries of V_H and V_L genes. Individual bacteriophages display copies of a specific antibody on their surface, and the phage library can be screened for the antibody of a defined specificity using immobilized antigen ("panning"). Large libraries displaying antibodies formed from more than 10^{12} different V_H and V_L combinations can be constructed; this provides a rich source of antibodies with high affinity.

ANTIGEN-ANTIBODY BINDING

Binding Forces

The strength of the binding of an antigen to an antibody depends on several forces acting cooperatively. These include van der Waals-London dipole-dipole interaction, hydrophobic interaction, and ionic coulombic bonding.[2]

Van der Waals-London Dispersion Forces

Van der Waals-London binding is caused by the attraction between atoms when they are brought together in close proximity. These interactions are basically electrostatic and are applicable to polarizable, noncharged molecules whose structure allows the electron cloud around the molecule to be distorted by outside forces in such a way that a transient charge separation (dipole) is produced. These forces operate over short distances (4 to 6 nm) and are more significant for larger molecules. Because polarizability varies inversely with temperature, the attractive force is inversely proportional to the temperature.

Hydrophobic Interaction

Hydrophobic interactions result because the association of nonpolar groups is energetically favored in aqueous or other polar solutions. In proteins, hydrophobic interactions bend and fold a molecule in a way that brings nonpolar groups inside to the less polar interior; polar groups are oriented outside toward the more polar aqueous environment. Thus hydrophobic bonding forms an interior, hydrophobic protein core, in which most hydrophobic side chains can closely associate and weakly bind. Hydrophobic interaction enhances or stabilizes antigen-antibody binding but is not necessarily the major force in such binding.

Coulombic Bonds

Coulombic bonding results from the attraction between charged groups on the antigen and the antibody, primarily carboxylate (COO^-) and ammonium (NH_4^+). The attraction between the charged groups is greatest in a medium with a low dielectric constant caused by reduced interaction of the solvent or other solute (salts) with the macromolecular ions. In a medium of high dielectric constant (aqueous solutions containing added salt), a diffuse double layer of charged particles will tend to shield the attraction of the charged species in the reactive sites of the antigen and antibody. This inhibition under certain circumstances can considerably reduce the binding constant for many antigen-antibody systems.

Given these forces, one would predict that changing pH, temperature, and ionic strength of the reaction medium should influence the binding of antigen and antibody. However, given a lower and upper limit of pH of 6.0 and 8.0 and an incubation temperature between 25 and 35°C, these variables have only minimal effect on the rate of association and immune complex formation.[3] However, extremes in pH (<4.0 and >8.0) can cause inhibition of binding or dissociation of already formed antigen-antibody complexes. In addition, changes in ionic strength will produce a significant effect on the rate of binding of antigen and antibody. This concept is studied further in the following sections.

Reaction Mechanism

The binding of antigen to antibody is not static but is an equilibrium reaction that proceeds in three phases. The initial reaction (phase 1) of a multivalent antigen (Ag_n) and a bivalent antibody (Ab) occurs very rapidly in comparison with subsequent growth of the complexes (phase 2) and is depicted by the following equation:

$$Ag_n + Ab \underset{k_{-1}}{\overset{k_1}{\rightleftharpoons}} Ag_n Ab \underset{k_{-2}}{\overset{k_2}{\rightleftharpoons}} Ag_a Ab_b \qquad (26.1)$$

where $k_1 >> k_2$, n is the number of epitopes per molecule, and a and b are the numbers of antigen and antibody molecules per complex. Phase 3 of the reaction involves precipitation of the complex after a critical size is reached. The speed of these reactions depends on electrolyte concentration, pH, and temperature and on antigen structure and antibody class and the binding affinity of the antibody. The concentration of sodium chloride (NaCl) is important, and in most cases saline (NaCl, 0.15 mol/L) is used. Higher concentrations of NaCl can lead to smaller amounts of precipitate; this is due not to increased solubility of the antigen-antibody complex, but to an equilibrium shift causing a given amount of antigen to combine with smaller amounts of antibody. Decreasing the NaCl concentration can lead to increased precipitation of other proteins.

It is best to use dilute Ab and Ag solutions for determining the influence of such factors as (1) ionic species, (2) ionic strength, and (3) pH. Use of dilute solutions slows the growth of antigen-antibody complexes; this results in more stable and homogeneous complexes.

Factors Influencing Binding

Factors that influence the strength of binding between an antigen and an antibody include ion species, ionic strength, and polymers used in the solution.

Ion Species and Ionic Strength Effects

Cationic salts produce an inhibition of the binding of antibody with a cationic hapten.[4] The order of inhibition by various cations is cesium (Cs^+) > rubidium (Rb^+) > ammonium (NH_4^+) > potassium (K^+) > sodium (Na^+) > lithium (Li^+). This order corresponds to the decreasing ionic radius and the increasing radius of hydration. Similar results are observed with anionic haptens and anionic salts. For example, the order of inhibition of binding for anionic salts is thiocyanate (CNS^-) > nitrate (NO_3^-) > iodide (I^-) > bromide (Br^-) > chloride (Cl^-) > fluoride (F^-), which again is in the order of decreasing ionic radius and increasing radius of hydration. If the competition theory as suggested by these experiments is correct, the degree of inhibition would be expected to be a concentration-dependent phenomenon, and indeed the rate of formation of immune complexes is slower in normal saline (NaCl, 0.15 mol/L) than the same reaction carried out in deionized water. Given the previous observation, F^- should be the anion of choice for immunochemical reaction buffers. In fact, F^- does provide a modest improvement over Cl^-, but the advantage is so small that laboratories rarely substitute toxic fluoride ion for innocuous chloride ion in buffer solutions.

Polymer Effect

In general, the solubility of a protein in the presence of different linear polymers is inversely proportional to the MW of the polymer (i.e., the higher the MW of the polymer, the lower is the solubility of the protein). For example, in the presence of Dextran 500, the solubility of α-crystalline < fibrinogen < γ-globulin < albumin << tyrosine.[5] Laurent thus proposed a steric exclusion mechanism to explain the effects of polymers on protein solubility. Assuming a fixed total volume (V_T) of solvent being occupied by both polymer and protein and defining the volume occupied by polymer as V_E (excluded volume; i.e., volume not accessible to proteins) and the volume occupied by protein as V', then the relation

$$V_T = V' + V_E \qquad (26.2)$$

implies that any increase in V_E caused by an increase in number or size of polymer molecules forces a decrease in V' and an effective increase in the concentration of protein molecules. Hence, as V_E is increased the effective protein concentration is increased, the probability of collision and self-association of protein molecules is increased, and large insoluble aggregates are formed.

Studies have provided support for the steric exclusion model[6] and have demonstrated that (1) the composition of the immune complex formed is not affected by the presence of a polymer; (2) no complex is formed between the polymer and the antigen, antibody, or immune complex; (3) the polymer effect depends on the MW of both antigen and polymer; and (4) the use of polymer in a reaction mixture can increase the precipitation of an immune complex with low-avidity antibody. Addition of polymer to a mixture of antigen and antibody causes a notable increase in the rate of immune complex growth, especially during the early phase of the reaction. Numerous polymer species have been tested (e.g., polyethylene glycol [PEG], dextran) for applications in immunochemical methods. The most desirable characteristics of the polymer are high MW, a high degree of linearity (minimal branching), and high aqueous solubility. Most investigators have found the polymer PEG 6000, in concentrations of 3 to 5 g/dL to be most useful in promoting immune complex formation.

Types of Reactions

Types of antigen-antibody reactions that are of analytical importance include the precipitin reaction and those noted at a solid-liquid interface.

Precipitin Reaction

If the number of antibody-combining sites is notably greater than the antigen-epitope sites ([Ab] >> [Ag]), then antigen-binding sites are quickly saturated by antibodies before cross-linking can occur, along with the formation of small insoluble antigen-antibody complexes (Fig. 26.2A). When an antibody is in moderate excess (i.e., [Ab] > [Ag]), the probability of cross-linking of Ag by Ab is more likely and hence large insoluble complex formation is favored (see Fig. 26.2B). When [Ag] is in great excess, large complexes would be less probable (see Fig. 26.2C). This model describes the results observed when antigens and antibodies are mixed in various concentration ratios. The curve shown in Fig. 26.3 is a schematic diagram of the classic precipitin curve. Although the concentration of total antibody is constant, the concentration of free antibody $[Ab]_f$ (i.e., not bound to antigen) and free antigen $[Ag]_f$ varies throughout the range for any given Ag/Ab ratio. A low Ag/Ab ratio exists in A of see Fig. 26.3 (zone of antibody excess). Under these conditions, $[Ab]_f$ exists in solution but $[Ag]_f$ does not. As total antigen increases, the size of the immune complexes increases up to equivalence (see Fig. 26.3B), in which little or no $[Ab]_f$ or $[Ag]_f$ exists. This is the zone of maximum immune complex size. This equivalence zone does not represent a ratio of exact molar equivalence of reactants but is the optimal combining ratio for cross-linking in the particular system under evaluation. As Ag/Ab increases (see Fig. 26.3C), the immune complex size will decrease and $[Ag]_f$ will increase (zone of antigen excess). No $[Ab]_f$ should exist in this area of the curve. However, for a given Ag/Ab ratio, the population of immune complexes formed at equilibrium will be heterogeneous with respect to size and composition.

Reactions at a Solid-Liquid Interface

If the antigen or antibody of interest is bound to a solid phase such as a synthetic particle (polystyrene or cellulose), the protein will exist in a microenvironment that is different from that of a protein in free solution. Water surrounding the protein is more highly ordered near the surface of the solid phase, and the condition that results is more favorable for van der Waals-London dispersion forces and coulombic bonding. This situation favors the formation of both low- and

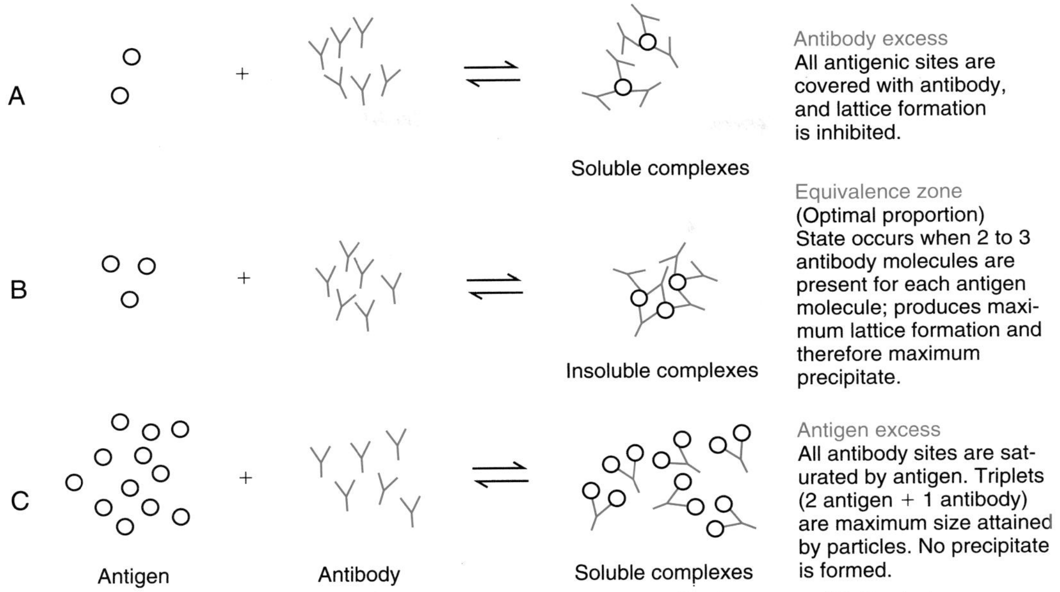

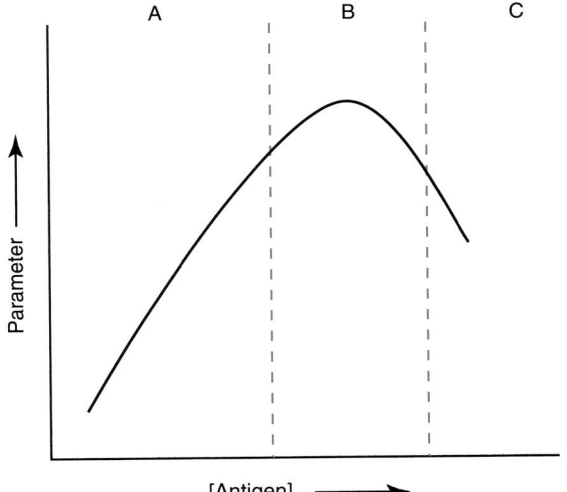

FIGURE 26.2 Schematic diagram for precipitin reaction. (A) Antibody excess. (B) Equivalence zone. (C) Antigen excess.

Antibody excess
All antigenic sites are covered with antibody, and lattice formation is inhibited.

Equivalence zone
(Optimal proportion) State occurs when 2 to 3 antibody molecules are present for each antigen molecule; produces maximum lattice formation and therefore maximum precipitate.

Antigen excess
All antibody sites are saturated by antigen. Triplets (2 antigen + 1 antibody) are maximum size attained by particles. No precipitate is formed.

FIGURE 26.3 Schematic diagram of precipitin curve illustrating zones of antibody excess (A), equivalence (B), and antigen excess (C). The parameter measured may be the quantity of protein precipitated, light scattering, or another measurable parameter. Antibody concentration is held constant in this example.

high-avidity antigen-antibody complexes and hence can provide lower detection limits for analytical applications.

Because of the exquisite specificity and the high affinity of antibodies for specific antigens, thousands of immunoassays have been developed to detect and measure a wide variety of biological analytes. In the next two sections, qualitative and quantitative immunotechniques are discussed.

QUALITATIVE METHODS

Various types of immunotechniques have been used for qualitative purposes; these include passive gel diffusion, IEP, and Western and dot blotting.

Passive Gel Diffusion

Many qualitative and quantitative immunochemical methods are performed in a semisolid medium, such as agar or agarose. The primary advantage of using a gelatinous medium is that visualization of precipitin bands is allowed for qualitative and quantitative evaluation of the reaction. Antigen-to-antibody ratio, salt concentration, and polymer enhancement have the same influence on the antigen-antibody reaction in gels that they have on reactions in solution.

The initial concentration of antigen and antibody is critical. Each molecule in the system will achieve a unique concentration gradient with time. When the leading fronts of antigen and antibody diffusion overlap, the reaction will begin, but formation of a precipitin line will not occur until moderate antibody excess is achieved (Fig. 26.3B). A precipitin band may form and be dissolved many times by an incoming antigen before equilibrium is established and the position of the precipitin band becomes stable. Because heavier molecules diffuse more slowly, the position of the precipitin band is in part a function of the molecular masses of both antigen and antibody. The precipitin band acts as a specific barrier; neither specific antigen nor antibody can penetrate without being precipitated by the other, but unrelated molecules can cross the band of precipitation freely. Basic approaches to passive diffusion include simple diffusion and double diffusion. With simple diffusion, a concentration gradient is established for only a single reactant. Single immunodiffusion usually depends on diffusion of an antigen into agar impregnated with antibody. A quantitative technique based on this principle is RID, which is discussed later. The second approach is double diffusion, in which a concentration gradient is established for both reactants (antigen and antibody).

Double immunodiffusion in two dimensions is a historical immunotechnique known as the Ouchterlony method. It allows direct comparison of two or more test materials and provides a simple method for determining whether the

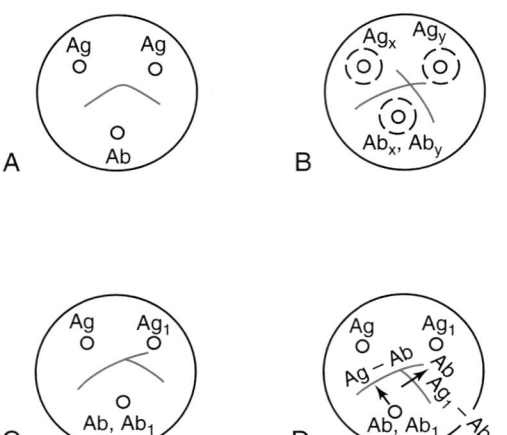

FIGURE 26.4 Double immunodiffusion in two dimensions by the Ouchterlony technique. (A) Reaction of identity; (B) reaction of nonidentity; (C) reaction of partial identity; (D) scheme for spur formation. *Ab,* Antibody; *Ag,* antigen.

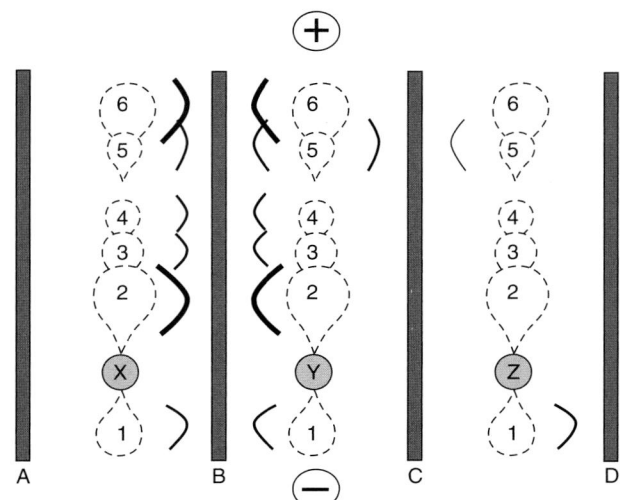

FIGURE 26.5 Configuration for immunoelectrophoresis. Samples fill the circular wells (X, Y, Z) punched into the agar and/or agarose gel. Electrophoresis separates the proteins in the sample. The six separated proteins of interest are indicated by the dashed lines. The vertical troughs (A, B, C, D) are loaded with antisera and the gel is incubated. Trough A is a negative control that does not contain relevant antibodies. Trough B contains antibodies to all six proteins. Trough C contains antibodies only specific for protein 5. Trough D contains antibodies only specific for protein 1. The precipitin lines are indicated by the solid curved lines of varying thickness.

antigens in the test specimens are identical, cross-reactive, or nonidentical.

The simplest method uses an agar dish or slide with holes cut as shown in Fig. 26.4. When the same antigen is in adjacent wells, the lines of precipitation fuse and are continuous—this is a reaction of identity (see Fig. 26.4A). When the precipitin bands cross each other, this is a reaction of nonidentity (see Fig. 26.4B); if the two antigens are related but are not identical, a reaction of partial identity is observed (see Fig. 26.4C). Here the cardinal point is that the precipitate serves as a barrier that does not block unrelated diffusing reactants. As shown in see Fig. 26.4D, when the two related antigens Ag and Ag_1 are in separate wells and the respective antibodies, Ab and Ab_1, are in the third well, an AgAb precipitate forms on one side and blocks further diffusion of Ab from the antibody well. However, on the other side, the Ag_1Ab_1 precipitate does not stop Ab from migrating further and forming an AgAb spur.

Note that a negative reaction does not necessarily imply absence of antibody or antigen. A negative reaction can result from using amounts of material too small for the detection limit of the method, or the antibody may be nonprecipitating.

Immunoelectrophoresis

If several antigens of interest exist in a solution (e.g., spinal fluid or serum), the various protein species can be separated and identified by IEP. This technique has been used extensively for the study of antigen mixtures and evaluation of the specificity of antiserum.[7,8]

The procedure is performed using an agarose gel medium poured onto a thin plastic sheet. The sample to be analyzed is placed in a reservoir in the gel, and an electrical field is applied across the gel surface. During electrophoresis, the proteins in the serum are separated according to their electrophoretic mobilities (Fig. 26.5). After electrophoresis, an antiserum against the protein of interest is placed in a trough parallel and adjacent to the electrophoresed sample. Simultaneous diffusion of the antigen from the separated sample and the antibody from the trough leads to the formation of precipitin arcs, whose shape and position are characteristic of

individual separated proteins within the specimen. By comparison with a known control separated on the same plate, individual proteins can be tentatively identified.

Crossed Immunoelectrophoresis

This technique, also known as two-dimensional IEP, is a variation of IEP in which electrophoresis is also used in the second dimension to drive the antigen into a gel containing antibodies specific for the antigens of interest. This technique is more sensitive and produces higher resolution than IEP.

Counterimmunoelectrophoresis

With CIE, two parallel lines of wells are punched in the agar. One row is filled with antigen solution, and the opposing row is filled with antibody solution (Fig. 26.6). If the solutions were allowed to passively diffuse, a precipitin line would form between the opposing wells in 18 to 24 hours. With CIE, this process is accelerated by applying a voltage across the gel so that the antigen and the antibody move toward each other. Qualitative information (i.e., identification of antigen) is provided within 1 to 2 hours. Historically, this method has found application in the detection of bacterial antigens in blood, urine, and cerebrospinal fluid (CSF).

Immunofixation

This technique has gained widespread acceptance as an immunochemical method for identifying proteins.[9] As in IEP and crossed radioimmunoelectrophoresis (CRIE), a first-dimension electrophoresis is performed in agarose gel to separate proteins in the sample. Subsequently, antiserum spread directly on the gel causes the protein(s) of interest to

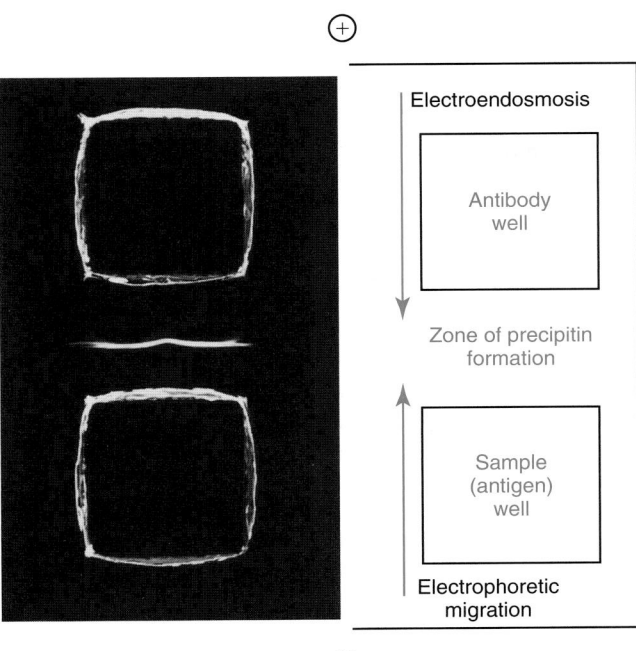

FIGURE 26.6 Counterimmunoelectrophoresis showing positive reaction between anti–*Haemophilus influenzae* B *(upper well)* and a cerebrospinal fluid sample containing *H. influenzae* B *(lower well)*. The white precipitin line forms in the zone between the square antibody and square sample wells. Each well has a white colored border that is an artifact from the creation of the wells.

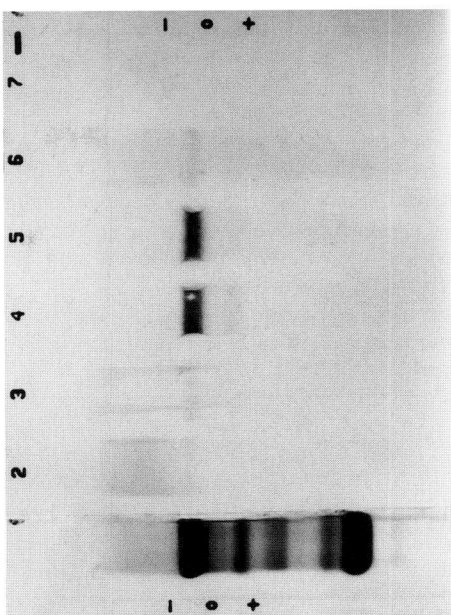

FIGURE 26.7 Immunofixation of a serum containing an immunoglobulin (Ig)M kappa paraprotein. *Lane 1,* Serum electrophoresis stained for protein; *lane 2,* anti-IgG, Fc piece specific; *lane 3,* anti-IgA, α-chain specific; *lane 4,* anti-IgM, μ-chain specific; *lane 5,* anti-κ light chain; *lane 6,* anti-λ light chain. (Courtesy Katherine Bayer, Protein Laboratory, Hospital of the University of Pennsylvania, Philadelphia, PA.)

precipitate. The immune precipitate is trapped within the gel matrix, and all other nonprecipitated proteins are removed by washing the gel. The gel may then be stained for identification of the proteins. Immunofixation is technically more efficient than IEP or CRIE, and it produces patterns that are interpreted more easily. The usefulness of immunofixation, which is now widely used for the evaluation of monoclonal gammopathies (e.g., multiple myeloma) is illustrated in Fig. 26.7.

Immunosubtraction Electrophoresis

A newer alternative method to immunofixation uses the "substraction" of specific immunoglobulin classes using class specific antibodies bound to Sepharose beads.[10] Serum depleted with antibody is then subjected to capillary zone electrophoresis. The electrophoretic pattern is then examined for a decrease in the appearance of the monoclonal protein.

Western Blotting

The techniques discussed previously use direct evaluation of the immunoprecipitation of the protein(s) in a gel. However, certain media, such as polyacrylamide, do not lend themselves to direct immunoprecipitation, nor is there always sufficient antigen concentration to produce an immunoprecipitate that will be retained in the gel during subsequent processing. Under these circumstances, Western blotting can be used. This technique involves an electrophoresis step followed by transfer of separated proteins onto an overlying strip of nitrocellulose or a nylon membrane by the process of

electro-blotting. Once the proteins are in the membrane, they can be detected using antibodies labeled with probes, such as radioactive isotopes or enzymes. When such probes are used, the limits of detection can be 10 to 100 times lower than when direct immunoprecipitation and staining of proteins are conducted. This technique is analogous to Southern blotting (electrophoresed DNA blotted onto a membrane), and Northern blotting (electrophoresed RNA blotted onto a membrane).

Protein transfer and immobilization after separation by electrophoresis, isoelectric focusing, sodium dodecyl sulfate polyacrylamide electrophoresis, or other methods provide a powerful tool for analytical study of proteins present in low concentrations in cell culture or body fluids. When applied to antigen assays, concentrations of antigen as low as 500 ng/mL or 2.5 ng/band in the gel can be detected by this method. The detection limit of the technique can be lowered to approximately 100 pg by using chemiluminescent labels on the antibody.[11]

Dot Blotting

A technique similar to Western blotting that bypasses the electrophoretic separation step is known as dot immunobinding (or dot blotting). A sample containing the protein to be analyzed (e.g., a viral protein) is applied to a membrane surface as a small dot and dried. The membrane is then exposed to a labeled antibody specific for the test antigen contained in the dotted protein mixture. After washing, bound labeled antibody is detected with a photometric or chemiluminescent detection system.

QUANTITATIVE METHODS

Several immunochemical techniques have been used to quantify analytes of clinical interest. They include RID and electroimmunoassays, turbidimetric and nephelometric assays, and labeled immunochemical antibody assays.

Radial Immunodiffusion and Electroimmunoassay

Historically, the two most commonly encountered gel-based methods for quantitative immunochemical studies were RID immunoassay and electroimmunoassay ("rocket" technique), but these methods have been mostly supplanted by other types of immunodetection techniques.

Radial Immunodiffusion Immunoassay

With this technique, a concentration gradient is established for a single reactant, usually the antigen. The antibody is uniformly dispersed in the gel matrix. Antigen is allowed to passively diffuse from a well into the gel, and immune precipitation occurs until antibody excess exists. The antigen-antibody interaction is manifested by a defined ring of precipitation around the antigen well, and ring diameter will increase with increased antigen concentration. Calibrators are run at the same time as the sample, and a calibration curve of ring diameter versus concentration is plotted. Under equilibrium conditions, a linear relationship exists between antigen concentration and the square of the precipitin ring diameter. In addition, the precision of the measurement of the ring diameter is better when equilibrium is established. However, quantitative data also can be derived by reading the ring diameter before equilibrium is established. This approach obviously is less precise. Antigen concentrations

are calculated in both the pre-equilibrium and equilibrium methods by plotting the square of the precipitin ring diameter against calibrating antigen concentrations. RID can be made more sensitive by using PEG to enhance precipitin line formation or by using [125]I- or enzyme-labeled reagents.

Electroimmunoassay

In electroimmunoassay, as in RID, a single concentration gradient is established for the antigen, but in this case, an applied voltage is used to drive the antigen from the application well into a homogeneous suspension of antibody in the gel (Fig. 26.8).[12] Unlike RID, this produces a unidirectional migration of antigen and results in a lower limit of detection for electroimmunoassay methods. The height of the resulting rocket-shaped precipitin line is proportional to the antigen concentration. Quantitation is enabled by using calibrators on the same plate and estimating the concentrations of unknowns from the heights of the "rockets" obtained from calibrators of known concentration. The calibration curve is linear only over a narrow concentration range, so samples may have to be diluted or concentrated as necessary. Electroimmunoassay methods produce the best results, with antigens having a strong anodic mobility and intermediate to low MW. Proteins such as transferrin, C3, or IgG, with low anodal mobility or virtually no net charge at pH 8.6 (the most common pH used for the method), can be modified by carbamylation or can be run at a lower pH to make their measurements by electroimmunoassay feasible.

Turbidimetric and Nephelometric Assays

Turbidimetry and nephelometry are convenient techniques for measuring the rate of formation of immune complexes in vitro. The reaction between antigen and antibody begins within milliseconds and continues for hours and both turbidimetric and nephelometric immunochemical methods using rate and pseudoequilibrium protocols can be devised for proteins, antigens, and haptens. In rate assays, measurements are usually made within the first few minutes of the reaction, when the largest change in intensity of scattered light *(Is)* with respect to time occurs *(dIs/dt)*. For so-called equilibrium assays, it is necessary to wait 30 to 60 minutes. For the purpose of this discussion, such conditions are referred to as pseudoequilibrium because true equilibrium is not reached within the time allowed for these assays. Measurement of the rate of immune complex formation also can be used for quantitative immunochemical studies. Either *dIs/dt* or the time required to reach peak rate can be related to antigen concentration in a manner analogous to any other rate

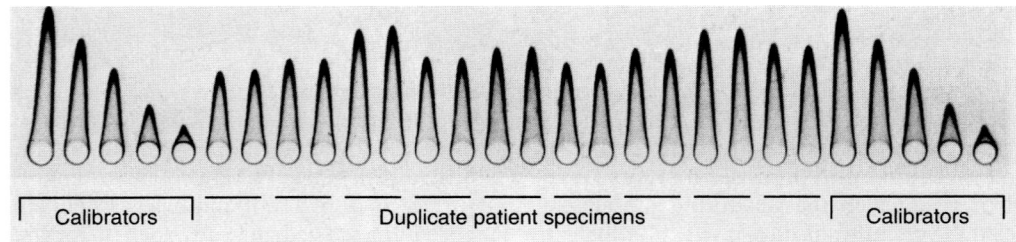

FIGURE 26.8 Rocket immunoelectrophoresis of human serum albumin. Patient samples were applied in duplicate. Standards were placed at opposite ends of the plate.

methodology. Rate nephelometric assays have the advantage that blank correction is not required and that several samples can be assayed in a few minutes instead of the 30 to 60 minutes required for pseudoequilibrium methods.[13] The analytical performance of nephelometric or turbidimetric assays can be significantly improved by increasing the reaction rate by adding water-soluble linear polymers. This allows the use of much lower reactant concentrations and results in more stable immune complexes.

Nephelometric methods in general are more sensitive than turbidimetric assays when measuring smaller particles and have an average lower limit of detection of 0.1 to 10 mg/L for a serum protein. Lower detection limits are obtained in CSF and urine because of their lower lipid and protein concentrations, resulting in a better signal-to-noise ratio. For both nephelometry and turbidimetry, assay detection limits can be lowered using a latex-enhanced procedure based on antibody-coated latex beads.

Nephelometric and turbidimetric assays also have been applied to the measurement of drugs (haptens). An example of this type of assay is the particle-enhanced turbidimetric inhibition immunoassay (PETINIA) (Fig. 26.9), which measures decreasing agglutination in the presence of increasing concentrations of analyte (e.g., digoxin).[14] The reagents comprise an antibody to the analyte of interest and a reagent containing the analyte of interest linked to a particle (latex bead). In the absence of analyte in a specimen, reagent antibody binds to the reagent containing the analyte linked to the latex bead, resulting in increased turbidity. When a specimen with high analyte concentrations is added to the reagent mixture, the reagent antibody is bound by the analyte in the specimen and not to the reagent containing the analyte linked to the latex bead. Thus the presence of specimen analyte results in less turbidity.

POINTS TO REMEMBER

- Turbidimetric (turbidity) and nephelometric (light scattering) immunoassays provide simple and rapid nonseparation (homogeneous) format immunoassays.
- Particle-enhanced turbidimetric inhibition immunoassays (PETINIA) use an antigen attached to a latex microparticle and are used for measurement of small molecules.

Label-Free Immunoassay: Surface Plasmon Resonance–Based Immunoassay (Immunosensor)

An important type of label-free immunoassay is based on surface plasmon resonance (SPR), an optical phenomenon that enables detection of unlabeled reactants in real time based on changes in the index of refraction at the surface where the binding interaction occurs. The assay is conducted on an electrically conducting gold-coated glass slide mounted on a prism. The binding agent is immobilized on the gold surface, over which reactant is flowed. Polarized light is directed underneath the glass slide and interacts with the gold surface to produce electron charge density waves called plasmons at the sample and gold surface interface. This results in a reduction in the intensity of the reflected light. Slight changes in the refractive index at the interface lead to a change in the signal, thus facilitating real-time detection of surface molecular interactions (e.g., association and dissociation of biomolecules with the binder immobilized on the gold surface). SPR assays (e.g., Biacore, Marlborough, Massachusetts) are used to characterize biomolecular interactions, such as antibody affinity, kinetics, and cross-reactivity.[15] Lower limits of detection range from 10^{-9} to 10^{-13} M.

Labeled Immunochemical Assays

The previously discussed methods rely on immune complex formation as an index of antigen-antibody reaction. As demonstrated previously in Eq. (26.1), the overall reaction occurs in sequential phases and only the final phase is the formation of the immune complex. However, the initial binding of the antibody and antigen has been demonstrated to be very useful analytically and has been used with labeled antigens and antibodies to develop many sensitive and specific immunochemical assays. The reaction describing this initial binding and the kinetic constant for the overall reaction are shown in Eqs. (26.3a) and (26.3b), respectively:

$$Ab + Ag \underset{k_{-1}}{\overset{k_1}{\rightleftharpoons}} AbAg \qquad (26.3a)$$

$$K = \frac{[AbAg]}{[Ab][Ag]} \qquad (26.3b)$$

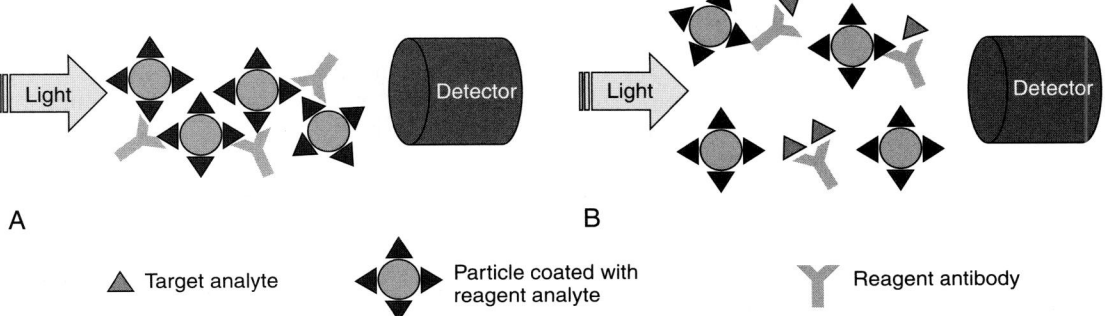

A   B

▲ Target analyte   Particle coated with reagent analyte   Y Reagent antibody

FIGURE 26.9 PETINIA (particle-enhanced turbidimetric inhibition immunoassay). PETINIA measures decreased agglutination in the presence of increasing analyte. In the *left panel* there is an absence of analyte which results in agglutination of the reagent particles and antibodies. The agglutination results in decreased light transmission to the detector (A). In the *right panel*, target analyte is introduced which binds the reagent antibody; there is less agglutination of the reagent particles and therefore decreased turbidity with increased light transmission (B).

TABLE 26.1   Labels Used for Nonisotopic Immunoassay

Type of Label	Examples
Chemiluminescent	Acridinium ester, sulfonyl acridinium ester, isoluminol
Cofactor	Adenosine triphosphate, flavin adenine dinucleotide
Enzyme	Alkaline phosphatase, marine bacterial luciferase, β-galactosidase, firefly luciferase, glucose oxidase, glucose-6-phosphate dehydrogenase, horseradish peroxidase, lysozyme, malate dehydrogenase, microperoxidase, urease, xanthine oxidase
Fluorophore	Cyanine dye, fluorescein, lanthanide chelate (europium, terbium), phycoerythrin
Free radical	Nitroxide
Inhibitor	Methotrexate
Metal	Gold sol, selenium sol, silver sol
Particle	Bacteriophage, carbon, erythrocyte, latex bead, liposome, magnetic nanoparticle, nanorod, nanotube, quantum dot
Phosphor	Upconverting lanthanide-containing nanoparticle
Polynucleotide	DNA
Substrate	Galactosyl-umbelliferone

where

k_1 = the rate constant for the forward reaction

k_{-1} = the rate constant for the reverse reaction

K = the equilibrium constant for the overall reaction

As would be predicted from the law of mass action, the concentration of Ab, Ag, and AbAg will depend on the magnitude of k_1 and k_{-1}. For polyclonal antiserum, the average avidity of the antibody populations will determine K (typically 10^8 to 10^{10} L/mol) and the magnitude of k_1 compared with k_{-1} will determine the ultimate limit of detection attainable with a given antibody population.

The original immunochemical assays used radioactivity for labeling but concerns about safe handling and disposal of radioactive reagents and waste have led to the development of alternative nonisotopic labels (Table 26.1).[16] In this section, the methodologic principles on which these assays are based and the factors that affect their analytical sensitivity are discussed. In addition, specific examples of these assays and the types of labels that are used in them are evaluated.

Methodologic Principles

To exploit the exquisite specificity and enhanced sensitivity that are possible with immunochemical assays, various methodologic principles have been applied in their development. These include competitive and noncompetitive reaction formats and different processing schemes for performing the assays.

Competitive versus noncompetitive reaction formats. The two major reaction formats that are used in immunochemical assays (Fig. 26.10) are termed *competitive* (limited reagent

Competitive (limited reagent)

Simultaneous

Ab + Ag + Ag − L ⇌ Ab:Ag + Ab:Ag − L
(free)   (bound)

Sequential

Step 1 Ab + Ag $\underset{k_{-1}}{\overset{k_1}{\rightleftharpoons}}$ Ab:Ag + Ab

Step 2 Ab:Ag + Ab + Ag − L ⇌ Ab:Ag + Ab:Ag − L + Ag − L

Noncompetitive (excess reagent, two-site, sandwich)

FIGURE 26.10 Immunoassay designs. *L,* Label.

assays) and *noncompetitive* (excess reagent, two-site, or sandwich assays).

Competitive Immunoassays. In a competitive immunochemical assay, all reactants are mixed together simultaneously or sequentially. In the simultaneous approach, the labeled antigen (Ag*) and the unlabeled antigen (Ag) compete for binding to the antibody. Under these conditions, the probability of the antibody binding the labeled antigen is inversely proportional to the concentration of unlabeled antigen; hence bound label is inversely proportional to unlabeled antigen concentration. Any differences in the avidity of the antibody for the labeled and unlabeled antigen do not present an issue as long as the calibrators are comparable to the patient samples.

In a sequential competitive assay, unlabeled antigen is first mixed with excess antibody and binding is allowed to reach equilibrium (see Fig. 26.10, *step 1*). Labeled antigen is then sequentially added *(step 2)* and is allowed to equilibrate. After separation, the bound labeled antigen is determined and is used to calculate the unlabeled antigen concentration. Using this two-step method, a larger fraction of the unlabeled antigen is bound by the antibody than in the simultaneous assay, especially at low antigen concentrations. Consequently, this strategy provides a twofold to fourfold improvement in the detection limit, provided $k_1 >> k_{-1}$. This improvement results from an increase in AgAb binding (and thus a decrease in Ag* binding), which is favored by the sequential addition of Ag and Ag*. If $k_1 >> k_{-1}$, dissociation of AgAb becomes more likely, resulting in increased competition between Ag* and Ag. A typical competitive immunochemical assay binding curve is shown in Fig. 26.11.

Noncompetitive Immunoassays. In a noncompetitive immunochemical assay, a capture antibody first is passively adsorbed or covalently bound to the surface of a solid phase. However, this can lead to some loss of antibody-binding capacity because of steric factors or attachment of the antibody via its Fab region. To protect the binding properties of the antibody, more complex sequences have been devised. For example, the solid support is coated with an antispecies antibody, and then the antispecies antibody is used to immobilize the capture antibody via an antigen-antibody reaction.

In the first stage of the assay, the antigen from the sample is allowed to react with the solid phase, capture antibody;

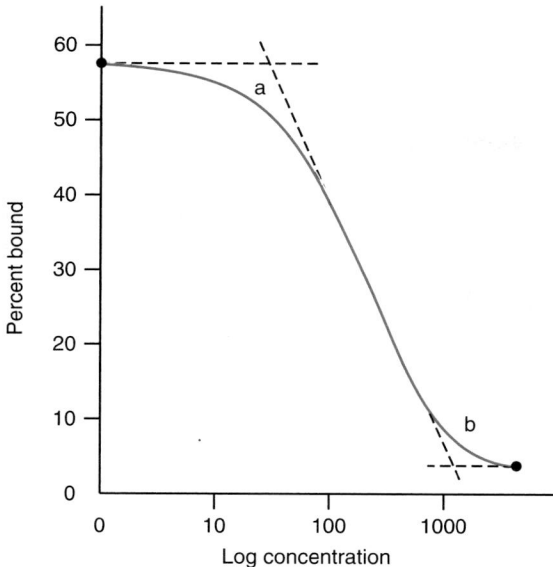

FIGURE 26.11 A schematic diagram of the dose-response curve for a typical competitive immunoassay. The analytically useful portion of the curve is bracketed by points *a* and *b*.

other proteins are washed away, and a labeled antibody (conjugate) is added that reacts with the bound antigen through a second and distinct epitope. After washing again, the bound label is determined and its concentration or activity is directly proportional to the concentration of the antigen.

In noncompetitive assays, the capture and labeled antibody can be polyclonal or monoclonal. If monoclonal antibodies having specificity for distinct epitopes are used, it is possible to incubate the sample and conjugate simultaneously with the capture antibody, thus simplifying the assay protocol.

Noncompetitive immunoassays are performed in a simultaneous (one-step) or sequential (two-step) mode. However, in the simultaneous mode, a situation can occur in which a high concentration of analyte can saturate both capture and labeled antibodies. When this occurs, the calibration curve of the assay exhibits a "hook effect," in which the assay response drops off at high analyte concentrations. Under these conditions, the analyte is present in such high concentrations that it reacts simultaneously with the capture antibody and the labeled antibody. This reduces the number of complexes formed and produces a falsely low result. Assays for analytes for which the normal pathologic concentration range is very wide (e.g., tumor markers) are particularly prone to this problem. Dilutions of a sample are usually reanalyzed to check for this type of analytical interference. One way of minimizing or eliminating the hook effect is to either ensure that the concentrations of capture and labeled antibody are sufficiently high to cover analyte concentrations over the entire analytical range of the assay or add a wash step before the addition of the labeled antibodies. Sequential noncompetitive immunoassays are not prone to this problem. Unfortunately, with modern automated immunoassays, hook effects may occur silently and can be undetectable. Immunoassays cleared by the US Food and Drug Administration typically define an analyte concentration up to which the assay is not affected by the hook effect.

Noncompetitive immunoassays rely on different epitopes on a large analyte molecule so as to provide a binding site for both the capture antibody and for the labeled antibody. In the past, a small molecule could not be measured using the conventional sandwich format because a small molecule had too few epitopes. Various strategies have been developed to expand the scope of the sandwich assay to small molecules.[17] A strategy, exemplified by a 25-hydroxyvitamin D assay (25OH-D), has made small molecules amenable to a routine sandwich immunoassay format. In this commercial assay format, 25OH-D binds to an immobilized capture antibody and a second antibody (an antimetatype antibody) specifically recognizes the immunocomplex formed between the 25OH-D molecule and the capture antibody, hence facilitating a sandwich assay design.[18]

Heterogeneous versus homogeneous immunochemical assays. Immunochemical assays that require separation of free from bound labels are termed *heterogeneous;* those that do not are called *homogeneous.*

Heterogeneous Assays. Heterogeneous assays implicitly assume that $k_1 \gg k_{-1}$ and that a variety of physical separation techniques are used to separate the free-label (Ag*) from the bound-label antigen (Ag*Ab). The most widely used of these techniques are precipitation and solid-phase adsorption.

Precipitation of the bound labeled antigen (Ag*Ab) from the reaction mixture can be achieved chemically by the addition of a protein-precipitating chemical, such as $(NH_4)_2SO_4$, or immunologically by the addition of a second, precipitating antibody. In the latter approach, if the primary antibody was obtained from rabbit antiserum, the precipitating antibody would be contained in a goat or sheep antiserum raised against rabbit globulin. This approach has the advantage that it can be used for practically any assay; however, it has the disadvantage that it usually requires longer assay times and additional processing steps.

Solid-phase adsorption is the separation technique that currently is the most popular and widely used in both manual and automated heterogeneous immunoassays. In this technique, the binding and competition of labeled and unlabeled antigens for the binding sites of the antibody occur on the surface of a solid support onto which the capture antibody has been attached by physical adsorption or covalent bonding. Several different types of solid support have been used, including the inner surface of plastic tubes or wells of microtiter plates and the outer surface of insoluble materials, such as cellulose or magnetic latex beads or particles. With the tubes and microtiter plates, the solid surface containing the attached antibody and the bound antigen is washed in place and indicator reagents are subsequently added to complete the assay. When beads or particles are used, they are added directly to the reaction mixture and after incubation are removed by centrifugation or magnetic separation. After the supernatant has been removed by siphoning or decanting, the beads or particles are washed, and indicator reagents are subsequently added to complete the assay.

Homogeneous Assays. The development of homogeneous assays that do not require separation of bound and free labeled antibody or antigen was a major advance in the field of immunochemical analysis. In this type of assay, the activity of the label attached to the antigen is directly modulated by antibody binding, with the magnitude of the modulation being proportional to the concentration of the antigen or antibody being measured. Consequently, in practice it is necessary to incubate only the sample containing the analyte antigen with the labeled antigen and antibody and then to directly measure the activity of the label in place, thus making these assays technically easier and faster. The original homogeneous immunoassay was developed for drug analysis and used a nitroxide spin label; this was termed a *free radical immunoassay technique*. The electron spin resonance spectrum of this label was modulated when the nitroxide-labeled drug was bound by a drug-specific antibody. This procedure was quickly superseded by homogeneous immunoassays that used enzyme labels and could be performed on spectrophotometric analyzers (see subsequent descriptions of enzyme-multiplied immunoassay technique [EMIT] and cloned enzyme donor immunoassay [CEDIA]).

A homogeneous sandwich format chemiluminescent immunoassay also has been developed that expands the scope of homogeneous assays to large molecules (see subsequent description of LOCI). In addition, a diverse range of homogeneous fluoroimmunoassays based on fluorescence energy transfer (FRET) between fluorescent donor and acceptor dye-labeled assay components represents a further expansion of the scope of homogeneous immunoassays (see subsequent descriptions of FRET).

Analytical and Functional Sensitivity

The analytical detection limits (sensitivity) of competitive and noncompetitive immunoassays are determined principally by the affinity of the antibody and the detection limit of the label used, respectively.[19] Calculations have indicated that a lower limit of detection of 10 fmol/L (i.e., 600,000 molecules of analyte in a typical sample volume of 100 μL) is possible in a competitive assay using an antibody with an affinity of 10^{12} L/mol. Table 26.2 illustrates theoretical detection limits for isotopic and nonisotopic labels. A radioactive label, such as ^{125}I, has low specific activity (7.5 million labels necessary for detection of 1 disintegration/s) compared with enzyme labels and chemiluminescent and fluorescent labels. Enzyme labels provide an amplification (each enzyme label produces many detectable product molecules), and the detection limit for an enzyme can be improved by replacing the conventional photometric detection reaction

by a chemiluminescent or bioluminescent reaction. The combination of amplification and an ultrasensitive detection reaction makes noncompetitive chemiluminescent immunoassays among the most sensitive types of immunoassay. Fluorescent labels also have high specific activity, and a single high-quantum yield fluorophore can produce 100 million photons/s. A detection limit as low as 2 fmol (~1,200,000,000 molecules) can be achieved with chemiluminescent immunoassays. In practice, several factors degrade the detection limit of an immunoassay; these include background signal from the detector, assay reagents, and nonspecific binding of the labeled reagent.

Secondary labels, such as biotin, can be used to introduce amplification into an immunoassay. The binding constant of the biotin-avidin complex is extremely high (10^{15} L/mol); capitalizing on this system allows immunoassay systems to be devised that are even more sensitive than simple antibody systems. A biotin-avidin system uses a biotin-labeled soluble antibody. Biotin can be attached to the antibody in relatively high proportion without loss of immunoreactivity. When an avidin-conjugated label is added, a complex of Ag:Ab-biotin:avidin label is formed. Further amplification can be achieved by a biotin:avidin:biotin linkage, because the binding ratio of biotin:avidin is 4:1. If the label is an enzyme, large numbers of enzyme molecules in the complete complex provide a large increase in enzymatic activity coupled with the small amount of antigen being determined, and the assay is correspondingly more sensitive.

Immunoassays are often categorized by their functional sensitivity (limit of quantitation), which is defined as the lowest concentration of an analyte that can be reliably detected and is defined in terms of the total error goal of the assay[19] (for further information on definitions of various measures of sensitivity including limit of detection and lowest limit of quantification, refer to Chapter 2). This is used to establish a more realistic and robust detection limit for an assay used in patient care. Functional sensitivity is associated with concept of assay generations, each successive generation representing a 1-log concentration improvement in sensitivity (e.g., for a thyroid-stimulating hormone [TSH] immunoassay first generation 1 mIU/L, second generation 0.1 mIU/L, third generation 0.01 mIU/L, etc.). See Chapter 57 for additional discussion on TSH testing.

TABLE 26.2   **Detection Limits for Isotopic and Nonisotopic Immunoassay Labels Based on Commonly Used Detection Methods**

Label	Detection Limit in Zeptomoles[a] (10^{-21} Moles)	Method
Alkaline phosphatase	50,000	Photometry
	300	Time-resolved fluorescence
	100	Fluorescence
	10	Chemiluminescence
β-D-Galactosidase	5,000	Chemiluminescence
	1,000	Fluorescence
Europium chelate	10,000	Time-resolved fluorescence
Glucose-6-phosphate dehydrogenase	1,000	Chemiluminescence
Horseradish peroxidase	2,000,000	Photometry
	1	Chemiluminescence
Iodine-125	1,000	Scintillation
Ruthenium (II) tris(bipyridyl)	20	Electrochemiluminescence

[a]One zeptomole = 10^{-3} attomoles or 10^{-6} femtomoles.

Examples of Labeled Immunoassays

In the decade after the pioneering developments of Yalow and Berson for insulin measurement,[20] all competitive and noncompetitive immunoassays used a radioactive label in a competitive assay format. Since the introduction of enzyme immunochemical assays in the 1970s, a vast array of sophisticated immunochemical assays have evolved; some of the major types are discussed in the following sections.

Radioimmunoassay. Radioimmunoassays (RIAs) were developed in the 1960s and used radioactive isotopes of iodine (^{125}I, ^{131}I) and tritium (^3H) as labels.[20] Labeled antibody noncompetitive assays (immunoradiometric or sandwich assay) have the advantage of not requiring a quantity of purified antigen because the antigen does not have to be labeled. This also obviates potential problems that may be caused by iodination of labile antigens. Antibodies are relatively stable proteins that are less difficult to label without damaging the function of the protein. Combinations of labels (e.g., cobalt [^{57}Co] and ^{125}I) have been used for simultaneous assays of vitamin B12 and folate, as well as lutropin and follitropin (LH and FSH).[21]

Enzyme immunoassay. Enzyme immunoassays (EIAs) use the catalytic properties of enzymes to detect and quantify immunologic reactions. In practice, enzyme-labeled antibodies or antigens (i.e., conjugates) are first allowed to react with ligands. Bound label is then separated, and enzyme substrates are subsequently added. Measurement of the resultant increase in product concentration is used to detect or quantify the antigen-antibody reaction. Alkaline phosphatase, horseradish peroxidase, glucose-6-phosphate dehydrogenase, and β-galactosidase enzyme labels predominate in EIAs.[16]

Various detection systems have been used to monitor and quantify EIAs. Assays that produce compounds that can be monitored photometrically are very popular because compact, high-performance photometers are available. However, EIAs that use fluorescent- or chemiluminescent-labeled substrates or products are often preferred to photometry-based assays owing to the inherent sensitivity of fluorescent and chemiluminescent measurements (see Table 26.2). Immunoassays that incorporate horseradish peroxidase as a label can be assayed by chemiluminescence using a mixture of luminol, peroxide, and an enhancer such as *p*-iodophenol (Fig. 26.12A)[22] or by using an acridan derivative.[23] A very sensitive assay for alkaline phosphatase labels uses a chemiluminescent adamantyl 1,2-dioxetane aryl phosphate substrate (see Fig. 26.12B). The enzyme dephosphorylates the substrate, which decomposes with a concomitant long-lived glow of light (detection limit for alkaline phosphatase using this assay is 10 zeptomoles [10^{-20} moles]).[24]

Types of enzyme-linked immunoassay include enzyme-linked immunosorbent assay (ELISA), EMIT, and CEDIA.

Enzyme-linked immunosorbent assay. ELISA is a heterogeneous EIA technique used in clinical analyses. In this type of assay, one of the reaction components is nonspecifically adsorbed or covalently bound to the surface of a solid phase, such as a microtiter well, a magnetic particle, or a plastic bead. This attachment facilitates separation of bound and free labeled reactants. In the most common approach to using the ELISA technique, an aliquot of sample or calibrator containing the antigen to be quantitated is added to and allowed to bind with a solid-phase antibody. After washing, enzyme-labeled antibody is added and forms a "sandwich

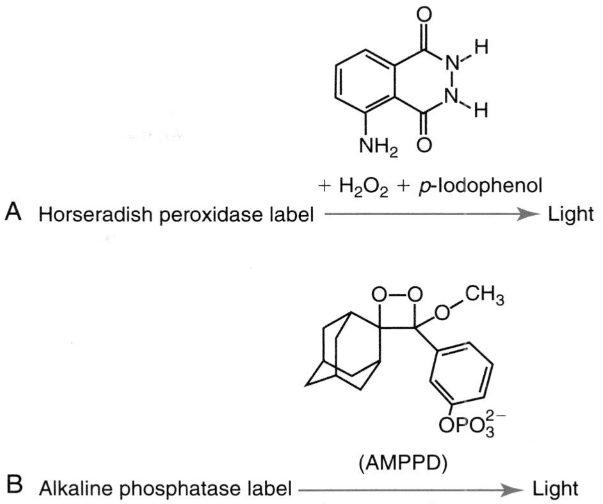

FIGURE 26.12 Ultrasensitive assays for horseradish peroxidase and alkaline phosphatase labels. (A) Chemiluminescent assay for horseradish peroxidase label using luminol. (B) Chemiluminescent assay for an alkaline phosphatase label using 3-(2′-spiroadamantyl)-4-methoxy-4-(3″-phosphoryloxy)-phenyl-1,2-dioxetane (AMPPD).

complex" of solid-phase Ab-Ag-Ab enzyme. Unbound antibody is then washed away, and enzyme substrate is added. The amount of product generated is proportional to the quantity of antigen in the sample. Specific antibodies in a sample also can be quantified using an ELISA procedure in which antigen instead of antibody is bound to a solid phase and the second reagent is an enzyme-labeled antibody specific for the analyte antibody. In addition, ELISA assays have been used extensively for detection of antibodies to viruses and autoantigens in serum or whole blood. In addition, enzyme conjugates coupled with substrates that produce visible products have been used to develop ELISA-type assays with results that can be interpreted visually. Such assays have been found very useful in screening, point-of-care, and home testing applications.

Enzyme Multiplied Immunoassay Technique. EMIT is a homogeneous EIA that is very widely used in clinical analyses, an illustration of which is shown in Fig. 26.13. Because EMIT does not require a separation step, it is simple to perform and has been used to develop a wide variety of drug, hormone, and metabolite assays. Because of their operational simplicity, EMIT-type assays are easily automated and are included in the repertoire of many automated clinical and immunoassay analyzers. In this technique, antibody against the analyte drug, hormone, or metabolite is added together with substrate to the patient's sample. Binding of the antibody and analyte occurs. An aliquot of the enzyme conjugated to exogenous analyte is then added as a second reagent; the enzyme-analyte conjugate binds with the excess antibody, forming an antigen-antibody complex. This binding of the antibody with the enzyme-analyte conjugate affects enzyme activity by physically blocking access of the substrate to the active site of the enzyme or by changing the conformation of the enzyme molecule and thus altering its activity. To complete the assay, the resultant enzyme activity is measured. The relative change in enzyme activity resulting from the formation of the antigen-antibody complex is proportional

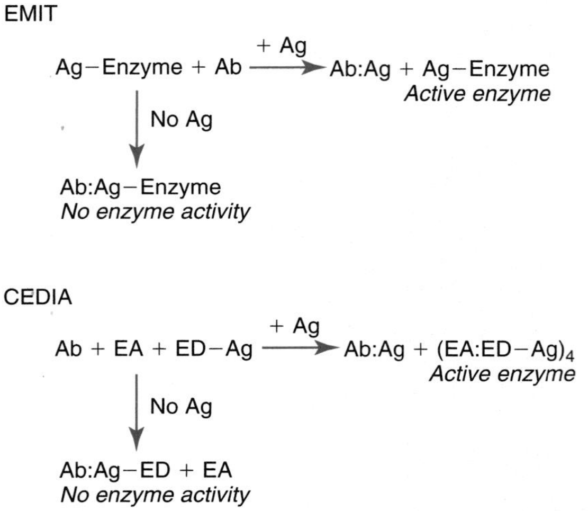

EMIT

$$\text{Ag--Enzyme + Ab} \xrightarrow{\text{+ Ag}} \text{Ab:Ag + Ag--Enzyme}$$
Active enzyme

↓ No Ag

Ab:Ag--Enzyme
No enzyme activity

CEDIA

$$\text{Ab + EA + ED--Ag} \xrightarrow{\text{+ Ag}} \text{Ab:Ag + (EA:ED--Ag)}_4$$
Active enzyme

↓ No Ag

Ab:Ag--ED + EA
No enzyme activity

FIGURE 26.13 Enzyme multiplied immunoassay technique *(EMIT)* and cloned enzyme donor immunoassay *(CEDIA)* homogeneous immunoassays. *EA,* Enzyme acceptor; *ED,* enzyme donor.

to the analyte concentration in the patient's sample. Concentration of the analyte is calculated from a calibration curve prepared by analyzing calibrators that contain known quantities of the analyte in question.

Cloned enzyme donor immunoassay. As shown in see Fig. 26.13, CEDIA is a homogeneous EIA; it was the first EIA designed and developed using genetic engineering techniques. Inactive fragments (the enzyme donor and acceptor) of β-galactosidase are prepared by manipulation of the Z gene of the *lac* operon of *Escherichia coli.* These two fragments spontaneously reassemble to form active enzyme even if the enzyme donor is attached to an antigen. However, binding of antibody to the enzyme donor-antigen conjugate inhibits reassembly and no active enzyme is formed. Thus competition between the antigen and the enzyme donor-antigen conjugate for a fixed amount of antibody in the presence of the enzyme acceptor modulates the measured enzyme activity (high concentrations of the analyte antigen result in the least

inhibition of enzyme activity; low concentrations result in the greatest inhibition). CEDIA assays have been used for measurement of a variety of small molecules. Some disadvantages of CEDIA assays include the selection of antibodies that inhibit enzyme complementation, as well as the time required for the reaction.

Fluoroimmunoassay. Examples of fluorophores that are used as labels in fluoroimmunoassay and their properties are listed in Table 26.3. Initially, background fluorescence from drugs, drug metabolites, and protein-bound substances, such as bilirubin, limited the usefulness of this technique. However, this problem has largely been overcome by the use of rare earth (lanthanide) chelates and background rejection (time-resolved) procedures.[25] Fluorescent emissions from lanthanide chelates (e.g., europium, terbium, samarium) are long lived (greater than 1 μs) compared with the typical background fluorescence encountered in biological specimens. In a time-resolved fluoroimmunoassay, a europium chelate label is excited by a pulse of excitation light (0.5 μs), and the long-lived fluorescence emission from the label is measured after a delay (400 to 800 μs). The measurement after the delay ensures that any short-lived background signal has decayed.

FPIA is a type of homogeneous fluoroimmunoassay previously used to measure drugs and other small molecules (Fig. 26.14). The polarization of the fluorescence from a fluorescein-antigen conjugate is determined by its rate of rotation during the lifetime of the excited state in solution. When the fluorescein-antigen conjugate is bound to the large antibody molecule, the fluorophore is constrained from rotating in the time between absorption of the incident radiation and emission of fluorescence; hence the fluorescence emission is still highly polarized. In contrast, when the fluorescein-antigen conjugate is free in solution it can rotate more rapidly and the emitted light is depolarized. Thus binding to antibody modulates polarization, and a homogeneous assay is possible.

Förster or fluorescence resonance energy transfer (FRET) is the distance-dependent transfer of energy from a fluorescent donor dye to a fluorescent acceptor dye. Distances at which there is 50% transfer efficiency are typically 1 to 10 nm,

TABLE 26.3	Properties of Fluorescent Labels			
Fluorophore	**Excitation (nm)**	**Emission (nm)**	**Fluorescence Quantum Yield[a]**	**Lifetime (ns)**
Cy3 (cyanine dye)	550	570	0.15	—
Cy5 (cyanine dye)	650	670	0.28	—
Europium (β-naphthoyl trifluoroacetone)	340	590, 613	—	500,000
Fluorescein isothiocyanate	492	520	0.0−0.85	4.5
NN382	778	806	0.59	—
	550−620	580−660	0.5−0.98	—
Rhodamine B isothiocyanate	550	585	0.0−0.7	3.0
Umbelliferone	380	450	—	—

[a]Fluorescence quantum yield: fraction of molecules that emit a photon.

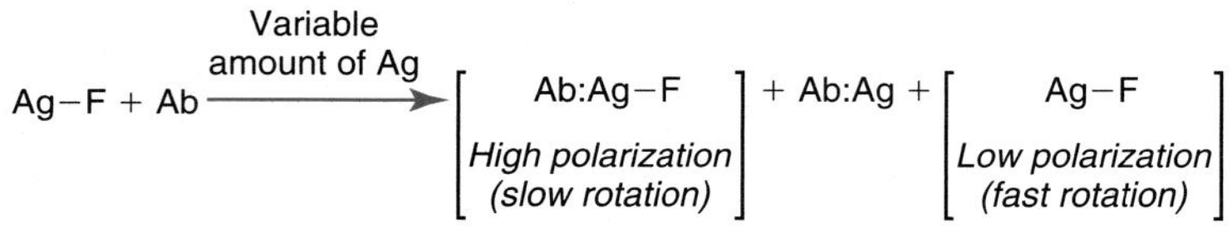

$$\text{Ag--F + Ab} \xrightarrow{\substack{\text{Variable} \\ \text{amount of Ag}}} \left[\begin{array}{c} \text{Ab:Ag--F} \\ \textit{High polarization} \\ \textit{(slow rotation)} \end{array} \right] + \text{Ab:Ag} + \left[\begin{array}{c} \text{Ag--F} \\ \textit{Low polarization} \\ \textit{(fast rotation)} \end{array} \right]$$

FIGURE 26.14 Homogeneous polarization fluoroimmunoassay. *F,* Fluorescein.

but up to approximately 20 nm is possible for some donor-acceptor pairs (e.g., lanthanide chelate–quantum dot).[26] For example, in a sandwich FRET immunoassay format used in the time-resolved amplified cryptate emission (TRACE) assays, an antibody labeled with a europium chelate (donor) is matched with an antibody labeled with an allophycocyanin dye (XL665; acceptor). The two antibodies form a sandwich immunocomplex with the antigen and after irradiation with excitation light (337 nm) energy transfer occurs from the donor europium chelate to the XL665 acceptor. In the absence of immunocomplex formation, the XL665 fluorescence is short lived (nanoseconds). However, with immunocomplex formation, the europium chelate provides energy to prolong the normally short-lived fluorescence of the XL665 dye (microseconds). Intensity of the 665-nm emission is proportional to antigen concentration. Another strategy used in the Triage system (Alere, Waltham, MA) for cardiac markers uses an antibody-coated latex particle containing a donor dye (a silicon [IV] phthalocyanine bis[7-oct-1-enyldimethylsilyloxide]) and a second antibody-coated latex particle containing an acceptor dye (2¹,2⁶,12¹,12⁶-tetraphenyldinaphtho [b,1]-7,17-dibenzo[g,q]-5,10,15,20-tetraazoporphyrinato] silicon bis(7-oct-1-enyldimethylsilyloxide). Analyte in the sample binds to create donor particle:analyte:acceptor particle complexes. Excitation at 670 nm excites the donor dye, and energy transfer to the acceptor dye occurs as a result of the proximity of the two different types of particle. The acceptor particle then emits light at 760 nm (long wavelength in the red portion of the spectrum). An advantage of this red emission is that scattering and fluorescence from blood plasma is minimized.[27] Other examples of donor-acceptor pairs include Cy3-Cy5, fluorescein-gold or Cy3-gold nanoparticles, blue fluorescent protein–green fluorescent protein, lanthanide chelate–quantum dot, europium cryptate–allophycocyanin, and upconverting phosphor–B-phycoerythrin.

Multiplexed fluoroimmunoassays can be achieved using fluorophores with different fluorescent emissions (e.g., lanthanide chelates). Multiplexing is also possible using quantum dot labels. A quantum dot is a nanometer-sized highly fluorescent nanocrystal composed of cadmium selenide (CdSe), cadmium sulfide (CdS), zinc selenide (ZnSe), indium phosphide (InP), or indium arsenide (InAs) or a layer of zinc sulfide (ZnS) or CdS on, for example, a CdSe core. Multiplexing is possible with these labels because their emission properties can be modulated by changing the size and composition of the nanocrystal (e.g., CdS emits blue light, InP emits red light).[28]

Phosphor immunoassay. A phosphor is a material that emits light (phosphorescence) over a relatively long time scale after exposure to excitation energy (see Chapter 16). A particular type of phosphor, an upconverting phosphor nanoparticle, can be used as a label for immunoassay.[29] In one application, the upconverting phosphor nanoparticle (200- to 400-nm diameter) was a crystalline lanthanide oxysulfide. This nanoparticle absorbs two or more photons of infrared light (980 nm) and produces light emission at a shorter wavelength (anti-Stokes shift). The phosphorescence is not influenced by reaction conditions (e.g., temperature, buffer), and no upconverted signal is received from biological components in the sample (low background). Multiplexing is possible because different types of particles produce different wavelengths of phosphorescence (e.g., yttrium/erbium oxysulfides are green [550 nm], yttrium/thulium oxysulfide particles are blue [475 nm]).

Chemiluminescent and bioluminescent immunoassays. Chemiluminescence is the name given to light emission produced during a chemical reaction. Isoluminol and acridinium esters are important examples of labels used in chemiluminescent immunoassay. Oxidation of isoluminol by hydrogen peroxide in the presence of a catalyst, such as microperoxidase, produces a relatively long-lived light emission at 425 nm, and oxidation of an acridinium ester by alkaline hydrogen peroxide in the presence of a detergent (e.g., Triton X-100) produces a rapid flash of light at 429 nm. Acridinium and sulfonyl acridinium esters are high-specific activity labels (detection limit for the label is 800 zeptomoles) that can be used to label both antibodies and haptens (Fig. 26.15A).[30]

Luminescent oxygen channeling immunoassay (LOCI) is a particularly important type of chemiluminescent immunoassay. It is one of the few homogeneous immunoassays that operate in a noncompetitive (sandwich) format and can be used to assay large molecules. LOCI uses two reagent particles (sensitizer and chemiluminescer particles) that form a complex with the analyte of interest.[31] The presence of analyte links the two reagent latex particles in close proximity. The first particle contains a photosensitizer (e.g., phthalocyanine) and in the presence of light converts oxygen to singlet oxygen. The second chemiluminescer particle contains a chemiluminescent agent (e.g., olefin) that reacts with singlet oxygen to

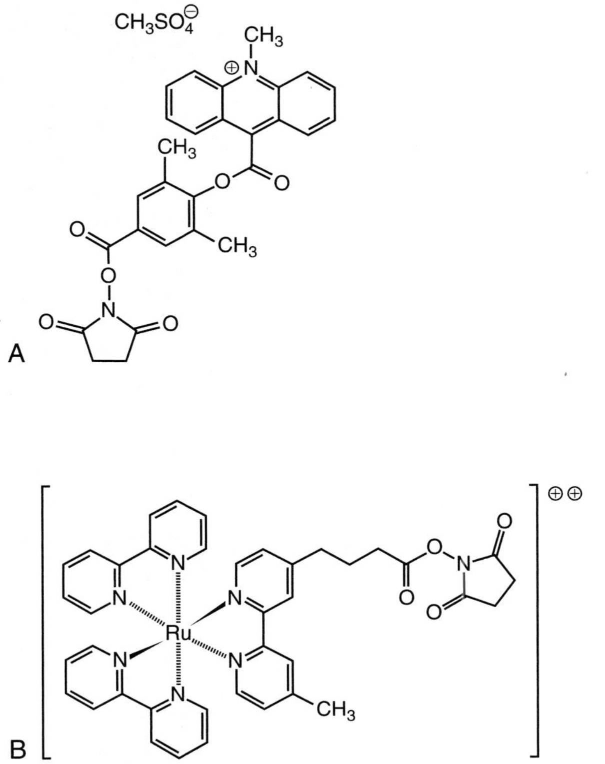

FIGURE 26.15 Luminescent labels. (A) Chemiluminescent acridinium ester label. (B) Electrochemiluminescent ruthenium (II) tris(bipyridyl) NHS ester label. (From Law S-J, Miller T, Piran U, Klukas C, Chang S, Unger J. Novel poly-substituted aryl acridinium esters and their use in immunoassay. *J Biolumin Chemilumin* 1989;4:88–98. Reprinted by permission of John Wiley & Sons.)

form a dioxetane that decomposes and emits light. This reaction occurs only if the two particles are in close proximity and the singlet oxygen can diffuse efficiently from the sensitizer particle to the chemiluminescer particle. Singlet oxygen does not react with unbound chemiluminescer particles because of the short lifetime of this transient species in an aqueous environment. An example of a LOCI assay for TSH is illustrated in Fig. 26.16. TSH binds to a biotinylated anti-TSH antibody, and this complex links the streptavidin-coated sensitizer particle to the anti-TSH antibody–coated chemiluminescer particle. Exposure of light results in emission of singlet oxygen from the photosensitive particle. The singlet oxygen activates the chemiluminescent particle to emit light that is then measured.

Components of bioluminescent reactions (light-emitting reactions that occur in living organisms) have also been exploited as labels. One example is the use of native or recombinant apoaequorin (from the bioluminescent jellyfish *Aequorea*) as a label. This protein is activated by reaction with coelenterazine, and light emission at 469 nm is triggered by reaction with calcium ions (calcium chloride).[32]

Electrochemiluminescent immunoassay. Ruthenium (II) tris(bipyridyl) (see Fig. 26.15B) undergoes an electrochemiluminescent reaction (620 nm) with tripropylamine at an electrode surface, and this chelate is now used as a label in competitive and sandwich electrochemiluminescence immunoassays. Using this label, various assays have been developed using magnetic beads as the solid phase. Beads are captured by a magnet at an electrode surface in a flow cell, and unbound label is washed out of the cell by a wash buffer. Label bound to the bead undergoes an electrochemiluminescent reaction, and the light emission is measured by an adjacent photomultiplier.[33]

Magnetic particle immunoassay. A magnetic particle has found application as a label in immunoassay. In one immunoassay design, a superparamagnetic particle (300-nm diameter) is used as the label and is detected by its magnetic properties using a giant magnetoresistance sensor.[34] A magnetic particle also can be detected based on its reflective and light-scattering properties (optomagnetic immunoassay). The assay is performed in a flow-through cartridge having a localized region with surface-immobilized capture antibodies. Magnetic nanoparticles coated with detection antibody bind to captured antigens. The bound magnetic particle labels are detected using frustrated total internal reflection. In the absence of binding, light projected onto the capture region is reflected at full strength and detected using a camera. Binding of the magnetic particle labels causes reflection and scattering of the light and the intensity of the light arriving at the camera is reduced in proportion to the number of the magnetic particle bound. An advantage of this assay format is speed (external fields are used to manipulate the magnetic particles), and it has been applied to a fast-turnaround intraoperative parathyroid hormone assay.[35]

Nuclear magnetic resonance (NMR) detection of magnetic particle labels facilitates a homogeneous immunoassay design. The assay uses magnetic nanoparticles (~20-nm diameter) coated with antibody that bind to and cluster around analyte in solution. A consequence of the binding and clustering is that the microscopic environment of water in the reaction mixture is altered, and this can be detected by NMR as a change in the T2 relaxation signal (Fig. 26.17).[36]

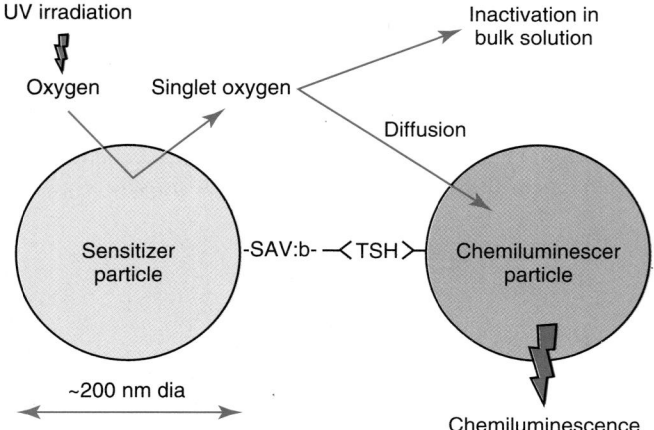

FIGURE 26.16 Example of luminescent oxygen channeling immunoassay (LOCI) for thyroid-stimulating hormone (TSH). In this assay, TSH links two latex microbeads—one containing a photosensitive reagent and the other a precursor of a chemiluminescent reagent. *UV,* Ultraviolet.

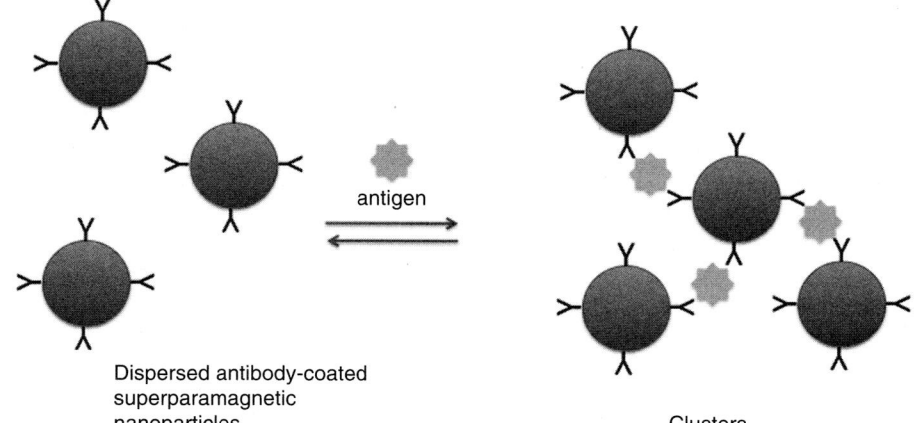

FIGURE 26.17 Magnetic particle immunoassay. Antigen binds to magnetic nanoparticles (~20-nm diameter) coated with antibody. The binding and resulting clustering of the particles alters the microscopic environment of water in the reaction mixture, and this can be detected by nuclear magnetic resonance (change in the T2 relaxation signal).

An advantage of this type of immunoassay is that the signal is unaffected by the sample matrix (e.g., opacity), and this allows direct detection in various types of specimens, such as whole blood and sputum.

Immuno–polymerase chain reaction and bio-barcode immunoassay. DNA has been used in a number of different immunoassay designs. Immuno-PCR (Innova Biosciences, Cambridge, United Kingdom) is a heterogeneous immunoassay in which a piece of single- or double-stranded DNA (dsDNA) is used as a label for an antibody in a sandwich assay.[37] Bound DNA label is amplified using PCR. The amplified DNA product is separated by gel electrophoresis and quantitated by either densitometric scanning of a gel or quantitative PCR.

In the bio-barcode assay, capture antibody immobilized on a magnetic particle binds to the analyte (e.g., a protein) and the bound analyte is reacted with a gold particle (30-nm diameter) decorated with detection antibody and barcode dsDNA (Fig. 26.18; refer to the figure legend for details). After complex formation and washing, one strand of the barcode, dsDNA is released from the gold particle. Next, the released barcode dsDNA is hybridized to an immobilized capture DNA probe and to a gold particle–labeled detection probe. The bound gold particle–labeled detection probe is first decorated with silver and then detected scanometrically. This type of assay has achieved very low detection limits, for example, the picogram per milliliter range for serum prostate-specific antigen.[38]

Multiplexed immunoassays and protein microarrays. Simultaneous multianalyte immunoassays in which two or more analytes are detected in a single assay (multiplex) improve the efficiency of detecting multiple analytes.

Protein microarrays are one example. Arrays of hundreds or thousands of micrometer-sized dots of antigens or antibodies immobilized on the surface of a glass or plastic chip are emerging as an important tool in proteomic studies and in assessing protein-protein interactions. This format facilitates simultaneous multianalyte immunoassays using, for example, enzyme- or fluorophore-labeled conjugates. The arrays are made by printing or spotting 1-nL drops of protein solutions onto a flat surface, such as a glass microscope slide. In a typical sandwich assay, the array on the surface of the slide is incubated with sample and then with conjugate. Bound conjugate is detected with chemiluminescence or fluorescence using a scanning device. The pattern of the signal provides information on the presence and amount of individual analytes in the sample or the reactivity of a single analyte with the range of proteins arrayed on the surface of the slide.[39]

Another type of microarray is the liquid array format known as multiplexed microsphere-based suspension array platform (Luminex xMAP; Austin, Texas). This assay is based on collections of microbeads optically coded with fluorescent dyes, each with a unique spectral identity.[40] Each type of fluorescent bead is coated with a different antibody or antigen. After addition of the sample, a labeled antibody forms an immunocomplex on each bead, which is assessed using flow cytometric or fluorescence imaging principles (Fig. 26.19). Up to 500 different signatures can be created, allowing multiplexing of up to 500 different assays in a single assay vessel. This technology has many applications for multianalyte detection such as cytokine, autoantibody, and allergen profiling, as well as molecular diagnostics. A common use

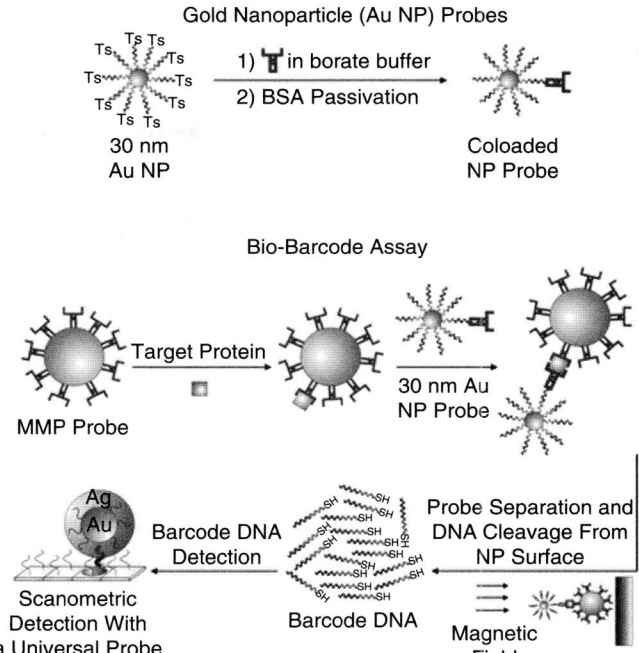

FIGURE 26.18 Bio-barcode assay for a protein target. Barcode DNA-functionalized gold nanoparticles *(Au-NP)* (30-nm diameter) are conjugated to target protein-specific antibodies (via tosyl [Ts] groups) to generate the coloaded target protein Au-NP probes that are then passivated with bovine serum albumin. The next steps in the sandwich immunoassay are reaction of the target protein with magnetic microparticle probes *(MMPs)* (1-μm diameter) coated with monoclonal antibodies to target protein, washing to remove excess serum components, and then reaction with the *Au-NP.* After magnetic separation and wash steps, the target protein-specific DNA barcodes are released into solution and detected using the scanometric assay (includes an Au-NP catalyzed silver enhancement step). Approximately half of the barcode DNA sequence is complementary to the universal scanometric Au-NP probe DNA, and the other half is complementary to a surface immobilized DNA sequence that is responsible for sorting and binding barcodes complementary to the target protein barcode sequence. (From Thaxton CS, Elghanian R, Thomas AD, Stoeva SI, Lee J-S, Smith ND, et al. Nanoparticle-based bio-barcode assay redefines "undetectable" PSA and biochemical recurrence after radical prostatectomy. *PNAS* 2009;106:18437–42 [with permission]).

for this technology in clinical laboratories is human leukocyte antigen (HLA).

Simultaneous immunoassays can also be enabled by combinations of labels such as europium (613 nm; emission lifetime, 730 μs) and samarium (643 nm; emission lifetime 50 μs) chelates. These two chelates have different fluorescence emission maxima and different fluorescence decay times and thus can be easily distinguished by making measurements at 613 nm, delay time 0.4 ms (europium), and 643 nm, delay time 0.05 ms (samarium). Apart from fluorophores, many other label combinations have been developed for simultaneous and multiplexed assays, including different radioisotopes, and nano-sized objects such as quantum dots, and other particles of different shapes and sizes.[41]

Digital immunoassay. A long-cherished goal in immunoassay has been single molecule sensitivity. A new digital

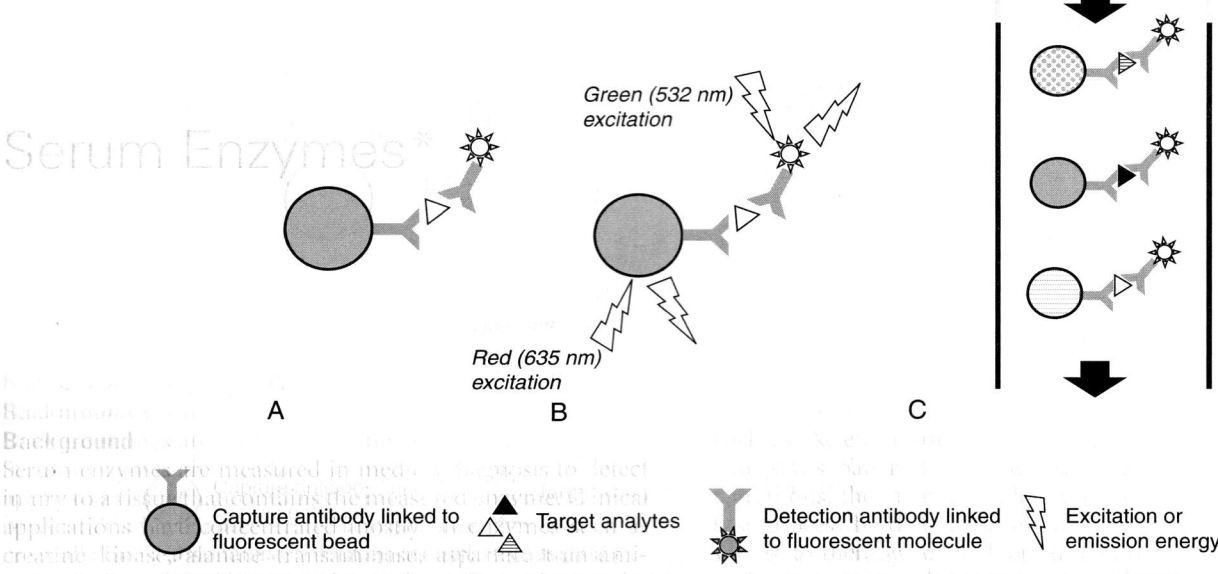

Green (532 nm) excitation

Red (635 nm) excitation

A   B   C

Capture antibody linked to fluorescent bead   Target analytes   Detection antibody linked to fluorescent molecule   Excitation or emission energy

FIGURE 26.19 Multiplexed Microsphere-Based Suspension Array Platform (xMAP). Luminex xMAP is a liquid phase method comprised of a 5.6-μm fluorescent bead linked to a capture antibody and a fluorescent molecule linked to a detection antibody; these create a "sandwich" with an analyte of interest (A). The beads contain varying ratios of two fluorophores so that each capture antibody has an associated bead with a unique spectral identity when excited with a 635-nm *(red)* laser (B). The detection antibody's fluorescent molecule is excited by a 532-nm *(green)* laser. In practice, a patient sample is examined for multiple analytes simultaneously. A complex of antibodies and analyte is formed, and then the complex is injected into a channel where each complex is excited by both the red and green lasers. The emission of the red laser gives the identity of the bead, whereas the emission of the green laser is for counting analyte bound into the "sandwich" (C).

immunoassay design (Simoa, Quanterix, Lexington, MA) led to dramatic improvements in sensitivity (Fig. 26.20). This ELISA type of assay is performed on small antibody-coated paramagnetic microbeads. At the end of the incubation of the capture antibody-coated beads with sample and β-galactosidase–labeled antibody, the beads, in the presence of a fluorogenic substrate, are distributed into an array of 216,000 wells (one bead per well), each with a volume of 40 fL. A single target molecule captured onto the bead in a femtoliter-sized well generates sufficient fluorescence signal for detection. The signal from the array of wells is imaged using a charge-coupled device camera and the number of fluorescent wells is counted (a digital read-out), thus counting the number of molecules in the sample. At the 10:1 bead-to-molecule ratio used in the assay the number of beads that carry a labeled immunocomplex follows a Poisson distribution, such that at low protein concentrations each bead will capture one labeled immunocomplex or none. The combination of the sensitive label detection method and the low background achieved by the signal counting leads to protein assays with femtogram per milliliter sensitivity.[42]

Fluoroimmunoassays also can be operated in a digital mode as exemplified by the Erenna Immunoassay System (Singulex, Alameda, California). This system combines a magnetic microparticle-based sandwich fluoroimmunoassay and single-molecule counting technology. It integrates capillary flow, laser-induced fluorescence, and a highly sensitive detection optics module for sample analysis. On completion of sandwich formation, the fluorescent dye–labeled detection antibody is released from the captured antigen and eluted into a very small volume (20 μL) for counting. Fluorescence detection occurs in a flow system in a very small interrogation space (5 μm) that is illuminated by a laser. Signals greater than the background are counted as digital events, and the sum of the digital events is related to the original concentration of the analyte in the sample.[43]

Simplified immunoassays. Integration of the technical advances made in molecular immunology with those made in the material and processing sciences has resulted in the development of simplified immunoassays for use in physicians' offices or the home (i.e., the point-of-care market, see Chapter 30). Early efforts were directed toward pregnancy and fertility testing and were based on agglutination and inhibition of agglutination using labeled red blood cells or latex particles in a slide format. Subsequently, sandwich immunoassays have been adapted for similar applications.

These tests require only the addition of sample, thus simplifying the assay protocol and minimizing possible malfunction resulting from operator error. Numerous one-step pregnancy tests are now available.[44] For example, one popular test device uses an absorbent strip that contains colored beads attached to an anti–human chorionic gonadotropin (hCG) monoclonal antibody. As urine moves by capillary action through the strip, labeled antibodies are mobilized and move up the test strip, which contains regions of immobilized antibodies. If hCG is present at a concentration of 25 mIU/mL or greater, a line becomes visible in the test region window. This region remains clear if hCG is not present in the urine specimen. The appearance of a control line indicates a valid test result in the control region of the result window to show the test is

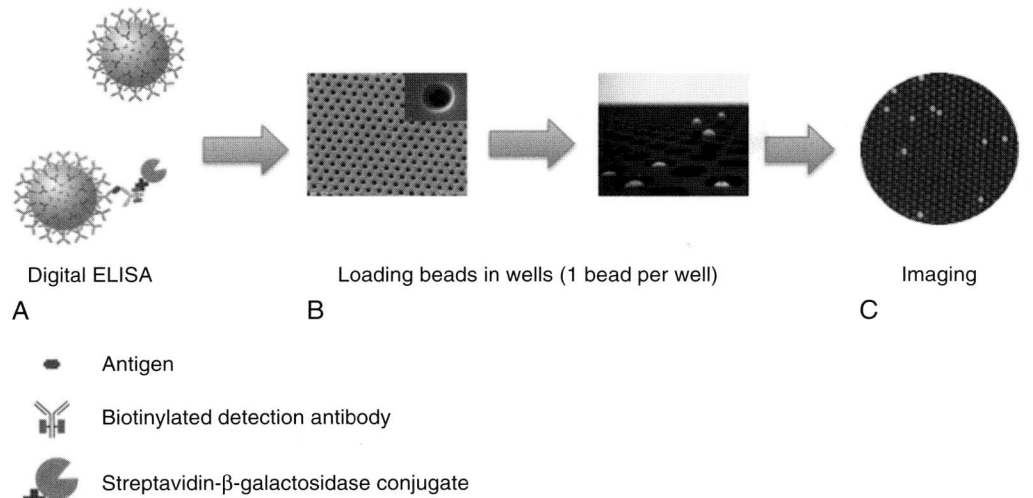

Digital ELISA   Loading beads in wells (1 bead per well)   Imaging

A   B   C

🦠 Antigen

🔱 Biotinylated detection antibody

🧩 Streptavidin-β-galactosidase conjugate

FIGURE 26.20 Design of a digital immunoassay (Simoa). (A) Reaction of the antigen with capture antibody-coated magnetic beads and biotinylated detection antibody. This is then followed by reaction of the bound complex with streptavidin-β-galactosidase conjugate to form single immunocomplexes of the magnetic beads. (B) The beads are loaded into wells, one bead per well and then treated with a fluorometric substrate for β-galactosidase and fluorescence from the beads in the array of wells imaged. *ELISA,* Enzyme-linked immunosorbent assay. (Images used with permission of Quanterix, Lexington, MA.)

complete and has worked correctly without degradation of antibodies or labels (see Chapter 30.)

Lateral flow assays are available in more sophisticated formats for their use in point-of-care settings. The Triage drug screen point-of-care device (Alere) allows for simultaneous detection of multiple analytes through a competitive lateral flow immunoassay. In one format, colorimetric detection of multiple drug metabolites is achieved using discrete test zones on a small piece of nylon membrane.[45] Each test zone consists of antibodies for a specific drug metabolite immobilized on the membrane surface. The reagents include each drug of interest bound to a colloidal gold particle, monoclonal antibodies specific for each drug of interest, and buffer. When mixed with a patient's urine sample containing one or more drug, some of the reagent antibody will bind to the free drug, leaving some of the corresponding reagent drug on the colloidal gold particle exposed. The exposed reagent drug can then be captured by the immobilized antibody in the corresponding test zone (see Chapter 30).

POINTS TO REMEMBER

- The most commonly used nonisotopic labels in immunoassay are:
  - Enzyme labels: Alkaline phosphatase, horseradish peroxidase, β-galactosidase
  - Fluorophore labels: Fluorescein
  - Chemiluminescent labels: Acridinium esters
  - Electrochemiluminescent labels: Ruthenium chelates
- The major types of nonseparation (homogeneous) immunoassays based on modulation of signal from the label are:
  - CEDIA: Cloned enzyme donor immunoassay
  - EMIT: Enzyme multiplied immunoassay technique
  - FPIA: Fluorescent polarization immunoassay
  - LOCI: Luminescent oxygen channeling immunoassay

Interferences in Immunoassays

Immunologic assays are prone to interferences, despite the use of highly specific antibodies for molecular recognition of the analyte. Falsely low results can occur because of the hook effect at high antigen concentrations (see earlier discussion). False-negative or false-positive results are encountered if the sample contains anti–animal immunoglobulin antibodies. For example, in a two-site sandwich assay for hCG based on mouse antibodies, human antimouse antibodies (HAMAs) present in the specimen may recognize the immobilized mouse capture, and mouse conjugate antibodies and will form a complex that is indistinguishable from an immobilized capture antibody:hCG:conjugate complex. This leads to a false-positive result. A false-negative result will be obtained if the HAMAs react with the capture antibody or the conjugate to such an extent that specific antibody binding to hCG is prevented. Many different types of circulating anti–animal immunoglobulin antibodies have been detected (e.g., human anti-goat, human anti-bovine antibodies) and shown to interfere in immunoassays. In most automated immunoassay platforms, this type of interference is minimized by including additives in the immunoassay reagents such as nonimmune serum or IgG from the species used to raise the antibodies used in the assay.

Other sources of interference with immunologic assays include antianalyte autoantibodies, therapeutic agents including animal antibodies and animal/recombinant proteins, as well as other exogenous agents or nutritional supplements.[46] For example, immunoassays that use streptavidin-biotin binding may be affected by interference from exogenous biotin present in a sample.[47] High doses of biotin supplements have resulted in clinically significant interference across a wide range of immunoassays. In practice, interferences can sometimes be uncovered by (1) clinical awareness, (2) performing dilution studies (nonlinear response), (3) testing on another assay platform that uses different reagents, or (4) from changes in values after incubation of the sample in a heterophile blocking tube or other binding agents.

CELL-BASED AND TISSUE-BASED IMMUNOCHEMICAL TECHNIQUES

Other analytical methods of clinical interest that use antibodies include immunohistochemistry and agglutination assays.

Immunohistochemistry

The use of labeled antibody reagents as specific probes for protein and peptide antigens allows the researcher and the pathologist to evaluate single cells or pieces of tissue for their synthetic capability and/or phenotypic identity. Immunohistochemistry has been rapidly expanded by immunoenzymatic methods, especially with regard to the use of horseradish peroxidase–labeled (immunoperoxidase) assays. Using enzyme labels provides several advantages over fluorescent labels. They permit the use of fixed tissue embedded in paraffin, which provides excellent preservation of cell morphology and eliminates the problem of autofluorescence from tissue. In addition, immunoperoxidase stains are permanent and only a standard light microscope is necessary to identify labeled features. The immunoperoxidase methods are also applicable to electron microscopy. Several approaches for immunoenzymatic assays have been used, including direct, indirect, peroxidase-antiperoxidase, and enzyme bridge methods.

Agglutination Assays

Agglutination assays have been used for many years for the qualitative and quantitative measurement of antigens and antibodies. In an agglutination method, the visible clumping of particulates, such as cells and latex particles, is used as an indicator of the primary reaction of antigen and antibody. Agglutination methods require stable and uniform particulates, pure antigen, and specific antibody. IgM antibodies are more likely to produce complete agglutination than are IgG antibodies because of the size and valence of the IgM molecule. Therefore when only IgG antibodies are involved, it may be necessary to use chemical enhancement or an antiglobulin agglutination method. As with all immunochemical reactions in which aggregation is the measured end point, the ratio of antigen to antibody is critical. Extremes in antigen or antibody concentration will result in inhibition of aggregation.

An incomplete agglutination reaction is one in which the primary reaction occurs, but no or only minimal aggregation of the particles occurs. Many particles, such as erythrocytes and bacteria in solution, have a net negative charge (zeta potential), which causes mutual repulsion. For successful agglutination, the antigen-antibody reaction must overcome this normal resistance. In the case of a weak antigen-antibody reaction, or one in which only IgG is involved, this mutual repulsion may be sufficient to inhibit agglutination completely or partially. In systems in which incomplete agglutination results, enhancement may be achieved by lowering the ionic strength or by introducing polymeric molecules, such as polymerized albumin (5 to 30%), dextran, hexadimethrine bromide (Polybrene, Santa Cruz Biotechnology), polyvinylpyrrolidone, or PEG.

Hemagglutination refers to agglutination reactions in which the antigen is located on an erythrocyte. Erythrocytes not only are good passive carriers of antigen; they also are easily coated with foreign proteins and can be easily obtained and stored.

Direct testing of erythrocytes for blood group, Rh, and other antigenic types is used widely in blood banks; specific antisera, such as anti-A, anti-C, and anti-Kell, are used to detect such antigens on the erythrocyte surface.

In indirect or passive hemagglutination, the erythrocytes are used as a particulate carrier of foreign antigen (and in some tests of antibodies); this technique has wide applications. Other materials available in the form of fine particles, such as bentonite and latex, also have been used as antigen carriers, but they are more difficult to coat, standardize, and store. In a related variation of this technique, known as hemagglutination inhibition, the ability of antigens, haptens, or other substances to specifically inhibit hemagglutination of sensitized (coated) cells by antibody is determined.

In general, agglutination methods are sensitive but are not as quantitative as other immunochemical methods discussed thus far. Nonisotopic immunoassays, especially EIAs, are as convenient as agglutination reactions and therefore are replacing agglutination methods in many laboratories.

NONANTIBODY BINDING AGENTS

This chapter has focused on antibodies as binding agents in assays. However, a variety of nonantibody alternatives are emerging, notably aptamers,[48] molecularly imprinted polymers (MIPs),[49] and boronates.[50] In addition, endogenous binding proteins are used in some competitive immunoassay formats as a capture agent (intrinsic factor and folate binding protein for vitamin B12 and folate measurement, respectively). See Chapter 39 for additional information.

Nucleic acid aptamers are single-stranded oligonucleotides (e.g., DNA, RNA) that bind to a specific target molecule. Aptamers against a specific target are identified by a selection process (e.g., systematic evolution of ligands by exponential enrichment [Selex]), in vitro selection). Binding properties of DNA aptamers can be improved by genetic alphabet expansion using unnatural bases (nucleotide triphosphates analogs). Aptamers with high affinity and specificity toward a wide range of target molecules have been developed and tested in various types of binding assays. These molecules can be multiplexed to quantify over a thousand proteins and are increasingly being used for biomarker discovery applications.[51]

MIP is a polymer that has been synthesized in the presence of a template molecule. During the polymerization process, complementary cavities are formed in the polymer and hence the resulting polymer (a "plastic antibody") has affinity for the template molecule. These synthetic binding agents represent an emerging type of alternative to an antibody as a binding agent.

Boronic acids have the property of binding to carbohydrates (cis-diols) and thus can serve as a binding agent for glycoproteins. An example of the use of a pair of boronate affinity reagents is shown in Fig. 26.21.[49] The assay used a solid-phase boronate affinity MIP array as the capture component and a boronic acid–coated silver nanoparticle as the detection reagent. The glycoprotein (e.g., α-fetoprotein) was

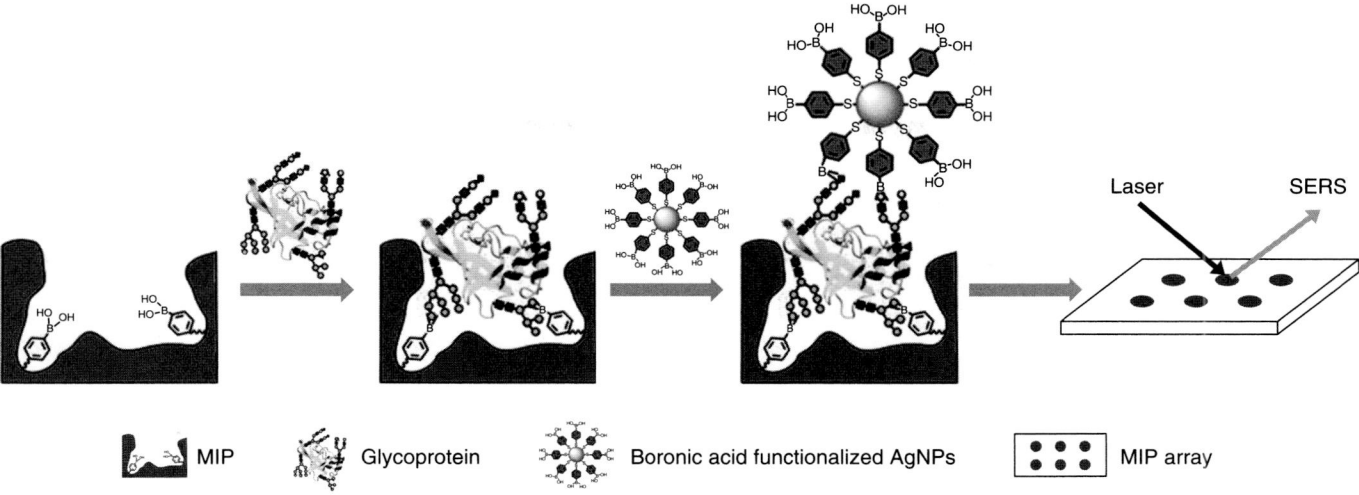

FIGURE 26.21 A boronate affinity sandwich assay for glycoproteins. At the *left* of the figure is a molecularly imprinted polymer *(MIP)*, which is a three-dimensional cavity synthesized from a 4-vinylboronic acid monomer; this cavity complements the structure of a specific glycoprotein. Next in the reaction, the glycoprotein of interest is bound by the MIP. A detection reagent based on a boronic acid and silver nanoparticles *(AgNPs)* is bound to the glycoprotein of interest. Finally, the binding of the AgNP detection reagent is detected by surface-enhanced Raman scattering *(SERS)*. (Reproduced with permission of John Wiley & Sons from Ye J, Chen Y, Liu Z. A boronate affinity sandwich assay: an appealing alternative to immunoassays for determination of glycoproteins. *Angew Chem Int Ed* 2014;53:10386–9.)

sandwiched between these two reagents (a boronate affinity sandwich), and after washing away unbound material the bound complex was detected via the surface-enhanced Raman scattering signal originating from the bound silver nanoparticles.

SELECTED REFERENCES

11. Kricka LJ. Chemiluminescent and bioluminescent techniques. Clin Chem 1991;37:1472–81.
13. Grange J, Roch AM, Quash GA. Nephelometric assay of antigens and antibodies with latex particles. J Immunol Methods 1977;18:365–75.
15. Safsten P, Klakamp SL, Drake AW, et al. Screening antibody-antigen interactions in parallel using Biacore A100. Anal Biochem 2006;353:181–90.
16. Weeks I, Kricka LJ, Wild D. Signal Generation and Detection Systems. In: Wild D, ed. The immunoassay handbook. 4th ed. Amsterdam: Elsevier; 2013:267-85.
18. Omi K, Ando T, Sakyu S, et al. Noncompetitive immunoassay detection system for haptens on the basis of antimetatype antibodies. Clin Chem 2015;61:627–35.
20. Yalow RS, Berson SA. Assay of plasma insulin in human subjects by immunological methods. Nature 1959;184:1648–69.
22. Thorpe GHG, Kricka LJ. Enhanced chemiluminescent reactions catalyzed by horseradish peroxidase. Methods Enzymol 1986;133:331–53.
24. Bronstein I, Edwards B, Voyta JC. 1,2-Dioxetanes: novel chemiluminescent enzyme substrates: applications to immunoassays. J Biolumin Chemilumin 1989;4:99–111.
31. Ullman EF, Kirakossian H, Switchenko AC, et al. Luminescent oxygen channeling assay (LOCI): sensitive, broadly applicable homogeneous immunoassay method. Clin Chem 1996;42:1518-26.
37. Maerle AV, Simonova MA, Pivovarov VD et al., Development of the covalent antibody-DNA conjugates technology for detection of IgE and IgM antibodies by immune-PCR. Plos One 2019; 14(1) e0209860.
40. Keij JF, Steinkamp JA. Flow cytometric characterization and classification of multiple dual-color fluorescent microspheres using fluorescence lifetime. Cytometry 1998;33:318–23.
42. Rissin DM, Fournier DR, Piech T, et al. Simultaneous detection of single molecules and singulated ensembles of molecules enables immunoassays with broad dynamic range. Anal Chem 2011;83:2279–85.
43. Todd J, Freese B, Lu A, et al. Ultrasensitive flow-based immunoassays using single-molecule counting. Clin Chem 2007;53:1990–5.
44. Braunstein GD. The long gestation of the modern home pregnancy test. Clin Chem 2014;60:18–21.
46. Park JY, Kricka LJ. Interferences in immunoassay. In: Wild D, ed. The immunoassay handbook. 4th ed. Amsterdam: Elsevier; 2013:403–16.

Microfabrication and Microfluidics and Their Application in Clinical Diagnostics*

Lindsay A.L. Bazydlo and James P. Landers

ABSTRACT

Background

Microfluidics is a burgeoning area of analytical chemistry that will impact many fields, including clinical diagnostics. The ability to miniaturize and expedite chemistry with smaller volumes presents the possibility for testing with expedited turnaround times at lower cost and possibly in a portable and handheld format.

Content

This chapter describes the basic concepts necessary to understand microfluidics at a fundamental level. This includes the methods and materials used for fabrication, both historically and currently, as well as aspects of microfluidic architecture necessary to carry out reactions, chemistry, labeling, and detection. The chapter highlights some of the basic developments associated with the microfluidic manipulation or analysis of diagnostically relevant analytes such as cells, nucleic acid (NA), proteins, and small molecules. It also presents some exemplary applications (e.g., circulating tumor cell capture and pathogen detection) that have paved the path for the development and adoption of microfluidics in clinical chemistry and molecular diagnostics.

---

*The full version of this chapter is available electronically on ExpertConsult.com.

Cytometry*

Howard M. Shapiro

ABSTRACT

Background

Cytometry, or "cell measurement," can describe any process by which individual biologic cells are counted or characterized, whether or not a human observer is involved. An apparatus used in the process is called a cytometer. From the 1950s on, cytometers, nearly all automated to some degree, have replaced microscopy in an increasing number of applications in both clinical and research laboratories. Some chemical assays can also be done using cytometers or similar instruments.

Flow cytometers, in which individual cells are measured as they pass through a series of optical or electronic sensors (or both), represent the majority of instruments now in use, and at least a plurality of clinical cytometric analyses is performed on cells from the blood and immune system. Apparatus, reagents, and other tools for cytometry now represent a multibillion-dollar market.

Although the sophistication and cost of high-end cytometers continue to increase, advances in optics and electronics during the past two decades could make cytometric technology affordable and applicable for a broader range of tasks worldwide within the next few years, including point-of-care assays for diagnosis and management of infectious diseases in both affluent and resource-poor countries.

Content

This chapter provides a historical overview of how cytometry evolved from microscopy; explains how cytometers work, with examples of what is measured and why; and considers some likely directions for future developments.

*The full version of this chapter is available electronically on ExpertConsult.com.

Automation in the Clinical Laboratory*

*Jonathan R. Genzen, Charles D. Hawker,
Carey-Ann D. Burnham, and Carl T. Wittwer*[a]

ABSTRACT

Background

Automation has dramatically changed both the analytical and nonanalytical aspects of clinical laboratory operations. Automation of laboratory test procedures began more than 50 years ago, but nonanalytical automation—including conveyor systems, interfaced analyzers, and automated specimen processing and storage—began in earnest in the 1990s. Today there is a wide selection of automation options designed to improve the quality, throughput, and efficiency of laboratory testing.

Content

This chapter covers automation from both nonanalytical and analytical perspectives. Historical contexts are provided. The discussion of preanalytical automation includes a review of labeling, barcoding, and portable wireless labeling systems along with the use of pneumatic tube systems and mobile robots for transport of specimens. Single-function robotic systems and multifunction systems for specimen processing are discussed. Some of these systems have pre- and postanalytical capabilities. Total laboratory automation (TLA) systems are discussed extensively. Several TLA systems include postanalytical functions; thus the chapter also addresses storage and retrieval systems. The second half of the chapter discusses automation from the analytical perspective, including specimen and reagent handling on analytical instrumentation, as well as common measurement approaches used by automated analyzers. The chapter concludes with area-specific considerations of how analytical automation has impacted all subdisciplines of laboratory medicine.

---

*The full version of this chapter is available electronically on ExpertConsult.com.

[a]The authors would like to acknowledge the original contributions of Ernest Maclin, PE; Donald S. Young, MB, PhD; and James C. Boyd, MD, upon which portions of this chapter are based.

Point-of-Care Testing

Ping Wang, Maurice O'Kane

ABSTRACT

Background

Point-of-care testing (POCT) is essentially any form of laboratory testing that takes place outside of the conventional or central laboratory setting and encompasses a wide variety of locations. Use of POCT has steadily increased over the 40 or so years since its introduction, principally driven by technology developments and changes in health care delivery that are aimed at delivering less costly and more effective care closer to the patient.

Content

This chapter describes the various POCT technologies, including those currently in use and those developed more than several decades ago such as glucose strips and lateral flow technologies. The succeeding years have seen these technologies refined and improved to deliver easier-to-use devices with incremental improvements in analytical performance. Other major technological developments include miniaturization and co-developments in consumer electronics. The developments have enabled what are essentially laboratory instruments to be reduced in both size and complexity so that they can be used in point-of-care locations. Thus the menu of tests that can be measured with POCT devices has grown to include many of the commonly requested analytes. Developments in information technology and informatics are described that make management of POCT devices easier and allow the generation of accurate and timely results. The importance of careful implementation of POCT is also discussed with various case histories to show the clinical and cost-effectiveness of POCT compared with central laboratory testing.

INTRODUCTION

Point-of-care testing (POCT) can be simply defined as "medical testing at the site of patient care", with the implication that appropriate and prompt decisions are made, leading to improved health outcomes. Many other terms have been used to describe POCT, including *bedside*,[1] *near patient*,[2] *physician's office*,[3] *extralaboratory*,[4] *decentralized*,[5] *offsite, satellite, kiosk, ancillary,* and *alternative site* testing.[6] In defining POCT, some may think that true POCT is testing carried out only by nonlaboratory personnel and should not include testing carried out by laboratory staff but in locations outside of the central laboratory. An example of the former is activated clotting time (ACT) measurements, which are usually performed in the operating room (OR) by nonlaboratory staff. In contrast, an example of the latter is intraoperative parathyroid hormone (PTH) measurements, which are often performed in the OR by laboratory personnel. For the purposes of this chapter, we take a broad view and define POCT as any testing done outside of the central laboratory, regardless of who performs it. POCT also includes "self-testing" in which the patient performs the tests himself or herself, and in fact, self-monitoring for blood glucose and prothrombin time (PT) or international normalized ratio (INR) together form the largest segment of the POCT market.

The first diagnostic or medical tests were performed at the bedside, then in the ward side-room, and then transferred to dedicated laboratory areas. This reflects a similar evolution in medical care that commenced in people's homes and then to a range of different locations that can be classified as primary, secondary, and tertiary care. These developments came about through advances in science and technology being applied to the understanding and practice of medicine. Further developments in science and technology, as reflected in the advances in POCT technology, have now enabled health care providers and patients to make choices about where testing is conducted. Box 30.1 shows the diversity of locations involved. The most prominent example of this diversity is glucose testing, which can be measured in the home by the patient, at numerous locations in the community, at the bedside by caregivers, or in the central laboratory. Currently, advances in a range of technologies and manufacturing processes, such as thin-film sensors, semiconductor engineering, plastic molding, microfluidics, nanotechnology, and consumer electronics, make it possible to adapt most of the methods used in the laboratory to the point-of-care setting.[7]

Several authors have suggested that we may be seeing the beginning of a movement of testing away from the central laboratory to the point of care.[8–10] Such a trend would clearly support the demand for improved access to health care that is closer to home and a general aim of limiting lengths of stay in hospital. There are a number of reasons for these trends, including clinical, sociologic, and economic arguments.[11] The need to limit the increasing cost of health care

---

BOX 30.1   Environments Where Point-of-Care Testing Might Be Used

Primary Care
Home
Community pharmacy
Health centers (general practice, primary care)
Workplace clinic
Physician's office and community clinic
Diagnostic and treatment center
Paramedical support vehicle (ambulance, helicopter, aircraft)

Secondary and Tertiary Care
Emergency department
Admissions unit
Ambulatory diagnostic and treatment center
Operating room
Intensive care unit
Ward
Outpatient clinic

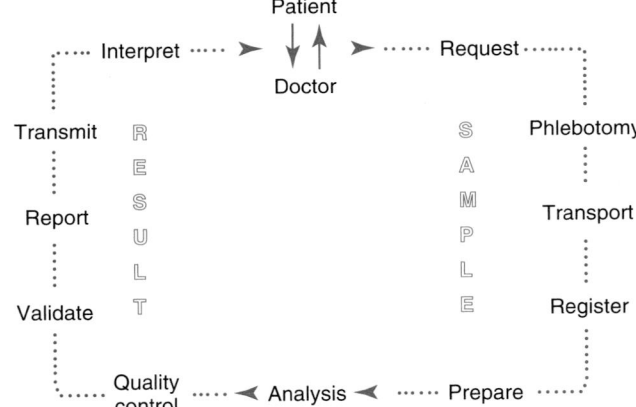

FIGURE 30.1 Schematic representation of the key steps in requesting, delivering, and using a diagnostic test result.

BOX 30.2   Potential Advantages and Disadvantages of Point-of-Care Testing

Advantages
Reduced turnaround time for test results
Improved patient management; improved engagement between patient and caregiver
Improved patient morbidity and mortality rates
Reduction in the administrative work associated with test requesting and reporting
Reduced risk of workflow-associated errors
Reduction in clinic visits
Reduction in hospital admissions
Decreased overall cost of care

Disadvantages
Increase in administrative work associated with training and certification of operators
Caregiver required to perform test
Increased risk of errors if tests performed by untrained operators
Increased cost of testing
Increased waste associated with single-use disposable tests

---

has prompted Christensen and colleagues to call for a radical change in the way that health care is delivered, a process he has called disruptive innovation.[12] In discussing how such changes can be brought to health care, he believes that POCT is one of the key enablers of disruptive innovation, citing as an example the major changes to diabetes care that have come about through the ability of patients to monitor their own glucose concentrations. The growth of telemedicine has further fueled the growth of POCT.[13]

Although POCT can be viewed as a means of delivering results rapidly to where they are needed (clinical need), it can also be seen as a means of reducing the complexity of the process associated with obtaining a test result (process need). Clinical needs met by POCT can include one of clinical urgency and one of improving the engagement between the patient and the clinician or caregiver to achieve greater patient empowerment and the potential to improve the clinical outcome. Similarly, process needs met by POCT can be improving the immediate patient-clinician-caregiver interaction, as well as reducing the longer process of the whole patient journey, improving the patient's experience and decreasing health care resource use. An example of the latter is INR testing, either by the patient or by the family doctor or general practitioner, in which the test results are integrated into the consultation process. Improving both clinical and process outcomes has the potential to reduce the errors and waste of resources while also reducing the cost of care and increasing societal gain. This argument can be applied simply to the testing process (Fig. 30.1) or to the wider aspects of the whole patient journey. See Box 30.2 for examples of the potential advantages of POCT.

The following sections of this chapter describe the technology available for POCT, how POCT should be managed from a quality perspective, an overview of the evidence for the effectiveness of POCT, and finally how POCT should be adopted and implemented.

TECHNOLOGY ASPECTS

The technology used to measure analytes outside of the conventional laboratory setting has come about partly through the long-term trend of miniaturization, including both analytics and electronics miniaturization. Also important have been advances in information and communications technologies. Starting with instruments to measure electrolytes, blood gases, and glucose, it is now possible to measure many other analytes using increasingly smaller devices. Accompanying the process of miniaturization has been the development of dry, stable reagents that can be incorporated in disposable unit-dose devices. Although the throughput of tests for these devices is low, the time required to produce the results is usually short.

Required Features of Point-of-Care Testing Devices

As with any device, it is important that designers first consider the needs of users, and these depend to some extent on the clinical setting or application. Some simply stated but critical requirements are:
1. Devices should be simple to use.
2. Reagents and consumables must be robust over extended periods of time.

3. Results from POCT devices should be concordant with established laboratory methods.
4. The device together with its associated reagents and consumables must be safe to use.

Design criteria become more specific for particular clinical settings. For example, criteria exist for devices designed for use in the developing world for sexually transmitted diseases, a major unmet medical need that is just beginning to be addressed effectively. Provided by the World Health Organization (WHO), the so-called ASSURED criteria[14] are as follows:

- **A**ffordable: for those at risk of infection
- **S**ensitive: minimal false negatives
- **S**pecific: minimal false positives
- **U**ser friendly: minimal steps to carry out test
- **R**apid and **r**obust: short turnaround time (TAT) and no need for refrigerated storage
- **E**quipment free: no complex equipment
- **D**elivered: to end users

In addition, target product profiles (TPPs) (scope, performance, operational characteristics, and price) have been developed to guide and support the development of POCT diagnostic tools for several infectious diseases such as tuberculosis and hepatitis C.[15–18]

There is, of course, a challenge in meeting all of these needs, and the final product inevitably is a compromise. Hsieh and colleagues have described the importance of understanding user needs in relation to testing for human immunodeficiency virus (HIV) and chlamydia to arrive at the best possible compromise of sensitivity versus TAT versus price.[19] Clinical needs assessment exercises such as this should be conducted and revisited throughout the entire product development process in other areas of POCT to produce devices that better meet user needs.[13]

Some of the requirements of POCT in the developed world are likely to be different than those in the ASSURED criteria. For example, connectivity to information systems, including the patient health record, is a growing requirement in modern health care systems. Although technology exists to do this, it comes at a cost, which is often difficult to recover in the usual business model in which POCT instrumentation is often supplied at no or low cost, with revenue being generated through reagent or consumable sales.

A more recent design challenge is the need to simultaneously measure multiple analytes in the same cartridge, so-called multiplexing. This is driven by the desire to measure a wider range of analytes on the same sample, avoiding the use of multiple devices. The Piccolo chemistry analyzer (Abaxis, Union City, CA) and blood gas or critical care analyzers are examples of such technologies.

Design

There is a great diversity of devices being used for POCT (Table 30.1), although it is interesting that by far, the majority of them rely on technologies devised more than 2 decades ago. Many of the devices use the same analytical principles as those found in conventional laboratory analyzers, but newer technologies are starting to appear, some of which will be described later in this chapter.

Irrespective of the type of technology, all POCT devices should have several key components, which include (1) the operator interface, (2) barcode identification systems, (3) sample and reagent delivery mechanisms, (4) reaction cell, (5) sensors, (6) control and communications systems, and (7) data management and storage. The main objectives of the design are to (1) enable the required reaction to take place that facilitates recognition of the analyte of interest, (2) ensure reliable performance of the device over a period of time, and (3) minimize the risk of error in the use of the device and within a wide range of environmental settings (e.g., temperature, humidity).

Operator Interface

The operator or user interface for a POCT device should (1) require minimal operator interaction, (2) guide the user through the operation, (3) indicate whether any key steps

TABLE 30.1 Classification of Types of Point-of-Care Testing Instruments and Devices

Type of Technology	Analytical Principle	Analytes
Small handheld, single-use POCT devices	Reflectance	Urine and blood chemistry
	Lateral-flow or flow-through immunoassays	Infectious disease agents, cardiac markers, hCG
Small handheld, single-use POCT devices with a monitoring device	Reflectance	Glucose
	Electrochemistry	Glucose
	Reflectance	Blood chemistry
	Light scattering or optical motion	Coagulation
	Lateral-flow, flow-through, or solid-phase immunoassays	Cardiac markers, drugs, CRP, allergy, and fertility tests
	Immunoturbidimetry	HbA$_{1c}$, urine albumin
	Spectrophotometry	Blood chemistry
	Electrochemistry	pH, blood gases, electrolytes, metabolites, infectious agents
	Fluorescence, electrochemistry with PCR	
Larger cartridge-type and bench-top POCT devices	Electrochemistry	pH, blood gases, electrolytes, metabolites
	Fluorescence	pH, blood gases, electrolytes, metabolites
	Multiwavelength spectrophotometry	Hemoglobin species, bilirubin
	Time-resolved fluorescence	Cardiac markers, drugs, CRP
	Electrical impedance	CBC
	Polymerase chain reaction	Bacteria and viruses

CBC, Complete blood count; *CRP,* C-reactive protein; *HbA$_{1c}$,* glycated hemoglobin; *hCG,* human chorionic gonadotrophin; *PCR,* polymerase chain reaction; *POCT,* point-of-care testing.

have not been completed correctly, and (4) include identifying the (a) operator, (b) patient, (c) test to be measured, and (d) reagent lot number and date/time of testing.

Advances in information technology (IT) and consumer electronics have had a major impact on this area. Other forms of user interface include keypads, barcode readers, and possibly a printer. In some devices, the display is the only means to show the result, but many POCT devices are taking advantage of developments in mobile telephone and computing technology displays and are rapidly adding more sophisticated touch screens that can be used for many different functions.

Barcode Identification Systems

Many POCT devices incorporate barcode reading systems for a number of purposes. These include (1) identifying the reagent package to the system (whether it is a single-use disposable or a multi-use reagent pack–based system), (2) incorporating factory calibration data, and in some cases (3) programming the instrument to process a particular test or group of tests. Some POCT devices use magnetic strips as a way of storing similar information, such as lot-specific calibration data. Other functions of the barcode reader include the capability to identify both the operator and the patient sample to the system. This provides traceability to the person who performed the test and links the results to the correct patient. The latter has assumed increasing importance as part of patient safety initiatives. All of this information can then be combined with the information on date and time when the test was performed to give the full identity of the specimen when the results are transmitted back to the patient record.

Sample Types and Sample Delivery

The vast majority of POCT devices to date have used whole blood or urine specimens; in the case of blood, this commonly involves a capillary or fingerstick sample. In this way, the sample can be introduced to the POCT device directly. Alternatively, a venous specimen can be collected and a small sample removed for POCT; in some cases, especially with critical care analyzers, the blood collection tube can be inserted directly into the POCT machine. Many POCT urinalysis devices can be dipped into the specimen, but this is much less common for POCT blood devices.

Looking to the future, there are devices that are designed for use with tears and interstitial fluid specimens. Sample access and delivery of the sample to the actual sensing component of the strip, cassette, cartridge, or fluidic cell are also key interactions of the user—and an opportunity for errors to be made. Ideally, after the addition of the sample, there should be no further need for operator intervention,[20] and devices are now available that minimize the degree of interaction to the point where a closed tube has simply to be placed in a holder and the instrument automatically performs all other functions.[21]

Reaction Cell

The design of the location where the analytical reaction takes place varies from a simple porous pad to a microfluidic cartridge or surface within a cartridge. An example of a cartridge type of design is shown in Fig. 30.2, which shows a cross-section through the Siemens DCA cartridge that measures

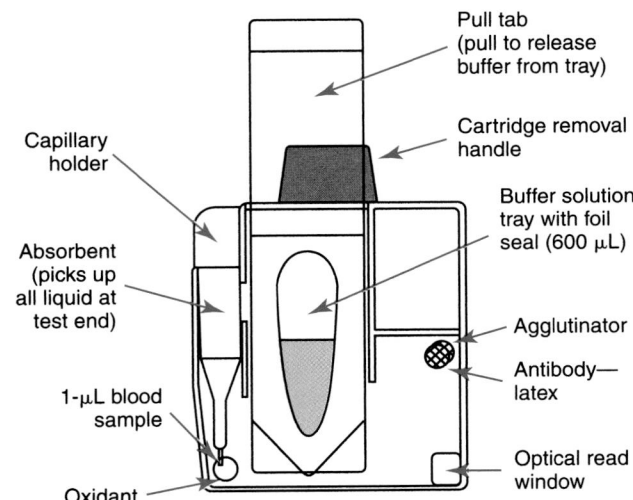

FIGURE 30.2 Schematic diagram of the Siemens DCA 2000 HbA$_{1c}$ immunoassay cartridge. (Courtesy Siemens Healthcare.)

glycated hemoglobin. To simplify the user interface, it is often necessary to design complexity into the reaction chamber. Advances in fluidics and fabricating techniques have been critical to the development of POCT devices[22] (for additional information, refer to Chapter 27). As analytical reactions have increased in complexity, more reaction cells or zones have been added. Thus in the case of molecular tests, different reaction zones may be required for DNA extraction, the amplification reaction, and product detection. In some situations, it may be necessary to remove some of the reaction constituents downstream from each zone before reaching the next reaction zone. There may also be differing reaction temperature requirements for each reaction zone. Another consideration in the design of reaction cells is to ensure that the requisite mixing of sample and reagents occur, which may be critical when using very small volumes.

Sensors

Much of the development focus in POCT devices has been concerned with the advances in sensor design of which there are various types.[23] A chemosensor is one where the analyte has an intrinsic property, such as electrochemistry, that enables it to be detected without a recognition element. More commonly, chemosensors used in many POCT devices have a transducing element such as a chemical indicator or binding molecule that recognizes the analyte to be measured and produces a signal, usually electrical or optical. A biosensor is distinguished from a chemosensor by having a biological or biochemical component as the recognition element. Enzymes are the most common biological element used followed by antibodies and nucleotides; transduction typically is via an optical or electrical signal. More detail about sensor design can be found in Chapter 17.

Control and Communications Systems

In even the smallest device, there is a control subsystem that coordinates all the other systems and ensures that all the required processes for an analysis take place in the correct order. Operations that require control include (1) insertion or removal of the strip, cartridge, cassette, or reagent;

(2) temperature control; (3) sample injection or aspiration; (4) sample detection; (5) reagent addition, especially in a fluidic-based system (6) mixing; (7) timing of the detection process; (8) detection of measurement signal; and (9) waste removal. Fluid movement is often accomplished by mechanical means through pumps or centrifugation and by fluidic properties, such as surface tension; the latter is often a critical element in the design of the simple strip tests and in microfabricated systems.[22]

Data Management and Storage

IT is as crucial to POCT devices as sensing technology. IT includes data management of calibration curve data and quality control (QC) limits and patient results. In some systems, data transfer and management take place when the meter or reader is linked to a small bench-top device called a docking station, but more commonly these days, devices use wireless technology to communicate. These and other devices include communication protocols that allow data to be transferred to other data management systems, to electronic medical records, and to other mobile computing devices.[24–26]

Manufacturing of Point-of-Care Testing Devices

Because many POCT devices are single use and discarded, reproducibility of manufacture is a key requirement so that consistent performance extends across a large number of strips or devices. The manufacturing process includes steps that are taken to ensure that the devices are reproducible and remain stable during transit and storage for the stated period of time.[27]

Types of Existing Point-of-Care Testing Technology

For the purposes of this review, POCT devices are classified into (1) small, quantitative handheld devices that often use qualitative or quantitative strips or similar technology but with a reader device and (2) larger bench-top devices that are often variants of ones used in conventional laboratories. This classification is somewhat arbitrary because there is no sharp demarcation between the types. There are gradations in both size and internal complexity of devices, although differentiation can sometimes be made on the need for external power. The clear trend is for devices becoming smaller and more capable. All the technologies described here are established commercially, sometimes for several decades, but the concluding section briefly mentions some emerging technologies that are likely to become commercial products.

Small Handheld, Single-use Point-of-Care Testing Devices

Many POCT devices fall into this category, including (1) single-pad or multipad tests that are read visually by reflectance photometry or electrochemically, (2) more complex pads that use light reflectance for measurement, and (3) fabricated cassettes or cartridges that incorporate methodologies such as immunochromatography, and are used as immunosensors. All of these devices are truly portable, and for that reason, the way they are used operationally, often immediately by the patient, is different to larger bench-top devices (e.g., devices that require application of a whole blood sample such as a glucose strip often obviate the need for sample containers, labeling, or transport compared with larger POCT instruments, which may be some distance from

the patient). Although avoiding these additional steps is convenient, there is the potential for error, and procedures need to be designed to reduce the risk of such errors.

Single-pad and multipad strip tests. Strip tests are single-pad or multipad devices that can measure up to 10 different analytes using reflectance technology. They are relatively simple in construction and are composed of a pad of porous material, such as cellulose, that is impregnated with reagent and then dried.[28] Samples are added to the device either by dipping (as, typically, in the case of urine analysis) or by spotting (as, typically, in the case of blood glucose analysis). In the latter case, there has been a gradual transition from optical to electrochemical detection, avoiding the need to wipe the strip to remove the red cells before measurement. A critical operator factor when spotting the sample on to the pad is the need to apply a sufficient but not superfluous amount of sample. In addition, because assay readout is sensitive to reaction timing, it is necessary to time the period between placing the sample on the pad and reading the result. The timing issues can be overcome in some instances with internal timer in the device.

Multilayer pads. More complex pads are composed of several layers, the uppermost of which is a semipermeable membrane that prevents red blood cells (RBCs) from entering the matrix. Again, with these devices, a critical operator factor is the need to cover the whole pad with the sample. In addition, because the reactions often do not proceed to completion, it is necessary to time the period between placing the sample on the pad and comparing the resulting color with a color chart. Developments of these single-stick devices include the inclusion of two pads. These are used for measurement of (1) different concentrations of the same analyte, such as hemoglobin and glucose,[28] and (2) both albumin and creatinine (semiquantitative) to provide an albumin-to-creatinine ratio.[29] Table 30.2 lists some of the tests performed by single-pad and multipad dipsticks and the chemistry used for analysis.

Immunostrips. These are biologic sensors in which the recognition agent is an antibody that binds to the analyte. Detection of the binding event or signal transducer is usually via an optical mechanism, either reflectance or fluorescence spectrophotometry, although visual inspection has also been used. Immunosensors usually use solid phase technologies in conjunction with (1) flow-through or (2) lateral-flow (also often referred to as immunochromatography) processes. In the flow-through format, a heterogeneous immunoassay takes place in a porous matrix cell that acts as the solid phase, capturing the bound label as the reaction mixture (sample and reagents) passes *through* the matrix.[30] In lateral flow, the separation stage takes place as the reaction mixture (sample and reagents) passes *along* the porous matrix.[31] In all of these different formats, uniform and predictable flow of the sample through or along the solid phase matrix is a major determinant of the reproducibility of the technique. Therefore the choice of matrix and how it interacts with the sample are of particular importance, and advances in the understanding of solid phase and surface chemistry technology have made major contributions to the development of immunosensors.[32]

An example of immunosensor technology is shown in Fig. 30.3. In this device, the blood sample is added and first flows through a glass fiber fleece, which separates the plasma

TABLE 30.2	Examples of Single-Pad or Multipad Stick Tests	
Test	**Sample**	**Chemistry**
Acetaminophen	Whole blood	Aryl acylamide amidohydrolase
Alanine aminotransferase	Whole blood	Alanine/glutamate
Albumin	Whole blood, urine	Dye binding
Cholesterol	Whole blood	Cholesterol oxidase
Creatinine	Whole blood, urine	Copper complexation
Glucose	Whole blood	Glucose oxidase
Lactate	Whole blood	Lactate dehydrogenase
Uric acid	Whole blood	Uricase
Alcohol	Urine	Alcohol dehydrogenase
Bilirubin	Urine	2,4-Dichloroaniline
Hemoglobin	Urine	Peroxidase activity
Leukocyte esterase	Urine	Pyrrole amino ester hydrolysis
Ketones	Urine	Sodium nitroprusside reaction
Nitrite	Urine	p-Arsanilic acid reaction
pH	Urine	Double-indicator principle
Protein	Urine	Protein error of indicators
Specific gravity	Urine	Polyacid pH change
Urobilinogen	Urine	Ehrlich's reaction

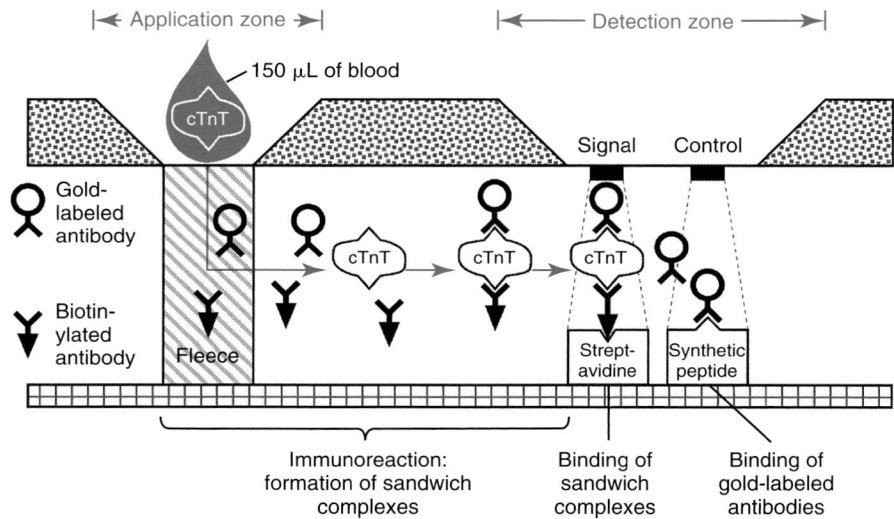

FIGURE 30.3 Schematic diagram of a lateral flow immunoassay strip for cardiac troponin T (cTnT). (Courtesy Roche Diagnostics International Limited Copyright.)

from whole blood. Simultaneously, two monoclonal antihuman cardiac troponin T (cTnT) antibodies, one conjugated to biotin and one labeled with gold particles, bind to the troponin T in the sample. The antibody-troponin complex then flows in a lateral direction along the cellulose nitrate test strip until it reaches the capture zone, which contains streptavidin bound to a solid phase. The biotin in the antibody-troponin complex binds to the streptavidin and immobilizes the complex. The complex is then visualized as a purple band by the gold particles attached to one of the antibodies. The unreacted gold-labeled antibody moves farther down the strip, where it is captured by a zone containing a synthetic peptide consisting of the epitope of human cTnT and is visualized as a separate but similar colored band. The presence of this second band serves as an important quality indicator because it

shows that the sample has flowed along the test strip and the device has performed correctly.[33,34]

Although the majority of quantitative lateral flow immunoassay devices measure only a single analyte at a time, some can measure a panel of analytes, such as (1) cardiac markers,[35] (2) fertility tests,[36] and (3) drugs of abuse.[37] In these devices, a mixture of antibodies is immobilized at the origin, and complementary antibodies for the various analytes are immobilized at varying positions along the porous strip. In the case of drugs of abuse, devices are designed such that positive responses are obtained only if the concentration is greater than a precalibrated cutoff value.[37] Another design variation is to take advantage of the competition between the target analyte and an analyte conjugate for antibodies. In this case, the analyte conjugate is immobilized close to the origin, and the specimen is mixed with antibodies before being applied to the strip. This design is well suited for semiquantitative applications with well-defined cutoff concentrations.[38]

Small Handheld, Single-use Point-of-Care Devices With a Monitoring Device

Glucose measurement. Clinically, POCT is most frequently used to measure glucose. These devices are biosensors because they all use an enzyme as the recognition agent, which is glucose oxidase (GO), hexokinase (HK), or glucose dehydrogenase (GDH), with photometric (reflectance) or now increasingly electrochemical detection.[39]

In general, all modern glucose strips are a form of what is called *thick-film* technology in that the film is composed of several layers each having a specific function. These are shown diagrammatically for a reflectance-based strip in Fig. 30.4. When blood is added to a strip, plasma passes into the film or analytical layer. For some photometric systems, erythrocytes must be excluded, and these processes are achieved by what is called the spreading or separating layer that contains various components, including glass fibers, fleeces, membranes, and special latex formulations. In photometric systems, a spreading layer is also important for the fast homogeneous distribution of the sample; electrochemical strips use capillary fill systems. The support layer is usually a thin plastic material that in the case of reflectance-based strips may also have reflective properties. Additional reflectance properties have been achieved through the inclusion of substances such as titanium oxide, barium sulphate, and zinc oxide.

Glucose strips are produced in large batches, and, after extensive quality assurance procedures, each batch is given a code that is stored in a magnetic strip on the underside of each test strip. This code describes the performance of the batch, including the calibrating relationship between the photometric or electrochemical signal and the concentration of glucose. More recently, strips that do not require coding have become more commonplace, and this advance has been facilitated by the development of electrochemical glucose strips. These are composed of an Ag-AgCl reference electrode and a carbon-based active electrode, both manufactured using screen printing technology with the ferrocene or its derivatives contained in the printing ink.[40] The conversion of glucose is accompanied by the reduction of ferrocene and the release of electrons (Fig. 30.5). Continuing innovations such as this have also facilitated the production of smaller meters, nonwipe strips, less need to clean instrument optics, more rapid results, and smaller sample volumes.

Although electrochemical systems have enabled the design of strips that are less subject to interferences, problems still persist. Strips that use GO are more substrate specific but are affected by oxygen tension and high partial pressure of oxygen (PO_2), leading to falsely low results.[41] Blood oxygen tension does not affect GDH-based strips, and genetically engineered GDH strips are free from interference by maltose, which plagued earlier versions. Hematocrit is another important interference, the effects of which have been reduced by some newer strip designs. Many different factors can lead to inaccurate glucose results from strip tests; a comprehensive review of them is provided by Tonyushkina and colleagues.[42]

The ubiquitous application of glucose meters has led to the publication of guidelines stipulating the required accuracy of meters as compared with laboratory results. This is particularly important when meters are being used to guide insulin regimens and achieve tighter glycemic control. Data by Karon and colleagues[43] show how insulin dosing errors can arise from inaccurate meters, and this has led to calls for tighter accuracy standards to prevent such errors occurring. Although it is possible that continuing innovation will lead to meters and strips that can meet these more demanding goals, it should also be recognized that tight glycemic control itself remains controversial.

International normalized ratio measurement. Another common meter type device used by patients at home and by health care providers in clinics is that used to monitor warfarin or Coumadin therapy and measure PT reported as INR

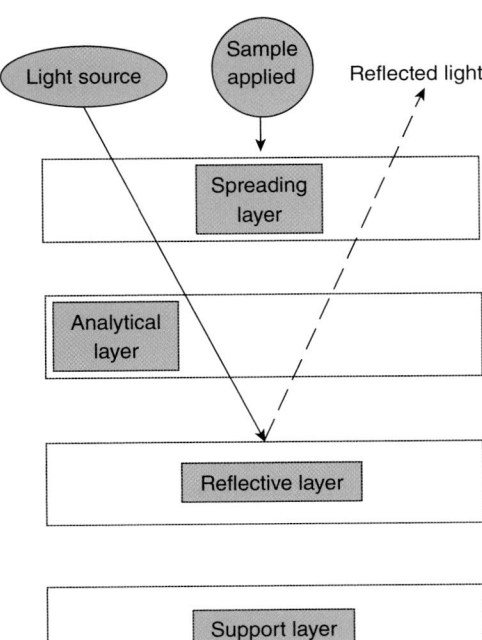

FIGURE 30.4 Schematic diagram of the components which make up a typical reflectance-based glucose strip.

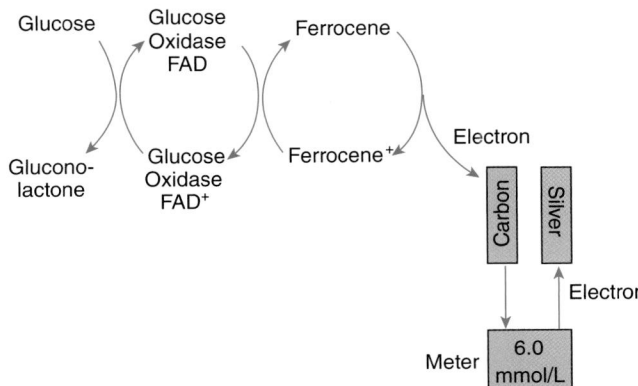

FIGURE 30.5 Schematic diagram of the reactions taking place in a MediSense electrochemical glucose strip. *FAD,* Flavin adenine dinucleotide. (Modified from Henning TP, Cunningham TP. Biosensors for personal diabetes management. In: Ramsay G, ed. *Commercial Biosensors.* New York: John Wiley & Sons: 1998:3–46.)

values. First devised some 2 decades ago, a number of different technologies have been developed to measure INR at point of care, including optical and electrochemical detection. Innovation has been applied both to the strip, where a drop of blood is placed, and to the meter into which the strip is placed. Historically, early systems used magnets to detect the decrease in sample flow or movement that results from the clotting process, but this required careful timing and a large blood sample while an alternative technology used optical sensors to monitor the decrease in sample speed flowing through a sample channel as the clot forms. Speckle detection technology has also been used to measure (1) PT, (2) activated partial thromboplastin time (APTT), and (3) ACT. In this approach, the instrument contains an infrared light source that directs a coherent light beam onto the oscillating sample. The movement of the RBCs in the blood results in the refraction of the light to produce an interference or "speckle" pattern that is recorded by the photodetector. This "speckle" pattern changes when the capillary flow slows as the sample clots. The time it takes for this to happen is a measure of the clotting time.

Newer detection technologies use electrochemical measurements. In the HemoSense device (Alere, Waltham, MA), clotting is detected by change in impedance (Fig. 30.6),[44] and in a Roche device (Roche Diagnostics, Basel, Switzerland), a change in current is detected.[45] Both devices incorporate inbuilt QC systems that are activated when a patient sample is placed on the strip. In the case of HemoSense, the strip has three channels, one for the patient test and the other two for different concentrations of internal QC material. All of these innovations have improved the reliability of these devices to the extent that a systematic review of the literature on the quality assessment of devices for self-monitoring indicated that they generally provide comparable results to laboratory-generated INR values.[46]

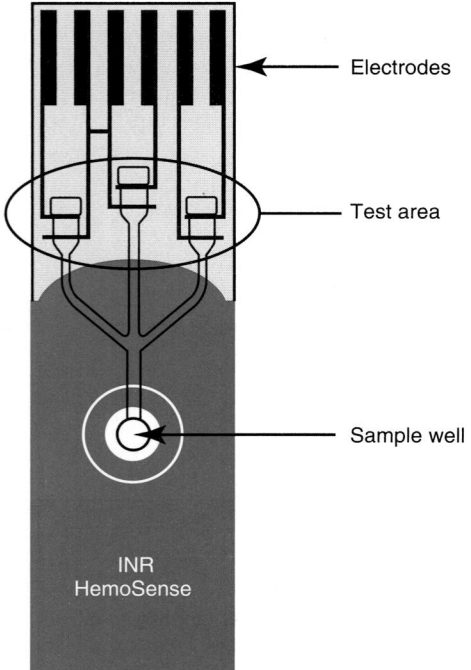

FIGURE 30.6 Schematic diagram of the HemoSense prothrombin time trip. *INR,* International normalized ratio. (Courtesy Alere.)

Handheld integrated cartridge technology. The prime example of this type of technology is the i-STAT analyzer (Abbott Point of Care, Princeton, NJ), a handheld device originally designed to measure blood gases but now with a considerably extended menu that includes electrolytes, glucose, creatinine, coagulation parameters, and cardiac markers.[47] In contrast to the thick-film technology described earlier, the single-use sensors in this device are constructed using *thin-film* technology. The latter involves microlithographic processes to deposit thin layers of 1 to 10 μm thick (as opposed to 10- to 50-μm thick layers in thick film technology) similar to the construction of computer chips and other silicon-based devices. The techniques such as sputtering or chemical vapor deposition that are used to make these devices including the electrodes and sensors of the i-STAT device are highly reproducible but require sophisticated and expensive manufacturing facilities.[48] Each single-use i-STAT cartridge contains an array of electrochemical sensors for a set of particular analytes, and it is operated in conjunction with a handheld reading device. Because the sensor layer is very thin, blood permeates this layer quickly, and the sensor cartridge, when it reaches room temperature if it has been refrigerated, can be used immediately after it is unwrapped from its packing. This is an advantage over some thick-film sensors that require an equilibration or wet-up time before they are used to measure blood samples. With the extended menu through the provision of different cartridges, this device has proven popular because its operation is similar for all analytes, thus avoiding the inconvenience and potential errors that may occur with multiple different instruments. Furthermore, it represents a potentially economical solution to the need for providing low sample numbers of critical analytes.

A disadvantage of thin-film technology is that manufacturing costs are high because of the need for special clean air facilities. Thus more recent technology to measure blood gases and related parameters uses less costly, so-called smart card technology. Fig. 30.7 shows two views of the Epoc test card, which is manufactured on a 35-mm tape on reel format; on the right is the top view of the test card showing the sample entry port, the sealed calibrator reservoir, and the sensor module at the top; on the left is the bottom view of the card with the sensor module where measurements take place, and below this are details of the test panel. The Epoc system (Siemens Healthineers, Ottawa, Canada) is used in conjunction with a handheld analyzer, and it also can provide a range of critical care tests, including immunoassay measurement,[49] with the advantage of operators having to be familiar only with the use of a single device.

Larger Cartridge Type and Bench-top Point-of-Care Testing Devices

This section includes a wide range of devices that are all quantitative and not handheld but vary considerably in size. The smaller ones typically incorporate small, compact detectors, such as a charge-coupled device (CCD) camera that is a multichannel light detector, similar to a photomultiplier tube in a spectrophotometer, but it detects much lower signals at low levels of light. This type of technology enables quantitative measurements of lateral-flow immunoassay strips and is incorporated in the many different POCT devices of this type that are available on the market.

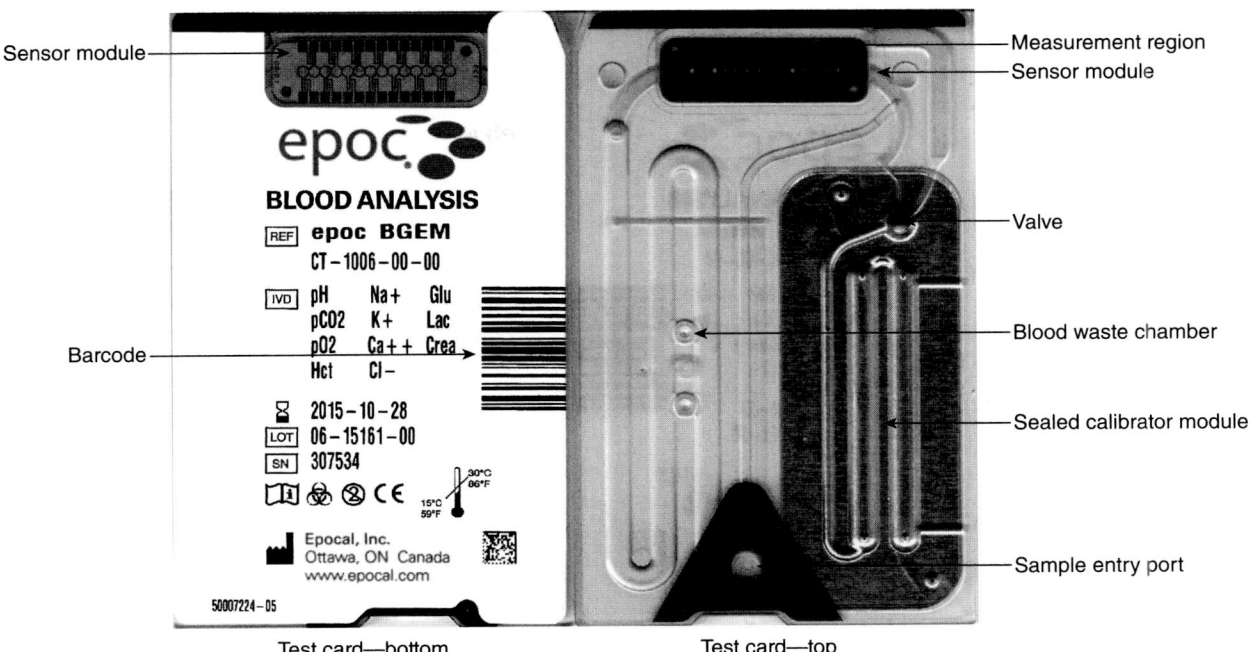

FIGURE 30.7 Epoch test card for blood gas analysis. (Courtesy Alere.)

Cartridge-type devices. A number of single-use, quantitative POCT devices are available that use a cassette or cartridge design rather than lateral-flow strips. Several cassette-based systems have been developed for measurement of hemoglobin. In one such system, RBCs are lysed in a minicuvet, hemoglobin is converted to methemoglobin, and the methemoglobin is measured at 570 nm; turbidity is corrected for by an additional measurement at 880 nm.[50]

Another type of cartridge design uses a light-scattering immunoassay to measure glycated hemoglobin (HbA_1c), together with a photometric assay for total hemoglobin. The cartridge is a relatively complex structure that contains all the reagents required for the immunoassay and lysing reagents and potassium ferricyanide reagent for measurement of total hemoglobin (see Fig. 30.2). Agglutination takes place between the latex-bound antibody and a synthetic polymer that contains the immunoreactive portion of HbA_1c, which leads to increased scattering of light. Addition of HbA_1c in the patient sample reduces the agglutination by competing for the latex bound antibody, and the reduction in light scattering is proportional to the concentration of HbA_1c.

Measurement takes place when the cartridge is placed into a temperature-controlled reader, and the analytical performance of the Siemens DCA device (Siemens Healthineers, Munich, Germany) is sufficient for quantitative monitoring of glycemic control and can also be used for measurement of urinary albumin and creatinine.[51] Increasingly more diabetes care is being delivered closer to the patient in various health care settings outside of the hospital, and this has driven the production of other POCT devices that can measure diabetes-related analytes. In addition to the Siemens DCA, there is the Affinion (Abbott Point of Care, Princeton, NJ) which has a similar menu to the DCA, and adds C-reactive protein (CRP)[52] and more recently the Roche Cobas b101 (Roche Diagnostics, Basel, Switzerland), which can measure HbA_1c and lipids.[53] The three devices share common features such as a simple user interface that enables easy application of whole blood to the reagent cartridge or discs. After placement into the instrument, the analysis proceeds without further involvement of the operator. Several evaluations have shown that all three instruments meet the required analytical performance for both HbA_1c and lipid monitoring.[51–53] The most recent of these instruments is also considerably smaller and that trend is likely to continue, facilitating their use in a variety of locations where space is often at a premium.

Small desktop instruments. A typical example of these is the Piccolo (Abaxis, Union City, CA), which can measure a wide range of general chemistry analytes on a very small sample volume. It uses a small disposable rotor that contains all the required reagents and diluents to perform a battery of common chemistry tests such as the Comprehensive Metabolic Panel.[54] The rotor also serves to centrifuge and separate whole blood samples, which are then mixed with reagent beads. The instrument monitors reaction products spectrophotometrically to calculate and print the results.

The Radiometer AQT 90 (Bronshoj, Denmark) bench-top, random access immunoassay analyzer uses a proprietary dry-chemistry concept and a detection method based on europium nonenhanced time-resolved fluorescence (TRF) technology. The AQT 90 has a unique, walk-away, closed-tube sampling device (Fig. 30.8) from which the instrument dispenses sample into a cup containing dried reagents including antibodies to the analytes of interest and europium lanthanide chelate as the signal reagent.[57] The europium-based chelates have certain natural advantages that allow sensitive and rapid detection methods. Analysis takes place in a small reagent cup on which are immobilized biotinylated capture antibodies and streptavidin and europium-labeled tracer antibodies. After addition of the patient sample and incubation, an antibody-antigen-antibody "sandwich" complex is formed, and after washing and drying, the europium response to excitation light is measured, the amount of which

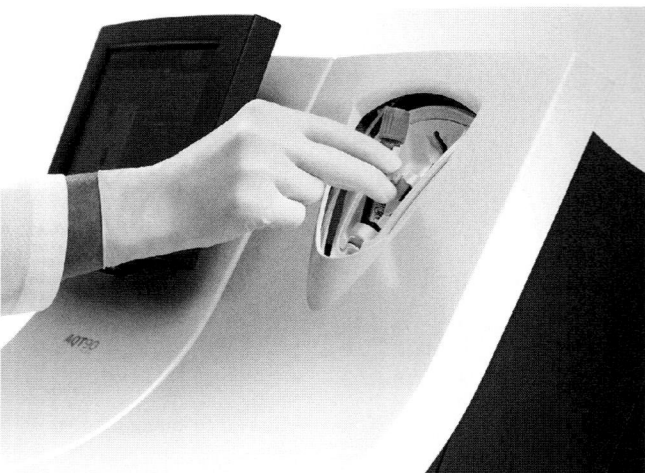

FIGURE 30.8 Touchscreen and sample port of the Radiometer AQT Flex analyzer. (Courtesy Radiometer, Copenhagen.)

is directly proportional to the antigen present. The menu includes troponin, brain natriuretic peptide (BNP), D-dimer, β-human chorionic gonadotropin (hCG), and CRP.

Critical care testing analyzers. These remain the most commonly used type of POCT bench-top analyzers with their expanded menu of analytes with the potential for use in many clinical areas. These devices use the same type of thick-film sensors or electrodes in strips as described earlier, but in this case, the sensors are designed to be reusable.[58] They are manufactured from thick films of paste and inks using screen-printing techniques to produce individual or multiple sensors for metabolites, blood gases, and electrolytes. Further details of the analytical principles behind these sensor technologies can be found in Chapter 17. The sensors have been incorporated with reagents and calibrators into a single cartridge or pack, which is placed in the body of a small- to medium-sized, portable critical care analyzer. Each pack contains reagents sufficient to measure a certain number of samples during a certain time period, after which it is relatively simple to replace. An example of such a device is the GEM Premier 4000 (Instrumentation Laboratory, Bedford, MA), and Fig. 30.9 shows the components and the fluid and patient sample pathways within this instrument. Evaluations of several different cartridge-based devices are available in the literature.[59–62]

These devices can also measure the various hemoglobin species and perform co-oximetry determinations. The latter relies on multiwavelength spectrophotometry in which light absorption by hemolyzed blood is measured at up to 60 or more wavelengths to determine the concentration of the five hemoglobin species.[63] Multiwavelength spectrophotometry can be extended to measure bilirubin directly in whole blood.[64] Details of the analytical principles of co-oximetry are given in Chapter 37.

Other key developments in critical care instruments include liquid calibration systems that use a combination of aqueous base solutions and conductance measurements to calibrate the pH and PCO_2 electrodes, with oxygen being calibrated with an oxygen-free solution and room air.[65] In addition, automated QC packages are integrated into these analyzers that ensure that QC samples are analyzed at regular intervals. These include packs or bottles of QC material that are contained within the instrument and sampled at predetermined intervals with on-board software interpreting the results and generating alerts, if necessary. Such devices also have the capability to be remotely monitored and programmed to respond to problems on instruments located long distances from the central laboratory.[66] Box 30.3 shows the various features that are incorporated into a critical care analyzer that contribute to its ease of use and reduce the potential for errors.

Hematologic and immunologic testing analyzers. Small bench-top devices are currently available to perform hematologic and immunologic analysis at the point of care. Again, they are often scaled-down versions of laboratory instruments, but these modified instruments have also been reduced in complexity, thus also reducing the risk from misoperation by nontechnically trained staff. The range of hematology instruments include ones that measure just hemoglobin and white cell counts to the Sysmex pocH-100i (Sysmex, Lincolnshire, IL), which can report up to 17 parameters.[67] An instrument with similar capabilities is the QBC Star (Drucker Diagnostics, Port Matilda, PA), which is a so-called dry hematology system, using dry reagents as opposed to bulky wet reagents, thus lending its use to POCT locations. The instrument can produce a nine-parameter blood count using a special hematocrit tube system. A recent evaluation showed comparable measurements with that of a conventional laboratory analyzer, and it was deemed suitable for use outside of the laboratory.[68]

Another relatively new product is the PIMA device (Abbott Point of Care, Princeton, NJ), which is small enough to be used for POC measurement of T-helper cells, or CD4 counts. The PIMA uses the same imaging and cell counting technology used in laboratory instruments but redesigned into a smaller, more compact instrument, which is simple to operate. These measurements are essential to guiding antiretroviral therapy for HIV and monitoring the course of immunosuppression. All of the required reagents including labeled antibodies to CD3 and CD4 antigens are contained in a small disposable cartridge to which is added 5 μL of whole blood, with the cartridge then being inserted into a small battery-powered desktop instrument. After mixing of the sample with the reagents and incubation, fluorescence is measured in the stained sample by a CCD camera, and the results are displayed on the screen. Several evaluations both in developed and emerging markets show that this instrument in the hands of non–laboratory-trained personnel provides a comparable quality of results with those obtained from the central laboratory.[69,70] By providing CD4 results at point of care, there is the potential to significantly improve treatment by offering prompt therapy to those in need.

Molecular diagnostic analyzers. The so-called Lab on a Chip (LOC) concept has been translated into devices for targeted measurement of nucleic acids at the point of care, particularly for detection of infectious agents. LOC devices have grown from the microelectronics industry through techniques of miniaturization and microfabrication,[71] incorporate features such as microfilters, microchannels, microarrays, micropumps, microvalves, and bioelectronics chips, and perform analysis at microscopic scales (i.e., 1 to 500 μm).[71]

One such device commercially available is the Cepheid GeneXpert system (Cepheid, Sunnyvale, CA). Although a

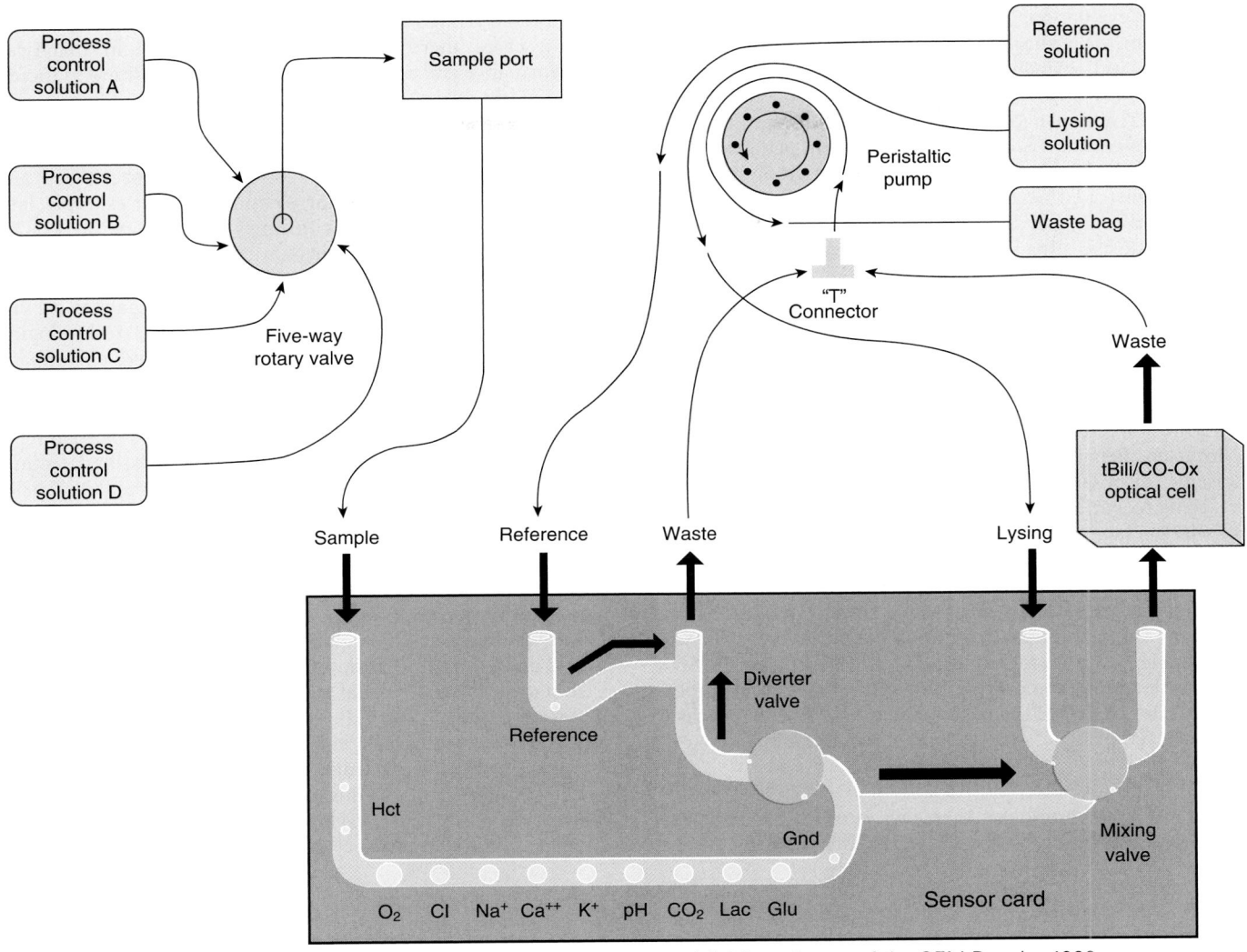

FIGURE 30.9 Schematic diagram of the components and fluidic pathways of the GEM Premier 4000 critical care analyzer. *Gnd,* Ground; *Hct,* hematocrit; *Lac,* lactate; *Glu,* glucose. (Courtesy Instrumentation Laboratory.)

BOX 30.3   Features of Critical Care Analyzers That Contribute to Ease of Use and Reduce the Risk of Errors

Long-life, maintenance-free electrodes or disposable sensor packs
Touch screens as the user interface
Software that can demand user and patient identification
Built-in barcode scanners
Sample aspiration instead of injection
Reduced sample sizes
Clot detection within analysis chamber
Sample detection to prevent short samples
Liquid calibration systems instead of gas bottles
Automated calibrations
Automated quality control sampling
Sophisticated quality control programs, including interpretation of data
Connectivity to information systems, allowing remote monitoring and control
Training videos incorporated

---

sizeable benchtop device, its ability to perform real-time quantitative polymerase chain reaction (PCR) in approximately 90 minutes with minimal operator interaction means that it offers the potential to perform rapid molecular testing in situations when the need for results is urgent.[72] The system uses single-use cartridges that each contain multiple chambers to hold the sample; various purification and elution buffers, and all the PCR reagents, including enzymes. In addition, all waste is retained within the cartridge. Attached to the cartridge is a PCR tube around which are heating and cooling tubes together with optical blocks that perform the amplification and fluorescence-based detection of the products. Within the cartridge is a syringe body designed in such a way to virtually eliminate sample contamination. Through a series of valves in the syringe, sample is moved through the various stages of the PCR process using the reagents stored in the cartridge and culminating in real-time detection of the amplified products.[73] Due to the sensitivity conferred by nucleic acid amplification, molecular diagnostic analyzers are able to overcome the limited sensitivity of traditional lateral flow assays, which is an advantage for some clinical applications, including infectious disease detection.

Several evaluations have been performed of the GeneXpert system for a number of clinical applications, including infectious and sexually transmitted diseases, using various sample types. Thus Spencer and colleagues[74] showed the GeneXpert system had 100% sensitivity and specificity for methicillin-resistant *Staphylococcus aureus* in pediatric specimens, and Buchan and colleagues[75] tested stool specimens and demonstrated near perfect sensitivity and specificity for *Clostridioides difficile* detection. An economic-based analysis of tuberculosis testing showed that the GeneXpert system was also cost effective.[76]

More molecular diagnostic point-of-care analyzers have been commercialized in recent years, such as the binx io (Binx Health, Trowbridge, Wilts, United Kingdom), Alere i (Abbott Point of Care, Pricenton, NJ), Roche Cobas Liat (Roche Diagnostics, Basel, Switzerland), Biofire FilmArray (Biofire Diagnostics, Salt Lake City, UT), and Biocartis Idylla (Biocartis, Mechelen, Belgium). The binx io system consists of a test-specific disposable cartridge containing all the necessary reagents to perform the test (Fig. 30.10) and uses a number of electrochemical labels.[77,78] Most of these platforms still require electricity and are best suited for the physician's office or central laboratory setttings. There are also platforms that are powered by batteries or laptops/tablets and target in-field POC use. Some examples include GeneXpert Omni (Cepheid, Sunnyvale, CA), and QuantuMDx Q-POC (QuantuMDX, Newcastle upon Tyne, United Kingdom). Isothermal amplification instead of PCR is used in some of these platforms to decrease temperature cycling control requirements.

Newer and Emerging Point-of-Care Testing Technologies

Many of the technologies that have been discussed earlier were devised several decades ago. The intervening time has seen them refined and packaged into smaller devices, and, in many cases, there has been an improvement in analytical performance and a reduced risk of error. That trend in incremental improvements will continue because no device is risk free, and, in some cases, there remains a need for better analytical performance. In addition, the search for fundamentally different technologies continues because there are known limitations to existing technologies. For example, lateral flow strip technology continues to dominate the POCT market, but lateral flow strips have a number of limitations, including inadequate sensitivity and difficulty with multiplex or measurement of more than two or three analytes on the same strip. Some emerging and growing POCT technologies are summarized in a review (Table 30.3).[13] These encompass innovations in multiple aspects, including specimen types and acquisition method, testing methods, fabrication, detection technologies, connectivity and integration of analyzers, choice of materials, data processing methods, and testing menu. The overall trend of the innovations in the POCT field is to facilitate more convenient, accurate, and cost-efficient measurement of a broader range of analytes near the patient. Another notable trend is to transition from in vitro and snapshot-based analysis to more continuous and real-time monitoring. Continuous glucose monitoring systems are already available in which glucose measurements in interstitial fluid are fed back to a monitor linked to an insulin pump.[82] Contact lens sensors that detect glucose in tears have also been described,[83] and other promising technologies include tattoo-based sensors[84] and smart holograms.[85] Clearly, changes in analyte concentrations may vary in different body fluid compartments, so this will have to be taken into account when designing and developing analytical technologies, as well as performing clinical validation studies.

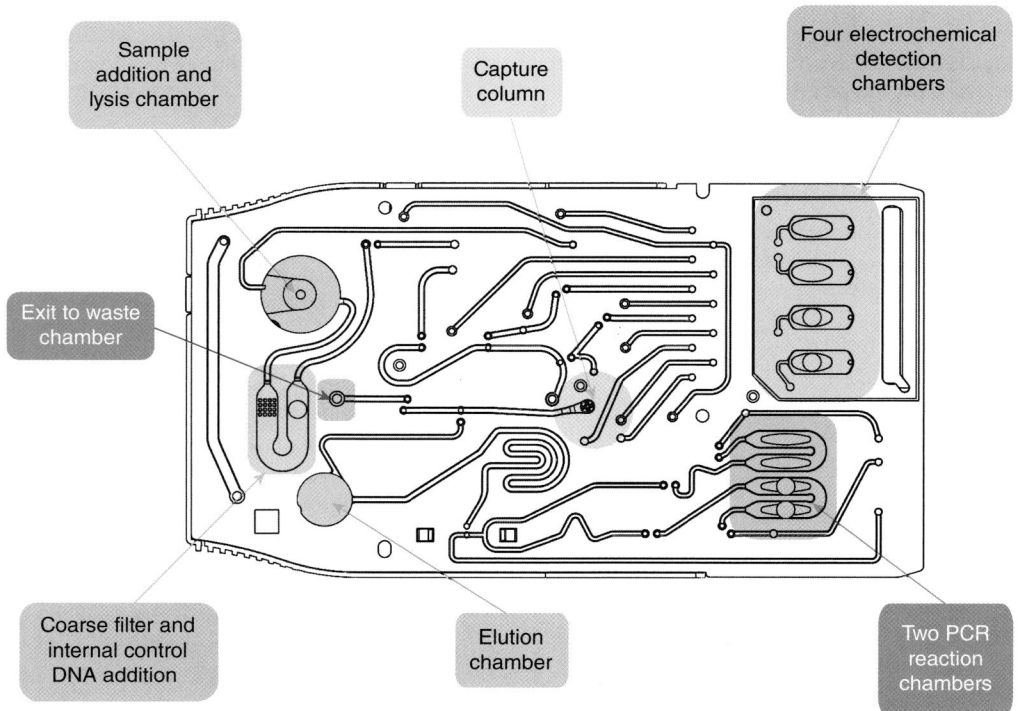

FIGURE 30.10 Schematic diagram of a microfluidic card using a molecular test for *Chlamydia trachomatis*. *PCR,* Polymerase chain reaction. (Courtesy Atlas Genetics Ltd., Bristol, United Kingdom.)

TABLE 30.3 Point-of-Care Testing Growth Points and Emerging Trends

Specimen	
Type	Breath (volatolomics), interstitial fluid
Acquisition	Painless sampling
Testing	
Noninvasive	Infrared-based testing
Invasive	Micro-needle devices
Continuous monitoring	Wearables, implantables, insertables
Multiplexing	Multiple detection zones, multiple labels, label-free
Analyzer	
Fabrication	3D printing
Fluidics	Digital microfluidics
Detection technologies	Nanopores, nanoelectronics, rapid PCR, nuclear magnetic resonance, mass spectrometry, ultrafast gas chromatography
Connectivity	Wireless enabled
Integration	Plug-in devices for smartphones, tablets, smart watches
Disposables	
Paper-based tests	2D and 3D μPads, Bluetooth-enabled lateral flow
Data	
Processing	Apps, Artificial intelligence, Cloud, telemedicine
Menu	
Expansion	Nucleic acid sequencing and targeted testing, marijuana in breath, sperm count and motility

From Wang P, Kricka L. Current and emerging trends in point-of-care technology and strategies for clinical validation and implementation. *Clin Chem.* 2018;64(10):1439–1452.

Informatics and Point-of-Care Testing

Most analytical devices used in clinical laboratories are directly linked or connected via an electronic interface to a laboratory information system (LIS). In this progression, many different informatics functions are used, including the electronic transfer of data from the analyzers to the LIS and ultimately into a patient's electronic medical record. This provides health care professionals with quick, accurate, and appropriate access to the patient's medical history and information.

Considerable effort has been expended to incorporate these same processes into POCT devices because of the vital importance of capturing analytical data in a patient's medical record to avoid the errors associated with manual transcription of data.[86] Thus newer POCT devices have addressed this problem by incorporating the prerequisite hardware and software into their designs, and in the past decade, so-called connectivity standards have also been introduced that facilitate linking devices to information management systems.

These standards are incorporated in a Clinical and Laboratory Standards Institute (CLSI) approved standard "Point-of-Care Connectivity: Approved Standard—Second Edition. CLSI Document POCT01-A2,"[87] and the potential benefits of POCT connectivity and what users should look for in POCT01-A2–compliant devices have been described by the CLSI in POCT02-A.[25] Adherence to these connectivity standards ensures that POCT devices meet critical user requirements, such as (1) bidirectionality, (2) device connection commonality, (3) commercial software interoperability, (4) security, and (5) QC or regulatory compliance.

Improved connectivity has enabled two major trends. First, and primarily because of demand from those responsible for the management of POCT, there has been the development of a range of commercial and specialized products for data management of POCT results with software devoted to ensuring compliance with procedures and managing data.[88] These systems offer a range of features and benefits, which include the ability of central laboratories to both monitor and remotely control their instruments in locations outside of the main laboratory (e.g., real-time control of approved operators, reagent, and QC lot information).[89] Although these systems are designed to interface primarily to the vendors' particular instruments, some systems can also incorporate competitive products.

The second trend is that connectivity standards, together with less expensive network technology, widespread access to the internet, and smart mobile phones, have provided the capability to establish POCT networks across major secondary and tertiary care institutions and perhaps more importantly to incorporate data collected in the community and in primary care into the those same POCT networks of major institutions. The structure of such a typical community POCT network is shown in Fig. 30.11. Nurses and other caregivers working within a clinic can enter test requests via a computer workstation; POCT devices interfaced to the same computer workstation can then combine the results with the test request and patient demographics that are received from a central patient management system. The data are uploaded to a POCT portal website, which provides a central repository of all results and patient details that can be accessed for review and audit as required. It also contains all of the quality data that are required to ensure that the network meets the required accreditation standards. The portal also sends completed results back to the patient management system that is responsible for delivering results into individual patient records. Caregivers can access the results via a computer workstation or other handheld device such as a smart phone or tablet computer. Networks similar to the one discussed earlier now exist in many places and have been described in the literature.[90–92]

The most important benefit of connectivity remains that of facilitating the transfer and capture of patient POCT and quality-related data into permanent medical records. Additional benefits include provision of alerts of abnormal results particularly those that may be critical. However, the increasing ability to interface devices more easily to other information systems should also enable the development of applications that add value to patient data such as the use of decision support software to assist with interpretation and therapy. One such example is the use of dosing software in combination with POCT INR measurements to manage patients taking warfarin.[93]

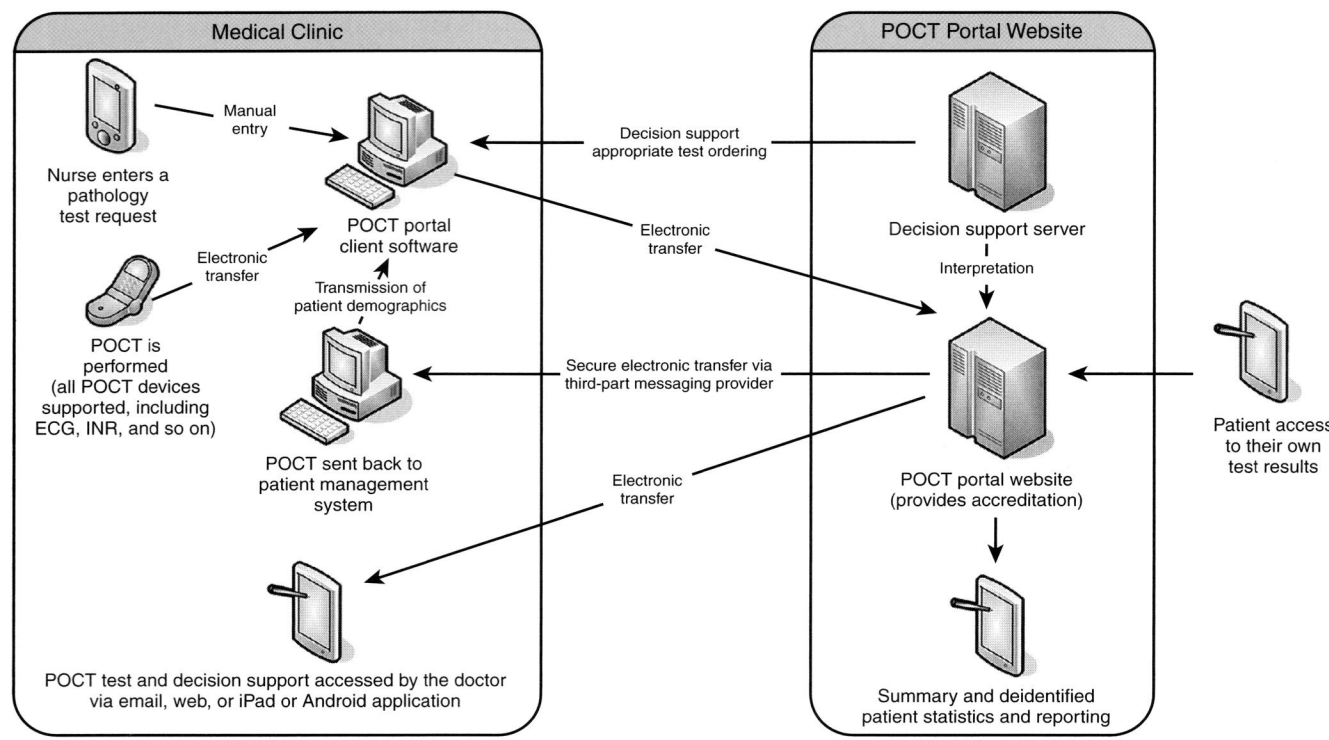

FIGURE 30.11 Schematic diagram of a point-of-care testing *(POCT)* network showing the relationships between the user, POCT device, other health information systems and the patient's caregiver. *ECG,* Electrocardiography; *INR,* international normalized ratio. (Courtesy R. Tirimacco, ICCNET.)

QUALITY MANAGEMENT

Management and maintenance of a POCT service in any health care facility require planning, oversight, inventory control, and assurance of the reliability of test results through adequate training and QC. Several guidelines document these requirements as based on the ISO standard 22870: 2016 ("Point-of-Care Testing [POCT]; Requirements for Quality and Competence")[94] and are available from various professional laboratory organizations.[24] Key aspects of quality management are described next.

Establishment of Need

As with centralized laboratory testing, the decision to implement a POCT service requires (1) establishment of the unmet need, which may be clinical, operational, or economic in origin; (2) critical appraisal of the evidence supporting the claimed clinical, operational, and economic benefits; and (3) examination of the costs and changes in the clinical process involved. This will form the foundation on which an implementation plan is built, together comprising the business case (see later in chapter).

Addressing the questions listed in Box 30.4 is useful for establishing the requirement for a POCT service.[11] Answering them will help to identify the test itself but should also explain why the current service is not meeting the needs of the patient or the clinician. A risk assessment should also be conducted that will focus primarily on the procedures and processes that have to be put in place to ensure the maintenance of a high-quality service.[95]

> **BOX 30.4** **Assessing the Need for a Point-of-Care Testing Service**
>
> Which tests are required?
> What is the turnaround time required?
> What clinical question is being asked when requesting this test?
> What clinical decision is likely to be made on receipt of the result?
> What action is likely to be taken on receipt of the result?
> What outcome should be expected from the action taken?
> Why isn't the laboratory able to deliver the required service?
> Will POCT provide the required accuracy and precision of result?
> Are there staff available to perform the test?
> Are there adequate facilities to perform the test and store the equipment and reagents?
> Will you abide by the organization's POCT policy?
> Are there operational benefits to this POCT strategy?
> Are there economic benefits to this POCT strategy?
> Will a change in practice be required to deliver these benefits?
> Is it feasible to deliver the change in practices that might be required?
>
> *POCT,* Point-of-care testing.

Organization and Implementation of a Point-of-Care Testing Coordinating Committee

When organizing and implementing a POCT service, it is important to consult with all of the stakeholders. ISO 22870:2016 states that the governing body of the health care organization should task a health professional grouping (e.g., a Medical Advisory Committee) with the responsibility of defining the scope of POCT to be made available within the organization.[94] The laboratory director should establish a multidisciplinary POCT management group that is charged with managing the whole process of delivering a high-quality POCT service. Membership of the POCT management group should include representatives from the laboratory, clinical services, and the organization's management team. Laboratory representatives should have expertise in the delivery of diagnostic and therapy services close to the patient. Representatives from clinical services may include physicians, physician assistants, family nurse practitioners, nurses, other health care providers, and patients. Typically, a laboratory professional will chair the management group because it is the laboratory that will provide the necessary backup if there is a service failure; furthermore, the laboratory professional will have had training and expertise in the analytical issues that are likely to arise. The POCT management group should have a formal reporting line within the health care organization; typically this would be to the medical director or other senior executive officer. The POCT management group should designate members who will take responsibility for the evaluation and selection of POCT devices, overseeing the training and accreditation of all POCT operators and for QC and quality assurance. The work of the management group should be governed by the organization's policy on POCT.

Point-of-Care Testing Policy and Accountability

Implementation of a POCT service requires a POCT policy that establishes all of the procedures required to ensure the delivery of a high-quality service, together with the responsibility and accountability of all staff associated with the POCT.[94] This may be (1) part of the organization's total quality management system,[95] (2) part of its clinical governance policy,[95] and (3) required for accreditation purposes.[94,95] The elements of a POCT policy are listed in Box 30.5.

Equipment Procurement and Evaluation

After establishing the requirement for POCT, establishing the POCT management group and writing the organization's POCT policy, the next stage in the process is equipment procurement. This involves first identifying candidate POCT equipment having the prerequisite analytical and operational capabilities to meet the clinical requirements of a POCT service. A CLSI protocol (CLSI Document POCT09-P. Selection Criteria for Point of Care Testing Devices) describes the features of the evaluation process,[96] and further guidance can be sought from other evaluations described in the literature.[97] In addition, the educational and certification requirements of the device operator also have to be identified and the potential for operator error determined. Independent validation of these analytical and operational characteristics is obtained from (1) the manufacturer, (2) published evaluations performed by government agencies, (3) reports in the peer-reviewed literature, and (4) discussions with colleagues who are operating similar equipment. When reviewing performance data, particular attention should be paid to the precision and accuracy of measurement, including the concordance between the results produced by the POCT device and by the routine laboratory method used at the same institution, because patients are likely to be managed using both analytical systems.

> ## BOX 30.5 Elements of a Point-of-Care Testing Policy
>
> Document information—
> - Approved by
> - Scheduled review interval
> - Original distribution
> - Related policies
> - Further information
> - Policy replaces previous one
>
> Introduction and background
> - Definition
> - Accreditation of services
> - Audit of services
>
> Laboratory services in the organization—location
> - Logistics
> - Policy on diagnostic testing
>
> Management of point-of-care testing—management group and accountability
> - Officers
> - Committee members
> - Terms of reference
> - Responsibilities
> - Meetings
>
> Equipment and consumable procurement—criteria for procurement
> - Process of procurement
>
> Standard operating procedures
> - Training and certification of staff—training
> - Certification
> - Recertification
>
> Quality control and quality assurance—procedures
> - Documentation and review
>
> Health and safety procedures
>
> Bibliography

This concordance may be difficult to assess, and it may be necessary to seek endorsements from current users of the systems and possibly conduct some form of internal trial.

An economic assessment of the planned POCT service, including the cost of consumables and servicing, should also be made.[24,96] This is likely to be a comparative exercise between the various point-of-care systems under consideration. Any comparison of costs with the laboratory service will be demonstrating only the cost per test, which will not give an accurate assessment of the cost-effectiveness of the system; details of the latter exercise are described later in the chapter. However, it is helpful at this point to have a good assessment of the relative staff costs associated with different systems because these are likely to be key aspects in the decision-making process. It is probable that the chosen system will be operated by staff already performing a wide range of other duties involving the care of patients, and therefore the amount of time required to operate the device may be critical (i.e., will they have sufficient time to perform the testing as required?).

After the comparison data have been obtained, tabulated, and interpreted, a POCT device is selected. It is then recommended that the laboratory professional conduct a short evaluation of the equipment to gain familiarization with the system. This evaluation will help to determine the content of the training routine that will have to be subsequently developed and what sort of problem troubleshooting may be required. Such an evaluation should document the concordance between the results generated with the device and those provided by the laboratory. All of this information should then be recorded in a logbook associated with the equipment. In addition, the organization may wish to undertake some form of safety check (e.g., electrical safety). All POCT devices should be added to a local inventory of POCT equipment, including serial number and unique identification, manufacturer/supplier, purchase date, and service history.[94] It should be noted that the processes described may differ among countries and organizations, particularly in relation to the order in which they are carried out and the relative emphasis on in-house evaluation compared with performance data available in the literature or from other users.

Training, Competency, and Certification

The confidence of the clinician, caregiver, and patient in the results generated by a POCT device depends on the performance and robustness of the instrument and the competence of the operator. Many of the agencies involved in the regulation of health care delivery now require that all personnel associated with the delivery of diagnostic results demonstrate their ongoing competence through a process of local accreditation (certification of competence), and this applies equally to POCT personnel. Typically, health care professionals involved in POCT will not have received training in the use of analytical devices as part of their core professional training but may be called upon to operate a number of what might be relatively complex pieces of equipment.

The elements of a training program are listed in Box 30.6. Clearly, the extent of this program will, to a certain extent, depend on how well the complexity of the analytical method has been engineered to minimize operator requirements. In practice, such a program is tailored to meet the needs of the individual and the organization. These may include formal presentations to groups or on a one-to-one basis, self-directed learning using agreed documentation, or computer-aided learning. For example, several of the current models of blood gas and electrolyte analyzers have on-board computer-aided

---

BOX 30.6   The Main Elements of a Point-of-Care Testing Training Program

Understanding the context of the test—pathophysiologic context
- Clinical requirement for the test
- Action taken on basis of result
- Nature of test and method used

Patient preparation required—relevance of diurnal variation
- Relevance of drug therapy

Sample requirement and specimen collection
Preparation of analytical device—machine or consumables
Performance of test
Performance of quality control
Documentation of test result and quality control result
Reporting of test result to appropriate personnel
Interpretation of result and sources of advice
Health and safety issues (e.g., disposal of sample and test device, cleaning of machine and test area)

---

training modules. Whatever the training strategy is used, it is important to document the satisfactory completion of training and that the individual has been tested and found competent with a combination of questions concerned with understanding and practical demonstration of the skills gained.[24] The latter may be achieved by performing tests on a series of QC materials and repeat testing of patient samples that have recently been analyzed in the laboratory or on another device—so-called parallel testing. Finally, the operator should be directly observed through the whole POCT procedure (i.e., the pre-examination, examination, and postexamination phases of testing).[24]

Competence on a long-term basis is maintained through regular practice of skills and continuing education, and it is important to build these features into any education and training program. Regular review of performance in QC and quality assurance programs will provide a means of overseeing the competence of operators. However, this is not always sufficient, particularly when operators are employed on irregular shifts or may not always be called on to perform POCT. In this latter situation, it may be necessary to create specific arrangements for individuals to undertake tests on QC material. The error log may also highlight when problems are arising. However, it is important to encourage an open approach to the assessment of competence so that operators themselves seek help if they believe that problems are occurring. Such an open approach should be supported with audit and performance review meetings during which problems are aired and developments discussed. The regular assessment of competence should be built into a formal program for recertification that will be a requirement of most accreditation programs, and web-based technology allows competency and other QA programs to be delivered to operators who are remote from the laboratory.[98] POCT connectivity allows real-time control of approved operators and can ensure that operators who have not completed recertification are locked out.

Infection Control

POCT has been associated with patient-to-patient transmission of infection (e.g., hepatitis B) (with recorded fatalities) through contaminated equipment or the contaminated hands of operators.[99] Training of POCT operators should cover appropriate hygiene steps such as hand hygiene, changing gloves between patients, instrument decontamination, safe practice to prevent needlestick injuries, and handling/disposal of infectious waste.[24]

Quality Control, Quality Assurance, and Audit

QC, external quality assurance (EQA), and audits provide a formal means of monitoring the quality of a service. The QC program is a relatively short-term view and typically compares the current performance of a device with that of the last time the analysis was made. EQA is a more comprehensive process that includes comparing testing performance of different sites or different pieces of equipment or methods. An audit is a more retrospective form of analysis of performance and, furthermore, takes a more holistic view of the whole process. However, the foundation to ensuring good quality remains a successful training and certification scheme.

Classically, quantitative QC involves the analysis of a sample for which the analyte concentration is known and the mean and range of acceptable results is quoted for the method used. There are several challenges to the classical approach with POCT. The first concerns are the frequency of testing—should a QC sample be analyzed every time that (1) a sample is analyzed, (2) a new operator uses the system, (3) a new lot number of reagents is used, or (4) the system is recalibrated? There is no consistent agreement on the correct approach, and one should be guided by the reproducibility and overall analytical performance of the system, workload, and type of test performed,[24] but it should never be less than what is recommended by the manufacturer. The approach used is also influenced by local circumstances, such as the number and competence of the operators, together with the frequency with which the system is used. For a bench-top or multitest analyzer, two different concentrations of QC samples should be run at a minimum of once per shift, or typically three times a day. Critical care analyzers (e.g., for blood gas and electrolyte measurements) are generally programmed to perform an automated QC check at intervals set by the manufacturer or those responsible for the device with automatic user lockout if the QC fails to meet prespecified targets.

For single-use POCT disposable devices, the aforementioned strategy does not completely monitor the quality of the test system. For example, when conventional QC material is analyzed on a unit-use or single-test POCT system, only that testing unit is monitored.[100] Thus it is impossible to test every unit with control material because, by definition, these are single-test systems, and it is not possible to analyze both control material and a patient sample with the single unit. Under these circumstances, there is greater dependence placed on the manufacturing reproducibility of the devices to ensure a good-quality service. Some single-test systems contain internal/procedural checking devices. For some systems the manufacturer supplies an electronic simulator device that acts as a check on electronic circuitry, optics, and signal reading. As with conventional QC, any electronic process checks should not be less than those recommended by the manufacturer. However, such checks do not test the whole process.[101] They should therefore be used in conjunction with the analysis of QC solutions to monitor the stability of reagents in cartridges and test strips (CLSI POCT04 2.8.4.9).[24] Different strategies may be adopted for the frequency of QC testing—for example the analysis of one QC sample during each shift or whenever there is a change to the testing system, such as a different batch of testing materials or a different operator. A 2002 CLSI guideline (CLSI, Document EP18-A, Quality Management for Unit-Use Testing: Approved Guideline) describes quality management procedures for unit-use testing from both a manufacturer's and a user's perspective.[100]

EQA is a systematic approach to QC monitoring in which blinded samples are analyzed by multiple laboratories to assess comparability of results. In this approach, the operator has no knowledge of the analyte concentration, and therefore it is considered closer to a "real testing situation." The results are transmitted to a central authority, who then prepares a report and returns a copy to each participating laboratory. The report will identify the acceptable range of results obtained for the complete group of participants and may be classified according to the different methods used by participants in the scheme. The scheme may encompass both laboratory and POCT users, which gives an opportunity to compare results with laboratory-based methods. In practice,

EQA is used in POCT to determine and document long-term performance. However, EQA samples and results generally cannot be used to establish concordance between POCT and central laboratory results because such samples do not behave in the same way as patient samples (refer to Chapter 6 for additional information on matrix effect of EQA samples). Analysis of the latter is required to determine to what degree POCT results compare with those from the central laboratory. It is also possible to operate an EQA scheme within a hospital or organizational setting; such a scheme would typically be run by qualified laboratory personnel. This provides the opportunity to compare the results being reported by both the laboratory and other POCT sites within the same organization. This is important when patients are managed in several departments or when machines break down and samples are taken to other sites for testing. When deteriorating or poor performance is identified in one of these schemes, it is important to document the problem and then provide and document a solution. It may be necessary as part of this exercise to review some of the patients' notes to ensure that incorrect results have not been reported and inappropriate clinical actions taken. In addition, if the solution highlights a vulnerable feature of the process overall or for one particular operator, then a process of retraining must be instituted. More details of QC and quality management as applied to POCT can be found in Chapter 6.

Maintenance and Inventory Control

The implementation and maintenance of a POCT service require that a supply of devices and associated consumables be maintained at all times and a formal program for doing so used. The key points in this process are to (1) adhere to the recommended storage conditions, (2) be aware of the stated shelf-life of the consumables, and (3) ensure that stocks are released in time for any preanalytical preparation to be accommodated (e.g., thawing). When multiple sites are using the same materials, then a central purchasing, supply, and inventory control system should be implemented. This will maximize the benefit from bulk purchasing and ensure that individual systems are not supplied unknowingly with different batches of consumables.

The complexity in the maintenance of reusable devices will vary from system to system, but clear guidelines will be available from the manufacturer and should be adhered to rigorously. Issues that usually require particular vigilance include expiration dates, biocontamination, electrical safety, maintenance of optics, and inadvertent use of inappropriate consumables.

Documentation

The documentation of all aspects of a POCT service continues to be a major issue. The documentation should extend from the standard operating procedure(s) for the POCT systems to records of training and certification of operators and internal QC and quality assurance data, together with error logs and any corrective actions taken. The requirements for documentation are outlined in CLSI POCT04.[24] The documentation of POCT results on individual patients in the laboratory or hospital information systems is too often limited or inconsistent. Thus it is critically important to keep an accurate record (in the medical record) of the (1) test request, (2) result, and (3) action taken. Some of these challenges are now being resolved with the advent of the patient electronic record, electronic requesting, and better connectivity of POCT instrumentation to information systems and the patient record (see earlier discussion).

Accreditation and Regulation of Point-of-Care Testing

The features of the organization and management of POCT described earlier are the same as those for the accreditation of any diagnostic services.[95] Accreditation of POCT should be part of the overall accreditation of laboratory medicine services or indeed as part of the accreditation of the full clinical service, as has been the case in many countries, including the United States and the United Kingdom, for a number of years. Thus the Clinical Laboratory Improvement Amendments of 1988 (CLIA) legislation in the United States stipulates that all POCT must meet certain minimum standards.[102–104] In the United States, the Centers for Medicare & Medicaid Services, the Joint Commission (formerly the Joint Commission on Accreditation of Healthcare Organizations), and the College of American Pathologists are among those responsible for inspecting sites, and each is committed to ensuring compliance with testing regulations for POCT.

EVIDENCE OF EFFECTIVENESS

The objective of using POCT is to enable clinical decisions to be made at the time of the consultation with the patient; these decisions may relate to screening, diagnosis, treatment, or monitoring. The outcomes of these decisions should lead to clinical, operational, or economic benefits if implementation is to be considered. At the level of the patient-caregiver interaction, POCT will help in the dialogue between patient and caregiver and improve both the efficiency and effectiveness of the assess-decide-act cycle (Fig. 30.12) (e.g., INR testing in the primary care setting[105] or antidiabetes medication adjustment for HbA_{1c} testing).[106] Typically, those involved in the management decisions to implement POCT will look for evidence of clinical and cost-effectiveness; those involved in implementation will, in addition, look for evidence of operational effectiveness as that evidence will inform the implementation plan. It follows therefore that the evidence of effectiveness that is used in making the case for adoption of POCT and the supporting business cases and implementation plan must address the needs of all of the stakeholders involved in delivering the care package being addressed.[107,108]

This can be challenging because stakeholder perspectives may differ across a care pathway (e.g., the current desire to shift care closer to home may have an adverse impact on the revenue received by the secondary care facility).

Clinical Effectiveness

The core outcome measures of clinical effectiveness are morbidity and mortality; however, these can be challenging to document and quantify. More commonly, surrogate or intermediate outcome measures are used for evidence of effectiveness in both the generation of evidence and in performance management and audit. Other important outcome measures include diagnostic accuracy and patient satisfaction with both the diagnostic or treatment phases of care. Some examples of outcome measures are given in Table 30.4. The generation of evidence of clinical effectiveness in the field of diagnostics including POCT is challenging primarily because (1) delivery of a result alone does not lead to improved outcomes, (2) variability can occur with both the decisions taken on receipt of the result and the quality of the clinical care delivered, and (3) it is difficult to design studies on diagnostics that minimize the generally accepted risks of introducing bias (e.g., operator bias; see Chapter 10 on evidence-based laboratory medicine). The latter is particularly the case with POCT when attempting to blind the operator (in this case, the "user of the result," e.g., a clinician) to the use of POCT or the comparator (the central laboratory service). For this reason, alternative approaches have been considered, including (1) observational studies in which appropriate outcome metrics are collected over a period of current practice (i.e., using the laboratory service) and then compared with the same outcome metrics using the point-of-care service, over the same time period; (2) comparison between a care provider using POCT and a care provider using a laboratory service (as current practice). One approach that is currently being increasingly used in health technology assessment for diagnostic studies is the use of "linked evidence." This approach evaluates the clinical utility of tests in the absence of direct clinical trial evidence by linking systematically acquired evidence from the separate components of the test-treatment pathway (i.e., diagnostic accuracy of the test, impact on clinical decision making, and the effectiveness of consequent treatment options).[109] However, this may not be appropriate for POCT as the key is changing the practice across the whole assess-decide-act cycle.

In the following paragraphs, examples of the clinical effectiveness of POCT are given for a range of test utilities, including the limitations of the evidence. In some instances when the benefits are more of an operational or economic nature, the studies, particularly those in a diagnostic setting, may appear in the section on cost effectiveness.

Rapid Diagnosis of Chlamydia Infection

There are two primary reasons for considering POCT for the detection of chlamydia infection: (1) improving patient access to screening programs and (2) reducing the number of patients lost to follow-up after the specimen is collected. The key clinical outcome measures are the incidence of the infection and its complications. It has been established that screening for chlamydia helps to identify more individuals with the infection while reducing the complications associated with the infection.[110] Both modeling and expert views

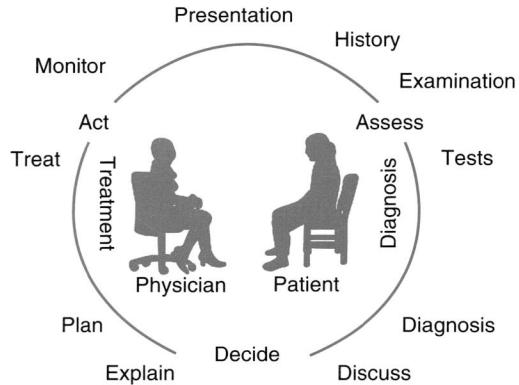

FIGURE 30.12 Schematic diagram of the patient-physician interaction and the steps of assess-decide-act.

TABLE 30.4 Outcome Measures Used to Assess Point-of-Care Testing Technologies

Test	Application	OUTCOME MEASURE	
		Clinical	Process
Urinalysis	Rule out UTI	Reduce antibiotic use	Reduce the need for laboratory tests
Urine albumin creatinine ratio	Rule out albuminuria	Early detection of renal disease	Advise the patient at the clinic visit
Natriuretic peptide	Rule out a diagnosis of heart failure	Faster and earlier diagnosis	Reduced clinic visits Use of echocardiography
Chlamydia	Screening for infection	Reduced complication rate	Reduced nonattendance at the clinic Reduced clinic visits
INR	Self-monitoring Self-dose adjustment	Increased period within the therapeutic window Reduced complication rate	Reduced clinic visits Reduced hospitalization
HbA$_{1c}$ in primary care	Primary care management of diabetes	Improved glycemic control indicated by HbA$_{1c}$	Reduced clinic visits
Troponin I or T in ED	Rule out acute coronary syndrome	Faster triage to therapeutic intervention	Reduced length of stay in ED
D dimer in primary care	Rule out DVT	Faster diagnosis and treatment	Reduced clinic visits

DVT, Deep vein thrombosis; *ED,* emergency department; *HbA1c,* glycated hemoglobin; *INR,* international normalized ratio; *UTI,* urinary tract infection.

suggest that the use of POCT will help in improving outcomes.[111] Modeling studies have suggested that higher sensitivity tests based on nucleic acid amplification rather than antigen based tests will offer the greatest benefits in improving outcomes.[112] Although one large study in a remote care setting using molecular POC for chlamydia showed a significant reduction in time to treatment,[113] there are no robust studies published as yet to show that POCT improves clinical outcomes.

Ruling out a Diagnosis of Deep Vein Thrombosis

The diagnosis of deep vein thrombosis (DVT) can be challenging because the symptoms are often mild and nonspecific, which could be one of the reasons why primary care physicians in several countries put it high on their list of POCT requirements.[114] In a diagnostic meta-analysis, Geersing and colleagues[115] concluded that POCT for D-dimer in the outpatient or physician office setting could safely rule out a diagnosis of DVT in low-risk patients. They also found that quantitative assays performed better than the semiquantitative assays. Van der Helde and colleagues[116] demonstrated that the use of POCT D-dimer testing together with a clinical decision rule in a primary care setting could rule out the need to refer patients for further investigations in 45 to 49% of cases. The data demonstrate the potential for reliable rule out of a diagnosis at the time of presentation. In turn, this has the potential to reduce pressure on emergency rooms, reduce patient costs, and increase patient satisfaction with care.

Managing Warfarin Treatment With International Normalized Ratio Self-monitoring

There is now substantial evidence to demonstrate that self-testing with INR with or without self-dosing guided by a treatment algorithm leads to improved patient outcomes, including reduction in thromboembolic episodes without an increased risk of major bleeding events, more time spent in the therapeutic range, and evidence from some studies of

improved mortality rates with a 26% reduction in death.[93,105] There is some evidence that the best outcomes are obtained in patients younger than 55 years of age, which may reflect operator ability.[117] Improvements in connectivity and network technology also offer the possibility of capturing home testing results into the patient's electronic health care record.

Managing Patients With Diabetes Using HbA$_{1c}$

A systematic review of randomized controlled trials (RCTs) found an "absence of evidence from clinical trials data for the effectiveness for POCT of HbA$_{1c}$."[118] However, the analysis was compromised by the use of different surrogate outcome measures, as well as a limited amount of information on stratification of patients at the time of selection and action taken when the HbA$_{1c}$ result was produced.[106] On the other hand, there was a more positive message from observational studies, including one conducted over a significantly longer period of time demonstrating the benefit of POCT HbA$_{1c}$, as shown by a reduction in the mean HbA$_{1c}$ value in the population being monitored.[119] A narrative review of 11 studies concluded that POCT HbA$_{1c}$ improved patient quality of life and contributed to greater compliance with HbA$_{1c}$ testing frequency requirements.[120] The use of POCT HbA$_{1c}$ in facilitating more timely treatment changes is recognized in the American Diabetes Association (2019) "Standards of Medical Care in Diabetes" guidelines.[121]

Cost-effectiveness

Economic assessment is becoming more important because of the growing debate around so-called value for money in health care; consequently, health care economics is seen as an integral part of evidence-based practice. Economic assessments often encompass both the operational efficiency and assessment of resource utilization, generally equated to the cost. However, it is important to consider each element as management decisions based on this information will require attention be given to process change and resource utilization. In the examples given later in this section, both aspects will be identified. Drummond and colleagues[122] define economic evaluation as the comparative analysis of alternative courses of action in terms of both costs and consequences. Thus an economic assessment of POCT would ask the question: "What are the complete consequences and costs of using POCT compared with testing done in the centralized laboratory?" The consequences would include any operational changes involved with introducing POCT. To obtain the best level of evidence, the study would be conducted as an RCT. A decision on whether to implement POCT would require full quantitation of the consequences and costs in both arms of the trial, and this is possible by a number of techniques.[122] The reality is that relatively few studies of economic assessment have been conducted in this way for laboratory tests and even fewer for POCT. More recently, attention has been given to alternative approaches to obtaining evidence of effectiveness such as the linked evidence approach.[109] This may be more appropriate, not only for obtaining evidence of clinical effectiveness but also for cost effectiveness and particularly when the process of care changes significantly, as in the case of POCT. Such an approach is similar to the technique of time-driven activity-based costing, a technique that estimates the cost of all of the processes involved in delivery of a care intervention.[124] Thus if POCT was used to enable a clinical decision and action to be taken in one visit, rather than two, there would be a net cost saving if the additional cost of the POCT was less than the cost of the second visit. This approach is often used in quality improvement studies.

Instead of robust economic studies, there has been a focus in the past on simplistic comparisons of the cost of POCT technology with that used in the central laboratory without any consideration of the patient outcomes from using the tests. Thus many studies in the literature are of the cost minimization type and, not surprisingly, have shown that POCT is more expensive than the central laboratory in which economies of scale can deliver obvious efficiencies. However, this situation is changing to one that moves beyond a comparison of testing costs to one that includes assessment of the complete process of patient care and identification of the economic outcomes that can be achieved with POCT.[125] Some of the economic benefits may result from a clinical impact on the patient, but others may be what are sometimes called operational benefits such as more rapid treatment or reduction in length of stay.

There are various types of economic analysis, but it is beyond the scope of this chapter to describe these in detail, and they can be found in the literature.[122,123,125] One of the more common forms of economic evaluation of diagnostic tests is cost-effectiveness analysis (CEA).[124] For example, if applied to the diagnosis of heart failure, it would compare the costs of two or more interventions, such as POCT BNP versus central laboratory BNP testing; the effectiveness could be calculated from the number of heart failure cases diagnosed by the two tests. From CEA analysis, it is possible to calculate another key economic parameter called the incremental cost-effectiveness ratio (ICER). The ICER compares the net difference in the cost of two interventions *a* and *b* (POCT BNP vs. central laboratory BNP) with the net difference in effectiveness (cases of heart failure diagnosed) as:

$$ICER = \Delta C/\Delta E$$
$$= Costs_a - Costs_b/Effectiveness_a - Effectiveness_b$$

Ideally, the measure or indicator of effectiveness would be one that could be compared across studies such as quality-adjusted life years (QALYs), which combines both length and quality of life into a single outcome and where 1 is perfect health and 0 is death. When QALYs are used as the clinical effectiveness measure, the analysis is sometimes referred to a cost-utility analysis.

Because of the difficulty of applying the QALY measure in relation to tests, both POC and central laboratory, it is more common to compare effectiveness in terms of other measures. For example, Laurence and colleagues,[126] in an RCT of POCT compared with laboratory testing of a number of analytes, used the proportion of patients within the therapeutic range for each analyte at the end of the trial as the clinical outcome indicator. More details of this study can be found in the cases section of this chapter.

The difficulty of performing RCTs of testing strategies has led to less robust but nevertheless informative assessments, including those of modeling.[127] Modeling tools generate decision trees that map out all the possible consequences or outcomes that can flow from all of the alternative testing options. Each of the consequences has a mathematical probability of occurrence, and such data are usually available in the literature from a variety of reported sources. The probabilities in each arm of the decision tree must sum to 1.0. There will also be a payoff or cost associated with each consequence, and the expected value of a particular strategy can be calculated from the probabilities and costs. The overall validity of modeling is dependent on several factors, one of which is the quality or robustness of the data that are input into the model. These data include test performance, such as sensitivity and specificity, the prevalence of the disease and its complications in the population on whom the model is being used, and accurate treatment costs. Some of the limitations of decision tree modeling can be addressed by Markov models, which take into account the effect of time on disease progression and treatment effects.[128] By way of example, Huntington and colleagues describe the challenges of modeling-based evaluations of POC multipathogen testing for sexually transmitted infections (STIs).[129]

A recent review of economic studies of POCT concluded that, although there was high-quality evidence to support POCT including RCTs, the number of studies was relatively few and the quality variable.[125] Appraisal of published studies can be facilitated by the use of checklists that highlight the key attributes that should be contained within any economic assessment (e.g., Consolidated Health Economic Evaluation Reporting Standards [CHEERS] statement).[130] Additional insight in how to interpret economic evidence of testing is contained in the paper by Goodacre and colleagues,[131] which reviews some of the challenges in conducting studies of the cost-effectiveness of newer cardiac markers such as troponin in the diagnosis of acute coronary syndrome. In the following paragraphs, several specific examples are given of the cost-effectiveness of POCT, with an emphasis on the operational changes required and the potential associated operational savings that can help to fund, or perhaps even more than offset, the required changes in the care pathway and processes.

Use of C-reactive Protein in Primary Care to Reduce Antibiotic Prescribing

Inappropriate prescribing of antibiotics wastes resources and drives antimicrobial resistance. Butler and colleagues investigated

CRP measurement by POCT in patients presenting to primary care with an acute exacerbation of chronic obstructive pulmonary disease: CRP-guided treatment was associated with a 20.4% reduction in antibiotic use without any evidence of detriment.[132] This study backed up the findings of previous studies such as Cals and colleagues,[133] who investigated the impact of CRP measurement by POCT and physician communication skills training in primary care on the amount of antibiotic prescribing in patients presenting with suspected lower respiratory tract infections. They found a significant reduction in antibiotic prescribing with all combinations of the two interventions (i.e., single or combined), from 68% to as low as 23%. The authors did not take into consideration the potential long-term economic effects of the development of antibiotic resistance, currently a topic of considerable interest at a societal level. However, the adoption of point-of-care CRP remains variable, with lower levels of adoption in the United States than in Europe, and there have been calls for robust cost-effectiveness data that would facilitate greater uptake.[134]

Managing Long-term Conditions in Primary Care

Policymakers in many parts of the world who are seeking to move care of long-term conditions into the community and shorten or eliminate the time to travel to distant health care facilities have focused on POCT use to improve accessibility and patient experience and to contain costs. The largest study of this topic has been the Australian POCT in General Practice Trial.[126] The study found that the cost of POCT for urine albumin creatinine ratio (ACR) was less that of the central laboratory, but that for INR, HbA$_{1c}$, and lipids was more expensive, although none was significant. On the other hand, POCT led to less cost incurred by patients and their families compared with current practice. The ICER was unfavorable for INR and favorable for urine ACR, with uncertainty in the data regarding HbA$_{1c}$ and lipid testing.

Improving Triage in the Emergency Department

Numerous studies have demonstrated a reduction in TAT for a range of analytes commonly measured in the emergency department (ED) (e.g., pregnancy testing, D dimer, lactate).[135] This resulted in reduced waiting times, reduced length of stay in ED, more rapid treatment decisions, and a reduction in the number of patients leaving without being seen. POCT troponin studies have demonstrated a reduction in the TAT for cardiac results for patients presenting with acute chest pain, together with a consequent reduction in the length of stay and a reduction in resource use.[136,137] The advent of high-sensitivity troponin assays which currently are available only as laboratory-based tests has allowed the implementation of 1-hour rule-out strategies[138]; however, this is not possible at present with current POCT troponin assays. For lactate measurement in patients with suspected sepsis, the use of POCT was associated with a reduced time to administration of intravenous fluids and a reduction in mortality.[139] Despite this substantial evidence of benefit, there is as yet relatively limited evidence of cost-effectiveness.

Improving the Efficiency and Effectiveness of Sexually Transmitted Infection Services

The ability to undertake the test-and-treat cycle in a single visit through using POCT, albeit with a slightly longer consultation, offers the possibility to reduce the resources required for each patient diagnosis and treatment. It can also reduce costs associated with other issues, such as reduction in patients lost to follow-up, improved morbidity and mortality, and reduction in patient overtreatment, as well as facilitating more efficient and effective screening programs. Turner and colleagues[140] undertook an economic simulation of the introduction of a molecular POCT-based service for chlamydia and gonorrhea for a population of 1.2 million individuals. The simulation indicated that there would be a 10% reduction in baseline costs, a 9.5% avoidance of inappropriate treatments, and a possible prevention of 189 case of pelvic inflammatory disease. Simulation modeling of a multipathogen POCT panel incorporating chlamydia, gonorrhea, *Trichomonas vaginalis,* and *Mycobacterium genitalium* testing compared with standard care also demonstrated significant cost savings, fewer clinic attendances, fewer onward STI transmissions, and inappropriate treatments.[128]

Intraoperative Testing

There is currently considerable use of POCT in the OR; much of this is for monitoring vital parameters with reflexive treatment to maintain body and organ functions. One of the alternative POCT strategies that has radically altered the way that patients are treated has been in the use of intraoperative POCT measurement of PTH.[141] Primary hyperparathyroidism is caused by a solitary adenoma in 85% of cases, with multiple adenomas (multiglandular disease) occurring in 15% of cases. Patients with a solitary adenoma may be suitable for focused surgery through minimally invasive parathyroidectomy (MIP); other patients may require bilateral parathyroid exploration. Although preoperative imaging is sensitive in identifying solitary adenomas, it is much less sensitive in identifying multiglandular disease. Intraoperative PTH monitoring during MIP following removal of an image identified abnormal parathyroid gland provides assurance that multiglandular disease is not being missed and is associated with high cure rates of 97 to 99% (i.e., a reduced requirement for further surgery, shorter postoperative stays, and better cosmetic outcomes).[141] Conversely, if during MIP, PTH monitoring suggests residual hypersecretion, surgery can be converted to bilateral parathyroid gland exploration. PTH is measured at baseline and then at 10 to 20 minutes following excision of the suspected adenoma; a reduction in PTH concentration of greater than 50% from baseline is considered to indicate confirmation of a solitary adenoma as the etiology of the hyperparathyroidism and that this has been successfully removed.

ADOPTION AND IMPLEMENTATION

The adoption of POCT into routine clinical practice is often very slow and patchy. This may reflect gaps in the evidence base for its clinical and cost-effectiveness and broader impact but also organizational challenges in adoption and implementation.[142,143]

The potential benefit of using POCT is to satisfy unmet needs associated with improving both the effectiveness and the efficiency of the care of individual patients. A generic description of the interaction between patient and care provider is described in the assess-decide-act cycle (see Fig. 30.12), in which the care provider makes an assessment of the patient presentation (and that may involve the use of medical tests) followed by a decision about the nature of the problem and then takes appropriate action.[11] Adoption of POCT therefore by definition, implies that the process of care, as well as the resource utilization and outcomes, will change compared with current (non-POCT–mediated) practice. As indicated earlier, the demonstration of effectiveness is primarily directed at policymakers, but the translation of this evidence into practice can be challenging because it has an impact on a number of stakeholders.[10] Any technological innovation is likely to reflect similar challenges, as outlined earlier, which may explain the many observations on the sluggish nature of technology adoption in health care.[142] Although adoption can be considered as the transition from aspiration to intention, implementation is the transition from intention to outcome. The basis of the aspiration is that there is a recognized unmet need in a particular setting, and an informed aspiration is one in which it has been demonstrated that the unmet need can be met—in the case of this discussion, through the use of POCT. This can be achieved through the development of a value proposition for the technology and the delivery of a different process of care.[107]

Implementation involves the development of a plan comprising four phases: (1) establishment of the unmet need, which may be clinical, operational, or economic in origin; (2) critical appraisal of the evidence supporting the claimed clinical, operational, and economic benefits; (3) examination of the costs and changes in the clinical process involved; and (4) a detailed implementation plan, including responsibilities, time frames, and performance metrics.[1119] This can be summarized in the steps identified in Box 30.7.

A crucial feature of implementation is audit to support performance management of the implementation phase. A set of metrics that represent the process, resource utilization, and outcomes (clinical, operational, and economic) from the current and revised practices, with particular attention being given to the changes that are part of the value proposition. A crucial part of this activity is to adopt a care pathway–wide approach to the changes in performance metrics. One field in which this has proved to be particularly challenging is in the areas of investment and disinvestment in resources.[107] Thus in the case study featured in Box 30.7, the major investments will be in the activities associated with operating POCT in primary care, such as training, operation, and QC, as well as the POCT system. The disinvestments will be primarily in the use of the laboratory service and approximately 50% of the ultrasonography contract and associated clinic visits. The challenges and approaches to disinvestment will depend on the resource, as well as the approach to reimbursement or payment for services in the overall health economy. Clearly, it is not possible to disinvest in large pieces of equipment or estate or even a service in a fully integrated health system, but it is fairly straightforward when using outsourced services. In these situations, other ways may have to be found to achieve the expected disinvestment. Individual solutions may have to be found for each health economy.

CONCLUSIONS

The technological vehicles to deliver diagnostic tests outside of the laboratory currently exist, and there is also evidence to demonstrate that this technology can deliver improved

---

> **BOX 30.7**   **Key Elements of the Business Case for Point-of-Care Testing to Inform the Adoption and Implementation (Plan) Using the Example of D-Dimer Testing in Primary Care**
>
> - Unmet need: triage of patients presenting in primary care with suspected DVT
> - Evidence of effectiveness of proposed intervention: POCT for D dimer is an effective in the context of a decision support tool, for ruling out DVT
> - Expected benefits associated with introduction of new intervention: reduction in number of patients referred to secondary care for ultrasonography, reduction in contracted requirement for ultrasonography, improved patient experience
> - Proposed change in care pathway process: POCT at presentation to primary care, with decision to refer within 30 min
> - Resource utilization in current pathway and proposed revision of that pathway: investment in POCT in primary care setting; disinvestment in a proportion of referrals to secondary care
> - Metrics to enable implementation and adoption according to the business case expectations: number of patients presenting to primary care, number of D-dimer tests, number of referrals, number of negative ultrasound investigations compared with baseline, follow-up of patients for 6 months to determine any missed cases, financial measures to match current and revised pathway (e.g., time in primary care, cost utilization of primary and secondary care visits, including cost of relevant diagnostics)

DVT, Deep vein thrombosis; *POCT,* point-of-care testing.

---

clinical and economic outcomes. Furthermore, it is now becoming increasingly evident that there is a desire of both patients and policymakers to develop more care closer to home and to encourage more patient involvement in the delivery of care.

However, there remains the need to produce devices that are more user friendly and reduce the risk of errors. In addition, devices are being developed that provide alternatives to fingerstick blood collection. Two examples are mentioned in the chapter, (1) with the use of tattoo-based noninvasive glucose monitoring and (2) the use of tear fluid for glucose monitoring and providing an alternative noninvasive approach for continuous monitoring. Furthermore, it is also important that any technology delivers the required analytical and clinical performance when operated by a person with no previous technical experience. It is important to stress the importance of clinical performance as we enter an era when analysis may be undertaken on alternative biologic fluids or compartments to those on which our knowledge base in laboratory medicine has been developed.

The trends described in this chapter illustrate the potential opportunities to disrupt longstanding and inefficient practices of delivering health care and provide the means to deliver more patient-centered care, including patients being more involved in their own care and health decision making. However, this may represent the greatest challenge because the adoption of new technologies, particularly POCT, is undoubtedly slow. This may, in part, be due to limited data on the health economics of diagnostic testing, but it is also because of the challenges involved in delivering a more integrated and personalized style of care.

POINTS TO REMEMBER

- POCT is testing performed closer to the patient with the expectation of making quicker decisions on patient care than might occur as a result of laboratory testing.
- The majority of current POCT is performed using well-established technologies such as glucose sensors and lateral flow immunoassays that have been refined over the years to improve analytical and clinical performance.
- Molecular diagnostic technologies have been adopted at the point-of-care for predominantly infectious disease testing.
- Emerging technologies have the potential to improve the performance and convenience of POCT, further expand the test menu, and provide more clinical and economic values.
- All POCT must be applied using quality management techniques that ensure that the results are appropriate for patient care.
- Measurement of both clinical and economic patient outcomes of POCT are required to ensure its overall effectiveness.

SELECTED REFERENCES

7. Kricka LJ. Point-of-care technologies for the future: technological innovations and hurdles to implementation. Point of Care 2009;8:42–4.
9. Price CP, Kricka LJ. Improving healthcare accessibility through point-of-care technologies. Clin Chem 2007;53:1665–75.
11. Price CP, St John A. Point-of-care testing. Making innovation work for patient-centred care. Washington, DC: AACC Press; 2012. p. 2.
12. Christensen C, Grossman J, Hwang J. The innovator's prescription. A disruptive solution to health care. New York: McGraw Hill; 2009.
13. Wang P, Kricka L. Current and emerging trends in Point-of-Care technology and strategies for clinical validation and implementation. Clin Chem 2018; 64:1439–52.
15. World Health Organization. Target product profiles and priority digital health products for TB. 2015. http://www.who.int/tb/areas-of-work/ digital-health/target-product-profiles/en/
16. World Health Organization. High-priority target product profiles for new tuberculosis diagnostics: report of a consensus meeting. 2014. http:// apps.who.int/iris/bitstream/10665/135617/1/WHO_HTM_TB_2014.18_eng. pdf?ua=1&ua=1
17. Ivanova Reipold E, Easterbrook P, Trianni A, et al. Optimising diagnosis of viraemic hepatitis C infection: the development of a target product profile. BMC Infectious Diseases 2017; 17(Suppl 1):707.
18. Chen H, Liu K, Li Z et al. Point of care testing for infectious diseases. Clin Chim Acta 2019;493:138–47.
19. Hsieh YH, Gaydos CA, Hogan MT, et al. What qualities are most important to making a point of care test desirable for clinicians and others offering sexually transmitted infection testing? PLoS ONE 2011;6:e19263.
94. Point-of-care testing (POCT) – Requirements for quality and competence. ISO 22870:2016. Geneva, Switzerland: International Organization for Standardization; 2016.
97. Harris J, Abdel Wareth LO, Lari S et al. Setting up a point-of-care testing service in a greenfield quaternary hospital. Arch Pathol Lab Med 2018;142:1223–1232
105. Sharma P, Scotland G, Cruikshank M et al. Is self–monitoring an effective option for people receiving long-term vitamin K antagonist therapy? A systematic review and economic evaluation. BMJ Open 2015;5:e007758.
106. Price CP, St John A. The value proposition for point-of-care testing in healthcare: HbA1c for monitoring in diabetes management as an exemplar. Scan J Clin Lab Invest 2019;79:298–304
112. Rönn MM, Menzies N, Gift TL et al. Potential for point-of-care tests to reduce chlamydia-associated burden in the Unites States: a mathematical modelling analysis. Clin Infect Dis 2019;70:1816–23.
113. Guy RJ, Ward J, Causer LM et al. Molecular point-of-care testing for chlamydia and gonorrhoea in Indigenous Australians attending remote primary health services (TTANGO): a cluster –randomised controlled crossover trial. Lancet Infectious Diseases 2018;18:1117–1126.
120. Schnell O, Crocker JB, Weng J. Impact of HbA1c testing at point of care on diabetes management. J Diabetes Sci Technol 2017;11:611–17.
129. Huntington SE, Burns RM, Harding-Esch E et al. Modelling-based evaluation of the costs benefits and cost-effectiveness of multipathogen point-of-care tests for sexually transmitted infections in symptomatic genitourinary medicine clinic attendees. BMJ Open 2018;8:e020394.
132. Butler C, Gillespie D, White P et al. C-reactive protein testing to guide antibiotic prescribing for COPD exacerbations. N Engl J Med 2019;381:111–20.
135. Rooney KD, Schilling UM. Point-of-care testing in the overcrowded emergency department—can it make a difference? Crit Care 2014;18:692–699.

SECTION III

Clinical Chemistry-Analytes

Exam questions, case studies, and additional resources are available on ExpertConsult.com.
*Full versions of these chapters are available electronically on www.ExpertConsult.com.

Amino Acids, Peptides, and Proteins*

Dennis J. Dietzen and Maria Alice Vieira Willrich[a]

ABSTRACT

Background
Amino acids are not only the building blocks of proteins, but they also play diverse roles in the provision of energy and the formation of a number of other important biomolecules, including hormones, neurotransmitters, and signaling molecules. The polymers of amino acids, peptides and proteins, orchestrate and control the vast array of human physiologic and biochemical processes. The catalog of amino acids, peptides, and proteins in various biological fluids is a target-rich environment for the detection of pathologic states.

Content
This chapter first describes the chemistry, metabolism, transport, and analysis of amino acids. Polymers of amino acids may be relatively short (peptides) or long (proteins). The human genome contains the information to dictate formation of approximately 20,000 polypeptides, but the actual diversity of the human proteome and peptidome is manifold more expansive. Proteome diversity arises from linear amino acid sequence and an array of modifications that include acylation, phosphorylation, glycosylation, and isoprenylation. Systems of short peptides, larger protein monomers, and multimeric protein complexes are the tools that orchestrate and control human physiologic and biochemical processes. Proper synthesis, folding, subcellular targeting, and catabolism of proteins and peptides are therefore essential for human health. Analytic exploitation of biologic fluids including blood, urine, and cerebrospinal fluid using chemical, immunologic, and mass spectrometric methods enables informed diagnosis and therapy in a multitude of disease states.

---

*The full version of this chapter is available electronically on ExpertConsult.com.

[a]The authors gratefully acknowledge the preceding foundation for this chapter laid by Glen L. Hortin and A. Myron Johnson, as well as generous assistance from Carl H. Smith on the topic of amino acid transport.

32

Serum Enzymes*

Mauro Panteghini

ABSTRACT

Background

Serum enzymes are measured in medical diagnosis to detect injury to a tissue that contains the measured enzyme. Clinical applications have concentrated mostly on enzymes such as creatine kinase, alanine transaminase, aspartate transaminase, alkaline phosphatase, γ-glutamyltransferase, lactate dehydrogenase (LDH), lipase, and (pancreatic) amylase.

Content

This chapter describes the use of the clinically most important enzymes as preferred markers in various disease states such as skeletal muscle disease, hepatocellular damage and cholestasis, pancreatitis, bone disorders, and cancer. In many conditions, they may provide a unique insight into the disease process by diagnosis, prognosis, and assessment of response to therapy. As the literature on the use of enzymes in various clinical conditions has accumulated, the scope of this chapter is to provide a comprehensive and updated analysis of this relevant topic, summarizing the evidence supporting the clinical usefulness of these biomarkers and highlighting all testing aspects (including pre- and postanalytical factors) that may influence their correct application.

*The full version of this chapter is available electronically on ExpertConsult.com.

Tumor Markers*

Catharine Sturgeon

ABSTRACT

Background

Tumor markers are substances present in and produced by a tumor or produced by the host in response to a tumor. Measured qualitatively or quantitatively by chemical, immunologic, genomic, or proteomic methods, tumor markers can be used to identify the likely presence of a cancer and/or to differentiate a tumor from normal tissue. Tumor markers can contribute to cancer management as screening tests for malignancy in asymptomatic patients, diagnostic aids, prognostic indicators, therapy predictors, and/or post-treatment monitoring. Reflecting the heterogeneous nature of cancer, tumor markers encompass a variety of tumor-derived or tumor-associated molecular species. Tumor markers can be produced by different tumor types. Few are organ-specific and few are specific for a particular malignancy. Tumor markers range from simple molecules (e.g., catecholamines) through relatively well-characterized proteins (e.g., hormones, enzymes, and gene products) to very large heterogeneous glycoproteins and mucins (e.g., CA125), which may be defined by the antibodies used to measure them, and the growing number of deoxyribonucleic acid (DNA) based markers for gene mutations or amplifications (e.g., HER2, EGFR). Although their structures vary widely, the same general principles apply to all tumor markers currently used in clinical practice.

Content

This chapter provides a brief overview of cancer, highlighting its variability and some of the current clinical challenges this important family of diseases poses to laboratory medicine. These are linked with chronological developments in tumor marker applications, from the early recognition of the importance of Bence Jones proteins in myeloma through to molecular and genetic assessment of mutations in solid tumors. Requirements of the "ideal" tumor marker are considered before reviewing the general principles that guide the effective use of tumor markers (i.e., requirements that must be met in the preanalytical, analytical, and postanalytical phases of laboratory service provision). The tumor markers most frequently used in routine practice are reviewed, and requirements for provision of an optimal tumor marker service are considered.

---

*The full version of this chapter is available electronically on ExpertConsult.com.

34

Kidney Function Tests*

Edmund J. Lamb and Graham Ross Dallas Jones

ABSTRACT

Background

The functional unit of the kidney is the nephron. Because glomerular filtration is the initiating phase of all nephron functions, quantitative or qualitative assessment of the glomerular filtration rate (GFR), or some variable that bears a reasonably constant relationship to it, together with assessment of the integrity of the filtration barrier, generally provide the most useful indices to assess the severity and progress of kidney damage.

Content

This chapter will describe tests that have proved the most practical and useful for screening for and diagnosing impaired kidney function in clinical laboratories and for assessing the severity and monitoring the course and management of chronic kidney disease (CKD) and acute kidney injury (AKI). Diagnosis and classification of CKD is primarily based upon measures of GFR and proteinuria/albuminuria and of AKI upon serum creatinine and urine output. This chapter describes the contemporary use of kidney function tests to facilitate diagnosis and classification, including their biochemistry and physiology, analytical procedures, and clinical utility.

*The full version of this chapter is available electronically on ExpertConsult.com.

35

Carbohydrates*

David B. Sacks[a]

ABSTRACT

Background
Carbohydrates are widely distributed in plants and animals. They perform numerous functions, ranging from structural components of deoxyribonucleic acid to serving as sources of energy. Glucose is derived from breakdown of carbohydrates in the diet and in body stores. In addition, glucose can be synthesized from protein or triglyceride.

Content
This chapter describes the chemistry and metabolism of carbohydrates. Carbohydrates in the diet are digested and absorbed in the gastrointestinal tract. Blood glucose concentration is regulated by the action of several hormones, including insulin. Measurement of glucose, one of the most commonly performed analytical procedures, is described in detail. Hyperglycemia, which is caused by diabetes mellitus, is the most frequent disorder of carbohydrate metabolism. Hypoglycemia is uncommon except in patients with diabetes. Inborn errors of carbohydrate metabolism and glycogen storage diseases are also addressed.

*The full version of this chapter is available electronically on ExpertConsult.com.
[a]The author gratefully acknowledges the original contributions by Drs. Wendell T. Caraway and Nelson B. Watts on which portions of this chapter are based.

Lipids and Lipoproteins

Jeffrey W. Meeusen, Masako Ueda, Børge G. Nordestgaard, and Alan T. Remaley

ABSTRACT

Lipids are essential sources of energy, structural components of cell membranes, and precursors of hormones, vitamins, and bile acids. Some of them are important in the pathogenesis of atherosclerotic cardiovascular diseases (ASCVD). Notably, cholesterol in low-density lipoproteins (LDL cholesterol) plays a causal role and has become a prime therapeutic target for the prevention of ASCVD. Other clinically established measures of lipid and lipoprotein metabolism include triglycerides, high-density lipoproteins (HDL) cholesterol, non–HDL cholesterol, apolipoproteins A-I and B, and lipoprotein(a).

This chapter first describes the basic pathways in lipid and lipoprotein metabolism, as well as genetic and acquired disorders in lipoprotein metabolism. Next, the pathophysiology of the development of ASCVD, in regard to lipoprotein metabolism and inflammation, is discussed, as well as how the various lipid and lipoprotein tests can be used in both adult and pediatric populations for predicting and monitoring ASCVD risk. Issues related to the measurement and the standardization of various lipid and lipoprotein biomarkers are reviewed, as well as other cardiovascular risk biomarkers, such as C-reactive protein.

HISTORICAL PERSPECTIVE

Much attention has been focused on certain lipids and the lipoproteins that transport them in the circulation, mainly because of their strong association with atherosclerotic cardiovascular disease (ASCVD) including coronary heart disease (CHD), cerebrovascular disease, peripheral vascular disease, and other atherosclerosis-related diseases. In the early 1980s, the landmark Coronary Primary Prevention Trial (CPPT) first demonstrated that treatments that lower plasma cholesterol reduce the incidence of ASCVD. Subsequently, a multitude of primary and secondary prevention trials, using diet or pharmacologic agents to lower blood cholesterol, have also shown a reduction in ASCVD, cardiovascular death, and in some studies even reduced death from any cause.

Based on these trials and other evidence, the National Heart, Lung, and Blood Institute in the 1980s established the National Cholesterol Education Program (NCEP) to increase public awareness about cholesterol, devise strategies for the diagnosis and treatment of hypercholesterolemia in adults, children, and adolescents, and improve the laboratory measurement of lipids. Many other international and US organizations have subsequently established similar programs to address these issues. Worldwide interest in 3-hydroxy-3-methylglutaryl coenzyme A reductase inhibitor (statin)-based prevention of ASCVD exploded after the landmark 1994 Scandinavian Simvastatin Survival Study (4S) demonstrated a significant reduction in ASCVD and all-cause mortality by lowering of cholesterol.

Initially, only the measurement of plasma total cholesterol (TC) and triglycerides (TG) was used clinically. Emerging evidence from statin trials subsequently shifted the focus toward low-density lipoprotein (LDL) cholesterol (LDL-C). For a period, high-density lipoprotein (HDL) cholesterol (HDL-C) and its main protein apolipoprotein A1 (apoA-I) also attracted interest, but randomized trials failed to show that raising HDL-C prevents cardiovascular events.

In 2022, three lipoproteins are of particular importance in the prevention of CVD. Multiple lines of evidence including randomized clinical trials and genetic studies support LDL-C, remnant lipoproteins, and lipoprotein(a) [Lp(a)] as independent and causal factors for ASCVD and/or aortic valve stenosis.[1–3] These three lipoprotein fractions are integrated by non–HDL cholesterol (non–HDL-C) or apolipoprotein B (apoB). Additionally, plasma TG can be used to assess the risk of acute pancreatitis in patients with hypertriglyceridemia (Table 36.1).[4]

LIPIDS

The general term "lipid" applies to a class of hydrophobic molecules that are synthesized by the condensation of coenzyme A-thioesters or isoprene units, which are soluble in organic solvents but nearly insoluble in water. Chemically, lipids are usually enriched in carbon and hydrogen and, after hydrolysis, typically yield fatty acids or complex alcohols. Some lipids, however, are more complex, containing other chemical groups, such as sialic, phosphoryl, amino, or sulfate groups. The presence of these charged or polar groups makes these lipids amphipathic, which gives them the property of having an affinity for both water and organic solvents at two opposite ends, which is an important feature in their ability

TABLE 36.1 Minimal, Standard, and Expanded Lipid Profiles for Clinical Use

Measurement	Lipid	Lipo-protein	Apolipo-protein	Used to Estimate Risk for	Minimal Lipid Profile	Standard Lipid profile	Expanded Lipid Profile	Not Advised as Single Measurement	Additional Measurements
Advantage					Inexpensive	Low cost	Relatively low cost	None	None
Disadvantage					No lipoprotein measurements	None	None	Cannot identify elevated triglycerides and remnant cholesterol	Expensive and largely unnecessary
Triglycerides	✓			ASCVD & pancreatitis	✓	✓	✓		
Total cholesterol	✓			ASCVD	✓	✓	✓		
LDL-C[a]		✓		ASCVD		✓	✓	✓	
HDL-C		✓		(ASCVD)[d]		✓	✓	✓	
Remnant cholesterol[b]		✓		ASCVD		✓	✓		
Non–HDL-C[c]		✓		ASCVD		✓	✓		
Lp(a)		✓		ASCVD & aortic stenosis			✓		
ApoB			✓	ASCVD			(✓)		✓
ApoA-I			✓	ASCVD					✓
Lipoprotein subfractions			✓	ASCVD					✓
Other apolipoproteins			✓						✓
Metabolomic phenotyping	✓								✓

[a] LDL-C with direct measurement at triglyceride concentrations ≥400mg/dL (4.5mmol/L).
[b] Remnant cholesterol (i.e., TG-rich lipoprotein cholesterol) is calculated as total cholesterol minus LDL-C minus HDL-C, using random, nonfasting, or fasting lipid profiles.
[c] Non–HDL-C is calculated as total cholesterol minus HDL-C and is equivalent to LDL-C and remnant cholesterol combined.
[d] Elevated triglycerides/remnant cholesterol together with low HDL-C indicate increased ASCVD risk. HDL-C is used to calculate LDL-C and non–HDL-C.
ApoB, Apolipoprotein B; ApoA-I, apolipoprotein A-I; ASCVD, atherosclerotic cardiovascular disease; HDL-C, high-density lipoprotein cholesterol; LDL-C, low-density lipoprotein cholesterol; Lp(a), lipoprotein(a).

BOX 36.1 Classification of Clinically Important Lipids

Sterol Lipids
Cholesterol and cholesteryl esters
Steroid hormones
Bile acids
Vitamin D
Noncholesterol sterols

Fatty Acyls
Short chain (2 to 4 carbon atoms)
Medium chain (6 to 10 carbon atoms)
Long chain (12 to 26 carbon atoms)
Prostaglandins

Glycerolipids
Triglycerides, diglycerides, and monoglycerides (acylglycerols)

Glycerophospholipids
Phosphoglycerides

Sphingolipids
Sphingomyelin
Ceramides
Glycosphingolipids

Prenol Lipids
Vitamin A
Vitamin E
Vitamin K
Saccharolipids
Polyketides

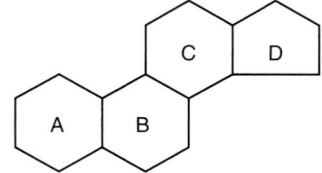

Perhydrocyclopentanophenanthrene
(sterane) skeleton

Cholesterol

FIGURE 36.1 Structure of cholesterol.

to form cell membranes and surfaces of lipoproteins. Lipids are broadly subdivided into eight classes based on their chemical structures (Box 36.1).[5]

Cholesterol

Every living organism has been found to contain cholesterol or cholesterol-like molecules such as phytosterols (plants) and ergosterols (fungi). Cholesterol is a sterol that has a tetracyclic perhydrocyclopentanophenanthrene skeleton and contains one unsaturated carbon double bond and one primary alcohol, thus making it an amphipathic lipid. Altogether it contains 27 carbon atoms ($C_{27}H_{46}O$), numbered as shown in Fig. 36.1. Knowledge of its structure and numbering system is important not only to clinical chemists but also to practicing clinicians because cholesterol is a precursor for many different metabolic pathways. These include pathways for the synthesis of vitamin D (see Chapter 54), steroid hormones (see Chapter 38), and bile acids (see Chapter 51). In addition, because enzymes that modify cholesterol or its derivatives are known by the location of the reaction on the sterol backbone and type of reaction (e.g., 21-hydroxylase in cortisol synthesis), the nomenclature of many diseases (e.g., 21-hydroxylase deficiency in congenital adrenal hyperplasia) depends on knowledge of the structure of cholesterol.

Cholesterol Absorption

Cholesterol enters the intestinal lumen from three sources: the diet, bile, and the intestine. Animal products—especially meat, egg yolk, seafood, and dairy products—provide the bulk of dietary cholesterol. Although dietary cholesterol intake varies considerably, the average American diet contains approximately 300 to 450 mg of cholesterol per day and 200 to 250 mg of phytosterols.[6,7] A much larger amount of cholesterol enters the gut from biliary secretion (3 to 10 times higher than dietary sources).[8] Additional quantities arise from the turnover of intestinal mucosal cells (~300 mg) and from direct intestinal secretion.[9] Practically all cholesterol in the intestinal lumen is present in the unesterified or free form. Esterified cholesterol, which accounts for approximately 15 to 20% of dietary cholesterol, is rapidly hydrolyzed in the lumen of the intestine to free cholesterol and free fatty acids by cholesterol esterases secreted from the pancreas and small intestine. Because the majority of the intestinal pool of cholesterol is from endogenous rather than exogenous sources, there is not a close relationship between dietary cholesterol intake and coronary atherosclerosis.[10] Consistent with this observation, since 2013 the American Heart Association (AHA) and American College of Cardiology (ACC) guidelines on the treatment of blood cholesterol have stated that there is insufficient evidence that lowering dietary cholesterol has a major impact on plasma cholesterol levels.[11]

To be absorbed, unesterified cholesterol must first be solubilized by emulsification. This occurs through the formation of mixed micelles that contain unesterified cholesterol, phytosterols, stanols (saturated sterols), fatty acids, monoacylglycerides (derived from dietary TG), lysophospholipids, and conjugated bile acids. Formation of mixed micelles promotes cholesterol absorption in the brush border of the proximal small intestine by both solubilizing cholesterol and facilitating its transport to the surface of the luminal cell, where it is absorbed by an active process involving an enterocyte membrane sterol influx protein called Niemann Pick C1 Like 1 protein (NPC1L1).[12] Loss of function of the *NPC1L1* gene is associated with both reduced plasma cholesterol concentrations and reduced risk of CHD.[13,14] NPC1L1, which is also

CHAPTER 36 Lipids and Lipoproteins 357

expressed at the hepatobiliary border, is the drug target for the cholesterol absorption inhibitor ezetimibe.[12–14] Because of their strong detergent-like effects, bile acids are the most important factor in micelle formation. In the absence of bile acids, digestion and absorption of both cholesterol and TG are severely impaired, leading to fat malabsorption. In healthy individuals, the degree of cholesterol absorption can vary widely, but on average about 50% of intestinal cholesterol is absorbed while the remainder leaves the body via stools.[15]

Absorption of cholesterol and phytosterols is limited by the presence of a sterol efflux transporter called the ATP binding cassette (ABC) transporter G5/G8, which is a heterodimer of G5 and G8. The ABCG5/G8 transporter is located at the luminal and biliary borders of enterocytes and hepatocytes, respectively, and facilitates sterol and stanol efflux from the body back into the gut lumen or biliary tree for return to the gut. Polymorphisms that cause partial loss of function of ABCG5 or ABCG8 result in hyperabsorption of cholesterol and mild to moderate degrees of phytosterolemia. Total loss of function of either ABCG5 or ABCG8 results in an autosomal recessive familial sitosterolemia, also termed *phytosterolemia* or *xenosterolemia*. It is characterized by a marked increase in plasma and tissue concentrations of cholesterol and phytosterols, such as sitosterol, campesterol, and stigmasterol, and an increased risk of cardiovascular disease (CVD).[15]

The ability of cholesterol to form micelles is also influenced by the quantity of dietary fat but not by its degree of saturation. Increased amounts of fat in the diet results in expansion of mixed micelles, which in turn allows more cholesterol to be solubilized and absorbed. As lipid absorption occurs in the small intestine, the micelles eventually break up, and the bile acids are either reabsorbed at the ileum or excreted.[16] Any cholesterol not absorbed is excreted either as free cholesterol or as coprostanol or cholestanol after conversion by gut microbes.

After its absorption into enterocytes, cholesterol and phytosterols have several possible fates. Acyl-coenzyme A:cholesterol acyltransferases (ACAT) may esterify cholesterol to cholesteryl ester (CE).[16] Free sterols can also be effluxed or pumped out of enterocytes by the ATP binding cassette transporters A1 (ABCA1) onto small HDL particles. In fact, about a third of plasma HDL cholesterol is formed by the gut during this process. In addition to acting as a lipid absorption organ, the intestine can also act as a secretory organ by returning excess esterified cholesterol, stanols, phytosterols, and free cholesterol back to the gut lumen via ABCG5/G8 transporters. Because of the combined actions of NPC1L1 and ABCG5/G8 transporters, relatively small amounts of phytosterols and stanols ever reach the systemic circulation. This allows absolute concentrations of phytosterols and stanols or their ratios to TC to be used as biomarkers of cholesterol absorption.[17,18]

Lipids, including TGs, phospholipids (PL), free and unesterified sterols, and a number of specific apolipoproteins, with the help of microsomal transfer protein (MTP) and apolipoprotein B-48 (apoB-48), are assembled into large lipoproteins called chylomicrons.[16] Patients with a rare deficiency in this process develop a disease called chylomicron retention disorder, which is characterized by excessive lipid accumulation in enterocytes and fat malabsorption.[19] Chylomicrons are secreted into the lymphatics and eventually enter

the thoracic duct, which connects to the systemic venous circulation at the junction of the left subclavian vein and the left internal jugular vein.

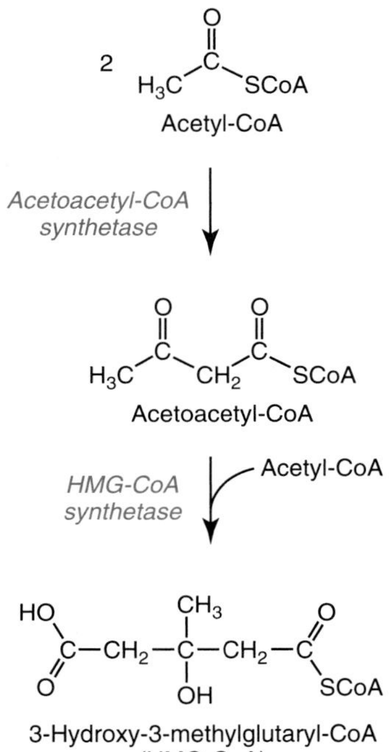

Cholesterol Synthesis

In addition to dietary sources, cholesterol can be synthesized by all tissues from acetyl-CoA (Fig. 36.2). Knowledge of this biochemical pathway, which took decades to elucidate, has acquired great significance, because the most commonly used drug agents for lowering plasma cholesterol (statins) act on the rate-limiting step in this pathway—namely, 3-hydroxy-3-methyl-glutaryl-CoA (HMG-CoA) reductase. Bempedoic acid is another cholesterol-lowering drug that inhibits adenosine triphosphate-citrate lyase (ACL), an enzyme upstream of HMG-CoA reductase. The necessity for understanding the fundamental biochemistry of this pathway was originally underscored by the triparanol disaster of 1960. Triparanol is a drug that inhibits the final step in the endogenous cholesterol synthetic pathway—the conversion of desmosterol to cholesterol—but it does not inhibit HMG-CoA reductase (see Fig. 36.2). When triparanol was used to treat hypercholesterolemia, the drug caused tissue accumulation of desmosterol, resulting in the development of cataracts, alopecia, and accelerated atherosclerosis.[20]

Although both the liver and the small intestine play a major regulatory role in cholesterol homeostasis, all cells have the capacity to synthesize cholesterol from acetate. Extrahepatic tissues are responsible for greater than 80% of TC production.[21] Cholesterol biosynthesis can be conceptualized as occurring in three stages (see Fig. 36.2 through Fig. 36.4). In the first stage, acetyl-CoA, a key metabolic intermediate that can be derived from carbohydrates, amino acids, and fatty acids, forms the six-carbon thioester HMG-CoA. In the second stage, HMG-CoA is reduced by HMG-CoA reductase to mevalonate, which is then decarboxylated to form a

FIGURE 36.2 Cholesterol biosynthesis (stage 1).

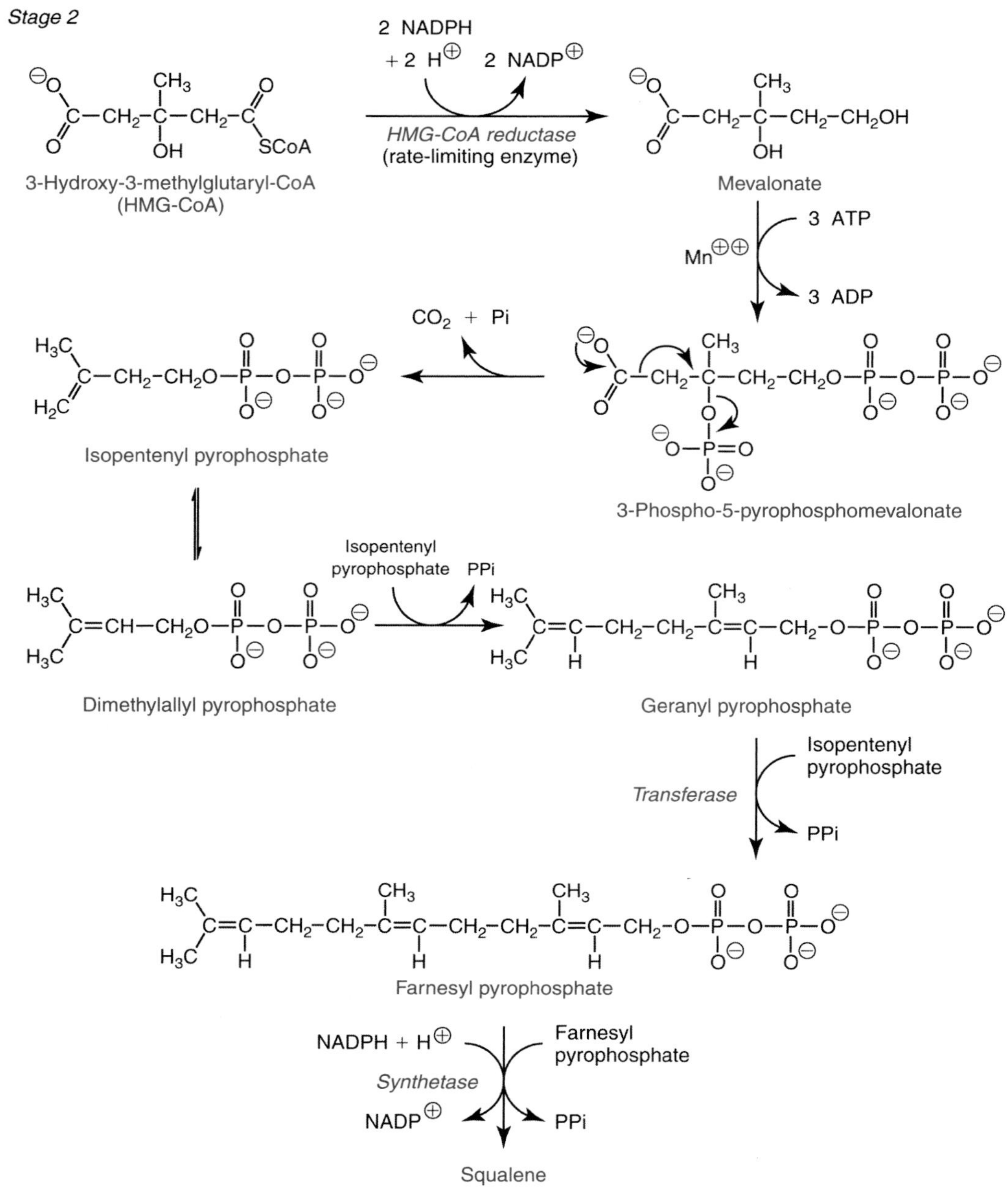

Stage 2

FIGURE 36.3 Cholesterol biosynthesis (stage 2).

five-carbon isoprene structure. These isoprenes are condensed to form first a 10-carbon (geranyl pyrophosphate) and then a 15-carbon intermediate (farnesyl pyrophosphate). Two of these C_{15} molecules combine via the enzyme squalene synthetase to form the final product of the second stage: squalene, a 30-carbon acyclic hydrocarbon. The second stage is important because it contains the regulatory enzyme HMG-CoA reductase, as well as the enzyme geranyl transferase, the second important site of cholesterol regulation. At this step, there is the regulated diversion of farnesyl pyrophosphate from the synthesis of cholesterol for the production of other physiologic lipids, such as dolichol or the modification (prenylation) of important membrane anchored proteins, such as Ras with farnesyl or geranylgeraniol groups.

The third and final stage of cholesterol synthesis occurs in the endoplasmic reticulum, with many of the lipid intermediate products being bound to a specific carrier protein. Squalene, after initial oxidation, undergoes cyclization to form lanosterol, a four-ring, 30-carbon intermediate. Lanosterol then undergoes several transitions either by the Kandutsch-Russell or Bloch pathways to become cholesterol with lathosterol and desmosterol, respectively, as the penultimate intermediates. The enzyme that dictates which pathway to be used is determined by the stage at which the double bond at position C24 of the aliphatic side chain is reduced.[22] Defects of enzymes in these pathways can lead to desmosterolosis, lathosterolosis, Smith-Lemli-Opitz, and other malformation syndromes.[23] The most common biomarkers used to assess cholesterol synthesis are absolute

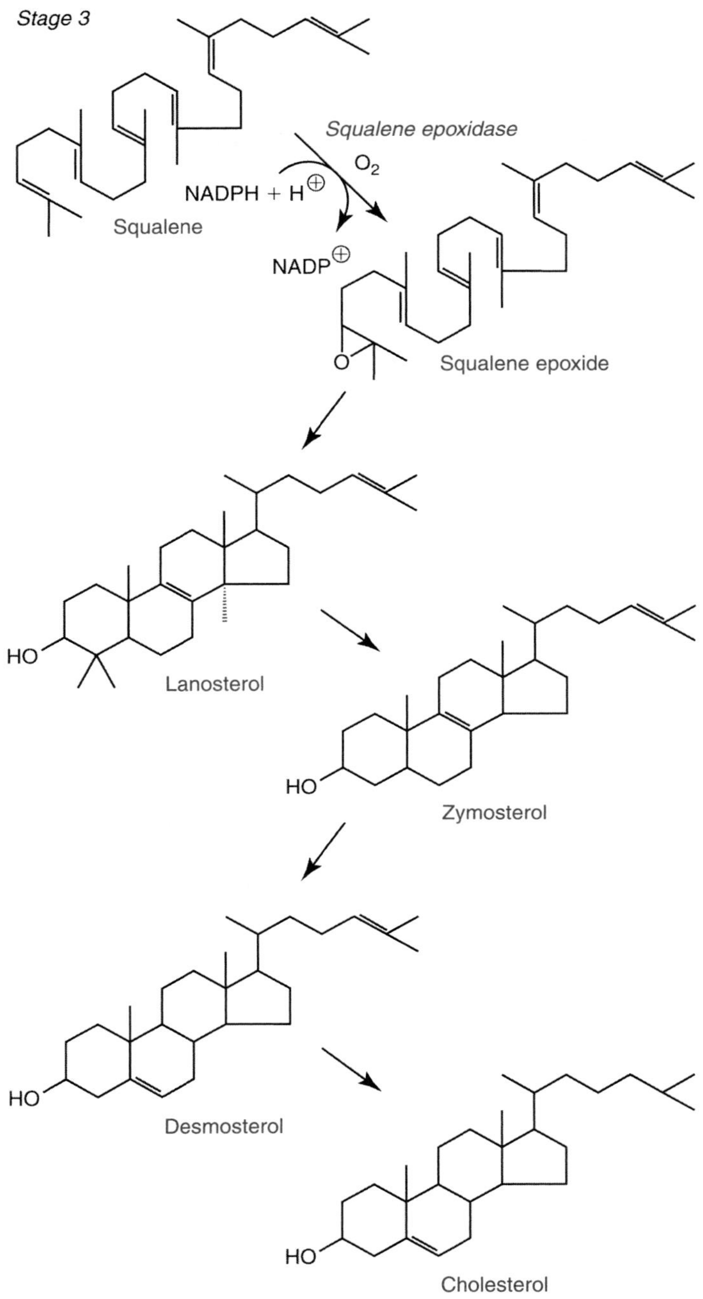

FIGURE 36.4 Cholesterol biosynthesis (stage 3; Bloch pathway).

concentrations of desmosterol and lathosterol or their ratios to TC.[24]

Cholesterol Esterification

The majority of cholesterol in the body is stored in cells or is transported in lipoprotein cores as hydrophobic CE molecules. The fatty acids most frequently esterified to the hydroxyl group of cholesterol are the 16-carbon unsaturated palmitic acid or the 18-carbon monounsaturated oleic acid, creating cholesteryl palmitate or oleate, respectively. Several intracellular enzymes (esterases) exist that can convert CE back to free cholesterol.

Almost all of the cholesterol in plasma is bound to lipoproteins, such as very-low-density lipoprotein (VLDL),

intermediate-density lipoprotein (IDL), LDL, Lp(a), or HDL. The major apolipoprotein found in VLDL, IDL, LDL, and Lp(a) is apoB-100, a large protein that contains over 4500 amino acids. The apoB-48 protein is a truncated version of apoB-100 found on chylomicrons and chylomicron remnants. It is produced in the intestine by a post-transcriptional editing step, which introduces a stop codon in the middle of the apo B-100 messenger ribonucleic acid (mRNA) transcript, thus resulting in a protein that is about 48% the length of the full-length apoB-100 protein.

The esterification of cholesterol is critical because it serves to enhance the lipid-carrying capacity of lipoproteins and prevents intracellular toxicity by free cholesterol. In the plasma, the reaction is catalyzed by lecithin-cholesterol

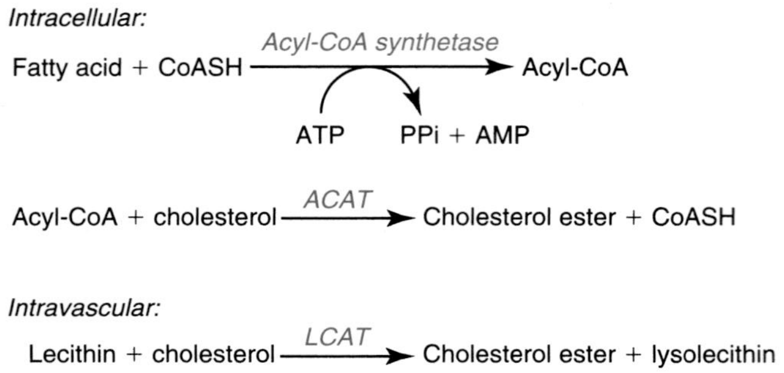

Intracellular:

$$\text{Fatty acid} + \text{CoASH} \xrightarrow[\text{ATP} \quad \text{PPi} + \text{AMP}]{\textit{Acyl-CoA synthetase}} \text{Acyl-CoA}$$

$$\text{Acyl-CoA} + \text{cholesterol} \xrightarrow{\textit{ACAT}} \text{Cholesterol ester} + \text{CoASH}$$

Intravascular:

$$\text{Lecithin} + \text{cholesterol} \xrightarrow{\textit{LCAT}} \text{Cholesterol ester} + \text{lysolecithin}$$

FIGURE 36.5 Intracellular and intravascular esterification of cholesterol mediated by acyl-CoA:cholesterol acyltransferase (ACAT) and lecithin:cholesterol acyltransferase (LCAT).

acyltransferase (LCAT) and in cells by acylcholesterol acyltransferase (ACAT). ACAT is an energy-requiring enzyme, and the initial reaction (Fig. 36.5) involves activation of a fatty acid with thio-coenzyme A (CoASH) to form an acyl-CoA, which in turn reacts with cholesterol to form CE. In contrast, the LCAT reaction does not require CoASH and transfers a fatty acid from the second carbon position of phosphatidylcholine (lecithin) to the hydroxyl group on the A-ring of cholesterol. CEs account for about 70% of the TC in plasma, and LCAT is responsible for the formation of most, with the residual being produced by ACAT that was released into the circulation during the secretion of lipoproteins. Two different LCAT activities have been described, with α-LCAT esterifying the free cholesterol of HDL and β-LCAT activity occurring on apoB-containing lipoproteins.[25] LCAT is synthesized in the liver and released into the circulation; it primarily resides on HDL and to a lesser degree on LDL and is activated by apoA-I. The esterification of cholesterol by LCAT on the polar hydroxyl group of cholesterol makes CE more hydrophobic than cholesterol. This esterified cholesterol partitions into the more hydrophobic core of lipoproteins, where TGs are also stored. This is important in the maturation or enlargement of HDL particles, allowing the surface to accommodate more free cholesterol from cellular efflux.

Cholesterol Catabolism

Once a lipoprotein enters a cell, its CEs and glycerol esters (most importantly TGs and PL) are hydrolyzed in lysosomes by lysosomal acid lipase (LAL), which is encoded by the gene *LIPA*. Partial or complete lack of this enzyme results in a lysosomal storage disorder, resulting in the intracellular accumulation of CEs and TGs, particularly in the liver. The partial loss of LAL results in the late-onset form of the disease and produces a clinical disorder known as *cholesteryl ester storage disease* (CESD).[26] CESD should be suspected in adults with dyslipidemia associated with elevated transaminases and LDL-C, and with reduced HDL-C. Unlike other forms of dyslipidemia, less than 50% of patients with this disease have increased plasma TG levels. The almost complete loss of activity of this enzyme presents usually shortly after birth as *Wolman disease*, which often results in liver failure from lipid accumulation. A recombinant human LAL known as Sebelipase alfa is approved as a therapy.[26]

Cholesterol reaching the liver may be secreted unchanged into bile as free cholesterol, metabolized to bile acids, or incorporated into and secreted back into the circulation on lipoproteins. Approximately one-third of the daily production of cholesterol (about 400 mg/day) is converted into bile acids (Fig. 36.6). Conversion of cholesterol to cholic and chenodeoxycholic acids, the major bile acids in humans, involves shortening of the cholesterol sidechain and hydroxylation of the sterol nucleus. The first step, which is also the rate-limiting step, is hydroxylation of the 7-position, catalyzed by the enzyme 7α-hydroxylase. The bile acids are made even more polar after conjugation with glycine or taurine and then are excreted into the bile, where they play an active role in fat absorption, as discussed previously. Some of the bile acids are deconjugated by bacteria and converted into secondary bile acids. Cholic acid is converted to deoxycholic acid, and chenodeoxycholic acid is metabolized to lithocholic acid. Except for lithocholic acid, about 90% of the bile acids are reabsorbed in the lower third of the ileum and returned to the liver in the portal vein by the enterohepatic pathway (see also Chapter 51).

A significant amount of cholesterol and phytosterols are also excreted from enterocytes and hepatocytes via the ABCG5/G8 transporter back into the gut lumen or bile, where they are resolubilized with bile salts and PL. If the amount of cholesterol in bile exceeds the capacity of these solubilizing agents, the excess cholesterol can precipitate, forming cholesterol gallstones, which account for about 80% of gallstones in Western societies. It is important to note that except for the liver and a few endocrine tissues (adrenal glands and gonads), most cells cannot further catabolize or modify cholesterol. Because of this and its limited aqueous solubility, cholesterol tends to accumulate, triggering cellular apoptosis or forming extracellular crystals, both of which can contribute to the development of atherosclerosis. As discussed below, cells have the ability to rid themselves of excess cholesterol to HDL via active sterol efflux pumps or by free diffusion to lipoproteins, erythrocytes, or albumin.[27]

Fatty Acids

Fatty acids, the simplest lipid-type molecules, are often indicated by the chemical formula RCOOH, where "R" stands for an alkyl chain. Fatty acid chain lengths vary and are commonly classified according to the number of carbon atoms present. Four somewhat arbitrarily defined groups of fatty acids are those containing 2 to 4 carbon atoms (short chain), 6 to 12 carbon atoms (medium chain), 14 to 26 carbon atoms (long chain), and greater than 26 carbon atoms (very long chain). Those of greatest importance in human nutrition and metabolism are long-chain fatty acids and typically contain an even number of carbon atoms.

Fatty acids are further classified according to their degree of saturation. Saturated fatty acids have no double bonds between carbon atoms, whereas monounsaturated fatty acids contain one double bond, and polyunsaturated fatty acids contain more than one double bond (Fig. 36.7). The double bonds in polyunsaturated fatty acids of both animal and plant origin are usually 3 carbon atoms apart. Some fatty acids from marine fish living in deep, cold waters (e.g., salmon), which form liquid oils at room temperature, possess numerous (up to 6) unsaturated bonds and are typically more than 20 carbon atoms in length. Polyunsaturated fatty acids are prone to oxidation, which occurs at the sites of unsaturation.

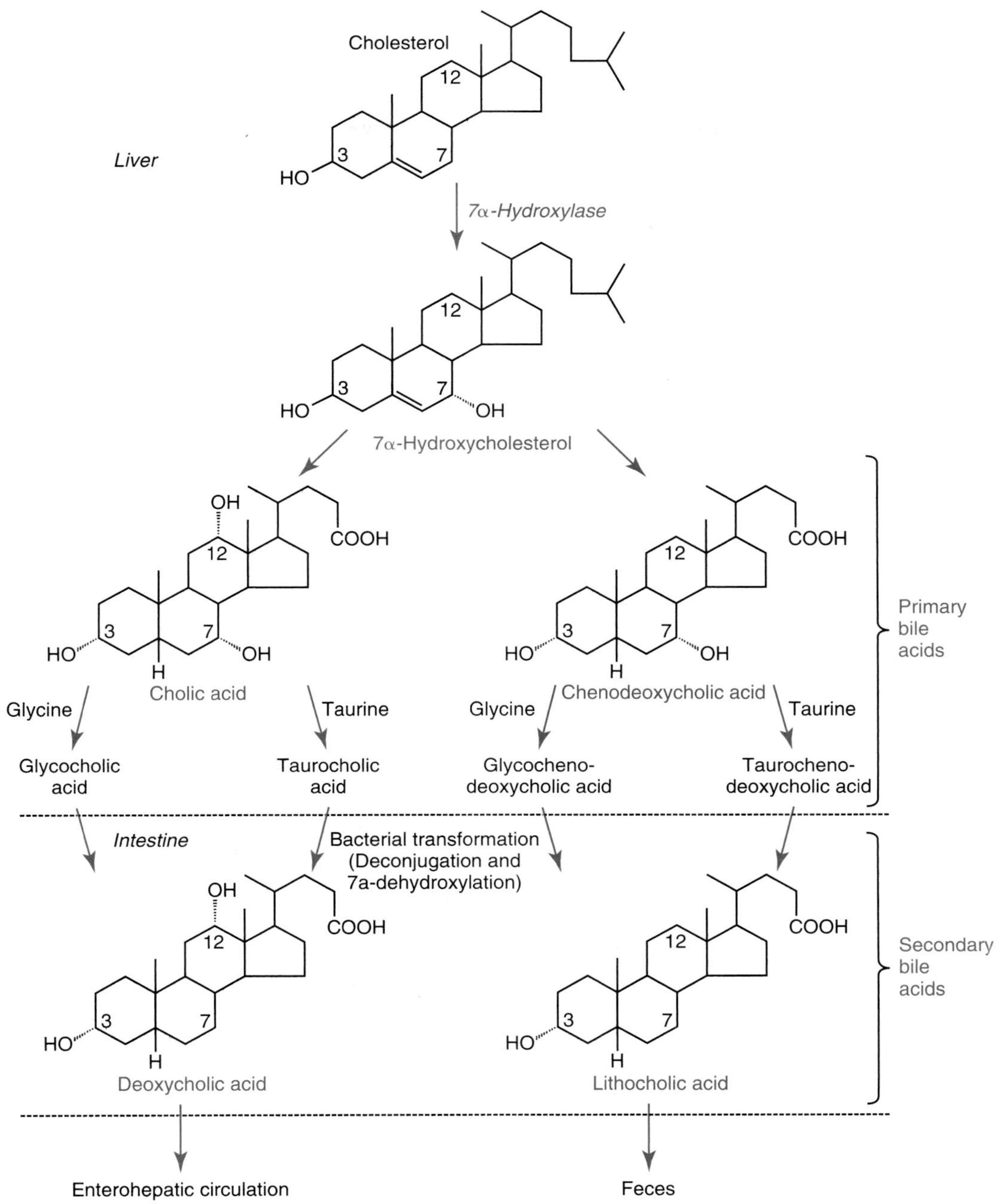

FIGURE 36.6 Bile acid synthesis.

In saturated fatty acids, the alkyl chain is extended and flexible (i.e., the carbon atoms rotate freely around their longitudinal axis), and each internal carbon atom is fully saturated or, in other words, is covalently linked to two hydrogen molecules. Cis-unsaturated fatty acids have a fixed 30-degree bend in their acyl chains at each double bond because two hydrogen molecules are missing from the same side of the carbon double bond. Lipids containing cis-unsaturated fatty acids, such as TGs or PL, have more complex spatial structures and lower melting points because these lipids cannot pack and interact as tightly by Van der Waals interactions. As a consequence, lipids containing *cis*-unsaturated fatty acids, such as olive oil and other plant oils, are usually liquids at room temperature.

In mammals, all naturally occurring unsaturated fatty acids are of the *cis* variety. *Trans* unsaturated fatty acids result from a chemical process called *catalytic hydrogenation,* which is used to "harden" unsaturated fats from plant sources in the manufacture of certain foods, such as margarine. Trans fats are artificially altered alkyl-molecules where cis-dienes are chemically hydrogenated into a trans-diene configuration, creating fatty acid isomers with very different physical properties. Although trans fatty acids are still unsaturated, one hydrogen is missing from each side of the carbon double bond, making these fatty acids resemble more the linear configuration of the alkyl chain of saturated fatty acids. This accounts for why lipids made with trans fatty acids form solids at room temperature, just like saturated fatty acids.

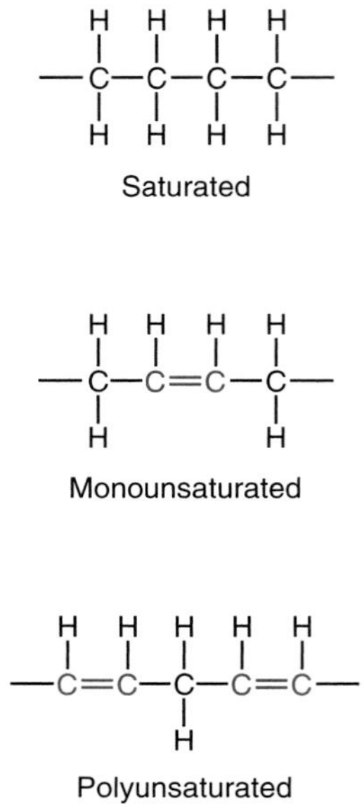

Saturated

Monounsaturated

Polyunsaturated

FIGURE 36.7 Structure of saturated and unsaturated fatty acids.

Epidemiologic and experimental studies have shown that *trans* fatty acids may promote ASCVD,[28] and thus the use of catalytic hydrogenation has been reduced in recent years in food processing in order to lower the overall consumption of *trans* fatty acids.[29] A number of countries have even banned use of *trans* fatty acids for human consumption.

The average diet in Western societies contains up to 40% fat, 90% of which is in the form of fatty acids conjugated to glycerol (e.g., TGs, PL) or to cholesterol (CE). Humans can synthesize most fatty acids, including saturated, monounsaturated, and some polyunsaturated fats. In contrast, linoleic acid, a plant-derived fatty acid, and linolenic acid cannot be readily synthesized and must be obtained from the diet.[30] These are thus termed *essential fatty acids*. Linoleic acid is converted to arachidonic acid, which has an important role in prostaglandin synthesis and in myelination of neurons.

The fatty acid carboxyl group has a pK_a of approximately 4.8, so free fatty acid molecules in both plasma and intracellular fluid exist primarily in an ionized form. Although most fatty acids in plasma are esterified, relatively small amounts are also transported as free fatty acids bound to albumin.[31] The normal concentration of free fatty acids in human blood is relatively low at 0.30 to 1.10 mmol/L, or about 8 to 31 mg/dL of plasma. The flux, however, of free fatty acids through the plasma is very large and is sensitive to physiologic energy demands (exercise and physical work), the availability of blood glucose, and psychological stresses that cause the liberation of epinephrine, which promotes intracellular lipolysis and the release of fatty acids from adipocytes.

Fatty Acid Catabolism

Long-chain fatty acids are oxidized in the mitochondria and produce cellular energy by a series of reactions that operate in a repetitive manner to sequentially shorten the fatty acid chain by two carbon atoms at a time from the carboxy (—COOH) terminus in a process known as β-oxidation. For example, 1 mole of C_{16} fatty acid is converted to 8 moles of acetyl-CoA. Acetyl-CoA does not accumulate in the cell but is enzymatically condensed with oxaloacetate, derived largely

from carbohydrate metabolism (Fig. 36.8), to yield citrate, a major component of the tricarboxylic acid cycle or *Krebs cycle*. The Krebs cycle serves as a common pathway for the final oxidation of nearly all food material, whether derived from carbohydrate, fat, or protein. It is important to note that the efficiency of the Krebs cycle depends on the availability of sufficient oxaloacetate to serve as an acceptor for acetyl-CoA.

Complete oxidation of a single fatty acid molecule produces a relatively large quantity of energy. For example, the complete oxidation of 1 mole of palmitic acid produces 16 moles of CO_2, 16 moles of H_2O, and 129 moles of adenosine triphosphate (ATP), or 2340 Calories (Cal). The unit used in discussing the energy value of food is the Calorie (Cal), equal to 1000 calories or 4.19 joules. Thus the standard free energy for oxidation of palmitic acid is 2340 Cal, whereas the free energy liberated by hydrolysis of 129 moles of ATP is only 940 Cal, indicating that the efficiency of energy conservation in fatty acid oxidation is approximately 40% under standard conditions.

By means of suitable enzyme reactions, the chemical energy stored in fatty acids can be released for metabolic processes or stored in the form of high-energy compounds, such as ATP or creatine phosphate. TGs are an efficient storage form for metabolic energy. The amount of energy produced by metabolizing 1 mole of palmitic acid (16 carbon atoms) is approximately twice that produced by metabolizing a similar mass (2.5 mole) of glucose (6 carbon atoms per molecule). Carbohydrate storage also requires a lot of water for hydration; TG storage does not. In addition to their high intrinsic energy content, the storage of TGs in subcutaneous fat deposits provides insulation for the body.

Ketone Formation

During prolonged starvation, or whenever carbohydrate metabolism is severely impaired, as in untreated type 1 diabetes mellitus (see Chapter 47) or intentionally induced nutritional ketosis from carbohydrate restriction, the formation of acetyl-CoA exceeds the supply of oxaloacetate. The abundance of acetyl-CoA results from excessive mobilization of fatty acids from adipose tissue and their conversion by β-oxidation in the liver.[32] The resulting excess acetyl-CoA is diverted to an alternative pathway in the mitochondria to form acetoacetic acid, β-hydroxybutyric acid, and acetone—three compounds known collectively as *ketone bodies*. Increased ketone bodies are a frequent finding in uncontrolled type 1 diabetes mellitus, but much lower levels can also result from nutritionally induced ketosis.[33] As shown in Fig. 36.9, the first product, acetoacetyl-CoA, condenses in the mitochondria with a third molecule of acetyl-CoA to yield HMG-CoA. This pool of HMG-CoA in the mitochondria is distinct from the pool in the cytosol, which is used for cholesterol biosynthesis. The HMG-CoA produced in the mitochondria is cleaved enzymatically to yield acetoacetate and acetyl-CoA. Some of the acetoacetate formed in liver cells is reduced to β-hydroxybutyrate. Because acetoacetate is unstable, a further portion decomposes to form carbon dioxide and acetone, the third ketone body found in high concentrations in pathologic ketotic states. Ketosis, therefore develops from excessive production of acetyl-CoA because the body attempts to derive energy from stored fat in the absence of an adequate supply of carbohydrate metabolites (see Chapter 35). In nutritional ketosis, the ketones serve as a physiologic energy supply and have been reported to increase LDL-C.[34]

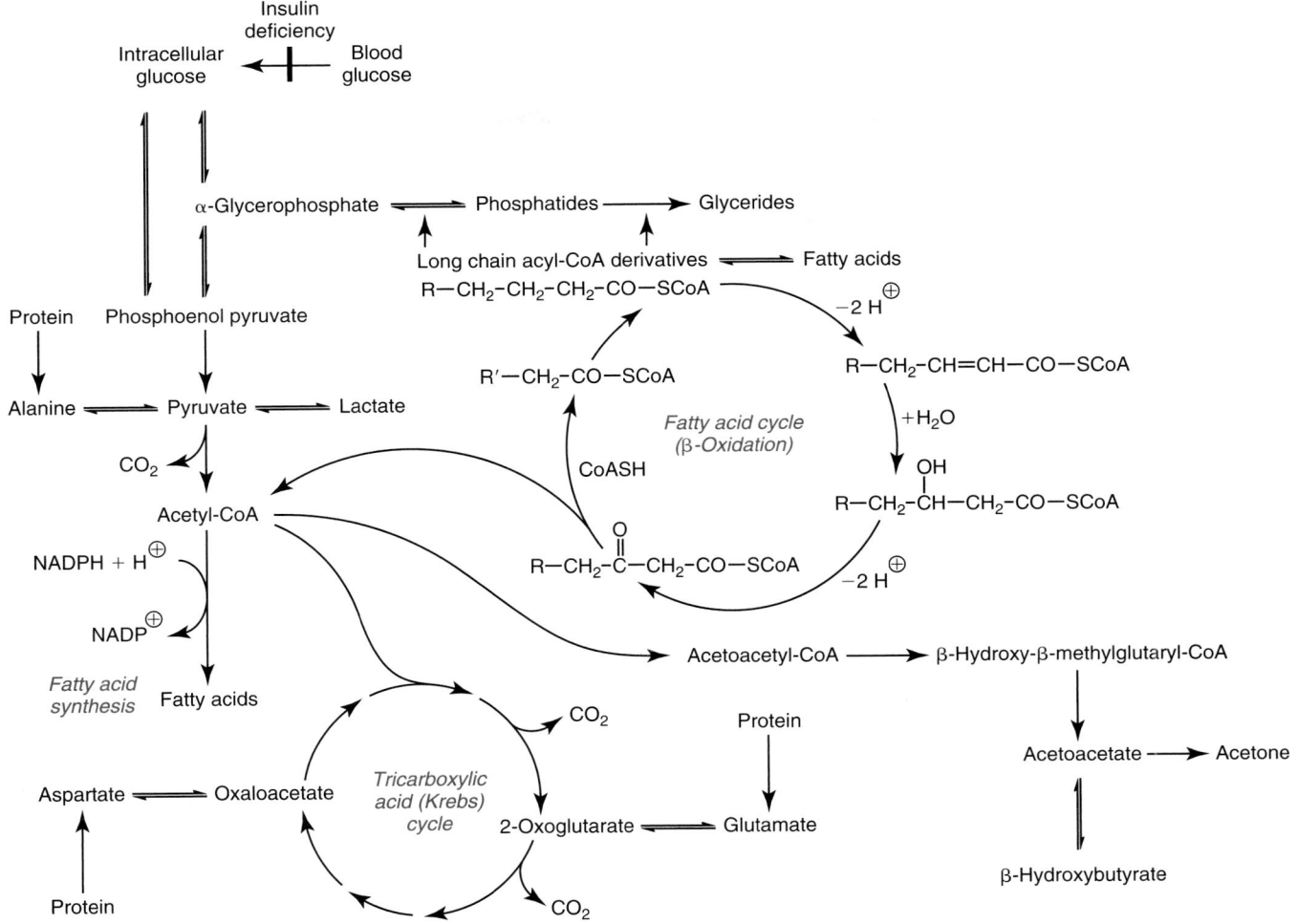

FIGURE 36.8 Metabolic relations among intermediates of carbohydrate, fat, and protein metabolism. Note that acetyl-CoA is produced from both carbohydrate and fat. The glucogenic amino acids, derived from protein metabolism, enter glycolytic paths as a-keto acids. Ketogenic amino acids enter as acetyl-CoA.

Inadequate incorporation of acetyl-CoA into the Krebs cycle may be further aggravated by inhibition of the oxaloacetate-generating enzyme system through excess accumulation of palmitic-CoA and other long-chain fatty acid–CoA derivatives in the liver. Skeletal muscle and the heart (and the brain in prolonged fasting) use ketone bodies by resynthesizing their CoA derivatives and subsequently oxidizing them for the production of energy. Although liver cells are largely responsible for generating ketones, they cannot metabolize acetoacetate because the liver lacks 3-ketoacid CoA transferase, the enzyme required for transferring CoA from succinyl-CoA.

The entire process of pathologic ketosis is reversed by restoring adequate metabolism of carbohydrate. In starvation, restoration consists of adequate carbohydrate ingestion. In diabetic ketoacidosis (DKA), ketosis can be reversed by insulin administration, which permits circulating blood glucose to be taken up by the cells. With restored concentrations of oxaloacetate, acetyl-CoA can then enter the Krebs cycle, thus restoring the normal pathway for energy metabolism. Eventually, the release of fatty acids from adipose tissue slows down and is finally reversed. A graphic view of these metabolic reactions is outlined in Fig. 36.8, which shows the overall interrelationship between carbohydrate, fatty acid, and protein metabolism.

Prostaglandins

Prostaglandins and related compounds are derivatives of long chain fatty acids, such as arachidonate. This group consists of prostaglandins, thromboxanes, some hydroperoxy—and hydroxy—fatty acid derivatives, and leukotrienes. There remains a paucity of widespread clinical application for prostaglandin diagnostics at this time.

Glycerolipids

As already described, almost all complex lipids contain fatty acids, and in most cases they are covalently linked to a backbone containing an alcohol. One of the most common alcohols found in lipids is glycerol, a three-carbon molecule containing three hydroxyl groups. The two terminal carbon atoms in the molecule are chemically equivalent and are designated α and α'. The center carbon is labeled β. A common alternative labeling system uses the stereospecific numbering system with sn-1, sn-2, and sn-3, respectively, relating the numeral 1 for the α-carbon, 2 for the β-carbon, and 3 for the α'-carbon. Glycerolipids can contain a single fatty acid, (monoglycerides), two fatty acids (diglycerides), or three fatty acids (TG). In a monoglyceride, the fatty acid may be linked to any of the three carbon atoms. By convention, the

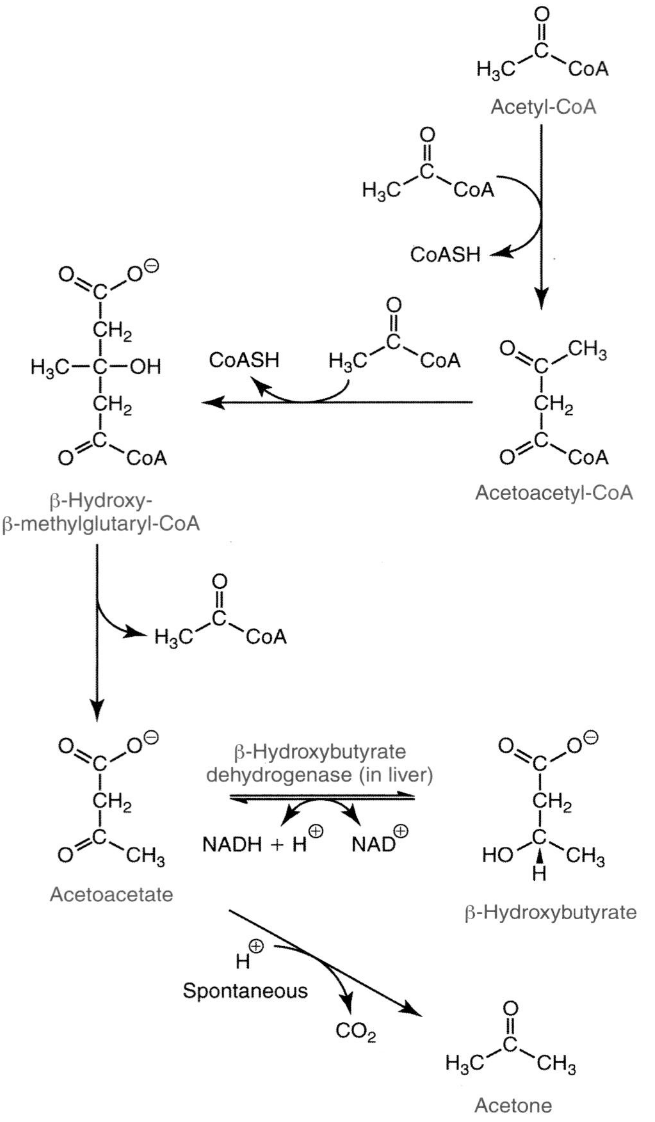

FIGURE 36.9 Formation of ketone bodies.

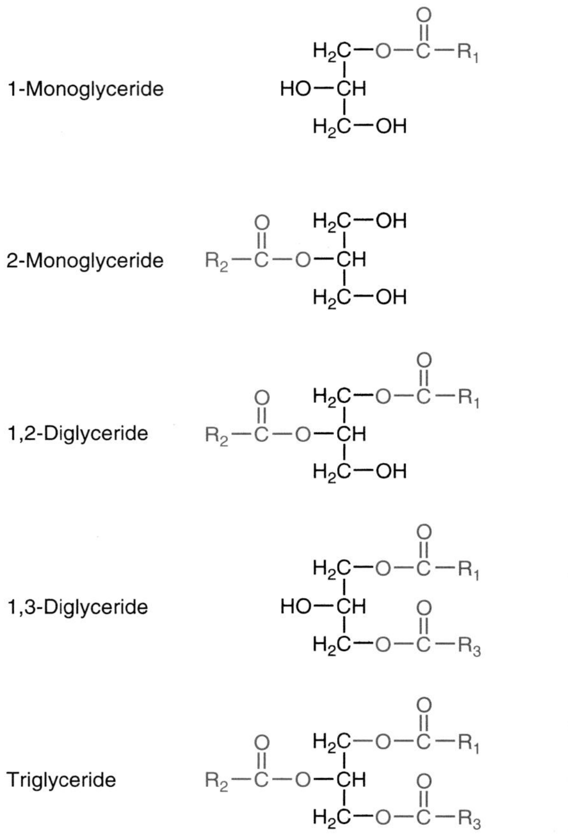

FIGURE 36.10 Structure and classification of glycerol esters (acylglycerols). R_1, R_2, and R_3 are fatty acids of varying chain length.

number system is used to indicate the carbon position (e.g., 1-monoglyceride indicates a fatty acid attachment to the α- or sn-1 carbon). This numbering system applies to all acylglycerols, including the phosphoglycerides, as shown later. Diglycerides may be 1,2- or 1,3-diglycerides (Fig. 36.10).

TGs are the most prevalent glycerol esters encountered in the body and constitute 95% of tissue storage fat; they also form a core lipid component of lipoproteins and are the predominant form of glyceryl ester found in plasma.[35] The types of fatty acids found in monoglycerides, diglycerides, or TGs vary considerably and include combinations of long-chain fatty acids. Limiting to just five different fatty acids, TG can exist as 105 different molecular TG species and with a wide variety of molecular weights. TGs from plants (e.g., olive, corn, sunflower seed, safflower oils) tend to have large quantities of *cis*-unsaturated fatty acids, such as linoleic acid, and are liquid at room temperature. TGs from animals, especially ruminants, tend to have saturated fatty acids and are solids at room temperature. Rarely, some plant TGs, such as palm and coconut oil, are highly saturated and form solids at room temperature.

Dietary TGs are digested (hydrolyzed) in the duodenum and the proximal ileum. Through the action of pancreatic and intestinal lipases and in the presence of bile acids and colipase, which activate lipases, they are hydrolyzed to glycerol, monoglycerides, and fatty acids. After absorption, TGs are reassembled from glycerol, monoglycerides, and fatty acids in intestinal epithelial cells and are combined with cholesterol and apoB-48 to form chylomicrons.

Glycerophospholipids

Glycerophospholipids (PL) are the main component of cell membranes, as well as the surface of lipoproteins keeping hydrophobic TGs and cholesterol esters in solution in the water phase of plasma.[36,37] PLs contain phosphoric acid at the third (α′) carbon atom (Fig. 36.11). In their simplest form, the A group is an H atom, so the molecule is called a glycerophosphate. Usually, however, the A is an alcohol-derived group, such as choline, serine, inositol, or ethanolamine (see Fig. 36.11). If A is choline, the molecule is referred to as phosphatidylcholine; if it is ethanolamine, it is referred to as phosphatidylethanolamine; and so on. The term lecithin, which is an older designation, is still commonly used for phosphatidylcholines. Because of the wide variety of fatty acid residues at positions R_1 and R_2 (see Fig. 36.11), many different types of PL can be formed. These PL are named according to the fatty acid acyl ester attached at C-1 and C-2 of the glycerol.

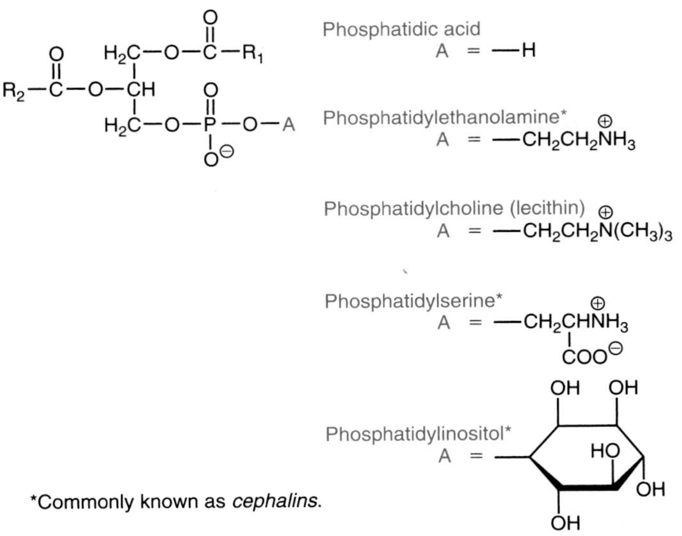

FIGURE 36.11 Structures of glycerophospholipids and common alcohol groups associated with them. R_1 and R_2 are fatty acid(s) of varying carbon atom lengths.

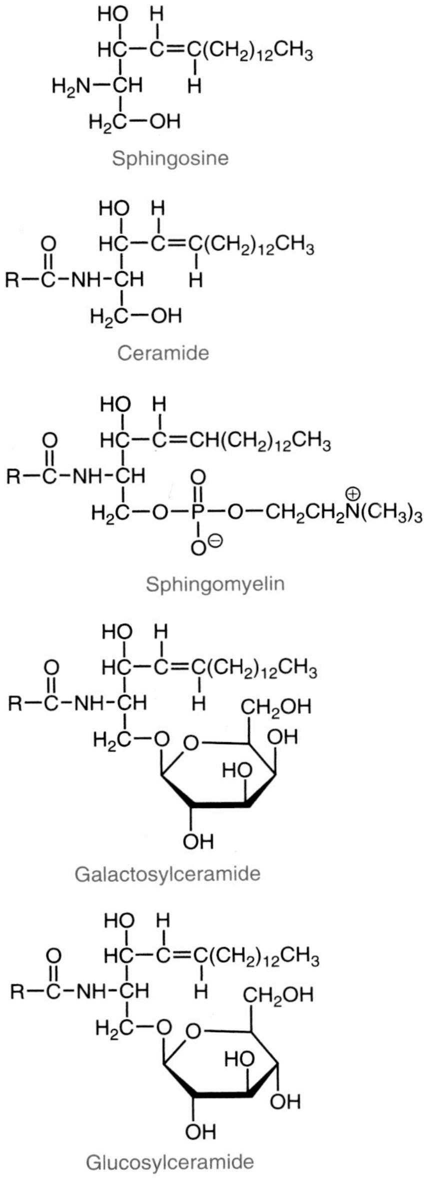

FIGURE 36.12 Structures of sphingolipids.

Saturated fatty acids are typically attached to the C-1 position, whereas (poly)unsaturated fatty acids are often present at the C-2 position. A PL that has lost one of its O-acyl groups is called a lysophospholipid. In inner mitochondrial membranes, more complex phosphoglycerides known as *cardiolipins* can be found.[38] They are derived from two phosphoglyceride molecules joined by a glycerol bridge. Enzymes that hydrolyze PL are termed *phospholipases* or *lysophospholipases*.

Sphingolipids

Sphingolipids, a fourth class of lipids found in humans, are derived from the amino alcohol sphingosine (Fig. 36.12).[36] This dihydric 18-carbon alcohol contains an amino group at C-17. A fatty acid containing 18 or more carbon atoms can be attached to the amino group through an amide linkage to form *ceramide*. Ceramides are an intermediary step in the formation of three important sphingolipids: sphingomyelin, galactosylceramide, and glucosylceramide (see Fig. 36.12). The sugar-containing ceramides can also have a sulfate group attached (usually on the 2-position of the galactose residue) to form the sulfatides. The glycosyl ceramides can have additional monosaccharide moieties, such as galactose, *N*-acetylgalactosamine, and *N*-acetylneuraminic acid to form complex globosides and gangliosides. These complex sphingolipids form the major lipids of cell membranes, particularly in the central nervous system. Gangliosides, for example, are particularly prevalent in the gray matter of the brain, whereas membrane glycosphingolipids have major roles in cellular interactions, growth, and development. Some glycolipids on red cells form blood group antigens, while others have been found to be tumor antigens. Sphingolipids like sphingomyelin tend to be enriched in lipoproteins that can induce atherosclerosis, and are known to lead to the aggregation of LDL when they are converted to ceramides.[39]

Prenol Lipids

Terpenes (vitamins A) and quinones (vitamins E and K) are subclasses of prenol lipids covered in Chapter 39.

LIPOPROTEINS

Lipids, whether synthesized or absorbed from the diet, must be transported to various tissues to accomplish their metabolic functions. Because of their relative aqueous insolubility, they are transported in the plasma in macromolecular complexes called *lipoproteins*. Lipoproteins are typically spherical particles with more hydrophobic nonpolar lipids (TG and CE) in their core, and more polar or amphipathic lipids (PL and free cholesterol) oriented on their surface as a single monolayer like a micelle. They also contain one or more specific proteins, called apolipoproteins, which usually are also located on their surface (Fig. 36.13).[40] This arrangement of core lipids with the overlying PL, cholesterol, and a protein coat is stabilized by noncovalent forces, mostly through hydrogen bonding and Van der Waals forces. This binding is loose enough to allow the rapid spontaneous exchange of free cholesterol, which is more water soluble than the other lipids, between plasma lipoproteins and cell membranes, including erythrocytes. The other more hydrophobic lipids require specific transfer proteins to exchange between lipoproteins, such as cholesteryl ester transfer protein (CETP), which exchanges TGs and CEs between lipoproteins. Another important

transfer protein is the PL transfer protein (PLTP), which promotes the transfer of PL between lipoproteins.

Lipoproteins have different physical and chemical properties (Table 36.2) because they contain different proportions of lipids and proteins (Table 36.3). Historically, lipoproteins have been categorized on the basis of their hydrated densities, as determined by ultracentrifugation or electrophoretically by their charge and size. The major lipoprotein fractions include chylomicrons, VLDL, IDL, LDL, HDL, and Lp(a). Among these major lipoproteins, they can be further subdivided, depending on the technology used, to even more subclasses.

Lp(a) is a unique lipoprotein (see Table 36.2) that is structurally related to LDL, containing one apoB-100 per particle and a similar lipid composition.[41] Lp(a) also contains a carbohydrate-rich protein called apolipoprotein (a) [apo(a)], which is covalently bound to apoB-100 through a disulfide linkage. Apo(a) has significant sequence homology with plasminogen, but unlike plasminogen, it is not an active protease. Apo(a) contains a high degree of variation in its polypeptide chain length because of a variable number of kringle domains (Fig. 36.14). Plasminogen contains five kringle domains, but apo(a) only contains kringle types 4 and 5. There are 10 distinct classes of kringle 4–like domains in apo(a) that differ from one another in amino acid sequence. Kringle 4 type 1 and kringle 4 types 3 to 10 are present as a single copy, but kringle 4 type 2 is present in variable numbers of repeats

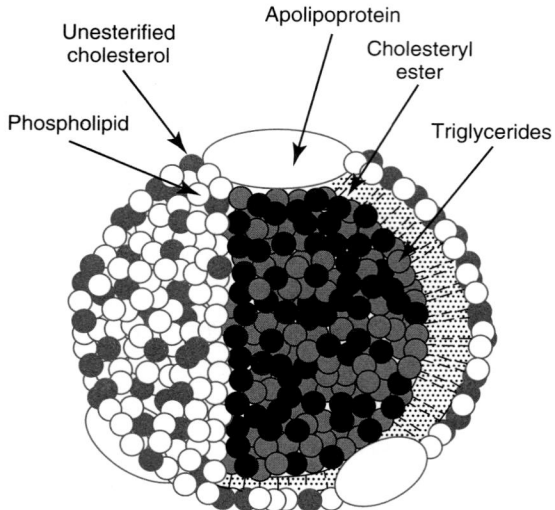

FIGURE 36.13 Structure of a typical lipoprotein particle.

TABLE 36.2 Characteristics of Human Plasma Lipoproteins

Variable	Chylomicron	VLDL	IDL	LDL	HDL	Lp(a)
Density, g/mL	<0.95	0.95–1.006	1.006–1.019	1.019–1.063	1.063–1.210	1.040–1.130
Electrophoretic mobility Approximate	Origin	Pre-β	Between β and pre-β	β	α	Pre-β
Molecular weight, Da	$0.4–30 \times 10^9$	$5–10 \times 10^6$	$3.9–4.8 \times 10^6$	2.75×10^6	$1.8–3.6 \times 10^5$	$2.9–3.7 \times 10^6$
Diameter, nm	>70	27–70	22–24	19–23	4–10	27–30
Lipid-lipoprotein ratio	99:1	90:10	85:15	80:20	50:50	75:27–64:36
Major lipids	Exogenous triglycerides	Endogenous triglycerides	Endogenous triglycerides, cholesteryl esters	Cholesteryl esters	Phospholipids	Cholesteryl esters, phospholipids
Major apolipoproteins	A-I	B-100	B-100	B-100	A-I	(a)
	B-48	C-I	E	—	A-II	B-100
	C-I	C-II	—	—	—	—
	C-II	C-III	—	—	—	—
	C-III	E	—	—	—	—

HDL, High-density lipoprotein; *IDL,* intermediate-density lipoprotein; *LDL,* low-density lipoprotein; *Lp(a),* lipoprotein(a); *VLDL,* very-low-density lipoprotein.

TABLE 36.3 Chemical Composition (%) of Normal Human Plasma Lipoproteins[a]

	SURFACE COMPONENTS			CORE LIPIDS	
	Cholesterol	Phospholipids	Apolipoproteins	Triglycerides	Cholesteryl Esters
Chylomicrons	2	7	2	86	3
VLDL	7	18	8	55	12
IDL	9	19	19	23	29
LDL	8	22	22	6	42
Lp(a)	8	25	29	8	30
HDL₂	5	33	40	5	17
HDL₃	4	25	55	3	13

[a]Surface components and core lipids given as percentage of dry mass.
HDL, High-density lipoprotein; *IDL,* intermediate-density lipoprotein; *LDL,* low-density lipoprotein; *VLDL,* very-low-density lipoprotein.

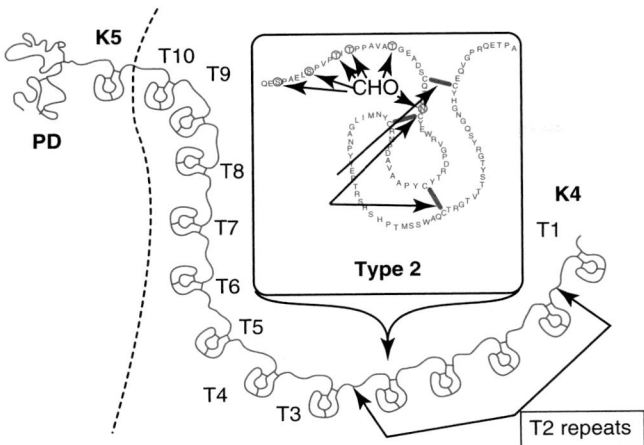

FIGURE 36.14 Structure of apolipoprotein(a). *K*, Kringle type; *T*, kringle subtype; *PD*, protease domain.

(1 to >40). Thus there are different-sized isoforms of apo(a) classically described as large, high molecular weight (HMW) or small, low molecular weight (LMW) forms. Paradoxically, due to ease of hepatic production and secretion of the LMW isoforms as compared to HMW isoforms, there can be a significant discordance between Lp(a) mass and Lp(a) particle concentrations (Lp(a)-P). At the same Lp(a) mass, those with LMW isoforms will have a higher Lp(a)-P concentration than those with HMW isoforms. It is believed that LMW isoforms are a more important cause of CVD than HMW isoforms, but this may be mostly related to their greater Lp(a)-P concentration than to anything inherent in the particle. Further confusing the picture is the codominant type of inheritance that occurs with Lp(a), with patients frequently having two different types of apo(a)-size isoforms expressed differently.[42] Due to the results of genome-wide association studies, Lp(a) is now widely recognized as one of the most important causal factors for ASCVD and aortic stenosis. It combines atherogenic features of LDL particles with prothrombotic impact

on fibrinolysis and the tissue factor pathway. Moreover, it is one of the main carriers of oxidized PL.[43]

Although all lipoproteins, even in the fasting state, transport some TGs, most plasma TGs are present in VLDL and their remnants IDL (see Table 36.3). In the postprandial state, chylomicrons and chylomicron remnants appear transiently and contribute significantly to the total plasma TG concentration. In contrast, LDL normally carries about 70% of total plasma cholesterol but relatively small amounts of TG (Table 36.3). HDL contains about 20 to 30% of plasma cholesterol and also only a small amount of TG. In states characterized by hypertriglyceridemia, both LDL and HDL, however, are enriched with TG. Their lipolysis promotes the generation of smaller, denser forms of LDL and HDL.

Lipoproteins can also be separated electrophoretically according to charge, size, or both, on agarose or on other solid support material, such as cellulose acetate, paper, or polyacrylamide gels. At a pH of 8.6, HDL migrates with the α-globulins, LDL with the β-globulins, and VLDL and Lp(a) between the α- and β-globulins, in the pre–β-globulin region. IDL forms a broad band between β- and pre–β-globulins. Chylomicrons typically, depending on their huge size, remain at the point of application. This forms the basis for the following common classification of lipoproteins: pre–β-lipoprotein, VLDL; β-lipoprotein, LDL; and α-lipoprotein, HDL.

Apolipoproteins

Apolipoproteins are the protein components of lipoproteins, and their physical characteristics and main functions are summarized in Table 36.4. Chylomicrons, VLDL, LDL, and Lp(a), each contain one molecule of apoB. HDL does not contain any apoB, but 2 to 5 molecules of apoA-I. Each class of lipoprotein contains additional apolipoproteins and other proteins in differing proportions. The proteome of LDL and Lp(a) is least diverse, the proteome of HDL is most diverse. ApoC-I, C-II, C-III, and E are present in various proportions in all lipoproteins and can rapidly exchange between lipoproteins. Apolipoproteins collectively have three major physiologic functions: activating/inhibiting important enzymes in the lipoprotein metabolic pathways, maintaining the

TABLE 36.4 Classification and Properties of Major Human Plasma Apolipoproteins

Apolipoprotein	Molecular Weight, Da	Chromosomal Location	Function	Lipoprotein Carrier(s)
ApoA-I	29,016	11	Cofactor of LCAT	Chylomicron, HDL
ApoA-II	17,414	1	Not known	HDL
ApoA-IV	44,465	11	Activates LCAT	Chylomicron, HDL
ApoB-100	512,723	2	Secretion of triglyceride from liver binding protein to LDL receptor	VLDL, IDL, LDL, Lp(a)
ApoB-48	240,800	2	Secretion of triglyceride from intestine	Chylomicron
ApoC-I	6,630	19	Activates LCAT Inhibits clearance of chylomicrons	Chylomicron, VLDL, HDL
ApoC-II	8,900	19	Cofactor of LPL	Chylomicron, VLDL, HDL
ApoC-III	8,800	11	Inhibits clearance of chylomicrons	Chylomicron, VLDL, LDL HDL
ApoE	34,145	19	Facilitates uptake of chylomicron remnant and IDL	Chylomicron, VLDL, LDL HDL
Apo(a)	187,000–662,000	6	Unknown	Lp(a)

HDL, High-density lipoprotein; *IDL,* intermediate-density lipoprotein; *LCAT,* lecithin cholesterol acyltransferase; *LDL,* low-density lipoprotein; *Lp(a),* lipoprotein(a); *LPL,* lipoprotein lipase; *VLDL,* very-low-density lipoprotein.

structural integrity of the lipoprotein complex, and facilitating uptake of lipoprotein into cells through their recognition by specific cell surface receptors. Besides these main apolipoproteins, lipoproteins carry a large number of other plasma proteins. For many of them, the relevance to lipoprotein metabolism and beyond is not fully understood at this time.

Apolipoprotein A Family

Most apolipoproteins, including those in the apoA family, contain a structural motif called an *amphipathic helix*. It is an α-helix with approximately half the amino acid residues comprising hydrophobic amino acids, which face toward the neutral lipid core when bound to a lipoprotein particle. The other side of the helix faces outward toward the surface of a lipoprotein particle and contains polar or charged amino acids. In general, the binding of amphipathic helices to lipoproteins is relatively weak, thus allowing apolipoproteins (except apo(a) and apoB) to readily exchange between different lipoproteins during their metabolism.

Together, apoA-I and apoA-II constitute about 90% of total HDL protein. The ratio of apoA-I to A-II in HDL is about 3:1.[44] In addition to being an important structural component of HDL, apoA-I is a ligand for the major cellular membrane sterol efflux protein, ABCA1.[45] It is also a cofactor for LCAT, the enzyme responsible for esterifying free cholesterol, a crucial step in the maturation and remodeling of HDL.[46] ApoA-I can be present from one to five copies per HDL particle, and it is the degree of twisting of apoA-I around the HDL particle surface that modulates particle size.[47] ApoA-I on spherical HDL particles has been proposed to exist in a trefoil configuration when three copies are present, but it can accommodate more copies in a similar structural arrangement.

The exact role of apoA-II is unclear, but there is some evidence that it inhibits hepatic lipase (HL).[48] ApoA-II can also delay the lipolysis of large TG-rich lipoproteins by interfering with lipoprotein lipase (LPL).[49] ApoA-IV, which is found in the apoA-I/C-III/A-IV gene cluster on chromosome 11, is synthesized in the intestine and is secreted as a component of chylomicrons. Chylomicrons may contain a variable number of apoA-IV proteins, which may allow them to exist in a wide spectrum of sizes. ApoA-IV may also contribute to the lipolysis of lipoproteins by facilitating the release of apoC-II from either HDL or VLDL.[50] Other potential functions of apoA-IV are activation of LCAT, promoting intestinal lipid absorption and satiety through a hypothalamic effect.

Another recently recognized apolipoprotein is apoA-V. It is relatively low in abundance compared with other apolipoproteins and appears to modulate TG concentrations by several mechanisms, including modulating VLDL secretion and enhancing LPL function. ApoA-V, as part of TG-rich lipoproteins, also traffics with the particle and binds to glycosylphosphatidylinositol-anchored HDL binding protein 1, thus facilitating its interaction with LPL. Several polymorphisms of apoA-V have been associated with hypertriglyceridemia.[51–53]

Apolipoprotein B

As already discussed, apoB exists in two forms: apoB-100 and apoB-48.[54] Most of the apoB in plasma is apoB-100. ApoB-100, a single polypeptide of more than 4500 amino acids, is the full-length translation product of the *APOB* gene. In humans, apoB-100 is made in the liver and is secreted into plasma as part of VLDL, IDL, Lp(a), or LDL.[55] ApoB-100 is also the major apolipoprotein of LDL and its measurement can serve as a surrogate for LDL particle concentration (LDL-P) when TG-rich lipoproteins and Lp(a) are not elevated.[56] Unlike other apolipoproteins, however, apoB-100 is not transferable and cannot move from one lipoprotein particle to another because in addition to amphipathic helices, it has β-sheets—a structural motif with much higher affinity for lipids.[57] It is for this reason that apoB-100 remains bound with VLDL and its lipolytic products IDL and LDL.

ApoB-48 contains 2152 amino acids and is identical to the amino-terminal portion of apoB-100. ApoB-48 results from post-transcriptional modification of internal apoB-100 mRNA, in which a single base substitution produces a stop codon corresponding to residue 2153 of apoB-100. ApoB-48 is made in the intestine and is the major apoB component of chylomicrons. Both apoB-100 and apoB-48 play important roles in the secretion of VLDL and chylomicrons, respectively. ApoB-100 is recognized by the LDL receptor (LDLR) in hepatic and peripheral tissues; it allows LDLR mediated internalization of LDL.[58] ApoC-III and apo(a) can camouflage the LDLR binding domain, hindering LDLR mediated clearance of apoC-III–containing particles and Lp(a), respectively.[55,59]

Apolipoprotein C Family

The apoC family mainly consists of three closely related proteins—apoC-I, apoC-II, and apoC-III—that are mostly made by the liver and, to a lesser degree, in the intestine. Another member of this family—apoC-IV—does not appear to be present in significant amounts in human serum. ApoC-I, the smallest of the C apolipoproteins with 57 amino acids, has been reported to activate LCAT and is also known to inhibit LPL, HL, phospholipase A2, and CETP.[60] In fact, it accounts for most of the CETP-inhibitory activity found in human plasma HDL. ApoC-II, consisting of 78 amino acids, plays an important role in the metabolism of TG-rich lipoproteins (VLDL and chylomicrons) by acting as an activator of LPL.[61,62] Because of differences in sialic acid content, apoC-III, a 79 amino acid glycoprotein, exists in at least three different isoforms termed 0, 1, and 2. ApoC-III$_1$ and apoC-III$_2$ correlate more strongly with TG levels than apoC-III$_0$. It is also associated with the generation of small LDL.[63] Recent studies reveal that apoC-III stimulates VLDL assembly and secretion and interferes with VLDL receptor, LDL receptor–related protein (LRP), and LDLR uptake of lipoproteins but does not, as previously thought, decrease lipolysis by direct inhibition of LPL.[64] In hypertriglyceridemia, most VLDL is secreted with apoC-III but without apoE, and such particles are not cleared until they lose apoC-III during lipolytic conversion to dense LDL.[55] LDLs that contain apoC-III are reportedly associated with ASCVD.[65,66] ApoC-III is also implicated in several inflammatory pathways. Mendelian randomization studies have shown loss-of-function mutations in *APOCIII* to be linked to favorable lipid profiles with low TG-rich lipoproteins and lower incidence of coronary artery disease. Antisense therapy with oligonucleotides that interfere with apoC-III synthesis are investigated by clinical trials,[67] and one such drug (Volanesorsen) has been approved in Europe to reduce TGs and risk of acute pancreatitis in individuals with the familial chylomicronemia syndrome (FCS).

Apolipoprotein E

ApoE is a 34-kDa plasma glycoprotein containing 299 amino acids. It is synthesized primarily by the liver but is also produced locally by many other tissues and cell types, such as in the brain and by macrophages. ApoE is found on all lipoproteins, but only a small amount is on LDL. Removal of apoE–bearing lipoproteins is mediated by several different cellular receptors that recognize a cluster of positively charged amino acids in a specific region of apoE. It regulates lipoprotein uptake in the liver through the interaction of a wide variety of receptors, such as the chylomicron remnant receptor, the LRP, and the LDLR. It also promotes the interaction of lipoproteins with proteoglycans.[68]

Three common apoE isoforms, designated E_2, E_3, and E_4, can be separated by isoelectric-focusing electrophoresis. These isoforms have amino acid substitutions at residues 112 and 158. ApoE$_2$ has cysteine residues in both positions, and apoE$_4$ has arginine residues in both positions, whereas apoE$_3$ has cysteine and arginine at positions 112 and 158, respectively. ApoE$_2$ has reduced binding affinity for the B and/or E remnant receptor compared with apoE$_3$, which can result in the accumulation of apoE–containing lipoproteins in the circulation. In contrast, apoE$_4$–containing lipoproteins are cleared more rapidly than those containing apoE$_3$. These isoforms are coded for by three alleles of the apoE gene: $\epsilon2$, $\epsilon3$, and $\epsilon4$. The $\epsilon3$ allele is most frequent, although relative proportions of the three alleles vary among populations.[69] These apoE alleles have been shown to contribute significantly to the variability of LDL-C and apoB concentrations within populations.[70] Individuals with at least one $\epsilon2$ allele tend to have lower concentrations of apoB and LDL-C than do those who are homozygous for the $\epsilon3$ allele, whereas individuals with at least one $\epsilon4$ allele tend to have higher concentrations of apoB and LDL cholesterol. This most likely occurs because increased hepatic uptake of lipoproteins in the presence of the $\epsilon4$ allele leads to an increase in hepatic cholesterol and downregulation of LDLR. ApoE$_4$ is also associated with increased cholesterol absorption. In the distant past, this may have offered a selective evolutionary advantage for humans on calorie-restricted and low-fat diets, but it now appears to be a disadvantage in regard to the development of atherosclerosis on our current high-fat diets. Statin hyporesponsiveness has often been noted in apoE4 carriers, which may be related to the lesser efficacy of statins in patients who hyperabsorb cholesterol.[71] A meta-analysis of 24 trials, however, suggested there was little clinical utility for APOE genetic testing for guiding treatment with statins.[72] Although the $\epsilon2$ allele is a strong genetic determinant of low Lp(a) concentrations, it does not modify the causal association of Lp(a) with myocardial infarction or aortic valve stenosis.[73,74]

Epidemiologically, the apoE$_4$ allele has been strongly associated with late onset Alzheimer disease and other neurologic diseases, but newer data suggest that risk is not only isoform dependent but also directly related to apoE concentration.[75] This association is likely related to the role of apoE in modulating lipid metabolism in the brain, but the exact connection between apoE$_4$ and neurologic disease is not known.

Lipoprotein Metabolism

The various pathways of lipoprotein metabolism are complex and intersect at several points. Through intestinal and hepatic pathways, lipoproteins transport lipids from dietary (exogenous) or hepatic (endogenous) origin (Fig. 36.15 and Fig. 36.16). Other key pathways are the intracellular LDLR pathway (Fig. 36.17) and the HDL-mediated l (reverse) cholesterol transport pathway (Fig. 36.18).

Intestinal (Exogenous) Pathway

The primary function of the intestinal pathway is the absorption of dietary lipids and delivery, particularly TG, to peripheral tissues and the liver. This pathway begins when nascent chylomicrons are assembled from dietary TG and cholesterol in the enterocytes and stored in secretory vesicles in the Golgi apparatus. Chylomicrons are then released by exocytosis into the extracellular space and enter the circulation by way of lymphatic ducts. The lipid content of nascent chylomicrons consists mainly of TG (90% by mass) and only a small amount of protein, mostly apoB-48 and various apoA isoforms (2% by mass). Shortly after secretion, these lipoprotein particles quickly acquire apoC-II and apoE from circulating HDL (see Fig. 36.15). ApoC-II on the surface of chylomicrons promotes lipolysis of TG by activation of LPL, which is mostly attached to the luminal surface of endothelial cells. The released free fatty acids generated by lipolysis associate with albumin and can be taken up by muscle cells as an energy source or by adipose cells for storage after conversion back to TG. Simultaneously, some of the PL on chylomicrons are transferred back to HDL during this process. The partially lipolyzed chylomicrons, called the chylomicron remnants, are smaller and contain 10 to 20% less TG than the original nascent chylomicron. Because of the presence of apoB-48 and apoE on their surface, chylomicron remnants are recognized by specific hepatic remnant receptors and are quickly internalized within hours by receptor-mediated endocytosis and are further hydrolyzed within the lysosomes. Proteoglycans in the hepatic sinusoids also contribute to the uptake of lipoproteins. Cholesterol that enters hepatocytes can be used in bile acid synthesis, incorporated into newly synthesized lipoproteins, effluxed to apoA-I particles, secreted directly into the bile, or stored as CE. Furthermore, cholesterol from chylomicron remnant uptake downregulates HMG-CoA reductase, the rate-limiting enzyme of cholesterol biosynthesis.

With respect to cholesterol, the vast majority (85 to 90%) of cholesterol that enters the intestinal lumen is from endogenous, not dietary (exogenous), sources. Large amounts of endogenously produced cholesterol enter the gut lumen via hepatobiliary delivery: direct intestinal secretion routes, termed *transintestinal cholesterol efflux* (TICE), or enterocyte membrane shedding of cholesterol.[76] After absorption, cholesterol is used in chylomicron formation or in the formation of nascent HDL by a process dependent on the ABCA1 transporter. Further complicating the issue about the source of cholesterol is that intestinally absorbed fatty acids of exogenous origin, which are first incorporated into enterocytes as TG in chylomicrons, start exchanging TG by CETP with other lipoproteins, immediately after entering the circulation. In this way the endogenously produced lipoproteins produced by the liver (VLDL, IDL, LDL, and HDL) rapidly acquire and traffic exogenous lipids as well.

Hepatic (Endogenous) Pathway

The hepatic pathway delivers lipids that are packaged in the liver to peripheral cells (see Fig. 36.16). As discussed previously, however, chylomicrons also deliver endogenously produced

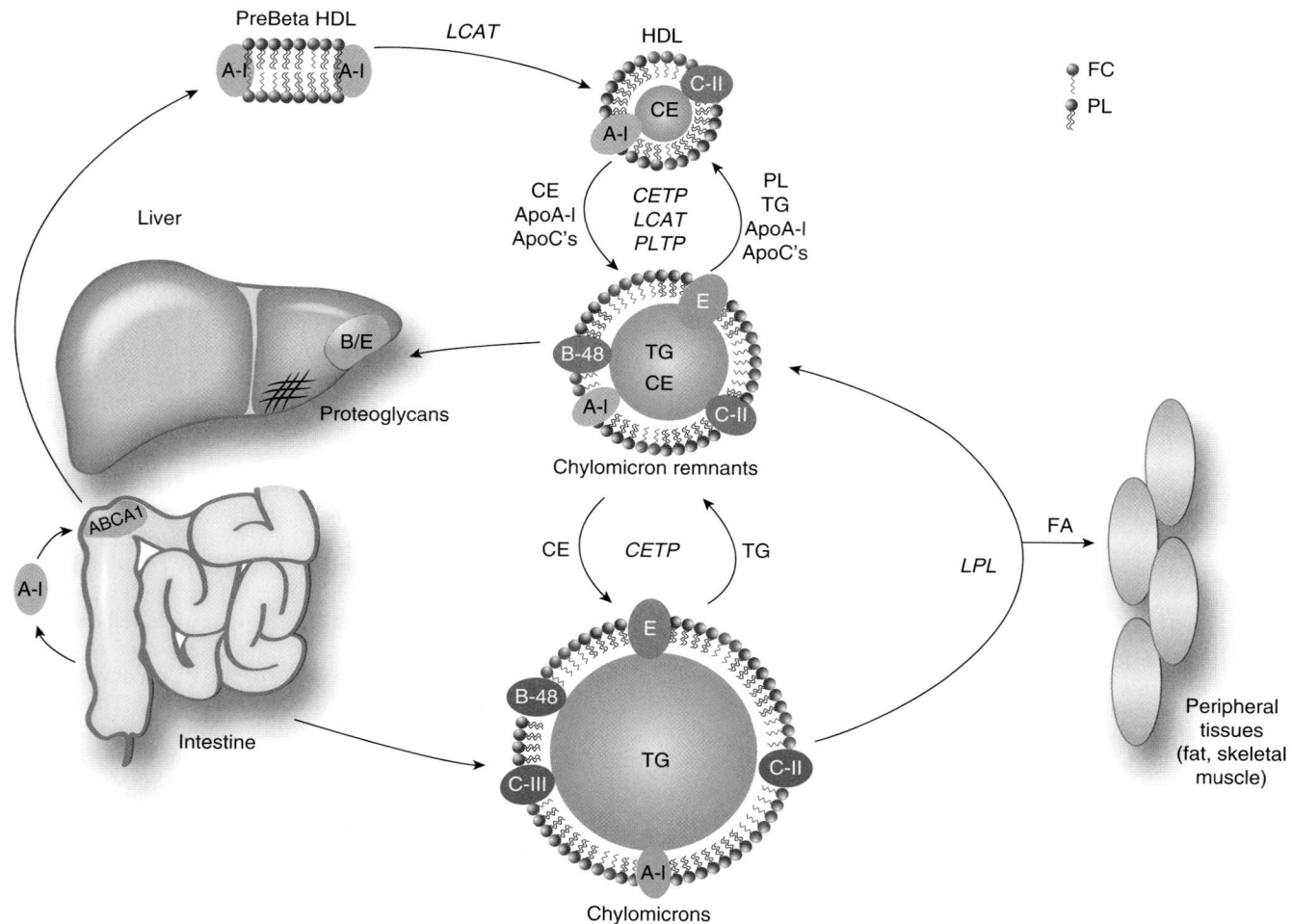

FIGURE 36.15 Intestinal (exogenous) lipoprotein metabolism pathway. *A-1*, Apolipoprotein A-I; *ABCA1*, ATP binding cassette transporter A1; *B-48*, apolipoprotein B-48; *B/E*, ApoB- and ApoE-dependent receptors; *C-II*, apolipoprotein C-II; *CE*, cholesterol ester; *CETP*, cholesterol ester transfer protein; *E*, apolipoprotein E; *FA*, fatty acid; *FC*, free cholesterol; *HDL*, high-density lipoprotein; *LCAT*, lecithin:cholesterol acyltransferase; *LPL*, lipoprotein lipase; *PC*, phosphatidylcholine; *PL*, phospholipid; *PLTP*, phospholipid transfer protein; *TG*, triglyceride.

cholesterol, and much of the lipoprotein transport of lipids is not only delivered to peripheral cells but also back to the gut or liver. When dietary cholesterol acquired from the receptor-mediated uptake of chylomicron remnants is insufficient, hepatocytes can also synthesize their own cholesterol by increasing the activity of HMG-CoA reductase or acquire cholesterol via internalization of LDL particles or through the delipidation of HDL particles when it interacts with the scavenger receptor B1 (SR-BI). Endogenously made TG and acquired or synthesized cholesterol are packaged along with apoB-100 into VLDL particles in the endoplasmic reticulum of hepatocytes in a step involving the MTP. A total loss of function of the MTP results in the inability to secrete apoB–containing lipoproteins and leads to the condition called *abetalipoproteinemia*. VLDL is a TG-rich lipoprotein (55% by mass) that contains apoB-100 and variable amounts of apoE and apoC apolipoproteins. The liver may also directly secrete a small amount of IDL and LDL with or without apoE and apoC-III.[55] Additional apoC apolipoproteins may be transferred from HDL to VLDL after it enters the circulation. Similar to chylomicron metabolism, apoC-II present on the surface of VLDL activates LPL on endothelial cells, which leads to the hydrolysis of VLDL TGs and the release of free fatty acids. During lipolysis, the particle decreases in size, and excess surface PL may be removed by PLTP and transferred to HDL. It is important to note, however, that the rate of hydrolysis of VLDL TG is significantly slower than that of chylomicron TG. The much larger chylomicrons have many more copies of apoC-II and apoE per particle than do VLDLs, thus enhancing their binding to LPL and clearance. The average residence time of TG in VLDL is 15 to 60 minutes, compared with only 5 to 10 minutes in chylomicrons.

During lipolytic catabolism of VLDL, as surface PL and core TG are hydrolyzed, and CETP mediates the exchange of core TG for CE with other lipoproteins, VLDL reduces in size allowing the apoCs and other apolipoproteins to be transferred to HDL, resulting in smaller CE-rich remnant VLDL. Then, VLDL remnants can be taken up by the liver or continue down the lipolytic cascade where they are converted to smaller, denser IDL particles, which can be removed by hepatic remnant receptors that recognize apoE. Alternatively, VLDL remnants can be removed from the circulation after

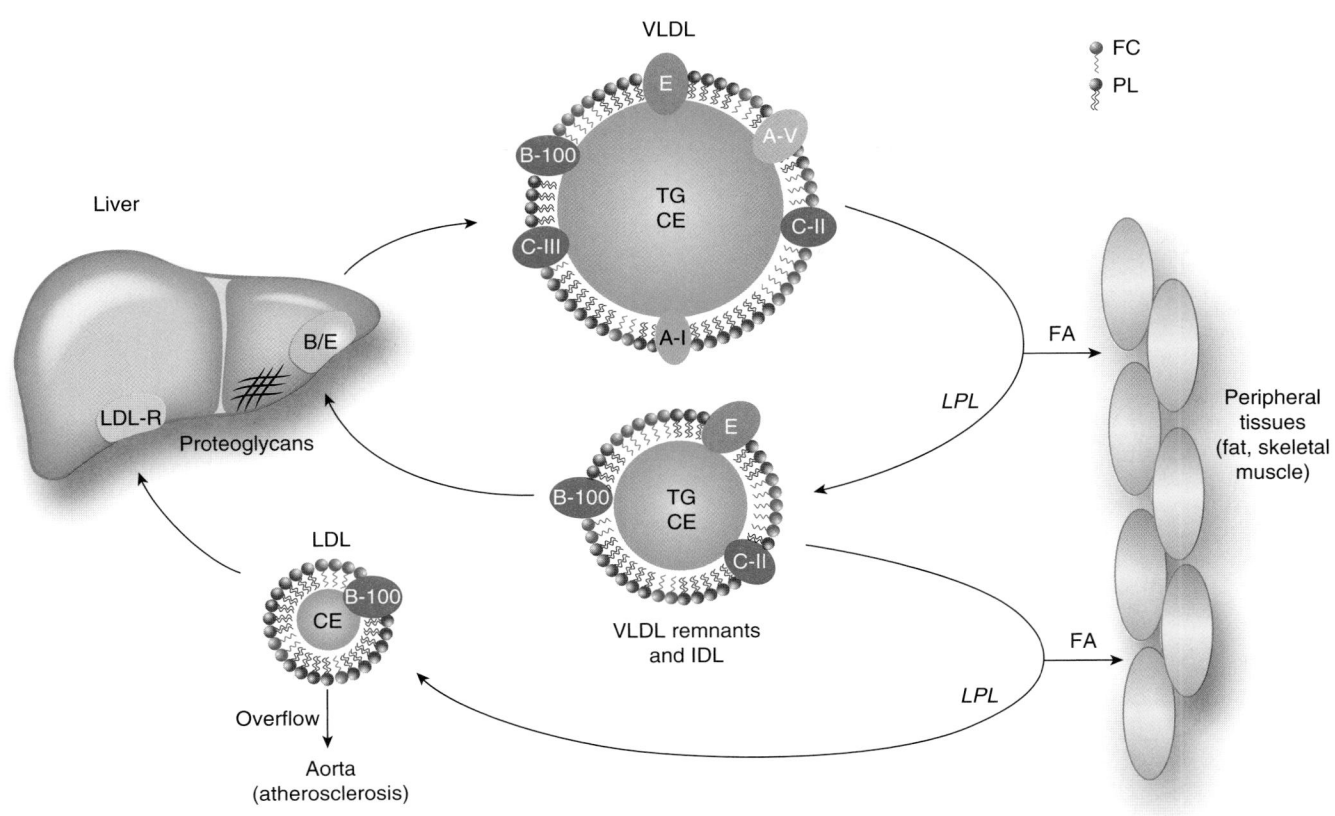

FIGURE 36.16 Hepatic (endogenous) lipoprotein metabolism pathway. *A-1,* Apolipoprotein A-I; *A-V,* apolipoprotein A-V; *B-100,* apolipoprotein B-100; *B/E,* ApoB- and ApoE-dependent receptors; *C,* apolipoprotein C-II; *CE,* cholesterol ester; *E,* apolipoprotein E; *FA,* fatty acid; *FC,* free cholesterol; *HDL,* high-density lipoprotein; *IDL,* intermediate-density lipoprotein; *LCAT,* lecithin cholesterol acyl-transferase; *LDL,* low-density lipoprotein; *LDLR,* low-density lipoprotein receptor; *LPL,* lipoprotein lipase; *PL,* phospholipid; *TG,* triglyceride; *VLDL,* very-low-density lipoproteins.

interaction with hepatic proteoglycans, either by direct internalization or indirectly after transfer to hepatic remnant receptors. Both VLDL remnants and IDL contribute to the return of cholesterol to the liver in a process termed *indirect reverse cholesterol transport.* The lipolytic fates of VLDL and IDL are highly dependent on their content of apoC-III and E.[55] As VLDL and IDL are depleted of core TG, excess surface components, such as PL, free cholesterol, and apolipoproteins, are transferred to existing HDL or are used in the generation of de novo HDL particles when they form complexes with lipid-free apoA-I.

CE molecules are also transferred from HDL to LDL by CETP in exchange for TG and this exchange can be inhibited by lipid transfer inhibitor protein or apolipoprotein F.[77] This transfer of neutral lipids from apoA-I to apoB particles is termed *heterotypic exchange* in contrast to the homotypic exchange that occurs between different apoA-I particles or between different apoB particles. The net result of the coupled lipolysis and CE exchange reaction is the replacement of much of the TG core in the original VLDL with CE. In humans, about half of IDL is removed by the liver, and the other half undergoes further TG hydrolysis, leading to the generation of LDL. Most LDL and its cholesterol content are eventually returned to the liver or intestine by the LDLR or by

non–receptor-mediated clearance.[78] When LDL particles are present in excess, independent of size, they can infiltrate into the vessel wall, where their accumulation can contribute to the development of atherosclerosis.

Low-Density Lipoprotein Receptor Pathway

The mechanism by which LDL is removed from the circulation is reasonably well understood and primarily occurs via both LDLR and nonreceptor pathways. Compared with VLDL and chylomicrons, LDL has a relatively long residence time in the circulation of about 3 days. Specific receptors present on plasma membranes recognize and bind apoB-100 or apoE when present on LDL (see Figs. 36.16 and 36.17). LDL in the circulation can acquire a hepatic secreted protein called proprotein convertase subtilisin kexin type 9 (PCSK9). LDL particles (with or without PCSK9) bind to membrane-expressed LDLR via the LDLR binding domain on apoB-100 and then are internalized in clathrin-coated pits and fuse with endosomes, which are mediated by a protein called the LDL receptor adaptor protein 1 (LDLRAP1), also known as autosomal recessive hypercholesterolemia (ARH) clathrin adaptor protein. If PCSK9 is present on the complex, it directs the LDLR to a catabolic pathway, and the receptor is degraded. Without PCSK9, the LDL particles are catabolized,

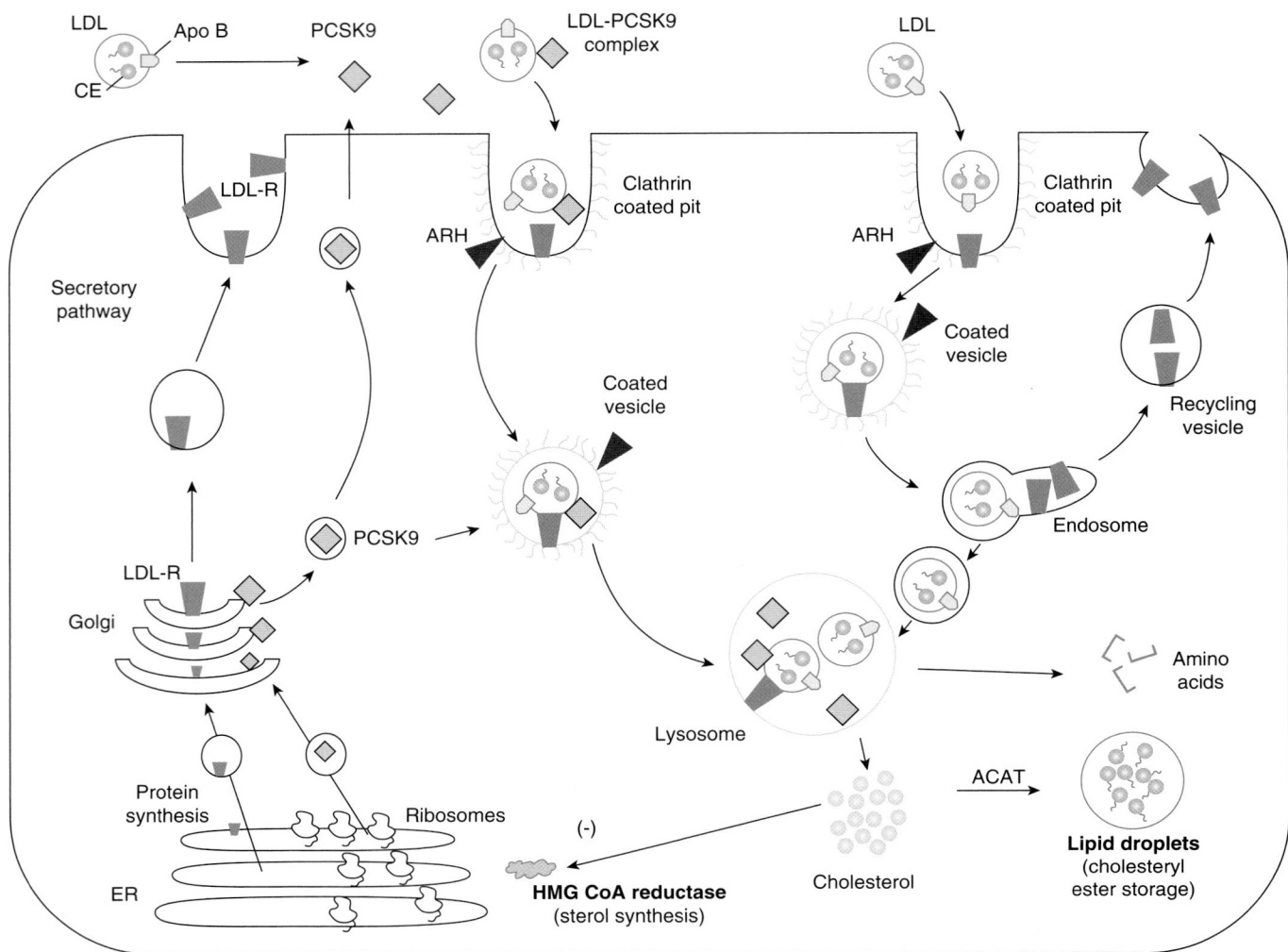

FIGURE 36.17 Low-density lipoprotein receptor pathway. *ACAT,* Acyl-CoA cholesterol acyltransferase; *ApoB,* apolipoprotein B-100; *ARH,* autosomal recessive hypercholesterolemia adaptor protein, *HMG-CoA reductase,* 3-hydroxy-3-methylglutaryl coenzyme A reductase; *LDL,* low-density lipoprotein; *LDL-R,* low-density lipoprotein receptor; *PCSK9,* proprotein convertase subtilisin/kexin type 9.

but the LDL-receptor protein is recycled back to the cell membrane, allowing for more efficient removal of LDL from the circulation.[79] Once LDL is delivered to the lysosome, apoB-100 is degraded into small peptides and amino acids. CE is hydrolyzed to free cholesterol, making it available for the synthesis of cell membranes, steroid hormones in endocrine tissues, or bile acids in hepatocytes.

Cells have multiple pathways for regulating their cholesterol content, most likely because of the cytotoxicity of excess free cholesterol. Excess unesterified cholesterol (1) decreases the rate of endogenous cholesterol synthesis by inhibiting the rate-limiting enzyme HMG-CoA reductase; (2) increases the formation of CE from unesterified cholesterol, catalyzed by ACAT; and (3) inhibits the synthesis of new LDLR by suppressing transcription. Many different intracellular pathways are also available for coordinated gene regulation of cholesterol metabolism, but the sterol regulatory element-binding protein (SREBP) transcription factors, which sense intracellular cholesterol concentrations, appear to play the most central role.[80]

Under normal circumstances, some LDL is taken up by extrahepatic tissues, mostly steroidogenic tissues and adipocytes, through LDLR, SR-B1, or non–receptor-mediated pinocytosis. Non–receptor-mediated uptake becomes important as plasma LDL concentrations increase, as in familial hypercholesterolemia (FH) when LDL penetrate from plasma across endothelial cells into the arterial intima. Non–receptor-mediated uptake is not saturable, is not regulated, and is probably largely due to the interaction of LDL with hepatic proteoglycans. Scavenger receptor A is also unregulated, and some recognize LDL that has been modified in various ways, such as oxidized LDL. Scavenger receptors A are largely found on macrophages, and this probably plays a role in the accumulation of lipid in the atherosclerotic plaque development. Macrophages that become engorged with CEs are called *foam cells* that are found in xanthomas and in atherosclerotic plaques.

High-Density Lipoprotein–Mediated Trafficking of Cholesterol

The traditional concept of the reverse cholesterol transport (RCT) pathway has recently undergone radical rethinking and might be better described as HDL-mediated trafficking of cholesterol. Historically, RCT was thought to help the body

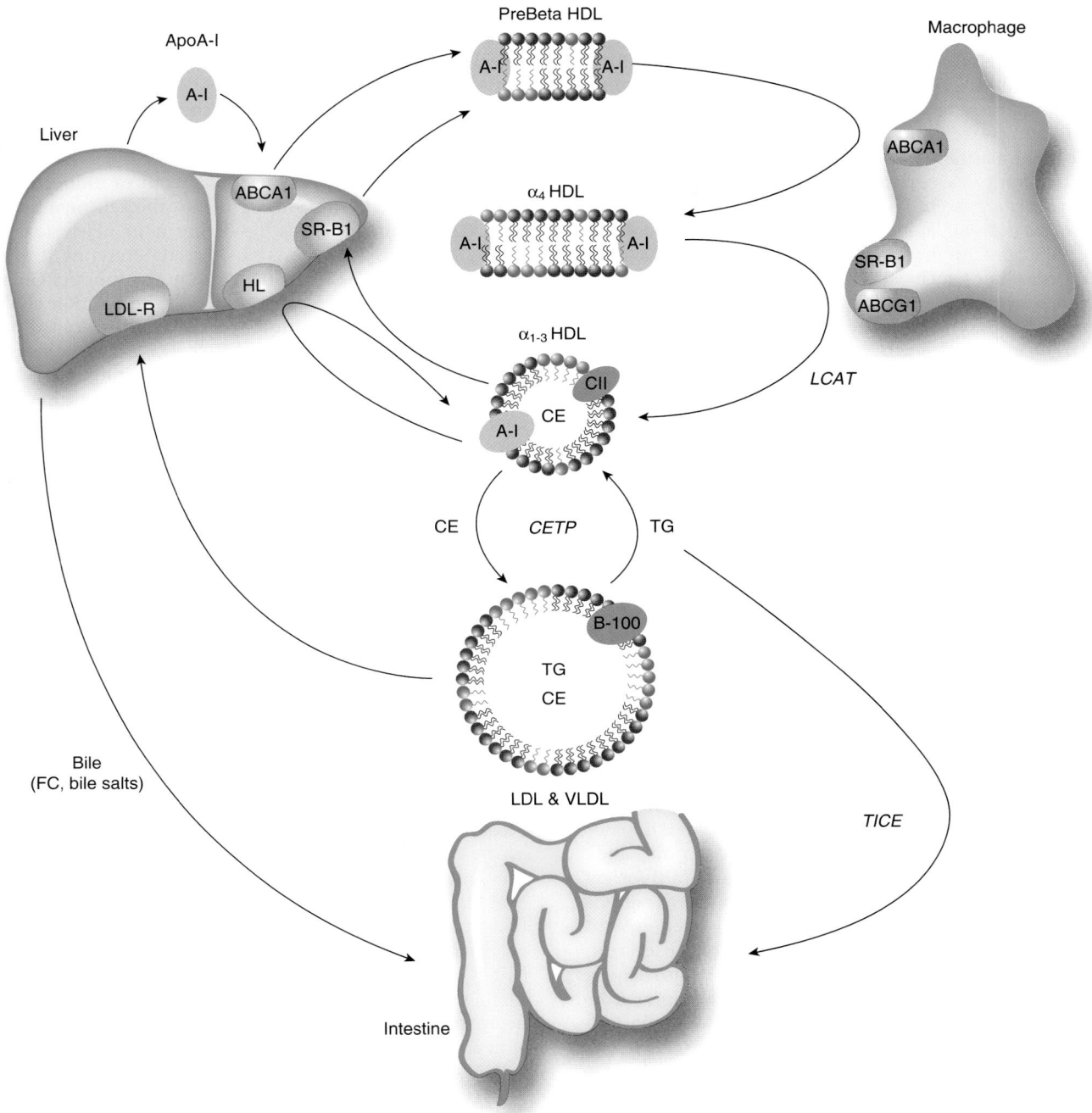

FIGURE 36.18 Reverse-cholesterol transport pathway. *ABCA1*, ATP binding cassette transporter A1; *ABCG1*, ATP binding cassette transporter GI; *A-I*, apolipoprotein A-1; *B*, apolipoprotein B-100; *CE*, cholesterol ester; *CETP*, cholesteryl ester transfer protein; *FC*, free cholesterol; *HL*, hepatic lipase; *HDL*, high-density lipoprotein; *LCAT*, lecithin cholesterol acyltransferase; *LDL*, low-density lipoprotein; *LDL-R*, LDL receptor; *SR-B1*, scavenger receptor B-I; *TG*, triglyceride; *TICE*, trans-intestinal cholesterol excretion; *VLDL*, very-low-density lipoproteins.

maintain cholesterol homeostasis by removing excess cholesterol from peripheral cells and delivering it to the liver for excretion. The focus most often was on removal of cholesterol from the atherosclerotic plaque; however, the existence of such a process has never been documented *in vivo* in humans. It was believed to be mediated mostly by HDL, thus accounting for its suggested "antiatherogenic" property. However, recent evidence shows that this pathway is a much more complicated and dynamic process involving other lipoproteins, including LDL, multiple pools of cholesterol, the intestine, and other organ systems.[27] Total RCT is the sum of direct and indirect pathways, which ultimately relocates or eliminates excess sterols from the body.[81]

This pathway begins when lipid-poor apoA-I is secreted from the liver or the small intestine. This lipid-free apoA-I is named pre–β-HDL based on its electrophoretic migration. ApoA-I rapidly acquires PL and cholesterol from cells by the ATP binding cassette transporter 1 (ABCA1). ABCA1 is believed to pump excess cholesterol and other lipids to the outer surface of the plasma membrane, where apoA-I, in a detergent-like extraction process, removes PL and nonesterfied cholesterol and forms nascent HDL. The form of HDL produced in this process is discoidal in shape and forms a flat PL disc in a bilayer-like configuration because it is relatively depleted in neutral core lipids such as TG and CE (see Fig. 36.18). Two molecules of apoA-I stabilize nascent HDL by wrapping around the surface of the PL bilayer. Although the majority of HDL formed by this process occurs in the liver and intestine, ABCA1 is also present in peripheral cells, and it enables them to efflux excess cholesterol to HDL. This is believed to result in the generation of a larger discoidal species of HDL called α_4-HDL. Because the majority of cholesterol within HDL is of hepatic origin, the concept has recently emerged that HDLs traffic cholesterol in numerous directions and help the body equilibrate cholesterol among the various tissue pools beyond cholesterol back to the liver via RCT. HL and SR-BI are also believed to be responsible for regenerating smaller spherical forms of HDL and pre–β-HDL, respectively, from mature alpha$_{1-3}$-HDL to restart this cycle.

As HDL acquires cholesterol, lecithin-cholesterol acyltransferase (LCAT-α) esterifies cholesterol by transferring fatty acids from the sn-2 position of neighboring PL, generating lysophospholipid and much more hydrophobic CE.[46] CE then moves to the core of HDL, thereby transforming it from a discoidal to a spherical shape, which is the shape found in mature HDL. Lysolecithin is removed from the surface of lipoproteins by binding with albumin. The larger spherical forms of HDL, which are sometimes called α_{1-3}-HDL based on their electrophoretic migration, can also acquire additional cholesterol by other cellular membrane transporters, such as by ABCG1 and the bidirectional sterol membrane CE transporter, SR-B1. As it matures, HDL can also acquire surface PL via PLTP, and smaller HDL particles can fuse, creating even larger species. Large HDL particles can also acquire unesterified cholesterol from cells via free diffusion or from other lipoproteins, erythrocyte membranes, or albumin-trafficked cholesterol.[82] During this process, numerous (>100) serum proteins and other lipid moieties can also attach to various subsets of HDL particles, which may potentially contribute to their function.[81]

Circulating cholesterol-rich, PL-rich, TG-poor HDLs have several options in dispensing their lipid cargo. CE can be transferred to other lipoproteins in exchange for TG via CETP. In this process, HDL particles can transfer CE to apoB–containing particles in a process called *heterotypic exchange* or to other HDL species in a process called *homotypic exchange*. Because they are by far the most numerous apoB–containing particles, much of the CE-TG exchange occurs between HDLs and LDLs. Potent CETP-inhibitors, which not only dramatically raise HDL-C but also significantly reduce LDL-C, suggest that a substantial number of the cholesterol molecules within LDLs are transferred from HDLs.[83]

After receiving CE from HDL, LDL and other apoB–containing particles can traffic it to the liver or intestine in a pathway called indirect RCT. Additional options for HDL trafficking of cholesterol include direct delivery by SR-B1–mediated uptake by the liver, steroidogenic tissues, or adipocytes, which serve as cholesterol storage organs. HDL particles may also participate in direct RCT by other putative hepatic-located receptors, such as the holoparticle or mitochondrial-produced ATP synthase β-subunit,[84] or by apoE receptor–mediated removal.

The liver has many options for "directly or indirectly" acquiring cholesterol: integrating it into the cell membranes, converting it to bile acids, lipidating it in newly forming VLDL, effluxing it to apoA-I, or directly excreting it to the biliary system via ATP binding cassette transporters G5 and G8 (ABCG5, ABCG8). The intestine can also promote cholesterol excretion or elimination by a new pathway called *transintestinal cholesterol efflux* (TICE).[76] The exact pathway by which TICE promotes cholesterol excretion into the intestine is not known, but is thought to involve the direct transfer of cholesterol from either HDL or apoB–containing lipoproteins to the enterocyte, which then excretes it into the intestinal lumen.

As mature HDLs acquire TG via CETP exchange, they are subject to increased lipolysis by HL and endothelial lipase. In this process, the larger HDLs are converted to smaller subspecies, which can break apart releasing apoA-I, leading to its renal catabolism by the megalin-cubilin complex.[85] Smaller HDLs can then re-enter the lipidation cycle. Although LDL is the major ultimate product from the lipolysis of VLDL, surface materials from TG-rich particles are transferred to the small circulating HDL$_3$ and subsequently esterified by LCAT to generate the larger CE–rich HDL$_2$. HDL$_2$ contains twice as many cholesterol molecules per unit of apolipoproteins as does HDL$_3$. HDL$_2$ can also be converted back to HDL$_3$ by HL.[86]

HDL nomenclature has been continually evolving and can be quite confusing. As preβ-HDL species mature, they may evolve into what a recent expert committee has labeled as very small, small, medium, large, and very large HDL particles. Historically, the small particles have been called HDL$_3$ (subtypes a, b, and c, with a being the largest), and the large particles have been called HDL$_2$ (subtypes a and b, with b being larger). NMR spectroscopic separation also refers to small, medium, and large particles called H1 to H5, with H5 being the largest. Two-dimensional electrophoretic separation with apoA-I staining classifies HDLs into preβ and α species, with α-4 being the smallest and α-1 being the largest.[86]

Previous research on HDL focused on a possible role in atherosclerosis and ASCVD prevention through RCT;[87] however, genetic studies and failures with therapies aimed at increasing HDL-C now question the role and function of HDL in human health and disease.[88–90] HDL is the most abundant lipoprotein in plasma of most species,[91] pointing to an important role of HDL in humans. Recent observational studies have shown that extreme elevations of HDL-C are associated with increased mortality,[92–102] leading to speculations that HDL could in some instances be harmful. In addition, evidence from observational and some genetic studies suggest that HDL concentration might be associated with the development of other major non-cardiovascular diseases such as infectious disease,[103] autoimmune disease,[104] and cancer.[105]

Because of the CE for TG *heterotypic exchange* between HDL and TG-rich lipoproteins, low HDL-C is a stable marker of average high TG and remnant cholesterol.[106] This suggests that low HDL-C can be used to monitor long-term average high TG and remnant cholesterol, analogous to high HbA1c as a long-term monitor of average high glucose levels.

REFERENCE LIPID, LIPOPROTEIN CHOLESTEROL, AND APOLIPOPROTEIN CONCENTRATIONS

At birth, the typical plasma cholesterol concentration is about 66 mg/dL (1.7 mmol/L) and is roughly equally distributed among LDL and HDL, with only a small amount in VLDL. Typical TG concentration in newborns is only about 36 mg/dL (0.41 mmol/L). Cord blood apoA-I, apoB, and Lp(a) have mean concentrations of about 80, 33, and 4 mg/dL, respectively.[107] Lipid, lipoprotein cholesterol, and apolipoprotein concentrations then rise sharply during the first few months of life, with LDL becoming the predominant carrier of plasma cholesterol, and remain relatively unchanged until puberty. Some data suggest LDL-C and HDL-C decrease during puberty while TG increases.[108] After puberty, TG, LDL-C, and apoB-100 all increase in both sexes. HDL-C and apoA-I are strongly influenced by androgen levels and are usually lower in men. After puberty, lipid levels continue to increase throughout adult life, with TC, LDL-C, and apoB being higher in men than in women up to age 55.[109] Thereafter, women have higher TC, LDL-C, and apoB levels than their age-matched male counterparts. In contrast to the other lipid parameters, Lp(a) concentration increases slowly and gradually to reach Lp(a) adult values after the third decade of life.[107] In women, as estrogen levels fall during menopause, Lp(a) levels can further increase.

The primary clinical indication for lipid and lipoprotein measurement is CVD risk assessment. There exists a continuum of risk associated with serum lipid concentrations even within the traditional reference intervals (i.e., 5th to 95th percentiles). For this reason, clinical decision limits with descriptions of desirable, borderline, or high have become standard practice when reporting serum lipids (Tables 36.5 and 36.6).[110–113] Plasma

TABLE 36.5 Recommended Clinical Decision Points for Lipids and Lipoproteins in Children and Adolescents

Lipid (mg/dL)	Acceptable	Borderline	Abnormal
Total cholesterol, mg/dL (mmol/L)	<170 (<4.3)	170–199 (4.3–5.1)	≥200 (≥5.1)
LDL-C, mg/dL (mmol/L)	<110 (<2.8)	110–129 (2.8–3.3)	≥130 (≥3.4)
Non–HDL-C, mg/dL (mmol/L)	<120 (<3.1)	120–144 (3.1–3.7)	≥145 (≥3.7)
TG, 0–9 years, mg/dL (mmol/L)	<75 (<0.8)	75–99 (0.8–1.1)	≥100 (≥1.1)
TG, 10–19 years, mg/dL (mmol/L)	<90 (<1.0)	90–129 (1.0–1.5)	≥130 (≥1.4 mmol/L)
HDL-C, mg/dL (mmol/L)	>45 (>1.2 mmol/L)	40–45 (1.0–1.2 mmol/L)	<40 (<1.0)
ApoB, mg/dL	<90	90–109	≥110

ApoB, Apolipoprotein B; *HDL*, high-density lipoprotein; *LDL*, low-density lipoprotein; *non–HDL-C*, non–high-density lipoprotein cholesterol; *TG*, triglycerides.

lipid and lipoprotein distributions based on the US National Health and Nutrition Examination Survey (NHANES) population are presented in Tables 36.7 through 36.14.[114]

Total plasma cholesterol can be split into HDL and non–HDL-C (Equation 36.1), and the latter into LDL-C and remnant cholesterol (TG-rich lipoprotein cholesterol).

$$\text{non–HDL-C} = \text{TC} - \text{HDL-C} \qquad (36.1)$$

Lp(a) cholesterol is part of total, non–HDL-C, and LDL-C, but not of remnant cholesterol. Because NHANES was designed to reflect the US population, data for the distribution of these apolipoproteins in the main American ethnic groups are available (Table 36.15).[114] Using this information, an apoB above 130 mg/dL is considered elevated and associated with increased risk similar to an LDL-C above 160 mg/dL[110] and apoB risk mitigation goals are less than 65, 80, and 100 mg/dL for very-high-, high-, and moderate-risk people, respectively.[111]

Until Lp(a) assays are better standardized, the development of absolute reference intervals for Lp(a) is problematic, and instead, cut points are often based on the 80th percentile population distribution for a given assay.[1,3,115] Based on data from different US studies, Table 36.16 shows Lp(a) values in nmol/L for different percentiles in different ethnicities. The population values are highest in blacks followed by whites and lowest in Asians. In whites, numerous studies show that risk of ASCVD and aortic stenosis increases markedly above the 80th percentile (100 nmol/L, 50 mg/dL). It is likely that these risks also increase above the same Lp(a) concentrations in other ethnicities; however, the evidence is less strong in blacks and Asians compared with in whites.

CLINICAL SIGNIFICANCE OF LIPIDS AND LIPOPROTEINS

The clinical significance of lipid and lipoprotein testing is primarily related to risk of ASCVD of the aorta and coronary, intra- and extracranial, renal, intestinal, and peripheral arteries. Major morbidities associated with the development of atherosclerosis include myocardial infarction, angina pectoris, stroke, claudication, and ultimately heart failure. Clinical significance also relates to risk of acute pancreatitis and aortic valve stenosis.

Association With Atherosclerotic Cardiovascular Disease

In 2022, the combined evidence from epidemiologic studies, causal, genetic Mendelian randomization studies, and randomized trials (latter for LDL-C mainly) unequivocally document that each of elevated LDL-C, elevated remnant cholesterol (i.e., cholesterol in TG-rich lipoproteins), and elevated Lp(a) are causally related to increased risk of ASCVD.[116–121] Based on data from the Copenhagen General Population Study,[2] a 39 mg/dL (1 mmol/L) increase in LDL-C was associated with a 1.3-fold higher risk of myocardial infarction (MI) (according to observational data) and causally with a 2.1-fold higher risk of MI (according to lifelong genetic data) (Fig. 36.19).[2] A 39 mg/dL (1 mmol/L) increase in remnant cholesterol corresponded to a 1.4-fold (observational) and 1.7-fold (genetic, causal) higher risk of MI, whereas a 39 mg/dL (1 mmol/L) increase in Lp(a) cholesterol corresponded to a 1.6-fold (observational) and 2.0-fold (genetic, causal) increased risk of MI.

TABLE 36.6	Clinical Decision Limits for Lipid and Lipoproteins Measured in Adults				
Lipid	Desirable	Above Desirable	Borderline High	High	Very High
Total Cholesterol, mg/dL (mmol/L)	<200 (<5.2)	–	200–239 (5.2–6.2)	≥240 (>6.2)	–
Non–HDL-C, mg/dL (mmol/L)	<130 (<3.4)	130–159 (3.4–4.1)	160–189 (4.1–4.9)	190–219 (4.9–5.7)	≥220 (>5.7)
LDL-C, mg/dL (mmol/L)	<100 (<2.6)	100–129 (2.6–3.3)	130–159 (3.4–4.1)	160–189 (4.1–4.9)	≥190 (>4.9)
Remnant cholesterol, mg/dL (mmol/L)	<30 (<0.8)	30–39 (0.8–1.0)	40–49 (1.0–1.3)	50–79 (1.3–2.10)	≥80 (≥2.1)
HDL-C, mg/dL (mmol/L)	≥40 men (≥1.0) ≥50 women (≥1.3)	–	–	–	–
TG, mg/dL (mmol/L)	<150 (<1.7)	–	150–199 (1.7–2.3)	200–499 (2.3–5.7)	≥500 (>5.7)
Lp(a), mg/dL (nmol/L)	<50 (105)				>180 (430)
ApoB, mg/dL	<90	90–119	120–129	>130	–

ApoB, Apolipoprotein B; *HDL*, high-density lipoprotein; *LDL*, low-density lipoprotein; *Lp(a)*, lipoprotein(a); *non–HDL-C*, non-high-density lipoprotein cholesterol; *TG*, triglycerides.

TABLE 36.7	Serum Total Cholesterol Distribution in the United States[a]													
	MALE								**FEMALE**					
		PERCENTILES								**PERCENTILES**				
Age, y	5	10	25	50	75	90	95	Age, y	5	10	25	50	75	90	95
6–17	113	121	134	148	171	191	203	6–17	113	123	137	155	178	197	209
18–29	125	133	151	172	195	224	245	18–29	124	135	150	172	197	223	247
30–39	144	154	171	199	226	254	274	30–39	130	142	162	185	206	234	249
40–49	137	151	178	197	224	259	281	40–49	141	153	174	197	219	249	262
50–59	129	144	168	200	229	258	276	50–59	148	159	182	209	235	264	277
60–69	119	134	153	179	209	238	265	60–69	135	150	175	203	227	266	281
≥70	110	121	140	170	197	224	240	≥70	134	142	170	199	226	257	274

[a]Values presented in mg/dL. To convert to mmol/L, multiply by 0.0259. Data from NHANES Survey 2015–2016.

TABLE 36.8	Serum Triglycerides Distribution in the United States[a]													
	MALE								**FEMALE**					
		PERCENTILES								**PERCENTILES**				
Age, y	5	10	25	50	75	90	95	Age, y	5	10	25	50	75	90	95
6–17	30	36	50	79	126	201	267	6–17	35	42	55	72	106	159	188
18–29	38	46	67	101	151	237	347	18–29	35	42	57	81	121	174	241
30–39	54	64	96	152	230	352	489	30–39	41	47	70	103	168	238	297
40–49	57	65	89	165	262	399	497	40–49	48	58	77	113	176	281	343
50–59	51	66	95	151	248	352	495	50–59	50	63	90	141	209	291	359
60–69	49	61	83	125	202	314	405	60–69	62	70	94	139	209	296	362
≥70	48	60	83	122	183	275	323	≥70	58	73	98	136	188	230	283

[a]Values presented in mg/dL. To convert to mmol/L, multiply by 0.0113. Data from NHANES Survey 2015–2016.

TABLE 36.9 Serum LDL-C Distribution in the United States[a]

	MALE								FEMALE						
Age, y	PERCENTILES							Age, y	PERCENTILES						
	5	10	25	50	75	90	95		5	10	25	50	75	90	95
6–17	44	53	65	79	99	117	126	6–17	47	56	68	85	103	122	133
18–29	54	64	80	100	121	145	158	18–29	58	64	79	95	119	142	160
30–39	69	79	96	117	143	169	180	30–39	61	73	87	103	125	148	166
40–49	60	74	96	118	140	162	186	40–49	66	77	92	114	134	163	177
50–59	57	66	89	117	141	166	178	50–59	61	74	95	121	145	169	185
60–69	47	60	79	100	128	153	171	60–69	58	68	89	111	136	165	183
≥70	42	51	69	90	119	145	157	≥70	55	65	83	109	134	161	182

[a]Values presented in mg/dL. To convert to mmol/L, multiply by 0.0259. Data from NHANES Survey 2015–2016.

TABLE 36.10 Serum HDL-C Distribution in the United States[a]

	MALE								FEMALE						
Age, y	PERCENTILES (mg/dL)							Age, y	PERCENTILES						
	5	10	25	50	75	90	95		5	10	25	50	75	90	95
6–17	34	38	45	54	64	73	81	6–17	36	40	46	53	63	73	79
18–29	29	34	41	48	58	68	75	18–29	36	40	46	57	69	79	87
30–39	28	31	36	44	54	67	77	30–39	33	37	45	54	66	78	86
40–49	29	32	38	45	54	67	72	40–49	33	37	45	54	66	82	90
50–59	27	31	37	45	58	72	81	50–59	37	40	47	57	70	83	96
60–69	28	32	39	46	59	75	80	60–69	35	39	46	57	72	87	92
≥70	30	32	39	48	60	72	82	≥70	39	42	50	60	74	88	98

[a]Values presented in mg/dL. To convert to mmol/L, multiply by 0.0259. Data from NHANES Survey 2015–2016.

TABLE 36.11 Serum Non–HDL-C Distribution in the United States[a]

	MALE								FEMALE						
Age, y	PERCENTILES							Age, y	PERCENTILES						
	5	10	25	50	75	90	95		5	10	25	50	75	90	95
6–17	61	68	80	96	115	135	145	6–17	63	69	83	99	116	135	148
18–29	69	78	95	117	147	174	196	18–29	70	76	89	109	131	159	185
30–39	90	102	122	150	180	207	228	30–39	74	84	103	125	148	180	194
40–49	84	101	127	148	177	210	227	40–49	84	93	110	135	159	190	206
50–59	80	91	119	148	176	206	229	50–59	87	96	118	143	173	198	219
60–69	72	84	103	128	155	189	216	60–69	78	91	115	138	165	194	222
≥70	63	71	92	115	141	169	184	≥70	75	86	106	132	158	188	200

[a]Values presented in mg/dL. To convert to mmol/L, multiply by 0.0259. Data from NHANES Survey 2015–2016.

TABLE 36.12 Serum Remnant Cholesterol Distribution in the United States[a]

	MALE								FEMALE						
Age, y	PERCENTILES							Age, y	PERCENTILES						
	5	10	25	50	75	90	95		5	10	25	50	75	90	95
6–17	8	8	11	15	22	34	46	6–17	8	10	12	14	19	27	32
18–29	9	10	13	18	27	42	62	18–29	8	9	11	15	21	31	41
30–39	10	12	17	27	41	60	90	30–39	9	10	13	18	29	42	52
40–49	11	12	16	29	45	69	87	40–49	9	11	14	20	31	49	59
50–59	9	12	17	27	43	65	83	50–59	9	11	16	24	37	51	60
60–69	10	12	15	22	34	55	67	60–69	11	13	17	24	35	53	63
≥70	10	12	16	22	32	46	56	≥70	11	13	17	24	32	40	49

[a]Values presented in mg/dL. To convert to mmol/L, multiply by 0.0259. Data from NHANES Survey 2015–2016.

TABLE 36.13 Serum ApoB Distribution in the United States[a]

Age, y	MALE PERCENTILES							Age, y	FEMALE PERCENTILES						
	5	10	25	50	75	90	95		5	10	25	50	75	90	95
6–17	42	49	56	65	79	94	105	6–17	46	48	57	68	80	89	99
18–29	50	54	67	79	99	116	135	18–29	49	55	64	76	92	104	123
30–39	67	71	85	104	121	136	147	30–39	56	62	70	87	101	116	139
40–49	60	70	83	100	121	140	151	40–49	62	67	80	93	111	133	142
50–59	57	67	81	100	116	134	148	50–59	63	71	83	99	118	133	143
60–69	57	64	76	88	106	129	144	60–69	61	67	79	93	109	130	140
≥70	50	56	68	85	100	115	119	≥70	57	64	76	91	105	129	143

[a]Values presented in mg/dL. Data from NHANES Survey 2015–2016.

TABLE 36.14 Serum ApoA-I Concentrations in Persons Aged ≥4 Years by Sex and Age

Age, y	MALE PERCENTILES							Age, y	FEMALE PERCENTILES						
	5	10	25	50	75	90	95		5	10	25	50	75	90	95
4–5	109	112	122	132	149	159	172	4–5	104	111	118	130	140	155	163
6–11	111	117	126	141	150	168	177	6–11	110	117	125	135	145	157	166
12–19	99	106	116	128	141	153	165	12–19	105	111	120	132	146	165	180
≥20	106	111	121	133	147	164	176	≥20	113	120	132	147	166	186	202
20–29	105	112	121	132	145	164	173	20–29	111	117	128	143	164	185	209
30–39	105	111	122	132	145	161	173	30–39	110	115	126	143	160	173	189
40–49	103	108	119	133	149	164	178	40–49	115	122	134	145	165	181	195
50–59	107	111	121	134	147	167	173	50–59	117	123	134	152	173	199	211
60–69	111	116	123	136	153	172	184	60–69	120	125	138	154	171	191	205
≥70	109	114	122	134	150	167	180	≥70	118	124	137	153	171	189	199

TABLE 36.15 Age-adjusted[a] Mean ApoA-I and ApoB by Ethnicity, mg/dL

Age, years	MEAN (SEM)[b] CONC, mg/dL					
	APOA-I			APOB		
	White	Black	Mexican American	White	Black	Mexican American
Males						
All	134	145	135 (2)	99	96	101
4–11	140 (2)	145	139 (2)	79	79	79
12–19	127	139 (2)	131 (3)	78	78	79
≥20	135	146	135 (2)	106	102	109
Females						
All	146	151	144 (2)	97	96	98
4–11	133	142 (2)	132	82	82	81
12–19	122 (2)	144 (2)	140 (4)	80	82	83
≥20	151	154	147 (2)	103	101	105

[a]Age-adjusted by the direct method to the 1980 US Census population.
[b]All SEMs were 1 mg/dL unless otherwise indicated. To convert to μmol/L: for APOA-I, divide by 2.81; for APOB, divide by 55.0.

Lp(a), nmol/L	10th	50th	75th	80th	90th	95th
Whites	1	20	73	100	154	209
Blacks	16	75	130	148	199	234
Asians	3	19	40	49	75	103

TABLE 36.16 Lp(a) by Ethnicity, nmol/L

Data from the Framingham Heart Study, the Coronary Artery Risk Development Study, and the Honolulu Heart Study. Modified from Marcovina SM, Albers JJ. Lipoprotein (a) measurements for clinical application. *J Lipid Res* 2016;57(4):526–537.

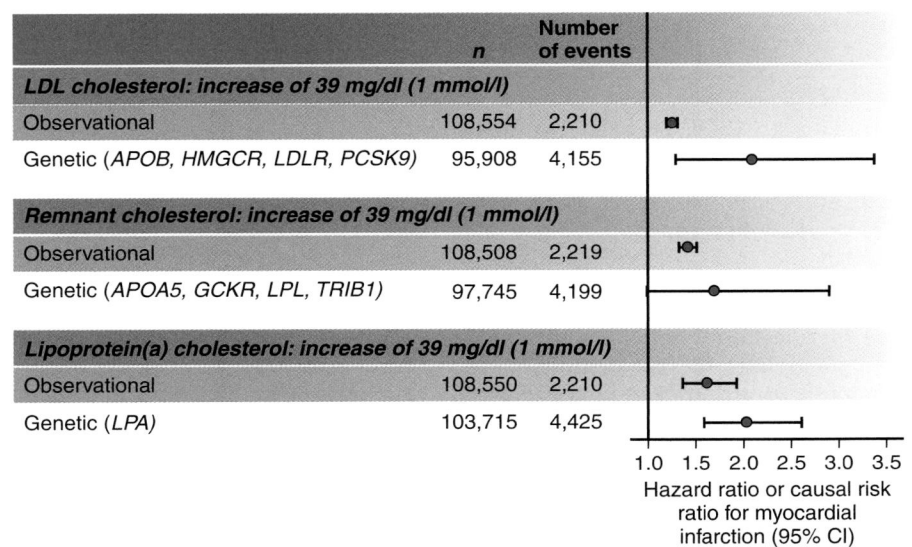

FIGURE 36.19 Comparison of risk of myocardial infarction with increasing levels of LDL cholesterol, remnant cholesterol (cholesterol in triglyceride-rich lipoproteins), or lipoprotein(a) cholesterol according to observational and causal, genetic study data in individuals in the Copenhagen General Population Study.[2]

As early as 1910, Windaus first described cholesterol in the lesions of diseased arteries. Subsequently, many studies confirmed that free and esterified cholesterol accumulate in the aorta, coronary arteries, and cerebral vessels, and the rate of accumulation seems to vary among individuals. The association between elevated serum cholesterol and atherosclerosis in humans was first suggested in 1938 when Muller and Thanhauser both demonstrated familial aggregation of hypercholesterolemia and CHD in the disease later named FH. Additional studies showed that when the TC concentration is high, the incidence and prevalence of CHD are also high, although the association with total mortality is not as strong. In the 1960s, Fredrickson and colleagues noted that lipid disorders (hyperlipidemia and dyslipidemia) could be classified into distinct lipoprotein phenotypes (e.g., hyperbetalipoproteinemia, increased LDL-C; hypoalphalipoproteinemia, low HDL-C). At the time, this provided a better mechanistic explanation of lipid-related disorders than did total lipid concentrations.

The overall relationship between cholesterol and atherosclerotic coronary disease is curvilinear. According to the Multiple Risk Factor Intervention Trial (MRFIT), if a risk ratio of 1.0 is arbitrarily assigned at a TC value of 200 mg/dL (5.2 mmol/L), the risk ratio increases to 2.0 at 250 mg/dL (6.5 mmol/L) and to 4.0 at 300 mg/dL (7.76 mmol/L) (Fig. 36.20).[122] Pathologic studies have helped to explain this curvilinear relationship. When 60% of the surface of coronary arteries is covered with plaque, a critical phase is reached in which any further increase in serum cholesterol will markedly increase CHD risk. Results of the Lipid Research Clinics (LRC)- CPPT have shown that use of the concentration at the 95th percentile of a population distribution is inappropriate to define hypercholesterolemia.[123] Data from this and other studies suggest that risk disproportionately increases as cholesterol concentrations increase; at concentrations of 200 to 240 mg/dL (5.2 to 6.2 mmol/L), the risk begins to accelerate at a greater rate. On average, each 1% reduction in cholesterol (2 to 3 mg/dL) (0.05 to 0.08 mmol/L) results in about a 2% reduction in CHD incidence—a relationship of considerable clinical and public health significance.[124] In addition, statin studies utilizing intravascular coronary ultrasound have shown that individuals with pre-existing disease may actually show some reversal of existing atherosclerosis, if they are aggressively treated with cholesterol lowering therapy.[125]

Many epidemiologic and clinical studies have shown that other lipids and lipoproteins, including LDL-C and HDL-C, are also useful for predicting ASCVD risk. In the case of LDL-C, some studies have suggested that small, dense LDL-C subfractions correlate with ASCVD risk.[126,127] However, to date, most studies have failed to show independent predictive utility beyond that of "standard" risk factors.[128]

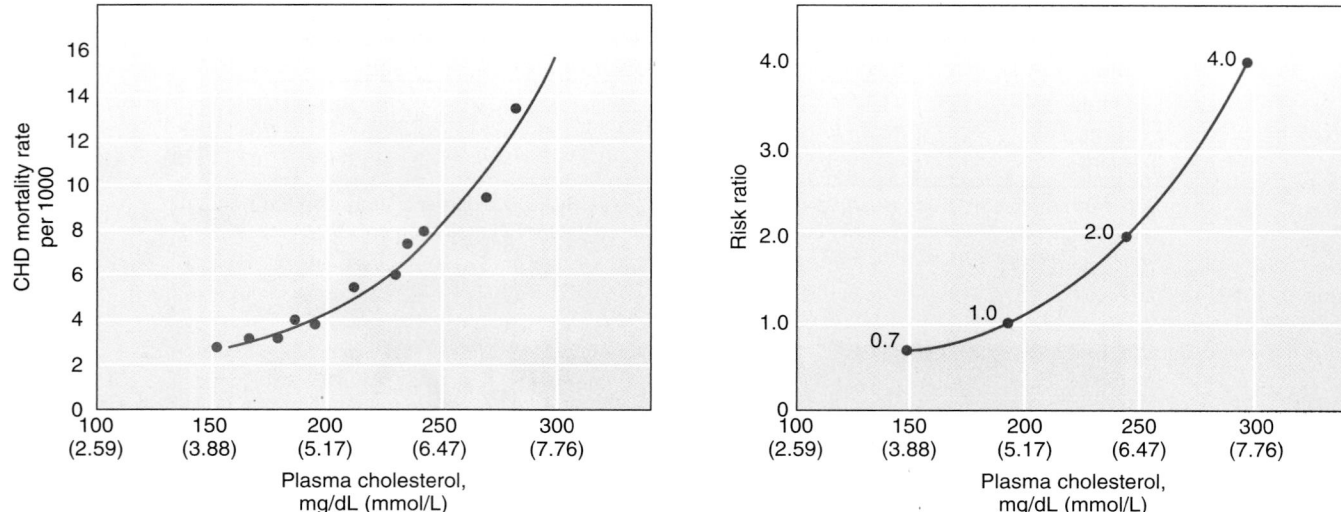

FIGURE 36.20 Relationship between cholesterol concentration and coronary heart disease mortality, expressed by yearly rate per 1000 and risk ratios (Multiple Risk Factor Intervention Trial [MRFIT] participants).[122]

TG are also considered a risk factor for ASCVD. Chylomicron and VLDL remnants and IDL, the products of the breakdown of TG-rich lipoproteins, are now also increasingly recognized as important players in atherogenesis and may account for the stronger association of nonfasting TG with cardiovascular events compared to fasting TG.

Any LDL-C reduction using statins, ezetimibe, and PCSK9 inhibitors have in randomized controlled trials documented reduced ASCVD and all-cause mortality, even when LDL-C is reduced to below 70 mg/dL (1.8 mmol/L).[129–132] Reduction of TG-rich lipoproteins associate similarly with reduced ASCVD in post hoc analyses of fibrate trials among those with elevated TG at study entry and in trials using icosapent ethyl (an ethyl alcohol derivative of eicosapentaenoic acid EPA).[119,133] No randomized trial has yet documented benefit of Lp(a) reduction; however, a phase 3 trial is underway.

Association With Acute Pancreatitis

Increasing elevations of plasma TG are associated with increasing risk of acute pancreatitis.[134] At concentrations above 500 mg/dL (5.7 mmol/L) and above 880 mg/dL (10 mmol/L) according to US and European guidelines, TG-lowering therapy is advised to prevent acute pancreatitis[110,111]; however, no randomized trials document this effect.

Association With Aortic Valve Stenosis

Based on observational and genetic data, elevated Lp(a) is a causal factor for aortic valve stenosis.[121,135,136] Similar recent data show that this is also the case for elevated TG-rich lipoproteins,[137] whereas the evidence for elevated LDL is less clear. There is no guideline advice to prevent aortic valve stenosis through lowering of lipids and lipoproteins.

Nonfasting Lipid Assessment

Clinical practice guidelines from most major cardiology societies and expert consensus statements have concluded that nonfasting blood samples are acceptable for routine lipid assessments.[1,110–112,138,139] Fasting samples were historically preferred in order to reduce the variability observed in measures of TG. The shift to nonfasting lipid assessment is supported by multiple lines of evidence.

First, studies have found that a significant number of patients do not fast despite being asked to do so.[140] Additionally, data show that observed TG increases due to nonfasting are clinically negligible in most cases. In fact, nonfasting TG concentrations remain less than 200 mg/dL in most patients.[141–143] This relatively normal concentration of TG in the nonfasting state contributes to the clinically insignificant impact observed by nonfasting lipid screening and subsequent LDL-C estimation.[4,142] Multiple studies have suggested that nonfasting lipid assessments are comparable and possibly superior at-risk CHD prediction.[144–146]

Another argument in favor of nonfasting lipid assessment is patient safety. As many as 20% of patients undergoing routine lipid assessment are at risk of fasting-evoked en route hypoglycemia.[147] Finally, random nonfasting compared to fasting lipid profiles represents a simplification for patients, clinicians, and laboratories alike.

Apolipoproteins and Patient Management

In the early 1970s, Alaupovic first suggested that apolipoproteins could be considered as risk markers when the contribution of lipids and lipoproteins to the development of atherosclerotic disease is evaluated.[148] Several studies showed that in people with CHD, changes in serum concentrations of apoA-I and apoB are similar to those for HDL-C and LDL-C, respectively. ApoB values were increased and apoA-I values were decreased in people with CHD compared with those without disease. In several studies, apoA-I and apoB were better discriminators of people with CHD than the cholesterol concentration of the corresponding lipoprotein.[54,149] Furthermore, apoA-I and apoB were shown to correlate better with the degree of coronary stenosis than LDL-C and HDL-C.[150] It has been shown that only 14.5% of patients with myocardial infarction younger than the age of 60 years have LDL-C above the 95th percentile. In contrast, 35% of these patients have apoB above the 95th percentile.[151] The measurement of apoB provides information regarding the number of apoB–containing particles because only one apoB molecule is present per lipoprotein particle. If the concentration of LDL-C is low, normal, or slightly increased, but apoB or total LDL-P is greatly increased, it is likely explained by cholesterol-depleted particles—either small LDL, Lp(a), or TG-rich, CE-depleted LDL of any size. Increased serum apoB and decreased apoA-I concentrations were also found in children of parents with premature atherosclerotic disease.[152] Overall, these and other findings suggest that apolipoproteins and other measures of particle number may be superior as cardiovascular risk markers. In 2022, many international cardiovascular prevention guidelines and consensus papers recommend the use of apoB measurements together with measurement of LDL-C and non–HDL-C under certain conditions, particularly if TG are increased; however, none recommend the use of apoA-I measurements.[110,111,153]

Cholesterol Lowering Early in Life

Although ASCVD is often not manifested clinically until the fourth decade of life, atherosclerosis is a process that begins early in life and progresses silently for many decades. Genetic disorders—for example, loss of function of PCSK9 or loss of function of NPC1L1—result in only modest reductions in LDL-C, but they are lifelong and result in marked reductions in CVD.[116] Autopsies performed on young American soldiers killed in action in Korea and Vietnam revealed the presence of subclinical atherosclerotic lesions. Coronary artery lesions were also found in aortas of children as young as the age of 3 years and in 10-year-olds in the International Atherosclerosis Project.[154–157] In the Pathobiological Determinants of Atherosclerosis in Youth (PDAY) study, intimal lesions appeared in all examined aortas and in more than half of the right coronary arteries of the youngest age group (15 to 19 years); they increased in prevalence and extent with age through the oldest age group (30 to 34 years). This study also showed that

some regions of the arteries were lesion prone and others were lesion resistant, and the propensity to develop raised or advanced lesions differed among right coronary artery, abdominal aorta, and thoracic aorta.[158] Findings from the Bogalusa Heart Study showed a correlation between systolic blood pressure, higher TC and LDL-C, and lower HDL-C concentrations and the degree of coronary and aortic atherosclerosis in children and adolescents.[159] In the PDAY study, postmortem cholesterol and thiocyanate, a marker for cigarette smoking, predicted the extent of coronary and aortic atherosclerosis, respectively, in autopsies of those aged 14 to 34.[160]

Therefore a direct relationship between determinant risk factors and the extent of atherosclerotic lesions in youth seems to exist and suggests that the identification and treatment of children and young adults who may be at high risk for developing CHD offers the possibility of preventing or delaying development of atherosclerotic disease. This is particularly relevant for children with heterozygous FH, where statin therapy should generally be initiated at 8 to 10 years of age if LDL-C is high.[161] Children with homozygous FH should receive aggressive LDL-C reducing therapy ideally in the first year of life and thereafter lifelong.[162]

Disorders of Lipoprotein Metabolism

Defects which result in marked abnormalities in plasma lipid and lipoprotein concentrations may be caused by increased or decreased production of lipoproteins, abnormal enzymatic processing (e.g., hydrolysis of TG), and/or increased or decreased catabolism and clearance (e.g., defective uptake of lipoproteins). Lipoprotein phenotypes reflecting lipoprotein disorders were originally classified into six patterns, by Fredrickson and colleagues, based on an electrophoretic separation scheme (Table 36.17).[163] Fredrickson phenotypes for dyslipidemia focused on the main classes of apoB-containing lipoproteins: LDL, IDL, VLDL, and chylomicrons. Nearly all

TABLE 36.17 Dyslipidemia Phenotypes and Genetic Causes

Dyslipidemia	Fredrickson Phenotype	Abnormal Lipoprotein(s)	Cholesterol, mg/dL (mmol/L)	TG, mg/dL (mmol/L)	Known Related Genes
Exogenous hyperlipemia (Familial chylomicronemia syndrome)	Type I	↑Chylomicrons	Any	>10,000 (>114)	LPL, APOC2, GPIHBPI, LMF1, APOA5
Familial hypercholesterolemia	Type IIa	↑LDL	>300 (>7.8)	<250 (<2.8)	LDLR, APOB, PCSK9
Hyperlipoprotein(a)	—	↑Lp(a)	Any	Any	LPA
Combined hyperlipidemia	Type IIb	↑LDL & VLDL	>200 (>5.2)	>250 (>2.8)	Polygenic
Dysbetalipoproteinemia (remnant hyperlipidemia)	Type III	↑IDL (a.k.a. b-VLDL)	Any	Any	APOE
Hypertriglyceridemia	Type IV	↑VLDL	Any	>250 (>2.8)	Polygenic
Polygenic chylomicronemia	Type V	↑Chylomicrons ↑VLDL	Any	>1,000 (>11.4)	Polygenic
Hyperalphalipoproteinemia	—	↑HDL	>200 (>5.2)	Any	CETP
Hypoalphalipoproteinemia	—	↓↓HDL	Any	Any	APOA1, ABCA1, LCAT
Hypobetalipoproteinemia	—	↓LDL, ↓VLDL	<100 (<2.6)	<50 (<0.6)	MTTP, APOB, SAR1B, ANGPTL3

HDL, High-density lipoprotein; *LDL*, low-density lipoproteins; *VLDL*, very-low-density lipoprotein.

possible permutations for elevations in these lipoproteins, taken one or two at a time, comprise the Fredrickson classification system of type I, IIa, IIb, III, IV, and V dyslipoproteinemias. However, not all lipid disorders are categorized by this classification system. Most importantly disturbances in HDL metabolism and elevations of Lp(a) are not captured by this classification.

Primary versus Secondary Dyslipoproteinemias

When dyslipidemia is first identified, it should be determined whether it is a primary or secondary lipoprotein disorder. Secondary influences include diet, alcohol intake and lifestyle, other diseases, as well as numerous pharmacologic agents, such as steroids, isotretinoin, β-blockers, and antiretroviral agents. The diagnosis of a primary disorder of lipoprotein metabolism is made after secondary causes have been ruled out (Table 36.18),[164] or when the underlying genetic etiology is identified.

Polygenic and Monogenic Lipoprotein Disorders

Most lipoprotein disorders have polygenic or multifactorial causes with small culmulative contributions by many genes or susceptible genes which might have been influenced by environmental factors and familial factors. Through

genome wide association studies, a great number of genes have been identified that are associated with various lipid abnormalities.

Monogenic disorders are typically rare, and caused predominantly by variations in a single gene with a large effect. They often have a recognizable familial inheritance pattern. To diagnose monogenic disorders, family history is important, not only for diagnosis, but also for family screening to clearly identify family members at risk. Recent advances in genetic technologies, with expanding availability and decreasing costs, have enabled and increased the ability to identify disease-causing mutations. Therefore it has become feasible to categorize these disorders according to their underlying genetic etiologies.

Familial Chylomicronemia Syndrome (Fredrickson Type I)

FCS(OMIM: 238600) is a group of genetically heterogenous and autosomal recessive disorders with five known causal genes: LPL,[165] apoC-II (APOC2),[166] glycosylphosphatidylinositol-anchored HDL-binding protein 1 (GPIHBP1),[167] lipase maturation factor 1 (LMF1),[168] or apoA-V (APOA5).[53,169]

All known FCS-causal genes are essential in proper LPL function. LPL is the main enzyme critical for the hydrolysis of TG. It requires apoC-II as an essential cofactor. Its action releases monoglyceride and fatty acids. By this process, chylomicrons are converted to chylomicron remnants. LMF1 is a chaperone protein of LPL, required for maturation and transport, and GPIHBP1 is an important protein for the transport of LPL through the endothelial cells from the adipose tissue and muscle to the luminal site of capillaries. ApoA-V functions as a stabilizing cofactor of LPL and apoC-II, and also a modulator of hepatic TG metabolism. FCS is extremely rare, and the incidence is thought to be one per million individuals, but over 200 mutations have been reported in LPL (Human Gene Mutation Database).[170] Acquired LPL deficiency has also been described, which commonly occurs later in life than FCS, due to the formation of inhibitory autoantibodies.

The typical onset of FCS is in childhood to adolescence, but it has been described in infants and older adults. Arriving at the clinical diagnosis of FCS is often delayed, and is generally only considered after recurrent episodes of acute pancreatitis. Acute pancreatitis is the most serious manifestation and the main morbidity of FCS and can be fatal. It is important to note that individuals with FCS do not appear to be predisposed to atherosclerotic disease because chylomicrons are too large to enter into the arterial intima.[171]

Other notable clinical manifestations include eruptive xanthomas, lipemia retinalis, and hepatosplenomegaly. Eruptive xanthomas are dermatologic features of severe hypertriglyceridemia: localized or wide-spread small yellowish papules with erythematous bases of 3 to 5 mm due to TG accumulation in subcutaneous macrophages on the torso, elbows, or buttocks.[172] Lipemia retinalis is a milky appearance of retinal vessels loaded with viscous lipemic plasma. Hepatosplenomegaly results from TG-rich lipoproteins which were taken up by macrophages in the reticuloendothelial system.

FCS plasma appears milky and turbid due to markedly elevated chylomicrons. TG measurement is typically over 1000 mg/dL (11.3 mmol/L) and can be higher than 10,000 mg/dL (113 mmol/L). TC can vary considerably (150 to 890 mg/dL; 3.88 to 23 mmol/L). VLDL cholesterol can also be elevated, while the

TABLE 36.18 Secondary Causes of Hyperlipemia and Dyslipoproteinemia

Secondary Factor	Triglycerides	LDL-C	HDL-C
Diabetes Mellitus (type 1 or 2)	↑↑	↑	↓
Obesity	↑↑	↑	↓
Nonalcoholic Fatty Liver Disease	↑↑		↓
Bile duct obstruction[a]		↑↑↑↑	↓↓
Immunologic disease (rheumatoid arthritis, lupus, gammopathy)	↑	↑	
Hypothyroidism		↑↑	
Nephrotic syndrome	↑	↑↑	
Glucocorticoids (prednisone, hydrocortisone)	↑↑	↑	↑
Oral estrogens (ethinyl estradiol)	↑	↑	↑
Anabolic steroids (depo-testosterone, oxandrolone)	↑	↑	↓
Estrogen receptor blockade (tamoxifen)	↑		
Retinoids	↑		↓
Diuretics (chlorothiazide, diuril)	↑↑		↓
Alcohol	↑		↑

[a]Elevated cholesterol associated with bile duct obstruction is measured as LDL-C by most methods but is actually LpX.

HDL-C, High-density lipoprotein cholesterol; LDL-C, low-density lipoprotein cholesterol; LpX, lipoprotein X.

From Benuck I, Wilson DP, McNeal C. Secondary hypertriglyceridemia. In: KR Feingold, B Anawalt, A Boyce, et al., eds. Endotext. South Dartmouth (MA): MDText.com, Inc.

concentrations of HDL-C and LDL-C cholesterol are usually very low. Furthermore, plasma apoA-I, A-II, and B-100 concentrations are also decreased, whereas apoB-48, apoC-III, and apoE concentrations can be elevated.

Historically, FCS diagnosis has relied on LPL enzyme activity analysis, which is not standardized and is only offered at specialized centers. LPL activity is measured by collecting two sets of plasma, before and after an intravenous heparin bolus (60 U/kg body weight) that releases LPL tethered to the endothelium into the circulation. Absent or markedly reduced LPL activity after excluding HL activity in the postheparin plasma is diagnostic for LPL or apoC-II deficiency. Then, apoC-II deficiency is delineated by restoration of LPL activity upon addition of apoC-II or "normal" plasma. LPL activity can also be assessed in adipose tissue biopsies. For apoC-II deficiency, the absence of apoC-II can be recognized by using an immunoassay for apoC-II. However, the latter approach may not differentiate nonfunctional forms of apoC-II.

A clinical diagnosis of FCS may be suspected with the finding of TG/TC ratio of greater than 5 in mg/dL (>2.2 in mmol/L) or TG/apoB ratio ≥8.8 in mg/dL (≥10 in mmol/L/ g/L).[173,174] Moreover, a low apoB (<75 mg/dL) can aid in distinguishing FCS from type V hyperlipoproteinemia in which high apoB is found. A recently developed FCS scoring system using clinical information may also be helpful in screening for FCS.[175] However, due to overlap of TG levels in FCS and polygenic chylomicronemias, and a lack of standardized assays for LPL activity and apoC-II, molecular diagnosis using single- or multi-gene panels targeting FCS-associated genes may be the more favored and practical approach.

Currently, medical nutrition therapy is the mainstay of treatment, aiming for less than 15% of fat in the diet. No US FDA-approved treatments are available for FCS; however, in Europe the apo-CIII antisense drug Volanesorsen is approved for this indication. There is an urgent need to develop more new and safe therapies for FCS. Therapeutic plasma exchange, especially with fresh frozen plasma which can provide exogenous apoC-II, can be used urgently to lower TG levels and to curtail pancreatitis, especially in apoC-II deficiency. ApoC-II mimetics are being developed, and would represent the most specific therapy for patients with apoC-II deficiency. Other novel biologics using antibody, antisense oligonucleotide inhibition, and small interfering RNA technologies for the treatment of hypertriglyceridemia may also be effective for FCS in the future.[2]

Hypercholesterolemia (Fredrickson Type IIa)
Familial Hypercholesterolemia
Familial Hypercholesterolemia (FH, OMIM: 14390) is genetically heterogeneous, and mutations in three genes, LDL receptor (*LDLR*), apoB (*APOB*), and/or proprotein convertase subtilisin/kexin type 9 (*PCSK9*) are autosomal dominant causes of FH, among which mutations in *LDLR* are most common.[176] Heterozygous FH is the most common metabolic disorder leading to premature CHD and death if untreated. Recent meta-analyses estimate a prevalence of 1 in 313 in the general population; however, no prevalence estimates are available for 90% of all countries in the world.[177,178] Homozygous FH is very rare with the prevalence of about one in 400,000 persons (estimated from a heterozygous prevalence

of 1 in 300). Increased use of genetics has enabled delineation of compound heterozygote FH from clinically diagnosed homozygous FH.[179]

FH is characterized by increased plasma concentrations of TC and LDL-C and results in progressive atherosclerotic plaque deposition in coronary and other vascular systems with an increased risk of CHD and other forms of vascular disease in early age. Xanthomas and xanthelasmas are dermatologic manifestations of cholesterol depositions mostly on tendons of the hands, elbows, knees, and feet (e.g., Achilles) and around the eyelids, respectively. Arcus corneae describes half or full opaque or whitish arcs around the corneas of the eyes.

Mean plasma LDL-C of heterozygous FH in children and adults is usually two to three times that of normal, whereas mean plasma LDL-C of homozygous FH is four to six times that of normal because of inadequate removal of LDL particles by LDLR. Although the number of LDL particles is increased in these patients, their lipid composition and lipid-to-protein ratio are usually not altered.[180] ApoB-100 is increased in proportion to LDL-C. TG concentration may be normal or only slightly increased, and HDL-C concentration is slightly decreased in both FH heterozygotes and homozygotes. Elevations of Lp(a) are common, especially in those with CVD and are associated with aortic calcification and stenosis.[181,182] Of all individuals diagnosed with clinical FH, elevated Lp(a) explains 25% of diagnoses.[183]

In FH, hypercholesterolemia is present at birth in most individuals, and persists throughout life. Cutaneous xanthomas can develop in early infancy and sometimes even at birth in homozygous FH. ASCVD complications including CHD beginning during childhood, and if left untreated, death from myocardial infarction and stroke can occur by the third decade or even earlier. In heterozygous FH, xanthomas may appear late in the second decade of life, and atherosclerotic CHD can appear during the fourth decade. If untreated, men are at a 50% risk for a fatal or nonfatal coronary event by age 50 years; untreated women are at a 30% risk by age 60 years.[184] However, the outlook for individuals with FH has improved greatly with the recent implementation of aggressive lipid-lowering therapy.[185,186]

All FH-causal genes encode for proteins associated with the LDLR pathway primarily in the liver. As already mentioned, the LDLR is a cell surface receptor and is responsible for the recognition and removal of LDL particles from the circulation.[187] Historically, molecular defects had been grouped into five classes—class I: null alleles, class II: transport defective alleles, class III: binding defective alleles, class IV: internalization defective alleles,[58] and class V: recycling defective alleles.

Mutations in *LDLR* are most common, and more than 2000 different loss-of-function (LOF) mutations have been reported.[188] FH-causal mutations in *APOB* are mostly limited to the LDLR binding regions that alter its affinity to the LDLR. Gain-of-function (GOF) mutations which enhance the function of PCSK9 cause FH. The identification of PCSK9 and its biological function has become the basis for new monoclonal antibody and small interfering RNA based therapies with success surpassing statins at LDL-C reduction.[2] ARH or *LDLRAP1* encodes for a chaperone protein that is necessary for proper recycling of the LDLR and is a rare cause of recessive homozygous FH.[189]

Since there is much phenotypic overlap between heterozygous FH and polygenic or common hypercholesterolemia, especially in adults, the finding of increased plasma LDL-C is often not sufficient to make the diagnosis of FH although incorporating family history may be helpful. There are three well established criteria for the clinical diagnosis of FH: (1) US MEDPED program, (2) Simon-Broome Registry, and (3) Dutch Lipid Clinic Network.[190]

The US MEDPED criteria uses age-specific and relative specific criteria for TC and LDL-C. Cut-off levels of TC in patients with first-, second-, or third-degree relatives with FH compared with the cut-off levels for the general population are different. The Simon-Broome criteria take cholesterol levels, clinical characteristics, genes, and family history into consideration in arriving at FH diagnosis. The Dutch criteria for the diagnosis of FH are similar to the Simon-Broome criteria, but in addition, the Dutch criteria use a point system to place more weight on molecular defects known to cause FH.

Facilitated with declining costs and increasing availability of FH genetic testing, molecular studies to definitively diagnose FH are becoming a more favored approach,[191,192] especially when insurance companies and national health care systems require these results to determine whether to cover for more expensive interventions. Genetic test findings can also facilitate familial cascade screening to conclusively identify additional family members with FH, and to implement therapy at an earlier age.

Polygenic or Common Hypercholesterolemia

Lipoprotein levels can be influenced by age, diet, and lifestyle. As individuals age, non–HDL-C concentrations tend to be increased and influenced by underlying genetics. Elevated levels of TC and LDL-C are associated with an increased incidence of CHD, but the disease typically appears later in life and presents less aggressively than in FH. TG and HDL-C concentrations are not usually affected. Since familial clustering can be observed in polygenic hypercholesterolemia, it is often difficult to differentiate polygenic hypercholesterolemia from heterozygous FH; however, the familial pattern is less discrete in polygenic hypercholesterolemia. Nonetheless, the medical management of these two disorders is similar.

Hyperlipoprotein(a)

Elevated lipoprotein(a) (Lp(a), OMIM: 152200) is a genetic disorder leading to ASCVD and aortic valve stenosis.[120,121] One in five with Lp(a) concentrations above the guideline endorsed cutoff of 50 mg/dL (100 nmol/L) have increased risk of these diseases with an up to threefold higher risk being seen at the highest concentrations. However, individuals with concentrations of 30 to 50 mg/dL (62 to 105 nmol/L) also display increased disease risk.[193] Elevated Lp(a) accounts for up to 25% of patients with putative FH due to elevated LDL-C.[194]

Lp(a) plasma concentrations are 80 to 90% genetically determined, largely due to kringle IV type 2 (KIV-2) present from 1 to greater than 40 copies on each allele.[195] The more KIV-2 copies the lower plasma Lp(a), and *vice versa*. Lifestyle intervention and statin use do not reduce plasma Lp(a) concentrations.[2,120] Niacin and PCSK9 inhibitors reduce Lp(a) by 20 to 30%; however, such reductions by these drugs are not documented to reduce the risk of ASCVD or aortic valve stenosis. Gene silencing using antisense oligonucleotides injected once monthly can reduce Lp(a) by 80% and a phase 3 randomized trial to reduce ASCVD is underway. Small interfering RNA technology is also being developed with the aim of reducing Lp(a).

Combined Hyperlipidemia (Fredrickson Type IIb)

A combination of lifestyle and genetic variants increasing both LDL-C and TG-rich lipoproteins will lead to combined hyperlipidemia. LDL-C is typically elevated around 190 mg/dL (4.91 mmol/L), while TG concentrations are also increased to between 200 and 400 mg/dL (2.26 and 4.52 mmol/L), but can be significantly higher. HDL-C is often low, particularly in the presence of hypertriglyceridemia. Xanthomas and other clinical features of hyperlipidemia are not common, and if present, suggest an alternative diagnosis. The onset of lipid disturbance or the diagnosis of combined hyperlipidemia is often delayed until adolescence, although younger children of families with premature CHD can sometimes present with elevated TC or TG, or both.[185]

Combined hyperlipidemia is often associated with obesity and with overproduction of VLDL and apoB-100. Kinetic studies have shown that the rate of flux of apoB from VLDL is approximately twice that of normal subjects. This leads to an increase in apoB levels, even in subjects with normal LDL-C.[196]

Dysbetalipoproteinemia (Fredrickson Type III)

Dysbetalipoproteinemia or remnant hyperlipidemia (Fredrickson Type III) is a very unique condition that manifests in a small portion of individuals (<5%) who are homozygous carriers of apo ε2 alleles. It is found in less than 1% of the population, and the presence of apo ε2/ε2 is not sufficient to cause this disease on its own. In addition, the condition has also been reported with rare bi-allelic mutations in *APOE*.[197] Phenotypic manifestation of dysbetalipoproteinemia is thought to require a "second hit" such as obesity, diabetes, hypothyroidism, renal disease, or the use of exogenous estrogen or alcohol.

The lipoprotein phenotype is characterized by increased plasma levels of both TC and TG, and their concentrations often approximate to the same level when expressed in milligrams per deciliter (mg/dL). The β-VLDL or floating β-lipoprotein present in type III has been shown to contain both apoB-100 and B-48, indicating that these TG-rich lipoprotein remnants are from both hepatic and intestinal sources. However, neither apoB levels nor LDL-P are found to be high because the condition is characterized by elevated remnants. An algorithm to facilitate the diagnosis of type III has been developed using lipid and apoB concentrations.[174,198,199]

As mentioned, apoE, present on the surface of lipoprotein remnants, interacts with specific hepatic receptors and facilitates the removal of lipoproteins from the circulation. Defective apoE cannot bind to the hepatic receptors, leading to inefficient removal of lipoprotein remnants of both intestinal and hepatic origin.[68] These particles are cholesterol enriched with a density less than 1.006 g/mL and are commonly referred to as β-VLDL or floating β-lipoprotein.[200]

Dysbetalipoproteinemia has a late onset and is rarely manifested in childhood. The most distinctive clinical feature is the presence of palmar xanthomas, which are yellow deposits that occur in the creases of the palms. This finding is pathognomonic. Tuberous and tuberoeruptive xanthomas also occur, but they are not unique to this condition. Premature atherosclerotic disease develops in up to half of these patients, particularly in the lower extremities. Because of the familial nature of this disorder, and the predisposition of these patients to premature atherosclerotic disease, family members should be carefully evaluated. The disorder has a fairly high frequency (0.2% in adult women and 0.4 to 0.5% in adult men), but it is often missed due to lack of awareness and infrequent use of definitive diagnostic tests, such as genetic testing or lipoprotein electrophoresis.[197]

In dysbetalipoproteinemia, the ratio of VLDL-C to plasma TG, expressed in terms of mass is 0.3 or higher while it is 0.2 or lower in normal samples and in those from patients with other lipoprotein disorders. This is because of the presence of β-VLDL, and the elevated ratio can persist even after treatment. In addition, a β-VLDL band is observed on agarose gel electrophoresis of the density less than 1.006 g/mL fraction because it migrates electrophoretically with LDL rather than VLDL (see Fig. 36.21). The VLDL-C to TG ratio of greater than 0.3 and the observation of β-VLDL in the ultracentrifugal supernatant are considered diagnostic characteristics of the type III dysbetalipoproteinemia.

Hypertriglyceridemia (Fredrickson Type IV)

A combination of lifestyle and genetic variants increasing TG-rich lipoproteins will lead to hypertriglyceridemia without LDL-C elevation.[201] Overproduction of VLDL in the liver, and overload of LPL lipolytic capacity result in TG accumulation. The cholesterol content of VLDL is also increased, but plasma LDL-C and apoB concentrations are usually normal, suggesting that the conversion of VLDL to LDL is not increased in these patients. The cause of overproduction of VLDL-TG is unknown, but obesity is commonly found in many of these patients. Furthermore, plasma HDL-C in hypertriglyceridemia is often dramatically decreased, probably secondary to elevated TG.[106] Administration of estrogen and corticosteroids are known to aggravate hypertriglyceridemia and can sometimes lead to acute pancreatitis.[202]

Polygenic Chylomicronemia (Fredrickson Type V)

Polygenic chylomicronemia, also known as mixed hyperlipemia (Type V), is also a heterogeneous group of hypertriglyceridemia-related disorders characterized by an increase in chylomicrons and VLDL. It has an incidence of about 1 in 600, and a parent to offspring transmission has been observed.[203] It is commonly a transient phenotype and is frequently associated with diabetes mellitus. Although the exact molecular cause of this disorder is not known, the metabolic defect appears to be

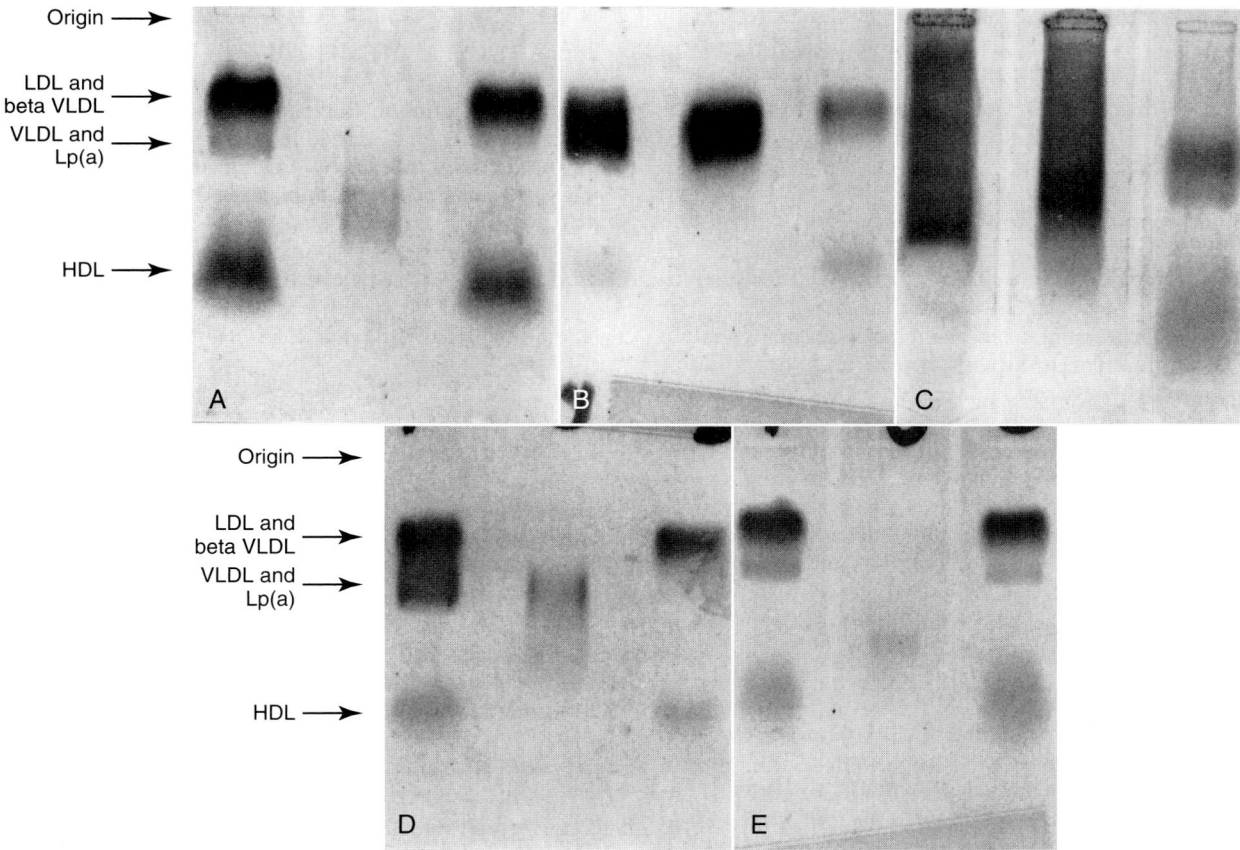

FIGURE 36.21 Agarose gel electrophoresis of plasma lipoprotein. In each photograph, the samples were applied in the following order, reading from left to right: unfractionated plasma, ultracentrifugal density 1.006 g/mL supernatant solution, ultracentrifugal infranatant solution. (A) Pattern seen in normal samples and samples with high LDL cholesterol concentrations. (B) Type III hyperlipoproteinemia pattern. (C) Severe hypertriglyceridemia, triglyceride = 3840 mg/dL. Note chylomicrons at origin. (D) Pattern observed in samples with moderately elevated triglyceride, triglyceride = 281 mg/dL, LDL cholesterol = 145 mg/dL. Note absence of chylomicrons. (E) Pattern observed in patients with high concentrations of Lp(a). Note presence of Lp(a) in infranatant solution. This sample had an Lp(a) concentration of 77 mg/dL. *LDL,* Low-density lipoprotein; *Lp(a),* lipoprotein(a); *HDL,* high-density lipoprotein; *VLDL,* very-low-density lipoprotein.

increased production or decreased removal of chylomicrons, or a combination of both. The activity of LPL in these patients may be normal or low, and the plasma concentration of apoC-II is normal.[185]

Although polygenic chylomicronemia does not typically manifest in childhood, several affected preadolescents have been described.[131] Clinical presentations in adults include eruptive xanthomas, lipemia retinalis, pancreatitis, and glucose intolerance with hyperinsulinism.

A causal molecular basis for primary mixed hyperlipidemia has been found in less than 5% of cases. Furthermore, no genetic susceptibility component has been proven reproducible in secondary cases.[204] However, not everyone with equivalent exposure to secondary factors develops equally severe dyslipidemia, which suggests a role for primary monogenic, or polygenic susceptibility with other genetic modifying influence.

Disorders of High-Density Lipoprotein Metabolism
Cholesteryl Ester Transfer Protein Deficiency

Cholesteryl Ester Transfer Protein feficiency (CETP deficiency, OMIM: 143470) is an autosomal recessive condition due to mutations in *CETP*, whose protein product facilitates the transfer of cholesterol esters from HDL to apoB-containing lipoproteins in exchange for TG, resulting in elevated levels of HDL-C, often above 150 mg/dL (3.9 mmol/L). Individuals with CETP deficiency have high HDL-C and low LDL-C. Heterozygotes have moderately elevated HDL-C. The condition was originally described in Japan and is associated with low incidence of CVD.[205]

Hypoalphalipoproteinemia

A clinical diagnosis of hypoalphalipoproteinemia can be made by finding the unique clinical features, but for a definitive diagnosis, molecular studies are necessary. There are several known molecular defects which can lead to hypoalphalipoproteinemia. This group of disorders is characterized by extremely reduced levels of HDL-C (<20 mg/dL) and occurs more frequently among men (1 in 300) compared to women (1 in 1000).[206] Hypoalphalipoproteinemia and its association with CHD is still being investigated due to conflicting reports. Low HDL is also associated with increased risk of infectious disease, diabetes, chronic kidney disease, autoimmune disease, and all-cause mortality.[96,104,207,208] There are no FDA-approved medications for disorders of HDL-C; therefore better understanding of the role of HDL in health and disease, as well as novel therapy for these conditions is needed.

Tangier Disease

Tangier disease, so named because the first case was observed in Tangier Island in Chesapeake Bay (Eastern United States), is characterized by severely reduced plasma HDL-C, abnormal HDL subfraction distribution, and an accumulation of cholesteryl ester (CE) in many tissues throughout the body. Tangier disease is an inherited condition due to mutations in ATP-binding cassette, subfamily A, member 1 (*ABCA1*: OMIM 600046).[209]

The notable clinical manifestations of Tangier disease are hyperplastic orange tonsils enriched in CE, splenomegaly, hepatomegaly, and peripheral neuropathy. Severely reduced HDL-C and enlarged orange tonsils (mostly seen in children) are pathognomonic for this condition. Deposition of CE is found in various tissues in the body. Some evidence suggests that these patients may have an increased incidence of CHD,

but they are seemingly less affected than would be expected for the reduced level of HDL-C. This may be attributed to the concurrently reduced concentrations of LDL.[210]

In homozygotes, plasma HDL-C and apoA-I concentrations are often undetectable, and apoA-II is present at less than 10% of its normal concentration and is often found in apoB-100–containing lipoprotein.[211] Heterozygotes are characterized by half-normal concentrations of HDL-C, apoA-I, and apoA-II. TC is typically low, around 70 mg/dL (1.8 mmol/L) in homozygous compared to about 160 mg/dL (4.14 mmol/L) in heterozygous individuals. On the other hand, TG can sometimes be modestly increased, depending on the diet.

The ABCA1 transporter is a key protein for the efflux of cholesterol from hepatocytes, enterocytes, and peripheral cells, particularly from macrophages and is important in the biogenesis of HDL. ApoA-I facilitates lipidation of nascent HDL particle by interacting with ABCA1 to allow efflux of cholesterol. Interestingly, kinetic studies have demonstrated that increased catabolism of HDL, rather than a defect in biosynthesis, is the cause of low HDL particles in Tangier disease.

Apolipoprotein A1 Deficiency

Rarely, patients can have mutations in the apolipoprotein A1 (apoA-I) (*APOA1*; OMIM 107680) gene, the main protein component of HDL, which can lead to profoundly low concentrations of HDL. ApoA-I facilitates the efflux of cholesterol and phospholipids (PL) out of cells, and the formation of mature HDL particles. Other clinical features include corneal clouding and xanthomas. About half of the normal concentrations of HDL-C and apoA-I have been observed in heterozygotes. Mutations such as a rearrangement at the apolipoprotein gene locus that inactivates both apoA-I and apoC-III, deletion of the entire locus, and an insertion in the apoA-I gene have all been described.[207]

ApoA-I Milano (R173C) and apoA-I Paris (R151C) are natural variants of human apoA-I that cause no deleterious health effects and may even improve cardioprotection despite abnormally low levels of plasma apoA-I and HDL and high levels of HDL-triacylglycerides in heterozygous mutation carriers.[212–214] Notably, mutations in apoA-I can also be causative of acquired or familial amyloidosis. These mutations often lead to apoA-I and HDL-C concentrations lower than normal reference populations. ApoA-I amyloid deposition occurs over time in peripheral organs, such as heart, liver, and kidneys.[215]

Lecithin-Cholesterol Acyl Transferase Deficiency

Mutations in the gene lecithin-cholesterol acyltransferase (*LCAT*: OMIM 606967) leads to defects in LCAT which lack the ability to esterify cholesterol and results in hypoalphalipoproteinemia. In LCAT deficiency, the primary form of HDL, pre–βHDL, and the nascent discoidal form of HDL, which is PL-rich and cholesterol-poor, cannot form the mature HDL. Because of their small size, these immature HDL particles are rapidly catabolized. There are two phenotypic forms: familial or complete LCAT deficiency (FLD), and partial LCAT deficiency or fish-eye disease (FED), which is associated only with cloudy corneas due to cholesterol deposition.[207]

Individuals with FLD have complete absence of LCAT activity on both HDL and LDL, cloudy corneas, and also mild hemolytic anemia, splenomegaly, and glomerulosclerosis associated with progressive proteinuria and renal failure, which is the main cause of morbidity. It is believed that proteinuria develops because of the presence of lipoprotein X (LpX).

Lipoprotein X

LpX is an abnormal lipoprotein particle that accumulates in the plasma of patients with obstructive jaundice, cholestasis, or other liver disease. LpX is enriched with unesterified cholesterol and often presents with acute elevations of cholesterol and LDL-C. Cholesterol associated with LpX cannot be distinguished from LDL-C. However, LpX can be readily identified by qualitative lipoprotein electrophoresis.[216]

LpX appears to be trapped within mesangial cells in the glomerulus, leading to lipid deposition and eventual development of glomerulosclerosis. Unlike other lipoprotein particles, which have a single layer of PL on their surface, LpX has a PL bilayer–like structure and can even form multilamellar vesicles with an aqueous core. It is believed that such structures are formed when availability of neutral lipid, such as CE, is insufficient to form the neutral lipid core in lipoproteins.[216]

Apolipoprotein B-Containing Lipoprotein Deficiencies

Abetalipoproteinemia, Homozygous Hypobetalipoproteinemia, and Chylomicron Retention Disease

Abetalipoproteinemia (ABL; OMIM: 200100), homozygous hypobetalipoproteinemia (OMIM: 615558), and chylomicron retention disease (CRD; OMIM: 246700) are extremely rare autosomal recessive disorders associated with very low levels of TC and LDL-C, and undetectable apoB. They are due to mutations in the microsomal TG transfer protein (*MTTP*), apoB (*APOB*), and Secretion-associated RAS-related GTPase 1B (*SAR1B*). Mutations in these genes lead to defective biogenesis and secretion of apoB-containing chylomicrons from the intestine and VLDL from the liver. Heterozygous carriers of a *MTTP* or *SAR1B* mutation typically do not have low TC and LDL-C, whereas carriers of a hypobetalipoproteinemia *APOB* mutation have lower TC and LDL-C than noncarriers in the same family.

These three disorders have similar clinical features of intestinal TG malabsorption, and intestinal and hepatic steatosis. A common first sign is intolerance to breast milk or infant formula that leads to failure to thrive with poor weight gain, associated with diarrhea and steatorrhea. ABL and homozygous hypobetalipoproteinemia are virtually indistinguishable. Patients with CRD may have a normal level of TG, and less severe reduction of TC, LDL-C, and HDL-C, compared to the other two disorders. Arriving at the correct diagnosis may be delayed due to clinical similarities to celiac disease, cystic fibrosis, lactose intolerance, or food allergies that are more prevalent in infancy.

TG accumulation within the intestinal wall may be visualized as "gelee blanche" on endoscopic evaluation, and with oil red O staining on histopathological slides. Hepatic steatosis presents as transaminase elevations. Development of micronodular cirrhosis has rarely been documented with implementation of medium-chain triglyceride (MCT) supplementation. Acanthocytosis describes the finding of abnormally spiculated erythrocytes due to altered membrane lipid composition that are observed in the peripheral blood smear.

Serious clinical manifestations of ABL and related disorders are the consequence of essential fatty acid and (vitamins A, D, E, and K) deficiencies, reflecting the critical role of lipoproteins in their absorption and transport. Inadequate consumption of essential fatty acids retards growth and development. Fat-soluble vitamin deficiencies lead to severe neurological abnormalities, including cerebellar dysfunction and ophthalmological abnormalities, including retinitis pigmentosa. Other features of these disorders may include coagulopathy and bone abnormalities.

Currently, no FDA-approved medications are available for these conditions. Fat-soluble vitamin supplementation and medical nutrition therapy with essential fatty acids and other nutrients are critically important in ameliorating devastating manifestations.

Familial Hypobetalipoproteinemia (Familial Combined Hypolipidemia)

Familial combined hypolipidemia (OMIM: 605019) is a recently identified rare autosomal recessive condition associated with low levels of TC, TG, HDL-C, and LDL-C, as well as of apoA-I and apoB. Nonsense mutations in the *ANGPTL3* gene have been identified in individuals with combined hypolipidemia, and frame-shift mutations have been identified in individuals with low levels of LDL-C. Familial hypobetalipoproteinemia is associated with reduced risk for CVD.

Other Monogenic Disorders Manifesting in Lipid Abnormalities

Sitosterolemia (Phytosterolemia or Xenosterolemia)

Sitosterolemia, (OMIM: 210250), formerly known as pseudo-FH, is an autosomal recessive disorder due to mutations in ATP-binding cassette, subfamily G, members 5 (*ABCG5*) or 8 (*ABCG8*). The *ABCG5* and *ABCG8* encode for sterolin-1 and sterolin-2, respectively. They are mainly expressed in the intestine but are also expressed in the liver. Sterolins are involved in eliminating plant sterols which cannot be utilized by humans, but excess plant sterols absorbed can be incorporated into lipoproteins due to the similarity to animal cholesterol. Since the phenotypic presentation of sitosterolemia is highly dependent on diet, the full spectrum and incidence of sitosterolemia is not fully understood.

Similar to FH, xanthomas or tuberous xanthomas can be found at the tendons of knees, elbows, and the Achilles, as well as on the buttocks. In addition, premature atherosclerosis and aortic valve abnormalities that can lead to myocardial infarction and sudden death are serious manifestations. Joint pain in childhood is often mistaken for juvenile rheumatoid arthritis. Hemolytic anemia, abnormally shaped erythrocytes (stomatocytes), and large platelets (macrothrombocytopenia) are other features, and they may be the initial presentation.

The clinical diagnosis of sitosterolemia can be made by measuring plant sterol levels by gas-liquid chromatography (GLC), gas chromatography/mass spectrometry (GC/MS), or high-pressure liquid chromatography (HPLC). A definitive diagnosis can be made by finding mutations in *ABCG5* and *ABCG8*. Treatment options for sitosterolemia include a diet with reduced plant sterols, and ezetimibe has been shown to effectively reduce plant sterols in this condition. Other clinical features may require symptomatic intervention.

Lysosomal Acid Lipase Deficiency

Lysosomal acid lipase deficiency (LALD; OMIM: 278000) is an autosomal recessive disorder due to mutations in the lysosomal acid lipase A gene (*LIPA*). LAL facilitates hydrolysis of CE and TG in lysosomes; therefore this defect results in

CE and TG accumulation in lysosomes. There are two main phenotypic presentations of LALD, the infantile-onset form (Wolman disease) and the late-onset CESD.

Wolman disease is characterized by malabsorption that results in malnutrition, and accumulation of CE and TG in hepatic macrophages, manifesting as hepatomegaly and fatty liver disease. Adrenal gland calcification develops which is pathognomonic for Wolman disease and associated with adrenal cortical insufficiency.

CESD presents in childhood in a manner similar to Wolman disease, or later in life with serum lipid abnormalities, hepatosplenomegaly, and/or elevated liver enzymes long before a diagnosis is made. Complications of late-onset CESD include atherosclerotic vascular disease (e.g., CHD or stroke), liver disease (e.g., abnormal liver function ± jaundice, steatosis, fibrosis, cirrhosis, liver failure, and esophageal varices), manifestations of secondary hypersplenism (e.g., anemia and/or thrombocytopenia), and malabsorption. However, LALD are not fully understood since dyslipidemia and mild LFT elevations may be the only notable features in people that they are not identified as having LALD. In the United States it is likely that many with LALD have not been identified because they may be just treated for dyslipidemia, and mild elevations of LFT are so common that many clinicians are probably not paying close attention.

The diagnosis of LALD can be made by finding a reduced lysosomal acid lipase A or *LIPA* mutations. Historically, infants with Wolman disease did not survive beyond one year unless they were successfully treated with hematopoietic stem cell transplantation (HSCT). However, the development of sebelipase alfa, an enzyme replacement therapy, has changed the outlook of these patients.

Hepatic Lipase Deficiency

HL deficiency (OMIM: 614025) is an autosomal recessive condition caused by mutations in the HL (*LIPC*) gene. HL facilitates the conversion of VLDL and IDL to LDL, and its deficiency leads to increased levels of TC and TG. HL deficiency is associated with premature CHD.

Glycerol Kinase Deficiency

Glycerol kinase deficiency (GKD; OMIM: 307030) is a rare X-linked recessive condition characterized by hyperglycerolemia and glyceroluria. There are three clinically distinct forms: (1) infantile form, (2) symptomatic juvenile form, and (3) benign adult form. The latter two forms are also known as "isolated" GKD.

The infantile form or GK complex deficiency is an Xp21 contiguous gene deletion syndrome involving multiple genes including nuclear receptor subfamily 0, group B, member 1 (*NR0B1*), alternatively known as the *DAX1* gene associated with congenital adrenal hypoplasia, and/or dystrophin (*DMD*) gene associated with Duchenne muscular dystrophy. The isolated forms of GKD are due to a mutation in *GK* gene alone. The juvenile form may be asymptomatic or symptomatic with a wide variability from asymptomatic hyperglycerolemia to a severe metabolic disturbance associated with growth and neurologic abnormalities. The adult form presents as an incidental finding of hyperglycerolemia that is often identified as hypertriglyceridemia.

Since most commercial laboratories determine TG levels by measuring glycerol, after hydrolyzing TG with bacterial lipase and releasing fatty acids, individuals with GKD are often mistaken as having hypertriglyceridemia. Glycerol-blanking is required to reveal the actual TG in these patients.

Inherited Lipodystrophy

Lipodystrophy (LD) is a group of heterogeneous disorders characterized by paucity or abnormal adipose tissue distribution and is associated with various metabolic derangements, including hypertriglyceridemia, diabetes mellitus, insulin resistance with/without acanthosis nigricans, and fatty liver (steatosis to cirrhosis), as well as other organ involvement including cardiac, renal, and immune systems. Generalized lipodystrophy is associated with the virtual absence of adipose tissue, and partial lipodystrophy is associated with selective paucity and abnormal distribution of adiposity.

Many genes have been identified with various types of LD, and some are inherited as autosomal dominant while others are autosomal recessive (*AGAT2, BSCL2, PTRF, LMNA, PPARG, AKT2, CAV1*, etc.). The prevalence of LD is estimated to be approximately one in 1 million but is likely underdiagnosed.

HTG and low HDL-C are often seen in LD. Severe HTG of greater than 10,000 mg/dL has been reported. However, the underlying mechanisms of dyslipidemia have not been well understood. Currently, leptin (metreleptin), therapy is the only disease-specific FDA-approved therapy for generalized lipodystrophy. Leptin therapy has been shown to ameliorate diabetes mellitus and fatty liver. It can also reduce severe HTG, but the reciprocal relationship between HTG and low HDL-C upon treatment as the effect of TG-lowering therapy has not been observed. Other clinical features are treated symptomatically. Currently, the use of leptin for partial lipodystrophy is being evaluated.

Smith-Lemli-Opitz Disease

Smith-Lemli-Opitz syndrome (SLOS; OMIM 270400) is an autosomal recessive multiple malformation syndrome associated with low TC levels. SLOS is due to mutations in the 7-dehydrocholesterol reductase (*DHCR7*) gene that encodes the last enzyme in the cholesterol synthetic pathway, reaffirming the importance of endogenous cholesterol synthesis in development. More information is available in Chapter 59.

SCREENING FOR AND DIAGNOSIS OF LIPOPROTEIN DISORDERS

In adults, a standard lipid profile that will identify most hyper- and dyslipidemias should include plasma cholesterol and TG together with LDL-C, HDL-C, and non–HDL-C (Table 36.19).[1,4,115] Plasma cholesterol, TG, and HDL-C are measured, while LDL-C and non–HDL-C can be calculated from the 3 measured values. LDL-C can also be measured directly using homogeneous assays at additional cost.

An expanded lipid profile should include Lp(a) and apoB, both recommended by many guidelines including the 2018 US and the 2019 European dyslipidemia guidelines that recommend measurement of Lp(a) once in all individuals.[110,111] When cost is a limiting factor, plasma measurement of cholesterol and TG are advised as this will diagnose many lipid disorders without overlooking severe hypertriglyceridemia putting the individual at high risk of acute pancreatitis (see Table 36.1). For this reason, measurement of either plasma cholesterol or LDL-C alone should be avoided. Additional measurements like apoA-I, lipoprotein subfractions, or yet other apolipoproteins are offered by specialty laboratories, but at present do not advance diagnosis of hyper- and dyslipidemias in most patients.

In children, the American Academy of Pediatrics recommends all children between ages 9 and 11 years old be screened

TABLE 36.19 Major Eligibility Criteria for Lipid Lowering Medications According to Atherosclerotic Cardiovascular Disease (ASCVD) Prevention Guidelines

UK 2016 NICE	Canada 2016 CCS	Europe 2019 ESC/EAS	US 2018 ACC/AHA
Secondary Prevention			
Most ASCVD	Most ASCVD	ASCVD LDL-C ≥55 mg/dL ≥1.4 mmol/L	Most ASCVD
Primary Prevention			
Lipid Based (Likely Familial Hypercholesterolemia)			
LDL-C >190mg/dL >4.9 mmol/L Or TC >290 mg/dL >7.5 mmol/L	LDL-C ≥193 mg/dL ≥5 mmol/L	LDL-C ≥190 mg/dL ≥4.9 mmol/L Or TC >309 mg/dL ≥8 mmol/L	LDL-C ≥190 mg/dL ≥4.9 mmol/L
Diabetes based			
Most diabetes	Most diabetes	Most diabetes	Most diabetes
Chronic Kidney Disease (CKD) Based			
Non–dialysis-dependent CKD	CKD (age ≥50 years) and eGFR <60 mL/min/1.73 m²	Non–dialysis-dependent CKD and eGFR <60 mL/min/1.73 m²	CKD used as risk enhancer, not as indication by itself
Absolute 10-Year Risk Based			
Age 40–75 years QRISK2 ≥10% predicted 10-year risk of any ASCVD	Age 40–75 years FRS ≥20% predicted 10-year risk of any ASCVD Or Age 40–75 years FRS 10–19% predicted 10-year risk of any ASCVD LDL-C ≥135 mg/dL[a] ≥4.3 mmol/L	Age 40–75 years LDL-C ≥100 mg/dL ≥2.6 mmol SCORE 5–9.9% predicted 10-year risk of fatal ASCVD Or Age 40–75 years LDL-C ≥70 mg/dL ≥1.8 mmol/L SCORE ≥10% predicted 10-year risk of fatal ASCVD	Age 40–75 years PCE ≥7.5% predicted 10-year risk of any ASCVD LDL-C 70–189 mg/dL 1.8–4.9 mmol/L

[a]Or non–HDL-C ≥166 mg/dL, or men aged ≥50 and women aged ≥60 with LDL-C < 135 mg/dL but with a CVD risk factor.
ACC, American College of Cardiology; *AHA,* American Heart Association; *ASCVD,* atherosclerotic cardiovascular disease; *CCS,* Canadian Cardiovascular Society; *EAS,* European Atherosclerosis Society; *ESC,* European Society of Cardiology; *FRS,* Framingham Risk Score; *LDL-C,* low-density lipoprotein cholesterol; *NICE* National Institute for Health and Care Excellence; *PCE,* pooled cohorts equations; *TC,* total cholesterol.

for high cholesterol.[110,217] Children between 2 and 10 years old whose parents have a history of premature heart or vascular disease (men age ≤55 and women age ≤65), whose parents or grandparents have TC ≥240 mg/dL, whose family history is unknown (adoption), or whose medical history includes high risk conditions (hypertension, obesity, diabetes mellitus) should be screened. The US National Heart Lung and Blood Institute (NHLBI) also recommends universal screening for dyslipidemia by the age of 9 to 11 years and subsequently at an age of 17 to 21 years. Lipid screening should be performed with either a fasting or a nonfasting lipid panel.

"High cholesterol" in children and adolescents are concentrations greater than the 95th percentile for TC and LDL-C in their age group (see Table 36.5). "Borderline" TC and LDL-C concentrations are defined as values between the 75th and 95th percentiles.

The Bogalusa Heart Study found that by using the selective screening approach, only 50% of white children and only 20% of black children with high LDL-C concentrations (>95th percentile) were identified.[218] Furthermore, it has been shown that self-reported cholesterol values among parents are an ineffective means of identifying children with high cholesterol.[219] In fact, more than 90% of children with TC greater than the 75th or 95th percentile were missed when physicians relied on cholesterol values reported by the parents. The universal screening approach is now advised for children based on these findings.

MANAGEMENT OF LIPOPROTEIN DISORDERS:

Management of Hypercholesterolemia in Adults

On the basis of findings from many different randomized controlled trials using statins, ezetimibe, and PCSK9 inhibitors, hypercholesterolemia in adults is recognized by all guidelines as the major causal risk factor for ASCVD.[116,117] In recent years, major cholesterol and dyslipidemia management guidelines in

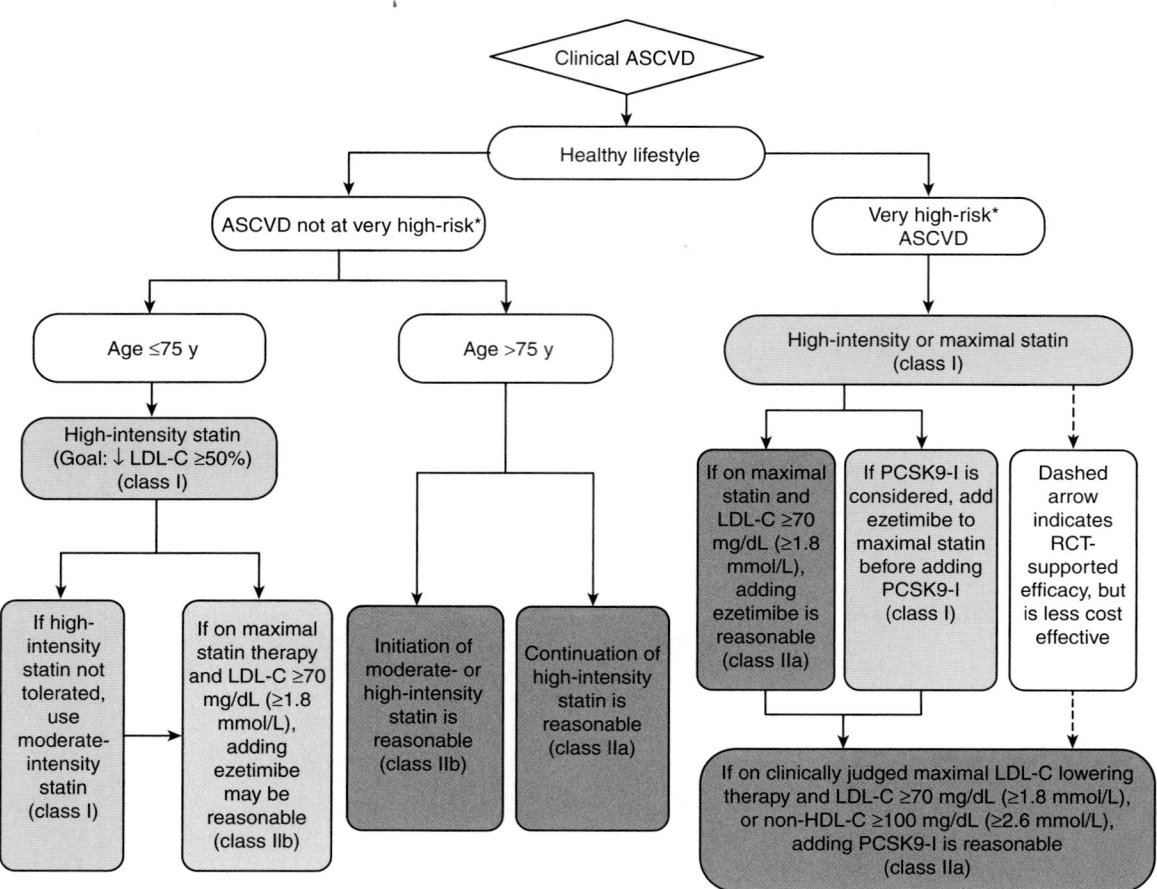

FIGURE 36.22 Secondary prevention in patients with clinical ASCVD. Colors correspond to Class of Recommendation: Gray Class I (Strong); Dark pink Class IIa (Moderate); Light pink Class IIb (Weak). Clinical ASCVD consists of ACS, those with history of MI, stable or unstable angina or coronary other arterial revascularization, stroke, transient ischemic attack (TIA), or peripheral artery disease (PAD) including aortic aneurysm, all of atherosclerotic origin. Very high-risk includes a history of multiple major ASCVD events or 1 major ASCVD event and multiple high-risk conditions. *ACS*, Acute coronary syndrome; *ASCVD*, atherosclerotic cardiovascular disease; *LDL-C*, low-density lipoprotein cholesterol; *HDL-C*, high-density lipoprotein cholesterol; *MI*, myocardial infarction; *PCSK9-I*, PCSK9 inhibitor.[110]

the United States, Europe, Canada, and the United Kingdom have been cooperatively published by multiple medical societies.[110–112,220] All patients with or at risk of ASCVD should be advised to adopt a healthy lifestyle. This should include dietary recommendations to lower cholesterol concentrations (Fig. 36.22 and Fig. 36.23).[110] Pharmacologic LDL-C lowering therapy is advised to most patients with ASCVD in secondary prevention, and for primary prevention in most with FH, diabetes, and chronic kidney disease (see Table 36.19).[110–112,220] For other patients, current guidelines endorse the use of risk calculators for treatment initiation decisions based on predicted ASCVD morbidity or mortality, that is, from CHD, stroke, and peripheral vascular disease. The absolute 10-year predicted risk of fatal ASCVD (Europe) and fatal or nonfatal ASCVD (United States, Canada, UK) together with LDL-C thresholds then determine whether patients should be offered statins or other LDL-C lowering therapy (see Table 36.19). The newer risk calculators also adjust the estimated risk based on the patient's race.

US, European, Canadian, and UK guidelines all advise on the use of high-intensity statin therapy for most patients aged 40 to 75 at high risk or with ASCVD.[110–112,220] This entails ≥50%

LDL-C reduction in most cases and depending on risk levels, goals of LDL-C to less than 55, less than 70, or less than 100 mg/dL (<1.4, <1.8, or <2.6 mmol/L) (Table 36.20).[110–112,220] Some guidelines have additional goals for non–HDL-C and apoB if TG are elevated. Each guideline offers specific diagnosis and treatment algorithms, differing slightly from guideline to guideline. Figs. 36.22 and 36.23 illustrate such algorithms for the 2018 US guidelines.[110] Guidelines also offer specific advice on when and in whom to use moderate-intensity statins, high-intensity statins, other LDL-C lowering therapy like ezetimibe and PCSK9 inhibitors, and TG-lowering drugs.

The percentages of individuals free of ASCVD but eligible for statins or other LDL-C lowering therapy in individuals aged 40 to 75 according to US, European, Canadian, and UK guidelines are shown in Fig. 36.24.[221,222] Based on individuals in the contemporary Copenhagen General Population Study, all four guidelines suggest that a higher and higher fraction of individuals in primary prevention setting (according to criteria in Table 36.19) should be offered statins from ages 40 to 75, and the proportion should approach 100% at age 70 to 75.[221,222] In addition, most guidelines present a list of risk-enhancing factors that if present will make even more individuals

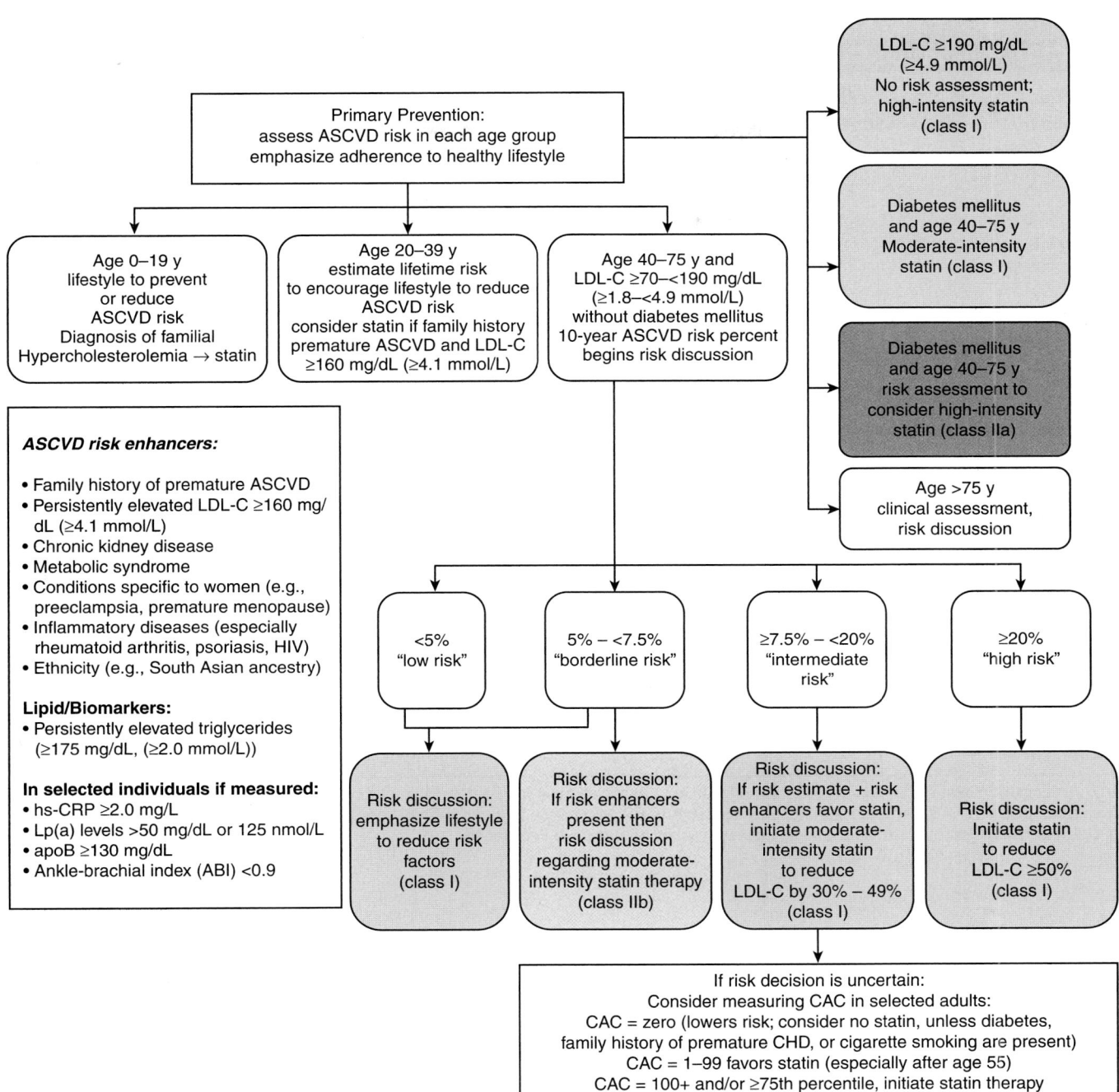

FIGURE 36.23 Primary ASCVD prevention strategy. Colors correspond to Class of Recommendation: Gray Class I (Strong); Dark pink Class IIa (Moderate); Light pink Class IIb (Weak). *apoB,* Apolipoprotein B; *ASCVD,* atherosclerotic cardiovascular disease; *CAC,* coronary artery calcium; *HIV,* human immuno-deficiency virus; *hsCRP,* high-sensitivity C-reactive protein; *LDL-C,* low-density lipoprotein cholesterol; *Lp(a),* lipoprotein (a).[110]

eligible for statin therapy. As exemplified for the 2018 US guidelines,[110] such risk enhancers are given in Box 36.2.

Management of Hypercholesterolemia in Children and Adolescents

To lower serum cholesterol concentration in children and adolescents, current pediatric guidelines have adopted strategies that combine two complementary approaches: a population approach and an individualized approach.

Population Approach

The population approach attempts to lower the mean cholesterol concentration by instituting population-wide modifications in nutrient intake and eating habits. Genetic studies have shown that even a modest decrease in mean cholesterol concentration in children and adolescents, if carried into adulthood, is likely to have a significant impact on lowering the incidence of ASCVD. The population approach is also critical from a public health standpoint because the focus of

TABLE 36.20 Lipid Reduction Goals According to Atherosclerotic Cardiovascular Disease (ASCVD) Prevention Guidelines

Target	UK 2016 NICE	Canada 2016 CCS	Europe 2019 ESC/EAS	US 2018 ACC/AHA
Secondary Prevention: ASCVD				
LDL cholesterol	≥50%	>50% or <77 mg/dL <2.0 mmol/L	≥50% & <55 mg/dL <1.4 mmol/L	≥50% & <70 mg/dL <1.8 mmol/L
Non–HDL cholesterol		<100 mg/dL <2.6 mmol/L	<85 mg/dL <2.2 mmol/L	<100 mg/dL <2.6 mmol/L
Apolipoprotein B		<80 mg/dL	<65 mg/dL	
Primary Prevention: Familial Hypercholesterolemia				
LDL cholesterol	≥50%	>50%	≥50% & <55 or <70 mg/dL <1.4 or <1.8 mmol/L	≥50%
Primary Prevention: Diabetes or Chronic Kidney Disease				
LDL cholesterol	≥40% ≥50% if ↑non–HDL-C	>50% or <77 mg/dL <2.0 mmol/L	≥50% & <55 or <70 mg/dL <1.4 or <1.8 mmol/L	≥30% or ≥50%
Non–HDL cholesterol		<100 mg/dL <2.6 mmol/L	<85 mg/dL <2.2 mmol/L	
Apolipoprotein B		<80 mg/dL	<65 mg/dL	
Primary Prevention: Absolute 10-year Risk Based				
LDL cholesterol	≥40% ≥50% if ↑non–HDL-C	>50% or <77 mg/dL <2.0 mmol/L	≥50% & <55, <70, or <100 mg/dL <1.4, <1.8, or <2.6 mmol/L	≥30% or ≥ 50%
Non–HDL cholesterol		<100 mg/dL <2.6 mmol/L	<85 mg/dL <2.2 mmol/L	
Apolipoprotein B		<80 mg/dL	<65 mg/dL	

ACC, American College of Cardiology; *AHA,* American Heart Association; *ASCVD,* atherosclerotic cardiovascular disease; *CCS,* Canadian Cardiovascular Society; *EAS,* European Atherosclerosis Society; *ESC,* European Society of Cardiology; *HDL,* high-density lipoprotein cholesterol; *LDL,* low-density lipoprotein; *NICE,* National Institute for Health and Care Excellence.

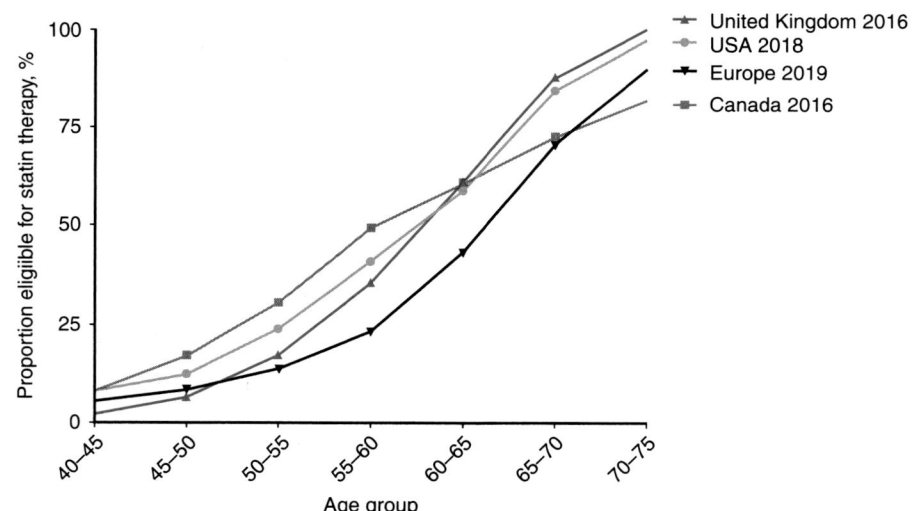

FIGURE 36.24 The percentage of individuals free of atherosclerotic cardiovascular disease but eligible for statins or other LDL cholesterol lowering therapy in individuals aged 40 to75 according to US, European, Canadian, and UK guidelines stratified by 5-year age groups, in the Copenhagen General Population Study. Statin eligibility percentage was calculated as statin-eligible persons divided by all persons × 100.[221,222]

BOX 36.2 Atherosclerotic Cardiovascular Disease Risk-Enhancing Factors[110]

- Family history of premature ASCVD (males, age <55 years; females, age <65 years)
- Primary hypercholesterolemia (LDL-C, 160–189 mg/dL [4.1–4.8 mmol/L]; non–HDL-C 190–219 mg/dL [4.9–5.6 mmol/L])
- Metabolic syndrome (3 or more of the below criteria):
  - Increased waist circumference
  - Elevated triglycerides (>150 mg/dL)
  - Elevated blood pressure
  - Elevated glucose
  - Low HDL-C (<40 mg/dL in men; <50 in women mg/dL)
- Chronic kidney disease (eGFR 15–59 mL/min/1.73 m² with or without albuminuria; not treated with dialysis or kidney transplantation)
- Chronic inflammatory conditions (e.g., psoriasis, rheumatoid arthritis, or HIV/AIDS)
- History of premature menopause (before age 40 years) and history of pregnancy-associated conditions that increase later ASCVD risk such as preeclampsia
- High-risk race/ethnicities (e.g., South Asian ancestry)
- Biomarkers
  - Hypertriglyceridemia (≥175 mg/dL)
  - High-sensitivity C-reactive protein (≥2.0 mg/L)
  - Lp(a): ≥50 mg/dL or ≥125 nmol/L
  - ApoB ≥130 mg/dL

From Grundy SM, Stone NJ, Bailey AL, et al. AHA/ACC/AACVPR/AAPA/ABC/ACPM/ADA/AGS/APhA/ASPC/NLA/PCNA Guideline on the Management of Blood Cholesterol: Executive Summary: A Report of the American College of Cardiology/American Heart Association Task Force on Clinical Practice Guidelines. *Circulation* 2019;139:e1046–e81.

treating most aggressively those patients at the greatest risk for ASCVD does not take into account the fact that the majority of patients who do go on to develop ASCVD are in the middle of the distribution for TC or LDL-C and may not appear to be at high risk, using the guidelines developed for the individualized approach.

The population approach in Western countries appears to have been successful, as non–HDL-C has decreased significantly in these countries.[223] Using data pooled from 1127 population-based studies that measured blood lipids in 103 million individuals aged 18 years and older, a global repositioning of cholesterol-related risk has been observed from 1980 through to 2018, with nonoptimal cholesterol shifting from a distinct feature of high-income countries in northwestern Europe, North America, and Australasia to one that affects countries in east and southeast Asia and Oceania.

Regarding children with hypercholesterolemia, it is thought that intake of total fat can be safely limited to 30% of total calories. It is recommended that saturated fat intake be limited to 7 to 10% of calories and that dietary cholesterol be limited to 300 mg/day. However, fat intake for infants younger than 12 months should not be restricted without medical indication.[217]

Individualized Approach

The latest NHLBI guidelines in 2011 for the management of children at risk for CVD are aimed at primary care physicians and are integrated guidelines that make age-specific recommendations on the multiple risk factors that contribute to CVD. An algorithm on how to use these guidelines is shown in see Fig. 36.25.[217] Unlike previous pediatric guidelines, which largely recommended identifying at-risk children based on family history of CHD or dyslipidemia, the current guidelines recommend universal screening by lipid testing at specific ages. Because it is more convenient, particularly for children, a nonfasting sample is adequate for screening, and criteria based on non–HDL-C, which is simply TC minus HDL-C, is used for making the initial decisions on management. If non–HDL-C is greater than 145 mg/dL (3.8 mmol/L), a fasting sample should be analyzed for lipids. Children with a TG of 500 mg/dL (5.7 mmol/L) or higher, or an LDL-C of 250 mg/dL (6.5 mmol/L) or higher, likely have a genetic lipid disorder and should be referred to a lipid specialist.

Like adults, recommended interventions for children are calibrated to the degree of CHD risk, and lifestyle changes are the first line of therapy for all patients. The most common type of dyslipidemic pattern in children is a moderate to severe increase in TG, with a moderate increase in LDL-C and low HDL-C. This type of dyslipidemia is often found in obesity and typically shows a good response to dietary changes and weight loss. Because there is less long-term safety and effectiveness data on drug therapy for children than adults, there is greater concern with using drugs, like statins, in this population. Nevertheless, it is well understood that the process of atherosclerosis often begins at an early age and that CHD risk factors in children, such as dyslipidemia and obesity, often persist into adulthood.

For children with heterozygous FH, earlier treatment has clearly been shown to lead to reduced CVD.[186] Statin therapy is advised for those aged 8 to 10 years or older with an LDL-C of 190 mg/dL (4.9 mmol/L) or greater after a 6-month trial of lifestyle management according to US guidelines (see Fig. 36.25) and with a target of LDL-C less than 130 mg/dL (<3.5 mmol/L) according to European consensus advice.[161] As described in Fig. 36.25, children with an LDL of 130 to 189 mg/dL (3.4 to 4.9 mmol/L) may also be candidates for statin therapy, depending on their other risk factors and family history. If children are placed on statin therapy, unlike adults, they should be started with the lowest possible dose, and hepatic transaminases and creatine kinase should be carefully monitored.

Management of Hypertriglyceridemia

Elevated TG-rich lipoproteins are causally related to ASCVD, just like elevated LDL and Lp(a) (Fig. 36.19). Such an elevation will be recognized via elevated plasma TG, elevated non–HDL-C and apoB while LDL-C is relatively low, and via elevated remnant cholesterol (i.e., cholesterol in TG-rich lipoproteins)[1,4,115] (see Table 36.6).

Evidence-based findings support TG to be an independent risk factor for CHD in both men and women and current guidelines place greater emphasis on management of patients with TG disorders.[110] Cardiovascular-related risk for TG begins at concentrations greater than 100 mg/dL (1.1 mmol/L) and becomes substantial at levels around 150 to 200 mg/dL (1.7 to 2.26 mmol/L).[119,224] Risk of acute pancreatitis likewise increases above 100 mg/dL (1.1 mmol/L) with higher risk accompanying higher TG concentrations.[134] Different organizations classify elevated TG somewhat differently, with the US AHA listing levels greater than 200 mg/dL (2.26 mmol/L) as high and greater than 500 mg/dL (5.66 mmol/L) as very high, whereas the US Endocrine Society lists moderate

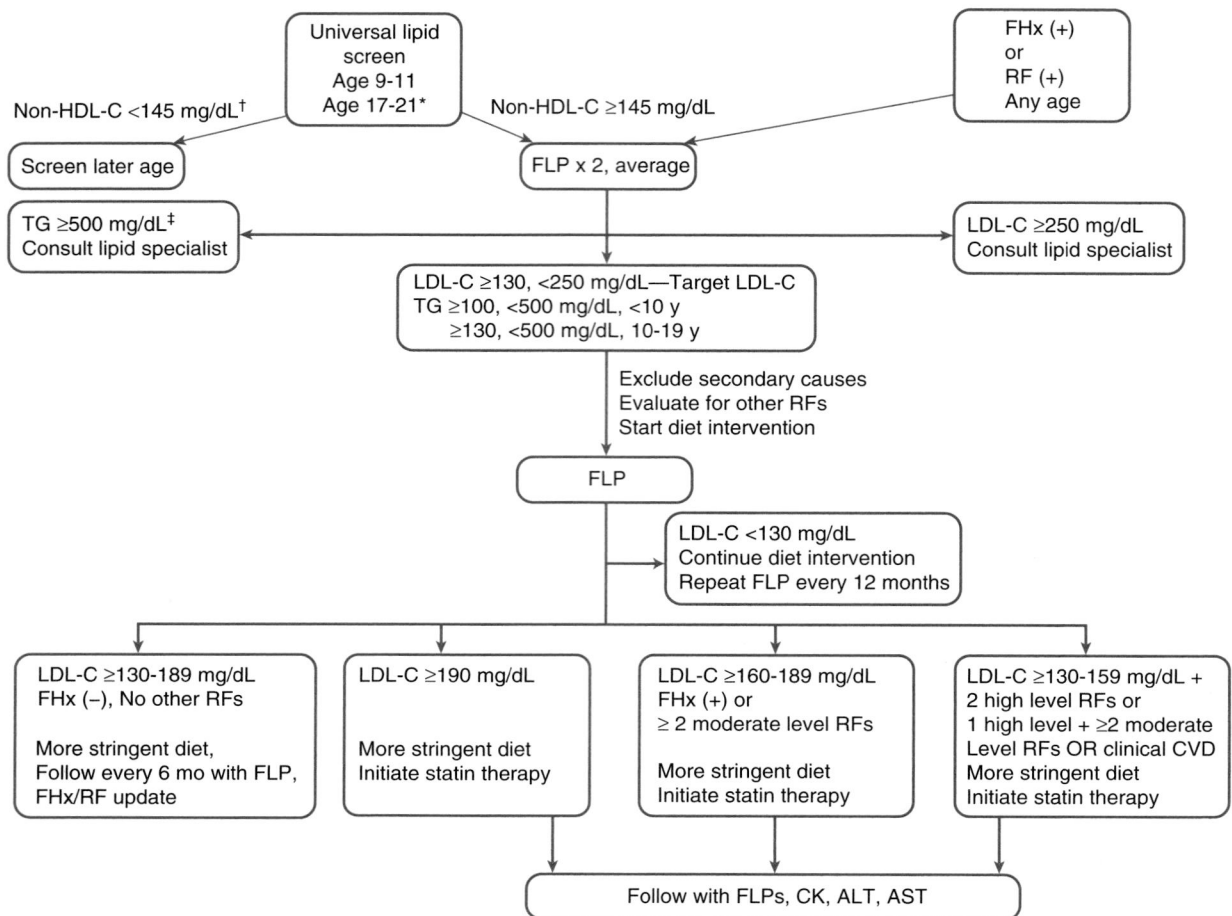

FIGURE 36.25 Algorithm for the assessment of coronary heart disease (CHD) risk in children based on lipid screening. [a]For ages 19 to 21, non–HDL-C greater than 90 mg/dL is the recommended cut point. [b]For HDL-C and LDL-C, to convert to mmol/L, divide by 38.66. [c]To convert to mmol/L, divide by 86.96. *FHx(+)*, Positive family history; *RF*, risk factor; *FLP*, fasting lipid profile; *ALT*, alanine aminotransferase; *AST*, aspartate aminotransferase; *CK*, creatine kinase.[217]

concentrations as 200 to 999 mg/dL (1.7 to 11.3 mmol/L), severe as 1000 to 1999 mg/dL (11.3 to 22.6 mmol/L), and very severe as greater than 2000 mg/dL (22.6 mmol/L). The European dyslipidemia guidelines recognize TG greater than 150 mg/dL (>1.7 mmol/L) as elevated entailing increased ASCVD risk.[111] Table 36.6 summarizes the 2020 US and European classification of desirable and high lipid values.

In the general population, several conditions and factors are associated with increased TG concentrations, including obesity, pregnancy, physical inactivity, and excess alcohol intake, as well as several diseases (e.g., type 2 diabetes, chronic renal failure), drugs (e.g., corticosteroids, estrogens, retinoids, antipsychotics, antiretroviral agents), and polygenetic and monogenic disorders (e.g., dysbetalipoproteinemia, FCS). NCEP ATP-III emphasized that TG is often associated with the metabolic syndrome in association with reduced HDL-C, insulin resistance, hypertension, fatty liver, and increased waist size (Box 36.2). TG-rich lipoproteins, which include remnant lipoproteins, are currently recognized to be atherogenic. In practice, VLDL-C or remnant cholesterol (measured or calculated as TG/5 in mg/dL and TG/2.2 in mmol/L) is often used as a measure of these atherogenic lipoproteins.

ATP III suggested the addition of non–HDL-C (Equation 36.1) as an indicator for all atherogenic lipoproteins (LDL, remnants, and Lp(a)).[225] Non–HDL-C is the primary treatment target in the United Kingdom and a secondary target of therapy after LDL-C targets are met in 2016 Canadian, 2018 US, and 2019 European guidelines (see Table 36.20). The goal for non–HDL-C in those with increased TG is 30 mg/dL (0.8 mmol/L) above what is set for LDL-C.

The treatment of hypertriglyceridemia depends on the cause of the increase and the severity. Those with TG less than 200 mg/dL (2.3 mmol/L) are treated with weight reduction and increased physical activity; for those at 200 to 499 mg/dL (2.3 to 5.6 mmol/L), drug therapy is also considered (high-intensity statins, fibrates, specifically fenofibrate, and icosapent ethyl). In the latter group, the non–HDL-C goal becomes a secondary target of therapy (see Table 36.20).

Those with TG greater than 500 mg/dL (5.65 mmol/L) are usually at increased risk of pancreatitis and may be treated with a low-fat diet (≤15% of calorie intake), weight reduction, increased physical activity, and TG-lowering drugs (high-intensity statins, fibrates, high-dose omega-3 fatty acids) if TG are up to 1000 mg/dL (11 mmol/L).

MEASUREMENT OF LIPIDS, LIPOPROTEINS, AND APOLIPOPROTEINS

Lipoproteins and their lipid and apolipoprotein constituents have become increasingly important in characterizing the risk of CVD and acute pancreatitis and in the diagnosis and management of lipoprotein disorders. In recent decades, our knowledge of such disorders has evolved from an essentially descriptive association between elevated plasma lipids and increased risk for CVD to a much broader understanding of the underlying biochemistry, physiology, and genetic interactions. Remarkable advances have also been made in our understanding of the contribution of lipoproteins to the development and progression of arterial lesions. Advances have also been made in the analytical techniques and methods used for measuring lipids, lipoproteins, and apolipoproteins. In this section, we begin with a brief historical perspective on the development of measurement technology, which is followed by a more detailed discussion of pertinent methods.

Historical Perspective and Background

The causal relationship between increased plasma concentrations of LDL and risk of CHD and the efficacy of LDL lowering to reduce risk was widely acknowledged by the mid-1980s. Awareness of the importance of intervention emphasized the necessity for a uniform means of defining hyperlipidemia and CHD risk. Previous practice had been to use cutoffs based on prevailing lipid and lipoprotein concentrations in the general population or in local populations of "normal patients." The relative nonspecificity of early chemical methods for cholesterol measurement and the different types of methods then in use allowed significant biases to sometimes exist between values obtained in different laboratories. Quantitation of the relationship between TC or LDL-C concentration and risk for CHD, demonstration of the efficacy of treatment, and development of reference methods and Centers for Disease Control (CDC) and Prevention standardization programs for lipids and lipoproteins made possible the use of risk-related cutoff points used in the earlier ATP-III guidelines. This led to the necessity for uniform definitions of hyperlipidemia based on commonly accepted risk-based lipid and lipoprotein cutoffs and the availability of accurate lipid and lipoprotein measurements.[226,227]

Consensus Guidelines From Expert Panels

Beginning in the mid-1980s, the NCEP convened several expert panels to develop guidelines for diagnosis and treatment of hypercholesterolemia and for reliable lipid and lipoprotein measurements. Two laboratory panels issued recommendations for blood lipids and lipoproteins. The first, the NCEP Laboratory Standardization Panel, focused on measurement of TC; the second, the NCEP Working Group on Lipoprotein Measurement, addressed measurements of TG, HDL-C, and LDL-C. In 2009, expert recommendations for apoB and LDL-P were published.[56] Here we summarize the principal considerations and recommendations for clinical lipid and lipoprotein measurements.

In developing recommendations for lipid and lipoprotein measurement, the different NCEP panels considered several basic issues. First, most of the large-scale clinical and epidemiologic studies that established (1) relationships between lipids and lipoproteins, (2) risk for CHD, and (3) efficacy of cholesterol lowering, measurements were made in standardized laboratories in which the accuracy of measurements was traceable to CDC reference methods. This included studies such as the National Diet Heart Study in the 1960s, various LRC program studies (early 1970s to 1990), Specialized Centers of Research in Atherosclerosis studies (early 1970s to the present), and several NHANES studies conducted between 1960 and 1994.[227,228]

Second, various methods used in laboratory or nonlaboratory settings should be capable of similar accuracy (i.e., the reliability of the measurements should be independent of how, where, or by whom they were performed). Ideally, it should be possible to consider all lipid measurements made in the United States (and eventually globally) as if they had been made in a single laboratory. This premise does *not* require that all laboratories use the same methods, but it does require methods that are capable of providing values equivalent to those on which the relationships between lipids, lipoproteins, and the risk for CHD were established.

Third, as new methods are developed, particularly those that may be more accurate and precise for various lipoproteins or lipoprotein subfractions, the particular lipoprotein included in the measurement should be specified. This is done to ensure that new methods can be linked to those that were used to establish the known lipoprotein–CHD risk relationships. To achieve these aims, development of reference methods that could be used as accuracy targets for lipid, lipoprotein, and apolipoprotein measurements was required; also, guidelines for analytical performance were established.

Analytical Challenges

Plasma lipoproteins are heterogeneous and polydisperse macromolecular complexes that vary considerably in size, composition, and function, and consequently, present exceptional analytical challenges (see Tables 36.2 and 36.3). Traditionally, lipoprotein concentrations have been expressed in terms of their cholesterol content. This approach simplified the methods used to determine lipoproteins because the lipoprotein fractions of interest have only to be separated from one another; the other plasma proteins do not have to be removed. Analytically, cholesterol has a known molecular structure and can be accurately and precisely measured with appropriate chemical or biochemical methods. Cholesterol exists as free and esterified forms; however, before measurement all cholesterol molecules are typically converted to the free form.

TG and the lipoproteins themselves, however, are not unique chemical entities (e.g., TG consist of many possible fatty acyl groups covalently attached to three positions on a glycerol backbone through ester linkages) (see Fig. 36.10). Fatty acyl groups vary in chain length and degree of saturation, leading to a mixture of TG of different molecular weights. Consequently, TG analysis usually measures the glycerol backbone, and TG concentration is then stated only in terms of molar concentration. In the United States, however, lipids have been traditionally expressed in terms of mass concentration (milligrams per deciliter), which is an approximation requiring an assumption about the average molecular weight of TG. Because palmitate, stearate, and oleate are the major fatty acids in plasma TG and have similar molecular weights, the conversion between molar and mass concentration usually assumes an average TG molecular weight of 885 Da, the molecular weight of tri-oleyl glycerol (triolein).

The situation is even more complicated for accurately measuring LDL and HDL. For example, LDL consists of a population of multiple subparticles with varying size and lipid composition, each containing apoB-100 as the major apolipoprotein component. Thus LDL has neither a unique molecular weight nor consistent lipid or protein composition. Adding to the complexity, Lp(a) cholesterol is co-measured with LDL-C. HDL is even more heterogeneous, consisting of at least 12 subclasses, differing in composition, function, and even CHD risk relationships.[229] Because of these complex characteristics, the exact concentration and composition of a fraction identified as LDL or HDL may vary, depending on how the fraction is isolated. Once isolated, however, the cholesterol content can be measured accurately. A major consideration, therefore was to define the lipoproteins in a uniform way to afford a common basis for standardization and the accurate assessment without compromising the development of new methods or necessitating the use of same methods in all laboratories.

Analytical Approach

For more than 50 years, the CDC has maintained reference methods for TC, TG, and HDL-C and has provided standardization programs targeted for the research laboratories. In addition, these reference methods were used to establish the accuracy of lipid and lipoprotein measurements in several population studies, including the LRC and CPPT studies, and several NHANES studies conducted by the National Center for Health Statistics since the 1960s.[230,231] From these studies, cut points for risk characterization in patients were derived. Because the standardization programs were already accepted as authoritative by the general laboratory and research communities, the NCEP laboratory panels recommended the CDC reference methods as the basis for defining "accuracy" in the context of recommendations for reliable lipid and lipoprotein measurements. Use of this approach had several advantages. First, it established the same basis for accuracy that had been used in developing the relationships between lipid and lipoprotein concentration and CHD. Second, it provided a reference point by which the accuracy of existing or newly developed methods could be assessed. By 2020, the CDC was developing reference methods for other lipid values, including for Lp(a) in collaboration with European Federation of Clinical Chemistry and Laboratory Medicine (EFLM).

Lipid and Lipoprotein Measurements

Various technologies have been used to separate and measure plasma lipids, lipoproteins, and lipoprotein subfractions, including enzymatic, immunochemical, and chemical precipitation reagents, and physical methods, such as ultracentrifugation, electrophoresis, column chromatography, and others. Moreover, although different methods of lipoprotein separation may produce similar lipoprotein fractions, they usually do not produce identical fractions, giving rise to systematic biases among methods that purport to measure the same component. The present discussion focuses primarily on accepted reference methods and procedures commonly used in clinical practice for lipid and lipoprotein measurements.

Reference Methods

Reference methods are the "gold standards" or accuracy targets that have been developed for the more common analytes,

such as TC, TG, and LDL-C and HDL-C. The reference method for cholesterol is fully validated and credentialed through the Joint Committee for Traceability in Laboratory Medicine. The other methods, although not formally credentialed, have been accepted by consensus.

Cholesterol. The original CDC reference method for cholesterol is based on a chemical method devised by Abell and colleagues.[231–233] The method exhibits an approximate 1.6% positive bias compared with isotope dilution MS, which is considered to be the highest-order method for cholesterol and was developed and applied by the National Institute of Standards and Technology.[231] Cholesterol may be expressed in terms of molar (millimoles per liter) or mass (milligrams per deciliter) concentration. Molar concentration is converted to mass concentration using the following equation:

$$\text{Cholesterol mg/dL} = \text{Cholesterol mmol/L} \times 38.7 \quad \textbf{(36.2)}$$

The CDC reference method, demonstrated to be readily transferable to other laboratories, has been widely adopted by reference laboratories and diagnostic manufacturers as the accuracy target, and it is the basis for calibration in cholesterol measurements.

Triglycerides. As with cholesterol, the original CDC reference procedure for TG was a chemical method.[227] It depended on extraction and alkaline hydrolysis to produce glycerol, which was then oxidized with periodate and reacted with chromotropic acid to generate a chromogen (see Fig. 36.26).

Results may be expressed in terms of molar concentration (millimoles per liter) or mass concentration (milligrams per deciliter). The following equation is used to convert mmol/L to mg/dL:

$$\text{TG mg/dL} = \text{TG mmol/L} \times 88.7 \quad \textbf{(36.3)}$$

The equation assumes an average molecular weight of 885 g/mol (triolein) for plasma TG. To facilitate standardization of TG measurements, a designated comparison method (DCM) has been developed by the Cholesterol Reference Method Laboratory Network (CRMLN), involving similar extraction steps followed by more robust enzymatic quantitation of the TG-derived glycerol. This DCM, established in other reference laboratories, is expected to become the secondary accuracy target for TG. More recently, a new reference method was developed for TG based on gas chromatographic isotope dilution mass spectrometry (GC-IDMS).[234,235] In this new method, all glycerides (TG, diglycerides, and monoglycerides), as before, are chemically reduced to glycerol, which then is measured by GC-IDMS.

High-density lipoprotein cholesterol. The CDC reference method uses a combination of ultracentrifugation and polyanion precipitation to isolate HDL.[236] The cholesterol in this fraction is then quantified using the CDC reference method for cholesterol. In this method, VLDL and chylomicrons, if

TG + KOH ⟶ Fatty acids + Glycerol

Glycerol + Periodate ⟶ Formic acid + Formaldehyde

Formaldehyde + Chromotropic acid ⟶ Chromogen

FIGURE 36.26 CDC reference method for triglyceride measurement.

present, are first removed by ultracentrifugation of an accurately measured volume of serum for 16.2 hours at 33,700 rpm in a Beckman-type 50.4 rotor. Under these conditions, VLDL and any chylomicrons accumulate as a floating layer at the top of the ultracentrifuge tube ($d = 1.006$ g/mL). A tube-slicing technique is used to remove the VLDL fraction. The infranatant, which contains IDL, LDL, Lp(a), HDL, and the other serum proteins, is recovered quantitatively. The apoB–containing lipoproteins in 2 mL of this fraction are precipitated by adding 80 μL of injectable heparin (5000 USP units/mL of 0.15 mol/L NaCl in water) and 100 μL of 1.0 mol/L manganese chloride to water. The precipitate is removed by centrifugation, and cholesterol in the supernatant is measured. HDL-C may be expressed in molar or mass concentration; molar concentration is converted to mass concentration using Eq. (36.2).

Heparin-$MnCl_2$ was selected as the precipitation reagent primarily for historical reasons because it was the method most commonly used in early studies to establish the relationship between HDL-C concentration and risk for CHD. The ultracentrifugation step was included to prevent interference with sedimentation of the apoB–containing lipoproteins by the lighter TG-rich lipoproteins, VLDL, and chylomicrons.

Only a few routine diagnostic laboratories have an ultracentrifuge and the experience required to reliably perform the CDC reference method for HDL-C. Furthermore, ultracentrifugation is expensive and necessitates obtaining an impractically large specimen volume, typically 5.0 mL. As a practical alternative, the CRMLN laboratories developed and validated a modified dextran sulfate (50,000 Da) procedure as a DCM to provide results approximately equivalent to those of the CDC reference method (RM), while avoiding ultracentrifugation.[237] The $MgCl_2$ concentration in the precipitant reagent was decreased slightly from that used in the previously published primary method to increase HDL-C values slightly, achieving closer agreement with the CDC reference method.

Low-density lipoprotein cholesterol. The CDC has also defined a reference method for LDL-C based on the similar techniques already described for HDL-C.[238] β-quantification follows the procedure adopted from the NIH Laboratory that was first used in the LRC Program, combining preparative ultracentrifugation and polyanion precipitation. An accurately measured aliquot of plasma at a native density of 1.006 g/mL is first ultracentrifuged at 105,000 × g for 18 hours at 10 °C. VLDL and, if present, chylomicrons and/or β-VLDL float over the infranatant containing primarily LDL and HDL, plus any IDL and Lp(a) that may be present. The floating layer, removed with the aid of a tube slicer, is sometimes analyzed as a check on recovery and may be saved for electrophoretic analysis to determine the presence of β-VLDL. The infranatant solution is remixed and reconstituted to known volume, and its cholesterol content is measured. Afterward, HDL can be determined following precipitation by heparin and manganese (Mn^{2+}), as described previously. After measurement of cholesterol in the d greater than 1.006 g/mL fraction and in the heparin-Mn^{2+} supernatant solution, LDL-C is estimated by calculating the difference. VLDL-C and LDL-C are calculated as follows:

$$(VLDL\text{-}C) = (TC) - (d > 1.006 \text{ g/mLchol}) \quad \textbf{(36.4)}$$

$$(LDL\text{-}C) = (d > 1.006 \text{ g/mLchol}) - (HDL\text{-}C) \quad \textbf{(36.5)}$$

LDL-C measured in this way is unaffected by the presence of chylomicrons or other TG-rich lipoproteins, or by β-VLDL. VLDL-C is usually calculated from Equation 36.4 rather than measured directly in the ultracentrifugal supernatant because it can be difficult to recover this fraction quantitatively, particularly when TG concentrations are high.

Lipoproteins included in the "LDL cholesterol" measurement. In this context, the term LDL-C includes cholesterol in IDL and Lp(a) fractions, as well as the core LDL. Although IDL and Lp(a) cholesterol usually contribute only a few mg/dL of the "total LDL-C" measurement, their contributions can be significant in patients with high IDL or Lp(a) concentrations. For example, assuming that cholesterol (i.e., sterol nucleus) constitutes about 30% of the mass of Lp(a), it can be calculated that the Lp(a) cholesterol concentration would contribute about 12 mg/dL (0.31 mmol/L), or about 12%, to the LDL-C measurement in a patient with an Lp(a) concentration of 40 mg/dL and an apparent LDL-C concentration of 100 mg/dL (2.59 mmol/L). This fraction can be substantially larger at very high Lp(a) concentration up to 400 mg/dL or when LDL-C is reduced maximally using statin, ezetimibe, and PCSK9 inhibitor treatment simultaneously.

It has been suggested that a more specific measure of LDL-C could be obtained by correcting the measured LDL-C value for the contribution of Lp(a) cholesterol, and a similar argument might be made for IDL. However, both IDL and Lp(a) contribute to increased risk for CHD (see section on Lp[a]); therefore although such correction will increase the specificity of methods for LDL-C, *per se*, it might also give LDL-C values that underestimate cardiovascular risk. Moreover, this might occur more frequently in patients with CHD or those who are at risk for CHD, based on their "LDL-C" concentrations. Consequently, the NCEP Working Group on LDL Cholesterol Measurement suggested that LDL-C values should *not* be corrected for the contribution of other atherogenic lipoproteins; this group also recommended that further research should be conducted to establish the individual contributions of IDL, Lp(a), and LDL-C to CHD risk.[225] NCEP guidelines published in 2001 expanded on this concept by introducing the term *non–HDL cholesterol*, which includes all of the apoB–containing atherogenic lipoproteins, including not only cholesterol on Lp(a) and IDL but also VLDL, remnant lipoproteins, and chylomicrons for nonfasting samples.

Application of Reference Methods to Standardization

Background. Early efforts in the mid-1980s to achieve general standardization of methods used by clinical laboratories began with a fairly traditional approach with secondary reference materials provided to the laboratory community. The reference materials consisted of lyophilized serum pools with target values assigned on the basis of replicate measurements, using the reference methods. However, problems were recognized with this approach, primarily from the confounding effects of matrix changes in the reference materials, making them noncommutable with native clinical samples. Secondary reference materials prepared from pooled serum spiked with artificial analytes and subjected to freezing and freeze-drying are not always commutable and did not behave like fresh patient specimens with some routine methods. Diagnostic manufacturers used the secondary reference materials to assign presumably reliable targets to their calibrators but subsequently found that results on patient specimens became inaccurate. The problem was compounded by national proficiency testing programs, which in an attempt to improve accuracy, began to report reference method target values with similarly prepared survey materials. Laboratories were adjusting calibration to achieve apparent accuracy on the survey materials; however, in some instances, results on actual patient specimens became inaccurate.

Recognition of these problems focused attention on the issues of "analyte" and "matrix" effects in reference materials.[239] Procedures commonly used in preparing secondary reference materials were inducing changes in the analytes themselves and in the other constituents. The fluids that surrounded the analytes made the analyses no longer comparable to the measurements in the authentic fresh specimens. After considerable study and reassessment, the conclusion was reached that the only universally reliable means of transferring accuracy from the reference methods to diagnostic manufacturers and individual laboratories was through direct comparison studies on fresh, representative patient specimens.[240] As a consequence, the CDC and other groups cooperated to organize a network of reference laboratories to provide the reference methods and fresh sample comparison studies.

The cholesterol reference method laboratory network. Because the CDC standardization laboratory maintaining the reference methods did not have the capacity to perform all necessary comparison studies directly, it was obvious that the reference laboratory capability would have to be expanded to accommodate the needs of the industry and the laboratory community. To this end, the CDC and several other interested laboratories cooperated to establish the CRMLN. Each participating network laboratory underwent stringent protocols to transfer the CDC reference methods and to maintain comparability with the CDC. In turn, the network laboratories performed comparison studies using fresh patient sera with the diagnostic manufacturers and with individual laboratories. Throughout the 1990s, the network was large and active to accommodate the demands of comparison studies. As standardization has steadily improved in subsequent years, the concentration of activity has declined, and the number of domestic US network laboratories has decreased. However, at the same time, the network laboratory program has expanded to include additional international laboratories.

The network offers protocols, based on Clinical and Laboratory Standards Institute guidelines, whereby diagnostic manufacturers ensure accuracy by completing comparison studies using the reference methods. A measurement system qualifies for certification by demonstrating agreement within specified limits for TC, HDL-C, LDL-C, and TG. Based on comparison results, calibrator set points are adjusted, if necessary, to bring performance into agreement with the reference methods. Diagnostic manufacturers, distributors, and instrument partners are encouraged to certify their systems at least every 2 years and to ensure that every production lot is calibrated to maintain traceability to the accuracy targets; this can be accomplished through ongoing participation in the CDC and/or CRMLN program. The CDC website provides details of the program, protocols for comparison studies, contact information for the CDC and/or CRMLN, and a listing of qualified commercial methods for certification.[241]

In 2020, the network has focused its attention on accurate measurement of LDL-C at very low concentrations, as this has become clinically relevant after introduction of PCSK9 inhibitors that, in combination with high-intensity statins, can lower LDL-C by 80%.

Routine Methods

Reference methods are complex, typically time-consuming, and at least partially manual, and they require a high degree of expertise for reliable operation. Consequently, simpler and more practical methods have evolved for routine clinical use.

Cholesterol. Enzymatic methods for cholesterol measurement are precise, accurate when calibrated appropriately, and easily adapted for use with modern analyzers. Commercially available cholesterol reagents commonly combine all the enzymes and other required components into a single photometric reagent. The reagent is usually mixed with a few microliters of serum or plasma and incubated under controlled conditions for color development, and absorbance is measured in the visible portion of the spectrum, generally at about 500 nm. The reagents typically use a bacterial CE hydrolase to cleave CE followed by cholesterol oxidase to generate peroxide which is used to enzymatically generate chromophore (Fig. 36.27).

These methods may be subject to interference from other colored compounds or those that compete with the oxidation reaction or react with peroxide, such as bilirubin, ascorbic acid, and hemoglobin. Assays are usually linear up to about 1000 mg/dL (25.9 mmol/L). Reagents have been refined by adding substances, such as bilirubin oxidase and dual-wavelength readings, to minimize the effects of hemolysis; interference from bilirubin is generally not an issue now in concentrations below 5 mg/dL (85.5 μmol/L). Enzymatic reagents are not entirely specific for cholesterol because β-hydroxy sterols and plant sterols (e.g., sitosterol) can also react. In human serum or plasma, however, this is not a major problem because these interfering sterols are generally present in relatively low concentrations.

In practice, reagent formulations vary from manufacturer to manufacturer. In most cases, the reagent from a particular manufacturer will have been optimized for use with one

$$CE + H_2O \xrightarrow{\text{Cholesteryl ester hydrolase}} \text{Cholesterol + Fatty acid}$$

$$\text{Cholesterol} + O_2 \xrightarrow{\text{Cholesterol oxidase}} \text{Cholest-4-en-3-one} + H_2O_2$$

$$H_2O_2 + \text{Phenol} + 4\text{–Aminoantipyrine} \xrightarrow{\text{Peroxidase}} \text{Quinoeimine dye} + 2H_2O$$

FIGURE 36.27 Clinical enzymatic method for cholesterol measurement.

or several specific instruments and calibration materials—usually those sold by that manufacturer. Over the past few years, most manufacturers have been supplying calibration materials with assigned values that are traceable to the CDC reference method; this has helped to reduce interlaboratory variations. Thus cholesterol analysis methods are best thought of as "measurement systems" composed of reagent, calibrator (cholesterol standard), and instrument. When a reagent-calibrator-instrument system from a single manufacturer is used, cholesterol measurements in the laboratory usually are accurate to within 1 to 3% of reference values, and such systems are routinely operated with coefficients of variation less than 2.5%. In some cases, however, a reagent from one manufacturer might be used with an instrument from another manufacturer. In this instance, the responsibility is on the user rather than the manufacturer to ensure that reagent and sample volumes, time and temperature of incubation, and the calibration produce precise and accurate measurements. Although the cholesterol oxidase reagent described previously in this chapter is by far the most common, reagents have been developed for using cholesterol dehydrogenase, which may have advantages in some instances.[242] In addition, other highly sensitive enzymatic methods have been described for specialized applications.[243] Free or unesterified cholesterol can be readily quantified by removing the cholesterol esterase from the reagent.

Triglycerides. TG are also commonly measured with enzyme reagents directly in plasma or serum. Reagents combining all required enzymes, cofactors, and buffers are available from various manufacturers. As within cholesterol, such reagents are optimized for use with particular instrument-calibrator systems. Several different enzyme reactions have been used (Fig. 36.28).

Enzymatic TG methods are fairly specific in that they do not detect glucose or PL. Most are linear in the concentration range up to about 1000 mg/dL (11.3 mmol/L), and when automated, they are operated with coefficients of variation up to approximately 3%. The methods are usually calibrated with reference solutions of pure glycerol or with serum-based secondary calibrators. However, because all methods measure the glycerol component, any free glycerol in the sample contributes to the apparent amount of TG. The NCEP Working Group on Lipoprotein Measurement originally recommended the use of glycerol blanking for TG measurement, but at this time, it is not a common practice because only a limited number of commercial assays are available. With routine methods, the decision must be made whether to correct for free glycerol by using a method that corrects for the free glycerol blank.

Triglyceride blanks (Correction for endogenous glycerol). Glycerol concentrations in freshly collected serum or plasma in healthy subjects are usually less than 5 to 10 mg/dL (543 to 1086 μmol/L). Because this small amount is clinically insignificant, the TG blank is usually ignored. Glycerol, however, can be higher in samples with increased TG concentrations and from patients with conditions such as diabetes or those receiving total parenteral nutrition, but even in these conditions, the free

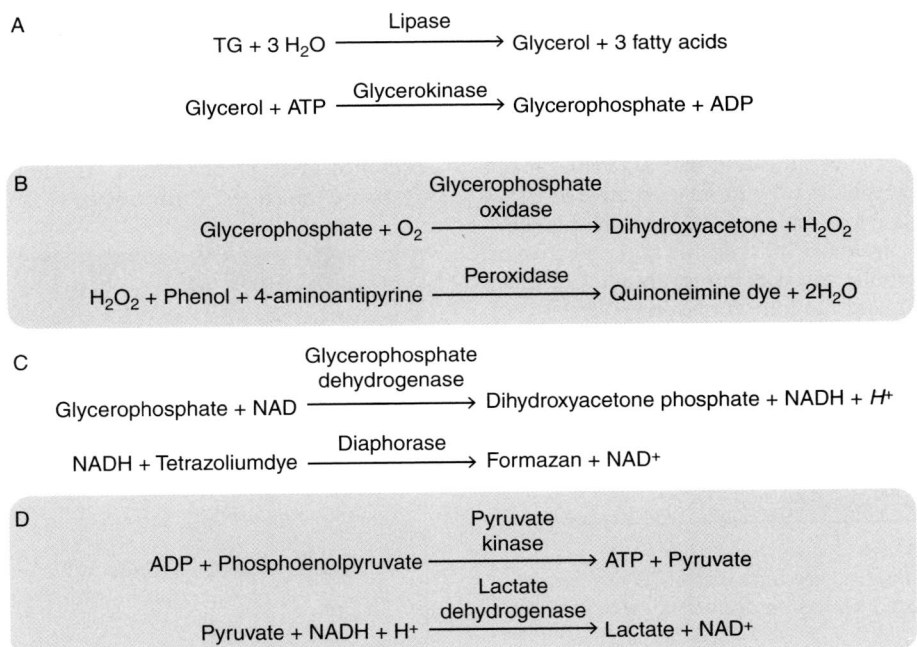

FIGURE 36.28 Clinical enzymatic methods for triglyceride measurement. (A) In all methods, the first step is the lipase-catalyzed hydrolysis of TG to glycerol and fatty acids followed by glycerol phosphorylation in an ATP-requiring reaction catalyzed by glycerokinase. (B) In the most commonly used methods, glycerophosphate is then oxidized to dihydroxyacetone and H_2O_2 in a glycerophosphate oxidase–catalyzed reaction, and the H_2O_2 formed in the reaction is measured following the reaction with 4-Aminoantipyrine to form the chromophore quinoneimine. (C) Alternatively, glycerophosphate can be measured in a reduced form of nicotinamide-adenine dinucleotide (NADH)-producing reaction, and NADH is measured by a spectrophotometer set at 340 nm or in a diaphorase-catalyzed reaction to create formazan whose absorbance is measured at 500 nm. (D) Other methods measure the ADP produced by conversion to pyruvate and monitoring the enzymatic reduction of NADH at 340 nm.

glycerol concentration does not generally substantially affect the interpretation. Rarely, glycerol can be markedly increased by 50- to 100-fold in a rare disorder called *hyperglycerolemia,* which is the result of a deficiency in glycerol kinase. This is sometimes called pseudohypertriglyceridemia and can result in improper CV risk assessment and treatment.[244]

Although TG blanks in most cases can be ignored in clinical measurements, they can dramatically affect conclusions about method accuracy. TG blanking usually requires a separate analysis of glycerol, expressed in terms of equivalent TG concentration, and the measured blank value is subtracted from the total TG measurement. Free glycerol can be measured enzymatically using reactions such as those shown in Fig. 36.28 with a reagent that is identical to the TG reagent, but lacking lipase—an approach designated as *two-cuvette blanking.* An alternative to the two-step approach carried out in a single cuvette first consumes any free glycerol to produce a colorless product in a preliminary reaction before a lipase enzyme is added to cleave and measure the TG-derived glycerol.

TG blanking by either of these approaches increases the time and cost of TG analysis. A more common practice, designated *calibration blanking,* which is used by some manufacturers, involves adjusting calibrator set points to compensate for the average amount of free glycerol in specimens. This is accomplished through a comparison study on actual patient specimens versus the reference method or an accurate equivalent. The calibration blanking approach will underestimate the blank in a few specimens but will provide a better and reasonably reliable estimation for most specimens.

Traditionally, TG concentrations have been determined on fasting samples obtained from patients after a 10- to 12-hour fast—a practice based on the historical practice in epidemiology studies to achieve a uniform metabolic state. However, patients do not routinely present to physicians' offices in the fasting state, and studies have suggested that TG values measured on nonfasting samples may be more predictive of CHD risk.[1] Postprandial collections are more likely to include remnant lipoproteins that are more atherogenic and reflective of the patient's usual metabolic state. US, European, and Canadian guidelines now recommend random nonfasting collections of lipid profiles as the screening sample[1,4,110–112,138,139,245,246]; this is particularly relevant in children and in those with diabetes to avoid episodes of hypoglycemia.

POINTS TO REMEMBER

Triglycerides
- Elevated triglycerides (TG) are a marker of TG-rich lipoproteins, causally related with atherosclerotic cardiovascular diseases (ASCVD).
- The higher TG, the higher the risk of both ASCVD and acute pancreatitis.
- At extremely high TG above roughly 500 mg/dL (5.7 mmol/L) the risk of acute pancreatitis is very high.
- TG are mostly transported in VLDL and their remnants, and in the postprandial phase additionally in chylomicrons and their remnants.
- Total TG can be measured in plasma or serum, using enzymatic assays.

High-density lipoprotein cholesterol. Under current recommendations for characterizing the CVD risk in patients, measurement of the two major cholesterol-carrying lipoproteins, HDL and LDL, is critical for CVD risk assessment. HDL-C is part of many risk calculators including the Pooled Cohort Equation for risk assessment,[247] and is used to calculate non–HDL-C by subtraction from TC. Low HDL-C can be a long-term marker of elevated TG-rich lipoproteins,[106] liver disease, amyloidosis, inborn errors of metabolism, and other diseases.[248] HDL is classically defined in terms of its density range (1.063 to 1.21 g/mL) obtained by ultracentrifugation, which has been used as the standard by which the accuracy of other HDL methods is determined. However, the density range of Lp(a) (1.04 to 1.13 g/mL) overlaps that of HDL (see Table 36.2), so in patients with high Lp(a) concentrations, ultracentrifugation at 1.063 g/mL would overestimate the true HDL-C concentration. As a consequence, the CDC reference method, described previously, uses precipitation to separate HDL, similar to the approach used for many research determinations. Most routine laboratories now use the newer direct or homogeneous assays, which became available beginning in the early 1990s. The homogeneous assays have advantages in terms of efficiency and convenience because they are capable of full automation. However, homogeneous assays have been shown to lack specificity, especially on specimens from patients with unusual lipoprotein distributions (see later). Because pretreatment precipitation methods were the standard for decades and preceded the currently more common homogeneous assays, these methods will be reviewed first.

Precipitation methods. In earlier years, HDL-C was most commonly measured (Box 36.3) in supernatant solutions after precipitation of the apoB–containing lipoproteins (VLDL, IDL, Lp(a), LDL, and, when present, chylomicrons) directly from plasma or serum, using agents such as polyanions in the presence of divalent cations. As indicated earlier, LDL and HDL are the largest contributors to TC in most people, with

BOX 36.3 Methods for High-Density Lipoproteins Separation/Quantification

Precipitation (First Generation)
Heparin-Mn^{2+}
  0.46 mmol/L (LRC method)
  0.92 mmol/L (recommended for EDTA plasma)
Dextran sulfate (50 kDa) Mg^{2+} (AACC Selected Method and DCM)
Phosphotungstate-Mg^{2+}

Facilitated Separation (Second Generation)
Magnetic with/dextran sulfate-Mg^{2+}

Homogeneous (Third Generation)
Antibody four-reagent method (International Reagents Corp.)
Polyethylene glycol modified enzymes w/cyclodextrin (Kyowa Medex)
Synthetic polymer/detergent (Daiichi)
Antibodies (Wako)
Catalase (Denka Seiken)

AACC, American Association for Clinical Chemistry; DCM, Designated comparison method; EDTA, ethylenediaminetetraacetic acid; LRSCs, Lipid Research Clinics.

LDL accounting for about two-thirds and HDL for about one-third of TC. In many individuals, IDL and Lp(a) each account for a smaller fraction of TC, although their concentrations can be considerably higher in some individuals. Polyanions bridge positively charged groups on lipoproteins, and their action is facilitated in the presence of divalent cations, which interact with negatively charged groups, forming aggregation and precipitation. Precipitation is usually complete within 10 to 15 minutes at room temperature; at 2 to 4 °C, a 30-minute incubation period is preferred. The precipitate is then sedimented by centrifugation, typically for 45,000 g-min (i.e., the equivalent of 1500 × g for 30 minutes). Centrifugation at higher g-forces (e.g., 10,000 × g) accelerates sedimentation and can improve complete removal of apoB–containing particles. HDL-C is then enzymatically measured in the clear supernatant.

Of several polyanion-divalent cation combinations, heparan sulfate with $MnCl_2$ was the most common and was eventually used in the CDC reference method. With the transition to enzymatic cholesterol assays, residual Mn^{2+} was found, however, to interfere, giving artifactually high results. Techniques were then devised to reduce this interference, but additional manipulations were required, making them inconvenient for routine use (e.g., the chelator ethylenediaminetetraacetic acid [EDTA] added to the cholesterol reagent to complex residual manganite), or carbonate was added in a second precipitation step to precipitate excess Mn^{2+}. Most laboratories avoided these tedious approaches and adopted alternative precipitants, such as dextran sulfate or phosphotungstate with Mg^{2+}. A method that used dextran sulfate with molecular weight of 50 kDa was developed during the 1980s and became the most commonly used precipitation reagent.[249]

The precipitability of lipoproteins with polyanions and divalent cations depends on the lipid and protein compositions of the particles. Thus various precipitants differ in their ability to precipitate apoB–containing lipoproteins while leaving HDL in solution, resulting in potential biases among reagents. With modern reagent-instrument-calibrator systems, conditions are generally optimized to produce values that closely approximate and are traceable to reference method values. Also, the precipitation methods can be inaccurate under certain conditions, such as with high concentrations of TG-rich lipoproteins. Any residual turbidity in the supernate indicates inadequate sedimentation of the apoB–containing lipoproteins, resulting in overestimation of HDL-C. Samples with high TG concentrations (generally those above 400 mg/dL [4.5 mmol/L]) frequently produce turbid supernatants because TG reduce the density of the lipoprotein-precipitating reagent complex to the point that some of the complex remains unsedimented.

In cases of extremely high TG concentrations, some of the precipitate may even form a floating layer over a clear or turbid supernatant, in addition to the usual precipitate at the bottom of the centrifuge tube. Such supernates require additional treatment with one of several techniques. Before precipitation, the sample can be ultracentrifuged and the TG-rich lipoproteins removed as described previously for the reference method. Alternatively, a turbid supernatant can sometimes be cleared by centrifuging for a longer time or at higher g-forces. More commonly, the sample can be diluted twofold with saline to reduce the concentration of TG-rich lipoproteins before the precipitant is added. A fourth approach is to pass the turbid supernatant through a 0.45-μm filter to remove the unsedimented precipitate before cholesterol in the filtrate is measured.

HDL-C determination can also be affected by sample matrix effects, which arise from the unusual nature of the sample itself, processing effects, or the addition of anticoagulants or preservatives. For example, HDL-C measurements can be inaccurate and are usually more variable when obtained from lyophilized samples than from fresh or frozen sera. Additives including anticoagulants, such as citrate and fluoride, can have large osmotic effects that cause water to shift from the cells to the plasma. This dilutes the lipoprotein by 10% or more and produces erroneously low values. EDTA, the past preferred anticoagulant for lipoprotein measurements has been used because it also inhibits certain oxidative and other changes that can affect some lipoprotein or apolipoprotein measurements despite causing a slight dilution. Lipid and lipoprotein concentrations in EDTA plasma tend to be about 3% lower than in serum. EDTA, however, complexes some of the Mn^{2+} in the heparin-Mn^{2+} method, and it has been found necessary to use a higher concentration of $MnCl_2$ (0.092 mol/L, final concentration in the reaction system) when the procedure is used with EDTA plasma than with serum (0.046 mol/L). Heparin, by virtue of its HMW, and when present in concentrations used for anticoagulation, has no measurable effect on lipid or lipoprotein concentration, and it does not affect HDL-C measurements.

Homogeneous assays. A major breakthrough in HDL determination was so-called homogeneous methods for lipoproteins (Box 36.3).[250] Compared with earlier precipitation methods requiring manual pretreatment steps, homogeneous methods were much better suited for the automated systems used in the modern clinical laboratory. Elimination of manual pretreatment was timely because laboratories were under pressure to reduce operating costs. The fully automated homogeneous methods also improved precision through more consistent pipetting of smaller specimen volumes, and precise temperature control and reaction timing, which facilitated achieving the NCEP analytical performance goals.

The first homogeneous assay for HDL-C required four successive reagent additions (International Reagents Corp., Kobe, Japan). The first reagent contained polyethylene glycol, resulting in aggregation of the apoB–containing chylomicrons, VLDL, IDL, Lp(a), and LDL. The second reagent protected or blocked the aggregated lipoproteins with antibodies to apoB and apoC. The cholesterol reaction enzymes (cholesterol esterase, cholesterol oxidase, and peroxidase) were added in the third reagent, which acted only on the unprotected HDL-C. The fourth reagent stopped the color reaction and solubilized the aggregates with guanidine salts, clearing the reaction mixture for measurement of color.

This breakthrough method, even though not suited for all analyzers because of the multiple reagent additions, was capable of full automation, paving the way for subsequent simpler two-reagent homogeneous methods that used sulfated α-cyclodextrins together with Mg^{2+} to selectively block but not precipitate apoB-containing lipoproteins, providing selectivity without the necessity for precipitation.[250] Second, covalently linked polyethylene glycol molecules enhanced the specificities of the enzymes cholesterol esterase and cholesterol oxidase toward the cholesterol in HDL. Polyethylene glycol having a MW of 6000 Da was thought to optimize the specificities at concentrations lower than those used previously to precipitate lipoproteins, implying that modified enzymes were able to distinguish lipoprotein classes on the basis of their size and/or charge. The result was a fully automated homogeneous assay with only two reagent additions applicable for general use. The original kit included the second enzyme-containing reagent in lyophilized form, necessitating reconstitution, but a modification introduced in mid-1998 included both reagents in liquid form. A third modification decreased the Mg^{2+} concentration, apparently to reduce carryover in pipetting.

A synthetic polymer, together with a polyanion to block the non-HDL lipoproteins, was used in a third homogeneous assay (Daiichi Pure Chemicals Co., Tokyo, Japan; Genzyme Corp., Cambridge, MA).[251] A detergent was added that exposes only cholesterol in HDL to the enzymes, giving specificity for HDL-C. This method required two reagent additions: the first with the polyanion and polymer-blocking agents and the second with detergent, enzymes, and substrates. A subsequent modification provided both reagents in liquid form with other changes to improve specificity and decrease potential interference. A third modification without Mg^{2+} has been reported.

A fourth early homogeneous assay was based on immuno-inhibition and included two reagents (Wako Pure Chemicals Industry, Osaka, Japan). The first reagent contained an antibody to human apoB that reacted with apoB–containing lipoproteins, chylomicrons, VLDL, IDL, Lp(a), and LDL, blocking their reaction to enzymes added in the second reagent. The more current formulation included both reagents in liquid form.

A fifth homogeneous method (Denka Seiken Co., Niigata, Japan; Polymedco Inc., Cortlandt Manor, NY; Randox Laboratories Limited, Crumlin, United Kingdom) allowed cholesterol esterase and oxidase to react with lipoproteins other than HDL, generating peroxidase, which in turn was scavenged by the enzyme catalase. An inhibitor of catalase and a surfactant in a second reagent specifically reacted with HDL-C, producing color through the usual peroxidase sequence. In subsequent years, the various homogeneous reagents have undergone many additional modifications in attempts to improve their convenience and specificity. Currently, at least seven separate reagent formulations are available.

At least one instrument application for each of the homogeneous assays discussed previously in this chapter has qualified for certification by the CRMLN, implying at minimum the capability to achieve agreement with the reference method. However, conditions, and especially calibration, may be different on various instrument applications, and many have not been evaluated. Thus certification for the reagents cannot be considered universally applicable to all distributor versions, instrument applications, and lots. Similarly, published evaluation studies have confirmed that these methods can be accurate but may not be so in every commercial application scenario. Laboratories choosing to adopt homogeneous assay applications that have not been certified by the CRMLN are encouraged to confirm that their particular systems are accurate. In addition, an evaluation of all current homogeneous HDL-C and LDL-C assays revealed that many of them lack ruggedness because of lack of lipoprotein specificity, especially on specimens with unusual lipoprotein composition.[252]

Specificity and interference. The accuracy of measuring HDL-C in each individual specimen is a function not only of mean bias or overall inaccuracy of a method related to calibration, but also its specificity for HDL-C and absence of interference by other lipoproteins and constituents of the specimen matrix. CRMLN certification studies and many published evaluation studies undertaken to assess accuracy included only samples from relatively normal subjects. Most studies did not determine performance in samples from patients with extreme hyperlipidemias, such as type III or other conditions such as liver and kidney disease, which often result in unusual lipoproteins with atypical separation characteristics. Only a few studies have included such extreme specimens and have raised questions about the specificity of the homogeneous reagents.[253] Most studies of interference have used fairly traditional spiking designs; they have been relatively modest in scope and have not properly addressed abnormal lipoprotein composition. Of note, hemoglobin below 2 g/L and bilirubin less than 10 mg/dL (1086 μmol/L) do not seem to interfere appreciably with any of the homogeneous methods.

Considerations in choosing a high-density lipoprotein method. Laboratories have had to consider the pros and cons in deciding whether to replace a conventional pretreatment method with a homogeneous reagent: improved efficiency on the one hand versus occasional discrepant results on the other. Routine clinical laboratories tend to choose the fully automated methods because of unavoidable pressures to improve efficiency. Laboratories performing research and supporting lipid clinics, on the other hand, often choose to retain a conventional precipitation method. An important factor in the latter choice is that a laboratory supporting long-term studies cannot tolerate potential changes and shifts in results that may occur because of frequent modifications to the homogeneous reagents.

POINTS TO REMEMBER

High-Density Lipoproteins
- Epidemiologic studies have shown that HDL-C is inversely related to ASCVD risk.
- Randomized trials and genetic studies document that HDL-C is not causally related to ASCVD.
- Reference methods involve precipitation of non–HDL lipoproteins.
- HDL-C can be directly measured using a homogeneous assay.
- ApoA-I is the main protein in HDL.

Low-density lipoprotein cholesterol. Methods for LDL-C generally quantitate a so-called broad-cut fraction, including not only the primary LDL species in the 1.019 to 1.063 g/mL density range but also IDL, density 1.006 to 1.019 kg/L, and Lp(a). LDL-C can be measured using both indirect and direct methods, and either approach has been used in major studies that established the relationship between LDL-C concentration and risk for CHD.[254]

Indirect methods. Indirect methods for measuring LDL-C are based on measuring a number of lipid-related analytes, followed by their use in calculating the LDL-C content of a specimen. This includes use of various equations for calculating LDL-C and the β-quantification method.

Friedewald equation. In the most widely used indirect method (Box 36.4), TC, TG, and HDL-C are measured and LDL-C is calculated from primary measurements using the following empirical equation developed by Friedewald and colleagues:

$$LDL\text{-}C = TC - HDL\text{-}C - \frac{TG}{5} \qquad (36.6)$$

where all concentrations are given in mg/dL (TG/2.22 when units are expressed in mmol/L).[255] The factor (TG)/5 is an estimate of VLDL-C and is based on the average ratio of TG to cholesterol in VLDL.

In practice, the Friedewald calculation is reasonably accurate, but Friedewald and colleagues outlined several well-known conditions in which it cannot be used. First, the calculation is precluded in samples that have TG concentrations above 400 mg/dL (4.5 mmol/L) or in those that contain increased quantities of chylomicrons (nonfasting specimens). At high TG concentrations, the factor (TG)/5 as an estimate of VLDL-C is not appropriate because such samples also contain chylomicrons, chylomicron remnants, or VLDL remnants, all of which have higher TG/TC ratios. Under these circumstances, use of the factor (TG)/5 overestimates VLDL-C and therefore underestimates LDL-C. The Friedewald equation has been found to be most accurate in samples with TG concentrations below 200 mg/dL (2.26 mmol/L), and the

error becomes unacceptably large at TG concentrations greater than 400 mg/dL (4.52 mmol/L).[256] That said, for the majority of random nonfasting samples the Friedewald equation works equally well as when using fasting samples.[1]

The opposite error can occur if the Friedewald equation is used in patients with type III hyperlipoproteinemia, which is characterized by the presence of β-VLDL not normally present in the blood. Biochemically, as its name implies, β-VLDL occurs in the VLDL density range but has β mobility on electrophoresis and is much richer in cholesterol than usual VLDL, with a ratio of TG to TC of the order of 3:1. Application of the factor (TG)/5 in patients with type III hyperlipidemia would underestimate VLDL-C and overestimate LDL-C. Fortunately, both of these conditions are uncommon. The 95th percentile for fasting plasma TG in the United States is below 300 mg/dL (3.4 mmol/L), indicating that only a small percentage of specimens will exceed the 400 mg/dL (4.5 mmol/L) cutoff. Plasma from fasting subjects usually does not contain any chylomicrons; even if present, chylomicrons can be observed visually as a floating "cream" layer in samples that have been allowed to stand undisturbed at 4 °C overnight. Finally, the prevalence of type III hyperlipoproteinemia in the general population is only about 1 to 2 per 1000 persons. On the other hand, as treatments for hyperlipidemia become more effective and more common, patients with very low concentrations of cholesterol are increasingly encountered. In this instance, LDL-C is severely underestimated.[256,257] Recent guidelines have acknowledged these limitations of Friedewald estimated LDL-C and endorsed the use of newer calculations for LDL-C.

Martin-Hopkins equation. Analysis of greater than 1.3 million fasting patient samples with TG less than 400 mg/dL reported a median TG to VLDL-C ratio of 5.2 (IQR 4.7 to 6.0).[258] The range of ratios spanned from 0.4 to 145 and were dependent on both TG and non–HDL-C concentrations. The Martin-Hopkins equation is similar to the Friedewald equation, but it substitutes a variable in the denominator for estimating the VLDL-C.

$$LDL\text{-}C = TC - HDL\text{-}C - \frac{TG}{X} \qquad \textbf{(Eq. 36.7)}$$

The value for X is determined by an empirically derived table with 180 cells which adjusts for TG values up to 400 mg/dL and non–HDL-C between 100 and 220 mg/dL. Using many different VLDL-C factors provides slightly more accurate LDL-C estimations. However, the VLDL-C and LDL-C values used to derive the equation were measured using a vertical auto-spin method, which is known to underestimate TG-rich lipoprotein cholesterol.[259,260] Overall, the Martin-Hopkins equation is an improvement over the Friedewald equation, but does not fully correct for the inaccuracies attributable to estimated LDL-C.[261] Nevertheless, some clinical laboratories have acquired licenses to use this proprietary equation.

Sampson-NIH equation. Another recently published equation was derived using samples measured by ß-quantification with a high frequency of extremely elevated TG. After mathematically fitting the VLDL-C as a function of TG and non–HDL-C, the new equation was able to replicate the empirically defined table on which the Martin-Hopkins equation is based. However, the use of a continuous equation with non–HDL-C and TG as inputs avoids disjointed values occasionally observed using the 180-cell table. A more generalizable estimate was developed by the National Institutes of Health (NIH) using this approach.[262]

$$LDL\text{-}C = \frac{TC}{0.948} - \frac{HDL\text{-}C}{0.971} - \left(\frac{TG}{8.54} + \frac{TG \times non\text{-}HDL\text{-}C}{2140} - \frac{TG^2}{16,100} \right) - 9.44$$

(36.8)

The use of continuous variables rather than a delimited table provides the NIH equation superior comparability to measured LDL-C methods at TG concentrations up to 800 mg/dL (9.1 mmol/L) and at LDL-C less than 70 mg/dL (<1.8 mmol/L).

It should be noted that, historically, all calculated LDL-C was derived using the Friedewald equation. However, some laboratories provide additional values calculated by other equations. Therefore estimated LDL-C results from different institutions can no longer be assumed to be identical.

Following the approaches used with homogeneous methods for HDL-C, similar homogeneous assays have also been developed to measure LDL-C. For example, at least seven homogeneous LDL-C methods are commercially available (see Box 36.4), which differ by containing different detergents and other chemicals, allowing specific blocking or solubilization of lipoprotein classes to achieve specificity for LDL. Most suppliers offer kits with two reagents which are readily adaptable to most clinical chemistry analyzers.[254]

Sugiuchi and colleagues developed the first homogeneous method for measuring LDL-C, a reagent distributed by Kyowa Medex (Tokyo, Japan) and Roche Diagnostics (Indianapolis, Indiana, USA). With this method, LDL-C was directly measured by suppressing the other lipoproteins (other methods suppressed LDL first and then reacted with other lipoproteins before determining LDL-C). The method was formulated in two reagents. The first had $MgCl_2$, dye, buffer (pH 6.75), and α-cyclodextrin sulfate, which has a highly concentrated negative charge to mask cholesterol in chylomicrons and VLDL in the presence of Mg ions. The second reagent included the enzymes cholesterol oxidase and cholesterol esterase, peroxidase, dye, buffer (pH 6.75), and a polyoxyethylene-polyoxypropylene polyether (POE-POP) to block cholesterol, especially in HDL. The molecular mass of POP in the POE-POP molecule and the hydrophobicity index determine its selectivity to LDL; 3850 Da was demonstrated to be optimum.

A second method by Sekisui Medical Co. (Tokyo, Japan; formerly Daiichi Pure Chemicals) was also a two-reagent system. The first reagent, containing ascorbic acid oxidase, 4-aminoantipyrine, peroxidase, cholesterol oxidase, cholesterol esterase, buffer (pH 6.3), and a detergent, solubilizes all non-LDL lipoproteins, and allows reaction of their cholesterol with the esterase and oxidase enzymes, forming a colorless product. The second reagent, containing N,N′-bis-(4-sulfobutyl)-m-toluidine Na_2 (DSBmT), buffer (pH 6.3), and a detergent, specifically releases LDL-C. Hydrogen peroxide generated is reacted with N,N′-bis-(4-sulfobutyl)-M-toluidine disodium salt to yield a colored product.

A third method (Wako Pure Chemicals) consists of a reagent containing Good's buffer (pH 6.8) (N-[2-hydroxy-3-sulfopropyl]-3,5-dimethoxyaniline, sodium salt), cholesterol esterase, cholesterol oxidase, catalase, polyanions, and amphoteric surfactants that selectively protect LDL from enzymatic reaction. The non–LDL-C reacts with esterase and oxidase, producing hydrogen peroxide, which is consumed by catalase.

The second reagent includes Good's buffer (pH 7.0), 4-aminoantipyrene, peroxidase, sodium azide, and a deprotecting reagent which allows the protecting agent from LDL, and enables its cholesterol to react with cholesterol esterase and cholesterol oxidase, producing hydrogen peroxide and a blue color complex.

Non–LDL-C is removed by a fourth method (Denka Seiken, Niigata, Japan; Polymedco Inc., Cortlandt Manor, NY) via a selective reaction with cholesterol oxidase and cholesterol esterase, with the resulting peroxide by-product eliminated by reaction with catalase (CAT). In this two-reagent method, the first reagent contains $MgCl_2$, cholesterol esterase, cholesterol oxidase, catalase, N-(2-hydroxy-3-sulfopropyl)-3,5-dimethoxyaniline sodium salt, and Emulgen 66 (polyoxyethylene compound; Kao) and Emulgen 90 (both nonionic surfactants) in Good's buffer (PIPES; 100 mmol/L; pH 7.0). Its second reagent contains peroxidase, 4-aminoantipyrine, sodium azide (to inhibit the catalase), and Triton X-100 in Good's buffer. The hydrophilic/lipophilic balance of the detergents is adjusted to obtain appropriate selectivity to the lipoproteins.[263]

In a fifth method (International Reagents Corp., Kokusai-Kobe, Japan), its first reagent contains the detergent calixarene, which converts LDL to a soluble complex. Cholesterol esters of HDL-C and VLDL-C are preferentially hydrolyzed by a cholesterol esterase (chromobacterium), cholesterol oxidase, and hydrazine, which transforms the accessible cholesterol to cholestenone hydrazone. A second reagent with deoxycholate breaks up the LDL-calixarene complex, allowing LDL-C to react with the esterase, a dehydrogenase, and β-NAD to yield cholestenone and β-NADH.

Analytical performance of low-density lipoprotein-cholesterol methods. Evaluations of LDL-C homogeneous assays indicate that the coefficient of variations (CVs) are generally less than 3% and consistently within the NCEP performance target of less than 4% CV (Table 36.21).[253,263] By contrast, the CV for the Friedewald calculation has been estimated to approximate 4% in expert laboratories but may be higher in routine clinical laboratories. With regard to accuracy, all of the homogeneous assays have qualified for certification through the CRMLN program, suggesting agreement with reference methods, at least in relatively normal specimens. Nevertheless, as indicated previously for HDL-C methods, many different instrument applications are available, and not all have been evaluated for bias. Factors, such as lot-to-lot differences, unique calibrations by distributors, different calibrations from country to country, and reformulations of reagents might affect actual biases. More importantly, method-dependent biases have been reported for all commercially available assays in dyslipidemic samples.[253,263]

Current homogeneous assays for LDL-C work relatively well on normolipidemic samples but are reported to be frequently discordant compared with the reference β-quantification procedure for patients with dyslipidemias.[253,264] Overall, these studies suggest that homogeneous assays interact unequally with different components of the "broad-cut LDL": LDL subclasses, IDL, Lp(a), and Lp-X.[54] A 2002 study of two homogeneous reagents using isolated lipoprotein fractions confirmed the lack of specificity for VLDL and LDL subclasses.[263] The two homogeneous methods included about 20% of isolated VLDL. Also, the reagents missed about 30% of IDL and up to 50% of isolated LDL fractions, especially the smaller subclasses. Through compensating errors, the inclusion of some VLDL could offset the

TABLE 36.21 Analytical Performance of Homogeneous Low-Density Lipoprotein Cholesterol Assays

| | Imprecision, CVs | Dynamic Range, mg/L | RECOVERY, % | | | ACCURACY | |
			LDL-C	VLDL-C	IDL-C	Bias, %	Bias, mg/L
Kyowa	0.7–3.1	2–4,100	97–105	16	52–64	0.8–11.2	−60 to −80
Daiichi	<3.1	4–10,000	87	19	31–47	3.9–5.1	−48 to −80
Wako	≤1.2	10–3,000	—	—	—	0.4	215
Denka	<1.8	70–5,500	95	10	31	—	—
IRC	≤0.6	?–4,000	—	—	—	—	—

CV, Coefficient of variation; *IDL-C*, intermediate-density lipoprotein cholesterol, *LDL-C*, low-density lipoprotein cholesterol; *VLDL-C*, very-low-density lipoprotein cholesterol.

loss of LDL fractions, so the overall lack of specificity may not be obvious in relatively normal specimens. However, lack of specificity for lipoprotein subclasses and differences among reagents can cause substantial errors in some specimens, depending on the particular lipoprotein profile and the particular reagent characteristics.

Spiking studies, in which potential interfering substances are added to a sample, have demonstrated that these methods are not subject to significant interference from bilirubin and hemoglobin. However, higher concentrations of TG have been shown to interfere, thus increasing apparent LDL-C; this is not surprising given the reported lack of specificity for LDL and the inclusion of some VLDL in the measurement. On the other hand, the sulfated α-cyclodextrin used in the Sugiuchi assay to block VLDL-C appeared to cause underestimation of LDL-C.[265]

An often-cited advantage of homogeneous methods may be the ability to use nonfasting specimens. Results, judged by mean differences between paired fasting and nonfasting specimens, were promising, but patient classifications were inaccurate with nonfasting specimens.[266] Lipoprotein composition is affected by recent diet; changes have been observed even with the more robust ultracentrifugation method. However, as stated elsewhere in this chapter, the impact of nonfasting does not alter estimated LDL-C to a clinically significant degree.

Other considerations in adopting an LDL-C method. Clinical laboratories are faced with the decision of whether to implement fully automated homogeneous methods for LDL-C, either replacing all measurements or supplementing estimated LDL-C in samples with TG above 400 mg/dL (4.5 mmol/L; Friedewald and Martin-Hopkins equations) or 800 mg/dL (9.1 mmol/L; NIH equation). The considerations are certainly not as compelling for homogeneous LDL methods as for HDL. Substantially better analytical performance, cost-effectiveness, or patient care have yet to be shown for homogeneous LDL methods, particularly when considering the new estimations that allow for nonfasting specimens and elevated TG.

Lipoprotein subclasses. Several approaches have been used to quantitate lipoprotein subclasses. Density-based subfractionation by analytical ultracentrifugation was among the earliest methods for characterization of lipoprotein subclasses.[267] However, the method is tedious and is not widely used except for research purposes. Importantly, no gold-standard method for lipoprotein subclassification, nor consensus

POINTS TO REMEMBER

Low-Density Lipoproteins
- LDL is a causative factor of ASCVD.
- ApoB-100 is the main protein in LDL.
- LDL is removed from circulation by LDLR.
- LDL-C concentrations are typically estimated but can be directly measured using homogeneous methods.
- HMG-CoA reductase inhibitors (statins) have been the most commonly used and effective drugs in reducing LDL-C concentrations.
- Ezetimibe added to statins further reduces LDL-C.
- Proprotein convertase subtilisin/kexin type 9 (PCSK9) inhibitors have shown to be very effective in reducing LDL-C concentrations, alone or when added to statins +/− ezetimibe.

nomenclature defining small versus large lipoproteins exists. Despite these limitations, several methods are commercially available and often used by lipid experts to determine treatment strategies.

Adequate resolution for determination of lipoprotein subclasses can be achieved in polyacrylamide gradient gels. Separation of LDL by polyacrylamide gradient gel electrophoresis was one of the first widely available methods to quantitate small versus large LDL particles.[268,269] Electrophoresis separates primarily on size (and to a lesser extent by charge), which deviates from the benchmark ultracentrifugation method separated on density. However, gel-electrophoresis is readily implemented in clinical laboratories allowing commercialization of kit-based systems. Gel electrophoresis techniques claimed to distinguish up to seven unique size categories for LDL.[270] In practice however, most labs only report a binary, small or large, classification system. According to the seminal work by Austin and Krauss in 1986, subjects with a majority of LDL particles migrating at bands ≥25.5 nm were considered Pattern A. Subjects with smaller LDL particles were considered Pattern B.[271]

Lack of standardization among commercial gel electrophoresis systems resulted in a wide variation of classification patterns of a given patient depending on the LDL subfractionation method used. Classification according to Pattern A or B was discrepant in as many as 76% of cases; the definition of small LDL varied between less than 25.5 nm and less than 26.8 nm for different methods.[272,273]

Density gradient ultracentrifugation is also used to characterize lipoprotein subclasses; it is performed in a vertical rotor with measurement of cholesterol continuously in fractions eluted from the gradient.[260] Mathematical curve deconvolution derives the component lipoprotein profiles and allows calculation of their concentrations in terms of cholesterol or other constituents. The method can determine the concentrations of cholesterol in VLDL, IDL, LDL, Lp(a), and HDL. LDL-C subclasses can be expressed separately or can be combined to obtain a measurement like that provided by the Friedewald equation or by β-quantification. A disadvantage may be that the procedure is technically demanding and requires instrumentation not usually available in routine clinical laboratories.

Nuclear magnetic resonance (NMR) spectroscopy detects protons in lipoprotein-associated fatty acyl methyl or methylene groups. Signals from subfractions of VLDL, IDL, LDL, and HDL vary by particle size and can be resolved mathematically through deconvolution based on calibration samples with values reported in terms of numbers of lipoprotein particles. A sample can be analyzed quickly using a small volume of serum or plasma. Several commercial manufacturers now offer systems for clinical laboratory lipid analysis. The different-size lipoprotein fractions can be aggregated to calculate LDL-P and HDL-P, which in several studies have been shown to be superior to using LDL-C and HDL-C as CVD risk biomarkers.[274]

Recently, a new MS technique based on airborne ion mobility has also been developed for measuring total lipoprotein subfractions.[275] An automated method for determining the small, dense fraction of LDL has also been described.[276] This homogeneous direct method for small, dense LDL-C is the first FDA-approved method for small LDL.[277,278]

Univariate analysis suggests some of these methods to be superior to conventional lipid and lipoprotein tests for ASCVD risk prediction. However, lack of independent predictive information when considered in models with TC or LDL-C has been repeatedly cited in many consensus documents.[128,270,279]

No medical society has endorsed the use of lipoprotein subfractions. The National Lipid Association, the National Academic of Clinical Biochemistry, the ACC, and the AHA have all published guidelines specifically recommending against the routine use of LDL subfractions.[280–282] The guidelines cite a lack of sufficient evidence to support LDL subfraction measurement for initial clinical assessment or on-treatment management decisions.

Remnant cholesterol (TG-rich lipoprotein cholesterol) Remnant lipoproteins include the lipolytic products of catabolism of the TG-rich lipoproteins, VLDL and chylomicrons, occurring in the VLDL density range. Since LPL begins degrading TG in both chylomicrons and VLDL immediately as they enter the plasma, all TG-rich lipoproteins in the plasma of most individuals can be considered remnants. Remnant lipoprotein cholesterol (RC), also referred to as TG-rich lipoprotein cholesterol (TRL-C) can be calculated as:

$$RC = TRL\text{-}C = TC\text{-}HDL\text{-}C - LDL\text{-}C \qquad (36.9)$$

These measures can all be based on directly measured TC, HDL-C, and LDL-C. LDL-C can also be calculated as described in Eqs. (36.6, 36.7, or 36.8). Elevated calculated remnant cholesterol is causally associated with increased risk of ASCVD (Fig. 36.19) and all-cause mortality, independent of LDL-C and Lp(a) concentrations.[224,283–285]

Corresponding to calculated remnant cholesterol, an assay for directly measured remnant cholesterol was recently devel-

oped by Denka Seiken.[286] This automated homogeneous assay uses a two-step process where first LDL and HDL are degraded and second the cholesterol content of the remaining remnants is measured. The assay is traceable to the cholesterol content in the ultracentrifugation density fraction less than 1.019 g/mL contained in the nonfasting state chylomicron remnants, VLDL, and IDL. Using this assay of remnant cholesterol, elevated concentrations were associated independent of LDL-C with increased risk of ASCVD.[277]

POINTS TO REMEMBER

Remnant Cholesterol
- Remnant cholesterol is defined as cholesterol carried in TG-rich lipoproteins.
- Remnant cholesterol is causally related to ASCVD.
- Remnant cholesterol is all the cholesterol *not* contained in HDL, LDL, and Lp(a).
- Remnant cholesterol can be calculated as total cholesterol minus HDL and LDL-C (latter includes Lp(a) cholesterol).
- A direct homogeneous assay for remnant cholesterol (TG-rich lipoprotein cholesterol) has been developed.

Sources of Variation in Lipid and Lipoprotein Measurements

Lipid and lipoprotein concentrations vary within individuals when measured on several occasions over time. Sources of variation can be broadly categorized as analytical and physiologic or preanalytical. Analytical variations are inherent in the measurements themselves and arise from sample collection procedures, volume measurements, instrument function, reagent formulations, uncertainty in the assignment of values to calibration materials, and other such factors. Normal physiologic variation occurs independently of analytical error and reflects actual changes in concentration that occur through the course of normal, day-to-day living. Such variations result from factors such as change in posture, which causes the redistribution of water between vascular and nonvascular spaces, thereby changing the concentrations of nondiffusible plasma components.[287]

Recent food intake produces transient increases in plasma TG up to 50% or greater and decreases of up to 10 to 15% in LDL-C and HDL-C, depending on the fat content of the meal.[288] However, fasting for more than 8 hours, as previously required for lipid profiles, normally only occurs a few hours before breakfast. In contrast, the nonfasting state predominates most of a 24-hour cycle and better captures the amount of atherogenic lipoproteins in plasma.[1,4] The maximal mean changes for random, nonfasting versus fasting concentrations are +26 mg/dL (0.3 mmol/L) for TG, −8 mg/dL (0.2 mmol/L) for TC, −8 mg/dL (0.2 mmol/L) for LDL cholesterol, +8 mg/dL (0.2 mmol/L) for remnant cholesterol, and −8 mg/dL (0.2 mmol/L) for non–HDL-C, while Lp(a), apoB and HDL-C are largely unaffected.[1]

Seasonal changes in lipids and lipoproteins have also been observed, probably resulting from changes in dietary and exercise patterns throughout the year.[289] Normal physiologic variations tend to occur in both directions, causing lipid or lipoprotein concentrations to vary somewhat about a mean value for a particular patient. Other kinds of physiologic conditions cause changes from the patient's usual steady-state concentrations—for example, acute illness, stress, pregnancy, or dietary changes that result in weight loss or gain, changes in saturated fat intake, or the effects of treatment with lipid-lowering medications. In these cases, changes tend to occur in one direction, and they are not considered normal physiologic fluctuations. Lipoprotein concentrations eventually return to original steady-state concentrations when the patient recovers, or a new steady state is achieved.

Because normal physiologic variations occur, it is difficult to evaluate a patient based on a single measurement that applies only to the current sample or status. It is more appropriate to consider the patient's usual range of concentrations and his or her average steady-state concentration. From the laboratory's standpoint, the aim is to provide accurate measurements in the particular sample being measured. For this reason, the laboratory is primarily concerned with minimizing analytical error. From the physician's standpoint, however, the goal is to establish the patient's usual range of concentrations during a 24-hour period for determining the diagnosis and the effects of therapy. This aim is affected primarily by physiologic variation because this variation contributes the larger proportion of the sample-to-sample variation observed in serial samples collected from the same patient. Some sources of physiologic variation, such as posture during blood sampling, can be controlled; other factors that cannot be controlled, such as pregnancy, should be considered in interpreting laboratory results.

Analytical Variation

Table 36.22 illustrates the current overall variation of lipid and lipoprotein measurements in more than 100 laboratories participating in an accuracy-based survey conducted by the College of American Pathologists. In this survey, fresh frozen serum is sent to participating laboratories, and the results are compared with the reference method when available. The results of TC meet the NCEP error goal for bias and imprecision. The average bias was in the range of −1.18 to 0.29%, and CVs less than 3%. These numbers represent the sum of within- and among-laboratory components of variation and suggest that reliable cholesterol measurements can be provided by most clinical laboratories. Similarly, the overall bias and precision of various TG assays were relatively good. For HDL-C, most participants used one of the current direct assays, and the average bias slightly exceeded the NCEP-recommended bias of 5% or less; the mean CV of the assays also slightly exceeded the 4% or less goal for imprecision. Results for LDL-C were not presented because freezing the serum was found to affect the commutability of the material, but the performance of the direct LDL-C assay is comparable with that of the direct HDL-C assay, suggesting the need for improvement. It is important to note that the performance of direct HDL-C and LDL-C assays may not be as good in patients with dyslipidemias or other conditions that may affect the specificity of assays for the lipoprotein being measured.

Physiologic Variation

The normal physiologic component of variation is calculated from the total variation of measurements in serial specimens from the same patients, after adjustment for analytical variation. Such estimates differ somewhat from study to study, but after

TABLE 36.22 Analytical Variation of Lipid and Lipoprotein Measurements[a]

Analyte	ABL-01/2009	ABL-02/2009	ABL-03/2009
Cholesterol			
Number of laboratories	135	135	134
Mean, mg/dL	150.8	179.2	244.9
CV, %	2.1	2.2	1.8
CDC value	152.6	180.0	244.2
% Bias	−1.18	−0.44	0.29
HDL-C			
Number of laboratories	134	133	135
Mean, mg/dL	31.7	56.6	49.2
CV, %	4.6	3.8	4.7
CDC value	33.9	56.8	49.3
% Bias	−6.49	−0.35	−0.20
	ABL-04/2008	ABL-05/2008	ABL-06/2008
Triglyceride			
Number of laboratories	142	141	142
Mean, mg/dL	88.8	204.8	225.7
CV, %	3.2	2.4	2.3
CDC value	91	202.5	223.6
% Bias	−2.42	1.14	0.94

[a]Bias calculated as: (Test mean − CDC value/CDC value) × 100.
CDC, Centers for Disease Control and Prevention measurement done with reference method; CV, coefficient of variation; HDL-C, high-density lipoprotein cholesterol.
Data from College of American Pathologists Chemistry Survey, Northfield, Ill, 2009.

TABLE 36.23 Physiologic Variation in Lipid and Lipoprotein Concentrations in Serial Specimens from the Same Individual

Component	Physiologic Variation, % CV	Percentage of Variance Contributed by Physiologic Variation[a]
Total cholesterol	6.5	91
Triglyceride	23.7	98
HDL cholesterol	7.5	69
LDL cholesterol	8.2	81

[a]Assuming the following analytical CVs: total cholesterol, 2%; triglyceride, 3%; HDL cholesterol, 5%; LDL cholesterol, 4%.
CV, Coefficient of variation; HDL, high-density lipoprotein; LDL, low-density lipoprotein.

an extensive review of the literature, the NCEP panels concerned with lipid and lipoprotein measurement assumed average physiologic CVs (Table 36.23). A wide variety of factors contribute to physiologic variations (Table 36.24).[290] Physiologic variations observed for cholesterol, HDL-C, and LDL-C are similar. Physiologic variation for TG is considerably higher because fasting TG concentrations can vary widely in an individual. Because the analytical CVs for these assays are relatively small, it can be calculated, and on average, physiologic variations contribute about 70 to 98% of the overall variance of

TABLE 36.24   Representative Preanalytical Sources of Variation (Including Biological)

	TC	HDL-C	TG	LDL-C
Intraindividual biological variation of healthy individuals (coefficient of variation)	6.5%	7.5%	23.7%	8.2%
Sampling				
Nonfasting	NC	−	++	−
Prolonged total fasting	++	−	+	+
Posture from standing to:				
Supine	−	− −	− −	− −
Sitting	−	−	−	−
Anticoagulants from serum:				
Plasma	−	−	−	−
Behavioral				
Diet				
Saturated fatty acids (palmitic acid)	+	NC	+	+
Monounsaturated fatty acids	−	NC	−	−
Polyunsaturated fatty acids	− −	−	NC	− −
Cholesterol intake	+	NC	NC	+
Fish oil	NC	NC	−	NC
Obesity	+	−	++	+
Smoking	+	−	++	+
Exercise (strenuous)	−	+	−	−
Alcohol intake	+	+	++	−
Clinical Sources				
Myocardial infarction				
24 hours	NC	NC	NC	NC
6 weeks	−	−	NC	−
Stroke	−	NC	NC	−
Hypertension	+	−	++	+
Nephrosis	++	NC	++	++
Diabetes (insulin resistance)	+	−	++	++
Infections	−	−	++	−
Pregnancy, second trimester	+	NC	++	+
Transplantation				
Cyclosporine	++	−	+	++
Prednisone	+	−	++	+

HDL-C, High-density lipoprotein cholesterol; *LDL-C,* low-density lipoprotein cholesterol; *NC,* essentially no change or trend; *TC,* total cholesterol; *TG,* triglycerides; +, minimal to moderate increase; ++, moderate to high increase; −, minimal to moderate decrease; − −, moderate to high decrease.

TABLE 36.25   National Cholesterol Education Program Recommendations for Analytical Performance of Lipid and Lipoprotein Measurements

	Total Error, %	NCEP Bias, %	NCEP CV, %	CDC Bias,[a,b]	CDC CV[b]
Cholesterol	8.9	≤±3	≤3	≤±3	≤3
Triglycerides	≤15	≤±5	≤5	≤±5	≤5
HDL-C	≤13	≤±5	≤4[c]	≤±5	≤4
LDL-C	≤12	≤±4	≤4	—	—

[a]With respect to reference values.
[b]Maximum allowable.
[c]When HDL-C <42 mg/dL, the NCEP CV criterion is SD ≤1.7.
CV, Coefficient of variation; *HDL,* high-density lipoprotein; *LDL,* low-density lipoprotein.

least 1 week apart should be used; two to three serial specimens are recommended, if feasible, for TG, HDL-C, and LDL-C.

The NCEP goals for analytical performance differ slightly from CDC standardization criteria because NCEP goals are stated in terms of total error, which reflects both bias and imprecision, whereas CDC standardization criteria consider each of them separately.[239] NCEP and CDC recommendations for total error are shown in Table 36.25.

These guidelines were established after considering degrees of accuracy and imprecision that are achievable in well-controlled research and clinical laboratories. A laboratory can approximate its conformance to the total error recommendations using the following equation:

$$\text{Total error} = \% \text{ Bias} + 1.96 \times (\text{CVa}) \quad \textbf{(36.10)}$$

where % bias is the mean laboratory difference between the measured value for a commutable serum control pool and the reference value for the pool, and CVa is the overall analytical CV for the pool, including within- and among-run variations, and calculated as follows:

$$\frac{\text{Standard deviation}}{\text{Laboratory mean}} \times 100 \quad \textbf{(36.11)}$$

Bias should be calculated as the difference from reference values rather than from manufacturers' stated values when these differ.

The individual biases and CVs shown in Table 36.25 should be viewed as examples of conditions under which the total error criteria can be met. A laboratory with less bias can tolerate slightly greater imprecision without exceeding the total error criteria. Conversely, imprecision must be lower if bias increases. For example, a laboratory operating with a bias of 3% and a CV of 3% for cholesterol would have a total error of 3% + (1.96 × 3%), or 8.9%. If, however, bias is only 1%, the CV could be as high as 4% without exceeding the criteria for total error [1% + (1.96 × 4%) = 8.8%]. (In practice, many laboratories can achieve total errors under 6%, assuming a bias of 2% and a CV of 2%.) It is important to note that the NCEP panel considered that the physicians usually do not distinguish between lipid and lipoprotein measurements on the basis of the method used to make the measurements. For this reason, NCEP guidelines do not distinguish among

lipid and lipoprotein concentrations (see Table 36.23). For this reason, a patient's usual lipid or lipoprotein concentration cannot be reliably established from a single measurement. NCEP guidelines recommend that for cholesterol, the average of measurements in two serial samples obtained at measurements made in the laboratory and those made in alternative settings with desktop analyzers or other methods.

As mentioned previously, CDC standardization criteria consider bias and imprecision separately. For this reason, each of the two criteria must be met to achieve standardization. Current CDC standardization criteria are shown in Table 36.25. NCEP guidelines are directed primarily to laboratories and users of laboratory measurements. Importantly, NCEP recommended that assay manufacturers calibrate their methods to traceable reference method values. Many manufacturers are now doing this, which probably accounts for the relatively small interlaboratory biases for TC and HDL-C, as reflected in Table 36.24.

Apolipoproteins

Apolipoproteins are measured by a wide variety of immunoassays, including ELISA, immunoturbidimetric assay, and immunonephelometric assay. The concentration of a particular apolipoprotein usually determines the technique used for its measurement.

Immunoturbidimetry and immunonephelometry are widely used to measure apoA-I and apoB, which are present at relatively high concentrations. According to the CAP Proficiency Testing Survey, all clinical laboratories in the United States that measure apoA-I and apoB use one of these two approaches. Alternatively, more sensitive techniques, such as ELISA, are perhaps more suitable for those apolipoproteins present at much lower concentrations, such as apoC-I and apoC-II. Additional considerations in apolipoprotein methods include distribution across lipoproteins, reactivity within lipoproteins, and allelic heterogeneity.[291]

ApoB, for example, is present on LDL, IDL, VLDL, and Lp(a) particles, which vary significantly in size and composition. To accurately determine the concentration of total apoB, the anti–apoB antibody used must be able to recognize apoB present on various lipoprotein classes equally and must display similar kinetic patterns with all of them.[292] Furthermore, the antigenic sites of apolipoproteins are often covered by lipids.[293,294] To have a maximal antigen-antibody interaction, these epitopes must be unmasked. Nonionic detergents are usually added to the assay buffer to disrupt the lipoprotein particles and make all of the antigenic sites on the apolipoproteins accessible to the antibodies.

Polyclonal antibodies are widely used in clinical laboratories for the measurement of plasma protein concentrations; however, immunoassays are often sensitive to the nature of the antibody used. The development of polyclonal antibodies is affected by several factors, such as the purity and dose of the antigen used, the species of host animal, and the immunization procedure. Monoclonal antibodies are viewed as a viable alternative to alleviate these problems. However, expression of particular epitopes varies with the lipoprotein particles and among individuals; in addition, the apolipoproteins themselves are polymorphic in nature. Therefore a single monoclonal antibody might not detect a particular variant. If a monoclonal antibody is used to determine an apolipoprotein, it should be directed to an epitope that is expressed on all polymorphic forms of that particular apolipoprotein. Furthermore, the epitope should be equally reactive to the antibodies, regardless of which lipoprotein class it is contained within. Alternatively, a mixture of monoclonal antibodies directed at different epitopes

of the apolipoprotein may be used. Such mixtures are referred to as *panmonoclonal* antibodies.

Finally, to standardize a particular protein, a purified form of that protein is necessary as a primary calibrator. However, the purified preparation must express the same immunoreactivity as the native protein. Unfortunately, once removed from its natural milieu, apoB is insoluble in aqueous buffers. This phenomenon is attributed to the very hydrophobic nature of apoB. An LDL preparation with density of 1.030 to 1.050 g/mL, often referred to as *narrow-cut* LDL, is generally used as the primary standard for apoB. The protein concentration of the purified preparation is determined by amino acid analysis. In contrast, freshly purified apoA-I is soluble in aqueous buffers and is suitable as a primary standard.

Considerable effort has been expended over the past decade by national and international organizations in overcoming the problems of apoA-I and apoB analysis standardization.[295] The Committee on Apolipoproteins of the International Federation of Clinical Chemistry (IFCC) embarked on an ambitious international collaborative study aimed at developing secondary serum reference materials that can be used, without influence of matrix bias effects, as master calibrators for all current commercial assays.[296] This program has now been successfully completed. A lyophilized serum preparation for apoA-I, designated SP1-01, and a liquid-stabilized serum preparation for apoB, designated SP3-07, have been approved as international reference materials by the World Health Organization (WHO). An apoA-I value of 150 mg/dL was assigned to SP1-01 by a highly standardized RIA calibrated with purified apoA-I for which the mass value had been determined by amino acid analysis. An accuracy-based apoB value of 122 mg/dL was assigned to SP3-07 using a nephelometric method that was calibrated with freshly isolated LDL, for which the apoB-100 mass value was determined by a standardized sodium dodecyl sulfate–Lowry protein procedure.

The WHO and the IFCC have appointed the CDC to be the repository for the WHO-IFCC First International Reference Reagents for apoA-I and apoB-100. Northwest Lipid Research Laboratories (NWLRL) in Seattle uses an IFCC calibration protocol to conduct the standardization and distribution program for manufacturers of instruments and reagents. This protocol involves establishing the linearity of dose response, the parallelism of kinetic responses of standards and calibration sera, the equality of intercepts for the reference materials, and an analysis of fresh frozen sera. NWLRL can be contacted for standardization services and the distribution of apolipoprotein reference materials. These reference materials are also available for reference laboratories in countries where standardized commercial methods are not readily available. It has been shown that through the use of these international reference materials, the analytical performance of apoA-I and apoB measurement, in terms of accuracy and precision, is superior to that of HDL-C and LDL-C. This effort has demonstrated that the use of certified reference materials can significantly reduce the bias of apoA-I and apoB measurements by different immunotechniques. However, an external quality assurance program using fresh or fresh frozen samples and WHO-IFCC–based value assignments is indispensable in monitoring the performance of clinical chemistry laboratories and manufacturers to ensure that accurate apolipoprotein measurements are made. The NWLRL conducts a quarterly standardization program or

Reference Lipoprotein Analysis Basic Survey, which provides the accuracy base for TC, TG, HDL-C, LDL-C, and apoA-I and apoB. To minimize matrix effects, the survey uses fresh human serum and leads to certification of traceability to the national reference system for cholesterol and to the WHO-IFCC International Reference Reagents for apoA-I and apoB-100.

Apolipoprotein measurements have been shown to further aid in the assessment of ASCVD risk and the diagnosis of hyperlipoproteinemia. For example, measurement of apoB provides a reliable clinical tool by which to identify subjects with increased risk for CHD who may not be readily identified by conventional cholesterol or lipoprotein cholesterol measurements (e.g., subjects with a borderline elevation of LDL-C, subjects with hypertriglyceridemia without an LDL-C elevation).[297] In addition, apoB measurements can assess whether lipid-lowering drugs are effective in reducing the number of atherogenic apoB–containing lipoproteins.[298] However, for apolipoprotein measurements to be used in routine clinical practice, clinically meaningful cutoff values for clinical decision making need to be established, and more information regarding their clinical utility is needed. The use of cutoff values for apoA-I and apoB-100, similar to those recommended by the NCEP for HDL-C and LDL-C, respectively, has been suggested. An apoA-I concentration less than 120 mg/dL may be associated with increased risk of CHD, whereas apoA-I of 160 mg/dL or greater may be protective. Current guidelines endorse an apoB cut point of 130 mg/dL, approximately corresponding to the LDL-C cut point of 160 mg/dL, which falls at approximately the 75th percentile.[110] Canadian and European guidelines use apoB less than 80 mg/dL and less than 65 mg/dL, respectively, as secondary treatment goals after achieving LDL-C goals (see Table 36.20).[111,112]

Lipoprotein(a)

The structural heterogeneity of Lp(a) as a consequence of apo(a) size heterogeneity has important implications for the accurate measurement of Lp(a) in human plasma.[43] Repeated antigenic determinants are present in variable numbers in different Lp(a) particles, and the immunoreactivity of the antibodies directed to these repeated epitopes can vary as a function of apo(a) size. As a consequence, immunoassays using polyclonal antibodies or monoclonal antibodies specifically directed to kringle 4 type 2 epitopes will tend to underestimate apo(a) concentration in samples with apo(a) of smaller size than the apo(a) present in the assay calibrator and will tend to overestimate the apo(a) concentration in samples with larger apo(a). A detailed evaluation of the effect of apo(a) size heterogeneity on measurement of Lp(a) has been reported.[299,300] Monoclonal antibody–based assays have the theoretical advantage that the antibodies can be immunochemically characterized and preselected on the basis of their specificity to single epitopes (e.g., those not located in kringle 4 type 2 domain).

Assays are used to measure Lp(a) in turbidimetric, nephelometric, radiometric, and enzymatic methods. Most of these assays, except for enzyme immunoassay (ELISA), are based on the use of polyclonal antibodies from various animal species. Commercially available, direct-binding, sandwich-type ELISAs are usually based on the use of a combination of monoclonal and polyclonal antibodies. One approach takes advantage of the presence of both apo(a) and apoB in Lp(a) particles. In this approach, Lp(a) particles are "captured" using a polyclonal or monoclonal antibody to apo(a), and an enzyme-conjugated antibody to apoB is used as the detection antibody. An ELISA method based on this approach has been described and is commercially available.[301]

In another approach, both capture and detection antibodies are specific for apo(a). At present, it is not clear which approach would be better with respect to estimating the risk for CHD or stroke because the pathogenic mechanisms involved have not yet been elucidated. Thus it is not known whether the risk is associated simply with an increased number of Lp(a) particles in the circulation (as measured using an anti–apoB antibody) or is also related to the presence of polyforms of a particular size (as might be detected more readily with anti-apo(a) detection antibodies). It is likely that both factors influence the risk.

Historically, Lp(a) concentrations have been reported in terms of total Lp(a) particle mass or, alternatively, in terms of Lp(a) protein. If the aim is to provide Lp(a) values that are independent of apo(a) size, it is recommended that the Lp(a) assay use antibodies directed to an apo(a) domain other than kringle 4 type 2 or to the apoB component of Lp(a). This would allow the values to be expressed in nanomoles per liter (nmol/L). Pan-monoclonal mixtures of antibodies to kringle 4 type 2 may be preferred if particular sizes of polyforms contribute to the risk.[43]

At present, Lp(a) measurements are not well standardized, and most Lp(a) assays have not been evaluated for their apo(a) size sensitivity. As a result, Lp(a) values reported in clinical studies are difficult to compare. Despite this, a value of about 30 mg/dL of total Lp(a) particle mass has traditionally been used as a cutoff, above which elevated concentrations of Lp(a) are associated with increased risk of CHD. Lp(a) concentrations can also be expressed in terms of particle number and mass of apo(a), apoB, or Lp(a) cholesterol. At present, Lp(a) values are most commonly expressed in terms of total Lp(a) mass.

In view of the current lack of reference methods or standardization procedures for Lp(a), it is difficult to define precise cutoffs that can be used to make clinical decisions. Although less than ideal, one approach would be to establish a reference interval for each assay and report individual results in terms of percentile values within these intervals. In whites, patients with Lp(a) values above the 80th percentile can be considered at increased risk for coronary atherosclerosis. However, because Lp(a) values can vary among ethnic groups, reference values need to be population based. Furthermore, such cutoffs may have to be racially specific. For example, African Americans in general have significantly higher Lp(a) concentrations than whites, but they may not manifest a higher incidence of CHD. An IFCC committee, using an approach similar to that of the apoA-I and apoB committee, developed reference materials that can be used with all commercially available Lp(a) methods. As expected, the use of a common calibrator led to improved harmonization of Lp(a) results but not complete standardization. Only when appropriate antibodies are used can standardization be achieved.

Virtually all retrospective case-control studies, large prospective population-based studies, and large genetic studies in whites have reported a strong association between increased Lp(a) and the risk of CHD (Fig. 36.19), aortic valve stenosis, and even all-cause mortality.[120,121,193,302] As such, elevated Lp(a) is considered a causal risk factor for ASCVD just like elevated LDL and remnant cholesterol.

Several studies have suggested that apo(a)-size isoforms may be related to a high prevalence of CHD (see earlier discussion). The procedure with the greatest resolution and sensitivity for determination of apo(a) phenotypes involves separation of apo(a) on agarose gel electrophoresis, immunoblotting with a specific antibody, and detection with radiolabeled protein A. This approach identifies at least 34 apo(a) polymorphs. It can be used to express apo(a) size in terms of kringle number and is consistent with observations on the size variation of the apo(a) gene obtained by pulsed-field gel electrophoresis and genomic blotting.[303] Using DNA-based methods, the sum of kringle 4 type 2 on the two alleles can also be used based on real-time polymerase chain reaction (PCR) methods.[304]

POINTS TO REMEMBER

Lipoprotein(a)
- Lp(a) is largely genetically determined where 20% of Whites have values above 50 mg/dL.
- Blacks have higher Lp(a) values than Whites, while Hispanics and south Asians have intermediate values and east Asians have values similar to Whites.
- Elevated Lp(a) is a causal risk factor for ASCVD, aortic stenosis, and all-cause mortality.
- Lp(a) is traditionally measured in mg/dL while ideally it should be measured in nmol/L due to large interindividual size heterogeneity from kringle IV type 2.

Apolipoprotein E

As discussed earlier, homozygosity for apoE$_2$ is characteristic of type III familial hyperlipoproteinemia. Homozygosity for apoE$_2$ is a necessary factor but is not solely sufficient for expression of the clinical phenotype of type III hyperlipoproteinemia (a.k.a. remnant hyperlipidemia or dysbetalipoproteinemia); a second gene defect or condition appears to be required to cause the characteristic hyperlipidemia. Heterozygosity for some rare apoE mutants may also be associated with type III hyperlipoproteinemia. The study of apoE variants has assumed greater importance in the last few years because of the association between the apoE$_4$ allele and dementia.[305]

Traditionally, the determination of apoE isoforms was assessed by isoelectric focusing (IEF) techniques. However, current genotyping techniques readily and accurately identify variations in the nucleotide sequence of the apoE gene and have become standard of care, despite some reported discrepancies between results of phenotyping.[305]

OTHER CARDIAC RISK FACTORS

Despite the strong association of lipid concentrations with CHD risk, it has long been recognized that half of all myocardial infarctions occur among individuals without overt hyperlipidemia. In the Women's Health Study (WHS), for example, 77% of future cardiovascular events occurred among those with LDL-C concentrations less than 160 mg/dL (4.1 mmol/L), and 46% occurred among those with LDL-C less than 130 mg/dL (3.4 mmol/L).[306] Furthermore, in another analysis of more than 120,000 patients, approximately 20% of all coronary events occurred in the absence of any of the major classical risk

factors: hyperlipidemia, hypertension, diabetes, and smoking.[307] Another large study showed that 85 to 95% of participants with CHD had at least one conventional risk factor, but so too did those participants without CHD, despite follow-up for as long as 30 years.[308] Part of the discordance between lipid concentrations and events can potentially be explained by measuring other markers such as apoB and LDL-P, and thus raises the question whether only traditional risk factors are adequate to identify all individuals at increased risk of CHD.

A wide variety of nonlipid biochemical markers has also been suggested in an effort to better identify those individuals at increased CHD risk, including markers of fibrinolytic and hemostatic function (tissue-type plasminogen activator antigen, plasminogen activator inhibitor-1, fibrinogen, von Willebrand factor, d-dimer, thrombin-antithrombin III complex, and factors V, VII, and VIII), homocysteine, and markers of inflammation (high-sensitivity C-reactive protein [hsCRP], lipoprotein-associated phospholipase A2 [Lp-PLA$_2$], myeloperoxidase, serum amyloid A, interleukins, adhesion molecules, heat shock proteins, and matrix metalloproteases). NT-proBNP and high-sensitivity troponin I have all emerged as predictors of risk, even in primary prevention settings (see Chapter 48). Most of these markers provide limited clinical value for one or more of the following reasons:
1. Lack of standardization among available methods
2. Inconsistent findings regarding their ability to *independently* predict future CHD risk
3. Inability to significantly improve prognostic value when added to traditional lipid screening or existing global risk prediction algorithms, such as the pooled cohort ASCVD risk score
4. Lack of appropriate interventions to modulate the concentration of the biomarker and also reduce the associated risk

A 2009 expert panel of the National Academy of Clinical Biochemistry (NACB) stated in its report on Laboratory Medicine Practice Guidelines for Emerging Biomarkers for Primary Prevention of Cardiovascular Disease that among all examined novel markers, only hsCRP met the previously mentioned criteria for acceptance as a biomarker of risk in the primary prevention setting.[282] These recommendations were consistent with those stated in the earlier report of the AHA and the CDC (AHA/CDC).[280,281] For this reason, hsCRP is the only nonlipid biomarker endorsed by the US multisociety guidelines for cardiovascular risk management.[110]

High-sensitivity C-Reactive Protein

Chronic inflammation is an important component in the development and progression of atherosclerosis, and numerous epidemiologic studies have demonstrated that increased serum CRP concentrations are positively associated with the risk of future CVD. It has also been shown to be predictive of future events in patients with acute coronary syndromes and in those with stable angina and coronary artery stents.[309–311]

The use of CRP for these purposes requires the use of high-sensitivity "hs"-CRP assays that have detection limits less than 0.3 mg/L. Several automated immunoturbidimetric and immunonephelometric assays are commercially available and are capable of sensitive and precise measurements at low concentrations of CRP. The analytical performance of several of these assays has been evaluated.[312] Additional information on CRP is presented in Chapter 31.

Because hsCRP values minimally correlate with most lipid concentrations, and lipid parameters account for less than 3 to 5% of the variance in hsCRP measurement, hsCRP values do not replace but instead complement the evaluation of lipids and other classical CHD risk factors in primary prevention strategies. Furthermore, elevated TG and remnant cholesterol, but not elevated LDL-C or Lp(a), are causally related to increased plasma hsCRP,[284,313,314] while elevated hsCRP *per se* is not causally related to CHD.[315] Large population studies have reported that hsCRP adds prognostic information at all concentrations of LDL-C and across risk calculated by age, sex, hypertension, and cholesterol.[316] However, newer meta-analyses cast doubt on the clinical significance of hsCRP improvements in measures of calibration, discrimination, and reclassification of patient risk.[317]

The Role of High-sensitivity C-Reactive Protein in Disease Intervention

Many behavioral interventions known to reduce the risk of clinical cardiovascular events have been linked to lower hsCRP values. Recently, a randomized clinical trial specifically targeted hsCRP values without influencing lipid biomarkers using canakinumab, a monoclonal antibody inhibitor of interleukin-1ß.[318] The trial demonstrated that lowering of hsCRP reduced vascular events independent of lipid-lowering. While it should be pointed out that there was no association between baseline hsCRP and treatment success, patients achieving on-treatment hsCRP less than 2 mg/L realized the greatest cardiovascular benefit.[319]

JUPITER was a clinical trial specifically designed to test the efficacy of statins in reducing clinical cardiovascular events among persons with hsCRP of 2 mg/L or greater and LDL-C less than 130 mg/dL (3.4 mmol/L), who make up an estimated 25% of the US population.[320] Approximately 18,000 subjects with such a phenotype were randomized to 20 mg of rosuvastatin per day or placebo and followed for a period of 4 years for the occurrence of myocardial infarction, stroke, arterial revascularization, hospitalization for unstable angina, or death from CVD (primary end point). However, the safety and efficacy board of the trial terminated it ahead of schedule because its continuation was deemed unethical based on the overwhelmingly positive results. Findings revealed a reduction in the primary trial end point of 44% in those who received rosuvastatin compared with those on placebo (Fig. 36.29).[320] The number of subjects with this phenotype who have to be treated with statin to prevent a single coronary event was 25, a number that is similar to those seen in hyperlipidemia trials. Furthermore, using hsCRP less than 2 mg/L and LDL-C less than 70 mg/dL (1.8 mmol/L) as dual target goals for statin therapy, a reduction of 65% in cardiovascular events was seen; a reduction of 80% in cardiovascular events was noted in those who achieved that concentration of LDL-C with hsCRP less than 1 mg/L (see Fig. 36.29).[321] The concept of dual target goals, using both LDL-C and hsCRP, to optimize statin therapy in patients with acute coronary syndrome has been explored and has been shown to be beneficial (see Fig. 36.29). Use of hsCRP as a risk enhancer for patient management decisions is endorsed by the US multi-society guideline.[110] Furthermore, a risk score utilizing hsCRP has been proposed and demonstrates performance comparable or superior to the ASCVD pooled cohort calculator.[322] However, citing weak reclassification data the US Preventive

Services Task Force claims that the incremental benefit of hsCRP for risk prediction is uncertain,[317] and the European guidelines review the literature without concluding any recommendation.[111]

POINTS TO REMEMBER

C-REACTIVE PROTEIN
- CRP is an acute-phase plasma protein (acute-phase reactant) and can be markedly increased in various infections and inflammatory diseases.
- Modest increases in CRP may also occur with low-level chronic inflammation such as that which occurs in ASCVD.
- High-sensitive CRP (hsCRP) assays allow for measurement within the "normal range" and are endorsed by multiple societies for evaluation CVD risk.

High-sensitivity C-Reactive Protein Analytical Considerations

Dozens of hsCRP assays are commercially available. In a study of nine such assays, all achieved a lowest detection limit of 0.3 mg/L or less, and five had within-laboratory analytical imprecision less than 10% (i.e., reproducibilities greater than 90%).[312] Agreement among hsCRP methods is essential because an individual patient's result will be interpreted within the context of nationally established cut points. A standardization program led by the CDC was initiated in 2002 to address this issue. A common calibrator identified from this initiative was shown to harmonize patients' results in most commercially available assays.[325]

Despite being an acute-phase reactant, hsCRP exhibits a relatively low degree of intraindividual variability in clinically stable patients. The incremental clinical benefit provided by serial assessment of hsCRP is uncertain. However, most studies in healthy clinically stable populations suggest that biological variability is comparable to that of serum cholesterol. Provided that a value less than 10 mg/L is obtained, multisociety guidelines recommend the use of two hsCRP measures taken 2 or more weeks apart (same as for lipid panels), prior to changing therapy. Because hsCRP may reflect subclinical infection, values greater than 10 mg/L should be disregarded initially and the test repeated when the patient has stabilized. Furthermore, because hsCRP values are unaffected by food intake and exhibit almost no circadian variation, measurements can be made without regard for fasting status or time of day.[326]

High-sensitivity C-Reactive Protein Reference Values

Most studies have reported only a modest relationship between age (range, 18 to 88 years) and serum hsCRP concentrations. Data from several large US and European cohorts indicate that the distribution of circulating hsCRP concentrations appears comparable among men and women who are not on postmenopausal hormone replacement therapy (HRT), with the 50th percentile for both genders being about 1.5 mg/L (Table 36.26).[327,328] hsCRP concentrations are higher in women who use oral HRT than in women who do not, and increased hsCRP from oral HRT has been associated with an increased risk of thrombotic events.[329]

Information on the distribution of hsCRP concentrations in nonwhite populations is sparse. In the nationally representative NHANES data set, no significant differences were noted in the

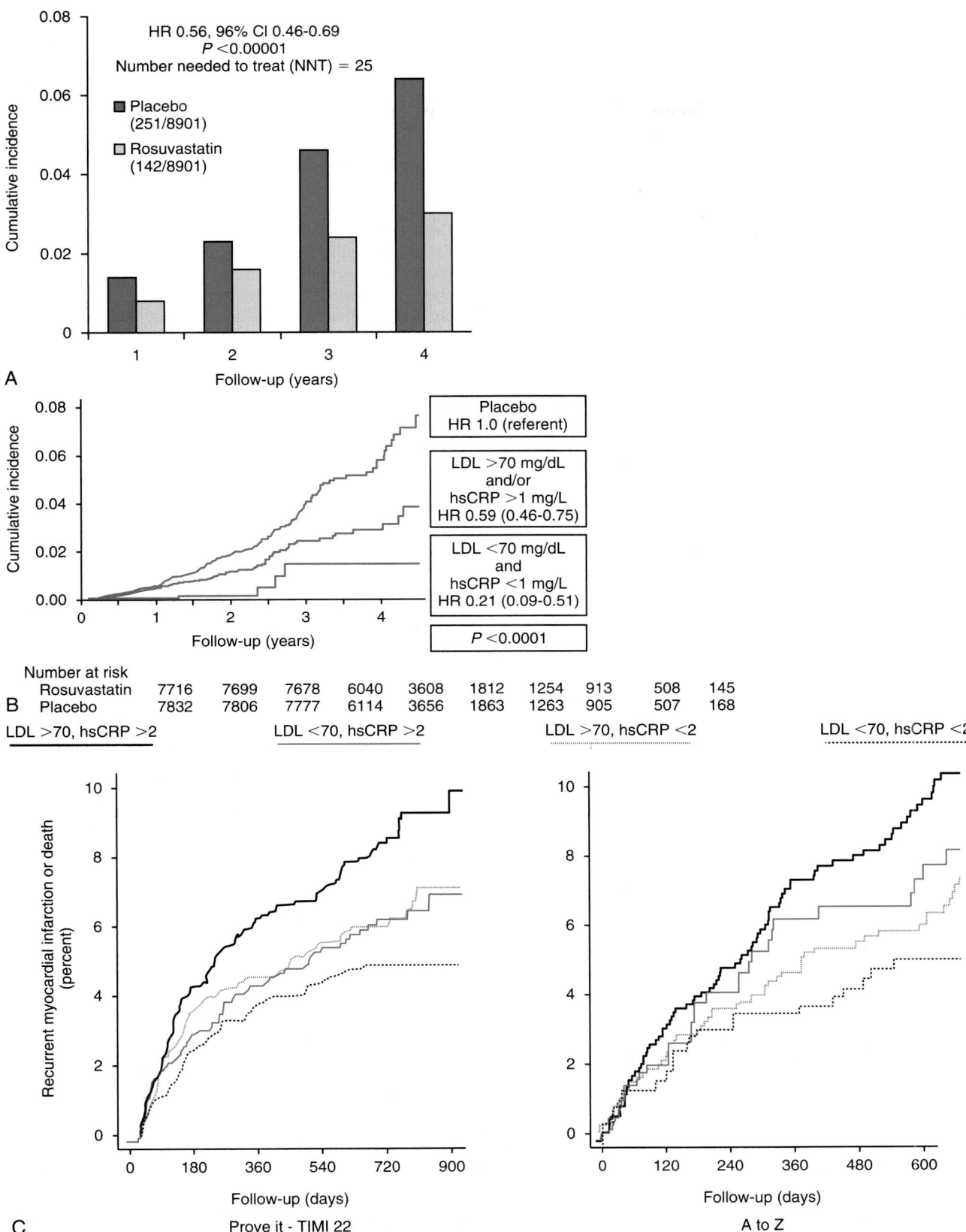

FIGURE 36.29 (A) Cumulative incidence of cardiovascular events in the JUPITER trial.[320] (B) Cumulative incidence of cardiovascular events in JUPITER in placebo and statin groups according to achieved LDL cholesterol and hsCRP.[321] (C) Cumulative incidence of cardiovascular events in PROVE IT and A to Z in placebo and statin groups, according to achieved LDL cholesterol and hsCRP.[323,324]

TABLE 36.26 Population Distributions of C-Reactive Protein, mg/L

Population	PERCENTILE						
	5th	10th	25th	50th	75th	90th	95th
American women[a]	0.2	0.3	0.6	1.5	3.5	6.6	9.1
American men	0.3	0.4	0.8	1.5	3.2	6.1	8.6
European women[a]	0.3	0.4	0.9	1.7	3.4	6.2	8.8
European men	0.3	0.6	0.8	1.6	3.3	6.5	8.6

[a]Only women not taking hormone replacement therapy.

TABLE 36.27 Distributions of C-Reactive Protein Among Men, mg/L

	PERCENTILE						
	5th	10th	25th	50th	75th	90th	95th
White American	0.2	0.4	0.7	1.6	3.4	6.7	12.3
African American	0.1	0.2	0.7	1.7	3.9	8.2	13.2
Mexican American	0.2	0.4	0.6	1.6	3.2	6.3	9.8
Japanese	—	<0.3	0.4	1.6	3.5	7.8	—

distribution of hsCRP concentrations among White, Black, and Mexican-American men (Table 36.27).[330,331] Moreover, a comparable hsCRP distribution was seen in Japanese men.[331] Although additional studies on the distribution and prognostic ability of CRP in non-White populations are clearly necessary, existing data are insufficient to support the exclusion of any racial or ethnic group from current guidelines for CRP testing.

SELECTED REFERENCES

1. Nordestgaard BG, Langsted A, Mora S, et al. Fasting is not routinely required for determination of a lipid profile: clinical and laboratory implications including flagging at desirable concentration cutpoints-a joint consensus statement from the european atherosclerosis society and european federation of clinical chemistry and laboratory medicine. Clin Chem 2016;62:930–46.
3. Nordestgaard BG, Langlois MR, Langsted A, et al. Quantifying atherogenic lipoproteins for lipid-lowering strategies: consensus-based recommendations from eas and eflm. Atherosclerosis 2020;294:46–61.
4. Nordestgaard BG. A test in context: Lipid profile, fasting versus nonfasting. J Am Coll Cardiol 2017;70:1637–46.
40. Rifai N. Lipoproteins and apolipoproteins. Composition, metabolism, and association with coronary heart disease. Arch Pathol Lab Med 1986;110:694–701.
43. Tsimikas S, Fazio S, Ferdinand KC, et al. Nhlbi working group recommendations to reduce lipoprotein(a)-mediated risk of cardiovascular disease and aortic stenosis. J Am Coll Cardiol 2018;71:177–92.

54. Meeusen JW, Donato LJ and Jaffe AS. Should apolipoprotein b replace ldl cholesterol as therapeutic targets are lowered? Curr Opin Lipidol 2016;27:359–66.
56. Contois JH, McConnell JP, Sethi AA, et al. Apolipoprotein b and cardiovascular disease risk: position statement from the aacc lipoproteins and vascular diseases division working group on best practices. Clin Chem 2009;55:407–19.
86. Rosenson RS, Brewer HB, Jr., Chapman MJ, et al. Hdl measures, particle heterogeneity, proposed nomenclature, and relation to atherosclerotic cardiovascular events. Clin Chem 2011;57:392–410.
88. Keene D, Price C, Shun-Shin MJ, et al. Effect on cardiovascular risk of high density lipoprotein targeted drug treatments niacin, fibrates, and cetp inhibitors: meta-analysis of randomised controlled trials including 117,411 patients. BMJ 2014;349:g4379.
110. Grundy SM, Stone NJ, Bailey AL, et al. 2018 aha/acc/aacvpr/aapa/abc/acpm/ada/ags/apha/aspc/nla/pcna guideline on the management of blood cholesterol: executive summary: a report of the American College of Cardiology/American Heart Association task force on clinical practice guidelines. Circulation 2019;139:e1046–e81.
111. Mach F, Baigent C, Catapano AL, et al. 2019 esc/eas guidelines for the management of dyslipidaemias: lipid modification to reduce cardiovascular risk. Eur Heart J 2020;41:111–88.
112. Anderson TJ, Gregoire J, Pearson GJ, et al. 2016 canadian cardiovascular society guidelines for the management of dyslipidemia for the prevention of cardiovascular disease in the adult. Can J Cardiol 2016;32:1263–82.
113. Jacobson TA, Ito MK, Maki KC, et al. National lipid association recommendations for patient-centered management of dyslipidemia: Part 1–executive summary. J Clin Lipidol 2014;8:473–88.
115. Langlois MR, Chapman MJ, Cobbaert C, et al. Quantifying atherogenic lipoproteins: current and future challenges in the era of personalized medicine and very low concentrations of ldl cholesterol. A consensus statement from eas and eflm. Clin Chem 2018;64:1006–33.
117. Boren J, Chapman MJ, Krauss RM, et al. Low-density lipoproteins cause atherosclerotic cardiovascular disease: Pathophysiological, genetic, and therapeutic insights: a consensus statement from the european atherosclerosis society consensus panel. Eur Heart J 2020;41:2313–30.
129. Cholesterol Treatment Trialists C, Baigent C, Blackwell L, et al. Efficacy and safety of more intensive lowering of ldl cholesterol: a meta-analysis of data from 170,000 participants in 26 randomised trials. Lancet 2010;376:1670–81.
133. Bhatt DL, Steg PG, Miller M, et al. Cardiovascular risk reduction with icosapent ethyl for hypertriglyceridemia. N Engl J Med 2019;380:11–22.
143. Sathiyakumar V, Park J, Golozar A, et al. Fasting versus nonfasting and low-density lipoprotein cholesterol accuracy. Circulation 2018;137:10–9.
221. Mortensen MB and Nordestgaard BG. 2019 vs. 2016 esc/eas statin guidelines for primary prevention of atherosclerotic cardiovascular disease. Eur Heart J 2020.
253. Miller WG, Myers GL, Sakurabayashi I, et al. Seven direct methods for measuring hdl and ldl cholesterol compared with ultracentrifugation reference measurement procedures. Clin Chem 2010;56:977–86.
319. Ridker PM, MacFadyen JG, Everett BM, et al. Relationship of c-reactive protein reduction to cardiovascular event reduction following treatment with canakinumab: a secondary analysis from the cantos randomised controlled trial. Lancet 2018;391:319–28.

Electrolytes and Blood Gases*

Mark Kellogg, John Benco, and Mark A. Cervinski

ABSTRACT

Background
Electrolyte balance within the human body is essential for maintenance of health. Dysregulation of electrolytes affects water homeostasis and acid-base status and often results in overt clinical signs and symptoms. The laboratory is tasked with aiding the clinician by providing accurate, timely results to narrow or confirm a diagnosis. In challenging cases in which the clinical context is lacking or conflicting, it is even more important for the laboratory to provide reliable data.

Content
This chapter compares analytical methods and describes their advantages, disadvantages, and pitfalls in the analysis of electrolytes (including detailed discussions on sodium [Na^+], potassium [K^+], chloride [Cl^-], and bicarbonate [HCO_3^-])

and blood gases. Sweat Cl^- quantification, which plays a central role in the diagnosis of cystic fibrosis (CF) and is known to be technically challenging, is also discussed.

Maintenance of water homeostasis is vital to life for all organisms. In humans, the maintenance of water homeostasis in various body fluid compartments is primarily a function of the four major electrolytes, Na^+, K^+, Cl^-, and HCO_3^-. These electrolytes also have a role in acid-base balance, heart and skeletal muscle function, and as cofactors for enzymes. Abnormal electrolyte concentrations may be the cause or the consequence of a variety of medical disorders. Because of their physiologic and clinical inter-relationships, this chapter discusses analysis of (1) electrolytes, (2) osmolality, (3) sweat Cl^-, (4) blood gases and pH, and (5) oxygen hemodynamics.

*The full version of this chapter is available electronically on ExpertConsult.com.

38

Hormones*

Timothy J. Cole

ABSTRACT

Background

Hormones are a diverse group of compounds that circulate in body fluids at very low and variable concentrations. Hormones perform important signaling and communication roles between cells and tissues of the body. Accurate measurement of hormone concentrations in patient samples is critical for accurate clinical diagnosis of acute illness and chronic disease.

Content

Endocrine hormones are chemical messengers that communicate between cells and tissues. They regulate development of the embryo, energy balance and integrated cellular metabolism, maintenance of homeostasis, cognition, and reproductive processes throughout life. Hormones are classified into three major groups: polypeptide hormones, amino acid-derived hormones, and steroid and other lipid-derived hormones. The synthesis and release of hormones from specialized endocrine cells and organs are tightly controlled. Each hormone is released for a specific purpose, has a defined half-life in the circulation, and can feed back to regulate subsequent hormone synthesis and release. Hormones act on target cells by binding to and activating specific protein receptors that are either embedded in the cell plasma membrane or reside intracellularly. The two largest groups of cell surface receptors are the G-protein-coupled receptors (GPCRs) and the enzyme-coupled receptor (ENZCR) families of proteins. Intracellular hormone receptors comprise the nuclear receptor (NR) superfamily. Receptor activation by hormone binding initiates intracellular signal transduction pathways that result in hormone-directed cellular and physiologic change. Accurate monitoring of systemic hormonal status is critical for the clinical diagnosis of illness and disease caused by abnormal hormone concentrations or defective receptor-signaling interactions.

*The full version of this chapter is available electronically on ExpertConsult.com.

Vitamins and Trace Elements*

Ravinder Sodi[a]

ABSTRACT

Background

An adequate supply of vitamins and trace elements is critical in maintaining optimum health. Measurements of vitamin and trace element concentrations are frequently helpful in nutritional assessment and may be a requisite in suspected deficiency or toxicity, and in the management of patients with cystic fibrosis (CF), bariatric surgery, and for those on nutritional support in the intensive or critical care units. There is also great public interest in and many misconceptions about vitamins and trace elements.

Content

This chapter describes the chemistry, dietary sources, absorption, transport, metabolism, excretion, functions, and recommended intakes of the essential vitamins and trace elements required in humans. These include the fat-soluble vitamins A, E, K with the exception of D; the water-soluble vitamins B_1, B_2, B_6, B_{12}, C, folate, biotin, niacin, and pantothenic acid; and the trace elements chromium (Cr), cobalt (Co), copper (Cu), iodine (I), manganese (Mn), molybdenum (Mo), selenium (Se), and zinc (Zn). Free radicals, their measurement, and the trace elements fluoride (F), boron (B), silicon (Si), and vanadium (V) are briefly discussed. The causes and effects of vitamin and trace element deficiency and toxicity are outlined and the laboratory assessment of status, preanalytical variables effecting the methods, and suggested reference intervals are critically evaluated. Some illustrative cases are included. For methodologic details, readers are invited to access the given original references provided in this chapter.

*The full version of this chapter is available electronically on ExpertConsult.com.
[a]The author gratefully acknowledges the contributions of Norman B. Roberts, Andrew Taylor, and Alan Shenkin in previous editions of this chapter.

40

Iron Metabolism*

Dorine W. Swinkels

ABSTRACT

Background

Iron plays an essential role in many biochemical processes, in particular in the production of heme for incorporation in hemoglobin and iron-sulfur clusters, which serve as enzyme cofactors. Measurement of iron and other indicators of body iron are helpful in the assessment of some of the world's most prevalent disorders: iron deficiency, iron overload, and iron distribution disorders.

Content

This chapter describes the processes involved in systemic and cellular iron metabolism. These processes can be disrupted by an inadequate body iron supply or excessive losses, lack or disruption of systemic or cellular iron regulatory mechanisms, defects in cellular iron acquisition or release, or defects in iron transport, handling, and storage proteins.

Defects in these processes that become manifest in clinical iron disorders are described. They include inherited or acquired iron deficiency anemias, iron distribution, and iron overload disorders.

Reliable analytical methods for the measurement of the analytes involved were among the first to be developed for routine use in the clinical laboratory. More recently, as a result from important discoveries in the underlying biological processes, new iron biomarkers were further added to this laboratory toolbox. This chapter illustrates that laboratory analysis has contributed significantly to our understanding of the physiologic and pathologic roles of these analytes and has allowed the design of novel algorithms and diagrams for the management of these disorders. Challenges ahead are described and include the determination of iron status when concomitant liver diseases, infection, and inflammation are present and further standardization of parameters, to increase their utility for both public health and clinical practice.

---

*The full version of this chapter is available electronically on ExpertConsult.com.

Porphyrins and the Porphyrias*

Michael N. Badminton, Sharon D. Whatley,
Caroline Schmitt, and Aasne K. Aarsand[a]

ABSTRACT

Background

The porphyrias are a group of rare, mainly inherited metabolic disorders that result from decreased or, in one rare form of erythropoietic protoporphyria, increased, activities of the enzymes of heme biosynthesis. Each porphyria is defined by the association of characteristic clinical features with a specific pattern of heme precursor accumulation that reflect the buildup of substrates upstream of the enzyme that is partially deficient, or of a secondarily rate-limiting enzyme.

Content

This chapter describes the metabolic pathway and regulation of heme biosynthesis, the excretion of heme precursors, the different porphyrias, and abnormalities of porphyrin metabolism not caused by porphyria. Porphyrias can be classified as hepatic or erythropoietic according to the main site of overproduction of heme precursors. From a clinical viewpoint, porphyrias are usually classified as acute, in which acute neurovisceral attacks occur, or as nonacute. Acute porphyrias include 5-aminolevulinate dehydratase deficiency porphyria (ADP), acute intermittent porphyria (AIP), variegate porphyria (VP), and hereditary coproporphyria (HCP). The nonacute porphyrias encompass porphyria cutanea tarda (PCT), congenital erythropoietic porphyria (CEP), erythropoietic protoporphyria (EPP), and X-linked erythropoietic protoporphyria (XLEPP). This chapter also covers the diagnostic approaches, with detailed information on biochemical and genetic analysis, and clinical management of the various forms of porphyrias.

*The full version of this chapter is available electronically on ExpertConsult.com.

[a]The authors gratefully acknowledge the contributions of George H. Elder and Allan C. Deacon on which this chapter is based.

Therapeutic Drugs and Their Management

Michael C. Milone and Leslie Michael Shaw[a]

ABSTRACT

Background

Therapeutic drug monitoring (TDM) is the traditional term used for the activity of measuring drug concentrations to tailor the dose of the medication to an individual. The use of monitored drug therapy is generally reserved for drugs with a narrow therapeutic index (TI), with variable pharmacokinetic behavior, and for which the efficacy or toxicity is difficult to measure or detect early during therapy.

Content

In this chapter, we review the rationale for TDM, the fundamental principles of pharmacokinetics that are required to effectively utilize drug concentration data, and analytical factors affecting concentration measurement. We also provide a broad overview of a selected group of commonly monitored drugs that includes some of the challenges and pitfalls to their monitoring.

INTRODUCTION

The Rationale for Monitoring Therapeutic Drugs

The ability of medicines to both heal and hurt has been recognized since ancient times. Immortalized by the writing of the Renaissance Swiss-German physician, Paracelsus, over 500 years ago:[1]

All things are poison and nothing is without poison, only the dose makes that a thing is not a poison.

The challenge in medicine is therefore to determine the optimal dose of medicine that will help a patient with limited associated harm.

Studies in the 1990s identified that adverse events associated with drug therapy rank within the top 10 causes of death in the United States.[2] While many of the severe or fatal events may not be preventable, more than a third appear to be preventable.[3] In addition to the tragic life and death consequences of adverse drug events (ADEs), failed drug therapy also has a significant economic impact. The estimated cost of ADEs ranges from $17 to 29 billion in the United States alone.[4] Just examining hospital-associated ADEs, the average cost of treating each preventable event is estimated to be greater than $3000 in addition to the increased length of stay.[5] The causes of preventable drug-related adverse events vary; however, inadequate monitoring of therapy represents major sources of preventable ADEs contributing to as much as 40% of these events.[2] Improving monitoring strategies is therefore likely to have an important impact on both health and its associated cost.

Drug therapy may be monitored in many ways. Clinical signs and symptoms of toxicity are often an effective way to detect toxicity or treatment failure. β-Blockers represent a typical example. Blood pressure and heart rate monitoring can be used to assess efficacy and toxicity of these drugs. Both are also easily measurable in the clinical setting and even at home. As a result, there is little need to perform monitoring beyond these straightforward clinical assessments.

The efficacy and toxicity of some drugs, however, can be much more difficult to monitor on clinical signs and symptoms alone. Insulin treatment in diabetes represents a case in point. The consequences of inappropriate insulin treatment are insidious, potentially life threatening, and very difficult to detect. Excessive insulin can lead to an acute decrease in blood glucose culminating in coma, permanent brain injury, and death. Inadequate insulin dosing, although not as acutely life threatening, leads over time to vascular disease, end-stage renal failure, blindness, and neuropathy that results in significant morbidity and mortality. Laboratory testing of blood glucose, a direct biomarker of insulin's mechanism of action, provides an ideal means to monitor insulin therapy and prevent these complications. It is so important in diabetes therapy that it has driven the commercial development of simple, point-of-care devices that patients can use to routinely monitor their therapy at home. Biomarkers of drug efficacy or toxicity such as blood glucose, while highly desirable, are not always available. In the absence of a useful biomarker of drug effect, measuring the drug itself provides a potential surrogate.

Therapeutic drug monitoring (TDM) is the traditional term used for the activity of measuring drug concentrations to tailor the dose of the medication to an individual. There is an implicit assumption in TDM of a relationship between drug concentrations and efficacy or toxicity outcomes. The use of TDM and *applied pharmacokinetics* to guide drug

---

[a]The authors gratefully acknowledge the contributions by Christine L.H. Snozek, Gwendolyn A. McMillan, and Thomas P. Moyer on which this chapter is based.

therapy began in the 1960s, coincident with the development of robust analytical techniques.[6–9] Since this time, TDM has become the standard of care for monitoring therapy with many drugs, including antiepileptic drugs (AEDs), immunosuppressive drugs (ISDs), and antibiotics. TDM is a complex process that involves several members of the health care team, including pharmacists, laboratory professionals, and physicians. To justify the costs associated with TDM, it must improve clinical outcome and reduce the overall cost of drug therapy. Prospective, randomized, concentration-controlled trials (RCCTs) of TDM are limited; however, some of these RCCTs show that concentration control can improve efficacy and reduce toxicity of drug therapy.[10–17] Cost-effectiveness of TDM is lacking for most drugs, but TDM has been shown to improve the costs of aminoglycoside therapy.[18] TDM may also aid in the detection of nonadherence to drug therapy,[19–21] which represents a frequent and important cause of preventable ADEs.[3,22] This benefit may even extend to drugs not routinely monitored by traditional blood concentration monitoring.[23]

This chapter will focus on the general principles of pharmacology and their application to TDM with a discussion of the pharmacology and TDM of some commonly monitored drugs. It is difficult to provide a comprehensive review of TDM in a single chapter. Readers are therefore referred to textbooks dedicated to the subject of TDM and applied pharmacology for more in-depth information.

FUNDAMENTAL PRINCIPLES OF APPLIED PHARMACOKINETICS

Basic Concepts and Definitions

Pharmacology comprises the body of knowledge surrounding chemical agents and their effects on living processes. This is a broad field, and it has traditionally been confined to drugs that are useful in the prevention, diagnosis, and treatment of disease. *Pharmacotherapeutics* is the part of pharmacology concerned primarily with the application or administration of drugs to patients for the purpose of prevention and treatment of disease. For this aspect of medical practice to be effective, the *pharmacodynamic* and *pharmacokinetic* (PK) properties of drugs should be understood. *Toxicology* is the subdiscipline of pharmacology concerned with adverse effects of chemicals on living systems. Toxic effects and mechanisms of action may be different from therapeutic effects and mechanisms for the same drug. Similarly, at the high dose of drugs at which toxic effects may be produced, rate processes are frequently altered compared with those at therapeutic doses. For these reasons, the terms *toxicodynamics* and *toxicokinetics* are now applied to these special situations.

Pharmacodynamics

Pharmacodynamics encompasses the processes of interaction of pharmacologically active substances with target sites, and the biochemical and physiologic consequences leading to therapeutic or adverse effects. For many drugs, the ultimate effect or mechanism of action at the molecular level is poorly understood, if at all. A pharmacologic effect (i.e., the therapeutic or toxic response to a drug) may be elicited by direct interaction of the drug with the receptor controlling a specific function or by a drug-mediated alteration of the physiologic

process regulating the function. For most drugs, the intensity and duration of the observed pharmacologic effect are proportional to the concentration of the drug at the receptor. In a given tissue, the site at which a drug acts to initiate events leading to a specific biological effect is called the site of action of the drug.

The mechanism of action of a drug is the biochemical or physical process that occurs at the site of action. Drug action is usually mediated through a receptor. Cellular enzymes, as well as structural or transport proteins, are important examples of drug receptors. Nonprotein macromolecules also may bind drugs, resulting in altered cellular functions controlled by membrane permeability or DNA transcription. Some drugs are chemically similar to important natural endogenous substances and may compete for binding sites. In addition, some drugs may block formation, release, uptake, or transport of essential substances. Others may produce an effect by interacting with relatively small molecules to form complexes that actively bind to receptors. These and other examples of receptor binding are more completely discussed in pharmacology texts.[24–29]

Although the exact molecular interactions that give rise to the mechanism of action for many drugs remain obscure, numerous theoretical models have been developed to explain drug action. One concept postulates that a drug binds to intracellular macromolecular receptors through ionic and hydrogen bonds and van der Waals forces. This theoretical model further postulates that if the drug-receptor complex is sufficiently stable and able to modify the target system, an observable pharmacologic response will occur. As Fig. 42.1 illustrates, the response is concentration dependent until a maximal effect is reached. The plateau may be due to saturation at the receptor or overload of a transport process.

The utility of monitoring drug concentration is based on the premise that pharmacologic response correlates with the concentration of the drug at the site of action (receptor). Although attempts have been made to measure the concentration of drugs at the receptor site in a patient,[30] in general, this approach is technically impractical, if not impossible for most drugs. Studies have shown that for many drugs, a strong correlation exists between the serum drug concentration and

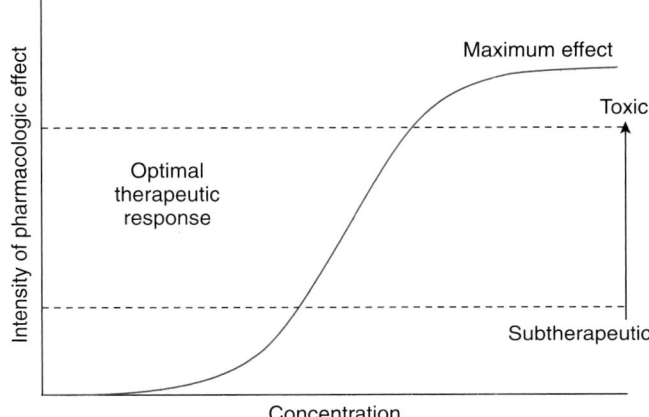

FIGURE 42.1 The dose-effect relationship. The probability of increasing pharmacologic response and risk for toxicity parallels concentration for most drugs. The plateau (maximum effect) is likely due to saturation at the receptor.

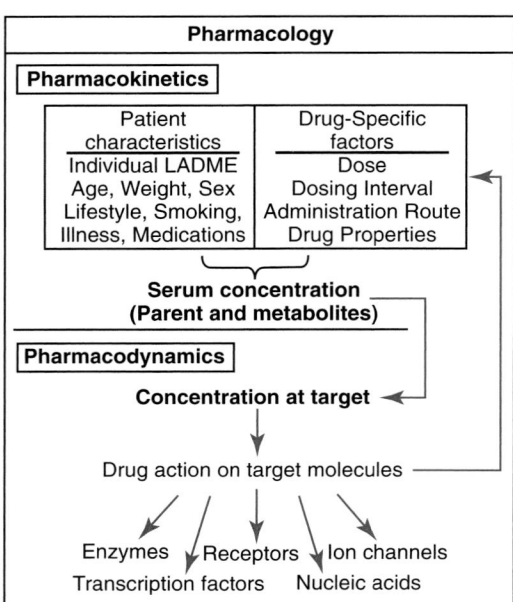

FIGURE 42.2 Conceptual relationship between pharmacodynamics and pharmacokinetics. Many drug- and patient-specific factors determine both the serum concentration of a therapeutic compound and its metabolites. Serum concentration in turn is related to the amount of drug present at the target site, resulting in effects on a variety of molecules (several examples shown) to induce a pharmacologic response. The efficacy and degree of response provide feedback to allow optimization of the dosing regimen for an individual patient. *LADME,* Liberation, absorption, distribution, metabolism, elimination.

the observed pharmacologic effect. In addition, years of relating blood concentrations to drug effects have demonstrated the clinical utility of drug concentration information. One must nevertheless always keep in mind that a serum drug concentration does not necessarily equal the concentration at the receptor but rather merely reflects it.

Pharmacokinetics

Pharmacokinetics describes the processes of uptake of drugs by the body, the distribution of the drugs into tissue, the biotransformations (i.e., metabolism) they undergo, and the elimination of the drugs and their metabolites from the body. Applied pharmacokinetics is the discipline that uses the principles of pharmacokinetics to enhance safety and effectiveness of a drug in an individual patient. It is this aspect of pharmacology that most strongly influences the interpretation of TDM results and that is dealt with in more detail in this chapter. Fig. 42.2 illustrates the conceptual relationship between pharmacodynamics and pharmacokinetics and the many factors affecting drug concentration and pharmacologic response.

Constant Change of Drugs in the Body

A large number of factors are now recognized to have a profound influence on the pharmacokinetics of drugs and consequently on a patient's pharmacologic response (Box 42.1). For example, the consideration of the patient's history, with particular emphasis on his or her pathophysiologic state and adjunct drug therapy, is essential at the initiation of drug therapy and TDM because these important factors may affect absorption, distribution, metabolism, and excretion of a drug.

BOX 42.1 Factors That Affect Drug Distribution in Humans

Demographic Factors
Age
Weight
Gender
Race
Genetics (e.g., metabolic enzyme polymorphisms)

Health-Related Factors
Liver disease (cirrhosis, hepatitis, cholestasis)
Kidney disease
Thyroid disease (hypothyroidism or hyperthyroidism)
Cardiovascular disease (arrhythmias, congestive heart failure)
Gastrointestinal disease (e.g., sprue or other malabsorption, peptic ulcer disease)
Cancer
Surgery
Burns
Volume status (e.g., dehydration)
Nutritional status (cachectic or anorexic)
Pregnancy or other factors affecting plasma proteins or body composition

Extracorporeal Factors
Hemodialysis
Peritoneal dialysis
Cardiopulmonary bypass
Hypothermia or hyperthermia

Chemical and Environmental Factors
Absorption of Drug
Food or coadministered drug affecting extent or rate of absorption
Immediate- or extended-release formulation

Distribution of Drug
Coadministered drugs affecting protein binding to plasma proteins or tissue

Metabolism of Drug
Food, herbs, or drugs competing for metabolism
Coadministration of drugs that induce metabolic enzymes (e.g., phenobarbital)
Coadministration of drugs that inhibit metabolic enzymes (e.g., cimetidine)

Excretion of Drug
Coadministration of drug competing for renal tubular secretory pathways (e.g., probenecid, penicillin)
Coadministration of drugs enhancing renal tubular reabsorption

Absorption

Most drugs administered chronically to patients are administered extravascularly. Although intramuscular and subcutaneous routes are used, the oral route accounts for most of the extravascular doses administered. The absorption process depends on the drug's dissociating from its dosing form, dissolving in gastrointestinal fluids, and then diffusing across biological membrane barriers into the bloodstream. The rate and extent of drug absorption may vary considerably depending on the nature of the drug itself (e.g., solubility, pK_a), on the matrix in which it is present, and on the physiologic environment (e.g., pH, gastrointestinal motility, vascularity).

The fraction of a drug that is absorbed into the systemic circulation is referred to as its bioavailability. The bioavailability (*f*) of a given drug is usually calculated by comparing, in the same subjects, the area under the plasma concentration–time curve (AUC) of an equivalent dose of the intravenous form and oral form:

$$f = \frac{\text{AUC}_{\text{oral}}}{\text{AUC}_{\text{iv}}} \qquad (42.1)$$

The bioavailability of a particular drug, if the drug is to be useful, must generally be great enough so that the active component can pass in sufficient amount and in a desirable time from the gut into the systemic circulation. Bioavailability of greater than 70% is most desirable for drugs to be orally useful. An exception would be a case in which the lumen of the gastrointestinal tract is the site of drug action (e.g., antibiotics used to sterilize the gut such as oral vancomycin). Low bioavailability would then be considered advantageous.

Some drugs that are rapidly and completely absorbed nevertheless have low bioavailability to the systemic circulation. This is true of drugs with a high *hepatic extraction rate*. After oral administration, drugs that are absorbed in the lumen of the small intestine are carried by the portal vein directly to the liver. The liver may extensively metabolize a drug with a high hepatic extraction rate before it reaches the systemic circulation, leading to low oral bioavailability. This phenomenon is the first-pass effect.

In addition to the extent of absorption, the rate of absorption is also important. The absorption of a drug is generally considered a first-order process, and the absorption rate constant of a drug is usually much greater than its elimination rate constant. Efforts are now being made in the pharmaceutical industry to decrease the apparent rate of absorption of many drugs by manipulating their formulations (e.g., theophylline, tacrolimus) to produce slow-release or sustained-release products. Formulations that provide sustained release permit drugs taken orally to be taken at less frequent intervals. Conditions that may influence the extent or rate of drug absorption include abnormal gastrointestinal motility, diseases of the stomach and of the small and large intestine, gastrointestinal infections, radiation, food, and interaction with other substances in the gastrointestinal tract. One should be particularly aware of coadministered drugs that directly affect gut absorption, such as antacids, kaolin, sucralfate, cholestyramine, and antiulcer medications.

Distribution

After a drug enters the vascular compartment, it interacts with various blood constituents and is carried by various transport processes to different body organs and tissues. The overall process is referred to as *distribution*. The factors determining the distribution pattern of a drug are binding of the drug to circulating blood components, binding to fixed receptors, passage of the drug through membrane barriers, and the ability to dissolve in structural or storage lipids. Molecular weight, pK_a, lipid solubility, and other physical and chemical properties of the drug are important determinants of distribution.

Once a drug enters the systemic circulation, it distributes and comes to equilibrium with many of the blood components, such as plasma proteins. An equilibrium exists between free and protein-bound drug. It is generally believed that only the free fraction of the drug is available for distribution and elimination. In addition, only the free drug is available to cross cellular membranes or to interact with the drug receptor to elicit a biological response. Therefore changes in the protein-binding characteristics of a drug can have a profound influence on the distribution and elimination of a drug, as well as on the manner in which total plasma or serum steady-state concentrations are interpreted. Each drug has its own characteristic protein-binding pattern that depends on its physical and chemical properties. As a general rule, however, acidic drugs are bound primarily to albumin and basic drugs primarily to globulins, particularly α_1-acid glycoprotein (AAG). Some drugs bind to both albumin and globulins.

Depending on its affinity for plasma proteins, a drug may be either tightly or loosely bound. A weakly bound drug can be displaced from its protein sites by a drug with a greater affinity for the plasma protein–binding sites. For example, phenytoin and valproic acid, drugs that are frequently coadministered for epilepsy, compete with each other as they bind to albumin. Because valproate is present at higher concentration, its mass causes a significant shift of phenytoin from bound to free form. Protein binding of a drug also depends on the physical characteristics of the plasma proteins and on the presence or absence of fatty acids or other drugs in the blood. Fatty acids can displace a drug from its protein-binding sites; tightly bound drugs are not displaced, but a weakly bound drug can be displaced quite rapidly by free fatty acids present in increased concentrations. It is important to recognize that even though the total drug concentration may remain unchanged, displacement of a drug from its plasma protein-binding sites increases free drug concentrations and can result in clinical toxicity. Remember that the free fraction is the form that crosses biological membranes and is available to bind to the receptor, so increasing the free fraction can produce significant toxicity.

Anything that alters the concentration of free drug in the plasma ultimately alters the amount of drug available to enter the tissues and interact with specific receptor systems. Disease states can alter free drug concentrations. For example, in uremia, the composition of plasma is altered by an increase in nonprotein nitrogen compounds, by acid-base and electrolyte imbalances, and often by a decrease in albumin; free drug concentrations are frequently increased. Patients may experience adverse effects that are a direct consequence of the increased free drug concentrations, especially if only total plasma drug concentration is monitored in these patients. For example, phenytoin is 90% bound and 10% free in healthy subjects. In uremic patients, 20 to 30% of the total plasma concentration of phenytoin may be free. In a healthy patient who has a total plasma phenytoin concentration of 15 μg/mL, the free phenytoin concentration is likely to be 1.5 μg/mL. If a uremic patient has a total concentration of 15 μg/mL, the free drug concentration may be 4.5 μg/mL. A free phenytoin concentration of 4.5 μg/mL is sufficient to precipitate severe phenytoin side effects, including lethargy and increased seizure frequency. In uremic patients, it is advisable to quantitate free phenytoin concentrations and adjust the drug dose to maintain free phenytoin concentration at approximately 2.0 μg/mL.

Alteration of protein concentration in response to acute stress can alter free drug concentration. For example, after myocardial infarction, there is a rapid rise in AAG concentration. Lidocaine is a commonly employed drug for control of arrhythmias secondary to acute myocardial infarction, but lidocaine is a basic drug that is highly bound to AAG. Doses of lidocaine adequate to control arrhythmia immediately after infarction are likely to become ineffective 48 to 72 hours later because the higher concentration of AAG that occurs after infarction diminishes the amount of free drug available to tissue.[31] The arrhythmia reappears and because the total lidocaine plasma concentration necessary to control the arrhythmia seems to be in the toxic range, the lidocaine dose is decreased when in reality it should be increased to maintain the optimal free concentration.

Some drugs exhibit saturation of the available plasma protein–binding sites at optimal total drug concentrations. For example, disopyramide binding is concentration dependent and varies widely among patients. Consequently, its total concentration and the observed clinical responses vary markedly among patients. Valproic acid is also a drug that shows saturation at concentrations greater than 100 μg/mL. Thus an increase of total plasma valproate concentration from 100 to 125 μg/mL represents a significant increase in the free valproate concentration.

Any change in normal physiologic status can alter free drug concentrations and thus change the distribution of drugs between plasma and tissue. Geriatric patients often exhibit hypoalbuminemia with a marked decrease in protein-binding sites for drugs. In the elderly, the classic signs of drug intoxication usually are not apparent; instead, the clinical symptoms of drug intoxication are manifested as impaired cognitive function—particularly confusion, which is a common symptom in patients with dementia. Reduction of drug dose to decrease the free drug concentrations may result in dramatic improvements in cognitive function and behavior in these patients.

Estimation of the free drug concentration will continue to be of interest to TDM. Equilibrium dialysis represents the gold-standard method for measuring the free, unbound concentration of a drug. However, this method typically requires 16 to 18 hours of incubation to achieve equilibrium, which severely limits the turnaround time for testing. Ultrafiltration techniques are useful alternatives that usually can be accomplished in a fraction of the time. In ultrafiltration, a sample of serum or plasma is forced through a filter membrane with a low molecular weight cutoff value, typically by centrifugation, to yield a protein-free sample. Provided this process is done rapidly and under appropriate temperature control, ultrafiltration can provide a useful estimate of the free drug concentration in circulating blood.[32,33] Sample drawing, processing, and storage can modify dissociation equilibria for some drugs affecting both equilibrium dialysis and ultracentrifugation measurements. Measurement of drugs in oral fluid (i.e., saliva) has been advocated as an alternative to plasma or serum testing because of the ease of collection and correlation with free drug concentration for some drugs. Despite these drawbacks, free drug estimations by ultrafiltration are superior to estimations of free drug concentration based on measurements in saliva. Few drugs show a strong correlation between salivary concentration and free drug concentration in plasma.[34] In addition, collection of saliva from acutely ill patients is often more difficult than blood collection.

Metabolism

The rate of the enzymatic process to metabolize a drug is usually characterized by the Michaelis-Menten equation (see also Chapter 25)

$$\frac{dC}{dt} = \frac{V_{max} \times C}{K_m + C} \tag{42.2}$$

where V_{max} is the maximum velocity of the reaction; K_m, the Michaelis-Menten constant, is the drug concentration at which the rate of metabolism is half of the maximum; and C is the drug concentration in blood.

Drugs are usually administered to achieve concentrations in the blood well below the K_m of a particular drug. Therefore if K_m is much greater than C, Eq. (42.2) can be simplified to

$$\frac{dC}{dt} = \left(\frac{V_{max}}{K_m} \right) \times C \tag{42.3}$$

and V_{max}/K_m can be written as the constant, K, such that

$$\frac{dC}{dt} = KC \tag{42.4}$$

where K is a simple first-order rate constant for the metabolic elimination. In other words, the rate of drug elimination from blood is proportional to the concentration of drug. *First-order kinetics* are characteristic of the metabolism of most drugs.

In the event that concentrations significantly exceed the K_m for a particular drug, the rate of elimination of the drug becomes independent of concentration and thus descriptive of a *zero-order* process in which Eq. (42.2) can be approximated by:

$$\frac{dC}{dt} = V_{max} \tag{42.5}$$

Several drugs, notably phenytoin, salicylates, ethanol, and theophylline, cannot be characterized by simple first-order kinetics. Instead, the rate of metabolism of these compounds is said to be *capacity-limited* or *nonlinear*, meaning clearance or the apparent half-life changes with changes in concentration. Fig. 42.3 shows how the kinetics of elimination is linear (first order) until the capacity of clearance pathways is reached, which occurs at concentrations that approach the K_m of the enzymatic pathways mediating metabolism. At this point, the relationship between dose and steady-state concentration becomes nonlinear. It should be evident, therefore that important clinical considerations arise when a patient is treated with a drug that displays nonlinear kinetics. First, changes in dosing result in disproportionate changes in steady-state drug concentrations so that titration to appropriate serum concentrations must be approached conservatively. Second, because both clearance and apparent half-life of the drug change with increasing drug concentration, the length of time required to reach a new steady-state concentration is prolonged.

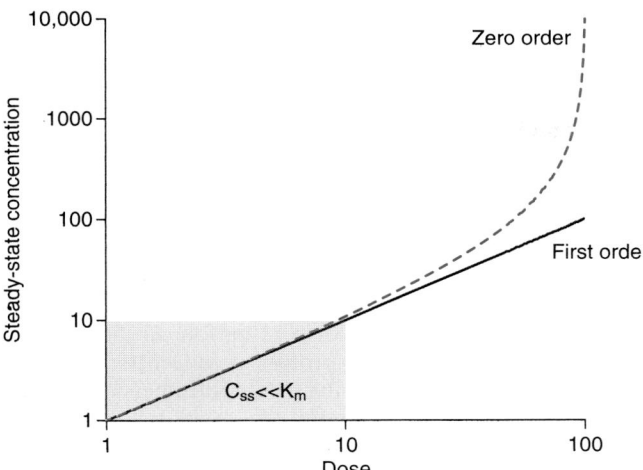

FIGURE 42.3 Nonlinear response to dose changes. Drugs with first-order kinetics *(solid black line)* display serum steady-state concentrations *(C)* that vary proportionately with dose. In contrast, for drugs with zero-order kinetics *(dotted red line),* an increase in dose may result in a disproportionate increase in serum steady-state concentrations.

All of the equations previously described for predicting dose or concentration assume linear kinetic systems; they are therefore not adaptable to treatment with drugs that display nonlinear kinetics. Methods for predicting phenytoin dose and concentration and using a linearized Michaelis-Menten equation have been developed and applied to individualize drug dosing regimens.

Biotransformation

The liver is the principal organ responsible for xenobiotic metabolism. One of its major roles is to convert lipophilic nonpolar molecules to more polar water-soluble forms. The drug molecule (a xenobiotic) can be modified by phase I reactions, which alter chemical structure by oxidation, reduction, or hydrolysis; or by phase II reactions, which conjugate the drug (glucuronidation or sulfation) to water-soluble forms. Typically, both phase I and phase II reactions occur. Most drug metabolism takes place in the microsomal fraction of the hepatocytes, where many environmental chemicals and endogenous biochemicals (xenobiotics) are also processed and by the same mechanisms.

Enzymes of the hepatic microsomal system can be induced or inhibited. Enzyme induction and inhibition have greatest significance for drugs with low to moderate hepatic extraction fractions.

Microsomal enzyme induction leads to an increase in the activity of enzymes present, most commonly through increases in the quantity of the oxidizing enzymes. The many isoenzymes of cytochrome P450 are affected variably by different enzyme-inducing drugs. Two classic and clinically relevant enzyme inducers can be contrasted.

First, phenobarbital represents the type of enzyme inducer with broad induction effects. After a latency period, production of cytochrome P450, cytochrome P450 reductase, and related enzymes is increased. In addition, liver weight, hepatic blood flow, bile flow, and production of hepatic proteins also increase. This induction apparently increases the P450 isoenzyme mass for which debrisoquine is a substrate because the hepatic clearance of debrisoquin is increased after phenobarbital administration. This enzyme system is referred to as cytochrome P450-2D6. Phenobarbital induction has little effect on theophylline clearance, suggesting a different isoenzyme for theophylline metabolism.

Theophylline and polycyclic hydrocarbons in tobacco smoke (3-methylcholanthrene) represent a second type of enzyme inducer with broad induction effects. They induce cytochrome P45-1A in which no change in P45 reductase occurs, and a different terminal oxidase appears. After this type of induction, the clearance of theophylline but not that of antipyrine is increased. These substances have served as prototypes for the classification of enzyme inducers. Obviously, when patients are on a drug with a narrow TI, their dosing regimen would need to be adjusted should a known enzyme-inducing drug be added to or deleted from their therapy.

Because the drug-metabolizing enzymes of the liver are nonspecific and interact with a wide variety of endogenous and exogenous substances, it is not surprising that the presence of one drug inhibits the metabolism of a second drug that is coadministered. Several general mechanisms have been proposed to describe these events. They include substrate competition, competitive or noncompetitive inhibition, product inhibition, and repression (where the amount of enzyme is reduced by either decreased synthesis or increased degradation). Most drug-drug interactions probably fall into the categories of substrate competition or competitive or noncompetitive inhibition. Examples of drugs that have been shown to significantly inhibit drug metabolism include chloramphenicol, cimetidine, valproic acid, allopurinol, and erythromycin. As with enzyme inducers, the addition or deletion of an inhibitory drug in a patient's drug therapy requires appropriate TDM and dose adjustment of the affected drug. TDM allows one to monitor these processes and adjust dosing accordingly.

The role of TDM becomes particularly apparent for drugs that undergo hepatic metabolism. Wide variability in the rate of metabolism of any given drug exists not only in different patients in the general population but also in the same patient at different times and in different circumstances. This variability is due to factors such as age, weight, gender, genetics, exposure to environmental substances, diet, coadministered drugs, and disease. Furthermore, unlike kidney function, in which creatinine provides a useful biomarker of function, there is no acceptable endogenous biochemical marker by which hepatic function, and consequently hepatic capability for drug clearance, can be routinely assessed before drug therapy is initiated.

The biotransformation of drugs may produce metabolites that are pharmacologically active. In such instances the metabolite should also be measured because it is contributing to the effect of the drug on the patient. Primidone and procainamide are examples of such drugs. If the metabolite is inactive, it need not be measured, but steps should be taken to ensure that it does not interfere in the analytical process. The latter problem of metabolite interference can cause significant problems for monitoring certain patients such as transplant patients receiving the ISDs cyclosporine or tacrolimus that have numerous active and inactive metabolites, which cross-react to varying degrees with the antibodies used in immunoassays for these drugs.[35]

Excretion

Excretion of drugs or chemicals from the body can occur through biliary, intestinal, pulmonary, or renal routes. Although each of these represents a possible mechanism of drug elimination, renal excretion is a major pathway for the elimination of most water-soluble drugs or metabolites and is important in TDM. Alterations in renal function may have a profound effect on the clearance and apparent half-life of the parent compound or its active metabolite(s); decreased renal function causes increased serum drug concentrations and increases the pharmacologic response.

Kidney function, in contrast to liver function, is readily and reliably evaluated by estimation of creatinine clearance. Creatinine is a metabolic product of muscle metabolism and is produced at a constant rate by the body. It is primarily eliminated from the body by the kidneys through the glomerular filtration mechanism. Renal clearance of creatinine at 120 mL/min approximates the glomerular filtration rate of 90 to 130 mL/min (see Chapter 34). Therefore measurement of creatinine clearance on a routine basis provides an effective tool to evaluate kidney function. A strong correlation has been shown to exist between creatinine clearance and the total body clearance or elimination rate constant of those drugs primarily dependent on the kidneys for their elimination. Examples of drugs whose therapeutic use is adjusted to account for changes in creatinine clearance include gentamicin, tobramycin, amikacin, digoxin, vancomycin, cyclosporine, and tacrolimus.

CHARACTERIZING DRUG EXPOSURE WITH MINIMAL ASSUMPTIONS: THE NONCOMPARTMENTAL ANALYSIS OF CONCENTRATION DATA OVER TIME

In pharmacokinetics, mathematical approaches are used to predict or describe certain events, usually for calculating a dosing regimen or predicting the serum drug concentration after a given drug dose. The mathematical tools most often used in clinical pharmacokinetics are compartmental models and model-independent relationships.

Model-independent relationships are becoming increasingly popular in clinical pharmacokinetics. The main advantages of model-independent relationships are fewer relationships to remember, fewer restrictive assumptions, a more general insight into elimination mechanisms, and easier computations. However, model-independent relationships are not without disadvantages; conceptualization of compartments or physiologic spaces may be lost, specific information that may be clinically relevant or pertinent to mechanisms of distribution or elimination can be lost, and the difficulty in constructing profiles of concentration versus time can be increased requiring greater numbers of samples to be collected.

The most frequently used model-independent, noncompartmental analysis approach for characterizing drug exposure uses algorithms to estimate the AUC after dosing of a drug. One of the simplest methods to estimate the AUC from timed concentration data uses the linear trapezoidal rule to divide the concentration-time curve of a drug into a series of trapezoids, the sum of which represents the AUC as diagrammed in Fig. 42.4. Accurate AUC estimation using the trapezoidal rule usually requires intense blood sampling during the dose interval.

In TDM, we are rarely concerned with a drug administered as a single, one-time intravenous bolus. Drugs are administered repetitively in the usual therapeutic situations. Fig. 42.5 shows that a drug repetitively administered at a fixed dosing interval will accumulate in the body until a steady-state condition exists. Note that a typical dosing cycle is once each half-life. *Steady state* can be defined as that point in the dosing scheme when the amount entering the circulation (governed by dosing rate) equals the amount eliminated (governed by elimination rate).

Theoretically, the AUC for the first dose of drug when time is extrapolated from time of zero to infinity should be equal to the AUC for a dose interval (τ) at steady state (see Fig. 42.4). The average drug concentration at steady state (C_{ss})

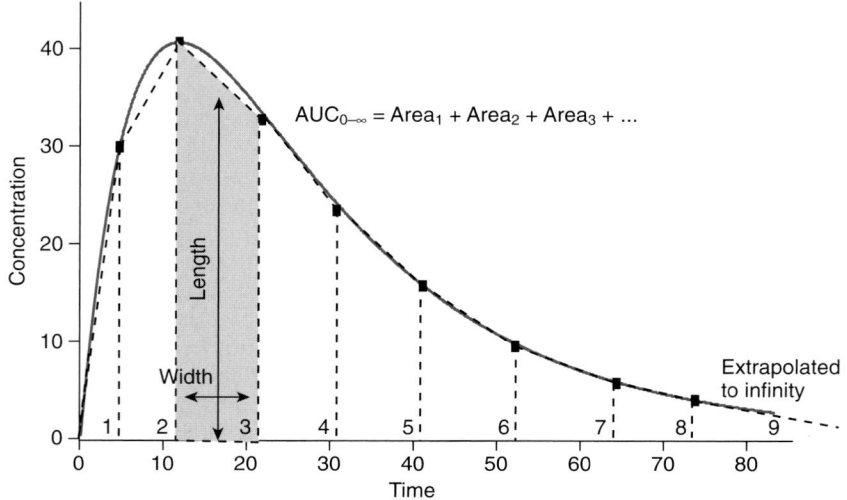

FIGURE 42.4 Determination of area under the curve (*AUC*) using the model independent trapezoidal rule for the extravascular (oral) route of administration.

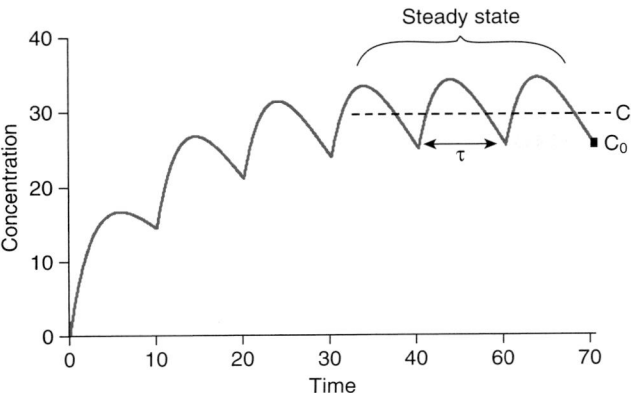

FIGURE 42.5 Concentration versus time curve for successive doses of a medication administered at constant dose interval (τ). At steady state the dose-time curves replicate.

is a frequent concentration reported for many drugs, and may be calculated using the formula

$$C_{ss} = \frac{AUC}{\tau} \qquad (42.6)$$

where τ represents the time duration of the dose interval. The maximum concentration (C_{max}) and minimum concentration (C_{min}) of a drug during a dose-interval are also frequently of interest because these concentrations may be associated with efficacy and/or toxicity of a drug. For most drugs, the C_{min} at steady state (also frequently referred to as the trough concentration) is the concentration obtained immediately before the dose at time of zero minutes (referred to as C_0); however, although generally the case, it is important to recognize that the C_{min} does not have to be equivalent to the C_0 concentration.

Clearance

Knowing the AUC of a drug after a defined dose allows calculation of the model-independent parameter of clearance, which provides a useful picture of the body's ability to eliminate a drug. Total body clearance (Cl_T or simply Cl) is defined as the theoretical total volume of blood, serum, or plasma completely cleared of drug per unit of time. It is usually expressed in units of mL/min, L/h, mL/min/kg, or L/h/kg. Cl is the sum total of all the clearances contributed by each elimination route (i.e., $Cl = Cl_{kidney} + Cl_{liver} + Cl_{biliary} + \ldots$). Cl is typically calculated from the AUC using the formula

$$Cl = \frac{D_0 \times f}{AUC_{0 \to \infty}} \qquad (42.7)$$

where AUC_0n_∞ is the AUC for the first dose integrated over time from zero to infinity. The variable f represents the bioavailable fraction of the drug, which is not generally known for orally administered drugs in a particular patient. Thus an apparent oral clearance (Cl_a) of a drug is calculated using

$$Cl_a = \frac{D_0}{AUC_{0 \to \infty}} \qquad (42.8)$$

Although Cl is model independent, it can be related to model-dependent parameters such as the volume of distribution and

elimination rate in a first-order, one-compartment model, as discussed in greater detail in the following section.

Hepatic Clearance

For drugs dependent solely on hepatic elimination, total body clearance (Cl_T) equals hepatic clearance (Cl_H). When the liver is considered from a purely physiologic perspective, the hepatic clearance is determined by the hepatic blood flow (Q) and the hepatic extraction fraction (E).

$$Cl = Q \times E \qquad (42.9)$$

The hepatic extraction fraction of a drug reflects the affinity of a particular drug for hepatic microsomal enzymes; E can be found experimentally or calculated by the equation

$$E = \frac{C_a - C_e}{C_a} \qquad (42.10)$$

where C_a is the concentration of the drug in blood entering the liver and C_e is the concentration of the drug in the hepatic venous effluent. For drugs that possess a high extraction fraction, hepatic clearance approaches hepatic blood flow (Q). The total body clearance of highly extracted drugs primarily depends on hepatic blood flow for their elimination. These drugs usually have low bioavailability because of the first-pass effect described earlier. Lidocaine is an example of such a drug. The clearance of low-extracted drugs is less dependent on blood flow and more dependent on the quantity and quality of the hepatic microsomal enzymes. Total body clearance of these drugs is affected by hepatic function, enzyme inducers and inhibitors, and changes in free drug concentration. Readers should recognize that this is a superficial view of a complex process. Several excellent reviews on this subject are available.[24,27,36]

PREDICTING DRUG CONCENTRATIONS USING A COMPARTMENTAL MODEL

Compartmental models are deterministic; that is, the drug concentration in blood and time data determine or define the model. The number and values of compartments assigned to the model have no true physiologic meaning or anatomic reality. The intravascular fluid compartment (blood) usually is the anatomic reference compartment. The advantage of intravascular fluid as the reference compartment is the ease with which it may be sampled to provide a definitive profile of blood concentration of drug versus time. The actual number of compartments can be quite extensive. However, for the sake of simplicity, one-, two-, and three-compartment models are most often used.

One-Compartment, First-Order Kinetic Model

In the simplest compartment model, the body is considered as a single compartment, as shown schematically in Fig. 42.6. It is assumed that after introduction of a drug, the substance is rapidly and uniformly distributed throughout the body, or said to be *kinetically homogeneous* within the compartment. Such a model is frequently applied to water-soluble antibiotics such as gentamicin. Fig. 42.7 illustrates graphically the relationship between log of concentration within the compartment and

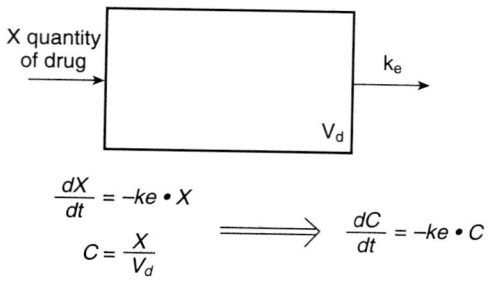

$$\frac{dX}{dt} = -ke \cdot X$$

$$C = \frac{X}{V_d} \implies \frac{dC}{dt} = -ke \cdot C$$

FIGURE 42.6 Schematic one compartment model and mathematical representation as discussed.

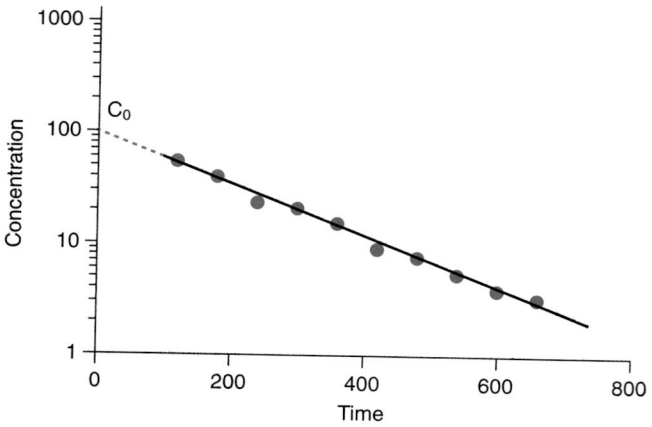

FIGURE 42.7 Semi-log plot of drug concentration (C) versus time extrapolated to time = 0 at which time, C = C_0, the theoretical initial concentration after a bolus administration.

time for a single-bolus injection of a drug. In the simple model of first-order elimination, the instantaneous change in quantity of drug within the compartment is proportional to the quantity (X) by the equation

$$\frac{dX}{dT} = -k_e X \qquad (42.11)$$

Integration of this equation using Laplace transformation yields the equation

$$X_t = X_0 \times e^{-k_e t} \qquad (42.12)$$

where X_0 is the initial quantity of the drug within the compartment, X_t is the blood concentration of the drug as a function of time, and k_e is the first-order elimination rate constant. From a practical perspective, the quantity of drug within the blood compartment cannot be easily measured. Instead, the concentration of drug within the compartment is the measured quantity. Dividing both sides of Eq. (42.12) by a volume of distribution (V_d) term converts this equation to

$$C_t = C_0 \times e^{-k_e t} \qquad (42.13)$$

where C_0, the initial concentration after bolus administration (which cannot be easily measured), is estimated by extrapolating the line shown in Fig. 42.7 to zero time. From knowledge of C_0 and k_e, one can theoretically predict the concentration at

any time (C_t). As shown later, most drugs are administered in repetitive doses rather than in a single bolus.

Volume of Distribution

For a drug that is assumed to be administered intravenously as a rapid bolus into a single, kinetically homogenous compartment, the C_0 is related to the compartment volume as follows:

$$C_0 = \frac{Dose}{V_d} \qquad (42.14)$$

V_d is called apparent *volume of distribution* because it is not a real volume in the physiologic sense, but instead is a proportionality constant to translate the absolute amount of drug present in the compartment (X) into its concentration relative to a volume. The V_d for an orally administered drug can be determined easily from concentration data using the one-compartment model after correction for bioavailability, f by

$$V_d = \frac{Dose \times f}{C_0} \qquad (42.15)$$

The units of V_d are usually liters (L). Although V_d is a mathematical term and not a real physiologic parameter, it is useful for contrasting degrees to which different types of drugs distribute. For instance, the polar hydrophilic drug gentamicin has a V_d = 0.2 L/kg of body weight, whereas the nonpolar lipophilic drug desipramine has a V_d = 34 L/kg of body weight. Gentamicin is concentrated in the blood, whereas desipramine is predominantly distributed into tissue.

Linear Kinetics of Elimination

Using the same assumptions of a one-compartment model as described earlier for calculation of the V_d, the first-order elimination rate constant can be determined by log transformation of Eq. (42.13) to give the natural logarithmic function:

$$\ln(C_t) = \ln(C_0) - k_e t \qquad (42.16)$$

Given a zero-time blood drug concentration (C_0), a non-zero time concentration (C_t), and a defined time (t), then k_e can be readily determined either algebraically or graphically. For example, in a plot of ln C_t versus t, the slope of the linear relationship is $-k_e$. The elimination rate constant k_e represents the fraction of drug removed per unit time and has units of reciprocal time (minute^{-1}, hour^{-1}, or day^{-1}).

Elimination Rate Constant and Half-Life

The elimination rate constant k_e can be related to another parameter, *half-life* $(t_{1/2})$, by the equation:

$$t_{1/2} = \frac{0.693}{k_e} \qquad (42.17)$$

where $t_{1/2}$ is usually defined as the time required for the amount of drug in blood to decline to half of a measured value. The constant, 0.693, in the equation represents the natural logarithm of 2. Fig. 42.7 demonstrates how the half-life can be rapidly determined from a semi-log plot of drug concentration versus time. As few as two successive concentrations

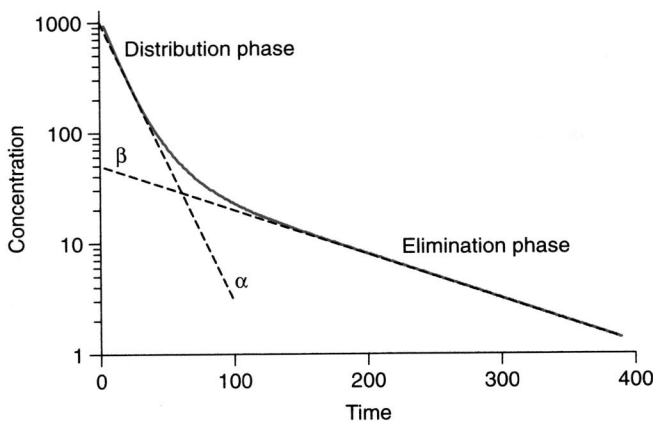

FIGURE 42.8 Drug concentration in plasma after administration of a dose for a two-compartment model. Decline from the original concentration (C_0) is affected by both the distribution phase (characterized by the constant α) and the elimination phase (characterized by the constant β) as described in the Fundamental Principles of Applied Pharmacokinetics section.

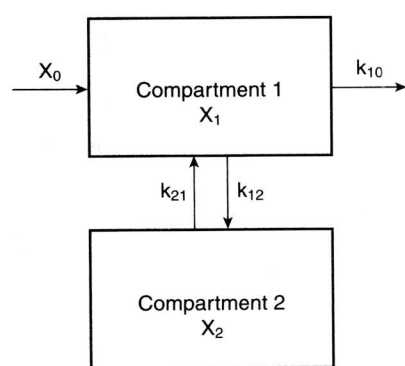

FIGURE 42.9 Two-compartment pharmacokinetic model. k_{21} and k_{12} are distribution rate constants, and k_{10} is the elimination rate constant for the central compartment, compartment 1 in this diagram.

collected at times t_1 and t_2 are required for the estimate of k_e using the equation

$$k_e = \ln(C_{t1}) - \ln\left(\frac{C_{t2}}{t_2}\right) - t_1 \qquad (42.18)$$

As discussed previously in the section on model-independent characterization of pharmacokinetics, Cl is a useful derived parameter for describing the elimination of a drug from the body. For a drug described well by a one-compartment, first-order kinetic model, Cl is mathematically related to V_d and k_e by the following relationship:

$$Cl = V_d \times k_e \qquad (42.19)$$

It is important to recognize that the previous equations are relevant only in the context of intravenous bolus administration of a drug. More prolonged infusions of drugs and oral administration require additional model terms to characterize the infusion rates, duration, or absorption lag time into the pharmacokinetic models presented. Details on these more complex one-compartment models can be found in textbooks dedicated to pharmacokinetics.[36]

Two-Compartment and Multicompartment Models

Fig. 42.8 illustrates the more complex kinetics demonstrated by a two-compartment model. The curve is described by the following equation:

$$C_t = Ae^{-\alpha t} + Be^{-\beta t} \qquad (42.20)$$

where the rate constant α is the slope of the curve during the phase in which the drug is being distributed, referred to as the *distribution phase*. β is the slope of the curve during the phase in which the drug is being eliminated by metabolism and excretion (assuming that distribution is complete) and is derived by extrapolating the *elimination phase* of the curve in Fig. 42.8 to time = 0 that would have existed if distribution had been immediate and complete. A is an estimate, using the method of residuals, of the theoretical plasma concentration

at time = 0, immediately after intravenous injection of a bolus of the drug. B is derived by extrapolation of the terminal slope of the distributive phase line to time = 0. From a physiologic perspective, the two-compartment model described earlier accounts for the initial decline of drug concentration in the reference compartment (i.e., the sampled plasma compartment) into a vascularized tissue compartment (the second compartment). A three-compartment model mimics a system like the two-compartment model with a third reservoir, such as adipose tissue or cellular nuclei, in which the drug resides over the long term. Fig. 42.9 depicts a two-compartment model, after an intravenous bolus administration of a drug. In these figures, X_0 represents the drug dose given and therefore the amount of drug in the system at zero time, X_1 the amount of drug in the central or reference compartment, and X_2 the amount of drug in the peripheral compartment in the case of the two-compartment model. k_{10} represents the elimination rate constant; that is, the rate at which the drug leaves the reference compartment and is lost from the system. k_{12} and k_{21} are transfer rate constants describing, for the two-compartment model only, rates at which the drug is exchanged between compartments within the system. Which model is the best for a particular drug is somewhat empirical and based on model-fitting statistics. For a more detailed discussion around model fitting, readers are referred to textbooks devoted to the subject.[37–40]

GENERAL CONSIDERATIONS FOR THE CLINICAL USE OF THERAPEUTIC DRUG MONITORING

There is no universal set of rules that determine whether a drug might benefit from TDM; however, numerous characteristics of a drug contribute to the need for TDM. TDM is most valuable when the drug in question is used chronically, has variable pharmacokinetics, and has a narrow TI. For drugs with a narrow TI, there is little if any window between blood (or serum for those drugs routinely measured in serum) concentrations associated with efficacy and those associated with toxic effects. The immunosuppressive calcineurin inhibitor drug tacrolimus provides a good example of a narrow TI drug with a wide variability in PK as shown in Fig. 42.10. The concentrations of tacrolimus that are associated with efficacy (i.e., freedom from graft rejection) and those associated with kidney toxicity overlap considerably.

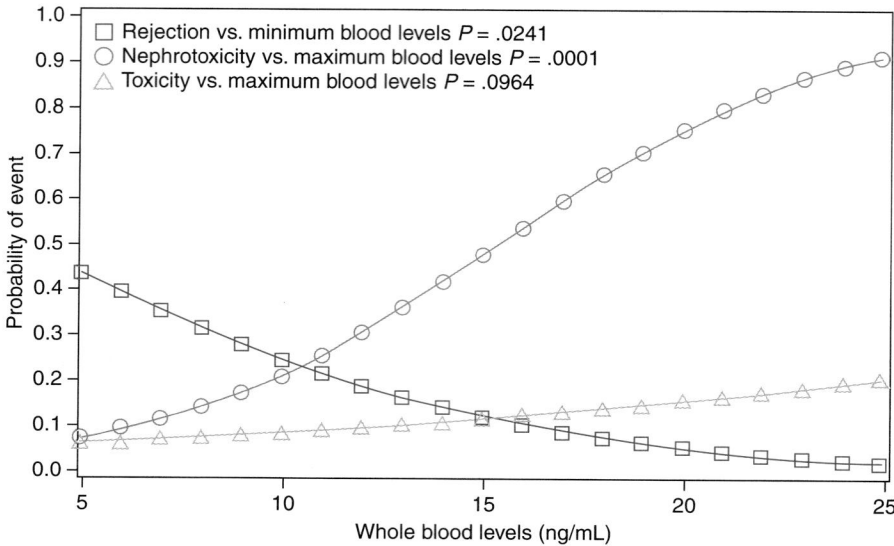

FIGURE 42.10 The pharmacodynamics of tacrolimus in renal transplantation. (Reprinted with permission from Venkataramanan R, Shaw LM, Sarkozi L, et al. Clinical utility of monitoring tacrolimus blood concentrations in liver transplant patients. *J Clin Pharm* 2001;41[5]:542–51 with permission.)

TDM helps navigate this tightrope. By itself, however, narrow TI is not necessarily sufficient to warrant TDM. Many narrow TI drugs are routinely used without monitoring, such as most cancer chemotherapy drugs. Additional factors therefore contribute to the need for TDM, such as the severity of failed drug therapy (e.g., antimicrobials) or toxicity (e.g., ISDs). Difficulty in recognizing efficacy or toxicity with use of these drugs can be life threatening. Many patients, especially those with chronic disease, also require prolonged drug therapy. The problem of compliance is particularly evident with patients who are characteristically free of pain or unusual discomfort, as with epilepsy, asthma, hypertension, mild heart disease, and transplantation. Patients may develop a sense that their disease has been cured and they no longer need the drug. The end result of noncompliance is exacerbation of the existing disorder and treatment failure. Drug concentration values provide positive feedback to physicians regarding complying and noncomplying patients.

For TDM to be useful, the concentration data must be accurate and precise. Numerous factors affect the measurement of drugs in blood. These factors, if not recognized, may lead to erroneous decision making that could negate any benefits of monitoring and might even lead to more harm than good from TDM.

Preanalytical Factors That Affect Therapeutic Drug Monitoring Results

To interpret a TDM result, it is critical that the dose of drug given to the patient is known. Dosage uniformity standards exist for drugs approved by the US Food and Drug Administration (FDA). Although most drug formulations are fairly consistent, the actual dose of a drug in a single tablet, suspension, or vial may vary. US Pharmacopeia (USP) standards dictate that the mean dose contained in a tablet must be within ±10% of the product labeling and no tested sample may fall outside of 75 and 125% of the mean. As a result, the dose content for a single dose theoretically could vary by as much as 25% and still fall within acceptable USP content

uniformity limits. This is further compounded by inaccuracies introduced by manipulation of the dose (e.g., splitting of scored tablets) or failure to administer or consume the entire dose (e.g., from vomiting). Drugs also may degrade over time or by storage method, leading to further inaccuracy of dose.

Beyond dose accuracy, pharmacokinetics is inherently time-based. Accurate timing of sample collection is often an important factor, especially when timed samples such as peak or trough samples are the primary means of monitoring. Specimen timing for routine TDM should therefore be as close as possible to the timing of collection used in clinical studies that support TDM use for a specific drug. Vancomycin trough samples provide an example in which collection immediately before the next dose is recommended because of the relatively short half-life of this drug (~6 to −12 hours).[41] Premature sampling in the context of rapidly changing concentration may lead to falsely increased concentrations if trough sampling is assumed, and this could alter decision-making given the generally narrow therapeutic range for this drug. In contrast, drugs with slow distribution but long half-life, such as digoxin, are optimally sampled in the postdistributive phase of longer than 6 hours after dosing. Sampling during steady state (generally more than four doses) is also an important assumption made for monitoring of many drugs, such as vancomycin.

Variation in collection and handling of samples for TDM also can affect the quality of concentration data. Although serum is the preferred sample for monitoring of many drugs, different collection tubes are available for generating serum that include plain glass or plastic tubes without additive (e.g., red-stoppered BD Vacutainer tubes [Becton, Dickinson, Franklin Lakes, NJ]), as well as specialized serum separator tubes (e.g., yellow-stoppered BD Vacutainer tubes) that contain a gel that separates serum from the cellular components after centrifugation. The latter tube may affect drug concentration because of adsorption of drug by the gel after prolonged contact. The adsorptive effects vary across drugs and have been shown to significantly reduce the concentration of some drugs such as phenytoin, particularly when the collection tubes are under-filled.[42]

The importance of preanalytical factors in the accuracy and precision of TDM results should not be underestimated. TDM laboratories are part of a larger health care system. It is imperative that laboratories engage and work with the many parts of this system, including pharmacists, nursing staff, and the phlebotomy team. Each individual plays an important role in TDM, and the effective control of the many factors that affect TDM accuracy are key to success of this complex feedback control system.

POINTS TO REMEMBER

Preanalytic Factors Affecting Therapeutic Drug Monitoring Results
- Dose accuracy
- Appropriate sampling time
- Specimen collection and handling
- Physiologic changes in the patient (e.g., serum albumin concentration)

Analytical Factors That Affect Monitoring Results

The laboratory, of course, plays a central role in the TDM process. Beyond the preanalytical factors affecting TDM results, analytical factors are important considerations in the interpretation of drug concentration data. Notable challenges in the analytical field include the availability of standardized reference material and the selectivity of methods for the drug of interest.

Analytical error falls into two general categories, random error and systematic error. Random error is generally inherent to a particular method. Efforts to characterize and limit random error are a mainstay of the development and validation of most analytical methods. In contrast, systematic error or bias is often insidious. Determining whether a method gives accurate results over the long term and across laboratories is often a difficult task. This is generally accomplished by either comparing the results of testing against a definitive analytical method or using a certified reference material. The International Union of Pure and Applied Chemistry defines a definitive method as[43]:

A method of exceptional scientific status, which is sufficiently accurate to stand alone in the determination of a given property for the certification of a reference material. Such a method must have a firm theoretical foundation so that systematic error is negligible relative to the intended use. Analyte masses (amounts) or concentrations must be measured directly in terms of the base units of measurements, or indirectly related through sound theoretical equations. Definitive methods, together with Certified Reference Materials, are primary means for transferring accuracy—that is, establishing traceability.[43]

Definitive methods generally employ very time-consuming and expensive techniques (e.g., isotope dilution mass spectrometry) to establish material purity and quantity that are not practical for general use in most clinical laboratories. The availability of certified reference material (also frequently referred to as standardized reference material) to which methods may be compared is a critical factor in helping control systematic error. Early studies of method comparability for AEDs demonstrated that concentrations varied greatly across laboratories and within laboratories over time. These data led to the development in the early 1980s by the National Institute for Standards and Technology (NIST) of a standard reference material of sufficient purity and accuracy to allow standardization of AED monitoring methods across different laboratories and manufacturers.[44] Unfortunately, this type of standardized reference material is unavailable for other monitored drugs.

The ability of a given method to detect a compound of interest among many potential substances present in a sample (referred to as method selectivity) represents another potential source of systematic error. Selectivity is particularly important for TDM tests because many drugs are structurally related, including to some endogenously produced compounds. Most drugs are also extensively metabolized through a number of different pathways of biotransformation. These metabolites are often similar to the parent compound in structure, but pharmacologic activity is variable. Tacrolimus provides a useful example. Antibodies directed against tacrolimus that are used for immunoassays demonstrate similar reactivity toward tacrolimus along with two of its metabolites, 15-desmethyl-tacrolimus and 31-desmethyl-tacrolimus. Although both metabolites are detected equally, the 15-desmethyl metabolite exhibits little immunosuppressive activity, whereas the 31-desmethyl metabolite exhibits immunosuppressive activity similar to that of tacrolimus. These metabolites are generally low in abundance in most patients; however, alterations in metabolism secondary to liver dysfunction can lead to their accumulation, resulting in a systematic error that complicates test interpretation.[45,46] Since selectivity often differs greatly across analytical platforms, this important performance characteristic must be recognized when interpreting testing, especially when done by different laboratories that employ different testing methods (e.g., immunoassay vs. liquid chromatography–tandem mass spectrometry (LC-MS/MS)).

The Concept of a Therapeutic Range

The relationship between serum drug concentration and clinical outcome forms the basis for TDM, as depicted in Fig. 42.1. One of the most common interpretative errors encountered regarding TDM is the presumption that a concentration within a reported therapeutic range will ensure treatment success in the absence of toxicity, and concentrations outside this range will not. In reality, the probability of success and toxicity are a continuum across the concentration range. These probabilities are maximized and minimized, respectively, within the therapeutic range. Nevertheless, therapeutic success can certainly occur at concentrations below the therapeutic range. More importantly, success also may be achieved by concentrations above the therapeutic range without associated toxicity in some patients. Experienced users of TDM often recognize these relationships and weigh the risks and potential benefits of drug concentrations in the context of the clinical situation using the therapeutic range as a guide.

Similar to a reference interval for any laboratory test, therapeutic ranges are based on population data from drug therapy trials and in some instances confirmed or established by RCCTs. The application of these population-based ranges to an individual therefore assumes similarity to the target population. Differences in metabolism, physiology, and/or the underlying disease process can alter these relationships, leading to unexpected and undesirable results. Phenytoin used for seizure control illustrates this limitation. A fairly good relationship between serum phenytoin concentration and seizure control exists. However, several factors have been shown to alter the dose-response relationships for phenytoin that might have an impact on the utility of defined therapeutic ranges. The presence of concomitant liver disease significantly alters the pharmacokinetics of phenytoin because of its high degree of binding to albumin, a protein that is significantly altered with moderate to severe liver disease. As a result, individuals with liver disease are at significantly higher risk for toxicity at total serum phenytoin concentrations that are otherwise appropriate for individuals without liver disease. The recognition of this problem led to the development of methods for measuring phenytoin that is unbound to albumin in serum (also known as free phenytoin) which also correlates with seizure control. Nevertheless, this example illustrates the need for caution in applying population-based relationships to individual patients who may not be represented by the population used for defining the therapeutic range. Another common challenge is the application of a therapeutic range defined for a drug typically used in combination where the individual TDM situation is not the same drug combination used in the clinical study in which the range was originally defined.

Beyond Empiric Dosing: Model-Based Dosage Adjustment

Use of a single measured drug concentration such as a trough concentration to forecast drug dose is one of the most commonly employed approaches to dose adjustment because of the simplicity of obtaining this in a clinical setting. In the simplest method of applying concentration data in the clinic, a provider adjusts a dose empirically based on these single concentrations in an attempt to achieve the desired concentration at the next measurement. This approach, which is generally based on a model (e.g., linear kinetics of elimination) and experience of the provider, will eventually yield the desired concentration in most patients; however, it may take long periods of monitoring to ultimately achieve the desired control. Beyond the costs, time is sometimes critical to treatment success such as with the use of antibiotics to treat life-threatening infections.

One of the major pitfalls to the use of a single, timed drug level for the adjustment of drug dosing is the potential error associated with an individual result. Patients are often treated with drugs during times when physiology is quite variable, such as the critically ill patient with an infection receiving an aminoglycoside antibiotic. Under these circumstances, a single concentration measurement usually does not possess sufficient information content to assess the adequacy of exposure or forecast future drug concentrations with dose changes.

To improve the precision of dose estimation based on a monitored drug concentration, several pharmacokinetic-based methods have been developed to estimate patient-specific pharmacokinetic parameters using two or more drug concentrations. The first described and most simple of these methods, often referred to as the Zaske-Sawchuk method,[47] was developed in the context of therapy with aminoglycoside antibiotics. In this method, multiple concentrations are obtained to estimate pharmacokinetic parameters for a specific patient that can be used to guide dosing.

Although the Zaske-Sawchuk method significantly improved the precision of therapy with aminoglycoside antibiotics and other drugs, numerous limitations still exist. Multiple concentration measurements are required for adequate confidence in parameter estimation. More importantly, they ignore prior information regarding parameter estimates that have been derived from population-based studies that could assist in the initial dosing of the patient. These methods also discard prior studies performed in a patient under evaluation that provide useful information regarding PK variability within an individual patient.

Improved methods of parameter estimation that use the Bayes theorem have therefore been developed in an attempt to overcome some of these limitations. Although beyond the scope of this chapter, the Bayes theorem provides a theoretical framework to relate the parameter estimates that are made from a set of concentration data to any prior information about these parameters. As a result, Bayesian methods permit incorporation of prior concentration and parameter information into the estimation process. Numerous studies have demonstrated the improvement in precision of concentration control for many drugs, often with less available data; however, the question of whether Bayesian methods improve clinical outcomes over simpler approaches remains.

POINTS TO REMEMBER

Analytical Factors That Affect Therapeutic Drug Monitoring Results
- Method selectivity for the target drug versus its metabolites
- Method precision relative to the desired therapeutic target range
- Availability of standardized reference material
- Interfering substances in the sample (e.g., antibodies that react with assay reagents)

THERAPEUTIC DRUG MONITORING OF SPECIFIC DRUGS IN COMMON CLINICAL USE

This section will discuss therapeutic drugs commonly monitored in clinical practice. It should be noted that the drug concentrations and ranges provided in this section serve as a general guide. Laboratories should verify that these ranges are appropriate for use in their own settings as ranges may depend upon analytic methodology, the patient population, and other factors such as concomitant drug therapy.

Antiepileptic Drugs

A number of AEDs are used to treat seizures (Table 42.1). Most can be measured by chromatographic methods or individually analyzed by immunoassay. The advantage of chromatographic methods such as gas chromatography–mass chromatography (GC-MS) or LC-MS is the ability to simultaneously analyze multiple AEDs in a single assay, with some methods reported to detect more than 20 individual compounds.[48] Immunoassay procedures are less labor intensive and are usually quicker to perform than chromatographic methods for measuring a single analyte. As a result, immunoassays are the mainstay of monitoring for these drugs in most clinical laboratories.

TABLE 42.1   Pharmacokinetic Parameters of Antiepileptic Drugs

Drug	RECOMMENDED THERAPEUTIC RANGE[a]		Mean Time to Steady State (d)	Observed Range of Half-Life in Adults (h)	Mean Volume of Distribution (L/kg)	Mean Oral Bioavailability (%)	Protein Binding (%)	Important Metabolizing Enzymes
	μg/mL	μmol/L						
Brivaracetam	0.2–2	1–10	1–2	7–8	0.5	100	35	Amidase, CYP2C9, CYP2C19
Carbamazepine	4–12	17–51	2–4	8–12	1.4	70	75	CYP3A4
Clonazepam	0.015–0.060	0.048–0.190	3–10	17–56	3.2	>90	85	CYP3A4
Eslicarbazepine Acetate[b]	3–35	12–139	3–4	13–20	2.7	<90	44	Esterases; glucuronidation of eslicarbazepine (10-hydroxycarbazepine)
Ethosuximide	40–100	283–708	7–10	30–60	0.7	>90	0	CYP3A4
Felbamate	30–60	126–252	3–4	14–21	0.8	>90	25	CYP3A4
Gabapentin	2–12	12–70	1–2	5–9	0.9	Variable	0	NA
Lamotrigine	2.5–15	10–59	3–6	20–30	1.2	>90	55	NA
Levetiracetam	12–46	70–270	1–2	6–8	0.6	>90	0	NA
Oxcarbazepine[c]	3–35	12–139	2–3	8–15	0.75	100	40	Glucuronidation of primary active metabolite (10-hydroxycarbazepine)
Phenobarbital	10–40	43–172	12–24	70–140	0.7	>90	50	CYP2C19
Phenytoin	10–20 (free: 1.0–2.0)	40–79	5–17	30–100	0.6	80	90	CYP2C9, 2C19
Primidone	5–10	23–46	2–4	3–22	0.7	>90	20	CYP2C9, 2C19
Topiramate	5–20	15–59	4–5	20–30	0.7	80	15	NA
Valproic acid	50–100	346–693	2–4	11–20	0.2	>90	90	CYP2C9,2C19, 2B6, 2E1, 2A6
Zonisamide	10–40	47–188	9–12	50–70	1.4	65	50	CYP2C9, 3A4

[a]Laboratories should verify that these ranges are appropriate for use in their own settings as ranges may depend upon analytic methodology, the patient population, and other factors such as concomitant drug therapy.

[b]All values refer to the active metabolite eslicarbazepine (10-hydroxycarbazepine).

[c]The recommended therapeutic range is that quoted for the active metabolite of oxcarbazepine, which is 10-hydroxycarbazepine.

Phenytoin

Phenytoin (diphenylhydantoin), most commonly available as Dilantin but also available in generic form, is used in the treatment of primary or secondary generalized tonic-clonic seizures, partial or complex-partial seizures, and status epilepticus. The drug is not effective for absence seizures. Phenytoin likely has many targets, but the most well-described mechanism of action is the modulation of voltage-gated sodium channels through prolonging channel inactivation, which reduces the ability of the neuron to respond at high frequency.[49,50] The physiologic effect of this action is reduction in central synaptic transmission, aiding in control of abnormal neuronal excitability.

Phenytoin is not readily soluble in aqueous solutions. When administered by intramuscular injection, most of the dose precipitates at the site of injection and is then slowly absorbed. A prodrug called fosphenytoin (Cerebyx) was introduced as a therapeutic form of phenytoin to improve phenytoin's pharmacology. Fosphenytoin has increased aqueous solubility for intramuscular injection.[51] After injection, it is rapidly converted to phenytoin. Absorption of oral phenytoin is slow and sometimes incomplete. Variations in the drug preparation have been blamed for low bioavailability. Once absorbed, the drug is tightly bound to protein (90 to 95%). As with all drugs, the pharmacologic effect of phenytoin is directly related to the amount present in the free (unbound) state. Only free phenytoin is available to cross biological membranes and interact at biologically important binding sites. The degree of protein binding can be reduced by the presence of other drugs, anemia, and hypoalbuminemia, which can occur in the elderly. In these conditions, an increased effect is observed at the same total drug concentration as in plasma from normal patients.

The optimal therapeutic concentration for seizure control without side effects is 10 to 20 µg/mL (40 to 79 µmol/L). In a large population study, Buchthal and colleagues[52] found a 50% response rate in patients with plasma concentrations greater than 10 µg/mL (40 µmol/L) and an 86% suppression of seizure activity at concentrations exceeding 15 µg/mL (59 µmol/L). These concentrations also serve as reasonable guidelines when the drug is used as a cardiac antiarrhythmic agent. Free phenytoin concentration in the range of 1 to 2 µg/mL (1 to 8 µmol/L) is frequently considered optimal. This free phenytoin reference interval[b] is based largely on studies of total serum phenytoin and an assumed 10% unbound drug fraction; however, the free fraction of phenytoin has been reported to vary considerably in otherwise healthy individuals from as low as 3% to as high as 37% in some patients.[53] Total phenytoin concentrations in excess of 20 µg/mL (79 µmol/L) do not usually enhance seizure control and are often associated with nystagmus and ataxia. Total phenytoin plasma concentrations in excess of 35 µg/mL (139 µmol/L) have been shown to actually precipitate seizure activity. A side effect of phenytoin not related to plasma concentration is development of gingival hyperplasia.

Phenytoin is metabolized by hepatic microsomal hydroxylating enzymes. The principal metabolite is 5-(p-hydroxyphenyl)-5-phenylhydantoin, which is excreted principally as a glucuronide ester. Other minor metabolites are of minimal clinical importance. Hepatic metabolism of phenytoin may become saturated within the therapeutic range. Once metabolism is saturated, small dose increments result in large changes in blood concentration (see Fig. 42.10); this phenomenon partially explains the wide variation in dose among patients that is required to accomplish a therapeutic effect.[54] Because of this saturation phenomenon, first–order kinetics do not generally apply to total phenytoin at blood concentrations in excess of 5 µg/mL (20 µmol/L).

The time to collect the specimen is dictated by the reason for monitoring. If a patient displays any symptoms of intoxication, the peak blood concentration is of interest. This specimen is collected 4 to 5 hours after the dose, although the peak level may be delayed up to 8 hours if the drug is given in conjunction with substances that increase stomach acidity. If the principal question at hand is adequate therapy, the trough concentration is more useful and the specimen is collected just before the next dose is given.

A number of drug interactions result in alteration of the disposition of phenytoin. Alcohol, barbiturates, and carbamazepine induce oxidative enzymes; this induction results in increased metabolism of phenytoin, reduced serum concentration of both total and free phenytoin, and reduced pharmacologic effect. Drugs such as chloramphenicol, cimetidine, disulfiram, isoniazid, and dicumarol compete with phenytoin metabolism, resulting in increase of both total and free phenytoin concentrations and enhancement of the pharmacologic effect. Salicylate, valproic acid, phenylbutazone, sulfisoxazole, and sulfonylureas compete with phenytoin for serum protein-binding sites. The end result is diminished total serum concentration of phenytoin while the free phenytoin concentration and pharmacologic effect remain approximately the same. The interest in monitoring the free phenytoin concentration is in response to these altered disposition states.

Carbamazepine

Carbamazepine (Tegretol) is used in the treatment of generalized tonic-clonic, partial, and partial-complex seizures. It is also used for the treatment of pain associated with trigeminal neuralgia and as a mood-stabilizing drug in bipolar disorder. Like phenytoin, carbamazepine modulates the synaptic sodium channel, which prolongs inactivation, reducing the ability of the neuron to respond at high frequency.[50] The physiologic effect of this action is reduction in central synaptic transmission, aiding in control of abnormal neuronal excitability. The mechanisms of action in mood stabilization are less clear, but appear to work through effects on inositol metabolism and glycogen synthase kinase 3-b (GSK3-b), which is an essential part of the Wnt/b-catenin pathway.[55] This latter pathway has been shown recently to play a critical role in neuronal adhesion, plasticity, and survival, as well as brain development.[56] In addition, GSK3-β appears critical to the action of dopamine and serotonin on the brain affecting behavior,[57] likely explaining many of the effects of mood-stabilizing drugs such as carbamazepine that inhibit this pathway.

After oral administration, carbamazepine is slowly and erratically absorbed with wide individual variability. The drug is highly protein bound (80%). The elimination half-life early in therapy is approximately 24 hours. With chronic therapy, the enzymes responsible for metabolism are induced, and the elimination half-life is reduced to 15 to 20 hours. Because hepatic metabolism is the principal means by which

---

[b]Laboratories should verify that these ranges are appropriate for use in their own settings.

drug is eliminated from plasma, any reduction in liver function results in drug accumulation.

The therapeutic concentration range for optimal pharmacologic effect of carbamazepine is a trough concentration between 4 and 12 μg/mL (17 to 51 μmol/L); however, this range depends on concomitant use of other AEDs. Toxicity associated with excessive carbamazepine ingestion occurs at plasma concentrations in excess of 15 μg/mL (63 μmol/L) and is characterized by symptoms of blurred vision, paresthesia, nystagmus, ataxia, drowsiness, and diplopia. Side effects unrelated to plasma concentration include development of an urticarial rash, which usually disappears on discontinuation of the drug, and hematologic depression (leukopenia, thrombocytopenia, and aplastic anemia).

The active metabolite of carbamazepine is carbamazepine-10,11-epoxide. This metabolite has been found to accumulate in children to concentrations equivalent to carbamazepine. It may contribute to symptoms of intoxication in children who have a therapeutic plasma concentration of the parent drug. Because carbamazepine is metabolized through the hepatic oxidative enzyme system, drugs that induce this system (phenytoin, phenobarbital) increase the rate of clearance of carbamazepine.

Coadministration of phenobarbital, phenytoin, or valproic acid increases the rate of metabolism of carbamazepine, reducing the blood concentration. Erythromycin and propoxyphene interfere with metabolism, increasing carbamazepine concentrations.

Trough concentration monitoring is the generally recommended sample for carbamazepine TDM; however, in the case of suspected mild intoxication, the peak value of the plasma concentration correlates more closely with toxicity. The peak specimen should be collected 4 to 8 hours after the oral dose in the setting of immediate-release formulations of carbamazepine.

Oxcarbazepine

Oxcarbazepine, trade name Trileptal, is an antiepileptic used to treat both focal and generalized seizures. It is also used both as solo therapy and add-on in patients with bipolar disease resistant to treatment with other therapeutics. Oxcarbazepine is a structural derivative of carbamazepine, wherein a ketone replaces the carbon-carbon double bond of the dibenzaprine ring at the 10 position. This structural modification of carbamazepine reduces the risk of hepatotoxicity by reducing production of the toxic 10,11 epoxide metabolite. Both oxcarbazepine and its primary metabolite, 10-hydroxycarbazepine act mainly by blocking voltage-sensitive sodium channels similar to the mechanism of action of carbamazepine.

Although oxcarbazepine has 100% bioavailability and is pharmacologically active, it has a very short half-life with a low, often undetectable plasma concentration. Following oral absorption of oxcarbazepine, it is rapidly converted to 10-hydroxycarbazepine (mostly as the (S)-(+) stereoisomer). As most of the pharmacologic activity of oxcarbazepine is attributable to 10-hydroxycarbazepine, this primary metabolite is currently the target compound used for TDM. The 10-hydroxycarbazepine metabolite exhibits linear pharmacokinetics with a time to maximal concentration (Tmax) of 3 to 6 hours. It is 40% bound to plasma proteins and has a therapeutic range of 3 to 35 μg/mL (12 to 139 μmol/L)(see Table 42.1).[58]

Eslicarbazepine Acetate

Eslicarbazepine acetate, brand name Zebinix, is a pro-drug, whose primary metabolite is the (S)-(+) stereoisomer of 10-hydroxycarbazepine, the same primary active metabolite of oxcarbazepine. Since the therapeutic range for this drug is also based upon the pharmacologically active metabolite 10-hydroxycarbazepine (see Table 42.1), no further discussion will be provided here. As is the case for oxcarbazepine, very little to no detectable parent drug is present in trough samples, and therefore the active 10-hydroxycarbazepine metabolite is the recommended monitored analyte.[58]

Valproic Acid

Valproic acid (Depakene or Depakote) is used for treatment of absence seizures. It also has been shown to be useful against tonic-clonic and partial seizures when used in conjunction with other AEDs such as phenobarbital or phenytoin. Beyond its use in the treatment of epilepsy, valproate also has mood-stabilizing effects that make it a useful agent, and alternative, in the treatment of bipolar disorder. The drug inhibits the enzyme γ-aminobutyric acid (GABA) transaminase, resulting in an increase in the concentration of GABA in the brain. GABA is a potent inhibitor of presynaptic and postsynaptic discharges in the central nervous system. Valproic acid also modulates the synaptic sodium channel by prolonging inactivation, which reduces the ability of the neuron to respond at high frequency.[50,59] Additional mechanisms of action have been reported, such as effects on inositol metabolism and GSK-3 activity that might explain its utility in mood disorders.[55,60,61]

Valproic acid is rapidly and almost completely absorbed after oral administration. Peak concentrations occur 1 to 4 hours after an oral dose. The principal metabolite, 2-n-propyl-3-ketopentanoic acid, has anticonvulsant activity comparable to that of valproic acid, although this metabolite does not accumulate in plasma. The single-dose half-life is 16 hours in healthy adults, but this reduces to 12 hours on chronic therapy and may be as short as 8 hours in children. In neonates and in hepatic disease, when metabolism is reduced, the half-life becomes prolonged. Valproic acid is highly protein bound (93%). In circumstances when competition for protein binding increases, such as in uremia, cirrhosis, or concurrent drug therapy, the percent of free valproic acid increases.

The minimum effective therapeutic concentration of valproic acid is 50 μg/mL (346 μmol/L). Concentrations in excess of 100 μg/mL (693 μmol/L) have been associated with hepatic toxicity and acute toxic encephalopathy.

Clearance of valproic acid is rapid, presenting a dosing dilemma. The dose must be adequate to provide a plasma concentration greater than 40 μg/mL (277 μmol/L) while avoiding concentrations in excess of 100 μg/mL (693 μmol/L). The ideal specimen for monitoring the blood concentration is that drawn just before the next dose, usually early in the morning, to confirm that an adequate dose has been prescribed before bedtime. Dosing is particularly problematic in young children, who might sleep for more than one complete half-life of the drug.

Valproic acid modulates the action of various other common AEDs. It inhibits the nonrenal clearance of phenobarbital, resulting in increased phenobarbital concentrations. It competes with phenytoin for protein-binding sites. The free phenytoin concentration remains approximately the same, but the total phenytoin in the plasma decreases. Because the free phenytoin concentration remains unchanged, the pharmacologic effect is retained. Other common AEDs that induce hepatic oxidative enzymes result in increased valproic acid clearance; this increased clearance rate requires a higher dose to maintain effective therapeutic concentrations.

Ethosuximide

Ethosuximide (Zarontin) is used for the treatment of absence seizures characterized by brief loss of consciousness. Ethosuximide reduces the flow of calcium through T-type calcium channels in the synapse of thalamic neurons; because thalamic neurons are the main source of 3-Hz spike-wave rhythms in absence seizures, reduction of calcium flow slows the rate of these seizure-inducing pulses.

Ethosuximide is readily absorbed from the gastrointestinal tract. The drug is cleared mainly by metabolism as either the hydroxyethyl compound or the glucuronide ester of the hydroxyethyl metabolite with a half-life of approximately 33 hours, although this may be prolonged in adults. The trough specimen yields the most useful information regarding therapeutic efficacy. The optimal therapeutic concentration of ethosuximide is 40 to 100 μg/mL (283 to 708 μmol/L). Toxicity related to an excessive blood concentration of ethosuximide is rare. Symptoms of gastrointestinal distress, lethargy, dizziness, and euphoria may be encountered early in therapy, but patients usually become tolerant to these symptoms.

Topiramate

Topiramate (Topamax) is a sulfamate-substituted monosaccharide anticonvulsant also approved for use in migraine headache therapy. The mechanisms by which topiramate exerts these effects is not clearly established. It is proposed that several effects may contribute to topiramate's pharmacologic activity, including blockage of voltage-dependent sodium channels, augmentation of the neurotransmitter γ-aminobutyrate action at some of the subtypes of the GABA-A receptor, antagonism of the AMPA/kainite subtype of glutamate receptors, and inhibition of isozymes II and IV of carbonic anhydrase.[62]

Topiramate is indicated as initial monotherapy or in combination with other anticonvulsants in patients 2 years of age and older with partial-onset or primary generalized tonic-clonic seizures, and also is effective in patients with seizures associated with Lennox-Gastaut syndrome and was originally approved for use as an anticonvulsant by the FDA in 1996.[63]

Topamax is generally well and rapidly absorbed after oral administration with a usual T_{max} between 2 and 4 hours and bioavailability of up to 95%. Coingestion of food can delay absorption by approximately 2 hours without effect on T_{max}. Average steady-state serum concentrations can fall by approximately 50% when either phenytoin or carbamazepine are co-administered.[64] The metabolism of topiramate is not well understood or described, but renal clearance of unchanged drug has been reported to account for the majority of clearance in the absence of co-administered inducing drugs like phenytoin or carbamazepine. In the presence of the latter, the contribution of hepatic clearance increases. Thus upon introduction of one of these inducing drugs into the regimen, or withdrawal, closer monitoring of serum concentrations of topiramate is warranted. In the presence of significant renal disease, lowering the dosage and judicious

use of TDM is recommended. Topiramate is only weakly bound to plasma proteins such that circumstances that alter drug binding in serum do not affect topiramate clearance or steady-state concentrations.

Based on retrospective studies and a concentration-controlled study, the usual range of concentrations is 5 to 20 μg/mL (15 to 59 μmol/L). The majority of seizure patients treated with topiramate are maintained with good safety and efficacy at concentrations in the middle of this target range.[65,66]

Lamotrigine

Lamotrigine (Lamictal) is not a GABA analog but binds to the GABA receptor; it is therefore considered a GABA-receptor agonist. Lamotrigine acts like phenytoin and carbamazepine, blocking repetitive nerve firings induced by depolarization of spinal cord neurons. Lamotrigine was approved by the FDA in 1994 for adjunctive therapy of partial seizures in adults. It has yet to be approved for use in children. Studies also suggest lamotrigine is effective against absence seizures.[67–69]

Lamotrigine is well tolerated and completely absorbed from the gastrointestinal tract after oral administration. It is 60% bound to plasma proteins. Optimal response appears to occur with blood concentrations in the range of 2.5 to 15 μg/mL (~10 to 60 μmol/L). However, dizziness, ataxia, diplopia, blurred vision, nausea, and vomiting are signs of toxicity that may occur when the blood concentration exceeds 10 μg/mL (40 μmol/L). Half-life ranges from 15 to 35 hours with monotherapy.[65] Elimination occurs through hepatic metabolism; the primary metabolite is the glucuronide ester. Coadministration with cytochrome P450–inducing drugs such as phenobarbital, phenytoin, or carbamazepine results in reduced lamotrigine concentrations—dosage increases of approximately 30% are required to maintain optimal blood concentrations.

Chromatographic methods for analysis of lamotrigine have been reported.[70] Commercially available immunoassays for lamotrigine have also been recently introduced.

Levetiracetam

Levetiracetam (Keppra) is an anticonvulsant drug approved in the United States for adjunctive therapy in patients with partial seizures. Levetiracetam belongs to the lactam class of molecules (racetams) that share a five-member pyrrolidone ring, which includes piracetam and ethosuximide. The mechanism of action for levetiracetam, although not fully understood, appears to be by binding to the synaptic vesicle protein SV2A, which appears to be a master regulator of synaptic vesicle and neurotransmitter trafficking within the neural synapse; however, the exact mechanism by which binding of this drug to SV2A modulates seizure activity is unknown.[71]

Levetiracetam, available in both oral and intravenous formulations, is mostly absorbed (>95%) within the gastrointestinal tract. Food intake causes a modest delay in absorption with reduced peak serum concentrations; however, overall bioavailability is unaffected. Levetiracetam is metabolized to the inactive acetamide form by hydrolysis (~27 to 34%), with the majority of the drug excreted by the kidneys unchanged into urine. Clearance of the drug is therefore affected by kidney disease. An increase in levetiracetam clearance has been observed during the third trimester of pregnancy; however, this change in clearance is variable. Because there is no significant hepatic metabolism of levetiracetam, liver function does not affect the pharmacokinetics of this drug.[72]

Serum concentrations of levetiracetam appear to correlate linearly with dose within the typical dosing range. Although the optimal target range for serum concentration has not been fully defined, retrospective analysis of data from clinical trials of levetiracetam suggest that concentrations within the range of 12 to 46 μg/mL (70 to 270 μmol/L) are associated with efficacy.[73]

Brivaracetam

Brivaracetam, sold under the trade name *Briviact*, is one of the newer AEDs approved in the US in 2016 as adjunctive therapy for focal (partial-onset) seizures in adults. Structurally, it is also racetam drug with a pyrrolidone nucleus related to levetiracetam. Brivaracetam was selected for its selective binding to the synaptic vesicle protein, SV2A, the target receptor for related levetiracetam with a greater than 10-fold higher affinity.[74]

Brivaracetam exhibits close to 100% bioavailability, is highly lipid-soluble, and rapidly crosses the blood-brain barrier. Similar to levetiracetam, it is highly metabolized to inactive metabolites by an amidase and CYP2C9 and CYP2C19 with the vast majority of the drug (92%) excreted as metabolite in the urine. Clearance is therefore reduced in individuals with hepatic impairment resulting in higher exposure necessitating dose reduction. Due to the low renal clearance of active drug, there is little impact of renal impairment on parent drug PK.

There are limited study data on the relationship between clinical effects and steady-state trough concentrations. Brivaracetam is a generally well tolerated anticonvulsant drug with most commonly reported side effects including somnolence, dizziness, fatigue, and headache. Serum concentration values ranging from 0.2 to 2 μg/mL are associated with efficacy based on retrospective analysis of data from clinical trials of brivaracetam.[58]

Felbamate

Felbamate (Felbatol) was approved by the FDA in 1993 for primary or adjunctive therapy of partial seizures. Its use is limited to patients who fail other drug treatments, because felbamate carries with it a substantial risk for aplastic anemia and liver failure that is not related to blood concentration. Biweekly monitoring of complete blood count, serum aminotransferases, and bilirubin is recommended to detect early onset of these side effects. Felbamate is particularly effective in control of Lennox-Gastaut syndrome.

Felbamate is completely absorbed from the gastrointestinal tract. The drug is 30% bound to plasma proteins, and optimal blood concentrations for felbamate, while poorly defined, has been suggested to range from 30 to 60 μg/mL (126 to 252 μmol/L).[75] It is eliminated by hepatic metabolism, with its half–life ranging from 14 to 21 hours. Felbamate saturates metabolism when the concentration exceeds 120 μg/mL (504 μmol/L); at that concentration, metabolism converts from first order to zero order. There are currently no commercially available immunoassays for felbamate. HPLC[76] and capillary electrophoresis[77] have been reported for felbamate analysis.

Phenobarbital

Phenobarbital is used in the treatment of all seizures except absence seizures and is known by a wide variety of proprietary names and found in combination with many other drugs. It is particularly useful for treatment of generalized tonic-clonic, partial, focal motor, temporal lobe, and febrile seizures. It is also known to reduce synaptic transmission, resulting in decreased excitability of the entire nerve cell and a consequent sedating effect. Phenobarbital potentiates synaptic inhibition through action on the GABA-A receptor by increasing the duration of chloride flow into the synapse.[25] The end result is an increase in seizure threshold and inhibition of the spread of discharges from the epileptic foci.

Absorption of oral phenobarbital is slow but complete. The time at which peak plasma concentrations are reached is widely variable and ranges from 4 to 10 hours after the dose. Phenobarbital is 40 to 60% bound to plasma proteins. The elimination half-life is from 70 to 100 hours and is age dependent (children average 70 hours, geriatric patients 100 hours). Because hepatic metabolism is one of the prime routes of elimination, reduced liver function results in prolonged half-life.

The optimally effective therapeutic concentration of phenobarbital is between 15 and 40 μg/mL (66 to 177 μmol/L).[78] The predominant side effect observed in adults at blood concentrations greater than 40 μg/mL (177 μmol/L) is sedation, although tolerance to this effect develops with chronic therapy. Because of the long elimination half-life of phenobarbital, the blood concentration does not change rapidly. Therefore a serum specimen collected late in the dose interval (postabsorptive) is representative of the overall effect. Results from specimens collected prior to 4 hours after the dose should be avoided due to the slow absorption.

Phenobarbital is metabolized in the liver to *p*-hydroxy phenobarbital, which is largely excreted as the glucuronide or sulfate ester. When renal and hepatic functions are decreased, patients experience decreased clearance of the drug. Elimination of phenobarbital may be decreased in the presence of valproic acid and salicylate if reduction in urinary pH occurs. During chronic administration of either valproate or salicylate, the concentration of phenobarbital may increase 10% to 20% and a dose adjustment may be necessary to avoid intoxication. Phenobarbital induces mixed-function oxidative enzymes, resulting in increased metabolism of other xenobiotics after approximately 1 to 2 weeks of therapy.

Primidone

Primidone (Mysoline) is effective in the treatment of tonic-clonic and partial seizures. The mechanism of action of this drug is similar to that described for phenobarbital, and the therapeutic effect is due partially to the accumulation of its major metabolite, phenobarbital. A second metabolite of primidone, phenylethylmalonamide, also has some antiepileptic activity.

Primidone is rapidly and completely absorbed after oral administration. Once absorbed, it is not highly protein bound and has a half-life of approximately 10 hours. Disposition of the drug is not known to be significantly altered by other disease states or other drugs.

The optimal therapeutic concentration of primidone has been established as 5 to 12 μg/mL (23 to 55 μmol/L). Because phenobarbital is an active metabolite of primidone, concurrent analysis of phenobarbital is required for complete result interpretation. The previously defined therapeutic range for phenobarbital applies to adequate primidone therapy. The phenobarbital concentrations rise gradually over a period of 1 to 2 weeks after therapy is initiated. Toxicity secondary to accumulation of primidone occurs at serum concentrations in excess of 15 μg/mL (69 μmol/L) and is usually associated with symptoms of sedation, nausea, vomiting, diplopia, dizziness, ataxia, and a phenobarbital concentration greater than 40 μg/mL (177 μmol/L). Specimen collection is dictated by the same rules that apply for phenobarbital; the trough concentration is most useful.

Coadministration of acetazolamide with primidone results in decreased gastrointestinal absorption of primidone and subsequent diminished plasma concentrations. Primidone administered in association with phenytoin produces a modest increase in the ratio of phenobarbital to primidone because phenytoin competes with the hepatic hydroxylating enzymes associated with phenobarbital's metabolism. Coadministration of valproic acid, for the same reasons outlined for phenobarbital, causes a modest increase in both primidone and phenobarbital serum concentrations.

Zonisamide

Zonisamide is the generic name used in the United States for a widely used seizure medication whose common brand name is Zonegran. The FDA approved zonisamide use in 2000 with the suggestion that it be used together with other anticonvulsants in the treatment of partial seizures in adults.[79] Mechanism of action studies in various in vitro neuronal culture systems indicate that zonisamide blocks repetitive firing of voltage-sensitive sodium channels and reduces voltage-sensitive T-type calcium currents without affecting L-type calcium currents, thereby suppressing overall excitation of nerve cells.[79]

Orally administered zonisamide is generally well absorbed, with little to no effect of concomitant food consumption, and this drug is only weakly bound to plasma proteins. Zonisamide is extensively metabolized by oxidative, acetylation, and other pathways and has essentially linear pharmacokinetics resulting in linearity for doses ranging from 10 to 15 mg/kg/day.[65] Concomitantly administered inducing drugs such as phenytoin or carbamazepine cause increased metabolism-based clearance and therefore a need for dose adjustment that can be aided by TDM of zonisamide. When concomitant therapy with an inducing drug is being withdrawn, adjustment of dosing of zonisamide using TDM is warranted.

A target TDM range of 10 to 40 μg/mL (47 to 188 μmol/L) has been recommended, based largely on retrospective studies, and, as with all other anticonvulsants, there is significant overlap of serum zonisamide concentrations between seizure-free patients and patients who do not respond to therapy with this drug and between patients who encounter side effects and those who do not. Thus finding an optimal therapeutic concentration within the individual patient is an essential need, not simply titrating the patient to be within the target therapeutic range.[79]

Antibiotics

Antibiotics that require TDM include aminoglycosides, chloramphenicol, sulfonamides, vancomycin, trimethoprim, β-lactams, and tetracyclines. Pharmacokinetic details of these antibiotics are summarized in Table 42.2.

TABLE 42.2 Pharmacokinetic Parameters of Commonly Monitored Antibiotics

Drug	Therapeutic Targets[a] μg/mL (μmol/L)	Half-Life (h)	Volume of Distribution (L/kg)	Oral Bioavailability (%)	Protein Binding (%)
Aminoglycosides					
Amikacin	C_{max}: 25–35 (43–60) C_{min}: 1–8 (1.7–13.7)	2[b]	0.2–0.4	NA	<11
Gentamicin	C_{max}: 5–12 (10.5–25) C_{min}: <1 (<2)	2[b]	0.2–0.4	NA	<30
Tobramycin	C_{max}: 5–12 (11–25.7) C_{min}: <1 (<2)	2[b]	0.2–0.4	NA	<15
Glycopeptides					
Vancomycin	C_{min}: >10–15 (>6.9–10.4)	6–12[c]	0.4–1	<1[d]	10–50
Other					
Chloramphenicol	C_{max}: 10–25 (31–77) C_{min}: 1–8 (3–25)	Adults: 1.5–4.1 Newborn: ≥24[e]	0.2–3.1 mean: 0.6–1.0	70–80[f]	60

[a]Target blood concentrations depend on the infection (e.g., tissue compartment), organism, and its sensitivity to the antibiotic (i.e., minimum inhibitory concentration). Laboratories should verify that these ranges are appropriate for use in their own settings.
[b]Clearance of aminoglycoside antibiotics depends on kidney function.
[c]Vancomycin best conforms to a multicompartment (two- or three-compartment) pharmacokinetic model.
[d]Absorption of vancomycin from the gastrointestinal tract leading to toxic concentrations has been observed in individuals with pseudomembranous colitis.
[e]Chloramphenicol clearance is reduced in neonates because of limited glucuronide conjugating activity of the liver.
[f]Bioavailability of chloramphenicol depends on the chemical form (succinate or palmitate).
NA, Not applicable.

Aminoglycosides

Aminoglycosides are polycationic agents that kill aerobic gram-negative bacteria. They act by binding to the 30S ribosomal subunit of bacterial mRNA, thereby inhibiting protein synthesis. They are inactive under anaerobic conditions because an oxygen-dependent active transport mechanism is involved in the transfer of aminoglycosides across the bacterial cell wall. The aminoglycoside class of drugs includes amikacin, gentamicin, kanamycin, neomycin, netilmicin, sisomicin, streptomycin, and tobramycin.

The aminoglycosides are a very polar group of compounds and are thus poorly absorbed from the intestinal tract. They are routinely administered intravenously or intramuscularly to achieve a high degree of bioavailability. When administered directly into the blood, they rapidly distribute to the extracellular fluid but do not cross cell membranes or bind to plasma proteins; this behavior is consistent with their unusually low volume of distribution. Most tissues and nonrenal or hepatic secretions contain very small concentrations of aminoglycosides, the exceptions being the renal cortex, where the drug is concentrated, and bile, because of active hepatic secretion. The drugs are mainly excreted by glomerular filtration. Elimination half-lives are short, ranging from 2 to 3 hours. Because clearance is highly dependent on renal function, any impairment of glomerular filtration causes accumulation of these drugs.

Therapy with antibiotic agents such as the aminoglycosides differs from the approach used for most other drugs discussed in this chapter. The goal is to achieve a concentration in plasma such that the bacteria are killed but the host remains undamaged. Because the organisms treated are variable and can become resistant to certain drugs, treatment with specific aminoglycoside agents should always be directed by susceptibility testing.

Numerous studies, summarized by Schentag,[80] Zaske,[81] and Mandell and colleagues,[82] recommend a limit to the blood concentration of aminoglycosides, although considerable variability is reported regarding the relationship of blood concentration to later onset of toxicity. Renal tubular necrosis and degeneration of the auditory nerve are the side effects most frequently experienced after exposure to high concentrations of aminoglycosides.[83] Both peak and trough specimens are required to monitor toxicity. Table 42.2 identifies target maximum peak and trough serum concentrations; in this mode of monitoring, the intent of therapy should be to dose the patient in such a manner that the peak concentration does not exceed these limits. In a large surgical patient survey in which dosing was carried out under controlled conditions, limited nephrotoxicity was experienced when the peak serum concentration of gentamicin was maintained below 8 μg/mL (17 μmol/L).[81] Using similar guidelines, Keys and colleagues[83] reported a 40% incidence of mild nephrotoxicity using a sensitive index of renal clearance (iothalamate clearance) when trough values regularly exceeded the limits defined in Table 42.2.

Dose corrections must be made in patients with compromised renal function because these patients have prolonged half--life and slower elimination.[84,85] This should then be followed by quantification of the blood concentration and dose adjustment following the method outlined by Gilbert.[86]

Toxicity associated with aminoglycosides manifests as delayed-onset vestibular and cochlear sensory cell destruction and acute renal tubular necrosis. The degree and severity of cell damage are variable among the different drugs, but they all cause cell damage if the concentrations are high. Unfortunately, the therapeutic concentration guidelines identified in Table 42.2 do not guarantee the avoidance of toxicity; a small number of patients experience toxic effects regardless of the concentration. Fortunately, most patients reverse the toxic effects without direct intervention if the toxicity is associated with reasonable blood concentrations. Irreparable loss of vestibular, cochlear, or renal function usually correlates with administration of one of the aminoglycosides at increased blood concentrations for periods longer than 2 weeks.

In certain patients with adequate renal function (generally glomerular filtration rate >30 mL/min), an alternative dosing schedule of once-daily, high-dose aminoglycoside therapy can be used. This dosing schedule is based on the concentration-dependent antimicrobial effect of these drugs, in which peak concentrations achieved rather than the time above the minimum inhibitory concentration (MIC) is most closely correlated with antimicrobial effect.[87–89] Unlike efficacy, toxicity of aminoglycoside antibiotics appears to be correlated with both peak and trough concentrations.[90,91] Peak concentrations at or above the therapeutic target based on MIC are generally with the once-daily strategy, and trough level concentration monitoring is used to reduce risk for toxicity. Based on several studies comparing once-daily dosing with conventional dosing with multiple-daily dosing and TDM, once-daily dosing appears to be equally as effective as multiple-daily dosing. The incidence of nephrotoxicity with once-daily dosing appears equal or lower compared to conventional dosing; however, the incidence of ototoxicity is less clear, with at least one study showing an increased risk for ototoxicity in pediatric patients using a once-daily regimen.[92–94]

Heparin has been implicated as a deactivator of gentamicin by formation of an inactive complex.[95] This complex, although biologically inactive, retains some structural resemblance to the initial aminoglycoside and cross-reacts with antibodies to the specific aminoglycoside. Heparin concentrations encountered in therapeutic antithrombotic therapy are less than 3 units/mL, making an in vivo complication unlikely. However, specimen collection tubes containing heparin (1000 units/mL) may lead to complex formation, a phenomenon that could interfere with some immunoassay procedures.

Before the 1980s, aminoglycoside antibiotics were analyzed by the bioassay technique. This method is variable and subject to significant interference by numerous drugs. Such assays should now be considered obsolete. Liquid chromatographic and immunochemical methods are available with enzyme immunoassay, fluorescence polarization immunoassay, or similar nonisotopic immunoassays, which are now considered the methods of choice for aminoglycoside analysis.

Chloramphenicol

Chloramphenicol (e.g., Chloromycetin) is used as a bactericidal agent. It acts by binding to the 50S ribosomal subunit of bacteria mRNA and inhibits protein synthesis in prokaryotic organisms. Use of this drug depends on its relative toxicity against the microorganism versus the host. The drug is used against gram-negative bacteria such as *Haemophilus influenzae, Neisseria meningitidis, Neisseria gonorrhoeae, Salmonella typhi,* all *Brucella* species, *Bordetella pertussis, Vibrio cholerae,* and *Shigella.* These organisms all are susceptible to a concentration of 6 μg/mL (19 μmol/L). Organisms that require higher concentrations of 12 μg/mL (37 μmol/L) are *Escherichia coli, Klebsiella pneumoniae, Pseudomonas pseudomallei, Chlamydia,* and *Mycoplasma.*

Chloramphenicol is rapidly absorbed in the gastrointestinal tract. Peak serum concentrations occur 1 to 2 hours after the oral dose. In plasma, chloramphenicol is approximately 50% protein bound and is cleared with a half-life of 2 to 3 hours. Peak serum concentrations after administration of chloramphenicol palmitate or succinate occur 4 to 6 hours after the dose. Chloramphenicol distributes to all tissues, and it concentrates in the cerebrospinal fluid. The drug is actively metabolized by the liver by *N*-acetylation and glucuronidation. Thus chloramphenicol accumulates in cases of hepatic disease. Renal disease does not dramatically reduce clearance.

Host toxicity displayed after chloramphenicol therapy includes hematologic toxicity and cardiovascular collapse; both show a modest relationship to blood concentration. The blood concentration–related hematologic toxicities include anemia, characterized by maturation arrest in the marrow; cytoplasmic vacuolation of early erythroid and myeloid cells; reticulocytopenia; and increases in both serum iron and serum iron-binding capacity. These symptoms are associated with serum concentrations in excess of 25 μg/mL (77 μmol/L). Development of idiosyncratic aplastic anemia also has been observed, but this complication appears unrelated to dose or blood concentration and necessitates frequent monitoring of complete blood counts. Cardiovascular collapse, which occurs primarily in newborns, has been related to a total serum chloramphenicol concentration in excess of 50 μg/mL (155 μmol/L). An oral dose of 50 mg/kg per day results in an optimal peak serum concentration of 10 to 25 μg/mL (31 to 77 μmol/L) in a healthy adult.

Procedures for the determination of chloramphenicol concentrations in blood serum include high-performance liquid chromatography (HPLC) and immunoassay. Methods for chloramphenicol determination must be able to differentiate between the prodrug forms, chloramphenicol palmitate or succinate, and their active metabolite, chloramphenicol.

Vancomycin

Vancomycin is a glycopeptide that is bactericidal against gram-positive bacteria and some gram-negative cocci. Vancomycin is used because of its activity against methicillin-resistant staphylococci and corynebacteria. It has thus become popular for treatment of endocarditis and sepsis caused by these organisms.

Although the drug is generally poorly absorbed when given orally (making it useful for treating *Clostridium difficile* infection), absorption leading to toxicity has been observed in patients with pseudomembranous colitis.[96] A 1-g dose given intravenously every 12 hours usually results in a peak blood concentration of 20 to 40 μg/mL (14 to 28 μmol/L) and a trough concentration of 5 to 10 μg/mL (4 to 7 μmol/L). It has an average elimination half-life of 5 to 6 hours. Blood concentration–related toxicity involves the auditory nerve. Concentrations less than 30 μg/mL (21 μmol/L) are rarely associated with this development.[97] Toxicities not related to dose or blood concentrations include fever, phlebitis, and pain at the infusion site. Erythema or flushing of the face, neck, and upper torso occurring within approximately 5 to 10 minutes after vancomycin infusion (sometimes referred to

as "red man syndrome" or "red neck syndrome") also has been observed. This syndrome is due to acute, non–immunoglobulin E–mediated mast cell degranulation and is generally controlled by slow infusion and administration of antihistamines. In patients with impaired renal function, the serum concentration may increase to toxic concentrations because of reduced clearance. Immunoassay is the standard approach to monitoring concentrations; HPLC methods to monitor the serum concentration are available.

Antifungal Antibiotics

Over the past decade, increasing evidence has accumulated to support the use of TDM to enhance the therapeutic safety and efficacy of antifungal medicines. The azole class of antifungals has the most data supporting concentration monitoring. Data supporting the monitoring of flucytosine are limited. Studies of TDM for other classes of antifungal medicines, including the echinocandins (i.e., caspofungin) and the polyenes (e.g., amphotericin B), have generated data showing either no or limited value to monitoring these drugs.

HPLC and LC-MS methods for detection of multiple azoles have been described and represent the predominant methods used for clinical testing by reference laboratories. Although these methods are generally highly specific, it should not be assumed that results are transferable across laboratories. A recent review of proficiency testing data that evaluated 5 years of data from 57 different laboratories around the world demonstrated that a wide variation in results, especially at low concentrations, is common, leading to results that can deviate by more than 20%.[98] New immunoassays for voriconazole and posaconazole have been described, but experience with these is limited. The availability of reliable immunoassays for these antifungals could foster more widespread experience in the effectiveness of their monitoring. Metabolism of the drugs also can affect interpretation of concentration data as discussed in more detail later.

Antifungal Azoles

The azoles represent an important class of drugs with broad-spectrum antifungal activity toward both pathogenic yeast and dimorphic fungi such as *Aspergillus* species. These drugs consist of two main structural families, the imidazoles and triazoles. The former class, which includes clotrimazole and ketoconazole, while active after systemic administration, are currently used primarily in topical formulations because of their poor oral absorption and the significant toxicity associated with their systemic use. The safer, triazole class, which includes fluconazole, itraconazole, voriconazole, and posaconazole, are the primary azoles in use systemically for the treatment of serious, invasive fungal infections, and these are the drugs described further below. All of the azoles mediate their antifungal activity by preferentially inhibiting fungal 14α-demethylase (a cytochrome P450 enzyme), which is critical for the generation of ergosterol required for cytoplasmic membrane synthesis.

Fluconazole. Fluconazole is available in both intravenous and oral formulation. It is frequently used in prophylaxis against invasive candidiasis and in the treatment of invasive fungal infections by *Cryptococcus neoformans,* coccidiomycosis, and candidiasis. Fluconazole shows high bioavailability of approximately 90%, and this absorption appears unaffected by food or gastric pH. It shows low serum protein binding with wide tissue distribution required for its use in treating invasive systemic fungal infections. Fluconazole is primary cleared by the kidney with an average half-life of approximately 32 hours.[99]

Due to the predominantly renal clearance of fluconazole, dosing requires adjustment according to estimated glomerular filtration rate.[100] There appears to be a pharmacodynamics dose-response relationship between exposure to fluconazole as assessed by the ratio of dose to the MIC of the organisms and efficacy.[101] Despite this relationship, TDM has not been generally recommended for fluconazole because of its linear pharmacokinetics[102] and generally good safety profile in adults and children.[103] There is, however, evidence to suggest that critically ill adults and children may not achieve adequate exposure based upon commonly recommended doses. This may be particularly challenging in patients with central nervous system disease or patients with infections caused by organisms with a high MIC. Monitoring may therefore be warranted in some patients but applying TDM to these settings is challenging because of the lack of appropriately defined target concentrations, which is likely to be affected significantly by the MIC of the organism.

Itraconazole. Itraconazole is a broad-spectrum antifungal agent with activity toward most clinically relevant organisms, including *Candida, Cryptococcus,* and *Aspergillus* species. Itraconazole is available in oral and intravenous (outside the United States) formulations. Unlike fluconazole, itraconazole exhibits much more variable bioavailability that appears to depend on the specific formulation used. Absorption is influenced by food and gastric pH for some formulations.[104,105] Itraconazole also displays nonlinear pharmacokinetics with slow clearance.[106–108] Due to the pharmacokinetic properties of itraconazole along with the appreciable gastrointestinal, neurologic, and liver toxicity,[109] TDM generally has been recommended for this drug.[110–113] The optimal target concentration for itraconazole will likely depend on the organism, its MIC, and its infection site, as suggested by experimental model systems[114,115]; however, retrospective studies suggest that concentrations above 0.5 μg/mL (0.7 μmol/L) are associated with the lowest risk for invasive fungal infections when used as prophylaxis in the setting of neutropenia.[116–118] Data on serum concentrations associated with efficacy in the treatment of invasive fungal infections is very limited, but most responding patients have concentrations greater than 0.6 to 1.0 μg/mL (0.9 to 1.4 μmol/L) on day 7 of treatment, suggesting that this may be a useful threshold to ensure efficacy.[119,120] The association between itraconazole concentration and toxicity also has been explored. Unfortunately, although a pharmacodynamic relationship appears to exist, these studies were performed using a bioassay for itraconazole that detects both the parent drug and the biologically active hydroxyitraconazole metabolite making it difficult to interpret the data when compared to concentrations obtained by HPLC or LC-MS, which are the methods generally used in the clinical setting.[121,122] Specific measurement of itraconazole alone also markedly underestimates the biologic activity of itraconazole in serum because of the presence of the hydroxyitraconazole metabolite, which may contribute as much as 80% of the biological activity in serum.[123]

Voriconazole. Voriconazole is a second-generation triazole with broad-spectrum antifungal activity, including enhanced potency against *Aspergillus* species, and is approved by the FDA for treatment of invasive aspergillosis, candidemia in non-neutropenic patients, esophageal candidiasis, disseminated candidiasis, and as salvage therapy for fungal infections caused by *Scedosporium apiospermum* and *Fusarium* species.

Therapy with voriconazole is generally initiated with a protocol-guided loading dose followed by empirically guided maintenance dosing. For patients who improve clinically from this treatment and who can tolerate orally administered drugs, empirically guided conversion to oral dosing of this antifungal can be achieved. The conversion from intravenous to oral voriconazole is made possible and effective as a result of the high bioavailability shown for adults[124]; however, bioavailability has been reported to vary significantly, especially in children,[125,126] with reported bioavailability as low as 60%.[127] Voriconazole, like itraconazole, displays saturable, nonlinear kinetics with variable clearance because of genetic and nongenetic variation in CYP450 metabolism, making prediction of concentration from dose difficult.

Based on the observed nonlinear pharmacokinetics and wide intersubject and intrasubject variability, the poor dose versus serum concentration relationship, narrow TI, and frequent drug-drug interactions, TDM has been advocated for voriconazole as a way to improve upon both efficacy outcomes and toxicity.[128,129] Based on mostly retrospective study data, it has been recommended that voriconazole trough concentrations be maintained between target of 1 to 2 μg/mL (3 to 6 μmol/L) on the low end and 5 to 6 μg/mL (15 to 17 μmol/L) on the upper end to maximize efficacy and limit neurologic and possibly hepatotoxicity.[128] In order to provide stronger support for instituting TDM for these medicines, the conduct of scientifically rigorous randomized, prospective concentration-controlled trials is optimal to verify the results of retrospective study data. Fortunately, a recent prospective, concentration-controlled study of voriconazole dosing to achieve serum concentrations in the 1 to 5 μg/mL (3 to 15 μmol/L) range on day 4 of therapy demonstrated both an improvement in efficacy and reduction in toxicity of voriconazole therapy when compared with standard, fixed dosing.[130] These data lend excellent support to the benefits of TDM for voriconazole and further validate the retrospectively defined target range for monitoring.

Posaconazole. Posaconazole is a broad-spectrum antifungal with structural similarity to itraconazole and activity toward *Candida, Aspergillus, Cryptococcus,* and *Mucor* species. It is currently available only in oral form. It is used in the treatment of invasive fungal infections and increasingly in the prophylaxis against infection in neutropenic patients. Posaconazole exhibits variable bioavailability. Absorption appears saturable and significantly affected by food and gastric pH. Administration with a high-fat meal increases exposure by as much as two fold to threefold compared with the fasting state.[131]

Posaconazole exhibits linear pharmacokinetics with a half-life of approximately 24 to 37 hours depending on the formulation. Due to the long half-life of this drug, steady-state concentrations are generally not reached until the end of the first week of dosing. The long elimination time also means that the concentrations change little over the typical 12-hour dose interval. Based on the variable pharmacokinetics observed with this drug, the presence of a concentration-response relationship in retrospective data[132–134] and the risk for treatment failure, TDM has been advocated for posaconazole. No prospective data are available to guide selection of a therapeutic concentration range; however, a minimum concentration of 0.7 μg/mL (1 μmol/L) has been suggested for prophylaxis, based largely upon analysis of phase 3 clinical trial data.[110] The minimum concentration for patients with invasive aspergillosis is suggested to be 1 μg/mL (1.4 μmol/L) based upon the pharmacodynamics relationships identified in the retrospective analysis of concentrations in clinical trials[134]; however, as for the other antifungals, the organism and its sensitivity to the posaconazole and the tissue sites will likely influence the efficacy. Although hepatotoxicity has been observed with posaconazole, the pharmacodynamics relationship between serum concentration and toxicity, if any, is unclear.

5-Flucytosine

One of the first antifungals developed, the pyrimidine analog 5-fluocytosine, is a broad-spectrum agent that is coadministered with another fungicidal drug (typically amphotericin B) to prevent the emergence of resistant pathogen populations. Toxicity of 5-flucytosine is well correlated with serum concentrations greater than 100 μg/mL (775 μmol/L) and manifests with myelosuppression (e.g., thrombocytopenia) or hepatic dysfunction evidenced by increased transaminases.[135]

5-Flucytosine bioavailability is excellent, but its renal elimination is variable and may be affected by nephrotoxicity associated with amphotericin B. 5-Flucytosine dose is therefore adjusted according to renal function as typically assessed by creatinine clearance.[135] Based on the seriousness of toxicity and the well-documented concentration-response relationships, TDM has long been recommended for this drug to prevent toxicity. Because of its short half-life, the drug is administered in multiple doses daily. It is recommended to draw TDM samples at peak serum concentrations, roughly 2 hours after a dose, and the first measurement should be made within the first 72 hours after initiation of treatment. Target concentrations for efficacy appear to vary with the pathogen and the extent of infection, and the relationships to efficacy have been much less defined. Based on the strong evidence that the risk for myelotoxicity rises significantly with peak serum concentrations above 100 μ/mL (775 μmol/L), peak concentrations of 50 to 100 μg/mL (388 to 775 μmol/L) have been recommended for most patients to minimize toxicity.[110]

Antineoplastic Agents

Methotrexate

Methotrexate (MTX) has proved useful in the management of acute lymphoblastic leukemia in children; choriocarcinoma and related trophoblastic tumors in women; carcinomas of the breast, tongue, pharynx, and testes; maintenance of remission in leukemia; and treatment of severe, debilitating psoriasis. High-dose MTX administration followed by leucovorin rescue is effective in treatment of carcinoma of the lung and osteogenic sarcoma. Intrathecal administration is effective in treating meningeal leukemia or lymphoma. Table 42.3 lists pharmacokinetic parameters for MTX.

MTX inhibits DNA synthesis by decreasing availability of pyrimidine nucleotides. MTX competitively inhibits the enzyme dihydrofolate reductase, thus decreasing the concentrations of the tetrahydrofolate essential to the methylation of the pyrimidine nucleotides and consequently the rate of pyrimidine nucleotide synthesis. Leucovorin, a folate analog, is used to rescue host cells from MTX inhibition; as a synthetic substrate for dihydrofolate reductase, leucovorin administration allows resumption of tetrahydrofolate-dependent synthesis of pyrimidines and reinitiation of DNA synthesis. MTX is a nonspecific cytotoxin, and prolongation of blood concentrations appropriate to killing tumor cells may lead to severe, unwanted cytotoxic effects such as myelosuppression, gastrointestinal mucositis, and hepatic cirrhosis.

Serum concentrations of MTX are commonly monitored during high-dose therapy (>50 mg/m^2) to identify the time at which active intervention by leucovorin rescue, typically begun at 24 to 36 hours from the start of MTX, can be safely stopped. Blood concentrations are generally monitored at 24, 48, and 72 hours after the MTX dose and leucovorin is administered until the MTX concentration is below 0.05 to 0.1 μmol/L.[136,136a]

The route of elimination for MTX is primarily renal excretion. During the period of high blood concentrations, particular attention must be paid to maintaining output of a large volume of alkaline urine. The pKa of MTX is 5.5; thus small decreases in urine pH result in significant reduction in its solubility. Keeping urinary pH alkaline diminishes the risks for intratubular precipitation of the drug and obstructive nephropathy during the treatment period. Monitoring blood concentrations therefore provides the basis for decisions for timing of initiation and continuance of leucovorin treatment and for managing urinary pH.

TABLE 42.3	Pharmacokinetic Parameters for Commonly Monitored Antineoplastic Drugs					
Drug	Minimum Effective Concentration	Minimum Toxic Concentration	Mean Half-Life (h)	Mean Volume of Distribution (L/kg)	Mean Protein Binding (%)	Metabolizing Enzymes
Busulfan, 6 hr dosing	AUC: 900 μmol × min/L	AUC: 1350 μmol × min/L	2.6	0.99	10	SULT
Busulfan, 24 hr dosing	AUC: 2400 μmol × min/L	AUC: 6000 μmol × min/L	2.6	0.99	10	SULT
Methotrexate						
At 24 hr	<10 μmol/L	>10 μmol/L	1.8	0.55	46	None
At 48 hr	<1 μmol/L	>1 μmol/L	8.4	0.55	46	None
At 72 hr	<0.1 μmol/L	>0.1 μmol/L	>10	0.55	46	None

MTX has been measured in biological specimens using a wide variety of techniques. RIA and the folate reductase inhibition techniques have been used, but nonisotopic immunoassays are now the method of choice. Liquid chromatographic procedures have also been developed to allow for co-analysis of the drug and its metabolites.[137]

Busulfan

Busulfan is a DNA alkylating agent available in both oral and intravenous formulation. High-dose busulfan is often used as part of the myeloablative preparative regimen for hematopoietic stem cell transplantation (HSCT). Clinical use of busulfan is complicated by significant interpatient variability in pharmacokinetic behavior with reported coefficients of variation (CVs) of 23%[138] and 25%[139] for the oral and IV formulations, respectively. Age, obesity, underlying disease, and organ dysfunction also exert a significant influence on observed clearance for busulfan. Children under the age of 6 typically display more than twice the average clearance of 2.5 mL/min/kg reported for adults.[140,141] The observed variability in the pharmacokinetic behavior of busulfan is relevant because several studies have identified a pharmacodynamic relationship between exposure to busulfan and both its toxicity and efficacy. Exposure to busulfan is typically estimated by measurement of several plasma concentrations over a 6-hour dose interval. This exposure is generally expressed as either the AUC in μmol $\times$ min/L or mean steady-state concentration ($\bar{C}_{ss}$), which is easily derived from the AUC (in ng $\times$ min/mL) by dividing this quantity by the dose interval in minutes *(t)*. The risk for toxicity caused by busulfan (venoocclusive disease or pulmonary toxicity) appears to rise significantly with a $\bar{C}_{ss}$ greater than 900 to 1025 ng/mL (3.65 to 4.16 μmol/L).[142–145] In contrast, the risk for relapse in patients undergoing HSCT for chronic myelogenous leukemia rises substantially with a $\bar{C}_{ss}$ of less than 917 ng/mL (3.72 μmol/L), indicating that a very narrow therapeutic range of exposure exists for this drug.[146] Table 42.3 shows pharmacokinetic parameters for busulfan.

Control of busulfan exposure within the apparent tight therapeutic range requires an accurate and precise estimate of exposure. To achieve this level of accuracy and precision, a pharmacokinetic study using extensive sampling is typically performed. Early approaches used noncompartmental analysis with estimation of AUC using the trapezoidal rule, which is required for the complex kinetics observed with oral busulfan. Although this approach was effective and can be used with intravenous formulations of busulfan, fitting the concentration data to a one-compartment, first-order pharmacokinetic model by nonlinear regression has become the preferred method for estimating the $\bar{C}_{ss}$ or AUC for a dose interval when using intravenous dosing of busulfan. Dosing schemes for busulfan vary, but once daily or every 6 hours over 4 days for a total of 4 or 16 doses, respectively, are commonly used. A study is typically performed after the first dose, and the results are promptly reported to effect a dose adjustment as early as possible in the course of the treatment regimen; however, the completion and reporting of a busulfan pharmacokinetic study is not a simple task. A variety of chromatographic methods are used for measurement of busulfan in plasma, with GC-MS and LC-MS/MS generally the preferred methods. Given the complexity of the analytical methodology, onsite testing is not always available. Sample extraction and analysis also usually require several hours to complete for a single patient. Nevertheless, using the previously described TDM approach with dose adjustment, exposures that are within less than 10% of the target exposure are possible and toxicity can be avoided without a compromise in efficacy.[142,143,145–147]

Thiopurines

Originally developed in the 1950s for their potent cytotoxic activity, the thiopurine drugs, 6-mercaptopurine (6-MP), azathioprine (AZA) (an azo precursor to 6-MP), and 6-thioguanine (6-TG), represent a class of drugs used today to treat cancer (e.g., acute lymphoblastic leukemia), rheumatologic disease, inflammatory bowel disease (IBD), and solid organ transplant rejection. These agents derive their potent pharmacologic activity from the dependence of normal and malignant lymphocytes on purine metabolism for proliferation and function. After the bioactivation of 6-MP and 6-TG through phosphoribosylation via hypoxanthine-guanine phosphoribosyltransferase (HGPRT) and conversion to 6-TG nucleotides, these thiol-containing nucleotides are readily incorporated into DNA. Cell death by apoptosis results secondary to failure of base mismatch repair induced by the false nature of these thioguanine nucleotides. Incorporation into RNA and inhibition of purine biosynthesis are likely to further contribute to the cytotoxic effect of these compounds.[25]

Myelosuppression represents the most pronounced toxicity associated with the thiopurine drugs. The dose-dependence of myelosuppression is well recognized; however, some individuals are much more sensitive to the myelosuppressive effects of 6-MP and AZA than others. The pharmacokinetic behavior of 6-MP and AZA is characterized by poor oral bioavailability (<25%) with a relatively short half-life ($t_{1/2}$) of approximately 50 minutes. The clearance of 6-MP is variable and is mediated primarily via two enzymatic pathways: (1) oxidation to thiouric acid by xanthine oxidase and (2) S-methylation via thiopurine S-methyltransferase (TPMT). Xanthine oxidase contributes significantly to the poor bioavailability of 6-MP and AZA through first-pass metabolism within the intestines and liver. Inhibition of xanthine oxidase via allopurinol leads to a fivefold increase in 6-MP bioavailability. In contrast, allopurinol exhibits little effect on 6-MP pharmacokinetics in plasma, suggesting that the contribution of xanthine oxidase to metabolism once the drug is absorbed is negligible.[148]

The large interindividual variability in sensitivity to toxicity noted with these drugs has led to the search for genetic factors that might contribute to the pharmacokinetics and pharmacodynamic variation of these drugs. TPMT-mediated metabolism appears to be the principal mechanism for plasma clearance of 6-MP. Studies in the 1980s demonstrated that white individuals could be classified into three categories of TPMT activity based on enzymatic assays of TPMT in red blood cell (RBC) lysates with frequencies suggestive of a monogenic inherited trait in Hardy-Weinberg equilibrium.[149] Individuals with the lowest TPMT activity, approximately 0.3% of whites, exhibit approximately 10-fold higher erythrocyte 6-TG nucleotide concentrations than the majority of individuals with wild-type enzymatic activity after 6-MP therapy.[150] All individuals with the lowest TPMT phenotype experience toxicity associated with doses of 6-MP derived from population-based pharmacokinetics and pharmacodynamics studies. Individuals with intermediate activity (~11% in white populations) also demonstrate higher erythrocyte 6-TG nucleotide concentrations that are intermediate between those of individuals with wild-type and low activity. The pharmacodynamics effects of this intermediate phenotype are still relevant, with 30 to 60% of heterozygous individuals experiencing significant 6-MP–associated toxicity requiring dose reductions.[150,151] These findings support the importance of TPMT as the principal mechanism for 6-MP and AZA clearance, and they further indicate that pretreatment recognition of individuals in the reduced metabolism category will benefit from a dose-reduction in 6-MP or AZA. Although TPMT activity explains much of the toxicity associated with these drugs, TPMT may explain only approximately a third of the toxicity.[152] Additional polymorphisms in genes such as inosine triphosphate phosphorylase also appear to contribute to the toxicity of these drugs.[153]

The dependence of 6-TG on TPMT for methylation leading to inactivation suggests that 6-TG pharmacokinetics should be well correlated with TPMT phenotype.[154] Despite the expectation that 6-TG nucleotide concentrations should be correlated with clinical efficacy and toxicity, the results of clinical studies exploring this relationship in patients with IBD are mixed.[155–159] This in part may be explained by the complex nature of the metabolic pathways involved. In a study of IBD patients resistant to thiopurine therapy, Dubinsky demonstrated that patients who respond to an increase in 6-MP/AZA dose show a significant rise in 6-TG nucleotide concentrations.[160] Furthermore, those who failed to respond to dose escalation also failed to show a significant rise in 6-TG nucleotide concentrations. Instead, a skewing toward TPMT metabolism with a rise in 6-methylmercaptopurine (6-MMP) ribonucleotide concentrations was noted, and this is associated with increased risk for hepatotoxicity.[160,161] These data suggest serial monitoring of 6-TG nucleotide and 6-MMP concentrations alone may be able to identify patients at risk for therapeutic failure, perhaps as a result of preferential metabolism by TPMT. Based on a meta-analysis of studies in IBD, the suggested optimal concentrations of 6-TG nucleotide fall within the range of 230 to 260 pmol/8 $\times 10^8$ RBC with concentrations above 400 pmol/8 $\times 10^8$ RBCs associated with increased toxicity.[162,163] Measurement of 6-TG nucleotide concentrations may play their most useful role in identifying patients with poor adherence to thiopurine therapy.[164] This is relevant since Mantzaris et al. reported that most patients with IBD exhibit some degree of therapy nonadherence.[165] The role of monitoring 6-TG nucleotide concentrations in other settings such as other autoimmune diseases, transplantation, and oncology are less clear.

Immunosuppressive Drugs

Tacrolimus

Tacrolimus (Prograf), formerly called FK-506, is a macrolide antibiotic isolated from a strain of *Streptomyces tsukubaensis* that has significant immunosuppressant properties.[166] Tacrolimus mediates its immunosuppressive action by entering the lymphocyte and binding to a receptor known as FK506–binding protein (FKBP). Once bound to FKBP, this drug-receptor complex interacts with, and blocks, the calcium-dependent phosphatase, calcineurin, which is critical for the translocation of nuclear factor of activated T cells (NFAT) to the nucleus,

where the latter regulates the transcription of cytokines and other genes important for T-cell activation, proliferation, and function. Calcineurin inhibition therefore leads to marked suppression of T cell–mediated immune responses such as those involved in solid organ transplant rejection and graft-versus-host disease after bone marrow transplantation. NFAT plays a role in other cell types, likely contributing to the toxic effects of tacrolimus.

Tacrolimus is administered predominantly orally in capsule form (Prograf) containing 0.5, 1, or 5 mg of the drug. A sterile solution containing the equivalent of 1 mg/mL of tacrolimus for intravenous administration and an ointment containing 0.1 or 0.03% for topical use on skin are also available. Rapid but incomplete absorption is characteristic of standard oral tacrolimus formulations, with an average time to peak concentration of 1.6 to 2.3 hours and average oral bioavailability of 17 to 22%.[167] Several prolonged-release formulations of tacrolimus have been developed, with the first, Advagraf, now available commercially.[168] Extended-release formulations afford delayed maximal concentrations with improved bioavailability leading to a slight reduction in dose to achieve equivalent AUC.

There is a fairly good correlation between tacrolimus trough concentration, graft rejection, and toxicity.[169] The target range for tacrolimus blood concentrations depends on the concomitant use of other ISDs, the transplant type, and the time after transplantation. An example of the immunosuppressive regimens used at our institution with the associated tacrolimus target ranges are shown in Table 42.4. Recent trends have aimed toward reducing the exposure for the calcineurin inhibitors tacrolimus and cyclosporine A (CsA) because of the increased recognition of long-term nephrotoxicity associated with their use in all solid organ transplant types.[170] Neurotoxicity is another notable adverse effect of tacrolimus. Like nephrotoxicity, the severity of neurologic toxicity generally correlates with trough concentration, with most significant neurologic events occurring with tacrolimus concentrations above 15 ng/mL (19 nmol/L).[171] Since the application of IDSs to transplantation is continuously evolving and the pharmacodynamics relationships depend on concomitant ISDs, the target concentration ranges for tacrolimus must be regularly reviewed to ensure they reflect current standards of practice.

Recent studies relating to target TAC concentrations have used as a surrogate endpoint de novo donor-specific antibodies (dnDSAs)—believed to be good predictors of long-term renal damage—to help determine and refine the lower end of the target range associated with renal allograft injury and the impact of time within the target range on risk of developing dnDSAs.[172,173] Such studies may help to improve upon previous studies, most of which relied on acute rejection rather than dnDSAs, for optimization of TAC dosing within individual patients.

The steady-state trough concentration of tacrolimus per unit of dose varies widely within and among patients.[169,174,175] The between-subject variability of dose-normalized tacrolimus has been estimated to be fivefold.[174] Factors known to contribute to this variability are many and include hematocrit; plasma albumin concentration; patient age; genotypes of metabolizing enzyme CYP3A5; drug-drug, herb-drug, and food-drug interactions; and disease.[167,176] The influence of one or more of these factors in transplant patients explains

TABLE 42.4 Immunosuppressive Regimens and Associated Tacrolimus Target Ranges Used at the Author's Institution

Organ	Immunosuppressive Regimen	Time After Transplant	TACROLIMUS THERAPEUTIC RANGE[a]	
			µg/L	nmol/L
Kidney	Tacrolimus + MMF	0–1 mo	8–12	10.4–15.6
		2–3 mo	7–10	9.1–13
		4–6 mo	6–8	7.8–10.4
		7–12 mo	5–7 (6–8 for higher risk)	6.5–9.1 (7.8–10.4 for higher risk)
		>12 mo	4–6 (5–7 for higher risk)	5.2–7.8 (6.5–9.1 for higher risk)
Heart	Tacrolimus + MMF	0–3 mo	10–12	13–15.6
		4–6 mo	10	13
		6–12 mo	8–10	10.4–13
		>12 mo	5–8	6.5–10.4
Liver	Tacrolimus + steroids ± azathioprine or MMF	0–3 wk	8–12 (6–8 with renal insufficiency)	10.4–15.6 (7.8–10.4 with renal insufficiency)
		4–6 wk	6–10 (6–8 with renal insufficiency)	
		7 wk–9 mo	5–8	7.8–13 (7.8–10.4 with renal insufficiency)
		10 mo–2 yr	4–6 (6 for AIH; 3–4 with renal insufficiency if also on an antiproliferative agent)	6.5–10.4
		>3 yr	3–4 (6 for AIH)	5.2–7.8 (7.8 for AIH; 3.9–5.2 with renal insufficiency if also on an antiproliferative agent)
				3.9–5.2 (7.8 for AIH)
Lung	Tacrolimus + MMF + steroids	0–12 mo	8–12	10.4–15.6
		>12 mo	6–8	7.8–10.4
Bone marrow	Tacrolimus		5–15	6.5–19.5

[a]Laboratories should verify that these ranges are appropriate for use in their own settings as ranges may depend upon analytic methodology, the patient population, and other factors such as concomitant drug therapy.
AIH, Autoimmune hepatitis; *MMF,* mycophenolate mofetil.

the wide within- and between-subject variability of tacrolimus concentrations. This, taken together with the narrow TI and the requirement of contemporary practice to lower the tacrolimus dosing and target trough concentration during the first transplant year and beyond to limit nephrotoxicity, is the basis for the need for close concentration monitoring of this drug.

Due to the high binding of tacrolimus to FK506-binding proteins within cells, including erythrocytes, the plasma concentration of tacrolimus is typically 1.5 to 8% of whole blood. Methods for quantitative analysis of this drug therefore generally begin with cell lysis and protein precipitation of whole blood to liberate cell-bound tacrolimus to allow measurement of the total drug present within whole blood. The lysis step is most commonly performed as a manual step using a water-miscible solvent (e.g., methanol) solution containing zinc sulfate ($ZnSO_4$) followed by centrifugation. Performance of this initial step is one of the critical points in tacrolimus analysis, and it represents an important source of potential error if not performed correctly or consistently.

Interferences in the measurement of tacrolimus include metabolites of the drug and other substances present in human blood such as antibodies that react with components of the assay (for additional discussion on interference in immunoassay, refer to Chapter 26).[177–179] The former represents the more frequent and challenging interfering substance. Tacrolimus undergoes extensive metabolism by the liver and gastrointestinal cytochrome P450 (CYP) enzyme system with less than 0.5% of the parent drug excreted unchanged in the feces and urine.[167] The CYP3A isoenzymes are the principle

CYP enzymes involved in tacrolimus metabolism with more than 15 different metabolites described. However, significant variability in metabolism has been reported because of both genetic factors and physiologic factors such as liver dysfunction.[180] Interference by metabolites represents a significant problem for the immunoassay methods. Evaluation of cross-reactivity for the most abundant metabolites of tacrolimus demonstrate that the M2 (31-desmethyl tacrolimus) and M3 (15-desmethyl tacrolimus) metabolites yield as much as 80% cross-reactivity with the antibodies used in some immunoassays.[181] M2 displays immunosuppressive activity equal to that of the parent compound, tacrolimus, in vitro, whereas M3 has minimal immunosuppressive activity. Hematocrit, and to a lesser extent albumin, have a significant impact on the measured concentration of tacrolimus. Several studies have demonstrated that a low hematocrit (<33%) leads to an increase in measured tacrolimus (upward bias) when compared with LC-MS/MS reference methods.[182,183] This bias is inversely related to the hematocrit, with as much as a 50% increase at a hematocrit of 20%. A similar bias is observed when albumin concentrations fall below 3 g/dL (4.4 µmol/L).

Cyclosporine

Cyclosporine (Sandimmune [Cyclosporin A or CsA] and Neoral) is a cyclic peptide composed of 11 amino acids, some of novel structure, isolated from the fungus *Trichoderma polysporum.* The compound has been shown effective in suppressing solid organ allograft rejection, graft-versus-host disease, and bone marrow transplantation. CsA is approved for use in renal, cardiac, hepatic, pancreatic, and bone marrow transplants.

CsA acts by a mechanism that is very similar to that of tacrolimus. After entry into the cell, CsA forms a complex with cytoplasmic receptors termed *cyclophilins* that are molecularly distinct from FKBP. These cyclosporine : cyclophilin molecular complexes interact with and inhibit the calcineurin phosphatase, preventing NFAT activation that is critical for lymphocyte proliferation and function.

Absorption of CsA in the form of Sandimmune is highly variable, ranging from 5% to 40%. There is a poor relationship between dose and blood concentration; however, the whole-blood concentration of CsA correlates with the degree of immunosuppression and toxicity.[184] A microemulsion form of CsA, Neoral, has more reproducible absorption, averaging 40%, and exhibits better correlation among dose, blood concentration, and clinical response.[185,186]

Immunosuppression requires trough whole–blood concentrations of at least 100 ng/mL (83 nmol/L).[184] Kahan and colleagues[187] found that trough whole–blood concentrations exceeding 600 ng/mL (499 nmol/L) were associated with hepatic, renal, neurologic, and infective complications. Shaw and colleagues have discussed strategies for reducing the toxicity of CsA and other ISDs.[188]

Therapeutic trough blood concentrations of CsA for renal transplants are 100 to 300 ng/mL (83 to 250 nmol/L), whereas 200 to 350 ng/mL (166 to 291 nmol/L) is used as the target concentration for cardiac, hepatic, and pancreatic transplants[184,189]; however, concomitant immunosuppression used in combination therapy, similar to combined drug therapy in other situations such as AED therapy in epilepsy, significantly affects the range of concentrations that are effective. Simultaneous immunosuppression with low-dose prednisone and either AZA or mycophenolate mofetil (MMF) allows the patient to enjoy a good response to CsA at lower concentrations; some renal transplant patients obtain a satisfactory response with trough CsA concentration of 70 ng/mL (58 nmol/L).

CsA is slowly absorbed, and peak concentrations are reached in 4 to 6 hours. Like tacrolimus, CsA is also highly (~90%) protein bound and concentrated in erythrocytes.[190] The degree of concentration in erythrocytes is temperature dependent in vitro; thus measurement of plasma concentration requires strict attention to specimen temperature if reproducible results are to be obtained.[191] Because of this effect, the best specimen for analysis is whole blood. The elimination profile of CsA is biphasic. An early elimination phase with an apparent half-life that typically ranges from 3 to 7 hours is followed by a slower elimination phase with an apparent half-life ranging from 18 to 25 hours. The volume of distribution is 17 L/kg. Many of the 31 known metabolites of CsA are inactive.[192] One of the major metabolites, hydroxylated at the number 1 amino acid, retains approximately 10% of the immunosuppressive activity of the parent compound.

Several drugs alter the disposition of CsA. Ketoconazole, erythromycin, melphalan, amphotericin B, and aminoglycoside antibiotics all prolong metabolism of CsA sufficiently to increase the risk of nephrotoxicity.[193] Co-administration of phenytoin, phenobarbital, carbamazepine, and rifampin results in induction of cytochrome P450 enzymes, which increase the rate at which CsA is metabolized.[184] Intravenous administration of sulfadimidine and trimethoprim decreases CsA concentrations.

The first procedure available for analysis of CsA was an RIA developed by Sandoz Pharmaceuticals (Princeton, NJ), the producer of the drug. This immunoassay, like most antibody-based assays for CsA, exhibited cross-reactivity with inactive metabolites. Currently, nonisotopic immunoassays performed on whole blood are the most commonly employed methods for measurement of CsA; however, many laboratories use HPLC and LC-MS/MS methods, which are more specific and less subject to metabolite interference. Methods for simultaneous detection of multiple ISDs have been reported.[194–196] It is important to ensure consistency with TDM by following individuals with the same method over time and to interpret results within the context of the method used.

Sirolimus

Sirolimus, also known as rapamycin, is a macrocyclic antibiotic that is a fermentation product of the actinomycete *Streptomyces hygroscopicus* that was isolated from soil samples collected on Rapa Nui (Easter Island) after a search for novel antifungal agents. Structurally, sirolimus is a lipophilic macrocyclic lactone comprising a 31-membered macrolide ring. It demonstrates antifungal, antitumor, and immunosuppressive activity in animal model studies and is approved in the United States for the prophylaxis of acute rejection in renal transplant patients.

The complex of sirolimus and the intracellular immunophilin, FKBP12, modulates the immune response by combining with the specific cell-cycle regulatory protein called the mammalian target of rapamycin (mTOR) and inhibiting its activation. This inhibition results in suppression of cytokine-driven T-lymphocyte proliferation, inhibiting the progression from the G_1 to the S phase of the cell cycle.[197]

The metabolism of sirolimus by the human body is driven by oxidative metabolism via CYP3A in the gastrointestinal tract and liver. There are at least seven metabolites characterized as 41-O- and 7-O-demethyl; several hydroxy, hydroxy-demethylated; and didemethylated sirolimus.[198–200] Total sirolimus metabolites accounted for 48 to 70%, and no single metabolite accounted for more than 10% of sirolimus in trough whole blood from stable renal transplant patients[201]; however, the immunosuppressive activity of individual metabolites is reported to be lower than that of the parent drug.[202]

Sirolimus is available as both an oral solution and a tablet. It is rapidly absorbed from the gastrointestinal tract, with the average time to reach maximal concentration in whole blood of approximately 2 hours.[203,204] The average bioavailability of sirolimus is low, at 15%, and attributable to extensive intestinal and hepatic metabolism by CYP3A and counter-transport by the multidrug efflux pump P-glycoprotein in the gastrointestinal tract. This absorption barrier varies considerably across patients and within-patient. It is also the site of clinically important drug-drug and drug-food interactions.[205]

Sirolimus distributes extensively into blood cells as reflected by the average blood to plasma ratio of 36:1 in renal transplant patients. Approximately 95% distributes into RBCs, 3% in plasma, and 1% each in lymphocytes and granulocytes.[198] The extensive and avid binding of sirolimus to the ubiquitously distributed intracellular FKBP12 accounts for the high blood to plasma sirolimus concentration ratio. Approximately 2.5% of the sirolimus within the plasma fraction is unbound with the remainder bound to plasma proteins.[205]

The relationship between sirolimus whole-blood trough concentrations has been investigated in renal transplant patients who received concomitant full-dose CsA and corticosteroid therapy. According to these analyses, the minimum effective sirolimus concentration below which there is a significant increase in risk for acute rejection is 4 to 5 μg/L (4.4 to 5.5 nmol/L).[205,206] The threshold concentration of 13 to 15 μg/L (14 to 16 nmol/L) was identified, above which the risks for the concentration-related side effects are thrombocytopenia (<100,000 platelets/mm³), leukopenia (<4000 leukocytes/mm³), and hypertriglyceridemia (>300 mg/dL or 3.4 mmol/L serum triglycerides).[206] More studies are needed to define these relationships for other transplant populations and for different concomitant immunosuppressants.

Several chromatographic (i.e., LC-MS, LC-MS/MS, HPLC) detection methods have been validated and are in use in laboratories worldwide,[207–212] including methods for simultaneous detection of multiple ISDs.[194–196] A commercial, automated immunoassay also has been developed. This latter assay, while showing high precision, exhibits modest bias because of metabolite interference (~25%) when results are compared to chromatographic methods.[213]

Everolimus

In April 2010, everolimus, a more water-soluble analog of sirolimus, was approved for use in CsA-sparing regimens, including the requirement for adjusting everolimus doses using target trough blood concentrations in renal transplant patients. The target ranges were established from earlier retrospective studies[214–217] and used prospectively to demonstrate equivalent acute rejection rates compared to the combination of standard dose CsA and empirical dose MMF.[218] More recently, the use of everolimus has expanded with approval in liver transplantation in combination with low-dose tacrolimus.[219] Recent studies have focused on the use of TDM to assure achievement of therapeutic target everolimus blood concentrations in concert with reduction or withdrawal of concomitant calcineurin inhibitor therapy in renal or heart transplant recipients.[220,221]

The mechanism of action and pharmacodynamic effects of everolimus are comparable to those for sirolimus. Similar to the other ISDs, wide pharmacokinetic variability of everolimus has been observed.[222] This variability is driven by the variable metabolism via CYP3A4/5 and p-glycoprotein along with frequent drug-drug interactions that are comparable to that observed for sirolimus. Everolimus trough concentrations show a significant, linear correlation with overall drug exposure as assessed by AUC with a coefficient (r^2) of 0.79. Similar degrees of correlation between everolimus trough concentration and thrombocytopenia, leucopenia, hypertriglyceridemia, or hypercholesterolemia have been observed in an investigation of 54 stable renal transplant patients (18 to 68 years).[223] Based upon the robust correlation between trough concentration and both efficacy and toxicity, a trough concentration of 3 to 8 ng/mL (3.1 to 8.3 nmol/L) has been suggested as the optimal target range.[224]

The bioanalytical method used for measurement of everolimus concentration in the pharmacokinetic assessments and prospective TDM protocols of many clinical investigations is a validated LC-MS/MS method.[214,218] Use of this bioanalytical methodology provides for sensitive and selective measurement of everolimus, and this attribute is important for reliable measurement of blood concentrations at the low end of the recommended target concentration range (3 ng/mL [3.1 nmol/L]) in currently used immunosuppression protocols.[218,225] In the future, we can anticipate the availability of immunoassays for everolimus, and it will be essential to understand the comparison between these methods and the current chromatographic methods.

Mycophenolic Acid

Mycophenolic acid (MPA) is a product of *Penicillium* species that exhibits antitumor, antiviral, antifungal, antibacterial, and immunosuppressive activity. MPA is administered as its morpholinoethyl ester, MMF. MMF, also known as RS-61433, is considered a prodrug because its immunosuppressive activity is expressed only after its hydrolysis to MPA in the body. MPA inhibits inosine monophosphate dehydrogenase, an important enzyme in the purine metabolic pathway. T lymphocytes rely on this pathway for purine synthesis, whereas other cells use the hypoxanthine–guanosine ribosyl transferase salvage pathway for purine biosynthesis. Thus MPA selectively inhibits purine synthesis, and thus transcription, in T lymphocytes.[226] MPA is of interest clinically because it has immunosuppressive activity similar to the thiopurine, AZA, but without many of its side effects.

MMF is completely absorbed and rapidly and completely metabolized to MPA, the active metabolite. The latter is metabolized in the liver by phase II enzymes to form the major metabolite, mycophenolic acid glucuronide (MPAG). The elimination half–life of MPA averages 18 hours, the volume of distribution averages 4 L/kg, and typical serum concentrations range from a peak of 12 μg/mL (37.4 μmol/L) to a trough value of 2 μg/mL (6.24 μmol/L).[227] Studies of MPA pharmacokinetics have shown that exposure correlates poorly with the dose of the drug, and many patients on standard fixed dosing have subtherapeutic concentrations of MPA.[228–231] It has therefore been suggested that monitoring serum concentrations of MPA is useful to overcome the variable pharmacokinetic behavior of this drug.[232,233] A prospective, randomized concentration-controlled study in kidney transplant patients demonstrated a positive correlation between AUC and acute rejection.[234] This same study, however, failed to reveal a correlation between AUC and gastrointestinal toxicity, the primary adverse effect of MPA. Subsequent prospective studies exploring the utility of TDM in MMF therapy have had mixed results, which may in part be a result of differing study designs. In particular, one of the studies failing to show a benefit used trough concentration monitoring. Unfortunately, trough concentrations, although simpler to collect, show a relatively poor correlation to AUC, likely limiting their utility. Limited sampling strategies that use three or four concentrations during the first few hours after dosing have shown improved correlation with dose interval AUC, and these strategies may be a better alternative to trough monitoring when full dose interval sampling is not feasible for AUC determination. Based on the available studies, the optimal immunosuppression for MPA appears to be achieved with target AUCs in the range of 30 to 60 mmol·min/mL range. Although poorly correlated, this is approximated by trough serum concentrations in the range of 2 to 4 μg/mL (6.24 to 12.5 μmol/L).[235]

Various methods for measurement of MPA have been developed. Most clinical studies have used a reference HPLC or

LC-MS/MS method. Commercial immunoassays for MPA determination are also available. These latter assays have slight positive bias, especially in patients with low glomerular filtration rate, likely the result of recognition of both MPA and its glucuronide-conjugated metabolite

Cardiac Glycosides

Digoxin

Digoxin (Lanoxin) is one of a group of cardiac glycosides obtained from digitalis plants (e.g., *Digitalis lanata*). Although used with substantially less frequency than in the past because of newer drugs, digoxin is still used for treatment of supraventricular arrhythmias such as atrial fibrillation because of its activity on atrioventricular nodal conduction. Digoxin also acts as an inotropic agent restoring the force of cardiac contraction in congestive heart failure. However, this use has decreased substantially. The drug binds to the extracytoplasmic side of the α-subunit of membrane-bound Na^+,K^+-ATPase, inhibiting both cellular Na^+ efflux and K^+ influx in myocardial cells. This reduces the sodium/potassium gradient in the Purkinje fibers of the atrial, junctional, and ventricular myocardium, resulting in a decreased transmembrane potential. Inhibition of Na^+, K^+-ATPase is postulated to enhance movement of calcium ions in the cell, increasing calcium ion availability and improving cardiac contractility. In addition to direct effects on the excitable tissues within the heart through the Na, K-ATPase, digoxin also has been shown to alter autonomic activity within the heart to promote parasympathetic activity, which may further contribute to its mechanism of action.[236–238]

At low concentrations, digoxin causes the atrium to be less electrically excitable. Moderate concentrations of digoxin are required to reduce the rate of depolarization in the spontaneously depolarizing conductive fibers (Purkinje fibers), and toxic concentrations of digoxin are necessary to diminish depolarization of the ventricular myocardium. Disagreement over the clinical value of digoxin measurements and the failure of the digoxin concentration to correlate with clinical toxicity are usually related to aberrations in serum and tissue concentrations of sodium, potassium, magnesium, and calcium. Increased sensitivity to digoxin can be noted in states of hypokalemia, hypomagnesemia, and hypercalcemia, which make establishment of the true therapeutic concentration of digoxin difficult because all parameters are interactive.

Absorption of digoxin is variable and dependent on the drug formulation. The USP requires more than 65% of digoxin in tablet form to dissolve in 60 minutes. In plasma, digoxin is 25% protein bound. Digoxin is concentrated in tissues, and at steady state the concentration of digoxin in cardiac tissue is 15 to 30 times that of plasma. Accumulation of digoxin in tissue lags behind the plasma concentration; that is, although the peak plasma concentration is reached 2 to 3 hours after the oral dose, the peak tissue concentration occurs 6 to 10 hours after an oral dose. Although pharmacologic effects and toxicity correlate with tissue concentration rather than plasma concentration, the safe therapeutic plasma concentration of digoxin has been reported to range from 0.8 to 2.0 ng/mL (1 to 2.6 nmol/L).[239] This range is not determined at the peak plasma concentration but rather at the time of peak tissue concentration.[240] Thus to ensure a correlation between plasma concentration and tissue concentration, the appropriate time to collect the specimen is 8 hours or more after the dose, at which time serum digoxin has reached distributional equilibrium with the drug in tissues. Results from specimens collected earlier than 8 hours after the dose are misleading because high concentrations may be misinterpreted as toxic concentrations, whereas they are more likely due to incomplete distribution.

Digoxin toxicity is characterized by nonspecific symptoms of nausea, vomiting, anorexia, and predominance of green/yellow visual distortion. Cardiac symptoms of intoxication include multiform premature ventricular contractions, ventricular bigeminy, ventricular tachycardia, and ventricular fibrillation. Combinations of decreased conduction and increased automaticity may result in paroxysmal atrial tachycardia with atrioventricular node block and nonparoxysmal junction tachycardia. These symptoms are frequently observed when the blood concentration exceeds 2 ng/mL (2.6 nmol/L) in adults. Children can tolerate higher concentrations and do not usually exhibit toxicity until the digoxin concentration exceeds 4 ng/mL (5.2 nmol/L).[241]

Significant controversy has surrounded the use of digoxin in the heart failure setting. A large prospective study of concentration-controlled digoxin in the 0.8 to 2 ng/mL (1 to 2.6 nmol/L) target range for the treatment of heart failure (the Digitalis Intervention Group [DIG]) demonstrated that the cohort of patients receiving digoxin therapy experienced a higher overall mortality compared to a placebo control, arguing against the use of digoxin in this setting.[242] A retrospective analysis of the DIG study data demonstrated that the overall mortality was correlated with serum digoxin concentration. The mortality in the patients with serum digoxin concentrations in the 0.5 to 0.8 ng/mL (0.6 to 1 nmol/L) range was in fact lower than in patients receiving the placebo control. Significantly increased mortality was observed in patients with serum digoxin concentrations greater than 1.2 ng/mL (1.5 nmol/L). This result indicates that the target concentration range of 0.8 to 2 ng/mL (1 to 2.6 nmol/L), suggested by the earlier pharmacodynamics studies of toxicity, is not optimal for balancing the effectiveness of digoxin with its toxicity in the heart failure population; lower concentrations of digoxin may be required to balance safety and efficacy.[243]

Elimination of digoxin follows first–order kinetics; 50 to 70% is excreted unchanged or in the form of digoxigenin monosaccharides or disaccharides in the urine. A small amount is metabolized to dihydrodigoxin and also excreted by the kidneys. The remainder is found in the stool as digoxigenin and its saccharides. As a result, digoxin toxicity develops more frequently and lasts longer in patients with renal impairment. Dose requirements are decreased in patients with renal disease. Bresnahan and Vlietstra[240] present a simple method for calculating dose, which is based on creatinine clearance. Co-administration of cyclosporine,[244] quinidine,[245] or verapamil[246] prolongs the rate of clearance of digoxin, requiring dose adjustment.

Decreased gastrointestinal absorption occurs with sprue and small intestinal resections, high-fiber diets, hyperthyroidism, and situations of increased gastrointestinal motility. Although seldom used, when quinidine is added to digoxin in the treatment of atrial fibrillation to convert patients to normal sinus rhythm, the concomitant administration of quinidine typically causes serum digoxin concentrations to increase twofold to threefold. The increase is probably due to decreased renal and extrarenal clearance. Studies have provided evidence that the p-glycoprotein multidrug transporter, responsible for export of digoxin from renal tubules to tubular lumen, is inhibited by drugs such as quinidine and verapamil.[247–249]

Currently, immunoassays remain the most widely used method for measurement of digoxin in serum and biological fluids.[250] For routine measurement of digoxin concentrations, several commercially available immunoassays are widely used, including RIA, fluorescence polarization, chemiluminescence, and enzyme immunoassays. The rich history of digoxin measurement methods and the overall improvements made over the past two decades has been reviewed and is beyond the scope of this chapter. More details can be found in the article by Jortani and Valdes.[251] Use of Digibind (GlaxoSmithKline, Middlesex, United Kingdom) or DigiFab (Protherics, West Conshohocken, PA), digoxin-specific Fab fragments that neutralize the drug and are used in the setting of acute toxicity, can significantly interfere with digoxin measurement by many immunoassays. Results of digoxin monitoring after administration of Digibind should therefore be interpreted with a high degree of caution.[252] Methods to eliminate the interference by therapeutic antidigoxin Fab therapy using ultrafiltration of serum to isolate free drug and remove the interfering Fab have been described, but these methods lack standardization.[253,254]

Drugs Used in Psychiatry

Lithium

Lithium (e.g., Eskalith, Lithane, Lithonate) is administered as lithium carbonate and used for the treatment of the manic phase of affective disorders, mania, and manic-depressive illness. The mechanism of action for lithium is not entirely clear. Early research suggested that it acts by enhancing reuptake of catecholamines, thereby reducing their concentration in the neuronal junction and producing a sedating effect on the central nervous system. More recently, lithium along with other mood-affecting drugs, such as valproic acid, carbamazepine, and the tricyclic antidepressants (TCAs), have been shown to inhibit GSK3-β, a protein central to the Wnt/β-catenin signaling pathway that affects gene expression involved in many aspects of cellular behavior, neuronal polarity, plasticity and survival, and brain development.[56] GSK3-β appears critical in the action of dopamine and serotonin on the brain in affecting behavior.[57] At least two mechanisms account for lithium's effects on GSK3-β. Lithium directly competes with magnesium, which is an important cation for GSK3-β activity. It also indirectly affects GSK3-β by inhibiting a critical phosphatase normally required for its activation.[255] Although other mechanisms of action cannot be excluded, the mechanisms described previously are likely to account for many of lithium's effects on mood.

Absorption of lithium from the gastrointestinal tract is complete, with peak plasma concentration reached 2 to 4 hours after an oral dose. This cation does not bind to protein. Lithium elimination is biphasic; during the first phase, 30 to 40% of the dose of lithium is cleared, with an apparent half-life of 24 hours. During the second phase, the remainder of lithium incorporated into the cellular ion pool is cleared, exhibiting a half-life of 48 to 72 hours. Clearance is predominantly a function of the kidneys, where active reabsorption occurs. Reduced renal function causes prolonged clearance times.

The optimal therapeutic response to lithium has not been related to a specific serum concentration; however, toxicity is related to serum concentration. Serum lithium concentrations are monitored to ensure patient compliance and avoid intoxication. It is recommended that a standardized 12-hour postdose serum lithium concentration be used to assess adequate therapy.[256] The interval of 1 to 1.2 mmol/L was identified as the optimal trough therapeutic concentration. Concentrations of 1.2 to 1.5 mmol/L signifies a warning range, and a concentration in excess of 1.5 mmol/L in a specimen drawn 12 hours after the dose indicates a significant risk for intoxication. Early symptoms of intoxication include apathy, sluggishness, drowsiness, lethargy, speech difficulties, irregular tremors, myoclonic twitching, muscle weakness, and ataxia. These symptoms, although not life threatening, are uncomfortable for patients and indicate that life-threatening seizures are imminent.

Lithium excretion parallels that of sodium. It readily passes the glomerular membrane and is reabsorbed in the proximal convoluted tubules. In situations in which patients are vulnerable to dehydration (fever, watery stools, vomiting, loss of appetite, hot weather), the potential for lithium intoxication is increased. In dehydration, the proximal tubular response to reabsorption of sodium (and lithium) is reduction of clearance. Increased reabsorption of lithium leads to increased blood concentration of lithium. Severe intoxication, characterized by muscle rigidity, hyperactive deep tendon reflexes, and epileptic seizures, is usually associated with lithium concentrations in excess of 2.5 mmol/L.

The concentration of lithium in serum, plasma, urine, or other body fluids can be determined by several methods, including flame emission photometry, atomic absorption spectrometry, ion-selective electrode, or inductively coupled plasma–mass spectrometry (ICP-MS) or optical emission spectrometry (ICP-OES). In contemporary clinical practice, automated methods are primarily used for routine measurement of lithium in serum using a chromophore (e.g., a substituted porphyrin) that forms a colored product readily detected spectrophotometrically upon binding to lithium.[257] The availability from NIST of a Standard Reference material (NIST SRM 3129a) provides manufacturers with the opportunity to prepare traceable calibrators and improve standardization of assays.[258]

Tricyclic Antidepressants

While TCAs were originally developed in the 1950s and a number of newer antidepressant drugs have been developed such as the selective serotonin reuptake inhibitors (SSRIs), TCAs continue to remain useful in the treatment of depression and anxiety disorders and chronic pain. TCAs work primarily by blocking the serotonin and norepinephrine transporters that mediate reuptake, resulting in increased synaptic concentrations of these neurotransmitters.[259] In addition to blocking serotonin and norepinephrine reuptake, TCAs have also been shown to bind and block a variety of neurotransmitter receptors with high affinity including members of the 5-HT receptor family,[260,261] alpha-adrenergic receptors,[260] and NMDA receptors.[262] These interactions likely contribute to both the beneficial actions of TCAs and their side effects.

TCAs are nearly completely absorbed from the gastrointestinal tract but undergo first-pass hepatic metabolism, so their ultimate bioavailability is variable. Because these drugs slow gastrointestinal activity and gastric emptying, their absorption also may be delayed, further contributing to variability. Once absorbed, they are highly protein and tissue bound, resulting in large apparent volumes of distribution. Peak plasma concentrations are reached from 2 to 12 hours after the oral dose. Metabolism is by *N*-demethylation and aromatic ring hydroxylation, followed by conjugation with glucuronic acid. If the drug administered is the tertiary tricyclic amine (amitriptyline, doxepin, imipramine), metabolism causes accumulation of the respective secondary amine (nortriptyline, nordoxepin, desipramine). These substances have generally equal pharmacologic activity and accumulate to concentrations approximately (but variably) equal to that of the parent drug. The hydroxylated metabolites have little pharmacologic activity. Taking these factors into consideration (i.e., variable bioavailability, high volume of distribution, variable metabolic activity, and generation of pharmacologically active metabolites), it is not surprising that patient response to these drugs is widely variable. Determining the serum concentration gives the physician the assurance that a patient has been properly dosed.

Drugs such as cimetidine, chloramphenicol, haloperidol, methylphenidate, and phenothiazines inhibit hepatic oxidative enzymes. Inhibition of end-product metabolism of the tertiary TCAs results in a greater accumulation of the secondary amine metabolite (amitriptyline is metabolized to nortriptyline, doxepin to nordoxepin, imipramine to desipramine), because conversion to the aromatic ring hydroxylated metabolites is blocked. Coadministration of perphenazine with a TCA causes accumulation of the secondary amine to concentrations two to four times normal, with onset of toxicity occurring at the expected blood concentrations.

TCAs show a good correlation between therapeutic response and serum concentration. A linear relationship between clinical improvement and serum concentration is noted for most of these drugs, the exception being nortriptyline, which has a specific therapeutic window. A serum concentration of nortriptyline below or above the concentration range of 50 to 150 ng/mL (0.19 to 0.57 μmol/L) correlates with worsening of moods. The other antidepressants do not display this effect; the upper limit of the optimum blood concentration for these other antidepressants is limited by the onset of toxicity. Toxicity is expressed as dry mouth and perspiration, signs that may also occur with depression. Thus it is difficult to differentiate between mild toxicity from the drug and the disease that is being treated. More serious toxicity is expressed as atrioventricular node block, characterized by a widening of the electrocardiographic QRS interval. Onset occurs at serum concentrations ranging from 800 to 1200 ng/mL (3.0 to 4.6 μmol/L), and the severity of intoxication is related to the serum concentration.[263] The relationship between serum concentration and cardiac toxicity diminishes with time after intoxication as the drug is absorbed into tissues. Despite this toxicity, the TCAs remain useful drugs in the treatment of depression.

Numerous methods have been published for analysis of TCAs. These drugs present various problems to the clinical laboratory: (1) the therapeutic serum concentration is 10 to 100 times lower than that of other commonly monitored drugs, and thus to be clinically useful the method must be able to measure serum concentrations below 25 ng/mL

($\sim$0.09 μmol/L); (2) these drugs have metabolites that also must be measured; and (3) they are structurally similar to common sleep inducers, antihistamines, and many over-the-counter medications used for appetite suppression, which are potential interferences. Of the many hundreds of methods published, only a few have satisfactorily overcome these obstacles. Analysis by gas-liquid chromatography (GLC)-MS, using selected ion monitoring, was the historical reference method, using either the electron impact mode[264] or the chemical ionization mode.[265] HPLC with photodiode array detection has also been successfully used for analysis of TCAs[266]; however, LC-MS/MS is the preferred reference method because of the ability to measure multiple TCAs and their metabolites simultaneously.[267,268]

Antipsychotics

Antipsychotic drugs are primarily used in the management of acute psychosis and its prevention in patients with schizophrenia. Earlier drugs including haloperidol and thioridazine were effective antipsychotic agents but were associated with significant incidence of extrapyramidal adverse effects including dystonia, tremor, and tardive dyskinesia. Second generation antipsychotics, commonly referred to as atypical antipsychotics include clozapine, risperidone, olanzapine, quetiapine, paliperidone, and aripiprazole. Antagonism of dopamine, serotonin, and adrenergic receptors within the CNS is central to the mechanism of action of these drugs. Although all antipsychotics appear to mediate their effects, both positive and negative, through attenuation of dopamine signaling via antagonism of the dopamine receptors, the atypical antipsychotics produce less extrapyramidal symptoms (EPS), which is hypothesized to be a result of altered binding kinetics to dopamine D2 receptors. The atypical antipsychotics have become the main agents employed for management of schizophrenia. Although they exhibit less EPS, especially tardive dyskinesia, the atypical antipsychotics are still associated with significant adverse effects including metabolic, cerebrovascular, and cardiovascular effects that complicate therapy and may lead to discontinuation. The requirement for TDM in the management of patients on antipsychotic drug therapy is still debated; however, it is widely used with some of the agents, most notably clozapine due to high variability in pharmacokinetics and adherence to therapy. An in-depth review on the clinical pharmacokinetics of the broad array of atypical antipsychotics can be found in Mauri et al.[269]

Clozapine

Clozapine remains one of the mainstays of atypical antipsychotic therapy for patients with schizophrenia. In addition to its antipsychotic effects, clozapine has also been shown to improve negative symptoms and cognitive deficits in schizophrenia along with prevention of suicidal ideation. Although clozapine shares the primary adverse effects associated with atypical antipsychotics including sedation and metabolic derangement that appear concentration-dependent, agranulocytosis represents a rare but important adverse effect of this drug that is unrelated to dosing and requires monitoring of white blood count during therapy.

Clozapine is well absorbed after oral administration, but it exhibits extensive first pass metabolism resulting in a less than 50% oral bioavailability. Clozapine is highly protein bound in the serum, binding primarily to alpha-1 acid gly-coprotein with a plasma half-life of 9 to 17 hours. Metabolism is mediated by both cytochrome P450 demethylation and oxidation and UDP-glucuronidation. CYP1A2 metabolism appears to be the most important and variable, influenced by tobacco and caffeine use necessitating the monitoring of their use during therapy with this drug. As a result of high genetic variability in metabolic pathways, clozapine exposure displays a very poor relationship to dose. Although interindividual variability in PK is high, intraindividual variation in exposure is much lower, estimated at approximately 20%.

Metabolism of clozapine produces two active metabolites, norclozapine (produced by CYP1A2) and clozapine-N-oxide (produced by CYP3A4). Norclozapine is the predominant metabolite with concentrations in plasma that can range from 50 to 90% of clozapine. While active, the norclozapine metabolite does not appear to possess much antipsychotic activity, but it may contribute to some of the adverse drug responses noted with clozapine use. Despite the variable metabolism and production of active metabolites, the antipsychotic effects and the adverse effects of clozapine are correlated with the plasma and serum concentration. It should be noted that serum concentrations are reported to be 10% lower than plasma concentrations.

There is still much debate regarding the optimal plasma or serum concentration range for clozapine. A 350 to 600 ng/mL range has been proposed; however, a randomized, concentration-controlled study of clozapine in patients with schizophrenia demonstrated comparable symptom control with serum concentrations in the 200 to 300 ng/mL target range versus a higher 350 to 450 ng/mL target range, suggesting that concentrations greater than 250 ng/mL may be adequate in many patients.[270] Toxicity also increases with exposure, most notably sedation, which has been reported to be twice as frequent with concentrations above 350 ng/mL compared with patients maintained below this concentration. An association between serum and plasma clozapine concentration, electroencephalogram (EEG) changes, and onset of seizure have also been reported, but the correlation may not be very predictive as seizure activity has been described in patients with clozapine concentrations below 450 ng/mL.[271] A 1000 ng/mL toxic threshold requiring provider alert has been suggested for this drug; however, the data supporting this threshold is limited and relatively weak. Importantly, as the intraindividual variation in clozapine blood concentrations are generally lower than 20%, highly variable concentrations within a patient suggest nonadherence to drug therapy, which is not infrequent in patients with schizophrenia.

Others

Theophylline

Theophylline, available under many proprietary names, relaxes bronchial smooth muscles to relieve or prevent asthma. The therapeutic effect of theophylline is likely due to antagonism of adenosine receptors in smooth muscle, whereas the toxic effects are due to inhibition of cyclic nucleotide phosphodiesterase. With increased use of β-adrenergic agonists, and because of the considerable toxicity associated with it, theophylline is now considered a second–level approach used only in treatment of persistent asthma.[272]

Theophylline is readily absorbed after oral, rectal, or parenteral administration. If the drug is taken orally without food, the blood concentration peaks within 2 hours. If it is administered with food or as a slow-release formula, peak concentrations occur 3 to 5 hours after the dose. Once absorbed, it is 50% protein bound. The drug is rapidly cleared in adolescents and in adults who smoke because of its higher rate of metabolism secondary to increased levels of CYP1A2. In these individuals, the half-life ranges from 3 to 4 hours. Nonsmoking adults in good health have an elimination half-life of approximately 9 hours. The half-life in neonates and in adults with congestive heart failure can be prolonged to 20 to 30 hours, depending on the degree of liver immaturity or loss of liver function. Coadministration of cimetidine, ciprofloxacin, and ticlopidine leads to reduced clearance of theophylline.

The relationship between serum concentration and prevention of symptoms of chronic asthma has been well documented.[273] There is a proportional relationship between forced expiratory volume and theophylline concentration, with the optimum therapeutic effect occurring at concentrations ranging from 8 to 20 μg/mL (44 to 111 μmol/L). Suppression of exercise-induced bronchospasm in asthmatic patients occurs at concentrations exceeding 10 μg/mL (56 μmol/L) and is optimal at 15 μg/mL (83 μmol/L). Neonatal apnea treated with theophylline responds to slightly lower concentrations, ranging from 5 to 10 μg/mL (28 to 56 μmol/L).[274] Relaxation of bronchial smooth muscle is directly proportional to blood concentration and continues at concentrations greater than 20 μg/mL (111 μmol/L). When the blood level exceeds 20 μg/mL (111 μmol/L), the secondary side effects become significant.

Theophylline typically exhibits first-order kinetics of elimination when used in most patients with serum concentrations in the range of 5 to 15 μg/mL (28 to 83 μmol/L); however, at serum concentrations greater than 20 μg/mL (111 μmol/L), theophylline exhibits zero-order pharmacokinetics with small dose increases leading to disproportionately large increases in serum concentration and intoxication. Symptoms of theophylline toxicity include nausea, vomiting, headache, diarrhea, irritability, and insomnia. Transient central nervous system stimulation occurring at initial administration is not directly related to blood concentration. This effect diminishes with chronic use. Serious toxicity characterized by cardiac arrhythmias and seizures is usually associated with serum concentrations in excess of 30 μg/mL (167 μmol/L). Once seizure activity begins, the final prognosis is very poor. Morbidity is reported in nearly all patients, and mortality can be as high as 50%.[275]

Immunoassay is the standard method for determination of theophylline concentration. Theophylline, caffeine, and dyphylline can be measured simultaneously by HPLC.

Caffeine

A minor metabolite of theophylline in adults, caffeine has been shown to accumulate to significant concentrations in neonates. Caffeine itself is an effective inhibitor of apnea,[276] which may explain the lower therapeutic concentration required for control of neonatal apnea. Therapy with caffeine alone also has been demonstrated as effective in the treatment of neonatal apnea; it is gaining popularity because of caffeine's long half-life in neonates (>30 hours). The optimal therapeutic concentration of caffeine in this situation ranges from 8 to 14 μg/mL (41 to 72 μmol/L). Caffeine can be measured by HPLC or immunoassay.

Biologics: Entering the New Frontier of Monoclonal Antibody Therapeutic Drug Monitoring

Biologic drugs (also called biopharmaceuticals) represent a varied group of therapeutic agents that are distinct from traditional small molecule pharmaceuticals in both their generally larger size that can range from a peptide or protein to a whole cell and origins that often require complex production methods using living cells (i.e., biotechnology). Monoclonal antibody (mAb)-based therapeutics represent one of the most rapidly expanding areas of biologic drug development. Beginning in 1983 with the US FDA approval of muromonab-CD3 for the treatment and prevention of kidney transplant rejection, over 79 mAbs have achieved regulatory approval in the United States and over 180 mAbs were in phase 3 development as of April 2019. MAb-based drugs represented seven of the 10 best-selling drugs worldwide in 2017 due in large part to their high cost. Infliximab (IFX; sold under the trade name Remicade) or its biosimilar (sold under the trade names Inflectra) can cost as much as $45,000 a year for patients with Crohn disease. Therapeutic monitoring of mAb-based therapeutics like IFX, in addition to potentially enhancing their efficacy and safety, may also contribute substantially to a reduction in the economic impact, or as some have termed "financial toxicity," of these revolutionary yet expensive drugs.

The pharmacology of mAbs is quite distinct from small molecule drugs. As proteins with a large molecular size (150 kD), mAbs cannot efficiently cross the plasma membranes of cells. Parenteral administration, primarily intravenous infusion, is therefore required with an initial volume of distribution that generally reflects the intravascular blood volume. The secondary distribution into tissues is dependent on the target antigen presence and density and the vascularity. Metabolism and elimination of mAbs are also quite distinct from small molecules. Uptake into cells via nonspecific pinocytosis or receptor-mediated endocytosis represent the principal modes of elimination. Receptor-mediated endocytosis of mAb through Fc-receptors (FcRs) present throughout the reticuloendothelial system is a primary mode of clearance especially when complexed with its target antigen. Upon internalization of mAb into the endosomal compartment, the mAb is degraded by proteolytic enzymes within the lysosome. Target antigen burden is an important factor affecting mAb clearance. Host antibodies can also form against mAb, especially those derived from other species, and these anti-drug antibodies (ADAs) can further enhance clearance. However, not all FcR-mediated internalization leads to degradation. Neonatal FcR (FcRn), which was originally identified in placenta and binds IgG and albumin, is expressed across a wide range of cells including endothelium, hepatocytes, gastrointestinal epithelium, and kidney glomerular and tubular cells.[277] FcRn mediates recycling of antibody and albumin within the endosomal compartment of cells, protecting these proteins from degradation contributing to the approximately 20-day half-life of antibody. FcRn also plays important roles in IgG transcytosis such as across the gastrointestinal epithelium, which further contribute to mAb clearance. Due to the variety of mechanisms of antibody clearance and the impact of ADAs, mAb concentrations can vary widely in relationship to dose.[278]

TDM has been advocated for many therapeutic mAbs. Although evidence for utility for most mAb therapeutics is absent, TDM is common for the anti–tumor necrosis factor (TNF) antibodies. As the number of therapeutic antibodies continues to rise, it is likely to be an expanding area of TDM.

Infliximab

IFX is a chimeric monoclonal antibody with antigen binding, variable domains derived from a mouse monoclonal antibody grafted onto a human IgG1 κ antibody framework. IFX binds to TNF α, and neutralizes the activity of this important inflammatory cytokine as its primary mechanism of action. IFX was initially approved for the treatment of Crohn IBD where it induces significant clinical improvement in 60 to 90% of patients with initial therapy. It is now approved for the treatment of multiple moderate to severe inflammatory disorders including both adult and pediatric IBD, rheumatoid arthritis, psoriatic arthritis, plaque psoriasis, and ankylosing spondylitis.

Although many factors influence the response to IFX therapy including the variable role of TNF-α in disease, pharmacokinetics has been shown to play a significant role in response to therapy. Several recent studies have demonstrated a pharmacodynamic relationship between IFX concentration and clinical response in both Crohn disease (CD) and ulcerative colitis (UC).[279–281] IFX concentrations in blood are influenced by body weight, and weight-based dosing of IFX is the standard approach. IFX exposure as measured by AUC is lower in subjects with higher C-reactive protein. The exact mechanism for this relationship is unknown but could be due to increased TNF concentrations that binds IFX forming immune complexes that accelerate its clearance. In UC, the gastrointestinal protein loss associated with intestinal inflammation may lead to IgG loss increasing IFX clearance. Albumin concentration has also been shown to correlate with IFX clearance, perhaps due to the association with FcRn for both molecules.[282] ADAs are thought to be the dominant factor mediating loss of therapeutic response, and these ADAs can affect response through both direct neutralization of IFX function and accelerating IFX clearance. Although changing therapy to another agent such as adalimumab, a fully human anti-TNFα mAb, may be necessary, some ADA resistance may be overcome by changes in dosing.

Based upon the apparent pharmacodynamic relationship between IFX concentrations and disease response, TDM for IFX has been advocated. Prospective and many retrospective studies have shown that trough concentrations of IFX above 1 mg/mL are needed to achieve an optimal response to therapy. The American Gastroenterology Association has recommended reactive TDM defined as measurement of trough and ADAs in response to new or continual active IBD during initial therapy. This group has proposed a 5 μg/mL trough threshold concentration as a guide to dose escalation in the setting of poor response. In addition, although dose escalation in response to symptoms alone without TDM may be an effective strategy for achieving maximal response, TDM has been shown to improve the decision making and decrease cost by 15% to 30%, which is significant in the context of the high cost of IFX.[283]

Several methods are available for measuring IFX concentrations in blood.[284] Immunoassays provide a simple method for IFX quantitation, representing one of the earliest methods available. These methods are subject to interference by ADAs, and it is therefore imperative that screening for ADAs is included in the testing algorithm. Alternative approaches that indirectly monitor IFX concentrations through their binding to labeled TNF-α that shift chromatographic mobility (Prometheus Anser IFX) or neutralization of TNF-α activity in a biologic assay (offered by ARUP Labs) are also available. More recently, LC-MS/MS-based methods for IFX measurement have been described that have the advantage of avoiding interference by ADAs.[285] Nevertheless, screening for ADAs is still an essential part of IFX TDM even with LC-MS/MS methods as the presence of ADA is important to decision making around dosing and switching to alternative therapies such as the fully human adalimumab.

SUMMARY AND CONCLUSION

The development of analytical techniques for drug measurement over the decades since TDM largely began in the 1970s has dramatically increased our understanding of pharmacokinetics and the ways in which drugs are used, especially those with low TI. Although understanding pharmacokinetics is critical to successful drug therapy, it is also important to not forget the variation in the pharmacodynamics effects of many drugs. Laboratory tests for inosine-5'-monophosphate dehydrogenase (IMPDH) activity, the enzyme targeted by the ISD, MPA, illustrate the potential of combined pharmacokinetic-pharmacodynamic modeling of drug therapy.[286] New technologies in the area of genomics and proteomics set the stage for increasing our understanding of the pharmacokinetic and pharmacodynamic behavior of many drugs. It is anticipated that TDM over the next decade will progress from traditional pharmacokinetic approaches to more integrated pharmacokinetic-pharmacodynamic monitoring approaches that fine tune a drug regimen through incorporation of newly identified genetic and protein biomarkers. The goals will remain the same: finding the right drug and regimen for a patient. The tools are simply evolving.

SELECTED REFERENCES

18. Touw DJ, Neef C, Thomson AH, et al. Cost-effectiveness of therapeutic drug monitoring: a systematic review. Ther Drug Monit 2005;27(1):10–7.
24. Gibaldi M, Prescott LF. Handbook of clinical pharmacokinetics. New York: ADIS Health Science Press; 1983.
25. Goodman LS, Brunton LL, Blumenthal DK, et al. Goodman & Gilman's the pharmacological basis of therapeutics. New York: McGraw-Hill Medical; 2011. p. 1 online resource (xvi, 2084).
26. Carruthers SG, Melmon KL. Melmon and Morrelli's clinical pharmacology: basic principles in therapeutics. 4th ed. New York: McGraw-Hill; 2000.

27. Rowland M, Tozer TN, Rowland M. Clinical pharmacokinetics and pharmacodynamics: concepts and applications. 4th ed. Philadelphia: Lippincott William & Wilkins; 2009.
28. Bauer LA. Applied clinical pharmacokinetics. 3rd ed. New York: McGraw-Hill; 2014.
29. Atkinson AJ. Principles of clinical pharmacology. 3rd ed. San Diego: Academic Press, Elsevier; 2012.
33. Wright JD, Boudinot FD, Ujhelyi MR. Measurement and analysis of unbound drug concentrations. Clin Pharmacokinet 1996;30(6):445–62.
41. Rybak MJ, Lomaestro BM, Rotschafer JC, et al. Vancomycin therapeutic guidelines: a summary of consensus recommendations from the infectious diseases Society of America, the American Society of Health-System Pharmacists, and the Society of Infectious Diseases Pharmacists. Clin Infect Dis 2009;49(3):325–7.
65. Patsalos PN, Berry DJ, Bourgeois BF, Cloyd JC, et al. Antiepileptic drugs—best practice guidelines for therapeutic drug monitoring: a position paper by the subcommission on therapeutic drug monitoring, ILAE Commission on Therapeutic Strategies. Epilepsia 2008;49(7):1239–76.
80. Schentag JJ. Aminoglycosides. In: Evans WE, Schentag JJ, Jusko WJ, editors. Applied pharmacokinetics: principles of therapeutic drug monitoring. San Francisco: Applied Therapeutics; 1980. p. xii, 708.
110. Ashbee HR, Barnes RA, Johnson EM, et al. Therapeutic drug monitoring (TDM) of antifungal agents: guidelines from the British Society for Medical Mycology. J Antimicrob Chemother 2014;69(5):1162–76.
136a. Ferrari S, Sassoli V, Orlandi M, et al. Serum methotrexate (MTX) concentrations and prognosis in patients with osteosarcoma of the extremities treated with a multidrug neoadjuvant regimen. J Chemother 1993;5(2):135–41.
146. Slattery JT, Clift RA, Buckner CD, et al. Marrow transplantation for chronic myeloid leukemia: the influence of plasma busulfan levels on the outcome of transplantation. Blood 1997;89(8):3055–60.
180. Jusko WJ, Thomson AW, Fung J, et al. Consensus document: therapeutic monitoring of tacrolimus (FK-506). Ther Drug Monit 1995;17(6):606–14.
197. MacDonald A, Scarola J, Burke JT, Zimmerman JJ. Clinical pharmacokinetics and therapeutic drug monitoring of sirolimus. Clin Ther 2000;22(Suppl B):B101–21.
219. Keating GM, Lyseng-Williamson KA. Everolimus: a guide to its use in liver transplantation. BioDrugs 2013;27(4):407–11.
227. Staatz C, Tett S. Clinical pharmacokinetics and pharmacodynamics of mycophenolate in solid organ transplant recipients. Clin Pharmacokinet 2007;46(1):13–58.
256. Bettinger TL, Crismon ML, Lithium. In: Burton ME, editor: Applied pharmacokinetics & pharmacodynamics: principles of therapeutic drug monitoring. Philadelphia: Lippincott Williams & Wilkins; 2006. p. 789–812.
278. Keizer RJ, Huitema AD, Schellens JH, Beijnen JH. Clinical pharmacokinetics of therapeutic monoclonal antibodies. Clin Pharmacokinet 2010;49(8):493–507.

Clinical Toxicology*

Loralie J. Langman, Laura K. Bechtel, and Christopher P. Holstege

ABSTRACT

Background

Toxicology is a broad, multidisciplinary science where the goal is to determine the effects of chemical agents on living systems. Innumerable potential toxins can inflict harm, including pharmaceuticals, herbals, household products, environmental agents, occupational chemicals, drugs of abuse, and chemical terrorism threats. Each year millions of human exposure cases are reported worldwide.[1-4] The Centers for Disease Control and Prevention (CDC) has reported that poisoning (both intentional and unintentional) is one of the leading causes of injury-related death in the United States in all adult age groups.[5] From the beginnings of written history, poisons and their effects have been well described. Paracelsus (1493–1541) correctly noted that "Alle Dinge sind Gift, und nichts ist ohne Gift; allein die Dosis macht, daß ein Ding kein Gift sei," which means, "Everything is a poison; there is nothing which is not. Only the dose differentiates a poison." As life in the modern era has become more complex, so has the study of poisons, their identification, and their treatments.

Content

This chapter provides a general overview of clinical toxicology and the laboratory services necessary to support the care of poisoned patients. Because a comprehensive discussion of all aspects of toxicology is beyond the scope of this chapter, the clinical significance and toxicity of only a select number of common drugs, drugs of abuse, and other chemicals are discussed.

*The full version of this chapter is available electronically on ExpertConsult.com.

Toxic Elements*

Frederick G. Strathmann and Lee M. Blum

ABSTRACT

Background

Elements have been recognized as toxins for centuries. Many elements are essential for life but if an individual's exposure exceeds a certain threshold, toxicity may develop. When identified early, disease caused by elemental exposure is readily treatable with good outcomes. Conversely, if exposure is not identified and reduced, serious and sometimes irreparable damage to the nervous, renal, and cardiovascular systems can occur. The laboratory plays a key role in this process and appropriate specimen collection coupled with accurate analysis can make a major difference in correct diagnosis.

Content

This chapter explores toxic elements and the role of the clinical laboratory in diagnosing and monitoring toxicity associated with exposure. A general overview of diagnostic and treatment options for the exposed patient is followed by detailed descriptions for 23 elements commonly associated with toxicity. Each section highlights the following areas: (1) sources of exposure, (2) toxicokinetics and toxicodynamics, (3) clinical presentation and treatment, (4) preanalytical and analytical aspects, (5) regulatory and occupational exposure aspects, and (6) areas of research. Each section concludes with recommendations for appropriate use and interpretation of test results.

---

*The full version of this chapter is available electronically on ExpertConsult.com.

Body Fluids*

Darci R. Block and Christopher M. Florkowski

ABSTRACT

Background
Body fluids are collected and analyzed either to gain insight into the processes that contribute to the accumulation of that fluid within a body compartment or to provide diagnostic information to investigate pathophysiologic processes.

Content
In the preanalytical phase, the route, equipment, and mechanism for obtaining and transporting the body fluid specimen (including required collection device, volume, temperature, and timeliness of transport to the laboratory) should be communicated and standardized.

In the analytical phase, body fluid testing often does not have manufacturer's performance claims or laboratory-developed test validation criteria. Such fluids include pleural, peritoneal, pericardial, and synovial fluids, as well as amniotic fluid and cervicovaginal secretions, saliva, sweat, semen, stool, pancreatic cyst fluid, fine needle aspiration biopsy (FNAB) washings, and cerebrospinal fluid. These alternative specimen types may contain matrix interferences that may unknowingly produce inaccurate results that could negatively affect patient outcomes. Recommendations are under development for more robust validation approaches in many of these areas.

In the postanalytical phase, decision limits are often available (e.g., Light's criteria for discriminating a pleural exudate from a transudate),[1] although the major limitations are the paucity of methodologic detail from historical studies and the fact that such criteria may not be applicable across all fluid types. For a clear understanding of how body fluid tests may leverage important decisions, it is critical that there is a good clinician-laboratory interface to communicate the limitations of body fluid analysis and that those results should always be interpreted in full clinical context.

---

*The full version of this chapter is available electronically on ExpertConsult.com.

Clinical Chemistry-Pathophysiology

Exam questions, case studies, and additional resources are available on ExpertConsult.com.
*Full versions of these chapters are available electronically on www.ExpertConsult.com.

46

Nutrition: Laboratory and Clinical Aspects

Ruth M. Ayling and Martin Crook

ABSTRACT

Background

Nutrition is relevant to every specialty within overall medical practice. Adequate nutrition, both qualitatively and quantitatively, is essential for normal development, growth, function, and health. Both excessive and insufficient intake of individual nutrients can have adverse consequences. Also, patients with many pathologic conditions who have free access to a good diet may benefit from nutritional supplementation or restriction.

Content

This chapter describes all the dietary components that are considered essential to human life, their sources and function, and the consequences of under- or oversupply. It discusses screening methods for malnutrition and the detailed assessment of nutritional status, emphasizing that none of the available techniques for the latter is on its own ideal and that clinical observation remains of paramount importance. The indications for and techniques of nutritional support are described in detail, with particular emphasis on the role of laboratory investigations in assessing its safety and efficacy. The neuroendocrine mechanisms of appetite control are discussed in detail as a preliminary to a discussion of the causes, consequences, and management of obesity, arguably the most important nutritional disorder of our age in developed (and increasingly developing) countries. The metabolic consequences of anorexia and bulimia nervosa are described, and reference is made to the many conditions in which nutritional manipulation may benefit conditions not primarily of nutritional origin, ranging from kidney and liver disease to inherited metabolic diseases, many of which are discussed in detail elsewhere in this book.

INTRODUCTION: THE SCOPE OF CLINICAL NUTRITION

Adequate nutrition—the intake of adequate sources of energy, the components or precursors of all the body's tissues, and water—is essential to normal life, growth, development, reproduction, and function. Inadequate nutrition is a potential direct cause of disease (and in many countries of the world is a major cause of disease). It ranges from deficiency of specific nutrients (e.g., vitamin A, deficiency of which remains a major cause of blindness worldwide) to generalized, or protein-energy, malnutrition. The United Nations Food and Agriculture Organisation (FAO) estimated that in 2018 more than 820 million people in the world were hungry, and over 2 billion did not have access to safe, nutritious, and sufficient food.[1] Children are particularly at risk with nearly half of all deaths in those under 5 years attributable to malnutrition.[2] In addition, malnutrition puts children at increased risk of succumbing to infectious diseases, particularly infective diarrhea, measles, malaria, and pneumonia. Although malnutrition-related morbidity and mortality primarily affect the inhabitants of less well-developed countries, undernutrition continues to occur in developed countries, particularly in older people in the context of acute or chronic illness.

Current production of crops has been estimated to be sufficient to provide enough food for the predicted world population of 9.7 billion in 2050. However, significant changes to both diet and socioeconomic conditions will be necessary for this to be achieved.[3]

Excess intake of nutrients is also harmful. For example, there is abundant evidence linking a high sodium intake with hypertension and a high intake of certain fats with a predisposition to hypercholesterolemia and thus to coronary heart disease. A high fat intake is associated with an increased risk of breast cancer and a high intake of red meat with colorectal cancer.[4] Obesity, which is rapidly increasing in prevalence throughout the world, is ultimately caused by an intake of energy substrates greater than the body's energy expenditure. The worldwide prevalence of overweight (body mass index [BMI] > 25 kg/m^2) in 2016 was estimated at approximately 38.9%, representing 2 billion people.[1] In 2018, 40.1 million children less than 5 year were overweight or obese. In children, the burden of both undernutrition and overweight is greatest in Africa and Asia where, in 2018, 9 out of 10 of all wasted children and nearly three quarters of the world's overweight children reside.[1]

We obtain our nutrients from food, and all components of all foods ultimately derive from sunlight-driven photosynthesis together with elements (e.g., nitrogen, phosphorus, and trace elements) derived from the air, soil, or water. Animals are incapable of photosynthesis, with the result that animal nutrition is ultimately entirely dependent on plants.

Foodstuffs are complex mixtures comprising both nutrients and non-nutrients (substances that do not contribute to the supply of energy or metabolic "building blocks"), and a broader definition of nutrition might include the processes involved in food production and intake, absorption, metabolism, and utilization. It thus encompasses geographic, economic, cultural, social, and religious aspects.

It should be noted that few foodstuffs contain only one nutrient (table sugar, comprising pure sucrose and table salt [sodium chloride] are two of the few examples). Most foods contain a variety of nutrients, although one may be predominant.

Food may contain harmful substances. Thus aflatoxin, produced by a mold that grows on peanuts, is a potent carcinogen; other non-nutrients may have pharmacologic effects (e.g., fungal-derived ergot alkaloids causing ergotism), and dietary components can interfere with the absorption of drugs. Cooking and food processing may have harmful effects, an example being the use of nitrites to preserve meat; these can lead to the production of carcinogenic nitrosamines. Food can be a vehicle for the transmission of infection, including food poisoning, but also systemic conditions such as typhoid fever. Exposure to some foods leads to adverse reactions, ranging from mild abdominal symptoms to potentially fatal anaphylaxis.

Nutrition is thus a hugely complex topic, and for the purposes of this chapter, we will adopt a narrow definition and discuss the major and minor nutrients and their pathophysiology, the assessment of nutritional status, the major nutritional disorders (under- and overnutrition) and their causes and management, and the role of nutritional manipulation in the management of conditions that do not have a nutritional basis.

NUTRIENT REQUIREMENTS

Various terms are used to quantify the desirable intake of nutrients. These include *dietary reference value, recommended daily intake or amount, estimated average requirement, reference nutrient intake,* and others. Unless otherwise stated, the figures quoted in this chapter are the dietary reference intakes (estimates of average requirements) for healthy men and women published by the US Food and Nutrition Board.[5] Values may be different in children and during pregnancy and lactation. In general, requirements tend to be higher in disease, for a variety of reasons, including an increased metabolic rate, a catabolic state, and increased losses. Energy requirements are greatly affected by the level of physical activity.

A CLASSIFICATION OF NUTRIENTS

The three major sources of energy are carbohydrates, fats, and proteins. Proteins are also the major source of nitrogen. These three comprise the "macronutrients." Minerals include those required in relatively large quantities (e.g., sodium, potassium, calcium, and magnesium) and the inorganic "micronutrients" (e.g., zinc, iron, copper). Micronutrients are required in only milligram (in some cases, microgram) quantities per day, and because such small quantities are required, the status of some purported inorganic micronutrients remains uncertain. The category of organic micronutrients comprises the vitamins—essential, and mostly complex—molecules that the body cannot synthesize (or synthesize in

sufficient quantities). These are conventionally divided into the water-soluble and fat-soluble vitamins, although this classification has no relation to their function. In addition, although often ignored in textbooks of nutrition, the body has an absolute requirement for water, and death may occur in the absence of water intake in less than 1 week. The roles of individual nutrients are summarized in Table 46.1. And although not conventionally regarded as a nutrient, humans' dependence on an adequate supply of oxygen is absolute. With the additional exception of water, deficiency in any of the nutrients discussed in this chapter only becomes life threatening after a period of weeks or even months. Deprivation of oxygen leads to brain death within a few minutes.

POINTS TO REMEMBER

Nutrients
- Nutrients are conventionally classified as being macronutrients (carbohydrate, fat, protein, and the major minerals) and micronutrients (vitamins and trace elements).
- The majority of vitamins and trace elements act as cofactors for enzyme-catalyzed reactions or as prosthetic groups for enzymes.
- Some vitamins and trace elements have important antioxidant properties.
- Both excessive and inadequate intake of nutrients may have harmful consequences.

MACRONUTRIENTS

Carbohydrate

Function and Sources
Carbohydrates of nutritional value include poly-, oligo-, and monosaccharides. The most abundant polysaccharide is starch, a linear polymer of glucose with α1–6 linkages that is widely distributed in plant products, including pulses, grains (cereals), and fruit. The major dietary disaccharide is sucrose (glucose–fructose), present in many processed foods, carbonated drinks, confections, and other products. Carbohydrates are not essential components of the diet but typically provide more than 50% of its energy content (4 kcal/g [16.8 MJ/g]) except in Inuits, whose major energy source is fat.

Homeostasis
The evolutionary importance of secure energy homeostasis both in times of plenty and of famine is undoubtedly the basis of the complex interaction of neural and hormonal mechanisms that controls appetite and in health adjusts food intake to the body's requirements. This topic is considered in detail later in this chapter, but it is salutary to consider that an average healthy man may consume food providing some 9×10^5 kcals (56.6×10^5 MJ) of energy per year, equivalent to approximately 130 kg of nonaqueous body mass, yet maintain the same body weight year after year. In the short term, the provision of sufficient energy substrates for normal function is primarily dependent on blood glucose homeostasis, a topic that is considered in detail in Chapter 47.

Deficiency
Because carbohydrates are not essential dietary components, there is no specific carbohydrate deficiency syndrome.

TABLE 46.1 **A Summary of Nutrients, Their Sources, Function(s), and Recommended Daily Intakes for Adult Males**

Nutrient	Source	Principal Function(s)	Daily Requirement
MACRONUTRIENTS			
Carbohydrate	Starchy vegetables	Energy source	Sufficient to provide 2000–2600 kcal (8.4–10.9 MJ)
Fat	Animal products, oily vegetables	Energy source; some fatty acids are essential (see text)	
Protein	Animal products, legumes, pulses	Source of essential and nonessential amino acids	40–60 g (also contributes to energy requirement)
Water	Various	Essential for maintenance of all body functions	1.0–2.0 L but dependent on ambient temperature and exercise
MAJOR MINERALS			
Calcium	Widespread, especially dairy products	Structural, second messenger, control of cellular excitability	1.0 g (25 mmol)
Chloride	Widespread	Principal intra- and extracellular anion	1.86 g (65 mmol)
Magnesium	Green vegetables	Structural, coenzyme	420 mg (18 mmol)
Phosphate	Widespread	Energy transformations	700 mg (22 mmol)
Potassium	Widespread, especially fruit and vegetables	Principal intracellular cation	4.7 g (120 mmol)
Sodium	Widespread	Principal extracellular cation	2.8 g (65 mmol)
Sulfur	Widespread (in sulfur-containing amino acids)	As component of essential amino acids; connective tissue	None available
TRACE ELEMENTS			
Chromium	Grains, nuts, yeast, liver	Cofactor in cellular glucose uptake	35 μg (0.7 μmol)
Cobalt	Animal and bacterial products only	Sole function is as component of vitamin B_{12}	See vitamin B_{12}; not required separately
Copper	Grains, nuts, liver, yeast	C-factor for several enzymes	1.2 mg (0.7 μmol)
Fluorine	Tea, fish consumed whole	Probably not essential but has positive effects on dental health	4 mg (210 μmol)
Iodine	Seafood, dairy products	Essential component of thyroid hormones	150 μg (1.2 μmol)
Iron	Animal products, especially red meat	Component of all heme pigments and enzyme activator	Men: 8 mg (142 μmol) Women: 18 mg (320 μmol)
Manganese	Grains, nuts, leafy vegetables	Enzyme cofactor	2.3 mg (42 μmol)
Molybdenum	Animal products, grains, legumes	Enzyme cofactor	45 μg (47 nmol)
Selenium	Animal products, grains, fish	Enzyme cofactor	60 μg (76 nmol)
Zinc	Animal products, poultry, eggs	Enzyme cofactor	10 mg (150 μmol)
VITAMINS			
A	Oily fish, eggs, dairy products	Vision, epithelial differentiation	900 μg
B_1 (thiamin)	Wheat germ, eggs, yeast	Enzyme cofactor	>1.4 mg
B_2 (riboflavin)	Milk, dairy products, green vegetables, yeast, offal	Component of flavoproteins	Men: 1.3 mg Women: 1.1 mg
B_3 (nicotinic acid)	Widely distributed	Component of NAD^+ and $NADP^+$	Men: 16 mg Women: 14 mg
B_5 (pantothenic acid)	Widely distributed	Component of coenzyme A	5 mg
B_6 (pyridoxine and derivatives)	Widely distributed	Enzyme cofactor	1.3 mg
B_7 (biotin)	Widely distributed	Enzyme cofactor in 1-C transfers	No recommendation
B_9 (folic acid)	Leafy vegetables, yeast, eggs	Cofactor in 1-C transfers; essential for purine and hence nucleic acid synthesis	400 μg
B_{12} (cobalamin)	Animal and bacterial sources only	Cofactor in 1-C transfers; essential for purine and hence nucleic acid synthesis	1 μg

TABLE 46.1 A Summary of Nutrients, Their Sources, Function(s), and Recommended Daily Intakes for Adult Males—cont'd

Nutrient	Source	Principal Function(s)	Daily Requirement
C (ascorbic acid)	Vegetables, fruit (especially citrus)	Antioxidant; electron donor in various enzyme-catalyzed reactions	Men: 90 mg
			Women: 75 mg
D (calciferol)	Oily fish; dietary provision usually insufficient for normal requirements	Stimulates absorption of dietary calcium and phosphate; essential for bone health.	600 IU (15 mg)
E	Vegetable oils, cereals	Antioxidant	15 mg as α-tocopherol
K	Green leafy vegetables	Synthesis of Gla proteins (including coagulation factors)	120 μg

Actual requirements may be modified considerably by physiologic and pathologic factors. NB molar units are not in general use for vitamins in the context of recommended daily allowances but are included for minerals to aid comparison with reference plasma concentrations.

However, because carbohydrates provide the major source of energy in most diets, a deficiency of dietary carbohydrate is virtually always a major contributor to generalized starvation. During starvation, even in the short term, when glycogen reserves have been depleted (see later discussion), there is some limitation of exercise capacity.

Excess

An intake of carbohydrate greater than that needed to satisfy the body's energy requirements inevitably leads to net fat synthesis, weight gain, and, if uncorrected, to obesity. Obesity is associated with insulin resistance, the metabolic syndrome, and type 2 diabetes, but there does not appear to be a causal relationship between these and a high carbohydrate intake per se.[6,7]

The World Health Organization recommends that free sugar intake should not provide more than 10% (and possibly even less) of total energy intake.[8]

Assessment of Status

There are no laboratory tests for the assessment of carbohydrate status. Energy reserves are typically measured by techniques to determine overall protein-energy nutritional status, which are discussed later in this chapter. Only the liver and muscle can store significant amounts of carbohydrate (in the form of glycogen). Hepatic, but not muscle, glycogen can be converted into glucose for delivery to the bloodstream. If no carbohydrate is ingested, hepatic glycogen stores can provide glucose for 18 to 24 hours, after which blood glucose is supplied by gluconeogenesis. Although fasting blood glucose falls by 10% to 20% in the first 72 hours of a fast,[9] it remains constant thereafter for several weeks until limited by the supply of protein during the terminal phase of starvation. The blood glucose concentration therefore provides no information about the body's carbohydrate stores.

Dietary Fiber

All foods of vegetable origin contain complex carbohydrates that cannot be digested in the small intestine; these are collectively termed *dietary fiber* or *nonstarch polysaccharides*.[10] They can be classified as water soluble and water insoluble. The former (pectins, gums, and mucilages) can be metabolized by colonic bacteria to form small molecules such as propionic acid (which can be absorbed and contribute to the

body's metabolism) and gases such as methane, hydrogen, and carbon dioxide. Water-insoluble fibers include lignin (noncarbohydrate), celluloses, and hemicelluloses. Lignin, but not celluloses, can be metabolized by the colonic biota.

Although dietary fiber is not an essential component of the diet, it plays an important role in the normal function of the gastrointestinal (GI) tract, for example, by stimulating intestinal transport and suppressing appetite. Dietary fiber can also affect the rate of absorption of other dietary components; soluble fiber reduces plasma total and low-density lipoprotein (LDL) cholesterol concentrations without affecting high-density lipoprotein (HDL) cholesterol. Dietary fiber intake correlates inversely with the risk of cardiovascular disease, including coronary heart disease.[11] There is a suggestion that a diet high in fiber might reduce the risk of several conditions including colon cancer.[12]

Fat

Function and Sources

Fat is a major dietary energy source, providing 9 kcal/g (56.6 MJ/g). For the most part, dietary fat comprises long-chain triglycerides (strictly, triacylglycerols) (e.g., the esters of glycerol with palmitic acid [16C] and stearic acid [18C]). In most triglycerides of mammalian origin, the fatty acids are saturated, but in fats derived from fish and vegetables, they tend to be variably unsaturated (fat derived from coconut is an exception, being mostly saturated). In unsaturated vegetable fats, ω6 fatty acids (see later discussion) predominate, but fish (particularly oily fish) have a higher content of ω3 fatty acids. Dietary fat also includes cholesterol esters and the fat-soluble vitamins (vitamins A, D, E, and K), which are discussed later in this chapter.

Homeostasis

It is beyond the scope of this chapter to describe in any detail the complex relationships and control mechanisms that ensure that sufficient energy substrates are made readily available to meet the body's requirements and that any excess is stored. Unlike those of carbohydrate, the body's fat stores are considerable; even in a lean man, 15% of total body weight may comprise fat, with a potential energy of 136 Mcal (570 MJ).

Deficiency

Because there is no specific requirement for dietary fat (except for fat-soluble vitamins and essential fatty acids [EFA]), there is no specific deficiency syndrome. However, during starvation, fat reserves become depleted, and there is loss of lean body mass as a result of the proteolysis required for gluconeogenesis.

Excess

As with carbohydrate, intake of energy in the form of fat in excess of the body's requirements promotes fat storage and obesity. It has been recommended that fat should not comprise more than 20% to 35% of total energy intake with no more than one third of the fat being saturated,[5] but the scientific basis of this advice has been challenged.[13] Furthermore, in practice, given the high fat content of many popular/processed foods, achieving less than 35% is difficult.

Assessment of Status

Fat stores can be assessed by a variety of clinical and physiologic methods ranging from the simple (e.g., skinfold thicknesses) to the complex (e.g., dual energy X-ray absorptiometry [DEXA]) (see later in this chapter). There are no reliable laboratory tests for fat stores, although correlations between plasma leptin concentrations and fat stores have been demonstrated.[14]

Essential Fatty Acids

The vitamins apart, the only essential fatty components of the diet are the EFA, α-linolenic acid (C18:3, ω3,6,9) and linoleic acid (C18:2, ω6,9). (The first figure indicates the number of carbon atoms, the second the number of unsaturated bonds, and the ω-number the position of the unsaturated bonds counting from the methyl end; an alternative nomenclature uses the symbol Δ to indicate the position of the double bonds starting with the carboxyl carbon). The EFA are precursors of prostanoids. EFAs were originally collectively known as vitamin F. Arachidonic acid (C20:4, ω 6,9,12,15) is also essential for prostanoid synthesis; although it is not able to be synthesized de novo in the body, it can be produced from linoleic acid. These entities are illustrated in Fig. 46.1.

Other functions of EFAs include maintenance of the epidermal barrier to infection and normal immune function, and a structural role in cell membranes. Features of EFA deficiency include skin rashes, hair loss and thrombocytopenia.[15,16] The recommended adequate intake of linoleic acid is 11 g for females and 15 g for males and for linoleic acid is 1.1 g and 1.6 g respectively.[5] Previously, ω3 fatty acids had been thought to have considerable benefit in the prevention of cardiovascular disease. More recent evidence suggests that, while they have an effect in reducing triglycerides any reduction in cardiovascular events or mortality is slight.[17,18]

EFA in plasma are measured by liquid chromatography coupled to tandem mass spectrometry. However, measurements in tissues (e.g., red blood cell membranes) may be more reliable indicators of EFA status. In EFA deficiency, where α-linoleic and linolenic acids are reduced, there is decreased production of arachidonic acid (tetraene) and oleic acid is preferentially metabolized to Mead acid (triene). An elevated triene:tetraene ratio is consistent with EFA deficiency.

Other Fats

Fat soluble vitamins are discussed later in this chapter. Although cholesterol and its esters are also present in dietary

SATURATED FATTY ACIDS

$CH_3(CH_2)_{14}COOH$
Palmitic (hexadecanoic) acid (C16:0)
$CH_3(CH_2)_{16}COOH$
Stearic (octadecanoic) acid (C18:0)

MONOUNSATURATED FATTY ACIDS

$CH_3(CH_2)_5 CH=CH(CH_2)_7 COOH$
Palmitoleic (Δ^9 hexadecenoic) acid (C16:1)
$CH_3(CH_2)_7 CH=CH(CH_2)_7 COOH$
Oleic (Δ^9 octadecenoic) acid (C18:1)

POLYUNSATURATED FATTY ACIDS

ω-6
$CH_3(CH_2)_4 CH=CHCH_2 CH=CH(CH_2)_7 COOH$
Linoleic ($\Delta^{9,12}$ octadecadienoic) acid (C18:2)

ω-3
$CH_3 CH_2 CH=CHCH_2CH=CHCH_2 CH=CH(CH_2)_7 COOH$
α linoleic ($\Delta^{9,12,15}$ octadecatrienoic) acid (C18:3)

ω-6
$CH_3(CH_2)_4 CH=CHCH_2 CH=CHCH_2 CH=CHCH_2 CH=CH(CH_2)_3COOH$
Arachidonic ($\Delta^{5,8,11,14}$ eicosatetraenoic) acid (C20:4)

FIGURE 46.1 Molecular structure of some fatty acids. (From Marshall WJ, Lapsley M, Day AP, Ayling RM. *Clinical biochemistry: metabolic and clinical aspects.* 3rd ed. Edinburgh: Elsevier; 2014.)

fat, cholesterol is synthesized in the body and is not an essential dietary component. Plasma cholesterol concentration is influenced by dietary cholesterol intake (although the intake of saturated fat has a greater influence). It was previously recommended that dietary cholesterol intake should not exceed 300 mg/day, but more recently focus has tended to be more on healthy eating patterns involving relatively low amounts of dietary cholesterol, rather than setting a numerical target.[19] Naturally occurring unsaturated fatty acids have *cis*-configuration double bonds. Dehydrogenation of saturated fats creates *trans*-unsaturated fatty acids. These are associated with an increased risk of cardiovascular disease, and the intake of foods containing them (e.g., margarines) should be limited. Indeed, in the United States, the Food and Drug Administration has ruled that partially hydrogenated oils, the primary dietary source of artificial trans fat in processed food, is removed from products intended for human consumption by 2021.[20]

Protein

Function and Sources

Protein is not an essential dietary component per se but is the major source, in the form of amino acids, of nitrogen. Proteins have numerous functions in the body, including structural (e.g., spectrin in RBC membranes, collagen in connective tissues), transport (e.g., hemoglobin, plasma hormone-binding proteins), the maintenance of plasma oncotic pressure (largely albumin), humoral (immunoglobulins), and as enzymes and receptors. Many amino acids can be synthesized in the body, but others cannot and must be included in the diet. The essential amino acids are isoleucine, leucine, lysine, methionine, phenylalanine, tryptophan, threonine, and valine. Histidine is an essential amino acid in infants but not adults.

All animal and most vegetable foodstuffs contain proteins, but on the whole, animal proteins have a greater content of essential amino acids. The recommended minimum dietary protein intake in adults is usually expressed in terms of nitrogen, using a factor of 6.25 g protein to g nitrogen, and is approximately 0.66 g/kg body weight/day. However, protein requirements are influenced by many factors, including the type of protein (and hence essential amino acid content) and the needs for growth, reproduction, tissue repair after trauma, and so on. The energy equivalent of the carbon skeletons of amino acids is approximately 4 kcal/g (16.7 MJ/g).

Homeostasis

As with the control of energy production and expenditure, the complex processes involved in the provision of amino acids to synthesize proteins is beyond the scope of this book (additional discussion on this topic can be found in Chapter 51). There are no specific body stores of protein, but under some circumstances, particularly acute inflammation, catabolism of albumin can provide amino acids for the synthesis of more essential (at least in the short term) proteins.[21] In starvation, protein catabolism is decreased, but some is required to provide glucose to tissues with an obligate requirement for glucose as a source of energy (RBCs, intestinal epithelial cells, and the renal medulla).

Deficiency

Inadequate protein intake can cause one of three major clinical syndromes: marasmus (effectively, cachexia, or chronic starvation, with generalized wasting) caused by a lack of protein and energy substrates; kwashiorkor, in which edema is a major clinical feature in affected people (usually children); and marasmic kwashiorkor, combining features of both conditions. Kwashiorkor tends to be seen in underdeveloped countries and has classically been associated with weaning and the transfer to a diet in which a low intake of protein, rather than energy, predominates, although loss of fat stores and lean body mass is also apparent. This nutritional edema is frequently associated with infection. It has been suggested that an important contributory factor may be the generation of toxic reactive oxygen species and other free radicals in combination with reduced availability of natural antioxidants, for example, vitamins A, C, and E and selenium. Oxidative damage to cell membranes might lead to increased capillary permeability and decreased synthesis of plasma proteins to hypoalbuminemia (a relatively late feature of "simple" starvation), which also contributes to the edema. However, supplementation of the diet with antioxidants has not been shown to decrease the risk of kwashiorkor in children at risk of the condition.[22]

Excess

There are no clinical syndromes of excessive protein intake, but amino acids in excess of requirement are deaminated with the carbon skeletons for the most part becoming substrates for gluconeogenesis and nitrogen being converted to urea and excreted. A high protein intake increases the requirement for the kidneys to excrete urea and may exacerbate renal failure. There is evidence that reducing protein intake (although not below a level required to meet normal requirements) can slow the rate of progression of renal disease, although patients on renal replacement treatment may require protein supplementation to reduce losses caused through dialysis or filtration. Protein restriction (possibly with supplementation of branched chain amino acids) may be of benefit in patients with encephalopathy caused by advanced chronic liver disease, but chronic liver disease is anorexigenic, and supplementation may be required earlier in the condition to prevent malabsorption.[23]

Assessment of Status

The management of patients with or at risk of malnutrition would be helped immensely by the existence of a reliable means of assessing the body's protein status. Numerous laboratory, physiologic, and clinical tests have been described, but all have their limitations. Although widely promoted as an index of protein status, plasma albumin concentration is of little value, except in monitoring (otherwise well) patients requiring nutritional support over the long term. Other plasma proteins are little better. This is because of the numerous factors other than nutritional status that can affect plasma protein concentration, not least the acute phase reaction seen in inflammation and sepsis, which can cause rapid decreases in the concentrations of some proteins but increases in others.[24]

Water
Function and Sources

Water is often not mentioned in scholarly accounts of nutrition, but it is arguably more important to health than conventional nutrients because complete water deprivation usually causes death within 7 to 10 days and sooner if there are excessive losses.

All body fluids are aqueous solutions, and water is also required for the excretion of waste products in the urine. On a normal diet, given minimum insensible losses (in sweat, expired gas, and feces), water loss is approximately 10 mL/kg body weight/24 hours. The figure in children is higher because of the greater ratio of surface area to body weight and higher still in newborns because of comparative renal immaturity and poorly keratinized skin. Latent heat released by the evaporation of water from the skin in sweat is an important component of temperature control; insensible losses in sweat can be considerably increased when the ambient temperature is high and during exercise. Water loss in feces is considerably increased in diarrheal illnesses, and they are a major source of morbidity and mortality, particularly in less well-developed areas of the world.

Small amounts of water (up to ≈300 mL/24 hours, more in catabolic patients) are produced by the oxidation of hydrogen in carbohydrates and fats; some is present in food, but the greater part of intake is as fluids. For most individuals in the developed world, safe water is freely available, but there are many areas where this is not the case, where the supply is either limited or contaminated with toxins, infectious agents, or both.

Homeostasis

Disturbances of water homoeostasis are encountered frequently in clinical practice.[26] Water homeostasis is a function of the hypothalamus, which contains osmoreceptors that sense plasma osmolality and respond by stimulating or suppressing the sensation of thirst and the secretion of vasopressin (antidiuretic hormone), which controls renal water excretion.

Increasing osmolality stimulates thirst and the release of vasopressin; decreasing osmolality has the opposite effect. Vasopressin acts by stimulating the insertion of aquaporins (water channels) into the otherwise water-impermeable luminal membranes of the cells of the renal collecting ducts, thus allowing water to be reabsorbed in response to the concentration gradient generated by the countercurrent system. These controls are exquisitely sensitive and in health maintain plasma osmolality in the range of 285 to 295 mmol/kg. Hypovolemia can also stimulate thirst and vasopressin secretion, and if severe, can override the osmolal control.

Water can move freely between the intra- and extracellular compartments if their relative osmolalities change. Any tendency for water to be lost from the extracellular compartment increases its osmolality and water moves from the intracellular compartment in response, lessening the effect on extracellular fluid (ECF) volume. With an increase in extracellular water, the reverse occurs. Thus both deficits and excesses of water are shared by the whole-body water compartment.

In most free-living people who have ready access to water, fluid intake is determined more by habit and social factors than physiologic controls, but lack of water, unconsciousness, confusion, inability to communicate, disability, and physical restraint are all threats to adequate hydration, so too are hypothalamic conditions affecting the thirst center.

Deficiency

Pure water deficiency (i.e., without concomitant loss of sodium) causes hypernatremia and indeed is its most frequent cause. Clinical features include thirst, dryness of mucous membranes, decreased salivation, dysphagia, and oliguria with a highly concentrated urine (unless uncontrolled renal water loss is the cause, as in diabetes insipidus). Because the loss of water is borne by the whole-body water compartment, the effect on ECF volume is less obvious than with combined water and sodium loss. Other causes of hypernatremia and its investigation are discussed in Chapter 50.

Excess

Healthy adult kidneys can excrete large amounts of water (>1 L an hour over short periods), and water excess usually occurs either when renal water excretion is impaired (as in renal failure) or if the normal inhibition of vasopressin secretion by a fall in plasma osmolality fails, as can occur acutely with stress or chronically in the syndrome of inappropriate antidiuresis. Hyponatremia is invariable. Clinical features relate mainly to cerebral overhydration as a consequence of an increased osmotic gradient with plasma and include impairment of consciousness, confusion, and convulsions. Other causes of hyponatremia and its investigation are discussed in Chapter 50.[25]

Assessment of Status

The assessment of hydration depends on both clinical examination and laboratory investigation (particularly measurement of plasma sodium concentration and osmolality). Dehydration is easier to diagnose clinically than overhydration. Accurate assessment can be a particular challenge in critical care patients.[26] Fluid balance charts (if kept accurately) are a valuable tool, as are short-term changes in body weight. Total body water (TBW) can be measured for research purposes using isotope dilution techniques.[27]

Sodium

Function and Sources

Sodium is the major extracellular cation; whereas the concentration in ECF is approximately 140 mmol/L, it is 14 mmol/L in intracellular fluid. Cell membranes are normally relatively impermeable to sodium, the difference in concentration being maintained by the energy-requiring Na^+,K^+-ATPase pump. The opening of sodium channels in the membranes of excitable tissues leads to sodium influx and membrane depolarization and initiates the action potential. The absorption of some nutrients from the gut is linked to the absorption of sodium; this fact provides the basis for the use of oral rehydration solutions containing glucose and sodium.[27]

Sodium is widely distributed but in general is present in higher quantities in animal products than vegetable. Common salt (sodium chloride) is used in many manufactured foods as a preservative and, supposedly, as a flavor enhancer. Many people add salt to food during cooking and at the table. The kidneys are able to produce a virtually sodium-free urine, and in health, in a temperate requirement, sodium balance can be maintained in adults on an intake of less than 50 mmol/day a maximum intake of 100 mmol/day (equivalent to 2.3 g/day of sodium or 5.8 g of salt) is recommended.[5]

Homeostasis

Sodium and water homeostasis are intimately related because sodium is the major cation contributing to plasma osmolality, which is maintained through effects on renal water excretion (see earlier discussion). As a result, body sodium content is the major factor determining ECF volume. There are obligatory losses in sweat (which can increase considerably with excessive sweating and are higher in patients with cystic fibrosis, who have a high sweat sodium content) and feces (increased in diarrheal illnesses), but sodium balance is maintained primarily through control of renal excretion. The most important factor is aldosterone, which increases sodium reabsorption in the distal nephron in response to activation of the renin–angiotensin axis by stimuli that reflect a decrease in body sodium.[28] Other factors involved include atrial natriuretic peptide (more important pathologically, e.g., in cardiac failure, than physiologically; see Chapter 48), sympathetic activity, and Starling forces in the peritubular capillaries. This topic is discussed in detail in Chapter 50.

Deficiency

Because of the wide availability of sodium, decreased intake is a rare cause of deficiency; this is more frequently a result of increased loss through the kidneys, through the GI tract, or from the skin (e.g., in burn patients). Sodium is never lost without water, and isotonic loss causes an early decrease in ECF (and thus plasma) volume, leading to peripheral circulatory insufficiency and a risk of acute kidney injury. Clinical features include hypotension, tachycardia, and cold peripheries. Small decreases in ECF volume do not increase vasopressin secretion (although this can increase massively with increases >5%), and plasma sodium concentration may be normal. In contrast to water deficiency, there are early increases in plasma urea and creatinine concentrations (urea often before creatinine). Except in renal injury or when diuretics have been used, urinary sodium concentration becomes very low and is a reliable guide to the presence of sodium depletion.

Excess

Sodium overload is usually iatrogenic and occurs in the context of decreased capacity of the kidneys to excrete sodium. In health, a high sodium intake causes thirst, ECF volume tends to increase, and the kidneys respond by excreting the excess. The most frequent cause of sodium overload is increased secretion of aldosterone, either primary or secondary to increased renin secretion. Hypernatremia may be present, particularly if the excess is acute, but most patients with sodium excess are normo- or even (paradoxically) hyponatremic. A high sodium intake predisposes to hypertension; there is a huge literature on this topic and the public health implications of a decrease in dietary sodium intake.[29]

Assessment of Status

Plasma sodium concentration reflects the relative amounts of sodium and water in the ECF. Particularly with mild sodium deficit or excess, plasma sodium concentration is often normal.

Plasma sodium concentration must be considered alongside the results of clinical assessment (of signs of abnormal ECF) or physiologic measurements (e.g., of central venous blood pressure). However, in practice, clinical assessment may be difficult because of confounding factors, particularly in critically ill patients. The value of urinary sodium measurement has been referred to earlier. Total body sodium can be measured using isotope dilution techniques, but this is never required in routine clinical practice.[30]

Potassium
Function and Sources

Potassium is the major intracellular cation. It is widely available in food of vegetable and animal origin. Hyperkalemia increases the excitability of nerve and muscle cells, hypokalemia having the opposite effect. The tendency of potassium ions to move down their concentration gradient from the intra- to extracellular compartment is countered by the action of Na^+,K^+-ATPase. There is considerable evidence that a high dietary potassium intake protects against hypertension, and as a result, the recommended intake is far greater than minimum requirements at 4.7 g (120 mmol/L).[31]

Homeostasis

Potassium homeostasis is complex and mainly occurs through the control of renal potassium excretion, which has reciprocal links to both sodium and hydrogen ion excretion. Aldosterone stimulates sodium reabsorption in exchange for potassium in the distal nephron, and its secretion is directly stimulated by hyperkalemia and through the actions of renin and angiotensin II. The kidneys are less able to conserve potassium than sodium, and obligatory renal losses in health are of the order of 30 mmol/24 hours, with small losses in sweat and feces. Because most of the body's potassium is intracellular, plasma concentration does not necessarily reflect total body potassium status (see later).

Deficiency

Potassium deficiency in free-living healthy subjects on a normal diet is very rare. It can be a feature of generalized malnutrition, but it is frequently iatrogenic, secondary to treatment with diuretics or a consequence of increased loss from the gut in patients with diarrheal illness. Potassium deficiency is not synonymous with hypokalemia, although most patients with hypokalemia are potassium deficient.[32] The causes, investigation, and diagnosis of hypokalemia are discussed in Chapter 50.

Excess

In health, potassium excess is rare and usually iatrogenic. However, high dietary intakes can lead to hyperkalemia in the presence of renal impairment. Potassium retention is most frequently a consequence of acute kidney injury or chronic kidney disease and is usually, but not always, associated with hyperkalemia.[32] Hyperkalemia can occur in the absence of an excess of potassium as a result of loss of intracellular potassium to the intracellular compartment either in vivo or in vitro (hypokalemia can occur with the reverse, but this is less common). The causes, differential diagnosis, and investigation of hyperkalemia are discussed in Chapter 50. Severe hyperkalemia (>6.5 mmol/L) is a medical emergency.

Assessment of Status

For the reasons outlined, plasma potassium concentration is on its own an unreliable guide to body potassium status, although the interpretation of an abnormal potassium concentration may be aided by the results of other investigations (e.g., of renal function or by clinical information, including a drug history). Total-body exchangeable potassium can be measured for research purposes by an isotope dilution technique.[30]

Chlorine
Function and Sources

Chlorine is present in many foods as sodium and potassium chloride; chloride ions are the major extracellular anion in the body. It thus has a role in the maintenance of ECF volume but does not appear to have a specific role in this regard independent of sodium. Chloride is secreted together with hydrogen ions into the lumen of the stomach; gastric acid is largely hydrochloric acid and can have a pH of as low as 1.00. The recommended minimum intake is 65 mmol/day.

Homeostasis

In general, chloride homeostasis is maintained by the mechanisms responsible for sodium and potassium homeostasis, and plasma chloride concentration tends to parallel that of sodium. The exceptions are states of abnormal acid–base balance when the concentration of bicarbonate, the other major extracellular anion, is abnormal. This topic is discussed in detail in Chapter 50.

Deficiency

Deficiencies of sodium and potassium are usually accompanied by deficiency of chloride, although this has no specific features. Two conditions are characterized by primary loss of chloride: loss of unbuffered gastric acid (e.g., in patients with vomiting and pyloric stenosis or with prolonged drainage of gastric secretion) and chloride-losing diarrhea (a rare inherited condition). These are both associated with a metabolic (nonrespiratory) alkalosis (see Chapter 50).

Excess

Chloride excess is usually associated with sodium excess and has no specific features. It is noteworthy, however, that the administration of intravenous (IV) 0.9 (g/v) % aqueous sodium chloride (often erroneously called "physiological" or "normal"; it is neither) can cause a hyperchloremic acidosis. This fluid is widely used in support of ECF volume but contains equimolar amounts (154 mmol/L) of sodium and chloride, and the plasma concentrations are of the order of 140 and 100 mmol/L, respectively. Overuse of this fluid can increase plasma chloride concentration at the expense of bicarbonate, causing acidosis.[33] This "dilutional acidosis" is the reverse of the "contraction alkalosis" sometimes seen in edematous patients treated with diuretics.[34]

Assessment of Status

Plasma chloride concentration reflects the relative amounts of water and chloride in the ECF and may not accurately reflect total body chloride status. In hypochloremia, a low urinary chloride concentration (<10 mmol/L) reliably indicates chloride deficiency unless this is a result of excessive renal excretion of chloride.

Phosphorus
Function and Sources

Phosphates are present in many foodstuffs, and isolated dietary deficiency is very rare. High-energy phosphates, particularly adenosine triphosphate (ATP), are generated by metabolism and drive the body's energy-dependent processes. Many metabolic processes are controlled by the activation and inactivation of enzymes through their phosphorylation and dephosphorylation. Phosphate is an essential structural component of bone mineral and tooth enamel, and phospholipids are key components of cell membranes. Phosphates are also important buffers of hydrogen ions in the urine. The recommended daily intake is 700 mg (22 mmol) as phosphorus. If dietary intake is low, calcitriol synthesis increases, triggering mechanisms that tend to raise the plasma concentration.

Homeostasis

Plasma phosphate concentration is maintained by the actions of parathyroid hormone and calcitriol acting on renal phosphate reabsorption. These processes are discussed in detail in Chapter 54.

Deficiency

As stated, dietary phosphate deficiency is exceedingly rare, but deficiency can occur in patients being fed artificially, particularly when nutritional support is provided to a malnourished individual (refeeding syndrome; see later discussion). Hypophosphatemia is a common and potentially dangerous metabolic abnormality. Its causes and investigation are discussed in Chapter 54.

Excess

Healthy kidneys can excrete phosphate readily, but phosphate overload, leading to hyperphosphatemia, is a frequent feature of renal impairment (see Chapters 34 and 49).

Assessment of Status

Total-body phosphorus can be measured by neutron activation analysis but is not required in clinical practice, where measurements of plasma concentration and urine excretion provide more relevant information.

Sulfur
Function and Sources

Sulfur is the third most abundant mineral in the human body (after calcium and phosphorus). It is present in foodstuffs, mainly in proteins in the amino acids cysteine and methionine, and to a lesser extent as inorganic sulfate and in other compounds. Disulfide bonds play an important role in maintaining the structure of proteins and peptide hormones (e.g., insulin), and sulfur is a component of many glycosaminoglycans (e.g., heparin sulfate). Sulfur has a key role in detoxication mechanisms. Many fat-soluble xenobiotics are rendered water soluble (and thus amenable to excretion) by sulfation, and the antioxidant function of glutathione is dependent on its sulfhydryl group. The oxidation of sulfur-containing amino acids generates sulfuric acid, which is excreted in the urine and comprises the bulk of fixed acid excretion. There are no recommendations concerning dietary intake.

Homeostasis, Deficiency, and Excess

There appears to be no specific homeostatic mechanism for sulfur or sulfate. No syndrome of excess has been described, and it remains uncertain whether there is a specific entity of sulfate deficiency, given that it is only likely to occur as part of overall protein deficiency.[35] There have been suggestions that sulfur deficiency, secondary to inadequate intake of sulfur-containing amino acids, may impair oxidative stress defense mechanisms and contribute to aging.[36]

Assessment of Status

Sulfate and the individual sulfur-containing amino acid concentrations can be measured in plasma, but there is no indication to do so in standard clinical practice.

Calcium
Function and Sources

Calcium is present in many foodstuffs but particularly dairy products and fish that are eaten whole (e.g., sardines, whitebait). It has many essential functions: structural, in bone and teeth (these tissues contain 99% of the body's calcium); in the control of membrane excitability; muscle contraction; neuromuscular transmission; blood coagulation; and as a second messenger. Even if there is an adequate dietary supply of calcium, its absorption may be limited by the presence of other dietary components, such as oxalate; phytates, which combine with it to form insoluble complexes; or inadequate calcitriol, which stimulates the absorption of calcium ions. The recommended calcium intake is 1000 mg/day (25 mmol/day). Greater quantities are required during pregnancy and lactation.

Homeostasis

Although the bulk of the body's calcium has a structural role, homeostatic mechanisms primarily control the concentration of free (ionized) extracellular calcium. Factors involved include calcitriol and parathyroid hormone. Calcitonin, although regarded as a calcimimetic hormone, appears to have only a minor physiologic role. Calcium homeostasis is described in detail in Chapter 54.

Deficiency

Adequate dietary calcium intake in childhood and adolescence is an important determinant of peak bone mass (typically attained at age 20 to 25 years), itself a determinant of the risk of osteoporosis. Plasma calcium concentration can, however, be maintained over a wide range of dietary intakes because the homeostatic mechanisms will sacrifice bone calcium to maintain the ECF concentration, if required, and excesses are usually readily excreted.

Excess

A high calcium intake may predispose to renal calculus formation, although it is rarely the sole cause. The milk-alkali syndrome, a cause of renal failure associated with a high intake of calcium-containing alkaline antacids, is now rare.[37] There has been considerable research into the relationship between calcium intake and cancer risk. Although the results of studies have not always been in agreement, it does appear that maintenance of the recommended intake does have a modestly beneficial effect on the risk of colorectal cancer.[38] There is evidence linking a high calcium intake with increased risk of cardiovascular disease.[39] Syndromes of hypercalcemia are discussed in Chapter 54.

Assessment of Status

For reasons alluded to already, plasma calcium concentration does not reflect total body calcium status, which is most relevantly assessed by measurements of bone mineral density.

The most frequent measurements made in clinical practice are of plasma calcium concentration and urinary excretion. The effect of protein binding on total calcium concentration and the indications for measurement of ionized calcium concentration are discussed in Chapter 54.

Magnesium
Function and Sources

Magnesium is the fourth most abundant cation in the human body. The majority is present in bone and muscle, with only approximately 1% being present in the ECF. Magnesium is a cofactor in more than 300 enzyme-catalyzed reactions. These include many responsible for energy metabolism (it is an obligate cofactor in reactions involving ATP) and the synthesis of proteins and nucleic acids. It controls various transmembrane ion channels and membrane excitability. Magnesium is widely distributed in foodstuffs, green vegetables being a particular rich source because it is a component of chlorophyll. The recommended daily intake is 420 mg (18 mmol) in men and 320 mg (10 mmol) in women.

Homeostasis

Magnesium absorption from the gut is to some extent controlled by the body's requirements, but the major organs of homeostasis are the kidneys; magnesium absorption is increased by hypomagnesemia (see Chapter 54).[40]

Deficiency

Isolated magnesium deficiency is uncommon; it is usually associated with loss of other cations either from the gut (e.g., with diarrhea) or the kidneys (frequently drug induced).[40]

Hypomagnesemia can cause hypokalemia (through adverse effects on Na^+,K^+-ATPase) and hypocalcemia (parathyroid hormone release is dependent on magnesium), and these may be responsible for some of its clinical manifestations (see Chapter 54).

Excess

A high intake of magnesium rarely causes hypermagnesemia if renal function is normal because any excess can be readily excreted. Hypermagnesemia is, however, a frequent complication of renal failure. The causes and investigation of hypermagnesemia are discussed in detail in Chapter 54.

Assessment of Status

Measurements of plasma magnesium concentration do not necessarily reflect total body magnesium status but are relevant in most clinical situations. Measurement of ionized magnesium, RBC magnesium, and assessment of deficiency using a parenteral loading test have all been proposed, but none is ideal.[41]

VITAMINS

Vitamins are organic substances, essential for normal function, which cannot be synthesized in the body (vitamin D is an exception). They are classified as micronutrients, being required (with the exception of vitamin C) in quantities of less than 10 mg/day. They are classified as either fat soluble (A, D, E, K) or water soluble, but this distinction has no relevance as far as their function is concerned. As understanding of their structure and function advanced, the original simple alphabetical nomenclature proved inadequate, so many (particularly what used to be called vitamin B) are now known by a letter and a number or, in some cases, by their trivial chemical name alone. Gaps in the alphabetical classification relate to substances no longer regarded as vitamins or otherwise classified. For example, what used to be known as vitamin H was later classified as a B vitamin (B_7) but is now called by name (biotin).

Because water-soluble vitamins can be excreted unchanged in the urine, they have low or negligible toxicity in excess (pyridoxine is an exception). Fat-soluble vitamins are less readily excretable, and toxicity can occur with excessive intake. Here we discuss the pathophysiology of vitamins; the determination of their status, either by direct or indirect techniques, is alluded to but discussed in detail in Chapter 39.

Vitamin A
Nature, Function, and Sources

This fat-soluble vitamin has the trivial name "retinol" and is an unsaturated long-chain alcohol attached to a β-ionone ring (Fig. 46.2). Retinol and related substances have three main functions in the body.[42]
- As a component of visual pigments (see later)
- As a cofactor for the synthesis of mannose-containing glycoproteins (retinyl phosphate)
- For controlling the differentiation and growth of epithelial cells, bone cells, and others, and maintaining normal mucin secretion (retinoic acid) (see later)

In the eyes, 11-*cis*-retinal is a component of rhodopsin in rods and iodopsins in cones. Light falling on the retina causes conversion to the *trans*-isomer and its release from its opsin protein. This in turn triggers changes in membrane potentials that are transmitted to the visual cortex and perceived as light. An isomerase then converts the *trans*-isomer back to the *cis*-form, which recombines with its opsin.

The actions related to growth and differentiation are mediated through binding to nuclear receptors, of which there

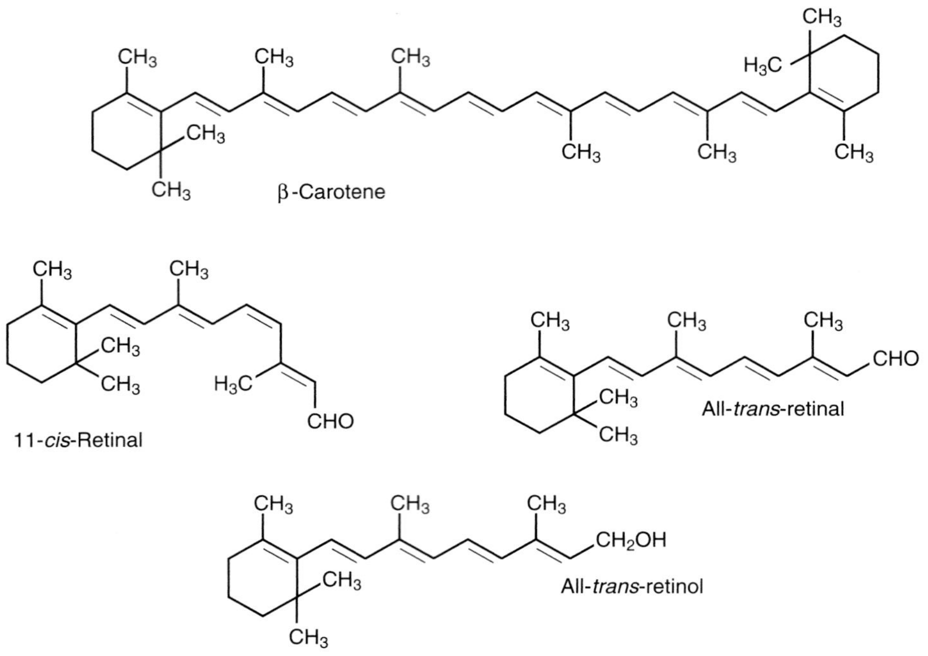

FIGURE 46.2 Vitamin A and related substances. (From Marshall WJ, Lapsley M, Day AP, Ayling RM. *Clinical biochemistry: metabolic and clinical aspects.* 3rd ed. Edinburgh: Elsevier; 2014.)

are two types: retinoic acid receptors (RER), which bind primarily all-*trans*-retinoic acid and retinoid X-receptors (RXR), which bind 9-*cis*-retinoic acid. These receptors must form heterodimers before they can bind to vitamin A-responsive regions in DNA. RXRs can also form heterodimers with other receptors (e.g., the vitamin D receptor and thyroid hormone receptor) and bind to regions of DNA not responsive to vitamin A.

Vitamin A is transported in the blood bound to retinol-binding protein (RBP), which complexes with thyroid-binding prealbumin. The vitamin is stored in the liver and it is notable that in protein-energy malnutrition, a functional vitamin A deficiency may develop even with adequate hepatic stores because of reduced synthesis of the binding protein. The recommended daily intakes of vitamin A are 900 μg in men and 700 μg in women.

Oily fish, eggs, and dairy products are good sources of vitamin A. In some countries, breakfast cereals and margarines are fortified with the vitamin. Carotenoids, present in green vegetables, carrots, and other yellow and red fruits, are also a source of retinoids, typically providing up to 25% of vitamin A in developed countries. The major dietary carotenoid, β-carotene, is cleaved in intestinal mucosa by a dioxygenase to form retinal, which can be reduced to retinol. However, the recovery of retinol is incomplete, and 6 μg of carotene is equivalent to only 1 μg of retinol.

Deficiency and Toxicity
Vitamin A deficiency is the commonest preventable cause of blindness in the world. The earliest feature is night blindness; this is reversible, but the other ocular manifestations are not. Decreased mucin secretion causes xerophthalmia, characterized by keratinizing squamous metaplasia of the conjunctivae, leading to the formation of areas of white, thickened epithelium (Bitot spots). Similar changes in the cornea lead

to softening and ulceration (keratomalacia), which, both directly and indirectly through predisposing to infection, cause blindness. Other less dramatic manifestations include increased susceptibility to infections, particularly respiratory, presumed to be related to the decreased mucin secretion. The absorption of vitamin A from the gut requires the formation of mixed micelles, and a functional deficiency may occur in severe malabsorption despite an adequate dietary supply of the vitamin.

Vitamin A is toxic in excess; acute ingestion of large quantities can cause raised intracranial pressure, with headache, nausea, and vomiting. Chronic excessive intake can cause bone damage, with loss of mineral from bone, increased susceptibility to fracture, and hypercalcemia. Retinol is teratogenic, and dietary supplementation must be avoided during pregnancy. Carotenoids have low toxicity, but a high intake may impart an orange hue to the skin. Carotenes are an antioxidant, and supplements have been tested as a means of reducing the risk of coronary heart disease. Not only are they ineffective,[43] but they also increase the risk of lung cancer.[44]

Assessment of Status
Vitamin A can be measured by high-performance liquid chromatography (HPLC). Normal plasma concentrations are 0.5 to 2.0 mg/L (1.75 to 7.0 μmol/L), but plasma concentrations are an unreliable reflection of tissue status. For additional information on the measurement of vitamin A, refer to Chapter 39.

Vitamin B₁ (Thiamin)
Nature, Function, and Sources
Thiamin pyrophosphate (Fig. 46.3A; also known as thiamin diphosphate) is a cofactor in several enzyme-catalyzed reactions, including the conversion of pyruvate to acetyl-CoA (pyruvate dehydrogenase complex), 2-oxoglutarate to

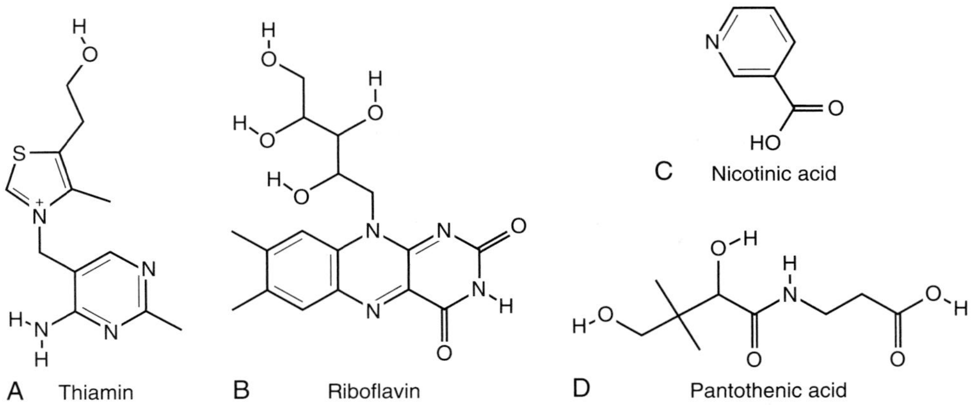

FIGURE 46.3 Thiamin (A), riboflavin (B), nicotinic acid (C), and pantothenic acid (D).

succinyl-CoA (2-oxoglutarate dehydrogenase complex), and two reactions in the pentose phosphate pathway catalyzed by transketolase: D-xylulose 5-phosphate with D-ribose 5-phosphate to form sedoheptulose 7-phosphate and glyceraldehyde 3-phosphate and D-xylulose 5-phosphate with erythrose 4-phosphate to form fructose 6-phosphate and glyceraldehyde 3-phosphate. It also has a role in the catabolism of branched chain amino acids and is involved in the synthesis of acetylcholine and γ-aminobutyric acid.[45]

Thiamin is essential for the metabolism of all living organisms but is synthesized only in plants, bacteria, and fungi. The best sources of the vitamin are wheat germ and the outer parts of other grains (thiamin deficiency used to be common in areas where rice is the staple and was consumed as polished rice, i.e., with the husk removed), yeast, and eggs. The recommended daily intake is not less than 1.4 mg, the requirement being higher with carbohydrate-rich than fat-rich diets and in men compared with women. The body's stores of thiamin are more limited than those of most other vitamins, and manifestations of deficiency may arise within 30 days of inadequate intake. Acute thiamin deficiency has been reported in starved individuals refed with a high carbohydrate intake, for example patients given parenteral nutrition (PN), in those with significant weight loss after bariatric surgery, with significant hyperemesis and after prolonged intensive care. Thiamin deficiency is associated with a high alcohol (ethanol) intake because this interferes with its absorption from the gut and because of reduced storage, which may reflect decreased hepatic capacity or poor intake or a combination of both. Patients on renal replacement treatment have increased requirements (and those of other water-soluble vitamins) because of increased losses.

Deficiency and Toxicity
There are three principal manifestations of thiamin deficiency: beriberi (wet and dry) and an encephalopathy (Wernicke-Korsakoff syndrome). The latter used to be thought to be two separate conditions (Wernicke encephalopathy and Korsakoff psychosis), but it is now clear that the encephalopathy is the acute (but to some extent reversible with thiamin treatment) manifestation that, if untreated, develops into a chronic psychosis that does not respond to provision of the vitamin.[46]

Wernicke encephalopathy is a medical emergency. The features are ophthalmoplegia, nystagmus, ataxia, and stupor.

Although resolution of the ophthalmoplegia and ataxia may be complete, up to 80% of patients develop features of psychosis, of which a retrograde amnesia and confabulation are the most notable features.

Beriberi is characterized by a peripheral neuropathy more prominent distally, muscle weakness, and fatigue; this is dry beriberi. In the wet form, the patient also develops edema and heart failure, possibly in part because of concomitant protein deficiency. Partial resolution occurs within 24 hours of starting thiamin treatment, but full recovery may take months. An infantile form of wet beriberi may occur in infants of subclinically deficient mothers and is rapidly fatal if untreated.

There are rare genetically determined disorders causing impairment of thiamin transport and metabolism. Mutation of the SLC19A2 gene leads to diabetes mellitus, megaloblastic anemia, and sensineural hearing loss. SLC19A3, SLC25A19, and TPR-1 related disorders are associated with recurrent encephalopathy, dystonia, and severe disability.[47]

Thiamin has low toxicity and can be given in large doses (typically 10 mg intravenously) in suspected deficiency, although there are reports of anaphylaxis occurring as a rare complication. No specific syndrome of toxicity has been reported.

Assessment of Status
A functional index of thiamin status is provided by measurement of RBC transketolase activity, with and without the addition of thiamin to the reaction mixture. However, thiamin can be better measured directly in blood by HPLC and by tandem mass spectrometry (for additional information on measurement, refer to Chapter 39). In practice, treatment should be instituted on the basis of clinical suspicion, and the response often provides a retrospective diagnosis.

Vitamin B₂ (Riboflavin)
Nature, Function, and Sources
Riboflavin (formerly known as vitamin G) (see Fig. 46.3B) is a constituent of the flavin mononucleotide (FMN) and flavin adenine dinucleotide (FAD), which are electron carriers in numerous essential biological oxidoreduction systems, including reactions in the tricarboxylic acid cycle and the mitochondrial electron transport chain. FAD is also a coenzyme for fatty acyl-CoA dehydrogenase and glutathione reductase; it is required for the conversion of retinol to retinoic acid (see

the earlier discussion of vitamin A) and for the synthesis of niacin from tryptophan (see later discussion of vitamin B_6). As a component of cryptochromes, the blue light–sensitive pigments in the eye, it has a role in the setting and maintenance of circadian rhythms. Other roles have been postulated but not substantiated.[48]

Riboflavin is present in milk and dairy products, green vegetables, yeast, offal, and mushrooms. Although cereals have a relatively low riboflavin content, they are an important source of the vitamin in areas where cereals are a staple. Milling removes the vitamin, and in some countries, including the United States, flour is fortified with riboflavin. The recommended daily intake is a minimum of 1.3 mg for men and 1.1 mg for women. There is a marked increase in requirements during pregnancy and lactation. Riboflavin is light sensitive, and solutions for parenteral administration (e.g., as part of a parenteral feeding regimen) must be protected from light.

Deficiency and Toxicity

Clinical riboflavin deficiency is uncommon; riboflavin is highly conserved in the body and can be reused. The features of experimentally induced riboflavin deficiency are primarily cutaneous (and not obviously related to the known functions of the vitamin). They include angular oral and glossal stomatitis, cheilosis, vascularization of the cornea, and a seborrheic rash of the genitalia. The patient may have anemia, thought to be related to decreased iron absorption, although it is usually normochromic and normocytic.

Riboflavin is poorly soluble in water, and its absorption is limited at high intakes, and excess is rapidly excreted in the urine. In consequence, no syndrome of toxicity has been reported.

Assessment of Status

Riboflavin can be measured directly in blood but indirect assessment by measuring the activity of glutathione reductase in the presence and absence of added FAD is preferred (see Chapter 39), because it provides an index of tissue riboflavin status. The normal plasma concentration is 3.8 to 72 nmol/L.

Vitamin B_3 (Niacin)

Nature, Function, and Sources

The term *niacin* is variably used as a synonym for nicotinic acid, nicotinamide, or the two together. The parent vitamin is nicotinic acid (see Fig. 46.3C), which is active in the form of its amide, principally as a component of nicotinamide adenine dinucleotide (NAD^+) and nicotinamide adenine dinucleotide phosphate ($NADP^+$). Both are involved in numerous oxidoreductase reactions, notably NAD in the transfer of electrons from metabolic intermediates to the mitochondrial electron transport and NADP as a reducing agent in numerous synthetic pathways, including cholesterol and fatty acids.[49]

Both forms of the vitamin are widely distributed in foods, including offal, eggs, yeast, and various fruit and vegetables. It is noteworthy that although both forms are present in maize, they have limited bioavailability. The recommended daily intakes are 16 mg/day for men and 14 mg/day for women. A small but potentially important amount of nicotinic acid is synthesized in the body in a minor pathway of tryptophan metabolism, with 60 mg of dietary tryptophan being regarded as equivalent to 1 mg of nicotinic acid.

Kynurenine is an intermediate in the pathway, and because kynureninase and kynurenine hydroxylase are dependent on pyridoxine and riboflavin, respectively, deficiencies of these vitamins can reduce endogenous nicotinic acid synthesis and precipitate clinical deficiency in borderline dietary deficiency. Two other conditions that are associated with potential nicotinic acid deficiency are Hartnup disease (in which there is a defect in the absorption of tryptophan from the gut) and the carcinoid syndrome (in which diversion of tryptophan to the synthesis of 5-hydroxytryptamine reduces the amount available for nicotinic acid synthesis).[49]

Nicotinic acid (but not nicotinamide) has a role in the management of dyslipidemias, the basis of which is unconnected with its function as a vitamin.[50] It acts at various points in lipid metabolism with a net effect of modestly reducing plasma LDL cholesterol concentration and increasing HDL cholesterol concentration. In contrast to previous studies, more recent trials have suggested lack of efficacy and it is no longer available for management of dyslipidemia in United States and Europe but remains in use in some other countries. There remains interest in its action as a potential moderator of NAD^+/sirtuin-mediated control of metabolism.[50]

Deficiency and Toxicity

The classic disease of nicotinic acid deficiency is pellagra (remembered by generations of doctors as the "four Ds"—dermatitis, diarrhea, dementia, and death). As alluded to earlier, it is particularly associated with areas where maize is the staple food, but it can occur in developed countries as part of generalized malnutrition and in chronic alcoholism. Some features of nicotinic acid deficiency are nonspecific—weakness, fatigue, irritability, depression, and diarrhea—but the dermatologic manifestations are more specific, with pigmented lesions in sun-exposed areas (and particularly of the neck, or Casal collar) and inflammation of the mouth and tongue. Untreated, patients become delirious, and death supervenes.[51]

Nicotinic acid can cause flushing, glucose intolerance, hyperuricemia, and hepatotoxicity when given in pharmacologic doses.[51]

Assessment of Status

Nicotinic acid can be measured in blood, but a better indication of tissue status is provided by the measurement of urinary metabolites (e.g., N'-methylnicotinamide and N'-methyl 2-pyridone 5-carboxamide; see Chapter 39).

Vitamin B_5 (Pantothenic Acid)

Nature, Function, and Sources

Pantothenic acid (see Fig. 46.3D) is a component of coenzyme A and thus is involved in numerous essential metabolic pathways. A pantothenic acid derivative is required for the activity of acyl-carrier protein, an enzyme involved in fatty acid synthesis.[52] Pantothenic acid is widely available in foodstuffs, including cereals, meat, egg yolk, milk, and vegetables. The recommended daily intake is 5 mg.

Deficiency and Toxicity

Isolated, spontaneous deficiency of pantothenic acid has not been unequivocally described although experimental deficiency leads to fatigue, apathy, and numbness and painful paresthesia ("burning heels"). Toxicity has not been described.

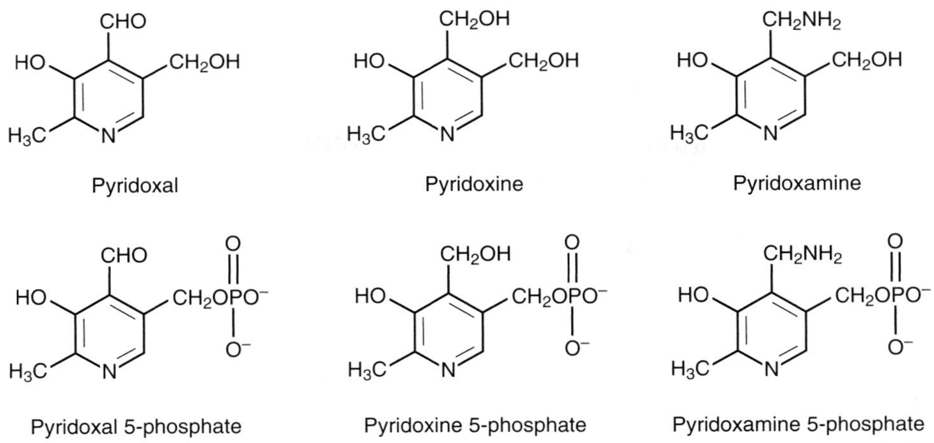

Pyridoxal   Pyridoxine   Pyridoxamine

Pyridoxal 5-phosphate   Pyridoxine 5-phosphate   Pyridoxamine 5-phosphate

FIGURE 46.4 Structures of the various forms of vitamin B_6. (From Marshall WJ, Lapsley M, Day AP, Ayling RM. *Clinical biochemistry: metabolic and clinical aspects*. 3rd ed. Edinburgh: Elsevier; 2014.)

Assessment of Status

Pantothenic acid can be measured in plasma by bacteriologic assay (see Chapter 39), but in practice, this is rarely required in a clinical setting.

Vitamin B_6 (Pyridoxine)

Nature, Function, and Sources

Three interconvertible compounds have vitamin B_6 activity: pyridoxine phosphate, pyridoxamine phosphate, and pyridoxal phosphate (Fig. 46.4).[53] Pyridoxal phosphate is a coenzyme for numerous reactions, including some involving amino acids (aminotransferases, cystathionine synthase, cystathionase, and the formation of nicotinic acid from tryptophan), monoamine neurotransmitter synthesis, carbohydrate metabolism (glycogen phosphorylase), and fat metabolism (sphingolipid synthesis, heme pigment synthesis [δ-aminolevulinate synthase]), and in the regulation of gene expression.[53] The vitamin is widely distributed in foodstuffs, including vegetables, grains, offal, and yeast. The recommended daily intake is 1.3 mg.

Deficiency and Toxicity

Because of its wide availability and because some is provided by the gut biota, dietary deficiency of vitamin B_6 is rare. The features of experimentally induced pyridoxine deficiency include seborrheic dermatitis, glossitis, angular stomatitis, conjunctivitis, somnolence, neuropathies, and sideroblastic anemia.

Pyridoxine has been used therapeutically in numerous conditions, in the great majority of instances without convincing evidence of benefit. An exception is certain forms of sideroblastic anemia[54] and of rare inherited metabolic diseases (e.g., type 1 hyperoxaluria).[55] Some drugs (e.g., isoniazid, penicillamine) interfere with the metabolism of pyridoxine, and supplementation is required in patients treated with them.[56,57] There is no evidence that a high dietary intake of pyridoxine is harmful, but high doses of supplements may cause a peripheral sensory neuropathy. Various upper limits for daily intake have been recommended; in the United States, it is 100 mg.

Assessment of Status

The various forms of the vitamin can be measured in plasma using liquid chromatography–mass spectrometry. The normal

FIGURE 46.5 Biotin.

plasma concentration of pyridoxal phosphate, the major circulating form, is 7 to 52 μg/L in men and 2 to 26 μg/L in women. Further details are provided in Chapter 39.

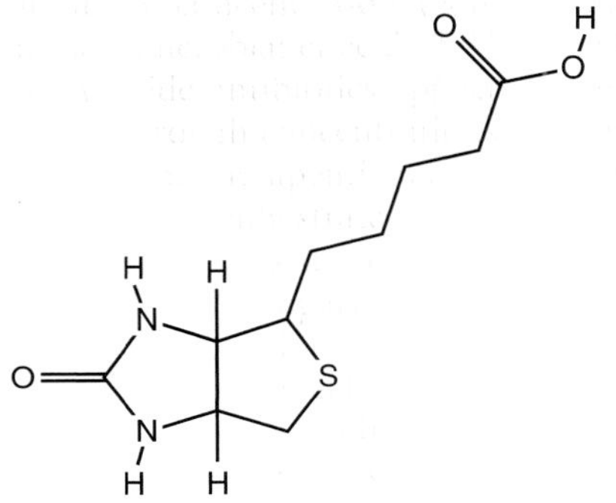

Vitamin B_7 (Biotin, Vitamin H)

Nature, Function, and Sources

Biotin (Fig. 46.5) is essential for several single-carbon transfer reactions. The reactions have two stages, first the ATP-dependent carboxylation of a biotin prosthetic group to form N-1′-carboxybiotin followed by carboxylation of the substrate (e.g., pyruvate carboxylase; pyruvate $\rightarrow$ oxaloacetate) and acetyl Co-A carboxylase (acetyl Co-A $\rightarrow$ malonyl CoA).[58] The first is a step in gluconeogenesis and an anaplerotic reaction that sustains the tricarboxylic acid cycle; the second is a key reaction in lipogenesis. It is also involved in the catabolism of branched chain amino acids.

Biotin is widely distributed in foodstuffs, with offal, eggs, and milk being particularly rich sources. Biotin is synthesized by the gut biota, but this appears to have limited availability. There is no recommended daily intake.

Deficiency and Toxicity

Isolated clinical biotin deficiency has been described only in the context of PN and in individuals who consume large quantities of raw eggs; egg white contains a protein called avidin, which binds biotin tightly and prevents its absorption. Avidin is denatured by cooking. Clinical features of deficiency include alopecia, dermatitis, and conjunctivitis. Subclinical biotin deficiency in pregnancy has been suggested as a potential cause of congenital malformations.[59] Two metabolic disorders are characterized by defects in biotin-related enzymes. These are biotinidase deficiency and holocarboxylase synthetase deficiency (HCSD) and both result in multiple carboxylase deficiency (MCD). In biotinidase deficiency MCD develops because biotinidase is required for the release and thus absorption of protein-bound dietary biotin whereas in HCSD it is a result of defective carboxylation even in the presence of adequate biotin.[60]

Assessment of Status

Biotin status can be assessed by measurement of propionyl CoA activity in lymphocytes, the urinary excretion of biotin (both decreased in deficiency), or the urinary excretion of 3-hydroxyisovaleric acid (increased) (see also Chapter 39).

Vitamin B₉ (Folic Acid, Vitamin M)

Nature, Function, and Sources

Folic acid (pteroyl L-glutamic acid) is the parent compound of a group of substances that have an essential role in a variety of metabolic processes, notably one-carbon transfers and methionine metabolism. The principal naturally occurring folates are tetrahydrofolate (THF), 5-methyl THF and 10-formyl THF, all of which contain variable numbers of glutamate residues (Fig. 46.6). The major circulating form is 5-methyl THF. Folic acid per se comprises less than 1% of normal dietary folate intake. The major dietary sources are green leafy vegetables, yeast, and nuts. The recommended daily intake is 400 µg. Normal body stores are approximately 10 mg, so the clinical consequences of deficiency may not become manifest for several weeks.

Folate derivatives can act as both a single-carbon donor (in purine, thymine, and glycine synthesis and in the conversion of homocysteine to methionine) and acceptor (conversion of serine to glycine and breakdown of histidine; Table 46.2). Its role in purine and thymine synthesis results in its being essential for the synthesis of DNA and RNA and explains the major effect of deficiency, a megaloblastic anemia (see Chapter 76).[61]

Deficiency

Folate deficiency can arise as a result of dietary insufficiency, malabsorption, increased utilization (e.g., pregnancy, hemolytic anemias) or loss (e.g., dialysis, inflammatory conditions, dermatoses), or the use of certain drugs. Pyrimethamine, methotrexate, and trimethoprim are all folate antagonists; phenytoin can decrease the intestinal absorption of folates, and ethanol both decreases absorption and increases excretion. (Macrocytosis is a frequent finding in individuals with a high ethanol intake.) Body stores of folate in adults are about 10 mg, sufficient for about 4 months at a normal rate of utilization, so the effects of deficiency may not be seen immediately when folate status is threatened by one of the mechanisms described. Deficiency responds rapidly to folate replacement.[62]

Folate antagonists are used therapeutically in chemotherapy and as antimicrobials; they act by competing for the enzyme dihydrofolate reductase, reducing the formation of 5-THF. When used as in chemotherapy, methotrexate is infused intravenously so as to achieve a high plasma concentration for a short time, the rationale being that this maximizes the damage to cancer cells but spares other tissues. However,

bone marrow is particularly susceptible, and the finding of a high concentration of methotrexate (e.g., >5.0 µmol/L [>2.5 mg/L] at 24 hours, >0.5 µmol/L [>0.25 mg/L] at 48 hours, but protocols vary) after an infusion is an indication for giving folinic acid (folinic acid "rescue"). This is not a complication of the use of antimicrobial folate antagonists (e.g., trimethoprim) because these act selectively on bacterial enzymes.

It is now routine practice to recommend dietary folate supplements (400 µg/day) from conception to the 12th week of pregnancy; such supplementation has been proven to reduce the incidence of neural tube defects.[63] If there is a family history of neural tube defects, the dose should be 5 mg. At least some parents of children with neural tube defects have a partial deficiency of the enzyme methylene tetrahydrofolate reductase (MTHRF).[64] Folate supplementation is also recommended for patients with increased folate requirements (e.g., those with hemolytic conditions).[61]

Assessment of Status

Folate status can be assessed by measurement of RBC or plasma folate concentrations. The former may give a better indication of total body status because the latter may be affected by recent intake. Plasma concentration may increase in vitamin B₁₂ deficiency, owing to reduced conversion of methyl-THF (the major circulating form; see earlier) to THF. However, RBC folate concentration tends to fall in vitamin B₁₂ deficiency. Further details of the assessment of folate status are provided in Chapter 39. Normal plasma folate concentration in adults is 3.0 to 13 0 µg/L (68 to 290 pmol/L), and normal RBC folate is 140 to 630 µg/L (30 to 140 nmol/L). Genetic variation in MTHFR is common and may affect RBC folate concentrations.

Vitamin B₁₂

Nature, Function, and Sources

Vitamin B₁₂ is structurally the most complex vitamin (and unique in containing cobalt; see later). It is a cobalamin, a family of substances consisting of a planar cobalt-containing tetrapyrrole (corrin) ring with a ribonucleotide set at right angles linked through the purine residue to the cobalt ion (Fig. 46.7). The major form of the vitamin in plasma is methylcobalamin (also present in cytoplasm); others include hydroxocobalamin and 5′deoxyadenosylcobalamin (the major form found in mitochondria). The latter has a role in the conversion of methylmalonyl-CoA to succinyl-CoA; methylcobalamin is a cofactor for the conversion of homocysteine to methionine, an essential step (also involving folate) in the pathway that provides methyl groups in DNA synthesis (Fig. 46.8).

Vitamin B₁₂ is synthesized by microorganisms and does not occur in the vegetable kingdom.[65] It is present in most foodstuffs of animal origin, with liver being a particularly rich source. Daily requirements are very small (~1 µg/day), and because the body stores 2 to 3 mg, the effects of deficiency may not become manifest for several years.

Whereas most vitamins are absorbed by passive or facilitated diffusion in the proximal small intestine, the absorption of vitamin B₁₂ is a complex process that involves both the stomach and the ileum, the actual site of absorption. Only about 50% of dietary vitamin B₁₂ is absorbed. Gastric acid is required to release dietary vitamin B₁₂ from proteins; it initially binds to the protein haptocorrin (transcobalamin I),

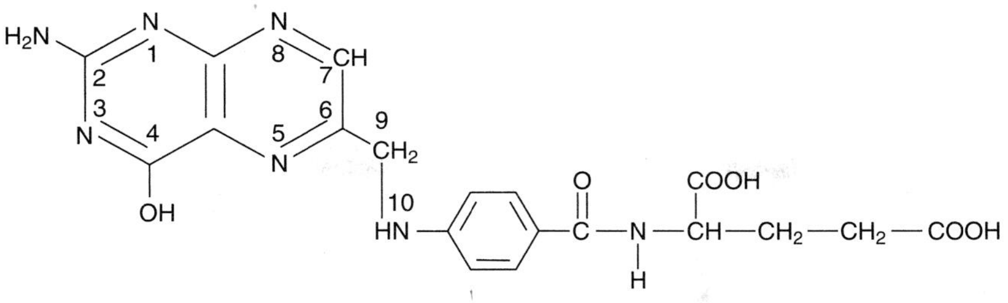

Pteridine *para*-Aminobenzoic acid Glutamic acid

Pteroyl glutamic acid

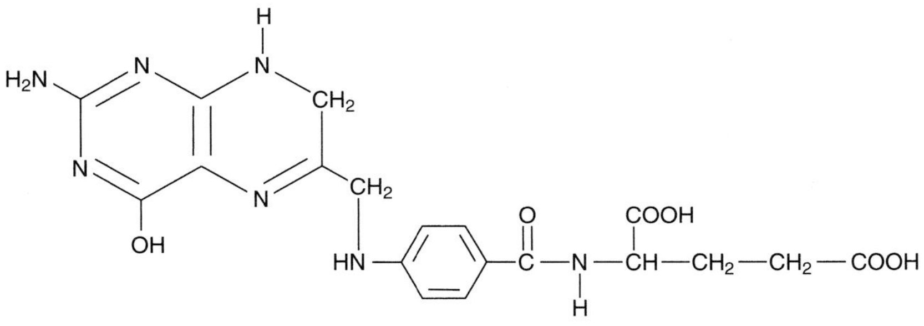

Dihydropteroyl glutamic acid
(dihydrofolate)

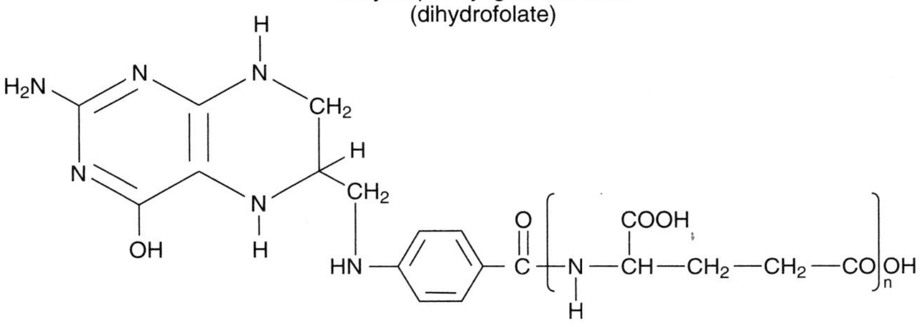

Tetrahydropteroyl glutamic acid
(tetrahydrofolate)

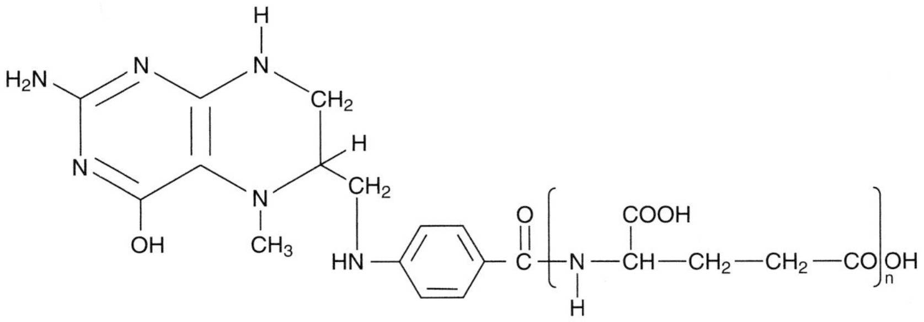

5-Methyl tetrahydrofolate

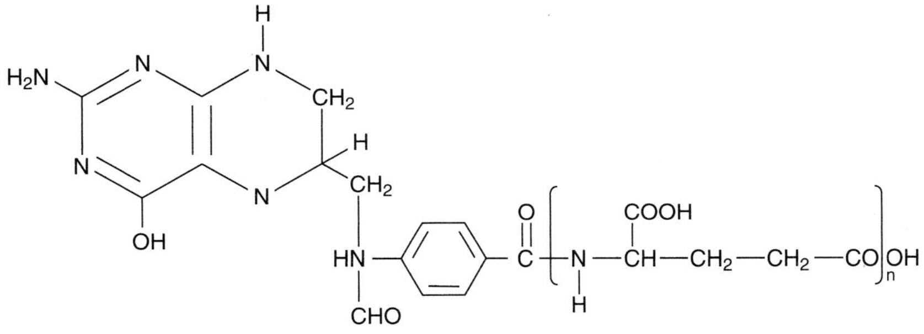

10-Formyl tetrahydrofolate

FIGURE 46.6 Pteroylglutamic acid (folic acid) and its derivatives. (From Marshall WJ, Lapsley M, Day AP, Ayling RM. *Clinical biochemistry: metabolic and clinical aspects*. 3rd ed. Edinburgh: Elsevier; 2014.)

but this complex is cleaved in the duodenum whereupon the vitamin binds to intrinsic factor (IF), a glycoprotein secreted by the gastric parietal cells. The vitamin B_{12}–IF complex is resistant to proteolysis; when it reaches the ileum, it binds to cubilin, a protein expressed on the surface of ileal enterocytes, and is internalized. Within the enterocytes, vitamin B_{12} is released, binds to transcobalamin II (TC II), and is released into the bloodstream. The vitamin B_{12}–TC II complex is termed *holotranscobalamin*.[66] Vitamin B_{12} is readily released

from this complex to bone marrow and other tissues. The complex is also referred to as "active B_{12}" to distinguish it from complexes with transcobalamin I and III, which bind the vitamin tightly and do not release it to tissues. Because of this, assays that measure total vitamin B_{12} may give a misleading indication of the amount of vitamin available to tissues, and "active B_{12}" assays are now available. However, "active B_{12}" measurements require interpretation accordingly to appropriately defined criteria.[67]

Deficiency

Deficiency can arise because of a lack in the diet (a risk for vegans but otherwise very uncommon), decreased gastric acid secretion (e.g., gastrectomy), ileal disease (e.g., Crohn disease, ileal resection), intestinal bacterial overgrowth, infestation with the fish tapeworm *Diphyllobothrium latum*, which binds cobalamin and prevents its absorption, and pernicious anemia. Pernicious anemia, the most common cause, is an autoimmune disease in which absorption is compromised by decreased production of IF (with autoantibodies to gastric parietal cells in the majority of cases) or the development of antibodies to IF; these latter antibodies can either prevent the formation of vitamin B_{12}–IF complexes (binding antibodies) or their absorption (blocking antibodies).[68]

Vitamin B_{12} deficiency causes two clinical syndromes: a megaloblastic anemia, discussed in detail in Chapter 76, and a neurologic disorder characterized by peripheral neuropathy, dysfunction of the posterior columns of the spinal cord (hence the term "subacute combined degeneration") and, in severe cases, psychosis and dementia.

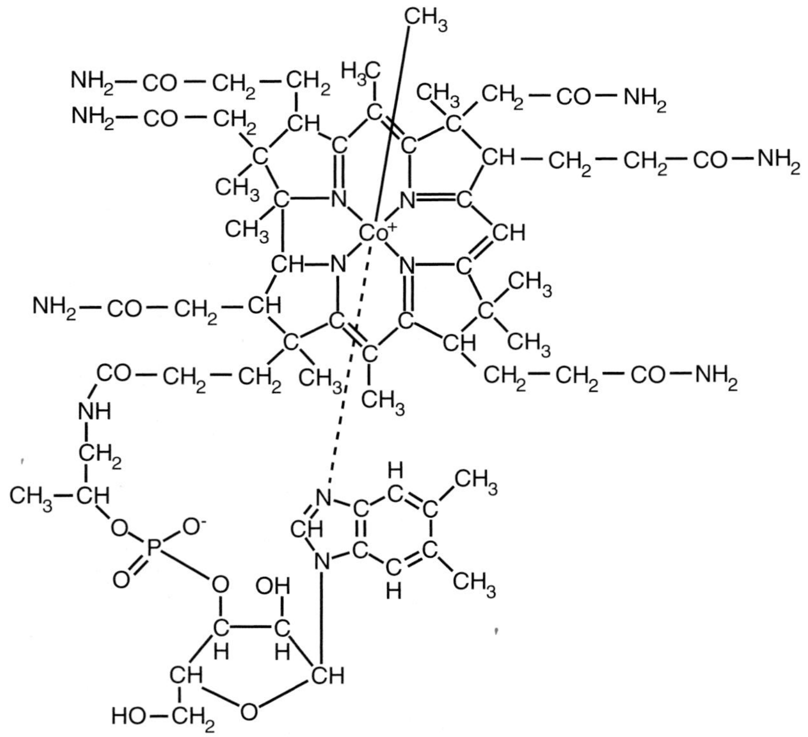

TABLE 46.2 Reactions in Which Folate Derivatives Are Involved

Folate Derivative Involved as	Reaction
Single-Carbon Donor	
10-formyl THF	Purine synthesis
5,10-Methylene THF	Thymine synthesis
5,10-Methylene THF	Synthesis of glycine from CO_2 and NH_4^+
5-Methyl THF	Homocysteine → methionine
Single-Carbon Acceptor	
THF (forms 5,10-methylene THF)	Serine → glycine
THF (forms 5-formimino THF)	Breakdown of histidine

THF, Tetrahydrofolate.
From Marshall WJ, Lapsley M, Day AP, Ayling RM. *Clinical biochemistry: metabolic and clinical aspects*. 3rd ed. Edinburgh: Elsevier; 2014.

FIGURE 46.7 Methylcobalamin, the major circulating form of vitamin B_{12}. Note the cobalt ion at the center of the planar ring, linked covalently to the purine component of the nucleotide above, and a methyl group below the ring. (From Ayling RM, Marshall WJ. *Nutrition and laboratory medicine*. London: ACB Venture Publications; 2007.)

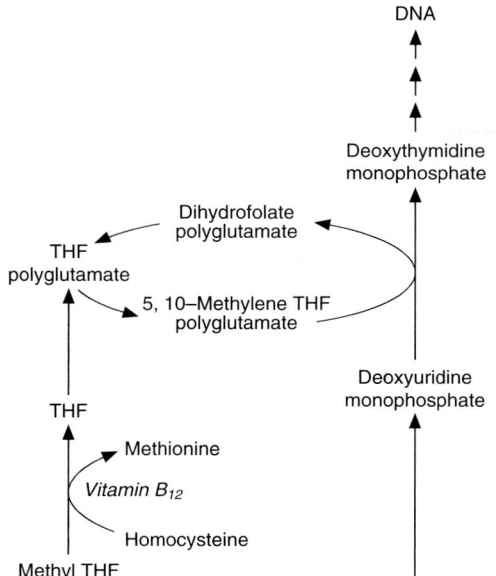

FIGURE 46.8 The link between folate and vitamin B_{12} deficiency in megaloblastic anemia. 5,10-Methylene tetrahydrofolate *(THF)* polyglutamate is required for a rate-limiting step in DNA synthesis, the conversion of deoxyuridine monophosphate to deoxythymidine monophosphate. Vitamin B_{12} is required in one of the reactions converting the main circulating form of folate, 5-methyl THF, to 5,10-methylene THF. (From Marshall WJ, Lapsley M, Day AP, Ayling RM. *Clinical biochemistry: metabolic and clinical aspects.* 3rd ed. Edinburgh: Elsevier; 2014.)

Assessment of Status

This is discussed in detail in Chapter 39. Serum vitamin B_{12} can be measured by immunoassay but is not specific because a low concentration may occur in folate deficiency. Increased plasma concentrations of methylmalonate and homocysteine are found in vitamin B_{12} deficiency but are not specific to it. Antibodies to IF are present in 90% of patients with pernicious anemia but may occur in up to 15% of healthy individuals. The finding of antibodies to IF is more specific but less sensitive. Normal total plasma vitamin B_{12} concentration is 300 to 900 ng/L (0.16 to 0.74 nmol/L). For information regarding measurements and reference intervals, refer to Chapter 39 and the Appendix, respectively.

Vitamin C (Ascorbic Acid)

Nature, Sources, and Function

Two substances comprise vitamin C: L-ascorbic acid and L-dehydroascorbic acid (Fig. 46.9). Both have biologic activity. They are interconvertible, but L-ascorbic acid is the major form in animal tissues. Most animals can synthesize vitamin C; humans and some other primates, guinea pigs, and some bats are among the exceptions.

Vitamin C functions as an electron donor in several enzyme reactions, including three that are essential in collagen synthesis (lysyl hydroxylase and two prolyl hydroxylases) and hence in wound healing and the maintenance of the health of skin, bone, and cartilage. It also has roles in carnitine synthesis (and hence in the transport of fatty acyl moieties into mitochondria, where they can be oxidized) and the synthesis

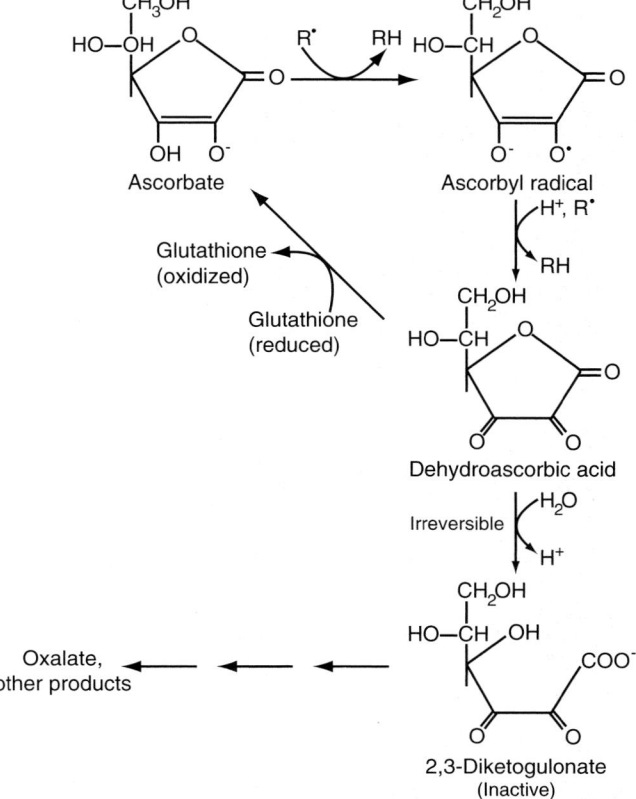

FIGURE 46.9 Ascorbic acid (vitamin C) and its role in scavenging free radicals. Dehydroascorbic acid can be metabolized to oxalate or reduced to ascorbate by glutathione. *R,* Free radical. (From Ayling RM, Marshall WJ. *Nutrition and laboratory medicine.* London: ACB Venture Publications; 2007.)

of monoamine neurotransmitters. It is an important antioxidant and scavenger of free radicals and facilitates the intestinal absorption of nonheme iron by maintaining iron in the Fe^{2+} (ferrous) form.[69]

Its major sources are fruit, particularly citrus fruits, and vegetables. Potatoes have a relatively low content but are an important source of the vitamin in regions where they are the major source of carbohydrate. It is highly labile; heat, light, metal ions, oxygen, and alkaline conditions destroy vitamin C. The recommended daily intake is 90 mg in men and 75 mg in women with a maximum of 2000 mg.

Deficiency and Toxicity

Deficiency of vitamin C causes scurvy, a particularly well-characterized and well-understood vitamin deficiency disease, with many of the manifestations relating directly to known functions of the vitamin. Manifestations include perifollicular hemorrhages and hemorrhage from mucous membranes, poor wound healing, and anemia. The anemia is multifactorial; potential causes include bleeding and reduced iron absorption. Behavioral changes may be a manifestation of disturbed neurotransmitter synthesis.[70]

Vitamin C has low toxicity, but high doses may cause indigestion and diarrhea (an effect linked to ascorbic acid per se and not such a problem with its calcium or sodium salts), and the high doses advocated by some for unproven indications (see later) are unlikely to be harmful. It has long been believed that a high intake may predispose to the formation of oxalate-containing renal calculi, but this remains controversial.[71]

High doses (e.g., 1000 mg/day) of vitamin C have been advocated as reducing the risk of a variety of conditions, including cancers, cardiovascular disease, and the common cold. Extensive research has failed to validate such claims except under some circumstances for the common cold.[72–74]

Assessment of Status

Measurement of plasma ascorbate reflects recent input. A more reliable indicator of tissues store is provided by measurement of ascorbate in leukocytes (reference interval, 1.1 to 2.8 mol/10^6 cells, 20 to 50 mg/10^8 cells) or of urinary ascorbate excretion after an oral loading dose, excretion being lower in deficiency. Individuals replete in ascorbate will excrete virtually all of a 500-mg oral dose over the following 6 hours.[75] For information regarding measurements and reference intervals, refer to Chapter 39 and the Appendix, respectively.

Carnitine

Carnitine is a quaternary ammonium compound that is involved in the transport of long-chain fatty acyl-CoA molecules from cytosol into mitochondria, an essential step in the generation of energy from fat. It is synthesized in the liver and kidneys. Carnitine is transported across the placenta mainly in the third trimester of pregnancy, and carnitine deficiency has been reported in such infants.[76] Carnitine is frequently added to PN prescriptions for premature infants, but there is no clear evidence of benefit from doing so.[77]

Choline

Similar to carnitine, choline is a quaternary ammonium compound. It is involved in neurotransmission (acetylcholine) and is a component of cell membranes (phosphatidylcholine) and the S-adenosylmethionine methylation pathway. Choline

is synthesized in the body, but it appears that endogenous synthesis may be inadequate to supply requirements in some groups, in particular, pregnant women and premature infants.[78] There appears to be wide variation in dietary choline requirements among individuals. Experimentally induced choline deficiency causes fatty liver and renal damage, both reversible with supplementation, but there is no clear evidence that deficiency occurs in a natural setting. Milk is an important dietary source of choline, and in the United States, infant formula feed made from other than cow's milk is required to have added choline.

Vitamin D
Nature, Sources, and Function

Vitamin D includes two chemically similar substances (both secosterols; Fig. 46.10): ergosterol (D_2) and cholecalciferol (D_3). The substance originally named vitamin D_1 was later shown to be a compound of ergocalciferol with lumisterol, and the term is no longer used. Ergosterol is semisynthetic, the form of the vitamin that is added to certain foodstuffs as a dietary supplement, and is also present in some fungi. Cholecalciferol is present in oily fish, dairy products, and egg yolk, but most of the body's cholecalciferol (~90%) is synthesized in vivo, through the action of ultraviolet B radiation on 7-dehydrocholesterol in the skin. Ergocalciferol and cholecalciferol appear to behave similarly in the body; for this reason, the term *vitamin D* is used in this chapter to refer to both substances.

Vitamin D has no biologic activity per se. It undergoes 25-hydroxylation in the liver in an unregulated reaction to form the major circulating and storage form, 25-OH vitamin D (calcidiol or calcifediol in the case of D_3). This has little biologic activity. In the plasma, it circulates bound to a specific binding protein. It undergoes further hydroxylation in the kidneys to form 1,25-dihydroxyvitamin D (calcitriol), a powerful calcium-regulating hormone. 1-Hydroxylation is stimulated by parathyroid hormone and hypophosphatemia and inhibited by the product of the reaction (see Chapter 54).

Calcitriol stimulates the synthesis of calbindins, proteins that mediate intestinal calcium absorption, and stimulates intestinal phosphate absorption. In both the liver and the kidneys, it stimulates the formation of inactive derivatives of 25-OH vitamin D. Its action to promote bone mineralization is mediated through its role in the control of extracellular calcium concentration. Although it has been demonstrated to promote osteolysis in vitro, the physiologic relevance of this observation is uncertain.

The vitamin D receptor, which binds calcitriol and mediates its action, is present in many tissues, and vitamin D appears to have a role in cellular differentiation, particularly in the immune system. The relevance of this to vitamin D deficiency is discussed later.

At higher latitudes, the amount of ultraviolet light reaching the earth's surface is insufficient to promote significant synthesis of vitamin D. Even where there is adequate ultraviolet light, many factors may result in inadequate endogenous synthesis (see later), and the recommended dietary intake is 600 IU/day (15 µg/day).[5]

Deficiency

The classic vitamin D deficiency diseases are rickets in children and osteomalacia in adults. In both there is inadequate

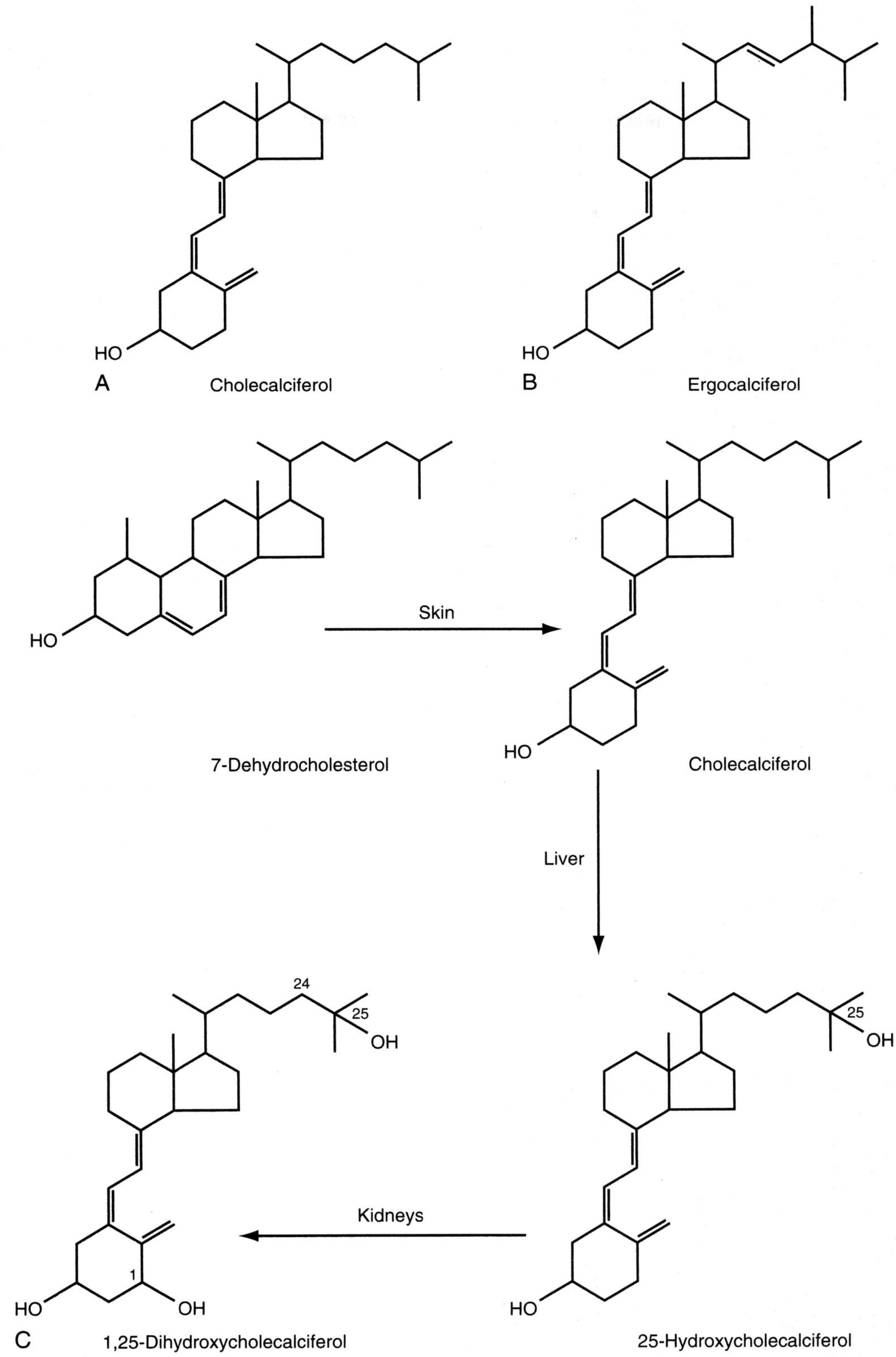

FIGURE 46.10 Vitamin D. (A) Cholecalciferol (vitamin D₃). (B) Ergocalciferol (vitamin D₂). (C) The formation of cholecalciferol from 7-dehydrocholesterol and its subsequent conversion to calcitriol by 25-hydroxylation in the liver and 1-hydroxylation in the kidney. (From Ayling RM, Marshall WJ. *Nutrition and laboratory medicine*. London: ACB Venture Publications; 2007.)

mineralization of bone, leading to deformity (especially in children) and increased risk of fracture; myopathy is frequently present. Hypocalcemia may be present but is often prevented by increased synthesis of parathyroid hormone (secondary hyperparathyroidism). Vitamin D deficiency is particularly likely to occur in very young individuals (especially premature infants and particularly if their mothers were deficient because vitamin D is only transferred across the placenta in the last trimester), elderly people, people with pigmented skins, and people who do not expose their skin to sunlight (e.g., those living in institutions). Also at risk are patients with malabsorption and people taking anticonvulsant drugs, which may interfere with the uptake of vitamin D from the gut or alter its metabolism (see Chapter 54).

There is considerable observational evidence that has been interpreted as implicating vitamin D deficiency in a wide range of conditions, including cardiovascular disease, type 2 diabetes, autoimmune diseases, and certain malignancies,[79,80] but a causative relationship has not been demonstrated, and there is scant evidence of benefit with regard to these conditions from supplementation in individuals at risk of vitamin D deficiency[81,82] except in the case of falls in elderly individuals.[83]

Rickets can also be caused by defective synthesis or action of calcitriol. Defective synthesis is most frequently seen in patients with chronic kidney disease, but there are two syndromes of vitamin D resistant rickets in which there is an inherited deficiency of the 1-hydroxylase enzyme. These should not be confused with the several conditions collectively termed *vitamin D–dependent rickets* in which there is an inherited renal tubular phosphate leak.

Excess

Excessive intake of vitamin D (achievable only through the misuse of supplements and in individuals taking 1-hydroxylated derivatives of vitamin D) can cause loss of mineral from bone and hypercalcemia. Emerging evidence links potential adverse effects to high concentrations, particularly greater than 150 nmol/L.[84] Patients being treated with 1-hydroxylated derivatives should have regular assessments of calcium concentration.

Assessment of Status

Vitamin D status is assessed by measurement of the 25-hydroxylated metabolites of D_2 and D_3 either together, as with most immunoassays, or separately, using liquid chromatography–mass spectrometry (see Chapter 39). There may be considerable variation in results using different immunoassays,[85] and the latter is the preferred technique.

Because many apparently healthy people may have borderline (subclinical) deficiency of the vitamin, it is more appropriate to refer to reference intervals based on lowest risk of adverse concentrations (low or high) than the values obtaining in the population at large. A concentration of less than 30 nmol/L (<12 μg/L) indicates unequivocal deficiency, 30 to less than 50 nmol/L (12 to <20 μg/L) indicates inadequate stores, putting the individual at risk of bone disease, ≥50 nmol/L (≤20 μg/L).[84]

Vitamin E

Nature, Sources, and Function

The term *vitamin E* includes a group of 10 closely related substances, each having a 6-chromanol ring structure and a side chain (Fig. 46.11). Whereas the tocopherols have saturated side alkane side chains, the tocotrienols have alkene side chains, with unsaturated bonds at the 3, 7, and 11 positions. About 90% of vitamin E in the body is α-tocopherol; the other tocopherols and the tocotrienols contribute little to the overall biologic activity of the vitamin. The most important dietary sources are vegetable oils and cereals. Animal products, including cow's milk (unlike human milk), are poor sources, and formula feeds are routinely supplemented with (a water-soluble derivative of) vitamin E. The recommended daily intake in adults is 15 mg/day as α-tocopherol. The higher the dietary content of polyunsaturated fatty acids, the higher the requirement for vitamin E, but foodstuffs rich in the former (e.g., vegetable oils) tend to have high vitamin E contents.

The most important action of vitamin E appears to be as an antioxidant.[86-88] Being fat soluble, it is present in cell membranes and acts to prevent lipid peroxidation by scavenging hydroxyl free radicals. In doing so, tocopheryl radicals are formed, which are then reduced back to the native state by hydrogen donors such as ascorbic acid. Other physiologic metabolites of vitamin E have been recognized, for example tocotrienols, α-tocopherol phosphate, and long chain metabolites resulting from ω-hydroxylase activity of cytochrome P450. Potential actions of these metabolites include effects on gene transcription, inflammation, and neuronal and hepatic cells.[89,90]

Deficiency and Excess

Vitamin E deficiency was first described in premature infants, in whom it is now largely preventable thanks to the supplementation of formula milk. Also susceptible are individuals with malabsorption and with abetalipoproteinemia. (Apolipoprotein B is required for the transfer of fat-soluble vitamins from enterocytes to the plasma.) Features of deficiency include spinocerebellar ataxia, myopathy, hemolytic anemia, and pigmentary degeneration of the retina. These can be prevented by supplementation and, in the case of established

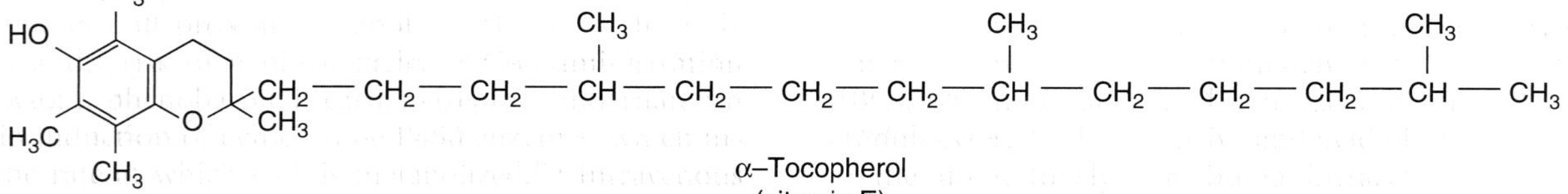

FIGURE 46.11 Structure of α-tocopherol (vitamin E). It is an alcohol of empirical formula $C_{29}H_{50}O_2$, with a long alkyl tail, which confers fat solubility. The hydroxyl group gives it its characteristic antioxidant properties. (From Marshall WJ, Lapsley M, Day AP, Ayling RM. *Clinical biochemistry: metabolic and clinical aspects.* 3rd ed. Edinburgh: Elsevier; 2014.)

deficiency, may in part reverse them. A similar clinical picture occurs in ataxia with vitamin E deficiency, in which a deficiency of hepatic α-tocopherol transfer protein limits the availability of the vitamin to tissues despite an adequate dietary supply.

There has been considerable interest in the possibility that vitamin E supplementation may have a beneficial effect preventing diseases in which autooxidation has been proposed as a causative factor, and in particular, cardiovascular disease. There is, however, no firm evidence to support this notion.[91,92]

A high intake of vitamin E can antagonize vitamin K and potentiate anticoagulant activity, leading to a bleeding diathesis. Because of this, it is recommended that the maximum daily intake should not exceed 1000 mg.[5]

Assessment of Status

Vitamin E can be measured by HPLC with electrochemical, fluorometric, or electron capture detection. Mass spectrometric–based methods can be used to measure the individual components. Because they bind principally to LDLs, their concentration may be more usefully expressed as a ratio to cholesterol concentration. For information regarding measurements and reference intervals, refer to Chapter 39 and the Appendix, respectively.

Vitamin K
Nature, Sources, and Function

Vitamin K comprises two naturally occurring naphthoquinone derivatives: phylloquinone (phytomenadione or vitamin K_1) and menaquinone (vitamin K_2); vitamin K_3 (menaquinone) is a synthetic compound and is the form used therapeutically (Fig. 46.12). There are several subtypes of vitamin K_2, differing by the number of isoprenoid residues in their side chains. Green leafy vegetables are the major source of vitamin K_1, which has a role in photosynthesis. The major form present in animals is vitamin K_2, much of which is derived from metabolism of vitamin K_1 by colonic bacteria.[93]

Vitamin K is a cofactor for the carboxylation of glutamic acid residues in certain calcium-binding proteins, notably the precursors of the so-called Gla proteins (Fig. 46.13). This process generates two adjacent carboxyl groups, to which calcium can bind, thereby conferring physiologic activity on the previously inactive proteins. Gla proteins include six

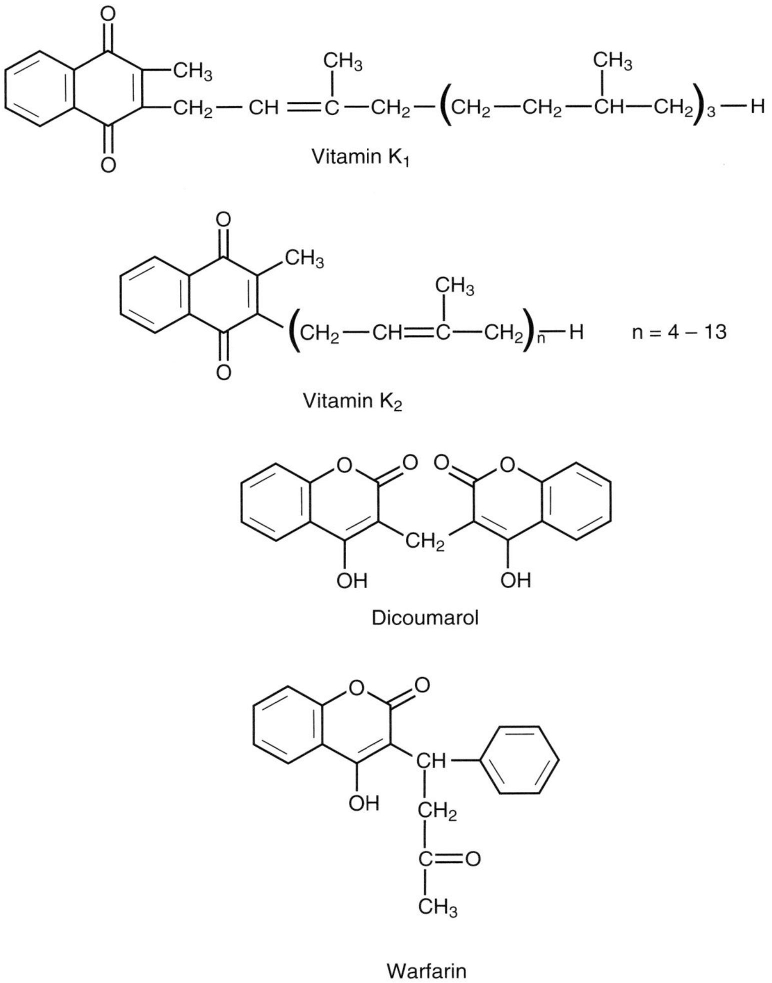

FIGURE 46.12 Structure of vitamin K_1 (phytomenadione) and vitamin K_2 (menaquinone), together with two vitamin K antagonists that have anticoagulant properties. (From Marshall WJ, Lapsley M, Day AP, Ayling RM. *Clinical biochemistry: metabolic and clinical aspects*, 3rd ed. Edinburgh: Elsevier; 2014.)

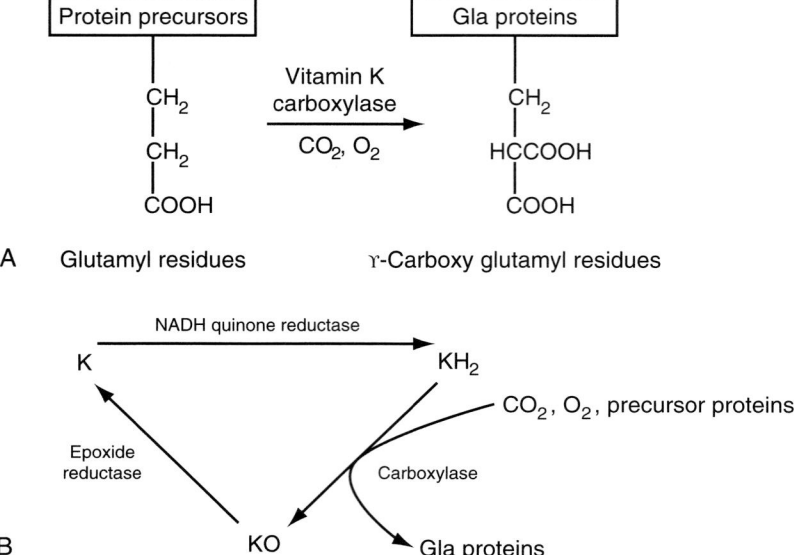

FIGURE 46.13 (A) The γ-carboxylation of glutamate residues in proteins. (B) The reactivation of vitamin K. (From Ayling RM, Marshall WJ. *Nutrition and laboratory medicine.* London: ACB Venture Publications; 2007.)

proteins involved in blood coagulation: factors II (prothrombin), VII, IX, and XI and the inhibitory proteins C and S. Vitamin K thus has an essential role in the initiation and regulation of blood clotting. Warfarin, a widely used anticoagulant, has structural similarities with vitamin K; its action is due to its inhibition of the reductase enzymes involved in the regeneration of reduced vitamin K. The carboxylation reaction results in the conversion of vitamin K to an epoxide, which is reduced back to reduced (active) vitamin K by the successive actions of an epoxide reductase and an NADH-dependent quinone reductase (see Fig. 46.13).

Other Gla proteins include several present in osteoblasts: osteocalcin (the most abundant Gla protein in the body), periostin, matrix Gla protein, and Gla-rich protein. All are involved in bone mineralization, but defective mineralization is not a feature of even severe vitamin K deficiency, and although there is some evidence suggesting that vitamin K supplementation can reduce the risk of osteoporosis, it is not recommended for this purpose in the United States or United Kingdom.

The recommended intakes are 90 μg/day in women and 120 μg/day in men. Newborn babies (particularly if premature) have lower (by ≈50%) plasma concentrations of vitamin K. In many countries, newborn infants are routinely given intramuscular vitamin K (0.5 to 1.0 mg) as prophylaxis against hemolytic disease of the newborn.

Deficiency and Excess

Dietary deficiency of vitamin K is uncommon in people eating a normal diet containing green vegetables. Functional deficiency can occur in malabsorption syndrome and patients with chronic liver disease in whom the synthesis of clotting factors may be decreased. (The distinction between true deficiency and functional deficiency can be made by assessing the response to parenteral vitamin K; the prothrombin time should respond within 24 hours of a parenteral dose of vitamin K in patients with defective synthesis of clotting

factors.) Transient deficiency may occur in patients treated with broad-spectrum antibiotics because of their effect on the gut biota.

Acute vitamin K deficiency tends to be manifest as a bleeding tendency because of inadequate vitamin K–dependent coagulation factors; this can be treated with phytomenadione. More long-term subacute deficiency of vitamin K dependent proteins may be associated with osteoporosis[94] and cardiovascular disease.[95]

Vitamin K toxicity has not been reported.

Assessment of Status

Coagulation assays, such as prothrombin time, will indicate significant vitamin K deficiency (see Chapter 81). Phylloquinone can be measured in serum, a concentration of less than 0.15 μg/L suggesting deficiency. However, measurement may reflect recent dietary intake. An indication of subclinical vitamin K deficiency can be obtained by measurement of undercarboxylated vitamin K–dependent proteins, of which PIVKA-II (protein induced by vitamin K absence) is the most commonly used.[96]

Other Organic Micronutrients

A variety of other substances have been suggested to be essential dietary components in humans. Even more are sold through retail pharmacists, websites, and health food outlets with no scientific evidence of benefit. These include coenzyme Q (ubiquinone), pangamic acid ("vitamin B_{16}"), and orotic acid ("vitamin B_{13}").

INORGANIC MICRONUTRIENTS

Chromium

Although chromium appears to be an essential micronutrient, the precise form in which it acts and the mechanism of its action remain uncertain. Its most well-accepted function is as a component of a poorly defined, low-molecular-weight chromium-binding substance called chromomodulin to potentiate the action of insulin by activating a tyrosine kinase domain within the insulin receptor, leading to increased tissue glucose uptake and storage.[97]

Other functions have been suggested but not proven.[99] Dietary sources include whole grains, yeast, liver, mushrooms, and nuts. The recommended daily intake is 35 μg/day (0.7 μmol/day). The normal plasma concentration is less than 0.3 μg/L (0.06 nmol/L), but special collection conditions are required to avoid contamination from syringes and blood tubes. For information regarding measurements and reference intervals, refer to Chapter 39 and the Appendix, respectively.

Chromium deficiency has been observed (and authenticated) in patients receiving PN who developed glucose intolerance that did not respond to insulin and a neuropathy but has not otherwise been observed.[98] Experimentally induced deficiency in animals causes hypercholesterolemia, but there is no clear evidence of this in humans nor evidence that chromium deficiency is an etiologic factor in diabetes.[99] Chromium supplements are marketed as being of potential benefit and have been reported to have glucose-lowering and cholesterol-lowering properties. Evidence suggests they may have some benefit without adverse side effects.[100] Chromium toxicity may arise from prosthetic joints and has been described in association with excessive dietary intake.[101]

Cobalt

The only known function of cobalt in the body is as a constituent of the cobalt–corrin ring in vitamin B$_{12}$. There is no indication for measuring plasma cobalt concentration specifically except in the context of suspected toxicity. Possible toxic effects of environmental cobalt and cobalt released in vivo from prosthetic joints and other sources are discussed in Chapter 44.

Copper

Function and Sources

Copper is a component of numerous metalloenzymes, including superoxide dismutase (which catalyzes the conversion of superoxide to hydrogen peroxide), tyrosinase (melanin synthesis), cytochrome c oxidase (the terminal step in the mitochondrial electron transport chain), dopamine hydroxylase (synthesis of norepinephrine [noradrenaline]), lysyl oxidase (essential to the crosslinking of the polypeptide chains in collagen and elastin), and ceruloplasmin (oxidation of iron [$Fe^{2+} \rightarrow Fe^{3+}$] in plasma).[102] The recommended daily intake is 1.2 mg (19 μmol); copper is toxic, and ingestion of as little as 20 mg can cause nausea, vomiting, and dizziness.

Copper is present in many foods, with nuts, shellfish, and offal being particularly rich sources, although not all dietary copper is available for absorption, and a high zinc intake reduces the copper absorption. Copper is transported to the liver bound to albumin and there is incorporated into ceruloplasmin (six copper ions per molecule), which accounts for approximately 90% of circulating copper. Copper is excreted in the bile and is retained in cholestasis. The normal total plasma concentration of copper is 64 to 140 μg/dL (10 to 25 μmol/L), but interpretation of plasma results is confounded by ceruloplasmin's being an acute phase protein. For information regarding measurements and reference intervals, refer to Chapter 39 and the Appendix, respectively.

There are two principal inherited metabolic diseases that involve copper metabolism: Wilson disease, in which reduced incorporation of copper into ceruloplasmin leads to increased free copper and accumulation of the metal in tissues, and Menkes disease, a condition in which there is a defect in the distribution of copper into tissues. These conditions are discussed elsewhere in this book (see Chapter 61).

Deficiency

Copper deficiency is rare; it has been described in children with severe malnutrition or severe malabsorption and individuals dependent on total parenteral nutrition (TPN) when provision has been inadequate. The principal clinical features are a microcytic anemia unresponsive to iron, and myeloneuropathy; some evidence suggests that subclinical copper deficiency may be a risk factor for cardiovascular disease.[103]

Fluorine

The average adult human body contains about 1 g of fluorine, of which almost all is in bone and teeth. It is certainly biologically active but is not strictly an essential nutrient in that no specific deficiency syndrome has been described. A low fluorine intake is undoubtedly a risk factor for the development of dental caries (and fluorine supplementation by fluoridation of drinking water during tooth development is protective,[104] as is the use of fluoride-containing toothpastes and varnishes after eruption) but is not a cause per se.[105,106] A low fluoride intake has been suggested to be a risk factor for osteoporosis, particularly in elderly individuals, but the evidence is inconsistent, and any effect is likely to be small.[107] Although fluoride has been used therapeutically with benefit in patients with osteoporosis, the dosage considerably exceeds the amount provided by fluoridation.

The best dietary sources of fluorine are tea and fish that are eaten whole (e.g., whitebait). An adequate intake of fluorine is 4 mg/day (210 μmol). An excessive intake can cause fluorosis (pitting and discoloration of the teeth in children), but protection against dental caries is not compromised. Normal plasma fluoride concentration in men is 0.3 to 1.5 μmol/L (5.7 to 28 μg/L) as measured by ion-specific electrode, but there is no indication for its measurement in ordinary clinical practice.

Iodine

Iodine has only one known function in humans, as a component of the thyroid hormones thyroxine and triiodothyronine (see Chapter 57). The major dietary sources are seafood, dairy products, eggs, and meat. Vegetables in general are a poor source, except in coastal areas where they grow in soil exposed to spray from seawater (which contains iodine). The recommended intake is 150 μg/day (1.2 μmol/day).

Iodine deficiency results in decreased synthesis of thyroid hormones, causing increased synthesis of thyrotrophin and in turn thyroid hypertrophy (clinically manifest as goiter). The increased thyroid mass and hence synthetic capacity may be sufficient to prevent clinical hypothyroidism. Nevertheless, iodine deficiency is the most common cause of hypothyroidism worldwide. It is particularly prevalent in mountainous areas (endemic goiter) where the iodine content of soil is low, but the addition of iodine to table salt or bread has reduced the prevalence of the condition. Dietary selenium deficiency may also be a contributory factor because selenoenzymes are involved in thyroid hormone synthesis.[108] Even with apparently adequate dietary intake of iodine, apparent deficiency may be a result of impaired utilization of iodine by the thyroid by "goitrogens." These include thiocyanates that can be formed from glucosinolates during the digestion of some foods (brassicas, plants of the Cruciferae family are particularly implicated) and cyanogenic glycosides, present in cassava. The adverse effects of some drugs used therapeutically on iodine metabolism and thyroid hormone synthesis are discussed in Chapter 57.

Iodine is readily excreted in the urine and toxicity is rare, even in individuals with high intakes as a result of consuming seaweed extracts to provide supplemental iodine.

Measurement of urinary iodine excretion provides the best index of dietary iodine intake[109]; sufficiency is indicated by a concentration of greater than 100 μg/L (>0.79 μmol/L).

Iron

Sources and Function

Iron is an essential component of heme, the active (oxygen-binding) center of hemoglobin and myoglobin. Heme is also a component of cytochromes and peroxidases, in which the iron acts as an electron donor and acceptor. Nonheme iron is an activator of several enzymes, including succinate dehydrogenase, phosphoenolpyruvate carboxykinase, and ribonucleotide reductase. Total body iron is about 4 g, of which two thirds is present in hemoglobin. Only about 0.1% is present in the plasma, where it is almost entirely bound to transferrin. Free iron is highly toxic, through its ability to generate free radicals.[110]

The major dietary source of iron is animal products (particularly red meat), in which it is present as heme. Iron in vegetables is mainly inorganic. Heme iron is more readily absorbed; the bioavailability of inorganic iron is reduced by binding to dietary phytates and oxalate; ferrous (Fe II) iron is more readily absorbed than ferric (Fe III) iron. About 30 mg of iron is required each 24 hours to fuel hemoglobin synthesis, but iron is highly conserved. The recommended daily intakes of iron are 8 mg (142 μmol) in men and 18 mg (320 μmol) in women. Typical intakes are higher than this, but iron is relatively poorly absorbed. In men, absorption of approximately 1 mg/day is required to maintain iron balance. Absorption is increased by vitamin C and organic acids, which promote the conversion of Fe III to Fe II.

The absorption of iron is a complex process involving various proteins that regulate absorption such that this is increased when there is increased demand for iron (e.g., increased erythropoiesis after hemorrhage) or body stores are reduced. The key protein is hepcidin, synthesis of which is stimulated by iron and inflammation and inhibited by deficiency, hypoxia, and an increase in erythropoiesis. The iron–hepcidin complex combines with ferroportin, a protein required for the export of iron from enterocytes, and prevents this export. Hereditary (genetic) hemochromatosis is a disorder in which iron absorption is increased to greater than requirements, resulting in iron deposition in tissues and consequent tissue damage.[111] See Chapter 51 for a more comprehensive discussion of this topic.

Deficiency and Toxicity

Iron deficiency is the most common cause of anemia worldwide. It is particularly common in women of childbearing years as a consequence of menstrual blood (hence iron) loss and transfer of iron to the fetus during pregnancy. Other causes related to blood loss include hookworm infection (common in developing countries) and celiac disease. The anemia is characteristically hypochromic and microcytic.[112]

Iron poisoning is more common in children (who may ingest their mothers' iron pills) than adults. It causes necrosis of the GI epithelium, with bleeding and fluid loss, which may lead to acute kidney injury. Hepatic failure may also occur. Treatment is with enteral desferrioxamine, which chelates iron in the gut, preventing absorption, and in the bloodstream, facilitating its excretion. Chronic iron toxicity occurs with genetic hemochromatosis (see earlier) and with chronic iron overload (e.g., from repeated transfusions in patients with thalassemia). These conditions are all discussed in detail in Chapter 51.

Assessment of Status

Various tests are available for assessing iron status. Serum iron concentration alone is of limited value (except in diagnosing poisoning) because it varies considerably in normal individuals. Serum ferritin concentration reflects iron stores, but the protein is an acute phase reactant, and concentrations may be normal in iron-deficient individuals with coexistent inflammation. Total iron binding capacity (TIBC) reflects transferrin concentration and is raised in iron deficiency. Transferrin saturation ([iron]/TIBC) is low (<15% in iron deficiency) and raised (>55% in men and >50% in women) in iron overload. Other tests for iron status include measurement of serum transferrin receptor (increased in iron deficiency but not, importantly, in the anemia of chronic disease). The definitive test is staining of a bone marrow aspirate for iron. Further details are provided in Chapters 39 and the Appendix.

Manganese

Manganese is a constituent or activator of a number of enzymes. It is present in pyruvate carboxylase, mitochondrial superoxide dismutase, and arginase, so it is involved in gluconeogenesis, protection of mitochondria against oxygen free radicals (such as are produced during ATP synthesis), and ammonia detoxication and urea synthesis. It is also an activator of numerous enzymes (although not essential to their activity), including phosphoenolpyruvate carboxykinase (also involved in gluconeogenesis), glutamine synthetase in the brain (hence having a role in the synthesis of neurotransmitters), glycosyltransferases (important in the synthesis of collagen), and others. The major dietary sources are whole (i.e., unrefined) grains, nuts, leafy vegetables, and tea. Dietary tannins, phytates, and oxalate reduce manganese absorption, but even in their absence, only approximately 5% of dietary manganese is absorbed. Excretion is mainly via the bile. The adequate daily intake is 2.3 mg for men and 1.8 mg for women.[5] Normal blood concentration (most manganese in blood is contained within RBCs) is 4.7 to 18.3 μg/L (85 to 330 nmol/L).

Although manganese deficiency has been well described in animals, with a variety of consequences, including poor growth and reproductive function, neurologic deficits, and impaired glucose tolerance, few cases of probable manganese deficiency occurring other than in an experimental setting have been described. One was a child receiving TPN who developed defective bone mineralization and impaired growth that were corrected by manganese supplementation.[113] Other features described include dermatoses and hypocholesterolaemia.[114] Of more concern has been manganese toxicity, both in manganese miners and patients on parenteral feeding.[114] This is discussed further in Chapter 44.

Molybdenum

A compound of molybdenum with a pterin (molybdenum cofactor) is a cofactor for four enzymes: sulfite oxidase, xanthine oxidase, aldehyde oxidase, and the recently described mitochondrial amidoxime reducing component. Sulfite oxidase is responsible for the oxidation of sulfite to sulfate, a reaction of importance in the metabolism of the sulfur-containing amino acids cysteine and methionine. Xanthine oxidase is involved in the conversion of purines to uric acid and aldehyde oxidase in various hydroxylation reactions; both of these enzymes are involved in the metabolism of xenobiotics.[115,116] The function of mitochondrial amidoxime-reducing component has yet to be fully elucidated, but it has a role in the detoxication of mutagenic N-hydroxylated bases.[117] The recommended daily intake is 45 μg. Plasma concentrations reflect intake and vary widely in healthy people.

Molybdenum is present in many foods, including meats, grains, and legumes, and isolated dietary deficiency has not been reliably described, although a case has been described in an individual on long-term parenteral feeding.[118] Symptoms included fatigue, headache, and mental disturbance. As might be expected from the known functions of molybdenum cofactor, the patient had hypouricemia and a low plasma sulfate concentration.

The rare inherited condition molybdenum cofactor deficiency, in which there is a defect in the synthesis of the cofactor, presents with neurologic abnormalities and severe mental retardation and is typically fatal within a few months of birth. These are thought to be caused by a toxic effect of sulfite. Other features include hypouricemia and xanthinuria. Supplementation with molybdenum has no effect on the condition, but daily injections of cyclic pyranopterin monophosphate, a precursor of molybdenum cofactor have been shown to be effective.[119] Molybdenum has low toxicity. Occupationally exposed workers may develop hyperuricemia and have an increased tendency to gout. There is an authenticated report of toxicity as a result of a high supplementary intake of molybdenum.[120]

Selenium

Selenium is an essential cofactor for at least three enzymes, including glutathione reductase, which is an important component of the body's defenses against oxidative stress.[121] The others are thioredoxin reductase, involved in nucleic acid synthesis, and through its action to reduce disulfide bonds, also having an antioxidant action, and iodothyronine deiodinase, responsible for the conversion of thyroxine to triiodothyronine. Two other selenoproteins have been described (selenoproteins P, found in plasma, and M, found in muscle), but their function is unknown.

Dietary selenium is mainly provided in the form of selenomethionine and selenocysteine in cereals, meat, and fish. The content in cereals is dependent on the selenium content of soil and that of animals in turn on the content in their feed. Endemic deficiency occurs in some areas of China where the soil content is low and is responsible for a potentially fatal cardiomyopathy (Keshan disease) that can be prevented (but is not cured) by selenium supplementation.[122] Skeletal myopathy may also occur. Concomitant infection with Coxsackie virus is also involved in the pathogenesis of this condition. There is also some evidence that a low selenium intake is associated with an increased incidence of cancer, and in some parts of the world, selenium is added to fertilizers for arable crops. Selenium deficiency has also been reported in patients with intestinal failure receiving long-term PN, although selenium is now typically provided in the feeds. It is also a risk in patients on restrictive diets for inherited metabolic diseases (e.g., phenylketonuria) and selenium status should be monitored in such patients.[123] The recommended daily intake varies from country to country but is of the order of 60 μg/day (760 nmol/day). Selenium status is most reliably assessed either by the measurement of RBC glutathione reductase activity or the plasma concentration of selenoprotein P. For information regarding measurements and reference intervals, refer to Chapter 39 and the Appendix, respectively.

Zinc

Sources and Function

Zinc is a cofactor for numerous enzymes covering a wide range of functions. Examples include alkaline phosphatase (a low plasma activity of this enzyme is a feature of zinc deficiency), carbonate dehydratase (carbonic anhydrase), thymidine kinase, and carboxypeptidase. It also has a role in various nonenzymic proteins, including the family of zinc finger proteins.[124] This is a large group of proteins involved in mediating the binding of smaller ligands to large molecules, in particular nucleic acids. Poultry, meat, eggs, and some shellfish are good dietary sources of zinc. Although present in cereals, its bioavailability is limited by the phytates that these contain, which bind zinc. The recommended daily intake is 10 mg (150 μmol).

Zinc is absorbed in the proximal small intestine, but its release into the plasma is controlled by metallothionein. Synthesis of this protein is increased (limiting its absorption) when zinc intake is high. Metallothionein also binds copper (and with a higher affinity), with the result that a high intake of zinc can reduce the absorption of dietary copper. Zinc is widely distributed in the body, particularly to skeletal muscle. In the blood, 80% is present in RBCs. Zinc in plasma is largely protein bound to albumin (loosely) and α_2-macroglobulin (tightly).[124]

Deficiency and Toxicity

Dietary deficiency of zinc is uncommon but has been well characterized. Inadequate provision of zinc during PN and increased loss of zinc from the body are important potential causes. Zincuria is a feature of the acute inflammatory response. The manifestations of zinc deficiency are protean, as might be expected from its wide range of functions. They include dermatitis, hair loss, poor wound healing, growth retardation, depressed immune function, anorexia, ageusia, and anosmia. Acrodermatitis enteropathica is an autosomal recessive disorder affecting intestinal zinc absorption. Affected children present with a scaly dermatitis (which often becomes secondarily infected), diarrhea, and impaired growth. These all respond to high doses of oral zinc.[125]

Zinc is relatively nontoxic, but poisoning has been reported in individuals drinking large amounts of water stored

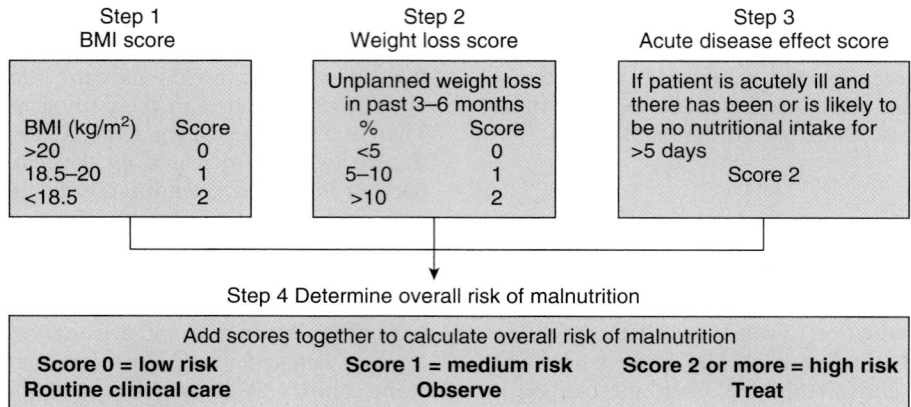

FIGURE 46.14 Malnutrition universal screening tool (MUST). *BMI,* Body mass index. (The "Malnutrition Universal Screening Tool" [MUST] is reproduced here with the kind permission of BAPEN [British Association for Parenteral and Enteral Nutrition]. For further information on MUST see www.bapen.org.uk. Copyright BAPEN 2012.)

in galvanized containers. A chronically high intake can lead to the development of features of copper deficiency (see earlier).

Zinc status is typically assessed by measuring plasma concentrations, but the influence of changes in plasma protein concentration must be borne in mind in interpreting the results. For information regarding measurements and reference intervals, refer to Chapter 39 and the Appendix, respectively.

Other Postulated Inorganic Micronutrients

With the exception of fluorine, the essential status of the micronutrients discussed is unequivocal. Each has a well-understood functional role and clinical features that have been reversed by supplementation suggest that these features are manifestations of deficiency.

Several other elements have been postulated as being essential but without unequivocal evidence. They include arsenic, boron, nickel, tin, and vanadium. They have been collectively described as "ultratrace" elements. If any of them is a true essential nutrient, the required intake to maintain health is likely to be very small indeed, and deficiency is unlikely to be observed in free-living subjects and impracticable to prove experimentally. None of these substances is included routinely in regimens for long-term TPN, with no apparent detriment to the patients. Interested readers may wish to consult the cited references for more information.[126,127]

THE ASSESSMENT OF NUTRITIONAL STATUS

Malnutrition has been defined as an acute, subacute, or chronic state of nutrition in which varying degrees of over- or undernutrition, with or without inflammatory activity, have led to a change in body composition and diminished function.[128] Malnutrition often goes unrecognized, and nutritional care can be suboptimal, in part because of a lack of designated responsibility and integration within complex health care settings. Because malnutrition may be associated with adverse clinical outcomes, it is advantageous for all patients to undergo a process of nutritional screening to identify those who are or who may be at risk of malnutrition and in whom formal nutritional assessment would be advantageous.

Nutritional Screening

Nutritional screening is different from nutritional assessment but complementary to it. Nutritional screening is a simple process and an essential part of the patient care process intended to identify those at specific nutritional risk or to document malnutrition and thus to facilitate referral for detailed nutritional assessment. Various nutritional screening tools have been identified. An example is the Malnutrition Universal Screening Tool (Fig. 46.14), which explores the patient's current condition and whether it is clinically stable, together with the likelihood of further deterioration and any contribution of underlying disease process to malnutrition.[129]

The tool is easy and practical to use and has proven reliability and validity.[130] However, future work optimizing specific tools for use in particular patient groups may be advantageous.

Nutritional Assessment

Nutritional assessment seeks to identify an individual's nutritional status. Ideally, any assessment would evaluate body composition and function and protein, energy, mineral, and micronutrient status. For clinical purposes, this is generally not practical, but information sought from assessment is useful to identify those at risk of malnutrition-related complications in whom the provision of nutrition support might be beneficial.[131] The available techniques are summarized in Box 46.1.

Dietetic Methods

Enquiry about a patient's diet should be concerned with any potential deviation from predicted requirements. It should

---

BOX 46.1   Techniques for Nutritional Assessment

Dietetic methods
Clinical assessment
Functional indices
Laboratory studies
Calorimetry
Measurement of body composition

include details of current intake and whether there has been any recent change and should attempt to reveal any factors contributing to undernutrition, for example, loss of appetite, factors affecting eating such as dental or swallowing problems, or difficulties in buying or preparing food because of mobility or socioeconomic issues.

Formal dietetic assessment is concerned with estimating food intake and can be broadly divided into methods that record current intake, recall past intake, and estimate typical intake.[132] Recording current intake can be achieved quantitatively by weighing or measuring all food before consumption typically for a 5- to 7-day period, but this is obviously inconvenient for patients and may cause them to select foods that can be most easily measured. Qualitative recording, by describing the amount of food eaten to a dietician, is a simpler process, and use of a photographic atlas of portion sizes can be used to assist accuracy. Past intake can be evaluated by asking patients to recall everything they have eaten in a time period, usually the previous 24 hours. Although it tends to lack accuracy and to underestimate energy intake, such dietary recall can often highlight areas of major deficiency requiring further assessment. To examine typical food intake (e.g., vegetable intake in middle-aged women), food frequency questionnaires are useful; these evaluate how often subjects eat food from different groups over a longer period.

Clinical Assessment
The standard clinical history and examination provide important information as to an individual's nutritional status. The history may reveal increased nutritional requirements (e.g., burns or sepsis), increased nutrient loss (e.g., vomiting, fistula, renal excretion), or decreased absorption (e.g., diarrhea, pancreatitis, intestinal resection). On examination, there may be signs of general nutritional depletion (evidence of recent weight loss, e.g., loose-fitting clothes, lax skin, loss of subcutaneous fat, muscle wasting or edema), or specific nutrient deficiency (e.g., anemia).

Subjective Global Assessment
This is a clinical method that assesses nutritional status using five clinical features of the history and clinical examination as shown in Box 46.2.

Subjective global assessment is relatively time consuming to perform, and patients may not always be able to supply the required information or to do so with sufficient accuracy. However, it has been demonstrated to be accurate in predicting the risk of complications associated with undernutrition.[134]

Anthropometry
Body weight is a useful parameter for nutritional assessment, but particularly in sick hospital patients, there may be changes in body weight that do not reflect nutritional status but are the result of over- or underhydration, edema, or ascites. Height measurements to enable evaluation of growth are an important part of nutritional assessment in children. In people of the same height, variation in weight is mostly due to differences in body fat, so height can be combined with body weight to calculate the BMI (Table 46.3).

Cut-off values defining obesity and underweight may need to be defined for specific reference populations. Proportions of body fat vary during childhood, so age-specific centiles should be used to interpret BMI in children; adult

BOX 46.2 Features Contributing to Subjective Global Assessment

History
Weight change: kilogram and percentage losses
Dietary intake: change and duration
Gastrointestinal symptoms
- Nausea
- Vomiting
- Diarrhea
- Anorexia
Disease and relation to metabolic demand
Physical examination
Loss of subcutaneous fat
Muscle wasting
Ankle edema
Sacral edema
Ascites
Subjective global assessment rating[133]
  A. Well nourished
  B. Moderately (or suspected of being) malnourished
  C. Severely malnourished

TABLE 46.3 Body Mass Index in Adults

Body Mass Index = Weight/Height^2 (kg/m^2)

Whites		South Asians[135]
<18.5	Underweight	
18.5–24.9	Normal weight	18.5–22.9
25–29.9	Overweight	23–27.8
≥30	Obese	≥27.8

BMI cut-off values should not be used. Although BMI is useful, it does not distinguish between fat and lean mass and so may be misrepresentative in patients with relatively little fat but a large muscle mass (e.g., some athletes). It may be hard to obtain accurate measurements in frail, immobile patients, but sitting scales and weigh beds are available. When patients are unable to stand and measurement of height proves difficult, alternative measurements such as arm span, demi-span, and knee height can be taken and nomograms used to predict actual height.[136]

Because body fat is stored subcutaneously, it can be assessed by measurement of skinfold thickness using specially designed calipers. The triceps skinfold (TSF), measured midway between the shoulder and the elbow, is most often used for this purpose because it is the most easily accessible, although biceps, subscapular, and suprailiac skinfolds are other potential sites. The technique is liable to both inter- and intraobserver error, and because weight loss of several kilograms is required before change is detected, it is not useful for short-term assessment.

Measurement of midarm circumference (MAC), measured midway between the shoulder and elbow, reflects fat, muscle, and protein. It can be used in conjunction with measurements of TSF to calculate muscle and hence protein stores.

$$\text{Arm muscle area} = \frac{\left[\text{MAC}-\left(\text{TSF}\times\pi\right)\right]^2}{4\pi}$$

Although it is a potentially useful and easily available assessment tool, MAC suffers from the same limitations as measurement of skinfolds alone.

Functional Indices

Malnutrition is associated with functional impairment (e.g., changes in immune function and ergonometer performance), as demonstrated by handgrip strength, and has been shown to be associated with postoperative complications.[137] Methods of nutritional assessment using handgrip strength, respiratory muscle strength, and muscle function by electrical stimulation have been developed. However, although muscle function is an index of protein status and can predict risk of complications, it is not clear how best to incorporate such assessment into routine clinical practice.

Laboratory Studies

Laboratory tests are often requested in patients whose nutritional status is suboptimal. However, their use in this setting is highly limited.

Nitrogen Balance

Improvement in nitrogen balance has been proposed to be the nutritional parameter most consistently associated with improved outcome, although loss of protein does not always correlate with function, particularly in critical illness.[138] However, accurate laboratory determination of nitrogen balance is not easily achievable. Assessment of nitrogen balance by measurement of urinary nitrogen or urinary urea requires 24-hour urine collection and estimation of nitrogen loss from all other sources (e.g., feces, skin) and hence tends to be inaccurate.

Plasma Proteins

Any protein used as a marker of nutritional assessment should, ideally, have a short half-life, relatively small body pool, rapid rate of synthesis, and constant rate of catabolism. In addition, changes in the plasma concentration of the marker should reflect the entire protein compartment status and should be responsive only to protein and energy restriction. The proteins most commonly measured for this purpose are albumin, prealbumin, retinol binding protein, transferrin, and, less often, insulin-like growth factor (IGF), but none is ideal (Table 46.4).

The value of all the proteins in current use as nutritional markers is greatly limited because factors other than nutritional status can influence their concentration. In sick, hospitalized patients, it may be particularly difficult to differentiate the effect of malnutrition on plasma proteins from that of the acute phase reaction, which tends to have effects on protein concentration by increasing capillary permeability, increasing protein catabolism, and decreasing hepatic protein synthesis.[139]

Albumin is frequently measured as part of nutritional assessment. Although its concentration in plasma is a good predictor of outcome,[140] change occurs slowly and is affected by fluid shifts and acute phase reactions. Likewise, transferrin is also subject to the potential confounding effects of changes as a result of the acute phase or in iron status. Prealbumin has been suggested as a nutritional marker,[141] and its value has been proposed to be greater if two measurements are made several days apart, together with C-reactive protein (CRP) to assist evaluation of any acute phase reaction. However, evidence analysis has indicated that prealbumin does not change consistently with weight loss, caloric restriction, or nitrogen balance.[142] Methods of assessment based on the evaluation of multiple biochemical variables, including CRP, are sometimes used, such as the prognostic inflammatory and nutritional index (which requires prealbumin, α_1-acid glycoprotein, CRP, and albumin). However such tools lack sensitivity and were originally conceived as tools for assessment of prognosis of critically ill patients rather than for nutritional assessment.[143]

Nutrition is a key regulator of plasma IGF-1 concentration, and the decrease during caloric restriction is independent of pituitary growth hormone secretion. It has been found to be a more sensitive indicator of malnutrition than albumin, prealbumin, transferrin, or RBP,[144] but IGF-1 is affected by the acute phase and by hepatic disease, because the liver is the main source of synthesis. There is also wide variation in response among individuals, and relative changes may be more meaningful than a single concentration.

POINTS TO REMEMBER

Nutritional Screening and Assessment
- Generalized malnutrition is common; all patients should be screened on admission to the hospital for preexisting malnutrition or to detect a high risk of developing malnutrition.
- Patients thus identified should be subject to formal nutritional assessment to determine their appropriate management.
- There are numerous techniques for nutritional assessment, including clinical, imaging, functional, and laboratory tests. Laboratory tests are widely used for this purpose, but their results must be interpreted with caution, owing to the existence of numerous confounding factors.

TABLE 46.4 Plasma Proteins Used for Nutritional Assessment

Protein	Half-Life	Body Pool Size	Concentration ↑ by	Concentration ↓ by
A	20 days	+++++	Dehydration, acute phase response	Overhydration, liver disease, burns, cardiac failure
PA	2 days	+++	Renal failure	Liver disease, acute phase response
TFN	8–10 days	++++	Iron deficiency, pregnancy, estrogens	Liver disease, renal failure, aminoglycosides
RBP	12–24 h	++	Renal failure	Liver disease, vitamin D deficiency, zinc deficiency, hyperthyroidism
IGF-1	2–4 h	+	Growth hormone	Liver disease, acute phase response, hypothyroidism

A, Albumin; *IGF-1,* insulin-like growth factor; *PA,* prealbumin; *RBP,* retinol-binding protein; *TFN,* transferrin.

Calorimetry

Energy utilization results in heat production. In direct calorimetry this heat is measured, and in indirect calorimetry, it is derived from measurement of oxygen consumption and carbon dioxide production (or oxygen consumption and an assumed respiratory quotient). Direct calorimetry requires sophisticated equipment and is not appropriate for routine clinical use. Indirect calorimetry can be performed at the bedside using a "metabolic cart," but this equipment is expensive and requires trained staff for operation. More recently, handheld devices have become available, which, although less accurate than other methods, may have a role in clinical settings. Basal energy expenditure can also be assessed from prediction equations (see later). However, assessment of energy expenditure does not necessarily equate with energy requirements, particularly in malnourished patients who are likely to require sufficient intake to replete their energy stores.

Assessment of Body Composition

Evaluation of body composition is an important aspect of nutritional assessment, for example, because loss of fat has different significance from loss of lean tissue. It is possible to use a two-compartment model of assessment, with the body divided into body fat and fat-free mass (FFM).[145] However, the development of more sophisticated methods of analysis has enabled evaluation using multicompartment models in which the FFM can be divided into water and protein and mineral content. Assessment of specific tissues and organs is possible with some techniques. Various models involve different combinations of the methods described next.[146]

Two-Compartment Models

Bioimpedance. Bioimpedance analysis measures impedance of the body to a small electric current by placing electrodes on the wrist and ankle. Because aqueous tissues are the major conductors of an electric current, it is possible to predict TBW and from that estimate FFM. Bioimpedance is of limited accuracy and is influenced by age and by clinical factors such as edema.

Densitometry. In this technique, total body density is measured (body mass/body volume), and FFM and fat mass are distinguished on the basis of their specific densities. Underwater weighing is considered to be the gold standard technique. It involves weighing the subject in air and then under water, applying a correction for residual air in the lungs. Air displacement plethysmography is an alternative method. Densitometry is potentially inaccurate in situations in which the lean mass may be abnormal, for example, with fluid retention or reduced bone mineralization.

Isotope dilution. TBW can be measured by isotope dilution, usually using tritium-, deuterium-, or ^{18}O-labeled water. From knowledge of the water–isotope–dilution volumes, fat-free body mass and fat (i.e., body weight minus fat-free body mass) can be predicted. However, the relationship between TBW and other body-composition components may change with disease, which may limit use of this method in some patient groups.

Multicompartment Models

Whole-body counting and neutron activation. Potassium occurs predominantly as an intracellular cation, particularly in muscle and viscera, with only very small amounts present in ECF. Measurement of total body potassium can therefore be used as an indicator of body cell mass and of fat-free cell mass. A small amount of body potassium exists as the ^{40}K isotope that emits high-energy radiation; hence, total body potassium can be estimated with the use of a whole-body spectrometer. When an atom captures a neutron, the atom is raised to another nuclear energy level, and the excess energy is released. In neutron activation analysis, the body is bombarded with neutrons, and the subsequent release of γ-rays is detected. Neutron activation can be used to assess a number of elements and hence give information about specific tissues or organs (e.g., calcium for evaluation of bone and iodine for the thyroid).

Computed tomography. Computed tomography (CT) is an imaging method for body composition analysis at the tissue and organ levels.[146] In this method, x-ray attenuation is measured, cross-sectional images are constructed, and numerical values are assigned based on tissue attenuation. The radiation dose from CT is high, so the technique is unsuitable for repeated measurements. However, scans used as part of routine management may be used opportunistically for evaluation of body composition, and the third lumbar vertebra has been suggested as a suitable level for assessment.[147]

Magnetic resonance imaging. Protons within tissues spin to produce tiny, randomly aligned magnetic fields. Magnetic resonance imaging (MRI) involves the application of a strong magnetic field, which causes these magnetic axes to align. If energy in the radiofrequency range is then applied, the axes of the protons momentarily align against the field and then relax. The release of energy is analyzed and recorded as digital images. This technique is of particular use in the evaluation of adipose tissue and skeletal muscle.[148] Because MRI does not use ionizing radiation, it is safe for use in all age and patient groups and could be used for serial monitoring. However, its use is limited by the high cost and the technical expertise required for analysis.

Dual energy x-ray absorptiometry. DEXA uses x-rays of two different energy levels and a photon detector that measures the amount of energy absorbed by soft tissue and bone; soft tissue can be further divided into fat and lean. The accuracy of the technique depends on the patient's body thickness and technical issues, but it has been shown to be reliable particularly for assessment of fat mass in a variety of disease states.[149]

In summary, nutritional assessment is an essential part of the evaluation of every patient. However, for clinical purposes, such assessment is predominantly based on patient history and examination. Although laboratory tests may be useful in the evaluation of specific nutrient deficiencies and to monitor for complications of nutrition support, they have little place in the diagnosis of malnutrition.

NUTRITION SUPPORT

Malnutrition has been defined as any disorder of nutrition status, including disorders resulting from a deficiency of nutrient intake, impaired nutrient metabolism, or overnutrition. However, the term *malnutrition* is commonly used to refer to undernutrition.[150] The prevalence of undernutrition among hospital inpatients has been shown to be as high as 40%, and recent studies suggest that this figure has changed little since the problem was first quantified more than 40 years ago.[151]

TABLE 46.5   Effects of Malnutrition in Hospital Inpatients

Effect	Consequence
Impaired immune response	Infection
Decreased muscle strength	Falls
	Inactivity: pressure sores, thromboembolism
	Poor respiratory effort: chest infection
Impaired wound healing	Infection
	Delayed fracture healing
Impaired thermoregulation	Hypothermia
Reduced psychosocial functioning	Apathy, depression
Specific nutrient deficiencies	Anemia
In childhood and adolescence	Growth failure
	Delayed puberty
	Impaired neurocognitive development

TABLE 46.6   Prediction Equations Used to Estimate Energy Requirements

Schofield Equation

Age (year)	Male BMR (kcal/24 h)	Female BMR (kcal/24 h)
19–30	15.0W + 690	14.8W + 485
31–60	11.4W + 870	8.1W + 842
>60	11.7W + 585	9.0W + 656

Harris-Benedict Equation

Male basal energy expenditure = 66.5 + (13.8W) + (5H) − (6.8A) (kcal/24 h)

Female basal energy expenditure = 665 + (9.6W) + (1.8H) − (4.7A) (kcal/24 h)

A, Age in years; *BMR*, basal metabolic rate; *H*, height in centimeters; *W*, weight in kilograms.

Malnutrition is a determinant of clinical outcome,[152] its effect on outcome depends on factors such as its extent, the patient's age, and the nature of their underlying illness, but even in young, previously healthy patients (e.g., admitted after trauma), it is associated with increased morbidity and mortality and prolonged hospital stays (Table 46.5). Patients who are undernourished or at risk of becoming so need to be identified and referred for further assessment.

Any decision to administer nutrition support needs to consider the patient's preexisting nutritional status, the effect of any underlying disease process on the patient's current or anticipated future intake, and whether nutrition support is likely to improve clinical outcome or quality of life. Nutrition support should certainly be considered for patients defined as being malnourished by any of:
- BMI below 18.5 kg/m²
- Unintentional weight loss of more than 10% within the past 3 to 6 months
- BMI below 20 kg/m² and unintentional weight loss of more than 5% within the last 3 to 6 months
  and for those defined as being at risk of malnutrition by
- having eaten little or nothing for more than 5 days
- and/or likely to eat nothing for at least a further 5 days
- Having poor absorptive capacity
- and/or high nutrient losses
- and/or increased nutritional needs (e.g., from catabolism)[153]

Nutritional Requirements

In adults, energy requirements are about 25 to 35 kcal/24 hours. Requirements can be matched more specifically to the needs of individual patients, for example, using calorimetry or prediction equations (Table 46.6).[154] The results of calculations from prediction equations should be adjusted to predict extra energy requirements in specific clinical circumstances (e.g., sepsis or burns), which can be achieved using nomograms or subjective addition of a stress factor.

Protein requirements in healthy adults average about 0.8 g/kg/24 hours, although hospitalized patients' requirements are likely to be increased and may be as high as 1.5 g/kg/24

hours in severe sepsis or after significant trauma. Protein is the only nitrogen-containing macronutrient; hence, requirements are sometimes expressed in grams of nitrogen. Approximately 16% of protein is nitrogen, and so calculations of protein requirements as grams of protein can be estimated by multiplying grams of nitrogen by 6.25. Both energy and protein requirements are higher in infants and children, owing to the needs for growth.

Nutritional Supplementation

Consumption of a standard diet should result in intake of sufficient energy and nutrients for the majority of people and should be encouraged, if possible, before considering any form of nutritional support. Many patients require assistance to eat because of non-nutritional difficulties such as impaired dexterity, cognitive impairment, or poor vision. A "protected mealtimes" policy, in which routine clinical activities are stopped, facilitates a quiet environment for patients to enjoy their meals and ensures staff are best able to assist. Dietary intake may also be improved by addressing other problems, for example, offering antiemetics for nausea; ensuring soft food for patients with swallowing difficulties; and resolving constipation, which, untreated, can cause anorexia and abdominal pain. Nutritional intake can be increased by providing snacks between meals and by food enrichment measures such as the addition of butter to potatoes and grated cheese or cream to soups.

If it is not possible to achieve sufficient energy intake with standard diet alone, nutritional supplements are available that are intended to be taken in addition to food. Their exact content and flavor differ among manufacturers. Modular supplements typically contain just one macronutrient and are supplied as powders that can be added to drinks or soups and to foods such as puddings or mashed potatoes. They are particularly useful for patients who require additional protein or energy and whose ability to take food orally is not impaired.

Nutritionally complete supplements are available in a range of flavors, presented as milkshakes or savory soups; they usually provide about 300 kcal/carton. Juice-style products are available and may be more palatable to some patients, but they tend not to be nutritionally complete.

Enteral Nutrition

Patients who are unable to achieve optimal nutritional status by oral feeding and those who cannot or will not eat are candidates for enteral nutrition support (Box 46.3). Enteral feeding involves the provision of nutrients directly into the GI tract via a feeding tube. The only absolute contraindication to enteral feeding is mechanical obstruction of the GI tract.

There are various routes for enteral feeding. Considerations for site of delivery include how long feeding is likely to be required and whether gastric emptying is delayed. Access to the GI tract through the nose using a nasogastric, nasoduodenal, or nasojejunal tube are options when feeding is likely to be required for less than about 4 weeks. For longer-term feeding, the use of a semipermanent tube placed directly into the gut is preferred. This is most commonly achieved by percutaneous endoscopic gastrostomy; the anterior gastric wall is punctured with a cannula, and a guidewire placed through it. Using endoscopy, the guidewire is retrieved, and the feeding tube is passed over it into the stomach (Fig. 46.15).

Composition of Enteral Feeds

It is possible to administer puréed, strained food through nasogastric tubes, but because of concerns about tube blockage and contamination, commercially prepared feeds are used in preference. Many are available, and they can be broadly classified into polymeric, disease-specific, immune-modulating, and elemental feeds. Standard polymeric feeds are nutritionally complete, containing vitamins and trace elements, and are usually isotonic. Most contain intact protein, glucose polymers or maltodextrin, and long-chain triglycerides. Feeds containing fiber are available and tend to reduce the occurrence of constipation associated with long-term enteral feeding. Disease-specific feeds are tailored to the requirements of particular patient groups, for example, high-energy feeds can be useful for those with high requirements or whose fluid intake is restricted. Feeds for patients with renal failure have reduced amounts of sodium, potassium, and phosphate but increased water-soluble vitamins to compensate for losses caused by dialysis. Immune-modulating enteral formulas containing nutrients such as glutamine, arginine, and ω-fatty acids, either alone or in combination, have been developed, but the situations when they may be of benefit are not fully determined.[155] Elemental feeds contain nitrogen as individual amino acids and fat as medium-chain triglycerides. Such feeds therefore confer advantages in patients in whom absorptive capacity is impaired (e.g., severe inflammatory bowel disease, acute pancreatitis).

Complications of Enteral Feeding

Enteral feeding is effective and safe in the majority of patients, but it is not without complications (Table 46.7).

Malposition of a feeding tube can result in its siting in the bronchial tree, or occasionally intracranially, and it is essential the position is checked before the introduction of feeding. This can be achieved by radiography or, for a tube sited in the stomach, by ensuring that the aspirate is acidic (pH of 5.5) using pH paper.[156]

Diarrhea is common in patients receiving enteral feeding, but such patients may, because of the nature of their illness, be receiving other preparations such as antibiotics or nonabsorbable carbohydrate (e.g., sorbitol in medications) that may be the cause. Aspiration of stomach contents into the lungs may occur, resulting in pneumonitis or asphyxia; the

---

BOX 46.3 Indications for Enteral Feeding

Malnutrition
Impaired swallowing (e.g., motor neuron disease)
Inability to eat (e.g., critical illness)
Upper gastrointestinal obstruction (e.g., esophageal stricture)
High requirements (e.g., burns, trauma)
Loss of appetite (e.g., anorexia nervosa)

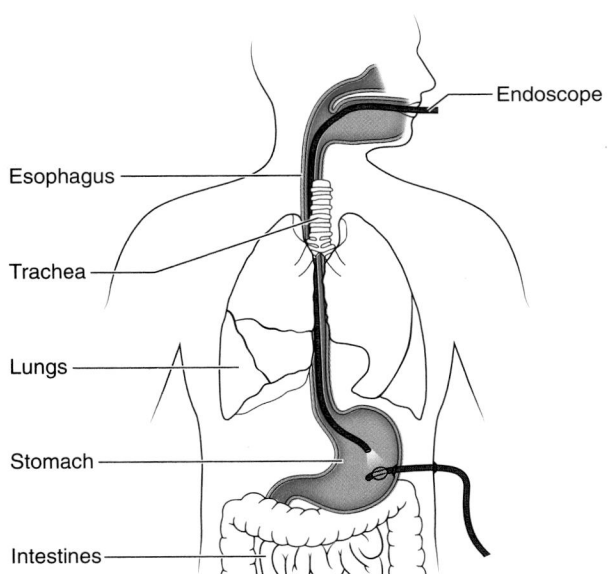

FIGURE 46.15 Placement of a percutaneous endoscopic gastrostomy tube.

TABLE 46.7 Complications of Enteral Feeding

Type	Complication
Insertion	Nasal damage
	Bronchial placement
	Intracranial placement
	Perforation
Postinsertion	Blockage
	Local physical damage
	Displacement
Gastrointestinal	Reflux
	• Esophagitis
	• Aspiration
	Intolerance
	• Nausea
	• Bloating
	• Abdominal pain
	• Diarrhea
Metabolic	Refeeding syndrome
	Hyperglycemia
	Electrolyte abnormalities
	Fluid overload

BOX 46.4 Indications for Parenteral Nutrition

Intestinal obstruction
Paralytic ileus
Surgical resection or short bowel
Fistulae
Dysmotility
Inflammatory bowel disease

BOX 46.5 Complications of Central Venous Catheterization

Air embolism
Arterial puncture
Pneumothorax
Mechanical problems
- Occlusion
- Displacement
- Fracture
Infection
Thrombosis

---

risk of this occurring is reduced by nursing patients receiving enteral feed with the bed head elevated by at least 30 degrees. Biochemical complications can occur during enteral feeding (see later) but less commonly than during PN.

Parenteral Nutrition

PN refers to the administration of nutrition support directly into the blood using a venous catheter. PN has been shown to be delivered most effectively by a multidisciplinary nutrition support team whose members may include a clinician, nutrition specialist nurse, dietician, pharmacist, and chemical pathologist or clinical biochemist. The term *total parenteral nutrition* is sometimes used synonymously with *parenteral nutrition*, but the latter may be supplementary to enteral feeding and does not need to provide a patient's total nutritional requirements.

Indications

PN is reserved for patients who are unsuitable for enteral feeding because of the presence of GI dysfunction that limits the absorption of nutrients (Box 46.4).

It may be difficult at the outset to predict how long PN will be required. For the majority of patients, PN is administered in hospital for less than 2 weeks, with oral or enteral feeding then being reintroduced. However, for some patients, the nature of their underlying pathology is such that their requirement for PN is lifelong. Such patients generally self-administer their feed at home, often at night, and may be able to continue with the activities of daily living relatively unencumbered.

Route of Administration

PN can be administered via catheters placed into peripheral or central veins. A potential advantage of peripheral PN is the ease of establishing access, which may prevent a delay in initiating nutrition support. However, the infusion of a large volume or of a solution of high osmolarity is likely to cause phlebitis. It can be challenging to formulate a feed suitable for peripheral administration that is still able to meet nutritional requirements, and this route is not generally recommended. Central venous access for PN may be achieved using a peripherally inserted central catheter (PICC) or nontunneled central venous catheter (suitable for short-term use) or a tunneled catheter or implantable device (for long-term feeding). The insertion of central venous catheters involves placement of the tip in the jugular vein or superior vena cava and is not without potential complications (Box 46.5).

Composition of Parenteral Feeds

PN solutions contain carbohydrate, amino acids, fat, vitamins, trace elements, and water. Delivery can be accomplished using a single "all-in-one" bag, although the fat emulsion may

---

TABLE 46.8 Typical Content of a Typical Parenteral Feed for an Adult Male Patient

Constituent	Amount
Nitrogen	12–14 g
Glucose	250 g
Fat	100 g
Sodium	80 mmol
Potassium	60 mmol
Calcium	5 mmol
Magnesium	10 mmol
Phosphate	25 mmol
Micronutrients	see Table 46.9
Total energy (non-nitrogen)	2000 kcal
Total volume	2500 mL

---

be infused separately out of preference or for reasons of stability. Feeds can be compounded individually in a suitable sterile production facility. However, various solutions are commercially available, and for the majority of patients, one of these can be selected with minor additions made to the electrolyte content according to specific requirements (Table 46.8).

The feed should meet the patient's energy needs, but carbohydrate and lipid should not exceed 7 and 2.5 g/kg/24 hours, respectively, to minimize adverse metabolic sequelae. Carbohydrate is provided as glucose, protein as a mixture of essential and nonessential amino acids, and fat as fatty acids. Previously, fat was supplied as long-chain triglyceride from a soya bean emulsion. However, concerns about impairment of the immune system by long-chain triglycerides have led to use of structured lipids, a combination of long- and medium-chain fatty acids, which tends to maintain a more favorable plasma LDL-to-HDL ratio, and ω3-fatty acids (fish oils), which have been shown to have beneficial effects on eicosanoid production. To prevent EFA deficiency, 1 to 2% of daily energy requirements should be derived from linoleic and about 0.5% from α-linolenic acid. The nitrogen component is supplied as a mixture of L-amino acids, essential amino acids comprising about 40% of the total. Enrichment with particular amino acids may be helpful in particular circumstances, for example, cysteine, which is considered to be conditionally essential in preterm neonates, and the branched chain amino acids leucine, isoleucine, and valine, which may be beneficial in hepatic encepahalopathy.[157] Glutamine is not an essential amino acid (strictly, an amine), but it may become so during metabolic stress. There is evidence to suggest that glutamine supplementation may improve outcome in certain groups of patients (e.g., those with critical illness as a result of burns or trauma), but its use is not recommended in critically ill patients with shock and multiorgan failure.[158]

The electrolyte content of a typical parenteral feed is shown in Table 46.8, although individual requirements vary, particularly if there are ongoing losses such as from vomiting, diarrhea, stoma, drains, or fistulae.

Early studies establishing micronutrient requirements were based on enteral rather than parenteral feeding, and the control of absorption of some vitamins and trace elements is exerted at the level of the gut. The initiation of long-term PN led to recognition of deficiencies and toxicities of some micronutrients, from which their parenteral requirements have been better defined. Further modification of current commercial preparations is suggested to meet the current recommendations (Table 46.9).

Choline is a quaternary amine, endogenously synthesized from methionine. It is technically not a vitamin but is considered an essential nutrient. There is evidence of benefit from its inclusion in PN solutions, but at present, no suitable preparations exist.

Monitoring Nutrition Support

Patients receiving nutrition support by enteral or parenteral routes require careful monitoring (e.g., for vomiting, diarrhea and gastric distension, and of fistula output) to ascertain their ability to tolerate diet and the presence of potential complications (e.g., nasal erosion from enteral tubes, infection or thrombophlebitis associated with IV lines). Their dietary requirements should be reviewed and the actual amount of feed administered noted. Fluid balance should be assessed from charted information, and clinical signs of dehydration or fluid overload should be sought. Particularly in patients on long-term feeding, measurement of body weight and skin folds, and in children, assessment of growth, should be part of monitoring.

For PN, biochemical monitoring should be performed, initially daily and then (when it is obvious that the patient is stable) less often. One suggested monitoring scheme is shown in Table 46.10; for patients receiving enteral or oral nutrition support, biochemical monitoring may be used selectively, particularly in those who are at high risk of refeeding syndrome (see later) or metabolically unstable.

TABLE 46.9   Current Recommendations for Adult Daily Parenteral Micronutrient Requirements

Micronutrient	Requirement
FAT-SOLUBLE VITAMINS	
Vitamin A	990 μg (3300 IU)
Vitamin D	5 μg (200 IU)
Vitamin E	10 mg (10 IU)
Vitamin K	150 μg
WATER-SOLUBLE VITAMINS	
Vitamin B$_1$ (thiamin)	6 mg
Vitamin B$_2$ (riboflavin)	3.6 mg
Vitamin B$_3$ (niacin)	40 mg
Vitamin B$_5$ (pantothenic acid)	15 mg
Vitamin B$_6$ (pyridoxine)	6 mg
Vitamin B$_{12}$ (cyanocobalamin)	5 μg
Vitamin C (ascorbic acid)	200 mg
Folate	600 μg
Biotin	60 μg
TRACE ELEMENTS[a]	
Copper	0.3–0.5 mg
Chromium	10–15 μg
Manganese	0.06–0.1 mg
Selenium	20–60 μg
Zinc	2.5–5 mg

[a]Fluoride (0.57 to 1.45 mg), iodine (10 to 130 μg), iron (1 to 1.95 mg), molybdenum (10 to 25 μg), and cobalt (0 to 1.67 μg) are routinely added to parenteral nutrition solutions in Europe but not in the United States.
Vanek VW, Borum P, Buchman A, et al. ASPEN Position Paper Recommendations for changes in commercially available parenteral multivitamin and multi-trace element products. *Nutr Clin Pract* 2012;27:400–91.

TABLE 46.10   Protocol for Laboratory Monitoring of Nutrition Support

Parameter	Frequency
Sodium, potassium, urea, creatinine	Baseline Daily until stable; then 1–2 times a week
Glucose	Baseline 1 or 2 times a day (or more if needed) until stable Then weekly
Magnesium, phosphate	Baseline Daily if risk of refeeding syndrome, 3 times a week until stable, then weekly
Liver profile, including INR	Baseline Twice weekly until stable; then weekly
Calcium, albumin	Baseline Then weekly
C-reactive protein	Baseline Then 2 or 3 times a week until stable
Zinc, copper	Baseline Then every 2–4 weeks depending on results
Selenium	Baseline if risk of depletion Subsequent frequency dependent upon baseline
Full blood count	Baseline 1–2 times a week until stable; then weekly
Iron, ferritin	Baseline Then every 3–6 months
Folate, vitamin B$_{12}$	Baseline Then every 2–4 weeks
Manganese	Every 3–6 months if on home PN
Vitamin D	Every 6 months if on long-term PN

INR, International normalized ratio; *PN,* parenteral nutrition.
From National Institute for Health and Care Excellence (2016) NICE Pathways: Nutrition support in adults London: NICE. Available from https://pathways.nice.org.uk/pathways/nutrition-support-in-adults. Reproduced with permission.

Laboratory markers can be used as part of nutritional assessment but have a limited role in ongoing monitoring of patients receiving nutritional support.

Complications of Parenteral Nutrition

In addition to problems secondary to the use of IV catheters, there are various complications of PN, as summarized in Box 46.6.

Fluid and electrolyte imbalance. It is important to ensure that PN includes sufficient fluid to avoid dehydration but excess fluid, particularly in patients with co-existing comorbidities, may lead to overhydration with edema or congestive cardiac failure. Accurate fluid balance charts and regular weight measurement are essential to support assessment of hydration status.

Mild electrolyte disturbance is common in patients receiving PN, particularly when potential pathophysiologic changes in electrolytes were not anticipated at the time of prescription of the feed (e.g., the development of renal failure leading to hyperkalemia). Hypokalemia may occur when replacement is insufficient to cover losses from fistula or kidneys or in patients who become anabolic after a period of catabolism. Mild hyponatremia in patients receiving PN is often multifactorial and may not require additional sodium, but supplementation should be given in patients with obviously high losses, (e.g., from a fistula or drain). Hypernatremia may be the result of sodium excess or water deficiency. Hypocalcemia may occur, particularly in the presence of hypomagnesemia.

The amount of calcium and magnesium that can be included in PN solution may be limited by the potential formation of insoluble precipitates with phosphate. This is dependent upon the concentration added and on the final pH of the solution and may vary with the amino acid source used. Other causes of hypomagnesemia include GI loss and secondary to drugs (e.g., diuretics and proton pump inhibitors). Hypophosphatemia tends to occur most often at the initiation of feeding as a consequence of rapid cellular uptake.

Refeeding syndrome. The refeeding syndrome describes the characteristic metabolic abnormalities that can occur when malnourished individuals are aggressively refed. It has been described after oral, enteral, and parenteral refeeding but is most commonly described with IV administration. Excess fluid and sodium intake may lead to volume expansion manifest clinically as heart failure and biochemically as hyponatremia. Carbohydrate administration increases demand for intracellular phosphate to synthesize intermediates in the glycolytic pathway (e.g., fructose 1-6-biphosphate and ATP), leading to hypophosphatemia and neuromuscular, cardiovascular, and respiratory sequelae. Carbohydrate metabolism may also increase the demand for magnesium and thiamin, precipitating deficiency.[159]

Recent consensus recommendations give the criteria for diagnosis of refeeding syndrome as a decrease in the concentration of at least one of phosphate, potassium, or magnesium of 10 to 20% (mild), 20 to 30% (moderate), or greater than 30% and/or organ dysfunction resulting from a decrease in any of these and/or due to thiamin deficiency (severe) and occurring within five days of initiating the feeding intervention.[160]

It is important to anticipate, and therefore avoid, the refeeding syndrome by identifying patients at particular risk of refeeding syndrome before starting nutrition support (Box 46.7). In such patients, nutrition support, both enteral and parenteral, should be initiated cautiously, for example, 100 to 150 g dextrose or 10 to 20 kcal/kg for the first 24 hours, increasing to meet target requirements over several days. The recommended daily allowance of thiamin is included in enteral and parenteral solutions but, for those at risk of refeeding

---

BOX 46.6   Complications of Parenteral Nutrition

Electrolyte imbalance
Refeeding syndrome
Hyperglycemia
Hypoglycemia
Hyperlipidemia
Hepatobiliary disease
Bone disease

BOX 46.7   Patients at Particular Risk of Refeeding Syndrome

	Moderate Risk (Two Criteria Needed)	Significant Risk (One Criterion Needed)
Body mass index	16–18.8 kg/m^2	<16 kg/m^2
Weight loss	5% in 1 month	7.5% in 3 months or >10% in 6 months
Calorie intake	None/negligible for 5–6 days or <75% of estimated energy requirements for >7 days during an acute episode or <75% of estimated energy requirements for >1 month	None/negligible for >7 days or <50% of estimated energy requirements for >5 days during an acute episode or <50% of estimated energy requirements for >1 month
Abnormal prefeeding serum potassium, phosphorus or magnesium concentrations	Minimally low concentration or currently normal but recently lower necessitating minimal or single-dose supplementation	Moderate or significantly low concentrations or currently normal but recent lower necessitating significant or multi-dose supplementation
Loss of subcutaneous fat	Evidence of moderate loss	Evidence of severe loss
Loss of muscle mass	Evidence of mild or moderate loss	Evidence of severe loss
Higher-risk comorbidities (e.g., AIDS, cancer, chronic alcohol and drug use disorder, postbariatric surgery etc.)	Moderate disease	Severe disease

syndrome, additional thiamin (100 mg) should be given prior to initiation of feeding or glucose-containing fluids. Additional supplementation of 100 mg for 5 to 7 days is recommended for those patients with severe starvation, chronic alcoholism, or other high-risk factors and/or clinical features of deficiency.[160]

Hyperglycemia. Hyperglycemia is a relatively frequent occurrence in patients receiving PN, particularly in elderly adults and those with sepsis or preexisting glucose intolerance. The stress of critical illness acts to increase endogenous glucose production, with a tendency to insulin resistance. The dextrose of PN may fail to suppress gluconeogenesis and further contributes to hyperglycemia.[161] It should be treated using IV insulin, aiming for strict glycemic control.

Hypoglycemia. Rebound hypoglycemia can occur if PN is terminated abruptly. However, it occurs less frequently now that lipid-containing "all-in-one" bags are used.

Hypertriglyceridemia. Hypertriglyceridemia may occur in patients receiving PN, particularly those with intercurrent diabetes mellitus, renal failure, hepatic disease, or pancreatitis.

Hepatobiliary disease. After several weeks of PN, it is common to find abnormalities of plasma bilirubin concentration and liver enzyme activities. Particularly in infants and children, prolonged PN may be associated with more marked changes, including steatosis, fibrosis, and cirrhosis; rarely, these are of sufficient severity that liver transplantation is required. The pathogenesis of such PN-associated liver disease includes a reduction in the secretion of regulatory hormones from the gut, leading to cholestasis, which in turn may facilitate accumulation of toxic substances such as methionine and trace elements that contribute to hepatotoxicity. Polyunsaturated fatty acids, as found in soybean emulsion, tend to lead to the accumulation of lipid particles in the liver and high plasma concentrations of potentially toxic polysterols. Lipid restriction was used in the past to reduce the extent of exposure and attempt to attenuate the deleterious effects. It is hoped that the newer lipid substrates now available will be beneficial. Parenteral fish oil is thought to be of benefit by inducing signaling pathways that inhibit de novo lipogenesis and stimulate β-oxidation of fatty acids.[162]

Metabolic bone disease. Metabolic bone disease is a complication of long-term PN and may present with bone pain, as evidence of demineralization on imaging, or as biochemical abnormalities. Etiologic factors include malnutrition, vitamin and mineral deficiencies (e.g., of vitamin D), toxic contaminants in PN solutions (e.g., aluminum, fluoride), and

related medications. Illness severe enough to necessitate PN may be associated with factors predisposing to bone disease (e.g., low body weight, immobility, and amenorrhea). In patients with ulcerative colitis or Crohn disease, the inflammatory process itself has been implicated as a factor in metabolic bone disease.[163]

OBESITY

Obesity is a major public health problem. It is commonly defined in adults using BMI, that is, weight (kg) divided by the square of height (m). Those with a BMI in the range of 25 to 29.9 kg/m^2 are termed overweight, those with a BMI of 30 to 39.9 kg/m^2 are classified as obese, and those with a BMI of 40 kg/m^2 or greater are classified as severely obese. This index is simple to obtain and has been used in the majority of studies evaluating the health effects of obesity. However, it is independent of distribution of body fat and does not allow for variation with ethnic group, age, or gender. Obesity may also be defined in terms of an increased percentage of body fat (>25% in men; >33% in women). Measurement of waist circumference provides a marker of abdominal fat stores that gives an indicator of long-term health risk, particularly cardiovascular disease and diabetes mellitus.[164] In children, obesity is usually defined as a BMI of the 95th centile or above for age.

Prevalence

Worldwide, the prevalence of obesity has nearly tripled since 1975. In 2016, it was estimated that more than 1.9 billion adults were overweight, and of them, 650 million were obese. Over 340 million children and adolescents were overweight or obese in 2016 and, in 2019, 38 million children less than 5 years were overweight or obese.[165]

Regulation of Energy Intake

Body weight tends to remain relatively constant despite variations in daily energy expenditure and food intake. Regulation of appetite is central to the pathophysiology of obesity and involves two-way communication between the central nervous system (CNS) and peripheral tissues, principally the GI system and adipose stores. In the brain, the hypothalamus is the area that is integral to the control of energy balance and acts to coordinate input from hormones, neural stimuli (e.g., from gastric distension), and input from the cerebral cortex (e.g., from the sight and smell of food) (Fig. 46.16).

Areas of the Brain Involved in Feeding Behavior

The hypothalamus contains a number of discrete neuronal areas, including the arcuate nucleus (ARC), paraventricular nucleus (PVN), lateral hypothalamic area (LHA), ventromedian nucleus, and dorsomedial nucleus. The ARC is adjacent to the median eminence, one of the areas of the brain characterized by extensive vasculature and deficient blood–brain barrier. Within the ARC, there are two distinct populations of neurons: One expresses the orexigenic (appetite-stimulating) factors neuropeptide Y (NYY) and Agouti-related protein (AgRP); the other expresses the anorectic (appetite-suppressing) factors cocaine-and-amphetamine-regulated transcript (CART) and pro-opiomelanocortin (POMC). The anorexigenic peptide α-melanocyte–stimulating hormone (α-MSH) is the result of post-translation modification processing of

---

POINTS TO REMEMBER

Nutrition Support
- Techniques for nutrition support range from the provision of general or specific supplements taken by mouth through various techniques of enteral feeding to parenteral feeding (i.e., IV, bypassing the gut).
- Enteral techniques should always be considered before providing PN.
- Complications of artificial nutrition relate both to the means of delivery (i.e., placement of feeding tube or provision of IV access) and the feed itself (e.g., refeeding syndrome and other metabolic disturbances). Infection is a major potential complication, but it should be preventable with scrupulous adherence to management techniques.

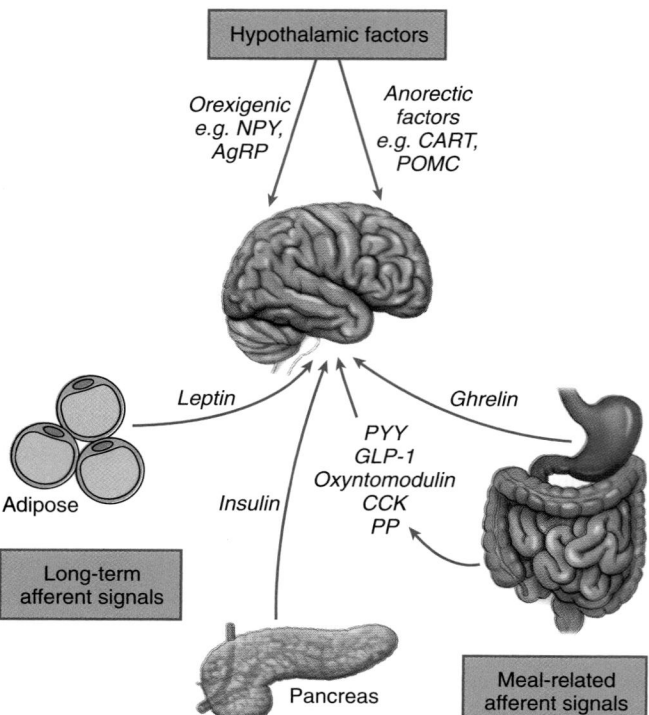

FIGURE 46.16 Regulation of food intake. *CART*, Cocaine-and-amphetamine-regulated transcript; *GLP*, glucagon-like peptide; *POMC*, pro-opiomelanocortin; *PYY*, peptide YY. (Illustrations adapted from Elsevier Image Collection.)

POMC. It binds to melanocortin-3 and -4 (MC3R and MC4R) receptors, which leads to reduced food intake and increased energy expenditure. Serotonin acts on POMC neurons through 5HT-2C receptors to cause anorexia. Peptides secreted from the PVN have a net catabolic effect, and this area of the hypothalamus also sends sympathetic signals to peripheral tissues, resulting in increased lipolysis and fatty acid oxidation.[166]

The ventromedial hypothalamic nucleus (VHN) receives neuronal projections from the ARC and projects axons to the brainstem, ARC, DMN, and LHA. It contains neurons able to sense glucose and leptin and is thus important in detection of satiety and in glucose homeostasis. In contrast, the LHA contains neuronal populations producing the orexigenic peptides melanin-concentrating hormone (MCH) and orexins (also called hypocretins). The effect of orexins on food intake is thought to be via a generalized increase in arousal because deficiency is associated with daytime somnolence, but MCH is believed to act centrally as an endogenous orexigen.[167,168] Other hypothalamic factors include endocannabinoids, which increase food intake, and nesfatin-1, which decreases it.

The brainstem is also important in the regulation of food intake. Satiety signals from the GI tract relay to the nucleus of the tractus solitarius (NTS) via the vagus nerve. The NTS is close to the area postrema, which, similar to the median eminence, has a deficient blood–brain barrier and is well placed for integrating hormonal and neural signals. There are extensive connections between the PVN and the NTS.

The midbrain is concerned with the desire to eat for pleasure, so-called hedonic feeding. The intake of palatable food elicits release of dopamine with activation of further neural pathways.

Peripheral Signals Regulating Food Intake

A number of circulating factors play a part in the regulation of food intake. Leptin is the product of the *Lep* (formerly *ob*) gene. It is produced by adipocytes in proportion to body mass. Circulating leptin enters the brain and binds to receptors in the ARC, bringing about increased activity of POMC/CART neurons and decreased activity of NPY/AgRP neurons with consequent reduction in food intake and energy expenditure. Leptin is also produced in the stomach, where it acts to amplify local satiety signals and has an effect on the threshold of sweet taste perception.[169]

Insulin is secreted from the pancreas postprandially, and fasting plasma insulin concentrations are related to fat mass. In the brain, insulin binds receptors in the ARC neurons with activation of POMC neurons and inhibition of NPY/AgRP neurons.

Appetite-regulating Gastrointestinal Hormones

In addition to the regulation of glucose homeostasis, insulin has anorectic effects within the CNS. Gut hormones are important in the regulation of energy intake, as well as for digestion and absorption of nutrients. Ghrelin is secreted from the stomach in response to fasting and acts via stimulation of NPY and AgRP neurons in the hypothalamus to increase food intake. Satiety hormones secreted from the gut include peptide YY (PYY), pancreatic polypeptide, cholecystokinin, and glucagon-like peptide-1 (GLP-1). Nutrients themselves are also important for satiety. Glucose, lipids, particularly long-chain fatty acids and amino acids, specifically leucine, have all been implicated.[170]

Pathogenesis

For obesity to develop, there must be an imbalance between energy intake and energy expenditure, and various mechanisms may contribute to this (Table 46.11).

Mealtimes are increasingly a focus of social and pleasurable activity rather than being seen purely for nutritional purposes, and this, coupled with a generalized reduction in physical activity, is likely to have contributed to the increase in obesity, particularly in children. Family studies have been used to investigate the genetic contribution to body weight and have estimated a heritability of 40 to 70%. Environmental factors, such as dietary change, may interact in patients

TABLE 46.11   Mechanisms of Development of Obesity

Mechanism	Example
Genetic	Monogenic disorders, e.g., MC4R mutation leptin deficiency, POMC deficiency
	Syndromes: Prader-Willi, Bardet-Biedl, Alstrom
Psychosocial	Alcohol, depression, eating disorders
Neurologic	Brain injury, brain tumor, post-cranial irradiation, hypothalamic obesity
Endocrine	Cushing syndrome, hypothyroidism, growth hormone deficiency
Drug induced	Antipsychotics, anticonvulsants, glucocorticoids, oral contraceptives
Infection	Adenovirus 36

BOX 46.8 Complications Associated With Obesity

Type 2 diabetes mellitus
Hypertension
Dyslipidemia
Heart disease
- Coronary artery disease
- Heart failure
- Atrial fibrillation
Cerebrovascular disease
Respiratory disease
- Asthma
- Obstructive sleep apnea
Gastrointestinal system:
- Gallstones
- Nonalcoholic fatty liver disease
- Gastrointestinal reflux
Cancer: breast, endometrium, colon
Osteoarthritis
Obstetrics and gynecologic problems
- Gestational diabetes
- Pregnancy-induced hypertension
- Polycystic ovarian syndrome
- Infertility
Psychosocial dysfunction

BOX 46.9 Considerations in the Management of Obese Patients

Screening for chronic conditions associated with obesity (e.g., type 2 diabetes mellitus, hypertension)
Identification of any medications potentially contributing to obesity (e.g., antipsychotics, some antiepileptics)
Identification of contributing factors (e.g., educational, socioeconomic)
Screening for secondary causes of obesity if clinically indicated (e.g., hypothyroidism)
Adherence to national cancer screening guidelines because of increased risk of malignancy in obesity

with an underlying polygenic trait. Monogenic causes of obesity have also been described. Rare abnormalities include mutations of the leptin gene and its receptor and of POMC. Mutations of the melanocortin receptor MC4R have been found in 1 to 2.5% of people with a BMI greater than 30 kg/ m^2, making it one of the most common genetic conditions. Obesity is also part of various syndromic disorders, often in association with dysmorphism, learning disability, and organ-specific abnormalities (e.g., Down and Prader-Willi syndromes). It may be that there is a role for inflammatory and infectious agents in obesity. The prevalence of certain viruses and concentrations of inflammatory markers has been found to be elevated in obese individuals.[171]

Complications

Significant obesity (BMI > 35 kg/m^2) has been linked to higher mortality, but the association with lesser degrees of obesity with mortality is less clear.[172] Complications of obesity are shown in Box 46.8. Not all obese people develop complications, and the age of onset of obesity, physical activity and fitness, distribution of body fat, and insulin resistance may be relevant to their occurrence. It has been estimated that the share of total health care spending on obesity-related illness in the United States rose from 20.6% in 2005 to 28.2% in 2013,[173] and if the trend in obesity continues, costs could rise by up to $66 billion a year by 2030.[174]

Treatment

Ideally, obesity should be prevented. When obesity has developed, modest weight loss is relatively easy to achieve in the short term; a relatively small reduction in body weight of only 3 to 5% that is maintained can produce clinically relevant health improvement, while larger amounts of weight loss can reduce additional risk factors for cardiovascular

disease.[175] However, long-term maintenance of weight loss is challenging.

In addition to offering treatment for the obesity itself, other considerations should form part of the management of obese patients (Box 46.9).

Public health programs may have a place in both prevention and to assist in management. Various approaches have been recommended, which include taxing food products deemed to be unhealthy; limiting advertising of such products, particularly to children; and providing nutritional information as part of food packaging using a "traffic-light" system.[176]

Given the magnitude of the health problem posed by obesity, there is perhaps scope for leaders from public health, industry, academia, and decision makers to consider legislative changes that will promote lifestyle changes to reduce obesity.

There are three main modalities for targeting obesity: dietary and lifestyle modification, pharmacotherapy, and bariatric surgery. Recent clinical practice guidelines recommend that diet, exercise, and behavioral modification should be included in all obesity management programs with pharmacotherapy used as an adjunct in those with a BMI greater than 30 kg/m^2 ($\geq$27 kg/m^2 with comorbidity) and bariatric surgery in those with patients with a BMI greater than 40 kg/m^2 (or BMI $\geq$ 35 kg/m^2 with comorbidity).[177]

Dietary and Lifestyle Measures

Very-low-calorie diets ($\leq$800 kcal/24 hours) are sometimes used and with success, but the requirement for medical supervision means they are rarely economical, and weight is usually regained. The effect of dietary macronutrient composition has been studied extensively but is probably less important than total energy restriction in achieving weight loss. At present, further evidence is needed before very low carbohydrate (ketogenic) diets can be recommended for weight loss.[178] Caloric restriction leads to loss of lean tissue and a reduced basal metabolic rate. Exercise can counteract this. Regular exercise is a predictor of maintenance of weight loss, and the percentage of weight lost as fat and reduction in abdominal and visceral fat is greater with exercise than diet.[179]

A number of commercial and proprietary weight loss programs are available. Some, such as Weight Watchers and Jenny Craig, have proven long-term results; others lack outcome data or show attenuation of effect after 6 months when reported.[179]

Increasingly, the Internet is being used for the delivery of weight loss intervention programs (including Weight Watchers). Such applications potentially overcome many of the barriers to weight loss by providing low-cost, targeted programs with facilities for online support. However, the most effective ways to use modern technologies to support individuals to achieve and maintain weight loss and the long-term efficacy of such strategies is not yet established.[180]

Pharmacotherapy

As already described, the control of appetite involves multiple and complex pathways whose function is integral to survival. Therefore apart from rare patients with genetic defects within specific parts of these pathways, it seems unlikely that a single agent would be able to be completely successful in the treatment of obesity.

Various drugs previously marketed for the treatment of obesity have been withdrawn from clinical use owing to adverse side effects. These include amphetamine (associated with addiction, hypertension, and myocardial toxicity); sibutramine (a monoamine reuptake inhibitor linked to major cardiovascular events); and rimonabant, an endocannabinoid receptor blocker (which precipitated psychiatric disorders).[181]

At present there are differences in the antiobesity drugs approved for use in the United States and Europe, with fewer drugs approved for use in Europe. Orlistat is widely available, on prescription as Xenical, and at a lower dose over the counter as Alli. It is an inhibitor of gastric and pancreatic lipase and acts by reducing dietary fat absorption.[182] Side effects include flatus, steatorrhea, oily spotting, and fecal incontinence; these tend to be worse after the consumption of fatty foods and may assist adherence to diet.

The centrally active agent phentermine is frequently prescribed for short-term use for obesity treatment. Doses higher than 30 mg are not approved, although they are readily available online.

For longer-term use, a number of agents that act as serotonin reuptake inhibitors (e.g., fluoxetine and sertraline) have potential to produce weight loss but are not marketed for this purpose. However, the selective serotonin 2C receptor lorcaserin is approved for the treatment of obesity. Its structure is similar to that of dexfenfluramine, an antiobesity agent that was withdrawn owing to associated cardiac valvulopathy, but the selectivity of lorcaserin is thought to protect against such adverse effects. The combination of phentermine and topiramate (marketed as Qsymia) uses an immediate-release form of phentermine, which is an adrenergic agonist causing appetite suppression, together with a slow-release form of topiramate. Topiramate is also used as an antiepilepsy drug and for prophylaxis of migraine and is thought to cause weight loss by a combination of increased energy expenditure, reduced energy efficiency, and appetite suppression.[183]

The combination of naltrexone and bupropion is known as Contrave (US) and Mysimba (EU). Naltrexone is an opioid antagonist with high affinity for the μ-opioid receptor; bupropion is an atypical antidepressant that inhibits reuptake of dopamine and norepinephrine and is a weak nicotinic acetylcholine receptor antagonist. In combination, these drugs stimulate POMC activity and remove β-endorphin inhibition of POMC.[184]

Liraglutide (Victoza, Saxenda) is a GLP-1 agonist, originally licensed for treatment of type 2 diabetes and now available for treatment of obesity. It binds to GLP-1 receptors in the ARC and activates NPY/AgRP neurons suppressing appetite.[185] In the future, it may prove a successful therapeutic strategy for those without diabetes. Setmelanotide, a MC4R agonist, has been shown to be effective in weight loss trials in patients with POMC or leptin receptor (LEPR)-deficient obesity and is now approved for use.[186]

Bariatric Surgery

The first bariatric procedure to be introduced was jejunal bypass, later abandoned because of its tendency to cause extreme malabsorption. In the past 20 years, there has been a significant increase in the number of patients referred for bariatric surgery, in parallel with advances in operative techniques. The operations used tend to be described according to the anatomic nature of the surgery (Fig. 46.17), but as the sequelae of these operations are becoming better understood, it is becoming clear that they have more wide-reaching effects on physiology. Careful clinical, metabolic, and psychological assessment is essential before surgery is undertaken.

Restrictive procedures. Procedures that were performed in the past include horizontal gastroplasty and vertical banded gastroplasty (VBG), but these have been abandoned with the advent of more modern, laparoscopic procedures. Laparoscopic adjustable gastric banding (LAGB) involves placing a horizontal band around the proximal part of the stomach. The band is inflated using a subcutaneous port. Vertical sleeve gastrectomy involves a vertical gastric resection, leading to creation of a long, narrow gastric reservoir. More recently, intragastric balloons have been developed which can be placed endoscopically or swallowed prior to inflation. These are being offered to some patients prior to definitive surgery. The procedure has potential advantages over surgery with respect to simplicity and cost, but further work is required to define long-term effects.

Combined restrictive and malabsorptive procedures. Roux-en-Y gastric bypass (RYGB) comprises construction of a proximal gastric pouch that empties into a segment of jejunum brought up to the pouch as a Roux-en-Y limb. Biliopancreatic diversion (BPD), with or without duodenal switch, combines a subtotal distal gastrectomy with alteration to the path of the intestines.

Effectiveness. Within the selected population in which it is performed, bariatric surgery is successful in producing weight loss and in reducing the complications and mortality associated with obesity.[187,188] Systematic review has calculated weighted mean excess weight loss of 56.7% for VBG, 45.9% for LABG, 74.1% for BPG, and 58.3% for sleeve gastrectomy.[189] Remission of diabetes has been observed in more than 50% of patients after RYGP and in nearly 20% of those who have had LAGB, with additional patients being able to reduce hypoglycemic therapy and stop insulin administration.[190]

Weight loss plays a role in the amelioration of complications after bariatric surgery, but many of the metabolic changes are evident soon after operation before significant weight loss has occurred. The various surgical procedures lead to different alterations in gut hormones (Table 46.12).

One explanation for the postoperative metabolic effects is a proximal gut hypothesis, which attributes the effect to the

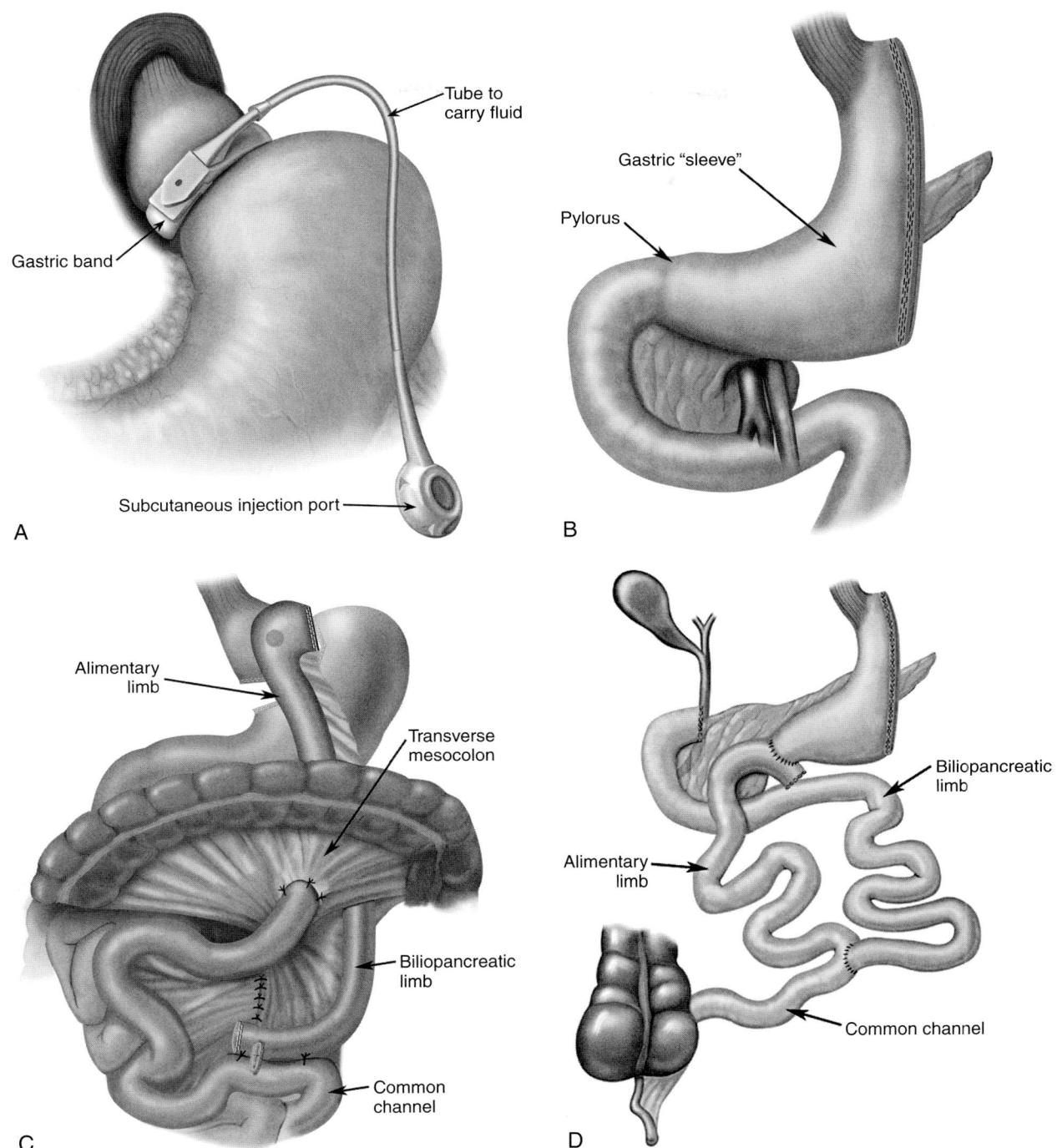

FIGURE 46.17 Common types of bariatric surgery procedures. (A) Adjustable gastric band. (B) Sleeve gastrectomy. (C) Roux-en-Y gastric bypass. (D) Biliopancreatic diversion with duodenal switch. (Reprinted with permissions from *Atlas of metabolic and weight loss surgery* published by Cine-Med, Inc., 2010, http://www.cine-med.com.)

bypassing of the upper GI tract. An alternative distal gut hypothesis proposes faster delivery of nutrients to the distal GI tract, leading to increased enteral hormone secretion.[191] Other contributory factors may include alteration in bile acids, hormones from adipose tissue, and gut flora.[192]

Complications. The average perioperative mortality rate after bariatric surgery has improved with time; short-term mortality after surgery has been estimated to be 0.18%,[193]

with increased adiposity being associated with poorer outcome.[194] Complications of bariatric surgery can be divided into those that occur early (e.g., anastomotic leak or postoperative bleeding) and those that occur later (e.g., nausea and vomiting, small bowel obstruction, band issues, fistulae, strictures, nutritional deficiencies, and dumping syndrome).

Postoperative monitoring. It is important that patients are monitored after bariatric surgery to ensure that they are

TABLE 46.12 Changes in Gut Hormones after Bariatric Surgery

	LAGB	LSG	RYGB	BPD	BPD-DS
GLP-1	→←	↑	↑	↑	↑
GIP	→←	?	↓	↓	↓
PYY	→←	?	↑	↑	↑
Ghrelin	→←	↓↓	↓	→←	↓↓

BPD/DS, Biliopancreatic drainage/duodenal switch; *GIP,* gastrointestinal polypeptide; *GLP-1,* glucagon-like peptide-1; *LAGB,* laparoscopic adjustable gastric band; *LSG, laparoscopic* sleeve gastrectomy; *PYY,* peptide YY; *RYGB,* Roux-en-Y gastric bypass.

meeting their nutritional requirements and to detect any nutritional deficiencies arising secondary to the procedure. All patients should receive multivitamin and mineral supplements postoperatively, the regimen being tailored according to the procedure performed and the patient's requirements. Similarly, postoperative monitoring of biochemical parameters must be performed and may differ according to the nature of the surgery that has been carried out. Various recommendations on postoperative management of bariatric surgery patients have been produced,[195,196] and suggestions for biochemical monitoring are shown in Table 46.13.

TABLE 46.13 Recommended Monitoring After Bariatric Surgery

Investigation	LAGB
Full blood count Biochemistry profile	Monitor annually or more frequently if there are concerns regarding nutritional intake
HbA$_{1c}$ in patients with preoperative diabetes mellitus	Monitor as appropriate
Lipid profile	Monitor in those with dyslipidemia
Vitamin D	Routine monitoring not required Measure if symptoms of vitamin D deficiency
24-h urine calcium excretion	Annually
Bone density (DEXA scan)	At 2 years

Investigation	LSG	RYGB	BPD/DS
Full blood count Biochemistry profile Ferritin, folate, vitamin D, PTH	3, 6, and 12 months in first year Then annually		
HbA$_{1c}$ in patients with preoperative diabetes mellitus	Monitor as appropriate		
Lipid profile	Monitor in those with dyslipidemia		
Vitamin B$_{12}$	6 and 12 months in first year Then annually *No need to monitor if patient receiving IM B$_{12}$ injections*		
Vitamin A	Routine monitoring not required	Measure if there are concerns about steatorrhea or deficiency (e.g., night blindness)	Annually; may need to measure more frequently in pregnancy
Vitamin E	Routine monitoring not required	Measure if concerns re deficiency (e.g., unexplained anemia, neuropathy)	
Vitamin K	Routine monitoring not required	Consider measuring INR if excessive bruising or coagulopathy	
Copper, zinc	Routine monitoring not required	Annually	
Selenium	Routine monitoring not required	Measure if the patient has unexplained fatigue, anemia, metabolic bone disease, chronic diarrhea, or heart failure	
Thiamin	Routine monitoring not required Clinicians should be aware that patients with prolonged vomiting can develop acute thiamin deficiency, which requires urgent treatment		
24-h urine calcium excretion	6 months Then annually		
Bone density (DEXA scan)	At 2 years		

BPD/DS, Biliopancreatic drainage/duodenal switch; *DEXA,* dual energy x-ray absorptiometry; *HBA$_{1c}$,* hemoglobin A$_{1c}$; *IM,* intramuscular; *INR,* international normalized ratio; *LAGB,* laparoscopic adjustable gastric band; *LSG,* laparoscopic sleeve gastrectomy; *PTH,* parathyroid hormone; *RYGB,* Roux-en-Y gastric bypass.

POINTS TO REMEMBER

Obesity

- Obesity is a major, and increasing, public health problem.
- Obesity has numerous adverse consequences, including increased risk of cardiovascular disease, type 2 diabetes, cancer, osteoarthritis, low self-esteem, and social isolation.
- Although obesity is ultimately a result of an energy intake higher than energy expenditure, the factors that contribute to this are complex and involve genetic, cultural, and behavioral factors.
- Dietary and lifestyle changes are fundamental to the successful management of obesity.
- The control of appetite is multifactorial, involving complex neuroendocrine mechanisms, making it unlikely that a single pharmacologic agent will be found to be effective as treatment.
- Bariatric surgery has the greatest long-term success rate in the management of severe obesity and is increasingly the treatment of choice. Techniques can be either restrictive (with the aim of reducing food intake) or involve bypassing a length of gut (reducing absorptive capacity) or a combination of both. Patients are at risk of developing various short- and long-term complications and require long-term follow-up.

ANOREXIA NERVOSA AND BULIMIA NERVOSA

These conditions[197] and their variants are not primarily nutritional disorders but can have profound nutritional consequences. Anorexia nervosa is characterized by low body weight (typically a BMI <17.5 kg/m^2), with weight loss sustained by techniques, including avoidance of food, increased exercise, and purging. The onset is usually in adolescence, and females are more frequently affected than males. Patients have a distorted body image, perceiving themselves to be overweight despite being the opposite.

Numerous endocrine disturbances may occur (Box 46.10). The suppression of the hypothalamo–pituitary–ovarian access in women causes amenorrhea and imposes a risk of osteoporosis. Perhaps surprisingly, specific nutrient deficiencies are uncommon; patients often consume sufficient protein and micronutrients, and the cessation of menstruation removes a major potential cause of iron deficiency. Patients with anorexia nervosa have been noted to have raised total and low-density cholesterol concentrations. Possible mechanisms include increased lipolysis and reduced endogenous cholesterol synthesis with a reduction in LDL clearance.[198] However, there are no definite data to support this being a risk factor for atherosclerosis in the condition.

Management requires input from a psychiatrist and dietician and often a family therapist and other staff. Artificial nutrition may be indicated in the most severe cases but needs to be provided with considerable care as there is a high risk of refeeding syndrome.

Bulimia nervosa is a distinct condition (although it may occur in conjunction or follow anorexia) in which binge eating alternates with self-induced vomiting, purging, and avoidance of food. Weight loss (if present at all) is less than in anorexia, and any endocrine abnormalities are less severe.

BOX 46.10 Neuroendocrine Disturbances in Anorexia Nervosa

The Hypothalamo–Pituitary–Adrenal Axis
- Increased plasma concentrations of cortisol
- Increased cortisol production rate
- Decreased metabolic clearance of cortisol
- Abnormal dexamethasone suppression test (either failure of suppression or "early escape")
- Increased 24-h urinary excretion of free cortisol

The Hypothalamo–Pituitary–Gonadal Axis
- Secondary amenorrhea
- Low plasma estradiol concentrations
- Low plasma LH and FSH concentrations
- Normal LH/FSH response to GnRH after priming

Other Hormonal Abnormalities
- Exaggerated GH response to GHRH
- Reduced GH response to apomorphine; abnormal release of GH in response to TRH
- GH response to a glucose load may show a paradoxical rise
- GH response to insulin hypoglycemia may be blunted
- Low plasma-free T_4 and free T_3 concentrations
- High plasma reverse rT_3 concentrations
- Delayed TSH response to TRH
- Subnormal AVP response to increased plasma sodium concentrations

AVP, Arginine vasopressin; *FSH*, follicle-stimulating hormone; *GH*, growth hormone; *GHRH*, growth hormone–releasing hormone; *GnRH*, gonadotrophin releasing hormone; *LH*, luteinizing hormone; *rT3*, triiodothyronine; *T$_4$*, thyroxine; *TRH*, thyrotrophin-releasing hormone; T$_3$, triiodothyronine; *TSH*, thyroid-stimulating hormone. From Marshall WJ, Lapsley M, Day AP, Ayling RM. *Clinical biochemistry: metabolic and clinical aspects.* 3rd ed. Edinburgh: Elsevier; 2014.

Metabolic consequences include severe potassium and magnesium depletion secondary to the use of diuretics and laxatives.[199,200]

OTHER ASPECTS OF CLINICAL NUTRITION

Nutrition affects every specialty in medical practice, and comprehensively exploring the relationships is beyond the scope of this chapter. Many are referred to elsewhere in this book.

Excess intake of nutrients can be as harmful as inadequate intakes; besides the obvious association between a high energy intake and obesity, excessive ingestion of certain nutrients can predispose to a variety of conditions, including hypertension and other cardiovascular diseases and cancer. The management of some conditions may include dietary manipulation that can have potentially harmful effects on the body as a whole, for example, restriction of protein intake in patients with chronic kidney disease (and it may be noted that patients on dialysis may have increased requirements for micronutrients, which are removed during dialysis). This is particularly true of some inherited metabolic diseases. An example is phenylketonuria, in which phenylalanine intake must be greatly restricted but not excluded entirely because it is an essential amino acid, and additional tyrosine must be provided because less can be synthesized from phenylalanine. Nutritional manipulation may be only one aspect of the management of a particular condition, as it is with chronic kidney and liver disease, chronic pancreatitis, and the short bowel syndrome. And the coexistence of two conditions may provide particular nutritional challenges, type 1 diabetes and cystic fibrosis being important examples.

Food intolerance (e.g., lactase deficiency), food allergies, and celiac disease all require input from the laboratory for their diagnosis. And food does not just contain nutrients. Preservatives, flavor enhancers, and other substances are absorbed into the body and have the potential to give rise to adverse effects. So, too, do contaminants, whether inorganic (e.g., mercury in shellfish), organic (e.g., aflatoxin, a potent carcinogenic mycotoxin), or living (e.g., microorganisms causing food poisoning or systemic infections).[201]

AT A GLANCE

Adequate nutrition is essential for normal health, growth, development, and reproduction. Its provision depends on numerous factors, including economic, biological, climatic, geographical, and societal, in addition to the ability of the body to absorb and use specific nutrients.

Nutrients are conventionally classified as macronutrients (e.g., carbohydrate, fats, protein, and major minerals) and micronutrients (vitamins and individual elements). Both excess and inadequate provision can be harmful: thus the provision of excessive energy substrates results in obesity and a high sodium intake contributes to hypertension while deficiencies can lead to generalized malnutrition and specific deficiency syndromes. Foodstuffs can also be a source of harm if they are contaminated with microorganisms or toxins.

It is recommended that all individuals interacting with health care be screened to ascertain their nutritional status. This is essential for patients admitted to hospitals and care facilities. Individuals with inadequate nutrient intake require nutritional support. With specific deficiencies, this can be achieved through supplementation of the nutrient in question. With generalized undernutrition, support should be provided enterally whenever possible, often as an adjunct to oral food intake; in patients with intestinal failure, parenteral support is required. Although often required for short periods in patients with acute illnesses, PN may be required in the long term, notably in patients with short gut syndrome as a result of surgical resection or generalized malfunction of the small intestine.

Knowledge of nutrient requirements is essential in the provision of nutritional support. This includes basal requirements sufficient to support normal function plus additional requirements arising as a result of the underlying illness. The delivery of nutritional support should be supervised by a multidisciplinary team of health care professionals, including physicians, dietitians, nurses, and laboratory staff.

Obesity is a common and increasingly prevalent condition throughout the world but particularly in so-called "developed" and "developing" countries. It imposes major threats to health, including increased risks of cancer, cardiovascular disease, type 2 diabetes, and social isolation. The causes are complex. Genetic factors are important, but the underlying cause is an energy intake in excess of energy expenditure. The regulation of appetite is a complex neuroendocrine process, but its elucidation is identifying possible targets for pharmacologic intervention. At present, however, the most successful treatments are surgical, including restrictive procedures (essentially reducing the size of the stomach), malabsorptive procedures (reducing the digestion or absorption of food), or a combination of both.

Anorexia nervosa and bulimia nervosa are neuropsychiatric disorders of perception of body image but can cause severe, and sometimes fatal, nutritional disorders.

SELECTED REFERENCES

1. Food and Agriculture Organization of the United Nations. The state of food security and nutrition in the world. 2019. Available from: www.fao.org/3/ca5162en/ca%162en.pdf. Accessed May 2019.
2. Unicef. The state of the world's children 2019: children, food and nutrition. Available from: www.unicef/data/resources/stateoftheworldschildren2019. Accessed May 2020.
5. National Acadamies of Sciences, Engineering and Medicine. Dietary reference Intervals. The National Acadamies Press. Available from http://ods.od.nih.gov/health.information/Dietary_Reference_Intervals.aspx. Accessed May 2020.
8. World Health Organisation. Sugars intake for adults and children. 2015. Available from http://www.who.int/nutrition/publications/guidelines/sugars_intake/en/. Accessed May 2020.
11. Veronese N, Solmi M, Caruso MG, et al. Dietary fibre and health outcome: an umbrella review of systematic reviews and meta-analyses. Am J Clin Nutr 2018;107:436–44.
19. Eckel RH, Jakicic JM, Ard JD, et al. 2013 AHA/ACC guidelines on lifestyle management to reduce cardiovascular risk. A report of the American College of Cardiology/American Heart Association Task Force on Practice Guidelines. Circulation 2014;129(S2):S76–99.
84. National Institute of Health. 2019 vitamin D fact sheet for health professionals. Available from http://ods.od.nih.gov/factsheets/VitaminD-HealthProfessional/. Accessed May 2020.
127. A Report of the Panel on Micronutrients, Subcommittees on Upper Reference Levels of Nutrients and of Interpretation and Uses of Dietary Reference Intakes, and the Standing Committee on the Scientific Evaluation of Dietary Reference Intakes, Food and Nutrition Board, Institute of Medicine. Dietary reference values for vitamin A, vitamin K, arsenic, boron, chromium, copper, iodine, iron, manganese, molybdenum, nickel, silicon, vanadium, and zinc. Washington DC: National Academies Press; 2015.
129. BAPEN. Malnutrition universal screening tool. 2003. Available from: www.bapen.org.uk/pdfds/must/must_full.pdf. Accessed May 2020.
139. Keller U. Nutritional laboratory markers in malnutrition. J Clin Med 2019;8:775. doi:10.3390/jcm80607775.
151. Butterworth CE. The skeleton in the hospital closet. Nutr Today 1974;9:4–8.

153. National Institute for Health and Care Excellence. Nutrition support in adults. Clinical guideline 32 2006 (Updated 2017) NICE London. Available from: www.nice.org.uk/guidance/cg32. Accessed May 2020.

156. Boullata JI, CarreraAL, Harvey L, et al. ASPEN Safe practices for enteral nutrition therapy. J Parent Ent Nut 2017;41:15–103.

160. da Silva J, Seres DS, Sabino K, et al. ASPEN Consensus recommendations for refeeding syndrome. Nutr Clin Pract 2020;35:178–95.

165. World Health Organization. Obesity and overweight. April 2020. Available from: www.who.int/news-room/fact-sheets/detail/obesity-and-overweight. Accessed May 2020.

173. Briener A, Cawley J, Meyerhofer C. The high and rising costs of obesity to the US health care system. J Gen Intern Med 2017;32:6–8.

185. Kim BY, Kang SM, Kang JH, et al. Current long term pharmacotherapies for the management of obesity. J Obes Metab Syndr 2020;29(2):99–109.

189. O'Brien PE, Hindle A, Brennan L, et al. Long term outcomes after bariatric surgery: a systematic review and meta-analysis of weight loss at 10 or more years for all bariatric procedures and a single centre review of 20 years outcomes after adjustable gastric banding. Obes Surg 2019;29:3–14.

196. O'Kane M, Parretti H, Pinkney J, et al. British obesity and metabolic surgery society guidelines on perioperative and postoperative biochemical monitoring and micronutrient replacement for patients undergoing bariatric surgery—2000. Obes Rev 2020;21:e13087.

201. Ayling RM, Marshall WJ. Nutrition and laboratory medicine. London: ACB Venture Publications; 2007.

47

Diabetes Mellitus

David B. Sacks

ABSTRACT

Background

Diabetes mellitus is a common disorder in which patients develop hyperglycemia due to inadequate insulin secretion, defective insulin action, or both. There are two major forms of diabetes, namely type 1 and type 2. The estimated global prevalence of diabetes in adults is ~460 million. Many patients with diabetes develop severe debilitating complications, including blindness, renal failure, peripheral vascular disease, myocardial infarction, and stroke.

Content

The pathophysiology of the different forms of diabetes is addressed. Hormones that regulate blood glucose concentrations include insulin and the counterregulatory hormones glucagon, epinephrine, and cortisol. Insulin synthesis, mechanism of action, and promotion of glucose uptake into fat and muscle are described. Several analytes that are measured in patients with diabetes are discussed in detail. These include glucose (in central laboratories, with hand-held meters, and by continuous glucose monitoring [CGM] devices), glycated proteins (such as hemoglobin A_{1c}, fructosamine, and glycated albumin), islet autoantibodies, and urine albumin. The clinical indications, analytical methods, and sample handling are covered. The essential role of clinical laboratories in the diagnosis and management of patients with diabetes is emphasized.

Diabetes mellitus is a group of metabolic disorders characterized by hyperglycemia resulting from defects in insulin secretion, insulin action, or both.[1] Some patients may experience acute life-threatening hyperglycemic episodes, such as ketoacidosis or hyperosmolar coma. Acute life-threatening hypoglycemic episodes may occur as a result of therapy. As the disease progresses, patients are at increased risk for the development of specific complications, including *retinopathy* leading to blindness, *nephropathy* leading to renal failure, and *neuropathy* (nerve damage), collectively known as microvascular complications, as well as *atherosclerosis,* which is considered a *macrovascular complication.*[2,3] The last may result in stroke, gangrene, or coronary artery disease.

Diabetes is a common disease, although the exact prevalence is unknown. The number of people with diabetes has increased dramatically worldwide. It is estimated that ~460 million adults currently have diabetes, and by 2045 this number is predicted to reach 700 million, 80% of whom will live in low- and middle-income countries.[4] In the United States, the prevalence in 1999 to 2002 was 9.3%, 30% of whom were undiagnosed.[5] Analysis of the 2011 to 2016 National Health and Nutritional Examination Survey (NHANES) by fasting glucose, oral glucose tolerance testing (OGTT), or hemoglobin A_{1c} shows a prevalence of diabetes in the United States in persons 20 years of age and older of 14.6%.[6] Similarly, the prevalence of diabetes in Asian populations has increased rapidly in recent decades,[7] with China and India ranked first and second, respectively, among countries with the largest diabetes populations. Analysis in Chinese adults suggests that in 2010 the estimated prevalence of diabetes and prediabetes was 11.6 and 50.1%, respectively, which is equivalent to 113.9 million persons with diabetes and 493.4 million with prediabetes.[8] The prevalence varies widely among countries, reaching as high as 25% in the Middle East and 30% in the Western Pacific. Information about individual countries, for example, number of patients, prevalence, and deaths, are compiled by the International Diabetes Federation (IDF) and can be found at https://diabetesatlas.org/data/en/ (accessed August 2020).

Diabetes has been described as "one of the main threats to human health in the twenty-first century."[9] It is estimated that ~50% of individuals with diabetes worldwide remain undiagnosed.[4] The absolute number of undiagnosed diabetes patients in the United States has remained fairly stable; thus the proportion of total diabetes cases that are undiagnosed decreased to 11% in 2006 to 2010.[10] The prevalence of diabetes mellitus increases with age, from 1.4% in adults aged 20 to 24 years to ~15% by the age of 50 years.[4] In the United States, more than 20% of the population older than 65 years have diabetes.[11,12] A racial predilection has been noted; 22.1, 20.4, 19.1, and 12.1% of Hispanics, blacks, Asians, and whites, respectively, in the United States have diabetes.[6] In 2017, diabetes was estimated to be responsible for $327 billion in health care expenditures in the United States.[13] This figure is an increase of 25% over 2012, and diabetes accounts for 1 in 4 health care dollars in the United States. The direct costs were $237 billion, with 59% of that total incurred by those

65 years and older. The estimated economic burden for undiagnosed diabetes, prediabetes, and gestational diabetes mellitus in 2017 was $77 billion, producing a total economic burden of ~$404 billion.[14] The IDF estimates that worldwide diabetes generated at least $760 billion in health expenditures in 2019,[4] though others claim costs that are twice as high, being $1.3 trillion in 2015.[15] Through its complications, diabetes is the fourth most common cause of death in the developed world.

CLASSIFICATION

Historical

Diabetes was initially diagnosed by the oral glucose tolerance test (OGTT). Values greater than two standard deviations (SDs) above the mean of the value found in a selected population of healthy volunteers without a family history of diabetes mellitus were accepted as diagnostic. This criterion led to the identification of large numbers of asymptomatic people with abnormally high 1-to-2-hour postload glucose values, but normal fasting blood glucose. They were presumed to have early or mild diabetes. In 1975 it was estimated that more than half the population older than 60 years was abnormal. Follow-up of these individuals indicated that most of them with lesser degrees of glucose intolerance did not manifest definite evidence of diabetes in the next 10 years, and a large percentage returned to normal glucose tolerance.

Most populations have plasma glucose values that exhibit a unimodal, log-normal distribution (a distribution curve that is skewed to the high end but becomes bell shaped on a logarithmic axis). Ethnic groups with a high prevalence of diabetes, such as the Pima Indians and Nauruans, exhibit bimodal blood glucose distributions.[16] Optimal distinction between normal and diabetes individuals in these groups occurs at a fasting glucose around 140 mg/dL (7.8 mmol/L) and glucose concentrations greater than 200 mg/dL (11.1 mmol/L) 2 hours after an oral glucose load. Furthermore, the specific microvascular complications of diabetes were believed to be rare in patients with fasting or 2-hour postprandial plasma glucose concentrations less than 140 or 200 mg/dL (7.8 or 11.1 mmol/L), respectively. These observations formed the basis for the criteria proposed in 1979 by a workgroup of the National Diabetes Data Group[17] and later endorsed by the World Health Organization (WHO) Committee on Diabetes.[18] Lower diagnostic values are used currently.

The 1979 classification scheme recognized two major forms of diabetes: type I (insulin-dependent) diabetes mellitus (IDDM) and type II (non–insulin-dependent) diabetes mellitus (NIDDM).[17] The terms *juvenile-onset* and *adult-onset diabetes* were abolished. To base the classification on cause rather than on treatment, the American Diabetes Association (ADA) established a workgroup in 1995 to re-examine the classification and diagnosis of diabetes mellitus. The revised classification, published in 1997,[1] eliminates the terms *insulin-dependent diabetes mellitus* and *non–insulin-dependent diabetes mellitus,* which now are termed *type 1* and *type 2 diabetes,* respectively (see Box 47.2). Furthermore, the categories of previous abnormality of glucose tolerance and potential abnormality of glucose tolerance have been eliminated.

Type 1 Diabetes Mellitus

Approximately 5 to 10% of all cases of diabetes mellitus are included in this category.[14] Patients usually have abrupt onset

---

BOX 47.1 Clinical Utility of Insulin, Proinsulin, C-Peptide, and Glucagon Assays

Insulin
Evaluation of fasting hypoglycemia
Evaluation of the polycystic ovary syndrome
Classification of diabetes mellitus
Prediction of diabetes mellitus
Assessment of β-cell activity
Selection of optimal therapy for diabetes
Investigation of insulin resistance
Prediction of the development of coronary artery disease

Proinsulin
Diagnosis of β-cell tumors
Familial hyperproinsulinemia
Cross-reactivity of insulin assays

C-Peptide
Evaluation of fasting hypoglycemia
  β-Cell tumors
  Factitious
Classification of diabetes mellitus
Assessment of β-cell activity
Obtaining insurance coverage for insulin pump
Monitoring therapy
  Pancreatectomy
  Transplant (pancreas-islet cell)
  Immunomodulation of type 1 diabetes

Glucagon
Diagnosis of α-cell tumors

---

of symptoms (e.g., polyuria, polydipsia, rapid weight loss) and ~30% present with diabetic ketoacidosis (DKA).[19] They have insulinopenia (a deficiency of insulin) caused by destruction of pancreatic islet β-cells and are dependent on insulin to sustain life and prevent ketosis. Most patients have antibodies that identify an autoimmune process (see later discussion). The peak incidence occurs in childhood and adolescence. Approximately 75% acquire the disease before the age of 18, but onset in the remainder may occur at any age. Age at presentation is not a criterion for classification. Three distinct stages of type 1 diabetes can be identified.[20] Stage 1: patients are normoglycemic but have multiple islet autoantibodies; Stage 2: patients have dysglycemia (IFG and/or IGT) with multiple islet autoantibodies; and Stage 3: hyperglycemia with clinical symptoms. In addition, there is increasing awareness of considerable disease heterogeneity in type 1 diabetes.[21]

Type 2 Diabetes Mellitus

This group accounts for approximately 90% of all cases of diabetes.[14] Patients have minimal symptoms, are not prone to ketosis, and *are not dependent on insulin* to prevent ketonuria. *Insulin concentrations may be normal, decreased, or increased,* and most people with this form of diabetes have impaired insulin action. *Obesity* is commonly associated, and weight loss alone usually improves hyperglycemia in these persons. However, many individuals with type 2 diabetes may require dietary intervention, oral anti-hyperglycemic agents, insulin, or other injectable drugs to control hyperglycemia. Most patients acquire the disease after age 40, but it may occur in younger people. Type 2 diabetes in children and adolescents is an emerging, significant problem, especially as the prevalence of obesity in this age group rises.[9,22] In Hong Kong, 90% of youth-onset diabetes is type 2, 60% in Japan, and 50% in Taiwan.[22] Some individuals cannot be classified at the time of diagnosis into type 1 or type 2 diabetes. Future classification schemes for diabetes are likely to focus on the pathophysiology of underlying β-cell dysfunction.[23]

Specific Types of Diabetes Mellitus Due to Other Causes

This subclass includes uncommon patients in whom hyperglycemia is due to a specific underlying disorder, such as genetic defects of β-cell function; genetic defects in insulin action; diseases of the exocrine pancreas (e.g., cystic fibrosis); endocrinopathies (e.g., Cushing syndrome, acromegaly, glucagonoma); administration of hormones or drugs known to induce β-cell dysfunction (e.g., dilantin, pentamidine) or to impair insulin action (e.g., glucocorticoids, thiazides, β-adrenergics); infection; uncommon forms of immune-mediated diabetes; or other genetic conditions (e.g., Down syndrome, Klinefelter syndrome, porphyria; see American Diabetes Association[24] for a detailed list) (see Box 47.2). This was formerly termed *secondary diabetes.* (Additional details can be found in Tuomi et al.[25])

Gestational Diabetes Mellitus

This was defined for many years as any degree of glucose intolerance (i.e., hyperglycemia) *with onset or first recognition during pregnancy*[26] (i.e., women with diabetes who become pregnant are not included in this category). Estimates of the frequency of abnormal glucose tolerance during pregnancy have ranged from less than 1 to 28%, depending on the population studied and the diagnostic tests employed[27] (discussed in more detail later in this chapter). In 2019, 15.8% (~20 million) live births were estimated to be affected by hyperglycemia in pregnancy.[4] In the United States, gestational diabetes mellitus (GDM) occurs in 6 to 8% of pregnancies (≈270,000 cases annually). The prevalence of GDM

BOX 47.2 Classification of Diabetes Mellitus

I. Type 1 diabetes
  A. Immune mediated
  B. Idiopathic
II. Type 2 diabetes
III. Other specific types
  A. Genetic defects of β-cell function
  B. Genetic defects in insulin action
  C. Diseases of the exocrine pancreas
  D. Endocrinopathies
  E. Drug or chemical induced
  F. Infections
  G. Uncommon forms of immune-mediated diabetes
  H. Other genetic syndromes sometimes associated with diabetes
IV. Gestational diabetes mellitus

From the American Diabetes Association. Diagnosis and classification of diabetes mellitus. *Diabetes Care* 2014;37(Suppl 1):S81–90.

---

is increasing, at least in part, due to the considerable increase in obesity. Women with GDM are at significantly greater risk for the subsequent development of type 2 diabetes mellitus, which ultimately occurs in 30 to 67%.[28] At 4 to 12 weeks postpartum, all patients who had GDM should be evaluated for diabetes using nonpregnant OGTT criteria. If diabetes is not present, patients should have lifelong screening for diabetes or prediabetes at least every 3 years.[20]

Categories of Increased Risk for Diabetes

People who have blood glucose concentrations above normal, but less than those required for a diagnosis of diabetes mellitus, have been recognized for many years. In 1979, this intermediate category was termed impaired glucose tolerance (IGT). It was defined as a 2-hour postload plasma glucose following an OGTT of 140 to 199 mg/dL (7.8 to 11.0 mmol/L).[17] An OGTT is required to assign a patient to this class. In order to avoid an OGTT, the category of impaired fasting glucose (IFG) was added in 1997 by the ADA[1] and by the WHO in 1999.[29] IFG is diagnosed by a fasting glucose value between those of normal and diabetic individuals, namely, between 100 and 125 mg/dL (5.6 and 6.9 mmol/L). (Note that the WHO and a number of other diabetes organizations define the lower cutoff for IFG at 110 mg/mL [6.1 mmol/L]).[30] In 2009, hemoglobin A_{1c} (HbA_{1c}) was added as a criterion to diagnose type 2 diabetes.[31] People with HbA_{1c} values below the cutoff for diabetes that is, 6.5% (48 mmol/mol), but above the reference interval (4 to 6%; 20 to 42 mmol/L), are at high risk of developing diabetes.[32] For example, the incidence of diabetes in people with HbA_{1c} between 6.0 and less than 6.5% (42 and 48 mmol/mol) is more than 10 times that of people with lower concentrations. Prospective studies reveal a 5-year cumulative incidence of diabetes ranging from 12 to 25% (threefold to eightfold higher than the general population) for people with HbA_{1c} of 5.5 to 6.0% (37 to 42 mmol/mol).[32]

Individuals with IFG and/or IGT and/or intermediate HbA_{1c} (5.7 to 6.4%; 39 to 46 mmol/mol) have been referred to as having "prediabetes" as they are at high risk for progressing to diabetes. Moreover, they are at increased risk for the development of cardiovascular disease.[33,34] Nevertheless, there is considerable controversy surrounding prediabetes.[35] For example, IFG, IGT, and HbA_{1c} do not always identify the same individuals.[31] There is also lack of agreement on the cutpoints for IFG and HbA_{1c}. This is due, in large part, to the continuous nature of the risk for the development of diabetes complications and the concentration of glucose or HbA_{1c}.[31]

HORMONES THAT REGULATE BLOOD GLUCOSE CONCENTRATION

During a brief fast, a precipitous decline in the concentration of blood glucose is prevented by breakdown of glycogen stored in the liver and synthesis of glucose in the liver. Some glucose is derived from gluconeogenesis in the kidneys.[36] These organs contain glucose-6-phosphatase, which is necessary to convert glucose 6-phosphate (derived from gluconeogenesis or glycogenolysis) to glucose. Skeletal muscle lacks this enzyme; muscle glycogen therefore cannot contribute directly to blood glucose. With more prolonged fasting (>42 hours), gluconeogenesis accounts for essentially all glucose production. In contrast, after a meal, the absorbed glucose is converted to glycogen (for storage in the liver and skeletal

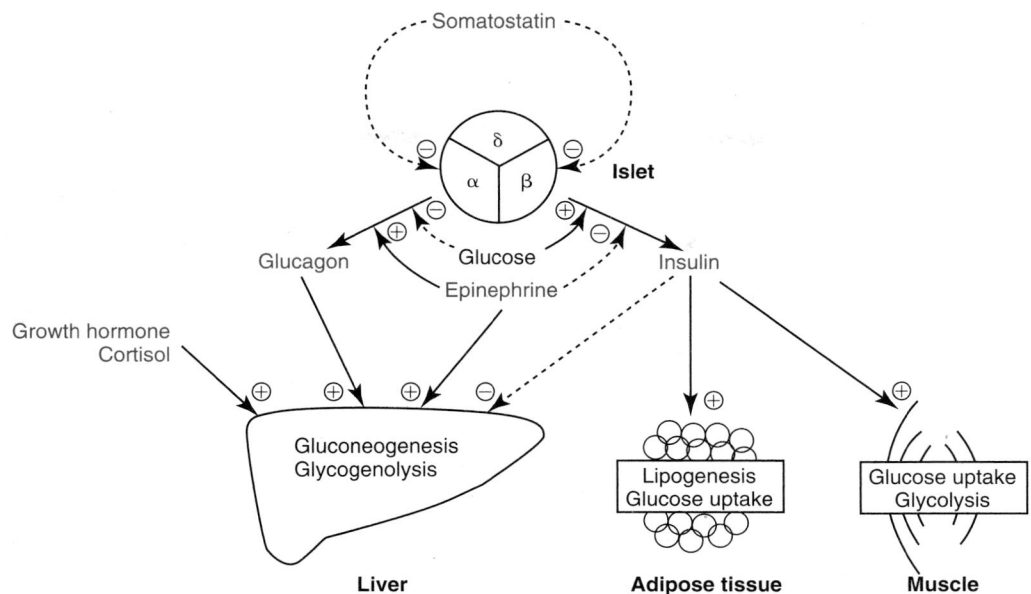

FIGURE 47.1 Hormonal regulation of blood glucose. +, stimulation; −, inhibition. Cortisol, growth hormone, and epinephrine antagonize the effects of insulin.

muscle) or fat (for storage in adipose tissue). Despite large fluctuations in the supply and demand of carbohydrates, the concentration of glucose in the blood is normally maintained within a fairly narrow range by hormones that modulate the movement of glucose into and out of the circulation. These include insulin, which decreases blood glucose, and the counter-regulatory hormones (glucagon, epinephrine, cortisol, and growth hormone), which increase blood glucose concentrations (Fig. 47.1).[36] Normal glucose disposal depends on (1) the ability of the pancreas to secrete insulin, (2) the ability of insulin to promote uptake of glucose into peripheral tissue, and (3) the ability of insulin to suppress hepatic glucose production. The major insulin target organs are liver, skeletal muscle, and adipose tissue. These organs exhibit some differences in their responses to insulin. For example, the hormone stimulates glucose uptake through a specific glucose transporter—GLUT4—into muscle and fat cells, but not into liver cells.

Insulin

Insulin is a protein hormone produced by the β-cells of the islets of Langerhans in the pancreas. Insulin was the first protein hormone to be sequenced, the first substance to be measured by radioimmunoassay (RIA), and the first compound produced by recombinant DNA technology for clinical use. It is an anabolic hormone that stimulates the uptake of glucose into fat and muscle, promotes the conversion of glucose to glycogen or fat for storage, inhibits glucose production by the liver, stimulates protein synthesis, and inhibits protein breakdown.

Chemistry

Human insulin (molecular weight [MW] 5808 Da) consists of 51 amino acids in two chains (A and B) joined by two disulfide bridges, with a third disulfide bridge within the A chain. The amino acid sequence of human insulin differs slightly from insulin of other species, but the carboxyl terminal region of the B chain (B23 to B26), which appears crucial

for the biological actions of insulin, is highly conserved among species. Insulin from most animals is immunologically and biologically similar to human insulin, and in the past, patients were treated with insulin purified from beef or pig pancreas. The most commonly used forms now are recombinant human insulins.

Synthesis

Preproinsulin, a protein of about 100 amino acids (MW 12,000 Da), is formed by ribosomes in the rough endoplasmic reticulum of the pancreatic β-cells (Fig. 47.2). Preproinsulin is not detectable in the circulation under normal conditions because it is rapidly converted by cleaving enzymes to proinsulin (MW 9000 Da), an 86 amino acid polypeptide. This is stored in secretory granules in the Golgi complex of the β-cells, where proteolytic cleavage to insulin and connecting peptide (C-peptide) occurs.[37] Cleavage of proinsulin is catalyzed by two Ca^{2+}-regulated endopeptidases: prohormone convertases 1 and 2 (PC1 and PC2).[38] PC1 (sometimes designated PC3) hydrolyzes the molecule on the C-terminal end of Arg-31 and Arg-32 (at the BC junction) to yield split-32, 33-proinsulin (Fig. 47.3). PC2 cleaves proinsulin on the C-terminal side of dibasic residues Lys-64 and Arg-65 (at the AC junction) to generate split-65,66-proinsulin. Each enzymatic hydrolysis reaction is rapidly followed by the removal of two newly exposed C-terminal basic amino acids by carboxypeptidase-H to produce insulin and C-peptide.

The split proinsulin intermediates are rarely detected in patient samples because of the relatively high quantity of carboxypeptidase-H. This enzyme produces the more commonly observed proinsulin intermediates, des-31,32-proinsulin and des-64,65-proinsulin (see Fig. 47.3). Most proinsulin processing is sequential. Intact proinsulin is initially hydrolyzed by PC1 or carboxypeptidase-H. The resultant des-31,32-proinsulin is converted by PC2 and carboxypeptidase-H to insulin and C-peptide. Less than 10% of proinsulin is metabolized via des-(64-65)-proinsulin, which is present in negligible

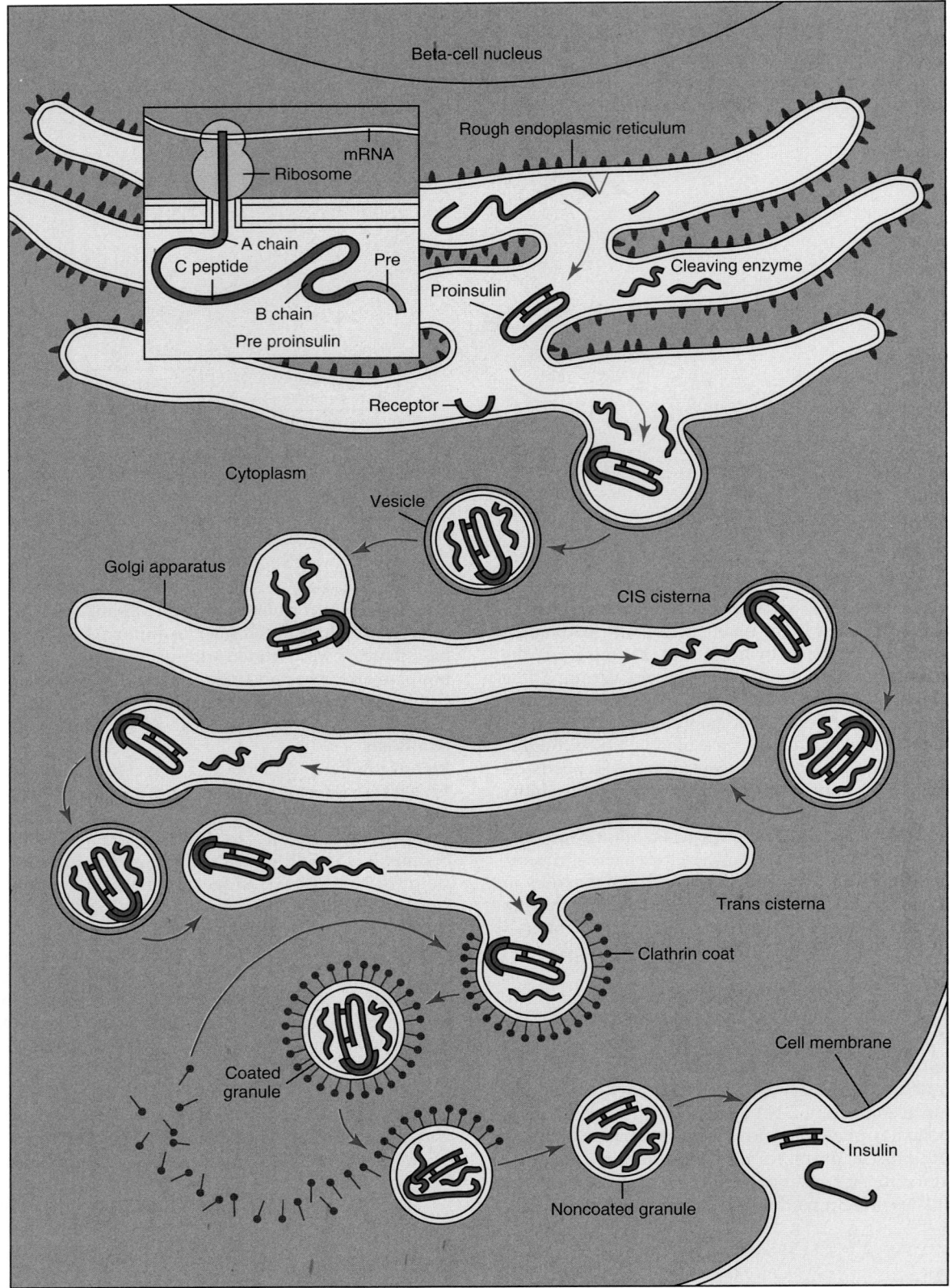

FIGURE 47.2 Insulin synthesis and release from the pancreatic β-cell. (From Orci L, Vassalli J-D, Perrelet A. The insulin factory. *Sci Am* 1988;259:85–94.)

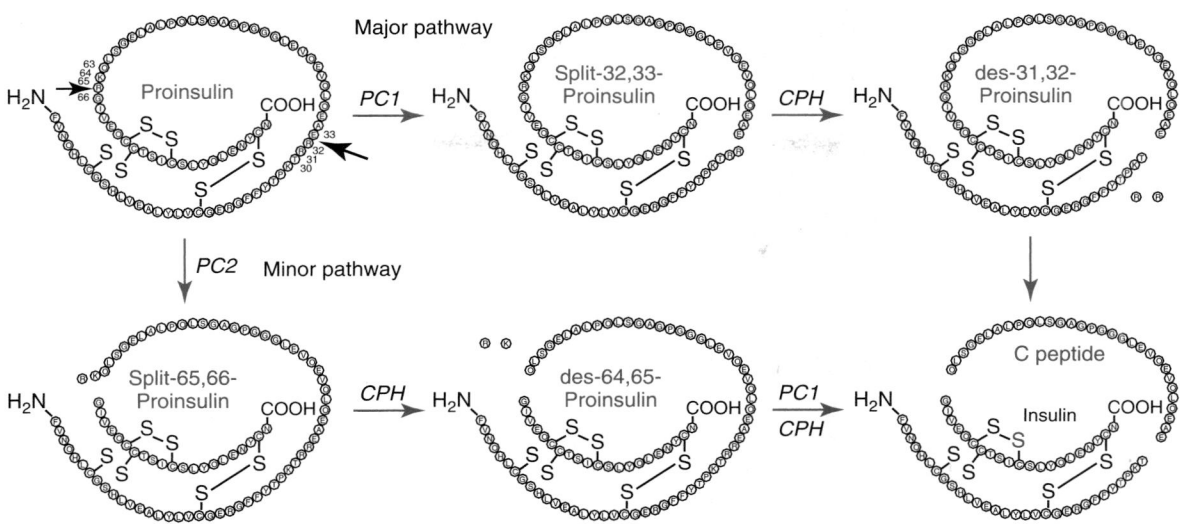

FIGURE 47.3 Processing of proinsulin. The enzymes prohormone convertase 1 and 2 (*PC1* and *PC2*) act on proinsulin to form the appropriate split proinsulins. Carboxypeptidase-H *(CPH)* removes the two exposed basic amino acid residues *(circles)*.

amounts in humans. Des-31,32-proinsulin is the major proinsulin conversion intermediate.[39] Glucose regulates biosynthesis of both proinsulin and PC1, but has no effect on PC2 or carboxypeptidase-H. At the cell membrane, insulin and C-peptide are released into the portal circulation in equimolar amounts. In addition, small amounts of proinsulin and intermediate cleavage forms enter the circulation.

Release
Glucose is the most important physiologic secretagogue for insulin.[40] An increase in blood glucose concentration stimulates insulin secretion within minutes. Insulin release is potentiated by substances such as the incretin hormones glucagon-like peptide 1 (GLP-1) and glucose-dependent insulinotropic polypeptide (GIP), as well as cholecystokinin, peptide YY, and oxyntomodulin, released from the gut in response to food.[40,41] Insulin release is inhibited by hypoglycemia, somatostatin (produced in the pancreatic δ-cells), and various drugs (e.g., α-adrenergic agonists, β-adrenergic blockers, diazoxide, phenytoin, phenothiazines, nicotinic acid).[42] In healthy individuals, insulin is secreted in a pulsatile fashion, with glucose and insulin the main signals in the feedback loop. Glucose elicits the release of insulin from the pancreas in two phases. The first phase begins 1 to 2 minutes after intravenous injection of glucose and ends within 10 minutes. This phase, illustrated by the sharp spike in Fig. 47.4A, represents the rapid release of stored insulin. The second phase, beginning at the point where the first phase ends, depends on continuing insulin synthesis and release and lasts until normoglycemia has been restored, usually within 60 to 120 minutes. With progressive failure of β-cell function, the first-phase insulin response to glucose is lost, but other stimuli such as glucagon or amino acids may be able to elicit this response. Although the second-phase insulin response is preserved in most patients with type 2 diabetes mellitus, both the first-phase response (Fig. 47.4B) and normal pulsatile insulin secretion[17] are lost. In contrast, patients with type 1 diabetes mellitus exhibit minimal or no insulin response (Fig. 47.4C).

Degradation
On the first pass through the portal circulation, approximately 50% of the insulin is extracted by the liver, where it is degraded. Because the amount extracted is variable, plasma insulin concentrations may not accurately reflect the rate of insulin secretion. Additional insulin degradation occurs in the kidneys. Insulin is filtered through the glomeruli, reabsorbed, and degraded in the proximal tubules. The basal insulin secretory rate is about 1 U (43 μg)/h, with total daily secretion of about 40 U. The half-life of insulin in the circulation is between 4 and 5 minutes.

Proinsulin
Proinsulin, which has relatively low biological activity (approximately 10% of insulin potency), is the major storage form of insulin.[43] Normally, only small amounts (about 3% of the amount of insulin, on a molar basis) of proinsulin enter the circulation. However, the hepatic clearance rate for proinsulin is only 25% of that for insulin, and the half-life of proinsulin is 30 minutes. Therefore in the fasting state, circulating proinsulin concentrations are approximately 10 to 15% of insulin concentrations.

C-peptide
Proinsulin is cleaved to a 31 amino acid connecting (C) peptide (MW 3600 Da) and insulin (see Fig. 47.3). C-peptide was initially thought to be devoid of biological activity and was necessary only to ensure the correct structure of insulin.[44] More recent evidence reveals that C-peptide has biological activity, but its possible physiologic significance remains controversial.[45] Although insulin and C-peptide are secreted into the portal circulation in equimolar amounts, fasting C-peptide concentrations are fivefold to tenfold higher than those of insulin owing to the longer half-life of C-peptide (≈35 minutes). The liver does not extract C-peptide, which is removed from the circulation by the kidneys and degraded, with a fraction excreted unchanged in the urine.

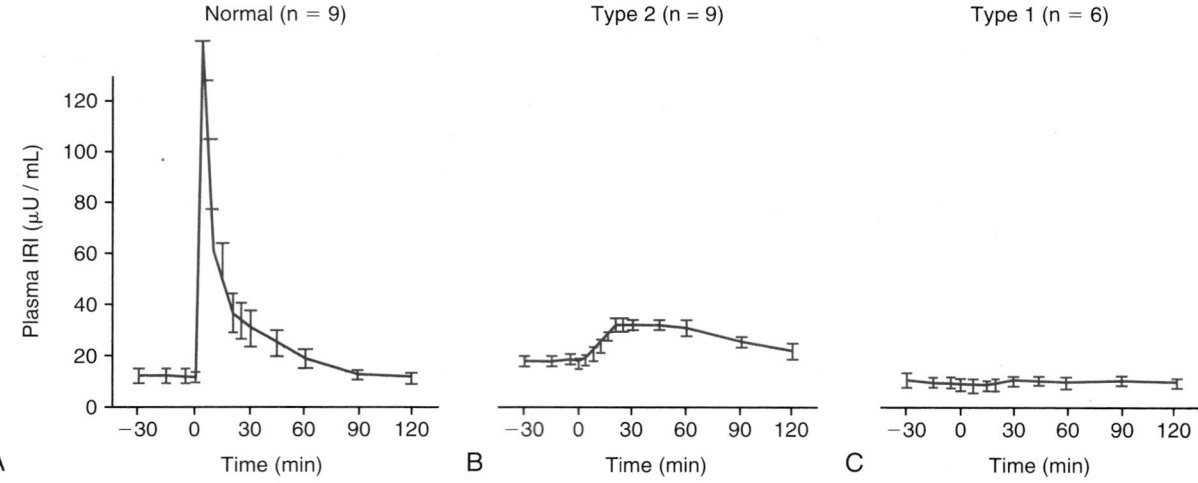

FIGURE 47.4 Response of plasma insulin to glucose stimulation. A 20-g glucose pulse is given intravenously at time 0. *A,* Healthy subjects. *B,* Patients with type 2 diabetes mellitus (NIDDM). *C,* Patients with type 1 diabetes mellitus (IDDM). *IRI,* Immunoreactive insulin. Values before time 0 represent baseline. (From Pfeifer MA, Halter JB, Porte D Jr. Insulin secretion in diabetes mellitus. *Am J Med* 1981;70:579–88.)

Antibodies to Insulin

Antibodies to insulin develop in almost all patients who are treated with exogenous insulin.[46] Note that these antibodies are distinct from insulin autoantibodies (IAAs), which are present in some patients with type 1 diabetes before they receive insulin (see Pathogenesis of Type 1 Diabetes Mellitus later in this chapter). Insulin antibodies rarely produce adverse effects. On rare occasions (usually in insulin-treated patients with type 2 diabetes), high titers of insulin antibodies may cause insulin resistance; this tends to be self-limited.[47] Patients who use inhaled insulin have significantly increased concentrations of insulin antibodies.[47] A quantitative estimate of the concentration of circulating insulin antibody does not appear to be of significant benefit.[48]

Insulin autoimmune syndrome (Hirata disease) is a rare condition found predominantly in Japan. Insulin-naïve patients present with fasting hypoglycemia and high IAAs. Although the condition usually resolves spontaneously, life-threatening hypoglycemia may require plasmapheresis.[47]

Although rare, patients with antibodies to the insulin receptor have been described.[49] On binding the receptor, these antibodies act as antagonists, producing hyperglycemia (e.g., in patients with acanthosis nigricans), or agonists, resulting in hypoglycemia.

The Mechanism of Insulin Action

Although the metabolic effects produced by insulin are well known, the molecular mechanism of insulin action remains incompletely understood.[50,51] It is generally accepted that the initial event is the binding of insulin to specific receptors in the plasma membrane (Fig. 47.5). The human insulin receptor, which is well characterized, is a heterotetramer, comprising two α- and two β-subunits. The α-subunit (MW 135,000 Da) is located on the outer surface of the plasma membrane and contains the site where insulin binds. The β-subunit (MW 95,000 Da) extends intracellularly through the plasma membrane and contains an intrinsic tyrosine kinase. Binding of insulin to the α-subunits induces a conformational change

in the receptor, resulting in activation of the tyrosine kinase, which catalyzes the phosphorylation of several proteins on tyrosine residues. One of the major substrates for this tyrosine kinase is the receptor itself, which is phosphorylated on multiple tyrosine residues. Insulin elicits two main functional effects, metabolic and mitogenic.

In addition to phosphorylating itself, the insulin receptor catalyzes the tyrosine phosphorylation of various specific intracellular proteins (Fig. 47.5). These include the four members of the family of insulin-receptor substrate (IRS) proteins (termed IRS-1, IRS-2, IRS-3, and IRS-4), Src homology 2 domain-containing (Shc), and growth factor receptor-bound protein 2 (Grb2).[52] The phosphorylated tyrosines on these target proteins act as docking sites for selected intracellular signal transducer proteins.[50] Most of these transducer proteins contain one or more Src homology 2 (SH2) domains. The SH2 domain is a sequence of approximately 100 amino acids that recognizes phosphotyrosine.[53] Sequence differences in the SH2 domain dictate the specificity of binding. SH2-containing proteins depicted in Fig. 47.5 include those labeled phosphatidylinositol 3-kinase (PI3K) and growth factor receptor–bound protein 2 (Grb2), both of which mediate downstream signal transduction events. The mitogenic effects of insulin are propagated by Shc and Grb2 via Ras which stimulates the mitogen-activated protein (MAP) kinase cascade. Metabolic signaling is mediated by PI3K, which activates Akt via 3-phosphoinositide dependent protein kinase-1 (PDK1).[52]

The effects produced by insulin differ among tissues. In skeletal muscle and adipose tissue, Akt regulates glucose transport by promoting translocation of GLUT4 (the insulin-sensitive glucose transporter; see below) to the plasma membrane. In the liver, Akt phosphorylates and inactivates GSK-3β (glycogen synthase kinase 3β), thereby enhancing glycogen synthesis. Akt also suppresses gluconeogenesis and activates lipogenesis in the liver. Some of these events are listed in Fig. 47.5. The pathways are elaborate with multiple feedback loops. While several components have been identified, there remain considerable gaps in our knowledge and understanding. Investigations have clarified

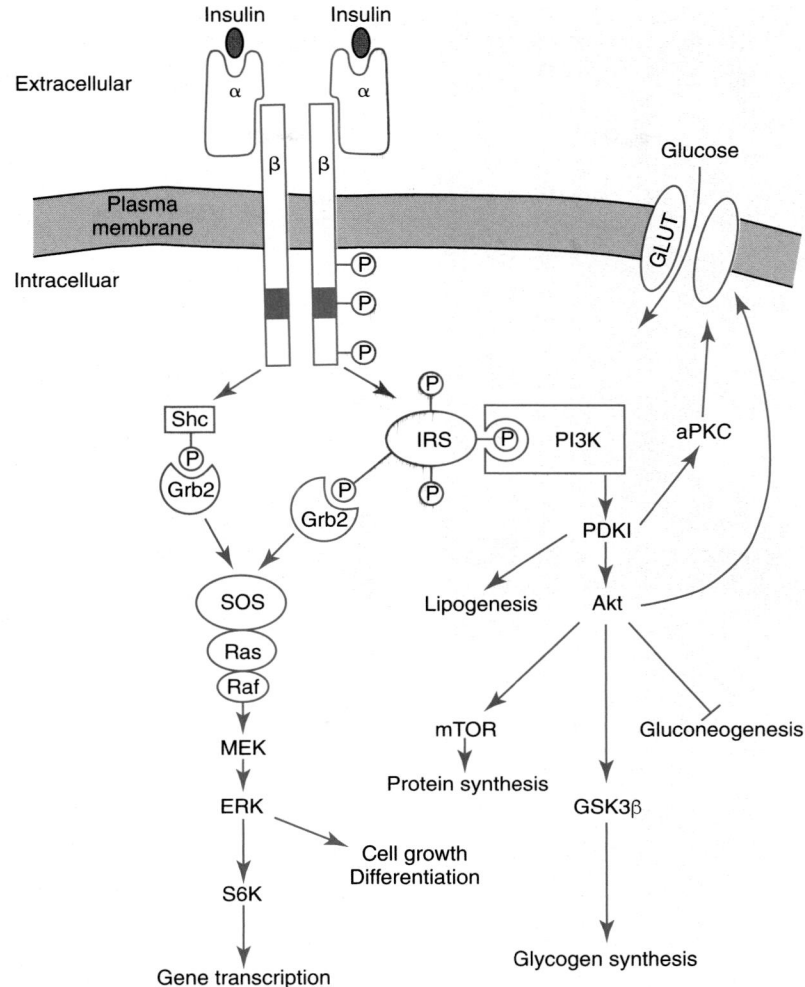

FIGURE 47.5 Mechanism of insulin action. Binding of insulin to the extracellular α-subunit of the in-sulin receptor induces autophosphorylation of the β-subunit of the receptor and phosphorylation of selected intracellular proteins, such as Shc and the insulin-receptor substrate *(IRS)* family. These latter phosphoproteins interact with other targets, thereby activating phosphorylation cascades, which result in glucose uptake (into adipose tissue and skeletal muscle), glucose metabolism, synthesis (of glyco-gen, lipid, and proteins), enhanced gene expression, cell growth, and differentiation. *aPKC,* Atypical protein kinase C; *p,* protein phosphorylation. See text for details.

a fundamental concept—that insulin-mediated signaling events are highly degenerate. For example, when two key insulin-signaling molecules, IRS-1 and GLUT4, were knocked out in transgenic mouse experiments, the resulting animals had minor metabolic defects rather than overt diabetes.[54] Similarly, mice with selective knockout of insulin receptors from only skeletal muscle do not develop diabetes.

Glucose Transport

The transport of glucose into cells is modulated by two fami-lies of proteins.[55] The sodium-dependent glucose transporters (SGLTs) use the electrochemical sodium gradient to transport glucose against its concentration gradient. SGLTs promote the uptake of glucose and galactose from the lumen of the small bowel and their reabsorption from urine in the kidney. In-hibitors of SGLT2 (e.g., canagliflozin and empagliflozin) are now used to treat patients with type 2 diabetes. These drugs increase glucose excretion in the urine by suppressing glucose

reabsorption in the kidney, thereby reducing blood glucose. Members of the second family of glucose carriers are called *facilitative glucose transporters* (GLUT), a family of membrane proteins that are encoded by the SLC2 genes (Table 47.1).[56] These transporters are designated GLUT1 to GLUT14, based on the order in which they were identified.[56,57] Eleven have been shown to transport glucose. Many also transport other hexoses, such as galactose, fructose, mannose, and xylose.[56] They can be divided into three classes, based on sequence similarities and characteristics. The best characterized are class I (GLUT1 to GLUT4). Less is known about those in classes II and III. GLUT1 is widely expressed and provides many cells with their basal glucose requirement. GLUT1 in the blood-brain barrier and GLUT3 in neuronal cells provide the constant high concentrations of glucose required by the brain. GLUT1 is responsible for mediating materno-placental trans-fer of glucose. GLUT2 is expressed in hepatocytes, β-cells of the pancreas, and basolateral membranes of intestinal and

TABLE 47.1 Facilitative Human Glucose Transporters

Name	Class	Tissue	Function
GLUT1	I	Erythrocytes, brain, blood-brain barrier, fetal tissues	Basal glucose transport, particularly in erythrocytes, brain, and placenta
GLUT2	I	Liver, β-cells of pancreas, small intestine, kidney, brain	Non–rate-limiting glucose transport
GLUT3	I	Brain (neurons), testis	Glucose transport in neurons
GLUT4	I	Skeletal muscle, cardiac muscle, adipose tissue (white and brown)	Insulin-stimulated glucose transport
GLUT5	II	Small intestine, kidney	Transports fructose (not glucose)
GLUT6	III	Brain, spleen, leukocytes	
GLUT7	II	Small intestine, colon, testis, prostate	
GLUT8	III	Testis, brain, adrenal gland, liver, spleen, brown adipose tissue, lung	
GLUT9	II	Kidney, liver, small intestine, placenta, lung, leukocytes	Transports urate
GLUT10	III	Heart, lung, brain, liver, pancreas, placenta, kidney	
GLUT11	II	Heart, skeletal muscle	
GLUT12	III	Heart, prostate, skeletal muscle, placenta	
HMIT (GLUT13)	III	Brain, adipose tissue	Transports *myo*-inositol (not glucose)
GLUT14	I	Testis	

renal epithelial cells. It is a low-affinity, high-capacity transport system that allows non–rate-limiting movement of glucose into and out of these cells. GLUT2 is the major glucose transporter of hepatocytes. GLUT3 is the primary mediator of glucose transport into neurons. GLUT4 catalyzes the rate-limiting step for glucose uptake and metabolism in skeletal muscle, the major organ of glucose consumption. GLUT4 is also present in adipose tissue.

When circulating insulin concentrations are low, most of the GLUT4 is localized in intracellular compartments and is inactive. After eating, the pancreas releases insulin, which stimulates the translocation of GLUT4 to the plasma membrane, thereby promoting glucose uptake into skeletal muscle and fat. Insulin-stimulated glucose transport into skeletal muscle is defective in type 2 diabetes mellitus, but the mechanism has not been established. Exercise also activates glucose entry into skeletal muscle, independently of insulin. Muscle contraction leads to GLUT4 translocation to the plasma membrane via a signaling pathway which differs from that stimulated by insulin.[58]

GLUT9 was initially thought to transport glucose or fructose, but it is established that GLUT9 transports urate. It is required for urate reabsorption in the kidney and appears to be associated with gout. GLUTs 6, 7, 10, 11, 12, and 14 were identified as a result of sequencing the human genome and their physiologic roles remain unclear.[56]

Insulin-like Growth Factors

Insulin-like growth factors 1 and 2 (IGF-1 and IGF-2) are polypeptides structurally related to insulin.[59] These hormones (previously referred to as *nonsuppressible insulin-like activity* or *somatomedin*) exhibit metabolic and growth-promoting effects similar to those of insulin. Accumulating evidence implicates the IGF axis in the development of several common cancers.[60] IGF-1 (previously known as somatomedin C) is an important mediator of growth hormone action and is one of the major regulators of cell growth and differentiation. Synthesis of IGF-1 depends on growth hormone and occurs predominantly in the liver. In addition, many other cells produce IGF-1 that

does not enter the circulation but acts locally. IGF-2 is expressed mainly in early embryonic and fetal development.[61] In adults, IGF-2 is produced in the liver and epithelial cells lining the brain. Circulating IGF-1 concentrations are approximately 1000-fold higher than insulin concentrations, and the hormone is kept inactive by binding to a family of at least six specific binding proteins.[62] These proteins regulate IGFs by protecting the ligands in the circulation and delivering them to their target tissue. In contrast to insulin, which is unbound in the circulation, less than 10% of total serum IGF-1 is free. The biological actions of IGF are exerted through specific IGF receptors or the insulin receptor. The IGF-1 receptor is closely related to the insulin receptor in structure and biochemical properties. In contrast, the IGF-2 receptor is quite different; it lacks tyrosine kinase activity, and its physiologic relevance is not understood. The IGF-1 receptor has a high affinity for both IGF-1 and IGF-2, but a low affinity for insulin. The IGF-2 receptor has high, low, and no affinity for IGF-2, IGF-1, and insulin, respectively. The insulin receptor binds insulin with high affinity and IGF-1 and IGF-2 with low affinity.

The significance of IGFs in normal carbohydrate metabolism is not known. Exogenous administration produces hypoglycemia, whereas a deficiency of IGF-1 results in dwarfism (pygmies and Laron dwarfs). IGFs, particularly IGF-2, may be produced in excess by extrapancreatic neoplasms, and patients may have fasting hypoglycemia.[63,64] The high concentrations of both IGF-2 protein in the blood and IGF-2 messenger RNA (mRNA) in tumor extracts have led to the proposal that IGF-2 is the humoral mediator of non–islet cell tumor–induced hypoglycemia.[65] Measurement of plasma IGF-1 concentration may be useful in evaluating growth hormone deficiency and excess (acromegaly), and in monitoring response to nutritional support.

Counter-Regulatory Hormones

Several hormones have actions opposite to those of insulin. These counter-regulatory hormones are catabolic and increase hepatic glucose production initially by enhancing the breakdown of glycogen to glucose (glycogenolysis), and later by stimulating the synthesis of glucose (gluconeogenesis).[36,66] The initial response (within minutes) to low blood glucose is an increase in glucose production, stimulated by glucagon and epinephrine. Over time (3 to 4 hours), growth hormone and cortisol increase glucose mobilization and decrease glucose use (Fig. 47.1). Evidence also suggests that glucose production by the liver is an inverse function of ambient glucose concentration, independent of hormonal factors (glucose autoregulation). The role of other hormones or neurotransmitters is not clear but appears relatively unimportant. Multiple counter-regulatory hormones exhibit both redundancy and hierarchy. Glucagon is the most important, and epinephrine becomes critical when glucagon is deficient. The other factors have lesser roles. These hormones, briefly described here, are discussed further in Chapters 38, 52, 55, and 56.

Glucagon

Glucagon is a 29 amino acid polypeptide secreted by α-cells of the pancreas. It is derived from proglucagon, which is hydrolyzed by PC2.[67,68] The major target organ for glucagon is the liver, where it binds to a specific G protein-coupled receptor, which is expressed abundantly in liver and kidney, and to a lesser extent in other tissues, including heart, adipose, pancreas, and brain. Glucagon stimulates the production of glucose in the liver predominantly by glycogenolysis. Gluconeogenesis is also activated and glycogenesis is inhibited. Glucagon secretion is regulated primarily by plasma glucose concentrations, with low and high plasma glucose being stimulatory and inhibitory, respectively. Long-standing diabetes mellitus impairs the glucagon response to hypoglycemia, resulting in an increased incidence of hypoglycemic episodes. Stress, exercise, and amino acids induce glucagon release. Insulin inhibits glucagon release from the pancreas and decreases glucagon gene expression, thereby attenuating its biosynthesis. Increased glucagon concentrations, secondary to insulin deficiency, contribute to the hyperglycemia and ketosis of diabetes. In addition to its effects on glycemia, glucagon directly regulates triglyceride, free fatty acid, and bile metabolism. For example, it enhances fatty acid oxidation and ketogenesis in the liver.

Proglucagon is also produced in the distal gut by enteroendocrine L cells and neurons in the nucleus of the solitary tract. In the intestinal L cells, proglucagon is cleaved by PC1/3 to GLP-1, GLP-2, oxyntomodulin, glicentin, and intervening peptide 2 (IP2).[68] Food ingestion stimulates secretion of GLP-1, which acts on β-cells of the pancreas to stimulate insulin gene transcription, potentiate glucose-induced insulin secretion, and inhibit glucagon secretion. GLP-1 and GIP (synthesized in and secreted from the duodenum and proximal jejunum) are incretin hormones that are responsible for up to 70% of postprandial insulin secretion.[69] GLP-1 receptors are widely expressed and GLP-1 also regulates glucose concentration through extrapancreatic mechanisms, including inhibiting glucose production and food intake. For these reasons, both GLP-1 receptor agonists and dipeptidyl peptidase 4 (DPP-4) inhibitors (which increase circulating GLP-1 and GIP) are used in the treatment of type 2 diabetes.[70,71]

Epinephrine

Epinephrine (also called adrenaline), a catecholamine secreted by the adrenal medulla, stimulates glucose production (glycogenolysis) and decreases glucose use, thereby increasing blood glucose concentrations. It also stimulates glucagon secretion and inhibits insulin secretion by the pancreas (see Fig. 47.1). Epinephrine appears to have a key role in glucose counter-regulation when glucagon secretion is impaired (e.g., in type 1 diabetes mellitus). Physical or emotional stress increases epinephrine production, releasing glucose for energy. Tumors of the adrenal medulla, known as pheochromocytomas, secrete excess epinephrine or norepinephrine and produce moderate hyperglycemia as long as glycogen stores are available in the liver.

Growth Hormone

Growth hormone is a polypeptide secreted by the anterior pituitary gland. It stimulates gluconeogenesis, enhances lipolysis, and antagonizes insulin-stimulated glucose uptake.

Cortisol

Cortisol, secreted by the adrenal cortex in response to adrenocorticotropic hormone (ACTH), stimulates gluconeogenesis and increases the breakdown of protein and fat. Patients with Cushing syndrome have increased cortisol production owing to tumor or hyperplasia of the adrenal cortex and may become hyperglycemic. In contrast, people with Addison disease have adrenocortical insufficiency caused by destruction or atrophy of the adrenal cortex and may exhibit hypoglycemia.

Other Hormones Influencing Glucose Metabolism

Thyroxine

Thyroxine, secreted by the thyroid gland, is not directly involved in glucose homeostasis, but it stimulates glycogenolysis and increases the rates of gastric emptying and intestinal glucose absorption. These factors may produce glucose intolerance in thyrotoxic individuals, but patients usually have a fasting plasma glucose concentration within the reference interval.

Somatostatin

Somatostatin, also called growth hormone–inhibiting hormone, is a 14 amino acid peptide found in the gastrointestinal tract, the hypothalamus, and the δ-cells of the pancreatic islets. Although somatostatin does not appear to have a direct effect on carbohydrate metabolism, it inhibits the release of growth hormone from the pituitary. In addition, somatostatin inhibits secretion of glucagon and insulin by the pancreas, thus modulating the reciprocal relationship between these two hormones.

CLINICAL UTILITY OF MEASURING INSULIN, PROINSULIN, C-PEPTIDE, AND GLUCAGON

Box 47.1 lists the clinical conditions in which hormones that regulate glucose, namely, insulin, proinsulin, C-peptide, and glucagon, have been measured. Although there is interest in the possible clinical value of measurement of the concentrations of insulin and its precursors, the assays are useful primarily for research purposes. There is no role for routine testing for insulin, proinsulin, or C-peptide in most patients with diabetes mellitus.[48,72] Measurement of C-peptide is sometimes necessary in the United States for patients to obtain insurance coverage for continuous subcutaneous insulin infusion pumps. Occasionally, C-peptide measurements may help distinguish type 1 from type 2 diabetes in ambiguous cases (e.g., patients who have type 2 phenotype, but present with ketoacidosis). It must be emphasized that the diagnostic criteria for diabetes mellitus do not include measurements of hormones, which remain predominantly research tools.

Insulin

The primary clinical application of insulin measurement is in the evaluation of patients with fasting hypoglycemia (discussed in more detail in Chapter 35). Measurement of circulating insulin could be helpful in evaluating insulin resistance and insulin secretion. Insulin determination has also been proposed to be of value in selecting the optimal initial therapy for patients with type 2 diabetes mellitus. In theory, the lower the pretreatment insulin concentration, the more appropriate might be insulin or an insulin secretagogue as the treatment of choice. Although intellectually appealing, no evidence suggests that knowledge of the insulin concentration leads to more efficacious treatment. Evidence indicates that increased concentrations of insulin in nondiabetic individuals are an independent predictor of the development of coronary artery disease.[73,74] Nevertheless, it is not clear whether the increased insulin is responsible for the risk of coronary disease, and the clinical value of measuring it in this context is questionable.[48] In the past, measurement of insulin was advocated by some in the evaluation and management of patients with polycystic ovary syndrome.[48,72] Women with this condition have insulin resistance with androgen excess and abnormal carbohydrate metabolism that may respond to oral antihyperglycemic agents. However, it is not clear whether assessing insulin resistance by measuring insulin concentrations affords any advantage over clinical signs of insulin resistance (body mass index, acanthosis nigricans), and the American College of Obstetrics and Gynecology (ACOG) does not recommend routine measurements of insulin.[75] Although a few investigators have advocated measuring insulin along with glucose during an OGTT as an aid to the early diagnosis of diabetes mellitus, this approach is not recommended.[48,72] Insulin measurements do not add significantly to diabetes risk prediction generated with traditional clinical and laboratory measurements.[76]

Proinsulin

High proinsulin concentrations are usually noted in patients with benign or malignant β-cell tumors of the pancreas. Most patients with β-cell tumors have increased insulin, C-peptide, and proinsulin concentrations, but occasionally only proinsulin is increased[77] because the tumors have defective conversion of proinsulin to insulin. Despite its low biological activity, proinsulin production may be adequate to produce hypoglycemia. In addition, a rare form of familial hyperproinsulinemia, produced by impaired conversion to insulin, has been described. Measurement of proinsulin can be useful to determine the amount of proinsulin-like material that cross-reacts in an insulin assay. Patients with type 2 diabetes have increased proportions of proinsulin and proinsulin conversion intermediates,[78] high concentrations of which are associated with cardiovascular risk factors.[79] Even relatively mild hyperglycemia produces hyperproinsulinemia, with values greater than 40% of insulin concentration in type 2 diabetes.[78] Similarly, women with GDM have higher concentrations of proinsulin and split-32,33-proinsulin than pregnant normoglycemic control subjects. An increased ratio of proinsulin-like molecules to insulin-like molecules at screening may be a better predictor of GDM than age, obesity, or hyperglycemia.[80] Interestingly, recent evidence reveals that almost all individuals with long-standing type 1 diabetes retain the ability to synthesize proinsulin.[81] Increased proinsulin concentrations may also be detected in patients with chronic renal failure, cirrhosis, or hyperthyroidism.

Accurate measurement of proinsulin has been difficult for several reasons: the blood concentrations are low; antibody production is difficult; most antisera cross-react with insulin and C-peptide, which are present in much higher concentrations; the assays measure intermediate cleavage forms of proinsulin, and reference preparations of pure proinsulin are not readily available. However, a more sensitive nonequilibrium RIA method for measuring proinsulin was developed by adsorbing the initial antiserum with biosynthetic human C-peptide coupled with agarose to eliminate cross-reactivity with C-peptide.[82,83] An enzyme-linked immunosorbent assay (ELISA) has been described that employs an antibody to C-peptide as the coating antibody and anti-insulin antibody for detection.[84] The detection limit is 0.25 pmol/L.[85]

C-Peptide

Measurement of C-peptide has several advantages over insulin measurement. Because hepatic metabolism is negligible, C-peptide concentrations are better indicators of β-cell function than is peripheral insulin concentration.[86] Furthermore, C-peptide assays do not measure exogenous insulin and do not cross-react with insulin antibodies, which interfere with the insulin immunoassay.

Fasting Hypoglycemia

The primary indication for measuring C-peptide is for the evaluation of fasting hypoglycemia. Some patients with insulin-producing β-cell tumors, particularly if hyperinsulinism is intermittent, may exhibit increased C-peptide concentrations with normal insulin concentrations. When hypoglycemia is due to surreptitious insulin injection, insulin concentrations will be high but C-peptide values will be low[87]; this occurs because C-peptide is not found in commercial insulin preparations and exogenous insulin suppresses β-cell function.

Insulin Secretion

Basal or stimulated (by glucagon or glucose) C-peptide concentrations provide estimates of a patient's insulin secretory capacity and rate. For example, diabetes patients with C-peptide concentrations greater than 1.8 ng/mL (0.60 nmol/L) after stimulation with glucagon behave clinically like patients with type 2 diabetes, and those with low peak C-peptide values (<0.5 μg/L; <0.16 nmol/L) behave like patients with type 1 diabetes.[88] In rare cases, this strategy may be helpful before discontinuation of insulin treatment (e.g., in an obese adolescent). Urine and fasting serum C-peptide concentrations appear to be of some value in differentiating patients with type 1 diabetes from those with type 2 diabetes.[89] In addition, patients who have type 1 diabetes but who have no C-peptide response are usually more labile than those with some residual β-cell function. Despite these observations, C-peptide measurement has a negligible role in the routine management of patients with diabetes. Medicare patients in the United States must have low C-peptide concentrations to be eligible for insurance coverage of insulin pumps.[48,72]

Monitoring Therapy

Measurement of C-peptide is used to monitor patients' response to pancreatic surgery. C-peptide should be undetectable after a radical pancreatectomy and should increase after a successful pancreas or islet cell transplant. In addition, C-peptide concentration is used as an endpoint in immunomodulatory trials for the prevention of type 1 diabetes.[90]

Measurements of urine C-peptide are useful when continuous assessment of β-cell function is desired, or when frequent blood sampling is not practical. The 24-hour urine C-peptide content (in the absence of renal failure, which produces increased concentrations) correlates well with fasting serum C-peptide concentration or with the sum of C-peptide concentrations in sequential specimens after a glucose load. However, the fraction of secreted C-peptide that is excreted in the urine exhibits high intersubject and intrasubject variability, limiting the value of urine C-peptide as a measure of insulin secretion.[91] Some have advocated C-peptide to creatinine ratio in a single urine sample to avoid the problems associated with 24-hour urine collection.[92]

Glucagon

Very high concentrations of glucagon are seen in patients with α-cell tumors of the pancreas called glucagonomas. Patients with this tumor frequently have weight loss, necrolytic migratory erythema, diabetes mellitus, stomatitis, and diarrhea.[93] Skin lesions often occur first and are frequently overlooked. Most tumors have metastasized when finally diagnosed. Low glucagon concentrations are associated with chronic pancreatitis and long-term sulfonylurea therapy.

METHODS FOR THE MEASUREMENT OF SPECIFIC HORMONES

Insulin

Although insulin has been assayed for over 60 years, no highly accurate, precise, and reliable procedure is available to measure the amount of insulin in a patient sample. Many insulin assays are commercially available.[94–96] The techniques most widely used are immunometric.[95,96] Bioassays, although of greater physiologic relevance because they measure biological activity, are labor intensive and are rarely used. A stable isotope dilution mass spectrometry (IDMS) assay yields lower values than an immunoassay.[97]

Patients treated with exogenous insulin may develop circulating anti-insulin antibodies, which compete with antibodies in the immunoassay. Endogenous antibodies and their bound insulin can be precipitated from serum with polyethylene glycol (PEG), and free insulin measured by immunoassay. Total insulin can be quantified by eluting antibody-bound insulin with hydrochloric acid (HCl), precipitating the antibody with PEG, and performing an immunoassay. The bound insulin is the difference between total and free insulin. A recent study comparing five commercial insulin assays observed substantial differences among the methods after PEG precipitation; gel filtration chromatography was found to be more sensitive than PEG in identifying anti-IAAs.[98]

Comments

General comments on the measurement of insulin include the following:

1. The term *immunoreactive insulin* is used in reference to assays that may recognize, in addition to insulin, substrates that share antigenic epitopes with insulin. Examples include proinsulin, proinsulin conversion intermediates, and insulin derivatives produced by glycation or dimerization.

2. Various insulin preparations, including human insulin, have been used as insulin calibrators. The insulin calibrator is expressed in terms of international units (IU). One IU of insulin is equal to approximately 43 μg of the WHO First International Reference Preparation (1st IRP) Code 66/304 (National Institute of Biological Standards and Control, South Mimms, Potters Bar, Hertfordshire, United Kingdom), which is 100% human insulin.

3. Antisera raised against insulin show some cross-reactivity with proinsulin but not with C-peptide. Specificity is not a problem in healthy individuals because the low proinsulin concentrations do not appreciably affect the absolute values of insulin. In certain situations (e.g., islet cell tumors and individuals with diabetes), proinsulin is present at higher concentrations, and direct assay of plasma may falsely overestimate the true insulin concentration. Because proinsulin has very low activity, incorrect conclusions regarding the availability of biologically active insulin may be reached in patients with diabetes. The magnitude of the error depends on the concentration of proinsulin and the extent of cross-reactivity of the antiserum with proinsulin.

4. A stable IDMS assay has been developed to measure insulin, proinsulin, and C-peptide.[97] The difference in mass among the three analytes allows specific measurement of each protein. Comparison of patient samples revealed that most, but not all, results were higher by immunoassay than by mass spectrometry.[97] Thus immunoassays may overestimate insulin, particularly at low concentrations. The high protein concentration in the serum requires extraction of proteins (e.g., by immunoaffinity) and purification by high-performance liquid chromatography (HPLC) before quantification by mass spectrometry. This method is not suitable for routine laboratory analysis but is the best higher-order measurement procedure available and can be used as a candidate reference measurement procedure.

5. The ADA appointed a task force to standardize the insulin assay.[46] Evaluation of unknown samples by 17 different laboratories revealed a wide range in insulin values, with interlaboratory variation up to threefold.[46] Large differences were observed even among laboratories using the same assays. Characteristics of some assays, including commercial kits, were unacceptable. The task force judged available proficiency and certification programs for insulin to be inadequate, and recommended the establishment of a central laboratory to provide certification for insulin assays.

6. In 2004, the ADA convened an international workgroup to establish guidelines for acceptability of insulin assays and to develop a standardization program that can be used to achieve uniform accuracy-based values.[99] Evaluation of ten commercial insulin methods from nine manufacturers

revealed within-assay CVs ranging from 3.7 to 39%, and seven assays had a CV ≤ 10.6%.[99] Interassay CVs ranged from 12 to 66%. A common insulin reference preparation failed to improve harmonization of results. The workgroup concluded that not all commercial insulin assays have acceptable performance characteristics. A study in the United Kingdom published at the same time[96] compared 11 commercially available insulin assays and made analogous observations. Insulin values among the different assays varied up to twofold.

The ADA workgroup later compared results of 10 commercial insulin assays against IDMS. Four methods were within 32% of the IDMS concentration.[95] Most methods had bias greater than 15.5%. Bias was reduced by calibration with serum pools but remained high for many methods at low insulin concentrations (<60 pmol/L; <10 μIU/mL).

7. Based on biological variability, desirable measurement bias of ±15%, imprecision of 10.6% CV, and total analytical error of 32.0% have been proposed for a single insulin measurement.[99]

8. Patient samples with high values should be diluted with the zero calibrator.

9. The workgroup recommended that insulin concentrations be reported in SI units: pmol/L.

10. The presence of antibodies to insulin produces spuriously increased or decreased (depending on the method used) insulin values.

11. Commercial immunoassays fail to detect commonly prescribed insulin analogues, which are modified forms of insulin with altered pharmacologic properties.[100] These need to be measured by mass spectrometry.

Reference Intervals

Reference intervals vary among assays, and each laboratory should ideally establish its own reference intervals. After an overnight fast, insulin concentrations in healthy, normal, nonobese people vary from 12 to 150 pmol/L (2 to 25 μIU/mL).[a] More specific assays that have minimal cross-reactivity with proinsulin reveal a fasting plasma insulin concentration of less than 60 pmol/L (<10 μIU/mL). Concentrations up to 1200 pmol/L (200 μIU/mL) can be reached during a glucose tolerance test. Representative values for insulin concentrations after glucose are shown in Fig.47.4. Fasting insulin values are higher in obese, nondiabetic people and lower in trained athletes.

Insulin Antibodies

When there is a clinical suspicion of insulin antibodies, insulin should be measured before and after the sample is diluted. Nonlinear values are highly suggestive of assay interference. Assays to identify insulin antibodies involve the separation of free insulin from bound insulin, followed by measurement of insulin by immunoassay. Separation can be achieved by precipitation with PEG or by gel filtration chromatography, which separates molecules on the basis of molecular mass. The latter is reported to be more sensitive.[98] These are discussed in greater detail in Reeves.[101]

---

[a]The conversion factor of 6.0 used to convert μIU/mL (or mIU/L) of insulin to pmol/L is based on an MW of insulin of 5807.58 and specific activity of 30 IU/mg.

Proinsulin
Principle

Accurate measurement of proinsulin has been difficult for several reasons: the blood concentrations are low; antibody production is difficult; most antisera cross-react with insulin and C-peptide, which are present in much higher concentrations; the assays measure intermediate cleavage forms of proinsulin; and reference preparations of pure proinsulin were not readily available.[102] The availability of biosynthetic proinsulin allowed the production of monoclonal antibodies to proinsulin[39,103] and has provided reliable proinsulin calibrators and reference preparations. An International Reference Preparation for human proinsulin (code 84/611) is available from the National Institute of Biological Standards and Controls (Potters Bar, UK). Immunometric methods have been developed[104] and assays that measure either intact or total proinsulin are commercially available. Earlier assays may have overestimated proinsulin concentrations.[105]

Reference Intervals

Reference intervals for proinsulin are highly dependent on the method of analysis, the degree of cross-reactivity of the antisera, and the purity of proinsulin calibrators. Each laboratory should establish its own reference intervals. Reference intervals in healthy, fasting individuals reported in the literature range from 1.1 to 6.9 pmol/L to 2.1 to 12.6 pmol/L (see Reference[104] and references therein). Proinsulin is stable in EDTA at room temperature for at least 24 hours.

C-Peptide
Principle

C-peptide undergoes minimal liver metabolism, and, in contrast to proinsulin, assays are not affected by anti-insulin antibodies. However, several methodologic problems produce large between-method variation. These difficulties include variable specificity among different antisera, variable cross-reactivity with proinsulin, and various types of C-peptide preparation used as a calibrator. The NIH formed a committee in 2002 to harmonize C-peptide measurements. Comparison of 40 serum samples using nine commercial C-peptide assay methods showed within- and between-run CVs ranging from less than 2 to greater than 10%, and from less than 2 to greater than 18%, respectively.[106] Some methods had high imprecision, with between-run CVs exceeding 15%. IDMS methods for measuring C-peptide have been developed.[107,108] Calibrating C-peptide measurements to a reference method using mass spectrometry increased comparability among laboratories.[106] However, by 2015 there were three different pure materials under evaluation by harmonization efforts in several different countries.[109] Better collaboration among these organizations is necessary to achieve standardization.

Reference Intervals

Fasting serum concentrations of C-peptide in healthy people range from 0.78 to 1.89 ng/mL (0.25 to 0.6 nmol/L). After stimulation with glucose or glucagon, values range from 2.73 to 5.64 ng/mL (0.9 to 1.87 nmol/L), or three to five times the prestimulation value. Urine C-peptide is usually in the range of 74 ± 26 μg/L (25 ± 8.8 μmol/L). C-peptide is excreted primarily by the kidney, and concentrations in the serum are increased in renal disease.

Glucagon

Principle

A competitive RIA is available for measuring glucagon. ^{125}I-labeled glucagon competes with glucagon in the patient specimen for binding to the polyclonal glucagon antibody. Bound glucagon is separated from free glucagon by the use of PEG and a second antibody. Bound radioactivity for the patient specimen is compared with that of glucagon calibrators. Calibrator values are assigned at the manufacturer using the WHO glucagon international standard (69/194). Immunoassays that do not use radioactivity have been developed. A recent comparison of ten commercially available assays reveals that some show cross-reactivity with other peptides from proglucagon, and all lack sensitivity at low glucagon concentrations.[110]

Reference Intervals

Fasting plasma concentrations of glucagon vary depending on the method, ranging from 0 to 20 to 135 ng/L (0 to 5.7 to 38.7 pmol/L). Values up to 500 times the upper reference limit may be found in patients with autonomously secreting α-cell neoplasms.

PATHOGENESIS OF TYPE 1 DIABETES MELLITUS

Type 1 diabetes mellitus results from cellular-mediated autoimmune destruction of the insulin-secreting cells of pancreatic β-cells.[111,112] In the vast majority of patients, destruction is mediated by T cells. This is termed type 1A or immune-mediated diabetes (Box 47.2). The α-, δ-, and other islet cells are preserved. The islet cells have a chronic mononuclear cell infiltrate, called insulitis. The autoimmune process leading to type 1 diabetes begins months or years before the clinical presentation, and an 80 to 90% reduction in the volume of β-cells is required to induce symptomatic type 1 diabetes. The rate of islet cell destruction is variable and is usually more rapid in children than in adults.

Antibodies

The most practical markers of β-cell autoimmunity are circulating antibodies, which have been detected in the serum years before the onset of hyperglycemia. Currently autoantibodies are not used in the routine management of patients with diabetes. The best characterized islet autoantibodies are as follows[48,112,113]:

1. *Islet cell cytoplasmic antibodies* (ICAs) react with a sialoglycoconjugate antigen present in the cytoplasm of all endocrine cells of the pancreatic islets. These antibodies are detected in the serum of 0.5% of normal subjects and 75 to 85% of patients with newly diagnosed type 1 diabetes. The antibodies are detected by immunofluorescence microscopy on frozen sections of human pancreatic tails. Results are compared with standard serum of the Immunology of Diabetes Workgroup[114] and are expressed in Juvenile Diabetes Foundation (JDF) units. Although not universal, many laboratories use 10 JDF units on two separate occasions or a single result of greater than or equal to 20 JDF units as a significant titer. The ICA assay is cumbersome, labor intensive, and difficult to standardize. Few clinical laboratories have implemented this assay, which has marked interlaboratory variability in sensitivity and specificity.[48]

2. *Insulin autoantibodies* IAA are present in ~80 to 90% of children who develop type 1 diabetes before age 5, but in less than 40% of individuals who develop diabetes after age 12. Their frequency in healthy people is similar to that of ICA. A radioisotopic method that calculates the displaceable insulin radioligand binding after the addition of excess nonradiolabeled insulin is recommended for IAA. Results are positive when concentrations exceed the 99th centile or the mean + 2 (or 3) SDs in healthy controls. Proficiency evaluation revealed poor concordance for IAA among laboratories.[115] Immunoassays that do not use radiolabel are available.[116] Insulin antibodies develop rapidly (<2 weeks) after initiation of insulin therapy. Therefore IAA should not be measured in insulin-treated patients as assays do not distinguish insulin antibodies from IAA.

3. *Antibodies to the 65 kDa isoform of glutamic acid decarboxylase* (GADA)[117] have been found up to 10 years before the onset of clinical type 1 diabetes and are present in ≈60% of patients with newly diagnosed type 1 diabetes. GADA may be used to identify patients with apparent type 2 diabetes who will subsequently progress to type 1 diabetes. Several different assay formats have been used for the measurement of GADA, including enzymatic immunoprecipitation assay, radiobinding assay, ELISA, immunofluorescence, and Western blotting.[118] Considerable variability among laboratories has been significantly reduced by the Second International GADAb Workshop.[118] A monoclonal antibody, MICA 3, was suggested as a reference standard. A dual micromethod and RIA performed with ^{3}H-labeled human recombinant GAD65 in a rabbit reticulocyte expression system is used by many laboratories. Methods for immunoassays for GADA without radiolabel are now commercially available.

4. *Insulinoma-associated antigens* (IA-2A and IA-2βA), directed against two tyrosine phosphatases, have been detected in ~40 to 60% of newly diagnosed type 1 diabetes patients. The frequency is highest in the young and decreases with age. A widely used method to measure IA-2A uses ^{35}S-labeled recombinant IA-2 in a dual micromethod and RIA. Concurrent analysis of IA-2 and GADA in a single assay has been reported.[119]

5. *Zinc transporter ZnT8* was identified in 2007 as a major autoantigen in type 1 diabetes.[120] ZnT8 is the least characterized of the autoantibodies in diabetes. Initial analysis identified ZnT8 in 60 to 80% of patients with new-onset type 1 diabetes compared with less than 2% of controls and less than 3% of individuals with type 2 diabetes. Importantly, antibodies to ZnT8 are detected in ~26% of patients with type 1 diabetes who are negative for other islet autoantibodies.[113]

Most islet autoantibodies are measured by quantitative radiobinding assays.[121] Radiolabeled recombinant insulin, GAD65, or IA-2 is incubated with patient's serum and the amount of radioactivity in the precipitated complex is proportional to the antibody concentration. Nonradioactive ELISA methods have become available for IAA, GADA, IA-2, and ZnT8 (the last was approved by the FDA in 2014 for use in the United States). While RIA remains the most widely used technique for patient samples and clinical studies, recent evidence reveals that some nonradioactive assays exhibit better performance than RIA,[122] and ECL assays for IAA and GADA are reported to be more sensitive and specific than RIA.[123] Newer strategies, such as plasmonic chip-based assays,[124,125] may also replace the requirement for radiolabel in the future.

The Centers for Disease Control and Prevention (CDC) and the Immunology of Diabetes Society established in 2000 the Diabetes Autoantibody Standardization Program (DASP). The major goals of DASP are: to assist laboratories in improving methods, to organize workshops for harmonization of antibody testing for type 1 diabetes, and to provide reference materials.[115,126] DASP provides serum from 50 patients with newly diagnosed type 1 diabetes and from 50 to 100 control individuals. DASP was subsequently replaced by the Islet Autoantibody Standardization Program (IASP), which is supported by the Immunology of Diabetes Society and the NIH. A WHO standard for GAD65 and IA-2A has been established and allows laboratories to express results in common units.[126] Several workshops have been held. The first assay proficiency evaluation revealed poor performance for IAA among 23 laboratories,[115] and most laboratories continue to have less than acceptable sensitivity and/or specificity.[113] By contrast, good concordance among laboratories was observed for GADA and IA-2A,[126] and comparable (though are not identical) results have been obtained with subsequent comparisons.[122,127] Ongoing harmonization is likely to enhance assay performance.

Autoantibody markers of immune destruction are present in 85 to 90% of individuals with immune-mediated diabetes when fasting hyperglycemia is initially detected.[1] Approximately 5 to 10% of white adult patients who have the type 2 diabetes phenotype also have islet cell autoantibodies, particularly GADA. This condition has been termed latent autoimmune diabetes of adulthood (LADA) (previously termed type 1½ diabetes or slow-onset diabetes in adults).[128] Up to 1 to 2% of healthy individuals have a single autoantibody and are at low risk of developing immune-mediated diabetes. Because the prevalence of immune-mediated diabetes is low (~0.3% in the general population in most countries), the positive predictive value of a single autoantibody will be extremely low. The presence of multiple autoantibodies is associated with a high risk of type 1 diabetes. A large study measured IAA, GADA, and IA-2 in 13,387 children who were at high risk for type 1 diabetes and followed them for 15 years.[129] The number of autoantibodies predicted development of type 1 diabetes, ranging from 10% for 1 autoantibody to almost 100% if multiple autoantibodies were present. Autoantibodies were not required for diabetes as 0.2% of autoantibody-negative children progressed to type 1 diabetes. The time interval from seroconversion to onset of disease varied from weeks to 18 years.[129] Screening for islet autoantibodies is controversial[48,121] because no acceptable therapy has been documented to reliably prevent or delay the clinical onset of diabetes in islet autoantibody-positive individuals.[112]

Although several agents can prevent or reverse type 1 diabetes in mouse models, these approaches have not been successful in humans.[130] Nevertheless, many clinical trials to intervene in the natural history of type 1 diabetes are being actively pursued[131,132] (for a recent review, see Warshauer et al.[133]). Primary prevention is directed at individuals with increased risk who have no signs of disease. At the time of writing, the only successful human prevention trial showed in 2019 that a single course of teplizumab (an Fc receptor-nonbinding anti-CD3 monoclonal antibody) delayed by 2 years the progression to clinical type 1 diabetes in a high-risk population.[134] Secondary prevention is targeted at individuals with persistent islet autoantibodies. Most strategies focus on immunosuppressive therapy to attenuate the autoimmune response. These can be divided into autoantigen-specific therapies (such as insulin [oral or nasal]), alum-formulated recombinant GAD65 or HLA peptides and nonautoantigen-specific therapies (such as Bacillus Calmette-Guerin [BCG] vaccine, cyclosporine, and monoclonal antibodies to CD3 or CD20). Tertiary prevention, or intervention, trials recruit patients newly diagnosed with type 1 diabetes where the objective is to preserve residual β-cell function (assessed by measuring C-peptide concentrations in the blood). Strategies include autoantigen-specific therapies, e.g., proinsulin peptide, and nonautoantigen-specific therapies, e.g., daclizumab (humanized IgG1 that binds to IL-2 receptor on T cells), rituximab, anakinra (IL-1β receptor antagonist), abatacept (fusion protein of cytotoxic T-lymphocyte protein 4 and immunoglobulin [CTLA4-Ig]) or antithymocyte globulin. Unfortunately, none of the secondary prevention or intervention trials or any of the immunosuppressive agents has preserved β-cell function in the long term. Some experts posit that monotherapy will be insufficient and therapies which combine immunomodulation using an autoantigen with immunosuppressive therapy are necessary.

Genetics

Susceptibility to type 1 diabetes is inherited,[135] but the mode of inheritance is complex and has not been defined. It is a multigenic trait, and the major locus is the major histocompatibility complex on chromosome 6. At least 11 other loci on 9 chromosomes also contribute, with the regulatory region of the insulin gene INS on chromosome 11p15 being an important locus. The human leukocyte antigen (HLA)-DQ and -DR genetic factors are by far the most important determinants for risk of type 1 diabetes.[48,136,137] The concordance rate between identical twins is approximately 30%. Approximately 95% of whites with type 1 diabetes express HLA-DR3 or HLA-DR4 histocompatibility antigens. However, up to 40% of the nondiabetic population also express these alleles. In contrast, the HLA-DQB1*0602 allele significantly decreases the risk of type 1 diabetes. HLA typing can indicate absolute risk of diabetes.[48] The risk of a sibling developing diabetes is 1, 5, and 10 to 20% if the number of haplotypes shared is none, one, and two, respectively. However, only 10% of patients with type 1 diabetes have an affected first-degree relative. Overall, more than 40 non–HLA-susceptibility gene markers have been confirmed, but these have smaller effects than HLA.[136] Non-HLA genetic factors that increase risk include the insulin gene (INS), cytotoxic T-lymphocyte-associated protein 4 (CTLA4), and protein tyrosine phosphatase nonreceptor type 22 (lymphoid) (PTPN22).[48,136,137] The multiplicity of independent chromosomal regions associated with a predisposition to type 1 diabetes suggests that other susceptibility genes will be identified. Routine measurement of genetic markers is not of value at this time for the diagnosis or management of patients with type 1 diabetes.[48]

Environment

Environmental factors are involved in initiating diabetes. Viruses, such as rubella, mumps, enterovirus, and Coxsackievirus B, have been implicated.[133,138] It seems likely that autoimmunity to β-cells is initiated by a viral protein (that shares amino acid sequence with a β-cell protein) or some other environmental insult. Genetic susceptibility and other host factors (e.g., HLA type) determine the progression of the β-cell destruction. Epidemiologic studies have implicated early exposure to cow's milk as a trigger of type 1 diabetes. This model is contentious and has been debated for decades.[139] A recent study of 2159 neonates at risk for development of type 1 diabetes who were followed for a median of 11.5 years observed no effect of cow's milk on the development of diabetes.[140] Environmental trials have failed to show a meaningful impact on the natural course of type 1 diabetes.[133]

PATHOGENESIS OF TYPE 2 DIABETES MELLITUS

At least two major identifiable pathologic defects have been reported in patients with type 2 diabetes.[141,142] One is a decreased ability of insulin to act on peripheral tissue. This is called *insulin resistance* and is thought by many to be the primary underlying pathologic process. The other is β-*cell dysfunction,* which is an inability of the pancreas to produce sufficient insulin to compensate for the insulin resistance. Thus a relative deficiency of insulin occurs early in the disease and absolute insulin deficiency late in the disease. The debate over whether type 2 diabetes is due primarily to a defect in β-cell secretion or to peripheral resistance to insulin, or to both, has been raging for decades. Data are available to support the concept that insulin resistance is the primary defect, preceding the derangement in insulin secretion and clinical diabetes by as much as 20 years.[141,143] Despite the lack of consensus, it is clear that type 2 diabetes mellitus is an extremely heterogeneous disease, and no single cause is adequate to explain the progression from normal glucose tolerance to diabetes. The fundamental molecular defects in insulin resistance and insulin secretion result from a combination of environmental and genetic factors.

Loss of β-Cell Function

Increased β-cell demand induced by insulin resistance is ultimately associated with progressive loss of β-cell function that is necessary for the development of fasting hyperglycemia.[144] The major defect is a loss of glucose-induced insulin release (see Fig. 47.4), which is termed *selective glucose unresponsiveness.* Hyperglycemia appears to render the β-cells increasingly unresponsive to glucose (called glucotoxicity), and the degree of dysfunction correlates with both glucose concentration and duration of hyperglycemia. Restoration of euglycemia rapidly resolves the defect. Increased free fatty acids in serum have also been implicated in β-cell failure (lipotoxicity).[145] Other insulin secretory abnormalities in type 2 diabetes include disruption of the normal pulsatile release of insulin and an increased ratio of plasma proinsulin to insulin.[78] The number of β-cells is also reduced in patients with type 2 diabetes.

Insulin Resistance

Insulin resistance is defined as "a decreased biological response to normal concentrations of circulating insulin"[146]; it is found in obese, nondiabetic individuals and in patients with type 2 diabetes. The underlying pathophysiologic defect(s) has (have) not been identified, but insulin resistance is usually attributed to a defect in insulin action. Systematic

inflammation, indicated by increased concentrations of proinflammatory cytokines (e.g., interleukin-6 and tumor necrosis factor) in the blood and inflammatory cells in adipose tissue and liver, contributes to insulin resistance.[147,148] Measurement of insulin resistance in a routine clinical setting is difficult, and surrogate measures, such as fasting insulin concentration or the euglycemic insulin clamp,[149,150] are used to provide an indirect assessment of insulin function. The euglycemic clamp is performed in hospital under close supervision. The subject receives a constant intravenous infusion of insulin in one arm with concurrent intravenous infusion of variable amounts of glucose in the other arm to maintain blood glucose at a normal fasting concentration. This provides a measure of sensitivity to insulin. A simpler, but indirect, approach (termed homeostasis model assessment [HOMA]) is a calculation derived from fasting glucose and insulin concentrations.[150] A broad clinical spectrum of insulin resistance ranges from euglycemia (with marked increase in endogenous insulin) to hyperglycemia (despite large doses of exogenous insulin). Several rare clinical syndromes are also associated with insulin resistance. The prototype is the type A insulin resistance syndrome, which is characterized by hyperinsulinemia, acanthosis nigricans, and ovarian hyperandrogenism.

The insulin resistance syndrome (also known as syndrome X, or the metabolic syndrome) is a constellation of associated clinical and laboratory findings, consisting of insulin resistance, hyperinsulinemia, obesity, dyslipidemia (high triglyceride and low high-density lipoprotein [HDL] cholesterol), and hypertension.[151] Individuals with this syndrome are at increased risk for cardiovascular disease. Several different definitions of the metabolic syndrome have been proposed by different organizations. Some consensus was reached in 2009, except for waist circumference. The metabolic syndrome is diagnosed if an individual meets three or more of the following criteria[152,153]:
- Increased waist circumference population- and country-specific, for example, Europe, Canada, and the United States: greater than 35 inches (>88 cm) (women) or greater than 40 inches (>102 cm) (men)
- Triglycerides greater than 150 mg/dL (>1.7 mmol/L)
- HDL cholesterol less than 51 mg/dL (<1.3 mmol/L) (women) or less than 39 mg/dL (<1.0 mmol/L) (men)
- Blood pressure greater than or equal to 130/85 mm Hg
- Fasting plasma glucose ≥100 mg/dL (≥5.6 mmol/L)

The concept of the "metabolic syndrome" has been questioned by several experts, including the person who first described it[154] and influential clinical diabetes organizations.[155] A WHO Expert Consultation concluded that while the metabolic syndrome may be useful as an educational concept, it has limited practical utility for diagnosis and management, and further efforts to redefine it are inappropriate.[156]

Environment

Environmental factors, such as diet and exercise, are important determinants in the pathogenesis of type 2 diabetes. Convincing evidence links obesity to the development of type 2 diabetes, but the association is complex. Although 60 to 80% of patients with type 2 diabetes are obese, diabetes develops in less than 15% of obese individuals. In contrast, virtually all obese subjects, even those with normal carbohydrate tolerance, have hyperinsulinemia and are insulin resistant. Other factors, such as family history of type 2 diabetes (genetic predisposition), the duration of obesity, and the distribution of fat, are important. Nevertheless, the rising prevalence of diabetes is believed to be a consequence of the increase in obesity (defined as a body mass index ≥ 30 kg/m^2), the prevalence of which was reported to be 39.6% in US adults in 2016[157] and is predicted to reach 48.9% by 2030.[158] Evaluation of 84,941 healthy women after 16 years in the Nurses' Health Study revealed that obesity was the most important predictor of type 2 diabetes.[159] Compared with women with body mass indices less than 23, the relative risks of developing diabetes were 20.1- and 38.8-fold with body mass indices 30 to 34.9 and ≥ 35, respectively. It is important to note that intervention can delay or prevent the onset of type 2 diabetes. Two randomized studies in the early 2000s documented that lifestyle changes (weight reduction and exercise) in individuals with IGT reduced the incidence of type 2 diabetes.[160,161] Although the weight loss was modest (5 to 7%), the rate of progression to type 2 diabetes was reduced by 58% in both studies. This observation has been validated by several other studies (reviewed in Schellenberg et al.[162]).

An inverse relationship has been noted between the degree of physical activity and the prevalence of type 2 diabetes. For every 500 kcal increase in daily energy expenditure, a 6% decrease in age-adjusted risk of type 2 diabetes occurs.[163] This effect is independent of both body weight and a parental history of diabetes. The mechanism of the protective effect of exercise is thought to be increased sensitivity to insulin in skeletal muscle and adipose tissue.

Type 2 Diabetes Susceptibility Genes

It is widely acknowledged that genetic factors contribute to the development of type 2 diabetes.[143] For example, the concordance rate for type 2 diabetes in identical twins approaches 100%. Type 2 diabetes is 10 times more likely to occur in an obese person who has a parent with diabetes than in an equally obese person without a family history of diabetes. However, the mode of inheritance is unknown, and type 2 diabetes has been described as a "geneticist's nightmare."[164] Many less common diseases (e.g., cystic fibrosis, Duchenne muscular dystrophy) are caused by mutations at a single locus. More common diseases, such as diabetes mellitus, schizophrenia, atherosclerosis, hypertension, and osteoporosis, are not inherited according to simple Mendelian rules. These conditions are genetically more complex, and multiple genetic factors interact with exogenous influences (such as environmental factors) to produce the phenotype.

Multiple factors complicate the search for susceptibility genes in type 2 diabetes.[141] A variety of approaches have produced several genes that are associated with type 2 diabetes. Recent genome-wide association studies (GWAS) have substantially contributed to our understanding of the genetic architecture of type 2 diabetes, with more than 240 genetic loci and 400 genetic variants now identified.[165] Most of these genetic loci are associated with the insulin secretion pathway, rather than with insulin resistance. Despite considerable effort to identify the genetic basis of type 2 diabetes mellitus, genetic defects identified to date account for only 5% of patients with type 2 diabetes. Moreover, the risk alleles in these loci all have relatively small effects (odds ratios, 1.1 to 13). Combined analysis of 48 different type 2 risk loci did not significantly affect the time from diagnosis to prescription of the first drug.[166]

Numerous mutations of the insulin receptor gene, *INSR*, have been identified.[146] Many patients with these defects have extreme insulin resistance, but the mutations are exceptionally rare and usually are found in only one patient or a single family. A small number of patients have been identified with mutations of substrates for the insulin receptor (e.g., IRS-1) that cause diabetes. Few mutations have been described in other potential candidate genes, including those coding for GLUT4 and glycogen synthase.

Monogenic Diabetes Mellitus

Mutation of a single gene that results in β-cell dysfunction accounts for ~2% of diabetes. At least 40 genes have been identified that cause monogenic diabetes. (A comprehensive list can be found in Carmody et al.[167]) The ADA recommends that monogenic diabetes should be considered in diabetes diagnosed within the first 6 months of life, "atypical diabetes" (without typical features of type 1 or type 2 diabetes, especially with a strong family history of diabetes), or in children with mild hyperglycemia, especially if nonobese.[20] Monogenic diabetes is usually separated into two categories on the basis of age of onset of hyperglycemia.

Neonatal Diabetes Mellitus. Persistent hyperglycemia occurring before the age of 6 months is termed neonatal (or congenital) diabetes. Genetic testing has identified monogenic etiology in ~85% of these patients.[168] The ADA recommends that all children diagnosed with diabetes in the first 6 months of life should have immediate genetic testing for neonatal diabetes. Accurate diagnosis is important as some patients require insulin while others can be managed with oral hypoglycemic agents. Some forms are transient, and insulin-requiring diabetes may resolve spontaneously between 6 and 18 months of age.[167]

Maturity-onset Diabetes of the Young. Maturity-onset diabetes of the young (MODY[169,170]) phenotypically resembles type 2 diabetes but occurs in young (usually <25 years) nonobese patients who have a family history of diabetes. Inheritance is autosomal dominant, and patients have no autoantibodies for type 1 diabetes. The clinical spectrum of MODY is broad, ranging from asymptomatic hyperglycemia to an acute presentation. Thirteen genes on different chromosomes are associated with this disorder. The most common form (estimated prevalence 1 in 1000), MODY2, results from mutations in the gene that encodes glucokinase (an enzyme that catalyzes the phosphorylation of glucose in the β-cell), leading to partial deficiency of insulin secretion. Patients have mild fasting hyperglycemia and glucose lowering therapy is rarely needed. Most of the other MODYs are caused by mutations in the genes that encode transcription factors that regulate expression of genes in pancreatic β-cells, resulting in impaired insulin synthesis or secretion or a reduced β-cell mass. MODY mutations have substitution, deletion, or insertion of nucleotides in the coding regions of the genes. These mutations are detected by PCR. OGTT, islet autoantibodies, and C-peptide may be helpful in differentiating MODY from type 1 or type 2 diabetes,[170] but genetic testing, now widely available, is required to establish the diagnosis of MODY. Genetic testing for MODY should be performed in those diagnosed in childhood or early adulthood with diabetes that is not characteristic of type 1 or type 2 diabetes that occurs in successive generations.

DIAGNOSIS

For many years the diagnosis of diabetes mellitus was dependent solely on the demonstration of hyperglycemia. For type 1 diabetes, the diagnosis is usually easy because hyperglycemia appears abruptly, is severe, and is accompanied by serious metabolic derangements. Diagnosis of type 2 diabetes may be difficult because hyperglycemia often is not severe enough for the patient to notice symptoms of diabetes. Nevertheless, the risk of complications makes it important to identify people with the disease.

The diagnostic criteria recommended in 1979 were:

- Classic symptoms of diabetes with unequivocal increase in plasma glucose,
- FPG greater than or equal to 140 mg/dL (7.8 mmol/L) on more than one occasion, or
- A 2-hour and one other postload glucose concentration greater than or equal to 200 mg/dL (11.1 mmol/L) during an OGTT.[17]

These criteria were widely adopted but are imperfect. The OGTT is more sensitive for diagnosis than fasting glucose early in the course of type 2 diabetes, resulting in lack of equivalence between fasting and 2-hour glucose values. Virtually all persons with an FPG concentration ≥140 mg/dL (≥7.8 mmol/L) have 2-hour glucose ≥200 mg/dL (≥11.1 mmol/L) in an OGTT. In contrast, in persons without previously identified diabetes, fasting glucose ≥140 mg/dL (≥7.8 mmol/L) is present in only 25% of those who have 2-hour glucose ≥200 mg/dL (≥11.1 mmol/L). To address these and other discrepancies, the diagnostic criteria were revised in 1997.[1,171] The major modification was lowering the diagnostic threshold for fasting glucose from 140 to 126 mg/dL (7.8 to 7.0 mmol/L) to better identify individuals at risk of retinopathy and nephropathy. The lower cutoff was suggested to provide earlier diagnosis of diabetes, with consequent earlier therapeutic intervention.[171]

Hemoglobin A_{1c}

A major change in the diagnosis of diabetes was recommended in 2009.[31,172] An International Expert Committee advised that HbA_{1c}, which reflects long-term blood glucose concentrations,[31] could be used for the diagnosis of type 2 diabetes (see Box 47.3). An HbA_{1c} value ≥6.5% (≥48 mmol/mol) was selected as the decision point, based on the prevalence of retinopathy.[31] This recommendation has been endorsed by the ADA[173] and several other influential clinical organizations, including the WHO, the IDF, and the European Association for the Study of Diabetes, and has been widely (albeit not universally) accepted. HbA_{1c} concentrations 5.7 to 6.4% (39 to 46 mmol/mol) indicate subjects at high risk of developing diabetes. Note that some organizations define high risk as HbA_{1c} concentrations of 5.5 to 6.4% (37 to 46 mmol/mol),[174] while others recommend 6.1 to 6.4% (43 to 46 mmol/mol). HbA_{1c} was also recommended as an alternative to glucose for screening for diabetes. This last recommendation has also been accepted by the ADA[173] and other clinical organizations.

Fasting Plasma Glucose

FPG concentrations of 126 mg/dL (7.0 mmol/L) or greater on more than one occasion are diagnostic of diabetes mellitus (see Box 47.3). Some investigators believe that fasting

---

BOX 47.3 Criteria for the Diagnosis of Diabetes Mellitus

Any one of the following is diagnostic:
1. Hemoglobin A_{1c} (HbA_{1c}) ≥6.5% (≥48 mmol/mol)[a] OR
2. Fasting plasma glucose (FPG) ≥126 mg/dL (≥7.0 mmol/L)[b] OR
3. 2 hr plasma glucose ≥200 mg/dL (≥11.1 mmol/L) during an oral glucose tolerance test (OGTT)[c] OR
4. In a patient with classic symptoms of hyperglycemia or hyperglycemic crisis, a random plasma glucose ≥200 mg/dL (≥11.1 mmol/L)

In the absence of unequivocal hyperglycemia, diagnosis requires two abnormal test results from the same sample or in two separate test samples.

[a]The test should be performed in a laboratory using a method that is NGSP-certified and standardized to the DCCT assay. Point-of-care assays should not be used for diagnosis.
[b]Fasting is defined as no caloric intake for at least 8 hours.
[c]The OGTT should be performed as described by the World Health Organization (WHO), using a glucose load containing the equivalent of 75 g of anhydrous glucose dissolved in water.
From the American Diabetes Association. Classification and diagnosis of diabetes: *Standards of medical care in diabetes—2020. Diabetes Care* 2020;34(Suppl 1):S14–31.

---

hyperglycemia may be a relatively late development in the course of type 2 diabetes, delaying the diagnosis and leading to underestimation of the prevalence of diabetes mellitus in the population.[175] Readers should be aware of the limitations of FPG in diabetes diagnosis, including the requirement that the patient fast ≥8 hours, large biological variation (even in a single individual on different days), and the risk of glycolysis in the test tube (for a review, see Sacks[176]).

Oral Glucose Tolerance Test

Serial measurement of plasma glucose before and after a specific amount of glucose given orally should provide a standard method by which to evaluate individuals and establish values for healthy and diseased subjects. Although more sensitive than FPG determinations, glucose tolerance testing is affected by multiple factors that result in *poor reproducibility* (Box 47.4).[48,177] Moreover, approximately 20% of OGTTs fall into the nondiagnostic category (e.g., only one blood sample exhibits increased glucose concentration).[48] Unless results are grossly abnormal initially, some organizations recommend that the OGTT should be performed on two separate occasions to establish the diagnosis of diabetes.

The following conditions should be met before an OGTT is performed: discontinue, when possible, medications known to affect glucose tolerance; perform in the morning after 3 days of unrestricted diet (containing at least 150 g of carbohydrate per day) and activity, and perform the test after a 10- to 16-hour fast only in ambulatory outpatients (bed rest impairs glucose tolerance), who should remain seated during the test without smoking cigarettes. Glucose tolerance testing should not be performed on hospitalized, acutely ill, or inactive patients. The test should begin between 7:00 am and 9:00 am. Venous plasma glucose should be measured fasting and then 2 hours after an oral glucose load. For nonpregnant adults, the recommended load is 75 g, which may not be a maximum stimulus[17]; for children, 1.75 g/kg up to 75 g maximum is given. The glucose should be dissolved in 300 mL of water and ingested over five minutes. A commercial, more palatable form of glucose may be ingested, but whether the anhydrous or monohydrate form of glucose should be used is still in question.[178]

An OGTT is rarely used in clinical practice for the diagnosis of diabetes in the US and many other countries owing to its lack of reproducibility and inconvenience. The sensitivity of FPG concentrations is lower than the OGTT for diagnosing diabetes, and some authors claim that the OGTT better identifies patients at risk for developing complications of diabetes. An FPG value less than 100 mg/dL (<5.6 mmol/L) or a random glucose concentration less than 140 mg/dL (<7.8 mmol/L) is sufficient to rule out the diagnosis of diabetes mellitus. An OGTT is indicated in the following situations.

- Diagnosis of gestational diabetes (GDM, discussed later).
- Initial postpartum screening of women with GDM for type 2 diabetes (discussed later).
- Diagnosis of IGT. This remains controversial. Individuals with IGT have increased risk of cardiovascular disease, but many of them do not have IFG by ADA criteria.[72]
- Evaluation of a patient with unexplained nephropathy, neuropathy, or retinopathy, with random glucose concentration less than 140 mg/dL (<7.8 mmol/L). Abnormal results in this setting do not necessarily denote a cause-and-effect relationship, and other diseases must be ruled out.
- Population studies for epidemiologic data.

A detailed comparison of the advantages and disadvantages of FPG, the OGTT, and HbA$_{1c}$ has been published.[176]

Intravenous Glucose Tolerance Test

Poor absorption of orally administered glucose may result in a "flat" tolerance curve. Some patients are unable to tolerate a large oral carbohydrate load or may have altered gastric physiology (e.g., after gastric resection). In these patients, an intravenous glucose tolerance test (IVGTT) may be performed to eliminate factors related to the rate of glucose absorption. In addition, measurement of the first-phase insulin response can identify the subgroup of individuals with increased concentrations of multiple autoantibodies who are at greatest risk of progression to type 1 diabetes.[179] The IVGTT is also used in a research setting to evaluate pancreatic β-cell function.[150]

Preparation of patients is the same as for the OGTT. The dose of glucose is 0.5 g/kg of body weight (maximum 35 g), given as a 25 g/dL solution. The dose is administered intravenously over 3 minutes ± 15 seconds, and blood is collected every 10 minutes after the mid-injection time for 1 hour. A single forearm vein cannula may be used for infusion and sampling, but it should be flushed with saline after the glucose is infused, and dead space should be cleared with several volumes of blood before each sample is drawn. In some cases, insulin and/or C-peptide assays are performed. Blood glucose concentrations decrease in an exponential manner, and the rate of glucose disappearance can be calculated from the formula $K = 70/t_{1/2}$, where $t_{1/2}$ is the number of minutes required for the blood glucose value to decrease to one half of the 10 minutes value, and K is the rate of disappearance of blood glucose, expressed as %/min. The glucose values are plotted on a log scale versus time on the abscissa. The best-fitting straight line is drawn through the points, and the time (in minutes) for the glucose concentration to decrease by 50% ($t_{1/2}$) is read. In healthy individuals, K usually exceeds 1.5%; values less than 1.0% are considered diagnostic of diabetes. Similar to oral glucose tolerance, intravenous glucose tolerance deteriorates with age.

In the formula $K = 70/t_{1/2}$, the value of 70 is derived from the logarithmic nature of the decrease in glucose concentration over time. The concentration of glucose at 10 minues will be twice that of the value obtained from the plot $t_{1/2}$. Using natural logarithms, the rate of decrease in glucose concentration, expressed as %/min (K), is given by

$$K = 100 \, (\ln 2 - \ln 1)/t_{1/2} = 69.3/t_{1/2} \cong 70/t_{1/2}$$

The main indication for the intravenous glucose tolerance test is in clinical research to evaluate the first-phase insulin response to glucose (see Fig. 47.4).[180] The test is performed as described earlier, but samples are drawn as follows: two baseline samples 5 minutes apart (the latter immediately before infusion) and samples 1, 3, 5, and 10 minutes after the end of the glucose infusion. The first-phase insulin release is usually measured by the sum of the insulin concentrations 1 and 3 minutes after the glucose bolus. Alternatively, the 0- to 10-minute incremental insulin area may be used. Analogous to the OGTT, the intravenous glucose tolerance test has poor reproducibility. It is important to appreciate that the insulin response during the IVGTT is nonphysiologic.[150]

GESTATIONAL DIABETES MELLITUS

For many years GDM was defined as any degree of glucose intolerance with onset or first recognition during pregnancy.[26] This can include women with preexisting, but undiagnosed, diabetes. Due to the increasing prevalence of obesity and type 2 diabetes, the number of pregnant women with undiagnosed type 2 diabetes has increased.[181] Therefore several organizations (including the ADA and WHO) now recommend that women with risk factors for type 2 diabetes should be screened at the first antenatal visit using standard diagnostic criteria (see Box 47.3).[20,32] Women diagnosed with diabetes by this approach should receive a diagnosis of diabetes in pregnancy. Other women should be rescreened for GDM at 24 to 28 weeks of gestation using the criteria in Table 47.2.

Normal pregnancy is associated with increased insulin resistance, especially in the late second and third trimesters.

TABLE 47.2 Screening for and Diagnosis of Gestational Diabetes Mellitus

I. One-step

1. Perform at 24–28 weeks of gestation in pregnant women not previously diagnosed with diabetes.
2. Perform in the morning after an overnight fast of at least 8 h.
3. Measure fasting venous plasma glucose.
4. Give 75 g of glucose orally.
5. Measure plasma glucose hourly for 2 h after glucose is given.
6. At least one value must meet or exceed the following:

Glucose Concentration	
Fasting	92 mg/dL (5.1 mmol/L)
1 h	180 mg/dL (10.0 mmol/L)
2 h	153 mg/dL (8.5 mmol/L)

II. Two-step

A. Step 1 (screening)

1. Perform at 24–28 weeks of gestation[a] in pregnant women not previously diagnosed with diabetes.
2. Give 50-g oral glucose load without regard to time of day or time of last meal.
3. Measure venous plasma glucose at 1 hour.
4. If glucose is ≥130, 135, or 140 mg/dL (7.2, 7.5, or 7.8 mmol/L), proceed to step 2 and perform a 100-g glucose tolerance test.

B. Step 2 (diagnosis)

1. Perform in the morning after an overnight fast of at least 8 hours.
2. Measure fasting venous plasma glucose.
3. Give 100 g of glucose orally.
4. At least two[b] of the values must meet or exceed the following:

Glucose Concentration	
Fasting	95 mg/dL (5.3 mmol/L)
1 h	180 mg/dL (10.0 mmol/L)
2 h	155 mg/dL (8.6 mmol/L)
3 h	140 mg/dL (7.8 mmol/L)

[a]The WHO states that this test can be performed at any time during pregnancy.
[b]The American College of Obstetricians and Gynecologists states that one increased value can be used for diagnosis (Committee on Practice Bulletins—Obstetrics. Practice Bulletin No. 190: Gestational Diabetes Mellitus. *Obstet Gynecol* 2018;131:e49–64.)

From the American Diabetes Association. Classification and diagnosis of diabetes: *Standards of medical care in diabetes—2020. Diabetes Care* 2020;34(Suppl 1):S14–31.

Euglycemia is maintained by increased insulin secretion, with GDM developing in those women who fail to augment insulin sufficiently. Risk factors for GDM include a family history of diabetes in a first-degree relative, obesity, advanced maternal age, glycosuria, and selected adverse outcomes in a previous pregnancy (e.g., stillbirth, macrosomia). Recommendations for screening and diagnosis were formulated in 1984 at the Second International Workshop-Conference on Gestational Diabetes Mellitus,[182] and were refined at the Third, Fourth, and Fifth International Workshop-Conferences in 1990, 1998, and 2007,[26] respectively. Despite these workshops, there is considerable disagreement regarding the approaches for screening and diagnosing GDM,[183] with wide variation among countries and often between diabetes and obstetric organizations in a single country.[184] Recommendations for screening range from none (i.e., do not screen) to selective (i.e., screen only high risk women) to universal.[183] In addition, screening is performed by measuring glucose fasting, random (regardless of the time of the last meal), or after (usually 1 hour) ingesting oral glucose. An OGTT is usually used to establish the diagnosis. Most criteria for diagnosis of GDM are based on the 1964 O'Sullivan and Mahan recommendations, which were derived from 752 women who had a 3 hours OGTT.[185] If two or more of these values exceeded 2SDs above the mean, GDM was diagnosed. The criteria are arbitrary and not related to adverse outcomes of the pregnancy; they predict postpartum development of diabetes. While the cutoffs have been altered in response to modifications in glucose measurements,[183,186] numerous influential clinical organizations continue to promulgate some form of these criteria. However, considerable differences are present among the recommendations. The major items of contention are the amount of the glucose load (75 or 100 g), the duration of the test (2 or 3 hours), the specific cutoffs, and the number of high values necessary (1 or 2) (See Table 47.1 in[183]).

A notable flaw in the GDM diagnostic criteria is that they have been based on the risk of future hyperglycemia, not on clinical sequelae. The Hyperglycemia and Adverse Pregnancy Outcome (HAPO) study was designed in order to address this deficiency. The objective of the HAPO study was to determine the relationship between maternal blood glucose concentrations and adverse pregnancy outcomes. The prospective, randomized multinational study included 23,316 women who had a 75-g OGTT at 24 to 32 weeks of gestation.[187] Primary outcomes were birth weight greater than the 90th centile (macrosomia), primary cesarean section delivery, clinical neonatal hypoglycemia, and cord C-peptide greater than the 90th centile (fetal hyperinsulinemia). The findings revealed that the risk of adverse maternal, fetal, and neonatal events increased continuously as a function of maternal glycemia, even within ranges previously considered normal for pregnancy.[187] Similar associations were observed between glycemia and secondary outcomes of the study, namely preterm birth, shoulder dystocia, preeclampsia, and intensive neonatal care.[187] There were no thresholds at which risk increased (i.e., no convenient cutoffs) and each of the three values in the OGTT (0, 1, and 2 hours) had an independent contribution to adverse outcome.

In order to translate the HAPO results into clinical practice, the International Association of Diabetes and Pregnancy Study Groups (IADPSG) sponsored a workshop to develop recommendations for the diagnosis and classification of hyperglycemia in pregnancy.[188] The panel suggested that a 75-g OGTT be performed and a diagnosis of GDM be made if one or more of the following values is equaled or exceeded: FPG (92 mg/dL; 5.1 mmol/L), 1 hour (180 mg/dL; 10.0 mmol/L), and 2 hours (153 mg/dL; 8.5 mmol/L) (Table 47.2, one step). Because only one increased glucose value is required (as opposed to two for prior recommendations), the prevalence of GDM in the United States would rise from ~7 to ~18% (~250,000 to ~640,000 women per year). Similar increases are anticipated for other countries.

Although they are the first large-scale evidence-based guidelines for GDM that correlate maternal glucose concentrations to outcomes, the IADPSG recommendations are controversial. While adopted in several countries, including Canada, Germany, Italy, Japan, China, and Australia, and by the WHO,[189] in the United States it has been accepted by the ADA and Endocrine Society, but not by ACOG. Moreover, in 2013 an NIH Consensus Development Conference panel supported the continuation of the two-step approach.[190] The main reasons proffered for not switching to the IADPSG criteria are lack of evidence that the additional women identified will have improved outcomes (the HAPO study was observational) and the considerable cost to society incurred by the large increase in the number of individuals with GDM. Universal criteria to diagnose GDM remain elusive.[183]

Multiple studies have evaluated other markers to diagnose GDM. Although conceptually appealing (as neither fasting nor drinking a glucose load is necessary), markers of long-term glycemia (e.g., HbA_{1c}, fructosamine, or glycated albumin) have not shown adequate sensitivity or specificity. An area of considerable recent interest is GDM in early pregnancy, i.e., the first trimester (1 to 12 weeks).[191] The most rapid fetal development occurs in the first trimester, more than 4 months before GDM screening is conducted. Questions that require answers include: Which analytes should be used to identify GDM in early pregnancy? Is diagnosis of GDM early in pregnancy of clinical value? Will identification and/or treatment of GDM in early pregnancy improve outcomes for mother and baby? Several clinical studies are underway to address these questions.[191]

While GDM is usually asymptomatic and not life-threatening to the mother, it is associated with an increased incidence of neonatal mortality and morbidity, including hypoglycemia, macrosomia, and hypocalcemia.[192,193] Maternal hyperglycemia causes the fetus to secrete more insulin, resulting in stimulation of fetal growth and macrosomia. Recognition is important because therapy can reduce perinatal morbidity and mortality.[194] Maternal complications include a high rate of cesarean delivery and hypertension. In addition, mothers with GDM are at significantly increased risk of subsequent diabetes, predominantly type 2. A meta-analysis and systematic review published in 2009 indicated that women with GDM have a sevenfold increased risk of developing type 2 diabetes compared with those who had a normoglycemic pregnancy.[195] The largest single study observed a 12.6-fold increased risk. The cumulative incidence of type 2 diabetes varies among populations, ranging from about 40 to 70%.[196] It rises markedly in the first 5 years and reaches a plateau after 10 years.

Distinct from GDM is pregnancy in a patient with preexisting diabetes (≈19,000 per annum in the United States). This is associated with an increased incidence of congenital malformation, but meticulous glycemic control during the first 8 weeks of pregnancy can significantly decrease the risk of congenital malformation.[197] Tight control results in an increased incidence of maternal hypoglycemia, which is teratogenic in animals but does not cause malformation in humans.[198]

Women with GDM should be screened for diabetes 4 to 12 weeks postpartum using nonpregnant OGTT criteria (see Box 47.3). (HbA_{1c} is not recommended because of the antepartum therapy for hyperglycemia.) If glucose values are normal, glycemia should be reassessed at least every 3 years using either glucose or HbA_{1c}.

CHRONIC COMPLICATIONS OF DIABETES MELLITUS

Pathogenesis

Patients with both type 1 and type 2 diabetes are at high risk for the development of chronic complications.[2,3] Diabetes-specific microvascular pathology in the retina, renal glomeruli, and peripheral nerves produces retinopathy, nephropathy, and neuropathy, respectively. As a result of these microvascular complications, diabetes is the most frequent cause of new cases of blindness in the industrialized world in persons between 25 and 74 years and the leading cause of end-stage renal disease. Diabetes is also associated with a marked increase in atherosclerotic macrovascular disease involving cardiac, cerebral, and peripheral large vessels. The consequence is that patients with diabetes have a high rate of myocardial infarction (the major cause of mortality in diabetes), stroke, and limb amputation. Prospective clinical studies document a strong relationship between hyperglycemia and the development of microvascular complications.[199,200] Both hyperglycemia and insulin resistance appear to be important in the pathogenesis of macrovascular complications.[200–202]

Progress has been made in our understanding of the molecular mechanisms underlying derangements produced by hyperglycemia.[2,201,203] Several hypotheses have been proposed to explain how hyperglycemia causes the neural and vascular pathology. These include increased aldose reductase (or polyol pathway) flux; enhanced formation of advanced glycation end products (AGE); activation of protein kinase C; production of superoxide and other reactive oxygen species (ROS) by the mitochondrial electron transport chain; endoplasmic reticulum stress; increased hexosamine pathway flux; and activation of Src homology-2 domain-containing phosphatase-1 (SHP-1).[201,203] Inhibitors of each of these have been shown to ameliorate diabetes-induced abnormalities in cell culture and animal models.[201] Overproduction of superoxide by the mitochondrial electron transport chain integrates these four apparently disparate mechanisms.[201] Clinical trials are under way using novel therapies specifically directed at the signaling molecules (such as protein kinase C) or employing anti-inflammatory agents.[204]

Effects of Intensive Therapy
Type 1 Diabetes

Although it had been theorized for many years that better glycemic control would decrease rates of long-term complications of diabetes mellitus, it was not until the publication of the Diabetes Control and Complications Trial (DCCT) in 1993[199] that this hypothesis was verified. The DCCT was a multicenter, randomized trial that compared the effects of intensive and conventional insulin therapy on the development and progression of complications in 1441 patients with type 1 diabetes. During the study period, which averaged 6.5 years, intensively managed patients maintained significantly lower mean blood glucose concentrations than those on conventional treatment. Compared with conventional therapy, intensive therapy reduced the risk of retinopathy, nephropathy, and neuropathy by 40 to 75%.[199] Intensive therapy delayed the onset and slowed the progression of these three complications, regardless of age, gender, or duration of diabetes. The absolute risks of retinopathy and nephropathy were proportional to the mean HbA_{1c} (discussed later in the chapter). Although intensive therapy also reduced the development of hypercholesterolemia, major cardiovascular and peripheral vascular diseases were not significantly decreased in the initial assessment. However, analysis after 17 years of follow-up showed that the incidence of cardiovascular disease was 42% lower in the intensively treated group.[205] This landmark study has had a considerable impact on therapeutic goals and comprehension of the pathogenesis of complications of diabetes.

At the conclusion of the DCCT, 95% of participants enrolled in the long-term follow-up study, termed the Epidemiology of Diabetes Interventions and Complications (EDIC). Five years after the end of the DCCT, no difference in metabolic control (assessed by HbA_{1c} measurements) was noted between the former conventional and intensively treated groups. Nevertheless, further progression of retinopathy, neuropathy, and nephropathy was significantly lower in the former intensive group, demonstrating that the beneficial effects of intensive treatment persisted for at least 19 years beyond the period of strictest intervention.[206-208] The molecular mechanism responsible for this effect, termed "metabolic memory," has not been identified.

Type 2 Diabetes

The role of hyperglycemia in the development of complications in individuals with type 2 diabetes was established in the United Kingdom Prospective Diabetes Study (UKPDS).[200] The UKPDS was a major randomized, multicenter clinical study that included 5102 patients with newly diagnosed type 2 diabetes who were followed for an average of 10 years. Analogous to the findings of the DCCT, the UKPDS demonstrated in patients with type 2 diabetes that intensive treatment diminishes by approximately 10 to 40% the development of microvascular complications.[209] Intensive treatment decreased the rate of occurrence of macrovascular complications. Although the reduction was not statistically significant initially, follow-up 10 years after the study ended showed a significant reduction in myocardial infarction among patients who had received intensive therapy.[210] Similar to the EDIC findings, long-term benefits for microvascular complications were observed with follow-up of patients in the UKPDS despite loss of glycemic separation between intensive and standard cohorts after the study ended.[210] An important caveat of both the DCCT and the UKPDS was that intensive therapy produced a threefold increase in the incidence of severe hypoglycemia.[199,200]

ROLE OF THE CLINICAL LABORATORY IN DIABETES MELLITUS

The clinical laboratory has a vital role in both the diagnosis and management of diabetes mellitus.[48] Some of the important variables assayed are outlined in Table 47.3. In 2002, the National Academy of Clinical Biochemistry (referred to as the NACB) published evidence-based guidelines for laboratory analysis in diabetes mellitus.[72] These guidelines were reviewed by the Professional Practice Committee of the ADA and were consistent in those areas where the ADA also published recommendations. Specific recommendations for laboratory testing based on published data or derived from expert consensus are presented.[72] An updated version of these guidelines was published in 2011.[48] The revised guidelines were also published as a Position Statement by the ADA.[48,211] A new version of the guidelines is in preparation with publication anticipated after this book goes to press. A brief overview is presented here.

Diagnosis

Preclinical (Screening)

Type 1 diabetes. Multiple studies indicate that measuring islet autoantibodies in persons genetically at risk for type 1 diabetes identifies individuals who may develop type 1 diabetes.[212] The risk of type 1 diabetes increases as the number of autoantibodies detected increases.[129] Therefore the ADA recommends screening of first-degree relatives of patients with type 1 diabetes by measuring a panel of islet autoantibodies in the setting of a research trial.[20] Until effective intervention therapy becomes available, screening for islet autoantibodies is not recommended outside of prospective clinical studies.[48]

Some experts have proposed that testing for islet autoantibodies may be useful in the following situations: to identify a subset of adults initially thought to have type 2 diabetes but who have islet autoantibody markers of type 1 diabetes and progress to insulin dependency; to screen nondiabetic family members who wish to donate a kidney or part of their pancreas for transplantation; to screen women with GDM to identify those at high risk of progression to type 1 diabetes; and to distinguish type 1 from type 2 diabetes in children to institute insulin therapy at the time of diagnosis.[48,72] Wide variability in clinical practice has been noted regarding the use of islet autoantibodies. Proponents argue that the results of autoantibody assays are clinically useful, whereas others point to lack of evidence. Although some clinicians, particularly those who treat pediatric patients, use autoantibody assays, clinical studies are necessary to provide outcome data to validate the clinical use of autoantibody assays.

Genetic screening by determining HLA type is not currently warranted, except in research studies.[48] For selected diabetes syndromes, e.g., neonatal diabetes, valuable information can now be obtained with definition of disease-associated mutations.[48]

A decrease in glucose-stimulated insulin secretion is the first functional abnormality in both type 1 and type 2 diabetes. Nevertheless, tests of insulin secretion are not currently recommended for routine clinical use.

Type 2 diabetes. Screening of asymptomatic individuals for type 2 diabetes has been the subject of much controversy,[213] but is now recommended by the ADA and several other clinical organizations. The ADA, which previously did

TABLE 47.3 Role of the Laboratory in Diabetes Mellitus

Diagnosis

Preclinical (Screening)	Immunologic markers (autoantibodies)
	  ICA
	  IAA
	  GADA
	  Protein tyrosine phosphatase
	    antibodies (IA-2)
	  Zinc transporter ZnT8 antibodies
	Genetic markers (e.g., human leukocyte
	  antigen [HLA])
	Insulin secretion
	  Fasting
	  Pulses
	  In response to a glucose challenge
	Blood glucose (fasting)
	Oral glucose tolerance test (OGTT)
	Hemoglobin A_{1c} (HbA_{1c})

Clinical	Blood glucose (fasting) Oral glucose tolerance test (OGTT) HbA_{1c} Ketones (urine and blood) Other (e.g., insulin, C-peptide, stimulation tests)

Management

Acute	Glucose
	  Blood
	  Urine
	Ketones
	  Blood
	  Urine
	Acid-base status (pH [H^+],
	  bicarbonate)
	Lactate
	Other abnormalities related to cellular
	  dehydration or therapy (e.g.,
	  potassium, sodium, phosphate,
	  osmolality)

Chronic	Glucose
	  Blood (fasting, random, continuous
	    monitoring)
	  Urine
	Glycated proteins
	  HbA_{1c}
	  Fructosamine
	  Glycated albumin
	1,5-Anhydroglucitol (1,5-AG)
	Urinary protein
	  Albuminuria (previously termed
	    "microalbuminuria")
	  Proteinuria
	Evaluation of complications
	  (e.g., creatinine, cholesterol,
	  triglycerides)
	Evaluation of pancreas transplant
	  (C-peptide, insulin)
	Eligibility for insulin pump
	  (C-peptide)

not support screening, now advocates screening of high-risk individuals for diabetes.[1,213,214] All asymptomatic individuals over the age of 45 years should be screened by HbA_{1c}, FPG, or the 2-hour OGTT.[20] If HbA_{1c} is less than 5.7% (<39 mmol/mol) or FPG is less than 100 mg/dL (<5.6 mmol/L), testing should be repeated at three-year intervals. Testing may be considered at a younger age or may be carried out more frequently in individuals at increased risk of diabetes (e.g., family history, members of certain ethnic groups, overweight or obese adults).[20,215] Patients with prediabetes (HbA_{1c} ≥ 5.7% [39 mmol/mol], IGT, or IFG) should be tested annually.[20]

Rationales for screening are that ~33% of individuals with type 2 diabetes are undiagnosed, complications are often present by the time of diagnosis, and treatment delays the onset of complications.[213] Notwithstanding these recommendations, no rigorous clinical trials have been performed to determine if treatment based on screening has value. However, a systematic review published in 2015 identified 16 trials that consistently found that treatment of IFG or IGT was associated with delayed progression to diabetes.[216] Moreover, computer simulation modeling suggests benefit from early diagnosis and treatment of hyperglycemia and cardiovascular risk factors in type 2 diabetes.[20]

The rising incidence of type 2 diabetes in adolescents has led to the recommendation for screening overweight youths (BMI >85th centile) with any one of the following risk factors:
- Family history of type 2 diabetes in first- or second-degree relative
- Belong to certain race and/or ethnic group
- Signs of insulin resistance or conditions associated with insulin resistance (e.g., hypertension, dyslipidemia, polycystic ovary syndrome)
- Maternal history of diabetes or GDM during the child's gestation.[20,72]

Testing should be done every 3 years starting at 10 years of age (onset rarely occurs before onset of puberty[22]).

Clinical

The laboratory diagnosis of diabetes is made exclusively by the demonstration of hyperglycemia, by measuring venous plasma glucose or HbA_{1c}. Although other tests (e.g., C-peptide, insulin analysis) have been proposed to assist in the diagnosis and classification of the disease, these do not at present have a role outside of research studies.[48]

Management

Acute Complications

The clinical laboratory has an essential role in both the diagnosis and monitoring of therapy in patients with DKA,[217] hyperosmolar hyperglycemic nonketotic syndrome (HHNS),[218] and hypoglycemia.[217] Several analytes are frequently measured to guide clinicians in treatment regimens to restore euglycemia and correct other metabolic disturbances. A brief overview of DKA and HHNS is provided below. Hypoglycemia is covered in detail in Chapter 35. The AACC/ADA guidelines[48] also provide information on the tests that are used.

Diabetic ketoacidosis. DKA is due to insulin deficiency plus increased concentrations of counter-regulatory hormones (glucagon, catecholamines, cortisol, and growth hormone). Together these hormonal changes increase hepatic glucose production and reduce insulin sensitivity in tissues, producing hyperglycemia. In addition, ketone body production is accelerated. Patients with DKA have hyperglycemia, ketonemia, and metabolic acidosis. The diagnostic thresholds differ among organizations. Cutoffs are plasma glucose greater than 200 or 250 mg/dL ($>$11 or 13.9 mmol/L), pH less than 7.3, bicarbonate less than 18 or 15 mEq/L ($<$18 or 15 mmol/L), and β-hydroxybutyrate greater than 31 mg/dL ($>$3 mmol/L). (See Ketone section below for further discussion of ketones.) The ADA classifies patients into mild, moderate, or severe based on laboratory criteria and the patient's mental status. DKA is most common in children and young adults with type 1 diabetes but can occur in type 2 diabetes. Patients who present with DKA are either newly diagnosed with diabetes, have an infection, or omitted insulin. More recently, DKA has been observed in patients treated with a new class of oral agents, sodium glucose transporter 2 (SGLT2) inhibitors. Patients with DKA usually have polyuria (increased urine output), polydipsia (thirst), and weakness, and may have nausea, vomiting, and abdominal pain. Initial laboratory evaluation includes blood glucose, electrolytes, creatinine, urea nitrogen, ketone bodies (plasma or urine), osmolality, pH (venous or arterial), and blood count. During therapy, capillary glucose should be measured every 1 to 2 hours and blood electrolytes, glucose, urea nitrogen, creatinine, and pH analyzed every 4 hours. Treatment comprises insulin, intravenous fluids (NaCl), and potassium. Some clinicians give bicarbonate if the pH is less than 6.9. Before the discovery of insulin, virtually all patients with DKA died. Mortality rates now are less than 1% in most cases.

Hyperosmolar hyperglycemic nonketotic syndrome. The HHNS (also termed hyperglycemic hyperosmolar state [HHS]) is characterized by hyperglycemia and hyperosmolality, but patients do not have ketoacidosis. The diagnostic criteria are plasma glucose greater than 594 to 600 mg/dL ($>$33 to 33.3 mmol/L), pH greater than 7.3, bicarbonate greater than 15 mEq/L ($>$15 mmol/L), β-hydroxybutyrate less than 31 mg/dL ($<$3 mmol/L), and serum osmolality greater than 320 mOsm/L. HHNS is most common in older patients with type 2 diabetes and comorbidities. Approximately 60% of HHNS is precipitated by infection (pneumonia or urinary tract infection). Patients usually present with altered mental status and dehydration. Laboratory evaluation is the same as outlined for DKA in the paragraph above. The first line of treatment is intravenous fluids, with replacement of potassium and insulin, as well as treating the underlying cause, also important. While HHNS is far less common than DKA (accounts for $<$ 1% of all diabetes-related hospital admissions), mortality rates range from 5 to 20%.

Chronic Complications

The DCCT[199] and UKPDS[200] studies documented a correlation between blood glucose concentrations and the development of long-term complications of diabetes. Measurement of glucose and glycated proteins provides an index of short- and long-term glycemic control, respectively (see section on glycated proteins later in the chapter). Detection and monitoring of complications are achieved by assaying serum creatinine and lipids, and urine for albumin. The success of newer therapies, such as islet cell or pancreas transplantation, can be monitored by measuring serum C-peptide or insulin concentrations.

SELF-MONITORING OF BLOOD GLUCOSE

Diabetes patients, especially those who need insulin therapy, require careful monitoring to maintain control of blood glucose. This has become particularly important with the results of the DCCT[199] and the recommendation that patients use intensive insulin therapy to achieve nearly normal glycemia. These regimens include multiple daily insulin injections, insulin pumps, and continuous subcutaneous insulin injections. Estimating blood glucose concentrations by monitoring urine glucose concentrations—a simple and convenient method—is undesirable for the following reasons.

1. The renal threshold (the blood glucose concentration above which glucose appears in the urine) averages 160 to 180 mg/dL (8.9 to 10.0 mmol/L) but varies widely among individuals. It may increase in long-standing diabetes or with age and may be lower in pregnancy or childhood. A decreased threshold ($\pm$100 mg/dL; 5.6 mmol/L) is known as *renal glycosuria*.
2. Monitoring of urine glucose concentrations lacks sensitivity and specificity. For example, one study demonstrated that patients with plasma glucose concentrations in the range 150 to 199 mg/dL (8.3 to 11.1 mmol/L) exhibited normal urine test results 75% of the time. Furthermore, 9% of patients with plasma glucose concentrations less than 149 mg/dL ($<$8.3 mmol/L) had glycosuria.[219]
3. A negative test result does not distinguish between hypoglycemia, euglycemia, and mild or moderate hyperglycemia.
4. Urine testing, which uses a color chart, is not accurate.
5. Other factors (e.g., fluid intake, urine concentration, ingestion of salicylates or ascorbic acid, urinary tract infections) may influence test results.

Testing urine for glucose is therefore not adequate for monitoring patients on insulin therapy.[220] Although some evidence suggests that it may be effective for monitoring type 2 diabetes,[221] the ADA states that limitations of urine testing make blood glucose measurements the preferred method of assessing glycemic control.[222]

Glucose Meters

Portable meters for measurement of blood glucose concentrations are used in three major settings: (i) in acute and chronic care facilities; (ii) in physicians' offices; and (iii) by patients at home, work, and school. The last, self-monitoring of blood glucose (SMBG) was performed in the United States in 1993 at least once a day by 40 and 26% of individuals with type 1 and 2 diabetes, respectively.[72] In 2006, the overall rate of daily SMBG had increased to 63.4% among all adults with diabetes in the United States and 86.7% among those treated with insulin.[48,223]

Patients measure their own blood glucose concentration and modify their insulin dose based on this glucose value. It is impractical for patients themselves to perform glucose determinations by the methods used in clinical laboratories, but a large number of simple test strips that are available permit rapid measurements on a drop of whole blood.[220] These use the same methodology as described earlier for glucose analysis—predominantly glucose oxidase or glucose dehydrogenase. In many strips, a dye is colored by the glucose oxidase-peroxidase chromogenic reaction. The reagents are combined in dry form on a small surface area of a test strip, and the colors that develop may be evaluated visually by comparison with a color chart (rarely used any more) or quantified in a specially designed meter. Visual reading with a color chart is not accurate enough for most clinical circumstances.

At least 75 different blood glucose meters are commercially available in the United States (numbers differ in other countries). These meters vary in size, weight, calibration method, minimum blood volume, and other features. They are reviewed annually in the ADA magazine *Diabetes Forecast.*

To perform the measurement, a sample of blood (usually from a fingerstick, but anticoagulated whole blood collected in ethylenediaminetetraacetic acid [EDTA] or heparin may also be used) is placed on the test pad, which is attached to a plastic support. The test strip is then inserted into the meter. (In some devices, the strip is inserted into the meter before the sample is applied.) After a fixed period of time, the result appears on a digital display screen. These meters use reflectance photometry or electrochemistry to measure the rate of the reaction or the final concentration of the products. Reflectance photometry measures the amount of light reflected from a test pad containing reagent. In electrochemical systems, the enzymatic reaction in an electrode incorporated on the test strip produces a flow of electrons. The current, which is directly proportional to the concentration of glucose in the sample, is converted to a digital readout. Large variability has been noted among meters as to the volume of blood required (0.3 to 1.5 μL), test time (5 to 45 seconds), and the claimed reading range (30 to 500 mg/dL [1.7 to 27.8 mmol/L] to 0 to 600 mg/dL [0 to 33.3 mmol/L]). Calibration is automatic on some devices, whereas others use lot-specific code chips or strips. Manufacturers supply control solutions. Advances in technology facilitate data analysis and sharing. Some meters have Bluetooth capabilities (enabling transmission of data to a smartphone or computer), cellular connections that automatically send data to the "cloud," USB ports, and/or communication with an insulin pump. Strict adherence to the instructions is necessary to obtain accurate results. Some meters have a porous membrane that separates erythrocytes, and analysis is performed on the resultant plasma. Whole blood glucose concentrations are approximately 10 to 15% lower than plasma or serum concentrations, but meters can be calibrated to report plasma glucose values, even when the sample is whole blood. An International Federation of Clinical Chemistry and Laboratory Medicine (IFCC) working group recommended that glucose meters measuring whole blood glucose be harmonized to report the concentration as a plasma glucose equivalent using a factor of 1.11×, irrespective of the original sample type or technology.[224]

Analytical Goals

Multiple analytical goals have been proposed for the performance of glucose meters. In 1987, the ADA recommended a goal of total error (in the hands of users) of less than 10% at glucose concentrations of 30 to 400 mg/dL (1.7 to 22.2 mmol/L) 100% of the time.[225] The recommendations promulgated in 2002 by the Clinical and Laboratory Standards Institute (CLSI) (previously called the National Committee for Clinical Laboratory Standards [NCCLS])[226] are that 95% of results should fall within 20% of laboratory-measured glucose concentrations when ≥75 mg/dL (>4.2 mmol/L) and within 15 mg/dL (0.83 mmol/L) of a laboratory glucose measurement if the glucose concentration is less than 75 mg/dL (<4.2 mmol/L). The 2003 International Organization for Standardization (ISO)[227] recommendations are identical. In both CSLI and ISO guidelines, 5% of these results can be considerably outside these limits. Note that the CLSI guideline is for meter use in acute and chronic care facilities (mainly hospitals), while the ISO guidelines pertain to meters

for self-testing (i.e., SMBG). Several experts believed these acceptance criteria to be too wide. Therefore the CLSI and ISO documents were revised in 2013, with tightening of acceptance criteria. The current CLSI guideline POCT12-A3 indicates that for 95% of the samples, the difference between meter and laboratory measurement be less than 12.5% when the laboratory glucose value is ≥100 mg/dL (≥5.6 mmol/L) and less than 12 mg/dL (<0.67 mmol/L) when the glucose concentration is less than 100 mg/dL (<5.6 mmol/L). In addition, no more than 2% of results can differ by greater than 20% at ≥75 mg/dL (≥4.2 mmol/L) and by greater than 15 mg/dL (>0.83 mmol/L) when the glucose concentration is less than 75 mg/dL (<4.2 mmol/L). The revised ISO goals are that for 95% of the samples, the difference between meter and laboratory measurement should be less than 15% when the laboratory glucose value is ≥100 mg/dL (≥5.6 mmol/L) and less than 15 mg/dL (<0.83 mmol/L) when the glucose concentration is less than 100 mg/dL (<5.6 mmol/L). Moreover, 99% of results must be within zones A and B of the consensus error grid (see following paragraph). In the United States, the FDA issued draft guidance in 2018 for glucose meters. Two separate documents were released, one for home (SMBG) use, the other for hospitals. The FDA stated that the ISO criteria are not sufficient to adequately protect lay-users using SMBG. The FDA standards for SMBG[228] recommend that, in the useable range of the meter, results for 95% of samples should be within 15% of laboratory glucose and 99% be within 20%. The FDA criteria for meters for hospital use are appropriately more stringent[229]; the meter should meet the following standards: For samples with glucose concentrations ≥75 mg/dL (≥4.2 mmol/L), 95% of results are within 12% of the comparator method and 98% are within 15% of the comparator method; similarly, below 75 mg/dL (<4.2 mmol/L), 95% of results are within 12 mg/dL (<0.67 mmol/L) of the results of the comparator method and 98% are within 15 mg/dL (>0.83 mmol/L).

A different method was proposed by Clarke,[230] who developed an error grid that attempts to define clinically important errors by identifying fairly broad target ranges. The error grid was subsequently modified to reflect current medical practice.[231]

In addition, an approach using simulation modeling reached the conclusion that meters that achieve both a CV and a bias less than 5% rarely lead to major errors in insulin dosing.[232] The lack of consensus on quality goals for glucose meters reflects the absence of agreed-upon objective criteria. When biological variation criteria are used, glucose measurement (on central laboratory analyzers) should have analytical imprecision ≤ 2.3%, bias ≤ 1.8%, and total error ≤ 5.5%.

Glucose meters are also used to calculate insulin dosage in patients without diabetes on tight glucose control protocols in intensive care units (ICUs). Evidence in 2001[233] showed that intensive insulin therapy significantly reduced the mortality and morbidity of critically ill patients in the surgical ICU. A subsequent meta-analysis of multiple randomized control trials failed to identify improved outcomes but did detect increased incidence of hypoglycemia.[234] It is important to emphasize that the 2001 study used accurate blood gas analyzers and collected arterial blood samples,[233] whereas subsequent studies often used glucose meters and capillary blood samples. Many factors, such as hypoxia, shock, and low hematocrit, are common in patients in ICUs and can compromise glucose analysis in capillary blood samples.[235] The use of glucose meters in these settings has been questioned by some experts.[236]

Performance of Glucose Meters

The most common errors in SMBG, such as proper application, timing, and removal of excess blood, have been reduced by advances in technology but can still occur. Additional innovations that reduce operator error include systems that abort testing if the sample volume is inadequate; built-in programs that simplify quality control; and automatic commencement of timing. The increased memory allows the instrument to store up to several hundred glucose readings that can be downloaded into a computer.

Several factors affect the accuracy and reproducibility of SMBG. These include user variability—up to 50% of values may vary by more than 20% from reference values[220]; hematocrit—the presence of anemia (false increase) or polycythemia (false depression) may result in up to 30% variability; and defective reagent strips or instrument malfunction (rare). Other variables include changes in altitude, environmental temperature, or humidity; hypotension; hypoxia; and high triglyceride concentrations. In addition, these assays are unreliable at very high and very low glucose concentrations (<60 and >500 mg/dL; <3.3 and >27.8 mmol/L). Because intravascular volume depletion, a common feature of DKA, greatly increases blood viscosity, inaccurately low blood glucose results may be obtained. Several drugs interfere, but not with all meters.[237] Another important factor is the lack of correlation among meters, even from a single manufacturer, caused by different assay methods and architecture. Moreover, results from 2 meters of the same brand have been observed to differ substantially.[238] Patient factors are also important, particularly adequacy of training. Recurrent education at clinic visits and comparison of SMBG with concurrent laboratory glucose analysis improved the accuracy of patients' blood glucose readings.[239] In addition, it is important to evaluate the patient's technique at regular intervals.

The performance of different meters varies widely. Note that the performance of glucose meters achieved by medical technologists is better than that achieved by patients. A 1998 study that evaluated meter performance in 226 hospitals by split samples analyzed simultaneously on meters and laboratory glucose analyzers revealed that 45.6, 25, and 14% differed from each other by greater than 10%, greater than 15%, and greater than 20%, respectively.[240] Comparison with laboratory values of almost 22,000 measurements of capillary glucose by patients using meters revealed no significant improvement in meter performance between 1989 and 1999.[241] While performance of newer meters has improved, imprecision remains high. An analysis in 2012 revealed that only 18 of 34 (53%) glucose meters approved for use in Europe fulfilled the minimum accuracy requirements of the 2013 ISO standard.[242] A study in 2017 found that only 2 of 17 meters for SMBG use met the ISO standard when their performance was tested with challenging sets of samples.[243] Similarly, a 2018 study of 18 commercially available glucose meters concluded that meters do not always meet the requirements for regulatory clearance.[244] The imprecision of meters precludes their use from the diagnosis of diabetes and limits their usefulness in screening for diabetes.[48]

Indications and Frequency of Self-Monitoring of Blood Glucose

The indications and frequency of self-monitoring vary among patients. SMBG should be performed by all patients treated with insulin. The role of SMBG in patients with type 2 diabetes not treated with insulin has not been defined.[48] A consensus statement by the ADA[220] recommended the following specific indications for SMBG:

- Patients undergoing intensive insulin treatment programs (in this group, glucose should be measured at least four times a day to achieve glycemic control)
- Prevention and detection of hypoglycemia, especially in people who are asymptomatic or unable to recognize the early warning signs
- Avoidance of severe hyperglycemia, particularly in situations of increased risk (e.g., medications that alter insulin secretion or action, intercurrent illness, elderly people)
- Adjusted pharmacologic therapy in response to changes in lifestyle, such as exercise or altering food intake
- Determination of the necessity for initiating insulin therapy in GDM. *Glucose meters should not be used to diagnose diabetes mellitus,* and their role in screening remains uncertain.[72]

Current ADA recommendations[20] are that all insulin-treated patients with diabetes who use intensive insulin regimens (multiple daily injections or insulin pump therapy)—and who are not using CGM (see next section)—should perform frequent SMBG. (For patients using CGM, meters should be used to calibrate the CGM (as directed by the CGM manufacturer) and to monitor performance of the CGM.) SMBG should be performed six to eight times per day, i.e., before meals and snacks, occasionally postprandially, at bedtime, before exercise, when they suspect low blood glucose, after treating hypoglycemia, and before critical tasks such as driving. A reduced frequency of SMBG results in deterioration of glycemic control.[245–247] Published studies revealed that self-monitoring is performed by patients much less frequently than recommended.[248] Subsequent evidence shows a gradual increase in use, with 63.4% of patients with diabetes reported in 2008 to monitor blood glucose at least once daily.[249] Guidelines on the recommended frequency and timing of SMBG vary among international diabetes associations.[250] Recommendations suggest that the frequency and timing of SMBG should be dictated by the particular needs and goals of the individual patient.[20,250]

The value of SMBG for patients with type 2 diabetes not on insulin therapy is controversial owing, in part, to the lack of well-designed studies. A meta-analysis of SMBG in non–insulin-treated patients with type 2 diabetes showed that SMBG slightly improved glycemic control up to 6 months after initiation and subsides after 12 months.[251] However, many studies in this analysis included patient education, and the contribution of SMBG to glucose control in non–insulin-treated patients remains contentious.[249] A recent open-label randomized trial, conducted in 15 primary care practices, evaluated use of SMBG in patients with type 2 diabetes not using insulin.[252] The study found no significant differences at 1 year in glycemic control (as assessed by HbA$_{1c}$) or health-related quality of life between patients who performed SMBG and those who did not. Despite controversy in the literature, a survey conducted in 14 countries in 2007 revealed unexpectedly high SMBG use in non–insulin-treated patients, with up to 75% of patients performing SMBG.[253] However, the evidence is insufficient to recommend routine use of SMBG for patients when diabetes is treated without insulin.

CONTINUOUS GLUCOSE MONITORING

Major limitations to performing SMBG are that it is painful and inconvenient. Since the 1960s, attempts have been made to develop a painless method for monitoring blood glucose concentrations. The concept underlying these methods is that the concentration of glucose in the interstitial fluid correlates with the blood glucose concentration. The Gluco-Watch G2 Biographer (Cygnus, Inc, Redwood City, CA) used a minimally invasive approach that applied a low-level electric current to the skin. This induces movement by electro-osmosis of glucose across the skin, where it is measured by a glucose oxidase detector.[254] The GlucoWatch, which was designed to measure glucose three times per hour for up to 12 hours, could be used to detect unsuspected hypoglycemia. Clinical studies revealed reasonable correlation of the GlucoWatch with SMBG.[254] Notwithstanding approval by the FDA in 2002, the device was withdrawn from the market 6 years later.

Several implanted biosensors with detection systems based on enzymes, electrodes, or fluorescence[255,256] have been developed. The most widely used method is an electrochemical sensor that is implanted subcutaneously. The devices, termed continuous glucose monitors (CGM), use glucose oxidase to measure glucose every 5 to 15 minutes. The measurement range is 40 to 400 mg/dL (2.2 to 22.2 mmol/L) or 20 to 500 mg/dL (1.1 to 27.8 mmol/L). CGMs can conveniently be divided into three types: (1) Real-time CGM, which transmits glucose values to a receiver or smart phone in real time; (2) Intermittently scanned (or flash) CGMs, which display readings only when the user swipes a reader or smart phone over the sensor; and (3) Professional CGMs, which store results that are downloaded later in the physician's office. CGM systems, which became widely available in the early 2000s, have become more accurate, smaller, and easier to use.[257] Some alert users to current or impending high or low glucose. These devices are subject to some limitations. An important caveat is that changes in glucose concentration in the interstitial fluid occur 4 to 20 minutes later than in the blood. Implantation of a needle type of sensor into the subcutaneous tissue induces inflammatory responses in the host that alter the sensitivity of the device. Therefore devices need to be replaced every 7 to 14 days. A sensor that is surgically implanted under the skin has a 90- to 180-day life. Until 2017 all sensors were used only as an adjunct to SMBG; meters were still required to adjust insulin dose. Newer CGMs can be used instead of meters. Another improvement is factory calibration. Older systems required calibration by the user every 12 hours with a glucose meter and were subject to the imprecision of the meter. This requirement has been eliminated from some new CGMs, which are factory calibrated.[257]

Another strategy uses microdialysis which measures glucose outside the body. Fluid is pumped from a storage bag through a microfiber under the skin. The solution carries the glucose sample back to a biosensor, which measures glucose every second and stores an average value every 3 minutes. This device, which is available in parts of Europe but not in the United States, can be worn for 14 days.

A randomized study published in 2008 of 322 patients with type 1 diabetes showed that adults aged 25 and older using intensive insulin treatment and real-time CGM had better long-term glycemic control than patients using intensive insulin therapy and SMBG.[258] Newer features, such as automated suspension of insulin delivery for up to 2 hours when glucose concentrations reach a preset low threshold, significantly reduce the rate of hypoglycemia[259] and improve HbA$_{1c}$[260] in patients with type 1 diabetes. CGM may be particularly useful in patients with hypoglycemic unawareness or frequent episodes of hypoglycemia. The potential use of CGM in pregnant women with diabetes is under investigation. Automated closed-loop insulin delivery systems (also termed the "artificial pancreas") are a focus of intense research.[261,262] The system employs a control algorithm that modulates insulin delivery according to real-time interstitial glucose measured by a CGM. Closed-loop systems have been shown to be superior to conventional insulin pump therapy and are likely to become used more widely in the near future.

Noninvasive Glucose Monitoring

Noninvasive in vivo monitoring of glucose, that is, without implanting a probe or collecting a sample of any type,[48] has been an area of active investigation for many years.[263] The approaches most widely evaluated involve passing a beam of light through a vascular region and analyzing the resulting light. Near-infrared spectroscopic devices measure the absorption or the reflection of light from subcutaneous tissue. Although glucose has a specific absorption at 1035 nm, many substances interfere. A computer, individually calibrated, screens out interfering information to obtain the glucose result. Alternative approaches include Raman scattering spectroscopy and photoacoustic spectroscopy. Notwithstanding the investment of considerable resources, no noninvasive sensing technology is approved for glucose measurement in patients. Major technological hurdles must be overcome before noninvasive sensing technology will be sufficiently reliable to replace existing portable meters, implantable biosensors, or minimally invasive technologies.[48]

KETONE BODIES

The development of ketosis requires changes in both adipose tissue and the liver. The primary substrates for ketone body formation are free fatty acids from adipose stores. Normally, long-chain fatty acids are taken up by the liver, re-esterified to triglycerides, and stored in the liver or incorporated in very low-density lipoproteins and returned to the plasma. In contrast to other tissue, the brain cannot use free fatty acids for energy. When glucose is unavailable, ketone bodies supply the vast majority of the brain's energy. After a 3-day fast, ketone bodies provide 30 to 40% of the body's energy requirements.[264] In uncontrolled diabetes, the low insulin concentrations result in increased lipolysis and decreased re-esterification, thereby increasing plasmafree fatty acids. Increased counter-regulatory hormones also augment lipolysis and ketogenesis in fat and liver, respectively. For example, glucagon enhances oxidation of fatty acids to ketones in the liver. Together, the increased hepatic ketone production and decreased peripheral tissue metabolism lead to acetoacetate accumulation in the blood. A small fraction undergoes spontaneous decarboxylation to form acetone, but most of it is converted to β-hydroxybutyrate. (Strictly speaking, β-hydroxybutyrate is not a ketone body, but it is considered to be equivalent to one as it is reversibly formed from acetoacetate.)

The relative proportions in which the three ketone bodies are present in blood vary, depending on the redox state of the cell. In healthy people, β-hydroxybutyrate and acetoacetate—which are present at approximately equimolar concentrations[264–266]—constitute virtually all the serum ketones. Acetone is a minor component. In severe diabetes, the ratio of β-hydroxybutyrate to acetoacetate may increase up to 6:1 owing to the presence of a large concentration of nicotinamide adenine dinucleotide (NADH), which favors β-hydroxybutyrate production.

None of the commonly used methods for the detection and determination of ketone bodies in serum or urine reacts with all three ketone bodies. Gerhardt's ferric chloride test reacts with acetoacetate only. Importantly, assays using nitroprusside are at least 10 times more sensitive to acetoacetate than to acetone, and give no reaction at all with β-hydroxybutyrate.

Most of the assays for ketosis essentially detect or measure acetoacetate only. This may produce a paradoxical situation. When a patient initially presents in ketoacidosis, the test results for ketones may be only weakly positive. With therapy, β-hydroxybutyrate is converted to acetoacetate, and the ketosis appears to worsen.

Traditional tests for β-hydroxybutyrate are indirect; they require brief boiling of the urine to remove acetone and acetoacetate by evaporation (acetoacetate first breaks down spontaneously to acetone), followed by gentle oxidation of β-hydroxybutyrate to acetoacetate and acetone with peroxide, ferric ions, or dichromate. The acetoacetate thus formed can be detected with Gerhardt's test or by one of the procedures in which nitroprusside is used.

Specific determination of β-hydroxybutyrate in urine is not considered to be a routine procedure. A paper strip for semiquantitative measurement of β-hydroxybutyrate in serum and urine has been described[267] but has not gained general acceptance. Quantitative enzymatic assays for β-hydroxybutyrate that can be performed directly on blood, plasma, or serum have become commercially available. Originally available as a bench-top analyzer (KetoSite, GDS Diagnostics, Elkhart, IN), the assay can now be performed on many automated chemistry instruments. In addition, hand-held devices that measure β-hydroxybutyrate from fingerstick capillary

blood samples are available from several manufacturers (e.g., Precision Xtra, Abbott Diagnostics, Abbott Park, IL; Nova Max Plus, Nova Biomedical, Waltham, MA and STAT-Site M B-HB, EKF Diagnostics-Stanbio, Boerne, TX).[268] Low-carbohydrate/high-fat diets (also termed ketogenic or Banting diets) often increase serum ketones to 10 mg/dL (1 mmol/L).[269] The wide popularity of these diets for weight loss, athletes, or management of diseases, including epilepsy, cancer, and diabetes,[270,271] has increased the home use of meters to measure β-hydroxybutyrate in the blood. Some blood glucose meters can also measure β-hydroxybutyrate with an appropriate test strip.

Clinical Significance

Excessive formation of ketone bodies results in increased blood concentrations (ketonemia) and increased excretion in the urine (ketonuria). This process is observed in conditions associated with reduced availability of carbohydrates (such as starvation or frequent vomiting) or decreased use of carbohydrates (such as diabetes mellitus, glycogen storage disease type I (von Gierke disease), and alkalosis). The popular high-fat, low-carbohydrate diets are ketogenic and increase ketone bodies in the circulation. Diabetes mellitus and alcohol consumption are the most common causes of ketoacidosis in adults. (Hyperglycemia is not usually present in the latter condition.) Ingestion of isopropyl alcohol and salicylate poisoning can also produce ketoacidosis. Urine ketone test results are positive in ≈30% of first morning void specimens from pregnant women. Measurement of β-hydroxybutyrate in blood is more accurate than determination of ketone bodies in urine in the treatment of DKA. Although not always excreted in proportion to blood ketone concentrations, because of convenience and cost, urine ketones are widely used by patients with type 1 diabetes for early identification of ketosis. The ADA states that ketone testing is an important part of monitoring by patients with diabetes, particularly those with type 1 diabetes, pregnancy with preexisting diabetes, and GDM.[222] Patients with type 1 diabetes should test for ketones during acute illness or stress, with consistent increases in blood glucose (>300 mg/dL; >16.7 mmol/L), during pregnancy, or when symptoms of ketoacidosis are present.[222] Patients treated with SGLT2 (sodium glucose transport) inhibitors are at increased risk of ketoacidosis and should check ketones at any sign of illness.

DKA is a potentially life-threatening acute complication of diabetes. Patients have hyperglycemia (glucose >200 mg/dL [11 mmol/L]), increased ketones (the concentration is not specified), and metabolic acidosis (pH < 7.3 with serum bicarbonate <15 mEq/L [15 mmol/L]).[272,273] Measurement of ketones by either a semiquantitative nitroprusside assay (on urine or serum) or quantification of β-hydroxybutyrate in the blood is acceptable for diagnosis of DKA. Accumulating evidence suggests that β-hydroxybutyrate in the blood is better than urine ketones in patients with type 1 diabetes, reducing frequency of hospital admission and shortening time to recovery from DKA.[274]

Determination of Ketone Bodies in Body Fluids

Although quantitative determination of individual ketone bodies is possible, these methods are not used as routine tests. The semiquantitative AimTab (Germain Laboratories, Inc, San Antonio, TX) or Ketostix (Bayer Health Care, Pine Brook, NJ) are frequently used but are insensitive to β-hydroxybutyrate.[275]

It is important to bear in mind, therefore that a negative nitroprusside test result does not rule out ketoacidosis.

Detection of Ketone Bodies by AimTab

AimTab ketone tablets contain a mixture of glycine, sodium nitroprusside, disodium phosphate (for optimum assay pH), and lactose. Acetoacetate or acetone (to a lesser extent) in the presence of glycine forms a lavender-purple complex with nitroprusside. β-Hydroxybutyrate does not react with nitroprusside. The disodium phosphate provides an optimum pH for the reaction, and lactose enhances the color.[276]

Detection of Ketone Bodies by Ketostix

Ketostix is a modification of the nitroprusside test in which a reagent strip is used instead of a tablet. The Ketostix test gives a positive reaction within 15 seconds with a specimen containing at least 50 mg of acetoacetate per liter. The accompanying color chart gives readings for ketone concentrations of 50, 150, 400, 800, and 1600 mg/L. Acetone also reacts, but the test is less sensitive to it.

Determination of β-Hydroxybutyrate

A 1995 short report on patients with DKA indicated that β-hydroxybutyrate correlated better than acetoacetate with changes in acid-base status.[277]

In this test, β-hydroxybutyrate in the presence of nicotinamide adenine dinucleotide (NAD$^+$) is converted by β-hydroxybutyrate dehydrogenase to acetoacetate, producing NADH. Diaphorase catalyzes the reduction of nitroblue tetrazolium (NBT) by NADH to produce a purple compound, and its absorbance is read at 505 nm. The assay can be performed on serum or plasma on open-channel automated chemistry analyzers and on whole blood with hand-held meters. Evidence indicates that β-hydroxybutyrate measurements with meters are less accurate at concentrations greater than 3 mmol/L.[273]

$$\beta\text{-Hydroxybutyrate} \underset{NAD^{\oplus}}{\overset{\beta\text{-Hydroxybutyrate dehydrogenase}}{\rightleftharpoons}} \underset{NADH + H^{\oplus}}{} \text{Acetoacetate}$$

$$NADH + NBT \overset{Diaphorase}{\rightleftharpoons} NAD^{\oplus} + \text{Reduced NBT}$$

Determination of Ketone Bodies in Urine

Test strips such as AimTab, Ketostix, Ketosis Test Strips (LW Scientific, Lawrenceville, GA), and TRUEplus Ketone Test Strips (Trividia Health, Ft. Lauderdale, FL) are suitable for detecting ketone bodies in urine. The sensitivity and specificity of these tests are the same as outlined for serum.

Reference Interval

Serum β-hydroxybutyrate values vary from 0.21 to 2.81 mg/dL (0.02 to 0.27 mmol/L) in healthy people after an overnight fast, while values of 30 to 40 mg/dL (3 to 4 mmol/L) can be reached in people on a ketogenic diet. Patients with DKA usually have β-hydroxybutyrate concentrations greater than 30 mg/dL (>3 mmol/L).

GLYCATED PROTEINS

Measurement of glycated proteins, primarily glycated hemoglobin (GHb), is effective in monitoring long-term glucose control in people with diabetes mellitus. It provides a retrospective index of integrated plasma glucose values over an extended period of time and is not subject to the wide fluctuations observed when blood glucose concentrations are assayed. GHb concentrations therefore are a valuable and widely used adjunct to blood glucose determinations for monitoring long-term glycemic control. In addition, GHb has recently been recommended for the diagnosis of diabetes and is a measure of risk for the development of microvascular complications of diabetes.

Glycated Hemoglobin[b]

Glycation is the nonenzymatic addition of a sugar residue to amino groups of proteins. Human adult hemoglobin (Hb) usually consists of HbA (97% of the total), HbA$_2$ (2.5%), and HbF (0.5%). HbA is made up of four polypeptide chains, two α- and two β-chains. Chromatographic analysis of HbA identifies several minor hemoglobins, namely, HbA$_{1a}$, HbA$_{1b}$, and HbA$_{1c}$, which are collectively referred to as HbA$_1$, fast hemoglobins (because they migrate more rapidly than HbA in an electrical field), glycohemoglobins, or GHbs (Table 47.4). The Joint Commission on Biochemical Nomenclature of the International Union of Pure and Applied Chemistry recommends the term neoglycoprotein for such derivatives and the term glycation to describe this process. Therefore although glycosylated and glucosylated have been widely used in the literature, the term glycated is preferred. HbA$_{1c}$ is formed by the condensation of glucose with the N-terminal valine residue of each β-chain of HbA to form an unstable Schiff base (aldimine, pre-HbA$_{1c}$; see Fig. 47.6). The Schiff base may dissociate or may undergo an Amadori rearrangement to form a stable ketoamine, HbA$_{1c}$. HbA$_{1a1}$ and HbA$_{1a2}$, which make up HbA$_{1a}$, have fructose 1,6-diphosphate and glucose 6-phosphate, respectively, attached to the amino terminal of the β-chain (see Table 47.4). The structure of HbA$_{1b}$, identified by mass spectrometry, contains pyruvic acid linked to the amino terminal valine of the β-chain, probably by a ketamine or enamine bond. HbA$_{1c}$ is the major fraction, constituting approximately 80% of HbA$_1$.

---

[b]The terms *glycated hemoglobin, glycohemoglobin, "glycosylated"* (which should not be used, as it refers to proteins in which carbohydrates have been attached enzymatically) *hemoglobin, HbA$_1$,* and *HbA$_{1c}$* have all been used to refer to hemoglobin that has been modified by the nonenzymatic addition of glucose residues. However, these terms are not interchangeable. The set of glycated hemoglobins includes HbA$_1$ and other non-enzymatically formed hemoglobin-glucose adducts; HbA$_1$ is made up of HbA$_{1a}$, HbA$_{1b}$, and HbA$_{1c}$. To eliminate this confusing nomenclature, and to remove mention of hemoglobin, which is confusing to patients as it has no obvious relation to diabetes or glucose, the term *A1c test* has been suggested. As described in the text, most of the available studies on the effects of metabolic control on complication rates (at least for DCCT and UKPDS) used assay methods that quantified HbA$_{1c}$ specifically, as do most clinical laboratories. In this chapter, the term *glycated hemoglobin* is used to refer to the set of all glycated hemoglobins, including glycated forms of hemoglobins other than hemoglobin A such as hemoglobin S and C.

Glycation may also occur at sites other than the end of the β-chain, such as lysine residues, or the α-chain. These GHbs are, in sum total, referred to as glycated HbA₀ or total GHb (see Table 47.4). Unlike at the end of the β-chain, glycations at these other sites cannot be separated from nonglycated hemoglobin by methods based on charge but are measurable by boronate affinity chromatography.

Formation of GHb is essentially irreversible, and the concentration in the blood depends on both the lifespan of the red blood cell (RBC; average lifespan is 120 days) and the blood glucose concentration. Because the rate of formation of GHb is directly proportional to the concentration of glucose in the blood, the GHb concentration represents integrated values for glucose over the preceding 8 to 12 weeks. This provides an additional criterion for assessing glucose control because GHb values are free of the influence of day-to-day glucose fluctuations and are unaffected by recent exercise or food ingestion.[176] It is important to realize that the contribution of the plasma glucose concentration to GHb depends on the time interval, with more recent values providing a larger contribution than earlier values. The plasma glucose in the preceding 1 month determines 50% of the HbA_{1c}, whereas days 60 to 120 determine only 25%.[278] After a sudden alteration in blood glucose concentrations, the rate of change of

HbA_{1c} is rapid during the initial 2 months, followed by a more gradual change approaching steady state 3 months later.

Labile intermediates (pre-HbA_{1c}, Schiff base) may be included in measurements of HbA_{1c}, especially in the common ion-exchange methods,[279] and produce misleadingly high results. The labile fraction changes rapidly with acute changes in blood glucose concentration and thus is not an indicator of long-term glycemic control. Pre-HbA_{1c} amounts to 5 to 8% of total HbA_1 in healthy individuals and ranges from 8 to 30% in patients with diabetes, depending on the degree of control of blood glucose concentration at or near the time of blood sampling.[280] If the analytical method measures both fractions, the labile pre-HbA_{1c} should be removed first, to prevent falsely increased results. In the absence of glucose, pre-HbA_{1c} reverts to glucose and HbA (see Fig. 47.6). This provides the basis for some procedures to eliminate the labile fraction by incubating washed red blood cells in saline. In some boronate affinity methods, the assay conditions favor rapid dissociation of the Schiff base.

Clinical Utility

Diagnosis of diabetes. As mentioned earlier in this chapter, since 2010 HbA_{1c} has been accepted as a criterion to diagnose diabetes. Advantages of HbA_{1c} (over glucose) include subject need not be fasting, very low biological variability, sample is stable, and the concentration predicts the development of microvascular complications of diabetes.[48,176] Point-of-care devices for HbA_{1c} should not be used for screening or diagnosis of diabetes.

Monitoring diabetes. HbA_{1c} has been firmly established as an index of long-term blood glucose concentrations and as a measure of the risk for the development of microvascular complications in patients with diabetes mellitus.[222] Most influential clinical diabetes organizations recommend that HbA_{1c} should be measured routinely in all patients with diabetes to document their degree of glycemic control and to assess response to treatment.[48] HbA_{1c} was a cornerstone of the DCCT.[199] (To prevent assay variability [see section on assay standardization later in this chapter], all GHb assays in the DCCT were done in a single laboratory that measured HbA_{1c} by HPLC.) The DCCT documented an exponential relationship between blood glucose concentrations (assessed by HbA_{1c}) and the risk for development and progression of microvascular complications.[199] The absolute risks of retinopathy and nephropathy were directly proportional to the mean HbA_{1c} concentration. Subsequent analysis revealed that the mean HbA_{1c} was the dominant predictor of retinopathy progression, and a 10% lower HbA_{1c} concentration was associated with a 45% lower risk.[281] Importantly, follow up over 30 years in the Epidemiology of Diabetes Interventions and Complications (EDIC) study reveals that HbA_{1c} is the

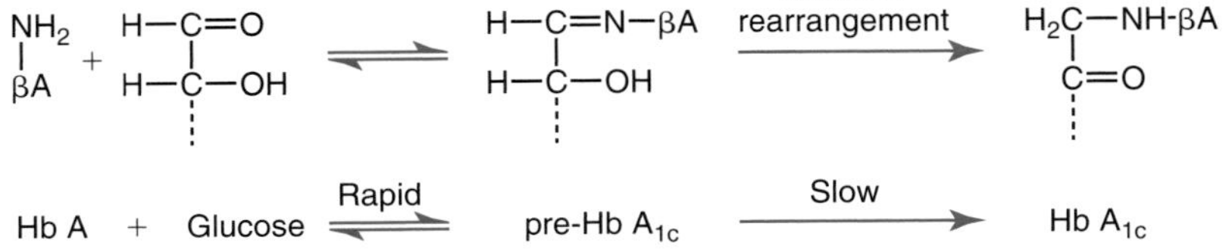

TABLE 47.4 Nomenclature of Selected Hemoglobins

Name	Component(s)
HbA	Constitutes ≈97% adult hemoglobin
HbA_0	Synonymous with HbA
HbA_{1a1}	HbA with fructose 1,6-diphosphate attached to the N-terminal valine of the β-chain
HbA_{1a2}	HbA with glucose 6-phosphate attached to the N-terminal valine of the β-chain
HbA_{1a}	Comprises HbA_{1a1} and HbA_{1a2}
HbA_{1b}	HbA with pyruvic acid attached to the N-terminal valine of the β-chain
HbA_{1c}	HbA with glucose attached to the N-terminal valine of the β-chain
Pre-HbA_{1c}	Unstable Schiff base (aldimine); a labile intermediary component in the formation of HbA_{1c}
HbA_1	Consists of HbA_{1a}, HbA_{1b}, and HbA_{1c}
Total glycated hemoglobin[a]	Consists of HbA_{1c} and other hemoglobin-carbohydrate adducts

[a]Also termed glycated hemoglobin or glycohemoglobin.
Hb, Hemoglobin.

FIGURE 47.6 Formation of hemoglobin A_{1c}.

strongest risk factor for the progression of retinopathy.[282–284] Since the risk of microvascular complications varies exponentially with HbA_{1c}, there is no HbA_{1c} concentration below which the risk is eliminated.

Analogous correlations between HbA_{1c} and complications were observed in patients with type 2 diabetes in the UKPDS trial.[200] To ensure that HbA_{1c} results in the UKPDS were comparable to the DCCT findings, an ion-exchange HPLC method calibrated to that in the DCCT was used. Mean HbA_{1c} values for the intensively treated and conventionally treated groups were 7.0 and 7.9% (53 and 63 mmol/mol), respectively.[200] Despite the relatively small difference in HbA_{1c}, microvascular complications were reduced by ≈25%. Each 1% reduction in HbA_{1c} (e.g., from 8 to 7% [64 to 53 mmol/mol]) was associated with risk reductions of 37% for microvascular disease, 21% for death related to diabetes, and 14% for myocardial infarction.[200] In patients without diabetes, HbA_{1c} is directly related to cardiovascular disease. In the European Prospective Investigation into Cancer and Nutrition (EPIC-Norfolk) study, an increase of 1% in HbA_{1c} was associated with a 28% increase in the risk of death.[285] Based on the DCCT and the UKPDS, major clinical diabetes organizations recommend that the goal for most patients with diabetes should be HbA_{1c} less than 6.5 to 7% (48 to 53 mmol/mol).[286] The more frequent use of this test in the management of patients is reflected in the increased number of laboratories participating in College of American Pathologists (CAP) GHb surveys. In 1985, 1990, 2003, 2009, and 2014 approximately 300, 700, 2000, 3250, and 3500 laboratories, respectively, were enrolled in the GHb surveys.

Methods for the Determination of Glycated Hemoglobins

More than 250 different methods have been described for the determination of GHbs. Most methods separate GHb from nonglycated hemoglobin using techniques based on charge differences (ion-exchange chromatography, HPLC, electrophoresis, and isoelectric focusing) or structural differences (affinity chromatography and immunoassay).[287] Chemical analysis (enzymatic, photometry, and spectrophotometry) has also been used. Recently, methods have become commercially available that use capillary electrophoresis or an enzymatic assay that specifically measure HbA_{1c}. Regardless of the method used, the result is expressed as a fraction of total hemoglobin. Analysis by gel electrophoresis, isoelectric focusing, or photometry is rarely used now and is not addressed further here. (Interested readers are referred to earlier editions of this book.) The selection of a method by a laboratory is influenced by several factors, including sample volume, patient population, and cost. It is advisable to consult clinicians in this process. The ADA recommends that laboratories use only HbA_{1c} assays that are certified by the NGSP (previously termed the National Glycohemoglobin Standardization Program) as traceable to the DCCT reference.[222] These assays are listed on the NGSP Website (www.NGSP.org/ accessed February 28, 2020) and are updated several times a year.

The evolution of GHb assays most widely used in the United States are depicted in Table 47.5. These data are based on results from 1947, 2396, and 3193 laboratories participating in quality control surveys conducted by the CAP in 1995, 2009, and 2019, respectively. The results demonstrate that by 2009, virtually all laboratories used immunoassay or ion-exchange chromatography. HbA_{1c} was measured by more

than 99% of laboratories (see Table 47.5). Total GHb and HbA_1 measurements had essentially disappeared. These results reflect considerable changes from the methods used in 1995, when affinity chromatography was the most common analytical method (see Table 47.5). Also, only 60% of laboratories reported HbA_{1c} in 1995. In addition, variation among mean values—both between and within methods—and imprecision were substantially lower in 2009 and continued to improve in 2019. Note that the CAP samples are prepared from human whole blood, which allows direct comparison among different methods and instruments. It should be borne in mind that these data refer only to these CAP surveys and are weighted to laboratories that participate (~15% of participants are from outside the United States). All of the methods described are commercially available from several different manufacturers.

High-performance liquid chromatography. HbA_{1c} and other hemoglobin fractions can be separated by HPLC, which employs cation-exchange chromatography.[288] Several fully automated systems are commercially available. Some assays require only 5 μL of whole blood, and fingerstick samples can be collected in a capillary tube for analysis. Anticoagulated blood is diluted with a hemolysis reagent containing borate. Samples are incubated at 37 °C for 30 minutes to remove the Schiff base and are inserted into the autosampler. (Some instruments have a shorter preincubation step, and others separate labile A_{1c} chromatographically, eliminating the step to remove the Schiff base.[289]) A step gradient using three phosphate buffers of increasing ionic strength is passed through the column. Detection is performed at both 415 and 690 nm, and results are quantified by integrating the area under the peaks. Analysis time is as short as 3 to 5 minutes. All HPLC methods had CVs less than 3.0% in a 2019 CAP survey (see Table 47.5). HbA_{1c} by HPLC was used for analysis of all patient samples in the DCCT.[288]

Chemically modified derivatives of hemoglobin occur when the charge on hemoglobin is altered by the attachment of noncarbohydrate moieties, as in uremia (carbamylated hemoglobin), alcoholism, lead poisoning, or chronic treatment with large doses of aspirin (acetylated hemoglobin). Hemoglobin variants (e.g., HbS, HbC, etc.), if present, can also be glycated in the same way as HbA. Variants or chemically modified hemoglobins that elute separately from HbA and HbA_{1c} usually have little effect on HbA_{1c} measurements. If the modified hemoglobin (or its glycated derivative) cannot be separated from HbA or HbA_{1c}, spuriously increased or reduced results will be obtained.[290] A variant that elutes with HbA_{1c} will yield a gross overestimation of HbA_{1c}, and a variant that coelutes with HbA will underestimate HbA_{1c}. Note that a single variant may falsely increase or decrease HbA_{1c}, depending on the method used.[290]

Immunoassay. Assays for HbA_{1c} have been developed using antibodies raised against the Amadori product of glucose (ketoamine linkage) plus the first few (four to eight) amino acids at the N-terminal end of the β-chain of hemoglobin.[291] A widely used assay measures HbA_{1c} in whole blood by inhibition of latex agglutination. The agglutinator, a synthetic polymer containing multiple copies of the immunoreactive portion of HbA_{1c}, binds the anti-HbA_{1c} monoclonal antibody that is attached to latex beads. This agglutination produces light scattering, measured as an increase in absorbance. HbA_{1c} in the patient's sample competes for the antibody on

TABLE 47.5 Methods of Glycated Hemoglobin Analysis[a]

Method	Component Reported	Year: 1995 (n = 1947)[b]				2009 (n = 2396)				2019 (n = 3193)			
		Number[c]	% of Total	Mean %[d]	CV, %[d]	Number[c]	% of Total	Mean %[e]	CV, %[d]	Number[c]	% of Total	Mean %[e]	CV, %[d]
Charge													
Ion exchange	HbA₁c	279	15	4.9–5.7	4.4–13.8	832	35	6.0–6.3	1.3–3	798	26	6.3–6.6	1.2–2.7
	HbA₁	22		6.5	15.2	—[f]							
Electrophoresis[g]	HbA₁c	138	12	4.9	16.5	0		—	—	70	2	6.3	1.6
	HbA₁	99		6.4–7.8	9.6–12.7	—							
Structure													
Affinity	HbA₁c	642	66	6.5	8.1	12	<1	5.9	2.3	222	7	6.2–6.5	1.8–2.0
	Total GHb	638		5.9–7.9	6.9–9.3	0		—	—	—			
Immunoassay	HbA₁c	129	7	5.7	3.5	1552	65	5.7–6.2	2.7–8	1805	57	6.3–6.6	1.7–3.7
Enzymatic	HbA₁c									259	8	6.4	1.6

[a]Results are based on 1995 CAP Survey, Set EC-B, Specimen GH-03; 2009 CAP Survey, Set GH2-A, Specimen GH2-02 and 2019 CAP Survey, Set GH5-C, Specimen GH2-12 (Copyright, 1995, 2009 and 2019 College of American Pathologists; data used with permission). See text for discussion of methods.
[b]n is the number of laboratories that participated in the survey.
[c]Indicates how many laboratories use the indicated method.
[d]Where more than one value is listed, the data vary among commercial assays. The range is presented.
[e]The NGSP values in 2009 and 2019 were 6.0 and 6.4%, respectively.
[f]Number of participants was too low to permit statistical analysis.
[g]Original methods used agar gel electrophoresis. Current (2019) method uses capillary electrophoresis.
CV, Coefficient of variation; GHb, glycated hemoglobin; Hb, hemoglobin.

the latex, inhibiting agglutination, thereby decreasing light scattering. Enzyme immunoassays using monoclonal antibodies are commercially available, and most exhibit reasonable imprecision (see Table 47.5). These assays are generally calibrated to give values that match and correlate with HPLC values. The antibodies do not recognize labile intermediates or other GHbs (such as HbA_{1a} or HbA_{1b}) because both ketoamine with glucose and specific amino acid sequences are required for binding. Similarly, several hemoglobin variants, such as HbF, HbA_2, HbS, and carbamylated hemoglobin, are not detected.[290] The procedure has been adapted for capillary blood samples using a bench-top analyzer with reagent cartridges designed for use in physicians' office laboratories.

Affinity chromatography. Affinity gel columns are used to separate GHb, which binds to the column, from the nonglycated fraction. *m*-Aminophenylboronic acid is immobilized by cross-linking to beaded agarose or another matrix (e.g., glass fiber). The boronic acid reacts with the *cis*-diol groups of glucose bound to hemoglobin to form a reversible five-member ring complex, thus selectively holding the GHb on the column (Fig. 47.7). The nonglycated hemoglobin does not bind. Sorbitol is then added to elute the GHb. Absorbance of bound and nonbound fractions, measured at 415 nm, is used to calculate the percentage of GHb.

A commercial assay is performed on an automated analyzer that uses a soluble reagent consisting of dihydroxyboronate coupled with high molecular weight polyacrylic acid.[292] GHb binds to the boronate. The polyanionic-glycated hemoglobin affinity complex attaches by electrostatic interactions to the cationic surface of the solid-phase matrix (ion capture). Nonglycated hemoglobin does not bind and is removed in a wash step. GHb is quantified by measuring quenching by hemoglobin of the fluorescence of an added fluorophore, 4-methyl-umbelliferone. Total hemoglobin is determined by fluorescence quenching of a second sample containing sorbitol. The sorbitol competes for boronate binding sites, and both nonglycated hemoglobin and GHb contribute to inhibition of the quenching. The fluorescence measurements are converted to glycated and total hemoglobin concentrations from separate stored calibration curves.

The major advantages of affinity chromatography are that there is no interference from nonglycated hemoglobins and there is negligible interference from the labile intermediate form of HbA_{1c}. It is unaffected by variations in temperature and has reasonably good precision. Hemoglobin variants such as HbS, HbC, HbD, or HbE produce little effect. Affinity methods measure total GHb. This includes components other than HbA_{1c} because the assay detects ketoamine structures on lysine and valine residues on both α- and β-chains of hemoglobin.

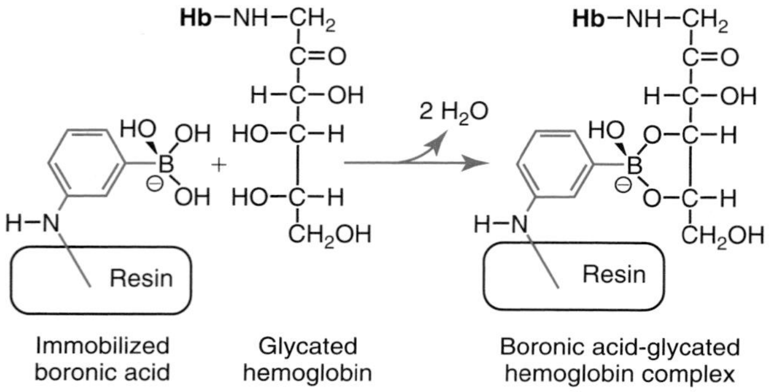

Although the method detects all GHbs, most commercially available systems are calibrated to report a standardized HbA_{1c} value. The value is derived from an equation obtained from linear regression between total GHb and HbA_{1c} analysis by HPLC.[292] A linear relationship has been demonstrated, and standardized HbA_{1c} values are thus comparable to values obtained by methods specific for HbA_{1c}. Columns and reagents are commercially available.

Capillary electrophoresis. HbA_{1c} was first identified in 1968 on agar gel electrophoresis at pH 6.2.[293] With development of better alternatives, electrophoretic methods disappeared from use (Table 47.5). The development of capillary electrophoresis has generated renewed interest in the technique. Advantages of capillary electrophoresis include high resolving ability (due to the high voltage that can be applied) and small sample volume (discussed in more detail in Chapter 18[294]). Briefly, charged molecules are separated by their electrophoretic mobility in an alkaline buffer (pH 9.4), as well as by electrolyte pH and electroosmotic flow. Hemoglobins are detected by absorption spectroscopy at the cathodic end of the capillary. An automated liquid-flow capillary electrophoresis method to measure HbA_{1c} is commercially available and has been approved by the FDA in the United States.

Enzymatic. Enzymatic assays to measure HbA_{1c} have been developed recently based on a method in which fructosyl peptide oxidase catalyzes the oxidative deglycation of *N*-(deoxyfructosyl)-Val-His.[295] Erythrocytes are lysed and sodium nitrite is added to oxidize total hemoglobin to methemoglobin. Addition of sodium azide produces azidomethemoglobin, which is quantified on a spectrophotometer at 476 nm.[296] Neutral protease is added to release fructosyl dipeptide [i.e., *N*-(deoxyfructosyl)-Val-His] from the N-terminal of the β-chain of HbA_{1c}. Fructosyl peptide oxidase hydrolyzes the fructosyl dipeptide, releasing hydrogen peroxide, which reacts with a chromogen in the presence of peroxidase, and the color is measured by absorbance at 660 nm. The procedure has been adapted for analysis on a high throughput automated analyzer[296] and the method has been approved by the FDA for use in the United States.

Removal of Labile Glycated Hemoglobin From Red Blood Cells

The concentration of the labile form of HbA_{1c} (Schiff base) fluctuates rapidly in response to acute changes in plasma glucose concentrations and should be removed before analysis by charge-based assays. This may be accomplished by incubating red blood cells in saline[297] or in buffer solutions at pH 5 to 6,[298] or by dialysis or ultrafiltration of hemolysates. Most kits for column assays contain reagents to remove this labile component.

Assay Standardization

Clinical laboratories measure GHb with diverse assays that use multiple methods and quantify different components. The DCCT results accentuated the need for accurate GHb measurement and provided a strong impetus for standardization of GHb assays. At the end of the DCCT, it was noted that absence of both a reference method and a single GHb standard had generated confusion.[299] Interlaboratory comparisons were

FIGURE 47.7 Reaction of glycated hemoglobin (GHb) with immobilized boronic acid.

not possible, and even a single quality control sample analyzed by a single method exhibited interlaboratory CVs as high as 16.5%. Similar large variability among laboratories was observed in Europe.[300] Committees were established under the auspices of the American Association for Clinical Chemistry (AACC) in 1993 and the IFCC in 1995 to standardize GHb assays.[301]

The NGSP was established in 1996 to implement the protocol developed by the AACC to calibrate GHb results to DCCT-equivalent values. Employing a network of reference laboratories, the NGSP interacts with manufacturers of GHb methods to help them calibrate their methods and trace values to the DCCT.[302] Manufacturers apply for certification by performing precision testing according to CLSI EP5-A guidelines and report results in DCCT-equivalent HbA_{1c} values. This calibration effort has markedly improved harmonization of results and has reduced imprecision.[301–303] Results obtained using NGSP-certified assays can be compared directly with results of the DCCT and UKPDS, allowing alignment with clinical outcomes data. The ADA recommends that clinical laboratories use only assays certified by the NGSP and participate in a proficiency testing program that uses fresh whole blood samples, for example, offered by the CAP. The CAP GHb survey uses pooled whole blood specimens at several HbA_{1c} concentrations. Target values are assigned by the NGSP network. Thus individual laboratories can directly compare their HbA_{1c} results with those of the DCCT and UKPDS.

A different approach was adopted by the IFCC. A working group was established to devise a reference system for standardization based on HbA_{1c}. The IFCC group developed a mixture of purified HbA_{1c} and HbA_0 as primary reference material.[304] Two candidate reference methods, namely, electrospray ionization mass spectrometry (ESI-MS) and capillary electrophoresis, were proposed.[304] These specifically measure the glycated N-terminal valine of the β-chain of hemoglobin. Analysis is performed by digesting the hemoglobin molecule with endoproteinase Glu-C, which cleaves the β-chain between Glu-6 and Glu-7, releasing the N-terminal hexapeptide. Glycated and nonglycated hexapeptides are separated and quantified by HPLC-ESI-MS or by HPLC-capillary electrophoresis.[304] HbA_{1c} is measured as the ratio between glycated and nonglycated N-terminal hexapeptides. The IFCC Working Group established a network of laboratories to implement and maintain the reference system.[305] Comparisons between IFCC and NGSP reference methods (and reference systems from Japan and Sweden) indicate a close and stable relationship and allow manufacturers to calibrate their instruments to a higher-level reference method.[305] However, HbA_{1c} results obtained using IFCC reference methods are 1.5 to 2% absolute HbA_{1c} units lower than those of the NGSP (and lower than other reference systems). The difference is probably due to measurement of glycated components other than HbA_{1c} by HPLC. The IFCC method is a higher order reference method and is not designed to be used for routine analysis of patient samples.

Test Limitations
Interpretation of HbA_{1c} depends on red blood cells having a normal lifespan. Patients with hemolytic disease or other conditions with shortened red blood cell survival exhibit a substantial reduction in HbA_{1c}.[290] Similarly, individuals with

recent significant blood loss have falsely low values owing to a higher fraction of young erythrocytes. One study has suggested that the differences in mean red cell lifespan may explain most of the interindividual variability in the relationship between average glucose and HbA_{1c} concentrations.[306,307]

The effects of hemoglobin variants (such as HbF, HbS, and HbC) depend on the specific method of analysis used.[290,308] Depending on the particular hemoglobin variant and assay, results may be spuriously increased or decreased. Boronate affinity chromatographic methods are minimally affected by hemoglobin variants. Visual inspection, or an automated report, of the chromatogram from HPLC and capillary electrophoresis methods can alert the laboratory to a variant. Most manufacturers of HbA_{1c} assays have modified their assays to eliminate interference from the most common hemoglobin variants. Therefore accurate measurement of HbA_{1c} is possible by selecting an appropriate instrument, provided the erythrocyte lifespan is not altered (see www.NGSP.org for additional information).

Race influences HbA_{1c} concentration. Published evidence suggests that HbA_{1c} concentrations in blacks, Asians, and Hispanics are higher than in whites. A 2017 meta-analysis in individuals without diabetes showed significantly higher HbA_{1c} concentrations in blacks (0.26%, 2.8 mmol/mol), Asians (0.24%, 2.6 mmol/mol), and Latinos (0.08%, 0.9 mmol/mol) than in whites.[309] Nevertheless, whether these differences have clinical relevance remains controversial.[310,311] For example, race did not modify the association between HbA_{1c} and adverse cardiovascular outcomes or death.[34] Moreover, all measures of long-term glycemia, namely, HbA_{1c}, fructosamine, glycated albumin, and 1,5-anhydroglucitol (1,5-AG), were higher in blacks than in whites and had similar associations with risk for nephropathy, retinopathy, and cardiovascular disease in the different races.[312] Clinical studies are ongoing to resolve the question.

Carbamylated hemoglobin is formed by the covalent attachment of isocyanic acid, which is derived from urea, to hemoglobin. Renal failure is common in diabetes patients and results in high concentrations of urea in the blood. While carbamylated hemoglobin interfered in older methods, it does not influence most modern methods of HbA_{1c} analysis.[313] High HbA_{1c} concentrations have been reported in iron deficiency anemia.[313] The mechanism is unknown, but increased glycation by malondialdehyde has been proposed.[314] Other factors that have been reported to interfere with some methods include hyperlipidemia and selected medications. Most of the interferents produce relatively small effects, and for the vast majority of patients with diabetes, HbA_{1c} can be measured accurately.

Reporting HbA_{1c}
HbA_{1c} is reported as a percentage of total hemoglobin in the NGSP system. These values, which are equivalent to those reported in the DCCT and the UKPDS, represent the most widely used reporting system in patient care and the published literature. The IFCC method reports HbA_{1c} as mmol/mol (HbA_{1c}/total Hb).[315] Comparison between the IFCC and NGSP networks produced a master equation that permits conversion between the two reference systems.[316] For example, an HbA_{1c} result of 7% (in NGSP/DCCT/UKPDS units) is equivalent to 53 mmol/mol (in IFCC units). Calculators that convert units are freely available at several websites, for

example, http://www.ngsp.org/convert1.asp. Many journals now require that HbA$_{1c}$ values be reported in both NGSP/DCCT and SI units.[315]

A multinational, prospective study (termed A$_{1c}$ Derived Average Glucose [ADAG]) evaluated the relationship between HbA$_{1c}$ concentrations and long-term glucose values.[317] A linear correlation was observed, permitting estimated average glucose (eAG) to be calculated from the HbA$_{1c}$ measurement. The regression equations are as follows: eAG mg/dL = 28.7 × HbA$_{1c}$ − 46.7, and eAG mmol/L = 1.59 × HbA$_{1c}$ − 2.59. For example, an HbA$_{1c}$ value of 7% (53 mmol/mol) translates into an eAG of 140 mg/dL. Some clinicians and many diabetes educators believe that the eAG will facilitate communication with patients.[318] The ADA and the AACC recommend that laboratories report both HbA$_{1c}$ and eAG. Nevertheless, the concept of expressing HbA$_{1c}$ in terms of average glucose is not accepted by all.[319,320]

Performance Goals

Some expert groups have proposed goals for HbA$_{1c}$ assay accuracy and precision, and these have tightened over the years. Intraindividual variation of HbA$_{1c}$ is low, with CVs less than 2%. The last ADA guidelines, published in 2011, recommend an intralaboratory CV less than 2% and an interlaboratory CV less than 3.5%.[48] Based on the performance of modern methods, desirable specifications for HbA$_{1c}$ measurement currently achievable are intralaboratory CV less than 1.5% and an interlaboratory CV less than 2.5%.

Specimen Collection and Storage

Patients need not be fasting. Venous blood should usually be collected in tubes containing EDTA or oxalate together with fluoride. Sample stability depends on the assay method used.[48] Whole blood may be stored at 4 °C for up to 1 week. Above 4 °C, HbA$_{1a+b}$ increases in a time- and temperature-dependent manner, but HbA$_{1c}$ is only slightly affected.[321] Storage of samples at −20 °C is not recommended for ion-exchange methods.[322] For most methods, whole blood samples stored at −70 °C or colder are stable for at least 18 months,[323] with reports of stability up to 14 years.[324] Repeated freeze-thaw cycles of stored samples should be avoided. Heparinized samples should be assayed within 2 days and may not be suitable for some methods of analysis (e.g., electrophoresis).

Reference Intervals and Targets

Values for HbA$_{1c}$ are expressed as a percentage of total blood hemoglobin. In the past, one of three major HbA$_{1c}$ species, namely, HbA$_1$, HbA$_{1c}$, or total GHb, was usually measured. The United States and many other countries, including Canada, Australia, New Zealand, and the United Kingdom, now report all results as HbA$_{1c}$. Reference intervals vary, depending on the HbA$_{1c}$ component measured. The reference interval for HbA$_{1c}$ (using an NGSP-certified method) is often quoted as 4 to 6% (20 to 42 mmol/mol).

The effects of age on reference intervals are controversial.[48] Some studies show age-related increases (≈0.1% per decade after age 30), whereas other reports show no increase in nondiabetic individuals.[325–327] It is not known whether these small, but statistically significant, increases in HbA$_{1c}$ concentrations with age have any clinical significance. Results are not affected by acute illness. Intraindividual variability is minimal (CV~1%).[328]

In patients with poorly controlled diabetes mellitus, values may extend to twice the upper limit of the reference interval or more, but rarely exceed 15% HbA$_{1c}$. Values greater than 15% (140 mmol/mol) or less than 4% (20 mmol/mol) should prompt additional studies to determine the possible presence of variant hemoglobin.[290] HbA$_{1c}$ should be repeated, if possible using a method with an analytic principle different to the initial assay. (In some low-income countries, HbA$_{1c}$ concentrations as high as 20% [195 mmol/mol] may be seen due to poor glycemic control.)

Target values derived from the DCCT and UKPDS and recommended by the ADA and other organizations, not the reference values, are used to evaluate metabolic control in diabetes patients. There is no specific value of HbA$_{1c}$ below which the risk of diabetes complications is eliminated completely. The ADA states that the goal of treatment in general should be to maintain HbA$_{1c}$ at less than 7% (53 mmol/mol).[214] (Some organizations recommend an HbA$_{1c}$ target of less than 6.5% [<48 mmol/mol].) HbA$_{1c}$ goals should be individualized. Pregnant women with preexisting diabetes should aim for HbA$_{1c}$ less than 6.5% (48 mmol/mol) to protect the fetus from congenital malformations and the baby and the mother from complications. These target values are applicable only if the assay method is certified by the NGSP as traceable to the DCCT reference. Assay precision is important because each 1% absolute change in HbA$_{1c}$ represents an approximate 30 mg/dL (1.7 mmol/L) change in average blood glucose.

No consensus has been reached on optimum frequency of testing. The ADA recommends that HbA$_{1c}$ should be routinely monitored at least every 6 months in patients meeting treatment goals (and who have stable glycemic control).[214] These recommendations are for patients with type 1 or type 2 diabetes. An analysis of greater than 79 000 patients revealed that the optimum testing frequency to maximize reduction in HbA$_{1c}$ was every 3 months; testing less frequently was associated with deteriorating control.[329]

POCT HbA$_{1c}$

Several small or hand-held devices are available to measure HbA$_{1c}$ at the point of care. Although many of these devices are NGSP-certified, published evaluations reveal that most POC devices for HbA$_{1c}$ do not exhibit adequate analytical performance to meet clinical needs.[330,331] A meta-analysis of 13 devices in 61 studies found nine devices with negative mean bias and four with positive bias; mean CVs were greater than 2% at HbA$_{1c}$ less than 6%.[332] Importantly, the test is waived in the United States and so proficiency testing is not mandated. Therefore minimum objective information is available concerning their performance in the hands of those who measure HbA$_{1c}$ in patient samples.[333] For these reasons, the ADA advises that POCT devices for HbA$_{1c}$ should not be used for diagnosis or screening for diabetes.[20] While some advocate that immediate feedback of HbA$_{1c}$ results at the time of the patient visit improves glycemic control,[334] not all studies support this premise.[335] Moreover, a systematic review and meta-analysis concluded that there is insufficient evidence of the effectiveness of POCT HbA$_{1c}$ in the management of diabetes.[336]

Glycated Serum Proteins

In selected patients with diabetes mellitus (e.g., GDM, change in therapy), assays may be needed that are more sensitive than HbA_{1c} to shorter-term alterations in average blood glucose concentrations. Nonenzymatic attachment of glucose to amino groups of proteins other than hemoglobin (e.g., serum proteins, membrane proteins, lens crystallins) to form ketoamines also occurs. Because serum proteins turn over more rapidly than erythrocytes (the circulating half-life of albumin is about 14 to 20 days), the concentration of glycated serum albumin reflects glucose control over a period of 2 to 3 weeks. Therefore both deterioration of control and improvement with therapy are evident earlier than with HbA_{1c}. In addition, glycated serum proteins are not influenced by changes in erythrocyte lifespan and can be used to monitor glycemia in patients with conditions (e.g., hemolysis, blood transfusion) that alter HbA_{1c} independently of glycemia.

Fructosamine

Clinical Significance

Fructosamine is the generic name for plasma protein ketoamines and the common name for 1-amino-1-deoxy-D-fructose (for reviews, see Refs.[337,338]) The name refers to the structure of the ketoamine rearrangement product formed by the interaction of glucose with the ϵ-amino group on lysine residues of albumin. Analogous to HbA_{1c}, measurement of fructosamine may be used as an index of the average concentration of blood glucose over an extended period of time, but one that is about 1/4 as long as the time examined with HbA_{1c}.

Because all glycated serum proteins are fructosamines and albumin is the most abundant serum protein, measurement of fructosamine is thought to be largely a measure of glycated albumin, but this has been questioned by some investigators.[339] Although the fructosamine assay is easily automated and cheaper than HbA_{1c}, there is a lack of consensus on its clinical utility. For example, evaluation of 65 studies led the authors to conclude that fructosamine determination is not a reliable test, and it has not been evaluated sufficiently for routine clinical use.[340] In contrast, a review of essentially the same data concluded that fructosamine could provide information useful in the management of diabetes.[337] Early work using the original assay, introduced in 1983,[341,342] indicated that fructosamine concentrations were significantly higher in diabetes individuals than in healthy subjects. Over the succeeding decade, the assay underwent numerous modifications because several artifacts were identified that rendered data from the first-generation fructosamine assay difficult to interpret. These include apparent lack of specificity for glycated proteins (up to 60% of the value was due to non-fructosamine reducing substances), lack of standardization among laboratories, difficulty in calibrating the assay, and interference by urates and hyperlipidemia.[343] Substantial modifications produced second-generation assays that contain uricase and higher detergent concentrations and are calibrated with glycated lysine.[344] In addition, an industry standard was adopted. These improvements resulted in average fructosamine values in nondiabetic individuals that are approximately 10% of those obtained with the first-generation assay. Modern assays show strong correlation with HbA_{1c} and prognostic value for the development of diabetes and microvascular complications. An important limitation is the lack of long-term prospective studies with clinical outcomes.[345] Therefore no agreed target for optimum glycemic control exists. The clinical value of fructosamine has not been firmly established, and further studies are required to determine whether it is useful for routine monitoring of patients' glycemic control.[48]

Because fructosamine determination monitors short-term glycemic changes different from HbA_{1c}, it may have a role in conjunction with HbA_{1c} rather than instead of it. In addition, fructosamine may be useful in patients in whom HbA_{1c} is of limited value, for example, decreased erythrocyte lifespan. Gross changes in protein concentration and half-life may have large effects on the proportion of protein that is glycated. Thus fructosamine results may be invalid in patients with nephrotic syndrome, cirrhosis of the liver, or dysproteinemias, or after rapid changes in acute-phase reactants. Initial reports indicated that, in the absence of significant alterations in serum protein concentrations, fructosamine results were independent of protein concentrations.[346] However, this observation has been questioned by other investigators who recommend that fructosamine values be corrected for protein concentrations. This issue remains to be resolved. It is generally accepted that the assay should not be performed when serum albumin is less than 30 g/L. Although it was initially postulated that the fructosamine assay would replace the OGTT, there is no role for the fructosamine assay in the diagnosis of diabetes mellitus. A few studies have evaluated fructosamine in identifying women with GDM.[347] Most of these include few patients and use different GDM diagnostic criteria and fructosamine thresholds. Measurement of fructosamine should not be used to screen patients for GDM.[347]

Determination of Fructosamine

Methods for measuring glycated serum proteins include: affinity chromatography using immobilized phenylboronic acid (similar to the HbA_{1c} assay)[348]; HPLC of glycated lysine residues after hydrolysis of the glycated proteins[349]; a photometric procedure in which mild acid hydrolysis releases 5-hydroxymethylfurfural—proteins are precipitated with trichloroacetic acid and the supernatant is reacted with 2-thiobarbituric acid[350]; other procedures using phenylhydrazine and ϵ-N-(2-furoylmethyl)-L-lysine (furosine). None of these assays is popular because they are not suitable for routine clinical laboratories. The development of monoclonal antibodies to glycated albumin,[351] although theoretically advantageous, has not yet resulted in the widespread availability of commercial assays. It should be noted that prolonged storage at ultra-low temperatures ($-96\,°C$) prevents in vitro glycation of serum proteins.[352]

The most widely used method for the measurement of fructosamine is a modification[344,353] of the original method of Johnson and colleagues.[342] This method is conducted under alkaline conditions and results in fructosamine undergoing an Amadori rearrangement with the resultant compounds having reducing activity that can be differentiated from other reducing substances. In the presence of carbonate buffer, fructosamine rearranges to the eneaminol form, which reduces NBT to a formazan (Fig. 47.8). Absorbance at 530 nm is measured at two time points, and the absorbance change is proportional to the fructosamine concentration. A 10-minute preincubation is necessary to allow fast-reacting interfering reducing substances to react. It is unnecessary to remove endogenous glucose from patients' samples because a pH greater than 11 is required for glucose to reduce NBT. The assay is easily automated and has excellent between-batch analytical precision. Hemoglobin (>100 mg/dL) and bilirubin (>4 mg/dL) may interfere; therefore moderate to grossly hemolyzed and icteric samples should not be used. Ascorbic

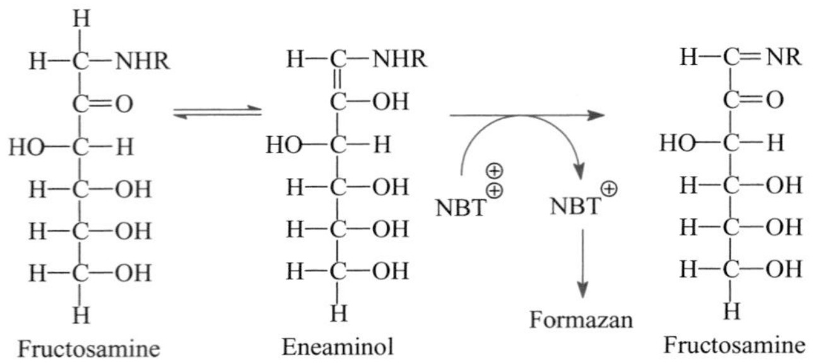

FIGURE 47.8 Reaction of fructosamine with nitroblue tetrazolium (NBT).

acid concentrations greater than 5 mg/dL may cause negative interference. Kits are commercially available (Roche Diagnostics, Indianapolis, IN).

Enzymatic methods have also been described.[354] Samples are incubated with proteinase K, which cleaves serum proteins into smaller fragments. The next step is addition of the enzyme fructosaminase, which catalyzes the oxidative degradation of the glycated peptides, resulting in the release of H_2O_2, which is quantified. The assay, which can be run on an automated analyzer, is commercially available (GlycoGap, Diazyme, Poway, CA) and has been approved by the FDA for use in the United States. Unlike the NBT assay, the fructosaminase assay is reported to have no significant interference at up to 7.5 mg/dL (128 umol/L) bilirubin and 200 mg/dL (124 mmol/L) hemoglobin. An assay that measures fructosamine by oxidizing the ketoamine bond using ketoamine oxidase, with release of hydrogen peroxide that is quantified by a photometric reaction, is also commercially available (Randox, Antrim, UK).

Reference Intervals
Values in a healthy reference population of 1799 individuals are 195 to 258 μmol/L using a colorimetric assay.[355] The reference interval for the enzymatic assay is reported to be 151 to 300 μmol/L.

Glycated Albumin
Albumin, which comprises ~60% of total serum protein, makes up ≥80% of total glycated serum proteins.[356] The N terminus and 59 lysine residues are potential glycation sites and it is not known how many of these are glycated in vivo. Analysis of human plasma by HPLC tandem mass spectrometry and $[^{13}C_6]$glucose labeling identified 35 different glycation sites on albumin.[357] Assays that measure only glycated albumin, rather than all glycated serum proteins (i.e., fructosamine), are commercially available.

The clinical use of glycated albumin is limited by the same caveats that apply to fructosamine, namely limited evidence relating it to the complications of diabetes and lack of long-term prospective studies with clinical outcomes. Nevertheless, accumulating published evidence suggests that glycated albumin may be useful for predicting diabetes and its microvascular complications. For example, a prospective cohort analysis of the Atherosclerosis Risk in Communities (ARIC) study showed that glycated albumin was strongly associated with incident diabetes, retinopathy, and chronic kidney disease.[358] Glycated albumin was also a risk factor for mortality and morbidity in patients on hemodialysis.[359] A case-cohort

analysis of a subpopulation of the DCCT revealed that glycated albumin and HbA_{1c} had similar associations with retinopathy and nephropathy, which were strengthened when both analytes were considered together.[360] Interestingly, HbA_{1c}, but not glycated albumin, was significantly associated with cardiovascular disease in the same study. Additional evidence for the combined use of glycated albumin and HbA_{1c} was obtained in the Africans in America study. In a population of self-identified healthy African immigrants to the Unite States, HbA_{1c} and glycated albumin had diagnostic sensitivities for prediabetes (diagnosed by an OGTT) of 50 and 42%, respectively.[361] Combining HbA_{1c} with glycated albumin increased the sensitivity to 78%. A subsequent analysis of a larger cohort of the African immigrants documented that glycated albumin identified prediabetes not detected by HbA_{1c} in nonobese subjects; in the obese, HbA_{1c} was a significantly better diagnostic assay than glycated albumin (64 vs. 16%).[361] Ongoing studies are anticipated to more clearly define the clinical value of glycated albumin in diabetes.

Determination of Glycated Albumin
Several different methods have been used to quantify glycated albumin.[356,362,363] These include: a colorimetric procedure in which mild acid hydrolysis releases 5-hydroxymethylfurfural—proteins are precipitated with trichloroacetic acid and the supernatant is reacted with 2-thiobarbituric acid[350]; RIA using beads coated with antibody to albumin and ^{125}I-labeled antibody directed against glucitol-lysine epitopes of glycated albumin previously reduced by sodium borohydride ($NaBH_4$) to reduce the Schiff base[364]; ELISA in which glycated albumin binds to a monoclonal antibody coated on a plate, followed by incubation with an enzyme-linked anti-human albumin antibody (Exocell, Philadelphia, PA); enzyme-linked boronate immunoassay where boronic acid-HRP conjugate binds to the cis-diols of glycated albumin, which is immobilized by an anti-human albumin antibody coated onto microtiter plate[365]; affinity chromatography using immobilized phenylboronic acid, followed by elution and measurement of albumin[348]; boronate affinity chromatography; HPLC with anion exchange chromatography to separate albumin, followed by boronate affinity chromatography to separate glycated from nonglycated albumin[366]; enzymatic assay using ketoamine oxidase[367]; and mass spectrometry.[368]

Probably the most widely used method globally is enzymatic. The assay has two steps. In the first, endogenous glycated amino acids are eliminated by oxidation with ketoamine oxidase.[367] In the second step, glycated albumin is hydrolyzed by an albumin-specific proteinase to glycated amino acids, which are subsequently oxidized by ketoamine oxidase to glucosone, producing hydrogen peroxide (Fig. 47.9). This is quantified with the chromogen 4-aminoantipyrene by measuring absorbance at 546/700 nm. Total albumin is measured with bromocresol purple and glycated albumin is expressed as a percentage of total albumin. The assay is commercially available (Lucica GA-L, Asahi Kasei Pharma Corporation, Tokyo, Japan) and has been used in numerous published studies. It was approved by the FDA in 2018 for use in the United States and can be performed on many automated analyzers.

Analogous to fructosamine, the evidence relating glycated albumin to clinical outcomes is limited. Further studies are required to determine its clinical value in diabetes.[48,369]

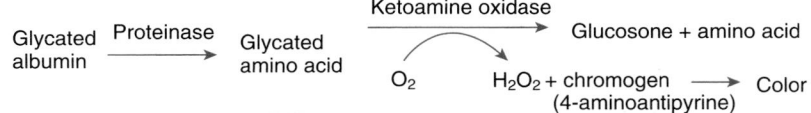

FIGURE 47.9 Hydrolysis of glycated albumin.

Reference Intervals

Reference intervals vary considerably, depending on the method, ranging from 0.8 to 1.4% to 18 to 22%.[356,362] The reference interval for the enzymatic assay, which is expressed as a percentage of total albumin, is 11.9 to 15.8%.[362] In a healthy reference population of 1799 US adults, the reference interval was 10.7 to 15.1%.[355]

Concentrations in women are slightly higher than in men. There is an inverse association with BMI (body mass index); glycated albumin is lower at higher BMI.[355,370] The reason for this is unknown. Values in blacks are significantly higher than in whites.[355,362] Intraindividual variation is low (CV 2.1%), but between-subject variation is reported to be 10.6%.[371] In patients with poorly controlled diabetes, values may increase by up to fivefold. Factors that influence albumin metabolism have been reported to alter glycated albumin independently of glycemia. These include the nephrotic syndrome, thyroid disease, cirrhosis of the liver, smoking, hyperuricemia, and hypertriglyceridemia.[356] Samples can be stored as long as 23 years at −70 °C.[372]

Advanced Glycation End Products

The molecular mechanism by which hyperglycemia produces toxic effects is unknown, but glycation of tissue proteins may be important. Nonenzymatic attachment of glucose to long-lived proteins, lipids, or nucleic acids produces stable Amadori early-glycated products. These undergo a series of additional rearrangements, dehydration, and fragmentation reactions, resulting in stable *advanced glycation end products* (AGEs). A series of distinct biochemical reactions produce multiple heterogeneous AGEs,[373,374] with greater than 20 identified, for example, N-(carboxymethyl)lysine (CML), pentosidine, pyrraline, and glyoxal lysine dimer. The amounts of these products do not return to normal when hyperglycemia is corrected, and they accumulate continuously over the lifespan of the protein. Hyperglycemia accelerates the formation of protein-bound AGE, and patients with diabetes mellitus thus have more AGE than healthy subjects. Through effects on the functional properties of protein and extracellular matrix, AGE may contribute to the microvascular and macrovascular complications of diabetes mellitus.[201,375] There is evidence that AGE in the diet contributes to AGE accumulation in tissues.

Measurement of AGEs in the circulation has also been used as a biomarker to monitor the complications of diabetes.[373] However, the diverse structures and composition of AGEs has resulted in assay difficulties. Analysis by ELISA has lacked standardization, yielding variable results.[376] The development of stable isotope dilution analysis liquid chromatography-tandem mass spectrometry, in conjunction with careful pre-analytic sample preparation, shows potential to resolve these problems.[374] However, this approach requires expensive, specialized equipment and the lack of isotope-labeled standards precludes assay standardization.[369] Some AGE products fluoresce, which forms the basis of noninvasive measurement of skin autofluorescence with a portable reader. Some studies have revealed a positive association of skin autofluorescence with complications of diabetes,[377] but adjustment for HbA$_{1c}$ rendered associations nonsignificant.[378] Limitations of skin autofluorescence measurements include lack of specificity for AGE and most AGEs are not fluorescent.[374]

Some of the family of heterogeneous AGEs can activate the receptor for AGE (RAGE) to induce intracellular signaling that leads to enhanced oxidative stress and the production of proinflammatory cytokines.[373,375] RAGE is a member of the immunoglobulin superfamily and is expressed on the surface of several cells, including endothelial and kidney. A truncated form of RAGE, termed soluble RAGE (sRAGE), is produced mainly by proteolysis of RAGE and is found in serum.[373] An ELISA is commercially available to measure sRAGE. However, the relationship between sRAGE concentrations and adverse outcomes in diabetes is contentious, with some published studies claiming increased sRAGE,[379] while others observe decreased sRAGE.[369,380] Further studies are required to clarify the association between sRAGE and health outcomes.

Promising findings have been obtained in studies of recombinant sRAGE in animals, suggesting this may be a therapeutic approach in humans. Similarly, inhibitors of AGE formation, such as aminoguanidine, have been shown to prevent several of the complications of diabetes in experimental animal models. While initial clinical trials in patients failed to show a significant benefit of anti-AGE therapy, this continues to be an area of active research.[373]

1,5-ANHYDROGLUCITOL

Another marker of long-term glycemia is 1,5-anhydroglucitol (1,5-AG), which reflects glucose concentrations over the preceding 2 to 14 days.[381,382] It is a 1-deoxy form of glucose that originates predominantly from the diet, with the vast majority (>99.9%) normally being reabsorbed from the glomerular filtrate by the SGLT4 SGLT. When blood glucose concentrations exceed the renal threshold (usually ~180 mg/dL [~10.0 mmol/L]), reabsorption of 1,5-AG decreases, leading to a rapid reduction in serum 1,5-AG concentrations. Therefore low 1,5-AG indicates hyperglycemia, correlating particularly with postprandial blood glucose concentration.[382] An automated assay is commercially available (and FDA-approved for use in the United States) (GlycoMark, Nippon Kayaku, Tokyo, Japan). The two-step colorimetric assay uses glucokinase initially to convert all the glucose in the sample to glucose 6-phosphate, to prevent it from interfering in the second step. Then, pyranose oxidase oxidizes the C-2 hydroxyl group of 1,5-AG, generating hydrogen peroxide, which is detected by colorimetry using peroxidase. The reference interval is 10.7 to 32.0 µg/mL (males) and 6.8 to 29.3 µg/mL (females). Blacks have higher 1,5-AG than whites.[355] Several factors unrelated to glycemia may alter 1,5-AG values, including diet, medications, renal disease, and liver disease.[382] Importantly, SGLT2 inhibitors, which are now used to treat type 2 diabetes, spuriously alter 1,5-AG concentrations as they increase glycosuria. A recent study found a significant association between low 1,5-AG concentrations and the risk of retinopathy and chronic kidney disease in patients with diabetes.[383] Nevertheless, there is limited evidence linking it to outcomes and the clinical value of measuring 1,5-AG remains to be established.

ALBUMINURIA

Clinical Significance

Patients with diabetes mellitus are at high risk of developing renal damage. End-stage renal disease requiring dialysis or transplantation develops in approximately one third of patients with type 1 diabetes,[384] and diabetes is the most common cause of end-stage renal disease in the United States and Europe.[385] Although nephropathy is less common in patients with type 2 diabetes, approximately 60% of all cases of diabetic nephropathy occur in these patients because of the considerably higher incidence of this form of diabetes. Early detection of diabetic nephropathy relies on tests of urine excretion of albumin. Persistent proteinuria detectable by routine screening tests (equivalent to a urine albumin excretion rate [AER] >200 μg/min or >300 mg/24 hours) indicates overt diabetic nephropathy. This is usually associated with long-standing disease and is unusual less than 5 years after the onset of type 1 diabetes. Once diabetic nephropathy occurs, renal function deteriorates rapidly and renal insufficiency evolves. Treatment at this stage can retard the rate of progression without stopping or reversing the renal damage. Preceding this stage is a period of increased AER not detected by routine dipstick methods. This range of 20 to 200 μg/min (or 30 to 300 mg/24 hours) of increased AER has been called microalbuminuria.[c] Note that it is not defined purely in terms of urine albumin concentration, although the ratio of the urine albumin concentration to the urine creatinine concentration (albumin-to-creatinine ratio [ACR]) in an untimed urine specimen can be used as a substitute for albumin measurements in a timed collection of urine, as described later. The term "microalbuminuria," although widely used, is misleading. It implies a small version of the albumin molecule rather than an excretion rate of albumin greater than normal but less than that detectable by routine methods. Use of the term is discouraged.[386]

The presence of increased AER denotes an increase in the transcapillary escape rate of albumin and, therefore is a marker of microvascular disease. Persistent AER greater than 20 μg/min represents a 20-fold greater risk for the development of clinically overt renal disease in patients with type 1 and type 2 diabetes. Prospective studies have demonstrated that increased urine albumin excretion precedes and is highly predictive of diabetic nephropathy, end-stage renal disease, cardiovascular mortality, and total mortality in patients with diabetes mellitus.[385,387] The DCCT and the UKPDS showed that intensive diabetes therapy can significantly reduce the risk of development of increased AER and overt nephropathy in individuals with diabetes.[199,200] In addition, increased AER identifies a group of nondiabetic subjects at increased risk for

coronary artery disease.[84,388] Interventions, such as control of blood glucose concentrations and blood pressure, particularly with angiotensin-converting enzyme (ACE) inhibitors, slow the rate of decline in renal function.[385]

Methods for Measuring Albuminuria

There are several methods for collecting a urine sample for measuring albumin. Variations in urine flow rate in a person may be corrected by expressing albumin as a ratio to creatinine (i.e., ACR). AER is increased transiently by physiologic and other factors (e.g., exercise within 24 hours, posture, diuresis), infection, fever, marked hyperglycemia, and sustained hypertension. Samples should not be collected after exertion, in the presence of urinary tract infection, during acute illness, immediately after surgery, or after an acute fluid load. All the following urine samples are currently acceptable: 24 hours collection; overnight (8 to 12 hours, timed) collection; 1 to 2 hours timed collection (in laboratory or clinic); and first morning sample for simultaneous albumin and creatinine measurement. Only results for timed specimens can be reported as mg albumin excreted per hour, but the AER is more practical and convenient for the patient and is the recommended method.[48] A first morning void sample is best because it has lower within-person variation for the albumin-to-creatinine ratio than a random urine sample[48,389]; this is the recommended sample. At least three separate specimens, collected on different days, should be assayed because of high intraindividual variation (CV of 30 to 50%) and diurnal variation (50 to 100% higher during the day). The ACR in the first morning void sample has a within-person CV of 31%.[390] Urine should be stored at 4 °C after collection. Alternatively, 2 mL of 50 g/L sodium azide can be added per 500 mL of urine, but preservatives are not recommended for some assays. Bacterial contamination and glucose have no effect. Specimens are stable in untreated urine for at least a week at 4 or −20 °C and for at least 5 months at −80 °C. Freezing samples has been reported to decrease albumin,[391] but mixing immediately before assay eliminates this effect. Neither centrifugation nor filtration is necessary before storage at −20 or −80 °C. The albumin concentration decreases by 0.27%/day at −20 °C.[48]

Screening tests should be positive in greater than 95% of patients with albuminuria.[48] Patients who screen positive should have quantitative measurement of urine albumin in an accredited laboratory.[48] The analytical CV of methods to measure albuminuria should be less than 15%.[48] Most quantitative assays achieve this target.[48] An estimated glomerular filtration rate (eGFR) should also be calculated from serum creatinine in patients who have a positive screening test. Serum creatinine and eGFR should be performed at least annually in all adults with diabetes as some patients have decreased GFR without albuminuria.[32]

Semiquantitative Assays

Several semiquantitative assays are available for screening for albuminuria. These test strips, most of which are optimized to read "positive" at a predetermined albumin concentration, have been recommended for screening programs. In view of the wide variability in AER, it must be borne in mind that a "normal" value does not rule out renal disease. Because these assays measure albumin concentration, dilute urine may yield a false negative test result. Refrigerated urine samples should be allowed to reach at least 10 °C before analysis.

---

[c]Current nomenclature has eliminated the terms "microalbuminuria" and "macroalbuminuria."

Chemstrip Micral (Roche Diagnostics Indianapolis, IN) uses a monoclonal anti-albumin IgG labeled with colloidal gold. The albumin in the urine binds to the antibody-gold conjugate in a zone on the test strip. Excess conjugate is retained in a separation zone containing immobilized human albumin, and only albumin bound to the antibody–enzyme immunocomplex diffuses to the reaction zone. The test strip is dipped into the urine for five seconds, and the intensity of the color after one minute is proportional to the urine albumin concentration. Direct visual comparison is made with printed color blocks, with 0, 20, 50, and 100 mg/L. No interference is observed with drugs (except oxytetracycline), glucose, urea, or other proteins. Urine samples with albumin concentrations greater than 100 to 300 mg/L may be diluted and reassayed. The assigned concentration of the color block is multiplied by the dilution factor to obtain the concentration in the sample. These semiquantitative assays have been recommended for screening only.

A number of strips that measured only albumin, for example, Microbumintest, AlbuScreen, and AlbuSure, are no longer commercially available; some have been replaced by point-of-care tests that measure both albumin and creatinine, and report an ACR. Clinitek Microalbumin (Siemens Healthineers, Deerfield, IL) measures albumin by dye-binding with bromophenol blue and creatinine with an enzyme assay using peroxidase. The strips are read in a reflectance meter. Results are reported as less than 30, 30 to 300, or greater than 300 mg/g (<3.4, 3.4 to 33.9, or >33.9 mg/mmol). Hemoglobin, myoglobin, contamination of the urine (e.g., with soaps, detergents, antiseptics or skin cleansers), and certain drugs (e.g., cimetidine, pyridium, or nitrofurantoin) may interfere. The assay is stated to detect albumin and creatinine at concentrations of 20 to 40 and 10 mg/dL (0.9 mmol/L), respectively. Aution (Arkray, Kyoto, Japan) also uses a small reflectometer to measure albumin and creatinine on a test strip.[392] Automated readers are more accurate than manual visual assessment of reagent strips.

Currently available dipstick tests do not have adequate analytical sensitivity to detect albuminuria.[48] This conclusion was confirmed in a recent systematic review of the diagnostic accuracy of point-of-care tests for detecting albuminuria.[393] The authors observed that results of individual studies vary widely, with sensitivities ranging from 18 to 92.9% and specificities of 60 to 100%. Pooling data yielded a sensitivity of 76% and specificity of 93% for semiquantitative tests.[393] The negative likelihood ratio was 0.26, indicating that a negative test does not rule out albuminuria.

Quantitative Assays

All sensitive, specific assays for urine albumin use immunochemistry with antibodies to human albumin. Four methods are available: RIA, ELISA, radial immunodiffusion, and immunoturbidimetry.[394] Each method has advantages and disadvantages. The immunoturbidimetric assay is the most reliable and should be considered the standard for comparison.[48] Detection limits range from 16 µg/L for RIA to 2 to 5 mg/L for the other methods.[48] Although dye-binding[395] and protein precipitation[396] assays have been described, these are insensitive and nonspecific and should not be used. The international standard reference material for serum albumin measurement was adopted as the standard reference material for urine albumin measurement.[397] The sensitivity and specificity for detecting albuminuria are 96 and 98%, respectively.[393] The negative likelihood ratio of 0.04 meets performance standards,[48] and quantitative assays can be used to exclude albuminuria.

Radial immunodiffusion. Radial immunodiffusion has not gained wide acceptance because it requires long incubation and a high level of technical skill and cannot be automated. The antibody is incorporated into an agar gel. Aliquots of samples and calibrators are added to wells and are allowed to diffuse into the agar. The antigen-antibody complexes precipitate at equilibrium, and after staining, the distance of migration is measured.

Radioimmunoassay. Standard RIA methods have been described[398] with ^{125}I-labeled albumin and anti-albumin antiserum, but reagents are radioactive and have a short shelf life. Commercial kits are available.

Enzyme-linked immunosorbent assay. Both competitive and "sandwich" ELISAs are available.[399,400] Although the competitive ELISA is faster because it uses only one incubation with an antibody, it is reported to be less sensitive and exhibits large imprecision. ELISA can be performed on a microplate reader, allowing semiautomation. In the sandwich assay, the primary antibody (anti-albumin antiserum) is fixed on the plastic plate, which is then washed. Samples, controls, and calibrators are added, and the complexes are detected and quantified by a second antibody conjugated to an enzyme label.

Immunoturbidimetry. Albumin in the urine sample forms an insoluble complex with antibodies to human albumin. PEG accelerates complex formation. The turbidity caused by these complexes is measured by a spectrophotometer at 340 or 531 nm and is a measure of albumin concentration. The background absorbance of the initial urine sample is subtracted automatically. This method is simple and less expensive than RIA, and rapid analysis of large numbers of samples is possible. Assays may be performed as kinetic or equilibrium reactions. Kits are commercially available for use with automated analyzers (Roche Diagnostics, Siemens). A point-of-care device that uses a cartridge which measures albumin and creatinine, and reports an ACR, is commercially available (DCA Vantage, Siemens).

Reference Intervals

		ALBUMINURIA		
		mg/day	mg/g creatinine	mg/mmol creatinine
Normal		<10	<10	<1
Mildly increased (mild)		10–29	10–29	1.0–2.9
Normal to mildly increased (normal to mild)	A1	<30	<30	<3
Moderately increased (moderate)	A2	30–300	30–300	3–30
Severely increased (severe)	A3	>300	>300	>30

The ADA position statement[20] recommends initial albuminuria measurement in patients with type 1 diabetes who have had diabetes for 5 years or longer, and in all type 2 diabetes patients. Because of the difficulty involved in dating the onset of type 2 diabetes, screening should commence at diagnosis. Analysis should be performed annually in all patients who have a negative screening result. Screening may be performed with a semiquantitative assay. If the screening result is positive, albuminuria should be evaluated by a quantitative assay.[48] Diagnosis requires the demonstration of albuminuria in at least two of three samples measured within a 3- to 6-month period.

If the confirmatory test result is positive, treatment with an ACE inhibitor or an angiotensin-receptor blocker should be initiated. ACE inhibitors delay progression to overt nephropathy, and the National Kidney Foundation recommends their use in both normotensive and hypertensive type 1 and 2 diabetic patients.[401] The role of monitoring albuminuria in patients on ACE inhibitor therapy is less clear, although many experts recommend continued surveillance.[20] Untreated, the albuminuria would increase by 10 to 30% per year, whereas the albumin-to-creatinine ratio in patients on ACE inhibitors should stabilize or decrease by up to 50%.

The mean value for AER (5 to 10 mg/day) in young healthy adults generally increases with age.[386] Several factors are associated with a higher AER. These include large body size, upright posture, pregnancy, exercise, fever, and activation of the renin-angiotensin system.[386] Diurnal and day-to-day variation are large. Urine ACR in untimed spot urine correlates well with AER in timed specimens.[48,402] An early morning sample is optimal as it has lower within-person variation.[48] Subjects should be fasting. Clinical laboratories should measure creatinine when urine albumin (or total protein) is requested and express the results as ACR (or protein to creatinine ratio) in addition to total albumin (or protein) concentration.[386]

POINTS TO REMEMBER

HbA1c
- Glycated hemoglobin is formed by nonenzymatic attachment of glucose to hemoglobin.
- HbA_{1c} has glucose attached to the N-terminal Val of the beta chain of hemoglobin.
- The concentration of HbA_{1c} depends on the concentration of glucose in the blood and the erythrocyte lifespan.
- The average erythrocyte lifespan is 120 days, and HbA_{1c} therefore reflects the average blood glucose concentration over the preceding 8–12 weeks.
- Any condition that substantially changes erythrocyte lifespan will alter HbA_{1c}.
- HbA_{1c} is used to diagnose diabetes, monitor glycemic control, evaluate the need to change therapy, and predict the development of microvascular complications.

POINTS TO REMEMBER

Glucose
- Hyperglycemia results from defects in insulin secretion and/or insulin action.
- Blood glucose homeostasis is regulated by several hormones, including insulin, glucagon, epinephrine, and cortisol.
- Blood glucose concentrations fluctuate widely during the day, depending on food ingestion, exercise, and other factors (e.g., stress).
- Self-monitoring of blood glucose using portable meters in patients with diabetes who require insulin has been shown to improve patient outcomes.
- Self-monitoring of blood glucose in non–insulin-treated patients is not yet proven to be effective.
- The use of continuous glucose monitoring systems (CGMS), which use subcutaneously implanted glucose sensors, by type 1 diabetes patients is increasing considerably.

POINTS TO REMEMBER

Type 2 Diabetes
- Type 2 diabetes is the most common form of diabetes, accounting for ~90% of all cases.
- The onset is insidious and patients have minimal symptoms.
- Many patients have irreversible complications at the time of diagnosis.
- Patients exhibit both insulin resistance and inadequate insulin secretion.
- Insulin resistance is very difficult to measure and at diagnosis patient may have normal, increased, or decreased insulin concentrations.
- The molecular defects are a consequence of both genetic and environmental factors.
- The gene (or genes) that cause the common forms of type 2 diabetes have not been identified.
- Obesity is linked to the development of type 2 diabetes, and lifestyle changes (weight loss and exercise) can delay the onset of the disease.

AT A GLANCE

Diagnosis of Diabetes

Diabetes is diagnosed if at least one of the following criteria is met:

- Fasting plasma glucose (FPG) ≥126 mg/dL (7.0 mmol/L)
- 2-h plasma glucose ≥200 mg/dL (11.1 mmol/L) during an oral glucose tolerance test
- HbA$_{1c}$ ≥6.5% (48 mmol/mol)

In the absence of unequivocal hyperglycemia, diagnosis requires two abnormal test results from the same sample or in two separate test samples.

In individuals with classic symptoms of hyperglycemia, diabetes can be diagnosed if random plasma glucose ≥200 mg/dL (11.1 mmol/L); repeating the assay is unnecessary in symptomatic individuals.

Glucose should be measured in venous plasma.

Glycolysis should be minimized by placing the tube immediately after collection in an ice-water slurry and separating plasma from cells within 30 minutes. If that cannot be achieved, blood should be collected in a tube containing a rapidly effective glycolysis inhibitor, for example, citrate buffer.

Plasma glucose and HbA$_{1c}$ should be measured in an accredited laboratory; point-of-care devices are not suitable for screening or diagnosis.

HbA$_{1c}$ analysis should be performed using a method that is NGSP-certified and standardized to the DCCT assay.

SELECTED REFERENCES

4. International Diabetes Federation. IDsF diabetes atlas. 9th ed. Brussels, Belgium: International Diabetes Federation; 2019.

20. American Diabetes Association. 2. Classification and Diagnosis of Diabetes: Standards of Medical Care in Diabetes—2020. Diabetes Care 2020;43:S14–31.

48. Sacks DB, Arnold M, Bakris GL, et al. Guidelines and recommendations for laboratory analysis in the diagnosis and management of diabetes mellitus. Clin Chem 2011;57:e1–47.

112. Atkinson MA, Eisenbarth GS, Michels AW. Type 1 diabetes. Lancet 2014;383:69–82.

133. Warshauer JT, Bluestone JA, Anderson MS. New Frontiers in the treatment of type 1 diabetes. Cell Metab 2020;31:46–61.

147. DeFronzo RA, Ferrannini E, Groop L, et al. Type 2 diabetes mellitus. Nat Rev Dis Primers 2015;1:15019.

176. Sacks DB. A1C versus glucose testing: a comparison. Diabetes Care 2011;34:518–23.

187. Metzger BE, Lowe LP, Dyer AR, et al. Hyperglycemia and adverse pregnancy outcomes. N Engl J Med 2008;358:1991–2002.

199. Diabetes Control and Complications Trial Research Group. The effect of intensive treatment of diabetes on the development and progression of long-term complications in insulin-dependent diabetes mellitus. N Engl J Med 1993;329:977–86.

200. U.K. Prospective Diabetes Study (UKPDS) Group. Intensive blood-glucose control with sulphonylureas or insulin compared with conventional treatment and risk of complications in patients with type 2 diabetes (UKPDS 33). UK Prospective Diabetes Study (UKPDS) Group. Lancet 1998;352:837–53.

203. Rask-Madsen C, King GL. Vascular complications of diabetes: mechanisms of injury and protective factors. Cell Metab 2013;17:20–33.

217. Umpierrez G, Korytkowski M. Diabetic emergencies - ketoacidosis, hyperglycaemic hyperosmolar state and hypoglycemias. Nat Rev Endocrinol 2016;12:222–32.

233. van den Berghe G, Wouters P, Weekers F, et al. Intensive insulin therapy in the critically ill patients. N Engl J Med 2001;345:1359–67.

236. Scott MG, Bruns DE, Boyd JC, Sacks DB. Tight glucose control in the intensive care unit: are glucose meters up to the task? Clin Chem 2009;55:18–20.

244. Klonoff DC, Parkes JL, Kovatchev BP, et al. Investigation of the accuracy of 18 marketed blood glucose monitors. Diabetes Care 2018;41:1681–8.

257. Beck RW, Bergenstal RM, Laffel LM, Pickup JC. Advances in technology for management of type 1 diabetes. Lancet 2019;394:1265–73.

290. Bry L, Chen PC, Sacks DB. Effects of hemoglobin variants and chemically modified derivatives on assays for glycohemoglobin [Review]. Clin Chem 2001;47:153–63.

303. Little RR, Rohlfing C, Sacks DB. The National Glycohemoglobin Standardization Program: over 20 years of improving hemoglobin A1c measurement. Clin Chem 2019;65:839–48.

369. Welsh KJ, Kirkman MS, Sacks DB. Role of glycated proteins in the diagnosis and management of diabetes: research gaps and future directions. Diabetes Care 2016;39:1299–306.

397. Miller WG, Bruns DE, Hortin GL, et al. Current issues in measurement and reporting of urinary albumin excretion. Clin Chem 2009;55:24–38.

48

Cardiac Function

Fred S. Apple, Peter A. Kavsak, and Allan Stanley Jaffe

ABSTRACT

Background

Increases in cardiac biomarkers of myocardial injury and particularly cardiac troponin (cTn), in the absence of analytical confounders, define the presence of myocardial injury which in the proper clinical situation can lead to the diagnosis of acute myocardial infarction (AMI). Other biomarkers such as natriuretic peptides (NPs) facilitate the diagnosis and/or exclusion of heart failure (HF). These and other important biomarkers improve patient management by leading to an earlier diagnosis, facilitating triage, helping to define treatments, and allowing for an expedited assessment of short- and long-term outcomes. Not only is patient care enhanced but with proper use, costs are constrained.

Content

Concepts and definitions of myocardial anatomy and physiology of the heart are briefly described, along with structural changes that occur during the onset and progression of heart disease. Analytical and biochemical characteristics of cardiac troponin I (TnI), cardiac troponin T (TnT), b type natriuretic peptide (BNP), and the NTproBNP fragment (NT-proBNP) and the assays used to measure them are discussed. The clinical use of cTn is discussed in helping to diagnose and rapidly exclude AMI. Modern-day high-sensitivity assays can also aid in both primary and secondary prevention. Outcome studies are reviewed to demonstrate the role of cTn in risk stratification and appropriate selection of treatments. The clinical role of BNP/NT-proBNP in diagnosing acute and chronic HF, their emerging role in predicting the development of HF, and their use in distinguishing dyspnea of a pulmonary origin from that due to myocardial dysfunction are highlighted. The use of NP assays in defining prognosis and identifying possible treatment options is addressed. Finally, novel biomarkers for detecting myocardial injury, hemodynamic stress, inflammation, plaque rupture, and ischemia are discussed.

Although the heart is an efficient and durable pump, a variety of pathologic processes are known to diminish cardiac function, leading to a multiplicity of dysfunctional clinical states, some subtle and incipient and some overt. Acute ischemic heart disease, mostly AMI, is the most common cardiac disease. Advances in treatment over the years have blunted the extent of damage done during an MI and thus its negative impact on mortality. This and the increasing longevity in developed nations such as the United States are in part responsible for an increase in the frequency of the heart failure (HF) syndrome.[1] Other processes can also lead to HF and often are associated with abnormal biomarkers.

The term acute myocardial infarction (AMI) refers to a situation in which death of myocytes is due to an imbalance between myocardial oxygen supply and demand.[2] When the blood supply to the heart is interrupted, first apoptosis and then necrosis of the myocardium results. Such extensive damage is most often associated with a thrombotic occlusion superimposed on coronary atherosclerosis. Initially, it was thought that the population of myocytes was fixed; however, it is now believed that the migration of a variety of precursor stem cells has the potential at least to replace some of the damaged myocytes although the mechanisms for these effects are controversial.[3,4] It is now thought that the process of plaque rupture or erosion and thrombosis is one of the ways in which coronary atherosclerosis progresses, and that we recognize only more severe events.[5,6] Total loss of coronary blood flow results in a clinical syndrome associated with what is known as ST segment elevation AMI (STE AMI).[2] Partial loss of coronary perfusion, if severe, can lead to necrosis as well, which is generally less severe and is known as non–ST elevation myocardial infarction (NSTEMI).[2] Other events of still lesser severity may be missed entirely or may be called angina, which can range from stable to unstable. With the increasing sensitivity of cardiac troponin (cTn) measurements, the frequency of unstable angina (UA) is disappearing and smaller NSTEMIs are being diagnosed more frequently, but UA is not totally gone.[7,8]

Key facts about cardiovascular disease.[1]

1. The age-adjusted death rate attributable to cardiovascular disease (CVD) in the United States, based on 2017 data, is 219.4 per 100,000.
2. On average, someone dies of CVD (AMI, stroke, HF, etc.) every 37 seconds in the US. There are 2353 deaths from CVD each day, based on 2017 data.
3. On average, someone dies of a stroke every 3.59 minutes in the United States. There are about 401 deaths from stroke each day, based on 2017 data.

4. CVD deaths have increased from 2303 each day in 2016. Stroke deaths increased from 389.4 per day in 2016.
5. A total of 116.4 million, or 46% of US adults have hypertension, based on 2013 to 2016 data.
6. Only 1 in 4 adults, or 24.3% of US adults, reported achieving adequate leisure-time aerobic and muscle-strengthening activities to meet the physical activity guidelines, based on 2017 data.
7. One in six males and one in eight females in the United States are current smokers, based on 2017 data.
8. By 2035, 45.1% of the US population is projected to have some form of CVD. Total costs of CVD are expected to reach $1.1 trillion in 2035, with direct medical costs projected to reach $748.7 billion and indirect costs estimated to reach $368 billion.

Coronary heart disease causes over 25% of all deaths in the United States. Historically, most deaths caused by ischemic heart disease were acute, but as our therapeutic abilities have increased, the disease is becoming more chronic. Deaths that occur acutely result from ventricular arrhythmias or pump dysfunction and congestive heart failure (CHF) with or without cardiogenic shock. Death rates increase sharply with age, both during hospitalization and in the year after infarction.[1]

Before the advent of coronary care units, treatment of AMI was directed toward allowing healing of the infarcted area. The concept that infarctions evolve over time and that their size can be moderated led to rethinking of this passive philosophy.[9] We now know that reestablishment of perfusion reduces the extent of myocardial injury and is an important determinant of prognosis.[10] Today the management of AMI suggested by most guidelines is aggressive and invasively oriented in the hope of reducing the extent of myocardial damage and thus improving prognosis.[10,11] In addition, prevention is finally being recognized as a key element in the long-term treatment of patients with atherosclerosis. Recently, different types of MI have been recognized. Those not related to acute plaque rupture events particularly deserve consideration and they less often require invasive management.[2,11]

BASIC ANATOMY

The average human adult heart weighs approximately 325 g in men and 275 g in women and is 12 cm in length. The heart is a hollow muscular organ, shaped like a blunt cone, and is approximately the size of a human fist. It is located in the mediastinum, between the lower lobes of each lung, and rests on the diaphragm. It is enclosed in a sac called the pericardium. The cardiac wall is composed of three layers: the epicardium, which is the outermost layer; a middle layer; and an inner layer, called the endocardium. The heart has four chambers. The two upper chambers are termed the right and left atria, and the two lower chambers are termed the right and left ventricles (Fig. 48.1). Under normal circumstances, the atria are compliant structures, so that intracavitary pressure is low. When anatomy is normal, each atrium is connected to its ventricle through an atrioventricular (AV) valve, which opens and closes (see discussion later in this chapter). The valve on the left side is called the mitral valve and the one on the right side, the tricuspid valve. The right ventricle is banana shaped and pumps blood into the pulmonary artery through a trileaflet pulmonic valve. The left ventricle pumps blood into the aorta through a trileaflet aortic valve. The ventricles, especially the left ventricle, are thicker and less compliant in keeping with the need to generate higher pressures than the right ventricle, and intercavitary pressures are much higher than in the atria. Under normal conditions, the conduction or electrical system of the heart coordinates the sequential contraction of first the atria and then the ventricles. Given that they are connected, each side can affect the other. This sequence of activation optimizes the interaction and thus the efficiency of cardiac function.

The right and left coronary arteries originate from two of three cusps of the aortic valve. They provide blood flow and thus nutritive perfusion to the heart. The largest vessels are on the epicardium, and these can be accessed therapeutically fairly easily. Subsequent smaller branches divide to supply the remaining myocardium. The endocardium is the layer most susceptible to ischemia because its perfusion relies on the smallest vessels.

The myocardium contains bundles of striated muscle fibers, each of which is typically 10 to 15 mm in diameter and 30 to 60 mm in length. The work of the heart is generated by the alternating contraction and relaxation of these fibers. The fibers are composed of the cardiac-specific contractile proteins actin and myosin and regulatory proteins called troponins. They also contain a variety of enzymes and proteins that are vital for energy use, such as myoglobin, creatine kinase (CK), and lactate dehydrogenase (LD), some of which can be used as markers of cardiac injury.[2]

PHYSIOLOGY

Cardiac Cycle

A typical cardiac cycle consists of two intervals known as systole and diastole (Fig. 48.2). During diastole, oxygenated blood returns from the lungs to the left atrium via the pulmonary veins and deoxygenated blood returns from other parts of the body to fill the right atrium. During this period, the AV valves are open, allowing passive filling of the ventricle. At the end of diastole, the atria contract, forcing additional blood through the AV valves and into the respective ventricles. During systole, the ventricles contract. This closes the AV valves when ventricular pressure exceeds atrial pressure, and the pulmonary and aortic valves are opened when ventricular pressure exceeds pressure in the pulmonary arteries and/or the aorta, and blood flows into those conduits. During systole, a normal blood pressure in the aorta is typically 120 mm Hg; during diastole, it falls to about 70 mm Hg. At rest, the heart pumps between 60 and 80 times/min. Stroke volume (i.e., the amount of blood expelled with each contraction) is roughly 50 mL, so cardiac output per minute is roughly 3 L. Typically, values are corrected for body surface area and are usually in the range of 2.5 to 3.6 L/min/m^2. Measurements of cardiac output and ventricular filling pressures are the standards for assessing cardiac performance and function. Furthermore, therapeutic intervention in patients with heart disease often includes assessment of cardiac output and ventricular pressures.

Cardiac Conducting System

The cardiac cycle is tightly controlled by the cardiac conducting system, which initiates electrical impulses and carries

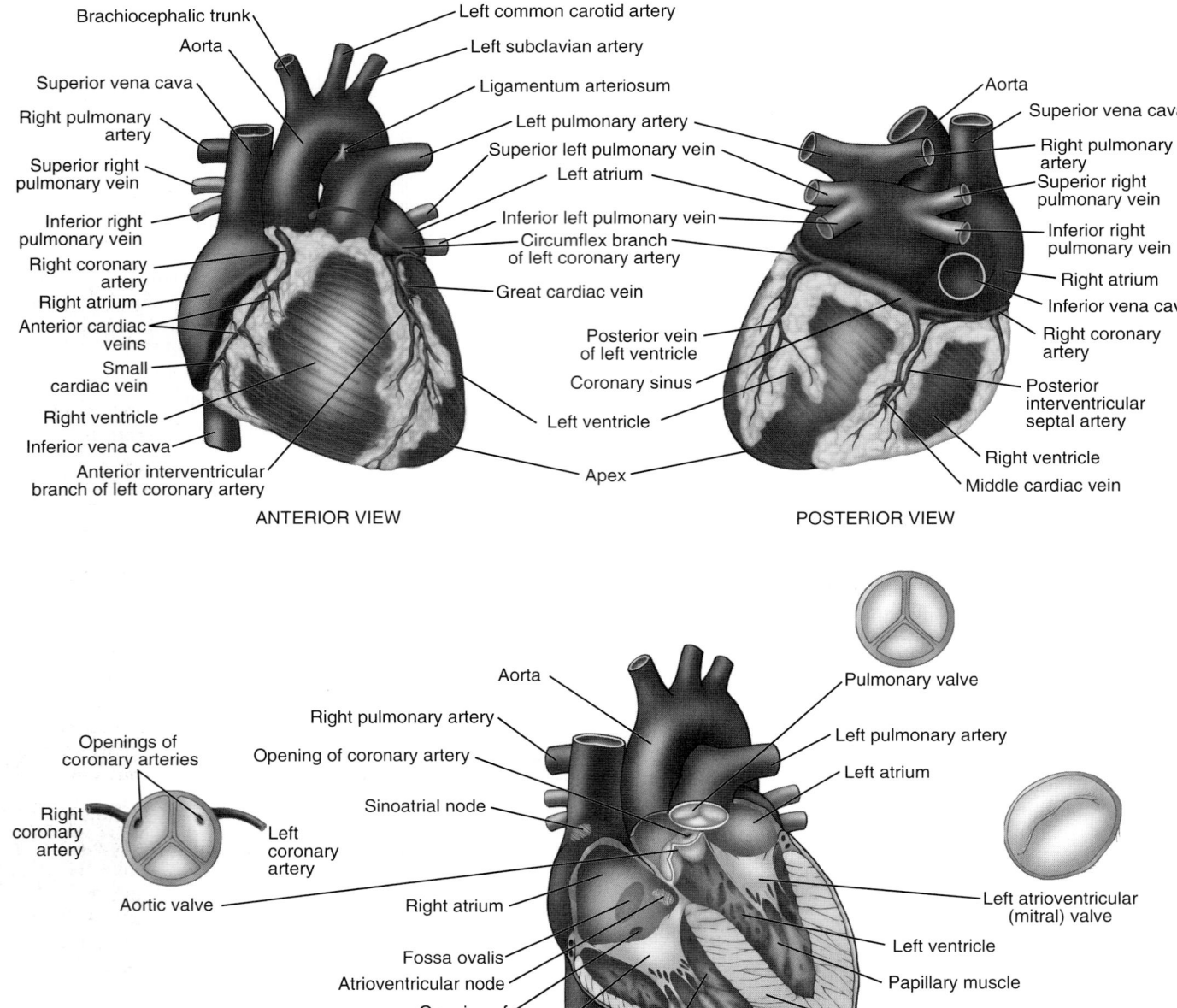

FIGURE 48.1 Anatomy of the heart. (From Elsevier. *Dorland's illustrated medical dictionary.* 32nd ed. Philadelphia: Saunders; 2011, Panel 18.)

them via a specialized conducting system to the myocardium. The surface electrocardiogram (ECG) records changes in potential and is a graphic tracing of the variations in electrical potential caused by excitation of the heart muscle and detected at the body surface.[12] Clinically, the ECG is used to identify (1) anatomic, (2) metabolic, (3) ionic, and (4) hemodynamic changes in the heart. The clinical sensitivity and specificity of ECG abnormalities are influenced by a wide spectrum of physiologic and anatomic changes and by the clinical situation.

Under normal circumstances, cardiac cycles are similar and each includes three major components (Fig. 48.3): atrial depolarization (the P wave), ventricular depolarization (the QRS complex), and repolarization (the ST segment and T wave). Atrial depolarization, which is depicted by the P wave, produces atrial contraction. Ventricular depolarization,

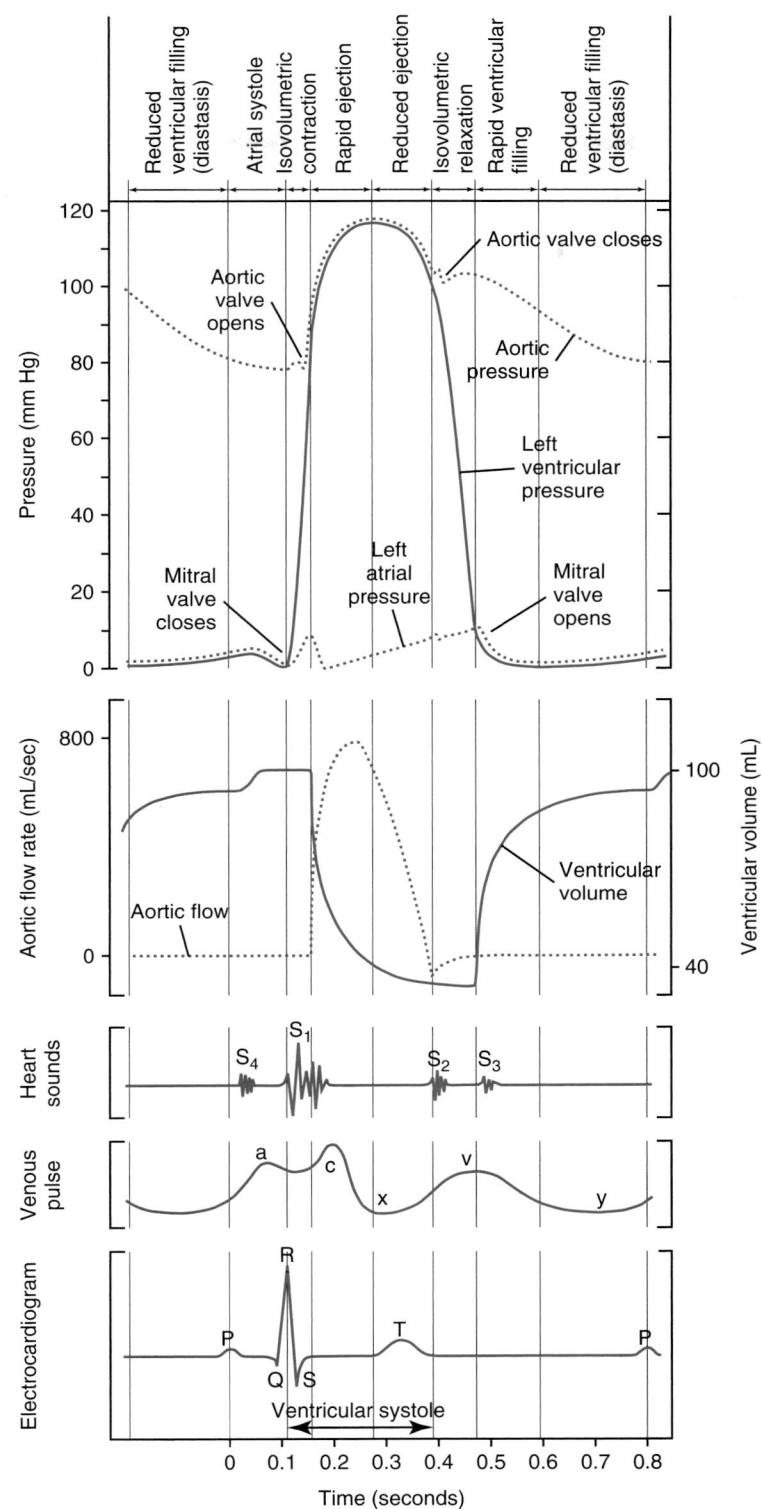

FIGURE 48.2 The cardiac cycle. (From Elsevier. *Dorland's illustrated medical dictionary.* 30th ed. Philadelphia: Saunders, 2003, with permission from the National Kidney Foundation.)

marked by the QRS complex, produces contraction of the ventricles. It is composed of as many as three deflections: (1) the Q wave, which when present is the first negative deflection; (2) the R wave, which is the first positive deflection; and (3) the S wave, which is a negative deflection after the R wave. On occasion, there is an R′, which is a second positive deflection. Whether each of these occurs depends on the path of depolarization of the ventricles, as does the significance. Thus not every QRS complex will have discrete Q, R, and S waves. The ST segment and the T wave are produced by

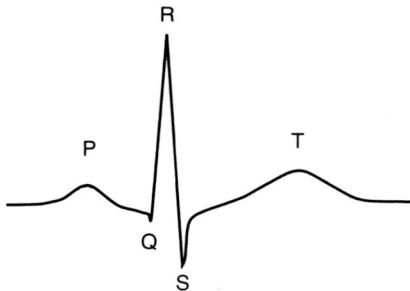

FIGURE 48.3 Electrocardiogram, serial tracing of a normal single heartbeat. Each beat manifests as five major waves: P, Q, R, S, and T. The QRS complex represents the ventricular contraction.

electrical recovery of the ventricles, and their mean electrical vector is under normal circumstances concordant (i.e., in roughly the same direction) with the mean QRS vector.

A routine ECG is composed of 12 leads. Six are called limb leads (I, II, III, aV_R, aV_L, and aV_F) because they are recorded between arm and leg electrodes; six are called precordial or chest leads (V_1, V_2, V_3, V_4, V_5, and V_6) and are recorded across the sternum and left precordium. Each lead records the same electrical impulse but in a different position relative to the heart. Areas of abnormality on the ECG are localized by analyzing differences between the tracing in question and a normal ECG in the 12 different leads.

CARDIAC DISEASE

Cardiac disease occurs in many forms. This chapter briefly covers HF, including CHF and acute coronary syndromes (ACSs), such as AMI. The vast number of other cardiac diseases are not discussed in depth here because of the smaller role of clinical laboratory tests in these disorders.

Congestive Heart Failure

CHF is a syndrome characterized by ineffective pumping of the heart, often leading to an accumulation of fluid in the lungs. At least half comes as a result of the loss of the function of the cardiac tissue and is called heart failure with reduced ejection fraction (HFREF). The other half is due to increased stiffness of the cardiac muscle. This type of HF is referred to as heart failure with preserved ejection fraction or HFPEF.[13] Other forms include those related to valvular heart disease and so-called high-output HF. The condition is one in which there is an abnormality of cardiac function such that the heart cannot pump sufficient blood to satisfy the requirements of metabolizing tissues, which are abnormally high.

Epidemiology

In the United States, CHF is the only CVD with an increasing incidence. The National Heart, Lung, and Blood Institute estimates current prevalence at 4.8 million Americans and 23 million worldwide with CHF.[14] There are approximately 580,000 new cases each year, with approximately 1 million admissions to hospitals for CHF per year.[14] CHF is the leading cause of hospitalization in individuals 65 years of age and older.

Therapeutic options for patients with HFPEF are more limited than for those who have systolic abnormalities.[15,16]

Current prognosis depends on disease severity, but overall it is poor. Mortality at 5 years is approximately 50%, and 10-year mortality is 90%.[14] These poor outcomes are not without substantial cost, estimated at $24 billion per year in the United States.

Currently, CHF patients are staged with the New York Heart Association (NYHA) functional classifications I to IV. Class I patients are generally considered asymptomatic, with no restrictions on physical activity; class IV patients are often symptomatic at rest, with severe limitations on physical activity. The problem with this classification system is that much of it is based on subjective criteria. Thus patients with co-morbidities that reduce their activities are hard to classify. In addition, dyspnea, which is the primary symptom in many of these individuals, has many causes. Finally, many patients with ventricular dysfunction modify their activities to accomplish activities of daily living and thus lack overt symptoms until late in their disease. Therefore patients with CHF often go undiagnosed and untreated early in their disease or are misdiagnosed because of conditions such as pulmonary disease. Initiating treatment in the more advanced disease state (higher degree of irreversible cardiac function and patient deconditioning) is challenging and more expensive (often requiring extended inpatient stay) and leaves patients with considerable morbidity on a daily basis. Obviously, misdiagnoses often lead to patient morbidity. That is the reason why natriuretic peptides (NPs) have been such an important advance in facilitating the diagnosis of HF[17,18] and if used properly help with treatment.[19]

Acute Coronary Syndrome

The term ACS encompasses patients who present with unstable ischemic heart disease.[11] If they have ST segment elevation, their events are called ST elevation myocardial infarctions (STEMI) (Fig. 48.4). Usually, but not always, these individuals develop Q waves on their ECGs, hence the term Q-wave MI. If patients do not have STE but have biochemical criteria for cardiac injury, they are called non-STEMI (NSTEMI), and most do not develop ECG Q waves. Those who have unstable ischemia and do not manifest necrosis are designated patients with UA. Most of these syndromes occur in response to an acute event in the coronary artery, when circulation to a region of the heart is obstructed for some reason. If the obstruction is high grade and persists, necrosis usually ensues. Because necrosis is known to take some time to develop, it is apparent that opening the blocked coronary artery in a timely fashion can often prevent some of the death of myocardial tissue. This is clearly the case with STEMI. With NSTEMI (American Heart Association [AHA]/American College of Cardiology [ACC] guidelines), early but not immediate intervention is advocated, because most often the infarct-related coronary artery is not totally occluded, and thus immediate intervention is less necessary. These syndromes are usually but not always associated with chest discomfort (see discussion later in this chapter).[10,11]

The major cause of ACS is atherosclerosis, which contributes to significant narrowing of the artery lumen and a tendency for plaque disruption and thrombus formation.[2] Myocardial ischemia and infarction are usually segmental diseases. In up to 90% of patients with these diseases, focal occlusion of only one of the three large coronary vessels or branches occurs. The resulting impaired contractile performance of

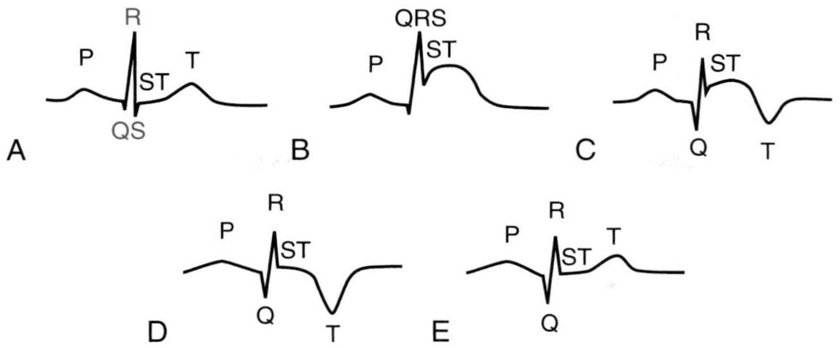

FIGURE 48.4 Electrocardiogram, serial tracing of a patient with an acute myocardial infarction. The sequence is *A*, normal; *B*, hours after infarction, the ST segment becomes elevated; *C*, hours to days later, the T wave inverts and the Q wave becomes larger; *D*, days to weeks later, the ST segment returns to near normal; and *E*, weeks to months later, the T wave becomes upright again, but the large Q wave may remain.

that segment occurs within seconds and is initially restricted to the affected segment(s). Myocardial ischemia and subsequent infarction usually begin in the endocardium and spread toward the epicardium.[19] The extent of myocardial injury reflects (1) the extent of occlusion, (2) the needs of the area deprived of perfusion, and (3) the duration of the imbalance in coronary supply. Irreversible cardiac injury consistently occurs in animals when the occlusion is complete for at least 15 to 20 minutes. Most damage occurs within the first 2 to 3 hours. Restoration of flow within the first 60 to 90 minutes evokes maximal salvage of tissue, but benefits of increased survival are possible up to 4 to 6 hours. In some situations, the restoration of coronary perfusion even later is of benefit.[10,11] The percentage of tissue at risk for necrosis (infarct size) depends on the amount of antegrade flow, the existing collateral flow, which is highly variable and difficult to predict, and the metabolic needs of the tissue.[12]

In almost all instances, the left ventricle is affected by AMI. However, with right coronary and/or circumflex occlusion, the right ventricle also can be involved, and there is a clinical syndrome in which damage to the right ventricle predominates and is the major determinant of hemodynamics. Coronary thrombi will undergo spontaneous lysis, even if untreated, in approximately 50% of cases within 10 days. However, for patients with STEMI, opening the vessel earlier with clot-dissolving agents (thrombolysis) and/or percutaneous intervention (PCI) can often save myocardium and lives. At present, immediate PCI with stenting is the preferred therapy for STEMI. However, many hospitals cannot or do not offer urgent PCI 24 hours per day, 365 days per year. Thus clot-dissolving medications still play a major role in the treatment of these patients. In addition, it is now apparent that urgent but not necessarily immediate invasive revascularization benefits those with NSTEMI.[20] These individuals usually have only partial coronary occlusion and smaller amounts of cardiac damage acutely. However, untreated, repetitive episodes often eventually damage larger amounts of myocardium, leading to increased morbidity and mortality over time. Treatments such as newer anticoagulants and antiplatelet and anti-inflammatory agents, in conjunction with coronary revascularization, save lives in this group.

The prognosis for patients with ischemia but without necrosis is far better. Some studies based on biomarkers would suggest that in patients with no troponin elevation, interventional therapies may be harmful.[21,22] Many of these patients are women who are known to have lower levels of cTn. With high-sensitivity assays, they will require different cutoff values, but the use of such assays will identify more women who are at risk.[23,24] A major determinant of mortality and morbidity is the amount of myocardial damage that occurs. With STEMI, most damage is acute, whereas with NSTEMI, damage may evolve as the result of repetitive events over many months; thus interrupting the process improves survival.

Precipitating Factors
In many patients with AMI, no precipitating factor can be identified. Studies have noted the following patient activities at the onset of AMI: (1) heavy physical exertion, 13%; (2) modest or usual exertion, 18%; (3) surgical procedure, 6%; (4) rest, 51%; and (5) sleep, 8%. Exertion before infarction is somewhat more common among patients without preexisting angina than in those who have a history of angina.[25]

Causes of infarction other than acute atherothrombotic coronary occlusion have been identified. For example, prolonged vasospasm can induce infarction, and spontaneous dissection is becoming more commonly appreciated in women, many of whom have fibromuscular dysplasia.[26] In addition, it is now clear that some patients, particularly women, can have acute infarction with normal-appearing angiographic coronary arteries.[27] Other conditions (Box 48.1) can cause the death of cardiomyocytes, leading to a biochemical signal (such as increased circulating concentrations of cTns) of myocyte damage, but these conditions should not be confused with MI.[2] Pulmonary embolism (PE) is another common cause of biochemical elevations that is secondary to right ventricular damage related to acute increases in wall stress and reduced subendocardial perfusion.[28,29]

Chronobiology
There is a pronounced periodicity for the time of onset of STE AMI.[25,30] Often an AMI occurs in the morning hours soon after rising; this is a period of (1) increasing adrenergic activity, (2) increased plasma fibrinogen levels, (3) increased inhibition of fibrinolysis, and (4) increased platelet adhesiveness. Studies have demonstrated that the early morning peak in MI parallels the peak incidence of death from ischemic heart disease, which occurs at approximately 8 am to 9 am.

A second peak has been noted at approximately 5 pm. Diurnal differences affect many physiologic and biochemical parameters; the early morning hours are associated with rises in plasma catecholamines and cortisol and increases in platelet aggregability. Tissue plasminogen activator (t-PA) activity is low and plasminogen activator inhibitor (PAI) activity is high during the early morning hours. Thus it is possible that some cyclic aspects of combined vasospastic, prothrombotic, and fibrinolytic factors, in the setting of preexisting atherosclerosis, lead to AMI.[25] NSTEMI does not exhibit this diurnal pattern.

Prognosis

STE and non-STE infarctions have distinctly different short-term prognoses. STE AMI is associated with higher early and in-hospital mortality.[10] It is said that mortality associated with STE AMI can occur up to 6 months after the event, but the vast majority (at least two-thirds) occurs during the first 30 or 40 days. It is this risk that coronary recanalization seems to benefit. NSTE AMI is associated with lower acute mortality and complication rates but a longer period of vulnerability to reinfarction and death. As a result, 1- to 2-year survival rates are similar to those for STEMI.[11] This is why intervention has been so effective in this group.

There is an additional subset of patients who have what are known as type 2 MI. Type 1 MI is the typical one due to acute atherothrombotic plaque disruption.[2] Type 2 MI is due to supply-demand imbalance leading to ischemia. Coronary artery disease (CAD) may or may not be present but changes in oxygen demand and, usually concomitantly, myocardial supply can lead to acute ischemia and if severe enough to acute myocardial injury (an increased cTn value with a rising and/or falling pattern). An example might be severe anemia where there is reduced oxygen carrying capacity along with compensatory increases in systemic volume and with these, increased myocardial work. Type 2 MI events can have ST segment elevation, ST segment depression, or even normal ECGs.[31] The prognoses of these patients in terms of mortality and cardiovascular events is at least as adverse as that of those with type 1 events.[31] A similar process can occur with supply-demand imbalance or direct myocardial injury due to circulating toxins such as carbon monoxide which can cause the same pattern of cTn release. However, if ischemia is not present, the proper term for this situation is "acute myocardial injury."[31] Acute myocardial injury can also occur after coronary interventions and cardiac bypass surgery. Criteria for MI exist in both those situations.[2] The key to being able to make the diagnosis is having a normal baseline cTn value.[32]

Clinical History

The clinical history remains of substantial value.[8] A prodromal history of angina is elicited in 40 to 50% of patients with AMI. Among patients with AMI who present with prodromal symptoms, approximately one-third have had symptoms from 1 to 4 weeks before hospitalization; in the remaining two-thirds, symptoms predate admission by a week or less, with one-third of patients having had symptoms for 24 hours or less. In most patients the pain of AMI is severe, but it is rarely intolerable. The pain may be prolonged, lasting up to 30 minutes. The discomfort is described as constricting, crushing, oppressing, or compressing; often the patient complains of something sitting on or squeezing the chest. Although usually described as a squeezing, choking, viselike, or heavy pain, it may be characterized as a stabbing, knifelike, boring, or burning discomfort. The pain is usually retrosternal in location, spreading frequently to both sides of the chest, and favoring the left side. Often the pain radiates down the left arm. Some patients note only a dull ache or numbness in the wrists in association with severe substernal discomfort. In some instances, the pain of AMI may begin in the epigastrium, simulating a variety of abdominal disorders; this often causes MI to be misdiagnosed as indigestion. In other patients, the discomfort of AMI radiates to the shoulders, upper extremities, neck, and jaw, again usually favoring the left side. In patients with preexisting angina, the pain of infarction usually resembles that of the angina pain with respect to features and location. However, it is generally much more severe, lasts longer, and/or is not relieved by rest and nitroglycerin.

Older individuals, patients with diabetes, and women often present atypically. For example, among individuals older than 80 years, less than 50% of those with AMI will have chest discomfort at the time of AMI.[33] Sometimes these patients will present with shortness of breath, fatigue, or even confusion. The pain of AMI may have disappeared by the time a physician first encounters the patient (or the patient reaches the hospital), or it may persist for a few hours.

Myocardial Changes After Acute Myocardial Infarction

Fig. 48.5 shows the temporal sequence of early biochemical, histochemical, and histologic findings after the onset of AMI. On gross pathologic examination, AMI can be divided into subendocardial (nontransmural) infarctions and transmural infarctions.[34] In the former, necrosis involves the endocardium, the intramural myocardium, or both without extending all the way through the ventricular wall to the epicardium. In the latter, myocardial necrosis involves the full thickness of the ventricular wall. The histologic pattern of necrosis may differ: contraction band injury occurs almost twice as often in nontransmural infarctions as in transmural infarctions. Unfortunately, the pathologic changes correlate poorly with clinical, ECG, and biochemical markers of necrosis, which is why those terms are no longer used clinically. Statistically, patients are more apt to have STE MI Q waves on the ECG and larger biochemical signals when the infarction is transmural pathologically.

Ultrastructural (electron microscopic) changes in myocardium. In experimental infarction, the earliest ultrastructural changes in cardiac muscle after occlusion of a coronary artery, noted within 20 minutes by electron microscopy, consists of reduction in the size and number of glycogen granules, intracellular edema, and swelling and distortion of the transverse tubular system, the sarcoplasmic reticulum, and the mitochondria. These early changes are partially reversible. Changes after 60 minutes of occlusion include myocardial cell swelling; mitochondrial abnormalities, such as swelling and internal disruption; development of amorphous, flocculent aggregation and margination of nuclear chromatin; and relaxation of myofibrils. After 20 minutes to 2 hours of ischemia, changes in some cells become irreversible, and progression of these

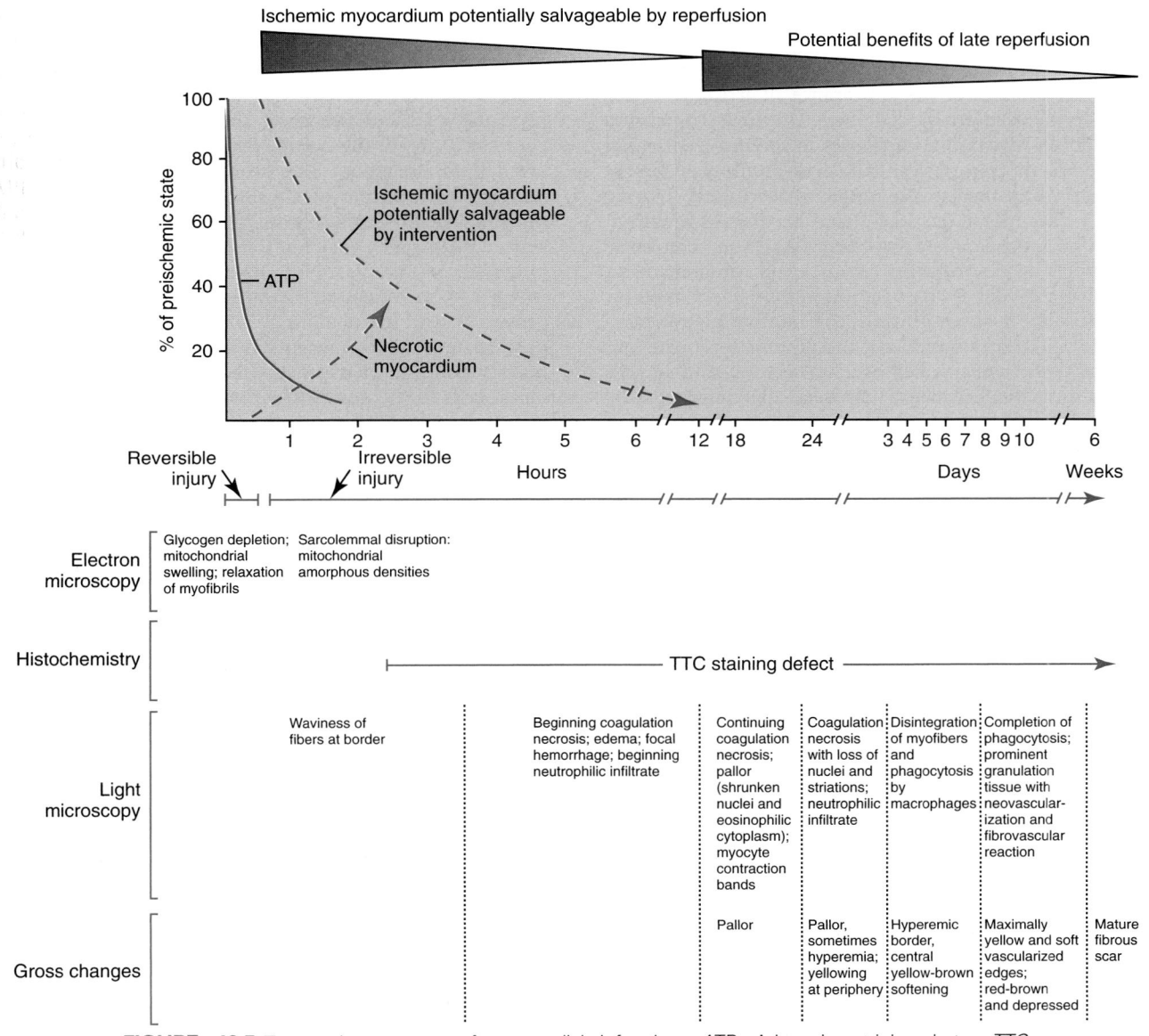

FIGURE 48.5 Temporal sequence of myocardial infarction. *ATP,* Adenosine triphosphate; *TTC,* 2,3,5-triphenyltetrazolium chloride. (From Antman EM, Braunwald E. Acute myocardial infarction. In: Braunwald E, editor. *Heart disease: a textbook of cardiovascular medicine,* 5th ed. Philadelphia: WB Saunders; 1997:1189.)

alterations occurs; additional changes include swollen sacs of the sarcoplasmic reticulum at the level of the A band, greatly enlarged mitochondria with few cristae, thinning and fractionation of myofilaments, disorientation of myofibrils, and clumping of mitochondria. Cells irreversibly damaged by ischemia are usually swollen, with an enlarged sarcoplasmic reticulum. Defects in the plasma membrane may appear, and the mitochondria are fragmented. Many of these changes become more intense when blood flow is restored.

Histologic (light microscopic) changes in myocardium. Although it was previously believed that no light microscopic changes could be seen in infarcted myocardium until 8 hours after interruption of blood flow, in some infarcts a pattern of wavy myocardial fibers may be seen 1 to 3 hours after onset, especially at the periphery of the infarct.[34] After 8 hours, edema of the interstitium becomes evident, as do increased fatty deposits in the muscle fibers, along with infiltration of neutrophilic polymorphonuclear leukocytes and red blood cells.

By 24 hours, clumping of the cytoplasm and loss of cross-striations are seen, with the appearance of irregular cross-bands in the involved myocardial fibers. The nuclei sometimes even disappear. Myocardial capillaries in the involved region dilate, and polymorphonuclear leukocytes accumulate, first at the periphery and then in the center of the infarct. During the first 3 days, the interstitial tissue becomes edematous. Generally, on approximately day 4 after infarction, removal of necrotic fibers by macrophages begins, again commencing at the periphery. By day 8, the necrotic muscle fibers have become dissolved; by about 10 days, the number of polymorphonuclear leukocytes is reduced, and granulation tissue first appears at the periphery. Removal of necrotic muscle cells continues until the fourth to sixth week after infarction, by which time much of the necrotic myocardium has been removed. This process continues, along with increasing collagenization of the infarcted area. By the sixth week, the infarcted area usually has been converted to a firm connective tissue scar with interspersed intact muscle fibers.

Gross changes in myocardium. Gross alterations of the myocardium are difficult to identify until at least 6 to 12 hours after the onset of necrosis.[34] However, several histochemical approaches have been used to identify zones of necrosis that can be observed after only 2 to 3 hours. Initially, the myocardium in the affected region may appear pale and slightly swollen. By 18 to 36 hours after onset of the infarct, the myocardium is tan or reddish purple (because of trapped erythrocytes). These changes persist for approximately 48 hours; the infarct then turns gray, and fine yellow lines, secondary to neutrophilic infiltration, appear at its periphery. This zone gradually widens and during the next few days extends throughout the infarct.

Eight to 10 days after infarction, the thickness of the cardiac wall in the area of the infarct is reduced as necrotic muscle is removed by mononuclear cells. The cut surface of an infarct of this age is yellow and is surrounded by a reddish-purple band of granulation tissue that extends through the necrotic tissue by 3 to 4 weeks. Over the next 2 to 3 months, the infarcted area gradually acquires a gelatinous, gray appearance, eventually converting into a shrunken, thin, firm scar that whitens and firms progressively with time. This process begins at the periphery of the infarct and gradually

moves centrally. In addition, more hemorrhage is seen in the area of damage because of the use of potent thrombolytic and anticoagulant agents.

Development and Progression of Atherosclerosis

Intrinsic to modern-day understanding of ischemic heart disease and to the intense interest in the development of markers of inflammation is the concept that atherosclerosis is a chronic inflammatory disease.[35] The concept is that some event damages the endothelium of blood vessels, which facilitates the egress of lipid into the subendothelial space. Putative injurious stimuli include turbulent flow in a blood vessel, which could occur for example because of hypertension or a noxious metabolite from a lipid fraction. This damage tends to occur at branch points of blood vessels. Regardless of the initial stimulus, once damaged, low-density lipoprotein (LDL) can cross into the vessel wall more easily in a nicotinamide adenine dinucleotide phosphate (NADPH) oxidase–mediated fashion. Whether minimal oxidation facilitates that egress or it occurs once the LDL is within the vessel wall is unclear, but a minimal degree of oxidation once in the vessel wall facilitates the egress of smooth muscle cells from the media of the vessel and macrophages that ingest cholesterol, hence the rationale for the measurement of oxidized lipids in blood. The process of atherosclerosis progresses slowly, with involvement of lymphocytes, monocytes, macrophages, and smooth muscle cells. The dynamic within a given plaque may vary, but there clearly is an inflammatory milieu, in part mediated by substances such as CD40 ligand, which can be measured directly or indirectly as C-reactive protein (CRP). Interleukins (IL)-1, IL-6, IL-8, and IL-18 also participate to various extents as part of this chronic inflammatory process. This process involves adherence of white blood cells to the damaged endothelial surface, with subsequent degranulation and elaboration of myeloperoxidase (MPO). A procoagulant component is due predominantly to the presence of tissue factor, which is localized immediately under the cap of the plaque. Intermittent instability is noted because of inflammatory products within the plaque that release chemicals, such as metalloproteinases. Initially the plaque expands by stretching the adventitia through a process of small ruptures with release of procoagulant and proinflammatory materials and then remodeling over time as anti-inflammatory and anticoagulant and thrombolytic substances are elaborated. This process of stretching the adventitia preserves the lumen such that by the time luminal encroachment occurs, there is a very large plaque burden.[36]

A categorization of plaques has been proposed to facilitate identification of those at risk for rupture that could lead to an acute event. It is acknowledged that the propensity for a plaque to rupture probably reflects a systemic predilection rather than a local one. Thus for a given patient at risk, there likely are many plaques that are metabolically at risk for rupture at any given time.[5,6] High-risk plaques have the following:

1. an active inflammatory environment that not only may be intrinsic but may be stimulated additionally by systemic infection;
2. a thin fibrous cap on the endothelial surface with a large lipid core that is filled with procoagulant substances, predominantly tissue factor;
3. endothelial denudation and fissuring caused by the elaboration of metalloproteinases;

4. local high shear stress, usually because they are severe, at branch points in the vessel.

Events likely occur because of superimposed thrombosis. This can be the result of erosions on the surface of the plaque or more often rupture of the plaque at its edges, where the cap is thinnest and most of the metalloproteinases reside. If rupture induces total thrombotic occlusion, the event is usually a STE AMI. If lesser degrees of occlusion occur, an NSTE AMI or UA may ensue. One of the causes that may participate in subtotal occlusive plaque rupture involves platelets and abnormal coronary vasomotion. It is known that diseased coronary arteries respond atypically to many stimuli, often constricting rather than dilating. Because the cross-sectional area of a vessel is related to the square of the radius, even modest amounts of constriction can markedly increase the extent of occlusion. Whether constriction occurs first, leading to changes of coronary flow and platelet aggregation on the plaque, or whether platelets stick and cause the aggregation, is not certain, but these processes reinforce one another. Platelets secrete vasoconstricting substances in response to a denuded area, which expresses cell adhesion molecule (CAM) receptors. This, in addition to stagnant blood flow, will cause platelets and white blood cells to adhere to the surfaces of vessels. It appears likely that platelets adhere and enhance vasoconstriction and then break off, causing small vessel emboli, sometimes in association with plaque debris and sometimes without. These processes, in addition to a reduction in flow, can lead to necrosis or at least recurrent ischemia. It is apparent that the process that eventually leads to acute events involves a systemic propensity to platelet aggregation and inflammation, because effluent flowing from the nonculprit vessel (distant from the putative coronary lesion causing the acute event) elaborates inflammatory mediators (e.g., MPO) similar to those observed from the affected vessel. This pathophysiology has recently been supported by the Cantos trial where inhibition of the interleukin one beta inflammasome was shown to reduce ischemic events.[37] Of interest, the antibody therapy used also reduced the incidence of lung cancer. A separate trial of low-dose methotrexate was null.[38] Finally, necrosis when present stimulates an acute-phase reaction and inflammation. Given this pathophysiology, many therapies are now oriented toward inhibition of thrombosis, fibrinolysis, platelet aggregation, and inflammation. Many inflammatory markers are used diagnostically and for assessment of therapeutic efficiency.

The more recent appreciation of the high frequency of type 2 MI has changed some of the thinking in regard to MI. Type 1 events which depend on acute atherosclerosis are benefited by invasive intracoronary interventions.[11] Type 2 events[39] due to supply-demand mismatch often do not require mechanical interventions even when coronary heart disease is present. In many instances, the coronary arteries may be normal or at least not badly diseased.[31] This entity has also resulted in rethinking which has moved those studying atherogenesis in multiple additional directions.[35]

Diagnosis of Acute Myocardial Infarction

The diagnosis of AMI established by the World Health Organization in 1986 included biomarkers as an integral part of the disorder and required that at least two of the following criteria be met: (1) a history of chest pain, (2) evolutionary changes on the ECG, and/or (3) elevations of serial cardiac

---

BOX 48.2 Criteria for the Definition of Acute Myocardial Infarction

1. Detection of a rise and/or fall of cardiac biomarker values (preferably cardiac troponin) with at least one value above the 99th percentile upper reference interval and with at least one of the following.
   a. Ischemic symptoms
   b. ECG changes of new ischemia (new ST-T changes or new left bundle branch block)
   c. Development of pathologic Q waves in the electrocardiogram
   d. Imaging evidence of new loss of viable myocardium or new regional wall motion abnormality
   e. Identification of an intracoronary thrombus by angiography or autopsy
2. Pathologic Q waves with or without symptoms in the absence of nonischemic causes
3. Imaging evidence of a region of loss of viable myocardium that is thinned and fails to contract in the absence of a nonischemic cause
4. Pathologic findings of a prior myocardial infarction.
5. Evidence of an imbalance between myocardial oxygen supply and demand unrelated to acute atherothrombosis meets criteria for type 2 MI.

Modified from Thygesen K, Alpert JS, Jaffe AS, Chaitman BR, Bax JJ, Morrow DA, et al. Fourth universal definition of myocardial infarction. *J Amer Coll Cardiol* 2018;72:2231–64.

---

markers to a level two times the normal value. However, over time, it became rare for a diagnosis of AMI to be made in the absence of biochemical evidence of myocardial injury. A 2000 European Society of Cardiology (ESC)/ACC consensus conference[40] updated in 2007 and 2012 (Global Task Force)[41,42] codified the role of markers by advocating that the diagnosis should be regarded as evidence of myocardial injury based on markers of cardiac damage in the appropriate clinical situation (Box 48.2).[2] The guidelines thus recognized the reality that neither the clinical presentation nor the ECG had adequate sensitivity and specificity. This guideline does not suggest that all elevations of these biomarkers should elicit a diagnosis of AMI—only those associated with appropriate clinical and ECG findings (see discussion later in this chapter). When elevations that are not caused by acute ischemia occur, the clinician is obligated to search for another cause for the elevation.[2] In the 2007 revision of the guidelines, several types of AMI were recognized, including the spontaneous type, which is associated with plaque rupture or erosion, and the type associated with fixed or transient coronary abnormalities but not thrombotic occlusion. These are discussed in greater detail in the following paragraphs. It is also recognized that one can have a classic AMI and succumb before markers are obtained or become elevated, and cardiac injury can occur in association with cardiac procedures.[2] In addition, criteria for different types of MI, including after coronary interventions and bypass surgery were suggested (Box 48.3).

Electrocardiography findings. At one time, the initial ECG was thought to be diagnostic of AMI in approximately 50% of patients.[2] As the frequency of STE AMI has diminished

BOX 48.3 Clinical Classification of Myocardial Infarction Types

Type 1: Spontaneous Myocardial Infarction
Related to atherosclerotic plaque rupture, ulceration, fissuring, erosion, or dissection with resulting intraluminal thrombosis in one or more of the coronary arteries leading to decreased myocardial blood flow or distal platelet emboli with ensuing myocyte necrosis. The patient may have underlying severe coronary artery disease (CAD) but on occasion nonobstructive or no CAD.

Type 2: Myocardial Infarction Secondary to Ischemia Imbalance
Myocardial injury with necrosis in which a condition other than CAD contributes to an imbalance between myocardial oxygen supply and/or demand, for example, coronary endothelial dysfunction, coronary artery spasm, coronary embolism, tachyarrhythmia, bradyarrhythmia, anemia, respiratory failure, hypotension, and hypertension with or without left ventricular hypertrophy.

Type 3: Myocardial Infarction Resulting in Death When Biomarker Values Are Unavailable
Cardiac death with symptoms suggestive of myocardial ischemia and presumed new ischemic electrocardiogram (ECG) changes or new left bundle branch block (LBBB), but death occurring before blood samples could be obtained or before cardiac biomarkers could rise; in rare cases cardiac biomarkers were not collected.

Type 4a: Myocardial Infarction Related to Percutaneous Coronary Innervation (PCI)
Myocardial infarction (MI) associated with percutaneous coronary innervation (PCI) is arbitrarily defined by elevation of cardiac

troponin (cTn) values greater than 5×99th percentile upper reference interval in patients with normal baseline values (<99th percentile upper reference interval) or a rise of cTn values above 20% if the baseline values are elevated and are stable or falling. In addition, (1) symptoms suggestive of myocardial ischemia; (2) new ischemic ECG changes or LBBB; (3) angiographic loss of patency of a major coronary artery or a side branch or persistent slow- or no-flow or embolism; or (4) imaging demonstration of new loss of viable myocardium or new regional wall motion abnormality are required. Postmortem demonstration of a procedure-related thrombus in the culprit artery, or a macroscopically large, circumscribed area of necrosis with or without intramyocardial hemorrhage meets the type 4a MI criteria.

Type 4b: Myocardial Infarction Related to Stent Thrombosis
MI related to stent thrombosis is detected by coronary angiography or autopsy in the setting of myocardial ischemia and with a rise and/or fall of cardiac biomarker values, with at least one value above the 99th percentile upper reference interval.

Type 5: Myocardial Infarction Related to Coronary Artery Bypass Grafting
MI associated with coronary artery bypass grafting (CABG) is arbitrarily defined by elevation of cardiac biomarker values greater than 10×99th percentile upper reference interval in patients with normal baseline cTn values (<99th percentile upper reference interval). In addition, (1) new pathologic Q waves or new LBBB, (2) angiographic documented new graft or new native coronary artery occlusion, or (3) imaging evidence of new loss of myocardium or new regional wall motion abnormality.

Modified from Thygesen K, Alpert JS, Jaffe AS, Chaitman BR, Bax JJ, Morrow DA, et al. Fourth universal definition of myocardial infarction. *J Amer Coll Cardiol* 2018;72:2231–64.

and the diagnosis has been made with increasingly greater sensitivity, this percentage has been greatly reduced. Serial tracings are helpful for STE AMI but not for what is now almost 70% of AMIs that are known as non-STE (NSTE) AMIs. The classic ECG changes of a STE AMI is ST segment elevation, which often evolves to the development of Q waves if intervention is not provided (see Fig. 48.4). Pericarditis, some normal variants, and transient causes that may result in myocardial injury such as myocarditis are well described and on occasion can mimic the changes of AMI. Most NSTE AMIs manifest as ST segment depression, with or without T-wave changes, as T-wave changes alone, or on occasion in the absence of any ECG findings. Those with ST segment change have a substantially worse prognosis.[2]

In some patients, the clinical history and ECG may be definitive. In others, they may not be as clear. Many other clinical aspects might suggest acute ischemia as the origin of a given biomarker elevation. For example, the finding of significant coronary obstructive lesions, especially in a pattern suggestive of recent plaque rupture, is highly suggestive. At times, a positive stress test with or without imaging may be what helps in making the diagnosis. However, if the clinical situation is not suggestive, other sources for cardiac injury should be sought.

The most recent Universal Definition[2] while providing similar operational metrics as the third iteration did increase

the emphasis on the concept that an elevated cTn value was a marker of myocardial injury and that myocardial injury was an entity in and of itself. If there are changes in values over time, the myocardial injury is deemed acute. If there are not changes over time, the myocardial injury is chronic. This clarification became important as higher-sensitivity cTn assay became available and it was clear that the largest percentage of increases were not associated with ischemia.[43] This does make the clinical triage of an increased cTn value more difficult and clinicians have in the past wished that all increases might be attributable to MI.[2,43]

BIOMARKERS IN ACUTE CORONARY SYNDROME

Analytical Considerations

Myocardial injury/damage detected by increases of cTn above the sex-specific 99th percentile upper reference limit (URL) is almost invariably associated with adverse clinical outcomes. This statement summarizes more than 30 years of analytical and clinical investigations pertaining to the clinical utility of cTnI and cTnT. This section of the chapter will focus on cTn biochemistry; the analytical aspects of assays used to measure cTn in whole blood, serum, and plasma; preanalytical and analytical specifications that manufacturers of cTn assays need to strive to optimize; 99th percentile

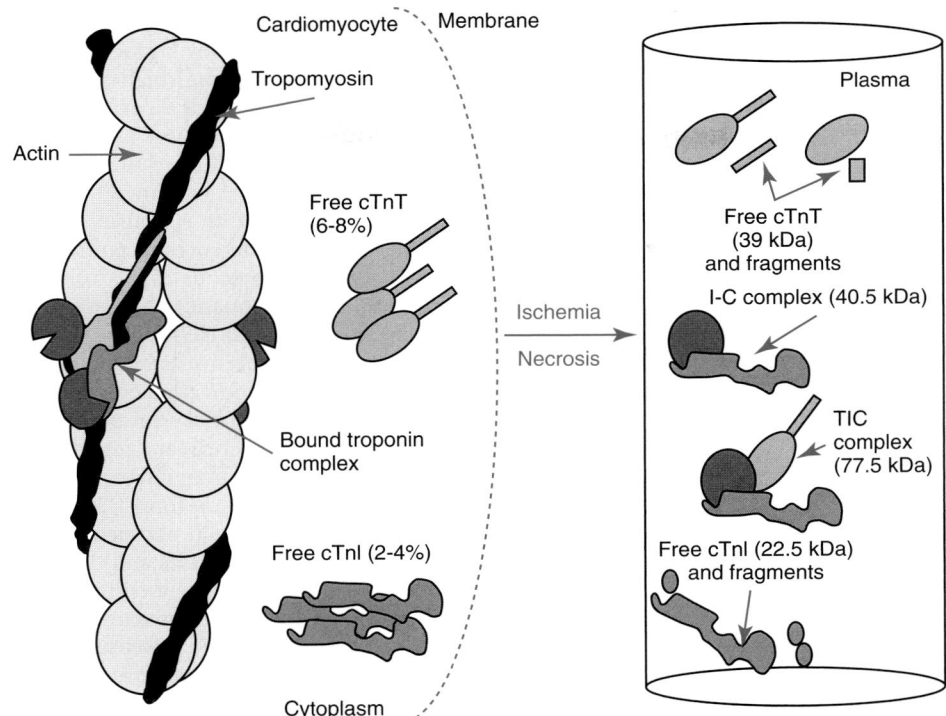

FIGURE 48.6 Structure of cardiac troponin *(cTn)* complex and troponin forms released after myofibril necrosis. *cTn1,* Cardiac troponin I; *cTnT,* cardiac troponin T. (From Gaze DC, Collinson PO. Multiple molecular forms of circulating cardiac troponin: analytical and clinical significance. *Ann Clin Biochem* 2008;45:349–59. Figure courtesy Paul Collinson.)

(normal) URL determinations; central laboratory and point-of-care (POC) testing strategies; recommendations for implementation of high-sensitivity cTn assays for appropriate (cost) utilization recommendations in clinical practice to assist in early ruling in and ruling out AMI.

Biochemistry

The contractile proteins of the myofibril include the three troponin regulatory proteins (Fig. 48.6).[44] The troponins are a complex of three protein subunits: troponin C (the calcium-binding component), TnI (the inhibitory component), and TnT (the tropomyosin-binding component). The subunits exist in a number of isoforms. The distribution of these isoforms varies between cardiac muscle and slow- and fast-twitch skeletal muscle. Only two major isoforms of troponin C are found in human heart and skeletal muscle. These are characteristic of slow- and fast-twitch skeletal muscle. The heart isoform is identical to the slow-twitch skeletal muscle isoform, thus the reason why cTnC was never developed as a cardiac-specific biomarker. Isoforms of cardiac-specific troponin T (cTnT) and cardiac-specific troponin I (cTnI) have been identified and are the products of unique genes.[45–48] Troponin is localized primarily in the myofibrils (94 to 97%), with a smaller cytoplasmic fraction (3 to 6%).[49] Some experts in the field think that 100% of cTn is myofibril bound and that the cytoplasmic fraction represents a more easily mobilizable fraction, rather than representing a different cellular localization.

cTnI and cTnT have different amino acid sequences from the skeletal isoforms and are encoded by unique genes. Human cTnI has an additional 31-amino-acid residue on the

amino terminal end compared with skeletal muscle TnI, giving it complete cardiac specificity. Only one isoform of cTnI has been identified. cTnI is not expressed in normal, regenerating, or diseased human or animal skeletal muscle.[45] cTnT is encoded for by a different gene than the one that encodes for skeletal muscle isoforms. An 11-amino-acid amino-terminal residue gives this marker unique cardiac specificity. However, during human fetal development, in regenerating rat skeletal muscle, and in diseased human skeletal muscle, small amounts of immunoreactive cTnT are expressed as one of four identified isoforms in skeletal muscle.[46,50–52] In humans, cTnT isoform expression has been demonstrated in skeletal muscle specimens obtained from patients with neuromuscular diseases, including muscular dystrophy, polymyositis, and dermatomyositis, as well as end-stage renal disease.[46,53–57] Thus care is necessary to choose antibody pairs for the cTnT assay that do not detect these reexpressed isoforms or the immunoreactive proteins expressed in neuromuscular skeletal diseases that show cross-reactivity to the commercial (Roche) cTnT assays. This may result in positive cTnT findings in the blood from noncardiac tissue (diseased skeletal muscle), that indicates a false-positive myocardial injury indication (as discussed later).[56–59] Recently, a POC hs-cTnT assay (Pylon, ET Healthcare) was approved in China (by cFDA) for clinical use that does not have skeletal muscle interference, as their antibodies capture and detect different epitopes compared to the Roche antibodies.[60] A substantial body of evidence shows that after myocardial injury or because of genetic disposition, multiple forms of cTn are elaborated both in tissue and in blood (Fig. 48.7).[40,48,60] These include the T-I-C ternary complex, IC binary complex, and free I; multiple modification of these three forms can occur, involving oxidation, reduction, phosphorylation, and dephosphorylation, as well as both C- and N-terminal degradation. Depending on the selection of antibodies used to detect cTnI, different antibody configurations can lead to a substantially different recognition pattern.[42] This was recently demonstrated in a study describing cTnI and cTnT forms released after MI and how the ability to measure different post-translation cTn forms varies depending on the antibody selection used in immunoassay, as shown in Fig. 48.8. The conclusions derived from these observations are that assays need to be developed in which the antibodies recognize epitopes in the stable region of cTnI and, ideally, demonstrate an equimolar response to the different cTnI forms that circulate in the blood. At present, standardization of cTnI assays has not been obtained.[61,62]

Immunoassays

Cummins and coworkers were the first to develop a radioimmunoassay (RIA) to measure cTnI, using polyclonal anti-cTnI antibodies.[47] The first of many monoclonal enzyme-linked

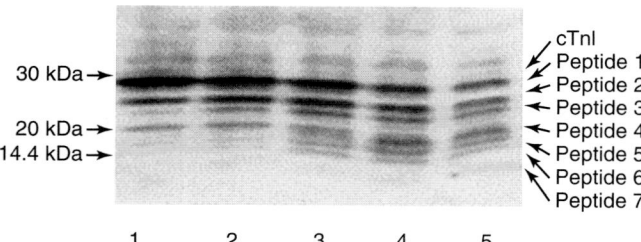

FIGURE 48.7 Western blot analysis of endogenous cardiac troponin I *(cTnI)* proteolysis in human heart tissue visualized with monoclonal anti-cTnI antibody. Protein extracts from tissue samples were incubated at 37 °C for 0 hour (lane 1), 2 hours (lane 2), 5 hours (lane 3), 8 hours (lane 4), and 20 hours (lane 5), separated by 10 to 20% gradient sodium dodecyl sulfate (SDS)-gel electrophoresis, transferred to a nitrocellulose membrane, and visualized by MAb 19C7. The apparent molecular masses and peptides are marked by *arrows*. (From Katrukha AG, Bereznikova AV, Filatov VL, Esakova TV, Kolosova OV, Pettersson K, et al. Degradation of cardiac troponin I: implication for reliable immunodetection. *Clin Chem* 1998;44:2433–40.)

immunosorbent assays, an anti-cTnI antibody–based immunoassay was described by Bodor and colleagues.[42,64–75] Current contemporary, POC, and high-sensitivity (hs-cTn) assays in the marketplace are well described on the IFCC Committee on the Clinical Application of Cardiac Biomarkers (C-CB) website that is updated 2 to 3 times a year, as shown for hs-cTn assays in Table 48.1. A timeline of hs-cTn assay regulatory approvals are shown in At A Glance. The tables demonstrate the similarities and differences in capture and detection antibodies in the heterogeneous assays used in clinical practice. In addition to these quantitative assays, several less frequently used qualitative (positive/negative) assays are also marketed as shown for representative assays in Table 48.1.[76]

Nonstandardization challenges do prevent the ease of switching from one assay to another in clinical practice or research.[77] First, no primary reference cTnI material is currently available for manufacturers to use in standardizing cTnI or cTnT assays. Second, cTn concentrations fail to be consistently harmonized between assays because cTnI circulates in its numerous forms and the different antibodies used in assays recognize different epitopes of cTnI, even for different assays and instruments marketed by the same manufacturer, as shown in the IFCC website. The cTnI Standardization Subcommittee of the American Association for Clinical Chemistry (AACC) in collaboration with the National Institute of Standards and Technology (NIST) did develop a cTnI reference material (SRM 2921), a TnC-cTnI-cTnT complex purified from human heart under nondenaturing conditions.[78] A cTnI value was assigned by a combination of reversed-phase liquid chromatography with ultraviolet detection and amino acid analysis. However, it appears to be of limited value, at best used for the potential of harmonization or possible use for cTnI traceability but was not helpful as a common calibration material for either cTnI or cTnT. Further, it appears this material is now out of stock. For complete standardization for cTnI assays, manufacturers would need to agree to use the same capture and detection antibodies showing similar specificity for the many cTnI molecules circulating in the blood. This would also overcome matrix effects that a current IFCC working group is investigating based on a serum-based common reference material for calibration, a process that will unlikely solve any of the above

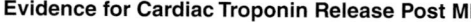

Evidence for Cardiac Troponin Release Post MI

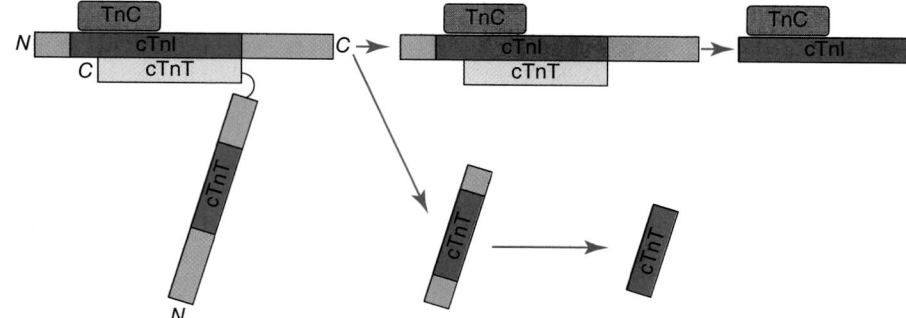

FIGURE 48.8 During progression post myocardial infarction *(MI)* the amount of ITC complex decreases, with no full-size cardiac troponin T *(cTnT)* or cardiac troponin I *(cTnI)* found, and how antibodies are chosen are important to detect maximum amount of cTn circulating. What is not clear is whether these processes occur in the myocardium only and or in blood. (From Vylegzhanina AV, Kogan IA, Katrukha IA, Koshkina EV, Bereznikova AV, Filatov VL, et al. Full size and partially truncated cardiac troponin complexes in the blood of patients with acute myocardial infarction. *Clin Chem* 2019;65:882–92.)

TABLE 48.1   Analytical Characteristics of Commercial and Research High-Sensitivity Cardiac Troponin I and T Assays as Stated by Manufacturer

Company/Platform/ Assay	LoD (µg/L)	99th % (µg/L)	%CV at 99th	10% CV (µg/L)	Risk Stratification	Epitopes Recognized by Antibodies	Detection Antibody Tag
Contemporary Assays							
Abbott ARCHITECT	<0.01	0.028	15	0.032	No	C: 87–91, 24–40; D: 41–49	Acridinium
Beckman Coulter Access 2	0.01	0.04	14	0.06	Yes	C: 41–49; D: 24–40	ALP
Roche E170	0.01	<0.01	18	0.03	Yes	C: 125–131; D: 136–147	Ruthenium
Siemens Centaur Ultra	0.006	0.04	10	0.03	Yes	C: 41–49, 87–91; D: 27–40	Acridinium
Siemens Dimension RxL	0.004	0.07	20	0.14	Yes	C: 27–32; D: 41-56	ALP
Siemens VISTA	0.015	0.045	10	0.04	Yes	C: 27–32; D: 41–56	Chemiluminescent
Tosch AIA II	0.06	<0.06	8.5	0.09	No	C: 41–49; D: 87–91	ALP
Ortho Vitros ECi ES	0.012	0.034	10	0.034	Yes	C: 24–40, 41–49; D: 87–91	HRP
Point-of-Care Assays							
Abbott i-STAT	0.02	0.08	16.5	0.10	Yes	C: 41–49, 88–91; D: 28–39,62–78	ALP
LSI Medience PATHFAST	0.008	0.029	5.1	0.014	No	C: 41–49; D:71–116, 163-209	ALP
Quidel/Alere Triage True hs-cTnI	1.9	26/14 (M/F)	6.5	8.4	No	NP (not provided)	Fluorophore
Radiometer AQT90 cTnI	0.009	0.023	17.7	0.039	NA	C: 41–49, 190–196; D: 137–149	Europium
Radiometer AQT90 cTnT	0.01	0.017	20.0	0.03	NA	C: 125–131; D:136–147	Europium
Response Biomedical RAMP	0.03	<0.1	18.5	0.21	No	C: 85–92; D: 26–38	Fluorophore
Roche Cardiac Reader	<0.05	<0.05	NA	NA	No	C: 125–131; D:136–147	Gold particles
Siemens Stratus CS	0.03	0.07	10.0	0.06	Yes	C: 27–32; D: 41–56	ALP
Siemens Atellica VTLi hs-cTnI	1.6	27/19 (M/F)	6.1	6.7	No	C: 41–49; D: cTnC, 2 antibodies in 20-100 range	Gold nanoparticles

High-Sensitivity Assays	ng/L	M/F (ng/L)		ng/L	% Normals Measurable		
Abbott ARCHITECT hs-cTnI	1.2	34/16	<6.0	3	96	C: 24–40; D: 41–49	Acridinium
Beckman Coulter Access hs-cTnI	2.1	11/9	<5.0	3.3	80	C: 41–49; D: 24–40	ALP
Ortho Vitros hs-cTnI	1.0	19/16	<5.0	6.5	75	C: 24–40, 41–49; D: 87–91	HRP
Roche E170 hs-cTnT (Gen 5 USA)	5	20/13	<8.0	13	25	C: 136–147; D: 125–131	Ruthenium
Siemens Atellica hs-cTnI	1.6	54/34	<4.0	<6	No	C: 41–50; C: 41–50, 171–190; D: 29–34	Gold nanoparticles

Sex-specific 99th percentiles.
F, Female; *hs-cTnI,* high-sensitivity cardiac troponin I; *LOD,* limit of detection; *M,* male;

limitations.[62] Several adaptations of the Roche cTnT immunoassay have been described over the years.[74,75,79,80] The current Roche FDA-cleared assay available in the United States (Gen 5) and the assay used worldwide outside the United States (designated hs-cTnT by Roche) involve two monoclonal, anti-cTnT antibodies. During one of those alterations, the negative effects of heparin were eliminated. Although skeletal muscle TnT itself may appear to be a potential interferent, recent studies in patients with neuromuscular disease have described false-positive cTnT findings in plasma, proposed to be an immunoreactive protein that does cross-react with both cTnT assays.[55–57] Because of calibration differences between the 4th generation, high-sensitivity (hs-TnT), or what is called Gen 5 in the USA by Roche, and POC assays or cTnT, minor differences in measured cTnT concentration have been shown between instruments.[59,71,73,81] Further, the two different hs-cTnT assays from ET Healthcare and Roche, as for cTnI assays, are not standardized or harmonized.

Assay Specifications

In 2001 and 2004 the IFCC Committee on Standardization of Markers of Cardiac Damage (C-SMCD) recommended quality specifications for contemporary cTn assays.[82,83] These specifications were intended for use by the manufacturers of commercial assays and by clinical laboratories using cTn assays. The overall goal was to attempt to establish uniform criteria so that all assays could be evaluated objectively for their analytical qualities and clinical performance. Both analytical and preanalytical factors were addressed. With the increasing conversion rate of contemporary assays to the hs-format, expert consensus recommendations were published by the AACC Academy in collaboration with the International Federation of Clinical Chemistry and Laboratory Medicine Task Force on Clinical Applications of Bio-Markers (IFCC TF-CB).[66] The document focused on clinical laboratory practice recommendations for hs-cTn assays utilizing expert opinion class of evidence to focus on the following 10 topics (Box 48.4): *(a)* quality control (QC) utilization, *(b)* validation of the lower reportable analytical limits, *(c)* units to be used in reporting measurable concentrations for patients and QC materials, *(d)* 99th percentile sex-specific URLs to define the reference interval; *(e)* criteria required to define hs-cTn assays, *(f)* communication with clinicians and the laboratory's role in educating clinicians regarding the influence of preanalytical and analytic problems that can confound assay results, *(g)* studies on hs-cTn assays and how authors need to document preanalytical and analytical variables, *(h)* harmonizing and standardizing assay results and the role of commutable materials, *(i)* time to reporting of results from sample receipt and sample collection, and *(j)* changes in hs-cTn concentrations over time and the role of both analytical and biological variabilities in interpreting results of serial blood collections. Publications have also attempted to provide guidance to regulatory agencies, health care providers, and laboratories.[76,84–86] A meeting between US laboratory medicine, emergency medicine, and cardiology biomarker experts and the FDA resulted in an opinion/perspective article with the objective of providing guidelines for uniform analytical and clinical standards for 510k studies being performed by manufacturers seeking cTnI and cTnT 510k assay clearance. Recommendations provided to the FDA addressed the following points: (1) the number of reference

---

> **BOX 48.4** **Clinical Laboratory Practice Recommendations for Use of Cardiac Troponin in Acute Coronary Syndrome: Expert Opinion From Academy of the AACC and the Task Force on Clinical Applications of Cardiac Bio-Markers of the IFCC**
>
> 1. Quality control (QC) utilization
> 2. Assay limits validating the lower reportable analytical limits (LOD)
> 3. Units to use in reporting measurable concentrations for patients and QC materials
> 4. 99th percentile sex-specific upper reference limits defining the reference interval
> 5. Criteria required to define hs-cTn assays
> 6. Communication with clinicians and laboratory role in educating clinicians on the influence of preanalytic and analytic issues that confound assay results
> 7. Authors/manuscripts need to document preanalytical/analytical variables on hs-cTn assays
> 8. Harmonizing and standardizing assay results and role of commutable materials
> 9. Time to reporting of results from sample receipt and sample collection
> 10. Changes in hs-cTn concentrations over time and role of both analytical and biological variabilities in interpreting results of serial blood collections

AACC, American Association for Clinical Chemistry; *LOD,* limit of detection.

individuals for determination of a 99th percentile upper reference interval, (2) limit of quantification, (3) total imprecision requirements, (4) enrollment of subjects for diagnostic studies, (5) patient adjudication processes, and (6) clinical end points and time limits to assess outcomes. A primary focus was to ensure that the suggested protocols also apply to hs-cTn assays. Unfortunately, the expert recommendations were not endorsed by the FDA.

Defining 99th Percentile Normal Reference Intervals for Cardiac Troponin Assays

Advancements in cTn assay technology have challenged clinicians and laboratory scientists to better understand the analytical characteristics of cTn assays to determine which assays are best for optimal patient care. International guidelines have defined an increased cTn above the 99th percentile URL as an abnormal result, as described in the clinical section.[2,11,65,87,88] Whether a clinical laboratory defines an abnormal result above the 99th percentile as a critical value needs to be assessed and determined by each individual laboratory. What has been lacking until recently was a uniform approach to define the 99th percentile across the heterogeneity of assays.[73] A review article has addressed the vast literature regarding defining normality, on a global basis.[89] Guidance is now proposed by experts (cardiology, emergency, laboratory medicine) by the joint AACC Academy and IFCC C-CB publication.[65] Despite evidence-based literature demonstrating that cTn concentrations tend to increase in individuals older than 60 years, likely because of unrecognized comorbidities, 99th percentiles are often determined across wide age ranges using subjects as old as 80 years (convenience samples).[64,73,74,90,91] Further frustrating the problem of selecting relevant reference subjects is the fact that in clinically defined normal individuals without known CVD, increased cTn concentrations are indicative of a significantly higher risk for death.[92,93] Given such problems, most laboratories (1) accept the manufacturer's reference interval from the package insert, (2) perform an underpowered normal study to establish a reference interval, or (3) accept a URL cutoff value published in the literature, which vary for the same assay between studies depending on the populations studied. Implementation of the 99th percentile URL, especially by sex-specific URLs, has not been globally accepted by laboratories, most likely because of pressures by clinicians who have been concerned that the imprecision of assays at the 99th percentile does not always meet the Fourth Universal Definition of MI (2018) recommendation of a 10% CV at the 99th percentile; analytical noise around the 99th percentile could result in a false-positive increase of cTn in patients without myocardial injury. However, the Universal Definition does clearly state that assays are clinically usable with up to a 20% CV at the 99th percentile. At least two serial samples are required to demonstrate a rising or falling cTn pattern.[2]

A recent study has attempted to define how to select healthy reference subjects in deriving 99th percentiles for cTn assays.[73] Its goal was to determine overall and sex-specific 99th percentile URLs in 9 hs-cTnI and 3 hs-cTnT assays using a universal sample bank (USB). The USB comprised healthy subjects, 426 men and 417 women, screened using a health questionnaire. Hemoglobin A1c (>URL 6.5%), NT-proBNP (>URL 125 ng/L), and eGFR (<60 mL/min) were used as surrogate biomarker exclusion criteria along with statin use. 99th percentiles were determined by nonparametric, Harrell-Davis bootstrap, and robust methods. Subjects were ages 19 to 91 years, Caucasian 58%, African American 27%, Pacific Islander/Asian 11%, other 4%, Hispanic 8%, and non-Hispanic 92%. The overall and sex-specific 99th percentiles for all assays, before and after exclusions ($n = 694$), were influenced by the statistical method used, with substantial differences noted between and within both hs-cTnI and hs-cTnT assays. Men had higher 99th percentiles (ng/L) than women, as shown in Fig. 48.9. The Roche cTnT and Beckman and Abbott cTnI assays (after exclusions) did not measure cTn values at ≥ the limit of detection (LOD) in ≥ 50% women. Representative histograms for the current hs-cTnI and hs-cTnT assays used worldwide demonstrate substantial differences in their abilities to measure concentrations greater than LOD especially in females, as shown in Fig. 48.10. The findings have important clinical implications in that sex-specific 99th percentiles varied according to the statistical method and hs-cTn assay used, not all assays provided a high enough percentage of measurable concentrations in women to qualify as a hs-assay, and the surrogate exclusion criteria used to define normality tended to lower the 99th percentiles.

Guideline-Supported Recommendations

Consensus guidelines from the Fourth Universal Definition of Myocardial Infarction (2018), the joint laboratory medicine AACC Academy and International Federation of Clinical Chemistry (IFCC) C-CB, the ACC/AHA and Epidemiology groups, the ACC Foundation, and the European Clinical and

Laboratory groups have recommended that, in patients who present with ischemic symptoms, a rising or falling serial pattern with at least one cTn concentration higher than the sex-specific 99th percentile URLs, during the first 24 hours after onset of symptoms indicates myocardial injury/necrosis/cell death. Fig. 48.11 shows a representative profile of the rise and fall pattern of cTn for type 1 MI, type 2 MI, and chronic myocardial injury patients. If this elevation occurs in the clinical setting of ischemia consistent with MI, that diagnosis should be made (see Box 48.2). It is recommended that cTn assays with appropriate QC and optimal total imprecision (CV ≤ 10%) at the 99th percentile URL are preferred.[82,85] Better imprecision at low cTn concentrations, based on high-sensitivity assays, appears to improve the value of interpreting cTn as an early rule out and rule in diagnostic tool and risk indicator (within 3 hours of baseline sampling), as will be discussed in the clinical section. Use of contemporary or POC cTn assays with intermediate imprecision (10 to 20% CV) at the 99th percentile, however, is deemed clinically acceptable and does not lead to patient misclassifications when serial cTn results are interpreted.

A challenge that needs to be considered as hs-cTn assays with improved analytical sensitivity become increasingly incorporated in laboratory practice is determining how these new assays compare with the older contemporary assays. In essence, as will be discussed below, the hs-assays improve clinical practice for diagnostics and risk assessment for more rapid (early) and improved patient management and care. Diagnostic clinical sensitivities using specimens collected serially from presentation for detection of MI have improved from 15 to 35% for the initial generations of cTn assays, to 50 to 75% for current contemporary assays, and to more than 80% for hs-assays, as shown in Fig. 48.12. To exclude an AMI with contemporary assays, the Global Task Force originally recommended a 6-hour period for assessing the optimal negative predictive value (NPV) for ruling out AMI. With hs-cTn assays, the timing for ruling out an AMI with greater than 99.5% NPV and 99% clinical sensitivity has decreased to less than 2 to 3 hours from the time of baseline/first blood draw, better defining the clinical playing field for hs-assays used to assist in the diagnosis of MI, rule out MI, and better stratify patients for risk of adverse events. The basis for these early approaches was that these early signals anticipated that eventually the criteria proposed by the Universal Definition of MI would be met.[2] Further, studies consistently now show by using hs-assays that in patients presenting with a low clinical likelihood of ACS, both hs-cTnI and hs-cTnT baseline concentrations below an assay's LOD with a nonischemic ECG can be used to rule out AMI, as will be discussed later in the chapter. Measurable cTn concentrations but less than the sex-specific 99th percentile URL or less than overall 99th percentile URL and without a significant delta (change) value (assay dependent) 1, 2, or 3 hours after the baseline sample, can also provide an NPV greater than 99.5% for early rule out in a substantial number of patients, as will be discussed later in the clinical section that addresses the caveat of early presenters at less than 2 hours following the index event onset. As the use of hs-cTn assays grows in the USA, having already done so worldwide outside the USA, triage of patients in the emergency department (ED) will be significantly improved, allowing for more rapid triage to an appropriate level of care or earlier discharge home, with minimal risk for an adverse event, with substantial financial savings to the health care

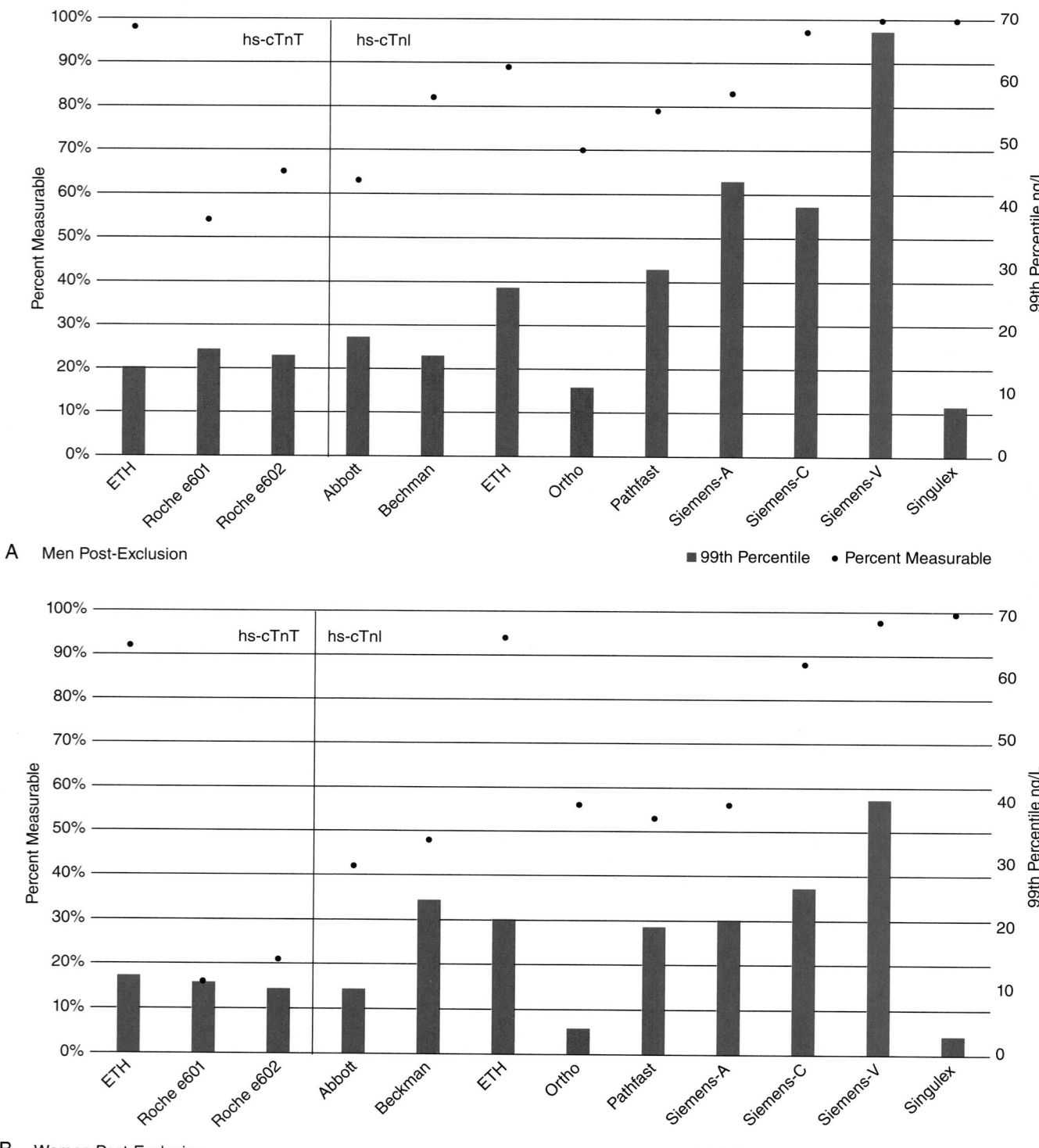

A Men Post-Exclusion

■ 99th Percentile ● Percent Measurable

B Women Post-Exclusion

■ 99th Percentile ● Percent Measurable

FIGURE 48.9 Comparison of both 99th percentile values *(boxes)* and percent measurable concentrations *(circles)* in a presumably healthy population for high-sensitivity cardiac troponin assays for males (A) and females (B). *cTnI,* Cardiac troponin I; *cTnI,* cardiac troponin T; *ETH,* ET healthcare. (From Apple FS, Wu AHB, Sandoval Y, Sexter A, Love SA, Myers G, et al. Sex-specific 99th percentile upper reference limits for high sensitivity cardiac troponin assays derived using a universal sample bank. *Clin Chem* 2020;66:434–44.)

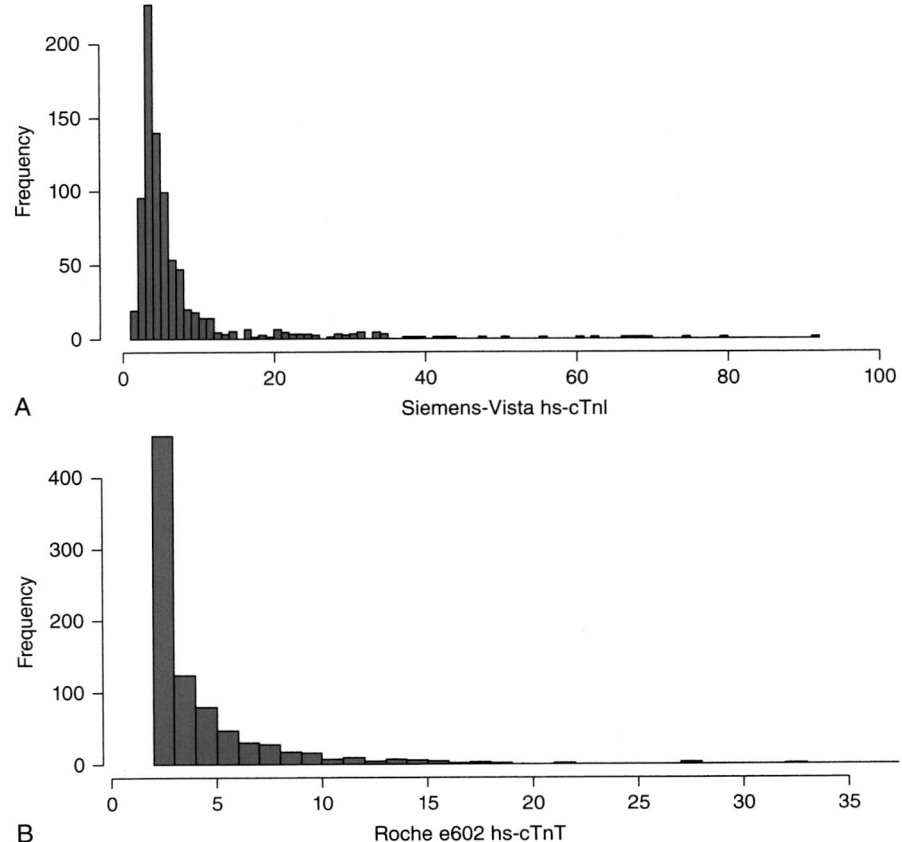

FIGURE 48.10 Representative histograms for (A) hs-cTnI and (B) hs-cTnT assays of plasma specimens from apparently healthy individuals. *cTnI,* Cardiac troponin I; *cTnI,* cardiac troponin T. (From Apple FS, Wu AHB, Sandoval Y, Sexter A, Love SA, Myers G, et al. Sex-specific 99th percentile upper reference limits for high sensitivity cardiac troponin assays derived using a universal sample bank. *Clin Chem* 2020;66:434–44.)

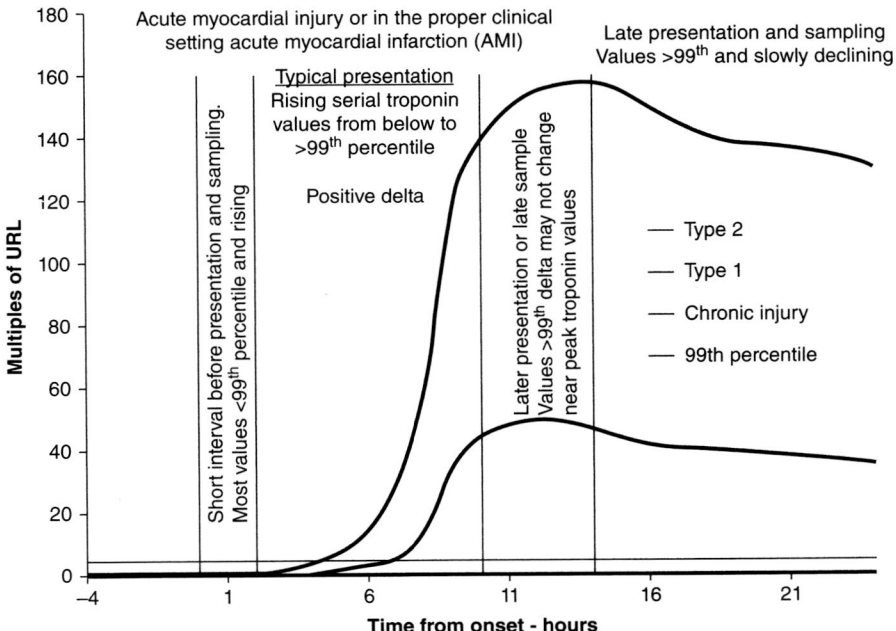

FIGURE 48.11 Representative profile of the rise and fall pattern of cardiac troponin for type 1 MI, type 2 MI, and chronic myocardial injury patients. (Courtesy IFCC C-CB, prepared by Paul Collinson).

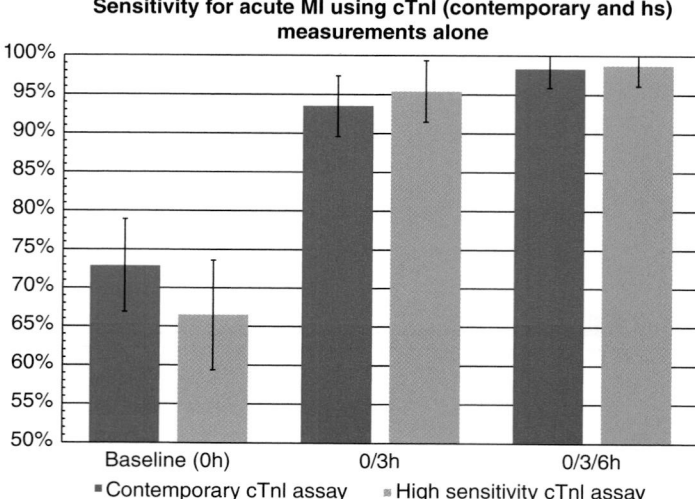

FIGURE 48.12 Diagnostic clinical sensitivities using specimens collected serially from presentation for detection of myocardial infarction *(MI)* comparing a high-sensitivity and contemporary cardiac troponin I assay *(cTnI)*. (From Sandoval Y, Smith SW, Thordsen SE, Bruen CA, Carlson MD, Dodd KW, et al. Diagnostic performance of high sensitivity compared to contemporary cardiac troponin I for the diagnosis of acute myocardial infarction. *Clin Chem* 2017;63:1594–604.)

system/hospital. Ongoing analytical and clinical development is underway to validate hs-POC cTn assays.

Defining Reference Populations

To address the conundrum of concentration differences across assays that have been shown for contemporary cTn assays, appropriate-sized, population-based, direct comparisons of hs-cTn assays have been carried out. Only the IFCC C-CB and the AACC Academy have provided an international group of experts that have published their opinion or guideline that defines an "apparently healthy population."[65] This approach suggests the use of a common normal reference population within a focused, healthy, age-defined group similar in age to patients presenting with symptoms suggestive of ACS to establish 99th percentile URLs, with the use of surrogate biomarkers to exclude silent pathophysiologies. Multiple studies using first-generation, contemporary, and hs-cTn assays have demonstrated that the cTn 99th percentile strongly depends on selection of individuals to be included in the reference population. Examining multiple contemporary and POC assays, the percent of measurable concentrations below the 99th percentile concentration were all less than 50%. Further, the 99th percentile URL variability among assays is substantial, further exemplifying the lack of cTnI and cTnT assay standardization. hs-cTn assays in comparison have demonstrated near-Gaussian distributions (see Fig. 48.10; assay dependent), with sex-specific URL differences that are not observed with contemporary and POC assays because of their lack of analytical sensitivity.

Defining Assays Analytical Characteristics

A two-tiered system of analysis using both 99th percentiles and imprecision values at the 99th percentile, based on a younger, healthy reference population that is diversified by sex, race, and ethnicity, has been proposed.[64] This approach has been challenged because (1) it does not provide an age-matched normal cohort matching the ACS patient population

that typically presents to rule out an AMI and (2) it is not based on clinical diagnostic or outcomes data at the 99th percentile URL.[93] The scorecard approach was based on a published scorecard concept to capture the essence of which assays are acceptable for use in clinical practice and to facilitate the transition to hs-cTn assays; based on designations of the total imprecision (% CV) of each assay at the 99th percentile and how many specimens from normal individuals have cTn concentrations that are actually measurable below the 99th percentile.[64] The ultimate goal is to have all assays be level 4 guideline acceptable. A point of controversy does exist regarding the way Roche has commercially designated their cTnT assay as high-sensitivity; the evidence-based literature does not support its designation as an hs-assay because the assay consistently measures less than 50% of normal female subjects above the LOD (see Fig. 48.9); as such they have designated their FDA-cleared assay as Gen 5 (even though it is the same assay designated high sensitivity for sale outside the USA). The likely clinical effects of using hs-assays rated by the scorecard as "guideline acceptable" (≤10% CV) or contemporary "clinically usable" (11 to 20% CV) include: (1) all providers will more accurately detect patients within the normal range and with minor myocardial injury, independent of the pathophysiologic mechanism; (2) emergency medicine physicians will achieve improvements in triage through earlier ruling out (improved NPV and sensitivity) and ruling in (improved positive predictive value [PPV] and specificity) of patients with MI; (3) cardiology, internal medicine (hospitalists), and family practice physicians will see improved outcomes for both inpatients (hospitalized, short-term risk) and outpatients (posthospitalization, long-term risk) because of the ability to detect injury earlier, and manage patients accordingly, compared to other diagnostic tools; (4) other medical specialty physicians will be better able to identify patients early at presentation, often without clinical symptoms, who may be at risk of cardiac-related adverse outcomes; and (5) clinical trial investigators will be able to identify appropriate and optimal patient reenrollment and outcome measures.

Optimal discrimination between a small amount of myocardial injury and analytical noise requires assays that have low limits of quantitation (LOQ; lowest concentration at 20% CV) and LOD, and require low imprecision at low cTn concentrations. Efforts to improve the imprecision of cTn assays are always warranted. Irrespective of how the testing is performed, whether in the central laboratory or at the bedside using POC assays, manufacturers need to define the imprecision profile (i.e., the scatter graph showing the %CV versus increasing cTn concentrations obtained using the Clinical and Laboratory Standards Institute [CLSI] EP5-A2 protocol) by assessing pools of human samples containing different cTn concentrations.[83] In particular, at least two cTn concentrations that cover the range between the LOD and the 99th percentile URL of the assay are recommended to be included; one around the LOD and one around the female and or male 99th percentile URL. Imprecision characteristics, including the 10 and 20% CV concentrations, the LOD, and 99th percentile data from current commercially available assays for contemporary, POC, and hs-cTn assays need to be addressed. It is concerning in the context of clinical practice that there still is some variability for an individual patient's cTn concentration caused by different lots of calibrators and different antibodies that do not recognize the same epitopes when the same sample is measured using the same manufacturer's assay in different laboratories. Such discrepancies highlight the need for local analytical validation whenever feasible. Laboratories at a minimum should determine total imprecision at the LOD and at each sex-specific URL and should continue to monitor assay performance over time using internal QC materials that include the lowest concentration corresponding to the 10 and 20% CVs, as well as at the 99th percentile if different from the 10% CV concentration. Patient specimen comparisons such as regression analysis and bias assessment should be performed according to CLSI guidelines and as outlined by AACC Academy and IFCC C-CB.

Many organizations, including the AACC Academy, IFCC C-CB, Global Task Force, and Cardiology and Epidemiology Societies have outlined analytical recommendations for cTn (as well as for other biomarkers of ACS). The most current recommendations by the AACC Academy and IFCC C-CB for the appropriate implementation and utilization of cardiac biomarkers, specifically for hs-cTn assays, to aid in the early rule-in and rule-out diagnosis of MI, complementing the quality specifications for contemporary cTn assays previously published, follow (see Box 48.4).[11,65]

Recommendation 1: For hs-cTn assays, laboratories should measure at least three different concentrations of QC materials at least once per day. For contemporary cTn assays, at least two different concentrations of QC materials must be assessed at least once per day. Before patient testing can be initiated, the values for acceptable imprecision must be, at a minimum, consistent with those specified by the manufacturer.

A. QC concentrations for hs-cTn assays (ng/L units with one decimal place):
   (1) Concentration 1: a concentration between the LOD and the lowest sex-specific 99th percentile.
   (2) Concentration 2: a concentration that is higher than but close (within 20%) to the highest sex-specific 99th percentile URL.
   (3) Concentration 3: a concentration that challenges the upper analytical range of reportable cTn results (e.g., multiples above the 99th percentile concentration).
B. QC concentrations for contemporary (pre-hs assays) cTn assays (ng/mL or µg/L units) with three decimal places:
   (1) Concentration 1: a concentration at or close to (within 20%) the overall 99th percentile.
   (2) Concentration 2: a concentration that challenges the upper analytical range of reportable cTn results (e.g., manufacturer).

Recommendation 2: During initiation of hs-cTn testing, clinical laboratories should validate the LoB, LOD outside the United States, or LoQ as applicable per FDA regulations in the United States. These analytical parameters should be validated minimally on an annual basis or more frequently as deemed necessary.

Recommendation 3: Report hs-cTn in whole numbers, using ng/L without decimal points. For reporting QC values, we recommend one decimal point. For contemporary cTn assays, units are reported in ug/L to two significant figures, with QC values reported to three significant figures.

Recommendation 4: Use a defined reference population to report 99th percentile concentrations according to sex-specific cutoffs for hs-cTn assays. This recommendation is not relevant for contemporary cTn assays. A minimum of 300 men and 300 women per group of healthy individuals is required for appropriate statistical determination for the 99th percentile (the robust statistical method is not recommended) of a normal reference URL for both cTn and CK-MB.

Recommendation 5: We recommend that assays unable to detect cTn at concentrations at or above the LOD in at least 50% of healthy men and women be labeled as contemporary cTn assays.

Recommendation 6: Laboratories should communicate with clinicians on the influence of preanalytic and analytic problems that confound hs-cTn assays. For institutions or health systems using 2 or more cTn assays, differences in the sensitivity of the various cTn assays should be explained to assist clinicians in understanding discrepancies when patients are transferred from other facilities

Recommendation 7: Authors of studies using cardiac biomarkers, including hs-cTn, should document preanalytical and analytical variables important to the study and be explicit concerning their postanalytical interpretative approaches.

Recommendation 8: Commutable materials should be developed for use in harmonizing and standardizing cTn measurements.

Recommendation 9: cTn results should be reported within 60 minutes or less of when a sample is received. There should be continued efforts to improve this to a time of 60 minutes from when the sample was collected.

Recommendation 10: The laboratory should help educate clinicians on the importance of specific metrics by which true clinical changes in cTn concentrations can be distinguished from analytical and biological variabilities.

Point-of-Care Testing

Laboratory Medicine Practice Guidelines for non–hs-cTn POC testing in ACS will be updated in 2021 by the AACC Academy and IFCC C-CB. Current guidelines address administrative issues, cost-effective usage, and clinical and technical performance of cardiac biomarkers in the ED. Eleven proposed elements of the guidelines are as follows:

1. Members of EDs, primary care physicians, cardiologists, hospital administrators, and clinical laboratory staff should work collectively to develop an accelerated protocol for the use of biomarkers in the evaluation of patients with possible ACS.
2. This protocol should be applied to facilitate the diagnosis of MI in the ED or to continue the diagnosis at other locations in the hospital.
3. Quality assurance measures should be used with monitoring to reduce medical errors and improve patient treatment.
4. Blood collection should be referenced to the time of presentation in the ED and, if available, to the reported time of symptom onset.
5. The interdisciplinary team should include personnel who are knowledgeable about local reimbursement.
6. The laboratory should perform biomarker testing with a maximum turnaround time (TAT) of 1 hour and optimally 30 minutes. The TAT is defined as the time from blood collection to reporting of results to the provider.
7. Institutions that cannot consistently provide a 1-hour TAT should consider POC testing assays if clinically necessary.
8. Performance specifications and characteristics for central laboratory and POC testing assays should not differ.
9. Laboratory personnel must be involved in selection of POC assays, training of individuals to perform the analysis (whether laboratory or nonlaboratory personnel), maintenance of POC equipment, oversight of proficiency and competency of operators, and compliance with requirements of regulatory agencies.
10. POC assays should provide quantitative results.
11. Manufacturers are encouraged to work closely with professional organizations to develop structured committees and establish quality performance specifications for new biomarkers.

No hs-cTn assays are available in a POC assay format for use in the USA.[94,95] Globally, POC testing is available for both hs-cTnI and hs-cTnT in China (ET Healthcare both cleared by cFDA). Some companies claim using plasma their POC assays to be hs,[96] however, evidence-based studies are lacking for whole blood and their ability to detect greater than 50%

of normal subjects for females. For both POC and central laboratory testing, and for practical considerations, anticoagulated whole blood or plasma appears to be the optimal specimen for rapid emergent processing. This eliminates the extra time needed for clotting and additional sample handling. Differences have been described among different plasmas, whole blood, and serum specimens for cTnI concentrations measurement by an individual assay. Both ethylenediaminetetraacetic acid (EDTA) and heparin are known to interfere with cTnI and cTnT antibody-binding affinity, as well as produce some matrix effect differences.[97,98] It is not recommended that different sample types are mixed during an individual's work-up when serial, timed samples are being drawn to rule in or out an MI. The interfering effect of blood tube additives has been extensively described in the Chapter 5.

Although clinicians and laboratorians continue to publish guidelines supporting TATs of less than 60 minutes for cTn, most studies demonstrate that TAT expectations are not being met in a large proportion of hospitals. While no recent studies have examined this question, as an example, the College of Pathologists (CAP) Q-Probe Survey study of 7020 cTn and 4368 CK-MB determinations in 159 hospitals demonstrated that median and 90th percentile TATs for troponin and CK-MB were as follows: 74.5 minutes, 129 minutes; and 82 minutes, 131 minutes, respectively.[99] Less than 25% of hospitals were able to meet the less than 60-minute TAT, representing the biomarker order-to-report time. However, data have shown that implementation of POC cTn testing can decrease TATs to less than 30 minutes in cardiology critical care and short-stay units.[95,100–105]

With the implementation of hs-cTn testing, which has been shown to provide early rule-out and early rule-in protocols within 3 hours of baseline blood sampling (discussed later in the chapter), the role of POC testing will need to be better defined. In medical centers where acceptable TATs are not being meet, where contemporary cTn assays are still utilized, the role of POC, especially in rural settings, may still be important whether a contemporary or hs assay is used. The following example, while 10 years old, demonstrates how an institution that addressed a poor TAT problem for a contemporary cTn assay improved laboratory services through cross-department cooperation.[101,106] Based at a 400-bed county hospital with 120,000 patient presentations per year through the ED, approximately 30,000 cTn orders per year were tested for both outpatients and the 1800 to 2000 patients admitted for short- or long-term care. A 2-month survey of the TAT for cTn showed a 90% TAT of 118 minutes. To better meet the published guideline of 60 minutes 100% of the time, the laboratory medical director, the emergency medicine staff whose primary responsibility involved ACS MI presentations, and the cardiology medical director who was responsible for the 11-bed cardiac 24- to 48-hour observation unit (cardiac short-stay unit [CSSU]), 28-bed telemetry unit, and 8-bed cardiac care unit (CCU) met and designed an ACS triage protocol. POC cTnI assay systems (using whole blood) were placed in the small ED laboratory, staffed by the clinical laboratory around the clock, in support of the hospital's level 1 trauma center. Additional POC assays were placed in the CSSU, in which 42 nurses were trained by the laboratories' POC coordinators. The flow of specimens was such that initial presentation cTnI requests ordered through the ED were analyzed in the ED laboratory, approximately 6000 to 8000 per year. TAT from the time of blood draw to the provider result report was less than 18 minutes, 100% of the time. The use of POC testing eliminated the additional time needed to transport and process specimens that would have been needed to analyze specimens in the central laboratory. Patients admitted to the hospital to rule in or rule out MI who were at low risk were admitted to the CSSU, where staff nurses provided less than 20-minute TAT 100% of the time from blood draw to results to provider. In the CSSU, in compliance with the hospital protocol that at least a 6-hour post-presentation sample had to remain normal for cTnI, two blood specimens, in addition to the ED presentation sample, were measured at 4 and 8 hours. The uniform timed ordering protocol for ruling out MI included four timed draws at 0, 4, 8, and 12 hours. In patients admitted to the telemetry unit or the CCU, a dedicated blood draw was tubed to the central laboratory, where specimens were given priority-testing status, and thus met a TAT of less than 60 minutes 98% of the time. During this process, it was recognized that POC testing was not cost-effective for patients in telemetry or CCU units. These were mostly patients at moderate to high risk in whom a clinical diagnosis had already been made; thus urgent cTn values were less necessary. The CSSU was successful in decreasing the length of stay in the unit by 0.8 day through implementation of POC testing, allowing triage to lower levels of care and/or discharge on a 24/7 basis. Although the direct cost per assay reagent increased from $3.83 (central laboratory) to $10.51 (POC testing), the overall cost to the patient decreased by more than $4000 per admission, primarily based on decreased bed charges from a costlier cardiac bed to a less expensive general medicine bed or to discharge. These data highlight the continued need for laboratory services and health care providers to work together to develop better processes to meet a TAT less than 60 minutes, as requested by physicians. A list of POC testing assays and manufacturers' analytical claims is found on the IFCC C-CB website.

It has been shown that a less-sensitive POC assay may miss a positive cTn value that would be detected as increased by a more-sensitive contemporary assay, as noted in Fig. 48.13. Further, POC cTnI assays also suffer from the lack of assay standardization. Fig. 48.14 shows that in a representative patient presenting with an evolving AMI, serial cTnI concentrations vary substantially between three POC assays versus a contemporary assay, with substantial variability in clinical sensitivities between assays. Contrary to the poor analytical sensitivity of POC assays, Fig. 48.15 shows that for an hs-cTnI assay, rising values are detected earlier even compared to a contemporary cTnI during the early course of an AMI. These data point to the need for clinical laboratories to replace contemporary cTn assays with hs-cTn assays.

Appropriate Use of Cardiac Troponin for the Diagnosis of Myocardial Infarction

With the increasing number of hs-cTnI and hs-cTnT assays cleared for clinical use globally (see IFCC website tables) numerous early rule-out and rule-in protocols are being used in clinical practice, including a recently published machine learning algorithm.[107] The Fourth Universal Definition of Myocardial Infarction (2018) provides an excellent expert consensus resource for navigating both the pathophysiology of myocardial infarction (MI) and the role of cTn monitoring,

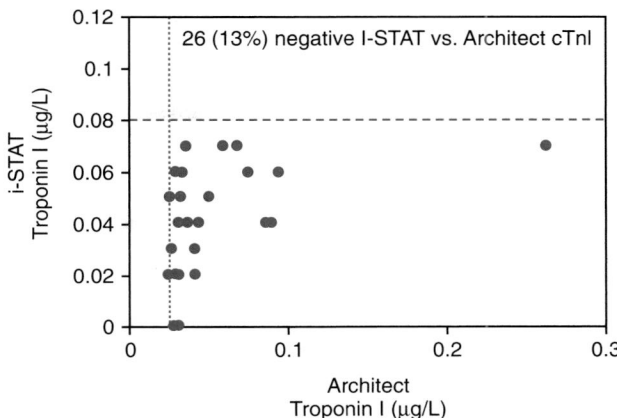

FIGURE 48.13 Scatterplot of i-STAT–negative and Architect-positive samples. The *dotted line* represents the 99th percentile cutoff for each instrument. *cTnI,* Cardiac troponin I. (Courtesy Jasbir Singh. From Singh J, Akbar MS, Adabag S. Discordance of cardiac troponin I assays on the point-of-care i-STAT and Architect assays from Abbott Diagnostics. *Clin Chim Acta* 2009;403: 259–60.)

complementing the IFCC-C-CB and AACC Academy analytical guidelines. The guideline provides new and updated information addressing the following pertinent to our chapter.

New:
1. Differentiation of MI from myocardial injury.
2. Highlighting peri-procedural myocardial injury after cardiac and noncardiac procedures as discrete from MI.
3. Use of cardiovascular magnetic resonance to define etiology of myocardial injury.
4. Use of computed tomographic coronary angiography in suspected MI.

Updated:
1. Type 1 MI: Emphasis on the causal relationship of plaque disruption with coronary atherothrombosis.
2. Type 2 MI: Settings with oxygen demand and supply imbalance unrelated to acute coronary atherothrombosis.
3. Type 2 MI: Relevance of presence or absence of CAD to prognosis and therapy.
4. Differentiation of myocardial injury from type 2 MI.
5. Types 4–5 MI: Emphasis on distinction between procedure-related myocardial injury and procedure-related MI. The need for a normal baseline value is a key element.
6. cTn: Analytical issues for cTns.
7. Emphasis on the benefits of high-sensitivity cTn assays.
8. Considerations relevant to the use of rapid rule-out and rule-in protocols for myocardial injury and myocardial infarction.
9. Issues related to specific diagnostic change ("delta") criteria for the use of cTns to detect or exclude acute myocardial injury.

International guidelines have suggested general times that cTn testing should be used to evaluate ruling in or out an AMI after a patient presents to an ED. It is not atypical for the laboratory to receive excessive cTn test orders well after a patient has been ruled in or ruled out for an MI, at a considerable unnecessary expense to the health care system. There is a substantial diversity across hospitals within the United States and internationally on how cTn testing is ordered, ranging from a hospital-wide serial order set such as at

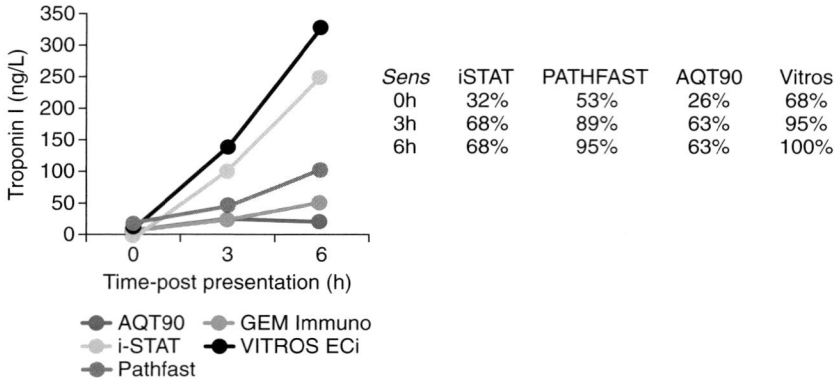

FIGURE 48.14 Serial cTnI findings for a representative myocardial infarction patient plotted as a function of time (hours) versus cTnI concentration for 5 cTnI assays; respective clinical sensitivities shown at baseline for assays. (From Palamalai V, Murakami MM, Apple FS. Diagnostic performance of four point of care cardiac troponin I assays to rule in and rule out acute myocardial infarction. *Clin Biochem* 2013;46:1631–5.)

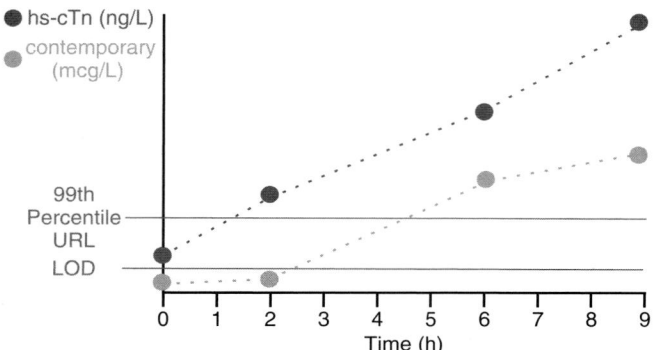

FIGURE 48.15 Cardiac troponin I kinetics comparing high-sensitivity and contemporary assays in a patient presenting with 30 minutes of an acute myocardial infarction. *hs-cTn,* High-sensitivity cardiac troponin; *LOD,* limit of detection; *URL,* upper reference limit.

presentation, 3, 6, and 12 hours for contemporary assays compared to 0/1 hour, 0/2 hours, 0/3 hours, and 6 hours for hs-cTn assays or to the ability to order cTn as a single test order at any time without any uniformity across a hospital/medical center. These orders are often complicated within teaching hospitals where both attending physicians and resident physicians may place multiple order sets, with substantial duplication and excessive cTn testing. Studies have made interesting observations in this regard.[110–112] First, in a monitored telemetry unit staffed by attending and resident physicians, an excessive number of cTnI tests were ordered after the diagnosis of both an MI (48% over testing) and no-MI (39% over testing) already had been established, with an average of approximately 6 to 7 cTn tests per diagnosis. Second, in the course of reviewing approximately 6000 cTn orders over 2 months in a 420-bed primary care hospital, providers (42% of whom were residents) acknowledged and overrode an electronic alert 97% of the time after a second set of serial cTn orders was placed, with 93% in non–ACS-related patients. Third, among patients with cTn increases, cardiologists are less likely than emergency medicine physicians to classify cTn orders as appropriate; discordance in appropriateness occurred most frequently when the diagnoses were

myocardial injury or type 2 myocardial infarction, and perceived appropriateness of cTn testing is influenced by subspecialty, diagnoses, and symptoms, with more research and guidance needed to refine the use of the test.

Overall, better education and monitoring of cTnI orders in the diagnosis or exclusion of MI is needed, with the need for electronic ordering review and/or electronic hard stop or manual discontinuation to be implemented when excessive testing is recognized. Proactive test use by laboratory professionals regarding cTn orders, working in concert with their clinical colleagues and information technology counterparts, should become a high priority in clinical laboratory practice to assist in health care savings.

Clinical Use of Cardiac Troponin

History

cTns have been available for clinical use since 1995, when the first cTn T (cTnT) assay was regulatory approved outside the USA. Since that time, enhanced diagnostics and particularly improved sensitivity in females led to more frequent and more accurate diagnosis of cardiovascular abnormalities, especially with the growing implementation of high-sensitivity cTn assays. Initial use of these assays was influenced in large part by CK-MB. CK-MB is substantially less sensitive and less cardiac specific than cTn, but because of its long use, it became entrenched in the thinking of clinicians and laboratorians. For this reason, perhaps, the first set of guidelines by the National Academy of Clinical Biochemistry (NACB) attempted to compromise between the use of these CK-MB and cTn using two cutoffs.[94] One cutoff was selected to be equivalent to values of CK-MB in the clinical identification of patients. This cutoff, known as the receiver operating characteristic (ROC) curve–derived cutoff value, considered CK-MB the standard. However, this cutoff did not take advantage of the increased analytical sensitivity of cTn values. A second cutoff was recommended for use at a lower level, the 97.5th percentile of a normal patient population, from subjects who were poorly clinically defined, above which patients were considered to have cardiac injury. But even patients with a classic history of AMI were designated as having "unstable angina with minimal myocardial necrosis." The guidelines followed extensive research demonstrating large numbers of patients with chest pain (roughly an additional

33%) whose prognoses in terms of subsequent frequency and timing of events were identical, and who had increased cTn values but normal CK-MB values.[113] These findings were documented despite the fact that the initial version of cTn assays was relatively insensitive compared with contemporary assays.

This concept of using prognosis to confirm diagnosis rapidly became the paradigm not only for cTn but for the validation of most other markers as well. It was not until 1999, when a task force empaneled by the ESC/ACC took issue with these guidelines, that the concept of using only one cutoff value was initiated. ESC/ACC guidelines suggested the use, not of the 97.5th percentile of a reference population but the 99th percentile, in recognition of increased sensitivity of cTn that led to many elevations that were difficult to explain. This had the potential benefit of reducing the overlap to 1% between those with disease and normal individuals.[38] It was conceptually important because even by this time, it was clear that enhanced sensitivity of cTn was leading to the identification of a substantial number of patients in whom the pathophysiologic cause of cardiac injury (see later sections) could not be determined. This is often the case when one moves from a relatively insensitive measure to one that has substantially greater sensitivity (i.e., when one uncovers new diagnostically and prognostically important increases).[113–115] Nonetheless, clinicians had difficulty understanding this because such elevations had not been described previously and the pathophysiology was obscure. This problem has been revisited today as hs-cTn assays become increasingly sensitive and replace contemporary cTn assays. The ESC/ACC biochemical group at that time also recommended that the 99th percentile should be measurable with excellent imprecision and suggested, not mandated, a criterion of a total 10% CV or less at the 99th percentile. The group did not, however, recommend that if assays did not reach that level of precision, the decision values should be raised above the 99th percentile value. Unfortunately, this was the extrapolation of some, and it led to even greater heterogeneity in how cTn values were interpreted.

Some individuals persisted in using the NACB recommendations, some used the ESC/ACC recommendations, and some because of fear of false-positive results caused by imprecision employed a value higher than the 99th percentile, usually at the level of the 10% CV value. Add to this the fact that local laboratories often felt the need (appropriately) to validate the assays in their own hands and come up with different values, and one can see how the use of cTn values became fragmented and idiosyncratic. This problem also led to tremendous heterogeneity in the published literature and confusion on the part of clinicians.[116–118]

It is now very clear that normal hs-cTn values are substantially lower than concentrations that are being reported for healthy individuals by contemporary assays. The reported concentrations in healthy individuals often represent "noise" (<LOD) in the contemporary assays. hs-cTn assays are growing worldwide, including in the United States, to have the ability to measure healthy individuals' low concentrations accurately. For the past 2 years, the IFCC C-CB has posted and revised quarterly updates provided by manufacturers, current hs-cTn assays, along with POC and contemporary assays. A wealth of clinical information has made it clear that for contemporary assays, the 99th percentile value is the key value to use when measuring cardiac cTn.[70,119–125] Any value above the 99th percentile should be considered abnormal,

indicative of myocardial injury. Concerns about false-positive results induced by such criteria should be minimal because assuming adequate quality assurance of the assays, even reduced imprecision should not lead to false-positive results provided cTn is measured in two serial samples. Usually reduced imprecision simply impairs the sensitivity of the assay. Statistical modeling of this issue suggests that the clinical impact of using even an imprecise assay is negligible with regard to false-positive results.

For this reason, along with the clinical data, the criteria in all guideline papers now include use of the 99th percentile, revised in 2018 from an overall URL to the use of individual, sex-specific 99th percentile URLs for males and females.[65] Although some studies have suggested a return to the use of the 97.5th percentile value for high-sensitivity cTn assays, this is unlikely to occur unless important clinical reasons for such a change can be demonstrated.[2,84,126] Once one recognizes that the 99th percentile is the only criterion for abnormality, one can progress to understanding how to use hs-cTn assays with sex-specific URLs in a variety of clinical situations for early rule out, early rule in, and risk assessment. Numerous publications have clearly demonstrated this point, which will be discussed in the following section.

Use of Cardiac Troponin for the Diagnosis of Acute Myocardial Infarction

AMI is a state characterized by abnormalities between nutrient perfusion and myocardial oxygen consumption. It is usually diagnosed when abnormalities in coronary flow at least in part contribute to the pathogenesis of cardiac injury. Because of the high sensitivity and specificity of cTn for the heart, cTn has become the cornerstone of the diagnosis of MI (see Boxes 48.2 and 48.3). As shown in Fig. 48.16 high-sensitivity cTn assays eliminate the noise of contemporary (and POC) assays, providing greater reliability of true measurement of cTn at the 99th percentile upper reference interval, and is now the standard assay of use in all clinical and research laboratories if available. An increased concentration of cTn greater than the 99th percentile URL is required in the

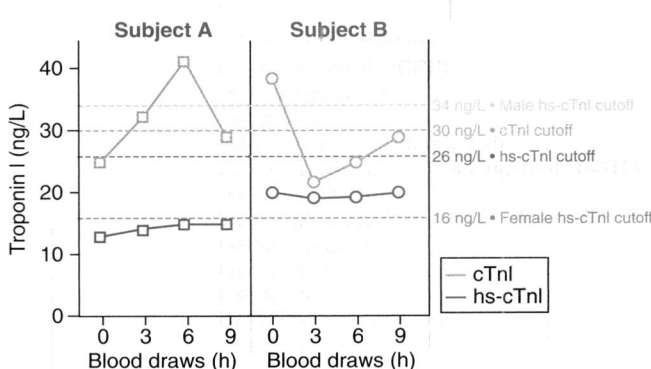

FIGURE 48.16 Representative serial cardiac troponin I *(cTnI)* concentrations in two patients measured by a contemporary and a high-sensitivity cTnI *(hs-cTnI)* (with sex-specific cutoffs) assay demonstrating analytical "noise" of the contemporary assay. (From Sandoval Y, Smith SW, Schulz KM, Murakami MM, Love SA, Nicholson J, Apple FS. Diagnosis of type 1 and type 2 myocardial infarction using a high-sensitivity cardiac troponin I assay with gender-specific 99th percentiles based on the Third Universal Definition of Myocardial Infarction classification system. *Clin Chem* 2015;61:657–63.)

appropriate clinical setting along with a rising or falling pattern for the diagnosis of AMI. With the growing use of high-sensitivity assays, earlier and more accurate diagnoses for ruling in and ruling out MI are being made within 1 to 3 hours of first blood draw compared to contemporary and POC assays. At A Glace 3 shows schematics of representative strategies to consider for early rule in and rule out based on implementation of hs-cTnI testing. Specifics of the MI definition are as follows.

The clinical substrate (usually risk factors for AMI in the patient) is key. An increased cTn value is not synonymous with the diagnosis of MI. First, risk factors and the presentation (most often chest discomfort) must be compatible with the diagnosis. At times, imaging, whether performed at the time of intervention by angiography or thereafter, may provide proof of the substrate.[2,78,87,127] Many clinical situations can mimic AMI,[128–132] the most common of which is myocarditis. Apical ballooning is another. Because of the increased sensitivity of cTn, clinicians need to be astute to the possibility that a given elevation in cTn, even with a rising pattern suggesting that it is acute, may not be due to ischemic heart disease (see Box 48.1). In addition, many groups such as women, the elderly, and diabetics can present atypically so interdigitating the biomarker information with the clinical is essential.[2] This is conceptually difficult for some clinicians because when CK-MB, which was reasonably insensitive, was used, most substantive elevations were associated with coronary heart disease, albeit not all.

Acute events leading to cardiac injury (see Box 48.1) usually will manifest a changing pattern of values.[2,132–138] The rationale for this is that as assays have become more analytically sensitive, it has become clear that elevations of cTn can exist chronically.[56,139–149] The most overt case of this is seen in patients with renal failure.[139] This is also the pattern manifest when artifactual increases occur as the result of analytical problems caused by interferences from human anti-mouse antibodies and heterophilic antibodies in the blood of some patients.[150,151] However, hs-cTn assays do not appear prone to as many analytical problems as early generations of assays. Nevertheless, a list of assay interferences involving hemolysis and biotin as potential interferents that is assay dependent is available on the IFCC C-CB website.[152] Although patients with chronic elevations (not those with artifactual causes) are at long-term high risk, they are not necessarily at high risk over the short term. For this reason, the guidelines groups have advocated the need for a rising pattern of cTn values in patients who present early after the onset of symptoms, because such increases usually are indicative of an acute process. However, the acute process may not be AMI. Whether AMI is present is a clinical decision. When cTn values are not rising, one might seriously question whether acute disease of any kind is present or whether the elevations are of a more chronic nature. Care is necessary to ensure that one does not miss individuals who come in late after the onset of symptoms, whose cTn values may be near peak values, or whose values are on the long persistent tail of the time-concentration curve. They may appear not to have a changing pattern of values because they are near the peak (that can range from 12 to 48 hours) of the time-concentration curve or on the gradual downslope. This may occur in greater than 20% of patients.

With hs assays, there will be more AMIs that are not due to plaque rupture (so called supply-demand type 2 AMI, which has its own ICD-10 code) because these usually elaborate less

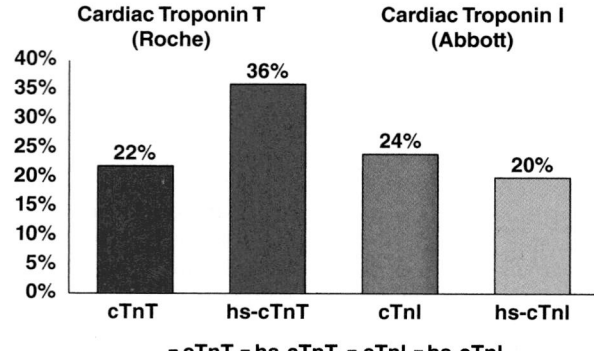

FIGURE 48.17 Expected measurement impacts from change from a contemporary to high-sensitivity assays in clinical practice. (Modified from Reichlin T, Cullen L, Parsonage WA, Greenslade J, Twerenbold R, Moehring B, et al. Two-hour algorithm for triage toward rule-out and rule-in of acute myocardial infarction using high-sensitivity cardiac troponin T. *Am J Med* 2015;128:369–79 (cTnT) and Sandoval Y, Smith SW, Thordsen SE, Bruen CA, Carlson MD, Dodd KW, et al. Diagnostic performance of high sensitivity compared to contemporary cardiac troponin I for the diagnosis of acute myocardial infarction. *Clin Chem* 2017;63:1594–604.)

cTn than plaque rupture events (type 1 AMI).[93,153–156] However, the criteria for a rising and/or falling pattern do not differ.[156] These will occur more frequently in women than in men. There are good data that the use of sex-specific cutoff values with hs-cTnI assays (limited data for hs-cTnT assays) improve the diagnosis of these patients.[124] While switching from a contemporary cTnT (fourth generation) to the hs-cTnT or Gen 5 cTnT assays is associated with an increased number of patients with the diagnosis of MI, this is not the case for replacing a contemporary to a hs-cTnI assay, as shown in Fig. 48.17.

The guidelines distinguish five types of MI (see Box 48.3); two will be considered here because they both manifest with chest discomfort and increased biomarkers. One (type 1 MI) is the so-called spontaneous, or "wild type," in which acute plaque rupture leads to some degree of thrombosis, or an episode in which platelet accretion occurs on a plaque, leading to thrombosis.[2,87] The second type (type 2 MI) includes coronary abnormalities with possible supply-demand imbalance, vasospasm, or endothelial dysfunction, which provides evidence of myocardial injury.[156,157]

Individuals with spontaneous AMI can have STEMI or non-STEMI as indicated by the ECG pattern they manifest.[2,19,28] Data indicate that immediate treatment aimed at opening the occluded artery is mandatory for patients with STEMI. This should be done based on the ECG pattern alone, even before biomarker values become available to assist with diagnosis. Opening of the artery is currently done with primary PCI and/or thrombolytic agents. The former is preferred when the two are available in similar time frames. With prompt coronary recanalization, the amount of myocardium lost is minimized and mortality is reduced.[18] It should be noted that coronary recanalization increases the rapidity of biomarker release, and thus the rate of rise of the time-concentration curve is increased and the time to peak values is shortened.

A non-STEMI is less often associated with total coronary occlusion and usually is identified by ECG changes, which show not ST segment elevation but rather ST segment depression or T-wave changes. Given the sensitivity of hs-cTn for this diagnosis, the ECG is even at times totally normal. Patients who present with chest pain as a result of CAD should have risk factors, an appropriate presentation, or imaging evidence of this syndrome. Patients with an increased cTn, and the recommended 99th percentile URL are known to have more severe coronary heart disease than individuals without increased cTns. Likely for this reason they also have more procoagulant activity. Multiple intervention studies have shown that these patients benefit from aggressive anticoagulation, including heparin (the data for low-molecular-weight heparin are much stronger than the data for unfractionated heparin), glycoprotein IIb/IIIa antiplatelet agents, and an early invasive strategy consisting of PCI or coronary artery bypass grafting (CABG). Use of these strategies in patients without increased cTn values has been shown to be of no benefit and, in some trials, has actually proved detrimental.[23] For these patients, expeditious but not necessarily immediate coronary interventions are suggested.[18] Studies using hs-cTn assays have demonstrated that within the sex-specific reference interval for hs-cTn assays (Fig. 48.18A and B) as has been documented

for patients above the 99th percentiles Fig. 48.19, increasing levels of risk are associated with increasing cTn concentrations.[92] However, given the increased frequency of type 2 MIs, it is unclear that invasive intervention will be necessary in all such patients. However, it is now well documented that among patients presenting to the EDs with an increased cTn, those with type 2 MI and myocardial injury from non-MI pathophysiology are at greater risk of adverse outcomes compared to type 1 MIs (Fig. 48.20).[93] Importantly, although patients with nonSTEMI who have an increased cTn value benefit from an invasive strategy, those who do not, as a group, do worse.[22,31]

Not all patients have easily identifiable culprit lesions in which to intervene, and this explains some apparent spontaneous AMIs without severe CAD.[27,128,138,157–160] These patients, often women, may have endothelial dysfunction, coronary vasospasm, coronary dissection, or some other transient process that has resolved before investigation. These patients have type 2 MI according to the guidelines. This group might also include those individuals who have fixed but stable CAD but have some degree of damage as a result of excessive

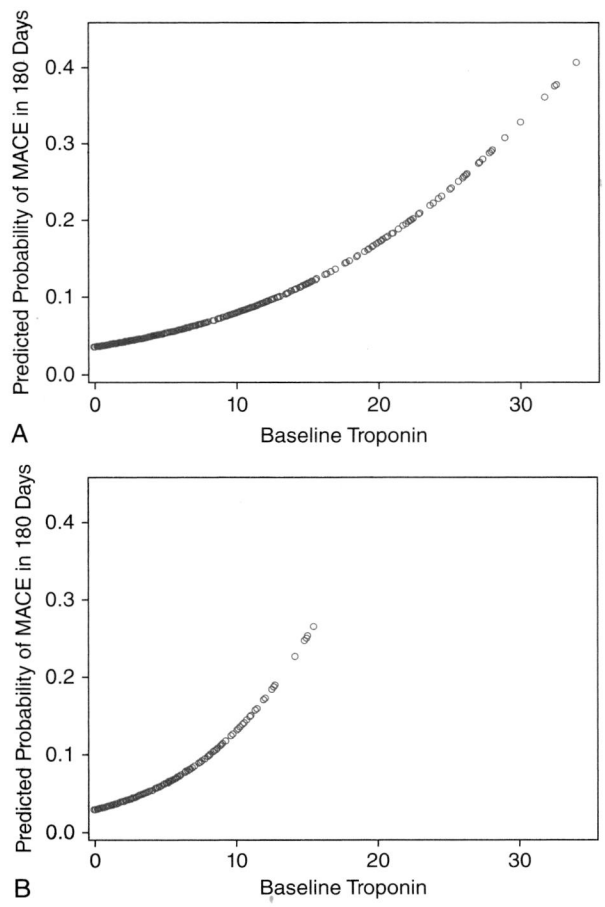

FIGURE 48.18 Predicted probabilities of 180-day MACE in relationship to baseline hs-cTnI concentrations as a continuous variable in relationship to 180-day major adverse cardiac event (MACE) for men (A) and women (B). (From Sandoval Y, Smith SW, MD, Sexter A, Gunsolus IL, Schulz K, Apple FS. Clinical features and outcomes of emergency department patients with high-sensitivity cardiac troponin I concentrations within normal sex-specific reference intervals. *Circulation* 2019;139:1753–5.)

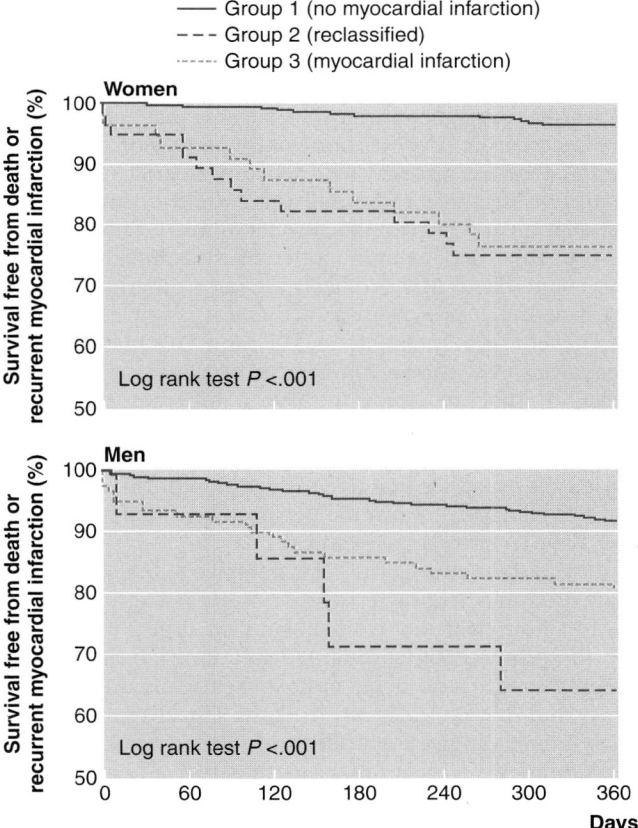

FIGURE 48.19 Survival free from death or recurrent myocardial infarction (MI) in women and men with suspected acute coronary syndrome. Outcomes are shown for women and men with no MI *(solid line)* and with MI *(dashed red line)*, in which both assays were concordant, and for those reclassified as having MI using the high-sensitivity assay with sex-specific thresholds *(dashed pink line)*. (From Shah AS, Griffiths M, Lee KK, McAllister DA, Hunter AL, Ferry AV, et al. High sensitivity cardiac troponin and the under-diagnosis of myocardial infarction in women: prospective cohort study. *BMJ* 2015;350:g7873.)

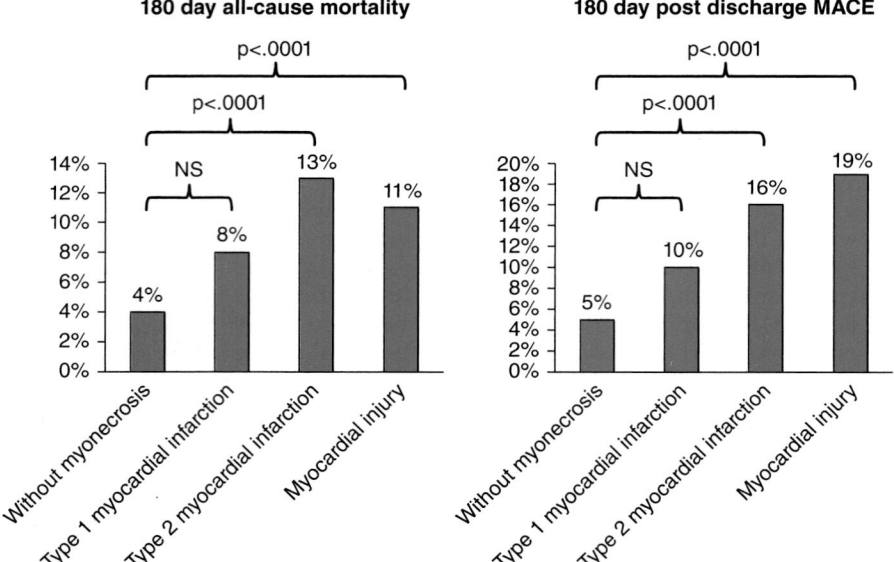

FIGURE 48.20 Adverse 2-year outcomes compared in patients with type 1 MI, type 2 MI, non-MI myocardial injury patients, and patients without myocardial injury; with increased cardiac troponin in about 1/3 of patients. *MI*, Myocardial infarction; *NS*, not significant. (From Sandoval Y, Smith SW, Thordsen SE, Bruen CA, Carlson MD, Dodd KW, et al. Type 1 and 2 myocardial infarction and myocardial injury: clinical transition to high-sensitivity cardiac troponin I. *Am J Med* 2017;130:1431–9.)

myocardial oxygen consumption, such as that caused by severe tachycardia, hypotension, or hypertension. Coronary arteries that are diseased tend to vasoconstrict rather than dilating in response to stimuli that would normally evoke vasodilation and increases in coronary flow.[159] These patients are probably fundamentally different from individuals who have spontaneous MIs and likely are not a subgroup that has nearly as much procoagulant activity; it is unclear whether they benefit from interventional therapy. This may be one of the reasons why women who tend to have more severe endothelial dysfunction seem to have a different profile.[27,158] Nonetheless, depending on the specific study reviewed, 10 to 30% of patients may not have an identifiable lesion that has caused the event, leading to consideration of this alternative pathophysiology.[159] From the perspective of diagnosis, however, the cTn criteria are identical.

Distinctions among the MI types have to be made on the basis of clinical characteristics and other diagnostic studies. It is now clear that women can have type 2 MI secondary to spontaneous coronary dissection.[26] It used to be thought that this occurred almost exclusively during pregnancy, but that is clearly not the case. This diagnosis can be easily missed angiographically and is associated in at least half of patients with coronary tortuosity[161] and evidence of fibromuscular dysplasia in other vascular beds.[162] Preliminary data suggest that unless these patients are hemodynamically compromised or have total coronary occlusion, a strategy of watchful waiting rather than intervention may be preferred.[163]

Other types of MIs are recognized.[2] First, one type does not use biomarkers at all. This includes patients who may present classically with both chest pain and ECG changes but succumb either before blood tests can be obtained or before enough time has elapsed for the circulating concentration of cTn to exceed the 99th percentile. Two other types of MIs have been designated; these are related to PCI and CABG and will be covered later under "Special Situations."

Operationalization of a Changing Pattern of Cardiac Troponin Values

This can be a challenging area but has been substantially resolved with early measurements using hs-cTn assays that eliminate small changes in values due to analytical causes. In general, two values are different if they differ by more than 2.77 standard deviations (SDs) (assuming the variances are comparable at the two concentrations).[120] Ideally, both analytical and biological variation would be included in calculation of the SDs.[77,164] Unfortunately, analysis of biological variation requires studies of stable subjects, and only hs-cTn assays can provide data on healthy people. Most analysis has focused on the use of data on analytical (total) imprecision alone. At high concentrations greater than 99th percentiles of cTns, the CV are 5 to 7%, so a difference of 20% is unlikely to be attributable to measurement imprecision. But as values begin to approach the low concentrations between the LOD and the 99th percentile, analytical %CV increases with contemporary assays, making the relative difference between two consecutive values prone to increases by random error alone.[120] Local analysis of imprecision should be used to guide interpretation of differences in results for consecutive samples, with larger percentage changes necessary to suggest real change at very low levels of cTn. Defining a consistent period for analysis is also key to an accurate approach to this analysis. High-sensitivity assays improve this problem; their excellent imprecision at low cTn concentrations (10 to 20% CV at or above the LOD) make it possible to calculate a reference change value (RCV).[77,120,164,165] hs-cTn assays show RCV values (biological variation) ranging from 50 to 85% (as

AT A GLANCE

Strategies for ruling in and ruling out acute MI with contemporary and high-sensitivity cTn assays.

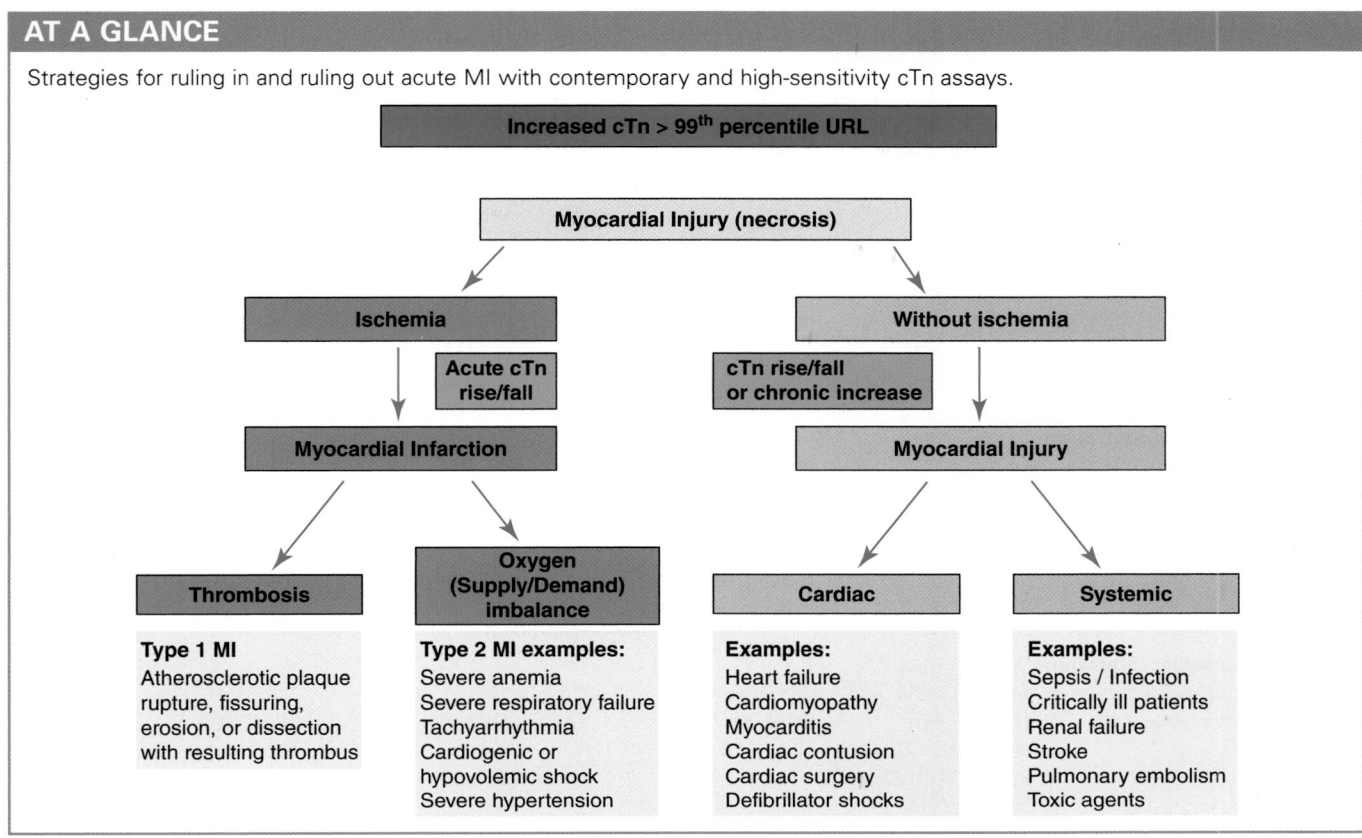

TABLE 48.2 Short-Term Analytical and Biological Variation of High-Sensitivity Cardiac Troponin Assays

	Abbott	Beckman	Roche (E170)	Siemens	Singulex
CV_A (%)	13.8	14.5	7.8	13.0	8.3
CV_I (%)	15.2	6.1	15.0	12.9	9.7
CV_G (%)	70.5	34.8	NA	12.3	57
Index of individuality	0.22	0.46	NA	0.11	0.21
RCV (%)	NA	NA	47.0	NA	NA
RCV increase (%)	69.3	63.8	NA	57.5	46.0
RCV decrease (%)	−40.9	−38.9	NA	−36.5	−32.
Within-subject mean (ng/L)	3.5	4.9	NA	5.5	2.8

CV_A, Analytical variation; CV_G, between-subject biological variation; CV_I, within-subject biological variation; *hs-cTnI*, high-sensitivity cTnI; *NA*, not available; *RCV*, increase and decrease percentages refer to nonparametric data and are log-transformed; *RCV*, percentage applies to the parametric data; *RCV*, reference change value.
From Apple FS, Collinson PO. Analytical characteristics of high-sensitivity cardiac troponin assays. *Clin Chem* 2012;58:54–61.

shown in Tables 48.2 and 48.3).[77,166] Although it is now clear that these values may work well when the baseline value is near the 99th percentile URL, when the baseline value is elevated, these values are less sensitive. Accordingly, for example, a recommendation (expert opinion) has been made for hs-cTnT to use a 50% change near the 99th percentile upper reference interval and a 20% change when the baseline value is elevated.[167] Similar percent change recommendations are now available for hs-cTnI assays, but can differ by assay as they are not standardized, as it appears different studies for different hs-assays may use different percent changes. Others have advocated for the use of absolute concentration change criteria if examining changes within the reference limits. In general, these are similar to percentage criteria when baseline values are near the 99th percentile URL but are much lower when the baseline values are elevated. It appears that these values provide better accuracy, especially when the baseline value is elevated, compared to percent criteria.[121,152,168–170] What is known is that individual hs-cTn assays will need to develop their own change values because there will not be a universal value that will be applicable to all hs-cTnI assays. Early clinical studies in this area often used convenience cohorts that may have had incomplete sample sets, used insensitive gold standards, and lacked early patients.

TABLE 48.3 **Use of Single hs-cTnI at Presentation Alone and in Combination With a Normal 12-Lead ECG for the Diagnosis of Acute Myocardial Infarction, Overall and by Type 1 and 2 MI**

Parameter	LOD (1.9 ng/L)		High-STEACS (<5 ng/L)	
	Baseline hs-cTnI < LOD	Baseline hs-cTnI< LOD and Normal ECG	Baseline hs-cTnI <5 ng/L	Baseline hs-cTnI <5 ng/L and Normal ECG
Acute Myocardial Infarction				
Proportion qualifying	444/1631 (27)	254/1631 (16)	812/1631 (50)	406/1631 (25)
Proportion of missed MIs	2/170 (1.2)	1/170 (0.6)	9/170 (5.3)	2/170 (1.2)
NPV	99.6 (98.9–100)	99.6 (98.8–100)	98.9 (98.2–99.6)	99.5 (98.8–100)
Sensitivity	98.8 (97.2–100)	99.4 (98.3–100)	94.7 (91.3–98.1)	98.8 (97.2–100)
PPV	14.2 (12.2–16.1)	12.3 (10.5–14.0)	19.7 (16.9–22.4)	13.7 (11.8–15.6)
Specificity	30.3 (27.9–32.6)	17.3 (15.4–19.3)	55.0 (52.4–57.5)	27.7 (25.4–30.0)
Type 1 Myocardial Infarction				
Proportion qualifying	443/1529 (29)	254/1529 (17)	807/1529 (53)	405/1529 (27)
Proportion of missed MIs	1/68 (1.5)	1/68 (1.5)	4/68 (5.9)	1/68 (1.5)
NPV	99.8 (99.3–100)	99.6 (98.8–100)	99.5 (99.0–100)	99.8 (99.3–100)
Sensitivity	98.5 (95.7–100)	98.5 (95.7–100)	94.1 (88.5–99.7)	98.5 (95.7–100)
PPV	6.2 (4.7–7.6)	5.3 (4.0–6.5)	8.9 (6.8–10.9)	6.0 (4.6–7.3)
Specificity	30.3 (27.9–32.6)	17.3 (15.4–19.3)	5.5 (5.2–5.8)	27.7 (25.4–30.0)
Type 2 Myocardial Infarction				
Proportion qualifying	443/1563 (28)	253/1563 (16)	808/1563 (52)	405/1563 (26)
Proportion of missed MIs	1/102 (0.98)	0/102 (0)	5/102 (4.9)	1/102 (0.98)
NPV	99.8 (99.3–100)	100 (100–100)	99.4 (98.8–99.9)	99.8 (99.3–100)
Sensitivity	99.0 (97.1–100)	100 (100–100)	95.1 (90.9–99.3)	99.0 (97.1–100)
PPV	9.0 (7.3–10.7)	7.8 (6.3–9.2)	12.9 (10.5–15.2)	8.7 (7.1–10.4)
Specificity	30.3 (27.8–32.6)	17.3 (15.4–19.3)	55.0 (52.4–57.5)	27.7 (25.4–30.0)

Values are number percentage or percent, with 95% CI.

ECG, Electrocardiogram; *High-STEACS,* high-sensitivity troponin in the evaluation of patients with suspected acute coronary syndrome; *LOD,* limit of detection; *MI,* myocardial infraction; *NPV,* negative predictive value; *PPV,* positive predictive value.

From Sandoval Y, Smith SW, Love SA, Sexter A, Schulz K, Apple FS. Single high-sensitivity cardiac troponin I to rule out myocardial infarction. *Am J Med* 2017;130:1076–83.

Special Situations With Acute Myocardial Infarction

After Percutaneous Coronary Intervention

It has long been appreciated that interventions done on the coronary arteries can result in the release from heart muscle of biomarkers indicative of cardiac injury.[2,171] For this reason, a variety of criteria have been promulgated, starting years ago with CK-MB. It was shown initially that elevations of CK-MB that occurred after the procedure were highly predictive of adverse events over the long term. These findings were difficult to explain because the amount of injury involved often was very minor but was nonetheless easy to document with sophisticated techniques such as cardiac magnetic resonance imaging (cMRI). However, controversy about the mechanisms continued and a large number are being hypothesized. The advent of cTn biomarkers has rendered this issue far less complex. Patients who have elevations of circulating cTn and who present with acute coronary problems have much more severe abnormalities in coronary anatomy than those who do not have cTn elevations.[172] In recent studies, the baseline cTn value has been added to the analysis of these post-PCI elevations.[2,173–175] This was done for many years, but not with assays that measured cTn concentrations even close to the 99th percentile. Accordingly, it is only recently that the data have confirmed several important conceptual issues.

The first concept is that a vast majority of patients with significant elevations (threefold to fivefold increase in CK-MB

or cTn) that in the past were associated with an adverse prognosis are those with increased cTn values at baseline. This usually (although not always) is indicative of an acute presentation and therefore a rising pattern of values. In the setting with a rising pattern of values, it is hard to know whether one should attribute the increases to the PCI or to the initial insult.[175] Nonetheless, when one incorporates the baseline value into the analysis, most of the prognostic significance of the post procedure cTn values is ablated.[173–175] Data suggest that it is only at an elevation of cTn at baseline that marked post-procedure elevations in cTn are apt to be frequently found, suggesting that in most instances at least a blend of the two processes occurs. These issues have been confounded not only by failure to use appropriate cutoffs for cTn, but by the use of insensitive cTn assays. More recent guidelines clarify this circumstance substantially by indicating that if one has an increased cTn at baseline before PCI, the diagnosis of post-PCI injury is confounded and cannot be made.[2] Thus a normal baseline cTn is required in almost all instances to identify procedure-related myocardial injury. If the baseline cTn is increased, subsequent increases may or may not be able to be attributable to the procedure itself and a diagnosis of post-PCI injury cannot be made with absolute confidence.

Marked elevations, as indicated previously, are uncommon but can occur. When they do occur, they are rarely of cardiovascular importance, in the sense that the more marked elevations are easily presaged by clinical information at the time of the procedure. Thus post-PCI cTn values add very little that is new. In addition, it is unclear whether patients have an adverse cardiovascular prognosis over time. In the most recent analysis done by using the most appropriate cut-off values and contemporary cTn assays, borderline statistical significance was attributed to post-PCI elevations.[174] However, most events that did occur were noted during procedures in patients who had severe underlying noncardiac comorbidities and therefore underwent palliative procedures. The event rate, if patients with non–cardiac-related subsequent complications are excluded, would not have been of statistical importance, even if their inclusion were of only borderline significance. Thus it now appears that collection of this information after PCI is not necessary. Recent data suggest that values even modestly below the 99th percentile upper reference interval have important prognostic significance, presaging in our opinion the likelihood that with hs-cTn assays, this effect will be strengthened and the prognostic impact of post-PCI values attenuated still further.

Nonetheless, criteria still exist for these occasional patients who may have post-PCI injury. The appropriate cutoff cTn value is unclear, but it is clear that very few patients will reach the marked fivefold elevation previously advocated if the baseline cTn is not increased.[2,173] This is likely to change, however, with hs-cTn assays. If cTn is increased post-PCI more than fivefold, with a normal baseline cTn value assumed, the patient can be diagnosed as having had a periprocedural MI if they have had symptoms or have ECG changes and/or had complications of the procedure.[2] No specific therapy is mandated. Regarding biomarker changes that occur after reperfusion of an occluded vessel after PCI or thrombolytic therapy in AMI patients, greater than twofold increases in biomarkers occur within 90 minutes of reperfusion, the rate of increase of biomarkers within the first 4 hours separates reperfused from nonreperfused patients, and after myocardial reperfusion in AMI patients, washouts of all biomarkers parallel each other.[176–180] However, increased washout does not define the level of reperfusion and cannot be used to define a post-PCI AMI.

One unique subset needs to be considered, and that is the small group of patients who may have chronic preprocedural elevations in cTn. These individuals will manifest a rising pattern, albeit from an increased baseline, when they have events, including post-PCI events. Accordingly, what has been suggested is that the criteria used for reinfarction of an increased value of 20% or more should be used to define post-PCI infarction in this group.[87]

Post–Coronary Artery Bypass Graft Myocardial Infarction

Abundant data indicate that after cardiac surgery patients have elevations in cardiac cTn. Indeed, in the vast majority of studies, such elevations are of prognostic importance—the higher the elevation, the worse the prognosis.[181–183] However, the underlying propensity for elevation is moderated in part by the details of the procedure. For example, procedures that are done off cardiopulmonary bypass evoke less cTn release,[181] as might be expected, because they cause less direct cardiac injury. In addition, a relationship has been noted between the duration of cross-clamp time and the amount of biomarker elaborated, the temperature of the cardioplegia, and the duration of the procedure. Most of the injury as assessed from cMRI studies is subendocardial and often apical. Higher post-CABG biomarker

values are associated with transmural injury.[184,185] Thus procedures that are longer, such as those that include valve replacement, are very likely to evoke more cardiac damage than those that are shorter. Accordingly, finding a single value that separates all of these different subsets is impossible. Therefore most recent guidelines have elected not to try to define separate criteria for subsets of these procedures, but instead have preferred to define a single cutoff that can be used for all the situations already described for which ancillary criteria need to be employed. Most recent guidelines support a ten-fold increase in cTn after the procedure and add additional criteria such as ECG changes, changes with imaging, and the development of new regional wall-motion abnormalities.[2]

The value of such an approach is that it allows use of a single cTn cutoff. The downside of the approach is that this cutoff lacks some precision when it comes to the types of procedures performed. It might be better to devise specific criteria for each subset of the procedures. This is an extensive task because of multiple variations in the way in which cardiac surgery is done. Nonetheless, the key concept is that the prognostic impact of increased cTn concentrations is related to the magnitude of the increase. Unfortunately, because of the complexity of these considerations, no one has been able to define a value at which increases in cTn can be attributed to a specific coronary-related event such as graft or native vessel occlusion.[186] Thus although the aggregate amount of marker that is released is prognostic (for both CK-MB and cTn), it does not distinguish the mechanism of injury. The guidelines nonetheless recommend the diagnosis of post-CABG AMI if there is a 10-fold increase in cTn in conjunction with additional imaging or clinical features of AMI.[2] Similar criteria are recommended for other invasive procedures such as transcatheter aortic valve replacement.

Pediatrics

Pediatricians are often asked to assist in evaluation of a baby or child with a cTn increase. The first question is what clinical rationale was used to obtain a cTn measurement. Studies have shown that measurements of cTn can be higher during the first 2 weeks of age and throughout adolescence, in comparison to established 99th percentile upper reference intervals for adults.[187,188] Whether this reflects evidence of cardiac necrosis is not always clear. However, acute injury should be able to be determined with confidence if rising cTn concentrations are documented with serial draws and the increased cTn concentrations fit the clinical presentation. An isolated single increase or chronic increases that may not show rising or falling values need to be clinically evaluated carefully because results may suggest that in children the 99th percentile may not be a reliable index of silent cardiac disease but rather may be indicating low-grade intercurrent illness. Additional studies are needed in this clinical area as hs-assays become more prevalently used in pediatric practice.

Evaluating Possible Acute Myocardial Infarction
Evaluating Possible Acute Myocardial Infarction: The Importance of Clinical Context With Monitoring High-Sensitivity Cardiac Troponin in Low-Risk, Intermediate-Risk, and High-Risk Patients

The clinical presentation of patients with possible AMI can be highly variable, as indicated earlier, and the interpretation of an elevated cTn value is very different in low-risk patients than in high-risk patients. Implementation of hs-cTn assays in clinical practice impart several important clinical improvements to the triage, management, and risk assessment of patients presenting with symptoms suggestive of ACS and or myocardial injury, as the following reviews.

First, recent findings from a randomized, controlled trial evaluated the effect of implementing hs-cTn testing and the recommendations of the Universal Definition of Myocardial Infarction. The study demonstrated that implementation of hs-cTn testing leads to a disproportionate increase in type 2 MI and myocardial injury. The authors opined that (a) clinicians should consider investigations to define coronary or structural heart disease in patients with type 2 myocardial infarction and myocardial injury, and (b) the risk of future cardiovascular events should be evaluated on an individual patient basis using all available clinical information, and that secondary prevention therapies should be considered on a case-to-case basis with the aim of reducing future cardiovascular risk even though the findings were not associated with consistent increases in treatment or improved outcomes.[189]

Second, hs-cTn assays are extremely sensitive for myocardial injury, and that myocardial injury does not always equate acute MI. Using a machine learning tool designated MI3 that incorporates variations in cTn concentrations by age, sex, and time between samples in patients with suspected MI has been shown to improve the assessment of risk for individual patients and objective assessment of the likelihood of MI, which can be used to identify low- and high-risk patients who may benefit from earlier clinical decisions.[190]

Third, a major role for hs-cTn testing is to assist in early identification of patients unlikely to have acute MI ("rule-out"), and to help identify patients with acute myocardial injury, in whom the diagnosis of acute MI is possible ("rule-in"). Strategies and/or pathways have been developed to help identify, among those in whom MI has been excluded, those whose risk of adverse events during follow-up is very low.[191]

Role of Single Baseline hs-cTn Measurement Predicated on the Limit of Detection

Numerous studies have shown that a single hs-cTn measurement less than LOD identifies patients unlikely to have acute MI. These studies have mainly been focused on both hs-cTnI and hs-cTnT assays. In a systematic review involving 19 international cohorts, Chapman and colleagues[192] reported that a single hs-cTnI (Abbott) measurement less than LOD (2 ng/L) offered an NPV of 99.8% and diagnostic sensitivity of 100%, with about 14% identified as low risk. Similarly, using hs-cTnT (Roche), in a collaborative meta-analysis involving 11 cohorts and 9241 patients, Pickering and colleagues[193] reported that a nonischemic ECG plus a single hs-cTnT less than LOD (5 ng/L) classified ~31% of patients as low risk with a pooled diagnostic sensitivity of 98.7% and NPV of 99.3%. Similar data has emerged for other assays, with a single baseline hs-cTnI less than 2 ng/L measured with the Access hs-cTnI, (Beckman Coulter) showing excellent diagnostic sensitivity and NPV.[194] For strategies using a single measurement, timing of the onset of symptoms and caution in early presenters is warranted, with a 2nd measurement recommended in those that present very early after symptom onset.[195–197] The Limit of Detection of Troponin and ECG Discharge (LOD) (ISRCTN86184521) study is an ongoing

multicenter, randomized controlled trial (primary endpoint: successful early discharge from hospital within 4 hours of arrival without major ad verse cardiac events within 30 days) that should provide further insights about the safety and cost-effectiveness of this approach.

In the United States the FDA cleared the Gen 5 cTnT assay (same assay as hs-cTnT) to allow reporting at 6 ng/L (LoQ) as the lowest reportable value, raising concern about whether using this slightly higher value is safe. McRae and colleagues[198] examined this question in a retrospective analysis of 7130 emergency room patients with suspected cardiac chest pain and reported that a hs-cTnT less than 6 ng/L had a 30-day diagnostic sensitivity and NPV greater than 99% for acute MI; however, at 30 days the diagnostic sensitivity for MACE was only 95% which was deemed unacceptably low.

Only one prospective, observational cohort study using a hs-cTnI assay (Abbott) in an unselected, heterogeneous population presenting to an inner city ED, in whom cTnI measurements were obtained on clinical indication, has been carried out in the USA to determine whether a single hs-cTnI measurement at presentation with concentrations below the LOD (1.9 ng/L) could rule out acute myocardial injury.[199] Myocardial injury was defined as any hs-cTnI concentration above the sex-specific 99th percentile (Use of Abbott High Sensitivity Troponin I Assay In Acute Coronary Syndromes [UTROPIA], NCT02060760). A total of 1647 patients were included. In patients with hs-cTnI concentrations less than LOD at presentation, regardless of ECG findings, the NPV and diagnostic sensitivity for acute myocardial injury was 99.1 and 99.0%, respectively. The NPV for AMI or cardiac death at 30 days was 99.6%. Only 4 patients had acute myocardial injury (0.9%, 4/448), of whom 2 had an AMI and none had a cardiac death at 30 days (0.45%, 2 out of 448) corresponding to a miss rate of 1 in 224. In the same UTROPIA cohort, acute MI occurred in 170 patients (10.4%), including 68 (4.2%) type 1 MI and 102 (6.3%) type 2 MI.[200] For hs-cTnI less than LOD (27%), the NPV and sensitivity for acute MI were 99.6% and 98.8. Using the High-STEAC model of hs-cTnI less than 5 ng/L (50%), the NPV and sensitivity for acute MI were 98.9 and 94.7%. In combination with a normal ECG, 1) hs-cTnI less than LOD had an NPV of 99.6% (98.9 to 100%) and sensitivity of 99.4% (98.3 to 100%); and 2) hs-cTnI less than 5 ng/L had an NPV of 99.5% (98.8 to 100%) and sensitivity of 98.8% (97.2 to 100%). The NPV and sensitivity for the safety outcome were excellent for hs-cTnI less than LOD alone or in combination with a normal ECG, and for hs-cTnI less than 5 ng/L in combination with a normal ECG.

In another USA study, using the Atellica IM TnIH and ADVIA Centaur TNIH hs-cTnI assays (Siemens Healthineers) among 2212 patients, acute MI occurred in 12%.[201] The limits of detection resulted in excellent sensitivities, range 98.6 to 99.6%, and NPVs, range 99.5 to 99.8%, for acute MI or death at 30 days across both assays. An optimized threshold of less than 5 ng/L identified almost one-half of all patients as low risk, with sensitivities of 98.6% and NPVs of 99.6% for acute MI or death at 30 days across both assays.

Role of Single Baseline hs-cTn Measurement Predicated on Data-Derived Cutoff

Another risk-stratification approach relies on data-derived cutoffs that use a single measurement based on the highest possible concentration threshold that permits a safe rule-out (based on metrics such as NPV and/or sensitivity) with the goal of identifying the largest possible proportion of patients in whom such strategy can be used. This approach was tested in the High-STEACS study using the hs-cTnI (Abbott) assay in which a single concentration less than 5 ng/L was shown to identify a substantial proportion of patients as low risk with an excellent NPV for the composite of index type 1 MI or type 1 MI or cardiac death at 30 days.[202] This strategy was subsequently examined in a pooled patient-level meta-analysis involving cohorts with varying prevalence of MI and showed to have a NPV of 99.5% for the primary outcome of type 1 MI or cardiac death at 30 days.[192] This approach is being tested as part of a pathway involving serial testing for those that present early or those with values between 5 ng/L and the 99th percentile URL in the High-Sensitivity Cardiac Troponin on Presentation to Rule Out Myocardial Infarction (HiSTORIC) stepped-wedge cluster randomized trial (NCT03005158).

Role of Early Serial hs-cTn Measurements

Accelerated serial sampling algorithms using hs-cTn assays are also used for ruling out MI.

Because hs-cTn assays permit more precise quantification of smaller concentration changes, numerous triage algorithms have been proposed to rule out AMI and to risk-stratify patients within 3 hours. The ESC guidelines have endorsed such algorithms with a class I indication for several years, including in 2011 for the 0/3 hours algorithm (class IB) that was largely based on the use of the 99th percentile,[203] and subsequently in the year 2015 for a 0/1 hour algorithm.[204] These algorithms incorporate baseline hs-cTn concentrations and/or absolute changes (deltas) on serial testing. Most of the literature using hs-assays has explored the use of the 0/1-hour algorithm[205–210]; however, algorithms exist for 0/2-hour.[211–213] Almost all are predicated on using hs-cTnT as the gold standard. Unfortunately, hs-cTnT and hs-cTnI correlate only modestly.[214] These algorithms have been studied extensively and for the most part have been shown to be safe and effective in chest pain populations, with some potential limitations such as in early presenters and at values where imprecision can cause misclassification of patients when very small changes in values are relied on. The RAPID-TnT study likely unmasked this fact as 13% of those in the 1-hour group returned for evaluation. It may well be that in other studies, excellent outpatient follow-up diminished the frequency of these problems. This is a critical area that requires additional scrutiny.[215]

Identification of Patients at High Risk and Rule-in Acute Myocardial Infarction

At presentation, if there is a reasonably high pretest probability of acute ischemic heart disease (*i.e.*: clinical history suspicious for ACS) and in the absence of other factors that could influence results such as critical illness or renal disease, marked increases in hs-cTn concentrations manifest a high diagnostic specificity and PPV for acute MI. Reichlin and colleagues showed that in patients with chest pain a baseline concentration of 100 ng/L using the hs-cTnT assay had a diagnostic specificity and PPV for acute MI of 99.3 and 89.3% respectively.[216] Observations are assay-dependent and the magnitude of concentration associated with an increased risk for MI will vary by assay and will also depend on the studied

population. A recent analysis based on the UTROPIA (USA) cohort demonstrates that a baseline hs-cTnI greater than 200 ng/L identifies a subset of patients at high risk for acute MI, due to the relationship between PPVs and type1 MI.[217] This threshold is approximately fourfold higher than the 52 ng/L rule-in threshold endorsed by the ESC,[204] likely because of differences in assays and the populations studied.

Serial Change Criteria (Deltas) Used to Facilitate the Identification of Patients at Both Low and High Risk

The presence or absence of significant serial change criteria (deltas) can be used to facilitate the identification of patients at both low and high risk. Several accelerated algorithms emphasize the absence of significant changes to identify patients at low risk. Conversely, those with significant concentration changes on serial sampling have acute myocardial injury and thus are more likely to have acute MI in the appropriate clinical setting. Deltas are assay-specific and the higher the absolute change the higher the likelihood for acute MI. For hs-assays, absolute changes (ng/L) have been shown to be superior to relative changes (%).[216] While the presence of marked changes increases the likelihood of acute MI, such deltas can also be seen with other conditions such as myocarditis and critical illness. Further, deltas are not able to distinguish type 1 from 2 MI.[218]

Interpretation will always require incorporation of pretest probability and consideration of the clinical presentation/history. Critically, timing of the onset of symptoms is of essence when interpreting cTn results in those with suspected acute MI. In those that present very early, a change may not be seen within the first two samples and a third sample may be necessary. In those that present late after symptom onset, cTn concentrations may appear stable ("flat") on serial sampling over short periods of time. This may be because of the plateau and slower downslope in the cTn time-concentration curve. In this situation, if there is high pretest probability of AMI, subsequent sampling may be necessary to confirm a fall in cTn, which would be indicative of an acute event. In one study, up to 26% of patients with NSTEMI failed to demonstrate a significant change in cTn concentrations on serial sampling mostly for this reason.[219]

OTHER CAUSES OF ACUTE CARDIAC TROPONIN ELEVATION IN THE ABSENCE OF ACUTE ISCHEMIC HEART DISEASE

Many acute diseases are associated with elevated cTns (see Box 48.1), and the frequency of such elevations will increase with the advent of hs-cTn assays. This can occur for many reasons, including direct trauma to the heart, implantable cardioverter-defibrillator (ICD) firings, biopsies, and cardioversions. Also, some patients may have type 2 MI, as indicated previously. Critically ill patients often have tachycardia, hypertension, or hypotension with or without drugs that may be given therapeutically, such as catecholamines, which in and of themselves can directly damage myocardium. In some instances this condition could be called type 2 AMI.[31] On the other hand, in the absence of at least some coronary artery abnormality to negatively affect perfusion, these episodes would not be designated as type 2 AMI. Patients in the absence of CAD who have very severe supply-demand imbalance may have elevated cTn, and these individuals should be diagnosed as having AMI if ischemia is present.[2] Direct toxic effects of circulating cytokines and catecholamines can also cause severe myocardial toxicity. Such is the case in sepsis. Finally, viruses, as experienced in the ongoing pandemic of COVID-19, have been implicated as a direct toxin to the myocardium. Thus consideration of each mechanism for a given elevation is important. A representative tabulation is provided here.

COVID-19/SARS-CoV-2 Virus[220–223]

An increased cTn above the 99th percentile URL, detecting myocardial injury, is not uncommon among patients with acute respiratory infections, including COVID-19, and is correlated with disease severity. Studies describing the clinical course during the pandemic outbreak, initially detected in Wuhan China in the fall of 2019 of this highly infectious and highly contagious COVID-19/ SARS-CoV-2 virus have shown detectable and increased hs-cTnI and hs-cTnT concentrations with frequencies of 7 to 28%, with significantly increased concentrations in more than half of the patients at high risk of death. Mortality rates are higher in hospitalized patients with myocardial injury (51.2 versus 4.5%). The risk of death starting from the time of symptom onset was more than four times higher in patients with evidence of myocardial injury on admission (hazard ratio 4.26; 95% CI 1.92 to 9.49). Differences in frequency of cTn elevations may be due to use of differing troponin assays and differences in patient populations. COVID-19 patients who showed signs of cardiac injury at presentation tended to be over the age of 50 years and have more comorbidities, such as a history of coronary heart disease and hypertension. The mechanisms explaining myocardial injury in patients with COVID-19 infection are not fully understood. Causes of myocardial injury in patients with COVID-19 include myocarditis (which may have a pseudo-infarct presentation with normal coronary arteries), hypoxic injury, stress cardiomyopathy, ischemic injury caused by cardiac microvascular damage or epicardial CAD (with plaque rupture or demand ischemia), and systemic inflammatory response syndrome (cytokine storm), with a direct ("noncoronary") myocardial damage likely the most common cause. The presence of abundant distribution of ACE2, the binding site for the SARS-CoV-2 in heart cells, has been postulated that myocarditis might explain increased hs-cTn in some cases, particularly as acute left ventricular failure. Both acute type 1 MI based plaque rupture triggered by the infection and type 2 MI–based on supply-demand inequity need to be considered but type 1 events appear to be unchanged or even diminished. Initial cardiology expert opinion for the clinical role of cTn monitoring advised only to measure cTn when clinical presentation was suggestive of MI on clinical grounds. However, with the evolving complications and adverse risk outcomes associated with increased cTn, a single cTn measurement upon presentation is more routinely being checked in patients hospitalized with COVID-19 to assist in patient management. However, most recently, rather than encouraging avoidance of cTn testing, other experts have suggested clinicians "must harness the unheralded engagement from the cardiovascular community due to COVID-19 to better understand the utility of this essential biomarker and to educate clinicians on its interpretation and implications for prognosis and clinical decision making."[223] Citing a cohort of 191 patients with confirmed COVID-19 based on SARS-CoV-2 RNA detection, the univariable odds ratio for death when hs-cTnI concentrations were above the 99th percentile URL was 80.1 (95% confidence interval [CI] 10.3 to 620.4, $P < .0001$). Patients were more likely to require invasive or noninvasive ventilation (22 versus 4%, and 46 versus 4%), and to develop acute respiratory distress syndrome (59 versus 15%) or acute kidney injury (9 versus 0%). Thus early recognition could facilitate appropriate triage to a high-intensity or critical care area, improve our understanding of the systemic consequences of COVID-19, and inform the use of inotropes, vasopressors, and diuretics in those with significant cardiac dysfunction. cTn testing in patients with COVID-19 could increase the need for cardiology consultation and downstream testing, including bedside echocardiography and angiography. However, recognition of a normal or modestly elevated cTn could conversely reduce the need for cardiac imaging and minimize the risk of exposure to cardiac physiology staff.

Atrial Fibrillation[224–226]

hs-cTnT was observed to be detectable in over 90% of patients with atrial fibrillation (AF) who have at least one clinical risk factor for stroke. Biomarkers have been studied for risk stratification in patients with AF. cTnI and NT-proBNP predict risk of stroke, systemic embolization, mortality, and bleeding. The Prevention of Stroke in Subjects with Atrial Fibrillation (ARISTOTLE) trial evaluated the association between baseline hs-cTnT and outcomes and found that increased baseline hs-cTnT predicted increased risk of stroke, myocardial infarction, cardiac mortality, total mortality, and bleeding. Patients with a hs-cTnT greater than 16.7 ng/L had double the risk of stroke compared with less than 7.5 ng/L. There was an increased risk of stroke in patients with smaller hs-cTnT levels (>11.0 ng/L). The lowest risk of stroke was in patients with a low CHA_2DS_2VASc score (<2) and low hs-cTnT (<11 ng/L). An elevated risk of stroke was identified in those with a low CHA_2DS_2VASc score (<2) and increased hs-cTnT. hs-cTnT was shown to provide better outcomes assessment regarding cardiac mortality, MI, and major bleeding compared to the CHA_2DS_2VASc score, with limited utility of the CHA_2DS_2VASc score in predicting events other than stroke in AF. Adding hs-cTnT level to the CHA_2DS_2VASc score predicted risk of events better compared to using either variable alone. Use of baseline hs-cTn can potentially aid in the shared decision-making process regarding anticoagulation. These studies support using baseline hs-cTn levels for risk assessment in AF patients. Similar results were noted in patients with AF already on chronic anticoagulation. The use of hs-cTnT, however, has not been shown to aid in predicting the safety or efficacy of treatment with specific anticoagulants.

Cardiotoxicity/Anthracycline[227,228]

Early identification of anthracycline-induced cardiotoxicity (e.g., doxorubicin) can potentially be reversed, whereas late identification may be permanent. Echocardiography lacks the sensitivity required to diagnose early cardiotoxicity, although newer data with strain are intriguing. Measurement of cTn may help predict those at higher risk of such cardiotoxicity. Comparing serial hs-cTnI in patients receiving anthracycline-based regimens to patients receiving non–anthracycline-based regimens a significant increase in hs-cTnI after five cycles of treatment in the anthracycline group (absolute delta increase of 30.7 ng/L) compared to no significant change in hs-cTnI in the non-anthracycline group which they conclude indicates subclinical cardiomyocyte damage. In a randomized trial, Cardinale and colleagues demonstrated that ACE inhibitor treatment reduced cTn increases and prevented cardiotoxicity.[228] hs-cTn may identify those who are at greater risk of developing chemotherapy cardiotoxicity and who would need earlier discontinuation of therapy or require closer cardiac monitoring.

Trauma

Contusion, slow potential cardiac ablation, pacing, ICD firings, cardioversion, myocardial biopsy, and closure after a variety of interventional procedures commonly cause elevations in cTn and should be expected. These elevations are usually modest. More marked elevations should engender suspicion of additional processes.

Congestive Heart Failure[229–233]

HF can cause acute cTn elevations, and elevations have been noted during long-term monitoring of patients as well. In both circumstances, they are markedly adverse prognostic signals and indicate more severe HF and an increased proximate likelihood of mortality. Such patterns can be rising but need not be, especially with more chronic HF. The prognostic significance of cTn is additive to that of the NPs. Elevations are usually modest. With hs-cTn assays, these increases will be more frequent but potentially more informative as well. Acutely, increases will be common and preliminary information suggests that the patterns of these elevations may be prognostically important, with hs-cTn assays providing better prognostic information and a better way to monitor treatment. Although many patients with HF have CAD, the cTn elevations observed occur in patients both with and without coronary heart disease, so they should not be used to include the diagnosis of AMI absent additional findings to suggest acute ischemic heart disease.

Severe Valvular Heart Disease

Severe valvular heart disease with volume or pressure overload can be associated with elevations in cTn. Elevations may be more apt to occur with cTnI for volume overload via a calpain-mediated mechanism and may be more common with cTnT with left ventricular hypertrophy (LVH).

Hypertension[21]

Hypertension in and of itself can cause LVH or cardiac enlargement, which increases wall stress and reduces nutritive perfusion, causing increases in cTn. LVH is associated with reduced subendocardial perfusion caused by increased wall stress; therefore subendocardial injury may occur in response to severe hypertension. Obviously, because hypertension is a risk factor for CAD, these processes may be exacerbated by each other, but this is not necessary for elevations to be observed. Elevations most often are modest. With hs-cTn assays, it is now appreciated that individuals with LVH (most often a consequence of hypertension) who have elevated hs-cTn values are at very high risk for both HF and mortality.

Hypotension and Tachycardia

Hypotension and tachycardia can be synergistic with underlying coronary abnormalities or may occur independently.

Nonetheless, at some point their severity can be sufficient to cause some degree of cTn release, usually modest.

Postoperative Noncardiac Surgery Patients[234–237]

Data indicate that elevations of cTn postoperatively are negatively prognostic. Many of these events are probably due to type 2 MI, but obviously not all of them. Indeed, autopsy studies suggest that half of those events that result in mortality are type 1 MIs. In vascular surgery patients, which is the group best studied, these cTn elevations seem to be related to underlying coronary heart disease in association with an abnormality in acute myocardial oxygen consumption, usually hypertension or hypotension and/or tachycardia, anemia, and the like. This is an area of expanding interest because it has become clear that an increasing number of non–cardiac surgery patients suffer events in the hospital, and it is likely that a more diverse group of patients will soon be elucidated. Causes of observed elevations may differ among the groups involved and may include, for example, PE, which is common in postoperative patients. Implementation of hs-cTn assays will benefit this area substantially. Preliminary data suggest that up to 45% of postoperative patients will have cTn elevations. There will be a desire to suggest all of these individuals have ischemic heart disease, but the data for that have not been developed. However, AMI should be considered only if there is a rising and/or falling pattern of hs-cTn. Solitary elevations should evoke a search for possible causes. For that reason, a baseline value is suggested. To emphasize, increases of cTns do not automatically suggest AMI but are associated with myocardial injury. Not only will it help in detection of a rising pattern of values, indicative of an acute event, but it will also identify high-risk patients. Mortality, even in patients undergoing noncardiac surgery, is higher in patients with myocardial injury presenting with post procedure cTn increases than in patients with a cTn in the normal range.

Patients With Renal Failure[238–242]

Patients with end-stage renal failure often have elevations in cTn that are highly prognostic. Elevations occur more frequently with cTnT than with cTnI, perhaps because processing of the two proteins is different in renal failure. Nonetheless, elevations are highly prognostic in this group, but not necessarily for CAD. A large percentage of renal failure patients die of sudden cardiac death. One should not presume that all cTn elevations occur in such groups, although this group does have an increased prevalence of CAD. The diagnosis of AMI still can be easily made using the presence of a rising and/or falling pattern. Almost all patients with end-stage disease will have elevations using the hs-cTnT assay, but only approximately 30% with an hs-cTnI assay. In addition, it is now clear that the distribution of hs-cTn values is increased with even lesser degrees of renal dysfunction.

Critically Ill Patients[243]

These individuals may or may not have underlying coronary heart disease, which is negatively synergistic with their acute illness, but they often have reasons for very substantial increases in myocardial oxygen consumption. Elevations in cTn are common and usually modest but nonetheless are highly negative prognostically in the short and long term. In patients with acute respiratory failure, elevations of cTn are strongly related to short- and long-term outcomes. In those with sepsis, the association is less strong short term but very powerful during long-term follow-up. Elevations of hs-cTn seem best related to abnormalities in diastolic function and right ventricular dysfunction. Patients with gastrointestinal bleeding are not at greater risk short term, and there is no signal that invasive evaluation is a problem. However, they are at substantial long-term risk.

Drug Toxicity[244–246]

Carbon monoxide poisoning is an archetypical example of drug toxicity. Increased cTn in response to drug toxicity, such as Propofol and cocaine as examples, have prognostic significance. Snakebite venom can be another cause. A far larger number of drug toxicities have been documented.

Inflammatory Heart Disease[247]

Myocarditis, when acute, commonly causes elevations of cTn. Myocarditis also can cause coronary vasospasm and is a common mimicker of ACSs. Elevation in this circumstance can be very high, even higher than that associated with acute infarction, or very modest, depending on whether patients have acute or chronic conditions. Approximately 50% of the patients in whom AMI is suspected but in whom coronary anatomy is deemed to be normal have myocarditis confirmed by magnetic resonance imaging.

Pulmonary Embolism

In general, the degree of cTn elevation is related to the degree of right ventricular dysfunction and therefore to the severity of pulmonary hypertension induced. Increased cTn defines a patient who is at high risk; some have advocated that it should be used as an indication for the use of thrombolytic therapy of PE. This recommendation is premature at the present time. Elevations that occur with PE usually resolve within 40 hours. If they do not, recurrent emboli or another cause should be considered, along with or independent of PE.

Sepsis[248,249]

Severe septicemia with hypotension probably has multifactorial causes for increases in cTn. Such increases are often related to elaboration of toxic cytokines such as tumor necrosis factor alpha (TNF-α) and heat shock proteins. Initially a relationship was noted between the magnitude of cTn elevation and the extent of myocardial depression associated with cTn elevation that was above that associated with a modest increase in cTn. Some of this may be due to the use of catecholamines, which are directly myocardial toxins, to treat these patients and may contribute to the supply-demand imbalance associated with type 2 AMI. It has been reported that hs-cTn elevations seem best related to abnormalities in diastolic function and right ventricular dysfunction.

Burns[250]

Only when they are severe are elevations observed; this probably reflects the marked hemodynamic changes associated with severe burns.

Acute Neurologic Disease[251,252]

Increases probably represent reflex stimulation from the central nervous system. A very substantial literature suggests that such is the case and that such increases seem to be related to insults in the midbrain; they are particularly prominent with subarachnoid bleeds. Such elevations are highly prognostic but not necessarily for coronary heart disease. Seizures can also cause elevations.

Rhabdomyolysis[245]

Rhabdomyolysis, which primarily is recognized as a skeletal muscle concern, can also occur systemically with associated direct and indirect injury to the heart.

Transplant Vasculopathy

Monitoring of cTn has not been useful as an early marker, but elevations do occur with both transplant vasculopathy and rejection.

Vital Exhaustion/Exercise[253–258]

Severe exercise has been shown to cause release of cTn. Whether this implies an element of minor myocardial injury or whether this could be release of cTn from a proposed cytoplasm pool is a difficult challenge to be definitive on. Nonetheless, studies suggest that patients, despite some having cMRI evidence of cardiac injury, do well and do not require emergency hospitalization.

Chronic Elevations of Cardiac Troponin[259,260]

Any chronic cardiac comorbidity, whether it is CAD, LVH, HF, or diabetes, can be associated with elevations in cTn. In general, these patients are the ones who have the most severe disease and poorest prognosis. Recent data suggest that patients with chronic heart disease at risk for subsequent events can be identified simply by looking at whether a cTn is detectable or not. This ability to predict those at risk is even better with hs-cTn. In addition, LVH and HF, both of which can cause increased wall stress and reduced subendocardial myocardial perfusion, are known to be associated with elevations in cTn. With hs-cTn assays, these elevations are substantially prognostic. The prognostic significance of elevations in older individuals is clear. It is also the case that elevations of hs-cTn in patients with putatively stable heart disease define a high-risk group. How to improve management of this group is unclear.

Hypothyroidism[261]

Hypothyroidism is a rare cause of cTn elevation. Usually, hypothyroidism in the modern era is detected fairly early and treated, and it seems to take fairly severe hypothyroidism for elevations in cTn to occur. This is in contrast to previous literature, which suggested a high frequency of elevated CK-MB. Given the cTn data, it is likely that CK-MB elevations were due to skeletal muscle abnormalities, rather than cardiac problems, as some might have initially surmised.

Infiltrative Diseases[262]

Amyloid and cardiomyopathies such as hemochromatosis are capable of causing increased cTns. In general, elevations are modest but very negatively prognostic.

Clinical Use of Myocardial-Bound Creatine Kinase[113,263–267]

Considering CK-MB an obsolete test has continued to be met with some resistance, in part because of difficulty clinicians have had in understanding how to use cTn measurements. This has been fueled in part by heterogeneity in the cTn assays available, diversity in the cutoffs intermittently advocated, and difficulty in understanding how to respond to elevations in cTn that are seen with cTns but not with CK-MB, because cTn is diagnostically and analytically more sensitive, as cTn is myocardial tissue specific compared to CK-MB which is not. Nonetheless, several groups have advocated that CK-MB assays should be eliminated. The major push for this comes from the thought that not only do they add expense while not adding clinical value but because clinicians who continue to rely on CK-MB often do patients a disservice. In addition, these assays retard clinicians' ability to learn how to use cTn measurements properly, which would be more efficacious in almost every situation. Accordingly, serious consideration should be given by laboratories to discontinuing the use of CK-MB. Testing is not essential even for skeletal muscle disease in which total CK is appropriate, but it does eliminate a source of what some would argue is confusion for clinicians. This position has been well articulated, and its use is now discouraged in recent guidelines.

Those who advocate continued use of CK-MB point to a small number of instances that are worthy of consideration. The first is the most controversial, which is the area of recurrent infarction after an index AMI. When initial guidelines for the use of cTn were developed, how well one would do in diagnosing recurrent injury with cTn was called into question because cTn elevations persist for so long. The data now confirm that cTn values detect acute recurrent injury very well (Fig. 48.21) and that new elevations occur with sufficient robustness that they can be detected promptly. Second, from principles related to sensitivity and specificity (see earlier), some would argue that cTn would be clearly superior in this area. Nonetheless, the diagnosis of reinfarction is common after non–Q-wave MI, and because CK-MB was initially used to unmask this, people have retained some enthusiasm for its use. This occurred in part because in the past, if individuals had chest pain, this did not trigger a rapid evaluation. Thus because CK-MB was thought to return to normal earlier, its elevation was helpful. However, this is not the case with contemporary and hs-cTn assays. Third, in modern practice, most patients with ACS are seen when chest pain is present and serial values are obtained. Thus in the series by Apple and Murakami, every patient identified had normal values of CK-MB, which subsequently increased to reach an abnormal threshold (see Fig. 48.21). Accordingly, with serial samples measured for both cTnI and CK-MB, CK-MB possessed no characteristics that would make it superior to cTn.

Fourth, when patients have recurrent chest discomfort, most immediately go back for coronary angiography to evaluate whether the chest pain is indicative of a problem with the area that has undergone intervention (e.g., stent thrombosis) or whether severe diminution in flow is present in that vessel. Thus the only patients who are really held for evaluation are those in whom there is uncertainty about the diagnosis, and for this group, one needs to wait for serial samples. Indeed, this is the recommendation of the ACC/AHA committee on the management of patients with UA and non–Q-wave MI and does still problematically include CK-MB. Fifth, the other major indication that some advocate using CK-MB for is in patients who undergo PCI. The problems with this approach are indicated earlier, in the section on post-PCI AMI. Therefore very few to no indications exist to justify the use of CK-MB, except when cTn measurements

are unavailable. This is a rare circumstance in the United States and in most of Western Europe but probably does occur elsewhere in the world, perhaps in countries with a much lower incidence of MI or countries that are resource poor and cannot afford the equipment needed to measure cTn. In this circumstance, most countries would rely on total CK, moving back even another step. In addition, immunoassays for cTn and CK-MB are reasonably comparably priced and use similar types of equipment. Nonetheless, if CK-MB is to be used, mass assays are considered far preferable. This is due to the fact that they are more sensitive and less prone to artifactual elevations. Increases in CK-MB from skeletal muscle injury clearly confound this measure and need to be considered. Use of the relative index (CK-MB divided by total CK), which used to be advocated by some because the percentage of CK-MB in cardiac muscle is so much higher than that in skeletal muscle, was discredited during the initial evaluation of cTn assays. The specificity of diagnosis is clearly improved when the index is used, but because so much CK is present in skeletal muscle, modest concurrent cardiac injury does not provide an adequate signal, so that sensitivity is lost.

Differences between males and females in reference intervals for CK-MB are likely related to differences in body mass. Thus if CK-MB is used, gender-specific reference intervals must be used, which improves the sensitivity. This will correct in part for the relative lack of sensitivity of CK-MB, particularly in women. When used, the same criteria as with cTn should be employed (i.e., a rising and/or falling pattern of results with at least one value above the 99th percentile of a normal reference population). However, very clear data indicate that elevations of CK-MB when cTn is normal identify patients who have skeletal muscle injury and not cardiac injury, as suggested strongly by the fact that these individuals do extremely well prognostically and do not appear to have an increased incidence of subsequent cardiovascular events.

Normal skeletal muscle, depending on its location, contains very little CK-MB. Percentages as high as 5 to 7% have been reported, but values less than 2% are much more common. Some differences are related to slow- versus fast-twitch muscle and thus also to race. Severe skeletal muscle injury after trauma or surgery can lead to absolute elevations of CK-MB to above the upper reference interval for CK-MB in serum. However, the percent CK-MB in serum would be low (percentages advocated vary, but in comparisons of activity versus activity, a percentage less than 5% is often used, and when CK activity is compared with CK-MB mass, a percentage less than 2.5% is usually advocated). Increases in serum total CK and CK-MB in several patient groups present a diagnostic challenge to the clinician. Persistent elevations of serum CK-MB resulting from chronic muscle disease occur in patients with muscular dystrophy, end-stage renal disease, or polymyositis and in healthy subjects who undergo extreme exercise or physical activity. The increase in serum CK-MB in runners, for example, may be related to adaptation by skeletal muscle during regular training and after acute exercise, resulting in increased CK-MB tissue concentrations.

Copeptin[268–270]

Copeptin is the preform of arginine vasopressin (AVP). It is cleaved from vasopressin and has a longer half-life, making measurement much easier. It correlates well with AVP, which is cleared very rapidly from the blood. Because AVP is a stress

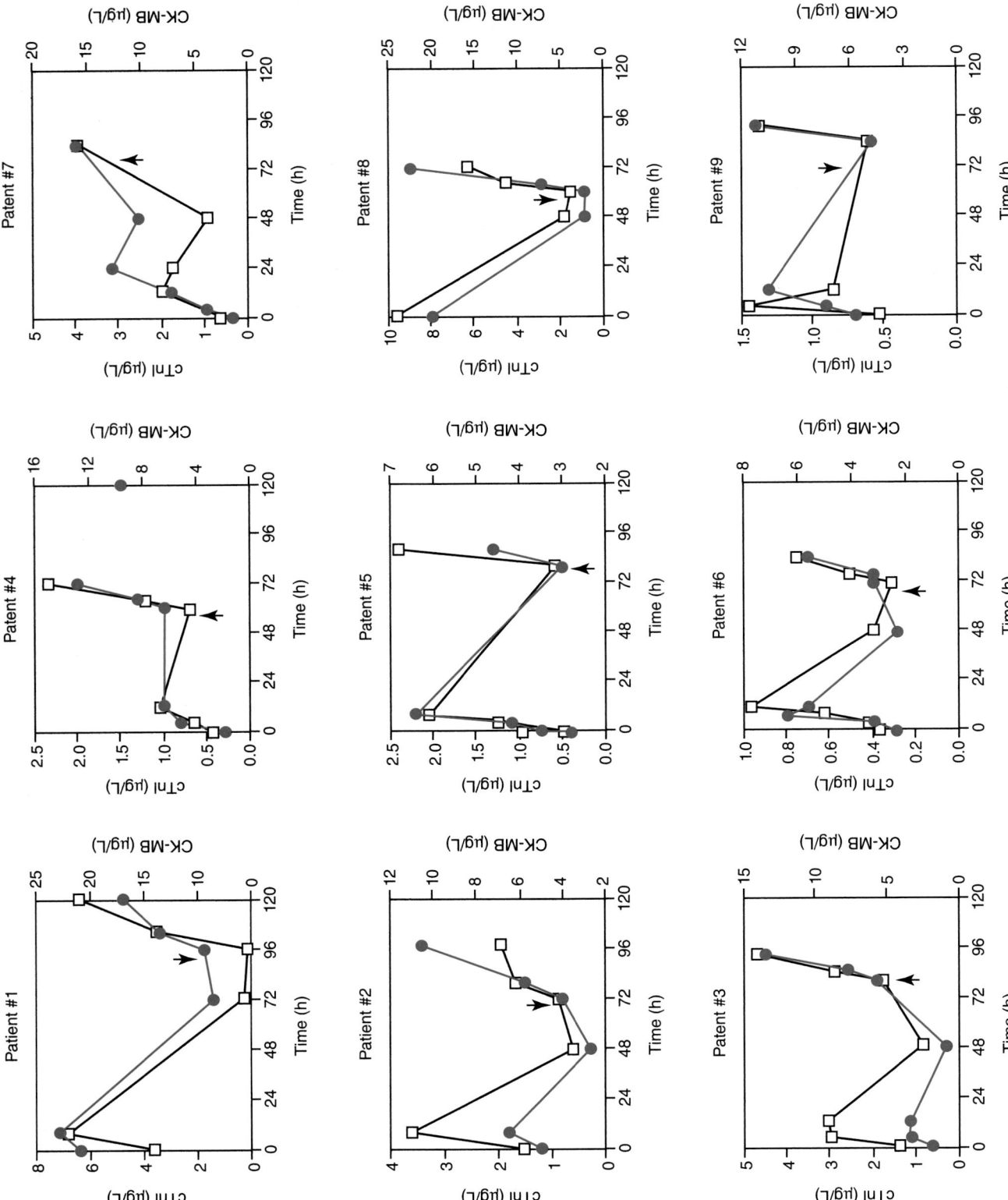

FIGURE 48.21 Time course of changes in biomarker concentrations in nine myocardial infarction patients who experienced reinfarction during hospitalization. *Red closed circles*, CTnI; *black open squares*, CK-MB, myocardial-bound creatine kinase; *CTnI*, Cardiac troponin I. (From Apple FS, Murakami MM. Cardiac troponin and myocardial-bound creatine kinase monitoring during in-hospital myocardial reinfarction. *Clin Chem* 2005;51:460–3.)

hormone, copeptin has been used to define hemodynamic stress in two clinical situations: possible AMI and patients with HF. The assay itself is robust. The first generation had a cutoff value of 14 ng/mL, but a more sensitive iteration is now available with a cutoff value of 10 ng/mL. Copeptin rises very rapidly in response to hemodynamic stress and falls rapidly as well. Its clinical use to rule out AMI has been predicated on its rapid increase. Thus elevations may precede those of cTn even in patients who present very early after the onset of AMI. Thus a normal copeptin value has been touted to provide accurate exclusion of AMI. The initial studies were done with conventional assays using well-defined cTn cutoff values to make the gold standard diagnosis of AMI. However, many of the subsequent clinical trials used local cTn assays with variable cutoff values, leading to questions about its role in the early diagnosis of AMI. Nonetheless, accuracy has been shown for the ruling out of AMI on the initial sample at the time of presentation. This would then in theory allow for a substantial number of patients with possible AMI to be discharged based on values from the first sample, an attractive characteristic. However, there have been several concerns about the use of copeptin. One has been that many studies have not been as rigorous as would be ideal in making the diagnosis of AMI. In addition, many studies have not included large numbers of patients presenting early after the onset of AMI. In addition, it is likely that this strategy will work only in patients who present without other major comorbidities that would evoke a stress response. Thus such strategies will need to compete with those that have been developed to exclude AMI with hs-cTn. In those sorts of studies, the relative yield of copeptin has been markedly diminished. Whether the small incremental yield with copeptin justifies the use of another biomarker, with its associated costs, with hs-cTn measurements is much less clear. Finally, it is clear that in some studies, the predictive accuracy of copeptin has been less than ideal but has been rescued by the judgment of the clinicians involved in the study.

In HF patients, AVP is thought to be an important neurohormonal compensation that becomes dysregulated. However, trials of AVP inhibitors have thus far shown no benefit. Increasing values of copeptin are prognostic both at baseline and during follow-up, especially in patients with hyponatremia. This raises the possibility that the marker may allow for the identification of patients who are in need of AVP inhibition and allow for more focused use of this therapy.

Recent findings regarding combined testing of hs-cTnT and copeptin at presentation provide, although still not ideal, a high NPV for the early rule out of AMI. A recent study examined whether a second copeptin measurement at 1 hour might further increase the NPV in a prospective diagnostic multicenter study where samples were taken at both presentation and at 1 hour in 1439 unselected patients presenting to the ED with suspected AMI. The study concluded that a 1-hour copeptin increased neither the safety of the rule-out process nor the NPV in the intermediate-risk setting. In contrast, the incremental value of 1-hour hs-cTnT was substantial in both settings.

Biomarkers No Longer of Clinical Use

Because of the lack of clinical utility compared to cTn the following biomarkers will not be discussed: CK isoenzymes, CK muscle type (CK-MM) (CK-1), and CK brain type (CK-BB) (CK-3); CK isoforms of CK-MM and CK-MB, myoglobin, AST, and LD isoenzymes LD1, LD2, LD3, LD4, and LD5.

CONGESTIVE HEART FAILURE

Natriuretic Peptides: Analytical Considerations

An endocrine phenotype of the heart muscle was suggested by anatomical findings half a century after the principal discovery of endocrine substances by Drs. Starling and Bayliss.[271] In the 1960s, electron microscopy revealed granules in the cytoplasm of atrial myocytes, which structurally resemble secretory granules in known peptide hormone–producing cells.[272,273] In 1981 the Canadian physiologist Adolfo de Bold and colleagues[274] reported that infusion of atrial tissue extracts elicits renal excretion of sodium and water. Moreover, a rapid decrease in blood pressure and increase in blood hematocrit was observed and the substance was named atrial natriuretic factor. This f-factor was then purified and identified as a peptide comprising 28 amino acid residues and renamed atrial natriuretic peptide (ANP).[275,276] The discovery paved the way for identification of two structurally related peptides in the porcine brain: brain natriuretic peptide (BNP) and C-type natriuretic peptide (CNP).[277–280] However, BNP is mainly expressed in the heart and the name "brain" NP is now replaced with B-type NP (Fig. 48.22).[279,280] CNP is expressed in the invertebrate heart and can be considered the ancestor gene for the NP family.[281] Nevertheless, the CNP gene is not expressed to the same extent in mammalian hearts and should not be considered a cardiac-derived hormone in humans, in which the gene dominantly is expressed in other tissues, including the vasculature and the male reproductive glands.[282,283] Other members of the NP family include Dendroaspis natriuretic peptide (DNP) and urodilatin. In addition, there is interest to develop designer therapeutic peptides that are chimeras between various NPs and therapeutics that modulate their concentrations. This chapter will focus on ANP and BNP predominantly because they are the only NPs used diagnostically.

The endocrine heart gained clinical interest when it was reported that patients with cardiac disease display increased concentrations of ANP in plasma.[284,285] In parallel, BNP circulates in highly increased concentrations in patients with CHF.[286,287] The concept of a quantitative plasma marker in the HF syndrome was thereby introduced and has been intensely pursued with a dominant focus on clinical applications. In addition to the bioactive end products, N-terminal fragments from the precursor peptides (proANP and proBNP) were also shown to circulate in HF plasma and provided new molecular targets for biochemical detection.[281,284,288–290] Currently, proBNP-derived peptides have become the preferred routine markers in HF diagnostics and prognosis because of the available automated assays, and the clinical relevance of peptide measurement is still being extensively reviewed.[291–298] In contrast to the clinical focus on the diagnostic possibilities, less is known concerning the biosynthesis of proANP and proBNP-derived peptides.[298–300] The post-translational phase of gene expression and the cellular secretion are areas of continuing research. The first data on the molecular composition in tissue and plasma suggested a simple cellular maturation with only one endoproteolytic cleavage before secretion. However, cardiac myocytes possess

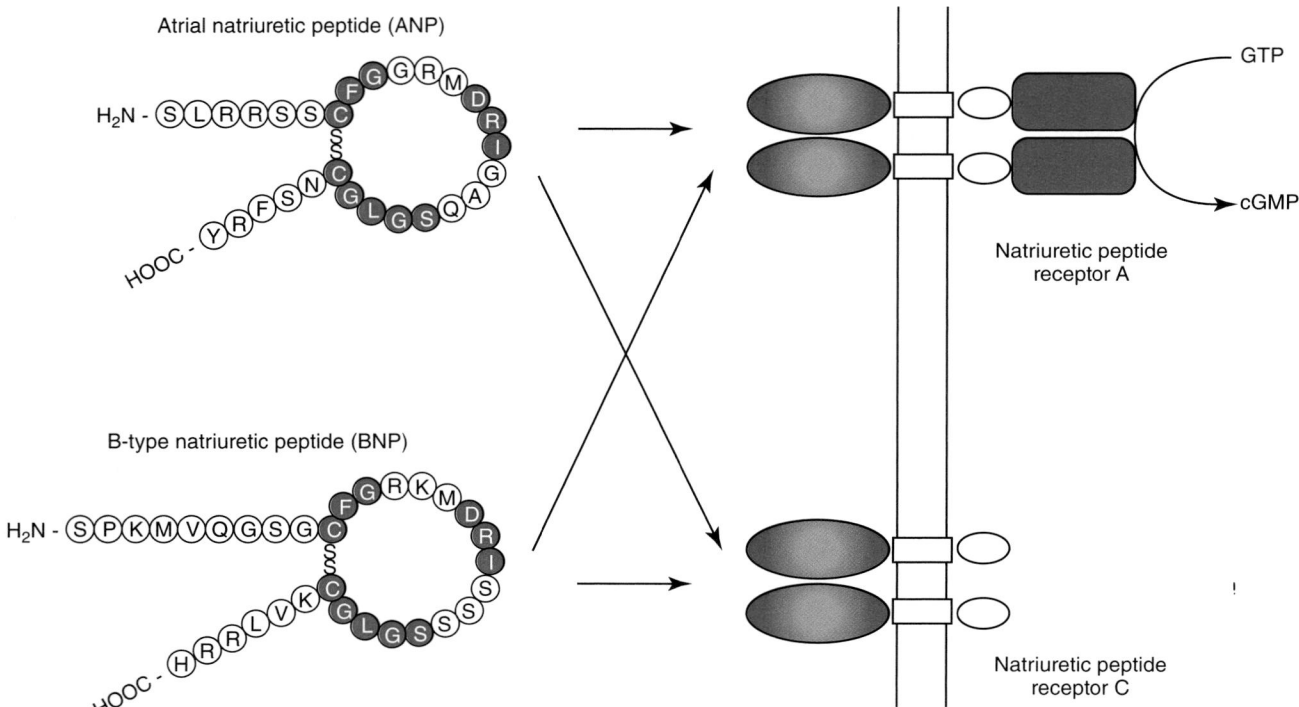

FIGURE 48.22 Schematic presentation of human atrial and B-type natriuretic peptides with their principal receptors. Homolog amino acid residues between the natriuretic peptides are marked in *bold circles*. The natriuretic peptide receptor *(NPR)*-A mediates atrial natriuretic peptide *(ANP)* and brain natriuretic peptide *(BNP)* signal transduction through induction of cyclic guanosine monophosphate *(cGMP)*. The NPR-C receptor lacks the intracellular domain and has been classed primarily as a clearance receptor. *GTP,* Guanosine triphosphate.

a biosynthetic apparatus, including several enzymes for propeptide processing, and cardiac prohormone maturation has proved much more complex than initially assumed. Clinical studies have revealed that plasma concentrations of the different proBNP-derived peptides vary greatly, which suggests that cardiac myocytes may not always release biosynthetic products on a simple equimolar basis.[301,302]

Peptide Nomenclature and Biosynthesis

Some confusion has arisen because of the incoherent nomenclature of cardiac NPs. In some ways, this confusion reflects the underlying lack of knowledge of the biosynthetic products, which has led researchers to apply nonspecific terms for the measured substances. A stringent nomenclature is, however, essential for a uniform understanding of peptide structure and function.[303] If the measured peptide is not readily distinguishable by its name, simple comparisons of reported concentrations may confuse and at worst lead to incorrect decisions. For instance, some of the abbreviations used do not identify the measured peptide(s), which should be the primary goal with the name. A common abbreviation— NT-proBNP—is used for one particular analytical method; it refers to the measurement of nonglycosylated proBNP 1-76, against which the immunoanalysis is calibrated. But the abbreviation does not provide specific information on the primary structure that is actually measured, which includes the intact precursor (proBNP 1-108) and with some cross-reactivity to the glycosylated forms (see later discussion). Other investigators have used broader terms for plasma

measurement, such as N-BNP, which refers to measurement of intact proBNP 1-108 and its N-terminal fragment(s). However, this abbreviation leaves the less astute user with the impression that it is the N terminus of BNP that is measured. The use of abbreviations such as BNP 77-108 is simply incorrect (BNP only includes 32 amino acid residues). Thus BNP-32 is synonymous with proBNP 77-108. A rational nomenclature needs to be structurally informative and should see the name in relation to its origin, that is, with insight in and reference to biosynthesis of the precursor. If this information is not available, then that should be stated. In the following section, a nomenclature based on these premises will be provided.

The Pretranslational Phase of B-Type Natriuretic Peptide Gene Expression

Human atrial (ANP) and B-type (BNP) natriuretic peptide are encoded by genes located on chromosome 1.[304,305] In rodents, the genes are located on chromosome 4 (mouse) or chromosome 5 (rat). The overall gene structure is simple and resembles other peptide hormone genes in size and composition with three exons separated by two introns. For both ANP and BNP, the major part of the coding sequence resides in exon 2. Genetic polymorphisms and mutations have been reported in both genes and in the NP receptor genes.[306] Although the impact of genetic variation in the ANP and BNP systems remains to be fully established, it seems reasonable to suspect that it may affect the plasma concentrations in a heritable manner, which in fact has been reported in the general population.[307] However, associations between mutations and risk for disease are of more clinical interest. Genetic variance in cardiac NPs may thus be involved in the pathophysiology of metabolic disorders.[294] To complicate matters further, diabetes mellitus induces increased risk for the development of CVD with concomitant changes in cardiac NP expression.[308] In addition to the promoter polymorphism, a frame shift mutation in the ANP gene has been reported in heritable AF. The frame shift introduces a C-terminally extended ANP peptide.[309]

The mature ANP and BNP transcripts consist of approximately 500 to 700 base pairs. Intracellular regulation of natriuretic gene transcription is extensive and has been reviewed elsewhere,[310–313] but both genes seem regulated by the same transcriptional factors including p38 mitogen-activated protein kinase (MAPK). p38 MAPK activates the transcription factor nucleic factor-κB (NF-κB) and subsequently ANP and BNP gene transcription.[314] Vasoactive substances such as catecholamines and angiotensin II increase natriuretic gene transcription in a p38 MAPK–dependent manner. Myocyte stretching increases the intracellular calcium concentration and modulates calcium-binding proteins that regulate downstream modulators, including calcineurin, which stimulates myocyte natriuretic gene expression.[315] Thus cardiac natriuretic gene expression can be modulated by blocking the p38 MAPK and the calcineurin pathways. Finally, the hypoxia inducible transcription factor (HIF) 1-α activates both ANP and BNP transcription, which is of importance in ischemic heart disease.[316,317] One scenario in which the ANP and BNP genes seem not to be co-regulated is in inflammation driven by specific cytokines, in which BNP gene expression increases and ANP gene expression is unaffected.[318] This differential gene expression has led to the suggestion that ANP and BNP gene products might be clinically useful when measured in concert during conditions with both hemodynamic changes and a proinflammatory drive on the cardiac myocytes, as seen after cardiac transplantation.[319]

One feature of ANP and BNP mRNA regulation should be reiterated. Although gene expression is regulated at the transcriptional level, another relevant mechanism is change in mRNA stability and the half-life of the transcripts. This RNA regulatory mechanism has been demonstrated for BNP mRNA through stimulation of α-adrenergic receptors.[320,321] The BNP mRNA stabilization is thought to be mediated though the elements in the 3′ untranslated region, which are not present in the ANP gene. Consequently, mRNA stabilization seems only to involve BNP and not ANP mRNA.

The Primary Structure of ProBrain Natriuretic Peptide

Human proBNP comprises 108 amino acid residues (see Fig. 48.22). The primary structure is slightly shorter in the mouse but with a similar C-terminal region, including the receptor binding motif. Mammalian precursor sequences have been deduced from complementary DNA (cDNA) sequences that encode the entire preprostructure.[322–325] Amino acid homology among species is largely confined to the amino- and carboxy-terminal regions, whereas the remaining prostructure varies considerably among animals. Moreover, the principal motifs for amino acid modifications and enzymatic prohormone processing are not well conserved across species.

In addition to proBNP, human preproBNP contains an N-terminal hydrophobic signal peptide of 26 amino acid residues (Fig. 48.23). As with most regulatory peptides, this sequence is removed during translation before synthesis of the C-terminal part of the precursor is completed. Interestingly, a fragment stemming from the signal peptide has been identified in cardiac tissue and in plasma from patients with cardiac disease.[326] However, preproBNP is not detectable in the blood. On the other hand, proBNP is an existing polypeptide, which has been demonstrated by chromatographic profiling and sequence-specific immunoassays.[281,289,290,327,328] The precursor molecule remains to be purified, together with the processing intermediates thereof, apart from the C-terminal 32 amino acid cleavage product, that is, BNP-32, and the N-terminal region of the precursor.[329–333] Thus whenever the primary proBNP structure is mentioned, it should be remembered that it refers to the cDNA-deduced preprosequence combined with antibody-based data from chromatographic elution, Western blotting, or immunoassays.

The Post-Translational Phase of B-Type Natriuretic Peptide Gene Expression

Post-translational BNP processing has become a subject of increasing interest. One factor contributing to this may relate to the troublesome lack of useful in vitro cellular models. Although neonatal atrial myocytes can be cultured for short periods, they do not anatomically or functionally resemble differentiated atrial, or for that matter ventricular, myocytes. Moreover, only a few immunoassays have been available for characterizing the molecular heterogeneity of the processing

---

cDNA-Deduced proBNP Sequences in Four Mammals

```
Cat    HPLGGPGPAS--EASAIQELLDGLRDTVSELQEAQMALGPLQQGHSPAESWEAQEEPPAR 58
Dog    HPLGGPGPAS--EASAIQELLDGLRDTVSELQEAQMALGPLQQGHSPAESWEAQEEPPAR 58
Man    HPLGSPGSASDLETSGLQEQRNHLQGKLSELQVEQTSLEPLQESPRPTGVWKSREVATEG 60
Mouse  YPLGSPSQSP--EQFKMQKLLELIREKSEEMAQRQLLKD---QG--------LTKEHPKR 47

Cat    VLAPHDNVLRALRRLGSSKMMRDSRCFGRRLDRIGSLSGLGCNVLRRH 106
Dog    VLAPHDNVLRALRRLGSSKMMRDSRCFGRRLDRIGSLSGLGCNVLRRH 106
Man    IRGHRKMVLYTLRAPRSPKMVQGSGCFGRKMDRISSSSGLGCKVLRRH 108
Mouse  VLRSQGSTLRVQQRPQNSKVTHISSCFGHKIDRIGSVSRLGCNALKLL 95
```

FIGURE 48.23 The primary structure of proBNP (pro-brain natriuretic peptide) in four mammals. The human proBNP sequence comprises 108 amino acid residues. The precursor sequence is evolutionary and is conserved in the C-terminal region that makes up the bioactive natriuretic peptide. In contrast, the cleavage site corresponding to position 73 to 76 in the human sequence is not well conserved. Amino acids are indicated by their single-letter codes.

intermediates. Recent advances through mass spectrometry combined with the development of sequence-specific antibodies have nevertheless revealed a complex cardiac biosynthesis of cardiac NPs.

Disulfide Bond Formation

The proBNP structure appears simple (see Figs. 48.22 and 48.23). In humans, it is divided into two principal regions by a cleavage site in position 73 to 76 (Arg-Ala-Pro-Arg). The first region is the N-terminal fragment proBNP 1 to 76, and the second region is the C-terminal BNP-32 (proBNP 77 to 108). In contrast to other prohormones, proBNP does not contain a C-terminal flanking region. The C-terminal region contains a ring structure formed by a disulfide bond between the cystyl residues in position 86 and 102, respectively (see Fig. 48.22). The ring formation is essential for receptor binding and biological activity.[334] This crucial modification in ANP and BNP synthesis takes place in the endoplasmic reticulum and may be considered the first step in post-translational processing. The protein disulfide isomerase family and thioldisulfide oxidoreductases are likely candidate enzymes involved in cardiac myocyte disulfide bond formation. Interestingly, cardiac expression of the protein disulfide isomerase transcript has been reported to be upregulated in cardiac disease.[335] Cellular experiments in vitro further suggest a direct cardioprotective effect of this regulation. It may be that not all cardiac NPs are activated through this enzymatic process, which introduces the earliest possible regulatory step in NP biosynthesis and hormone activation. Regulation of protein disulfide isomerase has been classified as endoplasmic reticulum stress, which is a hallmark of several pathologic disorders, including diabetes mellitus, neurodegenerative disorders, and ischemic heart disease.[336]

Glycosylation

Larger forms of BNP than the purified BNP-32 were first suspected from gel filtration studies of cardiac tissue extracts and plasma from patients with severe cardiac disease.[289,290,337,338] Some data even suggested molecular forms larger than the predicted precursor. Independently, several groups observed immunoreactive forms with molecular masses of 25 to 45 kDa in cardiac tissue and plasma (Fig. 48.24). Intact proBNP, however, has an expected mass of approximately 11 kDa based on the primary structure. Whether the peculiar elution patterns were in vitro artifacts or represented peptide binding to other molecules was put aside when it was shown that human proBNP exists as an O-linked glycoprotein.[339] In the precursor structure, the midregion (proBNP 36 to 71) contains seven seryl and threonyl residues, where O-linked glycosylation occurs either fully or partially (Fig. 48.25). This major modification of a polypeptide apparently does not affect the overall structure of the precursor.[298] However, the presence of carbohydrate groups clearly affects immunodetection if the epitope recognition resides within this region.[340] No specific immunoassay has yet been developed against the glycosylated forms, and the ratio between glycosylated and nonglycosylated proBNP products can be deduced only from assays that measure the nonglycosylated forms or cross-react with both forms. Whether O-linked glycosylation is an "unlimited" post-translational modification or is affected by increased BNP gene expression, as in heart disease, will be an important question for future

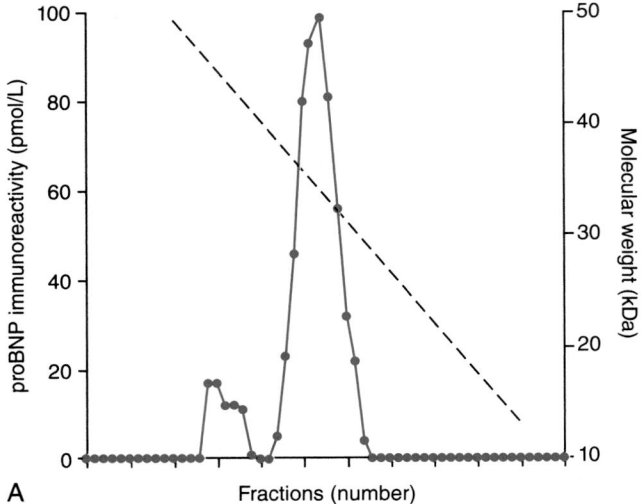

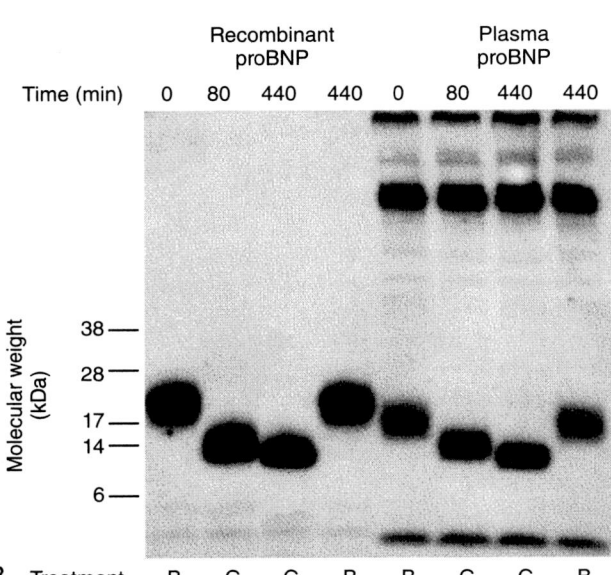

FIGURE 48.24 (A) Chromatographic profile of pro-brain natriuretic peptide *(proBNP)* immunoreactivity in human atrial tissue. Cardiac tissue extract was subjected to size exclusion high-performance liquid chromatography. Molecular size calibrators, eluted in a separate run, were used in determining molecular sizes *(dashed line)*. The proBNP immunoreactivity eluted in positions approximately three times higher than the theoretical molecular weight of intact proBNP. (B) Western blotting of recombinant *(left)* and patient *(right)* proBNP in buffer *(B)* or after deglycosylation *(G)*. The incubation time is also listed. (Modified from Schellenberger U, O'Rear J, Guzzetta A, Jue RA, Protter AA, Pollitt NS. The precursor to B-type natriuretic peptide is an O-linked glycoprotein. *Arch Biochem Biophys* 2006;451:160–6, with permission.)

studies. It should also be noted that the ANP precursor also may be subject to glycosylation.[341] In addition, the proBNP sequence varies considerably across species in the midregion (see Fig. 48.23), which probably makes glycosylation a species-specific modification. Finally, it is not known whether atrial and ventricular myocytes possess the same capacity to glycosylate natriuretic precursor peptides.

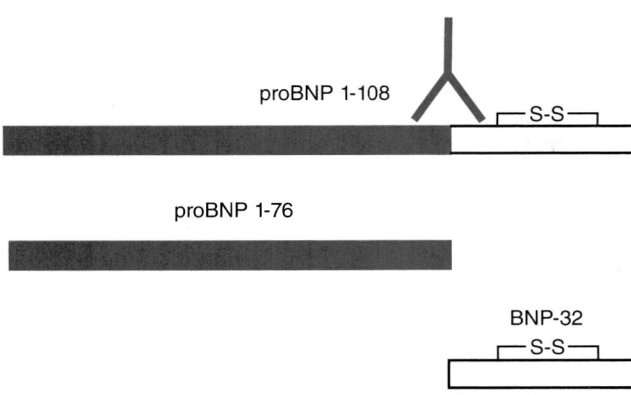

FIGURE 48.25 Immunoassay for detection of unprocessed human pro-brain natriuretic peptide *(proBNP)*. The assay uses antibody recognition of an epitope spanning the Arg-Ala-Pro-Arg site (proBNP74-76) thought to be cleaved by corin. *S-S,* Disulfide bond.

Glycosylation could perhaps be a biochemical target for diagnostic applications if the modification is affected by cardiac disease and/or reflects changes in BNP gene expression. Most interesting, however, is the potential impact of early biosynthetic glycosylation on cellular sorting and the subsequent precursor processing. Because O-linked glycosylation can occur close to the principal maturation site in position 74 to 76 (on the threonyl residue in position 71), the presence of carbohydrate groups can affect processing and hormonal maturation.[342] In turn, this modification could regulate prohormone cleavage by either blocking or guiding endoproteolytic enzymes, which may leave the propeptide with reduced or no biological activity. In fact, recent data has indicated a relationship between obesity and glycosylation at this site.[343]

Endoproteolysis and Exoproteolysis

Human proBNP was first suggested to be cleaved by the ubiquitous endoprotease furin; furin and the BNP gene are coexpressed in cardiac myocytes.[344,345] The Arg-Ala-Pro-Arg motif in position 73 to 76 in human proBNP has been shown to be a target for furin-mediated cleavage. In fact, endoproteolytic processing can be blocked in vitro by inhibition of furin, and furin has been shown to be essential for maturation of the structurally related CNP. Novel proteases designated corin and furin have been identified from human heart cDNA.[346,347] Corin is a serine protease that can cleave both proANP and proBNP in vitro, presumably at a similar cleavage site.[348–351] Corin contains a transmembrane domain anchored in the cell membrane and is thought to cleave the precursors on secretion. The enzymatic activity, however, does not require the transmembrane domain because a mutant soluble form also is capable of processing proANP.[352] A role of corin in the processing of cardiac NPs in vivo has been further substantiated by genetic coupling of corin mutations to clinical phenotypes that can be explained by reduced ANP and BNP bioactivity in circulation such as hypertension.[353,354] Corin thus seems to be a relevant candidate for cardiac processing of NPs generating the N-terminal processing fragments and C-terminal bioactive peptides.[351] Moreover, atrial post-translational processing of proANP and proBNP is likely to differ from ventricular processing because isolated atrial granules have been reported to contain both unprocessed

proANP and mature BNP-32.[355] Corin activity alone can therefore not fully explain the endoproteolytic maturation of cardiac natriuretic propeptides. It should be mentioned that the putative corin site in the BNP precursor is not conserved between mammals.

A well-established family of intracellular processing enzymes deeply involved in prohormone maturation is the proprotein/prohormone convertases (PCs). In addition to the already mentioned furin, the subtilisin-like endoproteases PC1/3 and PC2 are also expressed in the mammalian heart,[356,357] and PC1/3 expression has been demonstrated in both normal and pathologic human cardiac tissue.[358] Atrial myocytes transfected with an adenoviral vector expressing PC1/3 processes proANP to both mature ANP and to a truncated form.[359] Although the precise cleavage site was not established and the processing capacity was somewhat inefficient, this singular report does underscore the possibility that proteases other than furin and corin may be involved in the post-translational endoproteolysis of proANP and proBNP. PC1/3 is active in secretory granules and could therefore be an important regulator of atrial proBNP processing. Cardiac PC1/3 expression has been reported to be upregulated at the transcriptional level in heart disease.[360] Unfortunately, there are no data on other proBNP-derived fragments stemming from endoproteolytic processing. This may reflect the lack of specific tools for identifying such peptide fragments, which requires antibodies directed at epitopes other than the ones used so far for biochemical identification. Sandwich-based immunoassays are usually not ideal for this type of experiment. The precursor sequence contains several basic amino acid residues that potentially could represent cleavage sites for the PCs, and the molecular characterization may not be complete when it comes to identifying processing intermediates from the NP precursors.

N-terminal trimming of proBNP-derived peptides seems to be a biological feature because both the N terminus of the biosynthetic precursor and the C-terminal bioactive BNP product contain an amino acid motif for aminopeptidase recognition and cleavage. Both the N terminus of proBNP and BNP-32 (proBNP 77 to 108) contain a prolyl residue in position 2 (His-Pro and Ser-Pro, respectively). Although prolyl residues are important for peptide structure and folding, they also can be involved in exoproteolytic trimming when located near the N terminus.[361] N-terminal trimming has in fact recently been demonstrated for BNP in vitro.[288] Synthetic BNP-32 (proBNP 77 to 108) incubated in the presence of the dipeptidyl peptidase (DPP) IV removes the N-terminal Ser-Pro residues. DPP-IV is an enzyme located mainly on endothelial cells and in the circulation with a preference for cleaving N termini with either prolyl or alanyl residues in the second position.[362] Thus this DPP-IV cleavage in BNP-32 cannot per se be considered as a part of the biosynthetic maturation but is rather related to the elimination phase. An N-terminally trimmed form of proBNP lacking the His-Pro residues in position 1 to 2 also has been reported in HF patients.[363] This report disclosed that a truncated proBNP 3 to 108 form circulates in increased concentrations in HF patients. In this context, it is noteworthy that the initial report on glycosylated proBNP in a recombinant expression system (CHO cells) also identified a truncated proBNP 3-108 form in cell extracts.[339] Although this finding may be explained by experimental handling of extracts and medium, it could also imply that N-terminal exoproteolysis is a biosynthetic event. There are several enzymes which contribute to the production of BNP fragments including neprilysin (NEP) producing BNP 5-32aa, dipeptidyl peptidase IV (DPP-IV) producing BNP 3-32aa, corin (producing BNP 4-32 aa) and insulin degrading enzyme (cleavage of BNP at various positions).[364,365] In mammalian cells, intracellular aminopeptidase has been reported in compartments different from the lysosomes, suggesting N-terminal trimming as a possible part of the biosynthetic peptide maturation.[366,367] Whether the trimming of BNP and its molecular precursor serves an actual regulatory function in cardiac NP physiology remains an open question. It could be speculated that aminoterminal trimming affects the metabolic fate of the peptides and thus their turnover in circulation. There are, however, limited data available on an actual biological relevance of these trimmings.

Cellular Storage and Secretion

BNP gene expression is a feature of both atrial and ventricular myocytes. In the normal heart, the main site of BNP expression is in the atrial regions.[368,369] Ventricular BNP gene expression increases drastically in cardiac disease that affects the ventricles (e.g., CHF).[370] The observation of ventricular BNP gene expression in ventricular disease may have given rise to the common statement that BNP is predominantly a ventricular hormone. Atrial and ventricular myocytes, however, differ considerably with respect to their endocrine phenotypes, and it is reasonable to expect major differences in peptide storage and secretion patterns.[371,372] For instance, it is well established that atrial myocytes contain intracellular granules for peptide storage and maturation, which actually contributed to the primary hypothesis of the endocrine heart.[272,273] Atrial granules contain both intact precursors and biosynthetic end products, that is, bioactive ANP-28 and BNP-32. In contrast, normal ventricular myocytes do not seem to express such granules and normal ventricular myocytes do not contain proBNP-derived peptides.[368] A few reports have observed granules and proBNP-derived peptides in ventricular myocytes sampled from pathologic hearts.[373–375] Thus ventricular myocytes not only regulate the BNP gene at the transcriptional and post-translational level but also seem to be able to differentiate with respect to the biosynthetic apparatus per se. An acidic protein class involved in granule formation is the chromogranins.[376] Chromogranins, or just granins, comprise at least three proteins (A, B, and C) that possess aggregation characteristics suggesting a function in the formation of secretory granules. Cardiac expression of chromogranin A and B has been established.[377–379] The focus on cardiac chromogranins, however, has mainly been on the potential biological activity of chromogranin-derived fragments (the vasostatins) or on plasma measurement for diagnostic purposes.[380] Whether cardiac chromogranins are involved in the biosynthesis of ANP and BNP through formation of granules remains an area for future studies. It should be stated that chromogranin A–deficient mice do not reveal obvious changes in granule formation in, for instance, adrenal chromaffin cells.[381] Cardiac chromogranin B also has been suggested to be directly involved in BNP gene expression through a Ca^{2+}-dependent induction of the BNP promoter.[377] Further in vitro experiments targeted at proANP and proBNP maturation in cardiac cell systems devoid of chromogranin A and B may thus reveal a specific role for the granins in storage and secretion of NPs.

ProBNP-Derived Peptides in Plasma

ProBNP-derived peptides are secreted by cardiac myocytes and circulate in plasma. Their molecular heterogeneity has primarily been characterized by chromatography in combination with sequence-specific immunoassays. Much of our present conception of the cellular synthesis is in fact derived from the plasma phase, which represents the sum of secretion and metabolism. The picomolar concentrations in plasma limit the possibilities for full biochemical identification and underscore a careful understanding of epitope recognition by the immunoassays. With this in mind, it is established that bioactive BNP is secreted from the heart and circulates without binding to plasma proteins.[382] Synthetic BNP-32 (proBNP 77 to 108) is trimmed when incubated in whole blood, generating BNP forms lacking N-terminal amino acid residues.[338,383] As mentioned earlier, this molecular form can be generated in vitro by enzymatic trimming by DPP-IV and possibly other aminopeptidases.[288] Further processing of plasma BNP seems to involve degradation with a loss of bioactivity though disruption of the ring structure mediated by neutral endopeptidase (neprilysin, NEP 24.11) or by receptor-mediated cellular uptake. Although this has been known for some time, the therapeutic potential of inhibiting neprilysin with increased plasma concentrations of "beneficial" NPs is an appealing strategy.[384] The metabolic fate of BNP-32 has been reported to be 13 to 20 minutes.[385,386] Immunoreactive BNP is also excreted in urine, but the precise contribution of renal excretion to renal metabolism is not yet clarified. A minor degree of hepatic clearance also has been shown, which is not significantly altered in patients with liver failure.[387]

In addition to bioactive BNP, other proBNP-derived fragments circulate in plasma.[388,389] These fragments are commonly referred to as N-terminal proBNP, but the molecular heterogeneity also includes the intact precursor, in particular in HF patients.[290,302,390] Cardiac secretion of proBNP and its N-terminal fragments has been demonstrated by blood sampling from the coronary sinus. The molar ratio of secreted proBNP 1 to 76 to intact proBNP is not yet fully clarified but is likely to depend on cardiac status, that is, more unprocessed precursor compared to biosynthetic cleavage products in severe HF (Fig. 48.26). In the metabolic phase, there are still major discrepancies in the suggested half-life of N-terminal precursor fragments, which at least partially reflect the epitope recognition in the assays. Theoretically, the half-life of proBNP 1 to 76 in circulation should be approximately 25 minutes[391] and thus not differ greatly from the established metabolism of BNP-32 (proBNP 77 to 108). One report, however, suggested a considerably longer half-life (<90 minutes after cardiac pacing), which would fit well with the higher plasma concentrations of N-terminal proBNP fragments compared to bioactive BNP in healthy individuals and in cardiac patients. As our perception of the molecular heterogeneity in plasma has changed radically over the last several years, there is an urgent need for new pharmacokinetic experiments to separate the biosynthetic phase from the peripheral elimination.

Biosynthesis and Assay Calibration

Elucidation of cardiac NP biosynthesis has disclosed a complex post-translational maturation that produces a variety of peptides targeted for cellular secretion (see Fig. 48.26). The different phases of gene expression are not only region-specific

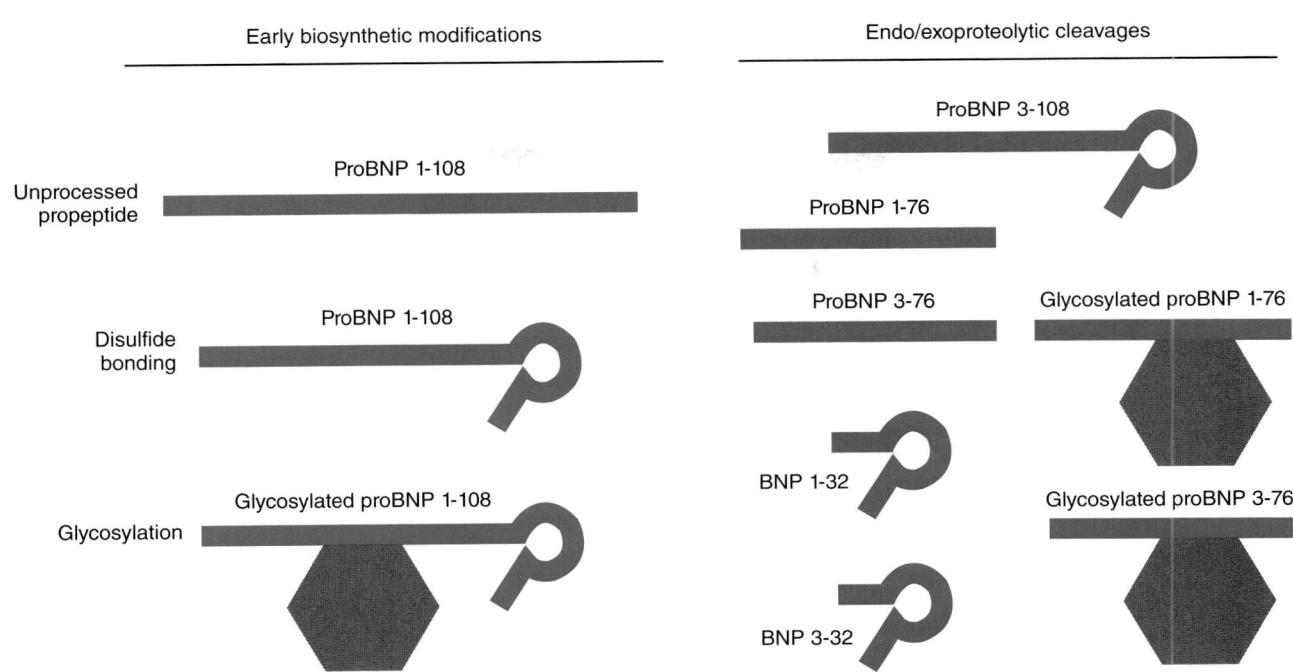

FIGURE 48.26 Schematic presentation of possible pro-brain natriuretic peptide *(proBNP)*-derived peptide products. Note that most peptides are not chemically identified but rather are suggested by biochemical methods that rely on antibody recognition. Carbohydrate is indicated by the *hexagons*.

but also depend on changes within the secretory apparatus in cardiac myocytes. The main clinical applications of the peptides today strongly relate to plasma measurement in cardiovascular diagnostics and prognosis. The immunoassays thus need to be designed with insight into the biosynthesis of the peptides. Another defining aspect of immunoassay measurement is the choice of calibrator. This aspect has so far not been scrutinized by researchers apart from the observation of disturbingly large discrepancies across the different assays.[392] On the other hand, it has not been possible to raise meaningful assay calibration issues before now, until the existence of a complex molecular heterogeneity has been established. One way of bypassing this lack of information has been introduced as a "processing-independent assay," which in principle quantifies one in vitro cleavage product that represents all the secreted precursor molecules. This assay then can be calibrated with the specific cleavage product and assay measurement performed on a stoichiometrically correct basis. If one is to choose a proBNP-derived calibrator peptide for plasma measurement, it becomes more complex. As the ratio of bioactive BNP to intact precursor shifts toward less processed biosynthetic products, the dominant "disease" form might be chosen over the more prevalent forms in healthy individuals. However, large comparative studies still have not revealed major differences between BNP or proBNP measurements in terms of overall clinical performance. One report on assay calibration has shown that assays directed at the C-terminal BNP region do not really cross-react with the larger biosynthetic products.[392] Plasma measurement based on assays directed against the N-terminal proBNP fragment is, however, greatly influenced by the degree of O-linked glycosylation. Clearly, this issue is far from settled and our present perception of "normal" concentrations of the different biosynthetic products may still have to be redefined.

Inefficient Prohormone Maturation in Heart Failure

HF patients display highly increased plasma concentrations of bioactive ANP and BNP. With a dramatic upregulation of the gene expression and concomitant high concentrations of immunoreactive ANP and BNP in plasma, it seems reasonable to expect increased natriuresis. The common presentation of HF, however, is congestion, sodium retention, and edema. Although HF is a complex syndrome with both activation and inhibition of multiple neurohumoral systems, the paradoxical lack of ANP and BNP bioactivity is still compelling. HF patients respond to intravenous administration of chemically synthesized ANP and BNP, which has led to the introduction of a BNP-32 analog, nesiritide.[393] This peptide is a potent drug in HF, which raised serious concerns regarding patient safety by causing unwanted hypotension.[394] Experts have further explored the possibilities of NP drugs by constructing structurally related peptides that possess natriuretic effects but without the undesirable hypotension.[395] Obviously, this research area could prove of major relevance to medical therapy because all the different physiologic effects of NPs could have specific roles in modern treatment of HF and other cardiovascular pathologic processes.

The endocrine paradox of sodium and water retention in HF, in which the gold standard biomarkers are the cardiac NPs, relates to insufficient post-translational maturation of the biosynthetic precursors.[396] A well-established analogy to this phenomenon is enhanced secretion of proinsulin over mature insulin in patients with type 2 diabetes. In the early stages of the disease, selective proinsulin measurement is therefore a valuable tool in evaluating pancreatic β-cell dysfunction. A shift toward secretion of unprocessed precursors in cardiac disease also may represent early involvement of ventricular expression and secretion because efficient precursor maturation seems to dominantly be an endocrine feature of atrial biosynthesis. In support of this explanation, the intracellular processing enzymes involved in ANP and BNP maturation are dominantly expressed in atrial myocytes. Moreover, the ventricular myocytes do not, at least in the early stages of disease, contain secretory granules for peptide storage and maturation. The post-translational processing of ventricular precursors may not be efficient in the production of needed natriuretic potency, although immunoassays cross-react to various degrees with the unprocessed biosynthetic products. Though speculative, there may be large individual differences in the heart's ability to process the precursor peptides, which could help explain the highly variable HF phenotypes. The ratio of mature BNP to unprocessed proBNP might be of diagnostic relevance in parallel with the present application of proinsulin to insulin measurement. These considerations are consistent with recent data that suggest that with acute HF, there is less perturbation of the NP system and specifically less glycosylation at threonine 71, which allows for more efficient conversion of proBNP to NT-proBNP and bioactive BNP.[13] This might explain why some studies have shown a rapid change in BNP values with diuresis in patients who present acutely.[14] With more chronic HF, glycosylation is more prominent, and thus there is less active BNP and the system likely requires more time and a greater degree of change to manifest clinical significance.

If specific assays for the various forms are applied together, it may be possible to define an early endocrine hallmark of the HF syndrome that could aid clinicians in tailoring diuretic therapy according to the patient-specific ability to ameliorate congestion through secretion of bioactive natriuretic hormones.

ANALYTICAL CONSIDERATIONS OF BIOMARKERS ASSAYS IN HEART FAILURE

In 2005 and 2007, IFCC committees provided recommendations on analytical and preanalytical quality specifications for NP assays, which was further updated in 2019.[397] The 2019 document by the IFCC Committee on Clinical Applications of Cardiac Bio-Markers (C-CB) was an educational document which highlighted the important biochemical, analytical, and clinical aspects pertinent to NP testing. The focus was related to NPs in HF with an assessment of previous laboratory recommendations regarding NP testing. As BNP and NT-proBNP become more integrated into clinical practice as diagnostic and prognostic biomarkers, understanding differences among individual assay characteristics is extremely important. The influence of clinical, analytical, and preanalytical factors on the increasing number of BNP and NT-proBNP assays is evident (see Table 48.4 as an example, as well as on the IFCC C-CB website: https://www.ifcc.org/ifcc-education-division/emd-committees/committee-on-clinical-applications-of-cardiac-bio-markers-c-cb/).[364,397,398] Thus there is a need for better understanding by clinicians on how to interpret findings of different studies predicated on BNP or NT-proBNP concentrations monitored by different assays.[397–400] The laboratory community must also work closely with the in vitro diagnostics companies to assist in defining the numerous assay characteristics.[401] When BNP or NT-proBNP assays are used as biomarkers for diagnosis, therapy decisions, and prognosis, or used in clinical trials or studies, they should be well characterized, as suggested in the list of recommendations that follows. It is further recommended that when designing studies using BNP or NT-proBNP, investigators should review the Standards for Reporting Diagnostic Accuracy[402] initiative for both assay characterization issues and for clinical and patient enrollment issues when monitoring BNP or NT-proBNP levels.

A growing diversity of BNP and NT-proBNP assays are used worldwide,[397,398] emphasizing the need for both analytical and clinical validation of all commercial assays to support definite clinical acceptance of these new biomarkers. At present (see C-CB website for most up to date list: https://www.ifcc.org/ifcc-education-division/emd-committees/committee-on-clinical-applications-of-cardiac-bio-markers-c-cb/), more companies have regulatory approved NT-proBNP assays as compared to BNP assays. Some assays are suitable for whole blood and thus can be used in the point-of-care setting (examples of companies with whole blood as an acceptable sample type include Abbott i-STAT, ET Healthcare, Medience, Radiometer, Roche, Siemens). Preliminary data from research assays for proBNP have been described but none to date have regulatory approval.[392] Furthermore, Thermo-Fischer-BRAHMS has the only regulatory approved assay for mid-range (MR)-proANP, and is equivalent to BNP as a biomarker to rule out and confirm HF.[397] As the number of assays for the different NP biomarkers grows, it is even more essential that appropriate clinical and analytical assay criteria are uniformly adapted. The accurate clinical performance of each NP assay, which may serve as the basis for life-and-death medical decisions, sets the stage to establish assay criteria as indispensable. Limited clinical data are available for MR-proANP, but it has been recommended as a biomarker in the ESC guideline.[397,403,404]

BNP and NT-proBNP are determined by a number of different immunoassays using antibodies directed to different epitopes located on the antigen molecules (see Table 48.4). For BNP one antibody binds to the ring structure and the other antibody to either the carboxy- or amino-terminal end. Degradation of BNP (amino acids [a.a.] 77 to 108) is known to occur by proteolytic cleavage of serine and proline residues in vivo and in vitro (see Fig. 48.26).[337,397,405] This degradation may affect antibody affinities and thus be responsible for differences in stabilities of BNP-32 monitored by different commercial BNP assays. For NT-proBNP (a.a. 1 to 76) monitoring, an improved understanding of potential cross-reactivity with split products of the N-terminal portion of NT-proBNP and proBNP itself are needed. For both assays, BNP and NT-proBNP, minimizing interferents from heterophilic antibodies and rheumatoid factor, for example, needs to be optimized. The influence, stabilizing or destabilizing, of anticoagulant additives, as well as the type of collection tube, have been well described.[337,406] For BNP, EDTA-anticoagulated whole blood or plasma appears to be the only acceptable specimen choice. For NT-proBNP, serum, heparin plasma, and EDTA plasma appear acceptable; however not all manufacturers and NT-proBNP assays have all three matrices listed so evaluation may be needed in selecting or switching the sample type. Plastic blood collection tubes are necessary for BNP, while for NT-proBNP, either glass or plastic is acceptable.

In the clinical setting,[348,407–410] BNP and NT-proBNP assay characteristics need to be better understood or better established for optimal consideration as diagnostic and prognostic

TABLE 48.4 Analytical Characteristics of Commercially Available Natriuretic Peptide Assays per the Manufacturer

Assay	Capture Antibody	Detection Antibody	Standard Material	Claim
BNP				
Abbott Architect, iSTAT	NH2 terminus and part of the ring structure (Scios), murine MAb, aa 5–13	COOH terminus, murine MAb, aa 26–32	Synthetic BNP 32	Assist in diagnosis of HF; assess severity of disease
Alere[a] Triage BNP	NH2 terminus and part of the ring structure (Scios), murine MAb, aa 5–13	BNP (Biosite), murine omniclonal AB, epitope not characterized	Recombinant BNP	Aid in diagnosis and severity assessment of HF; risk stratification of patients with ACS and HF; FDA cleared
Beckman Coulter[a] Access, Access 2, DxI	BNP (Biosite), murine Omniclonal AB, epitope not characterized	NH2 terminus and part of the ring structure (Scios), murine MAb, aa 5–13	Recombinant BNP	Diagnosis HF; assess severity HF; risk ACS; risk HF
Siemens (Bayer) ACS 180, Advia Centaur, Advia Centaur CP	COOH terminus (BC–203) (Shionogi), murine MAb, aa 27–32	Ring structure (KY-hBN-PII) (Shionogi), murine MAb	Synthetic BNP	Aid in diagnosis and assessment of severity of HF; predict survival and likelihood of future HF in ACS patients
Siemens (Dade Behring) Dimension VISTA, Dimension ExL	Ring structure (KY-hBNPII) murine MAb, aa 14–21	COOH terminus (BC-203), murine MAb, aa 27–32	Synthetic BNP 32	Aid in diagnosis and assessment of severity of HF; predict survival and likelihood of future HF in ACS patients; pending FDA clearance
Shionogi	COOH terminus (BC–203), murine MAb, aa 27–32	Ring structure (KY-hBN-PII), murine MAb	Synthetic BNP	Not FDA cleared
Tosoh ST AIA-PACK BNP	COOH terminus (BC–203), murine MAb, aa 27–32	Ring structure (KY-hBN-PII), murine MAb	Synthetic BNP	Not FDA cleared
NT-proBNP				
Alere Triage NT-proBNP	Murine MAb, aa 27–31	Sheep MAb, aa 42–46	Synthetic NTproBNP 1–76	Aid in diagnosis of HF; risk stratification of patients with ACS and HF; assessment of increased risk of cardiovascular events and mortality in patients at risk for HF who have stable CAD; not currently available in the US
bioMérieux NT-proBNP1 VIDAS	NH2 terminus polyclonal sheep AB, aa 1–21	Central molecule, polyclonal sheep AB, aa 39–50	Synthetic NTproBNP 1–76	Diagnosis HF
NT-proBNP2 VIDAS	Murine MAb, aa 27–31	Sheep MAb, aa 42 –46	Synthetic NTproBNP 1–76	Not FDA cleared
Mitsubishi Chemical PATHFAST	NH2 terminus polyclonal sheep AB, aa 1–21	Central molecule, polyclonal sheep AB, aa 39–50	Synthetic NTproBNP 1–76	Aid diagnosis of CHF; assess severity CHF; risk stratification in ACS and stable CAD
Nanogen LifeSign DXpress Reader	Monoclonal (mouse) and polyclonal (goat) Abs	Polyclonal sheep AB	Synthetic NTproBNP 1–76	Diagnosis HF
Ortho Clinical Diagnostics Vitros ECi	NH2 terminus polyclonal sheep AB, aa 1–21	Central molecule, polyclonal sheep AB, aa 39–50	Synthetic NTproBNP 1–76	Aid diagnosis of CHF; risk stratification of ACS and CHF; risk assessment of CV events and mortality in patients at risk for HF with stable CAD; assess severity in HF
Radiometer AQT90 FLEX NT-proBNP	NH2 terminus polyclonal sheep AB, aa 1–21	Central molecule, polyclonal sheep AB, aa 39–50	Synthetic NTproBNP 1–76	Diagnosis HF; risk stratification of patients with ACS and HF; not FDA cleared

TABLE 48.4   Analytical Characteristics of Commercially Available Natriuretic Peptide Assays per the Manufacturer   cont'd

Assay	Capture Antibody	Detection Antibody	Standard Material	Claim
Response Biomedical RAMP	Murine MAb, aa 27–31	Central molecule, polyclonal sheep AB, aa 39–50	Synthetic NT-proBNP 1–76	Diagnosis HF; assess severity HF
Roche NT-proBNP I Elecsys, E170	NH2 terminus polyclonal sheep AB, aa 1–21	Central molecule, polyclonal sheep AB, aa 39–50	Synthetic NT-proBNP 1–76	Diagnosis HF; assess severity HF; risk ACS; risk HF
NT-proBNP II Elecsys, E170	MAb, aa 27–31	Sheep MAb, aa 42–46	Synthetic NT-proBNP 1–76	Treatment monitoring in LVD
Siemens (Dade Behring) Dimension RxL, Stratus CS, Dimension VISTA, Dimension EXL with LM	NH2 terminus monoclonal sheep AB, aa 22–28	Central molecule, Sheep MAb, aa 42–46	Synthetic NT-proBNP 1–76	Aid in the diagnosis of CHF and assessment of severity; risk stratification of patients with ACS and HF
Siemens (DPC) Immulite 1000, 2000 2500	NH2 terminus polyclonal sheep AB, aa 1–21	Central molecule, polyclonal sheep AB, aa 39–50	Synthetic NT-proBNP 1–76	Not FDA cleared
Assay MR-proANP				
Thermo Fisher Scientific KRYPTOR	Polyclonal sheep AB, aa 50–72 of NT-proANP	Monoclonal rat AB, aa 73–90 of NT-proANP	Synthetic NTproANP 50–90	Not FDA cleared

aBoth the Alere and Beckman systems use the same two antibodies but due to their different assay formats, designation of the monoclonal and omniclonal antibodies as capture and detection antibody is not absolute. (Modified with permission from IFCC-International Federation of Clinical Chemistry and Laboratory Medicine, website http://www.ifcc.org and see IFCC C-CB https://www.ifcc.org/ifcc-education-division/emd-committees/committee-on-clinical-applications-of-cardiac-bio-markers-c-cb/ website for most recent updates)
aa, Amino acids; *AB,* antibody; *ACS,* acute coronary syndrome; *BNP,* b-type natriuretic peptide; *CAD,* coronary artery disease; *CHF,* congestive heart failure; *CV,* cardiovascular; *FDA,* US Food and Drug Administration; *HF,* heart failure; *LVD,* left ventricular dysfunction; *NA,* not available; *NP,* natriuretic peptide; *NT-pro BNP,* N-terminal pro-BNP. *MR-proANP,* midregional pro-ANP.
From Vasile VC, Jaffe AS. Natriuretic peptides and analytical barriers. *Clin Chem* 2017;63:50–8.

biomarkers, as discussed later. Further, recent observations that proBNP, the precursor peptide that splits into BNP and NT-proBNP, appears to have cross-reactivity with both BNP and NT-proBNP assays may have substantial implications regarding clinical usage.[327] Indeed, some would argue most of what is measured in HF patients is proBNP. The influence of age, gender, ethnicity, and non-HF pathologic processes has been shown to substantially influence what may otherwise be considered a normal reference concentration.[397,411] Renal impairment has been shown to substantially increase NT-proBNP concentrations and BNP to a lesser extent.[397,412–416]

For BNP a single cutoff at 100 ng/L (pg/mL) has been designated, likely driven by the FDA clearance at this value as the ROC curve value optimized for diagnostic accuracy. However, as shown in Fig. 48.27, values in normal subjects older than 75 years appear to be either falsely increased or are not normal, with the 100 pg/mL cutoff detecting occult pathologic processes. For NT-proBNP, most assays use cutoffs that are age-based for younger than 75 years (example, 125 ng/L cutoff) and older than 75 years (example 450 ng/L cutoff). Again, these cutoffs appear to misclassify many normal subjects, as shown in Fig. 48.28. Clinical studies (proBNP Investigation of Dyspnea in the Emergency [PRIDE]) have

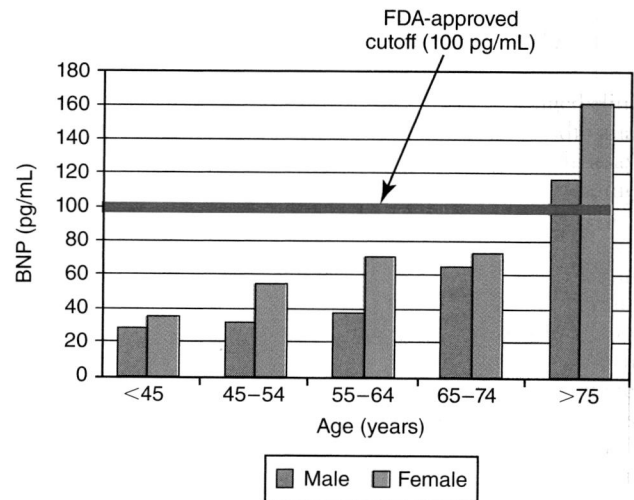

FIGURE 48.27 Representative brain natriuretic peptide *(BNP)* concentration distributions in normal males and females by decade (years) with indication of the US Food and Drug Administration *(FDA)*-cleared 100 pg/mL (ng/L) cutoff value.

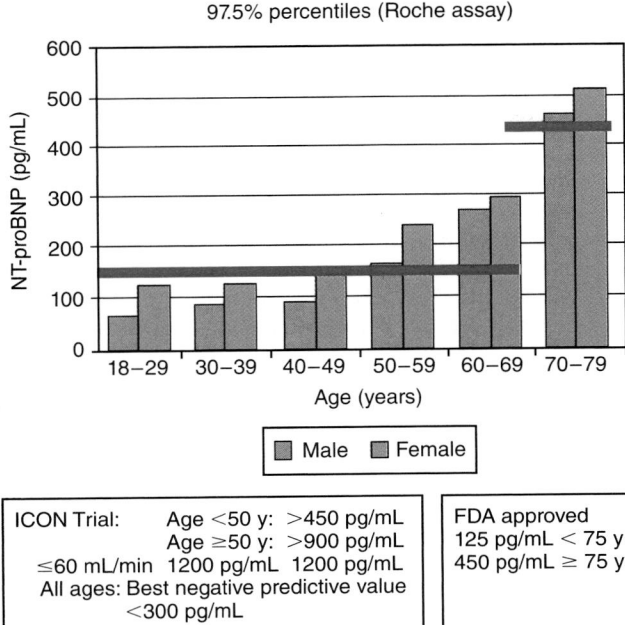

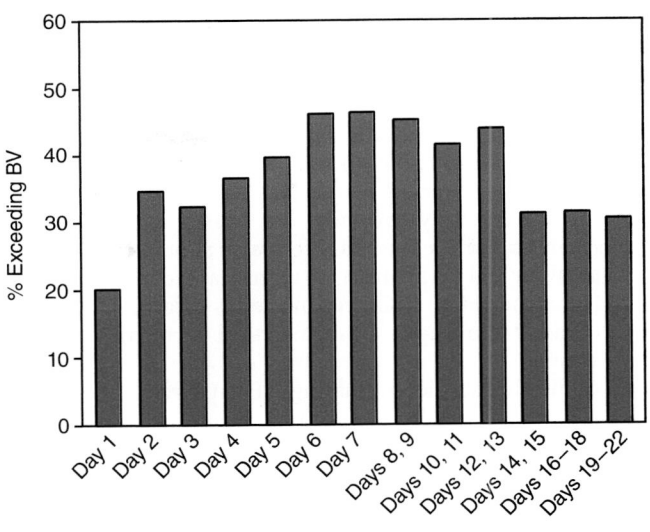

97.5% percentiles (Roche assay)

ICON Trial: Age <50 y: >450 pg/mL
                Age ≥50 y: >900 pg/mL
≤60 mL/min   1200 pg/mL   1200 pg/mL
All ages: Best negative predictive value
                <300 pg/mL

FDA approved
125 pg/mL < 75 y
450 pg/mL ≥ 75 y

FIGURE 48.28 Representative N-terminal pro-brain natriuretic peptide (NT-proBNP) concentration distributions in normal males and females by decade (years) with indication of the US Food and Drug Administration (FDA)-cleared age-related cutoff values compared with those recommended by the International Collaborative on NT-proBNP (ICON) trial determined by age and renal function.

64   62   58   54   59   87   69   80   66   69   69   56   31
Percent of changes that decreased

FIGURE 48.29 Variability of brain natriuretic peptide concentrations by day from initial admission order, with demonstration that more than 50% exceed biological variability (BV) (100% change) over a 2-week period. (From Wu AH, Smith A, Appel FS. Optimum blood collection intervals for B-type natriuretic peptide testing in patients with heart failure. *Am J Cardiol* 2004;93:1562–3, with permission from Excerpta Medica.)

more appropriately defined age-derived and renal function–derived cutoffs as also shown in Fig. 48.28, designated by 50 years of age and estimated glomerular filtration rate (eGFR) at 60 mL/min per 1.73 m², with an optimal NPV at less than 300 pg/mL that is age, gender, and eGFR independent. Obesity also has been shown to have an association with BNP and NT-proBNP measurements,[343,417–419] with an inverse relationship between increased BMI and BNP decrease in CHF patients. Also, HF patients who received the drug nesiritide (human recombinant BNP) for therapy and management may have had confounding BNP results because nesiritide is molecularly identical to endogenous BNP; however, it would not have confounded the NT-proBNP measurements. Finally, a lack of understanding of the physiologic and biological variability of BNP and NT-proBNP in HF patients may cause clinicians to misinterpret changing (increasing or decreasing) BNP and NT-proBNP concentrations in the context of establishing the success or failure of therapy. It has been shown that both BNP and NT-proBNP exhibit a within-subject biological variability of 35 to 45%.[420] Thus when considering what is significantly different between serial BNP or NT-proBNP values, a RCV of 80% is necessary, yet many HF trials use 30% change.[397] This is what has been documented in patients with chronic HF. A small study has demonstrated that in HF patients monitored for BNP over at least two periods during 2 weeks for BNP, that less than 50% of concentrations were found to be outside the expected biological variability (Fig. 48.29). However, it may be that the benefit in outcomes reported reflects the fact that those with reductions will continue to have their values decrease more substantially and thus become for a larger percent of patients beyond

the reference change interval. This implies that BNP or NT-proBNP monitoring may be overused and reemphasizes its role as a confirmatory biomarker and not a test that clinicians should solely rely on to manage HF patients.

Data have indicated low diagnostic concordance and correlation between BNP and NT-proBNP concentrations, especially among patients with chronic kidney disease using commercially available technology.[421] In addition, the literature is scattered with reports of home-brewed BNP and NT-proBNP assays that may add to the confusion of clinicians when interpreting and comparing data from different studies, whether in diagnosing or ruling out HF, managing HF, screening for asymptomatic left ventricular dysfunction, or for risk stratification and prognostication for patients with HF, ACS, or other pathologic processes. One must consider the assay used, the clinical evidence available based on the individual assay, and the aim of the biomarker-based studies. No peer-reviewed literature has demonstrated that the two assays are analytically equivalent at present.[421] Thus until large studies are available, caution is suggested before the conclusions based on one particular BNP or NT-proBNP assay are translated to another assay.

The following laboratory practice recommendations from the IFCC C-CB committee are provided in regard to NPs and HF.[397]

1. Using different NP assays in clinical practice is not recommended due to the complex nature of NP processing and cleavage and difference in what assays measure. Clinicians should be aware that different assays will provide different concentrations in any given clinical situation. Extrapolation from one assay concentration to another can be confounding.

2. NP assays require extensive characterization prior to implementation in clinical practice.
3. URLs for NP assays should be stratified by age and sex.
4. Development of higher order reference methods and commutable standards for BNP and NT-proBNP are strongly recommended, with standardization efforts to consider differences in the NP fragments detected and the impact of glycosylation.
5. Analytical imprecision of NP assays should be improved to allow for refinement of significant clinical changes. Here, the IFCC C-CB recommends a target CV of less than 10% to improve the analytical performance of NP assays.
6. Additional studies evaluating NPs in diverse ethnic populations are needed especially in regard to target-derived cutoffs.
7. Age-stratified cutoffs for BNP to rule in acute HF should be validated.
8. A specific BNP/NT-proBNP biomarker-guided strategy cannot be recommended at this time.
9. Comorbidities that influence NPs must be addressed when interpreting NP values and determining medical decision limits.
10. Additional studies are required to validate recent data that suggest that both BNP and NT-proBNP retain their long-term prognostic utility in patients receiving therapy with NEP inhibitors.

In summary, laboratorians and clinicians must be cognizant of the numerous considerations inherent in the NPs as markers for management of cardiology patients, including the form of the biomarker itself (BNP or NT-proBNP); the lack of standardization of immunoassays; that reference and medical decision limits are dependent on age and gender; that biological variation of NPs in individuals is inherently high; the diagnostic time window (admission or monitoring trends over time); the clinical setting in which NPs are used (e.g., general practice, emergency room, and coronary care unit); the patient subset being tested (i.e., renal failure, sepsis); and whether the application is for diagnostic use, prognostic use, or for a future potential application of therapeutic guidance. All of these aspects must be taken into consideration with the implementation of biomarkers such as NPs to avoid the possibility for misinterpretation of a result for patient care.

Clinical Use of Natriuretic Peptides

BNP, NT-proBNP, and novel NP assays that are being developed have proved of assistance to clinicians in the evaluation of patients with impaired left ventricular function, with or without CHF and those with coronary heart disease.[421-427] On the other hand, the more we have learned about NPs, the more complicated the biology of these biomarkers has become (see previous discussion).

Use in the Diagnosis of Congestive Heart Failure

The initial validation of NPs was done based on the ability to improve the diagnosis of CHF. The situations chosen to test this hypothesis were not in sophisticated cardiology offices but in the ED and primary care practices.[16,17] The emergency setting is an extremely busy environment in which there is often a severe press for time, making cautious and careful evaluation more difficult. In addition, ED physicians are generalists having to triage problems related to trauma, infectious disease, and a variety of other complaints relating to almost any organ system. Some are and some are not very sophisticated in regard to cardiovascular issues and the presenting symptoms and cardiovascular examination associated with HF. Accordingly, some have objected to the use of this as the primary testing ground for the use of NPs for the diagnosis of HF. General internists are in a similar position, especially in the outpatient setting where these evaluations are done where they have limited resources and a heterogeneity of expertise related to this particular diagnosis. Thus the relatively marginal improvement in diagnostic yield (74 to 81% in the Breathing Not Properly [BNP] trial and 92 to 96% in the PRIDE trial) is not terribly impressive in one sense. However, in parsing the data, it is clear that the majority of the benefit of the use of NPs for diagnosis resides in the triage of patients in whom clinicians are ambivalent, as recently documented.[428] When patients have a very low risk for HF, it is not clear that NPs help at all, and, similarly, when they have a classic presentation, they have such a high frequency of HF and such a high pretest probability that NPs are unlikely to be helpful. However, there is a group of patients with dyspnea in whom the clinician is ambivalent and it is this group in which NPs are helpful. Of importance in the interpretation of NPs in this situation is that marginal values often are not helpful. The BNP trial suggested the use of one cutoff value at 100 ng/L to make the diagnosis of HF. This value could have been altered to increase either sensitivity or specificity (Fig. 48.30).[429] However, 26% of the population had values between 100 and 500 ng/L. One-third of this group did not have CHF according to subsequent adjudication, and two-thirds did, but unfortunately, there was no cutoff value that distinguished these groups. For this reason, a group of investigators (ICON) analyzed their data with NT-proBNP looking to generate values that will help to both include and exclude disease.[430] This is an extremely valuable approach. They report that a value for NT-proBNP less than 300 ng/L effectively excludes CHF. Values over 450 ng/L in individuals who are younger than 50 years rules in HF, and values above 900 ng/L diagnose HF in patients who are over the age of 50. As is clear, there are gaps between these values describing the fact that clinical judgment addressing additional diagnostic investigation is still importantly necessary in the use of NPs. It is for this reason that most guidelines groups have not suggested the routine use of NPs for diagnosis in every patient who presents with dyspnea.[29,431,432] Instead, they recommend the judicious use in patients in whom the diagnosis is not clear. It is axiomatic to suggest that consideration of gender, age, and weight (see previous discussion) in interpreting such values is advised. In addition, it is clear that the worse the clinical class of the HF, the higher is the NP levels (Fig. 48.31). The diagnosis may be problematic, especially in patients who have other comorbidities.[39,433,434] Chronic obstructive pulmonary disease and CVD frequently overlap, and it is in these sorts of patients in whom the optimal use of NPs for diagnosis likely resides. Other disease processes (Box 48.5) can cause elevations and must be taken into account by including the clinical situation into interpretation of the NP values. It should be noted that the MR-proANP assay (listed above) is equivalent to BNP and NT-proBNP for the diagnosis of HF in the ED.[404]

PRIDE

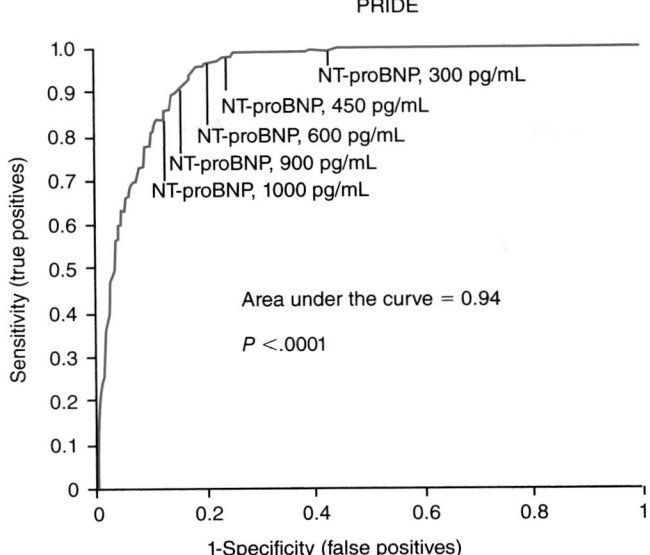

Cut point	Sensitivity	Specificity	Positive predictive value	Negative predictive value	Accuracy
300 pg/mL	99%	68%	62%	99%	79%
450 pg/mL	98%	76%	68%	99%	83%
600 pg/mL	96%	81%	73%	97%	86%
900 pg/mL	90%	85%	76%	94%	87%
1000 pg/mL	87%	86%	78%	91%	87%

Breathing Not Properly

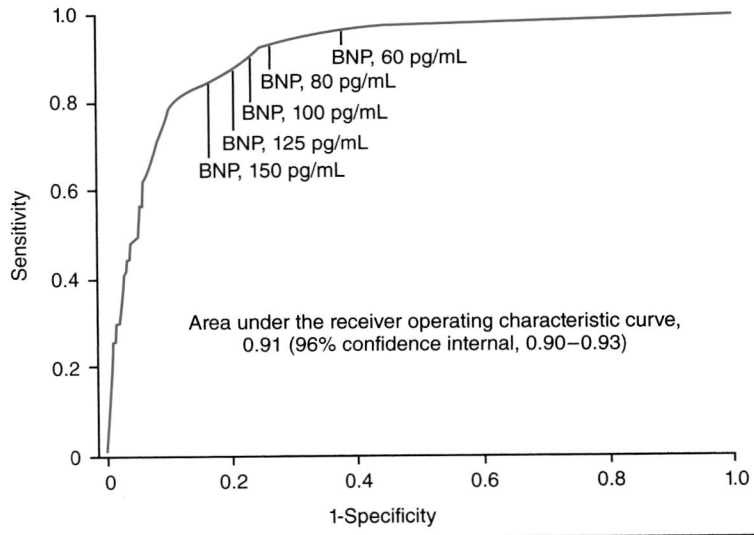

BNP pg/mL	Sensitivity (%)	Specificity (%)	Positive predictive value (%)	Negative predictive value (%)	Accuracy (%)
50	97 (98-98)	62 (60-66)	71 (68-74)	96 (94-97)	79
80	98 (91-96)	74 (70-77)	77 (76-80)	92 (89-94)	83
100	90 (88-92)	76 (73-78)	79 (78-81)	92 (87-91)	83
125	87 (86-90)	79 (78-82)	80 (78-83)	87 (84-89)	83
150	86 (82-88)	83 (80-86)	83 (80-86)	85 (83-88)	84

FIGURE 48.30 Receiver operating characteristic (ROC) analysis for brain natriuretic peptide *(BNP)* and N-terminal pro-brain natriuretic peptide *(NTproBNP)* for the diagnosis of acute heart failure. (From Tang WH, Francis GS, Morrow DA, Newby LK, Cannon CP, Jesse RL, et al. National Academy of Clinical Biochemistry Laboratory Medicine practice guidelines: clinical utilization of cardiac biomarker testing in heart failure. *Circulation* 2007;116:e99–109.)

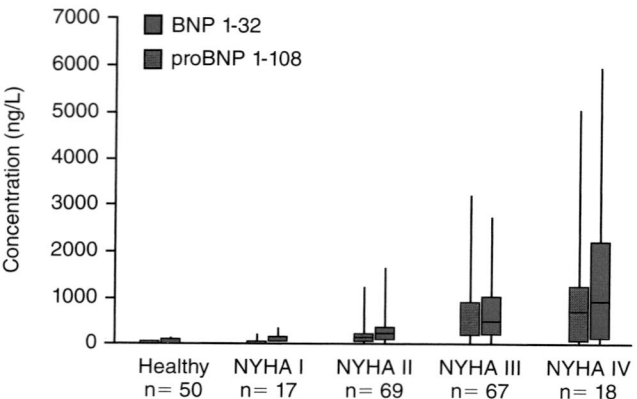

FIGURE 48.31 Relationship between pro-brain natriuretic peptide *(NTproBNP)* 1-108 and New York Heart Association *(NYAC)* classifications. *BNP,* Brain natriuretic peptide. (From Giuliani I, Rieunier F, Larue C, Delagneau JF, Granier C, Pau B, et al. Assay for measurement of intact B-type natriuretic peptide prohormone in blood. *Clin Chem* 2006;52:1054–61.)

BOX 48.5 Causes of Increased Natriuretic Peptides

1. Acute or chronic systolic or diastolic heart failure
2. Left ventricular hypertrophy
3. Inflammatory cardiac disease
4. Systemic arterial hypertension with left ventricular hypertrophy
5. Pulmonary hypertension
6. Acute or chronic renal failure
7. Ascitic liver cirrhosis
8. Endocrine disorders (e.g., hyperaldosteronism, Cushing syndrome)
9. Sepsis

BOX 48.6 Special Situations of Elevated Natriuretic Peptides

1. Well heart failure patients
2. Heart failure secondary to diastolic dysfunction
3. Acute mitral regurgitation
4. Pulmonary edema less than 1 hr old
5. Constrictive epicarditis
6. Other cases "upstream" from
   a. Left ventricle
   b. Mitral stenosis
   c. Atrial myxoma

Modified from van Kimmenade RR, Januzzi JL, Jr. Emerging biomarkers in heart failure. *Clin Chem* 2012;58:127–38.

Special Situations

Several additional caveats are necessary clinically. There is an increasing prevalence of HF with preserved ventricular function (Box 48.6). Controversy exists concerning the mechanisms for this clinical entity and some even question its existence, but a stiff, noncompliant left ventricle is clearly an important contributor. Unfortunately, the therapeutic modalities used for treatment have been shown to be ineffective.[15] In addition, because NPs are predominantly released in response to

end systolic wall stress, values are much lower in this disease state. Thus NPs provide aid in the inclusion or exclusion of HF secondary to systolic dysfunction, but do not provide similarly robust triage in patients with diastolic dysfunction, also known as heart failure with preserved systolic function (HEFPEF). The presence of primary or secondary valvular abnormalities that increase the pressure of volume overload, and particularly the latter, will cause increases in NP values because they increase wall stress and may be useful diagnostically to define severe disease and/or decompensation. Thus the presence of these abnormalities must be taken into account when interpreting NP values. Additionally, the presence of AF defines a group of patients with underlying CVD. NPs both in the presence and absence of HF will be higher in this setting, and this needs to be taken into account in interpreting values for diagnostic purposes. Finally, abnormalities in right ventricular function, even when the result of volume overload that will cause increases in wall stress, are associated with a blunted NP response, likely because of the smaller mass of myocardium involved. The constricted pericardium inhibits increases in wall stress, and thus NP values often are not elevated despite overt HF unless the constrictive process is superimposed on prior cardiac disease.[435]

Screening for Ventricular Dysfunction

The use of NPs for screening to identify patients with impaired ventricular function or those in whom the development of HF if likely has been proposed. The sensitivity and specificity of such an approach is far less than that of the acute circumstance, and for that reason most groups have not advocated the use of this analyte in that area, but as the criteria for diagnosis improve as more specific assays are developed, this may be an area in which NPs will be of value, especially if confined to high-risk groups. Two trials have shown a reduction in clinical events in response to treatment using such screening.[436–439]

Prognostic Use of Natriuretic Peptides

Some have argued for the ubiquitous use of NPs in all patients with dyspnea. The logic for such an approach is related to the fact that individuals with higher NP values have a more adverse prognosis (Fig. 48.32) in general than those with lower levels when they present either acutely or chronically.[410,430,440–448] There may be an exception to the idea that higher levels are always more negatively prognostic.[449] There is a report that in the extremely ill end-stage patient lower values are observed, which could reflect exhaustion of the NP system, but these observations remain to be confirmed. Thus one could argue that obtaining a NP value at the time of admission to hospital in a patient who has suspected CHF is valuable from the perspective of determining eventual risk. Indeed, it is well established that values obtained in this circumstance are highly prognostic with very high risk ratios and with higher values by and large being associated with worse disease. Maximal prognostic significance usually is associated with the value at the time of discharge. Thus a reasonable strategy would be to obtain one level at the time of admission and one at the time of discharge. Recent data suggest that if NP values are reduced substantially during hospitalization, patients tend to do better. However, most of the reductions that have been reported are modest compared to the biological variability (see earlier discussion). Thus it is

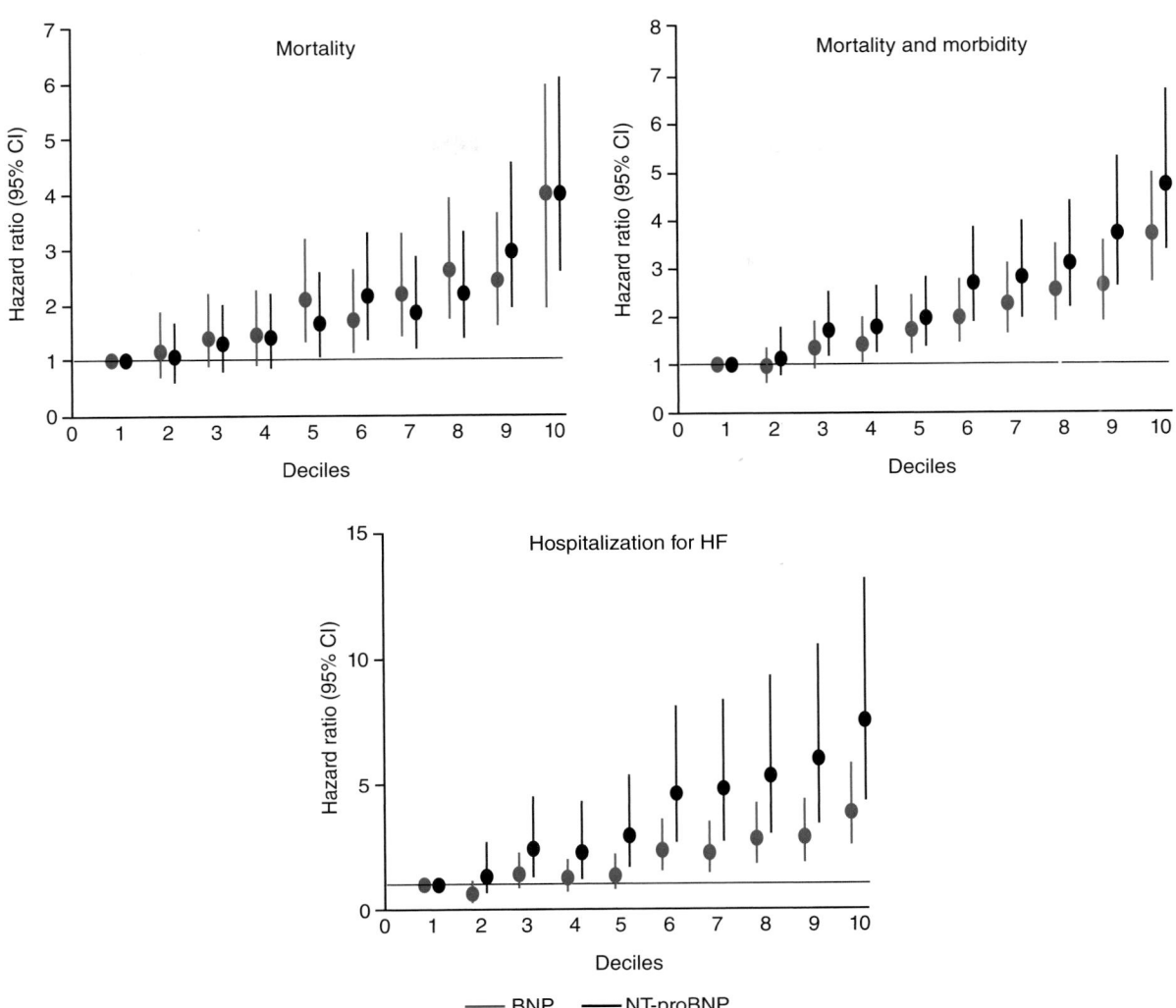

Covariates for adjustment: age, gender, NYHA class, ischemic etiology, LVEF, LVIDd, serum creatinine and bilirubin, randomized treatment, prescription of β-blockers, digitalis and diuretics, presence of AF or diabetes at study entry.

FIGURE 48.32 Relationships of brain natriuretic peptide *(BNP)* and N-terminal pro-brain natriuretic peptide *(NT-proBNP)* values and outcomes. *AF,* Atrial fibrillation; *HF,* heart failure; *LVEF,* left ventricular ejection fraction; *LVIDd,* left ventricular internal diameter end diastole; *NYHA,* New York Heart Association. (From Anand IS, Fisher LD, Chiang YT, Latini R, Masson S, Maggioni AP, et al. Changes in brain natriuretic peptide and norepinephrine over time and mortality and morbidity in the Valsartan Heart Failure Trial [Val-HeFT]. *Circulation* 2003;107:1278–83.)

hard to know how to interpret these changes, especially in individual patients. Recent data in the outpatient setting suggest that changes needed to overcome biologic variability of 80% or greater (see Fig. 48.32) are necessary to see substantive alterations in prognosis.[450,451] Nonetheless, in the clinical perspective, there probably are differences between those individuals with more chronic disease and those with only acute disease. Those with more chronic disease have a chronically induced NP system that probably responds more slowly than individuals who have simply an acute diathesis in whom NP levels may respond somewhat more rapidly. Accordingly, some degree of sub-classification of these patients in regard to these parameters is key. Unfortunately, there are no good studies defining what to do if NP levels do not respond rapidly and aggressively to change. It would be important if one could show that keeping patients in the hospital, for example,

would mitigate some of these problems, but that information is simply not available at present. Some studies have actually claimed benefit in reducing costs, but at times those studies have included very long hospital stays.[452] Thus management decisions cannot be made based solely on these values. In addition, extreme care is necessary because of the subset of patients who may have low levels if they are quite chronically ill and the heterogeneity of values associated with differences in body physiognomy likely related to the clearance of the NPs.

Use of Natriuretic Peptides to Guide Therapy

Perhaps the most interesting use of these markers is in the patient with HF with the hope of finding the ability to titer therapy more efficaciously in these individuals.[453–458] The logic of this approach suggests that many individuals are not as astute as they could be to their symptoms and that having an objective measure may be helpful. This has recently been tested in several randomized controlled trials. The first, Systolic Heart Failure Treatment Supported by BNP (STARS-BNP), suggested benefit to such an approach, but subsequent trials have not confirmed those findings. Most recently, the Guiding Evidence Based Therapy Using Biomarker Intensified Treatment in Heart Failure (GUIDE-IT) trial was terminated early for futility as in each arm, 37% of subjects (biomarker guided versus standard of care) reached the primary endpoint of cardiovascular death/HF hospitalization.[458] The negative results have been attributed to over-treatment of the control-arm (no biomarker testing) with arguments that in many of the trials a large percentage of the patients have been elderly and the thought is that elderly patients may not tolerate the increased doses of therapeutic agents used in the management protocols predicated on NPs. Indeed, if those older than 75 years of age are excluded, there is substantial benefit to this strategy.[459]

New challenges have been posed by the development of neprilysin inhibitors, which in theory inhibit the degradation of bioactive BNP. They have been linked to angiotensin receptor blockers (ARBs) in an agent called LCZ696, which is a combination of valsartan and the inhibitor named sacubitril.[460,461] Sacubitril has been combined with an ARB because neprilysin also degrades bradykinin among multiple other proteins and the association of this effect with ARBs exacerbates angioedema. The combination has been shown to markedly improve prognosis in patients with modest (mostly class 2) HF. One possible mechanism suggested has been that the agent works by reducing the degradation of BNP, and in the index randomized controlled trial the agent resulted in increases in BNP values and decreases in NT-proBNP values. It is likely given the complexity of the NP system that this is over simplistic and that the agent may work by its effects on multiple proteins, most likely ANP and adrenomedullin, and possibly bradykinin, substance P, endothelin 1, and/or angiotensin 2.[397] It is unclear how/if the effects shown in the recent trial will affect the use of NP measurements, however measurement of NT-proBNP may cause less diagnostic confusion early after initiation of neprilysin inhibition. A novel assay for neprilysin has been developed, and the values appear to have important prognostic significance.

Other Situations
Several investigations suggest that NPs can be used to determine when to intervene in patients with aortic stenosis and mitral regurgitation.[462–465] Unfortunately, usually only one value has been used and those values (corrected for differences in the assays) tend to be quite low. Using values relative to what a normal value might be has proven much more successful in a variety of situations. However, it is likely that using changes in NPs over time might provide a better paradigm. In some severe situations, changes in NPs can be associated with severe CHF in the absence of elevated levels of NPs. These include very acute HF before the stimulus to produce increased levels of NPs has had time to occur. In addition, cases in which the abnormality is above the ventricle, such as atrial myxoma or with mitral stenosis, can present with HF and normal NP values. Finally, constrictive pericarditis is associated with low values because increases in wall stress are precluded by the constricting pericardium.

Other situations in which NPs are elevated include any disease that increases blood volume and thus wall stress, such

as sepsis, anemia, renal dysfunction, Cushing syndrome, and/or hyperaldosteronism, hypertension with LVH, and cirrhosis. Some have suggested that values can be used to assess prognosis in patients with renal failure, albeit using higher cutoff values, and it does appear that the mechanisms for release are still the same.[374] However, mixing values between GFR groups is likely to be fraught with confusion. Using values within groups (e.g., those with severe disease on or off chronic dialysis) appears much more productive.[399,466]

Ischemic Heart Disease
Several investigations have suggested that NPs can be used to assess prognosis in patients who present with ACS and normal cTn values.[4,467–476] Most of these studies have used relatively insensitive cTn assays or higher cutoff values, but such assays and cutoff values are still in common use. If so, the finding of an elevated NP level may be helpful. In one study, such patients benefited from an invasive strategy.[23] The subgroup involved was mostly female, and it appears that women may have lower cTn levels than men. However, if this strategy is to be used, a relatively low cutoff value has been advocated. Whether these low values will allow adequate discrimination in large groups of patients is unclear. However, it is clear that the use of NPs may be helpful after the acute episode in predicting the subsequent risk for events. Indeed, over time in some studies they appear to be even more prognostic than troponin.[477] Thus eventually, it is likely that NPs may become part of a long-term risk stratification panel. NPs are also elaborated, albeit to a modest extent in those with positive treadmill stress tests.[478] Some of this release comes directly from the coronary arteries. Elevations also occur in those with diastolic abnormalities.[479] The changes appear too small to be used diagnostically. Recent data has also demonstrated the utility of preoperative NT-proBNP measurement for predicting cardiovascular events after noncardiac surgery.[476]

Novel Biomarkers Used in Prognosis
ST2
ST2 is a new biomarker that has potential utility in patients with HF and perhaps acute ischemic heart disease as well. It has been known as an inflammatory biomarker for years, but it was the discovery that the soluble form also was released by stretch of cardiomyocytes and macrophages that led to investigations concerning its utility in CVDs.[480] ST2 has three isoforms. One is within the cell, and binding by IL33 to that transmembrane receptor results in antihypertrophic and antifibrotic effects. It also works through intracellular nuclear transcription regulatory processes, which evokes inflammatory cytokines and an immune response. Its aggregate effects are thought to be protective. However, in response to stretch and inflammation, the soluble form is secreted and binds to IL33 and by doing so prevents binding to the transmembrane receptor and thus abrogates these protective effects.[481] There have been assays for ST2, but one has been developed that is more sensitive and is FDA approved.[482] It has good analytic characteristics with an LOD of 1.3 ng/mL and an LOQ of 2.4 ng/mL. However, there likely are multiple requisite forms (those bound to IL33 and others that are free). Normal values ought to be sex specific, but the FDA has suggested a cutoff value of 35 ng/mL and has not required sex-specific values. ST2 has only modest biological variation.[483] Clinically, increased values do not add diagnostically to other markers.

Thus in HF, ST2 is less valuable as a diagnostic marker than BNP. However, it is more prognostic for death and/or HF exacerbations[484] and in most studies it remains prognostic despite other biomarkers and often reduces or eliminates the prognostic impact of those other markers, including BNP.[485,486] This may be because it integrates both inflammatory and stretch-related processes in its prognostic approach. Importantly, ST2 is reduced by therapies known to have a positive impact on clinical outcomes such as β-blockers[487] and mineralocorticoid antagonists.[488] In comparative HF studies, it fares better than other markers thought to look at fibrotic pathways.[489,490]

In patients with acute ischemic heart disease, ST2 levels increase to peak approximately 6 to 18 hours after symptom onset. Levels in the upper quartile independently doubled the risk for cardiovascular death and HF.[491,492] Weaker associations occur with nonSTEMI.[493] ST2 predicts short-term (30-day) and long-term (>1 year) death and HF independent of clinical indicators, but not when NT-proBNP and the GRACE score are included in models.

This is a promising marker that has a chance to become important clinically if and when the proper studies are done.

POINTS TO REMEMBER
Measurement of BNP or NT-proBNP

- Most useful in ruling out heart failure (HF) in the emergency department and primary care.
- Confirms diagnosis of HF in patients with suggestive clinical symptoms.

Galectin-3

Galectin-3 is an interesting marker that plays a central role in the fibrotic process. In response to cellular injury, the inflammatory and wound healing responses evoke the egress of macrophages into the injured area. These macrophages release galectin-3, which is a β-galactoside–binding lectin that stimulates myofibroblasts to stimulate collagen formation and thus scar formation.[494] Experimental models are robust in supporting this role in multiple tissues, but particularly the heart and the kidney, and supporting the concept that mineralocorticoid antagonists and modified citrus pectin inhibit the process.[495–497] Galectin-3 also mediates cell-cell and cell–extracellular matrix adhesion, cell growth and differentiation, cell cycle regulation, apoptosis, angiogenesis, tumor genesis, tumor growth, metastasis, and immune reactions. Gene knockout experiments confirm the central role of this protein. Thus it is thought that elevated galectin-3, once stimulated, remains elevated and marks individuals who are prone to develop fibrosis.

The original assay had reasonable analytical characteristics with a normal range from 3.8 to 21.0 ng/mL[498] but that rises modestly in the presence of cardiovascular comorbidities.[498] Values do not change markedly over time,[499] but biological variation is substantial. Clinically, elevated galectin-3 is associated with an increased incidence of adverse outcomes after AMI and in community patients, as well as even when controlled for other important covariates. Such data have been shown in patients with acute[500] and chronic HF[501] and patients with diastolic HF.[502] In the Heart

Failure–A Controlled Trial Investigating Outcomes of Exercise (HF ACTION) registry, it was markedly prognostic.[503] It is also prognostic for the development of HF in patients who present with ACS.[504] Several of these studies have also suggested that elevated values in patients hospitalized with HF can predict readmissions.[505] However, the suggestion was made that a 15% change should/could be used as a criterion. This is substantially less than biological variation. Recently, it has been reported that changes in renal function cause systemic increases in galectin-3. This fact could explain part of its prognostic accuracy in patients with HF[506] but also complicate the use of the marker. In head-to-head comparisons with ST2, galectin-3 has been knocked out of the prognostic models.[489,490] Galectin-3 is a promising marker, but much better data and particularly treatment-related information are required before it will be useful as a routine clinical marker.

The Future

The potential future use of NPs, as indicated in the analytical sections, is growing as we understand more about the biochemistry and mechanisms of NP release. It appears that CHF is in part a clinical syndrome characterized by abnormalities in how the NP system works. The system synthesizes and releases large amounts of protein, but much of the protein is poorly functional. Whether this is because it is inadequately cleaved or whether it is due to glycosylation or other biochemical processes has yet to be determined. However, what is clear is that very little circulating active BNP is present in patients with HF.[389] Most of what appears to circulate is proBNP that is uncleaved, suggesting probable abnormalities in corin and furin that are indigenous to the pathophysiology of CHF. If one could manipulate these systems to facilitate the presence of active BNP or of other fragments that might have biological importance, one might substantially improve CHF. These are some of the approaches currently being pursued in the hope of improving therapy for this very large group of patients.

In addition, novel biomarkers (Table 48.5 and Box 48.7) have the potential to contribute substantially to this work. Recent data suggest that intact proBNP can be measured directly, which may lead to better understanding of underlying pathophysiology. As with other NPs, its circulating concentration tracks with the clinical class of HF (see Fig. 48.31).[140] In addition, a new test for ANP has been developed (MR-proANP) that may have some advantages. Preliminary data suggest that it is equivalent to other NPs in its ability to diagnose acute HF.[415] Such testing might allow the more rapidly responding atrial peptide and the slower to respond B-type NP to be used synergistically. Again, additional research is necessary.

NPs may be of additional value in several different intriguing areas that are being explored. One is sudden cardiac death. Several studies have associated elevated NP values with mortality and/or ICD discharges.[507,508] A second area involves the follow-up of patients who received cardiac resynchronization therapy devices. It appears that higher values help define a group apt to benefit, and although it takes some time for NPs to fall, their reduction is associated with clinical benefit over time.[418] Finally, several suggestions have indicated that BNP may be useful in helping diagnose PEs when they occur and to determine prognosis. Unfortunately, levels often

TABLE 48.5 Biomarkers in Heart Failure

Pathophysiology	Biomarker
Inflammation[a–c]	C-reactive protein
	Tumor necrosis factor-α
	Fas (APO-1)
	Interleukins-1, -6, and -18
Oxidative stress[a,b,d]	Oxidized low-density lipoproteins
	Myeloperoxidase
	Urinary biopyrrins
	Urinary and plasma isoprostanes
	Plasma malondialdehyde
Myocyte injury[a,b,d]	Cardiac-specific troponins I and T
	Myosin light-chain kinase I
	Heart-type fatty acid protein
	Myocardial-bound creatine kinase
Myocyte stress[b,d,e]	BNP
	NT-proBNP
	MR-proANP
	ST2
Extracellular matrix remodeling[a,b,d]	Matrix metalloproteinases
	Tissue inhibitors of metalloproteinases
	Collagen propeptides
New biomarkers[b]	Chromogranin
	Galectin 3
	Osteoprotegerin
	Adiponectin
	Growth differentiation factor 15
Neurohormones[a,b,c]	Norepinephrine
	Renin
	Angiotensin II
	Arginine vasopressin
	Endothelin

[a]Biomarkers in this category aid in elucidating the pathogenesis of heart failure.
[b]Biomarkers in this category provide prognostic information and enhance risk stratification.
[c]Biomarkers in this category can be used to identify subjects at risk for heart failure.
[d]Biomarkers in this category are potential targets of therapy.
[e]Biomarkers in this category are useful in the diagnosis of heart failure and in monitoring therapy.
BNP, b type natriuretic peptide.
Modified from Braunwald E. Biomarkers in heart failure. *N Engl J Med* 2008;358:2148–2159.

BOX 48.7 Biomarkers in Acute Coronary Syndrome

Serologic Biomarkers of Arterial Vulnerability
Lipid profile
- Apo B
- Lp(a)
- LDL particle number
- CETP
- Lp-PLA₂
- Inflammation

hs-CRP
sICAM-1
IL-6
IL-18
SAA
MPO
sCD40
- Oxidized LDL
- GPX1 activity
- Nitrotyrosine
- Homocysteine
- Cystatin C
- Natriuretic peptides
- ADMA
- MMP-9
- TIMP-1

Structural Markers of Arterial Vulnerability
Carotid IMT
Coronary artery calcium

Functional Markers of Arterial Vulnerability
Blood pressure
Endothelial dysfunction
Arterial stiffness
Ankle-brachial index
Urine albumin excretion

Serologic Markers of Blood Vulnerability
Fibrinogen
d-Dimer

Decreased Fibrinolysis
TPA/PAI-1

Increased Coagulation
von Willebrand factor

Structural Markers of Myocardial Vulnerability
Exercise stress echo
PET

Serologic Markers of Myocardial Injury
Cardiac troponins

ADMA, Asymmetric dimethylarginine; *Apo*, apolipoprotein; *CETP*, cholesterol ester transfer protein; *hs-CRP*, high-sensitivity C-reactive protein; *IL*, interleukin; *IMT*, Intimal-medial thickness; *LDL*, low-density lipoprotein; *Lp(a)*, lipoprotein a; *Lp-PLA₂*, phospholipase A2; *MMP*, matrix metalloproteinase; *MPO*, myeloperoxidase; *PET*, positron emission tomography; *SAA*, serum amyloid A; *sCD40*, soluble CD40 ligand; *sICAM*, soluble intracellular adhesion molecule; *TIMP*, tissue inhibitor of metalloproteinase; *TPA/PAI*, tissue plasminogen activator/plasminogen activator inhibitor-1.

are not markedly elevated, but with time this indication may be developed more fully.

Another area that needs to be discussed involves multimarker testing. It is clear that for ischemic heart disease, the addition of NPs to other markers in a multimarker strategy improves risk stratification, especially over the long term.[485,486] It also appears that benefit may be derived from the prediction of events in older, less acutely ill individuals. Recently, a group from Uppsala reported a rather striking improvement in the prediction of events (changes in the κ coefficient statistic from 0.644 to 0.766) with the use of a multimarker panel that included NPs. The panel included cTn, NT-proBNP, cystatin C, and CRP. If confirmed, this approach may become more widely used for risk prediction.

BIOMARKERS OF INTEREST (ALTHOUGH THEY ARE NOT CURRENTLY USED ROUTINELY)

Fig. 48.33 portrays a biochemical profile in coronary vascular disease that correlates staging of biomarker release into the circulation with various pathophysiologic mechanisms of ACS and HF. As shown in Table 48.5 and Box 48.7, numerous biomarkers have been studied and used for different clinical reasons, and other promising novel biomarkers are becoming established alongside cTn and NPs as routine clinical tools. We highlight some characteristics of several of these here. This list is not meant to be all inclusive.

C-Reactive Protein

CRP is an acute-phase reactant that was initially developed to evaluate patients with infection.[127,507–510] It now appears that concentrations below those seen in infection but above healthy values (as measured by high-sensitivity CRP [hsCRP] assays) can be a marker of the atherosclerotic process because both chronic and acute atherosclerotic processes involve an inflammatory component (see Chapter 36). Recent interventional data have confirmed that inhibition of the IL-1 beta inflammasome reduces acute coronary events, proving this inflammatory hypothesis.[37] Low-dose methotrexate did not.[39] Among the ligands that can stimulate CRP are TNF and IL-1, which are thought to stimulate IL-6, which then causes the elaboration of CRP from the liver. It is now clear that CRP itself can enhance the inflammatory and prothrombotic response. A large number of assays for hsCRP are available, as is a standard protocol for their reporting.

For primary prevention, values greater than 3 mg/L are considered high risk. Recent data suggest that using hsCRP data with the calculated LDL is a potent way to predict risk. For risk stratification in primary prevention the use of routine hsCRP is not recommended by the AHA/CDC panel. When used, less than 1 mg/L is considered low risk, 1 to 3 mg/L intermediate risk, and more than 3 mg/L high risk.

In patients who present with ACS, the initial value for hsCRP has prognostic significance. Whether it is short or long term depends on the study. In most studies, the influence of cTn measurements is the predominant short-term prognostic factor, and hsCRP adds to long-term prognosis.

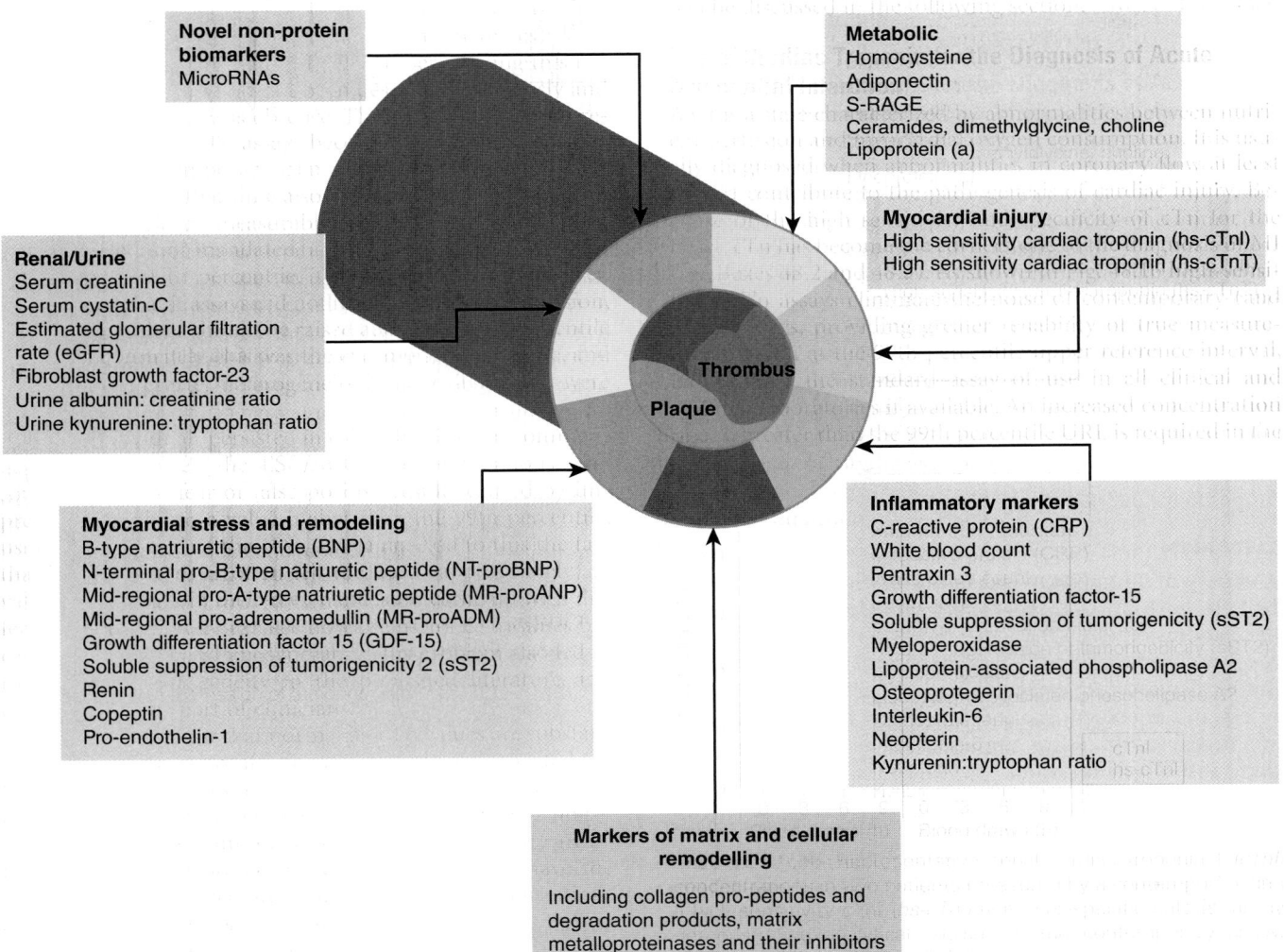

FIGURE 48.33 Selected cardiovascular biomarkers associated with prognosis in coronary artery disease. (From Omland T, White HD. State of the art: blood biomarkers for risk stratification in patients with stable ischemic heart disease. *Clin Chem* 2017;63:165–76.)

However, this is not always the case. Of interest, hsCRP measurements, similar to BNP, seem to predict death, but not recurrent infarction. This could be true because of the effect of mortality, which can confound multivariable models, but it is different from the data related to cTn (see discussion in this chapter).[122] It should be appreciated that once necrosis has occurred, hsCRP values rise and the ability to use them prognostically is attenuated.

Serum Amyloid Protein A

Serum amyloid protein A, an acute-phase protein and an apolipoprotein, has been used with hsCRP in cross-sectional studies. It can be synergistic with hsCRP but is much less commonly used. At present, no standardized assays, reference interval studies, nor consistent assay validations are available.

sCD40 Ligand [512]

CD40 ligand is a transmembrane protein related to TNF. It has multiple prothrombotic and proatherogenic effects. What is usually measured is the soluble form of the receptor, sCD40 ligand, which has been shown to be a predictor of events after acute presentation. At present, standardized assays, reference interval studies, or consistent assay validations are not available. Recent data raise substantial questions about the analytical stability in the samples that have been used to evaluate this particular marker.

Growth/Differentiation Factor 15 [513–515]

Growth/differentiation factor 15 (GDF15) was first identified as Macrophage inhibitory cytokine-1 or MIC-1. It is part of the transforming growth factor beta super family. It is in high concentrations in lung, liver, and heart. The function of GDF-15 is not fully understood but it seems to have a role in regulating inflammatory pathways and is involved in regulating apoptosis, cell repair, and cell growth. It also interdigitates the glucose-insulin pathways. In primary prevention populations, it seems to predict CVD and mortality. It seems to have similar prognostic abilities in those with ACS, and both STEMI and non-STEMI. Recent data suggest that in patients with AF that it helps to predict bleeding. For that reason, the ABC score which uses hscTn, NPs, and GDF-15 has been proposed for use in patients with AF.

Cytokines[31,37]

A variety of stimulatory and inhibitory interleukins (TNF, IL-1, IL-6, IL-8, IL-12, IL-18) are thought to help mediate the elaboration of CRP and the development of atherosclerosis and acute events. These cytokines may stimulate or inhibit leukocytes, often through T cell–mediated processes and effects on monocytes, which are indigenous to atherogenesis. In some studies, IL-6 is more prognostic than hsCRP. Inhibition of the IL6 pathway with canakinumab reduced atherosclerotic events in the Cantos trial. Thus one might expect more plaque rupture events with their elaboration in Covid 19. That has not been observed. These cytokines often have inhibitors and/or binding proteins that modulate their effects. At present, standardized assays, reference intervals studies, and consistent assay validations are not available. The interdigitation of these powerful inflammatory peptides with the cardiovascular system with the Covid pandemic has suggested their important role in CVD.

MYELOPEROXIDASE

MPO is released when neutrophils aggregate; this may indicate an active inflammatory response in blood vessels. It has been shown to be elevated chronically when chronic CAD is present.[516] It is increased when patients present with ACS.[517,518] Initial prognostic studies were encouraging but were done without adequate consideration of other analytes and specifically cTn. A multibiomarker study has shown that MPO as a prognostic tool depended on the outcomes studied (cardiac death) and the demographics of the patient population enrolled.[519] Accordingly, additional studies are needed. At present, no standardized assays, reference interval studies, nor consistent assay validations are available. Further, it has been demonstrated that the type of specimen collected is critical for the stability and accurate measurement of MPO.[520] For further information on this enzyme, see Chapter 32.

Lipoprotein-Associated Phospholipase A$_2$

Phospholipase A2 (Lp-PLA$_2$) is a phospholipase associated with LDL that is thought to be an inflammatory marker. It was previously known as platelet-activating factor acetyl hydrolase. It is synthesized by monocytes and lymphocytes and is thought to cleave oxidized lipids to produce lipid fragments that are more atherogenic and that increase endothelial adhesion. An FDA-approved assay for this analyte includes obligatory reference intervals. It has been shown to be predictive of events in a primary prevention cohort, even when hsCRP is present in the model, suggesting that it measures something different from what is measured by the acute-phase reactants associated with hsCRP.[521,522] Unfortunately, recent trials with inhibitors have been null.[523–526]

Pregnancy-Associated Plasma Protein A

Pregnancy-associated plasma protein A (PAPP-A) is a metalloproteinase that is thought to be expressed in plaques that may be prone to rupture. It is most often bound to mature basic protein. The literature in this regard is mixed at present concerning its use.[527–529] At present, standardized assays, reference interval studies, and consistent assay validations are not available. Recent data suggest that heparin administration in MI patients is associated with increased PAPP-A concentrations; this may limit its prognostic role. Recent attempts to develop assays for the IGF fragments that may be more representative of free PAPP-A have been associated with variable results as well.[530,531]

Oxidized Low-Density Lipoprotein

Oxidized LDL has been attributed a key role in the development of atherosclerosis (see Chapter 36). Several methods have been used to measure it, but they yield potentially different data. Some have correlated malondialdehyde LDL with the development of atherosclerosis and short-term events.[532] Direct identification with antibodies suggests that oxidized LDL may be released from vessels and may colocalize with lipoprotein a (Lp[a]) after acute events.[533]

Placental Growth Factor

Placental growth factor is an angiogenic factor related to vascular endothelial growth factor (VEGF), which stimulates smooth muscle cells and macrophages.[534,535] It also increases TNF and monocyte chemoattractant protein-1 (MCP-1). An assay for this analyte is thought to provide additional prognostic information on patients who present with ACS.[536] At present, standardized assays, reference interval studies, and consistent assay validations are not available.

Matrix Metalloproteinases

Matrix metalloproteinases (MMPs) can degrade the collagen matrix in coronary artery or myocardium. They are integral to remodeling of the coronary artery and/or the heart after acute events. Elaboration of MMP-9, a gelatinase, is thought to be important in plaque destabilization; thus some have tried to measure it as a prognostic index.[536] Other MMPs participate in the elaboration of extracellular matrix in the heart. Many MMPs also have inhibitors (tissue inhibitors of metalloproteinase [TIMPs]) that modulate their effects. At present, standardized assays, reference interval studies, and consistent assay validations are not available. Recent data suggest that this marker along with others may be helpful for evaluating patients with HF with preserved ejection fraction.[537]

Monocyte Chemotactic Protein

Monocyte chemotactic protein (MCP-1) is a chemokine that is thought to be responsible for the recruitment of monocytes into atherosclerotic plaque. It has been reported to be elevated in patients with ACS and to have long-term predictive value.[538] However, at present, standardized assays, reference interval studies, and consistent assay validations are not available.

Tissue Plasminogen Activator Antigen and Plasminogen Activator Inhibitor-1

t-PA is the body's physiologic fibrinolytic activator. Plasminogen activator inhibitor-1 (PAI-1), its endogenous inhibitor, binds to t-PA (see Chapter 79). Inhibition of fibrinolysis has been suggested to be a reason for recurrent infarction; the fact that maximal inhibition usually occurs in the early morning hours provides a potential explanation for the circadian variability of AMI.[539] It may also be the reason why persons with diabetes have such unstable disease; the growth factor properties of insulin stimulate increases in PAI-1.[540] An accurate assessment of this system includes both t-PA and PAI-1, along with some assessment of bound versus free levels.

Isoprostanes

Isoprostanes are the end breakdown products of lipid peroxidation, and urinary levels have been used to assess the level of oxidative stress.[541,542] It is thought that oxidation of LDL is essential for the development of atherosclerosis, and that high-density lipoprotein (HDL) and other antioxidants work by antagonizing this oxidative stress. Urinary isoprostanes give some assessment of this critical process. The most commonly measured are F_2-isoprostanes, but a large number of others are available for measurement. It does appear that they will eventually be helpful in assessing oxidative stress.

Urinary Thromboxane

Urinary thromboxane is the end metabolite of thromboxane A2, which is a measure of platelet aggregation. Urinary levels are elevated in patients with unstable coronary disease, in keeping with the known participation of platelets in the pathogenesis of CAD. This level is difficult to ascertain, and collecting urine in the acute situation is at times problematic. Recent data with a mass spectrometry assay that eliminates the measurement of the 2'3' component correlates far less well with ischemic heart disease, leading to questions about the value of this marker.

Adhesion Molecules

Adhesion molecules are a wide variety of molecules that can potentially be measured as a way of assessing the adherence of leukocytes, platelets, or other adhesive proteins to the endothelial matrix.[543] Some are receptors. Examples include platelet-endothelial adhesion molecule 1 (PECAM-1), P-selectin, E-selectin, and VCAM-1 (vascular CAM 1). At times, the receptor itself is measured, but often it is a soluble portion that circulates that is measured. At present, standardized assays, reference interval studies, and consistent assay validations are not available.

Choline

Choline is released after stimulation by phospholipase D and has been touted as a test of prognosis in patients with chest discomfort.[544] At present, standardized assays, reference interval studies, and consistent assay validations are not available.

Unbound Free Fatty Acid

Unbound free fatty acid (uFFA)[536] has been touted as a marker of ischemia. Most fatty acid is bound, and ischemia is thought to increase the small unbound fraction. Initial studies have reported mixed results. At present, standardized assays, reference interval studies, and consistent assay validations are not available.

Nourin

Nourin I is a small protein released rapidly by stressed myocytes. It induces changes in a variety of inflammatory cytokines and attracts neutrophils. Preliminary studies have been done to attempt to validate its use. At present, standardized assays, reference interval studies, and consistent assay validations are not available.

Fatty Acid Binding Protein[545]

Heart-type fatty acid-binding protein (H-FABP) is a small (15 kDa) cytoplasmic protein involved in lipid homeostasis. It is abundant in heart muscle with approximately 5- to 10-fold lower concentrations found in skeletal muscle, with concentrations in the kidney, liver, and small intestine even lower. After myocardial damage, H-FABP (measured by immunoassays) does appear in the bloodstream within 2 to 4 hours. However, its diagnostic performance during the first 4 hours after myocardial injury, including myocardial infarction, does not provide added value to cTnI or cTnT, as it lacks cardiac tissue specificity. Furthermore, clinical studies have demonstrated that H-FABP is inferior to the clinical sensitivity and clinical specificity necessary to detect MI significantly earlier than do cTn, especially with hs-cTn assays.

SELECTED REFERENCES

2. Thygesen K, Alpert JS, Jaffe AS, et al. Fourth universal definition of myocardial infarction (2018). J Am Coll Cardiol 2018;72:2231–64.

24. Shah AS, Anand A, Sandoval Y, et al. High-sensitivity cardiac troponin I at presentation in patients with suspected acute coronary syndrome: a cohort study. Lancet 2015;386(10012): 2481–8.

31. Sandoval Y, Jaffe AS. Type 2 myocardial infarction: JACC review topic of the week. JACC 2019;73:1846–60.

35. Libby P. The vascular biology of atherosclerosis. In: Libby P, Zipes DP, Bonow RO, Mann DL, Tomaselli GF, editors: Braunwald's heart disease: a textbook of cardiovascular medicine. 11th ed. Philadelphia, PA: Elsevier Inc.; 2019. p. 859–75.

62. Apple FS. Counterpoint: standardization of cardiac troponin I assays will not occur in my lifetime. Clin Chem 2012;58:169–71.

66. Wu AHB, Christenson RH, Greene DN, et al. Clinical laboratory practice recommendations for the use of cardiac troponin in acute coronary syndrome: expert opinion from the academy of the American Association for Clinical Chemistry and the task force on clinical applications of cardiac bio-markers of the International Federation of Clinical Chemistry and Laboratory Medicine. Clin Chem 2018;64:645–55.

74. Apple FS, Wu AHB, Sandoval Y, et al. Sex-specific 99th percentile upper reference limits for high sensitivity cardiac troponin assays derived using a universal sample bank. Clin Chem 2020;66:434–44.

94. Sandoval Y, Smith SW, Sexter A, et al. Type 1 and 2 myocardial infarction and myocardial injury: clinical transition to high-sensitivity cardiac troponin I. Am J Med 2017;130: 1431–9.

190. Than MP, Pickering JW, Sandoval Y, et al., on behalf of the MI³ collaborative. Machine learning to predict the likelihood of acute myocardial infarction. Circulation 2019;140(11): 899–909.

199. Sandoval Y, Smith SW, Shah ASV, et al. Rapid rule-out of acute myocardial injury using a single high-sensitivity cardiac troponin I measurement. Clin Chem 2017;63: 369–76.

222. Sandoval Y, Januzzi J, Jaffe AS. J Amer Coll Cardiol 2020; Troponin for the diagnosis and risk-stratification of myocardial injury in Coronavirus disease 2019 (COVID-19). Accepted.

397. Kavsak PA, Lam CSP, Saenger AK, et al. Educational recommendations on selected analytical and clinical aspects of natriuretic peptides with a focus on heart failure: a report from the IFCC Committee on Clinical Applications of Cardiac Bio-Markers. Clin Chem 2019;65:1221–7.

430. Januzzi JL, van Kimmenade R, Lainchbury J, et al. NT-proBNP testing for diagnosis and short-term prognosis in acute destabilized heart failure: an international pooled analysis of 1256 patients: the International Collaborative of NT-proBNP Study. Eur Heart J 2006;27:330–7.

432. Tang WH, Francis GS, Morrow DA, et al. National Academy of Clinical Biochemistry Laboratory Medicine practice guidelines: clinical utilization of cardiac biomarker testing in heart failure. Circulation 2007;116:e99–109.

510. Ridker PM. Clinical application of C-reactive protein for cardiovascular disease detection and prevention. Circulation 2003;107:363–9.

49

Kidney Disease

Michael P. Delaney and Edmund J. Lamb

ABSTRACT

Background

The kidneys play a central role in homeostasis, and reduced renal function strongly correlates with increasing morbidity and mortality. Laboratory investigations are central to the diagnosis and management of kidney disease and investigations of kidney function constitute a significant element of the workload of most clinical laboratories.

Content

This chapter describes the basic anatomy and physiology of the kidneys as a foundation for understanding the pathophysiology of disease and the rationale for diagnostic and management strategies in disease. Classification and management of both acute and chronic kidney diseases are described including detailed examination of the major complications (cardiovascular, mineral and bone, electrolyte, anemia) and causes (genetic, diabetes, hypertension, renovascular, glomerular and tubular diseases, myeloma, nephrolithiasis) of kidney disease. The chapter ends with a detailed description of renal replacement therapy (dialysis and transplantation). Wherever possible, throughout the chapter statements are based on latest clinical trial evidence or published expert guidelines and national registry data.

INTRODUCTION

The kidneys play a central role in the homeostatic mechanisms of the human body, and reduced renal function strongly correlates with increasing morbidity and mortality. Laboratory investigations are an important part of the clinician's diagnostic armamentarium, and investigations of kidney function constitute a significant element of the workload of most laboratories. The aim of this chapter is to ensure that the clinical chemist/biochemist understands the perspective of the nephrologist when dealing with laboratory investigations for patients with kidney disease. The basic anatomy and physiology of the kidneys are described as a foundation for understanding the pathophysiology of disease and the rationale for diagnostic and management strategies in kidney disease. Key analytical methods employed during the investigation of kidney disease are dealt with in Chapter 34.

ANATOMY

The kidneys form a paired organ system located in the retroperitoneal space. They extend from the level of the lower part of the eleventh thoracic vertebra to the upper portion of the third lumbar vertebra, with the right kidney situated slightly lower than the left. The adult kidney is about 12 cm long and weighs about 150 g (Fig. 49.1). The kidneys have both sympathetic and parasympathetic nerve supplies, whose function appears to be predominantly associated with vasomotor activity. The renal lymphatic drainage includes fine lymphatics in the glomerulus, some in close proximity to the juxtaglomerular apparatus (JGA[a]), which are associated with removal of material from the glomerular mesangial cells.

Blood Supply

In most cases, each kidney receives its blood supply from a single renal artery derived from the abdominal aorta. However, multiple renal arteries occur commonly. The renal artery divides into posterior and anterior elements, and ultimately into the afferent arterioles, which expand into the highly specialized capillary beds that form the glomeruli (Fig. 49.2). These capillaries then rejoin to form the efferent arteriole that then forms the capillary plexuses and the elongated vessels (the *vasa recta*) that pass around the remaining parts of the nephron, the proximal and distal tubules, the loop of Henle, and the collecting duct, providing oxygen and nutrients and removing ions, molecules, and water, which have been reabsorbed by the nephron. The efferent arteriole then merges with renal venules to form the renal veins, which merge into the inferior vena cava.

In adults, the kidneys receive approximately 25% of the cardiac output, about 90% of which supplies the renal cortex, maintaining the highly active tubular cells. Maintenance of renal blood flow is essential to kidney function, and a complex array of intrarenal regulatory mechanisms ensure that it is maintained across a wide range of systemic blood pressures (see discussion later in this chapter). The renal glomerular

---

[a]See a list of abbreviations used in this chapter in Resources.

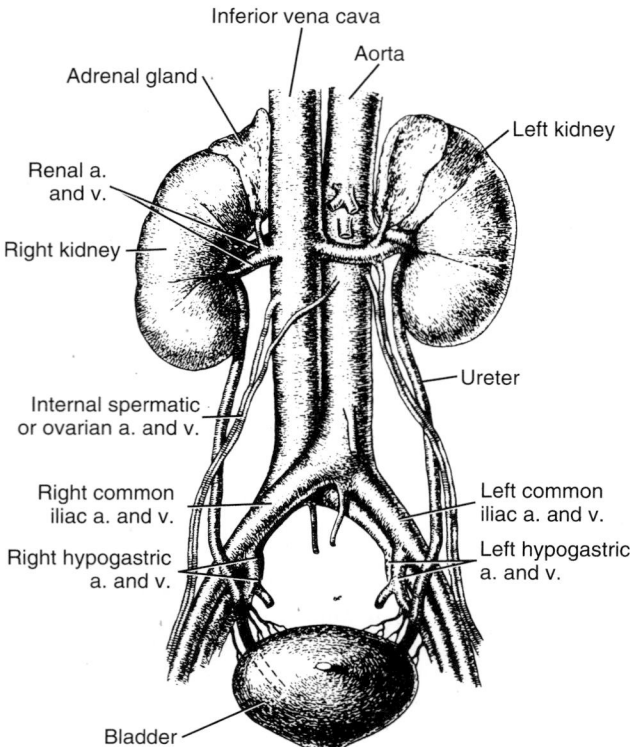

FIGURE 49.1 Vascular and anatomic relationships of the kidneys in man. (From Leaf A, Cotran RS. *Renal pathophysiology.* 3rd ed. Oxford: Oxford University Press, 1985. Reproduced by permission of Oxford University Press.)

perfusion pressure is maintained at a constant 45 mm Hg across systemic pressures between 90 and 200 mm Hg.

Nephron

The functional unit of the kidney is the *nephron.* Each kidney has been reported to contain between 600,000 and 1.5 million nephrons.[1] The number of nephrons that an individual is born with (the "nephron dose") may determine that individual's susceptibility to renal injury. The nephron consists of a glomerulus, proximal tubule, loop of Henle, distal tubule, and collecting duct (see Fig. 49.2). The collecting ducts ultimately combine to develop into the renal calyces, where the urine collects before passing along the ureter and into the bladder. The kidney is divided into several lobes. The outer, darker region of each lobe, the cortex, consists of most of the glomeruli and the proximal and distal tubules. The cortex surrounds a paler inner region, the medulla, which is further divided into a number of conical areas known as the renal pyramids, the apex of which extends toward the renal pelvis, forming papillae. Medullary rays are visible striations in the renal pyramids that connect the kidney cortex with the medulla. They are composed of descending (straight proximal) and ascending (straight distal) thick limbs of Henle and collecting ducts and associated blood vessels (the vasa recta). The central hilus is where blood vessels, lymphatics, and the renal pelvis (containing the ureter) join the kidney.

Glomerulus

The glomerulus is formed from a specialized capillary network. Each capillary develops into approximately 40 glomerular loops around 200 μm in size and consisting of a variety of different cell types supported on a specialized basement membrane (Fig. 49.3, *top*). Some endothelial and epithelial cells act in concert with the specialized glomerular basement membrane (GBM) to form the glomerular filtration barrier, in addition to mesangial cells.

The *capillary endothelial* cells are about 40 nm thick and are in contact with each other. However, in contrast to the continuous endothelial linings seen elsewhere in the body, circular fenestrations (pores) with diameters of approximately 60 nm collectively constitute 20 to 50% of the glomerular endothelial surface.[2] The endothelium permits virtually free access of plasma and small solutes to the basement membrane. However, although the fenestrations are far larger than the diameter of albumin (3.5 nm), it is thought that permselectivity to such larger molecules begins at the level of the endothelium because of the endothelial surface lining—a glycocalyx coating of negatively charged glycoproteins, glycosaminoglycans, proteoglycans, and absorbed plasma proteins, including orosomucoid and albumin. Estimates of the thickness of this layer vary depending on the visualization and preparation techniques used, but it may be between 200 and 400 nm thick.[2]

The *basement membrane* (see Fig. 49.3, *bottom*) of the glomerular capillaries is much thicker (approximately 300 nm) than that of other vascular beds and consists of three distinct electron-dense layers: the *lamina rara interna*, the *lamina densa*, and the *lamina rara externa*. The lamina densa consists of a close feltwork of fine, mainly type IV, collagen fibrils (each 3 to 5 nm thick) embedded in a gel-like matrix of laminin, nidogen/entactin, glycoproteins, and proteoglycans such as agrin and perlecan. The lamina densa forms the main size discriminant barrier to protein passage into the tubular lumen. The other two layers of the basement membrane are rich in negatively charged polyanionic glycoproteins, such as heparan sulfate; these may form a charge discriminant barrier to the passage of proteins, although the importance of the GBM in charge discrimination is still uncertain.[2]

The *epithelial cells* of the glomerulus line the outside of the glomerular capillaries, thus facing Bowman's capsule and the primary urine (see Fig. 49.3, *top*). These cells are called *podocytes* and have an unusual octopus-like structure in that they have a large number of cytoplasmic extensions or foot processes that are embedded in the basement membrane. Foot processes are anchored to the GBM via integrin molecules and dystroglycans and are divided into primary and secondary. The secondary processes between adjacent cells interdigitate to form filtration slits, which are 25 to 60 nm wide.[2] The podocytes are covered by a complex diaphragm ("slit diaphragm"), some of the molecular components of which (e.g., nephrin) appear crucial for the maintenance of larger proteins within the circulation. The resulting structure is relatively impermeable to most proteins above 60 kDa, but passage of proteins is modulated by their charge and shape. Podocytes are also covered by a glycocalyx of sulfated molecules, including glycosaminoglycans and glycoconjugates (e.g., podocalyxin). The surface anionic charge helps to maintain the foot process structure and the distance between the parietal and visceral epithelial cells constituting Bowman's space.[2]

The final cellular components of the glomerulus are the *mesangial cells,* which are found in the central part ("stalk")

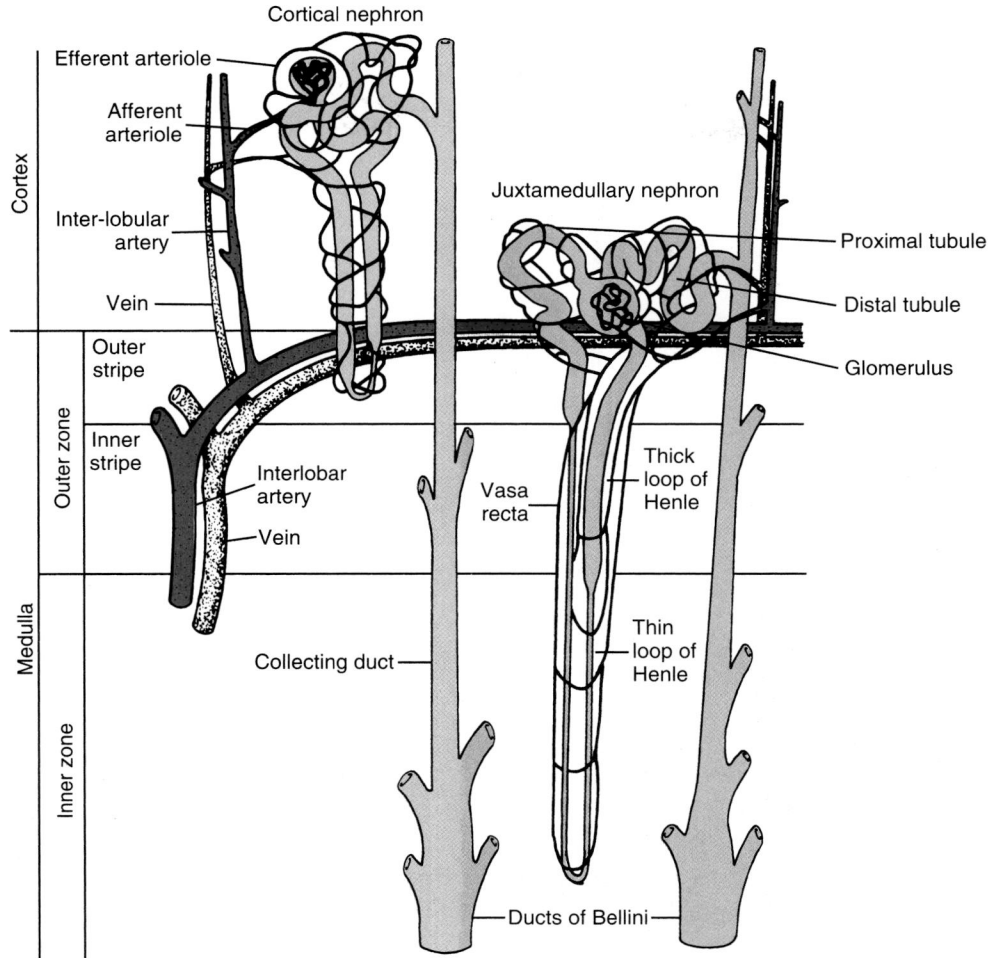

FIGURE 49.2 Diagrammatic representation of the nephron, the functional unit of the kidney, illustrating the anatomic and vascular arrangements. (From Pitts RF. *Physiology of the kidney and body fluids.* 3rd ed. Chicago: Year Book Medical Publishers, 1974.)

of the glomerulus between and within the capillary loops suspended in a matrix that they synthesize. They are in direct contact with glomerular endothelial cells and the inner layer of the GBM (lamina rara interna) and also with the extraglomerular mesangium and the JGA (see Fig. 49.3, *top*). Mesangial cells have the characteristics of smooth muscle cells (pericytes), in that they are rich in microfilaments and respond to and produce a variety of stimuli (e.g., angiotensin II [AII] and arginine vasopressin [antidiuretic hormone, ADH]).[3] Mesangial matrix is rich in collagens and proteoglycans but is different in composition from the matrix of the GBM. Its composition and volume are tightly regulated in health but can be markedly altered during certain diseases (e.g., diabetic nephropathy, immunoglobulin (Ig)A nephropathy). Mesangial cells have both structural and housekeeping functions. They have anchoring filaments to GBM opposite the podocytes and their contractile properties enable them to alter intraglomerular capillary flow and glomerular ultrafiltration surface area, and thereby single nephron glomerular filtration rate (GFR). The cells appear to respond to capillary stretch by generating soluble factors such as vascular endothelial growth factor and transforming growth factor-β (TGF-β), and by activating intracellular signaling pathways.

Mesangial cells also have specific and nonspecific mechanisms for removing macromolecules that reach the mesangial and subendothelial space, preventing their accumulation. These mechanisms include phagocytosis and degradation by the cells and trafficking along the mesangial stalk to the juxtaglomerular region, followed by elimination via the renal lymphatics, or by regurgitation into the glomerular capillary.

Proximal Tubule
Bowman's capsule forms the beginning of the tightly coiled, proximal convoluted tubule (*pars convoluta*), which on its progress toward the renal medulla becomes straightened and is then called the *pars recta*. The proximal tubule is about 15 mm long. The epithelial cells lining the convoluted section are cuboidal/columnar cells with a luminal brush border consisting of millions of microvilli, which expand the surface area for absorption of tubular fluid. The proximal tubule is the most metabolically active part of the nephron (Table 49.1).

Loop of Henle
The pars recta drains into the descending thin loop of Henle, which after passing through a hairpin loop becomes first the thin ascending limb and then the thick ascending limb. The

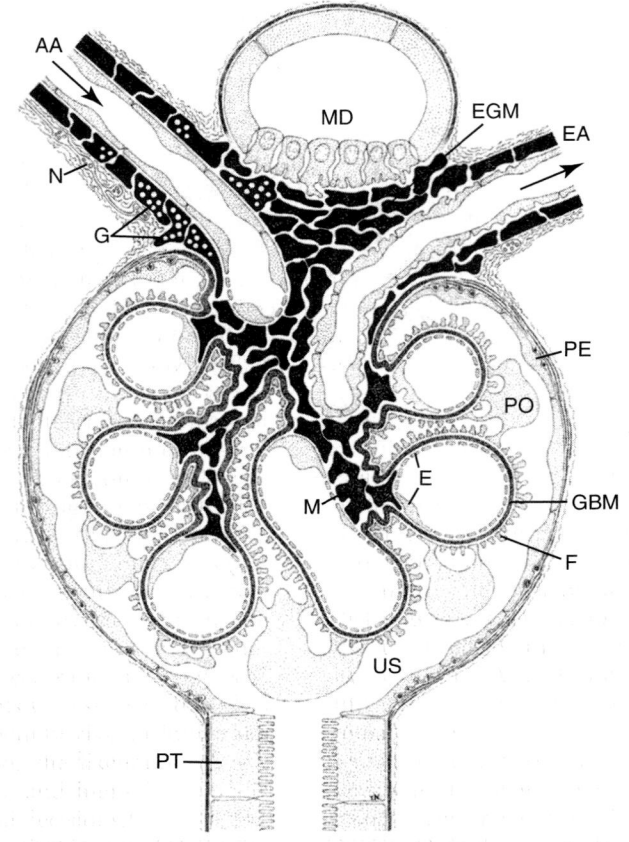

A

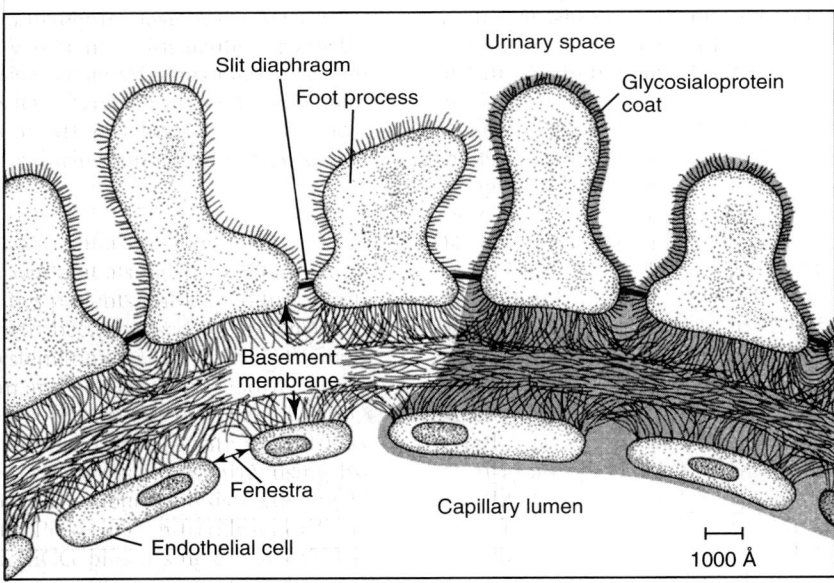

B

FIGURE 49.3 The glomerular cells and the glomerular filtration barrier. *Top,* Longitudinal section through a glomerulus and its juxtaglomerular apparatus. The capillary tuft consists of a network of specialized capillaries, which are outlined by a fenestrated endothelium (E). At the vascular pole, the afferent arteriole (AA) enters, branching into capillaries immediately after its entrance; the efferent arteriole (EA) is established inside the tuft and passes through the glomerular stalk before leaving at the vascular pole. The capillary network and the mesangium are enclosed in a common compartment bounded by the glomerular basement membrane (GBM). Note that there is no basement membrane at the interface between the capillary endothelium and the mesangium. The glomerular visceral epithelium consists of highly branched podocytes (POs), which, in a typical interdigitating pattern, cover the outer aspect of the GBM. At the vascular pole, the visceral epithelium and the GBM are reflected into the parietal epithelium (PE) of Bowman's capsule, which passes over into the epithelium of the proximal tubule (PT) at the urinary pole. At the vascular pole, the glomerular mesangium is continuous with

FIGURE 49.3 cont. the extraglomerular mesangium (EGM), which consists of extraglomerular mesangial cells and an extraglomerular mesangial matrix. The EGM and the granular cells (G) of the afferent arteriole, along with the macula densa (MD), establish the juxtaglomerular apparatus. All cells that are suggested to be of smooth muscle origin are shown in black. *US,* Urinary space; *F,* foot processes; *N,* sympathetic nerve terminals; *M,* messenger cells. (From Elger M, Kriz W. The renal glomerulus—the structural basis of ultrafiltration. In: Cameron JS, Davison AM, Grunfeld JP, Kerr D, Ritz E, eds. *Oxford textbook of clinical nephrology* [vol. 1]. 2nd ed. Oxford: Oxford University Press, 1998 [Chapter 3.1]. Reproduced by permission of Oxford University Press.) *Bottom,* Glomerular capillary wall. In glomerular filtration, filtered fluid is believed to traverse the capillary wall via an extracellular route, that is, through endothelial fenestrae, basement membrane, and slit diaphragms. Circulating polyanions (e.g., albumin) are thought to be retarded by the rich distribution in inner barriers of negatively charged sialylated glycoproteins (*shaded area* in schematic diagram) and by the slit diaphragms formed from adjacent interdigitating podocyte cells (see main text). (From Brenner BM, Beeuwkes R, III. The kidney in health and disease: III. The renal circulations. *Hosp Pract* 1978;13:35–46.)

TABLE 49.1   Metabolic Functions of the Different Parts of the Nephron

Molecule	PROXIMAL R	PROXIMAL S	LOOP OF HENLE R	LOOP OF HENLE S	DISTAL TUBULE R	DISTAL TUBULE S	COLLECTING DUCT R	COLLECTING DUCT S
Urea	+			(+)				
Proteins	+							
Peptides	+							
Phosphate	+							
Sulfate	+							
Organic anions			+					
Urate	+	+						
Sodium	+		+		+		+	
Chloride	+		+		+		+	
Water	+		+				+	
Potassium	+		+	(+)		+	+	
Hydrogen ion		+		+		+	+	+
Bicarbonate	+		+		+		+	+
Ammonium		+	+					+
Calcium	+		+		+		+	

R, Reabsorption; *S,* secretion; + indicates function; *(+)* indicates partial function.

cells of the thin ascending limb are very similar to those in the descending (with little brush border, flattened and interdigitated), but important differences are evident in their permeability to water and in their capability for active transport. The thick ascending limb is lined with cuboidal/columnar cells similar in size to those in the proximal tubule, but they do not possess a brush border. At the end of the thick ascending limb, near where it reenters the cortex and closely associated with the glomerulus and the efferent arteriole, a cluster of cells known as the *macula densa* is present (Fig. 49.4, see later). The main role of the loop of Henle is to assist in generating concentrated urine, hypertonic with respect to plasma: it also has several other functions (see Table 49.1).

Distal Convoluted Tubule

The distal convoluted tubule begins at a variable distance beyond the macula densa and extends to the first fusion with other tubules to form the collecting ducts. The cells of the distal convoluted tubule are cuboidal and contain numerous mitochondria. Na, K-ATPase activity is higher than in any other segment of the nephron, being located in the basolateral membrane and providing the main driving force for ion

transport. Reabsorption of sodium and chloride, with passive reabsorption of water, is the main function of the distal convoluted tubule (see later).

Collecting Duct

The collecting ducts are formed from approximately six distal tubules. These are successively joined by other tubules to form ducts of Bellini, which ultimately drain into a renal calyx. Two main cell types are found in the collecting duct: principal (light) cells and intercalated (dark) cells. Intercalated cells have a dark granular cytoplasm with high carbonic anhydrase activity but no Na, K-ATPase activity.

Juxtaglomerular Apparatus

Where the thick ascending limb of the loop of Henle passes very close to the glomerulus of its own nephron, the cells of the tubule and the afferent arteriole show regional specialization (Fig. 49.4). The tubule forms the macula densa; the arteriolar cells are filled with granules (containing renin or its inactive precursor, prorenin) and are innervated with sympathetic nerve fibers. This area, called the JGA, plays an important part in maintaining systemic blood pressure through

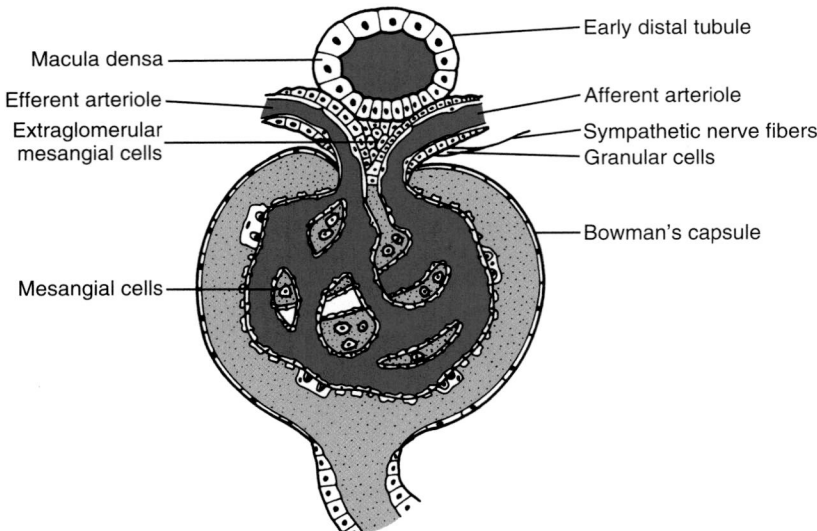

FIGURE 49.4 The juxtaglomerular apparatus. The beginning of the distal tubule (i.e., where the loop of Henle re-enters the cortex) lies very close to the afferent and efferent arterioles, and the cells of both the afferent arteriole and the tubule show specialization. The cells of the afferent arteriole are thickened, granular (juxtaglomerular) cells that are innervated by sympathetic nerve fibers. The mesangial cells are irregularly shaped and contain filaments of contractile proteins. Identical cells are found just outside the glomerulus and are termed extraglomerular mesangial cells or Goormaghtigh cells. (From Lote CJ. *Principles of renal physiology.* 4th ed. London: Kluwer Academic Publishers, 2000 [Chapter 2].)

regulation of the circulating intravascular blood volume and sodium concentration via the renin-angiotensin-aldosterone system (RAAS). The proteolytic enzyme renin is released primarily in response to decreased afferent arteriolar pressure and decreased intraluminal sodium delivery to the macula densa. Renin is an enzyme of the hydrolase class that catalyzes cleavage of the leucine-leucine bond in angiotensinogen to generate angiotensin I. Renin release from the macula densa is also influenced by nitric oxide, renal cortical prostaglandins (predominantly PGI2), and the sympathetic nervous system. Angiotensin I is converted in the lungs by angiotensin-converting enzyme (ACE) to the potent vasoconstrictor and stimulator of aldosterone release, AII. Vasoconstriction and aldosterone release (with increased distal tubular sodium retention) act in concert with the other action of AII to increase the release of vasopressin (see later), and to increase proximal tubular sodium reabsorption, intravascular volume, and pressure. AII also has an inhibitory effect on renin release as part of a negative feedback loop.

Renal Interstitium

In a normal renal cortex, the interstitium is sparse (7 to 9% by volume) because the tubules lie very close together. The interstitium contains a variety of cell types including lymphocytes and fibroblast-like cells.[4]

The medullary interstitium contains a further specialized cell, lipid-laden interstitial cells, which are arranged in a characteristic ladder-like pattern across the loops of Henle and the capillaries. The extracellular space is rich in glycosaminoglycans, resulting in a gelatinous matrix that contains various poorly characterized osmolytes, osmotically active molecules that help stabilize the high osmotic gradient essential to the countercurrent mechanism involved in the generation of hyperosmotic urine. The interstitium becomes very important

TABLE 49.2	**Important Components of Kidney Function**
Filtration	Preparation of an ultrafiltrate
Reabsorptive	Glucose, amino acids, electrolytes, proteins
Homeostatic	Extracellular volume, acid-base status, blood pressure, electrolytes
Metabolic	Synthetic: glutathione, glyconeogenesis, ammonia
	Catabolic: hormones, cytokines
Endocrine	Erythropoietin synthesis, activation of vitamin D, renin release

in a variety of kidney diseases, and its expansion, as a consequence or cause of nephron loss, plays an important part in progressive kidney disease. Interstitial expansion includes cellular infiltration and increased interstitial matrix synthesis and interstitial fibrosis.

KIDNEY FUNCTION AND PHYSIOLOGY

The kidneys regulate and maintain the constant optimal chemical composition of the blood and the interstitial and intracellular fluids throughout the body—the internal milieu—through integration of the major renal functions, namely filtration, reabsorption, and excretion. Mechanisms of differential reabsorption and secretion, located in the tubule of a nephron, are the effectors of regulation (Table 49.2).

Excretory and Reabsorptive Functions

The *excretory function* of the kidneys serves to rid the body of many end products of metabolism and of excessive inorganic substances ingested in the diet. Waste products include the nonprotein nitrogenous compounds urea, creatinine, and uric acid; a number of other organic acids, including amino acids, are excreted in small quantities. Dietary intake contains a variable and usually excessive supply of sodium, potassium, chloride, calcium, phosphate, magnesium, sulfate, and bicarbonate. The efficiency of the homeostatic role of kidney function is illustrated by the way the sodium content of the body is maintained essentially constant, regardless of whether daily sodium intake is 1 or 150 mmol or more. Daily intake of water is also variable and may, on occasion, greatly exceed the requirements of the body. Under such circumstances, water becomes additional waste material requiring excretion. To achieve excretion of metabolic wastes and ingested surpluses without disrupting homeostasis, the kidneys must exercise both their *excretory* and *reabsorptive* functions.

Mechanisms for the regulation of electrolytes, nitrogenous wastes and organic acids are similar although not identical. For all except potassium and hydrogen ions and a few organic acids, the maximal excretory rate is limited or established by their plasma concentrations and the rate of their filtration through the glomeruli. Bulk transfer of substances from blood to glomerular filtrate determines the initial mass on which the nephron must operate to produce and excrete urine. Thus the maximal amount of substance excreted in urine does not exceed the amount transferred through the glomeruli by ultrafiltration except in the case of those substances capable of being secreted by tubular cells. Depending on the activity of the renal tubular epithelial cells and their several reabsorptive capacities, excreted amounts of urinary constituents are in general less than the amounts filtered. Because of this general behavior, for many substances an estimate of the excretory capacity of the kidneys can be obtained by measuring the GFR or some variable that is closely related to it. The primary objective in evaluating renal excretory function is to detect quantitatively the degradation of normal capacities or the improvement of impaired ones.

Definitions
Urine is defined as a fluid excreted by the kidneys, passed through the ureters, stored in the bladder, and discharged through the urethra. In health, it is sterile and clear and has an amber color, a slightly acid pH (approximately 5.0 to 6.0) and a characteristic odor. In addition to dissolved compounds it contains a number of cellular fragments and complete cells, derived from normal turnover of tubular cells, casts, and crystals (formed elements). Urinary casts are cylindrical proteinaceous structures formed in the distal convoluted tubule and collecting ducts, which dislodge and pass into the urine, where they can be detected by microscopy.

Urination, also termed *micturition*, is the discharge of urine. In normal adults adequate homeostasis is maintained with a urine output of 400 to 2000 mL/day. Alterations in urinary output are described as *anuria* (<100 mL/day), *oliguria* (<400 mL/day), or *polyuria* (>3 L/day or 50 mL/kg body weight/day). The most common disorder of micturition is altered frequency, which may be associated with increased urinary volume or with partial urinary tract obstruction (e.g., in prostatic hypertrophy).

Formation of Urine—An Overview
The first step in urine formation is filtration of plasma water at the glomeruli. A net filtration pressure of about 17 mm Hg in the capillary bed of the tuft drives the filtrate through the glomerular membrane. The filtrate is called an *ultrafiltrate* because its composition is essentially the same as that of plasma, but with a notable reduction in molecules of molecular weight exceeding 15 kDa. Each nephron produces about 100 µL of ultrafiltrate per day. Overall, approximately 170 to 200 L of ultrafiltrate passes through the glomeruli daily. In the passage of ultrafiltrate through the tubules, reabsorption of solutes and water in various regions of the tubules reduces the total urine volume.

Transport of solutes and water occurs both across and between the epithelial cells that line the renal tubules. Transport is both active (energy requiring) and passive, but many of the so-called passive transport processes are dependent upon or secondary to active transport processes, particularly those involving sodium transport. All known transport processes involve receptor or mediator molecules, the activity of many of which is regulated by phosphorylation facilitated by protein kinase C or A. Their renal distribution has been shown to correlate with known regional functional activities, but the same transporters, or isoforms of them, can be found in other tissues, particularly the digestive tract. For instance, at least five independent proximal tubular transport processes may be noted for amino acids, including those for (1) basic amino acids plus cystine, (2) glutamic and aspartic acid, (3) neutral amino acids, (4) imino amino acids, and (5) glycine.[5] Inherited disorders of tubular transporters, discussed later in this chapter, may occur, as well as a well-known generalized disorder affecting all of the transport processes, causing Fanconi syndrome (see later) and resulting in decreased reabsorption of electrolytes and nutrients (e.g., glucose, amino acids).

Direct coupling of adenosine triphosphate (ATP) hydrolysis is an example of an active transport process. The most important enzymatic transporter in the nephron is Na, K-ATPase, which is located on the basolateral membranes of the tubuloepithelial cells. Na, K-ATPase accounts for much of renal oxygen consumption and drives more than 99% of renal sodium reabsorption (Fig. 49.5). Other examples of primary active transport mechanisms include a Ca-ATPase, an H-ATPase, and an H, K-ATPase. These enzymes establish ionic gradients, polarizing cell membranes and thus driving secondary transport processes.

Many renal epithelial cell membranes also contain proteins that act as ion channels. For example, there is one for sodium that is closed by amiloride and modulated by hormones such as atrial natriuretic peptide (ANP). Ion channels enable much faster rates of transport than ATPases but are relatively fewer in number e.g., approximately 100 sodium and chloride channels versus 10^7 Na, K-ATPase molecules per cell.

Different regions of the tubule have been shown to specialize in certain functions. The proximal tubule facilitates the reabsorption of 60 to 80% of the glomerular filtrate volume—including 70% of the filtered load of sodium and chloride, and most of the potassium, glucose, bicarbonate, calcium, phosphate, sulfate, and other ions—and secreting 90% of the hydrogen ion excreted by the kidney (see Table 49.1). Uric acid is reabsorbed in the proximal tubule by a passive sodium-dependent mechanism, but there is also an active secretory mechanism. Creatinine is secreted but only to a small extent, approximately 2.5 µmol/min.

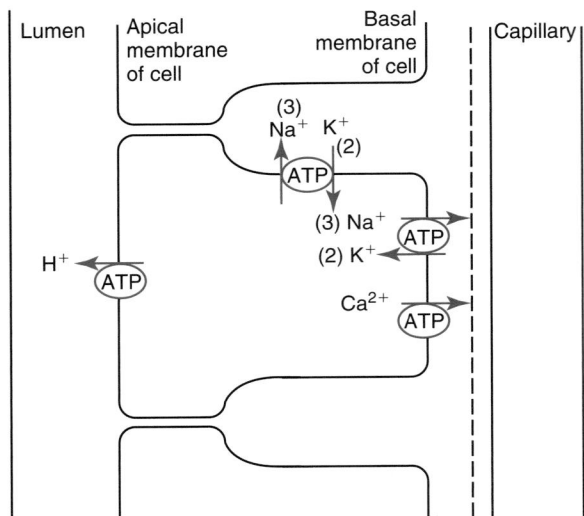

FIGURE 49.5 Tubular reabsorptive mechanisms: the major primary active transport processes in the proximal nephron. The renal tubular epithelium consists of a single layer of cells. At the luminal side, adjacent cells are in contact (the tight junction), whereas toward the basal side of the cells, there are gaps between adjacent cells (lateral intercellular spaces). (From Lote CJ. *Principles of renal physiology.* 4th ed. London: Kluwer Academic Publishers, 2000 [Chapter 4].)

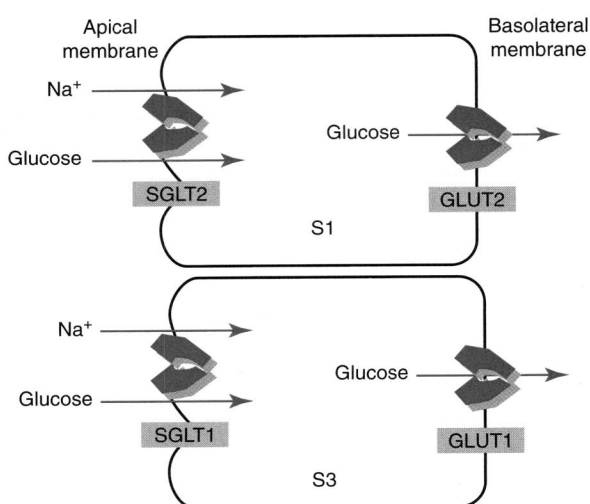

FIGURE 49.6 Glucose transport pathways across proximal tubule cells. Glucose is reabsorbed in conjunction with sodium at the apical membrane. The major mechanisms for glucose entry into the cells are the sodium-glucose cotransporters (SGLT1 and SGLT2). Glucose moves outward from the proximal tubule cells via the GLUT1 and GLUT2 transporters found in the S3 and S1 regions of the proximal tubule respectively. (From Lee YJ, Lee YJ, Han HJ. Regulatory mechanisms of Na+/glucose cotransporters in renal proximal tubule cells. *Kidney Int Suppl* 2007;72:S27–35).

Glucose is virtually completely reabsorbed, predominantly in the proximal tubule by a transport process that is saturated at a blood glucose concentration of about 180 mg/dL (10 mmol/L). On the apical membrane of the proximal tubule cells sodium/glucose cotransporters (SGLTs) are responsible for the transport of glucose, in conjunction with sodium, into the cells. The two main transporters involved are SGLT2, a low-affinity–high-capacity transporter expressed on the apical membranes of the convoluted proximal tubule cells (S1 and S2), and SGLT1, a high-affinity–low-capacity transporter found on the apical membranes of the straight proximal tubule (S3) cells. Approximately 90% of glucose is reabsorbed by SGLT2 with SGLT1 scavenging the remainder in the later (S3) portions of the proximal tubule. Glucose is returned to the circulation following transport out of the proximal tubule cells through the actions of basolateral sugar transporters GLUT2, located in the S1 segment of the tubule, and GLUT1, located in the S3 segment of the tubule (Fig. 49.6).[6]

Certain nonbiological compounds such as phenolsulfonphthalein and *p*-aminohippurate are secreted by the proximal tubule and have been used for the evaluation of renal tubular secretory capacity. When blood concentrations of creatinine increase above normal, creatinine is secreted in this region of the nephron. In the loop of Henle, chloride and more sodium without water are reabsorbed, generating dilute urine. Water reabsorption in the more distal tubules and collecting ducts is then regulated by vasopressin. In the distal tubule, secretion is the prominent activity; organic ions, potassium ions, and hydrogen ions are transported from the blood in the efferent arteriole into the tubular fluid.

Tubular epithelial cells synthesize a vast range of growth factors and cytokines in response to a variety of stimuli that can have both autocrine and paracrine effects. All cells secrete a range of cell adhesion molecules that are essential for cellular attachment to the tubular basement membrane.

Regulatory Function
Electrolyte Homeostasis
A complex interplay has been noted between the tubular transport systems regulating individual electrolytes. For simplicity, we have considered each electrolyte individually and have restricted our discussion to the systems of major physiologic, pharmacologic, and pathologic significance.

Sodium. Sodium reabsorption is required for the reabsorption of water and many solutes. The proximal tubule is highly permeable to sodium, and the net flux of reabsorption from the tubular lumen is achieved against a high backflux, particularly from paracellular[b] movement. Approximately 60% of filtered sodium is reabsorbed in the proximal tubule in an energy-dependent manner, driven by basolateral Na, K-ATPase pumps (see Fig. 49.5). Approximately 80% of sodium entering proximal tubular cells does so in exchange for hydrogen ion secretion, facilitated by apical Na-H exchangers. This process in turn permits bicarbonate reabsorption via carbonic anhydrases that are present in both the brush border and the intracellular compartment. A variety of apical sodium cotransporters also allow for reabsorption of other organic and inorganic solutes (e.g., chloride, calcium, phosphates, bicarbonate, sulfates,[7] glucose, urea, amino acids). Sodium transport activity is regulated by many factors, including protein kinase–dependent phosphorylation, which can increase both activity and channel numbers.

---

[b]Paracellular transport is that occurring between tubular epithelial cells and occurs by passive diffusion or by solvent drag.

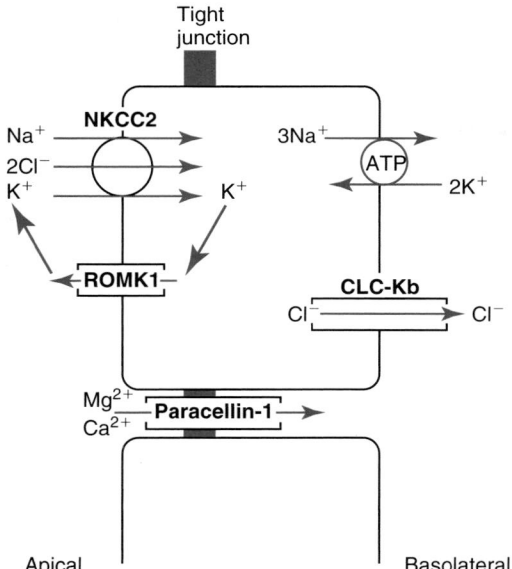

FIGURE 49.7 Schematic diagram showing the major pathways of solute reabsorption in the thick ascending limb of the loop of Henle. Sodium chloride is reabsorbed by the apical NKCC2 transporter. This electroneutral transport is driven by the low intracellular sodium and chloride concentrations generated by the basolateral Na, K-ATPase and the basolateral chloride channel CLC-Kb. The availability of potassium is rate-limiting for NKCC2, so potassium entering the cell is recycled back to the lumen via the ROMKI potassium channel. This potassium movement is electrogenic and drives paracellular resorption of Mg^{2+} and Ca^{2+} via paracellin-1. Mutations in NKCC2, ROMK1, or CLC-Kb cause Bartter syndrome. Mutations in paracellin-1 lead to disruption of this paracellular pathway and the tubular disease known as hypomagnesemic hypercalciuric nephrolithiasis. (From Alexander RT, Hoenderop JG, Bindels RJ. Molecular determinants of magnesium homeostasis: insights from human disease. *J Am Soc Nephrol* 2008;19:1451–8; Sayer JA, Pearce SHS. Diagnosis and clinical biochemistry of inherited tubulopathies. *Ann Clin Biochem* 2001;38:459–70).

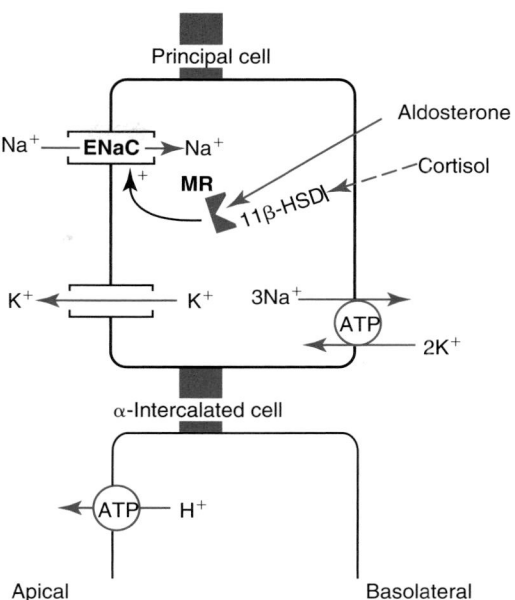

FIGURE 49.8 Schematic diagram showing the major pathways of solute reabsorption in the collecting duct. In principal cells, sodium reabsorption occurs through the amiloride-sensitive epithelial sodium channel (ENaC). Sodium reabsorption is influenced by the actions of aldosterone on the mineralocorticoid receptor (MR), with hyperaldosteronism producing an increase in channel activity. Cortisol, if permitted, will also bind to the MR, but a degree of specificity is maintained by 11β-hydroxysteroid dehydrogenase (11β-HSD), which inactivates cortisol to cortisone. Sodium uptake drives potassium secretion from principal cells and proton secretion from α-intercalated cells. In Liddle syndrome, mutations lead to an increase in ENaC activity, with increased sodium reabsorption and consequent potassium and proton loss. In pseudohypoaldosteronism type Ia, loss-of-function mutations inactivates ENaC, whereas in pseudohypoaldosteronism type Ib there are MR abnormalities. Both lead to reduced sodium entry via ENaC, causing salt wasting and decreased secretion of potassium and protons. Licorice causes hypertension and a hypokalemic metabolic alkalosis by inactivating 11β-HSD, allowing cortisol to act as a mineralocorticoid. (From Sayer JA, Pearce SHS. Diagnosis and clinical biochemistry of inherited tubulopathies. *Ann Clin Biochem* 2001;38:459–70).

A further 30% of filtered sodium is reabsorbed in the thick ascending limb of the loop of Henle, where it is achieved by an apical, bumetanide-sensitive, 130 kDa, electroneutral, Na-K-2Cl cotransporter (NKCC2), itself driven by a favorable inward gradient generated by the basolateral Na, K-ATPase pump (Fig. 49.7). NKCC2 is a kidney-specific member of a class of such channels found throughout secretory epithelia. Activation of these cotransporters appears, in part, to be a result of cell shrinkage. The distal tubule reabsorbs 5 to 8% of sodium via the apical thiazide-sensitive Na-Cl cotransporter (NCCT). Final sodium balance is achieved in the collecting duct via selective amiloride-sensitive, apical sodium channels (ENaCs) in exchange for potassium. ENaCs are controlled in part by the effects of aldosterone on the mineralocorticoid receptor (Fig. 49.8).

Potassium. Approximately 90% of daily potassium loss occurs via renal elimination. Potassium is freely filtered across the glomerulus and normally is almost completely reabsorbed in the proximal tubule. However, further regulation occurs in the loop of Henle, the distal tubule, and the collecting duct. Indeed, urinary losses can exceed filtered load, indicating the importance of distal secretion. Determinants of

urinary potassium loss are dietary intake of potassium and plasma potassium concentration, acid-base disturbances (acidosis reduces potassium secretion and vice versa), circulating vasopressin concentration (vasopressin increases potassium loss[8]), tubular flow rate (increased flow rate increases potassium loss[9]), and aldosterone secretion (enhances potassium loss and increases sodium retention).[10] Potassium ions are actively accumulated within tubular cells as a result of basolateral Na, K-ATPase activity, resulting in increase of intracellular potassium concentration to above its electrochemical equilibrium. Several types of potassium channels exist that have a range of functions: (1) maintenance of a negative resting cell membrane potential, (2) regulation of intracellular volume, (3) recycling of potassium across apical and basolateral membranes to supply NKCC2 and enable sodium reabsorption, and (4) potassium secretion in the cortical collecting tubule.[11] As mentioned previously, potassium is reabsorbed with sodium by NKCC2 in the thick ascending limb of the loop of Henle, but is recycled back into the lumen by renal outer medullary potassium-secreting channel 1 (ROMK1), thus generating an electrical gradient that drives passive paracellular reabsorption of calcium and magnesium down their electrochemical gradient (see Fig. 49.7).[12] ROMK1 is a pH-sensitive, membrane-spanning protein with several serine residues. At least two of these residues require phosphorylation by protein kinase A for the channel to be active.[11]

In the principal cells of the collecting duct, sodium reabsorption via ENaC is accompanied by movement of potassium into the lumen through potassium channels or through a K-Cl symporter (Fig. 49.8).[c]

Chloride. Approximately 60% of chloride is reabsorbed in the proximal tubule. In the early part of the proximal tubule, avid reabsorption of sodium in combination with glucose and amino acids occurs, creating a lumen-negative potential difference. The negative potential difference drives chloride reabsorption by diffusion through the paracellular pathway. Preferential reabsorption of glucose, amino acids, and bicarbonate in association with sodium in the early proximal tubule causes an increase in the luminal chloride concentration. This high chloride composition heralds the second phase of proximal chloride (and sodium) reabsorption: passive diffusion of sodium chloride via the paracellular pathway, and active reabsorption involving several antiporter[d] systems, by which chloride is exchanged for secretion of other anions (e.g., bicarbonate, formate, oxalate). In the thick ascending limb of the loop of Henle, further chloride reabsorption occurs in association with sodium via NKCC2. The concentration gradient is maintained by a basolateral chloride channel (CLC-Kb) (see Fig. 49.7).[13]

Calcium. Approximately 98% of filtered calcium is reabsorbed: 60 to 70% in the proximal tubule (predominantly via a paracellular pathway), 20% in the thick ascending limb of the loop of Henle, 10% in the distal convoluted tubule, and, finally, 5% in the collecting ducts. Although the distal nephron is only responsible for a small percentage of calcium reabsorption, it is the predominant site at which calcium excretion is regulated.[14] Calcium reabsorption is predominantly a passive process linked to active sodium reabsorption. In the proximal tubule the majority of calcium absorption occurs passively via a paracellular route: a small amount is reabsorbed actively via a transcellular pathway, with parathyroid hormone (PTH) and calcitonin regulating this process. No reabsorption occurs in the thin segments of the loop of Henle but in the thick ascending limb of the loop of Henle there is both paracellular and transcellular reabsorption of calcium. Paracellular calcium transport is driven by the potential difference created by ROMK1. The calcium sensing receptor (CaSR), located in the basolateral membrane of the thick ascending limb cells, also influences active calcium transport in this region. The CaSR controls expression of proteins known as claudins, which affect paracellular movement of divalent ions.[14]

Active processes, particularly in the distal tubule, tightly regulate the final amount of calcium excreted. Here, calcium reabsorption is exclusively transcellular, occurring against the existing electrochemical gradient, and being stimulated by PTH. Following entry into the cell from the lumen via an apical calcium channel (transient receptor potential vanilloid 5, TRPV5: previously called epithelial calcium channel 1, ECaC1), calcium binds to calbindin-D and is delivered to the basolateral membrane. Here it is extruded by a plasma membrane calcium-ATPase 1b (PMCA1b) and a Na-Ca exchanger (NCX1).[14] Transcription of messenger RNA coding for both TRPV5 and calbindin is stimulated by calcitriol (1,25(OH$_2$) D$_3$), possibly synthesized locally in the distal nephron and acting in a paracrine and autocrine fashion. A functional vitamin D response element has been identified in the promoter region of the calbindin-D gene, along with a putative site in the TRPV5 gene. TRPV5 is a pH-sensitive, 83-kDa protein with six transmembrane-spanning domains. Activation of the ion channel probably involves protein kinase C phosphorylation. Evidence indicates that stimulation of the renal CaSR by calcium in the tubular lumen can directly affect tubular reabsorption of calcium, independent of the effects of calciotropic hormones.[15]

Phosphate. Reabsorption of phosphate occurs predominantly (85%) in the proximal tubule and is mediated by a secondary active transport mechanism.[14] Three families (NPT2a, NPT2c, and PiT-2) of sodium-dependent, phosphate cotransporters have been identified, located in the apical plasma membrane. In humans, NPT2a (SLC34A1) and NPT2c (SLC34A3) are thought to be equally physiologically important. All phosphate cotransporters use the energy derived from the transport of sodium down its gradient to move inorganic phosphate from the luminal filtrate into the cell. NPT2a sodium-phosphate transporter is electrogenic (i.e., involves the inward flux of a positive charge), with three sodium ions and one divalent phosphate ion being transferred. NPT2c transport is electroneutral (involving two sodium ions and one divalent phosphate ion). Acute regulation of transport is achieved primarily by an alteration in the amount of cotransporter protein present in the apical membrane, with longer-term changes also involving increased transcription of the protein. Apical membrane levels of phosphate cotransporter proteins are controlled by a variety of dietary, hormonal, and environmental stimuli (e.g., PTH, fibroblast growth factor 23 [FGF-23], 1,25(OH)$_2$D$_3$, metabolic acidosis, hypertension).[14] Regulation predominantly involves internalization of the protein. Increased intracellular movement of the channel from the plasma membrane to the lysosomes is believed to follow both protein kinase A and C phosphorylation initiated by PTH receptor binding.[16] Transport of phosphate from the renal proximal tubule to the peritubular capillaries occurs via an unknown basolateral transporter.[14]

FGF-23 is a 32 kDa phosphate-regulating peptide, largely produced by bone cells in response to increased plasma phosphate concentration and/or phosphate ingestion. It was discovered during the 1990s following studies of severe hereditary osteomalacia characterized by severe hypophosphatemia and inappropriate phosphaturia.[17] Its major action is to inhibit sodium-phosphate coupled reabsorption in the renal proximal tubule, causing phosphaturia. Autosomal dominant hypophosphatemic rickets is due to a mutation in the FGF-23

---

[c]A symporter is an integral membrane protein that is involved in movement of two or more different molecules or ions across a phospholipid membrane such as the plasma membrane in the same direction, and is therefore a type of cotransporter.

[d]An antiporter (also called exchanger or counter-transporter) is an integral membrane protein which is involved in secondary active transport of two or more different molecules or ions (i.e., solutes) across a phospholipid membrane such as the plasma membrane in opposite directions.

gene that results in a hyperstable form of this protein.[18] FGF-23 interacts with fibroblast growth factor receptor 1 in the kidney via a transmembrane protein, klotho, thereby inhibiting sodium-coupled phosphate cotransporter activity. FGF-23 also inhibits 1α-vitamin D hydroxylase leading to reduced calcitriol production. These effects will reduce plasma phosphate concentrations. In addition, FGF-23 suppresses PTH synthesis, although the parathyroid glands are believed to become resistant to FGF-23 as kidney disease progresses.[14]

Normally less than 20% of the filtered load of phosphate is excreted into the urine, but above a plasma phosphate concentration of approximately 3.6 mg/dL (1.2 mmol/L), increments in urinary phosphate excretion increase linearly with the filtered load, suggesting that there is T_m (tubular maximal uptake) for phosphate. The T_m for phosphate is decreased by increases in the circulating PTH concentration and the ratio of T_m for phosphate to GFR (T_mP/GFR). T_mP/GFR has been used as a test in the differential diagnosis of hypercalcemia. Although superseded in this context by modern PTH assays, it may be useful in the investigation of inherited disorders of tubular phosphate handling.[19]

Magnesium. Approximately 96% of filtered magnesium is reabsorbed in the nephron: 10 to 30% in the proximal tubule; 40 to 70% in the thick ascending limb of the loop of Henle; and 5 to 10% in the distal convoluted tubule. A variety of coordinated transport processes are involved (see reference Blaine et al.[14] for further details), mutations of which cause a variety of electrolyte disorders (see later).

Bicarbonate and hydrogen ion. The kidney plays a central role in the maintenance of acid-base homeostasis through reabsorption of filtered bicarbonate and secretion of ammonium and acid. The tubular mechanisms underlying these processes are discussed in Chapter 50.

Water Homeostasis

Approximately 180 L glomerular filtrate is formed each day. The unique physiology of the kidney enables approximately 99% of this to be reabsorbed in the production of urine with variable osmolality (between 50 and 1400 mOsmol/kg H_2O at extremes of water intake). Plasma membranes of all human cells are water permeable but to variable degrees. In the kidney, different segments of the nephron show differing permeability to water, enabling the body to both retain water and produce urine of variable concentration. Water reabsorption occurs both isosmotically, in association with electrolyte reabsorption in the proximal tubule, and differentially, in the loop of Henle, distal tubule, and collecting duct in response to the action of vasopressin. Absorption of water depends on the driving force for water reabsorption (predominantly active sodium transport) and the osmotic equilibration of water across the tubular epithelium. The generation of concentrated urine depends upon medullary hyperosmolality: this in turn requires low water permeability in some kidney segments (ascending limb of the loop of Henle), whereas in other kidney segments (e.g., proximal tubule) there is a requirement for high water permeability. Differing permeability and facilitation of hormonal control appears to be partly achieved by differential expression along the nephron of a family of proteins known as the aquaporins (AQPs), which act as water channels.

At least 11 different mammalian AQPs have been identified, of which 7 (AQP1, -2, -3, -4, -6, -7, -8) are expressed in the kidney.[20,21] Many of these have extrarenal expression sites as well (e.g., AQP1 may be important in fluid removal across the peritoneal membrane). Two asparagine-proline-alanine sequences in the molecule are thought to interact in the membrane to form a pathway for water translocation. AQP1, which is found in the proximal tubule and the descending thin limb of the loop of Henle, constitutes almost 3% of total membrane protein in the kidney. It appears to be constitutively expressed and is present in both the apical and basolateral plasma membranes, representing entry and exit ports for water transport across the cell, respectively. Approximately 70% of water reabsorption occurs at this site, predominantly via a transcellular (e.g., AQP1) rather than a paracellular route. Water reabsorption in the proximal tubule passively follows sodium reabsorption, so that fluid entering the loop of Henle is still almost isosmotic with plasma.

Urinary concentration is partly achieved by countercurrent multiplication in the loop of Henle, where approximately 5% of water reabsorption occurs (Fig. 49.9). The descending thin limb is very permeable to water, but the ascending limb and the collecting duct are not (the collecting ducts are also poorly permeable to urea). Fluid entering the loop of Henle is isotonic to plasma but is hypotonic on leaving it. The ascending limb has active sodium reabsorption driven by Na, K-ATPase with electroneutralizing transport of chloride, a combined process that can be inhibited by the so-called loop diuretics (e.g., furosemide, see later). In this section of the nephron, sodium reabsorption is not accompanied by water, creating a hypertonic medullary interstitium and facilitating water reabsorption from the anatomically adjacent descending limb. The descending limb cells are permeable to sodium chloride, which is cycled from the descending limb back to the ascending limb. Countercurrent multiplication is responsible for generating approximately half of the maximal medullary concentration gradient (1200 mOsmol/kg H_2O), the remainder being generated by urea recycling (see later).[22]

A further 10% of water reabsorption occurs in the distal tubule, with the remainder (>20 L/day) reabsorbed in the collecting ducts. Entry of water into the collecting duct cells occurs via apical AQP2 channels, with exit probably occurring via basolateral AQP3 (cortical and outer medullary collecting ducts) and AQP4 (inner medullary collecting ducts). AQP2 appears to be the primary target for vasopressin regulation of water reabsorption. Vasopressin (Mr 1080) is a cyclic nonapeptide synthesized in the posterior hypothalamus and stored in the posterior pituitary. It is mainly released into the circulation in response to rising plasma osmolality, detected by osmoreceptors in the anterior hypothalamus, but other important stimuli include pain, acidosis, vomiting, hypoxia, hypotension and hypovolaemia.[23] AQP2 is stored in subapical vesicles in the collecting duct cells. Following vasopressin stimulation, these vesicles are cycled through, and inserted into, the plasma membrane by a cytoskeletal, dynein-mediated transport process. Stimulation occurs following binding of vasopressin to a V_2 receptor in the basolateral plasma membrane of the principal cells of the collecting duct, which promotes a cyclic adenosine monophosphate (cAMP)/protein kinase A cascade, resulting in phosphorylation and activation of AQP2. Vasopressin regulates the acute cellular water-retaining response (AQP2 trafficking) and its longer-term regulation via a conditioning effect on AQP2 gene transcription. The

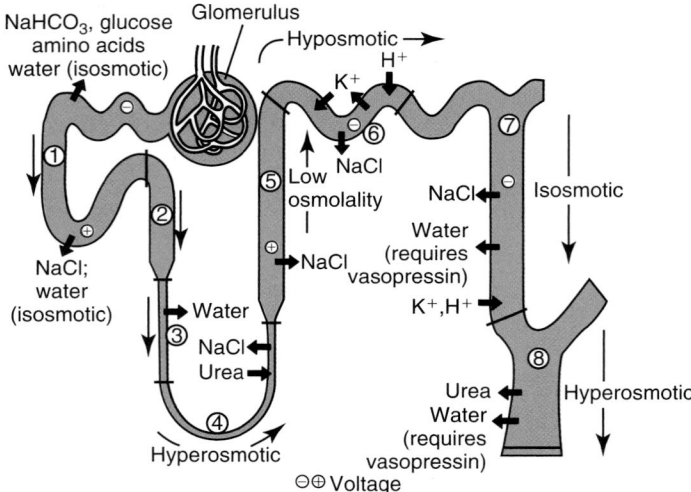

FIGURE 49.9 Countercurrent multiplication mechanism: schematic representation of the principal processes of transport in the nephron. In the convoluted portion of the proximal tubule (1), salts and water are reabsorbed at high rates in isotonic proportions. Bulk reabsorption of most of the filtrate (65 to 70%) and virtually complete reabsorption of glucose, amino acids, and bicarbonate take place in this segment. In the pars recta (2), organic acids are secreted and continuous reabsorption of sodium chloride takes place. The loop of Henle comprises three segments: the thin descending (3) and ascending (4) limbs and the thick ascending limb (5). The fluid becomes hyperosmotic, because of water abstraction, as it flows toward the bend of the loop, and hypoosmotic, because of sodium chloride reabsorption, as it flows toward the distal convoluted tubule (6). Active sodium reabsorption occurs in the distal convoluted tubule and in the cortical collecting tubule (7). This latter segment is water impermeable in the absence of antidiuretic hormone (ADH), and the reabsorption of sodium in this segment is increased by aldosterone. The collecting duct (8) allows equilibration of water with the hyperosmotic interstitium when ADH is present. For additional details, see text. (From Burg MB. The nephron in transport of sodium, amino acids, and glucose. Hosp Pract 1978;13:100. Adapted from a drawing by A. Iselin.)

AQP2 gene has a cAMP response element that is involved in the long-term upregulation of AQP2 expression by vasopressin. It is likely that there are also vasopressin-independent regulatory pathways of AQP2 expression (e.g., oxytocin).[22] Membrane insertion of AQP2 allows water to pass into the collecting duct cells under the influence of medullary hyperosmolality. Maintenance of medullary hyperosmolality depends upon efficient fluid removal, which is the function of the ascending *vasa recta*, a specialized medullary vasculature, and the close anatomic relations of all medullary constituents (see Fig. 49.2). AQP2 expression is decreased in a variety of polyuric conditions (e.g., diabetes insipidus, lithium treatment, hypokalemia, hypercalcemia, urinary obstruction) and is increased in some water-retaining states (e.g., heart failure, cirrhosis, and pregnancy).[21,24] A variety of V_2 receptor antagonists have been designed that block the actions of vasopressin. In contrast to diuretics, these agents promote the excretion of electrolyte-free water and have exciting therapeutic potential in water-retaining states.[24]

Vasopressin also increases the permeability of collecting duct cells to urea, which is the major osmotically active component of luminal fluid in the distal tubule. Fluid of high urea concentration therefore enters the deepest layers of the medullary interstitium, passing down its concentration gradient, contributing to medullary hyperosmolality.

Endocrine Function

The *endocrine functions* of the kidneys may be regarded as primary because the kidneys are endocrine organs producing hormones, or as secondary, because the kidneys are a site of action for hormones produced or activated elsewhere. In addition, the kidneys are a site of degradation for hormones such as insulin and aldosterone. In their primary endocrine function, the kidneys produce erythropoietin (EPO), prostaglandins, and thromboxanes, $1,25(OH_2)D_3$ and renin. The importance of renin in the maintenance of systemic blood pressure was discussed earlier (see "Juxtaglomerular Apparatus").

Erythropoietin

EPO is a large glycoprotein hormone (Mr 34 kDa) containing 165 amino acids responsible for stimulating erythroid progenitor cells within the bone marrow to produce red blood cells. It is secreted chiefly by renal peritubular capillary endothelial cells in the adult and by the liver in the fetus. Physiologically, reduced oxygen delivery to the kidneys initiates a process coordinated by hypoxia inducible factor-2 resulting in release of EPO, thereby stimulating erythropoiesis.[25] Conversely, with a surplus of oxygen in blood traversing the kidneys, as in some forms of polycythemia, the release of EPO into blood is diminished. The use of recombinant human erythropoietin (rhEPO, epoetin) in the management of anemia of kidney disease is discussed later.

Prostaglandins and Thromboxanes

Prostaglandins and thromboxanes are synthesized from arachidonic acid by the cyclooxygenase (COX) enzyme system. The COX system is present in many parts of the kidney and has an important role in regulating the physiologic action of other hormones on renal vascular tone, mesangial contractility, and tubular processing of salt and water. Prostaglandins have a critical role in renal hemodynamics, control of tubular function, and renin release. The major renal vasodilatory prostaglandin is PGE_2, which is synthesized predominantly in the medulla. The major vasoconstrictor prostaglandin is thromboxane A_2, which is produced primarily within the renal cortex.[26] PGE_2 increases renal blood flow rate, inhibits sodium reabsorption in the distal nephron and collecting duct, and stimulates renin release.[26] These actions promote natriuresis and diuresis. In patients with chronic kidney disease (CKD), renal PGE_2 production is increased, representing a compensatory response to loss of nephron mass.[27] Vasodilatory prostaglandins are synthesized following stimulation with renal sympathetic adrenergic and AII-dependent mechanisms to offset or modulate vasoconstriction.[28] In the tubule, prostaglandins act as autocoids, exerting their effects locally, near the site of synthesis.

In pathophysiologic circumstances, including various forms of acute kidney injury (AKI), thromboxane A_2 and various prostaglandins may have a significant role in inflammation and alteration of vascular tone. The effects of nonsteroidal anti-inflammatory drugs (NSAIDs) on renal prostaglandin metabolism are considered later. The lipoxygenase pathway, which leads to formation of leukotrienes, is also present within the kidneys, although the major source of leukotrienes in inflammatory disease of the kidneys is infiltrating white cells and macrophages.

1,25(OH$_2$)D$_3$

The kidneys are primarily responsible for producing $1,25(OH_2)D_3$ from 25-hydroxycholecalciferol as a result of the action of the enzyme 25-hydroxycholecalciferol 1α-hydroxylase found in proximal tubular epithelial cells. Regulation of this system is considered in Chapter 54. The management of renal mineral-bone disorders is considered later.

Glomerular Filtration Rate

The GFR is considered to be the most reliable measure of the functional capacity of the kidneys and is often thought of as indicative of the number of functioning nephrons. As a physiologic measurement, it has proved to be the most sensitive and specific marker of changes in overall renal function. Measurement of GFR is discussed in Chapter 34.

The rate of formation of glomerular filtrate depends on the balance between hydrostatic and oncotic forces along the afferent arteriole and across the glomerular filter. The net pressure difference must be sufficient not only to drive filtration across the glomerular filtration barrier but also to drive the ultrafiltrate along the tubules against their inherent resistance to flow. In the absence of sufficient pressure the lumina of the tubules will collapse. This balance of forces can be expressed as follows:

$$\text{Rate of Filtration} = K_f((P_{GCap} + \Pi_{BC}) - (P_{BG} + \Pi_{GCap})),$$

where

K_f = (hydraulic permeability $\times$ surface area)
P_{GCap} = glomerular-capillary hydrostatic pressure
Π_{BC} = oncotic pressure in Bowman's capsule
P_{BC} = hydrostatic pressure in Bowman's capsule
Π_{GCap} = oncotic pressure in the glomerular capillary

Because the oncotic pressure in Bowman's capsule (Π_{BC}) can be considered to be negligible (protein concentration is usually 10 to 100 mg/L), this equation becomes:

$$\text{Rate of Filtration} = K_f(P_{GCap} - P_{BC} - \Pi_{GCap})$$

Changes in K_f can be caused by drugs and by glomerular disease, but it is also physiologically regulated. Mesangial cell contraction, which is thought to be the main mechanism, causes a reduction in K_f, tending to reduce GFR. Net P_{GCap} represents a balance between renal arterial pressure and afferent and efferent arteriolar resistance. Although an increase in arterial pressure will tend to increase P_{GCap}, the magnitude of the change is modulated by differential manipulation of afferent and efferent tone, which can result in minimal change to the P_{GCap}. When the renal blood flow is low, oncotic pressure can change as the plasma passes along the renal capillaries. As filtrate is removed, the oncotic pressure rises, and by the end of the capillary the net filtration rate may become zero; thus GFR falls, and this limits the amount of filtrate that can be obtained from a given volume of plasma. The average ($P_{GCap} - P_{BC} - \Pi_{GCap}$) or net filtration pressure is about 17 mm Hg. This pressure is sufficient to drive the filtration of 180 L of fluid per day since the K_f for glomerular capillaries is several orders of magnitude greater than for nonrenal capillaries.

Regulation of Glomerular Filtration Rate

The factors involved in regulation of GFR are listed in Table 49.3. Autoregulation of renal blood flow and GFR is widely thought to be explained by the *myogenic theory*. This theory is based on the principle that an increase in wall tension of the afferent arterioles, brought about by an increase in perfusion pressure, causes automatic contraction of arteriolar smooth muscle, thus increasing resistance and keeping the flow constant despite the increase in perfusion pressure.

The *tubuloglomerular feedback mechanism*, involving the *macula densa* and release of the vasodilator adenosine, must also be considered. Although not fully understood, this mechanism appears to regulate GFR, with changes in renal

TABLE 49.3 Summary of Factors That Influence the Glomerular Filtration Rate		Effect on GFR
K_f	Increased glomerular surface area due to relaxation of mesangial cells	Increase
	Decreased glomerular surface area due to contraction of mesangial cells	Decrease
P_{GCap}	Altered renal arterial pressure	
	Afferent dilation	Increase
	Afferent constriction	Decrease
	Efferent constriction	Increase
	Efferent dilation	Decrease
P_{BC}	Increased intratubular pressure (e.g., tubular obstruction)	Decrease
$\Pi GCap$	Altered plasma oncotic pressure: increased	Decrease
	Altered renal blood flow: decreased	Decrease

(See text for explanation of terminology)
GFR, Glomerular filtration rate.

TABLE 49.4   Factors Altering Renal Artery Tone and Renal Blood Flow

	EFFECT ON		EFFECT ON	
Factor	Afferent Arteriole	Efferent Arteriole	RBF	GFR
Adenosine	Constriction	Dilation	N	N→NE
Angiotensin II	Constriction	Constriction	N	N
Epinephrine/norepinephrine	Constriction	Constriction	N	N→NE
Vasopressin	Constriction	Constriction	NE	N→NE
Endothelin	Constriction	Constriction	NE	N→NE
Leukotrienes	Constriction	Constriction	NE	N→NE
Thromboxane A_2	Constriction	Constriction	NE	N→NE
Prostaglandins (PGE_2, PGI_2)	Dilation	Dilation	NE	NE
Nitric oxide	Dilation	Dilation	N	N
Atrial natriuretic factor	Dilation	Constriction	N	N→P
Dopamine	—	Dilation	N	N

GFR, Glomerular filtration rate; *N*, negative; *NE*, negligible; *P*, positive; *RBF*, renal blood flow.

blood flow as a secondary consequence. For individual nephrons, evidence indicates that each single nephron GFR is influenced by the composition of the tubular fluid in the distal tubule, which in turn is influenced by the filtration rate. The *macula densa* is thought to sense the distal tubular sodium chloride content, its osmolality, or the rate at which sodium chloride is transported. The *macula densa* then signals the JGA via an uncertain mechanism to cause the release of adenosine and possibly AII and prostaglandins, which in turn affects vascular resistance.[e]

The result of the combination of myogenic mechanisms and tubuloglomerular feedback is that the net filtration pressure or P_{GCap} is kept reasonably constant over a wide range of systemic arterial pressures. It should be noted that renal blood flow and GFR change across this range of systemic pressures but to a significantly smaller extent than would be predicted if these autoregulatory mechanisms were not in place.

Other factors influencing renal blood flow are indicated in Table 49.4. The afferent and efferent arterioles are richly supplied with renal sympathetic nerves. Epinephrine acts via α-adrenergic receptors, leading to constriction of both arterioles and causing a decrease in renal blood flow.

Nitric oxide (NO) has been identified as an important vasodilator produced by vascular endothelial cells. NO is synthesized from L-arginine and oxygen by nitric oxide synthase (NOS), of which three isoenzymes are differentially located and regulated. Within the kidney are eNOS (endothelial) and iNOS (inducible) isoenzymes. Activation of NOS has been shown to occur as a result of shear stress (e.g., increased arteriolar tone). A variety of physiologic vasoconstrictors are present, including acetylcholine, bradykinin, endothelin, and serotonin; a rise in intracellular ionized calcium is required for the vasoconstrictors. NO synthesis is now known to play an important role in the regulation of human vascular tone and has a crucial role in control of blood pressure and kidney function.[29]

Age and the Kidney

Kidney function varies throughout life. In utero, urine is produced by the developing fetus from about the ninth week

of gestation. Nephrogenesis is complete by approximately 35 weeks gestation, although kidney function remains immature during the first 2 years of life. The kidney of the term infant receives approximately 6% of the cardiac output, compared with 25% in adults. Renal vascular resistance is relatively high and the low renal blood flow is particularly directed to the medulla and inner cortex. The gradual increase in renal blood flow that occurs with increasing age is directed mainly to the outer cortex and is mediated by local neurohormonal mechanisms.[30] The GFR at birth is approximately 30 mL/min/1.73 m².[31] It increases rapidly during the first weeks of life to reach approximately 70 mL/min/1.73 m² by age 16 days.[31] Normal adult values are achieved by age 14 years. Tubular functions, including salt and water conservation, are also immature at birth. Birth is associated with rapid changes in kidney function, with a switch to salt and water conservation mediated by catecholamines, the renin-angiotensin system, vasopressin, glucocorticoids, and thyroid hormone.[31] The immaturity of the neonatal kidney contributes to the relatively common problems of water and electrolyte disturbances in infants. These disturbances are more likely to occur in premature infants, particularly those born before 35 weeks gestation.

Aging is associated with a range of microscopic, macroscopic, and molecular changes in the kidney, which begin in early middle-age, including decreasing kidney weight, decreasing number of glomeruli, with the cortical glomeruli being particularly affected, GBM thickening, increased prevalence of renal cysts, parenchymal calcifications, and cortical scars. There is also glomerular sclerosis, tubular atrophy, interstitial fibrosis, and arteriosclerosis; collectively this tetrad of abnormalities is termed nephrosclerosis. At a molecular level, these changes are accompanied by cellular senescence, telomere shortening, and apoptosis.[32]

Structural change is accompanied by functional changes, which in many respects are the reverse of those seen in early life. On average, GFR declines with age by approximately 1 mL/min/1.73 m²/yr over the age of 40 years.[33–35] Renal blood flow, particularly to the cortical area, also decreases with age at a rate of approximately 10%/year from the fourth to fifth decade onward, while the filtration fraction (i.e., GFR/renal plasma flow)[33] and renal vascular resistance[36] increase. Tubular function, such as the ability to concentrate

---

[e]Vascular resistance is the resistance to flow that must be overcome to push blood through the circulatory system.

urine, retain sodium, and excrete water and salt load, is decreased, and nocturnal polyuria is common. These changes in part account for the increased risk of dehydration and AKI observed in older individuals.[32] The prevalence of albuminuria rises over the age of approximately 40 years.[37,38]

It is a moot point whether these changes are the result of a normal aging process (i.e., involutional) or whether they are caused by the interplay of pathology and age. Cumulative exposure to common causes of CKD such as (1) atherosclerosis,[39] (2) hypertension,[40] (3) heart failure,[41] (4) diabetes,[42] (5) obstructive nephropathy, (6) infection, (7) immune insult, (8) nephrotoxins such as lead,[43] and (9) dietary protein[44,45] increases with age and it is difficult to separate these effects from those of "healthy" aging. In the absence of these and other identifiable causes of kidney disease, many individuals have stable GFR as they age.

Loss of kidney function with aging appears to be heterogeneous and is not inevitable.[46,47] Kidney function may be well preserved in healthy older people, and assumptions with respect to GFR based solely on age could be erroneous. Furthermore, attention to the common causes of CKD could preserve function in older people.[48] Kidney disease is more common among older people. Studies from England,[49] France,[50] and Iceland[51] have demonstrated a near exponential rise in CKD with age. Data from the United States show the prevalence of GFR between 30 and 60 mL/min/1.73 m^2 to be 4.3% of the total noninstitutionalized population overall, but this rises to 25% among those over 70 years.[52] The prevalence may be even higher among institutionalized older people (e.g., 82% of a residential home population were identified as having a GFR <60 mL/min/1.73 m^2).[53] The incidence of AKI also increases with age.[54]

GLOMERULAR AND TUBULAR PROTEIN HANDLING

Glomerular Sieving

Approximately 10 kg/day of protein is presented to the glomerular filtration barrier, with only approximately 1 g passing into the proximal tubule.[55] Glomerular permselectivity to proteins is a function of the integrated actions of endothelial cells, the GBM, and the podocytes, although the exact contribution and importance of each is still a matter of some debate.[55,56] A variety of methods have been used to study the permeability of the glomerular barrier, including urinalysis in vivo, micropuncture of single nephrons, isolated perfused kidneys, isolated glomeruli, isolated GBMs, and artificial membranes. All of these techniques have contributed to knowledge of glomerular permeability characteristics, and all also have advantages and disadvantages. For example, micropuncture techniques may damage the barrier, and animal models may differ from human—permselectivity characteristics vary even between different rat species.[57] These issues have been reviewed by Haraldsson and associates.[2] Additionally, a range of different markers, including endogenous and modified proteins, dextran, and Ficoll polymers have been used to study glomerular permeability.[2] The glomerular permeability of a molecule is expressed in terms of its glomerular sieving coefficient (GSC). Molecules smaller than inulin (approximate Mr 5 kDa) are freely filtered. Therefore inulin, urea, creatinine, glucose, and electrolytes all have a

GSC = 1.0. Classic experiments in the 1970s used linear dextran chains of varying molecular weight and charge to study glomerular filtration characteristics. However, linear carbohydrate chains do not necessarily behave in the same manner as a globular protein of equal molecular weight or charge. For example, neutral dextran chains of 15 kDa (diameter 2.4 nm) have GSC = 1.0 whereas the smaller β_2-microglobulin (11.8 kDa, diameter 1.6 nm) has GSC = 0.7.[58] Linear molecules have higher GSC than globular proteins, and hence theoretical glomerular pore dimensions based on dextran studies were overestimated. More recently, Ficoll polymers were used. These are neutral, heavily cross-linked, sucrose-epichlorohydrin copolymers that behave as rigid hydrated spheres and are thought to behave more like globular proteins in their sieving behavior.[2]

As a result of such studies, some general conclusions can be drawn with respect to glomerular protein handling. The glomerulus acts as a selective filter of the blood passing through its capillaries, restricting the passage of macromolecules in a size-, charge-, and shape/configuration-dependent manner. Sieving coefficients (i) decrease as molecular size increases; (ii) are lower for anionic proteins than for neutral proteins of equivalent size; and (iii) are lower for globular rather than elongated proteins. Examples of the GSC for major urinary proteins are listed in see Table 34.2.

The protein concentration in the glomerular filtrate has been measured in several animal models by direct glomerular puncture. The concentration of total protein found is in the range of several hundred mg/L (approximately 1% of plasma), with albumin concentrations ranging from less than 40 to a few hundred mg/L. The filtered load of protein depends on the product of the GSC and the free plasma concentration: therefore the albumin load per nephron is much greater than that of the other filtered proteins.[58,59] In general, proteins larger than albumin (66 kDa, diameter 3.5 nm, charge −23) are retained by the healthy glomerulus and are termed high molecular weight proteins. However, lower molecular weight proteins are also retained to a significant extent.

Tubular Reabsorption

The final urinary concentration of proteins depends on the filtered load, but also on the efficiency of the proximal tubular reabsorptive process, in addition to any contribution of tubular secretion. Proteins are reabsorbed by receptor-mediated, low-affinity, high-capacity processes. Megalin (600 kDa) and cubilin (460 kDa) are endocytic, multiligand receptors that are important in protein reabsorption. Megalin belongs to the low-density lipoprotein (LDL) receptor family whereas cubilin is identical to the intestinal intrinsic factor-vitamin B12 receptor. In the kidney, both are localized in clathrin-coated pits in the apical brush border of renal proximal tubular cells and bind filtered proteins in a calcium-dependent process. This apparatus is found throughout the proximal tubule although there are notably fewer clathrin-coated pits and vesicles in the S3 segment. Megalin appears capable of both binding and internalizing its ligands whereas the cubilin-ligand complex requires megalin to be internalized. Some proteins such as albumin will bind to either receptor, whereas others are specific (e.g., transferrin binds to cubilin only, retinol-binding protein [RBP] and α1-microglobulin to megalin only).[60]

Once proteins have been internalized, they are transported by the endocytic vesicle and fuse with lysosomes. Proteolysis occurs, and the resultant amino acids are released into the tubulointerstitial space across the basolateral surface of the tubular epithelial cell. The membrane vesicles are then recycled to the brush border to complete the reabsorption cycle. Some small peptide fragments of proteins may be released back into the urinary space. An alternative reabsorptive pathway involves interaction with MHC-related Fc receptor (FcRN), leading to dissociation of albumin from megalin/cubilin and subsequent transcytosis of albumin i.e., transport of intact reabsorbed albumin across the tubular epithelial cell and back into the circulation. The quantitative significance of this mechanism remains unclear.[60] In health, the reabsorptive mechanism removes the majority of the filtered protein, thus retaining most of the essential amino acid constituents for reuse.[58] Capture of filtered transport proteins is also important in conserving vitamin status (e.g., vitamin A associated with RBP).

The tubular reabsorptive process is saturable. Any increase in the filtered load (caused by glomerular damage, increased glomerular vascular permeability [e.g., inflammatory response], or increased circulating concentration of low molecular weight proteins) or decrease in reabsorptive capacity (caused by tubular damage) can result in increased urinary protein loss (*proteinuria*).

Tubular secretion of proteins also contributes to urinary total protein concentration. In particular, in health, uromodulin (also known as Tamm Horsfall glycoprotein, THG) accounts for ~50% of urinary total protein. Uromodulin (200 kDa), a highly glycosylated acidic protein, is secreted into the tubular fluid only by the thick ascending limb and the early distal convoluted tubule and is thought to play a role in inhibiting kidney stone formation.[58,61] It is a major constituent of renal tubular casts along with albumin and traces of other proteins. Investigation for proteinuria is mandatory in any patient with suspected kidney disease and was considered in Chapter 34.

Consequences of Proteinuria

Experimental data indicate that proteinuria is not just a marker of, but contributes directly to, progression of kidney disease.[62,63] The accumulation of proteins in abnormal amounts in the tubular lumen may trigger release of profibrogenic and proinflammatory molecules (see later), which in turn contribute to tubulointerstitial structural damage and expansion, and progression of kidney disease.[64] Increasing evidence suggests that megalin may not just be a scavenger receptor for albumin, but that it may have signaling functions that regulate cell survival. Evidence gathered from in vitro studies suggests that glomerular filtration of abnormal amounts or types of protein induces mesangial cell injury, leading to glomerulosclerosis, and that these same proteins can have adverse effects on proximal tubular cell function. Excessive quantities of albumin in the tubular lumen may downregulate proximal tubular megalin expression, increasing cell sensitivity to apoptosis.[65]

Numerous studies have demonstrated that proteinuria is a potent risk marker for progression of renal disease in both nondiabetic[66–70] and diabetic[71–73] kidney disease. Furthermore, reducing proteinuria slows the rate of progression of proteinuric kidney disease. This effect has been observed in

clinical trials in patients treated with ACE inhibitors, angiotensin II receptor blockers (ARBs), and mineralocorticoid receptor antagonists, given alone or in combination.[68,74,75] Reduction of proteinuria has been proposed as a therapeutic target,[76,77] although this view is not universally held.[78]

PATHOPHYSIOLOGY OF KIDNEY DISEASE

Despite the diverse initial causes of injury to the kidney, progression of kidney disease leading to loss of function and ultimately to kidney failure is a remarkably monotonous process characterized by early inflammation, followed by accumulation and deposition of extracellular matrix, tubulointerstitial fibrosis, tubular atrophy, and glomerulosclerosis. Proteinuria is thought to be one of the most important risk factors for progression of kidney diseases (see earlier). Nephrons are also lost via toxic, anoxic, or immunologic injury that initially may occur in the glomerulus, the tubule, or both together. Glomerular damage can involve endothelial, epithelial, or mesangial cells, and/or the basement membrane.

The RAAS plays a pivotal role in many of the pathophysiologic changes that cause kidney injury and is an important therapeutic target (Fig. 49.10).[79] Renal cells are able to produce AII in a concentration that is much higher than in the systemic circulation, and AII generates potentially toxic reactive oxygen species within renal cells affecting signal transduction. In addition, many profibrogenic and proinflammatory mediators are induced within the kidney by AII. Aldosterone has been reported to enhance profibrogenic processes. Inflammatory mediators released include cytokines, chemokines, and growth factors, such as TGF-β, monocyte chemoattractant protein-1 (MCP-1), interleukin-6 (IL-6), interferon-γ, and tissue necrosis factor-α (TNF-α); these inflammatory factors activate resident lymphocytes and macrophages and recruit additional cells from the peripheral circulation. Thus cellular infiltration is a common but not universal finding in renal biopsy specimens. These activated cells can cause T cell–mediated cell lysis, activation, and proliferation of interstitial fibroblasts. Fibroblast activity results in increased extracellular matrix synthesis and eventually in glomerular and tubular fibrosis. Extracellular matrix expansion causes disruption of local blood flow, exaggerating regional ischemia, and a vicious cycle of inflammation, fibrosis, and cell death is propagated.

Elucidation of this common pathway is incomplete but is the focus of considerable research interest because novel therapies are required to reduce progression and ideally to reverse fibrosis.[80] A strong relationship has been described for proteinuria and MCP-1-mediated interstitial damage in a prospective study of patients undergoing kidney biopsy for CKD.[81] In rodent models, anti-MCP-1 gene therapy reduced interstitial inflammation and fibrosis.[82] Increased production and activity of TGF-β have also been demonstrated in glomerular disease: this acts as a key mediator, along with AII, of fibrogenesis.[83] Data support the hypothesis that during tubulointerstitial fibrosis α-smooth muscle actin-expressing mesenchymal cells might derive from the tubular epithelium via epithelial-mesenchymal transition (EMT) under the influence of TGF-β.[84] Strategies to block the process of EMT are being explored for future therapeutic targets in CKD. For example, an endogenous antagonist of TGF-β-induced EMT has been identified as bone morphogenic

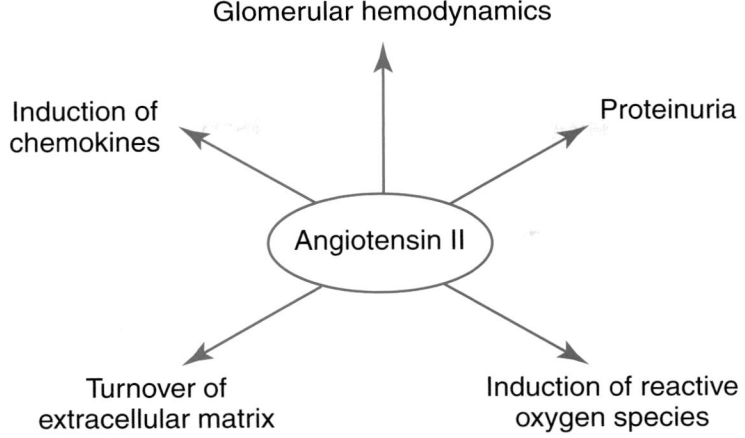

FIGURE 49.10 Angiotensin plays a pivotal role in kidney pathology in addition to classical hemodynamic effects.

protein-7, a member of the TGF-β superfamily. Systemic administration of bone morphogenic protein-7 repaired severely damaged tubular cells in mice and reversed renal injury.[85]

The kidneys have considerable ability to increase their functional capacity in response to injury. Thus a significant reduction in functioning renal mass (50 to 60%) may occur before the onset of any significant symptoms or even before any major biochemical alterations appear. The most sensitive and specific measure of functional change, the GFR, can be reduced to less than 60 mL/min/1.73 m² before signs and symptoms of kidney disease will be observed. This increase in workload per nephron is thought to be an important cause of progressive renal injury.[86] A well-recognized hypothesis suggests that independent of primary renal injury, a point is reached in the decline in nephron number when further loss becomes inevitable and progressive as a consequence of a common pathway leading to interstitial fibrosis.[87]

Overview of Kidney Disease and Its Clinical Manifestations

Most often kidney disease is detected opportunistically by measurement of blood pressure and urine and blood testing in asymptomatic individuals. Such testing can occur in the primary care setting or for health clearance purposes for insurance. Typical findings include isolated hematuria and isolated proteinuria. Kidney disease may also present with macroscopic hematuria, swollen ankles, headaches and visual disturbances due to severe hypertension, or as a manifestation of systemic disease such as in the vasculitides and systemic lupus erythematosus (SLE) (specific kidney diseases are discussed in greater detail later). Symptoms suggestive of advanced kidney disease include fatigue, nausea, vomiting, poor appetite, shortness of breath, fluid retention, poor memory, loss of libido, and itching. Unfortunately, many individuals present very late in their disease and may require urgent dialysis with no previous experience with the specialist nephrology service. These patients have a poor prognosis compared with patients who have been cared for in a multidisciplinary specialist environment for at least

1 year. Therefore early recognition of kidney disease is of paramount importance to outcome.

Detection and diagnosis of kidney disease requires a detailed history to include current symptoms, past medical and family history, social history, and a full drug history. A focused examination may identify potential causes of kidney disease such as obstructive uropathy in which the bladder is easily palpable or may indicate vascular disease associated with narrowing of the arteries supplying the kidneys (renal artery stenosis), systemic disease, or de novo kidney disease. Blood pressure measurement and urinalysis (see Chapter 34) are crucial baseline assessments. Examination of the skin may reveal evidence of advanced kidney disease with excoriations due to the intense itch that can occur. Signs of fluid overload can be seen in the ankles or effusions may be noted in the chest. Abdominal examination may detect a palpable bladder, renal bruits, or enlarged kidneys. Fundoscopic examination is performed in hypertensive and diabetic patients to identify microvascular damage to the retina.

Kidney disease may present with heavy blood and protein detected in a sample of the urine—a so-called "active urinary sediment." An acute "nephritic" syndrome may occur as the result of postinfectious glomerulonephritis, for example, following a streptococcal throat or skin infection. The patient presents with poor urine output, edema, hypertension, and brown discolored urine. This pattern of acute nephritis is commonly seen in the developing world and is relatively unusual in developed countries.

Proteinuria may be the only indicator of kidney disease in many people. Proteinuria, particularly if in excess of 1 g/day, is indicative of glomerular disease. Most cases of glomerular disease are chronic and patients may be followed for many years with monitoring of GFR and quantification of proteinuria.

Kidney disease presenting as nephrotic syndrome is characterized by the triad of heavy proteinuria (typically defined as exceeding an arbitrary threshold of 3 g/day), hypoalbuminemia, and edema. It is almost always caused by glomerular disease as opposed to tubular proteinuria. Several distinct pathologic entities that may cause nephrotic syndrome include minimal change nephropathy, focal segmental glomerular sclerosis, and membranous nephropathy; these are discussed later. Nephrotic syndrome can also be a manifestation of diabetic kidney disease (diabetic nephropathy).

Kidney disease often accompanies systemic diseases such as diabetes mellitus, vasculitis, SLE, and plasma cell dyscrasias. The whole spectrum of kidney involvement may be seen including an active urinary sediment, isolated proteinuria or hematuria, nephrotic syndrome, and rapidly progressive kidney failure.

Imaging of the renal tract to include kidneys, ureters, bladder, and prostate gland is very important in many kidney diseases and provides useful information. It is mandatory in all cases of new AKI (see later) to identify size and symmetry of kidneys and to exclude obstruction to urine flow anywhere within the tract. Renal ultrasound, the imaging technique of choice in most cases, gives reliable data on the size of kidneys and evidence of obstruction where present. Additionally, underlying structural abnormalities such as polycystic kidneys, renal cysts and tumors, and anatomic and congenital malformations may be demonstrated. Renal ultrasonography is easy, cheap, noninvasive, and without risk. Computed tomography (CT) imaging of the kidney-ureter-bladder has largely superseded intravenous pyelography in identifying kidney stones and structural diseases of the urinary tract. Invasive investigations of the urinary tract, particularly in patients with obstruction and hematuria, include cystoscopic examination of the bladder lining under direct vision, which allows for selective cannulation of each ureteric orifice and imaging with x-rays following injection of radiocontrast medium (retrograde study). The level of the lesion in an obstructed kidney can be ascertained by percutaneous insertion of a catheter into the kidney via a nephrostomy and subsequent injection of contrast via the nephrostomy tube, with x-rays taken as the contrast is drained from the kidney into the ureter and bladder (antegrade study).

Nuclear medicine scintigraphy is used to identify scars or cortical defects within kidneys and to assess the differential function of each kidney relative to the other. In addition, patients with well-preserved kidney function who are suspected of having renal artery stenosis can be challenged with an ACE inhibitor, such as captopril. This investigation assesses whether the flow of the radioisotope alters significantly following captopril administration. Radioisotopes are also utilized in some cases when obstruction is suspected but cannot be reliably demonstrated on ultrasound scanning, or when the collecting system with the kidney is dilated to assess whether there is a functional obstruction. Excretion of the radioisotope is tested following the administration of the loop diuretic furosemide.

In patients with suspected renal artery disease, examination of the blood supply is necessary. Noninvasive imaging is preferred for diagnosis and modalities include contrast enhanced CT angiography and magnetic resonance angiogram following intravenous gadolinium contrast injection. In cases requiring confirmation, or when an intervention to open the artery is proposed, selective renal angiography under x-ray screening can be performed following cannulation of the arterial tree via the femoral artery in the groin or an upper limb artery.

Despite all these investigations it is occasionally necessary to perform a kidney biopsy. Biopsy typically is indicated in patients with either nephrotic syndrome, moderate proteinuria in the presence of hematuria, rapidly progressive disease, and AKI, and in patients with CKD (see below) that is progressive despite attention to treatments targeted to preserve kidney function. A biopsy is taken from one kidney only following injection of local anesthetic. To minimize the risk of bleeding, the lower pole of the kidney is chosen because the lower pole is away from the hilum, where the major blood vessels are present. The lower pole is identified using ultrasound scanning, and a semiautomatic needle device is placed on the capsule of the kidney and is released into the cortex and medulla. A sample of tissue is obtained, and light microscopy, immunofluorescence, or immunoperoxidase staining is performed, as well as electron microscopy (EM). It should be emphasized that although approximately 13% of the adult population is estimated to have CKD[88] only a minority of patients undergo a kidney biopsy. A kidney biopsy should be undertaken only for nonmalignant disease in a specialist nephrology setting. Histopathologic examination of the specimen confirms the diagnosis and gives some indication of prognosis and the need for specific treatment.

Terminology of Kidney Disease

The nomenclature associated with kidney disease has been amended and is clarified here.[89] Previously, renal failure was divided into either *acute renal failure* (ARF) and *chronic renal failure* (CRF). These terms indicate the rate at which damage occurs, rather than the mechanism by which it occurs. The term *renal* has largely been replaced by *kidney* when referring to *chronic* disease because it is more easily understood by patients and nonspecialists. The commonly used term, *acute renal failure*, has been replaced by *acute kidney injury*. Kidney failure is defined as a GFR of less than 15 mL/min/1.73 m².[90] Not all patients with kidney failure require renal replacement therapy (RRT, dialysis or transplantation) to sustain life. In the United States, *end-stage renal disease* (ESRD) is a federal government-defined term that indicates the need for long-term chronic RRT. Each patient with ESRD is registered through the Medical Evidence form (2728), submitted by all dialysis and transplant providers. The term now includes both Medicare and non-Medicare populations.

Classification of Chronic Kidney Disease

Earlier studies to identify the incidence, causes, and complications of CKD largely focused on advanced disease and kidney failure. The number of patients with ESRD continues to rise, with associated poor prognosis despite modern replacement therapies (e.g., 33% 5-year survival on dialysis) and large health care costs (e.g., $35.9 billion total Medicare spending on ESRD in the United States in 2017), accounting for 7.2% of overall Medicare paid claims.[91] This has promoted the recognition of CKD as an important public health problem, emphasizing the need for earlier identification and treatment. In addition to the cost of ESRD, CKD expenditure was $84 billion in the Unites States in 2017.[91] Historically, data obtained from epidemiologic surveys were compromised by lack of consistent surrogate markers of kidney function to identify established disease. For example, serum creatinine, calculated creatinine clearance, and measured creatinine clearance were variously used. Landmark guidelines developed in the United States by the National Kidney Foundation-Kidney Disease Outcomes Quality Initiative

TABLE 49.5 Classification of Chronic Kidney Disease Indicating Prognosis and Secondary/ Tertiary Care Referral Decision Making by Glomerular Filtration Rate and Albuminuria Categories

				PERSISTENT ALBUMINURIA CATEGORIES: DESCRIPTION AND RANGE		
				A1	A2	A3
				Normal to mildly increased <30 mg/g (<3 mg/mmol)	Moderately increased 30–300 mg/g (3–30 mg/mmol)	Severely increased >300 mg/g (>30 mg/mmol)
Glomerular filtration rate categories (mL/min/ 1.73 m²): description and range	G1	Normal or high	>90	55.6	1.9 Monitor	0.4 Refer[a]
	G2	Mildly decreased	60–89	32.9	2.2 Monitor	0.3 Refer[a]
	G3a	Mildly to moderately decreased	45–59	3.6 Monitor	0.8 Monitor	0.2 Refer
	G3b	Moderately to severely decreased	30–44	1.0 Monitor	0.4 Monitor	0.2 Refer
	G4	Severely decreased	15–29	0.2 Refer[a]	0.1 Refer[a]	0.1 Refer
	G5	Kidney failure	<15	<0.1 Refer	<0.1 Refer	0.1 Refer

[a]Referring clinicians may wish to discuss with their local nephrology service depending on local arrangements regarding referral and monitoring. Numbers within the cells show the proportion (in %) of the adult population in the United States.[565]
Color key. Green: low risk (if no other markers of kidney disease, no CKD); yellow: moderately increased risk; orange: high risk; red: very high risk. Kidney Disease Improving Global Outcomes. Clinical Practice Guideline for the Evaluation and Management of Chronic Kidney Disease. *Kidney Int* 2013;3:1–150.

(NKF-K/DOQI)[92] attempted to evaluate, classify, and stratify CKD. These guidelines were published in 2002 and were based upon categories of GFR. They have subsequently been revised and updated by Kidney Disease: Improving Global Outcomes (KDIGO)[90,93] and broadly adopted by other national organizations e.g., the National Institute for Health and Care Excellence (NICE) in the United Kingdom (Table 49.5).[94] The KDIGO 2012 guideline added a second dimension to the classification system with 3 identified levels of albuminuria,[90] acknowledging the powerful additional prognostic information imparted by the presence of proteinuria (see Chapter 34).[95,96]

In the 2012 KDIGO system CKD is *defined* as abnormalities of kidney structure or function, present for *at least* 3 months, with implications for health.[90] Abnormalities in kidney structure (damage) generally precede abnormalities in kidney function (Fig. 49.11). The most commonly observed abnormalities in function are decreased GFR and/or increased albuminuria, although urinary sediment abnormalities, pathologic/imaging abnormalities, genetic disorders, or a history of renal transplantation must also be considered. CKD is *classified* based on cause, GFR category, and albuminuria category. The KDIGO guideline stratifies GFR from category G1 (≥90 mL/ min/1.73 m²) through to G5 (GFR <15 mL/min/1.73 m²). A GFR less than 60 mL/min/1.73 m² (G3 to G5) is considered decreased. Category G3 is subdivided into G3A (GFR 45 to 59 mL/min/1.73 m²) and G3B (GFR 30 to 44 mL/min/1.73 m²), on the basis of the differing epidemiologic and prognostic significances of these GFR levels. Proteinuria is graded in albuminuria categories, from A1 (<30 mg/day) through A2 (30 to 300 mg/day) to A3 (>300 mg/day). For example, a patient with a GFR of 50 mL/min/1.73 m² and albumin loss of 200 mg/day would be classified G3a, A2. Although the cutoff levels between stages are somewhat arbitrary, the classification allows for

consistency in prevalence reporting for epidemiologic studies, facilitates undertaking of comparative studies and analysis and allowing focused treatment schedules for individual patients (see Table 49.5).[97]

Since the introduction of the classification system in 2002, the documented prevalence of CKD has increased, and recognition of the importance of CKD led to the introduction of new diagnostic codes during 2006 (ICD-9-CM diagnosis codes). These codes have subsequently been further revised (ICD-10-CM diagnosis codes). The importance of early diagnosis of CKD was highlighted by the recognition that 40% of patients commencing dialysis treatment in the United States during 2006 had not previously seen a nephrologist, nor received a serum creatinine measurement within the previous year.[98] More recent data suggests that 33% of incident patients in the United States during 2017 still did not receive nephrology care prior to needing renal support.[91] It is anticiated that early diagnosis of CKD in people at high risk should allow for treatment to ameliorate the progressive decline in kidney function, treat complications of CKD, and plan for ESRD modalities, including where necessary, end-of-life care.

One of the concerns regarding the classification is the high prevalence of CKD imposed by the system itself. In the United States, it is estimated that 27 million individuals have CKD, representing almost 1 in 7 adults.[88] Population samples from elsewhere indicate similar prevalence rates. Most individuals with CKD do not progress to ESRD with prevalence rates of patients in GFR category G3 10 to 20 times higher than the prevalence rates of GFR categories G4 and G5 (see Table 49.5).[99,100] There is some concern that many individuals being identified with G3 CKD are not at increased risk:[99,101] use of cystatin C to delineate risk in this population has been proposed (see Chapter 34).[90,94,102]

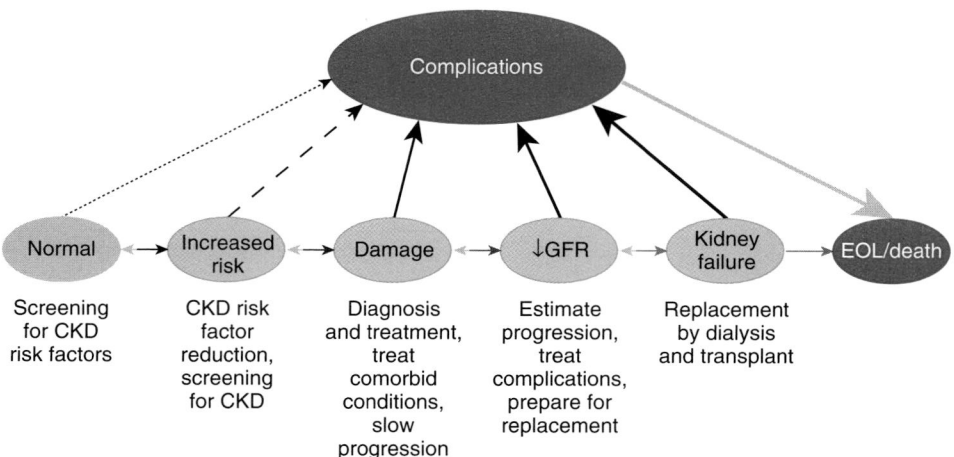

FIGURE 49.11 Conceptual model of CKD. Continuum of development, progression, and complications of CKD and strategies to improve outcomes. Horizontal arrows between circles represent development, progression, and remission of CKD. Left-pointing horizontal arrowheads signify that remission is less frequent than progression. Diagonal arrows represent occurrence of complications of CKD, including drug toxicity, endocrine and metabolic complications, cardiovascular disease, and others such as infection, cognitive impairment, and frailty. Complications might also arise from adverse effects of interventions to prevent or treat the disease. *CKD,* Chronic kidney disease; *EOL,* end-of-life care and/or conservative management; *GFR,* glomerular filtration rate. (Reproduced with permission from Levey AS, Stevens LA, Coresh J. Conceptual model of CKD: applications and implications. *Am J Kidney Dis* 2009;53:S4–16).

National data describing the incidence and prevalence of patients using RRT are available from the United States and the United Kingdom. The crude[f] annual acceptance rate for RRT continues to increase worldwide. However, standardized acceptance rates may have peaked. A recent United States Renal Data System (USRDS) annual report indicates a reduction in new, that is "incident," patients requiring RRT standardized to the age-sex-race distribution of the 2011 US population.[91] The reported crude incident rate in 2017 was 370.2 per million population (pmp) in the United States; the standardized rate was marginally down at 341 pmp, although much higher among African-Americans and Native Americans (Fig. 49.12).[91] In terms of absolute numbers it is pertinent to note that in excess of 120,000 people in the United States were taken onto RRT during 2017, representing a doubling over the past 25 years.[91] The annual acceptance rate onto RRT in the United Kingdom in 2017 was 121 pmp, compared to 118 pmp in 2016.[103] In the United Kingdom the median age of patients starting RRT was 63.7 years during 2017, but this was dependent on ethnicity (white 65.8 years, south Asian 61.1 years, and black 56.5 years).[103] It should be noted that the incidence of ESRD increases with age. Overall the crude prevalence rates of patients with ESRD are also increasing and reached 2203 pmp in 2017 in the United States, an increase of 65.0% since 2000.[91] The increase in prevalent patients is clearly dramatic with more than three quarters of a million people on RRT in the United States. The annual mortality rates have improved markedly over the past 20 years, and therefore people are living for a longer period of time with kidney failure. The crude mortality rate among all ESRD patients declined from 185.6 per 1000/year in 1996 to 137.2 per 1000/year in 2017, an absolute decrease of 48.4 per 1000/year.[91]

The main causes of CKD leading to kidney failure from 1980 to 2014 in the United States are indicated in Fig. 49.13. As indicated, diabetes mellitus is the largest single cause of advanced CKD and accounts for almost 50% of new dialysis patients in the United States. Hypertension is the underlying diagnosis in around 25% of new dialysis patients and is also particularly prevalent among African Americans. The myriad of kidney diseases, including glomerulonephritis, infective, hereditary, systemic, interstitial, and obstructive conditions, as well as those of unknown origin, account for the remainder. In the United Kingdom, during 2017 diabetic nephropathy as a primary renal disease was seen in approximately 29% of new patients.[103]

Ethnic origin also modifies risk of kidney disease.[104] The lifetime risk of developing ESRD in 20-year-old black men and women respectively has been estimated to be 7.3 and 7.8%, compared with 2.5% in white men and 1.8% in white women.[105] Family history of kidney disease is also a risk factor for developing ESRD. For example, a ninefold increased risk for ESRD has been noted in the African American community for those individuals with a first-degree relative with ESRD.[106] Therefore genetic influences may be involved in the development of kidney disease and the rate of progression to ESRD.

In summary, the presence of kidney disease can be easily identified through simple blood and urine testing. Subsequent diagnosis of the cause of kidney disease relies on medical history, examination, and laboratory and radiologic investigations and will be discussed in the relevant disease sections later in this chapter.

General Management of Chronic Kidney Disease

Complications of CKD that develop before the need for RRT are numerous and include cardiovascular disease, metabolic acidosis, bone disease, and anemia. There is a broad, and

---

[f]Crude rates are calculated by dividing the total number of cases in a given time period by the total number of persons in the population.

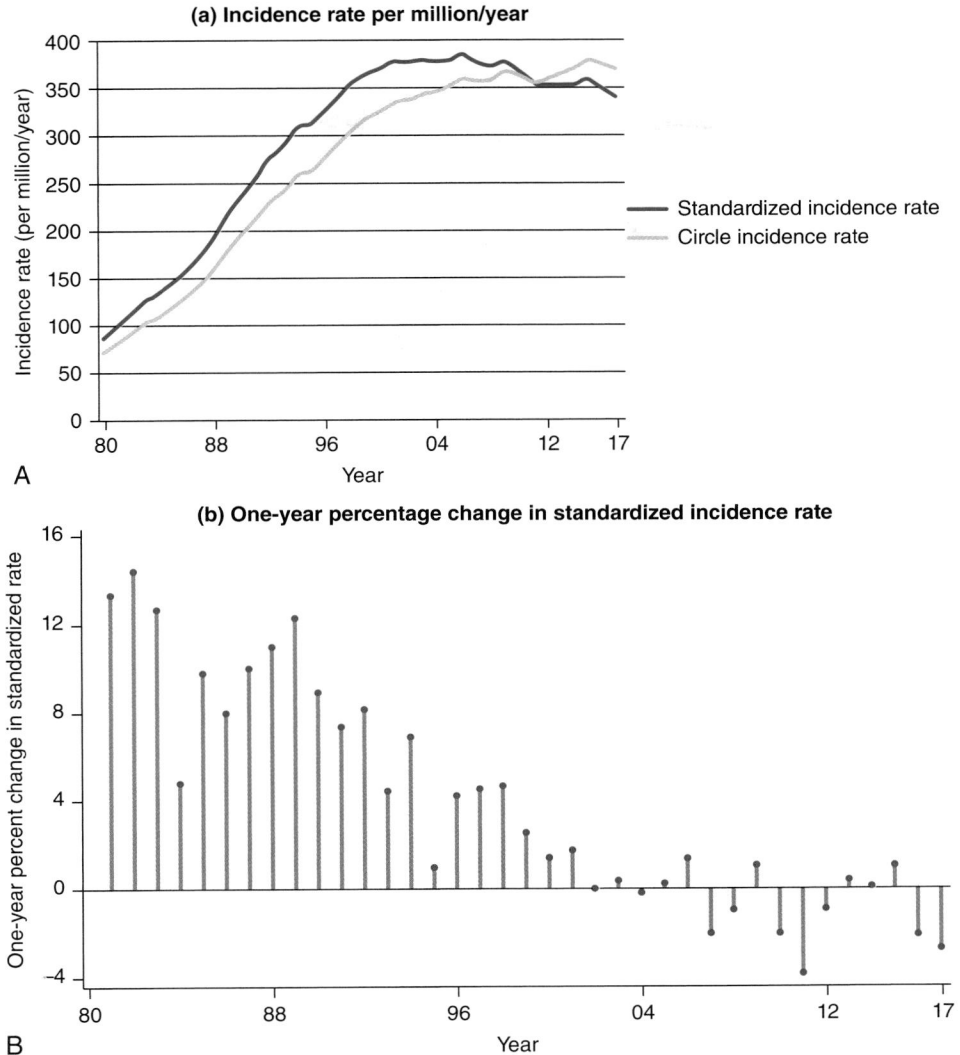

(a) Incidence rate per million/year

Standardized incidence rate
Circle incidence rate

A

(b) One-year percentage change in standardized incidence rate

B

FIGURE 49.12 Trends in the (A) crude and standardized incidence rates of end-stage renal disease (ESRD), and (B) the annual percentage change in the standardized incidence rate of ESRD in the US population, 1980 to 2017.[91] The number of incident (newly reported) ESRD cases in 2017 was 124,500. After a year-by-year rise in this number over three decades from 1980 through 2010, it now appears to have plateaued or declined slightly. The incidence rate of ESRD per million/year virtually plateaued beginning in 2000, and the adjusted incidence rate of 341 per million/year in 2017 is the lowest recorded since 1998.

often causal, relationship between the burden of illness and the level of GFR. Rate of progression of CKD, irrespective of underlying cause, is dependent on both nonmodifiable factors, such as age, gender, race, and level of kidney function at diagnosis, and modifiable characteristics, including proteinuria, blood pressure control, and smoking. Progression and specific treatment options for diabetic and hypertensive nephropathy are discussed separately later. The current discussion focuses on optimal treatment for nondiabetic CKD. Lowering blood pressure and reducing proteinuria have been shown to ameliorate the progression of CKD. The Modification of Diet in Renal Disease (MDRD) study compared the rates of decline in GFR in 840 patients with various causes of CKD versus a "usual" or "low" blood pressure goal.[107] Patients with type 1 diabetes were excluded. Outcome data suggest that a low blood pressure goal had some beneficial effect in

those patients with higher levels of proteinuria.[107,108] The study supported the concept that proteinuria is an independent risk factor for progression of kidney disease. For patients with proteinuria greater than 1 g/day the suggested target for mean blood pressure was 92 mm Hg (125/75 mm Hg).[69] The target blood pressure recommended by the eighth report of the Joint National Committee on Prevention, Detection, Evaluation, and Treatment of High Blood Pressure (JNC 8) is less than 140/90 mm Hg for patients with diabetes or kidney disease and the general population aged less than 60 years.[109] There is concern that lower blood pressures may be associated with worse outcomes in some patients. Hence target ranges in addition to thresholds are sometimes recommended. In the United Kingdom a target systolic blood pressure of less than 140 mm Hg (range 120 to 139 mm Hg) and diastolic blood pressure less than 90 mm Hg is recommended for

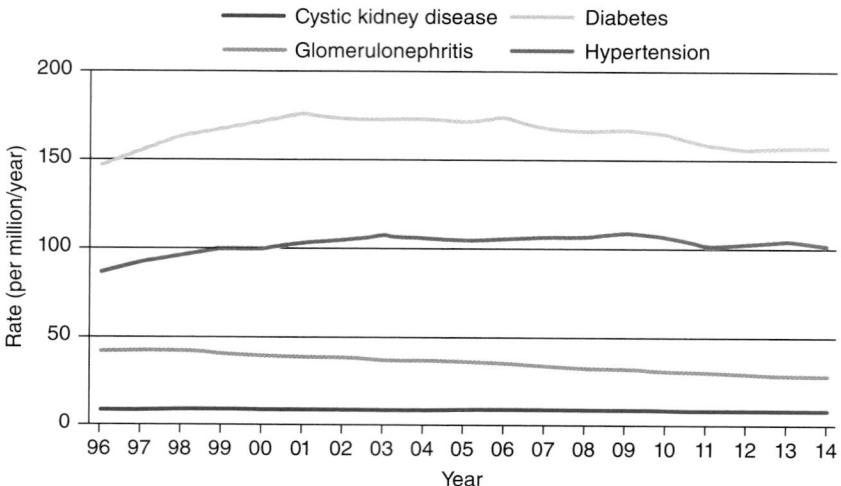

FIGURE 49.13 Trends in adjusted* ESRD incidence rate (per million/year), by primary cause of ESRD, in the US population, 1996 to 2014 *Adjusted for age, sex, and race. The standard population was the US population in 2011. *ESRD,* End-stage renal disease. The data show that diabetes as a cause of ESRD remains the most common diagnosis of new ESRD in the United States. The incidence of ESRD due to glomerulonephritis peaked in the mid-1990s.[256] Recent iterations of the US Renal Data System (USRDS) Annual Data Report (ADR) including the 30th report published in 2019 offer a note of caution regarding the validity of primary diagnosis data citing that physicians may over diagnose diabetes as a presumptive cause of ESRD, since very few patients with "diabetic" chronic kidney disease (CKD) will have a proven histologic diagnosis of diabetic nephropathy. (US Renal Data System. Annual Data Report: Epidemiology of Kidney Disease in the United States. 2019. Available at: https://www.usrds.org/2019/download/USRDS__ES_final.pdf. Accessed October 18, 2020.)

most patients with CKD.[94] A lower target systolic blood pressure of less than 130 mm Hg (target range 120 to 129 mm Hg) and diastolic target of less than 80 mm Hg is recommended in patients with an ACR greater than 70 mg/mmol (approximately equivalent to >1 g/day proteinuria) and/or diabetes.[94]

Data from the Third National Health and Nutrition Examination Survey (NHANES III, 1988 to 1994) reveal, that among hypertensive individuals with an increased serum creatinine concentration, 75% were on antihypertensive treatment, and only 11% had their blood pressure reduced to lower than 130/85 mm Hg.[110]

ACE inhibitors are more effective than other antihypertensive drugs in slowing the rate of progression of proteinuric CKD,[111–113] although they do induce a mild decrease in GFR (<10 mL/min/1.73 m^2). It should also be noted that the evidence base for ACE inhibitor use in the setting of CKD may not be generalizable to older (>70 years) nonproteinuric adults, who form the majority of patients with CKD.[114] The development of hypotension, AKI, or hyperkalemia (plasma potassium concentration >5.5 mmol/L) should prompt discontinuation of the drug until other causes have been excluded. Short-term studies show that ARBs have effects on blood pressure and proteinuria that are similar to those of ACE inhibitors.

Low-nitrogen (protein) diets have been advocated from the early years of treatment of severe chronic uremia.[115] The very-low-protein diets tested in the MDRD study were of marginal benefit in these well-supervised patients with very low renal function, but are not well adhered to in practice, may lead to negative nitrogen balance, and are not recommended. Protein intake is restricted spontaneously to approximately 0.6 to 0.8 g/kg/day by uremic patients not receiving dietary advice.[116] To prevent malnutrition, patients receive professional dietary advice, with diets containing an increased proportion of protein and a total calorie content of up to 35 kcal/kg/day. The NHANES III has confirmed an association with reduced GFR and malnutrition in noninstitutionalized individuals studied in a cross-sectional survey of more than 5000 participants stratified according to GFR.[117]

Although intuitively one might expect correction of renal acidosis to be beneficial, unanticipated secondary effects may impact on patient survival (e.g., increased vascular calcification following alkalinization or increased risk of heart failure).[118,119] A relatively small trial suggested that bicarbonate supplementation can slow the rate of progression of CKD[120] and further reports generally support this suggestion.[121,122] However, a pragmatic study (BiCARB) among older patients with CKD did not observe benefit from oral sodium bicarbonate supplementation in terms of improving physical function or reducing kidney function decline.[123]

Cardiovascular Complications of Chronic Kidney Disease

The spectrum of cardiovascular pathology predominant among patients with CKD (hypertensive cardiomyopathy, arrhythmias, heart failure, valvular disease, and peripheral vascular disease) differs from that predominant in the general population (atheromatous coronary artery disease).[124] The incidence of cardiovascular disease is 7- to 10-fold greater in patients with CKD than in non-CKD age- and gender-matched controls.[125] By the time patients develop the need for RRT, there is an approximately 17 times greater risk of cardiovascular death or nonfatal myocardial infarction among age- and sex-matched individuals without kidney disease.[124,126] Among patients treated by dialysis, the prevalence of coronary artery disease is approximately 40% and the prevalence of left ventricular hypertrophy (LVH) is

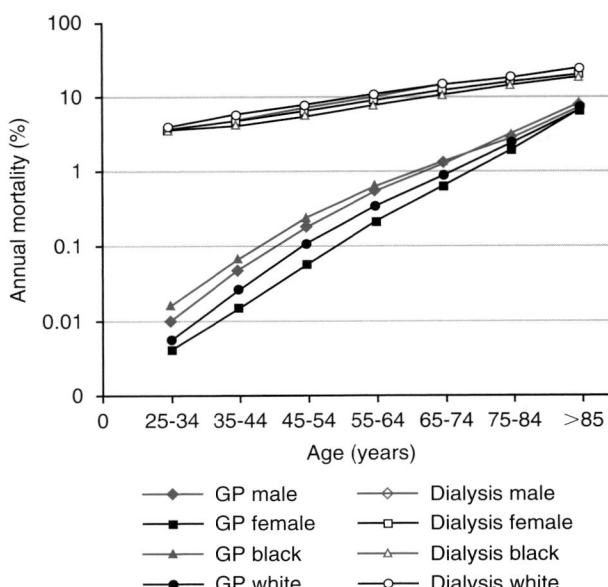

FIGURE 49.14 Cardiovascular disease mortality defined by death caused by arrhythmias, cardiomyopathy, cardiac arrest, myocardial infarction, atherosclerotic heart disease, and pulmonary edema in the general population (GP). Data from NCHS multiple cause of mortality data files compared with end-stage renal disease (ESRD) treated by dialysis. Data are stratified by age, race, and gender. (From Foley RN, Parfrey PS, Sarnak MJ. Clinical epidemiology of cardiovascular disease in chronic renal disease. *Am J Kidney Dis* 1998;32(suppl 3):S112–9, with permission from the National Kidney Foundation).

BOX 49.1   Traditional and Chronic Kidney Disease-Related Risk Factors for Cardiovascular Disease in Chronic Kidney Disease

Traditional Risk Factors for Cardiovascular Disease
Older age
Male gender
White race
Hypertension
Increased LDL cholesterol
Decreased HDL cholesterol
Smoking
Diabetes mellitus
Menopause
Sedentary lifestyle
Family history

CKD-Related Risk Factors for Cardiovascular Disease
Extracellular fluid overload
Left ventricular hypertrophy
Proteinuria
Anemia
Abnormal calcium and phosphate metabolism (vascular calcification)
Dyslipidemia
MIA syndrome
Infection
Thrombogenic factors
Oxidative stress
Increased homocysteine
Uremic toxins

LDL, Low-density lipoprotein; *HDL,* high-density lipoprotein; *MIA,* malnutrition inflammation atherosclerosis.

---

approximately 75%.[127,128] Cardiovascular mortality, defined as death caused by arrhythmias, cardiomyopathy, cardiac arrest, myocardial infarction, atherosclerotic heart disease, and pulmonary edema, has been estimated to be approximately 9% per year in dialysis patients, accounting for 50% of deaths of all patients with ESRD. Even after stratification by age, gender, race, and the presence or absence of diabetes, cardiovascular mortality in dialysis patients is 10 to 20 times higher than in the general population (Fig. 49.14).[129,130] Patients with ESRD should be considered in the highest risk group for subsequent cardiovascular events.

Risk factors for cardiovascular disease in CKD consist of a mixture of the traditional and CKD-specific factors. Traditional risk factors such as diabetes, hypertension, and dyslipidemia are more likely in CKD patients.[125] In addition, there are a number of CKD-related risk factors (Box 49.1).

Observational studies indicate that cardiovascular disease occurs at an early stage in CKD.[131] Thus among middle-aged men, increases in serum creatinine concentration (>1.5 mg/dL [>130 μmol/L]) are associated with an age-adjusted relative risk of 1.5 for coronary disease and 3.0 for stroke. Reduction of GFR is associated with increased risk of composite end points of cardiovascular death, myocardial infarction, and stroke.[132] Proteinuria has also been shown to be associated with increased risk of cardiovascular disease, cardiovascular mortality, and all-cause mortality.[133–135] These associations may arise because (1) CKD causes an increased level of cardiovascular disease, (2) cardiovascular disease causes CKD, or (3) some other factor, such as diabetes and hypertension, causes both CKD and cardiovascular disease. Significantly, there are

many more patients with category G3 than category G5 GFR (see Table 49.5). For example a longitudinal study of patients with G3/4 GFR in the United States reported an age-adjusted rate for development of ESRD of 0.67 per 100 person-years, compared to the rate for cardiovascular death of 5.25 per 100 person-years.[136]

Two large prospective randomized controlled studies reported significant reductions in cardiovascular morbidity and mortality associated with ACE inhibitor treatment among patients at high risk for future cardiovascular events.[137,138] The Prevention of Events with ACE Inhibition (PEACE) trial data revealed a higher risk of death among patients with an estimated GFR of less than 60 mL/min/1.73 m² at baseline, and a significant reduction in all-cause mortality associated with ACE inhibitor treatment in this subgroup.[139] Whereas none of the studies already mentioned specifically included patients with CKD, and all excluded patients with severe renal impairment, these data do provide support for the notion that ACE inhibitor treatment reduces cardiovascular risk in high-risk patients. Because cardiovascular disease remains the most important cause of death among CKD patients, it seems reasonable to recommend ACE inhibitor or ARB treatment for reduction of cardiovascular risk and for slowing of CKD progression. The use of ACE inhibitors must be tailored to the individual patient. Guidance in the United Kingdom is to use renin-angiotensin system antagonists in people with CKD and (1) diabetes and an ACR of 3 mg/mmol or more; (2) hypertension and an ACR of 30 mg/mmol or more; and (3) an ACR of 70 mg/mmol or more (irrespective of hypertension or cardiovascular disease).[94] There is the risk of a marked deterioration in kidney function in patients with cardiovascular disease and CKD during an acute, intercurrent illness: temporary discontinuation of ACE inhibitor/ARB treatment ("drug holidays") is recommended during such illnesses.[90] It is unclear how this message will be transferable to individual patients in practice.

Left Ventricular Hypertrophy

Among dialysis patients, the prevalence of congestive heart failure is approximately 40%. Both coronary artery disease and LVH are risk factors for the development of heart failure. In practice, it is difficult to determine whether cardiac failure reflects left ventricular dysfunction or extracellular fluid volume overload. LVH is demonstrable early in the course of CKD, with the proportion of patients with LVH increasing as kidney function declines. Univariate analysis of a single-center cohort of CKD patients in Canada revealed that age, systolic blood pressure, and hemoglobin were significantly different between the groups with or without LVH.[140] For each 5 mm Hg increase in systolic BP, the risk of LVH increased by 3%. A fall in blood hemoglobin concentration of 1 g/dL increased the risk of LVH by 6%. A large prospective multicenter study confirmed progressive increases in left ventricular mass index (LVMI) over a 12-month period, with the incidence of new LVH at 10% per year.[141] Again, lower hemoglobin concentrations and higher systolic blood pressures were associated with left ventricular growth. Anemia has both direct and indirect effects on left ventricular function and growth. Cardiac output increases because of a combination of increased cardiac preload and a reduction in afterload. Such changes lead to ventricular remodeling, with initial left ventricular dilation followed by subsequent hypertrophy. In ESRD other factors also contribute to LVH, including hypertension, volume expansion, and the metabolic consequences of uremia, to which may be added the effects of diabetes.[142]

Dyslipidemia in Chronic Kidney Disease

Various dyslipidemias are associated with CKD.[143] The pattern of dyslipidemia in CKD differs from that seen in non-CKD. It is characterized by an accumulation of partially metabolized triglyceride-rich particles (predominantly very low-density lipoprotein [VLDL] and intermediate-density lipoprotein [IDL] remnants), due mainly to abnormal lipase function. This causes hypertriglyceridemia and low high-density lipoprotein (HDL) cholesterol. Although total cholesterol concentration may be normal, there is often a highly abnormal lipid subfraction profile with a predominance of atherogenic small, dense LDL particles.[124] In a large cross-sectional analysis of 1047 hemodialysis (HD) patients in the Dialysis Morbidity and Mortality Study, only 20% of patients had low-risk lipid concentrations (i.e., LDL cholesterol <130 mg/dL [3.4 mmol/L], HDL cholesterol >40 mg/dL [1.0 mmol/L], and triglycerides <150 mg/dL [1.7 mmol/L]).[144] Low cholesterol was found to be associated with increased mortality, but this is probably a reflection of other conditions that lower cholesterol, such as inflammation and malnutrition ("reverse causality"). It is possible that other, nontraditional atherogenic lipoprotein abnormalities (e.g., lipoprotein [a] and oxidized LDL) are

present in HD patients.[145,146] Similar profiles are seen in peritoneal dialysis (PD) patients.

Lipoprotein (a) concentrations are also increased in CKD. Baseline data from the Chronic Renal Impairment in Birmingham (CRIB) study confirmed dyslipidemia in early CKD.[125] Patients had lower HDL and LDL cholesterol and higher triglyceride concentrations.

The challenge to the nephrology community is to establish whether interventions to modify the pattern of dyslipidemia with lifestyle changes and drug treatment will preserve kidney function and reduce cardiovascular morbidity and mortality. At present, no large, adequately controlled trials are testing the hypotheses that treatment of dyslipidemia preserves kidney function. There is a shortage of good trial data on which to base recommendations in CKD patients in general and more specifically among dialysis patients. The major trials of intervention with statins (3-hydroxy-3-methylglutaryl-Co-enzyme A [HMG-CoA] reductase inhibitors) in the general population and those with established cardiovascular disease have been limited with reference to CKD, because such patients have often been excluded from the trials as perceived to be at too high risk for inclusion.[147,148] The Heart Protection Study randomly allocated 20,536 adults with coronary artery disease, occlusive disease of noncoronary arteries, or diabetes to simvastatin (40 mg) or placebo.[149] In a subgroup analysis of more than 1300 patients with serum creatinine concentration between 1.2 and 2.3 mg/dL (110 and 200 µmol/L), fewer major vascular events were reported in the simvastatin group. The 4D Study investigated the use of atorvastatin in more than 1200 patients with type 2 diabetes mellitus undergoing HD and followed for a median period of 4 years. The study group concluded that atorvastatin had no statistically significant effect on the composite primary end point of cardiovascular death, nonfatal myocardial infarction, and stroke.[150] The AURORA study evaluated the use of rosuvastatin in subjects on HD and failed to demonstrate any beneficial effects of statins on cardiovascular outcomes despite markedly reduced lipid concentrations.[151] Although these studies have limitations, the most likely explanation for the lack of benefit associated with use of statins is that patients on dialysis have a different type of cardiovascular disease than individuals with earlier stages of CKD. The Study of Heart and Renal Protection (SHARP) evaluated the use of cholesterol lowering with simvastatin and ezetimibe in a broad range of more than 9000 patients with CKD, including 3000 dialysis patients. Benefit in terms of both cardiovascular risk reduction and amelioration of progression of CKD were studied. There were significant reductions in atherosclerotic end points including nonhemorrhagic stroke and arterial revascularization in the treated patients followed for a median of 4.9 years.[152]

Guidelines from the United Kingdom Renal Association[153] recommend that statins should be considered for primary prevention in all patients with CKD and GFR greater than 15 mL/min/1.73 m² and also for renal transplant patients if their 10-year risk of cardiovascular disease is calculated as greater than 20% according to the guidelines of the Joint British Societies.[154] The target total cholesterol should be less than 156 mg/dL (<4 mmol/L) or a 25% reduction from baseline, also a fasting LDL cholesterol of less than 78 mg/dL (<2 mmol/L), or a 30% reduction from baseline, should be achieved, whichever is the greatest reduction in all patients.[153] However, the

Joint British Societies risk calculations have not been validated in patients with kidney disease and lipid-lowering guidance remains controversial,[155] particularly in patients receiving dialysis. The KDIGO Lipid Working Group did not recommend specific lipid targets for patients with CKD due to safety concerns regarding the use of high-dose statins.[156] They recommend that statins, or statins with ezetimibe, be offered to adults aged greater than 50 years in the setting of GFR less than 60 mL/min/1.73 m^2 but not treated with renal replacement therapies (dialysis and transplantation).[156] With respect to patients commencing dialysis or changing RRT modality, the United Kingdom Renal Association recommends that statins should not be withdrawn from patients in whom they were previously indicated.[153]

Vascular Calcification

It has been known for many years that patients with kidney failure have vascular calcification. Serial x-ray studies and ultrasound imaging of large arteries confirm increased calcification in patients on dialysis over many years.[157] Studies have linked the presence of vascular calcification with reduced survival on dialysis.[158] Calcification of the major arteries occurs along the intimal lining of blood vessels in association with atheroma. However, in CKD, medial and adventitial calcification also occurs, reducing the compliance of the vessel. Reductions in vessel compliance can be observed by measuring pulse wave velocities along major arteries such as the aorta. The pulse wave velocity is increased in stiff (less compliant) vessels, causing the rebound pulse wave to return more quickly to the heart during the cardiac cycle. Early rebound of the pulse wave places extra strain on the heart, leading to LVH.[158] Vascular calcification has been studied in both CKD and non-CKD populations using electron beam CT imaging which acquires serial sections of the aortic arch, the coronary vessels, and the aorta. Areas of calcification can be identified and allocated a calcium score (Agatston score).[159] This approach cannot distinguish between intimal and medial calcification, but in non-CKD patients, the higher the calcium score, the more predictive it is of stenotic vascular disease.[160,161] Dialysis patients as young as 20 years exhibit vascular calcification, and calcium scores increase rapidly thereafter.[162]

Vascular calcification was previously thought to be a passive process caused by precipitation of mineral from the circulation. However, it is increasingly recognized that vascular calcification is a tightly regulated process with true bone marrow, osteo/chondrocytic cells, cytokines, matrix proteins, and matrix vesicles characteristic of mature bone-forming cells (osteoblasts) within calcified vascular lesions.[163] Mineralization-regulating proteins are deposited at sites of vascular calcification. The generation of a matrix gamma-carboxyglutamic acid (Gla) protein knockout mouse, which exhibits extensive and lethal calcification and cartilaginous metaplasia of the media of all elastic arteries, has refocused attention on the role of Gla-containing proteins in vascular calcification.[164] A number of proteins including matrix Gla protein, osteonectin, and osteoprotegerin are constitutively expressed by vascular smooth muscle cells in normal media but are downregulated in calcified arteries. In calcified plaques, vascular smooth muscle cells express osteoblast-like gene expression profiles, as demonstrated by in situ hybridization,[165] and are able to transdifferentiate into osteo/chondrocytic

cells in the arterial wall and to orchestrate bone formation and calcification in response to multiple factors such as hypertension, reactive oxygen species, advanced glycation end products (AGEs), lipids, and inflammatory proteins. Identification of natural inhibitors of calcification in plasma, such as human fetuin-A (α2-Heremans Schmid glycoprotein, AHSG) and matrix-Gla protein, suggests that the vascular endothelium may be continually subjected to calcification stresses and that regulatory systems break down in uremia. A cross-sectional study in HD patients demonstrated that AHSG concentrations were significantly lower in plasma of patients on HD than in healthy controls.[166]

The use of calcium-containing oral phosphate binders (see later) may be associated with increased risk of calcification.[162] The Treat to Goal study explored the use of a noncalcium, nonaluminum-containing phosphate binder, sevelamer hydrochloride, in 200 HD patients from Europe and North America.[167] This study demonstrated significant attenuation in the rate of calcification of vessels with sevelamer hydrochloride at 12 months. Patients were less likely to develop hypercalcemia and had lower plasma LDL cholesterol concentrations, but a tendency toward worsening acidosis was noted. Still other studies have identified a potential survival benefit for new ("incident") HD patients derived from treatment with sevelamer hydrochloride compared with calcium-based oral phosphate binders when treatment was provided for at least 18 months.[168] However, a study comparing sevelamer hydrochloride versus calcium-based binders in more than 2000 prevalent HD patients failed to show a significant difference between therapies in terms of all-cause mortality and cause-specific mortality.[169]

Disturbances in Calcium and Phosphate Metabolism

CKD is associated with complex metabolic disturbances in divalent ion and phosphate metabolism. Although this is commonly referred to as *renal osteodystrophy,* there has been a paradigm shift in terms of calcium, phosphate, and PTH management in patients receiving dialysis. The impetus for this change in approach has been recognition of the importance of the previously unheralded phosphate moiety in terms of increased risk of death in ESRD and the almost universal development of *cardiovascular calcification* (see earlier) that is seen in dialysis patients. It is likely that treatment of hyperphosphatemia in dialysis patients with calcium-based therapies may be contributing to vascular calcification; and therefore these two problems are intricately linked. In an effort to clarify the terminology of renal metabolic bone disease, KDIGO proposed that the term CKD-mineral and bone disorder (CKD-MBD) should be used to describe the syndrome of biochemical, bone, and extraskeletal calcification abnormalities that occur in patients with CKD, and that the term *renal osteodystrophy* should be used exclusively to define alterations in bone morphology, following bone biopsy, associated with CKD.[170] KDIGO published detailed international guidance on CKD-MBD in 2009 which was updated in 2017.[170,171]

As GFR declines, plasma phosphate concentration rises and ionized calcium concentration declines. The consequence of this is increased production of PTH by the parathyroid glands. PTH-producing cells are regulated tightly through complex feedback mechanisms to maintain normocalcemia (see Chapter 54). The CaSR is stimulated by calcium

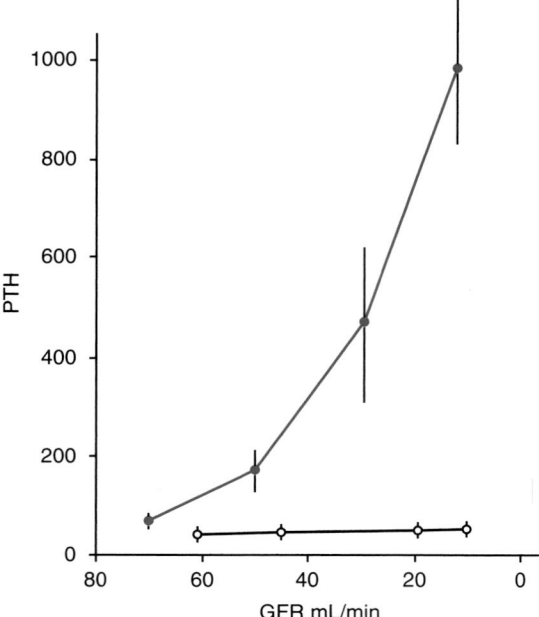

FIGURE 49.15 The relationship between parathyroid hormone (PTH) concentration and glomerular filtration rate (GFR) in two groups of dogs: those maintained on a normal phosphate diet (closed circles) and those maintained on a diet containing less than 100 mg of phosphate per day (open circles). The vertical lines represent ±1 SEM. Parathyroid hormone (PTH) is expressed in μEq/mL. (From Slatopolsky E, Caglar S, Pennell JP, Taggart DD, Canterbury JM, Reiss E, et al. On the pathogenesis of hyperparathyroidism in chronic experimental renal insufficiency in the dog. *J Clin Invest* 1971;50:492–9).

and has an inhibitory effect on PTH production.[172] In addition, phosphate has been reported to directly stimulate the production of PTH in vitro.[173] Elegant early experiments on dogs with varying levels of induced kidney failure confirmed the increase in PTH as GFR falls, with attenuation noted in animals fed a modified diet with very low levels of phosphate (Fig. 49.15).[174] FGF-23 concentrations increase markedly in CKD (between 10 and 600 times higher than the normal range) and are correlated with predialysis phosphate concentrations but not with bone mineral density.[175] Ongoing studies are evaluating the importance of FGF-23 in terms of skeletal resistance to PTH as seen in CKD patients.

In addition to hyperphosphatemia contributing to hypocalcemia, reduced 1α-hydroxylation of 25-hydroxycholecalciferol by the renal proximal tubular cells may lead to reduced production of calcitriol, the active form of vitamin D and a vitamin D receptor activator. Vitamin D is required in health to promote calcium and phosphate absorption from the gut. PTH-producing cells in the parathyroid gland have receptors for vitamin D (VDRs). The VDR is a 427 amino acid peptide that is widely found in tissues including parathyroid glands, intestine, and osteoblast-like cells. Binding of vitamin D to the VDR inhibits PTH production. The result of these complex metabolic disturbances is secondary hyperparathyroidism. Increased secretion of PTH stimulates resorption of calcium and phosphate from the major calcium reservoir, the bone. Problems can develop early, and patients with a GFR of less than 45 mL/min/1.73 m² should be evaluated for these

metabolic disturbances.[90] Secondary hyperparathyroidism classically causes bone changes consistent with osteitis fibrosa cystica. Bony erosions and intramedullary cysts are seen because of direct effects of PTH on osteoclasts and osteoblasts. Unchecked, this can lead to bone pain and fracture. Severe secondary hyperparathyroidism is associated with hyperplasia of the glands and ultimately with nodular hyperplasia. These grossly enlarged glands tend to be resistant to medical therapies of secondary hyperparathyroidism (see later), as they have significantly reduced expression of both the CaSR and VDR. Eventually, PTH secretion can become unhinged completely from feedback control; this autonomous production is called *tertiary hyperparathyroidism*. In this setting, medical treatment has failed and parathyroidectomy may be required,[170] although significant morbidity and mortality may be associated with this procedure with no improvement in fracture rate observed at 1 year postsurgery.[176]

A severe and often terminal manifestation of long-standing ESRD is calcemic uremic arteriolopathy ("*calciphylaxis*"). Calciphylaxis is characterized by calcium deposition within the arterioles of the microcirculation, leading to destruction of the vessel, and in turn causing necrosis of tissues, particularly the skin and adipose tissue on the legs and torso.[177]

Adynamic bone is characterized by low turnover and poor bone formation and is highly prevalent in CKD patients. It is commoner in older people and those with diabetes and malnutrition. Adynamic bone is associated with a low PTH concentration and abnormal calcium balance, hyperphosphatemia, and acidosis. Progression of CKD adds to the risk profile for adynamic bone because 1,25-dihydroxyvitamin D becomes markedly reduced in advanced CKD.[178] Diagnosis of adynamic bone is ultimately made on bone biopsy, but patients are reluctant to undertake this procedure. Unfortunately, PTH alone does not correlate with bone biopsy findings. However, serum bone-specific alkaline phosphatase measured using an immunoassay technique has good predictive value in separating high from low bone turnover, particularly in combination with PTH measurements.[179,180] Although adynamic bone has not proved to be associated with increased fracture risk in ESRD patients, dialysis patients with this condition are less able to incorporate calcium into bone and are at increased risk of vascular calcification.[181] Excessive use of vitamin D analogs including alfacalcidol (1α-hydroxyvitamin D3) and calcitriol is implicated in the high prevalence of adynamic bone in dialysis patients. KDIGO have advised that the use of these compounds should be largely avoided in adult patients with CKD categories 3A-5 who are not on dialysis.[171]

Bone disease in CKD is also complicated by the relatively high prevalence of hypogonadism in men on dialysis and the high prevalence of osteoporosis in postmenopausal women.

High concentrations of plasma phosphate are associated with increased mortality in HD patients.[182] In at least 50% of HD patients the serum phosphate is greater than 6.0 mg/dL (1.9 mmol/L) and in 25% of patients it is greater than 7.2 mg/dL (2.3 mmol/L). Higher corrected calcium and PTH concentrations are associated with death in HD patients. Patients with low phosphate concentrations are also at increased risk of death (relative risk of death increased by approximately 50% with phosphate <3 mg/dL) because low phosphate is associated with intercurrent illness and malnutrition. KDIGO recommend maintenance of serum phosphate within the normal range in CKD, and as close to the normal range as possible in patients receiving dialysis (Table 49.6).[171] The KDIGO update indicates a pragmatic approach to monitoring trends in CKD-MBD bone biomarker surrogates, rather than purely dictating target concentrations, representing a subtle paradigm shift in management.[171]

Strategies to reduce phosphate concentrations are employed routinely in the treatment of patients on dialysis. Inorganic phosphate within the blood accounts for less than 0.1% of total body phosphate. Clearance of phosphate on intermittent HD is approximately one third of that seen with urea and is subject to postdialysis rebound because of efflux from the intracellular to the extracellular space. Phosphate is present in many foods and is linearly associated with protein ingestion. The recommended allowance of phosphate is reduced for patients on dialysis to around 800 mg/day. Treatment with vitamin D analogs increases gut absorption of phosphate from approximately 65% to almost 85%. The use of phosphate binders, taken with meals, is almost universal in dialysis patients; treatment may include calcium-containing and non–calcium-containing binders (Table 49.7). Prescribing of phosphate binders should be individualized for each patient because each binder has pros and cons. Interest has focused on the increased propensity to vascular calcification

TABLE 49.6   The Kidney Disease: Improving Global Outcomes Target Guidelines for Plasma Calcium, Phosphate, and Parathyroid Hormone Concentrations in Chronic Kidney Disease Patients With Glomerular Filtration Rate Categories 3 to 5 Including Patients Receiving Dialysis (5D)

GFR Category	Phosphate	Calcium (Adjusted for Albumin)	Parathyroid Hormone
3–5	Laboratory reference intervals	Laboratory reference intervals	Target level unknown; however, if above upper limit of normal for the assay, assess vitamin D status and treat insufficiency and deficiency
5D	Maintain as close to laboratory reference intervals as possible	Laboratory reference intervals	Maintain within 2–9 times the upper limit of normal for the assay

GFR, Glomerular filtration rate.
Kidney Disease Improving Global Outcomes. KDIGO clinical practice guideline for the diagnosis, evaluation, prevention, and treatment of Chronic Kidney Disease-Mineral and Bone Disorder (CKD-MBD). *Kidney Int Suppl* 2009:S1–130.

TABLE 49.7   Examples of Available Oral Phosphate Binders

Phosphate Binder	Advantages	Disadvantages
Calcium carbonate	Aluminum free Moderate binding efficacy Relatively low cost Moderate tablet burden Chewable	Calcium containing—potential risk of hypercalcemia and ectopic calcification Parathyroid hormone oversuppression Gastrointestinal side effects Efficacy pH dependent
Calcium acetate	Aluminum free Higher efficacy than Calcichew/sevelamer Moderately cheap Lower calcium load than calcium carbonate Can be combined with magnesium to reduce calcium load	Calcium containing—potential risk of hypercalcemia and ectopic calcification, PTH oversuppression Gastrointestinal side effects Large tablets, nonchewable formulation
Sevelamer hydrochloride and sevelamer carbonate	Aluminum and calcium free No gastrointestinal absorption Moderate efficacy Reduces total and low-density lipoprotein cholesterol Powder for mixing with water available	Relatively costly High pill burden Large tablets Gastrointestinal side effects Binds fat-soluble vitamins
Lanthanum carbonate	Aluminum and calcium free Minimal gastrointestinal absorption High efficacy across full pH range Chewable formulation Low tablet burden Powder available to disperse on meal	Relatively costly Gastrointestinal side effects
Sucroferric oxyhydroxide	Calcium and aluminum-free Iron-based Low tablet burden Chewable tablet	High-cost drug Occasional diarrhea Feces discolored black on initiation of treatment

PTH, Parathyroid hormone.

noted in those dialysis patients receiving calcium-containing phosphate binders. These binders reduce phosphate absorption to 30 to 40% and decrease serum phosphate concentrations. However, a systematic review of randomized controlled trials concluded that no evidence suggests that phosphate binders reduce all-cause or cardiovascular mortality compared with placebo.[183] An updated meta-analysis comparing calcium-based with non–calcium based oral phosphate binders in patients with CKD, the majority of whom were receiving HD, concluded that there was a 22% risk reduction for all-cause mortality in those patients assigned a non–calcium containing binder.[184] This suggests that high exposure to calcium–containing phosphate binders is detrimental, contributing to a positive calcium balance, and reflecting physicians' historical practice of trying to compensate for the reduced production of activated vitamin D in these patients. There has been debate in the nephrology community since the late 1990s regarding the preferred oral phosphate binder to use to try to control serum phosphate concentrations in dialysis patients. In essence, the calcium-containing binders are well established and cheap, compared to the relatively novel non-calcium containing oral phosphate binders. The anticipated benefit in terms of cardiovascular protection by moving away from calcium-containing binders has not been realized. An observational study utilizing USRDS and Medicare claims data for example, showed no benefit for sevelamer carbonate compared to calcium acetate in older patients requiring HD.[185] Patients on conventional thrice weekly dialysis are in a net positive phosphate balance. Control of hyperphosphatemia can be regained following a kidney transplant. However, what more can be achieved in those patients maintained on HD? The Frequent Hemodialysis Network (FHN) Trial describes resolution of hyperphosphatemia in patients receiving six times per week HD.[186] In summary, while guidelines and target ranges relating to phosphate management exist, there is no definitive evidence that good phosphate control improves the length or quality of life of dialysis patients.[187]

Medical treatment strategies are designed to limit phosphate intake and normalize calcium. With the advent of vitamin D analogs it has been possible to supplement vitamin D, resulting in increased plasma calcium concentrations and switching off of PTH production. Unfortunately the commonly used analogs, such as 1α-hydroxyvitamin D3, also lead to increased absorption of calcium and phosphate from the gut. In the setting of aggressive treatment with vitamin D analogs, hypercalcemia may develop that is associated with low, suppressed concentrations of PTH. Alternative vitamin D receptor activators, such as paricalcitol, are associated with improved survival in United States dialysis patients and have a lower incidence of treatment-related hyperphosphatemia and hypercalcemia than calcitriol.[188,189] More information is needed on the use of "substrate" vitamin D supplementation in CKD and the results of the SIMPLIFIED trial (ISRCTN15087616) in the United Kingdom are awaited.

A further development in the management of CKD-MBD has been the generation of calcimimetic agents such as cinacalcet.[190,191] Calcimimetics can mimic calcium by directly stimulating the CaSR and can affect the molecular configuration of the CaSR to enhance its sensitivity to extracellular calcium.[191] Stimulation of the CaSR switches off

PTH production selectively with no risk of increased phosphate absorption. Use of cinacalcet has increased the proportion of patients who reach the biochemical management targets for CKD-MBD[192] and has reduced the need for parathyroidectomy in patients with secondary hyperparathyroidism[193]; a reduction in fracture rate has also been observed.[194] However, a major prospective randomized controlled trial (Evaluation of Cinacalcet HCL Therapy to Lower CardioVascular Events [EVOLVE]) in HD patients with moderate to severe secondary hyperparathyroidism did not demonstrate significant cardiovascular event or mortality reduction.[192]

Aluminum Toxicity

A causative factor for renal bone disease, historically, has been aluminum intoxication. Aluminum concentrations in dialysis fluids were previously high, but with modern dialysis facilities, this is no longer such a problem. Although aluminum accumulation, associated with the use of aluminum containing oral phosphate binders, is characterized by deposition along the mineralization surface of the osteoid and a low-turnover form of bone disease, this is likely to be of historical interest only since aluminum-based oral phosphate binders are no longer in manufacture.

Anemia

The World Health Organization (WHO) defines anemia, when the patient is at sea level, as a blood hemoglobin concentration of less than 13 g/dL (130 g/L) in adult men and less than 12 g/dL (120 g/L) in adult, nonpregnant women.[195] It is clearly established that anemia is inevitable as CKD progresses. Therapies are available to correct anemia; therefore it is mandatory that a patient with CKD should be assessed for anemia. The KDIGO 2012 Clinical Practice Guideline for the Evaluation and Management of CKD recommends that an estimated GFR of less than 60 mL/min/1.73 m^2 should be the cutoff value for determining the presence or absence of anemia and that, additionally, CKD should be considered as a possible cause of anemia when the GFR is less than 60 mL/min/1.73 m^2.[90] It is more likely to be the cause if the GFR is less than 30 mL/min/1.73 m^2 (<45 mL/min/1.73 m^2 in patients with diabetes) and no other cause (e.g., blood loss, folic acid or vitamin B$_{12}$ deficiency) is identified. The prevalence of anemia increases as GFR declines. In the NHANES III dataset the prevalence of anemia (defined as Hb less than 12 g/dL in men, Hb less than 11 g/dL in women) was 33% at a GFR of 15 mL/min/1.73 m^2 and 9% at a GFR of 30 mL/min/1.73 m^2.[52] CKD-related anemia occurs earlier in patients with diabetes and is highly prevalent among such patients.[196] In the United Kingdom the median hemoglobin of patients starting dialysis during 2016 was 9.9 g/dL.[103]

Detection is important because if left untreated, anemia causes many of the side effects of CKD, such as fatigue, breathlessness on exertion, intolerance to cold, and decreased exercise capacity. As indicated earlier, it is also a major factor in the high prevalence of cardiovascular disease in patients with CKD and contributes to the development of LVH. In patients on dialysis, large observational studies have clearly shown that anemia is associated with increased mortality rates and increased hospitalization.[197–200] In HD patients, hematocrit levels of 33 to 36% (corresponding to hemoglobin concentrations of 11 to 12 g/dL) were associated with the lowest risk for all-cause and cardiac mortality[199]; these patients also had the lowest risk of hospitalization.[200,201]

Etiology of anemia in chronic kidney disease . The etiology of anemia in CKD is multifactorial. A major cause, however, is the loss of peritubular fibroblasts within the renal cortex that synthesize EPO. Failure of EPO production in the kidney leads to inappropriately low concentrations within the blood for the concomitant hemoglobin concentration. Other causes of anemia include absolute or functional iron deficiency, folic acid and vitamin B_{12} deficiencies, infections, and chronic inflammation. Hepcidin, the main hormone responsible for iron metabolism, produced by the liver, and discovered in 2000, is upregulated in CKD, causing a reduction in the availability of iron for use in erythropoiesis.[202] Red cell survival may also be reduced. Hemodialysis patients tend to have more severe anemia than PD patients because of greater blood losses and hemolysis.

Several national and international organizations have published algorithms for the treatment of anemia in CKD and dialysis patients.[203–206] Concerns regarding the safety of treatment designed to *correct* anemia in CKD led to revision of guidelines, such that zealous attention to correction using the highest doses of erythropoiesis stimulating agents (ESAs) is avoided. The KDIGO recommendations include not intentionally increasing the hemoglobin above 11.5 g/dL.[203] The NICE guideline recommends that treatment should aim to maintain hemoglobin between 10.0 and 12.0 g/dL in adults.[204] Mainstays of treatment are iron supplementation and the use of ESAs. Warnings, indications, precautions, and instructions for dosing and administration of ESAs are available from national regulatory agencies, including the US Food and Drug Administration (FDA), and from product package inserts.

Assessment of iron and iron supplementation. Iron status is assessed by measurement of serum ferritin and transferrin saturation. Transferrin saturation gives an indication of iron "delivery." Ferritin is used to represent iron stores. In patients with CKD, a serum ferritin concentration less than 100 μg/L is considered to suggest iron deficiency, and a serum ferritin of 100 to 200 μg/L in association with transferrin saturation less than 20% represents "functional" iron deficiency. Treatment of anemia in CKD requires adequate iron stores. A very high concentration of ferritin (>800 μg/L) may suggest iron overload. However, these indices have limitations (e.g., a high ferritin concentration is also generated by an inflammatory process; transferrin varies with nutritional state and is also influenced by inflammation; high biological variation[207]). Clinical hematology laboratories may offer an automated estimate of the percentage of hypochromic red blood cells. A level above 10% is indicative of functional iron deficiency and the target is less than 2.5%.[205]

Iron deficiency (absolute or functional) was the main cause of ESA resistance in the United Kingdom, but this has been solved by iron replacement strategies. In HD patient populations, the inverse relationship between ESA dose and iron stores continues to maintain a linear relationship up to a mean ferritin of 500 μg/L. Parenteral iron is the treatment of choice for absolute and functional iron deficiency in HD patients because oral iron has low efficacy in CKD. Parenteral iron can easily be administered during dialysis in patients receiving HD. Hemodialysis patients have additional iron losses from gastrointestinal bleeding, blood tests, and losses in dialysis lines that result in iron supplementation requirements that outstrip the capacity of the gut to absorb iron. Maintenance intravenous iron in HD patients greatly reduces ESA requirements and costs.[208] High-dose iron sucrose administered proactively (400 mg monthly, unless serum ferritin concentration is greater than 700 μg/L or the transferrin saturation greater than or equal to 40%) has been shown to be superior to low-dose reactive iron dosing in a large open-label randomized controlled trial (PIVOTAL).[209] The outcome of the PIVOTAL trial has led to a change in anemia management guidance for HD patients.[210]

In non–dialysis-treated CKD, a randomized study of intravenous iron versus oral iron in predialysis patients demonstrated a greater improvement in hemoglobin outcome in those on intravenous iron but no difference in the proportion of patients who had to commence ESA after the start of the study.[211] Nevertheless, oral iron is easy and cheap to prescribe and can be used as first-line iron supplementation in nondialysis patients. It is appropriate to treat patients who have not responded to, or have been intolerant of, oral iron with intravenous iron every 6 to 8 weeks to maintain serum ferritin greater than 100 μg/L.

Use of erythropoiesis-stimulating agents. ESAs are human recombinant erythropoietin (rhEPO or epoetin), that is, synthetic versions of human EPO that are used to treat anemia. Following replenished iron stores and exclusion of other causes of anemia, the addition of ESAs is indicated for the treatment of CKD-related anemia. Measurement of serum EPO concentration is rarely indicated in the setting of renal anemia. The gene for human EPO was cloned in 1985, and epoetin was introduced into clinical practice shortly afterward.[212,213] ESAs are effective in correcting the anemia of CKD in 90 to 95% of patients. The most common side effect is hypertension; therefore blood pressure should be well controlled before treatment is introduced. Hypertension may develop or worsen in a quarter of patients. Failure to respond to treatment requires thorough investigation for many potential causes (Box 49.2). It is estimated that 3 million patients worldwide have received treatment with ESAs. A rare complication of ESA treatment is the generation of neutralizing antibodies to the ESA. These antibodies stop bone marrow erythroid cells from producing mature red blood cells, so-called pure red cell aplasia.[214] If a case of pure red cell aplasia is proven, then no additional recombinant ESAs are administered.

Many clinical benefits are derived from correcting anemia with ESAs, including (1) improved exercise capacity,[215]

BOX 49.2 **Causes of Failure to Respond to Erythropoiesis Stimulating Agents**	
Iron status	Patient adherence
Occult blood loss	Hypothyroidism
Vitamin B_{12} or folate deficiency	Primary disease activity
Infection and inflammation	Transplant rejection
Inadequate dialysis	Malignancy
Hyperparathyroidism	Pure red cell aplasia
Aluminum toxicity	Hepcidin upregulation

(2) improved cognitive function,[216] (3) better quality of life,[217,218] and (4) increased libido. Much of the evidence has been taken from studies in dialysis patients. In patients with advanced CKD not yet on dialysis, small nonrandomized studies have suggested that regression of LVH is possible with partial correction of anemia with epoetin.[219,220] Patients who receive an ESA consistently over the 2 years before commencement of dialysis may have improved survival,[221] although larger prospective randomized trials have not confirmed these observations. Two important studies focused on patients not yet on dialysis. The Correction of Hemoglobin and Outcomes in Renal Insufficiency (CHOIR) study showed no benefit of higher hemoglobin outcome (13.5 g/dL versus 11.3 g/dL) in CKD patients. Higher outcome target hemoglobin concentrations showed increased risk (using composite end points of death, myocardial infarction, and hospitalization for congestive cardiac failure) and no incremental improvement in quality of life.[222] The Cardiovascular Risk Reduction in Early Anaemia Treatment with Epoetin Beta (CREATE) study reported early correction of anemia to normal hemoglobin outcome (13.0 to 15.0 g/dL versus 10.5 to 11.5 g/dL) but did not reduce the risk of cardiovascular events in patients followed for 3 years.[223] Indeed the hazard ratio for primary end points of death from any cause or death from cardiovascular disease consistently (but not significantly) favored the lower hemoglobin target group. LVH remained stable in both groups, and quality of life was significantly better in the higher hemoglobin outcome group.

A large randomized controlled trial has tested the hypothesis that normalization of anemia would have benefits in terms of morbidity and mortality for HD patients with New York Heart Association (NYHA) heart failure stage I to III.[224] Patients were randomized to normalization of anemia (618 patients and target hemoglobin concentration of 14 g/dL) or to the control group (615 patients and target hemoglobin concentration of 10 g/dL). The study was terminated early because of a nonsignificant higher risk of death in the normalization group (relative risk 1.3, confidence interval [CI] 0.9 to 1.9). These studies have been instructive in setting the current hemoglobin target of 10.0 to 12.0 g/dL and in recommending ESA dose adjustments when hemoglobin is less than 10.5 or greater than 11.5 g/dL to balance benefit versus safety to patients. It is not recommended to begin treatment with an ESA in the setting of active malignancy or active stroke. Nondialysis CKD patients with a hemoglobin greater than 10 g/dL should not be commenced on an ESA.[203] In dialysis patients KDIGO recommend avoiding hemoglobin falling below 9 g/dL, and that the maintenance level in most patients should be below full correction. The United Kingdom Renal Registry reports that 59% of HD patients have a reported hemoglobin between the acceptable range of 10 to 12 g/dL.[103] Safety concerns outlined above have led to investigation of novel therapeutic approaches in anemia management. These new agents act by inhibiting enzymes (proly-4-hydroxylase domain enzymes) that degrade hypoxia inducible factors (HIFs), a family of oxygen-sensitive proteins that regulate the cellular response to hypoxia.[202] These orally active small molecules stimulate the body's response to hypoxia without any change to the partial pressure of oxygen in the blood or tissues. HIFs can be considered as "hypoxia mimetic agents" and several have been evaluated in phase III clinical trials. Indeed, Roxadustat (FG4592), for example, is currently licensed for treatment of anemia in CKD patients in China.[225] These novel drugs are not represented in national/international management guidelines at time of writing.

The Uremic Syndrome

Uremia is defined as the excess within the blood of urea, creatinine, and other nitrogenous end products of amino acid and protein metabolism that are normally excreted in the urine. The *uremic syndrome,* the terminal clinical manifestation of kidney failure, is the group of symptoms, physical signs, and abnormal findings on diagnostic studies that result from failure of the kidneys to maintain adequate excretory, regulatory, and endocrine function.

Classic signs of uremia include progressive weakness and easy fatigue, loss of appetite followed by nausea and vomiting, muscle wasting, tremors, abnormal mental function, frequent but shallow respirations, and metabolic acidosis. In patients with kidney failure (GFR <15 mL/min/1.73 m^2), signs and symptoms of uremia, or the need for RRT are generally present. The syndrome evolves to produce stupor, coma, and ultimately death unless RRT is provided. Regulation of body fluids is impaired in patients with uremia because of failure to excrete excess ingested fluid or to cope with fluid losses caused by vomiting or diarrhea. Patients also have difficulty excreting a salt load or retaining sodium when intake is low or vascular volume inadequate. Acid excretion is impaired, as is the ability to excrete nitrogenous metabolites from dietary sources. In addition to the consequences of reduced excretory, regulatory, and endocrine function of the kidneys, the uremic syndrome has several systemic manifestations, among them pericarditis, pleuritis, disordered platelet and granulocyte function, and encephalopathy that have been difficult to explain.

For longer than 200 years, scientists have been studying the nature of uremia, but no single retained molecule has yet qualified for the title "uremic toxin"; a variety of compounds are potential uremic toxins (Table 49.8). Approaching 100 organic compounds are known to be retained in uremia[226-228] and there is increasing evidence that some are not just markers of uremia but directly contribute to disease progression.[229] Many more still unidentified solutes are possibly retained and might exert systemic toxicity. Although urea was the first metabolite to be identified as increased in uremia, this does not appear to be responsible for the systemic manifestations of uremia. Urea is a 60-Da water-soluble compound that has the highest concentrations of presently known uremic retention solutes in uremic plasma. Although its removal by dialysis is directly related to patient survival, the effects of urea on biological systems are not clear. Urea removal by dialysis is not necessarily representative of other molecules retained in the uremic syndrome, particularly protein-bound solutes such as *p*-cresol, or higher molecular weight molecules such as PTH. Urea may be the source of other, more toxic moieties.[230] However, it is more likely that the syndrome is a result of the cumulative effect of many retained compounds, which may act as toxins and may have an effect on metabolism in general, for example, through enzyme inhibition or derangement in membrane transport. The decreased ability of the kidneys to degrade or eliminate hormones may also have a role.

TABLE 49.8 Potential Uremic Toxins

Toxin	Effect
Urea	At very high concentrations (>300 mg/dL [>50 mmol/L]) can cause headache, vomiting, and fatigue, carbamylation of proteins
Creatinine	Possibly affects glucose tolerance and erythrocyte survival
Cyanate	Causes drowsiness, hyperglycemia; a breakdown product of urea, it can cause carbamylation of proteins, altering protein function
Polyols (e.g., myoinositol)	Can cause peripheral neuropathy
Phenols	Can be highly toxic as they are lipid soluble and therefore can cross cell membranes easily
Middle molecules (e.g., atrial natriuretic peptide, cystatin C, delta sleep-inducing protein, IL-6, TNF-α, PTH)	Peritoneal dialysis patients clear middle molecules more efficiently than HD patients and show fewer signs of neuropathy than hemodialysis patients (many candidate molecules but none paramount)
β2-microglobulin	Causative agent in renal amyloid

HD, Hemodialysis; *IL-6,* interleukin 6; *TNF-α,* tumor necrosis factor alpha; *PTH,* parathyroid hormone.

Acute Kidney Injury

AKI has largely replaced the older term ARF and describes a sudden decline in kidney function over hours and days. AKI is an increasingly common and potentially catastrophic complication of systemic illness. Identifying the true incidence and prevalence of AKI has been difficult because of wide variation in the accepted definition of AKI. Several studies have reported multicenter experience with AKI in the intensive care unit (ICU) setting and note wide variation in practice and outcomes.[231,232]

In 2003, a new classification of AKI was proposed that was based on the combination of susceptibility, nature and timing of insult, biomarker response, urine output, and end-organ consequences.[233] In recognition of the potential clinical importance of small changes in kidney function and the need to standardize definitions of AKI for clinical and research purposes the RIFLE criteria were adopted by the Acute Dialysis Quality Initiative (ADQI), providing a graded definition of AKI severity.[234] The acronym RIFLE defines three grades of increasing severity of AKI (risk, injury, and failure) and two outcome variables (loss and ESRD). The grades of severity are established on the basis of change in serum creatinine concentration and decline in urine output from baseline. The most powerful tool to improve outcome in AKI is prevention and the advantage of the RIFLE criteria is the definition of "risk," where it is envisaged that intervention may prevent injury and failure. More recently the Acute Kidney Injury Network (AKIN) proposed three stages of increasing disease severity (Table 49.9).[235] This working group has modified the RIFLE criteria slightly to incorporate smaller changes in

TABLE 49.9 The Acute Kidney Injury Network Criteria for Acute Kidney Injury

AKIN Stage[a]	Serum Creatinine Criteria	Urine Output Criteria
1	↑ ≥0.3 mg/dL (≥26 μmol/L) or ↑ ≥150–200% from baseline	<0.5 mL/kg/h for >6 h
2	↑ >200–300% from baseline	<0.5 mL/kg/h for >12 h
3	↑ >300% (>3 fold) from baseline or ≥4 mg/dL (≥354 μmol/L) with an acute rise of ≥0.5 mg/dL (≥44 μmol/L) in ≤24 h or Initiation of renal replacement therapy (irrespective of stage at time of initiation)	<0.3 mL/kg/h for >24 h or Anuria for 12 h

[a]Only one criterion needs to be fulfilled to qualify for a stage.

serum creatinine concentration into the definition of risk, because it was appreciated that small changes in kidney function can affect outcome. In essence, the AKIN has provided the following diagnostic criteria for AKI: an abrupt (within 48 hours) reduction in kidney function currently defined as an increase in serum creatinine concentration of either 0.3 mg/dL (26 μmol/L) or greater; an increase of 50% or greater (1.5-fold from baseline); or a reduction in urine output (documented oliguria <0.5 mL/kg/h for >6 hours). The use of serum creatinine measurements to identify AKI is discussed in Chapter 34.

A prospective study of the initial hospital management of AKI confirmed that in almost 40% of cases AKI was iatrogenic or preventable.[236] In addition, a report by the National Confidential Enquiry into Patient Outcome and Death (NCEPOD: Adding Insult to Injury) published in 2009[237] found that opportunities were missed in the treatment of hospitalized patients that should have been rectified earlier and deaths of people with AKI were easily preventable. The report has driven the focus of care onto AKI risk, identification, treatment, and referral for specialist services, recently summarized in guidance from NICE.[238] Early identification of intravascular volume depletion, cessation of nephrotoxic drugs, and early diagnosis of causative conditions can prevent AKI. Therefore prompt administration of intravenous crystalloid solutions such as 0.9% sodium chloride and balanced salt solutions may prevent further deterioration of AKI in many cases. Patients at risk for AKI include older persons; those with preexisting CKD, sepsis, diabetes, and heart disease; and those taking nephrotoxic drugs, particularly in the setting of hypovolemia. Fluid replacement requirements need careful monitoring and review of the patient, with emphasis on restoring an optimal circulatory volume without developing signs of fluid overload such as pulmonary edema. Additional monitoring may include use of a central venous pressure (CVP) line. Insertion of a CVP line is a specialist skill that requires cannulation of the internal jugular vein, ideally utilizing ultrasonic guidance facilities. However, where hypovolemia is clinically apparent, the priority is to resuscitate the patient with fluid, rather than delay treatment, by establishing invasive monitoring. Severe AKI requiring RRT was particularly prevalent in hospitalized patients infected with severe acute respiratory coronavirus 2 (SARS-CoV-2) during the 2020 pandemic and carried a poor prognosis.[239] Although the precise etiology is not established, the importance of fluid management cannot be overstated.[240]

Clinical assessment of AKI should consider whether the precipitant is prerenal, intrarenal (intrinsic), or postrenal. Most commonly AKI is caused by ischemia, which initiates a complex sequence of hemodynamic changes, endothelial injury, epithelial cell injury, and immunologic mechanisms which underpin its initiation and extension.[241] Intrinsic AKI can be caused by primary vascular, glomerular, or interstitial disorders. It is therefore important that all patients presenting with AKI undergo urinalysis to test for infection, hematuria, and proteinuria. In most cases the kidney lesion seen on histology is referred to as acute tubular necrosis (ATN). ATN is caused by ischemic or nephrotoxic injury to the kidney. In 50% of cases of hospital-acquired AKI, the cause is multifactorial. (The term ATN is somewhat misleading, insofar as necrosis per se is seldom seen, rather tubular *damage* occurs.) Although the pathogenesis is uncertain, a well-recognized clinical pattern is associated with the development of ATN, with anuria or oliguria and abnormalities indicating tubular dysfunction (Fig. 49.16).[242] Necrosis of tubular cells need not be extensive, but obstruction by tubular casts, backleak of glomerular filtrate through gaps in the tubular epithelium caused by cellular denudation, and primary reductions in GFR caused by altered intrarenal hemodynamics, known as tubuloglomerular feedback may occur.[243] Direct vasoconstriction of glomerular capillaries in response to ischemic insults can also occur and may be mediated by AII, endothelin,[244,245] and serotonin.[246]

Laboratory tests and imaging are crucial in the management of AKI. Tests assist in establishing the underlying diagnosis and excluding obstruction as a cause. Specific investigations are requested if kidney function has not improved following volume correction (Table 49.10). Kidney biopsy is generally reserved for cases of AKI where an ultrasound scan has excluded obstructed kidneys, kidney sizes are maintained, the cause of AKI is otherwise unexplained, and an intrinsic pathology is suspected. Urinary electrolyte measurements are often undertaken in the investigation of AKI. However, in practice, since the treatment of prerenal AKI and ATN requires prompt and continued correction of hypovolemia, the urinary findings are generally unhelpful.

Metabolic acidosis is the most common acid-base disorder in patients with AKI. Reduced renal excretion of potassium and the effects of acidosis on the generation of extracellular potassium may lead to a very high plasma potassium concentration. Severe hyperkalemia (plasma potassium concentration >6.5 mmol/L) is associated with life-threatening cardiac arrhythmias. Emergency treatment of hyperkalemia should be instituted as necessary. Patients who have an abnormal electrocardiogram in the setting of high plasma potassium concentration, or a potassium concentration of 6.5 mmol/L or greater, should receive 10% calcium gluconate intravenously over 2 to 3 minutes through a large-bore peripheral venous cannula or a central line. This treatment stabilizes myocardial cells. However, calcium gluconate will not lower the potassium concentration. Infusion of high concentrations of glucose stimulates insulin secretion from the pancreas and uptake of potassium into the intracellular space. A fall in potassium concentration should be expected within 60 minutes. In addition, low-dose rapid-acting insulin can be administered with the glucose bolus. Blood potassium concentration should be monitored hourly until risk of a life-threatening cardiac event has passed and no evidence of potassium rebound is found. Blood glucose concentration should be monitored because hypoglycemia may occur following exogenous insulin. Again, care should be taken with 50% glucose infusions that good venous access is established, because extravasation can cause severe tissue necrosis. Cation exchange resins, such as sodium polystyrene sulfonate (SPS [Kayexalate, Covis Pharmaceuticals, Cary, NC]) in the United States and calcium polystyrene sulfonate (calcium resonium) in the United Kingdom, have been used for treatment of hyperkalemia for many decades. They are pH dependent and effective at binding potassium in the large bowel and rectum, and need to be given with laxatives, typically sorbitol in the United States.[247] There have been reports of serious

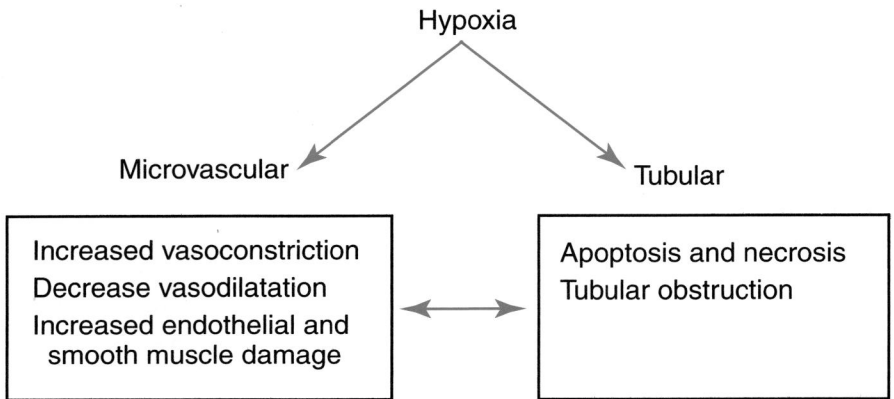

FIGURE 49.16 Pathogenesis of ischemic acute kidney injury, response to hypoxia.

TABLE 49.10   Investigation of Acute Kidney Injury

Test	Indication/Comments
Urine Testing	
Urine reagent strip ("dipstick")	Hematuria and proteinuria may indicate glomerular origin
Red cell casts on microscopy	(not available universally: may need bed-side microscope)
Urine microscopy and culture	Identify urinary tract infection
Urine protein electrophoresis and immunofixation	
Blood Tests	
Baseline Studies	
Urea, electrolytes and creatinine	Check previous laboratory reports: AKI or AKI with preexisting CKD
Calcium, phosphate, albumin	
Liver function tests	Suspected multiorgan involvement or abnormal coagulation
Acid-base studies	Arterial blood gas or venous plasma bicarbonate concentration
Full blood count	Anemia, hemolysis, thrombocytopenia
Coagulation studies	Evidence of intravascular coagulation; need to normalize if considering kidney biopsy and central line insertion
Selected Additional Investigations	
Blood culture	Any infection but especially endocarditis, severe pneumonia or urinary tract sepsis
Creatine kinase	Very high in cases of muscle inflammation and necrosis (rhabdomyolysis)
Lactate dehydrogenase	If high suspect renal infarction and consider hemolysis
Antineutrophil cytoplasmic antibodies	Vasculitides
Antiglomerular basement membrane antibody	Antiglomerular basement membrane disease
Antinuclear antibodies	SLE
Anti-dsDNA antibodies, extractable nuclear antigens	SLE
Low C3 complement	SLE, MPGN, C3 glomerulopathies
Low C4 complement	Systemic lupus erythematosus, atheroembolism, cryoglobulinemia, MPGN (immune complex positive)
Cryoglobulin	Cryoglobulinemia
Urate	Urate nephropathy
Serum protein electrophoresis	Myeloma
Virology studies	Hepatitis serology, human immunodeficiency virus
Other serology	Antistreptolysin O titer
Imaging	
Chest X-ray	Pulmonary edema, pneumonia, effusions, malignancy and granulomas
Abdominal X-ray (kidney, ureter and bladder)	Renal stones
Renal tract ultrasound scan	Identify size and symmetry of kidneys
	Evidence of an obstructed system
	Small shrunken kidneys in advanced CKD
Computed tomography scan	Anatomy and perfusion
Magnetic resonance imaging	Angiography to identify renovascular lesions
Formal angiography	Critical renal artery stenosis
Kidney Biopsy	
	Reserved for patients with unexplained AKI in whom acute tubular necrosis is not suspected. It is anticipated that additional therapy such as steroids, cytotoxic drugs and plasma exchange may be required.

CKD, Chronic kidney disease; *dsDNA,* double-stranded DNA; *MPGN,* membranoproliferative glomerulonephritis; *SLE,* systemic lupus erythematosus.

gastrointestinal complications from SPS particularly colonic necrosis. Patiromer is a synthetic polymer and is able to bind potassium in the colon and is licensed for treatment of hyperkalemia.[248] A further compound, sodium zirconium cyclosilicate (ZS-9), has also been introduced in the United Kingdom and is an effective treatment for acute hyperkalemia.[249] ZS-9 is a crystal, rather than a polymer, that is highly selective for potassium and ammonium ions, and is able to bind potassium throughout the gastrointestinal tract.[247] It is envisaged that these medications will be utilized in chronic hyperkalemia management among patients with comorbid cardiac failure requiring ongoing treatment with medications that typically increase serum potassium concentrations, including RAAS blockers and mineralocorticoid antagonists.[248,249]

When hyperkalemia persists despite appropriate medical measures, then RRT should be considered. Options for RRT include intermittent HD, PD, and continuous renal replacement therapies (hemofiltration [HF] and hemodiafiltration [HDF]) (see later). The continuous modalities are particularly appropriate for the ICU setting in cases of multiple-organ failure. Continuous therapies are useful in the treatment of septic shock, cardiac failure, pancreatitis, and acute respiratory distress syndrome. They also allow the use of supplementary feeding, which is important in the oliguric patient with established AKI, in whom fluid is restricted to avoid overload.

If the patient survives, recovery usually will occur within days or weeks following removal of the initiating event and requires ongoing careful monitoring. There is an initial polyuric phase, as glomerular function recovers before tubular function. This polyuric phase recedes after a few days to weeks. Uncomplicated AKI has a mortality rate of 5 to 10%,[250] although AKI complicating nonrenal organ system failure in the ICU setting is associated with mortality rates approaching 50 to 70%, despite advances in dialysis treatment.[233]

Serum creatinine is the most widely used parameter for everyday assessment of GFR, but it has poor sensitivity and specificity in AKI because it lags behind both kidney injury and recovery. Several urinary and serum biomarkers of early tubular injury are being studied to assess whether injury can be detected before GFR is decreased. These include urinary kidney injury molecule-1 (KIM-1), plasma and urinary neutrophil gelatinase-associated lipocalin (NGAL), and the product of tissue inhibitor of metalloproteinases-2 (TIMP-2) and insulin-like growth factor binding protein 7 (IGFBP7) (see Chapter 34).

Contrast-induced Acute Kidney Injury

Many procedures and tests that are undertaken within the hospital environment may contribute to the burden of AKI. In particular, intravascular administration of radiocontrast media during enhanced CT scanning and angiographic procedures has typically been reported as a cause of hospital-acquired AKI,[250] and preventative strategies are recommended for those at risk: in patients with diabetes mellitus, preexisting CKD, particularly in those with GFR of less than 40 mL/min/1.73 m^2, and in those who are dehydrated.[238]

Radiocontrast media are iodinated and may be ionic or nonionic. At concentrations required for angiography or CT scanning, the various agents used have differing osmolality. First-generation agents were ionic monomers with a very high osmolality with respect to plasma (e.g., 1500 to 1800 mOsmol/kg). Second-generation agents, such as iohexol are nonionic monomers with a lower osmolality, although still higher than that of plasma (e.g., 600 to 850 mOsmol/kg). An iso-osmolal agent, iodixanol, is also available (osmolality 290 mOsmol/kg). The use of low and iso-osmolar agents is associated with a lower incidence of adverse events, including AKI, compared to the older high osmolar compounds.[251,252] Nevertheless efforts to prevent AKI should be considered before a radiocontrast load is administered, regardless of the

agent used. If possible, alternative investigations should be performed. However, when radiocontrast is required, the patient should be adequately hydrated (intravascular volume expansion) to try to prevent AKI.[238] Typically this can be achieved by encouraging increased oral fluid. However, intravenous crystalloid solutions such as 0.9% sodium chloride, isotonic sodium bicarbonate, or balanced salt solutions should be considered in particularly high-risk groups. In the inpatient setting these include: patients with GFR below 30 mL/min/1.73 m^2; patients with a kidney transplant; when a large volume of contrast medium is being used; and if intra-arterial administration of contrast medium with "first-pass exposure" is being used.[238] Despite national guidance, a recent bench-marking exercise in the United Kingdom found that the majority of providers do not adopt intravenous volume expansion protocols for patients with severe CKD or kidney failure undergoing venography and fistulography (Delaney M, personal communication, available at: https://ukkw.wpengine.com/wp-content/uploads/2019/08/P007.pdf, accessed October 10, 2020). There is a dearth of advice relating to managing outpatients who fall into these categories. This is either based on an assumption that high-risk patients are admitted to hospital, or that guidance cannot be offered in an evidence-free arena. For example, major randomized trials, including the AMACING trial, did not include patients with an estimated GFR below 30 mL/min/1.73 m^2.[253] Although generally accepted, it should be noted that there has been a rebuttal of the dogma of iodinated contrast as an independent risk factor for AKI following CT scanning.[254] In this meta-analysis, conducted in the United States, risk of AKI, need for RRT, and mortality in patients following a CT scan did not differ between those who did and did not receive a contrast agent.

Gadolinium-based contrast agents are used in enhanced magnetic resonance scanning. These agents are typically non-nephrotoxic but can rarely be associated with a serious side effect, nephrogenic systemic fibrosis, in patients with advanced kidney disease including dialysis patients. Where there is no reasonable alternative to contrast-enhanced MRI then the lowest dose of the lowest-risk compounds can be administered even to those patients with advanced CKD.[251]

DISEASES OF THE KIDNEY

Diabetic Nephropathy

Diabetes mellitus is a state of chronic hyperglycemia sufficient to cause long-term damage to specific tissues, notably the kidney, retina, nerves, and arteries (see Chapter 47). Type 1 diabetes is due to autoimmune destruction of pancreatic islet β-cells, causing loss of insulin secretion. Type 2 diabetes is due to the combination of cellular resistance to insulin and β-cell failure. Tissue lesions are common to both types of diabetes, and chronic hyperglycemia (or a closely related metabolic abnormality) is responsible for diabetic complications including diabetic nephropathy. The WHO and national diabetes agencies have approved diagnostic criteria for diabetes based on venous plasma glucose concentrations, with subsequent guidance in 2011 confirming the acceptability of glycated hemoglobin for this purpose in certain situations (see Chapter 47). In 2014, the WHO estimated that 8.5% of adults aged greater than 18 years worldwide were affected by diabetes.

Background

Diabetic nephropathy is a clinical diagnosis based on the finding of proteinuria in a patient with diabetes and in whom there is no evidence of urinary tract infection (UTI). Overt nephropathy is characterized by protein loss greater than 0.5 g/day, approximately equivalent to albumin loss of greater than 300 mg/day or category A3 albuminuria. For a variety of reasons, it is preferable to assess proteinuria as albuminuria (see Chapter 34), and albumin has long been uniformly adopted as the "criterion standard" in evaluating diabetes-related kidney damage.[92,255] Category A_2 albuminuria, equivalent to urinary albumin loss of between 30 and 300 mg/day, was previously termed "microalbuminuria," although this terminology is no longer encouraged.[90] Diabetic nephropathy is the most common cause of ESRD in the United States: the number of incident patients with diabetes as the cause of ESRD exceeded 50,000 during 2010, but has fallen slightly since (see Fig. 49.13).[256] Almost 290,000 people receiving RRT in the United States in 2017 have diabetes as the cause of their ESRD, and this continues to rise steadily.[91] Among patients who require dialysis, those with diabetes have a 22% higher mortality at 1 year and a 15% higher mortality at 5 years than patients without diabetes. Diabetic nephropathy as a cause of ESRD in the United Kingdom is seen in approximately 28.6% of new patients—a lower percentage than that of the United States and Europe.[103] In the United States, a number of objectives were developed for reducing threats to the health of the nation as part of the Healthy People Initiative. One of the objectives of the Healthy People Initiative (HP 2010 Objective 4.7) was to reduce the incidence rate of ESRD caused by diabetes from 145 per million population in 2003 to 78 per million people by 2010.[257] However, the overall rate for new cases of ESRD caused by diabetes missed this target and was 157 pmp in 2011.[258] The Healthy People Initiative is ongoing and Healthy People 2020 is active, having been established in 2010. There are several important targets and aspirations related to CKD and ESRD within this program.[258] It is interesting to note that the HP2020 CKD 9.1 objective is to reduce kidney failure due to diabetes to the target of 152 pmp. The prevalence of diabetes as a cause of ESRD is variable among ethnic groups within the United States with whites having rates approximately 25% of those observed among African Americans.[258]

Diabetic nephropathy is clinically a very slowly developing condition, but ultrastructural evidence of glomerular damage has been found in renal biopsies taken from patients with type 1 diabetes within a few years of their diagnosis.[42,259,260] In type 1 diabetes, early macroscopic changes include kidney enlargement and pallor. With disease progression, the kidneys become smaller. Type 2 diabetes displays variable kidney contraction caused by associated ischemia. On histologic examination, glomerular changes include diffuse mesangial sclerosis with accentuation of matrix and irregularly thickened basement membranes; sclerotic, acellular mesangial nodules (so-called Kimmelstiel-Wilson lesions); hyaline fibrin cap lesions around peripheral capillary loops; capsular drop lesions located within Bowman's capsule; and hyalinosis of arterioles.

Clinical progression is defined in terms of changes in rate of urinary albumin loss and decline in GFR and blood pressure changes (Table 49.11). In type 1 diabetes, it is unusual to develop albuminuria within the first 5 years of diagnosis but it can occur anytime thereafter, and even after 40 years. Patients with type 1 diabetes and category A_2 albuminuria will progress to overt nephropathy at an average rate of 20% over 5 years.[261] Long-term follow-up data on albuminuric patients confirm that 30% regress to normoalbuminuria and the rest remain albuminuric at 10 years.[262] In Type 2 diabetes the UK Prospective Diabetes Study (UKPDS) has described the incidence of albuminuria (equivalent to A_2 albuminuria) as 6.5% and overt nephropathy (equivalent to A3 albuminuria) as 0.7% at diagnosis.[263] As albuminuria worsens and blood pressure increases, a relentless decline in GFR occurs.

Family studies of patients with type 1 diabetes have shown that diabetic siblings of patients with nephropathy have a fourfold risk of nephropathy compared with siblings without nephropathy. A family history of hypertension and cardiovascular disease may increase nephropathy rates.[264] Considerable work has been undertaken to look for genetic linkages with the development of nephropathy in diabetes.[265] However, the best available predictor for development of nephropathy is albuminuria.

Pathophysiology

Observational studies have shown that sustained poor glycemic control is associated with a greater risk for development of nephropathy in both type 1 and type 2 diabetes.[266-269] The exact mechanism for hyperglycemic tissue damage probably includes (1) glycation of proteins leading to the formation of

TABLE 49.11 Development of Diabetic Nephropathy

Stage	Designation	Characteristics	Structural Changes	Glomerular Filtration Rate (mL/min/1.73 m²)	Blood Pressure (mm Hg)
I	Hyperfunction	Hyperfiltration	Glomerular hypertrophy	>150	Normal
II	Normoalbuminuria	Normal albumin loss (<30 mg/day)	Basement membrane thickening	150	Normal
III	Incipient diabetic nephropathy	Increased albumin loss (30–300 mg/day)	Albumin loss correlates with structural damage and hypertrophy of remaining glomeruli	125	Increased
IV	Overt diabetic nephropathy	Clinical proteinuria (>300 mg/day)	Advanced structural damage	<100	Hypertension
V	Uremia	Kidney failure	Glomerular closure	0–10	High

AGEs, (2) overactivity of the polyol pathway, and (3) generation of reactive oxygen species.[270] Polyols are sugar alcohols formed from their respective sugars under the action of aldose reductase. Glucose is preferentially shunted through the polyol pathway under hyperglycemic conditions, generating sorbitol that accumulates within cells. A key step linking glucotoxicity to cell dysfunction in diabetic nephropathy is the excess of extracellular matrix within the glomerulus and interstitium. A number of genes encoding matrix proteins in hyperglycemic conditions have been identified.[271] For example, transcription of the gene for TGF-β is stimulated by hyperglycemia, AGE, AII, and reactive oxygen species.[272–274]

One important consequence of glucose-stimulated TGF-β transcription is upregulation of the insulin-independent GLUT-1 transporter in mesangial cells. Glucose is transported to the cells through GLUT-1 and is metabolized mainly by the glycolytic pathway. Increased de novo synthesis of diacylglycerol results in the activation of protein kinase C and mitogen-activated kinases. Activation of these enzymes can lead to stimulation of certain genes, including TGF-β. Activation of TGF-β can induce the expression of GLUT-1, and these signaling pathways induce the expression of extracellular matrix proteins. The formation of AGE also generates reactive oxygen species, which can activate latent TGF-β.[271] Studies employing neutralizing anti–TGF-β antibodies have provided evidence that the prosclerotic and hypertrophic effects of high ambient glucose in cultured renal cells are largely mediated by autocrine production and activation of TGF-β.[275,276] These antibodies can reverse established nephropathy in animal models.[277,278] Furthermore, glomerular TGF-β mRNA is markedly increased in kidney biopsy specimens from patients with proven diabetic kidney disease, and blood and urine sampling across the renal vascular bed confirms net renal production of TGF-β in diabetic patients.[279] Treatment with the ACE inhibitor captopril lowers circulating TGF-β concentrations in patients with diabetic nephropathy.[280] The receptor for AGE (RAGE) has been identified.[281] RAGE is selectively expressed in the glomerular epithelial cells (podocytes) and not in the mesangial cell or the glomerular endothelium.[282] Increased accumulation of AGE in diabetes engages podocyte RAGE and may lead to increased glomerular permeability.[283] Vascular hyperpermeability, a hallmark feature of diabetes, can be suppressed by inhibiting RAGE in the animal model of diabetes, the streptozotocin-treated rat.[284]

Studies of experimental diabetes in the rat suggest that hyperfiltration alone could cause glomerular changes; conflicting reports have described the effects in humans. Increased GFR could be a predictor of progression to albuminuria but is also a reflection of poor metabolic control. In the Diabetes Control and Complications Trial (DCCT),[266] no association was noted between hyperfiltration and subsequent development of albuminuria.[285] Systemic blood pressure is higher in patients with diabetes who subsequently develop albuminuria, although it is not clear which comes first. Tubulointerstitial fibrosis occurs in diabetic nephropathy, in addition to glomerulosclerosis. Decreased GFR correlates with interstitial and glomerular expansion.[286]

Treatment Strategies

The cornerstones of treatment for diabetic nephropathy consist of glycemic control, blood pressure control, particularly with drugs that block the RAAS, and management of cardiovascular risk.[266,269,287,288] Guidelines published by NICE recommend targeting glycated hemoglobin (HbA$_{1c}$) concentrations to 48 mmol/mol (6.5%) or lower, while acknowledging the need for individualized target setting in certain cases.[289–291] High blood pressure accelerates the progressive increase in albuminuria in patients with initially normal urinary albumin loss and accelerates loss of kidney function in those with overt nephropathy in type 2 diabetes.[292,293] The NKF Task Force on Cardiovascular Disease has recommended a target blood pressure of less than 125/75 mm Hg in diabetic kidney disease,[294] and in the United Kingdom a target blood pressure of less than 130/80 mm Hg is recommended for people with diabetes and CKD (see earlier).[94] ACE inhibitors and ARBs slow the progression of diabetic kidney disease[295–298] and prevent cardiovascular events.[137] In addition to lowered systemic blood pressure, patients receiving RAAS blockade have lowered glomerular capillary blood pressure and protein filtration.[299,300] ACE inhibitors and ARBs also reduce AII-mediated effects on glomerular permeability and cell proliferation and fibrosis[301,302] and should be incorporated into the treatment schedules of all patients with type 2 diabetes and those with type 1 diabetes and albuminuria. ACE inhibitors may exacerbate hyperkalemia in patients with advanced kidney disease and/or hyporeninemic hypoaldosteronism. In older patients with renal artery stenosis they may cause a rapid decline in kidney function. A low sodium diet potentiates the antihypertensive effect and antiproteinuric effect of AII blockade in type 2 diabetes.[303] Patients should be encouraged to stop smoking cigarettes because smoking increases the risk of albuminuria.[304] Dyslipidemias should be managed as outlined for nondiabetic proteinuric CKD. For many years the Steno Diabetes Center in Copenhagen, Denmark, has advocated multifactorial interventions in the management of type 2 diabetes. For example, intensified interventions including tight glucose regulation, use of RAAS blockers, aspirin, lipid-lowering agents, and lifestyle changes, were shown to reduce nonfatal cardiovascular disease among patients with type 2 diabetes[305] and subsequently beneficial effects with respect to vascular complications and on all-cause mortality.[306]

More recently, the novel drug class of SGLT2 (see earlier) inhibitors (gliflozines) have been introduced and are being investigated for protective effects in diabetic-kidney disease and nondiabetic kidney disease.[307] Although not initially licensed for patients with eGFR below 60 mL/min, these drugs are increasingly available at lower levels of kidney function. Gliflozines reduce blood sugar concentration by reducing the renal tubular reabsorption of glucose, increasing glycosuria. In addition to reports indicating cardiovascular benefits of these medications,[308] there has been signaling toward kidney protection effects.[309] The EMPA-KIDNEY study (ClinicalTrials.gov Identifier: NCT03594110) is an international study of 5000 randomized patients with mild to moderately reduced GFR (GFR 30 to 90 mL/min/1.73 m^2) at study entry, to assess progression of CKD and cardiovascular outcomes in patients identified as at risk of progressive CKD. These patients include those with diabetes and nondiabetic CKD. The study is likely to report in the mid-2020s.

Hypertensive Nephropathy

Hypertension is second only to diabetes as a primary diagnosis of ESRD for incident patients commencing dialysis in the

United States. (Fig. 49.13). The incidence is higher in older people and especially among the black population in the United States. Hypertension often develops as a consequence of CKD because of alterations in salt and water metabolism and activation of the sympathetic nervous and renin-angiotensin systems.[310,311] Hypertension can act as an accelerating force in the development of ESRD. As described earlier, treatment of hypertension to predefined target blood pressure values is critical in preventing progression to ESRD.[69,107,312] Various national and international guidelines on the treatment of hypertension have been published, although variability is evident among these recommendations. The JNC 7 report suggests that the risk of cardiovascular disease doubles for each increment in BP of 20/10 mm Hg beginning at 115/75 mm Hg. The report identifies 120/80 mm Hg as normotension. All patients with hypertension (>140/90 mm Hg) should receive lifestyle change advice and antihypertensive medication if necessary.[313]

Large vessel *renovascular disease* can cause hypertension. Primary diseases of the renal arteries usually involve the origin of the renal arteries at the aorta (ostial lesions). Secondary diseases with hypertension and CKD with small vessel and intrarenal disease are referred to as *ischemic nephropathy*. A complex interplay occurs between renal artery stenosis and ischemic nephropathy. Atherosclerosis accounts for more than 90% of renal artery stenosis. The disease is progressive and may cause renal artery occlusion.[314] Prevalence increases with age and is associated with refractory hypertension, low body mass index, smoking, diabetes, and established vascular disease elsewhere. In general, as a marker of established cardiovascular disease, atheromatous renal artery stenosis is associated with a poor prognosis.[315] Diagnosis requires a high index of suspicion and is guided by radiologic examination of the renal arterial anatomy. Patients who receive ACE inhibitors and ARBs may develop AKI in the setting of severe bilateral renovascular disease or severe disease to a single functioning kidney. Kidney function should be carefully monitored following the introduction of these drugs and a fall of GFR in excess of 15 to 20% should raise the suspicion of renovascular disease. The diagnosis is important to make because radiologic placement of intraluminal stents[316] is possible and surgical repair can be performed to prolong vessel patency.[317] Patients are at risk, however, of atheroembolism following intervention.[318] A correctable atherosclerotic renal artery stenosis (ARAS) lesion is found in less than 1% of all hypertensive patients, so investigation has to be targeted to high-risk groups. However, a note of caution: three large studies (ASTRAL, STAR, and CORAL) failed to confirm any benefit from radiologic interventions in patients with atheromatous renal artery stenosis.[319–321] The implication of these studies is that the disease should be managed medically with attention to traditional cardiovascular risk factor reduction strategies.

Renal artery stenosis in younger patients is characteristically due to fibromuscular dysplasia. The medial part of the artery is most commonly affected and presents radiologically as alternate bands of narrowing and dilatation, giving rise to a "string of beads" appearance. If the diagnosis is made then hypertension can be cured following balloon angioplasty to the artery in at least 50% of cases.

Noninvasive imaging is readily available and includes CT angiogram and MRI angiography with gadolinium-based contrast media. A rare but potentially fatal disease, nephrogenic systemic fibrosis, has been described in patients with advanced kidney disease receiving gadolinium-based contrast media during MRI. Because many patients who are investigated for ARAS will have CKD, the approach to investigation has changed. Nephrogenic systemic fibrosis was first described in 2000 as a cutaneous scleromyxedema-like disorder in patients with ESRD.[322] Gadolinium-based contrast media are not recommended for patients with advanced renal impairment, particularly those on dialysis.[323] The Royal College of Radiologists in the United Kingdom has published updated guidelines during 2015. These acknowledge that on occasions it is necessary for contrast-enhanced MRI to be used in patients with advanced CKD including those patients on dialysis (see earlier).[251]

Glomerular Disease

Glomerular disease is suggested clinically by the finding of blood and protein in the urine on reagent strip testing. Proteinuria of greater than 1 g/day (0.88 g/g creatinine; 100 mg/mmol creatinine) in the absence of an overflow-type proteinuria such as myoglobinuria or light chain-related disease is invariably glomerular in origin. Although a detailed discussion of each glomerular disease is beyond the scope of this book the most important diseases will be discussed to illustrate the spectrum of disease. For further information regarding clinical guidelines the reader is directed to the KDIGO Clinical Practice Guideline for Glomerulonephritis.[324] Whereas the incidence of kidney failure in the Western world has increased dramatically over recent years, in the United States the incidence rate due to glomerulonephritis has fallen (Fig. 49.13).[256] In the United Kingdom glomerulonephritis accounts for 14% of new cases of established renal failure.[325]

Primary Glomerular Disease

Glomerulonephritis can be primary (affecting only the kidneys) or secondary (in which the kidneys are involved as part of a systemic process). Histopathologic classification of glomerulonephritis may appear slightly cumbersome but is readily simplified by consideration of the glomerular structures and cells that may be involved and the presence or absence of immune complexes (Table 49.12). In essence, only three cell types are involved (endothelial, epithelial, and mesangial) plus the acellular GBM. The glomerular cells and the GBM have a limited range of response to injury, namely, proliferation, scarring (sclerosis), and GBM thickening. The term *focal* is used if fewer than half of the glomeruli are involved in the disease process as seen on light microscopy, whereas *diffuse glomerulonephritis* refers to cases in which all glomeruli are involved. Immune deposits identified following immunofluorescence or immunoperoxidase staining do not define whether a disease is focal or diffuse.

Immunoglobulin A Nephropathy

IgA nephropathy is an example of a focal glomerulonephritis with focal mesangial cell proliferation demonstrated by light microscopy. However, diffuse and global deposition of the Ig, IgA, can be demonstrated following immunostaining. It is the most common type of glomerulonephritis worldwide and has a particularly high prevalence around the Pacific rim where it is commonly reported as an incidental finding in

TABLE 49.12   Overview of Some Primary Glomerular Diseases

Disease	Histologic Findings	Clinical Spectrum	Treatment	Prognosis
IgA nephropathy	Focal mesangial cell proliferation on LM. IgA deposited within mesangial cells on IM	Variable: incidental finding; episodes of macroscopic hematuria; proteinuria and declining GFR. There is a male preponderance and the peak incidence occurs in the second and third decades of life. May be associated with systemic vasculitis in HSP	Generic treatment targeting blood pressure and RAAS blockade. Selected cases receive corticosteroids and cytotoxic drugs	Variable, but 30–40% progress to kidney failure over 20 years
Minimal change disease (MCD)	Little evidence of cellular involvement on LM. Podocyte foot process effacement demonstrated on EM. No immune deposits	Most common cause of nephrotic syndrome in children. Usually idiopathic. Relapsing and remitting course	Oral corticosteroids and cytotoxic drugs	Does not cause kidney failure. Significant side effects of immunosuppressant drugs.
Focal segmental glomerulosclerosis (FSGS)	Glomerular scarring, and nonspecific trapping of immune complexes in scarred areas	Common cause of nephrotic syndrome in adults. Congenital forms described. Secondary causes include collapsing variety seen in HIVAN	Idiopathic disease requires corticosteroids and cytotoxic drugs in selected cases	Nephrotic syndrome commonly refractory to treatment. 30–40% develop kidney failure at 10 years
Membranous nephropathy	Thickened GBM with immune deposits in subepithelial GBM. Classically "spikes" are seen along the GBM and represent new GBM squeezed between deposits	Common cause of nephrotic syndrome. Secondary causes in 20% of cases. Idiopathic or primary cause supported by PLA$_2$R antibody positivity	Treat underlying condition. Treat idiopathic membranous generically and if progressive add immunosuppressive drugs	Variable outcome: "Rule of thirds" (see text)

EM, Electron microscopy; *ESRD*, end-stage renal disease; *FSGS*, focal segmental glomerulosclerosis; *GBM*, glomerular basement membrane; *GFR*, glomerular filtration rate; *HIVAN*, human immunodeficiency virus-associated nephropathy; *HSP*, Henoch-Schönlein purpura; *IM*, immunofluorescence or immunoperoxidase microscopy; *LM*, light microscopy; *PLA$_2$R*, phospholipase A$_2$ receptor antibody; *RAAS*, renin-angiotensin-aldosterone system.

kidney biopsy specimens from potential kidney donors.[326] The disease tends to be slowly progressive (in terms of loss of kidney function) depending, as with most kidney diseases, on the degree of proteinuria, kidney function at time of diagnosis, and degree of interstitial fibrosis on kidney biopsy. Up to 50% of patients exhibit increased concentrations of serum IgA, and abnormal O-galactosylated IgA1 at mucosal surfaces indicates a defective mucosal immune system. The diagnosis of IgA nephropathy depends on kidney biopsy findings. Clinical presentation varies considerably from asymptomatic microscopic hematuria to macroscopic hematuria; proteinuria including nephrotic syndrome; and crescentic glomerulonephritis with kidney failure. Episodic macroscopic hematuria is seen in some patients at the same time as an upper respiratory tract infection. IgA nephropathy may also present with established proteinuria, renal impairment, and hypertension.

Treatment options range from tonsillectomy in patients with macroscopic hematuria associated with respiratory infection to no treatment in those with isolated microscopic hematuria or those with proteinuria of less than 1 g/day. In progressive disease, all patients are treated in a similar generic fashion as for most kidney diseases, including targeting blood pressure to less than 125/75 mm Hg and using comprehensive RAAS blockade to minimize proteinuria. Assessment of

the impact of immunosuppressive therapy is compromised by the heterogeneity of the disease and the duration of a randomized controlled study with sufficient numbers to allow a conclusion. Nevertheless, a large Italian study with more than 10 years of follow-up data demonstrated benefit from oral corticosteroids in high doses for 6 months.[327,328] In addition, a retrospective study reported benefit from corticosteroids.[329] Cytotoxic therapy can be considered for rapidly progressing or vasculitic IgA.[330] A recent trial has targeted mucosal immunity by delivery of the steroid budesonide to the distal ileum, and demonstrated reduced proteinuria after nine months of treatment.[331]

Nephrotic Syndrome

Nephrotic syndrome is defined as heavy proteinuria (>3 g/day), reduced serum albumin concentration, and edema. In comparison with nephritic syndrome, nephrotic patients may exhibit an otherwise bland urinary sediment with little hematuria. Nephrotic syndrome can occur at any age from neonate to elderly. Although the underlying kidney disease tends to vary with age, in all cases the lesion is within the glomerulus and is associated with damage to the specialized visceral epithelial cells, the podocytes (see earlier). Proteinuria is a consequence of a reduction in the charge-selective

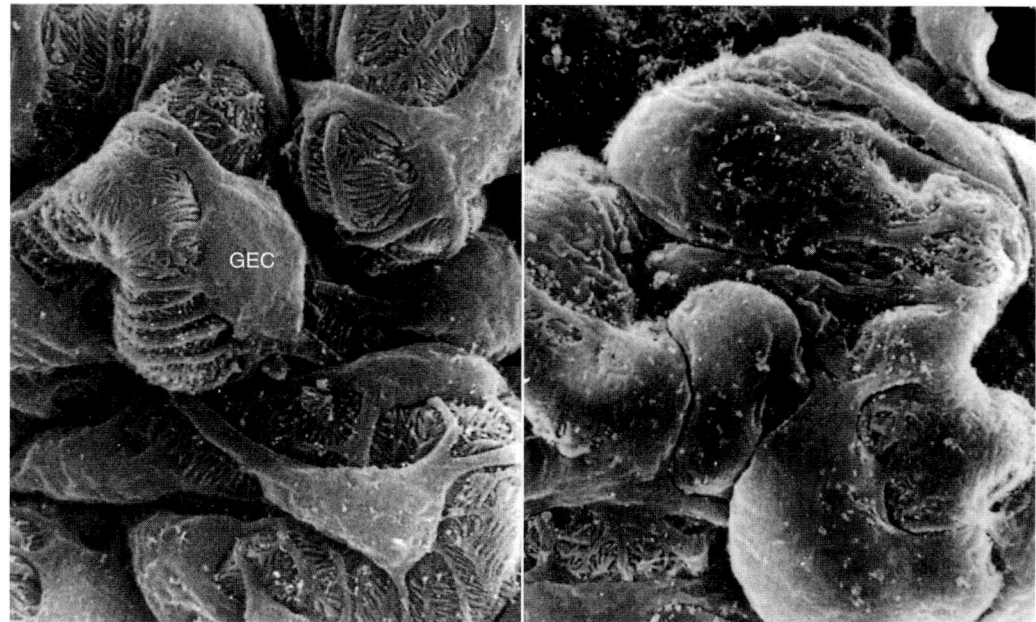

FIGURE 49.17 Graphic example of glomerular changes in nephrotic syndrome. Scanning electron microscopic view of glomerular epithelial podocytes from a vehicle-treated rat *(left)* and a puromycin aminonucleoside (PAN)–treated (180 mg/kg body wt) rat *(right)*. Note the extensive loss of podocyte foot processes, which occurs in response to PAN-induced nephrotic syndrome, and illustrates the major cellular changes that can occur in nephrotic syndrome. GEC, Glomerular epithelial cell. (From Ricardo SD, Bertram JF, Ryan GB. Antioxidants protect podocyte foot processes in puromycin aminonucleoside–treated rats. *J Am Soc Nephrol* 1994;4:1974–86).

properties of the filtration barrier, particularly the GBM, and of alterations in the slit diaphragms of interdigitating foot processes of adjacent podocytes (Fig. 49.17).[332,333] The primary glomerular diseases that cause nephrotic syndrome are termed *podocytopathies,* and a classification scheme has been proposed that will identify diseases based on both morphology and etiology.[334]

The most common causes of nephrotic syndrome are minimal change disease (MCD), focal segmental glomerulosclerosis (FSGS), and membranous nephropathy (see later). Secondary causes are discussed separately and include diabetic nephropathy, amyloidosis, and SLE. A kidney biopsy is generally undertaken in all adult patients who present with nephrotic syndrome. Nephrotic syndrome is associated with significant morbidity regardless of cause, and patients with the disease have increased cardiovascular disease as the result of marked hyperlipidemia and increased risk of infection and thromboembolic disease. Between 10 and 40% of patients with nephrotic syndrome develop evidence of arterial and venous thromboemboli, particularly deep vein and renal vein thrombosis. Renal vein thrombosis may be unilateral or bilateral and may extend into the inferior vena cava. However, most cases of renal vein thrombosis have an insidious onset and produce no symptoms. Infrequently, patients develop acute renal vein thrombosis and present with signs of renal infarction, including flank pain, and microscopic or gross hematuria. In addition, AKI may supervene in cases of nephrotic syndrome (Box 49.3), and prolonged proteinuria with a poor response to treatment may lead to kidney failure.

The management of nephrotic syndrome depends upon the underlying glomerular lesion, although general principles

---

BOX 49.3 Causes of Acute Kidney Injury in Nephrotic Syndrome

Acute tubular necrosis usually in MCD and patients >50 years of age

Minimal change disease with acute interstitial nephritis induced by NSAIDs

Tubular injury in collapsing FSGS either idiopathic or associated with HIV infection

Crescentic glomerulonephritis superimposed upon membranous nephropathy

FSGS, Focal segmental glomerulosclerosis; *HIV,* human immunodeficiency virus; *MCD,* minimal change disease; *NSAIDs,* nonsteroidal anti-inflammatory drugs.

---

apply in all cases (Box 49.4). In addition to general measures, specific treatment targeted at inducing remission from proteinuria usually requires a combination of immunosuppressive drugs, including corticosteroids and cytotoxic drugs.

MCD is the most common cause of nephrotic syndrome in children and young adults.[335] The incidence of MCD is estimated at 1 to 5 cases per 100,000 children per year. It typically presents with severe edema and hypoalbuminemia, and urine testing confirms heavy proteinuria. Kidney function is normal, with little evidence of a reduced GFR. MCD does not progress to kidney failure except in some cases of severe refractory disease that may be complicated by glomerular scarring lesions. Nephrotic syndrome in a noninfant child is assumed to be caused by MCD, and a kidney biopsy generally is not performed because the condition typically is responsive to a trial of corticosteroids with remission within 2 weeks. Following the disappearance of proteinuria, or 1 week after remission is induced, the corticosteroid dose can be reduced and tapered slowly. An attempt to stop treatment may be indicated after 8 weeks. Longer duration of corticosteroid therapy significantly reduces the risk of relapse, and many centers will treat for a minimum of 12 weeks, particularly with a first episode of steroid-responsive nephrotic syndrome. Around 60% of steroid-responsive patients experience multiple relapses. Some of these patients can be managed with low-dose corticosteroids given daily or on alternate days, but relapses do occur, especially if intercurrent infection is present. In addition to the comorbidity associated with nephrotic syndrome, the burden of long-term exposure to corticosteroids and cytotoxic drugs has to be considered. Cyclophosphamide, azathioprine, tacrolimus, and cyclosporin are reserved for refractory cases and can be used as corticosteroid-sparing agents with the aim of reducing relapse rates. Treatment with cyclophosphamide is limited to 8 to 12 weeks to reduce risk of gonadal toxicity.

The histologic lesion is by definition "minimal" when viewed on light microscopy. However, EM confirms disruption to the epithelial surface of the glomerular capillary. Podocyte foot processes are detached (effaced) from the GBM, conferring absence of the slit diaphragm, and therefore the final barrier to filtration fails (Fig. 49.17). The glomerular architecture is restored following prompt treatment with high-dose corticosteroids. In MCD, the onset of nephrotic syndrome is often preceded by an infection or allergic reaction, and it has been proposed that nephrotic syndrome may be the result of an exaggerated response to normal physiologic and immune mechanisms that increase proteinuria during infection. MCD does occur in adults who present with nephrotic syndrome. MCD occasionally complicates NSAID ingestion, and secondary MCD has been described in patients with malignancy (particularly Hodgkin lymphoma).

Focal segmental glomerulosclerosis (FSGS) is the most important cause of the nephrotic syndrome in adults and remains a frequent cause in children and adolescents, particularly in the United States, Brazil, and many other countries.[336] Genetic studies in children with familial nephrotic syndrome have identified mutations in genes that encode important podocyte proteins.[337,338] Nephrin was the first slit diaphragm protein identified, and mutations in this transmembrane protein cause congenital (Finnish-type) nephrotic syndrome which occurs with a frequency of 1/8200 live births in Finland. Among children with inherited nephrotic syndrome, mutations in other podocyte proteins (podocin, α-actinin 4, CD2-AP) have been described; all proteins are crucial to the interaction of the slit diaphragm with the podocyte cytoskeleton. Compelling evidence advocating a soluble permeability factor has been proposed as causing nephrotic syndrome in FSGS. Evidence includes experience in kidney transplantation, whereby FSGS may recur within hours of transplantation of a normal kidney into a recipient with FSGS.[339] The nature of the permeability factors remains unknown: candidate molecules include soluble urokinase-type plasminogen activator receptor and cardiotrophin-like cytokine-1.[340] The putative permeability factors can be removed by immunoabsorption to protein A and plasma exchange prior to transplantation.

Several disease processes lead to the description of FSGS on kidney biopsy and are shown in Box 49.5. Proteinuria in secondary FSGS, as in primary FSGS, reflects epithelial injury, although the mechanism is different. Following nephron loss, the remaining glomeruli undergo hypertrophy. Because podocytes are usually in a state of terminal differentiation and unable to replicate, the density of available foot processes to cover the enlarged glomerular surface is decreased. Focal areas of denudation from the GBM ensue, leading to proteinuria. Corticosteroids and other immunosuppressant drugs are not recommended for secondary forms of FSGS or for congenital forms. The treatment of primary disease-causing nephrotic syndrome is typically a course of high-dose corticosteroids given for at least 6 months as tolerated. Remission of nephrotic syndrome is characterized by absence of proteinuria, loss of edema, and normalization of serum albumin concentration.

Membranous Nephropathy

The term *membranous nephropathy* reflects the primary histologic change noted on light microscopy: basement membrane thickening with little or no cellular proliferation or infiltration. Immunostaining is typically positive to Igs and complement components. EM reveals electron-dense deposits within the GBM. Idiopathic membranous nephropathy is a common cause of nephrotic syndrome, accounting for approximately 30% of adult cases. The clinical features are variable and are classically described as follows ("rule of thirds");

(1) a third of cases undergo spontaneous remission of proteinuria and recovery of kidney function; (2) a third of cases have nonprogressive disease but evidence of ongoing proteinuria; and (3) a third of cases continue to exhibit nephrotic syndrome and are at high risk of progressive kidney failure.

The clinical course therefore is difficult to predict at the onset of the disease, although 40% of patients in the control arm of an immunosuppressive treatment trial developed kidney failure after 10 years.[341] Patients generally are observed for 6 months to assess the likely natural history of the condition and are treated generically. In progressive cases and in those who have evidence of nephrotic syndrome for at least 6 months, a course of immunosuppressive drugs is indicated. Typical immunosuppressive schedules include high-dose corticosteroids, calcineurin inhibitors such as cyclosporin, and cytotoxic drugs (chlorambucil and cyclophosphamide).[341,342] The immunosuppressive schedules are targeted at primary membranous nephropathy. A seminal paper from Debiec and others in 2002 described the discovery of an antibody to neutral endopeptidase (a human podocyte antigen) in antenatal cases of membranous nephropathy.[343] Target antigens for nephritogenic antibodies have since been further described. The M-type phospholipase A_2 receptor (PLA_2R) is the first podocyte antigen involved in membranous nephropathy to be described in adults.[344] Detection of autoantibodies directed to PLA_2R (anti-PLA_2R antibody) indicates primary disease rather than a secondary process and guides therapy. Biological agents directed at antibody formation, that is, against for example CD20 molecules, include rituximab, and are being used in the treatment of the disease.[345,346]

Secondary causes of membranous nephropathy are associated with a wide spectrum of diseases, including SLE, hepatitis B, falciparum malariae, malignancy, and drugs (e.g., gold, penicillamine, captopril). In comparison with idiopathic disease, the clinical outcome depends on the underlying disease process. Underlying malignancy has been thought to be responsible for up to 5 to 10% of cases of membranous nephropathy in adults; the risk is highest in patients older than 60 years of age. A solid tumor (such as carcinoma of the lung, colon, or prostate) is most often involved and usually is clinically obvious.[347]

Rapidly Progressive Glomerulonephritis

Rapidly progressive glomerulonephritis (RPGN) is a heterogeneous group of disorders characterized by a fulminant clinical course that leads to kidney failure in only weeks or a few months. The clinical picture of RPGN is often preceded by a systemic illness for several months associated with general malaise, weight loss, breathlessness, upper respiratory tract abnormalities, and skin changes. Clinical examination may reveal nailfold infarcts and palpable purple lesions on the skin of the legs. In severe cases, a renal-pulmonary syndrome supervenes with kidney failure and alveolitis with associated pulmonary hemorrhage. In some cases, the condition may be limited to the kidneys (renal-limited vasculitis).

These syndromes are often characterized by focal glomerulonephritis with glomerular ischemia, infarction, and tissue death (necrosis). Following release of inflammatory cytokines and chemokines from the necrotic capillaries there is proliferation of the epithelial cells of Bowman's capsule. The proliferated cells lie on top of adjacent cells and form a partial circle around the inner rim of Bowman's capsule that

is referred to as a *crescent*. Proliferating epithelial cells and macrophages eventually compress the glomeruli and obstruct the proximal convoluted tubules, thus severely compromising nephron function.

RPGN may be classified as idiopathic kidney disease or as a disease secondary to other conditions, such as infectious disease, multisystem disease, and occasionally an adverse reaction to medication. Anti-GBM antibodies may be present along the GBM in anti-GBM disease. Most commonly, however, there is no, or little, Ig deposition within the glomerulus (so-called "pauci-immune"). Approximately 80% of patients with active pauci-immune necrotizing and crescentic glomerulonephritis have been shown to possess antineutrophil cytoplasmic antibodies (ANCAs), irrespective of the presence or absence of a concomitant systemic vasculitis. This strong association has allowed serologic discrimination of this type of glomerulonephritis from other types of RPGN. Wegener's granulomatosis, microscopic polyangiitis, and Churg-Strauss syndrome are small-vessel vasculitides characterized by an association with ANCAs.

ANCAs were first reported in 1982 in patients with pauci-immune serologic glomerulonephritis.[348] Three years later, ANCAs were detected by indirect immunofluorescence on human neutrophils in patients with active granulomatosis and polyangiitis.[349] Since 1989, two subtypes of ANCA have been described: cytoplasmic (C-ANCA) and perinuclear (P-ANCA), reflecting the patterns observed by indirect immunofluorescence microscopy using alcohol-fixed neutrophils as a substrate.[350] C-ANCAs are directed toward a plasma proteinase (PR3) in neutrophil primary granules and are associated with granulomatosis with polyangiitis (GPA), whereas the P-ANCA target antigen is usually myeloperoxidase (MPO) and is associated with microscopic polyangiitis (MPA).[351,352] Vasculitis or angiitis is an inflammatory reaction in the wall of any blood vessel that can have diverse clinical presentations. The exact sequence of events that triggers perivascular inflammation leading to injury is unclear, but ANCAs have been identified that have at least diagnostic and prognostic usefulness. ANCAs appear in the plasma of almost all patients with active and generalized disease and are useful in diagnosis of the disease. However, false-positives and false negatives may occur necessitating histologic diagnosis where possible. The use of ANCA to predict relapse of disease is limited, and a response to treatment cannot rely on falling titers but must be assessed utilizing clinical parameters of inflammation.[353] Autoantibodies of other specificities in rheumatoid arthritis, SLE, and inflammatory bowel disease may mimic the P-ANCA pattern, and in isolation, the finding of P-ANCA has a low specificity for vasculitis. The "International Consensus Statement on Testing and Reporting of Antineutrophil Cytoplasmic Antibodies (ANCA)" was developed to optimize ANCA testing.[354] This two-stage process required that all sera were tested by indirect immunofluorescence examination of peripheral blood neutrophils and, where there is positive fluorescence, by immunoassays for antibodies against PR3 and MPO. However, during 2017, and in response to the European Vasculitis Study Group (EUVAS) evaluation of the value of this historic two-stage process,[355] an updated consensus statement was published.[356] The consensus statement indicates that modern high-quality immunoassays are the preferred screening method for patients that are suspected of having the ANCA-associated vasculitides

GPA and MPA, without the categorical need for indirect immunofluorescence. This is a welcome advance in the utility of ANCA testing.

RPGN accounts for 15% of patients presenting to specialist nephrology units for RRT and therefore is an important disease category to be aware of because if treatment is initiated early, independent kidney function can be restored, particularly if active lesions are seen on biopsy.[357] In addition to measurement of ANCA, C-reactive protein (CRP) is extremely helpful in assessment of the acute-phase reaction in active disease processes and is critical in helping to define disease remission. In patients in whom the CRP has returned to normal, disease remission is indicated; this prompts the clinician to reduce immunosuppressant treatment doses.[358]

Highly intensive immunosuppressive schedules are commenced in patients who present with RPGN. This *induction* phase of treatment is continued until the disease has remitted. Once remission is attained, a longer maintenance phase of treatment with less intensive schedules is commenced. In cases with a high index of suspicion on clinical grounds, treatment should begin empirically. Usually the diagnosis is made following a kidney biopsy and the result of an ANCA or anti-GBM antibody test. The mainstay of therapy has included high-dose oral prednisolone and oral or intravenous cyclophosphamide as standard baseline treatment. Adjunctive treatments that may be used routinely in severe cases include pulses of intravenous methylprednisolone (1 g/day for 3 days) or a series of plasma exchanges.[359] The rationale for these approaches is to switch off production of the antibody and attenuate the proinflammatory response to tissue damage. Because of the toxicity of existing protocols, major randomized intervention studies (e.g., PEXIVAS) have evaluated the use of adjunctive plasma exchange treatment and compared two regimens of corticosteroids in patients with severe disease.[360] The median duration of follow-up was 2.9 years and PEXIVAS demonstrated that plasma exchange did not reduce the incidence of death or ESRD. A reduced-dose regimen of corticosteroids was non inferior to standard-dose regimen, and associated with fewer infections.[360]

Patients are closely followed for many months for evidence of disease activity and signs of treatment-related toxicity. This involves monitoring of kidney function, full blood count, ANCA serology, and anti-MPO/PR3 titer, as well as CRP. Following remission of active disease, drug doses are tapered, and cyclophosphamide may be exchanged for azathioprine or mycophenolate mofetil (MMF). Serologic testing for ANCA and measurement of CRP are performed prior to immunosuppressant dose reduction to ensure that the disease activity has abated. Plans for long-term follow-up are made, and treatment is expected to be ongoing for at least 3 to 5 years. Relapses may occur as immunosuppression is reduced or withdrawn. The untreated mortality of ANCA-associated vasculitis is 90% at 1 year.[361] With current management strategies the mortality rate has fallen to 20 to 31%.[360] Older people are most susceptible both to the disease and to treatment-related morbidities, particularly infection. Patients who require dialysis or ventilatory support for pulmonary involvement have a higher mortality rate.

Anti-GBM disease (Goodpasture disease) affects 0.5 to 1 per million population per year in the United Kingdom.[362] Serologic detection of anti-GBM antibodies is helpful for assisting diagnosis in cases of RPGN. In this process, the antigens are well characterized and the antibody is directed at the α3 chain of type IV collagen. The disease is characterized by a relative lack of prodromal illness; a very rapid deterioration in kidney function; and a poor prognosis, with 0% renal survival at 12 months if oliguria or anuria should develop.[363] The kidney biopsy typically demonstrates crescents in all the glomeruli ("100% crescents") and each crescent is at a similar stage of development. The GBM stains positively in a linear pattern with anti-GBM antibodies. In addition to renal involvement, lung basement membrane can be affected, leading to pulmonary hemorrhage (Goodpasture syndrome). The environment plays a critical role in determining whether anti-GBM antibodies cause lung injury, because pulmonary hemorrhage occurs only in current cigarette smokers.

Systemic Lupus Erythematosus

SLE is a chronic inflammatory disease of unknown cause that can affect the skin, joints, kidneys, lungs, nervous system, serous membranes, and/or other organs of the body. Revised classification criteria for SLE, based on clinical and laboratory findings with positivity for antibodies to antinuclear antigens (ANA) as an entry criterion, have recently been endorsed.[364] The clinical course of SLE is variable and may be characterized by periods of remissions and chronic or acute relapses. Women, especially in their 20s and 30s, are affected more frequently than men. Renal involvement, termed *lupus nephritis*, occurs in up to 60% of adults with SLE. Lupus nephritis is especially common in black and Hispanic patients in the United States.[365] Lupus nephritis may present variably from incidental hematuria and proteinuria, nephrotic syndrome, or a fulminating RPGN. Most (75%) patients with SLE develop an abnormal urinalysis or impaired kidney function during the course of the disease. A pathologic description is required to stage the disease process in lupus nephritis. The classification of lupus nephritis has been revised, and treatment is targeted depending on the stage of disease.[366] In general terms, pathologic findings include a spectrum from focal mesangial proliferation to diffuse global necrotizing glomerulonephritis. Membranous nephropathy may also be present. Detection of lupus nephritis involves urine testing for blood and protein and tests of kidney function. In addition, serologic testing for autoantibodies to nuclear antigens and measurement of complement components C3 and C4 are undertaken (Table 49.13). Significant hypocomplementemia and increased anti-double stranded DNA (anti-dsDNA) titers suggest active disease. Combined use of corticosteroids and intravenous or oral cyclophosphamide has been the conventional treatment for diffuse proliferative lupus nephritis since the 1970s.[367] Treatment duration with cyclophosphamide is limited because of severe toxicity, including gonadal toxicity, hemorrhagic cystitis, bone marrow suppression, and carcinogenicity. Data suggest that MMF and corticosteroids can be as effective, but not superior to, intravenous cyclophosphamide for induction treatment for lupus nephritis.[368]

Acute Nephritic Syndrome

This disorder is characterized by rapid onset of hematuria, proteinuria, reduced GFR, and sodium and water retention, with resulting hypertension and localized peripheral edema. Congestive heart failure and oliguria may also develop. In a number of patients with the acute nephritic syndrome, the

TABLE 49.13   Laboratory Investigation of Vasculitic Syndromes

Disease	Serologic Test	Antigens	Associated Laboratory Features
SLE	ANA including antibodies to dsDNA and ENA (including SM, Ro [SSA], La [SSB] and RNP)	Nuclear antigens	Leukopenia, thrombocytopenia, Coombs test Complement activation: low serum concentrations of C3 and C4 Positive immunofluorescence using *Crithidia luciliae* as substrate Antiphospholipid antibodies, i.e., anticardiolipin, lupus anticoagulant, false-positive VDRL.
Goodpasture's disease	AntiGBM antibody	Epitope on noncollagen domain of type IV collagen	
Small Vessel Vasculitis			
Microscopic polyangiitis	P-ANCA	MPO	↑ CRP
Wegener granulomatosis	C-ANCA	Proteinase 3 (PR3)	↑ CRP
Churg-Strauss syndrome	P-ANCA in some cases	MPO	↑ CRP and eosinophilia
Henoch-Schönlein purpura	None		
Cryoglobulinemia			Cryoglobulins, rheumatoid factor, complement components, hepatitis C
Medium Vessel Vasculitis			
Classical PAN	None		↑ CRP and eosinophilia

ANA, Antinuclear antibodies; *ANCA*, antineutrophil cytoplasmic antibody; *C-ANCA*, cytoplasmic ANCA; *CRP*, C-reactive protein; *dsDNA*, double-stranded DNA; *ENA*, extractable nuclear antigens; *GBM*, glomerular basement membrane; *MPO*, myeloperoxidase; *P-ANCA*, perinuclear ANCA; *PAN*, polyarteritis nodosa; *RNP*, ribonucleoproteins; *SLE*, systemic lupus erythematosus; *VDRL*, Venereal Disease Research Laboratory.

pathologic process is related to recent group A β-hemolytic streptococcal infection of the pharynx or, less commonly, the skin. Only certain strains of streptococci are capable of inducing acute nephritis. A latent period averaging about 2 weeks exists between the time of streptococcal infection and clinical evidence of nephritis. In patients suspected of having acute poststreptococcal glomerulonephritis, evidence of recent infection may be found in increased titers of antibodies to streptococcal extracellular products: antistreptolysin O, antihyaluronidase, and antideoxyribonuclease-B. Serial measurements that document rising antibody titers against streptococcal antigens provide stronger evidence of recent infection than is provided by a single determination. Most patients have moderate reductions in total hemolytic complement activity (CH_{50}) and in the C3 component of the complement cascade. Typical poststreptococcal glomerulonephritis is now rare in developed countries, and a kidney biopsy may be performed in adult cases to establish the diagnosis pending serologic test results. A kidney biopsy of patients with poststreptococcal glomerulonephritis reveals diffuse involvement with enlarged hypercellular glomeruli infiltrated by polymorphonuclear leukocytes and monocytes. EM reveals deposits, presumably immune complexes, on the epithelial side of the GBM. Abnormal laboratory results are usually present early in the course of acute nephritis. Hematuria, which may be gross ("cola-colored" urine) or microscopic, and proteinuria, usually less than 3 g/day, are usually present. Red blood cell casts are highly suggestive of glomerulonephritis. These casts are commonly present in urine but are observed only if the specimen is fresh and acidic, centrifugation is light, and sediment (after decantation) is resuspended gently. Large numbers of hyaline and granular casts are common; waxy casts suggest a chronic process and should raise the possibility of acute exacerbation of a preexisting disease. Persistent and severe depression of C3 concentration should suggest membranoproliferative glomerulonephritis (MPGN, also known as mesangiocapillary glomerulonephritis [MCGN]), SLE, endocarditis, or other forms of sepsis. Although depressed levels of complement imply disease activity, they are not useful for grading the severity or determining the prognosis of the illness.

Other causes of acute nephritis include reactions to drugs, acute infection of the kidneys, systemic disease with immune complexes such as SLE, bacterial endocarditis, and finally disease in which the antigen is unknown but is possibly related to antecedent viral infection. These may manifest histologically as MPGN. The finding of immune complexes in these cases in kidney biopsy specimens subjected to immunofluorescence or immunoperoxidase staining should provoke a search for an underlying disease, typically either autoimmune (SLE, Sjogren syndrome), infection (hepatitis B and C), or a monoclonal gammopathy. In some cases complement reactants are present in the absence of immune complexes (immune complex negative MPGN), indicating an underlying C3 glomerulopathy,[369] and provoking a search for alternate pathway complement factor gene mutations and autoantibodies to C3 convertase.

Interstitial Nephritis (Tubulointerstitial Nephritis)

A variety of chemical, infectious, and immunologic injuries to the kidney may cause generalized or localized changes that primarily affect the tubulointerstitium rather than the glomeruli.[370] This group of disorders is characterized by alterations in tubular function that, in advanced cases, may cause secondary vascular and glomerular damage. Interstitial nephritis is also called tubulointerstitial nephritis and includes chronic pyelonephritis. *Pyelonephritis* is the term associated with a bacterial infection that causes this kind of damage and is a common cause of interstitial nephritis. Both acute and chronic types of pyelonephritis may occur; the acute type is most commonly associated with UTI. Acute pyelonephritis may develop into chronic pyelonephritis, usually as a result of a renal tract abnormality such as abnormal urethral valves. Interstitial nephritis is also associated with proteinuria that is less severe than in glomerular disease. In addition to conventional pyelonephritis, interstitial nephritis may present in acute and chronic forms and has many causes. Acute allergic interstitial nephritis presents with AKI and marked inflammation of the interstitium. Lymphocytes, polymorphonuclear cells, and eosinophils are prominent. The incidence is variable and depends on kidney biopsy practice. It may account for up to 7% of cases of AKI when an intrinsic kidney disease is diagnosed as opposed to purely toxic and/or ischemic acute tubular damage.[371] Higher values are likely in older people because of the increased incidence of drug reactions. A drug hypersensitivity reaction is the most common form of acute interstitial nephritis. Urinary findings may be normal, or low-level proteinuria and eosinophils may be seen on light microscopy. More than 100 different drugs have been implicated, but NSAIDs and β-lactam antibiotics are the drugs most commonly identified.[372] Nephrotic syndrome may accompany an acute interstitial nephritis associated with NSAIDs. Treatment is directed at removing any causative agent. Steroids are used to promote early resolution of the clinical course, although patients can develop chronic interstitial fibrosis.[373]

A relatively novel cause of tubulointerstitial nephritis, IgG4-related disease, was described in 2003.[374] The mean age at diagnosis is 60 years, and typically patients present with significant weight loss, along with single or multiple organ disease manifestations. The pathology of IgG4-related disease has been characterized, with typical features of a lymphoplasmacytic infiltrate, rich in IgG4-positive plasma cells, enmeshed within a twisted, so-called "storiform" fibrosis. Biomarkers are particularly helpful in diagnosis, and for monitoring response to treatment. Serum IgG4 concentration is increased in the majority of patients, indicating disease activity, and can be serially measured for assessment of the effectiveness of treatment and risk of relapsing disease. Additional laboratory tests should include serum complements C3 and C4 and serum IgE concentration. Active disease is associated with low serum C3 and C4 concentrations, and markedly high serum IgE concentrations. The kidneys are affected in several ways: (i) tubulointerstitial nephritis confirmed on kidney biopsy, causing a reduction in kidney function; (ii) nephrotic syndrome (membranous nephropathy); and (iii) atrophy of the kidneys as a consequence of blockage to urine flow within the ureters caused by retroperitoneal fibrosis (postrenal, obstructive nephropathy). Corticosteroids are the mainstay of treatment, targeting the immune system. Alternative treatments can be used to reduce the toxicity of a prolonged course of high-dose corticosteroids, and include cytotoxic and antiproliferative drugs, along with biological agents that deplete B cells, including rituximab. Outcome is dependent on the extent of organ damage at presentation, and relapse is described as treatment doses are reduced.

Sarcoidosis is a multisystem disorder associated with chronic granulomatous interstitial nephritis. Biochemical abnormalities include hypercalcemia, hypercalciuria, and increased serum ACE activity.[375] The condition may be effectively treated with steroids.

Prostaglandins and Nonsteroidal Anti-Inflammatory Drugs in Kidney Disease

Two isoforms of COX synthesize prostaglandins. COX-1 is a resident or constitutive form, and COX-2 is an inducible form that increases with disorders of inflammation.[376] Renal blood flow, particularly within the medulla, is dependent on systemic and local production of vasodilatory prostaglandins. NSAIDs are nonspecific inhibitors of both COX isoforms, hence blocking prostaglandin synthesis with resultant renal injury in susceptible individuals. Analgesic-related kidney damage is seen mostly within the medulla, with late changes causing papillary necrosis and interstitial fibrosis. Hyperkalemia can develop as a consequence of reduced GFR or secondary to hyporeninemic hypoaldosteronism. In addition, NSAIDs can rarely cause nephrotic syndrome and drug-related acute allergic interstitial nephritis.

Analgesic nephropathy is a common cause of incident kidney failure in many countries. In Australia, for example, it contributes around 10% of incident ESRD cases, despite awareness of the risk of kidney damage from chronic analgesic ingestion.[377] However, it is essentially a preventable condition for which monitoring of kidney function has proved useful. The incidence of this disease has decreased over the past decade as awareness has improved, and phenacetin was withdrawn from over-the-counter analgesic mixtures. In the United States, 1 in 5 citizens (50 million) report that they use an NSAID for an acute complaint.[378] Although most healthy individuals tolerate NSAIDs well, risks of kidney injury from exposure are higher in older people and those with preexisting CKD.[379]

Plasma Cell Disorders and Kidney Disease

Ig molecules are formed in secretory B cells (plasma cells) and consist of heavy chains, which denominate the antibody isotype, and either kappa (κ) or lambda (λ) light chains. The proportion of Ig containing κ versus λ is 3:2 in humans. The molecular weight of light chains is approximately 23 kDa. Excess production of light over heavy chains appears to be required for efficient Ig synthesis, resulting in the release of free light chains (FLCs) into the circulation. In normal individuals, the small quantity of circulating polyclonal light chains is filtered by the glomerulus, and 90% is reabsorbed in the proximal tubule and degraded by proteases.

Myeloma or multiple myeloma is a neoplastic proliferation of a clone of plasma cells that produce excessive amounts of a monoclonal (M) protein and FLCs. In multiple myeloma, complete monoclonal Igs (usually IgG or IgA) are accompanied in the plasma by variable concentrations of FLCs that appear in the urine as Bence Jones proteins (named after Henry Bence Jones who first described these in 1848). Immunoparesis, with reduction in non–M-protein Ig, is characteristic of myeloma. M-proteins and FLCs can be identified in the blood and/or the urine in 98% of patients with myeloma using protein electrophoresis and immunofixation. FLC immunoassays are now also used to detect monoclonal Ig in serum, to assess prognosis, and to monitor patients with myeloma.[380]

The kidneys are often affected in myeloma, with diverse clinical and pathologic presentations.[381] The three most common forms of monoclonal Ig-mediated kidney disease are cast nephropathy, monoclonal Ig deposition disease (MIDD), and AL amyloidosis. Evidence suggests that light chains are directly pathogenic.[382] The pattern of human renal injury associated with monoclonal light chains can be reproduced in mice injected intraperitoneally with large quantities of light chains isolated from patients with myeloma or light chain associated amyloid (AL-amyloid).[383] Increased concentrations of filtered light chains lead to alteration in the proximal tubule cells, including prominent cytoplasmic vacuolation, loss of the microvillous border, and epithelial cell exfoliation.[384]

Impairment of kidney function at presentation occurs in almost 50% of patients with myeloma.[381] Although most recover following treatment for other factors contributing to renal impairment (e.g., dehydration, hypercalcemia, infection, nephrotoxic drugs), about 10% have severe renal involvement caused by the effects of monoclonal FLCs on the kidney. Severe kidney failure may occur in myeloma following deposition of light chains within tubules—so-called cast nephropathy ("myeloma kidney"). Cast nephropathy can present acutely, again precipitated by dehydration, hypercalcemia, or NSAIDs, or de novo in the absence of these factors. It occurs when the reabsorptive capacity of proximal tubular cells is exceeded by overproduction of light chains. In myeloma, light chain excretion can exceed 20 g/day. Casts are large and numerous and are found predominantly in the distal convoluted tubule and collecting ducts, causing obstruction to urine flow. They have a hard and fractured appearance with lamination visible on histologic examination of kidney biopsy specimens. Immunofluorescence confirms that casts are composed of monoclonal FLCs and THG. Casts usually stain exclusively with either anti-κ or anti-λ antibodies demonstrating so-called "light chain restriction," indicative of a malignant process. At biopsy, there is often an interstitial inflammatory infiltrate, and fibrosis and tubular atrophy can be extensive. Not all light chains induce cast formation. The ability of light chains to form casts is based on binding to THG.[381] Light chains interfere with proximal tubule cell function, and this promotes delivery to the distal tubule. A specific binding site for light chains has been identified on THG, and light chains with high affinity appear to be more likely to produce obstructing intratubular casts.[385] Physicochemical determinants of binding of light chains to THG include the isoelectric point (pI) of the light chain. Those molecules with a pI above 5.1 (above the tubular fluid pH in the distal nephron) will have a net positive charge that may promote binding via charge interaction to anionic THG (pI, 3.2). Urinary alkalinization reduces binding of light chains to THG in animal models.[386] Nephrotoxicity may be determined by the ability of light chains to self-associate, leading to the formation of high molecular weight aggregates that are more likely to deposit in tissues, particularly in the setting of volume depletion. However, not all patients with excessive production of monoclonal Ig develop disease. Ig-independent mechanisms include dehydration, hypercalcemia, contrast medium, and NSAIDs.[381]

The clinical features of myeloma include a normochromic normocytic anemia, bone pain with pathologic fractures (back or chest rather than extremities), and hypercalcemia in 20% of patients. Severe kidney failure may dominate the clinical picture and 84% of patients studied retrospectively with severe renal impairment required dialysis.[387] Only 15% of these patients regained independent kidney function. Treatment has two main objectives: first, to reverse Ig-independent causes of AKI, and second to reduce the load of monoclonal Ig and free lights chains. In addition to chemotherapy protocols, plasma exchange was considered a useful adjunctive treatment to remove excess FLCs and reduce renal injury. However, a study from Canada of 104 patients presenting with myeloma and AKI, randomized to five to seven plasma exchange treatments, in addition to conventional treatment, showed no significant difference in the composite outcome of death, dialysis dependence, and GFR less than 30 mL/min/1.73 m^2 at 6 months.[388] Nevertheless, interest in direct removal of light chain has not abated, and other filtration technologies have been explored, notably extended hours dialysis with large pore membranes. This approach has been evaluated using high cutoff hemodialysis (HCO-HD) that can remove large quantities of FLCs per session. In the EuLite study, a randomized study in myeloma cast nephropathy, there was no benefit from HCO-HD over standard dialysis in those patients requiring dialysis at presentation.[389]

Excess production of monoclonal light chains (or rarely heavy chains) can cause disorders in which *fragments* are deposited in the kidney and other tissues. Amyloidosis is a condition characterized by extracellular deposition of fibrils in an antiparallel-pleated sheet arrangement. The type of amyloid is defined by the abnormal protein deposited. For example, in "primary amyloid" or "AL-amyloid," fibrils derived from the variable region of light chains are deposited in the tissue. Seventy-five percent are derived from the λ-light chain. Because it is the variable region that is deposited, it is often difficult to assess with immune reactants. Only 50% of AL-amyloid cases are stainable with commercially available antisera to κ and λ. The deposits are fibrillar in nature and bind to Congo red. Amyloid fibrils also bind to the serum amyloid P component, allowing noninvasive evaluation by radiolabeled serum amyloid P scanning.[390] The diagnosis of AL-amyloid can be suspected from the clinical findings of nephrotic range (>3.5 g/day) proteinuria and serum or urinary paraprotein. Amyloidosis is a relatively common cause of nephrotic syndrome in older people. However, 10 to 15% of patients with primary amyloid do not have a detectable serum or urinary paraprotein. Demonstration of a clonal excess of plasma cells on bone marrow biopsy may help with the diagnosis in those without detectable paraprotein. AL-amyloid has a poor prognosis, and mean survival is 18 months, with 50% of patients dying from cardiac failure. Treatment options are unsatisfactory, although prednisolone and melphalan may be tried.[391–393] Circulating FLCs can be detected by immunoassay in most patients with AL-amyloid, and patient outcome following treatment is improved if the concentration of FLCs can be reduced by 50%.[394]

The French Myeloma Group has published results of bone marrow or stem cell transplantation in AL-amyloid.[395] In a retrospective analysis of 21 patients treated with melphalan and stem cell transplantation, 43% died within 1 month, and the remainder had a favorable outcome.

Polycystic Kidney Disease

Autosomal dominant polycystic kidney disease (ADPKD) is the second most common inherited monogenic disease (after familial hypercholesterolemia), with an estimated incidence of 1:1000. It is by far the most common inherited kidney disease; 12.5 million people worldwide are affected.[396] In the United Kingdom, ADPKD is responsible for 11% of new ESRD in patients aged younger than 65 years and 4% of incident patients over age 65 years.[325] The prevalence of the disease ranges from 1 in 200 to 1 in 1000 of the population, but many cases, possibly up to 50%, remain clinically undiagnosed during life. Approximately 50% of ADPKD patients develop kidney failure by age 55 years.[397] It is therefore important to make the diagnosis in affected families and to monitor kidney function regularly. The intervals between estimations of GFR will depend on the stage of CKD, as with other progressive kidney diseases. An important clinical observation is the highly variable phenotype within families. The disease causes the development of multiple kidney cysts and extrarenal cysts occurring in the liver and pancreas. About 10% of ADPKD families have a strong family history of intracranial arterial aneurysm rupture. Hypertension is an early and frequent manifestation, and gross hematuria is a common presenting symptom. On the basis of effectiveness, cost, and safety, ultrasound is the imaging modality most commonly used to make the diagnosis. Screening for polycystic kidney disease is controversial, and age-dependent ultrasound diagnostic criteria for ADPKD have been developed. According to unified criteria, the presence of fewer than two renal cysts has a negative predictive value of 100% and is enough to exclude the disease in at-risk individuals who are 40 years of age and older.[398]

ADPKD is caused by mutations in the genes (*PKD1* and *PKD2*) that encode polycystin 1 and 2 which are located in primary cilia.[399] Mutations affecting *PKD1* are more prevalent than those of *PKD2* and tend to have a worse prognosis, with larger kidneys and earlier development of kidney failure. Genetic testing is not used routinely as a screening tool because current techniques identify only 70% of the hundreds of different PKD1 and PKD2 mutations.[400] The function of primary cilia is to act as flow sensors in the tubules, with flow-induced deformation resulting in calcium influx that leads to a proliferative cellular response mediated by intracellular cAMP. Animal model studies have demonstrated abnormalities in vasopressin and vasopressin receptors in ADPKD and these receptors have become therapeutic targets. Other mutations include the *PDK2* mutation on chromosome 4 (110 kDa) and *APKD3*, for which the gene product and the chromosomal location remain unknown.[401] *PKD2* appears to be a more slowly progressive form of the disease.[402] The median age of onset of ESRD with *PKD2* is 15 years later than with *PKD1*. Also, a rare (incidence 1/20,000) autosomal recessive form of the disease may present in childhood.

Generic treatment should include treatment of hypertension with ACE inhibitors and/or ARBs and maintaining a fluid intake of 2 to 3 L/day to reduce risk of kidney stone disease. Specific therapies are targeted at reducing cyst development and enlargement and delaying the onset of RRT. Estimates of cyst volume can be determined using MRI techniques and changes documented over a relatively short period of time.[403] This has allowed the performance of clinical trials of novel drugs such as the vasopressin V_2-receptor antagonist Tolvaptan. Tolvaptan has been shown in randomized, placebo-controlled clinical studies to slow the increase in size of the cysts, reduce pain associated with cysts and slow rate of

change in kidney function in early PKD with preserved kidney function,[404] and to slow rate of progression in more advanced cases.[405] Adverse events, primarily thirst and polyuria, due to anticipated increase in salt-free water excretion (aquaretic events), led to discontinuation of study drug in a small proportion of screened patients. In addition, abnormalities in liver function tests were reported and increases in serum alanine aminotransferase activity to more than three times the upper limit of normal range occurred in 5.6% of the tolvaptan-treated group: these abnormalities were reversible on cessation of the drug. Tolvaptan was approved by the FDA in 2018. Tolvaptan, under the trade name Jinarc, received its license (marketing authorization) during 2015 in the United Kingdom to slow progression of cyst development and renal insufficiency in ADPKD in adults with CKD and GFR $\geq$30 mL/min/1.73 m^2 at initiation of treatment with evidence of rapidly progressing disease.[406] It is also approved for treatment of ADPKD in Japan.[407]

Obstructive Uropathy

Benign prostatic hyperplasia (BPH) is one of the most common types of obstructive uropathy and is an almost universal finding in aging men.[408] For example, for men aged 50 years, the reported prevalence of BPH is 40%, and for men aged over 70 years, it is at least 75%.[409] No close relationship between the degree of enlargement and the symptoms experienced has been observed.[410] Among the most common symptoms are disorders of micturition, in particular increased frequency, and in many cases this can progress to bladder outflow obstruction. Between 10 and 40% of men with bladder outflow obstruction caused by BPH present in acute retention.[408] Approximately 5% of this group have high-pressure chronic retention of urine, which can result in upper urinary tract obstruction, and consequently CKD as a result of glomerular and tubular damage. Although medical treatments are available to decrease the rate of enlargement of the prostate, resection of the enlarged gland remains the most common surgical procedure performed on men. Urinary retention can be a chronic disorder, with acute exacerbations requiring bladder decompression by catheterization. If the obstruction is not removed by surgery, progressive kidney injury can occur as a result of backpressure along the urinary tract. It is important to identify those patients at risk of developing CKD, because failure to remove their enlarged gland can cause kidney failure. Obstruction can also occur because of kidney stones, which can cause bilateral or unilateral damage. In children, severe kidney damage can be caused by vesicoureteric reflux. One of the main complications of reflux, whether caused by obstruction or by an inherited defect, is the increased incidence of UTI. When the obstruction is relieved the kidney often regains some independent function. A tendency toward slower progression to kidney failure has been noted in obstructive uropathy compared with other kidney diseases.

Tubular Disease

Types of tubular disease discussed in this section include renal tubular acidoses (RTAs) and inherited tubulopathies.

Renal Tubular Acidoses

The RTAs constitute a diverse group of inherited and acquired disorders affecting the proximal or distal tubule. They are characterized by a hyperchloremic, normal anion gap, metabolic acidosis, and urinary bicarbonate or hydrogen ion excretion inappropriate for the plasma pH. They may result from failure to retain bicarbonate or from inability of the renal tubules to secrete hydrogen ion. Typically, the GFRs in RTAs are normal or slightly reduced, and there is no retention of anions, such as phosphate and sulfate (as opposed to the acidosis of kidney failure). Before attempting to understand the pathology of these conditions, the reader should ensure a good comprehension of normal renal acid-base (and ammonia) regulation (see Chapter 50).

Classification of RTAs is based on the biochemical expression and region of the defect, rather than on an understanding of the exact molecular defect. The three categories of RTA are distal (dRTA, type I); proximal (pRTA, type II); and type IV, which occurs secondary to aldosterone deficiency or resistance. (The term "type III RTA" [mixed proximal/distal defect] has been abandoned by some authors because it is not considered a separate entity.[411] It may arise as the result of a mutation in the gene coding for carbonic anhydrase type 2.[412])

Distal renal tubular acidosis (type I). Type I dRTA occurs most often in infants (sometimes transiently) and young children, but it may also be encountered in adults, in whom it is more common than pRTA. Clinical features generally include metabolic acidosis, muscle weakness, nephrocalcinosis (i.e., diffuse, fine, renal parenchymal calcification), and urolithiasis (i.e., the formation of calculi in the urinary tract). Biochemical features typically include hypokalemia, hypocitraturia, and low urinary ammonium ion. Several subtypes may be seen: urinary pH greater than 5.5 is a common feature.[411,413]

Classic Hypokalemic dRTA (Proton Secretion Defect).

Both inherited and acquired forms exist. There is increasing understanding of the genetic causes of dRTA.[414] Inherited forms are associated with mutations in proteins involved in hydrogen ion secretion, including defects of H+, ATPase and anion exchanger 1, or to mutations in carbonic anhydrase. Loss of function mutations affecting H+, ATPase are usually responsible for autosomal recessive forms of dRTA often associated with early or late sensorineural deafness. Medullary sponge kidney is also a primary cause of dRTA, related to the malformation of the distal tubules. Acquired impairment of the hydrogen ion secretion mechanism leading to dRTA may occur in association with a wide range of conditions, in particular a range of autoimmune disorders (e.g., SLE, Sjögren syndrome, primary biliary cirrhosis, thyroiditis). Some medications, such as topiramate and acetazolamide, can also inhibit carbonic anhydrase leading to dRTA. The pathogenesis of nephrocalcinosis and urolithiasis may be the result of decreased urinary citrate excretion secondary to cellular acidosis.

Back-Leak dRTA (Proton Gradient Defect)

Although the kidney tubule retains the ability to secrete hydrogen ions, the gradient is not maintained because of back-diffusion. Typically, this occurs in association with specific drug treatments (e.g., amphotericin B) that increase the permeability for protons of the apical membrane in the collecting duct, causing back-diffusion of secreted protons.

Voltage-dependent (Hyperkalemic) dRTA

This is due to failure to maintain an intraluminal negative potential and thus to promote hydrogen (and potassium) ion secretion, primarily due to reduced ENaC activity. Both genetic and acquired forms of reduced ENaC activity occur, with the latter being more common, for example in association with chronic urinary tract obstruction, CKD, and treatment with amiloride, cyclosporin, lithium, or triamterene. Voltage-dependent (hyperkalemic) dRTA has many features in common with type IV RTA (see later).

Incomplete dRTA

This is a less severe, normokalemic form, which may represent an early stage of overt dRTA. Some patients acidify urine at a submaximal rate, but at a rate that is generally sufficient to maintain acid-base balance. Potassium wasting, hypokalemia, and hyperchloremia are generally not present. However, when patients are stressed or are given an acid load test, their ability to excrete acid and to lower urine pH is suboptimal and urinary pH may exceed 5.5.

Proximal renal tubular acidosis (type II). In pRTA the primary defect is failure of proximal tubular bicarbonate reabsorption.[415] Proximal RTA may occur as: (1) an isolated defect (primary or sporadic type II pRTA) that occurs chiefly in infant males and, in its autosomal recessive form, is associated with growth retardation, ocular abnormalities, and mental retardation, or (2) as a disorder associated with a generalized proximal tubular disorder (Fanconi renal tubular syndrome [FRTS], see later).[416] Isolated proximal RTA is rare, except for iatrogenic forms associated with the use of carbonic anhydrase inhibitors (e.g., acetazolamide, topiramate). FRTS may be inherited (see later), secondary to nephrotoxic substances (e.g., heavy metal poisoning [lead, mercury, cadmium] and drugs [e.g., ifosfamide, valproic acid, tenofovir]), autoimmune diseases (e.g., Sjögren syndrome, renal transplantation), cancer (e.g., multiple myeloma), or in association with other multisystemic inherited disorders that affect the proximal tubule (e.g., cystinosis, tyrosinemia, galactosemia, hereditary fructose intolerance, Wilson disease, Lowe syndrome).[416] (Note that several of these disorders and agents also cause dRTA.) In pRTA the threshold for bicarbonate reabsorption is lowered (from a plasma concentration of 22 to 15 mmol/L).[411] Once plasma bicarbonate falls below this threshold, filtered bicarbonate is reclaimed, and urinary pH generally will be less than 5.5. In pRTA, contrary to dRTA, nephrocalcinosis and nephrolithiasis are rarely observed but metabolic bone disease is common.

Selective aldosterone deficiency (type IV renal tubular acidosis). In type IV RTA there is failure of distal potassium and hydrogen ion secretion, closely linked to disruption of the central role of aldosterone in acid-base regulation.[417] Type IV RTA results from either aldosterone deficiency (e.g., due to adrenalectomy or mutations in the gene CYP11B2 encoding for the enzyme aldosterone synthase), aldosterone resistance (e.g., due to inactivating mutations in the mineralocorticoid receptor), or from hyporeninemic hypoaldosteronism (e.g., due to diabetic nephropathy, tubulointerstitial disease, urinary obstruction, renal transplantation, or SLE). Hyperkalemia, although mild, is a usual manifestation.

Type IV RTA associated with pseudohypoaldosteronism type 2 (Gordon syndrome) may arise due to mutations in several genes, including *WNK*, which code for proteins that interact with electrolyte transport systems including ROMK and ENaC (Table 49.14).[418]

TABLE 49.14 Characteristics of Some Selected Inherited Tubulopathies

Disorder (OMIM Number)	Protein Defect (Gene)	Inheritance	Clinical Features/Notes	Biochemical Features
Proximal Tubule				
Fanconi renal tubular syndrome 1 (602360)	Glycine amidinotransferase (GATM)	AD	Polyuria, polydipsia, impaired growth, rickets, osteopenia and kidney failure.	Plasma: $\downarrow CO_2$, $\downarrow PO_4$, $\downarrow$uric acid Urine: $\uparrow$LMWP, $\uparrow$AA, $\uparrow PO_4$, $\uparrow$glycosuria
Fanconi renal tubular syndrome 3 (607037)	Enoyl-CoA hydratase and 3-hydroxyacyl CoA dehydrogenase, PBFE (EHHADH)	AD		
Fanconi renal tubular syndrome 4 (600281)	Hepatocyte nuclear factor-4 alpha, HNF-4 (HNF4A)	AD		
Lowe syndrome (oculocerebral dystrophy) (309000)	Inositol polyphosphate-5-phosphatase (OCRL1)	XR	hydrophthalmia, cataract, mental retardation, hypo-reflexia, hypotonia and progressive kidney failure: normotensive	Plasma: $\downarrow K$, $\downarrow CO_2$ Urine: $\uparrow$LMWP, $\uparrow$AA, $\uparrow PO_4$, $\uparrow K$
Wilson disease (277900)	ATPase, Cu++ transporting, beta polypeptide (ATP7B)	AR	liver disease ± neurologic symptoms, or both, Kayser-Fleischer rings, normotensive	Plasma: $\uparrow$free copper, abnormal LFTs Urine: $\uparrow$copper excretion, $\uparrow$LMWP, $\uparrow$AA, $\uparrow PO_4$, $\uparrow$Glycosuria
Dent disease (X-linked recessive hypophosphatemic rickets)(300009)	Chloride voltage-gated channel 5, CLC-5 (CLCN5)	XR	nephrocalcinosis, nephrolithiasis, rachitic and osteomalacic bone disease, progressive kidney failure, normotensive	Plasma: $\downarrow PO_4$, N/$\downarrow K$ Urine: $\uparrow$LMWP, $\uparrow$AA, $\uparrow K$, $\uparrow$Ca, $\uparrow PO_4$, $\uparrow$Glycosuria
X-linked dominant hypophosphatemic rickets (307800)	Phosphate regulating endopeptidase homolog, PHEX (PHEX)	XD	growth retardation, rachitic and osteomalacic bone disease, hypophosphatemia, and renal defects in phosphate reabsorption and vitamin D metabolism	Plasma: $\downarrow PO_4$, $\uparrow$ALP Urine: $\uparrow PO_4$
Loop of Henle				
Bartter syndrome type I (601678)	Solute carrier family 12 (Na/K/Cl transporter), member 1, NKCCT (SLC12A1)	AR	polyuria, polydipsia, muscle weakness, hypovolemia, normotensive or hypotensive (all types). Maternal polyhydramnios, premature birth, perinatal salt wasting, nephrocalcinosis and kidney stones (types I and II), milder phenotype with normocalciuria (type III), sensorineural deafness, motor retardation, renal failure (type IV),	Plasma: $\uparrow$renin, $\downarrow K$, $\uparrow CO_2$, mild $\downarrow Mg$ in some patients Urine: $\uparrow$Ca
Bartter syndrome type II (241200)	Potassium voltage-gated channel subfamily J member 1, ROMK (ROMK)	AR		
Bartter syndrome type III ("classic") (607364)	Chloride voltage-gated channel Kb, CLC-Kb (CLCKB)	AR		
Bartter syndrome type IVa (606412)	Barttin CLCNK type accessory beta unit, Barttin (BSND)	AR		
Bartter syndrome type IVb, digenic (602024)	Chloride voltage-gated channel Ka and chloride voltage-gated channel Kb, CLC-Ka and CLC-Kb (CLCNKA and CLCNKB)	DR		
Hypomagnesemic hypercalciuric] nephrocalcinosis (magnesium-losing kidney)(603959)	Claudin 16 (PCLN1)	AR	nephrocalcinosis, renal failure, ocular/hearing defects, polyuria, polydipsia, recurrent urinary tract infections, recurrent renal colic, normotensive	Plasma: $\downarrow Mg$, $\uparrow$PTH Urine: $\uparrow$Ca, $\uparrow Mg$

TABLE 49.14   Characteristics of Some Selected Inherited Tubulopathies—cont'd

Disorder (OMIM Number)	Protein Defect (Gene)	Inheritance	Clinical Features/Notes	Biochemical Features
Distal Tubule/Collecting Duct				
Liddle syndrome (600760)[a]	Sodium channel epithelial 1 beta subunit, ENaC (activating) (SCNN1B)	AD	early, and frequently severe, hypertension, stroke	Plasma: ↓renin, ↓K, ↓Mg, ↑CO_2, Urine: ↑K
Pseudohypoaldosteronism type Ia (600761)[a]	Sodium channel epithelial 1 gamma subunit, ENaC (inactivating)(SCNN1G)	AR	presents in infancy with salt-wasting and hypotension. Cough, respiratory infections	Plasma: ↑renin, ↓Na, ↑K, ↓CO_2 Urine: ↑K
Pseudohypoaldosteronism type Ib (177735)[a]	Nuclear receptor subfamily 3 group C member 2, mineralocorticoid receptor, MCR (NR3C2)	AD	presents in infancy with salt-wasting and hypotension. Milder than type 1a and remits with age	Plasma: ↑renin, ↓Na, ↑K, ↓CO_2, Urine: ↑K
Pseudohypoaldosteronism type II (Gordon syndrome)(145260)	Various mutations described (WNK4, WNK1, KLHL3,CUL3)	AD	hypertension (± muscle weakness, short stature, intellectual impairment). Correction of physiologic abnormalities by thiazide diuretics	Plasma: ↓renin, ↑K, ↓CO_2, ↑Cl Urine: ↓K
Gitelman syndrome (600968)	Solute carrier family 12 (Na/Cl transporter), member 3, NCCT (SLC12A3)	AR	hypotension, weakness, parasthesias, tetany, fatigue and salt craving. Presentation generally much later in life than in Bartter's and hypocalciuria is typical	Plasma: ↑renin, ↓K, ↓Mg, ↑CO_2, Urine: ↓calcium:creatinine excretion ratio (useful in distinguishing Gitelman and Bartter) (Note: biochemically can mimic thiazide use).
X-linked nephrogenic diabetes insipidus type I (304800)	Arginine vasopressin receptor 2 (ADHRV2R)	XR	hyperthermia, polyuria, polydipsia, dehydration, inability to form concentrated urine, mental retardation if diagnosis delayed. Symptoms in infancy	Hyperosmolar plasma, dilute urine
Nephrogenic diabetes insipidus type II (125800)	Aquaporin 2 (AQP2)	AD and AR	polyuria, polydipsia, dehydration, inability to form concentrated urine. Symptoms after first year of life	Hyperosmolar plasma, dilute urine

[a]See Figure 49.8

Note: This table is not an exhaustive list of the tubulopathies. Some of the material in this table has been adapted from Sayer JA, Pearce SHS,[421]Downie et al.,[423] and from Iancu D, Ashton E.[419] A useful resource for further information is the Online Mendelian Inheritance in Man (OMIM) Website that may be searched using the OMIM numbers given in the table (http://www.ncbi.nlm.nih.gov/entrez/query. fcgi?db=OMIM).

AA, Aminoaciduria; *AD*, autosomal dominant; *AR*, autosomal recessive; *DR*, digenic recessive; *LMWP*, low-molecular weight proteinuria; *XD*, X-linked dominant; *XR*, X-linked recessive.

Diagnosis of renal tubular acidosis. The finding of a hyperchloremic metabolic acidosis in a patient without obvious gastrointestinal bicarbonate losses (e.g., due to excessive diarrhea or small intestinal fistulas) and with no obvious pharmacologic cause should prompt suspicion of an RTA. The presence of suggestive clinical (e.g., nephrocalcinosis in dRTA) or biochemical (e.g., hypophosphatemia and hypouricemia as a result of proximal tubular wasting in pRTA) features should also be considered.

In addition to plasma electrolyte (including potassium) measurement, preliminary investigation should include measurement of urinary pH in a fresh, early morning urine sample. The finding of urine pH greater than 5.5 in the presence of systemic acidosis supports the diagnosis of dRTA, although it is not specific and will also be seen in types II and IV RTAs. If appropriate urinary acidification cannot be demonstrated, further investigation may involve assessing the ability of the kidneys to excrete an acid load (ammonium chloride load test) and to reabsorb filtered bicarbonate (fractional bicarbonate excretion). Additional details on the conduct and interpretation of these tests may be found in a review article.[411]

Treatment of renal tubular acidosis. Treatment of the RTAs is aimed at (1) correcting the biochemical disturbance and, where possible, underlying disorder, (2) improving growth in children, and (3) avoiding the development and progression of CKD. In both type I and II RTAs, bicarbonate is administered to correct the metabolic acidosis. Fludrocortisone and loop diuretics (see later) may be used to treat type IV RTA.

Inherited Tubulopathies

The inherited tubulopathies make up a heterogeneous group of disorders characterized by electrolyte disturbances and being caused by mutations in genes that encode transporter proteins (see Table 49.14). Many are eponymous and have been described clinically for many years, with Bartter and Gitelman syndromes representing the commonest examples. In addition to electrolyte disturbances (particularly of potassium), general reasons to suspect a tubulopathy include a familial disease pattern, renal impairment, nephrocalcinosis, and stone formation, especially if these should present at an early age. In cases in which a diuretic-sensitive channel is affected, these disorders may mimic the effects of diuretic use (see later), and exclusion of covert use of diuretics is important.

While enhanced understanding of the molecular biology of the tubular ion channel and transport pumps has delineated the mechanism of disease in many of these disorders, establishing a genetic diagnosis remains challenging for a variety of reasons. These include the variable clinical picture, overlapping phenotypes, insufficient exploration of the genome—especially of noncoding (intronic) areas, variable penetrance and expressivity of mutations, digenic inheritance patterns, or incomplete knowledge of the genes governing tubular function. Furthermore, acquired disorders may mimic genetic tubulopathies (e.g., a Gitelman-like syndrome as a rare consequence of Sjogren syndrome), large-scale genetic sequencing techniques may yield variants that are subsequently found to be nonpathogenic, disease expression may require the presence of environmental and genetic factors, and, for the rarer conditions, there are a limited number of patients available for study.[419] Variation in some genetic disorders may follow either an autosomal recessive or autosomal dominant pattern. Although phenotypically similar the disease mechanism in such cases may differ. For example, the autosomal dominant form of nephrogenic diabetes insipidus (see later) is caused by AQP2 mutations located toward the C-terminal end of the protein which exert a dominant negative effect.[419] In the United Kingdom, the NHS Genomics Medicine Service has signed off a panel for renal tubulopathies containing 59 genes, of which 43 are validated with high confidence (https://panelapp.genomicsengland.co.uk/panels/292/, accessed June 9, 2020).

Although they are individually uncommon or rare, an awareness of renal tubulopathies is critical for the clinical biochemist when considering the potential differential diagnoses in patients presenting with electrolyte imbalances. A brief description of these disorders follows; for more detailed information, the reader is referred to comprehensive reviews on this subject.[14,419-423] This section should be considered in conjunction with the description of tubular electrolyte handling (see earlier).

Fanconi syndrome. Biochemical features of FRTS include glycosuria, aminoaciduria, hypophosphatemia, hypouricemia, low molecular weight proteinuria, and bicarbonaturia. Patients may present with polyuria, polydipsia, impaired growth, rickets, and osteopenia. Three autosomal dominant forms are recognized; FRTS1, FRTS3, and FRTS4 (see Table 49.14). A fourth, autosomal recessive form (FRTS2) is still debated due to the small number of known cases. The genetic heterogeneity, combined with the many other secondary causes of FRTS, can delay diagnosis and management, increasing the risk of kidney failure which is a later feature of the condition.[419] Secondary causes of FRTS are discussed earlier.

Bartter syndrome. This group of autosomal recessive disorders is characterized by (1) renal salt wasting, (2) polyuria, (3) polydipsia, (4) impaired urinary concentrating ability, (5) a hyperreninemic, hypokalemic metabolic alkalosis, (6) low blood pressure, and (7) a mild hypomagnesemia in some patients. Biochemically, the effects resemble those of loop diuretic use, but clinically, the phenotype is highly variable. This variability arises because of the fact that the syndrome encompasses defects of several different transporters/channels in the loop of Henle. The biochemical effects are predictable from knowledge of the function of these transporters and channels (see Table 49.14; Fig. 49.7).

Mutations in the SLC12A1 and KCNJ1 genes encoding for NKCC2 (type I) or ROMK1 (type II) respectively are associated with the more severe phenotype, including polyhydramnios, premature birth, life-threatening salt wasting in the perinatal period, and hypercalciuria. Patients with ROMK1 defects tend to have less severe hypokalemia.

The milder ("classic," type III) Bartter syndrome is due to defects in the basolateral pump, CLC-Kb. Although the phenotype is extremely variable (neonatal, life-threatening presentations do occur), patients typically present in the first year of life with weakness and hypovolemia and normal urinary calcium excretion. Nephrocalcinosis and kidney stone formation usually are not features.

A fourth variant of Bartter syndrome (type IVa) is due to a mutation in the gene coding for Barttin. Barttin is an essential subunit of CLC-Kb that influences its function and expression in the cell membrane. Bartter syndrome type IV is characterized by severe, early-onset salt wasting, leading to polyhydramnios, premature birth, and inner-ear deafness.[13]

Bartter syndrome type IVb has been described where there is a digenic recessive inheritance pattern, with mutations in both CLCKA and CLCKB, or in both CLCKB and SLC12A3, the latter also being the gene affected in Gitelman syndrome (see later).[419]

Gitelman syndrome. This autosomal recessive disorder is characterized by a hypokalemic, hyperreninemic, hypomagnesemic, metabolic alkalosis. Presentation is generally much later in life than with Bartter syndrome, and hypocalciuria is typical. Clinical features include reduced blood pressure, weakness, paresthesia, tetany, fatigue, and salt craving.[424] The molar urinary calcium/creatinine excretion ratio can be useful in distinguishing between Gitelman (≤ 0.20) and Bartter (> 0.20) syndromes.[425] The molecular defect is in the thiazide-sensitive NCCT transporter (see Fig. 49.7), and the biochemistry can therefore mimic the effects of thiazide use (see later).

Liddle syndrome. This autosomal dominant disorder is characterized by a hypokalemic, hypomagnesemic metabolic alkalosis but, in contrast to Bartter and Gitelman syndromes, hypertension and hyperreninism also occur. The disease is due to mutations which prevent ENaC from being targeted for internalization: mutant channels hence remain at the cell surface resulting in enhanced sodium transport through the channel and consequent enhanced kaliuresis (Fig. 49.8).

Pseudohypoaldosteronism. This condition presents in infancy with salt wasting, hypotension, hyperkalemia, and significant hyperreninism and aldosteronism. Two different molecular mechanisms are causative. Type Ia (autosomal recessive) is caused by inactivating mutations of the ENaC gene, and type Ib (autosomal dominant) is caused by mutations in the mineralocorticoid gene. In both cases, sodium loss in the collecting duct is increased with consequent retention of potassium.

Dent disease. Dent disease is an X-linked condition characterized by hypercalciuria and kidney stone formation, low molecular weight proteinuria, aminoaciduria, hypophosphatemia, rickets, and progression to kidney failure.[426] The disease is most commonly (60% of cases) due to single-base change mutations in the gene coding for the tubular endosomal chloride channel CLC-5. CLC-5 has an important role in proximal tubular endocytosis, accounting for the low molecular weight proteinuria that is seen in Dent disease.[422,427] Reduced uptake of PTH by proximal tubular endocytosis results in increased activation of apical PTH receptors in later segments of the nephron, resulting in reduced phosphate reabsorption and phosphaturia. Increased concentrations of PTH also increase 1,25 dihydroxyvitamin D production, enhancing intestinal calcium absorption and ultimately leading to hypercalciuria which, together with phosphaturia, promotes stone formation.[422] Although X-linked, a mild form of the disease can be seen in females because of lyonization. The related syndromes (1) X-linked recessive nephrolithiasis, (2) X-linked recessive hypophosphatemic rickets, and (3) Japanese idiopathic low molecular weight proteinuria are also all related to defects in CLC-5.[428]

Phosphate disorders. Several disorders of tubular phosphate handling have been described, including X-linked dominant hypophosphatemic rickets (XLH; previously known as vitamin D resistant rickets), autosomal dominant hypophosphatemic rickets, and acquired oncogenic hypophosphatemic osteomalacia. Our understanding of the molecular biology of these and other renal phosphate transport disorders has advanced greatly in recent years.[16,429]

Many other tubulopathies are beyond the scope of this textbook. Features of some of these are described in Table 49.14.

Diuretics

Diuretics are among the most widely prescribed drugs. They are used predominantly to treat hypertension and/or disorders associated with fluid overload. All diuretics act by interfering with tubular reabsorption of sodium and/or chloride, thereby promoting water loss from the peripheral circulation. Diuretics are taken up by tubular cells across the basolateral membrane by specific anion- (e.g., furosemide, thiazides) or cation- (e.g., amiloride, triamterene) exchangers and then are secreted into the lumen through a process that has not been fully elucidated.[430] Different classes of diuretics act at different sites along the nephron. A basic understanding of these processes is helpful in understanding both the potency of different diuretic classes and their importance in the investigation

of electrolyte disorders, in particular hypokalemia. Many diuretics will cause hypokalemia to some degree, depending on potency, dose, duration of treatment, and the patient's underlying potassium balance.

Loop diuretics. Loop diuretics act largely by blocking sodium and chloride reabsorption in the ascending limb of the loop of Henle. Because this is a site at which 30% of sodium reabsorption normally occurs, these are considered potent diuretics. Loop diuretics specifically inhibit NKCC2; therefore they also have an effect on potassium handling in the ascending limb. Consequent changes in transepithelial potential result in a direct kaliuretic effect in this region,[10] causing hypercalciuria (see Fig. 49.7). Loop diuretics also paralyze the macula densa segment, stimulating renin secretion and subsequent aldosterone release, promoting sodium reabsorption and potassium loss in the distal tubule, and so further exacerbating the kaliuresis. Most significantly, blockage of loop sodium reabsorption results in enhanced delivery of sodium ions to the distal tubule, where sodium is reabsorbed in exchange for potassium secretion.[10] The affinity of loop diuretics for NKCC2 is bumetanide>torasemide>piretanide>furosemide>azosemide.[431] The net effect of loop diuretics is that increased sodium chloride with associated water is lost from the body: potassium loss as a result of the various mechanisms described here means that hypokalemia is a common side effect.

Thiazide diuretics. The benzothiadiazine group of compounds inhibits NCCT in the distal tubule. Because only 5 to 10% of sodium reabsorption occurs at this site, these agents are less potent than the loop diuretics, but hypokalemia is still common as a result of increased sodium delivery to the collecting duct. Thiazide diuretics also have secondary effects, resulting in increased calcium reabsorption, which may lead to hypercalcemia.[431]

"Potassium-Sparing" diuretics. These diuretics act by reducing sodium reabsorption in the collecting duct, hence increasing potassium retention. Spironolactone acts as a competitive antagonist of aldosterone, blocking its stimulatory effects on sodium reabsorption via the mineralocorticoid receptor. Both amiloride and triamterene inhibit ENaC. The danger associated with this group of diuretics is that they can induce hyperkalemia; this is particularly likely to occur in patients with kidney disease.

Diabetes Insipidus

Primary functions of the kidney include conservation of water and production of concentrated urine. A range of conditions are associated with disturbances of the renal concentrating mechanism, resulting in polyuria and an inability to produce hypertonic urine. General conditions giving rise to this picture include hypercalcemia, hypokalemia, and CKD. Specifically, diabetes insipidus is due to the absence of a vasopressin effect, caused by impaired or failed secretion (cranial or central diabetes insipidus) or lack of end-organ response to vasopressin (nephrogenic diabetes insipidus). A further disorder, psychogenic polydipsia, or compulsive water drinking can also present as diabetes insipidus. Polyuria is common to both diabetes insipidus and diabetes mellitus, but in diabetes insipidus, no hyperglycemia and no glycosuria are present. These individuals may fail to concentrate urine even in response to fluid restriction or synthetic vasopressin as a result of medullary "washout"; sustained fluid ingestion destroys the hyperosmolality of the medulla, which may take some time to recover. Differentiation and the pathology of these three conditions are discussed in Chapter 55. It should be noted that a vast diuresis can be induced by consumption of excessive fluid volumes (e.g., among heavy beer drinkers).

Congenital nephrogenic diabetes insipidus is associated with defects that have been characterized at the molecular level (Table 49.15).[432] Most (>90%) congenital nephrogenic diabetes insipidus patients have mutations in the AVPR2 gene, which codes for the arginine vasopressin receptor 2.

This results in an X-linked form of diabetes insipidus, with an estimated prevalence of 4 per 1 million males.[432] In less than 10% of cases, diabetes insipidus is caused by mutations in the AQP2 gene. This form of the condition can have both an autosomal dominant and an autosomal recessive inheritance pattern. Downregulation of AQP2 has been observed in a variety of acquired forms of diabetes insipidus, including lithium treatment, hypokalemia, hypercalcemia, ureteric obstruction, and, in animal models, chronic kidney failure.[21] Acquired forms of diabetes insipidus are more common than congenital forms.

TABLE 49.15   Toxic Nephropathy: Causes, Pattern, and Markers

Compound Category	Drug/Toxin	Type of Renal Injury/Pathology	Biomarkers/Notes
Antibacterial agents	Aminoglycosides (e.g., neomycin, gentamicin, tobramycin, amikacin)	Acute tubular necrosis and interstitial nephritis. Nonoliguric AKI	Plasma: ↓K, ↓Mg, ↓Ca urine: ↑LMWP, ↑Glycosuria nephrotoxicity major and common side effect
	Amphotericin	Initially distal tubular injury followed by medullary injury	Plasma: ↓K, ↑creatinine dRTA
Antiviral/antiprotozoal agents	Acyclovir	Nonoliguric AKI due to tubular obstruction and interstitial inflammation	Crystalluria and hematuria
	Pentamidine	Tubular toxicity	Plasma: ↓Mg, ↓Ca urine: ↑Mg, ↑Ca
	Indinavir	Nephrolithiasis, irreversible kidney failure in some patients	Crystalluria and hematuria
Radiocontrast agents	For example, iothalamate, iodixanol	Oliguric or nonoliguric AKI, generally reversible. Proximal tubular damage	↑Plasma creatinine after contrast administration
Antitumor drugs	Cisplatin	Irreversible dose-related and cumulative kidney failure. TIN with heavy proteinuria. Often AKI	Urine: ↑Mg, ↑PO₄, tubular casts and ↑LMWP in early stages
	Methotrexate	Nonoliguric AKI. Tubular atrophy and interstitial fibrosis	Only seen in association with high-dose therapy
	Interleukin-2	Reversible AKI due to ↓RBF	Observed in up to 90% of cases of high-dose therapy
Other drugs	ACE inhibitors	Dramatic ↓GFR due to ↓efferent arteriolar tone	Especially in the setting of bilateral renal artery stenosis ↑plasma creatinine and K
	5-aminosalicylic acid (e.g. mesalazine, olsalazine)	Occasional ATN and irreversible kidney damage	Tubular proteinuria
	Cyclooxygenase (COX)-2 inhibitors	Probably a similar pattern of renal injury to NSAIDs (see below)	
	Lithium	Distal tubular damage with nephrogenic diabetes insipidus + dRTA	
	Penicillamine	Membranous glomerulopathy with NS, occasionally AKI	Proteinuria
	NSAIDs	Several forms of nephropathy identified including (1) hemodynamically mediated AKI, (2) TIN + NS, (3) salt and/or water retention, (4) hyperkalemia, (5) CKD/ESRD (analgesic nephropathy)	Depends on type of effect
Heavy metals	Cadmium	Subtle but irreversible TIN	Fanconi syndrome with RTA. ↑urinary metallothionein
	Gold	Membranous glomerulopathy but normal GFR maintained	Proteinuria <3.5 g/24 h

TABLE 49.15 Toxic Nephropathy: Causes, Pattern, and Markers—cont'd

Compound Category	Drug/Toxin	Type of Renal Injury/Pathology	Biomarkers/Notes
	Lead	Proximal tubular atrophy with interstitial fibrosis	Reversible Fanconi syndrome in children with acute poisoning. In lead workers, urinary proteinuria <2 g/24 h in association with ↑plasma urate, hypertension + gouty arthritis
	Mercury	Proximal tubular damage with ATN	Urine: ↑LMWP
Other environmental agents	Hydrocarbons (e.g., paints, dry cleaning solvents)	ATN, chronic TIN, glomerulonephritis. Caused by renal cytochrome P450 metabolism of chloroform to toxic metabolites	Tubular proteinuria + ↑plasma creatinine
	Paraquat, diquat	ATN secondary to ↓RBF due to shock and direct toxic effects of paraquat. Intrinsic kidney damage due to production of reactive oxygen species	↑Plasma creatinine
Drugs used in transplantation	See Table 59.19		

ACE, Angiotensin converting enzyme; *AKI*, acute kidney injury; *ATN*, acute tubular necrosis; *CKD*, chronic kidney disease; *dRTA*, distal renal tubular acidosis; *ESRD*, end-stage renal disease; *LMWP*, low-molecular weight proteinuria; *NS*, nephrotic syndrome; *NSAIDs*, nonsteroidal anti-inflammatory drugs; *TIN*, tubulointerstitial nephropathy.
The list of agents shown is not exclusive but illustrates the range of compounds that may affect the kidney. For further information readers should consult: Palmer BF, Henrich WL. Toxic nephropathy. In: Brenner BM, editor. *Brenner and Rector's the kidney*. 7th ed. Philadelphia: Saunders; 2004 [Chapter 34].

Assessment of Renal Concentrating Ability: Urinary Osmolality

Urinary concentration can be quantified by measuring specific gravity or by measuring urinary osmolality. For most clinical purposes, measuring specific gravity is probably sufficient,[433] but urinary osmolality measurement is critical in the diagnosis of diabetes insipidus using the water deprivation test (see Chapter 55). Specific gravity may be misleading in certain situations (e.g., in the presence of proteinuria or radiocontrast dyes).

Urinary osmolality may vary widely, depending on the state of hydration. After excessive intake of fluids, for example, the osmotic concentration may fall to as low as 50 mOsm/kg H₂O, whereas in individuals with severely restricted fluid intake, concentrations of up to 1400 mOsm/kg H₂O can be observed. In individuals on an average fluid intake, values of 300 to 900 mOsm/kg H₂O are typically seen. If a random urine specimen has an osmolality of greater than 600 mOsm/kg H₂O (after 12 hours of fluid restriction), it generally can be assumed that the renal concentrating ability is normal.

In chronic progressive kidney disease, the concentrating ability of the tubules is diminished, and in ATN, the urinary osmolality, if there is urine output at all, approaches that of plasma.

Renal Calculi

Nephrolithiasis is the disease condition associated with the presence of renal calculi. Renal calculi, commonly termed *kidney stones*, occur in the renal pelvis, the ureter, or the bladder. In developed countries, bladder stones are now uncommon, because the causative factors of malnutrition and infection have been eliminated.[434] Calcification can also occur scattered throughout the parenchyma (nephrocalcinosis). Kidney stone formation is often considered to be a nutritional

or environmental disease, linked to affluence, but genetic or anatomic abnormalities are significant. Approximately 5 to 10% of the population of the western world are thought to have formed at least one kidney stone by the age of 70 years[434,435] and the prevalence of kidney stones is increasing.[436] A single stone former is defined as a patient who seeks advice for a single, solitary kidney stone episode and who has no other stones seen by imaging in the kidney. A recurrent calcium stone former is a patient with multiple kidney stones, which can occur at the same time or be temporally spaced.[437] For most stone types, there is a male preponderance. The passage of a stone is associated with severe pain called *renal colic*, which may last for 15 minutes to several hours and is commonly associated with nausea and vomiting.[438] Kidney stone formation contributes to the development of CKD[439,440] and has been associated with vascular calcification, a risk factor for cardiovascular disease, hypertension, obesity, and reduced bone mineral density.[441,442]

Background

Chemically, urine contains many mineral salts that are present in concentrations that approach their solubility products at body temperature. Anyone who has seen a urine sample before and after refrigeration has witnessed the consequences of this in the massive crystal deposits that can form on cooling. Crystals can form spontaneously if the salt concentrations are high enough or, alternatively, may bind to organic material, acting as a "seed": hyaluronic acid, a large glycosaminoglycan, has been suggested as one such promoter of crystal formation.[443] Human urine contains a number of promoters of stone formation and a variety of inhibitors, the concentrations of which can be influenced by dietary and metabolic factors (Fig. 49.18).

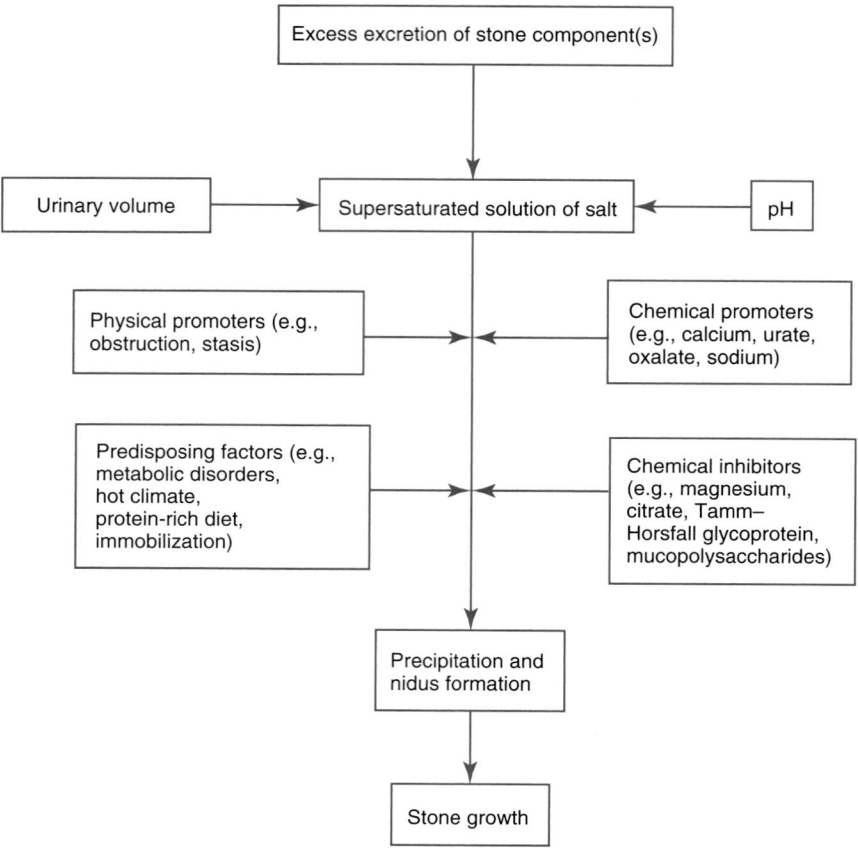

FIGURE 49.18 Diagrammatic representation of the interplay of factors involved in kidney stone formation. High or low pH may act as a promoter or inhibitor of stone formation depending on the stone type in question (e.g., calcium stone formation is favored by inadequate acidification, while urate is less soluble in acidic urine). Controversy exists as to whether formed stones become trapped as they pass through the nephron ("free particle theory"), or whether stone formation occurs at damaged sites on the tubule wall ("fixed particle theory").

Initial diagnosis and investigation of stones require radiologic investigation to explore the degree of intrarenal calcification and papillary damage. Plain x-rays are undertaken at initial presentation, although it should be noted that urate and other purine stones and some cystine stones are radiolucent. An intravenous urogram or spiral CT scan may be performed to establish the presence and extent of urinary tract obstruction, intrarenal reflux, and ureteric dilation. Further investigation of the patient with kidney stones or suspected of being a stone former involves analysis of blood, urine, and the stone itself, should one be obtained.[444]

Small stones (<5 mm in diameter) pass spontaneously in the urine as "gravel." Percutaneous nephrolithotomy (PCNL) is required to remove larger stones, while treatment of stones between 5 mm and 2 cm in diameter is generally undertaken using either retrograde intrarenal surgery (RIRS) or, most commonly, ultrasonic extracorporeal shock wave lithotripsy (ESWL). ESWL allows noninvasive destruction of stones but may be associated with higher recurrence rates than invasive treatment. There are advantages and disadvantages to each of these approaches and this remains an area of active debate. The European Association of Urology (EAU) recommended PCNL for large renal stones (>20 mm), ESWL or RIRS for small renal stones (<10 mm), and RIRS or PCNL for lower calyceal stones sized 10 to 20 mm with unfavorable factors for

ESWL.[445,446] Similar recommendations have been made by NICE.[447] PCNL may be required if ESWL fails. It is the preferred approach for removal of struvite stones[448] and may be required for the treatment of cystine stones, which are more resistant to ESWL than other stone types.[449]

After treatment and successful removal of a stone, follow-up monitoring is required: recurrence rates of 30[450] to 50%[451] are reported. The mechanisms responsible for multiple recurrences of kidney stones in only certain individuals are not completely understood. Factors involved include (1) urine flow (fluid intake); (2) excretion of excess quantities of stone components; (3) the relative absence of a substance, or substances, in the urine that inhibit stone formation; and (4) urinary pH (see Fig. 49.18). The predominant risk factor is poor hydration, with concentrated urine further increasing the concentrations of the mineral salts, predisposing to crystallization. Urinary concentration at least partially explains the increased incidence of kidney stone disease in hot climates, for example, in the Gulf States.

Kidney Stone Analysis

A majority of kidney stones found in the Western world are composed of one or more of the following substances: (1) calcium oxalate with or without phosphate (frequency 67%); (2) magnesium ammonium phosphate (12%); (3) calcium phosphate (8%); (4) urate (8%); (5) cystine (1 to 2%); and (6) complex mixtures of these substances (2 to 3%).[434] These poorly soluble substances crystallize within an organic matrix, the nature of which is not well understood.

When available, analysis of the chemical constituents of stones may be useful in establishing the cause and in planning rational therapy. Stone analysis complements and guides metabolic investigation of the patients and may be particularly useful in identifying rare stone types (e.g., xanthine, dihydroxyadenine), artifacts (e.g., Munchausen syndrome), or drugs precipitating in the urinary tract, such as triamterene[452] and indinavir.[453] Conversely, it has been argued that stone analysis is not useful clinically,[454] because the stone material that is passed often does not represent the initial metabolic derangement. This is a result of the phenomenon known as *epitaxy*, whereby nonspecific stone material, typically arising as a result of UTI (e.g., struvite), may accumulate on a preexisting "metabolic" nidus, the latter of which may not be detected during stone analysis. Clearly, for stone analysis to be useful, it must be accurate. A variety of techniques have been used over the years. Traditionally, stones were crushed and solubilized, and the resulting solution analyzed (at several dilutions when appropriate) with the use of conventional qualitative or semiquantitative chemical methods. Such techniques require relatively large amounts of stone, may miss rare and artefactual material, and analytically often perform poorly.[434] More sophisticated approaches including thermogravimetric analysis,[455] x-ray diffraction crystallography, and, particularly, infrared spectroscopy are preferred, a detailed description of which is beyond the scope of this chapter.[456–458]

Metabolic Investigation of Kidney Stone Formers

Ensuring adequate fluid intake remains the cornerstone of management of stone disease. Specific management of disease depending on the metabolic abnormality present is commonly undertaken, and a treatment rationale is emerging. However, with the exception of urate, there is little evidence to suggest that baseline biochemical evaluation predicts treatment efficacy.[459] Several misconceptions have arisen about the role of diet in stone formation, and optimal treatment at first may appear counterintuitive; some of these paradoxes are discussed here.

Further investigation of stone formers may be guided by knowledge of the type of stone formed. However, increasing use of lithotripsy means that often no stone material is available for analysis. Consequently, a management strategy that focuses on the cause of stone formation and is based on knowledge of blood and urinary composition is useful. Although historically, metabolic investigations have often been targeted at recurrent stone formers only, the increasing availability of simple assays for chemical risk factors and the health economic burden of renal colic suggest that metabolic investigation is likely to become more widespread: indeed a recent consensus conference has recommended metabolic investigation of single stone formers when they are deemed to be at high risk of recurrence (e.g., due to younger age or family history).[437] However, in some instances, it is not possible to demonstrate a biochemical abnormality in stone-forming individuals beyond a persistently small urine volume.

A variety of metabolic screening strategies have been proposed in stone-forming patients.[434,444,460,461] The chosen strategy should balance convenience for the patient and the laboratory against ability to intervene therapeutically. For example, although THG is known to inhibit stone formation, in the absence of a specific treatment, there is little merit in measuring it. A reasonable approach should probably include measurement of plasma sodium, potassium, chloride, bicarbonate, creatinine, calcium, phosphate, and urate, together with 24-hour urinary volume, calcium, magnesium, phosphate, oxalate, urate, creatinine, sodium, citrate, and microbiology (to exclude infection). Additionally, urinary pH and cystine should be measured on a fresh, early morning urine sample. Some investigators have proposed complex "supersaturation indices" that combine the information obtained from these studies in a numeric index.[462–464] Metabolic evaluation should be undertaken at least 6 weeks after the episode of renal colic and ideally should be done on several occasions.[460] Evaluation is most informative when undertaken on an outpatient basis with patients pursuing their normal diet and lifestyle. A brief description of the role of these risk factors is given here, with focus predominantly on the investigation of calcium stone formers. Methodologic approaches to the measurement of urinary oxalate, citrate, and cystine are discussed in Chapter 34.

Calcium. Most of the stones formed in the Western world are composed of calcium, often in association with oxalate, although calcium phosphate and urate may also be present, alone or in combination with calcium oxalate. As a consequence, urinary calcium measurement has been a central investigation. However, the significant role of oxalate is increasingly appreciated, and this has resulted in changes to the optimal management of hypercalciuria. As a rough guide, calcium oxalate stones tend to suggest hyperoxaluria as the main cause, while calcium phosphate stones implicate hypercalciuria and/or failure to adequately acidify urine.[434] A strict definition of hypercalciuria is difficult because of significant overlap between stone-forming and non–stone-forming individuals, but a cutoff of 4 mg/kg body weight (0.1 mmol/kg) is useful.[465,466] Excretion in excess of this, the most common metabolic abnormality seen in calcium stone formers, is observed in up to 50% of patients. The risk of crystal formation is clearly dependent on the concentration of calcium as opposed to its excretion rate.

Traditionally, some investigation strategies focused on whether patients demonstrated hypercalciuria while fasting (*renal hypercalciuria*) or in response to a calcium load (absorptive hypercalciuria)[438] This classification was the basis of an investigative and treatment strategy in patients with absorptive hypercalciuria who have abnormally high intestinal calcium absorption compared with non–stone formers (possibly because of a relative increase in $1,25(OH_2)D_3$ concentration and/or changes in intestinal vitamin D receptor activity). Treatment in these patients focused on dietary modification of calcium intake. Patients with renal hypercalciuria are now thought not to have a renal transport defect, but to have increased turnover of skeletal calcium, although management of such patients may involve pharmacologic modification of renal calcium handling (e.g., thiazide diuretics).[438]

However, convincing evidence questions the usefulness of this classification and these therapeutic approaches. In The Study of Osteoporotic Fractures, increased dietary calcium intake was observed to reduce the likelihood of nephrolithiasis in older women.[467] Dietary restriction of calcium now is generally regarded as ineffective, and actually counterproductive, as it results in an increase in intestinal oxalate absorption with consequent hyperoxaluria and increased risk of stone formation.[468,469] Further, patients with hypercalciuria are known to have reduced bone mineral density, and osteoporotic fractures are commoner in patients with nephrolithiasis:[470] dietary calcium restriction may exacerbate a tendency toward osteopenia and/or osteoporosis.[471,472]

A more useful approach is to classify hypercalciuric patients into hypercalcemic or nonhypercalcemic causes. The former is most commonly due to primary hyperparathyroidism, which is seen in approximately 5% of stone formers, although other causes of hypercalcemia should be considered (e.g., sarcoidosis, vitamin D excess). Treatment involves neck exploration and removal of the adenoma, although the risk of a stone recurring remains high for several years after parathyroidectomy.[473]

Nonhypercalcemic causes of hypercalciuria account for the majority of patients and, generally are classified as idiopathic (although causes such as RTA, high sodium intake, primary hyperoxaluria, enteric hyperoxaluria, chronic diarrhea, and prolonged immobilization should be excluded). It has been recommended that incomplete distal RTA as a cause should be excluded in recurrent calcium stone-forming patients with hypocitraturia and fasting urinary pH greater than 5.8.[437] Most patients with idiopathic hypercalciuria appear to have a generalized acceleration of calcium transport with increased absorption from the gut, increased mobilization from bone, and abnormal renal calcium conservation, all contributing to hypercalciuria.[466,474] In addition to increasing fluid consumption, idiopathic hypercalciuric patients appear to benefit from a diet that is low in animal protein and sodium.[475,476] Animal protein consumption increases the production of metabolic acids, increasing urinary calcium and uric acid excretion and decreasing urinary citrate (see later).[465] High sodium excretion as a result of high consumption inhibits tubular reabsorption of calcium, with a consequent increase in risk of calcium stone formation. Sodium is easily measured in urine and represents a modifiable risk factor. Other therapeutic maneuvers that may be useful include the use of thiazide diuretics or alkaline citrate, reducing oxalate, and increasing fiber intake.[461] Some of these factors are discussed in greater detail in the following sections. A recent systematic review of randomized controlled trial evidence concluded that there were grounds for recommending increased fluid intake for the prevention of recurrence in people who have formed a single calcium stone. For recurrent calcium stone formers the use of citrate, allopurinol, and thiazide diuretics further reduced recurrence risk.[459]

Magnesium. With calcium stone disease, magnesium is an inhibitor of stone growth. Magnesium forms complexes with oxalate that are more soluble than calcium oxalate. Increased urinary magnesium therefore inhibits stone formation.[477] Administration of magnesium has been shown to reduce enteral calcium absorption and has been proposed as a treatment for idiopathic hypercalciuric stone formers.[478] However, oral magnesium supplementation may have unpleasant side effects, and a positive benefit in terms of reducing stone recurrence has not been demonstrated.[461]

Urate. Some investigators believe that urate may potentiate calcium stone formation, although this has been questioned.[479] However, hyperuricosuria is common in calcium stone forming patients, termed hyperuricosuric calcium urolithiasis (HUCU), and treatment with allopurinol, possibly

by decreasing urate synthesis, reduces the rate of stone recurrence. Allopurinol treatment is therefore recommended for patients with HUCU.[437,461] Formation and management of pure urate stones are discussed in Chapter 34.

Oxalate. Hyperoxaluria is a powerful promoter of calcium oxalate stone formation; indeed, it is more significant in this respect than calcium itself.[434] Oxalate is an end product of metabolism, predominantly derived from breakdown of glyoxylate and glycine. The plasma concentration of oxalate is 1.0 to 2.4 mg/L (11 to 27 μmol/L), and it is excreted in the urine at a rate of 17.5 to 35.1 mg/day (200 to 400 μmol/day).[480] Day-to-day within individual variability in oxalate excretion has been reported to be approximately 16%.[481] Daily excretion is independently and positively associated with increased weight, BMI, vitamin C intake, and the presence of diabetes.[481]

Hyperoxaluria may occur as a result of excessive dietary intake, because of malabsorption and/or steatorrhea (enteric hyperoxaluria), or because of an inborn error of metabolism (primary hyperoxaluria). Enteric hyperoxaluria commonly occurs in association with inflammatory bowel disease and may contribute to an increased incidence of stone formation in such patients.[480] Fat malabsorption contributes to the formation of calcium fatty acid complexes ("soaps") in the intestine, increasing the enteric concentration of unbound oxalate that is absorbed through the damaged bowel wall. Primary hyperoxaluria may be type 1 (glycolic aciduria) or type 2 (L-glyceric aciduria). Patients with type 1 disease present in the first decade of life with recurrent calcium oxalate nephrolithiasis. Inheritance is autosomal recessive and survival is poor. Type 2 disease is rarer and has been claimed to run a milder course, despite the passage of similarly high concentrations of urinary oxalate. The urinary excretion of oxalate may increase to approximately 60 mg/day (700 μmol/day) when a diet containing an excess of oxalate-rich foods is taken, and to as much as 260 mg/day (3 mmol/day) in patients with primary hyperoxaluria.

A dietary history may be useful in the evaluation of calcium oxalate stone formers. Patients who are excreting large amounts of oxalate are often offered dietary advice to modify their risk of future stone formation. Foods rich in oxalate include spinach, beets, tea, sorrel, wheat bran, strawberries, rhubarb, blackcurrants, peanuts, and chocolate.[434,438,461] However, only 10 to 15% of urinary oxalate is derived directly from dietary sources[461] and the relationships between oxalate intake and both risk of nephrolithiasis[482] and urinary oxalate excretion[481] are weak. Furthermore, severe restriction of oxalate-rich foods would result in lower intakes of fruits, vegetables, and whole grains which are known to provide other major health benefits. Paradoxically, epidemiologic evidence has actually demonstrated a protective effect of high tea consumption.[469] This has been attributed to the low bioavailability of oxalate in tea and the inhibition of tubular vasopressin action by caffeine. It has been recommended that calcium-oxalate stone formers with hypercalciuria should maintain a dietary calcium intake not lower than 1000 mg/day, a sodium intake not higher than 2.4 g/day (or 6 g of salt), and a moderate intake of nondairy animal protein (i.e., 0.8 g/kg body weight or less).[437] Measurement of urinary oxalate is discussed in Chapter 34.

Citrate. Urinary citrate inhibits stone formation by forming soluble complexes with calcium. It is present in the diet in many fruits. Excretion (typically between 120 and 930 mg/day [0.6 and 4.8 mmol/day] for adult males and between 250 and 1160 mg/day [1.3 and 6.0 mmol/day] for adult females)[434] is reduced in the calcium stone forming population, with 50% of stone formers demonstrating hypocitraturia in one study.[450] Urinary citrate measurement may be of value in the assessment of stone-forming risk, particularly in the setting of distal RTA, where the reduction in filtered bicarbonate appears to increase tubular reabsorption of citrate with consequent hypocitraturia.[483] Inadequate urinary acidification compounds the increased risk of calcium stone formation. Treatment with carbonic anhydrase inhibitors (e.g., acetazolamide,[484] topiramate)[485,486] mimics distal RTA with a consequent increase in stone risk. Hypocitraturia may also be seen in malabsorption and UTI. Calcium-oxalate stone formers with low urinary citrate excretion should increase their intake of fruits and vegetables and limit nondairy animal protein.[437] Administration of oral alkaline citrate increases urinary citrate concentration by increasing the pH of tubular cells. It has been shown to be effective in the treatment of nephrolithiasis,[459] although side effects are reported and compliance is poor. Oral citrate treatment is indicated in recurrent calcium oxalate and calcium phosphate stone formers with: (1) low or relatively low urinary citrate excretion; (2) complete or incomplete distal RTA, chronic diarrheal states, drug induced or diet-induced hypocitraturia; and (3) osteopenia/osteoporosis.[437] Measurement of urinary citrate is discussed in Chapter 34.

Struvite stones. Struvite stones (also called *triple phosphate* or *infection stones*) are composed of magnesium ammonium phosphate hexahydrate. Struvite stones may form in the kidney or bladder. The formation of struvite stones requires UTI with urease-producing organisms, including both gram-negative and gram-positive species from the genera *Proteus, Staphylococcus, Pseudomonas, Providencia,* and *Klebsiella.*[448] When urease is present, water and urea are hydrolyzed to form carbon dioxide and ammonia, which then hydrolyze further to form ammonium and bicarbonate. If urinary pH is greater than 7.2 struvite will form from the product of ammonium and naturally occurring cations in urine such as magnesium and phosphate (carbonate apatite will form if the pH is 6.8 to 7.2).[448]

Struvite stones are more common in females and in certain patient populations (e.g., paraplegic individuals, people with congenital urinary tract malformation or stasis due to urinary tract obstruction).[448] The risk of progression to CKD appears higher in patients who develop infection stones than in those with other forms of stone disease.[439]

Cystinuria

Cystinuria is an inherited condition in which excessive urinary excretion of cystine results from a defect in proximal renal tubular reabsorption.[g] In the most common form of the disease, there is also excess excretion of the dibasic amino acids (lysine, ornithine, and arginine). These share the same renal tubular transporter, although their presence in excess in urine appears benign. More rarely, isolated cystinuria is seen. This phenotypic classification has been superseded by

increased understanding of the genetic basis of the disease. Mutations in either of the genes coding for two components of the dibasic amino acid transport system (SLC3A1 [Type A cystinuria] and SLC7A9 [Type B cystinuria]) cause cystinuria. More than 200 mutations have been reported. Type A is generally a recessive condition so affected individuals will have genotype AA, but some heterozygotes may develop cystinuria. Type B is usually a dominant condition, but with variable penetrance; both B and BB genotypes may develop cystinuria. Some patients have mutations in both genes (Type AB cystinuria). Occasionally there are more than two mutated alleles present (e.g., AAB or ABB).[487] A small percentage of patients with cystinuria do not have mutations in either of these genes.[449] There does not appear to be a clear genotype-phenotype association.[487]

The normal urinary excretion of cystine has been reported to be 5 to 48 mg/day (40 to 400 µmol/day).[434] Its relatively low limit of solubility, 18 mg/dL (1500 µmol/L),[438] is exceeded in many patients with cystinuria,[434] resulting in the formation of hexagonal crystals and, ultimately, cystine stones. Cystinuria may present at any age from infancy to old age, although presentation is most common in the second and third decades.[449,487] Cystinuria is often recurrent and associated with large kidney stones, including staghorn calculi and renal impairment.[487]

The finding of a cystine stone should prompt confirmation of cystinuria by urinary analysis.[434] It could be argued, however, that all stone formers should be screened for cystinuria; at least 10% of cystinuric individuals form stones in which cystine cannot be detected, presumably because of epitaxy.[488] The index of suspicion should be increased in patients who are relatively young (<30 years old) stone formers and in those with recurrent or bilateral stones or a positive family history.[449] Once a cystinuric patient is diagnosed, it is important to screen all members of the family, particularly to detect affected siblings.

Treatment of cystinuria is aimed at keeping cystine below its saturation point by maintaining high fluid intake (>3 L/day), particularly at night. Other treatments include reducing cystine (found in animal protein) and salt intake, urinary alkalinization (e.g., with potassium citrate—cystine is more soluble in alkaline urine) and chelation with thiol-binding drugs (e.g., D-penicillamine or –mercaptopropionylglycine [tiopronin]).[449] Quantitative analysis is an important adjunct for monitoring penicillamine therapy, which can be optimized on the basis of free cystine versus cystine/penicillamine disulfide. Penicillamine itself may cause glomerular damage; thus regular monitoring of urinary protein excretion is recommended. Measurement of urinary cystine is discussed in Chapter 34.

Toxic Nephropathy

A wide variety of nephrotoxins exist in the environment, in some cases associated with particular occupations (e.g., heavy metals, such as cadmium and lead). Both glomerular and tubulointerstitial damage may result from exposure to toxins; detection of both requires biochemical monitoring of GFR/serum creatinine concentration and tubular and glomerular proteinuria. Anatomic physiologic and biochemical features make the kidney susceptible to insult from a variety of medicinal and environmental agents. Factors contributing to the sensitivity of the kidney include its large blood flow, the

---

[g]The reader should note that cystinuria should not be confused with cystinosis, which is a condition associated with intracellular accumulation of cystine but not with excess urinary excretion of cystine.

TABLE 49.16 Laboratory Support for Dialysis Programs

Clinical Condition	Laboratory Tests
Acute Dialysis	
Dialysis disequilibrium	Urea and electrolytes, bicarbonate, calcium
Pyrexia	C-reactive protein, white cell count, blood cultures
Bleeding	Clotting screen, platelets
Chronic Dialysis Programs	
Anemia	Ferritin, transferrin saturation, B12, folate
	Blood film, PTH, C-reactive protein
Sepsis	C-reactive protein, blood, urine specimens for microscopy, culture and sensitivity.
Nutrition	Albumin, phosphate
Cardiovascular disease risk	Lipid profile
Dialysis-related amyloid	β_2-microglobulin (not routinely measured)
CKD-MBD	Predialysis plasma calcium, phosphate (monthly in hemodialysis patients; 3-monthly in peritoneal dialysis patients)
	Alkaline phosphatase
	PTH (at least every 3 months)
	Aluminum in patients receiving aluminum-based phosphate binders (3-monthly) (Historical as drug no longer manufactured)
Adequacy of hemodialysis as assessed by urea clearance	Predialysis and postdialysis urea
Sepsis, abdominal pain in peritoneal dialysis	Microscopy and culture of peritoneal dialysate
Adequacy of peritoneal dialysis as assessed by weekly small solute clearance	Dialysate creatinine, urea
Peritoneal membrane characteristics assessed by peritoneal equilibration test (PET)	Plasma and dialysate glucose and creatinine

CKD, Chronic kidney disease; *MBD,* mineral and bone disorder; *PTH,* parathyroid hormone.

concentration of filtered solutes during urine production, and the presence of a variety of xenobiotic transporters and metabolizing enzymes. Toxic nephropathy commonly occurs as a result of decreased renal perfusion, because of precipitation within the tubule, or because of direct toxic effects at the proximal tubule level. In some cases the conjugation of environmental chemicals (e.g., mercury, cadmium) to glutathione and/or cysteine targets these chemicals to the kidney, where inhibition of renal function occurs through a variety of mechanisms that are not completely understood. Although some drugs can cause kidney damage in the presence of normal renal function, a far greater variety of drugs can cause problems in patients with kidney disease, predominantly because of accumulation resulting from decreased renal elimination. A list of drugs and environmental toxins commonly known to cause kidney damage is given in Table 49.16.

RENAL REPLACEMENT THERAPY

RRT includes dialysis procedures such as HD, PD, continuous HF, and continuous HDF. These techniques are used to temporarily or permanently remove toxic substances from the blood when the kidneys cannot satisfactorily remove them from the circulation. In addition, kidney transplantation has become an effective form of RRT. Among prevalent ESRD patients in the United States in 2017, 63% used HD as their RRT, 7% used PD, and 30% had a functioning kidney transplant.[91] Extensive laboratory support is required by an RRT program (Table 49.16).

Background

In 1861, Thomas Graham Bell in Glasgow, Scotland, carried out the first dialysis experiments (and coined the term *dialysis*), separating crystalloids and colloids in a solution. Bell predicted that this technique could have medical application, but this was not realized until nearly 100 years later in the work of Willem Kolff and then Belding Scribner, who made HD a feasible treatment in the early 1960s. Since that time, HD and more recently PD have extended the lives of many people, sometimes for up to 20 or 30 years.

Dialysis

Dialysis is the process of separating macromolecules from ions and low molecular weight compounds in solution based on the difference in their rates of diffusion through a semipermeable membrane, through which crystalloids can pass readily but colloids pass very slowly or not at all. Two distinct physical processes are involved: diffusion and ultrafiltration.

The timing of initiation of dialysis treatment is controversial and requires judgment, taking into account the treatment of metabolic consequences of advanced CKD, the comorbidities of the patient, and the accepted impact of dialysis treatment on quality of life. No absolute recommendation of commencement of dialysis based on GFR alone can be made. KDIGO suggest that dialysis be initiated when one or more of the following are present: symptoms or signs attributable to kidney failure (serositis, acid-base or electrolyte abnormalities, pruritus); inability to control volume status or blood pressure; a progressive deterioration in nutritional status refractory to dietary intervention; or cognitive impairment. This often but not invariably occurs in the GFR range between 5 and 10 mL/min/1.73 m².[90] Not all individuals will be suitable for RRT and in this setting it is important that the multidisciplinary team facilitates care for people on the "conservative management" pathway.[90] The US Renal Data System reports that 14.1% of incident patients starting dialysis in 2016 had an estimated GFR below 5 mL/min.1.73 m², and during 2016 the mean estimated GFR at initiation of dialysis was 9.7 ml/min/1.73 m².[489]

Hemodialysis and Hemofiltration

HD is the method most commonly used to treat advanced and permanent kidney failure with 87% of incident patients requiring RRT in the United States in 2016 receiving HD (almost 10% received PD and fewer than 3% had a kidney transplant).[489] Clinically, it is considered the default therapy that is utilized in patients unsuitable for the alternate modalities of PD and kidney transplantation. Operationally, it involves connecting the patient to a circuit, into which his or her blood flows to and from a semi-permeable large surface area membrane, the hemodialyzer. After filtration to remove wastes and extra fluid, the cleansed blood is returned to the patient. This is a complicated and inconvenient therapy requiring a coordinated effort from a health care team that includes the patient, nephrologist, dialysis nurse, dialysis technician, dietitian, and others.

Description. HD utilizes diffusive and convective mass transfer across a semipermeable membrane. The driving force for diffusion is the concentration gradient between blood and dialysate. Smaller solutes with larger concentration gradients give increased diffusion. The concentration gradient is maintained by using countercurrent flows and high flow rates. Anticoagulated blood is pumped in one direction across the membrane, and the recipient fluid, the dialysate, flows at a rate of 500 to 800 mL/min in the opposite direction, as shown in Fig. 49.19. Water molecules and small

molecular weight molecules can cross the membrane, while larger proteins and cellular elements are retained in the vascular space. Convection is the bulk movement of solvent and dissolved solute across the membrane, down a transmembrane hydrostatic pressure gradient. The most important functional part is the dialyzer membrane. Biocompatibility of the dialyzer membrane is an essential requirement because of high surface areas and long contact times. Patients are dialyzed in home-based or hospital-based units, with dialysis usually performed three times a week for sessions lasting between 3 and 5 hours. This dialysis schedule is largely empirical, insofar as it reconciles adequate treatment with breaks between treatments to provide the patient with a reasonable quality of life. Approaches to increase the dose of dialysis have been explored. These include short daily HD that entails a 2- to 3-hour dialysis on 6 days per week.[490] Alternatively, slow overnight dialysis for 5 to 7 nights has been employed. These regimens have been reported to improve outcome.[490–492] The FHN Trial, in which patients received six HD sessions per week, demonstrated improved mortality, biochemical parameters, and LV mass.[186]

HD relies on good vascular access to the circulation of the patient to enable blood to be pumped around the extracorporeal circuit at a rate in excess of 300 mL/min. Suitable vascular access was not achieved until the 1960s. Although Kolff at Groningen Hospital in the Netherlands performed the first dialysis experiments in humans in 1943, the problem of dialysis support with long-term vascular access was not solved until Scribner developed the arteriovenous cannula in 1960. This advance was followed by the development of the surgically created arteriovenous fistula (AVF), introduced by Brescia and coworkers in 1966, which provided permanent vascular access. The Dialysis Outcomes Practice Patterns Study (DOPPS) confirmed a wide variation in how dialysis is achieved throughout the world. For example, most patients in Germany have an AVF as their main access, whereas in the United States a fistula was used for access in only 13% of

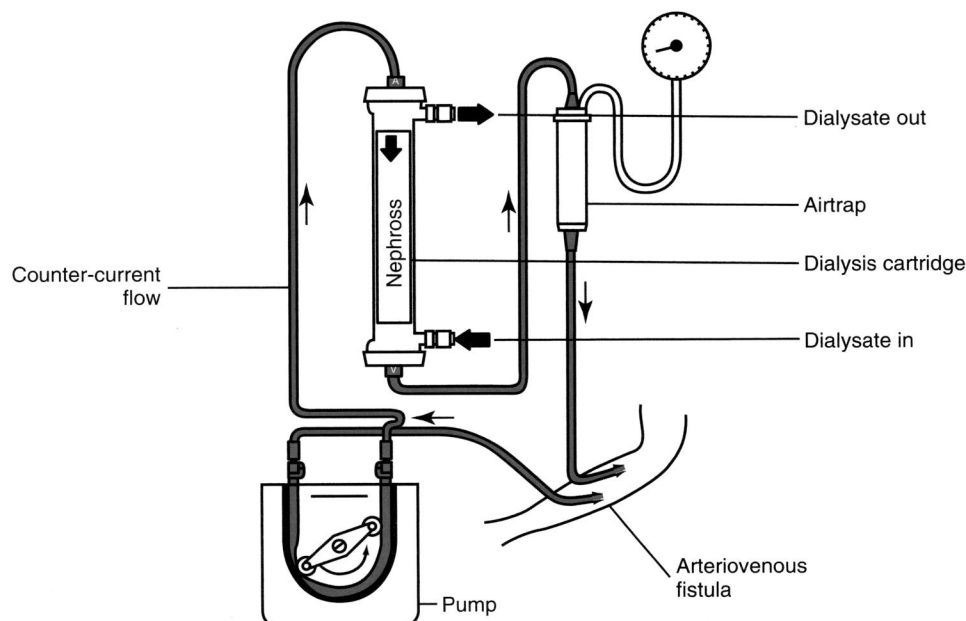

FIGURE 49.19 A hemodialyzer setup.

patients for their first dialysis in 2006,[98] reflecting suboptimal pre-ESRD care. AVF survival is longer in Europe than in the United States. However, recent coalition initiatives exemplified by the Fistula First Breakthrough Initiative (FFBI) and the K/DOQI Work Group have delivered service improvements with national AVF prevalent rates reported at 63% as of March 2015.[493] When used as a patient's first access, AVF survival is considered superior to arteriovenous grafts regarding time to first failure. It is of course salutary to note that 80% of patients in 2016 were using a central venous catheter at their first dialysis in the United States, indicating that few patients had viable definitive vascular access in preparation for starting RRT.[489]

Conventional HD uses low-flux dialyzers, allowing diffusive but little convective solute removal. Middle molecule clearance is poor. HF is a convective treatment. Although middle molecule clearances are improved, small molecule clearance is poor. HF is used for continuous treatment in ICU settings in the management of AKI. In addition, acute HD and continuous filtration in ICU are utilized in acute poisoning with for example, ethylene glycol and lithium. High-flux HD using biocompatible membranes allows convective and diffusive solute removal. The use of very pure water is crucial in high-flux modes because dialysis fluid is infused directly into the bloodstream by back-filtration. The Hemodialysis (HEMO) Study, a randomized clinical trial designed to determine whether increasing the dose of dialysis or using a high-flux dialyzer membrane alters major outcomes, concluded that patients undergoing HD thrice weekly derived no major benefit from a higher dialysis dose than that recommended by current United States guidelines, or from the use of a high-flux membrane.[494] However, subgroup analysis suggested benefit in patients maintained on dialysis for longer than 3.7 years and in those with diabetes.[495] The Membrane Permeability Outcome study group reported similar results[496] and the KDOQI recommends the use of high-flux membranes.[497]

HDF is HD in which fluid removal exceeds the desired weight loss, and fluid balance is maintained by the infusion of a sterile pyrogen-free solution. HDF offers the advantages of both HD and HF in a single therapy. The replacement fluid is generated "online" from concentrated bicarbonate, and 20 to 30 L of water is used per session.[498] The result is that HDF provides a 10 to 15% increase in urea clearance compared with HD along with increased middle molecule clearances. Water for online preparation of substitution solution should meet common standards for dialysis water regarding chemical contaminants but should be of higher quality regarding microbiological contaminants. Online HDF has been used extensively in continental Europe over the past 30 years or so.

After several years of HD, patients may develop carpal tunnel syndrome and evidence of amyloid deposition. The main constituent of dialysis-related amyloid is β_2-microglobulin. Circulating concentrations of β_2-microglobulin can be as high as 300 to 400 mg/L. Although no correlation is noted between circulating β_2-microglobulin concentration and risk of amyloidosis, evidence from the HEMO study indicates that concentrations are correlated with survival.[499] Retrospective data from Italy indicate that there is a 5% risk that carpal tunnel decompression surgery will be required after 8 years of extracorporeal therapy, and that a reduction in risk of 42% is seen in those patients treated by HDF and HF compared with conventional HD.[500] It is suggested that patients

on PD are less prone to developing amyloidosis. Although there is signaling that there is a survival advantage depending on modality, with improved survival in HDF treated patients,[501] it is uncertain whether this is genuine to the modality or represents bias from patient selection, since a good AVF is necessary to perform HDF efficiently. The High-volume Haemodiafiltration versus High-flux Haemodialysis Registry Trial (H4RT, available at: https://www.bristol.ac.uk/population-health-sciences/projects/h4rt-trial/, accessed April 17, 2020), is designed to answer this question.

Fluid management on HD is crucial for patient well-being and survival. Because conventional dialysis is based on a thrice weekly schedule, fluid is accumulated by the patient between dialysis sessions. Many patients are anuric or at least oliguric; therefore unrestricted fluid intake would result in fluid overload and complications of pulmonary edema and hypertension. Patients receiving HD are advised to restrict fluid intake to 1 L/day or so. This allowance is recommended to the individual patient by the dialysis nursing staff and the dietician to ensure that adequate nutrition is maintained. Nevertheless, many patients find the fluid restriction very difficult to maintain; therefore large weight gains between dialysis sessions are a common occurrence. During the dialysis session, the patient's "dry" or "target" weight is achieved. At dry weight, the fluid compartments are normal; this value is determined by gradually reducing weight until the patient is edema-free and reaches the point below which hypotension occurs on further fluid removal. The dry weight is difficult to reach in patients with abnormal cardiovascular responses, who may become hypotensive despite being relatively fluid replete.

When HD is begun, most patients have a small amount of residual renal function (RRF). This level of RRF may persist for many months and years; the volume of urine produced each day allows greater fluid intake and provides the benefit of reducing large fluctuations in body fluid volumes. RRF should be taken into consideration when dialysis prescriptions are adjusted. The K/DOQI Work Group 2006 updates include recommendations, as opposed to guidelines (opinion-based rather than evidence-based), for preserving RRF in patients receiving HD.[497]

Assessment of adequacy of hemodialysis. Assessment of adequacy of dialysis treatment for individual patients in the clinical setting includes consideration of the patient's well-being, cardiovascular risk, nutritional status, and degree of achievable ultrafiltration. It also includes estimates of a number of laboratory parameters such as hemoglobin, phosphate, and albumin, and clearance of the small solutes, urea and creatinine. Although a full description of adequacy is beyond the scope of this text, a brief outline will be provided. Urea removal is typically defined by the "Kt/V_{urea}." This ratio is a measure of the amount of plasma cleared of urea ($K \times t$, where t = time in hours) divided by the urea distribution volume (V). The urea distribution volume is considered equivalent to the total body water.[502] Kt/V during a dialysis session is calculated following determination of predialysis and postdialysis plasma urea concentrations, the time of the dialysis session, RRF, total clearance predicted from the dialyzer, and blood and dialysate flow rates. These variables are processed using computerized mathematical formulas. The Kt/V effectively describes the *power* of the dialysis session and continues to be valued as the most precise and accurate measure of dialysis.[497] A retrospective analysis of the National Cooperative Dialysis Study (NCDS) was the first study to identify a threshold in level of Kt/V and survival in HD.[503] In practice, a simple calculation may be performed to obtain an estimate of dialysis adequacy: the urea reduction ratio (URR). The URR is the percentage fall in plasma urea attained during a dialysis session and is measured as follows:

$$[(\text{Predialysis } \{\text{urea}\} - \text{postdialysis } \{\text{urea}\})/$$
$$(\text{predialysis } \{\text{urea}\})/(\text{pre})] \times 100\%$$

Observational studies in populations of dialysis patients have shown that variations in URR are associated with major differences in mortality.[504]

Following publication of the HEMO study,[494] the KDOQI Work Group 2006 update recommended that the target dose of delivered dialysis as calculated by Kt/V urea kinetic modeling was 1.4 per dialysis session. This dose is consistent with the target single pool Kt/V of approximately 1.4 set by the European Standards Group[505] and is roughly equivalent to a URR of 70% per dialysis for a patient receiving thrice weekly HD.

Peritoneal Dialysis

PD is a type of dialysis in which dialysate is passed into the patient's peritoneal cavity, with the peritoneum then employed as the dialysis membrane. It was first explored by Ganter in 1923 and initially showed poor results. The modern era of PD started in 1953, with intermittent irrigation of the peritoneal cavity with commercially prepared solutions and access achieved through a single disposable catheter (Fig. 49.20). Popovich and coworkers in 1976 introduced the concept of portable equipment; this approach led to the use of continuous ambulatory peritoneal dialysis (CAPD),[506] a type of PD performed in ambulatory patients during normal activities. Use of PD varies between countries depending on access to HD. For example, in the United Kingdom during 2017, at Day 90 19% of incident patients were receiving PD (compared to 65% receiving HD, and 10% with a functioning transplant: 6% had died or stopped treatment),[103] whereas in Mexico, 74% of patients receive PD.[507]

Description. Operationally, PD uses the patient's own peritoneal membrane (surface area approximately 2 m^2), across which fluids and solutes are exchanged between the peritoneal capillary blood and the dialysis solution placed in the peritoneal cavity. Fluid removal (ultrafiltration) is achieved by using dialysis fluids containing high concentrations of dextrose acting as an osmotic agent; as dextrose passes across the peritoneal membrane the concentration gradient diminishes and the rate of fluid removal decreases. Conventional therapies use four daily exchanges of approximately 2 L of fluid with approximately 10 L of spent dialysate generated (including ultrafiltration). RRF is critical to the success of PD because only a few milliliters per minute can contribute substantially to urea clearance and creatinine clearance (C_{Cr}), with each additional milliliter resulting in an extra 10 L of clearance per week. Practical reasons for opting for PD include (1) preservation of RRF and vascular access sites, (2) a home treatment facilitating increased patient autonomy, (3) flexibility as to where the treatment can be administered, and (4) ease of self-treatment, with lower capital costs involved. Blood pressure control and extremes of fluid shifts are not as problematic as those that occur on conventional HD.

Automated PD is now widely available. It requires a programmable machine to regulate flow, dwell time, and drainage, and it may be performed at night. Solute clearance can be increased by leaving fluid in the peritoneum during the day and by performing an additional daytime exchange.

The main disadvantage of PD is the risk of infection causing peritonitis. Incidence rates of peritonitis have decreased over the years with the introduction of disconnect PD systems, improved training of patients with regard to meticulous hygiene, and microbiological surveillance protocols. The International Society for Peritoneal Dialysis currently recommend reporting peritonitis rates as number of episodes per patient-year and that this should be no more than 0.5.[508]

Peritonitis typically presents with a cloudy dialysate effluent and abdominal pain. Additional features such as vomiting and a high temperature suggest serious infection. Blood and dialysate samples should be taken for urgent microbiological analysis and antibiotics administered via the dialysis catheter directly into the peritoneum. If antibiotic treatment fails, then the catheter is removed and the patient converted to HD. In the majority of cases, the episode of peritonitis responds to treatment and PD can continue, although it is likely that repeated episodes will cause scarring and fibrosis of the peritoneal membrane with permanent loss of ultrafiltration. Long-term serious complications may occur, such as sclerosing encapsulating peritonitis caused by adhesions and peritoneal thickening encasing the peritoneal contents and causing bowel obstruction. This unusual condition is associated with increased frequency of peritonitis episodes and longer duration of PD.[509]

Assessment of adequacy in peritoneal dialysis. Measures of PD solute removal (urea and creatinine) correlate with patient status and clinical outcome.[510–512] In particular, a multicenter prospective cohort study of 680 incident CAPD

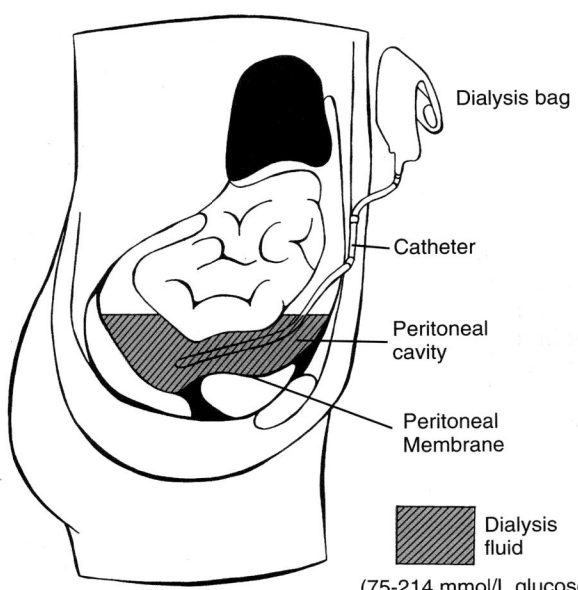

Dialysis bag

Catheter

Peritoneal cavity

Peritoneal Membrane

Dialysis fluid

(75-214 mmol/L glucose)

FIGURE 49.20 Diagrammatic sketch of peritoneal dialysis. (Redrawn from Nolph KD. Peritoneal anatomy and transport physiology. In: Maher JF, editor. *Replacement of renal function by dialysis.* 3rd ed. Kluwer Academic Publishers/Springer: Dordrecht, The Netherlands 1989 [Chapter 23].) To convert glucose concentration in mmol/L to mg/dL, multiply by 18.

patients (Canada-United States [CANUSA] Study) showed that a decrease of 0.1 in weekly urea clearance ratio (defined by Kt/V_{urea}) was associated with a 5% increase in the relative risk of death.[513] Similarly, a decrease of 5 L/wk/1.73 m^2 of total C_{Cr} was associated with a 7% increase in the RR of death. As a consequence of these studies, national guidelines from the United Kingdom[514] and the United States[515] have set standards of dialysis adequacy in terms of small solute removal. An estimate of adequacy is performed in all patients within 6 to 8 weeks of commencement of dialysis. Additional studies should be performed at least every 6 months.[514]

Obtaining the weekly Kt/V_{urea} requires measurement of the volume of spent dialysate and urine for a complete 24-hour period. The concentration of urea in dialysate (D) compared with plasma (P) is calculated (the D/P ratio), and this value is then multiplied by the volume of the drained effluent to obtain an estimate of Kt. The calculation of "V," or the volume of distribution of urea, is derived from an estimate of total body water.[516,517] An estimate of weekly Kt/V_{urea} is simply the daily clearance multiplied by a factor of seven. These equations are used for both peritoneal and renal clearance, and the total weekly clearance is obtained by addition. Calculation of C_{Cr} is based on the following clearance (C) formula:

$$C = [U (or\ D) \times V]/P$$

where U is the concentration of creatinine in urine or dialysate, V is the mean daily drain volume or urine volume (measured in liters), and P is the concentration of creatinine in the plasma. The daily clearances obtained for both urine and dialysate are added together and multiplied by seven for the total weekly C_{Cr}. Current recommendations from the United Kingdom Renal Association include a combined urinary and peritoneal Kt/V_{urea} greater than 1.7/wk or a creatinine clearance greater than 50 L/wk/1.73 m^2, which should be considered as reflecting minimal treatment doses. The dose should be increased in patients experiencing uremic symptoms.[514]

Compliance with complete collections is mandatory. To reduce sampling errors in patients who void infrequently, urine is collected over a 48-hour period. Dialysate sampling requires that all effluent bags obtained over a 24-hour period should be brought to the center renal unit; this can be difficult because the bags are heavy and bulky. Glucose concentrations in PD bags may reach 3852 mg/dL (214 mmol/L): it is important that glucose interference in the dialysate creatinine measurement is corrected for when Jaffe assays are used[518] or minimized by the use of an enzymatic creatinine method.[519] An adjunct to assessment of adequacy in PD patients is the peritoneal equilibration test (PET),[520] which assesses peritoneal membrane transport characteristics in terms of creatinine clearance, glucose absorption, and ultrafiltration. The results are used to select dialysis schedules appropriate to the transport characteristics of the patient.

Measurement of adequacy is burdensome, labor intensive, and prone to multiple measurement errors, particularly from volume measurements of urine and dialysate samples; laboratory errors in measurements of urea and creatinine in blood, urine, and dialysate; and finally adjustment of results to predict weekly clearance. Although dialysis center nursing staff and patients may collect the samples required for adequacy testing with the utmost diligence, the very complexity and number of measurements taken will lead to an accumulation of measurement errors. In the opinion of the authors of the NKF-K/DOQI Clinical Practice Guidelines for PD Adequacy, when properly performed, these measures are reproducible enough to be useful in routine clinical practice.[515] However, an alternative, simpler method for defining dialysis adequacy would be useful in practice.

Malnutrition in Dialysis Patients

Dialysis patients with ESRD tend to have a poor appetite. Protein metabolism is altered in the setting of chronic acidosis and low-grade inflammation. These factors in combination place patients at risk of protein and energy malnourishment. Nutritional screening is recommended in dialysis patients. Such screening may involve measurement of weight, a recent history of edema-free weight loss, the body mass index, and subjective global assessment.[153] Serum albumin is often used as a marker of malnutrition, even though it is a relatively poor nutritional marker.[521] However, good evidence indicates that the lower the albumin concentration, the worse is the long-term prognosis.[504,522,523] An albumin concentration of less than 3.5 g/dL (measured by a bromocresol green method) or less than 3.0 g/dL (bromocresol purple method) is indicative of undernutrition. Hypoalbuminemia is associated with increased markers of the acute-phase response, such as CRP.[524,525] Persistent increase of CRP is common in dialysis patients and may occur in the absence of detectable infection. Episodes of peritonitis in PD patients cause significant albumin losses as the result of membrane leakage.

Kidney Transplantation

Kidney transplantation is the most effective form of RRT, in terms of long-term survival and quality of life. In 2016, adjusted mortality rates for ESRD, dialysis, and transplant patients were 134, 164, and 29 per 1000 patient-years.[489] Data provided by the Organ Procurement and Transplantation Network reveal that, as of April 2020, 94,979 patients are on the waiting list for a kidney transplant and that more than 24,000 kidney transplants were performed in the United States during 2019 (see: http://optn.transplant.hrsa.gov/data/, accessed June 16, 2020), up from 17,000 in 2012. Median waiting time for a listed patient depends on his or her age. For example, for patients listed between 2003 and 2004, the median waiting time for a child aged 1 to 5 years was approximately 1 year, and for an adult aged 35 to 49 years, approximately 5 years. The median time for a white adult was 4.2 years in 2008. This was the last calculable median waiting time estimation as 2008 was the last listing year in which more than 50% of the waiting list underwent transplantation (see: https://srtr.transplant.hrsa.gov/annual_reports/2018/Kidney.aspx, accessed June 16, 2020}. Although patients with kidney failure should have equitable access to kidney transplantation, this is not always the case. In the United States there is marked variation in access to transplantation based on geography and proximity to a metropolitan transplanting center (donation service areas). The difference in regional waits for at least five years can vary between 10 and 80%. Only 23% of adult patients on dialysis in the United Kingdom are on the active renal transplant waiting list. Women have a lower chance of being added to the transplant list and, once added, a lower chance of receiving a transplant.[103] Patients in transplanting centers are more likely to be listed than those in nontransplanting centers, and more likely to receive a live donor transplant.[103] Waiting time spent on dialysis has been shown to be an important factor in determining mortality. In England and Wales, 45% of patients younger than 65 years were activated on the transplant list within 1 year of starting dialysis, and 66% were activated within 5 years. Evidence suggests that the very best outcomes are achieved using preemptive (i.e., before dialysis has become necessary) live donor transplant.[526] This has led to increased emphasis on preemptive transplantation, particularly in the United Kingdom following the National Service Framework for Renal Services, published in 2004.[527]

Since Joseph Murray in Boston performed the first successful transplant in 1954 from one twin to the other, progressive developments have occurred in this field of medicine. In 1959 Dameshek and Schwartz used 6-mercaptopurine (6-MP) in place of irradiation to precondition patients for bone marrow transplantation. Calne developed this work with the introduction of a safer derivative of 6-MP called azathioprine (AZA). By 1963, maintenance AZA and corticosteroids had become the standard regimen for kidney transplantation. Kidney transplant or "allograft" survival with these treatment protocols was approximately 40% at 12 months. In the late 1970s to early 1980s, cyclosporin was introduced and for many years was the mainstay immunosuppressive regimen in combination with AZA and corticosteroids. Cyclosporin-based protocols led to fewer episodes of acute rejection and improved graft survival at 12 months to 80 to 90%. Tacrolimus, MMF, sirolimus (Rapamycin), and everolimus (Ever) were developed for use in kidney transplantation in the mid- to late 1990s. Also, there has been progress on the development and use of biological agents (monoclonal or polyclonal antibodies directed against immune response cellular targets) to suppress the immune response to a graft in human transplant recipients. All these advancements have led to increases in graft and patient survival, with 1-year graft survival of approximately 90% being the norm.[528,529] By contrast, long-term graft survival remains a major problem, with half of transplants failing within 14 years, usually as a result of chronic allograft injury or death with a functioning graft. Transplantation medicine provides a constant challenge to balance the immunologic risk of damage to the allograft (rejection) versus the well-being of the recipient, while avoiding excess immunosuppression that increases the likelihood of opportunistic infection and malignancy. In addition, many of the powerful immunosuppressive drugs have idiosyncratic side effect profiles.

Preoperative Assessment
The criteria for acceptance into a transplant program differ slightly from center to center, and it is easier to consider reasons for exclusion (Box 49.6). Two important psychological issues remain to be considered: the concept of organ receipt and potential difficulty in complying with immunosuppressive therapies. Age is no longer a primary issue in an otherwise healthy individual, with almost 25% of the kidney transplant waiting list including potential recipients aged greater than 65 years (see https://srtr.transplant.hrsa.gov/annual_reports/2018/Kidney.aspx, accessed June 16, 2020). The median age of prevalent renal transplant patients in the United Kingdom has increased year-on-year and in 2017 was 54.8 years.[103]

> ### BOX 49.6 Exclusion Criteria for Consideration for a Kidney Transplant
>
> Serious concomitant illness (particularly if likely to shorten life expectancy or to be exacerbated by immunosuppressive treatment)
> Active malignancy[a]
> Inoperable ischemic heart disease
> Severe chronic lung disease
> Active systemic infection (e.g., tuberculosis)
> Active immunologic disease
> Severe irreversible hepatic disease
> Severe peripheral vascular disease
> Severe obesity (body mass index [BMI] > 40 kg/m^2)
> Lower urinary tract dysfunction not amenable to surgical repair
> Substance abuse
> Significant psychiatric disturbance
>
> [a]Malignancy that has been treated with no evidence of recurrence is not an exclusion provided the predefined remission period has elapsed.

Laboratory assessment includes indicators of general operative health (e.g., electrolytes, acid-base status, clotting profile, full blood cell count, cross-matching [Boxes 49.7 and 49.8]). In addition, a full screen for infectious diseases, particularly cytomegalovirus (CMV), Epstein-Barr virus, hepatitis B and C, varicella-zoster virus, and human immunodeficiency virus (HIV) status, is undertaken; these infections can be activated by immunosuppressive therapy.

The Operation
The donor kidney is usually placed extraperitoneally in the right or left iliac fossa. Anastomoses are constructed joining the transplant renal artery and vein to the recipient's respective iliac vessels. The ureter is joined to the bladder. The recipient native kidneys are left *in situ* in most cases. Living donor kidneys can be retrieved through open surgery or with the aid of laparoscopic techniques. The work-up for a live donor transplant is beyond the scope of this chapter.

Postoperative Assessment
During the initial postoperative phase of 1 to 2 weeks, careful monitoring of serum creatinine concentration and urine output is required to monitor graft function. Most transplanted kidneys (grafts/allografts) produce measurable amounts of urine within a matter of hours, and this is a clear sign of a functioning graft; however, in a certain proportion, perhaps 5 to 10% of cases, primary nonfunction is apparent. In this subgroup, continuing dialysis support is necessary. In some patients the condition resolves without treatment, but in others a percutaneous kidney biopsy may be necessary to establish whether the graft is still viable and what form of therapy should be initiated. In otherwise uncomplicated cases, the serum creatinine concentration falls rapidly postoperatively (Fig. 49.21). Early rejection episodes are suspected if the serum creatinine does not fall to the expected level, or if there is a rising creatinine concentration indicating allograft dysfunction. The differential diagnoses of graft dysfunction and complications that may ensue following transplant are summarized in Table 49.17. In the very early postoperative phase, in addition to rejection, graft dysfunction may be a

BOX 49.7   Immunologic Aspects of Transplantation

Although a detailed description of the immunologic aspects of transplantation is beyond the scope of this chapter, a brief discussion follows to highlight the close collaboration between clinicians and the tissue typing laboratory and to explore some of the recent advances in transplantation. The tissue type identifies an individual based on human leukocyte antigens (HLA) antigens expressed on cells. These antigens are coded by genes of the major (and minor) histo- (tissue) compatibility complex (MHC). Individuals who have received blood transfusions, previous transplants of nonidentical tissue, and females who have had pregnancies develop antibodies to nonself HLA. These antibodies can be detected by analyzing the recipient serum against a panel of cells containing various HLA types or more recently the introduction of antigen specific beads and flow cytometry. If a reaction is noted between donor cells/antigen beads and recipient serum in vitro then this is indicative of a potential positive crossmatch between donor organ and recipient at the time of transplantation. All recipients are tested regularly by the tissue typing service. Highly sensitized individuals form around 30% of those on the transplant waiting list in the United States, and have a number of antibodies or an antibody to a common HLA type resulting in a longer waiting time for a suitable donor kidney in the majority of cases.[563]

ABO blood group incompatibility and HLA crossmatch reactivity between donor organs and recipients result in an accelerated or "hyperacute" rejection of the nonself organ (allograft) and have been traditional barriers to transplantation. Recent developments have led to desensitization protocols to remove the preformed antibodies from the plasma of potential recipients and have permitted transplantation across ABO and HLA barriers. This has permitted previously unsuitable potential live donors to donate. The outcome for recipients of desensitization programs is very encouraging with 89% of allografts surviving at 22 months follow-up in a single center.[564] Following transplantation clinicians and the tissue typing laboratory must remain vigilant for the persistence or reappearance of antibodies that may mediate rejection of the allograft. Where desensitization schedules are deemed undesirable and too high-risk, organ-sharing schemes have been developed whereby the live donor-recipient pairs are matched in a run for suitability to be transplanted among a defined cohort of other listed donor-recipient pairs that cannot undergo transplantation directly.

BOX 49.8   Laboratory Assessment of Potential Kidney Transplant Recipient

Electrolytes, liver function tests, glucose, C-reactive protein
Acid-base status
Full blood cell count
Clotting profile
Cytomegalovirus (CMV)
Hepatitis B and C
Varicella-zoster virus (VZV)
Epstein-Barr virus (EBV)
Human immunodeficiency virus (HIV) 1 and 2
Toxoplasma
Syphilis serology
Blood group: ABO compatibility
Tissue typing: human leukocyte antigen (HLA)
Index of sensitivity to alloantigens: e.g. panel reactive antibodies (PRA) or cumulative frequency (CF) scores

Tests of cardiac disease, vascular disease and bladder function are also required in most cases.

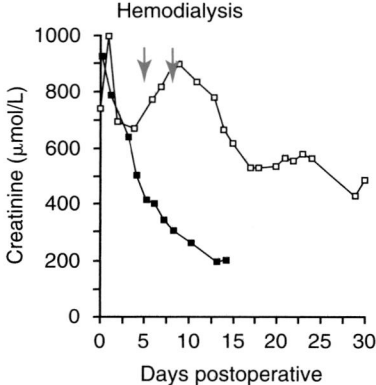

FIGURE 49.21 Post-transplantation biochemical profile. Open squares represent the course of a patient who experienced an early rejection episode (confirmed by biopsy, ↓) and requires initial hemodialysis support. Solid squares represent the typical profile of an uncomplicated transplant recipient. To convert creatinine concentration in μmol/L to mg/dL, multiply by 0.011.

consequence of delayed graft function, immunosuppressive drug toxicity, and acute tubular damage. Relative hypotension and dehydration may also contribute. Renal artery and venous thromboses are rare complications and ureteric obstruction can be readily diagnosed using ultrasonography. Histologic examination of a transplant biopsy is necessary to aid diagnosis and treatment adjustment. Regular monitoring of kidney function, drug concentrations, and viral polymerase chain reaction (PCR) (particularly for CMV viremia and polyoma viruses such as BK virus) is mandated following kidney transplantation in many centers.

Primary glomerular disease may recur following kidney transplantation, resulting in loss of the graft. An Australian study has confirmed the 10-year incidence of graft loss caused by recurrent glomerulonephritis as 8.4%.[530] Recurrence was the third most frequent cause of graft loss (chronic allograft nephropathy and death with a functioning graft were most common). As compared with the average for all recipients with a primary diagnosis of glomerulonephritis, FSGS (11.8%) and membranoproliferative glomerulonephritis ((MPGN), also known as mesangiocapillary glomerulonephritis (MCGN)) type 1 (10.2%) were most likely to recur causing graft loss. In contrast, graft loss due to recurrent IgA and pauci-immune crescentic glomerulonephritis occurred in only 2% of patients at 10 years follow-up.

Allograft rejection. The immune response to the foreign graft (allograft) is very brisk, and allograft rejection may occur in response to nonidentical HLA molecules. The majority of rejection episodes are asymptomatic, manifested by a rise in serum creatinine concentration above the baseline for the patient. However, biopsy of the kidney transplant is necessary to confirm the cause of graft dysfunction and to identify the

TABLE 49.17 Complications Following Kidney Transplantation

	Immediate Post Transplant	Early Post Transplant Period Until 3 Months	3–12 Months	After 1 Year	Comments
Surgical complications:	Renal venous thrombosis, arterial thrombosis Pelvic lymphocele adjacent to the transplanted kidney Ureteric obstruction			Ureteric obstruction, renal artery stenosis	Increased incidence of lymphocele reported with sirolimus
Kidney: (a) Immunologic (b) Recurrent disease	Acute tubular necrosis with delayed graft function				Dialysis treatment may need to be continued. Transplant usually recovers following adjustment of CNI doses. Electrolytes and creatinine should be measured daily
	Hyperacute rejection: occurs as a consequence of preformed antibodies in recipient serum to donor blood group or HLA antigens resulting in graft failure. Plasma exchange may be initiated but transplant nephrectomy likely	Acute rejection in 20–60% of patients. Associated with rise in serum creatinine concentration. Confirmed on biopsy. Pathologic description includes vascular and cellular infiltration by immune reactive cells. Requires urgent treatment with high dose corticosteroids	(a) Chronic allograft injury. Heralded by rising serum creatinine, proteinuria and hypertension. Common cause of graft failure in the long term. Complex pathogenesis with a combination of donor-specific and recipient influences. Humoral (antibody-mediated) rejection increasingly recognized as contributing to immunologic injury. Transplant biopsy may show peritubular capillary stain for complement degradation product C4d (b) Subclinical rejection not suspected from serum creatinine concentration. This is a pathologic diagnosis from transplant biopsy and is treated with high dose corticosteroids		Transplant centers may perform biopsy protocols at 3, 6 and 12 months to guide therapy Clinical episode of rejection considered if serum creatinine concentration increases from baseline Monitor recipient serum for antiHLA antibodies, particularly donor-specific antibodies Reduction in immunosuppression during maintenance phase of stable transplants
	Glomerular disease such as FSGS and MPGN may occur early and lead to graft failure		Risk of antiGBM disease in patients with Alport syndrome Familial hemolytic-uremic syndrome		Low risk of recurrent disease-causing graft failure in diabetes and IgA nephropathy
Infection	Chest infection Urinary tract infection Septicemia	Opportunistic infections: PCP, CMV infection and reactivation. High-risk cases include donor-positive and recipient-negative for prior exposure to CMV (D+/D−). Prophylactic antiviral drugs recommended in high-risk patients Varicella-zoster virus, polyoma virus (BK virus nephropathy), candidiasis	CMV viremia in high-risk cases following discontinuation of prophylactic antiviral medication		Increased risk of infection in all patients receiving immunosuppression. Patients advised to receive influenza vaccine annually and vaccination against pneumococcus Regular screening for viremia by PCR methodology Routine staining of transplant biopsy specimens for SV40 to identify BK virus nephropathy C-reactive protein, urine microscopy, cultures performed. Blood cultures Chest X-ray
Drug-related toxicity	See Table 48.19				

Continued

TABLE 49.17	**Complications Following Kidney Transplantation—cont'd**				
	Immediate Post Transplant	Early Post Transplant Period Until 3 Months	3–12 Months	After 1 Year	Comments
Lymphoproliferative		PTLD. Typically associated with EBV expression in patients exposed to highly potent immunosuppressive protocols	PTLD Includes non–EBV-related lymphoma	PTLD Includes non–EBV-related lymphoma	EBV-PCR CT/MRI scans of chest, abdomen and pelvis Tissue diagnosis mandatory from lymph node and bone marrow Serum lactate dehydrogenase activity increased
Malignancy	Increased risk of nonmelanotic skin malignancy and solid organ malignancy in all patients				
Cardiovascular disease	Increased incidence of cardiovascular disease following transplantation. Death with a functioning graft is a common cause of "graft failure"				
	The majority of transplant patients require treatment for hypertension and dyslipidemias				

CMV, Cytomegalovirus; *CNI*, calcineurin inhibitor; *EBV*, Epstein-Barr virus; *FSGS*, focal segmental glomerulosclerosis; *GBM*, glomerular basement membrane; *MPGN*, membranoproliferative glomerulonephritis; *PCP*, pneumocystis carinii pneumonia; *PCR*, polymerase chain reaction; *PTLD*, post-transplant lymphoproliferative diseases, *SV40*, simian virus 40 (cross-reacts with BK virus).

type of rejection that is occurring. A systematic classification system is employed ("Banff classification") to report transplant biopsy specimens.[531] The later updates from the Banff report have increasingly recognized the importance of humoral (antibody-mediated) rejection as a cause of allograft failure during the whole life of the transplant. Rejection has classically been divided into cellular and vascular types, and typically has been qualified by the speed of onset of graft dysfunction and the time since transplant. The recent classification builds on this but incorporates antibody-mediated rejection (acute or chronic), and T-cell-mediated rejection (again, acute or chronic). Advances in the diagnoses of humoral rejection have included identification of complement-fixing alloantibody along capillary walls within the transplant following the development of a stain for C4d product.[532] In addition, donor-specific anti-HLA antibodies can often be detected in the serum of the recipient during the course of the transplant and may predict graft dysfunction in some cases.[533,534] It is accepted that antibody and T-cell mediated rejection may coexist as causes of immunologic damage to the allograft. Allograft rejection typically is treated by escalating immunosuppression schedules, and treatment may include antithymocyte globulin and/or high-dose corticosteroids. Subclinical rejection is also described whereby there is no apparent rise in creatinine concentration, but rejection is diagnosed following a protocol biopsy.

Immunosuppression and therapeutic drug monitoring. As mentioned earlier, the introduction of immunosuppressive drugs in the 1970s led to vast improvement in the success rate of kidney transplantation. However, currently used drugs have potentially numerous and serious side effects that are summarized in Table 49.18.

Following the introduction of cyclosporin in the 1980s, a dramatic increase in 1-year graft survival resulted from the reduction in the number of acute rejection episodes.[535] However, a number of important side effects have been observed. Nephrotoxicity was soon apparent in early clinical trials[536] and remains a major clinical problem. During the 1990s, tacrolimus was introduced and 1-year graft and patient survival rates were equivalent to those achieved with cyclosporin therapy, although rates of acute rejection episodes were lower.[537–540] Five-year follow-up data suggest improved graft survival with tacrolimus compared with cyclosporin.[541]

Sirolimus, in contrast to cyclosporin, does not cause nephrotoxicity, gingival hyperplasia, or tremor. However, patients treated with sirolimus have a higher incidence of thrombocytopenia, hyperlipidemia, and lymphocele formation.[542] Sirolimus and MMF, both introduced during the late 1990s, have been studied in the setting of cyclosporin withdrawal and cyclosporin–free strategies in kidney transplantation,[528,543–547] the hypothesis being that withdrawal or avoidance of cyclosporin would improve long-term outcomes because there is no nephrotoxic stimulus. It has been shown in a multinational study that withdrawal of cyclosporin within 3 months of transplantation is feasible.[544] Studies have also shown that sirolimus in combination with MMF is safe and is associated with low rates of acute transplant rejection at 12 months.[528] Patients also received basiliximab, a monoclonal antibody to a specific target (CD 25) of T-cell activation that occurred in response to a nonidentical graft. However, the Cyclosporin Sparing with MMF, daclizumab and Corticosteroids in Renal Allograft Recipients (CAESAR) Study, found that use of MMF, corticosteroids, and daclizumab induction was associated with increased risk of rejection if cyclosporin was withdrawn by month 6 following the transplant, compared with continuation of low-dose cyclosporin.[546]

Cyclosporin is insoluble and is presented for clinical use as a microemulsion. It has a narrow therapeutic window, and in clinical transplantation it is important to monitor the blood concentration frequently. The most widely accepted practice is to monitor the "trough" concentration (C-0) just before the next dose. Accepted trough concentrations range from 100 to 300 μg/L (see Table 49.18). The highest concentrations are targeted during the induction phase of treatment for 2 to 3 months; subsequently, lower maintenance concentrations are desirable. The trough concentration within the blood may not provide a truly accurate guide to total drug exposure, because wide variation in absorption is seen over the

TABLE 49.18	Noninfectious Complications of Immunosuppressant Drugs		
Drug	**Drug Dose**	**Target Therapeutic Range[a]**	**Toxicity Profile**
Corticosteroids e.g., prednisone	Dose depends on weight of patient and time since transplant. Typically, 20 mg daily during first week and tapering to 5 mg at 3 months and withdrawal at 12 months	Not appropriate	Increase risk of developing diabetes mellitus Deterioration in diabetes control Osteopenia Osteoporosis Psychosis Fat redistribution Hypertension Dyslipidemia Cataracts Weight gain
Calcineurin Inhibitors Cyclosporin Tacrolimus	Variable Depends on weight, time since transplant and achieved drug concentration. Dose given in 2 divided doses and predose trough concentration measured in morning blood sample	200–300 µg/L for first 3–12 months. Thereafter aim for 100 µg/L	Nephrotoxicity Hypertension Neurotoxicity Hemolytic-uremic syndrome Tubular electrolyte abnormalities (hypophosphatemia, hypomagnesemia, hyperkalemia) Hirsutism Gingival hyperplasia Bone pains Dyslipidemia As for cyclosporin except no hirsutism or gingival hyperplasia Increased risk of diabetes mellitus Cardiomyopathy (children) Alopecia
Mycophenolate mofetil	Initially 2 g daily in divided doses	Not routinely measured	Abdominal pain Diarrhea Myelosuppression
Sirolimus	Dose depends on weight and achieved drug concentration. The drug is administered once daily	Level depends on time since transplant. Typical early (less than 3 months) target are 8–12 µg/L and thereafter 4–8 ug/L	Lymphocele (a fluid-filled collection near to transplanted kidney) Thrombocytopenia Hyperlipidemia
Azathioprine	Usual starting dose of 2 mg/kg body weight in a single daily dose	Levels not measured. Because the enzyme thiopurine methyltransferase (TPMT) metabolizes azathioprine; the risk of myelosuppression is increased in patients with low activity of the enzyme> Enzyme activity may be determined prior to commencing treatment and full blood counts are performed for several weeks following commencement of drug	Myelosuppression Severe interaction if used with allopurinol (treatment for gout)
Selected biological agents AntiCD25 monoclonal antibodies Basiliximab and daclizumab Polyclonal antithymocyte globulin (ATG) and antilymphocyte globulin (ALG), and monoclonal OKT3 Monoclonal antiCD52 antibodies: Alemtuzumab	Given at time of transplant and once thereafter Given in response to refractory rejection episodes in selected patients At induction in kidney and simultaneous kidney and pancreas transplant		Very well tolerated Increased risk of malignancy, post-transplant lymphoproliferative disease Hypersensitivity reactions

[a]These are not recommendations but are illustrative and will vary between centers.

first 2 to 4 hours following dosing.[548] This is important in that most of the pharmacodynamic effects of cyclosporin occur within 2 hours.[549] Studies from Canada suggest that trough concentrations do not reflect clinical outcomes in terms of acute rejection rates,[550] although high trough concentrations were associated with increased nephrotoxicity. A 2-hour drug (C-2) concentration correlated well with formal area under the curve measurements and is predictive of nephrotoxicity and acute rejection episodes. Among kidney transplant patients, the trough level of tacrolimus is correlated with acute rejection episodes and nephrotoxicity.[551] Trough concentrations also guide sirolimus therapy (see Table 49.18).[552]

MMF is morpholinoethyl ester of mycophenolic acid (MPA), a potent and reversible inhibitor of inosine monophosphate dehydrogenase isoform 2 (IMPDH) and has become the single most used immunosuppressant in solid organ transplantation. Excellent results have been obtained with a fixed-dose regimen. IMPDH is a target for immunosuppression because lymphocytes depend on the de novo guanosine nucleotide synthesis pathway for DNA synthesis and cell division.[553] MMF, because it is a prodrug of MPA, is rapidly absorbed following an oral dose and is de-esterified to MPA, which is highly protein bound. Free MPA concentrations determine the level of immunosuppressive activity, and this can be affected by hypoalbuminemia and renal insufficiency. Adverse events related to mycophenolate formulations include gastrointestinal disturbances, hematologic disorders (leucopenia and anemia), and infections.

Therapeutic drug monitoring of MPA is possible using HPLC and immunoassay techniques. However, it has not been universally accepted in kidney transplantation programs because prospective studies have given conflicting information of its value.[554] For example, in the Adaption de POsologie du MYcophénolate en Greffe REnale (APO-MYGRE) study a concentration controlled regimen based on MPA area-under-the-curve measurements was associated with fewer rejection episodes than use of a standard fixed dose of MMF.[555] The Fixed Dose–Concentration Controlled (FDCC) study compared a fixed-dose regimen of 2 g of MMF with a concentration controlled regimen based on abbreviated MPA area-under-the-curve measurements (target concentrations of 30 to 60 mg × h/L) in 901 patients who were treated with cyclosporin or tacrolimus.[556] An overall benefit could not be demonstrated in this large cohort over 12 months, despite an association with low MPA area-under-the-curve measurements and biopsy-proven acute rejection. In APOMYGRE and FDCC no correlation between MPA predose trough concentrations or area-under-the-curve measurements and MMF-related adverse events was observed in the first year after transplantation, despite differences in MPA exposure. A consensus report highlights that the use of imprecise definitions for adverse events, multicausality of adverse effects, including concomitant drugs, time elapsed between MPA measurement and event, assay used for MPA quantification, and associated toxicity profiles of concomitant immunosuppressive medications undermine the ability to demonstrate a relationship between drug exposure and toxicity.[554]

In summary, long-term graft failure is a major problem, and graft loss accounts for the return of increasing numbers of patients to dialysis. The most common cause of graft loss is death with a functioning graft. Kidney failure carries a considerable burden of cardiovascular morbidity. Although some risk factors, such as volume overload and anemia, are improved following transplantation, others, including dyslipidemia and hypertension, persist. The drugs used to prevent rejection can exacerbate these. Challenges to the nephrology community are complex and include improving access to transplantation, reducing side effects of the powerful drugs used to prevent rejection, and reducing in cardiovascular risk profiles for individual patients.

Simultaneous Pancreas-Kidney Transplantation

Patients with kidney failure and diabetes, predominantly type 1, but increasingly certain patients with type 2, and limited secondary complications of diabetes may be considered for simultaneous pancreas and kidney (SPK) transplantation. Patients tend to be younger than kidney only recipients (e.g., aged between 20 and 40 years). A 2011 analysis of 25,000 recipients of a pancreas transplant reported to the International Pancreas Transplant Registry (IPTR) in the United States since 1966 shows that the majority of recipients receive a simultaneous kidney and pancreas (75%), with 18% receiving a pancreas after kidney (PAK) and 7% pancreas only.[557] Patient survival now reaches over 95% at 1 year post-transplant and over 83% after 5 years. The data also show increasing age of the typical recipient and utilization of pancreas transplantation in C-peptide positive type 2 diabetic patients (from 2% in 1995 to 7% in 2010). These results compare favorably with those of cadaveric kidney only transplantation in diabetes. The main reason for the survival advantage of SPK over kidney only is the fact that younger donors and recipients are selected and the waiting time for the dual transplant is much shorter than for kidney-only transplants. In effect, the kidney-only "waiting-list" is a pool of patients with kidneys allocated primarily by tissue matching and age, whereas the SPK-listed patients are on a list, rather than in the pool. A separate prospective observational study examined the impact of SPK transplant in terms of quality of life.[558] At 3 years, SPK patients report greater improvements than kidney only recipients in physical functioning, bodily pain, general health, and perception of improvements to secondary complications of diabetes.

The surgical technique for SPK involves whole organ pancreas transplantation with the duodenal segment draining either into the urinary bladder through a duodenocystostomy, or more commonly now, enterically via an anastomosis between the graft duodenal segment and the recipient small bowel. The kidney is attached as usual to the iliac vessels, and the donor ureter is inserted into the bladder separately. Postoperatively, blood glucose concentrations are monitored closely and intravenous insulin is given as necessary. Exocrine pancreatic secretion can be measured in the urine for bladder-drained pancreas allografts. The major fear is rejection and a number of parameters are monitored, including plasma glucose, amylase, lipase, and 12- or 24-hour urinary amylase (again for bladder-drained allografts). For patients with bladder drainage, enteric conversion may be required for refractory problems, such as dehydration, metabolic acidosis, chronic urethritis caused by trypsinogen activation, UTI, and recurrent reflux pancreatitis. Because of high fluid, bicarbonate, and electrolyte losses into the urine in these patients, the need for supplementation is increased in SPK recipients.

There is a long-term need for high-dose oral sodium bicarbonate supplementation in bladder-drained pancreatic transplantation because of exocrine secretory losses. Hyperamylasemia is common postoperatively and may or may not signify allograft rejection. Immunosuppressive schedules vary between centers and include induction therapy with monoclonal or polyclonal anti-T-cell agents and a combination of the drugs outlined previously. Alemtuzumab (LEMTRADA), an anti-CD52 biological therapy with a profound lymphocyte depleting effect, has been increasingly utilized as induction therapy to permit corticosteroid-free protocols for SPK recipients with good outcome data.[559] The drug is unlicensed for this use but is available in the United Kingdom through a patient access program (see https://bnf.nice.org.uk/drug/alemtuzumab.html#unlicensedUse, accessed June 16, 2020) Diagnosis of pancreatic rejection in the absence of a simultaneous kidney transplant is very difficult. Signs of rejection include fever, pain, hematuria, reduction of urinary amylase, and unexplained hyperglycemia. Organ scanning and biopsy are also used. However, the function of the kidney in SPK mirrors the pancreas; therefore immunosuppression can be tailored to the requirements of the kidney.

ACKNOWLEDGEMENTS

We are grateful for data supplied by the US Renal Data System (USRDS). The interpretation and reporting of these data are the responsibility of the authors and in no way should be seen as an official policy or interpretation of the US Government. We are also grateful for data supplied by the U.K. Renal Registry. The interpretation and reporting of these data are the responsibility of the authors and in no way should be seen as an official policy or interpretation of the UK Renal Registry.

LIST OF ABBREVIATIONS

1,25(OH$_2$)D$_3$	calcitriol
11β-HSD	11β-hydroxysteroid dehydrogenase
99mTc-DMSA	technetium-99m-dimercaptosuccinic acid
99mTc-DTPA	99mTc-diethylenetriaminepentaacetic acid
99mTc-MAG3	99mTc-mercaptoacetlytriglycerine
AII	angiotensin II
ACE	angiotensin-converting enzyme
ADH	antidiuretic hormone
ADPKD	autosomal dominant polycystic kidney disease
ADQI	Acute Dialysis Quality Initiative
AE1	anion exchanger 1
AGE	advanced glycation end products
AHSG	α2-Heremans Schmid glycoprotein
AIN	acute interstitial nephritis
AKI	acute kidney injury
AKIN	Acute Kidney Injury Network
ALG	antilymphocyte globulin
ANA	antinuclear antibody
ANCA	antineutrophil cytoplasmic antibody
ANP	atrial natriuretic peptide
anti-GBM	anti–glomerular basement membrane
APD	automated peritoneal dialysis
AQP	aquaporin
ARAS	atheromatous renal artery stenosis
ARB	angiotensin receptor blocker
ARF	acute renal failure
ATG	antithymocyte globulin
ATN	acute tubular necrosis
AVF	arteriovenous fistula
AZT	azathioprine
BJP	Bence Jones protein
BP	blood pressure
BPH	benign prostatic hyperplasia
BSA	body surface area
CA II	carbonic anhydrase II
CA IV	carbonic anhydrase IV
cAMP	cyclic adenosine monophosphate
CAN	chronic allograft nephropathy
CAPD	continuous ambulatory peritoneal dialysis
CaSR	calcium-sensing receptor
CFU	colony-forming units
CHD	coronary heart disease
CI	confidence interval
CKD	chronic kidney disease
CKD-MBD	chronic kidney disease—mineral and bone disorder
CLC-Kb	chloride channel-Kb
CMV	cytomegalovirus
CNI	calcineurin inhibitors
COL4A5	A5 chain of type IV collagen
CO$_2$	carbon dioxide
COX	cyclooxygenase
CRF	chronic renal failure
CRP	C-reactive protein
CT	computed tomography
CVP	central venous pressure
DCCT	Diabetes Control and Complications Trial
dRTA	distal renal tubular acidosis
DTPA	99mTc-diethylenetriaminepentaacetic acid
DVT	deep vein thrombosis
ECaC1	epithelial calcium channel 1
EDTA	ethylenediaminetetraacetic acid
EM	electron microscopy
EMT	epithelial-mesenchymal transition
EMU	early morning urine
ENaC	apical sodium channel
EPO	erythropoietin
ERF	established renal failure
ESAs	erythropoiesis-stimulating agents
ESRD	end-stage renal disease
ESWL	extracorporeal shock wave lithotripsy
FcRN	MHC-related Fc receptor
FENa	fractional excretion of sodium
FGF-23	fibroblast growth factor-23
FRTS	Fanconi renal tubular syndrome
FSGS	focal segmental glomerulosclerosis
GBM	glomerular basement membrane
GFR	glomerular filtration rate
GN	glomerulonephritis
GSC	glomerular sieving coefficient
H$_2$CO$_3$	carbonic acid
HCO-HD	high cutoff hemodialysis
HD	hemodialysis

Continued

LIST OF ABBREVIATIONS—cont'd

HDF	hemodiafiltration	NOS	nitric oxide synthase
HDL	high density lipoprotein	NSAIDs	nonsteroidal anti-inflammatory drugs
HF	hemofiltration	PD	peritoneal dialysis
HIV	human immunodeficiency virus	PET	peritoneal equilibration test
HLA	human leukocyte antigen	pIgA	polymeric IgA
HOT	Hypertension optimal treatment	PKC-β1	protein kinase C- β1
HPLC	high-performance liquid chromatography	PMCA1b	plasma membrane calcium ATPase 1b
HUCU	hyperuricosuric calcium urolithiasis	pmp	per million population
ICU	intensive care unit	PRA	panel-reactive antibodies
IDL	intermediate-density lipoprotein	PR3	proteinase 3
ID-MS	isotope dilution mass spectrometry	pRTA	proximal renal tubular acidosis
Ig	immunoglobulin	PTH	parathyroid hormone
IL-6	interleukin-6	QOF	Quality and Outcomes Framework
IM	immunoperoxidase	RAAS	renin-angiotensin-aldosterone system
IVP	intravenous pyelography	RAGE	receptor for advanced glycation end products
IVU	intravenous urography	RBP	retinol binding protein
JGA	juxtaglomerular apparatus	rhEPO	recombinant human erythropoietin
JNC-VII	Joint National Committee on Prevention, Detection, Evaluation, and Treatment of High Blood Pressure	RIFLE	Risk, Injury, Failure, Loss, End-stage kidney disease
KDIGO	Kidney Disease Improving Global Outcomes	ROMK1	renal outer medullary potassium secreting channel 1
LDL	low density lipoprotein	RPGN	rapidly progressive glomerulonephritis
LM	light microscopy	RRF	residual renal function
LVH	left ventricular hypertrophy	RRT	renal replacement therapy
LVMI	left ventricular mass index	RTAs	renal tubular acidosis
MCD	minimal change disease	RVT	renal vein thrombosis
MCGN	mesangiocapillary glomerulonephritis	SAP	serum amyloid protein
MCP-1	monocyte chemoattractant protein-1	SIGN	Scottish Intercollegiate Guideline Network
MDRD	Modification of Diet in Renal Disease	SLE	systemic lupus erythematosus
MHC	major histocompatibility complex	SPK	simultaneous pancreas and kidney
MMF	mycophenolate mofetil	TGF-β	transforming growth factor β
6-MP	6-mercaptopurine	THG	Tamm Horsfall glycoprotein
MPA	mycophenolic acid	TIN	tubulointerstitial nephritis
MPGN	membranoproliferative glomerulonephritis	Tm	tubular maximal uptake
MR	mineralocorticoid receptor	TMB	tetramethyl benzidine
MRA	magnetic resonance angiography	TNF-α	tissue necrosis factor-α
MRI	magnetic resonance imaging	TPMT	thiopurine methyltransferase
NBC-1	Na-HCO$_3$ cotransporter	TRPV5	transient receptor potential vanilloid 5
Na, K-ATPase	sodium-potassium adenosine triphosphatase	UF	ultrafiltration
NAG	N-acetyl-β-D-glucosaminidase	UK	United Kingdom
NBC-1	Na-HCO$_3$ cotransporter	UKNEQAS	United Kingdom National External Quality Assessment Scheme
NCCT	Na-Cl cotransporter	UKM	urea kinetic modeling
NCXI	sodium calcium exchanger	UKPDS	United Kingdom Prospective Diabetes Study
NHANES III	Third National Health and Nutrition Examination Survey	UKT	UK transplant
NHE-3	Na-H exchanger	UNOS	United Network for Organ Sharing
NHS	National Health Service	URR	urea reduction ratio
NICE	National Institute for Health and Care Excellence	US	United States
NKCC2	Na-K-2Cl cotransporter	USRDS	United States Renal Data System
NKF-K/DOQI	National Kidney Foundation—Kidney Disease Outcomes Quality Initiative	UTI	urinary tract infection
NO	nitric oxide	VDR	vitamin D receptor
		VLDL	very-low-density lipoprotein

POINTS TO REMEMBER
Biochemical Characteristics of the Uremic Syndrome

Retained Nitrogenous Metabolites
Urea
Cyanate
Creatinine
Guanidine compounds
"Middle molecules"
Uric acid

Fluid, Acid-Base, and Electrolyte Disturbances
Fixed urine osmolality
Metabolic acidosis (decreased blood pH, bicarbonate)
Hyponatremia or hypernatremia
Hypokalemia or hyperkalemia
Hyperchloremia
Hypocalcemia
Hyperphosphatemia
Hypermagnesemia

Carbohydrate Intolerance
Insulin resistance (hypoglycemia may also occur)
Plasma insulin normal or increased

Delayed response to carbohydrate loading
Hyperglucagonemia

Abnormal Lipid Metabolism
Hypertriglyceridemia
Decreased high-density lipoprotein cholesterol
Hyperlipoproteinemia

Altered Endocrine Function
Secondary hyperparathyroidism
Osteomalacia (secondary to abnormal vitamin D metabolism)
Hyperreninemia and hyperaldosteronism
Hyporeninemia
Hypoaldosteronism
Decreased erythropoietin production
Altered thyroxine metabolism

Gonadal dysfunction (increased prolactin and luteinizing hormone, decreased testosterone).

POINTS TO REMEMBER
Causes of Acute Kidney Injury

Prerenal AKI:
  Hemorrhage
  Diarrhea
  Postoperative fluid and blood losses
  Sepsis
  Acute cardiac failure
Renal (intrinsic renal disease) AKI:
  Tubular
Any of the "prerenal" causes that are severe or that are not corrected promptly leading to ATN. Other causes of ATN
Drug nephrotoxicity
  NSAIDs, ACE inhibitors
  Aminoglycoside antibiotics
  Amphotericin
  Contrast nephropathy
Poisoning
TIN
  Allergic TIN associated with antibiotics and NSAIDs
  Sarcoidosis
  Pyelonephritis

Glomerular
  RPGN (ANCA-associated vasculitides, Goodpasture disease, SLE, other crescentic glomerulonephritides)
  Thrombotic microangiopathies
  Cryoglobulinemia
  Atheroembolism
Vascular
  Aortic dissection
  Renal vein thrombosis
Miscellaneous
  Rhabdomyolysis
  Urate nephropathy
  Hepatorenal syndrome
Postrenal AKI:
  Bladder outflow obstruction
  Benign and malignant prostate disease
  Invasive bladder carcinoma
  Bilateral renal calculi or calculi within a single kidney
  Retroperitoneal fibrosis

ACE, Angiotensin converting enzyme; *AKI*, acute kidney injury; *ANCA*, antineutrophil cytoplasmic antibody; *ATN*, acute tubular necrosis; *NSAIDs*, nonsteroidal anti-inflammatory drugs; *RPGN*, rapidly progressive glomerulonephritis; *SLE*, systemic lupus erythematosus; *TIN*, tubulointerstitial nephritis.

AT A GLANCE

At a Glance 1: Who Should Be Tested for Chronic Kidney Disease?

Monitor glomerular filtration rate (GFR) at least annually in people prescribed drugs known to be nephrotoxic, such as calcineurin inhibitors (for example, cyclosporin or tacrolimus), lithium and NSAIDs.

Offer testing for CKD using estimated GFR and urinary albumin to creatinine ratio (ACR) to people with any of the following risk factors:

- diabetes
- hypertension
- acute kidney injury
- cardiovascular disease (ischemic heart disease, chronic heart failure, peripheral vascular disease, or cerebral vascular disease)
- structural renal tract disease, recurrent renal calculi or prostatic hypertrophy
- multisystem diseases with potential kidney involvement—for example, systemic
- lupus erythematosus
- family history of kidney failure (GFR category G5) or hereditary kidney disease
- opportunistic detection of hematuria.

Do not use age, gender, or ethnicity as risk markers to test people for CKD. In the absence of metabolic syndrome, diabetes or hypertension, do not use obesity alone as a risk marker to test people for CKD.

National Institute for Health and Care Excellence. Chronic kidney disease. Early identification and management of chronic kidney disease in adults in primary and secondary care. 2014:http://www.nice.org.uk/nicemedia/live/13712/66658/.pdf. accessed 18/10/20.

AT A GLANCE 2

Defining and Classifying Chronic Kidney Disease

CKD is defined as abnormalities of kidney structure or function, present for ≥3 months, with implications for health.

Markers of reduced kidney function or damage include:

- Reduced glomerular filtration rate (GFR <60 mL/min/1.73 m²)
- Albuminuria (≥30 mg/24 h; ACR ≥30 mg/g [≥3 mg/mmol])
- Urine sediment abnormalities
- Electrolyte and other abnormalities due to tubular disorders
- Abnormalities detected by histology
- Structural abnormalities detected by imaging
- History of kidney transplantation

Assign GFR and albuminuria categories as described in Table 59.5.
Kidney Disease Improving Global Outcomes. Clinical Practice Guideline for the Evaluation and Management of Chronic Kidney Disease. *Kidney Int* 2013;3:1–150.

SELECTED REFERENCES

69. Peterson JC, Adler S, Burkart JM, et al. Blood pressure control, proteinuria, and the progression of renal disease. The Modification of Diet in Renal Disease Study. Ann Intern Med 1995;123:754–62.

91. United States Renal Data System. Annual data report: epidemiology of kidney disease in the United States. 2019. Available from: https://www.usrds.org/2019/download/USRDS__ES_final.pdf. Accessed October 18, 2020.

94. National Institute for Health and Care Excellence. Chronic kidney disease. Early identification and management of chronic kidney disease in adults in primary and secondary care. 2014. Available from: http://www.nice.org.uk/nicemedia/live/13712/66658/.pdf. Accessed October 18, 2020.

125. Wheeler DC, Townend JN, Landray MJ. Cardiovascular risk factors in predialysis patients: baseline data from the Chronic Renal Impairment in Birmingham (CRIB) study. Kidney Int Suppl 2003;(84):S201–3.

152. Baigent C, Landray MJ, Reith C, et al. The effects of lowering LDL cholesterol with simvastatin plus ezetimibe in patients with chronic kidney disease (Study of Heart and Renal Protection): a randomised placebo-controlled trial. Lancet 2011;377:2181–92.

171. Kidney Disease Improving Global Outcomes. KDIGO 2017 clinical practice guideline update for the diagnosis, evaluation, prevention, and treatment of Chronic Kidney Disease-Mineral and Bone Disorder (CKD-MBD). Kidney Int 2017;7:1–59.

209. Macdougall IC, White C, Anker SD, et al. Intravenous Iron in patients undergoing maintenance hemodialysis. N Engl J Med 2019;380:447–58.

210. United Kingdom Renal Association. Clinical practice guideline anaemia of chronic kidney disease. 2020. Avaialble from: https://renalorg/wp-content/uploads/2020/02/Updated-130220-Anaemia-of-Chronic-Kidney-Disease-1-1pdf. Accessed October 18, 2020.

227. Vanholder R, De Smet R, Glorieux G, et al. Review on uremic toxins: classification, concentration, and interindividual variability. Kidney Int 2003;63:1934–43.

238. National Institute for Health and Care Excellence. Acute kidney injury: prevention, detection and management. 2019. Available from: https://wwwniceorguk/guidance/ng148. Accessed October 18, 2020.

247. Sterns RH, Grieff M, Bernstein PL. Treatment of hyperkalemia: something old, something new. Kidney Int 2016;89:546–54.

306. Gaede P, Lund-Andersen H, Parving HH, et al. Effect of a multifactorial intervention on mortality in type 2 diabetes. N Engl J Med 2008;358:580–91.

344. Beck Jr LH, Bonegio RG, Lambeau G, et al. M-type phospholipase A2 receptor as target antigen in idiopathic membranous nephropathy. N Engl J Med 2009;361:11–21.

356. Bossuyt X, Cohen Tervaert JW, Arimura Y, et al. Position paper: Revised 2017 international consensus on testing of ANCAs in granulomatosis with polyangiitis and microscopic polyangiitis. Nat Rev Rheumatol 2017;13:683–92.

380. National Institute for Health and Care Excellence. Myeloma: diagnosis and management. 2018. Available from: https://wwwniceorguk/guidance/ng35/chapter/Recommendations. Accessed October 19, 2020.

399. Torres VE, Harris PC. Progress in the understanding of polycystic kidney disease. Nat Rev Nephrol 2019;15:70–2.

423. Downie ML, Lopez Garcia SC, Kleta R, et al. *Inherited tubulopathies of the kidney: insights from genetics.* Clin J Am Soc Nephrol 2021;16(4):620–30.

437. Gambaro G, Croppi E, Coe F, et al. Metabolic diagnosis and medical prevention of calcium nephrolithiasis and its systemic manifestations: a consensus statement. J Nephrol 2016;29:715–34.

514. United Kingdom Renal Association. Clinical practice guideline: peritoneal dialysis in adults and children. 2017. Available from: https://renalorg/guidelines/.

501. Grooteman MP, van den Dorpel MA, Bots ML, et al. Effect of online hemodiafiltration on all-cause mortality and cardiovascular outcomes. J Am Soc Nephrol 2012;23:1087–96.

50

Disorders of Water, Electrolytes, and Acid-Base Metabolism

Marc Berg, Joe M. El-Khoury, and Mark A. Cervinski

ABSTRACT

Background

A complex yet elegant system of chemical buffers together with highly specialized mechanisms of the lungs and kidneys continuously work in tandem to ensure a precise balance of water, electrolytes, and pH in both the intracellular and extracellular compartments of the human body. Although these systems display impressive resilience and responsiveness to perturbation by illness or injury, they do have limits, at which point medical evaluation and treatment are required.

Content

This chapter describes the various fluid compartments in the body and reasons for differences in composition between these compartments. Laboratory testing algorithms are used to investigate and treat perturbations of water and electrolytes in pathologic settings, including the role of such simple tests as urine electrolytes. Similarly, testing algorithms and mnemonic tools are presented to diagnose and manage disturbances in acid-base homeostasis. The clinical laboratorian needs to understand the nuances and pitfalls associated with these algorithms and associated tests to provide accurate and meaningful results to the clinician.

Adaptation to terrestrial life led to the evolution of physiologic systems to maintain the composition of the internal milieu of animals, including humans. These systems require the interaction of multiple organ systems such as the kidneys, lungs, heart, liver, brain, and lymphatics. In particular, a variety of chemical buffers and highly specialized mechanisms of the lungs and kidneys work together to regulate water, electrolytes, and pH between and within intracellular and extracellular compartments. Perturbations in the dynamic equilibria that exist for water, electrolytes, and pH may arise from external (e.g., trauma, changes in altitude, ingestion of toxic substances) or internal (e.g., normal metabolism, disease state) sources. Endogenous correction of these imbalances may not always be adequate; at these times, the clinical laboratory can provide valuable information for guiding therapy.[a]

TOTAL BODY WATER: VOLUME AND DISTRIBUTION

During gestation, $\approx$90% of fetal body weight is water.[1] Water is 70% of body weight for full-term infants. Water gradually decreases as percent of body weight, so that it accounts for 60% of body weight in adolescents and adult males[1] and $\approx$55% for adult females. As depicted in Fig. 50.1, approximately two-thirds of total body water (TBW) is distributed into the intracellular fluid (ICF) compartment, and one-third exists in the extracellular fluid (ECF) compartment. The ECF may be further subdivided into interstitial ($\approx$75% of ECF) and intravascular ($\approx$25% of ECF) compartments, which are separated by the capillary endothelium. The average adult has 5 L of blood volume (intravascular compartment) and a plasma volume of $\approx$3.0 L when the hematocrit is 40%. Although fluid from other clinically relevant ECF compartments (e.g., cerebrospinal fluid [CSF],[2] urine) may be analyzed in the clinical laboratory, most laboratory tests used to determine hydration, electrolyte, and acid-base status are performed on samples from the intravascular compartment.

The minimum daily requirement for water can be estimated from renal (1200 to 1500 mL in urine) and "insensible" losses ($\approx$400 to 700 mL) as a result of evaporation from the skin and respiratory tract. Activity, environmental conditions, and disease all have dramatic effects on daily water (and electrolyte) requirements. On average, an adult must take in $\approx$1.5 to 2.0 L of water daily to maintain fluid balance. Because primary regulatory mechanisms are designed to primarily maintain *intracellular* hydration status, imbalances in TBW are initially reflected in the ECF compartment. Table 50.1 lists common causes and clinical manifestations of expansion and contraction of the ECF compartment.

WATER AND ELECTROLYTES: COMPOSITION OF BODY FLUIDS

The primary cationic (positively charged) electrolytes are sodium (Na^+), potassium (K^+), calcium (Ca^{2+}), and magnesium (Mg^{2+}),

---

[a]Laboratories should verify that the values presented in this chapter, including the reference intervals are appropriate for use in their own settings.

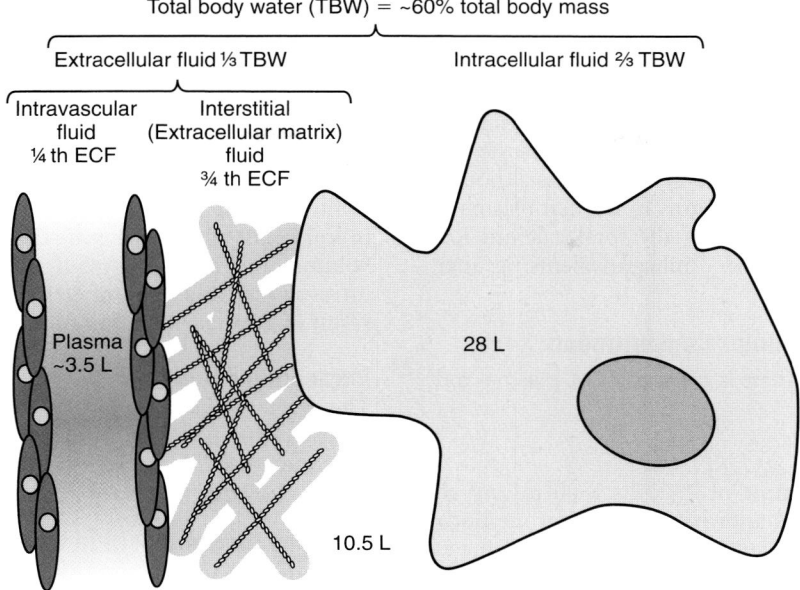

Total body water (TBW) = ~60% total body mass

FIGURE 50.1 Volume and distribution of total body water. Note that the intracellular and extracellular fluid compartments (intracellular fluid *[ICF]* and extracellular fluid *[ECF]*, respectively) are separated by cellular plasma membranes, and within the ECF, interstitial and intravascular fluids are separated by the capillary endothelium *(red cells)*. The volumes indicated represent water and not total volume. Endothelial cells = *red*; interstitial cell = *gray*; collagen matrix fibers = *black cables*.

TABLE 50.1 Causes and Clinical Manifestations of Changes in Extracellular Fluid Volume

	Clinical Manifestations	Causes
ECF loss	Thirst, anorexia, nausea, lightheadedness, orthostatic hypotension, syncope, tachycardia, oliguria, decreased skin turgor and "sunken eyes," shock, coma, death	Trauma (and other causes of acute blood loss), "third-spacing" of fluid (e.g., burns, pancreatitis, peritonitis), vomiting, diarrhea, diuretics, renal or adrenal (i.e., sodium wasting) disease
ECF gain	Weight gain, edema, dyspnea (secondary to pulmonary edema), tachycardia, jugular venous distention, portal hypertension (ascites), esophageal varices	Heart failure, cirrhosis, nephrotic syndrome, iatrogenic (intravenous fluid overload)

ECF, Extracellular fluid.

TABLE 50.2 Electrolyte and Water Composition of Body Fluid Compartments

Component	Plasma	Interstitial Fluid	Intracellular Fluid[a]
Volume, H$_2$O (TBW = 42 L)	3.5 L	10.5 L	28 L
Na$^+$	140	145	12
K$^+$	4	4	156
Ca^{2+}	2.4	2–3	0.3
Mg^{2+}	1	0.5–1	13
Trace elements	1	—	—
Cl$^-$	103	114	4
HCO$_3^-$	27	31	12
Protein$^-$	16	—	55
Organic acids$^-$	5	—	—
HPO$_4^{2-}$	1	—	—
SO$_4^{2-}$	0.5	—	—

[a]These values are derived from skeletal muscle.
All electrolyte values are expressed in millimoles per liter of *fluid*. Because the H$_2$O content of plasma is ≈93% by volume, the corresponding electrolyte concentrations in plasma water are ≈10% higher.
TBW, Total body water.

whereas the anions (negatively charged) include chloride (Cl$^-$), bicarbonate (HCO$_3^-$), phosphate (HPO$_4^{2-}$, H$_2$PO$_4^-$), sulfate (SO$_4^{2-}$), organic ions such as lactate, and negatively charged proteins. Electrolyte concentrations of the body fluid compartments are shown in Table 50.2. Na$^+$, K$^+$, Cl$^-$, and HCO$_3^-$ in the plasma or serum are commonly analyzed in an *electrolyte profile* because their concentrations provide the most relevant information about the osmotic, hydration, and acid-base status of the body. Although hydrogen (H$^+$) is a cation, its concentration is approximately 1 million–fold lower in plasma than the major electrolytes listed in Table 50.2 (10^{-9} versus 10^{-3} mol/L) and is negligible in terms of osmotic activity.

Any increase in the concentration of one anion is accompanied by a corresponding decrease in other anions or by an increase in one or more cations or both because total electrical neutrality must be maintained. Similarly, any decrease in the concentration of anions involves a corresponding increase in other anions, a decrease in cations, or both. In the case of polyvalent ions (e.g., Ca^{2+}, Mg^{2+}), it is important to distinguish between the substance concentration of the ion itself and the concentration of the ion charge. Thus although the concentration of total calcium ions in normal plasma is ≈2.5 mmol/L, the concentration of the total calcium ion *charge* is 5.0 mmol/L (also called 5 milliequivalents per liter [mEq/L]).

Extracellular and Intracellular Compartments

The extracellular compartment is composed of plasma and interstitial fluid.

Plasma

Plasma generally has a volume of 1300 to 1800 mL/m² of body surface and constitutes approximately 5% of the body volume (≈3.5 L for a 66-kg subject). Total body volume is derived from body mass by using an estimated body density of 1.06 kg/L. Table 50.2 describes the electrolyte composition of plasma. The mass concentration of water in normal plasma is approximately 0.933 kg/L, depending on the protein and lipid content (see "Electrolyte Exclusion Effect" in Chapter 37). Thus a concentration of sodium in the plasma of 140 mmol/L would correspond to a molality of sodium in plasma water of 150 mmol/kg H_2O (140 mmol/L divided by 0.933 kg/L). The concentration of net protein ions in plasma is ≈12 mmol/L.[3]

Interstitial Fluid

Interstitial fluid is essentially an ultrafiltrate of blood plasma (see Fig. 50.1). When all extracellular spaces except plasma are included, the volume accounts for about 26% (10.5 L) of the total body volume. Plasma is separated from the interstitial fluid by the endothelial lining of the capillaries, which acts as a semipermeable membrane and allows passage of water and diffusible solutes but not compounds of high molecular mass proteins. The exchange of water between the interstitial and intravascular compartments is governed by Starling forces, which demonstrates that the net movement of fluid across a capillary membrane is a function of membrane permeability and differences in hydrostatic and oncotic pressures on the two sides of the membrane.[1] The "impermeability" to proteins is not absolute, and in some pathologic conditions causing shock, such as bacterial sepsis, the permeability of the vascular endothelium increases dramatically, resulting in leakage of albumin, a reduction in the effective circulating volume, and hypotension. If not aggressively treated with intravenous fluids and/or vasopressors, this condition can result in death as the result of decreased cerebral perfusion.

Intracellular Fluid

The exact composition of ICF is difficult to measure. Therefore data for ICF (see Table 50.2) are considered only approximations. The ICF constitutes ≈66% of the total body volume (see Fig. 50.1).

Reasons for Composition Differences of Body Fluids

The composition of ICF can differ markedly from that of ECF because of separation of these compartments by the cell membrane. The composition differences are a consequence of both the Gibbs-Donnan equilibrium and active and passive transport of ions, as well as active transport of larger molecules.

Gibbs-Donnan Equilibrium

Two solutions separated by a semipermeable membrane will establish an equilibrium, so that all ions are equally distributed in both compartments, provided the solutes can move freely through the membrane. At the state of equilibrium, the total ion concentration and therefore the total concentration of osmotically active particles are equal on both sides of the membrane.

If solutions on two sides of a membrane contain different concentrations of ions that cannot freely move through the membrane (e.g., proteins), distribution of diffusible ions (e.g., electrolytes) at the steady state will be unequal, but the sum of the concentrations of ions in one compartment is equal to the sum of the concentrations of ions in the other compartment (Fig. 50.2). This is

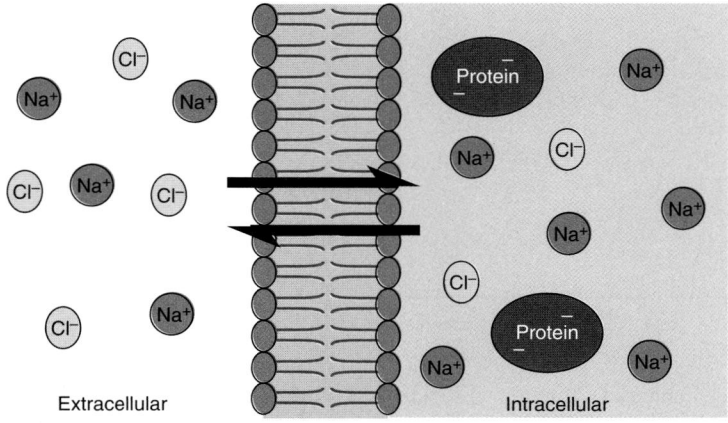

FIGURE 50.2 Schematic illustrating Gibbs-Donnan equilibrium across a cell membrane. The membrane is impermeable to the negatively charged proteins but permeable to the electrolytes (in this case sodium and chloride). To maintain electrical neutrality, the cations (sodium) move inside the cell, while the anions (chloride) move outside of the cell. This creates an uneven distribution of sodium and chloride across a permeable membrane, but electrical neutrality is maintained (total sum of ions on each side is the same).

referred to as Gibbs-Donnan equilibrium.[4] Importantly, the law of electrical neutrality must also be obeyed for both compartments. An example of the uneven distribution of an ion in two compartments with different protein content (nondiffusible ions) is the concentration of chloride ions in plasma and CSF. As a result of increased selectivity of the blood-brain barrier against proteins, Cl^- ions are $\approx$15% higher in CSF to establish electrical and osmotic equilibrium.[2] Cells, most notably those of the central nervous system (CNS), that contain nondiffusible protein anions can withstand only a limited and temporary difference in osmotic pressure across the cell membrane. Osmotic pressure is normally identical inside and outside the cells because the cell membrane can correct concentration differences by excluding some small ions through active, energy-requiring transport processes. If these processes cease, the cells will swell and eventually will burst (osmotic lysis).

Distribution of Ions by Active and Passive Transport

Examination of Table 50.2 reveals that the electrolyte compositions of blood plasma and interstitial fluid are similar and differ markedly from that of ICF. The major ECF ions are Na^+, Cl^-, and HCO_3^-, but in ICF, the main ions are K^+, Mg^{2+}, organic phosphates, and protein. This unequal distribution of ions is due to active transport of Na^+ from inside to outside the cell against an electrochemical gradient. An active sodium pump deriving its energy from glycolysis-generated adenosine triphosphate (ATP) is present in most cell membranes and frequently is coupled with transport of K^+ into the cell.

In addition to the Na^+/K^+-ATPase, a ubiquitous Na^+-H^+ exchanger (often referred to as an *antiporter*) actively pumps H^+ out of the ICF in exchange for Na^+.[5] This exchanger is critical for maintaining intracellular pH homeostasis. At least six different isoforms of this transmembrane protein have been identified.[5] Of particular importance is the role of this exchanger for acid-base regulation in renal tubular cells, as discussed later in this chapter.

Electrolytes

Disorders of Na^+, K^+, Cl^-, and HCO_3^- will now be separately considered, even though disorders of electrolyte and water homeostasis need a systematic evaluation rather than an individual review of each ion.[6]

Sodium

Disorders of Na^+ homeostasis can occur because of excessive loss, gain, or retention of Na^+, or as the result of excessive loss, gain, or retention of H_2O. It is difficult to separate disorders of Na^+ and H_2O balance because of their close relationship in establishing normal osmolality in all body water compartments.[7] As described in detail in Chapter 49, the primary organ for regulating body water and extracellular Na^+ is the kidney. As a brief introduction to this section, it is important to remind the reader of the functions of healthy kidneys.

The human body is in a dynamic state of flux as fluids and electrolytes are constantly being gained through mechanisms such as thirst and hunger and lost through processes such as sweating and urination. Homeostasis within a narrow window is necessary for life, and the body must defend against excessive gains or losses. Although certain behavioral adaptations are undoubtedly important (e.g., drinking when thirsty

to prevent water and volume loss) others may be more debatable (as in the case of dietary sodium restriction).[8] The kidney is responsible for not only clearing uremic toxins from the circulation but also in maintaining fluid balance and defending electrolyte homeostasis across a wide range of these gains and losses. In the proximal tubules, 70 to 80% of filtered Na^+ is actively reabsorbed, with H_2O and Cl^- following passively to maintain electrical neutrality and osmotic equivalence. In the descending loop of Henle, H_2O, but not electrolytes, is passively reabsorbed because of the high osmotic strength of interstitial fluid in the renal medulla. In the ascending loop of Henle, Cl^- is reabsorbed actively, with Na^+ following. At the level of the distal tubule, the first of the two primary Na^+/H_2O regulating processes occurs. Here, aldosterone stimulates the cortical collecting ducts to reabsorb Na^+ (with water following passively) and secrete K^+ (and to a lesser extent, H^+) to maintain electrical neutrality. Aldosterone is produced by the adrenal cortex in response to angiotensin II derived by the action of renin. The secretion of renin by renal juxtaglomerular cells is stimulated by low chloride, β-adrenergic activity, and low arteriolar pressure.[9] Thus when the kidneys are hypoperfused (as occurs when blood volume decreases, or when the renal arteries are obstructed), the distal tubules, under the influence of aldosterone, reclaim Na^+.

Further water regulation in the kidney occurs from the distal tubule through the collecting duct, where tubular permeability to H_2O is under the influence of vasopressin (also called antidiuretic hormone [ADH]) (see Chapters 49 and 55). Vasopressin is released by the posterior pituitary under the influence of baroreceptors in the aortic arch and hypothalamic chemoreceptors that are responsive to circulating osmolality, which is primarily a reflection of Na^+ concentration. When ECF volume is decreased, or when plasma osmolality is increased, vasopressin is secreted, tubular permeability to H_2O increases via aquaporins, and H_2O is reabsorbed in an attempt to restore blood volume or to decrease osmolality. In contrast, when ECF volume is increased or osmolality decreased, vasopressin secretion is inhibited, and more H_2O is excreted in the urine (diuresis).

Besides the kidney, the body's only other mechanism for restoring Na^+/H_2O homeostasis is ingestion of H_2O. Thirst is stimulated by decreased blood volume or hyperosmolality. It is important to remember that baroreceptors that influence renal handling of Na^+ and H_2O, and thirst, sense changes only in the intravascular blood volume and not the total ECF, whereas osmoreceptors in the brain, such as the organum vasculosum lamina terminalis (OVLT) neurons, sense the osmolality of the ECF surrounding the cells. Laboratory assessment of water and electrolyte disorders is made primarily from the blood volume (plasma); the clinician must assess the status of TBW and blood volume before interpreting laboratory values. The physical findings of these disorders are as important as the laboratory values in management of water and electrolyte disorders (see Table 50.1).

Hyponatremia

Hyponatremia is defined as a decreased plasma Na^+ concentration (generally <135 mmol/L) and is the most commonly encountered disorder of electrolytes, with incidences as high as 15 to 30% in acutely and chronically hospitalized patients.[10] Hyponatremia typically manifests clinically as nausea, generalized weakness, and mental confusion at values less

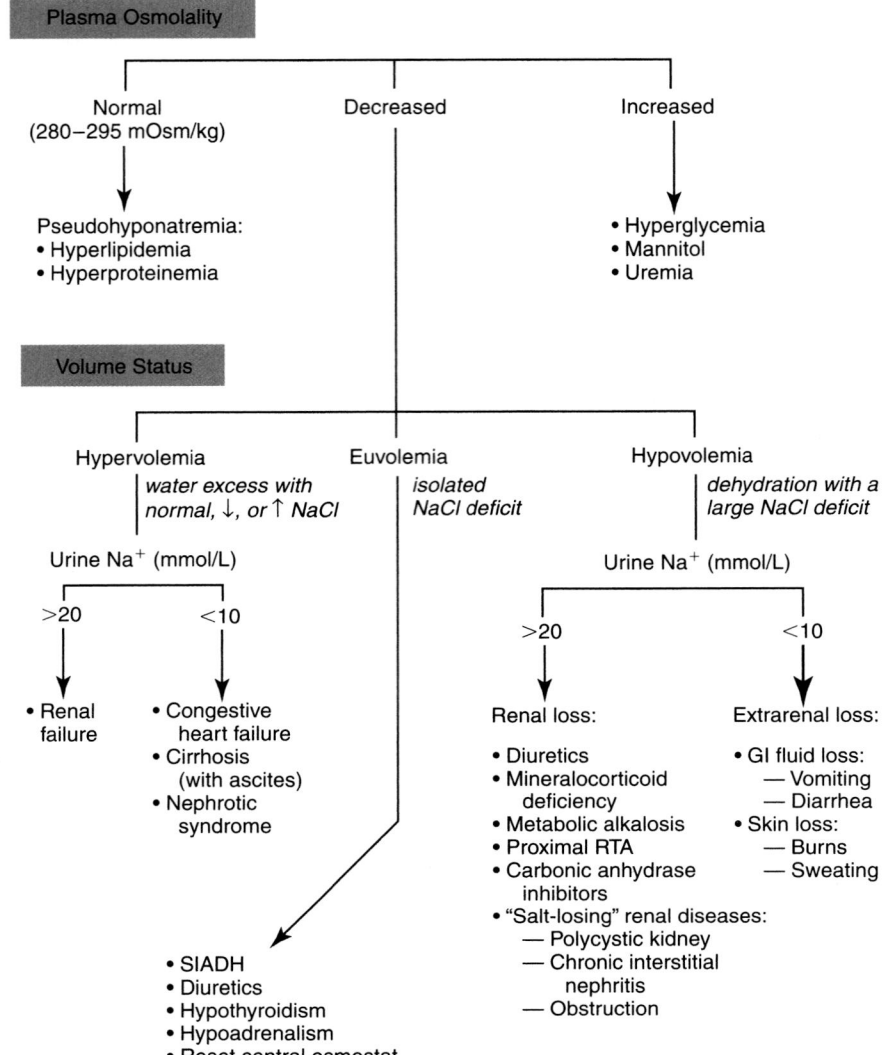

FIGURE 50.3 Algorithm for the differential diagnosis of hyponatremia. *GI*, Gastrointestinal; *RTA*, renal tubular acidosis; *SIADH*, syndrome of inappropriate secretion of antidiuretic hormone. (Modified from Kirkpatrick W, Kreisberg R. Acid-base and electrolyte disorders. In: Liu P, ed. *Blue book of diagnostic tests*. Philadelphia: WB Saunders; 1986:239–54.)

than 120 mmol/L and severe mental confusion plus seizures at less than 105 mmol/L.[11] The rapidity of development of hyponatremia influences the Na^+ concentrations at which symptoms develop (i.e., clinically apparent symptoms may manifest at higher Na^+ concentrations [≈125 mmol/L] when hyponatremia develops rapidly).[11] It is important to note that symptoms are due to changes in osmolality rather than to the Na^+ concentration per se. CNS symptoms are due to movement of H_2O into cells to maintain osmotic balance and subsequent swelling of CNS cells. These symptoms can occur more rapidly in children, so there is a need to be particularly vigilant in the pediatric population.

Hyponatremia can be hypo-osmotic, hyperosmotic, or iso-osmotic. Measurement of plasma osmolality is an important initial step in the assessment of hyponatremia. Of these, the most common form is hypo-osmotic hyponatremia, and it is important to distinguish it from the other two forms (hyperosmotic or iso-osmotic) because these represent situations

where hyponatremia does not need to be treated.[10] Fig. 50.3 describes an algorithm for laboratory measurements and physical examination findings in the differential diagnosis of plasma Na^+ less than 135 mmol/L.[12]

Hypo-osmotic hyponatremia. Typically, when plasma Na^+ concentration is low, calculated, or measured, osmolality will also be low. This type of hyponatremia can be due to excess loss of Na^+ *(depletional hyponatremia)* or increased ECF volume *(dilutional hyponatremia)*. Differentiating these initially requires clinical assessment of TBW and ECF volume by history and physical examination.

Depletional hyponatremia results from a loss of Na^+ from the ECF space that exceeds the concomitant loss of water. Hypovolemia is apparent in the physical examination (orthostatic hypotension, tachycardia, decreased skin turgor). If urine Na^+ is low (<10 mmol/L), the kidneys are properly retaining filtered Na^+ and the loss is extrarenal, most commonly from the gastrointestinal tract or skin (see Fig. 50.3). Preventing ongoing loss and restoring ECF volume with isotonic fluid is sufficient to correct hyponatremia in these situations.

Alternatively, if urine Na^+ is increased in this setting (generally >20 mmol/L), renal loss of Na^+ is likely. Renal loss of Na^+ occurs with (1) osmotic diuresis, (2) use of diuretics (which inhibit reabsorption of Cl^- and Na^+ in the ascending loop), (3) adrenal insufficiency (no aldosterone or cortisone prevents distal tubule reabsorption of Na^+), or (4) salt-wasting nephropathies, as can occur with interstitial nephritis and tubular recovery after acute tubular necrosis or obstructive nephropathy. Hypo-osmotic hyponatremia has also been attributed to cerebral salt wasting, a controversial diagnosis associated with subarachnoid hemorrhage (SAH) and other intracranial diseases/trauma. Despite being described in literature for $\approx$70 years, the condition remains controversial because the mechanism of the condition remains undefined.[13] If it is a physiologic condition, it is exceedingly rare as evidenced in a publication detailing a series of 100 patients with SAH. Of this population of 100 patients, 49 developed hyponatremia and the cause of the hyponatremia was ascribed to syndrome of inappropriate secretion of antidiuretic hormone (SIADH) in 71.4% patients. Of the remaining hyponatremic patients, 10.2% were incorrectly treated with hypotonic saline (0.45% saline), 10.2% were hypovolemic, and the remaining 8.2% had acute cortisol deficiency.[14]

Renal loss of Na^+ in excess of H_2O can also occur in metabolic alkalosis from prolonged vomiting, because increased renal HCO_3^- excretion is accompanied by Na^+ ions. In this case, urine sodium is increased (>20 mmol/L), but urine chloride remains low. In proximal renal tubular acidosis (RTA) type 2, bicarbonate is lost because of a defect in HCO_3^- reabsorption, and Na^+ is co-excreted to maintain electrical neutrality. As with extrarenal Na^+ loss, management of hyponatremia attributable to renal Na^+ loss is centered on the reversal of underlying cause and restoration of ECF volume.

Dilutional hyponatremia is a result of excess H_2O retention and often can be detected during the physical examination as edema. In advanced renal failure, water is retained because of decreased filtration and H_2O excretion. When ECF is increased but the circulating blood volume is decreased, as occurs in hepatic cirrhosis, heart failure, and nephrotic syndrome, a vicious cycle is established. The decreased blood volume is sensed by baroreceptors and results in increased aldosterone and vasopressin, even though ECF volume is excessive. The kidneys reabsorb Na^+ and H_2O in response to increased aldosterone and vasopressin in an attempt to restore the blood volume, resulting in further increases in ECF and further dilution of Na^+. In dilutional hyponatremia, the low serum sodium concentrations reflect the severity of the underlying disease process. Management should be focused on the treatment of the underlying disease, as correction of Na^+ concentrations alone have no effect on overall morbidity or mortality.[11]

In hypo-osmotic hyponatremia with a normal or euvolemic volume status, the most common causes are the syndrome of inappropriate ADH (vasopressin) (SIADH), primary polydipsia, and endocrine disorders such as adrenal insufficiency and hypothyroidism (see Fig. 50.3). Adrenal insufficiency causes hyponatremia through increased cortisol-releasing hormone, which stimulates vasopressin release,[15] while hypothyroidism impairs free H_2O excretion.

SIADH describes hyponatremia attributable to "inappropriate" vasopressin release, as from a malignancy, which stimulates excessive H_2O retention and increased urine osmolality.[16] Free water restriction is the mainstay of therapy in SIADH. However, in severe or symptomatic hyponatremia from any cause, the use of hypertonic saline solutions may be required to correct serum Na^+ concentrations.[11] In such cases, the hyponatremia must be corrected cautiously because too rapid correction can lead to brain demyelination (a condition known as osmotic demyelination syndrome). The pons is particularly sensitive to this, and rapid correction can lead to central pontine myelinolysis, a devastating condition characterized by dysarthria, dysphagia, weakness, and paralysis of the appendages, and, in the most serious cases, coma, paralysis of all voluntary muscles except those controlling the eye (locked-in syndrome), and death.[17] Current recommendations are to increase Na^+ by 0.5 to 2.0 mmol/L per hour and not to exceed a total increase in Na^+ greater than 18 over 48 hours.[18] For patients with severe symptoms, an easy-to-remember strategy called the "rule of sixes" is recommended (using the abbreviations six's for symptoms): "six a day makes sense for safety; so six [mmol/L] in 6 hours for severe sx's and stop."[10]

Finally, euvolemic hyponatremia also can be found in primary polydipsia when water intake is greater than the renal capacity to excrete excess H_2O. This can be the result of psychiatric illness, but diseases that cause hypothalamic disorders, such as sarcoidosis, also may cause polydipsia by altering the thirst reflex (see Fig. 50.3).

Hyperosmotic hyponatremia. Hyponatremia in the presence of increased quantities of other solutes in the ECF is the result of an extracellular shift of water or an intracellular shift of Na^+ to maintain osmotic balance between ECF and ICF compartments. The most common cause of this type of hyponatremia is severe hyperglycemia (see Fig. 50.3). As a general rule, Na^+ is decreased by $\approx$1.6 to 2.0 mmol/L for every 100-mg/dL (5.6-mmol/L) increase in glucose greater than 100 mg/dL (5.6 mmol/L).[18] Correction of hyperglycemia alone will restore normal blood Na^+. It also may occur when unmeasured solutes, such as mannitol, radiographic contrast agents, and glycine (surgical irrigant solutions), enter the intravascular fluid compartment. In these circumstances, plasma osmolality cannot be calculated accurately and it must be ascertained by direct measurement.

Isosmotic hyponatremia. If the measured Na^+ concentration in plasma is decreased, but measured plasma osmolality, glucose, and urea are normal, the most likely explanation is pseudohyponatremia caused by the electrolyte exclusion effect (see Chapter 37). This occurs when Na^+ is measured by an indirect ion-selective electrode (ISE) in patients with severe hyperlipidemia or, less commonly, hyperproteinemia. Hyperlipidemia, manifested primarily as hypertriglyceridemia, although a more common cause of pseudohyponatremia, is typically detected by visual or spectrophotometric screening of samples prior to analysis. Hypercholesterolemia, which in contrast, is not reliably detected by visual or spectrophotometric screening, may produce pseudohyponatremia. The common culprit in hypercholesterolemia-induced pseudohyponatremia is lipoprotein X, an abnormal lipid particle arising in the setting of cholestasis.[19] However, it is worth noting that high cholesterol concentrations are less likely to produce pseudohyponatremia, because the molecular mass of cholesterol is approximately 2.5 times lower than triglycerides and thus displaces a smaller amount of plasma water than triglycerides.[20]

Hyperproteinemia, the other common cause of pseudohyponatremia, also cannot be detected by visual or spectrophotometric inspection. As shown in a recent study, only 10.9% of sodium test orders included an order for total protein, and the prevalence of pseudohyponatremia due to hyperproteinemia (>7.9 g/dL) at a large academic medical center was 5.3%.[21] Of note, 36.6% of high total protein results in that study came from the hematology and oncology clinics, and many of the patients had restricted protein bands consistent with monoclonal disorders such as multiple myeloma or waldenstrom macroglobulinemia. Given that a high proportion of those patients with high total protein also had restricted peaks consistent with a plasma cell disorder, it is important to raise awareness of the potential for these patients to be at risk for pseudohyponatremia.

For laboratories serving a population with a high percentage of plasma cell disorders, the availability of a direct ISE method to help with the investigation of potential pseudohyponatremia cases is important because direct ISE methods are not subject to pseudohyponatremia.

Hypernatremia

Hypernatremia (defined as plasma Na^+ >145 mmol/L) is always hyperosmolar and is considerably less common than hyponatremia because a mild increase (1%) in serum osmolality increases thirst. However, hypernatremia occurs frequently in critically ill patients, where patients may be unable to drink water, and it is associated with very high mortality rates (40 to 60%) and prolonged length of intensive care unit (ICU) stay.[22] Symptoms of hypernatremia are primarily neurologic (because of neuronal cell loss of H_2O to the ECF) and include tremors, irritability, ataxia, confusion, and coma.[7,11] As with hyponatremia, the rapidity of development of hypernatremia will determine the plasma Na^+ concentration at which symptoms occur. Acute development may cause symptoms at 160 mmol/L, although in chronic hypernatremia, symptoms may not occur until Na^+ exceeds 175 mmol/L. In chronic hypernatremia, the intracellular osmolality of CNS cells will increase to protect against intracellular dehydration. Because of this, rapid correction of hypernatremia can cause dangerous cerebral edema because CNS cells will take up too much water if the ICF is hyperosmotic when normonatremia is achieved.[11]

In many cases, the symptoms of hypernatremia may be masked by underlying conditions. Hypernatremia rarely occurs in an alert patient with a normal thirst response and access to water. Most cases are observed in patients with altered mental status or infants, both of whom may not be capable of rehydrating themselves.

Hypernatremia arises in the setting of (1) hypovolemia (excessive water loss or failure to replace normal water losses), (2) hypervolemia (a net Na^+ gain in excess of water gain), or (3) normovolemia. Again, assessment of TBW status by physical examination and measurement of urine Na^+ and osmolality are important initial steps in establishing a diagnosis (Fig. 50.4).

Hypovolemic hypernatremia. Hypernatremia in the setting of decreased ECF is caused by renal or extrarenal loss of hypo-osmotic fluid, leading to dehydration. Thus once

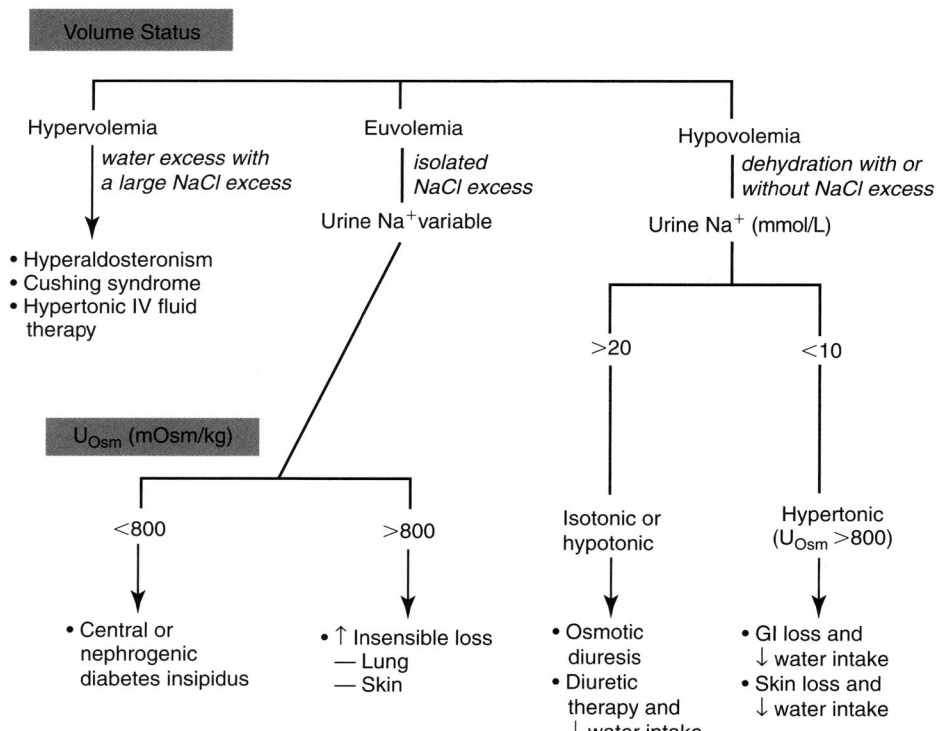

FIGURE 50.4 Algorithm for the differential diagnosis of hypernatremia. (Modified from Kirkpatrick W, Kreisberg R. Acid-base and electrolyte disorders. In: Liu P, ed. *Blue book of diagnostic tests.* Philadelphia: WB Saunders; 1986:239–54.)

hypovolemia is established by physical examination, measurement of urine Na^+ and osmolality is used to determine the source of fluid loss. Patients who have large extrarenal losses will have concentrated urine (often >800 mOsmol/kg) with low urine Na^+ (<20 mmol/L), reflecting a proper renal response to conserve Na^+ and water to restore ECF volume. Extrarenal causes include diarrhea, skin losses (burns, fever, or excessive sweating), and respiratory losses coupled with failure to replace the water. When gastrointestinal loss is excluded, and the patient has normal mental status and access to H_2O, a hypothalamic disorder (tumor or granuloma) inducing diabetes insipidus (DI) should be suspected.[11]

In patients with poorly controlled diabetes with glucose values greater than 600 mg/dL (33.3 mmol/L), an osmotic diuresis can occur that results in extreme dehydration and hypernatremia. This condition is referred to as hyperosmolar hyperglycemic nonketotic syndrome and occurs most commonly in elderly individuals with type 2 diabetes.

Normovolemic hypernatremia. Hypernatremia in the presence of normal ECF volume is often a prelude to hypovolemic hypernatremia. Insensible losses through the lung or skin must be suspected and are characterized by concentrated urine as the kidneys conserve water. Another cause of normovolemic hypernatremia is water diuresis, which is manifested by polyuria (see Fig. 50.4). The differential for polyuria (generally defined as greater than 3 L urine output/day) is a water or solute diuresis. Solute diuresis is exemplified by the osmotic diuresis of diabetes mellitus and generally is characterized by urine osmolality greater than 300 mOsmol/kg and hyponatremia (see previous discussion in this chapter). Water diuresis, a manifestation of DI, is characterized by dilute urine (osmolality <250 mOsmol/kg) and hypernatremia.[11] DI can be central or nephrogenic.[23] Central DI is due to decreased or absent vasopressin secretion resulting from head trauma, hypophysectomy, pituitary tumor, or granulomatous disease. Nephrogenic DI is due to renal resistance to vasopressin as a result of drugs (e.g., lithium, demeclocycline, amphotericin, propoxyphene); electrolyte disorders (e.g., hypercalcemia, hypokalemia); sickle cell anemia or Sjögren syndrome, which affect collecting duct responsiveness to vasopressin; or, more rarely, mutant vasopressin receptors.[24] When thirst and access to water are uncompromised, many patients with DI will remain normonatremic because their free water losses are offset by intake. Such patients display symptoms of only polyuria and polydipsia. However, overt hypernatremia can manifest with progression of underlying causes, impaired thirst, or restricted access to water. Administration of vasopressin can be used to treat central DI, although patients with nephrogenic DI may be resistant to it. Correction of underlying disorders or discontinuation of offending drugs may be required to normalize Na^+ concentrations in nephrogenic DI.[11]

Hypervolemic hypernatremia. The presence of excess TBW and hypernatremia indicates a net gain of water and Na^+, with Na^+ gain in excess of water (see Fig. 50.4). This rare condition is observed most commonly in hospitalized patients receiving hypertonic saline or sodium bicarbonate. It affects acute kidney injury (AKI) patients in the ICU at a high rate because these patients are often given large quantities of physiologic saline, leading to sodium and water retention (as evidenced by edema and substantial weight gain).[25] Hypernatremia then develops during the recovery of their renal function due to loss of water in excess of sodium and potassium. This type of hypernatremia can be prevented by paying close attention to the water and sodium balance in patients with large urine or stool outputs.[25]

Rarely, hypervolemic hypernatremia may also be the result of the intentional or accidental ingestion of large quantities of sodium rich fluids, otherwise known as salt poisoning. Ingestion of a concentrated salt (NaCl) solution may induce vomiting and had previously been used as an emetic. However, because a salt water solution may also produce life-threatening hyponatremia, the use of salt water as an emetic should be strongly discouraged.

The causes of salt poisoning also include inappropriately reconstituted oral rehydration solutions and infant formula, as well as the intentional ingestion of high-sodium solutions such as soy sauce, in suicide attempts.[26]

In contrast to other causes of hypernatremia, in which a rapid correction of hypernatremia may produce osmotic demyelination,[11] the rapid correction of acute salt poisoning with hypotonic solutions can prevent intracranial hemorrhage and neurologic sequelae.

Potassium

The total body potassium of a 70-kg subject is ≈3.5 mol (40 to 59 mmol/kg), of which only 1.5 to 2% is present in the ECF. Nevertheless, plasma K^+ is often a good indicator of total K^+ stores. Disturbance of K^+ homeostasis has serious consequences. For example, a decrease in extracellular K^+ (hypokalemia) is characterized by muscle weakness, irritability, and paralysis. Plasma K^+ concentrations less than 3.0 mmol/L are often associated with marked neuromuscular symptoms and indicate a critical degree of intracellular depletion. At lower concentrations, tachycardia and cardiac conduction defects are apparent on electrocardiogram (ECG) (flattened T waves) and can lead to cardiac arrest.[11]

High extracellular K^+ (hyperkalemia) concentrations may produce symptoms of mental confusion, weakness, tingling, flaccid paralysis of the extremities, and weakness of the respiratory muscles.[11] Cardiac effects of hyperkalemia include bradycardia and conduction defects evident on the ECG as prolonged PR and QRS intervals and "peaked" T waves. Prolonged, severe hyperkalemia greater than 7.0 mmol/L can lead to peripheral vascular collapse and cardiac arrest. Symptoms or ECG abnormalities are almost always present at K^+ concentrations greater than 6.5 mmol/L. Concentrations greater than 10.0 mmol/L in most cases are fatal, although fatalities can occur at significantly lower values.

Hypokalemia

Causes of hypokalemia (plasma K^+ <3.5 mmol/L) are classified as redistribution of extracellular K^+ into ICF, or true K^+ deficits, caused by decreased intake or loss of potassium-rich body fluids (Fig. 50.5).

Redistribution. Intracellular redistribution of K^+ is illustrated by the fall in plasma K^+ that occurs after insulin therapy for diabetic hyperglycemia. Insulin plays a crucial role in maintaining the intracellular distribution of K^+ through active cellular transport and glucose control. In alkalosis, redistribution hypokalemia occurs when K^+ moves from ECF into cells as H^+ ions are pumped out by the Na^+-H^+ antiporter. The resulting increase in intracellular Na^+ concentration from the action of the Na^+-H^+

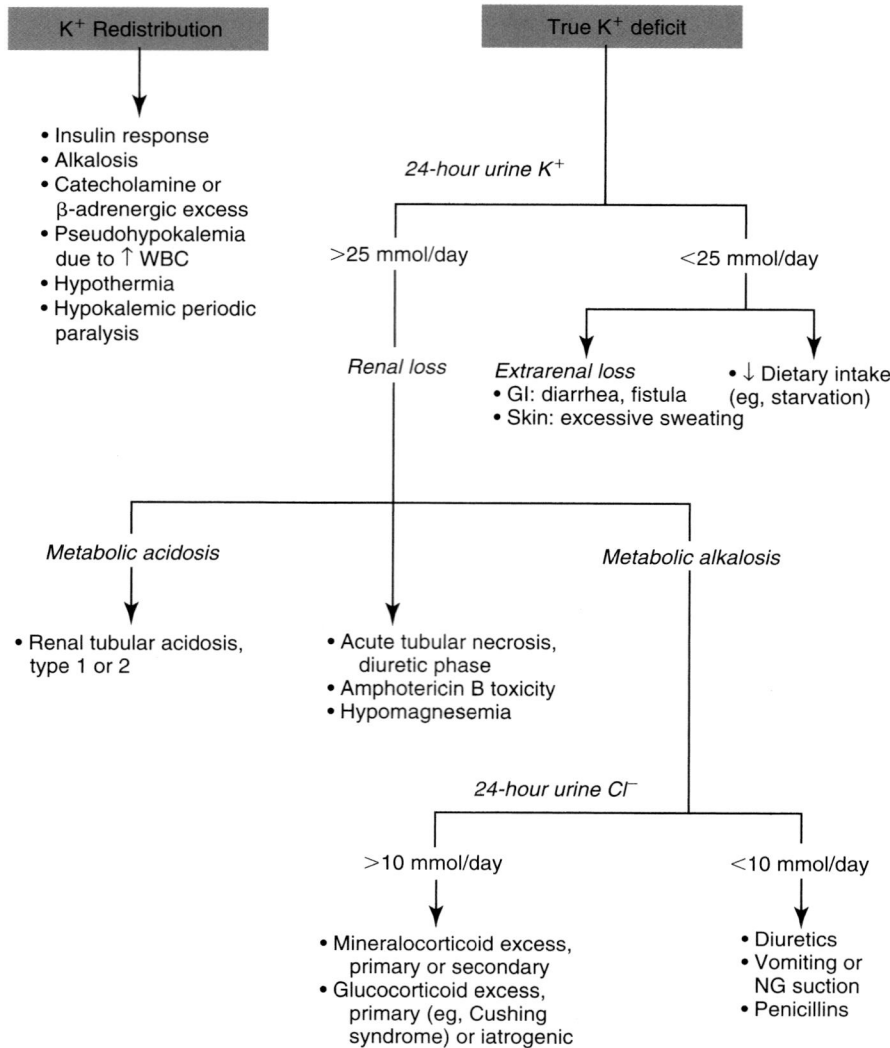

FIGURE 50.5 Algorithm for the differential diagnosis of hypokalemia. *GI,* Gastrointestinal; *NG,* nasogastric; *WBC,* white blood cell. (Modified from Kirkpatrick W, Kreisberg R. Acid-base and electrolyte disorders. In: Liu P, ed. *Blue book of diagnostic tests.* Philadelphia: WB Saunders; 1986:239–54.)

antiporter increases the activity of the Na$^+$/K$^+$-ATPase, resulting in a decrease in ECF K$^+$.[27] In addition, renal conservation of H$^+$ in the distal tubule occurs at the expense of K$^+$. Hypokalemia is not an uncommon condition in in patients with cancer, either due to effects of the tumor itself on adrenal or renal tissues or from side effects of the chemotherapeutic medications. However, it is important in this group to be sure that the hypokalemia is true hypokalemia and not due to pseudohypokalemia.

The risk of pseudohypokalemia is higher in patients with hematologic malignancies associated with acute leukemia. Pseudohypokalemia can arise when blood samples from patients with very high white blood cell counts are allowed to stand at room temperature prior to processing and analysis.[28] Pseudohypokalemia arises in this setting due to a time-dependent redistribution of K$^+$ from the plasma fraction into leukemic cells after the blood sample is collected. In addition, use of myelopoietic growth factors after chemotherapy can lead to rapid K$^+$ uptake by new cells.[29] In these settings, it is important to process the samples as quickly as possible.

Other causes of intracellular redistribution are listed in Fig. 50.5. Clinically, redistributive hypokalemia is generally a transient phenomenon that is reversed once underlying conditions are corrected. Therefore careful monitoring during treatment of these patients is essential to avoid overcorrection (termed "rebound hyperkalemia"), especially when considering that supplemental potassium is a common cause of hyperkalemia in hospitalized patients.[30]

True potassium deficit. Hypokalemia reflecting true total body deficits of K$^+$ because of potassium loss can be classified into renal and nonrenal losses, based on daily excretion of K$^+$ in the urine (see Fig. 50.5). If urine excretion of K$^+$ is less than 30 mmol/d, it can be concluded that the kidneys are functioning properly and are attempting to reabsorb K$^+$. The cause may be decreased K$^+$ intake or extrarenal loss of K$^+$-rich fluid. Causes of decreased intake include chronic starvation and postoperative intravenous fluid therapy with K$^+$-poor solutions. Gastrointestinal loss of K$^+$ occurs most commonly with diarrhea and loss of gastric fluid through vomiting.

Urine excretion exceeding 25 to 30 mmol/day in a hypokalemic setting is inappropriate and indicates that the kidneys are the primary source of K^+ loss. Renal losses of K^+ may occur during the diuretic (recovery) phase of acute tubular necrosis and during states of excess mineralocorticoid (primary or secondary aldosteronism) or glucocorticoid (Cushing's syndrome) production when the distal tubules increase Na^+ reabsorption and K^+ excretion. Renal loss of K^+ is also caused by thiazide and loop diuretics.[31] In addition to redistribution of K^+ into cells in an alkalotic setting, K^+ can be lost from the kidneys in exchange for reclaimed H^+ ions. This cause of true hypokalemia will be evident in low urine Cl^- and an alkaline urine. In patients with cancer, increased renal K^+ loss may be due to chemotherapy (e.g., cisplatin)-induced nephron and tubular damage.[29] Magnesium deficiency also can lead to increased renal loss of K^+, which is attributable to a reduction in the inhibitory effect of magnesium on luminal potassium channels.[32]

True potassium deficit requires replacement of potassium. Although there are dietary sources of potassium, such as potatoes and tomatoes, significant K^+ losses may require oral or intravenous supplementation with potassium chloride. The oral route is generally preferred, although intravenous correction should be pursued in patients with severe or symptomatic hypokalemia and those who are unable to take oral medication.[11] In individuals with ongoing sources of potassium losses, such as patients on diuretics, chronic supplementation with a daily regimen of oral potassium chloride is often used.

Hyperkalemia

Hyperkalemia (commonly listed as a plasma K^+ >5.0 mmol/L in adults) is a result of (singly or in combination) (1) redistribution, (2) increased intake, or (3) increased retention. In addition, preanalytical conditions—such as hemolysis, thrombocytosis (>500 × 10^9/L, when serum rather than plasma potassium is measured), and leukocytosis (>50 × 10^9/L together with delayed sample analysis)—have been known to cause marked pseudohyperkalemia, as described in detail in Chapter 37 (Fig. 50.6).[33]

Redistribution. The transfer of intracellular K^+ into ECF invariably occurs in acidemia as K^+ shifts outward as the result of pH-induced changes in Na^+/K^+-ATPase activity. In general, K^+ concentrations can be expected to rise 0.2 to 0.5 mmol/L for every 0.1-unit drop in pH. When acidemia is corrected, normokalemia will be restored rapidly. Extracellular redistribution of K^+ also may occur in (1) tissue hypoxia; (2) insulin deficiency (e.g., diabetic ketoacidosis); (3) massive intravascular hemolysis; (4) severe burns; (5) violent muscular activity, as in status epilepticus; (6) rhabdomyolysis; and (7) tumor lysis syndrome. Finally, important iatrogenic causes of redistribution hyperkalemia include digoxin toxicity and β-adrenergic blockade, especially in patients with diabetes or on dialysis.[11] Redistributive hyperkalemia can be corrected by reversing the aberrations that cause K^+ to shift out of cells. Insulin and sodium bicarbonate are commonly used and have a quick onset of action, particularly in the diabetic or acidemic setting. Drug-induced causes require cessation or dose reduction of the offending agent. Patients with digoxin toxicity should be given antibodies to digoxin as well,

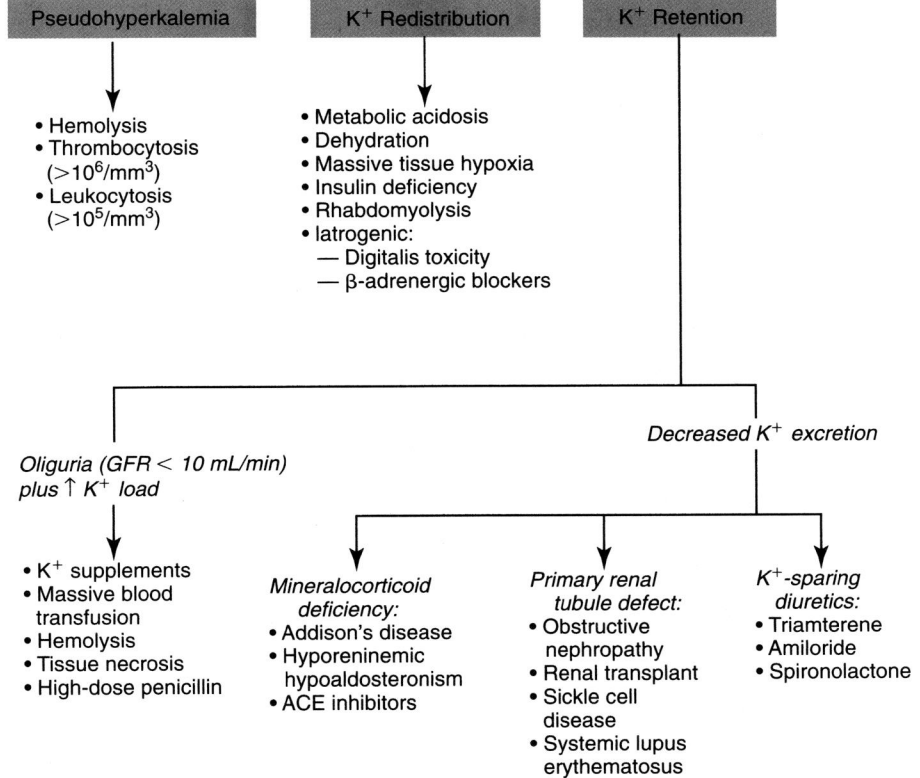

FIGURE 50.6 Algorithm for the differential diagnosis of hyperkalemia. *ACE,* Angiotensin-converting enzyme. (Modified from Kirkpatrick W, Kreisberg R. Acid-base and electrolyte disorders. In: Liu P, ed. *Blue book of diagnostic tests.* Philadelphia: WB Saunders; 1986:239–254.)

because of the high risk for mortality associated with hyperkalemia and supratherapeutic administration of digoxin.

Potassium retention. When glomerular filtration rate (GFR) or renal tubular function is decreased, hyperkalemia will often occur. In the absence of severe renal failure, hyperkalemia is seldom prolonged and may not even occur in some cases. Decreased excretion of K^+ in moderate and acute renal disease and end-stage renal failure (with oliguria or anuria) are the most common causes of prolonged hyperkalemia (see Fig. 50.6). Hyperkalemia occurs along with Na^+ depletion in adrenocortical insufficiency (e.g., Addison disease) because diminished Na^+ reabsorption results in decreased tubular K^+ secretion. Drugs that block the production of aldosterone, such as inhibitors of angiotensin-converting enzyme (ACE inhibitors; e.g., lisinopril), nonsteroidal antiinflammatory drugs, and angiotensin II–receptor blockers, may also cause hyperkalemia. Excess administration of potassium-sparing diuretics that block distal tubular K^+ secretion (e.g., triamterene, spironolactone) may also cause hyperkalemia.[31] In patients with cancer, hyperkalemia can be caused by adrenal insufficiency secondary to metastases to the adrenal glands, nephrotoxic chemotherapy agents (e.g., mitomycin-C, methotrexate, platinum compounds), postrenal obstruction, or tumor lysis syndrome.[29] Treatment of hyperkalemia includes agents that increase cellular uptake of K^+, such as glucose given with insulin, sodium bicarbonate, and β_2-adrenergic agonists. The rapid onset of these agents provides a quick reduction in ECF potassium concentrations, thus reducing the risk for immediate life-threatening cardiac effects of hyperkalemia.

In the setting of hyperkalemia, calcium salts are also frequently administered to counteract the depolarizing effects of high extracellular K^+. High K^+ concentration increases the resting membrane potential of the myocyte from approximately -90 to -80 mV, which is close to the depolarization threshold of -75 mV. This results in a greater likelihood of myocyte depolarization and arrhythmia. Infusion of calcium, in the form of $CaCl_2$ or calcium gluconate, rapidly increases extracellular Ca^{2+} concentrations, which raise the depolarization threshold to approximately -65 mV. Raising the depolarization threshold to -65 mV re-establishes the interval between the normal resting potential and normal depolarization threshold, in effect decreasing myocyte excitability.[34]

However, infusion of calcium does not contribute to the redistribution of extracellular potassium and should be combined with other treatment modalities. It is also important to note that treatments that increase intracellular redistribution of potassium are only temporizing measures when there is a true excess of potassium, and they need to be coupled with interventions that remove potassium from the circulation. To reduce the total body content of potassium, patients can be given K^+-losing diuretics, cation-exchange resins, and, finally, hemodialysis.[29] Stimulation of renal potassium excretion is preferred because the use of cation-exchange resins can be associated with bowel necrosis, particularly when given per rectum. Hemodialysis is an option of last resort, removing potassium through an extracorporeal circuit, which stimulates diffusion of potassium out of the circulating blood and into the discarded dialysate.

Chloride

In the absence of acid-base disturbances, Cl^- concentrations in plasma generally will follow those of Na^+. However, determination of plasma Cl^- concentration is useful in the differential diagnosis of acid-base disturbances and is essential for calculating the anion gap. Fluctuations in serum or plasma Cl^- were believed to have little clinical consequence and serving only as signs of an underlying disturbance in fluid or acid-base homeostasis. The specific replacement of chloride is rarely targeted at chloride deficit independently, but it is a cornerstone of management for metabolic alkalosis. This notion has been challenged in recent studies linking lower chloride levels with reduced loop diuretic response.[35] In addition, oral supplementation of sodium-free chloride in patients receiving high doses of loop diuretics saw increases in serum chloride levels and changes in cardiorenal parameters.[35]

Hypochloremia

In general, causes of hypochloremia (generally defined as Cl^- <98 mmol/L) parallel causes of hyponatremia. Persistent gastric secretion and prolonged vomiting result in significant loss of Cl^- and ultimately in hypochloremic alkalosis and depletion of total body Cl^- with retention of HCO_3^-. Respiratory acidosis, which is accompanied by increased HCO_3^-, is another common cause of decreased Cl^- with normal Na^+.

Hyperchloremia

Hyperchloremia (generally defined as Cl^- >107 mmol/L), similar to hypernatremia, occurs with dehydration, prolonged diarrhea with loss of sodium bicarbonate, DI, and overtreatment with normal saline solutions, which have a Cl^- content of 150 mmol/L. Mounting evidence suggests that use of 0.9% saline (NaCl) solution for maintenance, intraoperative, and resuscitative therapy can result in a host of hyperchloremia-induced side effects.[36] For these reasons, there is a movement toward more physiologic solutions such as lactated Ringer's solution that contain a lower concentration of chloride.[36] A rise in Cl^- concentration also may be seen in respiratory alkalosis because of renal compensation for excreting HCO_3^-.

POINTS TO REMEMBER

- Physical examination is important in assessing total body water (TBW) status and hyponatremic or hypernatremic disorders.
- Urine electrolytes are important to determine if the kidneys are functioning properly in disorders of electrolyte and water balance.
- Patient history can be important in assessing electrolyte disorders. Examples include medication use, vomiting, diarrhea, water deprivation, excess perspiration, anuria, diabetes, etc.

ACID-BASE PHYSIOLOGY

Normal metabolic processes result in the production of large amounts of carbonic acid and lower amounts of sulfuric, phosphoric, and other acids. For example, during a 24-hour period, a person weighing 70 kg disposes of approximately 20 moles of carbon dioxide (CO_2; the volatile form of carbonic acid) through the lungs and about 70 to 100 mmol (or ≈ 1 mmol/kg) of nonvolatile acids (mainly sulfuric and phosphoric acids) through the kidneys. These products of metabolism are transported to the lungs and kidneys via the

ECF and blood with no appreciable change in the ECF pH, and with only a minimal difference between arterial (pH 7.35 to 7.45) and venous (pH 7.32 to 7.38) blood. This is accomplished by the buffering capacity of blood and by respiratory and renal regulatory mechanisms.

Acid-Base Balance and Acid-Base Status

A description of acid-base balance involves an accounting of the carbonic (H_2CO_3, HCO_3^-, CO_3^{2-}, and CO_2) and noncarbonic acids and conjugate bases in terms of input (intake plus metabolic production) and output (excretion plus metabolic conversion) over a given time interval. The acid-base status of body fluids is typically assessed by measurements of total CO_2, plasma pH, and PCO_2, because the bicarbonate/carbonic acid system is the most important mammalian buffering system.

The following clinical terms are used to describe acid-base status. *Acidemia* is defined as an arterial blood pH less than 7.35, and *alkalemia* indicates an arterial blood pH greater than 7.45. *Acidosis* and *alkalosis* refer to pathologic states that often lead to acidemia or alkalemia. For example, in common acid-base disorders such as lactic acidosis and diabetic ketoacidosis, intermediate organic acids (lactic acid and β-hydroxybutyric acid, respectively), which normally are metabolized to CO_2 and water, may accumulate to a significant extent, resulting in acidemia. In addition, more than one type of pathologic process can occur simultaneously, giving rise to a mixed acid-base disturbance, in which the blood pH may be low, high, or within the reference interval.

Acid-Base Parameters: Definitions and Abbreviations

Acids are chemical substances that can donate protons (H^+ ions) in solution, and *bases* are substances that accept protons. Strong acids readily give up H^+, whereas strong bases readily accept H^+. Thus the conjugate base of a strong acid is a weak base and vice versa.

pH and pK. The pH of a solution is defined as the negative logarithm of the hydrogen ion activity (pH = $-\log_{10} aH^+$). *pH is a dimensionless quantity,* such that a decrease in one pH unit represents a 10-fold increase in H^+ activity. The average pH of blood (7.40) corresponds to a hydrogen ion concentration of 40 nmol/L, assuming an activity coefficient of 1. The relationship between hydrogen ion activity and pH is illustrated in Fig. 50.7. This relationship is inverse and logarithmic.

The pK (also, pK′ and pK_a) represents the negative logarithm of the ionization constant of a weak acid (K_a); that is, the pK is the pH at which an acid is half dissociated, existing as equal proportions of acid and conjugate base. Acids have pK values less than 7.0, whereas bases have pK values greater than 7.0. The lower the pK, the stronger is the acid, and the higher the pK, the stronger is the conjugate base. For example, the pK of lactic acid is ≈3.86, and that of ammonium ion NH_4^+ is 9.5. The high pK for the ammonium ion indicates that this species prefers to hold onto its proton, rather than dissociating into NH_3 and H^+.

The pH of plasma may be considered to be a function of two independent variables: (1) the PCO_2, which is regulated by the lungs and represents the acid component of the carbonic acid/bicarbonate buffer system, and (2) the concentration of titratable base (base excess or deficit, which is defined later), which is regulated by the kidneys. The plasma total

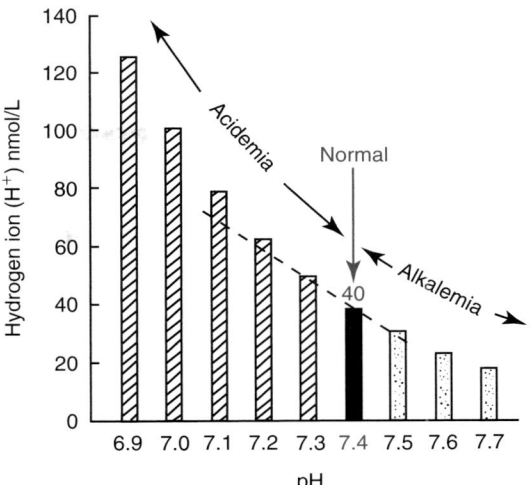

FIGURE 50.7 Relationship of pH to hydrogen ion concentration. A *broken line* is drawn to emphasize the (approximate) linear relationship between hydrogen ion concentration and pH over the pH range of 7.2 to 7.5. (From Narins RG, Emmett M. Simple and mixed acid-base disorders: a practical approach. *Medicine* 1980; 59:161–87.)

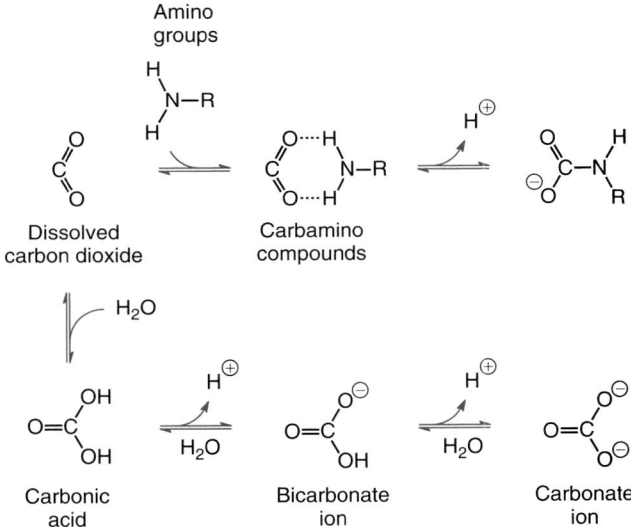

FIGURE 50.8 Reactions of carbon dioxide with water and amino groups. Hydrogen bonding is indicated by a *dotted line.* The carbamino acid is fairly strong ($-R-NH-COOH \rightarrow H^+ + R-NH-COO^-$).

CO_2 concentration generally is taken as a measure of the base excess or deficit in plasma and ECF.

Bicarbonate and dissolved carbon dioxide. Bicarbonate is the second largest fraction (behind Cl^-) of plasma anions. Conventionally, it is defined to include (1) plasma bicarbonate ion (HCO_3^-), (2) carbonate ion (CO_3^{2-}), and (3) CO_2 bound in plasma carbamino compounds (RCNHCOOH) (Fig. 50.8). Actual bicarbonate ion concentration is not measured in clinical laboratories. The analyte usually measured in plasma is total CO_2, which includes bicarbonate and dissolved CO_2 (dCO_2) but is often referred to as "serum bicarb." At the pH of the blood, the amount of dissolved CO_2 is 700 to 1000 times greater than the amount of carbonic acid

(H_2CO_3); therefore $cdCO_2$ is the term used to express their combined concentration. It is calculated from the solubility coefficient of CO_2 in blood at 37 °C ($\alpha = 0.0306$ mmol/L per mm Hg) multiplied by the measured PCO_2 in mm Hg. Thus at a PCO_2 of 40 mm Hg, $cdCO_2$ is 1.224 mmol/L (0.0306 mmol/L × 40 mm Hg). This $cdCO_2$ value can then be used, in the Henderson-Hasselbalch equation, to calculate the total bicarbonate concentration.

Henderson-Hasselbalch equation. The Henderson-Hasselbalch equation is described in detail in Chapter 37. However, it is important to review here because it enhances understanding of pH regulation of body fluids as it relates to compensatory mechanisms in acid-base disturbances. The equation derived in Chapter 37 can also be written as follows:

$$pH = 6.1 + \log\frac{cHCO_3^-}{cdCO_2}$$

where $cdCO_2$ is equal to α (0.0306 mmol/L per mm Hg) PCO_2 and 6.1 is the pK' for the carbonic acid/bicarbonate system. An alternative expression useful for approximating cH^+ in blood is as follows:

$$cH^+ = K \times \frac{PCO_2}{cHCO_3^-}$$

where $K = 24$ (nmol/L) (mmol/L) (mm Hg^{-1}).

The average normal ratio of the concentrations of bicarbonate (HCO_3^-) and $cdCO_2$ (dissolved CO_2 and $H_2CO_3^-$) in plasma is 25 (mmol/L)/1.25 (mmol/L) = 20/1. It follows then that any change in the concentration of bicarbonate or dissolved CO_2 relative to each other must be accompanied by a change in pH. Such changes in this important ratio can occur through a change in $cHCO_3^-$ (the renal component) or PCO_2 (the respiratory component). Clinical conditions characterized as *metabolic* disturbances of acid-base balance are classified as primary disturbances in $cHCO_3^-$. Those characterized as

respiratory disturbances are classified as primary disturbances in $cdCO_2$ (PCO_2). Various compensatory mechanisms attempting to reestablish the normal ratio of $cHCO_3^-/cdCO_2$ may result in changes in bicarbonate concentration, dissolved CO_2 concentration, or both. Application of the Henderson-Hasselbalch equation to human acid-base physiology can be illustrated by a lever-fulcrum (teeter-totter) diagram (Fig. 50.9).

Buffer Systems and Their Role in Regulating the pH of Body Fluids

A buffer is a mixture of a weak acid and a salt of its conjugate base that resists changes in pH when a strong acid or base is added to the solution. If concentrations of the acid and base components of a buffer are equal, the pH will equal the pK. In general, buffers work best at resisting pH changes in the interval ±1 pH unit of its pK and are more effective at higher molar concentrations. The action of buffers in the regulation of body pH can be demonstrated by using the bicarbonate buffer system as an example. If a strong acid is added to a solution containing $cHCO_3^-$ and H_2CO_3, the H^+ will react with $cHCO_3^-$ to form more H_2CO_3 and subsequently CO_2 and H_2O. The hydrogen ions are thereby bound, and the increase in the H^+ concentration will be minimal.

$$H^+ + HCO_3^- \Leftrightarrow H_2CO_3 \Leftrightarrow CO_2 + H_2O$$

Bicarbonate and Carbonic Acid Buffer System

The most important buffer of plasma is the bicarbonate/carbonic acid pair even though its pK is 6.1, and normal plasma pH is 7.4. The normal bicarbonate/dCO_2 ratio is 20:1, which is outside the 10:1 or 1:10 ratio at which buffers work best. However, the effectiveness of the bicarbonate buffer is based on the fact that the lungs can readily dispose of or retain CO_2, and it is present at higher concentrations than other buffers with the exception of hemoglobin (Hb). In addition, the renal tubules can increase or decrease the rate of reclamation of bicarbonate from the glomerular filtrate

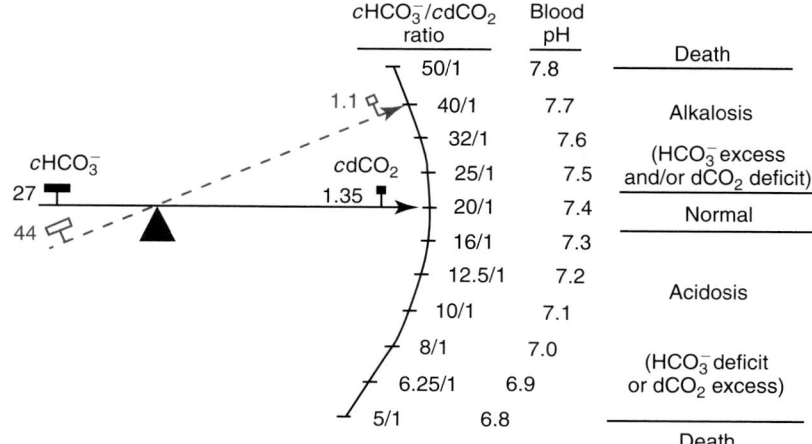

FIGURE 50.9 Scheme demonstrating the relation between pH and the ratio of bicarbonate concentration to the concentration of dissolved CO_2. If the ratio in blood is 20:1 ($cHCO_3^- = 27$ mmol/$cdCO_2 = 1.35$ mmol/L), the resultant pH will be 7.4, as demonstrated by the *solid beam*. The *dotted line* shows a case of uncompensated alkalosis (bicarbonate excess) with a bicarbonate concentration of 44 mmol/L and a $cdCO_2$ of 1.1 mmol/L. The ratio therefore is 40:1, and the resultant pH is 7.7. In a case of uncompensated acidosis, the pointer of the balance would point to a pH between 6.8 and 7.35, depending on the $cHCO_3^-/cdCO_2$ ratio. (From Weisberg HF. A better understanding of anion-cation ["acid-base"] balance. *Surg Clin North Am* 1959;39:93–120.)

(see Chapter 49). The importance of the relatively high concentration of bicarbonate (relative to H^+) becomes apparent when considering that at normal plasma pH, 5 mmol/L of lactate ($pK \approx 3.86$) generates ≈ 5 mmol/L of H^+ ion, which is remarkable given that a normal H^+ ion concentration is only 40 nmol/L. The buffer value (β) is defined as the amount of base required to cause a change in pH of 1 unit. The buffer value of the bicarbonate buffer in plasma is 55.6 mmol/L.[37]

Phosphate Buffer System

At a plasma pH of 7.4, the ratio $cHPO_4^{2-}/cH_2PO_4^-$ is 4:1 ($pK' = 6.8$). The total concentration of this buffer in both erythrocytes and plasma accounts for approximately 5% of the nonbicarbonate buffer value of plasma. However, organic phosphate in the form of 2,3-diphosphoglycerate (present in erythrocytes in a concentration of about 4.5 mmol/L), accounts for about 16% of the nonbicarbonate buffer value of erythrocytes.

The phosphate buffer reacts with acids and with bases as follows:

$$HPO_4^{2+} + H^+ \rightarrow H_2PO_4^+$$
$$H_2PO_4^+ + OH^- \rightarrow HPO_4^{2+} + H_2O$$

This system is most important in the titration and excretion of acids in urine.

Plasma Protein Buffer System

The buffer value (β) of the nonbicarbonate buffers of plasma totals approximately 7.7 mmol/L at pH 7.40 and a normal plasma protein concentration of 72 g/L. Proteins, especially albumin, account for the greatest portion (>90%) of the nonbicarbonate buffer value of plasma.

The significance of nonbicarbonate buffers of plasma can be illustrated by the chemical reactions during CO_2 equilibration:

$$CO_2 + H_2O \rightarrow H_2CO_3 \rightarrow HCO_3^- + H^+$$
$$HPr \rightarrow H^+ + Pr^-$$

where the HPr/Pr$^-$ system represents all nonbicarbonate buffers. Because the purpose of this buffer system is to maintain cH^+ constant, for each molecule of HCO_3^- generated, one molecule of nonbicarbonate buffer base disappears. Thus in alkalosis, the cH^+ from CO_2 equilibration falls and an excess of nonbicarbonate buffer base is the result. As follows, there is a consumption or negative excess of this buffer base in acidosis.

Hemoglobin Buffer System and Whole Blood Base Excess

The buffer value (β) of the nonbicarbonate buffers of erythrocyte fluid is approximately 63 mmol/L at pH 7.20, for an erythrocyte Hb concentration of 21 mmol/L (33.8 g/dL). Hb accounts for the major part (53 mmol/L), with the remainder attributable to 2,3-diphosphoglycerate (2,3-DPG). The imidazole groups of Hb are quantitatively the most important buffer groups with a pK = 7.3.

As in plasma, CO_2 equilibration of whole blood depends on the buffer value of nonbicarbonate buffers. Thus CO_2 equilibration in whole blood depends on Hb concentration and on pH and oxygenation status. It is possible to derive an approximate equation for whole-blood CO_2 equilibration and calculation of *whole-blood base excess* as follows:

$$\Delta cHCO_3^-(P) = -\beta \times \Delta pH(P) + \frac{\Delta cB'(B)}{\zeta}$$

where

$\Delta cHCO_3^-$ = measured plasma $cHCO_3^-(P) - 24.5$ mmol/L HCO_3^-

ΔpH = measured pH − the standard pH of 7.40

$\Delta cB'(B)$ = the *whole-blood base excess* (i.e., the concentration of titratable base when the blood is titrated with strong acid or base to pH = 7.40 at PCO_2 [Std] and 37 °C)

$\beta = \beta_mHb \times cHb(B) + \beta Pr$, where β_mHb is the molar buffer value of Hb (2.3 mol/mol), $cHb(B)$ is the substance concentration of Hb (Fe) in the blood (unit, mmol/L), and βPr is the buffer value of the plasma proteins (7.7 mmol/L): $\zeta = 1 - cHb(B)/c_{ref}$, where c_{ref} is an empirical parameter (43 mmol/L).

This equation for whole-blood base excess (known as the Van Slyke equation[38,39]), together with the Henderson-Hasselbalch equation, provides the simplest algorithm for calculation of various acid-base variables, and its clinical use is owed to Ole Siggaard-Andersen, an author of this chapter in the first two editions of this textbook.[38,39]

Isohydric and Chloride Shift

Because of continuous production of CO_2 within tissue cells, there is a concentration gradient for CO_2 from cells to plasma and thus to erythrocytes. Despite this, all buffer systems discussed previously interact through a phenomenon known as the isohydric Cl$^-$ shift, which keeps the $cdCO_2$ and cH^+ (pH) essentially constant between arterial and venous blood. A small portion of the CO_2 entering the plasma stays as dissolved CO_2, thus the slightly higher PCO_2 of venous blood. Most reacts with H_2O to form carbonic acid that dissociates into H^+ and HCO_3^-. The increased amount of H^+ is buffered by plasma buffers (Fig. 50.10, reaction 1). Another small portion combines with the amino groups of proteins and forms carbamino compounds (see Fig. 50.10, reaction 2). The normal concentration of carbamino compounds in the plasma is approximately 0.2 mmol/L. Most of the CO_2 enters erythrocytes and reacts with water to form carbonic acid. This reaction is catalyzed by the enzyme carbonic anhydrase and proceeds at a relatively high rate (see Fig. 50.9, reaction 3). Some CO_2 remains as dissolved CO_2, and some combines with Hb to form $HbCO_2$ (see Fig. 50.10, reaction 4).

The carbonic acid formed in Fig. 50.10, reaction 3 initially increases the H^+ concentration. However, the pH change is fully or partially compensated by the release of oxygen from O_2Hb, which involves the conversion of stronger acid (O_2Hb) into weaker acid (HHb) that then readily accepts the H^+. Furthermore, the HHb binds significantly more CO_2 in the form of carbamino-CO_2 than does oxyHb. The oxygen released from O_2Hb moves from the erythrocytes through the plasma into the peripheral tissue cells.

Remaining H^+ formed in reaction 3 are buffered by the nonbicarbonate buffers of the erythrocyte fluid, whereas the concentration of HCO_3^- increases to the same extent that the concentration of Hb anion falls. The transformations described so far (see Fig. 50.10, reactions 1 through 5) are

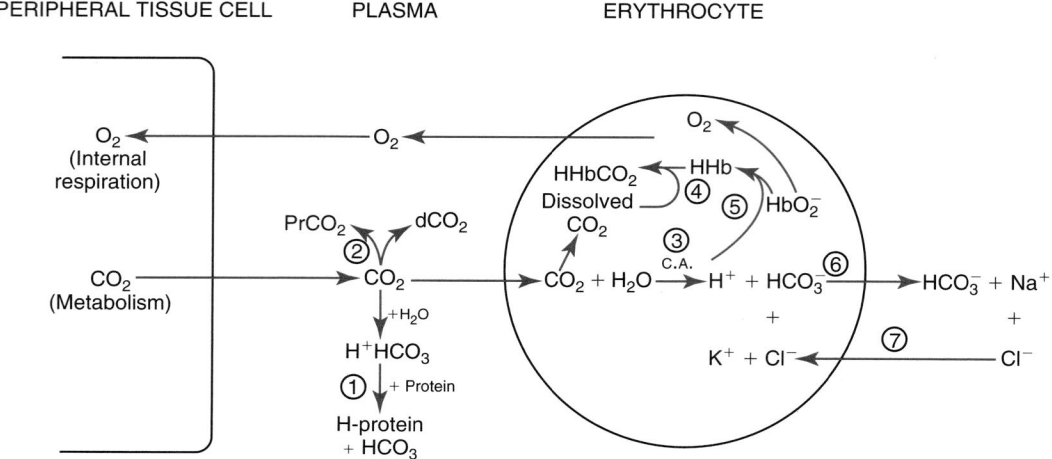

FIGURE 50.10 Scheme demonstrating the isohydric and chloride shift. The *encircled numbers* refer to the reactions described in the text. For details, see text discussion.

referred to as the isohydric shift (i.e., a shift in which the H^+ concentration remains unchanged).

However, the equilibrium between plasma and red cells has been disturbed by this isohydric shift. The concentration of HCO_3^- has increased relatively more in the erythrocytes than in the plasma; the pH of plasma has fallen relatively more than the pH of erythrocytes; and the nondiffusible ion concentration in the erythrocytes has fallen because of the increase in protonation of Hb. The membrane potential of the erythrocytes therefore becomes less negative, and the distribution of all diffusible ions must change with the new membrane potential. The ion shifts that occur rapidly include movement of HCO_3^- out of the erythrocytes and movement of Cl^- into the erythrocytes to provide electrochemical balance. This shift of chloride ions is referred to as the chloride shift (see Fig. 50.10, reactions 6 and 7). In the alveoli, low PCO_2 and high PO_2 cause a reversal of reactions 1 through 7, as shown in Fig. 50.10.

Respiration
Exchange of O_2 and CO_2 in the lungs between alveolar air and blood is called external respiration, in contrast to internal respiration, which occurs at the cellular level. During inspiration, muscular contraction expands intrathoracic volume, decreasing intrapulmonary pressure. Atmospheric air is drawn into the bronchial tree, which terminates at the alveoli, where the exchange of gases between alveolar air and pulmonary blood occurs. Expiration occurs passively as the elastic recoil of the lung tissue and chest wall shrinks thoracic volume.

Peripheral venous blood reaches the pulmonary circulation from the right ventricle of the heart and is arterialized in the capillaries of the alveoli by uptake of O_2 and loss of CO_2. Pulmonary venous blood then returns to the left ventricle by way of the left atrium and is pumped to the peripheral tissues.

In a resting state, the respiratory rate is normally 12 to 15 breaths/min for adults with a tidal volume of approximately 0.5 L. This yields a minute ventilation 6 to 8 L/min. Involuntary increases in rate and depth of respiration are regulated by the medullary respiratory center in the brainstem, which

is stimulated by central chemoreceptors located on the anterior surface of the medulla oblongata and by peripheral chemoreceptors located in the carotid arteries and aorta. Peripheral chemoreceptors are stimulated by a fall in pH caused by accumulation of CO_2 or a decrease in PO_2. Central chemoreceptors are stimulated only by a decrease in pH of the CSF.

Exchange of Gases in the Lungs and Peripheral Tissues
Diffusion of O_2 and CO_2 across alveolar and cell membranes is governed by gradients in the partial pressure of each gas (Fig. 50.11). Dry air inspired at a pressure of 1 atm (760 mm Hg) consists of 21% O_2 ($PO_2 \approx 160$ mm Hg), 0.03% CO_2 ($PCO_2 \approx 0.25$ mm Hg), 78% nitrogen, and $\approx 0.1\%$ other inert gases. As inspired air passes over the mucous membranes of the upper respiratory tract, it is warmed to 37 °C, becomes saturated with water vapor, and mixes with air in the respiratory tree, resulting in partial pressures of ≈ 150 mm Hg for O_2, ≈ 0.3 mm Hg for CO_2, ≈ 47 mm Hg for H_2O, and 563 mm Hg for nitrogen. Further mixing with alveolar air results in partial pressures at the alveolar membrane of ≈ 105 mm Hg for O_2, ≈ 40 mm Hg for CO_2, and ≈ 47 mm Hg for H_2O. Venous blood on the opposite side of the alveolar membrane has $PvO_2 \approx 40$ mm Hg and $PvCO_2 \approx 46$ mm Hg. Thus the gradient for O_2 is inward, toward the blood, and for CO_2, it is outward, toward the alveoli. CO_2 removal is so efficient that the PCO_2 in expired air is more than 100 times the PCO_2 in inspired air (see Fig. 50.11). In arterial blood, the PaO_2 is slightly lower than in alveolar air (90 to 100 versus 105 mm Hg) as the result of shunting of about 5% of blood that does not equilibrate.

At the arterial end of capillaries of peripheral tissues, the PO_2 at 95 mm Hg is substantially higher than the average PO_2 at the surface of tissue cells (20 mm Hg), and the PCO_2 at 40 mm Hg is substantially lower than that in the cells (50 to 70 mm Hg). Thus in the tissue capillary, the gradient for O_2 is inward to the cell; for CO_2, it is outward to the capillary blood. The arteriovenous difference in partial pressures is approximately 60 mm Hg for O_2 and 6 mm Hg or less for CO_2.

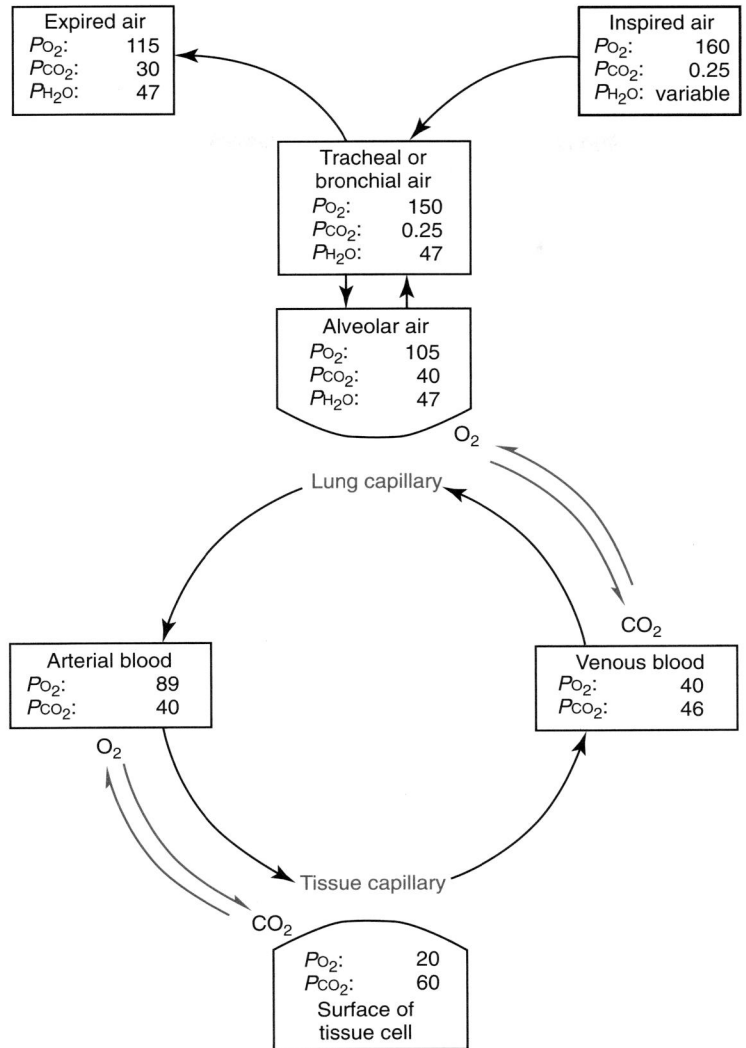

FIGURE 50.11 Partial pressures of oxygen and carbon dioxide in air, blood, and tissue. Values shown are approximations in mm Hg and are calculated assuming a 5% shunt. *Red arrows* show directions of gradients. (Modified from Tietz NW. *Fundamentals of clinical chemistry.* 3rd ed. Philadelphia: WB Saunders; 1987.)

Respiratory Response to Acid-Base Perturbations

Most metabolic acid-base disorders develop slowly, within hours in diabetic ketoacidosis and months in chronic renal disease. The respiratory system responds immediately to a change in acid-base status, but several hours may be required for the response to become maximal. The maximum response is not attained until both central and peripheral chemoreceptors are fully stimulated. For example, in the early stages of metabolic acidosis, the pH of blood decreases, but because H^+ ions equilibrate rather slowly across the blood-brain barrier, the pH in CSF remains nearly normal. However, because peripheral chemoreceptors are stimulated by the decreased blood pH, hyperventilation occurs, and PCO_2 is decreased. When this occurs, the PCO_2 of the CSF decreases immediately because CO_2 equilibrates rapidly across the blood-brain barrier, leading to a rise in pH of the CSF that inhibits the central chemoreceptors. As blood bicarbonate gradually falls because of acidosis, bicarbonate concentration, and pH in the CSF, will eventually fall. At this point,

stimulation of respiration becomes maximal from both central and peripheral chemoreceptors.

Renal Mechanisms in the Regulation of Acid-Base Balance

The average pH of plasma and the glomerular filtrate is ≈ 7.4, whereas the average urinary pH is ≈ 6.0, reflecting renal excretion of nonvolatile acids. Various functions of the kidneys respond to different alterations in acid-base status. In the case of acidosis, excretion of acids is increased and that of base is conserved; in alkalosis, the opposite occurs. The pH of the urine changes correspondingly and may vary in random specimens from pH 4.5 to 8.0. The ability to excrete variable amounts of acid or base makes the kidney the final defense mechanism against changes in body pH.

The various acids produced during metabolic processes are buffered in the ECF at the expense of HCO_3^-. Renal excretion of acid and conservation of HCO_3^- occur through several mechanisms, including (1) Na^+-H^+ exchange, (2) production

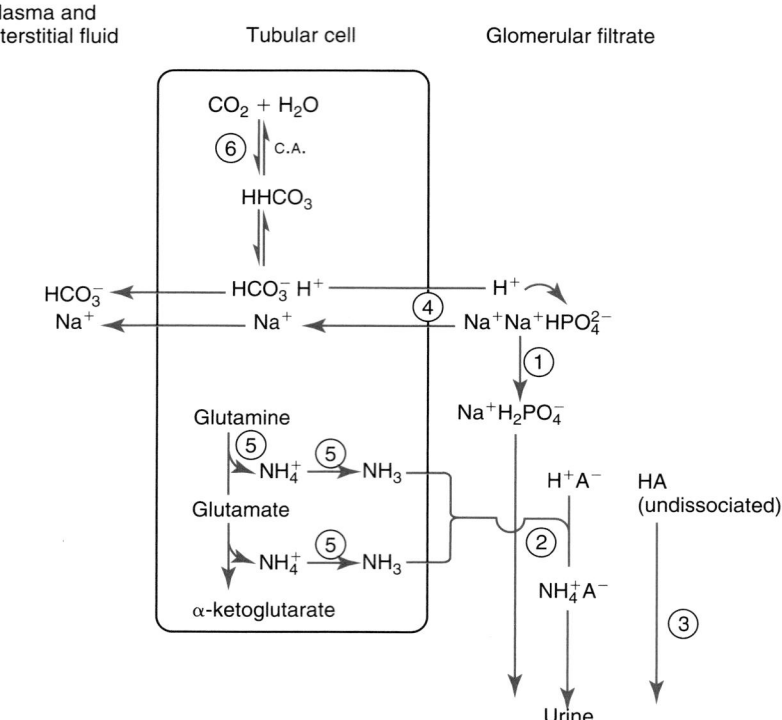

FIGURE 50.12 Hydrogen ion excretion, sodium hydrogen ion exchange, and ammonia production in the renal tubules. *1*, Conversion of HPO_4^{2-} to $H_2PO_4^{-}$; *2*, reaction of hydrogen ions with NH_3; *3*, excretion of undissociated acids; *4*, Na^+-H^+ exchange; *5*, NH_3 production; and *6*, synthesis of carbonic acid from CO_2.

of ammonia and excretion of NH_4^+, and (3) reclamation of HCO_3^-.

Na^+-H^+ Exchange

Nearly all mammalian cells contain a plasma membrane ATP-hydrolyzing protein capable of exchanging sodium ions for protons—the so-called Na^+-H^+ exchanger, of which there are six isoforms (Fig. 50.12).[5] In the renal tubules, two isoforms, NHE-1 and NHE-3, appear predominant. These isoforms extrude H^+ ions into the tubular fluid in exchange for Na^+ ions.

Na^+-H^+ exchange is enhanced in states of acidosis and inhibited in alkalosis. Both NHE-1 and NHE-3 are transcriptionally upregulated in response to acidotic states.[5] However, the proximal tubules cannot maintain an H^+ gradient of more than ≈ 1 pH unit, whereas the distal tubules cannot maintain more than ≈ 3 pH units. Thus maximum urine acidity is reached at $\approx$pH 4.4. In types 1 and 4 RTA, this exchange process is defective and may lead to a decrease in blood pH. In RTA type 1, an increase in urinary pH is often noted.

Potassium ions compete with H^+ in the renal tubular Na^+-H^+ exchanger. If the intracellular K^+ concentration of renal tubular cells is high, more K^+ and less H^+ are exchanged for Na^+. As a result, the urine becomes less acidic, thereby increasing the acidity of body fluids. If K^+ is depleted, more H^+ ions are exchanged for Na^+; the urine becomes more acidic and the body fluids more alkaline. Thus hyperkalemia contributes to acidosis and hypokalemia to alkalosis.

Renal Production of Ammonia and Excretion of Ammonium Ions

Renal tubular cells are able to generate ammonia from glutamine and other amino acids derived from muscle and liver cells according to the reaction in Fig. 50.13.

The ammonium ion produced dissociates into ammonia and hydrogen ions to a degree dependent on the pH (see Fig. 50.12). At normal blood pH, the ratio of NH_4^+/NH_3 is approximately 100 to 1. Ammonia is a gas that diffuses readily across the cell membrane into the tubular lumen, where it combines with hydrogen ions to form ammonium ions (see Fig. 50.12). At the acid pH of urine, the equilibrium between NH_4^+ and NH_3 shifts markedly to the left ($\approx$10,000 to 1), strongly favoring formation of NH_4^+. The NH_4^+ formed in the tubular lumen cannot easily cross cell membranes and thus is trapped in the tubular urine and excreted with anions such as phosphate, chloride, or sulfate. In normal individuals, NH_4^+ production in the tubular lumen accounts for the excretion of $\approx$60% (30 to 60 mmol) of the hydrogen ions. Finally, the α-oxoglutarate produced in this reaction is converted to bicarbonate (up to 270 mmol/day) that helps to replenish bicarbonate neutralized by metabolic acid production. The amount of H^+ excreted bound to NH_3 can be measured as NH_4^+. The H^+ required for NH_4^+ formation may be present in the glomerular filtrate or may be generated within tubular cells by carbonic anhydrase synthesis of carbonic acid from CO_2 (see Figs. 50.12 and 50.13). These H^+ ions are secreted into the tubular lumen through the Na^+-H^+ exchangers (see Fig. 50.12).

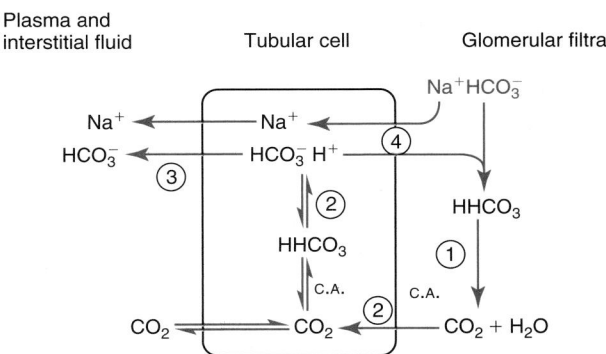

FIGURE 50.13 Generation of ammonia from glutamine by renal tubular cells.

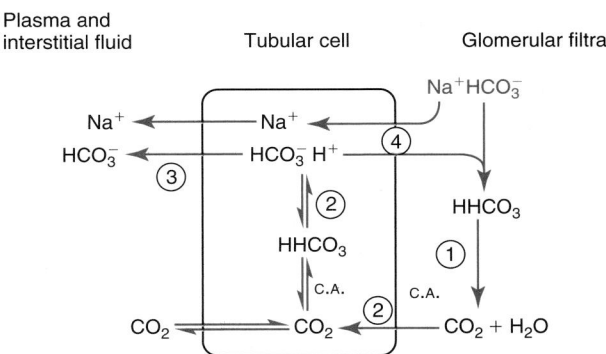

FIGURE 50.14 Reclamation of bicarbonate by tubular cells. *1*, Formation of CO_2 from bicarbonate in the tubular fluid; *2*, formation of H^+ and HCO_3^- from CO_2 in the tubular cell; *3*, new generation of HCO_3^-; and *4*, Na^+-H^+ exchange.

Excretion of Hydrogen as Dihydrogen Phosphate

H^+ secreted into the tubular lumen by the Na^+-H^+ exchanger also may react with hydrogen phosphate (HPO_4^{2-}) to form dihydrogen phosphate ($H_2PO_4^-$) (see Fig. 50.12). Under normal physiologic conditions, $\approx$30 mmol of H^+ is excreted per day as $H_2PO_4^-$. Acidemia increases phosphate excretion and thus provides additional buffer for reaction with H^+. A decrease in the GFR results in a decrease in $H_2PO_4^-$ excretion.

Reclamation of Filtered Bicarbonate

The unmodified glomerular filtrate has the same concentration of HCO_3^- as plasma does; however, with increasing acidification of proximal tubular urine, the HCO_3^- concentration is decreased. Excreted H^+ reacts with HCO_3^- (catalyzed by carbonic anhydrase, in the brush border of the proximal tubular cells) to form H_2CO_3 and subsequently CO_2 and H_2O (Fig. 50.14).

This increase in urinary CO_2 causes CO_2 to diffuse across the tubular cell membrane into the tubular cell, where it reacts with H_2O in the presence of cytoplasmic carbonic anhydrase to form H_2CO_3 and subsequently H^+ and HCO_3^- (see Fig. 50.14). Reclamation of bicarbonate consists of diffusion of CO_2 into tubular cells and its subsequent conversion to HCO_3^-. The increase in HCO_3^- helps to maintain or restore a normal pH in the circulation. Normally, $\approx$90% of filtered HCO_3^- (or $\approx$4500 mmol/day) is reclaimed in the proximal tubule, which parallels Na^+ reabsorption. Thus for each mmol H^+ secreted into the tubular fluid, 1 mmol Na^+ and 1 mmol HCO_3^- enter the tubular cell and return to the general

circulation. When plasma HCO_3^- concentration increases above $\approx$28 mmol/L, the capacity of the proximal and distal tubules to reclaim HCO_3^- is exceeded and HCO_3^- is excreted in the urine. RTA type 2 is caused by a decreased ability to reabsorb HCO_3^- in the proximal tubules, leading to a decrease in blood pH.

Conditions Associated With Abnormal Acid-Base Status and Abnormal Electrolyte Composition of the Blood

Abnormalities in acid-base status of the blood are always accompanied by characteristic changes in electrolyte concentrations in the plasma. H^+ ions cannot accumulate without concomitant accumulation of anions, such as Cl^- or lactate, or without exchange for cations, such as K^+ or Na^+. Consequently, the electrolyte composition of blood plasma is often determined along with measurements of blood gases and pH to assess acid-base disturbances.

Acid-base disturbances are traditionally classified as (1) metabolic acidosis, (2) metabolic alkalosis, (3) respiratory acidosis, or (4) respiratory alkalosis. In simple, straightforward acid-base disorders, the laboratory parameters observed for these groups are shown in Table 50.3. However, interpretation of laboratory values to classify these disorders is rarely straightforward because of compensatory responses by the respiratory and renal systems. Various heuristics methods to address this complexity are available to the clinician[40] and Table 50.3.

A logical approach to the classification of acid-base disorders is to consider that an acidosis can occur only as the result of one (or a combination) of three mechanisms: (1) increased addition of acid, (2) decreased elimination of acid, and (3) increased loss of base. Similarly, alkalosis occurs only by (1) increased addition of base, (2) decreased elimination of base, and (3) increased loss of acid.

Metabolic Acidosis (Primary Bicarbonate Deficit)

Metabolic acidosis is readily detected by decreased plasma bicarbonate (also represented as a negative extracellular base excess)—the primary perturbation in this acid-base disorder.[41] Causes include the following:

1. Increased production of organic acids that exceeds the rate of elimination (e.g., production of acetoacetic acid and β-hydroxybutyric acid in diabetic ketoacidosis). Bicarbonate is "lost" in the buffering of excess acid.
2. Reduced excretion of acids (H^+) as occurs in renal failure and some RTAs, resulting in an accumulation of acid that consumes bicarbonate.

TABLE 50.3 Classification and Characteristics of Simple Acid-Base Disorders

	Primary Change	Compensatory Response	Expected Compensation
Metabolic			
Acidosis	↓ $cHCO_3^-$	↓ PCO_2	$PCO_2 = 1.5\ (cHCO_3^-) + 8 \pm 2$
			PCO_2 falls by 1–1.3 mm Hg for each mmol/L fall in $cHCO_3^-$
			Last two digits of pH = PCO_2 (e.g., if PCO_2 = 28, pH = 7.28)
			$cHCO_3^- + 15$ = last two digits of pH ($cHCO_3^-$, pH = 7.30)
Alkalosis	↑ $cHCO_3^-$	↑ PCO_2	PCO_2 increases 6 mm Hg for each 10-mmol/L rise in $cHCO_3^-$
			$cHCO_3^- + 15$ = last 2 digits of pH ($cHCO_3^-$, pH = 7.50)
Respiratory			
Acidosis			
Acute	↑ PCO_2	↑ $cHCO_3^-$	$cHCO_3^-$ increases by 1 mmol/L for each 10-mm Hg rise in PCO_2
Chronic	↑ PCO_2	↑ $cHCO_3^-$	$cHCO_3^-$ increases by 3.5 mmol/L for each 10-mm Hg rise in PCO_2
Alkalosis			
Acute	↓ PCO_2	↓ $cHCO_3^-$	$cHCO_3^-$ falls by 2 mmol/L for each 10-mm Hg fall in PCO_2
Chronic	↓ PCO_2	↓ $cHCO_3^-$	$cHCO_3^-$ falls by 5 mmol/L for each 10 mm Hg fall in PCO_2

From Narins RG, Gardner LB. Simple acid-base disturbances. *Med Clin North Am* 1981;65:321–46.

TABLE 50.4 Conditions of Metabolic Acidoses With High and Normal Anion Gaps

Cause	Retained Acid(s)	Other Laboratory Findings
High Anion Gap (MUD PILES)		
Methanol	Formate	↑ Osmolal gap (>15 mOsmol/kg)
Uremia	Sulfuric, phosphoric, organic	↑ Urea and serum creatinine
Diabetes mellitus	Acetoacetate and β-hydroxybutyrate	↑ Plasma and urine glucose, hydroxybutyrate
Paraldehyde toxicity/Paracetamol (acetaminophen)	Acetate, chloracetate/pyroglutamate (5-oxoproline)	
Isoniazid, Iron, or Ischemia	Organic, mainly lactate	
Lactic acidosis	Lactate	
Ethylene glycol	Hippurate, glycolate, oxalate	↑ Osmolal gap (>15 mOsmol/kg), urine oxalate crystals
Salicylate	Salicylate	Respiratory alkalosis
Normal Anion Gap		
Gastrointestinal fluid loss/diarrhea	Primary loss of bicarbonate	Hypokalemia
Acetazolamide	Bicarbonate wasting	
Renal tubular acidosis		
Type 1	Decreased H^+ secretion	Hypokalemia
Type 2	Bicarbonate wasting	Hypokalemia
Type 4	Aldosterone deficiency or resistance	Hyperkalemia
Pancreatitis		
Pancreatic fistula	Bicarbonate wasting	

3. Excessive loss of bicarbonate secondary to increased renal excretion (decreased tubular reclamation) or excessive loss of duodenal fluid (as in diarrhea). In health care settings, provision of chloride anion, such as during large volume IV resuscitation with 0.9% sodium chloride, may create the same effect (i.e., urinary loss of bicarbonate in response to increased serum chloride). Similarly, if plasma $cHCO_3^-$ falls for any reason, the fall is associated with a rise in the concentration of inorganic anions (mostly chloride) to maintain electrical neutrality. Rarely a concomitant fall in the sodium concentration may be observed as well.

When any of these conditions exists, the ratio of HCO_3^-/cCO_2 is decreased because of the primary decrease in bicarbonate.

The resulting drop in pH stimulates respiratory compensation via hyperventilation, which lowers PCO_2 in order to raise (normalize) the pH. A recent expert panel review has created guideline recommendations on the diagnosis and treatment of metabolic acidosis.[42]

Increased Anion Gap Acidosis (Organic Acidosis)

Metabolic acidoses are classified as those associated with an increased anion gap or a normal anion gap (Table 50.4). The concept of the anion gap was originally devised as a quality control rule when it was noted that if the sum of Cl^- and HCO_3^- values was subtracted from the Na^+ values ($Na^+ - [Cl^- + HCO_3^-]$), the difference, or "gap," averaged 12 mmol/L

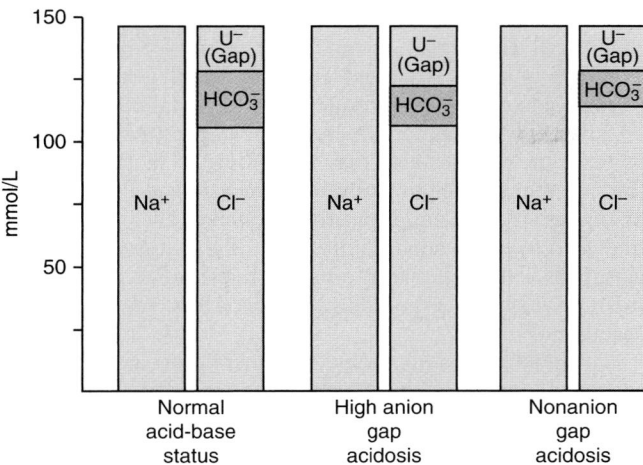

FIGURE 50.15 Simple "Gambelgram" depiction of normal gap, anion gap acidosis, and normal anion gap acidosis. Cations, Na^+ (and K^+, not shown here), are in *left bar* for each condition, whereas measured (Cl^- and HCO_3^-) and unmeasured (U^-) anions are in right bar.

BOX 50.1   A New Mnemonic for High Anion Gap Acidosis (GOLD MARK)

G   Glycols (ethylene and propylene)
O   Oxoproline
L   L-Lactate
D   D-Lactate (short bowel syndrome)
M   Methanol
A   Aspirin
R   Renal failure
K   Ketoacids

---

in healthy subjects (Fig. 50.15).[42] This apparent gap is due to unmeasured anions (e.g., proteins, SO_4^{2-}, $H_2PO_4^{2-}$) that are present in plasma. In reality, unmeasured cations (calcium, magnesium, organic cations) should be included in the equation with sodium and potassium, but their concentration in blood absent gross increases or decreases from the reference interval is relatively small compared with circulating sodium concentrations. Similarly, changes in protein concentration generally do not produce a noticeable effect on the anion gap value but can on occasion be associated with decreased or increased anion gaps that affect the accuracy of the anion gap (see Table 50.4).[43,44] In general, however, these extreme changes in unmeasured cations and proteins are not significant in the clinical utility of the anion gap. The anion gap is increased in most patients with a metabolic acidosis. The presence of an increased anion gap is often the first indication of a metabolic acidosis and should be assessed in the electrolyte profiles of all patients.[42]

All anion gap metabolic acidoses, besides inborn errors of metabolism, can be explained by one (or a combination) of eight underlying mechanisms listed here according to the common mnemonic device MUDPILES (see Table 50.4). The physiologic basis for the anion gap in these conditions is the consumption of bicarbonate in buffering excess acid. Cl^- values remain normal when the excess acid is any other than HCl, because lost bicarbonate is replaced by unmeasured anions. Alternative mnemonics for increased anion gap acidosis are available such as GOLD MARK (Box 50.1).[45]

Methanol. Although nontoxic itself, methanol is metabolized by the liver to formaldehyde and formic acid. Accumulation of this acid leads to metabolic acidosis with a high anion gap and to clinical symptoms of optic papillitis ("snow-field" blindness), retinal edema, and ultimately blindness caused by optic nerve atrophy, as well as neurologic defects that may lead to coma. Methanol and other ingested alcohols such as ethylene glycol, ethanol, and isopropanol will increase the osmolality of plasma. This "osmolal gap" (see Chapter 37) has been used in clinical medicine but its utility is in question, especially if the concentrations of the toxic alcohol are

low but within range where treatment should be initiated.[46] The calculation of the osmolal gap may also be misleading in cases in which the time of presentation and ingestion are separated by many hours.[46] Toxic alcohol ingestions are often treated with fomepizole, which competitively inhibits alcohol dehydrogenase and reduces the generation of toxic metabolites. Hemodialysis also may be required to remove high concentrations of accumulated alcohols directly from the bloodstream.

Uremia of renal failure. Loss of functional renal tubular mass results in decreased ammonia formation, decreased Na^+-H^+ exchange, and decreased GFR. All lead to decreased acid excretion (see Chapter 49). Acidosis usually develops if GFR falls below 20 mL/min. Serum creatinine and urea concentrations usually are increased and are used as an estimate of the degree of renal damage or, more appropriately, as an estimate of remaining functional renal capacity. Although the presence of mild acidosis alone can be managed conservatively in chronic kidney disease, the presence of other uremic symptoms, including intractable nausea, vomiting, fatigue, and altered mental status may be indications for hemodialysis.

Diabetic ketoacidosis. The pathogenesis of ketoacidosis is discussed in detail in Chapter 47. Ketoacids such as β-hydroxybutyrate and 2-oxoglutarate accumulate and represent the unmeasured anions. Accumulation of these ketone bodies causes a decrease in HCO_3^-, a normal serum chloride, and a high anion gap. Although the "D" in MUDPILES is listed as diabetic ketoacidosis, it is important to recall that ketoacids also accumulate in states of starvation, alcoholic malnutrition, and others. Treatment is directed at correcting the process responsible for the ketoacids, most commonly insulin deficiency, or starvation.

Paraldehyde or paracetamol (pyroglutamic acid) Paraldehyde toxicity is now included only for historical interest. It was used as a treatment for alcohol withdrawal, and metabolites from its chronic use led to an anion gap acidosis.

Chronic paracetamol (acetaminophen in the United States) use by patients with decreased glutathione stores can lead to an accumulation of pyroglutamic acid (5-oxoproline) that results in an anion gap.[47] Pyroglutamic acid is an intracellular intermediate in the γ-glutamyl cycle that is glutathione dependent. An anion gap acidosis usually develops only in chronic paracetamol users that have other comorbidities such as malnutrition, chronic renal failure, or liver disease. Cessation of the drug is mandatory.

Isoniazid, iron, or ischemia. These seemingly unrelated causes of high anion gap acidosis share a common feature: the accumulation of organic acids, with a predominance of lactic acid. Thus the "three Is" actually represent special cases in the general category of lactic acidosis. Both isoniazid, an antimycobacterial agent commonly used in the treatment or prophylaxis of tuberculosis, and iron toxicity involve the production of toxic peroxides that act as mitochondrial poisons and interfere with normal cellular respiration. In addition, isoniazid may be hepatotoxic, leading to significant liver damage and impairment of lactate clearance.[42] Tissue ischemia from many causes resulting in anaerobic metabolism with accumulation of primarily lactic acid.

Lactic acidosis. Lactic acid, present in blood as the lactate ion (pK = 3.86), is an intermediate of carbohydrate metabolism that is derived mainly from muscle cells and erythrocytes (see Chapter 35). It represents the end product of anaerobic metabolism and is normally metabolized by the liver. Therefore blood lactate concentration is affected by the rate of production and the rate of metabolism, both of which depend on adequate tissue perfusion. An increase in the concentration of lactate to greater than 3 mmol/L with the associated increase in H$^+$, and fall in pH, is considered lactic acidosis.[11,48]

Lactic acidosis is seen in severe anemia, shock, cardiac arrest, and pulmonary insufficiency and other conditions that result in tissue hypoxia. Severe oxygen deprivation of tissue blocks aerobic oxidation of pyruvic acid in the tricarboxylic acid cycle, resulting in the reduction of pyruvate to lactate. Extreme deterioration of the cellular oxidative process is associated with marked tachypnea, weakness, fatigue, stupor, and finally coma. Conditions at these later stages are frequently irreversible, even if treatment is instituted. If the source of lactate, most often shock, can be rectified, lactate is rapidly metabolized to CO$_2$, which then is eliminated by an intact respiratory system.

Lactic acidosis may also be caused by (1) drugs and toxins such as ethanol, methanol, isoniazid, metformin, and excess iron; (2) acquired and hereditary defects in enzymes involved in gluconeogenesis; (3) disorders such as uremia, tumors, and seizures; (4) anesthesia; and (5) abnormal intestinal bacteria producing D-lactate. Most common methods for lactate do not detect D-lactate acidosis; this form of lactic acidosis should be considered only in patients with short bowel syndromes or after other gastrointestinal surgeries resulting in "blind loops" where bacterial overgrowth may occur.[49] Treatment is directed toward the underlying cause of lactic acid accumulation. Conditions in which lactate clearance is impaired, most commonly hepatic insufficiency, are known as type-B lactic acidoses. The common use of continuous albuterol for status asthmaticus can create this condition.[50] Although some removal of lactate via dialysis is possible, the clearance rate is less than the production rate in shock and removal of lactate without correction of the underlying pathophysiology is not helpful.[51]

During vigorous, anaerobic exercise, lactate concentrations may increase significantly from an average normal concentration of ≈0.9 mmol/L to ≈12 mmol/L. However, under healthy conditions, the lactate is rapidly metabolized to CO$_2$, so the "acidosis" is only transient as hyperventilation eliminates the CO$_2$.

Lactate in spinal fluid normally parallels blood values. However, in cases of biochemical alterations in the CNS system, CSF lactate values change independently of blood values. Increased CSF lactate concentrations may be seen in intracranial hemorrhage, bacterial meningitis, epilepsy, and other CNS disorders.[2]

Ethylene glycol. Ingested ethylene glycol is metabolized primarily to glycolic and oxalic acids. Its metabolism leads to an acidosis with high anion and osmolal gaps. Accumulation of toxic metabolites also may contribute to lactic acid production that further contributes to the acidosis. Precipitation of calcium oxalate and hippurate crystals in the urinary tract may lead to acute renal failure. Clinically, patients develop a variety of neurologic symptoms that may lead to coma. Treatment of alcohol toxicities has been described previously (see "Methanol").

Salicylate intoxication. Acidosis generally occurs with blood salicylate concentrations greater than 30 mg/dL (2.1 mmol/L). Salicylate increases the anion gap in two ways. Salicylate is itself an unmeasured anion and further contributes to the anion gap by altering peripheral metabolism, leading to the production of various organic acids. Management of salicylate toxicity can be complex, both metabolic and respiratory acid-base disturbances occurring simultaneously. Salicylate toxicity can initially stimulate respiration leading to a respiratory alkalosis, followed by depression of respiration and subsequent respiratory acidosis. Early consultative input from critical care or toxicology is recommended, along with possible nephrology assessment for hemodialysis.

Normal Anion Gap Acidosis (Inorganic Acidosis)

In contrast to high anion gap acidoses, in which bicarbonate is consumed from buffering excess H$^+$, the cause of acidosis in the presence of a normal anion gap is the loss of bicarbonate-rich fluid from the kidney or the gastrointestinal tract (see Table 50.4). The anion gap does not develop in these situations, because the renal resorption of Cl$^-$ ions in conjunction with Na$^+$ is increased due to the loss of available HCO$_3^-$ ions that would normally accompany the resorption of Na$^+$ to maintain electroneutrality. The consequent increase in plasma Cl$^-$ is sufficient to balance the loss of anions (HCO$_3^-$) (see Fig. 50.15). Normal anion gap acidosis can be divided into *hypokalemic, normokalemic,* and *hyperkalemic* acidoses, which can be helpful in the differential diagnosis of this type of disorder (see subsequent section on RTA type 4).

Gastrointestinal losses. Diarrhea may cause acidosis as a result of loss of Na$^+$, K$^+$, and HCO$_3^-$. One of the primary exocrine functions of the pancreas is production of HCO$_3^-$ to neutralize gastric contents on entry into the duodenum. If the water, K$^+$, and HCO$_3^-$ in the intestine are not reabsorbed, a hypokalemic, normal anion gap metabolic acidosis will develop. The resulting hyperchloremia is due to replacement of lost bicarbonate with Cl$^-$ to maintain electrical balance.

Renal tubular acidoses. These syndromes are characterized by loss of bicarbonate secondary to decreased tubular secretion of H$^+$ (distal or type 1 RTA) or decreased reabsorption of HCO$_3^-$ (proximal or type 2 RTA).[52] Because the major urine-acidifying power of the kidneys rests in the distal tubules, proximal and distal RTAs may be differentiated by measurement of urine pH after administration of acid. In proximal RTA, urine pH becomes less than 5.5, whereas in distal RTA, the distal tubules are compromised and urine pH is greater than 5.5.[52] The seemingly paradoxically higher urine pH in the setting of acidosis (low blood pH) is the result of a failure to excrete H$^+$ in the distal convoluted tubule. RTA type 4 is due to decreased aldosterone or aldosterone resistance leading to decreased Na^+ reabsorption and thus decreased H^+ and K^+ secretion. It can be differentiated from type 1 by the increased K^+.[52]

Carbonic anhydrase inhibitors. Acetazolamide is the most commonly used drug in this class of therapeutic agents. It is used for urine alkalinization and in patients with open-angle glaucoma or acute mountain (altitude) sickness.[31] Inhibition of carbonic anhydrase causes wasting of Na^+, K^+, and HCO_3^- in the proximal tubules and represents a pharmacologically induced proximal RTA similar to type 2 RTA and subsequent metabolic acidosis.

Compensatory Mechanisms in Metabolic Acidosis

The buffer systems of the blood (mainly the bicarbonate/carbonic acid buffer) minimize changes in pH. In acidoses, the bicarbonate concentration decreases to yield a ratio of $cHCO_3^-/cdCO_2$ of less than 20:1. The respiratory compensatory mechanism responds to correct the ratio with increased minute ventilation, through both increased rate and depth of respiration, to eliminate CO_2. Table 50.3 depicts expected compensation in various cases of acidoses and alkaloses and corresponding laboratory intervals.

Respiratory compensatory mechanism. The decrease in pH in metabolic acidosis stimulates hyperventilation (Kussmaul respiration), which results in the elimination of carbonic acid as CO_2, a decrease in PCO_2 (hypocapnia), and thus a decrease in $cdCO_2$. There is also a decrease in $cHCO_3^-$ that is smaller than that in $cdCO_2$. For example, the ratio of $cHCO_3^-/cdCO_2$ may be 16:1.28 (12.5:1) for a pH of 7.2 before compensation, and 14.5:0.9 (16:1) for a pH of 7.30 after compensation (see Fig. 50.9).

Renal compensatory mechanism. If possible, the kidneys respond to restore the normal pH through increased excretion of acid and preservation of base (increased rate of Na^+-H^+ exchange, increased ammonia formation, and increased reabsorption of bicarbonate). When the renal compensating mechanisms are functioning, urine acidity and ammonium are increased. The total amount of H^+ excreted may be as great as 500 mmol/day. As a result, $cHCO_3^-/cdCO_2$ will increase, for example, to 22:1.1 (20:1) for a pH of 7.40. This is a fully compensated metabolic acidosis, because the pH has returned to normal; however, acidosis still exists because a process that consumes HCO_3^- persists.

Metabolic Alkalosis (Primary Bicarbonate Excess)

Alkalosis occurs when excess base is added to the system, base elimination is decreased, or acid-rich fluids are lost[41,53] (see At a Glance: Conditions Leading to Metabolic Alkalosis). Any of these can lead to a primary bicarbonate excess, such that the ratio of $cHCO_3^-/cdCO_2$ becomes greater than 20:1. For instance, a primary increase in bicarbonate to 48 mmol/L will alter the $cHCO_3^-/cdCO_2$ to 48:1.5 (32:1) for a pH of 7.6 (see Fig. 50.9). The patient will hypoventilate to raise PCO_2, thereby lowering the pH toward 7.4. However, the compensatory capacity of hypoventilation is limited by the hypoxia which accompanies hypovention. In practice, it is unusual for a patient to achieve a PCO_2 greater than 55 mm Hg for this reason. Greater than pH 7.55, tetany may develop due to increased binding of calcium ions by albumin and a resulting decrease in ionized calcium. Measurement of urine Cl^- can be helpful because causes of metabolic alkalosis fall into Cl^- responsive, Cl^- resistant, and exogenous base categories (see Fig. 50.5).

Conditions Leading to Metabolic Alkalosis

Chloride Responsive (Urine Chloride Less Than 10 mmol/L)
- Contraction alkaloses
  - Prolonged vomiting or nasogastric suction
  - Pyloric or upper duodenal obstruction
  - Prolonged or abusive diuretic therapy (loop diuretics)
  - Dehydration
- Posthypercapnic state
- Cystic fibrosis (systemic ineffective reabsorption of Cl^-)

Chloride-Resistant (Urine Cl^- Greater Than 20 mmol/L)
- Mineralocorticoid excess
  - Primary hyperaldosteronism (adrenal adenoma or, rarely, carcinoma)
  - Bilateral adrenal hyperplasia
  - Secondary hyperaldosteronism
  - Congenital adrenal hyperplasia (resulting from adrenal enzyme deficiencies in cortisol production (11β- or 17α-hydroxylase)
- Glucocorticoid excess
  - Primary adrenal adenoma (Cushing's syndrome)
  - Pituitary adenoma secreting adrenocorticotropic hormone (Cushing's disease)
  - Exogenous cortisol therapy
  - Excessive licorice ingestion
- Bartter syndrome (defective renal Cl^- reabsorption)

Exogenous Base
- Iatrogenic
  - Bicarbonate-containing intravenous fluid therapy
  - Sodium citrate excess (in massive blood transfusion)
  - Antacids
  - Cation-exchange resins in dialysis patients
  - High-dose carbenicillin or penicillin (associated with hypokalemia)
- Milk-alkali syndrome

Chloride-Responsive Metabolic Alkalosis

Most cases of Cl^--responsive metabolic alkalosis occur as a result of hypovolemia. When the ECF is severely depleted, the resulting acid-base disorder is often referred to as contraction alkalosis. Common causes of contraction alkalosis include prolonged vomiting or nasogastric suction, pyloric or upper duodenal obstruction, and the use of certain diuretics. After prolonged vomiting or gastric suction, excessive loss of hydrochloric acid from the stomach and hypovolemia occurs. In response to this hypochloremic, hypovolemic state the kidneys reabsorb Na^+ to restore vascular volume and in the absence of sufficient Cl^-, excess HCO_3^- is reabsorbed, to maintain electrical neutrality. The increased reabsorption of HCO_3^-, H^+, and K^+ are secreted in exchange for Na^+, potentially resulting in hypokalemia. In contraction alkalosis or chloride responsive alkalosis urine Cl^- will be less than 10 mmol/L (see Fig. 50.5). Treatment consists of correcting the underlying disorder leading to volume depletion, restoring the intravascular volume and carefully replacing depleted electrolytes.

Diuretic therapy. Prolonged administration of certain diuretics has been known to cause an alkalosis similar to that observed in a hypovolemic setting. The diuretics commonly associated with this phenomenon are those acting on the ascending limb of the loop of Henle (e.g., furosemide [Lasix]) that block sodium, potassium, and chloride reabsorption.[31] The resulting increase in Na^+ concentration reaching the distal convoluted tubule, particularly when combined with activation of the renin-angiotensin-aldosterone axis, leads to increased urinary excretion of K^+ and H^+. Loss of K^+ with furosemide is much greater than with thiazides. Continued abuse or unmonitored use of loop diuretics can lead to volume contraction and a contraction alkalosis. This is commonly seen among those abusing diuretics for the purpose of weight loss.

Chloride-resistant Metabolic Alkalosis

This condition is far less common than Cl^--responsive metabolic alkalosis and is almost always associated with an underlying disease (primary hyperaldosteronism, Cushing's syndrome, or Bartter's syndrome) or with excess addition of exogenous base. In these conditions, urine Cl^- will usually be greater than 20 mmol/L.

In states of adrenocortical excess (endogenous or pharmacologic, primary or secondary), K^+ and H^+ are "wasted" by the kidneys as a consequence of increased Na^+ reabsorption stimulated by increased aldosterone or cortisol. The attendant hypokalemia often further contributes to the alkalosis and should be treated with K^+ replacement therapy. The decreased tubular K^+ concentration stimulates ammonia production and thus renal H^+ excretion in the form of the ammonium ions, driving further alkalosis. This is accompanied by enhanced HCO_3^- reabsorption (see Figs. 50.4 and 50.13). Diseases in which endogenous mineralocorticoids, glucocorticoids, or both are increased include primary and secondary hyperaldosteronism, bilateral adrenal hyperplasia, pituitary adrenocorticotropic hormone (ACTH)-producing adenoma (Cushing's disease), and primary adrenal adenomas producing glucocorticoids (Cushing's syndrome) or aldosterone.

Finally, two rare causes of metabolic alkalosis. Black licorice ingestion may cause a form of Cl^--resistant alkalosis through inhibition of the enzyme 11-β-hydroxysteroid dehydrogenase (11βHSD) which normally catalyzes the conversion of cortisol to cortisone.[42] Inhibition of 11-βHSD by the glycyrrhizic acid in black licorice results in excess cortisol which binds to the mineralocorticoid receptor in the distal tubule leading to increased reabsorption of sodium with the concomitant loss of potassium as noted previously. In addition, several genetic (autosomal recessive) defects in Cl^- reabsorption within the thick ascending limb of the loop of Henle, conditions known collectively as Bartter's syndrome,[54] result in Cl^--resistant metabolic alkalosis.

Exogenous Base

Examples in this category include citrate toxicity after massive blood transfusion, aggressive intravenous therapy with bicarbonate solutions, and ingestion of large quantities of antacids in the treatment of gastritis or peptic ulcer (milk-alkali syndrome).[55] The latter is far less commonly seen since the introduction and now widespread use of H_2-receptor antagonists and proton pump inhibitors.

Compensatory Mechanisms in Metabolic Alkalosis

The compensatory mechanisms for metabolic alkalosis include both respiratory compensation and, if physiologically possible, renal compensation. The increase in pH depresses the respiratory center, causing retention of CO_2 (hypercapnia), which in turn causes an increase in cH_2CO_3 and $cdCO_2$. Thus the ratio of $cHCO_3^-/cdCO_2$, which was originally increased, approaches its normal value, although both $cHCO_3^-$ and $cdCO_2$ remain increased. The kidneys respond to the state of alkalosis by decreased Na^+-H^+ exchange, decreased formation of ammonia, and decreased reclamation of bicarbonate. However, this response is blunted in conditions of hypokalemia and hypovolemia.

Laboratory Findings in Metabolic Alkalosis

Plasma values for $cHCO_3^-$, $cdCO_2$, and PCO_2, and therefore the plasma total CO_2 concentration, are increased, and the ratio of $cHCO_3^-/cdCO_2$ is high. In uncomplicated metabolic alkalosis, the PCO_2 is increased by ≈ 6 mm Hg for each 10 mmol/L rise in $cHCO_3^-$. A higher-than-expected PCO_2 may indicate superimposed respiratory acidosis. The extent of increase in pH in uncompensated metabolic alkalosis can be estimated by adding 15 to the $cHCO_3^-$ to give the last two digits of the pH. For example, if the $cHCO_3^-$ were 35 mmol/L, the estimated pH would be 7.50 (35 + 15 = 50). In cases of prolonged vomiting, Cl^- (and sometimes K^+) concentrations are low because of loss of these ions through the vomitus. Plasma protein values may be increased as a result of dehydration, and if food intake is inadequate, formation of ketoacids may increase the organic acid fraction. In cases of excessive administration of $NaHCO_3$, Na^+ concentrations are increased.

In patients with adequate renal function, urinary pH values are usually increased as the result of decreased excretion of acid and increased excretion of bicarbonate. Urinary ammonium values are decreased because of decreased formation of ammonium in the tubules.

POINTS TO REMEMBER

- In determining the differential for an anion gap acidosis, mnemonic devices can be helpful (see Table 50.1 and Box 50.1).
- Volume depletion is very often accompanied by a hypochloremic metabolic alkalosis.
- Normal anion gap acidosis is due to loss of bicarbonate-rich fluid via the gastrointestinal tract (most often diarrhea) or the renal tubular acidoses.

Respiratory Acidosis

Any condition that decreases elimination of CO_2 through the lungs results in an increase in PCO_2 (hypercapnia) and dCO_2 (respiratory acidosis). Thus respiratory acidosis occurs only through decreased elimination of CO_2. Causes of decreased CO_2 elimination (See At a Glance: Conditions Leading to Respiratory Acidosis) are classified as acute or chronic. Alternatively, these conditions may be separated into those caused by factors that directly depress the respiratory center (e.g., centrally acting drugs, CNS trauma, or infection) and those that affect the respiratory apparatus or cause mechanical obstruction of the airways. Chronic obstructive pulmonary disease (COPD) is the most common cause. An increase in PCO_2 results in an increase in $cdCO_2$ (and thus H_2CO_3, which dissociates to H^+ and HCO_3^-), which in turn causes a decrease in the $c\text{HCO}_3^-/c\text{dCO}_2$ ratio (e.g., the ratio may be 28:1.7 [16:1] for a pH of $\approx$7.30; see Fig. 50.9). Doubling of $P\text{CO}_2$ will cause a fall in pH of approximately 0.23 when other factors remain constant.

AT A GLANCE

Conditions Leading to Respiratory Acidosis

Factors That Directly Depress the Respiratory Center
- Narcotics and barbiturates
- Central nervous system (CNS) trauma, tumors, and degenerative disorders
- Infections of the CNS such as encephalitis and meningitis
- Comatose states such as cerebrovascular accident secondary to intracranial hemorrhage
- Primary central hypoventilation

Conditions That Affect the Respiratory Apparatus
- Chronic obstructive pulmonary disease (COPD) (most common cause)
- Severe pulmonary fibrosis
- Status asthmaticus (severe)
- Disease of the upper airways such as laryngospasm or tumor
- Pulmonary infection (severe)
- Impaired lung motion secondary to pleural effusion or pneumothorax
- Acute respiratory distress syndrome
- Chest wall disease and chest wall deformity
- Neurologic disorders affecting the muscles of respiration
- Opioids

Others
- Abdominal distention, as in peritonitis and ascites
- Extreme obesity (pickwickian syndrome)
- Sleep disorders such as sleep apnea

Compensatory Mechanisms in Respiratory Acidosis

Compensation for respiratory acidosis occurs immediately via buffers, and over time via the kidneys and, if possible, the lungs. Excess carbonic acid present in blood is buffered to a great extent by the Hb and protein buffer systems (see Fig. 50.10).[3] The kidneys respond to respiratory acidosis similarly to the way they respond to metabolic acidosis, namely, with (1) increased Na^+-H^+ exchange, (2) increased ammonia formation, and (3) increased reclamation of bicarbonate. In a partially compensated chronic respiratory acidosis at steady state, the plasma pH is returned approximately halfway toward normal compared with the acute (uncompensated) situation. Renal compensation is not effective before 6 to 12 hours and is not optimal until 2 to 3 days. In chronic respiratory acidosis, such as occurs in patients with COPD, full renal compensation may be seen even in patients with very high $P\text{CO}_2$ ($>$50 mm Hg). However, patients with severe COPD often present with a superimposed metabolic alkalosis arising from a variety of causes, such as prolonged administration of diuretics.

The increase in $P\text{CO}_2$ stimulates the respiratory center, resulting in an increased respiratory rate and depth, provided that the primary defect is not in the respiratory center. Elimination of CO_2 through the lungs results in a decrease in $c\text{dCO}_2$; thus the ratio of $c\text{HCO}_3^-/c\text{dCO}_2$ and pH approach normal.

Laboratory Findings in Respiratory Acidosis

Plasma $c\text{dCO}_2$, $P\text{CO}_2$, $c\text{HCO}_3^-$, and therefore $c\text{tCO}_2$ are increased in respiratory acidoses. Because of an increase in $c\text{dCO}_2$, the ratio of $c\text{HCO}_3^-/c\text{dCO}_2$ is decreased, resulting in a decreased pH. In the acute phase, $c\text{HCO}_3^-$ will increase by $\approx$1 mmol/L for each 10 mm Hg rise in $P\text{CO}_2$. If respiratory acidosis persists, the change will be $\approx$3.5 mmol/L, mainly as a result of renal compensation. For every increase in $P\text{CO}_2$ of 25 mm Hg, pH decreases in the acute phase by $\approx$0.10 pH unit and in chronic conditions by slightly less than 0.05 pH unit. For example, if the $P\text{CO}_2$ increases acutely by 30 mm Hg, the pH drops to $\approx$7.28. The same $P\text{CO}_2$ increase in a chronic condition results in a pH of $\approx$7.31. The plasma chloride decreases as plasma bicarbonate increases. Hyperkalemia may occur but is not as predictable as in some forms of metabolic acidosis. For every 0.1-unit decrease in pH, there is generally an inverse change of 0.6 mmol/L in K^+. Urinary acidity and ammonium content are increased as the kidney attempts to compensate for the respiratory acidosis.

Respiratory Alkalosis

A decrease in $P\text{CO}_2$ (hypocapnia) and the resulting primary deficit in $c\text{dCO}_2$ (respiratory alkalosis) are caused by an increased rate and/or depth of respiration. Therefore the basic cause of respiratory alkalosis is excess elimination of acid (CO_2) by the respiratory route. Excessive elimination of CO_2 reduces the $P\text{CO}_2$ and causes an increase in the $c\text{HCO}_3^-/c\text{dCO}_2$ ratio. The latter shifts the normal equilibrium of the bicarbonate/carbonic acid buffer system, reducing the hydrogen ion concentration and increasing the pH. This shift also results in a decrease in $c\text{HCO}_3^-$, which somewhat ameliorates the change in pH. Analogous to causes of respiratory acidosis, causes of respiratory alkalosis can be classified as those with a direct stimulatory effect on the respiratory center and those resulting from effects on the pulmonary system. These and some additional conditions underlying respiratory alkaloses are listed in At a Glance: Factors Causing Respiratory Alkalosis.

POINTS TO REMEMBER

- Respiratory acidosis results in an increased $P\text{CO}_2$ secondary to the inability of the lungs to eliminate CO_2.
- Respiratory alkalosis is result of excess elimination of CO_2 via hyperventilation.
- Respiratory compensatory mechanisms in primary metabolic acidosis or alkalosis settings should not be interpreted as respiratory disorders.

Compensatory Mechanisms in Respiratory Alkalosis

The compensatory mechanisms respond to respiratory alkalosis in two stages. In the first stage, erythrocyte and tissue buffers provide H^+ ions that consume a small amount of HCO_3^-. The second stage becomes operational in prolonged respiratory alkalosis and depends on renal compensation as described for metabolic alkalosis (decreased reclamation of bicarbonate).

Laboratory Findings in Respiratory Alkalosis

In this condition, $c\text{dCO}_2$, $P\text{CO}_2$, $c\text{HCO}_3^-$, and thus total CO_2 concentration, all decrease. The ratio of $c\text{HCO}_3^-/c\text{dCO}_2$ is increased, causing an increase in pH. During the acute phase, $c\text{HCO}_3^-$ falls by 2 mmol/L for each decrease of 10 mm Hg in

AT A GLANCE

Factors Causing Respiratory Alkalosis

Nonpulmonary Stimulation of Respiratory Center
- Anxiety, hysteria
- Fever
- Sepsis (related to metabolic acidosis)
- Metabolic encephalopathy (e.g., secondary to liver disease)
- Central nervous system (CNS) infection such as meningitis and encephalitis
- Stroke
- Intracranial surgery
- Hypoxia (e.g., severe anemia, acute response to high elevation)
- Drugs and agents such as salicylates, catecholamines, and progesterone
- Pregnancy, mainly third trimester (increased progesterone?)
- Hyperthyroidism

Pulmonary Disorders[a]
- Pneumonia
- Pulmonary emboli
- Interstitial lung disease
- Large right-to-left shunt (PCO_2 <50 mm Hg)
- Congestive heart failure
- Respiratory compensation after correction of metabolic acidosis

Others
- Ventilator-induced hyperventilation

[a]The severe stages of some of these disorders may be associated with respiratory acidosis if elimination of CO_2 is severely impaired.

PCO_2 (e.g., if the PCO_2 falls by 20 mm Hg, $cHCO_3^-$ is decreased by 4 mmol/L). For the same decrease of 20 mm Hg in PCO_2, the (H^+) will decrease by 16 nmol/L. The resulting alkalosis (lower H^+) will result in a greater binding of Ca^{2+} by albumin and a lower free (ionized) Ca^{2+}, which can lead to hypocalcemic symptoms of tetany such as Chvostek's and Trousseu's signs (see Chapter 54).

If the original cH^+ was 40 nmol/L, it would now be 24 nmol/L ($40 - 16 = 24$), which corresponds to a pH of 7.61 (see Fig. 50.7). Finally, individuals living at high altitudes chronically hyperventilate because of hypoxia and have PCO_2 values lower than those seen at sea level.

SELECTED REFERENCES

1. Ruth JL, Wassner SJ. Body composition: salt and water. Pediatr Rev 2006;27:181–8.
2. Watson MA, Scott MG. Clinical utility of biochemical analysis of cerebrospinal fluid. Clin Chem 1995;41:343–60.
7. Adrogué HJ, Madias NE. Hypernatremia. N Engl J Med 2000; 342:1493–9.
10. Verbalis JG, Goldsmith SR, Greenberg A, et al. Diagnosis, evaluation, and treatment of hyponatremia: expert panel recommendations. Am J Med 2013;126:S1–42.
13. Verbalis JG. The curious story of cerebral salt wasting: fact or fiction? Clin J Am Soc Nephrol 2020;15(11):1666-8.
18. Verbalis JG. Hyponatremia and hypoosmolar disorders. In: National kidney foundation primer on kidney diseases 2017. p. 68–76.
21. Katrangi W, Baumann NA, Nett RC, Karon BS, Block DR. Prevalence of clinically significant differences in sodium measurements due to abnormal protein concentrations using an indirect ion-selective electrode method. J Appl Lab Med 2019;4:427–32.
23. Robertson GL. Diabetes insipidus. Endocrinol Metab Clin North Am 1995;24:549–72.
26. Metheny NA, Krieger MM. Salt toxicity: a systematic review and case reports. J Emerg Nurs 2020;46:428–39.
27. Aronson PS, Giebisch G. Effects of pH on potassium: new explanations for old observations. J Am Soc Nephrol 2011;22: 1981–9.
33. Ranjitkar P, Greene DN, Baird GS, Hoofnagle AN, Mathias PC. Establishing evidence-based thresholds and laboratory practices to reduce inappropriate treatment of pseudohyperkalemia. Clin Biochem 2017;50:663–9.
40. Baillie JK. Simple, easily memorised "rules of thumb" for the rapid assessment of physiological compensation for respiratory acid-base disorders. Thorax 2008;63:289–90.
45. Mehta AN, Emmett JB, Emmett M. GOLD MARK: an anion gap mnemonic for the 21st century. Lancet 2008;372:892.
46. Glaser DS. Utility of the serum osmol gap in the diagnosis of methanol or ethylene glycol ingestion. Ann Emerg Med 1996; 27:343–6.
49. Bianchetti DGAM, Amelio GS, Lava SAG, et al. D-lactic acidosis in humans: systematic literature review. Pediatr Nephrol 2018; 33:673–81.

51

Liver Disease

William Malcolm Charles Rosenberg, Tony Badrick,
Stanley F. Lo, and Sudeep Tanwar[a]

ABSTRACT

Background

The liver is the largest and most complex organ in the body. The anatomy of the liver is intricate, and its function is dependent on the close interaction of resident cell lineages; the arterial, venous, and portal vasculature; and the biliary system. The liver plays a central role in numerous biochemical processes, executing metabolic and catabolic functions that are vital for homeostasis and health. Biochemical tests can be used to determine the cause and prognosis and to monitor liver diseases.

Content

This chapter reviews the anatomy and physiology of the liver, the major causes of acute and chronic liver diseases, and the patterns of biochemical test results associated with these disorders.

The chapter describes how tests can be used to investigate the liver through the measurement of the enzymes and proteins it produces and the processes that it regulates. The chapter also explains how clinical chemistry can provide powerful insights into the health of the liver, the likely etiology of disease, and prognosis.

In chronic liver disease, inflammation initiates liver fibrosis, which can progress to cirrhosis and liver cancer. This chapter describes how biochemical markers of liver fibrosis can be used to determine the severity and prognosis of liver disease and monitor disease course.

This chapter covers the use of biochemical tests to help determine the etiology, chronicity, severity, and prognosis, as well as monitoring the course of a wide range of liver pathologies.

INTRODUCTION

The liver has a central and critical biochemical role in the metabolism, digestion, detoxification, and elimination of substances from the body. All blood from the intestinal tract initially passes through the liver, where products derived from digestion of food except lipids are processed, transformed, and (in some cases) stored. These include amino acids, carbohydrates, vitamins, (apart from fat-soluble vitamins D, A, K, and E) and minerals (see Chapters 31, 35, and 39, respectively). Most major plasma proteins (with the exception of immunoglobulins [Igs] and the von Willebrand factor) are mainly or exclusively synthesized in the liver. The liver responds to multiple hormonal and neural stimuli to regulate blood glucose concentrations. Not only does it extract glucose from blood for use in generating energy, but it also stores dietary glucose as glycogen for later use. The liver is also the major site for gluconeogenesis, which is critical for maintaining blood glucose concentration in the fasting state. The liver plays a major role in lipid metabolism; it is the principal site of cholesterol, triglyceride, and lipoprotein synthesis; it extracts and processes fatty acids that are generated through lipolysis in adipose tissue. It also removes cholesterol from the circulation by endocytosis of remnants of chylomicrons and very-low density lipoproteins (VLDLs) and low-density lipoproteins (LDLs) and by selective uptake from high-density lipoproteins (HDLs). Cholesterol and bile acids synthesized by the liver from cholesterol are secreted into the bile, which facilitates the absorption of dietary fat and fat-soluble vitamins. The liver is also the primary site of metabolism of both endogenous substances and exogenous compounds (e.g., drugs and toxins). This process, known as biotransformation, converts lipophilic substances to hydrophilic ones for subsequent elimination. The liver is a major site of catabolism of hormones, and thus participates in regulation of plasma hormone concentrations. The liver is also involved in hormone synthesis, producing such hormones as insulin-like growth factor 1, angiotensinogen, hepcidin, thrombopoietin, erythropoietin, and the prohormone 25-OH vitamin D. Many of these hepatic functions can be assessed by laboratory procedures to gain insight into the integrity of the liver.

As a large organ, the liver shares with many other organs the ability to perform its functions with extensive reserve capacity. In many cases, individuals with liver disease maintain normal function despite extensive liver damage. In such cases, liver disease may be recognized only by using tests that detect injury. Most commonly, this is accomplished by measuring plasma activities of enzymes found within liver cells, which are released in somewhat specific patterns with different forms of

[a]The authors gratefully acknowledge the original contributions by Drs. D. Robert Dufour, Keith G. Tolman, Robert Rej, and Basil T. Doumas, upon which portions of this chapter are based.

injury. Chronic liver injury often involves fibrosis in the liver; markers of the fibrotic process can indicate the degree of injury. Chronic damage is often due to chronic inflammation; cytokines alter the pattern of liver protein production, which allows detection of inflammation (although not necessarily that involving the liver). Some proteins are produced in increased amounts with liver regeneration and neoplasia; such markers may be useful in detecting liver cell proliferation.

The chapter begins by describing the anatomy and biochemical functions of the liver. Various disease states that involve the liver are then discussed. The chapter concludes with a discussion of the use of laboratory test results in recognizing and characterizing patterns of liver injury.

ANATOMY OF THE LIVER

The adult liver weighs approximately 1.2 to 1.5 kg. It is located beneath the diaphragm in the right upper quadrant of

the abdomen and is protected by the ribs and held in place by ligamentous attachments.

Gross Anatomy

The liver is divided into left and right anatomic lobes by the falciform ligament, an anterior extension of the peritoneal folds that connects the liver to the diaphragm and the anterior abdominal wall (Fig. 51.1). Two smaller lobes are found between the left and right lobes: the caudate lobe, situated on the posterior-superior surface of the right lobe, receiving blood supply from the left and right hepatic arteries and the portal vein, and the quadrate lobe that sits on the under surface of the medial segment of the left lobe. Riedel's lobe, an anatomic extension of the right lobe of the liver, consists of a projection that may feel like a mobile tumor in the right abdomen.

The liver has a dual blood supply. The portal vein, which carries blood from the spleen and nutrient-enriched blood

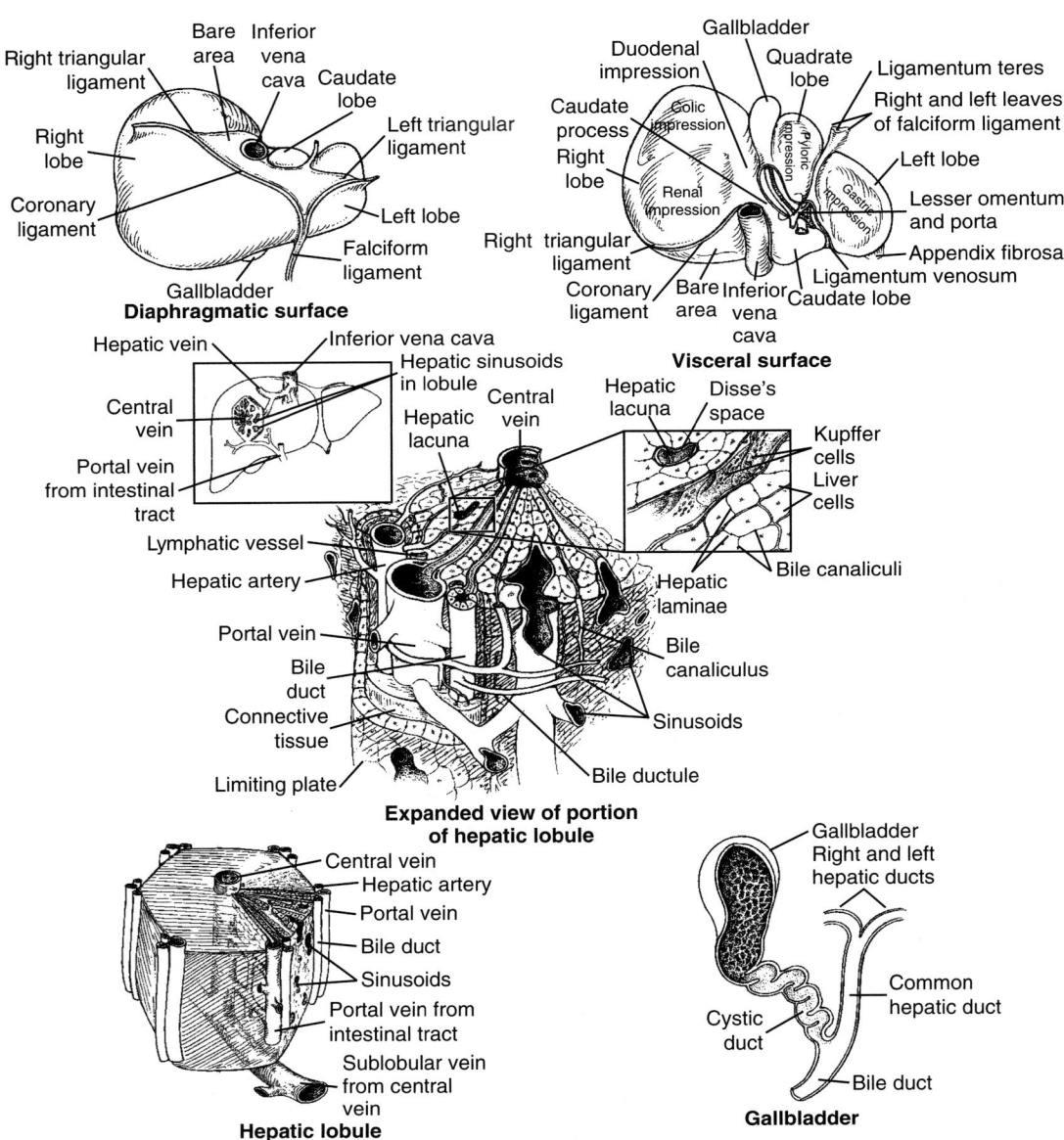

FIGURE 51.1 Structure of the liver. (From *Dorland's Illustrated Medical Dictionary*. 30th ed. Philadelphia: Saunders; 2003, plate 26.)

from the gastrointestinal (GI) tract, supplies approximately 70% of the blood supply; the hepatic artery, a branch of the celiac axis, provides oxygen-enriched arterial blood. Each supplies approximately half of the oxygen reaching the liver, making it highly resistant to infarction. Ultimately, these two blood supplies merge and flow into the sinusoids that course between individual hepatocytes. Venous drainage from the liver ultimately converges into the right and left hepatic veins, which exit on the posterior surface of the liver and join the inferior vena cava near its entry into the right atrium. The caudate lobe drains directly into the inferior vena cava and so may continue to function if the hepatic venous outflow is occluded (Budd-Chiari syndrome).

The liver is covered by an anterior reflection of the peritoneum known as Glisson capsule. Other extensions of the peritoneum form ligaments that hold the liver in place. Internal extensions of the capsule provide an internal supporting framework that divides the liver into lobules and ultimately surrounds blood vessels and nerves. One of the ligaments, the ligamentum teres, is the vestigial remnant of the umbilical vein; it connects the umbilicus to the inferior border of the liver. When portal hypertension occurs, the umbilical veins may reopen, leading to venous dilatation around the umbilicus (termed caput medusae).

The nerve supply to the liver comes from the vagus and phrenic nerves, and the sympathetic ganglia originating from cell bodies in the spinal cord that are located between the seventh and tenth thoracic vertebrae. These merge to accompany the hepatic arteries and bile ducts throughout the liver.

Biliary drainage originates at the bile canaliculi; these grooves between adjacent hepatocytes form ductules that merge to create the intrahepatic bile ducts, which ultimately join to form the right and left hepatic bile ducts, which exit from the liver at the porta hepatis and combine to form the common hepatic duct. The hepatic duct is joined by the cystic duct that drains the gallbladder to form the common bile duct (see Fig. 51.1). The common bile duct then enters the duodenum (usually with the pancreatic duct) at the ampulla of Vater. The duodenal portion of the common bile duct is surrounded by longitudinal and circular muscle fibers that form the sphincter of Oddi. This musculature relaxes when the gallbladder contracts, allowing bile to enter the duodenum; in its normally contracted state, the sphincter prevents reflux of acidic duodenal contents into the bile duct. The gallbladder, which is located on the undersurface of the right lobe of the liver, is the site for storage and concentration of bile, a complex mixture of bile salts and waste products. In the adult, it averages approximately 10 cm in length and has a capacity of 30 to 50 mL of bile. Hormonal stimuli initiated by food ingestion cause contraction of the muscular wall of the gallbladder, releasing bile salts into the intestine to facilitate digestion of fat.

Microscopic Anatomy

The functional anatomical unit of the liver is the acinus, which is adjacent to the portal triad (which consists of a branch of each of the portal vein, hepatic artery, and bile duct). Each acinus is a diamond-shaped mass of liver parenchyma that is supplied by a terminal branch of the portal vein and of the hepatic artery and is drained by a terminal branch of the bile duct. The blood vessels radiate toward the periphery, forming sinusoids, which perfuse the liver and ultimately drain into the central (terminal) hepatic vein (Fig. 51.2). The sinusoids are lined by fenestrated endothelial cells (which

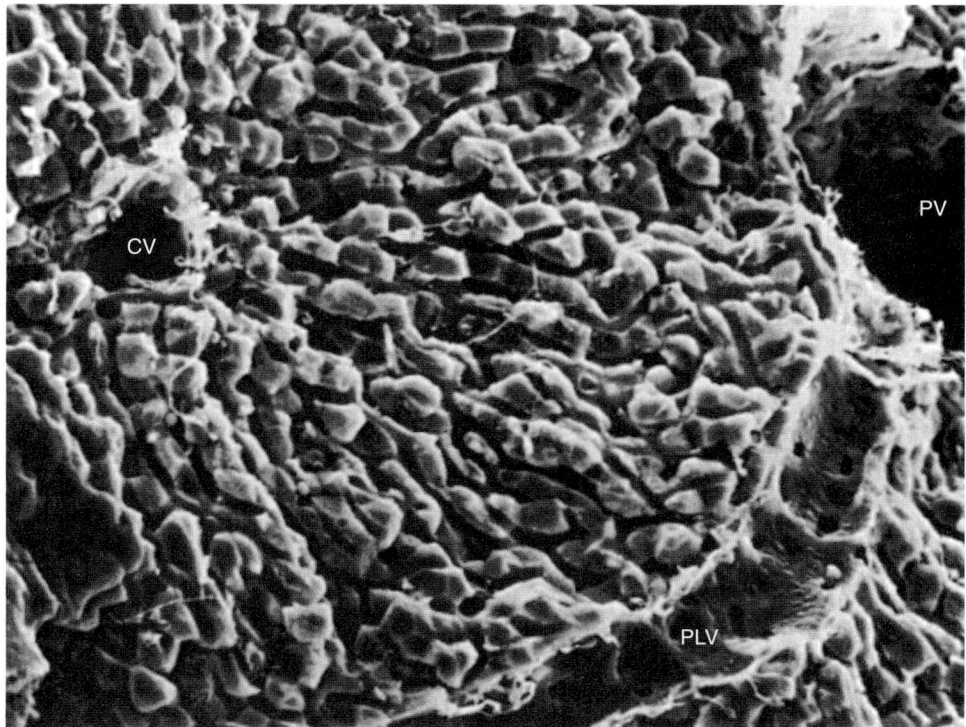

FIGURE 51.2 A low-magnification scanning electron micrograph depicting a portion of a liver lobule from a rat liver. *CV*, Central vein; *PLV*, perilobular venules; *PV*, portal vein. (From Zakim O, Boyer TD. *Hepatology: a textbook of liver disease.* 3rd ed. Philadelphia: WB Saunders; 1996. p. 9.)

allows free filtration of blood) and phagocytic Kupffer cells (see Fig. 51.1). The Kupffer cells are derived from blood monocytes. They contain lysosomes with hydrolytic enzymes that break down phagocytized foreign particles (e.g., bacteria). They also have Ig and complement receptors and are the main site for clearance of antigen–antibody complexes from blood. Kupffer cells secrete interleukins (ILs), tumor necrosis factor (TNF), collagenase, prostaglandins, and other factors involved in inflammatory responses.

Hepatocytes are the major functioning cells in the liver and are responsible for approximately 70% of liver mass. They perform most of the metabolic and synthetic functions of the liver. Two other cell types are found in small numbers within the liver. The stellate cells (sometimes referred to as Ito cells) are located between the endothelial lining of the sinusoids, and the hepatocytes are within a small cleft referred to as the space of Disse. In their normal, quiescent state, stellate cells serve as a site of storage for fat-soluble vitamins, particularly vitamin A. When stimulated, stellate cells are morphologically and functionally transformed. They synthesize collagen and are the cells responsible for fibrosis, and eventually, cirrhosis. They also synthesize nitric oxide, which helps to regulate intrahepatic blood flow. Oval cells, found near the portal areas around small bile passages, are believed to be liver stem cells involved in regeneration of hepatocytes and bile ducts after liver injury.[1]

The blood supply to each acinus consists of three zones (Fig. 51.3). Hepatocytes in zone 1, the area immediately adjacent to the portal tract, are enriched with lysosomes and mitochondria. Zone 1 appears to be involved in protecting the liver from external injury and providing a base for hepatic regeneration. Zone 2 predominantly contains hepatocytes that perform the major metabolic functions of the liver. The periphery of the acinus, zone 3, contains hepatocytes that are enriched with endoplasmic reticulum, are metabolically active, and have relatively low oxygen tension. This area is most susceptible to injury.

Ultrastructure of the Hepatocyte

Hepatocytes contain a well-developed organelle substructure (Fig. 51.4). Mitochondria, which constitute approximately 18% of hepatocyte volume, are the sites of oxidative phosphorylation and energy production. They contain enzymes involved in the citric acid cycle and in β-oxidation of fatty acids. The rough endoplasmic reticulum is the site of synthesis of many proteins, including albumin, coagulation factors, enzymes (e.g., glucose 6-phosphatase), and triglycerides. The smooth endoplasmic reticulum contains microsomes that are involved in bilirubin conjugation, detoxification (cytochrome P_{450}–dependent isoenzymes), steroid synthesis, cholesterol synthesis, and bile acid synthesis. Several microsomal enzymes, including γ-glutamyltransferase, are induced by many drugs and inhibited by others. γ-Glutamyl transpeptidase (GGT) catalyzes the transfer of the γ-glutamyl moiety from γ-glutamyl peptides to other peptides such as glutathione and to L-amino acids. GGT is present in the cell membranes of many tissues, with greatest activity in biliary epithelial cells, pancreatic acinar cells, renal tubular epithelial cells, and also in mammary glands in some species. It is believed that it is involved in amino acid transport across membranes as part of the γ-glutamyl cycle, although hydrolysis of glutathione may be a more important function. This is the site of most drug metabolism and many important drug interactions.

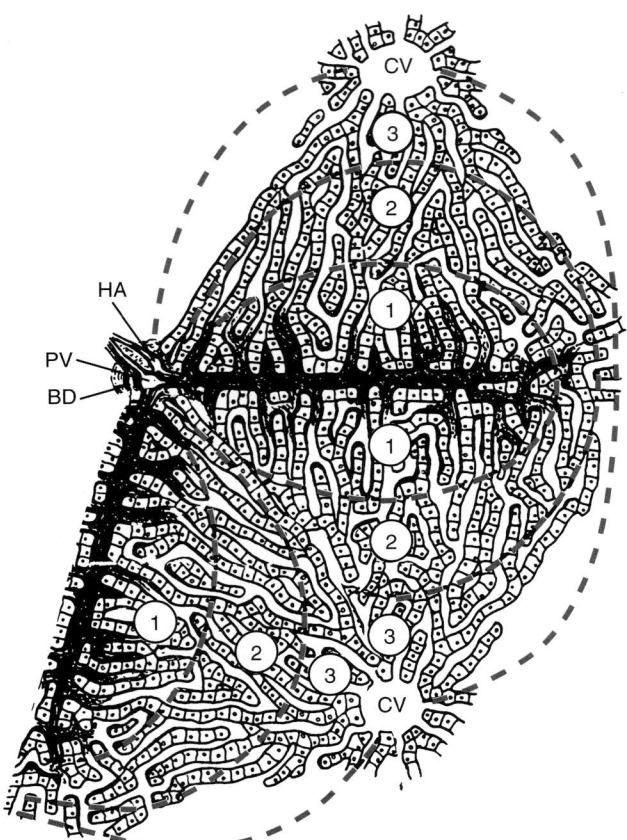

FIGURE 51.3 Blood supply of the simple liver acinus. Zones 1, 2, and 3 indicate corresponding volumes in a portion of an adjacent acinar unit. Oxygen tension and the nutrient level in the blood in sinusoids decrease from zone 1 through zone 3. *BD,* Bile duct; *CV,* central vein; *HA,* hepatic artery; *PV,* portal vein. (From Zakim O, Boyer TD. *Hepatology: a textbook of liver disease.* 3rd ed. Philadelphia: WB Saunders; 1996. p. 10.)

Peroxisomes are found near the smooth endoplasmic reticulum and contain oxidases that use molecular oxygen to modify a variety of substrates, leading to the production of hydrogen peroxide. They also contain catalase, which decomposes hydrogen peroxide. Peroxisomes catalyze the β-oxidation of fatty acids that have 7 to 18 chain lengths. Approximately 5 to 20% of the metabolism of ethanol also occurs in the peroxisomes. Lysosomes are dense organelles that contain hydrolytic enzymes that act as scavengers. Deposition of iron, lipofuscin, bile pigments, and copper occurs in the lysosomes. The Golgi apparatus lies near the canaliculus and is involved in the secretion of various substances, including bile acids and albumin.

Gut Microbiome

The human intestine is home to a variety of microbes (bacteria, archaea, fungi, and viruses). The gut contains approximately the same number of bacterial cells as there are human cells in the body, but the human microbiome contains over 3 million genes, compared with only around 23,000 in the human genome.[2,3]

The gut microbiota plays crucial roles in: the maturation and continued stimulation of the host immune response[4]; the maintenance of the intestinal barrier integrity, which limits

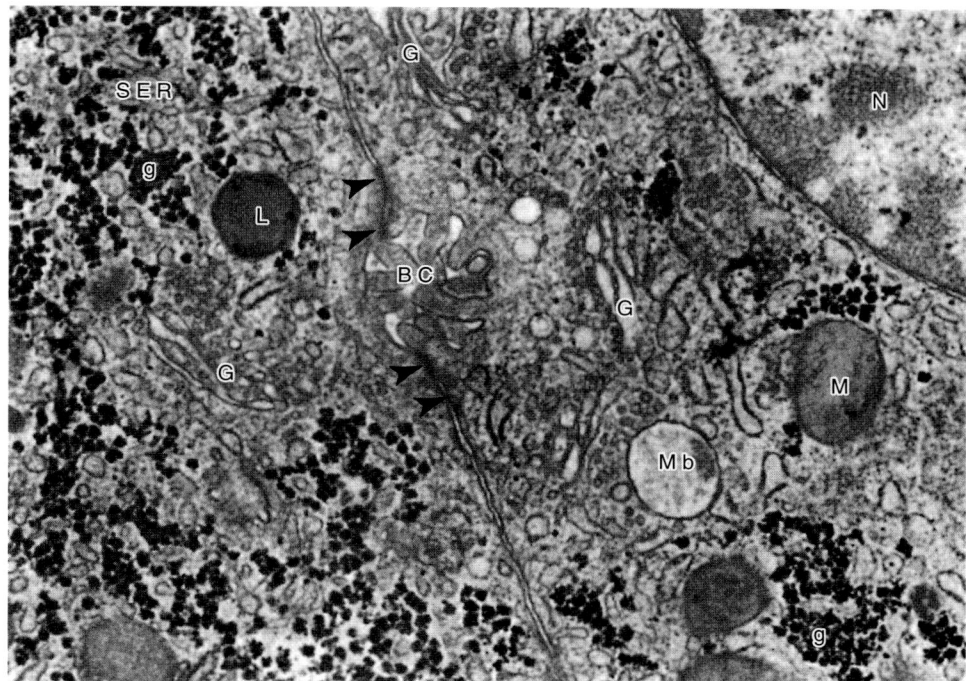

FIGURE 51.4 Portions of two human liver cells showing the relationship of the organelles and a typical bile canaliculus (BC). *Arrowheads* indicate light junctions. *G*, Golgi; *g*, glycogen; *L*, lysosome; *M*, mitochondria; *Mb*, microbody; *N*, nucleus; *SER*, smooth endoplasmic reticulum. (From Zakim O, Boyer TD. *Hepatology: a textbook of liver disease*. 3rd ed. Philadelphia: WB Saunders; 1996. p. 20.)

pathogen perpetuation in the gut; modulation of host-cell proliferation[5] and vascularisation[6]; and regulation of intestinal, neurologic,[7] and endocrine functions,[8] and bone density.[9] The human gut microbiota provides a source of energy[10]; helps in the synthesis of vitamins[11] and neurotransmitters; metabolizes bile salts[12]; reacts to or modifies specific drugs; and eliminates exogenous toxins.[13] In a healthy colon, the gut microbiota maintains a symbiotic relationship with the host and rapidly adapts to maintain eubiosis after an acute insult.[14]

The gut-liver axis refers to the bidirectional relationship between the gut and its microbiota, and the liver. There is a constant interchange generated by dietary, genetic, and environmental factors established via the portal vein that carries gut-derived products to the liver, and the liver feedback of bile and antibody secretion from the liver into the intestine via the biliary tree. The control of the microbial communities is critical to maintain the homeostasis of the gut-liver axis, and as a part of this two-way communication, the liver shapes intestinal microbial communities.

An altered microbiota or "dysbiosis," an impaired intestinal barrier, and endotoxemia are well-recognized features of advanced alcohol-related liver disease (ArLD).[15] Disturbances of the intestinal barrier can result in an increased portal influx of bacteria or their products to the liver where they can cause or worsen hepatic diseases and inflammation and potentiate disease. In alcoholic liver disease, the toxic effect of alcohol on hepatocytes, abnormal microbiota, and loss of intestinal function all contribute to the pathogenesis of the disease. Alcohol causes bacterial overgrowth and reduced bacterial diversity[16] and a reduction in the diversity of the mycobiome particularly influencing yeast and fungi and a reduced mycobiome (yeast and fungi).[17] These changes lead

to alterations in bile acid homeostasis increasing intestinal deconjugation of bile acids and exposure of hepatocytes to more toxic bile acids. Alcohol disrupts the intestinal microbiome, alters the intestinal barrier, and might affect various other intestinal functions such as mucosal immunity.[18] Although the role of the bacterial component of the gut microbiota in ArLD has been the major focus of research, the contribution of the mycobiota in this disease is of particular interest, given the increased risk of fungal infections in patients with ArLD. The mycobiota is also known to be altered in other diseases, including hepatitis B and inflammatory bowel disease.

In nonalcoholic fatty liver disease (NAFLD), bacterial overgrowth and changes in the microbiota population occurs and these changes correlate with increased intestinal permeability and features of the metabolic syndrome.[19,20]

In cirrhosis, there is marked impairment of the gut barrier that worsens as the disease advances. The gut microbiota in cirrhosis is characterized by reduced diversity, increased overgrowth of potentially pathogenic bacteria, and decreased abundance of beneficial bacteria.[21,22] Infections are the most common cause of death in these patients and with advanced liver cirrhosis which is associated with a profound dysbiosis. It is suggested that decompensation of liver events in cirrhosis and typical complications of advanced liver disease such as hepatic encephalopathy and bacterial peritonitis are substantially driven by the microbiota.[23]

Alteration of gut microbiota may play an important role in the development and progression of NAFLD. It was shown more than 20 years ago in animal models that changing the microbiota composition by using prebiotics such as inulin-type fructans reduces hepatic steatosis and de novo lipogenesis.[24] Feeding of prebiota was found to inhibit all lipogenic enzymes and thereby VLDL production so that plasma triglyceride concentrations are decreased. The fermentation of prebiotics by gut microbes increases the abundance of short-chain fatty acids in the caecum and also in the portal veinous blood, where the concentration of both acetate and propionate is doubled leading to a reduction in hepatic lipogenesis. In this way, the microbiota contributes to the regulation of de novo hepatic lipogenesis. Further, specific nutrients such as fat and alcohol change the composition of the microbiota in a harmful manner, whereas prebiotics may counteract these effects. Hepatic lipid metabolism is influenced by the innate immune system and xenobiotic metabolism control liver lipid metabolism via mechanisms involving bacterial components and metabolites. Thus hepatic innate immunity can influence the liver's production of bioactive lipids and contribute to switch from NAFLD to nonalcoholic steatohepatitis.[25]

Emerging work suggests that altered gut microbiota may contribute to the pathology of other liver diseases. There is a specific microbiome signature found in primary sclerosing cholangitis (PSC) with an increased population of *Veillonella* as is the situation with other human chronic inflammatory disorders. This microbiome signature is different than the one observed in patients with ulcerative colitis without liver disease.[23]

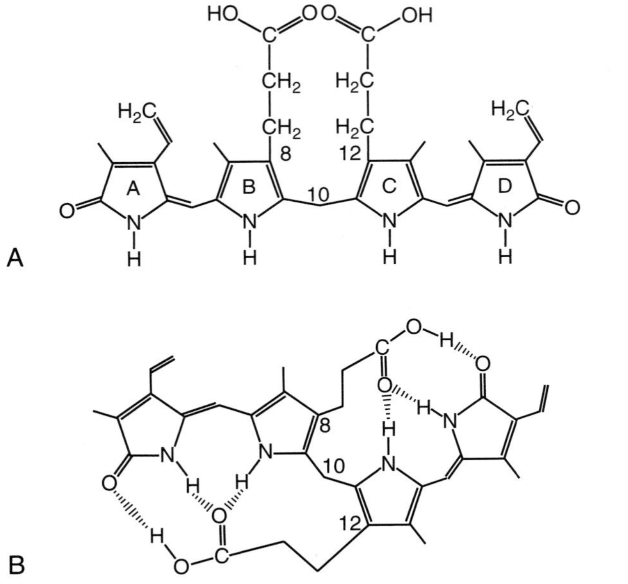

BIOCHEMICAL FUNCTIONS OF THE LIVER

The liver is involved in various excretory, synthetic, and metabolic functions. Clinical laboratories perform numerous tests that are useful in the biochemical assessment of these functions.

Hepatic Excretory Function

Organic compounds of both endogenous and exogenous origin are extracted from the sinusoidal blood, biotransformed, and excreted into the bile or urine. Assessment of this excretory function provides valuable clinical information. The most frequently used tests involve the measurement of plasma concentrations of endogenously produced compounds, such as bilirubin and bile acids. In specialist centers, these tests may be augmented by determination of the rate of clearance of exogenous compounds, such as aminopyrine, lidocaine, and caffeine.

Bilirubin

Bilirubin is the orange-yellow pigment derived from heme, which is mainly a product of red blood cell (RBC) turnover. It is extracted and biotransformed in the liver and excreted in bile and urine.

Chemistry

Bilirubin was discovered by Virchow in 1849 in blood extravasates; he called the yellow pigment "hematoidin." The term *bilirubin* was coined by Stadeler in 1864, and in 1874, Tarchanoff demonstrated the direct association of bile pigments with Hb. In 1942, Fisher and Plieninger synthesized bilirubin IXα and proposed the structure shown in Fig. 51.5A. This linear tetrapyrrolic structure of the bilirubin molecule was accepted for longer than 30 years. However, important chemical properties of the bilirubin molecule are its insolubility in water and

FIGURE 51.5 (A) A Linear Molecular Representation of Unconjugated Bilirubin. (B) The Preferred Structure of Unconjugated Bilirubin IXa, Z,Z Configuration. The folded ridge-tile structure is stabilized by six hydrogen bonds formed between the two carboxyl groups of the sidechains and the two carbonyl and four imino groups. The ridge involves carbon atoms 8 through 12. *CO*, Carbon monoxide; *Fe*, iron; *NADPH*, nicotinamide adenine dinucleotide phosphate reduced.

its solubility in a variety of nonpolar solvents. The solubility of bilirubin in nonpolar, lipid solvents is not predicted from this linear tetrapyrrole structure because the two propionic acid side chains would be expected to make the bilirubin molecule highly polar and, therefore water soluble. The overall chemical structure of bilirubin was established by x-ray crystallography.[26] According to this work, bilirubin assumes a ridge-tiled configuration stabilized by six intramolecular hydrogen bonds. Two additional important structural features have also been noted: (1) a so-called *Z-Z (trans)* conformation for the double bonds between carbons 4 and 5 and 15 and 16, and (2) an involuted hydrogen-bonded structure in which the propionic acid–carboxylic acid groups are hydrogen-bonded to the nitrogen atoms of the pyrrole rings (see Fig. 51.5B).[27] These bonds stabilize the *Z-Z* configuration of bilirubin and prevent its interaction with polar groups in aqueous media. When exposed to light, the *Z-Z* configuration is converted to the *E-E (cis)* conformation and to other combinations, namely, 4E-15Z and 4Z-15E. The *E-E* conformation and other *E*-containing isomers do not permit the degree of internal hydrogen bonding that occurs in the *Z-Z* conformation and, therefore are more water soluble than in the *Z-Z* conformation. Thus light-exposed forms of bilirubin are more water soluble and are readily excreted in the bile. This is the rationale for irradiating jaundiced newborns with 450-nm light.[28]

The bilirubin molecule in the crystalline state takes, as mentioned earlier, the form of a ridge tile rather than a linear tetrapyrrole, with the ridge being along the line C8-C10-C12. In this configuration, rings A and B lie in one plane and rings C and D in another, with a 98° angle between the two rings. The preferred conformation of bilirubin in aqueous solution at pH 7.4 is not known, but the occurrence of a hydrogen-bonded structure in aqueous solution would explain some of the unique chemical properties of bilirubin IXα. For example, the addition of hydrogen bond–breaking chemicals, such as caffeine, methanol, ethanol, urea, or surface active agents, is required for unconjugated bilirubin to react with diazo reagent. These reagents likely act by breaking the internal hydrogen bonds of the bilirubin molecule, allowing it to react with diazotized sulfanilic acid or other diazo compounds. In contrast, bilirubin IXα monoglucuronide and diglucuronide are soluble in water and react readily with diazo reagents. The bulky glucuronic acid moiety precludes conjugated bilirubin from undergoing internal hydrogen bond formation. Bilirubin glucuronides, which are water soluble, are readily excreted in the bile and urine, whereas unconjugated bilirubin is not.

Bilirubin derived from natural sources consists almost entirely (99%) of the isomer IXα. Bilirubins IXβ and IXδ, which arise from cleavage of the β- and δ-methene bridges, consist of less than 0.5% of bilirubin isolated from bile. However, bilirubin reference materials available from commercial sources and from the National Institute of Standards and Technology (Standard Reference Material 916a) contain variable quantities of IIIα and XIIIα isomers.[29] The two isomers are formed by cleavage of bilirubin IXα at the central methylene bridge; subsequent recombination of the two different dipyrrole units gives a mixture of the three isomers. This isomerization of bilirubin occurs in aqueous solution at acidic or neutral pH, but not when bilirubin is bound to albumin.[30]

Biochemistry

Bilirubin IXα is produced from the catabolism of protoporphyrin IX by a microsomal heme oxygenase.[31] The tetrapyrrolic product of the ring opening at the α-methene bridge is the green pigment biliverdin, which is subsequently reduced to bilirubin by the reduced form of nicotinamide adenine dinucleotide phosphate–dependent cytosolic enzyme biliverdin reductase (Fig. 51.6). For each mole of heme catabolized by this pathway, one mole each of carbon monoxide, bilirubin, and ferric iron is produced. Daily bilirubin production from all sources in humans averages from 250 to 300 mg. Approximately 85% of the total bilirubin produced is derived from the heme moiety of Hb released from senescent erythrocytes that are destroyed in the reticuloendothelial cells of the liver, spleen, and bone marrow. The remaining 15% is produced from RBC precursors destroyed in the bone marrow (so-called ineffective erythropoiesis) and from the catabolism of other heme-containing proteins, such as myoglobin, cytochromes, and peroxidases.

In blood, bilirubin is bound to albumin ($K_d \approx 10^{-8}$ mol/L) and is transported to the liver.[32] Bilirubin then dissociates from albumin by an unknown process at the sinusoidal membrane of the hepatocyte. It is transported across the membrane (Fig. 51.7).

It is theorized that the organic anion transport proteins (OATPs) 1A1 (OMIM*604843) and 1B3 (OMIM*605495), which are encoded on the solute carrier organic anion transporter (SLCO) superfamily of genes, are responsible for the uptake of bilirubin into the hepatocyte.[33] Once inside the liver cells, bilirubin is reversibly bound to soluble proteins known as ligandins or protein Y. Ligandins are cytosolic proteins of the glutathione-S-transferase gene family and include

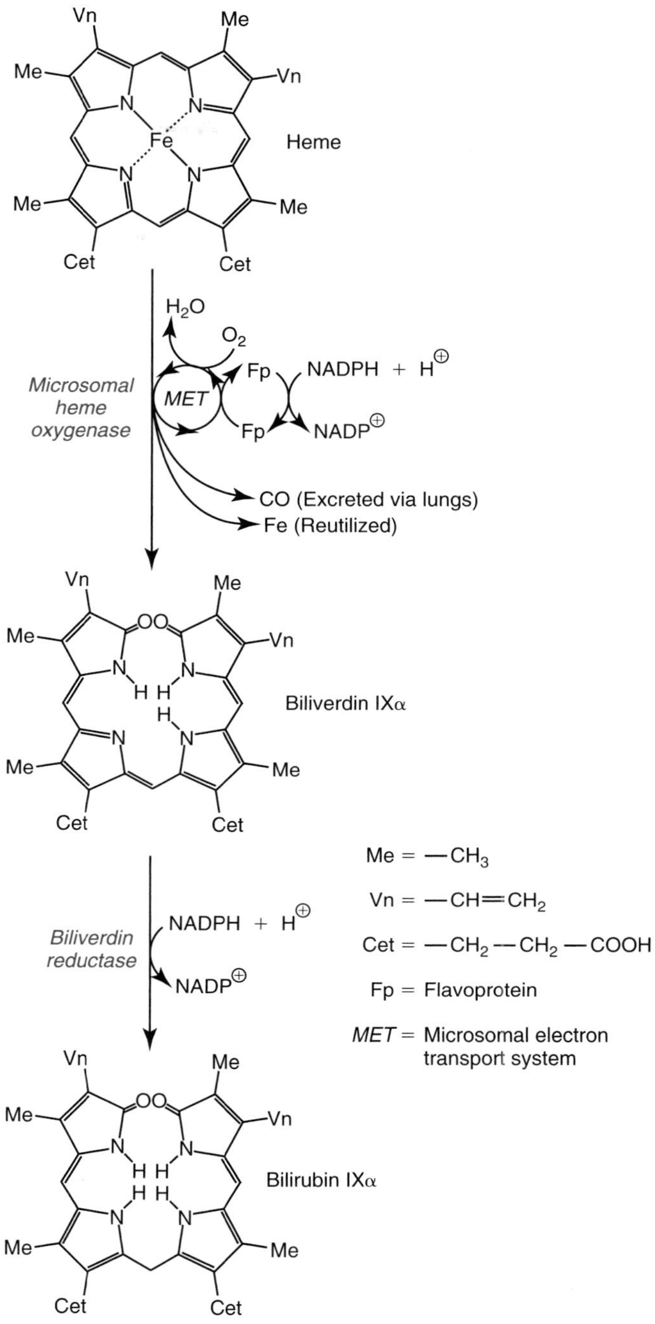

FIGURE 51.6 Catabolism of Heme to Bilirubin IXα. (Modified from Tenhunen R, Marver HS, Schmid R. The enzymatic conversion of hemoglobin to bilirubin. *Trans Assoc Am Physicians* 1969;82:363–71.)

approximately 5% of the total protein of human liver cytosol.[34,35] Ligandin also binds a variety of other compounds, such as steroids, bromsulphthalein (BSP), indocyanine green, and some carcinogens. Ligandin likely plays an important role in the processing of these compounds; it may increase the net efficiency of uptake by retarding the reflux of these substances back to plasma.

Inside the hepatocytes, bilirubin is rapidly conjugated with glucuronic acid to produce bilirubin monoglucuronide

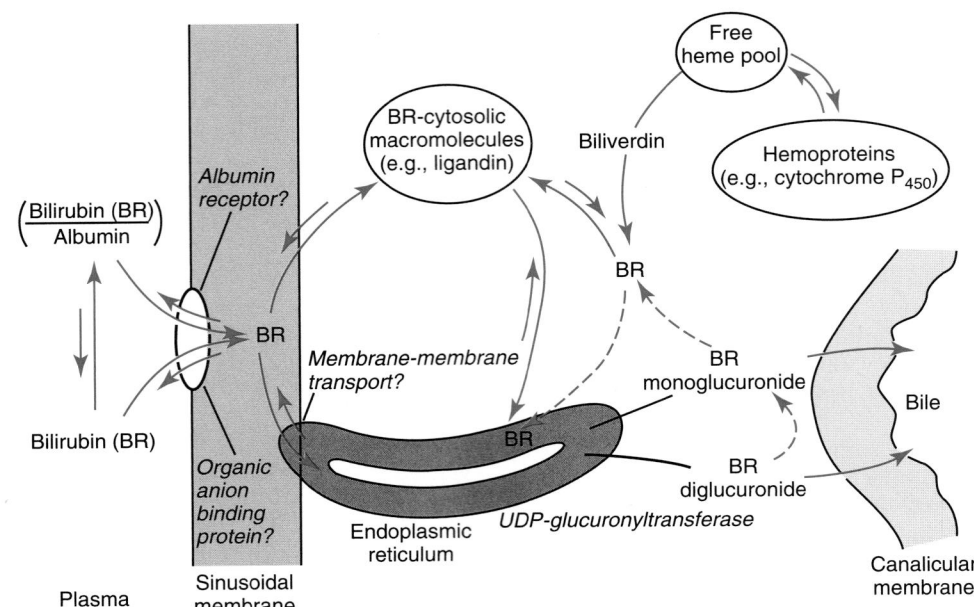

FIGURE 51.7 Bilirubin Uptake, Metabolism, and Transport in the Hepatocyte. (From Gollan JL, Schmid R. Bilirubin update: formation, transport, and metabolism. In: Popper H, Schaffner F, editors. *Progress in liver diseases*, vol. 7. Philadelphia: WB Saunders, 1982 [chapter 15].)

and diglucuronide, which then are excreted into bile (see Fig. 51.7). The enzyme bilirubin uridine diphosphate (UDP)–glucuronyltransferase 1A1 (OMIM*191740) is a tetramer that catalyzes the formation of bilirubin monoglucuronide and diglucuronide. This is a transmembrane protein primarily localized to the smooth endoplasmic reticulum. A specific binding site exists for bilirubin and glucuronic acid.[36] It is speculated that the monomer catalyzes monoglucuronide formation and the tetramer is required for the diglucuronide conjugate at the luminal surface of the endoplasmic reticulum.[37] The bilirubin diglucuronide returns to the cytosol, likely through a transporter, and binds to ligandin where it will diffuse to either the canalicular pole for secretion into bile or the sinusoidal pole for secretion back into plasma. The process is mediated by an adenosine triphosphate–binding cassette transporter ABCC2, which was previously named multidrug-related protein 2 (MRP2), at the canalicular pole. Although other transporters exist for this function, such as ABCG2, most are removed by MRP2/ABCC2. At the sinusoidal pole, an ABCC3 transporter returns bilirubin into plasma where reuptake is possible by the OATP1B1 and OATP1B3 transporters.[38]

In the presence of bilirubin monoglucuronide, albumin (and other proteins) can be postsynthetically modified by covalent attachment to lysine residues. In the case of albumin, this produces a protein-bound form termed biliprotein or δ-bilirubin. Increases in conjugated bilirubin or δ-bilirubin are highly specific markers of hepatic dysfunction (except in the presence of rare inherited disorders that impair excretion of conjugated bilirubin, such as Dubin-Johnson syndrome).

In adults, virtually all bilirubin excreted in bile is in the form of glycosidic conjugates; glucuronides account for approximately 95% of them, and glucosides and xylosides constitute the remainder. Of the glucuronides, diglucuronide is the major fraction (≈90%), and monoglucuronide is the minor fraction (≈10%).

Bilirubin glucuronides are not substantially reabsorbed in the intestine. Rather, they are hydrolyzed by the catalytic action of β-glucuronidase from the liver, intestinal epithelial cells, and bacteria. This unconjugated bilirubin is then reduced by anaerobic intestinal microbial flora to form a group of three colorless tetrapyrroles collectively called urobilinogens. In each of these three bilirubin reduction products, all bridge carbons are in the saturated (methylene) form. The urobilinogens differ from one another in the degree of hydrogenation of the vinyl sidechains and in the two end pyrrole rings. Urobilinogens contain 6, 8, or 12 more hydrogen atoms than does bilirubin and are named stercobilinogen, mesobilinogen, or urobilinogen, respectively. Up to 20% of the urobilinogen produced daily is reabsorbed from the intestine and enters the enterohepatic circulation. Most of the reabsorbed urobilinogen is taken up by the liver and is reexcreted in the bile; a small fraction (2 to 5%) enters the general circulation and appears in urine. In the lower intestinal tract, the three urobilinogens are spontaneously oxidized at the middle methylene bridge to produce the corresponding bile pigments stercobilin, mesobilin, and urobilin, which are orange-brown and the major pigments of stool. Approximately 50% of the conjugated bilirubin excreted in bile is metabolized to products other than the urobilinogens. The detailed structure of these metabolites has not been characterized.

Increased plasma bilirubin typically is classified as primarily indirect (an approximation of unconjugated bilirubin) or direct (an approximation of the sum of conjugated bilirubin and biliprotein). Increased indirect bilirubin indicates overproduction of bilirubin, which is usually caused by hemolysis, or decreased metabolism by the liver, which is primarily caused by congenital defects involving uridine 5-phosphate-glucuronyl transferase. The physiologic jaundice observed in neonates is due to increased indirect bilirubin caused by the delayed maturation of the conjugation process to remove it. With severe liver injury, which occurs with fulminant hepatic failure and end-stage cirrhosis, liver disease may cause primarily unconjugated hyperbilirubinemia. Increased urine urobilinogen occurs when bilirubin delivery to the intestinal tract is increased (as with hemolysis, or after recovery from hepatitis or obstruction) or when liver clearance is decreased, which occurs in portal hypertension.

Increased direct bilirubin generally results from functional or mechanical impairment in bilirubin excretion from the hepatocyte. Increased conjugated bilirubin is found in most cases of acute hepatitis and cholestasis (stoppage or suppression of the flow of bile); the percentage of direct bilirubin is similar in both types of liver disease. Urine bilirubin reflects increased plasma concentrations of conjugated bilirubin. With resolution of liver disease, conjugated bilirubin is rapidly cleared, and biliprotein may become the only form present; urine bilirubin is typically absent in such circumstances. Increased conjugated bilirubin is rarely seen with congenital defects in bilirubin excretion, such as Dubin-Johnson syndrome, and with impaired bilirubin excretion, which occurs in sepsis or other acute illness.

Bilirubin is known as a strong antioxidant and mild or moderately increased serum bilirubin seems to be beneficial[39]; the protective effects of bilirubin on atherogenesis and cancerogenesis have been demonstrated in both in vitro and in vivo studies.[40,41] However, high concentrations of unconjugated hyperbilirubinemia are toxic and cause bilirubin encephalopathy (kernicterus) which is due to inhibition of DNA synthesis and direct neurotoxicity causing mass destruction of neurons through apoptosis and necrosis.[42] Bilirubin may also uncouple oxidative phosphorylation and inhibit adenosine triphosphatase (ATPase) activity of brain mitochondria.[43] Bilirubin mediated inhibition of various enzyme systems, RNA synthesis and protein synthesis in the brain and liver, and/or alteration of carbohydrate metabolism in the brain can also contribute to its toxicity. The accumulation of bilirubin in plasma and tissues results in characteristic yellow discoloration of tissues known as icterus or jaundice.

Clinical Significance of Bilirubin

Jaundice is a condition characterized by hyperbilirubinemia and deposition of bile pigment in the skin, mucous membranes, and sclera, with a resulting yellow appearance of the patient; it is also called icterus. Defects in bilirubin metabolism resulting in jaundice can occur at each step of the metabolic pathway (see Fig. 51.7). The disorders are usually classified as inherited disorders of bilirubin metabolism and jaundice of the newborn. All of these disorders are characterized by increases in conjugated or unconjugated bilirubin in the absence of other abnormal liver tests. Bilirubin fractionation is clinically useful only for these disorders.

Patients are occasionally seen with isolated increases in bilirubin concentration. In most cases, this is due to inherited disorders of bilirubin metabolism, familial hyperbilirubinemia, or hemolysis. It is not difficult to establish hemolysis as the cause of hyperbilirubinemia because the patient with severe hemolysis will have many other disease manifestations. An algorithm for differentiating familial causes of hyperbilirubinemia is presented in Fig. 51.8.

Analytical Methods

Several analytical techniques are used to measure bilirubin and metabolites in serum, urine, and feces. Measurement of

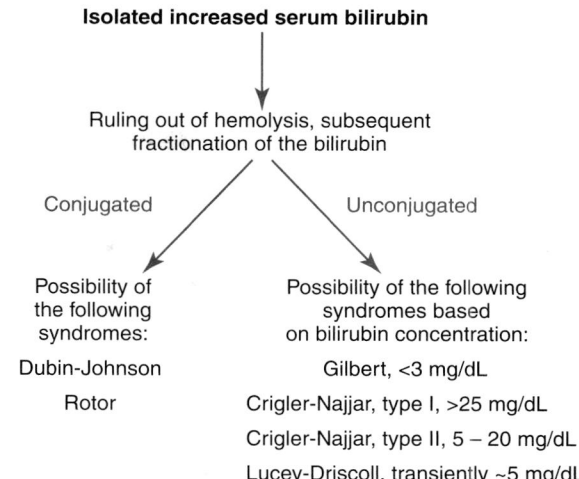

FIGURE 51.8 Algorithm for Differentiating the Familial Causes of Hyperbilirubinemia.

bilirubin in amniotic fluid is discussed in Chapter 45 on Body Fluids.

Serum Bilirubin

The reaction of bilirubin with diazotized sulfanilic acid, known as the diazo reaction, discovered by Ehrlich in 1883 and applied to the measurement of bilirubin in serum and bile by van den Bergh and Muller in 1916, is the basis of the most widely used methods for measuring bilirubin. These researchers observed, in sera from jaundiced infants, the reaction was slow and required an accelerator to proceed, and that it was rapid in bile and in adult sera without addition of ethanol, which led to the terms indirect and direct bilirubin, respectively. The chemical nature of direct and indirect bilirubins was elucidated by Billing and colleagues in the mid-1950s.[44] By using open-column, reversed-phase chromatography on siliconized kieselguhr (cellite or diatomaceous earth), investigators isolated three bilirubin fractions—unconjugated bilirubin (indirect reacting fraction) and bilirubin monoglucuronide and diglucuronide (direct reacting fractions). Kuenzle and colleagues[45] were the first to successfully use an open-column chromatography technique that did not involve a deproteinization step. They obtained four bilirubin fractions—unconjugated bilirubin (α-bilirubin), monoconjugated bilirubin (β-bilirubin), diconjugated bilirubin (γ-bilirubin), and a fraction bound strongly to protein (δ-bilirubin). The last fraction was clearly distinct from the albumin-bilirubin complex that exists in serum.

Diazo methods. The most widely used chemical methods for bilirubin measurement are those based on the coupling of bilirubin with a diazo compound.[46] In this reaction (Fig. 51.9), diazotized sulfanilic acid (the diazo reagent) reacts with bilirubin to produce two azodipyrroles (azopigments), which are reddish-purple at neutral pH and blue at low or high pH values. Van den Bergh and Muller[47] applied this reaction to the quantitation of bilirubin in serum. They described the fraction of bilirubin that reacted with the diazo reagent in the absence of alcohol as the direct bilirubin fraction and used the term indirect bilirubin for the difference between total bilirubin (found after the addition of alcohol to the reaction mixture) and the direct bilirubin fraction. Numerous variations of the

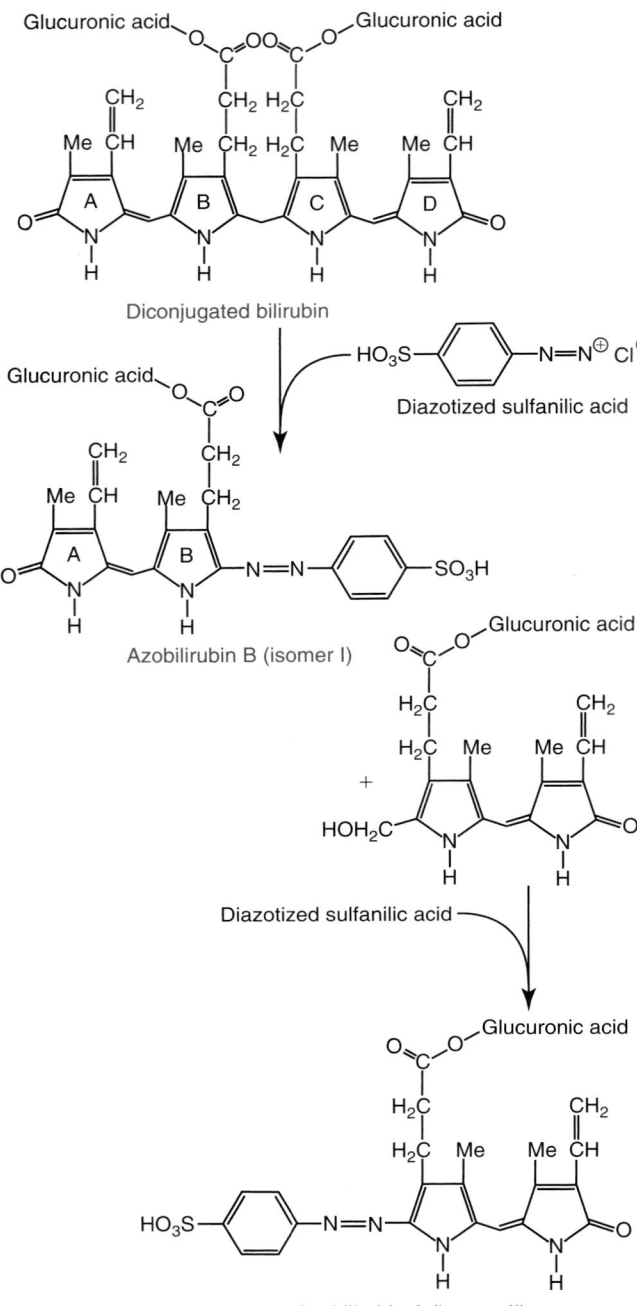

FIGURE 51.9 The Reaction of Bilirubin Glucuronide with Diazotized Sulfanilic Acid to Produce Isomers I and II of Azobilirubin B. Unconjugated bilirubin reacts in the same way to produce isomers I and II of azobilirubin A.

The diazo method described by Jendrassik and Grof in 1938[48] and later modified by Doumas and colleagues[52] gives results for serum total bilirubin that are reproducible and reliable.[53–55] In this procedure, an aqueous solution of caffeine and sodium benzoate serve as the accelerators. Studies on the mechanism by which the caffeine-benzoate solution facilitates the reaction of unconjugated bilirubin with the diazo reagent have provided strong, albeit indirect, evidence that caffeine, and perhaps benzoate, displaces unconjugated bilirubin from its association sites on albumin. This occurs by (1) formation of hydrogen bonds between bilirubin and caffeine,[56,57] thus making bilirubin water soluble, or (2) complex formation and disruption of the bilirubin internal hydrogen bonds. With the use of samples prepared by addition of unconjugated bilirubin and authentic human diconjugated (with glucuronic acid) bilirubin to low-bilirubin pooled sera—and a nuclear magnetic resonance technique—Lo and Wu[58] have shown that the modified Jendrassik-Grof total bilirubin assay detects unconjugated and diconjugated bilirubin quantitatively (as unconjugated bilirubin equivalents). This method has acceptable transferability among laboratories[53,55,59] and is currently the method of choice.

Other methods for determining bilirubin include direct spectrophotometric measurement of total bilirubin in serum using analysis of a two-component system by measuring absorbance at two wavelengths and solving a system of two simultaneous equations. This approach is applicable to sera from healthy neonates because only unconjugated bilirubin is present in such sera. Correction for oxyhemoglobin is necessary because it is invariably present in sera from neonates.

Calibrators for bilirubin measurements. A number of instrument manufacturers use bovine serum, instead of human serum, as the protein base for preparing fluids for calibrating methods for total and direct bilirubin; the protein base is enriched with unconjugated bilirubin or ditaurobilirubin or both. Unconjugated bilirubin in human serum reacts completely with the reference method and with diazo methods available in commonly used clinical analyzers; however, its reaction in bovine serum from commercial sources is incomplete and unpredictable.[60] That makes the assignment of accurate bilirubin values to calibrators virtually impossible, the protein base of which is commercial bovine serum. In human serum, ditaurobilirubin was underestimated by two of seven clinical analyzers tested; the calibrators of these two analyzers were made in bovine serum. Ditaurobilirubin in commercial bovine serum was underestimated by all analyzers and by the reference method; in human serum, it was underestimated by two analyzers only. The practice of using bilirubin calibrators in bovine sera should be abandoned because it compromises the accuracy of bilirubin measurements in jaundiced neonates. However, fresh bovine serum (obtained from a slaughterhouse) has only a small effect on the measurement of unconjugated bilirubin or ditaurobilirubin.

High-performance liquid chromatography. High-performance liquid chromatography (HPLC) methods have been developed for relatively rapid separation and quantification of the four bilirubin fractions. HPLC has been helpful in separating and detecting the various bilirubin photoisomers produced during phototherapy in newborns and thus in elucidating the mechanism by which phototherapy lowers the concentration of bilirubin in newborn blood.[57,61] Several HPLC methods are available for analysis of bilirubin fractions.

van den Bergh and Muller method have been developed. All use one of a variety of "accelerators," which, like alcohol, facilitate the reaction of unconjugated (indirect) bilirubin with the diazo reagent; the most commonly used accelerators are caffeine,[48] dyphylline,[49] and several surface active agents. The diazo method of Malloy and Evelyn,[50] which uses methanol as an accelerator, has substantial matrix effects, negative interference by Hb, turbidity due to protein precipitation by methanol, and a long reaction time.[51] This method, which has been virtually abandoned, is mentioned here for historical reasons only.

In the method of Blanckaert,[62] bilirubin conjugates, but not unconjugated bilirubin, are converted to the corresponding bilirubin methyl esters by base-catalyzed transesterification in methanol followed by extraction with chloroform. With this procedure, the α-, β-, and γ-bilirubin fractions are recoverable, but the δ-fraction (δ-bilirubin) remains in the denatured protein pellet that is produced by the chloroform extraction. In the HPLC method of Lauff and coworkers,[63] all four bilirubin fractions remain in solution after a step that involves salting out globulins with sodium sulfate. Both methods require the use of dim incandescent or yellow light to minimize photodegradation of the various bilirubin species. A simple and fast HPLC method has been published by Adachi and associates[64]; this method uses a Micronex RP-30 column (Sekisui Chemical Co., Mount Laurel, NJ), which does not require salting out of globulins or chemical transformation of bilirubin conjugates. This method separates serum bilirubin into five fractions; the fifth fraction eluted between the monoglucuronide and the unconjugated bilirubin is the Z,E or the E,Z photoisomer. The elution sequence is the same as in the procedure of Lauff and colleagues.[63] Osawa and associates have successfully developed an isocratic mobile phase.[65] The elution buffer includes 0.8% sodium ascorbate to maintain the stability of the bilirubin species. Isolation was improved with the addition of 1% Brij 35. This method strongly correlates with the HPLC method by Adachi and colleagues. Using the method by Osawa and colleagues, molar absorptivities for unconjugated bilirubin, bilirubin monoglucuronide, bilirubin diglucuronide, and δ-bilirubin were calculated at 450 nm, giving this method the potential for evaluating the accuracy of bilirubin assays.

Additional studies have indicated that the δ-bilirubin fraction consists of one or more bilirubin species that are covalently bound to albumin.[66] Existence of covalent linkage is supported by the fact that the associated bilirubin species are not released from the albumin fraction by treatment with strong acid or base, or a variety of strong denaturing agents, by hydrolysis with proteolytic enzymes, or by boiling in methanol. Delta-bilirubin reacts directly (without a promoter) with diazotized sulfanilic acid. The discovery of δ-bilirubin has solved the mystery of persistent high bilirubin concentrations that mostly direct react in patients with intrahepatic or obstructing jaundice long after hepatitis has subsided or obstruction has been relieved. It is the slowest fraction to clear from serum because it follows the catabolism of albumin, which has a half-life of approximately 17 to 19 days.

HPLC has been helpful in elucidating the nature of the bilirubin species that occur naturally in blood or are formed during phototherapy. Clinically, it offers little, if any, aid to the physician in the differential diagnosis of jaundice, because knowing the percentage of each of the bilirubin fractions in blood is of no diagnostic value. It cannot be considered as a reference method for measuring total bilirubin in blood because its accuracy and precision are inadequate. The method is calibrated with unconjugated bilirubin with the untested assumption that the other three bilirubin fractions have molar absorptivities identical to that of the calibrator,[67] when in fact this is not known. Furthermore, errors in measurement of the four species may be cumulative and may result in a large total error; also, the method is insensitive at total bilirubin concentrations of less than 1 mg/dL (17 μmol/L) and is too laborious

for routine clinical analysis. Some of the δ-bilirubin may be lost during pretreatment of samples.

A capillary electrophoresis method for measuring the different types of bilirubin has been developed by Wu and his associates.[68]

Enzymatic methods. Enzymatic methods for total and direct bilirubin and for bilirubin conjugates with glucuronic acid are based on the oxidation of bilirubin with bilirubin oxidase to biliverdin with molecular oxygen.[69] At a pH near 8, and in the presence of sodium cholate and sodium dodecylsulfate, all four bilirubin fractions are oxidized to biliverdin, which is further oxidized to purple and finally colorless products. The decrease in absorbance at 425 or 460 nm is proportional to the concentration of total bilirubin. Results obtained by the bilirubin oxidase method were in good agreement with those obtained by the Jendrassik-Grof procedure.[70] Direct bilirubin is measured at pH 3.7 to 4.5; at this pH range, the enzyme oxidizes bilirubin conjugates and δ-bilirubin, but not unconjugated bilirubin.[71,72] At pH 10, the enzyme selectively oxidizes the two glucuronides.[72,73] Delta-bilirubin is not oxidized at all, and only 5% of unconjugated bilirubin is measured as conjugates.[73]

Transcutaneous measurement of bilirubin. A noninvasive approach for measuring bilirubin was introduced in 1980 by Yamanouchi and colleagues.[74] The first bilirubinometer (icterometer) was a reflectance photometer, which used two filters to correct for the color of Hb and required measurements at eight body sites. Efforts to improve the accuracy of such measurements have been successful and led to the development of devices of acceptable performance. Reports indicate that at least one of these devices (Bili*Check* SpectR$_x$ Inc., Norcross, GA) provides results that are within ±2 mg/dL (34 μmol/L) of those obtained using a serum diazo procedure.[75,76] Another study found that the Bili*Check* underestimated serum bilirubin when its concentration was greater than 10 mg/dL (170 μmol/L).[77]

Although transcutaneous bilirubin measurements may not substitute for laboratory quantitative determinations, they provide instantaneous information, reduce the necessity for serum bilirubin determinations, spare infants the trauma of heelsticks, and save money.[78] Furthermore, they are useful in determining whether it is necessary to draw blood in a jaundiced infant before initiating treatment, such as phototherapy or exchange transfusion (currently, this is extremely rare). Another application is predicting those babies who require follow-up according to the "hour-specific" serum bilirubin nomogram developed by Bhutani and coworkers.[79]

Urine bilirubin. Because only conjugated bilirubin is excreted in urine, its presence indicates conjugated hyperbilirubinemia. The most commonly used method for detecting bilirubin in urine involves the use of a dipstick impregnated with a diazo reagent. Dipstick methods are capable of detecting bilirubin concentrations as low as 0.5 mg/dL (9 μmol/L).

A fresh urine specimen is required because bilirubin is unstable when exposed to light and room temperature, and it may be oxidized to biliverdin (which is diazo negative) at the normally acidic pH of the urine. If the test is delayed, the sample must be protected from light and stored at 2 to 8 °C for no longer than 24 hours. The reagent strip (Chemstrip, Roche Diagnostics, Indianapolis, IL; Multistix, Siemens Healthcare Diagnostics, Deerfield, IL) is immersed in the urine specimen for no longer than 1 second and is read

60 seconds later. During this time, bilirubin reacts with a diazo reagent, yielding a pink to red-violet color, the intensity of which is proportional to the bilirubin concentration. The reaction mechanism for urinary conjugated bilirubin is the same as that described in Fig. 51.9, except that 2,6-dichlorobenzene-diazonium-tetrafluoroborate is substituted for diazotized sulfanilic acid in the Chemstrip, and 2,4-dichloroaniline diazonium salt in the Multistix. Another commonly used test, more sensitive than the Multistix, is the Ictotest reagent tablet (Siemens Healthcare Diagnostics); in this semiquantitative procedure, the diazo reagent is *p*-nitrobenzenediazonium-*p*-toluenesulfonate.

Chemstrip and Multistix strips for bilirubin in urine are highly specific tests and have a low incidence of false-positive results. However, medications that color the urine red or that give a red color in an acid medium, such as phenazopyridine, can produce a false-positive reading. Large quantities of ascorbic acid or of nitrite also worsen the detection limit of the test. In practice, bilirubin is rarely measured in urine.

Measurement of Bilirubin

> **POINTS TO REMEMBER**
>
> 1. The most common method for measuring serum total bilirubin uses a diazo reagent.
> 2. Calibrators for bilirubin measurement use unconjugated bilirubin and ditaurobilirubin as a conjugated bilirubin surrogate.
> 3. The HPLC method is helpful in identifying different bilirubin species that naturally occur in blood; however, it is of limited use clinically.
> 4. While transcutaneous measurement of bilirubin has its advantages, it is not a substitute for quantitative bilirubin determinations.

Urobilinogen in Urine and Feces

The measurement of urobilinogen in urine is of no diagnostic value in the assessment of liver disease. The same applies to the measurement of urobilinogen in fecal 72- or 96-hour specimens. Both tests are obsolete and are not presented here.

Bile Acids

Regulation of bile acid metabolism is a major function of the liver. Alterations in bile acid metabolism are usually a reflection of liver dysfunction. Cholesterol homeostasis is in large part maintained by the conversion of cholesterol to bile acids and subsequent regulation of bile acid metabolism. Bile acids themselves provide surface-active detergent molecules that facilitate both hepatic excretion of cholesterol and solubilization of lipids for intestinal absorption. Bile acid homeostasis requires normal terminal ileum function to absorb bile acids for recirculation (enterohepatic circulation). Alterations in hepatic bile acid synthesis, intracellular metabolism, excretion, intestinal absorption, or plasma extraction are reflected in derangements of bile acid metabolism.

Chemistry. Four major bile acids are known. Cholic acid and chenodeoxycholic acid, the primary bile acids, are synthesized in the liver. The sequence of reactions involved in the synthesis of cholic acid from cholesterol is shown in Fig. 51.10. To date, nine inborn errors of bile acid synthesis have been identified; these can present with neonatal hepatitis,

fat malabsorption, or neurologic defects that can progress to chronic liver disease or liver failure and death.[80] The primary bile acids are metabolized (by bacterial 7α-dehydroxylase) in the intestinal lumen to the secondary bile acids—deoxycholic acid and lithocholic acid. Bile acids (through their carboxylate groups) are conjugated in the liver with the amino acid glycine or taurine. This decreases passive absorption in the biliary tree and proximal small intestine but permits conservation through active transport in the terminal ileum. Approximately 0.1 to 0.6 g of bile acids is lost in the feces daily.

Because they possess both polar and nonpolar regions, molecules of bile acids are able to solubilize biliary lipids. Such molecules align at water–lipid interfaces and reduce surface tension, acting as detergents. In an aqueous solution, bile acids aggregate to form small polymolecular aggregates approximately 5 nm in diameter called micelles, which are capable of incorporating cholesterol and phospholipids to form mixed micelles. Micellar solubilization of these water-insoluble constituents maintains cholesterol in solution. In the intestinal lumen, dietary cholesterol and the products of triglyceride digestion (predominantly free fatty acids and monoglycerides) are incorporated into mixed micelles. Micelles deliver lipolytic products to the mucosal surface. To carry out these functions, a critical micellar bile acid concentration of approximately 2 mmol/L is necessary. Bile acids are thus important for ensuring the solubility of cholesterol (a major component of most gallstones) in bile and dietary lipids (including fat-soluble vitamins) in the intestinal lumen.

Clinical significance of bile acids. In view of the multiple processes involved in bile acid synthesis, conjugation, and excretion, and in its hepatic and intestinal uptake, several potential sites for primary or secondary disturbances have been identified (Box 51.1). With hepatocyte dysfunction (which occurs in many liver disorders), decreased bile acid synthesis results in low primary bile acid concentrations and a decreased ratio of primary to secondary bile acids in plasma; in addition, decreased extraction from plasma often leads to increased concentrations of bile acids, particularly in the nonfasting state. With cholestatic disorders, decreased delivery of primary bile acids to the intestine with resulting decreased secondary bile acid production causes an increased ratio of primary to secondary bile acids, as well as increased total bile acid concentrations. With intestinal disease (including bypass operations that may be performed to treat obesity), increased fecal loss of bile acids leads to decreased concentrations of both primary and secondary bile acids and often a decrease in plasma cholesterol concentration caused by an increased need for bile acid synthesis. Although plasma bile acid concentrations are abnormal in many situations, their measurement adds little to standard tests of liver function, and they are rarely used in clinical medicine except in the investigation of unexplained pruritus. This is because of the wide biological variation due to changes in prandial state and due to diurnal rhythm which is independent of food intake.

The value of measuring total bile acid in serum or plasma for diagnosing intrahepatic cholestasis in pregnancy has been recently highlighted and endorsed by a number of scientific societies.[81–83] In particular, the guidelines of the UK Royal College of Obstetricians and Gynaecologists state that abnormal values of aminotransferases, GGT, and total bile acids are sufficient to support the diagnosis of obstetric cholestasis,[84]

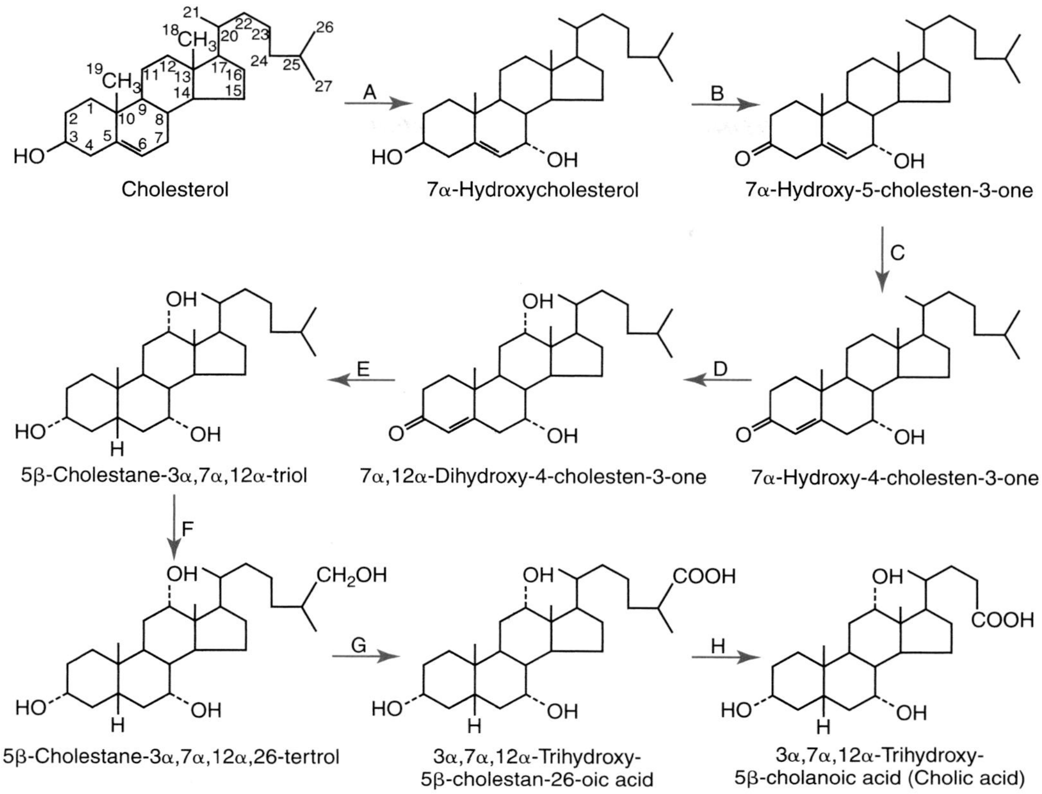

FIGURE 51.10 The biosynthetic pathways of cholesterol conversion to cholic acid. (A) 7-α-Hydroxyl-ation of cholesterol (addition of –OH group at position 7-α-configuration), the rate-limiting step in the biosynthetic pathway. (B) Oxidation of the 3-β-hydroxyl group (to form 3-oxo compound). (C) Isomeriza-tion of the 5-ene structure. (D) 12-α-Hydroxylation (for cholic acid only). (E) Saturation of the double bond and reduction of the 3-one group. (F) Hydroxylation of the side chain at C-26 position. (G) Side chain oxidation to cholestanoic acid. (H) Hydroxylation at C-24 and β-oxidation to reduce the length of the side chain. (From Balistreri WF, Setchel KDR. Clinical implications of bile acid metabolism. In: Silverberg M, Daum F, editors. *Textbook of pediatric gastroenterology.* 2nd ed. Chicago: Year Book Medical Publishers; 1988. p. 72–89. By permission of Mosby, Inc.)

BOX 51.1 Disturbances in Bile Acid Metabolism

Defective bile acid synthesis
Inherited defects in bile acid synthesis
Acquired defects in bile acid synthesis secondary to liver disease
Extrahepatic bile duct obstruction
Bile acid malabsorption
Effective uptake or altered intracellular metabolism

---

and also provide valuable therapeutic information for pre-venting fetal complications attributable to the toxic effects of bile salts. The reference range of total bile acids in the se-rum of pregnant women has been recently established at 0.3 to 10 μmol/L, whereas serum or plasma values greater than 40 μmol/L are diagnostic of severe obstetric cholestasis and were found to be strongly associated with impaired fetal outcome.[85]

Analytical methods. Analytical techniques used to quan-tify total or individual bile acids in biological fluids include gas-liquid chromatography, HPLC, enzymatic assay, radioim-munoassay, enzyme-linked immunosorbent assay (ELISA), and high-resolution tandem mass spectrometry.[86]

Hepatic Synthetic Function

The liver has extensive synthetic capacity and plays a major role in the regulation of protein, carbohydrate, and lipid me-tabolism (see Chapters 31, 35, and 36). A bidirectional flux of precursors and products, such as glucose, amino acids, free fatty acids, and other nutrients, occurs across the hepatocyte membrane. Normal blood glucose concentrations are main-tained during short fasts by the breakdown of hepatic glyco-gen and during prolonged fasts by hepatic gluconeogenesis. The primary sources of carbon atoms for gluconeogenesis are amino acids derived from muscle proteins. To a lesser extent, lactate (produced in skeletal muscle and erythrocytes) and glycerol (obtained from hydrolysis of triglycerides) also serve as substrates for gluconeogenesis. In humans, the oxidation of odd-numbered fatty acids yields propionyl-coenzyme A (CoA), which can be converted to glucose. However, the for-mation of glucose in this manner is not quantitatively sig-nificant. Protein, triglyceride, fatty acid, cholesterol, and bile acid synthesis also occur within the liver.

Protein Synthesis

The liver is the primary site of the synthesis of most plasma proteins (see Chapter 31). Synthesis occurs in the rough en-doplasmic reticulum of hepatocytes, followed by release into the hepatic sinusoids. Although disturbances of protein synthesis occur as a consequence of impaired hepatic function, a variety of other factors may affect plasma protein concentrations. These include decreased availability of amino acids (malnutrition, maldigestion, and malabsorption), catabolic states (hyperthyroidism, Cushing syndrome, burns, postsurgery recovery), protein-losing states (nephrotic syndrome and protein-losing enteropathy), actions of cytokines (decrease in transport proteins, such as albumin, transferrin, and lipoproteins, but an increase in inflammatory response modifiers such as α_1-antitrypsin [AAT], ceruloplasmin, and α_2-macroglobulin), action of hormones (such as growth hormone [GH], cortisol, estrogen, androgens, and thyroid hormones) to increase or decrease production of specific proteins, and congenital deficiency states (Wilson disease and AAT deficiency). In addition, the liver has a significant reserve capacity that prevents protein concentrations from decreasing unless liver damage is extensive. In addition, many liver proteins have relatively long half-lives, such as albumin, which lasts approximately 3 weeks. For this reason, the sensitivity and specificity of protein concentrations for diagnosis of liver disease are far from ideal.

The patterns of plasma protein alterations seen in liver disease depend on the type, severity, and duration of liver injury. For example, in acute hepatic dysfunction, there is usually little change in the plasma protein profile or the total plasma protein concentration; with fulminant hepatic failure or severe liver injury, concentrations of short-lived hepatic proteins (such as transthyretin and prothrombin) fall quickly and become abnormal, whereas those of proteins with longer half-lives are normal or minimally changed. In cirrhosis, concentrations of liver-synthesized plasma proteins and Igs decrease and increase, respectively. Serial determination of plasma proteins provides prognostic information; for example, worsening of prothrombin time (PT) during acute hepatitis suggests a poor prognosis.

Plasma proteins

Albumin. Albumin, the most commonly measured plasma protein, is synthesized exclusively by the liver. The rate of synthesis varies, depending on the hormonal environment, nutritional status, age, and other local factors. In inflammatory conditions, IL-6 inhibits albumin synthesis but induces synthesis of acute-phase response proteins (see Chapter 31). With liver disease, hypoalbuminemia is noted primarily in cirrhosis, autoimmune hepatitis (AIH), and alcoholic hepatitis. The mechanism is multifactorial. In cirrhosis, hepatic synthesis of albumin may be decreased, normal, or increased. Loss of albumin into ascitic fluid seems to be responsible for the decrease in albumin in many cases. There is a strong correlation between serum albumin and mortality risk in a wide range of diseases.[87]

One important consideration in measurement of albumin is the inaccuracy of dye-binding methods in patients with liver disease. Although bromocresol green measurements tend to overestimate albumin concentration at low concentrations,[88] bromocresol purple methods give falsely low values in patients with jaundice because of the interference of bilirubin at the site of binding.[89]

Transthyretin. This protein has a short half-life of 24 to 48 hours, making it a sensitive indicator of current synthetic ability. Transthyretin is typically decreased in cirrhosis (among other conditions) as a result of decreased synthesis.

It is more commonly used as a measurement of nutritional status.

Immunoglobulins. Plasma Ig concentrations are commonly increased in cirrhosis, AIH, and primary biliary cirrhosis (PBC), but they are normal in most other types of liver disease. IgG is increased in AIH and cirrhosis; IgM is increased in PBC. IgA tends to be increased in all types of cirrhosis. None of these findings are specific, and they are seldom used in the diagnosis of liver disease, but IgG concentrations can be used to track response to treatment and disease activity in AIH.

Ceruloplasmin. The concentration of this protein is decreased in Wilson disease, cirrhosis, and many causes of chronic hepatitis, but it may be increased by inflammation, cholestasis, hemochromatosis, pregnancy, and estrogen therapy. It is discussed in greater detail in the section on Wilson disease.

Alpha$_1$-antitrypsin. Concentrations of this protein, which is the major serine protease inhibitor (serpin) in plasma, is decreased in homozygous deficiency and cirrhosis, and is increased by acute inflammation. It is discussed in greater detail later in the section on Alpha$_1$-Antitrypsin Deficiency.

Alpha-fetoprotein. The concentration of this protein, a normal component of fetal blood, falls to adult values by 1 year of age. Mild increases are seen in patients with acute and chronic hepatitis and indicate hepatocellular regeneration. It is present at higher concentrations in hepatocellular carcinoma (HCC), and is discussed in greater detail later and in Chapter 33.

Coagulation proteins

The coagulation proteins that are synthesized in the liver are listed in Table 51.1. These proteins interact to produce a fibrin clot (see Chapter 79). Inhibitors of the coagulation system, including antithrombin, protein C, and protein S, are also synthesized in the liver. Some of the coagulation factors (II, VII, IX, and X) require vitamin K for post-translational carboxylation within the hepatocyte. Proteins C and S are also carboxylated by a vitamin K–dependent enzyme. Activated protein C in plasma inhibits coagulation by inactivating factors V and VIII. Parenchymal liver disease of sufficient severity to impair protein synthesis or obstructive

TABLE 51.1	**Blood Coagulation Factors**
Number or Abbreviation	**Name**
I	Fibrinogen[a]
II	Prothrombin[a,b]
III	Tissue factor
IV	Calcium (Ca^{2+})
V	Proaccelerin[a]
VI	—
VII	Proconvertin[a,b]
VIII	Antihemophilic factor
IX	Christmas factor[a,b]
X	Stuart-Prower factor[b]
XI	Plasma thromboplastin antecedent[a]
XII	Hageman factor[a]
XIII	Fibrin-stabilizing factor[a] (Laki-Lorand factor)
PK	Prekallikrein (Fletcher factor)[a]
HMWK	High-molecular-weight kininogen[a]

[a]Protein synthesized in liver.
[b]Synthesis requires vitamin K.

liver disease sufficient to impair intestinal absorption of vitamin K is, therefore a potential cause of bleeding disorders. Because of the great functional reserve of the liver, failure of hemostasis usually does not occur except in severe or long-standing liver disease.

PT depends on the activity of fibrinogen (factor I), prothrombin (factor II), and factors V, VII, and X. Because all of these factors are made in the liver, and several are vitamin K–dependent, a prolonged PT often indicates the presence of significant liver disease. In cholestasis, vitamin K deficiency may cause an increase in PT. In this case, the coagulation abnormality is corrected in 1 to 2 days by parenteral injection of 10 mg of vitamin K. In contrast, if PT is prolonged because of hepatocellular disease, factor synthesis is decreased, and administration of vitamin K does not typically correct the problem. PT is also prolonged in some patients with liver disease because of the presence of dysfibrinogenemia, an abnormal form of fibrinogen that does not clot normally, which may predispose patients to thrombosis.[90]

The method for reporting PT in liver disease remains controversial. PT measures the time for plasma to clot after exposure to tissue factor. Reagents differ in the amount of tissue factor present; in patients on warfarin, clotting times are more greatly prolonged when lower amounts of tissue factor and other reagents that stimulate clotting are in the reagents. This makes a reagent more sensitive to clotting factor abnormalities but makes standardization of results among laboratories difficult. The international normalized ratio (INR) was developed by the World Health Organization (WHO) and the International Committee on Thrombosis and Hemostasis for reporting the results of blood coagulation (clotting) tests. All results are standardized using the international sensitivity index (ISI) for the particular thromboplastin reagent and instrument combination used to perform the test. In practice, it requires determination of the ISI based on the slope of the relationship between PT using the reagent and that using a reference method in patients on warfarin. The INR is then calculated as follows:

$$INR = \left[\frac{PT\left(patient\right)}{PT\left(geometric\ mean\ of\ normal\right)} \right]^{ISI}$$

INR has been found to standardize interpretation of PT measurements among laboratories for those taking warfarin. Unfortunately, INR does not have the same relationship with impairment of clotting in individuals with liver disease.[91] The liver is responsible for the synthesis of nearly all clotting factors and their inhibitors. As a result, patients with chronic liver disease and cirrhosis experience a rebalancing of their hemostatic variables.[92] Patients with acute liver failure (ALF) likely experience minimal effects on their in vivo coagulation profiles as assessed with thromboelastography (TEG) despite mean INR values greater than 3.[93] Furthermore, these patients have significant rates of hypercoagulable (35%) and hypocoagulable (20%) states. To further complicate matters, the presence of a hypercoagulable state does not exclude the presence of a tendency toward increased bleeding risk, and conversely, increased bleeding risk does not rule out the development of a new thrombus. The apparent explanation lies in the mechanism of clotting factor deficiency in liver disease and warfarin administration. Although liver disease inhibits synthesis of clotting factors, warfarin impairs vitamin K–dependent carboxylation, which impairs the ability of the

factors to bind calcium. These noncarboxylated clotting factors (termed proteins induced by vitamin K absence [PIVKAs]) appear to act as inhibitors of coagulation; thus when lower amounts of tissue factor are present, clotting times are more prolonged.[94] In contrast, in liver disease, factor deficiency is due to impaired factor synthesis, and no PIVKAs are present (except in HCC, as discussed later in this chapter). This leads to lesser increases in PT in individuals with liver disease and an underestimation of the degree of clotting impairment when reagents with a low ISI are used. Studies have shown that calculation of a different ISI using plasma samples from patients with liver disease can standardize PT results with different reagents,[95,96] but to date, such liver ISI information is not readily available to laboratories.

Lipid and lipoprotein synthesis. The liver plays a key role in the metabolism of lipids and lipoproteins (see Chapter 36). On a daily basis, approximately 33% of the fatty acids originating from adipose tissue enter the liver, where they undergo esterification into triglycerides or are oxidized. Oxidation is favored in the fasting state and esterification is favored in the nonfasting state. Excessive esterification results in fatty liver, a disorder in which excess triglycerides are deposited in large vacuoles that displace other cellular components. Most cholesterol is synthesized endogenously, in the liver. The endogenously synthesized cholesterol and that of dietary origin enter the hepatic pool, where they are converted to bile acids, incorporated into lipoproteins, or used in the synthesis of liver cell membranes. The relative rates of secretion of bile acids, cholesterol, and lecithin are important factors in the pathogenesis of cholesterol gallstones.

Urea synthesis. Patients with end-stage liver disease may have low concentrations of urea in plasma (see Chapters 34 and 49). The rate of urea excretion in urine is lower in these patients than that in healthy individuals. In addition, plasma concentrations of urea precursors—ammonia and amino acids—are increased. In nonalcoholic steatohepatitis, the function of urea cycle enzymes may be affected, resulting in hyperammonemia and the risk of disease progression. In nonalcoholic steatohepatitis (NASH) animals, gene and protein expression of ornithine transcarbamylase (OTC) and carbamoylphosphate synthetase were reversibly reduced. Hypermethylation of urea cycle enzymes is a potential underlying mechanism. The functional changes of urea synthesis in NASH are associated with hyperammonemia. Hyperammonemia can cause progression of liver injury and fibrosis.

Hypermethylation of *Otc* gene promoters has been observed. Additionally, in animal models of NASH and in patients with NAFLD, OTC concentration and activity were reduced and ammonia concentrations were increased, which was further exacerbated in those with NASH. In primary hepatocytes, induction of steatosis was associated with *Otc* promoter hypermethylation, a reduction in the gene expression of *Otc* and *Cps1*, and an increase in ammonia concentration. These findings suggest that patients with liver disease have an impaired ability to metabolize protein nitrogen and to synthesize urea. The rate of hepatic urea synthesis also depends on exogenous intake of nitrogen and on endogenous protein catabolism.

Hepatic Metabolic Function

A recurring theme is the central importance of the liver in metabolic and regulatory pathways. The functional expression of the complex, integrated organelle structure includes the metabolism of drugs (activation and detoxification) and the disposal of exogenous and endogenous substances, such as galactose and ammonia. In addition, metabolic abnormalities due to specific inherited enzyme deficiencies can affect the liver. A classic example is galactosemia. In this condition, congenital absence of galactose 1-phosphate uridyltransferase allows accumulation of the toxic metabolite galactose 1-phosphate, which causes injury to the liver, brain, and kidneys.

Ammonia Metabolism

Biochemistry and physiology. Ammonia is a by-product of nitrogen metabolism, and its formation in the body is predominantly a consequence of the action of the enzyme glutaminase, located within enterocytes of the small intestine and colon, as well as the action of the vast number of urease-producing bacteria located in the gut. Plasma ammonia concentration in the hepatic portal vein is typically fivefold to tenfold higher than that in the systemic circulation. Under normal circumstances, most of the portal vein ammonia load is metabolized to urea in hepatocytes through the Krebs-Henseleit (urea) cycle during the first pass through the liver; this process includes intramitochondrial and cytosolic enzyme-catalyzed steps (Fig. 51.11).

Ammonia enters the tissue of the central nervous system by passive diffusion. The rate of entry increases in proportion to the plasma concentration and is dependent on pH. Ammonia crosses the blood–brain barrier more readily than the ammonium ion. As pH increases, the rate of entry of ammonia into the central nervous system tissue increases as the result of an increase in ammonia relative to ammonium. Because the acid dissociation constant (pK_a) of ammonia is 9.1 at 37 °C, approximately 3% of total blood ammonia is ammonia at the normal physiological pH of 7.4. An increase in pH to 7.6 produces an increase in ammonia to approximately 5% of total blood ammonia, which is a 67% increase in concentration.

Clinical significance. Animal and human studies have shown that an increased concentration of ammonia (hyperammonemia) exerts toxic effects on the central nervous system. Several causes, both inherited and acquired, of hyperammonemia are known. Inherited deficiencies of urea cycle enzymes are the major cause of hyperammonemia in infants.[97] The two major inherited disorders are those that involve the metabolism of the dibasic amino acids lysine and ornithine and those that involve the metabolism of organic acids, such as propionic acid, methylmalonic acid, isovaleric acid, and others (see Chapter 60). Insult to the liver, whether

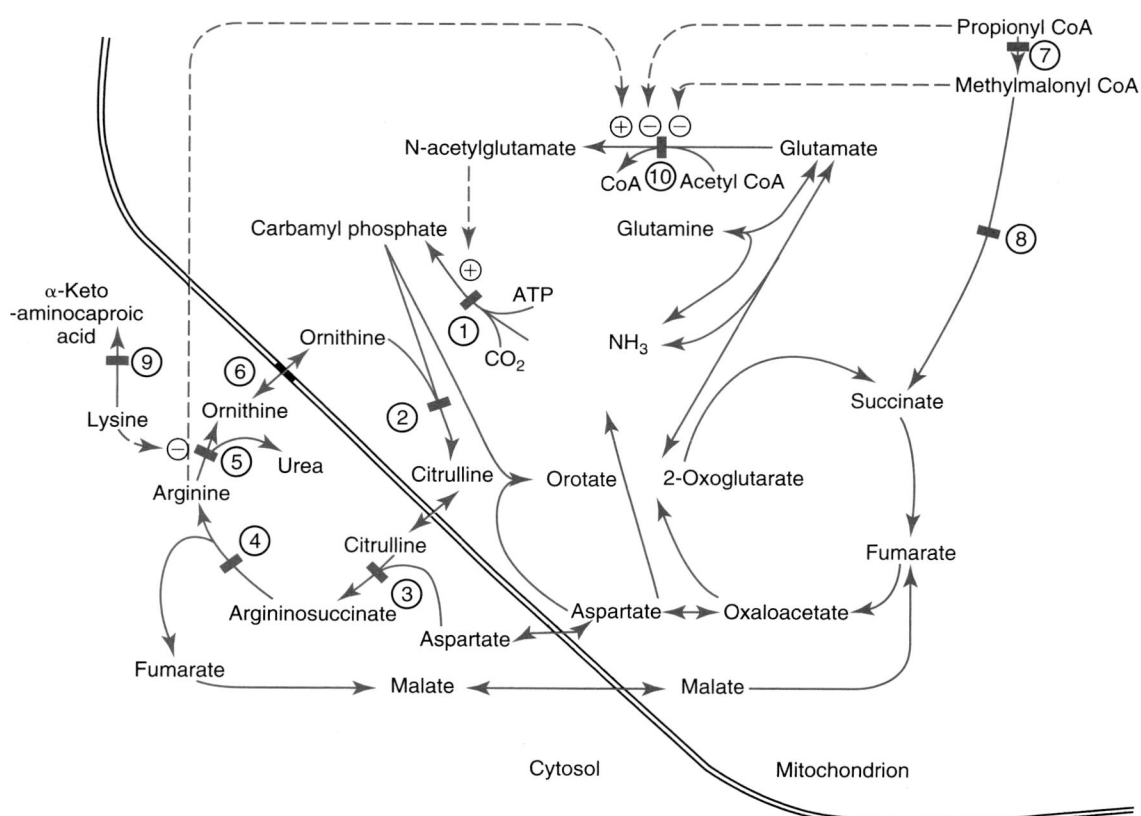

FIGURE 51.11 Major metabolic pathways for the use of ammonia by the hepatocyte. *Solid bars* indicate the sites of primary enzyme defects in various metabolic disorders associated with hyperammonemia: (1) carbamyl phosphate synthetase 1, (2) ornithine transcarbamylase, (3) argininosuccinate synthetase, (4) argininosuccinate lyase, (5) arginase, (6) mitochondrial ornithine transport, (7) propionyl coenzyme-A (CoA) carboxylase, (8) methylmalonyl CoA mutase, (9) l-lysine dehydrogenase, and (10) N-acetyl glutamine synthetase. *Dotted lines* indicate the site of pathway activation (+) or inhibition (−). (From Flannery OB, Hsia YE, Wolf B. Current status of hyperammonemia syndromes. *Hepatology* 1982;2:495–506.)

acute or chronic in nature, reduce its capacity to metabolize ammonia and this creates an ammonia burden on extrahepatic tissues which can result in hyperammonemia up to five times that of normal blood ammonia concentrations. The occurrence of hyperammonemia is not specific to liver dysfunction and can also be observed in various other disease states including, but not limited to, inborn errors of the urea cycle, Reye syndrome, and valproate poisoning.

The main acquired causes of hyperammonemia are advanced liver disease and renal failure. Severe or chronic liver failure (which occurs in fulminant hepatitis or cirrhosis, respectively) leads to significant impairment of normal ammonia metabolism. Reye syndrome, which is primarily a central nervous system disorder with minor hepatic dysfunction, is also associated with hyperammonemia. Hepatic encephalopathy in the cirrhotic patient is often precipitated by GI bleeding, which enhances ammonia production through bacterial metabolism of protein found in blood. Other precipitating causes of encephalopathy include excess dietary protein, constipation, infection, drugs (particularly central nervous system depressants and those that alter blood biochemistry such as diuretics), and electrolyte and acid-base imbalance (alkalosis). Because cirrhosis is accompanied by portosystemic shunting, ammonia clearance is impaired, leading to increased concentrations of blood ammonia. Impaired renal function also causes hyperammonemia. As blood urea concentration increases, more diffuses into the GI tract, where it is converted to ammonia.

The fasting venous plasma ammonia concentration is useful in the differential diagnosis of encephalopathy, when it is unclear whether encephalopathy is of hepatic origin.[98] It is especially helpful in diagnosing Reye syndrome and the inherited disorders of urea metabolism, as well as increased ammonia concentrations due to drugs such as salicylates or valproate. In acute liver injury, ammonia concentrations more than 200 μmol/L (340 μg/dL) are associated with cerebral edema and a poor prognosis,[99] and it has been suggested that ammonia concentrations should be used as part of the evaluation of prognosis in ALF.[100] However, plasma ammonia is not useful in patients with known chronic liver disease.[101] Although ammonia concentrations are higher as the degree of encephalopathy worsens, significant overlap between concentrations is seen in different stages of encephalopathy, and approximately 70% of those with cirrhosis without encephalopathy have increased ammonia concentrations.[102] Ammonia concentrations may actually better reflect the presence of shunting blood around the portal veins than the degree of liver dysfunction.[103] There is growing recognition of the complex and synergistic relationship between ammonia, inflammation (sterile and nonsterile), and oxidative stress in the pathogenesis of hepatic encephalopathy which develops in patients with liver dysfunction.[104]

Preanalytic issues. The concentrations of analytes may be affected by numerous factors that should be explored in order to establish ideal sampling conditions, processes, handling, and storage. These include diurnal variation, effects of feeding and fasting, donor position, sample containers, preservatives, sample handling, and sample processing and storage, including the influence of storage time, temperature, and freeze-thawing (see Chapter 5).

Analytical methodology. Both enzymatic and chemical methods are used to measure ammonia in body fluids. An enzymatic assay with glutamate dehydrogenase is the most frequently used method. Plasma ammonia measurement is particularly susceptible to contamination, leading to falsely increased concentrations. Common preanalytical problems are discussed in Chapter 4 on Specimen Collection and Processing.

Reference intervals. For the enzymatic method, the reference interval is 15 to 45 μg/dL (11 to 32 μmol/L). For more details on age-dependent values, see the Appendix on Reference Intervals. Laboratories should verify that these ranges are appropriate for use in their own settings.

Carbohydrate Metabolism

Because the liver is a major processor of dietary and endogenous carbohydrates, liver disease affects carbohydrate metabolism in a variety of ways (see Chapter 35). However, none of the conventional modes of evaluating carbohydrate metabolism has value in the diagnosis of liver disease. Because the liver is the major site of both glycogen storage and gluconeogenesis, hypoglycemia is a common complication in certain liver diseases, particularly Reye syndrome, fulminant hepatic failure, advanced cirrhosis, and HCC.

Xenobiotic Metabolism and Excretion

Xenobiotics are chemical substances that are foreign to the biological system. Biochemically, they are cleared and/or metabolized by the liver; some have been used as the basis of tests of liver function. Rates of metabolism of these compounds are sometimes referred to as quantitative liver function tests, to distinguish them from the more commonly used term, liver function tests, which is often used to refer to measurements of liver-associated enzymes. As liver disease progresses, quantitative liver function test results gradually worsen, but their measurement adds little to that obtained by widely used tests such as bilirubin, albumin, and INR measurement.[105] Even when these tests are used, significant overlap of values is noted in persons with cirrhosis and less severe degrees of liver scarring, which limits their usefulness.

Dye excretion tests. Dye excretion tests, such as BSP and indocyanine green clearance, were formerly used as indicators of liver disease. With the development of more sensitive and specific indicators of liver disease, dye excretion tests have become obsolete, although until the 1970s, BSP was the most frequently used dye excretion test. Because of reports of fatalities resulting from hypersensitivity and other adverse effects, BSP use has been discontinued. Indocyanine green clearance is still occasionally used[106] for investigating hepatic blood flow and for predicting clearance rates of drugs that undergo first-pass clearance by the liver, such as lignocaine. Typical indocyanine green clearance values in healthy subjects range from 6.5 to 14 mL/min/kg body weight.

Drug clearance tests. A variety of drugs that are metabolized by the liver have been used to study the action of various P_{450} (mixed-function oxidase) enzymes. Aminopyrine is demethylated to form carbon dioxide and aminoantipyrine. With the use of ^{13}C- or ^{14}C-labeled aminopyrine, the resulting isotopically labeled carbon dioxide is measured in breath as a reflection of functioning liver mass. Decreases in metabolism are common in persons with cirrhosis,[107] but metabolism is also affected by other factors such as cigarette smoking and use of drugs such as oral contraceptives; significant intraindividual variation in results has been noted.[108]

Overall diagnostic sensitivity is similar to that of other more routine laboratory tests.[109]

Caffeine clearance is altered during hepatic injury; it is prolonged in both chronic hepatitis and cirrhosis.[110] Caffeine is rapidly and nearly completely absorbed from the GI tract and then undergoes N-demethylation by the hepatic mixed-function oxidase system. A single dose of caffeine (3.5 mg/kg to a maximum dose of 200 mg, dissolved in water, fruit juice, or milk for oral administration) is administered. This caffeine dose is equivalent to that found in one cup of brewed coffee or in one can of a commercial soft drink.

Blood (or salivary samples) obtained before and at timed intervals after caffeine ingestion can be analyzed by reversed-phase HPLC or immunoassay. A close correlation is found between plasma and salivary caffeine concentrations. Caffeine half-life is approximately 5.5 hours in healthy adults and 3 hours in healthy children, with clearance of approximately 2 mL/min/kg in healthy adults and 10 mL/min/kg in healthy children. Caffeine clearance correlates with the aminopyrine breath test and has similar limitations, although it is less subject to effects of variables, such as smoking and oral contraceptive use.[108] Lidocaine undergoes N-deethylation in the liver by cytochrome P_{450} to form monoethylglycinexylidide (MEGX); the rate of appearance of MEGX in plasma reflects hepatic lidocaine clearance. Because lidocaine is highly extracted, its clearance is flow dependent. Thus alterations in hepatic blood flow also influence lidocaine elimination.[111] Lidocaine (1 mg/kg) is given by intravenous bolus; plasma is obtained at baseline and at 15 minutes for MEGX concentration (time of plateau concentration in healthy individuals). MEGX is most commonly measured using an immunoassay. Lidocaine clearance has been used to assess liver transplantation function, but its use is limited by the effect of hypoperfusion (which occurs in sepsis or volume depletion).[112]

Hepatic Storage Function

Because individual cells are unable to store a sufficient supply of energy-rich carbohydrate substrates, the liver serves as the major site for their storage. For example, hepatic storage of glycogen allows the release of glucose to other tissue when the need exists (e.g., when plasma concentrations of glucose decrease). Other tissues, such as muscle and adipose tissue, store proteins and triglycerides, respectively, and are capable of adaptation. Depending on the availability of oxidizable fuels, these tissues also switch from the storage mode to the synthesis or release mode during periods of decreased carbohydrate intake.

CLINICAL MANIFESTATIONS OF LIVER DISEASE

Various characteristics indicate the presence of liver disease, including peripheral signs such as jaundice and spider naevi; evidence of fibrosis and portal hypertension and evidence of abnormalities of renal function, drug metabolism, hemostasis, metabolic abnormalities, and release of enzymes into various body fluids.

Liver Fibrosis
Pathogenesis of Liver Fibrosis
As the first solid organ beyond the gut to process ingested antigens, the liver is constantly exposed to antigen-rich blood;

therefore it is a major line of defense against such antigens, especially microorganisms. Both the adaptive and innate immune systems of the liver are highly evolved to serve this function. Fibrosis should be considered as a normal component of the innate immune response to tissue injury, and as such, is controlled by the cells and products of the immune system.[113] Both the innate and adaptive immune systems play an important role in hepatic fibrosis modulation. For example, in the liver, type I collagen (which predominates in fibrotic scar) protects hepatocytes against toxic stimuli. Inflammation and tumorigenesis are tightly linked pathways impacting cancer development. Inflammasomes are key signaling platforms that detect pathogenic microorganisms, including hepatitis C virus (HCV) infection, and sterile stressors (oxidative stress, insulin resistance, lipotoxicity) able to activate pro-inflammatory cytokines IL-1β and IL-18. In the liver, this inflammation can be due to acute or chronic viral hepatitis, AIH, alcohol or bile salt exposure, or fatty liver disease. Hepatic dysfunction is caused by degeneration and necrosis of epithelial cells (hepatocytes and/or cholangiocytes), replacement of liver parenchyma by fibrotic tissues and regenerative nodules, and loss of liver function. In the liver, when the inflammatory insult becomes chronic, fibrosis can then lead to apoptosis and loss of the architectural integrity of the liver and cirrhosis. Regeneration of these epithelial cells is essential for architectural and functional recovery of the organ.

Hepatic fibrosis is a dynamic process characterized by the net accumulation of extracellular matrix (ECM), or scar, resulting from chronic liver injury of any etiology, including chronic viral infection, alcoholic liver disease, bile salt exposure, and NASH. Fibrosis is a physiologic response to a wide range of stimuli including the degeneration and necrosis of epithelial cells (hepatocytes and/or cholangiocytes) that leads to replacement of liver parenchyma by fibrotic tissues and regenerative nodules, and a resulting loss of liver function. The remaining liver parenchymal cells may proliferate within regenerative nodules. Although fibrosis can reverse after elimination of the cause of injury, chronic injury left unchecked can lead to cirrhosis, which is characterized by distortion of the hepatic architecture associated with abnormal blood flow and eventually portal hypertension. Decompensated liver disease is characterized by the onset of reduced hepatic function and disordered blood flow leading to portal hypertension and complications including ascites, hepatic encephalopathy, and variceal hemorrhage. Cirrhosis is a major cause of mortality world-wide and is associated with increased individual risk of HCC.

The process of hepatic fibrosis involves the activation of hepatic stellate cells (HSCs) (or portal fibroblasts in biliary disease), Kupffer cells, and an array of other cells, proteins, and signaling pathways. The complexities of these interactions are becoming better understood, and the currently known roles of the many players are summarized in the following.

Hepatic stellate cells. HSCs reside in the space of Disse, interposed between the endothelium and hepatocytes,[114] where they encircle the liver sinusoids. After liver injury, HSCs become activated by the products of apoptotic mesenchymal cells, which leads to the conversion of a resting vitamin A–rich cell (a quiescent HSC) to one that has lost vitamin A droplets by autophagy, which leads to increased proliferation and contraction, and the release of proinflammatory, profibrogenic, and promitogenic cytokines. The activated HSCs become contractile myofibroblasts that generate a scar that forms around the injury site.

HSC activation can be divided into two phases: initiation and perpetuation.[115] Initiation, which is also known as the preinflammatory stage, refers to early changes in gene expression and phenotype. It is the result of primarily paracrine stimulation from damaged parenchymal cells. Maintenance of these stimuli leads to a perpetuation phase that is regulated by autocrine and paracrine stimuli. Perpetuation involves at least six distinct changes in HSC behavior, including proliferation, chemotaxis, fibrogenesis, contractility, matrix degradation, and retinoid loss.[116]

Myofibroblasts. The profibrotic myofibroblasts are the master regulators of the fibrotic response because of their scar-producing, proliferative, migratory, contractile, immunomodulatory, and phagocytic properties. Myofibroblasts are the prototypical mesenchymal cell type that regulates repair after an injury in a range of tissues, including liver, kidneys, skin, lungs, and bone marrow, as well as the central nervous system.[117] Myofibroblasts, once activated, are capable of enhanced migration and deposition of ECM components.[117] Although HSCs are the primary source of this fibrogenic population in the liver,[118] other cells such as bone marrow–derived cells, portal fibroblasts, and epithelial-to-mesenchymal transition from hepatocytes and cholangiocytes also contribute to fibrogenesis, although their exact role in disease is not completely understood.

Role of the extracellular matrix. In the normal liver, the ECM provides structural and biochemical support to the surrounding cells and is composed mainly of a number of structural proteins (including collagens IV and VI), as well as a range of growth factors and matrix metalloproteinases (MMPs) that are specifically bound and preserved in latent forms.[119] The ECM can modulate the activation and proliferation of HSCs, angiogenesis, and the availability and activity of growth factors and MMPs. The ECM also provides cells with signals for polarization, adhesion, migration, proliferation, survival, and differentiation. ECM–cell interactions are determined largely by specific membrane adhesion receptors. The ECM may prevent apoptosis in the damaged liver and also prevent growth factor proteolysis.[120] Interactions between ECM and its surrounding cells are bidirectional. After injury, the fibrillary collagens I and III predominate together with fibronectin.[113] Liver fibrosis as a consequence of liver injury entails both qualitative and quantitative changes in ECM composition as a result of an imbalance between the rates of matrix synthesis and degradation. The ECM becomes progressively insoluble and resistant to protease digestion because of the thickening of fibrotic septae and increased cross-linking.[121,122]

Matrix metalloproteinases. MMPs, also known as matrixins, are the major family of calcium-dependent enzymes that degrade collagenous and noncollagenous ECM substrates. There are 25 members of this tightly regulated family, which are classified on the basis of their substrate specificity: interstitial collagenases, gelatinases, stromelysins, membrane types, and metalloelastases. MMPs are secreted as inactive proenzymes, have complex transcriptional control, and their action is inhibited by a family of endogenous proteinase inhibitors known as tissue inhibitors of metalloproteinases (TIMPs).[121–123] Four TIMP members bind reversibly to the active site of all

MMPs and have different affinities for specific MMPs. Thus TIMPs play an important role in preventing degradation of the accumulating matrix during liver injury by antagonizing the activity of MMPs. TIMP-1 also has an antiapoptotic effect on HSCs; it prevents clearance of activated HSCs during injury and promotes their survival through induction of B-cell lymphoma.[124] HSCs are a key source of MMPs, especially MMP-2, -3, -9, and -13. In chronic human liver disease and animal models of fibrosis, concentrations of MMP-1 and/or -13 do not change, but there is a progressive increase in TIMP-1 and -2 as fibrosis advances. TIMP expression can be detected soon (6 hours) after liver injury and may precede the induction of procollagen I.[125]

Cytokines. Fibrosis usually follows an inflammatory insult; therefore certain cytokines secreted by a range of cells, including Kupffer cells, HSCs, hepatocytes, natural killer cells, lymphocytes, and dendritic cells play a key role in the response. These include the chemokines (monocyte chemotactic protein-1, RANTES [Regulated on Activation, Normal T Expressed and Secreted; also known as CCL5 or C-C motif chemokine ligand 5], IL-8), interferons (IFN-α, IFN-γ), ILs (IL-1, IL-6, IL-10), growth factors, adipokines, and soluble neurohumoral ligands (endocannabinoids). Adipokines (adipose tissue cytokines) are polypeptides secreted mainly by adipocytes, and to a lesser extent, by stromal cells, including macrophages, fibroblasts, and infiltrating monocytes. Leptin and adiponectin are the main adipokines implicated in liver injury.[126,127]

Hepatocytes. The hepatocytes are the major cell type in the liver and are also involved in the process of fibrosis and cirrhosis. Normally, hepatocytes can regenerate removed liver tissue rapidly, but in chronic disease states they appear to become senescent with respect to this function; however, the HSCs become activated and are sufficient to regenerate the biliary and hepatocellular epithelium.[128]

Kupffer cells. Kupffer cells are specialized, self-renewing, long-lived macrophages located in the liver that line the walls of the sinusoids that form part of the reticuloendothelial system (RES). Their role is to regulate the local immune system in response to bacteria, bacterial toxins, and debris that are derived from the GI tract. Kupffer cell activation is responsible for early ethanol-induced liver injury, which is common in chronic alcoholics. Chronic alcoholism and liver injury involve a two-hit system. If the toxic effect of alcohol is considered to be the first "hit," the second hit is characterized by activation of the Toll-like receptor 4 and CD14, which are receptors on the Kupffer cells that internalize endotoxin (lipopolysaccharide). This activates the transcription of proinflammatory cytokines (TNF-α) and production of prooxidant superoxides. TNF then activates the HSCs, which leads to collagen synthesis and fibrosis. In response to hepatic injury, the liver macrophage populations change. During hepatic inflammation and fibrosis, the number of Kupffer cells decrease, and they are gradually replaced by monocyte-derived macrophages. The Kupffer cells have a key role in early response to injury and are replenished as the inflammation and fibrosis subsides. The macrophages secrete cytokines TNF-α and IL-1β, which stimulates the activation of HSCs and ECM synthesis. Hepatic macrophages are also involved in matrix remodeling and play an important role in matrix degradation through increased MMP-13 production during resolution of liver fibrosis.[128,129]

Lymphocytes. The relative balance of T-helper 1 (TH1) and T-helper 2 (TH2) cells has an impact on the outcome of fibrosis. TH1 cells are antifibrotic, whereas TH2 are strongly profibrotic. IL-13, which is associated with TH2, stimulates transforming growth factor (TGF)-β1 synthesis and upregulates MMP-9. TH1 cells are associated with IFN-γ, and IL-12 suppresses collagen deposition by regulating the balance of MMP and TIMPs. There are other T-cell subsets that may also play a role, including TH17, which stimulates Kupffer cells, HSCs, and cholangiocytes, and the secretion of proinflammatory cytokines, such as IL-1β, IL-6, TNF, and TGF-β. The influence of these different T-cell populations on the fibrosis process is probably dependent on the underlying cause of the injury. Innate natural killer T cells are proinflammatory and may have a role in initiating and perpetuating fibrosis, whereas γδ-T cells may be antifibrotic by promoting HSC apoptosis.

Crosstalk between hepatocytes and immune cells is also mediated by inflammasomes, large multiprotein complexes that sense intracellular danger signals via Nod-like receptors (NLRs) (e.g., NLRP3). Inflammasomes mediate the cleavage and activation of pro–IL-1β and pro–IL-18. Damaged hepatocytes can transfer their danger signals by regulating inflammasome activation in immune cells. In fact, molecules such as ATP and uric acid, which are released from injured hepatocytes, cause inflammasomes in liver Kupffer cells in murine models of ASH and NASH.[130,131]

Because the liver is exposed to gut-derived microbial products, liver inflammation is modified by the microbiota in the gut. Gut dysbiosis has been demonstrated in obesity, metabolic syndrome, diabetes, cardiovascular diseases, and NAFLD.[132,133]

Thus both endogenous ligands generated from injured cells and exogenous ligands generated from the gut microbiota activate inflammatory pathways.

Liver sinusoidal endothelial cells. The highly fenestrated liver sinusoidal endothelial cells (LSECs) constitute the sinusoidal wall or endothelium of the liver, where they act as a dynamic filter that facilitates the exchange of metabolites and fluids between the blood and the hepatocytes. Defenestration and capillarization of the LSECs can lead to impaired substrate exchange and hepatic dysfunction. However, differentiated LSECs promote reversion of activated HSCs to quiescence and thereby accelerate regression and prevent progression of fibrosis.

Platelets. Platelets have the features of inflammatory cells and release factors, such as platelet-derived growth factor (PDGF), vascular endothelial growth factor (VEGF), TGF-α, which induce angiogenesis, wound healing, liver regeneration, and metastasis.[134] In chronic hepatitis, blood platelet numbers gradually fall, which is reflected in liver fibrosis. The thrombocytopenia seen in chronic hepatitis has many causes, including increased splenic breakdown of platelets and pooling, and decreased marrow production. However, there may be a role for platelets in the pathogenesis of liver fibrosis and hepatic cell carcinoma. Platelets accumulate in noncancerous liver tissues of patients with cirrhosis and chronic hepatitis as blood platelet numbers drop. In chronic HCV infection, platelets accumulate in the sinusoidal space mediated by the activated RES involving Kupffer cells. HSCs express the PDGF receptor, which is the most basic mediator involved with platelet granules and is involved with fibrosis and malignancy. When HSCs

express this receptor, they are susceptible to PDGF contained in platelets, and this may be why platelets accumulate in patients with chronic hepatitis.[134] Platelets also accumulate in cancerous tissue in the blood space through a mechanism that involves Kupffer cells.

Reversibility of Fibrosis

Hepatic fibrosis is reversed or stabilized in up to 80% of patients in whom the underlying cause of the liver fibrosis is treated such as patients with ArLD who maintain abstinence, obese patients with NASH who lose weight, AIH treated with immunosuppression, hemochromatosis treated with venesection and following control or elimination of HBV or HCV respectively.[135–137]

Features of irreversibility are not firmly identified, but it remains likely that changes to the extracellular environment brought about by HSC activation contribute substantially. Thus further clarification of the contribution of HSCs to fibrosis at all stages could yield important insights relevant to not only chronic liver disease but also advanced cirrhosis.[138] Two key events in fibrosis resolution are the degradation of the fibrillar ECM and reduction in myofibroblast survival. TIMPs play an important role in preventing degradation of the accumulating matrix during liver injury by antagonizing the activity of MMPs and promoting survival of activated HSCs. In contrast, several mediators have been implicated in inducing apoptosis and clearance of HSCs. Similarly, p21 and p16 proteins can limit the fibrogenic response by promoting senescence of HSCs.

Jaundice

Jaundice (or icterus) is a physical sign characterized by a yellow appearance of the skin, mucous membranes, and sclera caused by bilirubin deposition. It is the most specific clinical manifestation of hepatobiliary dysfunction but is not present in many individuals with liver disease (especially chronic liver disease) and may occur in states of bilirubin overproduction (such as hemolysis). Jaundice is seen most easily in the sclera of the eyes, where yellow contrasts sharply with the usual bright white color. Jaundice is usually apparent clinically when the plasma bilirubin concentration reaches 2 to 3 mg/dL (34 to 51 μmol/L), although higher concentrations may be required when fluorescent lighting is used. When bilirubin clearance from the liver to the intestinal tract is impaired (as in acute hepatitis and bile duct obstruction), acholic (gray colored) stools may be noted. Bilirubin is the source of stercobilin, which produces the brown color of normal stools. Increases in plasma-conjugated bilirubin lead to orange-brown colored urine, because conjugated bilirubin is water soluble. Jaundice may also be due to disorders of bilirubin metabolism.

Portal Hypertension

The portal circulation handles all venous outflow of the GI tract, the spleen, the pancreas, and the gallbladder (Fig. 51.12). The portal vein is formed by the union of the splenic vein and the superior mesenteric vein. Portal flow is normally 1000 to 1200 mL/min, with pressure of 5 to 7 mm Hg. Portal hypertension occurs when portal flow is obstructed anywhere along its course. Causes of obstruction leading to portal hypertension are classified by site: presinusoidal, sinusoidal, and postsinusoidal. Presinusoidal portal

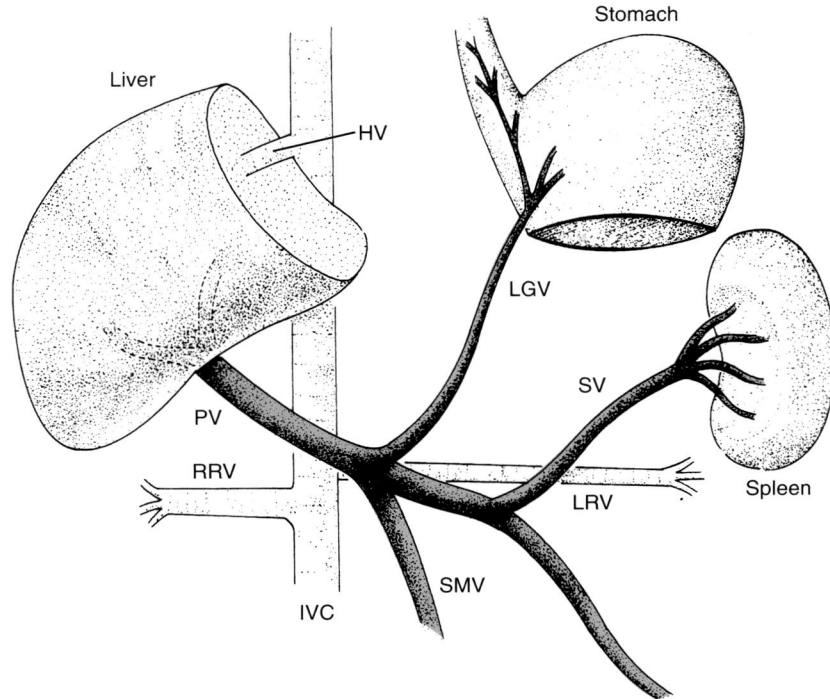

FIGURE 51.12 The portal-venous system. *HV*, Hepatic vein; *IMV*, inferior mesenteric vein; *IVC*, inferior vena cava; *LGV*, left gastric vein; *LRV*, left renal vein; *PV*, portal vein; *RRV*, right renal vein; *SMV*, superior mesenteric vein; *SV*, splenic vein. (From Zakim O, Boyer TD. *Hepatology: a textbook of liver disease.* 3rd ed. Philadelphia: WB Saunders; 1996. p. 721.)

hypertension is most commonly caused by portal vein thrombosis or schistosomiasis, but may also occur with increased portal flow, such as that occurs with Felty syndrome (a combination of chronic rheumatoid arthritis, splenomegaly, leukopenia, vasculitis that may be manifest by pigmented spots on the lower extremities, and sometimes other evidence of hypersplenism, such as anemia and thrombocytopenia). Sinusoidal hypertension is most commonly caused by cirrhosis but may occur transiently with acute and chronic hepatitis or acute fatty liver. The most important cause of postsinusoidal hypertension is hepatic vein occlusion or Budd-Chiari syndrome,[139] in which sudden obstruction or occlusion of the hepatic veins (associated with myeloproliferative disorders in one-half of cases) causes hepatomegaly, abdominal pain, severe ascites, mild jaundice, with acute portal hypertension, and may progress to long-standing portal hypertension and liver failure.[140] The most common cause of postsinusoidal hypertension is cardiac disease, most commonly congestive heart failure. Chronic congestive heart failure is usually associated with portal hypertension and ascites and may even lead to increased activities of aminotransferases.[141] Other causes include abscesses, membranous obstruction of the vena cava, and venoocclusive disease (as may be seen in patients after bone marrow transplantation). The causes of increased resistance to blood flow through the liver include the previously described static factors and may be compounded by the dynamic alterations in vascular and sinusoidal tone due to contraction of hepatic myofibroblasts and vasoactive compounds. These dynamic factors may cause acute rises in portal pressure, resulting in complications such as variceal hemorrhage. Although increased portal resistance

is the major factor that causes portal hypertension, it is often accompanied by decreased resistance to blood flow through other blood vessels, which enhances blood flow through the portal veins.

When portal pressure increases, the portal venous system becomes dilated and forms collateral connections to the systemic venous flow (Fig. 51.13), leading to portosystemic shunting. Initially, this is clinically silent, but as portal hypertension worsens, it compromises many of the metabolic functions of the liver. One such abnormality is altered estrogen metabolism, which increases the ratio of plasma estrogen to testosterone concentrations. Clinical consequences include spider telangiectasias and palmar erythema, gynecomastia in men, and abnormal vaginal bleeding and irregular menstrual periods in women. Impaired protein metabolic functions cause the accumulation of ammonia and abnormal neurotransmitters, ultimately leading to hepatic encephalopathy.[142] Because most nutrients arrive through the portal vein, synthetic functions are also impaired, leading to hypoalbuminemia (contributing to ascites), decreased clotting factors (predisposing to bleeding), and reduced thrombolytic factors, such as antithrombin (predisposing to venous thrombosis).

Bleeding Esophageal Varices

The most life-threatening consequence of portosystemic shunting is the development of varices (enlarged and tortuous veins), which can occur throughout the GI tract but are most common in the esophagus, stomach, and rectum, at sites of portosystemic anastomosis. Bleeding from varices is one of the leading causes of morbidity and mortality in patients with cirrhosis. Varices are present at the time of

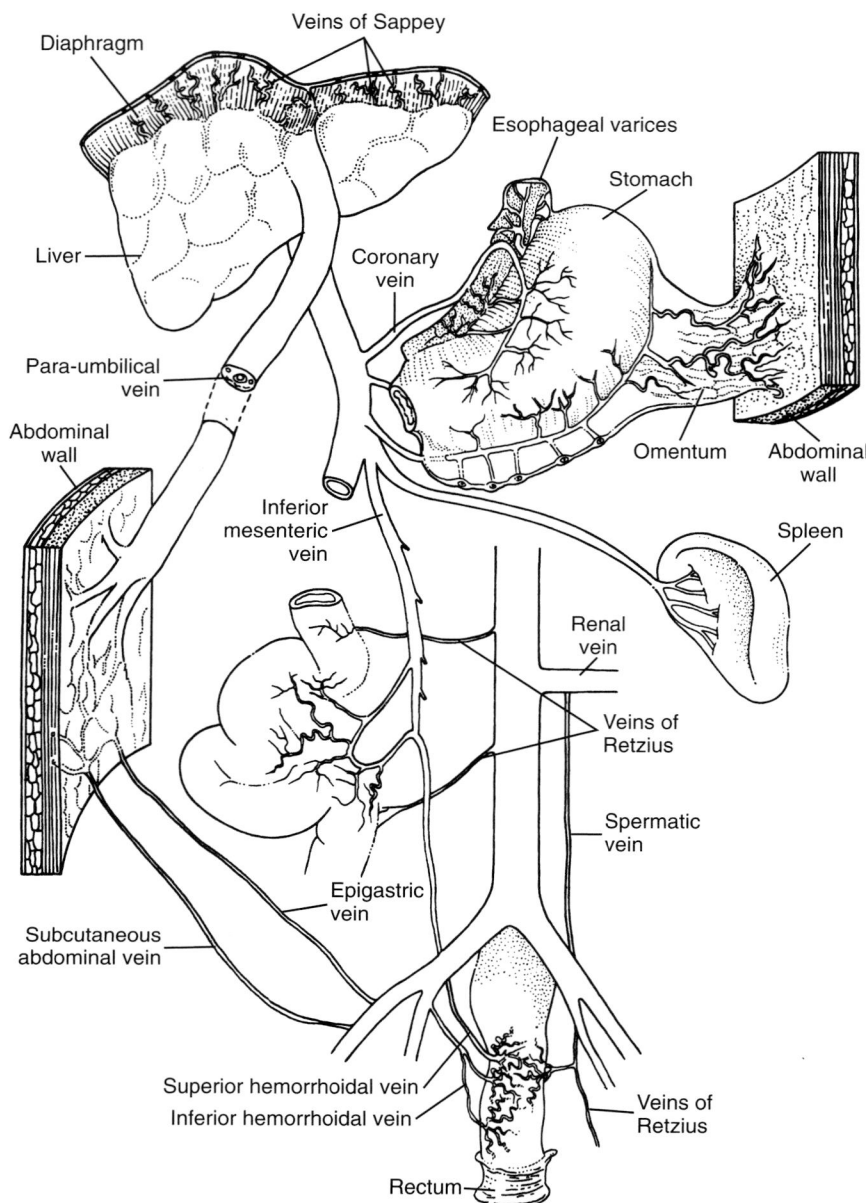

FIGURE 51.13 Sites of portosystemic collateral circulation in cirrhosis of the liver. (From Sherlock S, Dooley J, editors. *Diseases of the liver and biliary system.* 9th ed. London: Blackwell Scientific Publications; 1993. p. 134.)

diagnosis of cirrhosis in approximately 40% of patients and occur in an additional 6% per year.[143] Normal portal pressure ranges between 1 and 5 mm Hg. When the portal pressure exceeds 10 mm Hg, collateral portosystemic shunts may open, with an increased risk of bleeding once the portal pressure exceeds 12 mm Hg. The major consequences of varices are rupture and bleeding, usually presenting as hematemesis. Treatment of portal hypertension and varices is directed at obliterating the dilated blood vessels or reducing portal pressure. Pressure can be reduced by pharmacologic agents, such as nonselective β-adrenergic blockers, but if this is not effective, invasive procedures can be used, most commonly by putting rubber bands around large varices (banding), or if this is not successful, by placing a stent through the jugular and hepatic veins to connect to the portal vein (transjugular

intrahepatic portosystemic shunting).[144] Because portal flow is already significantly reduced before shunting, minimal change in liver function is usually seen, but the incidence of hepatic encephalopathy after the placement of shunts is markedly increased.

Ascites

Ascites is the effusion and accumulation of fluid in the abdominal cavity. Ascites is the most common clinical finding in patients with portal hypertension. Ascites itself is not life threatening, but it is uncomfortable and may compromise respiration (from upward displacement of the diaphragm and compression of the lungs). It predisposes individuals to spontaneous bacterial peritonitis (SBP), which is life threatening (see the following).

The pathogenesis of ascites is complex because of a number of simultaneously operating factors. Of these, the most important are increased hydrostatic portal venous pressure, with increased resistance to flow, decreased colloid osmotic (oncotic) pressure due to hypoalbuminemia, and leakage of protein-enriched fluid from the surface of the liver, which increases intraperitoneal colloid pressure. The primary event is probably peripheral vasodilation due to an imbalance of vasoactive factors, including endothelins. The net effect of these forces is shrinkage of the central blood volume, which decreases renal perfusion and leads to sodium retention through activation of the renin–angiotensin system. Sodium retention leads to water retention, but because of increased portal hydrostatic pressure and decreased intravascular colloid pressure, the fluid leaks into the so-called third space, causing ascites and edema.

There is a role for nitric oxide (NO)[145] as the primary mediator of vasodilation in cirrhosis. The possible factors responsible for the increased NO synthesis in cirrhosis include stimulation by endotoxin or other bacterial products, such as bacterial DNA from the GI tract, which are less efficiently cleared due to portal-systemic shunting and decreased reticuloendothelial cell function in cirrhosis.[144]

Ascites has many causes, and it is important to differentiate ascites secondary to portal hypertension from ascites due to other causes. This is done by analyzing ascitic fluid. The feature that best distinguishes portal hypertension is an increase in the serum/ascites albumin gradient. A gradient greater than 1.1 g/dL (11 g/L) is characteristic of ascites caused by portal hypertension,[147] but a high serum/ascites albumin gradient can also be seen in congestive heart failure or nephrotic syndrome. For more details on the biochemical tests in peritoneal fluid, refer to Chapter 45 on Body Fluids.

Ascites due to portal hypertension is managed by creating a negative sodium balance or by relieving portal hypertension. A negative sodium balance can be obtained by reducing sodium intake and enhancing sodium excretion using diuretics. In cirrhosis, activation of the renin-aldosterone axis (caused by a variety of factors) necessitates use of agents that act at the distal nephron as the primary diuretic used, but these can be combined with other diuretics that act more proximally. In patients who require more urgent treatment for relief of symptoms, or who do not respond adequately to diuretics, ascitic fluid may be removed with a catheter placed percutaneously through the abdominal wall (paracentesis). More than 10 L of fluid may be drained to relieve patient discomfort or respiratory compromise. Removal of more than 4 L of ascites requires concomitant plasma volume expansion to prevent renal failure; albumin is effective as an expander.[148] Portal hypertension can be managed with the insertion of mechanical porto-systemic shunts via the trans-jugular route. Trans-jugular porto-systemic shunts (TIPSS) have been shown to reduce bleeding from varices and the accumulation of ascites but may precipitate hepatic encephalopathy.[146]

Spontaneous Bacterial Peritonitis

Ascites predisposes to SBP, defined as peritoneal infection (typically Gram negative), in the absence of mechanical disruption of the bowel.[149] The condition usually presents in an individual with known cirrhosis and manifests by the development of abdominal pain, fever, or leukocytosis. The diagnosis is established by examination of the ascitic fluid; more than 250 neutrophils/mL (or >500 neutrophils/mL in the absence of a positive blood culture) is considered diagnostic. In contrast, secondary peritonitis is usually associated with higher neutrophil counts, along with high protein and low glucose in ascitic fluid. Several studies have suggested that dipsticks that detect the presence of leukocyte esterase could be used to identify increased leukocytes and to diagnose SBP; however, a recent review found poor sensitivity and frequent false-negative results in asymptomatic patients.[150,151] Unless cell counts are not available (e.g., in an office setting or in a remote site), use of dipsticks for leukocyte esterase is not recommended. Culture of ascites may be negative in up to 60% of cases, but infection should be treated empirically if symptoms and signs are indicative of SBP.

Hepatic (Portosystemic) Encephalopathy

Hepatic encephalopathy is a metabolic disorder characterized by a wide spectrum of neuropsychiatric dysfunction.[142,152] It may occur as an acute syndrome in patients with acute hepatic failure, or as a chronic, relapsing syndrome associated with cirrhosis. As implied by the synonym, chronic hepatic encephalopathy occurs in the setting of portosystemic shunting, usually as a result of cirrhosis. It may occur as the result of a range of metabolic disturbances, including dehydration, electrolyte imbalances, ingestion of excess protein, bleeding, sepsis, renal dysfunction, hypoxia, portosystemic shunting, increased demands on hepatic function (e.g., surgery), and commonly due to drugs, particularly those that act on the central nervous system (e.g., benzodiazepines).

The clinical syndrome is variable but follows a reasonably predictable course. Disturbed consciousness always occurs. It usually starts as hypersomnia and progresses to sleep reversal, in which the patient tends to sleep through the day and be awake at night. This is followed by decreased spontaneous movement, apathy, and gradually increasing levels of coma. Personality changes may be conspicuous, especially in patients with chronic disease. Irritability and disturbed social behavior may follow. Intellectual deterioration occurs and generally progresses to overt confusion. Neurologic abnormalities include slurred speech, a characteristic flapping tremor called asterixis, increased muscle tone, and abnormal reflexes. Disturbed gait may ensue. In chronic encephalopathy, these changes typically fluctuate over time and follow a waxing and waning course. Acute encephalopathy progresses rapidly, often within hours, and is characterized by cerebral edema, which may result in brainstem herniation and death.

The pathophysiology of hepatic encephalopathy is not completely understood but includes an increased sensitivity to dietary proteins. Ammonia concentrations are typically increased with acute encephalopathy[153] and are often but not invariably increased with chronic encephalopathy. A reduction in plasma ammonia concentration is often associated with symptomatic improvement. However, because plasma ammonia concentrations do not correlate with the severity of the encephalopathy, it has been suggested that other factors are involved.[154] It is recognized that a variety of neurotransmitter systems are dysfunctional in hepatic encephalopathy, but the exact cause of the changes is not known. One important contributor is the endogenous benzodiazepine agonist system.

The diagnosis of chronic hepatic encephalopathy is usually made on clinical grounds. Plasma ammonia concentrations are rarely helpful for diagnosis or for monitoring the patient's disorder; normal ammonia concentrations are helpful in excluding hepatic encephalopathy as a cause of cerebral dysfunction when the clinical picture is not clear. As alluded to earlier, ammonia is more helpful in acute encephalopathy in proving a hepatic cause and is of some prognostic importance in ALF.[100] Increased ammonia concentrations in this situation suggest acute hepatic failure or Reye syndrome. The most reliable diagnostic assessment is the electroencephalogram, which is usually abnormal in patients with symptomatic hepatic encephalopathy, with triphasic waves over the frontal lobes that oscillate at 5 Hz and δ-wave activity in the most advanced stages of the condition.[142]

Treatment is largely empirical, based on observations that intestinal bacteria and protein loads in the intestinal tract are important in the symptoms of hepatic encephalopathy. Lactulose has long been known to reduce symptoms in chronic hepatic encephalopathy. Antibiotic treatment with a nonabsorbable antibiotic (e.g., rifaximin) reduces the number of bacteria and is especially helpful in patients with GI bleeding. Patients with acute encephalopathy may require measures to reduce intracranial pressure, such as osmotic diuretics.

Hepatorenal Syndrome

Hepatorenal syndrome (HRS) is a severe complication of end-stage cirrhosis characterized by increased splanchnic blood flow, a hyperdynamic circulation, a state of decreased central volume, activation of vasoconstrictor systems, and extreme kidney vasoconstriction leading to decreased glomerular filtration rate (GFR). Portal hypertension is a common factor in all cases of HRS that develop in chronic liver disease, but HRS may also occur in ALF. Although formerly believed to be a rapidly progressing, terminal event in a person with end-stage liver disease, it is now recognized that HRS falls into two major varieties.[155] Type 2 HRS is more common; it represents a slowly progressive or stable decline in renal function that is due to peripheral vasodilation and renal vasoconstriction. Type 1, or classic HRS, represents rapidly declining renal function, which is usually seen in a person with preexisting type 2 HRS. Type 1 HRS usually develops in the setting of an acute decrease in blood pressure, which is often due to SBP or variceal bleeding.

A common feature in both forms of HRS is activation of the renin–angiotensin–aldosterone axis, which is caused by intravascular volume depletion.[156] As with other forms of prerenal azotemia (increased concentrations of urea, creatinine, and other compounds rich in nitrogen), HRS in the untreated patient is generally associated with increased antidiuretic hormone and with profound thirst. This leads to the development of hyponatremia, hypokalemia, metabolic alkalosis, low urine sodium, high urine potassium excretion, and high urine osmolality. Plasma urea and creatinine concentrations, and creatinine clearance are not reliable indicators of renal function in HRS.[157] Urea production by the liver is often decreased in advanced liver disease; it is also increased after upper GI bleeding, which is a common cause of worsening renal function in HRS. Creatinine production by muscle is reduced in cirrhosis, causing a misleadingly low plasma creatinine concentration and creatinine clearance. Although plasma cystatin-C concentration has better correlation with the measured GFR,[157,158] it has not been widely adopted for monitoring persons with cirrhosis, and one study has suggested that it may be misleading after liver transplantation.[159]

Despite its limitations, the most widely accepted criterion for diagnosis of HRS is an increase in plasma creatinine concentration or a reduction in estimated GFR. Because no specific clinical or laboratory features of HRS have been identified, diagnosis depends on the presence of severe liver disease, a rise in creatinine to more than 1.5 mg/dL (133 μmol/L), no evidence of other renal disease by urinalysis and clinical history, and lack of improvement in renal function with treatments that increase intravascular volume (such as stopping diuretics, or administration of fluids and/or albumin).[155] The latter two criteria are important because laboratory findings are similar to those of volume depletion, with low urine output, low urine sodium concentration, and increased urine osmolality.

Treatment of HRS is best accomplished by increasing systemic vascular resistance, using the vasopressin analog terlipressin, octreotide, and midodrine, in conjunction with intravascular volume expansion. The choice of agents remains controversial, but albumin infusion has been shown to reduce both the incidence of HRS and mortality. Measures that reduce portal venous pressure, such as a transjugular intrahepatic portosystemic shunt, may also be effective but may be contraindicated due to hepatic encephalopathy. Both approaches have shown promise in improving renal function in HRS.[160]

Altered Drug Metabolism

Because of the central role of the liver in drug metabolism and disposition, alterations in drug metabolism may occur in patients with liver disease. In general, this is reflected in delayed metabolism. Only patients with evidence of liver failure, such as encephalopathy, coagulopathy, or ascites, need alterations in dosing. In general, patients with liver disease are not more susceptible to drug-induced hepatotoxicity. However, those with alcoholic liver disease who continue to consume alcohol are susceptible to liver injury from acetaminophen, even at therapeutic doses.[161]

Nutritional and Metabolic Abnormalities

The intake and disposition of nutrients in patients with chronic liver disease are altered, which subjects them to nutritional imbalance. Severe metabolic and nutritional derangements have been observed in cirrhotic patients, including alterations in glucose metabolism caused by insulin resistance, and hypokalemia caused by secondary hyperaldosteronism. In addition, hypoalbuminemia is frequently present because of decreased production and sinusoidal leakage of albumin in patients with portal hypertension. Also, in patients with chronic cholestasis, impaired delivery of bile salts to the duodenum may result in malabsorption of lipids and fat-soluble vitamins, leading to deficiencies in vitamins A, D, E, and K (see Chapters 39 and 46). Vitamin A deficiency in association with liver disease may cause night blindness, but rarely progresses to serious visual impairment. Vitamin D deficiency causes osteopenia, and in severe cases, osteomalacia. Osteopenic bone disease may be one of the most crippling results of chronic cholestatic liver disease, such as PBC.[162] Vitamin E deficiency is of little clinical significance. Vitamin K deficiency leads to hypoprothrombinemia, with easy bruising and bleeding.

Disordered Hemostasis in Liver Disease

As discussed later and in Chapter 79, the liver manufactures most of the soluble clotting factors (the major exceptions being factor VIII and von Willebrand factor) and a number of inhibitors of clotting (proteins C and S, antithrombin III). The liver also clears activated clotting factors from the circulation. Bile acids are necessary for vitamin K absorption and are needed to produce the active forms of several clotting factors, as well as proteins C and S. Disorders of fibrinogen also occur in liver disease. For example, dysfibrinogenemia may be seen in both acute and chronic liver disease and leads to prolongation of the partial thromboplastin time.[163] Patients with AIH may have anticardiolipin antibodies and antibodies to platelets. The liver is the major source of thrombopoietin, which is needed to produce platelets. Portal hypertension results in splenomegaly, which often leads to thrombocytopenia. In addition, persons with liver disease often have evidence of platelet-associated antibodies,[164] although their contribution to low platelet counts in liver disease is questionable.[165]

Although these facts suggest that hemostatic problems are common in patients with liver disease, discordance is often noted between the degree of abnormality of laboratory tests of coagulation and clinical evidence of bleeding.[166–168] Even in patients bleeding from esophageal varices and who have prolonged clotting times, administration of blood components (including activated factor VII) has not been associated with any clinical difference in degree of bleeding or need for blood transfusions.[168]

Enzymes Released From Diseased Liver Tissue

Because hepatic function is often normal in many patients with liver disease, the plasma activities of several cytosolic, mitochondrial, and membrane-associated enzymes are measured because they are increased in many forms of liver disease. Because plasma enzyme measurements are discussed in greater detail in Chapter 32, only those factors relevant to an understanding of liver disease will be summarized here.

Reference Intervals for Alanine Aminotransferase

One area of significant concern is the reference intervals for liver-associated enzymes, particularly for alanine aminotransferase (ALT; EC 2.6.1.2). In most laboratories, reference intervals are based on samples of the apparently healthy population. For ALT, that upper reference interval is often approximately 40 to 45 U/L in men, but many laboratories have upper reference intervals of 65 to 70 U/L, depending upon the methods used.[169] These differences are greater than can be explained by analytical differences among methods.[170] Although ALT values are approximately 40% lower in females (a difference found even in children), not all laboratories have different reference intervals for the two sexes. For more information, refer to the Appendix on Reference Intervals and to the CALIPER database on pediatric reference intervals: http://www.sickkids.ca/Caliperproject/intervals/index.html.

However, population-based reference intervals may not be adequate for identifying persons with liver disease or for recognizing persons who may be at risk for metabolic syndrome or cardiovascular disease. Because many chronic liver disorders (e.g., HCV, alcoholic liver disease, NAFLD) are prevalent in the population, such reference intervals may include many persons with liver disease. A widely cited Italian study, which excluded persons with known or likely liver disease, suggested lowering reference intervals for ALT to approximately 30 U/L in males and 19 U/L in females.[171] However, racial and ethnic variations should be considered.

A study among dialysis patients (who had 25% lower aspartate aminotransferase [AST] and ALT compared with healthy controls) in Taiwan found that the optimal cutoff value for detecting viral hepatitis was 17 U/L.[172] In Korea, risk of development of liver steatosis increased with increasing serum ALT activity, even among those within its usual reference intervals,[173] which was also true with risk of death from cardiovascular disease.[174] A study using the Framingham study offspring in the United States found that risk of metabolic syndrome and cardiovascular disease increased significantly with ALT, which was above the lowest quartile of the normal reference intervals.[175] The National Academy of Clinical Biochemistry and the American Association for the Study of Liver Diseases (AASLD) guidelines on liver-related tests recommend that health-related reference intervals should be developed for ALT.[176] These data provide some preliminary information toward that end.

ALT values are affected by many factors, including lifestyle; reference interval determinations using apparently healthy individuals may contain individuals with undetected liver disease, such as HCV or NAFLD. Different methods for determining ALT activity also produce different results with the same population. Therefore the physician must be aware of the reference interval for a particular laboratory's method but also should be cautious in interpreting a normal ALT in a particular patient. The debate about the upper cutoff for ALT activity is ongoing and will require a reevaluation of the risk–benefit and cost-effectiveness of any change to the conventional model of using a population-derived upper reference interval.[177–179]

The interpretation of a test is usually based on a reference interval, a decision point (threshold or cutoff) or monitoring individual patient levels changes. Universal cutpoints for ALT have been suggested in a number of guidelines.[180,181] However, because of the analytical variation with ALT assays including the inclusion or not of pyridoxal-5-phosphate, there is a risk that individuals may be misclassified using these thresholds. This can lead to overdiagnosis and unnecessary additional testing.[182]

This problem applies to many measurands where there are fixed limits for interpretation but no standardization of the test using the principles of traceability.

Factors Affecting Plasma Enzyme Quantities

Because the pattern and degree of increase of enzyme activity vary with the type of liver disease, their measurement is extremely helpful in the recognition and differential diagnosis of liver damage. Several factors govern the ability of liver enzymes to assist in diagnosis, including their tissue specificity, subcellular distribution, relative activity of enzyme activity in liver and plasma, patterns of release, and clearance from plasma.

Tissue Specificity

Four enzymes—ALT, AST (EC 2.6.1.1), alkaline phosphatase (ALP; 3.1.3.1), and γ-glutamyltransferase (GGT; EC 2.3.2.2)—are commonly used to detect liver injury. ALT and GGT are present in several tissues, but increased plasma activities primarily reflect liver injury. AST is found in the liver and muscle (cardiac and skeletal), and to a limited extent in red cells. ALP is found in a number of tissues, but in normal individuals, it primarily reflects bone and liver sources. Thus based on tissue distribution, ALT and GGT would seem to be the most specific markers for liver injury.

Subcellular Distribution

Enzymes are found at different locations within cells. AST and ALT are cytosolic enzymes. As such, they can be released with cell injury and appear in plasma relatively rapidly. AST and ALT have both mitochondrial and cytosolic isoenzymes in hepatocytes and other cells containing these enzymes. In the case of ALT, the relative amount of mitochondrial isoenzyme is small, and its plasma half-life is extremely short, making it of no diagnostic significance. In the case of AST, the mitochondrial isoenzyme represents a significant fraction of total AST within hepatocytes. In contrast, ALP and GGT are membrane-bound glycoprotein enzymes. The most important location of both enzymes is on the canalicular membrane of hepatocytes.

Relative Activity in Liver and Plasma

For cytoplasmic enzymes, the relative amount of enzyme in the liver relative to plasma is an important determinant of diagnostic sensitivity. The activity of AST within hepatocytes is approximately twice that of ALT, although plasma activities are similar. The relative amount of enzyme in tissue is not necessarily the same in disease; in cirrhosis and malnutrition, and with alcohol abuse, greater decreases are seen in cytoplasmic ALT than in cytoplasmic AST.[183] In addition, other mechanisms may be responsible for this difference in enzyme activity. The development of immunoassays for measuring ALT has led to the observation of discordance between enzymatic activity and mass in several types of liver disease.[184] In chronic hepatitis and in healthy individuals, ALT activity and mass change in parallel. In acute hepatitis, activity is increased to a much greater degree than mass; the opposite pattern is seen in cirrhosis and HCC. Additional studies are necessary to confirm these findings, but these results suggest that poorly understood factors still affect enzyme activity.

Mechanisms of Release

Several mechanisms appear to be involved in the release of enzymes from hepatocytes. Cell injury, the simplest mechanism, appears to allow leakage of cytoplasmic enzymes from cells, but minimal release of other types of enzymes. Thus necroinflammatory disease leads to release of AST and ALT, but not of a mitochondrial isoenzyme of AST nor ALP or GGT. Alcohol appears to induce expression of mitochondrial AST on the surface of hepatocytes.[185]

The mechanism of release of membrane-bound enzymes such as GGT and ALP into the circulation is less well understood. Synthesis of GGT and ALP appears to be increased in the diseased human liver.[186] How this enhanced synthesis of tissue-bound enzymes translates into increased activity in plasma is not clear. However, fragments of hepatocyte membrane rich in GGT and ALP activity have been detected in the plasma of patients with cholestasis; this process may be a result of membrane fragmentation by bile acids. Furthermore, bile acids, which are detergents, could solubilize and release GGT and ALP from plasma membranes. In vitro studies of membranes treated with bile acids have shown that this possibility exists.[187]

Rate of Clearance of Enzyme From Plasma

Clearance of liver enzymes from plasma occurs at variable rates. The half-life of ALT is 47 hours and that of cytosolic AST is 17 hours; thus although more AST is released from the liver, the much longer half-life of ALT leads to higher activities of ALT than AST in most forms of hepatocellular injury. The half-life of the liver isoenzyme of ALP has been variously reported as from 1 to 10 days; the former figure appears to correspond better to changes seen with removal of gallstones. The half-life of GGT has been reported as 4.1 days. The mechanism by which enzymes are removed from the circulation is not completely known, although receptor-mediated endocytosis by liver macrophages is likely involved.

DISEASES OF THE LIVER

The liver has a limited number of ways of responding to injury.[188] Acute injury to the liver may be asymptomatic, but often presents as jaundice. The major acute liver disorders are acute hepatitis and cholestasis. Chronic liver injury generally takes the clinical form of chronic hepatitis; its long-term complications include cirrhosis and HCC. The discussion of liver disease will focus mainly on these patterns and on a few diseases that differ from this general pattern.

Mechanisms and Patterns of Injury

Cell death occurs by necrosis (death of cell) or apoptosis (programmed cell death) or both. The target cell determines the pattern of injury, with hepatocyte injury leading to hepatocellular disease and biliary cell injury leading to cholestasis. All cellular injury induces fibrosis as an adaptive or healing response, with the duration of injury and genetic factors determining whether cirrhosis and ultimately carcinoma occur (Fig. 51.14).

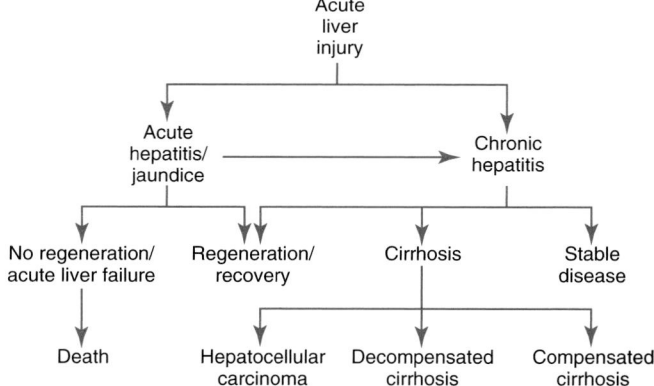

FIGURE 51.14 Natural history of liver disease. With acute injury to the liver, several outcomes are possible. In many individuals, damage is clinically inapparent and recovery occurs with clearance of the causative agent. In some, clinical acute hepatitis occurs. In most of these, clearance of the causative agent results in complete recovery; in a small minority, damage is so severe that acute liver failure (fulminant hepatitis) develops, which is usually fatal without liver transplantation. A variable percentage of persons with acute liver injury (dependent on the cause) progress to chronic hepatitis. In some, recovery eventually occurs naturally or following treatment of the underlying cause. Among those in whom chronic hepatitis persists, many will never progress to cirrhosis. Most of those who do will remain well for many years, but approximately 3% per year develop decompensated cirrhosis (bleeding varices, ascites, hepatic encephalopathy) or hepatocellular carcinoma. These are the most common causes of death from liver disease.

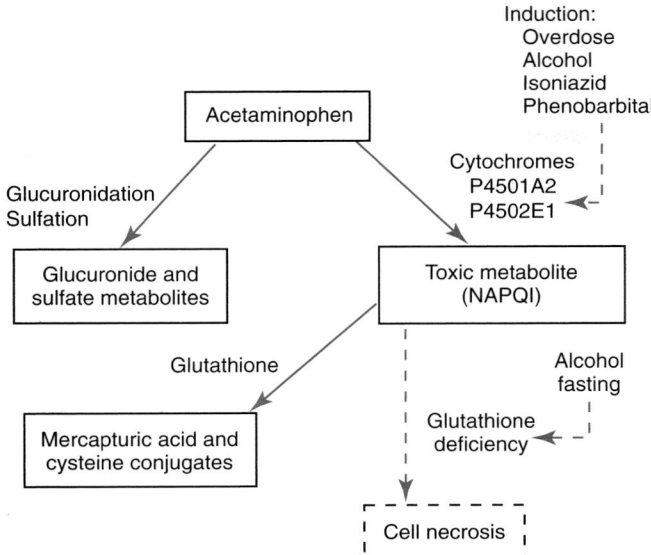

Induction:
Overdose
Alcohol
Isoniazid
Phenobarbital

Cytochromes
P4501A2
P4502E1

Acetaminophen

Glucuronidation
Sulfation

Glucuronide and
sulfate metabolites

Toxic metabolite
(NAPQI)

Glutathione

Alcohol
fasting

Glutathione
deficiency

Mercapturic acid and
cysteine conjugates

Cell necrosis

FIGURE 51.15 Metabolism of acetaminophen by the liver.

Cellular necrosis occurs as the result of an injurious environment and has been referred to as "murder." It is characterized by cellular swelling with loss of membrane integrity. Toxic injury from compounds such as carbon tetrachloride, aspirin, and acetaminophen (Fig. 51.15) occurs for the most part by necrosis. Apoptosis occurs as the result of accelerated programmed death in which the cell participates in its own demise and thus commits "suicide." It is characterized by cell shrinkage, with nuclear chromatin condensation and fragmentation forming apoptotic bodies. Regardless of the cause, cell death typically leads to leakage of cytoplasmic enzymes. Most forms of hepatitis are associated with apoptosis.

Laboratory tests are helpful in distinguishing between the pattern of injury (hepatocellular vs. cholestatic), the chronicity of injury (acute vs. chronic), and the severity of injury (mild vs. severe). In general, the aminotransferase enzymes and ALP are used to distinguish the pattern, the plasma albumin determines the chronicity, and the PT or factor V concentration determines the severity. Classically, liver fibrosis has been assessed using liver biopsy, but in recent years several noninvasive methods of assessment of liver fibrosis have been described and evaluated. Although liver biopsy yields incomparable information about the nature, severity, and chronicity of liver disease, noninvasive tests may provide more accurate assessment of liver fibrosis, and in particular, disease severity and prognosis.

Disorders of Bilirubin Metabolism
Inherited Disorders of Bilirubin Metabolism
Inherited disorders of bilirubin metabolism include Gilbert, Crigler-Najjar (types I and II), Lucey-Driscoll, Dubin-Johnson, and Rotor syndromes.

Gilbert syndrome. Gilbert syndrome is a benign condition manifested by mild unconjugated hyperbilirubinemia. This abnormality, which affects 3 to 10% of the population, is clinically important because it is often misdiagnosed as chronic hepatitis.[189] The serum concentration of bilirubin fluctuates between 1.5 and 4 mg/dL (26 and 70 μmol/L) and tends to increase with fasting. Hepatic glucuronyltransferase

activity is low (≈30% of normal activity) because of a mutation in the bilirubin-UDP-glucuronosyltransferase (*UGT1A1*) gene located on chromosome 2. In most patients, this mutation is a repeat in the promoter, so that there are seven rather than the "normal" six ATs. Occasionally, subjects are encountered with five or eight repeats; the transcription of the gene is inversely proportional to the number of repeats,[190] so that bilirubin concentrations tend to be higher in those patients with the largest number of repeats in the promoter. In Asia, Gilbert syndrome is sometimes found to be caused by a single point mutation in exon 1 of the *UGT1A1* gene.[191] The Framingham Heart Study population was studied for subjects homozygous for the insertion of seven TA repeats in the promotor region of the *UGT1A1* gene (designated UGT1A1*28; genotype 7/7) and discovered higher bilirubin concentrations strongly associated with a lower risk of cardiovascular disease.[192] These findings support the concept of bilirubin possessing a protective antioxidant effect that leads to the prevention of LDL oxidation, thus lowering cardiovascular risk.[193] Additional protective effects have been suggested for diabetes and metabolic syndrome.[194,195] Gilbert syndrome is easily distinguished from chronic hepatitis by the absence of anemia and bilirubin in urine, and by normal liver function tests. The condition is probably inherited as an autosomal recessive trait. Despite the fact that total biliary bilirubin is reduced, the ratio of bilirubin monoglucuronide to diglucuronide is increased, suggesting that a defect is also present in the conversion of bilirubin monoglucuronide to diglucuronide.

Patients with Gilbert syndrome may be predisposed to acetaminophen toxicity because acetaminophen is primarily metabolized by glucuronidation. The diagnosis is usually made by chance on routine medical examination or when jaundice occurs after an intercurrent infection or fasting. Special diagnostic tests are occasionally necessary and include demonstrating a rise in bilirubin on fasting and a fall in bilirubin upon taking phenobarbital. No treatment is needed, but patients must be reassured that they do not have liver disease.

Crigler-Najjar syndrome (type I). Crigler-Najjar syndrome type I (OMIM* 218800),[196] a rare disorder caused by complete absence of UDP-glucuronyltransferase 1A1, is manifested by high concentrations of unconjugated bilirubin often exceeding 20 mg/dL (340 μmol/L). Because no glucuronidation occurs, conjugated bilirubin is not detectable. It is inherited as an autosomal recessive trait. Most mutations have been identified to exist in exons 2 to 5, and result in truncated proteins or amino acid substitutions resulting in little to no enzyme activity.[197] Most patients die of severe brain damage caused by kernicterus (encephalopathy related to increased serum bilirubin that leads to permanent brain damage) within the first year of life. Phlebotomy and plasmapheresis can reduce the serum bilirubin, but encephalopathy usually develops. Early liver transplantation is the only effective therapy.

Crigler-Najjar syndrome (type II). Crigler-Najjar syndrome type II (OMIM*606785)[198] is a rare autosomal dominant disorder characterized by a partial deficiency of UDP-glucuronyltransferase 1A1. Enzyme activities are usually less than 10% of normal activity. Unconjugated bilirubin is usually 5 to 20 mg/dL (85 to 340 μmol/L). Unlike the Crigler-Najjar syndrome type I, type II responds dramatically to phenobarbital, and a normal life span is expected. Pregnant type II patients can be treated with phototherapy and phenobarbital without affecting either the mother or the fetus.[199]

Lucey-Driscoll syndrome. Lucey-Driscoll syndrome,[200,201] also known as maternal serum jaundice or transient familial hyperbilirubinemia, is a familial form of unconjugated hyperbilirubinemia caused by a circulating inhibitor of bilirubin conjugation. The hyperbilirubinemia is mild and lasts for the first 2 to 3 weeks of life.

Dubin-Johnson syndrome. Dubin-Johnson syndrome[202] is due to a rare autosomal recessive disorder and is characterized by jaundice with predominantly elevated conjugated bilirubin and a minor increase of unconjugated bilirubin. Excretion of various conjugated organic anions and bilirubin, but not bile salts, into bile is impaired, reflecting the underlying defect in canalicular excretion. At least 20 mutations in the *ABCC2* gene on chromosome 10 have been identified to result in the Dubin-Johnson phenotype.[203] The transporter ABCC2 is responsible for the active transport of many organic anions, in addition to conjugated bilirubin, into the bile canaliliculus.[204]

Intravenous cholangiography does not show the gallbladder, but a [99m]technetium-hepatobiliary iminodiacetic acid (HIDA) scan does. A derangement in the excretion of urinary coproporphyrin occurs, and the normal ratio of coproporphyrin I to III is reversed. The liver has a characteristic greenish black appearance, and liver biopsy reveals a dark brown pigment in hepatocytes and Kupffer cells that looks like lipofuscin but probably is melanin. Serum ALT and ALP are usually normal, and pruritus is absent. The condition is benign, although patients may develop jaundice during pregnancy or while taking oral contraceptives.

Rotor syndrome. Rotor syndrome[205–207] is another form of conjugated hyperbilirubinemia similar to Dubin-Johnson syndrome, but without pigment in the liver. Contrary to findings in Dubin-Johnson syndrome, the gallbladder is seen on intravenous cholecystography. Total urinary coproporphyrins are increased, with approximately two-thirds being coproporphyrin I. The prognosis is excellent.

Jaundice in the Neonate

Disorders that cause jaundice in the neonate are classified as unconjugated or conjugated hyperbilirubinemia (Box 51.2).[208,209]

Unconjugated hyperbilirubinemia. Unconjugated hyperbilirubinemia poses a risk for development of kernicterus (acute bilirubin encephalopathy), especially in low-birth-weight infants. Kernicterus refers to a neurologic syndrome that results in brain damage because of deposition of bilirubin in the basal ganglia and brain stem nuclei. In term infants, the early symptoms of kernicterus are poor feeding, lethargy, and vomiting; later, opisthotonos (backward arching of the trunk) and seizures; death may follow. Seventy percent of affected infants die within the first week, and those remaining have severe brain damage. This syndrome can be prevented by phototherapy and exchange transfusion in infants with increased unconjugated bilirubin concentrations.

Causes of unconjugated hyperbilirubinemia in the neonate are physiologic jaundice of the newborn, hemolytic disease, and breast milk hyperbilirubinemia.

Guidelines for assessing risk. In 2004, the Subcommittee on Hyperbilirubinemia of the American Academy of Pediatrics (AAP) issued new guidelines for the management of jaundice in the neonate.[209] These guidelines became necessary

---

BOX 51.2 Physiologic Classification of Jaundice

Unconjugated Hyperbilirubinemia
Increased Production of Unconjugated Bilirubin From Heme
Hemolysis
- Hereditary
- Acquired

Ineffective erythropoiesis
Rapid turnover of increased red blood cell mass (in the neonate)

Decreased Delivery of Unconjugated Bilirubin (in Plasma) to Hepatocyte
Right-sided congestive heart failure
Portocaval shunt

Decreased Uptake of Unconjugated Bilirubin Across Hepatocyte Membrane
Competitive inhibition
- Drugs
- Others

Gilbert syndrome
Sepsis, fasting

Decreased Storage of Unconjugated Bilirubin in Cytosol (Decreased Y and Z Proteins)
Competitive inhibition
Fever

Decreased Biotransformation (Conjugation)
Neonatal jaundice (physiologic)
Inhibition (drugs)
Hereditary (Crigler-Najjar)
- Type I (complete enzyme deficiency)
- Type II (partial deficiency)

Hepatocellular dysfunction
Gilbert syndrome

Conjugated Hyperbilirubinemia (Cholestasis)
Decreased Secretion of Conjugated Bilirubin Into Canaliculi
Hepatocellular disease
- Hepatitis
- Cholestasis (intrahepatic)

Dubin-Johnson and Rotor syndromes
Drugs (estradiol)

Decreased Drainage
Extrahepatic obstruction
- Stones
- Carcinoma
- Stricture
- Atresia

Sclerosing cholangitis
Intrahepatic obstruction
- Drugs
- Granulomas
- Primary biliary cirrhosis
- Bile duct paucity
- Tumors

because newborns are currently discharged between 36 and 72 hours after birth, and severe hyperbilirubinemia may not be present at discharge. The time-honored bilirubin concentration of 20 mg/dL (340 μmol/L), which was considered critical and required action (e.g., phototherapy, exchange transfusion), is now being abandoned and replaced by monitoring the increase in bilirubin concentration from the time of birth until the time of discharge from the hospital. In practice, it is now recommended that a plot of bilirubin concentration (milligrams per deciliter or micromoles per liter) versus time (hours) is constructed and compared with the Bhutani predictive nomogram for hyperbilirubinemia found in the AAP guideline.[79] The nomogram is easily searchable on the internet. Others have chosen to create a numeric chart that indicates multiple hours of age, total bilirubin concentration, and risk.[210] Alternatively, websites have been developed to provide the hour-specific risk as described in the 2004 AAP guidelines. For example, at http://bilitool.org, two options for determining risk are provided, each depending on the desired patient data for input. One requires the date and time of birth, date and time of draw, and the total bilirubin (milligrams per deciliter or micromoles per liter), whereas the other option requires the patient's age in hours and total bilirubin (milligrams per deciliter or micromoles per liter).

Interestingly, Trikalinos and colleagues and the US Preventative Services Task Force reported in 2009 that the benefits of implementing bilirubin screening did not provide evidence to decrease the incidence of kernicterus.[211,212] In contrast, a retrospective study by Kuzniewicz and colleagues of 360,000 term newborns showed a significant reduction in severe hyperbilirubinemia when bilirubin screening was implemented.[213] Consistent with these findings, a 5-year prospective study that involved more than 1 million infants showed universal bilirubin screening before discharge significantly reduced the incidence of severe hyperbilirubinemia with a small increase in phototherapy use.[214] Nevertheless, additional recommendations were made in 2009 that require universal predischarge bilirubin screening and a structured approach to management and follow-up based on the predischarge screening process.[215]

Clinical practice guidelines have been developed in several other countries, including Canada in 2001, the United Kingdom in 2008, Norway in 2011, and Australia in 2012.[216–219] Many recommendations are similar throughout these guidelines; however, there are notable differences.[220] For example, the United Kingdom guideline recommends interpreting bilirubin concentrations using a threshold table (not a nomogram) for infants at ≥38 weeks' gestation with hyperbilirubinemia. With the age determined in hours, and the bilirubin concentration, the table can be used to identify one of four follow-up procedures, such as repeating bilirubin measurement within 6 to 12 hours or starting phototherapy.

Physiologic jaundice of the newborn. Babies frequently become jaundiced within a few days of birth; this condition is known as physiologic jaundice of the newborn. Bilirubin concentrations reach a peak within 3 to 5 days of birth and remain increased for less than 2 weeks. Bilirubin is usually less than 5 mg/dL (85 μmol/L), with 90% unconjugated. Factors contributing to physiologic jaundice include (1) an increased bilirubin load in the newborn because the RBCs have a shortened life span; (2) the appearance of "shunt" bilirubin, which is bilirubin derived from ineffective erythropoiesis or

non-RBC sources; (3) decreased conjugation of bilirubin because of a relative lack of glucuronyl transferase (conjugating enzyme) in the first few days after birth; (4) increased absorption of bilirubin in the intestine caused by β-glucuronidase in meconium, which hydrolyzes bilirubin conjugates to unconjugated bilirubin that can be passively reabsorbed; and (5) exposure of breast-feeding infants to pregnanediol, nonesterified fatty acids, and other inhibitors of bilirubin conjugation present in breast milk.

Bilirubin concentrations of 13 mg/dL (222 μmol/L) or greater occurred in 6% of 2297 infants who weighed more than 2500 g.[221] Physiologic jaundice generally is not harmful, but bilirubin concentrations of more than 10 mg/dL (170 μmol/L), coupled with prematurity, low serum albumin, acidosis, and substances that compete for the binding sites of albumin (e.g., ceftriaxone, sulfisoxazole, aspirin), may increase the risk for kernicterus. Physiologic jaundice of the newborn is treated with phototherapy; the infant is exposed to light of approximately 450 nm that disrupts intramolecular hydrogen bonds in the bilirubin molecule and yields several photoisomers that are more water soluble than the Z,Z-isomer and thus are excreted in the bile.[199] Exchange transfusions are rarely necessary.

Hemolytic disease. Hemolytic disease of the newborn results from maternal–fetal incompatibility of Rhesus blood factors (Rh) in which the maternal Rh-negative blood becomes sensitized by a previous pregnancy with a Rh-positive fetus or a Rh-positive blood transfusion. The infant becomes jaundiced with unconjugated bilirubin in the first or second day of life and is susceptible to kernicterus. The diagnosis is confirmed by a Coombs test with Rh-positive blood in the infant and Rh-negative blood in the mother. Other rare, inherited hemolytic anemias, such as glucose-6-phosphate dehydrogenase deficiency, may also lead to unconjugated hyperbilirubinemia (see Chapter 78 on Enzymes of the Red Blood Cell for more detail.)

Breast milk hyperbilirubinemia. This type of hyperbilirubinemia affects approximately 30% of breast-fed newborns. It is due to α-glucuronidase in breast milk, which hydrolyzes conjugated bilirubin in the intestine. The unconjugated bilirubin, being more lipophilic, is passively absorbed. The condition lasts for a few weeks and is treated by discontinuation of breast-feeding.

Conjugated hyperbilirubinemias. These syndromes are characterized by hyperbilirubinemia in which conjugated bilirubin exceeds 1.5 mg/dL (26 μmol/L). The most important are idiopathic neonatal hepatitis and biliary atresia. Diagnosing the cholestatic syndromes may be difficult. The family history may be helpful in diagnosing α₁-antitrypsin deficiency, cystic fibrosis, galactosemia, hereditary fructose intolerance, and tyrosinosis. Serum tyrosine and α₁-antitrypsin concentrations should be obtained. If galactosemia is suspected, the diagnosis is confirmed by absence of the enzyme UDP galactose-1-phosphate uridyl transferase in cells and tissues, such as RBCs and liver. Serologic tests may be necessary for hepatitis A, B, and C, and for adenovirus, Coxsackie virus, cytomegalovirus (CMV), herpes simplex, rubella, and *Toxoplasma*. Liver biopsy may be performed, but the liver tends to look similar, with giant cells and extramedullary erythropoiesis dominating in hepatitis and cholestatic syndromes. The typical features of periportal red hyaline globules seen with periodic acid–Schiff stain that are characteristic for α_1-antitrypsin deficiency usually are not seen early in the course of the disorder. An HIDA isotope scan is essential for determining the patency of the biliary tree. Percutaneous or endoscopic cholangiography may be done in patients with equivocal HIDA scan results.

Conjugated hyperbilirubinemia is seen fairly often in the newborn as a complication of parenteral nutrition.

Idiopathic Neonatal Hepatitis

Approximately 75% of cases of hepatitis in the neonate are idiopathic giant cell hepatitis, a disorder of unknown origin characterized by cholestatic jaundice. A familial trend may reflect an autosomal recessive inheritance. Jaundice appears within the first 2 weeks. The child initially appears well and gains weight. The liver and spleen then become enlarged, and stools become pale. Serum aminotransferases are usually 400 U/L; the PT is prolonged. Liver biopsy reveals characteristic giant cells with hepatocyte acinar formation. Cholestasis is prominent. It is important to rule out extrahepatic biliary obstruction, such as occurs in biliary atresia, with an HIDA scan.

Treatment is supportive, with adequate nutrition and correction of hypoprothrombinemia. The prognosis is favorable, with 90% of infants surviving without sequelae.

Biliary Atresia

Biliary atresia is a heterogeneous group of acquired disorders that involve the extrahepatic or intrahepatic bile ducts. Possible causes include CMV, reovirus III, Epstein-Barr virus (EBV), rubella virus, α_1-antitrypsin deficiency, Down syndrome, and trisomy 17 or 18.

Extrahepatic biliary atresia may involve all or part of the extrahepatic biliary tree. Also termed neonatal hepatitis, it is the most common cause for neonatal cholestasis and considered the most common reason for liver transplantation, accounting for 40 to 50% of all pediatric liver transplantations.[222] Obstruction due to either inflammation, fibrosis, or a mixed source results in biliary atresia. The frequency of disease changes with geographic region from 1 in 5600 in Taiwan[223] to 1 in 13,700 live births in the United States. Females are slightly more affected than males.[224] Symptoms begin within the first few months of life. The gallbladder is usually absent. Involvement of the hepatic or common duct leads to the characteristic syndrome of severe cholestatic jaundice. It occurs in 1 in 10,000 births, with females more commonly affected than males. Jaundice and pruritus usually appear in the first week. Stools are pale, and the urine is tea colored. Jaundice is deep, but the aminotransferases are only mildly increased. If jaundice persists beyond 14 days of age, a direct or conjugated bilirubin measurement must be performed to exclude biliary atresia. If it is increased, the urine should be tested for bile and the stool color inspected; if the stool is not green or yellow, biliary atresia is likely. Early identification of this condition is essential if these infants are to benefit from the operation of portoenterostomy, which should be performed no later than 60 days after birth.[225] If portoenterostomy is not successful, liver transplantation is the treatment of choice. Children rarely live beyond 3 years unless the lesion is surgically correctable.

More recently, clinical phenotypes have been developed based on the combination of clinical, pathologic, and molecular features. The perinatal form is the most common clinical form. Approximately 80% of newborns fall into this phenotype. Characteristically, both jaundice and acholic stools develop after birth.[226] The embryonic form is found in 10% of affected newborns. Common features are associated with early onset injury, including the absence of extrahepatic bile ducts, and abnormalities of the spleen that may or may not be portal vein defects. When specific splenic and portal vein defects are observed, it is termed biliary atresia splenic malformation syndrome.[227] Patients with biliary atresia splenic malformation have poorer outcomes after hepatoportoenterostomy. Cystic biliary atresia is detected in approximately 8% of patients. In this phenotype, a cystic malformation is located near the obstructed site and has been correlated with improved bile drainage after hepatoportoenterostomy. Delaying portoenterostomy past 70 days of age will typically have a poorer response.[228,229] The last phenotype is CMV-associated biliary atresia. Several studies have indicated that the presence of CMV results in poor bile drainage and a high risk of death after hepatoportoenterostomy.[230] Staging of biliary atresia remains unclear because histopathology, molecular staging, and clinical outcome lack correlation. Numerous factors for the observed pathophysiology have been implicated, such as defective embryogenesis, genetic factors, environmental factors, viral infection, and autoimmunity. These factors have been classified into three broad categories of abnormal morphogenesis, environmental factors, and inflammatory dysregulation.[231] Research to improve the outcome of this disease has progressed substantially; however, much remains to be completed. Fortunately, large multicenter investigations will be facilitated by the European consortium of Biliary Atresia and Related Disease and the Childhood Liver Disease Research Network.[232,233] Intrahepatic biliary atresia is characterized by a paucity of intrahepatic bile ducts. Jaundice usually appears within the first few days of life. Serum bilirubin is increased, and serum cholesterol may be very high, leading to the formation of xanthomas. The hepatic histology is nonspecific, showing bile duct paucity, giant cells, inflammation, and fibrosis. Survival into adolescence is common, although growth is usually retarded.

A syndromic variant, Alagille syndrome,[234] has similar features, but it is an autosomal dominant condition with a characteristic triangular face, skeletal abnormalities, retinal pigmentation, and pulmonary stenosis.

Treatment of intrahepatic biliary atresia includes intramuscular replacement of vitamins A, D, and E. Medium-chain triglycerides that do not need bile acids for absorption provide calories in patients with partial atresia. Cholestyramine may relieve pruritus. Ursodeoxycholic acid (UDCA) reduces serum enzyme activities and relieves pruritus in some patients.

Hepatic Viral Infection

Five viruses (hepatitis A, B, C, D, and E) have been identified as causes of infections that primarily target the liver. In addition, certain other viruses may infect the liver as part of a more generalized infection, of which the more important causes include CMV, EBV, and herpes simplex virus (HSV). Several other viruses have been proposed as causes of liver injury; these include hepatitis G virus[235] (HGV; discussed later), transfusion-transmitted virus,[236] and the closely related SEN virus.[237] Although all three are blood-borne chronic viral infections, and in the case of transfusion-transmitted virus and SEN, have been known to replicate in the

TABLE 51.2 Types of Viral Hepatitis

	A	B	C	D	E	G
Type	RNA	DNA	RNA	Partial	RNA	RNA
Incubation period, days	45–50	30–150	15–160	30–150	20–40	Unknown
Transmission						
Fecal–oral	Yes	No	Minimal	No	Yes	No
Household	Yes	Min	Min	Yes	Yes	No
Vertical	No	Yes	Min	Yes	No	Yes
Blood	Rare	Yes	Yes	Yes	Unknown	Yes
Sexual	No	Yes	Min	Yes	Unknown	Yes
Diagnosis	Anti-HAV IgM	HBsAg, PCR, anti-HBc IgM	Anti-HCV, PCR	Anti-HDV	Anti-HEV	Anti-HGV
Carrier state	No	Yes	Yes	Yes	Yes	Yes
Risk of chronic hepatitis	No	Depends on age, immune status	50–70%	Yes	Rare[a]	No
Risk of liver cancer	No	Yes	Yes	No	No	No
Prevention						
Vaccine	Yes	Yes	No	Yes[b]	No	No
Immunoglobulin	Yes	Yes	No	Yes[b]	No	No
Response to interferon	Not used	30%	40–80%	Yes	Not used	Yes

[a]Only with severe immunosuppression.
[b]Vaccination and passive immunization against HBV protects against HDV infection.
HAV, Hepatitis A virus; *HBc*, hepatitis B core antigen; *HBsAg*, hepatitis B surface antigen; *HCV*, hepatitis C virus; *HDV*, hepatitis D virus; *HEV*, hepatitis E virus; *HGV*, hepatitis G virus; *IgM*, immunoglobulin M; *PCR*, polymerase chain reaction.

liver, none of these viruses appear to cause acute or chronic liver injury.[238–240] The various hepatitis viruses are outlined in Table 51.2.

Hepatitis A Virus

Hepatitis A virus (HAV) has historically accounted for approximately one-fourth to one-third of cases of clinical acute hepatitis in the United States and 20 to 25% worldwide. Since the mid-1980s, a vaccine has been available for HAV, and incidence has declined to its lowest ever in the United States.[241] Current recommendations are that all children should be immunized for HAV, along with adults at high risk for HAV,[242] as well as persons planning international travel and individuals exposed to HAV.[243] Although most commonly an infection in children and adolescents before the introduction of widespread immunization, the disease has now become more common in developed countries in adults than children; it is most common in young adult men, particularly in people exposed to sewage, those who eat raw seafood, people who inject drugs, and in men who have sex with men.[244] It tends to be most virulent in middle-aged and older people. Epidemics have been associated with waterborne and foodborne contamination. Ingestion of raw shellfish from contaminated waters has caused both sporadic and epidemic cases. Although not as common a cause of liver infection as HBV, it is more frequently associated with jaundice when it occurs in adults than HBV or HCV; an estimated 50 to 70% of infected adults develop jaundice, and mortality is almost 2% with infection in those older than 60 years of age.[241] In contrast, HAV infection in children is rarely associated with jaundice, and thus is usually not detected clinically. HAV may cause

severe hepatitis and death in those who have chronic hepatitis, particularly hepatitis B or C.[245]

HAV is caused by a 27-nm RNA picornavirus. It has four capsid proteins (VP1–4), but only one serotype has been identified. The virus is not cytopathic to hepatocytes but causes liver injury by stimulating both cellular and humoral immune responses. HAV occurs in sporadic and epidemic forms, with an incubation period of 15 to 50 days. The clinical course of acute HAV is usually that of a mild flu-like illness that lasts for a few days to a few weeks. There is no chronic form of HAV, but cholestasis (manifested by several weeks of jaundice and pruritus) may occur in some adults. Although a rare occurrence, relapse has been known to happen 1 to 3 months after the acute illness in up to 5% of patients. It resembles the acute illness and is associated with viremia, but recovery always ensues.

Although tests for HAV RNA are available for research purposes, diagnosis of HAV is based primarily on serologic tests for antibodies to HAV. Total anti-HAV is believed to be protective and occurs with natural exposure to HAV and to HAV vaccine. With natural exposure, HAV antibodies appear to persist for life.[246] IgM antibodies to HAV are always present at the time of diagnosis of acute HAV and generally remain present for 3 to 6 months, although they may persist for longer in approximately 14% of individuals.[247] With the falling prevalence of HAV, the number of cases of acute HAV reported to the Centers for Disease Control and Prevention (CDC) that are due to false-positive results exceeds the frequency of actual cases of HAV.[248] For this reason, IgM anti-HAV should be used only in the clinical setting of acute hepatitis.

Three types of effective vaccines are available. A monovalent vaccine against HAV, a combined HAV and HBV vaccine, and a combined HAV and typhoid vaccine. Vaccination followed by a booster at 12 months will provide immunity for up to 20 years.

Hepatitis B Virus

HBV is the most common cause of acute hepatitis, and the most common chronic viral infection worldwide. An estimated 350 million individuals are chronically infected with HBV, and several times as many individuals have been exposed to HBV. The frequency of chronic HBV infection varies worldwide, and it is highest in most of central and southeast Asia, central Africa, and southern Europe (prevalence >8% of the population) and intermediate (2 to 8%) in most of the rest of Asia, Africa, and South America. It occurs rarely among those born in North America and Europe[249]; one study found that 86% of US residents with chronic HBV were actually born outside the United States.[250] In endemic areas, the incidence of new infection has decreased markedly in those places where HBV vaccine has been introduced. HBV is transmitted through body fluids, primarily by parenteral or sexual contact; it can be transmitted from mother to child, usually at or after delivery (termed vertical transmission). In parts of the world with high rates of chronic infection, much of the transmission is vertical. The residual risk from transfusion is estimated to be 1 in 600,000.[251]

HBV is caused by a 42-nm DNA virus that is a member of the hepadnavirus family. The DNA is partially double stranded and contains 3200 nucleotides with overlapping coding regions, leading to several major open reading frames. The S gene codes for several different length variants of surface protein; the smallest form, HBV surface antigen (HBsAg), is produced independently of and in excess of the amount needed for viral replication; the largest form (S1) makes up the surface coat of circulating viral particles. The C gene encodes the HBV core antigen (HBcAg), which is part of the infectious core of the virus. The X gene codes for a transactivating factor that may be involved with viral replication and the development of malignancy. The precore and basal core promoter regions code for production of hepatitis B e antigen (HBeAg), which is a protein found only in those with (but separate from) circulating viral particles. The final major viral protein is a polymerase, which has several different enzymatically active sites. Hepadnaviruses are unusual among DNA viruses because they produce the first strand of DNA from a form of viral messenger RNA (mRNA), using the reverse transcriptase activity of HBV polymerase. This error-prone reproductive strategy, along with an extremely high rate of viral replication in chronically infected individuals, leads to a high rate of mutation in HBV. The significance of several mutants is described later.

Hepatitis B was first described in the 1960s by Blumberg and colleagues after discovery of a protein, termed the Australia antigen, which was initially believed to be a tumor marker for leukemia.[252] Subsequent studies confirmed it to be a marker for a form of hepatitis initially termed serum hepatitis. Later work established that this was HBsAg. The complete HBV virion (Dane particle) consists of a core containing DNA attached to DNA polymerase and HBcAg, surrounded by the S1 form of surface protein. HBsAg and other forms of surface protein contain a common determinant, a,

and four subdeterminants designated d, y, w, and r. These determinants are responsible for determining HBV genotypes; the eight major genotypes, termed A through H, have less than 92% homology with other types.[253] Geographic differences in genotype distribution have been noted; genotype A predominates among those infected in North America, whereas genotype C is the dominant form in those infected in Asia. Although not routinely determined at present, evidence indicates that genotype is an important predictor of the natural course of HBV and response to certain forms of treatment.[254] For example, genotypes A1 and F1 are associated with HCC in young adults and (in Alaska with genotype F1) children.[255] Genotype C has a higher risk of development of cirrhosis and HCC than is the case with most other genotypes. Genotype C has a low likelihood of response to INF treatment.

Several mutants of HBV may have clinical importance (see the following).

Pathogenesis of hepatitis B. The HBV is not directly cytopathic. The liver damage associated with HBV infection is mediated by the immune response to HBV with innate and adaptive inflammatory immune responses causing hepatocyte necrosis and apoptosis that is accompanied by wound healing response, which results in liver fibrosis. This results in the typical histologic picture of viral hepatitis characterized by hepatic inflammation with interface hepatitis and fibrosis. Recognition of the importance of the immune response to HBV has led to the classification of stages of chronic hepatitis based on the host immune response. In the early "immune-tolerant" phase of chronic infection,[256] the host mounts little in the way of an immune response to high levels of viral replication. This is characterized by high levels of viremia, normal ALT values, and eAg positive eAb negative serology. Once host immunity is activated, hepatitis ensues, characterized by falling levels of viremia, increased transaminases, and fluctuating serology. This phase is termed the immune-reactive phase. In most cases, this phase gives way to a prolonged period of immune control with inactive disease characterized by eAg negativity, eAb positivity, low or undetectable HBV viremia, and normal transaminases. In a minority of eAg negative patients, the emergence of replicative mutants results in rising HBV DNA titers that may be accompanied by immune activation and an HBVeAg negative hepatitis. In some cases, this pattern of disease may fluctuate with periods of activity and periods of inactive hepatitis, making diagnosis difficult and dependent on frequent blood tests. Both chronic eAg negative hepatitis and fluctuating eAg negative hepatitis are associated with progressive fibrosis and hepatocellular cancer, and should be looked for in patients with eAg negative disease. Normal blood tests for HBV DNA and ALT every 2 to 3 months over 12 months should exclude active hepatitis in more than 90% of cases.

Hepatitis B e antigen and hepatitis B e antigen mutants. Hepatitis B e antigen is a protein of uncertain function produced by viral mRNA. It is released into the circulation by infected hepatocytes and may be involved as a "decoy" that prevents the immune system from attacking HBV viral particles. The most common HBV mutations involve the regions that code for production of HBeAg. The highest frequency is for a mutation at nucleotide 1896 that inserts a stop codon in the mRNA, preventing production of HBeAg. Mutations in the precore promoter region, particularly at nucleotides 1762 and 1764, are associated with reduced production of normal HBeAg. Such mutants are associated with undetectable HBeAg and are usually found in patients with detectable levels of anti-HBe. Precore and core promoter mutants are found in most individuals chronically infected with HBV in areas with high rates of infection, such as Asia and Southern Europe. In North America, it is estimated that 10 to 20% of individuals with chronic HBV infection have such precore mutants.[257] Such mutants may be present at the time of infection or may develop during the course of disease. Although initially it was believed that individuals infected with such mutants were much more likely to have severe acute infection, the high prevalence of such mutants suggests that this is not the case. Infection with these mutant strains is associated with a higher risk of development of HCC, and risk is stronger for the basal core promoter mutations.[258]

Polymerase mutants. Treatment with antiviral agents that inhibit the reverse transcriptase domain of HBV polymerase is now the most widely used therapy for chronic HBV.[259] As with human immunodeficiency virus (HIV), specific amino acid substitutions have been linked to resistance with several of the commonly used agents, particularly lamivudine and adefovir. The longer these agents are used, the greater is the likelihood that resistant mutants will emerge. Testing to detect resistant mutants is becoming more widely performed, particularly in individuals who have been exposed to more than one reverse transcriptase inhibitor (such as those who also are infected with HIV). Nucleotide and nucleoside polymerase inhibitors that are highly potent and present a higher barrier to resistance (e.g., tenofovir and entecavir) are much less likely to select resistance and can be used long term to suppress viremia. However, it is mandatory that patients prescribed these drugs are checked regularly for adherence to treatment, therapeutic effectiveness, and for the emergence of mutants.

Hepatitis B surface antigen mutants. Mutations in the "a" determinant of HBsAg are the most important HBsAg mutants. Antibody to HBsAg, which is developed by natural exposure or by the HBV vaccine, is primarily directed against the "a" determinant. Exposure to strains that have mutations in this domain can result in infection despite the presence of protective titers of anti-HBs. In areas where HBV is endemic, up to 25% of cases of HBV in immunized infants are due to infection by such mutants.[260,261] In addition, the reagents used to detect HBsAg are antibodies to anti-HBs; therefore mutant strains can be missed by HBsAg assays.[262–264] The ability of reagents to identify these mutant strains differs, mainly because of the specific epitopes recognized by the antibody (or antibodies) used in the assay.[265] Use of assays with antibodies to multiple epitopes improves detection of such mutant strains.[266] At present, the importance of such mutant strains is unknown. Data suggest that most individuals infected with mutant strains have such viral particles at low titers, usually in the presence of larger amounts of wild-type virus. Thus most infected persons will be detected by the current assays for HBV. However, some infected individuals (perhaps more commonly those immunized for HBV) will be missed by some current assays.

Immunization. Hepatitis B may be prevented by passive (hepatitis B immune globulin [HBIG]) or active (hepatitis B recombinant vaccine) immunization. In the United States, current data suggest that more than 90% of children have been immunized against HBV infection, leading to a historically low incidence of acute HBV infection. Because infants born to HBsAg mothers have a high risk of developing chronic HBV infection, routine prenatal testing for HBsAg is needed to identify infants at risk. Infection occurs in only approximately 2% of infants before birth[267]; postexposure prophylaxis (typically used in infants of HBsAg positive mothers), which consists of passive immunization with 0.06 mL/kg of HBIG and the first dose of hepatitis B vaccine within 24 hours of birth is more than 95% effective in preventing infection.[268] A universal immunization program in Taiwan, where vertical transmission of HBV was endemic, has greatly reduced the death rate from HCC in young individuals.[269]

Diagnostic tests for hepatitis B. More diagnostic tests exist to measure HBV than any of the hepatitis viruses; consequently, interpretation of results is complicated. Testing currently primarily involves ELISA or related techniques to measure viral antigens or antibodies, but nucleic acid–based tests are becoming more widely used.

HBsAg, the most widely used marker for detecting current HBV infection, is detected by kits using antibody to HBsAg. Occasionally, false-positive results occur in testing, particularly during pregnancy; a neutralization assay is available. Low-level reactivity (as evaluated by the ratio of the signal from the sample to that of the cutoff for distinguishing positive and negative, termed the signal/cutoff [S/C] ratio) is highly predictive of samples that fail to confirm neutralization.[270] False-negative results can occur with mutants in the surface antigen (as previously described), and they occur more commonly in early HBV infection. Most assays are qualitative; quantitative HBsAg assays have been available in Europe for more than a decade. Some studies have shown a direct relationship (in untreated individuals) between quantitative HBV DNA and viral load[271]; others have not.[272] Declines in quantitative HBsAg during treatment have been found to be predictive of response to treatment for chronic HBV,[273,274] and lower levels of HBsAg may identify patients with HBeAg negative disease who do not require long-term treatment to maintain viral suppression.

Antibody to the HBV core antigen (anti-HBc) is the most commonly detected antibody against HBV. Two assays are usually used: IgM and total anti-HBc. IgM anti-HBc assays typically use a large dilution of plasma (1:100) before analysis to reduce the likelihood of positivity in individuals with chronic HBV. The total antibody assay measures both IgM and IgG antibodies. Anti-HBc appears to last longer than anti-HBs in natural infection and is still present in 97% of previously infected individuals more than 30 years after exposure.[275] Isolated anti-HBc is a relatively common finding, particularly in the setting of HCV coinfection,[276] but is also found in immunosuppressed individuals. Although this may represent a false-positive result, particularly as a transient phenomenon after influenza vaccination, current guidelines on hepatitis B recommend consideration of individuals with isolated anti-HBc as having been exposed to HBV.[277]

Antibody to the HBsAg (anti-HBs) is considered evidence of immunity to hepatitis B and is the only marker found in those who have received the hepatitis B vaccine. The WHO has developed reference material that contains 10 IU/mL of anti-HBs. Current guidelines suggest that immunocompetent individuals who achieve an anti-HBs of ≥10 IU/mL have life-long immunity to HBV.

The HBeAg and antibody to the e antigen (anti-HBe) are typically used only in the setting of chronic HBV infection. Although HBeAg typically appears at about the same time as HBsAg in acute hepatitis, it is rarely used as a marker for acute infection. In chronic infection, HBeAg has historically been used as a marker of persistence of infectious virus; its clearance and the appearance of anti-HBe have been used as indicators of conversion to the nonreplicating state and as goals of antiviral treatment. With widespread availability of HBV DNA assays with low detection limits, the discordance between HBeAg and the presence of infectious viral particles has become apparent. Although most untreated patients with HBV who are HBeAg positive have high viral loads (usually $>10^6$ IU/mL), detectable HBV DNA is also found (usually with lower viral load) in approximately 70% of those who are HBeAg negative. When HBeAg-positive individuals are treated with polymerase inhibitors, loss of HBV DNA occurs in the majority, and HBeAg usually remains detectable. Loss of HBeAg during treatment, with development of anti-HBe, indicates a high likelihood that viral suppression will be maintained after discontinuation of treatment.[259] In contrast, in those with HBV viremia who were HBeAg negative (and anti-HBe positive) before treatment, discontinuation of treatment usually leads to recurrence of viremia. Thus HBeAg remains an important marker for monitoring therapy, but has largely been replaced by HBV DNA for detection of those who harbor the infectious virus.

Hepatitis B viral DNA is now routinely measured using amplification techniques. The WHO has established an international reference material for HBV DNA, and results are typically reported in international units per milliliter[278]; conversion from copies per milliliter differs on the basis of viral load and is different for various assays. Because much older literature and some currently published papers still report HBV DNA in copies per milliliter, a rough conversion factor is 5 copies/mL = 1 IU/mL. Currently, assays that use amplification, particularly polymerase chain reaction (PCR) methods, have detection limits of 100 IU/mL, although nonamplified assays are still available. It is unclear what amount of HBV DNA represents clinically important viremia; however, data (primarily from Taiwan) have shown that risk of progression to cirrhosis or HCC increases at viral loads of more than 10,000 copies/mL (2000 IU/mL).[279] Current treatment guidelines suggest that this number should be used as one criterion in treatment decision-making.[280]

Hepatitis B mutants and genotypes are usually determined by direct sequencing or with the use of line probes.

Hepatitis C virus. The HCV is the cause of most cases previously known as non-A, non-B hepatitis. It was recognized in 1989[281] and fully characterized 2 years later.[282] It is the most common cause of chronic viral hepatitis in North America, Europe, and Japan, and is estimated to infect approximately 170 million individuals worldwide. Although HBV infection appears to have been present for a long time, evidence suggests that HCV is a more recently developing viral infection, because rates of HCV-related liver disease have been increasing in many parts of the world. Predictions are that HCV-related end-stage chronic liver disease will increase twofold to threefold over the next 20 to 30 years.[283] HCV infection primarily occurs through plasma; major risk factors are injection drug use and transfusion. For example, before the recognition of and availability of tests for HCV, the

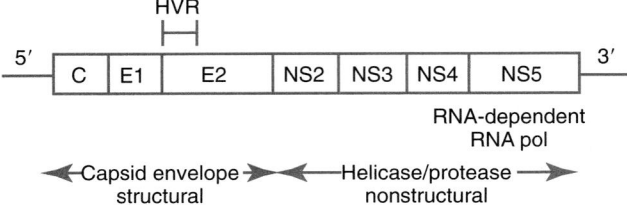

FIGURE 51.16 Structure of the hepatitis C genome.

frequency of post-transfusion hepatitis (mainly due to HCV) was 3.5%[284]; the risk of HCV transmission by transfusion is currently estimated at 1:2,000,000.[251] Because of its mode of spread, HCV infection is rare in children; the only common causes of pediatric infections are vertical transmission from an infected mother (estimated to occur in <5% of infected women[285]) and previous transfusion of infected blood products. In countries where standards of hygiene are suboptimal, unsterile medical and ritual practices continue to account for new infections.

HCV is a single-stranded enveloped RNA virus of the flavivirus family, which includes other hepatitis viruses (yellow fever virus) and viruses that cause unrelated disease (such as West Nile virus). HCV RNA contains one reading frame (Fig. 51.16). The resulting polypeptide is cleaved to core and envelope antigens, and a number of nonstructural proteins, including a polymerase, a protease, and an INF response element. As an RNA virus, HCV is subject to a high rate of spontaneous mutation, giving rise to large numbers of variants. This results in six major genotypes (<70% nucleotide homology), along with a number of subtypes (77 to 80% homology).[286,287] According to various global reviews, genotype 1 (G1) is the most common (46%; affecting ≈83 million cases, one-third of which are in East Asia), followed by G3 (22 to 31%; ≈54 million), G2 (13%; ≈22 million), and G4 (13%; ≈22 million).[288,289] In a chronically infected individual, numerous quasispecies (>90% homology) develop over time. These quasispecies seem to be important in establishing chronic infection[290] and appear to be related to the fluctuating nature of chronic inflammation in chronic HCV infection.[291] Quasispecies are unique to the individual infected; those infected from a common source show different patterns of mutation.[292]

Chronic HCV infection is associated with evidence of chronic liver injury in most cases. Increases in liver-associated enzymes, particularly ALT, are usually mild and fluctuate between normal and abnormal in most infected individuals. In an estimated 15 to 20% of cases, cirrhosis becomes evident an average of 20 to 30 years after exposure. HCC may develop once cirrhosis is present, at an average rate of 1.5 to 3 cases per year. In North America, Europe, and Japan, HCV is the most common risk factor in the development of HCC. Various extrahepatic manifestations of chronic HCV infection may be noted; the most common are cryoglobulinemia and porphyria cutanea tarda (see Chapter 41 on Porphyrias). Epidemiologic evidence has linked HCV to increased risk of lymphoma and type 2 diabetes mellitus.

Prevention. Prevention of HCV has proved more difficult than that of HAV and HBV. However, an 80% decrease in the incidence of acute HCV has occurred,[241] which is similar to what occurred with HAV and HBV; this is believed to be due to testing of blood donors for HCV and to safe injection practices that have been instituted to reduce the risk of HIV infection. Vaccine development has been difficult because of the many subspecies of virus and the presence of many quasispecies with different antigenic determinants. The dramatic evolution in treatments for HCV over the last two decades has culminated in the development of drugs capable of eradicating infection in more than 90% of cases of most genotypes of HCV.[293]

Diagnostic tests for hepatitis C. Measurement of the antibody to HCV (anti-HCV) is the principal screening test for HCV exposure. These tests, which use ELISAs and related microparticle chemiluminescence formats, detect the presence of antibodies to one or more HCV antigens (derived by recombinant technology from yeast cultures or through production of synthetic peptides). Although the initial assay detected only antibody to a single antigen, subsequent tests have used antigens from four different regions of the HCV genome. Second-generation assays become positive an average of 12 weeks after exposure, and third-generation assays become positive an average of 9 weeks after exposure. After comparison with a cutoff value, results are interpreted as positive or negative. As is true for HBsAg, samples with a low S/C ratio are often false positive, whereas false-positive results are rare in samples with a high S/C ratio.[294,295] Current CDC recommendations suggest use of an S/C ratio of less than 3.8 for both second- and third-generation ELISA assays, and an S/C ratio less than 8.0 for the chemiluminescence assay, to define low-positive results.[277] Samples with a low S/C ratio are recommended to be confirmed, ideally with the use of a recombinant immunoblot assay (RIBA).

RIBA is a technique similar in principle to Western blotting. HCV antigens used in anti-HCV assays are typically blotted onto a membrane as dots, and reactivity is detected after incubation with serum. Results are interpreted as negative if there is less than 1+ reactivity with any of the four antigens, indeterminate if there is 1+ or greater reactivity to only a single antigen (or to more than one antigen along with the nonspecific yeast marker superoxide dismutase), and positive with 1+ or greater reactivity to multiple antigens. Third-generation RIBAs have considerably fewer indeterminate results than second-generation RIBAs.

HCV RNA measurement has become the most widely used test to detect current HCV infection. Typical of RNA in general, HCV RNA is labile in whole blood because of the action of RNAses primarily found in blood cells. Rapid separation of serum from a clot is critical for accurate measurement of HCV RNA. If serum is separated from the clot by centrifugation within 1 hour, HCV RNA does not show an appreciable decline until 6 hours after collection. If serum is physically separated from cells within 1 hour, samples are stable at room temperature for 3 days, at refrigerator temperatures for 1 week, and indefinitely if frozen.[296] Samples collected in ethylenediaminetetraacetic acid (EDTA), which inhibits enzyme activity, are stable for 24 hours, even if plasma is not separated from red cells.[297]

Assays for HCV RNA historically were divided into qualitative and quantitative variants. An international reference material for quantification of HCV RNA has been developed,[298] and quantitative HCV RNA assay results are calibrated using this material and are reported in international units per milliliter. The relationship between international

units per milliliter and copies per milliliter differs significantly for different assays. Results expressed in international units per milliliter agree within 1 log in approximately 90% of samples, but discrepant results do occur.[299] Until recently, qualitative assays had significantly lower detection limits than quantitative assays, but quantitative assays using real-time PCR have equivalent or lower detection limits compared with qualitative assays. If assays with detection limits of 10 to 20 IU/mL are used (as is the case in many settings), qualitative assays are no longer needed.[300] One of the currently available real-time PCR assays tends to under-report viral load among 15% of individuals infected with genotype 2[301] and may cause falsely negative results with genotype 4.[302]

Hepatitis C core antigen (HCV Ag) is produced by the most constant part of the HCV genome. HCV Ag is one of the major targets of antibody formation, and most HCV Ag circulates bound to antibody. HCV Ag has a similar time course to that of HCV RNA in both acute and chronic HCV infection[303]; the currently available assay for HCV Ag becomes reliably positive when HCV RNA is 20,000 IU/mL or greater.[304] In one laboratory, experience with several thousand HCV RNA samples suggested that less than 5% of untreated HCV RNA–positive individuals had a viral load of less than 20,000 IU/mL. In contrast to HCV RNA, HCV Ag is stable in storage. Currently, no commercial HCV Ag assays are available in North America.

Hepatitis C genotype shows regional diversity and is an important parameter in the development of vaccines and for determining the length and intensity of antiviral therapy.[287–289] Several methods are currently used to determine the infecting genotype. Although serologic assays to detect antibodies to specific genotypes of HCV are available, their correlation with direct tests is approximately 90%,[305] and a significant minority of infected individuals have antibodies to more than one genotype.[306] However, detection of viral RNA of more than one genotype is exceptionally rare. The most reliable method involves direct sequencing of regions of the genome that show characteristic patterns with specific genotypes and subtypes. Commercial assays using the 5-untranslated region are the most widely used,[307] although assays using the NS5b region are now available. All currently available assays show good agreement on genotype, although they differ in their detection limits.[308] Sequencing methods have the advantage that they can be used to identify treatment resistance–associated variants that may develop under selection pressure from the new directly acting antiviral agents. Line probe assays are also widely used and show good agreement with direct sequencing assays.[309]

Hepatitis D Virus (Delta Agent)

Hepatitis D virus (HDV) is an incomplete, 36-nm RNA particle that cannot replicate on its own.[310] It is coated with HBsAg and is dependent on HBV for its activation. It is thus a satellite virus similar to that seen in plants. The D virus is a single-stranded antisense RNA virus. It is very infectious and strongly associated with intravenous drug use; approximately 10 million individuals have been infected worldwide, although the incidence is declining with the fall in incidence of HBV infection.[311] It occurs as simultaneous infection with HBV (coinfection) or as a superimposed infection in someone with chronic HBV (superinfection). Coinfection usually runs the same time course as acute HBV, and HDV is spontaneously cleared as the hepatitis B resolves, but the risk of fulminant hepatitis is higher than in HBV infection alone, and mortality is higher. Superinfection typically results in chronic HDV infection, suppression of HBV DNA replication, and more rapid progression to cirrhosis (estimated 4%/year) and HCC (estimated 3%/year).[312] It should be assessed in all patients with HBV infection due to the seriousness of coinfection and suspected in patients with HBV infection whose condition worsens.[313] Although it is traditionally diagnosed serologically by detection of anti-HDV (total or IgM) and/or HDV Ag,[314] HDV RNA measurements are often used as evidence of current infection.[315]

Hepatitis E Virus

Hepatitis E virus (HEV) is a 34-nm, single-stranded, unenveloped RNA virus. It accounts for sporadic and epidemic hepatitis in tropical and semitropical countries and in people returning from these areas.[316] Although considered to be rare in Europe and nontropical areas of North America, HEV RNA is frequently isolated from city sewage treatment plants in such nonendemic areas.[317] A number of small outbreaks have occurred in Europe over the past several years[318]; in one institution in England, HEV was responsible for approximately 10% of otherwise undiagnosed cases of acute hepatitis.[319] It is enterically transmitted, as is HAV, and viral RNA has been detected in plasma and in stools.[320] There is probably only one species, although four genotypes are known. Tests to detect an antibody to HEV have been developed; specificity for HEV is high only for assays that detect an antibody to the open reading frame 2 antigen.[321] The prevalence of antibodies to HEV is high in the United States, with 21% of randomly selected individuals having anti-HEV from 1988 to 1994.[322] HEV has been isolated from a number of animals, notably rats[323] and pigs[324]; the significance of this is unclear, although it has been speculated that HEV is a zoonotic disease.[325,326] In several countries, HEV has been linked to ingestion of pork,[318] and in the United States, to ingestion of liver (from unclassified species).[322]

As with HAV, IgM anti-HEV detection of antibodies has been considered diagnostic of acute infection by HEV, but false-positive results have been reported with hepatitis due to CMV and EBV.[327] The clinical course is similar to that of HAV infection, in that HEV typically infects young people, has a self-limited course, and has not been associated with chronicity. Recently, however, chronic infection with HEV has been documented in organ transplantation recipients.[328,329] A peculiar feature of this disease is its virulent course in late pregnancy in India, with mortality generally in the range of 20 to 25%, but rates as high as 50% have been reported.[330] Mortality during pregnancy is not increased in other parts of the world.[331] Mortality is increased among the elderly and in those with chronic liver disease.[319] The interested reader is referred to more recent reviews for further information on the epidemiology, diagnosis, and treatment of HEV infection.[332,333]

Hepatitis G Virus

HGV, also known as GBV-C, is an RNA virus of the flavivirus family and is closely related to HCV.[235] It is most commonly transmitted by plasma[334]; vertical transmission has also been reported.[335] Although it has a very high infection rate in recipients of contaminated blood (>90%), HGV infection appears to have no adverse consequences.[336] Although it has

been called a hepatitis virus, viral RNA cannot be isolated from the liver in chronic infection.[337] Coinfection with HCV and HGV is common, but coinfection has no effect on prognosis in HCV.[338,339] HGV and HIV coinfection is common; individuals coinfected with HGV and HIV have lower HIV viral loads and a better prognosis than those infected with HIV alone.[340–342] The pathogenesis of this presumed viral interaction is still unknown,[343] although stimulation of innate immunity may be involved.[344]

Acute Hepatitis

Acute hepatitis refers to an acute injury directed against the hepatocytes. The injury may be mediated directly, which occurs with certain drugs, such as acetaminophen or with ischemia, or indirectly, which occurs with immunologically mediated injury from most of the hepatitis viruses and most drugs, including ethanol. In direct injury, a typical rapid rise in cytosolic enzymes, such as AST, ALT, and lactate dehydrogenase (LD), is followed by a rapid fall, with rates of decline similar to known half-lives of the enzymes. With immunologic injury, a gradual rise in cytosolic enzymes occurs, followed by a plateau phase and gradual resolution of enzyme increase. Although jaundice is a key clinical finding in acute hepatitis, it is often absent (as discussed later under the various forms of viral infection). An increase in AST activity to greater than 200 U/L or in ALT activity to greater than 300 U/L has sensitivity and specificity greater than 90% for acute hepatitis.[345]

ALP usually is mildly increased and typically is less than three times the upper reference limit in 90% of cases of acute hepatitis.[345] Increased plasma concentration of bilirubin, when present, typically is predominantly due to direct reacting bilirubin; indirect bilirubin is higher than direct bilirubin in approximately 15% of cases.[38] The distribution of direct bilirubin percentage is identical in acute hepatitis and bile duct obstruction, making the relative amount of direct bilirubin inconsequential in the differential between hepatitis and obstruction.[38] Liver synthetic function usually is well preserved in most forms of acute hepatitis. These and other features that are helpful in the differential diagnosis of acute hepatitis are summarized in Table 51.3.

The outcome of acute hepatitis is variable. In most cases, complete recovery occurs, and liver regeneration leads to normal structure and function. With some viruses, failure to clear infection leads to development of chronic hepatitis. In a small percentage of cases, massive destruction of the liver leads to acute (fulminant) hepatic failure, which is associated with high mortality unless liver transplantation is performed.[346,347]

Acute Viral Hepatitis

All forms of acute viral hepatitis have similar pathology and a similar clinical course. They are all diagnosed on the basis of marked increases in serum aminotransferase activities, usually to between 8 and 50 times the upper reference intervals, with only slight increases in ALP and little or no effect on hepatic synthetic function. ALT is typically higher than AST because of slower clearance. Enzyme increases typically peak before peak bilirubin occurs and remain increased for an average of 4 to 5 weeks (longer for ALT than AST because of its longer half-life). Bilirubin increase is variable, as is discussed later. The incidence of acute viral hepatitis due to HAV, HBV, and HCV reached historically low levels by 2007.

TABLE 51.3 Laboratory Features of Different Forms of Acute Hepatitis

Type	AST/ALT	ALP	Bilirubin	PT (s)	Serology	Other
Viral	8–50× URL	<3× URL	5–15 mg/dL (86–256 µmol/L)	<15	Positive	
HAV					IgM anti-HAV	
HBV					HBsAg, IgM anti-HBc	
HCV					HCV RNA ± anti-HCV	
Alcoholic	<8× URL	>3× URL in 25%	5–15 mg/dL (85–256 µmol/L)	<15	Negative	AST > ALT
Toxic	>50× URL	Normal	<5 mg/dL (<85 µmol/L)	>15	Negative	Toxin usually detectable; acute renal failure common
Ischemic	>50× URL	Normal	<5 mg/dL (<85 µmol/L)	>15	Negative	Acute renal failure common
Drug induced	8–50× URL	>3× URL in 50%	5–15 mg/dL (85–256 µmol/L)	<15	Negative	Eosinophilia, skin rash common
Autoimmune	8–50× URL	<3× URL	5–15 mg/dL (85–256 µmol/L)	<15	Positive ANA or ASMA	Low albumin, high globulins
Wilson	8–50× URL	Low normal or decreased	5–15 mg/dL (85–256 µmol/L)	<15	Negative	Hemolytic anemia, renal failure, low ALP common; low ceruloplasmin often absent

ALP, Alkaline phosphatase; *ALT*, alanine aminotransferase; *ANA*, antinuclear antibody; *ASMA*, anti–smooth muscle (or antiactin) antibody; *AST*, aspartate aminotransferase; *HAV*, hepatitis A virus; *HBc*, hepatitis B core antigen; *HBsAg*, hepatitis B surface antigen; *HBV*, hepatitis B virus; *HCV*, hepatitis C virus; *IgM*, immunoglobulin M; *URL*, upper reference limit.

However, the incidence of these infections reported in the most recent report from the CDC in 2013 described an increase in acute cases of all three infections. This has been attributed in part to changes in methodology in 2011, but also to a large outbreak of HAV, inward migration of people carrying HBV, and better diagnoses of cases of HCV infection.[241] For more detailed information on acute viral hepatitis, the reader is referred to the practice guideline of the World Gastroenterology Organisation.[348]

Acute hepatitis A. In adults, approximately 70% of those with acute HAV infection develop jaundice much more commonly than those with HBV or HCV. In children, acute HAV infection typically goes unrecognized and is often considered to be a viral gastroenteritis or other viral disease, because only 10% of children become jaundiced. The disease is more prolonged and serious in individuals older than age 60 years, can cause liver failure in persons with chronic HCV[245] or cirrhosis,[349] and has high mortality. The specific etiologic diagnosis is made with serologic tests. An IgM antibody (anti-HAV IgM) appears early in the course of the illness and persists for an average of 2 to 6 months; rarely, IgM antibodies may remain positive for a year or longer. The presence of IgM anti-HAV has therefore been considered diagnostic of a recent HAV infection. No antigen tests are available for detection of hepatitis A in serum. Incubation of stool samples with labeled antibodies to hepatitis A and examination with an electron microscope have been used in the past to detect infectious viral particles. Amplification techniques (usually with reverse transcriptase PCR [rt-PCR]) have been used to detect virus in epidemiologic studies but are not routinely used to diagnose infection.

Acute hepatitis B. In most of the world, HBV is the most common cause of acute viral hepatitis. As with HAV, most infections in children are clinically silent. An estimated one-third of adolescents and adults with acute HBV infection develop jaundice. The outcome in acute HBV infection is strongly influenced by age and immune status. In healthy adolescents and adults, an estimated 1 to 3% of cases will progress to chronic infection. In a person with immunosuppression, the likelihood of chronic infection increases to 10%. Neonates infected with HBV have a 90% likelihood of chronic infection, and the risk falls gradually during the first 5 years of life.[350]

The serologic course of acute hepatitis B infection is illustrated in Fig. 51.17. HBsAg is the first serologic marker to appear, although HBV DNA may be detectable slightly earlier. HBsAg usually appears 1 to 2 months after infection and before the onset of clinical illness and is the last protein marker to disappear. HBV DNA replication is slower than that of HCV; doubling time averages 2 to 3 days.[351] Persistence of HBsAg for longer than 6 months beyond the onset of acute hepatitis indicates chronic infection. HBeAg appears at about the same time as HBsAg; however, because it is not usually measured except in the setting of chronic HBV infection, it usually is not helpful as a marker to document acute infection. The first antibody to appear, which usually coincides with the onset of clinical evidence of hepatitis 3 to 6 months after infection, is the anti-HBc. As with hepatitis A, an IgM antibody is the first to appear and usually persists for 3 to 6 months; it is usually considered diagnostic of acute hepatitis B infection. However, in chronic infection, the IgM antibody may become detectable with flares of severity of disease; thus it is not completely reliable in recognizing a recent infection.[352] The typical pattern at clinical presentation is positive serology for anti-HBc (both total and IgM), HBsAg, HBeAg (when measured), and negative anti-HBs. A small percentage of individuals have negative HBsAg and anti-HBs at the time of initial presentation, leaving IgM anti-HBc as the only commonly measured marker that is positive; this finding has been termed the core window. With current sensitive assays for HBsAg, it is rare to encounter individuals in the core window. Clearance of HBeAg with development of anti-HBe is the first sign of viral clearance and usually predates loss of HBsAg. Clinically, HBsAg clearance from serum is associated with recovery from acute hepatitis and has been believed to confer life-long immunity to HBV.

Accumulating evidence indicates that HBV remains dormant in the body and HBV DNA circulates in many to most individuals who have recovered from acute hepatitis as evidenced by clearance of HBsAg and acquisition of HBsAb. This has been termed occult HBV infection.[353] Several studies have demonstrated that HBV DNA is still present in low amounts, in both plasma and liver, in most individuals who have had past acute HBV infection and who were HBsAg negative and anti-HBc positive.[276,354,355] Viral loads typically consist of ≤100 copies/mL, and it has been estimated that the number of liver cells infected may be as low as 1%. Such individuals have been shown to transmit HBV infection if their organs are used for transplantation (if treatment to prevent this is not given). The significance of circulating HBV DNA for the individual infected or for others (in the absence of transplantation) seems to be minimal, however, in that liver enzymes are usually normal, and circulating HBV DNA is found mainly in immune complexes.

In recent years, the problem of reactivation of HBV has been increasingly recognized. Reactivation refers to return of viral replication, which is often accompanied by acute liver injury (and in a high percentage of cases, liver failure) in a person with HBsAg but who has inactive viral replication (sometimes also called seroreversion) or less often in patients with occult HBV. Typically, agents that suppress the immune system (chemotherapeutic agents, glucocorticosteroids, antilymphoid treatments) allow return of viral replication that was kept in check by the immune system.[356–359] Withdrawal of immune suppression (including immune restoration in persons with HIV[360]) leads to liver injury. Treatment with lamivudine (or other agents that suppress HBV replication) before immune suppression is highly effective in preventing such reactivation, and guidelines have recommended testing all patients who receive immune suppression for HBV, including testing for HBcAb, before such agents are used.[361,362]

Acute hepatitis C. Acute HCV infection is responsible for 10 to 15% of cases of acute hepatitis in the United States; an estimated 10 to 30% of those with acute infection develop jaundice. Increased aminotransferases usually develop approximately 6 to 8 weeks after infection. In those cases in which clinical acute hepatitis develops, jaundice typically begins approximately 2 to 3 months after exposure. HCV RNA and HCV Ag are detectable in plasma 2 to 4 weeks after initial exposure. Viremia increases rapidly (average doubling time, 17 hours) and plateaus at high viral loads (often > 10^7 IU/mL). In acute hepatitis C infection, anti-HCV is present in a little more than one-half of cases at the time of

presentation.[363,364] IgM anti-HCV assays are not commercially available, but in contrast to HAV and HBV, IgM antibodies are encountered in both acute and chronic HCV infection, making the test useless diagnostically.[365] HCV RNA and HCV Ag usually are both present at the time of diagnosis, and viral load is often significantly increased compared with values seen in chronic hepatitis. Diagnosis of acute HCV is likely if anti-HCV is absent but HCV RNA is positive. Diagnosis of acute HCV is also likely if the HCV RNA viral load is high and the anti-HCV titer is low or increases with time.[365,366] Viral load falls with development of antibodies to one or more HCV proteins, and may become transiently negative. HCV antibodies never appear or disappear in 30 to 50% of those who recover from acute HCV.[367,368] The importance of recognizing acute hepatitis C is that, if virus does not clear spontaneously, treatment is highly effective when given in the first 6 months after diagnosis.[369]

Other types of acute viral hepatitis. Numerous other viruses can affect the liver, causing acute hepatitis. The most common are EBV and CMV. Features are otherwise typical of viral hepatitis, although signs of systemic infection are often seen as well. HSV occasionally may cause severe hepatitis in adults.[370] Infection with each of these agents is more commonly associated with hepatitis in the neonatal period, during which it is part of the disseminated infection. Diagnosis of infection with these viruses involves serologic and nucleic acid tests; none are specific to the liver.

Sudden flares of activity in individuals with chronic hepatitis B may mimic acute hepatitis. An acute rise in cytoplasmic enzymes commonly occurs, often in association with jaundice and other clinical features, suggesting an acute liver disease. For example, development of an immune response that leads to clearance of HBeAg or HBsAg is often associated with clinical and enzymatic features of acute hepatitis.[254] Recognition of this cause of the clinical picture of acute hepatitis in a person with chronic hepatitis relies on demonstration of antigen loss and antibody development, along with absence of other causes of acute hepatitis.

Toxic Hepatitis

Toxic hepatitis refers to direct damage of hepatocytes by a toxin or toxic metabolite. Toxic reactions are usually predictable and are directly related to the dose of the agent ingested. Acetaminophen toxicity is the second most common cause of liver transplantation worldwide and the most common in the United States. It is responsible for 56,000 emergency department visits, 2600 hospitalizations, and 500 deaths per year in the United States. Fifty percent of these are unintentional overdoses.[371,372]

In North America and Europe, the most common cause of toxic hepatitis (and the most common cause of ALF) is acetaminophen, a widely used nonprescription pain reliever.[373] The metabolism of acetaminophen is affected by dose, induction of metabolic enzymes, and concentrations of glutathione (see Fig. 51.15). Acetaminophen is normally metabolized through glucuronidation and sulfuration, both of which occur in the liver. In an overdose, these pathways are saturated, and more acetaminophen is subsequently metabolized to *N*-acetyl-p-benzoquinoneimine (NAPQI) by cytochrome P450. NAPQI is a toxic substance that is safely reduced by glutathione to nontoxic mercaptate and cysteine compounds, which are then renally excreted. An overdose (the average lethal dose as a single ingestion is 15 g) depletes the stores of glutathione, and once they reach less than 30% of normal, NAPQI concentrations increase and subsequently bind to hepatic macromolecules causing hepatic necrosis. This is irreversible.[374]

When a large dose of acetaminophen is ingested (the average lethal dose as a single ingestion is 15 g), the metabolic pathways are overwhelmed, glutathione is depleted, and toxic intermediates accumulate, causing liver damage. When metabolic enzymes are induced (such as by ethanol) or glutathione is depleted (which occurs in alcoholism and with starvation), toxicity can occur with relatively small doses of acetaminophen (total doses of 2 to 4 g).[161] Toxicity can also occur with excessive cumulative doses of acetaminophen; such accidental overdoses appear to be responsible for approximately one-half of cases of toxicity.[375] Diagnosis is often based on history and increased acetaminophen concentrations; in patients who present later, and for whom a history cannot be obtained, measurement of acetaminophen-protein adducts allows diagnosis.[376] The first laboratory abnormality to appear is an increase in PT, followed by increased activity of cytosolic enzymes, with AST tending to be higher than ALT.[377] Peak activities (typically > 100 times the upper reference intervals) usually occur by 24 to 48 hours, followed by rapid clearance at rates approximating the known half-lives of the enzymes.[378] PT increases are typical and are more than 4 seconds above the control value in most cases. Prognosis is related most closely to the prolonged increase in PT[379]; persistent increase of PT 4 days after ingestion is associated with a poor prognosis.[380] Other markers of risk include development of acute renal failure and the presence of lactic acidosis, particularly if the pH is less than 7.30 ([H^+] > 50 nmol/L).

Ischemic Hepatitis (Shock Liver)

Hepatic hypoperfusion (ischemic hepatitis) is one of the most common causes of increased cytosolic enzymes; in hospital patients, it is the cause of most cases of acute hepatitis.[381,382] Ischemic hepatitis may follow any cause of shock; the most common causes are septic and cardiogenic shock (sometimes termed cardiac hepatopathy[141]). Not all patients with shock develop ischemic hepatitis; in one recent study, only 13.8% of those with septic shock did, but mortality was significantly higher in such patients.[383] Another study found that cardiac dysfunction, especially right heart failure, appeared necessary to cause the clinical picture of ischemic hepatitis.[384] Bilirubin increases typically are minimal, and they usually peak several days after enzyme activity reaches its greatest point.[385] Laboratory findings are similar to those seen in toxic hepatitis, and acute renal failure is a common complicating factor. Prognosis is primarily related to the underlying cause of hypotension[385]; individuals with prolonged increase of bilirubin appear to have a poor prognosis.[386]

Reye Syndrome

Acute encephalopathy in combination with fatty degeneration of the viscera was initially described by Reye and associates in Australia in 1963,[387] with nearly simultaneous case descriptions by Johnson and colleagues in the United States.[388] In most of these early cases, the disease was fatal. It most frequently strikes children aged 6 to 11 years and infants, although it may affect individuals of other ages. The syndrome is characterized by a prodromal, febrile viral illness (usually influenza B or varicella), followed by

approximately a week of protracted vomiting associated with lethargy and confusion, which may deteriorate rapidly into stupor and coma.[389] At the same time, the liver enlarges, increased aminotransferases and PT develop, and ammonia increases. A prolonged PT more than 3 seconds above normal (INR >1.2) and a plasma ammonia concentration more than 100 μmol/L (140 μg/dL) usually indicate a poor prognosis. Serum bilirubin concentration is typically normal or only mildly increased. Other laboratory features include hypoglycemia and hyperuricemia.

Only sporadic case descriptions of Reye syndrome were published until 1974, when 379 cases in the United States were reported to the CDC. The mortality rate in this series was 41%. The number of cases peaked in 1980 at 555.[390] At about the same time, articles began to appear linking Reye syndrome with aspirin treatment of viral illness[391]; these were followed by a case control study that strongly implicated salicylate in the pathogenesis of Reye syndrome.[392] Although CDC guidelines recommending avoidance of aspirin in children with febrile illness were not published until 1985,[393] a decline in salicylate use began before this time, and Reye syndrome has again become a rare disease. A 2008 review suggested that children who present with a clinical picture similar to Reye syndrome are actually much more likely to have inborn metabolic errors, particularly those involving the urea cycle or mitochondrial enzymes (see Chapter 60), and should be evaluated for those before a diagnosis of Reye syndrome is considered.[394]

Other Causes of Acute Hepatitis

Alcoholic hepatitis is discussed more fully in the Alcohol-Related Liver Disease section later in this chapter. Alcoholic hepatitis is often suspected by the combination of mild increases in enzymes (peak AST typically <300 U/L), AST/ALT ratio greater than 2, jaundice, and leukocytosis.[395] Drugs can cause liver injury through a number of mechanisms, but the most common is idiosyncratic, immune-mediated injury to hepatocytes. The most common pattern is similar to that of other types of acute hepatitis; cholestatic hepatitis, with increased aminotransferases and ALP, is more common in drug-induced hepatitis than with other causes of acute hepatitis, but it is present only in a minority of cases (40% in a 2008 US study).[396] Criteria used to recognize drug-induced liver injury include a temporal relationship between drug exposure and onset of hepatitis, exclusion of other known causes of hepatitis, the presence of extrahepatic hypersensitivity (especially skin rash, arthralgia, renal injury, and eosinophilia), the development of liver injury on rechallenge, and ideally, previously published reports of similar reactions.[397] Several standardized approaches for evaluation of possible drug-induced liver disease have been developed.[398–400] Hepatic drug reactions were reported to represent approximately 6% of all adverse drug reactions[401] in a Danish study and approximately 1% of cases of acute hepatitis in an Indian survey.[402] Although usually associated with prescription drugs, complementary and alternative products are becoming increasingly recognized as causes of acute hepatitis,[403,404] and in a US study, these products were responsible for 9% of all cases.[396] Although drug reactions typically develop soon after the start of treatment, several months may elapse between the time of initial exposure and development of acute hepatitis. Approximately 60% of cases cause severe acute hepatitis with jaundice; fatalities can occur,[405] although often death is not due to liver disease.[396] Serious reactions are more common in individuals who are continued on the medication.[406] In 15 to 30% of cases, liver injury persists and becomes chronic after cessation of the drug.[396]

Some of the disorders that usually produce chronic hepatitis (and are discussed more fully later) may occasionally present in an acute fashion. AIH has an acute component in up to 40% of cases. Clinically, it differs from other forms of acute hepatitis because it is characterized by decreased albumin, increased globulins, and a more protracted increase in aminotransferases.[407–409] Acute AIH is diagnosed by the absence of other causes of acute hepatitis and the presence of autoimmune markers (discussed in detail in the section on Chronic Hepatitis). Wilson disease is the result of deficiency of an intracellular adenosine triphosphastase[410–412] and typically presents in childhood with neuropsychiatric findings, which are almost always associated with chronic liver injury. Wilson disease may also present as acute hepatitis that is often associated with fulminant hepatic failure[413]; in one study, 8 of 14 patients who had hepatic injury due to Wilson disease had an acute presentation.[414] The classic biochemical findings of Wilson disease are often absent (low plasma ceruloplasmin, low plasma copper) or misleading (high urine copper is common to all forms of acute hepatitis) in the setting of acute Wilson disease.[414,415] However, in advanced liver disease or acute hepatitis, ceruloplasmin concentrations may be misleading and be in the normal range because of an acute inflammatory response. Additional features often suggest the diagnosis, including nonimmune hemolytic anemia, acute tubular necrosis, and a low ratio of serum ALP (in units per liter) to bilirubin (in milligrams per deciliter). One recent study found that if this ratio was less than 4, sensitivity was 94% and specificity was 96%, which is far superior to tests such as ceruloplasmin and plasma copper.[416]

Other Disorders With Laboratory Findings Similar to Acute Hepatitis

Several conditions mimic the laboratory picture of acute hepatitis. Hemolytic anemia can cause jaundice, increased plasma LD activity, and slight increases in AST and ALT. In contrast to hepatitis, the increase in bilirubin is predominantly (often >80%) indirect reacting. LD activity is increased to several times that of AST, and AST activity usually is several times that of ALT. Acute injury to skeletal or cardiac muscle may cause significant increases in AST, and to a lesser extent, ALT, but the ratio of AST/ALT activity is generally more than 3 at presentation (although, as with liver injury, the shorter half-life of AST will cause the ratio to become less than 1 with time, usually after 3 days).[417] Plasma bilirubin concentration is not usually increased, but mild increases in unconjugated bilirubin from metabolism of myoglobin may be seen in severe skeletal muscle injury. Acute bile duct obstruction, particularly when caused by gallstones, can resemble acute hepatitis. In the early stages of obstruction, transient increases in AST and ALT are common,[418] and their activities may rarely exceed 2000 U/L.[419,420] Increases in ALP develop more slowly than those of the aminotransferases, masking the presence of cholestasis early in the course. Increases in bilirubin are typically predominantly directly reacting, creating a presentation similar to that seen in acute

hepatitis. Even if obstruction persists, aminotransferase activity falls rapidly, with AST typically returning to normal within 8 days[421] and ALP activity gradually increasing. ALP activities more than 300 U/L in this setting strongly suggest the presence of obstructive jaundice.[422] Acute biliary obstruction by gallstones is often accompanied by acute pancreatitis; increased plasma amylase and lipase activities should suggest biliary tract obstruction as the cause of any noted liver abnormalities.

Approach to the Patient With Acute Hepatitis

Once a diagnosis of acute hepatitis has been established, additional laboratory testing is usually required to determine the cause. Although the incidence of acute viral hepatitis has decreased, serologic studies should be performed to rule out infectious causes. A typical panel of tests should include IgM anti-HAV, HBsAg, IgM anti-HBc, anti-HCV, and HCV RNA (or HCV core antigen, if available). Marked increases (>100 times the upper reference intervals) in AST or ALT, particularly if AST is higher than ALT, should suggest the possibility of toxic or ischemic liver injury. Minimal increases (<8 times the reference interval) in AST, with AST greater than ALT, in a patient with jaundice and leukocytosis indicate likely alcoholic hepatitis. Imaging studies of the biliary tract are appropriate to rule out obstruction in those who present with sudden onset of symptoms, especially if accompanied by right upper quadrant pain and tenderness, laboratory evidence of pancreatitis, or a history of gallstones. The presence of increased plasma globulin and decreased albumin concentrations, or the presence of hemolytic anemia and acute renal failure, should suggest the possibility of AIH or Wilson disease, respectively.

Follow-up of Acute Hepatitis

Important uses of laboratory tests in acute hepatitis are to identify individuals with fulminant hepatic failure, to document recovery, and to determine clearance of any infectious agents. The most important tests in determining the extent of injury are not plasma activities of cytosolic enzymes, but evidence of impaired liver function. The most important indicator of prognosis in acute viral hepatitis is impairment in synthetic function, with PT a widely accepted indicator. In acute viral or alcoholic hepatitis, a PT of more than 3 seconds above normal (INR >1.2) is associated with a poor prognosis,[379] whereas in toxic hepatitis, persistent increase more than 4 days after ingestion has prognostic importance.[380] Low concentrations of other markers of synthetic function, such as transthyretin or actin-free Gc globulin,[423] or of markers of hepatocyte regeneration, such as α-fetoprotein,[424] have been found to predict poor prognosis. In alcoholic hepatitis, bilirubin and INR are the most reliable predictors of prognosis; several indexes, discussed later in the section on Alcoholic-Related Liver Disease, have been used to predict risk of death and need for treatment.[395] Plasma activities of cytosolic enzyme decrease rapidly in ischemic and toxic hepatitis or obstruction, regardless of outcome, and fall more gradually in viral and alcoholic hepatitis, but are not helpful in evaluating outcome. With hepatitis B and C, cytosolic enzyme activities may return to normal even if viral replication persists[425,426]; serologic tests are the only reliable means to evaluate resolution of infection.

DIAGNOSTIC ALGORITHM OF VIRAL HEPATITIS THROUGH SEROLOGY

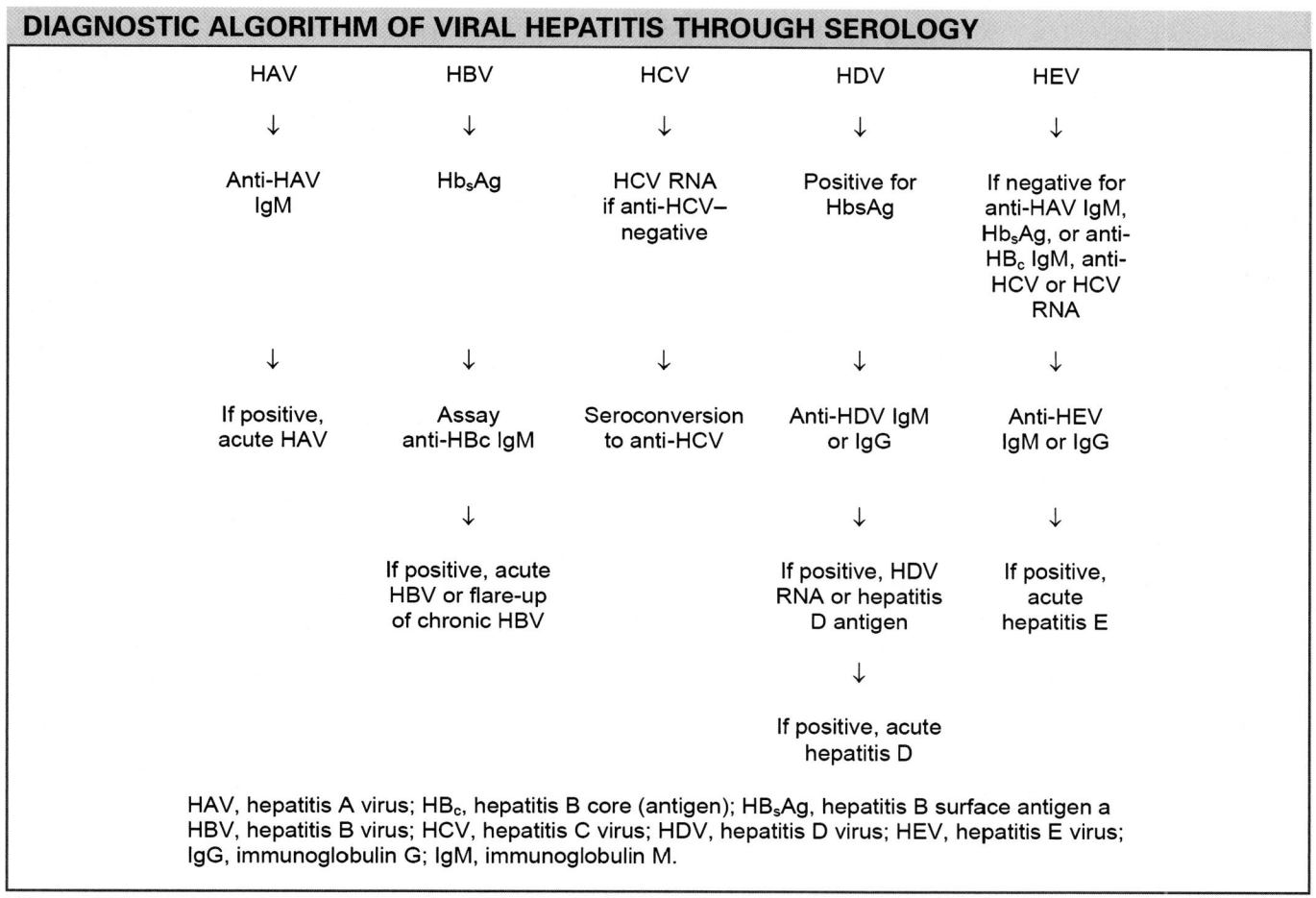

HAV	HBV	HCV	HDV	HEV
↓	↓	↓	↓	↓
Anti-HAV IgM	Hb$_s$Ag	HCV RNA if anti-HCV–negative	Positive for HbsAg	If negative for anti-HAV IgM, Hb$_s$Ag, or anti-HB$_c$ IgM, anti-HCV or HCV RNA
↓	↓	↓	↓	↓
If positive, acute HAV	Assay anti-HBc IgM	Seroconversion to anti-HCV	Anti-HDV IgM or IgG	Anti-HEV IgM or IgG
	↓		↓	↓
	If positive, acute HBV or flare-up of chronic HBV		If positive, HDV RNA or hepatitis D antigen	If positive, acute hepatitis E
			↓	
			If positive, acute hepatitis D	

HAV, hepatitis A virus; HB$_c$, hepatitis B core (antigen); HB$_s$Ag, hepatitis B surface antigen a HBV, hepatitis B virus; HCV, hepatitis C virus; HDV, hepatitis D virus; HEV, hepatitis E virus; IgG, immunoglobulin G; IgM, immunoglobulin M.

This serologic algorithm can be supplemented through the use of molecular tests for the presence, and quantitative measurement of viral RNA or DNA, but serologic tests will be sufficient in the majority of cases. (From the World Gastroenterology Organisation Practice Guidelines–Management of Acute Viral Hepatitis. December 2003. http://www.worldgastroenterology.org/guidelines/global-guidelines/management-of-acute-viral-hepatitis/acute-viral-hepatitis-english.)

Chronic Hepatitis

Chronic hepatitis is defined as chronic inflammation of the liver that persists for at least 6 months, or signs and symptoms of chronic liver disease in the presence of increased cytosolic enzymes.[427] It is characterized by ongoing inflammatory damage to hepatocytes, which are often accompanied by hepatocyte regeneration and scarring. Formerly, chronic hepatitis was subdivided into three forms (chronic persistent, chronic lobular, and chronic active) based on histologic characteristics. It was recognized that individuals often had each of these diseases at different points in time, and often in different areas of the liver in the same biopsy. Current classifications describe the cause and evaluate the severity of inflammatory injury (termed grade) and the extent of fibrosis

(termed stage). The importance of these findings will be discussed in detail later. Common causes of chronic hepatitis and tests used to make a specific etiologic diagnosis are listed in Table 51.4.

The clinical features of chronic hepatitis are highly variable. Most patients are asymptomatic, but nonspecific features, such as fatigue, lack of concentration, and weakness may be present. Most patients are diagnosed because of an unexplained abnormality in aminotransferase activities or detection of positive results on a screening test for a cause of chronic hepatitis. Moderate increases in plasma aminotransferase activities (an average of approximately twofold, and in most cases, less than fivefold) are characteristic, whereas results of most other tests are normal. Normal aminotransferase activities do not rule out histologic evidence of chronic hepatitis, especially in the presence of chronic viral hepatitis or NASH.[300,398,428,429] Characteristically, ALT is increased to a greater degree than AST,[430] although increases in both are common; reversal of the AST/ALT activity ratio to more than 1 suggests coexisting alcohol abuse or development of cirrhosis in patients with a variety of causes of chronic liver disease[431–434] (as discussed in greater detail later in this chapter). One study found that the AST/ALT ratio was significantly higher in women than in men[435]; however, in most studies in which the AST/ALT ratio was used, separate analyses were not done by sex. Although ALT is relatively specific for the liver, skeletal muscle sources for AST and ALT should always be considered, especially in physically active young individuals.[417,436,437] A finding of persistent increase of aminotransferase activity should lead to an evaluation for chronic hepatitis using the tests outlined in Table 51.4. A liver biopsy may be helpful in determining the cause, assessing severity, and following treatment. A specific etiologic diagnosis is essential because it dictates the treatment. The most common causes of chronic hepatitis are chronic HBV, HCV, and NASH, but a variety of other disease processes may cause chronic hepatitis.

Chronic Hepatitis B

Worldwide, HBV infection is the most important cause of chronic hepatitis.[438] According to the WHO, approximately 350 million individuals worldwide have chronic HBV infection; most cases are found in Asia, Africa, and southern Europe.

In most circumstances, HBV is not cytopathic because the injury results from an immune-mediated inflammatory attack against hepatocytes. Chronic hepatitis results when the immune response is incomplete and the virus is not eliminated from infected cells. This leads to a continuing cycle of viral replication, reinfection of regenerating hepatocytes, and immune damage to newly infected cells that is inadequate to clear infection. The details are not completely understood, but it appears that in normal circumstances, hepatocytes express surface markers (in this case, HBcAg and human leukocyte antigen [HLA] class 1 proteins).[439] Primed lymphocytes then attack the infected hepatocytes.[440] It appears that many chronic hepatitis B patients are deficient in or have an inadequate response to INF, and by inference, are unable to express HLA antigens that would attract an appropriate lymphocyte response.[441] The discovery of INF deficiency led to the successful use of IFN-α therapy in chronic HBV.

The clinical presentation may be complicated by various extrahepatic complications (which occur in 1 to 10% of those with HBV[351]), including polyarteritis, glomerulonephritis, polymyalgia rheumatica, cryoglobulinemia, myocarditis, and Guillain-Barré syndrome. These conditions are associated with circulating immune complexes containing HBsAg.[442] Immunocompromised persons, such as HBV/HIV coinfected individuals, typically have higher replication markers, less hepatic inflammation, and poorer survival than those with HIV alone.[443,444]

The natural history of chronic hepatitis B (defined by the persistence of HBsAg) varies.[254] Features of the different stages of chronic HBV are given in Table 51.5. It is convenient to divide chronic hepatitis B infection into two basic types—replicative and nonreplicative—although transitions between these stages are common. In the chronic replicative form, viral DNA is found in the cytoplasm of infected hepatocytes, and complete viral particles are produced and released into the circulation. In the replicating form of infection, viral loads in plasma are usually high ($>10^5$ copies/mL, often $>10^8$ copies/mL, or $>20,000$ IU/mL, often $>2 \times 10^7$ IU/mL; 1 IU/mL = 5.6 copies/mL). In those infected later in life who develop chronic hepatitis, evidence of hepatocyte injury (increased aminotransferase activity and inflammation in liver biopsy sections) is found in most cases (termed immune active[254] or chronic active phase). However, in those infected early in life, evidence of hepatocyte injury is often minimal; this has been referred to as the immunotolerant phase of chronic HBV. Those in the immune tolerant phase may

TABLE 51.4 Causes of Chronic Hepatitis and Diagnostic Strategies

Cause	Diagnosis
Hepatitis B	History, HBsAg, anti-HBs, anti-HBc, HBV DNA
Hepatitis C	Anti-HCV, HCV RNA by PCR
Autoimmune type 1	ANA, anti–smooth muscle antibody
Autoimmune type 2	SLA, anti-LKM1
Wilson disease	Ceruloplasmin
Drugs	History
AAT deficiency	AAT phenotype
Nonalcoholic fatty liver disease	Metabolic syndrome, liver ultrasound, liver biopsy
Idiopathic	Liver biopsy, absence of markers

AAT, α1-Antitrypsin; *ANA*, antinuclear antibody; *HBc*, hepatitis B core antigen; *HBsAg*, hepatitis B surface antigen; *HBV*, hepatitis B virus; *HCV*, hepatitis C virus; *LKM1*, liver-kidney microsomal antigen type 1; *PCR*, polymerase chain reaction; *SLA*, soluble liver antigen.

TABLE 51.5 Patterns of Chronic Hepatitis B Virus Infection

Type	AST/ALT	HBsAg	HBeAg	Anti-HBc	HBV DNA
Occult	Normal	Negative	Negative	Positive	Negative[a]
Immune control	Normal	Positive	Negative	Positive	Negative[a]
Immune tolerant	Normal	Positive	Negative/Positive	Positive	Positive
Immune active	Increased	Positive	Positive	Positive	Positive, viral load usually > 106 IU/mL
HBeAg-negative chronic hepatitis	Increased	Positive	Negative	Positive	Positive, viral load usually < 106 IU/mL

[a]May have very low level (usually <102 IU/mL) in serum.

ALT, Alanine aminotransferase; *AST*, aspartate aminotransferase; *HBc*, hepatitis B core antigen; *HBeAg*, hepatitis B e antigen; *HBsAg*, hepatitis B surface antigen; *HBV*, hepatitis B virus.

transition to the immune active phase, but do not always do so. In the nonreplicating form, circulating viral load is low or undetectable, and evidence of hepatocyte injury is usually absent. This variant has been termed the HBV carrier state, although current terminology describes this phase as the immune control phase. Traditionally, HBeAg had been used to differentiate replicative and nonreplicative types of chronic hepatitis, with negative HBeAg and positive anti-HBe believed to indicate the nonreplicating stage of infection. As discussed earlier, however, this distinction is inaccurate, and classification is based on HBV DNA concentrations, along with ALT activities and histology.[350] All of the three phases of chronic HBV are associated with the presence of HBsAg in serum. As mentioned earlier, occult HBV infection is present in many individuals previously exposed to HBV, but it is not associated with inflammation in the liver or increased aminotransferases.

In general, chronic HBV passes through stages in untreated persons. For those infected early in life, the immune tolerant phase is usually followed by an immune active phase that may vary in duration and may cause significant liver damage. This phase usually gives way to a protracted period of immune control, with HBsAg positivity or occult infection if HBsAg is cleared. For those infected individuals who go on to have chronic infection as older children or adults, the immune tolerant phase may be a short period or absent, leading straight into the immune active phase. Approximately 8 to 10% of persons per year will transition from the immune active to the immune control phase of chronic HBV.[259] A variable, but low, proportion of those in the immune control phase will revert to the immune active phase (mainly dependent on genotype).[350] Approximately 0.5 to 1% of persons per year will convert from HBsAg positive to HBsAg negative, entering the occult phase of infection (or, in a minority, resolved HBV). Each of these transitions can be associated with an acute rise in aminotransferase activities in a clinical picture that mimics acute viral hepatitis, as discussed earlier.

For individuals who have chronic replicating infection, the major risk is development of cirrhosis and HCC. An estimated 20 to 30% of individuals with chronic hepatitis B will develop cirrhosis over a 20-year follow-up period; the risk is directly related to the amount of HBV DNA, with risk progressively increasing at viral loads of more than 2000 IU/mL (10,000 copies/mL).[445] Once cirrhosis has developed, a 1.5 to 5% annual risk of development of HCC is noted. Although the risk of HCC is lower in individuals with HBV infection who do not have cirrhosis, risk is directly related to viral load and rises at quantities above 2000 IU/mL.[446] Even a person in the nonreplicating stage of infection has a 10-fold higher risk of HCC.[279] On a worldwide basis, hepatitis B infection is the most common cause of liver cancer.

Efficacy of treatment is typically measured by response of ALT and/or AST and HBV DNA; goals of treatment include normalization of ALT and suppression of HBV DNA below the limits of detection of assays, ideally with detection limits of approximately 20 to 50 IU/mL. With polymerase inhibitors, approximately 70 to 80% of patients will achieve these goals within 1 year of treatment. Duration of treatment is largely dependent on HBeAg status before the start of therapy, and for those who are HBeAg positive before treatment, the duration depends on the response of HBeAg on therapy. For those who are HBeAg negative, treatment typically is

continued indefinitely, as long as treatment is effective. For those who are HBeAg positive before treatment, loss of HBeAg and development of anti-HBe indicate a high likelihood of maintenance of HBV DNA control and normalization of ALT once treatment is stopped (after 6 to 12 months of further treatment once anti-HBe appears). With INF therapy, response rates to 1 year of treatment are somewhat lower than with polymerase inhibitors, but treatment requires only 6 to 12 months. Loss of HBsAg is uncommon; with most agents, the likelihood of loss of HBsAg usually is not higher than that in untreated persons, although it may be higher with INF and tenofovir.[259]

Chronic Hepatitis C

Approximately 170 million individuals worldwide have been diagnosed with chronic HCV infection; most cases are found in North America, Northern Europe, and Japan.[447] In contrast to HBV, the risk of chronic hepatitis does not appear related to age at exposure (although perinatal infection is uncommon with HCV), and the likelihood of chronic infection is much higher overall. Many studies state an approximate 80 to 85% likelihood of chronic infection by HCV; this interpretation is based on the frequency of finding HCV RNA on a chronic basis among those who are anti-HCV positive. However, as mentioned earlier, many individuals who clear HCV with acute exposure never develop or lose anti-HCV. Among persons followed prospectively after an acute HCV infection, chronic HCV infection actually developed in only about 50 to 70%.[369,448,449] Once viremia becomes established beyond 6 months after initial exposure, it essentially never resolves spontaneously; in one study of 320 patients followed serially for more than 3 years, only 6 patients with end-stage liver disease lost detectable HCV RNA.[450] HCV viral load fluctuates little over time; in most individuals, viral load differs by less than 0.5 log,[451,452] and gradually increases by an average of 0.2 to 0.3 log/year.[451,453] It is estimated that approximately 20 to 30% of patients with hepatitis C will progress to cirrhosis over a period of 20 years.[454] The frequency of progression appears to be increased by age older than 40 years at the time of infection, male sex, alcohol abuse,[455] and immunosuppression, but it is less than 5% after 20 years of infection in those infected during the first 20 to 30 years of life.[368,448,449,456] In those who develop recurrent HCV after liver transplantation, the response rate is lower, and the rate of progression to cirrhosis is faster than in primary infection. As with HBV, the likelihood of progression to HCC is between 1.5 and 5% per year in those with cirrhosis.[457]

The clinical picture of chronic HCV is similar to that of HBV in producing chronic hepatitis. Infection with HCV is characterized by fluctuating ALT activities over time. Only about one-third of those with chronic HCV have continually increased ALT, and many of these individuals show variation in ALT activity.[458] It is common for individuals with fluctuating values to have multiple normal ALT activity values interspersed with increased values.[426,459] Individuals with normal ALT tend to have milder fibrosis and less severe disease on liver biopsy, but a minority have advanced fibrosis.[300] In contrast to HBV, individuals with continually normal ALT activity have a similar rate of response to antiviral treatment.[300]

Dramatic advances in the treatment of chronic hepatitis C have revolutionized outcomes for patients and changed the requirements for laboratory testing in the management of patients

TABLE 51.6   Tests for Evaluating Chronic Hepatitis C Virus Infection and Its Treatment

Time of Testing	Test	Condition	Use/Interpretation
Pretreatment	HCV viral load	Detectable	Baseline (to compare with 12-week value)
	Genotype	2 or 3 vs. other	Length of treatment (24-week genotype if 2 or 3, 48-week if other genotype)
4 weeks on treatment	HCV viral load	Undetectable	Rapid virologic response—high likelihood of treatment success
12 weeks on treatment	HCV viral load	<2 log drop	Stop treatment (nonresponder)[a]
		>2 log drop	Continue treatment (on treatment responder)
End of treatment[b]	Sensitive HCV RNA[c]	Detectable	Nonresponder or breakthrough (if was previously undetectable)
24 weeks after completion	Sensitive HCV RNA[d]	Not detectable	Treatment responder
		Detectable	Relapser
		Not detectable	Sustained virologic responder

HCV, Hepatitis C virus.

[a]Less than 3% chance of sustained virologic response; some continue treatment to 24 weeks and reevaluate.
[b]Done at 24 weeks if genotype 2 or 3, done at 48 weeks if other genotypes; not all recommend evaluating end of treatment response.
[c]Lower detection limit less than 50 IU/mL.
[d]Done only if genotype not 2 or 3.

on treatment. Directly acting antiviral agents that target critical HCV proteins have been shown to cure infection in most patients. Tests for evaluating chronic HCV infection and its treatment are shown in Table 51.6. Although this remains a rapidly evolving field, it is highly likely that it will be possible to cure infection within the next decade[460] in any patient capable of adhering to a full course of treatment. HCV susceptibility to these drugs is determined by HCV genotype; therefore genotyping before treatment remains mandatory. This permits the treating clinician to select the most appropriate combination of drugs and the correct duration of therapy. Tests are used to monitor response to treatment by measuring serum HCV RNA concentrations during and 4 and 12 weeks after the end of treatment. Patients who have undetectable HCV RNA 12 weeks after the end of treatment are considered cured. The extent to which liver fibrosis reverses in patients who attain clearance of HCV still needs to be established, but studies of patients who have been cured using INF-based therapies suggest that the long-term risks of liver cancer and bleeding varices are reduced even in cirrhotic patients who attain clearance of HCV.[461]

Hepatitis B and C coinfection. Approximately 2 to 10% of individuals infected with HCV are coinfected with HBV; of those with chronic HBV, 15 to 20% are also HCV positive.[462,463] Clinical and laboratory features of coinfected patients are somewhat contradictory and differ from those in individuals infected with a single hepatitis virus. Coinfected patients have lower viral loads than do those with single infection.[464] In patients with chronic HBV who develop acute HCV infection, the likelihood of progressing to chronic HCV infection is low,[465] and acute infection with HBV can lead to clearance of HCV.[466] These features would suggest a beneficial effect of coinfection. In contrast, patients with chronic HBV/HCV coinfection have more rapid progression to cirrhosis.[467] Patients with acute coinfection have severe acute hepatitis more frequently.[463,468] Some studies suggest a high frequency of HBV DNA viral replication in the liver even in the absence of circulating HBsAg; such subclinically coinfected patients have more severe liver injury and a higher frequency of cirrhosis.[469,470] Despite some favorable findings, the outcome of hepatitis in coinfected patients seems to be worse than for those infected with only a single agent.

Nonalcoholic Fatty Liver Disease and Nonalcoholic Steatohepatitis

NAFLD is now a major cause of chronic liver disease and is increasing in prevalence.[471] Ludwig and colleagues first described patients who had histologic features identical to those of alcoholic hepatitis (including hepatocyte ballooning, presence of Mallory hyaline, and neutrophil infiltration), but who had no history of heavy alcohol intake and did not have AST values higher than ALT values.[472] They introduced the term NASH to describe this entity, which was more common in women than in men, and was usually associated with diabetes and/or obesity. (Because alcohol ingestion is common in the population, and alcoholic liver disease does not occur with daily ingestion of less than 20 g ethanol, this threshold has been suggested as the maximum alcohol intake compatible with a diagnosis of NAFLD.)[473,474] It is now recognized that NAFLD is associated strongly with the presence of the metabolic syndrome; almost half of individuals who meet the criteria for metabolic syndrome have NAFLD, and as many as 20 to 30% of the population in North America and Europe has NAFLD,[475] making it far and away the most common form of liver disease and an extremely common condition in the population in the developed world.[476] Approximately 10% of those with NAFLD have the more severe form, NASH. The frequency in obese or diabetic individuals is much higher, with NAFLD in 60 to 75% and NASH in 20 to 25%.[474,477] Prospective studies of patients with liver disease have confirmed that NASH is a common cause of increased liver enzymes in an unselected population of patients referred to gastroenterologists or seen in primary care settings.[478–480] The frequency of cirrhosis in NASH is not well established, but it has been suggested that NASH may be a major cause of cryptogenic cirrhosis, that is, cirrhosis for which no underlying cause can be determined. Because weight loss develops with chronic illness, fat may disappear from the liver, leaving only fibrosis.

Current evidence suggests that accumulation of fat in NAFLD is a consequence of insulin resistance. A variety of mechanisms may lead to insulin resistance, including genetic predisposition, increased concentrations of free fatty acids, and the presence of cytokines such as TNF-α. Because TNF-α is produced at a rate that correlates with body fat mass and is critical to development of insulin resistance in obesity, it may be a key factor in the development of NAFLD. However, the pathogenesis is likely to be more complicated because a variety of other factors lead to increased fat accumulation in the liver, including increased carbohydrate intake, certain drugs, and mutations in lipid synthesis, but they have not been associated with the development of NASH.

A clinical approach to the identification of patients with NASH typically involves a compatible clinical history and the presence of steatosis on imaging studies, exclusion of other causes of liver injury, and may include liver biopsy to confirm the diagnosis and determine the extent of injury (but not if patients improve clinically with weight loss and exercise). Although increased activities of liver enzymes are often used to distinguish NASH from other forms of NAFLD, the degree of necroinflammatory damage is not related to increases in AST or ALT activity, and the likelihood of significant liver damage is similar in those with normal or increased ALT.[429] The search for laboratory tests capable of identifying the minority of patients with NASH among the large numbers of individuals with NAFLD have highlighted CK18[481,482] and PIIINP[483] as potential serum markers of NASH.

Greater progress has been made in the identification and validation of blood tests for liver fibrosis in NAFLD with a variety of indirect and direct tests being validated for this purpose, including the NAFLD Fibrosis Score, BARD (calculated from body mass index, AST/ALT ratio and diabetes), and the Enhanced Liver Fibrosis (ELF) test.[483–486]

Of these, both the NASH Fibrosis Score and ELF tests have been shown to predict long-term outcomes in NAFLD. It remains to be seen if these tests either alone or in conjunction with other tests will be capable of accurately stratifying patients with NAFLD into those with NASH and those with fibrosis.

To date, major treatments for NAFLD have been aimed at lowering body weight and fat content. Loss of weight is often associated with decreased ALT values; in one study, a 1% decrease in weight was associated with an 8% decrease in ALT activity.[487] The association of NAFLD with insulin resistance has suggested treatment with antidiabetic medications, particularly those that increase insulin responsiveness (such as peroxisome proliferator-activated receptor-γ agonists and metformin); studies have not been conclusive as to the benefits of such treatment.[488]

Autoimmune Hepatitis

AIH represents a rapidly progressive form of chronic hepatitis, with up to 40% 6-month mortality in untreated individuals[489]; it is associated with the presence of autoimmune markers. It is relatively uncommon, with an annual incidence of 1.9 cases per 100,000 population in the United States,[490] but it is responsible for 3 to 6% of all liver transplantations[491]; the disease recurs in approximately 30% of patients after transplantation.[492] As with most autoimmune diseases, there is a strong female predominance. Forms of AIH have been found in individuals of all ages, with no racial or ethnic predilection. It has been associated with specific HLA haplotypes, notably DR3 and DR4, as is true for many other autoimmune diseases. Practice guidelines on autoimmune chronic hepatitis have been developed by the American Association for the Study of Liver Diseases or AASLD.[493]

AIH is associated with the presence of liver and nonliver autoantibodies in plasma. These are helpful in diagnosis but are not likely to be the cause of liver injury. The most important antibodies for diagnosis include antinuclear antibody (ANA), anti–smooth muscle (or anti-actin) antibody (ASMA), anti-liver–kidney microsomal antigen type 1, and antisoluble liver antigen (SLA), which is insensitive but highly specific. A variety of other autoantibodies are found frequently in AIH, some of which are found in other disorders. A summary of the most common autoantibodies, their associations, and their molecular targets (when known) is given in Table 51.7. Tests for these autoimmune markers initially used cell or tissue preparations studied by indirect immunofluorescence,

TABLE 51.7 Serologic Markers of Autoimmune Liver Disease

Antibody Name	Antigen Target	Associations
Antiactin	Actin	AIH type 1; more specific than ASMA, poor response to corticosteroids, early age of onset
Anti-asialoglycoprotein receptor	Transmembrane antigen binding protein	AIH, correlate with activity, disappear with successful treatment
Anti–LKM1	Cytochrome P450 2D6	AIH type 2; seen in only 4% of US cases; usually in children
Anti–liver-specific cytosol	Enzyme (possibly formiminotransferase cyclodeaminase or argininosuccinate lyase)	AIH in younger patients, often with anti-LKM1, primary sclerosing cholangitis; vary with activity of disease
Antimitochondrial antibody	Dihydrolipoamide acyltransferase	Primary biliary cirrhosis
Antineutrophil cytoplasmic antibodies	Bactericidal/permeability protein, cathepsin G, lactoferrin	PSC (50–70%), ulcerative colitis (50–70%), AIH; nonspecific
Antinuclear antibody	Multiple targets (centromere, ribonucleoproteins); may not be detected by ELISA	AIH type 1, some PSC cases
ASMA	Actin, tubulin, vimentin, desmin, skelitin	AIH type 1, seen in other autoimmune diseases in lower titers
Antisoluble liver antigen/ liver pancreas	UGA tRNA suppressor–associated transfer protein	AIH type 3; specific for AIH, correlate with relapse after corticosteroid withdrawal

AIH, Autoimmune hepatitis; *ASMA*, anti–smooth muscle antigen; *ELISA*, enzyme-linked immunosorbent assay; *LKM1*, liver-kidney microsome; *PSC*, primary sclerosing cholangitis.

but these have largely been replaced by assays that detect antibodies to purified proteins. Individuals who are negative for common autoantibodies, but who otherwise meet criteria for diagnosis, have a similar prognosis and response to treatment.[494]

Criteria for the diagnosis of AIH were developed by an international group[495] and subsequently revised[496]; a simplified scoring system has also been developed.[497] The simplified criteria include exclusion of viral hepatitis, increased plasma IgG concentration, positive autoantibodies, and compatible histologic features.

It is controversial whether AIH should be further divided into subtypes; the international group that codified diagnostic criteria does not recommend use of subtypes,[496] but many authorities recognize three different forms (types 1, 2, and 3). Although differences in epidemiology may be evident among the different forms, there do not seem to be differences in clinical course or response to treatment. Type 1, which is the most common form and the only one seen frequently in North America, is predominantly a disease of middle-aged women. It is characterized by ASMA or anti-actin (found in 87% of cases) and/or ANA (found in 67% of cases); one or the other is present in nearly 100% of cases. Because of the nonspecific nature of these antibodies, the strength of the antibody reaction (titer or immunoassay signal) is important in determining the likelihood of AIH. In children, the strength of the reaction is typically lower than in adults. Type 2 AIH, which characteristically occurs in children (although 20% occurs in adults), represents up to 20% of cases in Europe. It is associated with antibodies to liver–kidney microsomal antigen 1 or cytochrome P$_{450}$ 2D6 (CYP2D6).[498] Some cross-reactivity has been noted between this antibody and certain HCV antigens, leading to positive anti-CYP2D6 in individuals with HCV infection. The epitopes recognized by anti-HCV antibodies are different from those in persons with type 2 AIH.[499] Type 3 often lacks other autoimmune markers but is positive for antibodies to soluble liver antigen liver–pancreas. This antibody is directed against the UGA tRNA suppressor-associated antigenic protein.[500]

Immunosuppressive treatment using prednisone, alone or in combination with azathioprine, is effective in inducing clinical remission of disease in approximately 80% of cases; other immunosuppressants are now being used to reduce dependence on corticosteroids.[501] Because inherited differences in the activity of thiopurine methyltransferase affect approximately 10% of the population,[502] it has been recommended that pretreatment determination of enzyme activity should be used to reduce the likelihood of toxicity. Remission typically begins with improvement in symptoms, followed by normalization in laboratory abnormalities, and finally, histologic resolution. Laboratory remission generally does not occur until after at least 12 months of treatment, but it almost always occurs within 24 months in responders. Histologic remission is less common and usually requires at least 3 to 6 months longer than laboratory evidence of remission.[489] Sustained remission can persist off-treatment in 80% of those with normal histology after therapy, but relapse occurs in 50% within 6 months if inflammation persists in the liver biopsy.[503] Liver biochemistry and serum IgG concentrations can be used to identify patients in whom immunosuppression can be safely withdrawn.[504]

Inherited Liver Disease Presenting as Chronic Hepatitis

Inherited liver diseases that present as chronic hepatitis include hemochromatosis, Wilson disease, and AAT deficiency.

Hemochromatosis. Hereditary hemochromatosis (HH) is an autosomal recessive disorder of iron metabolism that results in excessive iron absorption and accumulation in tissues, specifically in the parenchymal cells of the liver, heart, pancreas, and other organs (see also Chapters 40 and 44). HH is caused by mutations that affect any of the proteins that control the entry of iron into the circulation. These proteins include hepcidin, HFE, transferrin receptor 2 (Tfr2), hemojuvelin (HJV) (these proteins all sense iron accumulation that hepcidin acts to correct), and the protein ferroportin (FPN), which is a cellular transporter of iron, normally downregulated by hepcidin. The transcription activity of the gene HAMP is the main regulator of hepcidin expression.[505] Hepcidin is believed to be the major regulator of dietary iron absorption and cellular iron release. It regulates iron by counteracting the function of FPN, the major cellular iron exporter in the membranes of macrophages, hepatocytes, and the basolateral site of enterocytes. Hepcidin induces the internalization and degradation of FPN, which results in increased intracellular iron stores, decreased dietary iron absorption, and decreased circulating iron concentrations. Patients with most forms of HH are unable to appropriately upregulate hepcidin synthesis in response to increased iron stores. This dysregulation is caused by defects in certain genes encoding positive regulators of hepcidin. *Hjv* and *hamp* are genes involved in the production of hepcidin, a peptide that regulates iron homeostasis by adjusting its absorption. *Hjv* and *hamp* mutations, therefore lead to decreased hepcidin concentrations, and consequently to iron overload in the body.[506]

Hemochromatosis is classified on the basis of the genetic abnormality as type 1 (*Hfe* C282Y homozygote), HJV-related (type 2A), HAMP-related (type 2B), or tfr2-associated (type 3) or type 4, which is hemochromatosis caused by mutations in SLC40A1 that lead to ferroportin gain of activity.[507]

HH Type 1 is primarily a disease in men and postmenopausal women with common clinical features, including lethargy and weakness, arthralgia, loss of libido, upper abdominal discomfort, hepatomegaly, grey/bronze skin pigmentation, testicular atrophy, and joint swelling and/or tenderness. Untreated, HH can lead to serious complications, including liver fibrosis and cirrhosis with HCC in approximately 30% of patients with cirrhosis, diabetes mellitus, and cardiomyopathy, and arrhythmias. Cardiac and endocrine cells are more susceptible to rapid iron loading because they have more mitochondria and less antioxidants.[508]

The gene for HH Type 1 has long been linked to chromosome 6, close to the genes for the HLA system; it has been definitively identified and termed the *Hfe* gene, which codes for a 343-residue type I transmembrane glycoprotein similar to the class I major histocompatibility complex (MHC) molecule.[509,510] The protein product of the *Hfe* gene is a 343-residue type I transmembrane glycoprotein that resembles the MHC class I protein molecules in sequence and three-dimensional structure (CC). Both the HFE and MHC class I proteins contain a membrane-bound heavy chain with three extracellular domains. HFE protein regulates iron uptake by binding to the transferrin receptor (TfR) on cell membranes and acts as an iron sensor that controls the release of hepcidin. Most cases of hemochromatosis are caused by alterations in the genes that regulate hepcidin synthesis, including *Hfe*, *Tfr2*, and *Hjv*. Deficiency of hepcidin activity in macrophages and enterocytes leads to unrestricted Fpn-mediated iron export into the circulation. Hepcidin secretion is part of the innate immune response induced by inflammation and infection. It serves to restrict the amount of iron available for use by invading pathogens.[508,511] In North America and Europe, more than 90% of individuals with HH are homozygous for a single point mutation that encodes a tyrosine instead of cysteine at residue 282 (termed the C282Y mutation).[511] Although it is a frequent genetic trait (estimated to be found in 1 in 8 persons of northern European ancestry carrying this mutation, with approximately 1 in 250 being homozygous), most individuals who are homozygous for this mutation do not develop evidence of iron overload. A large population-based study showed that only 28% of males and approximately 1% of females homozygous for the C282Y mutation develop HH.[512]

However over their lifetimes up to approximately 60 to 70% of C282Y homozygotes will develop iron overload even if they do not develop HH. Approximately 2% of people with HH are compound heterozygotes for two different mutations in *Hfe* with the C282Y gene mutation carried on one chromosome and the H63D mutation carried in *Hfe* on the chromosome inherited from the other parent. Clearly, the family members of individuals with HH, unaffected C282Y, compound heterozygotes, and C282Y heterozygotes may be at increased risk of having HH and should be advised to have the gene test and iron studies performed.[513,514]

Liver disease due to hemochromatosis is rare in younger individuals but becomes more common after the age of 30 years. Liver function tests are frequently normal in asymptomatic patients but may be abnormal in symptomatic patients. The most useful tests are fasting transferrin saturation and serum ferritin. The transferrin saturation reflects increased iron absorption, and a value more than 45% is the most sensitive marker of early iron overload, but neither a raised fasting transferrin saturation nor ferritin concentration is diagnostic of HH. Ferritin is also an acute-phase reactant and can be raised nonspecifically in the presence of alcohol consumption, inflammation, and other liver disease. Serum ferritin is considered to be abnormal when it is more than 250 μg/L in premenopausal women and more than 300 μg/L in men and postmenopausal women. If the fasting transferrin saturation or serum ferritin is increased on more than one occasion, HH should be suspected, even if there are no clinical symptoms or abnormal liver function tests. In this situation, the *Hfe* gene test should be requested. Iron studies may be normal in individuals with a genetic predisposition to HH who have not developed iron overload. Up to 40% of homozygotes have normal results in iron studies, which may be due to overt (blood donation) or covert (gynecologic or GI) blood loss. The likelihood of liver disease is related to serum ferritin concentrations. Follow-up of all patients with iron overload should occur regardless of the HFE gene test. It is suggested that if the patient is C282Y homozygous without iron overload, then iron studies should be repeated every 2 to 5 years. If the patient is C282Y homozygotic and has iron overload, then lifelong venesection is necessary, usually every 2 to 3 months after the results of iron studies have become normal. The patient should also reduce their red meat and

alcohol intake. Noncirrhotic patients who are treated early have a normal life expectancy. Cirrhosis is unlikely if the ferritin is less than 1000 μg/L, plasma AST activities are normal, and there is no hepatomegaly. Cirrhotic patients rarely regress to normal and have a lifelong risk of HCC.[513,514]

There are rarer forms of disease that also lead to iron accumulation in the liver which can lead to cirrhosis. Aceruloplasminemia is caused by homozygous mutations in the *Cp* (encoding ceruloplasmin) gene causing very low concentrations of plasma iron and transferrin saturation, which causes anemia, but patients have systemic iron excess. It is possible that this is due to the loss of the ferroxidase activity of ceruloplasmin, limiting iron release from macrophages into plasma.[515] Usually the spleen is not overloaded with iron, and the liver has iron deposition in hepatocytes, suggesting that the precise mechanisms governing organ iron distribution are not yet understood. The potential effect of anemia in favoring iron excess through the downregulation of hepcidin expression has been proposed. Whether compensatory ferroxidase activity by hephaestin has a role in ensuring iron export from macrophages despite low ceruloplasmin-related ferroxidase activity should be considered.[507] Aceruloplasminemia presents with very low ceruloplasmin concentrations and magnetic resonance imaging (MRI) and CT scans which are strongly suggestive of Wilson disease, which we describe next. It is often complicated by neuropsychiatric disease including movement disorders and dysarthria with iron deposition in the basal ganglia which can be visualized with MRI.

Wilson disease. Wilson disease is an autosomal recessive disorder of copper metabolism.[410] It has a gene frequency of 1 in 200 and a disease frequency of 1 in 30,000. It is due to 1 of more than 7700 mutations in a gene on chromosome 13 that codes for a copper-transporting adenosine triphosphatase (ATP7B).[411,412] (http://www.hgmd.cf.ac.uk/ac/index.php) This enzyme, found mainly in the liver, is involved in the movement of copper into bile and delivers copper for the synthesis of ceruloplasmin, the major copper-transporting protein in the body; deficiency leads to accumulation of copper in the liver and eventually in other tissues. Mutations in the ATP7B and inactivation of the QATP7B transporter in hepatocytes leads to failure to excrete copper in the bile which in turn leads to disturbances in copper homeostasis. Oxidative stress caused by reactive oxygen species is probably the cause of the liver damage associated with copper accumulation. This oxidative stress leads to damage to lipids, proteins, and DNA and RNA molecules. Copper toxicity may also lead to the induction of apoptosis via the activation of acid sphingomyelinase.[516] Pathologic changes include astrogliosis, demyelination, and tissue disintegration, most often seen in the basal ganglia, thalamus, cerebellum, and upper brainstem.[517] The rapid release of copper caused by mass hepatocyte necrosis in Wilson disease mimics copper toxicity and leads to nonautoimmune hemolytic anemia accompanied by rhabdomyolysis and renal tubular damage.

Guidelines on diagnosis and treatment of Wilson disease have been updated.[518]

Wilson disease usually manifests at age younger than 30 years,[519] and for reasons that are unknown, patients usually present either with the hepatic or the neuropsychiatric form of the disease. In children, hepatic involvement tends to predominate, whereas, in adolescents and adults, the neuropsychiatric form becomes more common. Patients presenting with neuropsychiatric manifestations commonly have advanced liver disease at the time of presentation, whereas those presenting with liver disease may have little in the way of neurologic damage. Hepatic manifestations include fulminant hepatitis (as discussed earlier), but more commonly, chronic hepatitis, with or without cirrhosis, is the presenting finding.[520,521] Studies attempting to find genotype-phenotype correlations have been unsuccessful.[522–527]

Studies involving homogeneous twins with Wilson disease who present with different phenotypes suggest that epigenetic mechanisms may be involved with the pathogenesis of the disease.[528–530] Environmental or nutritional factors may involve methionine metabolism as this has a regulatory effect on DNA methylation.[531,532] Occasionally, the features mimic those of AIH, with increased plasma globulins and positive ANAs.[533]

The classic clinical finding of increased copper deposition in the eye is the Kayser-Fleischer ring, caused by deposition of copper at the edge of the cornea. Although found in approximately 95% of patients with neurologic or psychiatric manifestations, it is present in only approximately one-half of patients with hepatic forms of Wilson disease[532] and is rarely present in children.[534] As mentioned earlier, hemolytic anemia and renal failure commonly accompany acute forms of Wilson disease; hemolytic anemia may be episodic even in chronic forms of Wilson disease.[518] Abnormal lipid metabolism is commonly associated with either copper overload or deficiency and is observed in Wilson disease, NAFLD, and diabetes mellitus. The assembly of chylomicrons, blood vessel formation, myelination of neurons, wound healing, and the immune response depend on copper homeostasis.[535]

Several laboratory tests are available for the diagnosis of Wilson disease; ceruloplasmin measurement is discussed in detail in Chapter 31 and copper measurement in Chapters 39 and 44. Test results are often affected by other conditions, sometimes making diagnosis difficult. Classic findings of Wilson disease include decreased plasma ceruloplasmin, decreased total plasma copper, increased plasma-free (or non-ceruloplasmin) copper, increased urine copper excretion, and increased hepatic copper content. Ceruloplasmin is a ferroxidase that typically is measured by enzymatic activity or by immunoassay. The controversy is ongoing over which assay format is preferable, and guidelines have not specified one type.[176,518] Plasma ceruloplasmin concentrations are low in infants, gradually rise to higher concentrations than adult concentrations in early childhood, then gradually decline to adult concentrations. The use of age-appropriate reference intervals is critical for diagnosis in children. Ceruloplasmin is an acute-phase protein, and its synthesis is induced by estrogen; concentrations may be falsely normal with acute illness or with high estrogen states. Low concentrations of ceruloplasmin are seen with malnutrition, in protein-losing states, and cirrhosis of any cause. These preanalytical variables cause ceruloplasmin to have low predictive value as a single test for Wilson disease; in one study of patients with chronic hepatitis, the positive predictive value was only 6%.[536] Ceruloplasmin is also decreased in approximately 20% of heterozygous carriers of the Wilson disease gene.[537] Because most plasma copper is bound to ceruloplasmin, total plasma copper is affected by factors that affect ceruloplasmin. Some experts recommend estimation of free (non-ceruloplasmin) copper as the difference between total copper

(micrograms per deciliter) and ceruloplasmin (3× mg/dL); values more than 25 μg/dL (3.9 μmol/L) suggest Wilson disease.[538] Measurement of urine copper excretion is the most specific noninvasive test for Wilson disease; 24-hour urine copper excretion is typically more than 100 μg/24 hours (15.7 μmol/24 hours) in Wilson disease. Unfortunately, the clinical sensitivity of copper excretion appears to be only 75 to 85%.[415,534] The diagnosis of Wilson disease is usually based on biochemical findings. If observed in combination with low ceruloplasmin concentrations, the presence of Kayser-Fleisher rings is almost pathognomonic. If timing during diagnostic testing is an issue and if the results from molecular genetic testing may not be available immediately, quantification of hepatic copper content (on biopsy) may be required. In this instance, molecular genetic testing is also strongly encouraged for confirmation.[535,539]

Treatment of active, symptomatic Wilson disease is aimed at increasing urine copper excretion to eliminate excess copper from the tissue. The primary therapy for Wilson disease usually involves chelating agents such as D-penicillamine and trientine, which is now more widely used because of its lower rate of side effects. Zinc (particularly zinc acetate) inhibits copper absorption from the intestinal tract; it is usually used for maintenance treatment after copper chelation, but it can also be used as initial therapy. Monitoring treatment (particularly with zinc) by annual measurement of urine copper excretion can be helpful in ensuring that excess copper is no longer being excreted.[518]

Alpha₁-antitrypsin deficiency. Alpha₁-antitrypsin is the most important of the serine protease inhibitors (collectively termed serpins; see also Chapter 31). As its name implies, AAT inhibits trypsin, but it also inhibits other proteolytic enzymes, including neutrophil-derived elastase, cathepsin G, and proteinase 3. It is produced principally in the liver but also in neutrophils, monocytes, and airway epithelial cells. The gene for AAT (originally called *PI*, but now called SERPINA1) is located on chromosome 14, is highly polymorphic, and over 150 alleles have been described. Several genetic variants of AAT (differing by a single amino acid) have been classified on the basis of their electrophoretic mobility; the slowest migrating of these was termed the Z variant. Some variants, particularly S and Z, form loop sheet polymers,[540] causing impaired release from the endoplasmic reticulum, hepatocytic inclusions of AAT, and reduced plasma concentrations. This disease is a hereditary, co-dominant autosomal disorder characterized by a high risk of developing emphysema at any age. The most severe forms of disease have been associated with homozygosity for the Z variant, which is found in 1 in 1000 to 2000 individuals in Europe and North America.[541] This variant is due to a point mutation that causes retention of the AAT within hepatocytes and other AAT producing cells. There is no detectable AAT in serum and the mutation which generally occurs is due to a premature stop codon. However, it is estimated that only approximately 10% of those with AAT deficiency develop clinical disease.[542] Lung disease in adults can manifest as early as the third decade of life and occurs mainly due to loss-of-function characterized by an inadequate protease protection of the lung. Circulating and intrapulmonary polymers of misfolded AAT, particularly the Z variant, as well as gain-of-function endoplasmic reticulum (ER) stress-related effects in monocytes and neutrophils play a role in the inflammatory manifestations of the disease.[543]

Liver disease in children and adults is associated with gain-of-function effects due to the accumulation of misfolded AAT protein within the ER of hepatocytes. Gain-of-function effects in liver manifest through two principal mechanisms: the perturbation of homeostasis within the lumen of the ER and the production of polymers of Z AAT within the circulation that can cause chemotaxis and activation of inflammatory cells.[543] The effects of AAT deficiency on the liver are controversial. In neonates, AAT deficiency is often associated with hepatitis; in one study, almost one-third of infants with prolonged jaundice were found to be AAT deficient.[544] Approximately 20% of AAT-deficient infants develop hepatitis,[545] with up to 25% 1-year mortality.[546] However, in those who survive the first year, evidence of liver injury diminishes and usually resolves by age 12 years.[547,548] At age 18 years, none of 183 individuals with AAT deficiency had clinical evidence of liver disease, none had increased plasma procollagen III peptide concentrations, and less than 20% had increased concentrations of liver-associated enzymes.[549]

Data on the association of AAT deficiency with liver disease in adults are somewhat contradictory.[550] In several studies, cirrhosis was present in one-third to one-half of those with AAT deficiency, and HCC was present in approximately one-third of those with cirrhosis.[551,552] The frequency was similar in those with heterozygous and homozygous presence of the PiZ variant.[552] In two studies of patients with cryptogenic liver disease, the frequency of the PiZ heterozygotes was significantly higher than that found in the general population.[553,554] However, two other studies found a similar frequency of liver disease in those with AAT deficiency and controls.[555,556] Some evidence suggests that AAT deficiency may increase risk of liver damage from other factors. In one study, most individuals with AAT deficiency and liver injury were also positive for anti-HCV; only 11% had no other liver risk factors.[557] In those with AAT deficiency and no evidence of liver disease (usually viral-related), life expectancy was no different from that of healthy controls. A 2007 research conference found evidence that defects in degradation of AAT underlie differences in protein accumulation, which is necessary for the development of liver disease.[558] It is likely that, as with hemochromatosis, the abnormal form of AAT is necessary, but perhaps not sufficient, to cause liver disease.

AAT is estimated by protein electrophoresis, in which it constitutes most of the α_1-globulin band; this was the original means by which AAT deficiency was recognized.[551] It can also be quantified by a variety of other techniques (see Chapter 31). AAT is an acute-phase response protein; misleadingly normal concentrations have been reported in approximately 40% of PiZ heterozygotes,[559] although rarely in PiZZ homozygotes. This is due to the acute-phase response increasing AAT concentrations into the reference range, a consequence that may affect other proteins produced by the liver, including ferritin and ceruloplasmin. Determination of phenotype was typically accomplished by isoelectric focusing and had been recommended as the diagnostic test of choice in one guideline,[176] but phenotyping cannot distinguish true homozygotes from heterozygotes who have a null genotype on the other *AAT* gene. Molecular tests are now available to determine *AAT* genotype.[560] Most laboratories provide genotype allele specific amplification of the most common alleles associated with deficiency, Z and S. Genotyping can be performed using DNA from using dried blood spots, saliva, or whole blood. Reflex testing for risk alleles is usually performed by PI typing using isoelectric focusing. S and Z alleles are present in greater than 95% of all AAT deficient individuals; approximately 5% will have a rare allele associated with reduced, dysfunctional, or no serum AAT. These rare alleles are not detected by routine methods and in order to identify them a combination of PI testing typing and next generation sequencing of the AAT gene is used.[561] Because the prognosis may vary between those who are actually homozygous for the Z variant and those with null phenotype, molecular testing of the SERPINA1 gene is considered preferable.[542]

Drug-induced liver injury. As discussed earlier, most cases of drug-induced liver injury (DILI) present as acute hepatitis. Less commonly, drugs have produced chronic liver injury in a pattern that mimics chronic hepatitis or other chronic liver injury (chronic cholestasis and hepatic granulomas).[562] The drugs most commonly linked to chronic hepatitis are nitrofurantoin, methyldopa, and hydroxy-3-methylglutaryl-CoA reductase inhibitors; however, a large number of drugs have been associated with liver injury,[563] and herbal medications have been linked to chronic hepatitis.[564,565] In individuals with increased activities of aminotransferases and no obvious cause, prescription drug use was significantly more likely to be present than in those with a known cause for increased enzyme activities.[566] As with acute drug reactions, establishing drugs as the cause of chronic hepatitis is difficult; temporal relationships to drug ingestion are not as clear as with acute hepatitis, and reactions can be seen first in those who have been taking the medication for many months.[567,568] Most chronic drug reactions resolve when administration of the drug is discontinued.[569,570] The National Institute of Diabetes and Digestive and Kidney Diseases (NIDDK) DILI network in the US provides an invaluable resource for investigating and reporting potential DILI (https://repository.niddk.nih.gov/studies/dilin/).

Significance of Chronic Hepatitis

In many cases, chronic hepatitis is a disease with minimal consequences. As mentioned earlier, an average of 20 to 30% of individuals with chronic HBV or HCV progress to cirrhosis over a 20-year period. However, cirrhosis was the sixth leading cause of death in the United States in 35- to 44-year-olds and the fourth leading cause of death in 45- to 54-year-olds in 2012 (the most recent year for which full data are available).[571] The frequency of cirrhosis and HCC has been increasing in much of the Western world,[572] mostly caused by the increase in cases related to HCV. The proportions of individuals with HCV with cirrhosis and HCC are expected to double by 2020, and the number of deaths caused by liver disease is expected to almost triple.[284] The ability to predict which patients are at increased risk for such late complications of chronic hepatitis would allow more appropriate treatment. Even with the advent of highly effective and well-tolerated treatments for HCV, it is likely to be decades before the burden of infection is brought under control sufficiently to reduce the incidence of complications of disease and the necessity for liver transplantation,[460] making the search for a prophylactic vaccine an imperative.

Fibrosis and necroinflammatory activity are the two major components of chronic hepatitis. The extent of fibrosis (stage) is strongly related to the risk of progression,[573–575] whereas necroinflammatory activity (grade) is correlated with progression in some,[575–577] but not all,[578,579] studies. Because ALT activity is strongly correlated with necroinflammatory activity,[580] it is also associated with risk of progression to cirrhosis in some, but not all, studies. Clinical variables are associated with risk of progression as well; these include age at infection, male sex, alcohol intake, and the presence of immunosuppression.[578,581–583]

The process of scar formation in the liver involves numerous factors and differs in some important ways from that in other sites in the body.[584,585] Increasing evidence suggests that the process of fibrosis is reversible, even when cirrhosis is histologically present.[137] For example, two studies found that successful treatment of HBV[586] and HCV[587] was associated with reversal of cirrhosis in 50 to 75% of cases. Although the principal component of hepatic scars is type III collagen, other components include type I and type IV collagen, laminin, elastin, and fibronectin. Proteoglycans, especially hyaluronate, are also involved in scar formation. Production of scar in the liver is affected by the rate of enzymatic degradation; a variety of MMPs are found in areas of scar formation, along with several TIMPs. MMPs are involved in degradation of the normal connective tissue of the liver (a necessary prequel to fibrosis), but they are also involved in breakdown and remodeling of collagen. HSCs are critical in this process; they produce both MMP and TIMP, as well as collagen and other matrix materials.[114,588] Recruitment and activation of stellate cells involve the action of a number of cytokines, particularly TGF-β, PDGF, and IL-6.[114] Evidence indicates that a variety of other cells also contribute to development of scar tissue within the liver.[589]

As discussed earlier in the chapter, the gold standard for evaluation of the extent of liver damage has been liver biopsy. Because the degree of injury is not uniform throughout the liver, the sample taken may not be representative of the extent of damage.[590] This has led to interest in the use of laboratory tests to predict the extent of fibrosis in the liver as described previously. Increasingly, these tests are being used to stratify and monitor patients with chronic liver disease.

Alcohol-Related Liver Disease

ArLD differs clinically and biochemically from other forms of hepatitis and liver disease.[591] It is a common cause of liver disease in the developed world, but the incidence of acute alcoholic hepatitis and death from alcoholic cirrhosis is declining in North America and Europe.[592,593] Risk factors for developing ArLD include the following.

1. *Duration and magnitude of alcohol ingestion.* As discussed later in the chapter, ArLD does not occur in all individuals with chronic ethanol intake; although there appears to be a threshold intake of 40 g/day in men and 10 g/day in women,[594] meta-analysis of published studies shows that risk increases even at intakes of less than 25 g/day.[595] Most individuals with ArLD ingest more than 80 g of alcohol per day.[596] Daily drinking appears to be riskier than intermittent drinking.

2. *Sex.* There is a greater likelihood of progression to cirrhosis in women.[597] Although some studies have suggested that this is due to lower activities of gastric mucosal alcohol dehydrogenase in women, 2002 data show that this is true only in younger women, and that older women actually have higher activities than older men.[598]

3. *Hepatitis B or C infection.* Both may increase the severity of liver damage in persons who drink heavily, and both correlate with degree of liver damage. For example, antibodies to HCV are several times more common in individuals with alcoholic hepatitis than in drinkers without hepatitis or in age- and sex-matched controls, suggesting a synergistic role for HCV.[599]

4. *Genetic factors.* As discussed later, an inherited predisposition to alcoholism has been clearly established. *Hfe* gene mutations are more common in people with alcoholism with liver disease than in those with no evidence of liver disease.[600]

5. *Nutritional status.* Protein-calorie malnutrition is extremely common among alcohol misusers. Malnutrition may be due not only to poor intake but also to abnormal nutrient metabolism. Although poor nutrition may contribute to the evolution of ArLD, adequate nutrition does not prevent its development. Studies suggest that obesity may be a risk factor (perhaps because of the presence of coexisting NAFLD).

Alcohol is metabolized to acetaldehyde by cytosolic alcohol dehydrogenase and microsomal enzymes (primarily CYP2E1). Acetaldehyde is subsequently metabolized to acetyl-CoA by aldehyde dehydrogenase. This is further broken down to acetate, which may be converted to carbon dioxide and water through the citric acid cycle to be converted to fatty acids. The latter is a major mechanism for induction of fatty liver by alcohol, but acetaldehyde is probably the primary toxin. It causes most of the injury to liver cells, as well as the induction of collagen synthesis leading to fibrosis, and ultimately, cirrhosis.

The mechanism for liver injury in alcohol misuse is still unclear. Only a minority of patients (less than one-third) who abuse alcohol develop ArLD,[601] and only 5% of the heaviest drinkers develop cirrhosis.[395] Acetylation of a variety of liver proteins occurs with alcohol misuse, leading to loss of function of affected proteins in many cases.[602] Antibodies to acetylated liver proteins have been detected in patients with ArLD.[603,604] Alcohol causes damage to intestinal epithelial cells, leading to release of lipopolysaccharide, which can also damage liver cells.[605] Activation of innate immunity, through either or both of these mechanisms, appears to be central to damage in ArLD.[606] A variety of other metabolic changes have been observed in ArLD, including changes in methionine metabolism and oxidative stress.[607]

Genetic factors seem to play a role in both alcohol abuse[608–610] and misuse and ArLD.[611] As much as 40 to 60% of alcohol misuse is due to inherited factors.[608] Much effort has been expended in finding specific genetic markers; some of the more commonly implicated specific genes are those coding for alcohol dehydrogenase and several brain receptors, including those for γ-aminobutyric acid and acetylcholine. Genetic variants in alcohol-metabolizing enzymes (including alcohol dehydrogenase, aldehyde dehydrogenase, and microsomal enzymes such as CYP2E1) are linked to alcohol misuse. However, most believe that multiple genes are involved in alcohol misuse. Genetic factors may also be important in determining which persons with alcohol misuse develop liver disease; as with alcohol misuse itself, as much as half of the risk of cirrhosis is due to genetic factors.[612] Similar genes may be involved; a 2009 study showed that heavy drinkers with cirrhosis were much more likely to have mutations in CPP2E1 and γ-aminobutyric acid receptors than heavy drinkers without cirrhosis.[613]

Acute alcoholic hepatitis clinically is an acute febrile illness[395] that is characteristically associated with leukocytosis[614] and increased plasma concentrations of acute-phase response proteins.[615] It causes mild increases in cytosolic enzymes; AST activity is typically more than two times greater than that of ALT,[616] and it is rare for AST to be more than eight times the upper reference interval.[612] Among the factors involved in causing the higher AST/ALT ratio in alcoholic hepatitis are damage to mitochondria, causing release of mitochondrial AST[617,618]; deficiency of pyridoxal 5-phosphate[618]; and a reduction in ALT content within the liver.[619] A cholestatic form of the disease, with increases in ALP activity to greater than three times the upper reference interval, is seen in up to 20% of cases; it is associated with higher mortality.[620] Increases in bilirubin are common, and reduced liver-synthesized protein concentrations are commonly present. Increased bilirubin, decreased albumin, and prolonged PT are poor prognostic markers in alcoholic hepatitis.[621] The Maddrey discriminant function ($4.6 \times$ (PT − Control PT)) + Plasma bilirubin (milligrams per deciliter)) value of more than 32 identifies individuals with a high mortality rate,[594] and a Model for End-Stage Liver Disease (MELD) score more than 11 has been found to have similar sensitivity and better specificity.[622]

A large number of biochemical markers have been proposed for the detection of excessive alcohol consumption.[623–625] Among routine laboratory tests, the most widely used are GGT and mean corpuscular volume (MCV). Serum GGT activity is commonly used as a screening test for alcohol misuse. However, GGT is an inducible enzyme that is increased by many drugs and a variety of other factors such as cigarette smoking and other forms of liver disease.[176] The threshold for positivity is approximately 2 drinks/day, and increase is more common in those who drink regularly than in binge drinkers. Although the clinical sensitivity of GGT for alcohol misuse is in the range of 70%, specificity is poor.[626] GGT remains increased for an average of 25 days after alcohol abstention.[627] MCV has similar clinical sensitivity, and specificity is low.[626]

Alcohol leads to production of isoforms of transferrin with low sialic acid content, termed carbohydrate-deficient transferrin (CDT; also called hyposialyl- and asialyltransferrin). The use of CDT for detecting problem drinkers has been reviewed.[628] CDT returns to a normal concentration in a mean of 10 days with abstention from alcohol,[627] and so is of particular use in confirming or questioning abstinence. In a pilot study, CDT was found to be the only test to reliably distinguish alcoholic hepatitis from NALFD.[629] It has been suggested that combining markers such as CDT and GGT will enhance accuracy in identifying problem drinkers.[626] CDT is frequently increased in persons with end-stage liver disease, regardless of cause.[630]

Other markers of alcohol misuse have been studied, but with fewer data than for the markers mentioned earlier. Fatty acid ethyl esters are formed with acute and long-term alcohol intake.[631] Similarly, alcohol metabolites combine with glucuronic acid, forming ethylglucuronides in patients who misuse alcohol.[632] Acetaldehyde adducts with serum[633] proteins and sialic acid[634] have also been evaluated as markers of alcohol misuse. Proteomic techniques have been used to try to identify additional markers,[635] with the suggestion that these will perform better than the currently used markers (e.g., GGT and CDT).

POINTS TO REMEMBER

Most Common Causes of Chronic Liver Disease
- Alcohol
- Fatty liver disease
- Chronic viral hepatitis B or hepatitis C

AT A GLANCE

Causes of Chronic Liver Disease
Often the cause of chronic liver disease is not immediately obvious. In this situation, a systematic approach to differential diagnosis should be taken, gathering history, and the findings of clinical examination, blood and urine tests, as well as imaging and biopsy.

The following categories of causes of chronic liver disease should be considered:
- Toxins: alcohol, drugs
- Viruses: HBV, HCV
- Metabolic liver diseases: fatty liver disease, hemochromatosis, AAT deficiency, Wilson disease
- Immune-mediated liver diseases: AIH, primary biliary cholangitis, primary sclerosing cholangitis
- Infiltration of the liver
- Tumors: benign and malignant (primary, secondary)

Cirrhosis

Cirrhosis, which is defined anatomically as diffuse fibrosis with nodular regeneration, represents the end stage of scar formation and regeneration in chronic liver injury. This response to injury occurs independently of the etiology and thus it is not possible, in most circumstances, to determine the cause of cirrhosis based on histology. Classically, cirrhosis has been classified as micronodular, macronodular, or mixed, based on the histology and gross appearance of the liver. However, this is considered inadequate for etiologic or prognostic purposes. Consequently, it is more common to classify cirrhosis on the basis of its presumed or known etiology. Common causes of cirrhosis and their therapies are listed in Table 51.8. Virtually all chronic liver diseases are known to lead to cirrhosis (see Fig. 51.14), but most cases of cirrhosis occur as a result of chronic hepatitis.

In the early stages of transition from chronic hepatitis to cirrhosis, termed compensated cirrhosis, no signs or symptoms of liver damage may be present. Laboratory abnormalities usually appear before clinical findings, such as ascites, gynecomastia, palmar erythema, and portal hypertension, begin to develop. Often cirrhosis is only suspected when laboratory abnormalities develop such as a fall in platelet count, an increase in PT, a decrease in the plasma albumin-to-globulin concentration ratio to less than 1, and an increase in the AST/ALT activity ratio to more than 1.[636,637] Generally, in those with documented cirrhosis, decompensation occurs slowly, at a rate of approximately 3% per year; 10-year survival with compensated cirrhosis is 90%.[637] However, once decompensation occurs, 10-year survival is only approximately 20%.[638] However, prognosis varies with etiology and may be influenced dramatically by response to treatment (as is the case in viral hepatitis B and C) or by abstinence from alcohol in ArLD. Jaundice is a late finding in decompensated

TABLE 51.8 Causes and Treatment of Cirrhosis

Cause	Treatment
Viral	
Hepatitis B	Administration of nucleoside or nucleotide HBV DNA polymerase inhibitors or pegylated α-interferon
Hepatitis C	Directly acting antiviral inhibitors of HCV and/or pegylated α-interferon with or without ribavirin
Toxic	
Alcohol	Abstinence, liver transplantation
Metabolic	
Hemochromatosis	Phlebotomy
Wilson disease	Penicillamine, zinc trientine
α1-Antitrypsin deficiency	Gene therapy, protein administration
Nonalcoholic fatty liver disease	Diet, exercise, insulin sensitizers
Biliary	
Primary biliary cirrhosis	Ursodeoxycholic acid
Primary sclerosing cholangitis	Liver transplantation
Autoimmune hepatitis	Corticosteroids, azathioprine, other immunosuppressants
Idiopathic	Consider immunosuppression
Advanced cirrhosis, irrespective of cause	Liver transplantation

HBV, Hepatitis B virus; *HCV,* hepatitis C virus.

TABLE 51.9 Child-Pugh System for Classifying Severity of Cirrhosis

Feature	1 Point	2 Points	3 Points
Encephalopathy	None	Grade 1–2	Grade 3–4
Ascites	None	Slight	Moderate-severe
Albumin, g/dL	>3.5	2.8–3.5	<2.8
Prothrombin time, seconds prolonged	<4	4–6	>6
Bilirubin, mg/dL (μmol/L)	<4 (<68)	4–10 (68–170)	>10 (>170)

Scoring: <7 points: class A; 7 to 9 points: class B; >9 points: class C.

cirrhosis. A variety of staging systems have been used to predict prognosis in cirrhosis. For many years, the most common classification system was the Child-Pugh class system, summarized in Table 51.9. Currently, the MELD score is used to identify patients with advanced cirrhosis who may be candidates for liver transplantation; it appears superior to the Child-Pugh scoring system in predicting short-term survival.[639–641] The MELD score is calculated as:

$$\begin{aligned} \text{MELD Score} &= (0.957 \times ln\,[\text{serum creatinine}]) \\ &+ 0.378 \times ln\,(\text{serum bilirubin}) \\ &+ 1.120 \times ln\,(\text{INR}) + 0.643 \\ &\times 10\ (\text{if hemodialysis, value for} \\ &\text{creatinine is automatically set to 4.0}) \end{aligned}$$

or in SI units as:

$$\begin{aligned} \text{MELD Score} &= 10 \times ([0.957 \times ln\,\{\text{creatinine}/88.4\}]) \\ &+ 0.378 \times ln\,[\text{bilirubin}/17.1]) \\ &+ 1.120 \times ln\,[\text{INR}]) + 0.643 \end{aligned}$$

Risk of death over 3 months is low in those with MELD scores less than 10, intermediate in those with scores of 10 to 20, and high in those with scores of more than 20.[642] Various modifications of the MELD score have been developed. Children younger than age 12 years should be assessed by the Pediatric End-Stage Liver Disease (PELD) Score. If a patient has had two or more hemodialysis treatments or 24 hours of continuous venovenous hemodialysis in the week before the time of the scoring, creatinine will be set to 4 mg/dL (353.6 μmol/L), the maximum creatinine concentration allowed in the model. For patients with HCC, the PELD/MELD score is increased according to an algorithm established by the United Network for Organ Sharing. Additional information about the MELD and PELD scores and web-based calculators can be found at http://optn.transplant.hrsa.gov/resources/by-organ/liver-intestine.

Laboratory findings in cirrhosis reflect ongoing liver injury and decreased hepatic function. Plasma activities of aminotransferases are variable in cirrhosis and reflect underlying necroinflammatory activity. If the cause of cirrhosis has been eliminated (as by abstinence from ethanol or successful treatment of viral hepatitis), aminotransferase activity is often within the reference interval. If aminotransferases remain increased, risk of development of HCC is increased.[643] As described earlier, the ratio of AST/ALT activity is often more than 1 in cirrhosis; this is usually a result of a fall in ALT and minimal change in AST activities. The mechanism for these changes is not clear, but there appears to be a decrease in the production

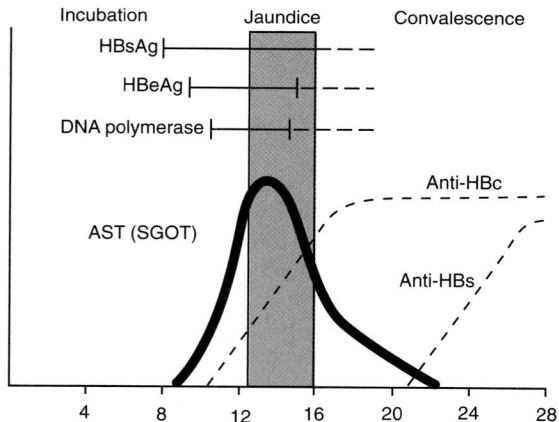

FIGURE 51.17 Course of acute type B hepatitis with recovery. *1,* Onset of hepatitis with jaundice 3 months after exposure; *2,* detection of hepatitis B surface antigen *(HBsAg)* 2 to 8 weeks after exposure, followed by appearance of its antibody *(anti-HBs)* 2 to 4 weeks after HBsAg is no longer detectable; *3,* detection of hepatitis B e antigen *(HBeAg)* shortly after HBsAg disappears (this is usually followed by the appearance of antibody to HbeAg *[anti-HBe],* which persists); *4,* detection of hepatitis B core antibody *(anti-HBc)* at the time of onset of disease 2 to 3 months after exposure. Anti-HBc immunoglobulin M will be detectable in high levels for approximately 5 months. (From Balistreri WF. Viral hepatitis: unique aspects of infection during childhood. *Consultant* 1984;24:131–153.)

of enzymatically active ALT in cirrhotic individuals,[644] along with a high ratio of immunoreactive to enzymatically active ALT in plasma.[184] Increases in AFP are common in cirrhotic patients, even in the absence of HCC.[645]

Acute on Chronic Liver Failure

Patients with compensated liver cirrhosis may experience decompensation due to a wide variety of precipitating factors, including infection, metabolic disturbance, bleeding, and protein overload. An international consortium of hepatologists has collected data on cirrhotic patients to identify markers of acute decompensation of cirrhosis that they have termed "Acute on Chronic Liver Failure" (ACLF).[646] This syndrome is characterized by acute decompensation (ascites, encephalopathy, GI hemorrhage, and/or bacterial infections), organ failure (liver, kidney, brain, coagulation, respiration, circulation), and high short-term mortality (i.e., 28-day mortality rate ≥ 15%).[101] The European Association for the Study of the Liver Chronic Liver Failure "CLIF Consortium" has derived the Chronic Liver Failure-Sequential Organ Failure Assessment score, which combines biochemical markers, including bilirubin, INR, and platelet count, with assessment of organ failure to derive a prognostic score that can be used to predict outcomes in patients with liver failure.[647] The use of the term ACLF in place of "decompensated cirrhosis" has been suggested as a means of highlighting the onset of acute liver dysfunction, which is often accompanied by other organ dysfunction due to an acute insult, in the context of cirrhosis, and to differentiate ACLF from decompensation due to gradual and progressive loss of liver function. The emphasis on determining other organ dysfunction may be clinically important, but the value of differentiating ACLF from decompensated cirrhosis remains controversial.

Hepatic Glycogenoses

The glycogenoses are a group of disorders that are characterized by excessive and/or aberrant glycogen storage in various tissues.[648] Most of these have deficient glucose production by the liver, leading to hypoglycemia. All are inherited by autosomal recessive transmission, except for type IV, which is sex linked. The hepatic glycogen storage diseases and their enzyme defects are listed in Table 51.10 and discussed in more detail in Chapter 35 on Carbohydrates. Most of these disorders are associated with growth retardation and hepatosplenomegaly. Mental development is usually normal. Hypoglycemia is a prominent feature in types I, III, and VI, and needs to be treated with continuous glucose feeding of uncooked cornstarch, which results in slow release of glucose. The diagnosis is based on the demonstration of excess glycogen in the liver biopsy and in vitro identification of the abnormal enzyme or aberrant glycogen. Prognosis and treatment vary with each entity (for more details, see Chapter 35).

Cholestatic Liver Disease

Cholestasis (stoppage or suppression of the flow of bile) is characterized by retention of bile within the excretory system. The term obstruction is often used inappropriately because cholestasis has been known to occur without mechanical obstruction to the biliary tract. Although intrahepatic cholestasis may be due to functional or mechanical problems, extrahepatic cholestasis is always due to physical obstruction of the bile ducts by gallstones, biliary strictures, and tumors. The major cholestatic diseases include mechanical obstruction of the bile ducts, primary biliary cholangitis (PBC), and PSC. Other cholestatic disorders include post–bone marrow transplantation cholangiopathy, post–liver transplantation cholangiopathy, drug-induced cholestasis, acquired immunodeficiency syndrome (AIDS) cholangiopathy, parenteral nutrition (see Chapter 46 on Nutrition), and bilirubinostasis of acute illness. Cholestatic hepatitis, which was discussed previously, may also cause cholestasis, but generally presents in a fashion similar to hepatitis. There are specific types of cholestasis that can occur in pregnancy; these are discussed in Chapter 59 on pregnancy-related disorders.

The clinical consequences of prolonged cholestasis are related to impaired biliary drainage. Deficiency of bile acids in the intestinal tract leads to malabsorption of fat and the fat-soluble vitamins A, D, E, and K (see Chapters 39, 46, 54, and 81, and the Bile Acids section of this chapter). Vitamin A malabsorption results in night blindness. Vitamin D malabsorption leads to calcium and phosphate malabsorption, causing rickets in children and osteomalacia in adults. Vitamin K malabsorption results in deficiency of coagulation factors II, VII, IX, and X, leading to prolonged clotting times, and sometimes bleeding. Lack of excretion of normal bile contents results in their accumulation in plasma. Bile acid retention leads to increased bile acid concentrations in plasma. Bilirubin retention leads to jaundice, dark urine, and pale stools. Increased bilirubin generally occurs only with

TABLE 51.10	Hepatic Glycogen Storage Diseases		
Type	**Eponym**	**Enzyme Defect**	**Involved Tissues**
0		Glycogen synthetase	Liver
I	von Gierke	Ia glucose 6-phosphatase	Liver, kidney, intestines
		Ib translocase for glucose 6-phosphatase	
		Ic phosphate/pyrophosphate translocase	
II	Pompe	Lysosomal acid α-1,4 glucosidase	Most tissues
III	Cori	Amylo-1,6 glucosidase debranching enzyme	Liver, muscle, WBCs
IV	Anderson	Amylo-1,4–1,6 trans-glucosidase (branching enzyme)	Most tissue
VI	Hers	Liver phosphorylase	Liver, WBCs
VII		Phosphorylase activation	Liver
IXa		Phosphorylase kinase	Liver, WBCs, RBCs

RBCs, Red blood cells; *WBCs,* white blood cells.

complete obstruction, and thus is more commonly seen with extrahepatic rather than intrahepatic cholestasis.

Laboratory features of cholestasis vary, depending on whether the process causes complete or partial impairment of biliary drainage. A common feature of all cholestatic disorders is an increase in plasma activities of canalicular enzymes, such as ALP and GGT. Because this process involves both increased synthesis of enzyme and release of enzyme from its membrane-bound forms, a short lag period is generally seen between the onset of cholestasis and the increase in plasma activities. In the early stages of an acute mechanical obstruction (especially from gallstones), transient increases may be noted in plasma activities of liver cytosolic enzymes, such as AST and ALT. Activities of plasma AST and ALT may exceed 400 U/L, and in 1 to 2% of cases are greater than 2000 U/L. Even in the presence of continued obstruction, AST and ALT activity gradually decreases, and AST is typically within the reference interval within 8 to 10 days. Increases in total bilirubin typically occur only with complete extrahepatic obstruction, although they may be seen with extensive intrahepatic cholestasis. Increases in direct bilirubin are more commonly seen, and direct bilirubin has been reported to be the most sensitive functional test for the presence of cholestasis. Prolonged PT is the most commonly detected coagulation abnormality. It usually is corrected by administration of parenteral vitamin K. Accumulation of cholesterol is associated with the development of an abnormal lipoprotein, termed lipoprotein-X,[649,650] which contains phospholipids, cholesterol, fragments of cell membrane (along with ALP),[651] and albumin; the lipid may deposit in connective tissue, producing xanthomas.[652] It is often measured as LDL cholesterol.[653,654]

Mechanical Bile Duct Obstruction

The most common cause of cholestasis is biliary tract obstruction by space-occupying lesions.[655] Extrahepatic bile duct obstruction occurs most commonly as the result of gallstones in the common bile duct or because of tumors in the head of the pancreas or duodenum. Other causes of extrahepatic obstruction include (1) bile duct strictures, (2) extrinsic compression of the bile ducts by enlarged lymph nodes, (3) congenital biliary atresia, and (4) PSC. Extrahepatic obstruction is commonly associated with jaundice, especially when obstruction is complete. Increase in canalicular enzymes is common, but is not present in all cases[656]; marked increases (>3× the upper reference limit) are more common with gallstones as a cause of obstruction.[422] Transient increases in aminotransferases are more common with choledocholithiasis than with other causes of extrahepatic obstruction.[657] Transient increases in CA 19-9 occur with bile duct obstruction[658]; this is an important consideration, because CA 19-9 is often used as a diagnostic test for pancreatic and bile duct carcinoma (for more details see Chapter 33 on Tumor Markers). A key feature of extrahepatic obstruction is dilation of more proximal and intrahepatic bile ducts, which can be visualized by imaging studies.

Intrahepatic cholestasis caused by mechanical obstruction is also common, but is rarely associated with jaundice or with visibly dilated ducts on imaging studies, although it may be associated with increased direct bilirubin. Jaundice typically occurs only with lesions that are large, or are located near the porta hepatis, where they may obstruct both hepatic ducts. Common causes of intrahepatic obstruction include tumors

(particularly metastases), granulomatous diseases (such as sarcoidosis and tuberculosis), and infiltrative processes (such as lymphoma, leukemia, and extramedullary hematopoiesis).

Primary Biliary Cholangitis

Primary biliary cholangitis, formerly known as primary biliary cirrhosis, is an uncommon chronic autoimmune disorder that targets the small intrahepatic bile ducts[659,660] with accompanying cholestasis.[490] Its prevalence is approximately 2 to 8 per 100,000 population in Northern Europe and North America, but is much lower in developing areas. The reported prevalence of PBC is appears to be stable. The median age at onset is 50 years, and the female-to-male ratio is approximately 10:1.[661,662] An association with HLA class II antigen DR8 has been noted in some populations. A family history of PBC is seen in 1 to 4% of cases with a reported sibling relative risk of 10%.[663] In up to 80% of cases, the condition is associated with other autoimmune processes, most commonly Sjögren syndrome and hypothyroidism (which often develops before the onset of PBC).[664]

PBC is an immune-mediated biliary disorder that is likely due to an interaction of host immunogenetic and environmental factors. The role of host immunogenicity is supported by studies in monozygotic twins and the identification of associated genetic loci in Genome Wide Association Studies (GWAS).[662,665] Case control studies have also confirmed that cigarette smoking and recurrent urinary tract infections are both strongly associated with PBC.[666] Mechanistically, it is known that destruction of the bile duct in PBC is mediated by T cells in the presence of upregulation of HLA class I antigens on hepatocytes and HLA class II antigens on biliary epithelial cells.[667] Although the target antigens of the T cells have not been identified, at least 95% of patients have antimitochondrial antibodies that react against the dihydrolipoamide acyltransferase component of the pyruvate decarboxylase complex.[668] Part of this complex is found on the apical surface of biliary epithelial cells, suggesting a role for this antigen as an immune target.[669] In individuals with coexisting Sjögren syndrome, the antigen is also expressed on the surface of salivary gland cells.[670]

PBC typically presents as a chronic asymptomatic increase of ALP, but may present with features of cholestasis, particularly pruritus or with fatigue.[671] Metabolic bone disease and xanthomas are common complications of PBC.[672] Occasionally, autoantibodies are detected (usually because of the presence of another autoimmune disease or because of a family history of PBC) before increase of ALP.[673] Aminotransferase activities are increased in 50% of cases, but are more than twice the upper reference limit in only 20% of cases.[674] Increased bilirubin is a late finding and is important in predicting decompensation.[675] Antibodies to mitochondria or to the recombinant pyruvate decarboxylase complex appear similar in sensitivity, although the latter are more specific.[676] An increased bilirubin is a late finding and is important in predicting decompensation.[673] A polyclonal increase of IgM is also characteristic of PBC.[677] Serologically, PBS is characterized by autoantibodies specific for mitochondrial, nuclear, and centromere antigens.[678] Antibodies to mitochondria or to the recombinant pyruvate decarboxylase complex (M2) appear similar in sensitivity, although the latter are more specific.[674] To diagnose PBC, the combination of cholestatic liver function tests and PBC serologic antibodies are highly accurate (sensitivity and specificity both >95%).[679] As such a liver biopsy is not required for diagnosis in most cases, but may be helpful in those with low titer antibodies or with a greater than twofold increase in aminotransferase activity.

The natural history of PBC is one of slow progression to portal hypertension, often without development of cirrhosis; the average time from diagnosis to death in untreated patients is 22 years.[671] Development of jaundice is the most important indicator of advanced disease and serves as the most important prognostic test.[672] Medical management of PBC consists of UDCA therapy; most evidence suggests that survival is improved in treated patients.[672]

Historically, UDCA was the only agent employed in the treatment of PBC. Under normal circumstances, UDCA accounts for 4% of bile acids but UDCA itself becomes the predominant bile acid while on treatment. Most evidence suggests that both biochemistry and survival is improved in PBC patients treated with UDCA.[670] With regard to dosing, UDCA at 13 to 15 mg/kg/day has been identified to be superior in efficacy than low-dose (5 to 7 mg/kg) or high-dose (23 to 25 mg/kg) strategies.[680] Overall, few adverse events have been noted with UDCA and it is deemed safe to use during pregnancy. An analysis of 3 large randomized controlled trials in PBC highlighted that the use of UDCA was associated with a one third reduction in death or the need for liver transplantation.

More recently, obeticholic acid (OCA), a semi-synthetic hydrophobic bile acid, has been licensed for use in PBC. OCA is highly selective for farnesoid X receptor (FXR) which itself regulates genes involved in bile acid synthesis, secretion, absorption, and detoxification. OCA has been used as an add-on treatment to UDCA. In a phase 3 trial in which patients who had not responded to UDCA after 12 months (as defined as ALP >1.67 upper limit of normal (ULN) and/or total bilirubin <2 ULN) the use of OCA at 2 doses (5 mg or 10 mg) together with UDCA resulted in a 46 to 47% biochemical response as compared to 5% in patients treated with placebo.[681] OCA treatment is associated with the development of pruritis and up to 10% of patients need to discontinue treatment because of this side effect. Dose adjustment and careful monitoring are required when using OCA in patients with advanced liver disease.

Although a rare complication, the relative risk of developing HCC is significantly increased in individuals with PBC.[682] Liver transplantation is the only definitive treatment, but even when it is performed, PBC may recur in the transplanted organ.[683]

Biochemical tests and direct markers of liver fibrosis have been studied as surrogate markers of disease severity and prognostic markers of survival in PBC. Of these, the ELF test (see section of this chapter on Direct Biomarkers of Liver Fibrosis) has been shown to be the most accurate in determining prognosis.[684]

Primary Sclerosing Cholangitis

PSC is a chronic inflammatory disease of the biliary tree that most commonly affects the extrahepatic bile ducts; involvement of intrahepatic ducts, with extrahepatic involvement or as an isolated finding, is also possible.[685,686] Primary sclerosing cholangitis (PSC) is an immune mediated chronic inflammatory disease of the intrahepatic and/or extrahepatic bile ducts.[683,684] Analogous to other etiologies of CLD, PSC can cause progressive hepatic fibrosis which may result in the development of cirrhosis and its complications including portal hypertension and decompensation.[687] Typically, the biliary tree in PSC when imaged (cholangiography) at MRCP (magnetic resonance cholangiopancreatography) or ERCP (endoscopic retrograde cholangiopancreatography) is abnormal and appears irregular and beaded. A variant of PSC known as small duct PSC is characterized by the same cholestatic biochemical and histologic features of PSC but with normal cholangiographic appearances.[688] PSC overlap/variant syndromes present with features of both PSC and other immune-mediated liver diseases including AIH. Patients with features of both PSC and AIH are typically younger; have higher aminotransferase activities; increased Igs; positive ANA, SMA, and or LKM antibodies; and histologically have features of both AIH and PSC.[689]

In contrast to PSC, secondary sclerosing cholangitis is not immune mediated and is instead secondary to another pathology. Regardless, the cholangiographic appearances of PSC and secondary sclerosing cholangitis can be identical. Causes of secondary sclerosing cholangitis include malignancy (cholangiocarcinoma), gallstone disease, hilar lymphadenopathy, infection, and bile duct injury.

In contrast to PBC, PSC has a male predominance (60 to 70%) and a younger median age at onset (30 years). In 70 to 90% of patients, PSC is associated with ulcerative colitis, which usually (but not always) precedes onset of PSC; conversely, only approximately 2 to 4% of patients with ulcerative colitis develop PSC.[685] This has led to speculation that bacterial antigens in portal blood might be involved in the pathogenesis of PSC.[690] An autoimmune component is likely because 97% of patients with PSC have one or more autoantibodies present in their plasma.[691] The prevalence of PSC is similar to that of PBC, but geographic differences in prevalence have been observed; it is most common in Northern Europe, where PSC accounts for 5% of liver transplants for cirrhosis.[692,693] A markedly increased prevalence of HLA antigens B8 and DR3 has been noted.[694]

The clinical presentation of PSC, similar to that of PBC, is typically an asymptomatic patient with increased ALP activities found during routine laboratory screening. Symptoms are ultimately present in most patients with PSC; the most common are pruritus and intermittent abdominal pain, but fever may also be present.[686] Treatment, with UDCA may improve both the results of laboratory tests and symptoms but does not improve long-term survival[695,696] and is not currently recommended.[693,694] Immunosuppressive treatment has not been shown to improve outcomes in PSC. Transplantation, the major treatment available for end-stage PSC, results in a high rate of long-term survival. Although PSC recurs after transplantation in approximately 20 to 35% of cases, it does not appear to affect survival.[697] Transplantation also appears to increase the severity of underlying ulcerative colitis, when present.[698] The major cause of death in individuals with PSC is cholangiocarcinoma, which ultimately develops in up to 40% of patients.[685,686] Transplantation in the presence of cholangiocarcinoma is contraindicated as it is associated with rapid development of metastatic disease and poor survival.[688,699] PSC also increases the likelihood of colon carcinoma in individuals with coexisting ulcerative colitis, although the risk is not affected by liver transplantation.[700]

Patients with PSC and AIH overlap syndromes may respond favorably to long-term immunosuppression with agents such as azathioprine and corticosteroids. At the time of diagnosis, most patients with PSC have increased ALP activities and other canalicular enzymes; bilirubin concentration is typically normal, although it may increase with acute exacerbations.

The diagnosis of PSC is based on the typical radiographic appearance of beading and irregularity of the bile ducts. By contrast, small duct PSC is diagnosed histologically in the context of chronic cholestasis. PSC overlap/variant syndromes will have features of both PSC and AIH. Antineutrophil cytoplasmic antibodies are present in approximately 80% of patients[701] but are not specific for PSC; they are also present in PBC and AIH. Typically, the antibodies have an atypical perinuclear pattern because they are located around the nucleus in formalin- and methanol-fixed preparations. Antigens include lactoferrin, bactericidal and/or permeability increasing protein, and cathepsin G.[691]

Because of the discontinuous nature of the histologic lesion in PSC, liver biopsy is of limited value in staging disease severity, but magnetic resonance cholangiopancreatography provides a view of the entire biliary tree. Similar to PBC, the ELF test, which is a combination of direct markers of liver fibrosis, has been demonstrated as the best prognostic biochemical marker for PSC.[702]

Patients with PSC are at increased risk of gallbladder malignancy. As such, international guidelines recommend that patients with PSC should undergo annual ultrasound surveillance with the aim of detecting gallbladder polyps prior to malignant progression.[703]

Drug-Induced Liver Injury

Drugs are a common cause of cholestasis, causing approximately 15% of cases.[704,705] Drug reactions are especially common in older individuals, among whom up to 50% of individuals have increased enzymes because of medications.[704] Nonmedicinal drugs are also increasingly recognized as a cause of cholestasis.[706] Drugs can cause a cholestatic picture by two major mechanisms.[707] In some cases, only conjugated bilirubin is increased, whereas canalicular enzymes are not increased. This picture, which is often seen with estrogen and anabolic steroids, appears to be due to inhibition of production of the multidrug resistance protein-2[708] an ABC transporter that transports drug-conjugates and divalent bile salt conjugates into bile. More commonly, drugs induce a cholestatic hepatitis, as discussed earlier. The National Institutes of Health website, http://livertox.nih.gov, and recent reviews provide further information and excellent support in the investigation of suspected drug-induced liver toxicity.[709,710]

Gallstones

Gallstones are solid formations in the gallbladder that are composed of cholesterol and bile salts. Although they vary in chemical composition, they generally contain a mixture of cholesterol, bilirubin, calcium, and mucoproteins. In the United States, 70 to 85% of all gallstones are predominantly cholesterol, and more than 10% of the adult population is affected.

Three major types of gallstones are cholesterol, pigmented, and the most common, mixed. These stones form whenever bile is supersaturated with cholesterol or unconjugated bilirubin. For these stones or cholesterol gallstones to form, bile must be supersaturated with cholesterol. Whenever an increase in cholesterol or a decrease in bile acids or lecithin occurs, bile becomes lithogenic and cholesterol may precipitate. Factors that predispose to cholesterol hypersecretion include obesity, aging, certain drugs such as clofibrate and nicotine, and certain hormones such as estrogen. Factors that decrease bile acid secretion include terminal ileal disease and cholestatic diseases, such as PBC, PSC, and cystic fibrosis. Genetic factors also appear to be involved. Within racial groups, women are more frequently affected than men. Diet may play a role because it appears that people who ingest diets high in polyunsaturated fats have a higher incidence, whereas those with a diet high in fiber have a decreased incidence.

Pigmented gallstones are associated with conditions in which the bilirubin concentration is increased, such as hemolytic anemia, or when bilirubin becomes insoluble (i.e., deconjugated), such as occurs in cholestasis or chronic biliary infection.

Rare Causes of Cholestasis

Several other disorders are associated with cholestasis. Because they occur in specific settings, they are often suggested by the clinical picture. Laboratory tests are of little help in establishing the correct diagnosis.

Cholestasis may develop following bone marrow transplantation because of a variety of factors. Acute graft versus host disease (GVHD) is a consequence of the infusion of allogeneic immunocompetent T-lymphoid cells into an immunocompromised host that cannot reject these cells.[711] Periductular epithelial cells are the primary targets of injury in both acute and chronic GVHD.[712] Clinical features of GVHD include skin rash, intestinal symptoms (nausea, vomiting, diarrhea, and abdominal pain), and cholestasis. The histologic appearance is characteristic, but a liver biopsy is somewhat hazardous in these patients; thus most cases are diagnosed on clinical grounds.

Although acute liver transplantation rejection is associated with necroinflammatory changes and increased aminotransferases, chronic rejection is often associated with cholestasis. The primary targets of immunologic injury are bile ductules and blood vessels.[713] Because of cholestasis, plasma bile acids are often increased early in the process of rejection. Increased numbers of canalicular membranes are often the first evidence of rejection.[713] Although eosinophilia is common in rejection,[714] it is also a common finding in drug-induced cholestasis and thus is not helpful in the differential diagnosis.

AIDS cholangiopathies are caused by organisms not previously known to infect the biliary tree; they have become less common with reduction in the frequency of immunosuppression because of combination antiretroviral treatment. Cryptosporidium is the most common organism. Microsporidium, CMV, *Mycobacterium avium* complex, and cyclospora have also been identified. The clinical presentation usually includes abdominal pain, diarrhea, and cholestasis manifested by threefold to tenfold increases in plasma ALP, mild increases in aminotransferases, and rarely, jaundice. Papillary stenosis at the ampulla of Vater is present in patients with pain, and the bile ducts have features of PSC. Cholangiography is needed for the diagnosis but is indicated only in patients with pain. Brushings and biopsies at the time of cholangiography will establish the diagnosis. Treatment is primarily endoscopic. Sphincterotomy will give pain relief in approximately 70% of patients.

Hepatic Tumors

The liver is host to a wide variety of benign and malignant primary tumors. It is the second most common site of metastases; metastatic tumors account for 90 to 95% of all hepatic malignancies. Primary tumors may arise from many cell lines in the liver, but they arise most commonly from parenchymal and biliary epithelial cells and from mesenchymal cells (Table 51.11). The two most important primary liver tumors are HCC and cholangiocarcinoma.

Hepatocellular Carcinoma

HCC is the fifth most common cancer worldwide and a leading cause of cancer death; more than 500,000 cases occur annually, with a similar number of deaths.[715] Wide geographic and ethnic variations are noted in the incidence, suggesting that both host and environmental factors are involved in its origin. For example, approximately 75% of HCC cases occur in Asia, with an annual incidence of HCC in China of approximately 30 cases per 100,000 males. Worldwide, the incidence is twofold to threefold higher among men than among women. The incidence of HCC has been increasing in the United States[716,717] and much of Europe because of the increasing frequency of cirrhosis caused by HCV; however, incidence has declined in many parts of the world because of the success in prevention of infection by HBV.[718,719] Although cirrhosis is present in most patients with HCC, it is absent in approximately 25 to 30% of cases, often in association with HBV.[720,721] More importantly, the presence of cirrhosis had been recognized before diagnosis of HCC in approximately one-third of cases.[721,722] Wide variations in the incidence of HCC are associated with different causes of cirrhosis. For example, HCC commonly occurs in cirrhosis caused by

TABLE 51.11	Classification of Hepatic Tumors	
Type	**Benign**	**Malignant**
Epithelial	Adenoma	Hepatocellular
	Bile duct adenoma	carcinoma
	Cystadenoma	Cholangiocarcinoma
	Carcinoid	Cystadenocarcinoma
	Focal nodular	Squamous
	hyperplasia	carcinoma
	Diffuse nodular	
	hyperplasia	
Mesenchymal	Cavernous	Hemangiosarcoma
tumors	hemangioma	Fibrosarcoma
	Fibroma	Leiomyosarcoma
	Leiomyoma	Hepatoblastoma
	Hematoma	
Metastatic	Colon	
tumors	Pancreas	
(most	Stomach	
common	Breast	
sources)	Lung	
	Unknown primary	

alcohol abuse, hemochromatosis, AAT deficiency, HBV, and HCV, but it is rare that it is caused by AIH and Wilson disease.

In most parts of the world, the major risk factors for development of HCC are infection with HBV or HCV. In Asia, Africa, and Alaska, the major risk factor is HBV infection. The presence of HBsAg and HBeAg is associated with a relative risk of HCC of 60, whereas the presence of HBsAg with negative HBeAg is associated with a relative risk of 10.[723] This is probably due to the lower viral loads in HBeAg negative chronic HBV; in all forms of chronic HBV, risk of HCC is directly related to viral load.[448] Once cirrhosis has developed, the rate of development of HCC is approximately 1.5 to 5% per year in both HBV and HCV[643,724]; the relative risk of HCC doubles in those coinfected with these viruses.[725] The risk of HCC is higher in those with cirrhosis who have increased aminotransferase activities than in those with normal ALT activity.[643,726] The mechanism of increased risk in HBV is believed to be related to integration of HBV DNA into the host genome, possibly caused by the action of the HBV X gene, which may block the activity of p53.[727,728] The mechanism of increased risk of HCC in HCV has not been identified, but may be related to ongoing injury.

Aflatoxin, a product of *Aspergillus flavus* contamination of grain, has been linked to risk of HCC; although it is harmless, it is metabolized to aflatoxin 8,9-epoxide. This reactive intermediate binds to guanosine bases in DNA, leading to mutagenesis. If the formed adduct is not repaired, G-to-T transversion occurs in codon 249 of the *TP53* gene (p53), causing an inactivating mutation.[729] Under normal circumstances, the mutagenic aflatoxin 8,9-epoxide is rendered harmless by glutathione-*S*-transferase, which converts it to a glutathione conjugate, which in turn is metabolized to 1,2-dihydrodiol by epoxide hydrolase.[730] However, both detoxifying enzymes are polymorphic in humans, and the mutant forms are less active. Patients with HCC are more likely to have the mutant forms of epoxide hydrolase and glutathione-*S*-transferase; this allows accumulation of the epoxide.[731]

The clinical presentation of HCC is variable and usually does not occur until late in the course of disease when the tumor is large and resection is impossible. In some cases, acute decompensation occurs in a patient with cirrhosis, but clinical presentation may include detection of a right upper quadrant mass, shock due to hemorrhage into the peritoneal cavity, or right upper quadrant pain. Nonspecific signs and symptoms, such as fever, malaise, anorexia, and anemia, are common, and jaundice may occur with central tumors that obstruct biliary drainage. In a small number of cases, paraneoplastic features, such as hypoglycemia, hypercalcemia (due to parathyroid hormone–related peptide production), or erythrocytosis (due to erythropoietin production), may be the initial presenting findings; such paraneoplastic findings occur in up to 20% of cases, usually in association with poor prognosis.[732,733] Laboratory findings include those of cirrhosis and cholestasis, and (except for tumor markers discussed later) are nonspecific.

Because treatment usually is not possible in individuals with clinically diagnosed HCC, much interest has focused on screening high-risk individuals. Most professional societies have not advocated screening for HCC in Europe or North America, although the AASLD has endorsed screening of high-risk patients every 6 to 12 months.[734] Although some data have suggested that screening is effective in detecting small, treatable tumors, other data have not been as supportive.

The most common screening programs have used plasma tumor marker concentrations or tumor markers plus imaging studies; the AASLD recommends imaging as the primary screening modality and recommends against using only tumor markers (although tumor markers were noted to be useful as an addition to imaging).[734] Ultrasound is typically used as the imaging modality for screening because of its low cost. The tumor marker most widely used for screening purposes is AFP; it is typically quantified using assays that measure its total concentration. Although it appears to be relatively sensitive,[735] increase of AFP is common in individuals with chronic hepatitis and cirrhosis, which is the group at highest risk for HCC. In our experience, AFP above the upper reference limit has a positive predictive value of only 16% for HCC. Use of higher cutoff values than the upper reference limit improves clinical specificity of total AFP, at the expense of clinical sensitivity; for example, at a cutoff of 20 ng/mL, approximately three times the upper reference limit, sensitivity is only 60%.[734] As discussed in Chapter 33 on Tumor Markers, modified forms of AFP are more specific for tumors, particularly the L3 isoform recognized by lens culinaris (lentil) lectin. The L3 isoform by itself has low sensitivity for HCC,[736] and it is the only positive tumor marker in only a small number of cases. In contrast, specificity and positive predictive value are significantly improved when the L3 isoform is combined with the AFP total.[736] An L3 isoform more than 15% of total AFP may be associated with more aggressive and less well-differentiated tumors.[737]

Des-γ-carboxy prothrombin (DCP)—also called PIVKA-2 (factor II PIVKA)—is the inactive form of prothrombin found in individuals taking warfarin or other vitamin K antagonists. Its plasma concentration was first found to be increased in HCC in 1984,[738] but its measurement was not widely used until the early 1990s. Initial studies found that DCP was increased in some patients who did not have increased AFP but was insensitive to small HCC that might be curable. DCP immunoassays with lowered detection limits have been developed and have shown increased sensitivity for small HCC, and DCP seems directly related to tumor size[739] and prognosis.[736] Pretreatment with vitamin K, to eliminate other causes of increased DCP, further improves specificity.[740] DCP is best used as an adjunct to AFP, because tumors often produce one or the other tumor marker.[741]

Treatment of HCC is dependent on the extent of the tumor. Small tumors are often treated by transplantation, after which there is a low rate of recurrence. Local techniques, such as ethanol injection, chemoembolization, and use of radiofrequency ablation, are increasingly used before transplantation or instead of transplantation. Larger tumors generally are not resectable but may be treated by chemoembolization if a single feeding vessel is identified. A novel approach to identifying micrometastases has been described using rt-PCR to amplify mRNA for AFP to detect recurrence or metastasis.[742]

Tumors of the Gallbladder and Bile Ducts

Benign lesions such as papillomas or adenomas may be seen as an incidental finding at cholecystectomy; malignant disease of the gallbladder is uncommon. Cholelithiasis may be an etiologic factor, because 85% of gallbladder carcinomas occur in patients with gallstones. However, less than 1% of patients with gallstones develop carcinoma. It has been suggested that a calcified gallbladder is especially prone to malignant transformation. Various pathologic forms exist, including papillary adenocarcinoma, squamous cell carcinoma, and anaplastic tumors. These tumors usually arise in the neck of the gallbladder and spread rapidly, causing obstruction and cholestasis. Physical examination reveals a hard, tender mass in the gallbladder fossa. These lesions are particularly difficult to treat, and most cases are inoperable at the time of diagnosis.

Cholangiocarcinoma, or primary carcinoma of the bile ducts, can arise at any point in the biliary tree, including the small intrahepatic bile duct radicals. This lesion is typically associated with underlying liver disease, such as PSC, congenital cystic lesions, or chronic infestation with *Clonorchis sinensis*. The clinical presentation is that of cholestasis, including jaundice, dark urine, tan-colored stool, and pruritus. This condition is differentiated from other cholestatic diseases by visualizing the biliary tree.

DIAGNOSTIC STRATEGY

Liver function tests are useful in detecting and diagnosing liver disease and dysfunction, as well as in evaluating severity, monitoring therapy, and assessing prognosis. They are also useful in directing further diagnostic workup. The array of tests useful for these purposes (Table 51.12) includes measurement in plasma of total and direct bilirubin, protein, and albumin concentrations, and the activity of enzymes such as the aminotransferases (AST and ALT), ALP, and GGT. By using a combination of these tests, it is possible to categorize broad types of liver disease, which can then be more accurately diagnosed through disease-specific tests. An algorithm for this process is presented in Fig. 51.18. It should be born in mind that all diagnostic tests should be applied after determining the pretest probability of disease and in the full knowledge of the test performance to derive a post-test probability of disease.[743]

TABLE 51.12   Tests of Hepatic Function and Injury

Test	Utility
Bilirubin	Diagnosing jaundice, modest correlation with severity
Alkaline phosphatase	Diagnosing disorders of metabolism and disorders of the newborn
Bilirubin fractionation	Diagnosing cholestasis and space-occupying lesions
AST	Sensitive test of hepatocellular disease; AST > ALT in alcoholic disease
ALT	Sensitive and more specific test of hepatocellular disease
Gamma-glutamyltransferase	Prognostic indicator for increased cardiovascular and all-cause mortality
Albumin	Indicator of chronicity and severity
Prothrombin time	Indicator of severity of cholestasis

ALT, Alanine aminotransferase; *AST,* aspartate aminotransferase.

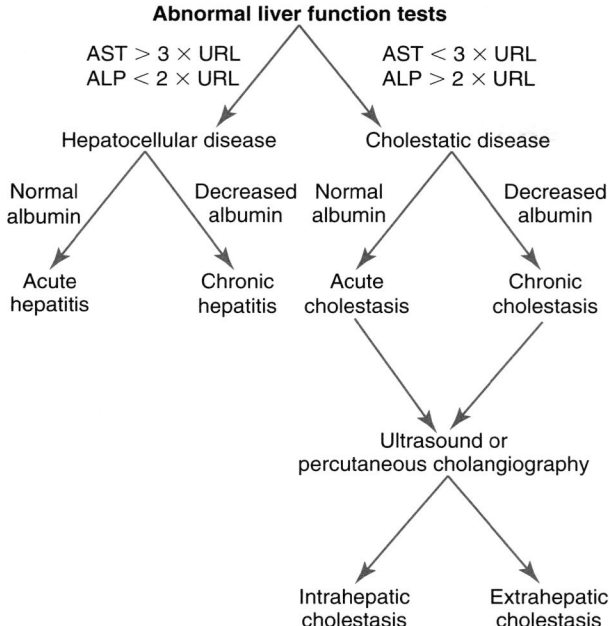

Abnormal liver function tests

FIGURE 51.18 Algorithm for using abnormal liver function tests to classify and diagnose various types of liver disease. Initial evaluation is best accomplished by examining the pattern of liver-associated enzymes. If elevation primarily affects one of the aminotransferases, then hepatocellular disease is likely; an increase primarily in alkaline phosphatase *(ALP)* suggests a cholestatic disorder. If only ALP is elevated, then it is appropriate to consider nonhepatic sources before further investigation (using measurement of other canalicular enzymes such as γ-glutamyl-transferase *[GGT]* or ALP isoenzymes). If the liver is the source of elevated ALP, then an imaging study to evaluate the ducts is the next test performed; dilated ducts establish a mechanical cause of obstruction, and normal ducts indicate intrahepatic cholestasis requiring further evaluation, as discussed in the text. Predominant increases in aminotransferases suggest hepatocellular injury; values more than 10× upper reference limit *(URL)* usually indicate acute hepatitis, and lower values are typical of chronic hepatitis. If aspartate aminotransferase *(AST)* is higher than alanine aminotransferase *(ALT)*, common causes include early hepatic injury, nonhepatic injury (such as muscle injury), and with mildly increased values, cirrhosis.

Plasma Enzymes

In practice, plasma aminotransferases and ALP are the most useful tests, because they allow differentiation of hepatocellular disease from cholestatic disease in most cases. The importance of this distinction cannot be overstated: failure to recognize cholestatic disease caused by extrahepatic biliary obstruction will result in liver failure if the obstruction is not quickly corrected. It is also important to recognize that there may be a grey zone of mixed hepatocellular and cholestatic disease wherein the tests do not distinguish one disease from the other. In this case, it is wise to assume that the problem is cholestatic and rule out biliary obstruction. In all cases, the use of imaging to look for evidence and causes of biliary obstruction must be a high priority, with ultrasound being the cheapest and mostly widely available imaging modality.

Patients are occasionally seen with isolated increases in ALP or aminotransferase enzyme activities. In practice, an isolated increase in ALP activity is difficult to interpret. In children, benign transient hyperphosphatasemia should always be considered. In adults, it is necessary to first confirm that the ALP is of hepatobiliary origin. This can be done by isoenzyme fractionation (see Chapter 32 on Serum Enzymes) or GGT, which tends to parallel the activity of ALP in cholestasis. The most important aspect of the workup is to rule out space-occupying lesions by visualizing the liver with computed tomography, and biliary tract disease by visualizing the biliary tree with ultrasound or magnetic resonance cholangiography.

Increased plasma activities of AST and ALT are common in many disorders. To determine whether this increase is liver related, administration of all drugs and alcohol intake (especially if AST is higher than ALT) should be discontinued. If the increase persists, ultrasound (looking for a nonalcoholic fatty liver) and HBV and HCV serology should be performed. More than 50% of isolated enzyme increases of liver origin will be caused by these disorders. A liver biopsy is often needed to allow a more specific diagnosis. No reliable test other than liver biopsy can be used to detect fibrosis. The investigation of the patient with isolated increases of liver enzymes in the absence of overt liver disease represents the investigation and differential diagnosis of all chronic liver disease. The common causes are described elsewhere in this chapter, but include alcohol, drugs, fatty liver disease, and viral, metabolic, and immune causes of liver disease; the investigation involves taking a thorough history, physical examination, and imaging.

Evidence is accumulating that GGT, as a marker of oxidative stress, is associated with increased cardiovascular and all-cause mortality.[744,745] It has shown prognostic value in assessing adverse outcomes after acute coronary syndrome and/or acute myocardial infarction and chronic cardiac disorders. Increasing GGT over time is associated with type 2 diabetes and the metabolic syndrome. These associations are weaker than that of cholesterol and smoking, and current evidence is limited that measuring GGT improves cardiovascular disease risk prediction beyond conventional risk factors.[744,745]

Albumin

Serum albumin measurements are useful in assessing the chronicity and severity of liver disease. For example, the plasma albumin concentration is decreased in advanced chronic liver disease. However, its usefulness for this purpose is somewhat limited because the plasma albumin concentration may also be decreased in severe acute liver disease and is lowered by many other disorders, and nonspecifically in acute illness. Serial measurements of plasma albumin can be used in chronic liver disease to assess deterioration in the patient's condition.

Prothrombin Time

PT measurements can be used to differentiate between cholestasis and severe hepatocellular disease. In practice, PT should be measured again after vitamin K injection, because cholestasis may cause a decrease in PT as the result of malabsorption of vitamin K. The patient has cholestasis if the PT corrects after vitamin K replacement (10 mg subcutaneously or intramuscularly, followed by PT measurement 24 hours later). Over time, if the PT does not return to normal, the patient has severe hepatocellular disease.

Bilirubin

Serial measurement of serum bilirubin concentration is helpful in assessing the severity of liver damage in several types of liver disease (e.g., alcoholic hepatitis, cirrhosis). In acute hepatitis, bilirubin peaks later than enzyme activities, and bilirubin remains increased for longer than urine bilirubin because of the presence of biliprotein (δ-bilirubin). Increases in bilirubin in most liver diseases are primarily due to an increase in conjugated bilirubin, which is usually detected as direct reacting bilirubin. An increase in unconjugated bilirubin usually is not due to liver disease, although severe acute hepatitis and cirrhosis are often associated with increases primarily of unconjugated bilirubin, and autoantibody negative hemolytic anemia is a feature of Wilson disease.

Patients are frequently seen with isolated increases in bilirubin concentration and normal activities of liver-associated enzymes. Increased unconjugated (indirect reacting) bilirubin in such situations is usually due to increased production of bilirubin (hemolysis, rhabdomyolysis, large hematomas), which is prehepatic or due to impaired conjugation (inherited decrease in activity of conjugation in Gilbert syndrome or Crigler-Najjar syndrome, drug-induced inhibition of enzyme activity by atazanavir, immaturity of liver in physiologic jaundice of the newborn; see earlier section of this chapter). Gilbert syndrome is the most common cause of isolated unconjugated hyperbilirubinemia, and concentrations of bilirubin characteristically increase with fasting or intercurrent illness. Increases in conjugated (direct reacting) bilirubin are common in seriously ill individuals (bilirubinostasis of sepsis) and are less common with inherited defects in excretion of conjugated bilirubin (Dubin-Johnson syndrome, Rotor syndrome). An algorithm for differentiating the familial causes of hyperbilirubinemia is presented in Fig. 51.19.

Liver Fibrosis Assessment

Chronic liver disease is characterized by progressive hepatic fibrosis, which over time culminates in the development of cirrhosis and its complications of portal hypertension, HCC, and liver failure.[746] The reference standard for staging liver

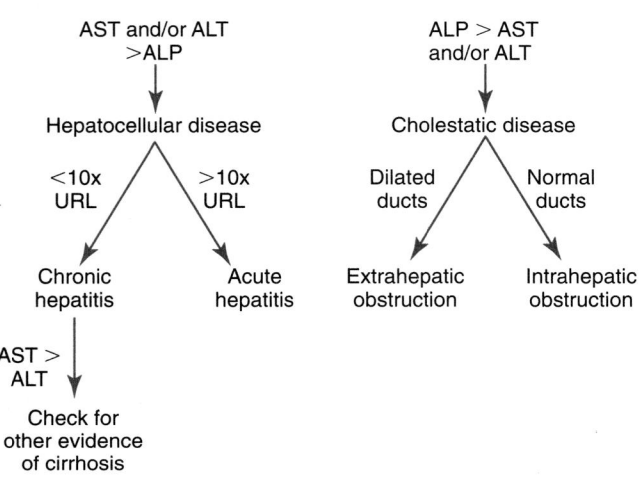

FIGURE 51.19 Algorithm for differentiating causes of abnormal liver-associated enzymes.

---

disease is the histologic staging of a liver biopsy specimen. Liver biopsy is invasive and resource-intensive even under optimal conditions, and it is far from a perfect reference standard. Even in experienced centers, biopsy is associated with complications such as pain (20%), serious morbidity (0.6%) (including bleeding that requires intervention), and even death (0.01%).[747] Aside from the hazards associated with the procedure itself, sampling variability may under or over stage fibrosis in as many of 20% of liver biopsies.[747] Moreover, the accuracy and reliability of liver biopsy is compromised by sampling error[748] and inter- and intraobserver variability.[749] For a confident histopathologic fibrosis stage to be assigned to a biopsy, the liver biopsy specimen must be of adequate size (e.g., 15 mm or five portal tracts). Nevertheless, at this size, a liver biopsy specimen represents only 1/50,000th of the liver, and it is well documented that liver histologic changes can vary within a particular liver segment or lobe. Accordingly, it has been argued that the maximum diagnostic accuracy of liver biopsy under optimal circumstances could be no more than 90%.[750] Because of the associated morbidity, the use of liver biopsy to perform longitudinal monitoring of liver disease raises ethical considerations and has contributed to the quest for noninvasive tests that can replace biopsy. The high reproducibility and low coefficients of variation associated with automated blood and biochemical tests have resulted in considerable interest in the use of blood tests to assess fibrosis. However, it should be recognized that liver histology generates more information than just assessment of liver fibrosis; therefore the place and importance of liver biopsy should not be underestimated. It should be recognized that even if it were possible to develop perfect blood tests, they would not replace histology and physical methods that estimate liver stiffness such as transient elastography provide no information about liver morphology and should not be thought of as having the potential to replace liver histology.

Biomarkers of Fibrosis

Due to the limitations of liver biopsy, several noninvasive methods have been developed to detect progressive liver fibrosis and stage liver disease. Over the past two decades, numerous serum markers or biomarkers have been identified and described. In contrast to a liver biopsy, biomarkers are less invasive, with minimal associated procedural morbidity. Serum biomarkers of fibrosis can be categorized into direct serum markers (measuring parameters directly related to both the fibrolytic and fibrogenic processes involved in liver matrix turnover) and indirect serum markers (combinations of serum parameters that are related to liver function, including AST and ALT).[746]

Candidate biomarker derivation. Typically in biomarker derivation studies, a "training set" of patients with defined severity of chronic liver disease is used, and putative candidate biomarkers are measured. The diagnostic performance of the biomarkers is then determined by measuring their ability to detect the stage of liver fibrosis determined by liver biopsy. Fibrosis stages are usually dichotomized into diagnostic targets, such as those with and without mild (e.g., meta-analysis of histologic data in viral hepatitis [METAVIR] F0-1), moderate (e.g., METAVIR F2-4), advanced (e.g., METAVIR F3-4) liver fibrosis, and cirrhosis (e.g., METAVIR F4). Thereafter, logistic regression modeling is used to derive a predictive algorithm that includes an individual biomarker or a combination of biomarkers. The diagnostic accuracy of a biomarker algorithm to correctly identify a particular stage of fibrosis can be examined by a receiver-operator characteristic curve (AUC), which plots sensitivity against $1 -$ specificity for all values of the biomarker as a continuous variable (see Chapter 2). The AUC ranges between 0 (a test with 0% sensitivity and 0% specificity) and 1 (a test with 100% sensitivity and 100% specificity). Typically, good diagnostic test performance is defined as an AUC of more than 0.8 by convention. However, it should be noted that if sampling error and inter- and intraobserver variability limit the sensitivity and specificity of the liver biopsy itself to 90%, then a truly perfect biomarker of fibrosis could obtain a maximum AUC of no more than 0.9.[751] Thereafter, biomarker algorithms derived from a training set are validated in an independent cohort of patients ("validation set"), and their AUCs calculated. For more information on how new biomarkers are developed and evaluated, refer to Chapter 2 on Statistical Methodologies in Laboratory Medicine and Chapter 10 on Evidence-Based Laboratory Medicine.

Direct biomarkers. Direct biomarkers exhibit biological plausibility because they represent alterations of ECM composition that occur during hepatic fibrosis. The most widely studied direct biomarker is hyaluronic acid (HA), a glycosaminoglycan that is synthesized by HSCs and degraded by liver sinusoidal cells.[752] Other direct biomarkers include terminal peptide of procollagen III,[607] TIMP-1,[753] type IV collagen,[754] and TGF-β.[755] As derived by logistic regression, panels of direct biomarkers have also been described. Combinations of direct biomarkers can result in superior diagnostic performance for the detection of fibrosis compared with their constituent components. The ELF[756] test is a combination of HA, TIMP-1, and procollagen III that has been validated for the detection of fibrosis in a variety of liver diseases, including viral hepatitis B[757] and C,[758] NAFLD in children[759] and adults,[486] and PBC[675] and PSC.[702] FIBROSpect (Prometheus, Mayo Medical Laboratories, Rochester, MN) is a combination of the direct biomarkers HA, TIMP-1, and α_2-macroglobulin.[760]

Indirect biomarkers. By contrast, indirect biomarkers reflect parameters that are altered because of changes in hepatic function that arise in the context of a particular stage of liver fibrosis. Indirect biomarkers include biochemical or hematologic variables that are synthesized or regulated by the liver (for example, clotting factors, cholesterol, and bilirubin), or indicate inflammation (for example, aminotransferases).

Hitherto, the AST-to-platelet ratio has been one of the most studied indirect biomarkers of liver fibrosis.[761] The AST-to-platelet ratio is calculated by dividing AST by the ULN of AST (for the sex of the patient) and the platelet count, and multiplying by 100. Another indirect biomarker is Fib-4, which is a combination of AST, ALT, age, and platelet count.[762] The Forns index is an indirect biomarker panel that consists of age, GGT, cholesterol, and platelet count.[763]

Hybrid biomarker. Indirect biomarkers can also be combined with direct biomarkers to form combination or hybrid biomarkers. Fibrometer is a hybrid biomarker that uses age, platelets, prothrombin index, AST, α_2-macroglobulin, HA, and urea.[764] Hepascore is a combination of bilirubin, GGT, HA, α_2-macroglobulin, age, and sex.[765] Fibrotest is a combination of GGT, bilirubin, haptoglobin, α_2-macroglobulin, apolipoprotein A1, age, and sex.[766]

Imaging modalities. Conventional imaging techniques including ultrasonography, CT, and MRI can detect liver cirrhosis by identifying and detecting characteristic morphologic changes that occur in the cirrhotic state, including liver surface nodularity and the presence of portal hypertension. These conventional imaging findings have an intermediate specificity but a low sensitivity for a diagnosis of compensated cirrhosis. Moreover, conventional imaging modalities perform poorly for the detection of lesser degrees of fibrosis. These failings of conventional imaging modalities to quantify liver fibrosis have driven the development of novel imaging technologies. Nevertheless, in contrast to serum markers, imaging modalities for fibrosis are time consuming and are more suited for use in a secondary care setting.

The most widely studied imaging modality for the detection of liver fibrosis is Transient Elastography (FibroScan, Echosens, France). In this modality, a specialized transducer emits painless mild amplitude, low-frequency vibrations into the liver, which propagates a shear wave. Assessment of the velocity of this shear wave allows interpretation of liver stiffness, and by inference, the degree of liver fibrosis. The results are available instantaneously, and the volume of liver assessed equates to a 1- by 4-cm cylinder, far exceeding the tissue volume reviewed by liver biopsy. Although its usefulness in obese patients has increased with the advent of new probes (XL probe), a failure rate of 1% with the XL probe and 15% with the standard M probe is still associated with the procedure.[767]

An alternative form of ultrasound elastography is the acoustic radiation force impulse (ARFI) imaging.[768] ARFI technology can be integrated into standard ultrasound units; it interrogates the mechanical properties of the liver tissue by evaluating the attenuation of propagated acoustic waves. In addition, because it is used in standard ultrasound apparatus, ARFI can localize areas of abnormality and perform a simultaneous abdominal and liver ultrasound.

Advances in magnetic resonance imaging technology have precipitated interest in magnetic resonance elastography.[769] Magnetic resonance elastography provides a uniform assessment of the overall liver, but is expensive, time-consuming, and limited in those with metallic implants and those who experience claustrophobia.

Detection of chronic liver disease in primary care. The current British Society of Gastroenterology (BSG) guidance advocates the use of a two-tier sequential testing strategy in primary care in which NAFLD patients with an indeterminate FIB4 score undergo an ELF test or elastography to determine the presence of F3-4.[770] Indeed this approach performs very well as evidenced by a large-scale evaluation of the use of FIB-4 and ELF to stratify NAFLD patients in primary care.[771] In this study, the overall PPV of this strategy was 30%. As compared to prior the use of standard LFTs to refer NAFLD patients the use of this pathway reduced unnecessary referrals by 80% and increased the detection of advanced fibrosis fivefold and cirrhosis threefold.

Prognosis and monitoring. Noninvasive tests have been shown to be better than liver biopsy at determining prognosis in chronic liver diseases,[772] and therefore may be a useful adjunct to liver biopsy when assessing a patient. A further advantage of noninvasive testing compared with liver biopsy is the readiness with which blood tests or imaging can be repeated to track changes in disease severity over time and in response to interventions. This use is proving particularly valuable in determining the impact of treatments for specific chronic liver diseases such as viral hepatitis and in monitoring responses to new antifibrotic therapies in clinical trials as part of drug discovery. For these reasons, noninvasive tests of liver fibrosis are gaining increasing acceptance as valuable additions to the repertoire of tests in the assessment and monitoring of patients with chronic liver disease.

LIVER TRANSPLANTATION

Clinical biochemistry plays an important role in the management of patients before and after transplantation. As described previously in this chapter, algorithms incorporating biochemical and other clinical parameters have been developed for the assessment of the need for transplantation in patients with acute and chronic liver disease. These include the formerly described Child-Pugh-Turcotte, MELD, and United Kingdom Endstage Liver Disease Score classifications. Post-transplantation, the main focus of management is on detecting graft failure, organ rejection, and monitoring the efficacy of immunosuppression (see Chapters 42 and 95). Laboratories are closely involved in monitoring the levels of liver enzymes, tests of hepatic synthetic function, therapeutic drug monitoring, and monitoring for viruses, including recurrence of HBV or HCV and CMV, which may complicate the course of recovery in immune-suppressed patients.

A detailed description of the interpretation of the results of these tests in the context of liver transplantation is beyond the scope of this text. The goal of the transplantation physician is to be alert for evidence of cellular rejection as indicated by increases of liver enzymes while monitoring the concentrations of immunosuppressive drugs and potential evidence of their toxicity, which is primarily indicated by renal impairment or leukopenia. Unfortunately, the current assays for cellular rejection are not sufficiently specific, and increases in liver enzymes may be the result of many other causes in patients who receive transplants. Furthermore, the currently widely used immunoassays of the major immuno-suppressive agents are inaccurate and do not permit precise prediction of therapeutic doses. This should be addressed by the introduction of LC-MS assays. Thus the monitoring and treatment of patients after transplantation remain the domain of expert and experienced clinicians working in close partnership with clinical chemists and other members of the multidisciplinary transplantation team.

SELECTED REFERENCES

52. Doumas BT, Poon PKC, Perry BW, et al. Candidate reference method for determination of total bilirubin in serum: development and validation. Clin Chem 1985;31:1779–89.

54. Lo SF, Jendrzejczak B, Doumas BT. Laboratory performance in neonatal bilirubin testing using commutable specimens: a progress report on a College of American Pathology study. Arch Pathol Lab Med 2008;132:1781–5.

101. Arroyo V, Fernandez J, Ginès P. Pathogenesis and treatment of hepatorenal syndrome. Semin Liver Dis 2008;28:81–95.

116. Friedman SL. Evolving challenges in hepatic fibrosis. Nat Rev Gastroenterol Hepatol 2010;7:425–36.

137. Friedman S, Bansa LM. Reversal of hepatic fibrosis—fact or fantasy? Hepatology 2006;43:S82–8.

176. Dufour D, Lott J, Nolte F, et al. Diagnosis and monitoring of hepatic injury. I. Performance characteristics of laboratory tests. Clin Chem 2000;46:2027–49.

209. Subcommittee on Hyperbilirubinemia. Management of hyperbilirubinemia in the newborn infant 35 or more weeks of gestation. Pediatrics 2004;114:297–316.

231. Asai A, Miethke A, Bezerra JA. Pathogenesis of biliary atresia: defining biology to understand clinical phenotypes. Nat Rev Gastroenterol Hepatol 2015;12:342–52.

254. McMahon B. The natural history of chronic hepatitis B virus infection. Hepatology 2009;49:S45–55.

281. Choo QL, Kuo G, Weiner A, et al. Isolation of a cDNA clone derived from a blood-borne non-A, non-B viral hepatitis genome. Science 1989;244:359–62.

293. Lam BP, Jeffers T, Younoszai Z, et al. The changing landscape of hepatitis C virus therapy: focus on interferon-free treatment. Therap Adv Gastroenterol 2015;8:298–312.

356. EASL. *Clinical Practice Guidelines. Management of chronic hepatitis B.* 2012; <http://www.easl.eu/research/our-contributions/clinical-practice-guidelines/detail/management-of-chronic-hepatitis-b-virus-infection>. (Accessed October 29, 2020).

373. Lee W. Acetaminophen-related acute liver failure in the United States. Hepatol Res 2008;38:S3–8.

395. Lucey M, Marthurin P, Morgan T. Alcoholic hepatitis. N Engl J Med 2009;360:2758–69.

414. Gow P, Smallwood R, Angus P, et al. Diagnosis of Wilson's disease: an experience over three decades. Gut 2000;46:415–19.

432. Fontana R, Lok A. Noninvasive monitoring of patients with chronic hepatitis C. Hepatology 2002;36:S57–S64.

471. Day CP. Non-alcoholic fatty liver disease: a massive problem. Clin Med 2011;11:176–8.

486. Guha IN, Parkes J, Roderick P, et al. Non-invasive markers of fibrosis in nonalcoholic fatty liver disease: validating the European Liver Fibrosis panel and exploring simple markers. Hepatology 2008;47:455–60.

497. Hennes E, Zeniya M, Czaja A, et al. Simplified criteria for the diagnosis of autoimmune hepatitis. Hepatology 2008;48:169–76.

508. Pietrangelo A. Hereditary hemochromatosis: pathogenesis, diagnosis and treatment. Gastroenterology 2010;139:393–408.

642. Kamath P, Wiesner R, Malinchoc M, et al. A model to predict survival in patients with end-stage liver disease. Hepatology 2001;33:464–70.

672. Lindor K, Gershwin M, Poupon R, et al. Primary biliary cirrhosis. Hepatology 2009;50:291–308.

704. Zimmerman H. Drug-induced liver disease. Clin Liver Dis 2000;4:73–96.

756. Rosenberg WM, Voelker M, Thiel R, et al. Serum markers detect the presence of liver fibrosis: a cohort study. Gastroenterology 2004;127:1704–13.

Gastric, Intestinal, and Pancreatic Function*

Roy Alan Sherwood and Natalie E. Walsham

ABSTRACT

Background

The stomach, intestinal tract, and pancreas are closely related both anatomically and functionally. The clinical manifestations, such as diarrhea or malabsorption, may be associated with disease of any of these organs. It is therefore appropriate to discuss them together. Advances in imaging techniques and improvements in endoscopic procedures have led to many traditional laboratory tests of gastrointestinal (GI) and pancreatic function becoming obsolete. However, in recent years, there has been a resurgence in the role of the laboratory in the investigation of the GI tract, particularly with the development of noninvasive biomarkers of GI tract inflammation and in the detection of pancreatic insufficiency.

Content

In this chapter, the anatomy and physiology of the GI tract and the normal processes of digestion and absorption are reviewed. Disorders of the stomach, pancreas, and intestine in which the laboratory plays a role in diagnosis and monitoring are discussed. The chapter concludes with an overview of GI regulatory hormones and neuroendocrine tumors in which GI symptoms are prominent, and with sections on strategies for the investigation of malabsorption and diarrhea.

*The full version of this chapter is available electronically on ExpertConsult.com.

Monoamine-Producing Tumors*

Graeme Eisenhofer

ABSTRACT

Background

Monoamine-producing tumors include neuroblastomas, pheochromocytomas, paragangliomas, and gastroenteropancreatic neuroendocrine tumors (GEP-NETs). Synthesis, storage, and secretion of biogenic amines and polypeptide hormones are characteristics of these tumors that both underlie their clinical manifestations and provide a means for laboratory diagnosis. The clinical features and related patterns and types of hormones produced by the tumors are highly heterogeneous and no single biomarker can reliably diagnose any tumor group. Heterogeneity not only reflects underlying genetic mutations and downstream tumorigenic pathways, but also susceptibility of progenitor cells to specific mutations from which the tumors develop and produce specific secretory products.

Content

This chapter describes the structure and function of peripheral monoamine systems and provides a comprehensive overview of laboratory diagnostic and clinical aspects of various monoamine-producing tumors. Neuroblastomas present in early childhood and develop from neural crest cells halted in their differentiation at the neuroblast stage and from which they can either spontaneously regress or follow an aggressive clinical course. Biochemical diagnosis depends mainly on measurements of urinary homovanillic acid and vanillylmandelic acid, biomarkers with limited diagnostic utility. Pheochromocytomas and paragangliomas, which develop from neural crest-derived chromaffin cells, are more readily detected by plasma or urinary normetanephrine, metanephrine, or methoxytyramine. Production of these metabolites varies depending on the underlying mutation. GEP-NETs secrete more variable products, requiring careful test considerations and interpretation according to clinical manifestations. Choice, interpretation, and development of biochemical tests can be facilitated by an understanding of the underlying biology of monoamine-producing tumors.

---

*The full version of this chapter is available electronically on ExpertConsult.com.

Bone and Mineral Metabolism*

William Duncan Fraser and David N. Alter[a]

ABSTRACT

Background

The skeletal system is one of the largest organs in the body and is one of the hallmarks that distinguishes vertebrates from invertebrates. It is the storehouse for 98 to 99% of the body's 1 kg of calcium. Bones are mineralized connective tissue in which type I collagen forms a network of flexible fibers. Mineralization of this network, or matrix, with calcium salts is required to produce the rigid skeleton. Bone is a living tissue that is constantly being remodeled by degradation of old tissue and replacement with new bone matrix. Osteoclasts and osteoblasts are the bone cells mainly responsible for remodeling. Osteocytes are important regulators of bone cell activity that can be estimated by laboratory methods.

Calcium is required for mineralization of bone and is a key regulator of many body processes. Calcium ions play critical roles in intracellular signaling, in regulation of events at the plasma membrane, and in the function of extracellular proteins such as those involved in blood coagulation. The circulating concentration of calcium ions is kept constant under the control of parathyroid hormone (PTH) and metabolites of vitamin D. Deviations of the concentration of free (ionized) calcium outside its very narrow reference interval can cause morbidity and mortality. The importance of the tight regulation of free calcium (ionized calcium) is underscored by the recognition that skeletal health is allowed to suffer markedly to allow physiologic processes in other organs to be maintained.

Phosphate is also important in bone mineralization and is a component of high-energy molecules. Fibroblast growth factor 23 (FGF23) is involved in regulation of phosphate in combination with PTH and vitamin D metabolites. Bone is increasingly recognized as having endocrine functions playing an important role in regulating metabolic processes.

Content

This chapter provides an overview of skeletal metabolism and then details the clinical chemistry of calcium and other ions, including phosphate and magnesium. Key molecules regulating these minerals in health and disease are described. Measurement of markers of bone metabolism, and the role of molecules involved in major disorders of bone and mineral metabolism are discussed.

*The full version of this chapter is available electronically on ExpertConsult.com.
[a]The authors gratefully acknowledge the contributions to previous editions by Drs. David B. Endres, Michael Kleerekoper, Juha Risteli, Leila Risteli, and Robert K. Rude, upon which portions of this chapter are based.

Pituitary Function and Pathophysiology

Daniel Thomas Holmes, Roger L. Bertholf, and William E. Winter[a]

ABSTRACT

Background

The anterior and posterior lobes of the pituitary gland control processes vital for survival of the individual and the species. Although growth in infancy and childhood depend on nutrition, genetics, and environment, thyroid hormone and growth hormone (GH) are essential contributors to growth. Thyroid hormone is a master regulator of the metabolic rate and neurologic development in utero, in infancy, and in childhood. The stress response requires the participation of cortisol. Together, cortisol and GH help maintain normal plasma glucose levels. Although prolactin is also a stress hormone, its role in lactation is evolutionarily required for the nutrition, hydration, and survival of the newborn and infant. The survival of the species is dependent upon reproduction and the gonadotropins, which regulate spermatogenesis and ovulation beginning during puberty. The posterior pituitary is no less important than the anterior pituitary. Antidiuretic hormone (ADH) is a key regulator of water balance. Because humans are 60% water (and infants and children have proportionately more total body water than adults), maintenance of intracellular and extracellular volumes is necessary for health and survival. Lastly, oxytocin is involved in breast feeding and parturition. Collectively, the most complex endocrine systems involve the cerebral cortex, hypothalamus, anterior and posterior lobes of the pituitary, pituitary hormones, and target organs and tissues.

Content

This chapter focuses on disorders of the anterior and posterior pituitary that produce deficient or excess hormone activity. In some instances, more specific details are provided in other chapters that concern specific hormone systems. By necessity this chapter provides specific numerical values for reference intervals and diagnostic cut-offs. However, decision thresholds, physiologic ranges, and reference intervals provided in this chapter serve as a general guide. Laboratories should verify that these ranges are appropriate for use in their own settings because values may vary depending on methodologies and other factors.

The pituitary gland (also called the hypophysis) regulates the endocrine system by integrating chemical signals from the brain with feedback from the concentration of circulating hormones to stimulate intermittent hormone release from target endocrine glands.[1,2] The pituitary serves as the master gland in maintaining homeostasis by orchestrating the many processes necessary for survival. There are also many important endocrine systems operating independently of the pituitary gland, such as the renin-angiotensin-aldosterone system (RAAS),[3] the calcium-parathyroid axis,[4] and the glucose-insulin axis.[5] Each of these systems and/or axes is far more complex than their simple names. For example, maintenance of normal plasma glucose concentrations involves multiple cells, tissues and organs (e.g., the islets of Langerhans [β, α, and δ cells], liver, adipose tissue, muscle, and intestine), hormones (e.g., insulin, glucagon, growth hormone [GH], cortisol, somatostatin, and the incretins), and various physiologic and biochemical events (e.g., nutrient absorption, glycolysis, glycogen synthesis, gluconeogenesis, glycogenolysis, lipid, and protein metabolism).

The hypophysis is composed of the adenohypophysis (the anterior lobe of the pituitary; ≈75% of the pituitary mass) and the neurohypophysis (the posterior lobe of the pituitary, ≈25% of the pituitary mass—also called the pars nervosa) (Fig. 55.1).[6] In turn, the adenohypophysis has three parts: (1) the pars distalis, where most hormone-producing cells are located; (2) the pars tuberalis, which is part of the hypophyseal stalk; and (3) the pars intermedia. The pars intermedia may be referred to as the intermediate lobe of the pituitary, although it is actually part of the adenohypophysis.

The biology of the adenohypophysis is distinctly different from that of the neurohypophysis; the adenohypophysis is controlled by the hypothalamus via releasing or inhibiting hormones, whereas the cell bodies of the neurohypophysis are anatomically located in hypothalamic nuclei, with oxytocin or ADH reaching the neurohypophysis through neurohypophyseal nerve axons.[7] Thus the neurohypophysis is not a discrete endocrine organ, but rather functions as a reservoir for these two hormones.

[a]The authors gratefully acknowledge the contributions of Ishwarlal Jialal, Mary Lee Vance, Ronald J. Whitley, A. Wayne Meikle, Nelson B. Watts, Laurence M. Demers, and Ann McCormack on which portions of this chapter are based.

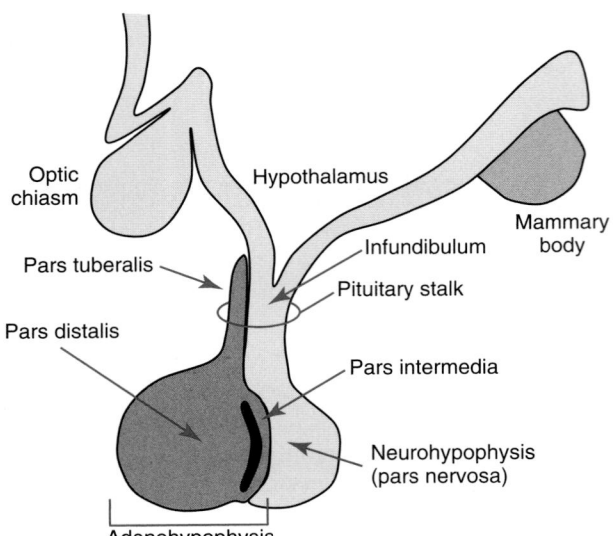

FIGURE 55.1 The Hypophysis (Pituitary Gland) Is Composed of the Adenohypophysis (the Anterior Lobe of the Pituitary) and the Neurohypophysis (the Posterior Lobe of the Pituitary; Pars Nervosa). The adenohypophysis has three parts: the pars distalis, where most of the hormone-producing cells are located; the pars tuberalis, which is part of the pituitary stalk; and the pars intermedia.

The roles of the various hormones secreted by the pituitary are exceedingly diverse and include regulation of (1) the body's response to stress (adrenocorticotropic hormone [ACTH or corticotropin] and GH), (2) the metabolic rate (thyroid-stimulating hormone [TSH or thyrotropin]), (3) growth (TSH and GH), (4) reproduction (luteinizing hormone [LH] and follicle-stimulating hormone [FSH]), (5) nourishment for the newborn and infant (prolactin), (6) parturition and milk letdown during breast feeding (oxytocin), and (7) fluid balance and blood pressure regulation in states of stress (ADH, or vasopressin, and cortisol).[8] Some of the pituitary hormones have specific targets (e.g., ACTH, TSH, LH, or FSH), whereas other hormones have multiple targets (e.g., GH, prolactin, oxytocin, and ADH). The action of the various hormones is dependent on the expression of the pertinent receptor in the target cell and associated second messenger systems.

A newly recognized product of the pituitary gland detected in some peri- and postmenopausal women is human chorionic gonadotropin (hCG).[9] Usually, hCG is associated with pregnancy or gestational trophoblastic disease. In early pregnancy, hCG doubles approximately every 48 hours, whereas the concentration of hCG originating from the pituitary or gestational trophoblastic disease is relatively stable and does not increase in concentration in the pattern seen in pregnancy. If an elevated hCG of 5 to 14 IU/L is detected in a postmenopausal woman, it is likely to be of pituitary origin if (1) the FSH is elevated (>45 IU/L), (2) the hCG is suppressed after 2 weeks of estrogen replacement, and (3) gestational trophoblastic disease has been excluded.

The placenta produces several hormones similar to pituitary hormones: hCG has functional and structural similarity to LH; human placental lactogen (hPL, or somatomammotropin) has actions similar to prolactin and GH; placental GH

becomes the predominant maternal GH during gestation; and placental corticotropin-releasing hormone (CRH) concentration rises in the fetus throughout gestation.[10] Placental GH (GH-V) differs from pituitary GH in 13 of 191 amino acids. Furthermore, GH-V exists in glycosylated and nonglycosylated forms, whereas pituitary GH is not glycosylated.

ANATOMY

The pituitary is located at the base of the brain and is protected anteriorly, inferiorly, and posteriorly by a depression in the sphenoid bone called the sella turcica. Inferior and anterior to the sella is the sphenoid sinus, which communicates with the nasopharynx. Neurosurgeons take advantage of the proximity of the sphenoid sinus to the pituitary using it as the preferred surgical access to the pituitary.

The pituitary weighs only 0.5 to 0.6 g. The gland is larger in women than in men; its size increases during pregnancy, and it is larger in multiparous women. At the completion of pregnancy, when the pituitary is largest, it is susceptible to infarction if hypovolemic shock develops from postpartum hemorrhage, producing a state of postpartum panhypopituitarism called Sheehan syndrome.[11]

If the pituitary is greatly reduced in size or is apparently absent on magnetic resonance imaging (MRI) studies, the sella is said to be "empty."[12] In the empty sella syndrome, the sella may be normal in size or enlarged. An incompetent diaphragma sella with compression of the pituitary gland by a herniating arachnoid can cause an empty sella, or the pituitary may be reduced in size as the result of previous apoplexy (i.e., spontaneous ischemic or hemorrhagic infarction) of a tumor, radiotherapy, or surgery.

Arterial blood is supplied to the pituitary via the superior and inferior hypophyseal arteries, both of which are branches of the internal carotid arteries. The superior hypophyseal arteries supply the anterior pituitary and hypophyseal stalk, whereas the inferior hypophyseal arteries supply the posterior pituitary.

Direct delivery of hypothalamic regulatory hormones to the adenohypophysis occurs through the hypothalamic-pituitary portal system, surrounding the adenohypophysis (pars distalis). A portal system is a vascular apparatus in which blood that initially passes through one capillary network (e.g. the hypothalamus) is collected into vessels that subsequently supply a second capillary network (e.g., the anterior pituitary). Anatomically, this is similar to the nephron where blood from glomerular capillaries is collected into the efferent arteriole to be distributed again to the peritubular capillaries or vasa recta. In this way, the hypothalamus controls the secretion of adenohypophyseal hormones via delivery of hypothalamic venous blood to the anterior pituitary gland. There is also retrograde flow from the pituitary to the hypothalamus via the portal system.

Pituitary venous drainage is moved to the cavernous and intercavernous sinuses via the lateral hypophyseal veins. The cavernous sinus drains to the superior and inferior petrosal sinuses, which join the transverse sinus to form the jugular vein. This anatomic relationship is clinically important because access to pituitary secretions can be afforded by cannulation of the inferior petrosal venous sinuses.[13] Usually, the neuroradiologist places catheters bilaterally into the femoral veins and passes them via the iliac veins, inferior vena cava, and superior vena cava to the jugular veins to enter the inferior petrosal sinus. Inferior petrosal sinus sampling (IPSS) is used to distinguish Cushing disease (i.e., anterior pituitary corticotroph adenoma) and Cushing syndrome caused by ectopic ACTH production. An important corollary of the plexiform venous drainage of the pituitary is that IPSS cannot be used to determine which side of the pituitary contains a corticotroph adenoma because left-side tumors can have venous drainage to the right and vice versa.

The internal carotid arteries are lateral to the pituitary. Above the pituitary is the diaphragma sellae, which comprises circular (intercavernous) sinuses containing venous blood. Anterior and superior to the pituitary is the optic chiasm. These relations are clinically important because pituitary neoplasms can invade or compress these structures, as well as the sella turcica. For example, superiorly expanding anterior pituitary adenomas can compress the optic chiasm, producing bitemporal hemianopsia, that is bilateral peripheral vision loss.[14]

PITUITARY EMBRYOLOGY

The adenohypophysis develops in utero from a dorsal evagination of the roof of the stomodeum, which becomes the Rathke pouch.[15] The superior portion of the Rathke pouch constitutes the pars tuberalis (see earlier), whereas the posterior portion of the Rathke pouch develops into the pars intermedia (or intermediate lobe). Transcription factors regulating the development of the anterior pituitary gland include HESX, FGFR1, LHX3, LHX4, SOX3, Pit-1, PROP1, RIEG, and GLI2.[16–18] Mutations in these transcription factors can cause various types of hypopituitarism, along with other conditions such as septo-optic dysplasia (SOD).[18,19] The pars intermedia, which is active only late in pregnancy and in utero, secretes α-, β-, and γ-melanocyte stimulating hormone (MSH), corticotropin-like intermediate lobe peptide, γ-lipotropin, and β-endorphin. MSH is believed to promote melanin synthesis. Lipotropins mobilize fat from adipose tissue, and endorphins are endogenous opioids.[20] The clinical significance of these intermediate lobe products as causes of disease is poorly understood.

Regulation of Function of the Adenohypophysis

The synthesis and release of the following anterior pituitary hormones are stimulated by hypothalamic-releasing hormones: ACTH, TSH, GH, LH, and FSH.[7] Prolactin is the sole anterior pituitary hormone whose release is predominantly regulated through suppression—specifically via dopamine. Corticotrophs secrete ACTH, thyrotrophs secrete TSH, somatotrophs secrete GH, gonadotrophs secrete both LH and FSH, and lactotrophs secrete prolactin. Except for LH and FSH, each hormone is normally produced by a unique cell type. However, some somatotroph adenomas, which cause pituitary gigantism and acromegaly co-secrete prolactin. The molecular composition of the anterior pituitary hormones is summarized in Table 55.1.

Multiple levels of control of the hypothalamic-pituitary-end organ-hormone axis are known (Fig. 55.2).[21] Except for prolactin and LH at the midpoint of the menstrual cycle, negative feedback controls secretion of the adenohypophyseal hormones. The long feedback loop involves suppression of the hypothalamic-releasing hormone and the anterior pituitary trophic hormone by the hormonal product of the target tissue. The major site of negative feedback for cortisol (regulated by ACTH), insulin-like growth factor-I (IGF-I; regulated by GH), and sex steroids and inhibins (regulated by LH and FSH) is the hypothalamus. In contrast, for thyroid hormone (regulated by TSH), the major site of negative feedback is the anterior pituitary. Retrograde flow from the pituitary to the hypothalamus via the portal system permits the existence of short negative feedback loops in which pituitary hormones suppress the secretion of hypothalamic-releasing hormones. Ultra-short feedback loops also exist in which pituitary hormones inhibit their own secretion.

TABLE 55.1 Hypothalamic-Releasing or -Inhibiting Hormones, Their Target Cells, and the Hormone That Is Regulated

Hypothalamic Hormone/Abbreviation	Amino Acids	Anterior Pituitary Target Cell	Hormone Regulated	Amino Acids	MW (kDa)
Corticotropin-releasing hormone (CRH)	41	Corticotroph	ACTH	39	4.5
Thyrotropin-releasing hormone (TRH)	3	Thyrotroph	TSH[a]	α: 92	28
				β: 118	
Growth hormone–releasing hormone (GHRH)	44	Somatotroph	GH	191	22
				176	20
Somatotropin release–inhibiting hormone (SRIH)[b]	14	Somatotroph	GH	176	20
Gonadotropin-releasing hormone (GnRH)	10	Gonadotroph	LH[a]	α: 92	32
				β: 121	
			FSH[a]	α: 92	30
				β: 111	
Dopamine	1	Lactotroph	Prolactin	199	22

ACTH, Adrenocorticotropic hormone; *FSH,* follicle-stimulating hormone; *GH,* growth hormone; *LH,* luteinizing hormone; *MW,* molecular weight.
[a]All α-glycoprotein chains are identical, including the α-chain of human chorionic gonadotropin.
[b]Also known as somatostatin.

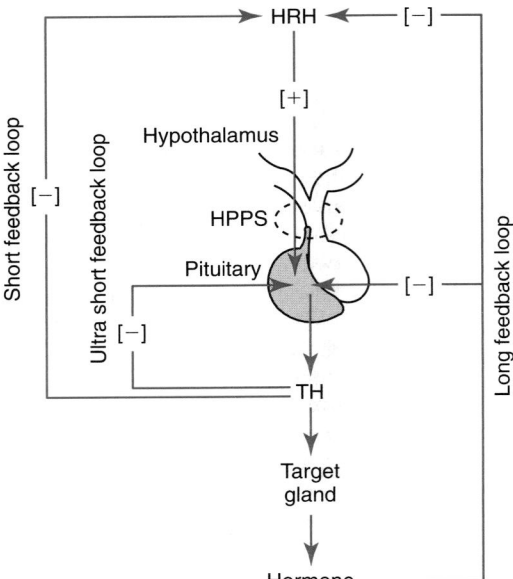

FIGURE 55.2 Many Anterior Pituitary Trophic Hormones (e.g., Adrenocorticotropic Hormone *[ACTH]*, Thyroid-Stimulating Hormone *[TSH]*, Growth Hormone *[GH]*, Luteinizing Hormone *[LH]*, Follicle-Stimulating Hormone *[FSH]*) Are Regulated by Hypothalamic Releasing Hormones *(HRHs)*. Releasing hormones secreted by the hypothalamus reach the pituitary via the hypothalamic-pituitary portal system *(HPPS)*. Long feedback loops involve negative feedback of the target cell hormone at the pituitary gland and hypothalamus. The short feedback loop involves the anterior pituitary trophic hormone feeding back at the hypothalamus, whereas the ultra-short feedback loop involves the anterior pituitary hormone feeding back at the anterior pituitary. *[+]*, Stimulation; *[−]*, suppression; *TH*, trophic hormone.

POINTS TO REMEMBER

- Most anterior pituitary hormones are predominantly regulated by stimulatory hypothalamic hormones. The exception is prolactin, which is tonically suppressed by dopamine.
- Pulsatile secretion of hypothalamic-releasing hormones is required for normal release of anterior pituitary hormones such as luteinizing hormone and follicle-stimulating hormone.
- Either hypo- or hyperfunction can develop from pathologic processes involving the hypothalamus, the hypothalamic-pituitary portal system, or the anterior pituitary.
- Reference intervals may depend upon age, gender, time of collection, menstrual cycle and menopausal status.

HYPOTHALAMIC REGULATION

The hypothalamus is a region of the brain producing hormones that control a number of bodily functions, including the release of hormones from the anterior pituitary gland. The hypothalamus is located in the middle of the base of the brain and encapsulates the ventral portion of the third ventricle.

The hypothalamic hormones regulating the anterior pituitary hormones are listed in Table 55.1. With the exception of CRH, these are structurally smaller than their pituitary counterparts.

CRH has wide distribution throughout the brain and brainstem.[22] In the hypothalamus, it is released by the paraventricular nucleus (PVN). CRH secretion is stimulated by systemic physiologic stress via (1) neurons of subfornical origin, (2) neurons of the nucleus tractus solitarius, (3) hypothalamic glutamatergic neurons, and (4) 5-hydroxytryptamine–secreting neurons of the raphe nucleus. Neurogenic stress to release CRH also acts via hypothalamic glutamatergic neurons. Stress inhibits hypothalamic GABAergic neurons of the PVN that otherwise would suppress CRH release. Gamma-aminobutyric acid (GABA) serves as an inhibitory neurotransmitter. GABAergic neurons innervating CRH-secreting neurons also originate from the lateral septum and the bed nucleus of the stria terminalis. ACTH release is stimulated by serotonin, endorphins, and acetylcholine but is suppressed by GABA. Physiologically, stress, inflammation, and hypoglycemia stimulate ACTH release.

Thyrotropin-releasing hormone (TRH) is a tripeptide product of the PVN of the hypothalamus.[23] TRH-secreting neurons in the PVN are innervated by axons that release (1) norepinephrine, (2) leptin, (3) neuropeptide Y, (4) agouti-related protein, (5) MSH, (6) CRH, or (7) somatostatin. Leptin is produced by adipose tissue and acts to reduce appetite and raise energy expenditure as body fat stores rise. Leptin receptors are expressed in the ventromedial nucleus of the hypothalamus. Leptin (*LPE* gene) deficiency and leptin receptor (*LEPR* gene) deficiency are rare causes of severe, early-onset genetic forms of obesity.[24] Neuropeptide Y and agouti-related protein promote food intake.

The energy state and temperature of the organism influence TRH secretion. In addition to TRH regulation of TSH, TSH secretion is suppressed by (1) thyroid hormones, (2) glucocorticoids, (3) estrogens, and possibly (4) GH. Acute inflammatory cytokines such as interleukin (IL)-1β, IL-6, and tumor necrosis factor (TNF)-α stimulate ACTH release but suppress TRH and TSH. Norepinephrine stimulates TSH release, whereas endorphins, serotonin, and dopamine suppress TSH.

GH–releasing hormone (GHRH) is produced by neurons in the arcuate nucleus of the medial basal hypothalamus. Stimulators of GHRH release include dopamine- and galanin-secreting neurons and brain stem neurons with catecholaminergic inputs.[25] Galanin is a neuropeptide that is widely expressed in the endocrine, central nervous, and peripheral nervous systems. There are three unique galanin receptors.[26] Hypothalamic somatostatin suppresses both GHRH release and anterior pituitary GH release. Leptin from adipose tissue and ghrelin from the stomach have the net effect of increasing GHRH secretion and directly increasing GH concentrations. However, the clinical relevance of these influences and of other GH-releasing peptides (e.g., GHRP-6) is not well understood. Ghrelin binds to GH secretagogue receptors, which increases food intake. Ghrelin and obestatin are derived from the ghrelin-obestatin preproprotein. The actions of obestatin may involve anxiety and thirst reduction, recall enhancement, sleep regulation, cell division, and augmented pancreatic enzyme secretion.[27] Hormones affecting GH secretion include estrogen, testosterone, and glucocorticoids. Physiologically, amino acids and hypoglycemia stimulate GH release. Glucagon stimulates both GH and cortisol release (which is why glucagon-stimulation tests are a clinical alternative to the insulin tolerance test [ITT]). In turn, the secretion of IGF-I in response to GH is influenced by nutrition, sex steroids, thyroid hormone, and the presence of chronic disease. Malnutrition, sex hormone deficiency in adolescents and adults, hypothyroidism and chronic disease all produce varying degrees of GH-resistance. Dopamine, endorphins, serotonin, and norepinephrine stimulate GH secretion.

Gonadotropin-releasing hormone (GnRH) regulation is complicated by the fact that GnRH must differentially control LH and FSH secretion, which vary greatly during the menstrual cycle in women.[28] GnRH-secreting neurons are not located in a discrete nucleus but are diffusely distributed throughout the hypothalamus. Embryologically, these neurons are unusual because they originate outside the central nervous system (CNS). GnRH secretion is stimulated by neurons that secrete (1) galanin-like peptide, (2) kisspeptin, (3) glutamate, (4) neuropeptide Y, and (5) norepinephrine. Kisspeptin, derived from *Kiss* 1 gene expression, is a neuropeptide that regulates puberty and reproduction. Hyperprolactinemia inhibits *Kiss* 1 gene expression and leads to diminution of GnRH and gonadotropin secretion. Neurons secreting GABA, β-endorphins, and CRH inhibit GnRH. Gonadotropin release is stimulated by norepinephrine, GABA, and acetylcholine, and is suppressed by endorphins, dopamine, and serotonin.

GnRH pulsatility is essential to gonadotroph responsiveness. Tonic release of GnRH downregulates GnRH receptors on gonadotrophs causing hypogonadism. Therapeutically, downregulation is accomplished with a long-acting GnRH agonist, such as leuprolide acetate in the treatment of central precocious puberty in children or the induction of hypogonadism in men with prostate cancer. Conversely, pulsatile GnRH administration is used to initiate puberty and to induce ovulation or spermatogenesis in states of GnRH deficiency. The rate of pulsatility may influence the relative secretion of LH and FSH. In primate studies, GnRH at one pulse per hour preferentially released LH, whereas one pulse every three hours caused a decline in LH and a mild rise in FSH.

Anterior Pituitary

In the anterior pituitary, (1) CRH receptors are expressed on corticotrophs, (2) TRH receptors are expressed on thyrotrophs, (3) GHRH receptors are expressed on somatotrophs, (4) GnRH receptors are expressed on gonadotrophs, and (5) prolactin-inhibiting hormone (PRIH, dopamine) receptors are expressed on lactotrophs. There are two CRH receptors

(CRHR1 and CRHR2) that are G-protein–coupled receptors.[29] The gene for CRHR1 is located on chromosome 17q21.31. The gene for CRHR2 is located on chromosome 7p14.3. The TRH receptor is also G-protein coupled. The gene for the TRH receptor is located on chromosome 8q23.1. Chromosome 7p14.3 is the location of the GHRH receptor gene. The gene for the G-protein–coupled GnRH receptor is chromosome 4q. In pathologically high concentrations, TRH stimulates the release of LH and prolactin which is why primary hypothyroidism is a cause of prolactin elevation. Otherwise, TRH does not appear to play a major role in regulating LH or prolactin secretion.

Corticotrophs are stimulated by high concentrations of proinflammatory cytokines, such as IL-1, IL-6, and TNF-α.[30] This emphasizes the interrelationship of the endocrine and immune systems in a hypothalamic-pituitary-adrenal-immune system axis. Through vasopressin type 3 receptors (also known as the arginine vasopressin receptor 1B, V1b receptors, gene location: chromosome 1q32), high concentrations of ADH stimulate corticotrophs to release ACTH.

The hormonal products of each anterior pituitary target cell (if applicable) are listed in Table 55.2 together with a summary of each system. Many of these hormones display circadian (daily), ultradian (more than daily), or infradian (less than daily) variation that reflects changes in hypothalamic control. Deficiency of an individual pituitary hormone is typically called hypopituitarism,[31-33] whereas deficiency of all anterior pituitary hormones is termed panhypopituitarism.

Growth Hormone and Insulin-like Growth Factors

Linear growth is the consequence of (1) genetic potential, (2) nutrition, (3) the presence or absence of disease, and (4) hormonal effects.[34] Many hormones influence growth, but the most important are GH, thyroid hormone, and sex steroids. Excess glucocorticoids can impair growth in children. GH deficiency can be symptomatic in adults, and so GH appears to be essential for health throughout life.

Growth Hormone–releasing Hormone

The *GHRH* gene is located on chromosome 20q11.2. Prepro-GHRH is a polypeptide chain of 108 amino acids (12.4 kDa). Removal of the 20 amino acid signal (leader) sequence peptide yields the 88 amino acid pro-GHRH. Cleavage of the 11 amino acid N-terminal pro-sequence and the 31 amino acid C-terminal pro-sequence, with release of two free amino acids (positions 76 to 77 with reference to prepro-GHRH),

TABLE 55.2 Hypothalamic-Pituitary-End Organ Physiology

Hypothalamic Hormone	Anterior Pituitary Hormone	Target Organ/Tissue	Target Hormone
CRH	ACTH	Adrenal cortex: zona fasciculata and zona reticularis	Cortisol
TRH	TSH	Thyroid follicular cell	Thyroxine (T$_4$) and 3,5,3′-triiodothyronine (T$_3$)
GHRH and SRIH	GH	Liver and many tissues of the body	IGF-I, IGFBP-3, and ALS
GnRH	LH, FSH	Gonad	Sex steroids and inhibins
Dopamine	Prolactin	Breast	Not applicable

ACTH, Adrenocorticotropic hormone; *ALS*, acid-labile subunit; *CRH*, corticotropin-releasing hormone; *FSH*, follicle-stimulating hormone; *GH*, growth hormone; *GHRH*, growth hormone–releasing hormone; *GnRH*, gonadotropin-releasing hormone; *IGFBP-3*, IGF binding protein-3; *IGF-I*, insulin-like growth factor-I; *LH*, luteinizing hormone; *MW*, molecular weight; *SRIH*, somatotropin release–inhibiting hormone; *TRH*, thyrotropin-releasing hormone.

TABLE 55.3   Biology of the Somatostatin Receptors

SSTR	Gene Location	Amino Acids/Molecular Weight	SST Binding	Distribution
SSTR1	14q1	391 aa 42.7 kDa	SST-14 >SST-28	Fetal kidney, fetal liver, adult pancreas, brain, lung, jejunum, stomach
SSTR2	17q2	369 aa 41.3 kDa	SST14 and SST-28	Cerebrum, kidney
SSTR3	22q13.1	418 aa 45.8 kDa	SST-14 and SST-28	Brain, pituitary, pancreas
SSTR4	20p11.2	388 aa 42 kDa	SST-14	Fetal and adult brain, lung, stomach, less in kidney, pituitary, adrenals
SSTR5	16p13.3	364 aa 39.2 kDa	SST-28 >SST-14	Adult pituitary, heart, small intestine, adrenal, cerebellum, fetal hypothalamus

aa, Amino acid.

produces the 44 amino acid mature GHRH. The terminal leucine of GHRH is amidated. Alternative splicing of the mRNA (isoform 2) produces a prepro-GHRH protein of 107 amino acids, which is missing amino acid 103.

Somatostatin

Somatostatin is also known as somatotropin release–inhibiting hormone (SRIH).[35] It is widely expressed throughout the body (CNS, gut, and δ-cells of the islets of Langerhans) and produces multiple physiologic effects. Somatostatin receptors are likewise widely distributed (see Table 55.3). Somatostatin functioning as SRIH is produced by the PVN of the hypothalamus. In pancreatic islets, somatostatin suppresses both glucagon and insulin secretion, whereas somatostatin release is stimulated by both of these hormones. In this way, δ-cell somatostatin modulates islet function by smoothing out extremes in the secretion of glucagon and insulin to maintain a stable blood glucose concentration. Somatostatin in the gut is found in highest concentration in the duodenum and jejunum.

The somatostatin gene is located on chromosome 3q2. Expression of the somatostatin gene produces the 116 amino acid polypeptide prepro-somatostatin. Cleavage of the signal sequence (24 amino acids) produces pro-somatostatin (92 amino acids), and subsequent cleavage of the N-terminal pro-sequence (64 amino acids) yields a 28 amino acid form of somatostatin (SST-28). SST-28 has an intrachain disulfide bond between amino acids 17 and 28. In many tissues, SST-28 undergoes cleavage to a 14 amino acid form (SST-14) through removal of the N-terminal 14 amino acid sequence by the enzymes prohormone convertase 1/prohormone convertase 2 (PC1/PC2) and carboxypeptidase E (CPE). SST-14 is the major form of somatostatin in the CNS and δ-cells, whereas SST-28 is the major form in the gastrointestinal tract. SST-28 is also the major circulating form of somatostatin. Therefore somatostatin measurements in peripheral blood do not reflect SRIH secretion. Somatostatin is highly conserved in nature; all vertebrates have the identical sequence for SST-14.[35]

In addition to GH suppression, somatostatin also suppresses TRH, TSH, CRH, and ACTH. However, the effect of somatostatin on the regulation of the adrenal cortical and thyroid axes is usually minor. In the gastrointestinal tract, somatostatin reduces the secretion of multiple hormones, including (1) gastrin, (2) secretin, (3) cholecystokinin, (4) vasoactive intestinal polypeptide, (5) motilin, (6) neurotensin, and

(7) pepsin, and reduces gastric pH, intestinal motility, ion and nutrient absorption, and proliferation of the mucosa (see Chapter 52). This motivates the clinical use of octreotide (a synthetic somatostatin analogue) in the medical management of VIPoma and glucagonoma.[36–38] Calcitonin, catecholamines, renin, and pancreatic exocrine function and insulin release are also suppressed by somatostatin. Indium-111 and gallium-68 labeled octreotide have been used for imaging, and lutetium-177 labeled octreotide has been used in radiotherapy of tumors expressing somatostatin receptors (e.g., neuroendocrine tumors).[39] For more information on neuroendocrine tumors, refer to Chapter 53.

Growth Hormone–releasing Hormone Receptor

The anterior pituitary somatotroph GHRH receptor (GHRHR) is a member of family B-III of the G-coupled receptor superfamily (the "secretin" family).[7] Receptors for (1) secretin, (2) vasoactive intestinal polypeptide, (3) parathyroid hormone (PTH), and (4) calcitonin share partial sequence identity with GHRHR.

Pre-GHRHR is a 423-amino-acid polypeptide that is converted to the mature 401-amino-acid form of GHRHR by removal of the 22-amino-acid signal peptide. The N-terminal extracellular domain is 110 amino acids. GHRHR has seven transmembrane domains and a 42-amino-acid cytoplasmic domain. Amino acid 50 may be glycosylated.

Somatostatin Release–inhibiting Hormone Receptor

Throughout the body, there are five receptors for somatostatin (SSTR1 through SSTR5; Table 55.3). Each receptor is encoded by a gene located on a separate chromosome. SSTR2 has two alternatively spliced isoforms. All of the SSTR receptors have seven transmembrane domains and are coupled with a pertussis toxin–sensitive G-protein. SSTR2, SSTR3, SSTR4, and SSTR5 are expressed in the pituitary.

Growth Hormone

Growth hormone has two disulfide bridges (amino acids 54 and 165, and amino acids 182 and 189).[40] Structurally, GH has four main α-helices, and within the connecting loops, it has three mini-helices. Two circulating forms of GH are present: a 22-kDa form that is a 191 amino acid chain (full-length GH) that represents 85 to 90% of circulating GH, and a 20-kDa GH that lacks amino acids 32 through 46.[41] The 20-kDa form of GH results from alternative splicing of the

GH mRNA transcript. In addition to the 22- and 20-kDa forms, circulating GH exists as aggregates and oligomers. "Big GH" is a dimer of GH monomers, and "big, big GH" is GH associated with its binding protein (GHBP). GHBP is the external domain of the GH receptor (GHR), which binds GH with high affinity and is produced by cleavage of the GHR. Approximately 55% of all circulating GH forms are monomeric; big GH and big, big GH represent approximately 27% and approximately 18% of circulating GH, respectively. Approximately 50% of GH is not bound to GHBP; approximately 45% is bound to GHBP, and the remaining 5% of GH is bound to low-affinity binding proteins. Considering the multiple forms of GH, it is not surprising that significant analytical biases were historically observed between different immunoassays for GH. With the availability of recombinant standardized reference materials, this problem is expected to improve.

The gene for GH (chromosome 17q24.2) is a member of the GH subfamily that includes (−5′ to 3′ direction) (1) GH (the GH1 gene), (2) a chorionic somatomammotropin (hPL) pseudogene designated CSHP, (3) a chorionic somatomammotropin-A designated CSH1, (4) the placentally produced 22-kDa GH variant (GH-V; gene designation GH2), and (5) chorionic somatomammotropin-B (gene designation CSH2).[42] Somatomammotropin (hPL) is a placental hormone with growth-promoting properties. Prolactin (199 amino acids) shares a homologous amino acid sequence with GH, but prolactin, encoded on chromosome 6p22, is not part of the GH complex on 17q24.2.

GH has both direct and indirect activity. Its direct actions will be described in the following sections.[43] The indirect activity of GH is mediated by IGF-I. To initiate its direct and indirect activity, GH binds to receptors (GHR) that appear to be expressed by all tissues.

Growth Hormone Receptor

The GHR is a member of the class 1 hematopoietic cytokine family.[44] Other members of this family include receptors for erythropoietin, granulocyte-macrophage colony-stimulating factor, and various interferons. Structurally, the GHR is a single-chain, 620-amino-acid protein (130 kDa). Pre-GHR includes an 18 amino acid leader sequence. The GHR structure includes an extracellular domain (246 amino acids), a transmembrane domain (24 amino acids), and a cytoplasmic domain (350 amino acids).[45] When the extracellular portion of the GHR is shed, the 55-kDa GHBP moiety is released into the circulation.

Four isoforms of the GHR are expressed by alternative splicing of the nascent mRNA. Isoform 1 is the full-length receptor. Isoform 2 differs in the sequence of amino acids 292 to 297 (with reference to pre-GHR) and lacks amino acids 298 to 638. Isoform 3 differs in the sequence of amino acids 292 to 294 and lacks amino acids 295 to 638. An alanine at position four is replaced by aspartic acid, and amino acids 25 to 46 are missing in isoform 4.

The GHR exists as a cell surface dimer in its inactive state (Fig. 55.3). When GH binds to the GHR, the receptor recruits or activates 120-kDa Janus-associated kinase enzymes (JAK2; a type of adapter tyrosine kinase). JAK2 then exerts tyrosine kinase activity by phosphorylating itself and the GHR.[46,47] Phosphorylation activates JAK2, which triggers several intracellular pathways involving (1) signal transducers and activators of transcription (STATs), (2) the insulin receptor substrate,

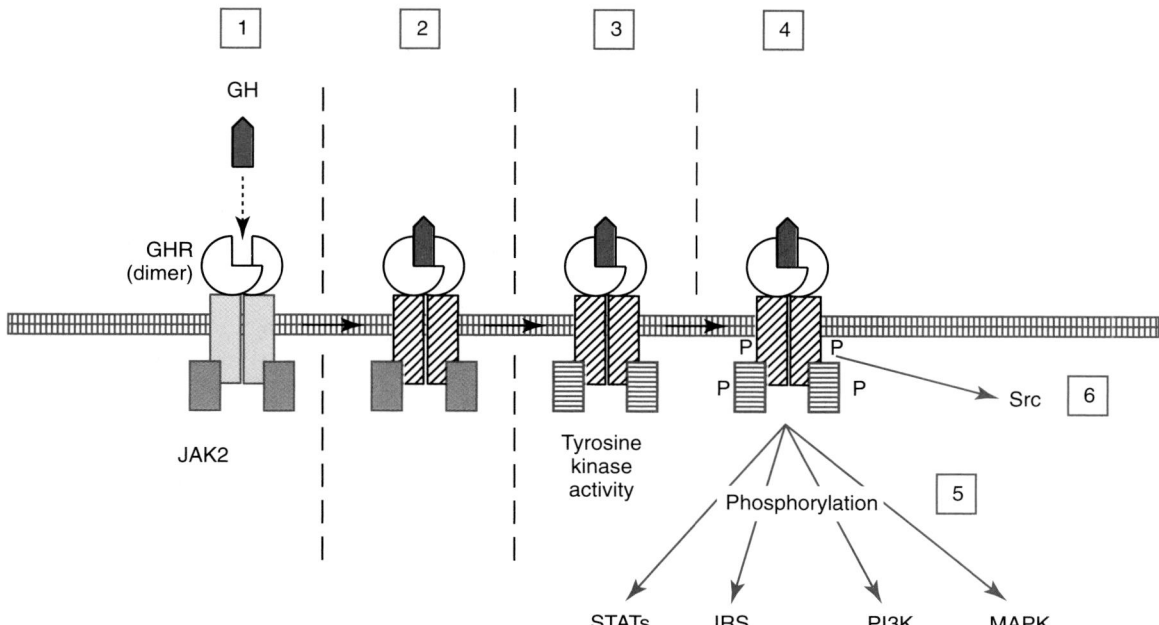

FIGURE 55.3 The Growth Hormone Receptor *(GHR)* Exists as a Cell Surface Dimer in Its Inactive State. With growth hormone *(GH)* binding to the GHR *(1)*, the GHR recruits or activates Janus-associated kinase enzyme *(JAK2) (2)*. JAK2 then achieves tyrosine kinase activity *(3)*, and JAK2 and the GHR are phosphorylated *(4)*. Activated JAK2 triggers several intracellular pathways involving signal transducers and activators of transcription *(STATs)*, the insulin receptor substrate *(IRS)*, phosphatidylinositol 3′-kinase *(PI3K)*, and a mitogen-activated protein kinase *(MAPK) (5)*. Independent of JAK2, GHR signaling can proceed via Src *(6)*.

(3) phosphatidylinositol 3′-kinase (PI3K), and (4) a mitogen-activated protein kinase (MAPK). Via receptor-associated kinases, members of the STAT family are phosphorylated to permit the formation of homodimers or heterodimers that act as transcriptional activators once they translocate to the cell nucleus.[48] STAT5b is involved, but it is unclear whether STAT5a is also involved.[49] In its role as a transcription factor, phosphorylated, dimerized STAT5b enters the nucleus to promote gene transcription. Independent of JAK2, GHR signaling can be effected via *Src*, which is a tyrosine kinase. (Note: *Src* is the Rous sarcoma virus protooncogene).

Insulin-like Growth Factors

IGF-I is a member of the insulin-related peptide family whose other members include IGF-II, insulin, and relaxin. Stimulated by hCG during pregnancy, relaxin is produced by the corpus luteum verum (the corpus luteum of pregnancy), the decidua (the uterine lining during pregnancy), and the placenta. Relaxin increases collagenase activity to soften and lengthen the cervix and pubic symphysis and facilitate parturition. Relaxin also reduces uterine contractility by inhibiting myosin kinase activity. In humans, there are three nonallelic relaxin genes: *RLN1, RLN2,* and *RLN3.*

Proinsulin, IGF-I, IGF-II, and relaxin are all composed of two domains (A and B) joined by a connecting domain. The connecting domains vary in sequence and length much more than the A and B domains. The connecting domain of proinsulin is cleaved to release C-peptide (connecting peptide), producing insulin A and B chains. Insulin, IGF-I, IGF-II, and relaxin have two disulfide bridges. IGF-I and IGF-II share 62% homology, and they each share 50% homology with insulin.

The 110 amino acid sequence of preproinsulin includes a signal peptide (amino acids 1 to 24), the insulin B chain (amino acids 25 to 54), C-peptide (amino acids 57 to 87), and the insulin A chain (amino acids 90 to 110). The two interchain disulfide bonds are between amino acids 31 and 96, and 43 and 109. The single intrachain disulfide bond is between amino acids 95 and 100.

Two forms of prepro–IGF-I are expressed as a consequence of alternative mRNA splicing: IGF-IA and IGF-IB. The IGF-IA preprohormone is 153 amino acids, including a signal peptide (amino acids 1 to 21), an N-terminal propeptide (amino acids 22 to 48), IGF-I (70 amino acids), and a C-terminal propeptide (the E domain, amino acids 119 to 153). The IGF-I polypeptide includes the B domain (amino acids 49 to 77), the C (connecting) domain (amino acids 78 to 89), the A domain (amino acids 90 to 110), and the D domain (amino acids 111 to 118). Three disulfide bonds are present between amino acids 54 and 96, 66, and 109, and 95 and 100. IGF-I is not glycosylated. A relatively common (~0.6%) single nucleotide polymorphism in IGF-I (A70T) has been identified in the screening population for acromegaly which is clinically relevant since some commercial immunoassays do not detect this variant form leading to factitiously decreased IGF-I concentrations.[50]

The 195 amino acid IGF-IB preprohormone is composed of a signal peptide (amino acids 1 to 21), a propeptide (amino acids 22 to 48), IGF-I (70 amino acids), and another propeptide region (the E domain, amino acids 119 to 195). Differences in the D domain of the prepro–IGF-I distinguish IGF-IA from IGF-IB; the tertiary structure of the IGF-I proteins and the placement of disulfide bonds are identical between IGF-IA and IGF-IB.

The IGF-II preprohormone comprises 180 amino acids. The first 24 residues constitute the signal peptide. After their removal, IGF-II is derived from pro–IGF-II after cleavage of the C-terminal E peptide (amino acids 92 to 180). Therefore amino acids 25 to 91 include the B region (amino acids 25 to 52), the C region (amino acids 53 to 64), the A region (amino acids 65 to 85), and the D region (amino acids 86 to 91) of IGF-II. Isoform I is the full-length prepro–IGF-II (180 amino acids). Formed by alternative splicing, isoform II lacks amino acid 25 (alanine) and is therefore 179 amino acids in length. IGF-II is glycosylated at amino acid 99 and has three intrachain disulfide bonds between amino acids 33 and 71, 45 and 84, and 70 and 75. A potential glycosylation site is amino acid 163.

Prorelaxin is a 185-amino-acid protein that contains a signal sequence (amino acids 1 to 22), a B chain (amino acids 23 to 53), a connecting propeptide (amino acids 56 to 158), and an A chain (amino acids 163 to 185). A–B interchain disulfide bonds can occur between amino acids 35 and 172, and 47 and 185. An additional disulfide bridge may occur between amino acids 171 and 176.

IGF-I and IGF-II circulate together with an IGF binding protein (IGFBP) (most importantly IGFBP-3), and the acid-labile subunit (ALS) to form a 150-kDa trimeric protein complex. Approximately 75 to 80% of IGF-I/IGFBP-3 complexes are trimeric; the remaining IGF-I/IGFBP-3 complexes are dimeric and may include other IGFBPs. Less than 1% of the total IGF-I is free (the biologically active form). The binding affinity of IGF-I for the insulin receptor is low (≈7% of insulin affinity) but circulating IGF-I concentrations exceed insulin by three orders of magnitude. Without binding proteins, therefore IGF-I could cause potentially devastating hypoglycemia.

The trimeric IGF-I-IGFBP-3-ALS complexes do not normally cross capillary membranes because of their size. However, the 50-kDa binary complex and free IGF-I are able to enter the interstitium, where binding to type I IGF receptors can occur.

Most of the circulating IGF-I is produced by hepatocytes.[51] However, IGF-I is also produced locally throughout the body and thus acts as a paracrine and an autocrine hormone. The possible endocrine (systemic) influence of IGF-I on growth is discussed later.

Similar to IGF-I, IGF-II does not normally produce hypoglycemia. However, tumors that secrete a larger than normal form of IGF-II have been described. These are usually more than 0.5 kg in size; nonislet cell tumors are most often of mesenchymal or hepatic origin.[52] Since big IGF-II does not bind normally to IGFBP-3, the free IGF-II concentration is greatly elevated, and the molar IGF-II to IGF-I ratio is greater than 10. As a result of IGF-II binding to the insulin receptor, the clinical syndrome is similar to that of hypoglycemia caused by hyperinsulinism (i.e., absence of ketonemia with no elevation of free fatty acids, lactate, or alanine), and insulin itself is suppressed because β-cells are normal. Physiologically, hypoglycemia stimulates the release of counter-regulatory hormones such as GH, but in this scenario IGF-II suppresses the GH axis. Removal of the tumor leads to the resolution of hypoglycemia.[53,54]

TABLE 55.4   Characteristics of Insulin-like Growth Factor Binding Proteins

IGFBP	Chromosome Gene Location	Amino Acids	Affinity for IGF-I vs. IGF-II	Specific Features
1	7p13	234	1 = 2	RGD sequence[a]
2	2q3	289	1 < 2	RGD sequence[a]
3	7p13	264	1 = 2	N-glycosylation
4	17q	237	1 = 2	Extra cysteines
5	2q3	252	1 < 2	Ternary complex with ALS
6	12q13	216	1 < 2	O-glycosylation
7	4q12	282	[b]	Stimulates prostacyclin production

[a]RGD sequence = arginine-glycine-aspartic acid.
[b]Binds IGF-I and IGF-II with low affinity.
ALS, Acid-labile subunit; *IGF,* insulin-like growth factor; *IGFBP,* insulin-like growth factor protein.

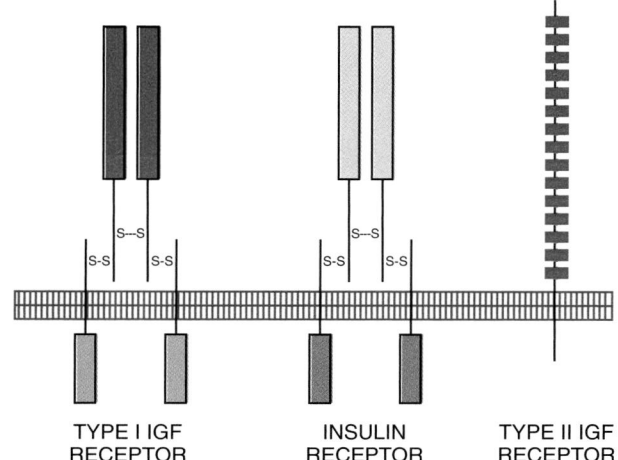

FIGURE 55.4 The Type I Insulin-like Growth Factor *(IGF)* Receptor Is Structurally Similar to the Insulin Receptor. The structure of the type II IGF receptor is similar to that of the epidermal growth factor receptor.

Insulin-like Growth Factor Binding Proteins

Because of their high affinity (K_d 10^{-10} to 10^{-11} M) for IGFs, IGFBPs are regarded as inhibitors of IGF action.[55] IGFBPs have higher affinity for IGFs than do the IGF receptors. IGFBP-3 has biological actions independent of the IGF/IGF-I receptor axis.[56] Receptors for IGFBPs have been described. Proteolysis of IGFBPs releases IGF-I; therefore IGFBP proteases can influence free IGF-I concentrations. Table 55.4 summarizes the features of the seven known IGFBPs. From a clinical standpoint, only IGFBP-3 has relevance as it is used as an adjunctive tool in addition to GH and IGF-I in the diagnosis of GH deficiency.[57]

Receptors for Insulin-like Growth Factors

Two types of receptors for IGFs have been identified: the type I IGF receptor and the type II IGF receptor (Fig. 55.4).[58] Structurally, the type I IGF receptor is similar to the insulin receptor. Because this receptor does not exclusively bind IGF-I, the terminology "IGF-I receptor" is not recommended. The type I receptor is derived from a single precursor protein of 1367 amino acids that include the 30 amino acid signal peptide. The 706 amino acid (130 kDa) α-chain is extracellular and is bound by a disulfide bond to the transmembrane 90-kDa (627 amino acids) β- chain. Cleavage of the α- and

β-chains releases a tetrapeptide (707 to 710: arginine-lysine-arginine-arginine). Beta-chain amino acids 906 to 929 form a transmembrane domain. The receptor exists as a homodimer (β-α-α-β) with the two α-chains bound to each other by two disulfide bonds. Similar to the type I IGF receptor, the insulin receptor is a homodimer of two 135-kDa α-chains and two 95-kDa β-chains.

Tyrosine kinase activity in the cytoplasmic portion of the type I IGF receptor β-chain results from binding of an IGF molecule to the cysteine-rich portion of the α-chains (amino acids 148 to 302), which causes conformational changes in both α- and β-chains. Intracellular signaling involves autophosphorylation and phosphorylation of the 185-kDa insulin receptor substrate 1, which is the predominant target of the active type I IGF receptor. The type I IGF receptor binds IGF-I with higher affinity than IGF-II, and affinity for insulin is lower than the affinity of the receptor for IGF-I or IGF-II. The affinities of the insulin receptor are the opposite: insulin ≫ IGF-II > IGF-I.

The type II IGF receptor is structurally dissimilar from the type I IGF receptor and the insulin receptor. The 270-kDa, 2451-amino-acid, type II IGF receptor is a monomeric protein that is similar to the epidermal growth factor (EGF) receptor. (Note: The leader sequence is 40 amino acids.) The EGF receptor itself is also known as ErbB1 or HER1. The external portion of the receptor is 2264 amino acids, the transmembrane domain is 23 amino acids, and the cytoplasmic domain is 164 amino acids. Beginning at the N terminus, there are 13 amino acid repeats of approximately 150 amino acids, and a 47 amino acid fibronectin type II domain, followed by 2 more repeats. Evidence indicates at least five glycosylation sites: amino acids 112 (with preference for the pre–type II IGF receptor), 581, 626, 747, and 1246. Two disulfide bonds are found between amino acids 1903 and 1927 and between amino acids 1917 and 1942.

Ligand binding to EGF receptors results in dimerization and tyrosine kinase activation. The external ligand-binding domain of EGFs is composed of numerous short amino acid repeats. The type II IGF receptor removes IGF-II from the circulation. The type II IGF receptor binds mannose-6-phosphate, in addition to IGFs, permitting the uptake and intracellular movement of mannose-6-phosphate–containing lysosomal enzymes. The binding sites for IGFs and mannose-6-phosphate are found on different parts of the receptor. The affinities of the type II IGF receptor are as follows: IGF-II ≫ IGF-I > insulin. Because this receptor does not exclusively bind IGF-II, the terminology "IGF-II receptor" is not recommended.

A hybrid receptor consisting of the α–β-chain of the insulin receptor and the α–β-chain of the type I IGF receptor has been described. It has been suggested that these hybrid receptors may allow cancers to respond to insulin.[59] In cancers, insulin is also thought to act through the insulin signaling pathway via insulin receptors and also probably acts through receptors that bind IGF-I. Thus IGF-I also plays a role in cancer biology. Increasing evidence suggests that IGF-I may enhance the growth of many tumors, and it is known that acromegaly confers increased risk for both colorectal and thyroid cancer.[60] Thus the casual use of IGF-I injections in children to enhance growth in short but otherwise normal children is problematic and potentially carcinogenic.

POINTS TO REMEMBER

- Growth hormone (GH) deficiency in children should be considered only when other causes of low growth-velocity short stature have been excluded.
- The diagnosis of GH deficiency usually requires stimulation testing, although some endocrinologists will diagnose GH deficiency based solely on the measurement of insulin-like growth factor-I (IGF-I).
- Defects in IGF-I generation and response are rare compared to GH deficiency.
- GH deficiency does occur in adults, and accordingly, they may benefit from GH replacement.
- GH excess produces the clinical syndrome of gigantism in children and acromegaly in adults.
- GH excess is diagnosed by elevated IGF-I levels and the failure of GH suppression after an oral glucose load.
- Reference intervals for IGF-I are influenced by methodology, age, sex, and pubertal stage.

Regulation of Growth Hormone Secretion

Growth hormone ultimately stimulates release of IGF-I, which negatively feeds back to regulate GH release via two hypothalamic hormones: somatostatin (or SRIH; from the hypothalamic PVN) and GHRH (from the hypothalamic infundibular nucleus) (Fig. 55.5). These hypothalamic GH-regulating hormones are carried to the anterior pituitary via the specialized hypothalamic-pituitary portal vascular system. Somatotrophs of the anterior pituitary gland have receptors for both hormones. Somatostatin inhibits GH release, whereas GHRH promotes the release of GH. However, GH release is the predominant hypothalamic effect because surgical interruption of the pituitary stalk with destruction of the hypothalamic-pituitary portal system leads to GH deficiency, not excess. In addition to its hypothalamic negative feedback effects, IGF-I directly suppresses pituitary release of GH.

Physiologically, GH secretion is episodic and pulsatile.[61] Consequently, random measurements can neither exclude GH deficiency nor confirm its excess; between pulses, GH concentrations can be quite low and do not distinguish GH insufficiency from normal production of the hormone. During daytime hours, the plasma concentration of GH in healthy adults remains stable and relatively low (<2 ng/mL; <2 μg/L) with several secretory spikes occurring approximately 3 hours after meals (particularly meals high in protein

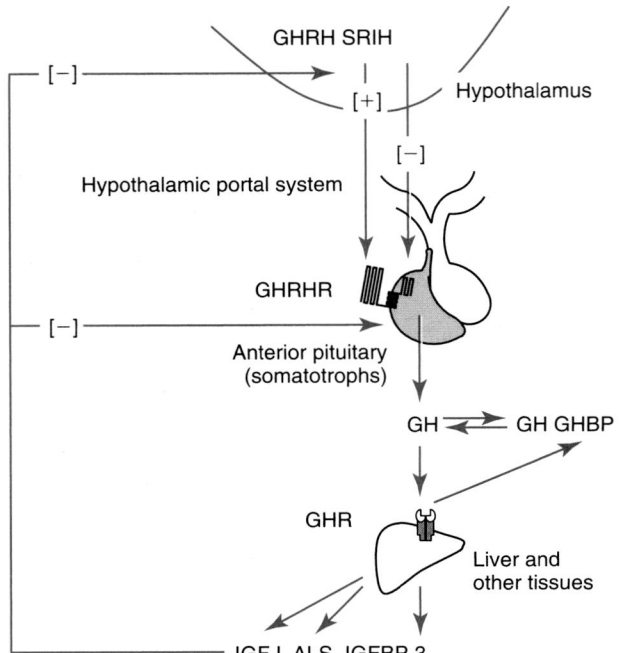

FIGURE 55.5 The Hypothalamus Secretes Growth Hormone–releasing Hormone *(GHRH)* and Somatotropin Release–inhibiting Hormone *(SRIH;* Somatostatin*)*, Which Regulate Growth Hormone *(GH)* Release. The receptor for GHRH *(GHRHR)* is illustrated because mutations in this receptor can cause some forms of inherited GH deficiency. GH circulates unbound and bound to its binding protein *(GHBP)*. GHBP is the extracellular domain of the GHR, which is cleaved from the GHR and circulates in the plasma. GH releases IGF-I, IGF binding protein 3 *(IGFBP-3)*, and the acid-labile subunit *(ALS)*. IGF-I negatively feeds back at the anterior pituitary somatotrophs and at the hypothalamus. Because transection of the pituitary stalk leads to GH deficiency, the predominant hypothalamic control of GH is stimulatory via GHRH.

and arginine) and after exercise. In contrast, during the evening hours, adults and children show a marked rise in GH secretory activity approximately 90 minutes after the onset of sleep; GH concentrations reach a peak value during the period of deepest sleep. This pattern of GH secretion may be important for anabolic and repair processes and for proper skeletal growth. GH is also increased by psychologic or physical stress and hypoglycemia. Normal GH secretion requires thyroxine and age-appropriate concentrations of testosterone or estrogen.

GH is suppressed by elevations in blood glucose. One of the tests for GH excess measures GH after an oral glucose load (e.g. 75 g in adults and 1.75 g/kg in children); the normal response is a GH concentration of less than approximately 0.4 ng/mL (0.4 μg/L) for a modern analytically specific chemiluminescent sandwich assay.[62,63] Some research further suggests that body mass index should be considered when interpreting GH results after a glucose load (Box 55.1).[63] GH also declines with increases in free fatty acid concentrations, rapid eye movement sleep, and aging. In the presence of abnormally high concentrations of glucocorticoids, GH secretion is suppressed. In addition, circulating GH is thought to influence the release of hypothalamic hormones through the short feedback loop. Other hypothalamic hormones, such as

BOX 55.1 Protocol for Glucose Suppression of Growth Hormone Test

Rationale

Normal subjects show suppression of serum growth hormone (GH) concentrations after oral administration of glucose. Subjects with acromegaly fail to exhibit appropriate GH suppression.

Procedure

The test should be performed after an overnight fast with the patient maintained at bed rest. After a baseline blood specimen is collected for GH and glucose measurement, a solution of 75 g of glucose is given orally (in children, 1.75 g/kg to a maximum dose of 75 g). Glucose and serum GH are measured again on specimens collected 30, 60, 90, and 120 min later.

Interpretation

Serum GH concentrations in normal individuals fall to less than 0.4 ng/mL (0.4 μg/L) using a modern chemiluminescent sandwich assay. Subjects with acromegaly fail to show this suppression and sometimes show a paradoxical increase in GH concentration. Patients with liver disease, uremia, or heroin addiction may have false-positive results with this test (failure to suppress serum GH concentrations after oral glucose load).

TRH and GnRH, do not affect GH release in normal subjects but may provoke GH release in patients with acromegaly.

Age-associated decline in GH production, as can be appreciated through age-dependent IGF-I reference intervals,[64] has spawned an industry of dietary supplements purported to "support" GH secretion.[65] These supplements are amino acid preparations that theoretically stimulate release of the subject's own GH. Such dietary supplements have no proven medical value. Use of GH by athletes to enhance strength or promote recovery from injury is prohibited in most sports.

The role of non-GHRH GH secretagogues in the physiologic control of GH and growth is highly debated.[66] One such secretagogue is ghrelin (28 amino acids, 3.4 kDa; gene name: GHRL; chromosome 3p2). Although ghrelin is produced in the hypothalamus, its highest concentration is found in gastric tissue. In addition, ghrelin is widely distributed in the rest of the gastrointestinal tract, heart, lung, and adipose tissue. Ghrelin appears to stimulate food intake and obesity.[67]

Ghrelin binds to the somatotroph GH-secretagogue receptor (gene name: GHSR; isoform 1A: 366 amino acids, 41 kDa; isoform 1B: 289 amino acids, 32 kDa; chromosome 3q26.31), which is distinct from the GHRHR. GHRL, the gene that encodes ghrelin, also encodes the 23 amino acid peptide obestatin. As noted previously, obestatin may decrease food intake and increase satiety, but this has been debated. Obestatin is a ligand for the orphan GPR39 receptor (453 amino acids, 51 kDa; chromosome 2q21). However, despite obestatin binding to the GPR39 receptor, receptor activation may not follow.[68]

Physiologic Actions

Growth hormone effects can be classified as indirect or direct.[69] GH directly raises blood glucose by stimulating gluconeogenesis and reducing insulin sensitivity. Also, it causes adipose tissue lipolysis, and the resulting GH-induced elevations in free fatty acids provide an alternative energy source that serves to spare glucose for CNS use. Therefore when glucose and free fatty acid concentrations are raised at times of stress, in partnership with epinephrine, glucagon, and cortisol, fuels for the fight-or-flight response are provided. GH has other effects on intermediary metabolism: GH stimulates the uptake of nonesterified fatty acids by muscle and accelerates the mobilization and metabolism of fat from adipose tissue to the liver.

At the epiphysis of growing bone, GH promotes epiphyseal prechondrocyte differentiation. GH directly stimulates the production of the ternary complex of IGF-I, IGFBP-3, and the ALS. In turn, after entering the interstitium, unbound IGF-I binds to type I IGF receptors.

Indirect effects of GH are mediated through IGF-I production, which (together with GH) is necessary for linear growth in childhood. IGF-I is mitogenic and antiapoptotic. Epiphyseal prechondrocyte differentiation stimulated by GH, along with the local effects of IGF-I (also under the control of GH), stimulates the clonal expansion of differentiating chondrocytes.

Thus the overall effect of GH is to promote growth in soft tissue, cartilage, and bone. This action results from stimulation of protein synthesis that is induced in part by an increase in amino acid transport through cell membranes. The effects of GH on bone and muscle are exerted both directly and through the effects of IGF-I under the influence of GH. Increased growth of soft tissue and the skeleton is accompanied by changes in electrolyte metabolism, including positive nitrogen and phosphorous balance, a rise in plasma phosphorous concentration, and a fall in blood urea and amino acid concentrations. Additional responses to GH include increased intestinal absorption of calcium and decreased urinary excretion of sodium and potassium. The metabolic changes most likely are caused by increased uptake of these ions by growing tissue.

IGF-I increases glucose oxidation in adipose tissue and stimulates glucose and amino acid transport into diaphragmatic muscle and heart muscle. Synthesis of collagen and proteoglycans is enhanced by IGF-I, which also has positive effects on calcium, magnesium, and potassium homeostasis. The insulin-like effects of this growth factor have been ascribed in part to its structural similarity to insulin.

Evidence indicates that the local effects of IGF-I (autocrine or paracrine) are predominant in stimulating growth when compared with the systemic effects of IGF-I produced by the liver. When the hepatic IGF-I gene was knocked out in mice (although nonhepatic tissues expressed IGF-I), growth was normal, and IGFBP-3 and ALS concentrations were low. IGF-II may function as a growth factor in utero; however, its secretion in utero is not under the control of GH.

In the absence of GH, IGF-I is not as effective a growth stimulant as it is when GH and IGF-I both are present. IGF-I treatment alone is not recommended as therapy for GH deficiency; IGF-I therapy is reserved for cases of GH resistance due to GHR deficiency (e.g., Laron syndrome).[47,70]

GH (through IGF-I) and insulin induce growth in a similar manner because both have protein anabolic effects and stimulate the transport of amino acids into peripheral cells. Their respective effects on glucose homeostasis, however, oppose one another—chronic GH excess induces diabetes mellitus. Most growth-promoting GH effects are delayed rather than immediate and are exerted primarily through IGF-I.

IGF-I concentrations vary widely with age and gender.[64] IGF-I rises during childhood, and during puberty, IGF-I concentrations can be two to three times the adult concentration. After adolescence, IGF-I concentrations show steep decline until age 30, followed by a gradual decline until old age.

GH is not the only determinant of IGF-I concentration in the circulation. Transformation of the GH stimulus to IGF-I production and secretion is modulated by (1) nutrition, (2) the presence or absence of chronic inflammation, (3) thyroid function, (4) glucocorticoids, and (5) sex steroids. IGF-I secretion is reduced by (1) malnutrition, (2) malabsorption (e.g. inflammatory bowel disease, celiac disease), (3) obesity (4) cystic fibrosis, (5) chronic disease, (6) sex hormone deficiency in adolescence. Therefore a decreased IGF-I concentration is not necessarily synonymous with GH deficiency.

In cases of acquired GH resistance and genetic GH resistance (GHR mutation or signaling disorder), GH concentrations will rise, and high concentrations of GH produce hyperlipidemia and hyperglycemia.[71] Cases of acquired GH resistance are not treated with GH or IGF-I, but instead are treated by addressing the underlying disorder.

The actions and regulation of IGF-II have been debated.[72] IGF-II is believed to be important for intrauterine growth. Mice display intrauterine growth retardation when the IGF-II gene is knocked out. Although IGF-II–producing tumors are rare, such tumors can produce hypoglycemia attributable to incompletely processed variant of IGF-II.[48,54] Both IGF-I and IGF-II are of great interest to oncology researchers; the reader is referred to the literature for a detailed discussion of this topic.

Clinical Significance

Diagnosis of clinically important states of GH excess or deficiency are uncommon and may go unrecognized for years.[73] GH concentrations vary widely under normal circumstances; therefore random measurements of GH, in general, are not diagnostically useful. A single GH measurement cannot distinguish between normal fluctuations and the low or high concentrations that are typical of various diseases. GH measurements are best determined as part of dynamic function testing: physiologic or pharmacologic provocative stimuli are used to help diagnose GH deficiency, whereas GH suppression (or lack thereof) following glucose administration is used to identify GH excess.[74] IGF-I concentrations often correlate better with the clinical severity of acromegaly than with glucose-suppressed or basal GH concentrations.[75]

In contrast to GH, a single measurement of IGF-I is considered to be an accurate reflection of GH-IGF-I production, irrespective of the time of the day or meals. IGF-I has a much longer half-life than GH and accordingly has more stable plasma concentrations. The half-life of GH is slightly longer than 15 minutes, whereas the half-life of the trimeric IGF-I-IGFBP-3-ALS complex is 17 to 22 hours. The half-life of unbound IGF-I is only 10 to 20 minutes, but the unbound form of the hormone accounts for less than 1% of the total concentration. Serum concentrations of IGF-I are influenced by (1) age, (2) sex, (3) degree of sexual maturity, (4) thyroid

status, (5) nutritional status, and (6) body mass index. As mentioned previously, IGF-I concentrations are low in GH deficiency and in patients with acute or chronic protein or caloric deprivation and, in the other extreme, obesity. In pediatric endocrinology, measurements of IGFBP-3 have been used in addition to IGF-I measurements to assess GH; however, the additional value of IGFBP-3 measurement over and above IGF-I measurement has not been firmly established. The diagnostic use of GH to stimulate IGF-I production is controversial and is not currently included in standard medical practice.[76]

Growth Hormone Excess

Acromegaly is the rare clinical syndrome in adults resulting from GH excess.[77,78] Even less common is pituitary gigantism, which results from GH excess in childhood. The clinical features of acromegaly involve overgrowth of the skeleton and soft tissue, producing (1) acral enlargement (enlargement of the extremities), (2) organomegaly (enlarged heart and/or liver), (3) facial coarsening, (4) intestinal polyposis and attendant increased risk of colorectal cancer, (5) premature cardiovascular disease, (6) hyperhidrosis (increased sweating), (7) skin tags, (8) bone and joint disorders, (9) myopathy with weakness, (10) insulin resistance, and often (11) diabetes mellitus. Premature cardiovascular disease is the most common cause of death in individuals with acromegaly. Gigantism is characterized by extreme tall stature, in addition to the clinical features of acromegaly, as pathologic GH excess occurs before epiphyseal fusion is complete (e.g., in children or adolescents).

Most cases of acromegaly ($\approx$95%) result from anterior pituitary GH-secreting tumors ("somatotroph adenomas" or "somatotropinomas").[79] Somatotropinomas are usually macroadenomas ($>$10 mm in diameter) by the time they come to clinical attention; the vast majority of these can be visualized by computed tomography (CT) or MRI. Some anterior pituitary tumors secrete both GH and prolactin (somatomammotropinomas). GH-secreting anterior pituitary adenocarcinomas are exceedingly rare. Approximately 5% of GH-secreting tumors are familial and caused by disorders such as multiple endocrine neoplasia type 1 syndrome, familial acromegaly, Carney syndrome, McCune-Albright syndrome, and familial isolated pituitary adenoma.[80] Rare causes of acromegaly include GHRH-secreting hypothalamic tumors, extrapituitary somatotropinomas, and GHRH-secreting islet cell tumors, or those of lung or breast.

In severe or advanced cases of GH excess, the diagnosis may be nearly certain on the basis of physical appearance alone. However, in less severe or early cases, the physical changes may be subtle and gradual, so careful attention to clinical findings is required to make an early diagnosis. The reversibility of tissue changes depends largely on the duration of the disease. In addition to soft tissue changes, acromegaly may cause severe disability or death from cardiac, pulmonary, and/or neurologic sequelae. The most important requirement for the diagnosis of acromegaly is the demonstration of inappropriate and excessive GH secretion.[81]

As many as 10% of patients with active acromegaly have random serum GH concentrations that fall within the reference interval. Essentially all patients with acromegaly have an abnormal GH response to an oral glucose load (see Box 55.1). Patients with acromegaly typically show modest or no change in their basal concentration of GH or demonstrate a paradoxical increase in GH[82]; in contrast, normal individuals show suppression of GH concentrations to less than 0.4 ng/mL (0.4 μg/L) after a 75-g oral glucose.[62,63] IGF-I is considered to be the most important diagnostic tests for the initial diagnosis of acromegaly.[83,84] Additionally, because of the development of GH-receptor antagonist therapies for acromegaly (e.g. pegvisomant), IGF-I is also the only clinical tool available for monitoring patients receiving these therapies.

Growth Hormone Deficiency and Growth Retardation

In children, short stature with a normal growth velocity (≥4 to 5 cm/year) results from (1) familial short stature, (2) primordial growth failure (prenatal-onset growth failure), or (3) constitutional delay in growth and adolescence (delayed maturation).[85] Short stature with a low growth velocity (<4 to 5 cm/year) results from genetic short stature, chronic illness, malnutrition, deprivation (nutritional or psychological), Turner syndrome, or endocrine disorders (e.g., hypothyroidism, disorders of the GHRH-GH-IGF-I axis, extremely poorly controlled diabetes, rickets, pseudohypoparathyroidism, pseudopseudohypoparathyroidism, and Cushing syndrome).[86]

Idiopathic short stature is the term that is used when children with short stature and a low growth velocity lack evidence of pathology. It has been increasingly recognized that 5 to 15% of these children have a mutation in the *SHOX* (short stature homeobox) gene located on chromosome Xp22.33. Forearm anomalies are common in such children, and they become more evident during puberty.[87]

GH deficiency is not a common cause of growth retardation. Approximately one-half of children evaluated for growth retardation have no specific organic cause; approximately 15% have an endocrine disorder, of which approximately half (approximately 8% of all children with short stature) have GH deficiency. Children with significantly reduced height and low growth velocities with no clear explanation should be screened for GH deficiency once other endocrine disorders have been excluded.

GH deficiency in children is characterized by (1) short stature, (2) low growth velocity, (3) immature facial appearance, (4) delayed bone age on radiologic examination, and (5) increased adiposity. In cases of congenital GH deficiency, size at birth is usually normal because in utero IGF-I does not appear to be under GH control. Micropenis is evident in some boys with congenital GH deficiency and will resolve with GH replacement in childhood. Micropenis suggests hypopituitarism, although there are other causes for micropenis.[88] Adults with GH deficiency experience (1) reduced muscle mass ("sarcopenia"), (2) increased central adiposity, (3) osteoporosis with decreased bone density, (4) increased fracture risk, (5) decreased quality of life, (6) dyslipidemia, and (7) increased risk of cardiovascular disease.[89] GH deficiency is probably the most common endocrine abnormality in adults with large (non-somatotroph) pituitary adenomas[90] and in patients who have undergone pituitary irradiation. Recovery of normal hormonal production after surgery for these types of pituitary adenomas occurs uncommonly. GH replacement therapy forms an important part of the clinical care of GH-deficient children. Whether GH therapy is required in GH-deficient adults remains controversial.

GH insufficiency can be a consequence of (1) hypothalamic disease, (2) disruption of the portal system between hypothalamic nuclei and the anterior pituitary, (3) GHRHR loss-of-function mutations, or (4) somatotroph disease. GH deficiency can occur in isolation (isolated GH deficiency) or together with other pituitary deficiencies (multiple pituitary hormone deficiencies [MPHDs] or combined pituitary hormone deficiencies [CPHD]). Patients with isolated GH deficiency should be followed clinically for the development of other pituitary hormone deficiencies because MPHD can evolve over time. Biochemical stimulation testing is necessary to establish the diagnosis of GH deficiency, GH resistance, or MPHD. In most affected children, the cause of GH deficiency is unknown (idiopathic GH deficiency).[91] An organic cause is identified in about one in four children with proven GH deficiency; half of these children will be diagnosed with a CNS tumor.[92]

Any type of hypothalamic disease or dysfunction can lead to or be associated with GHRH deficiency, including (1) tumors, (2) inflammation, (3) previous infection, (4) trauma (including previous surgery),[93] (5) hemorrhage, (6) irradiation, and (7) malformations (e.g., SOD).[19] Low-dose irradiation of the hypothalamus and/or pituitary can cause idiopathic GH deficiency, whereas higher doses of irradiation can cause MPHD. SOD is defined by the triad of (1) midline brain defects, such as agenesis of the septum pellucidum and/or corpus callosum, (2) hypoplasia of the optic nerve, and (3) anterior and/or posterior pituitary hormone abnormalities. A small number of cases of SOD are explained by mutations in HESX1, SOX2, and SOX3, all of which are transcription factors. HEXS1 (chromosome 3p14.3) is a paired-like homeobox gene, SOX2 (chromosome 3q26.3) is the SRY (sex-determining region on the Y chromosome) box 2 gene, and SOX3 (chromosome Xq27.1) is the SRY box 3 gene. Midline brain tumors, such as craniopharyngiomas, meningiomas, gliomas, germinomas, third ventricle colloid cysts, ependymomas, and optic nerve gliomas, also affect the hypothalamus. Disruptions in the hypothalamic-pituitary portal system can result from tumors, inflammation, previous infection, trauma (including previous surgery), and irradiation.

Congenital GH deficiency from pituitary disease has many causes, including GHRHR gene mutations (idiopathic GH deficiency type IB), GH1 mutations (idiopathic GH deficiency types IA, IB, II, and III, and bioactive GH), and transcription factor mutations (which usually cause MPHD: LHX3, LHX4, PROP1, Pit-1, RIEG) and malformations (anencephaly and holoprosencephaly) (Table 55.5).[86] Homozygous LHX3 mutations have caused panhypopituitarism, with the exception that ACTH was not affected.[94] Heterozygous LHX4 mutations have caused deficiencies of GH, TSH, and ACTH. PROP1 (name derived from PROphet of Pit-1; POU1F1; Pit-1 stands for "paired-like homeodomain transcription factor")[95] mutations cause deficiencies of GH, prolactin, TSH, and gonadotropins. ACTH deficiency has also occurred in some cohorts. PROP1 gene mutations are inherited as autosomal recessive traits. Pit-1 gene mutations cause GH, prolactin, and variable degrees of TSH deficiencies. These transcription factor mutations may be inherited as autosomal recessive or dominant traits. Heterozygous RIEG gene mutations (PITX2, a paired-like homeobox gene) are the cause of Rieger syndrome, which may include GH deficiency. Features of Rieger syndrome encompass developmental abnormalities of the teeth, the anterior chamber of the eye, and the umbilicus. Mutations in GLI1, GLI2, Shh, ZIC2,

TABLE 55.5	Growth Hormone Deficiency of Genetic Etiology	
Gene/Classification/Inheritance	Mutation	Phenotype
GH1; IA; AR	Deletion, FS, NS	Absent GH expression; immune resistance to GH treatment is common
GH1; IB; AR	Splicing?	Reduced GH; responds to GH treatment[a]
GHRHR; IB; AR	Possible MS	Reduced GH; responds to GH treatment[a]
GH1; II; AD	DN	Reduced GH; responds to GH treatment; MPHD is possible
Unknown; III; XLR	—	Reduced GH; responds to GH treatment; agammaglobulinemia is possible

[a]One third of heterozygotes may be short.
AD, Autosomal dominant inheritance; *AR*, autosomal recessive inheritance; *DN*, dominant negative; *FS*, frameshift; *GH*, growth hormone; *MS*, missense mutation; *NS*, nonsense mutation (stop codon); *XLR*, X-linked recessive; *?*, otherwise not defined.

SIX3, tgif, PATCHED1, DGF1, and FAST1 have variously been cited as causes of holoprosencephaly.[96] Children with midline facial clefts (cleft lip, cleft palate, or combined) or a single central incisor can exhibit GH deficiency. A number of GH1 gene mutations have been identified to cause bioinactive GH.[97] In these mutations, GH does not have full biological activity but may retain its immunoreactivity. Therefore in contrast to other forms of pituitary or hypothalamic disease, the measured GH concentration has been observed to be high. Reference laboratories can provide GHRHR, GH1, and GHR gene sequencing services.[98–100]

Acquired causes of pituitary disease include (1) tumors (anterior pituitary adenoma, craniopharyngioma), (2) congenital cysts (Rathke cleft cyst, arachnoid cyst), (3) infiltrative disease (amyloidosis, histiocytosis, hemochromatosis), (4) inflammation (autoimmune, granulomatous or IgG4-related hypophysitis), (5) infection, (6) trauma (including surgery), (7) bleeding, (8) irradiation, (9) infarction (from pituitary apoplexy and Sheehan syndrome). Hemochromatosis does not cause hypopituitarism until many decades have passed.[101] Some investigators believe that all patients with "idiopathic" hypopituitarism should be screened for hemochromatosis.[102]

Investigation of growth hormone deficiency. The diagnosis of GH deficiency in adults and children is different, the latter being a more complex topic.[103] In adults, initial screening is performed by the measurement of IGF-I and followed up with stimulation testing. A definitive diagnosis of GH deficiency in children usually requires the performance of a GH stimulation test, though biochemical testing is not always required for the diagnosis depending on the prior medical history. All forms of GH testing should be performed after the subject has fasted overnight. Common provocative agents include insulin, glucagon, clonidine, arginine, and L-dopa. However, the ITT requires both good communication skills and emotional resolve on the part of the patient, which are often lacking in children. This makes it a less popular option in pediatric settings. In peripubertal children, the likelihood of a falsely abnormal GH screening test can be reduced by pretreatment of both boys and girls with a short course of sex steroids (ethinyl estradiol [40 μg/m^2 daily] for 2 days before testing).[104] The mechanism of sex-steroid priming is unclear; however, sex steroids appear to play a major role in increasing the response of IGF-I to GH at the time of puberty. From clinical experience, GH deficiency is overdiagnosed in some peripubertal children who are tested without the benefit of sex hormone priming.

Exercise physiologically enhances GH release.[105] Typically, in the fasting state, the child exercises vigorously for approximately 20 minutes (e.g., running up and down stairs, running

---

BOX 55.2   Protocol for the Exercise Stimulation Test for Growth Hormone

Rationale
Brisk exercise normally causes an increase in serum growth hormone (GH) concentrations.

Procedure
The test is best performed in the morning after an overnight fast but may be done at any time. Vigorous physical exercise (running or calisthenics) is performed for 20 min. A venous blood specimen for determination of GH is drawn immediately after termination of exercise.

Interpretation
If the serum GH concentration is 7–10 μg/L or greater (depending on the specific GH immunoassay used), GH deficiency is unlikely in children. A normal response in adults is a GH concentration of ≥5 μg/L. In children, a single subnormal response is not diagnostic for GH deficiency and should be confirmed with a second provocative test.

---

on a treadmill). At the completion of the exercise, when the child is tachycardic and sweating, a venous sample is collected for GH measurement (Box 55.2). A baseline GH measurement is not required. A GH concentration may also be obtained 40 minutes after exercise, in case of a delayed GH release.

It has been argued that measuring GH during sleep is a physiologic assessment of the hypothalamic-somatotroph-GH axis. Some authorities suggest electroencephalographic monitoring with GH measured during deep sleep (e.g., stage III, stage IV). More simply, GH could be measured 1 hour after the onset of sleep. However, in reality, these types of sleep studies are cumbersome because they require hospitalization or overnight boarding in a sleep laboratory. In practice, they are rarely performed. Furthermore, the high cost of hospitalization or the sleep laboratory suggests that an exercise tolerance test or a simple pharmacologic stimulus would be a more cost-effective approach to initial GH testing.

As discussed, reference intervals for IGF-I and IGFBP-3 are age- and sex-dependent.[64,106] If IGF-I is squarely within its reference interval for age and sex in children, GH deficiency is excluded. If IGF-I is low, definitive GH testing is required. Because IGF-I concentrations can be depressed in states of (1) malnutrition/malabsorption, (2) obesity, (3) chronic disease, (4) hypothyroidism, and (5) sex hormone deficiency, a low IGF-I concentration does not confirm

GH deficiency. IGFBP-3 is less dependent on good nutrition to achieve normal concentrations, so it may have advantages over IGF-I measurement. However, one study failed to demonstrate that measuring IGFBP-3 alone or together with free IGF-I was superior to measuring IGF-I alone as a screening test for GH deficiency.[107] In another study, only approximately 50% of GH-deficient children had a low IGFBP-3 concentration; this finding calls into question its value as a sensitive screening test.[108]

Analytical advantages of IGFBP-3 measurements over IGF-I measurements include the following: (1) IGF-I must be separated from its binding proteins to be measured, whereas IGFBP-3 does not require a dissociation step; (2) IGFBP-3 is present in higher concentrations than IGF-I; and (3) less age dependency is seen for IGFBP-3 compared with IGF-I.[109] Because of stable concentrations, IGF-I and IGFBP-3 measurements may be obtained at any time of day. However, some researchers have concluded that IGFBP-3 measurements are too nonspecific to be used for the evaluation of GH deficiency.[110] Furthermore, reports indicate that IGF-I and IGFBP-3 exhibit imperfect sensitivity and specificity for the diagnosis of GH deficiency.[111]

IGF-I measurements in adults are often diagnostically unhelpful.[112] For reasons that are unclear, IGF-I concentrations can be normal in GH-deficient adults. Therefore a normal IGF-I does not rule out adult GH deficiency. If the IGF-I concentration is low and suspicion for GH deficiency is high (MPHD or childhood-onset severe GH deficiency), some experts would diagnose GH deficiency in the absence of GH testing.[113]

GH responses to insulin-induced hypoglycemia (ITT) (Box 55.3) and GH responses to centrally acting pharmacologic or biological agents (Box 55.4) are considered definitive tests. The stimuli can be sequential or administered on different days. The classical diagnosis of pediatric GH deficiency requires that GH responses to two different stimuli (Table 55.6) be deficient. Note that many variations of these protocols exist because endocrinologists often customize these tests.

Of children with appropriate stature for age, approximately 80% will have normal GH responses to one stimulus, and at least 95% will have normal GH responses to at least one of two stimuli. This is why two GH stimuli are generally recommended—to avoid overdiagnosis of GH deficiency, though in select clinical circumstances of major congenital malformation, tumor or previous irradiation, it has been recommended that no GH stimulation is required for the diagnosis of GH deficiency.[114]

A history of childhood GH deficiency, CNS disease, trauma, or irradiation is an indication to test adults for GH deficiency.[115,116] Retesting of adults with the diagnosis of childhood GH deficiency is necessary because not all adults with childhood GH deficiency remain GH deficient. In adults, a single abnormal GH response to a stimulus is diagnostic of GH deficiency if the deficiency is congenital or genetic, or if MPHDs are due to organic disease.

The ITT is considered the gold standard stimulus when hypoglycemia is achieved (glucose <40 to 45 mg/dL) (<2.2 to 2.5 mmol/L).[117] The risk associated with this type of test is that untreated severe hypoglycemia can be life threatening. Venous access for infusion of glucose is mandatory during the ITT. If vascular access is lost during the ITT, glucagon should be readily available for an intramuscular (IM)

BOX 55.3 Protocol for the Insulin-Induced Hypoglycemia Stimulation Test (Insulin Tolerance Test)

Rationale

The stress of insulin-induced hypoglycemia triggers the release of growth hormone (GH) and adrenocorticotropin hormone (ACTH) from the pituitary gland in normal subjects. The GH response is measured directly. Cortisol is measured as the indication of the ACTH response.

Procedure

The test is done after an overnight fast with the patient at bed rest. An indwelling intravenous (IV) line is inserted. Sampling begins after a 30-min rest period. Baseline samples are drawn for determination of glucose, GH, and cortisol. Regular insulin, 0.1–0.15 U/kg body weight, is injected intravenously. Samples are then obtained at +10, +20, +40, and +60 min for glucose, GH, and cortisol determinations. Optional time points are +30, +75, +90, and +120 min. To be confident that adequate stress has been applied, the patient must become symptomatic (exhibit sweating or tremor), or the glucose concentration must fall to less than 40–45 mg/dL (2.2–2.5 mmol/L). Additional IV insulin may be given if this has not occurred by 30 min, in which case sampling should be prolonged by 30 min. The physician should be in attendance throughout the test, and 50% dextrose for IV administration should be kept on hand to be used in the event of severe hypoglycemic reaction and after adequate hypoglycemia has been documented. Glucagon (1 mg) should be available for parenteral administration in case IV access is lost. The test is contraindicated in older adult patients and those with a seizure disorder, ischemic heart disease, or cardiovascular insufficiency.

Interpretation

The serum cortisol concentration should increase to a peak value of 15–20 μg/dL (414–552 nmol/L) or greater. The serum GH concentration should rise to a peak value of 5–7 ng/mL (5–7 μg/L) or greater. No response or inadequate response may be due to pituitary hormone deficiency or a hypothalamic lesion.

BOX 55.4 Protocol for the Arginine Stimulation Test for Growth Hormone

Rationale

In normal subjects, intravenous (IV) administration of arginine hydrochloride stimulates growth hormone (GH) release.

Procedure

The test should be done after an overnight fast with the patient maintained at bed rest. A 10% solution of arginine hydrochloride, 0.5 g/kg body weight (maximum dose = 30 g), is infused intravenously over 30 min. Blood samples are drawn for determination of GH before the infusion is started and 30, 60, and 90 min after the infusion is begun. Optional time points are +15 and +120 min.

Interpretation

The serum GH concentration should rise to a peak value of 5–7 ng/mL (5–7 μg/L) or greater. A subnormal response is seen in GH-deficient subjects, but a single subnormal GH response is not diagnostic for GH deficiency and should be confirmed with a second provocative test.

TABLE 55.6   Growth Hormone Stimuli

GH Stimulus	Dose	GH Sampling[a] (min)
Glucagon	0.03–0.1 mg/kg, IM, max 1 mg	0, 30, 60, 90, 120, 150, 180, ±240 (maximum response ≈2–3 h)
L-Dopa	500 mg/m^2 (15 mg/kg) max 500 mg (or) <15 kg: 125 mg 15–30 kg: 250 mg >30 kg: 500 mg	0, 40, 60, 90, 120
Clonidine	0.15 mg/m^2 <13.6 kg: 0.05 mg >13.6 kg: 0.1 mg (0.1 mg/tab)	0, 30, 60, 90
Arginine HCl	0.5 g/kg, max 30 g (10% solution IV over 30 min)	0, ±15, 30, 60, 90, ±120
Insulin tolerance test	0.1 U/kg (0.05–0.15) IV push insulin	0, 10, 20, ±30, 40, 60, ±75, ±90, ±120
Arginine-insulin tolerance test	Arginine: begin at time zero, give insulin at +60 min	0, 30, 60, 70, 80, 100, 120

[a]Experts may differ on the best interval of GH measurements; ± indicates an optional time point.
GH, Growth hormone; *HCl*, hydrogen chloride; *IM*, intramuscular; *IV*, intravenous.

injection (the dose of glucagon is 1 mg). If IV access cannot be ensured, stimuli other than insulin should be considered. In general, GH stimulation tests are not conducted by laboratory personnel because of the risks and complexities of testing. Arginine infusion presents the danger of acidosis and even death.[118]

Stimulated GH concentration less than 4 to 7 ng/mL (4 to 7 μg/L) defines GH deficiency in children.[119,120] The cutoff defining GH deficiency is method-dependent and subject to interpretation by clinicians and may vary between countries. The definition of GH deficiency also differs between adults and children. In adults, the threshold for defining GH deficiency differs by stimulus. For the ITT, deficiency is present when the stimulated GH is less than 5 ng/mL (5 μg/L), whereas a threshold of 3 μg/L has been recommended for glucagon stimulation. Still different BMI-specific thresholds are for GHRH plus arginine.[121]

Controversy continues as to what constitutes a normal GH response to stimuli because insulin-induced hypoglycemia is considered by some to be a nonphysiologic stimulus. Discordance between normal stimulated GH concentration and a deficient spontaneous rise in GH concentration has been described as neurosecretory GH deficiency.[122] Neurosecretory GH deficiency can result from CNS or hypothalamic disease. The diagnosis of neurosecretory GH deficiency requires overnight blood sampling with GH measurements every 20 minutes, which is a protocol that ordinarily requires hospitalization. The combined costs of GH assays, physician

fees, and inpatient services would exceed several thousand dollars.

The definition of partial GH deficiency is especially problematic because the definition of GH deficiency is itself controversial.[123,124] Eliminating GH stimulation testing has been proposed with the diagnosis of GH deficiency based on growth parameters, IGF-I, and IGFBP-3 measurements, neuroradiologic investigation, and genetic considerations.[125–127] There is increased pressure to diagnose GH deficiency because the clinical indications for GH therapy are expanding. Non-GH deficient conditions are also sometimes treated with GH (e.g., Prader-Willi syndrome, Turner syndrome, and chronic renal failure). There is concern about the long-term risks of GH therapy.[128]

Growth Hormone Resistance

In children with short stature and low growth velocity, if IGF-I is (1) below the reference interval for the child's bone age and gender, (2) if the GH concentration is normal or elevated, and (3) if non–GH-dependent causes of IGF-I deficiency (malnutrition, malabsorption, chronic disease, hypothyroidism, and sex hormone deficiency compared with the patient's bone age) have been excluded, GH resistance should be considered.[129] As uncommon as GH deficiency is in the general pediatric population (1 in 10,000 children), GH resistance as a primary problem is far less frequent.

GH resistance can be congenital, resulting from loss-of-function GHR mutations or GHR signaling defects (STAT5b mutations),[130,131] or from defects in the production of IGF-I itself. Most GHR mutations involve the extracellular domain that involves GH binding to the GHR. Some GHR mutations affect homodimerization. Loss of the intracellular GHR domain can result from splice-site mutations. GHR is not expressed on the cell surface if the transmembrane domain is defective. Recall that circulating GHBP is derived from the extracellular domain of the GHR. Most cases of GHR deficiency display low or absent concentrations of GHBP. STAT5b is necessary for normal GH-GHR signaling to the cell nucleus. These are autosomal recessive disorders. Size at birth is normal because in utero IGF-I production is independent of GH.

IGF-I gene–inactivating mutations or deletions are rare, and only two such mutations have been described. In contrast to GHR and signaling defects, when IGF-I itself cannot be produced because of intrinsic IGF-I gene mutations, intrauterine growth retardation will result in addition to extrauterine growth failure. Other consequences of IGF-I gene mutations include severe mental retardation, deafness, and micrognathia (mandibular hypoplasia).[132,133]

IGF-I and IGFBP-3 concentrations are low in rare cases of ALS deficiency, whereas baseline and poststimulation GH concentrations are normal.[134] Although adolescence was delayed, adult stature was nearly normal in persons with ALS deficiency.

Acquired GH resistance is far more common than congenital GH resistance. In cases of acquired GH resistance, the IGF-I is low (despite sufficient GH secretion) because of malnutrition, malabsorption, chronic disease, hypothyroidism, or sex hormone deficiency. An acquired form of GH resistance has also been observed in patients with idiopathic GH deficiency type I; they develop GH-inhibitory antibodies when treated with exogenous GH. Because GH is absent in this form of congenital GH deficiency, exogenous GH is seen by the immune system as foreign. Apparently, the resulting antibodies directed against exogenous GH bind to, and inactivate, the GH. This is reminiscent of the development of factor VIII antibodies in some boys with severe hemophilia A, who are treated with exogenous factor VIII.

A number of criteria for GH resistance have been proposed, including (1) height more than 3 SDs below the mean for age; (2) basal GH greater than 2.5 ng/mL (>2.5 µg/L); (3) basal IGF-I less than 50 ng/mL; (4) basal IGFBP-3 more than 2 SDs below the mean for age; (5) an increase in IGF-I of less than 15 ng/mL after 4 days of GH treatment (0.05 mg/kg/day); and (6) increase in IGFBP-3 of less than 0.4 µg/mL after GH treatment. The largest concentrations of subjects with GH resistance are found in Israel and southern Ecuador.[135]

Insulin-like Growth Factor-I Resistance

Even less common than GH resistance as a cause of growth failure is IGF-I resistance.[136,137] IGF-I resistance is characterized by growth failure despite elevations in GH and IGF-I. In contrast to GH deficiency and GH resistance states, and in common with IGF-I gene mutations, IGF-I resistance causes intrauterine growth retardation and growth failure in childhood. IGF-I resistance can result from mutations in the type I IGF receptor (IGFR) or from downstream signaling mutations.

Rare cases of familial short stature have been ascribed to hemizygosity for the type I IGF receptor gene.[138] Approximately 1 in 50 children with intrauterine growth retardation, short stature, and normal IGF-I concentrations have heterozygous type I IGF receptor mutations.

Measurement of Growth Hormone in Blood

A variety of isotopic and nonisotopic assays for GH are commercially available; most of the modern GH assays use mouse monoclonal antibodies and recombinant-derived GH as the competing (labeled) antigens, or as calibrators. A number of gravimetrically prepared international reference preparations (IRPs) have been offered but collaborative groups have recommended use of the recombinantly derived WHO IRP 98/574 to harmonize GH assays,[139,140] and some commercially available two-site noncompetitive immunoassays have been harmonized to this IRP.[141,142]

Noncompetitive two-site immunoassays for GH are widely available; most include monoclonal antibodies coupled to an enzyme, chemiluminescent, or fluorescent label. Sensitivity as low as 0.05 ng/mL (0.05 µg/L) has been reported for an electrochemiluminescent immunoassay.[142] Mass spectrometric methods for GH measurement have also been described.[143,144]

Analytical Challenges

GH is not a single molecular species, but instead exists in the circulation as a heterogeneous mixture of structural isoforms, including monomeric, dimeric, and oligomeric forms, as well as post-translationally modified monomers with molecular weights ranging from 20 to 22 kDa.[145]

Two genes on chromosome 17q code human GH: the product of one is designated GH-N (or GH1) and is expressed primarily in the pituitary; the other is designated GH-V (or GH2) and is derived from the placenta (see the

earlier discussion in this chapter). Both products are 22-kDa proteins, but they differ at 13 residues, and the GH-N isoform is susceptible to deletion of an internal 15 amino acid sequence, producing a 20-kDa GH isoform that accounts for 5 to 10% of the total GH; it has a propensity to dimerize. Normally, the human gene for GH that directs the synthesis of a monomeric 22-kDa protein accounts for most of the GH found in the circulation. The 20-kDa variant has less biological activity and does not react with some GH assays, but antibodies that specifically recognize the 20-kDa variant are available.[146] No clinical indications are known for measuring the 20-kDa form of GH, but it has been suggested that it can be used to detect GH doping in sports (see the following). Because recombinant GH is the 22-kDa isoform, and exogenous GH suppresses endogenous secretion of the hormone, administration of the recombinant hormone should suppress production of the 20-kDa variant; this effect has been demonstrated.[147] The immunoreactivity of the oligomeric (up to pentameric) isoforms of GH has not been well characterized, although it is known that they have reduced bioactivity and clearance.

Approximately one-half of circulating GH is bound to GHBP derived from the extracellular domain of the GH receptor,[148,149] and a small amount (5 to 8%) is bound to a low-affinity protein.[150] Generally, anti-GH antibodies have sufficiently higher affinity for GH to compete with GH-binding proteins when enough time is allowed for the GH-protein complexes to dissociate. Therefore immunoassays provide a good approximation of total hormone concentration. Assays for measuring unbound (free) GH have also been developed.[151] Free GH concentrations are proportional to total GH and are inversely proportional to GHBP, but the clinical usefulness of free GH measurements has not been established. Significant challenges remain in the harmonization of methods for GH measurements.[152,153]

Detecting Growth Hormone Doping in Athletes

Because GH promotes anabolic and lipolytic activities, it has been used by athletes to enhance their physical size, strength, and endurance. In response, the World Anti-Doping Agency has banned the use of GH by athletes competing in sanctioned events. Detecting GH use is challenging, however, because recombinant forms of the hormone are available that are identical to endogenous GH, and normal GH concentrations vary significantly because of the pulsatile nature of hormone release from the pituitary.[154] Although suppression of the 20-kDa GH isoform has shown some promise as a marker of GH doping, most current strategies focus on secondary markers, including IGF and IGFBP.[155–157]

Specimen Collection and Storage

The preferred specimen is serum; plasma with ethylenediaminetetraacetic acid (EDTA) or heparin added to prevent coagulation may also be used, but values are method dependent. Serum specimens should be stored at 2 to 8 °C if they are not to be tested within 8 hours. If specimens must be stored for longer periods, they should be frozen at −20 °C or colder.

Comments

A single basal or random concentration of GH provides limited diagnostic information. As discussed earlier in this chapter, secretion of GH by the pituitary gland is both episodic and pulsatile, and transient concentrations of up to 40 ng/mL (40 µg/L) have been observed in normal healthy subjects. Serum concentrations are low between pulses in healthy individuals, and some immunoassays are not sensitive enough to distinguish patients with abnormally low concentrations from healthy individuals who have concentrations that happen to fall in the low to normal reference interval. In some individuals, spontaneous low GH secretion is better monitored by using a continuous withdrawal pump or by drawing specimens for GH assay every 20 to 30 minutes over a 12- to 24-hour period (e.g., during evaluation of neurogenic GH deficiency).

Measurement of Insulin-like Growth Factors

The liver is the primary source of circulating IGF-I (somatomedin C), but autocrine and paracrine production of IGF-I (as controlled by GH) is responsible for growth.

IGF-I has a longer biological half-life than GH, so its measurement provides an integrated estimate of GH secretion; it is also a more sensitive measure of GH excess in acromegaly. IGF-II is a fetal GH, and the clinical usefulness of measuring IGF-II is limited to patients being investigated for a possible IGF-II–secreting tumor causing insulin-independent hypoglycemia.[54]

Current IGF-I methods should use a reference material that is traceable to the International Reference Preparation IGF-I 87/518, or the newer WHO First International Standard 02/254.[158] To avoid interference from IGF-binding proteins, many assays isolate IGF using a variety of extraction methods, including (1) gel filtration, (2) acid-ethanol precipitation, (3) cryoprecipitation, (4) C-18 column extraction, or (5) reversed-phase chromatography.[159] Direct (no extraction) procedures are also available, but extraction methods prevent the formation of complexes with carrier proteins and serum proteases. Moreover, extraction procedures are better able to discriminate between GH-deficient patients and age-matched controls. Commercial assays that include chemiluminescent labels are available for measuring IGF-I, usually with minimal cross-reactivity to IGF-II (0 to 3%). It is important to establish age- and sex-related reference intervals for IGF-I because of marked differences in hormone concentrations between adults and children and between males and females. Mass spectrometric methods for IGF-I have been described,[160] but those using trypsinization and measurement of a proteotypic peptide do not require an extraction. As with GH methods, harmonization of IGF-I assays remains a challenge.[161–163] IGFBP-3 is the major protein carrier of circulating IGF-I and is an indirect measure of GH activity. Measurement of IGF-I has become a staple in the evaluation of GH abnormalities, but problems with interassay agreement remain, mostly related to binding proteins,[161] and this has obvious consequences for reference value studies.[164]

Specimen Collection and Storage

Serum or plasma (with heparin or EDTA added to prevent coagulation) is used, depending on the assay method. Samples should be centrifuged within 1 hour of collection and stored frozen at −20 °C or colder for up to 30 days. Some procedures use dried whole blood or serum collected on filter paper.[165]

Prolactin

Prolactin is secreted by lactotrophs of the adenohypophysis.[166] Prolactin stimulates and sustains lactation in postpartum mammals after the mammary glands have been prepared by other hormones, including estrogens, progesterone, GH, corticosteroids, and insulin.

Biochemistry

The hypothalamic prolactin release inhibitory hormone is dopamine, which is a product of the tuberoinfundibular cells and the hypothalamic tuberohypophyseal dopaminergic system. In lactotrophs, dopamine binds to the type 2 dopamine (D2) receptor, one of five dopamine receptors. Dopamine receptors are located in the caudate putamen, nucleus accumbens, and olfactory tubercle, affecting (1) locomotion, (2) learning, (3) memory, (4) reward, and (5) reinforcement.

The gene for the D2 receptor is located on chromosome 11q2, contains 443 amino acids, and has a mass of 50.6 kDa. The extracellular domain is 37 amino acids, and seven transmembrane domains are present, along with a 14-amino-acid cytoplasmic domain. A large extracellular loop is evident between amino acids 211 and 373. Three potential sites of N-glycosylation have been noted: amino acids 5, 17, and 23. A disulfide bridge may occur between amino acids 107 and 182. Three isoforms of the D2 receptor have been identified: the full-length isoform is referred to as D2 (long); isoform 2 is D2 (short) and lacks amino acids 242 to 270; isoform 3, D2 (longer), contains a val → trp-glu substitution at position 270. Mutations in the D2 receptor cause dystonia type 11 (myoclonus dystonia, or alcohol-responsive dystonia).

The gene encoding prolactin was described in the section concerning the GH1 gene. Initially, preprolactin is synthesized (227 amino acids), and after cleavage of the leader sequence, the 199 amino acid prolactin hormone is liberated. Amino acid 59 is the site of putative N-glycosylation. Intrachain disulfide bonds are located between amino acids 32 and 39, 86 and 202, and 219 and 227.

Circulating prolactin exists in several forms: monomeric prolactin (23 kDa, "little" prolactin), dimeric prolactin (48 to 56 kDa, "big" prolactin), and polymeric prolactin (>100 kDa, "big, big" prolactin). Occasionally, and independent of the presence or absence of disease, IgG autoantibodies against prolactin can bind to prolactin, forming macroprolactin. The presence of macroprolactin elevates the total prolactin concentration, as the result of lower clearance, in the absence of excess prolactin secretion by the anterior pituitary lactotrophs. Failure to recognize macroprolactin can lead to the inappropriate diagnosis of hyperprolactinemia. In nature, many examples of macroproteins resulting from the complex of an antibody and a protein can be found, such as macro-troponin and macro-TSH.[167,168]

The gene for the prolactin receptor (PRLR) is located at chromosome 5p13.2. Pre-PRLR is 622 amino acids (69.5 kDa). Upon removal of the signal peptide, the full-length PRLR is released (598 amino acids). The first 210 amino acids of the receptor are extracellular, 24 amino acids are present in the transmembrane domain, and the cytoplasmic domain consists of 364 amino acids. Amino acids 27 to 121 (with reference to preprolactin) represent a fibronectin type III-1 domain, whereas amino acids 127 to 227 represent a fibronectin type III-2 domain. Amino acids 215 to 219 display a WSXWS motif, and amino acids 267 to 275 display a box 1 motif. The WSXWS motif is the tryptophan-serine-wild card-tryptophan-serine sequence located near the lipid bilayer. Box 1 motifs are expressed in the cytoplasmic domain of receptors that engage in JAK2 receptor signaling. Glycosylation may occur at amino acids 59, 104, and 233, and intrachain disulfide bonds occur between amino acids 36 and 46, and 75 and 86. The PRLR forms a homodimer upon binding prolactin.

Eight isoforms of the PRLR have been described. Isoform 1 is the full-length PRLR. In isoform 2, amino acids 24 to 124 are missing. In isoform 3, amino acids 229 (aspartate) and 230 (phenylalanine) are replaced, respectively, by alanine and tryptophan (amino acids 231 to 622 are missing; therefore this protein lacks a transmembrane domain, and the protein is soluble). This isoform has been reported as the product of a breast cancer cell line. Isoform 4 has changes in the amino acid sequence of amino acids 338 to 376, with the remaining amino acids deleted, and is nonfunctional. Because of a deletion of part of exon 10, and a frameshift mutation, the sequence of isoform 5 is altered among amino acids 337 to 349; thereafter, the remaining amino acids are absent. In isoform 6, amino acids 286 to 288 (lysine-glycine-lysine) are replaced, respectively, by valine, tyrosine, and proline, and the amino acids distal to 288 are absent; this receptor is nonfunctional. Isoform 7 is secreted with changes in amino acids 229 to 268, and amino acids 269 to 622 are absent. Last, isoform 8 begins at amino acid 72, and amino acids 286 to 288 are replaced, respectively, by valine, tyrosine, and proline; the amino acids distal to 288 are absent, as in isoform 6.

Physiology

In women, prolactin is necessary for lactation after delivery of the newborn. Recent work in animal models provides some evidence that the different prolactin isoforms may have independent biological functions. In addition, the discovery of extrapituitary sites of prolactin secretion has also provided insights into a wider function of this hormone.[169] Prolactin is stimulated by breast-feeding, chest wall disease, and stress. Although prolactin is higher during the day than at night, and a night-to-day prolactin ratio greater than 1:2 is considered normal, the ratio has no diagnostic value. Prolactin is measured in its basal state without stimulatory or suppressive manipulation. As with other adenohypophyseal hormones, the release of prolactin is episodic and varies predictably during the day, with lowest concentrations found at midday, and highest values found shortly after the onset of deep sleep.

Receptors for prolactin are located in the hypothalamus, breast, and ovaries. Breast development during puberty can occur in the absence of prolactin, but estrogen is required,

along with GH and GH-stimulated IGF-I. Fetal breast development is stimulated by parathyroid hormone–related peptide, which shares the N-terminal active domain of parathyroid hormone but is produced outside the parathyroid.

Prolactin secretion by lactotrophs is controlled predominantly through suppression by dopamine.[170] In addition, prolactin may provide feedback centrally to stimulate dopamine in a short negative feedback loop, but this has been difficult to confirm. An ultra-short feedback loop is present where prolactin suppresses its own release. In addition to high concentrations of TRH, other factors that may stimulate prolactin secretion include oxytocin, vasoactive intestinal polypeptide, basic fibroblast growth factor, EGF, hypothalamic prolactin-releasing peptide, galanin, and neurotensin. Identified in the hypothalamus, amygdala, basal ganglia, and dorsal gray matter of the spinal cord, neurotensin is a 13 amino acid peptide neurotransmitter. Neurotensin affects gastrointestinal function and has a role in pain perception.[171]

Estrogen increases prolactin gene transcription and secretion; this explains why prolactin concentrations are higher in women than in men. The upper limit of the prolactin reference interval for women is approximately 20 ng/mL (≈420 mIU/L), whereas in men it is approximately 10 ng/mL (≈210 mIU/L). Prolactin rises during pregnancy because of elevated concentrations of sex steroids (predominantly estradiol). The average serum prolactin during pregnancy is approximately 200 ng/mL (≈4200 mIU/L). Because of increased lactotrophs, the pituitary approximately doubles in size during pregnancy.

The breast is prepared for lactation during pregnancy through the actions of (1) estrogen, (2) progesterone, (3) prolactin, (4) GH-V, (5) hPL, and possibly (6) IGF-I.[172] As the visible size of the breast increases during pregnancy, many microscopic changes also occur in breast tissue. Typically, lactation is not active until after delivery when estrogen and progesterone concentrations have declined. Prolactin increases amino acid and glucose uptake by breast tissue, and synthesis of α-lactalbumin and β-casein, lactose, and milk fats is increased.

Postpartum, a positive feedback loop is seen between suckling and milk production. Transmitted via nerve fibers from the nipple to the CNS, suckling reduces dopamine, which increases prolactin release. With suckling, prolactin can rise by more than eightfold over baseline. The positive feedback loop of suckling, prolactin secretion, and milk production is a "stimulus-secretion" reflex. However, with continued breast-feeding, prolactin concentrations decline. One report observed mean prolactin concentrations of 162 ng/mL (≈3400 mIU/L) 2 to 4 weeks postpartum, 130 ng/mL (≈2730 mIU/L) 5 to 14 weeks postpartum, and 77 ng/mL (≈1620 mIU/L) 15 to 24 weeks postpartum. Suckling also stimulates oxytocin release, which is discussed in the section of this chapter concerning the posterior pituitary.

Because elevated prolactin concentrations reduce LH and FSH by inhibiting GnRH release (a short feedback loop between prolactin and the hypothalamus), breast-feeding delays the onset of menses after delivery.[173] Lactation amenorrhea is beneficial because it temporarily ensures that the mother can adequately breast-feed her newborn before she becomes pregnant again. It is understood that oligomenorrhea, amenorrhea, and infertility in hyperprolactinemic women, and impotence and oligospermia in hyperprolactinemic men, result from prolactin suppression of GnRH secretion. Prolactin has direct effects on prolactin receptors in the ovaries.

Hyperprolactinemia

Hyperprolactinemia is the most common hypothalamic-pituitary disorder encountered in clinical endocrinology.[174] Prolactin concentrations may be elevated in women who have only subtle alterations in fertility, such as (1) anovulation with or without menstrual irregularity, (2) amenorrhea and galactorrhea, or (3) galactorrhea alone. In men, prolactin excess usually manifests as a result of low serum testosterone, with reduced libido and central weight gain. Hyperprolactinemia can also cause galactorrhea in men. Additionally, men, more than women, present with prolactin-secreting macroadenoma with visual field disturbances.

An irregular menstrual period frequently reveals a microadenoma ($\leq$10 mm in diameter) in women. Elevated prolactin concentrations are observed in as many as 30% of women with polycystic ovarian syndrome and patients with clinically silent pituitary adenoma. If a borderline elevation of prolactin is found, it is advisable to repeat the measurement on at least two other occasions, taking care to obtain a morning specimen under conditions of minimal excitement or stress to the patient (i.e., no trauma and no breast stimulation). Ideally, the patient should not be on any medication that could stimulate prolactin release (discussed in more detail later in this section). The differential diagnosis of hyperprolactinemia is extensive (Table 55.7).

An extremely important cause of hyperprolactinemia is a prolactinoma.[175,176] The higher the prolactin concentration, the greater is the likelihood that hyperprolactinemia is the result of a prolactinoma. As a general rule, prolactin levels caused by medications and stalk-effect tend to be lower than those seen in prolactinoma per se, but there is certainly overlap. Hyperprolactinemia due to a prolactin producing macroadenoma (>10 mm in diameter) can produce prolactin concentrations into the tens of thousands (ng/mL). Prolactin concentrations greater than 200 ng/mL (approximately 4000 mIU/L) usually indicate a macroprolactinoma. Prolactinomas are diagnostically challenging. Because any degree of hyperprolactinemia can be seen in cases of prolactinoma, if hyperprolactinemia is otherwise not explained, a thorough search for a prolactinoma, including MRI imaging, should be undertaken. Idiopathic hyperprolactinemia does exist but is a

diagnosis of exclusion. Mass displacement effects from an anterior pituitary tumor include destruction of the sella turcica, invasion of other structures, compression of the stalk, or optic nerve compression causing bitemporal hemianopsia.

Early diagnosis of a prolactinoma is critical because therapy with dopamine agonists, such as bromocriptine or cabergoline, can reduce tumor size and control tumor progression.[177] Surgical excision of a prolactinoma usually is considered if there is tumor growth or failure to lower prolactin levels with dopamine agonist therapy (the "dopamine-resistant prolactinoma"), or where there is failure to quickly reverse any associated visual loss or in a patient intolerant of dopamine agonists.

Macroprolactin is a common cause of an elevated plasma prolactin concentration; this benign condition should be ruled out before additional diagnostic studies are performed.[178] Macroprolactinemia typically results from prolactin-immunoglobulin G complexes but can also be caused by high molecular weight forms of prolactin caused by glycosylation and aggregation of prolactin.[179] The molecular weight of macroprolactin (in the past referred to as "big big prolactin") is greater than 100 kDa, typically 150 to 170 kDa for the immunoglobulin complexes.[180]

These forms of prolactin lack biological activity; thus none of the sequelae associated with an elevated prolactin concentration (sexual dysfunction and galactorrhea) are present. In addition, macroprolactinemia is not associated with negative or positive feedback effects at the hypothalamus. Because macroprolactin is formed outside of lactotrophs, it is not found in pituitary tissue, and its size prevents entry into the cerebrospinal fluid. Therefore macroprolactin appears to be confined to the vascular compartment.

Macroprolactinemia, although asymptomatic, is troublesome for clinicians and the laboratory because it is detected by most prolactin immunoassays. In one report, almost 20% of patients who presented for a clinical workup for prolactinoma were found to have hyperprolactinemia attributable to macroprolactin.[181] However, the overall rate of macroprolactinemia in the testing population was approximately1.5%. Other studies seeking to estimate population-level prevalence of macroprolactinemia have found values closer to 4%.[179] For these reasons, clinical laboratories must be able to rule out the presence of a macroprolactin.[182] Macroprolactin can be precipitated by the addition of polyethylene glycol (PEG) to serum; this is the most common laboratory approach to detecting macroprolactin (see details in the section *Measurement of Prolactin*[183]).

Another diagnostic challenge in the investigation of hyperprolactinemia is the presence of a pituitary incidentaloma in a patient with elevated prolactin that could potentially lead to inappropriate medical or surgical treatment.[184,185] The presence of a lesion on MRI is not assumed to be the cause of prolactin elevation—some are merely incidental findings, referred to as "incidentalomas." Incidental pituitary adenomas are common, occurring in 10 to 20% of the population.[186] However, mild to moderate elevations in prolactin (50 to 200 ng/mL, 1100 to 4200 mIU/L) are possible when other anterior pituitary tumors compress the hypothalamic-pituitary portal system, impairing the delivery of dopamine to the lactotrophs. This phenomenon is referred to as the "stalk effect." Treatment with a dopamine agonist should lower prolactin concentrations in cases of a true prolactinoma but will not reduce prolactin concentration in the

TABLE 55.7	**Differential Diagnosis of Hyperprolactinemia**
Dopamine deficiency	Hypothalamic disease
	Interruption in the hypothalamic-pituitary portal system
Drugs	Dopamine antagonists
	Cholinergic antagonists
	Serotonergic antagonists
	Antipsychotic medication
Hormones	Estrogen, pregnancy
Neurogenic	Nursing (nipple stimulation)
	Chest wall disease
	Spinal cord injury
Other diseases	Hypothyroidism (pathologically elevated TRH can release prolactin)
	Chronic renal disease
	Cirrhosis

TRH, Thyrotropin-releasing hormone.

case of stalk effect. Prolactin measurements are also susceptible to a high-dose hook effect that may lead to a missed diagnosis of a macroprolactinoma,[187] although this has been mitigated by the wide analytical measuring range of modern commercial automated sandwich immunoassays. Nevertheless, if a macroadenoma is identified by MRI, but the prolactin is only modestly elevated, clinicians may request that the prolactin be remeasured at 1 to 10 and 1 to 100 dilution. If a hook effect is present, the concentration of the diluted sample will be significantly higher than that of the undiluted sample (see Chapter 26 for more detail).

MRI of the pituitary gland is performed as part of the clinical assessment when a prolactinoma is suspected. Because half of all prolactin-secreting microadenomas are too small to be detected by imaging methods, differentiating between a small pituitary tumor, prolactin-cell hyperplasia, and idiopathic hyperprolactinemia may not be possible.

Medications that stimulate prolactin release (through dopamine suppression) are the most common cause of hyperprolactinemia in otherwise healthy individuals.[188,189] When significant elevation of prolactin is confirmed, a careful history should rule out the possibility that medications are the cause. In addition to estrogens, dopamine receptor blockers (such as the phenothiazines) and dopamine antagonists (e.g., gastric motility agents such as metoclopramide and domperidone) cause significant increases in prolactin. Certain psychiatric drugs, including typical antipsychotics (e.g., haloperidol), atypical antipsychotics (e.g., risperidone) and selective serotonin reuptake inhibitors, monoamine oxidase inhibitors and some tricyclics may cause elevated prolactin. Antihypertensive agents (such as β-blockers and calcium channel blockers) and antihistamines (such as cimetidine and ranitidine) are associated with modest elevations in prolactin. TSH should be measured in patients suspected of a prolactinoma to rule out primary hypothyroidism; in rare cases of severe primary hypothyroidism, TRH will promote release of prolactin. A pregnancy test should be performed in women of reproductive age because pregnancy is a cause of hyperprolactinemia (see Table 55.7).

Prolactin Deficiency

Prolactin is of great clinical importance in the postpartum period because prolactin is required for lactation.[190] Without the availability of infant formulas or wet nurses, failure of maternal lactation can be fatal to the newborn. However, other than the necessity for breast-feeding, prolactin deficiency in humans is not known to have adverse consequences.

Measurement of Prolactin

Prolactin assays typically involve noncompetitive, heterogeneous "sandwich" techniques using two antibodies to recognize different epitopes on the prolactin polypeptide.[191]

Structural variations in circulating prolactin result in biases between immunoassays for this hormone. Monomeric prolactin accounts for more than 85% of the total circulating hormone, but glycosylated and aggregated forms constitute a significant fraction, and immunoreactivity to these forms is variable. Macroprolactin, usually caused by IgG-prolactin complexes, is a relatively common finding in healthy patients, and according to one study, may account for up to 10% of misdiagnoses in hyperprolactinemic patients[182] because renal clearance of the Ig-bound hormone is reduced.[192] IgG-bound prolactin can be separated by gel filtration chromatography, or more conveniently by precipitation of Ig complexes with the addition of PEG. PEG precipitation removes a fraction of monomeric prolactin as well but remains a useful strategy to distinguish clinical hyperprolactinemia from macroprolactinemia.[180,187,188,193] If the ratio of the precipitated prolactin to the total prolactin is 0.50 or greater, macroprolactinemia is said to be present,[194,195] though other strategies are described.[196]

Prolactin methods should be calibrated against reference materials with known international unit potency, such as the WHO IRP (now in its fourth iteration, IS 83/573), to allow assay-to-assay comparison. Despite the heterogeneity of prolactin, immunoassays correlate well with bioassay-validated prolactin standards. A method for measuring prolactin by liquid chromatography/multiple reaction monitoring mass spectrometry has been described.[197]

Specimen Collection and Storage

Prolactin is measured in serum or plasma, although individual assays may recommend serum only. Special handling procedures are not necessary; specimens can be stored at 4 °C for at least 24 hours, but should be frozen if analysis is delayed for longer than 24 hours. Emotional stress, exercise, ambulation, and a protein-rich diet all stimulate prolactin secretion; thus specimens collected after an overnight fast when the patient is resting provide the most reliable prolactin concentrations.

POINTS TO REMEMBER

- Cushing syndrome can be endogenous or exogenous from the excess administration of glucocorticoids.
- Endogenous Cushing syndrome can result from an anterior pituitary adenoma (i.e., Cushing disease), ectopic adrenocorticotropic hormone (ACTH) or corticotropin-releasing hormone secretion, or a cortisol-secreting adrenocortical tumor.
- ACTH deficiency produces cortisol deficiency, although aldosterone secretion remains intact.

Adrenocorticotropic Hormone and Related Peptides

ACTH (corticotropin) is secreted by adenohypophysis as a derivative of pro-opiomelanocortin (POMC).[198,199] ACTH acts primarily on the adrenal cortex, stimulating its growth and the secretion of corticosteroids (specifically cortisol). ACTH production is increased during physiologic or psychologic stress.

Biochemistry

The biochemistry of ACTH, with its origin from POMC and POMC-derived peptides, is described in detail in Chapter 56.

Regulation of Adrenocorticotropic Hormone Secretion

Many variables affect the secretion of ACTH, which is both pulsatile and circadian in nature. Thus regulation of pituitary secretion of ACTH by the hypothalamus is complex. The control of ACTH release by the pituitary is an integral part of the neuroendocrine regulation of stress homeostasis.

Cortisol is the major negative feedback hormone for the tonic inhibition of hypothalamic CRH and pituitary

ACTH secretion. However, endogenous opioids such as met-enkephalin and β-endorphin, which are produced by the adrenal glands, have a downregulatory effect on the hypothalamic-pituitary-ACTH axis as well. Regulation of ACTH is discussed at length in Chapter 56.

Clinical Significance

Because ACTH synthesis originates from the POMC precursor peptide, its production by the pituitary is closely linked with the secretion of endogenous opioid peptides, such as β-endorphin.[1] The physiologic effects of endogenous opiates include (1) sedation, (2) an increased threshold of pain, and (3) autonomic regulation of respiration, blood pressure, and heart rate. These peptides are also involved in modifying endocrine responses to stress and water balance, and may play a role in the regulation of reproduction and the immune system.

Gonadotropin secretion by the pituitary is under inhibitory control by opioid peptides, as is evident by the effects of β-endorphin analogs on the pulse frequency and amplitude of pituitary LH release. In contrast, β-endorphin antagonists (such as naloxone) can elicit an increase in the amount and pattern of gonadotropin secretion. ACTH secretion is similarly downregulated by endogenous opioid peptides; therefore naloxone causes an increase in plasma ACTH concentrations.

No diseases have been clearly associated with disordered metabolism of opioid peptides, but changes in their plasma concentrations may accompany other disorders, such as Cushing disease and depression (increased β-endorphin concentrations)[200] or pheochromocytoma (increased enkephalin concentrations; see Chapter 53). Altered concentrations of opioids in cerebrospinal fluid may reflect disorders such as chronic pain syndrome, schizophrenia, and depression.

In summary, the only POMC derivative that is measured in the diagnosis of certain human disease states is ACTH. Further discussion of adrenal disorders, including disorders of ACTH secretion, is found in Chapter 56.

Measurement of Adrenocorticotropic Hormone

Bioassays and receptor assays for ACTH are of historical interest only. Immunoassays are now used almost exclusively. Competitive binding radioimmunoassays (RIAs) have been developed for ACTH; they differ in (1) the choice of radioactive label (125 iodine is the most common), (2) separation system (charcoal adsorption, PEG, or second-antibody precipitation), (3) antibody (N-terminal or C-terminal specificity), and (4) whether preextraction of ACTH is required. Most polyclonal antibodies recognize a segment of the biologically active N-terminal portion of the molecule and react with intact ACTH (amino acids 1 to 39), N-terminal ACTH fragments (amino acids 1 to 24), and ACTH precursors (e.g., POMC and pro-ACTH).

Immunoradiometric ACTH assays that use labeled monoclonal antibodies in noncompetitive formats were also developed but are becoming historical. In these assays, two monoclonal antibodies (or a polyclonal/monoclonal combination) are directed toward different sites on the ACTH molecule (e.g., the N-terminal and C-terminal domains).[201] These sandwich immunoassays can detect ACTH concentrations of 1 to 4 pg/mL (0.22 to 0.88 pmol/L). Use of monoclonal antibodies have improved the analytical specificity for intact ACTH but may not recognize biologically active precursors and fragments.[202] Less specific ACTH immunoassays are sometimes used to detect the presence of these peptide fragments in patients with cancer-related syndromes (e.g., ectopic ACTH Cushing syndrome). Modern assays for ACTH are two-site chemiluminescent sandwich assays) and may afford divergent results due to the presence of ACTH precursors or fragments. These and other discrepancies can be investigated with mass spectrometric analysis.[203] Currently, manufacturers of commercial ACTH immunoassays usually calibrate their assays with ACTH preparations obtained from research centers, such as human purified ACTH 1-39 (MRC 74/555, 6.2 IU/25 μg), supplied by the National Institute for Biological Standards and Control (United Kingdom), or synthetic ACTH 1-39. For comparison between assays, the calibrators used in a particular assay system must be clearly specified.

Specimen Collection and Storage

Some precautions are necessary in the collection, transportation, and storage of specimens. ACTH is easily oxidized, adsorbs to glass surfaces, and is rapidly degraded by plasma proteases into nonreactive fragments during freezing and thawing of the specimen. Factors that influence plasma ACTH, such as previous administration of corticosteroids, the time of day at which the specimen is collected (diurnal variation), and stress from the venipuncture procedure, should be taken into account. To minimize these problems, it is recommended that blood specimens are collected into prechilled polystyrene (plastic) tubes containing EDTA, immediately placed on ice, and centrifuged at 4 °C. Some laboratories recommend the use of protease inhibitors, such as aprotinin (Trasylol). The plasma should be transferred to another plastic tube and frozen at −20 °C or colder if analysis is delayed. In chilled samples with the addition of EDTA and aprotinin, the plasma proteases that would otherwise degrade ACTH are inhibited, permitting freezing and thawing without substantial subsequent degradation. Antioxidants, such as mercaptoethanol, may be used to stabilize ACTH. Immediately before the ACTH assay is set up, frozen specimens should be thawed and centrifuged to remove any fibrin clots that can interfere with the assay.

Measurement of Endogenous Opioid Peptides

β-Endorphin is a cleavage product of POMC, which is also the precursor to ACTH and β-lipotropin. Both RIAs and immunoradiometric assays have been developed for measurement of β-endorphin. The concentration of β-endorphin is usually very low or undetectable in healthy subjects, and some analytical methods require extraction procedures to detect meaningful concentrations in plasma. The specificity of commercial antibodies for β-endorphin (relative to β-lipotropin) can be variable, and some assays cross-react as much as 50% with β-lipotropin. Assays based on polyclonal antibodies may produce spuriously high results as the consequence of cross-reactivity with serum IgG (e.g., in patients with an IgG myeloma).[204]

Met-enkephalin shares a 5 amino acid N-terminal sequence with β-endorphin but is thought to be derived from pro-enkephalin, rather than POMC. Measurement of met-enkephalin in plasma is difficult because of its very short half-life (2.5 minutes at 37 °C). Even if blood is immediately chilled on ice and centrifuged under refrigeration, approximately 50% of met-enkephalin is lost unless the specimen is collected in 23 mmol/L of citric acid. Commercial assays for met-enkephalin have been developed, and anti-enkephalin antibodies are available. Assays for endogenous opioid peptides maybe useful for research purposes but are not currently applicable for solving clinical endocrine problems.

Gonadotropins (Follicle-stimulating Hormone, Luteinizing Hormone)

LH and FSH are synthesized by gonadotrophs in the adenohypophysis. The actions of FSH are to (1) stimulate the growth and maturation of ovarian follicles, (2) stimulate estrogen secretion (estradiol), (3) promote, via estrogen, the endometrial changes characteristic of the first phase (proliferative or follicular) of the menstrual cycle, and (4) stimulate spermatogenesis in males.

LH and FSH act synergistically to promote ovulation and secretion of androgens (androstenedione) and progesterone. The actions of LH are to (1) promote and maintain the second phase (secretory or luteal) of the menstrual cycle; (2) in females, to assist in the formation of the corpus luteum; and (3) in males, to stimulate the development and functional activity of testicular Leydig cells that produce testosterone.

Biochemistry

Under the generic term gonadotropins, LH and FSH control the functional activity of gonads. In males and females, gonadotropin secretion is regulated via GnRH.[205] Pituitary gonadotropin secretion is controlled by feedback from the gonadotropic hormones. In females, estrogen and inhibin regulate LH and FSH secretion, respectively, and in males, testosterone and inhibin regulate LH and FSH release.

There are two GnRH genes: GnRH1, located at chromosome 8p21, and GnRH2, located at chromosome 20p13. Prepro-GnRH1 is a 92 amino acid, 10.4-kDa polypeptide with a 23 amino acid leader sequence. Removal of the leader sequence produces pro-GnRH1, which is 69 amino acids in length. Release of the C-terminal GnRH-associated peptide-1 yields GnRH1 (amino acids 24 to 33). Amino acid 24 is modified as a pyrrolidone carboxylic acid, and amino acid 33 is modified as a glycine amide.

GnRH2 is expressed in higher concentrations outside the CNS than within the CNS. GnRH2 is principally produced in the prostate, bone marrow, and kidneys. PreproGnRH2 is a 120 amino acid (12.9 kDa) polypeptide. Cleavage of the 23 amino acid leader sequence generates proGnRH2, which is 97 amino acids in length. Release of the C-terminal GnRH-associated peptide 2 yields GnRH2 (amino acids 24 to 33). Similar to GnRH1, amino acid 24 is modified as a pyrrolidone carboxylic acid, and amino acid 33 is modified as a glycine amide. GnRH2 has three isoforms: isoform 1 is the full-length protein; isoform 2 lacks amino acids 52 to 59; and isoform 3 is missing amino acids 52 to 58.

The receptor for GnRH (GnRHR) is expressed on anterior pituitary gonadotropic cells. The gene for GnRHR is located at chromosome 4q. GnRHR is a 328 amino acid protein; the first 38 amino acids are extracellular, and seven transmembrane domains are present. Only two amino acids are cytoplasmic. The GnRHR is possibly glycosylated at amino acids 18 and 102, and a disulfide bond is probably present between amino acids 114 and 196. Two isoforms of GnRHR are expressed: the full-length protein (isoform 1), and isoform 2, which differs in the amino acid sequence between residues 176 and 328. A putative second GnRHR (GnRH2R) exists, comprising 178 amino acids. However, the gene for GnRH2R (located on chromosome 1) has been identified as a pseudogene.

Both LH and FSH are secreted by gonadotrophs. Similar to TSH and hCG, LH and FSH are glycoprotein α-/β-heterodimers.[206] The α-chain is common among all four hormones. The glycoprotein α-chain gene is located on chromosome 6q1. The α-chain includes 116 amino acids and weighs 13.1 kDa, including a leader sequence of 24 amino acids; the secreted chain is 92 amino acids. Amino acids 76 and 102 in the α-chain are glycosylated. Five disulfide bonds are present at amino acids 31 to 55, 34 to 84, 52 to 106, 56 to 108, and 83 to 111.

The gene for the LH β-chain is located at chromosome 19q13.3. The leader sequence (amino acids 1 to 20) is followed by the 121 amino acid β-chain, which is the secreted form. The β-chain is glycosylated at amino acid 50, and six disulfide bonds are present at amino acids 29 to 77, 43 to 92, 46 to 130, 54 to 108, 58 to 110, and 113 to 120.

The gene for the FSH β-chain is located at chromosome 11p1. The 129 amino acid pre-FSH β-chain is 14.7 kDa, including an 18 amino acid leader sequence; the secreted FSH β-chain is 111 amino acids. FSH-β is glycosylated at amino acids 25 and 42 and contains six disulfide bonds at amino acids 21 to 69, 35 to 84, 38 to 122, 46 to 100, 50 to 102, and 105 to 112. Isolated α-subunits are devoid of biological activity; the β-subunit of FSH may have slight intrinsic biological activity, but full activity is attained when α- and β-subunits are recombined. This suggests that the presence of both α- and β-subunits is important for specific receptor recognition, and that the β-subunit is responsible for eliciting the specific biological response.

In men, the LH receptor (LHR) is expressed by Leydig cells, whereas in women, the LHR is expressed on theca cells and is induced by FSH on granulosa cells during the follicular phase of the menstrual cycle. The gene for the LHR is located at chromosome 2p21. The pre-LHR protein is 699 amino acids (78.6 kDa). After removal of the leader sequence, LHR is 673 amino acids long. The extracellular domain is 337 amino acids, followed by seven transmembrane domains and a cytoplasmic domain of 72 amino acids. Seven leucine-rich repeats are present at amino acids 48 to 71, 97 to 121, 122 to 147, 149 to 171, 172 to 196, 197 to 220, and 221 to 244. Cysteines at positions 643 and 644 are lipidated to S-palmitoyl cysteine. Potential glycosylation sites exist at amino acids 99, 174, 195, 291, 299, and 313. A disulfide bond is likely between amino acids 439 and 514. Two isoforms of LHR are expressed: the long isoform is the full-length LHR, and the short isoform lacks amino acids 227 to 289.

The FSH receptor (FSHR) is expressed on Sertoli cells in men and on granulosa cells in women. Following the 17 amino acid leader sequence is the 678 amino acid FSHR. The extracellular domain is 349 amino acids, with seven trans-membrane domains. The cytoplasmic domain is 65 amino acids. Ten leucine-rich repeats are present at amino acids 18 to 48, 49 to 72, 73 to 97, 98 to 118, 119 to 143, 144 to 169, 170 to 192, 193 to 216, 217 to 240, and 241 to 259. The FSHR has four proven or suspected sites of glycosylation at amino acids 191, 199, 293, and 318; two definitive disulfide bonds (amino acids 18 to 25 and 23 to 32); and one possible disulfide bond (amino acids 442 to 517). Two isoforms of the FSHR are expressed: isoform 1 is the full-length FSHR, and isoform 2 lacks amino acids 224 to 285.

Physiologic Activity

In men, LH stimulates testosterone synthesis and secretion by Leydig cells. In response to FSH, Sertoli cells nourish developing sperm during spermatogenesis.

Based on the two-cell model of estradiol and progesterone production by the adult ovary, androstenedione is produced by theca cells in response to LH stimulation (Fig. 55.6). Granulosa cells do not have direct access to the circulation;

therefore low-density lipoprotein (LDL) cholesterol is not readily available to granulosa cells in the follicular phase of the menstrual cycle. Consequently, granulosa cell synthesis of sex steroids is dependent on theca cell androstenedione. Granulosa cells initially respond to FSH, and later to FSH plus LH.

FSH has several effects on the ovary during the follicular phase of the menstrual cycle (see Chapter 58). When bound to granulosa cell FSHRs, FSH stimulates granulosa cell proliferation. As a result, a dominant follicle develops containing the ovum that will be expelled midcycle (ovulation) to be captured by the fimbriae of the fallopian tube. When this event is being stimulated by FSH, granulosa cells use theca cell androstenedione as the precursor for estradiol synthesis. FSH also stimulates the expression of LHRs on the granulosa cells. Estradiol and inhibins from the ovary provide negative feedback for hypothalamic release of GnRH.

At midcycle, as a consequence of the LH surge, the follicle ruptures with release of the ovum (ovulation). The corpus luteum of the ovary (Fig. 55.7) is formed from the remaining theca and granulosa cells. The theca cells (responsive to LH)

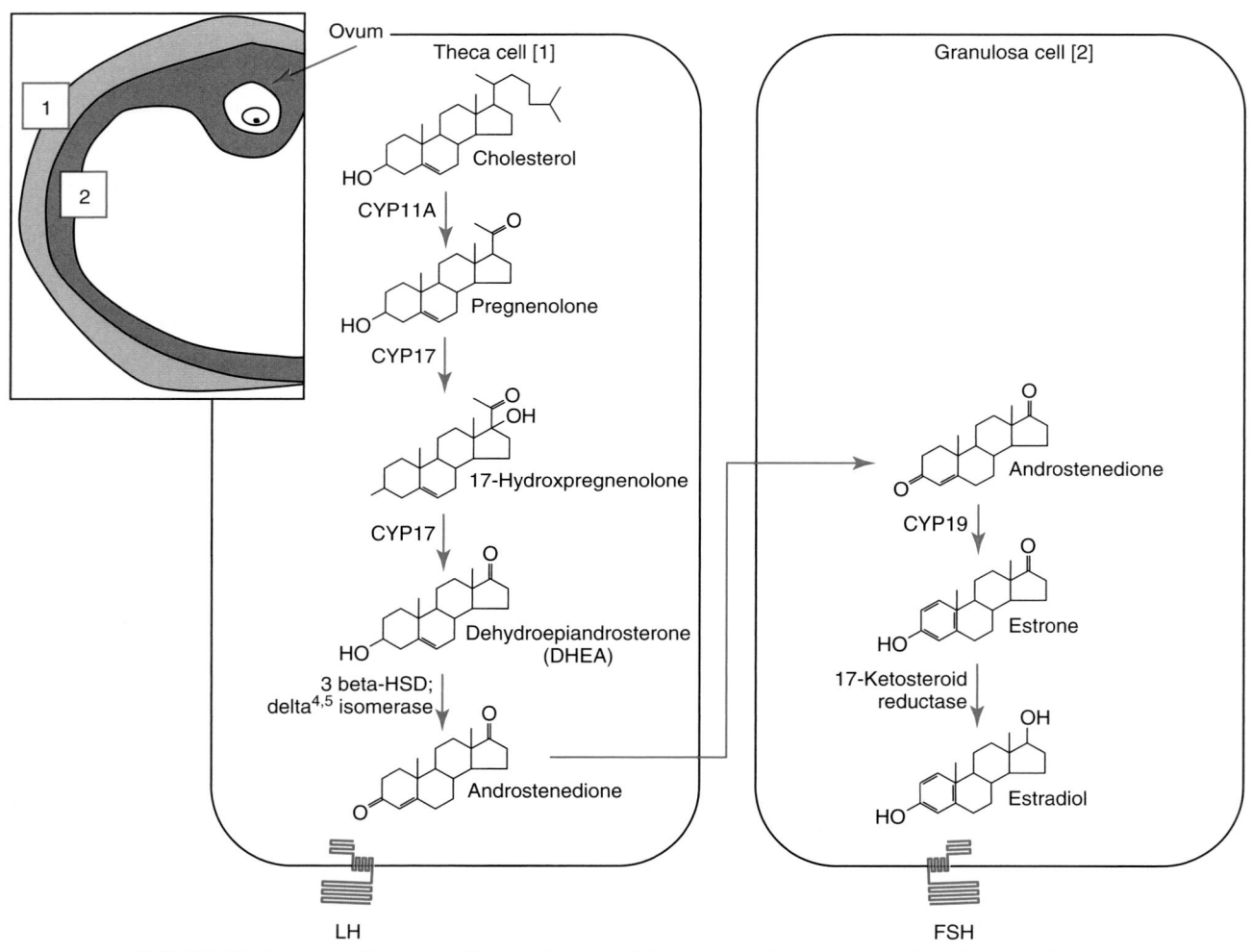

FIGURE 55.6 In the follicular (proliferative) phase of the menstrual cycle, under the influence of luteinizing hormone *(LH)*, Theca cells *(1)* Produce androstenedione from cholesterol (the intermediary steps are illustrated). Under the influence of follicle-stimulating hormone *(FSH)*, granulosa cells use the androstenedione produced by the theca cells to synthesize estradiol (the intermediary steps are illustrated) *(2)*. *3 Beta-HSD,* 3 Beta-hydroxysteroid dehydrogenase; *CYP11A,* 20,22 desmolase; *CYP17,* 17-hydroxylase activity; *CYP19,* aromatase.

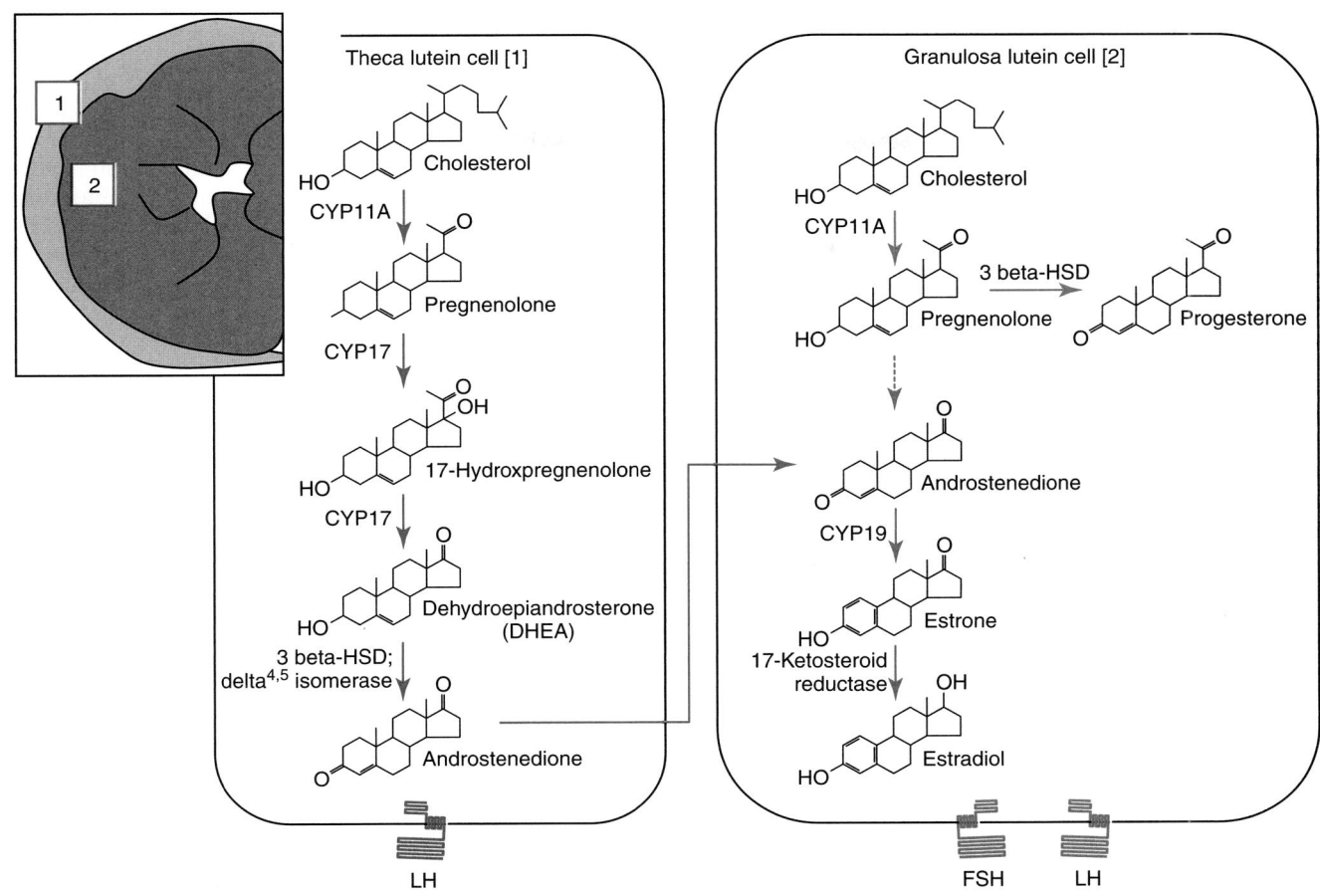

FIGURE 55.7 In the luteal (secretory) phase of the menstrual cycle after ovulation, under the influence of luteinizing hormone *(LH)*, Theca lutein cells *(1)* Produce androstenedione from cholesterol (the intermediary steps are illustrated). Under the influence of follicle-stimulating hormone *(FSH)* and LH, granulosa lutein cells use androstenedione produced by the theca cells to synthesize estradiol, and use cholesterol available from low-density lipoprotein *(LDL)* to synthesize progesterone (the intermediary steps are illustrated) *(2)*. *3 Beta-HSD,* 3 Beta-hydroxysteroid dehydrogenase; *CYP11A,* 20,22 desmolase; *CYP17,* 17-hydroxylase activity; *CYP19,* aromatase.

become the theca lutein cells, and the granulosa cells (now responsive to LH and FSH) are converted to the granulosa lutein cells, which now are vascularized and gain access to LDL cholesterol from the circulation. With an adequate supply of cholesterol from LDL, the granulosa lutein cells generate progesterone and estradiol. Estradiol and progesterone convert the proliferative endometrium of the first half of the menstrual cycle to the secretory endometrium of the second (luteal) half of the menstrual cycle.

In the absence of pregnancy (i.e., in the absence of hCG), progesterone concentrations decline, and menstruation occurs because the corpus luteum atrophies to become the corpus albicans. However, if a fertilized ovum implants in the uterine wall, the syncytiotrophoblast, via hCG, will maintain the corpus luteum, and menstruation is avoided because of continued secretion of estradiol and progesterone. The corpus luteum (supported by hCG) then becomes the corpus luteum of pregnancy.

Regulation and Clinical Significance
In hypogonadal patients, if gonadotropin concentrations are greatly elevated, hypergonadotropic hypogonadism is

diagnosed, indicating that gonadal (end-organ) failure has occurred.[207] Alternatively, if gonadotropin concentrations are consistently low in hypogonadal patients, the diagnosis of hypogonadotropic hypogonadism is likely. To ensure that the pituitary is unable to respond to GnRH, a GnRH stimulation test can be performed.[208,209] GnRH testing should be performed in children (especially boys) in whom hypogonadotropic hypogonadism versus constitutional delay in growth and adolescence (delayed puberty) is a diagnostic question; basal LH and FSH may also be low. If basal LH and FSH concentrations are low, but LH and FSH rise substantially after GnRH stimulation, constitutional delay in growth and adolescence is likely, and hypogonadotropic hypogonadism can be excluded. The therapeutic approach to these two conditions is different. Children with constitutional delay in growth and adolescence eventually will enter puberty (albeit later than their peers), whereas hypogonadotropic hypogonadism will require sex hormone replacement therapy for initiation of puberty. If hypogonadotropic hypogonadism is diagnosed, a thorough search for its cause (e.g., genetic, functional, structural, or neoplastic) is essential. Induction of fertility in patients with hypogonadotropic hypogonadism requires gonadotropin replacement. A protocol for performance of the GnRH test is discussed in the following section.

Hypogonadotropic hypogonadism has also been found to result from loss-of-function mutations in the GnRHR gene.[210] Isolated FSH deficiency can result from mutations in the FSH β chain. However, isolated FSH deficiency is a rare cause of infertility in men or women. Men with FSH deficiency (but LH sufficiency) will have normal testosterone concentrations because LH and responding Leydig cells are normal.

Gain-of-function mutations in the LHR cause a hypogonadotropic, familial, male precocious puberty, in which the testes autonomously and prematurely produce testosterone (testotoxicosis).[211] Leydig cell adenomas with LHR mutations can cause precocious puberty.

LHR loss-of-function mutations cause Leydig cell hypoplasia and inadequate virilization of males in utero, leading to ambiguous genitalia.[212] In females, LHR loss-of-function mutations cause oligomenorrhea, amenorrhea, or infertility. FSHR loss-of-function mutations in females result in ovarian dysgenesis.

Central precocious puberty occurs with early activation of the hypothalamic-pituitary-gonadal axis, leading to gonadotropin-driven early puberty (onset of breast development or pubic hair before age 8 years or menses before age 9.5 years in girls, and puberty onset in boys before age 9 years).[213] In most girls (≈95%), no specific cause is identified (idiopathic precocious puberty). Central precocious puberty is uncommon in boys. However, when central precocious puberty occurs in boys, the likelihood of CNS pathology is greater than that in girls.

Other details concerning the regulation and clinical significance of LH and FSH are discussed in Chapter 58.

Measurement of Luteinizing Hormone and Follicle-stimulating Hormone

The α subunit of LH and FSH is a member of the "cystine knot" superfamily of polypeptides that also includes GH, chorionic gonadotropin (hCG), and thyrotropin (TSH). Therefore analytical methods for measuring LH and FSH must recognize the unique β subunits of these hormones because the α subunit is shared among several homologous pituitary products and hCG.

Two-site (double antibody) heterogeneous immunoassays are currently the most common methods for measuring gonadotropins, and a wide variety of assays have been adapted to automated platforms. Some commercially available methods attach a capture antibody to the surface of test tubes or plastic beads, whereas others use a paramagnetic label or a microparticle to capture the antibody–antigen complexes. Numerous labels have been used for the second antibody, including radioisotopes, enzymes,[214] fluorophores,[215] and chemiluminescent molecules. The analytical sensitivity of LH assays is especially important in the evaluation of prepubertal children and patients with hypothalamic disorders because LH concentrations are very low.

Calibration of gonadotropin assays is difficult because LH and FSH undergo post-translational modifications producing a mixture of closely related compounds.[216] The earliest reference material used for calibration of LH and FSH assays was the second IRP for human menopausal gonadotropins, isolated from the urine of postmenopausal women. However, alterations during metabolism and excretion limited the

comparability of this preparation with circulating forms of the hormones, and subsequent calibrators were prepared from extracts derived from the human pituitary gland. Purified pituitary extracts, such as the first and second IRPs for FSH and LH, were available for many years but have been replaced by highly purified extracts that have minimal contamination with cross-reacting glycoproteins. Manufacturers of older immunoassays for LH and FSH used one or more pituitary-derived reference materials for their working calibrators, but recombinant gonadotropin calibrators are now available.

Biases in analytical results still exist between different immunoassay systems (most notably in LH assays), and results can differ by more than 50%, even when calibrated with the same reference preparation.[217,218] The most likely explanation for the bias is noncommutability of the reference material. Gonadotropic hormones are glycosylated, and this affects their antigenicity.[219] For example, LH immunoassays using monoclonal antibodies generate considerably lower LH concentrations than RIAs using polyclonal antibodies, presumably because of the greater specificity of monoclonal antibodies, which may recognize only a subset of LH isoforms and epitopes. Other factors that contribute to method-dependent biases include differences in calibration procedures and the assay matrix itself.

Specimen Collection and Storage

Serum is the preferred specimen for gonadotropin measurements. Hemolyzed, lipemic, and/or icteric specimens should not be used. Both hormones are stable for 8 days at room temperature, and for 2 weeks at 4 °C; for longer periods, the serum specimen should be frozen at or below −20 °C. Because of episodic, circadian, and cyclic variations in the secretion of gonadotropins, meaningful clinical evaluation of these hormones may require determinations in pooled blood specimens, multiple serial blood specimens, or timed urine specimens. Urine specimens should not contain preservatives; storage at or below −20 °C is recommended.

Measurement of Urinary Follicle-stimulating Hormone and Luteinizing Hormone

Clinically, the pulsatile and episodic release of gonadotropins makes a single blood measurement of FSH or LH difficult to interpret unless they are noted very low or very high in the presence of low end-hormone concentrations and a clinical presentation of hypogonadism. In adults, concentrations of gonadotropins in blood, particularly LH, may differ as much as threefold between blood specimens collected from the same individual 20 minutes apart. In addition, the lower detection limit of many FSH and LH immunoassays may be within the reference interval for these hormones in normal adults. In prepubertal children, most blood assays are not capable of measuring normal concentrations because they are so low. To improve detection limits for gonadotropin assays in children, urinary FSH or LH assays have been used.[220]

Thyroid-stimulating Hormone

TSH (thyrotropin), which is synthesized in thyrotrophs of the adenohypophysis, promotes the growth of thyroid follicular cells and sustains and stimulates the hormonal secretion of thyroid gland hormones 3,5,3′,5′ tetraiodothyronine (thyroxine; T4) and 3,5,3′-triiodothyronine (T3).[221]

Biochemistry and Physiology

TSH binds to TSH receptors (TSHRs) located on the surfaces of thyroid follicular cells.[222] TSH (1) stimulates growth and vascularity of the thyroid gland, (2) stimulates growth of thyroid follicular cells, (3) promotes thyroid hormone synthesis by increasing the uptake of iodine (via the sodium-iodide transporter), (4) promotes the organification (reduction) of iodine, (5) promotes the coupling of tyrosines, and (6) promotes the proteolytic release of stored thyroid hormone from thyroglobulin. TSH release is stimulated by TRH and is suppressed by thyroid hormone (principally, circulating T4).

TRH is a modified tripeptide produced by the hypothalamus. The thyroid-releasing hormone receptor (TRHR) is expressed on anterior pituitary thyrotrophs. TRHR is a 398 amino acid protein, and 28 of its amino acids constitute an extracellular domain. Seven transmembrane domains are present, along with a 79 amino acid cytoplasmic domain. Two possible glycosylation sites exist at amino acids 3 and 10, and a disulfide bridge is present between amino acids 98 and 179. Details of TRH and TRHR production are discussed in Chapter 57.

The glycoprotein α chain, shared with FSH, LH, and hCG, was described earlier in this chapter. The β-chain of TSH is encoded on chromosome 1p13. After removal of the 20 amino acid leader sequence, the pro-TSH β-chain consists of 118 amino acids. Cleavage of the six C-terminal residues released from the propeptide yields the TSH β-chain (112 amino acids). TSH is glycosylated at residue 43, and disulfide bonds are likely at amino acids 22 to 72, 36 to 87, 39 to 125, 47 to 103, 51 to 105, and 108 to 115.

Regulation, Clinical Significance, and Analytical Methods

Details concerning the regulation, clinical significance, and measurement of TSH are discussed in detail in Chapter 57.

Assessment of Anterior Pituitary Lobe Reserve

Evaluation of endocrine function is an important part of the management of patients with pituitary disease.[223,224] Detection of hormone deficiencies before and after treatment and recognition of hormone-producing tumors are the two objectives of testing of pituitary function in patients with pituitary disease.[225]

Assessment of anterior and posterior pituitary function in patients with a pituitary tumor is important in the identification of clinically significant hormone deficiency states caused by the tumor, and in the re-evaluation of patients after pituitary surgery or irradiation to detect hormone deficiencies that occur as a result of invasive treatment. Testing of pituitary function usually is performed under basal conditions, but it can be performed under provocative conditions to expose subtle or mild deficiencies observed in disorders of the adrenal gland or gonads. The primary relevance of prolactin deficiency relates to Sheehan syndrome, in which postpartum hemorrhage results in pituitary infarction and panhypopituitarism; this is still an important problem in developing countries. However, Sheehan syndrome can develop years after delivery.[226]

The lower detection limits of two-site immunoassays for the measurement of pituitary hormones make it possible to distinguish an abnormally low value from the lower end of the normal reference interval. Although assessment of a particular aspect of pituitary function should include clinical

---

BOX 55.5 Assessment of Pituitary Reserve in Surgical Patients

Before Pituitary Surgery
Adrenal function: measurement of morning serum cortisol concentration or 1 ug cosyntropin stimulation test:
- Thyroid function: thyroid-stimulating hormone with free T4
- Gonadal function: sex hormone determinations (estradiol in women and testosterone in men) and gonadotropins (luteinizing hormone and follicle-stimulating hormone) if sex steroids are low

Shortly After Pituitary Surgery (2–4 Days After Surgery)
- Adrenal function: morning serum cortisol concentration
- Monitor urine and sodium status to detect hyponatremia or diabetes insipidus
- Thyroid function: deferred
- Gonadal function: deferred

Six Weeks After Pituitary Surgery
- Adrenal function: cosyntropin stimulation test or insulin tolerance test
- Thyroid function: free T4
- Gonadal function: sex hormone determinations (estradiol in women and testosterone in men)

---

findings of hormone deficiency and measurement of hormones secreted by the pertinent endocrine gland (e.g., T4, cortisol, testosterone), newer ultrasensitive assays for TSH, FSH, LH, and ACTH may allow accurate distinction between a pathologically low result and a low-normal result. A scheme for testing of pituitary reserve is proposed in Box 55.5.

Hypothalamic-Pituitary-Adrenal Axis

A morning serum cortisol concentration in excess of 11 to 15 μg/dL (303 to 414 nmol/L) usually provides adequate evidence that the hypothalamic-pituitary-adrenal (HPA) axis is intact and is functioning properly though concomitant measurement of ACTH provides necessary corroboration. A typical reference interval for morning cortisol is 5 to 23 μg/dL (138 to 635 nmol/L). A morning cortisol result can fall within the reference interval, yet may not prove that the patient has a normal HPA axis.

If the morning cortisol is frankly low (<5 μg/dL; <138 nmol/L) or equivocal (5 to 15 μg/dL; 138 to 414 nmol/L), or if a strong clinical suspicion of adrenal insufficiency is present, the cosyntropin (Synacthen) stimulation test is helpful. Cosyntropin provocation of cortisol release is performed by obtaining a baseline blood specimen for cortisol followed by IV or IM administration of 250 μg of cosyntropin (an active ACTH analog). Blood specimens are collected 30 and 60 minutes after administration of cosyntropin (see Box 56.1 and Chapter 56 for more detail). A lower dose cosyntropin test (1.0 μg IV) has been proposed as a more sensitive test of impaired pituitary reserve, but its usefulness is still unclear and controversial.[227,228] The use of such testing in the setting of critical illness to assess adrenal function or direct steroid therapy is controversial.[229]

Tests of the entire HPA axis, such as the ITT (also called the insulin-induced hypoglycemia stimulation test; see Box 55.3), occasionally are abnormal in patients who have

(1) a normal morning cortisol result, (2) a normal response to cosyntropin, and (3) no signs of adrenal insufficiency. Although an abnormality in these sensitive tests suggests some diminution of ACTH reserve, the clinical significance is most relevant when the patient encounters a major stress, such as gastroenteritis. These tests should be reserved for patients who are strongly suspected of having adrenal insufficiency, or whose morning cortisol concentration or response to ACTH has been found to be abnormal. Standard protocols for the performance and interpretation of these tests have been published. The ITT in particular has a risk of inducing a hypoglycemic seizure, particularly if there is preexisting risk of seizure. Additionally, patients are likely to experience discomfort, so these tests must be performed under the direct supervision of an experienced physician in the inpatient setting. Certainly, good vascular access should be available for ITTs. Because glucagon administration stimulates ACTH, glucagon stimulation testing can be used as an alternative to ITT when there is a contraindication to hypoglycemia.

Measurement of ACTH in blood collected at baseline or after stimulation with insulin adds little to the utility of the tests discussed previously and generally is not performed. In patients who have undergone pituitary surgery, the cortisol negative feedback loop to ACTH secretion may take time to normalize. ACTH and cortisol measurements after administration of CRH potentially are a direct test of pituitary ACTH reserve. The insulin-induced hypoglycemia test is currently the definitive test of ACTH and/or cortisol reserve; however, this test is contraindicated in patients aged older than 70 years, those with a history of coronary heart disease, seizure disorder, or general debility.

Hypothalamic-Pituitary-Thyroid Axis

Because the current generation of TSH assays provide limits of detection extending to ≤ 0.01 mIU/L, which is sufficient to distinguish between low-normal and pathologically suppressed TSH secretion, TRH testing usually is not required for assessment of thyroid function.[230] Pharmaceutical TRH currently is not available in the United States.

While previously the TRH stimulation test found clinical use in a number of contexts, the advent of ultrasensitive TSH assays has made this test of limited value. It still finds some use in specific clinical contexts, namely: an adjunctive tool to distinguish TSH producing pituitary adenoma from thyroid hormone resistance, or to differentiate pituitary from hypothalamic forms of hypothyroidism.[231] In cases of TSH-secreting pituitary adenoma, patients present with increased free T4 and an inappropriately normal or elevated TSH.[232] In these patients, the TSH response to TRH is impaired, and elevations of the free α subunit may also be seen.

TRH testing involves the bolus IV administration of TRH (100 μg/m², or 500 μg total in adults), along with the measurement of TSH at baseline and at 30 minutes. (Note: Some protocols extend TSH measurements to 45 and 60 minutes.) The expected (normal) response is an increase in TSH concentration over the baseline of 5 to 30 mIU/L. Some sources report that a normal response to TRH is a fivefold to tenfold increase in serum TSH concentration within 60 minutes after TRH administration. A TSH change of less than 5 mIU/L indicates TSH suppression (primary hyperthyroidism) or the inability of the pituitary to respond (secondary hypothyroidism). TSH responses greater than 30 mIU/L are consistent with primary hypothyroidism. In tertiary hypothyroidism, TSH will rise slowly in a delayed response pattern.

Hypothalamic-Pituitary-Gonadal Axis

History and physical examination are extremely helpful in evaluating the status of the hypothalamic-pituitary-gonadal axis, particularly in women during their reproductive years.[233,234] Normal menstrual cycles usually indicate an intact hypothalamic-pituitary-gonadal axis in women of reproductive age. A serum progesterone concentration greater than 3 ng/mL (10 nmol/L) one week before the onset of the next menstrual cycle supports the diagnosis of ovulation.

Baseline laboratory assessment for hypothalamic-pituitary-gonadal dysregulation should include measurement of serum gonadotropins (LH and FSH) and sex steroids (estradiol in females and testosterone in males). Provocative testing of this axis with GnRH administration and measurements of FSH and LH (Box 55.6) are useful in selected patients. However, the definition of an appropriate response to GnRH is controversial and depends on the stage of sexual maturation of the subject. After GnRH injection, LH normally rises more than FSH. Two shortened variations of the GnRH test are available: in one variation, leuprolide (a GnRH agonist; 20 μg/kg) is injected subcutaneously, and LH and FSH are measured 3 hours later; in the other variant, 100 μg of GnRH is injected subcutaneously, and LH and FSH are measured 40 minutes later. However, these tests can be unreliable in differentiating pituitary disorders from hypothalamic dysfunction; the physician usually is dependent on an accurate determination of gonadotropins and sex steroids, along with clinical judgment, in differentiating hypothalamic from pituitary disease.

BOX 55.6   Protocol for the Gonadotropin-releasing Hormone Stimulation Test for Luteinizing Hormone and Follicle-stimulating Hormone Reserve

Rationale

The hypothalamic releasing hormone gonadotropin-releasing hormone (GnRH) stimulates the pituitary release of both luteinizing hormone (LH) and follicle-stimulating hormone (FSH) in normal individuals. Subnormal responses are seen in some patients with pituitary or hypothalamic disorders. However, the magnitude of LH and FSH responses to GnRH is usually predictable from basal LH and FSH concentrations. This test may be useful in patients in whom the clinical picture and basal gonadotropin measurements are inconclusive.

Procedure

The test may be performed without regard to previous feeding or time of day. After baseline specimens are obtained for LH and FSH measurement, 100 μg or 2.5 μg/kg (to a maximum of 100 μg) GnRH is given intravenously. Samples for LH and FSH determination should be drawn every 15–20 min for 1–2 h.

Interpretation

LH response should increase by 3 to 10-fold. The FSH response is of lesser magnitude (usually a 1.5- to 3-fold increase). Peak responses for both LH and FSH occur between 15 and 30 min.

AT A GLANCE

The pituitary is a master gland for many vital endocrine functions regulating growth (GH), thyroid function (thyrotropin), reproduction (LH, FSH, and prolactin), stress responses (corticotropin), parturition (oxytocin), and water balance (antidiuretic hormone). The most common pituitary disorders encompass over or under production of pituitary hormones, and pituitary tumors.

The hypothalamus regulates pituitary hormone release or is the site of synthesis of the posterior pituitary hormones. Like the pituitary, hypothalamic disease can involve over or under production of hypothalamic hormones.

Pituitary Assessment in Surgical Patients

Initial Assessment

Preoperative testing is indicated in patients with large pituitary tumors or specific clinical indications such as suspected ACTH deficiency, when glucocorticoids may be required preoperatively (see Box 55.5), but the gonadal axis may be compromised in patients with microadenomas as well. In addition to the history and physical examination, patients at risk for pituitary insufficiency should be evaluated for endocrine function before surgery is performed, including laboratory measurements of serum prolactin, free T4, LH, FSH, sex steroids (testosterone in males and estradiol in females), IGF-I, GH, serum sodium, and urine specific gravity (or serum and urine osmolality), and a morning serum cortisol or cosyntropin stimulation test.

Perioperative Assessment

The optimum time for retesting endocrine function after pituitary surgery is not known. Many protocols (often based on sparse data) explain how potential cortisol deficiency is managed in the perioperative period. Some neurosurgeons provide "stress" doses (high doses) of glucocorticoids immediately before, during, and after surgery. If the patient had ACTH deficiency preoperatively, IV glucocorticoids can be replaced with oral replacement doses (e.g., the equivalent of 12 mg/m^2 per day of hydrocortisone in children, or 20 to 30 mg in adults in two divided doses, 15 to 20 mg in the morning and 5 to 10 mg in the afternoon) after 2 to 3 days. If the patient had normal adrenal function preoperatively, exogenous glucocorticoids can be discontinued on the second or third postoperative day. Morning cortisol should be measured 24 hours later; if the result is less than 5 μg/dL (138 nmol/L), ACTH deficiency is likely, and glucocorticoid replacement is indicated. If the 24-hour postoperative cortisol is 10 μg/dL (276 nmol/L) or greater, the HPA axis is normal, and glucocorticoid replacement is not required. If cortisol is between 5 and 10 μg/dL (138 to 276 nmol/L), the patient should be treated with glucocorticoids until provocative testing can be performed (ITT or glucagon stimulation test) safely; the ITT can be used concurrently to assess GH deficiency. Many clinicians prefer to perform a cosyntropin test at least 6 weeks postoperatively as an alternative to evaluate the HPA axis.

Some neurosurgeons do not treat with glucocorticoids if preoperative adrenal function is normal,[235] preferring instead to assess postoperative morning cortisol concentration in the patient. If cortisol concentration is less than 5 μg/dL (138 nmol/L), ACTH deficiency is present and glucocorticoid treatment is necessary. If cortisol is greater than 15 μg/dL (414 nmol/L), ACTH deficiency is not present, and glucocorticoid treatment is not required. Provocative testing is required only for patients with a morning cortisol of 5 to 15 μg/dL (138 to 414 nmol/L); pituitary function in these patients can be evaluated with an ITT or glucagon stimulation test (or cosyntropin test at least 6 weeks postoperatively). These patients will be covered with glucocorticoid until diagnostic clarity can be established.[236]

In the first 6 weeks after pituitary surgery, the cosyntropin test may not be a reliable indicator of HPA axis integrity. During this period, the adrenal response to cosyntropin may be normal, yet endogenous ACTH may be insufficient in the basal state or at times of stress to avoid glucocorticoid insufficiency. Once the adrenal gland atrophies from a deficiency of endogenous ACTH (which may take 6 weeks), the cosyntropin challenge becomes abnormal, reflecting endogenous ACTH deficiency.

Postoperative Assessment

It is advisable to wait until 1 month or longer after surgery to evaluate thyroid function (TSH and free T4) and gonadal function (testosterone in males and estradiol in females; see Box 55.5). Early treatment of thyroid and gonadal deficiencies is not critical, and misleading test results might be observed in the early postoperative period. Adrenal function should be reassessed with a low dose (1-μg) or standard dose (250-μg) cosyntropin stimulation test 6 weeks after surgery even if immediate results are subnormal because ACTH deficiency after pituitary surgery may be transient. Periodic clinical follow-up and laboratory assessment should be tailored to individual circumstances.

Stimulation tests for the secretion of ACTH, GH, and GnRH can be combined. For example, the ITT can be combined with the GnRH stimulation test. The ITT assesses GH and ACTH secretion, whereas the GnRH stimulation test assesses the ability of the anterior pituitary to secrete gonadotropins in response to GnRH.

After pituitary irradiation, patients should be evaluated yearly with measurement of free T4, sex steroids, cortisol and IGF-I.

POINTS TO REMEMBER

- Antidiuretic hormone (ADH) and oxytocin synthesizing cells are located in the hypothalamus.
- ADH and oxytocin are released from axons in the posterior pituitary.
- There are no known diseases of oxytocin deficiency or excess.
- ADH deficiency or resistance causes diabetes insipidus with excess free water loss.
- ADH excess causes syndrome of inappropriate ADH, which results in excess free water retention.

Neurohypophysis

The neurohypophysis (posterior pituitary) is derived from the brain neuroectodermis. Embryologically, ventral evagination of the floor of the third ventricle forms the neurohypophysis.[237]

ADH (vasopressin) and oxytocin are secreted from the neurohypophysis, the cell bodies of which are located in hypothalamic supraoptic and paraventricular nuclei. These neurons are located in and travel through the median eminence and pituitary stalk, with nerve endings projecting to the posterior lobe of the pituitary gland.

Antidiuretic Hormone

Disorders of ADH involve excess hormone (syndrome of inappropriate ADH [SIADH]) or deficient ADH action (diabetes insipidus [DI]). DI can result from ADH deficiency, ADH resistance, or renal tubular disease; the latter two conditions are termed nephrogenic DI. Disorders of oxytocin secretion have not been described. However, the discovery that receptors for oxytocin are expressed on osteoblasts and osteoclasts opens the door for a role of oxytocin in bone physiology and bone disease.[238]

Biochemistry

Both ADH and oxytocin are nonapeptides consisting of a cyclic hexapeptide and a three amino acid side chain (Fig. 55.8). At the physiologic pH of plasma, ADH and oxytocin circulate mainly as unbound (free) hormones.

The *AVP* gene for ADH is located at chromosome 20p13. Prepro-ADH consists of 164 amino acids (17.3 kDa). The gene also encodes neurophysin 2 and copeptin. The first 19 amino acids of prepro-ADH are the leader sequence. Amino acids 20 to 28 constitute the ADH nonapeptide hormone; amino acids 32 to 124 represent neurophysin 2, and amino acids 126 to 164 represent copeptin (C-terminal provasopressin). The glycine residue at position 28 is amidated, and amino acid 131 is glycosylated. Disulfide bonds are definitive or possible at amino acids 20 to 25, 41 to 85, 44 to 58, 52 to 75, 59 to 65, 92 to 104, 98 to 116, and 105 to 110. The disulfide bridge at residues 20 to 25 is within ADH.

The ADH receptor in the renal tubules (specifically, the collecting ducts) is termed the arginine vasopressin receptor 2 (V2 receptor). The V2 receptor is a member of the seven-transmembrane domain G-protein–coupled receptor superfamily, whose other members include the V1a and V1b vasopressin receptors and the oxytocin receptor.

The gene for the V2 receptor is located on chromosome Xq28. The receptor has 371 amino acids (40.3 kDa), including a 38 amino acid extracellular domain, 7 transmembrane

domains, and a 43 amino acid cytoplasmic domain. Amino acid 22 may be glycosylated, and amino acids 341 and 342 are lipidated as S-palmitoyl cysteines. Two isoforms of the V2 receptor are known: isoform 1 is the full-length receptor, whereas isoform 2 varies in the sequence of amino acids 305 to 309, and amino acids 310 to 371 are absent.

The V1a receptor (V1 receptor) gene is located at chromosome 12q14. The protein has 418 amino acids and weighs 46.8 kDa. A 52 amino acid extracellular domain is present, along with 7 transmembrane domains and a 67 amino acid cytoplasmic domain. Glycosylation is possible at amino acids 27 and 196. Amino acids 365 and 366 may be lipidated as S-palmitoyl cysteines. A serine residue at position 404 may be phosphorylated to phosphoserine, and a disulfide bond is likely between amino acids 124 and 203.

The V1b receptor (V3 receptor) is encoded by a gene located on chromosome 1q32. The V3 receptor has 424 amino acids (47.0 kDa). A 35 amino acid extracellular domain is present, along with 7 transmembrane domains and an 83 amino acid cytoplasmic domain. The receptor is possibly glycosylated at amino acid 21, and a disulfide bond is likely between amino acids 107 and 186.

The action of ADH is to simulate the movement of aquaporin-2 from the cytoplasm to the basal plasma membrane. In this way, ADH allows the reabsorption of water from the collecting duct. Aquaporin-2 is a 271 amino acid protein (28.8 kDa).[239] The gene encoding aquaporin-2 is located on chromosome 12q1. The external domain contains 16 amino acids, along with 7 transmembrane domains and a 47 amino acid cytoplasmic domain. Phosphoserines are possible or definitive at amino acids 256, 261, and 264, and amino acid 123 is a possible site of glycosylation. Amino acids 68 to 70 and 184 to 186 are NPA (asparagine-proline-alanine) motifs.

Regulation of Antidiuretic Hormone Secretion

Antidiuretic hormone secretion is controlled predominantly by plasma osmolality (tonicity).[240] Plasma osmolality is sensed by osmoreceptors located in cell bodies in or near the magnocellular nuclei of the hypothalamus. Increased osmolality results in ADH release; even relatively small changes in osmolality affect ADH secretion. A 2% increase in extracellular fluid osmolality can stimulate the osmoreceptor to release ADH. Plasma osmolality above 280 mOsm/kg (mmol/kg) is thought to be the osmotic threshold for triggering ADH release.

In addition to the osmoreceptor mechanism of vasopressin release, physiologic regulation of ADH secretion involves a pressure–volume mechanism that is distinct from the osmotic sensor. High-pressure arterial baroreceptors of the aortic arch and carotid sinus, and low-pressure volume receptors in the pulmonary venous system and atria, also regulate ADH release. Therefore ADH is secreted in response to decreased circulating blood volume or decreased blood pressure. Other nonosmotic stimuli for ADH release include pain, stress, nausea and vomiting, sleep, exercise, and chemical agents, such as catecholamines, angiotensin II, opiates, prostaglandins, anesthetics, nicotine, and barbiturates.

The thirst center is regulated by many of the same factors that determine ADH release. This center has a higher set point than the osmoreceptors and responds to osmolalities above 290 mOsm/kg. Responses involving ADH, thirst, and renal reabsorption of sodium and water are coordinated in a

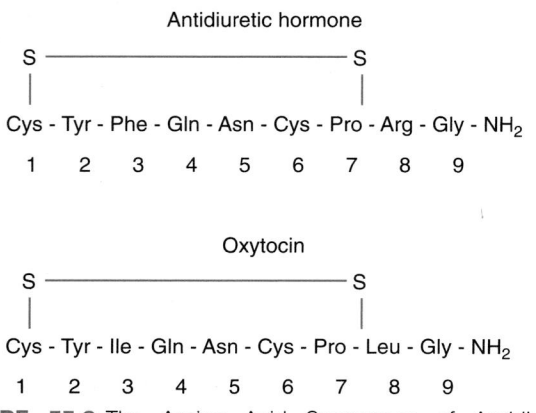

FIGURE 55.8 The Amino Acid Sequences of Antidiuretic Hormone *(ADH)* and Oxytocin Are Compared.

complex scheme that maintains plasma osmolality in healthy individuals within a narrow interval (~285 to ~295 mOsm/kg [mmol/kg]).

Physiologic Activity

Both ADH and neurophysin 2 are present in secretory vesicles that reach the terminal portion of the axon 12 to 14 hours after they are synthesized (this is also true for oxytocin and neurophysin 1). Upon nerve stimulation, release of neurohypophyseal hormones into the portal circulation occurs via calcium-dependent exocytosis. When a stimulus for secretion of ADH or oxytocin occurs, the stimulus acts on the appropriate magnocellular cell body in the hypothalamus, sending an action potential down the long axon to the posterior pituitary, causing an influx of calcium and the release of hormone from neurosecretory granules.

The exact role of the neurophysins is unclear, but their proper synthesis is necessary for ADH secretion. The biological role of copeptin is unknown. Copeptin is being investigated as a marker of myocardial infarction.[241] Because of analytical difficulties in measuring ADH, some investigators have suggested measuring copeptin as a surrogate for ADH because copeptin is secreted in amounts stoichiometrically equivalent to ADH, and copeptin is stable in plasma. Additionally, copeptin measurement after hypertonic saline infusion has been proposed as an alternative to the water deprivation test to distinguish primary polydipsia from DI, showing better sensitivity and diagnostic accuracy.[242] If copeptin measurement becomes more widely available, use of this provocative test may increase.

The actions of ADH are to conserve free water (via V2 receptors) and stimulate vasoconstriction (via V1a receptors).[243] These effects combine to maintain proper osmolality of the extracellular space (the major action of ADH) and blood pressure through maintenance of circulating blood volume and prevention of dehydration and excessive loss of water.

ADH increases the permeability of renal collecting ducts to water, thereby increasing water reabsorption and concentrating the urine to a higher specific gravity (Fig. 55.9).

An alternative name for ADH is vasopressin (or arginine vasopressin), which emphasizes the vasoconstrictive effects of high concentrations of ADH.[244] These vasoconstrictive effects are manifested when ADH binds to V1a receptors on arterial smooth muscle cells. Note that the major endocrine system regulating blood pressure is the RAAS. However, ADH is believed to play an important role in the maintenance of arterial blood pressure during blood loss. Release of ADH into the pituitary portal system also augments the release of ACTH from the adenohypophysis but does not appear to affect the release of other anterior pituitary hormones.

ADH binding to the V1a receptor stimulates the secretion of vascular endothelial growth factor. The V1a receptor may

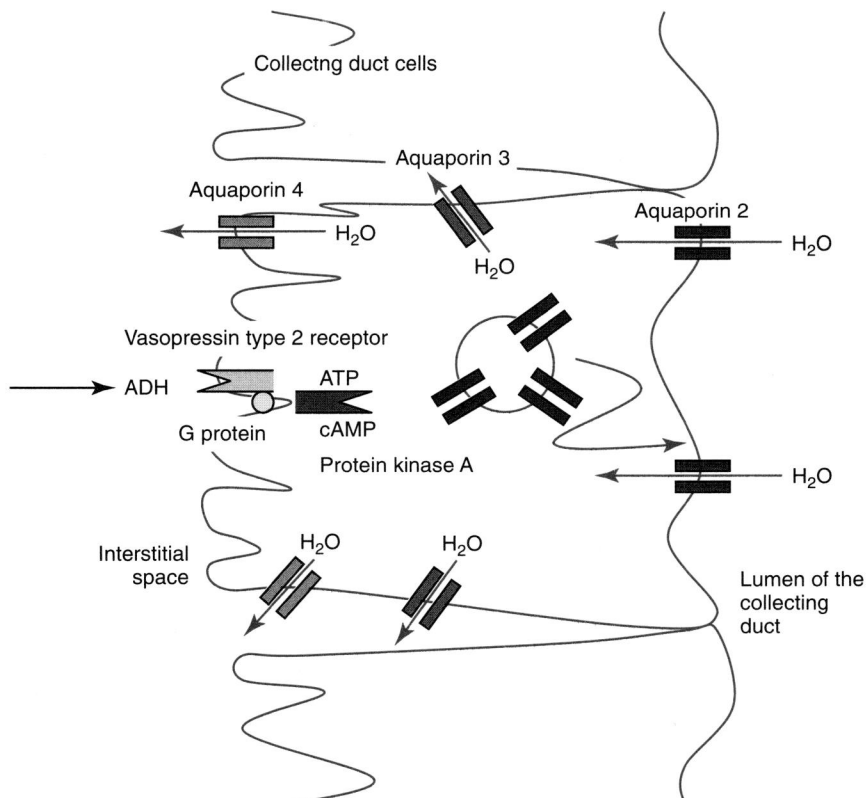

FIGURE 55.9 Vasopressin Type 2 Receptors on Collecting Duct Cells Bind Antidiuretic Hormone *(ADH)*. Via a G-protein system, adenosine triphosphate *(ATP)* is converted to cyclic adenosine 3′,5′-monophosphate (cAMP) via adenylate cyclase with protein kinase A activation. This leads to translocation of aquaporin-2 water channels from an intracellular pool to the apical plasma membrane, allowing free water uptake by cells of the collecting duct. Via the basolateral plasma membrane aquaporin-3 and aquaporin-4 water channels, free water then leaves these cells.

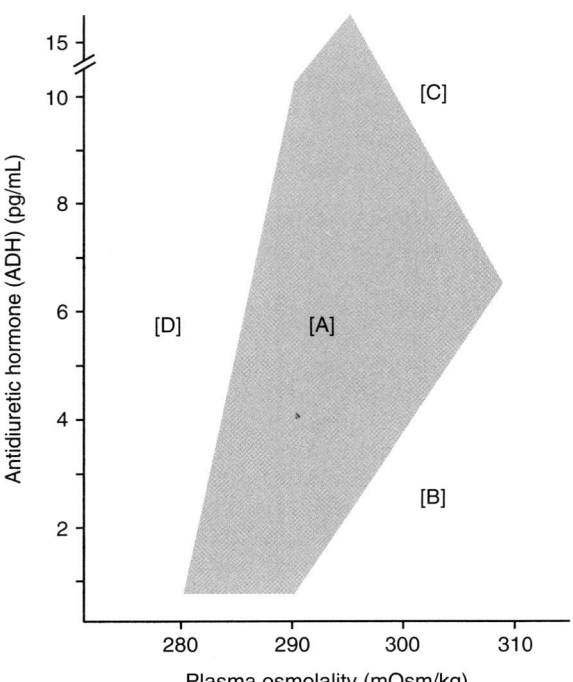

FIGURE 55.10 The Relationship of Plasma Antidiuretic Hormone *(ADH)* to Plasma Osmolality. Region *(A)* is the reference interval and the results observed in subjects with psychogenic polydipsia and excessive water intake. Region *(B)* represents findings in central diabetes insipidus, whereas region *(C)* represents findings in nephrogenic diabetes insipidus. Region *(D)* represents findings in the syndrome of inappropriate ADH *(SIADH)* secretion. (Modified from Zerbe RL, Robertson GL. A comparison of plasma vasopressin measurements with a standard indirect test in the differential diagnosis of polyuria. *N Engl J Med* 1981;305:1539–46.)

also affect platelet aggregation, coagulation factor release, and glycogenolysis by its expression on platelets and hepatocytes.

The V1b receptor (V3 receptor) is expressed in the CNS. In this way, ADH can release ACTH to aid in the response to stress. The V1b receptor also has been reported to be expressed in islet cells, influencing insulin secretion.

Clinical Significance

Disorders of ADH activity have been divided into hypofunction (DI) and hyperfunction (SIADH) (Fig. 55.10).[245,246]

Polyuric states and diabetes insipidus. Polyuric states are divided into two main categories: (1) deficient ADH action, producing DI, and (2) excessive oral water intake (psychogenic polydipsia).[247] Inadequate ADH activity can result from ADH deficiency or ADH resistance. Osmotic diuresis may also produce polyuria and polydipsia. Uncontrolled diabetes mellitus with a high glucose load to the kidney is a common cause of osmotic diuresis.

In DI, polyuria results from excessive loss of water into the urine.[248] Under normal circumstances, urine output is predominantly dependent on fluid intake; thus an arbitrary upper limit for normal urine output cannot be defined. When urine output is greater than 2.5 L/day, investigation is usually indicated. In the absence of ADH, urine output may approach 1 L/h. Increased osmolality normally stimulates thirst.

TABLE 55.8	**Causes of Central Diabetes Insipidus**
Congenital	Midline malformations: septo-optic dysplasia, holoprosencephaly, single central incisor, and cleft lip and/or palate
	Malformation of the pituitary (ectopia or hypogenesis)
	Diabetes insipidus-diabetes mellitus-optic atrophy syndrome (Wolfram syndrome)
	Familial diabetes insipidus (autosomal dominant and recessive forms)
Acquired	Tumors (craniopharyngioma, germinoma, pinealoma, optic glioma, pituitary adenoma, metastatic tumor, leukemia)
	Trauma (e.g., stalk section)
	Infarction (e.g., septic shock, Sheehan syndrome, hypoxic injury)
	Infiltrative disease (sarcoidosis, hypophysitis, histiocytosis)
	Cysts and aneurysms
	Drugs (opiates, alcohol, phenytoin, alpha-adrenergic agents, etc.)
	Infection
	Increased metabolism of ADH (vasopressinase in pregnancy)

ADH, Antidiuretic hormone.

Therefore if a patient with DI has an intact thirst mechanism and free access to water, excessive urinary loss of water should be matched by excessive intake of fluids. Patients will drink excessively according to their thirst. The major laboratory finding in DI is urine of inappropriately low osmolality relative to the serum sodium which is in the upper half of the reference interval with a corresponding high-normal serum osmolality. If water is not available, or the individual with DI is physically impaired or lacks a normal thirst mechanism, plasma osmolality rises, plasma sodium rises (producing hypernatremia), urine osmolality remains low, and polyuria continues. With dehydration, weight loss is acute (because of fluid loss), and blood pressure falls, inducing tachycardia.

Central DI can result from any destructive hypothalamic lesion or infundibular lesion (Table 55.8). DI resulting from such lesions can equally be termed hypothalamic, neurogenic, central, or cranial DI. Central DI is caused by failure of the posterior pituitary gland to secrete appropriate amounts of ADH in response to rising plasma osmolality. Increased fluid intake promoted by thirst mechanisms usually prevents dehydration in DI. When the thirst center is also abnormal, severe dehydration can occur. Destruction of 80% of ADH-secreting neurons is required to produce central DI. Surgical or traumatic injury to the neurohypophysis may cause transient or permanent DI.

The incidence of central DI is approximately 1 in 25,000 people. In 30% of patients, central DI occurs without apparent cause. The remaining cases are associated with (1) neoplastic disease, (2) neurologic surgery, (3) head trauma, (4) ischemic or hypoxic disorder, (5) granulomatous disease, (6) infection, or (7) autoimmune disorder. A hereditary form of the disorder is transmitted as an autosomal recessive or autosomal dominant trait.[249] Inborn errors in the ADH gene cause deficiency of the hormone. Individuals with familial neurohypophyseal diabetes insipidus (FNDI) are typically recognized before the age of 6 years and display worsening polyuria and compensatory polydipsia.[250] While FNDI comes in many forms, of those caused by mutations in the ADH gene, more than 70 mutations have been identified.[251] Although rare, DI can develop during pregnancy as a result of high circulating concentrations of the enzyme cysteine aminopeptidase (vasopressinase), which inactivates ADH.[252] The vasopressinase may be of placental origin.

DI can result from tubular diseases that affect the responsiveness of renal tubules to ADH (nephrogenic DI). In X-linked congenital DI, an inactivating mutation of the V2 receptor is noted.[253] Loss-of-function mutations in aquaporin-2 cause autosomal recessive and autosomal dominant forms of congenital nephrogenic DI.[254] Chronic hypokalemia and hypercalcemia produce a form of nephrogenic DI that results from downregulation of aquaporin-2 expression.[255]

In the broadest sense, any form of tubular injury with impaired water reabsorption, including (1) polycystic kidney disease, (2) medullary cystic kidney, (3) chronic pyelonephritis, (4) acute tubular necrosis, (5) obstructive uropathy, (6) sickle cell nephropathy, and (7) renal amyloidosis can cause nephrogenic DI. A large number of drugs can cause nephrogenic DI, including (1) lithium,[256,257] (2) various antimicrobials (amphotericin B, rifampin, methicillin, demeclocycline, and foscarnet), and (3) several antineoplastic drugs (cisplatin and ifosfamide). In psychogenic polydipsia (primary polydipsia), excessive water intake eventually begins to impair the concentrating ability of the kidney.

Investigation of polyuria. Assuming that diabetes mellitus is excluded, a differential diagnosis of polyuric states can be made using measurements of plasma and urine osmolality and plasma ADH concentrations (if the findings are equivocal).[256,258] A recommended strategy is shown in Box 55.7. A simple screening test for ADH sufficiency is the measurement of the urine specific gravity in the first morning-voided urine sample. The specific gravity should be 1.010 or greater in patients with adequate ADH secretion. Failure to demonstrate an appropriate urine specific gravity and response in a subject with a history of polyuria and polydipsia should trigger assessment of a basic metabolic panel, urinalysis, serum osmolality, and urine osmolality. Hyperglycemia or glycosuria with an elevated urine specific gravity would suggest diabetes mellitus (see Chapter 47).

Urine osmolality less than 300 mOsm/kg (mmol/kg) combined with serum osmolality more than 300 mOsm/kg (mmol/kg) (or with hypernatremia) is diagnostic for DI. If urine osmolality is above 600 mOsm/kg (mmol/kg), and serum osmolality is below 270 mOsm/kg (mmol/kg), DI is unlikely.

If the diagnosis of DI is unclear, a water deprivation test should be performed, although this is rarely needed.[257,259] Before a water deprivation test, uncontrolled diabetes mellitus should be corrected, and thyroid and adrenal function should be normal (or treated if deficient). Water deprivation testing should not be carried out if the subject is dehydrated at baseline or has renal insufficiency. The overnight water deprivation test is usually conducted in a hospital setting because of the immediate concerns of profound hypotension and possible mortality.[258–261]

The water deprivation test is usually begun on the morning after an overnight fast, unless the history describes large volumes of water ingested and urine produced, in which case the test should begin after breakfast. The subject remains fasting throughout the entire test. A heparin lock is inserted intravenously, so that serial blood samples are obtained easily. Baseline laboratory tests include (1) sodium, (2) potassium, (3) chloride, (4) serum carbon dioxide (CO_2), (5) urea (blood urea nitrogen [BUN]), (6) creatinine, (7) glucose, (8) calcium, and (9) serum osmolality. Potassium and calcium are measured to exclude hypokalemia and hypercalcemia as causes of nephrogenic DI (see later).

Measurements of serum or plasma sodium, chloride, CO_2, and urine pH provide an assessment of the patient's renal tubular acid-base function.[260,262] Renal function and hydration status are evaluated with creatinine and urea (BUN) measurements. A urine specimen is obtained for measurement of urine sodium, urine osmolality, and urine specific gravity. Body weight and vital signs at baseline are recorded. Thereafter, each hour, serum and urine tests are repeated with measurement of hourly urine output, body weight, and urine volume. If ADH measurements are requested, they can be performed at the beginning, middle, and completion of the test; however, ADH measurements are not required for making the diagnosis of DI. The test is continued for 8 to 10 hours unless the diagnosis of DI is confirmed before the full time has elapsed.

One approach that reduces laboratory testing is to perform serum and urine measurements every 4 hours until plasma osmolality reaches 280 mOsm/kg (mmol/kg), when the frequency is increased to every 2 hours. When plasma osmolality reaches 290 mOsm/kg (mmol/kg) or serum sodium exceeds 140 mEq/L (mmol/L), or weight loss nears 3%, the tests are performed hourly. During the water deprivation test, if urine osmolality exceeds 600 mOsm/kg (mmol/kg) on two samples 1 hour apart, or a single urine sample exceeds

---

BOX 55.7 Diagnosis of Diabetes Insipidus

Document polyuria (urine volume >2.5 L/day in adults) and exclude glycosuria. If desired, creatinine excretion can be measured as an estimate of the completeness of the urine collection. Substances that influence antidiuretic hormone (ADH) secretion should be avoided (e.g., nicotine, alcohol, caffeine). If plasma osmolality is more than 295 mOsm/kg (millimoles per kilogram), or if the serum sodium concentration is more than 145 mEq/L (millimoles per liter), primary polydipsia is unlikely. If the diagnosis of diabetes insipidus is unclear, proceed with the overnight water deprivation test (see text for a description of this test).

Overnight water deprivation test: if the ratio of urine to plasma osmolality is less than 1.5 at the end of the test, primary polydipsia is unlikely. Measure plasma and urine osmolalities, and plasma ADH concentrations at the end of the test; use these relationships to differentiate normal, nephrogenic, and hypothalamic diabetes insipidus, as well as psychogenic polydipsia. If urine osmolality is more than 400 mOsm/kg (millimoles per kilogram) at the end of the test, give 5 U of aqueous vasopressin subcutaneously (minimum, 1 U/m²). If urine osmolality increases by more than 10%, central diabetes insipidus is probable; if urine osmolality does not increase, nephrogenic diabetes insipidus is highly probable.

1000 mOsm/kg (mmol/kg), DI is effectively ruled out, and the test can be concluded. If urine osmolality is less than 600 mOsm/kg (mmol/kg), and serum osmolality is more than 300 mOsm/kg (mmol/kg), DI is diagnosed, and the test can be concluded. If serum osmolality does not exceed 300 mOsm/kg (mmol/kg), the test should be continued. If mental status changes or hypotension occurs, or weight loss exceeds 3%, the test should be terminated.

If DI is diagnosed during a water deprivation test, aqueous vasopressin is injected subcutaneously (1 U/m^2), or des-amino-d-arginine vasopressin (desmopressin) is given IV/IM (2 μg) or intranasally (20 μg). A decline in urine volume with doubling of urine osmolality over the next 1 to 2 hours identifies the DI as central in origin with the patient being ADH deficient. After exogenous ADH administration, some references define an increase in urine osmolality of 10% or greater over 60 minutes as evidence of ADH deficiency. Failure to respond to exogenous ADH defines nephrogenic DI. Most patients with psychogenic polydipsia have normal urine osmolality after water deprivation, but some fail to produce concentrated urine unless the water deprivation is prolonged. When psychogenic polydipsia is suspected, the patient should be given a minimum of 1 L of normal saline IV to re-establish the renal medullary concentrating gradient, so that the patient can respond appropriately to ADH.

The diagnosis of "partial" DI, in which test results fall between normal and frank DI, is difficult because no clear-cut boundaries are evident between normal and partial DI, or between partial DI and complete DI.[261,263] In some cases, measurement of ADH in plasma or urine may be required to reach the correct diagnosis. After water deprivation, patients with central DI have low or inappropriately normal plasma ADH concentrations relative to high plasma osmolality or low urine osmolality, whereas patients with nephrogenic DI have high plasma concentrations of ADH when plasma osmolality exceeds 300 mOsm/kg (mmol/kg), and urine osmolality is low. Patients with primary polydipsia have normal concentrations of ADH relative to their plasma osmolality. Because ADH concentrations are most discriminatory when plasma osmolality is high, in the past, ADH was measured after hypertonic saline was administered to the patient. However, this saline infusion test is not widely used by clinical endocrinologists, though recently investigated for use in combination with copeptin measurement.[242]

Syndrome of inappropriate antidiuretic hormone secretion. The autonomous, sustained production of ADH in the absence of recognized and appropriate stimuli (such as hyperosmolality) is termed SIADH.[262,264] In this syndrome, plasma ADH concentrations are "inappropriately" elevated relative to decreased plasma osmolality, and relative to normal or increased plasma volume.

SIADH may be the result of one of several factors (Table 55.9), including (1) production of ADH by a malignancy (such as small cell carcinoma of the lung), (2) the presence of acute or chronic disease of the CNS, (3) pulmonary disorders, or as (4) a side effect of certain drug therapies. In addition, as many as 10% of patients who undergo pituitary surgery have transient SIADH (for 2 to 3 days) approximately 8 to 9 days after surgery (typically when the patient is at home) that responds to water restriction and resolves spontaneously. This may represent the release of ADH from the posterior pituitary or hypothalamus after surgical trauma. A rare form of

TABLE 55.9 Causes of the Syndrome of Inappropriate Antidiuretic Hormone

CNS disease	Brain tumor
	Infection (e.g., meningitis, encephalitis, abscess)
	Prolonged seizure
	Psychiatric disease
	Stress (e.g., prolonged nausea)
Non-CNS tumor (e.g., leukemia)	
Pulmonary disease	Hypoxia (e.g., neonatal)
	Infection (e.g., pneumonia, emphysema)
Nonpulmonary infection (e.g. AIDS)	
Drugs	Drugs with CNS effects (anticonvulsants, antiparkinsonian drugs, antipsychotics, antipyretics, antidepressants)
	Angiotensin-converting enzyme inhibitors
	Antineoplastic drugs
	First-generation sulfonylureas

CNS, Central nervous system.

nephrogenic SIADH results from a gain-of-function mutation in the V2 receptor.[254,265,266]

In SIADH, primary excess of ADH, coupled with unrestricted fluid intake, promotes increased reabsorption of water by the kidney. The consequences are decreased urine volume and increased urine osmolality. The increase in intravascular volume causes hemodilution accompanied by dilutional hyponatremia and low plasma osmolality. Physiologically, hypo-osmolality in blood should result in dilute urine, but in SIADH urine osmolality is inappropriately high for the plasma osmolality. It is important to know that although osmoregulation is tightly controlled, volume regulation always takes precedence over osmoregulation when the intravascular volume changes by more than 10% (e.g., as is the case in SIADH due to fluid overload). Via suppression of the renin-angiotensin-aldosterone axis, volume expansion also decreases renal sodium reabsorption; thus the urine sodium concentration is typically 20 to 40 mEq/L (mmol/L) despite dilutional hyponatremia in blood. This hypervolemia-induced urinary sodium excretion, coupled with water loss, explains why patients with SIADH are euvolemic.

SIADH is a common cause of hyponatremia in hospitalized patients.[263,267] However, other disorders can cause dilutional hyponatremia and must be differentiated from SIADH. These conditions include (1) congestive heart failure, (2) renal insufficiency, (3) nephrotic syndrome, (4) liver cirrhosis, and (5) hypothyroidism. The mechanism of hyponatremia in congestive heart failure, and in nephrotic syndrome and liver cirrhosis is partly due to the compensatory secretion of ADH in response to decreased cardiac output and volume depletion.[264,268] These nonosmotic stimuli for ADH release, mediated through high (aortic arch and carotid sinus) and low (left atrial) pressure baroreceptors, increase the secretion of ADH at any plasma osmolality. Excessive administration of hypotonic fluids and treatment with drugs that stimulate ADH (chlorpropamide, vincristine, carbamazepine, nicotine, phenothiazines, and cyclophosphamide) can also cause dilutional hyponatremia. In addition, hyponatremia may occur from renal or extrarenal sodium loss (depletional hyponatremia) as a result of vomiting, diarrhea, excessive sweating, diuretic abuse, salt-losing nephropathy, or mineralocorticoid deficiency. In these latter conditions, plasma urea is generally increased. Hyponatremia is recognized as a marker of disease severity.[265,269] However, selectively increasing the patient's plasma sodium through fluid manipulation will not improve the outcome; it is the underlying disorder that most likely is responsible for the hyponatremia, as well as the poor clinical outcome.

Clinical manifestations of hyponatremia are nonspecific and include nausea, weakness, and apathy in mild cases, and CNS changes such as lethargy, coma, and seizures in more severe cases.[266,270] However, symptoms may be mild to absent in cases where hyponatremia has developed slowly and become chronic. No signs or symptoms are specific for SIADH. History, physical examination, and routine laboratory test results often suggest that hyponatremia is dilutional (decreased urea, hemoglobin, or albumin) or depletional (increased urea, hemoglobin, or albumin).

Measurements of sodium and osmolality in blood and urine, combined with clinical assessment of volume status, usually permit the appropriate differential diagnosis of hyponatremic conditions (Box 55.8). The diagnosis of SIADH is usually one of exclusion and is closely tied to the clinical context, the required laboratory studies discussed previously.[267,271] SIADH is diagnosed when hyponatremia (<135 mEq/L [mmol/L]) and reduced serum osmolality (<270 to 280 mOsm/kg [mmol/kg]) are present, together with an inappropriately concentrated urine (urine osmolality >100 mOsm/kg [mmol/kg]). Maximally dilute urine normally is 50 to 80 mOsm/kg, and this is expected in the setting of hyponatremia and hypo-osmolality. However, in SIADH, despite serum hypo-osmolality, urine osmolality is typically 250 to 1400 mOsm/kg (mmol/kg). It is important to point out that the urine osmolality does not need to exceed the serum osmolality for the diagnosis of SIADH to be made: the urine need only be inappropriately concentrated with respect to the serum. Urine sodium in SIADH is usually 40 to 60 mEq/L (mmol/L) or greater.

Patients with dilutional hyponatremia resulting from excess water intake (psychogenic polydipsia) have hypotonic plasma, an unremarkable urine sodium concentration (<20 mEq/L [mmol/L]), and a dilute urine (urine osmolality less than that of plasma).[268,272] Patients with depletional hyponatremia caused by extrarenal sodium loss have hypotonic plasma, a low urine sodium concentration (usually <10 to 20 mEq/L [mmol/L]), and urine osmolality greater than that of plasma. Patients with depletional hyponatremia caused by impaired renal sodium conservation have similar results, except that their urine sodium concentrations are inappropriately elevated in the setting of volume depletion. Urinary sodium wasting is evident in an elevated fractional excretion of sodium.

Water load testing is not recommended in cases of suspected SIADH because it may cause acute hyponatremia with significant adverse consequences. Acute oral water loading to excess can produce fatal hyponatremia and cerebral edema.[269,273]

Diagnostic Studies

ADH usually is not measured for diagnostic purposes because ADH excess and deficiency are evident in changes in serum and urine osmolality, serum sodium, and urine volume.[274] Less precise measures of fluid balance include clinical evaluation for dehydration, blood pressure (supine and upright), heart rate, and body weight. Hormone concentration is not measured in some endocrine disorders because the consequent metabolic abnormality is more important. The best example is diabetes mellitus. The diagnosis and management of diabetes mellitus center on measurement of glucose (and now glycated hemoglobin) and not on measurement of insulin or C-peptide.

Serum osmolality can be estimated from serum sodium, glucose, and urea (BUN), but is more reliably measured directly by freezing point depression. Vapor pressure osmometry is not as robust an analytical method as freezing point depression (see also Chapter 37). Various formulae are available for estimating serum osmolality; all are based on the fact that sodium represents approximately half of all the ions in serum (each sodium is balanced by an anion, and sodium accounts for almost 95% of all cations); among all nonionic solutes, only glucose and urea have high enough concentrations to substantially affect (alone) osmolality. Hence, osmolality can be estimated by adding together twice the sodium, the glucose, and the urea concentrations (in the United States, glucose and urea (BUN), measured in mg/dL, must be converted to mmol/L by dividing their concentrations by 18 and 2.8, respectively).

Several variations may be seen in the calculation of serum osmolality. The equation

$$\frac{mOsmol}{kg} = \left(2 \times \left[Na^{+}\right]\right) + \frac{\left[Glucose\left(\frac{mg}{dL}\right)\right]}{18} + \frac{\left[Urea\left(\frac{mg}{dL}\right)\right]}{2.8}$$

underestimates the true osmolality by 5 to 10 mOsm/kg (mmol/kg) because of the remaining constituents in serum that do not, individually, have significant concentrations, but when combined, they contribute approximately that amount.

BOX 55.8 Diagnosis of the Syndrome of Inappropriate Antidiuretic Hormone

Document plasma hypo-osmolality (≤275 mOsm/kg [millimoles per kilogram]) and hyponatremia (sodium concentration ≤130 mEq/L [millimoles per liter]). Use the history, physical examination, and appropriate laboratory tests to exclude cardiac, hepatic, renal, thyroid, or adrenal failure, along with the effects of pituitary surgery, diuretic therapy, or medications known to stimulate antidiuretic hormone [ADH] release. (Syndrome of inappropriate ADH [SIADH] cannot be diagnosed unless these factors are corrected.) Measure the urine sodium concentration and osmolality. Urine osmolality greater than plasma osmolality and without correspondingly low urine sodium concentration (usually >40–60 mEq/L [millimoles per liter]) indicates that SIADH is probable (see the text for details). If the cause of SIADH is unclear, consider measuring plasma ADH and plasma renin concentrations. SIADH is characterized by high ADH concentration and low renin concentration. If both plasma ADH and renin concentrations are low, a primary defect in renal water excretion is present.

Some laboratories provide a reference interval that accounts for the difference, whereas others add an average factor (often 8 or 9 mOsm/kg [mmol/kg]) (and use a different reference interval) to make the calculated osmolality a closer estimate of measured osmolality. The equation assumes that the activity coefficient for sodium (Na^+) is 1.0, and this is not really the case—nor is it the case for other osmotically active substances, like ethanol. Regression analysis of sodium versus measured osmolality produces a slope that corresponds to a factor of approximately 1.86, so some calculations of osmolality (particularly automated calculations) use that factor instead of 2, which results in a bias of approximately 5% between the two equations. As discussed in Chapter 37, the following equations are often recommended:

$$\frac{mOsmol}{kg} = \left(1.86 \times \left[Na^+\right]\right) + Glucose\left(\frac{mmol}{L}\right) + Urea\left(\frac{mmol}{L}\right) + 9$$

or

$$\frac{mOsmol}{kg} = \left(1.86 \times \left[Na^+\right]\right) + Glucose\left(\frac{mg}{dL}\right)/18 + Urea\left(\frac{mg}{dL}\right)/2.8 + 9$$

In the absence of proteinuria, hematuria, glycosuria, and other osmotically active substances (such as radiocontrast dyes), urine specific gravity generally reflects urine osmolality.

Measurement of Antidiuretic Hormone

Measurement of ADH typically requires extracting and concentrating the hormone from biological fluids because of its low (pmol/L) concentration and the presence of potentially interfering compounds. ADH can be extracted into acetone, petroleum ether, or ethanol,[275] or it can be chromatographically isolated using octadecyl silica (C-18) columns.[267,276,277] Although nonisotopic (enzyme) immunoassays have been described,[278,279] most laboratories measure ADH by RIA. Most ADH RIA methods are noncompetitive, and separation of bound and free ligand is commonly achieved using second-antibody precipitation techniques.

An ADH method described by Kluge and colleagues[267] extracts the hormone from 0.5 mL of acidified plasma onto a C-18 column preconditioned with methanol and water. After washing with 0.67 mol/L acetic acid, ADH is eluted from the column with 1.0 g/L trifluoroacetic acid in methanol. The extract is dried and reconstituted in 0.25 mL of phosphate buffer containing 2.5 g/L bovine serum albumin, 0.01 mol/L EDTA, and 1 g/L neomycin sulfate. A 100-μL aliquot of reconstituted extract is mixed with 25 μL of polyclonal ADH antisera, and after incubation for 24 hours at 4 °C, 125I-labeled ADH is added, followed by incubation for 16 hours. Antigen–antibody complexes are adsorbed on activated charcoal, and after centrifugation, radioactivity is measured in the pellet. This method had an average coefficient of variation of 3.4% over an analytical range of 0.25 to 5.1 ng/L and a minimum detectable concentration of 0.06 ng/L, determined by 3 SD above the mean result for an ADH-free calibrator. Methods for measuring ADH have been recently reviewed.[280]

Vasopressin (ADH) use is banned by the World Anti-Doping Agency, and liquid chromatography and tandem mass spectrometry has been used to detect vasopressin in urine.

Specimen Collection and Storage

Blood specimens for ADH should be collected into prechilled tubes containing EDTA as an anticoagulant. Most procedures recommend that specimens be delivered to the laboratory on ice and centrifuged at 4 °C within 30 minutes of collection. The plasma is then removed and stored or shipped frozen at −20 °C until analysis is performed. Random urine specimens may be collected without preservatives; alternatively, complete 24-hour urine specimens may be collected in 10 mL of 6 mol/L hydrochloric acid.[281] Significant deterioration of ADH occurs after prolonged storage.

Oxytocin

Oxytocin is a nonapeptide secreted by the magnocellular neurons of the hypothalamus and stored in the neurohypophysis along with ADH. It promotes uterine contractions and milk ejection and contributes to the second stage of labor.[282]

Biochemistry

The structure of oxytocin is similar to that of ADH (see Fig. 55.8), but with a phenylalanine → isoleucine substitution at residue 3, and an arginine → leucine substitution at residue 8.

The gene for oxytocin is located on chromosome 20p13. Prepro-oxytocin is 125 amino acids (12.7 kDa). Similar to the ADH gene, the oxytocin gene encodes two proteins: oxytocin and neurophysin 1. In contrast to prepro-ADH, prepro-oxytocin lacks a sequence analogous to copeptin in ADH. Following the leader sequence of 19 amino acids, the nonapeptide oxytocin is encoded, followed by the 94 amino acid C-terminal propeptide neurophysin 1. The glycine residue at position 28 is amidated. Suspected or definitive disulfide bonds are at amino acids 20 to 25 (within oxytocin), 41 to 85, 44 to 58, 52 to 75, 59 to 65, 92 to 104, and 105 to 110. ADH and oxytocin are highly conserved throughout a variety of species, suggesting that mutations in the genes that encode these proteins are likely to produce serious consequences.

Oxytocin receptors are expressed in the uterine myometrium and myoepithelial cells of the breast. More myometrial receptors are expressed toward the end of pregnancy. The gene for the oxytocin receptor is encoded on chromosome 3p25. Of its 389 amino acids (42.8 kDa), the first 38 amino acids are extracellular, followed by seven transmembrane domains and a 57 amino acid cytoplasmic domain. Three potential sites of glycosylation are known: amino acids 8, 15, and 26. A disulfide bond may be found between amino acids 112 and 187. Oxytocin receptors occur throughout the CNS, and it is thought that these receptors affect behaviors related to stress, socialization, and maternity.

Regulation of Oxytocin Secretion and Physiologic Activity

Oxytocin is present in both males and females, but its physiologic effects are known only for females.[283] Afferent nerve fibers from the uterus and cervix (and possibly the vagina) communicate with the paraventricular (PVN) and supraoptic nuclei (SON) in the hypothalamus; these are the sites of cell bodies that synthesize oxytocin. Near the conclusion of pregnancy, mechanical stimulation of the cervix by the growing fetus stimulates stretch mechanoreceptors that, in turn, promote oxytocin release from the hypothalamus. Next, uterine contractions during labor trigger additional release of oxytocin. The effect of oxytocin is to increase the strength of

TABLE 55.10 Disorders of Overproduction and Underproduction of Pituitary Hormones

Pituitary Hormone	Consequences of Hormone Excess	Consequences of Hormone Deficiency
ACTH	Cushing disease	Cortisol deficiency
TSH	Central hyperthyroidism	Central hypothyroidism
GH	Children: gigantism	Children: short stature
	Adults: acromegaly	Adults: adult GHD
LH, FSH	Alpha-chain overproduction	Hypogonadism
Prolactin	Galactorrhea, hypogonadism	Inadequate lactation or lactation failure in mothers after delivery
ADH	SIADH	DI

ACTH, Adrenocorticotropic hormone; *ADH*, antidiuretic hormone; *FSH*, follicle-stimulating hormone; *GH*, growth hormone; *LH*, luteinizing hormone; *SIADH*, syndrome of inappropriate ADH; *TSH*, thyroid-stimulating hormone.

uterine contractions, providing positive feedback to oxytocin release until the time of delivery of the fetus. For the myometrium to respond to oxytocin, it must be estrogen primed. Thus increasing responsiveness of the myometrium to oxytocin is noted near term. Increased sensitivity to oxytocin in the myometrium may reflect changes in oxytocin receptor number and/or responsiveness. Centrally, estrogens enhance the response of oxytocin to these stimuli. The influence of oxytocin on other parts of the brain has been reported. For example, emotional stress inhibits lactation.

With delivery of the newborn and placenta, declining concentrations of sex steroids allow prolactin to trigger active lactation. The role of oxytocin is to stimulate the smooth muscle cells of the breast to propel the milk toward the nipple. These smooth muscle cells (myoepithelial cells) surround the milk-producing cells. With suckling, afferent fibers that travel to the PVN and SON trigger oxytocin release. Contraction of the myoepithelial cells causes "milk let-down" (milk ejection), and milk can leak from the nipple if suckling is not continued.

In summary, oxytocin stimulates uterine smooth muscle contraction during labor and milk duct constriction during suckling that propels milk toward the nipple. Therefore oxytocin is critical for delivery of the newborn. Likewise, oxytocin is exceedingly important for nourishment and hydration of the newborn and infant.

Clinical disorders involving oxytocin have not been reported. However, oxytocin and its derivatives (pitocin) are used as pharmaceuticals to increase the intensity of uterine contractions during labor (e.g., as treatment for prolonged or failed labor) and to prevent or treat postdelivery uterine hemorrhage.

Measurement of Oxytocin
Immunoassays for measuring oxytocin in plasma or urine have been developed but are mostly of research interest because no clinical indications for measuring oxytocin are known. With most plasma oxytocin assays, a preliminary extraction procedure is required to concentrate the hormone and remove interfering substances.

SUMMARY OF PITUITARY-RELATED DISORDERS

Disorders that result from over- or underproduction of pituitary hormones are tremendously diverse (Table 55.10). Pituitary adenomas may be secretory or nonsecretory.[284]

Corticotropinomas secrete ACTH, somatotropinomas secrete GH, and prolactinomas secrete prolactin. Gonadotropinomas usually do not secrete intact LH and/or FSH but may secrete free α subunits.[285] Pituitary adenomas, whether functional or not, can lead to deficiencies of other pituitary hormones through compression and destruction of the adjacent pituitary cells. These topics are reviewed in depth in many chapters in this textbook. Understanding pituitary function and the various diseases that result from pituitary dysfunction is a fundamental and essential aspect of clinical and laboratory medicine practice.

SELECTED REFERENCES

4. Cooper MS. Disorders of calcium metabolism and parathyroid disease. Best Pract Res Clin Endocrinol Metab 2011;25:975–83.
31. Ascoli P, Cavagnini F. Hypopituitarism. Pituitary 2006;9:335–42.
34. Winter WE, Hardt NS. Laboratory evaluation of short stature in children. In: Winter WE, Sokoll L, Jialal I, editors. Handbook of diagnostic endocrinology. Washington DC: AACC Press; 2008. p. 139–74.
63. Schilbach K, Gar C, Lechner A, et al. Determinants of the growth hormone nadir during oral glucose tolerance test in adults. Eur J Endocrinol 2019;181:55–67.
76. Obara-Moszynska M, Kedzia A, Korman E, et al. Usefulness of growth hormone (GH) stimulation tests and IGF-I concentration measurement in GH deficiency diagnosis. J Pediatr Endocrinol Metab 2008;21:569–79.
85. Rogol AD, Hayden GF. Etiologies and early diagnosis of short stature and growth failure in children and adolescents. J Pediatr 2014;164:S1–14.
95. Mullis PE. Genetics of growth hormone deficiency. Endocrinol Metab Clin North Am 2007;36:17–36.
111. Rosenbloom AL, Connor EL. Hypopituitarism and other disorders of the growth hormone-insulin-like growth factor-I axis. In: Lifshitz F, editor. Pediatric endocrinology. New York: Informa Healthcare; 2007. p. 65–99.
128. Rosenfeld RG, Hwa V. New molecular mechanisms of GH resistance. Eur J Endocrinol 2004;151(Suppl 1):S11–5.
152. Wieringa GE, Sturgeon CM, Trainer PJ. The harmonisation of growth hormone measurements: taking the next steps. Clin Chim Acta 2014;432:68–71.
166. Goffin V, Binart N, Touraine P, et al. Prolactin: the new biology of an old hormone. Annu Rev Physiol 2002;64:47–67.

169. Bernard V, Young J, Chanson P, et al. New insights in prolactin: pathological implications. Nat Rev Endocrinol 2015;11:265–75.

184. Molitch ME. Pituitary tumours: pituitary incidentalomas. Best Pract Res Clin Endocrinol Metab 2009;23:667–75.

191. Wheeler MJ. The measurement of LH, FSH, and prolactin. Methods Mol Biol 2013;1065:105–16.

199. Winter WE, Harris NS. Laboratory approaches to diseases of the adrenal cortex and adrenal medulla. In: Winter WE, Sokoll L, Jialal I, editors. Diagnostic endocrinology. Washington, DC: AACC Press; 2008. p. 75–138.

207. Ciccone NA, Kaiser UB. The biology of gonadotroph regulation. Curr Opin Endocrinol Diabetes Obes 2009;16:321–7.

228. Cemeroglu AP, Kleis L, Postellon DC, et al. Comparison of low-dose and high-dose cosyntropin stimulation testing in children. Pediatr Int 2011;53:175–80.

240. Ball SG. Vasopressin and disorders of water balance: the physiology and pathophysiology of vasopressin. Ann Clin Biochem 2007;44:417–31.

251. Christ-Crain M, Bichet DG, Fenske WK, et al. Diabetes insipidus. Nat Rev Dis Primers 2019;5:54.

270. Douglas I. Hyponatremia: why it matters, how it presents, how we can manage it. Cleve Clin J Med 2006;73(Suppl 3):S4–12.

56

Adrenal Cortex*

Roger L. Bertholf, Mark Cooper, and William E. Winter

ABSTRACT

Background

The adrenal cortex produces three types of steroid hormones: mineralocorticoids, which regulate sodium and water balance; glucocorticoids, which stimulate glucose production and suppress immune function; and adrenal androgens, which influence sexual differentiation. All three types of adrenocortical steroids are synthesized from cholesterol, but regulation of production and secretion of the hormones involves several biosignaling mechanisms, some of which are unique to a particular hormone, and others that affect multiple biosynthetic pathways.

Content

Disorders of adrenocortical hormones can result from mutations causing deficiency in the enzymes that synthesize them, overproduction by hormone-secreting neoplasms, or impaired function due to inadequate tissue response to hormone activity. Laboratory assessment of adrenocortical dysfunction often involves multiple tests that measure responsiveness to the biochemical signals that normally regulate the production and secretion of steroid hormones.

*The full version of this chapter is available electronically on ExpertConsult.com.

57

Thyroid Disorders

Christina Ellervik, David John Halsall, and Birte Nygaard

ABSTRACT

Background

The ability to accurately diagnose thyroid disease using a blood test is arguably one of the greatest triumphs of modern clinical chemistry. Thyroid function tests are now among the most widely requested laboratory investigations. This is because of the relatively high incidence of thyroid disease, the symptoms of the disease often being nonspecific, and effective treatment options for the most common forms of thyroid disease being readily available. Despite the success of diagnostic and therapeutic interventions, both clinical chemists and clinicians need to be aware of the limitations of these strategies.

Content

This chapter describes the physiology of the normal and abnormal thyroid and the role of the thyroid hormones. This includes the importance of iodine in the correct functioning of the thyroid gland and the effect of common medications and nonthyroidal illness on thyroid function. Laboratory methods for thyroid function tests are critically reviewed. The clinical presentation of thyroid disease is described along with treatment options. This chapter includes sections on thyroid disease in pregnancy, subclinical thyroid disease, and the genetic basis of inherited thyroid diseases.

HISTORICAL LANDMARKS

A total of 213,515 publications on the entry word "thyroid" are registered in PubMed (by March of 2020), with the first registered in 1842. Up until 1945, the annual number of publications ranged from 1 to 35. After World War II, the number of publications has steadily increased every year, with 8000 publications in 2019. In Box 57.1, historical landmarks are listed in chronological order.[1-38]

ANATOMY

The thyroid consists of two lobes connected by an isthmus and is like a butterfly in shape with the right lobe being slightly larger than the left.[39] It is located in the front of the neck just above the trachea. The gland synthesizes thyroid hormones and calcitonin through two distinct cell types: the epithelial or follicular cells and the parafollicular (or C) cells, respectively.[40] The gland's name derives from its topographic relationship to the laryngeal thyroid cartilage, whose shape resembles a Greek shield or *thureos*.[39] The normal adult thyroid gland weighs 15 to 25 g, but in specific disease states, it can attain a weight of several hundred grams. The thyroid gland receives its blood supply from the carotid arteries, branches of the common carotid artery, and subclavian arteries.

The thyroid gland is composed of follicles or acini (Fig. 57.1). In the center of the follicle is the lacuna, which contains colloid composed predominantly of thyroglobulin (Tg). The parafollicular (or C) cells are usually located below the basement membrane but not adjacent to the lacuna of the follicle. The parafollicular cells produce the polypeptide hormone *calcitonin*.

Thyroid Morphogenesis and Dysmorphogenesis

Embryologically, the thyroid gland is formed by fusion of three anlagen that develop from the anterior foregut.[40] The primitive thyroid tissue descends to a pretracheal position (fourth to seventh weeks), and differentiates into a hormone-producing gland (the thyroid hormone producing follicular cells) by the end of the third month.[39,41] During its descent, the thyroid is remodeled into a bilobed organ.[40] The understanding of the complex morphogenesis has mainly come from animal models, but in the genetic era, understanding of the genetic basis of thyroid dysgenesis has further elucidated stages of normal human thyroid morphogenesis.[40] The molecular bases for many of the morphogenetic stages are still uncovered. Understanding how the thyroid reaches a position far from its origin will likely provide further detail on thyroid ectopia.[40]

Thyroid dysgenesis is a collective designation for thyroid agenesis (or athyreosis, i.e., the complete lack of thyroid tissue), hypoplasia, hemiagenesis (lacking one lobe), and thyroid ectopia (complete or coexisting with normal positioned tissue, i.e., the aberrant location of thyroid tissue along its embryologic descent).[39,40,42] The developmental defects have considerable phenotypic variations.[40] Ectopic tissue may coexist with a normally positioned gland.[39] It is important to localize ectopic thyroid tissue before thyroidectomy.[39]

Thyroid Hormones in Fetal Growth

Fetuses are dependent on thyroid hormones for normal growth and organ development, especially brain development and maturation.[41,43]

BOX 57.1 Historical Landmarks in Chronological Order

Circa 3600 bc, early Chinese medical writings described decreases in goiter size upon ingestion of seaweed and burnt sea sponge.[1]

Early 13th century, endemic cretinism was noted in alpine Europe.[2]

16th century, Paracelsus, physician and alchemist, was the first to mention coexistence of endemic goiter and cretinism in the Duchy of Salzburg.[3]

1786, Caleb Hillier Parry, a practitioner at Bath, England, was the first person to describe the features of hyperthyroidism (later known as Graves disease).[4]

1811, a French chemist, Bernard Courtois, described the chemical properties of an unknown substance, later known as iodine.[5] Joseph Louis Gay-Lussac, Andre Ampere, and Sir Humphry Davy continued his work but with some controversy on whom to credit for the discovery.[6]

1813, Gay-Lussac published the first paper presenting the new element iodine, termed after the Greek word *ioeides*, meaning violet colored.[6]

1819, Jean-Francois Coindet, a physician in Switzerland, published his observations that administration of iodine decreased goiter size.[7]

1833, the French chemist Boussingault was the first to hypothesize that salt fortification with iodine would prevent goiter.[8,9]

1835, Robert James Graves (Ireland), published a description of exophthalmic goiter.[10]

1840, Adolph von Basedow (Germany), described toxic goiter.[11]

1851, 10 iodine pharmaceutical companies showed iodine compounds publicly for the first time at an exhibition in London.[6]

1852, Adolphe Chatin, a French chemist, published the hypothesis that population iodine deficiency was associated with endemic goiter.[9,12]

1880, Ludwig Rehn (Germany) performed the first thyroidectomy on a patient with Graves disease.[13]

1888, on the basis of the work by Gull,[14] Ord,[15] Kocher,[16,38] and Reverdin,[18] the Clinical Society of London linked cretinism, myxedema, and the "cretinism-like" state after thyroidectomy to the same disease, later known as hypothyroidism.[19]

Furthermore, they also described delusions and hallucinations linked to the disease.

1891, treatment for hypothyroidism with sheep thyroid extract was first described by Murray.[20]

1896, Eugen Baumann reported the discovery of iodine within the thyroid gland.[21]

1909, Theodor Kocher was awarded the Nobel Prize in Physiology and Medicine for his work on the physiology, pathology, and surgery of the thyroid gland.[38]

1912, Hakaru Hashimoto, a Japanese medical doctor, first described Hashimoto thyroiditis.[22,152]

1915, Kendall described the crystallization of a compound, which he called thyroxin.[23]

1922, iodine fortification of table salt began in Switzerland.[9]

1927, Harington and Barger described the synthesis of thyroxin.[24]

1938, Hertz, Evans, and Roberts made the short-lived labeled ^{128}I for the first use of uptake of a labeled substance in animals.[25,26]

1939, Hamilton and Soley described two other labeled radioiodines, ^{130}I and ^{131}I, with longer half-lives, to study iodine physiology in humans.[27]

1943, Astwood described thiouracil to treat hyperthyroidism.[28]

1949, Asher revisited the psychiatric symptoms in myxedema and introduced the terminology "myxedema madness."[29]

1952, Carbimazole was introduced.[28]

1952, Triiodothyronine was discovered by Gross and Pitt-Rivers.[30]

1956, Roitt and colleagues reported the presence of circulating thyroid autoantibodies in Hashimoto thyroiditis.[31]

1963, Condliffe purified thyrotropin (thyroid-stimulating hormone).[32] Later the same year, Condliffe together with Odell and Utiger reported the first immunoassay for human thyrotropin.[33]

1970, Braverman, Ingbar, and Sterling described that endogenous triiodothyronine was generated from thyroxine.[34]

1971, Mayberry[35,36] and Hershman[37] independently described use of thyrotropin immunoassays for diagnosis of hypothyroidism.

1980, The World Health Organization published for the first time the global estimate on the prevalence of iodine deficiency or goiter to affect 20 to 60% of the world's population, mostly in developing countries.[9]

Courtesy Christina Ellervik.

Fetal thyroid hormone availability is dependent on placental permeability to maternal thyroid hormones in the first half of gestation and the bioavailability of the fetus' own production during the second half of gestation. Availability and concentrations of the thyroid hormones depend on development of the fetal hypothalamic–pituitary–thyroid (HPT) axis, the thyroid hormone transporters, the deiodinases, gestational age, nutrition, and other intrauterine endocrine conditions. Maturation of the HPT axis occurs by the middle of the second trimester, enabling the fetus to become responsible for its own production of thyroid hormones by 20 weeks gestation; the axis becomes fully mature and functional around the time of birth. In fetal and in adult life, hypothalamic thyrotropin-releasing hormone (TRH) stimulates thyrotropin (thyroid-stimulating hormone [TSH]), which in turn stimulates thyroid hormone synthesis, and the thyroid hormones control their production by negative feedback on the hypothalamus and pituitary. The synthesis of thyroid

hormones is dependent on active iodine transport across the placenta. By 10 weeks of gestation, fetal thyroid follicles and thyroxine synthesis are demonstrable (Fig. 57.2). Thyroxine-binding globulin (TBG) and thyroxine (T4) are first detectable in fetal serum at 8 to 10 weeks of gestation and increase thereafter until they plateau at 35 to 37 weeks. Deiodinases (see later) are responsible for the in utero conversion of T4 to the bioactive triiodothyronine (T3) or the relatively bioinactive reverse T3 (rT3). During most of the fetal life, T4 is primarily metabolized to rT3, and clearance of T3 is high because of the relative concentrations of different deiodinases in fetus and placenta. Toward term, these ratios change, resulting in a rise in fetal plasma T3, which is important for a range of maturational effects before birth such as pulmonary gas exchange, thermogenesis, hepatic gluconeogenesis, and cardiac adaption.

Within hours of birth, plasma TSH, T4, and T3 concentrations rise rapidly (Fig. 57.3).[44] It is believed that cold stress

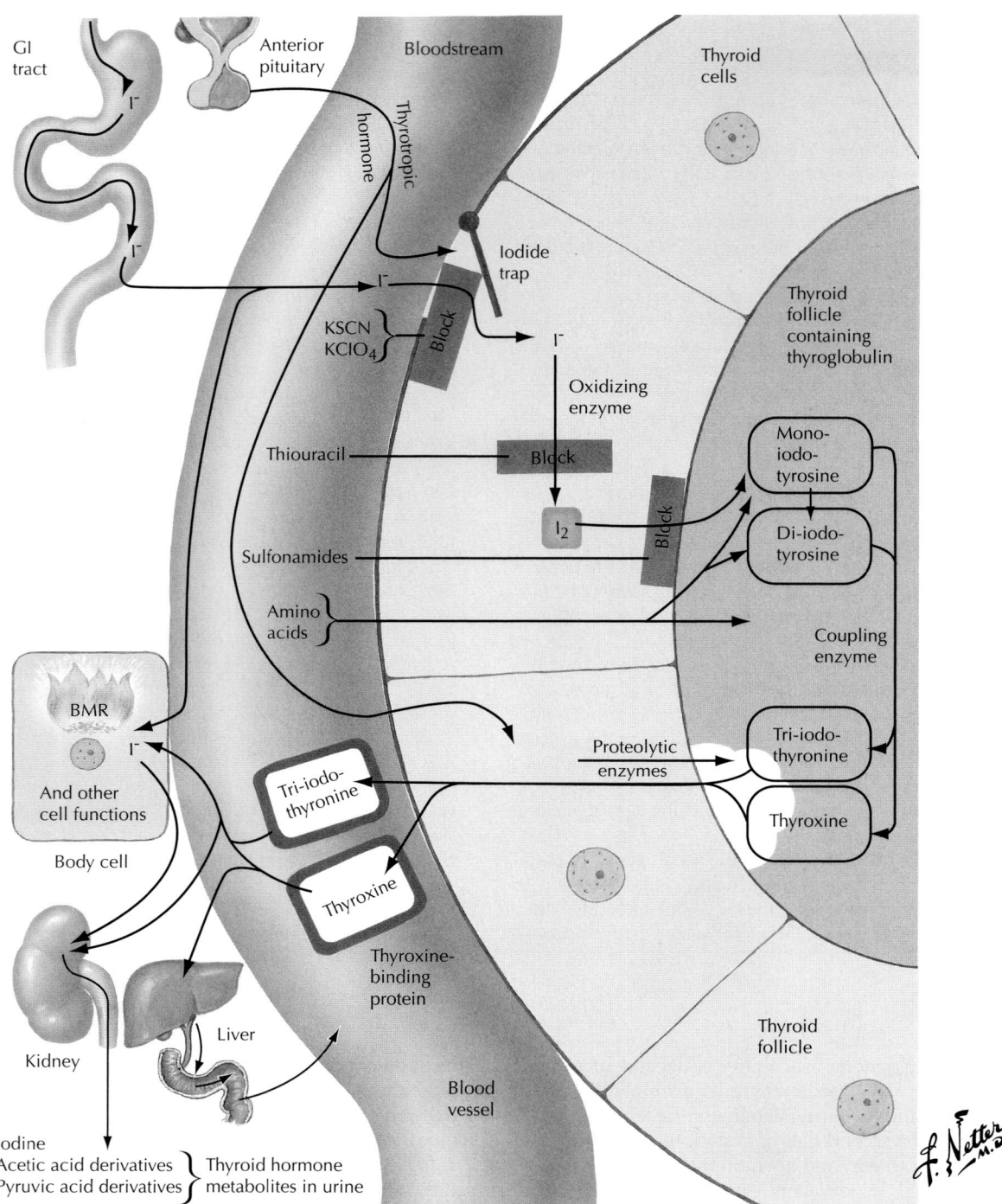

FIGURE 57.1 Physiology of Thyroid Hormones. *DIT,* Diiodotyrosine; *GI,* gastrointestinal; *MIT,* monoidotyrosine; *NIS,* sodium/iodide symporter; *THOX2,* thyroid oxidase 2; *TPO,* thyroid peroxidase; *TSH,* thyroid-stimulating hormone. (From Netter, FH, Young, WF. (2011). The Netter collection of medical illustrations: The endocrine system (2nd ed.). Philadelphia: Saunders.)

is responsible for the massive TSH surge. By 2 to 3 days, TSH concentrations fall. T4 falls to adult concentrations by 1 to 2 months of age.[45] The postbirth rise in T3 results from increased thyroid gland release in response to the rising TSH concentration and also increased conversion of T4 to T3 because of the maturation of type I deiodinase enzyme.

THYROID HORMONES

The thyroid gland secretes two hormones, thyroxine (3,5,3,5′-L-tetraiodothyronine) and triiodothyronine (3,5,3′-L-triiodothyronine), which are commonly known as T4 and T3, respectively, based on the number of iodine atoms in each molecule (Table 57.1; see Fig. 57.1).

Changes in Fetal Thyroid Function During Gestation

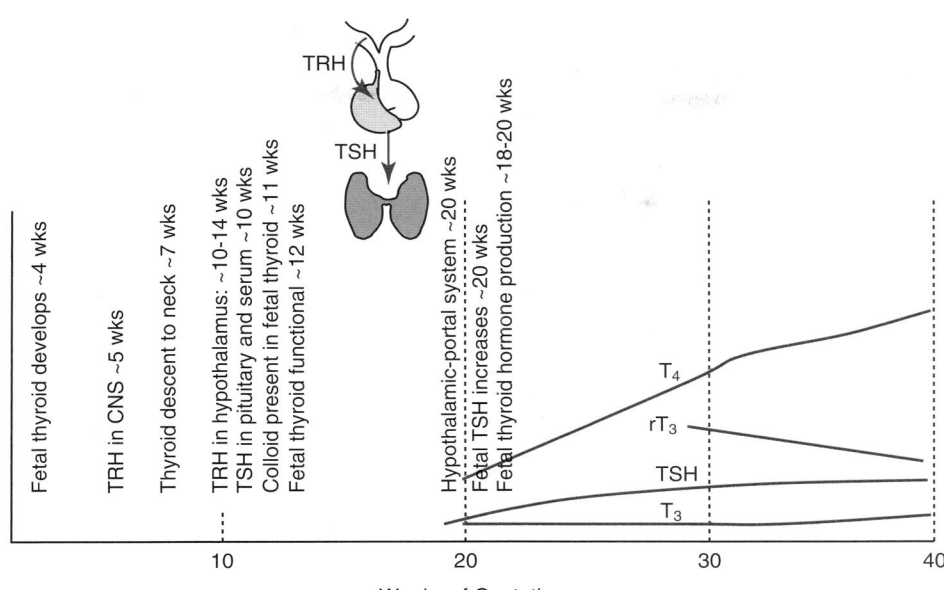

FIGURE 57.2 Changes in fetal thyroid function during gestation. During the first half of gestation, the fetus is dependent on transplacental passage of thyroid hormone. After midgestation, the fetus produces its own thyroid hormone. *CNS,* Central nervous system; *TRH,* thyrotropin-releasing hormone; *TSH,* thyroid-stimulating hormone.

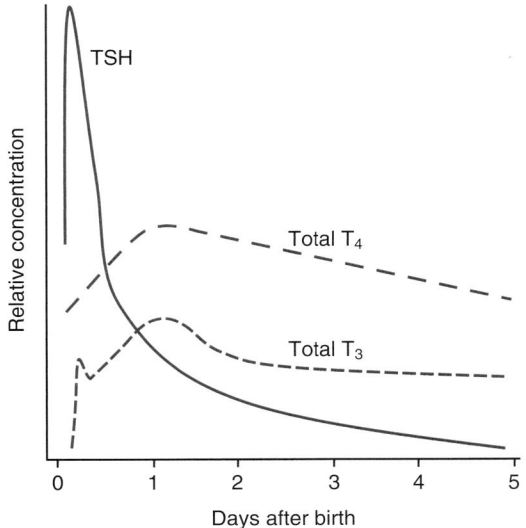

FIGURE 57.3 Concentrations of thyroid hormones for 5 days after birth. After birth, an immediate thyroid-stimulating hormone *(TSH)* surge peaks at about 30 minutes. Triiodothyronine *(T3)* and thyroxine *(T4)* rise rapidly, peaking at about 24 hours after delivery. The greater initial rise in T3 compared with T4 in the first 24 hours of life likely represents acutely increased conversion of T4 to T3. After their peak concentrations, T4 and T3 decline to stable concentrations.

Biological Function

The functions of thyroid hormones include (1) control of the basal metabolic rate and calorigenesis, (2) enhancement of mitochondrial metabolism, (3) stimulation of neural development and normal growth, (4) promotion of sexual maturation, (5) stimulation of adrenergic activity with increased heart rate and myocardial contractility, (6) stimulation of protein synthesis and carbohydrate metabolism, (7) increasing the synthesis and degradation of cholesterol and triglycerides, (8) increasing the requirement for vitamins, (9) increasing calcium and phosphorus metabolism, and (10) enhancing the sensitivity of adrenergic receptors to catecholamines. These effects are typically magnified in patients with either an overactive thyroid gland (such as in hyperthyroidism), or reduced in patients with reduced thyroid function (such as, hypothyroidism).

Physiology

The *hypothalamic-pituitary–thyroid axis* is a classic endocrine negative feedback loop.[46,47] *Thyrotropin-releasing hormone (TRH)*, which is produced in the paraventricular neurons on the hypothalamus, stimulates the release of *thyrotropin* (also called *thyroid stimulating hormone, TSH*), from the anterior pituitary cells known as *thyrotrophs*. TRH is delivered to the anterior pituitary gland via the hypothalamic-pituitary portal system. TSH is the principal regulator of thyroid hormone synthesis and secretion by the thyroid gland. TSH binding to the TSH receptor (TSHR) stimulates the thyroid gland to produce thyroid hormones.

TRH and TSH are inhibited by the negative feedback from thyroid hormones. This effect is mediated by the thyroid hormone receptor THRβ-2, although the effect on TRH in the hypothalamus is minor compared with the suppression of TSH in the pituitary. The negative feedback is such that TRH and TSH concentrations rise in thyroid hormone deficiency and decline when thyroid hormone is in excess.

Synthesis of Thyroid Hormones

Thyroid hormone synthesis occurs within the thyroid follicles. A follicle consists of thyroid follicular cells (thyrocytes) surrounding a lumen with colloid matrix. Dietary iodine is the basic element involved in the synthesis of thyroid hormones. It is normally ingested in the form of iodide. Iodide transport to the follicles is the first and rate limiting step in the synthetic process. The first step in this process is the active

transport of iodide into the follicular cells against an approximate 30-fold concentration gradient. This is performed by the basolateral transmembrane sodium-iodide (Na^+/I^-) symporter, NIS, which uses the sodium gradient generated by the Na^+/K^+-ATPase.[48] NIS is encoded by the *SLC5A5* gene. After active transport into the follicular cells, iodide is passively transported to the follicular lumen by the anion exchange protein pendrin and possibly by as yet unidentified ion channels.[49] Within the follicular lumen, iodide is oxidized to iodine and bound to tyrosine residues in the thyroid specific protein Tg catalyzed by the enzyme thyroid peroxidase (TPO). This reaction is dependent on hydrogen peroxide, which is produced by dual oxidase 2 (DUOX2).

Tg is produced in the follicular cells and secreted into the colloid matrix where it serves as a protein backbone for thyroid hormone synthesis. TPO catalyzes both iodination of tyrosyl residues and the coupling of monoiodotyrosines (MIT) and diiodotyrosines (DIT) to form the T3- and T4-iodothyronine Tg complexes (Figs. 57.4 to 57.6). The nomenclature of iodothyronines is based on the position of iodine on the four possible iodination sites at the meta position on the two tyrosine-derived phenyl rings. The 3 and 5 positions are on the inner or α ring and the 3′ and 5′ positions on the outer or β ring. T3 is 3,5,3-triiodothyronine and T4 is 3,5,3′,5′-tetraiodothyronine.

The follicular cells engulf colloid globules by endocytosis; these globules then merge with lysosomes in the follicular cells. Lysosomal proteases break the peptide bonds between iodinated residues of Tg, and MIT, DIT, T4, and T3 are released into the cytoplasm of the follicular cells. T4 and T3 are then exported to the circulation by the transporter monocarboxylate transporter 8 (MCT8; gene symbol *SLC16A2*). MIT and DIT undergo deiodination by the thyroidal enzyme iodotyrosine deiodinase 1 (DEHAL).[50] The freed iodide is then reused for thyroid hormone synthesis. One hundred percent of T4 is produced in the thyroid, whereas generation of T3 is largely produced outside the thyroid in the euthyroid state.[51] The adult human thyroid secretes on average 100 μg of T4 and 10 to 22 μg of T3 daily.[52]

Circulating Thyroid Hormone Binding Proteins

T4 and T3 are secreted as free hormones but as they are hydrophobic, they are bound reversibly and almost completely to carrier proteins in the circulation. These carrier proteins are (1) TBG, (2) transthyretin (TTR) also known as thyroxine-binding prealbumin, and (3) albumin (Table 57.2). TBG has the highest affinity for T4 and binds 75% of plasma T4. "Total" means bound, and collectively, these proteins bind 99.97% of total T4 and 99.7% of Total T3.[53,54] Thus only a very small fraction of each of these hormones is unbound and free for

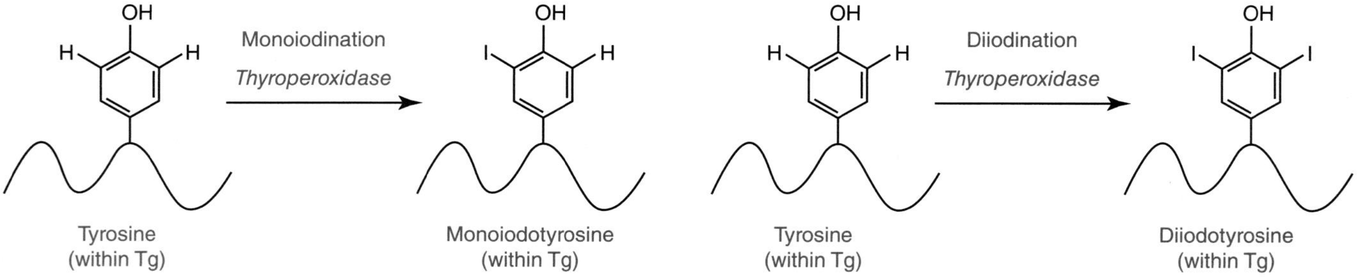

TABLE 57.1	Nomenclature and Abbreviations for Thyroid Tests
Name	**Abbreviation**
Hormones	
Total thyroxine	T4
Total triiodothyronine (3,5,3′-triiodothyronine)	T3
Free thyroxine	fT4
Free triiodothyronine	fT3
Thyrotropin (thyroid-stimulating hormone)	TSH
Reverse T3 (3,3′,5′-triiodothyronine)	rT3
Serum-Binding Proteins	
Thyroxine-binding globulin	TBG
Transthyretin (thyroxine-binding prealbumin)	TTR
Albumin	Alb
Tests for Autoimmune Thyroid Disease	
Autoimmune thyroid disease	AITD
Thyroglobulin autoantibodies	Anti-Tg
Thyroperoxidase autoantibodies	Anti-TPO
TSH receptor autoantibodies	Anti-TSHR
Anti-TSHR binding assay	TRAb
TSHR blocking antibodies	Anti-TSHRB
TSHR stimulating antibodies	Anti-TSHRS
Other Hormones, Thyroid-Related Proteins, and Conditions	
Thyroid peroxidase	TPO
Thyrotropin-releasing hormone	TRH
Thyroglobulin	Tg
Thyroid hormone receptor	THR
Deiodinase 1,2,3	D1, D2, D3
Iodotyrosine dehalogenase 1	DEHAL
Sodium/iodide symporter	NIS
TSH receptor	TSHR
Dual oxidase 1 and 2	DUOX1 and DUOX2
Thyroid hormone receptor-α	THRα
Thyroid hormone receptor-β	THRβ

FIGURE 57.4 Monoiodination and di-iodination of tyrosine.

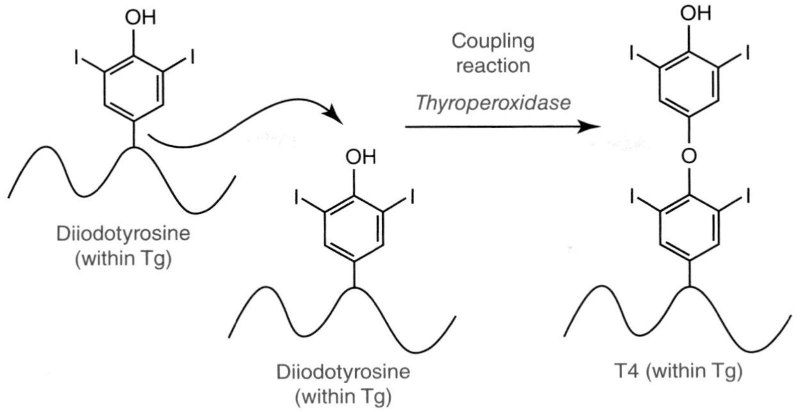

FIGURE 57.5 Chemical coupling of two molecules of diiodotyrosines to produce a molecule of thyroxine (T4). The reaction is catalyzed by thyroperoxidase.

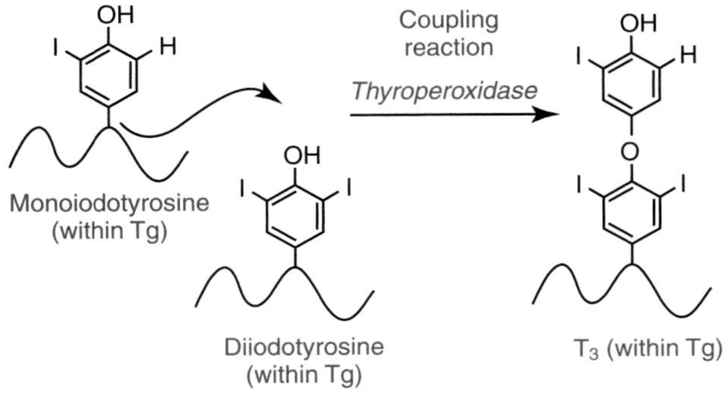

FIGURE 57.6 Chemical coupling of one molecule of monoiodotyrosine and one molecule of di-iodotyrosine to produce one molecule of T3. The reaction is catalyzed by thyroperoxidase.

TABLE 57.2 Thyroid Hormone Transport in Plasma			
Thyroid Binding Protein	**TBG**	**TTR**	**Albumin**
Concentration in plasma (mean normal, mg/L)	16	250	40,000
T4 capacity (μg/dL)	22	120	1000
Distribution			
T4	75%	20%	5%
T3	75%	<5%	20%
Approximate molecular mass (kDa)	54	55	66
Structure	Monomer	Tetramer	Monomer
Number of binding sites for T4 and T3	1	2	Several
Association Constant (M^{-1})			
For T4	1×10^{10}	2×10^{8a}	1.5×10^{6a}
For T3	1×10^{9}	1×10^{6}	2×10^{5}

[a]Value given is for the high affinity binding site only.
T3, Triiodothyronine; *T4,* thyroxine; *TBG,* thyroxine-binding globulin; *TTR,* transthyretin.
Modified from Feldt-Rasmussen U, Rasmussen ÅK. Thyroid hormone transport and actions. In: Krassas GE, Rivkees SA, Kiess W, editors. *Diseases of the thyroid in childhood and adolescence.* Basel: Karger; 2007:80–103.

biological activity. Because a wide variation exists in the concentration of thyroid hormone binding proteins, even under normal circumstances, a wide variation also exists in T4 concentrations among individuals with normal (euthyroid) thyroid function. Total T3 concentrations also vary with alterations in binding proteins, although usually to a lesser degree than T4 concentrations. As thyroid hormone enters target cells unbound, the free fraction of hormone in the plasma best represents the biologic activity of the thyroid hormones, the total amount being largely determined by the concentrations of binding proteins. Changes in concentrations or affinity of binding proteins are dependent on age, genetics, and medication. The functions of the binding proteins include limiting urinary loss of thyroid hormones, buffering fluctuations in thyroid output of hormones so free hormone concentrations are maintained, and acting as a reservoir of thyroid hormone, so the amount of free hormone can be kept constant. Many immunoassays for free thyroid hormones are affected by alterations in binding protein concentrations and return incorrect values, largely because of limitations in assay design rather than to a genuine change in free hormone concentration. Consequently, the clinical chemist needs to be aware that alterations in thyroid-binding protein concentrations are still a cause of abnormal thyroid function test results. Familial dysalbuminemic hyperthyroxinemia (FDH) causes a dramatic rise in total T4 (tT4) and affects many immunoassays for free T4 to varying degrees.[55]

Deiodination of Thyroid Hormones

Activation and inactivation of T4 to T3 and rT3 inside the cells is carried out by three iodothyronine deiodinases (DIO1, DIO2, and DIO3), which have different tissue distributions and physiologic roles (Table 57.3).[56–58] The deiodinases catalyze the removal of iodine atoms at the phenolic ring (activation pathway) or at the tyrosyl ring (inactivation pathway) of T4 and T3.[59] DIO1 catalyzes both phenolic (i.e., outer) and tyrosyl (i.e., inner) ring deiodination and DIO2 catalyzes only phenolic ring deiodination; thus T4 is converted to the active thyroid hormone T3 by two deiodinases, D1 and D2, by outer-ring deiodination (Fig. 57.7).[56,58]

TABLE 57.3   Characteristics of the Deiodinases

	D1	**D2**	**D3**
Source	Liver, kidneys, thyroid	Brain, pituitary, skeletal muscle	Brain, placenta, fetal tissues
Location	Plasma membrane	Endoplasmic reticulum	Plasma membrane
Substrates	rT3 >> T4 > T3	T4 > rT3	T3 > T4
Role	Plasma T3 production, rT3 clearance, clearance of hormone	Local T3 production, T3	T3 degradation, prevents exposure of fetus to T3
Half-life	Several hours	20 min	Several hours
Effect of hypothyroidism	Decrease	Increase	Decrease
Effect of hyperthyroidism	Increase	Decrease	Increase
Inhibition by propylthiouracil	Yes	No	No

D1, D2, D3, Deiodinase 1, 2, and 3, respectively; *rT3,* reverse triiodothyronine; *T3,* triiodothyronine; *T4,* thyroxine.

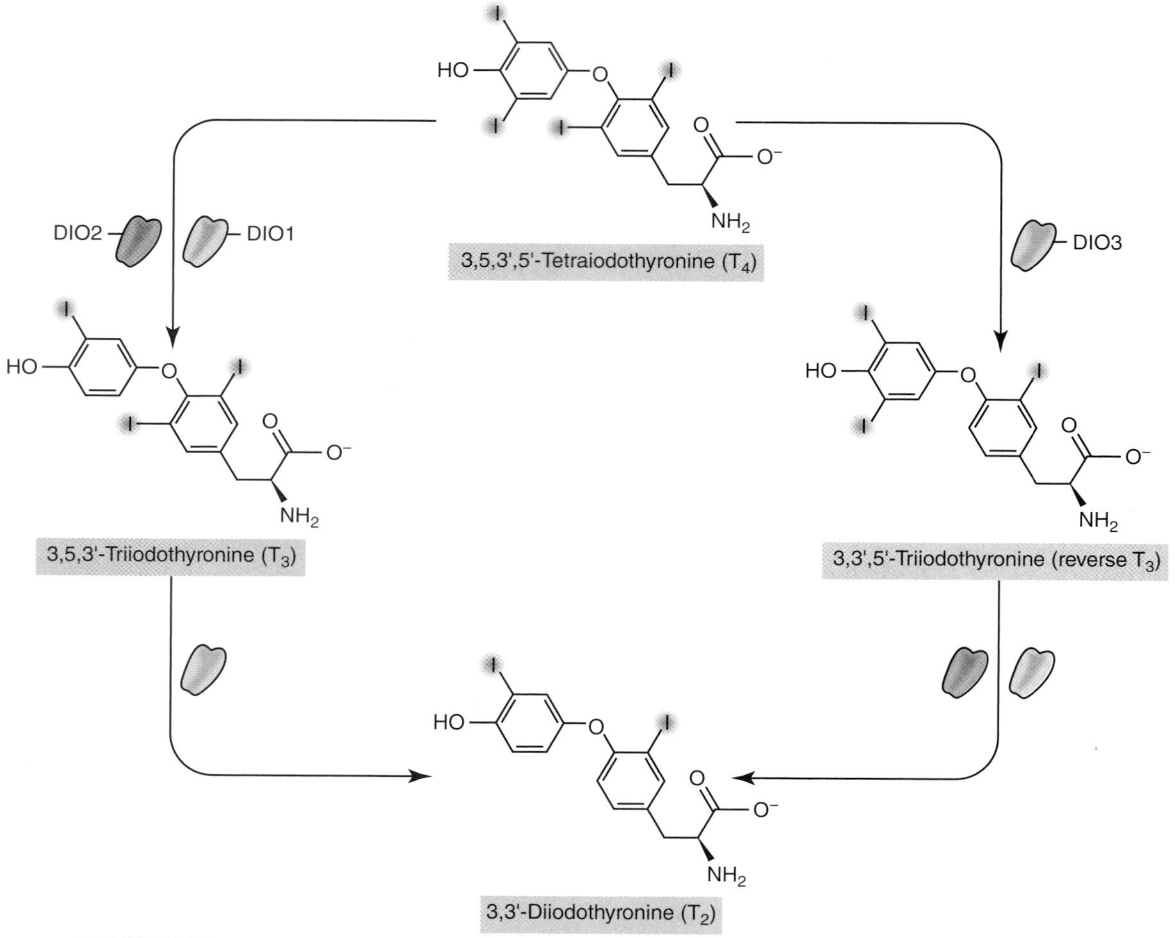

FIGURE 57.7 Chemical structures of thyroxine (T4), triiodothyronine (T3), and reverse T3 and deiodinase thyroid hormone action. (From Luongo C, Dentice M, Salvatore D. Deiodinases and their intricate role in thyroid hormone homeostasis. *Nat Rev Endocrinol.* 2019;15[8]:479–88.)

DIO3 inactivates both T3 and T4 through tyrosyl ring deiodination (Figure 57.7).[59]

Alternate pathways are also involved.[60] Approximately one third of secreted T4 is deiodinated in peripheral tissues by enzyme deiodinases to yield T3, and about 45% is deiodinated to yield rT3, a biologically inactive metabolite. At least 85% of T3 production and essentially all rT3 production is accounted for by peripheral deiodination of T4 rather than by direct secretion from the thyroid gland (see Fig. 57.7).

T3 is at least four to five times more potent in biological systems than T4, which is largely considered to be a prohormone for T3.

The deiodinase enzymes (see Table 57.3) are homologous homodimeric membrane selenoproteins of around 30 kDa.[56–58] The modified amino acid selenocysteine is critical for deiodinase function. Severe selenium deficiency or defects in the incorporation of selenocysteine into the enzymes are a rare cause of abnormal thyroid function tests.[61]

Thyroid Hormone Action

Thyroid hormones are imported into target cells via several described carrier proteins.[62] OATP1C1, MCT8, and MCT10 are likely to be the most important channels because they are most specific for thyroid hormones.[63] OATP1C1 may be involved in the transport of T4 across the blood–brain barrier. MCT8 and MCT10 are widely expressed. In the cell, T4 can be further activated to T3 by iodothyronine deiodinase action.

The molecular mechanisms of thyroid hormone action are both *genomic* and *nongenomic*.[64] Whereas thyroid hormones exert genomic actions via nuclear receptors, the nongenomic actions are exerted on the plasma membrane, in the cytoplasm, or on organelles such as the mitochondria. Genomic and nongenomic actions may overlap, such that hormonal actions outside the nucleus often result in nuclear transcriptional events regulated by intranuclear receptors and other nuclear transcription factors, and nongenomic actions may involve support of trafficking of transcriptional regulators from the cytoplasm to the nucleus.[65]

T3 exerts genomic effects within the nucleus by binding to one of the two nuclear hormone receptors (THRα and THRβ) to control gene expression.[66] Together with retinoid X receptor (RXR), thyroid hormone receptors bind to specific thyroid response elements that are located in the promoter region of thyroid responsive genes.[66] The widely expressed THRα and THRβ are tissue dependent and developmentally regulated.[66,67]

Nongenomic actions are more rapid compared with the genomic actions.[64,68] Nongenomic actions of thyroid hormones T4 and T3 begin at the hormone receptor the heterodimeric integrin αvβ3. T4 has a higher affinity for integrin αvβ3, but T3 has a higher affinity for the nuclear thyroid hormone receptors, THRα and THRβ. Other thyroid hormone metabolites have also been shown to bind the extranuclear thyroid hormone receptors, but the physiologic effect of these has not been fully elucidated.[69] Some tissues, particularly muscle, can respond to thyroid hormones more quickly than can be explained by genomic actions.[70] These effects are transcription independent. They may be coordinated by cytosolic THRs via interaction with the PI3 or cAMP kinase pathways or via alternative receptors such as the recently described plasma membrane integrin αvβ3 T4 receptor.

Thyroid Hormone Inactivation

In target tissues, both T4 and T3 are also inactivated by inner-ring deiodination by D1[56] but also more significantly by a third de-iodinase, D3.[57] T4 is metabolized to 3,3′,5′- triiodothyronine (reverse T3, rT3) and T3 to 3,3′-di-iodothyronine (3,3′-T2). The iodothyronine breakdown products of T3 and T4 may be further decarboxylated to generate thyronamines.[56-58] Iodothyronines, other than T3 and T4, and thyronamines, are called nonclassical thyroid hormones, and are present in plasma at much lower concentrations and have previously been considered inactive breakdown products, but recent research has shown that they may have relevant biologic effects. Thus 3,5 T2 is called a "hot" hormone because it increases thermogenesis, whereas 3T1 is called a "cold" hormone because it decreases thermogenesis.[69,71]

Selective and reciprocal activation or inactivation of T4 by peripheral deiodination is thought to represent a second, extra-pituitary regulation of thyroid hormone status, and explains the finding that while circulating fT3 concentrations are relatively constant, the tissue content of T3 can differ considerably.[72] Deiodination is a rapidly responsive mechanism of control for thyroid hormone balance. Acute or chronic stress or illness causes a shift in the direction of this deiodination, favoring formation of rT3 rather than T3. Various medications also shift deiodination toward the inactive product rT3.

Alternate pathways of thyroid hormone metabolism include conjugation (sulfation and glucuronidation) in the liver and kidney, thereby increasing water solubility (see Fig. 57.1). Glucuronidated thyroid hormones are secreted into the bile and either eliminated in the feces or deconjugated by gut microorganisms and recycled in the enterohepatic circulation. Typically, 20% of T4 produced is excreted in the feces. Sulfated thyroid hormone is deiodinated and eliminated in the urine or feces.[60]

IODINE

Iodine (or iodide [I⁻] in its ionized form) is a trace element and an essential nutrient. Iodine is an indispensable component of the iodothyronines and thyronamines, which are the only iodine-containing hormones in vertebrates. Without iodine, there is no biosynthesis of thyroid hormones. Thus thyroid function requires an adequate supply of iodine to the thyroid gland.

Geography and Iodine Supply

Iodide ions in seawater and coastal seaweed beds are oxidized to elemental iodine, which then volatilizes into the atmosphere and is returned to the soil by rain. This process (the iodine cycle) is slow and incomplete in many regions, thus leaving soils and drinking water iodine depleted. Crops grown in these soils are low in iodine, and animals consuming food grown in these soils become iodine deficient. The common iodine-deficient soils are found in mountainous areas such as the Alps, Andes, and Himalayas and areas of frequent flooding such as the Ganges River plain of northeastern India. Central Asia and Africa, Central and Eastern Europe, and the littoral of the Great Lakes of the United States and Canada are other areas of iodine deficiency.[73]

Various foods contain iodine.[74,75] Foods of marine origin, such as kelp and kombu seaweed, have the highest iodine content. Brown seaweeds contain a particularly high concentration of iodine and have been used as raw material for iodine production since the early 1800s.[76] Other sources include bread, soup, nonorganic milk, and fortified salt. Some vitamin preparations may also be fortified with iodine. The major source of iodine in industrialized countries is iodized salt, and if that is not available, then dairy products.[73] Natural (organic) milk contains very little iodine, but iodine supplements are often given to livestock and increase the iodine content of dairy products.[77] Also, many countries use iodized salt for cooking and seasoning of foods. Potassium iodate (KIO₃) is the recommended form of iodine in salt because it has increased stability in the presence of salt impurities, humidity, and porous packaging compared with potassium iodide (KI).[78,79]

The recommended dietary allowances by the World Health Organization (WHO)[78,79] are shown in Table 57.4. Pregnant and lactating women have higher demands for iodine because of an increase in maternal T4 production to maintain

TABLE 57.4 World Health Organization Recommendations for Iodine Intake by Age or Population Group

Group	Iodine Intake (μg/day)
Children 0–5 years	90
Children 6–12 years	120
Adults > 12 years	150
Pregnant women	250
Lactating women	250

Reproduced with permission from Zimmermann MB, Boelaert K. Iodine-deficiency disorders. *Lancet Diabetes Endocrinol* 2015;3: 286–95.

TABLE 57.5 Iodine Deficiency Disorders by Age Group

Age Groups	Health Consequences of Iodine Deficiency
All ages	Goiter
	Increased susceptibility of the thyroid gland to nuclear radiation
	In severe iodine deficiency, hypothyroidism
Fetus	Abortion
	Stillbirth
	Congenital anomalies
	Perinatal mortality
Neonate	Infant mortality
	Endemic cretinism
Children and adolescents	Impaired mental function
	Delayed physical development
Adults	Impaired mental function
	Reduced work productivity
	Toxic nodular goiter, hyperthyroidism

Reproduced with permission from Zimmerman MB, Boelaert K. Iodine-deficiency disorders. *Lancet Diabetes Endocrinol* 2015;3: 286–95.

maternal euthyroidism and also transfer of thyroid hormone to the fetus early in the first trimester.[80]

Cruciferous vegetables, such as cabbage, kale, cauliflower, and broccoli, contain glucosinolates, and their metabolites compete with iodine for thyroidal uptake.[81] Cassava, linseed, and sweet potato contain cyanogenic glucosides, which can be metabolized to thiocyanates and compete with iodine for thyroidal uptake.

Deficiencies of selenium, iron, or vitamin A exacerbate the effects of iodine deficiency.[82] Pregnant women, who are often iron deficient, and poor maternal iron status can predict both higher TSH and lower T4 concentrations during pregnancy in areas of borderline iron deficiency.[80]

Iodine-Containing Products and Goitrogens

Exposure to iodine can also occur from iodine containing products, such as disinfectants, amiodarone, radiology contrast agents, and topical antiseptics such as the surgical scrub povidone–iodine. The iodine content of these agents is several thousand-fold higher than iodine appearing in naturally occurring foods.[83] Iodine deficiency is the major cause of endemic goiter, but naturally occurring compounds and environmental pollutants may also be goitrogenic.[84,85] Goitrogens can be either agents acting directly on the thyroid gland or cause a goiter by indirect action. Interestingly, cigarette smoking is associated with high plasma concentrations of thiocyanate, which can compete with iodine for uptake into the thyroid.

Public Health Programs

There are two kinds of public health programs for securing optimal thyroid function. One is newborn screening for thyroid function (see section on congenital hypothyroidism); the other is iodization of salt.

It is estimated that 2 billion people worldwide have insufficient iodine intake.[86] In regions that are affected by iodine deficiency, the most effective way to control this is through salt iodization. In the 1910s and 1920s, studies by Swiss and American physicians demonstrated the efficacy of iodine prophylaxis in the prevention of goiter and cretinism. The Swiss surgeon Hans Eggenberger was the first person to promote a general public health measure by using salt iodization because it is effective, inexpensive, and safe.[87]

During the period from 1970 to 1990, controlled studies in iodine-deficient regions showed that iodine supplementation eliminated new cases of hypothyroidism, reduced infant

mortality rates, and improved cognitive function in the rest of the population. The new term *iodine-deficiency disorders* (IDDs) has gained recognition as a spectrum of related disorders affecting billions of people[79,88] (Table 57.5). Since 1990, elimination of the IDDs has been an important part of many national nutrition strategies. The WHO and the United Nations Children's Fund (UNICEF) are working closely with the International Council for Control of Iodine Deficiency Disorders (ICCIDD) and the salt industry.

The WHO, UNICEF, and ICCIDD recommend that iodine status of populations should be assessed by median urinary iodine concentration (UIC); however, they have also recently recognized increased Tg as a sensitive marker of iodine deficiency, at least in children.[89] Surveys of iodine intake have been performed in 152 countries, representing 98% of the world's population. People of 74% of the countries have sufficient iodine intake, 19% have insufficient intakes, and 7% have excessive intake.[79] However, only a few countries have done national UIC surveys in pregnant women to detect iodine deficiency.[90] Iodine deficiency is not only a problem in developing countries but also a problem in transitioning countries (e.g., Russia) and high-income countries (e.g., Denmark). Data from 128 member states in UNICEF have shown that overall, 70% of all households worldwide have access to adequately iodized salt[91,92]; about 30% of the member states have attained universal salt iodization, with at least 90% of households consuming adequately iodized salt; about 40% of the member states have coverage in 50 to 89% of households; and about 30% of the countries still have coverage in fewer than 50% of households. However, in Australia, the United Kingdom, and the United States, iodine intakes are falling. The current global push to reduce salt consumption to prevent chronic disease and the policy of salt iodization to control iodine deficiency do not necessarily conflict. Iodization methods can fortify salt to provide adequate iodine even if the intake of salt is reduced, providing that all salt produced is iodized.[93]

In systematic reviews, iodine supplementation has been shown to improve maternal thyroid indices and cognitive function in school-age children.[94] Global meta-analyses investigating the effects of salt iodization particularly are lacking on thyroid and iodine-deficiency endpoints,[95] but median UICs have improved.[96] Universal salt iodization reduced the prevalence of goiter in a period after the intervention, but the fact that the prevalence of goiter and toxic nodular goiter had increased recently suggests that both insufficient and excess iodine may be associated with goiter.[97]

Iodine Biochemistry

Dietary iodine controls its own absorption through post-transcriptional regulation of the intestinal Na^+/I^- symporter (NIS).[98] The thyroid gland has autoregulatory mechanisms to handle excess iodine intake involving the sodium iodide symporter.[48] Excess iodine has an inhibitory effect on thyroxine synthesis in intact thyroids.[99] In conditions of adequate dietary iodine supply, the healthy thyroid usually takes up less than 20% of absorbed iodine. However, in chronic iodine deficiency, this fraction can be more than 80%. The thyroid is thus able to adapt to low intakes of dietary iodine by marked modification of its activity. In most adults, if iodine intake falls below 100 μg/day, TSH secretion is increased. Iodine in plasma has a half-life of approximately 10 hours, but this can be less in iodine deficiency or hyperthyroidism. A healthy adult has up to 20 mg of iodine of which up to 80% is in the thyroid. The metabolism of circulating thyroid hormones in peripheral tissues releases iodine that enters the plasma iodine pool, which in turn can be taken up by the thyroid or excreted by the kidney. Approximately 90% of ingested iodine is excreted in the urine and approximately 10% in feces.[100]

Iodine Deficiency

Both deficient and excessive intakes of iodine can impair thyroid function.[79] The clinical presentations of iodine deficiency are largely age dependent (see Table 57.5).[79,101] In fetuses, deficiency may cause abortion, stillbirth, and congenital anomalies, and in neonates, deficiency may cause infant mortality and endemic cretinism. Deficiency may cause impaired mental function, and in children and adolescents also delayed physical development and low IQ. In severe, chronic iodine deficiency, iodine concentrations are too low to produce thyroid hormones, and overt hypothyroidism develops with increased TSH and decreased T4 and T3. Most affected individuals develop goiter.[79,102] Correction of iodine deficiency in adult populations, irrespective of severity, reduces thyroid size and the prevalence of diffuse goiter at all ages.[79]

Iodine Excess

Thyroid dysfunction may occur in vulnerable patients if exposed to excess iodine. These patients include those with preexisting thyroid disease, older adults, pregnant and lactating women, fetuses, and neonates.[83] Because iodine is present in medications, supplements, and iodinated contrast agents in much higher concentrations than are found in naturally occurring foods, iodine excess can result in adverse thyroidal effects after only a single exposure to these substances. Excess dietary iodine intake in pregnant and lactating women in iodine-replete areas may lead to an increase in plasma TSH concentrations and thus to subclinical hypothyroidism (SCH).[103,104]

EXTRATHYROIDAL FACTORS THAT AFFECT THYROID FUNCTION

Epidemiologic Factors

Concentrations of thyrotropin, thyroid hormones, thyroid antibodies, and thyroid-binding proteins are to varying degrees determined genetically[105–107] and by epidemiologic factors such as age,[45,108–114] gender,[108,109,111] ethnicity,[45,108–111] body mass index,[113] smoking,[115] pregnancy,[116] nutritional iodine,[79] season,[117] nonthyroidal disease,[118] radiation,[119] circadian rhythm,[120] and medication.[121] Despite these variations, reference intervals are mostly just stratified by age, gender, and pregnancy. The effect of age or gender is modest[122] on TSH concentrations apart from at the extremes of age. The TSH surge during the neonatal period is well described. TSH concentrations can reach in excess of 80 mIU/L but typically drop to below 20 U/L in the first day of life, falling into the adult reference limits during the first month. The effect of old age on the TSH reference interval is a topic of active debate because these ranges are used to define the prevalence of hypo- and hyperthyroidism in this group. Current consensus is that the TSH reference limits increase with age and that the use of age-specific reference intervals is appropriate.[123] TSH has a circadian rhythm with peak levels at around midnight and nadir in the morning through noon.[120] Sleep deprivation causes a rise in TSH. The circadian rhythm of TSH is lost during illness.

Drugs

Many drugs, other than those used for treatment of thyroid disorders, interfere with thyroid hormone homeostasis (Table 57.6) through actions on thyroid hormone synthesis, secretion, transport, metabolism, and absorption.[121,124,125]

Thyroid hormone homeostasis may be affected at different levels. In the gut, drugs may cause reduced thyroid hormone absorption. In the thyroid, the synthesis or secretion of thyroid hormones may be altered, leading to changes in the plasma concentrations of thyroid hormones. Drugs may also influence the binding of thyroid hormones by competing for hormone-binding sites. Some drugs may modify cellular uptake and metabolism of thyroid hormones or interfere with hormone action at the target tissue level. Some drugs may interfere simultaneously through many actions.

Drugs That May Affect Plasma Thyroid-stimulating Hormone Concentration

At the pituitary or hypothalamic level, drugs may affect TSH secretion.[125] Dopamine and dopamine agonists, such as

TABLE 57.6 Effects of Some Drugs on Thyroid Function

Cause	Drug	Effect
Inhibit TSH secretion	Dopamine L-dopa Glucocorticoids Somatostatin	↓T4; ↓T3; ↓TSH
Inhibit thyroid hormone synthesis or release	Iodine Lithium	↓T4; ↓T3; ↑TSH
Inhibit conversion of T4 to T3	Amiodarone Glucocorticoids Propranolol Propylthiouracil Radiographic contrast agents	↓T3; ↑rT3; ↓, ⇋, ↑T4 and FT4; ⇋, ↑TSH
Inhibit binding of T4/T3 to serum proteins	Salicylates Phenytoin Carbamazepine Furosemide NSAIDs Heparin (in vitro effect)	↓T4; ↓T3; ⇋, ↑FT4; ⇋TSH
Stimulate metabolism of iodothyronines	Phenobarbital Phenytoin Carbamazepine Rifampicin	↓T4; ↓FT4; ⇋TSH
Inhibit absorption of ingested T4	Aluminum hydroxide Ferrous sulfate Cholestyramine Colestipol Iron sucralfate Soybean preparations Kayexalate	↓T4; ↓FT4; ↑TSH
Increase in concentration of T4-binding proteins	Estrogen Clofibrate Opiates (heroin, methadone) 5-Fluorouracil Perphenazine	↑T4; ↑T3; ⇋FT4; ⇋TSH
Decrease in concentration of T4-binding proteins	Androgens Glucocorticoids	↓T4; ↓T3; =FT4; ⇋TSH

↓, Reduced serum concentration; ↑, increased serum concentration; ⇋ no change; *FT4*, free thyroxine; *NSAID*, nonsteroidal anti-inflammatory drug; *rT3*, reverse triiodothyronine; *T3*, triiodothyronine; *T4*, thyroxine.
Data obtained from Smallridge RD. Thyroid function tests. In: Becker KL, editor. *Principles and practice of endocrinology and metabolism.* 7th ed. Philadelphia: JB Lippincott; 1995:299–306.

bromocriptine and cabergoline used in patients with hyperprolactinemia, may suppress TSH through action on the dopamine D2 receptor. Somatostatin and its analogues may inhibit TSH secretion; these agents can be used clinically in patients with TSH-secreting pituitary adenomas. Other drugs that can suppress TSH secretion include glucocorticoids, metformin, and antiepileptics such as carbamazepine, valproic acid, and phenytoin.[126]

Drugs Affecting the Synthesis and Secretion of Thyroid Hormones

Lithium. Lithium, which is still a widely used drug for the treatment of bipolar disorder, is associated with subclinical and overt hypothyroidism in up to 34 and 15% of patients, respectively.[121,124,127] These may develop even after many years of treatment. Patients should have regular thyroid function tests, at least once or twice per annum. Lithium primarily inhibits thyroid hormone secretion, although it appears also to have effects on iodine trapping, release, and coupling.

Drugs Influencing the Metabolism of Thyroid Hormones

The cytochrome p450 complex consists of more than 100 isoenzymes. Some of these enzymes (CYP3A) can be induced by antiepileptic agents such as phenytoin, phenobarbital, and carbamazepine and the antituberculosis drug rifampicin.[124–126] Plasma thyroid hormone concentrations can decrease markedly in patients taking these drugs. The effect on TSH are, however, minor. Phenytoin has been shown to displace T4 and T3 from the binding site on TBG in vivo. Although this effect is compensated for in vivo by a reduction in tT4, it is compounded by a possible in vitro effect on fT4 immunoassays because this displacement effect can be reversed if the serum is diluted during analysis.[128] As the metabolic clearance rate and hepatic metabolism of T4 increases in patients taking phenytoin, it is likely that in normal subjects, thyroid secretion increases to compensate for the increased metabolism; hypothyroid subjects taking phenytoin need increased doses of levothyroxine.[129]

Rifampicin acts on intracellular thyroid hormone metabolism.[130–132] T4 kinetic data show that rifampicin increases the plasma clearance rate of T4; it has little effect on T3 metabolism. Thus drugs that enhance the activity of the hepatic p450 enzyme system result in a decrease in plasma tT4 concentrations because of an acceleration of hepatic metabolism of T4. As a result, the plasma half-life of T4 decreases, and its metabolic clearance rate increases. Euthyroid subjects have a slight increase in T4 production; thus T3 concentrations do not change, and plasma TSH may increase slightly but not significantly. Importantly, patients on levothyroxine replacement therapy started on treatment with any of these drugs are likely to require an increase in their dosage.

A number of environmental pollutants, such as organochlorine, pesticides, dioxins, and furans, can induce hepatic uridine diphosphonate glucuronyl transferase (UDPGT), resulting in a lower plasma T4 concentration.[133]

Drugs Inhibiting Monodeiodination of Thyroxine

Deiodinase type 1 is inhibited by several drugs, including propylthiouracil (PTU).[56] Dexamethasone and propranolol can also inhibit this enzyme.[134]

The β-receptor antagonist propranolol is used in the treatment of thyrotoxicosis to alleviate the manifestations of increased sympathetic activity, such as tremor. It is particularly useful in the treatment of thyrotoxic crisis. It can induce a modest reduction in plasma fT3 concentration and a small increase in rT3 concentration owing to the inhibition of hepatic monodeiodination, but the clinical benefit far exceeds what might be expected from the modest reduction in plasma T3 concentrations. This effect is unique to propranolol and is not shared with other β-receptor antagonists or mixed β- and α-receptor antagonists such as labetalol.[135]

Drugs Affecting the Transport and Action of Thyroid Hormones

Many drugs inhibit the binding of T4 and T3 to the binding sites on the plasma transport proteins in vitro. These effects often require high concentrations of such drugs.

Nonsteroidal anti-inflammatory drugs, including salicylate, inhibit T4 and T3 binding to both TBG and TTR.[136] Other nonsteroidals, such as fenclofenac, can displace T4 from its binding site.[137] Enoxaparin and heparin can displace T4 from its serum binding proteins and increase fT4 concentration. This has been shown to be an in vitro effect caused by nonesterified fatty acid production by lipoprotein lipase released in vivo by heparin. Consequently, this effect is exacerbated by delays in analysis.[138]

Drugs Acting at More Than One Site

Some drugs interfere with the thyroid hormone homeostasis at various sites.

Amiodarone. Amiodarone is a class III antiarrhythmic drug that comprises 37% iodine by weight and has structural similarities with thyroid hormones. The drug has a long half-life, large distribution volume, and wide tissue distribution.[121,139] The mechanisms of amiodarone injury are multifactorial and involve accumulation of iodine, formation of free radicals, and immunologic injury. The effects of amiodarone can be divided into effects occurring in everyone treated with amiodarone, resulting in changes in thyroid function tests ("obligatory effects"), and effects only occurring in some people treated with amiodarone ("facultative effects"), resulting in clinically overt thyrotoxicosis or hypothyroidism.

During metabolism of amiodarone, large amounts of iodine are released into the plasma, but renal iodine clearance does not change, resulting in urinary iodine excretion 100 times higher than for the recommended daily iodine intake.[121,139] The iodine excess causes the thyroid to initially inhibit iodine organification (the Wolff-Chaikoff effect), thereby decreasing T4 and T3 production with a resulting TSH increase.[121,139] This effect can be interpreted as an autoregulatory response of the thyroid gland to avoid excessive production of thyroid hormone when exposed to high doses of exogenous iodine. Later, the thyroid escapes the Wolff-Chaikoff effect, resulting in TSH returning to baseline values after 3 months. Amiodarone inhibits type 1 deiodinase, resulting in decreased T3 production and increased rT3, and inhibits T4 transport into the liver, resulting in decreased T4 metabolism and consequently increased plasma T4. The changes in T3 and T4 are observed early during the amiodarone treatment and are sustained during the treatment; therefore specific reference intervals should be used. In clinical practice, patients who are on long-term amiodarone should have TSH and thyroid antibodies measured at the beginning of therapy and fT4 and TSH at 6-month intervals. It may take several months for normalization of thyroid function tests after discontinuation of amiodarone treatment.[121,139]

Amiodarone-induced thyrotoxicosis (AIT) is particularly prevalent (10%) in iodine-deficient regions, in men, and in patients with underlying thyroid disease (e.g., nodular goiter or Graves disease). AIT may occur at any time during treatment. There are two types of AIT: type 1 is similar to classic iodine-induced excess of hormone synthesis in patients with preexisting thyroid abnormalities; type 2 resembles a subacute destructive thyroiditis with excess hormone release in patients with no previous thyroid disease, possibly owing to a direct cytotoxic effect of amiodarone. Color-flow Doppler sonography may be able to distinguish between the two types. High-dose thionamides should be initiated in type 1 AIT. Corticosteroids are effective in type 2 AIT.[121,139]

Amiodarone-induced hypothyroidism occurs primarily in iodine-sufficient regions and in women with preexisting anti-TPO antibodies.[121,139] Amiodarone-induced hypothyroidism develops early after starting treatment. It is thought this may be due to a direct inhibitory effect of the excess iodine supply leading to defective organification and subsequent hormone synthesis. If the patient has underlying disease (e.g., Hashimoto thyroiditis, Graves disease), escape from the Wolff-Chaikoff effect is less likely, and permanent hypothyroidism can develop. In addition, amiodarone and its main metabolite desethylamiodarone are weak antagonists of thyroid hormone actions. Treatment of amiodarone-induced hypothyroidism is often challenging because the drug has a long and varying half-life because of mobilization of the drug from lipophilic stores. The terminal half-life after cessation of therapy is approximately 40 ± 10 days for amiodarone and 57 ± 27 days for the main metabolite, desethylamiodarone. Patients should be managed jointly by a cardiologist and an endocrinologist. In patients with amiodarone-induced hypothyroidism, there is no need to stop the amiodarone, but the patient should be prescribed levothyroxine.[121,139]

Dexamethasone. Dexamethasone has multiple effects on the thyroid: It can suppress TSH secretion, reduce plasma T3 concentration, and increase rT3 production.[121,140] In Graves disease, it can reduce T4 secretion, either by a direct thyroidal effect or by increasing thyroid-stimulating immunoglobulin production. It can also markedly decrease plasma T3 concentrations.

Cytokines can alter thyroid hormone secretion and metabolism. Administration of interferons and interleukins may cause drug-induced thyroiditis.[121,141]

Tyrosine kinase inhibitors are promising new agents used in advanced papillary and medullary thyroid cancer (MTC) when there is resistance to conventional chemotherapy.[142] In addition to the effect on cancer growth, they also influence the thyroid gland, and patients treated with levothyroxine may need to increase their dosage. The potential mechanisms seem to be either impairment of enteral absorption, reduction of enterohepatic reabsorption, or increased deiodination and clearance of thyroxine.

Nonthyroidal Illness

Abnormal thyroid function test results are common in patients with both acute and chronic illness and in starvation.[118,143] They are features of a wider neuroendocrine response to illness and stress. The biochemical pattern is typically a low plasma fT3 concentration with raised rT3, so this condition is also known as the low fT3 syndrome. However, with more severe or longstanding illness, plasma fT4 can also be low with TSH concentrations that can be inappropriately normal or low, but generally are not reduced to the extent seen in hyperthyroidism. Whether fT4 is genuinely low in nonthyroidal illness (NTI) or is a consequence of assay interference caused by compounds released during illness that can affect the binding of T4 to its binding proteins remains controversial. Total T4 is typically low, but reduction in T4 binding protein concentrations and the possible cleavage of TBG by inflammatory proteases is a dominant contributor to this effect.

Reduced activity of hepatic D1 deiodinase is a major contributory factor to the low plasma fT3 concentration seen in NTI.[118,143] Hepatic D1 expression is regulated by cytokines and possibly leptin, which may contribute to the starvation response.

The changes in TSH and possible changes in fT4 are evidence of diminished hypothalamic function, which is well described in severe illness.[118,143] This is also likely to be mediated by cytokine effects, although the nature of these effects is currently poorly defined; a reduction in TRH secretion is a likely mechanism.

Whether the NTI syndrome confers any evolutionary benefit remains a topic of debate. This is more likely to be the case in acute illness or starvation, in which a reduction of energy expenditure may be beneficial but less plausible for the chronically ill patient and unlikely in critically ill patients. The magnitude of the change in thyroid function in NTI has prognostic value.[144] However, the use of thyroid hormone replacement in severely ill patients with NTI remains controversial.[118]

THYROID DISEASE

Autoimmune Thyroid Disease

Autoimmune thyroid disease (AITD) comprises two main diseases, Hashimoto thyroiditis and Graves disease.[145] The prevalence is estimated to be 5%, but the prevalence of thyroid antibodies in the general population is 10 to 20%.[146,147] AITD is a T cell–mediated disorder leading to an immune attack of the thyroid in an individual with genetic susceptibility accompanied by environmental factors.[145] Examples of factors that increase the risk of AITD include ethnicity, pollutants (smoking, radioiodine), dietary (iodine excess, selenium deficiency), endocrine (female gender, parity, postpartum, oral contraceptives), infections, drugs, and trauma.[148,149]

Pathologically, AITD is characterized by lymphocyte infiltrates within the thyroid. AITD is associated with other autoimmune diseases, either organ specific (autoimmune polyglandular syndromes) or systemic (type 1 diabetes, rheumatoid arthritis, systemic lupus erythematosus, Sjögren syndrome, systemic sclerosis, cryoglobulinemia, sarcoidosis, psoriatic arthritis)[145]; these associations reflect common genetic susceptibilities and common pathogenic mechanisms. Autoimmune disease is also associated with papillary thyroid cancer.[150,151]

Hashimoto Thyroiditis

Hashimoto thyroiditis was first described in 1912 by Hakaru Hashimoto, a Japanese physician.[22,152] Also known as chronic lymphocytic thyroiditis, Hashimoto thyroiditis is the most common type of thyroiditis and in iodine-sufficient areas also the most frequent cause of hypothyroidism and goiter. It leads to the destruction of thyroid follicular cells through a T-cell–mediated autoimmune process.[141,145] Histologically, the gland is infiltrated with lymphocytes and plasma cells, which can lead to the development of secondary lymphoid follicles within the gland which are similar to the secondary follicles observed in normal lymph nodes. The initial finding is usually a firm, symmetric goiter, but over time, the gland can atrophy, reflecting destruction of the gland. The gland may often be lobulated, which sometimes makes it difficult to distinguish from multinodular goiter.

The diagnosis of Hashimoto thyroiditis is supported by recognition of autoantibodies against TPO (anti-TPO) or Tg (anti-Tg).[141] Ninety percent of patients with chronic lymphocytic thyroiditis (the histologic description of Hashimoto thyroiditis) have anti-TPO at presentation, and 20% to 50% have anti-Tg autoantibodies, making these autoantibodies excellent markers for the condition.[141,153] The thyroid is hypoechogenic on ultrasound examination.

If overt hypothyroidism is present or SCH with high serum thyroid antibody concentrations, patients should be treated with levothyroxine with the goal of normalizing TSH. TSH-suppressing doses can be used short term to reduce goiter size.[141] TSH should be used for monitoring.

There is a strong association between Hashimoto thyroiditis and primary B-cell lymphoma of the thyroid, although this is a rare condition.[154] It is thought that prolonged stimulation of the intrathyroidal B cells results in the emergence of a malignant clone. In addition, the frequency of papillary carcinoma may be increased in chronic autoimmune thyroiditis, particularly in women.[155] Fine needle aspiration (FNA) biopsy or surgical biopsy may be required to distinguish between these conditions.

Graves Disease

Graves disease results from an autoantibody that binds to and activates the TSHR, producing excessive release of thyroid hormone and clinical hyperthyroidism.[156,157] In patients with Graves disease, the thyroid gland is no longer under the control of pituitary TSH but is constantly stimulated by the circulating antibodies with TSH-like activity. Both B and T lymphocytes are known to be directed at three well-characterized thyroid autoantigens, namely Tg, TPO, and TSHR. Most evidence, however, suggests that the TSHR is the primary autoantigen of Graves disease and that the immune response to the other two thyroid antigens is reflective of the resulting thyroiditis.

Graves ophthalmopathy has an autoimmune pathogenesis, with important genetic and environmental influences, particularly smoking.[158,159]

The diagnosis of Graves disease is based on laboratory demonstration of thyrotoxicosis, clinical features (particularly Graves disease–specific extrathyroidal manifestations, including ophthalmopathy, dermopathy, and [rarely] acropachy), and the presence of a moderate, diffuse, and soft goiter over which a vascular bruit may be detectable.[156,160] Ophthalmopathy, thyroid dermopathy, and acropachy (soft-tissue swelling of the hands and clubbing of the fingers) occur in 25, 1.5, and 0.3% of patients with Graves disease, respectively.[161] Patients with ophthalmopathy, who are also smokers, have a higher risk of developing or worsening of the condition.[159]

Thyroiditis

Thyroiditis means inflammation of the thyroid. Thyroiditis encompasses many thyroid disorders, some of which have an autoimmune etiology, including Hashimoto thyroiditis, painless sporadic thyroiditis, and painless postpartum thyroiditis.[141] The prevalence of individuals with high serum concentrations of thyroid antibodies varies with gender, age, and ethnicity[109]; the prevalence is higher in women, in people older than 60 years of age, and in whites. It has been suggested that dietary iodine deficiency may be protective against certain types of thyroiditis because of the geographical variations in incidence seen in Hashimoto thyroiditis, painless postpartum thyroiditis, and painless sporadic thyroiditis.[162,163]

The different types of thyroiditis may cause thyrotoxicosis, hypothyroidism, or both.[141] All types of thyroiditis may eventually progress to permanent hypothyroidism, and the risk is higher in patients with high serum thyroid antibody concentrations.[146,164,165] As thyroid function declines, TSH secretion increases, resulting in SCH (elevated TSH, normal T4 and T3), and later in overt hypothyroidism with clearly elevated TSH and a preferential expression of T3 but low T4, and finally, in thyroid failure also low T3.[141]

Painless Sporadic Thyroiditis, Painless Postpartum Thyroiditis, and Painful Subacute Thyroiditis

Painless sporadic thyroiditis (synonyms: silent sporadic thyroiditis, subacute lymphocytic thyroiditis), painless postpartum thyroiditis (synonyms: postpartum thyroiditis, subacute lymphocytic thyroiditis), and painful subacute thyroiditis (synonym: de Quervain thyroiditis) are pathologically characterized by lymphocytic infiltration in the first two and with giant cells and granulomas in the third.[141,166] The inflammatory destruction of the thyroid in these conditions leads to release of preformed thyroid hormones from the damaged gland, leading to a transient thyrotoxicosis. Subsequently, patients become euthyroid, but hypothyroidism may eventually develop as the thyroid hormone stores are depleted. An increased plasma concentration of Tg is an early biomarker of inflammatory thyroiditis.[167] The thyrotoxicosis is characterized by decreased TSH and, in contrast to Graves disease, a preferential increase in T4 in comparison with T3, reflecting the release of the stored thyroid hormone. The signs and symptoms of thyrotoxicosis in thyroiditis are usually mild. Painless sporadic thyroiditis and painless postpartum thyroiditis are similar except that the latter occurs following pregnancy.[141]

Painless Postpartum Thyroiditis

The term *postpartum thyroiditis* refers to destructive thyroiditis occurring in the first 12 months postpartum and *not* to Graves disease, although the two conditions may occur together. The immunologic damage to the thyroid is mediated by complement- and lymphocyte-associated mechanisms.[141] Approximately 4 to 9% of unselected postpartum women develop postpartum thyroiditis,[168,169] although the incidence varies with geographical location. Of women who are euthyroid in the first trimester of pregnancy but test positive for thyroid autoantibodies, 50% will develop postpartum thyroiditis. Furthermore, postpartum thyroiditis has been associated with specific human leukocyte antigen (HLA) haplotypes.[170]

Approximately 20% of women develop a triphasic pattern, 50% of women develop isolated hypothyroidism, and 30% develop isolated thyrotoxicosis.[141,168,169] There is an increased incidence of postpartum thyroiditis in women with Graves disease, type 1 diabetes, chronic viral hepatitis, systemic lupus erythematosus. The severity of symptoms varies. The thyrotoxic phase is relatively asymptomatic, although the patient may have palpitations and tachycardia. The hypothyroid phase may be more clinically apparent. Postpartum thyroiditis thyrotoxicosis is more common than Graves disease thyrotoxicosis postpartum. The presence of TRAb points toward

thyrotoxicosis caused by Graves disease and helps in differentiating it from postpartum thyroiditis thyrotoxicosis.[171] Because there is no excess thyroid hormone production in painless postpartum thyroiditis, antithyroid drugs are contraindicated, but if thyrotoxicosis is severe, it is treated with beta-blockers. Levothyroxine is indicated if plasma TSH is greater than 10.0 mIU/L.[172]

Although the thyrotoxicosis in postpartum thyroiditis always resolves, several long-term studies of the hypothyroid phase show persistence of hypothyroidism in up to 30% of cases.[169] It has been estimated that 50% of women who develop postpartum thyroiditis remained hypothyroid at 1 year after delivery.[173] Women with a previous history of postpartum thyroiditis should have TSH concentrations measured annually owing to the increased risk of developing permanent hypothyroidism.[174] Women who are TPO antibody positive should have TSH measured at 6 to 12 weeks of gestation and again at 6 months postpartum if not otherwise clinically indicated.[174]

Painful Subacute Thyroiditis

Painful subacute thyroiditis (synonyms: De Quervain thyroiditis, subacute thyroiditis) usually occurs (2 to 8 weeks) after a viral upper respiratory tract infection (Coxsackie virus, mumps, measles, adenovirus, and other viral infections).[141,175] Treatment is symptomatic. Clinical features may include neck pain, swelling, and fever, usually preceded by a prodromal phase with myalgias, pharyngitis, mildly elevated temperature, and fatigue. Approximately half of affected patients have thyrotoxicosis, followed by several weeks by hypothyroidism; the majority recover to normal thyroid function after 3 to 6 months, but late relapses sometimes occur. In severe cases, corticosteroid treatment is used.

Suppurative Thyroiditis

Suppurative thyroiditis is rare and caused by bacterial infection, fungal, or parasitic infections.[141] TPO antibodies are absent, and patients are usually euthyroid. Treatment is with drugs appropriate to the infection.

Riedel Thyroiditis

In this rare condition (also known as Riedel disease or chronic fibrous thyroiditis), the thyroid gland can become fibrotic with possible attachment to adjacent structures that can produce, for example, tracheal compression. Riedel thyroiditis occurs in 0.05% of people with thyroid disease.[141] Painful subacute thyroiditis can also lead to Riedel thyroiditis.[176] It is now believed that Riedel thyroiditis is part of the IgG4-related systemic sclerosing disease spectrum associated with multisystem fibrosis which is also related to Hashimoto thyroiditis.[177–179] The etiology of Riedel thyroiditis is uncertain, although an autoimmune basis has been suggested because of the presence of thyroid antibodies and histologic finding of lymphocytes and plasma cells.[178,180] At presentation, most patients are euthyroid, but they become hypothyroid as fibrosis replaces thyroid tissue. The diagnosis is by open biopsy. Treatment is surgical, but immunosuppressants may be effective in the early stages of disease.[141,178]

Hypothyroidism

Hypothyroidism is defined as a deficiency in thyroid hormone production or secretion producing a variety of clinical signs and symptoms of hypometabolism. The term *myxo-edema* is used in severe or complicated cases but strictly refers only to the appearance of the skin as it becomes infiltrated with glycosaminoglycans.[181]

Hypothyroidism is a common endocrine disorder that is frequently overlooked but often may present with serious signs and symptoms. The disorder is treatable with a good prognosis. Hypothyroidism is the commonest disorder of thyroid function.[182]

Hypothyroidism (Box 57.2) can be classified[181] according to age of onset (congenital or acquired), HPT level (*primary* with defect in the thyroid, or *secondary* with defect in the hypothalamus or pituitary gland, also called *central hypothyroidism*), severity (overt [clinical] or mild [subclinical]), and duration (permanent or transient).

Epidemiology

In a meta-analysis of European studies, the prevalence of undiagnosed hypothyroidism was about 5%, the prevalence of previously diagnosed hypothyroidism was about 3%, and the incidence rate of hypothyroidism was about 226 per 100,000 per year.[183] Worldwide, the most common cause of hypothyroidism is still iodine deficiency.[79] However, in developed countries where iodine fortification is widespread, the most common cause of primary hypothyroidism is Hashimoto thyroiditis. Hypothyroidism is more common in women than men, increases with age, and is higher in whites than in blacks or Hispanics.[109,182,184]

Etiology

Hypothyroidism has many etiologies (some of which are described in other sections of this chapter), including thyroiditis and in particular autoimmune thyroiditis, postpartum phase, drugs, previous thyroid injury, hypothalamic or pituitary disorders in central hypothyroidism, and iodine deficiency.[181] Congenital hypothyroidism is discussed in a separate section.

BOX 57.2   Causes of Hypothyroidism

Primary Hypothyroidism
Thyroid dysgenesis
Destruction of thyroid tissue
Chronic autoimmune thyroiditis: atrophic and goitrous forms
Thyroid ablation
Subtotal and total thyroidectomy
Infiltrative diseases of the thyroid (amyloidosis, sarcoid, lymphoma, hemochromatosis, scleroderma)
Defective thyroid hormone biosynthesis
Congenital defects in thyroid hormonal biosynthesis
Iodine deficiency
Drugs with antithyroid actions: lithium, iodine and iodine-containing drugs, radiographic contrast agents

Central Hypothyroidism (Secondary Hypothyroidism)
Pituitary disease
Hypothalamic disease

Transient Hypothyroidism
Silent (painless) thyroiditis including postpartum thyroiditis
Subacute thyroiditis (De Quervain syndrome)

POINTS TO REMEMBER

Hypothyroidism
- Hypothyroidism is the commonest disorder of thyroid function.
- It is more common in women, and the risk of developing hypothyroidism increases with age.
- Hypothyroidism is a known risk factor for cardiovascular disease.
- Excluding the newborn period and iodine deficiency, autoimmune thyroid disease is the most common cause of primary hypothyroidism.
- Central hypothyroidism (thyroid-stimulating hormone deficiency) is a rare cause of hypothyroidism.

Previous thyroid injury. Acquired primary hypothyroidism may be caused by previous thyroid injury as a result of surgery (thyroidectomy for thyroid cancer) or irradiation (for head and neck malignancy), radioactive iodine therapy for thyrotoxicosis (Graves disease or toxic nodular goiter), or environmental exposure to radioiodine.

Central hypothyroidism. Central hypothyroidism is caused by an insufficient stimulation by TSH of an otherwise normal thyroid gland.[185] The prevalence is estimated to be 1 in 20,000 to 1 in 80,000 in the general population, accounting for 1 in 1000 hypothyroid patients.[185,186] Neonatal screening programs have shown a prevalence of congenital hypothyroidism of central origin of 1 in 160,000.[187] In the Netherlands, the neonatal screening program using a combined TBG, TSH, and T4 strategy has shown that central hypothyroidism is diagnosed earlier with milder forms with an incidence of 1 in 16,000.[188] In countries that only use TSH for screening, central hypothyroidism will not be detected.

Central hypothyroidism may arise from pituitary disorders (secondary) or hypothalamic (tertiary) disorders including the pituitary stalk (Box 57.3). Tertiary hypothyroidism is a result of insufficient TSH stimulation by TRH. Anti-POU1F1 (anti-PIT-1) is a unique autoantibody against pituitary transcription factor PIT-1. It is detectable in patients with an acquired combined pituitary hormone deficiency characterized by specific defect in growth hormone (GH), prolactin, and TSH.[189]

Central hypothyroidism can be classified into invasive or compressive lesions, iatrogenic factors (e.g., cranial surgery or irradiation), injuries (e.g., head traumas), vascular accidents

---

BOX 57.3   Possible Causes of Central Hypothyroidism

Tumors: pituitary macroadenomas, craniopharyngiomas, meningiomas, gliomas, Rathke cleft cysts, metastases
Iatrogenic: cranial surgery or irradiation, drugs
Injury: head traumas, traumatic delivery
Vascular: postpartum necrosis (Sheehan syndrome), pituitary apoplexy, carotid aneurysms
Infiltrative diseases: sarcoidosis, hemochromatosis
Infectious disease: tuberculosis, syphilis, mycoses
Genetic: *TSHβ* mutations
Idiopathic
Malformations: Empty sella syndrome

(e.g., pituitary apoplexia, postpartum pituitary [Sheehan] syndrome), autoimmune disease (e.g., polyglandular autoimmune diseases), infiltrative lesions (e.g., iron overload, sarcoidosis), inherited diseases, and infectious diseases (e.g., tuberculosis).[181,185] Invasive or compressive lesions include pituitary macroadenomas, craniopharyngiomas, meningiomas or gliomas, Rathke cleft cysts, metastases, empty sella syndrome, and carotid aneurysms.[185] The inherited forms are rare and may include TSHβ mutations[190] or TRH receptor mutations[191] or pituitary transcription factor defects (mutations in *POU1F1, PROP1, HESX1, LHX3, LHX4,* or *LEPR*) with combined pituitary hormone deficiencies including TSH deficiency.[192,193]

Transient or reversible forms of central hypothyroidism can be observed with drugs affecting the neuroendocrine TSH regulation, such as somatostatin analogs, glucocorticoids, or dopaminergic compounds acutely inhibiting TSH secretion.[185] Transient or reversible forms may also occur during recovery from prolonged thyrotoxicosis or severe chronic diseases.[185] Transplacental passage to the fetus of TSH receptor-stimulating antibodies or thyroid hormones from a thyrotoxic mother or corticosteroids or dopamine given to mothers during complicated delivery may also transiently affect neonates' suppression of TSH secretion and central hypothyroidism.[185]

The clinical manifestations of central hypothyroidism (caused by either pituitary or hypothalamic disease) are like those of primary hypothyroidism but tend to be less severe (unless diagnosed in infancy). If a mass is taking up space in the cranium, headache, visual field disturbances, and hypopituitarism may develop. Nonthyroidal illness may have a similar picture as central hypothyroidism because of suppression of the hypothalamic–pituitary axis.[118] Undiagnosed central hypothyroidism in infancy leads to cretinism.

The laboratory diagnosis is based on demonstration of low, normal, or slightly elevated TSH concentrations combined with low tT4 or fT4 concentrations.[185] In neonatal screening programs, central hypothyroidism can only be identified if TSH and T4 are both measured.[185,194] The treatment of central hypothyroidism is the same as that of primary hypothyroidism (levothyroxine).[195]

Symptoms and Signs of Hypothyroidism

Thyroid hormones affect the function of most of the organs and tissues of the body (Box 57.4). The clinical features of thyroid hormone deficiency are therefore quite diverse and may involve multiple systems. The thyroid gland itself may be enlarged as a goiter; either firm or granular in texture; tender or nontender, or normal, small, or impalpable, depending on the etiology of the hypothyroidism.

Cardiovascular system. Hypothyroidism is a known risk factor for cardiovascular disease.[181] Atherosclerosis is most likely a result of the dyslipidemia and the hypertension that can occur with thyroid hormone deficiency.[196] There is an increase of 50 to 60% in peripheral vascular resistance in hypothyroid patients and a 30 to 50% decrease in resting cardiac output. A total of 20 to 40% of patients with hypothyroidism have hypertension, with the diastolic pressure being increased more than the systolic. This is primarily attributable to the increase in systemic vascular resistance. Importantly, all the changes in the cardiovascular function, as well as in lipid metabolism, in patients with hypothyroidism improve in response to treatment with levothyroxine or liothyronine.

BOX 57.4   Clinical Manifestations of Hypothyroidism

Symptoms

Fatigue
Lethargy
Sleepiness
Mental impairment
Depression
Cold intolerance
Hoarseness
Dry skin
Hair loss
Decreased perspiration
Weight gain
Decreased appetite
Constipation
Menstrual disturbances (typically menorrhagia) and infertility
Arthralgia
Paresthesia

Signs

Goiter (may be present)
Slow movements
Slow speech
Hoarseness
Bradycardia
Dry skin
Loss of outer lateral eyebrow
Nonpitting edema (myxedema) (caused by accumulation of glycosaminoglycans in subcutaneous and other interstitial tissue)
Carpal tunnel syndrome
Psychosis
Galactorrhea
Hyporeflexia
Delayed relaxation of reflexes
Myopathy
Congestive cardiac failure (severe hypothyroidism)
Coma (severe hypothyroidism)
Growth failure and mental retardation (undetected congenital hypothyroidism)
Prolonged jaundice (neonatal hypothyroidism) (as a result of immaturity of uridine diphosphonate glucuronyltransferase

---

Myocardial dysfunction, both systolic and diastolic, occurs with hypothyroidism. Hypothyroidism is also associated with congestive cardiac failure, particularly in individuals with severe thyroid hormone deficiency. Up to 50% of studied patients with thyroid gland failure have pericardial effusions; pericardial tamponade is rare but has been reported.[197]

Gastrointestinal system, liver, and pancreas. Despite reduced appetite, most individuals with hypothyroidism show moderate weight gain. This is primarily owing to fluid retention. Hypothyroidism reduces GI tract motility, often causing constipation. Thyroid hormone deficiency can lead to decreased bile flow because of gallbladder hypotonia and also alterations in bile composition. This is probably the underlying reason for the propensity for hypothyroid patients to have bile duct stone formation.[198] Importantly, hypothyroidism caused by Hashimoto thyroiditis is associated with an increase in autoimmune disorders of the GI tract such as pernicious anemia, gluten sensitivity, celiac disease, primary biliary cirrhosis, and autoimmune hepatitis.

Endocrine and metabolic dysfunctions. Primary hypothyroidism is also associated with types 1 and 2 diabetes. The relationship to type 1 may be shared autoimmune predisposition; the relationship to type 2 diabetes is more complex.[199] Thyroid hormones regulate thermogenesis and metabolic rate. In patients with hypothyroidism basal metabolic rate and thermogenesis are reduced causing cold sensitivity, whereas in patients with hyperthyroidism basal metabolic rate and thermogenesis are increased causing heat sensitivity.[200]

Central and peripheral nervous systems. Mental retardation and cretinism are well-recognized complications of endemic iodine deficiency and untreated congenital hypothyroidism. Adults with acquired hypothyroidism are more likely to develop entrapment neuropathies, such as carpal tunnel syndrome, metabolic polyneuropathies and, rarely, cerebellar ataxia. Psychiatric disturbances, particularly depression, are well-known features of hypothyroidism. Thyroid hormone deficiency has also been linked to other neuropsychiatric abnormalities, including poor concentration, impaired memory, cognitive dysfunction, paranoia, hallucinations, and schizophrenia.[201]

Musculoskeletal system. Arthralgia, myalgia, proximal muscle myopathy, and acute exertional rhabdomyolysis have been reported in patients with hypothyroidism.[202–204]

Skeletal muscles can show abnormal structure on microscopy with loss of striations, edema, swelling of fibers, and relative deficiency of type II fibers. Plasma creatine kinase activity is often increased.

Respiratory system. Abnormal respiratory muscle function may occur in patients with preexisting lung disease leading to exacerbation of any carbon dioxide retention. Upper airway obstruction can also occur from soft tissue enlargement or goiter leading to sleep apnea. They may also develop pleural effusions.

Skin and connective tissue. Hypothyroidism can have a marked effect on the epidermis, dermis, sweat glands, hair, and nails. *Myxedema* is the term describing the edema-like skin that results from deposition of glycosaminoglycans (e.g., hyaluronic acid) within the dermis. This appears as nonpitting cutaneous edema with firm texture and a pale waxy appearance. Facial puffiness, periorbital edema, and enlargement of the tongue can also occur. There may be associated anemia and hypercarotenemia through impaired conversion of beta carotene into retinol. This can make the skin look pale yellow. The hair becomes coarse, dry, and brittle with alopecia, and there may be thinning of the eyebrows, especially the lateral portion. Vitiligo can occur in patients with autoimmune pathogenesis.

Kidneys and electrolyte metabolism. Renal blood flow and glomerular filtration rates (GFRs) are both decreased, but total-body water has been shown to increase in patients with hypothyroidism owing to impaired renal excretion of water.[205] Although exchangeable body sodium is increased, the dilutional effect leads to a mild hyponatremia. Plasma vasopressin concentrations have been reported to be inappropriately increased in some patients.[206]

Reproductive system. Hypothyroidism leads to a reduction in libido and subfertility in men and women.

The frequency of menstrual disturbances, both oligo- and polymenorrhea, in hypothyroidism is approximately three times greater than in the normal population.[207]

Oligospermia can occur; it is thought to be owing to impaired luteinizing hormone secretion. Hypothyroidism leads to a reduction in plasma sex hormone–binding globulin concentration and subsequent reduction in total testosterone. Free testosterone is also reduced in around 60% of hypothyroid men. In hypothyroid men, the prevalence of hypoactive sexual desire, delayed ejaculation, and erectile dysfunction has been estimated to be 64% and of premature ejaculation 7%.[208]

Pituitary and adrenal disorders. Lack of thyroid hormone significantly reduces spontaneous nocturnal GH secretion and GH response to stimuli such as insulin-induced hypoglycemia and GH-releasing hormone.[209] In addition, hypothyroidism may inhibit the response of cartilage to insulin like growth factor 1. These abnormalities lead to significant growth failure and short stature in children with hypothyroidism.

With increased TRH release, patients with hypothyroidism sometimes exhibit hyperprolactinemia. Women may thus develop galactorrhea and amenorrhea, and it is imperative that these patients are identified as having primary hypothyroidism to avoid inappropriate treatment for hyperprolactinemia.

In hypothyroid patients, cortisol production rate and metabolic clearance are diminished. However, because both are decreased, the plasma cortisol concentrations remain relatively normal.

Hematology and hemostasis. Hypothyroid patients frequently have a mild normochromic, normocytic, or slightly macrocytic anemia. This is due to decreased erythropoiesis as a result of low plasma erythropoietin concentrations and possibly hypocellular bone marrow. Iron deficiency can occur as a result of either impaired intestinal iron absorption or associated achlorhydria or from menorrhagia. Megaloblastic anemia from vitamin B_{12} deficiency is seen in patients with associated pernicious anemia. Low plasma coagulation factor VIII concentrations and prolonged partial thromboplastin time may lead to easy bruising and to excessive bleeding after minor injuries or procedures or during menstruation.[210] Factor IX concentrations and platelet adherence may also be reduced.

Severity of Hypothyroidism

Importantly, hypothyroidism may be overt or subclinical. Overt hypothyroidism is defined by a high serum TSH concentration and low serum fT4; SCH is defined by a high serum TSH (but usually <10 mIU/L) and a normal serum fT4 concentration.

Subclinical Hypothyroidism

SCH, also called "compensated hypothyroidism," is classified as mild (TSH between 4 and 9.9 mIU/L) or severe (TSH ≥ 10 mIU/L) but with fT4 within the reference interval[211–213]; trimester and age-dependent cut-offs differ and should be applied as appropriate. The elevation in TSH should have persisted for 6 to 12 weeks or longer in the setting of fT4 concentrations that are repeatedly found within the reference interval.[214] The prevalence increases with age and is higher in women than in men. Population prevalence differs; in the United States, it is estimated to be 4 to 9% in individuals without known thyroid disease.[109,184]

The biochemical features of SCH may also be present in patients with overt hypothyroidism, who are inadequately treated, have poor compliance, or because of drug-interactions.[121,215] SCH is more common in iodine-sufficient regions, and iodine supplementation may increase the incidence in mild to moderate iodine-deficient regions.[79,215]

In meta-analyses of observational studies, SCH is not associated with increased fracture risk[216,217] or cognitive impairment[218] but is associated with risk of heart failure with TSH of 10 mIU/L or greater.[219] Meta-analyses and nationwide studies disagree on whether risk is increased for coronary heart disease, fatal coronary heart disease, and all-cause mortality.[220–223] Population studies suggest elevated lipoproteins in SCH.[196] However, the use of thyroid hormone therapy is not associated with improvements in general quality of life (QoL) or thyroid-related symptoms in nonpregnant women.[224]

Myxedematous coma. Patients with severe hypothyroidism may present with myxedematous (hypothyroid) coma, a syndrome of decreased consciousness, hypothermia, and other features of hypothyroidism.[225] This condition has a high mortality and requires aggressive treatment in a critical care facility with facilities for mechanical ventilation if required.

Laboratory Diagnosis of Hypothyroidism

Serum TSH is the first-line measurement with an age-dependent reference interval usually between 0.4 and 4.2 mIU/L (reference intervals vary according to methodology, see also Appendix). *Overt hypothyroidism* is defined as an increased TSH and low fT4. In this case, autoantibodies should also be measured, indicating an autoimmune etiology.

Patients diagnosed with SCH (defined as increased TSH but fT4 within the reference interval) should be followed up with repeat measurements together with measurement of TPO antibodies preferably after a 2- to 3-month interval.[213] The presence of antibodies indicates increased risk of progression to overt hypothyroidism. In patients with negative TPO antibodies and persistent increased s-TSH and no history of surgery, radioiodine therapy, or radiation, measurement of Tg antibodies or TSHR (blocking) antibodies could be measured to indicate autoimmunity. Other conditions in which TSH is elevated but fT4 is normal encompass recent institution of thyroid hormone replacement therapy (fT4 returns to normal before TSH declines), poor compliance with treatment in primary hypothyroidism, recovery from NTI, positively interfering heterophilic antibodies (e.g., human antimouse antibodies) in double-antibody immunoassays, autoimmune TSH-Immunoglobulin complexes ("macroTSH"), and thyroid hormone resistance.

In central hypothyroidism, the laboratory diagnosis is based on low, normal, or slightly elevated TSH combined with low tT4 or fT4 concentrations.[185]

Treatment of Hypothyroidism

Levothyroxine sodium (thyroxine) is the treatment of choice for hypothyroidism with few adverse events if used appropriately.[195] It is chemically stable with relatively modest product deterioration during storage. The American Thyroid Association (ATA) recommends against the routine use of combination treatment with levothyroxine and liothyronine replacement therapy in patients with primary hypothyroidism because evidence of superiority of combination therapy over monotherapy with levothyroxine is not consistently strong.[195]

Levothyroxine is absorbed in the proximal small bowel; it has a 7-day half-life in plasma because of protein binding and is metabolized to triiodothyronine in the tissues by deiodination. The bioavailability is 60 to 80% in healthy volunteers under fasting, with time to maximum concentration of about 2 hours. Absorption is delayed by food. In hypothyroidism, the time to maximum concentration may be prolonged (3 hours), and the bioavailability may be higher.[226] Optimal treatment is typically about 1.8 μg/kg/d but higher in infants and young children and lower in older adults (0.5 μg/kg/d), in patients with ischemic heart disease, and in patients with SCH.[181] Patients who are thyroidectomized tend to need higher doses than those who have autoimmune thyroiditis.[181] It is essential to appreciate that patients with central hypothyroidism may have concomitant central adrenal insufficiency; this must always be excluded before starting levothyroxine therapy because of the risk of precipitating an adrenal crisis.

The European Thyroid Association and ATA are generally in agreement with their recommendations for treatment in SCH.[213,227] Levothyroxine is recommended for younger patients (<65 to 70 years) with serum TSH levels greater than 10 mIU/L. In younger SCH patients (serum TSH < 10 mIU/L) with symptoms suggestive of hypothyroidism, levothyroxine replacement therapy should be considered. If symptoms fail to improve with treatment, levothyroxine should usually be stopped. In those 80 to 85 years or older with elevated serum TSH of 10 mIU/L or less, a wait-and-see strategy is recommended.

Initiation of treatment should start with a dose in the lower end of what is anticipated to be the optimal dosage. It is usually not recommended to start at a low dose with upward titration because this prolongs recovery, but it is essential to do so in patients with longstanding disease or evidence of ischemic heart disease.[181] Steady-state concentrations of the drug are reached by approximately 6 weeks after starting treatment or changing the dose. Patients are customarily advised to take levothyroxine sodium 0 to 60 minutes before breakfast because food and caffeine can have a minor interference with its absorption. Bedtime administration is equally effective and may be better suited to patients who take a number of other medications or to ensure compliance.

In primary hypothyroidism, the treatment goal is to have TSH within the reference interval. In the initial phase of titrating the appropriate dose, changes in TSH lag serum thyroid hormone levels; therefore TSH should be measured no earlier than 4 to 6 weeks after adjustment of thyroxine dosage. According to the ATA guidelines, TSH monitoring is then repeated after 4 to 6 months and then yearly when the patient has reached the optimal dose to maintain euthyroidism.[195] In central hypothyroidism, fT4 should be monitored, and the treatment goal is to maintain fT4 concentration toward the upper end of the reference interval to ensure adequate replacement and euthyroidism.[181]

Reasons for an elevated TSH in treated patients include suboptimal dosing (inadequate prescribed dosage, noncompliance), a decrease in endogenous thyroid production (autoimmune thyroiditis), reduced absorption (because of interactions with drugs [e.g., iron, calcium carbonate, cholestyramine, sucralfate] or diet [fibers, grapes, soybeans, papaya, and coffee], fasting, or compliance with therapy), comorbid conditions (malabsorption, small bowel surgery), pregnancy (caused by increased TBG, increased clearance, increased body mass), diet, and increased clearance (drug interactions [phenytoin, carbamazepine, phenobarbital, rifampicin], comorbid conditions [kidney disease]); in all of these conditions, an increased dose is required.[181,226] A multicenter study demonstrated that up to 50% of patients with long-term levothyroxine (L-T4) treatment have s-TSH values above the reference range due to poor compliance.[228] A decreased dose may be required in older adults and with increasing age.

The metabolism of other drugs can also be affected in hypothyroidism. Because of a smaller distribution volume,[229] plasma concentrations of drugs may be higher than is typical, and because of decreased metabolism, the doses of certain drugs may need to be lower. However, dosage adjustment will usually be needed when euthyroidism is restored.[181]

Adverse reactions include clinical or subclinical thyrotoxicosis with increased risk of bone loss and atrial arrhythmias. In patients with ischemic heart disease, thyroxine treatment may worsen myocardial ischemia.[181]

Factors to consider when initiating levothyroxine therapy are patient age, concurrent comorbidities and medication, and lean body mass.[195] In older adults, the TSH reference interval is higher than in younger individuals; therefore the TSH treatment target should also be higher compared with younger individuals. Older adults often have less lean body mass than younger individuals and thus decreased T4 turnover; therefore the dose needed to normalize the TSH is generally lower. The general recommendation by ATA for treatment with levothyroxine in older adults is that, regardless of known heart disease or risk factors for heart disease, levothyroxine should be initiated with low doses and the dose titrated slowly based on TSH.[195]

It is debated on whether and when to treat in SCH; however, if patients with a laboratory diagnosis of SCH have clinical signs and symptoms, treatment should be instituted. But results from meta-analyses of randomized clinical trials have not shown consistent beneficial effects of levothyroxine treatment on serum lipid concentrations, myocardial infarction, or all-cause mortality in patients with SCH.[220,230] Effect of L-T4 therapy in SCH on QoL and tiredness has also been debated, however meta-analysis showed no improvement in older patients (>65 years).[224]

Hyperthyroidism

The term *hyperthyroidism* refers to a sustained increase in thyroid hormone biosynthesis and secretion by the thyroid gland.[156] The term *thyrotoxicosis* refers to a condition with excess thyroid hormone. The term *thyrotoxicosis* relates to its clinical manifestations: a syndrome of hypermetabolism and hyperactivity resulting from an elevation of plasma T4 or T3 concentration (most usually both). The terms *thyrotoxicosis* and *hyperthyroidism* are not entirely synonymous. For example, thyrotoxicosis can occur as a result of excessive hormone release from the thyroid in the absence of increased synthesis, as may occur in thyroiditis. Excessive intake of thyroid hormones can also cause thyrotoxicosis but not hyperthyroidism. Box 57.5 summarizes the clinical manifestations of thyrotoxicosis.

Epidemiology

In a meta-analysis of European studies, the prevalence of undiagnosed hyperthyroidism was 1.72%, the prevalence of previously undiagnosed and diagnosed hyperthyroidism

---

BOX 57.5   Clinical Manifestations of Thyrotoxicosis

Symptoms

Nervousness, stroke, agitation or irritability
Fatigue, lethargy
Weakness
Increased perspiration
Heat intolerance
Tremor
Hyperactivity
Palpitation
Appetite change (usually increase)
Weight change (usually weight loss)
Increased bowel movement
Menstrual disturbances

Signs

Hyperactivity
Tachycardia or atrial arrhythmia
Systolic hypertension
Warm, moist, smooth skin
Stare and eyelid retraction
Tremor
Hyperreflexia
Muscle weakness
Goiter
Thyroid bruits (with Graves disease, exophthalmos, pretibial myxedema, onycholysis, thyroid acropachy)
Digital clubbing, swelling of digits and toes
Periosteal reaction at extremities of bones

---

combined was 0.75%, and the incidence rate of hyperthyroidism was about 51 per 100,000 per year.[183] The risk increases with age and is higher in women.[156,165]

The population prevalence of subclinical hyperthyroidism (i.e., low TSH but normal fT4) is 0.6 to 2% depending on the cut-off used for TSH concentration[109,215,231,232]; the prevalence is higher in women and increases with age, with prevalence reported to be 2% in people older than 65 years of age. In the National Health and Nutrition Examination Survey, 1.8% had TSH less than 0.4 mIU/L (4% in blacks and 1.4% in whites), and 0.7% had TSH less than 0.1 mIU/L.[109]

The incidence of thyroid storm has been estimated in Japan to be 0.2 persons per 100,000 per year (i.e., 0.22% of all thyrotoxic patients and 5.4% of thyrotoxic patients admitted to hospitals).[233]

Graves disease, the commonest cause of hyperthyroidism, affects approximately 0.4% of the US population and occurs more often in women than in men (5:1). Graves disease is associated with other autoimmune disorders.[234] There is a genetic susceptibility to Graves disease, as shown by a sibling occurrence risk of 11.6%[235] and a heritability of 75% in twin studies;[236,237] the rest is environmental with smoking being a significant risk factor.[158,159,238]

Thyrotropin–secreting anterior pituitary adenomas are very rare and account for about 1% of all pituitary adenomas.[239] TSH-secreting tumors may occur at any age and occur with equal frequency in men and women.[240,241]

Causes of Thyrotoxicosis

The causes of thyrotoxicosis are listed in Box 57.6. Thyrotoxicosis is usually associated with hyperthyroidism but not always.[156] Among common causes for thyrotoxicosis associated with hyperthyroidism[156] are (1) *production of abnormal thyroid stimulator* (TSHR-stimulating antibody) in Graves disease and (2) *thyroidal autonomy*, including toxic multinodular goiter and solitary toxic adenoma. Less common causes include (A) *conditions with production of thyroid stimulating hormones* (TSH-secreting pituitary adenoma, pituitary resistance to thyroid hormone, neonatal Graves disease [TSHR-stimulating antibody from the mother], choriocarcinoma [hCG secretion], and hyperemesis gravidarum [hCG secretion]), (B) *conditions with thyroidal autonomy* (e.g., congenital hyperthyroidism [activating mutations in the TSHR], struma ovarii), and (C) *drug-induced hyperthyroidism* (iodine, iodine-containing drugs [e.g., amiodarone], and radiographic contrast agents).[156]

Common causes for thyrotoxicosis *not* associated with hyperthyroidism include (1) *thyroiditis* (silent sporadic thyroiditis, postpartum thyroiditis, subacute thyroiditis) and (2) *excess exogenous thyroid hormone* (iatrogenic or factitious).[156] Less common causes include (A) *drug-induced thyroiditis* (e.g., amiodarone, interferon alpha, lithium, iodine containing contrast), (B) *acute infectious thyroiditis*, (C) *radiation thyroiditis*, (D) *infarction of thyroid adenoma*, and (E) *"hamburger" thyrotoxicosi*s (caused by ingestion of thyroid-contaminated food from animal sources).[156]

The prevalence of the causes varies with iodine intake, such that in iodine-sufficient areas, Graves disease is the most common cause of thyrotoxicosis, accounting for 60 to 90% of cases. But in iodine-deficient areas, thyroidal autonomy is more common.[242] Thyroiditis accounts for about 10% of all causes of thyrotoxicosis.[156] Iodine fortification induces a temporary, modest increase in the incidence of hyperthyroidism in mild to moderate iodine-deficient regions.[243]

BOX 57.6   Causes of Hyperthyroidism

Endogenous Thyroid Disorders

Autoimmune thyroid disease
Graves disease
Postpartum thyroiditis
Toxic multinodular goiter
Toxic adenoma
Struma ovarii
hCG-induced hyperthyroidism
    Gestational hyperthyroidism
    hCG-secreting tumors (trophoblastic tumor)
Atopic thyroid tissue
Secondary hyperthyroidism (pituitary tumor secreting TSH)

Exogenous Disorders

Thyroid destruction from viral or bacterial thyroiditis, e.g., de Quervain
Iodine-induced hyperthyroidism, e.g., amiodarone
Thyroid hormone ingestion (thyrotoxicosis factitia)

hCG, Human chorionic gonadotropin; *TSH,* thyroid-stimulating hormone.

Signs and Symptoms of Thyrotoxicosis and Hyperthyroidism

Thyrotoxicosis can affect any physiologic system in the body (see Box 57.5) with the frequency and severity of signs and symptoms varying considerably among patients. Some of the causes produce characteristic clinical signs, for example, orbital and cutaneous manifestations in Graves disease. The age of the patient and presence of concomitant disturbances may have an impact on the clinical features of hyperthyroidism, either exaggerating or diminishing them. For example, older patients may have less marked evidence of sympathetic activation such as anxiety, hyperactivity, or tremor and less weight loss but marked features of cardiovascular dysfunction such as congestive cardiac failure and atrial fibrillation.

Cardiovascular system. Cardiovascular symptoms and signs often predominate.[156,244–247] Of the many clinical manifestations of hyperthyroidism, cardiovascular complications represent the highest potential for morbidity and mortality; the rate of cardiovascular death is higher in patients with hyperthyroidism than in euthyroid subjects. Typical symptoms in thyrotoxicosis include palpitations, exercise intolerance, exertional dyspnea, angina, chest pain, and tachycardia. Typical signs include systolic hypertension, atrial fibrillation, cardiac hypertrophy, peripheral edema, pulmonary hypertension, and ultimately heart failure.

High circulating concentrations of thyroid hormone have a direct stimulatory effect on cardiac muscle. Heart rate and volume are increased at rest, and peripheral vascular resistance is reduced, which leads to a marked rise in cardiac output in patients who have no preexisting cardiac disease. This results in increased cardiac oxygen demand and risk of ischemia, increasing the risk of atrial arrhythmia (particularly atrial fibrillation) and promoting the development of congestive cardiac failure in susceptible individuals. In patients with preexisting ischemic heart disease, thyrotoxicosis may precipitate angina. Many of these symptoms and signs mimic those that occur in states of increased β-adrenergic activity. However, catecholamine metabolism is usually normal, and urinary excretion of catecholamine metabolites is also normal. Despite this, the adrenergic antagonists (e.g., propranolol) do mitigate or even prevent some of the ionotropic and chronotropic responses, particularly to T3.

Thyroid hormone increases the synthesis and secretion of renin and aldosterone. This contributes to the increase in renal sodium absorption and blood volume that occurs in thyrotoxicosis. Thyrotoxicosis can cause primarily systolic hypertension as a result of the tachycardia.

Metabolic and ischemic cerebrovascular events have both been described in patients with overt hyperthyroidism; embolic events resulting from atrial fibrillation is more common.

Gastrointestinal system and liver. Increased bowel motility leading to hyperdefecation is a frequent finding in patients with overt hyperthyroidism.[248] There is a shortened small bowel transit time, although true diarrhea does not usually result. Nausea and vomiting are not common but can precede the onset of a thyrotoxic crisis. Weight loss is a common feature of hyperthyroidism owing to increased basal metabolic rate.

Hepatic changes occur with thyroid hormone excess, typically with mild elevations of plasma aminotransferase activities, which may be a result of increased oxygen demand in the face of normal or diminished hepatic blood flow.[249,250] In severe hyperthyroid states, liver function can be markedly deranged with hypoalbuminemia; marked elevation of plasma aminotransferase and alkaline phosphatase activities can occur. The latter can be of mixed bone and liver origin.

Central and peripheral nervous systems. Tremor associated with thyrotoxicosis is usually most evident in the hands but can occur elsewhere (e.g., the lower extremities, trunk, and tongue). It is thought to be caused by β-adrenergic stimulation and responds well to β-adrenergic blocking agents such as propranolol.[251]

Seizures are a well-recognized component of thyroid storm but occur only in a minority (<1%) of patients with moderate hyperthyroidism.[251] The exact mechanism is unknown, but seizures and electroencephalogram abnormalities resolve with correction of thyroid hormone concentrations.

Mental and psychiatric disorders. Thyrotoxicosis may be associated with a number of neuropsychiatric symptoms, including restlessness; irritability; agitation; emotional lability; anxiety; depression; and, rarely, encephalopathy, psychosis, and coma.[251]

Musculoskeletal system. Some degree of myopathy occurs in the majority of patients with overt hyperthyroidism. It is usually proximal and involves the pelvic girdle and shoulder muscles. Advanced hyperthyroidism can lead to muscle wasting owing to its catabolic effect.[251]

Skeletal involvement includes loss of bone mineral density with increased bone turnover markers, including hydroxyproline, hypercalciuria, and, occasionally, hypercalcemia. There have been many studies demonstrating an increased risk of fracture in patients with a history of thyrotoxicosis.[252]

Eye involvement. Hyperthyroidism itself can cause a characteristic "staring" expression (eyelid retraction with sclera being seen above and below the iris). In addition, there is a tendency for the eyelid movement to lag that of the globe as patients look forward from a position of maximum upward gaze (eyelid lag).

In addition, specific orbital signs and symptoms occur in patients with Graves disease (Graves ophthalmopathy). This condition is characterized by periorbital and conjunctival edema and erythema (caused by compression of orbital veins, resulting in venous stasis), retraction of the upper eyelid (caused by sympathetic hyperactivity), and proptosis caused by the increased volume of orbital contents.[251] The last two can lead to corneal ulceration because of incomplete eye closure. The complaints include grittiness in the eyes, excess watering, photophobia, retro-orbital pain, gaze-provoked pain, and diplopia. Features of a myopathy in Graves ophthalmopathy include failure of relaxation of involved muscles, most commonly the levator palpebrae superioris and the inferior and medial recti. Risk factors for Graves ophthalmopathy include smoking and radioiodine therapy for hyperthyroidism (especially among smokers).[253,254] The onset of eye disease in Graves disease usually coincides with that of thyrotoxicosis, but it is not uncommon for the ophthalmopathy to precede or follow thyrotoxicosis by months or even years. It is usually bilateral but can be asymmetrical in up to 15% of cases.[255]

Respiratory system. Exertional dyspnea is a common manifestation of thyrotoxicosis. It is a result of respiratory muscle weakness, enhanced ventilatory drive, diminished lung compliance, and concurrent cardiovascular complications (e.g., congestive cardiac failure).[256,257]

Skin and hair. Diffuse hair loss is common with prolonged elevation of thyroid hormones.[258] The nails are brittle and may become elevated from the nail bed (onycholysis). The skin is warm, soft, and smooth, and there may be palmar erythema.

Graves disease is associated with unique extrathyroidal manifestations, including ophthalmopathy (see earlier discussion), thyroid dermopathy, and, rarely, acropachy.[161] Thyroid acropachy in patients consists of a triad of digital clubbing of fingers and toes, soft tissue swelling of the hands and feet, and a characteristic periosteal reaction of the distal metatarsals. Thyroid dermopathy presents with indurated purple skin lesions over the anterior tibia (pretibial myxedema); these contain large amounts of glycosaminoglycans.

Renal function and electrolytes metabolism. The GFR is increased owing to the increased renal blood flow that results from increased cardiac output and vasodilatation.[259] Thyrotoxic individuals often complain of increased thirst and mild polyuria even in the absence of an obvious cause such as hyperglycemia. Plasma sodium and potassium concentrations are usually normal, but there may be an increase in urinary magnesium excretion, leading to a low plasma magnesium concentration.

Reproductive system. Hyperthyroidism is associated with impaired reproductive function in both men and women. Menstrual abnormalities are common with either a scanty menstrual loss, an irregular cycle, or both. Although cycles usually remain ovulatory, fertility is reduced.[207,260]

In one study in men with hyperthyroidism, the prevalence of hypoactive sexual desire was 17.6%, erectile dysfunction was 2.9%, premature ejaculation was 50%, and delayed ejaculation was 14.7%.[208] Plasma sex hormone–binding globulin concentration is increased, leading to increased total testosterone and estradiol concentrations. Preferential metabolism of androgen to estrogens may be the reason for gynecomastia seen in a small proportion of men with hyperthyroidism.

Hematology. Anemia not attributable to other causes, such as iron deficiency or vitamin B_{12} deficiency, is a frequent finding in patients with Graves disease.[261] Relative neutropenia and lymphocytosis have also been described in patients with untreated Graves disease.[262] There is also some evidence to suggest that thyrotoxicosis is associated with a hypercoagulable state, but patients requiring anticoagulation appear to have a decreased warfarin dose requirement owing mainly to an increased rate of clotting factor degradation.[263]

Thyroid (thyrotoxic) storm. Thyroid storm (also known as thyrotoxic crisis) is a rare, severe, exaggerated, and life-threatening condition of thyrotoxicosis and is triggered by precipitating factors.[225,264] Thyroid storm is most often seen in the context of underlying Graves hyperthyroidism but can complicate thyrotoxicosis of any etiology. It is much less common today than in the past owing to earlier diagnosis and treatment of thyrotoxicosis. The results of laboratory tests are indistinguishable from those seen in patients with uncomplicated thyrotoxicosis; the diagnosis of thyroid storm remains a clinical diagnosis. The condition has a potentially high mortality rate, and it is thus often necessary to begin treatment without waiting for biochemical confirmation of the diagnosis.

Laboratory Diagnosis of Thyrotoxicosis
The laboratory diagnosis of thyrotoxicosis is based on a suppressed TSH and increased fT4 or increased fT3 or total T3.

TSH is the most sensitive biomarker. A total of 2 to 4% of patients with hyperthyroidism have increased concentration of fT3 or tT3 but normal concentration of fT4 (T3 thyrotoxicosis).[160]

However, low TSH can also be caused by other conditions relevant for the diagnosis, discussed elsewhere in the chapter.[156] Low TSH may also be drug induced (glucocorticoids and dopamine) or caused by NTI. If TSH is not reduced, then thyrotoxicosis can be excluded except for rare diagnoses such as pituitary adenoma (secondary hyperthyroidism = central hyperthyroidism), which secrete TSH, and thyroid hormone resistance syndrome (discussed below).

The presence of TRAb (TSHR-binding antibodies) effectively confirms a diagnosis of Graves disease in most cases.[265,266] Sensitivity and specificity for third-generation TRAb assays are high. A total of 75% of patients with Graves disease have TPO antibodies but in presence of TRAb measurements of TPO antibodies is not indicated as a routine.

Patients with Graves disease should have a baseline complete blood count, including white blood cell (WBC) count with differential, and a liver profile, including bilirubin and transaminases, before initiating antithyroid drug therapy for Graves disease.[267]

If the etiology of thyrotoxicosis is uncertain, a RAIU test should be performed; iodine uptake of the thyroid gland is low in thyroiditis and high in Graves disease and autonomous nodules (single or multiple). A thyroid scan should be added in the presence of nodularity;[267] technetium scintigraphy (TcO4) and ^{123}I scintiscan are both useful. Technetium scintigraphy uses pertechnetate that is trapped by the thyroid and not organified, resulting in a low range of normal uptake and high background activity, but total-body radiation exposure is less than for ^{123}I scintiscan. Ultrasonography should be used in the differential diagnosis of thyrotoxicosis when radioactive iodine is contraindicated (e.g., pregnancy or breastfeeding) or not useful (e.g., following recent iodine exposure). Absence of nodularity and high flow indicates Graves disease.

Treatment of Graves Disease

The natural history of the thyrotoxicosis of Graves disease in most patients is of successive relapse and remission over many years. In about 30% of patients, there is a single episode of hyperthyroidism lasting several months followed by prolonged remission and even the eventual development of hypothyroidism up to 20 years thereafter. The main treatment modalities recommended by ATA in association with the American Association of Clinical Endocrinologists (AACE) include: antithyroid drugs, thyroidectomy, radioiodine therapy (131I), and beta-blockers.[267]

Antithyroid drugs (thionamides) include carbimazole, methimazole, and PTU. They reduce symptoms. They act principally by inhibiting the action of TPO and therefore thyroid hormone synthesis. PTU, unlike methimazole, also decreases the conversion of T4 to T3 in peripheral tissues, inhibiting the activity of iodothyronine deiodinase 1 (D1). They are almost completely absorbed, and metabolism is hardly affected by liver or kidney disease.[268]

Before antithyroid drug treatment, patients should have a baseline complete blood cell count, including WBC count with differential, and a liver profile, including bilirubin and transaminases.[267]

Methimazole is the drug of choice for Graves disease, except during the first trimester of pregnancy when PTU is preferred, in thyroid storm, and in patients who experience minor adverse effects with methimazole. Treatment with methimazole is typically given for 12 to 18 months, but the subsequent relapse rate is high. TRAb titers should be measured before stopping antithyroid drug therapy because normal concentrations indicate a greater chance of remission. If hyperthyroidism persists after methimazole treatment, radioactive iodine or thyroidectomy should be considered as alternatives.[267] Treatment guidelines may differ in different countries. In USA, radioactive iodine has been the preferred treatment choice for patients above 40 years, whereas antithyroid drugs are preferred in Europe, Latina America, and Japan, no evidence are present to recommend between the two alternatives.[267]

Both methimazole and PTU are very (at least 90%) effective in controlling thyrotoxicosis caused by Graves disease. There have recently been concerns about PTU-related hepatotoxicity, and these have led the ATA and the US Food and Drug Administration to recommend that methimazole should be used instead of PTU as first-line therapy unless the patient has an adverse reaction or in the first trimester of pregnancy. Patients should be advised to consult a physician if they experience pruritic rash, jaundice, light-colored stools or dark urine, arthralgia, abdominal pain, nausea, fatigue, fever, or pharyngitis. If patients experience symptoms suggestive of agranulocytosis or hepatic injury, they should stop medication immediately and call their physicians because these are potential life-threatening conditions. If agranulocytosis is suspected (e.g., because of a febrile illness or pharyngitis), a WBC count should be performed. Liver function tests should be performed if the patient develops a pruritic rash, jaundice, light-colored stools or dark urine, joint pain, abdominal pain or bloating, anorexia, nausea, or fatigue. Antihistamine therapy may be used for minor cutaneous reactions without stopping the antithyroid drug. If minor side effects of antithyroid medication persist, the drug should be stopped and treatment changed to another antithyroid medication, radioactive iodine, or surgery. If patients experience serious allergic reactions, prescribing an alternative drug is not recommended. Methimazole is the recommended first-line therapy in children.[267]

Radioiodine therapy: Radioiodine therapy has been widely used for adults with thyrotoxicosis caused both by Graves disease and other common causes such as multinodular goiter. [131]I is the isotope of choice. It is effective, safe, and relatively inexpensive. It is administered orally as a single dose in a capsule or in water. It is rapidly and completely absorbed and is then concentrated, oxidized, and organified by thyroid follicular cells. It causes cellular necrosis, which in turn provokes an inflammatory response; patients may develop a mild thyroid tenderness in the few days after treatment. Others may develop transient worsening of their thyrotoxicosis caused by the leakage of stored T4 and T3 from disrupted follicles. Over time, chronic inflammation and fibrosis result in a substantial decrease in the size of the thyroid gland. [131]I therapy should be avoided in very young children.[156,267]

Pregnancy or the possibility of pregnancy is an absolute contraindication for radioiodine therapy. A negative pregnancy test result 48 hours before administration of radioiodine should be ensured. Pretreatment with β-adrenergic blockade and methimazole before radioactive iodine therapy should be instituted in patients with Graves disease who are at increased risk of complications because of worsening of hyperthyroidism (i.e., those who are extremely symptomatic or have fT4 concentrations two to three times the upper limit of normal). Furthermore, pretreatment for any comorbid conditions should be optimized.[267]

Hypothyroidism is a common dose-related side effect of radioiodine therapy in patients treated for Graves disease.[269] In nodular goiter the risk is smaller as the radioiodine is only taken up in the hyperactive nodules. Measurement of fT4 and tT3 should be done within the first 1 to 2 months after radioactive iodine therapy and be continued at 4- to 6-week intervals while the patient remains thyrotoxic. If hyperthyroidism persists after 6 months, retreatment with ^{131}I is recommended.[267]

Radioiodine treatment for hyperthyroidism is a risk factor for development of cancer of the small bowel and thyroid, but the standardized incidence risk is low (4.81 and 3.25, respectively).[270,271] Development or worsening of ophthalmopathy may be preventable by glucocorticoid therapy begun concurrently or immediately after radioactive iodine therapy.

Thyroidectomy: Surgery may be the treatment of choice in adolescents and pregnant women who are allergic to or noncompliant with antithyroid drugs, patients with large goiters or severe ophthalmopathy, and when patients prefer destructive therapy but are apprehensive about radioiodine therapy.[156,267] Thyroidectomy is highly effective for treating patients with Graves disease, but the patients must be rendered euthyroid before surgery, usually by using methimazole. Antithyroid drugs should be stopped at the time of thyroidectomy and patients weaned from β-adrenergic blockers after surgery. Potassium iodide can be given in the immediate preoperative period. In Graves disease, to avoid the risk of relapse and the requirement for repeat surgery, total thyroidectomy is undertaken rather than subtotal thyroidectomy. All patients are thus rendered hypothyroid postoperatively and have to be initiated on thyroid hormone replacement immediately postsurgery. Thyroidectomy in children should be chosen when definitive therapy is required and the child is too young for ^{131}I treatment. After thyroidectomy, serum calcium or intact parathyroid hormone concentrations should be measured, and oral calcium and calcitriol supplementation should be administered if required based on laboratory results.

Other medications: β-Adrenergic blockade should be considered in all patients with symptomatic thyrotoxicosis. Concurrent corticosteroids should be considered in patients with Graves disease and mild active ophthalmopathy who are also smokers or have other risk factors for Graves ophthalmopathy and who are to undergo radioactive iodine therapy.

Subclinical Hyperthyroidism

Subclinical hyperthyroidism is defined by a low serum TSH and a normal serum fT4 and T3 concentration.[215] Subclinical hyperthyroidism is classified as mild if TSH is in the range 0.1 to 0.4 mIU/L.[215]

Persistent subclinical hyperthyroidism may be caused by unintended overtreatment with levothyroxine or by endogenous causes as in primary hyperthyroidism such as Graves disease, toxic multinodular goiter, or solitary autonomous nodule.[215] Exogenous subclinical hyperthyroidism is the most common and is reversible by reduction of levothyroxine

dose. Transitory subclinical hyperthyroidism may be caused by treatment with radioiodine or antithyroid drugs in patients previously with overt hyperthyroidism or as part of thyroiditis. Transitory subclinical hyperthyroidism may develop into overt hyperthyroidism over time, particularly if TSH is suppressed.[215,272,273] The TSH progression over time also depends on the underlying disease; in patients with solitary autonomous nodules or multinodular goiter, the TSH is more likely to persist or progress, but in patients with Graves disease, TSH more often tends to revert to normal values.

Patients with subclinical hyperthyroidism have increased risk of ectopic beats,[274] carotid artery plaques and stroke,[275] atrial fibrillation,[276,277] osteoporosis, and fractures.[278] However, it is debated if cardiovascular and all-cause mortality are increased.[279–281]

The treatment of patients with asymptomatic hyperthyroidism is much more controversial than the treatment of those with asymptomatic hypothyroidism. In the absence of a clinically compatible cardiac arrhythmia or significantly reduced bone mineral density, there is little justification for treating a patient with subclinical hyperthyroidism with thionamide.[215] Current ATA and AACE guidelines state that when a TSH is persistently below 0.10 mIU/L, treatment of subclinical thyrotoxicosis should be strongly considered for patients older than the age of 65 years, in postmenopausal women who are not taking estrogens or bisphosphonates, and in patients with osteoporosis or cardiac risk factors.[267]

Other Forms of Hyperthyroidism

Toxic adenomas and toxic multinodular goiter. Toxic adenomas and toxic multinodular goiter are conditions in which the follicular cells function and produce thyroid hormones independently of thyrotropin (TSH) and TSHR-stimulating antibody. This autonomous secretion of thyroid hormones leads to TSH suppression and ultimately results in thyrotoxicosis. Such thyroid autonomy is a common finding in iodine-deficient areas, where it accounts for up to 60% of cases of thyrotoxicosis. However, thyroid autonomy is rare in regions with sufficient iodine supply (3 to 10% of cases with thyrotoxicosis).[282]

Gain-of-function mutations of the thyroid-stimulating hormone receptor. A familial autosomal dominant form of hyperthyroidism has been described that is caused by gain-of-function mutations in the TSHR. The gain-of-function mutation places the TSHR in the "on" position in the absence of ligand (TSH) binding. In infants homozygous for such mutations, neonatal thyrotoxicosis, so severe as to require emergency thyroidectomy, has been observed. Certain heterozygous mutations have been reported to cause infantile hyperthyroidism.[283]

Central hyperthyroidism. Central hyperthyroidism is rare but is most frequently caused by nearly always benign TSH–secreting pituitary adenomas. A total of 75% of the tumors are macroadenomas, having a diameter larger than 10 mm at the time of diagnosis, but microadenomas (diameter < 10 mm) are increasingly recognized owing both to early diagnosis and improvements in imaging techniques.[239]

TSH adenomas may show concomitant hypersecretion of other pituitary hormones (GH, prolactin, and less frequently follicle-stimulating hormone and luteinizing hormone) together with the hypersecretion of TSH.[239]

Patients with TSH-secreting tumors present with signs and symptoms of thyrotoxicosis, but extrathyroidal manifestations (i.e., ophthalmopathy, pretibial myxedema, and acropachy) are absent. Goiter is a common finding as a consequence of chronic TSH hyperstimulation. Patients may also have symptoms related to the mass effect of the pituitary adenoma such as visual field defects, headache, or loss of other anterior pituitary function (menstrual disorders, galactorrhea acromegaly).

The laboratory diagnosis is based on a nonsuppressed TSH in the presence of elevated concentrations of free thyroid hormones (fT3 and fT4).[239] Evidence of a pituitary mass using imaging techniques supports the diagnosis.[284] There are both clinical situations (in particular) and possible laboratory artefacts that may cause a biochemical profile similar to that characteristic of patients with TSH-secreting tumors; these include thyroid hormone resistance, binding protein abnormalities, falsely high fT4 results, and falsely high (given the high T4) TSH concentrations. Dynamic function tests such as the TRH test or T3 suppression tests or a trial of somatostatin analogue can aid the differential diagnosis as can the molar ratio of α-subunit:TSH,[285] however this later parameter must be interpreted with caution as it is affected by circulating levels of other pituitary glycoprotein hormones.[286] The molar ratio of α-subunit to TSH may serve as a useful tumor marker in the differential diagnosis of a TSH-secreting pituitary adenoma, in which the ratio of α-subunit to TSH concentrations is typically larger than 1 ng/mL, from thyroid hormone resistance syndrome, in which the ratio is less than or equal to 1 ng/mL.[240,241,287]

Transsphenoidal resection is the recommended therapy for TSH-secreting tumors.[288] Pharmacologic reduction of TSH secretion can be used as an adjunct to surgery or may be used postsurgery if some tumor still remains. Long-acting somatostatin analogues (e.g., octreotide, lanreotide) may reduce TSH secretion and tumor size in individual cases.[289] Dopaminergic agonists, such as bromocriptine and cabergoline, may also be effective in residual or recurrent tumors.[241] If surgery is contraindicated or declined, or in the case of surgical failure, pituitary radiotherapy may be considered. Ablative antithyroid therapy (e.g., with antithyroid agents) leads to control of the hyperthyroidism but does not deal with the primary problem and is thus generally not indicated.

Early diagnosis and treatment are essential for a good prognosis. The main prognostic factors are size and invasiveness of the tumor, duration of symptoms, and intensity of hyperthyroidism.[290]

Resistance to thyroid hormone. Resistance to thyroid hormone (RTHβ) is usually caused by mutations in the thyroid hormone receptor β (THRβ) gene.[66] The HPT axis is affected with impairment of the central T3 feedback loop. The typical clinical phenotype is of sinus tachycardia, attention deficit hyperactivity disorder, and goiter.[291] The phenotype reflects tissues expressing thyroid hormone receptor α-isoform being overstimulated and tissues expressing the thyroid hormone receptor β-isoforms 1 and 2 being resistant. The clinical phenotypes can be highly variable, and the pathogenic basis for this may be based on the degree of tissue responsiveness to elevated thyroid hormone levels in a given individual.

Only a few patients have been described with mutations in the thyroid hormone receptor α gene *(THRα)*. The HPT axis is minimally affected, and the central T3 feedback loop is not impaired. Laboratory results in patients with RTHα show plasma TSH concentration within the reference interval, slightly lowered concentrations of fT4, slightly elevated tT3,

and an abnormally low free T4:T3 ratio. The clinical phenotype is different from RTHβ, and symptoms and signs have been described as a variable degree of mental retardation, short stature, chronic constipation, and bradycardia.

Hyperthyroidism caused by human chorionic gonadotropin. Human chorionic gonadotropin–induced hyperthyroidism is observed in gestational transient thyrotoxicosis, resulting from TSHR sensitivity to (appropriately) high hCG concentrations during pregnancy and to hCG-secreting tumors.[292] Tumors that secrete hCG, such as choriocarcinoma, hydatidiform mole, and metastatic embryonal carcinoma, can cause hyperthyroidism through hCG stimulation of the TSHR.[293]

POINTS TO REMEMBER

Thyrotoxicosis
- Central hyperthyroidism (TSH-secreting tumors) is a very rare cause of thyrotoxicosis.
- Graves disease is the most common cause of thyrotoxicosis and most of the remaining causes are toxic nodular goiter and toxic adenoma.
- Of all clinical manifestations of thyrotoxicosis, cardiovascular complications represent the highest potential for morbidity and mortality.
- Antithyroid drugs (e.g., methimazole) remain the mainstay of treatment in Graves disease.
- [131]I may be the treatment of choice for multinodular goiter and toxic adenoma.
- [131]I treatment is absolutely contraindicated in pregnancy or the possibility of pregnancy.

Thyroid Disorders in Pregnancy and Postpartum

It is estimated that approximately 4% of pregnant women have a history of thyroid disease, develop thyroid disease during the pregnancy, or are for the first time diagnosed with thyroid disease within 5 years after a pregnancy.[294] Postpartum thyroiditis is discussed earlier in the section on thyroiditis.

Physiologic Changes

Plasma tT3 and tT4 concentrations increase during pregnancy owing to an increase in TBG concentration. This increase is caused by enhanced hepatic synthesis and reduced metabolism (a result of increased estrogen levels) early in pregnancy, resulting in a 1.5-fold increase in TBG by 6 to 8 weeks of gestation. TBG remains elevated throughout pregnancy.[169,295]

Placental hCG shares the same α subunit with TSH but has a unique β subunit and acts in early pregnancy as a TSH agonist by binding to TSHRs on the thyroid gland.[169,295] The physiologic consequences of the mild hCG stimulation of the thyroid in early pregnancy leads to a physiologic rise in T4 and T3, which, by the HPT axis feedback mechanism, inhibits TSH secretion, causing TSH to fall. The decrease in serum TSH in the first trimester is followed by a rise during the second and third trimesters when the hCG concentrations fall but do not exceed prepregnancy values. There is transient rise in fT4 during the first trimester owing to the relative high circulating concentration of hCG and a gradual fall of fT4 in the second and third trimesters.[296] Changes in fT3 concentrations are broadly parallel with those of fT4. TSH is higher in singleton pregnancies than in twin pregnancies.[297]

Hypothyroidism in Pregnancy

A total of 2 to 3% of all iodine-sufficient pregnant women have undiagnosed hypothyroidism, mostly SCH.[169,298] Overt hypothyroidism is estimated to occur in 0.5% of all pregnant women. Worldwide, the most common cause is endemic iodine deficiency. Two percent have isolated hypothyroxinemia (e.g., decreased thyroid hormone without plasma TSH elevation and without the presence of autoantibodies).[299] The exact implication of this is unclear.

The diagnosis of hypothyroidism in pregnancy is based, as in nonpregnant subjects, on the finding of an elevated serum TSH concentration with low concentrations of fT4, using trimester-specific reference intervals (see Appendix). Untreated overt maternal hypothyroidism is associated with adverse maternal and fetal outcomes.[169,300,301] There is an increased risk of miscarriage, preterm delivery, and preeclampsia in the mother. In the newborn, there is an increased risk of neonatal mortality caused by preterm delivery, risk of low for gestational age birth weight, and decreased IQ. The complications are similar in SCH but occur at a lower frequency. About 10 to 20% of women in the childbearing years have detectable autoantibodies (TPO or Tg autoantibodies).[302] Also, in euthyroid women positive for autoantibodies, there are increased risks of miscarriage, preterm delivery, and postpartum thyroiditis.[169]

Treatment and Monitoring

The ATA recommends levothyroxine treatment for all pregnant women with a TSH concentration above the trimester-specific reference interval with a decreased fT4, and those with a TSH concentration above 10.0 mIU/L irrespective of fT4 concentration or with TPO autoantibodies (Fig. 57.8).[169,172]

The treatment goal is TSH within trimester-specific reference intervals. In women with SCH who test positive for TPO autoantibodies, the ATA recommends levothyroxine treatment, but for those who test negative for TPO autoantibodies, evidence for treatment is insufficient.

In women with SCH in pregnancy who are not initially treated, the ATA recommends monitoring with TSH and fT4 every 4 weeks or so until 16 to 20 weeks of gestation and at least once between 26 and 32 weeks of gestation.

In euthyroid women not receiving levothyroxine who are TPO autoantibody positive, the ATA recommends monitoring for hypothyroidism during pregnancy. Serum TSH should be evaluated every 4 weeks during the first half of pregnancy and at least once between 26 and 32 weeks of gestation.

In women treated with levothyroxine, lower preconception TSH values within the nonpregnant reference interval reduce the risk of TSH elevation during the first trimester. When pregnant, TSH should be measured every 4 weeks until 20 weeks of gestation and at least once in the second half of pregnancy. The required dose of levothyroxine is typically higher in pregnancy and should be returned to the prepregnancy amount immediately postpartum. Six weeks postpartum, thyroid function tests should be performed again. At that time, TSH and thyroid hormones are no longer affected by the pregnancy. Isolated hypothyroxinemia should not be treated in pregnancy.

Thyrotoxicosis in Pregnancy

Graves disease occurs in 0.1 to 1% of all pregnancies.[169] Transient gestational hyperthyroidism usually occurs in the first trimester with a prevalence of 2 to 3% in Europeans.[303] The causes of thyrotoxicosis in pregnancy are the same as for thyrotoxicosis generally; however, transient gestational hyperthyroidism is pregnancy specific. Thyrotoxicosis may be present before pregnancy or be diagnosed in pregnancy or postpartum.

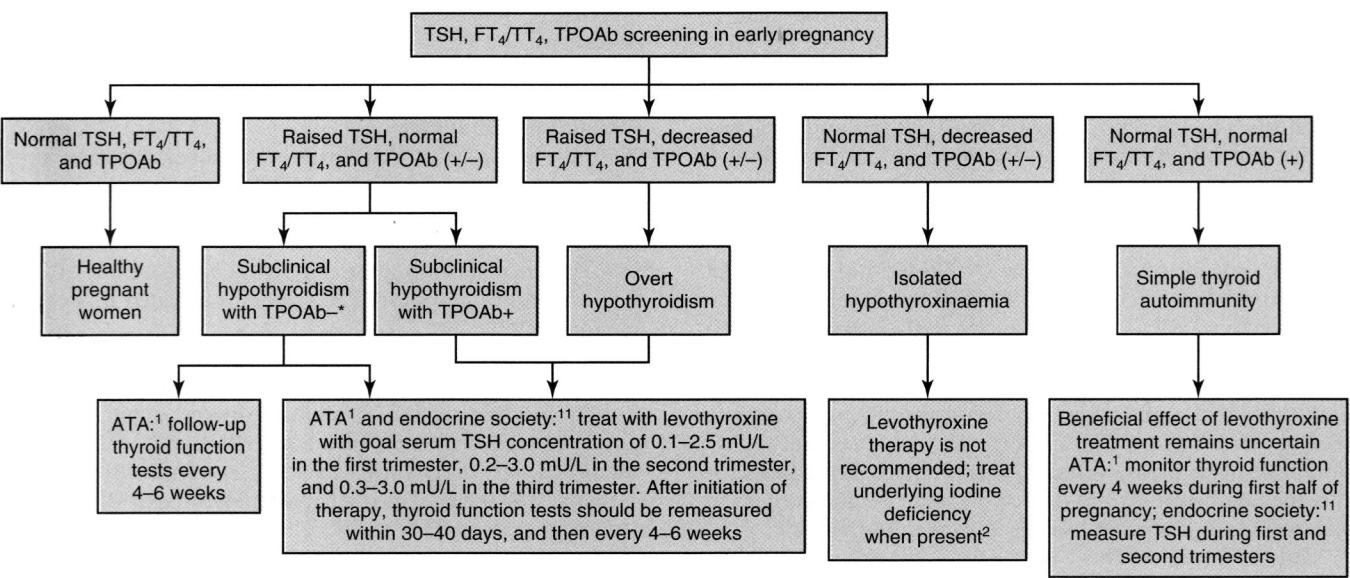

FIGURE 57.8 Screening, diagnosis, and management of hypothyroidism in pregnancy. *ATA*, American Thyroid Association; *FT*, free thyroid; *TSH*, thyroid-stimulating hormone. (Reproduced with permission from Teng W, Shan Z, Patil-Sisodia K, Cooper DS. Hypothyroidism in pregnancy. *Lancet Diabetes Endocrinol* 2013;1:228–37. Based on recommendations from American Thyroid Association [ATA] and The Endocrine Society.)

The diagnosis of thyrotoxicosis in pregnancy, as at other times, is made by finding a low plasma TSH concentration and elevated concentrations of fT3, fT4, or both using trimester-specific reference intervals. Subclinical hyperthyroidism in pregnancy is defined as a low plasma TSH concentration with normal concentrations of fT4 or fT3.[169] In patients with Graves disease, TSH and thyroid hormones should be measured every 4 to 6 weeks during pregnancy.[156]

Measurement of TSHR binding antibodies (TRAb) should be reserved for patients with Graves disease who become pregnant or if Graves disease is suspected during pregnancy. In the former, TRAb should be measured at diagnosis and at 24 to 28 weeks gestation because these antibodies can cross the placenta, starting in late second trimester.[169] Testing for other thyroid autoantibodies is not required, although these are typically present in high titers.

Graves disease in pregnancy. Uncontrolled, untreated Graves disease is associated with adverse pregnancy outcomes (fetal loss, preeclampsia, miscarriage, premature labor) and risk of maternal heart failure.[156,169,172,304,305] Risk for the fetus and neonate include hyperthyroidism caused by TSHR stimulating antibodies crossing the placenta (fetal tachycardia, accelerated bone maturation, fetal goiter, intrauterine growth restriction and signs of congestive heart failure, low birthweight for gestational age, poor Apgar scores, and respiratory distress syndrome), risk of hypothyroidism caused by treatment with antithyroid drugs, and congenital abnormalities caused by hyperthyroidism and the teratogenic effects of antithyroid drugs. Neonatal hyperthyroidism is infrequent and occurs in fewer than 1% of infants born to mothers with Graves disease (effectively 1 in 50,000 neonates). However, if it is not recognized and treated properly, the mortality rate can be as high at 30%.

If Graves disease is diagnosed before pregnancy, the aim should be to achieve a euthyroid state before conception. In patients with a diagnosis of Graves thyrotoxicosis for the first time in pregnancy, the symptoms often will have preceded conception by several months. Many signs and symptoms are commonly seen as normal features of pregnancy, such as mild palpitation, heat intolerance, and shortness of breath on exercise. Features such as a family history of thyroid disease or other autoimmune conditions, the presence of goiter, ophthalmopathy, vitiligo, tachycardia (pulse >100 beats/min), weight loss, or inability to gain weight should help make the diagnosis. TRAb are elevated in most patients with Graves disease but often disappear during the pregnancy.

In many pregnant women, Graves disease tends to become exacerbated in the first trimester, improves during later pregnancy, but relapses postpartum. As a result of the improvement during pregnancy, the dose of antithyroid drugs may be lowered or treatment even withdrawn.

In pregnant women with thyrotoxicosis, antithyroid drugs are the treatment of choice.[156,169,172,267,304,305] Because of the risk of hepatotoxicity, current guidelines recommend that PTU be used in the first trimester only and should be avoided in the second and third trimesters. The risk of embryopathy with PTU has previously been considered to be low in the first trimester. In the second and third trimesters, methimazole or carbimazole should be used, but these should be avoided during the first trimester (the period of fetal organogenesis) owing to risk of malformation. However, two meta-analyses have

shown increased risk of congenital anomalies using PTU, methimazole, or carbimazole, either alone or in switching regimens.[306,307]

Therefore guidelines suggest in mild hyperthyroidism to avoid antithyroid drugs during first trimester.[172] If moderate to severe hyperthyroidism, PTU should be used. Combined antithyroid drug and T4 therapy (block and replacement) is not recommended in pregnancy because it does not prevent neonatal hypothyroidism and usually requires the administration of higher doses of the antithyroid drugs than would otherwise be necessary. Pregnant patients with thyrotoxicosis require careful monitoring to keep the dose of the antithyroid drug to a minimum, especially during the last trimester, because these compounds cross the placenta and may render the fetus hypothyroid. The goal of therapy is to keep fT4 within or slightly above the trimester-specific reference interval.

Fetal thyroid gland suppression by thionamides is a concern when any pregnant woman with hyperthyroidism is treated. The size of the fetal thyroid gland can be monitored by ultrasonography. TSH and T4 can be measured in fetal blood obtained by cordocentesis (a high-risk procedure) or in the amniotic fluid.[308] Besides the analytical challenge of measuring the very low concentrations of these hormones in nonplasma body fluids, the choice of an appropriate reference interval can be difficult. Also, it is unlikely that many laboratories have validated measurements of thyroid hormone or TSH in amniotic fluid.

Thyroidectomy is rarely needed unless a larger goiter compresses the trachea. Subtotal thyroidectomy is an effective management and is usually performed in the second trimester, but there are very few indications.

Therapy with ^{131}I is contraindicated because it can produce fetal hypothyroidism. Subclinical hyperthyroidism does not require treatment in pregnancy.

Transient Gestational Hyperthyroidism and Hyperemesis Gravidarum

Transient gestational thyrotoxicosis is a nonautoimmune hyperthyroidism occurring in pregnant women with a spectrum ranging from no emesis, to emesis, to hyperemesis gravidarum (when dehydration could be so severe that intravenous fluid replacement may be required).[169,300,309–311] Gestational transient thyrotoxicosis occurs in 2 to 3% of all pregnancies and results from activation of TSHRs by hCG. It is important to distinguish between Graves disease and transient gestational thyrotoxicosis. In both conditions, palpitations, anxiety, hand tremor, and heat intolerance are common clinical manifestations. In transient gestational thyrotoxicosis, thyroid autoantibodies are negative; in Graves disease, diffuse goiter and ophthalmopathy may be present, and thyroid autoantibodies are positive.

Transient gestational thyrotoxicosis may occur in women with hyperemesis gravidarum, in twin or higher-order pregnancies, and in association with hydatidiform mole, all conditions in which hCG concentrations are high. Hyperemesis gravidarum occurs in 0.3 to 1% of pregnancies and is characterized by severe nausea and vomiting in the first trimester, leading to more than 5% weight loss, ketonuria, dehydration, and liver and electrolyte abnormalities (particularly hypokalemia). Serum hCG concentrations are positively correlated with the severity of nausea and vomiting. The thyrotoxicosis of hyperemesis gravidarum usually resolves spontaneously within several weeks as the vomiting disappears. The degree of hyperthyroidism is typically mild.

Most patients with hyperemesis gravidarum and transient gestational hyperthyroidism do not require antithyroid medication. Supportive treatment includes rehydration, replacement of electrolytes, and antiemetics.[172] Antithyroid drugs are not indicated. However, it is important to exclude concomitant Graves disease because it needs specific treatment.

Thyroid Autoantibodies in Euthyroid Pregnant Women

TPO antibodies and Tg antibodies can be detected in 10 to 20% of pregnant women, but most of the women are euthyroid.[302] The presence of the autoantibodies reflects an autoimmune process in the thyroid gland. A meta-analysis has shown that maternal thyroid autoantibodies are strongly associated with miscarriage and preterm delivery.[302] A randomized trial has also shown that treatment with levothyroxine reduces the risks[312] but is currently not recommended by any obstetric, thyroid, or endocrine society.[172]

Postpartum Thyroiditis

Postpartum thyroiditis may be difficult to differentiate from Graves disease. The differences between the two include the presence of goiter, ophthalmopathy, and thyroid receptor stimulating antibodies (TRAb) in Graves disease with high iodine or technetium uptake; these are not present in thyroiditis. Approximately 4 to 9% of unselected postpartum women develop postpartum thyroiditis, although the incidence varies with geographical location.[169,300] Postpartum thyroiditis is characterized by a short period of thyrotoxicosis due to a destruction of the thyroid follicles seen typically 2 to 6 months after pregnancy; hereafter the patient develops hypothyroidism, transient or permanent. Postpartum thyroiditis often recurs in subsequent pregnancies. Postpartum thyroiditis only requires beta-blockers for treatment.

Thyroid Function Testing in Pregnancy

During pregnancy, the TSH reference interval is shifted downward relative to the nonpregnant reference interval, with a reduction in both the lower and the upper limit of maternal TSH. The extent of the reduction varies between different racial and ethnic groups. ATA 2017 guideline recommends for TSH to use population-based trimester-specific reference intervals in pregnant women with no known thyroid disease, optimal iodine intake, and negative TPOAb, but if this is not possible then "the lower reference interval of TSH can be reduced by approximately 0.4 mU/L, while the upper reference interval is reduced by approximately 0.5 mU/L."[172]

The reliability of immunoassays for the measurement of fT3 and fT4 is decreased in pregnancy owing to higher TBG but lower albumin concentrations.[313-315] Liquid chromatography–tandem mass spectrometry combined with equilibrium dialysis or ultrafiltration methods are more reliable for both total and free hormone concentrations during pregnancy.[316,317]

Thyroid Screening in Pregnancy

Thyroid dysfunction during pregnancy may affect maternal health, fetal health, and obstetric outcome. Recommendations for screening for thyroid disorders in pregnancy vary among different clinical associations.[172,174,227] The controversies can be narrowed down to whether to screen universally or to use a targeted approach and what criteria should be used for targeted screening, such as age, previous pregnancy-related adverse outcomes, comorbid disease (especially autoimmune disease), presence of thyroid antibodies, obesity, family history of thyroid disease, goiter, medication, iodine availability in the area of living, and previous thyroid disease. The consequence of the different guidelines is different practices among physicians nationally and internationally.[318-321]

POINTS TO REMEMBER

Pregnancy

- Use trimester-specific thyroid reference intervals based on locally established population-based pregnancy reference intervals.
- Thyroid-stimulating hormone (TSH) may be misleading in the first trimester and fT4 values will give a more accurate estimate of clinical status.
- Late in gestation, TSH concentrations are more reliable, but T4 may fall, especially during the third trimester.
- In some cases, anti-thyroid peroxidase antibodies can provide further information; this can predict risk of hypothyroidism.
- Measurement of thyrotropin receptor autoantibodies is indicated in all women with active Graves disease or a history of this condition because transplacental transfer of this antibody can cause fetal hyperthyroidism.

Thyroid Neoplasia

The prevalence of palpable thyroid nodules in adults is about 5%, the prevalence of nodules found on ultrasonography is 13 to 30%, and the prevalence of nodules found on autopsy is 49 to 57%.[322] The prevalence of cancer in single nodules has been estimated to be 5% and may be less frequent in multinodular goiter.[323] Cancer risk depends on age, sex, radiation exposure, family history, and other factors.[324] A recent meta-analysis of observational studies showed that vegetables overall may have a protective effect on thyroid cancer incidence and likewise fish and shellfish in iodine-deficient areas, but no effects were observed in iodine-rich areas.[325]

Thyroid cancer is a rare cause of cancer death (<0.4% in the United States) because the incidence is low (~2%).[326] The female-to-male ratio is 3 to 1.[327] The incidence is increasing, but mortality rates from thyroid cancer have remained stable. Therefore it is debated whether this increase in cases is due to overdiagnosis, as a consequence of high-resolution imaging,[328] or a true increase caused by environmental factors such as radiation exposure.[329]

There are four main types of thyroid cancer[330] (listed from the most common to the least common): differentiated thyroid cancer (DCT), including (1) papillary and (2) follicular thyroid cancer, accounting for more than 90% of thyroid cancers in United States[324]; (3) MTC (<5%)[331,332]; and (4) anaplastic thyroid cancer, accounting for about 2%.[333] Follicular cells give rise to well-differentiated papillary and follicular carcinomas but also the poorly differentiated anaplastic carcinomas, which have a worse prognosis. Parafollicular or C cells secrete calcitonin and give rise to MTC, with an intermediate prognosis. MTC may be sporadic or hereditary, but most cases (80%) are sporadic (i.e., not genetically inherited and occur randomly).

The main role for the clinical biochemist is the monitoring of TSH suppression therapy, determination of cancer ablation, the detection of recurrence in patients given definitive treatment such as thyroidectomy, and prognosis.

Although the diagnosis of thyroid neoplasia is largely reliant on clinical, radiologic, and histologic investigations, serum TSH measurement is a key investigation in a patient presenting with a thyroid nodule. Suppressed TSH is in keeping with an autonomous nodule; these have a low risk of being malignant, but patients may need treatment for thyrotoxicosis. A normal or high TSH should prompt ultrasound investigations with FNA biopsy dependent on results.

Differentiated Thyroid Cancer

Patients with DTC have a favorable prognosis.[324,326,330] Evaluation and treatments for DTC are multimodal. Evaluation involves ultrasound, FNA biopsy, imaging, and blood tests. The goals of therapy are to remove the primary tumor and clinically significant lymph node metastases with thyroidectomy and local nodal dissection and to minimize the risk of disease recurrence and metastatic spread with adjuvant therapy radioactive iodine and TSH suppression. Routine TSH suppression therapy for benign thyroid nodules in iodine-sufficient populations is not recommended.

Biochemically, TSH and Tg are useful markers. Serum TSH should be measured during the initial evaluation of a patient with a thyroid nodule. A low or low within the reference interval TSH concentration is suggestive of the presence of some autonomous nodules in patients with multiple nodules.

Because TSH is a major trophic factor for thyroid carcinoma, suppression of TSH using exogenous thyroid hormone administration after surgery reduces the risk of recurrence and prevents hypothyroidism. Consequently, the routine measurement of serum TSH, fT4, and fT3 is required for patient follow-up. Free T3 analysis can provide reassurance that these patients have not been rendered overly hyperthyroid.

Serum Tg concentration can be elevated in many thyroid diseases and is not sensitive or specific for thyroid cancer; thus it is not recommended to measure serum Tg for initial evaluation of thyroid nodules or preoperatively. However, it is a useful marker for disease recurrence in thyroidectomized patients because it should be undetectable. Tg should not be used as a tumor marker in the presence of anti-Tg antibodies owing to measurement interference. TSH stimulation by either temporarily ceasing thyroid hormone replacement or by the administration of recombinant TSH greatly increases the sensitivity of Tg measurement, but this may not be necessary using more sensitive Tg assays. The optimal cut-off for Tg for predicting recurrence is not known. There is a general agreement that a stimulated Tg less than 1 ng/mL with no other radiologic or clinical evidence of disease and in the absence of autoantibodies suggests no evidence of disease, although recurrence has been described below this cut point. Tg should be measured 6 weeks to 3 months after surgery and then every 6 to 12 months, but there is no agreement on the ideal timing and frequency of testing. Persistently elevated Tg concentrations may indicate either recurrence or a thyroid remnant. Newer Tg assays have limits of detection of 0.1 ng/mL or less (compared to older assays with 1 ng/mL); this allows for earlier identification of recurrence and avoidance of the use of TSH stimulation.

About 20 to 30% of patients with DTC have Tg antibodies (TgAbs).[334,335] If Tg cannot be measured on a mass spectrometric method in the presence of Tg antibodies, then TgAbs themselves may be used as surrogate tumor marker instead of Tg.[336,337] Both the actual concentrations and values over time may be used. TgAbs should not be used within the first weeks after thyroidectomy because a transient rise may be caused by TgAbs reacting to released Tg. However, TgAbs have a role in long-term follow-up after thyroidectomy. Whereas a sustained high level or persistent rise suggests recurrence, a persistent fall suggests low risk of recurrence.

Immunometric assays used to measure Tg and TgAbs are prone to interferences.[324] The hook effect can cause falsely low values for Tg and TgAbs. Thus an apparent absence of TgAbs may be a result of antibodies not being detected, and in such instances, low Tg concentrations may be misleading. Furthermore, both Tg and TgAb immunometric assays may be affected by heterophilic antibodies, causing falsely elevated results. If TgAbs are absent on immunometric assays, but pathology shows Hashimoto thyroiditis, then the presence of TgAbs should be suspected. Serially measured Tg and TgAbs should be done on the same analyzer using the same assay.

Medullary Thyroid Cancer

The diagnosis of MTC is based on FNA biopsy, imaging, blood tumor markers, and genetic testing.[330,332] The standard treatment for patients with sporadic or hereditary MTC is total thyroidectomy and dissection of cervical lymph node compartments depending on serum calcitonin concentrations and ultrasound findings and subsequent replacement with levothyroxine.[331,332] Radiation or chemotherapy may be used as palliative measures but not as a cure. The prognosis depends on the spread of the cancer, with localized cancers having a good 10-year prognosis but cancers with peripheral metastases having a poor prognosis. Serum TSH and serum calcium should be measured postoperatively. The goal is to render patients euthyroid and to prevent hypocalcemia.

Calcitonin, produced by C cells, is a valuable blood tumor marker for MTC.[330,332] Calcitonin is a 32-amino-acid monomeric peptide that is the result of cleavage and posttranslational processing of procalcitonin, which is itself a product of preprocalcitonin. Serum calcitonin can be used as a screening test in patients with a family history of MTC,[332] who are at risk of developing the disease. The use of calcitonin as a screening marker in patients with nodular goiter and with no family history is debatable. Calcitonin is also used diagnostically as an immunohistochemical marker. Basal serum calcitonin and carcinoembryonic antigen (CEA) should be measured concurrently. CEA is not a specific biomarker for MTC and is not useful in the early diagnosis of MTC. However, CEA is useful for evaluating disease progression in patients with clinically evident MTC and for monitoring patients after thyroidectomy. All patients diagnosed with MTC should be tested for the genetic mutations associated with hereditary forms of the disease. A small number of patients with sporadic MTC can have RET gene mutations. To predict outcome and plan long-term follow-up in patients treated by thyroidectomy for MTC, TNM (tumor, node, metastasis) classification, the number of lymph node metastases, and postoperative serum calcitonin and CEA should be used. Genetic status also determines prognosis in patients with hereditary MTC.

Measurements of calcitonin may also be used to monitor for persistent or recurrent disease after surgery because the concentrations correlate with tumor burden. The MTC growth rate can be determined by measuring serum levels of calcitonin or CEA over multiple time points to determine the rate at which each marker's value doubles. Furthermore, serum TSH and serum calcium should be measured postoperatively. The goals are to get patients euthyroid and to prevent hypocalcemia.

Measurement of serum calcitonin. Blood samples should be drawn in the fasting state. Calcitonin has a low stability in serum at room temperature, so the sample must be immediately spun after coagulation and then frozen and transported on ice to the laboratory. Measurement of calcitonin is by immunoassay.[331] Historically, radioimmunoassays were used, but more recently, automated noncompetitive immunoassays (e.g., immunochemiluminometric assays [ICMAs]) have largely taken over owing to their low limit of detection and specificity for monomeric calcitonin and comparable analytical performances. With ICMAs, cross-reactivity with procalcitonin and other calcitonin-related peptides is largely eliminated. Measured concentrations of calcitonin may be falsely high (because of heterophilic antibodies) or falsely low (because of a hook effect, as can be seen in patients with a large tumor burden and very high concentrations), causing interpretation problems. Normal reference intervals are higher in men than in women, likely because of a higher C-cell mass. Because of intermethod differences pre- and post-thyroidectomy and during treatment, concentrations should be measured using the same assay and instrument in the same laboratory. Because reference intervals depend on the method used and gender and whether basal or stimulated (calcium and pentagastrin provocation) calcitonin is measured, each laboratory should determine its own reference intervals based on these criteria. Alternatively, manufacturers' recommendations or reference intervals from relevant literature may be used. Basal serum calcitonin concentrations greater than 100 pg/mL measured by ICMA are suggestive of MTC. The predictive value for MTC of an elevated basal calcitonin is increased by a positive stimulation test result. Simultaneous elevations of serum CEA and calcitonin concentrations in serial measurements indicate disease progression. Misdiagnosis or advanced dedifferentiation of the MTC indicating a poor prognosis should be suspected if patients with advanced MTC have normal or low serum concentrations of calcitonin and CEA.

Other than MTC, calcitonin may also be increased in nonthyroidal cancer, inflammation and sepsis, acute and chronic renal failure, hypercalcemia, pulmonary disease, and hypergastrinemia. Calcitonin may also be high during the first week of life and in low-birthweight children and premature infants.[332] Besides gender and age, growth in children and during pregnancy, and lactation may also influence circulating concentrations of calcitonin.[338] The relevance of calcitonin to bone and mineral metabolism is discussed in Chapter 54.

Anaplastic Thyroid Cancer

Anaplastic thyroid cancer (ATC) is the most infrequent but also the most lethal of the thyroid cancers.[330,333] There is no particular specific circulating biomarker for ATC.

Thyroid Disease in Children

Thyroid disease as described in this chapter can occur at any age; however, some characteristics in newborns, children, and adolescents are worth mentioning. The consequences of a hypofunctioning thyroid (see later) in developing and maturing children may be long lasting if not diagnosed and treated early.[339] Neonatal hyperthyroidism may be caused by transplacental passage of thyroid-stimulating maternal immunoglobulins[340] (due to active maternal Graves disease) or by activating TSHR mutations[341] (see subsequent text). In older children and adolescents, the most common cause of hyperthyroidism is Graves disease,[342] and the most common cause of hypothyroidism in iodine-replete areas is Hashimoto thyroiditis.[343]

Iodine Deficiency in Children

Iodine deficiency leads to reduced thyroid hormone synthesis, increased TSH secretion, which stimulates proliferation of thyroid cells, and consequently thyroid enlargement and goiter.[344] If the iodine deficiency is severe, thyroid hormone production will continue to fall, leading to hypothyroidism. Thyroid hormone plays a vital role in growth and neurodevelopment, and meta-analyses have shown that children living in iodine-deficient areas have IQs that are 6 to 12 points lower than children living in iodine-replete areas.[345,346]

Congenital Hypothyroidism

Before the introduction of newborn screening programs, the incidence of congenital hypothyroidism was estimated to be 1 in 7000 newborns.[339] However, recent surveys estimate the incidence to be 1 in 2000 to 1 in 4000 newborns[347,348]; the incidence is higher in Asians and Hispanics than whites and blacks. The incidence is higher in older compared with younger mothers and in preterm infants versus term infants. Incidence rates are dependent on TSH screening cut-offs.

Congenital hypothyroidism can be categorized into *permanent* and *transient* forms, which again can be divided into *primary* (thyroid disorder), *secondary* (i.e., central hypothyroidism; see earlier discussion), and *peripheral*.[194,347] Permanent congenital hypothyroidism (75 to 86%) needs lifelong replacement treatment, but transient forms resolve within weeks to months after birth.[349] Permanent primary congenital hypothyroidism may be caused by defects in thyroid development, thyroid dysgenesis (85%), or dyshormonogenesis (15%), a biosynthesis defect of thyroid hormone production in a structurally normal gland.[40,350] Thyroid dysgenesis may consist of either thyroid agenesis, failure of the gland to descend normally during embryologic development with or without ectopy, or hypoplasia of a normally localized gland. Central hypothyroidism occurs in 1 in 25,000 to 1 in 50,000 newborns.[339]

Transient congenital hypothyroidism is most commonly caused by inadequate maternal iodine intake in areas of endemic iodine deficiency.[339,347] Transient congenital hypothyroidism may also be caused by maternal antithyroid medication during pregnancy, transfer of maternal blocking antibodies, maternal iodine exposure (e.g., amiodarone), liver hemangiomas causing increased production of deiodinase 3, and genetic defects.

Unless born with thyroid agenesis, most newborns with congenital hypothyroidism have some thyroid function.[194,347] Many newborns, even those with thyroid agenesis, do not present with classic symptoms and signs of hypothyroidism owing to transplacental passage of maternal thyroid hormones. Early symptoms and signs of congenital hypothyroidism include a lethargic infant with increased sleep, prolonged jaundice, myxedematous facies, large fontanels, macroglossia, distended abdomen, hypothermia, and hypotonia. Later symptoms and signs include poor sucking effort leading to feeding difficulties, constipation, developmental delay with cognitive and growth retardation, myxedema, umbilical hernia, and decreased activity. Ten percent of children born with congenital hypothyroidism have other congenital birth defects, and, of those, 50% of them have congenital heart deects.[351]

Levothyroxine is the treatment of choice with treatment goals to raise serum T4 and normalize serum TSH.[352] Levothyroxine treatment can prevent mental retardation in most children (>90%) if commenced within the first 2 weeks of life.[194]

Laboratory diagnosis of congenital hypothyroidism. Newborn screening for congenital hypothyroidism is a successful public health program for secondary prevention of mental retardation.[194,347] Worldwide it is estimated that 25% of the newborn population undergoes a screening for congenital hypothyroidism.

Screening strategies differ between countries with some countries measuring TSH initially with a reflex T4 if TSH is abnormal. Others measure T4 as a first-line test and if T4 is below a certain cut-off reflex test for TSH or measure a combination of TSH, T4, and Tg to differentiate between primary and secondary causes. The disadvantage of screening programs only measuring TSH with a reflex T4 is the inability to detect central hypothyroidism. The initial screening occurs on the second to fifth day of life; children discharged from the hospital on the first day of life may have a sample taken at this time. Some programs routinely obtain a second specimen at 2 to 6 weeks of age. Some programs use cord blood at birth, and others use heel prick on filter paper after birth. Many programs now use initial TSH measurement from heel prick blood on filter cards. Filter cards are mailed to a central laboratory. Each program has its own cut-offs for test results. Thyroid hormone levels and TSH are higher in the first days of life but have usually fallen to concentrations typically seen in infancy within 2 to 4 weeks.

An abnormal result on screening should lead to a confirmatory test in a serum sample, but this should not delay treatment. Confirmatory testing includes TSH and free or total T4 and should be compared with appropriate age-dependent reference intervals (see Appendix for reference intervals). Further diagnostic tests may include radionuclide thyroid uptake and scanning, thyroid sonography, and serum Tg to determine the subtype of congenital hypothyroidism but should not delay the initiation of treatment.

False-positive elevations in TSH may be seen within the 2 first days of life but revealed after repeated testing on a confirmatory test. Transplacental transfer of TSH heterophile antibodies is well described as a false-positive interference in blood spot TSH and maternal thyroid function tests need to be checked in this context.[353] Preterm infants with immature HPT axis and acutely ill term infants may have a late rise in TSH and may not show elevated TSH on the first screening test; many programs have a second screening test for these babies. Dopamine used in the treatment of ill premature neonates can also attenuate TSH release. Seasonal variations in TSH occur with an increased false-positive rate of congenital hypothyroidism in the winter (0.9%) compared with the summer (0.6%);[117] this is in accordance with globally conducted previous studies that have identified an increased prevalence of suspected and confirmed cases of congenital hypothyroidism in the winter months.

GENETICS

Evidence from twin studies has shown that about 65% of baseline TSH and thyroid hormone concentrations are genetically determined,[354,355] with about 20% of the variability coming from common genetic variation at the population level.[105] This suggests a genetic basis for narrow intraindividual variation in these hormone concentrations. Several loci have been identified in genome-wide association studies (GWAS) for the circulating concentrations of TSH, thyroid hormones, thyroid autoantibodies,[356,357] and deiodinases.[106] Also, GWAS studies have identified common polygenic variations in DTC.[358,359]

Genetics in Autoimmune Thyroid Disease

Autoimmune susceptibility against the thyroid gland is estimated to affect 5% of the general population, and 80% of this susceptibility is estimated to be explained by genetic factors. The rest is explained by environmental triggers, including dietary iodine, stress, smoking, and infection.[107] Autoimmune susceptibility genes include thyroid-specific genes (Tg and TSHR) and immune-regulatory genes, which are shared with other autoimmune diseases.[149] Concordance for AITD is higher among monozygotic twins than among dizygotic twins.[360] Twin studies have estimated that 75% of Graves disease is heritable.[236,237]

Genetics in Congenital Hypothyroidism

Thyroid dyshormonogenesis is inherited in an autosomal recessive pattern.[349] Thyroid dysgenesis, on the other hand, is inherited in only approximately 2% of cases; the rest are sporadic. Monogenetic thyroid dysgenesis can be classified into syndromic and nonsyndromic forms. The sporadic cases of thyroid dysgenesis may also have a genetic component but not a classic Mendelian inheritance; rather, they have a polygenic or epigenetic inheritance.

Genes associated with *thyroid dyshormonogenesis* are involved in the steps of thyroid hormone synthesis,[194] including (1) iodine transport into the thyroid follicle through the sodium-iodine symporter NIS[361] and the anion exchange protein pendrin on the apical site of the follicular cells,[362] and (2) iodine incorporation into the nascent thyroid hormone, that is, the enzyme TPO,[363] DUOX,[364] and the matrix protein Tg.[365,366]

Nonsyndromic thyroid dysgenesis genes include inactivating mutations in the TSHR,[367] and the *syndromic thyroid dysgenesis* include genes for $G_s\alpha$ and for the transcription factors TITF-1, TITF-2, and PAX-8.[350]

Resistance to TSH that results from mutations in *TSHR* causes overt or subclinical congenital hypothyroidism.[367] It has been shown that heterozygous individuals experience stable thyroid hormone concentrations and only mild SCH not amenable to treatment, but homozygous individuals experience low fT4 over time requiring treatment with levothyroxine.[368]

Thyroid-stimulating Receptor Mutations and Resistance to Thyroid-stimulating Hormone

Cases of familial thyrotoxicosis with absence of evidence of autoimmunity and children with persistent isolated neonatal hyperthyroidism should be evaluated for familial nonautoimmune autosomal dominant hyperthyroidism (FNAH) and persistent sporadic congenital nonautoimmune hyperthyroidism (PSNAH) caused by rare germline mutations in the *TSHR* gene.[369] The mutation changes an amino acid in the transcript and results in a TSHR that is continuously activated with consequent overproduction of thyroid hormones. As a result, the thyroid gland enlarges (goiter) with symptoms of hyperthyroidism. The laboratory diagnosis shows hyperthyroidism confirmed by high serum concentration of fT4 and low TSH or subclinical hyperthyroidism with only suppressed TSH. Somatic mutations in autonomous adenomas reveal a similar phenotype.[341] Qualitatively, the activating mutations are similar in FNAH, PSNAH, and autonomous adenomas; however, the onset is different.

Thyroid Hormone Receptor Mutations and Resistance to Thyroid Hormone

Two different thyroid hormone receptors are known, thyroid hormone receptor α (THRα) and thyroid hormone receptor β (THRβ), encoded by the *THRA* and *THRB* genes, respectively.[66,291] THRα has three isoforms, the main form being THRα1, and THRβ has two main isoforms, THRβ1 and THRβ2, for mediating thyroid hormone action. The clinical phenotypes in patients with resistance to thyroid hormone α (RTHα) and resistance to thyroid hormone β (RTHβ) are different.

Patients with mutations in *THRB* present with resistance to thyroid hormone β (RTHβ) characterized by raised levels of thyroid hormone, normal or elevated levels of TSH, and goiter, suggesting a critical role for *THRB* in negative-feedback regulation.

Only a few patients with resistance to thyroid hormone α (RTHα) have been described.[290,370] Patients show features of hypothyroidism, typically growth and developmental retardation, skeletal dysplasia, and constipation caused by effects on the GI tract, skeletal muscle, and skeleton. However, these patients have near-normal concentrations of thyroid hormones and TSH, suggesting that the central T3 feedback loop is not impaired and that the HPT axis is only minimally affected. This contrasts with the clinical phenotype in patients with RTHβ.

EVALUATION OF THYROID FUNCTION

Serum or Plasma Measurements

The widespread availability of high-sensitivity serum TSH assays is arguably one of the most impressive achievements of modern clinical chemistry. Serum TSH can be accurately measured at picomolar concentration, with minimal cross-reactivity with other highly homologous pituitary hormones present in serum. Given the classic endocrine feedback loop, TSH concentrations change logarithmically when the thyroid axis is perturbed. Consequently, in most cases and given an intact hypothalamic-pituitary axis, a serum TSH measurement within the reference interval effectively excludes primary thyroid disease. Given the prevalence of thyroid disease and the often-nonspecific symptoms, it has become one of the most popular clinical chemistry investigations. Historically, there has been considerable debate concerning the utility of TSH assay alone as a "first-line" test to exclude thyroid disease because measurement of thyroid hormone is also often required to establish a secure diagnosis.[371,372] Robust automated fT4

assays, which estimate the biologically active fraction of circulating T4, are also widely available, and a combination of these two assays is a very powerful tool for minimally invasive investigation of the pituitary–thyroid axis. The performance of fT4 assays is equally impressive; these work in the picomolar (ng/dL) range and against a vast excess of bound thyroid hormone. However, the free hormone assay designs are complex and are based on theoretical and empirical assumptions. Clinical chemists and clinicians need to be aware of the limitations of these assays when interpreting thyroid function tests because overreliance on the numbers generated by these assays can be to the detriment of patient care, albeit in the minority of cases.[373–375]

Historical nomenclature for both TSH and fT4 assays is confusing and reflects serial improvements in assay design and performance. TSH assays have a "generational" nomenclature that describes improvement in limit of detection, which was required to establish the utility of the assay in hyperthyroid and hypothyroid patients. fT4 assays have an array of terms to describe assay architecture. At this stage in assay development, it is unlikely that any further reduction in the limit of detection for TSH assay will yield a proportionate gain in clinical utility but that there is scope to better harmonize the current TSH assays in clinical use.[376] It also seems unlikely that the "perfect" fT4 assay, which is truly independent of T4 binding proteins, can be designed.[377]

Thyroid-stimulating Hormone

Because TSH is used as the primary marker of thyroid function, serum TSH concentrations must be interpreted against relevant reference intervals. Within individuals, TSH concentrations are remarkably constant with intraindividual variation being at least less than half of the reference interval.[378] Depending on the clinical context in which the test is used, which can be screening, primary diagnosis, or therapeutic monitoring, the "reference interval" concept for TSH may need to be used with caution.[379,380]

Thyroid-stimulating Hormone Population Distribution

The distribution of plasma TSH concentrations in a healthy population is positively skewed. This may be due to "contamination" of the reference population with patients with AITD, which is evidenced by studies of autoimmune markers of thyroid disease in these participants. However, recent evidence suggests that physiologic heterogeneity and the presence of subclinical disease is also likely to contribute to this asymmetry.[381,382]

What can be concluded from both the relatively wide interindividual variation and the non-Gaussian nature of the reference interval is that a "binomial" approach to TSH reference intervals is too simplistic and that borderline TSH concentrations need to be interpreted in context with clinical findings. Clinically specific cut points for TSH concentration have been proposed, above which intervention for primary hypothyroidism is likely to be beneficial.[212] However, providing a useful sensitive cut point to exclude evolving hypothyroidism is more challenging. One attempt is to define the TSH concentration below which the incidence of thyroid autoantibodies no longer increases. However, using this threshold, many false diagnoses would be made in patients with no clinical evidence of AITD. Given indeterminate results, most authorities recommend repeat measurement of TSH.[212,213]

Measurement of Thyroid-stimulating Hormone

Most clinical laboratories use immunometric assays to measure TSH in serum, typically with chemiluminescent probes and solid phase capture antibodies, as this format gives the required analytical limit of detection. Limit of detection of TSH assays is a major issue because it is necessary to measure well below the population reference interval to differentiate primary hyperthyroidism from other causes of low serum TSH concentration. The previously used "generational" concept for TSH assays is now largely redundant because clinical guidelines now specify the appropriate limit of detection for TSH assays. In short, first-generation assays could only discriminate normal from hypothyroid subjects; second-generation assays could detect TSH below the reference interval but not well enough to reliably discriminate primary hyperthyroidism from other causes of low TSH. This can be achieved with third-generation assays.[383] All assays in clinical practice should be "third generation," that is the functional sensitivity (20% interassay coefficient of variation) should be at a concentration of 0.01 to 0.02 mIU/L.[384,385] It is beholden to the clinical chemist to be aware of and to monitor this aspect of the assay.

The specificity of TSH assays is largely of historical concern because modern assays show little cross-reactivity with the other highly homologous pituitary glycoprotein hormones despite sharing the common α-subunit.

Although the clinical performance of TSH assays is impressive, further challenges for the clinical chemist remain. This is because of the heterogeneity of the TSH molecule. The protein is 25% by mass glycosylated and the pituitary secretes a range of glycoforms that differ with thyroid status. This makes TSH assays difficult to standardize because a homogenous reference preparation will not accurately reflect all isoforms and glycosylation state is likely to affect relation between TSH immunoreactivity and biologic activity. This is of particular concern in the diagnosis of secondary (pituitary) thyroid disease as the pituitary can produce immunoreactive but biologically inactive TSH in this setting. However, work by the IFCC has shown that clinically used TSH assays can be substantially harmonized using common calibrants despite the lack of an established reference method procedure;[386] this may allow common reference intervals to be established.

Bioassays for serum TSH concentration are available, but these are complex and difficult to standardize and are rarely used in clinical practice.[387]

Both serum and plasma are acceptable substrates for TSH immunoassay. TSH is stable in serum for at least 5 days at 4 °C,[388] and at least 29 years at −25 °C.[389]

Free T4

Most authorities now subscribe to the "free hormone hypothesis," that is, that the measurement of non–protein-bound T4 in circulation (fT4) is a more accurate reflection of thyroid status than the total amount of T4 (free plus bound T4 or tT4). This is because tT4 concentrations are clearly influenced by changes in thyroid-binding proteins and HPT axis regulation. However, the measurement of fT4 presents both theoretical and practical challenges, which limit the utility of this assay.[390,391] Unbound fT4 is present in picomolar concentration in plasma and represents only about 0.03% of the total. fT4 must be measured despite this vast excess of bound hormone and in the presence of other iodothyronines

such as T3. All current methods represent varying degrees of compromise because it is difficult to separate bound from free hormone without perturbing the equilibrium between the two species. Several assay designs have been established that have been given confusing and often nonstandard nomenclature.[377] Pragmatically, immunoassays for fT4 have gained widespread popularity and clinical use, but an awareness of the limitations of these assays is required to prevent misdiagnosis.[392]

The first level of assay hierarchy is between "direct" methods, which use a physical separation of bound from free T4, such as equilibrium dialysis or ultrafiltration, and indirect methods that estimate fT4 in the presence of T4 binding proteins. Of the indirect methods, immunoassay methods are almost universally used in clinical chemistry laboratories. Immunoassays are further divided into one- and two-step methods depending on whether a wash step is included to remove serum constituents before the addition of the T4 immunoassay tracer. Modern immunoassay methods are also "analog" because chemically modified T4 probes are used rather than historic radiolabeled hormones.

Direct methods are conceptually easier to understand; fT4 is separated from protein bound T4 using a physical method such as dialysis or ultrafiltration. Competitive immunoassay methods were originally used to measure T4 in the protein-depleted fraction, but these methods are now being replaced with mass spectrometric methods.[393] Although direct methods have been proposed for routine clinical use, the complexity and expense of these methods compared with the easily automatable indirect immunoassay methods has prevented wide-scale implementation of direct fT4 assays. Dialysis has been proposed as the international conventional reference measurement procedure for fT4 analysis.[394] However even dialysis methods are not infallible and need to be used with caution as dialysis conditions will affect results. The conditions that determine the equilibrium between free and bound T4 in vivo must be carefully maintained during dialysis. Serum components that can displace T4 from its binding proteins represent a challenge because the relative concentration of these agents changes during the inevitable serum dilution that occurs during dialysis. Nonesterfied fatty acids are the best described displacing agent; these are particularly difficult because they can be generated ex vivo because of the continuing action of lipoprotein lipase.[138]

Indirect immunoassay methods assume that the fT4:tT4 equilibrium is maintained during immunoassay to such an extent that a clinically relevant estimation of fT4 can be returned. One-step methods incubate the assay antibody and tracer in the presence of all serum constituents. Two-step or "back-titration" methods allow T4 to equilibrate with the assay antibody in the presence of all serum components but wash away uncaptured components before back titrating with tracer. Although both methods sequester a significant amount of T4 from the serum pool during assay, the fT4:tT4 equilibrium is maintained sufficiently to provide a reliable estimate of fT4 under most conditions, however given the variety of methods used comparability can be poor. Both one- and two-step methods will fail when the nature or concentration of T4 binding proteins is significantly different in the analytical sample compared with the serum-based calibrator used. This is apparent in samples from patients with genetic abnormalities of thyroid-hormone binding proteins such as FDH or transthyretin (TTR).[395] These effects are assay dependent, with some assay designs more susceptible than others. Patients with autoantibodies generated against T4 are well described; these antibodies are particularly problematic for one-step assays because they can sequester the immunoassay tracer, giving false-positive results.[396,397] Two-step assays are more resistant to this class of interference because the autoantibody is removed before the immunoassay tracer is added. Both labeled tracer and labeled antibody methods are currently used in clinical practice. Although labeled antibody methods have theoretical advantages in terms of limit of detection susceptibility to anti T4 antibodies and binding protein abnormalities remain an issue. Harmonization initiatives by the IFCC aim to establish calibration traceability, particularly for free thyroid hormones[376] have demonstrated that the comparability of fT4 assays in current practice could be dramatically improved.

fT3

Analysis of fT3 presents similar challenges to that of fT4 and being present in serum at lower concentration. Like T4, the hormone is also extensively protein bound, although not to the same extent. Similarly, most clinical laboratories use competition immunoassay for the estimation of fT3. fT3 methods from different assay providers in current practice are poorly comparable, a situation that could be improved by better calibrant traceability.[392] Unlike fT4, to date a reference measurement procedure has not been established. Advances in mass-spectrometric methods allow the measurement of fT3 by direct methods such as equilibrium dialysis or ultrafiltration followed by tandem mass-spectrometry;[398] the use of these methods has brought into question the reliability of immunoassay methods.[399] However, direct methods are considerably more labor intensive than indirect immunoassay methods and so are not widely used in clinical laboratories. fT3 immunoassay methods are also susceptible to alterations in thyroid hormone binding proteins such as familial dysalbuminemic hyperthyroxinemia, albeit to a lesser extent.[400]

Total Thyroxine and Triiodothyronine

Total thyroid hormone measurements are now largely used to confirm the results of fT4 measurements when they are in doubt. Because total thyroid hormone is present in the serum in nanomolar concentrations, it is less of an analytical challenge than the measurement of free hormone. Mass spectrometric measurements are now the method of choice for total thyroid hormone analysis because this technique is relatively straightforward given the sensitivity and selectivity of modern mass spectrometers.[401,402] However, competitive immunoassay is still in widespread use. These methods include a displacing agent such as 8-anilino-1-napthalene-sulfonic acid to release thyroid hormone from high-affinity serum binding sites; this is less of an issue for tT3 methods owing to the weaker binding of T4 to serum thyroid hormone–binding proteins. The efficiency of this process for tT4 methods may contribute to relatively poor method comparisons both between immunoassay methods and between immunoassay and mass spectrometry.

Thyroid Hormone Metabolite Panels

Given the rapid improvement in the performance and the availability of high-resolution mass spectrometers it is now possible to measure profiles of thyroid hormone metabolites including T3 and reverse T3 but also other iodothyronine metabolites.[403] The clinical utility of these measurements is yet to be proven.

Thyroid Autoantibodies

The most common causes of both hyper- and hypothyroidism are autoimmune in nature. Consequently, detection of autoantibodies directed against the thyroid during autoimmune destruction of the gland in Hashimoto thyroiditis or activating antibodies directed against the TSHR in Graves disease can be useful diagnostic markers (Table 57.7). A variety of antithyroid antibodies have been used to diagnose Hashimoto thyroiditis with anti-TPO and anti-Tg antibodies proving to be the most effective. Anti-TPO is most often used in this context as it has high sensitivity (~95%) albeit rather lower specificity. Antithyroglobulin antibodies are also raised in Hashimoto hypothyroidism (sensitivity 60 to 85%) but are most frequently measured to raise awareness of the possibility of interference in Tg assays. These are used as a tumor marker for the detection of residual thyroid tissue in patients with therapeutic thyroidectomies as treatment for

TABLE 57.7	Thyroid Autoantibodies				
Autoantibody	Antigen	Prevalence in Autoimmune Hypothyroidism	Prevalence in Graves Disease	Action of Antibody	Principal Clinical Use
Anti-TPO	Thyroid Peroxidase	>95%[a]	>80%[a]	? cytotoxic[b]	Diagnosis and risk of developing autoimmune hypothyroidism
Anti-thyroglobulin	Thyroglobulin	60–80%[a]	50–60%[a]	Passive	Detection of possible antibody interference in thyroglobulin immunoassays
Anti-TSHR	TSH receptor	0–20%[a]	98%[c]	Stimulatory, inhibitory or apoptotic[d]	Diagnosis of Graves disease

[a]PMID: 28536577.
[b]PMID: 22259066.
[c]PMID: 11069209.
[d]PMID 32022598.
TPO, Thyroid peroxidase; *TSH*, thyroid stimulating hormone; *TSHR*, thyroid stimulating hormone receptor.

thyroid cancer. Antibodies directed against T4 itself have also been described in autoimmune hypothyroidism, which unfortunately have the potential to interference with 1-step fT4 competitive assays for fT4, as they can sequester the T4 trace and generate falsely high results. Antibodies directed against the TSH receptor (TRABs) can be inhibitory or stimulatory; also, they may have no effect (neutral) on T4 synthesis but stimulate thyrocyte apoptosis.[404] These antibodies can occasionally coexist making interpretation complex. The most well-established indication for their measurement is the diagnosis of Graves disease, where they offer virtually unparalleled diagnostic accuracy (>98%).[405]

Antithyroid Peroxidase

Anti-TPO assays are in widespread use as a marker of AIDH because their presence is widely accepted as a risk factor for developing hypothyroidism. Historically, TPO autoantibodies (anti-TPO) were detected as thyroid microsomal antibodies using agglutination or immunofluorescence methods. The principal autoantigen was found to be the membrane protein TPO as described earlier, which led to the development of specific immunometric methods that are more easily automated. Immunometric methods are in widespread use, but despite the availability of an international reference preparation, methods do not agree well.[406] Consequently, results from different assays cannot be compared.[407] Anti-TPO assay is a very sensitive marker for Hashimoto thyroiditis, and it has been implicated in the disease process.[408] Anti-TPO assay is a very sensitive, but less specific, marker for Hashimoto's thyroiditis, and it has been implicated in the disease process.[408] The specificity of the assay is dependent on the type of assay used and the population studied, being affected by age, gender, ethnicity, and iodine status.[409] Anti-TPO antibodies are also typically raised in Graves disease (>80% sensitivity),[406] but anti-TPO antibodies have been superseded by anti-TSHR antibodies for this application. Serial measurement of anti-TPO is of little value because the treatment is aimed at the thyroid dysfunction rather than the autoimmune process.[410]

Anti–Thyroid-stimulating Hormone Receptor Antibodies TRAb

T4 secretion from the thyroid is stimulated by TSH binding to the thyroidal TSHR. This receptor can also be stimulated or blocked by autoantibodies directed against the TSH receptor (TRAbs). The nomenclature to describe TRAbs is complex and is based on either the detection method used or the action of the antibody; also, a "generational" system based on limit of detection is in use.[411] The original TRAb assays utilized detergent solubilized TSHR preparations to capture competing radiolabeled TSH or TRAb from patient serum. As such, these assays were also called thyroid binding inhibitory immunoglobulin assays (TBII). These "first-generation" assays had detection limits around 2IU/L. To reduce limit of detection and simplify assay protocols "second-generation" assays using immobilized TSHR and chemiluminescent labeled TSH were developed which halved the limit of detection and allowed the development of automated TRAb assays. "Third-generation" assays use a high affinity monoclonal TRAb (M22) instead of TSH which further reduced the limit of detection to around 0.4 IU/L. Despite high diagnostic efficiency high levels of TRAb have been described in some patients with transient hyperthyroidism. However, typical features of Graves disease were absent

in these patients, necessitating a degree of caution when interpreting TRAb in this context.[412] While TRAb assays are extremely effective for the diagnosis of Graves disease they cannot distinguish between thyroid stimulatory antibodies, blocking antibodies, and "neutral" TRAb species.[413] There are some clinical scenarios when this can be restrictive. These include:

- The transplacental passage of TRAb: As either stimulatory or blocking antibodies can be transferred to the fetus, knowledge of the antibody class can predict fetal response and direct appropriate therapy,[414]
- "Class switching": Production of antibodies in patients with AITD can switch between stimulating and blocking antibodies. An awareness of antibody type can anticipate the need to modify therapeutic interventions[415]
- Differential diagnosis of Hashimoto hypothyroidism: A significant proportion of autoimmune hypothyroid patients (8%) have TSH blocking antibodies; this may represent a second etiology for autoimmune hypothyroidism or may precede the development of the T-cell meditated cell destruction that defines Hashimoto thyroiditis.[416] As to whether alternate therapies can be used based on the detection of blocking antibodies is the subject for further research.

More complex cell-based assays have been designed to discriminate stimulatory and blocking antibodies;[417] these are based on the generation of cellular cyclic adenosine monophosphate (cAMP) as the second messenger for TSH signaling. As well as discriminating antibody type, these assays have low limits of detection. Unfortunately, these assays are complex and unsuited to the routine clinical chemistry laboratory. Recently more accessible cell-based assays that incorporate a luciferase reporter construct have been developed;[418] these assays exceed the performance of TRAbs and have been recently FDA approved for clinical use. Given the complexity of the bioassays, attempts have been made to redesign the TSHR to be more specific for stimulating rather than blocking assays for use in the simpler competition immunoassay format.[419] This assay utilizes a genetical modified TSH/ LH receptor fusion and "bridging" technology which uses the TRAb to link the chimeric receptor to a reporter construct. While effective as a TRAb assay, the specificity of the assay for TSI alone (rather than blocking antibodies) is contested.[420] TRAbs may affect other functions of TSHR apart from stimulation of T4 secretion such as thyrotroph differentiation and apoptosis, the potential impact of this effect on the diagnosis and treatment of AITD is a topic which warrants further study.[421]

Thyroglobulin

Tg is detectable in the plasma and as such acts as a marker for the presence of active thyroid tissue. Tg concentrations are determined by thyroid mass; TSH stimulation; and thyroid manipulation, including surgery, FNA, or thyroid injury.[335] The primary use of serum Tg measurement is as a tumor marker in patients with DTC who have undergone thyroidectomy, although Tg levels cannot discriminate between malignant and nonmalignant thyroid tissue.[422] It is also used in the diagnosis of congenital hypothyroidism and may be of use in the differential diagnosis of factitious hyperthyroidism. Tg is notoriously difficult to measure owing to the heterogeneity of the molecule, largely because of different glycoforms and because of the prevalence of endogenous anti-Tg or antireagent antibodies that interfere with immunoassay. Current practice for thyroidectomized thyroid cancer patients is to withdraw thyroxine replacement to stimulate endogenous TSH secretion or to use recombinant human TSH to stimulate any residual or neoplastic thyroid tissue.[423] This can be inconvenient, unpleasant, or expensive. Consequently, a Tg assay with a limit of detection required to detect Tg in the absence of TSH stimulation (i.e., suppressed) is desirable.[424] Three methods are in current use, each with its own advantages and limitations.

- **Competitive immunoassay:** These methods are labor intensive and have higher limits of detection than immunometric assays (~5 ng/mL). However, they may be more robust to antibody interference than the immunometric assays.[425]
- **Immunometric assay:** While immunometric assays are highly sensitive ($\leq$0.1 ng/mL) and amenable to automation[426,427] they are prone to antibody interference.[335] Despite the availability of an international reference preparation[334] methods are poorly standardized and do not correlate well. To identify cases of possible antibody interference, immunometric Tg assays should be reported together with anti-Tg antibody results, and Tg should not be used as a tumor marker in the presence of anti-Tg antibodies.[335] Tg-antibody assays are also poorly standardized[428] and cut-offs used as indicative of assay interference need to be carefully considered.[429]
- **Peptide mass spectrometric assay**[430]**:** These assays are limited by the relatively high limit of detection and the low mass range available to current mass spectrometers. However, they offer the promise of robustness to antibody

interference. Proteolytic digestion is required to generate specific peptides small enough for analysis. Some form of immunoconcentration step, either of the parent protein[431] or the specific proteolytic peptide,[432] is required to provide the desired limit of detection. Sensitivities of 0.4 ng/mL are now achievable, which, although not as sensitive as immunometric assays, are sufficient for clinical use. Not surprisingly, method comparison between immunoassay and mass spectrometry is poor at low Tg concentration, which is likely to be due to a combination of assay interference with the immunoassays and the higher limit of detection of the mass spectrometric assays.[430] Whether the robustness to antibody interference confers any clinical benefit is still to be established. The measurement of Tg in fine-needle aspirate fluid has also been advocated as an adjunct to cytologic investigations.[433]

Assay Interference

Despite improvement in immunoassay design, the potential for interference, which may affect patient management, remains an ongoing challenge for the clinical chemist. This is particularly relevant for immunoassay-based thyroid function tests as they are widely used as a test for general malaise. Situations where the immunoreactivity of the analyte under assay conditions does not reflect its biological activity are a major cause of diagnostic error. Several classes of interference have been described (Fig. 57.9).[374,399]

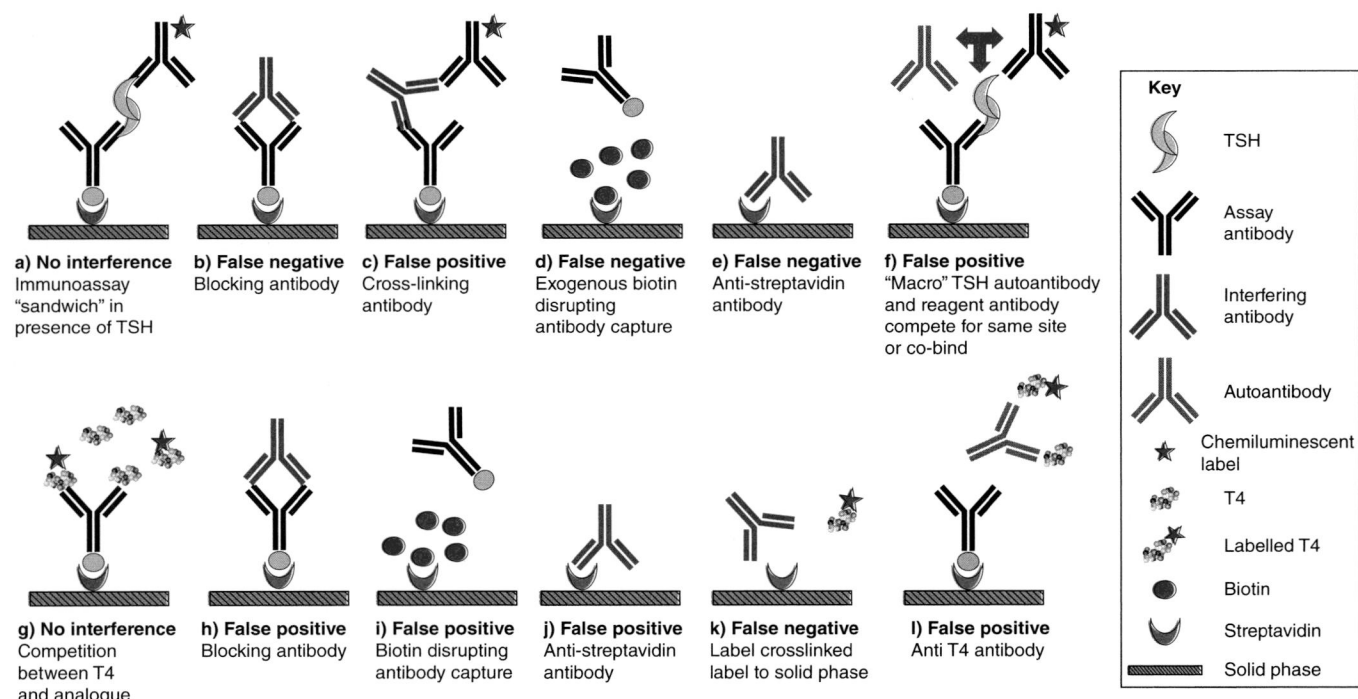

FIGURE 57.9 Mechanisms of antibody interference in thyroid immunoassay. Schematic to show how anti-reagent antibodies *(red)* and autoimmune antibodies *(grey)* can interfere with immunoassay. With immunometric designs *(a to f)* a positive signal occurs when the chemiluminescent signal is immobilized to the solid phase. In the competitive designs *(g to l)* a positive signal occurs when the chemiluminescent signal is displaced from the solid phase. With autoantibodies *(grey)* false-positive interference is caused by the presence of an immunoreactive but biologically ineffective hormone species. Anti-T4 antibodies can sequester the T4 analogue. Macro thyroid-stimulating hormone *(TSH)* antibodies are likely to compete with reagent antibodies but may bind simultaneously.

Interference Specific to Assay Design

The design of some clinical assays leaves them prone to interference from exogenous compounds such as therapeutics. Biotin interference in immunoassay is well reported and is because of the effect of exogenous biotin on the biotin-streptavidin linkage that is utilized by many immunoassay manufacturers to immobilize antibody reagents.[121] If biotin is present at high enough concentration in the patient sample, then immobilization of the reagent antibody can be impaired which can lead to false negative results in immunometric assays or false positive results in competitive designs. This can lead to an unfortunately plausible constellation of results for thyroid function tests giving a false negative TSH result with false positive results for thyroid hormone and thyroid stimulatory antibody tests leading to the erroneous diagnosis of Graves disease. High concentration biotin is an established treatment for multiple sclerosis and biotin–thiamine–responsive basal ganglia disease,[434] but biotin can also be present in over-the-counter medications at sufficient concentration to cause this effect. This presents a considerable challenge to the clinical chemist and physician as neither may be aware of the presence of the potential interferent.[121] While assay manufacturers are attempting to eliminate this class of interference by changing assay configurations, awareness of which assay designs are susceptible to this class of interference is key to managing this potential risk of misdiagnosis. Either rechecking samples using a biotin resistant method or re-sampling after the cessation of biotin therapy for 48 hours can eliminate this effect.

Antibody Interference—Anti-Analyte Antibodies

Antibodies directed against T4 are well described and are common during the destructive phase of Hashimoto thyroiditis. As described above, one-step fT4 assays are prone to this class of interference, as anti-T4 antibodies present in patient serum can bind the T4 analogue tracer and cause false positive results. The incidence of T4 autoantibodies has been reported at 1.8%, but the incidence of significant analytical interference is likely to be less.[435]

Autoantibodies directed against TSH have also been described. The TSH:Ig complex is commonly referred to as "macro-TSH" given the increase in apparent molecular mass of the TSH when analyzed by size exclusion chromatography.[436] In the presence of anti-TSH autoantibodies the relation between biologically active TSH and the immunoassay result is complex and method dependent, as the relevant epitopes affected and the relative affinity of the autoantibody and immunoassay antibodies during assay conditions both affect the amount of detectable TSH. Gel filtration methods, which separate the TSH immunoreactive species by size, have been proposed as gold standard methodology for quantifying macro-hormone complexes, but these methods are also flawed due to sample dilution during assay and the limitations of immunoassay as a detection method in the presence of anti-TSH antibodies. The prevalence of macroTSH may be as high as 0.8%,[437] and as anti-TSH antibodies can be transferred trans-placentally, can be a cause of false positive congenital hypothyroidism screening tests.

Anti-Assay Component Antibodies

Antibodies can also be directed against assay components;[374] these can be specific anti-animal antibodies or weak poly-specific antibodies usually referred to as heterophiles. When directed against the assay antibodies they can either block or cross-link antibodies depending on the assay design. Antibodies against assay components such as streptavidin which is often used to attach capture antibodies to solid phase components via the streptavidin biotin linkage have also been described.[438]

Most clinical free hormone assays are done using indirect competitive immunoassays. These assays assume that the equilibrium between free and bound hormone is maintained during assay conditions. As these assays are invariably calibrated against serum with "wild-type" binding proteins at expected physiologic concentrations and in the absence of drugs that may compete with the thyroid hormone binding sites, perturbation of this equilibrium is inevitable and a source of error to which all immunoassays in current clinical use are susceptible.[138] "Gold standard" direct methods such as equilibrium dialysis are not necessarily immune to this class of interference either as these methods invariably incur some sample dilution, so diluents must not show a differential effect between "normal" and "abnormal" binding proteins. Familial dysalbuminemic hyperthyroxinemia is perhaps the best described binding protein abnormality which affects fT4 and to a lesser extent fT3 assays. A gain of function mutation in albumin (most often at codon 218) causes increased affinity for T4. This effect is clinically benign but typically generates falsely high fT4 results in most assays. The frequency of FDH is estimated at 1:10,000 but varies with ethnicity. Inherited alternations in TBG and TTR have also been described, but at lower frequency.[439,440]

As the T4 binding sites on albumin are not specific T4 can be displaced by other endogenous metabolites or drugs. Two effects are commonly seen. The best characterized is that described above of the displacement of T4 by nonesterified fatty acids. This is typically an "in vitro" effect caused by heparin administration which releases lipoprotein lipase from tissue vascular beds, which continues to act postvenesection and can return dramatically elevated fT4 concentrations with tT4 results being unaffected.[138] The second effect is method dependent and is caused by re-equilibration of T4 and the displacing agent during assay conditions with unpredictable effects. Best described are the effects of the older antiepileptic agents, which often generate artefactually low fT4 results and inducing the enzymatic clearance of thyroid hormone.[441]

Laboratory Approaches for the Detection and Elimination of Assay Interference

While most thyroid function tests accurately reflect thyroid status a small minority can give misleading information. The laboratory is faced with two challenges: when to suspect assay interference and how to confirm its presence. Several methods have been proposed for the detection of immunoassay interference but unfortunately no one single method can detect all types of interference. Consequently, the clinical laboratory has a major role to play in raising awareness of the possibility of assay interference when clinical presentation and thyroid function test results are at odds.[442] Method comparison using a suitably orthologous method is a practical and effective method, and the availability of mass-spectrometric methods for free thyroid hormones and Tg has greatly facilitated this.[399,422] For analytes where mass-spectrometric methods are currently unavailable as an alternative to immunoassay methods that use different assay architecture (i.e., biotin resistant), antibodies from different species, or simple immunosubtraction methods such as PEG precipitation can be used good effect.

Algorithm for Laboratory Evaluation of Thyroid Function

Most thyroid function tests are easy to interpret and will confirm a clinical suspicion of hyper- or hypothyroidism or rule out thyroid disease with good accuracy (At a Glance). The relationship between TSH and fT4 has traditionally been described as log-linear, at least until TSH concentrations are greater than 23 mU/L,[443] although individual variation thyroid axis set point reduces the utility of these data (Fig. 57.10).[444] However, given the widespread use of these tests a significant number of results appear confusing, either because they are at odds with clinical findings or the TSH and fT4 results are discordant. Such results need careful consideration to prevent misdiagnosis.[374] Medications (see Table 57.6), intercurrent illness, and physiologic changes such as pregnancy can affect thyroid function tests. Assay interference should also be considered as a possible cause of incorrect results.[374] If these are excluded, the possibility of rare genetic and acquired disorders of the HPT axis such as resistance to thyroid hormone or thyrotropinoma (TSHoma) should be considered.

Some general principles are outlined:

1. A plasma TSH concentration within the appropriate reference interval excludes primary thyroid disease with good accuracy in most cases. However, TSH will not return an accurate assessment of the HPT axis in the following situations and should not be used alone without

a reasonable degree of confidence that these conditions do not exist:
   - Recent treatment for thyrotoxicosis (TSH may remain suppressed even when thyroid hormone concentrations have normalized.)
   - Nonthyroidal illness
   - Medications such as glucocorticoids, which will transiently depress TSH
   - Central hypothyroidism (e.g., hypothalamic and pituitary disorders)
   - TSH-secreting pituitary adenoma (TSHoma)
   - Resistance to thyroid hormone
   - Disorders of thyroid hormone transport or metabolism.
   It is worth considering the relatively wide between-subject variation in TSH and the effects of extremes of age when considering a reference interval with which to compare TSH results,[380] as discussed earlier.

2. TSH and fT4 concentrations in plasma have an approximately log-linear relation[443] (see Fig. 57.10); paired and consecutive results should be interpreted accordingly. Again, because of the wide interindividual variation of fT4,[444] comparison with previous results is likely to be more valuable than the use of generic reference intervals. In primary thyroid disease, TSH is likely to change before fT4 as the axis attempts to restore homeostasis; this leads to the diagnosis of subclinical disease in which TSH is out of the reference interval, but fT4 is not.[212]

3. Consider the use of additional tests. If TSH is undetectable in patients not on treatment, fT3 aids the diagnosis of T3 toxicosis; indeed some laboratories use fT3 rather than fT4 when TSH is found to be low. TRAb has a high sensitivity and specificity for Graves disease.

AT A GLANCE

Algorithm for Laboratory Evaluation of Thyroid Function

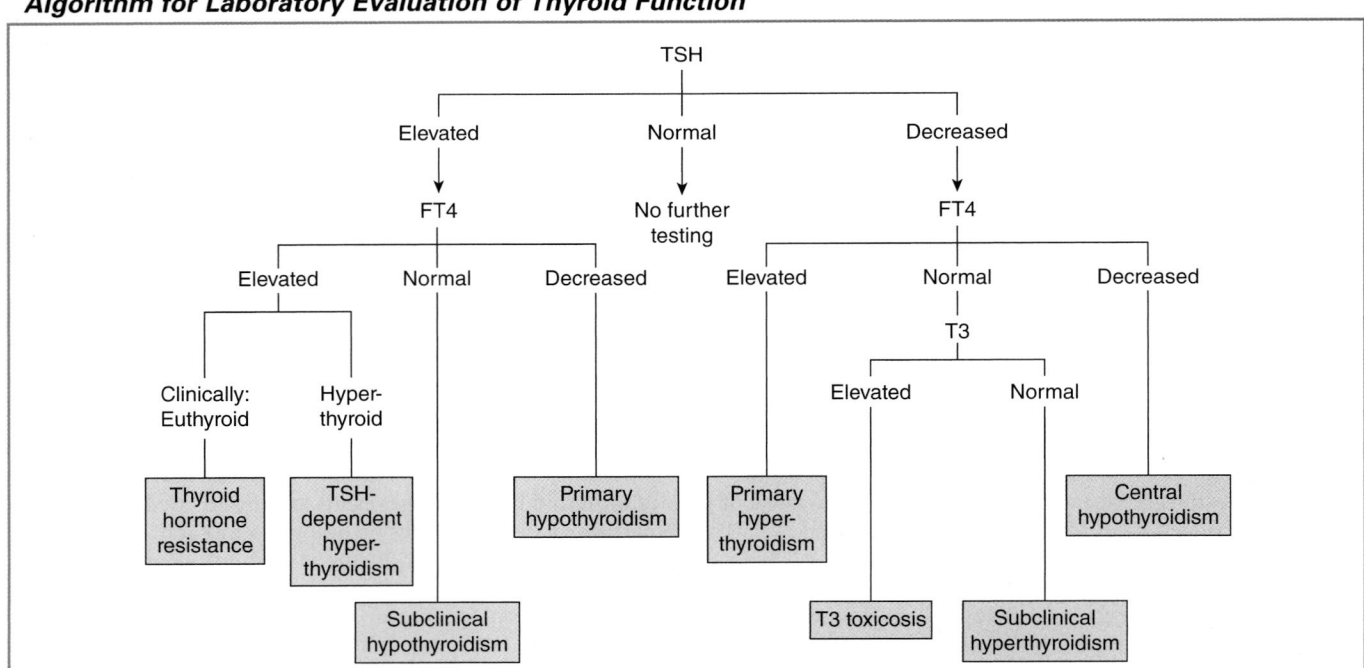

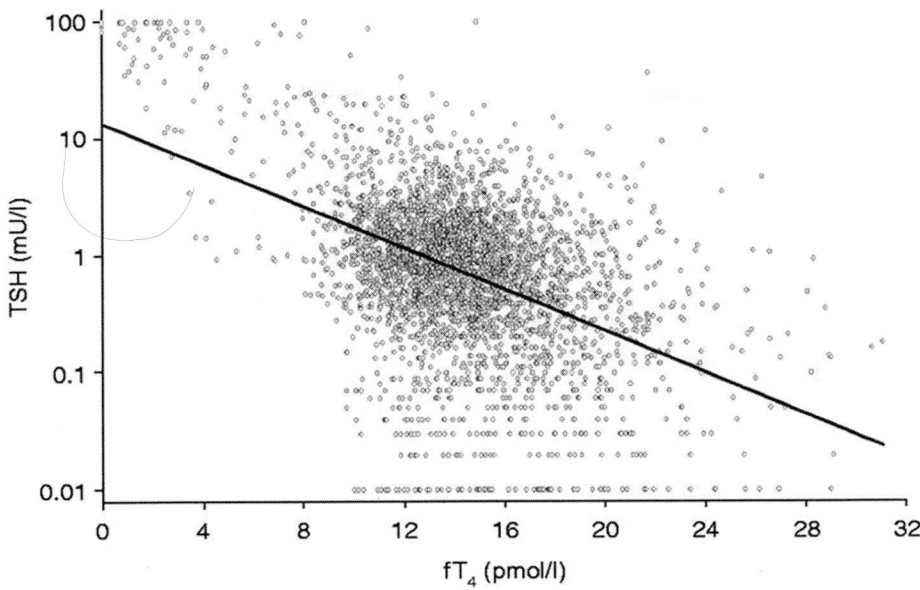

FIGURE 57.10 The log-linear relationship between thyroid-stimulating hormone *(TSH)* and free thyroxine *(fT4)* concentrations in plasma. The *lines* represent the linear regression fitted to the data points. (Modified from Hoermann R, Eckl W, Hoermann C, Larisch R. Complex relationship between free thyroxine and TSH in the regulation of thyroid function. *Eur J Endocrinol* 2010;162:1123–29.)

4. If TSH and fT4 are discordant, consider or reassess clinical findings and the *a priori* odds of relevant conditions.
5. The combination of a normal plasma TSH concentration with mildly elevated fT4 is commonly seen in patients on thyroid hormone replacement. In the absence of levothyroxine therapy, the differential diagnosis includes the genetic conditions FDH[395] and THR,[445] and also TSH-secreting pituitary tumors,[239] although assay interference is more common, and should be excluded before undertaking further investigation.[375,446]

Measurement of Urinary Iodine Concentration

The population status of iodine intake is best determined by measurements of UIC.[78,447–452] Because most of the body's iodine is excreted in urine, UIC is considered a reliable and valid biomarker of the iodine intake and iodine deficiency of the population. Secondary measurements for estimating iodine deficiency are thyroid size, TSH concentration, and thyroid hormones.

The gold standard is 24-hour urine collection. However, in large-scale epidemiologic studies, a random spot urinary measurement is preferred. This is considered to provide a reliable and valid estimate considering the costs, feasibility, and patient convenience. The iodine concentration can be expressed in relation to urinary creatinine excretion or as UIC per liter. Even though the UIC/Cr measurement corrects for the day-to-day variability in iodine intake, water consumption, and the equilibration time for iodine, the UIC per liter is the most widely used and internationally accepted form of expression of results. UIC show circadian rhythmicity independent of age, gender, and season with the lowest values in the morning between 8:00 and 11:00 AM increasing progressively between noon and midnight before falling and

with intermediate peaks 4 to 5 hours after main meals. The circadian rhythmicity of UIC is important to take into consideration in multinational population studies because morning measurements may not be directly comparable to measurements at other times of the day.

The laboratory tests are collectively called urinary iodine tests, although it technically is an assessment of urinary iodide anion concentration. The inductively coupled plasma mass spectrometry (ICPMS) methods have the best analytical performance but require complex instrumentation and qualified staff. More simple colorimetric methods are still in widespread use and are typically based on the Sandell–Kolthoff reaction in which urine is first acid digested under mild conditions and iodine is then determined by a catalytic reduction of ceric ammonium sulfate (yellow) to the colorless cerous form in the presence of arsenious acid.

Imaging the Thyroid

Radionuclide imaging and uptake studies of the thyroid gland were once frequently used in the investigation of thyroid disease but owing to the availability of ultrasound imaging and FNA and biopsy, they are now of less importance. However, there has been a considerable growth in the use of photon emission computed tomography (PECT) imaging to improve the detection and follow-up of thyroid cancers of a variety of types, especially PECT/computed tomography (CT) imaging with fluro-2-deoxy-D-glucose.

With the proliferation of imaging tests such as CT, magnetic resonance imaging (MRI), and carotid ultrasonography, as well as great availability of diagnostic ultrasound devices in primary care and endocrinology doctors' offices, there has been an increase in the detection of incidental nonpalpable thyroid nodules. A small but significant fraction of these nodules is malignant. There is much debate that some of these smaller cancers may not be clinically relevant.[453] Thyroid cancer incidence rates have increased nearly threefold in the past 20 years with much (but not all) of the increase being cancers smaller than 1 cm in diameter.

Thyroid ultrasonography can demonstrate the type of thyroid enlargement (diffuse or localized) and nature, solid or cystic, single or multiple, thyroid nodules. Benign nodules (thyroid adenomas, hyperplastic nodules) are hypoechoic relative to normal thyroid tissue, but so are thyroid carcinomas, and the two cannot be distinguished reliably based on size; degree of echogenicity; or presence of a sonographic halo, calcification, or vascularization. To do this requires FNA or biopsy of the nodule under ultrasound guidance.[454] A Thyroid Imaging Reporting and Data System (TIRADS) has been developed that summarizes low- versus high-risk features on ultrasonography.[455] The ATA in its 2015 Clinical Practice Guidelines recommends that "thyroid sonography with survey of the cervical lymph nodes should be performed in all patients with known or suspected thyroid nodules."[324] Risk factors for malignancy include history of childhood neck radiation, family history of MTC, and multiple endocrine neoplasia (MEN) II.[456]

Real-time ultrasound elastography is a technique to study the hardness and elasticity of nodules in an effort to differentiate malignant nodules from benign but cannot by itself differentiate between benign and malignant nodules. Most thyroid cancers (90%) are solid rather than cystic. Color-flow Doppler sonography is also increasingly being used to distinguish between type I (increased uptake as seen in benign nodules with an active thyroid hormone production and in malignant nodules) and type II (decreased or absent uptake, as seen in benign nodules).

The major nuclide imaging agents for thyroid disease have typically been radioactive iodine radioisotopes (^{131}I, ^{123}I, and more recently ^{124}I [PET tracer]).^{99m}Tc pertechnetate (TcO_4^-) is now used extensively. ^{99m}Tc is given intravenously as pertechnetate and is initially concentrated within the gland but is not organified into thyroid hormones and therefore diffuses out of the gland. This fact along with the short half-life of the isotope mean that large doses can be administered without delivery of a high radiation dose to the thyroid. The disadvantages of using ^{99m}Tc are that it cannot reliably be used to identify retrosternal glands, and it does not give information regarding iodine organification. A ^{99m}Tc can be useful in patients with suppressed s-TSH suspected of having a "hot" thyroid nodule as a positive scan would indicate an effect of ^{131}I therapy.

The use of radioisotopes of iodine (e.g., ^{123}I) bypasses this latter problem. ^{123}I delivers a much lower total radiation dose to the gland than the other iodine isotopes and is used when imaging the thyroid tissue in its normal site. The isotope ^{131}I has higher energy and a longer half-life and is useful when deep thyroid tissue is sought or when there is a need to detect functionally active metastatic thyroid carcinoma and treat it by irradiation.

Although quantitative radioactive iodine uptake (RAIU) studies have been superseded by biochemical tests of thyroid function, they may still be useful to identify some patients with hyperthyroidism and negligible uptake (painless thyroiditis) and hyperthyroid patients after treatment with amiodarone.

Perchlorate Discharge Test

Very rarely, hypothyroidism or goiter results from enzyme defects responsible for the incorporation of iodine into thyroid hormone. In such cases, iodine will be trapped within the follicular cells but not organified. The perchlorate discharge test can be used to detect defects in iodine oxidation or the iodination of Tg.[457]

Under normal circumstances, iodide ions are rapidly transported into the thyroid gland via NIS. The NIS also concentrates other anions within the thyroid gland, such as thiocyanate (SCN), pertechnetate (TcO_4^-), and perchlorate (ClO_4^-). After a dose of labeled perchlorate, if there is an enzyme defect, a supranormal amount of radioiodine is released from the thyroid gland, and the perchlorate discharge of radioiodine is increased. If there is a defect in the NIS (e.g., a loss of function mutation), the release of radioiodine is not increased after perchlorate because radioiodine was not initially taken up by the thyroid gland.

POINTS TO REMEMBER

Questions to Ask When Interpreting Thyroid Function Test Results
- Are the results consistent with clinical findings?
- Are the results typical for a particular thyroid disease?
- Any medications that may explain discordant results?
- Any physiologic or pathologic confounders?
- Consider the use of additional tests (e.g., fT3, TPOAb, TRAb).
- Consider assay interference or rare acquired or genetic pituitary or thyroid syndromes.

SELECTED REFERENCES

59. Luongo C, Dentice M, Salvatore D. Deiodinases and their intricate role in thyroid hormone homeostasis. Nat Rev Endocrinol 2019;15(8):479–88.
66. Ortiga-Carvalho TM, Sidhaye AR, Wondisford FE. Thyroid hormone receptors and resistance to thyroid hormone disorders. Nat Rev Endocrinol 2014;10:582–91.
79. Zimmermann MB, Boelaert K. Iodine deficiency and thyroid disorders. Lancet Diabetes Endocrinol 2015;3:286–95.
106. Dayan CM, Panicker V. Novel insights into thyroid hormones from the study of common genetic variation. Nat Rev Endocrinol 2009;5:211–8.
121. Burch HB. Drug effects on the thyroid. N Engl J Med 2019;381:749–61.
141. Pearce EN, Farwell AP, Braverman LE. Thyroiditis. N Engl J Med 2003;348:2646–55.
160. Bartalena L. Diagnosis and management of Graves disease: a global overview. Nat Rev Endocrinol 2013;9:724–34.
169. Stagnaro-Green A, Pearce E. Thyroid disorders in pregnancy. Nat Rev Endocrinol 2012;8:650–8.
181. Roberts CG, Ladenson PW. Hypothyroidism. Lancet 2004;363:793–803.
194. Gruters A, Krude H. Detection and treatment of congenital hypothyroidism. Nat Rev Endocrinol 2012;8:104–13.
215. Cooper DS, Biondi B. Subclinical thyroid disease. Lancet 2012;379:1142–54.

330. Fagin JA, Wells Jr SA. Biologic and clinical perspectives on thyroid cancer. N Engl J Med 2016;375:1054–67.

376. Thienpont LM, Van Uytfanghe K, Van Houcke S, et al. A progress report of the IFCC committee for standardization of thyroid function tests. Eur Thyroid J 2014;3:109–16.

386. Thienpont LM, Van Uytfanghe K, De Grande LAC, et al. Harmonization of serum thyroid-stimulating hormone measurements paves the way for the adoption of a more uniform reference interval. Clin Chem 2017;63:1248–60.

392. Thienpont LM, Van Uytfanghe K, Beastall G, et al. Report of the IFCC Working Group for Standardization of Thyroid Function Tests; part 2: free thyroxine and free triiodothyronine. Clin Chem 2010;56:912–20.

401. Thienpont LM, Van Uytfanghe K, Beastall G, et al. Report of the IFCC Working Group for Standardization of Thyroid Function Tests; part 3: total thyroxine and total triiodothyronine. Clin Chem 2010;56:921–9.

58

Reproductive Endocrinology and Related Disorders

Robert D. Nerenz and Benjamin Boh[a]

ABSTRACT

Background

The field of reproductive endocrinology encompasses the hormones of the hypothalamic-pituitary-gonadal axis and the adrenal glands that are crucial for reproductive function. Hypothalamic gonadotropin-releasing hormone (GnRH) directs the pituitary to synthesize and release follicle-stimulating hormone (FSH) and luteinizing hormone (LH), which in turn stimulate gonadal synthesis of the sex steroids that govern the development and maintenance of secondary sex characteristics. In states of reproductive health, serum concentrations of these hormones rise and fall in a tightly regulated and well-characterized pattern. In states of reproductive dysfunction, measurement of these hormones in the clinical laboratory often provides the necessary information to identify the underlying abnormality and guide appropriate treatment.

Content

Reproductive endocrinology encompasses the hormones of the hypothalamic-pituitary-gonadal axis, as well as the adrenal glands (see Chapters 55 and 56). These hormones are crucial for reproductive function and include gonadotropin-releasing hormone (GnRH), luteinizing hormone (LH),

follicle-stimulating hormone (FSH), and a multitude of sex steroids. The sex steroids are synthesized by the ovaries, testes, and adrenal glands and are responsible for the manifestation of primary and secondary sex characteristics. This chapter discusses the actions of these hormones in typical developmental and reproductive processes, disease states caused by hormone dysregulation, and current techniques used to measure these hormones in the clinical laboratory. The first section covers Male Reproductive Biology, with an emphasis on testosterone synthesis, activity, and transport and explains alterations in hormonal signaling that lead to common reproductive abnormalities. Similarly, the second section discusses Female Reproductive Biology and focuses on the activities of estrogens and progesterone in states of reproductive health and disease. The third section highlights important considerations for the evaluation and management of Transgender Endocrinology. The fourth section describes the clinical approach to evaluating both male and female Infertility. Finally, the fifth section summarizes analytical Methods used to measure reproductive hormones in the clinical laboratory, with particular attention given to the strengths, limitations, and ideal clinical applications of immunoassay- and mass spectrometry–based methods.

MALE REPRODUCTIVE BIOLOGY

The mature testes synthesize both sperm and androgens. The testes contain a structured network of tightly packed seminiferous tubules. The lumina of the seminiferous tubules are lined by maturing germ cells and Sertoli cells. Sertoli cells play a crucial role in sperm maturation and secrete *inhibin B*, a 32-kDa glycoprotein that inhibits the pituitary secretion of FSH. Surrounding the seminiferous tubules are the interstitial Leydig cells, the primary site of androgen production. The principal androgen in man is testosterone, which serves a central role in reproductive physiology. Testosterone is required for sexual differentiation, spermatogenesis, and promotion and maintenance of sexual maturity at puberty. At the cellular level, these effects are mediated by binding of

testosterone or its more potent metabolite dihydrotestosterone (DHT) to the androgen receptor or via aromatization to estradiol and subsequent binding to the estrogen receptor. Testicular function is under the control of the hypothalamic-pituitary-gonadal axis.

Hypothalamic-Pituitary-Gonadal Axis

Gonadotropin-releasing hormone (GnRH) is a decapeptide synthesized in the hypothalamus and transported to the anterior pituitary gland, where it stimulates the release of both FSH and LH (see also Chapter 55).

In adult men, GnRH and thus LH and FSH are secreted in pulsatile patterns. A circadian rhythm is present, with higher concentrations found in the early-morning hours and lower concentrations in the late evening.[1] LH acts on Leydig cells to stimulate the conversion of cholesterol to pregnenolone in the initial step in testosterone synthesis (Fig. 58.1). FSH acts on Sertoli cells and spermatocytes and is central to the initiation (in puberty) and maintenance (in adulthood) of

[a]The authors gratefully acknowledge the original contribution of R.J. Whitley, A.W. Meikle, and N.B. Watts, on which portions of this chapter are based.

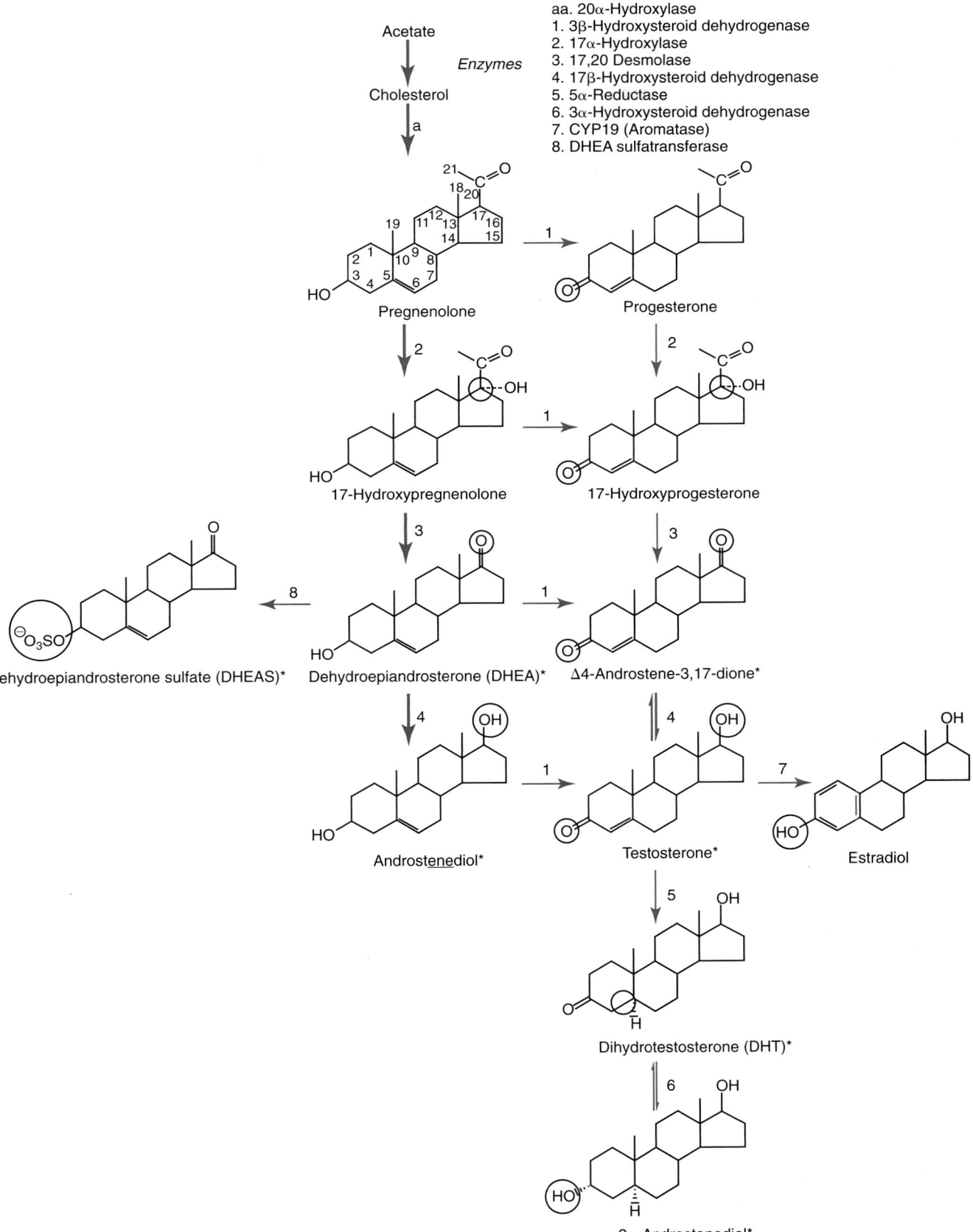

FIGURE 58.1 Biosynthesis of androgens (adrenal glands and testis). The heavy arrows indicate the preferred pathway. The enclosed area represents the site of chemical change. *Denotes androgens.

spermatogenesis. Sex steroids and inhibin B provide negative feedback control of LH and FSH secretion, respectively. LH secretion is inhibited by testosterone and by its metabolites: estradiol and DHT. FSH may be elevated in disorders in which Sertoli cell numbers (and thus inhibin concentrations) are reduced. Likewise, a reduction in the number of Leydig cells (and thus testosterone secretion) leads to increased LH concentrations.

Androgens

Androgens are a group of C-19 steroids (see Fig. 58.1) responsible for masculinization of the genital tract and development and maintenance of male secondary sex characteristics. Testosterone is the principal androgen secreted in men.

Biosynthesis of Testosterone

Testosterone is synthesized primarily by the Leydig cells of the testes (95%) and, to a lesser extent ($\approx$5%), via peripheral conversion from the precursors dehydroepiandrosterone (DHEA) and androstenedione, which are synthesized in the zona reticularis of the adrenal glands (for more information on adrenal androgen synthesis and regulation, refer to Chapter 56). Synthesis of androgens begins with mobilization of cholesterol derived from lipoprotein cholesterol or by de novo synthesis.[2,3] Cholesterol released from the lipid droplets migrates to the inner mitochondrial membrane, where pregnenolone formation is catalyzed by the cholesterol sidechain cleavage enzyme, CYP11A1. Conversion of cholesterol to pregnenolone is the rate-limiting step in testosterone synthesis; however, it is thought that the rate of steroidogenesis is determined not by the activity of CYP11A1, but rather by delivery of cholesterol to the enzyme in the inner mitochondrial membrane by the steroidogenic regulatory protein (StAR)—a process thought to be regulated by LH.[4] Following the formation of pregnenolone, four additional enzymatic steps are required to convert cholesterol to testosterone. The pathway for testosterone formation is shown in Fig. 58.1, with the preferred pathway defined by heavy red arrows.

Androgen Transport in Blood

Testosterone and DHT circulate in plasma freely (2 to 3%) or bound to plasma proteins. Binding proteins include the specific sex hormone–binding globulin (SHBG) and nonspecific proteins such as albumin. SHBG is an α-globulin that has low capacity for steroids but binds with very high affinity ($K_a = 1 \times 10^8$ to 1×10^9), whereas albumin has high capacity but low affinity ($K_a = 1 \times 10^4$ to 1×10^6).[5] SHBG has the highest affinity for DHT and the lowest for estradiol. In men, testosterone circulates bound 44 to 65% to SHBG and 33 to 50% to albumin, whereas in women testosterone is bound 66 to 78% to SHBG and 20 to 30% to albumin.[6]

The biologically active fraction includes free testosterone; some have suggested that albumin-bound testosterone may also be available for tissue uptake.[7,8] Therefore the bioavailable testosterone is equal to approximately 35% of the total quantity (free + albumin-bound). Whether albumin-bound testosterone dissociates sufficiently fast to enter tissues is controversial.[9,10] However, concentrations of bioavailable testosterone correlate with those of free testosterone.[11,12]

Testosterone and SHBG exhibit rhythmic variation in their circulating concentrations. Testosterone concentrations

peak at approximately 0400 to 0800 hours, and nadir concentrations occur at between 1600 and 2000 hours.[13] Daily variations in SHBG concentrations are similar to those of other proteins and albumin in serum, with major changes related to posture. Concentrations of SHBG are elevated with hyperthyroidism and in hypogonadal men.

Metabolism of Testosterone

Circulating testosterone serves as a precursor for the formation of two additional active metabolites: DHT and estradiol. In one pathway, 5α-reductase converts 6 to 8% of testosterone to DHT. Both testosterone and DHT bind the androgen receptor, but DHT binds with higher affinity. In an alternative pathway, testosterone and androstenedione are converted to estrogens ($\approx$0.3%) through aromatase (CYP19). DHT is formed in androgen target tissues such as the skin and prostate, whereas aromatization occurs in many tissues, especially the liver and adipose tissue. Peripheral aromatization occurs primarily in adipose tissue (of both men and women) because of the high concentration of aromatase in this tissue. The rate of extraglandular aromatization therefore increases with body fat.[14]

Dihydrotestosterone is metabolized to 3α-androstanediol (see Fig. 58.1) and then is conjugated to form 3α-androstanediol glucuronide. These metabolites have been used as markers of DHT production in peripheral tissues. Serum concentrations of 3α-androstanediol glucuronide or 3α-androstanediol reflect the production of DHT in peripheral tissues such as skin.[15,16] However, DHT may also arise from precursors other than testosterone. The reduction in serum 3α-androstanediol glucuronide concentrations noted in patients treated with glucocorticoids that suppress adrenal glucocorticoid and androgen production supports this conclusion.[17]

The main excretory metabolites of androstenedione, testosterone, and DHEA are shown in Fig. 58.2. Except for epitestosterone, these catabolites constitute a group of steroids known as *17-ketosteroids* (17-KS); they are excreted primarily in the urine.

Testosterone Concentrations

Testosterone is required for proper sexual development and function throughout all stages of life: fetal, pubertal, and adult (Fig. 58.3). Fetal testes produce testosterone around the seventh week of gestation, with peak serum concentrations of approximately 250 ng/dL (8.7 nmol/L) observed at the beginning of the second trimester, and with concentrations gradually returning to baseline by birth. Shortly after birth, the concentration of testosterone begins to increase, peaking again at approximately 250 ng/dL (8.7 nmol/L) at 2 to 3 months of age, and then falls to baseline again by 6 to 12 months. The function of this neonatal testosterone surge is not entirely clear, but it is thought to be important for bone growth and remodeling[18] and development of external male genitalia.[19] The concentration of testosterone remains low (<50 ng/dL, 1.7 nmol/L) until puberty, when the concentration of testosterone rises to 500 to 700 ng/dL (17.3 to 24.3 nmol/L). Testosterone remains elevated through adulthood until around the third to fourth decade.[20]

Men beyond 30 to 40 years of age experience an age-dependent decrease in circulating testosterone concentration. This has been demonstrated consistently in both cross-sectional and longitudinal analyses. Collectively these studies

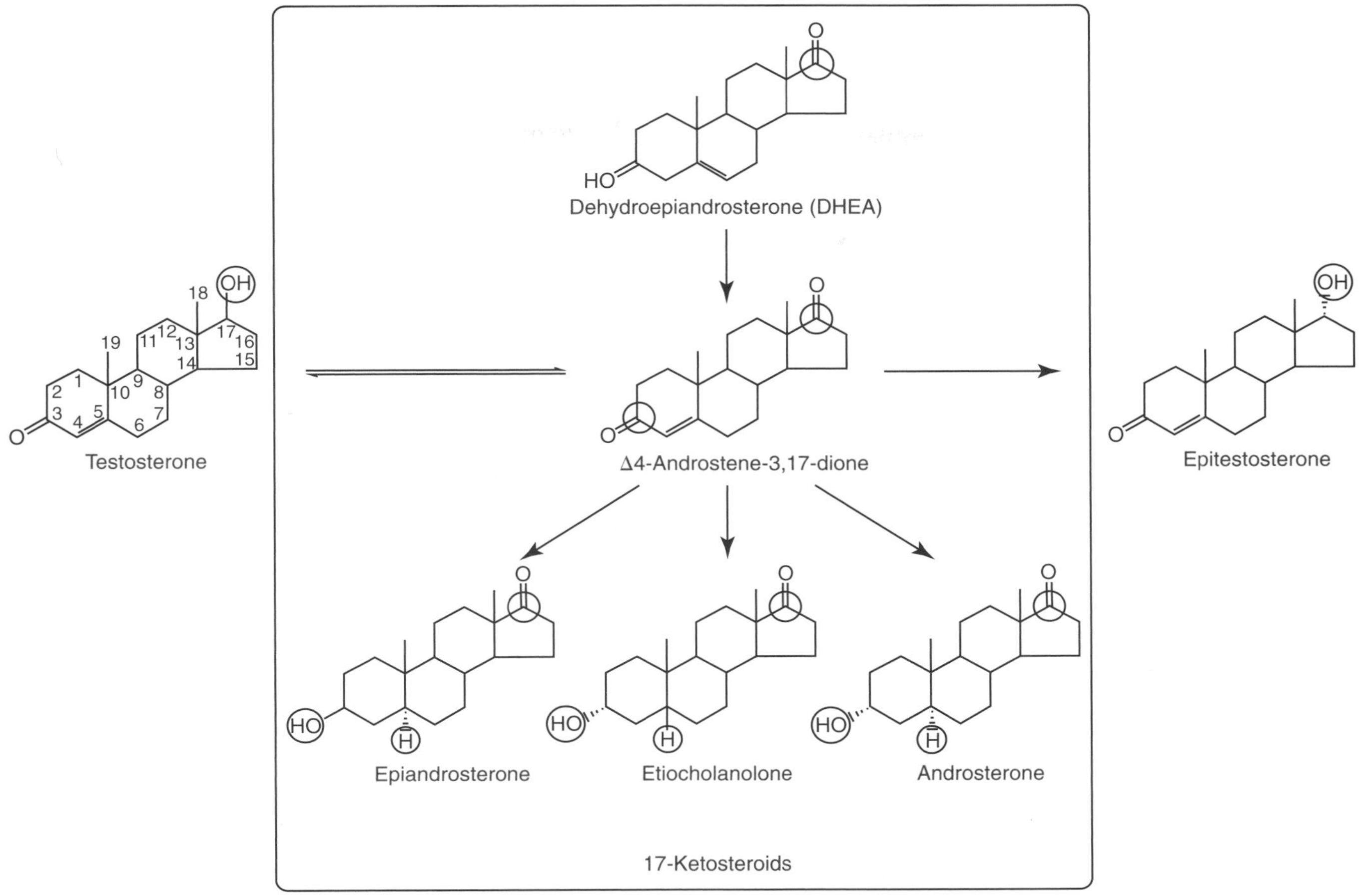

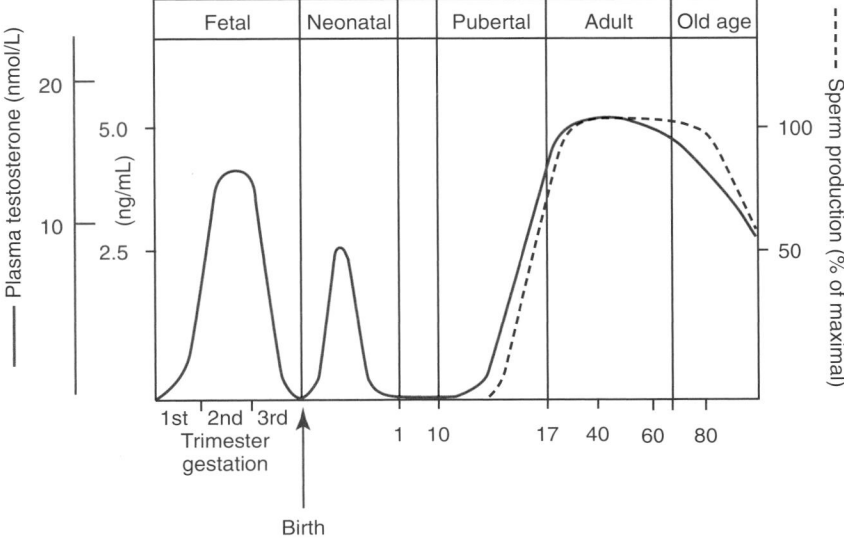

FIGURE 58.2 Catabolism of C19O2 androgens. The circled area represents the site of chemical change.

FIGURE 58.3 Schematic diagram of different phases of male sexual function during life as indicated by mean plasma testosterone concentration and sperm production at different ages. (From Griffin JE, Wilson JD. The testis. In: Bondy PK, Rosenberg LE, eds. *Metabolic control and disease*. 8th ed. Philadelphia: WB Saunders; 1980:1535–78.)

have shown a 0.5 to 2% decrease per year in total serum testosterone from about the fourth decade onward.[21–23] This decline in testosterone is thought to be due to (1) a decrease in Leydig cell numbers, (2) decreased GnRH pulse amplitude, and (3) increases in SHBG.[23] In the past, these decreases in circulating concentrations of testosterone were viewed as a normal part of the aging process. Now, however, these decreases, when accompanied by symptoms of decreased libido, sexual dysfunction, decreased energy levels, and decreased muscle mass, are regarded as a syndrome with a variety of names, such as androgen deficiency in the aging male (ADAM), partial androgen deficiency of the aging male (PADAM), late-onset hypogonadism (LOH), and, erroneously, andropause. The name *andropause* is inaccurate and misleading, given that in contrast to menopause in women, concentrations of sex steroids in men do not decrease sharply with secondary cessation of reproductive function. A name put forward more recently is *testosterone deficiency syndrome (TDS),* highlighting a specific deficit in testosterone as part of the clinical picture.[24,25]

Diagnosis of LOH (TDS) should be based on both clinical and laboratory assessment.[26] Clinically, patients should exhibit symptoms suggestive of testosterone deficiency, such as decreased libido, erectile dysfunction, decreased muscle mass and strength, decreased bone mineral density, and changes in mood. Patients should exhibit one to three of these symptoms with a concomitant low concentration of serum testosterone to fit various diagnostic criteria. Total serum testosterone is the most widely used biochemical parameter for assessment of hypogonadism; although there is no agreed-upon lower limit of normal, recently published consensus recommendations drafted by five professional andrology/urology societies concur that total testosterone above 350 ng/dL (12 nmol/L) does not require testosterone supplementation, whereas patients whose concentrations fall below 230 ng/dL (8 nmol/L) may benefit from testosterone replacement. This value is similar to the 200-ng/dL (6.9-nmol/L) intent-to-treat cutoff published in the 2002 practice guidelines of the American Association of Clinical Endocrinology.[27] The joint societies further recommend, for those patients falling in the gray zone between 230 ng/dL and 350 ng/dL (8 to 12 nmol/L), repeat measurement of serum total testosterone with measurement of SHBG to calculate free testosterone, or direct measurement of free testosterone by equilibrium dialysis (if available). Measurement of free or bioavailable testosterone should be considered when total testosterone is not diagnostic despite the clinical presentation of hypogonadism.[28]

This is particularly true in the setting of advanced age, where concentrations of SHBG have been shown to be elevated. High concentrations of SHBG may result in normal total testosterone but low free testosterone. Transient decreases in testosterone secondary to acute illness should be excluded during this assessment. Moreover, underlying chronic disease that lowers concentrations of testosterone should be taken into consideration and treated appropriately. To assess whether hypogonadism is primary or secondary, serum LH should be measured; a serum prolactin measurement is indicated when serum testosterone concentrations are lower than 150 ng/dL (5.2 nmol/L) or when secondary hypogonadism is suspected.[29] In sum, no absolute cutoffs or specific tests (total versus bioavailable versus free testosterone)

are recommended for the laboratory diagnosis of hypogonadism in the aging male. Each patient's laboratory results should be interpreted on an individual basis, with particular attention given to those parameters of the biochemistry of testosterone (e.g., obesity, age, comorbidities, medications) that may affect the findings.

Some patients may be candidates for treatment with testosterone replacement therapy (TRT). Considerable controversy surrounds TRT, primarily regarding potential adverse effects on prostate and cardiovascular health.[29] TRT in younger patients diagnosed with hypogonadism has been proven both safe and effective, but data from prospective randomized controlled trials regarding the efficacy and safety of TRT in the aged population are lacking. Despite this lack of evidence, TRT prescriptions are on the rise[30]; thus a sustained role for the laboratory in the diagnosis of LOH becomes evident, particularly given a growing aging population of males older than 65 years, projected to number some 31.3 million in the United States by the year 2030.[31]

The Endocrine Society's 2018 guidelines[32] recommend TRT only in men with consistent symptoms (fatigue, decreased muscle mass, osteopenia, diminished sexual function), unequivocally low serum testosterone, no personal or family history of prostate cancer, and the absence of poorly controlled heart failure. The recommendation to reserve a diagnosis of hypogonadism for only those men with both consistent signs and symptoms and unequivocal low serum testosterone is driven by studies questioning the utility of TRT in adults, arguing that underlying poor health rather than low testosterone is the true cause of symptoms for the majority of patients evaluated for LOH.[33–35] This is supported by the observation that many symptomatic men do not have low testosterone and many men with low testosterone do not have symptoms.[36] Furthermore, lifestyle changes that result in improved metabolic profiles are often associated with increases in serum testosterone concentrations in individuals with previously low testosterone.[37] Additional evidence suggests an increased risk of cardiovascular events in frail, elderly men or men with underlying cardiovascular disease who receive TRT.[38] In summary, despite the increasing number of patients receiving TRT, it has yet to be conclusively demonstrated that its benefits outweigh the potential risks for the majority of patients.

Male Reproductive Abnormalities

A wide variety of abnormalities affect the male reproductive system before birth, in childhood, or in adulthood. For the purposes of this chapter, they have been divided into categories of (1) hypogonadotropic hypogonadism, (2) hypergonadotropic hypogonadism, (3) defects in androgen action (Box 58.1), (4) erectile dysfunction, and (5) gynecomastia. The effects of these abnormalities on infertility are discussed later in this chapter.

Hypogonadotropic hypogonadism. Male hypogonadism is a condition caused by decreased function of the testes, which can lead to abnormalities in sexual development if manifested prepubertally. Hypogonadism is classified as *hypo*gonadotropic or *hyper*gonadotropic.

Hypogonadotropic hypogonadism occurs when defects in the hypothalamus or pituitary prevent normal gonadal stimulation. Causative factors include congenital or acquired panhypopituitarism, hypothalamic syndromes, GnRH deficiency,

BOX 58.1 Male Reproductive Abnormalities

Hypogonadotropic Hypogonadism

Panhypopituitarism (congenital or acquired)
Hypothalamic syndrome (acquired or congenital)
Structural defects (neoplastic, inflammatory, and infiltrative)
Prader-Willi syndrome
Laurence-Moon-Biedl syndrome
GnRH deficiency (Kallmann syndrome)
Hyperprolactinemia (prolactinoma or drugs)
Malnutrition and anorexia nervosa
Drug-induced suppression of luteinizing hormone (androgens, estrogens, tranquilizers, antidepressants, antihypertensives, barbiturates, cimetidine, GnRH analogs, and opiates)

Hypergonadotropic Hypogonadism

Acquired (irradiation, mumps orchitis, castration, and cytotoxic drugs)
Chromosome defects
Klinefelter syndrome (47, XXY) and mosaics
Autosomal and sex chromosomes, polyploidies
True hermaphroditism
Defective androgen biosynthesis
20α-Hydroxylase (cholesterol 20,22-desmolase) deficiency
17,20-Lyase deficiency
3β-Hydroxysteroid dehydrogenase deficiency
17α-Hydroxylase deficiency
17β-Hydroxysteroid dehydrogenase deficiency
Testicular agenesis
Selective seminiferous tubular disease
Miscellaneous
Noonan syndrome (short stature, pulmonary valve stenosis, hypertelorism, and ptosis)
Streak gonads
Myotonia dystrophica
Acute and chronic disease

Defects in Androgen Action

Complete androgen insensitivity *(testicular feminization)*
Partial androgen sensitivity
5α-Reductase deficiency

GnRH, Gonadotropin-releasing hormone.

hyperprolactinemia, malnutrition or anorexia, and iatrogenic causes. All of these abnormalities are associated with decreased testosterone and gonadotropin concentrations.

Kallmann syndrome, the most common form of hypogonadotropic hypogonadism, results from a deficiency of GnRH in the hypothalamus during embryonic development.[39] It is characterized by hypogonadism and anosmia (loss of the sense of smell) in male or female patients and is inherited as an autosomal dominant trait with variable penetrance. This syndrome arises from a defect in the migration of GnRH neurons to the hypothalamus. The pituitary disorders are characterized by isolated gonadotropin deficiency with or without growth hormone deficiency. Patients with isolated gonadotropin deficiency display sexual infantilism and long arms and legs; those with combined deficiency do not have long arms and legs. These patients must be distinguished from those with growth delay. In all of these patients, LH,

FSH, and testosterone concentrations are lower than normal. However, heterogeneity exists in the degree of gonadotropin deficiency; hence concentrations of LH, FSH, and testosterone have been shown to differ among affected patients.

Hypergonadotropic Hypogonadism

Hypergonadotropic hypogonadism results from a primary gonadal disorder. Patients with primary testicular failure have increased concentrations of LH and FSH and decreased concentrations of testosterone. Causes for primary hypogonadism are categorized as (1) acquired causes (irradiation, castration, mumps orchitis, or cytotoxic drugs), (2) chromosome defects (Klinefelter syndrome), (3) defective androgen synthesis (20α-hydroxylase deficiency), (4) testicular agenesis, (5) seminiferous tubular disease, and (6) other miscellaneous causes. Aging is associated with gonadal failure, specifically, decreased Leydig cell mass and reserve capacity with reduction in pulsatile secretion of GnRH by the hypothalamus, leading to decreased testosterone secretion.[40]

Defects in Androgen Action

The most common and severe defect in androgen action is *androgen insensitivity syndrome* (AIS), a disorder arising from mutations in the androgen receptor gene (AR). AIS may be classified as complete (CAIS) or partial (PAIS), depending on the amount of residual receptor function. Individuals with complete AIS (formerly known as testicular feminization) have a male karyotype (46, XY) with female external genitalia (labia, clitoris, and vaginal opening). The testes are present intra-abdominally, and because they produce anti-Müllerian hormone (AMH) (also known as Müllerian inhibitory substance), no uterus, fallopian tubules, or proximal vagina is present. The circulating concentration of testosterone in these patients is greater than or equal to that of a healthy male.[41] Concentrations of LH are increased, presumably because of resistance of the hypothalamic-pituitary system to androgen inhibition.

Males with *5α-reductase deficiency* (5-ARD), an autosomal recessive condition caused by inactivating mutations in *SRD5A2*, do not convert testosterone to the more potent DHT. Because DHT leads to masculinization of external genitalia in utero, males are born with ambiguous genitalia.[42] High ratios of the circulating concentrations of testosterone to DHT are indicative of 5-ARD. Moreover, evidence indicates that DHT formation is deficient in the tissues of the urogenital tract in these patients.[43]

In patients with cryptorchidism or ambiguous genitalia, identification of abdominal gonads is essential for proper diagnosis and treatment. The presence of testicular tissue has traditionally been detected by measurement of Leydig cell testosterone production after stimulation with hCG.[44] A growing appreciation of assessment of Sertoli cell function has been noted. Inhibin and AMH reflect Sertoli cell function and may offer a noninvasive evaluation of seminiferous tubular integrity.[45–48] In one study, the mean plasma AMH concentration in anorchid patients was 0.8 ng/mL (5.7 pmol/L), compared with 48.2 ng/mL (344.1 pmol/L) in patients with normal testes.[46] AMH concentrations are also elevated in boys with delayed puberty and partial androgen insensitivity. Inhibin B may be used as a basal serum marker for the presence and function of testicular tissue in boys with nonpalpable testes.[49–51]

Studies have shown that boys with anorchia have unde-tectable serum inhibin B concentrations.[51] Boys with severe testicular damage or gonadal dysgenesis also have undetect-able or very low concentrations of inhibin B, whereas normal serum inhibin B concentrations are observed among boys with abdominal "normal" testes.[51]

Erectile Dysfunction

Erectile dysfunction (formerly referred to as *impotence*) is the persistent inability to develop or maintain a penile erection that is sufficient for intercourse and ejaculation in 50% or more of attempts.[52] A wide variety of organic and psycho-logic abnormalities may cause changes in sexual drive and in the ability to have an erection or to ejaculate. Psychogenic erectile dysfunction is the most common diagnosis. Other causes include vascular disease, diabetes mellitus, hyperten-sion, uremia, neurologic disease, hypogonadism, hyperthy-roidism and hypothyroidism, neoplasms, and drugs. The physician must pursue a careful evaluation of possible psychologic factors, neuropathy, or vascular abnormalities that may be interfering with proper sexual function. If no obvious explanation for erectile dysfunction can be found, measurement of morning serum testosterone, LH, and thyroid-stimulating hormone (TSH) concentrations has been suggested.[53] Elevated gonadotropin concentrations indicate primary hy-pogonadism. Total and even free testosterone concentrations may be within normal reference intervals, yet still may be subnormal for a given patient if found in the presence of elevated LH or FSH. Hyperprolactinemia is an infrequent cause of erectile dysfunction but should be considered in unusual situations.

Sildenafil (sold under the trade names Viagra, Revatio, and others) was approved by the US Food and Drug Administra-tion (FDA) in April 1998 for use as an oral therapeutic agent for male erectile dysfunction.[54–56] This agent and the drugs tadalafil (Cialis) and vardenafil (Levitra) are selective inhibi-tors of phosphodiesterase 5 (PDE5).[56] By inhibiting PDE5 in the corpus cavernosum of the penis, these drugs block degra-dation of cyclic guanosine monophosphate (cGMP), which is increased during sexual arousal. Increased cGMP results in relaxation of vascular smooth muscle and increased inflow of blood. A high-performance liquid chromatography (HPLC) method for sildenafil has been developed.[57]

Gynecomastia

Gynecomastia, the benign growth of glandular breast tissue in men, is a common finding among males of varied ages.[58–60] Gynecomastia, which is associated with an increase in the estrogen/androgen ratio, is commonly associated with three distinct periods of life. First, transient gynecomastia can be found in 60 to 90% of all newborns because of high estrogen concentrations that cross the placenta. The second peak oc-curs during puberty in 50 to 70% of normal boys. It is usually self-limited and may be due to low serum testosterone, low DHT, or a high estrogen/androgen ratio. The last peak is found in the adult population, most frequently among men aged 50 to 80 years. Gynecomastia may be due to testicular failure, resulting in an increased estrogen/androgen ratio, or to increased body fat, resulting in increased peripheral aro-matization of testosterone to estradiol.[58–60]

Gynecomastia may also develop as the result of iatrogenic causes, hyperthyroidism, or liver disease. Liver disease impairs

estrogen clearance and SHBG production, leading to increased bioavailable estrogen and subsequent gynecomastia. Finally, germinal cell or nonendocrine tumors that produce the free beta subunit of human chorionic gonadotropin (β-hCG), as well as estrogen-producing tumors of the adrenal glands, the testes, or the liver, will cause gynecomastia. hCG stimulates testicular aromatase activity and estrogen production, result-ing in gynecomastia.[59] In cases of striking gynecomastia in which history and physical examination point to no specific disorder, measurements of hCG, plasma estradiol, testosterone, and LH concentrations are appropriate.[58] It is important to note that prolactin plays an important role in *galactorrhea* (milk production), but only an indirect role in gynecomastia.

POINTS TO REMEMBER

- GnRH stimulates LH and FSH release, which increase testosterone and sperm production, respectively.
- LH secretion is inhibited by testosterone, and FSH secre-tion is inhibited by inhibin.
- Testosterone is transported in blood tightly bound to SHBG and loosely bound to albumin.
- Free testosterone is biologically active and represents 2–3% of total testosterone.
- Pituitary defects result in hypogonadotropic hypogonadism.
- Primary gonadal defects result in hypergonadotropic hypo-gonadism.

FEMALE REPRODUCTIVE BIOLOGY

The ovaries produce ova and secrete the sex hormones progesterone and estrogen. Every healthy female neonate possesses approximately 400,000 primordial follicles, each containing an immature ovum. During the reproductive life span of an adult woman, 300 to 400 follicles will reach maturity.[61,62] A single mature follicle is produced during each normal menstrual cycle at approximately day 14. Surround-ing the oocyte of the mature follicle are three distinct cell layers: *theca externa, theca interna,* and *granulosa cells.* The theca interna cells are the primary source of androgens, which are transported to adjacent granulosa cells, where they are aromatized to estrogens.[63]

The mature follicle undergoes ovulation by the process of rupture, thereby releasing the oocyte into the proximity of the fallopian tubes. The follicle then fills with blood to form the corpus hemorrhagicum. The granulosa and theca cells of the follicle lining quickly proliferate to form lipid-rich luteal cells, replacing the clotted blood and forming the *corpus luteum* (yellow body). The luteal cells produce estrogen and proges-terone. If fertilization and pregnancy occur, the corpus luteum persists and continues to produce estrogen and progesterone. If no pregnancy occurs, the corpus luteum regresses, and the next menstrual cycle begins.

The uterine cavity is lined by the endometrium. The endo-metrium undergoes cyclic changes in preparation for implanta-tion and pregnancy in response to cyclic changes in estrogen and progesterone. During the follicular phase, the endometrial lining increases in thickness and vascularity in response to in-creasing circulating concentrations of estrogen; after regression of the corpus luteum, menstruation begins, and the endome-trium is shed in response to the withdrawal of progesterone.

Hypothalamic-Pituitary-Gonadal Axis

In adult women, a tightly coordinated feedback system exists among the hypothalamus, anterior pituitary, and ovaries to orchestrate menstruation. FSH serves to stimulate follicular growth, and LH stimulates ovulation and progesterone secretion from the developing corpus luteum. These actions are discussed in greater depth later in this chapter.

Estrogens

Estrogens are responsible for the development and maintenance of female sex organs and female secondary sex characteristics. In conjunction with progesterone, they participate in regulation of the menstrual cycle and of breast and uterine growth, and in the maintenance of pregnancy.

Estrogens affect calcium homeostasis and have a beneficial effect on bone mass. They decrease bone resorption, and in prepubertal girls, estrogen accelerates linear bone growth, resulting in epiphyseal closure. Long-term estrogen depletion is associated with loss of bone mineral content, an increase in stress fractures, and postmenopausal osteoporosis.

Estrogens also have well-established effects on plasma proteins that influence endocrine testing. They increase concentrations of SHBG, corticosteroid-binding globulin, and thyroxine-binding globulin. Hence, boys and girls have comparable concentrations of SHBG, but adult men have SHBG concentrations that are about one-half those of adult women. Concentrations of plasma proteins that bind copper and iron are also elevated in response to estrogen, as are those of high-density and very high-density lipoproteins. In addition, estrogens are believed to play a preventive role in coronary heart disease.[64]

Chemistry

The three most biologically active estrogens in order of potency are estradiol (E_2), estrone (E_1), and estriol (E_3) (Fig. 58.4). Structurally, estrogens are derivatives of the parent hydrocarbon *estrane*, which is an 18-carbon molecule with an aromatic ring A and a methyl group at C-13.[65] All estrogens possess a phenolic hydroxyl group at C-3, which gives the compounds acidic properties, and lack a methyl

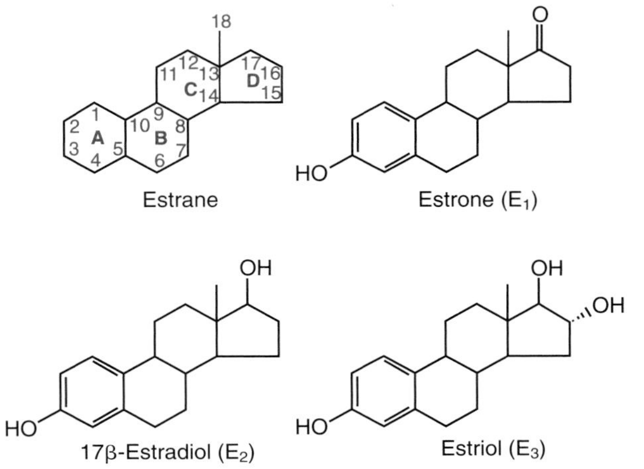

FIGURE 58.4 Biologically active estrogens. (Data from Nakamoto JM, Mason PW, eds. The Quest Diagnostics manual: Endocrinology, test selection and interpretation, 5th ed. Capistrano, CA.: Quest Diagnostics/Nichols Institute, 2012.)

group at C-10 (in contrast to other sex steroids). In addition, estrogens may possess a ketone (estrone) or hydroxyl group (estradiol) at position C-17. The phenolic ring A and the hydroxyl group at C-17 are essential for biological activity.

Biosynthesis

The biochemical pathway illustrating aromatization of testosterone to estradiol and androstenedione to estrone is shown in Fig. 58.5. The role of estrogens in normal and abnormal menstrual cycles is described later in this chapter.

Estrogens are secreted primarily in healthy women by the ovarian follicles and the corpus luteum and during pregnancy by the placenta. The adrenal glands and testes (in men) are also believed to secrete minute quantities of estrogens. The ovary synthesizes estrogens via aromatization of androgens. Synthesis of estrogens begins in the theca interna cells with the enzymatic synthesis of androstenedione from cholesterol. Androstenedione is then transported to the granulosa cells, where it is further metabolized directly to estrone (androstenedione → estrone), or first to testosterone and then to estradiol (androstenedione → testosterone → estradiol). These conversions are catalyzed by the enzyme aromatase. The healthy human ovary produces all three classes of sex steroids: estrogens, progestagens, and androgens; however, estradiol and progesterone are its primary secretory products. Because the ovary lacks both the 21-hydroxylase and 11β–hydroxylase enzymes, glucocorticoids and mineralocorticoids are not produced in the ovary.[66] More than 20 estrogens have been identified, but only 17β-estradiol (E_2) and estriol (E_3) are routinely measured clinically. The most potent estrogen secreted by the ovary is 17β-estradiol. Because it is derived almost exclusively from the ovaries, its measurement is often considered sufficient for evaluation of ovarian function.

Estrogens are also produced by peripheral aromatization of androgens, primarily androstenedione. In healthy men and women, approximately 1% of secreted androstenedione is converted to estrone.[67] Although the ovaries of postmenopausal women do not secrete estrogens, these women have significant blood concentrations of estrone originating from the peripheral conversion of adrenal androstenedione. Because a major site of this conversion is adipose tissue, estrone is increased in obese postmenopausal women, sometimes yielding enough estrogen to produce bleeding.[68]

Biosynthesis During Pregnancy

Research has shown that biosynthesis of estrogens differs qualitatively and quantitatively in pregnant women compared with nonpregnant ones. In pregnant women, the major source of estrogens is the placenta, whereas in nonpregnant women, the ovaries are the main site of synthesis.[68] In contrast to the microgram quantities secreted by nonpregnant women, the quantity of estrogens secreted during pregnancy increases to milligram amounts. The major estrogen secreted by the ovary is estradiol (E_2), whereas the major product secreted by the placenta is estriol (E_3). E_3 is formed in the placenta by sequential desulfation and aromatization of plasma dehydroepiandrosterone sulfate (DHEA-S). Except during pregnancy, measurements of E_3 have little clinical value because in nonpregnant women, E_3 is derived almost exclusively from E_2 (see also Chapter 59).

E_3 is the predominant hormone of late pregnancy. Maternal E_3 is almost entirely (90%) derived from fetal and placental

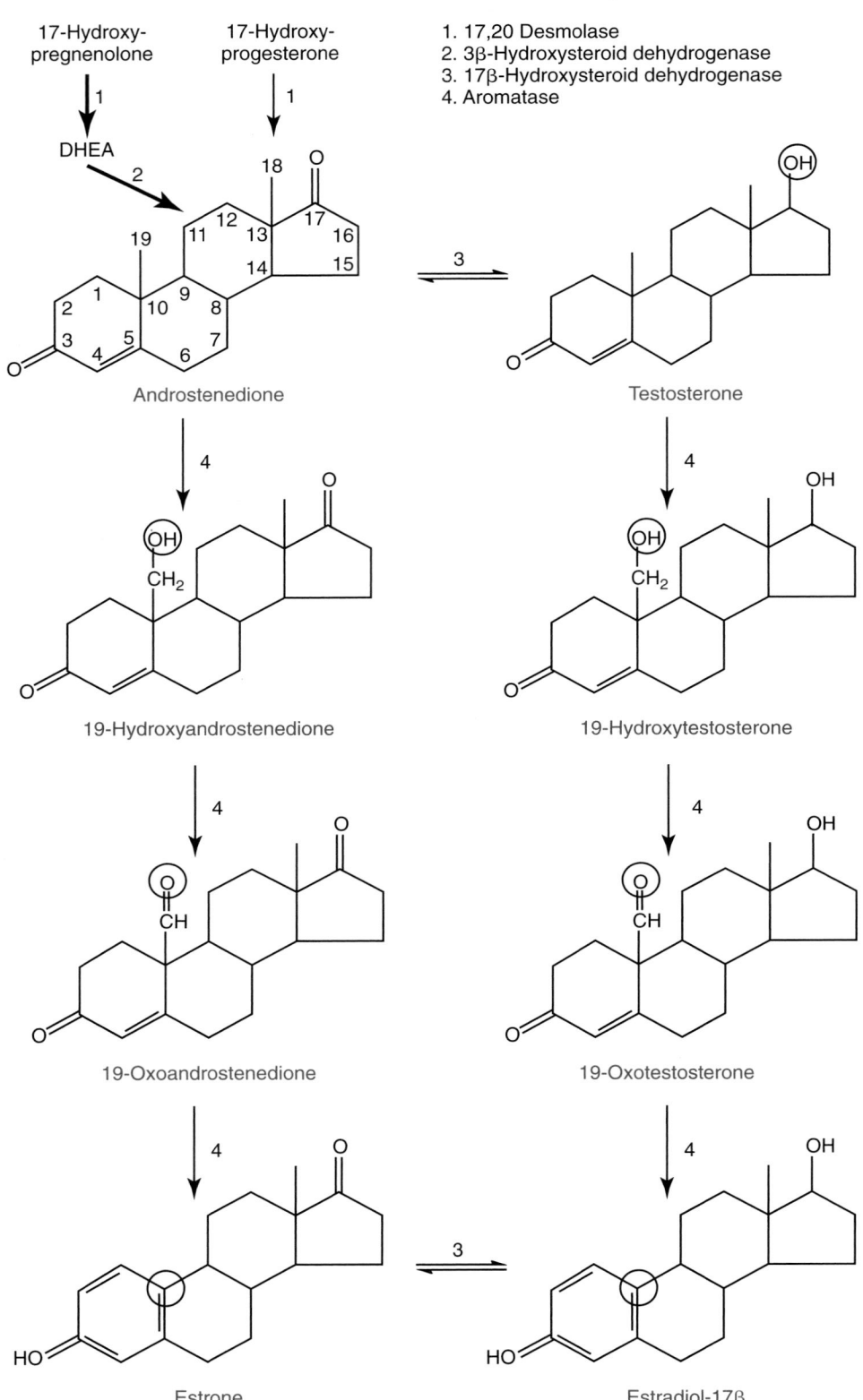

FIGURE 58.5 Biosynthesis of estrogens. Heavy arrows indicate the Δ5-3β-hydroxy pathway. The circled area represents the site of chemical change. See Fig. 58.1 for early synthetic steps. (Data from Nakamoto JM, Mason PW, eds. The Quest Diagnostics manual: Endocrinology, test selection and interpretation, 5th ed. Capistrano, CA.: Quest Diagnostics/Nichols Institute, 2012.)

sources. It is first detected during the ninth gestational week and gradually increases during the first and second trimesters. Plasma and salivary E_3 concentrations peak approximately 3 to 5 weeks before labor and delivery.[69] This characteristic surge in E_3 has been observed in term, preterm, and post-term pregnancies. Some reports have suggested utility in the measurement of salivary E_3 in the prediction of risk for spontaneous preterm birth.[70–75] This test has a high negative predictive value but a low positive predictive value. Consequently, the American College of Obstetricians and Gynecologists does not now suggest measuring salivary E_3 concentrations, except for research purposes.[76] Details regarding techniques used to determine serum and salivary E_3 concentrations are discussed later in the section on analytical methods. For further discussion of saliva formation, see Chapter 45.

Serum unconjugated E_3 measurements, along with alpha fetoprotein, hCG, and inhibin A, are commonly used as part of the "quad" maternal screens for Down syndrome–affected fetuses. On average, unconjugated E_3 is 0.72 times less than normal (median value at 16 weeks: 0.30 to 1.50 μg/L, 1.04 to 5.2 nmol/L) when fetal Down syndrome is present.[77–80] For more on maternal serum screening, see Chapter 59.

Transport in Blood

More than 97% of circulating E_2 is bound to plasma proteins. It is bound specifically and with high affinity to SHBG and nonspecifically to albumin.[6] SHBG concentrations are increased by estrogens and therefore are higher in women than in men. They are also increased during pregnancy, oral contraceptive use, hyperthyroidism, and administration of certain antiepileptic drugs such as phenytoin (Dilantin). SHBG concentrations may decrease in hypothyroidism, obesity, or androgen excess. In women, E_2 circulates bound 40 to 60% to SHBG and 40 to 60% to albumin. SHBG has a higher affinity for testosterone than E_2; therefore in men, E_2 circulates 20 to 30% bound to SHBG and 70 to 80% bound to albumin.[6] Only 2 to 3% of total E_2 circulates in free form in both men and women. In contrast, estrone and estrone sulfate circulate bound almost exclusively to albumin. As with testosterone, both free and albumin-bound fractions of E_2 are thought to be biologically available,[9] but measurement of this fraction has not been shown to be clinically important.

Diurnal variation in blood estrone concentrations occurs in postmenopausal women, presumably reflecting the variation in the androstenedione precursor that originates in the adrenal glands. However, no such diurnal rhythms have been demonstrated for E_2.

Metabolism

The metabolism of E_2 is chiefly an oxidative process dominated by three pathways, of which the fastest is oxidation of the β-hydroxy group at C-17 to a ketone (estradiol → estrone). This process is reversible; however, equilibrium favors the estrone species. Estrone is further oxidized along two pathways: the *2-hydroxylation pathway*, leading to formation of catechol estrogens (2-hydroxyestrone, 2-hydroxyestradiol, and 2-hydroxyestriol and their corresponding methoxy derivatives), and the *16α-hydroxylation pathway*, leading predominantly to formation of E_3 (Fig. 58.6).[81]

Normally, blood estrone concentrations parallel E_2 concentrations throughout the menstrual cycle, but at one-third to one-half their magnitude. Estrone metabolism is influenced by the metabolic state. For example, obesity and hypothyroidism

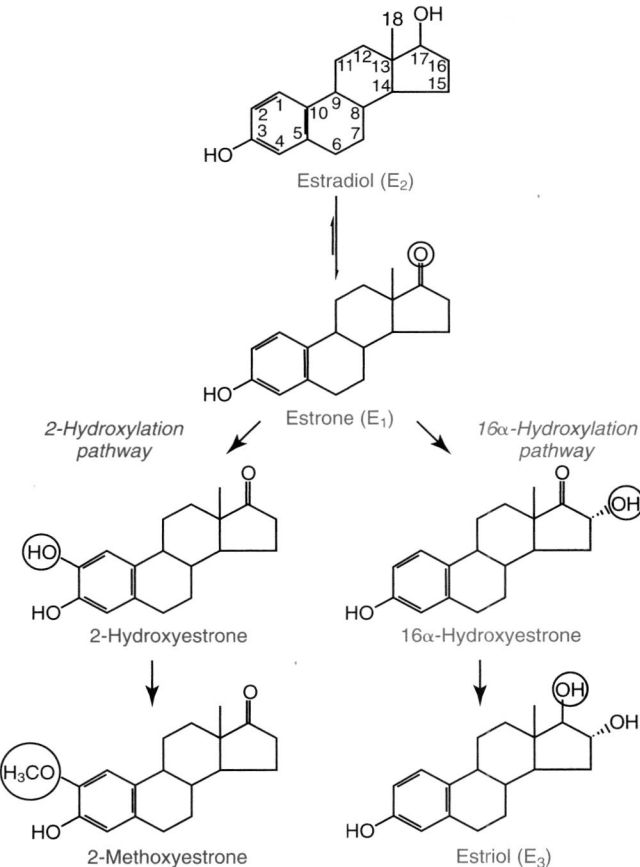

FIGURE 58.6 Main pathways of estradiol metabolism in humans. The circled area represents the site of chemical change. (Data from Nakamoto JM, Mason PW, eds. The Quest Diagnostics manual: Endocrinology, test selection and interpretation, 5th ed. Capistrano, CA.: Quest Diagnostics/Nichols Institute, 2012.)

are associated with an increase in E_3 formation, whereas low body weight and hyperthyroidism are associated with formation of catechol estrogens.[82] Although assays for catechol estrogen measurement are available,[83] they have no known current clinical value.

In addition to the oxidative pathways already described, formation of estrogen conjugates has been reported as a major route of estrogen metabolism. The most abundant circulating estrogen conjugates are the sulfates, followed by the glucuronides, with estrone sulfate circulating at concentrations 10-fold higher than unconjugated estrone.[84] Initially, it was thought that sulfate conjugation would lead to an increase in polarity, making the compound more readily excretable; however, estrogen sulfates actually exhibit a longer half-life than do parent estrogens.[84] These observations have led to the idea that estrone sulfate may serve as a precursor for the bioactive estrogens via desulfation and conversion to E_2 by 17β-hydroxysteroid dehydrogenase. In contrast to estrogen sulfates, glucuronidation of estrogens generally is accepted to serve a classic excretory role. Estrogen glucuronides are detectable in both urine and bile.

Progesterone

Progesterone, similar to the estrogens, is a female sex hormone. In conjunction with estrogens, it helps to regulate the accessory organs during the menstrual cycle.[85] This hormone

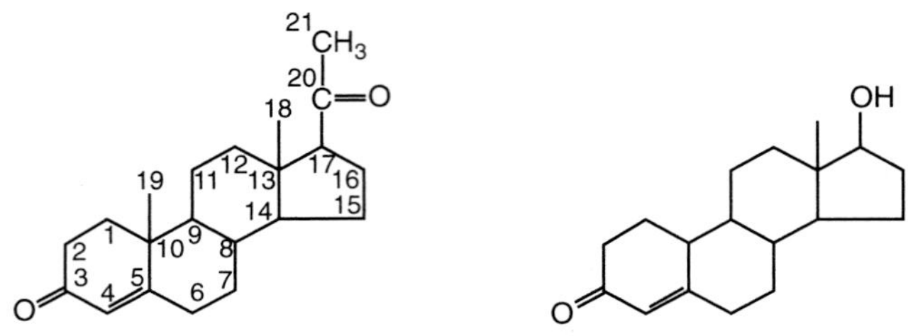

Progesterone
(Pregn-4-ene-3,20-dione)

Nortestosterone
(17β-Hydroxy-19-norandrost-4-en-3-one)

FIGURE 58.7 Structural formulas of progesterone and 19-nortestosterone. (Data from Nakamoto JM, Mason PW, eds. The Quest Diagnostics manual: Endocrinology, test selection and interpretation, 5th ed. Capistrano, CA.: Quest Diagnostics/Nichols Institute, 2012.)

is especially important in preparing the uterus for implantation of the blastocyst and in maintaining pregnancy. In nonpregnant women, progesterone is secreted mainly by the corpus luteum. During pregnancy, the placenta becomes the major source of this hormone. Minor sources are the adrenal cortex in both sexes and the testes in men.

Chemistry

The structural formula of progesterone, a C_{21} compound, is shown in Fig. 58.7. Similar to the corticosteroids and testosterone, progesterone (pregn-4-ene-3,20-dione) contains a keto group (at C-3) and a double bond between C-4 and C-5 (Δ^4); both structural characteristics are essential for progestational activity. The two-carbon sidechain (CH_3CO) on C-17 does not seem to be very important for its physiologic action. Indeed, the synthetic compound 19-nortestosterone (Fig. 58.8) and its derivatives, which are widely used as oral contraceptives, are more potent progestational agents than progesterone itself.

Biosynthesis

Biosynthesis of progesterone in ovarian tissues follows the same path from acetate to cholesterol through pregnenolone as it does in the adrenal cortex (see Fig. 58.1).[86,87] In luteal tissue, however, low-density lipoprotein cholesterol is thought to serve as the preferred precursor despite the potential of the corpus luteum to synthesize progesterone de novo from acetate. Initiation and control of luteal secretion of progesterone are regulated by LH and FSH.

Transport in Blood

Progesterone does not have a specific plasma-binding protein but is primarily bound to albumin with a smaller fraction bound to corticosteroid-binding globulin. Reported concentrations for plasma free progesterone vary from 2 to 10% of total concentration, and the percentage of unbound progesterone remains constant throughout the normal menstrual cycle. The production rate of progesterone during the luteal phase reaches as high as 30 mg/day (95 μmol/day), whereas the production rate of progesterone by the placenta during the third trimester of pregnancy is approximately 300 mg/day (950 μmol/day).

Metabolism

The important metabolic events leading to inactivation of progesterone are reduction and conjugation. The main metabolic pathway for the metabolism of progesterone is outlined in Fig. 58.8.

Metabolites of progesterone are classified into three groups based on the degree of reduction:
1. *Pregnanediones.* The C4-5 double bond is reduced, producing two compounds: pregnanedione (hydrogen atom at C-5 is in β-orientation) and allopregnanedione (hydrogen atom at C-5 is in α-orientation).
2. *Pregnanolones.* The keto group at C-3 is reduced, producing hydroxyl groups in α- or β-orientation. However, most urinary pregnanolones exist in the α-configuration.
3. *Pregnanediols.* The keto group at C-20 is also reduced. As in the previous case, metabolites containing the 20-hydroxyl group in α-orientation are quantitatively more important. In fact, urinary measurement of pregnanediol (5β-pregnane-3α,20α-diol) can be used as an index of endogenous production of progesterone because this metabolite is quantitatively very significant, and its concentration correlates with most clinical conditions.

Reduced metabolites are eventually conjugated with glucuronic acid and excreted as water-soluble glucuronides.

Female Reproductive Development

Reproductive development begins with anatomy during the fetal period, a postnatal period of adaptation to reduced maternal sex steroids, and finishes with sexual maturation during puberty. Normal females remain fertile and menstruating until menopause.

Fetal

In the genotypic female, a lack of both testosterone and AMH causes regression of the wolffian ducts and maintenance of the Müllerian ducts, thus forming the female reproductive tract. Gonadotropin activity in utero is suppressed because of negative feedback by high concentrations of placental steroids.[88]

Postnatal

When the placenta separates, concentrations of fetal sex steroids drop abruptly. Serum E_2 in neonates is decreased to basal concentrations within 5 to 7 days after birth and persists at this concentration until puberty. The negative feedback action of steroids is now removed, and gonadotropins are released.[88] Postnatal peaks of LH and FSH are measurable for a few months after birth, peaking at 2 to 5 months and then dropping to basal concentrations. During childhood, circulating concentrations of sex steroids and gonadotropins are low and are similar for both sexes. However, in patients with hypogonadism (Turner syndrome), LH and FSH concentrations are higher than in unaffected children.[89]

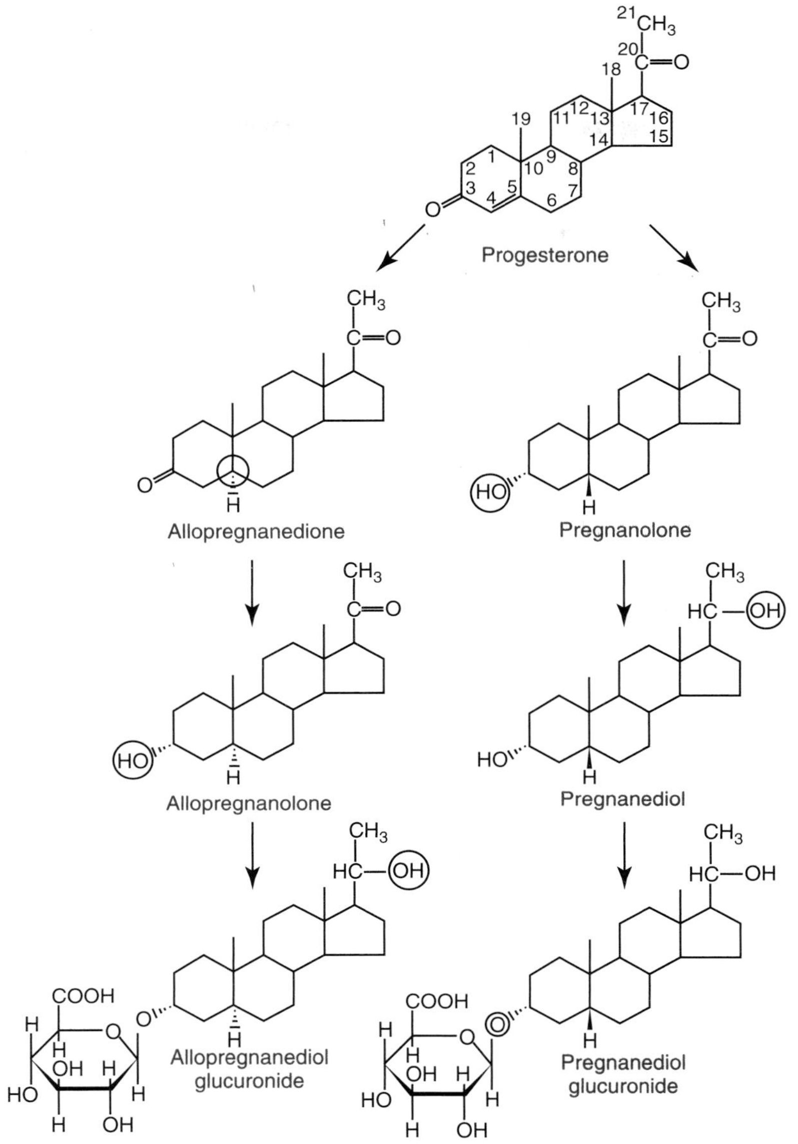

FIGURE 58.8 Metabolism of progesterone. The circled area represents the site of chemical change. (Data from Nakamoto JM, Mason PW, eds. The Quest Diagnostics manual: Endocrinology, test selection and interpretation, 5th ed. Capistrano, CA.: Quest Diagnostics/Nichols Institute, 2012.)

Puberty

The transition from sexual immaturity appears to begin with diminished sensitivity of the pituitary gland or hypothalamus, or both, to the negative feedback effect of sex steroids. The mechanism for this change is unclear. As puberty approaches, nocturnal secretion of gonadotropins occurs. Concentrations for LH, FSH, and gonadal steroids rise gradually over several years before stabilizing at adult concentrations when full sexual maturity is reached. In girls, puberty is considered precocious if onset of pubertal development (secondary sex characteristics) occurs before the age of 8 years (see later section on precocious puberty) and is considered delayed if no development has occurred by the age of 13 years or if menarche has not occurred by age 16.5 years.[89] It was reported in 2003 that the median age of menarche in the United States is 12.43 years, which is 0.34 year earlier than that reported in 1973.[90,91] This study also found that the median age at menarche of non-Hispanic black (12.06 years)

girls is significantly earlier than that of non-Hispanic white (12.55 years) and Mexican American (12.25 years) girls.[90]

Adrenarche precedes puberty by a few years. In girls, the rise in adrenal androgen concentrations (DHEA, DHEA-S, and androstenedione) begins at age 6 to 7 years.[92] This rise in adrenal androgen concentrations lasts until late puberty. A cortical androgen-stimulating hormone may contribute to the rise in adrenal androgens at puberty in both sexes but its existence has not been definitively proven and other structural mechanisms have been proposed.[93] In girls, puberty is associated with elevations in estrogen secretion by the ovary in response to gonadotropin concentrations that increase in response to GnRH. Estrogen secretion by the ovary increases, causing enlargement of the uterus and breasts. In the breast, estrogen enhances growth of ducts; progesterone augments this effect. As the breast develops, estrogen increases adipose tissue around the lactiferous duct system, contributing to the further enlargement of breast tissue.[94] These physiologic and physical processes associated with puberty in girls culminate in *menarche*—the beginning of menstrual function and the first menstrual period.

Normal Menstrual Cycle

During a normal menstrual cycle, a closely coordinated interplay of feedback effects occurs between the hypothalamus, the anterior lobe of the pituitary gland, and the ovaries. In addition, cyclic hormone changes lead to functional and structural changes in the ovaries (follicle maturation, ovulation, and corpus luteum development), uterus (preparation of the endometrium for possible implantation of the fertilized ovum), cervix (to permit transport of sperm), and vagina (Fig. 58.9).

Phases. The menstrual cycle is measured beginning on day 1 as the first day of menstrual bleeding. Each cycle consists of a follicular phase followed by ovulation and then a luteal phase.

Follicular phase. The *follicular phase*—that is, the selection and growth of the dominant follicle—actually begins during the last few days of the previous luteal phase and terminates at ovulation (see Fig. 58.9). During the early part of the follicular phase, concentrations of FSH rise and then decline up until ovulation (see Fig. 58.9). LH secretion begins to increase around the middle of the follicular phase. Just before ovulation, estrogen secretion by the follicle increases dramatically; this positively stimulates the hypothalamus and triggers the LH surge. The LH surge is a reliable predictor of

ovulation, with onset of the surge for 90% of women occurring 16 to 58 hours before, and the peak occurring 3 to 36 hours before, ovulation.[95] Ovulation occurs around day 14 in a 28-day menstrual cycle.

Luteal phase. The *luteal phase*, the last half of the cycle, is characterized by increasing production of progesterone and estrogen from the corpus luteum with consequent gradual lowering of LH and FSH concentrations. The concentration of progesterone reaches a peak at about 8 days after ovulation. If ovulation does not occur, the corpus luteum fails to form, and a cyclic rise in progesterone is subnormal. If ovulation and pregnancy occur, hCG maintains the corpus luteum, and progesterone continues to rise. In the absence of conception, the corpus luteum resolves, resulting in a decrease in estrogen and progesterone concentrations and a breakdown of the endometrium. The average duration of menstrual flow is 4 to 6 days, and average menstrual blood loss is 30 mL.[96]

Cycle variation. Healthy women display considerable variation in cycle length ranging from 26 to 34 days (29 days on average).[97] Much of the cycle variation can be attributed to variation in the length of the follicular phase while the length of the luteal phase remains relatively constant.[98]

Role of individual hormones. To explain further the intricacies of the normal menstrual cycle, fluctuations in each major hormone are discussed separately in the following sections with regard to control and effects (see Fig. 58.9).

Gonadotropin-releasing hormone. Gonadotropin-releasing hormone triggers the surge of LH that precedes ovulation.[99]

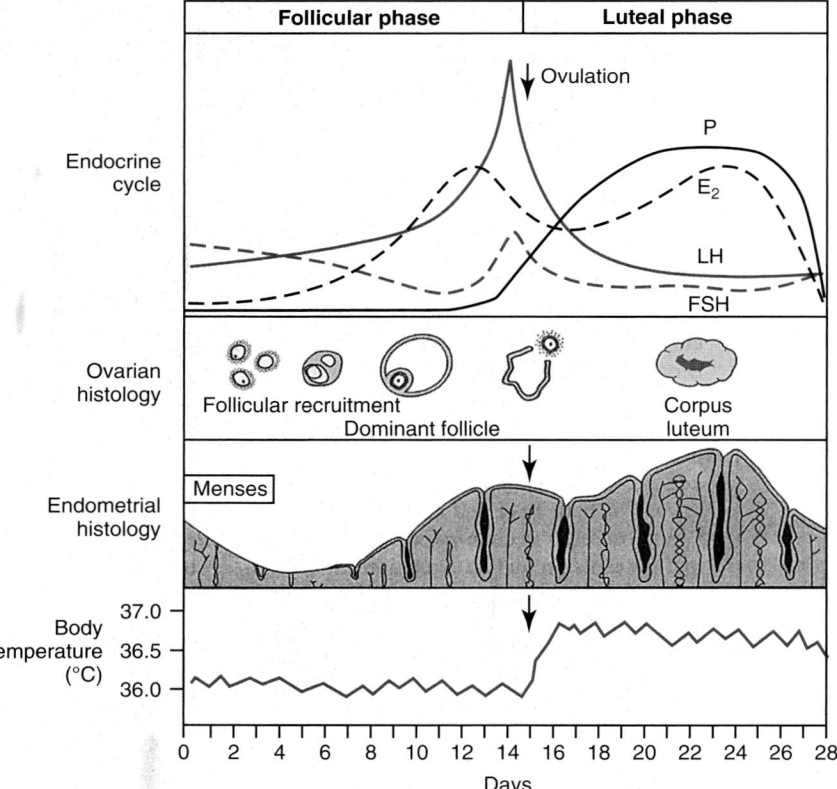

FIGURE 58.9 Hormonal, ovarian, endometrial, and basal body temperature changes throughout the normal menstrual cycle. (Data from Nakamoto JM, Mason PW, eds. The Quest Diagnostics manual: Endocrinology, test selection and interpretation, 5th ed. Capistrano, CA.: Quest Diagnostics/Nichols Institute, 2012.)

There appear to be two separate feedback centers in the hypothalamus: a tonic negative feedback center in the basal medial hypothalamus and a cyclic positive feedback center in the anterior regions of the hypothalamus. Low concentrations of E_2, such as those that are present during the follicular phase, affect the negative feedback center, whereas high concentrations of E_2, such as those seen just before the midcycle LH peak, trigger the positive feedback center. Progesterone, in combination with estrogen, affects the negative feedback center in the luteal phase. GnRH is released in a pulsatile fashion and has a self-priming effect; the first dose potentiates the effects of subsequent doses. The magnitude of the LH response to GnRH increases steadily through the follicular phase and is greatest at the time of the preovulatory surge of LH, after which it declines again.

Follicle-stimulating hormone. A few days before day 1 of the cycle, FSH begins to rise (see Fig. 58.9), probably triggered by a fall in E_2 concentration that briefly eliminates the negative feedback effect.[100] This rise in FSH initiates the growth of a cohort of ovarian follicles. LH and FSH release is pulsatile throughout the cycle; therefore the values shown in Fig. 58.9 represent integrated concentrations. As estrogen is released from the growing follicles, FSH concentrations fall again and remain low through the follicular phase. By days 5 to 7, a single, dominant follicle is selected for further growth and maturation. The effect of FSH on the maturing follicle is increased through estradiol-induced changes in FSH receptors. FSH, aided by E_2, acts on the cells of the follicle to increase the responsiveness of LH receptors by the time of the midcycle surge. FSH and LH receptors respond with an increase in their number or in their affinity for corresponding gonadotropin. A rise in FSH at midcycle is triggered by progesterone. The function of this peak is not entirely known, but it is thought to stimulate plasminogen activator and increase granulosa cell LH receptors.[101] During the luteal phase, FSH is suppressed by negative feedback from E_2 until a lesser FSH peak, occurring near the end of the cycle, starts off the follicular recruitment for the next cycle.

Luteinizing hormone. Luteinizing hormone secretion is suppressed in the follicular phase by negative feedback from E_2.[99,100] As E_2 production by the developing follicle increases, the effect of E_2 on the positive feedback center becomes important. Increasing release of GnRH from the hypothalamus and increasing the sensitivity of the anterior lobe of the pituitary gland to GnRH lead to the midcycle surge of LH. Ovarian follicle receptors for LH, sensitized by FSH and E_2, transmit the stimulus to enhance differentiation of the theca cell and production of progesterone by the developing corpus luteum. LH production is suppressed during the luteal phase by negative feedback from progesterone combined with E_2, but a low concentration of LH is probably necessary to prolong corpus luteum function.

Estradiol. E_2 production by the ovary decreases near the end of a cycle but begins to increase again under the influence of FSH (see Fig. 58.9).[101] E_2 enhances the FSH effect on a maturing follicle through changes in FSH receptors of the follicular cells, but it suppresses pituitary FSH and LH release during the follicular phase through negative feedback. Before the mid-follicular phase, estrogen concentrations are less than 50 pg/mL (183.5 pmol/L), but they increase rapidly as the follicle matures (Appendix – Reference Information for the Clinical Laboratory). E_2 production increases, reaching a midcycle peak at between 250 and 500 pg/mL (917.5 to 1835 pmol/L). E_2 concentrations decrease abruptly after ovulation but increase again as the corpus luteum is formed, reaching concentrations of approximately 125 pg/mL (458.8 pmol/L) during the luteal phase. Progesterone produced by the corpus luteum, combined with E_2, exerts a negative effect on the hypothalamus and anterior lobe of the pituitary gland. As a result, LH and FSH secretion is suppressed again during the luteal phase. E_2 is essential for the development of proliferative endometrium and is synergistic with progesterone for the development of changes in the endometrium that initiate shedding; the decrease in negative feedback from E_2 on the anterior lobe of the pituitary gland triggers the FSH surge that begins the development of an ovarian follicle for the next cycle.

E_2 is not the only estrogen produced; estrone secretion, mainly from peripheral sources, also is increased throughout the cycle. Estrogen and progesterone have visible effects on vaginal cytology and cervical mucus, and progesterone elevates body temperature (as discussed later). Changes in androgen production also occur during the menstrual cycle, with a peak at midcycle.

Progesterone. Progesterone is not produced in significant amounts until the midcycle LH surge and ovulation. LH enhances theca cell differentiation and progesterone production, which increase by a factor of 10 to 20 to a maximum about 8 days after the midcycle peak of LH. Progesterone is thought to stimulate the ovulatory peak of FSH and to promote the growth of secretory endometrium, which is necessary for implantation of the fertilized ovum.[85]

Ovulation. An intricate interplay of endocrine events contributes to follicular maturation. Growth of ovarian follicles appears to be continuous. How an individual follicle is singled out for each menstrual cycle is not known; however, the late-cycle peak in FSH concentration is likely important in this process. Once a follicle has been stimulated, E_2 production causes that specific follicle to be more receptive to effects of FSH. The high concentration of E_2 just before midcycle is responsible for triggering positive feedback in the hypothalamus that leads to the midcycle LH surge. After ovulation, LH is suppressed by progesterone and E_2, but the effect of LH on the corpus luteum is increased.[102] In the event of successful fertilization and implantation, corpus luteum function is sustained by hCG produced by trophoblastic cells of the developing embryo with high molecular homology to LH and is capable of binding and stimulating LH receptors. Otherwise, the declining concentration of E_2 leads to regression of the corpus luteum and to the late-cycle FSH peak that starts the process again.

Menopause

Menopause is defined as the permanent cessation of menstruation resulting from loss of ovarian follicular activity. It begins with the ovaries failing to produce adequate amounts of estrogen and inhibins A and B; as a result, gonadotropin production is increased in a continued attempt to stimulate the ovary (Fig. 58.10). The mean age of menopause in the United States is 51 years but varies considerably.[103] Ovarian failure may occur at any age, but menopause before age 40 years is considered premature.[104]

Hormonal changes begin about 5 years before the actual menopause, as the response of the ovary to gonadotropins

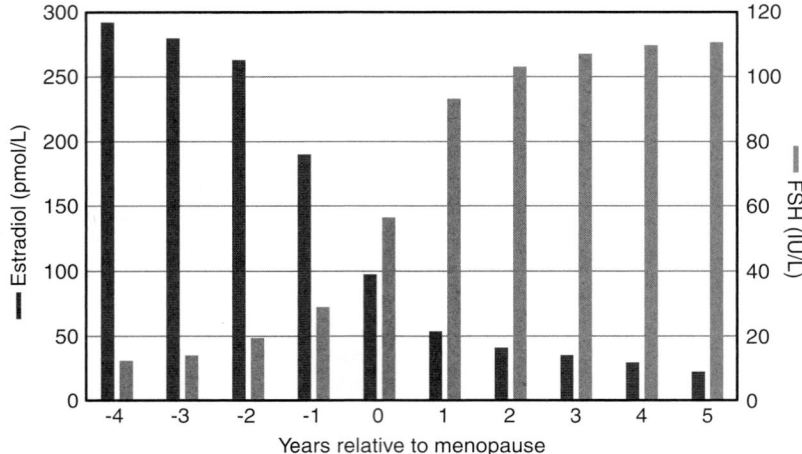

FIGURE 58.10 Geometric means for follicle-stimulating hormone *(FSH)* and estradiol in relation to the final menstrual period (FMP). The horizontal axis represents time (y) with respect to the FMP (0); negative (positive) numbers represent time before (after) the FMP. (Data from Nakamoto JM, Mason PW, eds. The Quest Diagnostics manual: Endocrinology, test selection and interpretation, 5th ed. Capistrano, CA.: Quest Diagnostics/Nichols Institute, 2012.)

begins to decrease and menstrual cycles become increasingly irregular.[105] The term *perimenopausal* refers to the time interval from onset of these menstrual irregularities to menopause itself. This transition phase will last from 2 to 8 years.[105] At this time, FSH concentrations increase and E_2 concentrations decrease, whereas LH and progesterone concentrations remain unchanged, indicating that menstrual cycles remain ovulatory. As estrogen continues to decline, an associated decrease in prolactin concentrations is noted. The decrease in estrogen concentrations gives rise to vasomotor instability and so-called "hot flashes."

After menopause, the ovary continues to produce androgens, particularly testosterone and androstenedione, as a result of increased LH concentrations. In addition, the adrenal gland continues to secrete androgens. The resulting decrease in the estrogen/androgen ratio is the cause of the hirsutism seen in some postmenopausal women.[106] In general, menopause may be diagnosed in women over the age of 45 on the basis of menstrual history and age without relying on laboratory test results, although serum FSH values may be helpful.[107,108] In women younger than 40 with menopausal symptoms and irregular menses, other causes of menstrual irregularities should be ruled out prior to making the diagnosis of primary ovarian insufficiency (POI) (previously known as premature ovarian failure [POF]). The etiology of POI warrants further investigation.

The issue of hormone replacement therapy (HRT) for vasomotor symptoms, osteoporosis, various cardiac problems, and other disorders has received a great deal of attention, and data concerning the benefits and risks have changed ideas about indications and contraindications. Current guidelines and consensus statements emphasize that each woman's individual medical history, symptoms, and goals for treatment should guide decisions regarding the type of HRT chosen, when treatment is initiated, how treatment is administered, and what dose is used.[109,110] In general, the benefits of HRT before age 60 or within 10 years of menopause are considered to outweigh the risks associated with treatment.

Relief of vasomotor symptoms remains the primary indication, but HRT also decreases the risk of osteoporosis-related fractures and modestly decreases the risk of coronary heart disease in women under 60 or within 10 years of menopause. HRT consisting of estrogen alone (ET) is associated with an increased risk of endometrial cancer and is contraindicated in women with an intact uterus or endometriosis. Because of the increased risk of uterine cancer associated with ET, HRT consisting of estrogen and a progestogen (EPT) is indicated in women with an intact uterus, but it is recommended that these women limit their duration of therapy because the risk of breast cancer increases after 3 to 5 years of EPT treatment. HRT is contraindicated in women with a history of either breast or endometrial cancer. For further details, the reader is directed to recent guidelines and position statements.[109–111]

It is important to note that perimenopausal and postmenopausal women secrete pituitary hCG.[112,113] Serum concentrations generally are low (<13 IU/L), but positive hCG results often cause confusion and can delay important diagnostic tests or treatments. Pituitary versus placental hCG can be confirmed by measuring serum FSH (concentrations of FSH > 45 IU/L are consistent with menopause and make pregnancy unlikely) or by 2 weeks of hormone replacement therapy (hormone replacement therapy should decrease LH, FSH, and hCG concentrations).[114,115]

Female Reproductive Abnormalities

A wide variety of abnormalities affect the female reproductive system and have been classified in a variety of ways. For the purposes of this chapter, they have been divided into categories of (1) 46, XX disorders of sex development (DSDs), (2) precocious puberty, (3) irregular menses, and (4) menopause. Infertility from the male and female perspective is discussed in a separate section.

46, XX DSDs

Individuals with 46, XX DSDs (formerly known as female pseudohermaphrodites) are genetically female but have varying degrees of male phenotypic characteristics. In neonates with a 46, XX karyotype and ambiguous genitalia, *congenital adrenal hyperplasia* (CAH) should be considered. CAH is a family of autosomal recessive disorders of adrenal steroidogenesis (see Chapter 56). Each disorder has a specific pattern of hormonal abnormalities, resulting in deficiency or excess of androgens. The molecular genetics of CAH is discussed in detail in several reviews.[116–119] In female fetuses, exposure to androgens before the 12th week of gestation causes ambiguous genitalia; after 13 weeks, it results in clitoral enlargement. Because androgen excess occurs before the 12th week of gestation in those with CAH, ambiguous genitalia are almost always present. Only deficiencies of 21-hydroxylase and 11β-hydroxylase are predominantly virilizing disorders. Deficiency of 3β-hydroxysteroid dehydrogenase is rare, but when it occurs, affected girls may exhibit virilization.

Diagnosis of *21-hydroxylase deficiency* is made in infants and children with elevated concentrations of plasma 17-hydroxyprogesterone and androstenedione.[118,120] However, sick and premature infants may have elevated concentrations of 17-hydroxyprogesterone and androstenedione.[118] Elevation of 17-hydroxyprogesterone concentrations in early infancy (>3000 ng/dL; 90.9 nmol/L) confirms the diagnosis of this disorder.[121] Additionally, molecular diagnostic testing is now available for detection of the mutations that account for most cases (80 to 90%) of 21-hydroxylase deficiency.[122]

An *11β-hydroxylase deficiency* is confirmed by finding elevated plasma concentrations of 11-deoxycortisol and deoxycorticosterone, increased concentrations of their metabolites in urine, and their suppression by glucocorticoid therapy (see Chapter 56). Plasma renin activity and aldosterone concentrations are low in this deficiency.[123,124]

Elevated plasma concentrations of 17-hydroxypregnenolone, DHEA, and DHEA-S are found in patients with *3β-hydroxysteroid dehydrogenase deficiency* (see Chapter 56). Plasma concentrations of 17-hydroxyprogesterone may be elevated as a result of peripheral conversion of 17-hydroxypregnenolone. The ratio of 17-hydroxypregnenolone to 17-hydroxyprogesterone is strikingly elevated in these patients.[125]

Precocious Puberty

Precocious puberty is the development of secondary sexual characteristics in girls younger than 8 years old and boys younger than 9 years old.[126,127] In 1999, the Lawson Wilkins Pediatric Society issued new recommendations to lower the age standards at which puberty should be considered precocious from 8 to 7 in white girls and to 6 in black girls.[128] These recommendations have been met with criticism because they are based solely on a single epidemiologic study performed by Herman-Giddens and collaborators in 1997.[129] Many argue that the decreased age standards will result in underdiagnosis of this condition.[130]

Despite the debate over the age of onset, pediatric endocrinologists agree that it is important to distinguish between benign advanced pubertal conditions and true precocious puberty.[131–134] Early puberty is manifested by the appearance of secondary sexual characteristics such as premature thelarche (premature breast development) for girls, or premature testicular enlargement for boys. When presented as isolated cases, these secondary sexual characteristics are not necessarily considered to be pathologic. However, if a child demonstrates progressive development of the characteristics and/or

increased rates of bone growth and maturation, causes of true precocious puberty must be considered.[135]

Precocious puberty has been classified as GnRH dependent or independent.[131–133,135] GnRH-dependent precocious puberty (also called *central precocious puberty*) is due to precocious activation of the hypothalamic-pituitary-gonadal axis. In girls, the cause is most commonly idiopathic (90%); however, idiopathic cases account for less than 10% of central precocious puberty in boys. Central nervous system tumors also have been known to cause central precocious puberty, the most common being hypothalamic hamartoma. Neurofibromatosis has been documented to lead to GnRH-dependent precocious puberty.

GnRH-independent precocious puberty (also called *pseudoprecocious puberty*) refers to precocious sex steroid secretion that is independent of pituitary gonadotropin release. Congenital adrenal hyperplasias (CAH) are a common cause of pseudoprecocious puberty. Classic forms of CAH present with virilization, growth acceleration, and accelerated bone maturation. Nonclassic or late-onset forms usually present in childhood or adolescence with premature adrenarche and acne. In fact, 5 to 10% of children who present with premature adrenarche have late-onset adrenal hyperplasia. Tumors of the adrenal gland, ovaries, and testes that secrete androgens or estrogens may result in GnRH-independent precocious puberty. Signs of puberty exhibited in males around 2 years of age are characteristic of testotoxicosis, a familial male-limited form of precocious puberty. This autosomal dominant disorder is due to activating mutations affecting LH receptors.[136] The McCune-Albright syndrome is due to mutation of the *GNAS1* gene, which is involved in the signaling of G-proteins associated with gonadotropin receptors.[137] The mutation causes the gonads to function as if both FSH and LH receptors are constitutively activated. Although this mutation results in GnRH-independent precocious puberty in both sexes, it is most common in girls. Precocious puberty, polyostotic fibrous dysplasia, and café au lait pigmentation are hallmarks for McCune-Albright syndrome. Severe hypothyroidism is also associated with GnRH-independent precocious puberty, likely caused by intrinsic FSH activity of high circulating concentrations of TSH. Unlike the other causes, hypothyroid-induced precocious puberty is associated with skeletal and growth delays.

Diagnosis of precocious puberty is based on clinical presentation, a thorough pubertal history, bone age determinations, and laboratory tests performed to assess gonadotropin concentrations and response to exogenous GnRH.[132] The GnRH stimulation test is the gold standard for diagnosis of GnRH-dependent precocious puberty. Pubertal responses of LH and FSH to GnRH stimulation are considered diagnostic of precocious puberty when chronological age is inappropriate for the hormone response. A diagnosis of GnRH-dependent precocious puberty can also be made without proceeding to the GnRH stimulation test if baseline plasma LH concentrations are greater than 5 IU/L. The GnRH stimulation test is also used to monitor the effectiveness of GnRH agonist therapy used to treat central precocious puberty.[138–140] Typically, an IV bolus of exogenous GnRH is administered (100 µg or 2.5 µg/kg, maximal dose 100 µg), followed by a single measurement (at 40 to 45 minutes) or serial measurements of LH and FSH concentrations.[132,141–143] A predominant LH response correlates with a pubertal pattern, and cutoffs vary depending on the assay, with sex differences noted. A typical pubertal response is characterized by a rise in LH to 8 IU/L or greater after IV administration of 100 μg GnRH. In girls, peak LH/FSH ratios (>0.66 to 1.0) have been proposed to be diagnostic of central precocious puberty.[144] Highly sensitive fluorometric[145] and chemiluminometric[146] immunoassays are now available, which have facilitated the use of basal LH concentrations instead of the GnRH stimulation test for diagnosis of central precocious puberty. A fluorometric assay resulting in a basal concentration of LH greater than 0.6 IU/L in either sex indicates a pubertal pattern and is consistent with precocious puberty. Values less than 0.6 IU/L have been seen with all forms of precocious puberty and require follow-up with a GnRH stimulation test.[145] A similar pattern is observed for immunochemiluminometric assays using a cutoff of 0.3 IU/L.[143,146]

Response to exogenous GnRH is suppressed, and LH and FSH concentrations are low in individuals with GnRH-independent precocious puberty. The diagnosis of GnRH-independent precocious puberty must exclude nonclassic adrenal hyperplasia (NCAH or NCCAH). Basal 17-hydroxyprogesterone concentrations of early-morning samples have been used to screen for 21-hydroxylase–deficient NCAH. A basal 17-hydroxyprogesterone concentration less than 200 ng/dL (6.0 nmol/L) almost always rules out 21-hydroxylase–deficient NCAH. Morning basal 17-hydroxyprogesterone concentrations as low as 82 ng/dL (2.5 nmol/L) have been documented in children with NCAH, but use of this lower threshold value resulted in suboptimal specificity and is not considered useful for routine clinical application.[147,148] Patients with intermediate (200–500 ng/dL; 6–15 nmol/L) basal 17-hydroxyprogesterone concentrations should undergo an ACTH stimulation test to confirm the presence of 21-hydroxylase–deficient NCAH. This is achieved by measuring the 17-hydroxyprogesterone response to ACTH stimulation. An exaggerated response is expected in cases of NCAH. The Endocrine Society Clinical Guidelines (2018) recommend a 17-hydroxyprogesterone diagnostic cutoff of greater than 1000 ng/dL (30 nmol/L).[149] However, some argue that the cutoff should be raised to greater than 1500 ng/dL (45 nmol/L) or 2000 ng/dL (60 nmol/L) because the value of 1000 ng/dL (30 nmol/L) was set before molecular genotyping became available, and studies have indicated that several nonaffected carriers exhibit 17-hydroxyprogesterone concentrations above 1000 ng/dL (30 nmol/L).[150]

Therapy for precocious puberty is dependent on the presenting symptoms and underlying causes.[151] Isolated premature thelarche or adrenarche does not require therapy. Patients with premature thelarche should be followed for 3 to 6 months and require further evaluation for precocious puberty. Cases of premature adrenarche should be evaluated for NCAH and/or polycystic ovary syndrome in girls with determined insulin resistance. GnRH-dependent precocious puberty is treated with GnRH agonists to inhibit normal gonadotropin release, thereby slowing pubertal progression. Therapy for GnRH-independent precocious puberty is determined by the underlying cause.

Estrogens and Breast Cancer

Suspicions of estrogen-based causes in the development of human breast cancer stem from epidemiologic and experimental observations.[152] Early menarche and later natural menopause are associated with increased risk of breast

cancer. A two-stage mechanism has been postulated: initiation of a precancerous state by ovarian activity during the early reproductive years and continuation of ovarian activity in later years as a promoting influence on already initiated tumor cells. Ovarian estrogen has been assumed to be the causative factor because administration of estrogen negates the protective effects of early oophorectomy. According to the theory, relative concentrations of individual estrogen fractions (E_1, E_2, and E_3) produced in the first decade or so after puberty are important determinants of a woman's lifetime risk of breast cancer.[153] In particular, pregnancy at a young age is associated with both favorable estrogen fraction ratios and decreased risk. Further discussion of the role of estrogen in the genesis of breast cancer can be found in monographs and review articles.[154–158]

Irregular Menses

Amenorrhea, the absence of menstrual bleeding, is traditionally categorized as primary (women who have never menstruated) or secondary (women in whom menstruation is present for a variable time and then ceases). Amenorrhea is a relatively common disorder, with an estimated prevalence of 5% in the general population and as high as 8.5% in an unselected adolescent postpubescent population.[159]

Primary amenorrhea. Primary amenorrhea is defined as failure to establish spontaneous periodic menstruation by the age of 16 years regardless of whether secondary sex characteristics have developed.[159,160] About 40% of phenotypic females who have primary amenorrhea (nearly always associated with absence of development of secondary sex characteristics) have *Turner syndrome* (45, X karyotype) or *pure gonadal dysgenesis* (46, XX or XY karyotype).[161] *Müllerian duct agenesis* or *dysgenesis* with absence of the vagina or uterus is the second most common manifestation, and the third most common is *androgen insensitivity syndrome* (androgen receptor deficiency and normal or elevated plasma testosterone concentrations if the patient is past puberty and is karyotype XY but has female sex characteristics).

A *17α-hydroxylase deficiency* is a rare form of CAH that is associated with delayed puberty, primary amenorrhea, and hypertension. Patients have a 46, XX karyotype with elevated gonadotropins, low sex steroids, hypertension, and hypokalemia.[162]

Another rare cause of amenorrhea is the so-called *resistant ovary syndrome*. This primary hypogonadal condition is associated with increased concentrations of plasma FSH and LH and ovaries that contain predominantly primordial follicles. It is thought to arise from a defect in FSH receptors.[163] This disorder can be diagnosed only by examination of an ovarian biopsy specimen, which will exhibit functioning ovarian follicles despite the presence of amenorrhea. Ovulation sometimes is induced in these patients with administration of high doses of gonadotropins.

As discussed earlier, *Kallmann syndrome* involves hypogonadotropic hypogonadism associated with anosmia or hyposmia and is caused by a defect in the formation and migration of GnRH neurons. Sexual infantilism is the prominent manifestation, and primary amenorrhea is common.[39] Finally, delayed pubertal development should be considered.

Evaluation of primary amenorrhea. When puberty is delayed in a girl, serum gonadotropins should be measured. Low concentrations may indicate pituitary failure, whereas concentrations elevated into the postmenopausal interval indicate definite gonadal failure.[159] In the latter case, chromosome studies are indicated. In the former case, pituitary function testing and radiography may be helpful. Patients with short stature without Turner syndrome but with primary amenorrhea may have multiple deficiencies of pituitary hormone secretion. In these patients, a craniopharyngioma or pituitary tumor should be suspected. In patients with normal development of secondary sex characteristics and a normal karyotype who experience primary amenorrhea, a structural abnormality blocking the outflow of blood should be suspected.

The diagnosis of *17α-hydroxylase deficiency* is made when the concentration of (1) serum progesterone is greater than 300 ng/dL (9.54 nmol/L); (2) 17α-hydroxyprogesterone is less than 20 ng/dL (0.6 nmol/L); (3) aldosterone is low; and (4) 11-deoxycorticosterone is elevated. Plasma concentrations of 11-deoxycortisol, testosterone, E_2, and DHEA-S are also low. Urinary steroid profiling (USP) may also provide helpful diagnostic information (high corticosterone metabolite to cortisol metabolite ratio). The diagnosis is confirmed with an *ACTH stimulation test* in which baseline concentrations of progesterone and 17α-hydroxyprogesterone are measured first, followed by administration of 0.25 mg ACTH. Diagnosis is made if serum concentrations of progesterone are significantly elevated and 17α-hydroxyprogesterone concentrations are unchanged at 60 minutes after ACTH administration.[162]

Secondary amenorrhea. Secondary amenorrhea is defined as absence of periodic menstruation for at least 6 months in women who have previously experienced menses.[164,165] *Oligomenorrhea* is infrequent menstruation that occurs fewer than eight times per year.[166] With few exceptions, the causes of primary and secondary amenorrhea overlap (Box 58.2). Pregnancy, the most common cause of secondary amenorrhea, must be considered first and ruled out.[159] Elevated concentrations of prolactin—iatrogenic or induced by a prolactin-secreting tumor—have been found to result in oligomenorrhea or amenorrhea. About one-third of women with no obvious cause of amenorrhea have elevated prolactin concentrations.[167] It is thought that hyperprolactinemia interferes with GnRH pulsatility, resulting in impaired release of LH and FSH. If hyperprolactinemia is identified, hypothyroidism should be ruled out because correction of hypothyroidism may lead to normalization of plasma prolactin concentrations. Additionally, both hyperthyroidism and hypothyroidism are associated with a variety of menstrual disorders because of their effects on metabolism and interconversion of androgens and estrogens.[168] In practice, it is

---

BOX 58.2   Causes of Amenorrhea

Primary Amenorrhea

Lower tract defects
- Vaginal aplasia
- Imperforate hymen
- Congenital vaginal atresia

Uterine disorders
- Congenital absence of the uterus
- Endometritis
- Müllerian agenesis (Mayer-Rokitansky-Kuster-Hauser syndrome)

Ovarian disorders
- XO gonadal and X dysgenesis and variants
- XX gonadal dysgenesis
- Turner syndrome
- 17-Hydroxylase deficiency of the ovaries and adrenal glands
- Autoimmune oophoritis
- Resistant ovary syndrome
- Polycystic ovary syndrome

Adrenal disorders (congenital adrenal hyperplasia)

Thyroid disorders (hypothyroidism)

Pituitary-hypothalamic disorders
- Hypopituitarism
- Constitutional delay in the onset of menses (physiologic)
- Nutritional disorders
- Kallmann syndrome

Secondary Amenorrhea

Pregnancy/lactation

Uterine disorders
- Post-traumatic uterine synechiae (Asherman syndrome)
- Progestational agents

Ovarian disorders
- Polycystic ovary syndrome (hypothalamic)
- Ovarian tumor

Primary ovarian insufficiency (idiopathic, autoimmune, chemotherapy, radiation, injury)

Antimetabolite therapy

Adrenal disorders
- Late-onset adrenal hyperplasia
- Cushing syndrome
- Virilizing adrenal tumors
- Adrenocorticoid insufficiency

Thyroid disorders
- Hypothyroidism
- Hyperthyroidism

Pituitary disorders
- Acquired hypopituitarism (trauma, tumor, Sheehan syndrome, lymphocytic hypophysitis)
- Physiologic or pathologic hyperprolactinemia

Hypothalamic disorders
- Tumor and infiltrative disease
- Nutritional disorders
- Hypophysitis
- Excessive exercise
- Stress

Iatrogenic
- Antipsychotics (phenothiazines, haloperidol, clozapine, pimozide)
- Antidepressants (tricyclics, monoamine oxidase inhibitors)
- Antihypertensives (calcium channel blockers, methyldopa, reserpine)
- Drugs with estrogenic activity (digitalis, flavonoids, marijuana, oral contraceptives)
- Drugs with ovarian toxicity (busulfan, chlorambucil, cisplatin, cyclophosphamide, fluorouracil)

helpful to separate patients with secondary amenorrhea into those with and without signs of estrogen production. Many other factors or conditions have been observed to cause secondary amenorrhea, including disorders of the ovary, uterus, pituitary, and hypothalamus and the use of drugs.

Disorders of the ovary, such as *primary ovarian insufficiency (POI)* (also referred to as premature ovarian failure [POF]) and loss of ovarian function, have been known to cause amenorrhea. POI has been defined as failure of ovarian estrogen production that occurs in a hypergonadotropic state at any age between menarche and 40 years.[104] If the patient is younger than 25 years or shorter than 5 feet tall, karyotyping or chromosomal microarray should be performed to rule out the presence of a variety of chromosomal abnormalities involving duplications or absence of the X chromosome or the presence of a Y chromosome. Screening for the fragile X premutation *(FMR1)* should also be performed. Patients with POI may present with symptoms of hypoestrogenism, including hot flashes and high gonadotropin concentrations. Autoimmune disorders have been associated with 20 to 40% of cases of POI that result in destruction of the ovary and in amenorrhea. Patients also may have antibodies to other endocrine and nonendocrine tissues. Other causes for ovarian failure include oophorectomy, cystic degeneration, trauma, infection, galactosemia, interference with blood supply, radiotherapy treatment, and treatment with cytotoxic chemotherapeutic agents. In rare patients, ovarian resistance to gonadotropins may be evident.

Secondary amenorrhea may also result from an issue with the outflow tract. The patient with a uterine problem is normal hormonally but does not menstruate. *Asherman syndrome*, or intrauterine adhesions, is the most common outflow tract abnormality that causes amenorrhea. Endometrial damage may occur in response to a dilatation and curettage and to infection of the endometrium. Pituitary dysfunction will also cause secondary amenorrhea. This is most often due to intrinsic pituitary tumors. However, Sheehan syndrome and pituitary apoplexy can result in panhypopituitarism. Empty sella syndrome has been reported in 4 to 16% of patients with amenorrhea and galactorrhea.

Evaluation of secondary amenorrhea. Evaluation of women with secondary amenorrhea should begin with a careful history that includes a complete description of menstrual patterns. In addition, the patient should be evaluated for galactorrhea, hot flashes, symptoms of hypothyroidism, hirsutism, prior abdominal surgery, pelvis or uterus trauma, medications prescribed, nutritional history, patterns of exercise, previous contraceptive use, weight changes, stress, and chronic disease. The physical examination should determine the visual fields, thyroid size and function, cushingoid appearance, galactorrhea, hirsutism, abdominal masses, pelvic masses, clitoral enlargement, and evidence of malnutrition. Serum or urine β-hCG should be measured to rule out pregnancy. Because both hypothyroidism and hyperprolactinemia have been known to cause amenorrhea, they are easily excluded by measuring concentrations of serum thyroid-stimulating hormone and prolactin.

A 24-hour urine sample for cortisol measurement or an overnight dexamethasone suppression test is performed in those patients suspected of having Cushing syndrome (see Chapter 56). On the basis of the preliminary assessment, MRI of the sella turcica should be performed in patients with evidence of pituitary or hypothalamic disease, or clinical hypoestrogenism. A GnRH stimulation test with measurement of LH and FSH concentrations in those patients with gonadotropin deficiency assists in differentiating hypothalamic disease from pituitary disease. For diagnosis of polycystic ovary disease (PCOS), see the section "Laboratory Evaluation of Hirsutism/Virilization" later in this chapter.

Progesterone challenge for evaluating amenorrhea. When the cause of amenorrhea is unclear after the initial assessment, relative estrogen status should be determined. Serum E_2 can be measured, but results must be interpreted with caution because serum E_2 fluctuates throughout the menstrual cycle. A *progesterone challenge* may be performed as a functional assessment of relative estrogen status.[169] Women with an estrogen-primed uterus have withdrawal vaginal bleeding after treatment with oral progestin (medroxyprogesterone acetate; Provera), 30 mg daily for 3 days, 10 mg daily for 5 to 10 days, or 100 to 200 mg of progesterone in oil given intramuscularly. If estrogen concentrations are adequate and the outflow tract is intact, menstrual bleeding should occur within a week of treatment. In patients with withdrawal bleeding, the plasma E_2 concentration is usually greater than 40 pg/mL (146.8 pmol/L). However, the progesterone challenge test is subject to false positives because up to 20% of normoestrogenic women with oligomenorrhea do not experience withdrawal bleeding, as well as false negatives because up to 40% of women with oligomenorrhea and reduced plasma E_2 experience withdrawal bleeding.[159] A pelvic ultrasound to evaluate the thickness of the uterine cavity may also be helpful.

If the patient demonstrates withdrawal bleeding after the progestin challenge test, this indicates that the ovaries are producing sufficient estrogen to cause endometrial proliferation and no anatomic obstruction is present. Most of these women have a history of progestin-containing contraceptive use (the progestin-dominant state can thin the endometrium), stress, weight loss, or excessive exercise.

If bleeding fails to occur after progestin challenge, then additional laboratory tests are indicated, including measurement of FSH to localize the problem to the follicle, pituitary, or hypothalamus. High FSH concentrations indicate that the ovarian follicle is not responding to gonadotropin stimulation. A single measurement of FSH greater than 50 IU/L is suggestive of ovarian failure or primary ovarian insufficiency in women younger than 40 years of age

Because of the association of *primary ovarian insufficiency* (POI) with thyroid, parathyroid, or adrenal insufficiency secondary to autoimmune disease, it has been suggested that patients younger than 40 years should be screened for thyroid antibodies.[170] Increasing evidence indicates that young women with spontaneous POI are at increased risk of developing autoimmune adrenal insufficiency.[171,172] It has been suggested that adrenal antibodies (21-hydroxylase antibodies or adrenal cortex autoantibodies) should be measured during the initial evaluation of women with spontaneous POI. Periodic monitoring for the development of antiadrenal antibodies should also be performed in women with idiopathic POI. Patients in whom antiadrenal antibodies have been detected and patients with signs and symptoms of adrenal insufficiency should be tested using a standard ACTH stimulation test. The differential diagnosis for evaluation of amenorrhea is listed in Table 58.1 and Box 58.2. As indicated by the clinical presentation, special additional testing may be required.

TABLE 58.1 Differential Diagnosis of Secondary Amenorrhea

Causes	FSH	LH	Estrogen (E₂)	Uterine Bleeding After Progesterone
Hypothalamic				
CNS—hypothalamic dysfunction				
Idiopathic	↓ or N	↓ or N	↓ or N	±
Secondary to medications	↓ or N	↓ or N	↓ or N	±
Secondary to stress	↓ or N	↓ or N	↓ or N	±
CNS—hypothalamic dysfunction or failure due to exercise	↓ or N	↓ or N	↓ or N	±
CNS—hypothalamic dysfunction or failure due to weight loss				
Simple weight loss	↓ or N	↓ or N	↓ or N	±
Anorexia nervosa	↓	↓	↓	—
CNS—hypothalamic failure				
Lesions	↓	↓	↓	—
Idiopathic	↓	↓	↓	—
CNS—hypothalamic–adreno-ovarian dysfunction (polycystic ovary syndrome) or hyperandrogenic chronic anovulation	N	↑*	N	+
Pituitary				
Destructive lesions (Sheehan syndrome)	↓	↓	↓	—
Tumor	↓	↓	↓	—
Ovarian				
Premature ovarian failure	↑	↑	↓	—
Loss of ovarian function (oophorectomy, infection, cystic degeneration, chemotherapy, radiation)	↑	↑	↓	—
Uterine				
Uterine synechiae (Asherman syndrome)	N	N	N	—

CNS, Central nervous system; *FSH*, follicle-stimulating hormone; *LH*, luteinizing hormone; *N*, value within normal reference interval; ↓, value below normal reference interval; ↑, value above normal reference interval; ↑*, >25 IU/L, less than menopausal concentration; ±, positive or negative bleeding response to progesterone.
From Davajan V, Kletzky OA. Amenorrhea. In: Mishell DR, Davajan V, Lobo RA, eds. *Infertility, contraception and reproductive endocrinology.* 3rd ed. Boston: Blackwell Scientific Publications, 1991:373.

Androgen excess. Amenorrhea due to androgen excess can be due to adult-onset CAH, corticotropin-dependent Cushing syndrome, or polycystic ovary syndrome (PCOS). Patients with androgen excess often will present with acne, obesity, and variable degrees of excess hair on the face, chest, abdomen, and thighs. Some individuals with 21-hydroxylase deficiency do not manifest any developmental abnormalities or salt wasting, but they present with signs of androgen excess. This clinical syndrome, referred to as *nonclassic, adult-onset,* or *late-onset CAH,* may be clinically indistinguishable from PCOS.[173,174]

PCOS is characterized by infertility, hirsutism, obesity (in approximately half of those affected), and various menstrual disturbances ranging from amenorrhea to irregular vaginal bleeding (Table 58.2). Metabolic abnormalities including insulin resistance are also observed in many women with PCOS, leading to an increased prevalence of diabetes and an increased risk for coronary heart disease. PCOS patients have substantial estrogen production because of the peripheral conversion of androgens to estrogens. Abnormal bleeding patterns seen in PCOS are due to chronic anovulation and lack of progesterone stimulation and withdrawal. Chronic estrogen exposure without progesterone may predispose patients to endometrial cancer. Although this syndrome is associated with polycystic ovaries, they often are not present in women

TABLE 58.2 Clinical Features of the Polycystic Ovary Syndrome*

Clinical Feature	Frequency (%)
Hirsutism	65
Acne	25
Obesity	35
Infertility	50
Amenorrhea	35
Oligomenorrhea	40
Regular menstrual cycle	20

*Data were compiled from three studies. Two used ultrasonography as the primary method of diagnosis, one used ovarian histology. Total *n* = 1935.
Modified from Franks S. Polycystic ovary syndrome. *N Engl J Med.* 1995;333:853.

with this syndrome. The name is actually a misnomer in that the ovaries are covered with follicles, not cysts.

PCOS occurs in 4 to 10% of premenopausal women, and the prevalence varies depending on the diagnostic criteria used. The Rotterdam Consensus Criteria define hyperandrogenism, oligomenorrhea or amenorrhea, and polycystic ovaries by ultrasound as the characteristic signs and symptoms and require the presence of two of the three for diagnosis of PCOS.[175] This definition has been criticized by the Androgen Excess Society, which requires the presence of hyperandrogenism in conjunction with either oligomenorrhea/amenorrhea or polycystic ovaries.[176,177] Despite these concerns, current Endocrine Society guidelines recommend the use of the Rotterdam Consensus Criteria.[178]

Because the pathophysiologic mechanism is unknown, PCOS remains a diagnosis of exclusion clinically defined by hyperandrogenism with chronic anovulation in women with no other cause.[179] Relatively low FSH and disproportionately high LH concentrations are common in PCOS, although this ratio should not be used in a routine PCOS workup. Some attempt has been made to link PCOS to *leptin*, a hormone that is secreted by adipocytes and is thought to play a role in regulating food intake and metabolism.[180] While animal studies provide suggestive evidence,[181,182] clinical studies have yet to conclusively demonstrate that leptin plays a role in PCOS, and it remains a subject of research interest only.[183,184] Other studies have reported higher serum AMH concentrations in women with PCOS relative to healthy women,[185,186] and ongoing work is evaluating the potential utility of including AMH measurement in PCOS diagnostic criteria.[187] Some have proposed a serum AMH cutoff of >35 pmol/L (5 ng/mL) as an alternative to antral follicle count (AFC) for the detection of polycystic ovarian morphology.[188] However, these same authors have documented discordance between AMH concentrations and AFC and highlight interindividual variation in AMH production per follicle as one contributing factor.[189,190] As a result, the 2018 International PCOS Network has recommended against using serum AMH measurement as an alternative for the detection of polycystic ovarian morphology or as a standalone test for the diagnosis of PCOS.[191]

Recent evidence has demonstrated that biochemical androgen excess in women with PCOS is associated with an increased risk of insulin resistance and other metabolic dysfunction[192,193] and that metabolic disease severity increases with increasing androgen excess.[194] Many women with PCOS have normal serum testosterone concentrations but demonstrate clinically apparent hyperandrogenism. In the presence of oligomenorrhea and/or polycystic-appearing ovaries on ultrasound, this is enough to make the diagnosis of PCOS. On the other hand, measurement of serum androstenedione has been advocated on the grounds that peripheral conversion of androstenedione to testosterone may explain clinical symptoms of hyperandrogenism in women with normal serum testosterone.[195] In a recent study, serum androstenedione detected androgen excess (as defined by either serum testosterone or androstenedione concentrations above the appropriate reference interval) in PCOS patients, fulfilling the Rotterdam consensus criteria with a sensitivity of 88.3% and specificity of 97.7% compared to 65.1 and 88.3% for testosterone.[194] As will be discussed below, routine measurement of androstenedione and testosterone will require widespread use of liquid chromatography-tandem mass spectrometry (LC-MS/MS) due to the limitations of immunoassays in the measurement of androgens in women. For women with clinically apparent virilization, DHEA-S should also be measured along with serum testosterone to rule out an androgen-secreting tumor (see below).

For PCOS patients who are not interested in conceiving, the mainstay of therapy is oral contraceptive pills for regulation of menstrual periods. In many cases, hirsutism is the primary focus of treatment and may be addressed by androgen receptor antagonists, androgen suppressing agents, or 5α-reductase inhibitors. For those who are overweight or obese, weight loss and exercise are advocated. For women with PCOS who wish to conceive, treatment is aimed at ovulation induction. Weight reduction helps to promote ovulation. Medications such as aromatase inhibitors and clomiphene citrate are useful.[179] Metformin may be a helpful adjuvant in women with documented glucose intolerance as measured by a 2-hour oral glucose tolerance test.

Ovarian hyperthecosis, a non-neoplastic lesion of the ovary characterized by the presence of islands of luteinized thecal cells in the ovarian stroma, is sometimes confused with PCOS. Features that distinguish it from PCOS include higher concentrations of testosterone, androstenedione, and DHT derived from ovarian secretion. Thus androgenization is greater than is usually observed in patients with PCOS. Both LH and FSH concentrations are low or low-normal. Insulin resistance and hyperinsulinism are present to a greater degree than in PCOS. Finally, patients with ovarian hyperthecosis fail to ovulate when treated with an antiestrogen such as clomiphene citrate.[196]

Hirsutism and virilization. Hirsutism is defined as excessive growth of terminal hair in women and children in a distribution similar to that occurring in postpubertal men.[197,198] True hirsutism, which is androgen responsive, has to be distinguished from hypertrichosis, which consists of excessive growth of vellus or non–androgen-responsive hair. Women with androgen-dependent hirsutism may have exposure to excess androgens or may have heightened sensitivity to normal circulating concentrations of androgen.

The causes of hirsutism are listed in Box 58.3. The estimated prevalence for idiopathic hirsutism ranges from 6 to 50% of women evaluated for hirsutism, depending on the definition.[199–201] Typically, idiopathic hirsutism is defined by normal physical and laboratory findings in hirsute women. Non-neoplastic forms of hirsutism are slow to progress and usually manifest at the time of puberty, when circulating concentrations of androgens increase, after a period of weight gain, or when oral contraceptives have been stopped.[198] Rapid onset of hirsutism suggests an iatrogenic cause or, if associated with virilization, a neoplastic source of androgens. The most common cause of androgen hypersecretion in women is PCOS; 70 to 80% of hirsute women are reportedly afflicted with this disorder.[201] Late-onset CAH (see Chapter 56), acromegaly, hyperprolactinemia, menopause (see earlier section "Menopause"), and ACTH-dependent Cushing syndrome have been observed to cause hirsutism.

Virilization is characterized by clitoral hypertrophy, deepening of the voice, temporal hair recession, baldness, increased libido, decreased body fat, and menstrual irregularities or amenorrhea. The 2018 Endocrine Society Clinical Practice Guideline observes that hirsutism is usually associated with normal or slightly elevated serum androgens, whereas virilization is associated with marked increases in ovarian or adrenal androgen production and is an indication for more intensive investigation.[202]

Laboratory evaluation of hirsutism/virilization. The two most important screening tests used in the evaluation of women for hirsutism and virilization are serum total or free testosterone and DHEA-S.[202,203] Elevation of DHEA-S

BOX 58.3 Causes of Hirsutism

Ovarian
  Severe insulin resistance
  Hyperthecosis, hilus cell or stromal cell hyperplasia
  Androgen-producing ovarian tumor
  Menopause
Adrenal
  Classic congenital hyperplasia
  21-Hydroxylase deficiency
  11-Hydroxylase deficiency
  3β-Hydroxysteroid dehydrogenase deficiency
  Adult or attenuated adrenal hyperplasia
  Androgen-producing adrenal tumor
Familial hirsutism
Endocrine disorders
  Polycystic ovary syndrome
  Hyperprolactinemia
  Acromegaly
  Cushing syndrome
Idiopathic hirsutism (includes increased skin sensitivity to
  androgens)
Iatrogenic
  Androgens
  Phenytoin
  Diazoxide
  Minoxidil
  Streptomycin
  Cyclosporine
  Danazol
  Metyrapone
  Phenothiazides
  Progestagens (19-nonsteroid derivatives)

concentration suggests an adrenal origin of androgens, whereas elevations in testosterone indicate an adrenal or ovarian source. Neoplastic disease is unlikely if the serum testosterone concentration is less than 200 ng/dL (6.9 nmol/L), the DHEA-S concentration is less than 700 μg/dL (19 μmol/L), or 17-KS concentrations are less than 30 mg/dL (1 mmol/L).[204] When other, more common causes have been excluded, 17-hydroxyprogesterone may also be measured (early morning; follicular phase) to evaluate the possibility of nonclassic CAH due to 21-hydroxylase deficiency.[202] If the result is less than 200 ng/dL (6.1 nmol/L), CAH can be excluded, although an estimated 2 to 11% of adult patients with NCAH will be missed using this approach.[149,205] Concentrations greater than 1500 ng/dL (45 nmol/L) in nonpregnant women are confirmatory. When basal concentrations between 200 and 1500 ng/dL (6.1 to 45 nmol/L) are found, an ACTH stimulation test should be performed. Patients with NCAH typically achieve a 17α-hydroxyprogesterone concentration greater than 1500 ng/dL (45 nmol/L), and classic CAH has a response over 2000 ng/dL (60 nmol/L).[149,198,203] Patients with attenuated forms of CAH usually have normal concentrations of FSH and LH. About one-half have elevated testosterone and androstenedione concentrations. Most of these patients also have increased concentrations of DHEA-S, and more than 90% have supranormal concentrations of androstanediol glucuronide, although this testing is not available in most clinical laboratories.[17,206]

Regardless of the source of excess androgen production, the androstanediol glucuronide concentration is elevated in more than 90% of women with hirsutism because it is a marker of excessive DHT production in skin. Concentrations of SHBG can be decreased in hirsute women, so there has been some debate over whether total testosterone or bioavailable testosterone (free and weakly bound testosterone) is more clinically informative in diagnosing hirsutism. The reader is directed to a review by Wheeler that discusses many of these issues.[207]

Polycystic ovary syndrome is primarily a clinical diagnosis, and few laboratory tests are needed. Provided that other causes of oligomenorrhea or amenorrhea have been ruled out (thyroid disease, hyperprolactinemia), given a history of androgen excess, the only condition that needs to be excluded is 21-hydroxylase–deficient nonclassic CAH (described above). Serum testosterone measurement is not necessary if clear hirsutism is present. Testosterone concentrations greater than 60 ng/dL (2 nmol/L) are consistent with PCOS.[179] FSH concentrations are often disproportionately normal or low. Patients with PCOS usually have E_2 concentrations greater than 40 pg/mL (147 pmol/L) and therefore experience withdrawal bleeding in response to a progestin challenge.

Other factors. Hypothalamic dysfunction consists of those disorders that disrupt the frequency or amplitude of GnRH. Rarely is this due to a lesion or tumor. However, most commonly, disruption occurs in response to psychological stress, depression, severe weight loss, anorexia nervosa, or strenuous exercise.[159] A syndrome known as the *female athletic triad* has been described. This syndrome is prevalent in women who exercise vigorously, and it is associated with amenorrhea, disordered eating, and osteoporosis. Competitive long-distance runners, gymnasts, and professional ballet dancers appear to be at highest risk. Although the mechanism for the disturbance is unclear, symptoms and laboratory profiles are similar to those of other forms of hypothalamic amenorrhea. LH and FSH concentrations are normal or low, and E_2 concentrations are low. As a result of chronic low estrogen, bone mineral content is low and the incidence of stress fractures is increased.[208]

Several hormone-producing tumors of the ovary, pituitary gland, and adrenal glands occur in combination with amenorrhea.[209,210] This amenorrhea may be confused with pregnancy if the tumors produce hCG. Choriocarcinoma of the uterus or ovary may produce large amounts of hCG that cause hyperthyroidism because of the slight thyrotropic action of hCG. Granulosa–theca cell tumors are usually associated with estrogen secretion that results in amenorrhea and irregular menses and, rarely, excessive androgen with associated virilization.[211]

Many drugs produce amenorrhea (see Box 58.2), particularly phenothiazines and other psychotropic drugs such as haloperidol, pimozide, or clozapine.[159] Phenothiazine-induced amenorrhea is usually associated with hyperprolactinemia and galactorrhea. Drugs that affect the normal pathway of dopamine secretion will produce amenorrhea by decreasing the secretion of norepinephrine. Because norepinephrine is important in controlling the synthesis and secretion of GnRH, any alteration in its synthesis or secretion will result in menstrual abnormalities.[212] Older formulations of oral contraceptive pills utilized higher doses of estrogen that were thought to have suppressive effects on the HPO axis.

This is no longer the case. Normal menses should resume shortly after the cessation of combined oral contraceptive pills.[213] If menses has not resumed after ceasing the oral contraceptive pill, evaluation is warranted. If other causes of amenorrhea are suspected, evaluation should not be delayed.

POINTS TO REMEMBER

- GnRH stimulates LH and FSH release, which control oocyte maturation and ovulation and increase estradiol and progesterone production.
- Estradiol is transported in blood tightly bound to SHBG and loosely bound to albumin, while progesterone is bound to corticosteroid binding globulin.
- Estradiol and progesterone both inhibit and stimulate LH and FSH release, with the type of regulation dependent on the stage of the menstrual cycle and the serum steroid hormone concentration.
- PCOS is defined by hyperandrogenism and oligo/anovulation and remains a diagnosis of exclusion based primarily on clinical evaluation.
- Pituitary secretion of hCG is often seen in postmenopausal women, and the pituitary origin can be confirmed by the presence of concurrent elevated serum FSH.

Transgender Medicine

Individuals who identify as transgender are those whose gender identity does not match their sex assigned at birth. Transgender individuals experience a difference between primary and secondary sexual characteristics and gender identity, which is termed gender incongruence. Gender dysphoria occurs when gender incongruence progresses to a sense of distress and unease with the lack of agreement between one's gender identity and designated gender. It should be noted, however, that not all individuals who experience gender incongruence also experience gender dysphoria. Transgender care dates back to the 1940s, when a pioneering endocrinologist named Harry Benjamin began treating individuals exhibiting gender dysphoria with sex hormones. Since that time, transgender individuals have become an increasingly visible part of society and there are now established guidelines for their care.[214]

It is important to recognize that transgender individuals constitute a diverse group with different goals and expectations and not all individuals seek medical or surgical intervention. For those who seek hormonal and/or surgical intervention to help align their sexual characteristics with their gender identity, these treatments are often referred to as gender-affirming hormone treatment and gender-affirming surgical procedures. The goal of masculinizing and feminizing hormone treatment is to develop the secondary sexual characteristics of the individual's affirmed gender. An equally important goal of gender-affirming hormonal treatment is to suppress the endogenous hypothalamic-pituitary-gonadal axis, which will facilitate the development of the desired feminizing and masculinizing features.

Transgender women. Transgender women are individuals that are assigned male at birth and have an affirmed female gender identity. In transgender women, the goals are typically to induce female secondary sexual characteristics and suppress androgen production. High serum androgen concentrations are typically undesired in transgender women, as elevated androgens promote male body hair distribution, maintain increased muscle mass and cause androgenic alopecia. Goals of feminizing treatment are breast development, development of a female body fat distribution, and softening of skin. Transgender women who elect gender-affirming hormonal treatment are prescribed 17β-estradiol, which is available in pill, transdermal patch, and injectable formulations. Risks of estradiol use include an increase in venous thromboembolic events (VTEs), hypertriglyceridemia, and cholelithiasis.[215,216] The thrombophilic properties of estradiol are thought to be due to first pass metabolism and direct stimulation of hepatic clotting factors. By eliminating first pass metabolism, transdermal estradiol is thought to carry a lower risk of VTE. A large analysis in the United Kingdom confirmed previous discoveries that estradiol patch use in postmenopausal women did not raise the risk of venous thromboembolic events.[217] Furthermore, oral estradiol carries a lower risk of VTE than oral conjugated equine estrogen.[217]

Hormonal treatment of transgender women with testes will typically require an anti-androgen, with spironolactone being the most common. In addition to spironolactone's antimineralocorticoid effect, it is an antagonist of the androgen receptor and reduces testosterone action.[218] Alternatives to spironolactone include androgen receptor blockers (bicalutamide) or medications that suppress gonadotropin production (leuprolide depot and cyproterone acetate [not available in the United States]). Progesterone may also be used to help suppress testosterone production and experimentally to augment breast development. The most common preparation is micronized progesterone, either taken orally or as a rectal suppository. Progesterone is typically administered at bedtime due to a mild sedating effect. Historically, irritability and negative mood changes have been reported with progesterone, however clinical data to support these effects are lacking. Transgender women who elect orchiectomy will no longer require treatment with an antiandrogen.

Laboratory monitoring of transgender women on gender-affirming hormones is required to ensure that therapeutic hormone concentrations are maintained and adverse drug effects are prevented. For adequate feminization, estradiol and total testosterone concentrations are typically maintained in the normal female range. The Endocrine Society Clinical Practice Guidelines recommend monitoring estradiol and total testosterone every 3 months.[214] Typically, estradiol doses are lowered when there has been adequate feminization. Hypertriglyceridemia is a known risk of oral estrogen use and rarely can be severe. Therefore an annual fasting lipid panel is recommended for all transgender women on gender-affirming hormones. Spironolactone use requires the measurement of serum creatinine and potassium at baseline, again within 1 week of initiation, and with each subsequent dose increase.

Transgender men. Transgender males are individuals who are assigned a female sex at birth and who identify as male. Transgender men who elect masculinizing hormone treatment can expect menstrual cessation, development of male body and facial hair distribution, drop in voice pitch, increased libido, clitoromegaly, acne, and increased skeletal muscle mass. The most commonly prescribed formulations of testosterone are parenteral and transdermal. Parenteral formulations are more common, due to the fact that transdermal formulations are costly and have the potential for transfer to female partners and children. Oral preparations of testosterone are contraindicated due to hepatotoxicity.[219] Injectable testosterone is formulated for deep intramuscular injection. However, small case series and widespread clinical use has demonstrated that weekly administration of testosterone via subcutaneous injection results in serum testosterone concentrations well within the normal male range and these concentrations remain relatively stable over the 7-day dosing interval.[220,221] Masculinizing hormone treatment in transgender men mimics the treatment of male hypogonadism, and therefore monitoring of transgender males should follow similar recommendations. The early stage of treatment requires more frequent testosterone dosing titration to ensure progression of male secondary sexual characteristics and therefore it is suggested to monitor total serum testosterone, luteinizing hormone (to assess for HPG axis suppression), estradiol, and a complete blood count every 3 to 4 months for the first year.[214] The most common adverse reaction of testosterone replacement in hypogonadal males is erythrocytosis.[222] If erythrocytosis is observed, subsequent investigation should be initiated to exclude an underlying cause such as untreated sleep apnea or tobacco use. After 1 year of treatment, monitoring of the previously mentioned analytes and a lipid panel should be performed on an annual basis. These recommendations are similar to The Endocrine Society Clinical Practice Guidelines for Endocrine Treatment of Gender-Dysphoric/Gender-Incongruent Persons.[214]

Interpretation of laboratory tests with sex-specific values. As discussed above, those who receive gender-affirming hormones require routine laboratory testing to monitor for complications and ensure dosing adequacy. In this patient population, it is essential to consider the sex-specific nature of many clinical laboratory tests in order to avoid misinterpretation of reported results, which often leads to unnecessary follow-up testing and/or misdiagnosis. To avoid diagnostic error, clinical laboratory tests with sex-specific reference intervals should be interpreted in the context of the interval that matches the sex of the gender-affirming hormone treatment. A frequently encountered example is the incorrect diagnosis of anemia in a transgender woman receiving 17β-estradiol, whose hemoglobin results are flagged as inappropriately low when interpreted in the context of a male reference interval. Complicating matters is the fact that the decision to change one's gender designation in the electronic medical record is personal and the timing is variable, with some individuals requesting a change to the medical record early in transition while others prefer to wait until they have completed gender-affirming medical therapies.

While there are limited published data on the effects of gender affirming hormones on laboratory values, clinical experience has demonstrated significant changes in hemoglobin, creatinine, LDL, and HDL. In transgender men, hemoglobin increases after starting testosterone, which is attributed to an increase in erythropoietin combined with the cessation of menses (which typically occurs within 6 to 9 months of starting testosterone). Conversely, transgender women have a reduction in hemoglobin concentration due to the dramatic reduction in serum testosterone.[223] As serum creatinine concentrations correlate with muscle mass, most transgender men will demonstrate an increase in serum creatinine. Serum creatinine levels in transgender women typically remain relatively stable.

Testosterone treatment typically increases LDL and decreases HDL while estrogen treatment has the opposite effect, but further work is required to conclusively establish the effects of gender-affirming hormone treatment on circulating lipids in transgender patients. Lastly, the effect of gender-affirming hormones on sex-specific laboratory values varies with treatment time as only modest changes are observed in the initial weeks after initiating treatment but values match the reference intervals associated with the new hormonal milieu with extended treatment.

POINTS TO REMEMBER

- Transgender individuals experience gender incongruence, defined as a difference between one's primary and secondary sexual characteristics and gender identity
- Transgender individuals constitute a diverse group with different treatment goals and expected outcomes
- Transgender women who pursue gender-affirming hormone treatment receive 17β-estradiol and an anti-androgen while transgender men undergoing gender-affirming hormone treatment receive testosterone
- Care should be taken to interpret sex-specific clinical laboratory test results from transgender individuals in the context of the appropriate reference interval

---

INFERTILITY

Infertility is defined as the inability to conceive after 1 year of unprotected intercourse.[224] It has been estimated that 93% of healthy couples practicing unprotected intercourse should expect to conceive within 1 year.[225] A specific cause of infertility is identified in approximately 80% of couples: one-third are due to female factors alone, one-third to male factors alone, and one-third to a combination of problems.

Primary infertility refers to couples or patients who have had no previous successful pregnancies. Secondary infertility encompasses patients who have previously conceived but are currently unable to conceive. These types of infertility generally share common causes.

Infertility problems often arise as a result of hormonal dysfunction of the hypothalamic-pituitary-gonadal axis. Measurements of peptide and steroid hormones in the serum are therefore essential aspects of the evaluation of infertility. This section focuses on hormonal and biochemical aspects of evaluating infertility.

Male Infertility

A list of the most common male infertility factors is given in Box 58.4. One algorithm for the evaluation of male infertility is shown in At a glance. Initial evaluation of male infertility should include a detailed history and physical examination. The physical examination should pay particular attention to (1) the external genitalia—for evidence of proper androgenization; (2) hair pattern—degree of virilization; (3) breast abnormalities—gynecomastia and or discharge; and (4) neurologic findings—sense of smell and visual impairments. The history must include (1) reproductive history, including living children and any pregnancies that resulted in miscarriage; (2) prescribed medications; (3) recreational and performance-enhancing drug and alcohol use; (4) systemic illness; and (5) potential toxin exposure. Sexual history should include

BOX 58.4 Male Infertility Factors

Endocrine Disorders
Hypothalamic dysfunction (Kallmann syndrome)
Pituitary failure (tumor, radiation, surgery)
Hyperprolactinemia (drug, tumor)
Androgen insensitivity syndrome (AIS)
Exogenous androgens
Thyroid disorders
Adrenal hyperplasia
Testicular failure

Anatomic
Congenital absence of vas deferens
Obstructed vas deferens
Congenital abnormalities of ejaculatory system
Varicocele
Retrograde ejaculation

Abnormal Spermatogenesis
Unexplained azoospermia
Chromosomal abnormalities
Mumps orchitis
Cryptorchidism
Chemical or radiation exposure

Abnormal Motility
Absent cilia (Kartagener syndrome)
Antibody formation

Psychosocial
Unexplained impotence
Decreased libido

Modified from Morell V. Basic infertility assessment. *Primary Care* 1997;24:195–204.

AT A GLANCE

Evaluating Male Infertility

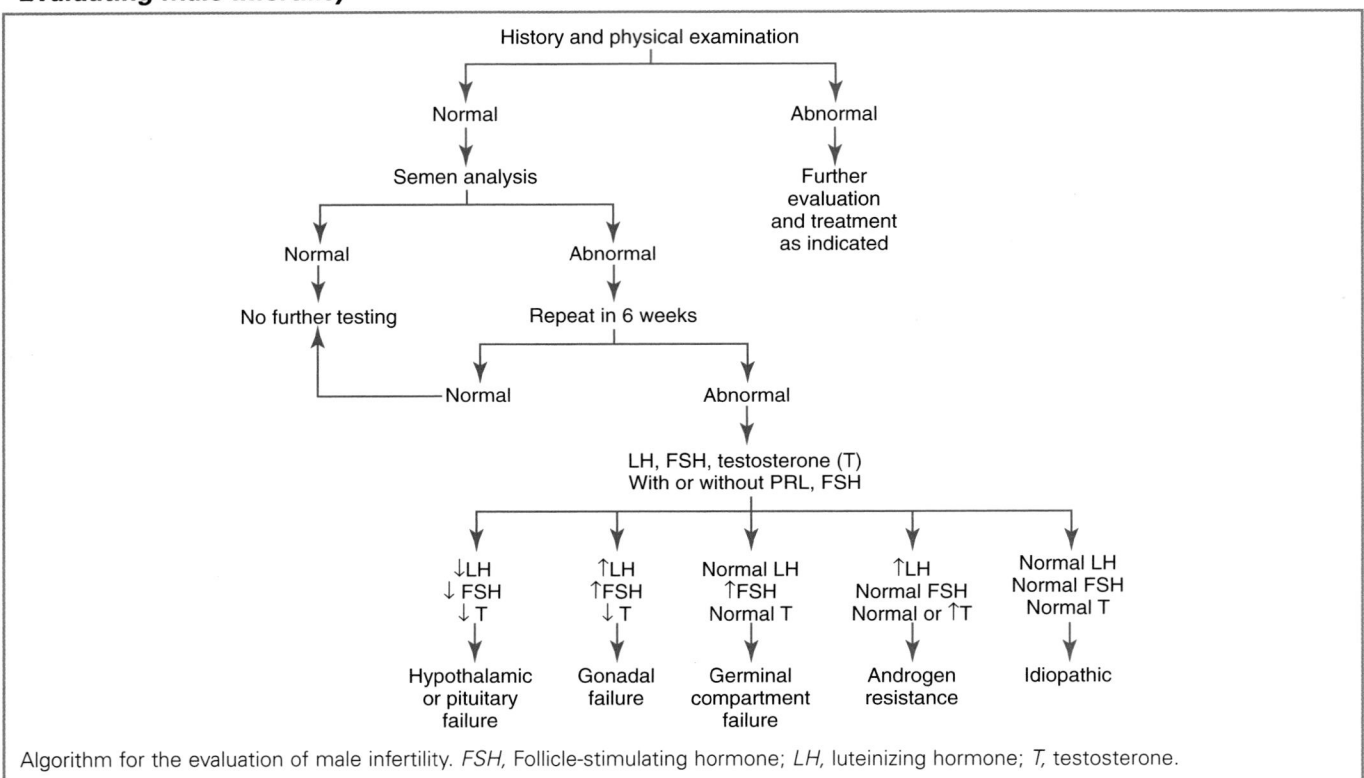

Algorithm for the evaluation of male infertility. *FSH,* Follicle-stimulating hormone; *LH,* luteinizing hormone; *T,* testosterone.

sexual technique, frequency of intercourse, and use of any lubricants. Issues of potency must be distinguished from those of infertility or subfertility. All abnormalities in the history and physical examination should be pursued. Testosterone should be measured, especially when the patient history or physical examination suggests deficient development of secondary sex characteristics. Laboratory evaluation of male infertility should begin with evaluation of semen, which should be followed by evaluation of endocrine parameters.

Evaluation of Semen

Semen analysis measures ejaculate volume, pH, sperm count, motility, forward progression, and morphology. Semen should be analyzed within 1 hour after collection. Although semen analysis is not a test for infertility, it is considered the most important laboratory test in the evaluation of male fertility. Controversy exists as to what constitutes a "normal" semen profile. With the exception of the *azoospermic* male (defined as no sperm in the ejaculate), the lines

TABLE 58.3   Normal Seminal Fluid Values

Parameter	Value
Ejaculate volume	>1.5 mL (1.4–1.7)[a]
Sperm density	>15 million/mL (12–16)[a]
Total sperm count	>39 million/ejaculate (33–46)[a]
Motility	>32% progressive motility (31–34); >40% total (38–42)[a]
Morphology	>4.0% normal (3–4)[a]
pH	7.2–8.0[a]
Color	Gray-white-yellow
Liquefaction	Within 40 min
Fructose	>1200 μg/mL
Acid phosphatase	100–300 μg/mL
Citric acid	>3 mg/mL
Inositol	>1 mg/mL
Zinc	>75 μg/mL
Magnesium	>70 μg/mL
Prostaglandins (PGE$_1$ + PGE$_2$)	30–200 μg/mL
Glycerylphosphorylcholine	>650 μg/mL
Carnitine	>250 μg/mL
Glucosidase	>20 mU per ejaculate

[a]Values from World Health Organization. Cooper TG, et al. World Health Organization reference values for human semen characteristics. *Hum Reprod Update* 2010;3:231.

between fertility and infertility are blurred and are intimately associated with the status of the female partner's reproductive function. However, clinical studies of infertile men and World Health Organization (WHO) guidelines have helped establish limits of adequacy (Table 58.3).[226] If semen analysis is normal, it is unlikely that other laboratory testing will be useful. If semen analysis is abnormal, it should be repeated in approximately 6 weeks. One approach to semen analysis for investigation of infertility uses a monoclonal antibody to sperm protein SP-10 as a proxy for sperm count. A version of the test is available to check the success of vasectomy.[227,228]

Evaluation of Obstruction

Obstruction of the male reproductive tract will result in male infertility, and analysis of specific semen parameters has proved a useful adjunct to physical examination in the evaluation of male reproductive tract obstruction. Testosterone produced after administration of hCG causes the seminal vesicles, epididymis, and prostate to increase the volume of ejaculate. An appropriate increase in serum testosterone without change in the ejaculate volume may indicate mechanical blockage. Absence of, or a decrease in, specific biochemical markers such as acid phosphatase and citric acid (from prostate), fructose, and prostaglandins (from seminal vesicles) can assist determination of the location of blockage.[229] Low seminal glucosidase concentrations in the presence of testes of normal size and consistency, normal semen volume, and normal serum FSH have been used as an indication of obstruction (usually in the epididymis) or congenital bilateral absence of the vas deferens (a condition associated with mutations of the *CFTR* gene in cystic fibrosis).[230]

Evaluation of Endocrine Parameters

If severe oligospermia or azoospermia is found, then measurement of serum testosterone, LH, and FSH concentrations is warranted, with or without measurement of prolactin and TSH. Hyperprolactinemia is a cause of secondary testicular dysfunction.[231] Prolactin excess likely causes hypogonadism by impairing GnRH release. It also leads to underandrogenization and erectile dysfunction (see earlier section "Erectile Dysfunction"). If hyperprolactinemia is found, it is imperative to check for hypothyroidism because elevated TRH concentrations can result in hyperprolactinemia. Pituitary adenomas and drugs such as anxiolytics, antihypertensives, serotonergics, and histamine H$_2$ receptor antagonists also increase serum prolactin.[232] Hyperthyroidism and hypothyroidism will alter spermatogenesis. Hyperthyroidism affects both pituitary and testicular function, with alterations in the secretion of releasing hormones and increased conversion of androgens to estrogens.

Patients with borderline or suppressed testosterone concentrations can be evaluated with an *hCG stimulation test.* With this test, an injection of 5000 IU hCG is administered intramuscularly following collection of a basal, early-morning testosterone sample. Serum testosterone is measured 72 hours later. Hypogonadal men show a depressed rise in testosterone concentration in response to this challenge. Doubling of testosterone concentration over baseline is consistent with normal Leydig cell function.[233] Failure to increase testosterone to greater than 150 ng/dL (5 nmol/L) indicates primary hypogonadism.[234] Alternatively, sperm counts may be evaluated before and after administration of clomiphene citrate or hCG. This represents more of a trial-and-error approach but is simpler to perform than a formal hCG stimulation test and is often preferred in clinical practice. Letrozole, an aromatase inhibitor, is also used to improve semen parameters is hypogonadal men.[235]

Testosterone is essential for normal sperm development (see Fig. 58.3). Therefore any disorder that results in hypogonadism (and thus low testosterone concentrations) results in infertility. Among the causes are hypogonadotropic and hypergonadotropic hypogonadism.

Hypergonadotropic hypogonadism. Measurement of the concentration of FSH is indicated in men with sperm count lower than 5 to 10 million/mL. Elevated concentrations of FSH indicate Sertoli cell dysfunction and, in azoospermic men, primary germinal cell failure, Sertoli cell–only syndrome, or genetic conditions such as Klinefelter syndrome.[226] Radiotherapy and gonadotoxic chemotherapy can also lead to testicular failure with azoospermia. Elevated FSH in the setting of decreased testosterone and oligospermia indicate primary testicular failure.

Hypogonadotropic hypogonadism. Decreased concentrations of testosterone (<200 ng/dL, 7 nmol/L) and decreased concentrations of FSH (<10 IU/L) are suggestive of hypogonadotropic hypogonadism. Administering GnRH may help to distinguish between gonadal insufficiencies caused by pituitary versus hypothalamic failure. Because the pituitary is sensitive to sex steroids for appropriate gonadotropin secretion, patients with long-standing hypogonadism should be given exogenous testosterone for 1 week before the GnRH stimulation test is administered. One approach to this test involves the intravenous injection of 100 μg of GnRH with measurement of FSH and LH concentrations at 0, 30, 60, 120, and 180 minutes after injection. Results of the GnRH test are classified as follows. An increase in serum gonadotropins of 10 IU/L or more over baseline is normal. If little to no increase in gonadotropins is seen, pituitary disease is likely. Patients with hypothalamic disease will demonstrate a delayed but significant increase of 7 IU/L or more within 180 minutes.[236] The most common cause of hypothalamic hypogonadism is *congenital idiopathic hypogonadotropic hypogonadism* (IHH) or its variant, Kallmann syndrome (see earlier section "Male Reproductive Abnormalities").[237] An adult-onset form of IHH has been recognized as a potentially treatable form of male infertility. Molecular diagnosis using fluorescence in situ hybridization (FISH) analysis is now offered to families with X-linked Kallmann syndrome. This is the most common type of testing performed, but it will detect only major deletions in the *KAL* gene. Genome microarray analysis and prenatal diagnosis also are now available.

Mutations in the X chromosome gene, *DAX1*, also have been known to cause hypogonadotropic hypogonadism in association with congenital adrenal hypoplasia. This gene encodes an orphan nuclear hormone receptor that has a critical role in development of the hypothalamus, pituitary, adrenal, and gonads.[238]

Y-Chromosome Microdeletions

Deletions in either of the azoospermia factor regions (*AZF1* and *AZF2*) on the long arm of the Y chromosome are associated with an inability to make sperm. In addition, genes such as *SRY* (sex-determining region Y) are on the short arm of chromosome Y. Y-microdeletions in the *AZF* regions are associated with azoospermia or, less frequently, oligospermia. The incidence of Y microdeletions was 5.0% in men with sperm concentrations 0-1 million/mL and 0.8% when sperm concentrations were 1-5 million/mL.[239] Testing for Y-chromosome microdeletions includes polymerase chain reaction (PCR) of specific regions of the Y chromosome to identify microdeletions. Tests should span *AZF1* (*AZFa*) and *AZF2* (*AZFb* and *AZFc*) and other regions thought to encode putative spermatogenesis genes.[240] The utility of testing for Y-chromosome microdeletions is to provide additional information as to whether or not sperm might be retrieved on a testicular sperm extraction procedure.

Immunologic Parameters

Antibodies to sperm surface antigens have been explored as a cause of infertility. They are thought to impair fertility by decreasing motility, increasing agglutination, and impairing the ability of sperm to penetrate human ova.[241] However, this is controversial, and laboratory testing for antisperm antibodies is rarely performed.[242]

Female Infertility

Evaluating female infertility is more complex than evaluating infertility of the male. A list of the most common female infertility factors is given in Box 58.5. One algorithm for the evaluation of female infertility is shown in At a glance. This evaluation should be considered after 1 year of unprotected intercourse in women with regular menses younger than 35. If a woman is over the age of 35 or if the woman or her partner has a history of issues that would contribute to infertility, this workup should ensue sooner. Examples of issues that would prompt earlier workup include irregular menses,

---

BOX 58.5   Female Infertility Factors

Ovarian or Hormonal Factors
Metabolic disease
  Thyroid
  Liver
  Obesity
  Androgen excess
  Polycystic ovarian syndrome
Hypergonadotropic hypogonadism
  Menopause
  Luteal phase deficiency
  Gonadal dysgenesis
  Primary ovarian insufficiency (autoimmune, cytotoxic, chemotherapy, radiation, tumor)
  Resistant ovary syndrome
Hypogonadotropic hypogonadism
  Hyperprolactinemia (tumor, drugs)
  Hypothalamic insufficiency (Kallmann syndrome)
  Pituitary insufficiency (tumor, necrosis, thrombosis, stress, exercise, anorexia)

Tubal Factors
Occlusion or scarring
Salpingitis isthmica nodosa
Infectious salpingitis

Cervical Factors
Stenosis
Inflammation or infection
Abnormal mucous viscosity

Uterine Factors
Leiomyomata
Congenital malformation
Adhesions
Endometritis or abnormal endometrium

Psychosocial Factors
Decreased libido
Anorgasmia
Iatrogenic
Immunologic (Antisperm Antibodies)

Modified from Morell V. Basic infertility assessment. *Primary Care* 1997;24:195–204.

---

history of pelvic inflammatory disease or sexually transmitted infection, and history of exposure to gonadotoxic agents.

Initial Evaluation of Female Infertility

The initial evaluation of female infertility should include a detailed history and physical examination. The physical examination should include evaluation of (1) the external genitalia and hair pattern (for signs of androgen excess, including clitoromegaly, hirsutism, and virilization), (2) the pelvis (for masses, nodularity, or tenderness), (3) the breasts (for signs of galactorrhea), (4) neurologic findings (sense of smell and visual impairments), (5) the thyroid (for enlargement or nodules), and (6) body mass index. All abnormalities in the history and physical examination should be pursued. A thorough medical and surgical history is also necessary, including an assessment of the patient's gravidity and parity,

AT A GLANCE
Evaluating Female Infertility

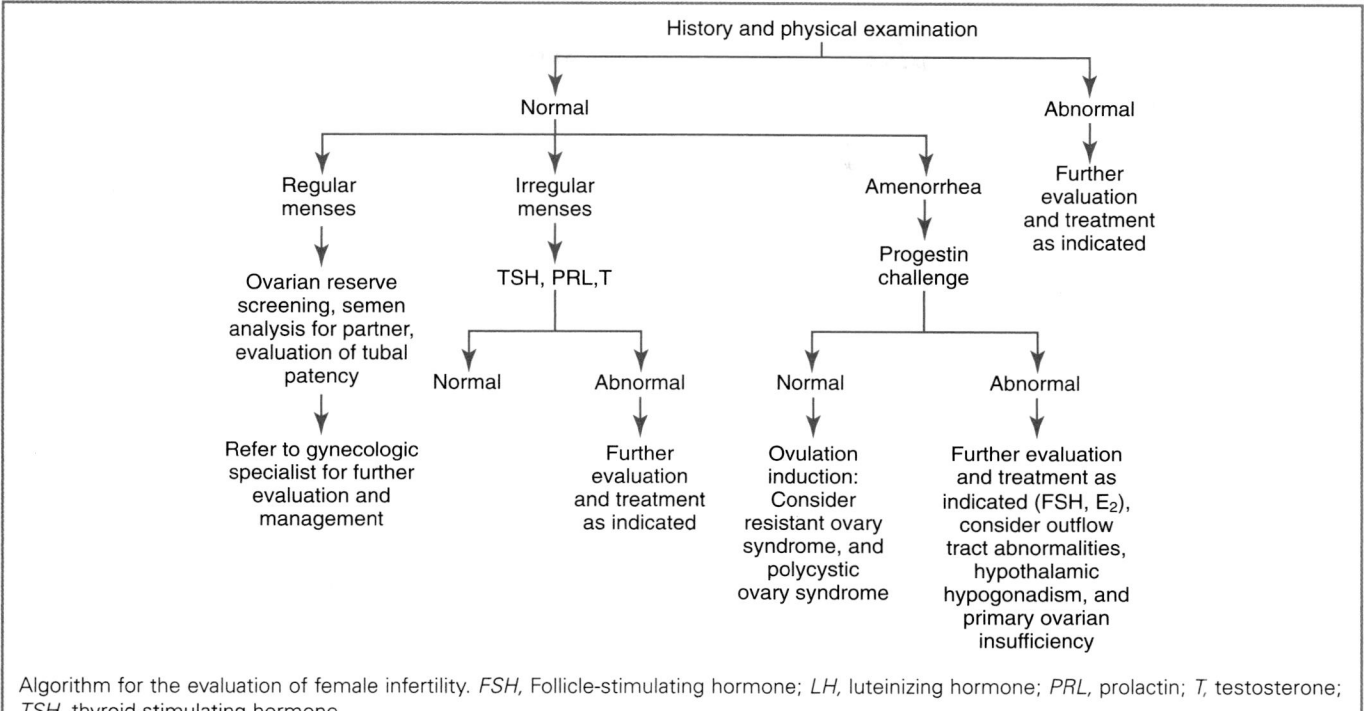

Algorithm for the evaluation of female infertility. *FSH*, Follicle-stimulating hormone; *LH*, luteinizing hormone; *PRL*, prolactin; *T*, testosterone; *TSH*, thyroid-stimulating hormone.

coital frequency, duration of infertility, and prior workup and treatment for infertility. History of sexually transmitted infections, assessment of previous cervical cytologic and human papillomavirus (HPV) testing and treatment, and a menstrual history also should be obtained. Concentrations of TSH, testosterone, and prolactin should be measured if menstrual cycles are absent or irregular or if signs of galactorrhea or thyroid abnormalities are present. Ovulation reserve testing as discussed here should be considered in cases where diminished ovarian reserve is suspected.

Evaluation of ovulation. In the menstruating woman, the next step would be to determine whether ovulation occurs. No current laboratory tests will confirm ovum release. However, measurement of the concentration of midluteal plasma progesterone does indicate that a corpus luteum was formed. Other methods, such as measurement of the LH surge (to predict ovulation) and basal body temperature (to detect a midcycle rise in progesterone), have been used to assess ovulation.

Progesterone measurement. Measurement of the concentration of serum progesterone is the primary assay used for the evaluation of ovulation.[243,244] It is important to note that an increase in progesterone concentration indicates that a corpus luteum has been formed, but it does not confirm that the oocyte was actually released. Beginning immediately after ovulation, serum progesterone concentrations rise (see Fig. 58.9); they peak within 5 to 9 days during the midluteal phase (days 21 to 23).[244] If ovulation does not occur, the corpus luteum fails to form, and the expected cyclic rise in progesterone concentration is subnormal. If pregnancy occurs, hCG maintains the corpus luteum, and progesterone production continues to rise. Midluteal progesterone concentrations

greater than 300 ng/dL (9.5 nmol/L) indicate that ovulation has taken place.[245]

Basal body temperature. Basal body temperature charts have long been accepted as simple, cost-effective indicators of ovulation. Ovulation is associated with a rapid rise in body temperature (by 0.2 to 0.5 °F, or 0.1 to 0.3 °C), which persists through the luteal phase. The rise in temperature is due to increased progesterone concentration. However, similar to progesterone, the rise in body temperature is evident only retrospectively and therefore does not predict imminent ovulation in a way helpful for timing intercourse.

Measurement of the luteinizing hormone surge. Luteinizing hormone appears in the urine just after the serum LH surge and 24 to 36 hours before ovulation (see Fig. 58.9). Measurement of LH does not confirm ovulation or provide insight into the cause of anovulation, but rather indicates when ovulation should occur and provides a guide with which to time intercourse. Methods for laboratory measurement of LH are given in Chapter 55.

Monoclonal technology has led to the use of *home LH kits* that not only provide accurate information as to the timing of ovulation but may reduce stress and costs associated with infertility programs because these tests are performed at home and are comparatively inexpensive.[246] Most home ovulation kits consist of a "dipstick" that uses a two-site, double monoclonal enzyme-linked immunoassay. Urine is applied to the test pad, and capillary action draws fluid across the pad. LH in the urine first is bound to an anti-LH antibody that is coupled to an enzyme conjugate, or colloidal gold. The LH-antibody complex then migrates to a region coated with a second anti-LH antibody. Once bound to this site, the substrate-enzyme reaction or colloidal gold complexes result in a color change that is proportional to the amount of LH present. A reference region is provided. A test result that matches or is darker in color than the reference region is considered a positive result, indicating that the LH surge is occurring. These tests effectively predict ovulation in 70% of women.[247] In one study of 26 normal women, home LH kits had a 92% positive predictive value for ovulation to occur within 48 hours of a positive urine LH screen.[248] The clinical utility of these devices is controversial, however,[249] and no studies have been performed to determine whether the use of home LH devices alters outcomes in women not being treated for infertility. A few studies have been published to look at outcomes in infertility patients, but the results are mixed when compared with serum LH testing or basal body temperature.[249] On the other hand, studies comparing urinary LH surge testing to ultrasound monitoring and human chorionic gonadotropin injections to monitor and trigger ovulation for intrauterine insemination have found no differences in chances of pregnancy between the two approaches, although the cost and time commitment to the latter option is clearly more involved.[250,251]

Evaluation of Endocrine Parameters

Disorders of the hypothalamus, pituitary, and ovary are endocrine causes of infertility.

Hypergonadotropic hypogonadism. Premature ovarian failure is indicated by repeatedly elevated basal FSH concentrations (>30 IU/L) or a single elevation of greater than 40 IU/L in a woman younger than 40 years. These patients are often hypoestrogenic (E_2 < 20 pg/mL, 73 pmol/L)[244] and do not respond to a progestin challenge because their endometrium is atrophic (see earlier section on evaluation of secondary amenorrhea). A pelvic ultrasound will reveal a thin endometrium. Basal serum FSH has been used as an indicator of relative ovarian reserve. Fig. 58.11 shows the relationship between rising serum FSH and the reduced rate of successful pregnancy. A precipitous drop occurs at concentrations greater than 20 IU/L.

Assessing ovarian reserve. Women in their mid to late 30s and early 40s with infertility constitute the largest portion of the total infertility population. These women are also at increased risk for miscarriage. This reflects a diminished ovarian reserve as a result of follicular depletion and a decline in oocyte quality. As women age, serum FSH concentrations in the early follicular phase begin to increase. It has been suggested that this is due to a decline in the number of small follicles secreting inhibin B.

The concomitant measurement of follicular phase serum FSH and E_2 is a popular screening test for assessing ovarian reserve. In general, day 3 FSH concentrations greater than 20 to 25 IU/L are considered to be elevated and associated with poor reproductive outcome.[252] Concomitant measurement of serum E_2 concentration adds to the predictive power of an isolated FSH determination. Early follicular phase E_2 concentrations greater than 75 to 80 pg/mL (275–294 pmol/L) may be associated with poor response to ovarian stimulation and pregnancy outcome, although these concentrations may also be slightly elevated in women with PCOS.[253]

More recently anti-Müllerian hormone (AMH) (also known as Müllerian-inhibiting substance [MIS]) has emerged as a helpful indicator of ovarian reserve. AMH regulates follicle development and maturation and E_2 production.[254] AMH is produced by small, growing follicles but ceases to be produced during FSH-dependent follicular growth or in atretic follicles.[255] Serum AMH remains relatively constant throughout the menstrual cycle and decreases with age,[256,257] leading to its promotion as a marker of ovarian reserve and reduced reproductive capacity.[258–260] However, additional reports have demonstrated noticeable intraindividual variation in serum AMH.[261,262] This observation, coupled with the lack of standardization of AMH assays or clearly defined reference intervals,[187] concerns about sample stability,[263,264] and successful pregnancy in childhood lymphoma survivors with low serum AMH,[265] has led to concerns regarding the use of AMH to classify a patient's ovarian status.

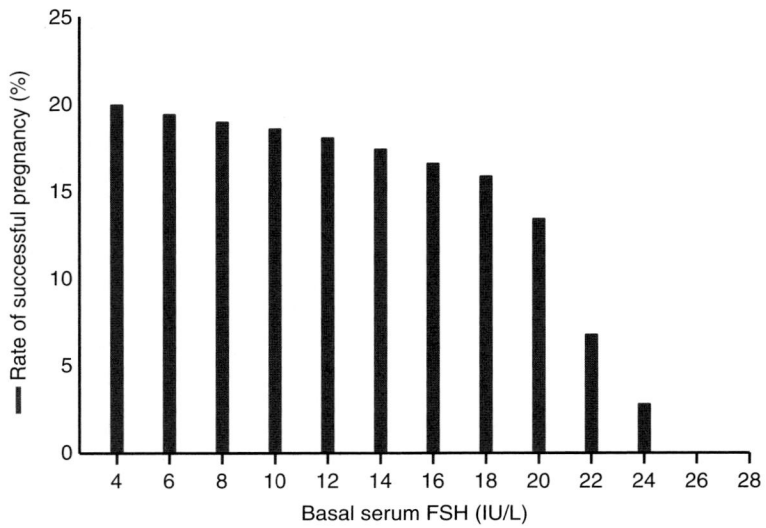

FIGURE 58.11 The relationship between increasing follicle-stimulating hormone *(FSH)* concentrations and decreased percentage of successful pregnancies. (Modified from Jones H, Toner JP. The infertile couple. *N Engl J Med* 1993;329:1710–5.)

Current literature suggests the most beneficial application of AMH measurement is not in AMH's ability to predict the chance of pregnancy but rather in predicting response to controlled ovarian stimulation used in assisted reproductive techniques.[266–269] Patients with elevated serum AMH concentrations are often "high responders" and are at risk of ovarian hyperstimulation syndrome (OHSS) if a standard ovarian stimulation protocol is used. As a result, these women may undergo a modified stimulation protocol to minimize the risk of OHSS. At the other end of the spectrum, women with low serum AMH concentrations are considered "low responders" and often require greater ovarian stimulation to ensure successful oocyte collection. Using AMH in conjunction with another screen of ovarian reserve (like ovarian antral follicle count [AFC] as measured by transvaginal ultrasound) can be quite helpful in optimizing the approach to ovarian stimulation for fertility treatment.

Inhibin B is produced by developing follicles, and concentrations peak during the follicular phase. Concentrations of inhibin B can be used in conjunction with serum FSH and E_2 to assess ovarian function. However, measurement of inhibin adds little to the more established use of serum FSH and E_2, AMH, and/or AFC. Measurement of inhibins, therefore remains of research interest only.

Hypogonadotropic hypogonadism. In hypogonadotropic hypogonadism, serum E_2 concentrations are less than 40 pg/mL (147 pmol/L); therefore there is no withdrawal bleeding with a progestin challenge because the endometrium is thin.[169] Decreased LH (<10 IU/L) and decreased FSH (<10 IU/L) are also present.[244] Hyperprolactinemia can cause hypogonadotropic hypogonadic infertility. The upper limit of normal plasma prolactin in an amenorrheic, hypoestrogenic, nonpregnant woman is 400 to 500 mIU/mL (20 to 25 ng/mL). If estrogen status is normal, maximum prolactin concentrations vary from 600 to 800 IU/L (30 to 40 ng/mL).[270] Thyroid-stimulating hormone should be measured to exclude hypothyroidism. Prolactin concentrations can be elevated in patients with PCOS and those taking medications such as antidepressants, cimetidine, and methyldopa, and in stressful conditions. Prolactin concentrations can be elevated if drawn later in the day or after a meal, so they should be drawn fasting, early in the day. In cases where hyperprolactinemia is noted, radiographic imaging of the pituitary is indicated to rule out pituitary adenoma or empty sella syndrome.

Ovulatory factors. Ovulatory dysfunction is difficult to diagnose because it will manifest in the presence or absence of normal menses. Metabolic diseases of many types affect ovulatory function, including those that result in androgen excess. PCOS, which results in androgen excess, is the most common cause of anovulation and was discussed in detail earlier in the chapter. In women with hirsutism, CAH should be considered. 21-Hydroxylase deficiency or 3-β-hydroxysteroid deficiency may be present in up to 26% of cases.[271] Elevated follicular phase serum 17-hydroxyprogesterone concentrations require further evaluation for these conditions. In addition, it is possible for ovulatory dysfunction to be secondary to liver or thyroid disorders.

As with male infertility, hypogonadism (hypergonadotropic or hypogonadotropic) results in female infertility. Causes of hypergonadotropic hypogonadism include primary ovarian insufficiency (POI), gonadal dysgenesis, resistant ovary syndrome, menopause, and luteal phase deficiency. Causes of hypogonadotropic hypogonadism include pituitary or hypothalamic insufficiency and hyperprolactinemia. Many of these pathologic states have been discussed in the earlier section "Irregular Menses."

Historically, ovulation with inadequate luteinization and reduced progesterone secretion during the luteal phase was termed *luteal phase deficiency*. Currently, luteal phase deficiency is defined as a short luteal phase defined by less than 10 days between ovulation and menses or less than 13 days between the LH surge and menses.[272] Decreased progesterone production is presumed to be responsible, but this may follow insufficient follicular phase FSH secretion, abnormal LH surge, or other endocrine abnormalities. While serum progesterone measurement or endometrial biopsy was used historically to diagnose luteal phase deficiency, it remains a clinical diagnosis defined by length of the luteal phase. It is often treated by using clomiphene citrate or aromatase inhibitors early in the follicular phase to improve follicular recruitment and subsequent luteal function, or with progesterone supplementation in the luteal phase. The clinical significance of luteal phase deficiency remains unclear.[273]

Postcoital test. The postcoital test has been used historically to evaluate infertility; however, it has been shown to have limited utility.[274]

Immunologic factors. Antisperm antibodies have been proposed to contribute to female infertility. However, this topic is controversial, and laboratory testing for antisperm antibodies is rarely performed.[242]

Assisted Reproduction

Couples with a multitude of infertility problems, including unidentified causes and persistent infertility despite standard treatments, may benefit from assisted reproductive techniques (ART). If no definable cause is identified, standard initial therapy consists of ovulation induction with intrauterine insemination for three cycles before progression to more aggressive techniques such as controlled ovarian hyperstimulation (COH) with inseminations or in vitro fertilization (IVF) with or without intracytoplasmic sperm injection (ICSI).[275] If very low sperm counts are present, it is often reasonable to proceed directly to IVF with ICSI (see below). Significant tubal pathology often warrants proceeding directly to IVF.

The laboratory plays an important role in the process of controlled ovarian hyperstimulation. The principle involves administration of gonadotropins to stimulate follicular growth, followed by hCG to stimulate follicular maturation and ovulation. Clinical, laboratory, and ultrasound monitoring of the treatment cycle is necessary to (1) identify the dose and length of therapy, (2) determine when or whether to administer hCG, and (3) obtain an adequate ovulatory response while avoiding hyperstimulation.[276]

Infertility treatments involve procedures that deliver a concentrated sperm sample directly to the uterus (intrauterine insemination) or assisted reproductive techniques. The latter are techniques that involve acquiring fertile ova using transvaginal ultrasound and assisting fertilization in the laboratory with conventional IVF or ICSI in the fallopian tubes using gamete intrafallopian transfer (GIFT) or zygote intrafallopian transfer (ZIFT).[245] IVF then requires embryo transfer back into the uterus. Very few GIFT or ZIFT procedures are performed today owing to the availability of improved embryo culture techniques. The latest successful techniques include direct ovum fertilization using direct micropipette ICSI of the sperm. This procedure provides hope to even the azoospermic man for whom testicular aspiration may yield a few nonmotile sperm. ICSI is widely used today for non–male factor infertility cases as well, and it is employed in about 50 to 60% of IVF cycles.

Despite these advances, the 2016 Centers for Disease Control and Prevention (CDC) surveillance summary of ART reported that only 52.4% (80,971 out of 154,439) of all embryo transfers performed in the United States resulted in a clinical pregnancy.[277] This represents a modest improvement relative to the 2012 CDC surveillance summary that reported a clinical pregnancy rate of 46.8% (62,977 out of 134,419).[278] Multiple embryos are often transferred during a single ART cycle to improve the chance of pregnancy, which frequently results in multiple-gestation pregnancies. In 2016, 32% of children born following an ART procedure were multiple-birth infants.[277] With an understanding of the risks associated with multiple-gestation pregnancies[279] and the pressures to improve the success rate of ART, substantial research effort is focused on selecting embryos with the highest probability of successful implantation and healthy development, leading ultimately to a single live birth.[280] More emphasis is placed on single-embryo transfer.[281] Noninvasive approaches beyond morphology have been evaluated for embryo selection, including sampling of embryo culture medium to evaluate glucose consumption and embryo selection using time-lapse imaging. However, neither of these has proven to be as good as preimplantation genetic screening (PGS) to identify euploid embryos or preimplantation genetic diagnosis (PGD) to detect genetic variants associated with selected inherited conditions.[282–286] The drawback of PGS is that it is invasive, and it often requires freezing the embryos because many clinics do not have the facilities to perform the analysis of the cells in time for a fresh transfer. Thus PGS often requires additional time and cost commitment to an IVF cycle. Work on improving IVF outcomes has also focused on assessing endometrial receptivity to facilitate embryo transfer during the relatively brief window of the menstrual cycle when the endometrium is most likely to support blastocyst implantation.[287–290] Large clinical trials are required to definitively prove the clinical benefit of any of these techniques, but it is hoped that further optimization and eventual concurrent use of multiple techniques will improve the success rate of ART, while minimizing the occurrence of multiple-gestation pregnancies.

POINTS TO REMEMBER
Facts About Infertility

- A specific cause of infertility is identified in 80% of infertile couples.
- Infertility often arises as a result of hormonal dysfunction of the hypothalamic-pituitary-gonadal axis.
- Laboratory measurement of serum hormone concentrations is an integral part of the workup of both female and male infertility.

ANALYTICAL METHODS FOR REPRODUCTIVE HORMONES

A variety of methods are available for measuring sex steroids in body fluids. Currently, the most common method is nonisotopic immunoassay. However, use of mass spectrometry to measure sex steroids is increasing. Some of the advantages and disadvantages are discussed in this chapter. Methods used for reproductive protein hormones are discussed in Chapters 55 and 59. Methods used for reproductive steroid hormones are discussed here.

Measurement of Sex Steroids by Mass Spectrometry

Although immunoassays are the predominant method for the detection and measurement of sex steroids (E_2, testosterone, progesterone, etc.), they are associated with considerable analytical problems. For example, automated testosterone immunoassays (nonisotopic) perform well in healthy adult males and estradiol immunoassays perform well in healthy premenopausal females but are unacceptable for use in children or adult patients with low hormone concentrations due to accuracy and imprecision problems at the low end of detectability. Studies by Wang and associates comparing testosterone measurement by the four most commonly used automated direct immunoassay platforms against an LC-MS/MS reference method indicate acceptable agreement only in the adult male range.[291] Immunoassay methods failed to accurately and precisely detect concentrations of testosterone below 100 ng/dL (3.47 nmol/L).[291] Because concentrations of testosterone in women, children, and hypogonadal men typically fall below 100 ng/dL (3.47 nmol/L), measurement by immunoassay is not recommended. In addition, there is a clinical demand for the measurement of low concentrations of E_2 (<25 pg/mL or < 90 pmol/L)—for example, in the setting of breast cancer risk assessment among postmenopausal women or following response to aromatase inhibitor treatment.[292] Again, these demands are not met by current automated immunoassays and call for a more sensitive approach.[293]

Mass spectrometry–based methods have been described for several of the sex steroids, including testosterone, DHT, E_2, and progesterone.[294–297] In addition, methods are available to measure precursors and metabolites, including DHEA, DHEA-S, androstenedione, and androstenedione glucuronide.[298–300] Tandem mass spectrometry coupled with liquid chromatography (HPLC) offers several advantages over traditional immunoassays, including lower limits of detection, enhanced specificity, small sample size, decreased lot-to-lot variability, and the possibility of analyzing multiple steroids within the same sample. This ability to simultaneously measure a variety of analytes provides the opportunity for steroid profiling, which may enhance diagnostic capabilities. Because of these advantages, the Endocrine Society suggested using extraction and chromatography followed by MS or MS/MS as a potential gold standard for measurement of testosterone.[301] For a more thorough discussion of tandem mass spectrometry and steroid analysis, the reader is directed to Chapters 20 and 56 and a review by Soldin and Soldin.[302]

However, this technology has some disadvantages, including the requirement for highly trained personnel, high costs of equipment and maintenance, and lack of standardization. Because testosterone and estradiol assays are not standardized, observations from clinical studies that demonstrate increased disease risk at a given steroid hormone concentration cannot be transferred to other institutions that utilize a different assay method.[303] As a result, generalized cutoffs associated with disease risk cannot be defined, universally accepted reference intervals and clinical decision points cannot be established, and patient care guidelines either do not exist or cannot be applied. These differences in assay performance are attributed to differences in assay accuracy, specificity, imprecision, and calibration that are most pronounced in steroid hormone immunoassays, but mass spectrometric assays also require standardization.[304,305]

To address these issues, the Centers for Disease Control and Prevention (CDC) has developed the Hormone Standardization (HoSt) program.[306,307] In the initial phase, 40 samples with known hormone concentrations established using the CDC reference method are distributed to participating laboratories to facilitate assay calibration. In the second phase, participating laboratories are issued quarterly challenges to ensure the established calibration remains accurate. Following implementation of the HoSt program, mean bias between participating mass spectrometric testosterone methods and the CDC reference method decreased by 50% from 2007 to 2011.[306]

Methods for Determination of Total Testosterone in Blood

Circulating testosterone comprises three different forms or pools: a non–protein-bound or "free" form, a weakly bound form, and a tightly bound form. The weakly bound form is associated with albumin, and the tightly bound form is associated with sex hormone–binding globulin (SHBG), which is also known as testosterone/estradiol-binding globulin. The term *total testosterone* refers to serum measurements of free testosterone, albumin-bound testosterone, and SHBG-bound testosterone. Bioavailable testosterone includes circulating free testosterone and albumin-bound testosterone. Testosterone bound to SHBG is not biologically active, whereas the free form is available for target cells. Albumin-bound testosterone is also available to target tissues because testosterone can dissociate from the albumin carrier and rapidly diffuse into target cells.[9]

Methods

A 2019 College of American Pathologists (CAP) survey reports that 1492 out of 1527 (98%) participating laboratories measure the concentration of circulating testosterone (both protein-bound and non–protein-bound forms) using nonisotopic enzyme immunoassays. The remaining 35 laboratories utilize mass spectrometry.[308]

Direct (no extraction required) immunoassay methods have been developed for the determination of testosterone in serum or plasma.[309] In these methods, the steroid must be displaced from its binding proteins (albumin and SHBG), and results of the assay depend on the effectiveness of the displacement. Methods used to release testosterone from endogenous binding proteins include use of salicylates, surfactants, pH alterations, temperature changes, and competing steroids such as estrone or estradiol. Most of the direct immunologic methods use antisera generated against a C_{19} testosterone-protein conjugate. These assays have

demonstrated variable precision agreement with mass spectrophotometry and established RIA methods.[310–312] However, most routine immunoassays are not sensitive enough to measure very low testosterone concentrations such as those found in women, children, or hypogonadal men. The Endocrine Society recommends use of a highly sensitive method such as a liquid chromatography/mass spectrometry/mass spectrometry (LC-MS/MS) method whenever low testosterone concentrations are suspected.[301]

Gas chromatography combined with mass spectrometry (GC-MS) remains the reference method for testosterone measurement, although LC-MS/MS reference methods are also in use.[313] Mass spectrometric reference methods are often used to assess the bias of routine immunoassay methods as discussed earlier.[310,314,315] Several other mass spectrometry–based methods have been described.[295,296]

Regardless of immunoassay type, almost all testosterone antisera show some degree of cross-reactivity with DHT (typically 3 to 5%) but show negligible cross-reactivity with other androgens. Assays that use antisera generated against the C-19 position provide maximum analytical specificity with respect to endogenous steroids. However, cross-reactions with 19-nonsteroids used in contraceptive preparations sometimes cause a problem. In most clinical situations, estimation of testosterone without prior separation of DHT is permitted because plasma concentrations of DHT are only 10 to 20% of those for testosterone. Moreover, testosterone and DHT are the two most important androgens in the systemic circulation; even when a method measures the concentrations of both, clinically useful information about the total androgen load is obtained. DHEA-S has been reported to cross-react in some testosterone assays.[316] If specific estimation of testosterone concentration is required, mass spectrometry is recommended.

Specimen collection and storage. Serum or heparinized plasma is used to measure total testosterone. Testosterone is subject to diurnal variation, reaching a peak concentration at between 0400 and 0800 hours. Therefore morning specimens are preferred. Serum/plasma samples are stable for up to 24 hours at room temperature, up to 1 week refrigerated, and up to 1 year frozen at $-20\,°C$.[317,318] DHEA supplementation should be avoided before testing.[319]

Reference intervals. Example reference intervals for total testosterone in serum are listed in Table 58.4.[b,320]

Comments. Estimation of SHBG in serum is useful for interpreting blood concentrations of total testosterone and for calculating androgen index and bioavailable testosterone. Immunoassays for measurement of SHBG in the routine laboratory have been developed.[321] SHBG concentrations are increased by estradiol and decreased by testosterone[322] and therefore change with age.[323]

Methods for the Determination of Free and Bioavailable Testosterone in Blood

In cases where SHBG concentrations are altered, as in women, aging men, and illness, it has been argued that measurements of free or bioavailable testosterone more accurately reflect androgen status. Excellent reviews of

---

[b]Laboratories should verify that these ranges are appropriate for use in their own settings.

TABLE 58.4 Reference Intervals for Total Testosterone in Serum

Testosterone (Method: LC/MS/MS)	ng/dL	nmol/L
Adults		
18–69 y, males	250–1100	8.7–38.2
females	2–45	0.07–1.6
70–89 y, males	90–890	3.1–30.9
70–94 y, females	2–40	0.07–1.4
1st-trimester pregnancy	20–135	0.7–4.7
2nd-trimester pregnancy	11–153	0.4–5.3
3rd-trimester pregnancy	11–146	0.4–5.1
Children		
Cord blood, males	17–61	0.6–2.1
females	16–44	0.6–1.5
1–10 d, males	≤187	≤6.5
females	≤24	≤0.8
1–3 mo, males	72–344	2.5–11.9
females	≤17	≤0.59
3–5 mo, males	≤201	≤7.0
females	≤12	≤0.4
5–7 mo, males	≤59	≤2.1
females	≤13	≤0.5
7–12 mo, males	≤16	≤0.6
females	≤11	≤0.4
1–5.9 y, males	≤5	≤0.2
females	≤8	≤0.3
6–7.9 y, males	≤25	≤0.9
females	≤20	≤0.7
8–10.9 y, males	≤42	≤1.5
females	≤35	≤1.2
11–11.9 y, males	≤260	≤9.0
females	≤40	≤1.4
12–13.9 y, males	≤420	≤14.6
females	≤40	≤1.4
14–17.9 y, males	≤1000	≤34.7
females	≤40	≤1.4
Tanner Stages		
I, males	≤5	≤0.2
females	≤8	≤0.3
II, males	≤167	≤5.8
females	≤24	≤0.8
III, males	21–719	0.7–25.0
females	≤28	≤1.0
IV, males	25–912	0.9–31.7
females	≤31	≤1.1
V, males	110–975	3.8–33.8
females	≤33	≤1.2

From Nakamoto JM, Mason PW, eds. *The Quest Diagnostics manual: endocrinology, test selection and interpretation*, 5th ed. Capistrano, CA: Quest Diagnostics/Nichols Institute, 2012. Prior to use, laboratories should verify the transferability of these reference intervals to their patient population following the methods described in Chapter 9.

TABLE 58.5 Reference Intervals for Free Testosterone in Serum

Free Testosterone (Method: Tracer Equilibrium Dialysis)	pg/mL	pmol/L	Free Fraction (% of Total)
Men			
18–69 y	35.0–155.0	121–538	1.5–2.2
70–89 y	30.0–135.0	104–468	1.5–2.2
Women			
18–69 y	0.1–6.4	0.4–22.2	0.5–2.0
70–89 y	0.2–3.7	0.7–12.8	0.5–2.0
Pregnancy			
1st trimester	0.5–6.0	1.7–20.8	0.15–0.66
2nd trimester	0.2–3.1	0.7–10.8	0.10–0.34
3rd trimester	0.2–4.1	0.7–14.2	0.15–0.51
Children, Males			
5–9 y	≤5.3	≤18.4	0.44–1.78
10–13 y	0.7–52.0	2.4–180	0.53–3.33
14–17 y	18.0–111.0	62–385	1.05–2.91
Children, Females			
5–9 y	0.2–5.0	0.7–17.4	0.28–1.81
10–13 y	0.1–7.4	0.3–25.7	0.36–3.16
14–17 y	0.5–3.9	1.7–13.5	0.41–2.34

From Nakamoto JM, Mason PW, eds. *The Quest Diagnostics manual: Endocrinology, test selection and interpretation*, 5th ed. Capistrano, CA: Quest Diagnostics/Nichols Institute, 2012. Prior to use, laboratories should verify the transferability of these reference intervals to their patient population following the methods described in Chapter 9.

2. Estimation of combined free and weakly bound (bioavailable) testosterone fractions by selective precipitation of the tightly bound form
3. Calculation of free and weakly bound testosterone concentrations by mathematical modeling

Methods not recommended for use in clinical practice include:

1. Estimation of free hormone using a direct (analog tracer) radioimmunoassay
2. Calculation of the androgen index using indices that reflect the ratios of testosterone pools

Each approach is discussed in turn in the following sections. Example reference intervals for free testosterone and percent free testosterone in serum are listed in Table 58.5 and those for bioavailable testosterone in Table 58.6.[c]

Equilibrium Dialysis/Ultrafiltration

Only a small fraction (1 to 2%) of unconjugated testosterone exists in the free state (non–protein-bound) in serum or plasma. None of the conventional assay methods, including RIA, is sufficiently sensitive to quantify free steroid directly in a protein-free ultrafiltrate of plasma. Instead, free steroid is

various methods used to measure this fraction of testosterone are available.[207]

The three methods routinely used in clinical practice include:

1. Estimation of the free testosterone fraction by equilibrium dialysis or ultrafiltration

[c]Laboratories should verify that these ranges are appropriate for use in their own settings.

TABLE 58.6 Reference Intervals for Bioavailable Testosterone in Serum

Bioavailable Testosterone (Method: Calculation)	ng/dL	nmol/L
Adults		
18–69 y, males	110–575	3.8–20.0
females	0.5–8.5	0.02–0.3
70–89 y, males	15–150	0.5–5.2
females	0.5–8.8	0.02–0.3
Children		
1–11.9 y, males	≤5.4	≤0.2
females	≤3.4	≤0.1
12–13.9 y, males	≤140	≤4.9
females	≤3.4	≤0.1
14–17.9 y, males	8.0–210	0.3–7.3
females	≤7.8	≤0.3

From Nakamoto JM, Mason PW, eds. *The Quest Diagnostics manual: Endocrinology, test selection and interpretation*, 5th ed. Capistrano, CA: Quest Diagnostics/Nichols Institute; 2012. Prior to use, laboratories should verify the transferability of these reference intervals to their patient population following the methods described in Chapter 9.

estimated in plasma by adding a known amount of radiolabeled compound to the sample and allowing labeled and unlabeled compounds to reach equilibrium in their competition for the same binding sites on proteins. Bound and free radiolabeled fractions are then separated, and the ratio of free labeled to total labeled compound is determined. At equilibrium, this ratio is taken as a measure of the free testosterone fraction. An estimate of serum free testosterone can be calculated by multiplying the free testosterone fraction by the total testosterone concentration. The reader is directed elsewhere for a detailed equilibrium dialysis procedure.[324]

Most of the problems with this procedure have involved tracer impurities and separation of bound and free labeled fractions. Several separation techniques have been used, including equilibrium dialysis, membrane ultrafiltration, and steady-state gel filtration. Deficiencies associated with these techniques include a requirement for a large sample volume, the need for complicated correction of sample volume changes that occur during the separation, and difficulties involved in collecting and measuring radioactivity in numerous fractions of each sample. Equilibrium dialysis has been used most often in the past, but serious errors often arise from the sample dilution required by this method.[325] Symmetric dialysis of undiluted samples is reported to be less susceptible to tracer contamination and dilution effects.[326] Ultrafiltration appears to overcome these problems and to obviate errors due to dilution.[327] Due to the labor-intensive nature of both equilibrium dialysis and ultrafiltration, these methods are used almost exclusively at reference laboratories.

Selective Precipitation
Selective precipitation of SHBG with ammonium sulfate is also used to measure bioavailable testosterone. With this technique, aliquots of serum or plasma are first incubated with radiolabeled testosterone. Testosterone bound to SHBG is then precipitated with 50% ammonium sulfate. The samples are centrifuged, and aliquots of the supernatant containing free and albumin-bound testosterone (also known as *non–SHBG-bound testosterone*) are radioactively counted. The percentage of radio label not bound to SHBG is subsequently multiplied by the total testosterone concentration to obtain the bioavailable testosterone.[207] Similar to equilibrium dialysis and ultrafiltration methods, performance of selective precipitation is generally limited to reference laboratories.

Calculated Free Testosterone
Methods based on mathematical modeling use algorithms to derive non–SHBG-bound testosterone. These algorithms assume that when concentrations of total testosterone, SHBG, and albumin and the constants for binding of testosterone to SHBG and albumin are known, free testosterone and bioavailable testosterone can be calculated. These calculations are based on a proper estimation of the association constant for binding of testosterone to SHBG and albumin. The reader is directed to other references for further details on this method.[207,328] Because automated assays are available for total testosterone, SHBG, and albumin, calculation-based methods of measuring free testosterone are inexpensive and suitable for routine use in nonreference labs. Calculation-based methods also generate results that correlate well with equilibrium dialysis.[12,329] However, various association constants for SHBG have been reported, and conditions resulting in abnormal plasma protein concentrations, such as nephrotic syndrome, cirrhosis, and pregnancy, require adjustments in the assumption for albumin concentration.

Several different algorithms based on concentrations measured with a gold standard technique have been proposed.[330-332] Algorithms for calculating bioavailable testosterone are available free online (http://www.issam.ch/freetesto.htm); however, these sources do not always provide a reference for which algorithm is being used.

While calculated free testosterone algorithms are convenient and correlate well with equilibrium dialysis, it should be noted that no consensus has been reached about their use. De Ronde and colleagues compared five algorithms and concluded that they are not transferable to samples from other laboratories unless revalidation using laboratory-specific assays has been performed.[332] Likewise, Giton and colleagues reported that instead of using theoretical association constants, optimal paired association constants should be determined for each studied population.[333] Because this is impossible for the average clinician to do, these authors suggest using ammonium sulfate precipitation. Finally, Dechaud and colleagues reported an age-associated discrepancy between calculated and measured bioavailable testosterone, suggesting that a simplified law of mass action cannot predict variations in steroid distribution in serum.[334] These authors state that consensus is needed regarding the proper measurement of bioavailable testosterone for therapeutic decisions.

Direct (Analog Tracer) Radioimmunoassay
Several RIA procedures have been described for the direct estimation of free testosterone.[11,207,309,335] These assays use a labeled derivative (analog) of testosterone that, in theory, retains the ability to react with exogenous antitestosterone antibodies but is restricted from interacting with testosterone-binding proteins in the serum sample. In practice, development of an analog that does not interact with endogenous proteins has been difficult to achieve.

Advantages of RIA analog methods include a small sample requirement, relatively rapid results, a simple procedure, and the option to measure free testosterone without the need to measure total testosterone.[11,12,309,335] However, some have reported that direct RIAs are grossly inaccurate, underestimating free testosterone concentrations by manyfold.[336,337] For example, one study in females revealed that free testosterone concentrations obtained by two different analog assays were 15 to 35% and 25 to 30% of those obtained by ultrafiltration.[338] As a result, direct RIAs are not recommended by the Endocrine Society,[32] and they have largely been replaced by calculation methods based on total testosterone, SHBG, and albumin concentrations.[339]

Androgen Index

This index is a ratio of testosterone and SHBG multiplied by 100.[207] Although this is only an indicator of free testosterone, some have found it to be useful in the evaluation of hirsutism.[340] Other reports have indicated that the free androgen index is not a reliable parameter of free testosterone because of its variability as a function of SHBG concentration.[11,12,341] Use of the androgen index remains primarily of research interest.

Methods for the Determination of Testosterone Precursors and Metabolites in Blood

Several biosynthetic precursors and metabolites of testosterone are measured using specific immunoassays (directly or after sample extraction), chromatography, or LC-MS/MS.[295,298-300] Examples include DHT, 3α-androstanediol glucuronide, and androstenedione. Example reference intervals for these analytes in serum are listed in Table 58.7.[d]

Methods for the Determination of Dehydroepiandrosterone and Its Sulfate

Measurements of DHEA or its sulfated conjugate, DHEA-S, in serum and plasma are important for investigations of adrenal androgen production, such as assessment of adrenal hyperplasia, adrenal tumors, adrenarche, delayed puberty, or hirsutism. DHEA-S in circulation originates primarily from the adrenal glands, although in men some may be derived from the testes; none is produced by the ovaries. DHEA is secreted almost entirely by the adrenal glands.

DHEA concentrations exhibit a circadian rhythm that reflects the secretion of ACTH; these concentrations vary during the menstrual cycle. DHEA-S concentrations, however, do not exhibit a circadian rhythm because of their longer circulating half-life.[342] Concentrations in serum are increased in cord blood and drop precipitously at birth. Concentrations in premature infants in general are much higher than those in full-term infants. Pregnancy and oral contraceptives induce a modest reduction, and glucocorticoids induce a marked decrease. Patients with polycystic ovary disease often have elevated concentrations of DHEA-S, suggesting an adrenal androgen contribution to the defect in this disorder.[343] Concentrations of DHEA-S are also elevated in CAH and with adrenal cortical tumors (concentrations higher with adrenal carcinoma than with adrenal adenoma).[344] However, concentrations are not elevated in women with virilizing ovarian tumors. Glucocorticoid administration for several days suppresses concentrations

TABLE 58.7 Reference Intervals for Dihydrotestosterone (DHT), 3α-Androstanediol Glucuronide, and Androstenedione in Serum

	ng/dL	nmol/L
Dihydrotestosterone (DHT) (Method: LC/MS/MS)		
Adult men	16–79	0.55–2.7
Adult women	5–46	0.17–1.6
3α-Androstanediol Glucuronide (Method: RIA)		
Men	260–1500	5.5–32
Women	60–300	1.3–6.4
Children		
Prepubertal	10–60	0.2–1.3
Tanner II–III		
Males	19–164	0.4–4.5
Females	33–244	0.7–5.2
Androstenedione (Method: LC/MS/MS)		
Men		
18–30 y	50–220	1.7–7.7
31–50 y	40–190	1.4–6.6
51–60 y	50–220	1.7–7.7
Women		
Follicular	35–250	1.2–8.7
Luteal	30–235	1.0–8.2
Postmenopausal	20–75	0.7–2.6
Children		
Premature infants (31–35 weeks)	≤480	≤16.8
Term infants	≤290	≤10.1
1–12 mo	6–78	0.2–2.7
1–4 y	5–51	0.2–1.8
5–9 y	6–115	0.2–4.0
10–13 y	12–221	0.4–7.7
14–17 y	22–225	0.8–7.9
Tanner II–III		
Males	17–82	0.6–2.9
Females	43–180	1.5–6.3
Tanner IV–V		
Males	57–150	2.0–5.2
Females	73–220	2.6–7.7

From Nakamoto JM, Mason PW, eds. *The Quest Diagnostics manual: endocrinology, test selection and interpretation*, 5th ed. Capistrano, CA: Quest Diagnostics/Nichols Institute; 2012. Prior to use, laboratories should verify the transferability of these reference intervals to their patient population following the methods described in Chapter 9.

in patients with adrenal hyperplasia. DHEA is commercially available in health food stores; therefore increased serum concentrations may be due to exogenous use.

Methods

According to a 2019 CAP survey, all participating laboratories used nonisotopic immunoassays for the measurement of DHEA-S.[308] Other methods include competitive protein-binding assays and GC-MS.[21,343] Immunoassays for DHEA-S demonstrate significant cross-reactivity with DHEA, androstenedione, and androsterone, yet the relative concentrations of these steroids have a minimal effect on assay performance.

---

[d]Laboratories should verify that these ranges are appropriate for use in their own settings.

Specimen collection and storage. Serum or plasma (preserved with ethylenediaminetetraacetic acid [EDTA]) is suitable for DHEA or DHEA-S immunoassays.[320] Early-morning collection, before 10:30 a.m., is preferred for DHEA. DHEA-S specimens are stable for at least 1 day at room temperature. Refrigerated serum/plasma samples (4 to 8 °C) are stable for up to 14 days, and those frozen at −20 °C are stable for longer than 1 year.[317,318]

Reference intervals. Example reference intervals for serum concentrations of DHEA-S and DHEA are listed in Table 58.8.[†,320]

Comments. Analysis of DHEA by immunoassay usually requires pretreatment of serum samples because the serum concentration of DHEA is 1000-fold lower than that of DHEA-S. While several extraction and chromatographic procedures have been suggested for this purpose, these have largely been replaced by LC-MS/MS methods performed at a reference laboratory.[299]

Determination of 17-Ketosteroids in Urine

The 17-ketosteroids (KS) are metabolites of steroids that contain a keto group at C-17 and include androsterone, epiandrosterone, etiocholanolone, DHEA, 11-keto- and 11β-hydroxyandrosterone, and 11-keto- and 11β- hydroxyetiocholanolone. In men, approximately one-third of total urinary 17-KS represents metabolites of testosterone secreted by the testes, whereas most of the remaining two-thirds is derived from steroids produced by the adrenal glands. In women, who normally excrete smaller quantities than men, total 17-KS concentrations are derived almost exclusively from the adrenal glands. Thus the main purpose of measuring these steroid metabolites is to assess adrenal androgen production.

Measurement of DHEA-S in serum serves as a more convenient marker for adrenal androgen production than does urinary 17-KS excretion because 24-hour urine collection is not required and because many drugs interfere with the 17-KS assay.[345] For these reasons, many clinicians now prefer concentrations for plasma DHEA-S to those for urinary 17-KS.

Methods for the Detection of Anabolic Steroids

Detection of exogenous steroids used to improve athletic performance poses a challenge for the laboratory, given the variety of exogenous anabolic steroids, which include both natural and synthetic testosterone analogs. Since the 1980s, GC-MS has been the method of choice to detect anabolic steroids.[346] The ratio of testosterone to epitestosterone (17 α-epimer) in urine has been used as a screening test for the detection of anabolic steroid abuse. A ratio of testosterone to

TABLE 58.8 Reference Intervals for Dehydroepiandrosterone Sulfate and Unconjugated Dehydroepiandrosterone in Serum

DHEA-S (Method: Immunochemiluminometric Assay)	µg/dL	µmol/L	DHEA-S (Method: Immunochemiluminometric Assay)	µg/dL	µmol/L
Men			female	≤92	≤2.5
18–29 y	110–510	3.0–14.0	10–13 y, male	≤138	≤3.7
30–39 y	110–370	3.0–10.0	female	≤148	≤4.0
40–49 y	45–345	1.2–9.4	14–16 y, male	38–340	1.0–9.2
50–59 y	25–240	0.7–6.5	female	37–307	1.0–8.3
≥60 y	≤204	≤5.5	Tanner stages		
			I, male	≤89	≤2.4
Women			female	≤46	≤1.2
18–29 y	45–320	1.2–8.7	II, male	≤81	≤2.2
30–39 y	40–325	1.1–8.8	female	15–113	0.4–3.1
40–49 y	25–220	0.7–6.0	III, male	22–126	0.6–3.4
50–59 y	15–170	0.4–4.6	female	42–162	1.1–4.4
≥60 y	≤145	≤3.9	IV, male	33–177	0.9–4.8
			female	42–241	1.1–6.5
Children			V, male	110–510	3.0–13.8
0–1 mo, male	≤316	≤8.6	female	45–320	1.2–8.7
female	15–261	0.4–7.1			
1–6 mo, male	≤58	≤1.6	**DHEA (Method: LC/MS/MS)**	**ng/dL**	**nmol/L**
female	≤74	≤2.0	Men	61–1636	2.1–56.4
7–12 mo, male	≤26	≤0.7	Women	102–1185	3.5–40.9
female	≤26	≤0.7	Children		
1–3 y, male	≤15	≤0.4	1–5 y	≤377	≤13.0
female	≤22	≤0.6	6–9 y	19–592	0.7–20.4
4–6 y, male	≤27	≤0.7	10–13 y	42–1067	1.4–36.8
female	≤34	≤0.9	14–17 y	137–1489	4.7–51.3
7–9 y, male	≤91	≤2.5			

DHEA, Dehydroepiandrosterone; *DHEA-S,* dehydroepiandrosterone sulfate.
From Nakamoto JM, Mason PW, eds. *The Quest Diagnostics manual: Endocrinology, test selection and interpretation,* 5th ed. Capistrano, CA: Quest Diagnostics/Nichols Institute; 2012. Prior to use, laboratories should verify the transferability of these reference intervals to their patient population following the methods described in Chapter 9.

epitestosterone greater than 6:1 suggests exogenous steroid use, and further testing should be performed for confirmation.[347,348] Others have suggested the ratio of testosterone to LH in the urine as an indication of testosterone doping. Detailed studies of these ratios are available.[349] Because hCG stimulates testosterone production by the testes, hCG has been placed on the World Anti-Doping Agency list of prohibited substances for male athletes. Measurement of intact hCG, free β subunit, and β-core fragment in the urine of male athletes is therefore an important consideration for antidoping laboratories.[350] For a more in-depth discussion of analytical considerations around drug monitoring in athletes, the reader is referred to the review by Bowers.[346]

Methods for the Determination of Estradiol in Blood

Both chromatography–mass spectrometry and immunoassay-based methods are used to measure estrogens in blood. GC-MS methods utilizing isotope dilution provide the most accurate and reliable measurement of E_2.[351–353] The main steps in these reference methods include solvent extraction, chromatographic fractionation, and chemical derivatization before analysis. Validation of immunoassay methods by this technique has become important in many external quality assurance programs.

Immunoassays consist of both indirect (extraction required) and direct (no extraction required) methods. The most common antigen used to prepare antibodies for E_2 assays is estradiol-6-(O-carboxymethyl) oxime conjugated to bovine serum albumin.[354] Cross-reactivity with other C-18 steroids is usually minor because the 3- and 17-hydroxyl groups are left free. A 2019 CAP survey reported that 1479 of 1490 participating laboratories utilized direct enzyme immunoassays for routine measurement of E_2 concentrations and the remaining 11 laboratories used mass spectrometry.[308] Evaluation of estrogen concentrations in men, women taking aromatase inhibitors, postmenopausal women, and children requires the use of mass spectrometry–based methods described earlier.

To measure E_2 directly without extraction and chromatography, the steroid must be displaced from its binding proteins. The displacing agents used in commercial methods often are not disclosed, but in some systems, effective displacement is achieved by adding 8-anilino-1-naphthalene sulfonic acid (ANS) or a large excess of a competing steroid such as dihydrotestosterone to the sample.[354]

Caution should be exercised when assaying samples from subjects who are receiving oral contraceptives or estrogen replacement therapy because cross-reacting steroids may cause elevated results. Most notably, cross-reactivity with estrone is as high as 10% for some assays, but much lower (<1%) for others. This is likely due to a difference in the specificity of the antibody used for E_2. Similar effects have been observed for metabolites conjugated at the 3 position, such as estrone-3-sulfate and estrone-3-glucuronide.[355,356]

Several immunoassays for E_2 have been developed and adapted for use on fully automated immunoassay systems.[357] All are heterogeneous assays (separation step needed), but most are direct assays and do not require preliminary extraction. Most procedures offer the convenience of solid-phase separation methods. For routine clinical applications, the greatest experience is with enzyme immunoassays. Most commercial enzyme immunoassays use alkaline phosphatase

to label E_2 antigens; enzyme activity is determined using a variety of fluorescent,[358] or chemiluminescent substrates.[359] A semiautomated "ultrasensitive" chemiluminescent immunoassay for E_2 has been described.[360] This method is advantageous because it is reportedly capable of accurately measuring low concentrations (<50 pmol/L) of E_2 observed in perimenopausal and postmenopausal women, healthy men, and children.

Taieb and colleagues compared detection limits and functional sensitivities of nine automated E_2 immunoassays.[361] They concluded that functional sensitivities, defined as the lowest concentration of analyte that can be measured with a run-to-run imprecision of 20%, were twofold to fourfold higher than detection limits of the tests. It is also important to note that none of the assays analyzed in this study had the functional sensitivity required for evaluation of serum E_2 measurements in men, menopausal women, and children.[362] Functional sensitivities ranged from 5.5 to 46 pg/mL (20 to 169 pmol/L). These assays have been optimized for clinical applications such as monitoring of ovarian stimulation for IVF, in which high E_2 concentrations are expected, but the values obtained depend on the method used.[363] The authors suggest that until E_2 assays are better standardized, reference intervals and cutoff points used as clinical decision criteria must be evaluated and modified, if necessary, for each assay.

Estradiol Assay Standardization

Specimen collection and storage. Serum and plasma (with EDTA or heparin as anticoagulant) have been used. Specimens should be centrifuged and separated within 24 hours. Serum/plasma specimens may be stored at room temperature for 1 day, refrigerated for 3 days, or frozen for up to 1 year.[317] Oral contraceptives have been known to alter E_2 concentrations.

Reference intervals. Example reference intervals for serum concentrations of E_2 are listed in Table 58.9.†

TABLE 58.9 Reference Intervals for Estradiol (E2) in Serum

Estradiol (Method: LC/MS/MS)	pg/mL	pmol/L
Men	≤29	≤106
Women		
Follicular	39–375	143–1377
Midcycle peak	94–762	345–2797
Luteal phase	48–440	176–1615
Postmenopausal	≤10	≤37
Children		
Prepubertal (1–9 y), males	≤4	≤15
females	≤16	≤59
10–11 y, males	≤12	≤44
females	≤65	≤239
12–14 y, males	≤24	≤88
females	≤142	≤521
15–17 y, males	≤31	≤114
females	≤283	≤1040

From Nakamoto JM, Mason PW, eds. *The Quest Diagnostics manual: Endocrinology, test selection and interpretation*, 5th ed. Capistrano, CA: Quest Diagnostics/Nichols Institute; 2012. Prior to use, laboratories should verify the transferability of these reference intervals to their patient population following the methods described in Chapter 9.

Methods for the Determination of Estriol in Blood

Except for purposes of fetal aneuploidy screening, measurement of E_3 has little clinical value because in nonpregnant women, E_3 is derived almost exclusively from E_2. A 2019 CAP survey reported that automated enzymatic immunoassay methods account for all unconjugated E_3 measurements.[308] Several of these assays have been validated for use in maternal serum screening.[364,365]

Specimen Collection and Storage

E_3 serum or plasma specimens are stable at room temperature for 24 hours; they can be refrigerated for 2 days and frozen at −20°C for up to 1 year.[318]

Methods for the Determination of Estrone in Blood

Estrone determinations have limited clinical utility. Normally, blood estrone concentrations parallel E_2 concentrations throughout the menstrual cycle, but at slightly lower concentrations. For a specific analysis of estrone, the interested reader is directed to other references.[366,367]

Methods for the Determination of Progesterone in Blood

A 2019 CAP survey reported that enzyme immunoassays accounted for all progesterone assays used by survey participants.[308] Initial immunoassays for serum progesterone measurement used organic solvents to remove the steroid from endogenous binding proteins such as corticosteroid-binding globulin and albumin. Direct (nonextraction) measurement of progesterone in serum or plasma is considered the method of choice for routine applications. Various antigens have been used to prepare antisera for progesterone assays. Cross-reactivity is most prominent with 5α-pregnanediol ranging from 6 to 11%.

Several immunoassays are available on fully automated immunoassay systems.[323,368–370] All are heterogeneous assays that require separation of free and antibody-bound fractions. Enzymes appear to be the most widely used nonradioactive label. Alkaline phosphatase and horseradish peroxidase coupled to progesterone or antiprogesterone antibodies are particularly popular. An assortment of photometric,[356] fluorescent,[370] and luminescent[371] substrates are available for monitoring the enzyme activity of the antibody-bound fraction. Direct time-resolved fluoroimmunoassays for progesterone have been described.[372]

Although automated immunoassays are less labor intensive than RIAs and yield results in less time without the need for radioactivity, these assays do not have adequate functional sensitivity for the measurement of low progesterone concentrations in men, postmenopausal women, and children. Taieb and colleagues analyzed the detection limits and functional sensitivities of eight automated progesterone methods.[361] They reported that functional sensitivities (10 to 45 ng/dL or 0.32 to 1.43 nmol/L), defined as the lowest concentration of analyte that could be measured with a run-to-run imprecision of 20%, ranged from twofold to fourfold higher than the manufacturer-stated detection limit (6 to 15 ng/dL or 0.19 to 0.48 nmol/L). Automated progesterone assays have been optimized for use in in vitro fertilization protocols as a rapid, cost-effective way to evaluate ovarian stimulation and monitor ovulation.

Double-isotope derivative methods[373] and competitive protein-binding assays have been applied to the measurement of serum progesterone, but these methods require extensive

TABLE 58.10 Reference Intervals for Progesterone in Serum

Progesterone (Method: LC/MS/MS)	ng/mL	nmol/L
Men		
18–29 y	≤0.3	≤1.0
30–39 y	≤0.2	≤0.6
40–49 y	≤0.2	≤0.6
50–59 y	≤0.2	≤0.6
Women		
Follicular phase	≤2.7	≤8.6
Luteal phase	3.0–31.4	≤100
Postmenopausal	≤0.2	≤0.6
Children		
5–9 y, male	≤0.7	≤2.2
female	≤0.6	≤1.9
10–13 y, male	≤1.2	≤3.8
female	≤10.2	≤32.4
14–17 y, male	≤0.8	≤2.5
female	≤11.9	≤38

From Nakamoto JM, Mason PW, eds. *The Quest Diagnostics manual: Endocrinology, test selection and interpretation*, 5th ed. Capistrano, CA: Quest Diagnostics/Nichols Institute, 2012. Prior to use, laboratories should verify the transferability of these reference intervals to their patient population following the methods described in Chapter 9.

purification of the steroid and are labor intensive. GC procedures using flame ionization, electron capture, or nitrogen detection have been used to improve the accuracy of progesterone analysis. However, these methods are time-consuming and often require solvent extraction, chromatography, and derivatization before the steroid is quantitated. GC-MS has been recommended as a reference method for progesterone determination. The GC-MS method of Thienpont and colleagues[374] uses heptafluorobutyric ester derivatives and 19-^{2}H$_3$-progesterone as internal standards.

Plasma concentrations of 17α-hydroxyprogesterone are measured to evaluate 21-hydroxylase deficiency. For specific methods regarding this analyte, the reader is referred to a review by Wallace.[121]

Specimen Collection and Storage

Serum or plasma (with heparin or EDTA as anticoagulant) is used and should be separated within 24 hours.[320] The patient need not be fasting, and no special handling procedures are necessary. Serum/plasma specimens may be stored at room temperature for 24 hours and refrigerated at 4 to 8 °C for up to 3 days or at −20 °C for up to 1 year.[317,318]

Reference Intervals

Example reference intervals for serum concentrations of progesterone are listed in Table 58.10.[e,320]

Measurement of Salivary Sex Steroids

Measurement of steroid concentrations in saliva has the potential to serve as a noninvasive and convenient procedure for the

---

[e]Laboratories should verify that these ranges are appropriate for use in their own settings.

assessment of "serum free" steroid concentrations. However, primarily because of rapid fluctuations in salivary concentration necessitating the collection of multiple samples, salivary testing for sex steroids is not commonplace. For further discussion of salivary steroid measurements, the reader is referred to a review by Wood.[375]

POINTS TO REMEMBER

- Measurement of total serum steroid hormone concentrations requires displacement of hormone from its binding proteins.
- Immunoassay remains the most common method of steroid hormone measurement, but mass spectrometry is becoming more widely used.
- Automated testosterone and estradiol immunoassays are acceptable for use in healthy adult men and women, respectively, but most lack sufficient accuracy and precision for use in children and adults with low steroid hormone concentrations.
- Mass spectrometry–based methods offer improved accuracy and a lower limit of detection but require highly trained personnel and increased equipment costs.
- Free testosterone is most accurately measured by equilibrium dialysis or ultrafiltration in a reference laboratory. Direct immunoassay measurement of free testosterone is not recommended.

SELECTED REFERENCES

11. Morley JE, Patrick P, Perry HM. Evaluation of assays available to measure free testosterone. Metabolism 2002;51:554–9.
30. Layton JB, Li D, Meier CR, et al. Testosterone lab testing and initiation in the United Kingdom and the United States, 2000 to 2011. J Clin Endocrinol Metab 2014;99:835–42.
32. Bhasin S, Brito JP, Cunningham GR, et al. Testosterone therapy in men with hypogonadism: an endocrine society clinical practice guideline. J Clin Endocrinol Metab 2018;103:1715–44.
38. Vigen R. Association of testosterone therapy with mortality, myocardial infarction, and stroke in men with low testosterone levels. JAMA 2013;310:1829.
95. Direito A, Bailly S, Mariani A, Ecochard R. Relationships between the luteinizing hormone surge and other characteristics of the menstrual cycle in normally ovulating women. Fertil Steril 2013;99:279–85.
99. Christian CA, Moenter SM. The neurobiology of preovulatory and estradiol-induced gonadotropin-releasing hormone surges. Endocr Rev 2010;31:544–77.
103. Greendale GA, Lee NP, Arriola ER. The menopause. Lancet 1999;353:571–80.
104. Nelson LM. Primary ovarian insufficiency. N Engl J Med 2009;360:606–14.
109. The NAMS 2017 Hormone Therapy Position Statement Advisory Panel. The 2017 hormone therapy position statement of The North American Menopause Society. Menopause 2017;24:728–53.
115. Gronowski AM, Fantz CR, Parvin CA, et al. Use of serum FSH to identify perimenopausal women with pituitary hCG. Clin Chem 2008;54:652–6.
175. Revised 2003 consensus on diagnostic criteria and long-term health risks related to polycystic ovary syndrome. Fertil Steril 2004;81:19–25.
187. Dewailly D, Andersen CY, Balen A, et al. The physiology and clinical utility of anti-Müllerian hormone in women. Hum Reprod Update 2014;20:370–85.
189. Alebic MŠ, Stojanovic N, Dewailly D. Discordance between serum anti-Müllerian hormone concentrations and antral follicle counts: not only technical issues. Hum Reprod 2018;33:1141–8.
191. Teede HJ, Misso ML, Costello MF, et al. Recommendations from the international evidence-based guideline for the assessment and management of polycystic ovary syndrome. Hum Reprod 2018;33:1602–18.
214. Hembree WC, Cohen-Kettenis PT, Gooren L, et al. endocrine treatment of gender-dysphoric/gender-incongruent persons: an endocrine society clinical practice guideline. Endocr Pract 2017;23:1437.
301. Rosner W, Auchus RJ, Azziz R, Sluss PM, Raff H. Utility, limitations, and pitfalls in measuring testosterone: An Endocrine Society position statement. J Clin Endocrinol Metab 2006;92:405–13.

Pregnancy and Its Disorders*

Robert D. Nerenz and Julie A. Braga[a]

ABSTRACT

Background

The clinical laboratory has an important role in monitoring pregnancy when an expectant mother is being treated. In contrast to most clinical situations in which a physician is caring for one patient, the physician must simultaneously care for both a mother and her fetus. The usual results for many clinical measurements no longer apply during pregnancy, further complicating the management of the patients.

Content

This chapter reviews the biology of pregnancy and discusses laboratory tests used to detect, evaluate, and monitor both normal and abnormal pregnancies. The physiologic changes associated with normal pregnancy are described along with a discussion of events surrounding conception and development of the fetus. Although most pregnancies progress without problems, complications can arise in the mother, placenta, or fetus. Diagnosis and management of maternal complications such as ectopic pregnancy, trophoblastic disease, preeclampsia, and liver disease, as well as fetal complications including hemolytic disease of the newborn (HDN) and vertically transmitted infections are highlighted. Laboratory testing is available to screen for and diagnose many fetal anomalies such as chromosomal abnormalities and neural tube defects. A detailed discussion of prenatal screening for fetal anomalies is provided. Lastly, this chapter will examine the chemistry, biochemistry, methods, and clinical significance of specific laboratory tests used in the management of pregnancy.

*The full version of this chapter is available electronically on ExpertConsult.com.
[a]The authors gratefully acknowledge the original contributions of George J. Knight, Edward Ashwood, David Grenache, and Geralyn Lambert-Messerlian, upon which portions of this chapter are based.

Exam questions, case studies, and additional resources are available on ExpertConsult.com.
*Full versions of these chapters are available electronically on www.ExpertConsult.com.

886

Newborn Screening and Inborn Errors of Metabolism*

Marzia Pasquali and Nicola Longo[a]

ABSTRACT

Background

Newborn screening can detect many metabolic disorders, allowing early initiation of treatment to prevent morbidity and mortality. The introduction of tandem mass spectrometry (MS/MS) has dramatically increased the number of conditions detectable at birth to include several inborn errors of amino acid metabolism, fatty acid oxidation, and organic acidemias.

Content

This chapter describes a range of metabolic disorders amenable to newborn screening. Amino acids and acylcarnitine are currently detected by MS/MS. The concentration of amino acids increases with inborn errors of amino acid metabolism (for example, phenylalanine in phenylketonuria). Acylcarnitine analysis can identify disorders of the intermediary metabolism of amino acids (organic acidemias) and disorders of the carnitine cycle and fatty acid oxidation. For each condition, the specific abnormal metabolites are indicated with the most appropriate way to confirm or exclude the diagnosis. In some cases, diagnostic metabolites disappear or are markedly reduced after the newborn period, so DNA testing is indicated for diagnostic purposes. Early identification of metabolic disorders allows prompt therapeutic intervention and improves long-term outcomes. Available therapies for metabolic disorders are also discussed in this chapter, along with the appropriate monitoring procedures.

*The full version of this chapter is available electronically on ExpertConsult.com.

[a]The authors gratefully acknowledge the contributions of Drs. Piero Rinaldo, Si Houn Hahn, and Dietrich Matern to the previous edition on which portions of this chapter are based.

Inborn Errors of Metabolism: Disorders of Complex Molecules*

Roy W.A. Peake, Olaf A. Bodamer, and Timothy Wood

ABSTRACT

Background

Inborn errors of metabolism (IEM) caused by defective processing of complex molecules comprise a specific subgroup of genetic disorders. Since these disorders are clinically heterogeneous, their diagnosis requires a high index of clinical suspicion combined with targeted laboratory testing.

Content

This chapter focuses on IEM arising from defective metabolism of "complex molecules." This IEM group is largely caused by defects in biological processes within intracellular organelles such as lysosomes and peroxisomes. Lysosomes are responsible for the breakdown of complex molecules such as glycosaminoglycans and sphingolipids. Deficiencies in enzymes required for the metabolism of these molecules result in intralysosomal substrate accumulation. Peroxisomes perform a large number of important functions within the cell, including the metabolism of complex molecules such as very long chain fatty acids. Peroxisomal disorders result from defects in their synthesis or in one of their essential catalytic functions. A large and growing number of IEM are caused by congenital defects of protein glycosylation. As such, this chapter describes the clinical and laboratory aspects of the three major types of IEM related to complex molecules: lysosomal storage disorders (LSDs), peroxisomal disorders (PDs), and congenital disorders of glycosylation (CDGs). Although these disorders are individually rare, they are considerably more prevalent as a collective and represent some of the most rapidly expanding IEM groups. The biochemical genetics laboratory plays a key role in the detection of LSDs, PDs, and CDGs. As with many other IEM, early recognition and treatment of these disorders are often associated with improved clinical outcomes. This is particularly true for LSDs, where new treatments such as enzyme replacement therapy have led to their inclusion in public newborn screening programs. Analytical methods used for the identification of these disorders are usually reserved for subspecialty biochemical genetics laboratories. For diagnosis of LSDs, enzyme activity measurement is used in combination with molecular testing. Biochemical screening for PDs requires the measurement of accumulated substrates, such as very long chain fatty acids, using techniques such as gas and liquid chromatography combined with mass spectrometry. Finally, for CDG identification, sophisticated approaches using high-resolution mass spectrometry in combination with molecular testing is often necessary. The diagnosis of IEM of complex molecules increasingly requires integration and correlation of biochemical data with clinical and molecular findings.

---

*The full version of this chapter is available electronically on ExpertConsult.com.

Molecular Diagnostics

Exam questions, case studies, and additional resources are available on ExpertConsult.com.
*Full versions of these chapters are available electronically on www.ExpertConsult.com.

Principles of Molecular Biology

John Greg Howe

ABSTRACT

Background

Molecular diagnostics and its parent field, molecular pathology, examine the origins of disease at the molecular level, primarily by studying nucleic acids. Deoxyribonucleic acid (DNA), which contains the blueprint for constructing a living organism, is the centerpiece for research and clinical analysis. Molecular pathology is an outgrowth of the enormous amount of successful research in the field of molecular biology that has discovered over the last seven decades the basic biological and chemical processes of how a living cell functions. The success of molecular biology, as noted by the large number of Nobel prizes awarded for its discoveries, is now used for clinical diagnosis and the development and use of therapeutics.

Content

The following chapters are devoted to describing this field and the specific applications currently being used to characterize and help treat patients with a variety of ailments, including hereditary genetic diseases, cancer neoplasms, and infectious diseases. In this chapter the fundamentals of molecular biology are reviewed, followed by the discussion of the techniques for isolating and analyzing nucleic acids in Chapters 63 and 64. Chapter 65 will focus on genomes and their variants, as well as massively parallel methods, while Chapter 66 discusses clinical genome sequencing in depth. The clinically important subdivisions of molecular diagnostics are then reviewed and include microbiology in Chapter 67, genetics in Chapter 68, solid tumors in Chapter 69, and hematopoietic malignancies in Chapter 70. Chapters 71 and 72 are devoted to the molecular diagnostic analysis of circulating tumor cells and circulating nucleic acids. Finally, pharmacogenetics is the focus of Chapter 73.

HISTORICAL DEVELOPMENTS IN GENETICS AND MOLECULAR BIOLOGY

Molecular diagnostics would not be possible without the many significant pioneering efforts in genetics and molecular biology. Earlier observations in genetics began with the discovery of the inheritance of biological traits made by Gregor Mendel in 1866 and the observation in 1910 that genes were associated with chromosomes by Thomas Morgan. The initial findings that contributed to determining that DNA was the transmittable genetic material were performed by Griffith in 1928 and Avery, McLeod, and McCarty in 1944.[1,2] The definitive studies, published by Hershey and Chase in 1952, demonstrated that radiolabeled phosphate incorporated into the DNA of a bacteriophage was found in newly synthesized DNA containing bacteriophage instead of radiolabeled sulfur in protein, which showed that DNA and not protein was the genetic material.[3]

Deciphering the structure of DNA required several crucial findings. These included the observation by Erwin Chargaff that the quantity of adenine is generally equal to the quantity of thymine, and the quantity of guanine is similar to the amount of cytosine[4] and the pivotal x-ray crystallography results produced by Rosalind Franklin and Maurice Wilkins.[5,6]

Molecular biology has historically traced its beginnings to the first description of the structure of DNA by James Watson and Francis Crick in 1953.[7,8] The description of the DNA structure initiated the dramatic increase in the knowledge of the biology and chemistry of our genetic machinery. The impact of the Watson and Crick discovery was so significant that it is considered one of the most important scientific discoveries of the 20th century.[9]

One reason the work of Watson and Crick had such a dramatic impact on scientific discovery was that they not only described the structure of DNA, but hypothesized about many of its properties, which took decades to confirm experimentally.[7,8,10] One of those properties was the replication of DNA, which was shown to be semiconservative by Meselson and Stahl[11] in 1958. At the same time, DNA polymerase, which replicates the DNA, was discovered by Arthur Kornberg.[12] Deciphering the genetic code was vital for understanding the information stored in DNA, and cracking the code in 1965 required many scientists, most prominently Marshall Nirenberg.[13] Additional studies described the transcription and translation processes and uncovered several startling findings. One finding was the isolation of reverse transcriptase, an enzyme that synthesizes DNA from ribonucleic acid (RNA), which demonstrates that genetic information can be transferred in part in a bidirectional manner.[14,15] Another finding showed that the eukaryotic gene structure was composed of alternating non–protein-encoding introns and protein-encoding exons.[16],[17] Along with the discovery of the basic biology of genes and their expression, many important techniques were invented. For example, the isolation of restriction enzymes[18] and DNA ligase allowed for the construction of recombinant DNA,[19] which could be transferred from one organism to another, leading to the cloning of DNA[20] and the emergence of genetic engineering. The Southern blot method, which identified specific electrophoretically separated pieces of DNA, participated in many discoveries and was one of the first molecular diagnostics methods to be used to test for genetic diseases.[21] DNA sequencing technologies were invented[22],[23] and further advances in these technologies led to the first large biological science research undertaking, the Human Genome Project. Along with DNA sequencing, further technical discoveries, including the polymerase chain reaction in 1986[24] and microarray technology in 1995,[25] became methodologic foundations for molecular diagnostics.

MOLECULAR BIOLOGY ESSENTIALS

Whether it is a bacterium, virus, or eukaryotic cell, the genetic material located in an organism dictates its form and function. For the most part the genetic material is DNA, which is composed of two strands of a sugar-phosphate backbone that are bound together by hydrogen bonds between two purines and two pyrimidines attached to the sugar molecule, deoxyribose, in a double helix (Figs. 62.1 and 62.2). DNA in human cells is wrapped around histone proteins and packaged into nucleosome units, which are compacted further to form chromosomes (Fig. 62.3). There are 23 pairs of chromosomes, two of which are the sex chromosomes, X and Y. Each chromosome is a single length of DNA with a stretch of short repeats at the ends called telomeres and additional repeats in the centromere region. In humans, there are two sets of 23 chromosomes that are a mixture of DNA from the mother's egg and father's sperm. Each egg and sperm is

therefore a single or haploid set of 23 chromosomes and the combination of the two creates a diploid set of human DNA, allowing each individual to possess two different sequences, genes, and alleles on each set of chromosomes, one from each parent. Each child has a unique combination of alleles because of homologous recombination between homologous chromosomes during meiosis in the development of gametes (egg and sperm cells). This creates genetic diversity within the human population. If a child has a random DNA sequence change or mutation, the child's genotype is different from that inherited from either of the parents (de novo variant). If the child's genotype leads to visible disease, the child has acquired a different phenotype from the parents.

Human cells have a limited lifespan and die through a process called apoptosis. Therefore most cells replace themselves as they progress naturally through their cell cycle. As a cell moves through phases of the cell cycle, its DNA doubles during the synthesis phase when the double-stranded DNA molecule separates. Each strand of DNA is used as a template to make a complementary strand by DNA polymerase in a process called DNA replication. Eventually during the cell cycle, two cells are created from one during the final mitotic phase.

DNA is composed of genes that code for proteins and RNA. For DNA to convert its store of vital information into functional RNA and protein, the DNA strands need to separate so that RNA polymerase can bind to the start region of the gene. With the help of transcription factors that bind upstream to promoters, the RNA polymerase produces single strands of RNA that are further processed to remove the introns and retain the protein-encoding exons. The mature, processed RNA molecule, the messenger RNA (mRNA), migrates to the cytoplasm, where it is used in the production of protein.

To start the process of protein synthesis or translation, the mRNA is bound by various protein factors and a ribosome,

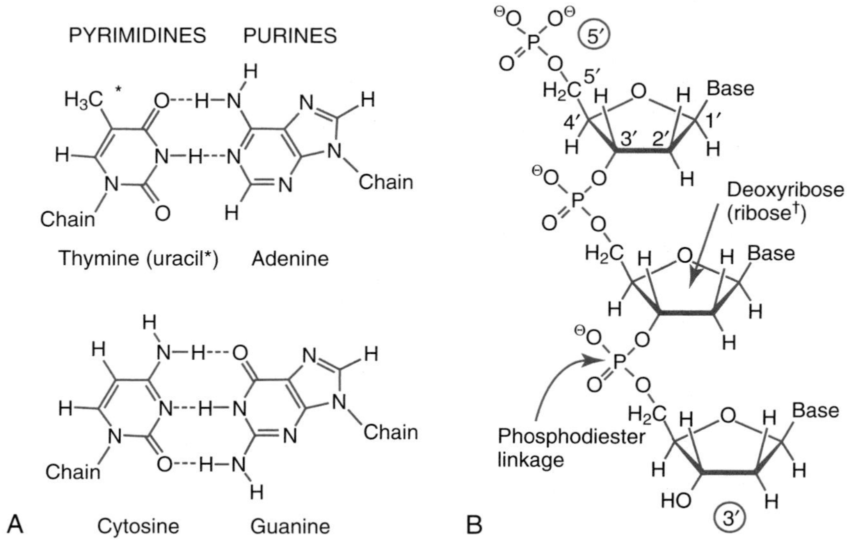

FIGURE 62.1 (A) Purine and pyrimidine bases and the formation of complementary base pairs. *Dashed lines* indicate the formation of hydrogen bonds. (*In RNA, thymine is replaced by uracil, which differs from thymine only in its lack of the methyl group.) (B) A single-stranded DNA chain. Repeating nucleotide units are linked by phosphodiester bonds that join the 5' carbon of one sugar to the 3' carbon of the next. Each nucleotide monomer consists of a sugar moiety, a phosphate residue, and a base. (†In RNA, the sugar is ribose, which adds a 2'-hydroxyl to deoxyribose.)

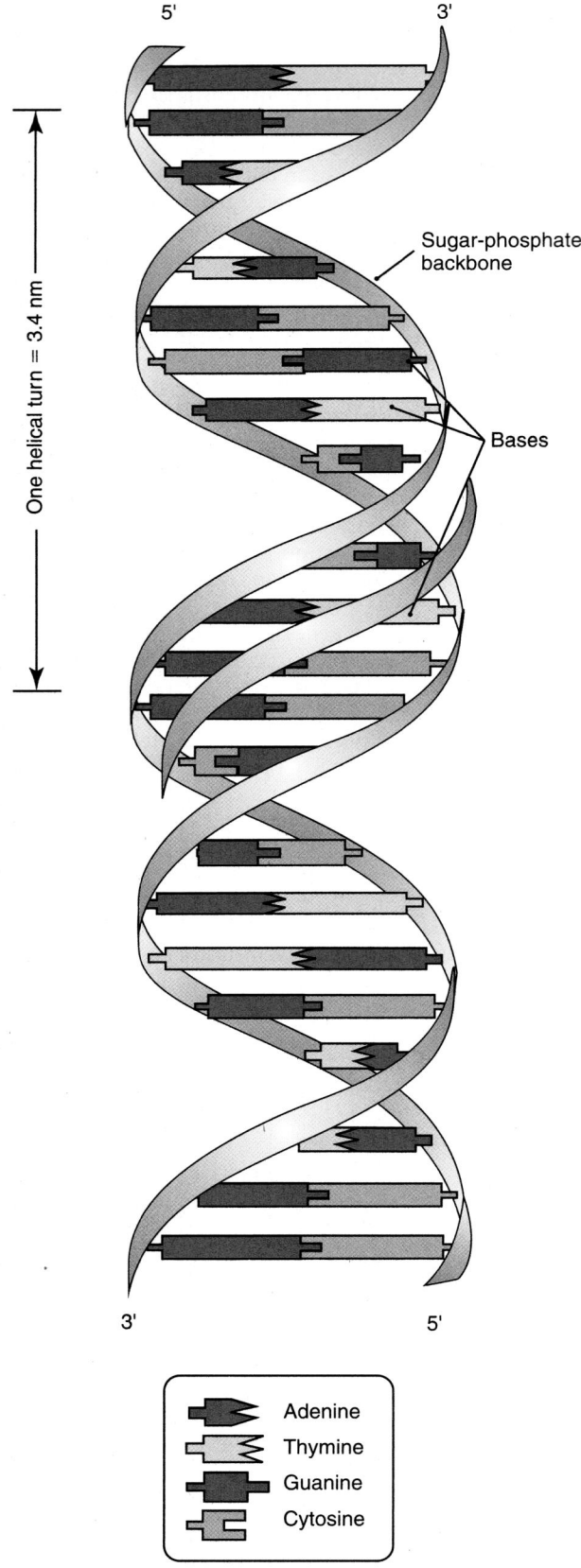

Sugar-phosphate backbone

Bases

One helical turn = 3.4 nm

Symbol	Base
	Adenine
	Thymine
	Guanine
	Cytosine

FIGURE 62.2 The DNA double helix, with sugar-phosphate backbone and pairing of the bases in the core-forming planar structures. (From Jorde LB, Carey JC, Bamshad MJ, editors. *Medical genetics.* 4th ed. Philadelphia: Mosby; 2010.)

which contains ribosomal RNA (rRNA) and protein. The mRNA-bound ribosome begins to produce a polypeptide chain by binding a methionine-bound transfer RNA (tRNA) to the mRNA's initiating AUG codon or triplet code. The conversion of the nucleic acid triplet code to a polypeptide is accomplished by the tRNA, which contains a nucleic acid triplet code (anticodon) in its RNA sequence that is specific for an amino acid bound to one end of the tRNA molecule. After synthesis, the protein migrates to its functional location and eventually is removed and degraded.

NUCLEIC ACID STRUCTURE AND FUNCTION

DNA is a rather simple molecule with a limited number of components compared to those of proteins. DNA is composed of a deoxyribose sugar, phosphate group, and four nitrogen-containing bases. Deoxyribose is a pentose sugar containing five carbon atoms that are numbered from 1′ to 5′, starting with the carbon that will be attached to the base in DNA and progressing around the ring until the last carbon that is not part of the ring structure. The bases consist of the purines, adenine and guanine and the pyrimidines, cytosine and thymine; an additional base, uracil, replaces thymine in RNA. A basic building block is the nucleotide, which consists of a deoxyribose sugar with an attached base at the 1′ carbon and a phosphate group at the 5′ carbon. The triphosphate nucleotide is the building block for making newly synthesized DNA. Newly synthesized DNA forms a polynucleotide chain that connects the individual nucleotides through the 5′ and 3′ carbons of each deoxyribose sugar via phosphodiester bonds.

Structure of Deoxyribonucleic Acid

DNA is double stranded, and the two strands bind to one another through hydrogen bonds between the bases on each strand. Hydrogen bonding is augmented by hydrophobic attraction (stacking) between bases on adjacent rungs of the DNA ladder. Both hydrogen bonds and base stacking are not covalent, but are weak bonds that can be broken and reestablished. This important property is exploited by many of the methods that are used in molecular diagnostics. The composition of DNA is equal quantities of guanine and cytosine and equal quantities of adenine and thymine, because, in general, guanine binds to cytosine and adenine binds to thymine.[4,7] There are two hydrogen bonds between adenine (A) and thymine (T) and three hydrogen bonds between cytosine (C) and guanine (G), and because of this difference in the number of hydrogen bonds, separating a guanine-cytosine (G-C) pair takes more energy than an adenine-thymine (A-T) pair (see Fig. 62.1).

Each of the two DNA strands is formed by an alternating phosphate sugar backbone that starts at the 5′ phosphate and ends at a 3′ hydroxyl group with the complementary bases binding to one another between the two phosphate sugar backbones. Each strand is therefore a polar opposite of the other (see Fig. 62.2). When the two strands are bound to one another they progress in opposite 5′ to 3′ directions in an antiparallel configuration. By convention, the DNA sequence is denoted in a 5′ to 3′ direction. As discussed later, both the replication of new DNA and the transcription of DNA to RNA progress in the 5′ to 3′ direction. In addition, the conversion of RNA to protein, a process called translation,

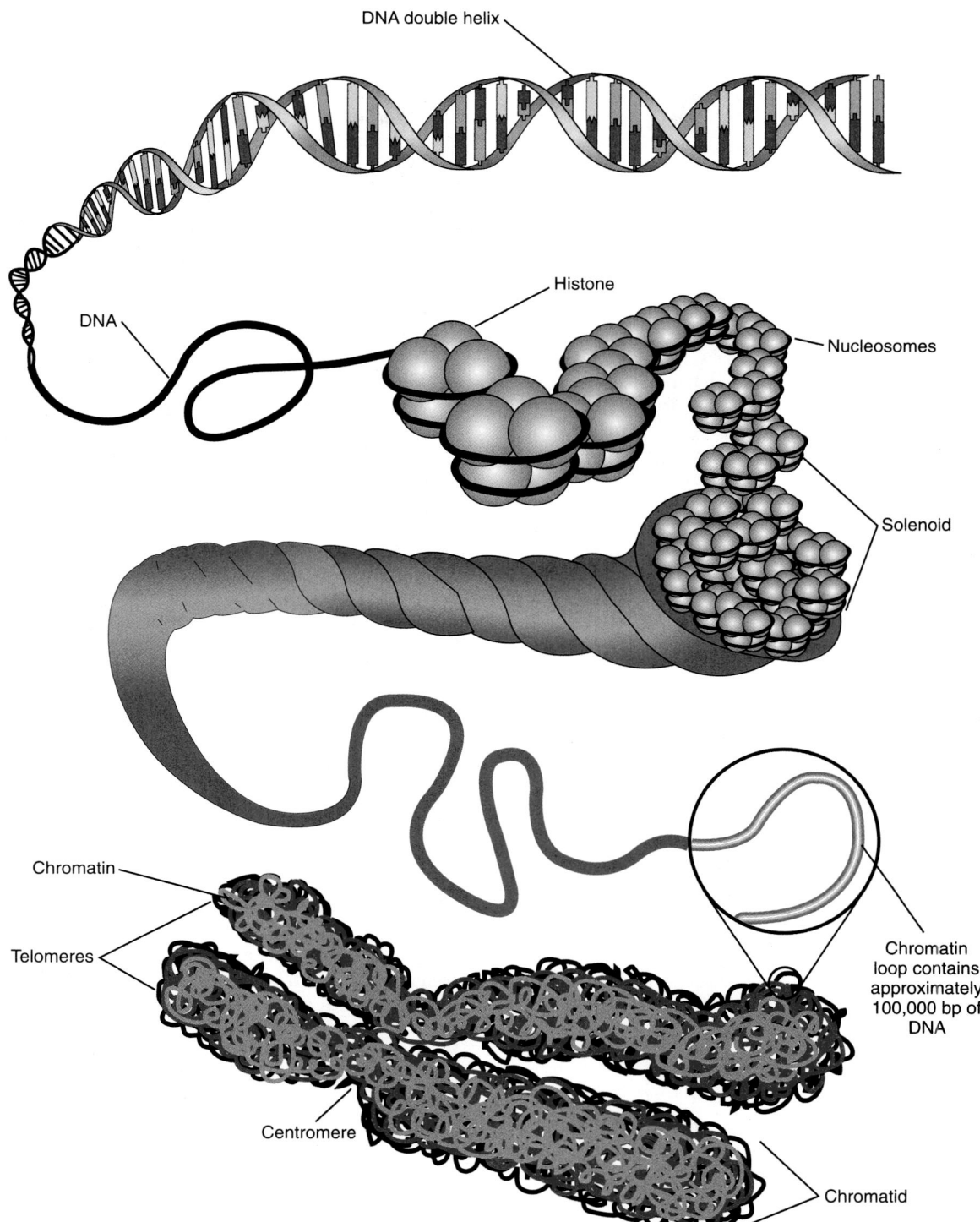

FIGURE 62.3 Structural organization of human chromosomal DNA. Double-stranded DNA is wound around the octamer core of histone proteins to form nucleosomes, which are further compacted into a helical structure called a solenoid. Nuclear DNA in conjunction with its associated structural proteins is known as chromatin. Chromatin in its most compact state forms chromosomes. The primary constriction of a chromosome is the centromere, and the chromosome's ends are the telomeres. (From Jorde LB, Carey JC, Bamshad MJ, editors. *Medical genetics*. 4th ed. Philadelphia: Mosby; 2010.)

proceeds from the 5′ end of the RNA to the 3′ end. The combination of the base pairing and the directionality of the two DNA strands allows for the deciphering of the DNA sequence on one strand of DNA when the other complementary strand sequence is known.

Types of Deoxyribonucleic Acid

Double-stranded DNA in living cells is generally found as the right-handed B-DNA helical structure, which has specific dimensions. Each turn of the helix is 3.4 nm long and consists of 10 bases. The DNA sugar-phosphate backbone is on the outside of the helix, and the bases of each strand are inside bound to their complement on the other strand by hydrogen bonds. Other conformational structures of DNA occur, mostly associated with DNA sequences that are repeated. These non-B DNA forms include a left-handed Z-form, A-motif, tetraplex G-quadruplex, i-motif, hairpin, cruciform, and triplex and are abundant in the human genome because a large percentage of the genome contains various repeats. Non-B DNA is associated with many biological processes, including transcriptional control. However, these structures also can create genetic instability, which can lead to various diseases such as neurologic disorders.[26]

Molecular Composition of Ribonucleic Acid

The composition of RNA is similar to that of DNA because it contains four nucleotides linked together by a phosphodiester bond, but with several important differences. RNA consists of a ribose sugar with a hydroxyl group at the 2′ carbon instead of the hydrogen atom in DNA. The bases attached to the ribose sugar are adenine, cytosine, and guanine, but not thymine because RNA uses another pyrimidine—uracil—as a substitute for thymine.

Structure of Ribonucleic Acid

One significant difference between DNA and RNA is that RNA does not normally exist as two strands bound to one another, although a single strand can bind internally to itself creating functionally important secondary structures. Although in the past several decades the complexity and number of different RNAs has greatly expanded, the majority of cellular RNA is composed of a rather small number of RNA types. These include mRNA, rRNA, and tRNA.

Ribonucleic Acids Associated With Protein Production

mRNA is the most diverse group of the three major types of RNAs but constitutes only a small percentage of the total RNA. mRNAs are transcribed from DNA that codes for proteins and therefore are used as the template for the translation of proteins. In the case of prokaryotes, the mRNA is colinear with the protein that is translated; however, in eukaryotes the mRNA begins as a precursor RNA called pre-messenger or heterogeneous nuclear RNA (hnRNA) that includes untranslated intron and translated exon regions. After transcription the hnRNA is spliced into mature mRNA lacking the introns. The mature mRNA contains only exons and can be further modified by the addition of a 7-methyl-guanosine cap at the 5′ end, which protects the mRNA from degradation, and a polyadenosine (polyA) sequence at the 3′ end. In eukaryotes the production and processing of the hnRNA to mRNA takes place in the nucleus, and the final form of the mRNA is then transported to the cytoplasm to be translated.

rRNA is associated with ribosomes, which are the primary structures that produce protein through the biological process of translation. rRNA, unlike mRNA, does not code for proteins. The ribosome is composed of two structures, the 50S and 30S subunits found in prokaryotes and the 60S and 40S subunits found in eukaryotes. The "S" stands for Svedberg units and is determined by the centrifugal sedimentation rate. The Svedberg unit measures the mass, density, and shape of an object. The ribosome is a mixture of RNA and protein. In eukaryotes there are four major rRNAs: the 18S rRNAs found in the 40S subunit and the 28S, 5.8S, and 5S rRNAs found in the 60S subunit. In prokaryotes, the 50S subunit contains the 23S and 5S rRNAs and the 30S subunit contains the 16S rRNA. Synthesis of eukaryotic rRNA occurs as a large 45S precursor RNA that is enzymatically cleaved to form all the rRNAs except the 5S RNA, which is transcribed separately. Ribosomal RNAs have secondary and tertiary structures that are well conserved with various loops, stem loops, and pseudoknots that contribute to their function. Ribosomal RNA and protein, as the components of ribosomes, function to carry out the translation of proteins. The sequence of the 16S rRNA has alternating conserved and divergent regions that can be used to identify microorganisms. The structure of the ribosome is now known, and the rRNA is more important than ribosomal proteins in ribosome functioning. The RNA acts as a catalytic agent called a ribozyme.[27,28]

Another important group of RNAs are the tRNAs, which function as key molecules that act as a bridge between the nucleic acids and the proteins. They have a unique cloverleaf secondary structure, with the 3′ end covalently attached to the amino acid by specific aminoacyl tRNA synthetases. In the middle of the tRNA structure is the anticodon sequence that binds to a specific homologous codon in the mRNA. Therefore the codon directs the binding of a specific tRNA linked to its corresponding amino acid. The genetic code, which consists of a 64 3-base code, specifies the appropriate amino acid to be attached to the growing polypeptide chain (see Figs. 62.7 and 62.8). There are several different classes of aminoacyl tRNA synthetases, but there is at least one aminoacyl tRNA synthetase for each of the 20 amino acids. There is also at least one tRNA for each amino acid; however, there can be more depending on the species.[29]

Besides the three major types of RNAs, other RNAs include nuclear, nucleolar, and cytoplasmic small RNAs, signaling RNAs, telomerase RNA, and micro-RNAs.[30] This list appears to be growing with each passing year. Some of the first characterized small RNAs, the nuclear and nucleolar small RNAs, are involved with the processing of precursor RNAs to mature RNAs, including splicing of hnRNA to mRNA and precursor rRNA to mature rRNAs. More recently a large number of microRNAs have been discovered that partly function in the regulation of translation. In addition, there are many other noncoding RNAs whose functions are just beginning to be understood.

Human Chromosome

Human double-stranded DNA that is contained in the sperm or egg is a single copy or haploid amount of DNA made up of approximately 3 billion base pairs (bp). To be more precise, the Human Genome Project consensus sequence of the human genome was 2.91×10^9 bp[31] and the first human to be sequenced, Craig Venter, had a genome size of 2.81×10^9 bp,[32] not including remaining gaps of highly repetitive sequences, many near centromeres and telomeres (see Chapter 65). The DNA in the cell is bound by many proteins to form chromatin (see Fig. 62.3). The proteins in chromatin consist of histones, which are bound in precise amounts per length of DNA, and other proteins called nonhistone proteins that are bound more irregularly and in widely varying amounts. The histone proteins consist of eight proteins (two copies each of H2A, H2B, H3, and H4) that bind as a unit to 147 bp of DNA to make up a nucleosome, and the protein, H1, that binds between the nucleosomes (Fig. 62.4). The nucleosomes are the basic structure to which many other proteins interact and modify to regulate gene expression. For example, the access to DNA by transcription factors is controlled by proteins that remodel the histone proteins through phosphorylation, acetylation, and methylation. The nucleosomes are condensed into filaments and even more compact structures to form a chromosome (see Fig. 62.3). There are 23 pairs of chromosomes: 22 autosomal chromosomes and 2 sex chromosomes, X and Y, with an XX pair denoting female and an XY pair denoting male. The DNA in chromosomes is continuous for each chromosome and can be as much as several hundred million base pairs in length for the largest chromosomes.

From a cytogenetic viewpoint, regions of the chromosomes can be classified by their transcriptional activity. The more condensed heterochromatin DNA is transcriptionally inactive and stains with Giemsa, a mixture of several dyes that bind to AT-rich regions of DNA. The less condensed euchromatin DNA is transcriptionally active and does not stain with Giemsa. The ends of the chromosomes, called telomeres, contain a repeat sequence, such as TTAGGG that is found in humans and shortens with age. The centromeres, at the center of most chromosomes, are important for linking sister chromatids during mitosis and contain various satellite

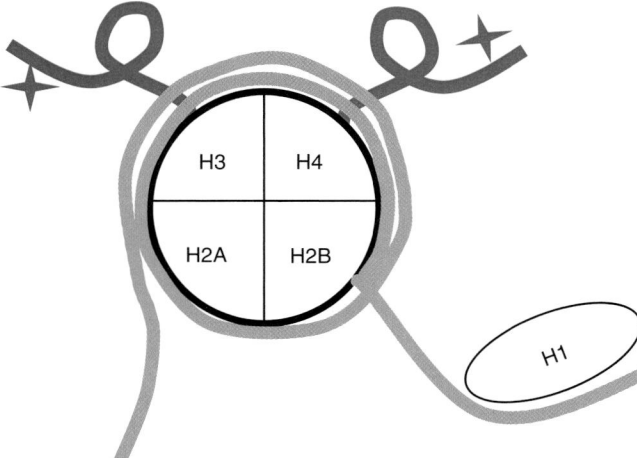

FIGURE 62.4 Schematic illustration of a nucleosome unit. A segment of DNA is wound around a nucleosome core particle consisting of an octamer of two each of the histone proteins H2A, H2B, H3, and H4. Tails with modifications (indicated by a *red star*) are shown to protrude from H3 and H4. Adjacent nucleosomes are separated by a segment of linker DNA and the linker histone, H1.

DNAs, such as α-satellite tandem repeats (171 bp) that are over several million base pairs (Mb) in length.

Surprisingly, most (98 to 99%) human DNA does not code for the expression of protein. As much as 50% of human DNA consists of many types of interspersed repeat sequences, such as satellites, telomeres, microsatellites, minisatellites, short and long interspersed nuclear elements (SINES, LINES), and retrovirus elements.[31] Like other eukaryotes, human genes are in pieces with the protein-encoding regions, exons, alternating with the introns, which do not code for protein sequence and occupy more than a quarter of the human DNA.[33] Other regions around the genes, such as the promoter regions and the 3′ untranslated regions are also not translated into proteins. After all the noncoding sequences are removed, the protein-coding DNA sequence spans only approximately 1.2 to 1.5% of human DNA. Even though most human DNA is not associated with protein-producing genes, the Encyclopedia of DNA Elements (ENCODE) project has shown that much of the non–protein-encoding DNA is transcribed into noncoding RNAs, most with unknown function.

CENTRAL DOGMA OF MOLECULAR BIOLOGY

Francis Crick originated the concept of the central dogma of biology, which describes the transfer of genetic information into functional macromolecules.[34] This was generally depicted to show the movement of genetic information from DNA to RNA via transcription using RNA polymerase and further translated from RNA into protein via ribosomes and various factors. This is a simplistic version of the original concept, which took into consideration every possible transfer of information even though no evidence existed at the time. However, since the original publication, a number of other postulated transfers have been described. DNA can enzymatically replicate itself by DNA polymerase, and RNA can be made into DNA using reverse transcriptase.[35] Many of these enzymes are used in molecular diagnostics assays.

Deoxyribonucleic Acid Replication

A general principle underlying the synthesis or replication of new DNA is that it uses one of the two DNA strands as a template to make a new homologous strand. This is termed semiconservative replication and was first theorized by Watson and Crick.[7] DNA replication begins at an adenine and thymine (AT)-rich structure called an origin of replication. In bacteria there is generally only one origin of replication, but in eukaryotic cells there are thousands. Since DNA can be supercoiled into more structures, a topoisomerase is required to first unwind this structure so that the DNA is accessible. A DNA helicase binds to the double-stranded DNA and separates the two strands, providing two single-stranded DNA templates. Replication progresses in a 5′ to 3′ direction; therefore one strand, the leading strand, is synthesized as one continuous strand using the 3′ to 5′ template and the other strand, called the lagging strand, is synthesized in small segments called Okazaki fragments from the 5′ to 3′ template. Because the DNA polymerase requires a primer, small RNA primers are made by a primase enzyme on the 5′ to 3′ template and the Okazaki fragments are synthesized starting from the primer. Okazaki fragments are finally linked by a ligase (Fig. 62.5).[36]

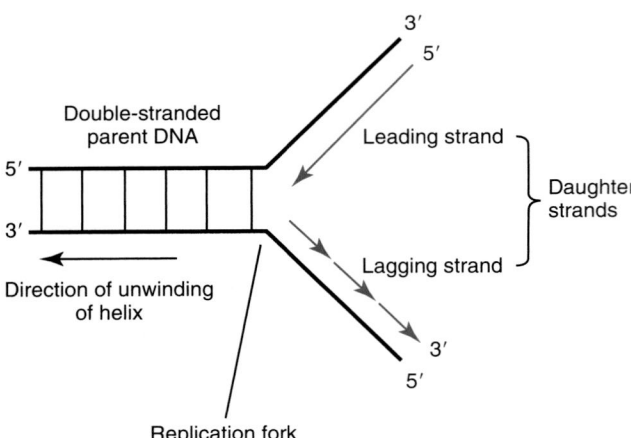

FIGURE 62.5 DNA replication. Double-stranded DNA is separated at the replication fork. The leading strand is synthesized continuously, whereas the lagging strand is synthesized discontinuously but is joined later by DNA ligase.

DNA polymerases of various types have been identified and they function in many different roles, the most important being the replication of new DNA and the repair of existing DNA. Using the template strand as a guide, the DNA polymerase binds a nucleotide triphosphate to the primer at a free 3′ hydroxyl group, releasing pyrophosphate. The specific nucleotide selected depends on the base on the template strand; for example, an adenine nucleotide is used if a thymine nucleotide is in the template strand. In summary, a complementary sequence is synthesized opposite the template strand. The insertion of the correct nucleotide does not always occur. Mistakes occur approximately every 100,000 nucleotides; therefore a major function of a DNA polymerase is error correction or proofreading and is accomplished by an intrinsic 3′ to 5′ exonuclease activity. DNA polymerases are important in molecular diagnostics because they are used in the polymerase chain reaction (PCR) and DNA sequencing.

DNA replication is part of the cell cycle and occurs during the synthesis phase. The rest of the cell cycle is the interphase, further divided into the first growth phase (G_1) and the second growth phase (G_2), along with the DNA replication or synthesis (S) phase that lies between G_1 and G_2. The mitosis phase, which involves the splitting of one cell into two cells, occurs after the G_2 phase. Mitosis is divided into six subphases: prophase, prometaphase, metaphase, anaphase, telophase, and cytokinesis.

At important control points in the cell cycle the cell will commit significant resources to proceed further. One of these control points is between the G_1 and S phase, just before it begins DNA replication. The G_1/S boundary control point is disrupted in many cancers. It is common for neoplasms to have mutations in the retinoblastoma gene *(RB1)*, whose protein product regulates cell cycle progression from G_1 to S. Another control point is between G_2 and M, just as the cell commits to creating two cells from one.

Deoxyribonucleic Acid Repair

The integrity of DNA is damaged in a variety of ways that culminate in changes or mutations in the DNA sequence. DNA bases may be damaged, removed, cross-linked, or incorrectly paired with one another, and single- or double-stranded

breaks may also occur.[37,38] When the cell senses that its DNA has become damaged, it stops the progression of its cell cycle and initiates DNA repair processes.[39] Cells repair these lesions by employing multiple DNA repair mechanisms that are specific for the type of DNA lesion and include base excision repair, nucleotide excision repair, mismatch repair, and homologous recombination repair.

Mechanisms

Base excision repair removes bases that are damaged by deamination, oxidation, and alkylation. Deamination of guanine, cytidine, and adenine converts them into structures that will incorrectly base pair, creating transition mutations, which are changes between similar nitrogenous bases such as a purine to a purine. A transversion mutation is a change from a purine to a pyrimidine or vice versa. DNA glycosylases, such as uracil-DNA-glycosylase, cleave the damaged base, and a 5′-deoxyribose phosphate lyase removes the nucleotide upstream of the removed base. DNA polymerase and ligase then add a new nucleotide repairing the damage. One of the inherited disorders associated with this repair process that leads to a predisposition to various neoplasms is caused by mutations in *MUTYH*, a DNA glycosylase gene.[38,40]

Nucleotide excision repair removes base modifications that change the helical structure of DNA, including bulky DNA distortions and covalently bound structures that may be created by ultraviolet radiation and certain cancer drugs. The damage is recognized by global and transcription-mediated repair processes. After the repair is initiated, the transcription factor, TFIIH, binds to a complex of proteins and makes an incision. The damaged DNA is unwound, and the gap is filled by DNA polymerase and finally sealed by DNA ligase. Mutations in the nucleotide excision repair genes cause xeroderma pigmentosum, which leaves affected individuals susceptible to specific tumors.[38,41]

Mismatch repair recognizes base incorporation errors and base damage. DNA polymerase has a 3′ to 5′ editing exonuclease with a proofreading function that is not completely effective and allows some mismatches to occur that can lead to mutations after DNA replication. The mismatched nucleotides must be repaired on the newly synthesized strand of DNA, which in prokaryotes is recognized by its unmethylated state. In eukaryotes the mechanism is different, and it is proposed that proteins associated with the replication apparatus, specifically the proliferating cell nuclear antigen protein determines the appropriate DNA strand for repair.[38] These mutations are corrected with DNA mismatch repair proteins, which identify the mismatches by their methylation patterns, excise the surrounding sequence, and then repair the excision with new sequence. Mutations in the human mismatch repair genes are associated with Lynch syndrome (hereditary nonpolyposis colorectal cancer).

Double-stand breaks are a very destructive form of DNA damage that destabilizes the genome, sometimes resulting in gross chromosomal changes, such as translocations that are frequently found in cancer. Double-stranded breaks are caused by several processes, including ionizing radiation and chemotherapy drugs, and are repaired by either homologous recombination or nonhomologous end joining.[38,41] The homologous recombination repair pathway is initiated by recognition of a double-stranded break, followed by resection using exonucleases to create a 3′ single-stranded overhang.

With the assistance of many proteins, RAD51 is bound to the single-stranded DNA, which invades the intact homologous double-stranded DNA of the sister chromatid and uses it as a template for new double-stranded DNA repair.[38]

DNA repair mechanisms operate independently to repair simple lesions. However, the repair of more complex lesions involves multiple DNA processing steps regulated by the DNA damage response pathway. When single- and double-stranded DNA breaks occur, a cascade of responses is initiated that culminates in either DNA repair, stopping the cell cycle, or programmed cell death. After DNA damage has occurred, the DNA damage response pathway activates the protein kinases ATM (ataxia telangiectasia mutated) and ATR (ataxia telangiectasia and Rad3-related protein) to phosphorylate signaling proteins, such as p53, which eventually leads to cell cycle arrest at the G_1/S boundary. This gives time for the DNA repair mechanism to repair the damaged DNA; however, if the damage is too extensive, the cell initiates apoptosis or cell death.[39]

Deoxyribonucleic Acid Modification Enzymes

There are two groups of nucleases, the endonucleases that cut through the sugar-phosphate backbone and exonucleases that digest the ends of DNA. The commercially important restriction endonucleases, which bacteria have acquired to protect themselves from viral infections, are used to cleave DNA at a specific nucleotide sequence or restriction sites.[42] Several thousand restriction endonucleases have been characterized and are used extensively to manipulate DNA in molecular biology and molecular diagnostics. Recent work has described new nucleases, such as the RNA-guided engineered nuclease, CRISPR/Cas system, that can precisely cleave genomic DNA.[43] Significant progress has been made with the CRISPR-Cas technology, which has not only advanced our knowledge of basic biology, but also created methods that will have a therapeutic impact on medicine. These methods include human genome editing of patients with hematopoietic genetic diseases, such as sickle cell disease, and immunotherapy using chimerism antigen receptor (CAR) T-cell therapy for patients with cancer, such as acute lymphoblastic leukemia.[44] The CRISPR-Cas technology has also been used for diagnostics as demonstrated by the development of the DETECTR method,[45] which was used to quickly develop a test for COVID-19 at the start of the pandemic.[46]

DNA glycosylases are a family of enzymes associated with base excision repair that are used in the first step of DNA repair to remove the damaged base, without disrupting the sugar-phosphate backbone. An important member of that family, uracil DNA glycosylase, repairs the most common mutation found in humans, the spontaneous deamination of cytosine to uracil, by removing the uracil base.

Gene Structure

The structure of prokaryotic genes is straightforward; almost all of the gene sequence is used to make protein; however, this is not the case with eukaryotic genes. One of the unique hallmarks of eukaryotic genes is that the protein-coding DNA is interspersed with regions that do not code for DNA, an observation made by Richard Roberts and Phillip Sharp in 1977. A mature mRNA retains only the protein-coding sequences called exons, and the sequences between the exons are non–protein-encoding sequences called introns that are removed during mRNA maturation (Fig. 62.6).[47]

In addition to introns and exons, eukaryotic genes consist of regulatory regions, such as promoters and enhancers, and 3′ regions that contain termination and polyadenylation signals. The regulation of the expression of eukaryotic genes can occur at all levels from transcription to splicing to translation to degradation; however, most gene regulation occurs at the initiation of transcription by various promoters and enhancers.[48] There are two groups of regulatory elements: one is close to the transcriptional start site and is made up of the core promoter and ancillary promoters slightly further away from the start of transcription. The other group of regulatory elements can be much further away, not only upstream but also downstream from the gene. This second group is made up of enhancers, silencers, insulators, and locus-specific control regions.[48,49] These regulatory elements contain specific sequences that bind to transcription factors that can upregulate or downregulate the expression of a gene. There are only several thousand human transcription factors, much less than the number of human genes; therefore each gene has many regulatory elements to provide the needed complexity to function in 200 different human cell types.[48]

A surprising property of human genes is that there are so few compared to less complex species. Humans have approximately 21,000 genes, many fewer than found in rice and

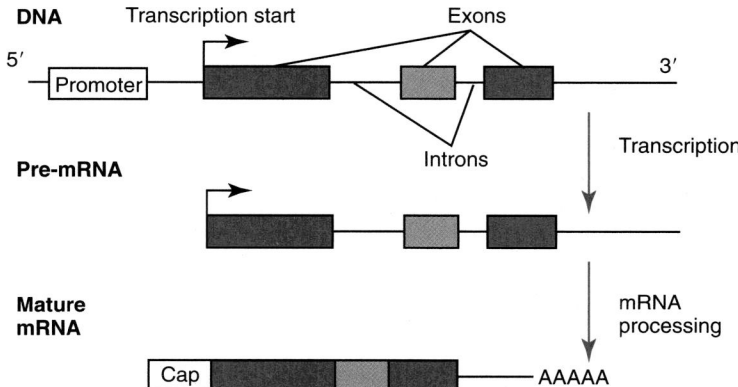

FIGURE 62.6 DNA transcription and messenger RNA processing. A gene that encodes for a protein contains a promoter region and variable numbers of introns and exons. Transcription commences at the transcription start site. Pre-messenger RNA or heterogeneous nuclear RNA (hnRNA) is processed by capping, polyadenylation, and intron splicing and becomes a mature messenger RNA.

only slightly more than found in the roundworm, *Caenorhabditis elegans*.[50-53] Results from the ENCODE project have challenged the concept of "one gene, one protein."[54] Their studies show that the exon of one gene can be spliced into the exon of another gene.[55] This result, along with alternative splicing, demonstrates that one gene can make multiple proteins and is one of the main reasons human genomes can display so much complexity despite having such a small number of genes.

Ribonucleic Acid Transcription and Splicing

RNA transcription involves synthesizing an RNA strand using DNA as a template. This requires many different proteins, the most important being the RNA polymerases, of which there are three types in eukaryotic cells. RNA polymerase I is specific for the rRNAs, 28S, 18S, and 5.8S, which are initially transcribed as a single primary transcript of 45S. RNA polymerase II transcribes all genes that encode proteins and the small nuclear RNA (snRNA) genes. RNA polymerase III transcribes a variety of small RNAs, including the 5S rRNA, and tRNA. Additional proteins called transcription factors function in combination to recognize and regulate transcription of different genes.[56]

The synthesis of RNA proceeds in a 5′ to 3′ direction using DNA as a template and a specific DNA sequence that acts as a transcription start site. Transcription progresses through three phases: initiation, elongation, and termination. The initiation phase includes the binding of transcription factors to promoters upstream from the start site, including the core promoter immediately upstream and the ancillary promoters further away. However, some of the small RNA gene promoters can be in the middle of a gene. Transcription factors binding to upstream promoters act as regulators of the transcription of genes. These factors generally bind in pairs or dimers and have several functional domains. One functional domain of the transcription factor binds to a specific promoter DNA sequence via several structures, such as the helix-turn-helix, zinc finger, and leucine zipper structures. Another domain binds to the other transcription factor of the dimer pair, and a third domain may bind to the RNA polymerase complex that carries out transcription.[49] Even though promoters and the transcription factors binding to them are far away from the transcription initiation complex, the promoter DNA folds back on itself to allow for the transcription factors to interact with the RNA polymerase complex.[57]

Important recurring sequences are found in the core promoter. For example, the core promoter of an RNA polymerase II gene contains a TATAAA sequence, called a TATA box located upstream 25 to 40 nucleotides from the transcriptional start site. Only 20 to 30% of eukaryotic promoters contain TATA boxes, but they are highly regulated compared to those without TATA boxes that are mostly housekeeping genes.[50,58,59]

The first step in mRNA transcription is the binding of transcription factor IID (TFIID) to the TATA box, which in turn promotes the binding of other transcription factors (TFIIA, TFIIB, TFIIE, TFIIF, and TFIIH), RNA polymerase II, and proteins attached to the upstream promoter sites. To form a functional transcription complex, the promoter region's doubled-stranded DNA separates and the transcription complex moves away from the core promoter region.[50] Once started, the RNA polymerase adds nucleotides to the 3′

free hydroxyl group in a manner similar to that of DNA replication. Transcription is eventually terminated by one of several termination mechanisms. In bacteria a termination factor bound to the RNA polymerase recognizes a DNA sequence termination signal. In the case of genes transcribed by RNA polymerase II, termination is coupled with the polyadenylation step (see Fig. 62.6).

Two post-transcriptional processing events are performed on the newly formed hnRNA, one at each end of the RNA. At the 5′ end, the hnRNA is capped with a 7-methyl guanosine molecule to help protect the hnRNA from degradation. At the 3′ end, a polyadenosine (poly A) stretch is added by poly A polymerase after the RNA sequence AAUAAA is synthesized. Some transcribed mRNAs are not polyadenylated, such as histone mRNAs.[60] An additional modification of mRNA is N^6-methyladenosine (m6A) methylation, which has been found throughout the life of the mRNA transcript. The m6A modification is used by the cell to coordinate transcript processing and translation during development. Cancer and human viruses have been shown to utilize m6A methylation.[61]

Transcription initially produces an hnRNA that contains both exons and introns, which needs to be processed or spliced into mature mRNA for it to be properly translated into protein. RNA splicing involves cleavage and removal of intron RNA segments and splicing of exon RNA segments. The process uses consensus splice site sequences located at both the 5′ (GU) and 3′ (AG) ends of the intron and an internal intron sequence. Splicing requires the effort of a number of proteins and small RNAs that come together to form a spliceosome, which directs the splicing of exons and removal of introns.[62] Splicing begins with the binding of the U1 small nuclear ribonucleic protein (snRNP) to the donor splice site and the U2 snRNP to the internal intron sequence, followed by the binding of U4, U5, and U6 snRNPs, resulting in excising the intron and joining (splicing) of the ends of the two exons on either side of the excised intron (see Fig. 62.6).[62] The spliceosome has been recently shown to be in close proximity to the RNA polymerase II. The speed at which the transcription process progresses determines the assembly of the spliceosome and its subsequent splicing of introns.[63]

An important modification of the splicing process, alternative splicing, allows for the generation of different mRNAs from the same primary RNA transcript by the cutting and joining of the RNA strand at different locations. Among the types of alternative splicing are exon skipping, alternative 3′ and 5′ splice sites, and intron retention. It is estimated that 92% to 95% of all human genes are alternatively spliced.[64,65]

The movement of cellular signals from the surface of a cell to the nucleus is called signal transduction, and one of the eventual targets is the modification (e.g., phosphorylation) of transcription factors, which can modulate the binding of other transcription factors to DNA and their dimerization, thereby controlling gene expression.[66] A common cascade of signaling begins with the activation of a receptor on the cell surface, such as a tyrosine kinase receptor. The tyrosine kinase receptor in the form of a dimer can be activated by binding to a hormone or growth factor, for example, which causes a dimerization and autophosphorylation of the tyrosine receptor protein kinase. This in turn activates a cytoplasmic protein, such as the guanine nucleotide exchange factor that activates the G-protein Ras, which can then modify another G-protein, Raf, which propagates the signal to a common signaling pathway, the mitogen-activated protein (MAP) kinases. The final enzyme in the pathway can then act on downstream targets, including other protein kinases, and transcriptional factors. Some mutations in the tyrosine kinase receptor or Ras protein switches them to an unregulated "on" position, which can lead to uncontrolled growth of the cell and eventually to cancer.[66]

Translation

The final phase of the transfer of information from DNA is to proteins, the structural and functional molecules that make up the majority of a living organism, such as the human body. Proteins are long single strands of various amino acids and are synthesized by a process called translation, which requires the functioning of many protein factors, tRNAs, and ribosomes.

Amino acids have a common structure consisting of a carbon atom bound to amino and carboxylic acid groups and a unique side chain. There are 20 amino acids each with a different side chain that give them their unique properties. The side chains can be divided into four types: nonpolar (hydrophobic), polar (hydrophilic uncharged), and negative and positively charged. Nonpolar (hydrophobic) amino acids include alanine, leucine, isoleucine, valine, proline, methionine, phenylalanine, and tryptophan. The uncharged polar (hydrophilic) amino acids include glycine, serine, threonine, cysteine, tyrosine, glutamine, and asparagine. The negatively charged (acidic) amino acids are aspartic acid and glutamic acid, and the positively charged (basic) amino acids are arginine, histidine, and lysine. A protein's amino acid makeup and sequence in the polypeptide chain determine the overall structure and function of the protein. Some amino acids have a more significant presence than others. For example, proline, which disrupts secondary structure, and cysteine, which can cross-link to another cysteine through disulfide bonds, can change the structure of a protein.

Protein structures are grouped into four different classes. The primary structure is the sequence of the amino acids in the protein. There are several common types of secondary structure, such as β-pleated sheets and α helixes. Proteins can be constructed with a combination of these different types of secondary structures. Tertiary structure applies to the folding of the polypeptide chain into a three-dimensional form. Quaternary structure is the structural relationship of more than one polypeptide/protein joining together, such as in immunoglobulin molecules, that contains light and heavy proteins bound together by cysteine residues.

Once proteins are synthesized, they can be modified in various ways. One of the most common modifications is phosphorylation of the amino acids serine, threonine, and tyrosine, which can regulate protein activity. Other modifications include proteolytic cleavage, such as removal of the signal transport sequence, and acetylation of the N terminus of most eukaryotic proteins that helps to prevent degradation. Glycosylation of secreted and membrane proteins on asparagine, serine, and threonine residues and formation of disulfide bonds via cysteine cross-linking are additional modifications.

Taking into consideration these post-translational modifications and alternatively spliced forms mentioned earlier, the total number of proteins in the more than 200 human cell types is estimated to range from 250,000 to several million.[67]

The genetic code, which was deciphered in the early 1960s, is required to convert a nucleic acid sequence into an amino acid sequence.[13] It was reasoned that if there are 20 amino acids, a code of at least three nucleotides was necessary to have enough combinations. A three-nucleotide code gives 64 combinations, and therefore one hallmark of the genetic code is that it is redundant, meaning that there are several codes for one amino acid. That is the case for most amino acids, but not all; for example, methionine and tryptophan have only one code. The redundancy is usually in the third base of the code. All of the 64 three-nucleotide codon possibilities code for an amino acid, except 3 that serve as stop codons (UAA, UGA, and UAG) (Fig. 62.7).

Protein synthesis or translation occurs in the cytoplasm and proceeds in three steps: initiation, elongation, and termination. The process requires tRNA and rRNA molecules, as well as ribosomes and initiation, elongation, and termination factors. One of the most important groups of molecules are the tRNAs, which are recognized by aminoacyl tRNA synthetase enzymes that attach amino acids to the 3′ end of specific tRNA molecules. Each tRNA has a three-base sequence (anticodon) that facilitates the specific recognition and interaction with a codon in the mRNA.

The initiation step of protein synthesis is the most complex and begins with the binding of initiation factor 4E to the cap structure on the 5′ end of the mRNA and binding of poly-adenosine–binding protein (PABP) to the 3′ PABP polyadenosine tail. The binding of initiation factor 4G to both initiation factor 4E and PABP circularizes the mRNA and prepares it for binding to the preinitiation complex containing the 40S ribosomal subunit, initiation factor 2, and methionine tRNA. The preinitiation complex then scans the mRNA until it finds a methionine start codon (AUG), at which point the 60S ribosomal subunit binds forming the 80S initiation complex and initiates translation elongation.[68] This is a simplistic description of the initiation process because over a dozen additional initiation and auxiliary factors are involved.

Ribosomes have at least three structural positions where tRNAs can bind, the acceptor (A), peptidyl (P), and exit (E) sites. The acceptor site binds the incoming aminoacyl-tRNA. The peptidyl site holds the peptidyl-tRNA that is covalently linked to the growing polypeptide chain, and the exit site binds to the outgoing empty tRNA that carries no amino acid.[68,69]

The first codon (AUG) always codes for methionine; therefore to initiate translation the methionine tRNA binds to the aminoacyl-tRNA binding site of the ribosome. The tRNA specific for the next three-base codon—for example, lysine—binds to the acceptor site of the ribosome and with the help of elongation factors (e.g., eEF2), the amino acid in the peptidyl site is bound to the amino acid in the acceptor site by the formation of a peptide bond. A peptide bond is created between the amino group of one amino acid and the carboxyl group of the next amino acid through condensation releasing water. At the same time the tRNA shifts positions, with the methionine tRNA shifting to the exit site and the tRNA containing the growing chain of amino acids shifting to the peptidyl site. Concurrently, the ribosome moves forward one codon and the next tRNA specific for the next codon through its anticodon binds in the acceptor site, and the process is repeated until a termination codon is reached (Fig. 62.8).

Second letter

		U		C		A		G		
U	UUU UUC	Phenyl-alanine	UCU UCC	Serine	UAU UAC	Tyrosine	UGU UGC	Cysteine	U C	
	UUA UUG	Leucine	UCA UCG		UAA UAG	Stop Codon Stop Codon	UGA UGG	Stop Codon Tryptophan	A G	
C	CUU CUC CUA CUG	Leucine	CCU CCC CCA CCG	Proline	CAU CAC	Histidine	CGU CGC CGA CGG	Arginine	U C	
					CAA CAG	Glutamine			A G	
A	AUU AUC AUA	Isoleucine	ACU ACC ACA ACG	Threonine	AAU AAC	Asparagine	AGU AGC	Serine	U C	
	AUG	Methionine			AAA AAG	Lysine	AGA AGG	Arginine	A G	
G	GUU GUC GUA GUG	Valine	GCU GCC GCA GCG	Alanine	GAU GAC	Asparatic Acid	GGU GGC GGA GGG	Glycine	U C	
					GAA GAG	Glutamic Acid			A G	

First letter (left axis) — Third letter (right axis)

FIGURE 62.7 The genetic code. The first, second, and third bases of an mRNA triplet code for one of the 20 amino acids *(white)* or a stop codon *(red)*.

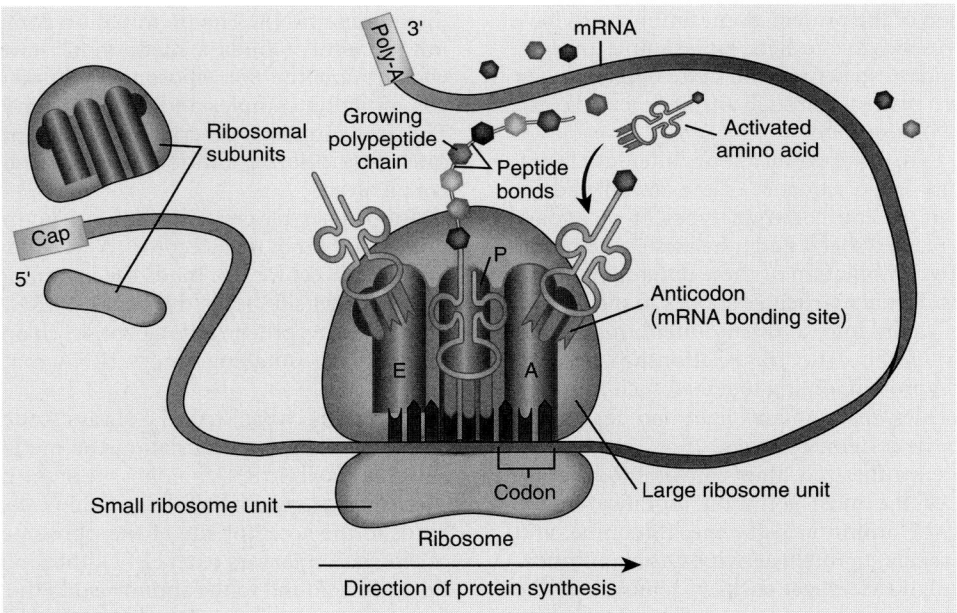

FIGURE 62.8 Translation of messenger RNA to amino acids during protein synthesis. Shown is a ribosome bound to a messenger RNA converting the messenger RNA triplet code (codon) via a specific amino acid–bound transfer RNA containing a complementary anticodon sequence. There are three transfer RNA positions. A new amino acid–bound transfer RNA first arrives on the ribosome at the *A* or acceptor site at the front of the moving ribosome and then moves to the *P* or peptidyl site where the amino acid on the newly arrived transfer RNA combines with the growing polypeptide chain. Finally, the now empty transfer RNA moves to the *E,* or exit site, where it prepares to leave the ribosome. (Modified from Huether SE, McCance KL. *Understanding pathophysiology.* 6th ed. St. Louis: Elsevier; 2017.)

Termination factors then bind and stop the translation process.[68] Protein synthesis occurs in the eukaryotic cytoplasm in the endoplasmic reticulum where multiple ribosomes called polyribosomes are involved in translating an individual mRNA.

Regulation of translation is not as extensive as that for transcription. However, there is global regulation of eukaryotic translation at the initiation step with phosphorylation of initiation factor 2B by four different protein kinases. This occurs when the cells are under stress, such as amino acid starvation or DNA damage.[70] In addition, mRNA-specific translational regulation can occur through binding to specific sequences located in the 5′ and 3′ untranslated regions. Furthermore, there are over 1000 microRNAs in humans,[71] many of which regulate transcription. The microRNA genes are transcribed as precursor RNA and then processed into a mature 22-nucleotide form by the processing enzymes Dicer and Drosha. The mature form of microRNAs can bind to specific sites on mRNA while associated with the Argonaute protein and either reversibly inhibit translation or degrade the mRNA.[68,72] For example, microRNAs Mir 15a/16-1 are deleted in chronic lymphocytic leukemia, thereby increasing Bcl2 expression and inhibiting apoptosis or cell death to prolong the life span of the cell.[73] Another interesting translational regulatory mechanism is ribosome heterogeneity where ribosomes specialize in the translation of specific transcripts and thereby regulate the expression of groups of genes.[74]

After proteins are synthesized there are two major processes to remove excess or damaged proteins. One process degrades the proteins ingested and uses nonspecific proteases, such as pepsin and trypsin, to digest proteins associated with foodstuff in the gut into amino acids so they can be absorbed. The second process digests extracellular and intracellular proteins by either general proteinases within lysosomes or by protein degradation via ubiquitination. With the latter mechanism, proteins are tagged for degradation by binding to ubiquitin, which is recognized by a large multiprotein structure, the proteasome that degrades the ubiquitinated proteins by proteolysis.[75]

EPIGENETICS

Although the original meaning of epigenetics encompassed all molecular pathways that affect the expression of genes, over time the definition has focused on the regulation of gene expression by heritable modifications that do not change the DNA sequence.[76] More recently this has been broadened to include nonheritable modifications.[76-80] Currently there are three major areas of epigenetic modifications or marks: (1) DNA methylation; (2) chromatin conformation regulation through histone modifications, including ATP-dependent remodeling enzymes and histone variants; and (3) noncoding RNAs.[81]

Deoxyribonucleic Acid Methylation

DNA methylation is a well-known epigenetic change that is important in X chromosome inactivation, gene imprinting (e.g., Prader-Willi, Angelman syndromes), and cancer. The most common methylation event is the methylation of cytosine to form 5-methylcytosine. DNA methylation typically occurs at cytosines directly upstream of guanines, or CpG dinucleotides. Cytosine is both methylated and demethylated by a variety of enzymes. The initial methylation state is catalyzed by one type of DNA cytosine-5-methyltransferase, whereas the maintenance of the methylated state is performed by another type of DNA cytosine-5-methyltransferase and occurs during each cell division after being established in early embryonic development.[82]

Demethylation involves three members of the ten-eleven translocation (TET) family of dioxygenases, which catalyze the conversion of 5-methylcytosine to other modified forms, such as 5-hydroxymethylcytosine during demethylation.[83] 5-Hydroxymethylcytosine is found in high amounts in neural cells and is postulated to regulate gene expression.[83]

Gene expression is altered by methylation via several mechanisms. The most direct effect is through altering the ability of transcription factors to bind to promoters. Methylation decreases the affinity of transcription factors to a DNA promoter and enhances the binding of methylation-specific transcription factors (Fig. 66.9). Additionally, methylation compacts the chromatin structure, thus reducing the access of transcription factors to a promoter.[84] Cancer is the most common human disease associated with aberrant DNA methylation.[85] Interestingly, the overall level of 5-methylcytosine in cancer cells is 60% less than in normal cells; however, certain promoter-specific CpG islands are hypermethylated.[85] Other human diseases that are associated with methylation include lupus and many neurologic diseases.

Chromatin Conformation Regulation

Many basic cellular functions require proteins to interact with DNA. However, DNA is generally not freely accessible but is wound around histones to form nucleosomes and further condensed or compacted into heterochromatin that decreases gene expression. The cell requires the DNA to be accessible to carry out DNA replication, repair, and transcription.[81,86] The chromatin, therefore is a very dynamic structure; at any one point in time portions of the DNA are being exposed and other portions are being covered. The mechanisms that control chromatin conformation include histone modifications, histone variants, and ATP-dependent remodeling enzymes.

Specific histones are reversibly and post-translationally modified at their N-terminal tails and globular regions to change the chromatin from a euchromatin state to a heterochromatin state and back (see Fig. 62.9). These modifications include acetylation of lysine residues at the N-terminal tails of H2A, H3, and H4 by histone acetyltransferases (HATs) and deacetylation by histone deacetylases (HDACs). Histone acetylation removes the positive charge on the lysine residue, leaving the lysine less attracted to the negatively charged DNA phosphate backbone and thereby opening the DNA.[84]

Histone methylation of lysine and arginine residues occurs mostly on histone protein H3, but also histone protein H4, and is carried out by histone methyltransferases (HMTs) and histone demethylases (HDMs). The effect of methylation on chromatin structure ranges from active to poised to repressed. Histone lysine and arginine residues can be mono-, di-, and tri-methylated, but the positive charge is unchanged.[39,86] Histone methylation is found associated with DNA transcription, replication, and repair.

Histones are phosphorylated at serine, threonine, and tyrosine residues and are associated with DNA repair and

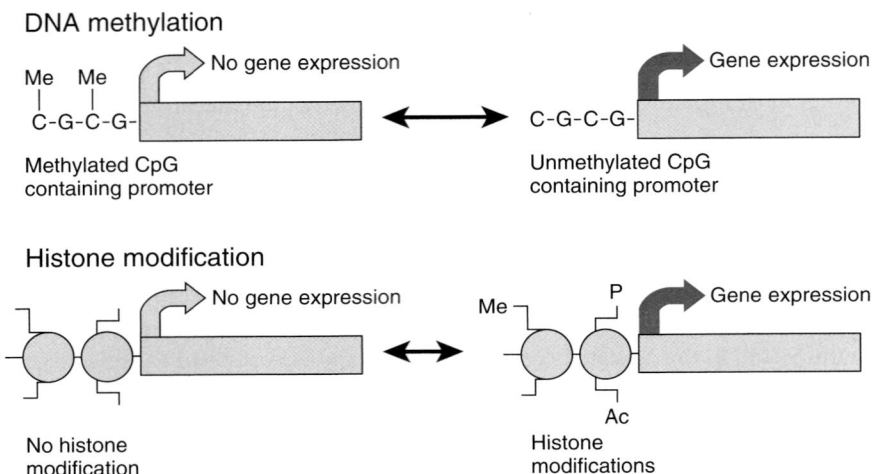

FIGURE 62.9 Epigenetics. *(Top)* DNA methylation of CpG island regions indicated by *Me* in and around gene promoters is associated with loss of gene expression and silencing of the gene. When *CpG* islands are unmethylated, shown by absence of *Me*, gene expression is unaffected. *(Bottom)* Modifications of the tails of histone proteins, such as methylation, acetylation, and phosphorylation, shown as *Me, Ac,* and *P,* respectively, can increase gene expression. (Modified from Zaidi SK, Young DW, Montecino M, van Wijnen AJ, Stein JL, Lian JB, et al. Bookmarking the genome: maintenance of epigenetic information. *J Biol Chem* 2011;286:18355–61.)

transcription. The addition of a negatively charged phosphate group to the histone will repel the histone away from the negatively charged DNA and loosen up the chromatin structure.[87] Other modifications include poly(ADP-ribosyl)ation, ubiquitination, SUMOylation, and glycosylation.[88]

Histone variants have been known for decades, but many of their functions are not well established. Histone protein variants H3.3 and H2A.Z are the most well known and are shown to function in regulation of gene expression.[89] Histone variant H3.3 incorporates into chromatin independent of replication and is associated with active chromatin.[90,91]

ATP-dependent remodeling enzymes use the energy from the hydrolysis of ATP to change the structure of chromatin.[91,92] ATP-dependent remodeling enzymes are grouped into four families including SWItch/Sucrose NonFermentable (SWI/SNF), imitation switch (ISWI), inositol requiring 80 (INO80), and chromodomain (CHD).[86,92]

The remodeling enzymes have similar properties, including (1) specific interaction with nucleosomes, (2) attraction to the modified histone tail residues found in nucleosomes, (3) contain an ATPase domain, (4) ATPase regulatory function, and (5) ability to interact with transcription factors and chromatin-associated proteins.[88,92] The primary role of the enzymes is to remodel the chromatin structure. The SWI/SNF proteins function in the sliding and ejecting of nucleosomes, but do not function in chromatin assembly. The IWSI family of enzymes changes the nucleosome spacing through sliding that is necessary after DNA replication. This family interacts with unmodified histone tails and functions to regulate transcription. The CHD family functions to slide and eject nucleosomes, by which it regulates transcription. The INO80 family of proteins has an insertion in the middle of its ATPase domain and functions in promoting transcription and DNA repair. A mammalian member of this family, SWR1, can exchange histones to facilitate DNA repair.[88,92–94]

At a less granular scale the chromosomes are arranged into configurations that allow them to be organized into functional compartments. The higher-order organization of chromatin consists of large compartments: A and B. Within these compartments of chromatin are topologically associating domains (TADs) and loop structures controlled by CCCTC-binding factor and cohesion that help to facilitate the interaction between enhancer and promoter and regulate gene expression.[95]

Noncoding Ribonucleic Acids

Most of the expressed RNA in a cell is not translated into protein. Only the mRNAs are translated into protein, and they represent only 1 to 5% of the total RNA depending on cell type. Much of this noncoding RNA is known and includes rRNA and tRNAs. However, over the last several decades two large groups of noncoding RNAs have been discovered, the short and long noncoding RNAs. The ENCODE project tested for DNA expression not associated with genes. Over 80% of the human DNA could be assigned a biochemical function, although biochemical function was liberally defined.[96] The bulk of the human genome is expressed into RNA.[97]

Recently, it was determined that there are approximately 21,000 noncoding transcripts, which is similar to the number of protein encoding genes.[53] The short noncoding RNAs consist of microRNAs, small interfering RNAs, and piwi interacting RNAs.[98,99] MicroRNAs regulate gene expression by binding to a specific sequence of the mRNA and inhibiting its translation. Small interfering RNAs (siRNA) inhibit translation by also binding to a region of the mRNA, but do so by initiating the degradation of the mRNA by the associated Argonaute protein. Piwi interacting RNAs (piRNA) function in the repression of transposons and are important in the development of gametes in many multicellular eukaryotic species.

The long RNAs are arbitrarily designated to be greater than 200 nucleotides while the short RNAs are between 20 and

200 nucleotides.[100] Only recently has the extent of long non-coding RNAs been appreciated.[97] The diversity of the long noncoding RNAs is predicted to be in the hundreds of thousands in vertebrates and their expression pattern is highly regulated during the development of an organism. A well-described example of a long noncoding RNA is XIST, which associates with the Polycomb group complex 2 and inactivates the X chromosome by inducing heterochromatin formation and repressing gene expression.[101] Examples such as XIST and a similarly acting protein, HotAir, have given rise to the possibility that the noncoding regions of the human genome have important functions.[100]

The function of most noncoding RNAs (ncRNAs) is unknown, but it is speculated that coding and noncoding RNAs, referred to as competing endogenous RNAs (ceRNAs), are in competition for shared microRNA binding sites in untranslated regions of mRNAs, thereby regulating their expression. Interestingly, the enhancers associated with the transcribing of genes are genes themselves that transcribe noncoding enhancer RNAs.[102] The ceRNA hypothesis proposes a new layer of regulation of gene expression that could help explain the function of the large percentage of the human genome that expresses non–protein-coding RNA.[103–105] An example of this regulation is found in breast cancer where several of the ceRNA networks between the ncRNAs are disrupted in the development of the disease. Understanding of the basic biology of this disruption could lead to the development of breast cancer biomarkers and therapeutics.[106]

UNDERSTANDING OUR GENOME

Genomics is recognized as a unique field since the first free-living organisms were completely sequenced in the 1990s. With the publication of the first draft of the human genome in 2001 and the final results of the Human Genome Project in 2004, the genomics field started to impart greater influence on biomedical research and its application to medicine.[31,107] Genomics is characterized by the comprehensive nature of its collection of data and the technical development necessary to obtain, analyze, store, and make available such large amounts of data. There are also ethical, legal, and social implications of the research and clinical application of genomics.[108]

Large research projects that were initiated during the latter years of the Human Genome Project produced comprehensive biological catalogs of genetic variants, important DNA functional sequences, and expressed products from not only humans but also many other organisms.[108]

Single nucleotide variants (SNVs) are the most common DNA differences found in the human population, and they number in the millions, with each individual differing on average by 1 in 1000 nucleotides. Human SNVs (including both benign polymorphisms and disease-causing variants) are cataloged in the SNP database (http://www.ncbi.nlm.nih.gov/SNP).

Genome-wide association studies employ microarray tests that use large numbers of SNVs to find associations between genetic variations and diseases. DNA variants are often clustered into regions by genetic recombination during the formation of sperm and eggs that are inherited as a unit, such that a unique SNV pattern or haplotype can be passed from generation to generation. The International HapMap Project also uses SNVs to investigate haplotype associations and disease.

The 1000 Genomes Project complements the previously mentioned projects by sequencing a large number of diverse human samples from around the world. The goal is to build a comprehensive catalog of the most common human genetic variants, which includes single nucleotide variants, as well as insertions, deletions, and copy number variants that are found in the population at greater than 1%. The Exome Aggregation Consortium (ExAC) has sequenced over 60,000 exomes to delineate common genetic variation within human exomes. Its follow-up program, the Genome Aggregation Database (gnomAD), has doubled the number of exomes (and ethnicities) and includes genomes. The SNP database, International HapMap Project, 1000 Genomes Project, ExAC, gnomAD, and genome-wide association studies have helped to define genetic variability within individuals and populations and have led to understanding the basis of many genetic diseases.[108,109]

A more fundamental biology project is the encyclopedia of DNA elements, or ENCODE, whose goal is a catalog of the functional elements of the genomes of humans and other species. The functional elements include the genes and all their expressed RNA forms and epigenetic modifications.[53] One of the most important findings is the discovery that much of the human genome is expressed into RNA.

With the introduction of the first massively parallel DNA sequencing instrument in 2005 and subsequent instruments from 2006 onward, the current technologic era of genomics has progressed over the last decade to make significant inroads into applying genomics to patient care.[110] Along with the technologic innovation in DNA sequencing, there has been innovation in bioinformatics, which is required to manage and interpret the large amount of information generated by massively parallel DNA sequencing instruments.

Although the Human Genome Project is a significant feat, it was not the first whole genome to be sequenced. Whole genome sequencing initially focused on infectious pathogens, because of their impact on human health and also their size. The first free-living organism to be sequenced was *Haemophilus influenzae* in 1995.[111] Subsequently, many species from a cross-section of living organisms have been sequenced. The first individual human to have their whole genome sequenced was Craig Venter, who led one of the two groups that first sequenced the human genome. The second person to have their whole genome sequenced was James Watson, whose genome was the first to be sequenced by using massively parallel DNA sequencing.

An important clinical application of genomics is cancer diagnostics (see Chapters 69 and 70); however, the diversity and complexity of cancer requires a significant amount of basic biological information to interpret molecular diagnostic testing results of patient samples. The first whole genome sequencing of a cancer was an acute myeloid leukemia in 2008,[112] and many others have subsequently been sequenced. The Cancer Genome Atlas project includes large numbers of the most common cancers to identify all their associated mutations. For example, a recent study describes mutational data for 12 of the most common cancers.[113] The significant amount of basic information now available on human cancers and the availability of new therapeutics targeting specific cancer-associated genes allows the clinical use of molecular profiling in cancer patients.[114]

With the increasing use of genetic and genomic information to characterize a patient's disease, an interesting convergence of electronic medical records and genomics is emerging. The implementation of electronic medical records throughout the United States will allow for greater access to the large amount of genomic data that will be available on patients, which will eventually be a source for scientific research and discovery. The Electronic Medical Records and Genomics Network is currently developing tools and conditions under which genomic research can be pursued using electronic medical records.[115]

The significant reduction in the cost of DNA sequencing has led to the development of additional DNA sequencing programs that target specific populations. These include the Newborn Sequencing in Genomic Medicine program, which explores how to use genomic sequence information to care for newborn babies; and large-scale sequencing programs, such as the Geisinger MyCode Community Health Initiative, and the Genomics England project that will sequence up to 5,000,000 genomes and will be used to care for patients.

The increase in patient DNA sequencing has led to programs to determine its clinical usefulness and include the Clinical Sequencing Evidence-Generating Research program and IGNITE pragmatic Clinical Trials that examine how genome sequencing can be used in clinical settings and determine whether it is cost effective; and the Clinical Genome Resource that will develop an accessible resource of annotated genes and variants from clinical specimens.[109]

All of the previously discussed advances have made the field of molecular diagnostics an important and exciting area that is going to have an even greater impact on medicine in the future. As an increasing number of diseases are characterized at the molecular (e.g., nucleic acid and protein) level, new therapeutics and diagnostics specifically targeting these molecular changes will continue to emerge.

POINTS TO REMEMBER
DNA and Genome Structure

- The two strands of DNA are bound together by hydrogen bonds and stacking forces that can be broken and reformed without permanent damage to the DNA. This property is exploited by many of the methods used in molecular diagnostics.
- The composition of DNA is equal quantities of guanine and cytosine and equal quantities of adenine and thymine, because, in general, guanine binds to cytosine and adenine binds to thymine.
- Only 1.2–1.5% of the human genome is translated into protein; however, much more of the genome is made into RNA.
- Even though human DNA has approximately 21,000 genes, this is far less than what would be expected given the number of proteins in a human cell. The higher number of proteins results from alternative splicing,
- There are two hydrogen bonds between adenine (A) and thymine (T) and three hydrogen bonds between cytosine (C) and guanine (G), and therefore separating a guanine-cytosine (G-C) pair takes more energy than an adenine-thymine (A-T) pair.

POINTS TO REMEMBER
Transcription and Splicing

- Transcription requires three types of RNA polymerases. RNA polymerase I is specific for the rRNAs, 28S, 18S, and 5.8S. RNA polymerase II transcribes all genes that encode proteins and the small nuclear RNA (snRNA) genes. RNA polymerase III transcribes a variety of small RNAs, including the 5S rRNA, and tRNA.
- Transcription progresses through three phases: initiation, elongation, and termination.
- Transcription produces hnRNAs that contains both exons and introns, which are spliced into mature mRNAs. RNA splicing involves cleavage and removal of intron RNA segments and splicing of exon RNA segments.
- Alternative splicing allows for the generation of different mRNAs from the same primary RNA transcript by the cutting and joining of the RNA strand at different locations. It is estimated that 92 to 95% of all human genes are alternatively spliced.

POINTS TO REMEMBER
Understanding the Genome

- The 1000 Genomes Project sequenced a large number of diverse human samples from around the world. The goal was to build a comprehensive catalog of the most common human genetic variants.
- Single nucleotide variants (SNVs) are the most common DNA differences found in the human population; they number in the millions and are cataloged in the SNP database.
- The goal of the encyclopedia of DNA elements, or ENCODE is to catalog the functional elements of the genomes of humans and other species.
- The goal of the Cancer Genome Atlas project is to identify all the associated mutations of the most common cancers.
- The Electronic Medical Records and Genomics Network develops tools and conditions under which genomic research can be pursued using electronic medical records.

SELECTED REFERENCES

7. Watson JD, Crick FH. Genetical implications of the structure of deoxyribonucleic acid. Nature 1953;171:964–7.
13. Nirenberg M, Leder P, Bernfield M, et al. RNA codewords and protein synthesis. VII. On the general nature of the RNA code. Proc Natl Acad Sci U S A 1965;53:1161–8.
31. Venter JC, Adams MD, Myers EW, et al. The sequence of the human genome. Science 2001;291:1304–51.
35. Crick F. Central dogma of molecular biology. Nature 1970;227:561–3.
36. O'Donnell M, Langston L, Stillman B. Principles and concepts of DNA replication in bacteria, archaea, and eukarya. Cold Spring Harb Perspect Biol 2013;5:a010108.
38. Iyama T, Wilson DM 3rd. DNA repair mechanisms in dividing and non-dividing cells. DNA Repair (Amst) 2013;12:620–36.
47. Sharp PA. The discovery of split genes and RNA splicing. Trends Biochem Sci 2005;30:279–81.

48. Maston GA, Evans SK, Green MR. Transcriptional regulatory elements in the human genome. Annu Rev Genomics Hum Genet 2006;7:29–59.

62. Wahl MC, Will CL, Luhrmann R. The spliceosome: design principles of a dynamic RNP machine. Cell 2009;136: 701–18.

65. Kornblihtt AR, Schor IE, Allo M, et al. Alternative splicing: a pivotal step between eukaryotic transcription and translation. Nat Rev Mol Cell Biol 2013;14:153–65.

68. Jackson RJ, Hellen CU, Pestova TV. The mechanism of eukaryotic translation initiation and principles of its regulation. Nat Rev Mol Cell Biol 2010;11:113–27.

75. Reinstein E, Ciechanover A. Narrative review: protein degradation and human diseases: the ubiquitin connection. Ann Intern Med 2006;145:676–84.

82. Schubeler D. Function and information content of DNA methylation. Nature 2015;517:321–6.

84. Zhang G, Pradhan S. Mammalian epigenetic mechanisms. IUBMB Life 2014;66:240–56.

96. ENCODE Project Consortium. An integrated encyclopedia of DNA elements in the human genome. Nature 2012;489:57–74.

97. Djebali S, Davis CA, Merkel A, et al. Landscape of transcription in human cells. Nature 2012;489:101–8.

98. Castel SE, Martienssen RA. RNA interference in the nucleus: roles for small RNAs in transcription, epigenetics and beyond. Nat Rev Genet 2013;14:100–12.

107. International Human Genome Sequencing Consortium. Finishing the euchromatic sequence of the human genome. Nature 2004;431:931–45.

108. Green ED, Guyer MS, National Human Genome Research Institute. Charting a course for genomic medicine from base pairs to bedside. Nature 2011;470:204–13.

110. Wheeler DA, Wang L. From human genome to cancer genome: the first decade. Genome Res 2013;23:1054–62.

Nucleic Acid Isolation*

Stephanie A. Thatcher and Linnea M. Baudhuin

ABSTRACT

Background
Effective isolation of nucleic acids (NAs) is important for sensitive and accurate clinical molecular methods that interrogate deoxyribonucleic acid (DNA) or ribonucleic acid (RNA). There are many different techniques and methods (including commercial kits) available for NA isolation, or sample preparation, and the choice often depends on the source of NA and downstream analytical method. The most common procedures in clinical and research laboratories utilize solid-phase NA separation, such as automated bead separation, or centrifugation filter techniques.

Content
Optimal NA isolation includes lysis from diverse sources such as human cells, viruses, bacterial spores, or protozoan oocysts, and purification of DNA or RNA. Techniques involve sample exposure to chemicals, enzymes, or binding matrices that reduce sample volume, variability, and complexity to achieve purity goals. The isolated NA should be efficiently separated from molecules that could act as potential inhibitors of a downstream molecular assay. The best preparation method depends on the requirements for a specific application. Goals may include flexibility for multiple sample types, large batch processing, speed, or high-purity NA. Consistent results for today's molecular methods can usually be obtained by the right combination of lysis, concentration, purification, and efficiency for NA isolation.

---

*The full version of this chapter is available electronically on ExpertConsult.com.

Nucleic Acid Techniques*

Gregory J. Tsongalis and Carl T. Wittwer

ABSTRACT

Background
Nucleic acid techniques as applied to molecular diagnostics have enabled the laboratorian to modify, amplify, detect, discriminate, and sequence nucleic acids with levels of sensitivity and specificity unparalleled by other laboratory techniques. Molecular diagnostic techniques continue to produce results that are faster, better, and cheaper, a trend that translates into better patient care and that fully supports precision medicine initiatives.

Content
Molecular diagnostic techniques typically require nucleic acid extraction and some type of target amplification followed by detection of the desired sequence. The polymerase chain reaction (PCR) remains the most common method of amplification for both research and clinical diagnostics, although similar isothermal methods like the recombinase polymerase assay (RPA) are becoming more common. The early replacement of radioactive detection methods with colorimetric or fluorescence detection and most recently electrochemical detection have advanced the field. The development of "closed" systems that amplify, detect, identify, and/or quantify based on real-time PCR and melting analysis with fluorescence have simplified the workflow and reduced turnaround times. Multiplexed methods go beyond single target queries, and can provide diagnostic data for more complex clinical syndromes. The simplicity and specificity of nucleic acid complementarity remains essential in probe- and primer-based methods. Microarrays, initially used for gene expression research, are now used to detect copy number variations with proven clinical utility in constitutional and somatic diseases. DNA and RNA sequencing methods have progressed from base termination fragments visualized by gel electrophoresis, through fluorescent labeled fragments detected by capillary electrophoresis, to the current workhorse of massively parallel methods.

---

*The full version of this chapter is available electronically on ExpertConsult.com.

Genomes, Variants, and Massively Parallel Methods

Jason Y. Park and Carl T. Wittwer

ABSTRACT

Background

One of the defining achievements of the early 21st century is the sequencing and alignment of more than 90% of the human genome. Of course, there is not a single human genome: individuals differ from each other by about 0.1% and from other primates by about 1%. Variation comes in many different forms, including single base changes and copy number differences in large segments of DNA. Even more challenging than sequencing the whole genome is documenting and understanding the clinical significance of human sequence variation. We are still very early in our understanding of the human genome.

Content

Beginning with a historical perspective, the structure of the human genome is described in detail, followed by comparison to other interesting species. Then, different types of genomic variation are covered, including single base changes (substitutions, deletions, insertions), copy number variations, translocations and fusions, short tandem repeats of different size and number, and larger repetitive segments, some of which can hop around the genome as transposons. The function of different genomic elements is considered, along with many different classes of RNA transcribed from the DNA. How to name all the different genes, variants, and elements is a daunting task, and accepted nomenclature is presented. Massively parallel methods for genomic analysis including microarrays and massively parallel sequencing are detailed. We end with a description of basic informatics tools that provide a pipeline from massive amounts of raw sequencing data to finished sequence, including variant annotations.

INTRODUCTION

It is easy to be carried away by the detectable peculiarities and to forget that much underlying variability is still hidden from view until some new technical device discloses the finer structure of chromosomes...

Lionel Penrose, Chicago, IL.
Third ISCN Consensus Conference, 1966[1]

In 1966 it was recognized that the effort to characterize human cytogenetic variation was only the tip of the iceberg in terms of our understanding of genetic detail and that many more types of variation would be revealed with advancing technology. Since the time when DNA was discovered as the major molecule for genetic inheritance, there has been a need to understand how DNA variations affect growth, development, and disease. Even after over 50 years of advances in DNA technology, many types of DNA variation have yet to be identified, named, cataloged, and studied.

HUMAN GENOME

The word *genome* signifies the collection of genes in an organism and is believed to have been coined by the German botanist Hans Winkler in the 1920s.[2] The human genome encompasses all of the information needed for growth, development, and heredity. This information is copied in the nucleus of every cell in the body.[3]

The determination of 46 chromosomes in humans occurred in 1956.[4] The following years were marked by increased activity in human cytogenetics, but it soon became apparent that there was no coordination of how findings were named or classified.[1] Beginning in 1960, a consensus meeting of laboratories (Denver Conference) established basic guidelines for naming large chromosomal variations. The findings from multiple subsequent consensus conferences were unified in a single document, "An International System for Human Cytogenetic Nomenclature (1978)."

Some of the basic concepts of chromosomes are described in ISCN 1978: autosomes are numbered from 1 to 22 in descending order of length. The sex chromosomes are named X and Y. The symbols p and q designated the short (p for "petit," meaning small in French) and long arms of the chromosomes, respectively. A chromosome band is the part of the chromosome that is clearly distinguishable from adjacent segments which are darker or lighter in appearance. G-bands are the bands resulting from Giemsa dye staining. In addition to describing the normal state of chromosomal features, ISCN 1978 considered the naming of chromosomal rearrangements such as inversions, deletions, and translocations.

In more recent times, the ISCN 2013 version introduced new features such as the term "hg" for "human genome build or assembly," and a chapter titled "Microarrays," which is devoted to naming changes identified by oligonucleotide microarrays. Of note, there is a separate consortium focused on microarrays knows as ISCA (The International Standard for Cytogenomic Arrays). ISCA is focused on microarray test quality improvement by projects such as variant databases linked to clinical data.[5]

Throughout the 1990s, there was an international effort to sequence the human genome. The first draft was released in 2001,[6,7] followed by a more complete version in 2004.[8] The 2004 version contains 2.85 billion nucleotides (bases) and was considered 99% complete for euchromatic DNA. The overall size of the genome, including both euchromatic and heterochromatic sequence (tightly compact DNA found at centromeres and telomeres), was estimated to be 3.08 billion nucleotides.

Thus the total overall genome was only 92.5% sequenced when it was first declared "essentially" complete. Within the 2.85 billion nucleotides of euchromatic DNA there were 19,438 known genes and an additional 2188 predicted genes. The total number of nucleotides encoding protein was approximately 34 million (1.2%) of the genome. This portion of the genome encoding proteins is also known as the *exome*. Genomic terms and definitions used in this chapter are given in Box 65.1.

The 2004 genome contained 341 gaps in heterochromatic regions.[9] These regions contain DNA that is difficult to sequence (e.g., repetitive elements, GC-rich sequence) or where

---

BOX 65.1 Genomic Terms and Definitions

Adapter: Oligonucleotides that are ligated to library fragments in order to provide consensus priming sites.

Annotation: Biologic information attached to genomic sequence.

Annotation track: Optional metadata in a genome browser that allows viewing of genes, exons, SNVs, repeats, etc.

Assembly: Reconstruction of short sequence reads on a scaffold of reference DNA.

Binary alignment map (BAM): After alignment to a reference genome, the aligned data for each read produces a sequence alignment map (SAM file). The BAM file is the binary equivalent of the SAM file, and allows for efficient random access of the data.

Browser extensible data (BED): A tab delimited text file that defines the data lines in an annotation track, including the chromosome name, the starting and the ending positions.

Contig: A linear stretch of consensus sequence assembled from smaller overlapping sequence fragments.

Copy number polymorphism (CNP): A copy number variant present at more than 1% in a population.

Copy number variant (CNV): A structural variant of a large region of the genome that has been deleted or duplicated.

Coverage: The percent of target bases that were sequenced at least a given number of times.

Deletion: A DNA sequence that is missing in one sample compared to another. Deletions may be as small as one nucleotide or as large as an entire chromosome.

De novo assembly: Formation of a contig without using a reference sequence.

DNA library: A collection of DNA fragments with ligated adapters that will be sequenced.

DNA microarray: An array of microscopic DNA spots attached to a solid surface or surface within a chamber. Each DNA spot contains of a specific DNA sequence, known as a probe. Probe-target hybridization is usually detected and quantified by detection of fluorescently labeled targets to determine the relative abundance of target nucleic acid sequences.

FASTA file: A nucleotide sequence text file.

FASTQ file: A text output file of sequencing reads in a run, along with the quality scores of each position.

Fusion: A translocation, inversion, large deletion, or large duplication resulting in a hybrid gene formed from originally separate genes.

Gb: Gigabase (1,000,000,000 bases).

Indel: Originally referred to a unique class of sequence variants that included both an insertion and a deletion usually (but not always) resulting in an overall change in the number of base pairs. Today more commonly refers to either insertions or deletions or a combination thereof.

Insert: Part of the original DNA that has been fragmented before ligation to adapters.

Insertion: An extra DNA sequence that is present in one sample compared with a reference sequence.

Heteroplasmy: A mixture of more than one type of mitochondrial sequence in one cell.

Intergenic: DNA sequence between genes.

kb: Kilobase (1000 bases).

Mate-pair sequence: Sequence obtained from both ends of a DNA fragment that is typically 5000–10,000 bases long.

Mb: Megabase (1,000,000 bases)

Missense: A nucleotide substitution that changes a codon to the code for a different amino acid. Although these sequence changes are commonly referred to as missense "mutations," this is strictly a misnomer because missense variants may be benign and cause no disease.

Mutation: A disease-causing sequence variation. Historically, the term has been interchangeable with variant to describe any change in DNA sequence regardless of relation to disease causation. For current clinical descriptions or reporting, the use of mutation is reserved for the scenario when disease causation is known. Many clinical laboratories no longer use the term "mutation" and instead favor "likely pathogenic variant" or "pathogenic variant."

Nonsense: A nucleotide substitution that results in a stop codon, prematurely terminating the protein.

Nonsynonymous: Nucleotide substitutions that are predicted to change the coding amino acid to a different amino acid (missense) or stop codon (nonsense).

Oligonucleotide: A short single-stranded polymer of nucleic acid.

Paired-end sequence: Sequence from both ends of a DNA fragment typically hundreds of bases long.

Phred score: Estimate of the error probability for a base called in DNA sequencing. It is represented as a Q-score; the higher the number, the higher the probability of a correct call.

Plasmid: An extrachromosomal ring of double-stranded, closed DNA found in bacteria.

Polony: A microscopic colony of clonal temples used in massively parallel sequencing. A polony may be generated by PCR, bridge amplification, or isothermal amplification.

Pseudogene: A genetic element that does not code for a functional gene product, usually because of accumulated sequence variations.

Sequence alignment map (SAM file): A file generated by alignment of sequence data to a reference genome. This file type is often converted to a BAM file to save space.

BOX 65.1   Genomic Terms and Definitions—Cont'd

Short tandem repeat (STR): A simple sequence repeat that is 1–13 bases long.

Simple sequence repeat (SSR): A sequence from 1 to 500 bases that is repeated end to end. If the repeat unit is 1–13 bases, it is a microsatellite or STR. If the repeat is 14–500 bases it is a minisatellite.

Single nucleotide polymorphism (SNP): A benign single nucleotide variant (substitution, deletion, or insertion) that occurs in a population at a frequency of at least 1%.

Single nucleotide variation (SNV): A single nucleotide variant (substitution, deletion, or insertion). SNVs may be benign or may cause disease.

Structural variation: A region of DNA greater than 1000 bases in size that is inverted, translocated, inserted, or deleted.

Synonymous variant: A nucleotide change that results in no change to the amino acid sequence. Although synonymous variants are typically considered to be benign since there is no protein coding change, there is the possibility of pathogenicity by changes in splicing, gene expression, or mRNA stability.

Transposon: A mobile genetic element that can delete and insert itself variably into the genome.

Variant call format (VCF): After aligning all reads onto a reference sequence, variants that are different from the reference genome at a given nucleotide position are stored in a text file in a specific format.

Variation: A change in DNA sequence. It may be benign or may cause disease.

---

no clone/template could be made. Commonly used DNA sequencing technologies require a scaffold on which sequence fragments are pieced together.[10] The first human reference sequences were assembled by the University of California at Santa Cruz (UCSC) and were numbered starting with "hg1" in May of 2000. The National Center for Biotechnology Information (NCBI) produced their own genome builds starting in December 2001 as NCBI build 28 (equivalent to hg10 from UCSC) as the genome was further refined. This led to the publicly available 2004 version of the human genome known as NCBI35/hg17. This template or reference sequence has subsequently undergone continuous improvement under the international Genome Reference Consortium (GRC),[10] producing GRCh37/hg19. In the future, only one designation will be given, such as the currently released GRCh38.[3]

Since the 2004 genome publication, there have been continuing efforts to create "Platinum Genomes" that address the missing information (gaps) and improve the quality of data.[11] Prior gaps have been sequenced by utilizing DNA from a haploid cell line.[12] Long-read sequencing technologies can create de novo assemblies that do not require the use of reference genomes.[13] Hybrid sequencing methods are emerging that combine the advantages of short-read sequencing for single nucleotide base accuracy with the advantages of long-read sequencing to further decrease gaps in human genome data and reveal new mechanisms of human variation. For example, the use of long-read sequencing technology has provided the first assembly of the highly repetitive centromere region of the Y-chromosome,[14] and all gaps in the entire human X chromosome have been removed.[15] Complete "telomere-to-telomere" genome sequencing of the malaria parasite, *Plasmodium falciparum*, has been accomplished.[16] Eventually, it is likely that all human chromosomes will be sequenced from telomere-to-telomere, including the repetitive centromeric regions.

Each human cell contains two copies of the 3.08-billion genome divided into 46 chromosomes. Table 65.1 summarizes statistics for the human genome and the types of variations that are important in clinical diagnostics. Three quarters of human DNA is intergenic or between genes. More than 60% of this intergenic sequence consists of "parasitic" DNA regions of mostly defective transposable elements 100 to 11,000 bases in length. Between 2 and 3 million of these "retrotransposons" are present in each copy of the genome.

They contribute to genetic recombination and chromosome structure and provide an evolutionary record of sequence variation and selection.

Segmental duplications constitute 5.3% of the human genome. They are over 1 kilobase (a thousand bases, or kb) in length, have a sequence identity of at least 90% and are not transposable. Segmental duplications are common in the human genome and are prone to deletion or rearrangements, often with medical consequences. Intergenic DNA also carries most of the simple sequence repeats (SSRs) present in the genome. A subset of SSRs, the short tandem repeats (STRs) have repeat units of 1 to several bases that may be repeated up to thousands of times. STRs have played a large role in genetic linkage studies and in forensic and medical identity testing. They are formed by slippage during replication and are highly polymorphic between individuals. The most common STRs are dinucleotide repeats, such as ACACAC and ATAT. On average, one STR occurs every 2000 bases.

Approximately 2% of DNA is required to maintain the structure of chromosomes and is located at chromosome centers (centromeres) and ends (telomeres) and makes up heterochromatic DNA. Centromeric DNA includes many tandem copies of nearly identical 171 base pair (bp) repeats encompassing 0.24 to 5.0 Mb per chromosome. Each chromosome end is capped with several kb of the telomeric 6 base repeat TTAGGG. Although intergenic DNA does not code for protein and was originally considered "junk," much of this DNA is transcribed to RNA, producing a complex "transcriptome" network of RNA control elements whose function and mechanics are active areas of investigation.[17]

There are about 20,000 genes that code for about 200,000 transcripts. Alternative splicing of exons produces many more transcripts than there are genes. The average gene covers 27,000 bases, but only about 1300 of these bases code for amino acids. The primary RNA transcript is processed by splicing to retain exons that are interspersed throughout the gene and have a higher GC content than noncoding regions. On average, 95% of a gene is excised as introns, retaining a mean of 10.4 exons, of which on average 9.1 are translated into proteins. Exons make up only 1.9% of the total genome, with 1.2% of the genome coding for proteins. Some important genes are present in many copies, so that overall protein expression is not affected if a chance variation occurs in one

TABLE 65.1 The Human Genome and Its Sequence Variation

The Human Genome

3.08 billion base pairs in 24 chromosomes

23 chromosome pairs (46–244 million base pairs per chromosome)

75% Intergenic Sequences

Transposable elements	45%
Segmental duplications	5%
Simple sequence repeat	3%
Structural (centromeres, telomeres)	2%
Other	20%

25% Genes That Code for Proteins

Introns	23%
Exons	1.9%
• Coding segments	1.2%
• Untranslated regions	0.7%
Number of genes	19,438 known
	2188 predicted
Average gene	27,000 base pairs
	10.4 exons
	9.1 transcribed exons
	1340 exonic bases
	446 amino acids

Sequence Variants

99.9% identity (one difference every 1250 bases between randomly selected haploid genomes)

Single-Nucleotide Variants (SNVs): Identified Every 75 Bases on Average

Noncoding	97%
Average number within a gene	126
Average number within the coding region of a gene	5

Copy Number Variants (CNVs): Involves 5–12% of the Genome

Disease-Causing Variants

SNVs	68%
• Missense (amino acid substitution)	45%
• Nonsense (termination)	11%
• Splicing	10%
• Regulatory	2%
Small insertions or deletions (or both)	24%
Structural variants (copy number variations, inversions, translocations, rearrangements, repeats)	8%

Epigenetic Alterations

Variable initiation and alternative splicing

Cytosine methylation

Histone phosphorylation, methylation, acetylation

Data from Lander et al.,[7] Venter et al.,[6] and the International Human Genome Sequencing Consortium.[8]

copy. If extra copies of genes lose their function, they are known as pseudogenes. At least as many pseudogenes as functional genes are present in the human genome. It is important to distinguish pseudogenes from functional genes because variants in pseudogenes are seldom of clinical importance, and they often complicate DNA diagnostic assays.

POINTS TO REMEMBER

Human Genome

- Contains approximately 3 billion base pairs per haploid genome
- Protein coding nucleotides are about 1% (30 million base pairs)
- Noncoding sequence has important regulatory roles

NONHUMAN GENOMES

Before the human genome was completed, other genomes of smaller size were sequenced, enabling advancements in technology and logistical organization to sequence the human genome.[18,19] The genomes of different species vary in size and the complexity can be surprising. One of the largest known genomes is the white spruce tree (*Picea glauca*) at 26.9 billion bases. On the opposite end of the spectrum is Porcine circovirus-1, a single-stranded DNA virus with a genome that is less than 2000 bases. There is overlap in the genome size of eukaryotes (animals, plants, fungi), viruses, and bacteria (Table 65.2 and Fig. 65.1).

Primates

Comparison of the chimpanzee genome with the human genome shows a genome-wide difference of only 1.23%.[20] This approximate 1% difference translates to 35 million nucleotides and 5 million insertion/deletion differences. There are also differences at the level of proteins between humans and chimpanzees. Only 29% of proteins are identical at the amino acid level, but proteins that are different only differ by an average of two amino acids.[20]

TABLE 65.2 *Homo sapiens* in Comparison to Other Genomes

Organism/Name	Group	Size (Mb)
Human (*Homo sapiens*)	Animals	3080
White spruce tree (*Picea glauca*)	Plants	26,900
Migratory locust (*Locusta migratoria*)	Animals	5760
Mouse (*Mus musculus*)	Animals	~2500
Rat (*Rattus norvegicus*)	Animals	~2750
Apple tree (*Malus domestica*)	Plants	742
Roundworm (*Caenorhabditis elegans*)	Animals	97
Aspergillus fumigatus	Fungi	~30
Baker's yeast (*Saccharomyces cerevisiae*)	Fungi	12.3
Haemophilus influenzae	Bacteria	1.8
Human immunodeficiency virus (HIV) 1	Viruses	0.0092
Porcine circovirus-1	Viruses	0.00173

Data from the National Center for Biotechnology Information (http://www.ncbi.nlm.nih.gov/genome).

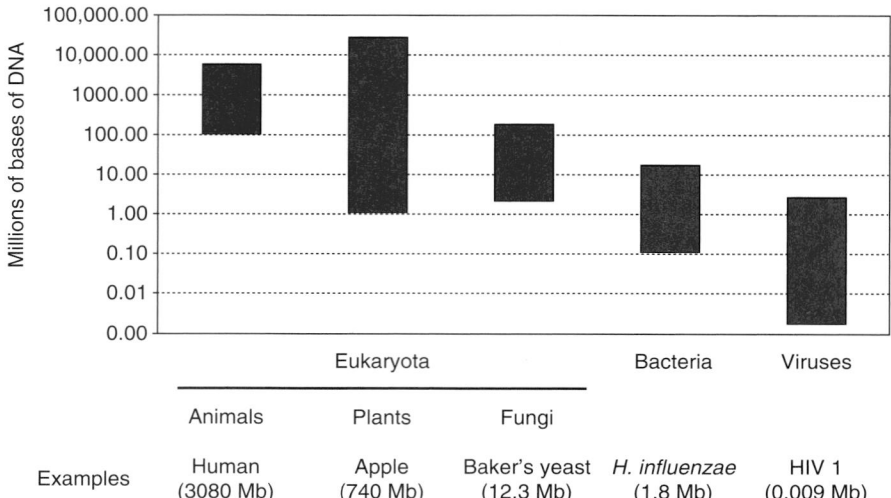

FIGURE 65.1 Range of genome sizes. Among different organisms, there is wide variation in genome size. In this plot of publicly available genomes, the *y*-axis is in megabases, and the *x*-axis lists various organisms: Eukaryota (animals, plants, fungi), bacteria, and viruses. On average, Eukaryota have larger genomes compared with bacteria and viruses; however, there are exceptions in which virus genomes are larger than bacteria or Eukaryota. The difference between the smallest and largest known genomes is more than six orders of magnitude. Several specific genome sizes are illustrated in Mb (megabases, million). (Data extracted from the National Center for Biotechnology Information: http://www.ncbi.nlm. nih.gov/genome.)

Two orangutan species have been sequenced.[21] Their genome sizes are similar to humans at 3 billion bases. During evolutionary development, the number of structural rearrangements in orangutans has been less than the Human and Chimpanzee branches.[21] For example, the number of genome rearrangements greater than 100 kb was 38 in the orangutan, but 85 and 54 in the chimpanzee and human, respectively.

An improved understanding of the ape genome was demonstrated by combining sequencing technologies including long-read DNA sequencing and cDNA sequencing.[22] Previous genomic analysis of apes relied to some extent on human genomic analysis. In this novel analysis, the genomes of two humans, one chimpanzee, and one orangutan were assembled independently without the use of reference genomes. This independent assembly of genomes improved the understanding of differences between human and ape genomic variation including approximately 17,789 structural variants predicted to disrupt 479 genes in humans. When DNA genomics were compared to RNA expression in neural progenitor cells, 41% of genes with downregulated expression in humans compared to chimpanzees had an associated disrupting structural variant. This type of loss of expression in humans compared to apes is supportive of a theory that human evolution involved the loss of neuronal gene expression.

An example of nonprotein coding variation between primates is the number and types of DNA insertions. A comparison of 5 primate genomes (chimpanzee, gorilla, orangutan, gibbon, and macaque) identified regions of human DNA that were absent in nonhuman primates.[23] More than 200,000 human-specific DNA insertions were identified; the majority of these were less than 10 nucleotides in length and were eliminated from further study. There were 5582 genes identified that contained larger insertions; 2450 of these genes were expressed in brain tissue. Many of the human-specific insertions were transposable elements and long terminal repeats.[23]

Rodents

The mouse genome is 14% smaller than the human genome (2.5 billion bases compared to the human size of approximately 3 billion bases).[24] In comparison, the rat (*Rattus norvegicus*) genome is in between the size of the human and mouse (2.75 billion bases).[25] The number of genes is similar between all three species. About 40% of the rat, mouse, and human genomes are in alignment. Another 30% of the rat and mouse genomes match each other but not the human genome.

Fungi

Fungi are eukaryotes and their genomes are less complex than the human genome. Common fungi that cause human disease have genome sizes of 7.5 to 30 million bases and 8 to 16 chromosomes, as well as mitochondrial genomes. Some fungi have diploid genomes, and others have haploid genomes. Many of their genes have introns. For instance, *Aspergillus fumigatus* (a fungus that causes allergic reactions and systemic disease with a high mortality rate) has a haploid genome of about 30 million bases with more than 9900 predicted genes on eight chromosomes. Its genes are smaller than human genes, with an average length of 1400 bp and 2.8 exons per gene.

The first eukaryotic genome sequenced was *Saccharomyces cerevisiae* (baker's yeast).[19] This fungal genome has 12 million bases arranged into 16 chromosomes. In addition to the importance of yeast in baking breads and brewing alcohol, yeast is an important model organism and pathogen. With the identification of the approximately 6000 genes within the *S. cerevisiae* genome, systematic alteration of each gene or combination of genes can now be explored to examine the role of genes in yeast and higher organisms.

Bacteria

Bacterial genomes are considerably less complex than human or fungal genomes. Common bacteria have only one chromosome, usually a circular DNA double helix of 4 to 5 million base pairs, about 1000 times less than the amount of DNA in a human cell. About 90% of the DNA in bacteria codes for protein. There are no introns, but there are multiple small intergenic regions of repetitive sequences that are dispersed throughout the genome. *Escherichia coli*, a common bacterium in the human intestinal tract has about 4300 genes.

In addition to the large circular chromosome that carries essential genes, bacteria also carry accessory genes in smaller circles of double-stranded DNA (dsDNA) known as plasmids. Plasmids range in size from 1000 to more than 1 million base pairs. Plasmids are important in the molecular diagnosis of bacterial infections because they often encode pathogenic factors and antibiotic resistance.

The bacterial repertoire of DNA can be altered by (1) gain or loss of plasmids; (2) single-base changes, small insertions, and deletions as in eukaryotic genomes; and (3) large segmental rearrangements, including inversions, deletions, and duplications. Some genes, such as those for ribosomal RNA, are present in many copies, making them good targets for molecular assays to identify species of bacteria. In addition, the intergenic repetitive sequences serve as multiple targets for oligonucleotide probes, enabling the generation of unique DNA profiles or fingerprints for individual bacterial strains.

The first genome sequenced by random fragmentation and computational assembly was the pathogenic bacteria, *Haemophilus influenza*.[18] Its genomic DNA was fragmented into 19,687 templates and inserted into plasmids and bacteriophages. A total of 24,304 sequences were successfully generated over 3 months. The sequencing data required 30 hours of computational time to be assembled. A total of 11 million bases of DNA were sequenced and used to generate the 1.8 million bases of the *H. influenzae* genome. In addition to being the first genome solved by shotgun sequencing, it was also the first bacterial genome sequenced. Multiple strains of *H. influenzae* have been subsequently sequenced. These additional genomes have revealed heterogeneity in the number of genes between different strains. Of the approximately 3000 genes identified, only 1461 are common to all strains.[26] The differences in genes between different strains may be associated with differences in the infectious pathogenicity of *H. influenza*.

Viruses

Viral genomes are considerably less complex than bacterial genomes. Common viruses that infect humans vary in size from about 5000 to 250,000 bases, or 20 to 1000 times less than the amount of nucleic acid in *E. coli*. Because viruses use the host's cellular machinery, they do not need as many genes as bacteria do. Small viruses may encode only several genes, but the larger viruses can encode hundreds. The viral genome consists of either DNA or RNA, and the nucleic acid may be single stranded or double stranded, linear, or circular with one or multiple fragments or copies per viral particle. As in bacteria, there are no introns. In fact, in some viruses the

exons overlap with different reading frames that code different products from the same nucleic acid sequence. Noncoding regions are usually present at the terminal ends of linear genomes. Repeat segments are often found as terminal or internal repeats and may be inverted.

Sequence alterations in viruses are common. Areas of high sequence variation may be interspersed between conserved domains. Higher frequencies of variation correlate with lower polymerase fidelity and may allow escape from antibody recognition and antiviral drugs. Common sequence variants in viruses include single base changes, insertions, and deletions. Sequence diversity within a viral species may be so great that consensus sequences for molecular typing are difficult to find.

DNA THAT CODES FOR RNA BUT NOT PROTEIN

Even though 99% of the human genome does not code for protein, most of it is transcribed into noncoding RNA. At least 93% of the genome is transcribed,[17] producing more than 10 times the amount of RNA that is produced from the coding segments of genes.[27] Both strands of DNA may be transcribed, and long noncoding transcripts may overlap coding regions, producing a complex transcriptome of functional RNA molecules that may variably regulate transcription of coding regions, RNA processing, mRNA stability, translation, protein stability, and secretion. In addition to long noncoding RNA, ribosomal RNA, and transfer RNA, specific classes of noncoding RNAs include small nuclear RNAs critical for splicing, small nucleolar RNAs that modify rRNA, telomerase RNAs for maintenance of telomeres, small interfering RNAs, and microRNAs (miRNAs) that regulate gene expression.[28–30] In a recent review on RNA, 54 different categories were identified.[31] Some of the more important types of RNA are listed in Table 65.3.

MicroRNAs (or miRNAs) are particularly interesting as potential markers for disease. For example, concentrations of specific, circulating miRNAs correlate with many different types of cancer.[32] MicroRNAs are noncoding but functional single-stranded RNAs that are 21 to 22 bases long and are expressed in a tissue-specific manner. They are initially transcribed as longer precursors that undergo two rounds of truncations as they are transported from the nucleus to the cytoplasm in the cell. The mature miRNA is then integrated into a protein complex called the *RNA-induced silencing complex*, which regulates translation of mRNA. MicroRNAs hybridize to a 6 to 8 base sequence in the 3′ untranslated region of target mRNAs and inhibit mRNA expression either by mRNA degradation if the bases are perfectly complementary, or by blocking of translation if they are imperfectly complementary. Currently for humans, there are 1917 precursor miRNA and 2654 mature miRNAs cataloged in miRBase.[33] Despite the promise of miRNAs as tumor markers, the literature is often contradictory and inconsistent with few accepted conclusions.[34]

VARIATION IN THE HUMAN GENOME

If the DNA of any two individuals is compared, on average one difference is noted every 1250 bases (i.e., approximately 99.9% of the sequence is identical between randomly chosen copies of the genome). However, copy-number variants involve a greater amount of the genome, with 0.5% of the genome differing on

TABLE 65.3   Some Common, Interesting, and Important Types of RNA

Abbreviation	Description
mRNA	Messenger RNA is translated to protein by the ribosome.
rRNA	Ribosomal RNA is a major component of ribosomes.
tRNA	Transfer RNA pairs an amino acid with its anticodon in protein synthesis.
ncRNA	Noncoding RNA is not translated to protein.
lncRNA	Long noncoding RNA is greater than 200 bases and is not translated to protein.
hnRNA	Heterogeneous nuclear RNA is the initial RNA transcript that includes introns.
Ribozyme	RNA that has catalytic activity.
Riboswitch	RNA that switches between 2 conformations under certain conditions (ligand exposure).
Telomerase RNA	Structural part of telomerase that also provides a hexamer template.
Xist RNA	X-inactive–specific transcript RNA inactivates one X chromosome in females.
snRNA	Small nuclear RNA is found in the eukaryotic nucleus.
snoRNA	Small nucleolar RNA are intron fragments essential for pre-rRNA processing.
siRNA	Small interfering RNA can cleave perfectly complementary target RNA.
gRNA	Guide RNA pairs with an RNA target and guides proteins for cleavage and so on.
miRNA	MicroRNA affects target mRNA regulation or decay.

average between two individuals when copy-number variants greater than 50 kb are considered.[35] Between individuals, at least five times as many bases are affected by copy number changes as by small sequence differences.

Most human genetic material is present in two copies, with the exception of the unpaired sex chromosome in males and mitochondrial DNA. The presence of only single gene copies on the X and Y chromosome in males leads to well-known sex-linked disorders. In contrast, the 16,500-bp mitochondrial genome is present in multiple copies per cell, constituting about 0.3% of human DNA, depending on the tissue source. Allele fractions may vary over a wide range when all mitochondria in a cell are considered. That is, sequence variations in mitochondrial DNA are heteroplasmic, meaning that the ratio of the wild-type allele to a variant allele can vary almost continuously, sometimes resulting in a wide range of symptoms even when only one sequence variant is involved.

Large-scale human genome sequencing projects have cast a wide net across many diverse populations. These projects have provided a wealth of knowledge of the genetic diversity that exists in humans. An alternative approach to human genetic diversity is to examine more homogenous populations. Several studies have examined the genetics of a large number of individuals from Iceland. A whole genome sequencing study of 2636 Icelanders observed 20 million single

nucleotide variants (SNVs) and 1.5 million insertions/deletions.[36] The data from this whole genome sequencing study were combined with a previous data set of 104,220 Icelanders who had been SNV typed at 676,913 locations. By applying whole genome sequencing data from only a small subset of individuals, the full genetics could be inferred for a larger set of over 100,000 individuals who had only had SNV typing.

Another interesting result of the Icelandic whole genome study was the identification of 6795 loss of function single nucleotide variants, insertions, or deletions in 4924 genes.[37] Loss of function changes (homozygous or compound heterozygous) were found in 7.7% of the individuals sequenced. In essence, this study identified a surprisingly high percentage of individuals with "knocked-out" or functionally silenced genes.

Any sequence change (compared to a reference sequence) is called a sequence variant or variation. Many variations do not affect human health and are benign or silent. For example, most (1) copy-number variations, (2) SNVs, and (3) STRs found between genes are seldom associated with disease.

Single Nucleotide Variants

The most common sequence variants are single nucleotide changes, known as SNVs. More than 40 million SNVs have been described, and many new SNVs continue to be reported. Some SNVs are common in the population, with allele frequencies of 0.1 to 0.5 (i.e., present in 10 to 50 of every 100 copies studied), but other single base changes are very rare. The vast majority of SNVs (97%) occur in noncoding regions; only 3% of SNVs are associated with exons. Similarly, most of the SNVs within introns, except for splicing and regulatory variants, are not known to affect gene function. In addition, some of the SNVs within exons are silent alterations that do not code for a change in amino acid sequence because of the redundancy in the genetic code. Still other SNVs in exons code for amino acid changes that do not affect protein function. However, some silent SNVs may affect DNA splicing, and others are of interest as genetic markers.

Examination of SNVs reveals thousands of variants in each gene, many of which do not cause disease. The international 1000 Genomes Project sequenced 2504 individuals representing 26 subpopulations from Europe, East Asia, South Asia, West Africa, and the Americas.[38] All participants were sequenced by both whole-genome sequencing and exome sequencing. Individuals had on average 4.1 to 5.0 million sites different from the human reference genome. Greater than 99% of single nucleotide variants occurred in greater than 1% of individuals examined. Importantly for clinical genetic studies, all participants were self-declared as healthy at the time of sample collection. The genome aggregation database (gnomad.broadinstitute.org) lists over 18 million variants found in 25,000 exomes (Fig. 65.2). Most were rare variants (found only once or twice) and less than 0.1% were known to be disease-associated.

In the current age of genomics, the lack of understanding of disease causation based on variant identification is referred to as an "interpretive gap." Disease classification of variants (e.g., benign or pathogenic) lags far behind our ability to discover these variants. Sequence alterations that are known to cause disease are often called *mutations, pathogenic variants,* or *disease-causing variants.* About 68% of known disease-causing variants involve only a single base change. Most of the remaining disease-causing variants (24%) are

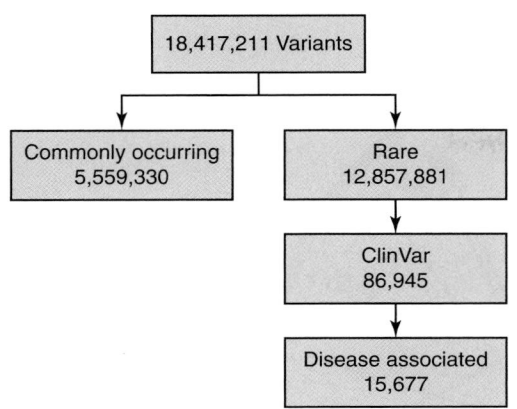

FIGURE 65.2 There are millions of variants in human genes. A population database (gnomAD v2.1.1, accessed February 2020) of over 25,000 exomes cataloged 18,417,211 variants that differ from the GRCh37 reference genome. Thirty percent of these occurred in at least three exomes. Conversely, 70% were rare and only occurred in one or two exomes. Among the rare variants, only 0.7% had a description in the public database, ClinVar. Only 18% of these had a disease association with a pathogenic or likely pathogenic interpretation. (Courtesy Eric Crossley, Advanced Diagnostics Laboratory, Children's Health, Dallas, TX.)

small insertions or deletions. The remainder (8%) includes more complex structural variations (see Table 65.1).

Most SNVs that cause disease are missense and result in amino acid substitutions; significantly fewer are nonsense variants that result in a termination codon and premature polypeptide chain termination. Approximately 10% of disease-causing variants are SNVs that affect splicing sites and result in altered concatenation of coding sequences. Finally, less than 2% of known disease-causing variants are SNVs that affect the regulatory efficiency of transcription by altering promoter or enhancer regions in introns or the stability of the RNA transcript.

Small insertion and deletion variants account for 24% of variants that cause disease. An insertion refers to the presence of extra bases, whereas deletion implies the absence of certain bases in comparison with a reference sequence. Insertions and deletions often cause a shift of the codon reading frame, resulting in altered amino acid sequence downstream of the variation—commonly followed by chain termination from a nonsense codon.

The remaining 8% of variants that relate to health and disease are mostly structural variants including (1) duplications or deletions of entire exons or genes; (2) gene fusions, including chromosomal translocations and inversions; (3) STR expansions (e.g., an increased number of trinucleotide repeats); (4) gene rearrangements (e.g., rearrangements of immunoglobulin genes in B cells that are required for production of antibodies); (5) complex polymorphic loci related to health and disease (e.g., human leukocyte antigens); and (6) copy number variants (CNVs).

Copy Number Variation (Gains and Losses)

Although SNVs are the most common sequence variant, CNVs cover more of the genome than SNVs. Examples of large gains or losses in genomic DNA have been known for many years in syndromic diseases. However, an examination of phenotypically normal individuals by array-based comparative genomic hybridization revealed an average of 12.4 large copy number variations per individual.[39] Some CNVs in phenotypically normal individuals involved 2 million bases of DNA. CNVs may be duplicated in tandem or may involve complex gains or losses of homologous sequences at multiple sites in the genome. CNV regions exist in every chromosome and involve 5 to 12% of the human genome.[35,40]

Higher resolution comparative genomic hybridization has now revealed the presence of deletions across hundreds of additional individuals.[41–44] In total, these studies have found over 1000 unique deletions. Some deletions are in regions without known genes; however, hundreds of known or predicted genes exist at the site of the observed deletions. Interest in CNVs in relation to disease has increased recently as the extent of variation has become clear.[45] CNVs can involve genes or contiguous sets of genes. When the normal dosage of the gene is two, but more than two functional copies of a gene are present, then the gene is "amplified." If a dosage-sensitive gene, such as HER2 (ERBB2) is amplified, it usually leads to overexpression of mRNA and protein, resulting in cellular abnormalities and possible progression to disease such as cancer. When the normal gene dosage is two, and loss of one of the functional copies of the gene occurs, disorders such as mental retardation and developmental delay may result. Structural variants can be determined by cytogenetic techniques, including karyotyping, fluorescent in situ hybridization, comparative genomic hybridization, and virtual karyotyping by SNV microarrays.

Fusions

Gene fusions arise by deletions, duplications, inversions, and translocations and are commonly found in cancer.[46] Often they arise by balanced translocations, whereby a chimeric protein is created by the fusion of two coding regions. Gene fusions promote tumor proliferation by either activating an oncogenic driver or inactivating a tumor suppressor. Although translocations are rare outside of cancer, massively parallel sequencing now allows insight into the myriad of translocations that occur in both hematologic and solid tumors. By identifying gene fusions that act as primary oncogenic drivers, the hope is that targeted therapies may be available for precision treatment. Fusions across the genome can be visualized on Circos plots,[47] where sequential chromosomes form arcs around a positional genomic circle. Intra- and interchromosomal fusions are indicated by curves connecting different genomic locations. Fig. 65.3 shows a Circos plot of a prostate cancer genome that includes many intrachromosomal fusions and several interchromosomal fusions.[48] Additional concentric circles on Circos plots can indicate additional tracts of data, such as copy number information, allowing related genomic metadata to be presented in a very condensed format.

Short Tandem Repeats

Short tandem repeats are DNA motifs that are defined by 1 to several bases that are repeated many times in tandem. STRs have been implicated in more than 40 genetic diseases.[49] In the case of Fragile X, there is an expansion of CGG repeats that results in disruption of protein expression of the *FMR1* gene. For Huntington disease, an expansion of a CAG repeat results in abnormal protein expression of the *HTT* gene. Many massively parallel sequencing platforms use short reads

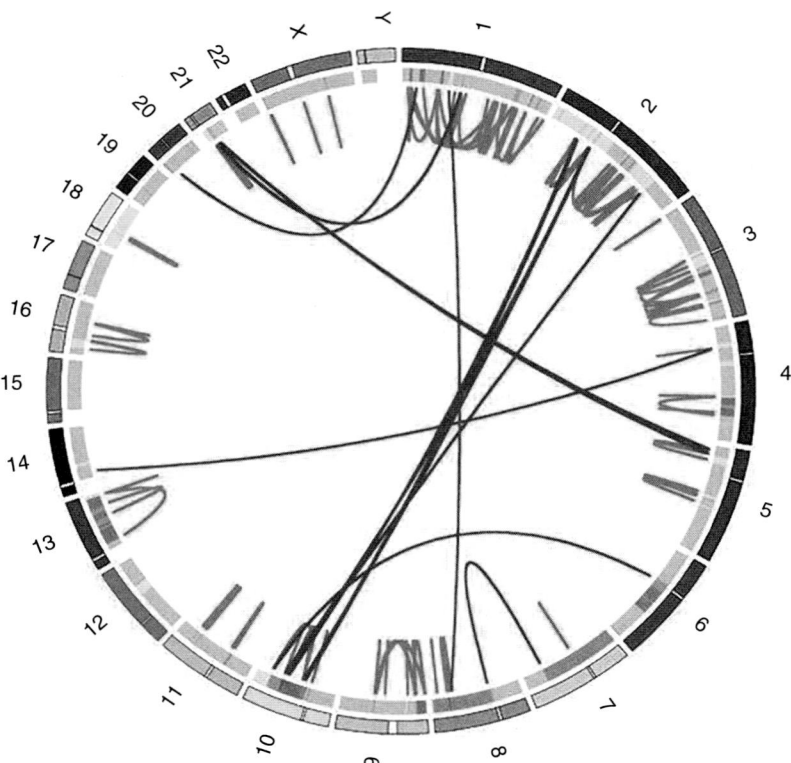

FIGURE 65.3 A Circos plot for graphical representation of genomic fusions and copy number changes. Chromosomes and their positions are indicated around the outside of the circle. Intrachromosomal fusions are indicated by short connections within chromosomes, while interchromosomal fusions cross through the interior of the circle. Copy number changes are indicated on an internal concentric circle by color and intensity. (Reprinted with permission from Berger MF, Lawrence MS, Demichelis F, et al. The genomic complexity of primary human prostate cancer. *Nature* 2011;470:214–20.)

of information that are less than 200 bases in length, and these short reads have made the analysis of repetitive sequences difficult.

One group proposes a "thesaurus" approach in which an extensive catalog of repetitive DNA elements is used within the existing analysis framework.[50] The catalog contains almost 3 billion entries that are representative of the variety of repetitive elements seen in a human genome. This approach was successful in detecting novel variants without extensive changes to typical analysis approaches. Massively parallel sequencing technology and informatics are limited in the amount of STR data that is sequenced and analyzed. A recent informatics tool, lobSTR, can accurately genotype STRs from massively parallel sequencing datasets.[51] When lobSTR was applied across whole genome datasets from the 1000 Genomes Project, 700,000 STR loci were catalogued, and 350,000 STR loci were found per individual.[49] Some STR loci were common with 300,000 having a mean allele frequency of greater than 1% and 2237 were located within 20 bases of an exon-intron junction.[49] The high frequency of STR loci and their proximity to coding DNA suggest a larger role for STR variants in influencing growth, development, and disease. A genome-wide study of 652 individuals compared whole genome sequencing to tissue-specific RNA gene expression across 17 different tissue types.[52] The study identified 28,375 STRs which were correlated with the expression of 12,494 genes. Future studies will examine the contribution of these STRs to human disease.

Transposable Elements and Their Genetic Fossils

Transposable elements are composed of repetitive DNA that could originally facilitate homologous recombination, or create deletions, duplications, inversions, and translocations.[53] Most of these elements are no longer active and are categorized as retrotransposons, including long terminal repeats (LTRs), long interspersed nuclear elements (LINEs), and short interspersed nuclear elements (SINEs). In a conservative estimate not including repeat-rich regions like centromeres, these elements comprised 30 to 50% of the total DNA in mammals. In comparison, the genomes of birds were less than 10% derived from transposable elements.[53]

In one human study, repetitive DNA including transposable elements and their nonfunctional descendants consumed 66 to 69% of the human genome.[54] In humans, active transposable elements include a subset of L1 LINEs and *Alu* (a type of SINE).[55] These active elements have *de novo* germline insertions ranging from 1 in 20 to 1 in 916 births. The insertion of these elements has multiple possible effects on the transcriptional regulation of genes including disruption of the open reading frame, creation of a novel promoter, alternative splicing, an alternative poly(A) tail, disruption of transcription factor bindings sites, and changes in small RNA regulation.[55] In a recent study on clinical exomes, mobile element insertions were investigated on 89,874 samples from 38,871 individuals.[56] Overall, 23,014 mobile element insertions were identified encompassing the mobile element types of L1, Alu, and SVA (SINE-R); an average of 12.2 insertions were detected per individual. Only 14 of the mobile element insertions were classified as clinically significant with an overall diagnostic yield of 0.15%. Common repeat sequences in the human genome are cataloged in Table 65.4. Their distribution in humans and other species is shown in Fig. 65.4.

Human Epigenetic Alterations[60]

In addition to the sequence variants considered above, epigenetic alterations, including alternative splicing and methylation, affect gene expression. Even though the number of genes may be limited to less than 25,000, variable transcription initiation and exon splicing produce about 200,000 unique mRNA transcripts and protein products.

Methylation of cytosine to 5-methylcytosine occurs frequently; about 70% of CpG dinucleotides in the human genome are methylated. Although not inherited, interest in this "fifth base" has increased as correlations with cancer have been reported. CpG islands are about 1000 bases in length and are often found near the 5' end of genes. These regions consist of clusters of CG dinucleotides that are usually not methylated in normal cells. However, CpG methylation correlates with condensed chromatin structure and promoter inactivation; an important example occurs in tumor-suppressor genes. Other epigenetic targets include nucleosome histone phosphorylation, acetylation, and methylation that can all affect gene expression.

ENCODE PROJECT

ENCODE (Encyclopedia of DNA Elements) is a project that was initiated by the National Human Genome Research Institute in 2003 to examine all functional elements in the human genome.[61] The functional elements defined were not only the discrete genomic areas that encode a product, such as protein, but any genomic area with a reproducible biological effect on processes such as transcription or chromatin structure. These genomic areas include both exons and nonprotein coding areas such as promoters, enhancers, and silencers. The genomic areas that do not encode protein have significant contributions to human variation.[62] From a survey of 150 genome-wide association studies using SNVs to identify

TABLE 65.4 Repeat Sequences in the Human Genome

Type	Abbreviations	Size	Copies (Thousands)	Genome (%)
Retrotransposons				
Long interspersed elements	LINEs	900 bp	850	21
	L1		516	16.9
	L2		315	3.22
	L3		37	0.31
Short interspersed elements	SINEs	100–400 bp	1500	13
	Alu	350 bp	1090	11
	MIR		393	2.2
	Ther2/MIR3		75	0.34
Long terminal repeats	LTRs	1.5–11 kb	450	8
	ERV		112	2.89
	ERV(K)		8	0.31
	ERV(L)		83	1.44
	MaLR		240	3.65
Segmental Duplications		>1000 bp		5.3
Structural Repeat and Gene Clusters				
	Centromeres	171 bp		3-6
	Telomeres	6 bp		<0.1
	Ribosomal			0.41
DNA Transposons		80–3000 bp	300	3
Simple Sequence Repeats	SSRs	1–500 bp		3
Short Tandem Repeats	STRs	1–13 bp		0.17
		1		0.53
		2		0.10
		3		0.34
		4		0.27
		5		0.14
		6		0.09
		7		0.11
		8		0.09
		9		0.16
		10		
Processed Pseudogenes		~1300	20	1.2

Data extracted from Lander et al.,[7] Venter et al.,[6] The International Human Genome Sequencing Consortium,[8] Richard et al.,[57] Stultz et al.,[58] and Torrents et al.[59]

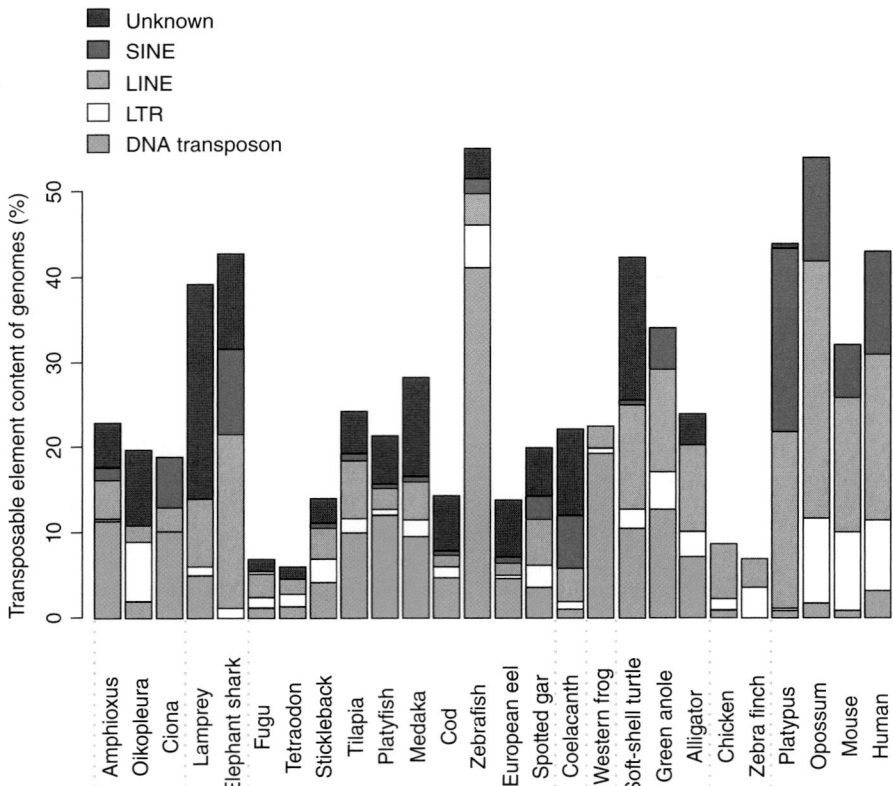

FIGURE 65.4 Transposable element diversity among species, including both retrotransposons and active transposons. The percentage of inactive retrotransposons (SINE, LINE, LTR) and active DNA transposons is shown for each organism. The organisms are grouped into invertebrates (e.g., Amphi-oxus), nonbony vertebrates (e.g., lamprey), actinopterygian fish (e.g., Fugu), lobe-finned fish (e.g., Coelacanth), amphibians (e.g., Western frog), nonbird reptiles (e.g., soft-shell turtle), birds (e.g., chicken), and mammals (e.g., platypus). In mammals, transposable elements contribute to more than 30% of the total genome. In comparison, in other organisms such as chicken and fugu, transposable elements are less than 10% of the genome. (Reprinted with permission from Chalopin D, Naville M, Plard F, et al. Comparative analysis of transposable elements highlights mobilome diversity and evolution in vertebrates. *Genome Biol Evol* 2015;7:567–80.)

genes linked to disease, 465 unique disease-associated SNVs were identified.[63] Of these 465 variants, 88% (*n* = 407) were present in the regions between genes (intergenic) or within introns. These results suggest the importance of noncoding variants in disease.

POINTS TO REMEMBER
Variations

- Small variants such as single nucleotide changes are the easiest to correlate to human disease.
- Most of the genome is repetitive, noncoding sequences with functions just now being uncovered by massively parallel sequencing.

NOMENCLATURE

Amino acid variations were associated with human disease long before DNA variation.[64] Amino acid variants were found first because techniques for amino acid sequencing matured prior to DNA sequencing. Advances in DNA technology

enabled the investigation of DNA variations associated with disease. For example, the characterization of amino acid variants in the globin gene products (*HBB* and *HBA*) preceded the descriptions of DNA variation in the globin genes.

Small Variants

More than 25 years ago, the need for a human database of genetic variants associated with disease was recognized. In 1996, the Mutation Database Initiative was sponsored by the Human Genome Organization (HUGO).[64] In 2001, the HUGO Mutation Database Initiative became the Human Genome Variation Society (HGVS).[65] In addition to the documentation and collection of variant information, the HGVS created a nomenclature system for standardizing the reporting of variations. An early recommendation proposed a hybrid model in which traditional disease alleles such as hemoglobin S for sickle cell disease and the Z allele for α1-antitrypsin deficiency would retain their historic nomenclature and new disease alleles would use the new nomenclature system.[66] Current HGVS nomenclature has features that can be found in this early proposed system (Box 65.2).[67] In the HGVS system, disease alleles are described at the DNA level

BOX 65.2   The Human Genome Variation Society Nomenclature for Naming Small Sequence Variants

The position of single nucleotide substitutions can be referenced to the genome (g.), amino acids in the protein (p.), or nucleotide bases in the cDNA transcript (c.). In all cases, the genome build and the sequence accession number should be specified.

For genomic coordinates, specify the chromosome and the base position followed by the base change. For example: GRCh37/hg19 Ch17: g.3424566C>T. Genomic coordinates are the only option for all intergenic variants, as well as deep intronic variants.

When the variant is within the protein coding region of a gene and protein coordinates are preferred, give the gene name followed by the number of the amino acid affected starting with the initiating methionine as 1. The wild-type amino acid is listed to the left of the number, and the variant amino acid is listed to the right. For example: *CYBB* p.T42R (or *CYBB* p.Tyr42Arg) for the one letter and three letter codes for amino

acids, respectively. The protein coordinates best specify the phenotype, but it is a challenge to convey the results of frameshifts and the exact nucleotide change is often ambiguous.

When the variant is in or near the exons of a gene, you can use the cDNA coordinates. In this case, give the gene name followed by the base number using the A in the ATG initiation codon as 1 and then the base change. For example: *CYBB* c.125C>G. If the base change is in an intron (e.g., a splice site mutation), you count from the nearest intron–exon boundary. For example: *CYBB* c.141+2T>C or c.142-12C>T. If the variant is 5′ of the ATG initiation sequence, you count back using negative numbers (*CYBB* c.-64C>T), or if it is 3′ of the last exon, you count up (*CYBB* c.*67G>A). With c. coordinates, you know the exact base change relative to a specific mRNA transcript.

Nomenclature for insertions and deletions are also specified by the Human Genome Variation Society.

TABLE 65.5   Describing Hemoglobin Variants by Different Systems

Traditional Name	Disease Associated	Gene	Amino Acid Change (Traditional)[a]	Amino Acid Change (HGVS)	HGVS Nucleotide Change (mRNA Transcript)[b]	Genomic Coordinate (GRCh37/hg19)[c]
Hemoglobin SS	Sickle cell anemia	*HBB*	Gln6Val	p.(Gln7Val)	c.20A>T hom (NM_000518.4)	Chr11:g.5248232T>A
Hemoglobin CC	Hemolytic anemia	*HBB*	Glu6Lys	p.(Glu7Lys)	c.19G>A hom (NM_000518.4)	Chr11:g.5248233C>T
Hemoglobin Austin	None	*HBB*	Arg40Ser	p.(Arg41Ser)	c.123G>T het (NM_000518.4)	Chr11:g.5247999C>A
Hemoglobin G Philadelphia	None	*HBA2*	Asn68Lys	p.(Asn69Lys)	c.207C>A het (NM_000517.4)	Chr16:g.223235C>A

[a]The amino acid change for hemoglobin diseases was characterized by amino acid sequencing before the advent of DNA sequencing. The first amino acid, methionine, was not included, so that the Gln to Val change in sickle cell anemia was described as the "6" position rather than the "7" position.

[b]The "c." annotation is based on a reference transcript (NM number).

[c]The HGVS nucleotide position is from 5′ to 3′ on the strand. However, the genomic coordinates are not oriented to the gene. The nucleotide position based on mRNA transcript may increase while the genomic position increases or decreases, depending on the orientation of the gene on the chromosome.

Data formatted according to den Dunnen JT, Antonarakis SE. Mutation nomenclature extensions and suggestions to describe complex mutations: a discussion. *Hum Mutat* 2000;15:7–12.

rather than as amino acid changes. Preferred terminology does not ascribe disease potential to the naming of a variant because all variants are not disease-causing mutations. The preferred terms include sequence variant, copy number variant, and single nucleotide variant. Hemoglobin variants were initially named by a combination of letters (Hemoglobin A, B, S, C, F) and the city of discovery. Hematologists continue to use the traditional or legacy nomenclature (Table 65.5) that does not distinguish between variants from β-globin (*HBB*) and α-globin (*HBA*). In addition to the hemoglobin genes, other genes have both a traditional/legacy nomenclature system and the HGVS nomenclature.

Naming Genes

As significant as the naming of DNA variants, the naming of genes has also become standardized over the past 30 years.[68]

The basic components of gene names include the gene name, which may include information on gene function, and the gene symbol, which is a short abbreviation in upper case Latin letters and Arabic numbers that are both italicized. The currently accepted gene naming system is by the HUGO Gene Nomenclature Committee (HGNC).[69] As with all standardization activities, there is a trade-off. The more familiar historic names are established in the literature and used by practitioners in the specialty concerned with that gene. However, for a particular disease-associated gene, communication outside of the specialized field of knowledge may by difficult and lead to errors. Especially in the current era with genomic tests examining hundreds to tens of thousands of genes, a common gene naming system is necessary. In reporting specific genes, a hybrid approach that uses both the consensus nomenclature and the traditional name may be useful. A current database of recommended gene names and symbols, as well as traditional names can be found on the HGNC online database. The HGNC database currently contains information on 19,320 protein-coding genes.

VARIANT DATABASES

Databases of DNA variations may focus on specific genes or diseases (e.g., hemoglobinopathy variants cataloged in HbVar)[70] or catalog variants throughout the genome. Some genomic databases target somatic variants found in cancer, including The Cancer Genome Atlas (TCGA)[71] and the Catalog of Somatic Mutations in Cancer (COSMIC).[72] Constitutional or germline variants that are passed from generation to generation are the focus of most genomic databases. Some of the most common are dbSNP (Database of Single Nucleotide Polymorphisms), HGMD (Human Gene Mutation Database), ClinVar (Clinical Genome Resource's variant database), gnomAD (Genome Aggregation Database), and OMIM (Online Mendelian Inheritance in Man).

A systematic catalog of SNVs including small insertions and deletions was created as the dbSNP in 1998 as a collaboration between the NCBI and the National Human Genome Research Institute (NHGRI).[73] The reference identifier for variants in dbSNP begins with the prefix "rs" and over 500,000,000 variants are currently cataloged.[74]

HGMD is a database of variants with reported disease associations.[75,76] The number of new reports of germline mutations was less than 250 per year through 1990, but throughout the 1990s reports grew into the thousands and now 275,716 disease-associated variants are cataloged in release 2019.4 of HGMD Professional, a privatized derivative of the originally public database. As databases grow, curation and the avoidance of errors become critical; incorrect annotations do arise from database issues or problems with the primary literature. At one point in time, 80% of the HGMD disease-causing variants from the 1000 Genomes Project dataset had an allele frequency of more than 5%[77]; however, rare diseases are expected to have allele frequencies much less than 5%.

The chief limitation of databases such as dbSNP and HGMD is that they rely on published reports. As new variants of known genes are discovered in research or clinical laboratories, they are rarely published. This recognition of the under representation of clinically significant variants resulted in the ClinVar project, which allows for the contribution of annotated variants by clinical laboratories, research laboratories, and the literature into a publicly available database.[78] The dataset combines submitter, variant, and phenotype and is

given an accession number with the prefix "SCV" (Submitted Clinical Variant). As of February 2020, ClinVar included over 677,341 unique variation records with classifications.

The application of massively parallel sequencing to human exomes and genomes continues to identify new variants at a rapidly accelerating pace. The Genome Aggregation Database (gnomAD) is an international coalition to aggregate and harmonize variant data from exome and genome sequencing.[79] Version 2 catalogs over 17 million variants from the exomes of 125,748 individuals and over 260 million variants from 15,708 unrelated genomes. Version 3 of this database adds an additional 71,702 genomes.

Instead of cataloging variants, OMIM is organized by disease state and is manually curated by a team of professionals located at Johns Hopkins University.[80] It was started by the geneticist Victor McKusick in the 1970s as "Mendelian Inheritance in Man," first a series of published books and later an online resource. By design, the OMIM is not a comprehensive catalog of every variant ever described with disease but rather a catalog of genes and variants representative of a disease type. As of February 2020, OMIM contained 4225 genes with mutations associated with phenotypes. Conversely, the number of phenotypes with a molecular basis catalogued in OMIM was 6594.

MASSIVELY PARALLEL METHODS

It is a daunting task to experimentally investigate the enormous complexity of biological genomes and their variants. Nevertheless, methods that interrogate entire genomes are now in common use. Perhaps the simplest genomic DNA analysis is using flow cytometry to quantify the total amount of DNA in cells. Somewhat more complex is the analysis of individual chromosomes by conventional cytogenetics. Even more detailed are nucleic acid microarrays, allowing SNV genotyping, gene expression analysis, and copy number quantification. Finally, the ultimate genomic analysis is whole genome sequencing, enabled today by massively parallel sequencing. In this section we focus on microarrays and massively parallel sequencing.

NUCLEIC ACID MICROARRAYS

Nucleic acid microarrays (also called DNA arrays, DNA chips, or oligonucleotide arrays) were introduced in the mid-1990s.[81] They function by nucleic acid hybridization, conceptually identical to low- and medium-density arrays discussed in the previous chapter (see Chapter 64) on Nucleic Acid Techniques. However, compared to medium-density arrays, spot sizes in microarrays are decreased to approximately 100 μm in diameter, such that one array contains thousands to millions of spots. This dimensional change requires (1) specialized detection equipment, (2) software, and (3) informatics to analyze the data. Because of their high density and information content, microarrays have attracted intense interest among researchers who wish to monitor the whole genome for (1) SNVs, (2) gene expression, or (3) copy number variation.

Because SNVs represent the most common genetic difference among individuals, much effort has focused on correlating SNV genotypes to phenotype and disease association. SNV microarrays have been used in many genome-wide association studies (GWAS). Microarrays that analyze human SNVs

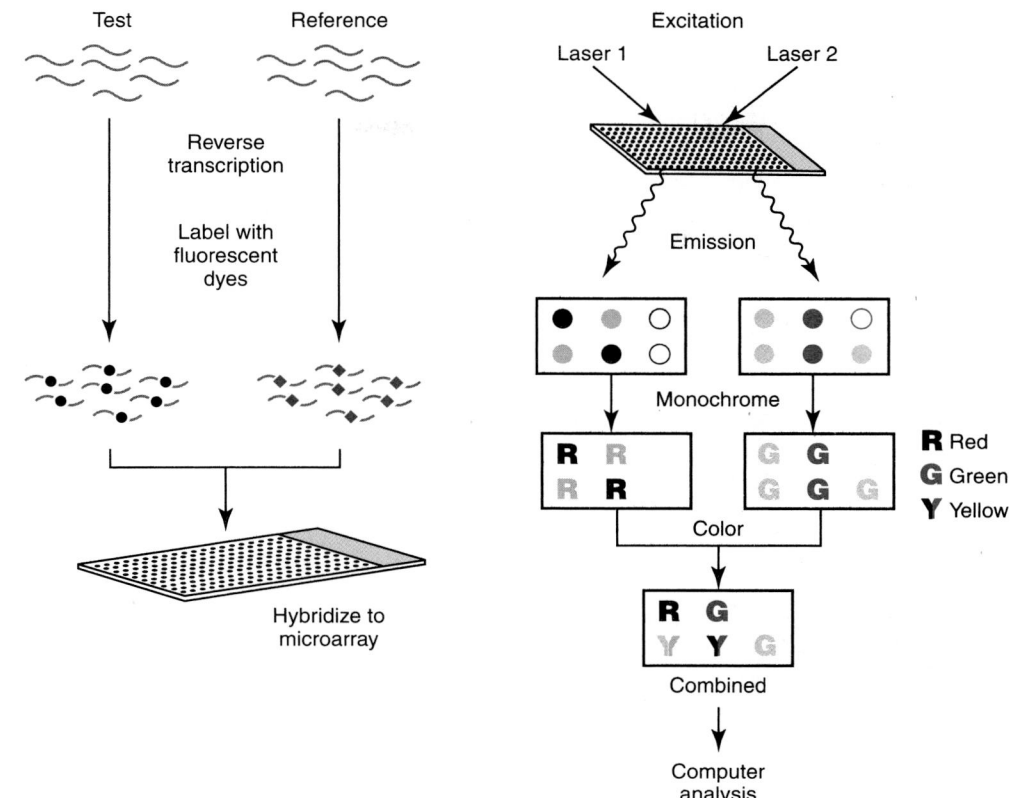

FIGURE 65.5 A two-color microarray experiment. An array of DNA oligonucleotides with sequences of messenger RNA are affixed to a glass slide. Messenger RNAs in the test and reference specimen are converted into differentially labeled cDNA by reverse transcription and incorporation of two different fluorescent dyes. The two samples are hybridized together onto the array. The array is washed, and the image is captured twice, each time with a laser of a wavelength that excites one of the dyes but not the other. The monochromatic images are then converted to two colors (green for the test sample [G], and red for the reference [R]), and the images are combined. If the abundance of cDNA is the same in each of the two samples, then the composite spot is yellow (Y). If one is in greater abundance, then that color will be preserved. Up-regulation and down-regulation of gene expression are then analyzed by software.

("SNV chips") provide the technology to genotype most frequent human SNVs in one experiment. Nearby SNV alleles tend to cluster together as haplotypes, so disease association by haplotype simplifies the analysis. Although some valuable markers have been found by these GWAS,[82] the yield of useful disease markers obtained by these methods has been disappointing,[83] and many difficulties remain, such as identifying adequate control populations.[84] SNV arrays can also be used to genotype SNVs of known association with disease and to assess copy number variation. Cytogenomic arrays, including SNV and comparative genomic hybridization (CGH) arrays, can analyze the entire genome, providing chromosome maps of copy number changes (large insertions and deletions) across each chromosome.

Gene expression microarrays quantify the relative amounts of different messenger RNAs in test and reference samples. An example of a two-color microarray for gene expression is shown in Fig. 65.5. Probes that hybridize to mRNA are usually directly synthesized on microarrays. Modern gene expression arrays have been used to measure the mRNA transcribed from all human genes in one experiment. They have been applied to almost every conceivable human circumstance, including (1) neoplastic, (2) inflammatory, and (3) psychiatric conditions. It is expected that application of this technology will lead to better (1) diagnosis, (2) molecular staging, (3) prognosis, and (4) therapy through understanding of disease pathogenesis. In oncology, gene expression microarrays have led to new diagnostic and prognostic markers in breast cancer,[85] bladder cancer,[86] leukemia,[87] and sarcoma,[88] among others. Molecular expression signatures often divide cancer into subtypes that respond differently to therapy. For example, Fig. 65.6 shows a "heat map" of 165 patients with bladder cancer and the relative expression of 768 genes for each patient. Four major subtypes are apparent by clustering the expression signatures, and one of the subtypes was more responsive to anti-PD-L1 immunotherapy.[89] Even with much progress, expression arrays are used directly in only a few clinical diagnostic and prognostic tests. Most arrays are used in marker discovery projects for selection of a smaller panel of expression targets that are then analyzed by other quantitative methods, such as real-time PCR, that provide greater precision and dynamic range.

Another important clinical application of microarrays is the genome-wide analysis of deletions and duplications,

Tissue samples (*n* = 165)

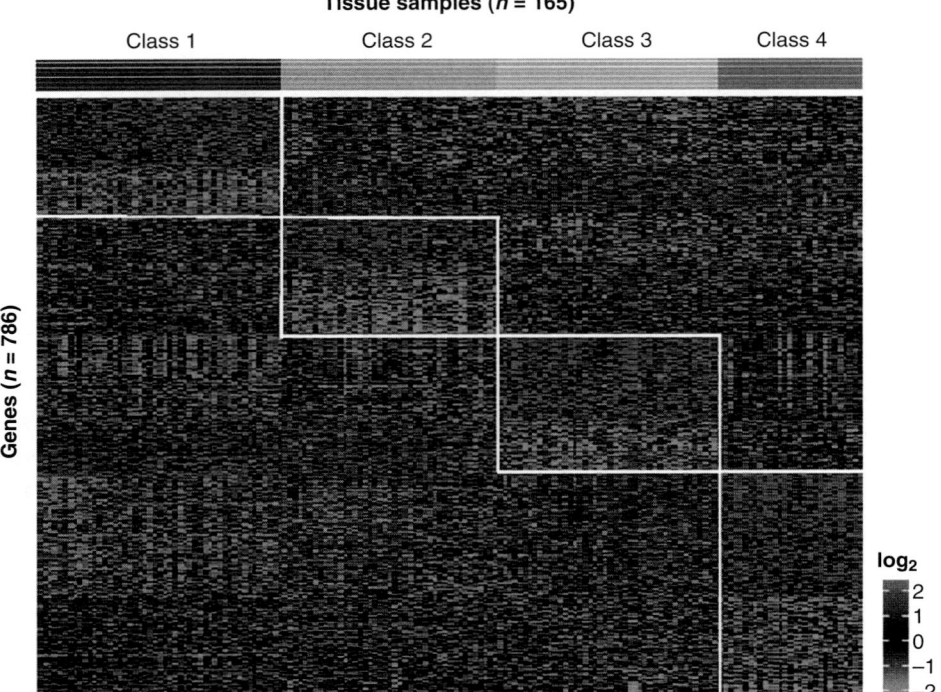

FIGURE 65.6 Heat map showing unsupervised hierarchal clustering of gene expression from 786 genes and 165 bladder cancer tissues. The molecular signature identifies four subgroups. Typically, underexpression is shown in red and overexpression is shown in green, with different intensity levels differing by log₂. (Modified with permission from Song BN, Kim SK, Mun JY, et al. Identification of an immunotherapy-responsive molecular subtype of bladder cancer. *EBioMedicine* 2019;50:238–45.)

referred to as copy number variants (CNVs). CNV analysis using microarrays is replacing traditional cytogenetic chromosome analysis (karyotyping) and fluorescence in situ hybridization (FISH) analysis for detection of genome-wide copy number alterations. Similar to gene expression arrays, many of the CNV arrays use two-color comparative hybridization to determine the gene dosage in a specimen compared with a normal reference genome (array comparative genomic hybridization [aCGH]). Arrays for CGH use oligonucleotide probes for very high resolution and data density. An example of CNV analysis using aCGH is shown in Fig. 65.7. SNV arrays also are used to detect copy number changes by loss of heterozygosity (this method is sometimes referred to as *virtual karyotyping*). Unlike aCGH, SNV arrays have the advantage of analyzing the specimen without the need to mix in a reference genome. SNV arrays are also able to detect copy number neutral changes caused by inversions or uniparental disomy that are not detected by aCGH methods. When a clinically significant copy number change is found, it can be verified by an orthogonal method such as FISH or high-resolution melting.[90]

Massively Parallel Sequencing[91–93]

The need to understand the full extent of genome-wide human variation led to the human genome project. Sequencing the human genome began with the orderly "conventional" sequencing of large (150-kb) fragments of DNA that were divided among members of the consortium and methodically sequenced. However, random "shotgun" sequencing proved to be faster and was an important tool for completing

the sequence of the first human genome. Massively parallel sequencing is the current technology used for genome sequencing. Fig. 65.8 contrasts these different sequencing approaches.

Massively parallel sequencing evolved out of earlier sequencing methods. When genomic DNA is sequenced by massively parallel sequencing, the basic steps include random DNA shearing (fragmentation), sequencing in parallel reactions, and data assembly (*left panel* of Fig. 65.8). The randomly sheared fragments are end-modified with oligonucleotides that aid in the identification, immobilization, and sequencing of the fragments; this step is referred to as library creation. In the case of whole-genome sequencing, this "library" of modified fragments is then sequenced. However, if only a subset of genes is of interest or if only the coding nucleotides are of interest (exome), the specific targets can be hybridized and "captured" after the library step. Targeted capture of regions of interest is a key step in exome sequencing. More than 1 million sequencing reactions occur in parallel, generating more than 100 bases of data per reaction. After sequencing, the short reads of DNA are assembled based on a reference genome (e.g., GRCh38).

In comparison, the conventional sequencing of genomes was the technology used for the initiation of the Human Genome Project (*middle panel* of Fig. 65.8). This method started with the genome cloned into large molecules such as Yeast Artificial Chromosomes (YACs) and later bacterial artificial chromosomes (BACs). These larger molecules, which carried genomic inserts greater than 150 kb in size, were then divided among the members of the genome sequencing consortium

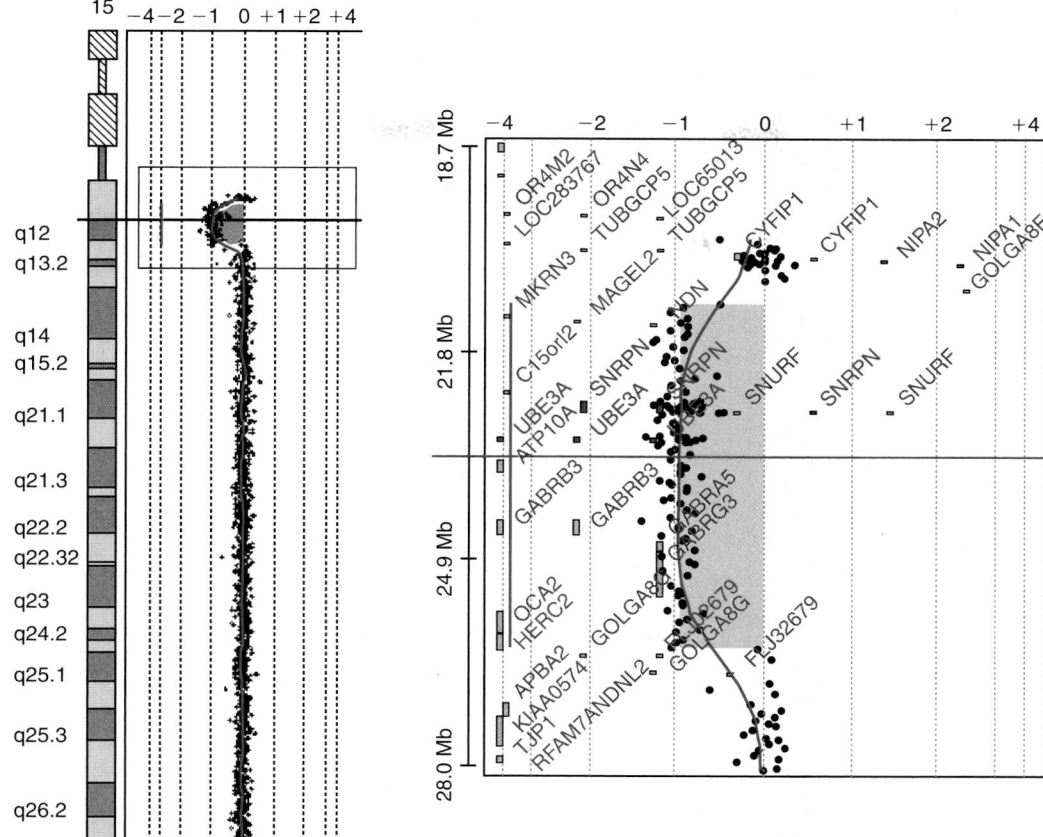

FIGURE 65.7 Copy number variation identified with a comparative genomic hybridization array made from oligonucleotides. DNA from a subject is fragmented, labeled with Cy5, and hybridized onto a microarray, together with Cy3-labeled reference DNA. On the array are 44,000 oligonucleotide probes, each about 60 bases long and tiled across the whole genome at an average spacing of 75 kb. Shown on the *left panel* are results of probes on chromosome 15 (all other chromosomes are analyzed in this assay but are not shown). Each *dot* represents a specific probe to which the subject's DNA hybridizes. Their positions (0, −1, +1, and so on) reflect the dosage of the subject's DNA relative to the reference DNA. A majority of the probes line up on "0," indicating no quantitative difference compared with the reference DNA. Probes in the 15q11 to 15q13 region, however, are on the "−1" line, indicating that the subject has a deletion of that region. A closer view of that region (*right panel*) shows that among the deleted genes are *UBE3A,* which causes Angelman syndrome, and *SNRPN,* which causes Prader-Willi syndrome. Because the method does not distinguish the methylation status of the deleted alleles, this result alone cannot determine which of the two disorders the subject has. (Courtesy Sarah South, PhD, ARUP Laboratories.)

and methodically sequenced in 700 base reactions. Each round of sequencing depended on the sequencing data from the prior round. The assembly of data is not as computationally intensive as massively parallel or shotgun sequencing.

Finally, shotgun sequencing was key to the speedy completion of the Human Genome Project (*right panel* of Fig. 65.8). Rather than methodically sequencing targets of interest, the method relied on random shearing of DNA and subcloning the fragments into plasmids. The plasmids were then sequenced in parallel (separate) reactions. The evolutionary roots of massively parallel sequencing technology originated in shotgun sequencing.

Compared with conventional dideoxy-termination sequencing, massively parallel sequencing generates up to 1 billion more bases of sequence data in one operation at 10,000 to 100,000 times lower cost per base. The method

continues to improve toward even higher throughput and lower costs. Much of the progress that has been made is dependent on advances in optical data processing, bioinformatics, and overall computer power. The cost and turnaround time of these methods continue to decrease, and their convenience continues to improve, leading to increased uptake in clinical laboratories. Clinical laboratory standards for massively parallel sequencing are published,[94,95] and there are practical guidelines for implementing massively parallel sequencing tests.[96] Clonal sequencing methods replicate a single DNA strand to form a clonal template in order to generate sufficient signal for detection. In contrast, single-molecule sequencing methods must be sensitive enough to detect single molecules of DNA. Characteristics of massively parallel sequencing methods are summarized in Table 65.6, from available recent reviews.[97,98]

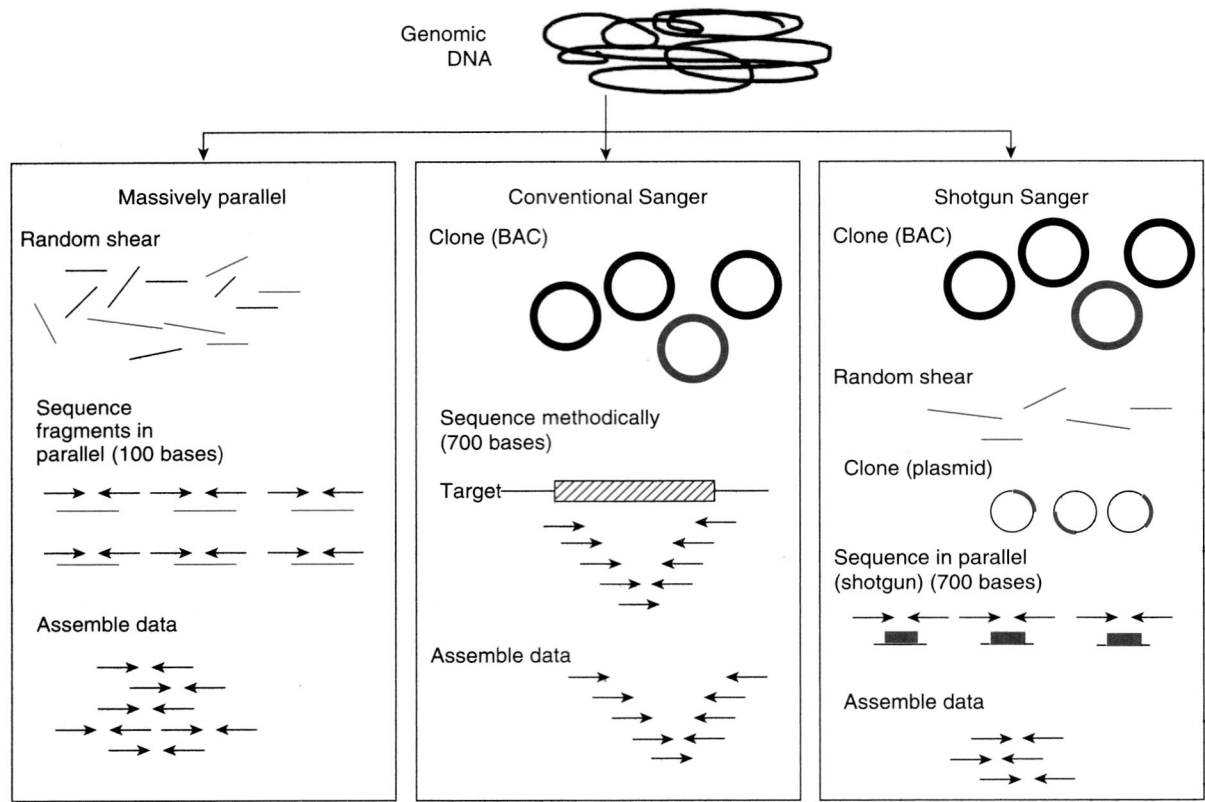

FIGURE 65.8 Genome sequencing approaches. Massively parallel sequencing *(left panel)* is the current technology used for genome sequencing, but it evolved out of earlier conventional Sanger *(middle panel)* and shotgun Sanger *(right panel)* sequencing methods. See text for details. *BAC,* Bacterial artificial chromosomes.

TABLE 65.6   Characteristics of Massively Parallel Sequencing Methods

Method	Principle	Detection	Clonal	Run Time	Output per Run	Read Length (bp)
Synthesis	Pyrophosphate Release	Chemiluminescence	Emulsion PCR	10–23 hours	40–700 Mb	400–700
Synthesis	pH Change	Electronic CMOS	Emulsion PCR	3–4 hours	1.5–10 Gb	125–400
Synthesis	Reversible Terminator	Fluorescence	Bridge Amplification	2.7–12 days	15–1000 Gb	200–600[a]
Synthesis	Reversible Terminator	Florescence	Rolling Circle replication	1–4.5 days	15–6000 Gb	100–300[a]
Single Molecule	Zero-Mode Waveguide	Fluorescence	No	2 days	5 Gb	10 kb
Single Molecule	Conductivity	Electronic	No	"Minutes to Days"	Depends	5 kb

[a]Includes both paired end reads (sequencing from both ends).

Sequencing From Clones

Clonal sequencing methods start with producing a random library of fragments that are typically 70 to 1000 bases in length, although some methods require 6- to 20-kb fragments or greater. The starting material may be genomic DNA, a hybridization capture-based subset of genomic DNA (as in exome sequencing and some gene panels for specific diseases), or PCR products that focus on limited regions of interest. Fragmentation is usually physical or enzymatic.[99] Common physical methods include sonication and acoustic shearing. Depending on the frequency and geometry of the sample and acoustic generator, fragments averaging from 100 to 20,000 bases can be produced. Hydrodynamic shearing can

also be obtained by compressed air to atomize the liquid into a fine mist (nebulization), forcing the solution through a fine-gauge needle, or through a French pressure cell. Enzymatic fragmentation can be from restriction endonucleases, nonspecific DNAses, or a transposase enzyme that simultaneously fragments and adds adapter sequences.[100] In each case, conditions can be modified to produce different fragment sizes.

Adapter sequences are typically added to each end of the random fragments. The primary role of these adapters is to provide common priming sites for each fragment to initiate massively parallel sequencing reactions. One primer set amplifies a massive array (beads or planer flow cell) of library

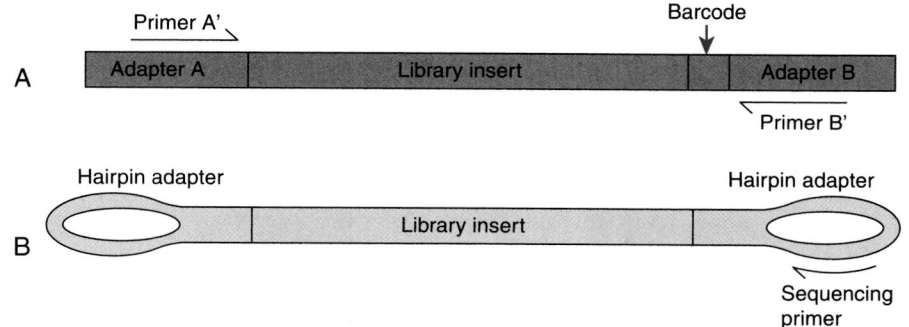

FIGURE 65.9 Diagram of different library designs used in massively parallel sequencing. (A) Two adapters that include consensus PCR priming sites are ligated onto each end of the library inserts produced by fragmentation. If multiplexing different samples is desired, a barcode is added so that each read can be assigned to a specific sample. (B) A library insert is bounded by hairpin adapters that allow primer binding to the single-stranded loops on each end for rolling circle amplification.

inserts. Adapters also facilitate initial capture of DNA fragments onto solid surfaces and spatially restrict clonal amplification products generated from the fragments onto beads or spots on an array surface. The fragment ends typically need to be "polished" by filling in any missing bases and optionally adding a single extra A to the 3'-ends to facilitate ligation to the adapters. If multiplexing of different DNA samples is desired, a sequence "barcode" is often added as well to identify which DNA sample the clone arose from. A typical library insert with adapters and a barcode is shown in Fig. 65.9A. The libraries are then partitioned according to size to select a band optimal for the downstream sequencing technology.

Clonal amplification for massively parallel sequencing is usually performed on single DNA molecules within microreactors. The partitions may be minute aqueous droplets in a water-in-oil emulsion *(emulsion PCR),*[101] PCR colonies *(polonies)* on a thin film of acrylamide gel,[102] clusters on the surface of a planar flow cell generated by bridge amplification,[103] or beads with clonally amplified template attached to their surface.[104–106] When amplification is observed in these massively parallel reactions, chances are that clonal amplification has occurred from a single template molecule. Clonal amplification is usually performed by either emulsion PCR or bridge amplification.

Emulsion Polymerase Chain Reaction

In emulsion PCR, one strand of a library element is captured on one bead and is clonally amplified inside a water-in-oil droplet, generating a bead covered with single-stranded PCR products (Fig. 65.10). The emulsion is formed by mixing beads (each covered with one primer), aqueous PCR components (including the other primer, polymerase, and dNTPs), and a mixture of oils under agitation to ideally form droplets that each contain only one bead and one library insert. The two primers are complementary to the adapters; one coats the bead surface, and one is free in solution. During emulsion PCR, all of the beads are amplified together in aqueous microdroplets dispersed in oil. The emulsion is amplified in a standard PCR thermal cycler. After PCR and denaturation, millions of copies of identical single-stranded PCR products are on each bead with each bead carrying distinct, oriented inserts flanked by the adapters. The emulsion is then broken and, after elimination of empty beads, is ready for sequencing.

Bridge Amplification

Bridge amplification generates clusters of single-stranded PCR products tethered to the surface of a planar flow cell (Fig. 65.11).[103] In contrast to the clonal bead generation of emulsion PCR, the amplification occurs on a flat surface. The primers, complementary to the adapters, are both attached to the surface, either randomly or in a fixed pattern. The library DNA is then denatured to form single strands that hybridize to the primers on the surface. After extension of the surface-bound primers, the original template strands are washed away under denaturing conditions. What follows is called bridge amplification, which is very similar to PCR except that both primers are bound to the surface, so that single strands bound to the surface must bend over to find their opposite primer, resulting in a double-stranded bridge after extension. Instead of denaturing with heat as in PCR, the flow cell is kept at 60°C, and a chemical denaturant is introduced to dissociate the two bridge strands, except now both strands are attached to the planer surface. When the flow cell is flushed with a polymerase and dNTPs under favorable extension conditions, both can find new primers to form additional bridges. The process repeats until about thousands of copies are formed. One of the bound primers can be designed to include a cleavable site (either chemical or enzymatic) so that one strand can be removed after denaturation. After capping the 3'-end of the single strands with ddNTPs (to prevent any undesired extension with the closely packed templates), the surface is ready for sequencing.

Sequencing by Synthesis

Sequencing by synthesis can be detected by (1) pyrophosphate release, (2) a pH decrease, or (3) the fluorescence of reversible terminators. The clonal amplification methods allow parallel observation of thousands to millions of strand extensions, greatly increasing the signal strength. However, the extensions must be controlled at each step because continuous strand extension would not remain synchronous between strands. This is achieved by immobilizing the clones into arrays so that reagents can be applied sequentially (no pun intended).

Pyrosequencing[104]

Pyrosequencing was used in the first massively parallel sequencing platform but has not remained competitive because

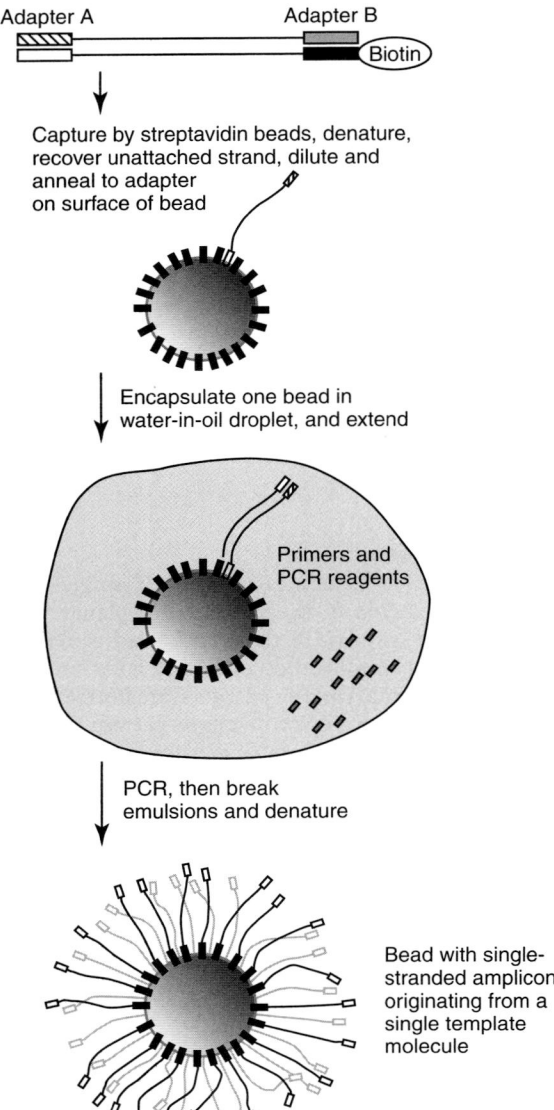

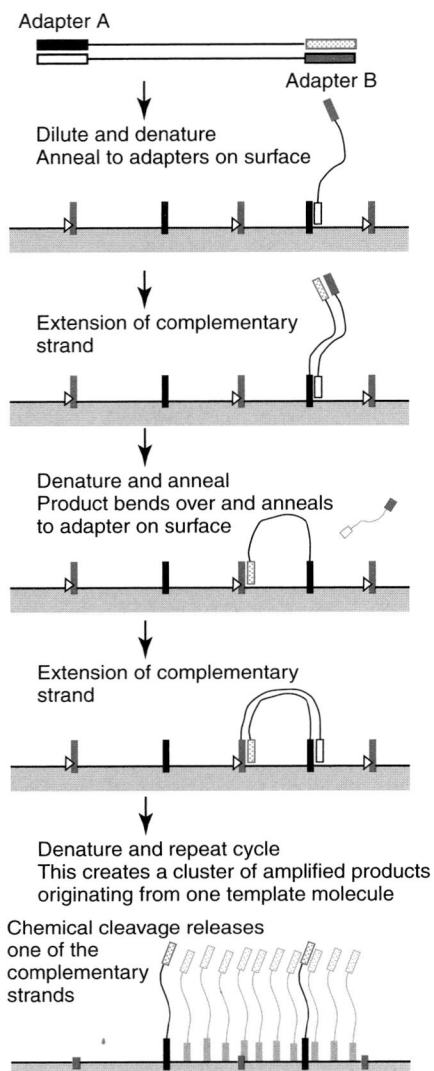

FIGURE 65.10 Emulsion polymerase chain reaction *(PCR)*. Two adapters *(adapters A* and *B)* are randomly ligated to DNA fragments. Adapter B has a biotin on its 5′ end. Fragments with adapter B on one or both ends are captured by streptavidin beads, while fragments with only adapter A are washed away (not shown). Then the fragments are denatured, and the free strand with adapter A and adapter B at each end is collected (fragments with adapter B on both ends will not be released from the streptavidin bead). One molecule of the single-stranded template is then captured on a bead coated with adapter and is encapsulated inside a water-in-oil droplet that contains PCR reagents and primers. After PCR, the emulsion is broken and the DNA is denatured. This generates a bead with a large number of clonal single strands tethered to it. The bead is then deposited into one of many wells on a fiberoptic slide, or onto a glass slide for sequence analysis (not shown).

FIGURE 65.11 Bridge amplification. Two adapters *(adapters A* and *B)* are ligated to a DNA template. After they are diluted and denatured into single strands, the template is captured onto a flow cell surface by annealing to one of the two surface-bound primers that share sequences with adapter A or B. The polymerase reagent introduced into the flow cell extends the primer and generates the complementary strand of the template. The denaturant (usually sodium hydroxide) is introduced to the flow cell to release the original template strand. The free end of the newly synthesized strand anneals to a nearby primer by bending over, and a second round of reagent addition catalyzes the synthesis of another complementary strand. By repeating many of these cycles, a clonal cluster that consists of 1000 to 30,000 copies of single-stranded template tethered to the surface is generated. This cluster is still a mixture of both complementary strands. One of the strands is selectively eliminated by treatment with periodic acid that cleaves the diol linkage present in one of the surface-bound primers *(open triangle on red primer)*. The cluster now contains only one of the template strands and is ready for sequence analysis.

of lower throughput and higher cost. Clonal beads were fit into picoliter reaction chambers formed in etched individual fibers of a fiberoptic cable. Solutions of dATPαS, dCTP, dGTP, or dTTP were passed over chambers one at a time under conditions that favor extension. If there was a base match, the nucleotide will be incorporated, and pyrophosphate will be

released. Pyrosequencing signal generation occurred by linked enzymatic reactions, leading to luciferase chemiluminescence (dATP was replaced with dATPαS to prevent interference, see Chapter 64). The light produced was captured by the individual light fibers and detected on a CCD. If more than one base occurs in a row (a homopolymer stretch), multiple bases of that nucleotide were incorporated, and the signal was proportionately higher. As the number of identical bases increased, it became harder to determine their exact number.

Semiconductor Sequencing[105]

Similar to pyrosequencing detection, clonal beads are used as a template. However, the beads are arrayed on semiconductor sensors modified to detect pH changes.[107] The chip does not detect light but a slight change in pH produced as a consequence of conversion of one of the dNTPs into pyrophosphates by the many clones on the bead. Similar to pyrosequencing, homopolymer stretches can be problematic. By leveraging semiconductor technology development, the chip has rapidly increased in performance by decreasing the size of the beads and sensor wells and increasing the size of the chip. Run times can be as short as 3 to 4 hours.

Reversible Terminators

After bridge amplification on a planar flow cell, one of four nucleotides is passed through the flow cell under conditions that favor extension. Unlike pyrosequencing and semiconductor sequencing, the nucleotides are fluorescent terminators so that only one base is incorporated, avoiding the problems with homopolymer stretches. Each nucleotide has a different fluorescent label so that each can be distinguished by color. Furthermore, the fluorescent terminators are reversible, which means that the blocked 3′-end can be regenerated by simple chemical means provided by the flow cell. Each cycle involves (1) adding polymerase and dNTPs as fluorescently labeled terminators under conditions that favor extension, (2) washing the flow cell, (3) imaging the fluorescence, (4) cleaving the fluorescent terminator, and (5) washing the flow cell. Output per run can be greater than 1000 Gb in 1 day.

Another type of reversible terminator sequencing ligates DNA fragments from a library into circular constructs which are then amplified by rolling circle replication. Each fragment is amplified into several hundreds of copies and forms a compact single-stranded structure termed a "DNA nanoball" which is bound onto a patterned flow cell. Sequencing of the DNA nanoballs is conducted with fluorescent reversible terminators as above, or nonfluorescent (cold) terminators can be used followed by base-specific antibodies that are fluorescently labeled. The base-specific antibodies may be added two at a time, simplifying the required optics.[108]

Single Molecule Sequencing

Single-molecule sequencing methods do not require template amplification. Base reads do not require syncing with other clonal strands because there are none. Sensitive optical or electronic methods are required to detect base sequence in a single molecule.[109] If long reads and high accuracy are achieved, advantages include efficient sequence assembly, analyses of repetitive sequences, de novo sequencing, mapping of chromosomal rearrangements, and fusions. In contrast, massively parallel sequencing methods usually generate short sequence reads (100 to 700 bases long) that have to be aligned and analyzed to derive a consensus, then stitched together, and compared with reference genome sequences.

Accurate assembly of sequence data relies on sufficient coverage and/or redundancy across the sequenced region.[110]

Real-Time Single Molecule Sequencing With Fluorescent Nucleotides[109]

Library preparation is unique for this method because fragmentation is tuned to provide about 10-kb or greater length inserts, and the adapters are designed as hairpins. The result is a double-stranded insert bounded by identical single-stranded loops on each end (see Fig. 65.9 B). Sequencing primers are annealed to the loop region and bound to a single polymerase molecule at the bottom of a zero-mode waveguide to form an active polymerase complex. The zero-mode waveguide allows single molecule detection of transient fluorescent labels that are covalently attached to the terminal phosphate of each dNTP. The four dNTPs are added to the wells with different labels that can be distinguished optically. When a fluorescent dNTP pairs with its complement near to the polymerase active site, it is in a perfect position for fluorescence detection. After being incorporated into the growing strand, the terminal fluorescent label (attached to pyrophosphate) diffuses away from the polymerase. The fluorescent signals are acquired continuously at high speed as the primer proceeds around the loop by rolling circle amplification. The process can be stopped after one loop or continued for multiple reads for error checking. Base reads of greater than 175,000 contiguous bases have been reported.

Nanopore Sequencing[111]

Another single-molecule sequencing approach that does not require amplification and uses electronic, rather than optical, detection is nanopore sequencing. Single DNA strands are channeled through nanopores formed by immobilized proteins. Passage of individual DNA bases through the protein nanopore generates characteristic electrical signals that can reveal the identity of the base (or combination of bases) traversing the nanopore. In essence, this is similar to a nano-sized Coulter counter that quantifies base differences on a single strand of DNA rather than cell size. Kilobases can be sequenced in a single read. The method is nondestructive and can discriminate methylated DNA bases and normal bases.[112] A number of nanopores are currently under study (α-hemolysin, *Mycobacterium smegmatis* porin A [MspA], and others), and solid-state nanopores are also being intensively investigated. Shorter and narrower nanopores that interrogate single bases would be ideal, but current material limitations allow about four bases within the nanopore at the same time. Ultra-long reads (>100 kb) have enabled the assembly and phasing of the entire 4 Mb major histocompatibility complex.[113]

APPLICATIONS ENABLED BY MASSIVELY PARALLEL SEQUENCING

Although human genome sequencing is the most obvious application of massively parallel sequencing, the impact of this technology goes far beyond the human genome. Hybridization capture of genomic subsets can reduce the sequencing burden greatly. For example, exome sequencing is a popular approach to identify disease variants that reduces the need for sequencing by almost 100-fold.[114] Sequencing of mRNA ("RNA-Seq") is achieved by conversion of message transcripts to double-stranded DNA by priming with poly-T oligonucleotides and reverse transcriptase, a method that has quantitative advantages over microarrays,[115] and can easily detect fusions. Variants that are traditionally hard to detect by sequencing, including copy number variants[116] and chromosomal rearrangements,[117] are becoming easier to identify with advances in bioinformatics. In "ChIP-seq," the readout of chromatin immunoprecipitation experiments that identify binding sites of transcription factors is greatly simplified.[118] The genomic landscape of accessible chromatin can be determined by "ATAC-seq," a method for in vitro transposition of sequencing adaptors into native chromatin.[119] Many of these methods can be performed on single cells, for example, "CITE-seq" (cellular indexing of transcriptomes and epitopes) combines RNA-Seq with protein identification by sequence-tagged antibodies that can simultaneously be analyzed on thousands of cells.[120] Although it might seem like genomic sequencing only needs to be performed once on any particular individual, this is not true in cancer. Single cell sequencing of neoplastic populations may identify resistant clones that may be therapeutically important.[121,122] The enormous complexity of life is being met with an equally enormous capacity for analysis.

INFORMATICS

The modern era of human genome sequencing is underpinned by massively parallel sequencing. As suggested by the name, both the method and the amount of data are massive. Fortunately, as the scale of sequencing has increased, tools have been developed to manage and analyze the information. Many recent reviews and evaluations of existing software tools are available.[123]

Both publicly available tools and commercial software are assembled into what is referred to as a pipeline. In the pipeline, the information is processed in a serial manner (Fig. 65.12). First, raw data (fluorescence, time, position) is analyzed by instrument-specific methods to generate serial base calls, each with an estimated uncertainty or quality of each base call. This information is saved in a text file, typically a FASTQ file. An example short sequencing read in FASTQ format is shown in Fig. 65.13. One FASTQ file typically contains data from millions of short sequencing reads, so the files are very big and not usually readable by standard text editors. Depending on the coverage required, there may be tens to thousands of sequencing reads at a single nucleotide position.

Different sequencing reads start and stop at different genomic positions, so an alignment program is used to register each sequencing read to the reference genome. An example alignment is shown in Fig. 65.14. After alignment, each base position is "called" or assigned depending on its quality from each read, the percentage of reads that are in agreement, and the total number of reads. At any nucleotide position, there may be more than one base, which is expected in the case of heterozygous variants (1:1 ratio), mitochondrial variants (variable ratios), or somatic variants in cancer (variant bases may be rare). After the bases are called at each nucleotide position, a variant call file (VCF) is generated and a quality or Q-score assigned (Box 65.3). The VCF only includes the nucleotide positions that differ from the reference genome and are tabulated by the genomic coordinate of the variant. A simplified VCF file with three entries is shown in Fig. 65.15.

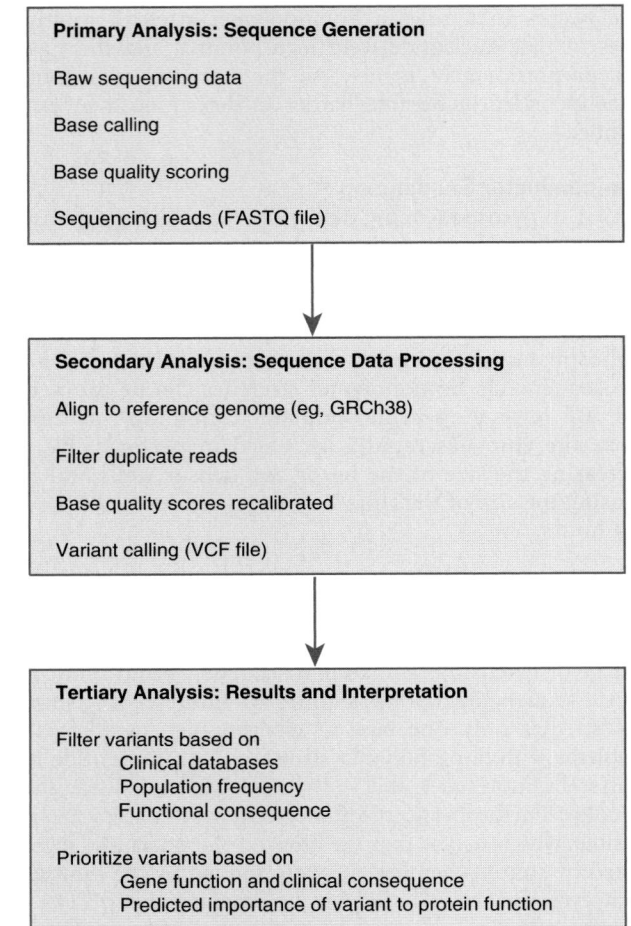

FIGURE 65.12 Bioinformatics pipeline. The analysis of data from massively parallel sequencing occurs in three phases. *Primary analysis:* The raw output (e.g., optical or electronic signals) from the sequencing instrument is transformed into data that describe the individual bases of DNA and the quality and confidence of the base call at each position. These reads of DNA are assembled into a FASTQ data file. *Secondary analysis:* The data file is then assembled onto a reference sequence. For human DNA sequencing, this is typically a reference genome such as GRCh38. If the fragments of DNA were prepared by randomly sheared fragments, then the sampling of a wide diversity of fragments improves quality and is ensured by sequencing that is from exact duplicates. When the fragments are assembled against the reference genome, the quality of each of the base calls at specific nucleotide positions can be determined. The variant at each position is then determined and reported in a single variant call file (VCF). *Tertiary analysis:* The variants are then queried against multiple databases that have information on population frequency and clinical significance. Based on these queries, the variants can be prioritized in terms of importance to the given scientific question or clinical scenario. (Modified with permission from Oliver GR, Hart SN, Klee EW. Bioinformatics for clinical next generation sequencing. *Clin Chem* 2015;61:124–35.)

Each VCF entry is then queried against existing knowledge, a process that is often both manual and automated. Because of the large number of variants that require analysis at this stage, some sort of automated database filtering is almost always performed. Consideration of population databases is a useful initial filter. A database minor allele frequency

```
@SEQ_ID
ACGGATATACTGCGACGTAGCTAGAGTGCTATCGGCATGCAT
+
!-3I [FFMNO|>/%%%A) ) . /834ff {} ** CCCC&& ==_) tB
```

FIGURE 65.13 The format of a FASTQ text file sequence entry. Each sequence entry uses four lines. The first line begins with "@" and a sequence identifier, followed by an optional description. The second line is the base sequence written 5' to 3', in this example, a short 42-bp sequence. The thrid line begins with "+" and optionally repeats the identifier and description of the first line. The fourth line contains the same number of characters as the sequence, identifying the sequence quality for each base in the second line. Quality characters vary from ASCII "!" (lowest quality) to ASCII "~" (highest quality).

greater than 5% is considered stand-alone evidence that a variant is benign. In contrast, identification of a nonsense, frameshift, or severe splice site variant is very strong, but not absolute, evidence of a pathogenic variant. Computational and predictive data for missense variants can also be automated. These predictive tools are not always accurate, but they may be helpful to prioritize the examination of a long queue of variants from a sequencing study. Finally, some manual curation is usually necessary and may include functional and segregation data from the literature, and parental testing to establish de novo variants or cis/trans relationships. Databases used for filtering are typically population frequency-based, evidence-based, or prediction-based.

In 2015, standards and guidelines for the interpretation of sequence variants were recommended by the American College of Medical Genetics and Genomics and the Association for Molecular Pathology.[127] Specific standard terminology for variant pathogenicity into five categories was recommended for Mendelian disorders: pathogenic, likely pathogenic, uncertain significance, likely benign, and benign. Criteria for classifying pathogenic (P) variants include very strong (PVS), strong (PS), and supporting (PP) criteria with combinatorial rules to establish pathogenic and likely pathogenic variants. Similarly, criteria for classifying benign (B) variants include stand-alone (BA), strong (BS), and supporting (BP) criteria with combinatorial rules to establish benign and likely benign variants. When the criteria and rules are insufficient to

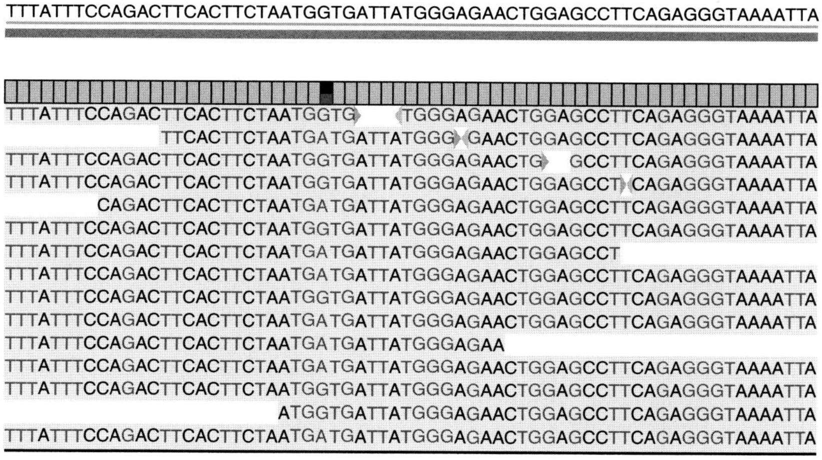

FIGURE 65.14 Sequence alignment of short reads from massively parallel sequencing. Multiple sequence reads are aligned to each other and the reference sequence *(top)*. The read starts and stops are variable, reflecting random library inserts. Most base positions are identical across reads, although at one position, two bases are present at a 50:50 ratio, suggesting a heterozygous base which differs from the reference sequence. Alamut Visual version 2.12 (SOPHiA GENETICS, Lausanne, Switzerland).

BOX 65.3 Phred Quality Score (Q-Score)[124–126]

In the 1990s, Phil Green at the University of Washington developed software to automatically read the fluorescent sequence chromatograms generated from Sanger sequencing. The original software, Phred (**Ph**il's **r**ead **ed**itor), used the following basic parameters:

1. Find the predicted location of peaks.
2. Find the observed location of peaks.
3. Match predicted and observed peaks.
4. Find missing peaks.

A component of Phred was an estimator of the error probability of a base call. A quality value (Q-score) was generated from the formula:

$q = -10 \times \log_{10}(p)$

q = quality value

p = estimated error for a base call

Some representative examples of quality value (*q*) scores:

Q-score of 30 (Q30): The probability (*p*) is 1/1000 of being incorrect.

Q-score of 20 (Q20): The probability (*p*) is 1/100 of being incorrect.

Q-score of 10 (Q10): The probability (*p*) is 1/10 of being incorrect. Although massively parallel sequencing does not generate a Sanger sequencing type chromatogram, the convention of a Phred Q-score is still used to calculate the quality (and accuracy) of a sequenced base. Under ideal conditions, current massively parallel sequencing can achieve more than 90% of bases at Q30.

```
##fileformatVCFv4.3
##fileDate=20200407
##reference=file:///seq/references/1000Genomes Pilot–NCBI36. fasta
.
.
.
```

#CHROM	POS	ID	REF	ALT	QUAL	FILTER	INFO
7	29611028	rs823375	T	C	17	q20	NS=39
1	115287199	.	T	C	26	PASS	NS=7
9	123994361	rs1973	C	A	38	PASS	NS=21

FIGURE 65.15 An example variant call format *(VCF)* text file with three entries. VCF files catalog sequence variants that are different from a reference sequence. Meta-information is listed first with each line proceeded by "##." Recommended keywords include fileformat, fileDate, and reference with additional common keywords of INFO, FILTER, and FORMAT (not shown). Next, a header line provides column headings for a table of variants, one to each subsequent line. For each variant the chromosome number (CHROM), genomic position (POS), dbSNP rs# (ID, if available), reference allele (REF), alternate allele (ALT), quality score (QUAL), any filters passed (FILTER), and optional additional information (INFO) are provided (e.g., NS is the number of reads with data).

establish any of these four categories, the variant is classified as that of uncertain significance. The intent for the likely pathogenic and likely benign categories is at least of 90 probability of being pathogenic or benign, respectively. These guidelines have been adopted internationally, adapted to copy number variants,[128,129] and refined for compatibility with Bayesian statistical reasoning.[130] Specific classification criteria and combinatorial rules are described in the next chapter on Clinical Genome Sequencing.

In 2017, standards and guidelines for the interpretation and reporting of sequence variants in cancer were jointly recommended by the Association for Molecular Pathology, the American Society of Clinical Oncology, and the College of American Pathologists.[131] Somatic sequence variants were categorized into tiers based on their clinical significance: variants with strong clinical significance, variants with potential clinical significance, variants of unknown clinical significance, and variants deemed benign or likely benign. Evidence for clinical significance is collected along 10 evidential lines, including FDA approval, professional guidelines, investigational studies, mutation type, variant frequency, presence in databases, predictive software, pathway involvement, and publications. The process has been semi-automated in software to standardize the interpretation.[132]

Massively parallel methods require informatics to process the enormous amount of data generated. Large laboratories often assign the different stages of the analysis pipeline to different specialists, including sequence analysts to extract the best sequence information, variant scientists to interpret the pathogenicity of variants, genetic counselors to draft reports and follow-up with clients, and medical directors to coordinate and take medical responsibility for the results.

SELECTED REFERENCES

6. Venter JC, Adams MD, Myers EW, et al. The sequence of the human genome. Science 2001;291:1304–51.
7. Lander ES, Linton LM, Birren B, et al. Initial sequencing and analysis of the human genome. Nature 2001;409:860–921.
8. International HGSC. Finishing the euchromatic sequence of the human genome. Nature 2004;431:931–45.
9. Finishing the euchromatic sequence of the human genome. Nature 2004;431:931–45.
17. Amaral PP, Dinger ME, Mercer TR, Mattick JS. The eukaryotic genome as an RNA machine. Science 2008;319:1787–9.
27. Carninci P, Kasukawa T, Katayama S, et al. The transcriptional landscape of the mammalian genome. Science 2005;309:1559–63.
31. Cech TR, Steitz JA. The noncoding RNA revolution-trashing old rules to forge new ones. Cell 2014;157:77–94.
38. Genomes Project C, Auton A, Brooks LD, et al. A global reference for human genetic variation. Nature 2015;526:68–74.
40. Redon R, Ishikawa S, Fitch KR, et al. Global variation in copy number in the human genome. Nature 2006;444:444–54.
49. Willems T, Gymrek M, Highnam G, Mittelman D, Erlich Y. The landscape of human STR variation. Genome Res 2014;24:1894–904.
56. Torene RI, Galens K, Liu S, et al. Mobile element insertion detection in 89,874 clinical exomes. Genet Med 2020;22(5):974–8.
62. A user's guide to the encyclopedia of DNA elements (ENCODE). PLoS Biol 2011;9:e1001046.
78. Landrum MJ, Lee JM, Riley GR, et al. ClinVar: public archive of relationships among sequence variation and human phenotype. Nucleic Acids Res 2014;42:D980–5.
83. Patron J, Serra-Cayuela A, Han B, Li C, Wishart DS. Assessing the performance of genome-wide association studies for predicting disease risk. PLoS One 2019;14:e0220215.
94. Rehm HL, Bale SJ, Bayrak-Toydemir P, et al. ACMG clinical laboratory standards for next-generation sequencing. Genet Med 2013;15:733–47.
97. Gao G, Smith D. Clinical massively parallel sequencing. Clin Chem 2020;66:77–88.
103. Bentley DR, Balasubramanian S, Swerdlow HP, et al. Accurate whole human genome sequencing using reversible terminator chemistry. Nature 2008;456:53–9.
105. Merriman B, Ion Torrent R, Team D, Rothberg JM. Progress in ion torrent semiconductor chip based sequencing. Electrophoresis 2012;33:3397–417.
106. Shendure J, Porreca GJ, Reppas NB, et al. Accurate multiplex polony sequencing of an evolved bacterial genome. Science 2005;309:1728–32.
120. Stoeckius M, Hafemeister C, Stephenson W, et al. Simultaneous epitope and transcriptome measurement in single cells. Nat Methods 2017;14:865–8.

Clinical Genome Sequencing*

Leslie Burnett and Elaine Lyon

ABSTRACT

Background
Soon after whole genome sequencing was developed, it was validated for use in a clinical setting, now known as clinical genome sequencing or cGS. Mostly cGS is used for rare, undiagnosed diseases, where the patient's symptoms and/or family history are consistent with an inherited disease. Although costs seem high, ending a diagnostic odyssey using cGS may be cost-effective in overall health care costs. While clinical exome sequencing (cES) of all known genes is a less expensive option, genome sequencing has the potential to improve diagnostic yield with more consistent coverage of the exome, as well as including nonexome regions containing variations that contribute to disease.

Content
This chapter focuses on the unique aspects of cGS as a diagnostic test. Special considerations of standard molecular genetics laboratory processes that apply to cGS will be presented. Current challenges, limitations and opportunities for future directions will be discussed.

*The full version of this chapter is available electronically on ExpertConsult.com.

67

Molecular Microbiology*

Heba H. Mostafa, Stefan Zimmerman, and Melissa B. Miller[a]

ABSTRACT

Background

Nucleic acid (NA) amplification techniques are now routinely used to diagnose and manage patients with infectious diseases. The growth in the number of US Food and Drug Administration–approved/cleared and European CE-IVD tests has facilitated the use of molecular technology in clinical laboratories. Technological advances in NA amplification techniques, automation, NA sequencing, and multiplex analysis have reinvigorated the field and created new opportunities for growth. Simple, sample-in, answer-out molecular test systems are now widely available that can be deployed in a variety of laboratory and clinical settings, including at the point of care. Molecular microbiology remains the leading area in molecular pathology in terms of both the numbers of tests performed and clinical relevance. NA-based tests have reduced the dependency of the clinical microbiology laboratory on more traditional antigen detection and culture methods and created new opportunities for the laboratory to impact patient care.

Context

This chapter reviews the molecular technology currently available in clinical laboratories to diagnose infectious diseases and emerging technology that may impact the field. The application of these technologies to diagnose health care–associated infections, syndromic infectious diseases, and infectious diseases at the point of care is reviewed while highlighting the unique challenges and opportunities that these tests present for clinical laboratories.

*The full version of this chapter is available electronically on ExpertConsult.com.

[a]The authors wish to acknowledge the contributions of Frederick S. Nolte who authored this chapter in the previous edition.

Genetics

Cindy L. Vnencak-Jones and D. Hunter Best

ABSTRACT

Background

The invention of the polymerase chain reaction (PCR) over 30 years ago along with the chemistry of fluorescently labeled molecules; high-density DNA single nucleotide polymorphism arrays; massively parallel sequencing (MPS) technology for exomes, genomes, and transcriptomes; chromosomal microarrays; the availability of public databases; and advances in bioinformatics have revolutionized the field of human genetics. The collective use of these technologies for nucleic acid analysis has facilitated disease discovery, enabled the identification of pathogenic variants for rapid prenatal and newborn diagnoses, and has sparked increased awareness and interest from the general population for genomic testing.

The age of personalized/precision medicine is upon us with exciting breakthroughs in all areas of medicine and with it comes unique discoveries yet new challenges.

Content

This chapter discusses recent advances in the field using some common inherited autosomal recessive, autosomal dominant, and X-linked diseases as examples. In addition, some common mitochondrial, imprinting, and complex disorders and inherited cancers are reviewed. For each disease, information regarding the clinical phenotype, gene, protein function, clinical testing techniques, and treatment are discussed with associated relevant ethical and genetic counseling issues.

DISEASES WITH MENDELIAN INHERITANCE

Autosomal Recessive Disorders

An individual with an autosomal recessive disease has inherited two abnormal alleles at a given locus by receiving one variant allele from each carrier parent; the disease-causing gene is on one of the autosomes (1 to 22) and not on a sex chromosome (X or Y). Typically, the carrier parent with one abnormal allele has no clinical features of the disease yet possesses a 50% risk of transmitting the variant allele to his or her offspring. Matings in which both partners are carriers of an abnormal allele have a 25% chance of having a child with both normal alleles, a 50% chance of having a child that has received only one abnormal allele, and a 25% chance of having an affected child with two variant alleles. The affected patient may be homozygous for a specific variant by inheriting the same variant from each parent or may be a compound heterozygote having inherited a different variant from each parent. The specific variants present influence the clinical severity of the disease and account for variability in the expression of the disease among different patients, referred to as genotype–phenotype correlation. Modifier genes and environmental factors also play a role in determining the patient's phenotype. Among pedigrees illustrating autosomal recessive disorders, males and females are equally affected, and for rare diseases, consanguinity is likely to be observed. Table 68.1 provides a list of some of the inherited autosomal recessive disorders commonly tested in clinical molecular diagnostic laboratories.

Cystic Fibrosis

Cystic fibrosis (CF) (Online Mendelian Inheritance in Man [OMIM] #219700) is one of the most common autosomal recessive diseases in people of Northern European ancestry with an estimated incidence in the United States of about 1 in 2500 to 3500 and a carrier frequency of about 1 in 25 to 30. Within other ethnic populations, the frequency of the disease varies with an estimated incidence of about 1 in 3500 Ashkenazi Jews, 1 in 8500 Hispanics, 1 in 17,000 African Americans, and 1 in 31,000 Asian Americans. CF is a multisystem disorder characterized by progressive pulmonary disease, pancreatic insufficiency, elevated sweat electrolytes, male infertility, and a predisposition to sinonasal disease.[1] The phenotypic expression of the disease is heterogeneous, ranging from meconium ileus and severe respiratory disease in infants to mild pulmonary symptoms and no evidence of gastrointestinal problems in adulthood. Atypical CF patients with a nonclassical presentation may have involvement of only one organ, as in congenital bilateral absence of the vas deferens (CBAVD), pancreatitis, rhinosinusitis, or nasal polyps. Variability in expression is explained by both allelic heterogeneity at the CF gene locus and genetic variation in modifier genes. Loss or decreased amounts of the disease-associated protein cause mucous accumulation and airway obstruction; recurrent infection with pathogens, such as *Pseudomonas aeruginosa* and *Staphylococcus aureus*; and excessive inflammation with progressive lung damage and ultimately respiratory failure.[2–4]

Originally considered a fatal childhood disease, according to the US Cystic Fibrosis Foundation, although most patients

TABLE 68.1 Examples of Autosomal Recessive Disorders

Disease	Gene	Location	OMIM Entry #	Incidence
α_1-Antitrypsin	SERPINA1	14q32.13	613490	1 in 5000–7000
Canavan disease	ASPA	17p13.2	271900	1 in 6400–13,400 Ashkenazi Jews (less common in other populations)
Friedreich ataxia	FXN	9q21.11	229300	1 in 25,000–50,000
Gaucher disease type I	GBA	1q22	230800	1 in 850 Ashkenazi Jews (less common in other populations)
Glycogen storage disease	G6PC	17q21.31	232200	1 in 100,000
Hereditary hemochromatosis	HFE	6p22.2	235200	1 in 200–350
Hurler syndrome: mucopolysaccharidosis type 1	IDUA	4p16.3	607014	1 in 100,000
Medium-chain acyl-coenzyme A dehydrogenase (MCAD) deficiency	ACADM	1p31.1	201450	1 in 4900–17,000
Niemann-Pick type C	NPC1	18q11.2	257220	1 in 100,000–150,000
Tay Sachs disease	HEXA	15q23	272800	1 in 3500 Ashkenazi Jews (less common in other populations)

OMIM, Online Mendelian Inheritance in Man.

(75%) are diagnosed by 2 years of age, more than 50% of CF patients are older than 18 years of age with the average life expectancy of 37.5 years.[5] The increase in survival age is due to organ transplantation, improved nutrition, respiratory therapies, antibiotics and new drug therapies. The disease is complex with clinical management of most patients at one of more than 130 specialized care centers in the CF Care Center Network. This approach provides widespread communication among health care providers who are experts in the care of patients with CF and enables monitoring of a large population of patients with respect to treatment outcome, health care, and disease-specific variables. The diagnosis of CF is based on multiple criteria including newborn screening (NBS) results, clinical symptoms, sweat chloride testing, and analysis of the cystic fibrosis transmembrane conductance regulator (*CFTR*) gene. In the United States, NBS for CF is conducted in all 50 states and the District of Columbia and is based on the measurement of immune reactive trypsinogen (IRT) from dried blood spots to detect elevated levels of this pancreatic enzyme. Interestingly, due to implementation of early screening, >50% of newly diagnosed patients may be asymptomatic or present with mild symptoms of disease. A positive NBS is generally followed by sweat chloride testing. By virtue of the intricacies of this test, it is recommended that these tests only be performed according to defined laboratory standards.[6] A sweat chloride concentration of 60 mmol/L or greater is considered diagnostic of CF and referral to a CF care center is indicated for early intervention and care.[7] In a small number of patients, an indeterminate or borderline value of 30 to 59 mmol/L or even a normal value of less than 30 mmol/L can be observed. A normal sweat chloride value makes CF less likely but cannot exclude the disease.

The severity and frequency of the disease led to an intensive search for the gene, which was eventually cloned in 1989.[8-10] The *CFTR* gene maps to chromosome 7q31.2 and has 27 exons encoding a transcript of approximately 6.5 kb. The CFTR has 1480 amino acids and is a member of the ATP-binding cassette (ABC) transporter superfamily of membrane transport proteins. CFTR consists of two transmembrane domains (TMDs), each containing six hydrophobic transmembrane sections and one hydrophilic intracellular nucleotide-binding domain (NBD).[9] The TMD/NBD segments are linked by a highly charged regulatory domain containing multiple sites for phosphorylation and activation. The molecule is unique among ABC proteins because it does not actively transport but rather serves as an ATP-gated chloride ion channel pore within the lipid bilayer, predominantly at the apical membrane of secretory epithelial cells. In addition to epithelial chloride conductance as an ion channel, CFTR mediates the passage of bicarbonate and other small ions, including sodium and potassium, from the intracellular compartment to the extracellular surface.[11-14] Whereas opening and closing of the channel requires ATP binding and hydrolysis (ATP-gated channel), channel activity requires phosphorylation of the cytoplasmic regulatory domain by protein kinase A. The wide clinical diversity of CF is based in part on the varying effects conferred on this protein with almost 2100 variants reported within this gene.[15]

Because CF is an autosomal recessive disorder, patients with CF must have two *CFTR* variant alleles (homozygous or compound heterozygous) to develop the disease. Some variants are "private" and unique to a family; others may be common among CF patients. More than half of all variants are missense (39%) or frameshift (16%) variants, with exon 14 containing the largest number of different disease-causing variants (8%).[16] The types of variants and frequencies of each differ significantly among populations.[17] Variants can be divided into six classes based on their effect on the protein (Table 68.2).[18] Class I variants result in no functional protein production and mostly include nonsense or frameshift variants that cause premature truncation of the protein, splice site mutations, and exon or gene deletions or rearrangements. Class II variants are the most common and are associated with defective processing of CFTR and the inability of the protein to reach the apical cell surface. Class II variants cause misfolding of the fully translated CFTR protein and result from an amino acid alteration such as a deletion or a missense variant. In the case of class I and II variants, CFTR is not present on the apical cell membrane, and as predicted, these variants are typically associated with a severe disease phenotype. Class III and IV variants are generally due to missense changes that result in full-length CFTR expression at

TABLE 68.2 American College of Obstetricians and Gynecologists/American College of Medical Genetics Recommended CFTR Variant Panel for Cystic Fibrosis Carrier Screening

		VARIANT FREQUENCY AMONG PATIENTS WITH CLINICALLY DIAGNOSED CYSTIC FIBROSIS (%)				
CFTR Variant	Variant Class	Ashkenazi Jewish	Non-Hispanic White	Hispanic White	African American	Asian American
p.Phe508del	II	31.41	72.42	54.38	44.07	38.95
p.Gly542Ter	I	7.55	2.28	5.10	1.45	0.00
p.Trp1282Ter	I	45.92	1.50	0.63	0.24	0.00
p.Gly551Asp	III	0.22	2.25	0.56	1.21	3.15
c.621+1G>T	I	0.00	1.57	0.26	1.11	0.00
p.Asn1303Lys	II	2.78	1.27	1.66	0.35	0.76
p.Arg553Ter	I	0.00	0.87	2.81	2.32	0.76
p.Ile507del	II	0.22	0.88	0.68	1.87	0.00
c.3849+10kbC>T	V	4.77	0.58	1.57	0.17	5.31
c.3120+1G>T	V	0.10	0.08	0.16	9.57	0.00
p.Arg117His	IV	0.00	0.70	0.11	0.06	0.00
c.1717-1G>T	I	0.67	0.48	0.27	0.37	0.00
c.2789+5G>A	V	0.10	0.48	0.16	0.00	0.00
p.Arg347Pro	IV	0.00	0.45	0.16	0.06	0.00
c.711+1G>T	I	0.10	0.43	0.23	0.00	0.00
p.Arg334Trp	IV	0.00	0.14	1.78	0.49	0.00
p.Arg560Thr	II	0.00	0.38	0.00	0.17	0.00
p.Arg1162Ter	I	0.00	0.23	0.58	0.66	0.00
c.3659delC	I	0.00	0.34	0.13	0.06	0.00
p.Ala455Glu	V	0.00	0.34	0.05	0.00	0.00
p.Gly85Glu	II	0.00	0.29	0.23	0.12	0.00
c.2184delA	I	0.10	0.17	0.16	0.05	0.00
c.1898+1G>A	I	0.10	0.16	0.05	0.06	0.00
Total		94.04	88.29	71.72	64.46	48.93

Modified from Watson MS, Cutting GR, Desnick RJ, et al. Cystic fibrosis population carrier screening: 2004 revision of American College of Medical Genetics mutation panel. *Genet Med* 2004;6:387–91.

the cell membrane. Class III variants are more severe, resulting in defective gating; class IV variants generally cause a milder phenotype with reduced conduction of ion flow (e.g., chloride and bicarbonate). Class V variants are associated with reduced amounts of CFTR at the cell membrane and are most often associated with abnormal splicing and decreased amounts of normal *CFTR* messenger RNA (mRNA). These variants may be associated with a severe phenotype (c.621 + 1G>T) or a mild phenotype (c.2789 + 5G>A). Lastly, class VI variants cause decreased stability of CFTR in the membrane.

The most common variant, p.Phe508del (c.1521_1523delCTT) (also known through legacy nomenclature as "deltaF508"), is a class II variant and is detected in about 70% of *CFTR* alleles in whites of Northern European descent. This CFTR protein is misfolded and not properly processed by the endoplasmic reticulum with the majority of the protein rapidly degraded.[19] Whereas common variants p.Gly542Ter and p.Trp1282Ter are class I variants and cause premature translation termination and premature truncation of the protein, variant p.Gly551Asp results in a full-length CFTR that reaches the apical membrane but improperly regulates the chloride channel.[20,21] Infertile males with only the genital form of CF—CBAVD—usually have a variant associated with a severe phenotype on one allele and a variant associated with a mild phenotype on the second allele. The most frequently reported *CFTR* genotype in this population is the 5T polymorphism in intron 8, c.1210-12T(5), which corresponds to a sequence of

five thymidines. This 5T variant is observed in about 5% of *CFTR* alleles and is less common than the 7T or 9T alleles, c.1210-12T(7) or c.1210-12T(9). The 5T variant affects mRNA splicing and can cause exon 9 to be deleted; without exon 9, the chloride channel is not functional.[22–24] An adjacent polymorphic TG dinucleotide sequence c.1210-34TG(9_13) regulates the efficiency of mRNA splicing, with the higher number of TG repeats c.1210-34TG(13) associated with decreased efficiency of splicing.[25] Thus the c.1210-12T(5) c.1210-34TG(12) or c.1210-12T(5) c.1210-34TG(13) allele is more commonly associated with an abnormal phenotype than is the c.1210-12T(5) c.1210-34TG(11) allele.

Understanding the effect of each variant on the CFTR protein is important for choosing the corrective drug therapy required for each patient.[26] Therapy for patients with class I or II variants is the most challenging because CFTR in most cases is absent or in reduced amounts. Gene therapy to deliver a functional CFTR protein is one effective way to treat these patients and is also applicable to CF patients with variants in classes other than I or II.[27] For patients with nonsense stop codon p.Gly542Ter, the drug ataluren, an orally administered small molecule that enables readthrough of the transcript, has been attempted. Unfortunately, aminoglycoside antibiotics frequently used by patients with CF can potentially inhibit this molecule, rendering it less effective in a subset of patients. For some class II and for all class III variants, the potentiator ivacaftor has been administered to increase the effectiveness of chloride transfer through the channel. This drug improves the clinical outcome of patients, especially for those with the common class III variant p.Gly551Asp and for 37 other class IV, V, and VI variants.[28] Ivacaftor has proven more effective in some class II variants, most notably the common p.Phe508del variant, in combination with a second small molecule, lumacaftor.[29] Lumacaftor, a CFTR corrector molecule, helps the misfolded p.Phe508del protein reach the cell surface. Tezacaftor (which has similar effects as lumacaftor, but with fewer drug-drug interactions) in combination with ivacaftor has also been given to patients homozygous for p.Phe508del. Most recently, a combination drug of tezacaftor, ivacaftor, and elexacaftor acts to bring p.Phe508del containing CFTR proteins to the cell surface and has been approved for patients 12 years of age or older. This drug benefits p.Phe508del CFTR proteins in addition to other abnormal CFTR proteins and may benefit up to 90% of CF patients.[28] Multiple additional drugs are in phase two clinical trials.[30] Antisense oligonucleotides have also been examined as a potential therapy for some CFTR variants.[27,31]

The CFTR genotype and clinical phenotype correlations are most closely related for pancreatic involvement rather than for pulmonary manifestations of the disease.[32] Most patients with two "severe" variants, which cause a "severe" CF phenotype, usually variants in classes I to III, have pancreatic insufficiency, but patients with one or two "mild" variants, which cause a "mild" CF phenotype, variants generally in classes IV to VI, have pancreatic sufficiency (PS) but have an increased risk of developing pancreatitis.[33] Furthermore, CF patients with PS generally have milder disease with longer overall survival, a later age of diagnosis, and lower sweat chloride levels. Although variants in CFTR confer susceptibility to pancreatitis, variants in several other genes inherited in combination with or without CFTR variants are seen in patients with chronic pancreatitis. In contrast, lung disease is more dependent on environmental factors (e.g., secondhand smoke and pathogens and genetic modifiers).[34,35]

DNA testing for the identification of CFTR variants is performed for a variety of reasons (Box 68.1). In the NBS and sweat chloride positive patient with symptoms of CF, CFTR testing identifies the DNA variants to determine the prognosis and guide therapy. In the patient with intermediate sweat chloride results (30 to 59 mmol/L) or normal (<30 mmol/L)

BOX 68.1 Referrals for CFTR Variant Analysis

Confirm diagnosis of cystic fibrosis
Determine prognosis
Screen patient with pancreatitis
Family member testing
Newborn screening
Preconception couples
Expectant couples
Prenatal testing—at-risk fetus
Prenatal testing—hyperechogenic bowel
Preimplantation genetic diagnosis
Infertile male with congenital bilateral absence of the vas deferens
Semen and oocyte donors

CFTR testing is performed to aid in the diagnosis. If two disease-causing variants are identified, the diagnosis of CF is confirmed in the absence of a sweat chloride test result of ≥ 60mmol/L. If one CFTR variant is detected and one variant of unknown significance is reported or only one CFTR variant is observed and no second disease-causing variant is identified, the diagnosis of CF can be made by demonstrating CFTR dysfunction using intestinal current measurement (ICM) or nasal potential difference (NPD).[7] If patients are NBS positive and have an intermediate sweat chloride, but no known CFTR variant or inconclusive CFTR variants they may be designated as CFTR-related metabolic syndrome or CF inconclusive. These patients should be monitored closely and may ultimately develop symptoms of CF.[36] In addition, CFTR gene screening can be performed if a diagnosis of CF is considered in a patient with a CFTR-related disorder such as chronic pancreatitis, CBAVD, or sinusitis. Importantly, regardless of the clinical scenario, when CFTR variants are identified in a proband, carrier or diagnostic testing for other at-risk family members can be performed.

CFTR testing in the symptomatic patient often begins with a core panel of the most common CF variants represented at frequencies of at least 0.1%.[37] However assays may also include additional variants to represent CFTR variants more common in other ethnic populations.[38] Massively parallel sequencing (MPS) enables a more comprehensive analysis of the gene and is used when clinical suspicion of CF exists but common CFTR screening panels are unable to identify two CFTR variants for confirmation of disease. MPS has been proposed as an alternative to CFTR screening panels for NBS.[39] In addition to CFTR gene testing for the symptomatic patient and their at-risk family members, CF carrier screening is also offered as a single gene-specific test or may be included within high-throughput large, expanded carrier screening panels that detect both common CFTR gene variants and targeted variants in other genes. CF carrier screening for preconception and expectant couples was first recommended in October 2001 by the American College of Obstetricians and Gynecologists (ACOG) in conjunction with the American College of Medical Genetics (ACMG). The carrier detection rate of the core panel is about 88% for non-Hispanic whites yet lower in other ethnic populations (see Table 68.2).[37] Although CF is more common in the white and Ashkenazi Jewish populations, the standard of care recommended by the ACOG is to make CF testing available to all preconception or expectant couples, especially because it is becoming more difficult to assign a single ethnicity to a patient to best determine their carrier risk. Counseling for CF carrier testing is complex and should include information about CF and CFTR-related disorders and the a priori likelihood of having a child with CF based on personal and family history and ethnicity.[40] Furthermore, it is important for the patient to understand the inability of the screening panel to detect all CF variants and the residual risk of being a carrier despite a negative test result (Table 68.3). This is especially important for patients in ethnic groups for which the CFTR gene variant detection level is reduced. The genetics professional should discuss the possibility of stigmatization or anxiety associated with being a carrier of a genetic disease and how knowing this information may affect her pregnancy. In addition, counseling should include that CF carriers themselves may be at an increased risk for cystic fibrosis-related

TABLE 68.3 Cystic Fibrosis Variant Carrier Risk

	Ashkenazi Jewish	Non-Hispanic White	Hispanic White	African American	Asian American
Detection rate of ACOG/ACMG 23 variant panel (%)	94	88	72	64	49
Estimated carrier risk in population	1/24	1/25	1/58	1/61	1/94
Estimated residual carrier risk after no variant detected on screening panel	1/380	1/200	1/200	1/170	1/180

ACMG, American College of Medical Genetics; *ACOG,* American College of Obstetricians and Gynecologists.
Modified from ACOG committee opinion no. 486: update on carrier screening for cystic fibrosis. *Obstet Gynecol* 2011;117:1028–31.

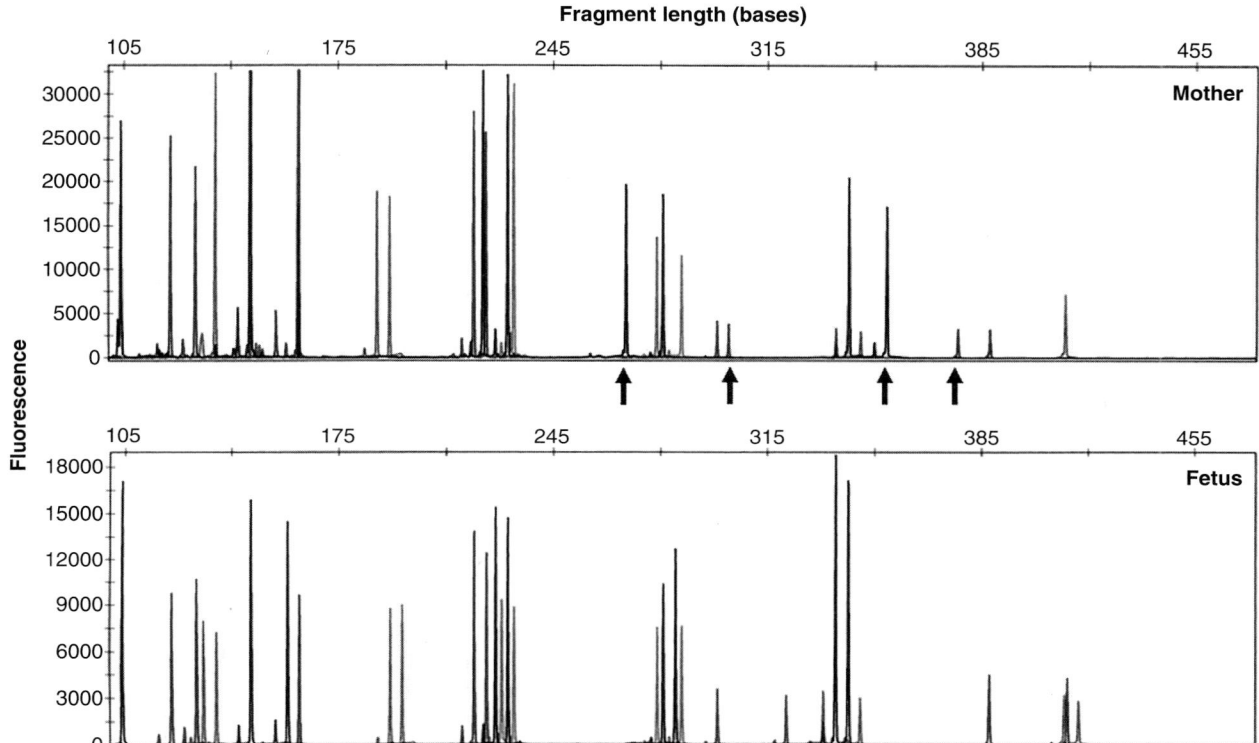

FIGURE 68.1 Electropherograms obtained after polymerase chain reaction *(PCR)* amplification of maternal *(upper panel)* and fetal *(lower panel)* DNA at 15 independently segregating loci and one gender-specific marker. Extracted maternal and fetal DNA were amplified by PCR using a multiplex PCR assay with fluorescent labeled primers (PowerPlex 16 HS System PCR Amplification kit, Promega Corporation, Madison, WI). Amplicons were detected after capillary electrophoresis on an ABI 3500*xl* Genetic Analyzer and were analyzed using GeneMapper software (Applied Biosystems). Amplicon sizes in bases are noted at the top of the figure (*x*-axis) and the relative amount of fluorescence detected for each amplicon is measured by the peak height (*y*-axis). *Arrows* in the *upper panel* denote several maternal alleles obviously absent in the *lower panel* corresponding to the fetal DNA specimen. The absence of both maternal alleles at informative loci signifies the absence of maternal DNA in the fetal sample. The X chromosome is associated with a PCR fragment size of 105 bases, whereas the Y chromosome is associated with a PCR fragment size of 110 bases. The presence of a single peak at 105 bases for both the mother and the fetus and the absence of a peak at 110 bases reveals that both samples are derived from female subjects.

conditions including but not limited to pancreatitis, male infertility, bronchiectasis, diabetes, and constipation.[41] After DNA testing, it is very important for the genetics professional to know relevant family history when interpreting and reporting the test results to the patient and reproductive partner to accurately assess the risk to the couple of having a child with CF.

In families at risk for a child with CF, prenatal testing of the fetus may be requested. With biopsy of chorionic villi or sampling amniotic fluid, there is a chance of maternal cell contamination (MCC) which can interfere with the interpretation of fetal test results. Thus prenatal samples should be screened for MCC. This is best performed by using the PCR amplification for highly polymorphic short tandem repeat loci coupled with capillary electrophoresis (Fig. 68.1).[42] In the case of prenatal *CFTR* gene testing with a maternal variant carrier, if the fetus actually has no variant *CFTR* allele but the extracted fetal DNA is contaminated with maternal DNA, the maternal *CFTR* variant could be detected, and the fetal DNA test result could be erroneously interpreted as a carrier of a *CFTR* gene variant. Furthermore, if the fetus inherited a paternal *CFTR* variant and maternal DNA contaminated the fetal DNA specimen, the fetal DNA test results could show the presence of two *CFTR* gene variants, and the fetal DNA test result could be erroneously interpreted as a compound heterozygote affected with CF.

CFTR gene testing is performed using a laboratory-developed test or one of a variety of commercially available platforms cleared by the US Food and Drug Administration (FDA). The number of variants detected by each assay is variable.[43] Furthermore, because the detection rate of the 23 variant gene panel is lower in some ethnicities, laboratories serving such populations often supplement the screening panel with additional variants analysis.[44]

Spinal Muscular Atrophy

The spinal muscular atrophies (SMAs) are a heterogeneous group of neurodegenerative disorders characterized by progressive loss of motor neurons in the spinal cord and lower brainstem with muscle weakness and atrophy. A wide clinical spectrum is observed with variability in age of onset, motor function impairment, and inheritance patterns. Survival of motor neuron (SMN)-related SMA, also known as SMA5q, is an autosomal recessive disorder that accounts for up to 95% of SMAs, has an incidence of 1 in 6000 to 10,000 births, and is a leading cause of death in infants. SMA5q is caused by variants in the survival motor neuron 1 gene *(SMN1)* and is divided into five types based on clinical presentation and age of onset.[45] Type 0 is one of the rarer forms of SMA and presents prenatally. It is associated with decreased fetal movement during gestation, severe neonatal hypotonia, and respiratory failure at birth.[46] Type 0 is uniformly fatal with patients typically living a few weeks to (rarely) 6 months. Type 1 (OMIM #253300) is the most common (representing 50% of SMA cases); it is associated with age of onset younger than 6 months and has a median survival time of less than 1 year. These children have profound hypotonia, no control of head movement, and are unable to sit. Intercostal muscle weakness leads to respiratory failure and tongue fasciculation, dysphagia, and fatigue, making feeding difficult, worsening the condition, and increasing the risk of aspiration pneumonia. SMA type II (OMIM #253550), representing about 20% of cases, has an age of onset between 7 and 18 months with median survival into the third decade of life. These children can sit, and some can stand, although none can walk independently. SMA type III (OMIM #253400) is seen in about 30% of cases and has an age of onset after 18 months. These patients have a mild phenotype with gradually progressive disease but a normal life expectancy. SMA type IV (OMIM #271150) is rare and is the mildest of all forms. This type is initially characterized by muscle weakness in the second or third decade of life. These patients are ambulatory and have a normal lifespan.

The gene for SMA, *SMN1*, was mapped to chromosome 5q11.2–13.3 in 1990 and cloned in 1995.[47–49] This gene contains 9 exons (numbered 1, 2a, 2b, and 3 to 8) spanning about 28,000 bases and encodes a 1.7 kb mRNA transcript producing a 38-kDa protein composed of 294 amino acids that is ubiquitously expressed in the nucleus and cytoplasm.[50] The SMN protein is one of nine core proteins in a multiprotein complex that also contains the proteins Unrip and Gemins 2 to 8.[51] This complex is enriched in the nucleus in size and number to form Gems.[52] The SMN-GEMINs is essential for the cytoplasmic assembly of small ribonucleoproteins (snRNPs) into the spliceosome, critical components for pre-mRNA splicing.[53] SMN is essential during embryogenesis, evidenced by embryonic lethality in *SMN1* knockout mice.[54] In the majority of cases, SMA results from homozygous deletions of *SMN1*. Some SMA cases result from gene conversion of *SMN1*, and in 2 to 5% of cases, patients are compound heterozygotes with an *SMN1* deletion on one allele and a pathogenic single nucleotide substitution or insertion/deletion variant on the second allele.[46,55] In rare cases, a pathogenic single nucleotide substitution or insertion/deletion variant in *SMN1* is present on both alleles.

SMN1 is contained within a large, inverted repeat sequence that contains the highly homologous *SMN2* gene. *SMN2* differs from *SMN1* by only five bases; it lies in the opposite orientation and is centromeric to *SMN1*.[48,56] Although the five bases that differ between *SMN1* and *SMN2* do not affect the amino acid sequence of the protein, a C-to-T transition in exon 7 of *SMN2* corresponding to codon 280 causes alternative splicing and the deletion of exon 7 in 90% of *SMN2* transcripts.[57] Without exon 7, SMN is unstable and is unable to efficiently oligomerize to form the SMN complex that drives snRNP assembly.[58] Thus even though most patients with SMA have intact *SMN2* genes, they still have disease because most *SMN2* transcripts do not contain exon 7 (SMAΔ7). Thus the pathogenesis of the disease in most patients results from no *SMN1* transcripts, few full-length *SMN2* transcripts, limited functional SMN protein, reduced snRNP assembly, and ultimately aberrant mRNA splicing.

The *SMN2* gene is a modifier of the severity of SMA, and its effect is based on the *SMN2* gene copy number.[46,59,60] Some *SMN1* deletion haplotypes also contain an *SMN2* deletion, but other *SMN1* deletion haplotypes may have two or even three copies of *SMN2*. In patients with milder forms of the disease, three or four copies of *SMN2* may be present.[46] Increased *SMN2* copies result in production of more *SMN2* transcripts, some of which translate to functional SMN protein, thereby providing some normal SMN protein for required cellular functions. Prior et al. described three unrelated individuals with *SMN1* homozygous deletions and 1 or 2 *SMN2* genes but an unexpected mild phenotype.[61] A single nucleotide variant in exon 7 of *SMN2* in these patients created an exonic splicing enhancer element and increased levels of full-length *SMN2* transcript to regain increased cellular levels of SMN protein despite the homozygous loss of *SMN1*. Although *SMN2* copy number or transcripts from *SMN2* are known to influence SMA severity, other uncharacterized factors appear to be contributory. Males with identical biallelic *SMN1* deletions and identical *SMN2* copy numbers appear to be more severely affected than females, and the SMA phenotype is variable even within families whose members share identical genotypes.[62]

Treatment for SMA is supportive for the management of respiratory insufficiency, nutritional deficiency, and orthopedic needs.[63] Because *SMN2* serves to modify the SMA phenotype, it can provide a therapeutic target for treatment by correcting aberrant splicing of *SMN2* using antisense oligonucleotides (ASOs) to allow for full-length transcription of SMN2 and a functional SMN protein. This approach has resulted in the FDA approved drug nusinersen (trade name Spinraza©). Nusinersen is approved for use in all types of SMA and has been shown to prevent disease in some patients while slowing progression in others.[64–67] Recently, a gene therapy drug (onasemnogene abeparvovec, trade name Zolgensma©) was approved by the FDA for the treatment of patients with type I SMA. Onasemnogene abeparvovec is administered as a single intravenous injection of an adeno-associated viral vector containing an intact copy of the *SMN* gene that ultimately results in increased levels of functional SMN protein in motor neurons.[68] Type I SMA patients that have been treated using this method have shown improved motor function and survival.[68]

DNA testing for SMA is performed using a variety of techniques.[69] Diagnostic or carrier testing for SMA can be complicated by (1) the polymorphic nature of the *SMN* locus, with alleles containing varying copy numbers of *SMN1* and/or *SMN2* genes; (2) the degree of homology between *SMN1* and *SMN2*; (3) a small percentage of affected alleles with single nucleotide variants rather than deletions within *SMN1*; and (4) a 2% rate of de novo cases, which most frequently occurs during paternal meiosis.[46,70] A common diagnostic assay for SMA includes multiplex ligation dependent probe amplification (MLPA) and capillary electrophoresis (Fig. 68.2).[71] This method is able to determine copy number for relevant exons in both *SMN1* and *SMN2* making it a quick and simple method capable of confirming a diagnosis or carrier status.

However, this method will not detect the rare SMA cases caused by sequence variants.

Population-based carrier screening for SMA has been endorsed by the ACMG.[72] With an early age of onset for most SMA patients and the prospects of therapeutic treatment of this disease, NBS for SMA allows early identification of patients and enables timely treatment intervention, thereby minimizing the severity of the disease. As of this writing, five states routinely test for SMA in newborns and an additional 13 are in the process of implementing testing for this disorder.

Nonsyndromic Hearing Loss and Deafness

More than 100 genetic loci have been linked to nonsyndromic hearing loss and deafness, and most demonstrate an autosomal recessive mode of inheritance.[73] The most common autosomal recessive nonsyndromic hearing loss and deafness locus is DFNB1 (DeaFNess autosomal recessive [B] locus 1), which in most cases is associated with congenital, nonprogressive moderate to profound impairment and no other clinical phenotypic findings.[74] DFNB1A variants occur in the gene gap junction protein beta-2 (*GJB2*) encoding the protein connexin 26 (OMIM #220290).[75] Also mapped to this region on chromosome 13q12.11 is the gap junction protein β-6 (*GJB6*) gene encoding the protein connexin 30, which is associated with DFNB1B autosomal recessive nonsyndromic hearing loss and deafness (OMIM #612645).

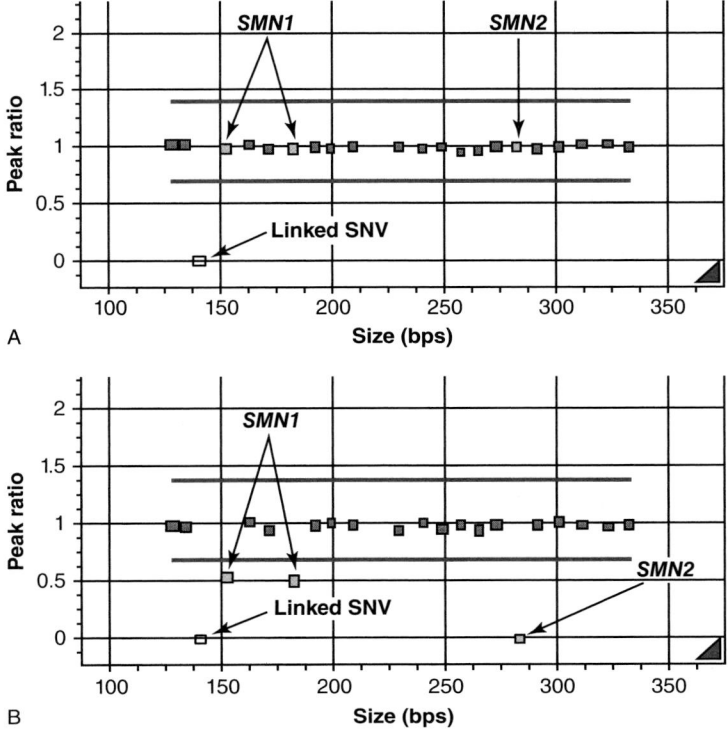

FIGURE 68.2 MLPA testing for spinal muscular atrophy. (A) Data from a noncarrier patient that has two copies (peak ratio = 1) of *SMN1* (both exons 7 and 8 are interrogated) and two copies of *SMN2*. Note that this assay also detects a common single nucleotide variant *(SNV)* that is linked to carrying two copies of *SMN1* on a single chromosome. This patient does not carry this SNV and is therefore less likely to carry both copies of *SMN1* in *cis*. All other data points are reference only. (B) In this patient only a single copy of *SMN1* exon 7 is present indicating that this patient is a carrier for SMA. Also note that this patient carries zero copies of *SMN2* exon 7.

The incidence of newborn or prelingual hearing loss is about two to three per 1000 births in the United States. Although the etiology is heterogeneous, including cytomegalovirus infection and other environmental causes, the primary cause of congenital hearing loss is genetic (50 to 60%) with a small percentage of CMV positive newborns having an underlying genetic cause for their hearing loss.[76,77] Because the presentation of deafness at this age is considered relatively common and early intervention (prior to 6 months) in these patients is associated with improved clinical outcomes, newborn hearing screening (NHS) programs are mandated across the United States. Newborns identified with a sensorineural loss in either ear are referred for audiologic confirmatory testing and, if a sensorineural loss is confirmed, are further referred for genetic evaluation, including a physical examination and pre- and postnatal history. If there is a strong suspicion of a genetic basis for hearing loss, DNA testing is ordered to make or confirm a diagnosis.[78] Passing the NHS does not exclude the risk of hearing loss, thus children who have passed NHS but have risk factors for hearing loss (e.g., family history of childhood hearing loss, developmental delay, in utero infections, head trauma among other things) should be monitored and reevaluated as needed at subsequent visits.[78]

The first linkage of a gene to autosomal recessive nonsyndromic hearing loss on chromosome 13q was by Guilford and colleagues in 1994.[79] In 1996, the connexin 26 gene (GJB2) was mapped to 13q11–q12, and the following year, variants in this gene were identified as disease-causing in Pakistani families with profound deafness.[80,81] The GJB2 gene encodes a member of the gap junction family of connexin proteins.[82] GJB2 is flanked by other gap junction proteins with GJB6 positioned 5′ to GJB2 and gap junction protein α-3 (GJA3) located 3′ to GJB2. Common to other connexin genes, although the 5510-bp gene has two exons, only the second exon contains coding sequences for this 26-kDa, 226-amino-acid protein. More than 20 genes encode the connexin proteins, which are expressed throughout the body, most notably in the skin, nervous tissue, heart, muscle, and ear. Each protein has four TMDs connected by two extracellular loops and one intracellular cytoplasmic loop, with the amino and carboxyl termini located in the cytoplasm.[83,84] Connexin proteins oligomerize to form a hexameric connexon or hemichannel of identical (homomeric) or different (heteromeric) connexin proteins dependent on the tissue.[82,85] The connexon formed in the plasma membrane of one cell aligns with the connexon from the plasma membrane of the adjacent cell to form gap junction channels in the extracellular space. These channels allow for the exchange of ions and small molecules between adjacent cells. Connexin 26 and connexin 30 are widely expressed in epithelial cells and interspersed hair cells of the cochlea and in the connective tissue, and to a lesser extent, connexins 29, 31, 43, and 45 have also been detected.[76,86,87] In the cochlea, normal hearing requires properly functioning gap junctions for the movement and homeostasis of potassium ions between these cells.

More than 200 GJB2 gene variants have been described with most associated with a loss of normal function of the connexin 26 protein.[88] The different GJB2 variants result in varying effects on connexin 26 and ultimately on gap function. Variants can affect the proper formation of the gap junction, a loss of function of the gap junction, or a loss of permeability of selected ions through the gap junction, or variants can cause a gain of function with abnormal opening and increased gap junction activity.[86] The most common variant, c.35delG, has a carrier frequency as high as 3 to 4% in some white populations and has the highest worldwide carrier rate of 1.5%.[89,90] This is a frameshift variant that leads to premature termination of the protein. The high relative frequency of this variant in multiple populations suggests that it is an ancestral founder variant. Other common GJB2 frameshift founder variants include c.167delT and c.235delC, which are common in the Ashkenazi Jewish and Asian populations, respectively.[91,92] The symptomatic patient can be homozygous for variant c.35delG or be a compound heterozygote with another GJB2 gene variant present on the second allele. In addition to GJB2 c.35delG, a less common variant frequently included in a first-tier genetic screening test for nonsyndromic autosomal recessive hearing loss is variant GJB6-c.-301126_443del.[93] This 342-kb deletion is one of over 100 GJB6 variants reported, and encompasses a portion of the GJB6 gene and the 5′ regulatory sequences of GJB2, thus disrupting normal expression of GJB2.[94] This variant is most commonly associated with GJB2 c.35delG in compound heterozygous patients with one copy of each variant on each allele.[95] Alternatively, this variant can be detected in a homozygous state in which it is present on both alleles of the patient. Although most GJB2 gene variants cause a loss of function and demonstrate autosomal recessive inheritance, some variants located in the first extracellular domain of the protein can create a dominant-negative effect on connexin 26 if present in a heterozygous state and can be linked to dominantly inherited deafness.[96] In these cases, the production and subsequent incorporation of an altered protein into the hexameric connexon structure results in abnormal function of the gap junction. These autosomal dominant nonsyndromic hearing loss GJB2 variants (OMIM#601544) and similar dominant GJB6 gene variants (OMIM#604418) define DFNA3 (DeaFNess autosomal dominant [A] locus 3) DFNA3A and DFNA3B, respectively.[97] Gap junctions are also important in the epidermis for intercellular communication, and connexin 26 and connexin proteins 30, 30.3, 31, and 43 are widely expressed at this site and are important for growth and differentiation of keratinocytes.[83] Some GJB2 gene variants demonstrating autosomal dominant inheritance patterns are associated with syndromic hearing loss and characteristic skin diseases such as Bart-Pumphrey syndrome (OMIM#149200), Vohwinkel syndrome (OMIM#124500), and others.[83,98]

Genetic testing to identify the pathogenic variant associated with hearing loss is important to families for diagnosis, determining recurrence risks, enabling subsequent targeted variant analysis for at-risk family members, and determining the likely degree of hearing impairment for the child (e.g., mild, moderate, severe or profound).[74] However, despite the presence of the same variant within family members, modifier genes and environmental factors influence the phenotype such that the degree of hearing impairment may be different between siblings.[74] After a thorough examination of the newborn by the clinical geneticist and a review of family and patient medical history, nonsyndromic autosomal recessive hearing loss may be

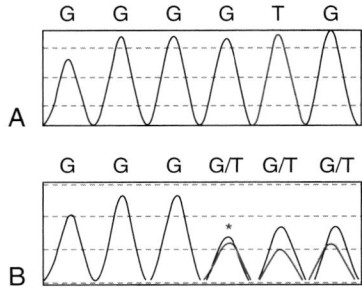

FIGURE 68.3 Sanger sequencing of the *GJB2* gene illustrating a wild-type sequence (A) and the common c.35delG variant (B, *asterisk*). This variant results in a frameshift and premature truncation of the protein.

suspected. Because up to 50% of these patients have *GJB2* gene variants, full-gene *GJB2* Sanger sequencing and *GJB6*-c.-301126_423del analysis is often performed (Fig. 68.3).[95] Because the etiology of hearing loss is heterogeneous, if no variant is detected or if the clinical suspicion of a *GJB2* gene variant is not high, MPS with targeted panels containing genes known to cause hearing loss is suggested.[99,100] In a multi-tiered approach, if MPS targeted panels do not identify a pathogenic disease-causing variant(s), if clinically indicated, whole-exome sequencing can be done to possibly identify pathogenic variants in novel candidate genes segregating in the family.[101–104] The algorithmic approach taken may be different between various clinical teams and laboratories offering this service. Regardless of the etiology of the hearing loss, these patients and their families require a multidisciplinary team of both health care professionals to manage the clinical needs of the patient and family support services to assist them in adjusting to these new and challenging circumstances.[105] Treatment for patients with hearing loss is dependent on the degree of impairment, and can include hearing aids or cochlear implantation. Early cochlear implantation surgery results in significant speech perception and language advantages.[106] Cochlear gene therapy targeting variants in genes associated with sensorineural hearing loss is ongoing with both progress and challenges while CRISPR/Cas9 technology for targeted genome editing is also underway.[107,108]

Autosomal Dominant Diseases

In autosomal dominant disorders, a single abnormal allele is sufficient to cause disease despite the presence of a normal allele. An individual with an autosomal dominant disease may have inherited an abnormal allele from an affected parent, or the variant allele may have arisen de novo as a new variant during gametogenesis in an unaffected parent. The disease-causing gene is on one of the autosomes (1 to 22) and is not on a sex chromosome (X or Y). An affected individual has a 50% risk of donating the variant allele to each offspring. Different variants within the gene may have varying effects on the protein, causing differences in clinical expression between patients who have pathogenic variants. In some instances, known variant gene carriers have no clinical symptoms of the disease, a phenomenon referred to as *reduced penetrance*; however, they still possess a 50% risk of donating the variant allele to each offspring. Differences in phenotypic expression of the disease between patients who share identical gene variants are commonly explained by the effects of modifier genes or environmental influences (or both). Among pedigrees illustrating autosomal dominant inheritance, both males and females are affected, and male-to-male transmission is observed (unlike X-linked inheritance). Table 68.4 provides a list of some of the inherited autosomal dominant disorders commonly tested in clinical molecular diagnostic laboratories.

Huntington Disease

Huntington disease (HD; OMIM#143100) is an autosomal dominant, late-onset neurodegenerative disorder with an incidence of about 3 to 10 per 100,000 in most populations but may be as high as 10 to 15 in some populations of Western European origin. First described by George Huntington in 1872, this progressive disease is characterized by choreic movement, cognitive decline, and ultimately dementia and psychiatric disturbances.[109,110] The mean age of onset is 45 years, but

TABLE 68.4 Examples of Autosomal Dominant Disorders

Disease	Gene(s)	Location	OMIM Entry #	Incidence
Achondroplasia	*FGFR3*	4p16.3	100800	1 in 26,000–28,000
CHARGE syndrome	*CHD7*	8q12.1-q12.2	214800	1 in 10,000
Familial hypercholesterolemia	*LDLR*	19p13.2	143890	1 in 200–500
Hereditary hemorrhagic telangiectasia	*ACVRL1*	9q34.11	187300	1 in 10,000
	ENG	12q13.13		
	GDF2	10q11.22		
	SMAD4	18q21.2		
Long QT syndrome	Numerous	—	192500	1 in 3000–7000
Myotonic dystrophy type 1	*DMPK*	19q13.32	160900	1 in 20,000
Neurofibromatosis type 1	*NF1*	17q11.2	162200	1 in 3000
Polycystic kidney disease 1 and 2	*PKD1*	16p13.3	173900	1 in 400–1000
	PKD2	4q22.1	613095	
Retinoblastoma	*RB1*	13q14.2	180200	1 in 15,000–20,000
Tuberous sclerosis	*TSC1*	9q34.13	191100	1 in 5800
	TSC2	16p13.3	613254	

OMIM, Online Mendelian Inheritance in Man.

subtle signs may be evident before clinical onset and diagnosis. Further, studies suggest that the pathogenesis of HD likely initiates with abnormal brain development during childhood and potentially even prenatally.[111] Approximately 25% of patients first display symptoms after the age of 50 years, and about 5 to 10% of patients have juvenile HD with the age of onset before 20 years. In addition, the disease presentation differs between various age groups.[112] The median survival time is 15 to 18 years after the onset of symptoms.[110] The duration of the disease is long with widespread symptoms involving motor, cognitive, psychiatric, and somatic categories. As such, international guidelines were established for health care providers to standardize care and improve the everyday life of these patients.[113] Early in the disease, primary symptoms include cognitive deficits; clumsiness; and mood disturbances such as depression, anxiety, irritability, and apathy. The next stage of the disease is associated with slurred speech (dysarthria), impairment of voluntary movements, hyperreflexia, chorea, gait abnormalities, and behavioral disturbances such as intermittent explosiveness and aggression. As the disease advances, bradykinesia, rigidity, dementia, dystonia, dysphagia, severe weight loss, sleep disturbances, and incontinence occur.[110] The HD phenotype is initially caused by selective loss of the medium spiny neurons in the striatum, but in later stages of the disease, there are cortical atrophy and widespread degeneration. The average age of death is 54 to 55 years.[114]

In 1983, Gusella and associates reported linkage between DNA marker D4S10, on the short arm of chromosome 4, and HD, based on studies of a large kindred in Venezuela.[115] Through an international collaborative effort, 10 years after its initial localization, the HD gene was cloned.[116] The molecular basis for HD was determined to be an expansion of a glutamine-encoding CAG trinucleotide repeat in exon 1 of the HD gene, *HTT*. This was confirmed in a worldwide study by the identification of expanded CAG-repeat alleles in HD patients from 565 families, representing 43 national or ethnic groups.[117] In this initial international study, the median CAG-repeat length was reported to be 44 in affected patients and 18 in control participants. Normal CAG repeat lengths range from 10 to 26, whereas repeats of 27 to 35 are considered intermediate or "mutable," repeats of 36 to 39 are considered HD alleles associated with reduced penetrance of the disease, and repeats of 40 or greater are diagnostic of HD (Fig. 68.4).

HD is one of over 30 trinucleotide repeat expansion diseases associated with neurologic and neuromuscular dysfunction.[118,119] In HD, the number of CAG repeats is inversely correlated with the age at onset of the disease. Patients with onset as early as 2 years of life have a repeat number approaching 100 or greater, and late-onset-disease patients have repeat numbers of 36 to 39.[120,121] Although the CAG-repeat number accounts for the majority of variance in age of onset for HD (~70%), the remainder of the variance comes from modifier genes and environmental factors.[122] While the CAG repeat number and polyglutamine length in the normal huntingtin protein (htt) is not considered a modifier of age of onset for HD, a G>A variant (rs13102260) in the *HTT* promoter can reduce transcription if present on the normal allele and lead to an earlier age of onset.[123,124] Most recently it has been reported that HD expanded CAG repeat alleles with

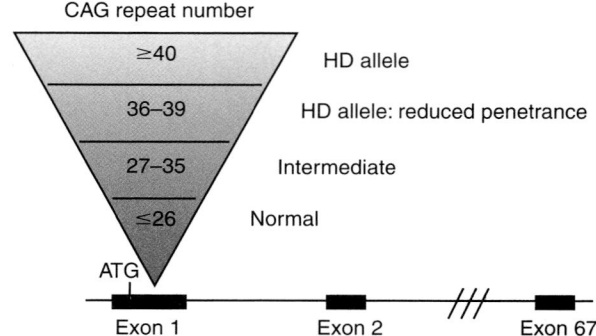

FIGURE 68.4 Schematic representation of the polyglutamine-encoding CAG repeat in exon 1 of the *HTT* gene and associated alleles. A CAG-repeat number of 26 or less is considered normal. CAG-repeat numbers of 27 to 35 are intermediate, and although they are not associated with an abnormal phenotype, these alleles are susceptible to meiotic expansion to a Huntington disease *(HD)* causing allele. CAG repeats of 36 to 39 have reduced penetrance, and both unaffected and affected patients have been reported with alleles of this size. CAG repeats of 40 or more are associated with HD with complete penetrance.

no interrupting CAA glutamine encoding repeats have a decrease in somatic stability and an earlier age of onset as compared to patients with the same number of expanded polyglutamine residues with CAA repeats.[125,126] In addition, genome wide association studies have identified multiple age of onset genetic loci which appear to accelerate or delay the age of onset.[127] Pathogenic variants in *HTT* causing HD in the absence of a family history occur from expansion of a CAG-intermediate allele, which occurs almost exclusively through paternal transmission, although maternal intermediate allele expansion has been reported.[128,129] Intermediate alleles are present in about 1% of the population. The instability of these alleles may be influenced by flanking DNA sequences, which may enhance the formation of hairpin loop structures and cause replication slippage.[130,131] Single sperm analysis studies have demonstrated 11% instability (9% expansions and 2.5% contractions) in CAG repeats of 30 compared with 0.6% instability (contractions only) seen in average-sized alleles of 15 to 18 repeats, indicating that CAG instability increases as the repeat number increases.[132] CAG repeats of 36 showed 53% instability, and CAG repeats from 38 to 51 had instability ranging from 92 to 99%. In families with HD, the onset of symptoms occurs at a progressively younger age in successive generations, a pattern referred to as *anticipation*. Anticipation is explained by meiotic expansion of the unstable CAG repeat during transmission by the affected parent, resulting in an even higher CAG-repeat number in the offspring and an earlier age of onset. In addition, although 69% of affected father–child pairs show expansion, only 32% of affected mother–child pairs demonstrate expansion. Furthermore, less than 2% of maternal expansions result in a change of more than five repeats, but up to 21% of paternal transmissions increase by more than seven repeats.[133] For this reason, the affected parent in most cases of juvenile-onset HD is the father. However, the largest reported CAG-repeat number of approximately 130 occurred via maternal expansion of 70 CAG repeats.[134] Expansions may also occur through mismatch repair defects. Previous studies in the HD mouse model have proposed that variants in mismatch repair genes may modify somatic CAG expansion and disease progression.[135,136] Recently, a variant in the mismatch repair gene MSH3 (p.Pro67Ala) was identified as a modifier of disease progression likely by reducing somatic expansion.[137]

The *HTT* gene contains 67 exons and encodes a novel protein, htt, with 3144 amino acids and a molecular mass of approximately 350 kDa.[138] Htt is ubiquitously expressed in both neural and nonneural tissue with highest levels in the brain.[139,140] Htt is required for neuronal development with the complete absence of htt being lethal in mice.[141] Htt is predominantly localized in the cytoplasm, but lesser amounts are also found in the nucleus.[142,143] The structure of htt includes the CAG encoded polyglutamine repeat, a proline-rich domain, and 3 HEAT repeats, which form a rodlike helical scaffold to which other components can attach and are involved in intracellular transport, and a nuclear localization domain at the C terminal end. The HEAT acronym is derived from four proteins found to also contain this amino acid sequence and unique structure: **H**untingtin, **E**longation factor 3, regulatory **A** subunit of protein phosphatase 2A, and **T**OR1. In neurons, htt is associated with synaptic vesicles and microtubules and is abundant in dendrites and nerve terminals. Huntingtin has more than 400 protein-protein interactions and is involved in intracellular trafficking and signaling, cytoskeletal organization, endocytosis, and transcription regulation.[144] Variant htt (vhtt) with expanded polyglutamine tracks are effectively transcribed and translated. Post transcriptional modification of vhtt and protease cleavage produces N terminal fragments with elongated polyglutamine (polyQ) sequences. These polyQ fragments have a gain of function property to self-assembly into aggregates.[142,145] These protein aggregates appear as intranuclear inclusions in the neuron and may sequester other cellular proteins preventing their normal function, thereby disrupting normal protein homeostasis and conferring neurotoxicity.[146] HD remains an incurable complex disease with current treatment primarily focused on improving the quality of life of these patients.[113] However, multiple therapeutic approaches are being evaluated.[147] A clinical trial investigating the use of ASOs to inhibit variant *HTT* (v*HTT*) messenger RNA (mRNA) did show a dose dependent reduction of v*HTT* mRNA in cerebral spinal fluid of treated patients as compared to patients receiving placebo.[148,149] RNA interference strategies and engineered zinc finger protein transcription factors to specifically target v*HTT* mRNA are also being investigated.[150–152] DNA testing for HD is performed using PCR to determine the CAG-repeat number.[153] The most common method includes PCR with fluorescently labeled primers coupled with capillary electrophoresis (Fig. 68.5).[154] Technical standards and guidelines for HD diagnostic testing for clinical laboratories have been developed by the American College of Medical Genetics and Genomics.[153]

Many ethical issues are associated with HD testing, primarily as they relate to presymptomatic testing (Box 68.2). The first policy statement on ethical issues related to predictive genetic testing for HD was adopted in 1989 at a joint meeting with representatives from the International Huntington Association and the World Federation of Neurology.[155] At that time, the gene had not yet been cloned, and predictive testing was performed using linkage studies and the at-risk patient was quoted only the likelihood of inheriting the mutant allele. These tests were less than perfect and provided, at best, results in only 60 to 75% of families. Moreover, the possibility of recombination resulted in an inaccurate carrier assessment.[153,156] In other families, living affected members were not available, or markers were not informative. After the gene was cloned and direct variant analysis was possible, previously quoted risk assessments were changed in a small percentage of patients.[157]

When determination of the CAG repeat number was possible, guidelines for predictive testing using direct variant analysis were established.[158,159] This model includes a multidisciplinary team involving neurology, psychiatry, and genetics specialists; pretest evaluation and counseling; individual support from family members or close friends; and post-test follow-up sessions.[160] Predictive testing should be performed for patients 18 years of age or older and only with informed consent. Informed consent implies that the patient has been thoroughly counseled and clearly understands both the advantages and the disadvantages of knowing the results. An advantage of having this test is the removal of uncertainty regarding whether patients have or have not inherited the variant allele and thus a feeling of relief for those who have not inherited a variant *HTT* allele. This knowledge can help patients plan their career goals and personal affairs involving marriage, children, and long-term care insurance. Disadvantages of knowing this information include, but are not limited to, (1) the feeling of "survivor's guilt" in those who learn that they have not inherited a variant allele while other family members have, (2) fear from learning that they have inherited a variant *HTT* allele and will develop this incurable disease, (3) potential risk of discrimination in employment, (4) concern for passing this gene on to their offspring, and (5) uncertainty of developing the disease if a variant *HTT* allele with 36 to 39 CAG repeats is identified.

When at all possible, the patient should be accompanied by a trusted friend or loved one throughout the counseling and testing procedure. This person can provide stability to the patient by being able to intimately speak to the patient about the situation and discuss the information shared at the counseling sessions. Most important, as a part of this process, the partner will be present when the results of testing are revealed and can provide comfort and support as needed both then and in the following days, weeks, or months. Ultimately, however, it is the patient's decision to proceed with this testing and to accept both the benefits and pitfalls of knowing this information. The patient's decision to proceed must be his or hers, without coercion from family members, clinicians, friends, or employers. Equally as important as the pretest counseling is a post-test counseling to convey the results to the patient.[161]

For at-risk individuals requesting genetic testing, their mental stability should be considered for the safety of the patient; a psychiatric assessment is often part of the testing protocol because HD test results can precipitate depression. Results of the psychiatric evaluation can influence the timing of the DNA test, postponing it until such time when the patient is considered mentally able to deal with the possibly devastating news. Suicidal tendencies are present in both at-risk patients and those with HD.[162,163]

Because HD is most often a delayed-onset disease, as the asymptomatic at-risk patient ages, the risk of testing positive

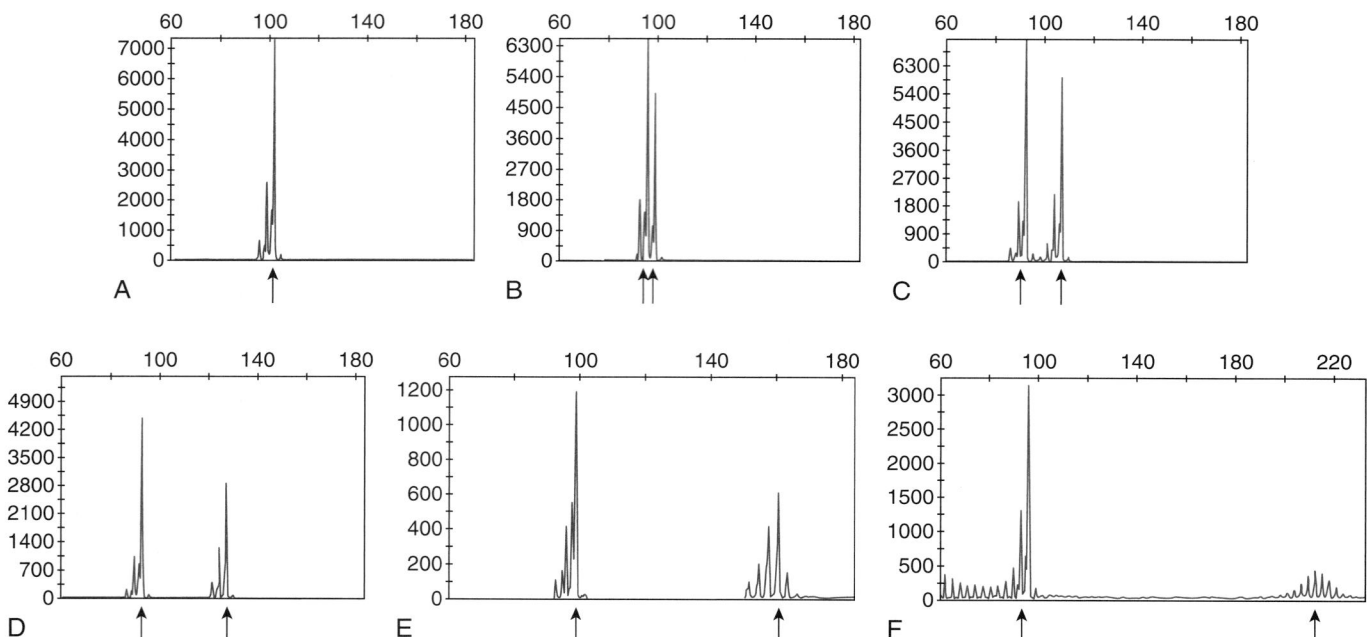

FIGURE 68.5 Electropherograms representing various patterns observed in patients referred for Huntington disease *(HD)* testing. The polyglutamine-encoding CAG repeat in exon 1 is amplified by polymerase chain reaction *(PCR)* using flanking oligonucleotide primers, one of which is labeled with a fluorescent dye. Amplicon sizes in bases are noted at the top of the figure (*x*-axis), and the relative amount of fluorescence detected for each amplicon is measured by the peak height (*y*-axis). *Arrows* indicate the predominant amplicons observed for each patient with the size of the amplicons corresponding to the CAG repeat number. Additional smaller peaks not indicated by arrows represent "stutter" peaks and result from strand slippage during PCR of repetitive sequences. (A) Amplicons 101 bp in length correspond to 20 CAG repeats on both HD alleles. (B) Amplicons 95- and 98-bp correspond to CAG repeats of 18 and 19. (C) Amplicons 92- and 107-bp represent CAG repeats of 17 and 22, respectively. The diagnosis of HD can be ruled out in these three patients. (D) Amplicons 92- and 128-bp correspond to CAG repeats of 17 and 29. The results would not support a diagnosis of HD. However, a CAG repeat of 29 is considered an intermediate allele and can undergo meiotic expansion to an HD allele during gamete formation. (E) CAG repeats of 19 and 39, as depicted by amplicons 98 and 158 bp in length. In a symptomatic patient, these results would support the diagnosis of HD. However, in a presymptomatic patient, the phenotype of an HD allele with reduced penetrance cannot be predicted with certainty. (F) CAG repeats corresponding to 18 and 57 with amplicons 95 and 212 bp in length. These results confirm the diagnosis of HD in this patient. Genetic counseling regarding the implications of HD DNA findings is indicated.

BOX 68.2   Ethical Issues Associated With Presymptomatic DNA Testing for Huntington Disease

Patients must be 18 years of age or older.

The decision to proceed with testing must be voluntary and informed.

Genetic counseling regarding the benefits and pitfalls of testing is required.

A support partner is needed for the patient for counseling and the testing process.

Diagnosis of Huntington disease in the family should be confirmed by DNA testing before presymptomatic testing.

Psychiatric assessment of patient is necessary before testing.

Follow-up genetic counseling is recommended after delivery of results.

Prenatal testing of fetuses is controversial; preimplantation diagnosis is available.

---

with an expanded CAG repeat decreases.[161] Thus if the patient elects not to have predictive testing, the genetic counselor can provide information regarding the probability that a HD CAG repeat expansion exists, which, based on the individual's age, may provide some comfort to the patient.[164] Some individuals may begin the multistep counseling process and then withdraw from the study without receiving test results. If possible, before presymptomatic variant testing, the diagnosis of HD should be confirmed in an affected member of the family to be certain that the disease segregating in the family is HD. It is important to note that a normal *HTT* CAG repeat number does not rule out a different, dominantly inherited neurodegenerative disease in the family for which the patient likely retains a risk of development.

Genetic counseling for HD may present with a variety of clinical scenarios and counseling in families with no prior family history of HD may be especially challenging when the expanded CAG repeat appears to be de novo

(Box 68.3). Without understanding the mechanism of a new variant in the affected individual, an *a priori* risk assessment for HD in at-risk family members may be inaccurate. Thus counseling for the risk of HD is only prudent after accurate DNA testing.

Prenatal testing for HD, another complicated issue associated with this disease, may not be provided in all laboratories that perform routine HD testing for several reasons. Ethical issues include possible pregnancy termination for a late-onset disorder, presymptomatic testing of the child if the parents choose not to terminate, and technical issues that may compromise testing of chorionic villus and amniocentesis samples. As an alternative for prenatal testing, preimplantation genetic diagnosis (PGD) can be performed.[165] In PGD, in vitro fertilization is used to produce embryos that then undergo a single cell biopsy for genetic analysis. After PCR testing has been used to determine the *HTT* CAG-repeat numbers, embryos with normal HD alleles are implanted. This method, which combines direct variant analysis and PGD, eliminates the necessity for subsequent prenatal testing to determine the HD status of the fetus. Exclusion testing whereby only embryos who have not inherited an affected allele are implanted without disclosing information regarding the *HTT* CAG repeat numbers in all tested embryos is an option for some families that do not wish to know the genotype of the asymptomatic at-risk parent.[166,167]

Marfan Syndrome

Marfan syndrome (MFS; OMIM #154700) is a relatively common autosomal dominant multisystem connective tissue disorder with primary manifestations involving the ocular, musculoskeletal, and cardiovascular systems with an estimated worldwide incidence of 1 in 3000 to 5000.[168–170] The most common ocular feature of MFS is myopia, but other associated features include unilateral or bilateral ectopia lentis (60%), or retinal detachment. In addition, patients with MFS are at increased risk for glaucoma and cataracts at a younger age as compared with the general population. Characteristic facial features may include a long narrow face, deep-set and downward-slanting eyes, flat cheek bones, and micrognathia. Skeletal abnormalities arise from bone overgrowth and joint hypermobility. MFS patients are tall with frequent clinical findings including pectus excavatum or pectus carinatum, caused by overgrowth of the ribs, which can interfere with pulmonary function and require surgery. Patients typically have an arm span-to-height ratio greater than 1.05 and a reduced upper body-to-lower extremity ratio. Scoliosis is present in about half of patients; it can be mild to severe and is

progressive. Morbidity and early mortality are linked to cardiovascular manifestations of the disorder, which are characterized by progressive dilation of the aortic root, predisposition to aortic dissection, mitral and tricuspid valve prolapse with or without regurgitation, and dilation of the proximal pulmonary artery. Wide phenotypic variability is observed, with some patients presenting as neonates with severe and progressive disease that is sometimes fatal, but others can remain undiagnosed until adulthood. Unfortunately, for undiagnosed patients, presentation may be sudden premature death caused by aortic dissection or rupture.[171,172] An early diagnosis is associated with an improved long-term outcome.[173–175] Additionally, as long-term survival of MFS patients increases it has become clear that a number of systems not previously thought to be associated with the disorder are likely involved.[176] It is therefore likely that our understanding of this disorder will likely continue to evolve over time.

The diagnosis of MFS is based on family history of the disease; however, as many as 25% of MFS cases are characterized by a new (de novo) variant and no family history.[169,177] In the absence of a documented family history of MFS, currently the clinical diagnosis of MFS is made using the revised Ghent diagnostics nosology with most of the emphasis on the presence of an aortic root aneurysm and ectopia lentis.[168] In the absence of one or both of these, a variant in the gene associated with MFS or manifestations in other MFS-related organ systems are required. Some MFS features may be isolated findings and not associated with MFS, and some overlap with other genetic syndromes.[168,170] Because most MFS clinical manifestations increase with age, these criteria may make diagnosis in the pediatric patient more difficult, and often these patients may carry a diagnosis of "potential" MFS and require periodic follow-up visits for reevaluation.[170]

MFS is associated with variants in the fibrillin-1 (*FBN1*) gene mapped to chromosome 15q21.1.[177–179] The gene spans 237,414 bp, is composed of 65 exons, and encodes a 10 kb mRNA, prefibrillin-1.[180] *FBN1* is ubiquitously expressed in connective tissue. The 320-kDa, 2871-amino-acid extracellular glycoprotein, fibrillin-1, self-assembles into macroaggregates to serve as the primary structural component of 10-nm-diameter microfibrils located throughout the basal lamina in both elastic and nonelastic tissue.[180–182] In elastin-expressing tissue, such as blood vessels, lung, and skin, microfibrils make up the scaffold for elastin assembly within the extracellular matrix (ECM). In nonelastic tissue, including the ciliary zonule of the eye and of basement membranes, they have an anchoring function and provide tensile strength.[183] In most cases in which sequence variation causes abnormal fibrilin-1 protein, a dominant negative effect occurs when fibrillin-1 is incorporated into the microfibril, resulting in functionally inferior connective tissue. In other cases, disease results from reduced protein production or haploinsufficiency. Fibrillin-1 contains several motifs, including 47 cysteine-rich epidermal growth factor-like (EGF) domains, most of which bind calcium.[184] These domains are interspersed with seven TGF-β binding protein-like (TB) domains, and there are two hybrid domains with sequences similar to both the EGF and TB motifs.[184] Latent TGF-β binding proteins interact with fibrillin-1 and together bind TGF-β to inactivate and thereby prevent signaling through the SMAD 2/3 pathway.[182,183,185,186] Dysregulation of TGF-β signaling affects the development of vascular smooth muscle and the integrity of the ECM.

Variants in *FBN1* are heterogeneous with almost 2000 reported throughout the gene.[187] Single nucleotide variants represent the largest category at 66%; 20% are small deletions or insertions, 11% are splice site variants, and the remainder represent large deletions or duplications. In all cases, increased TGF-β signaling is observed. Phenotype–genotype studies have shown that neonatal MFS or early onset and severe MFS is associated with variants spanning exons 24 to 32.[188,189] These patients also have an increased likelihood of developing ectopia lentis, ascending aortic dilation, mitral valve anomalies, scoliosis, and a reduced life expectancy. This region of the protein contains the longest stretch of EGF-like domains and is thought to be important for microfibril biogenesis. Traditionally, in-frame missense variants have been thought to result in more severe complications of MFS than variants predicted to cause premature truncation of the protein. However, recent studies indicate that this is not the case.[190,191] Because wide phenotypic variability is observed even for individuals harboring the same recurrent variant, modifier genes likely play a role in the MFS phenotype.[188] Interestingly, the phenotypic expression of MFS may be related in part to varying degrees of expression between the normal and variant allele, and these differences may also be tissue specific.[192] The lack of consistent genotype–phenotype correlations provides little prognostic value for individual patient management. Although variability in expression is observed, *FBN1* variants are considered highly penetrant.

Management of patients with MFS is similar to that of patients with other inherited multisystem disorders, involving a team approach with specialists in many areas of medicine including a cardiologist, ophthalmologist, orthopedist, and geneticist. Because the pathogenesis of MFS is due to dysregulation of TGF-β and increased TGF-β signaling, one pharmacologic treatment for MFS is the drug losartan, an angiotensin II type 1 receptor inhibitor used to inhibit excessive TGF-β signaling and slow aortic growth.[193,194] However, some studies suggest that this therapy may be more effective in patients with *FBN1* haploinsufficiency as opposed to dominant negative *FBN1* variants.[195] Other successful treatments for aortic aneurysms associated with MFS include β-blockers and statins or tetracycline to inhibit TGF-β signaling through inhibition of matrix metalloproteinase-2 and -9 and ERK inhibitors to inhibit ERK signaling.[193] Clinical trials investigating the best therapy to treat patients with MFS and other aortopathies are ongoing. Annual ophthalmologic and transthoracic echocardiographic imaging is important for monitoring, and prophylactic surgery for aortic root replacement is recommended when the aortic root reaches a critical diameter of 5.5 cm.[196,197] Lifestyle changes to limit physical activity to low-impact sports in order to prevent physical exhaustion are recommended to prevent high blood pressure and aortic wall stress.

FBN1 is one of the largest human genes and DNA sequencing has historically been considered the gold standard for genetic testing for MFS. This may be most effective in patients when the clinical diagnosis of MFS is likely.[198] After a *FBN1* variant has been identified within a family, predictive targeted *FBN1* variant specific testing for at-risk family members can be performed and enables early diagnosis and proper management in identified variant-positive family members. However, despite extensive *FBN1* analysis, 7 to 30% of MFS patients will have no variant detected. These cases could reflect patients with *FBN1* variants that are contained within regions of the gene that cannot be detected by current screening techniques.[199] Alternatively, these may be patients who have a phenotype suspicious for MFS but who do not meet the strict Ghent diagnostic criteria. MPS with a targeted panel of genes, which includes *FBN1* and other candidate genes associated with thoracic aortic aneurysms or aortic dissections, may be an efficient screening method. Associated syndromes and genes may include Loeys-Dietz (*SMAD3, TGFBR1, TGFBR2, TGFB2, TGFB3*) Ehlers-Danlos type IV (*COL3A1*), or genes associated with familial thoracic aortic aneurysm and dissections (*ACTA2, MYH11, MYLK, TGFBR1,* and *TGFBR2*).[200] Collectively, these disorders are described as aortopathies. Aortopathies are a common cause of morbidity and mortality in the United States. In fact, it is reported that aneurysm of the aorta is responsible for 1 to 2% of all deaths in the Western world.[196,201] MPS-based testing using an aortopathy gene panel is rapidly becoming the first-line diagnostic test for individuals who present with a phenotype that could fit any one of multiple disorders (e.g., MFS and Loeys-Dietz syndrome). Fig. 68.6 illustrates the identification of a variant in a Marfan patient using an MPS-based aortopathy panel.

Multiple Endocrine Neoplasia

Multiple endocrine neoplasia (MEN) is an autosomal dominant disorder characterized by the presence of tumors in two or more endocrine glands. There are two major types of MEN disease: type 1 (MEN1, which is also known as Werner syndrome) and type 2 (MEN2, which is also known as Sipple syndrome). Both MEN1 and MEN2 are clinically distinct and should be considered as independent disorders with separate genetic causes.

Multiple endocrine neoplasia type 1 (OMIM #131100) is a relatively common disorder with an estimated incidence ranging from 1 in 10,000 to 50,000.[202–204] MEN1 is characterized by the presence of any one of a number (>20) of tumor types, and a clinical diagnosis requires that an individual have at least two endocrine tumors that are parathyroid, pituitary, or gastroenteropancreatic in nature.[202,203] Parathyroid tumors are the most common tumors observed in MEN1 and occur in approximately 95% of patients.[205] Consequently, hyperparathyroidism resulting from overproduction of hormones by parathyroid tumors is a common early manifestation.[202,206] Parathyroid tumors also often cause hypercalcemia, which ultimately results in a multitude of medical issues (e.g., depression, nausea, vomiting, kidney stones, and hypertension, among others).[202] Pancreatic islet cell tumors are the second most common tumors observed in MEN1 with approximately 40% of patients developing a neoplasm of this area.[205,206] Pancreatic tumors are of particular importance in MEN1 because gastrinomas (Zollinger-Ellison syndrome) are the most common cause of morbidity in patients with this disease.[203,205] Pituitary tumors occur in 30% of patients with MEN1 and represent the third most prevalent tumor type. Of note, a multitude of non–endocrine-associated tumors (carcinoid, adrenocorticoid, facial angiofibromas, lipomas, meningiomas, among others) commonly occur in patients with MEN1.[202,203,205,206]

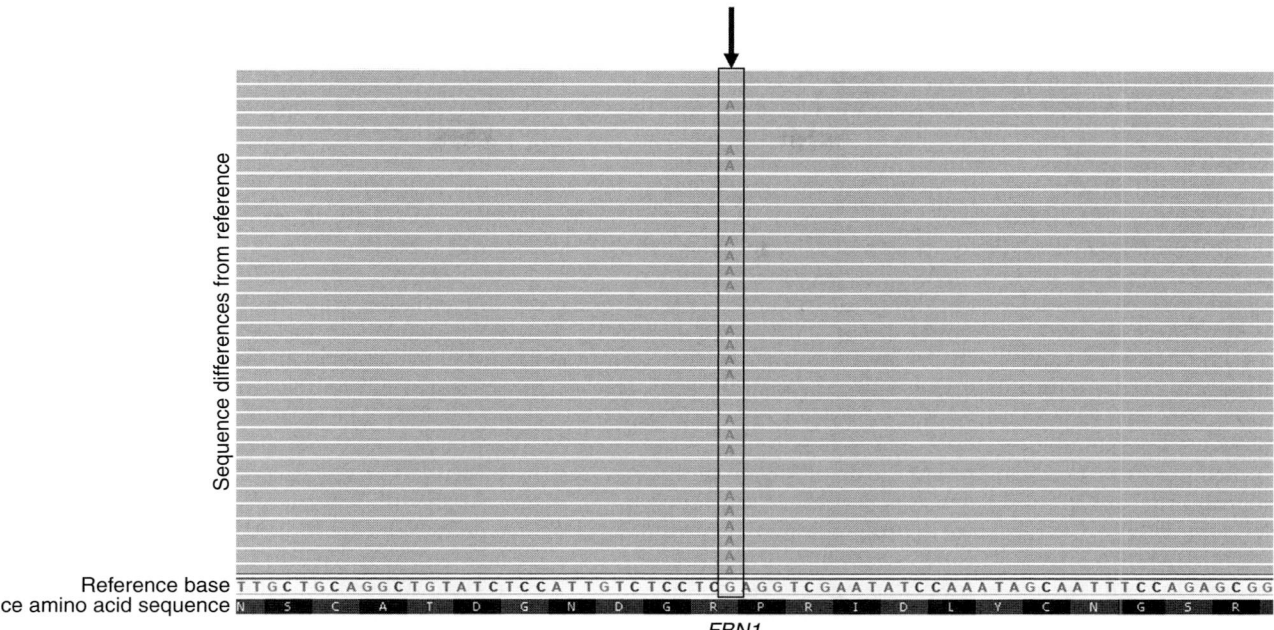

FIGURE 68.6 Massively parallel sequencing data visualization. This example shows numerous massively parallel sequencing reads visualized horizontally in the Integrative Genomics Viewer (IGV, https://igv.org). The reference sequence (both nucleotide and single letter amino acid code) of a segment of the *FBN1* gene is at the bottom. Additional aligned sequence reads are shown above the reference. Only differences from the reference sequence are shown, revealing that about half of the reads have an A instead of a G at one position *(arrow)*, indicating a heterozygous nucleotide variant (c.4621G>A, *arrow*). This nucleotide substitution results in a premature termination codon (p.Arg1541Ter) and is predicted to be causative for Marfan syndrome.

Using a combination of linkage analysis and deletion mapping techniques, investigators in several groups were able to identify a region on chromosome 11 (11q13) likely to contain the gene responsible for MEN1.[207–216] In 1997, the gene causative for MEN1 was identified and named multiple endocrine neoplasia I (*MEN1*).[217,218] The *MEN1* gene contains ten exons that encode a 610 amino acid protein known as menin.[217] Menin is a ubiquitously expressed protein that can localize to either the nucleus or cytoplasm.[219,220] However, other than clearly defined nuclear localization signals, menin lacks functional domains homologous to those observed in other proteins, making it difficult to predict how it functions.[221] Menin protein interactions suggest that it functions in transcriptional regulation, cell division and proliferation, and genome stability.[221–224] Based on loss of heterozygosity (LOH) patterns observed during gene identification, *MEN1* was considered a likely tumor suppressor gene. Several studies have since shown that overexpression of menin in vitro results in suppression of cellular proliferation.[225–227] Furthermore, the loss of menin results in immortalization of cells.[228] Taken together, these data support a tumor suppressor role for menin, but its specific function is not yet known.

To date, more than 500 unique disease-causing variants have been described in the *MEN1* gene.[223] Variants are located in all coding exons of the gene, and there are no significant mutational hot spots. The bulk of variants reported in *MEN1* are those that lead to truncated forms of the menin protein (e.g., frameshift, nonsense, gross deletions).[223] Most known

variants in *MEN1* result in the loss of nuclear localization, and loss of function appears to be the mechanism of disease.[202,223] However, there are no clear genotype–phenotype correlations in patients with MEN1. *MEN1* missense variants, which are unlikely to be loss of function, have been reported in individuals with familial isolated hyperparathyroidism (FIHP).[229–231] There have also been several truncating variants reported in FIHP that also occur in classic MEN1 disease.[223] It is therefore not possible to predict the course of disease based on genotype alone.

Molecular diagnosis of MEN1 typically involves Sanger sequencing of the entire coding region of the *MEN1* gene. This method detects disease-causing variants in 80 to 90% of familial cases and 65% of isolated cases.[202,232,233] Symptomatic individuals with negative Sanger sequencing results should be screened for gross deletions and duplications. Testing for large deletions and duplications (typically performed by MLPA) detects variants in an additional 1 to 4% of patients.[202,223,234–238] Combining both techniques, a causative variant is found in approximately 95% of familial MEN1 cases. After a causative germline variant is identified in a family, other at-risk family members should be offered targeted testing for the identified variant as soon as possible because the disease may begin to show manifestations as early as 5 years of age.[203,239] An MPS-based gene panel that includes the *MEN1* gene is another option for molecular diagnosis of this disease and should be considered in cases where an alternative endocrine tumor disorder is a possibility. Because MEN1 is autosomal dominant, the risk of MEN1 in the child of an affected individual is 50%. Approximately 10% of variants identified in *MEN1* are de novo, so recurrence risk is much lower in families where the proband is the child of individuals in which no *MEN1* gene variant has been identified and correct parentage has been confirmed.[223] However, all children of an individual with a de novo change have a 50% chance of inheriting the causative variant.

Treatment of MEN1 disease is largely driven by the presentation of disease in the individual patient. Surgical intervention is recommended to remove all functional tumors and those that are greater than 4 cm in size or demonstrate rapid growth.[239] In some cases in which pancreatic tumors become metastatic (or are inoperable), chemotherapy may be used.[239] Individuals with hyperparathyroidism may undergo a subtotal or total parathyroidectomy.[239] Thymectomy may be performed prophylactically to prevent the development of carcinoid tumors, but in most cases, it is performed after tumor development.[202,239] Surveillance in presymptomatic individuals with a known disease-causing variant in *MEN1* is recommended to begin as early as age 5.[203]

Multiple endocrine neoplasia type 2 is divided into three phenotypically distinct subtypes: MEN2A (OMIM #171400), MEN2B (OMIM #162300), and familial medullary thyroid carcinoma (FMTC, OMIM #155240). Unlike MEN1, tumors associated with MEN2 disease are highly malignant and life threatening. The MEN2A and MEN2B subtypes are both characterized by medullary thyroid carcinoma (MTC) and pheochromocytoma but also have unique distinguishing features. MEN2A is the most common form of MEN2 disease and accounts for approximately 55% of patients. It is characterized by MTC with pheochromocytomas in 50% of patients and parathyroid adenoma in approximately 20% of patients.[205,240,241] A clinical diagnosis of MEN2A requires the presence of both MTC and pheochromocytoma or a parathyroid adenoma (or parathyroid hyperplasia) in a single individual.[235] MEN2B is much less common, representing only 5 to 10% of MEN2 patients.[205,206,236,240,241] It is characterized by MTC with pheochromocytoma but very little risk for parathyroid adenoma. MEN2B patients also commonly have mucosal neuromas of the lips or tongue, marfanoid habitus, distinctive facies, intestinal autonomic ganglion dysfunction, and medullated corneal fibers.[205,240] A clinical diagnosis of MEN2B typically requires the presence of most of these features in addition to MTC. FMTC accounts for 35% of MEN2 cases and is characterized by MTC in the absence of other malignancies.[205,206] FMTC is clinically diagnosed in families with four or more individuals affected with MTC alone.[240] Interestingly, the onset of disease varies significantly between the subtypes of this disorder. The onset of MTC is typically observed in early adulthood in MEN2A, in early childhood in MEN2B, and often in middle age in FMTC patients.[240]

Using a combination of linkage analysis and gene mapping techniques the gene causative for MEN2A was located in a 480-kb region of chromosome 10q11.2.[242–245] The proto-oncogene *RET* was later identified as causative for MEN2A, FMTC, and MEN2B.[245–248] *RET* is a proto-oncogene containing 21 exons that encode an 1114-amino-acid protein called RET. RET is a receptor tyrosine kinase for members of the glial cell line–derived neurotrophic factor family (GDNF) of signaling molecules.[249–252] RET contains three functional domains: an extracellular ligand-binding domain, a TMD, and

a cytoplasmic tyrosine kinase domain.[253] It is involved in several signaling pathways during development that control proliferation, differentiation, survival, and migration of enteric nervous system progenitor cells.[253] Not surprisingly, *RET* gene variants that result in MEN2 disease are activating in nature.[254] Interestingly, variants that inactivate the *RET* gene result in Hirschsprung disease (OMIM #142623), a disorder characterized by the absence of neuronal ganglion cells in the large intestine.[255,256]

More than 100 variants have been described in the *RET* gene in association with the MEN2 phenotype with several variant hotspots.[257] In fact, variants at *RET* codon 634 account for more than 85% of familial MEN2A, and variants in three cysteine residues located at codons 609, 618, and 620 account for 50% of FMTC.[205,240] Similarly, a single variant resulting in a change from methionine to threonine at codon 918 (p.Met918Thr) in *RET* exon 16 accounts for 95% of MEN2B patients.[206] Because the bulk of MEN2-associated *RET* gene variants are limited to exons 10, 11, and 13 to 16, molecular testing is typically limited to Sanger sequencing of these regions. When a diagnosis of MEN2B is suspected, targeted testing for the p.Met918Thr variant is often performed first. All subtypes of MEN2 are inherited in an autosomal dominant manner, so any individual found to have a disease-causing *RET* variant has a 50% chance of passing the disease-causing allele to each of his or her offspring. Five percent of MEN2A-related and 50% of MEN2B-related *RET* gene variants are caused by a de novo change.[240] In these cases, the children of an individual with a de novo variant also have a 50% chance of inheriting the disease.

Treatment of MEN2 is dependent on the disease presentation. Individuals with MTC typically undergo thyroidectomy and lymph node dissection. Patients with pheochromocytoma have laparoscopic adrenalectomy.[206] Presymptomatic individuals with a disease-causing *RET* variant should be screened regularly to detect early manifestations of disease. These individuals may also elect to have prophylactic thyroidectomy to prevent MTC.

X-linked Diseases

In X-linked diseases, the variant allele resides on the X chromosome. In X-linked recessive diseases, females are heterozygous carriers of the disease with one normal and one variant allele and are typically not affected. Males receiving the variant allele from their mothers are considered hemizygous with one variant allele and no normal allele. All daughters of affected males are carriers of a variant allele. A carrier female has a 25% chance of transmitting her normal allele to a son, a 25% chance of having an affected son, a 25% chance of having a daughter who carries the variant allele, and a 25% chance of having a daughter who receives her normal allele. In the absence of a family history, an affected male can have a variant allele that arose de novo as a new variant during gametogenesis in the formation of the egg. Roughly one third of all cases of X-linked disorders represent de novo new variants with the absence of a family history. In these cases, the mother is not a carrier of a variant allele and is not at risk for having subsequent affected children. In pedigrees associated with X-linked recessive conditions, typically only males are affected, and male-to-male transmission of the disease is not seen. In less frequent, X-linked dominant diseases, one copy of the variant allele is sufficient to cause disease despite the

TABLE 68.5   Examples of X-linked Disorders

Disease	Gene	Location	OMIM Entry #	Incidence
Fabry disease	GLA	Xq22.1	301500	1 in 50,000 males
Hemophilia A	HEMA	Xq28	306700	1 in 4000–5000 males
Hemophilia B	HEMB	Xq27.1	306900	1 in 20,000 males
Hunter syndrome: mucopolysaccharidosis type II	IDS	Xq28	309900	1 in 100,000 males
Incontinentia pigmenti	IP	Xq28	308300	1 in 1,000,000 females
Lesch-Nyhan syndrome	HRPT1	Xq26.2-26.3	300322	1 in 380,000 males
Menkes disease	ATP7A	Xq21.1	309400	1 in 100,000 males
Ornithine transcarbamylase deficiency	OTC	Xp11.4	300461	1 in 14,000 males
Severe combined immunodeficiency	IL2RG	Xq13.1	300400	1 in 50,000–100,000 males
Wiskott-Aldrich syndrome	WAS	Xp11.23	301000	1 in 100,000 males

OMIM, Online Mendelian Inheritance in Man.

presence of a normal allele. In these disease processes, females are affected, and in males with only a single variant allele, these diseases are often lethal. Table 68.5 provides a list of some of the inherited X-linked disorders commonly tested in clinical molecular diagnostic laboratories.

Duchenne Muscular Dystrophy

Duchenne muscular dystrophy (DMD; OMIM #310200) is a fatal X-linked recessive disorder characterized by progressive skeletal muscle wasting. The incidence of DMD is about 1 in 5000 male births, making it the most common severe neuromuscular disease in humans. Classic DMD presents in early childhood, with delayed motor skills or an abnormal gait and has a mean age of diagnosis of 41 months.[258,259] This is followed by progressive muscle weakness, calf hypertrophy, and grossly elevated serum creatine kinase ($>10\times$ normal) caused by degenerating muscle fibers. Progressive weakness initially affects the lower extremities, causing most DMD patients to require wheelchairs between 10 and 15 years of age. Continual degeneration and regeneration and inflammation of muscle eventually lead to the replacement of muscle tissue by adipose and connective tissue and progressive disease. A muscle biopsy will show variation in fiber size, necrosis, inflammation, fibrosis, and fiber regeneration and may be required for confirmation of disease in about 5% of patients in whom no DNA variant is identified. Immunohistochemistry (IHC) staining using antibodies directed against different epitopes of the DMD encoded protein, dystrophin, shows complete or almost complete absence of carboxy-terminal antigens in the majority of DMD patients. Scoliosis is common and affects respiratory function. Chronic respiratory insufficiency develops in all patients. Cardiac disease is most commonly dilated cardiomyopathy (DCM) caused by cardiac fibrosis or rhythm and conduction abnormalities and is characterized by left ventricular dilation and ultimately congestive heart failure. Cardiorespiratory failure is the primary cause of death.[260] In some patients, however, only the heart is affected, causing DMD-associated X-linked DCM (OMIM #302045).[261] Additionally, many patients with DMD exhibit lower IQs and nonprogressive cognitive impairment with the degree of impairment possibly associated with the location of the variant within the DMD gene.[262,263] Clinical management of patients with DMD is complex, requiring a multidisciplinary team approach.[264,265] Glucocorticoids are used to slow muscle weakness, angiotensin-converting enzyme

inhibitors, β-blockers and diuretics for cardiac disease, and noninvasive ventilation for respiratory care. In addition to health care professionals in these respective areas, team members in the areas of psychosocial, gastrointestinal, pain, and speech and language are required. Elevated serum creatine kinase (CK) levels can be measured from newborn screening blood spots, enabling early identification of affected children and potential better outcomes from early intervention. A two-tiered pilot program performing both CK and DNA analysis on dried blood spots was successfully implemented in Ohio, screening 37,649 newborn males and identifying 6 affected patients.[266] As novel therapies for DMD continue to develop and the efficacy of targeted treatment for early intervention is validated, NBS for DMD may ultimately be adopted. Although NBS for DMD has not been implemented in the United States, a multidisciplinary team continues to move these efforts forward.[267]

Because DMD is an X-linked recessive disorder, most carrier females are asymptomatic. Similar to other X-linked diseases, the varying degree of clinical manifestations among carrier females depends on the degree of inactivation of the X chromosome harboring the variant DMD gene in various tissues where the DMD protein is expressed. Up to as many as 20% of female carriers can display some symptoms of DMD or of the less severe associated disease, Becker muscular dystrophy (BMD; OMIM#300376). The phenotypes most frequently observed in female manifesting carriers (MCs) include muscle weakness with elevated serum CK levels or cardiac involvement, including DCM or left ventricle dilation.[268] Females with severe disease most often result from skewed lyonization in carrier females or an X-autosome translocation involving the DMD gene.[269–272]

Cytogenetic abnormalities in DMD patients and DNA linkage studies localized the DMD locus to chromosome Xp21.[273–275] By mixing DNA enhanced for X-linked genes from a 49, XXXXY cell line with DNA from a patient with DMD and a cytogenetic deletion in Xp21, Kunkel and colleagues cleverly used subtraction hybridization to clone the DNA corresponding to the patient's deletion.[276] The DMD gene (Xp21.2) is complex and is one of the largest genes in the human genome, spanning 2.4 Mb. DMD contains 79 exons, representing less than 1% of the gene, and encodes a 14-kb mRNA.[277] The gene has multiple tissue-specific promoters that transcribe various full-length dystrophin isoforms differing in their amino terminal sequences. The full-length protein product, dystrophin, contains 3685 amino acids; has a molecular weight of 427 kDa; and contains four distinct domains, including an actin-binding domain, a central rod domain with spectrin-like repeats, a cysteine-rich domain, and a unique COOH-terminal domain. Dystrophin is predominantly expressed in skeletal, cardiac, and smooth muscle. Additional dystrophin isoforms transcribed from four internal promoters and splice variants are found in nonmuscle organs throughout the body.[278] Dystrophin is a rod-like cytoskeletal protein and is a critical component of the dystrophin-associated protein complex (DAPC).[279]

The DAPC interacts with a host of cytoskeletal, transmembrane, extracellular, trafficking, and intracellular signaling proteins. In skeletal muscle, DAPC plays a structural role by connecting the actin cytoskeleton to the ECM, stabilizing the sarcolemma of muscle fibers during repeated cycles of contraction and relaxation, and transmitting force generated in the muscle sarcomeres to the ECM.[279] The DAPC is also important for Ca^{2+} homeostasis. In the absence of normal dystrophin and the DAPC, the sarcolemmal integrity is compromised, allowing an influx of calcium, immune cells, and cytokines to occur, causing the activation of proteases and the breakdown of the ECM. Secondary morphologic findings including autophagy, necrosis, and fibrosis are associated with progressive muscle wasting.[280] Dysregulation of matrix metalloproteinases important for normal muscle repair may also contribute to the pathogenesis in muscle tissue. In addition, there is abnormal signaling of nuclear factor-κ β, mitogen-activated protein kinases (MAPK), and phosphatidylinositol 3 kinase/AKT pathways.[281]

DMD gene variants are heterogeneous.[282,283] Intragenic deletions encompassing one or more exons represent 65 to 70% of variants and affect the translational reading frame of the protein leading to a truncated and nonfunctional protein. Duplications of one or more exons are observed in about 5 to 10% of patients. Single nucleotide coding variants account for the majority of remaining variants, but small insertions, deletions, or splice site variants are also detected.

Becker muscular dystrophy is a milder and less common form of muscular dystrophy with an estimated incidence of 1 in 18,500 births. BMD is an allelic variation of DMD that is caused by different variants within the *DMD* gene that result in either reduced protein levels or a partially functional protein.[284] As such, BMD is associated with a milder phenotype, with only half of BMD patients displaying symptoms of disease by 10 years of age with the mean age of death in the mid-40s.[285,286] About 85% of BMD patients have deletions of one or more exons; 5 to 10% have duplications involving one or more exons; and 5 to 10% have a small insertion, deletion, or single base substitutions. The BMD phenotype is variable and is associated with the type of variant and the resulting effect on the corresponding structural characteristics of dystrophin.[287] Patients with deletions involving the distal rod domain of dystrophin (exons 45 to 60) show the mild BMD phenotype and in some cases remain free of symptoms until their 50s.[288] However, BMD patients with deletions involving the amino-terminal domain of dystrophin (exons 1 to 9) have a more severe BMD phenotype with an earlier age of onset and more rapid progression of disease.

Patients with DCM may have a variant at the dystrophin locus, resulting in *DMD*-associated X-linked DCM.[261,289,290] DCM is characterized by dilation of the left ventricle and

reduced left ventricular systolic function and is a rapidly progressive, fatal disease with an onset of symptoms early in the third decade of life.[291] The lack of the functional dystrophin isoform in the heart results from altered tissue-specific transcription or alternative splicing from variants involving the promoter region or exon 1, splice sites, or specific exonic duplications and deletions. Although variants in *DMD* can cause DCM, variants in other genes are also associated with this phenotype.[292]

DNA testing for DMD confirms the diagnosis, identifies pathogenic variants segregating in the family, and enables targeted analysis for carrier testing of at-risk females and prenatal or preimplantation testing as requested. A variety of techniques are used for genetic testing of patients and at-risk family members.[293] Deletion and duplication testing for all 79 exons is frequently performed by multiplex ligation-dependent probe amplification assay (Fig. 68.7).[294] This method determines whether each exon is present, deleted, or duplicated compared with control DNA. Alternatively, microarray-based comparative genomic hybridization can be used for deletion and duplication screening[295] or MPS for the *DMD* gene is a useful tool for the detection of variants not detected using other screening methods.[296] In <5% of DMD and BMD patients, the pathogenic DNA variant is not identified. Although a muscle biopsy can be used to confirm

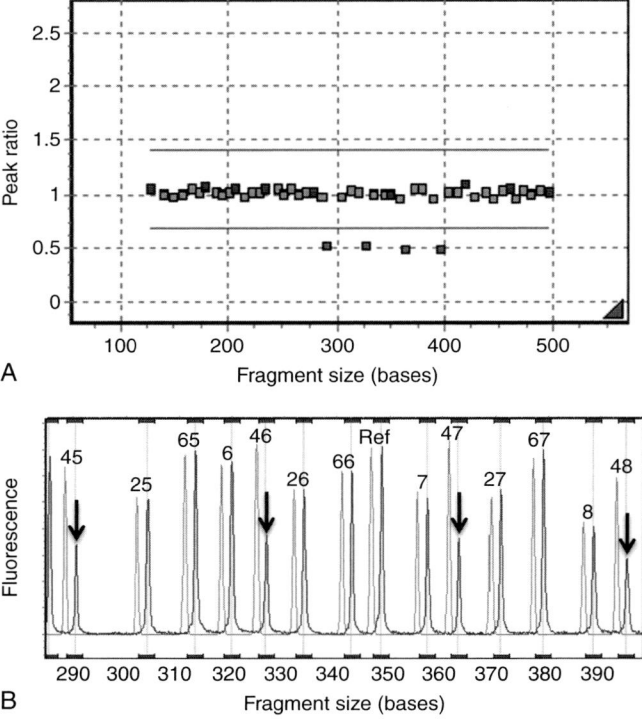

FIGURE 68.7 Deletion/duplication analysis of the *DMD* gene in a female patient by multiplex ligation-dependent probe amplification (*MLPA*). (A) Wild-type (normal) alleles demonstrate a peak ratio of about 1. In this example, the patient is positive for a deletion of 4 exons, shown with a peak ratio of approximately 0.5. Note that size does not correlate with exon number. (B) Electropherogram data showing the reduction in peak height (*y*-axis, relative fluorescence) for exons 45 to 48 (*arrows*) in one genotype (*grey peaks*) relative to the other control genotype (*black peaks*). Exons are denoted by numbers above the peaks.

the diagnosis, in the absence of the pathogenic variant, targeted *DMD* gene analysis is not possible for additional at-risk family members.

Particularly difficult are sporadic cases of DMD or BMD in which no other family member with DMD or BMD is known and no variant is identified in the proband. Generally, one third of sporadic cases are thought to represent a de novo variant in the mother's gamete from which that individual was derived.[292] In true sporadic cases, neither the mother nor female siblings are carriers, and the risk to the mother for a second affected son would be considered minimal. However, there are some apparent sporadic cases in which a female in these families could be a carrier who, although clinically asymptomatic, would be at risk of having an affected child.[297] Furthermore, carrier assessment can be complicated by the phenomenon of germline mosaicism, in which no *DMD* gene variant is present in lymphocyte DNA but a *DMD* disease causing gene variant is present in the germline tissue. These de novo variants occur during mitosis in germline proliferation and explain the report of multiple affected children of women whose lymphocyte DNA contains no *DMD* disease-causing variants. If no variant within the family is known, linkage analysis using intragenic and *DMD* flanking polymorphic markers can be used for carrier, prenatal, and pre-implantation genetic testing.[298]

Although no curative treatment for DMD is available, innovative therapies are emerging.[299,300] Clinical trials are in progress utilizing recombinant adeno-associated virus (AAV) vectors which can accommodate insertions of small amount of human dystrophin gene sequences.[301] This *micro-dystrophin* gene therapy has initially demonstrated successful delivery to skeletal muscle of patients. Suppression of variants causing premature truncation of the dystrophin protein generated by base pair substitutions in about 10 to 15% of patients can be accomplished with some success using the drug ataluren. Alternatively, for the majority of patients with gene deletions or duplications, exon skipping using antisense oligonucleotide therapy targeting specific exons has been successful for exon 51 using eteplirsen which has received FDA approval.[302] Alternative therapeutic approaches and new targets linked to the pathogenesis of the disease are being evaluated including use of the patient's stem cells and gene editing by homologous recombination (CRISPR-Cas9).[303–305]

Fragile X Syndrome

Fragile X syndrome (FXS) (OMIM #300624) is one of the most commonly inherited forms of intellectual disability, with an estimated incidence of approximately 1 in 4000 males and approximately 1 in 8000 females. The name of the condition reflects the cytogenetic abnormality of a breakpoint or fragile site in the X chromosome. The clinical syndrome was first described by Martin and Bell in 1943 in a family with sex-linked mental retardation in both males and females yet who had no dysmorphic features.[306] The disease was later redefined by Lubs, who noted the presence of a marker X chromosome in leukocytes of males incubated in cell culture media depleted of folate and thymidine and that segregated with mental retardation within the family.[307]

The chromosomal locus for this fragile site was later localized to Xq27.3.[308] Common clinical features associated with FXS are intellectual disability, delayed motor and speech development, macroorchidism, long face, prominent forehead

and jaw, large ears, flat feet, and abnormal behavioral characteristics (e.g., hyperactivity, hand flapping, temper tantrums, persevering speech patterns, poor eye contact, and autism spectrum disorder [ASD]).[309] FXS represents about 2 to 3% of patients with ASD.[310] The features of FXS are often milder in affected females than in affected males because of random X inactivation of the abnormal fragile X gene in females with the expression of the normal gene theoretically in half of their tissues.[311] The primary molecular basis of FXS includes expansion of the 5′ UTR (untranslated region) CGG repeat sequence coupled with hypermethylation and histone deacetylation of this region and the adjacent CpG island in the promoter region of the *FMR1* gene.[312–316] This results in transcriptional silencing of the gene and no production of the associated *FMR1* protein, FMRP. Males with full expansion alleles but incomplete methylation (methylation mosaic males) and mosaic males with a premutation allele in some tissues and a full expansion allele in others, have some production of FMRP and have higher cognitive function as compared to full mutation males with no FMRP.[317] It is important to note that FXS has been reported to be caused by other disease-causing variants in *FMR1* including single exon or large gene deletions and single nucleotide substitutions.[318,319]

As a sex-linked disease, FXS has a complicated inheritance pattern. Affected females are heterozygous for the expanded variant, and unaffected males can transmit the premutation allele to offspring in the family. For this reason, Sherman and colleagues proposed that FXS was an X-linked dominant disorder with reduced penetrance (79% for males and 35% for females), but the penetrance of the disease appeared to increase in subsequent generations within a family.[320,321] The mechanism of this "Sherman paradox" was resolved when the gene causing FXS, *FMR1* (Fragile X *m*ental *r*etardation 1), was cloned in 1991.[312,322–325] *FMR1* was the first gene discovered to cause disease through expansion of an unstable trinucleotide repeat sequence. The gene spans 38 kb, with 17 exons, and encodes a 4.4-kb mRNA transcript that contains 190 bp of the 5′UTR.[326] *FMR1* mRNA is expressed in neural and nonneural tissues during embryonic development and throughout life.[327] The primary *FMR1* protein, FMRP, is a ~80-kDa transacting RNA-binding protein with multiple domains for chromatin-binding, RNA-binding domains, and protein binding domains along with a nuclear localization signal and a nuclear export sequence.[328,329] FMRP is most abundant in the brain, testes, and ovaries, correlating with the two most prominent features of this disease, intellectual disability and macroorchidism. In the neurons, FMRP shuttles mRNAs from the nucleus to the cytoplasm, but it predominantly resides in postsynaptic spaces of dendritic spines, where it is associated with polyribosomes and plays a role in the regulation of translation of mRNAs important for synaptic plasticity.[330–332] Several models have been proposed to explain the process by which FMRP inhibits mRNA translation, including (1) blockage of translation initiation, (2) stalling of the polyribosome during translation, and (3) repression of translation via the RNA interference pathway.[330] Thus loss of function of FMRP in fragile X patients results in abnormal translation profiles and altered synapse structure and signaling. FMRP mRNA targets are large in number yet are specific, with binding occurring only to mRNA transcripts with specific motifs.[333] Most well characterized is FMRPs' normal steady-state repression of translationally upregulated mRNAs in response to stimulation of group 1 metabotropic glutamate receptors (mGluRs). Upon mGluR activation, FMRP is dephosphorylated, translation inhibition ceases, mRNA translation is enabled, and long-term depression of synaptic transmission occurs. In the absence of FMRP in fragile X patients, there is constitutive translation of these mRNAs in the absence of mGluR activation and excessive and prolonged synaptic long-term depression. However, clinical trials using GluR antagonists for patients with fragile X have been largely unsuccessful.[334] Treatment for patients is largely supportive to manage symptoms yet multiple therapeutic approaches for FXS are in consideration.[335–339] Possible strategies include gene replacement, CGG repeat deletion, *FMR1* reactivation, regain of translation efficiency, and correction of dysregulated pathways. In the 5' UTR of *FMR1*, blocks of CGG repeats are generally 7 to 13 repeats in length, and can be interspersed with single AGG repeats.[340,341] Allelic diversity results from the variable numbers and lengths of these CGG-repeat blocks. Normal alleles have 5 to 44 repeats; gray zone, intermediate, or borderline alleles have 45 to 54 repeats; premutation alleles have 55 to 200; and full expansion alleles contain more than 200 repeats (Table 68.6). Individuals with a normal number of CGG repeats do not have FXS, nor are they at risk of having an affected child. Individuals with 45 to 54 repeats represent alleles in the upper range of normal and are referred to as gray zone alleles. These individuals do not have FXS, yet some families may have a slightly increased risk of repeat instability and expansion to a *FMR1* premutation allele in their offspring. Premutation alleles, CGG repeats 55 to 200 repeats, are unstable and can expand to a full variant allele of >200 CGG repeats, and are associated with a risk of an offspring with FXS. However, a large expansion to a full variant is largely confined to maternal transmissions. Alternatively, premutation alleles can remain stable or increase to a larger premutation allele. Less commonly, a premutation allele can contract to a smaller premutation allele, a gray zone allele, or even to a normal allele.[342] The risk of CGG expansion from a premutation to a full variant allele is dependent on both *cis*- and *trans*-acting factors, including the number of pure uninterrupted CGG repeats, the number and position of interspersed AGG repeats, maternal age, haplotype background, and less well-characterized heritable factors.[343–348] As

the CGG-repeat length increases, the risk of expansion from a premutation to a full variant in premutation carrier females increases. A premutation carrier female with a premutation CGG repeat length of 55 to 59 has about a 5% risk of expansion to a full variant, a woman with a repeat length of 70 to 79 has a 31% risk of expansion, and a woman with a CGG-repeat length greater than 100 has close to a 100% chance of expansion.[349] Although CGG repeat length is the best predictor of maternal premutation expansion, AGG interruptions reduce the risk of transmission for CGG repeat lengths below 100. Nolin et al. examined 457 maternal transmissions, including intermediate (45 to 54) and small premutation alleles (55 to 69) and reported that 97% of premutation alleles with 0 AGG repeats were unstable, displaying an increase in CGG repeat number compared with only 19% of alleles with two interspersed AGG repeats. Only 9 of these 457 transmissions resulted in a full variant, which originated from a CGG repeat with no interspersed AGG repeats. This study supports the low frequency of full variant expansion from CGG repeat numbers below 65 and the relevance of AGG repeats for reducing the risk of expansion.[346] Thus the presence of AGG repeat numbers within CGG repeats can be incorporated into risk assessment for the premutation carrier patient at risk of having a child with FXS.[346,347]

Most CGG expansion occurs before zygote formation. CGG expansion that occurs after zygote formation will result in mosaicism with the presence of cells containing either a premutation or full variant *FMR1* allele. CGG repeat expansion occurs during DNA replication through either the incorporation of looped DNA intermediates on the nascent leading or lagging strand or stalling and restarting of the replication fork.[344,350] Alternatively, abnormal processes in DNA repair may be involved in the mechanism of expansion.[351] Premutation carriers do not have fragile X syndrome. Although *FMR1* is overexpressed in these individuals, FMRP is diminished, indicating reduced translation efficiency (see Table 68.6). The incidence of a premutation allele in females is estimated to be between 1 in 200 females.[341,352] About 20% of premutation carrier females have fragile X associated primary ovarian insufficiency (FXPOI) with cessation of menstrual periods before 40 years of age.[342,353] Interestingly, women with premutation alleles between 80 and 100 repeats have the highest risk

---

TABLE 68.6 FMR1 Alleles and Associated Fragile X (FX) Phenotype

CGG Repeat Number	Frequency	RNA	Protein	Phenotype
5–44 Normal	Predominant In Population	Normal expression	Normal amount	Normal
45–54 Gray zone	1/66 male 1/112 female	Normal expression	Normal amount	Normal
55–200 Premutation	1/800 male 1/200 female	Increased expression with gain of function (RNA toxicity)	Decreased amount	FX tremor ataxia syndrome (75% by age 80) Increased risk for neurodevelopmental problems FX primary ovarian insufficiency (20%) FX tremor ataxia syndrome (16%) Increased risk for mild cognitive impairment
>200 Full mutation	1/4000 male 1/8000 female	Absent	Absent	Intellectual disability, macroorchidism, delayed motor and speech development, long face, prominent forehead and jaw, large ears, autism spectrum disorder

of developing FXPOI. Toxicity from increased expression of premutation *FMR1* mRNA contributes to these clinical symptoms.[343,354] As expected, full variant carrier females with no *FMR1* mRNA do not develop ovarian dysfunction, thereby suggesting that decreased or absent FMRP is not contributory to this phenotype. In addition, premutation carrier females are at an increased risk for other medical, reproductive, psychiatric, and cognitive features compared with noncarrier control participants.[344,355]

Premutation carrier males are less common and are estimated at 1 in 800 males.[341,352] Although premutation carrier males do not have fragile X syndrome, they do have neurodevelopmental problems, including higher rates of attention deficit disorder, shyness, social deficits, and ASDs.[356] Further, as adults, about one third of premutation carrier males older than the age of 50 years exhibit fragile X–associated tremor and ataxia syndrome (FXTAS) with 17% of males between the ages of 50 and 59 years and as many as 75% of males older than 80 years of age affected.[357] FXTAS is a neurodegenerative syndrome characterized by progressive intention tremor, cerebellar gait ataxia, parkinsonism, neuropathy, cognitive decline, psychiatric features, and generalized brain atrophy.[358] Although predominantly in premutation carrier males, FXTAS can be seen in up to 16% of premutation carrier females. The lower incidence of FXTAS in females may be explained by the presence of a second X chromosome with a normal *FMR1* gene expressed in approximately half of all cells. The pathogenesis of FXTAS likely results from multiple factors, including (1) increased expression of *FMR1* mRNA, resulting in a gain-of-function through sequestration of specific proteins and a loss of their normal function; (2) translation of unique (CGG) proteins without an AUG start site; or (3) antisense transcription from the *FMR1* locus and decreased production of FMRP.[359]

DNA testing for FXS is primarily performed using triplet primed PCR.[360,361] This assay utilizes three primers, including a forward and reverse primer specific to this unique area within the genome and a third oligonucleotide complementary to the CGG repeat itself (Fig. 68.8). The methylation status of the CGG repeat in a full variant allele can also be assessed using PCR.[362] *FMR1* DNA testing for fragile X syndrome is often requested for children with (1) the fragile X phenotype, (2) developmental delay, (3) intellectual disability, (4) ASD, or (5) family members of individuals with a diagnosis of fragile X syndrome. Fragile X DNA testing is generally performed for carrier testing in at-risk pregnant or preconception female patients with a family history of fragile X or intellectual disability of unknown cause. Prenatal testing can be performed on chorionic villi tissue or cultured amniocytes for at-risk pregnancies. Preimplantation diagnosis for fragile X syndrome has been reported but can be complicated by ovarian dysfunction in premutation carrier females.[363] *FMR1* premutation allele testing is performed on patients with clinical suspicion of FXPOI or FXTAS. NBS for FXS, although feasible from blood spots as demonstrated from several pilot studies, is not currently included in NBS panels.[364,365] NBS enables early detection and intervention for the affected child but also identifies at-risk family members who did not consent to this test and may not wish to know personal health information regarding their own risk for late-onset disorders such as FXPOI and FXTAS. Educational resources and counseling programs regarding the

medical implications of the various *FMR1* alleles identified through NBS need to be established before implementation of such programs.

Rett Syndrome

Rett syndrome (OMIM #312750) is an X-linked dominant cause of inherited intellectual disability with an estimated incidence of 1 in 10,000 female births. This disorder was first described in a cohort of patients with identical wringing of their hands by Dr. Andreas Rett in 1966.[366] However, it was not until the 1980s when additional studies described similar patients that the syndrome was given its name. Rett syndrome is characterized by progression in stages with initial normal development up to age 18 months followed by a period of developmental inactivity and overall signs of failure to thrive (e.g., microcephaly, weight loss).[367,368] This stage is quickly followed by a period of rapid developmental regression and the loss of purposeful hand movement. It is during this period that patients exhibit signs of autism and profound intellectual disability. Rett syndrome is also marked by progressive motor deterioration that typically results in patients being wheelchair bound by their teens.[367,369] Although some patients have unexplained death,[370] many patients survive into the sixth or seventh decade of life. It should be noted that Rett syndrome is almost exclusively observed in females because *MECP2* variants in males are typically embryonic lethal.

Identification of the genetic cause of Rett syndrome was initially difficult because traditional linkage methods were ineffective due to the sporadic nature of the disease.[369] However, using exclusion mapping methods, it was determined that the causative gene for Rett syndrome was located at chromosome Xq28.[371–375] Systematic analysis of this region identified variants in the methyl-CpG binding protein 2 (*MECP2*) gene as causative for Rett syndrome in 1999.[376] The *MECP2* gene is composed of four exons that produce two different protein isoforms.[369,377] The protein produced by the *MECP2* gene is a chromosome binding protein expressed in all tissues that specifically targets 5-methyl cytosine residues.[378] MECP2 contains three functional domains: a methyl-CpG binding domain (MBD),[379] a transcriptional repression domain (TRD),[380] and a C-terminal domain (CTD).[381] The MBD specifically binds to methylated cytosine residues and shows a preference for binding to CpG dinucleotide sequences that are adjacent to A/T-rich motifs.[382] Downstream from the MBD is the TRD, which is critical in the interaction of MECP2 with histone deacetylases and other transcription corepressors.[369,376,377,380–383] Finally, the CTD enables MECP2 binding to the nucleosome core and allows the protein to bind to naked DNA.[369,377] All of these domains are essential for the MECP2 protein to properly function, and variants in each of these domains have been found in patients with Rett syndrome. However, the vast majority of disease-causing variants are found in either the MBD or TRD.[367]

MECP2 gene variants are identified in approximately 95% of patients with a classic Rett syndrome phenotype.[346] To date, more than 900 *MECP2* unique gene variants have been reported in the literature, and newly identified variants are regularly added to the RettBASE online variant database.[367,384,385] Described pathogenic *MECP2* gene variants include nonsense, missense, frameshift, and large deletions.[367,384,385] Interestingly, variants at eight common residues account for approximately

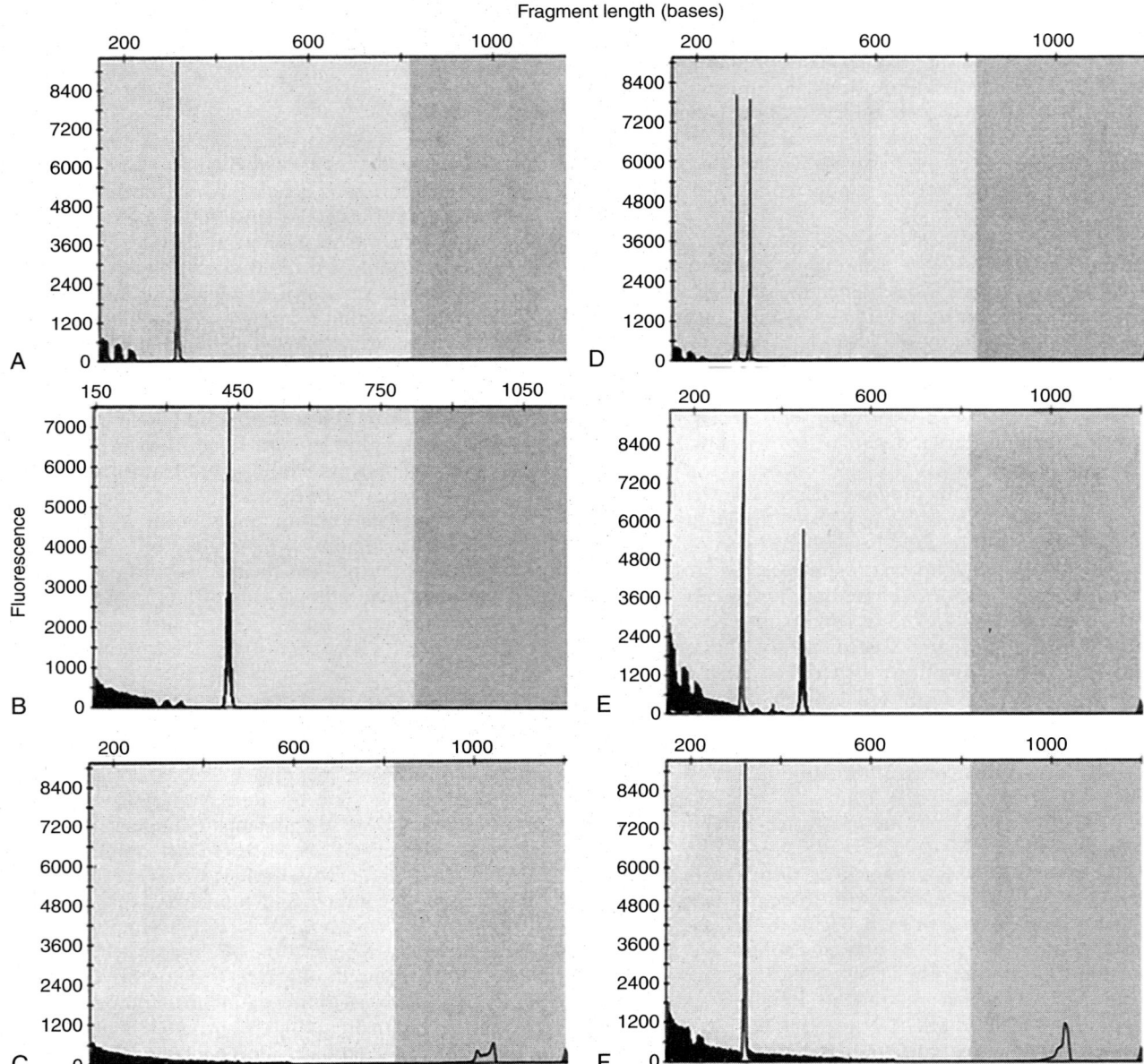

FIGURE 68.8 Electropherograms of PCR products of the CGG repeat number in exon 1 of the *FMR1* gene. Amplicon sizes in bases are noted at the top of the panels and the relative amount of fluorescence detected for each amplicon is measured by the peak height (*y*-axis). Results were generated using the AmplideX kit (Asuragen, Inc.). PCR products were amplified by using a primer pair flanking the CGG repeat of the *FMR1* gene and a 15-bp oligonucleotide as a primer within the CGG repeat itself. (A) A normal male with a CGG repeat number of 29 corresponding to an amplicon of 316 bp in length. (B) A premutation carrier male with a CGG repeat number of 67 and an amplicon 430 bp in length. (C) The characteristic full mutation pattern obtained from a male with fragile X syndrome with more than 200 CGG repeats. (D) A pattern from a normal female with CGG repeats of 20 and 30 corresponding to amplicons at 289 and 319 bp, respectively. (E) A premutation female with CGG repeats of 29 and 74 corresponding to amplicons of 316 and 454 bp, respectively. (F) A female affected with fragile X syndrome with both a normal *FMR1* allele with 31 CGG repeats corresponding to an amplicon of 322 bp, and a second *FMR1* allele with a full mutation with CGG repeats greater than 200 *(pink shaded area)*.

47% of all cases.[367] These common variants all occur in CpG dinucleotides and include p.Arg106, p.Arg133, p.Thr158, p.Arg168, p.Arg255, p.Arg270, p.Arg294, and p.Arg306 (Fig. 68.9). Because there is a large degree of phenotypic heterogeneity in patients with Rett syndrome, several studies have been performed to correlate genotype with phenotype. Truncating (nonsense or frameshift) variants cause a more severe phenotype than missense variants, and variants that occur in the CTD typically result in milder disease presentation.[367,369,386] The majority of variants in *MECP2* are de novo events.[387,388] However, there are cases in which variants are maternally inherited from an individual who is either unaffected or mildly

CHAPTER 68 Genetics **955**

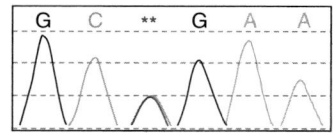

FIGURE 68.9 Sanger sequencing of the *MECP2* gene illustrating a common pathogenic variant (c.808C>T; p.Arg270Ter) *(asterisk)*. This C>T transition variant results in a stop codon *(TGA)* and premature truncation of the protein.

affected because of skewed X-inactivation. It is therefore important to establish whether a pathogenic variant is de novo or maternally derived as the recurrence risk in future pregnancies of variant-positive females with skewed X-inactivation approaches 50%.

Because of the heterogeneous nature of disease-causing variants in *MECP2*, clinical testing for confirmation of a diagnosis of Rett syndrome typically involves DNA sequencing of the entire *MECP2* gene coding region. If variants are not identified by sequencing analysis, large deletion and duplication analysis (typically MLPA) is performed. This combination detects approximately 95% of causative variants in patients with a clinical diagnosis of Rett syndrome. Recently, variants in the *CDKL5* and *FOXG1* genes have been shown to cause variant forms of Rett syndrome and should therefore be considered for follow-up testing in individuals not found to have variants in *MECP2*.[368,389–395] Alternatively, consideration may be given to an MPS-based gene panel that includes a number of genes associated with Rett (and Rett-like syndromes).[368] However, as noted elsewhere, the risk for uncertain results increases with the utilization of large gene panels. Although a number of Rett syndrome clinical trials have been conducted over the past few decades, none have resulted in updated therapeutic strategies.[367] Therefore Rett syndrome treatment is largely based on the manifestations of disease and therefore should be tailored to each individual patient.

Complex Diseases

A complex or multifactorial inheritance pattern suggests interaction of one or more genes in combination with lifestyles and one or more environmental factors. Multifactorial diseases can be prevalent in some families with several affected family members, but the disease does not follow typical Mendelian inheritance patterns. A disease may present in multiple family members because of the sharing of similar disease-predisposing alleles and often sharing of similar daily habits, routines, and diet. The specific genes, lifestyle habits, and environmental factors and their respective contribution in predisposition to disease vary among diseases and are difficult to elucidate. Twin studies are often used to determine the relative importance of each component. Among twins who were raised together, a greater concordance of disease among monozygotic (MZ) twins (who share all of their genes) than among dizygotic (DZ) twins (who share 50% of their genes) provides strong evidence of a genetic component of the disease. Conversely, disease concordance of less than 100% in MZ twins is strong evidence that nongenetic factors play a role in the disease process. Large genome-wide association studies (GWAS) are used to identify genes and genetic variants that play a role in the pathogenesis of common complex diseases. Examples of complex adult-onset diseases include type 1 diabetes, rheumatoid arthritis, multiple sclerosis,

osteoporosis, Parkinson disease, Alzheimer disease, hypertension, atrial fibrillation, alcoholism, schizophrenia, depression, obesity, and thrombophilia.

Thrombophilia

Thrombophilia is defined as an abnormality of hemostasis with a predisposition to thrombosis. A common complication of venous thromboembolism (VTE) is the development of a deep vein thrombosis (DVT) or a more serious, and potentially fatal, pulmonary embolism. Thrombophilia (OMIM #188050) is a multifactorial disorder resulting from the interaction of genetic, lifestyle, and environmental factors. Risk factors include the use of oral contraceptives, hormone replacement therapy, trauma, obesity, malignancy, surgery, immobility, pregnancy, and advanced age.[396]

Protein products of many genes are involved in the anticoagulation and coagulation pathway to regulate hemostasis. Hypercoagulability, or an alteration in the coagulation pathway that predisposes to thrombosis, can be caused by variants in genes encoding proteins involved in the coagulation pathway. Although familial thrombophilia can be attributed to mutations in genes encoding protein C, *PROC* (OMIM #176860); protein S, *PROS1* (OMIM #612336); or antithrombin III, *SERPINC1* (OMIM #107300), 50 to 60% of familial thrombophilia is associated with variants in genes encoding coagulation factor V, *FV* (OMIM #188055) or factor II, *F2* (OMIM #176930). In 1993, Dahlbäck reported that familial thrombophilia caused resistance to activated protein C (APC).[397] In 1994, Bertina and colleagues reported linkage of a common G-to-A base substitution at nucleotide 1691 (c.1691G>A) in exon 10 of the *FV* gene with the APC resistance phenotype.[398] This nucleotide change results in an arginine-to-glutamine substitution in the FV protein at codon 506 (p.Arg506Gln) and is commonly referred to as FV Leiden, named for the Dutch city where it was discovered. The c.1691G>A substitution is common in the white population of Northern European descent with a reported frequency of about 3 to 5%, but it is absent in other populations, including those in Africa and Southeast Asia.

The *FV* gene is localized to chromosome 1q24.2, is about 72 kb, contains 25 exons, and encodes a 330 kDa protein.[399] In the coagulation pathway, FV is converted to an activated form, FVa, by thrombin. FVa is a cofactor for activated factor X, FXa, and is required for the conversion of prothrombin (F2) to thrombin (F2a). Thrombin is essential for the last step of the coagulation cascade by catalyzing the conversion of fibrinogen to fibrin for clot formation. Activated FV is converted to an inactive form by APC. The arginine residue at codon 506 is one of three peptide bonds (Arg306, Arg506, and Arg679) cleaved by APC to inactivate FV and decrease the affinity to FXa, thereby reducing the conversion of prothrombin to thrombin.[400,401] Substitution of a glutamine residue at this site prolongs APC inactivation of FVa by approximately 10-fold, thereby shifting the balance of hemostasis to favor coagulation and increasing thrombin production.[402]

Heterozygous *FV* gene c.1691G>A carriers have a lifelong 5- to 10-fold increased relative risk of venous thrombosis compared with an increased relative risk for homozygotes as high as 10- to 20-fold.[403] However, FV Leiden does not confer increased risk for arterial thrombosis.[404] The mean age of onset of symptoms associated with thrombosis is 44 years for heterozygotes and 31 years for homozygotes.[405]

FV c.1691G>A carriers represent about 25% of patients with idiopathic VTE, 30 to 50% of patients with recurrent VTE, 20 to 60% of oral contraceptive–associated VTE, 20 to 40% of pregnancy-associated VTE, and 8 to 30% of patients with pregnancy loss.[406] Although *FV* gene variants are considered dominant (heterozygous variant carriers can be symptomatic), many heterozygous carriers remain asymptomatic because thrombophilia is a complex disease resulting from the interaction of genetic, lifestyle, and environmental factors.

Several years later, also in Leiden, Poort and coworkers described a genetic variant in the 3′ untranslated region of the *F2* gene present in 18% of patients with a documented family history of venous thrombosis.[407] The *F2* gene maps to chromosome 11p11.2, is ~21 kb in length, contains 14 exons, and encodes a 70-kDa protein.[408] The *F2* 3′ variant that segregated with disease, c.*97G>A, results in increased levels of plasma coagulation F2, prothrombin, and a 2.8-fold lifelong increased risk of venous thrombosis.[407] Inherited together, *FV* c.1691G>A and *F2* c.*97G>A convey a lifelong 20-fold increased risk for a VTE event, indicating an example of additive genetic effects associated with a complex disease.[404] The c.*97G>A variant allele is largely confined to white populations at a frequency of 1 to 2% and is rare in other populations. FII requires activation and conversion to thrombin by FXa and FVa to catalyze the conversion of fibrinogen to fibrin, the last step of blood clot formation. The G-to-A substitution does not alter the coding region of the protein; rather, it enhances prothrombin mRNA stability and ultimately results in increased production of both prothrombin and thrombin.[409]

Venous thromboembolism most often is classified as "provoked" with one or more predisposing risk factors. In 25 to 50% of cases, it is "unprovoked" with the precipitating cause not determined and an increased risk of reoccurrence compared to those with a provoked VTE.[410] The initial treatment of patients with VTE uses both heparin and vitamin K antagonists (e.g., warfarin). After several days, the heparin is discontinued, and warfarin therapy is continued. For "provoked" VTE, therapy is discontinued after 3 months for distal DVT and 6 months for proximal DVT or PE. Therapy may be altered based on the type of thrombotic event, the type of precipitating event, or the absence of a triggering cause. The recurrence risk is higher in "unprovoked" VTE and in patients with cancer, suggesting prolonged or indefinite anticoagulant therapy and D-dimer levels may identify patients for continued anticoagulation therapy.[411,412] Antithrombic agents may be most advantageous in the management of pregnancy VTE and associated thrombophilia.[413] To avoid the risk of bleeding with sometimes fatal complications, treatment is regularly monitored using prothrombin time reported as the international normalized ratio (INR) ideally achieving an INR of 2.0 to 3.0. Historically, anticoagulant therapy for thrombophilic patients has included warfarin or heparin, however, more recently FIIa and FXa inhibitors can be used that provide a lower risk of bleeding complications and appear to provide similar efficacy compared to standard treatment.[414]

Another genetic risk factor for predisposition to thrombophilia is a common 1-bp guanine deletion/insertion (4G/5G) polymorphism at c.-817dupG in the promoter region of the *SERPINE1* gene located on chromosome 7q22.1 (OMIM#173360).[415] This gene is approximately 12.2 kb in length with nine exons and encodes a mature 379-amino-acid protein with a molecular weight of about 42.7 kDa.[416-418] This protein, plasminogen activator inhibitor-1 (PAI-1), is a member of the serine protease inhibitor family and is released by endothelial cells to block the degradation of fibrin clots. Increased levels of PAI-1 can be associated with thrombophilia, and the *SERPINE1* 4G allele is associated with higher transcription levels than the 5G allele.[415,419,420] Patients with the 4G allele coupled with the FV variant had a higher risk of VTE.[421] A variety of DNA testing platforms have been used for the detection of *FV* c.1691G>A and *F2* c.*97G>A variants, including Invader chemistry, PCR coupled with restriction-endonuclease digestion and gel electrophoresis, exonuclease probe PCR, or real-time PCR followed by melting curve analysis with fluorescence resonance energy transfer probes (Figs. 68.10 and 68.11). The most common testing methods for the 4G/5G *SERPINE1* polymorphism involve the use of PCR and melting curve analysis or PCR coupled with capillary electrophoresis and fragment analysis. Any testing platform is acceptable for clinical use as long as the procedure has been properly validated in a CLIA-certified laboratory that follows appropriate regulatory and quality assurance guidelines.

DNA testing for factor V Leiden may be requested when a patient tests positive on the functional activated protein C resistance assay to both confirm the diagnosis and distinguish between *FV* c.1691G>A heterozygotes and homozygotes.[422] At many hospitals, screening for *FV* variants using the functional activated protein C resistance assay is the preferred method because it is cost effective, can be automated, and can easily be performed in hospitals that do not have a molecular diagnostic laboratory.[423] However, DNA testing should be ordered in place of the functional assay for patients taking FIIa or FVa oral inhibitors (e.g., argatroban, dabigatran, bivalirudin, or rivaroxaban) because these can interfere with the functional assay causing a falsely normal result. Similarly, inaccurate results can be obtained in patients with lupus anticoagulants.[422] The clinical utility of knowing the *FV* or *F2* genotype has been debated because it may not affect the clinical management of patients.[424] Yet testing for *FV* and *F2* variants is common in clinical practice, and most experts believe that testing is appropriate for targeted patients, including those with: (1) venous thrombosis or pulmonary embolism before 50 years of age; (2) venous thrombosis at an unusual site (hepatic, mesenteric, portal, or cerebral veins); (3) recurrent VTE; (4) VTE and a strong family history of thrombotic disease; (5) VTE in pregnancy, postpartum, or associated with contraceptive use or hormone replacement therapy; (6) unexplained recurrent pregnancy loss; or (7) patients with low activated protein C (APC) resistance activity.[425,426] In addition, screening may be considered for: (1) siblings of a *FV* or *F2* homozygous variant carrier, (2) female smokers < age 50 with a history of myocardial infarction, (3) pregnant females, (4) females that are considering pregnancy or the use of oral contraceptives who have a first-degree relative that had either an unprovoked VTE or a VTE during pregnancy or oral contraceptive use, or (5) if they have a first-degree relative who is a carrier of a *FV* or *F2* variant.[426] Routine screening before oral contraceptive use or hormone therapy is not recommended or cost-effective. Modifications to patient management after the identification of a *FV* or *F2* variant may involve length of treatment with anticoagulants

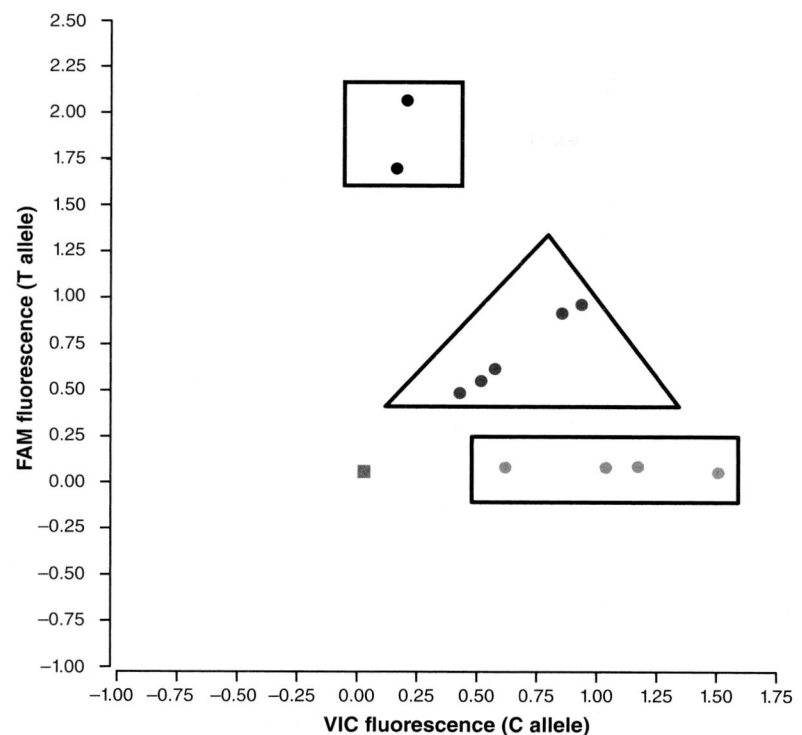

VIC C-reference	FAM T-variant	Genotype	Interpretation
0.586	0.608	C/T	Heterozygous
1.516	0.042	C/C	Normal
0.945	0.953	C/T	Heterozygous
1.047	0.069	C/C	Normal
0.170	1.697	T/T	Homozygous variant
1.180	0.069	C/C	Normal
0.864	0.908	C/T	Heterozygous
0.524	0.542	C/T	Heterozygous
0.622	0.071	C/C	Normal control
0.435	0.479	C/T	Heterozygous control
0.215	2.057	T/T	Homozygous variant control
0.035	0.051	N/A	Negative control

FIGURE 68.10 Genotype analysis for *FV* variant c.1691G>A using an exonuclease probe assay on a QuantStudio Real-Time PCR instrument (Thermo Fisher Scientific, Waltham, MA). Allelic discrimination data *(right)* with the corresponding scatter plot *(left)*. The *FV* single nucleotide polymorphism (SNP) genotyping assay contains two probes. Each probe contains a quencher molecule and a reporter molecule (either VIC or FAM). The DNA sequence of each probe is identical except at the position of the SNP. The probe complementary to the reference sequence c.1691G contains a C while the probe complementary to the variant c.1691G>A contains a T. The genotype is determined based on the amount of VIC and FAM measured for each sample *(right)*. A patient with both VIC and FAM detected in fairly similar amounts would be heterozygous for variant c.1691G>A. Samples with this genotype will cluster together as illustrated in the triangle on the scatter plot *(left)*. In this assay, a patient with only the VIC fluorochrome detected will be homozygous normal and these samples will cluster alongside each other as shown in the rectangle on the scatter plot. Samples homozygous for variant c.1691G>A will hybridize only to the probe with a T and the fluorochrome FAM and will have predominantly only this fluorochrome detected. These samples will cluster close to each other as demonstrated by the square on the scatter plot. The small square on the scatter plot represents the results obtained from the negative control specimen with no significant VIC or FAM fluorescence detected in that reaction tube.

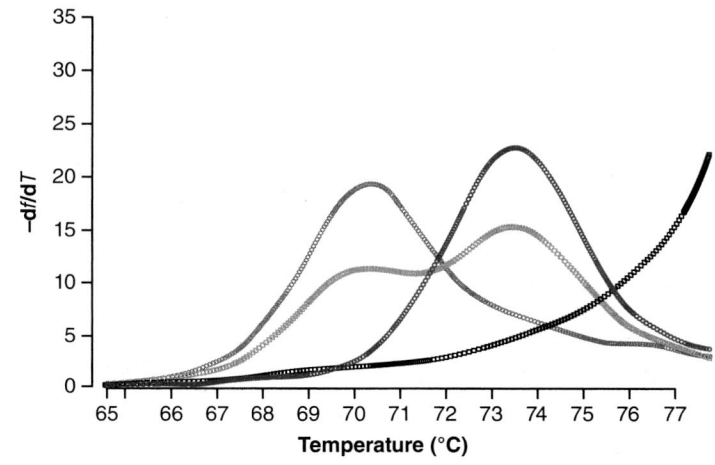

FIGURE 68.11 Interrogation of the common c.*97G>A variant in the *F2* gene by melting curve analysis. A perfectly matched probe is more tightly bound to the polymerase chain reaction (PCR) product and therefore will melt at a higher temperature than when there is a nucleotide mismatch between the probe and the PCR product. In this example, the probe perfectly matches the wild-type allele *(red)*. When the *F2* c.*97G>A variant is heterozygous, the probe binds to the variant allele imperfectly (with a lower melting temperature) and to the wild-type allele perfectly, resulting in the presence of two peaks *(pink)*. When a patient is homozygous for the c.*97G>A variant, only an imperfect match is possible, resulting in a single peak at the lower temperature *(gray)*. A no-template control is always included to rule out potential DNA contamination *(black)*. *Y*-axis denotes the negative derivative of fluorescence with respect to temperature $(-df/dT)$.

and management of other procoagulation risk factors. First-degree relatives of *FV* or *F2* variant positive patients are at a higher risk of related thrombotic events if the proband was younger and experienced an "unprovoked" thrombophilic event. DNA testing for *FV* or *F2* variants is not recommended for the general population, prenatal carrier screening, or NBS. In addition, variants at two other factor V arginine-cleavage sites have been reported, but these variants are rare and are not part of routine *FV* DNA testing.[427] Although *FV* or *F2* variants are present in 50 to 60% of families with inherited thrombophilia, defects in protein C, protein S, and antithrombin are detected in 10 to 15% of families with inherited venous thrombosis. These less common coagulation deficiencies are typically diagnosed through immunologic or functional assays that do not involve DNA testing. Furthermore, unlike *FV* and *F2* genes, no single common variants in *PROC*, *PROS1*, or *SERPINEC1* have been identified.

Hereditary Pancreatitis

Hereditary pancreatitis (HP; OMIM# 167800) occurs in approximately 1 in 300,000 individuals.[428] HP traditionally refers to the occurrence of pancreatitis in two or more individuals in two or more generations of a family.[428] Additionally, HP can refer to individuals with disease-causing germline variants in any of the genes associated with the disorder.[429] Individuals affected with HP are typically characterized by acute pancreatitis (disease with a duration of a few days to a few weeks) that eventually progresses to chronic pancreatitis (disease with a duration > 6 months) over a period of years.[429,430] The onset of symptoms is difficult to predict, but most individuals with HP are first affected with acute pancreatitis by 10 to 12 years of age and chronic disease by age 20 years.[428,431] Given the inflammatory nature of the disease, HP patients are also at higher risk for pancreatic cancer than the general population and should be routinely screened.[432] The complex nature of disease (and variable penetrance) indicates that although genetics is a risk factor for disease, several environmental factors (e.g., diet, tobacco use, alcohol consumption) also contribute to disease manifestations.[428,431] Variants in the protease, serine, 1 (*PRSS1*) gene (also known as cationic trypsinogen, located at chromosome 7q35) are the most common genetic cause of pancreatitis, accounting for >60% of HP families.[428] Cationic trypsinogen is the main isoform of trypsinogen in human pancreatic juice and is involved in facilitating zymogen activation.[433-435] Variants in the *PRSS1* gene cause a gain of function and typically result in the constitutive autoactivation of the cationic trypsinogen protein.[436-440] These variants are inherited in an autosomal dominant manner with variable penetrance.[441] In fact, several studies conducted using large HP patient cohorts have reported that the penetrance of *PRSS1* variants ranges between 40 and 96%[442-449]; therefore predicting disease progression in presymptomatic individuals who carry pathogenic *PRSS1* gene variants is not possible because symptoms and onset are extremely variable even among affected members of the same family.

Several additional genetic risk factors for pancreatitis have been identified.[450-452] In 1998, variants in the *CFTR* gene (located at chromosome 7q31.2) were reported as a genetic cause of pancreatitis.[451] As discussed in detail earlier, *CFTR* gene variants are causative for the multisystem autosomal recessive disorder CF. One of the most common features of CF is altered pancreatic function, so the discovery of genetic

variants in the *CFTR* gene in patients with isolated pancreatic disease is not surprising. However, unlike individuals with classic CF disease who carry two severe *CFTR* gene variants, pancreatitis patients often carry a severe pathogenic *CFTR* gene variant on one chromosome and a mild variant on the other (or a mild variant on both chromosomes).[451] About 30% of patients with pancreatitis remained idiopathic and did not have variants in *PRSS1* or *CFTR*. In 2000, autosomal recessive variants in the serine protease inhibitor, Kazal type 1 (*SPINK1*) gene (located at chromosome 5q32), were reported as an additional cause of HP.[452] In this study, 96 patients with chronic pancreatitis were tested for variants in the *SPINK1* gene, and 23% of the patients tested positive for variants.[452] Interestingly, a single variant in codon 34 (p.Asn34Ser) was the most common variant identified.[452] The *SPINK1* gene produces a protein (SPINK1) that prevents premature trypsinogen activation through the inhibition of trypsin activity in the pancreas.[453] Therefore *SPINK1* variants may cause a decrease in the ability of SPINK1 protein to inhibit trypsin.[452] However, functional studies have been inconclusive and the exact mechanism by which *SPINK1* variants cause pancreatitis remains unknown.

Variants in the chymotrypsin C (*CTRC*) gene (located at chromosome 1p36.21) are the most recently described genetic cause of HP.[450] An international team of investigators screened a large cohort of German pancreatitis patients ($n = 901$) for variants in the *CTRC* gene.[450] *CTRC* variants were identified in 3.3% of this patient group, and subsequent studies in an Indian population identified *CTRC* variants in 14.1% of affected individuals.[450] Given the overrepresentation of *CTRC* variants in patients with pancreatitis (compared with control populations), the authors were able to conclude that variants in the *CTRC* gene increase the risk for pancreatitis.[450] The *CTRC* gene produces a digestive enzyme called chymotrypsin C (CTRC) that promotes proteolytic inactivation of trypsinogen and trypsin and is essential for limiting intrapancreatic trypsinogen activation.[454,455] Functional studies indicate that variants in *CTRC* are loss of function, resulting in diminished secretion ability, impaired catalytic activity, and an inability to degrade trypsin.[454] Similar to *SPINK1*, variants in the *CTRC* gene are autosomal recessive and require the presence of two pathogenic variants to cause disease.

DNA testing for pancreatitis is most often performed stepwise with Sanger sequencing of the *PRSS1* gene as the first step. The identification of a single pathogenic *PRSS1* gene variant confirms a diagnosis of HP in symptomatic patients and indicates a substantial risk for the development of disease in an asymptomatic individual. If *PRSS1* analysis is negative, Sanger sequencing of *CFTR*, *SPINK1*, and *CTRC* can be considered. All three of these genes are inherited in an autosomal recessive manner, and therefore identifying two pathogenic variants is required to confirm a diagnosis in a symptomatic individual. The identification of a single pathogenic variant may increase the risk for pancreatitis but, by itself, is not causative for disease. Comprehensive testing of all four HP-associated genes by an MPS-based gene panel can be performed as the initial test in HP patients. However, this may increase the complexity of the results obtained (e.g., variants of uncertain significance), so patients should be counseled carefully before ordering such a panel.

Even with the advances over the past decade in our understanding of the genetics responsible for HP, cases remain that are not explained by variants in a single gene.[428,430] These individuals appear to have complex disease that involve a number of pathogenic variants in several genes (e.g., *CFTR*, *SPINK1* and others) suggesting that gene–gene interactions govern their disease.[428,430] In fact, as many as one third of pancreatitis cases (acute and chronic) result from complex inheritance patterns.[429,456] In some cases, environmental factors may play a more significant role than genetics in the development of this disease.[456] A number of recent studies have identified additional genes involved in trypsin regulation (e.g., *CASR*, *CLDN2*) that may increase the risk of development of HP when combined with the appropriate environmental stimulus.[428,430,457,458] However, additional studies are required to further elucidate their role in HP.

Treatment for HP varies between acute and chronic disease. Pain management is the primary focus for patients with acute pancreatitis.[429] Patients are also counseled to abstain from activities that will predispose them to future attacks (e.g., smoking, alcohol consumption).[459] Patients with chronic pancreatitis may be treated with pancreatic enzyme replacement therapy to aid with digestion.[459] In some severe cases, patients may undergo total pancreatectomy with islet autotransplantation.[459] Additional treatment should be based on manifestations of disease such as diabetes mellitus.

Hereditary Breast and Ovarian Cancer

Breast cancer is the most common cancer in women with about 1 in 8 developing invasive cancer during their lifetime.[460] Approximately 5 to 10% of breast cancers appear to be familial, exhibiting dominant inheritance. Inherited breast cancer is associated with multiple cases of breast or ovarian cancer within the family, an early age of disease onset, bilateral disease or multiple cancers in the same breast, and an increased prevalence of male breast cancer. Epithelial carcinoma of the ovary is the fifth leading cause of death in women with a woman's lifetime risk of 1 in 78.[461]

Most hereditary breast and ovarian cancer (HBOC) syndrome patients have variants in *BRCA1* (OMIM #113705) or *BRCA2* (OMIM #600185). While these two genes collectively represent the highest percentage of patients, a significant number of variants in other genes, at much lower frequencies, can lead to inherited breast and ovarian cancer.[462–467] Like *BRCA1* and *BRCA2*, the encoded protein products of most of these genes play a role in genome stability and maintenance, some of which interact directly with *BRCA1* and *BRCA2*. In addition to a predisposition to breast and ovarian cancer, *BRCA1* and *BRCA2* germline variant carriers are at an increased risk for pancreas cancer and male carriers are at an increased risk for prostate and male breast cancer.[468] The incidence of *BRCA1/BRCA2* variants in the United States is estimated to be between 1 in 300 to 500.[469] However, the combined frequency of two founder variants in *BRCA1* c.68_69delAG (185delAG) c.5266dupC (5382insC) and one in *BRCA2* c.5946delT (6174delT) account for up to 99% of variants seen in the Ashkenazi Jewish population with a carrier frequency as high as almost 3%.[470]

Although dominantly inherited, *BRCA1/BRCA2* variant carriers do not possess a 100% certainty of developing cancer. Rather, as tumor suppressor genes, inactivation of both alleles is required for tumorigenesis. In a patient who has inherited a variant *BRCA1* or *BRCA2* allele, the second normal allele is altered and most often deleted via somatic DNA alterations

as is common in Knudson's two hit hypothesis in cancer cells.[471] By the age of 70 years, *BRCA1* variant carriers have between a 46 and 87% risk of developing breast cancer, an 83% chance of developing contralateral breast cancer after an initial cancer is found, and a 39 to 63% possibility of developing ovarian cancer.[472] Slightly lower frequencies are observed for *BRCA2* variant carriers who have a 38 to 84% risk of developing breast cancer, a 62% chance of developing contralateral breast cancer, and a 16.5 to 27% possibility of developing ovarian cancer by 70 years of age.[472] Penetrance of the disease in *BRCA1/BRCA2* variant carriers is determined by both other genes and lifestyle and environmental factors. Identified susceptibility factors influencing development of disease include parity; body mass index; age at menarche, menopause, and first full-term pregnancy; breastfeeding; smoking; and oral contraceptive usage.[473,474] Additional genetic susceptibility factors include variants in multiple genes or genetic regions such as *FGFR2*, *TOX3*, *MAP3K1*, *LSP1*, *SLC4A7*, 2q35, and 5p12 for *BRCA2* germline variant carriers and variants in *TOX3* and genetic factors located at 2q35 for *BRCA1* germline variant carriers.[475] Understanding susceptibility factors, both environmental and genetic, aid in appropriate counseling for patients by either increasing or decreasing their overall risks for the development of cancer and help guide their clinical management decisions for surgical interventions. Although *BRCA1* and *BRCA2* clinical testing has been available for more than 20 years, only about 20% of patients with breast or ovarian cancer who meet guidelines for inherited cancer testing are tested.[476] To prevent disease in *BRCA1/BRCA2* variant carrier women, population-based testing for all women as routine medical care has been proposed.[477] This screening would identify germline variant carriers and enable appropriate clinical management to reduce their lifetime cancer risks. Recently, in a paper from the American Society of Breast Surgeons, they proposed their role in facilitating the uptake of germline genetic testing for patients in whom inherited cancer predisposition genes may exist.[478] Similarly, a United States preventive services task force recommends that primary care clinicians should be more engaged in *BRCA1* and *BRCA2* risk assessments for their patients.[479]

Interestingly, *BRCA1*- and *BRCA2*-variant positive breast tumors have distinct morphologic and histologic findings.[480] *BRCA1* positive tumors were most frequently invasive ductal carcinomas (80%), grade 3 (77%) with the majority of tumors (69%) triple negative (TN) for the expression of estrogen (ER), progestin (PR), and *HER2*.[480] In contrast, *BRCA2*-variant positive breast tumors likewise were predominantly invasive ductal carcinomas (83%) but with relatively equal numbers of grade 2 (43%) and grade 3 (50%) observed. However, unlike *BRCA1* variant–positive tumors, only 16% were TN. Medullary carcinomas were more frequent in *BRCA1* variant–positive tumors (9.4%) compared with *BRCA2* (2.2%), and invasive lobular was seen more frequently in *BRCA2* variant positive tumors (8.4%) compared with *BRCA1* variant positive tumors (2.2%). Interestingly, *BRCA1*-variant TN tumors were highest in patients with an earlier age of onset, but TN tumors were more common in tumors from *BRCA2*-positive carriers with an older age of onset. Both *BRCA1* and *BRCA2* variant–positive ovarian tumors were morphologically similar, with most serous (66 and 70%) and grade 3 (77 and 73%), respectively. Overall, about 15% of ovarian cancers are associated with germline variants in *BRCA1/BRCA2,* and up to 25% of high-grade serous tumors are positive for germline variants in one of these two genes.[481] Although the median age for ovarian cancer is close to 60 years, it is about 10 years earlier in patients with a genetic predisposition to this disease. Recently, it was reported that germline *BRCA* positive endometrial carcinomas have distinct clinicopathologic findings including most notably high grade (79%) with no LOH of the normal allele (40%) and overall less favorable outcome.[482]

Using DNA linkage studies, Hall and coworkers mapped the gene for early-onset familial breast cancer to chromosome 17q21.[483] In 1994, *BRCA1* was cloned; it was later confirmed by several other investigators as the susceptibility gene in breast and ovarian cancer kindreds.[484–486] The *BRCA1* gene on chromosome 17q21.31 spans over 81 kb and is composed of 24 exons; 22 encode the 7.8-kb mRNA that is translated into a protein of 1863 amino acids. Exon 11, encoding 60% of the protein, is alternatively spliced in a number of tissues. In families not linked to *BRCA1*, a second susceptibility locus at chromosome 13q12-13 was proposed, and in 1995, *BRCA2* was cloned.[487–489] The *BRCA2* gene, 13q12.3, spans over 84kb, contains 27 exons, encodes an 11.5-kb mRNA, and is translated into a protein of 3418 amino acids.

BRCA1 is a widely expressed multifunctional, tumor suppressor protein that maintains genomic stability in the repair of double-strand breaks in DNA via the homologous recombination pathway and cell cycle checkpoint control.[467,490,491] BRCA1 also plays a role in transcription regulation, chromatin architecture, apoptosis, mRNA splicing, and ubiquitination of multiple proteins. Although a distinctly different protein, BRCA2 is also important in the repair of double-strand DNA breaks and in transcription regulation.[492] Because BRCA1/BRCA2-deficient tumors have aberrant DNA repair pathways, they are more sensitive to treatment options causing DNA damage such as platinum-based chemotherapies cisplatin and carboplatin. PARP (poly ADP ribose polymerase) inhibitors for the treatment of patients with BRCA1/ BRCA2-deficient tumors have been effective.[493] PARP1 is required for base excision repair and repair of DNA single-strand breaks. When PARP1 inhibition occurs in BRCA1/BRCA2 tumors, both double- and single-strand DNA breaks are not repaired, and cell death occurs. However, similar to other targeted therapy, resistant clones develop, and the effectiveness of therapy diminishes.

Variants in *BRCA1* and *BRCA2* are heterogeneous and are located throughout each gene with founder variants identified in many different ethnic populations.[494] Most variants represent loss-of-function alleles, with more than 75% of the reported variants as deletions, nonsense variants, or insertions, with deletions representing the majority. Many pathogenic missense variants occur at critical BRCA1- or BRCA2-protein binding sites that are required for normal function. Although the majority of variants detected are obviously pathogenic (e.g., nonsense or frameshift variants causing premature truncation of the protein), some detected gene variations may be family specific and may not result in an obvious biologic functional change to the protein based on *in silico* analysis. These variants of unknown significance (VUS) are most often missense, splice site, or small in-frame insertions or deletions. These may be as common as 7 to 15% of the reported *BRCA* variants in individuals of European

ancestry and can be even higher for patients of other ethnicities for which common variants have not been well characterized.[495] Segregation studies confirming linkage of VUS with disease can be performed if archived tissue or DNA from multiple family members is available. Unfortunately, in many situations, DNA from an adequate number of family members to perform these studies is not possible. The clinical significance for some VUS may become clear by sharing data between laboratories; however, at some testing sites, these databases remain proprietary.[496]

In families in which the clinical history is suggestive of hereditary breast and ovarian cancer, DNA tests for *BRCA1* and *BRCA2* may be requested. Testing should be considered for a woman if (1) there are at least three cases in her family of breast, ovarian, or pancreatic cancer at an early age or aggressive prostate cancer; (2) she has breast or epithelial ovarian cancer and is younger than 45 years; (3) both breast and ovarian cancers are present in her or in a family member; (4) she has breast or ovarian cancer and is of Ashkenazi Jewish descent; (5) she has a male relative with breast cancer; (6) she has a family member with a known *BRCA1* or *BRCA2* variant; or (7) she has breast cancer and a family history of *BRCA1*- or *BRCA2*-related tumors.[497] In addition, *BRCA1* and *BRCA2* testing should be performed on any man with breast cancer. Nevertheless, *BRCA1* and *BRCA2* variants can be found in families that do not meet these criteria, and variants may not be found even when expected.

Before testing, a genetic professional should discuss the likelihood of a *BRCA1* or *BRCA2* variant, the types of variants that may be identified, and that offspring and other family members may also be at risk for having a variant. Mathematical models are available to determine the likelihood of *BRCA1* or *BRCA2* variants, and these models can be used to assist in counseling.[498,499] After a *BRCA* variant has been detected, on-line tools such as All Syndromes Known to Man Evaluator can be used to guide patient counseling with information including risks for other cancers for the patient based on the patient's age and gene identified in the HBOC family.[500,501] Subsequently, targeted variant analysis can be performed in presymptomatic family members at risk for inheriting the variant. Counseling for presymptomatic patients may include discussing psychological issues involving the fear of cancer or medical procedures and cancer surveillance and potential risk-reducing surgery options if a variant is identified. Management of presymptomatic *BRCA1* or *BRCA2* variant–positive women is complex. The National Comprehensive Cancer Network Clinical Practice Guidelines in Oncology has established surgical and surveillance guidelines to decrease the risk of disease in these women.[502] The patient may wish to have prophylactic mastectomy, salpingo-oophorectomy, or both. Alternatively, she may choose to use increased surveillance and prevention strategies for the early detection of breast and ovarian cancer. Surveillance for breast cancer in *BRCA1* or *BRCA2* variant–positive individuals should include annual mammography and breast magnetic resonance imaging beginning at 25 years of age. Surveillance for ovarian cancer should include transvaginal ultrasonography and CA-125 measurement every 6 months beginning at age 35 or 10 years earlier than the earliest age of onset in the family.[503] Clinical management for patients with a *BRCA1* or *BRCA2* VUS is challenging, and the use of risk-reducing surgeries is appropriately lower.[504] In these cases, because a VUS may ultimately be reclassified as pathogenic, likely pathogenic, or even benign, counseling is recommended depending on personal and family medical history rather than solely on *BRCA* variants.[505]

For presymptomatic patients with a family history but no prior DNA testing for breast or ovarian cancer, the genetic professional should explain before testing the possibility of a VUS result and continued anxiety and uncertainty. In addition, the patient should understand the possibility of

false-negative results because (1) not all possible *BRCA1* or *BRCA2* gene variants may be detected (2) there may be possible variants in another breast cancer susceptibility gene. Since not all familial breast and/or ovarian cancer is due to *BRCA* variants, MPS analysis for a panel of breast- and/or ovarian-related cancer predisposing genes may be more appropriate and more cost effective (Table 68.7). This strategy reduces the possibility of a false-negative result by increasing the variant detection rate by a small percentage. Appropriate

TABLE 68.7 Common Inherited Breast, Gynecologic, and Gastrointestinal Cancer Susceptibility Genes

Gene	Location	Name	Function	Associated Cancer	Disease
APC	5q22.2	Adenomatous polyposis coli	Control of cell proliferation	Colon, small bowel, thyroid, liver, pancreas	Familial adenomatous polyposis
ATM	11q22.3	Ataxia-telangiectasia mutated	Cell cycle control	Breast, ovarian, gastric, hematologic	Ataxia-telangiectasia
AXIN2	17q24.1	Axin 2	Assumed WNT signaling pathway regulator	Colon	Oligodontia-colorectal cancer syndrome
BARD1	2q35	BRCA1-associated ring domain 1	DNA repair, apoptosis, cell cycle arrest	Breast, ovarian, brain	Familial breast cancer
BMPR1A	10q23.2	Bone morphogenetic protein receptor, type IA	Cell signaling, proliferation, and differentiation	Colon, stomach, pancreas	Familial juvenile polyposis
BRCA1	17q21.31	Breast cancer 1, early onset	DNA repair	Breast, ovarian, prostate, pancreas	Hereditary breast and ovarian cancer
BRCA2	13q13.1	Breast cancer 2, early onset	DNA repair	Breast, ovarian, prostate, pancreas, brain, kidney, gastric	Hereditary breast and ovarian cancer
BRIP1	17q23.2	BRCA1-interacting protein C-terminal helicase 1	DNA helicase, DNA repair	Breast, ovarian, hematologic	Fanconi anemia type J, familial breast cancer
CDH1	16q22.1	E-cadherin	Cell signaling, adhesion, and proliferation	Gastric, breast, ovarian, endometrium, prostate	Hereditary diffuse gastric cancer
CDKN2A	9p21.3	Cyclin-dependent kinase inhibitor 2A	Cell cycle control	Pancreas, skin	Pancreatic cancer/melanoma syndrome
CHEK2	22q12.1	Checkpoint kinase 2	Cell cycle control	Breast, prostate, colon, bone	Li-Fraumeni syndrome
EPCAM	2p21	Epithelial cell adhesion molecule	Cell adhesion, signaling, proliferation, differentiation, and migration	Colon, endometrium, ovary, stomach, small bowel, hepatobiliary tract, urinary tract, brain, pancreas, sebaceous	Lynch syndrome
GREM1	15q13.3	Gremlin 1	Control of cell proliferation	Colon	Hereditary mixed polyposis syndrome
MLH1	3p22.3	MutL homolog 1	DNA mismatch repair	Colon, endometrium, ovary, stomach, small bowel, hepatobiliary tract, urinary tract, brain, pancreas, sebaceous	Lynch syndrome
MSH2	2p21	MutS homolog 2	DNA mismatch repair	Colon, endometrium, ovary, stomach, small bowel, hepatobiliary tract, urinary tract, brain, pancreas, sebaceous	Lynch syndrome
MSH6	2p16.3	MutS homolog 6	DNA mismatch repair	Colon, endometrium, ovary, stomach, small bowel, hepatobiliary tract, urinary tract, brain, pancreas, sebaceous	Lynch syndrome

Continued

TABLE 68.7 **Common Inherited Breast, Gynecologic, and Gastrointestinal Cancer Susceptibility Genes—cont'd**

Gene	Location	Name	Function	Associated Cancer	Disease
MUTYH	1p34.1	Mut Y homolog	DNA repair	Colon	MUTYH-associated polyposis
POLD1	19q13.33	Polymerase (DNA-directed), delta 1, catalytic subunit	DNA replication and repair	Colon, endometrium	CRC-polymerase proofreading-associated polyposis syndrome
POLE	12q24.33	Polymerase (DNA-directed), epsilon, catalytic subunit	DNA replication and repair	Colon	CRC-polymerase proofreading-associated polyposis syndrome
PALB2	16p12.2	Partner and localizer of BRCA2	DNA repair	Breast, pancreas	Familial breast cancer; Fanconi anemia type N
PMS2	7p22.1	PMS2 postmeiotic segregation increased 2	DNA mismatch repair	Colon, endometrium, ovary, stomach, small bowel, hepatobiliary tract, urinary tract, brain, pancreas, sebaceous	Lynch syndrome
PTEN	10q23.31	Phosphatase and tension homolog	Cell cycle control	Breast, thyroid, renal, endometrium, colon, skin, CNS	PTEN hamartoma tumor syndrome
RAD51C	17q22	RAD51 paralog C	DNA repair	Breast, ovarian	Familial breast and ovarian cancer
RAD51D	17q12	RAD51 paralog D	DNA repair	Breast, ovarian	Familial breast and ovarian cancer
SMAD4	18q21.2	SMAD family member 4	Cell signaling and control of proliferation	Colon, stomach, pancreas	Familial juvenile polyposis
STK11	19p13.3	Serine/threonine kinase 11	Cell signaling and control of proliferation	Breast, colon, ovary, stomach, lung, pancreas	Peutz-Jeghers syndrome
TP53	17p13	Tumor protein p53	DNA repair; cell cycle control	Breast, brain, renal, adrenal, hematologic	Li-Fraumeni syndrome

CNS, Central nervous system; *CRC,* colorectal cancer; *PTEN,* phosphatase and tensin homolog.

patient surveillance and management depend on the altered gene identified. However, while the detection of a variant may be increased by additional gene testing, variants in other genes are less well characterized and many more variants may result in a VUS classification. A VUS can be detected at a rate of about 0.008 variants per 1000 bases of exonic DNA that is sequenced.[506] Thus while providing more comprehensive testing to patients, the lack of certainty regarding clinical relevance of VUS will remain challenging for health care providers in the care and management of patients and may be particularly disconcerting among certain racial/ethnic groups with less characterized VUS.[507] In addition to the identification of the problematic VUS, expanded genetic testing also reveals variants in cancer susceptibility genes that are less well characterized than *BRCA1* and *BRCA2.* Many of these genes demonstrate reduced penetrance, making it difficult to translate the identification of a variant to a calculable cancer risk, and for many, clinical recommendations and guidelines have not yet been established.[508] Because founder gene variants are observed for some susceptibility genes, a specific gene test or cancer panel may be requested based on the ethnicity of the patient and the presence of that gene in a panel. If multiple cancers are reported in the family in addition to breast or ovarian cancer, a more comprehensive cancer susceptibility panel may be advised as a first-tier testing strategy. The

genetics professional must be ever mindful of the insurance coverage for the patient and the financial resources available to the patient for testing to be sure to maximize efficacy of the testing yet minimize unnecessary costs to the patient and carefully determine the appropriate first-tier test to order, whether it is a single gene test, small, targeted cancer-specific panel, or a larger comprehensive cancer panel. Regardless of the MPS cancer panel chosen, pathogenic variants are detected in only about 30% of cases suggestive of familial breast cancer.[509]

Inherited Colorectal Cancer

Colorectal cancer (CRC) is the fourth most common cancer in the United States with an overall lifetime risk of ~4% for both men and women. Annually there are 150,000 new cases of CRC and about 50,000 deaths attributed to this disease. Approximately 3 to 5% of CRC cases are associated with inherited gene variants linked to highly penetrant colon cancer syndromes.[510] In as many as 20 to 30% of cases, familial clustering is observed, thereby suggesting the involvement of less penetrant susceptibility genes and environmental factors. Environmental risk factors include obesity; lack of exercise; moderate to heavy alcohol use; smoking; increased consumption of red or processed meats; and reduced whole-grain fiber, fruits, and vegetables. About 85% of carcinomas arise from transformation of the normal mucosa to adenomas and then to carcinomas, and carcinoma arises through the serrated polyp pathway in 15%. The molecular basis of CRC is a complex multistep process that involves genetic and epigenetic alterations. The various molecular pathways of disease convey different clinical features, prognosis, treatment plans, and pathologic findings.

The microsatellite instability (MSI) pathway represents about 15 to 20% of CRC cases and is characterized by inherited, inactivating variants in genes involved in DNA mismatch repair (MMR) or by acquired epigenetic silencing of these genes. MMR is a ubiquitous DNA repair process that occurs in all dividing cells. Because of a dysfunctional MMR system, DNA replication errors within microsatellite repeats or short tandem repeat sequences of 1 to 6 base pairs in length remain uncorrected and accumulate throughout the genome. Expansion or contraction of the microsatellite-repeat number in noncoding areas of the genome is of little significance; however, the predisposition to CRC results when changes occur within coding microsatellites of the genome and specifically within targeted genes whose protein products are involved in cell growth (*TGFBR2*), apoptosis (*BAX*), or DNA repair (*MSH6*).

The chromosomal instability (CIN) pathway is observed in 75 to 80% of CRC cases and was first proposed more than 25 years ago.[511] The CIN pathway is characterized by inherited or somatic variants causing inactivation of the tumor suppressor gene *APC*, resulting in activation of the Wnt signaling pathway coupled with the acquired loss of chromosomal material as tumorigenesis progresses. These karyotypic changes most frequently involve the chromosomal regions of 5q, 18q, and 17p encompassing tumor suppressor genes *APC*, *DCC*, *SMAD2* and *SMAD4*, *TP53*, and adjacent DNA sequences at frequencies of 30 to 70%, 6%, 10 to 20%, and 40 to 50%, respectively.[512] Gain of function activating variants in codons 12, 13, and 61 of the *KRAS* proto-oncogene on chromosome 12p12.1 is also present in ~30 to 50% of these tumors. Collectively, this molecular profile results in unrestrained cell growth, proliferation, and loss of apoptosis. The tumors derived from the CIN pathway are most often microsatellite stable. The CpG island methylator phenotype (CIMP) is considered a subset of the MSI pathway by which CRC may arise.[513] As a subset of MSI tumors, these tumors are expectedly CIN negative, and CpG island hypermethylation occurs in a characteristic pattern of specific genes. These epigenetic changes cause silencing of the respective genes with no transcription; therefore ultimately no translation of the associated gene product.[514] CIMP tumors can be further classified based on the degree of methylation and the number of genes in which hypermethylation is observed.[515] CIMP tumors typically display MSI because the MMR gene, *MLH1*, is hypermethylated.

Lynch Syndrome

The most common CRC susceptibility syndrome is Lynch syndrome (LS; OMIM #120435), also referred to as hereditary nonpolyposis colorectal cancer (HNPCC), which represents about 3 to 5% of all CRC cases. This disorder has an incidence of about 1 in 500 and is named after Dr. Henry Lynch's observation of an autosomal dominant predisposition to early-onset CRC with stomach and endometrial tumors in two large Midwestern kindreds.[516] LS is a heterogeneous disorder caused by one of multiple genes, manifests a variable age of onset, demonstrates reduced penetrance with lifetime risks of CRC of 35 to 85%, and confers increased risks for other associated tumors including, but not limited to, endometrial, gastric, ovarian, prostrate, biliary, urinary, and glioblastoma (Fig. 68.12).[517] The risk of CRC-associated cancers increases with age but the overall lifetime risk is lowest with *PMS2*, 34% at age 75, and highest with *MSH2*, 84% at age 75. CRC in LS patients is distinguished by a few polyps that possess an accelerated transformation potential to carcinoma in as little as 2 to 3 years. This predisposing event is linked to germline variants in MMR genes that are associated with the MSI pathway. Both CRC tumors in LS families and sporadic tumors with MSI more commonly occur in the proximal part of the colon (right sided). These tumors are typically associated with a better prognosis but, in the absence of MMR proteins, have a poor response to adjuvant 5-FU–based chemotherapy.[518] Histologically, these tumors

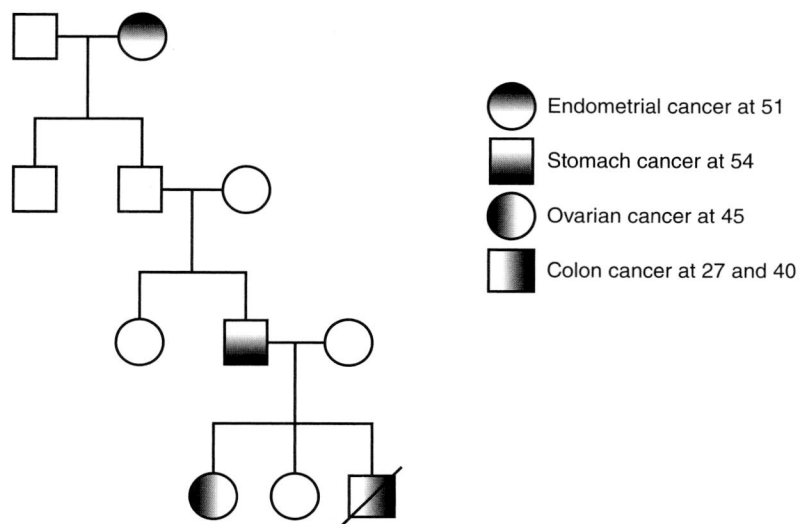

Endometrial cancer at 51

Stomach cancer at 54

Ovarian cancer at 45

Colon cancer at 27 and 40

FIGURE 68.12 Pedigree for a family with Lynch syndrome. Reduced penetrance and a highly variable presentation can often make it difficult to diagnose before several generations are affected.

display infiltrating lymphocytes, are mucinous with signet ring cells, and are poorly differentiated.

The first MMR gene was mapped to chromosome 2p15-16 using large LS kindreds.[519] Simultaneously, MSI was noted in a subset of sporadic CRC.[520,521] The MMR genes associated with LS include *MSH2* (2p15-16), *MSH6* (2p15-16), *MLH1* (3p21), and *PMS2* (7p22).[522,523] The majority of LS mutations are observed in *MSH2* (~35%) and *MLH1* (~45%).[524] A small percentage of patients with LS (1 to 3%) have germline deletions affecting a non-MMR gene, the epithelial cell adhesion molecule (*EPCAM*) gene (2p21), resulting in silencing of the downstream *MSH2* gene promoter and no translation of the associated MSH2 protein.[525]

Lynch syndrome–related *MMR* gene variants are diverse and are located throughout these genes. Almost all errors made during DNA replication are repaired through the proofreading 3′-to-5′ exonuclease activity of DNA polymerase. Uncorrected errors of mismatched bases between the two strands are repaired before cell division by the MMR proteins, a process that is critical for maintaining genomic stability.[518] In addition to providing the repair of a mismatched base–base pair, the MMR system repairs "loop outs" from small insertions or deletions, unmatched bases that can occur during replication of a microsatellite or small repetitive sequences. The repair process includes three steps: (1) recognition of the mismatch, (2) excision, and (3) resynthesis to restore the correct sequence. In the MMR process, the MLH1 and PMS2 proteins dimerize facilitating the binding of other proteins involved in MMR, and the MSH2 protein forms a heterodimer with the *MSH6* gene product to identify mismatches.[522,523,526] When the normal function of MMR proteins is altered through DNA variants, mismatched bases generated through DNA replication are not fixed, leading to strands of DNA with repeats of different lengths. In LS, a germline variant in an MMR gene is inherited, causing one allele to be nonfunctional. In the tumor tissue of these patients, the second allele is inactivated through a somatic variant or is deleted, a phenomenon referred to as loss of heterozygosity. Uncorrected somatic replication errors thus accumulate in noncoding and insignificant locations throughout the genome but also in the coding regions of genes involved in cell growth, signaling, and DNA repair. Approximately 15 to 20% of all CRC display MSI. In sporadic, non-LS associated CRC, MSI is attributed to epigenetic silencing of *MLH1* expression through biallelic methylation.[527]

To assist clinicians in identifying patients in LS kindreds, several criteria have been adopted, including the Amsterdam criteria first developed in 1990 and the more inclusive Bethesda criteria developed in 1998.[528,529] These recommendations have further evolved to maximize the identification of index cases in these families.[530] MSI testing should be performed on CRC tumor tissue if one of the following criteria is met: (1) age younger than 50 years; (2) regardless of age, synchronous or metachronous CRC or the presence of other LS-associated tumors, including the endometrium, ovary, stomach, hepatobiliary system, small bowel, ureter, renal, pelvis, and brain; (3) age younger than 60 with histology demonstrating a typical MSI pattern of tumor-infiltrating lymphocytes, Crohn-like lymphocytic reaction, mucinous–signet ring differentiation, or a medullary growth pattern; (4) the patient has one or more first-degree relatives with a LS-related tumor that was diagnosed before age 50 years; or

(5) there are two or more first- or second-degree relatives with CRC or LS-related tumors, regardless of their age. Despite these revised guidelines, some index cases are still not identified, so universal screening for all CRC has been recommended.[531–533] Equally important is screening for LS in patients with endometrial cancer (EC) because approximately 3% of patients with EC have an MMR gene variant. The lifetime risk of EC in LS women is 25 to 60% with a mean age at diagnosis between 48 and 62 years and lifetime risk for developing ovarian cancer at 4 to 12% with a mean age of 42.5 years.[534] Approximately 10 to 15% of hereditary ovarian cancer is due to LS. Synchronous tumors of the endometrium and ovary may be observed in as many as 20% of women with LS.[535] In many women with LS, EC often precedes CRC as their initial malignancy. Identification of the increased risks of LS-related tumors can be followed by increased surveillance, counseling, and testing for at-risk family members. For these reasons, universal screening for all newly diagnosed EC has been proposed because a significant percentage of LS patients are missed when relying on MMR-associated tumor morphology or patient indices such as age (<50 years) and history.[536–538]

Molecular testing for MSI can identify defects in MMR genes through germline or somatic changes, and IHC testing is performed to detect expression of MMR proteins.[539] MSI testing by PCR may be the preferred method in some facilities. Alternatively, IHC testing may be performed if MSI testing is not readily available or if there is a limited amount of tumor tissue. In some settings, however, both molecular MSI testing and IHC testing may be performed concurrently to account for possible false-negative results that may be obtained from either methodology.[540] At many institutions, a multidisciplinary team develops and agrees on a standard protocol for universal screening of suspected LS patients. Because mononucleotide microsatellite repeats are more susceptible to MMR errors, MSI testing is most often performed using a multiplex PCR for several mononucleotide loci and requires normal adjacent tissue for comparison (Fig. 68.13). MSI is characterized by the expansion or contraction of DNA sequences through the insertion or deletion of repeated sequences. If MSI is detected at two or more of five loci, or more than 30% of the loci analyzed, the tumor has a "high" frequency of MSI (MSI-H). If MSI is detected at one locus, or less than 30%, the tumor has a "low" frequency of MSI (MSI-L). If MSI is not detected at any locus, the tumor is considered to be microsatellite stable (MSS). MSI-L or MSS results greatly reduce the likelihood of LS.

If MSI-H is detected, it is necessary to determine whether the MSI results from an inherited inactivating germline MMR gene variant or from the more frequent somatic CpG methylation of *MLH1* seen commonly in sporadic CRC. Because somatic CpG methylation of *MLH1* is frequently associated with a somatic *BRAF* proto-oncogene p.Val600Glu variant, this test is often performed as a reflex test on tumor tissue DNA after MSI-H results are obtained (Fig. 68.14).[523,534] If a somatic *BRAF* p.Val600Glu variant is detected, LS is unlikely. If, however, no *BRAF* gene variant is detected, a germline MMR gene variant is more likely, and the testing algorithm continues with *MLH1* promoter hypermethylation studies of tumor tissue DNA. If epigenetic biallelic *MLH1* gene promoter hypermethylation is detected, a sporadic CRC tumor is the diagnosis. Conversely, the lack of *MLH1*

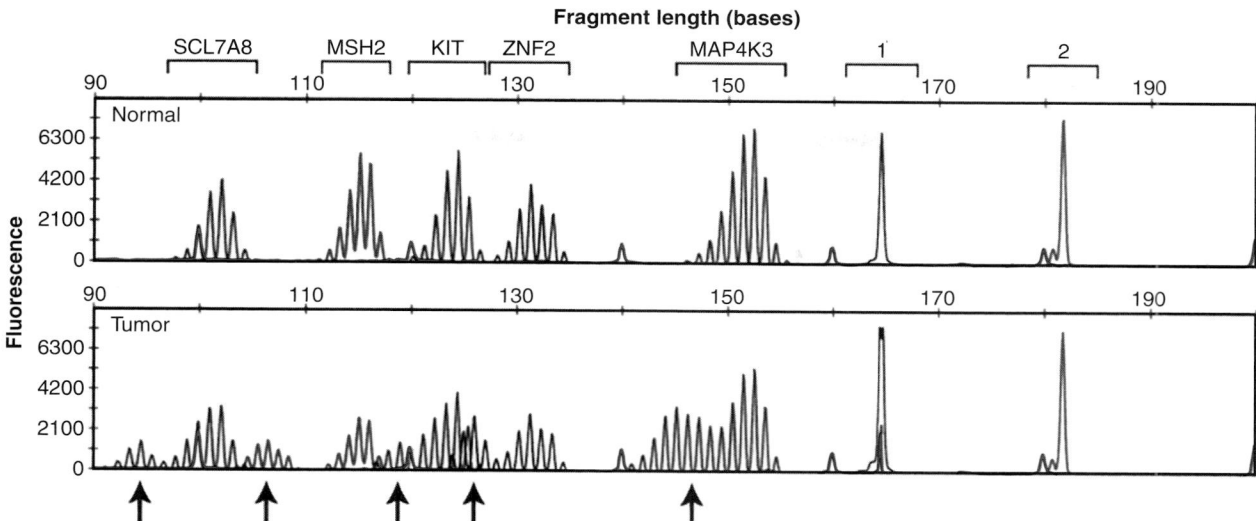

FIGURE 68.13 Electropherograms illustrating microsatellite instability *(MSI)* in tumor DNA. Patient DNA is extracted from peripheral blood or normal tissue and is compared with DNA extracted from tumor tissue. DNA is amplified in a multiplex PCR assay using fluorescent labeled primers corresponding to five mononucleotide loci *(SCL7A8, MSH2, KIT, ZNF2,* and *MAP4K3)* and two pentanucleotide loci (1 and 2) (Promega Corporation, Madison, WI). Amplicon sizes in bases are noted at the top of the figure, and the relative amount of fluorescence detected for each amplicon is measured by the peak height (*y*-axis). Multiple peaks seen at each locus represent "stutter" peaks and result from strand slippage during PCR of repetitive sequences. *Arrows* denote a shift in product size at five of five mononucleotide loci, indicating microsatellite instability. Identical patterns between normal and tumor DNA at the polymorphic pentanucleotide markers suggest that normal and tumor DNA are derived from the same individual.

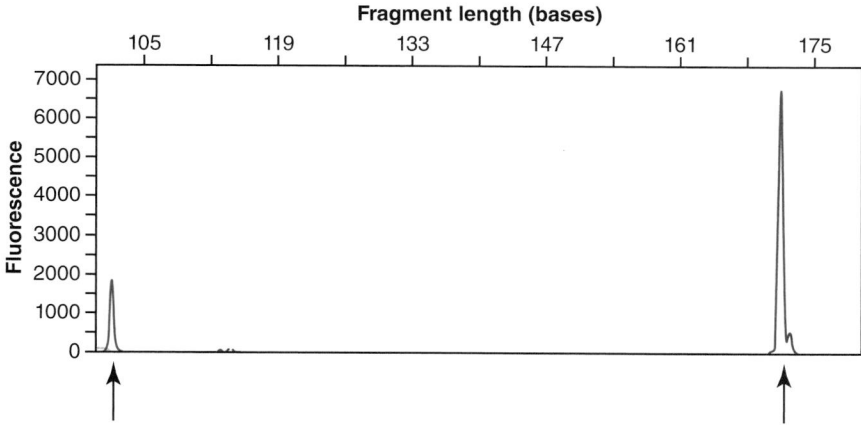

FIGURE 68.14 Detection of *BRAF* c.1799T>A (p.Val600Glu) by allele-specific polymerase chain reaction (PCR).[541] Amplicon sizes in bases are noted at the top of the figure, and the relative amount of fluorescence detected for each amplicon is measured by the peak height (*y*-axis). *BRAF* c.1799T>A can be detected using allele-specific PCR coupled with capillary electrophoresis. DNA was extracted from a paraffin-embedded MSI-H (microsatellite instability–high) colon tumor. An internal control 171-bp fragment was amplified using a primer pair flanking exon 15 with the 3' primer fluorescently labeled. In the same reaction, a 101-bp allele specific amplicon was generated with the same 5' forward primer and a second 3'-fluorescently labeled primer specific for *BRAF* c.1799T>A.[542] The *right arrow* points to the internal control, and the *left arrow* confirms the presence of *BRAF* c.1799T>A (p.Val600Glu) in the tumor, thereby suggesting that the MSI-H phenotype observed in the colon tumor is associated with sporadic colon cancer and not to variants in an *MMR* gene associated with Lynch syndrome.

promoter hypermethylation indicates the possibility of LS, and DNA sequence analysis of MMR genes from the patient's peripheral blood lymphocytes to identify a germline MMR gene variant is performed.

More recently, MSI has been detected with MPS. In these cases, the MSI status in addition to overall tumor mutational burden is often included in NGS-based multigene solid tumor panels for the molecular profiling of diagnostic tissue specimens.[543–546] This testing is required for choosing an appropriate treatment plan for the patient based on the presence or absence of specific gene variants in the tumor tissue (e.g., *KRAS, BRAF*). In many instances, tumor tissue

DNA is analyzed alongside normal tissue DNA from the patient to readily identify and report germline pathogenic variants and facilitate referral to genetic counseling services.[547,548] In addition this newer testing algorithm may facilitate the identification of more LS patients and their families and identify additional CRC predisposition genes.[517,549] Further, while MSI is typically associated with colon and endometrial cancer, submission of many different types of tumors for these panels demonstrates that it is a more common cancer phenotype. MSI-H results enables eligibility for immune checkpoint inhibitors such as pembrolizumab and nivolumab and conveys a better prognosis.[550–554] Lynch syndrome–associated gene variants are heterogeneous; most are nonsense or frameshift variants expected to result in premature truncation of the protein and loss of function.[524] The majority of germline variants occur in *MLH1* and *MSH2* and to a lesser degree in the *MSH6* gene. Variants in the *PMS2* gene are the least common. An inherent problem in DNA sequencing is the identification of sequence VUS, which are most often missense, intronic, or silent variants and for which no significant biologic function has been determined. Thus it is difficult to assign a pathologic role to these variants without functional assays to confirm their relevance in the disease process. Challenging, however, are "private" variants segregating within a single family and the associated uncertainty of characterizing those genotype–phenotype correlations and predictive risk assessments for specific variants based on the clinical findings in just one family. The best validation of pathogenicity of a VUS is segregation analysis within families with linkage of the variant to disease.

Overall genotype–phenotype correlations for MMR genes indicate that individuals with *MLH1* gene variants have the earliest age of onset and highest risk for developing CRC by age 70 years while *MSH2* gene carriers have the highest risk of extracolonic tumors.[555] *MSH6* gene variant carriers have the latest onset of cancers and *PMS2* gene variant carriers have the overall lowest penetrance of disease and are associated with the highest incidence of glioblastomas.[555,556] In addition, *MLH1* and *MSH2* variants have been identified in patients with Muir-Torre syndrome (MTS) at frequencies of <10 and 90% respectively with a median age of approximately 53 years of age. MTS is less common in *MSH6* and *PMS2* gene variant carriers.[557] In rare cases, patients with biallelic germline variants in an MMR gene result in constitutional mismatch repair deficiency syndrome (OMIM #276300) with early-onset CRC and childhood hematologic or brain tumors.

Once a germline variant has been identified in a proband, asymptomatic at-risk family members can be screened to determine their risk for LS. Both pre- and post-test genetic counseling is indicated. Before testing, similar to presymptomatic testing for other adult-onset disorders, the counseling session should include verification of the family history, discuss the clinical course of the disease in the family, include a prior risk of developing the disease and issues associated with disease management. Discussions should also include how the patient will act on both positive and negative results, feelings of survivor guilt or stigmatization, and the possibility of discrimination for insurance and employment. Post-test counseling includes disclosing the results and implications to the patient and his or her family members. The genetics professional should provide a management and surveillance plan

for the patient based on the MMR gene involved and the identified variant. If a germline variant is detected in the presymptomatic patient, a colonoscopy should be performed every 1 or 2 years beginning at age 20 to 25 years or 10 years younger than the youngest age of diagnosis in the family.[558] Surveillance for EC and ovarian cancer for at-risk women with LS should include transvaginal ultrasonography and endometrial biopsy every 1 to 2 years beginning at 30 to 35 years of age.[558] Furthermore, prophylactic hysterectomy and bilateral salpingo-oophorectomy can be considered for women who have completed childbearing. An approach to develop vaccines against neo-antigens generated from LS-CRC patients to treat relapse and prevent tumors in LS-gene carriers is under consideration.[556,559–561] If presymptomatic genetic testing is not pursued, relatives should begin an intensive screening program with colonoscopy every 1 to 2 years, starting between 20 and 30 years of age, and then annually after age 40 years. If no pathogenic MMR germline variant is detected in the proband despite MSI and IHC testing suggestive of an MMR germline variant and LS, presymptomatic DNA testing for family members is not possible. These variant-negative families or Lynch-like families may have (1) an MMR VUS that may eventually be reclassified, (2) an MMR gene variant in a region of the genome that is not screened, (3) a structural variant not detected by current methodologies, or (4) a germline variant in other yet to be determined MMR genes or genes that regulate MMR genes. Although detection of a variant in a family that meets LS criteria is not always possible, heightened surveillance of the proband and at-risk family members should be implemented.

Familial Adenomatous Polyposis

Familial adenomatous polyposis (FAP; OMIM #175100) is an autosomal dominant disorder with an incidence of about 1 in 8000 to 15,000 characterized by hundreds to thousands of adenomatous polyps throughout the colon and rectum. This disorder has a high penetrance, conveying a lifetime risk of CRC in untreated variant carriers of close to 100%. FAP accounts for 1% of CRC cases observed in the United States and is the second most common inherited colon cancer syndrome. Interestingly, in about 20 to 30% of cases, no family history exists, and the disease is the result of a de novo event. Polyps appear during the second decade of life in about half of the patients with almost all patients developing polyps by the age of 35.[562] Untreated, CRC develops approximately 10 to 15 years after the onset of polyposis most often on the left side of the colon (70 to 80%), with the median age of CRC about 40 years of age.[562,563] It is the sheer number of polyps in these patients that increases the likelihood that one will progress to cancer. For this reason, close surveillance of these patients is indicated, and colectomy is advised when multiple adenomas are observed or if high-grade histologic findings are reported. Furthermore, patients with FAP have an increased risk of developing other malignancies, including carcinoma of the small bowel, most often in the duodenum or periampulla; papillary thyroid carcinoma; hepatoblastoma; pancreatic cancer; and brain tumors.[564] In addition, these patients are at risk of developing extraintestinal manifestations of the disease, including adrenal or desmoid tumors, osteomas, congenital hypertrophy of the retinal epithelium, and dental abnormalities.[565] Desmoid tumors in vital areas have been reported as a cause of death in as many as 21% of patients with FAP.[566] Thus close clinical surveillance of FAP patients and at-risk family members is critical to reducing CRC and CRC-associated mortality and APC-associated complications.

Familial adenomatous polyposis is caused by germline variants in the adenomatous polyposis coli (*APC*) gene, which was cloned in 1991.[567–569] The *APC* gene, 5q22.2, has 15 exons, contains 8535 base pairs, and encodes a protein of 2843 amino acids and a molecular weight of about 310 kDa. The APC protein is a multidomain, multifunctional tumor suppressor protein with multiple binding partners that play key roles in regulating the β-catenin level and thus the Wnt, signaling pathway.[570,571] In this process, APC together with glycogen synthase kinase-3β and axin regulate the amount of β-catenin through the phosphorylation of cytoplasmic β-catenin for ubiquitin-dependent degradation. In the absence of functional APC, β-catenin is unregulated and accumulates in the nucleus, leading to ligand independent constitutive oncogenic Wnt signaling and transcription mediated by lymphoid enhancer-binding factor/T-cell factor (LEF/TCF) transcription factors, resulting in the upregulation of genes involved in proliferation.[572] For this reason, APC is commonly referred to as a "gatekeeper" of tumor progression. Similar to autosomal dominant inherited variants in other tumor suppressor genes, the normal allele must also be inactivated to manifest the disease phenotype for the classic Knudson's two hit hypothesis.[471] Therapeutic approaches targeting the Wnt pathway are under investigation.[570,573] This protein is also involved in other cellular processes, including cell adhesion and migration, DNA repair, apoptosis, FAK/Src signaling, microtubule assembly, and chromosome segregation.[570,574]

Collectively, Sanger and MPS DNA sequencing studies have identified well over 1700 germline variants in *APC*, most of which result in truncated proteins because of small frameshift or nonsense variants.[575] Gross rearrangements have been identified using MLPA.[576] Despite the heterogeneous nature of these variants, two hot spots occur with 10 and 15% of all variants found specifically at codons 1061 and 1309, respectively, with about 30% of additional variants occurring between these two sites.[575] Interestingly, the location of the germline variant determines the second somatic variant. Variants between codons 1194 and 1392 have a second hit as a loss of the normal allele, LOH.[577] Alternatively, germline variants outside of these regions are more often associated with second hit variants that result in protein truncation and occur between codons 1286 and 1513.[577] Genotype–phenotype correlations exist for some *APC* variants.[578] The AAAAG deletion at codon 1309 is associated with a younger age of onset, ~20 years.[579] FAP patients with variants between codons 168 and 1580, but excluding codon 1309, have an age of onset ~30 years of age, whereas variants 5' to codon 168 and 3' of codon 1580 have delayed onset of disease at ~52 years of age.[580] Attenuated FAP (AFAP) is seen in about 8 to 10% of patients with FAP and is associated with fewer colonic polyps (10 to 100) and an older age of onset for both the development of polyps and cancer, generally 50 to 55 years.[581–583] These patients typically have truncating variants at the extreme 5' end of the gene (codons 1 to 177), in exon 9 or at the carboxyl-terminal end of the gene.[580] Lifetime risk for CRC in AFAP patients with these variants is 70%. Intra- and interfamilial phenotypic variability exists even in the presence of identical variants and may be explained by a modifier gene or genes.[584,585]

If APC is suspected, full gene sequence analysis is recommended coupled with deletion and duplication analysis to detect about 10% of variants that may not be identified by Sanger or MPS. If the variant within the family can be identified, at-risk family members as young as 10 to 12 years of age may be referred for genetic counseling and presymptomatic DNA testing.[586] Although DNA testing on an asymptomatic minor is usually not endorsed by the genetic community, in this scenario, early identification of the variant in these patients will clearly affect their clinical management because intense screening programs and possible prophylactic colectomy may be initiated as early as the second decade of life. If a variant is detected in the family, endoscopy should be performed every 2 years and if adenomas are detected, colonoscopy should be performed every year until the colectomy is performed.[587] Annual thyroid and abdominal ultrasonography for detection of thyroid malignancy and desmoid tumors may also be included in the surveillance screening. Family members who test negative for the variant do not have increased risk of CRC, can avoid these intensive screening programs, and should follow the screening programs for the general population. If the variant in the family cannot be identified, screening with sigmoidoscopy is recommended every 2 years, starting as early as age 10 to 12 years. Furthermore, when repeatedly negative sigmoidoscopy results are obtained, the frequency of such examinations can be reduced in each subsequent decade of life, and frequent surveillance may be discontinued at age 50 years.[587] Because AFAP is associated with a later age of onset and most adenomas are in the right part of the colon, colonoscopy is the recommended screening method beginning at 18 to 20 years of age.

In 2002, *APC* variant-negative adenomatous polyposis patients were found to have biallelic mutations in the base excision repair gene *MUTYH*, a disorder known as *MUTYH*-associated polyposis (MAP; OMIM #604933).[588,589] This gene contains 16 exons, encodes a protein with 535 amino acids, is located on chromosome 1p34.3-p32.1, and encodes an adenine-specific DNA glycosylase involved in DNA base excision repair (BER). This protein removes adenine when it is inappropriately paired with guanine, cytosine, or oxidatively damaged DNA containing 8-oxo-7,8-dihydroguanine. If not repaired, these mispairings can result in G:C to T:A transversion variants in the *APC* gene, the *KRAS* gene, and others associated with CRC.[590] *MUTYH* gene variant–positive patients have CRC at a mean age of 51.7 ± 9.5 years.[591] Incomplete penetrance is observed, and the polyp burden is variable with typical patients having between 10 and 100 polyps. Close surveillance of these patients is recommended, similar to that provided for AFAP, with colonoscopy screening beginning as early as 25 to 30 years of age and colonoscopy performed every 2 years thereafter. Further, at age 30 to 35 an upper endoscopy and side viewing duodenoscopy is recommended.[592] These patients are also at an increased risk for ovary, bladder, breast, and endometrial cancer.[592] In addition, although this is an autosomal recessive condition, heterozygous carriers with only one *MUTYH* gene variant are at increased risk for CRC, thus indicating that close clinical surveillance may be indicated in this population as well.[591,593]

Variants in the *MUTYH* gene are heterogeneous and scattered throughout the gene with more than 300 unique variants reported.[594] Most variants cause amino acid substitutions in the gene, and ethnic-specific common variants are observed.[595] Patients can be homozygous for the same variant or compound heterozygotes with two different variants. Clinical presentation and personal and family history should be carefully reviewed when determining the most appropriate molecular testing to recommend. In some families, MPS using a targeted comprehensive panel of susceptibility genes for colon cancer may afford a higher likelihood for identification of the disease gene segregating in the family in a faster and more cost-effective manner (see Table 68.7).[596] Alternatively, DNA testing for MAP may include the *APC* gene and/or the *MAP* gene, depending on the observed phenotype, or be targeted to common variants within the *MAP* gene or be specific for a known variant segregating in the family.[597]

POINTS TO REMEMBER

Inherited Cancer

- Disease can result from the inheritance of a single activating variant in a proto-oncogene.
- Disease can result from the inheritance of a single loss-of-function variant in a tumor suppressor or mismatch repair gene followed by somatic inactivation of the second allele.
- Age of onset and type of tumor(s) observed within family members are variable.
- MPS-based disease-specific tumor panels are currently most often used to identify the gene variant segregating in the family.
- Routine clinical surveillance screening is initiated in variant-positive asymptomatic family members.
- Genetic counseling is an important component of patient care and management.

MITOCHONDRIAL DNA DISEASES

Mitochondria are organelles ubiquitous to the cytoplasm of all eukaryotic cells of animals, higher plants, and some microorganisms. Mitochondria generate energy for cellular processes by producing ATP through oxidative phosphorylation (OXPHOS); they are important in maintaining both calcium homeostasis and various intracellular signaling cascades, including apoptosis.[598–602] The matrix of the mitochondrion is surrounded by a cardiolipin-rich inner membrane, and both are enclosed by a second outer membrane. Within the matrix are copies of mitochondrial DNA (mtDNA). Each mitochondrion usually contains 2 to 10 copies of mtDNA, so with hundreds of mitochondria per cell, an estimated 10^3 to 10^4 copies of mtDNA exist within each cell, with brain, skeletal, and cardiac muscle having particularly high concentrations. Alterations in mtDNA copy number or variants in mtDNA are associated with both inherited and acquired diseases.[598,603–605] The mitochondrial genome is composed of a double-stranded, circular DNA molecule containing 16,569 base pairs that encodes 37 genes, including two ribosomal RNAs (rRNA), 22 transfer RNAs (tRNA), and 13 subunits required for the OXPHOS system, with 7 belonging to complex I, 1 to complex III, 3 to complex IV, and 2 to complex V.[599,606] Most subunits involved in the OXPHOS system are nuclear encoded,

as are several nuclear gene products that regulate mitochondrial gene expression. The mitochondrial genetic code is slightly different from the universal code. For example, in mtDNA, TGA codes for tryptophan rather than a termination codon, and all mitochondrial-translated mRNA contains codons requiring only 22 mitochondrial-encoded tRNA molecules for translation rather than the 31 predicted by Crick's wobble hypothesis.[607,608] The high copy number of mtDNA per cell coupled with a small genome and highly polymorphic sequence variations among individuals makes mtDNA sequence analysis an ideal tool for forensic studies.[609,610]

Mitochondria-related diseases have an incidence of 1 in 1000 to 5000 and can result from variants in nuclear DNA (85 to 90%) or, as first reported in 1988, from variants in the mitochondrial genome (10 to 15%).[599,611–613] Variants in mtDNA occur at a higher rate than nuclear DNA, probably because of differences in chromatin structure, lack of DNA repair machinery, and the continual generation of reactive oxygen species. Mitochondrial genetics is different from Mendelian genetics in several aspects. First, all mtDNA is maternally inherited, with mature oocytes having the highest mtDNA copy number per cell at 10^5 and with sperm having the lowest mtDNA copy number per cell at 10^2.[598] After fertilization, sperm mtDNA is selectively degraded so that only maternal mtDNA remains. Thus if a mother is carrying an mtDNA variant, it will be transmitted to all of her children, but only her daughters can transmit the disease to their offspring (Fig. 68.15). Although this is considered the rule, paternal mtDNA inheritance has been reported and may result from incomplete degradation of sperm mtDNA in early embryogenesis.[614,615] If a mtDNA variant arises, it will exist among a population of normal mtDNA. This coexistence of normal and variant mtDNA copies within the same cell is referred to as *heteroplasmy* and is the second unique feature of mitochondrial genetics. Third, during cell division, the proportions of normal and variant mtDNA can shift as mitochondria, and their accompanying genomes are partitioned into daughter cells. Thus in development and differentiation, the proportions of normal and variant mtDNA can vary among cells and tissues within the body. Last, the percentage

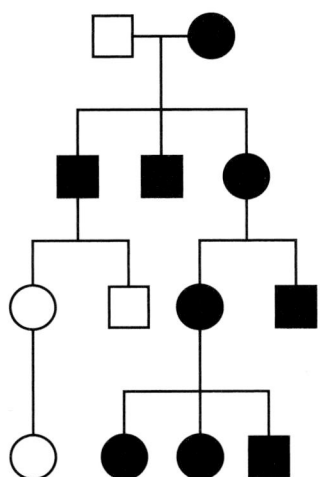

FIGURE 68.15 Mitochondrial disease pedigree. In all but the rarest cases, mitochondria are maternally inherited resulting in most offspring of an affected female also being affected. However, offspring of affected males do not inherit the disorder.

of variant mtDNA required within a cell, tissue, or organ system to produce a deleterious phenotype is referred to as the *threshold effect*. The threshold for disease varies among people, energetic requirements for tissue, and the mtDNA variant. Genetic counseling for families with mtDNA disorders is complicated by an inability to accurately predict phenotype caused by heteroplasmy and the threshold effect.

Two types of mtDNA variants exist: those that affect mitochondrial protein synthesis (tRNA and rRNA genes) and those within the protein-encoding genes themselves.[616,617] Traditionally, testing for mtDNA variants was performed by direct Sanger sequencing or by targeted variant testing for specific disease-related variants. Over the past several years, most clinical laboratories have moved to MPS-based testing for the detection of mtDNA alterations. Recently, the Mitochondrial Medicine Society released a consensus statement on the diagnosis of mitochondrial diseases.[618] This statement indicates that MPS-based testing of the entire mitochondrial genome is now the preferred method for the diagnosis of a suspected mitochondrial disorder and should be considered the first-line DNA-based test (as opposed to targeted variant analysis).[618] MPS-based testing for mtDNA variants usually involves a preliminary long-range PCR to amplify the entire mitochondrial genome.[619–621] After this step is complete, the amplified mtDNA is processed, sequenced, and then analyzed.[620] mtDNA variants identified by MPS-based methods are usually confirmed by a secondary method (e.g., Sanger sequencing). Using MPS-based testing and subsequent variant confirmation techniques, investigators have been able to reproducibly detect heteroplasmy levels of approximately 10%.[619,620] Because of the limitations in the detection of heteroplasmy using MPS-based methods, some laboratories are continuing to use PCR-based methods capable of detecting lower levels of heteroplasmy to target specific disease-causing mtDNA variants. Although mtDNA variants are now associated with a significant number of inherited diseases, acquired mtDNA deletions are associated with the aging process, and mitochondrial dysfunction is associated with neurodegenerative diseases and cancer.[605] Many somatic mtDNA variants occur via damage by oxygen free radicals produced as byproducts of aerobic metabolism.[622,623]

Clinical treatment of mitochondrial disorders is largely supportive in nature. Several treatment modalities are currently under investigation (e.g., antioxidant therapy, gene therapy/editing, stimulation of mitochondrial biosynthesis, among others).[599] However, these potential treatments remain largely experimental.

Leber Hereditary Optic Neuropathy

Leber hereditary optic neuropathy (LHON; OMIN #53500), the most common mitochondrial disease, was the first linked to maternal inheritance through a variant in the mtDNA.[612] LHON is characterized by acute or subacute bilateral loss of central vision caused by focal degeneration of the retinal ganglion cell (RGC) layer and, in some individuals, impairment of optic nerve function.[624] The specific nature of the disease in terms of RGC degeneration is unknown, but it could be caused by differences in superoxide regulation.[625] Age of onset is typically in the second to fourth decade of life, and after initial symptoms, both eyes are usually affected within 6 months. Approximately 50% of males and only 10% of females who possess an LHON mtDNA variant will develop

disease.[624] In addition, yet to be defined environmental factors, nuclear-encoded modifier genes that affect mtDNA expression, mtDNA products, or mitochondrial metabolism may modify the phenotypic expression of LHON. The explanation for differences in rates between genders has not been determined but could be related to genes on the X chromosome.[626–628] It has also been suggested that sex hormones may provide a protective effect in females. Experiments using LHON cybrid cell lines indicate that the presence of estrogens results in more efficient oxidative phosphorylation suggesting that hormones explain gender differences in LHON.[629] Genetic counseling in LHON is complicated because the amount of variant mtDNA transmitted by heteroplasmic females is not predictable. Furthermore, genetic testing does not predict which individuals will develop visual symptoms.[630] LHON can be confused with autosomal dominant optic atrophy (OMIN #165500), which shares a similar ocular phenotype but results from variants in the gene *OPA1* (3q28-29). It is interesting to note that OPA1 is a nuclear-encoded mitochondrial protein required for mitochondrial fusion, maintenance of cristae architecture, and regulation of apoptosis.[602]

Leber hereditary optic neuropathy is a disorder caused by OXPHOS deficiency. Although many variants have been associated with this disease, mtDNA variants m.3460G>A, m.11778G>A, and m.14484T>C represent 90% of those identified.[599,631] Variant m.11778G>A was the first described, is the most common, and accounts for at least 50% of cases. In most affected individuals, LHON variants appear to be homoplasmic, with only variant mtDNA detected, but in 15% of cases, the variants are heteroplasmic, with a mixture of both normal and variant mtDNA detected.[632,633] Each of the common variants affects a subunit of the nicotinamide adenine dinucleotide: ubiquinone oxidoreductase in complex I of the OXPHOS pathway. The mechanism by which these variants cause the LHON phenotype is not well understood.[634]

Leigh Syndrome

Leigh syndrome (OMIM #256000), or subacute necrotizing encephalopathy, is a progressive neurodegenerative disorder that most often leads to death before the age of 5 years. In contrast to LHON, most patients present within the first year of life with hypotonia, failure to thrive, psychomotor regression, ocular movement abnormalities, ataxia, and brainstem and basal ganglia dysfunction caused by severe dysfunction of mitochondrial energy metabolism. The clinical phenotype for Leigh syndrome is variable in patients with the same pathogenic mtDNA variant and results from differences in the percentages of variant mtDNA among organs and tissues within an individual.[635,636] However, it appears that heteroplasmy alone cannot explain the differences in phenotypic presentation because individuals with high levels of the common Leigh syndrome variant m.8993T>C present with other disease manifestations.[637]

Leigh syndrome exhibits extensive genetic heterogeneity, with disease-causing variants identified in both nuclear-encoded genes and mtDNA, making both Mendelian and maternal patterns of inheritance possible for this syndrome.[637] Variants in more than 80 genes have been described to cause Leigh syndrome.[599] The most common mitochondrial-encoded variant associated with Leigh syndrome is seen in the *MT-ATPase 6* gene (complex V) with a T>G transversion variant at nucleotide m.8993. The most common nuclear-encoded variant associated with Leigh syndrome is in the *SURF1* gene (9q34), which encodes a cytochrome oxidase assembly factor. Regardless of which gene is involved, the overall prognosis of these patients is generally poor, and treatment of mitochondrial disease is in its infancy.[638] Because of the lethality of Leigh syndrome, PGD can be considered and has been successfully performed with the implantation of a disease-free embryo.[639]

Mitochondrial Encephalomyopathy, Lactic Acidosis, and Stroke-like Episodes

Mitochondrial encephalomyopathy, lactic acidosis, and stroke-like episodes (MELAS; OMIM #540000) is a multisystem disorder characterized by generalized tonic-clonic seizures, recurrent headaches and vomiting, hearing loss, exercise intolerance, and proximal limb weakness.[640] Manifestations of MELAS routinely appear in early childhood, and the disease is commonly fatal by young adulthood.[641] As with other mitochondrial disorders, phenotypic presentation in MELAS is widely variable among individuals. In fact, it is not possible to predict the course of disease even among individuals with the same variant or in the same family.[603,641,642]

The disorder is primarily caused by variants in the mitochondrial tRNA encoding gene *MT-TL1*.[643] A single *MT-TL1* A>G transition variant located at nucleotide m.3243 is responsible for disease in approximately 80% of MELAS patients.[640] An additional two *MT-TL1* point variants (m.3271T>C and m.3252A>G) are responsible for disease in approximately 12% of patients.[640] Variants in a second mitochondrial gene (*MT-ND5*) that encodes the NADH-ubiquinone oxidoreductase subunit 5 are also a relatively common cause of MELAS.[644] Although several causative variants have been described in the *MT-ND5* gene, a single nucleotide variant, m.13513G>A, is by far the most common.[645] There are also rare cases in which causative variants have been identified in other mitochondrial (and some nuclear) genes.[640]

Myoclonic Epilepsy Associated With Ragged Red Fibers

Myoclonic epilepsy associated with ragged red fibers (MERRF; OMIM #545000) is characterized by myoclonus, epilepsy, ataxia, dementia, muscle weakness, hearing loss, short stature, and optic atrophy.[646] MERRF patients commonly undergo a period of normal development before showing manifestations of disease in childhood.[646] The "ragged red fibers" denote the hallmark finding of frayed muscle fibers observed in muscle biopsies from these patients. Although the clinical presentation of MERRF can vary widely, there are four key characteristics required for diagnosis: myoclonus, ataxia, generalized epilepsy, and ragged red fibers observed in the muscle biopsy.[646]

The disorder is caused by variants in mitochondrial tRNA genes that result in altered translational efficiency.[605,647] Variants in several tRNA genes have been described in this disorder, but the most frequently observed alteration (m.8344A>G) occurs in the *MT-TK* gene that encodes the tRNA^Lys and is causative for 80% of cases.[648] Three additional *MT-TK* gene variants (m.8356T>C, m.8361G>A, and m.8363G>A) are responsible for disease in an additional 10%.[646] Rare variants

in the *MT-TI*, *MT-TP*, *MT-TF*, and *MT-TL1* genes also result in MERRF. There is much heterogeneity in the presentation of MERRF patients. In fact, a large percentage of patients with the common m.8344A>G variant do not exhibit all four of the hallmark findings of MERRF,[649] suggesting further refinement of diagnostic criteria in the future.

Kearns-Sayre Syndrome

Kearns-Sayre syndrome (KSS; OMIM #530000) is a progressive multisystem disorder with onset occurring before age 20 years. KSS is defined by the presence of progressive external ophthalmoplegia and pigmentary retinopathy and at least one additional hallmark finding (cardiac conduction block, cerebrospinal fluid protein concentrations of > 100 mg/dL, or cerebellar ataxia).[604,605] Additional clinical findings of KSS may include ptosis, hearing loss, short stature, limb weakness, dementia, hypoparathyroidism, and others.[604] The disease often results in early adulthood death. Unlike most other mitochondrial disorders, KSS usually results from de novo alterations that likely occur in the maternal oocyte during germline development or embryogenesis.[604,650]

In the late 1980s, large deletions in mtDNA were identified as the cause of KSS.[613,651] The size of these deletions varies among individuals, but a common deletion approximately 4.9 kb in size is found in approximately 30% of KSS patients.[651] Studies indicate that regardless of the deletion size, the removal of critical tRNAs needed for protein synthesis results in the disease phenotype.[604] Additionally, the variable presence of deleted mtDNA in specific tissues results in the clinical phenotype of patients.[605] Patients with KSS often have partially deleted mtDNAs in all tissues examined, which is likely to explain the multisystem involvement of this disorder.[605]

Clinical DNA testing for KSS involves the use of deletion and duplication analysis performed by any number of testing modalities (e.g., CGH microarray, quantitative PCR, MLPA). Deletion and duplication testing detects disease-causing variants in 90% of patients affected with KSS.[604] Patients with a KSS phenotype that test negative for deletions may pursue MPS-based mitochondrial genome sequencing because rare single nucleotide variants can cause a KSS-like phenotype.

IMPRINTING

Imprinting refers to the differential marking or "imprinting" of specific paternally and maternally inherited alleles during gametogenesis, resulting in differential expression of those genes. Such imprints on the DNA during gametogenesis must be maintained through DNA replication in the somatic cells of the offspring, must be reversible from generation to generation, and must influence transcription. DNA methylation is the primary mechanism for genomic imprinting. The number of imprinted genes in the human genome is estimated to be fewer than 200, and most are clustered around imprinting control centers. Alterations in normal imprinting patterns can result in disease.[652]

Prader-Willi and Angelman Syndromes

Prader-Willi syndrome (PWS; OMIM #176270) is a complex multisystem, neurogenetic disorder with an incidence of 1 in 10,000 to 30,000. PWS, along with Angelman syndrome (AS), were the first reported human disorders resulting from imprinting. Prenatal features of PWS include diminished fetal movement (88%), polyhydramnios (34%), and small gestational age (65%).[653] PWS is associated with mild craniofacial anomalies and severe hypotonia at birth.[654,655] Small hands and feet, hypogonadism, and hypogenitalism are also observed. Hypotonia persists resulting in poor feeding and failure to thrive. Developmental delay is present for both motor skills and language, and continues throughout life, with a mean IQ of 60 to 70. Early in childhood, a unique and characteristic insatiable appetite, hyperphagia, that is hypothalamic in origin presents; obesity ensues with associated complications and is the major cause of morbidity, mortality, and sleep disorders.[656] In addition, patients have short stature and abnormal body composition characteristic of growth hormone deficiency and generally are started on growth hormone therapy a few months after birth. Management of this disease is complex with a spectrum of associated phenotypic findings requiring specialists for obesity; diabetes; behavioral and psychiatric disorders; bone complications such as scoliosis, osteopenia, and fractures; and in addition to growth hormone therapy, treatment for thyroid dysfunction, hypogonadism, and adrenal insufficiency.[657,658] Premature mortality in these patients is most often associated with comorbidities associated with obesity. A new drug, AZP-531 (Livoletide), an inhibitor of appetite stimulating hormone ghrelin, is in clinical trials with initial findings indicating improvement to hyperphagia for PWS patients.[659] Further, as an epigenetic disease, potential therapy could include treatment to reactivate the silenced maternal gene in these patients.[660,661]

Angelman syndrome (OMIM #105830) is a neurogenetic disorder with a similar incidence in the population as PWS. The AS clinical phenotype includes severe intellectual disability (IQ < 40), inappropriate bouts of laughter, absence of speech, gait ataxia, progressive microcephaly, dysmorphic facial features, and epilepsy.[662] Because these patients demonstrate bursts of laughter and smiling, AS is sometimes referred to as the "happy puppet syndrome." Unique electroencephalographic patterns are seen in most individuals with AS younger than 2 years of age and can be helpful in diagnosing the condition. As many as 6% of patients who display both intellectual disability and epilepsy may have AS. Some of the phenotypic features associated with AS can be nonspecific or can occur separately in other syndromes or nonsyndromic conditions; thus a constellation of findings with associated laughter, unique smiling, and happy demeanor of people with AS helps in the diagnosis.

Apparent from the characteristic physical findings, PWS and AS are clinically distinct syndromes, yet each results from different genetic alterations involving an imprinted segment within 8 million bases on chromosome 15q11.2-q13.[663] The genes at both ends of this region have biparental expression, but they flank genes that demonstrate exclusively paternal or maternal expression. The expression of either paternal or maternal genes is controlled by an imprinting center (IC) with the imprinting "reset" during gametogenesis between parent and offspring of a different gender. If paternally expressed genes in this region are missing, defective, or epigenetically silenced through DNA methylation and only an inactive, nonexpressed maternal allele remains, PWS is observed. Conversely, if maternally expressed genes in this region are not functional and only the inactive paternal allele remains, the clinical phenotype will be AS.

The most 5′ gene in the paternally expressed region is *MKRN3* that encodes makorin ring finger protein 3, with several zinc finger motifs and no introns and is involved in controlling the onset of puberty through the neurokinin pathway.[663,664] Adjacent to *MKRN3* are the structurally similar and intronless genes *MAGEL2* (alias *NDNL1*) coding melanoma antigen family L2 and *NDN*, a melanoma antigen family member, both are present in neurons.[663,665,666] This region also contains the locus *SNURF-SNRPN*, a bicistronic gene with two different proteins involved in a variety of functions including growth and differentiation and neuronal circuitry. *SNRPN* upstream reading frame (SNURF), which is found in the nucleus, contains 71 amino acids, may bind RNA, and has a C-terminal motif similar to ubiquitin and small nuclear ribonucleoprotein polypeptide N (*SNRPN*) that is involved in mRNA processing and formation of the spliceosomal A complex in splicing. Lastly there are multiple C/D box SNORNA genes, which are noncoding RNA molecules that modify both rRNA and snRNA by the methylation of the ribose 2′-hydroxyl group.[667,668] Sahoo et al. were the first to link the loss of paternal SNORNA genes to PWS in 2008.[669] The mechanism by which the absence of these genes results in the pathogenesis of PWS is not clearly understood. Nor is the mechanism by which human assisted reproductive technologies (ART) lead to abnormal methylation patterns of this region understood. Interestingly, the incidence of imprinting diseases is increased in ART pregnancies and there is a 3.44-fold higher risk of PWS in these pregnancies than in the general population.[670]

Loss of normally expressed paternal genes on chromosome 15q11-q13 resulting in PWS can occur by several mechanisms (Table 68.8). Most commonly, PWS (65 to 75%) results from a de novo deletion involving one of two common centromeric breakpoints (BP1 or BP2) and a telomeric breakpoint, BP3, on the paternal allele.[671] Deletions may be type 1 or type 2. The type I deletion is the larger of

TABLE 68.8	Molecular Mechanisms for Prader-Willi and Angelman Syndromes	
Molecular Mechanism of Disease	**Angelman Syndrome (Frequency)**	**Prader-Willi Syndrome (Frequency)**
Deletion of 15q11–13	Loss of maternal allele (70–75%)	Loss of paternal allele (65–75%)
Uniparental disomy	Two paternal chromosomes (3–7%)	Two maternal chromosomes (20–30%)
Imprinting center defect epimutations or microdeletions	Maternal allele (2–3%)	Paternal allele (2%)
UBE3A variant	10%	Not applicable
Rearrangement involving 15q11–13	Maternal allele (<1%)	Paternal allele (<1%)
Cause not identified	10%	Rare

the two and involves BP1 and BP3 while the smaller deletion involves BP2 and BP3. A small number of patients (~5%) will have breakpoints outside of these regions.[655,672] This renders the zygote monosomic for these genes, and the zygote possesses only the maternal copy of this region. Alternatively, 20 to 30% of cases of PWS are caused by uniparental disomy (UPD). In the case of PWS, although two copies of the genes located in 15q11.2-q13 exist, both are maternal in origin and in most cases arise from meiosis I nondisjunction followed by postzygotic mitotic loss of the third, paternally derived chromosome 15 via a process referred to as *trisomy rescue*. This mechanism rescues the zygote from trisomy 15, a condition that is incompatible with life.[673] Although the fetus is genetically complete with two chromosome 15s (disomy), both chromosomes have been received from the mother (uniparental), and no expression of paternally expressed genes occurs in this imprinted region. Not surprisingly, maternal age has been reported to be significantly higher in PWS patients resulting from UPD caused by maternal meiosis I nondisjunction than in PWS patients resulting from a de novo deletion.[674] Maternal UPD with two identical chromosome 15s from the mother due to nondisjunction in meiosis II can also occur and is referred to as isodisomy. Some cases of PWS result from microdeletions encompassing the paternal imprinting center (IC) or, in 2% of cases, from abnormal methylation at this site.[675] A variant involving the IC prevents this *cis*-acting control center from resetting the imprint in the germline. These variants will result in PWS because if they are present on the maternal chromosome of phenotypically normal fathers, they will be transmitted to offspring because now the paternal chromosome will maintain the maternal imprint and will be silenced. Finally, fewer than 1% of PWS cases are caused by chromosomal rearrangements disrupting the genes in the 15q11.2-q13 region.[676] Interestingly, differences in the phenotype of PWS patients resulting from a deletion has been noted when compared to PWS patients arising from UPD.[677]

The maternally expressed gene *UBE3A* is telomeric to the SNORNA genes and oriented in the opposite orientation on chromosome 15q11.2-q13.[678,679] The *UBE3A* gene encompasses 120 kb; contains 16 exons; and encodes E3 ubiquitin protein ligase, a multifunctional protein involved in the ubiquitin proteasome degradation pathway with both nuclear and cytoplasmic functions.[680,681] Three protein isoforms are produced from this gene by alternative splicing, and they differ at their N-termini.[682] Interestingly, in neurons, only the maternal *UBE3A* allele is expressed; however, both alleles are expressed in other tissues. Copy number variants due to duplications of this region have been associated with autism spectrum disorders.[683] Recent studies have associated UBE3A to the Wnt signaling pathway in early brain development.[681,684] A second gene, *ATP10A*, is upstream from *UBE3A* and is also contained within the AS region.[679] Similar to PWS, most patients with AS (70 to 75%) have a deletion of the critical 15q1.21-q13 region. However, unlike PWS, in AS, the disease-causing deletion occurs on the maternal allele. In 3 to 7% of AS patients, the syndrome is attributed to UPD from the inheritance of two paternally derived chromosome 15s; as a consequence, there is no transcription of *UBE3A*. An IC defect has been described in 2 to 3% of patients with AS; a chromosome rearrangement has

been reported in fewer than 1%; and in 10% of cases, a *UBE3A* variant has been detected. Most of the *UBE3A* gene variants are frameshift or nonsense variants and result in loss of function.[685] Using the AS mouse model, a possible treatment for this disease could be increasing expression of the normal paternal allele and silencing the variant transcript with antisense oligonucleotides.[686] In about 10% of AS cases, the molecular basis of the disease has not been determined. It is possible that these patients are misdiagnosed with AS and rather are similar to AS but clinically and molecularly separate.[687] Similar to PWS, phenotypic differences are observed depending on the molecular basis of the disease. AS with deletions are more likely to have hypopigmentation of skin, eye, and hair or microcephaly and are more likely to be severely affected.[688] In contrast, patients with AS arising from UPD have normal head circumference and are more often mildly affected.

Diagnostic testing for individuals suspected of having AS or PWS can involve a variety of laboratory techniques and testing algorithms. Methylation-specific PCR (msPCR) coupled with gel electrophoresis is one cost-effective approach (Fig. 68.16). In methylation-specific PCR, genomic DNA is treated with sodium bisulfite which converts unmethylated cytosine residues to uracil without altering the methylated cytosine residues (those which are silenced in the 15q11.2-13 region through imprinting). The subsequent PCR uses oligonucleotide primers complementary to DNA strands that contain uracil (from unmethylated cytosines) or cytosine (from methylated cytosines).[689] msPCR provides a rapid and reliable diagnostic test for PWS or AS. Fewer than 1% of PWS cases and about 20% of AS cases are not detected by this assay. Additionally, msPCR coupled with melting curve analysis or methylation-specific MLPA can be used.[690] Although msPCR is frequently the first tier of testing and can be used to diagnose PWS or AS, it cannot determine the molecular basis of disease. If the msPCR result is positive, chromosomal microarray analysis will identify chromosome deletions, and in UPD cases, the parental origin of both chromosomes can be determined.[672] Patients with PWS and patients with a chromosomal rearrangement disrupting the genes in this area will not be identified by these testing methods nor will AS patients with a *UBE3A* variant. Rather, in these cases, a routine karyotype or DNA sequence analysis is required for diagnosis. Early diagnostic testing for PWS or AS is critical to initiate intervention and achieve better outcomes for patients. Currently however, NBS for PWS/AS is not performed although testing is feasible from newborn bloodspots currently used for NBS.[691] Testing to identify the molecular mechanism of disease for PWS and AS is important for accurately determining recurrence risk to the family. For example, although variants causing AS can arise de novo (e.g., UPD with a <1% recurrence risk), other AS-causing variants can be silently transmitted through several generations. If a *UBE3A* variant arose de novo on a paternal allele transmitted to a son, the son could transmit the variant to a son or daughter to produce a normal phenotype. However, although this son could transmit the silenced *UBE3A* variant to his offspring, his sister could donate her altered *UBE3A* paternally derived allele to her offspring, and the child would have AS. The recurrence risk for her to have another affected child in this case would be 50%.

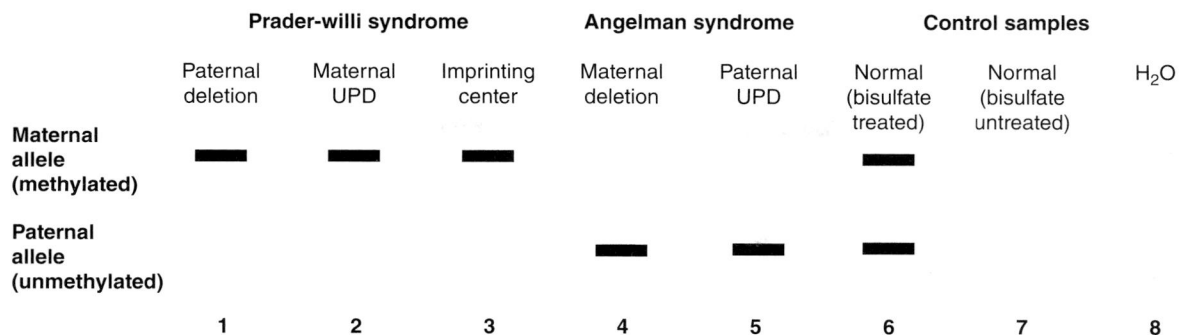

FIGURE 68.16 Schematic representation of methylation-specific polymerase chain reaction (*PCR*) for the diagnosis of Prader-Willi syndrome (*PWS*) and Angelman syndrome (*AS*). Extracted DNA is treated with sodium bisulfate before amplification using PCR and oligonucleotide primers specific for modified DNA. PCR products are subjected to gel electrophoresis. PWS patients show only the maternal allele, and AS patients show only the paternal allele. Normal individuals show two amplicons representing their methylated maternal allele and unmethylated paternal allele. Patient DNA with patterns diagnostic of PWS *(lanes 1–3)* and AS *(lanes 4 and 5)*. Control samples include normal DNA treated with and without bisulfate *(lanes 6 and 7,* respectively) and a negative control reaction in which no template DNA was added in *lane 8.* No amplification products are observed in unmodified normal control DNA *(lane 7),* illustrating the specificity of PCR primers prepared specifically for sodium bisulfate–modified DNA.[689]

POINTS TO REMEMBER

Inherited Diseases

- Mitochondrial and imprinting disorders follow non-Mendelian patterns of inheritance.
- Complex diseases result from the contribution of both genetic and environmental factors and do not follow Mendelian inheritance patterns.
- For most genes, pathogenic variants are located throughout the gene and are heterogeneous in nature.
- For some disease genes, the type of variant and effect on the encoded protein can predict the clinical phenotype and identify targeted therapy for patient care.
- Diagnostic DNA testing is complicated by genetic and allelic heterogeneity.
- Genetic counseling is an important component of patient care and management.

EXPANDED CARRIER SCREENING

Carrier screening refers to the use of genetic testing to determine individuals who are at risk of having a child affected with an autosomal recessive disorder. Carrier screening for disorders has long been a mainstay of genetic laboratories and has increased dramatically over the past decade. Carrier screening for some common lethal disorders (e.g., CF) is considered the standard of care in prenatal patients regardless of ethnicity.[692] For some ethnic groups, such as Ashkenazi Jews, the carrier frequency for several lethal disorders is relatively high.[693] As a result, screening for many of these disorders (e.g., Tay-Sachs, Canavan) has long been recommended to Ashkenazi Jewish couples during preconception and prenatal counseling.[693]

Conventional carrier screening used targeted variant panels (e.g., the ACMG *CFTR* 23 variant panel) that identify the majority of variant carriers for a single disorder. Over the past several years, carrier screening (particularly in preconception/prenatal care) has shifted toward new testing platforms that simultaneously screen for hundreds of common disease-associated base pair substitutions. With the advent of these new technologies many laboratories are offering expanded carrier screening (ECS) panels. Initially, ECS panels simply increased the number of variants that were tested in a single gene (e.g., *CFTR*). More recently, ECS panels have broadened to include known variants for a multitude (>100 in some cases) of inherited disorders in a single test.[694,695] The clear advantage of ECS panels is that they provide a cost-effective method to screen for multiple genetic disorders. In many cases, the cost of an ECS panel is less than screening for a single gene by traditional means. ECS panels also provide patients with carrier status data on additional disorders not routinely included on traditional carrier screening panels. However, ECS panels have come under criticism because of several drawbacks.

Traditionally, variants included on carrier screening panels were selected based on confirmed pathogenicity and the carrier frequency of the variant.[37] With the advent of ECS panels, some laboratories have included variants with reduced penetrance or mild clinical effects.[696,697] Some expanded CF screening panels include variants that are known to have variable clinical impact and in some cases result in no discernible phenotype.[697] The inclusion of such variants in a genetic screening assay can be confusing and lead individuals to make reproductive decisions without a complete understanding of the information provided.[697,698] Some disorders that have been selected for inclusion on commercially available ECS panels do not meet generally accepted criteria for carrier screening.[698,699] For example, some disorders are rare and have a reported incidence of less than 1 per million births.[699,700] Not surprisingly, the targeted variants in many of these rare disorders only account for a small fraction of those capable of causing disease. A negative screening result in an individual with a family history for a rare disorder may give a false sense of security. Because of this low sensitivity, if a variant is identified in one partner for a rare disorder, that individual's reproductive partner likely will undergo full gene sequencing for the causative gene, thus increasing the costs of screening dramatically.[699] ECS panels have also been criticized for including variants (and functional polymorphisms) of variable penetrance that are very common in certain ethnic groups or society at large (e.g., factor V Leiden, *HFE*-related hemochromatosis, MTHFR deficiency).[698] Typically, disorders with such high frequency in the population are not recommended for carrier screening because their clinical implications are uncertain. The identification of these variants in the context of preconception (or prenatal) counseling are especially controversial because fetal testing for some of these disorders (e.g., MTHFR deficiency) is not routinely offered in the United States.[698] The clinical validity of some of the variants that are included on prenatal screening panels is unclear.

Another aspect of ECS panels that merits mention is the inclusion of adult-onset disorders. Some disorders (e.g., familial Mediterranean fever, α_1-antitrypsin deficiency, *GJB2*-related nonsyndromic hearing loss, atypical CF) have variable ages of onset and disease manifestations. Carrier screening for variants that cause these disorders in individuals of reproductive age can provide an unexpected diagnosis of a disease that they have not yet developed. In one study, 78 of 23,453 individuals tested were identified as either compound heterozygous or homozygous for disease-causing variants.[700] Of the patients identified, only three patients reported a previous diagnosis or history of disease.[700] These data illustrate the complex counseling-related issues that ECS panels have created. Because traditional carrier screening has focused on severe, disease-causing variants, the likelihood of diagnosing an asymptomatic individual with disease was very low. The newer ECS panels require that all patients undergoing such screening be properly advised as to the potential testing outcomes.

To address the issues associated with ECS testing, in 2013 the ACMG released a position statement regarding prenatal and preconception ECS that outlined criteria for inclusion of diseases or variants on a carrier screening panel, including (1) a clearly defined clinical association; (2) most at-risk patients would choose fetal testing to aid in preconception or prenatal decision making; (3) a clearly defined residual risk for individuals that test negative; and (4) for any adult-onset disorder that may affect the individual being tested, pretest counseling and consent should be performed.[701] Subsequently, the ACOG released additional guidance regarding the criteria that should be used to determine the content of ECS panels.[702] ACOG suggests, among other things, that any disorder included should have a carrier frequency of at least 1 in 100, have a detrimental impact of quality of life, or require surgical or medical intervention.[702] Additionally, ACOG also released a statement to help guide physicians in offering, consenting, and counseling patients about ECS panels and their results.[703]

The clinical use of ECS panels is still in its infancy. As with any new technology and the increase in data that it provides, unforeseen ethical issues can arise. As the use of ECS panels becomes widespread and professional organizations develop formal guidelines, many of the issues outlined here will be resolved. However, preconception and prenatal genetic counseling will continue to be important in helping patients to understand the clinical implications of their screening results.

MASSIVELY PARALLEL SEQUENCING

Massively parallel sequencing (also referred to as next-generation sequencing) is a high-throughput DNA sequencing technology capable of generating data on a genomic scale in a short period of days (see Chapter 65). Not since the introduction of PCR in the 1980s has a technology revolutionized the field of molecular diagnostics like MPS has in the past decade. At the most basic level, MPS uses similar concepts to traditional capillary-based Sanger sequencing in that fluorescently labeled dNTPs are used to determine the template sequence. However, the distinct advantage of MPS is its ability to perform simultaneous sequencing reactions on millions of target sequences at a vastly lower cost per base than traditional Sanger sequencing. There are several different MPS methods, but most have similar sample preparation workflows. Typically, DNA fragmentation is followed by insert selection, library formation, and clonal amplification. Then sequencing by synthesis signals are acquired by measuring pyrophosphate release, generation of hydrogen ions, or the fluorescence of reversible terminators. This massively parallel clonal sequencing of library inserts generates anywhere from gigabases to terabases of sequencing data at a cost that is feasible for clinical testing. One drawback to such massive data generation is that bioinformatics filtering processes are required to efficiently interpret the numerous variants identified. Data filtering in MPS typically involves the utilization of publicly available variant databases (e.g., dbSNP; The Genome Aggregation Database (gnomAD), Exome Aggregation Consortium [ExAC], National Heart, Lung, and Blood Institute Exome Sequencing Project) to eliminate variants that occur at high frequency in the general population and therefore are likely benign. After the common variants have been filtered, locus-specific variant databases and *in silico* prediction programs (e.g., SIFT and PolyPhen2) can aid in the interpretation of potential disease-causing variants. Variants are then classified as pathogenic, likely pathogenic, uncertain significance, likely benign, or benign.[704] Data filtering systems are commercially available to help in the interpretation of MPS data, but many laboratories have chosen to develop their own software pipelines internally. Table 68.9 summarizes some of the resources commonly used in the analysis and interpretation of MPS data in more detail.

One of the most significant advantages of MPS for diagnostic testing is the ability to target all genes known to be associated with a specific diagnosis (or phenotype) in a single test that is comparable in price and turnaround time to that of Sanger sequencing for a single-gene analysis. These targeted gene panels are the most commonly ordered clinical tests using MPS technology (Table 68.10). Before development of MPS, testing patients for causative variants in multiple genes that cause a single syndrome was a very expensive and time-consuming process. For example, retinitis pigmentosa (RP, OMIM #268000) is a group of inherited degenerative ocular disorders that affects 1 in 3000 to 7000 people.[705] Locus heterogeneity is a hallmark of RP because variants in more than 60 genes have been reported to cause this disease. Using traditional Sanger sequencing to determine the underlying molecular alteration would be cost prohibitive for most

TABLE 68.9 Computational Aids Used in Sequence Variant Classification

Computational Aid	Description	Example
Data aggregation databases	Databases that compile large sets of genome/exome data and provide population frequency data. The available population frequency data helps to determine if a variant is rare or commonly occurring.	Genome Aggregation Database (gnomAD) https://gnomad.broadinstitute.org
In silico prediction software	Software programs that use proprietary algorithms to predict whether an amino acid change is likely to impact function.	PolyPhen-2 https://genetics.bwh.harvard.edu/pph2 SIFT https://sift.bii.a-star.edu.sg
ClinVar	A freely accessible archive of reports of DNA variants and their associated phenotype. Supporting evidence for variant interpretations is also provided and many genes are expertly curated.	https://www.ncbi.nlm.nih.gov/clinvar
Locus-specific variant databases	Expert curated databases that focus on a single gene or set of genes associated with a specific phenotype.	HbVar http://globin.cse.psu.edu/globin/hbvar RettBASE http://mecp2.chw.edu.au/#mutations

TABLE 68.10 Commonly Ordered Massively Parallel Sequencing–based Gene Panels

Panel Name	Included Disorders[a]	Targeted Patient Group
Aortopathy disorders	Ehlers-Danlos syndrome (I, II, and IV), Loeys-Dietz syndrome, Marfan syndrome, familial thoracic aortic aneurysm and dissection	Individuals with disease affecting any aortic section
Breast and ovarian hereditary cancer	Hereditary breast and ovarian cancer syndrome	Individuals with a strong family history of breast and ovarian cancer; individuals with early onset of breast or ovarian cancer
Cardiomyopathy disorders	Dilated cardiomyopathy, hypertrophic cardiomyopathy, arrhythmogenic right ventricular cardiomyopathy	Individuals with a suspected diagnosis of a hereditary cardiomyopathy disorder
Expanded carrier screening	Numerous (>100)	Individuals planning pregnancy or prenatal reproductive partners
Hearing loss	Keratitis–ichthyosis–deafness syndrome, nonsyndromic hearing loss, Usher syndrome	Individuals with a suspected diagnosis of either syndromic or nonsyndromic hearing loss
Hereditary endocrine cancer	Multiple endocrine neoplasia type 1, multiple endocrine neoplasia type 2, Von Hippel-Lindau disease	Individuals with a family history of endocrine cancer; individuals with a personal history of endocrine cancer
Hereditary gastrointestinal cancer	Familial adenomatous polyposis, juvenile polyposis syndrome, Lynch syndrome	Individuals with a personal or family history of gastrointestinal cancer
Noonan spectrum disorders	Cardiofaciocutaneous syndrome, Costello syndrome, Noonan syndrome	Individuals with a suspected diagnosis of Noonan syndrome or a related disorder
Periodic fever syndromes	Familial Mediterranean fever, Majeed syndrome, Muckle-Wells syndrome	Individuals with a suspected diagnosis of a periodic fever syndrome
X-linked intellectual disability	Rett syndrome, Duchenne muscular dystrophy, ornithine transcarbamylase deficiency	Individuals with intellectual disability inherited in an X-linked manner

[a]This is a selected list of commonly included disorders and is not comprehensive.

patients with RP, yet an MPS RP gene panel is cost effective and timely. RP is one example of how MPS implementation has advanced our ability to provide a molecular diagnosis for a genetically heterogeneous disorder. Table 68.8 lists some commonly ordered MPS-based gene panels. MPS also enables the sequencing of very large genes at a reasonable cost (e.g., the DMD gene that causes DMD and BMD). The flexibility of MPS selection and library preparation can provide a comprehensive test of more than 100 genes (e.g., an X-Linked Intellectual Disabilities Panel) or a more targeted panel that analyzes a handful of genes associated with a specific phenotype (e.g., a hereditary gastrointestinal cancer panel). Over the next few years it is likely that Sanger sequencing assays will further decline in use and sequencing technology will continue to evolve.

NONINVASIVE PRENATAL TESTING

Noninvasive prenatal testing (NIPT) is an MPS-based method that has revolutionized the field of prenatal screening. Unlike traditional prenatal testing methods that require the direct (and invasive) harvesting of fetal cells (i.e., amniocentesis),

TABLE 68.11 Benefits of Noninvasive Prenatal Testing Compared to Traditional Genetic Testing Methods

Noninvasive Prenatal Testing	Amniocentesis/ Chorionic Villi
• No risk to fetus • Performed on maternal peripheral blood • Quick turnaround time • Can be performed as early as 9 weeks of gestation • Can eliminate the need for invasive diagnostic testing	• ~1–3% risk of pregnancy loss • Invasive sample collection • Potentially prolonged turnaround time due to cell culturing needs • Typically performed between 10 and 13 weeks of gestation

NIPT is performed on circulating cell-free fetal DNA present in the maternal blood stream. NIPT has rapidly become the preferred method for screening for aneuploidies as it poses little risk to fetus or mother. It can also be offered as early as 9 weeks gestation leaving ample time for diagnostic testing in the event of an abnormal result. Many of the benefits of NIPT as compared to traditional prenatal diagnostic testing are highlighted in Table 68.11.

NIPT is typically performed using one of two methods: (1) the quantitative molecular counting method or (2) the SNP genotyping method. The quantitative counting method works under the premise that fetal DNA representing the entire genome of the fetus is present in the maternal circulation at a consistent relative proportion.[706,707] More specifically, this method uses MPS to indiscriminately sequence both maternal and fetal DNA. Millions of sequencing reads are generated and then they are mapped to the matching chromosomes.[706] The reads are then counted and when the proportion of fetal DNA that maps to a chromosome of interest (e.g., chromosomes 13, 18, or 21) exceeds what is expected (or is underrepresented), it is evidence that the fetus may have aneuploidy for that respective chromosome.[706,707] This method is not dependent on the presence of DNA polymorphisms and can be performed when only a relatively small amount of fetal DNA is present. It should be noted that this method is usually performed as a genome wide test and is therefore capable of identifying aneuploidy in all chromosomes (although not all are routinely reported clinically). However, this method is not capable of determining if these abnormalities are present in the fetus or maternal sample.[708]

The SNP genotyping method of NIPT is designed to look at commonly occurring DNA changes located only on the chromosomes of interest. Historically, the SNP method requires that DNA is extracted from both maternal plasma and maternal leukocytes. The plasma sample is expected to contain both maternal DNA and circulating fetal DNA while the maternal leukocyte sample is purely maternal DNA.[708] Targeted SNP amplification is then performed and sample genotypes are analyzed. Fetal genotype can be determined by comparing the genotype obtained from the plasma to the purely maternal sample.[708] Aneuploidy is determined by comparing the observed fetal SNP distribution to that expected.[709] Recent updates to computer algorithms now allow for the SNP-based method to be performed without analysis

of a separate maternal leukocyte sample. It should be noted that the SNP-based NIPT method is the only reliable method for determining parent of origin when aneuploidy is present or detecting triploidy. However, it cannot be used in scenarios where more than two genotypes are present in the plasma (e.g., egg donor pregnancy, twin pregnancy).[708]

Regardless of the methodology, the fetal fraction (the percentage of circulating DNA in the maternal plasma that is fetal in origin) is a critical component in determining the reliability of NIPT results.[710] Measurement of fetal fraction is important in any NIPT protocol as it guarantees that enough fetal DNA is present in a sample to effectively determine a fetal genotype.[710] Most laboratories set a minimum acceptable fetal fraction based on the performance characteristics of their test. As such, there is no industry standard fetal fraction cutoff but this value generally falls in the 2 to 4% range.[710] It is reported that most pregnancies between 10 and 20 weeks of gestation have an average fetal fraction of 10 to 15% but this is often impacted by several factors (e.g., maternal weight, ethnicity).[710,711] It is generally accepted that a higher fetal fraction results in higher confidence in the final NIPT result. As the fetal fraction declines the detection rate of the assay also decreases and may ultimately result in indeterminate findings.[710] However, NIPT is a robust assay and when performed on an appropriate sample it is an accurate and sensitive screening method. Studies have demonstrated that the sensitivity of NIPT for detecting trisomy 21 routinely surpasses 98% while specificity is >97%.[712] NIPT is therefore the most effective aneuploidy screening method currently available.

Although NIPT is currently used mainly as a screening tool for aneuploidies, there is a push to detect variants in single gene targets for diagnostic purposes. Noninvasive prenatal diagnosis (NIPD), like NIPT, would be preferable to traditional prenatal diagnostic testing as it poses little to no risk to the fetus. Many studies have been performed demonstrating that NIPD is possible but many technical challenges still remain.[713] It is likely that within the next several years we will see NIPD become part of routine clinical testing. NIPT and NIPD are further discussed in Chapter 72.

WHOLE-EXOME SEQUENCING

Whole-exome sequencing (WES) refers to an MPS-based DNA sequencing method that specifically targets the coding regions (exons) and directly adjacent intronic regions for the majority of the approximately 20,000 genes known to exist in the human genome. Although the exome only accounts for approximately 1% of the human genome, variants in gene encoding regions are responsible for the vast majority of human inherited diseases. On average, WES is able to identify an underlying genetic alteration anywhere from 8 to 100% of patients (depending on the inclusion criteria) with a median diagnostic yield of 33.2%.[714] This makes WES an effective diagnostic tool for patients with a phenotype that suggests an inherited disorder that does not fit the clinical characteristics of previously described syndromes.[715,716]

Most exome sequencing performed in clinical laboratories currently uses a hybridization-based capture method of tagged (biotinylated) probes targeted to specific areas of the fragmented template DNA.[717] These probes are bound to magnetic beads allowing a simple washing process to separate targeted DNA regions from the excess unwanted (intronic) DNA.[717]

After this enrichment process, the DNA is ready to be sequenced. Several exome capture kits are commercially available, making WES easily performed in most molecular diagnostic laboratories. Often, the limiting factor in implementing WES is the large amount of data produced; therefore a well-defined bioinformatics workflow is critical for the timely reporting of WES results. Several data analysis programs are commercially available to aid in the interpretation of WES data, and many publications describe informatics workflows.[718]

Clinical WES sequencing is often performed on both the symptomatic proband and their (typically asymptomatic) parents (often referred to as a trio). Sequencing parents helps with interpretation of sequence variants that are identified in the proband. For example, if a potentially pathogenic variant is identified in the proband but not observed in the parental samples, that variant is likely de novo (assuming confirmed paternity) and potentially causative. Likewise, if a potentially pathogenic variant is identified in a gene that is dominantly inherited but is also identified in an asymptomatic parent, it is less likely to cause the patient's phenotype. Parental samples can also be used to establish phase in the detection of two pathogenic variants in a gene inherited in an autosomal recessive manner. Use of familial samples to aid interpretation of WES results is a powerful tool capable of dramatically increasing clinical sensitivity of the test and should be pursued in all patients undergoing WES. Although the analysis method for WES will vary between laboratories, a general workflow for analysis of exome data is provided in Fig. 68.17.

WES has been implemented widely in clinical diagnostic laboratories in the United States, and thousands of patients have been tested by this method. WES should be considered in patients with a phenotype suspected to be caused by a variant in a single gene when known single-gene disorders have been eliminated.[715] Careful consideration should always be given to the patient's presentation before determining whether or not WES is the appropriate test for a given phenotype. Specifically, a detailed family history, a systematic characterization of the patient's phenotype, and a careful literature review is recommended before ordering WES.[715] Obtaining this information can help determine if the patient is actually affected by a previously described, but rare, syndrome with a known genetic cause that should be ruled out before proceeding to WES.[715] In many cases, a single gene test or a targeted MPS-based gene panel with multiple genes may be the appropriate first test to order. To aid clinicians in determining which molecular testing protocol is best for their patients, algorithms have been developed.[719,720] These testing algorithms suggest that individuals with multiple nonspecific clinical findings or with a clinical presentation associated with marked genetic heterogeneity (e.g., intellectual disability) are good candidates for WES.[719,720] Individuals with distinctive clinical features, family history of a specific disorder, or indicative findings for specific disorders should be counseled to pursue either single-gene or MPS-based gene panel testing.[719,720] Using these testing guidelines, approximately 50% of patients received a genetic diagnosis using "traditional" methods of diagnosis.[719] Single-gene or targeted MPS panel testing is therefore not obsolete because of WES but continues to be the appropriate diagnostic tool in many clinical cases.

Counseling for WES is highly complex because issues relating to test results must be considered. The risk of identifying a VUS exists in all sequencing-based genetic tests. However, the risk for the identification of a VUS increases dramatically for WES. Patient counseling for WES should always include a discussion of VUSs because these are likely to appear on any WES report even though the clinical implications of these findings are unclear.[720] Patients should be counseled on the possibility that incidental findings may include the identification of pathogenic variants in clinically actionable genes (e.g., BRCA1) that are unrelated to the patient's current phenotype. The return of incidental findings (IFs) in WES is a controversial topic and has resulted in the ACMG formalizing recommendations for which IFs should be returned to the patient.[721,722] The ACMG recommendations provide a list of 59 genes that represent the "minimum" IFs that should be reported to the clinician when a pathogenic variant is identified regardless of the clinical indication for testing.[722] The gene list generated by the ACMG was developed to include genes for conditions that are verifiable by other diagnostic methods and that cause highly penetrant disorders that would likely benefit from medical intervention.[721,722] The release of the ACMG recommendations was met by criticism because the guidelines were seen by some to violate existing ethical norms in genetic testing and the patient's right to autonomy by suggesting that IFs in the 59-gene list should be returned regardless of patient preference.[721–723] In response to criticism from its members, the ACMG released a statement in April 2014 revising its recommendations to allow patients to opt out of receiving incidental

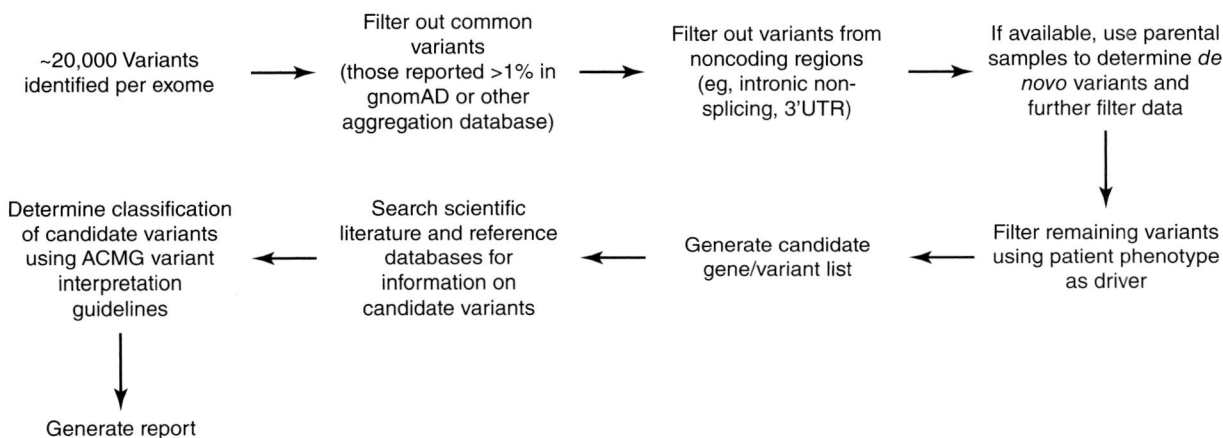

FIGURE 68.17 General workflow for exome sequencing analysis and interpretation.

findings. Even after this revision, debate continues among members of the ACMG and clinical geneticists regarding how IFs should be returned to patients.[724] Recommendations on the return of IFs likely will continue to evolve as WES genomic testing becomes more commonplace in clinics.[725]

Over the past several years, WES has proven to be an invaluable research tool in the discovery of the underlying genetic alterations for many Mendelian disorders.[726–728] In some cases, these discoveries identified the first known genetic cause of a disorder (e.g., Miller syndrome, Kabuki syndrome), and in others, additional genes were discovered to cause an already well-defined phenotype (e.g., RP, nonsyndromic hearing loss, osteogenesis imperfecta, intellectual disability, and many others).[729–735] WES studies also have elucidated alternative phenotypes caused by variants in genes already known to cause a genetic disorder.[736–738] The benefits of these discoveries in the clinical diagnosis and treatment of patients cannot be overstated. Identification of the underlying molecular alteration (and molecular pathogenesis) that results in a specific disease is the first step in developing treatment modalities. Because of the discoveries made by WES and the increased adoption of whole genome sequencing (discussed in detail in Chapter 66), the next decade will see a vast improvement in the treatment of many inherited disorders. Moreover, it is likely that in the next decade we will also see the discovery of the underlying cause for the vast majority of inherited genetic disorders.

CYTOGENOMICS

The term *cytogenomics* describes the application of molecular techniques to cytogenetics. In a broad sense, this applies to fluorescence in situ hybridization (FISH) analysis. In this molecular cytogenetic technique, a fluorescently labeled DNA molecule serves as a "probe" and is hybridized to metaphase chromosomes or interphase nuclei, and the fluorescent probes are visualized using a fluorescent microscope. In a more narrow sense, cytogenomics applies to the use of chromosome microarray (CMA) technology, including array comparative genomic hybridization (aCGH) and SNP arrays.[739] SNP and aCGH arrays have revolutionized the field of cytogenetics as important tools for both clinical diagnosis and disease discovery.[740–742] However, these technologies do not identify balanced translocations or inversions, both of which require routine karyotyping, FISH analysis, or both.[743,744]

Instrumentation and associated kits for aCGH and SNP arrays are commercially available. Platforms and methods vary, including the probe size, spacing between the probes on the array, copy number resolutions, and probe sensitivity.[739,745] In aCGH, the patient and control DNA are labeled with two different fluorochromes and co-hybridized to the array, but with a SNP array, no control DNA is used; rather, the fluorescent signals are measured against a reference pattern.[739] Both aCGH and SNP arrays can detect copy number variants (CNVs).[746] In addition, SNP arrays provide the genotype and determine if the patient is homozygous (AA, BB) or heterozygous (AB) for each SNP present on the array. SNP genotype analysis allows long stretches of homologous DNA sequences, also referred to as regions of homology (ROHs) or regions with an absence of heterozygosity (AOHs), to be identified. These segments of DNA are important to identify UPD in the diagnosis of imprinting disorders.[747,748] However, detection of an ROH or AOH could represent an

incidental or unexpected finding of parental relatedness or consanguinity. Depending on the degree of homozygosity, these findings could suggest incestral mating. Standards and guidelines for laboratory reporting of incidental findings suggestive of consanguinity have been developed by the ACMG, and care must be taken by clinicians in communicating these results to patients.[749,750]

CMA's clinical utility is in the diagnosis and management of patients referred for multiple congenital anomalies, dysmorphic features, neurodevelopmental disorders, developmental delay or intellectual disability, and ASDs.[741,742] The ACMG recommends CMA as a first-tier genetic test for patients with these conditions, and practice standards and guidelines for these applications have been established.[751] Prior to reporting CNVs of potential clinical significance, FISH, MLPA, or real-time PCR studies are often used for confirmation of novel aberrant CNV findings to prevent false-positive reporting (Fig. 68.18). Public databases (e.g., Database of Genomic Variants, National Center for Biotechnology Information) are used to determine the genes that are contained within the CNV and that may be either lost or gained.[752,753] Generally, the larger the CNV and the more genes contained within the DNA region of interest, the more the variant is likely to have a clinical consequence and the more likely a deletion is to be pathogenic compared with duplications. After careful review of various databases, the patient's clinical findings and peer-reviewed publications for the function of the genes involved in the CNV and their associated phenotype using ClinGen and OMIM) the significance of the CNV is reported using guidelines established by the ACMG.[541,754,755] Results may be reported as pathogenic or as a variant of uncertain clinical significance (VUS). Appropriate literature should be referenced, and the variant should be reported according to standard CNV nomenclature. To ascertain the significance of any VUS, parental specimens should be requested (see Fig. 68.18).

Chromosome microarray is the recommended first-line diagnostic test when abnormal ultrasound findings are observed.[756] Since CMA testing is unable to identify balanced rearrangements, low-level chromosomal mosaicism, or inversions, additional diagnostic testing may be required in CMA negative patients.[744] CMA testing can be performed on DNA extracted from cultured amniocytes or chorionic villi tissue. However, CMA testing in prenatal cases can be especially challenging if a VUS is identified as it may be difficult to predict the postnatal effect.[757,758] CMA analysis on DNA extracted from representative tissue of products of conception can be useful in determining the etiology of the pregnancy loss.[759,760]

In addition to using aCGH and SNP arrays to detect constitutional or germline changes associated with disease, these arrays are also used on hematologic and solid tumors.[761] In somatic tissue, the detection of copy number changes can define regions of DNA and specific genes involved in the pathogenesis of neoplastic processes. In addition, the ability of SNP arrays to determine genotype enables the identification of copy neutral LOH. Similar to constitutional UPD seen with imprinting disorders, copy neutral LOH is a somatic event and indicates two copies of the same chromosomal region. This may involve part of the chromosome or the entire chromosome, and most often, the region involved harbors a "driver" variant in a particular gene that promotes growth and proliferation for the neoplastic process.

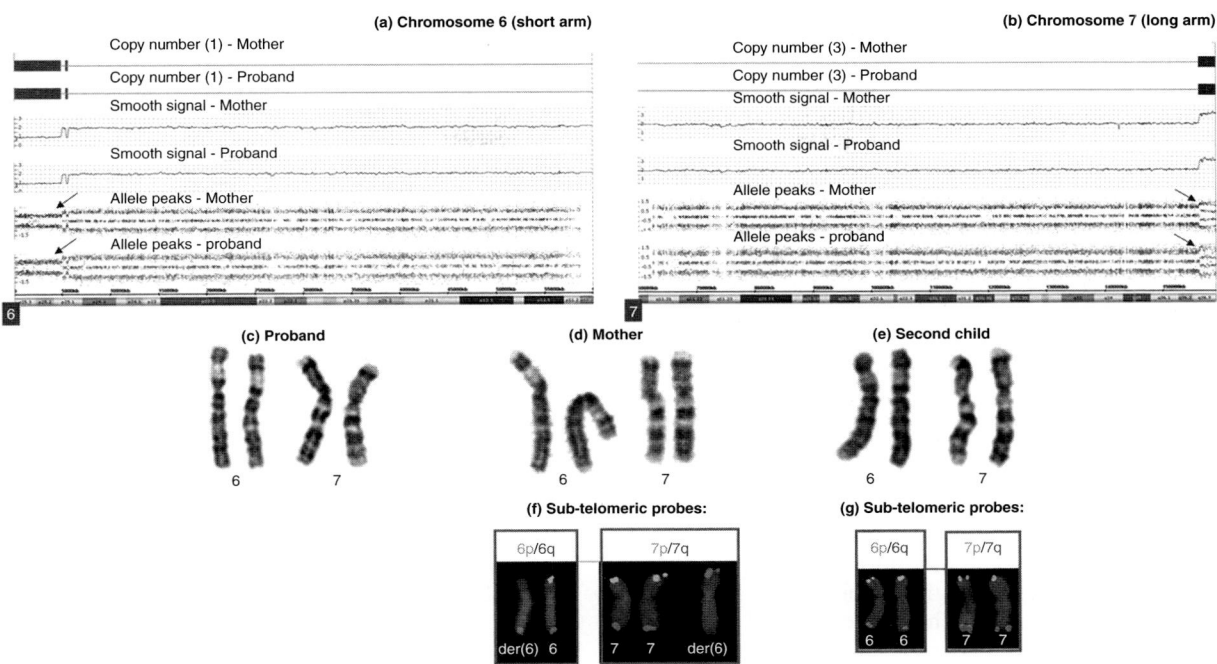

FIGURE 68.18 Cryptic familial unbalanced translocation detected using SNP/copy number microarray technology. The proband was referred for cytogenetic testing at 2 days of age due to eye abnormalities and other congenital malformations. Conventional GTG-banding was normal (image c) and reflex microarray testing was performed. The microarray study showed a 4820-kb deletion (one copy) of the distal short arm of chromosome 6 (6p25.3 to 6p25.1; panel a; left arrows), and a 2936-kb copy number gain (three copies) of the distal long arm of chromosome 7 (7q36.3; panel b; right arrow). When both a loss and gain involving two different chromosomes are present in a child, these imbalances may result from the malsegregation of a balanced translocation in a parent so parental chromosome studies are recommended. The GTG-banding analysis of the mother was also normal (image d). However, her microarray test showed the same imbalances as those seen in her infant (panels a and b). A FISH test (panel f), using subtelomeric probes specific for the short arm and long arm of chromosome 6 and chromosome 7 confirmed: (1) loss involving the distal short arm on one chromosome 6, and (2) gain involving the distal long arm of chromosome 7 on the short arm of the derivative chromosome 6 (for a total of three copies of 7q). Phenotypic traits correlated with the identified cytogenetic findings. The results from these studies enabled testing on a subsequent child and were normal (images e and g). (Courtesy Dr. Colleen Jackson-Cook, Director Cytogenetics Laboratory, Department of Pathology, Virginia Commonwealth University Health System.)

POINTS TO REMEMBER

Clinical Utility of Molecular Methods

- Targeted PCR amplification is most useful in the identification of common pathogenic point variants.
- msPCR is capable of determining the methylation status of DNA and is often used in the diagnosis of imprinting disorders.
- Full-gene Sanger sequencing is typically used to identify pathogenic base pair substitutions and small insertion or deletion variants in disorders associated with a single disease-causing gene.
- MPS is an ideal technology to use for the identification of point variants and small insertions or deletions when large genes, multiple genes, exomes, or full genome sequencing is desired.
- MLPA is most useful in the detection of large (exon level or bigger) deletions or duplications in three or fewer disease-causing genes.
- Array-based technology is most useful in the simultaneous detection of large deletions or duplications in numerous genes.

REPORTING OF TEST RESULTS

As the preceding pages show, DNA testing for inherited diseases is complex, and thoroughly conveying genetic test results is important. Results must be presented so they can be easily and accurately understood by a professional whose expertise may not be genetics because in many instances, primary care providers communicate test results to the patient. With the increasing clinical demand for genetic testing and the increasing numbers of laboratories performing such tests, uniformity and standardization in communicating these complex results to referring clinicians is important, and failure to include some pertinent information in these reports constitutes a deficiency in the molecular pathology laboratory inspection checklist of the College of American Pathologists (CAP).[762,763] A comprehensive genetic report should include the patient's name, medical record number or birth date, sex of the patient, ethnicity of the patient (if relevant), type of specimen and date received, specimen's laboratory identification number, laboratory test requested, name and address of laboratory performing the test, name and address of referring health care professional or hospital, date of the report, analytic interpretation of the results using standard nomenclature for all variants identified, detailed description of the method used (citing literature if needed), and sensitivity and specificity of the assay (e.g., number of variants analyzed, percentage of variants not detected, possibility of genetic heterogeneity, chance of genetic recombination, and any other limitations of the assay (e.g., deletion/duplication detection)). All sequence variants are classified as one of the following: pathogenic, likely pathogenic, uncertain significance, likely benign, or benign.[704] In silico tools such as PolyPhen2, SIFT, gene specific databases, MutationTaster, and a variety of online websites should be reviewed to determine significance of the variant (see Table 68.10). The DNA and protein change, if applicable, should be listed using guidelines of the Human Genome Variation Society.[764] The laboratory should include the reference sequence, genome build, genomic coordinates of the variant(s), and depth of coverage.[765] The report must also include a clinical interpretation of the findings as applicable. Although preparation of the clinical interpretation can be labor intensive, this section is vital to most genetic reports and is important for describing the clinical significance of the results as they apply specifically to the patient and his or her family. This section should include a brief clinical history of the patient (indicating the reason for testing) and may discuss recurrence risk, genotype–phenotype correlation or penetrance, associated disease or carrier risk calculations for other members of his or her family, and citations of literature as needed. Importantly, a statement that genetic counseling for the patient is indicated must be included. In addition, easy access to genomic testing results to both the patient and all health care providers involved in the care of the patient is essential for appropriate patient care and management.

Furthermore, because many assays performed in clinical DNA laboratories are laboratory-developed tests (LDTs) or procedures (LDPs) that have been well designed, developed, and validated by a specific laboratory and are not approved by the FDA, reports must include a disclaimer to state this fact. Class I analyte-specific reagents may be purchased from a vendor and sold for a specific test, or they may be independently purchased by the laboratory and assembled into a laboratory-designed test. An example of the disclaimer would state: "This test was developed and its performance characteristics determined by [laboratory name]. It has not been cleared or approved by the US Food and Drug Administration." In addition, the CAP recommends inclusion of these additional statements: "The FDA does not require this test to go through premarket FDA review. This test is used for clinical purposes. It should not be regarded as investigational or for research. This laboratory is certified under the Clinical Laboratory Improvement Amendments (CLIA) as qualified to perform high-complexity clinical laboratory testing."[762] Lastly, reports should be reviewed and signed by the laboratory director or a qualified designee.

LABORATORY REGULATION

Regulatory oversight of clinical laboratories is essential to maintaining consistency across testing centers. All molecular genetic laboratories offering clinical testing should be CLIA certified and be actively participating in proficiency testing. In most cases, molecular laboratories are accredited by the CAP, which is considered to be the gold standard. CAP accreditation requires that laboratories undergo biannual inspection by an outside team of laboratory scientists using a specified checklist of requirements.[762] Maintaining accreditation requires that any deficiencies identified during a CAP inspection must be corrected. Laboratories are required to perform proficiency testing, which covers the scope of the tests performed in the laboratory. CAP provides proficiency testing samples or packets for a number of commonly ordered tests (e.g., HD, fragile X). CAP also provides method-based proficiency testing to verify that a clinical laboratory using a general method (e.g., Sanger sequencing, MPS) reports results consistent with those of other clinical laboratories. For tests that are offered clinically but are not covered by CAP proficiency testing, other means of confirming test accuracy must be pursued. This can involve sample exchanges with other laboratories that offer a similar clinical test or can simply be internal proficiency testing whereby a sample is randomly selected and is anonymously retested (among other patient samples) to confirm that the same results are obtained. Regardless of the method used, adequate records of proficiency testing results must be kept, and any discrepancies among results must be investigated and addressed. More information on the CAP accreditation and proficiency testing process can be found at http://www.cap.org.

While most genetic testing conducted in the United States is ordered by health care providers (HCP) to diagnose, treat, or identify risks of disease, an increasing number of genetic tests are being performed as direct-to-consumer (DTC) testing. The rise of DTC testing can be associated with technological advances (e.g., MPS), thereby lowering overall costs for companies; ease of sample collection and shipment (e.g., saliva); wide availability of the internet with DTC companies providing interactive tools to review results and data share; social media providing increased marketing; and the concept of personalized/precision medicine spawning elective, nonmedically indicated DTC testing. DTC testing poses a number of challenging issues and ethical considerations.[766,767] Most importantly, DTCs are void of the involvement of a HCP to provide pretest counseling regarding the benefits, clinical utility, and scientific validity of genetic testing and post-test counseling for interpretation of results and recommendation of appropriate clinical treatment and management as needed.[768] DTC testing can burden the health care industry especially HCPs in genetics and increase health care costs.[767] While not initially involved in the DTC process, when patients present to genetic clinics with DTC results seeking explanations, HCPs are required to provide time-consuming interpretations on some DTC variants for which there may be inadequate scientific and clinical validity. In addition, they may be requested to order additional costly laboratory testing to support or refute DTC test results. Lastly and equally as important is the concern regarding the storage, security, and confidentiality of patients' data and the potential lack of understanding by patients of common commercialization policies of some of these companies.[769]

SELECTED REFERENCES

16. Brennan ML, Schrijver I. Cystic fibrosis: a review of associated phenotypes, use of molecular diagnostic approaches, genetic characteristics, progress, and dilemmas. J Mol Diagn 2016;18:3–14.

105. Alford RL, Arnos KS, Fox M, et al. American College of Medical Genetics and Genomics guideline for the clinical evaluation and etiologic diagnosis of hearing loss. Genet Med 2014;16:347–55.

147. Tabrizi SJ, Ghosh R, Leavitt BR. Huntingtin lowering strategies for disease modification in Huntington's disease. Neuron 2019;101:801–19.

175. Wagner AH, Zaradzki M, Arif R, Remes A, Muller OJ, Kallenbach K. Marfan syndrome: A therapeutic challenge for long-term care. Biochem Pharmacol 2019;164:53–63.

203. Kamilaris CDC, Stratakis CA. Multiple endocrine neoplasia type 1 (MEN1): an update and the significance of early genetic and clinical diagnosis. Front Endocrinol (Lausanne) 2019;10:339.

241. Thomas CM, Asa SL, Ezzat S, Sawka AM, Goldstein D. Diagnosis and pathologic characteristics of medullary thyroid carcinoma-review of current guidelines. Curr Oncol 2019;26:338–44.

293. Zhang K, Yang X, Lin G, Han Y, Li J. Molecular genetic testing and diagnosis strategies for dystrophinopathies in the era of next generation sequencing. Clin Chim Acta 2019;491:66–73.

330. Santoro MR, Bray SM, Warren ST. Molecular mechanisms of fragile X syndrome: a twenty-year perspective. Annu Rev Pathol 2012;7:219–45.

367. Gold WA, Krishnarajy R, Ellaway C, Christodoulou J. Rett syndrome: a genetic update and clinical review focusing on comorbidities. ACS Chem Neurosci 2018;9:167–76.

410. Connors JM. Thrombophilia testing and venous thrombosis. N Engl J Med 2017;377:1177–87.

428. Hasan A, Moscoso DI, Kastrinos F. The role of genetics in pancreatitis. Gastrointest Endosc Clin N Am 2018;28:587–603.

467. Nielsen FC, van Overeem Hansen T, Sorensen CS. Hereditary breast and ovarian cancer: new genes in confined pathways. Nat Rev Cancer 2016;16:599–612.

522. Hegde M, Ferber M, Mao R, Samowitz W, Ganguly A. ACMG technical standards and guidelines for genetic testing for inherited colorectal cancer (Lynch syndrome, familial adenomatous polyposis, and MYH-associated polyposis). Genet Med 2014;16:101–16.

523. Sinicrope FA. Lynch syndrome-associated colorectal cancer. N Engl J Med 2018;379:764–73.

565. Dinarvand P, Davaro EP, Doan JV, et al. Familial Adenomatous Polyposis syndrome: an update and review of extraintestinal manifestations. Arch Pathol Lab Med 2019;143:1382–98.

599. Mustafa MF, Fakurazi S, Abdullah MA, Maniam S. Pathogenic mitochondria DNA mutations: current detection tools and interventions. Genes (Basel) 2020;11:192.

663. Ehrhart F, Janssen KJM, Coort SL, Evelo CT, Curfs LMG. Prader-Willi syndrome and Angelman syndrome: visualisation of the molecular pathways for two chromosomal disorders. World J Biol Psychiatry 2019;20:670–82.

694. Gregg AR. Expanded carrier screening. Obstet Gynecol Clin North Am 2018;45:103–12.

704. Richards S, Aziz N, Bale S, et al. Standards and guidelines for the interpretation of sequence variants: a joint consensus recommendation of the American College of Medical Genetics and Genomics and the Association for Molecular Pathology. Genet Med 2015;17:405–23.

708. Skrzypek H, Hui L. Noninvasive prenatal testing for fetal aneuploidy and single gene disorders. Best Pract Res Clin Obstet Gynaecol 2017;42:26–38.

714. Smith HS, Swint JM, Lalani SR, et al. Clinical application of genome and exome sequencing as a diagnostic tool for pediatric patients: a scoping review of the literature. Genet Med 2019;21:3–16.

Solid Tumors[*]

Elaine R. Mardis and Gregory J. Tsongalis

ABSTRACT

Background

Once thought of as a simple clonal expansion of abnormal cells, cancer is now recognized as a complex, multifactorial, and polygenic syndrome. Many cancer types have been reclassified due to new understanding of molecular-based phenotypes and tumor-host interactions. Since the initial human genome reference sequence in 2004,[1] cancer genomics research has focused on using this reference as a template for characterizing the somatic genomic variants that underlie cancer development and those germline genomic variants that underlie human susceptibility to develop cancer. The Human Genome Project also promised to identify novel therapeutic targets for treating cancer, and we are seeing those efforts come to fruition with new targeted small molecule- and immunotherapies. Major advances in technology, including massively parallel sequencing, have provided a comprehensive somatic landscape of most major cancer types that informs our understanding of the numbers and types of variants in the cancer genome.[2–4]

Content

The diagnosis of human cancer is based mainly on the morphologic characteristics of tumor cells and some specific protein expression detected by immunohistochemical staining. More recently, genomic analyses have become an integral component of cancer patient management, guiding therapy selection based on somatic and/or germline variant profiles. This is possible due to the cumulative knowledge gained from large-scale cancer genomics discovery efforts in tens to thousands of human cancers across many tissues of origin using high complexity molecular-based technologies. This chapter will outline aspects of molecular assays of solid tissue malignancies in the clinical setting that have been informed by research-based discovery over the last 20 years.

[*]The full version of this chapter is available electronically on ExpertConsult.com.

982

Hematopathology*

Jay L. Patel and Devon S. Chabot-Richards

ABSTRACT

Background

The field of hematology has long been at the forefront in the use of histopathology combined with ancillary laboratory methods, including genetic testing, to improve clinical outcomes. The benefits of these efforts for patients with hematopoietic malignancies have been numerous. They include improved diagnostic accuracy, refined prognostication, and identification of potential new therapeutic targets. Molecular testing methods such as polymerase chain reaction (PCR), Sanger sequencing, and fluorescence in situ hybridization (FISH) have, for many years, been a routine part of the laboratory evaluation of these patients. However, like other areas of oncology, the last few years have seen further advances in the understanding of the genetic basis of these neoplasms, primarily due to the influence of new sequencing technologies. Massively parallel sequencing has made comprehensive genomic characterization of hematopoietic malignancies routine.

Content

In this chapter we cover the breadth of hematopoietic malignancies with a focus on molecular genetics and the modern diagnostic approach. We approach hematopoietic malignancies from a laboratory standpoint starting with structural chromosomal abnormalities and translocations and moving to smaller scale genetic changes found in single genes and finally to epigenetic changes. We compare and contrast the various laboratory methods used to query these abnormalities and highlight the utility of new and advancing technologies and platforms including array-based methods and massively parallel sequencing. Finally, the chapter ends with a discussion of lymphoid clonality testing, an area of hematology testing that is also benefiting from the influence of modern sequencing technology.

---

*The full version of this chapter is available electronically on ExpertConsult.com.

Circulating Tumor Cells and Circulating Nucleic Acids in Oncology

Catherine Alix-Panabières, Valérie Taly, and Klaus Pantel

ABSTRACT

Background
The analysis of circulating tumor cells (CTCs) and tumor cell products (DNA, RNA, extracellular vesicles) released into the blood may provide clinically relevant information as a "liquid biopsy" and provide new insights into tumor biology.

Content
CTCs are complementary to other liquid biopsy biomarkers such as circulating cell-free DNA (ctDNA), circulating microRNAs,[1] extracellular vessels, and tumor-educated platelets. Validation of liquid biopsy assays is essential and has been performed by the EU/IMI consortium CANCER-ID (www.cancer-id.eu), an activity sustained now by the European Liquid Biopsy Society (ELBS) consortium (www.elbs.eu).

Liquid biopsy analyses with validated platforms provide information on early detection of cancer, identification of cancer patients at risk to develop relapse (prognosis), and it may serve to track tumor evolution, therapeutic targets, or mechanisms of resistance on metastatic cells. Metastatic cells might have unique characteristics that can differ from the bulk of cancer cells in the primary tumor currently used for stratification of patients to systemic therapy. Moreover, monitoring of blood samples in the context of therapies might provide unique information for the future clinical management of the individual cancer patient and might serve as surrogate markers for response to therapy. Liquid biopsy analysis can be used to improve the management of individual cancer patients and contribute to personalized medicine.

Tissue biopsies, the current "gold standard" in cancer diagnostics, have some limitations which may be overcome by liquid biopsies (Figs. 71.1 and 71.2). The term *liquid biopsy* refers to testing of body fluids (e.g., blood, urine, saliva, cerebrospinal fluid [CSF])[2,3] derived mainly from circulating tumor cells (CTCs), circulating tumor DNA (ctDNA), circulating miRNAs, and extracellular vesicles (EVs) (see Fig. 71.1). Liquid biopsy offers a minimally invasive insight into a patient's cancer.[4-6] Currently the most promising role for liquid biopsy is the profiling of CTCs or ctDNA as a way to monitor patients in the course of therapy—particularly by using novel technologies for a better and earlier indication of either response or emerging resistance to a particular treatment (Fig. 71.3). The next logical step is to better understand the mechanisms of evolving resistance and hopefully to guide treatment strategies to overcome resistance. The utility of liquid biopsy is not just limited to being a mirror of tissue biopsy, but it is a potential tool that can detect unique and impactful information about a patient's cancer that tissue testing cannot. Just a few years ago, the liquid biopsy approach was limited to research studies, but it is now entering prospective clinical trials. It can be used for patients whose tumors are hard to access by biopsy or when the site of the primary tumor is unknown.[7] With respect to the clinical laboratory, the development of targeted molecular assays as companion diagnostics, for disease monitoring, and even for early cancer detection are all potential possibilities at various stages of development. It may in the future enable decisions for targeted therapies in patients who have failed treatment on a particular drug regimen.

Potentially, liquid biopsy may aid in the investigation of the evolution of subclonal cancer cell populations. Liquid biopsy may be a minimally invasive method for determining dominant clones to direct targeted therapies against. There is hope that this approach can illuminate strategies to combine drugs that affect the dominant mutated populations and also inhibit other subclonal populations from expanding. This approach may impact the definition of minimal residual disease[8,9] because it can change the clinician's ability to predict the risk of recurrence in early-stage cancer patients whose tumors have been surgically removed.

Liquid biopsy as a diagnostic, prognostic, and theranostic tool is appealing because it is minimally invasive and easily performed in a serial manner. However, there are several barriers to the routine clinical use of liquid biopsy. Numerous technologies are available for the detection and molecular characterization of CTCs and ctDNA (and other circulating cancer biomarkers), resulting in different test results even if the same blood samples are analyzed, which points to the urgent need for standardization of the preanalytical and analytical phase of the applied tests to obtain robust and reproducible results.[10] Moreover, well-designed comparison studies on large patient cohorts comparing the clinical relevance of liquid biopsy (CTCs and/or ctDNA) and tissue biopsy with defined clinical endpoints (e.g., progression-free or overall survival [OS]) are still needed to demonstrate clinical utility.[10] Liquid biopsy, tissue biopsy, and imaging may provide complementary information, which could lead to the establishment of a composite diagnostic panel with the highest accuracy and benefit for cancer patients. Thus the

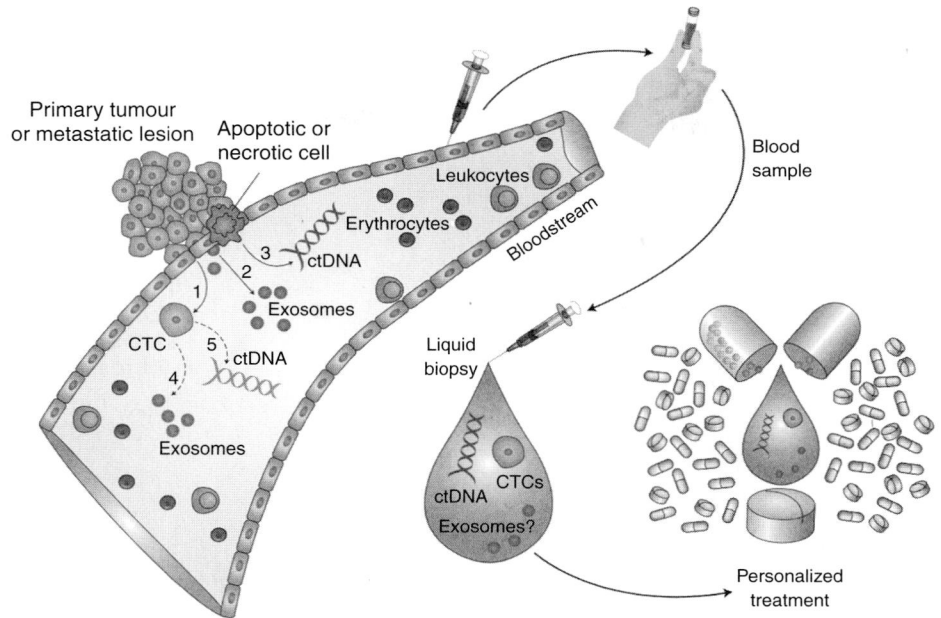

FIGURE 71.1 Circulating tumor cells (CTCs), circulating tumor-derived DNA (ctDNA) and exosomes as complementary blood-based biomarkers. A subset of aggressive tumor cells enters the bloodstream from the primary tumor and/or metastatic lesions (CTCs (1)). Exosomes are released by viable tumor and normal cells (2). Apoptotic or necrotic tumor cells release ctDNA into the bloodstream (3). CTCs can further contribute to the pool of circulating exosomes (4) and ctDNA (5). Repeated blood sampling can be performed to stratify patients, monitor therapeutic efficacy, identify therapeutic targets, and detect the emergence of resistance mechanisms and the progression of the disease to a metastatic form. (From Alix-Panabières C, Pantel K. Clinical prospects of liquid biopsies. *Nat Biomed Eng*, 2017;1:1–3.)

present over-competition between researchers working in different biomarker fields (e.g., ctDNA versus CTCs) appears to be counterproductive.

POINTS TO REMEMBER

Liquid Biopsy
- The liquid biopsy approach extracts molecular information from the tumor by detailed analysis of circulating tumor-derived genetic material in the bloodstream. The sources of this material are circulating tumor cells (CTCs), circulating tumor DNA (ctDNA), circulating miRNAs, and extracellular vesicles (EVs).
- Liquid biopsy can provide detailed information on tumor genome and transcriptome evolution over time through conventional peripheral blood sampling that can be used for serial monitoring of a patient.

CIRCULATING TUMOR CELLS

Circulating Tumor Cells: Historical Background

The presence of CTCs was first reported in 1869 by Thomas Ashworth (Fig. 71.4).[11] In 2005, the clinical importance of disseminated tumor cells (DTCs) in the bone marrow of breast cancer patients was shown.[12] However, analysis of DTCs in bone marrow is invasive and thus difficult to repeat. CTCs are rare cells that originate from primary and metastatic tumors that have managed to get into the circulation and that may extravasate to different organs (Fig. 71.5). Despite the assumption that only a small fraction of CTCs

will develop into metastasis,[13] the CTC counts at initial diagnosis and during the postsurgical follow-up period are tightly correlated to the risk of relapse in breast cancer and other solid tumors.[8] For example, in breast cancer the recurrence risk was increased more than six times in patients with 5 or more CTCs per 7.5 mL blood before receiving neoadjuvant therapy,[14] and the prognostic value was independent from the response of the primary tumor to neoadjuvant therapy.[15] Cancer metastasis is the main cause of cancer-related death, and dissemination of tumor cells through the blood circulation is an important intermediate step that also exemplifies the switch from localized to systemic disease.[16] Detection of CTCs has also been proposed as a companion diagnostic to identify glioblastoma multiforme patients with extracranial tumor cell spread, in order to exclude these patients as organ donors.[17] CTCs are therefore major players in the liquid biopsy approach and may provide important insights into the biology behind metastatic progression and real-time information on a patient's disease status.

Many advances have been made in the detection and molecular characterization of CTCs.[8] The presence of CTCs in peripheral blood has been linked to worse prognosis and early relapse in various types of solid cancers.[18] The FDA has cleared the CellSearch system for breast (2004), colorectal (2008), and prostate (2008) cancer based on the critical role that CTCs play in the metastatic spread of carcinomas.[19] Detection of CTCs is correlated with decreased progression-free survival (PFS) and OS in both operable breast cancer and metastatic breast cancer (MBC), and various studies on other tumor types have confirmed this prognostic relevance. This has led to the introduction of a new stage, cM0(i+),

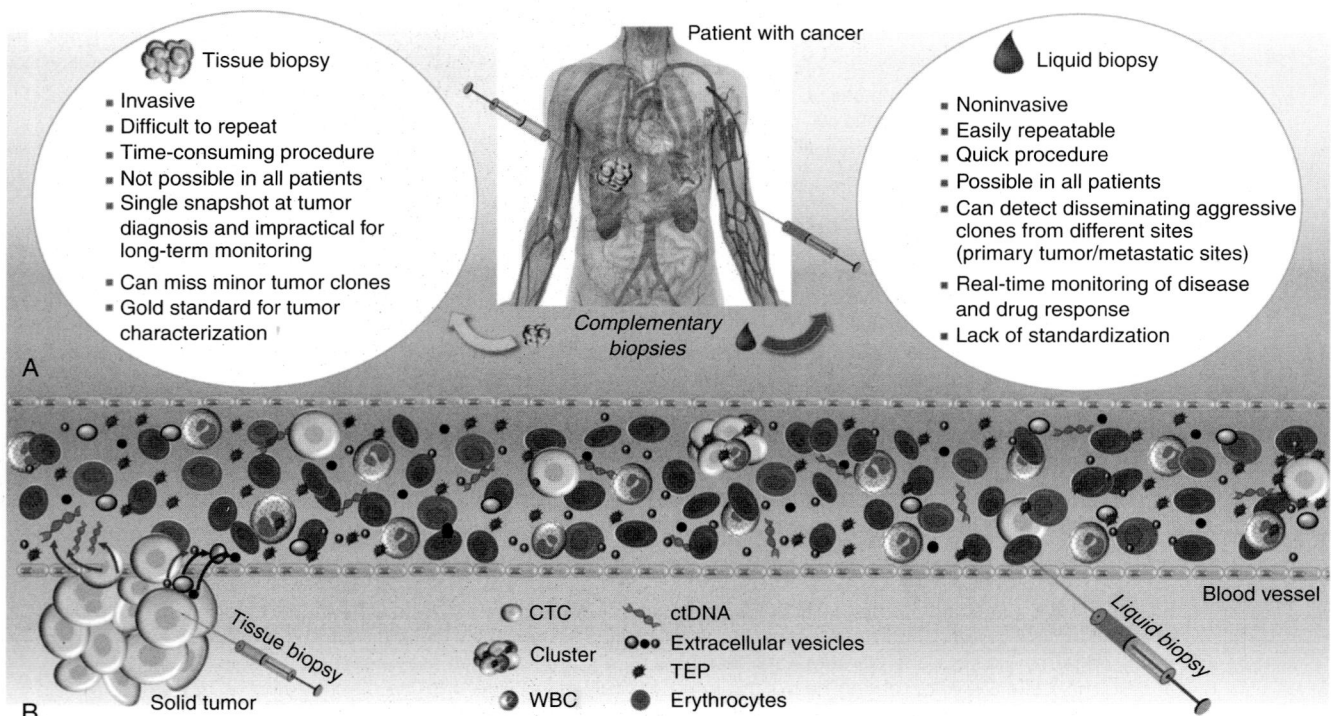

FIGURE 71.2 The potential of liquid biopsy for cancer monitoring. (A) Complementarity of tissue and liquid biopsies. (B) Overview of liquid biopsy biomarkers that represent tumor molecular heterogeneity and immunologic phenotype. The primary tumor and metastatic sites release different cells and biomolecules in the bloodstream. Circulating tumor cells (CTCs as single cells or clusters), circulating tumor DNA (ctDNA), extracellular vesicles (EVs), and tumor-educated platelets (TEPs) can be isolated from whole blood to obtain cancer genome, transcriptome, proteome, and secretome data in real time. Moreover, white blood cells (WBC) can give information on the immunity of the patient with cancer, mainly on their potential to eradicate cancer cells. All these biomarkers are complementary and can be used to build a precise index or an algorithm based on qualitative and quantitative data at different times during the disease course. (From Eslami-S Z, Cortés-Hernández LE, Cayrefourcq L, Alix-Panabières C. The different facets of liquid biopsy: a kaleidoscopic view. *Cold Spring Harb Perspect Med* 2020;10:a037333.)

characterized by the absence of clinical overt metastases (cM0) but the detection of isolated tumor cells (i+) in blood or other compartments, into the 2018 AJCC classification for breast cancer. Thus CTCs may qualify as a new tool to enrich for high-risk M0 patients, which may be used in future clinical studies assessing the clinical value of adjuvant therapies. Focusing on high-risk patients can speed up time-consuming and costly clinical studies in the adjuvant setting. Nevertheless, enumeration of CTCs might not be sufficient and further downstream analysis will provide more information on the biology of CTCs and their metastasis-initiating potential to extravasate and colonize distant sites. This information might further increase the diagnostic accuracy of CTC analyses. For example, in the analysis of the prognostic value of Bidard and colleagues[14] approximately 25% of breast cancer patients with detectable CTCs had no signs of relapse within the observation period of 70 months. On the other hand, approximately 20% of patients without detectable CTCs had experienced relapse, which points to the need of increasing the sensitivity of CTC analysis, for example, by the introduction of new markers targeting CTCs with nonepithelial phenotype or increasing the blood volume analyzed.

CTCs are targets for understanding tumor biology and tumor cell dissemination in humans. Their molecular characterization offers an exciting approach to understanding resistance to established therapies and elucidating the complex biology of metastasis.[20] Further research on the molecular characterization of CTCs should contribute to a better understanding of the biology of metastatic development in cancer patients and the identification of novel therapeutic targets, especially after elucidating the relationship of CTCs to cancer stem cells (CSCs). This approach may provide individualized targeted treatments and spare cancer patients unnecessary and ineffective therapies.[21]

CTCs are rare, and the amount of available sample is limited, presenting formidable analytical and technical challenges. Recent technical advancements in CTC detection and characterization include multiplex reverse transcription quantitative polymerase chain reaction (PCR) (RT-qPCR) methods, image-based approaches, and microfilter and microchip devices for their isolation.[8] However, direct comparison of different methods for detecting CTCs in blood from patients with breast cancer has revealed a substantial variation in the detection rates.[22,23] There is a lack of standardization in reference material, which hampers

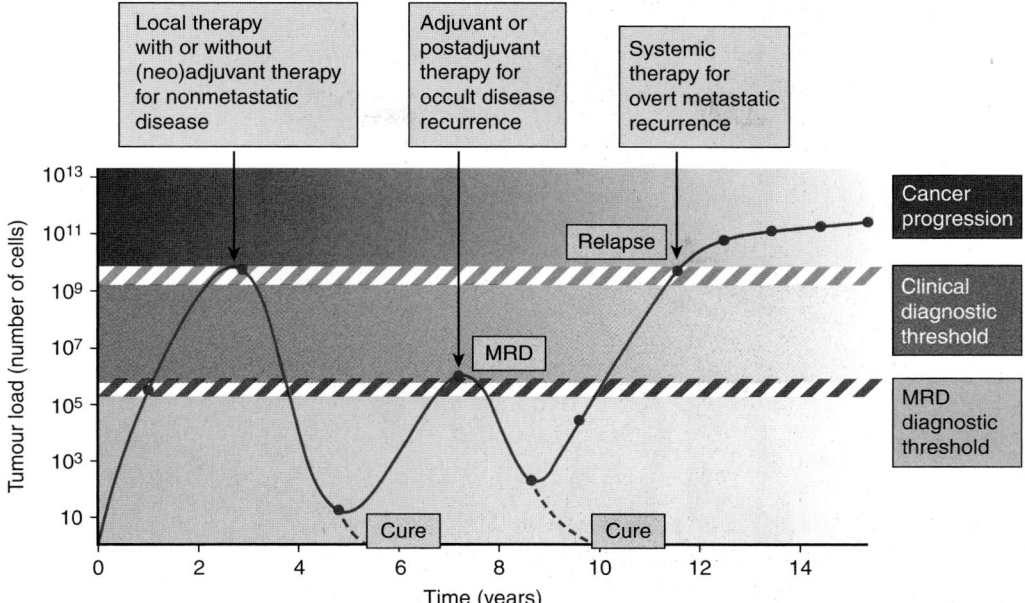

FIGURE 71.3 Therapy depends on dynamic changes in the tumor burden in patients with cancer. The graph illustrates the changes in tumor load over time in a hypothetical patient with cancer. When the tumor load reaches the diagnostic threshold for the first time, the primary tumor is detected and treated using local therapies (surgery and/or radiotherapy) and possibly neoadjuvant and/or adjuvant systemic therapy (for example, chemotherapy or endocrine therapy), which reduces the tumor burden to below the diagnostic level. In some patients, all disseminated tumor cells (DTCs) will be eradicated (*dashed lines*), resulting in cure, whereas other patients have residual DTCs that can expand and eventually increase the tumor burden to above the diagnostic threshold of circulating tumor cell (CTC) or cell-free tumor DNA (ctDNA) assays for minimal residual disease (MRD). At this point, postadjuvant therapy could be initiated to treat the occult metastatic or locoregional disease. In some patients, such interventions might lead to the eradication of all tumor cells (cure); however, in others, the tumor cells will become resistant, the disease burden will grow to reach the MRD level, and ultimately, clinical diagnostic thresholds (relapse), and systemic therapies will again be applied to treat overt metastatic disease. If therapy fails, the metastatic tumor burden will continue to increase. (From Pantel K, Alix-Panabières C. Liquid biopsy and minimal residual disease-latest advances and implications for cure. *Nat Rev Clin Oncol* 2019;16:409–24.)

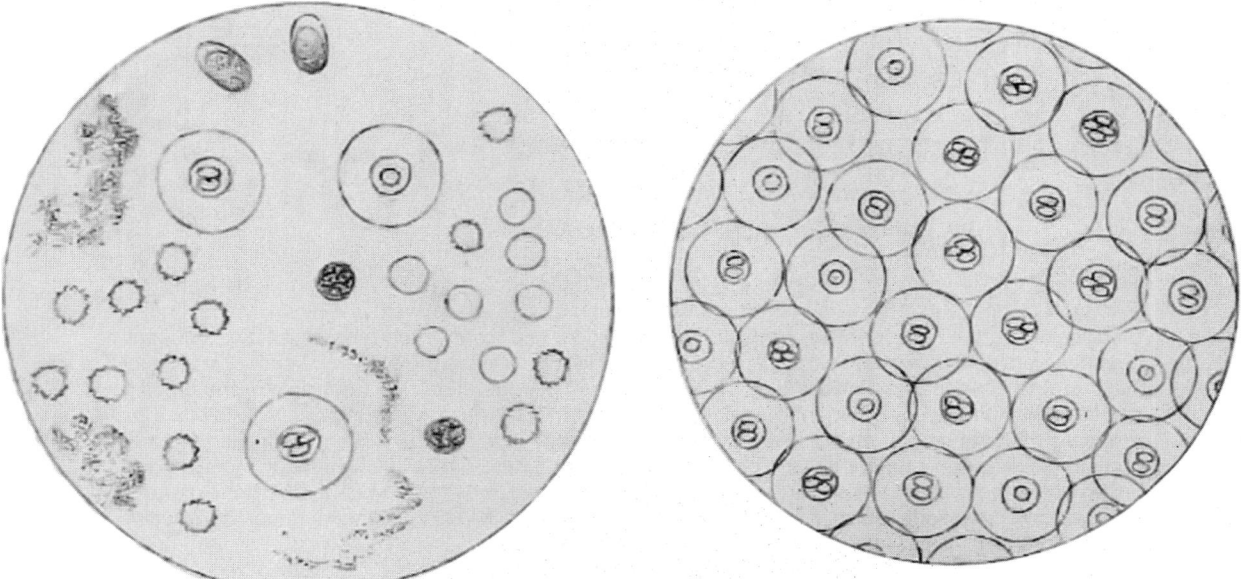

FIGURE 71.4 First description of "CTCs". Hand drawing by Ashworth to describe the similar microscopic appearance of tumor cells in the blood of a patient (*left side*) and in one of several tumor masses (*right side*). (Adapted from Ashworth T. A case of cancer in which cells similar to those in the tumours were seen in the blood after death. *Med J Aust* 1869;14:146–7.)

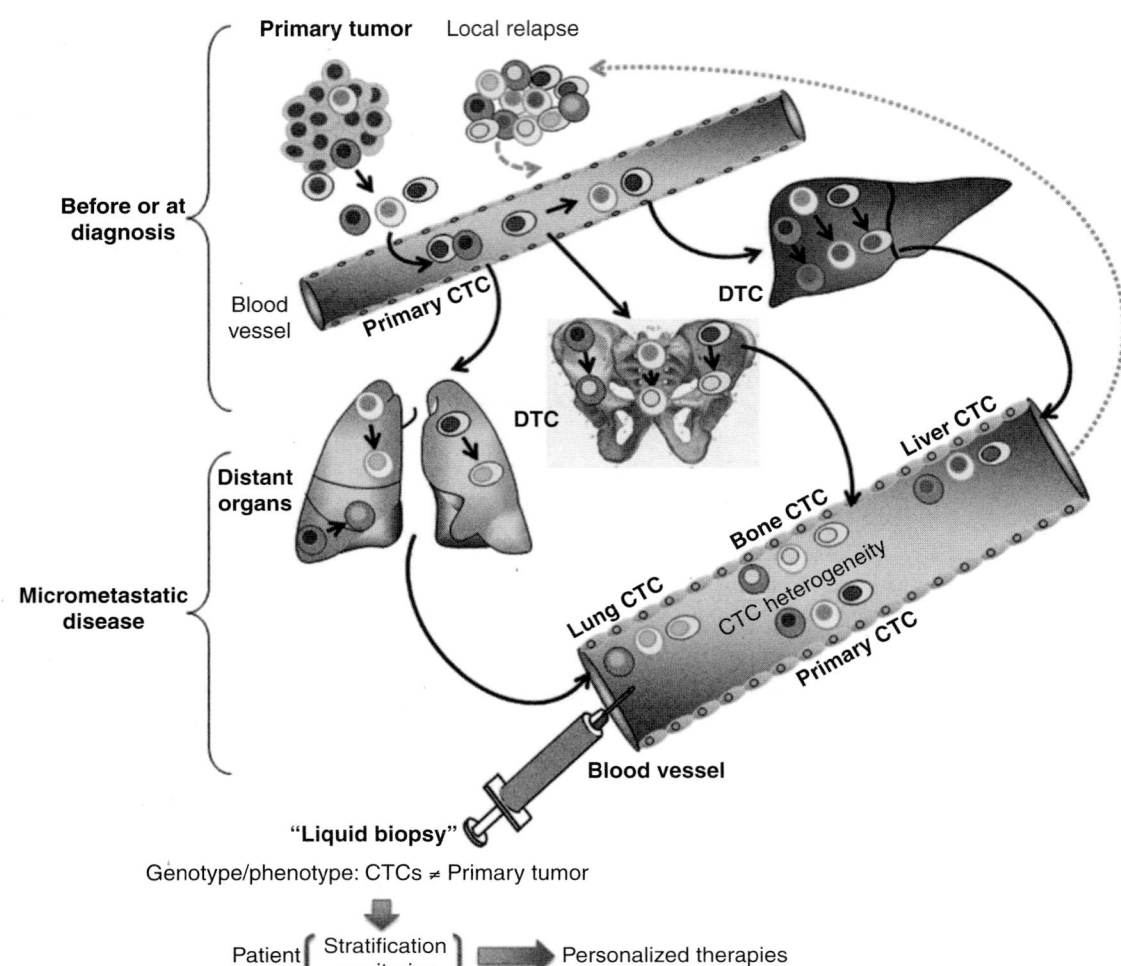

CTCs	Treatments
Proteins	
ER⁺	Endocrine therapy
HER2/*neu*⁺	Trastuzumab
DNA mutations	
KRAS mutations	EGFR-targeted therapies
PIK3CA mutations	HER2/*neu*-targeted therapies

FIGURE 71.5 Circulating tumor cells (CTCs) as a real-time liquid biopsy. CTCs can be derived from different sources (e.g., primary tumor or organs of metastasis, such as liver, lung, and BM) depending on disease stage. CTCs serve as a liquid biopsy of cancer and reveal important information on therapeutic targets and/or resistance mechanisms, which might be used in the future to stratify patients for such targeted therapies as inhibition of EGFR/HER2 or endocrine therapy and to monitor the efficacy of treatment and the development of resistance in real time. Disseminated tumor cells (DTCs) are tumor cells found in distant organs (e.g., BM). They can enter in dormancy, disseminate again to other organs including the primary site or initiate a metastasis. Usually, they are detected in the BM, an organ where they can hide in special niches considered as a reservoir for the DTCs. *BM,* Bone marrow; *ER⁺*, estrogen receptor positive. (From Alix-Panabieres C, Pantel K. Circulating tumor cells: liquid biopsy of cancer. *Clin Chem* 2013;59:110–8.)

the implementation of CTC measurement in clinical routine practice. Thus while the potential of CTC analysis is now widely recognized, many challenges remain.[24]

Circulating Tumor Cells: Technical Challenges

The enrichment and detection technologies for highly pure CTCs are challenging as these cells are extremely rare in the peripheral blood.[25] Indeed, CTCs occur at very low concentrations in the bloodstream, ranging between 1 and 10 cells per 10 mL in most cancer patients. Usually, CTCs are coisolated with normal peripheral blood mononuclear cells (e.g., leukocytes). Thus efficient enrichment of CTCs can be achieved by approaches that exploit differences between tumor cells and leukocytes, including the differential expression of cell surface proteins or distinct physical properties of the cells.

The combination of high-throughput and automated CTC isolation technologies with validated downstream detection assays are necessary for the routine use of CTC-based diagnostics in the clinical management of cancer patients. CTC analysis includes isolation/enrichment, detection, enumeration, and characterization. The main analytical systems used are described below, and an outline is presented in Fig. 71.6.

Strategies for Circulating Tumor Cell Enrichment

CTCs can be infrequent, depending on the cancer stage. One CTC may be present among 10^6 to 10^8 peripheral blood cells. CTC isolation and enrichment from peripheral blood are thus extremely challenging and very demanding. It is not only that these cells circulate at very low numbers, but they are heterogeneous even within the same patient. Highly standardized and robust isolation protocols are necessary for downstream CTC analysis and molecular characterization. Toward this goal, a lot of effort has focused on developing novel technologies for the isolation and enrichment of CTCs from peripheral blood.

A large spectrum of technologies is available to enrich CTCs from surrounding normal hematopoietic cells (see Fig. 71.6). These enrichment methods rely on different properties of CTCs that can be positively or negatively enriched on (i) label-dependent systems based on biological properties (e.g., surface protein expression) and (ii) label-independent systems based on physical properties (e.g., size, density, electric charges, and deformability).[8] In vivo methods for increasing CTC yield have also been developed. Moreover, CTC recovery from blood samples collected close to the tumor (i.e., in vessels located in the drainage area of the primary tumor or metastases) can considerably increase the chance to collect more CTCs (Fig. 71.7).[26,27] In colorectal cancer (CRC), the comparative analysis of CTCs obtained from the mesenteric and peripheral blood demonstrated a cascade of genomic events related to metastatic progression (Fig. 71.8).[28]

The most important systems for the isolation/enrichment of CTCs are discussed in the following text. In many cases, these technologies are complementary to each other because they target different properties of CTCs and may define different CTC populations.

Label-dependent circulating tumor cell enrichment systems. **Biological properties** are used in immunologic procedures with antibodies against either tumor-associated antigens (positive selection) or common leukocytes antigen CD45 (negative selection).

Positive enrichment should reach high cell purity, depending on the antibody specificity used in the assay. Among the current positive systems, most of the technologies target the epithelial cell adhesion molecule (EpCAM) antigen (e.g., FDA-cleared CellSearch system, the current gold standard). However, capturing CTCs that are not expressing EpCAM has pushed researchers to use panels of antibodies against various other epithelial cell surface antigens (such as epidermal growth factor receptor [EGFR], MUC1), tissue-specific antigens (such as PSA, human epidermal growth factor receptor 2 [HER2]), or mesenchymal/stem-cell antigens (such as Snail, ALDH1).[29] Positive selection of CTCs is possible because the phenotype of CTCs is well known. However, many CTCs are heterogenous. Any bias can be avoided by negative selection where CTCs are not targeted directly but the unwanted cells, such as leukocytes, are depleted from the samples. Indeed, negative enrichment targets and removes surrounding normal cells, using antibodies against CD45 (not expressed on cancer cells) and other leukocyte antigens (e.g., CD14, CD8, CD19). The advantages of negative enrichment are: (i) CTCs are not tagged with a difficult-to-remove antibody, (ii) CTCs are not activated or modified via an antibody-protein interaction, and (iii) antibody selection does not bias the subpopulation of CTCs captured. The leukocyte-depletion procedure has a high recovery rate; however, the samples are less pure than positive selection procedures; indeed, more remaining leukocytes are present.

Positive selection. Positive selection is the most widely used CTC isolation/enrichment system. This approach captures CTCs through specific monoclonal antibodies against epithelial cell surface markers that are expressed on CTCs but are absent from normal leukocytes. CTCs can be tagged using antibody-conjugated magnetic microbeads (diameter: 0.5 to 5 μm) or nanoparticles (diameter: 50 to 250 nm) that bind to a specific surface antigen. Intracellular antigens like cytokeratins can also be used as targets.[30] Immunomagnetic assays require a short incubation (~30 minutes) for antigen/antibody binding that couples the cells to magnetic beads, followed by isolation of the cells using a magnetic field.

Various antigens have been exploited for the positive immunomagnetic isolation of CTCs. Among these, EpCAM is the most common. This approach is well established in terms of proven clinical significance of the captured cells. However, capture with EpCAM has the disadvantage of missing some cells that are undergoing epithelial-mesenchymal transition (EMT; Fig. 71.9). We also now know that CTCs are highly heterogeneous, but one approach to partially overcome this issue is to use a "cocktail" of antibodies that targets multiple antigens.[31] Along these lines, several organ- or tumor-specific markers, such as carcinoembryonic antigen (CEA), EGFR, prostate-specific antigen, HER-2, cell surface–associated mucin 1 (MUC-1), ephrin receptor B4 (EphB4), insulin-like growth factor 1 receptor (IGF-1R), cadherin-11 (CAD11), and tumor-associated glycoprotein 72 (TAG-72), have been used to isolate CTCs.[32] The expression of vimentin by CTCs may also be a good marker for epithelial cancers undergoing EMT.[29] By using a specific monoclonal antibody against vimentin, EMT-CTCs were detected in patients undergoing postsurgery adjuvant chemotherapy for metastatic colon cancer.[33] These isolated EMT-CTCs were characterized further using EMT-specific markers, fluorescent in situ hybridization, and single-cell mutation analysis. This antibody

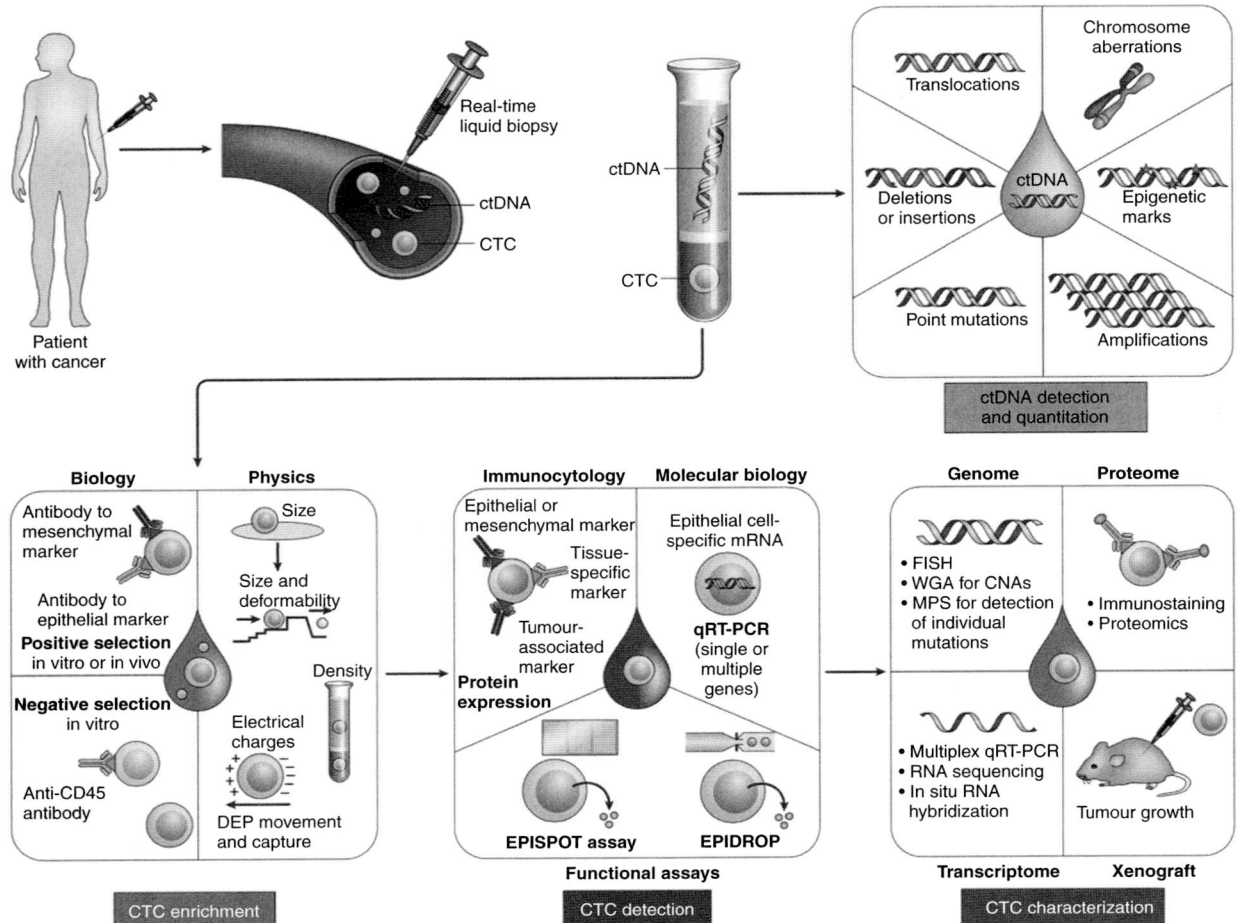

FIGURE 71.6 Overview of technologies for circulating tumor cell (CTC) and cell-free tumor DNA (ctDNA) enrichment, detection, and characterization. CTCs and circulating ctDNA can be isolated simultaneously from the same blood sample. Quantitative detection of ctDNA is based on the identification of various tumor-specific genetic aberrations or epigenetic markers in plasma cell-free DNA samples, primarily through DNA sequencing. CTCs in blood can be enriched using marker-dependent techniques: CTCs can be positively selected in vitro or in vivo using antibodies to epithelial and/or mesenchymal proteins (such as the epithelial cell adhesion molecule (EPCAM) and/or cytokeratins and mesenchymal vimentin or N-cadherin) or negatively selected for through depletion of leukocytes using anti-CD45 antibodies. Positive enrichment of CTCs can also be performed in vitro using assays based on CTC characteristics including size, deformability, density, and electrical charge. Following enrichment, the isolated CTCs can be identified using immunocytologic, molecular, or functional assays. With immunocytologic platforms, CTCs are identified by membrane and/or intracytoplasmic staining with antibodies to epithelial, mesenchymal, tissue-specific, or tumor-associated markers. Molecular technologies enable the identification of CTCs using RNA-based assays, such as quantitative reverse transcription PCR (qRT-PCR), RNA sequencing, or in situ RNA hybridization. Functional assays can be used to detect viable CTCs on the basis of their biological activities, for example, the fluoro-Epithelial ImmunoSPOT (EPISPOT) assay for certain proteins secreted or shed by CTCs and the related EPISPOT in a drop (EPIDROP) technology that enables the detection of single CTCs in microdroplets. The molecular characteristics of CTCs can be further explored at the DNA, RNA, and protein level, and the functional properties of CTCs can be investigated in vivo by injecting the cells into immunodeficient mice to form patient-derived xenograft models. *CNAs,* Copy number alterations; *DEP,* dielectrophoresis; *FISH,* fluorescence in situ hybridization; *MPS,* massively parallel sequencing; *WGA,* whole-genome analysis. (From Pantel K, Alix-Panabières C. Liquid biopsy and minimal residual disease-latest advances and implications for cure. *Nat Rev Clin Oncol* 2019;16:409–24.)

exhibited high specificity and sensitivity toward different epithelial cancer cells and was used to detect and enumerate EMT-CTCs from patients. The number of EMT-CTCs detected correlated with the therapeutic outcome of the disease. According to these results, cell surface vimentin is a promising marker for the isolation of EMT-CTCs from a wide variety of tumor types.

Another example of positive selection is the MagSweeper, an immunomagnetic cell separator.[34] In this device, magnetic beads are coated with an antibody targeting epithelial cell surface markers. These immunomagnetic beads are added into blood samples, and cancer cells are attached to the beads. This device gently enriches target cells and eliminates cells that are not bound to magnetic particles by using centrifugal

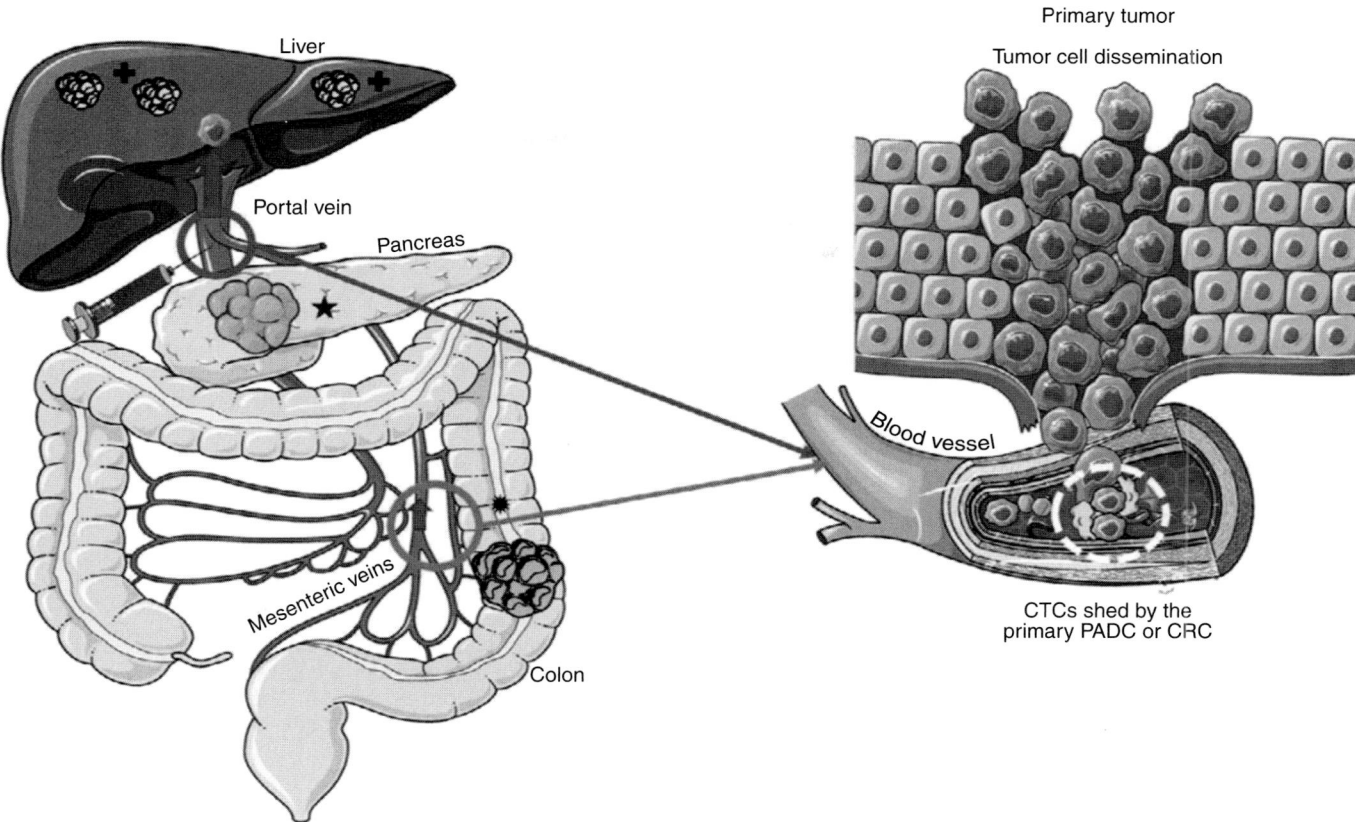

FIGURE 71.7 Circulating tumor cell (CTC) detection in the portal vein of patients with pancreatic or colorectal cancer. Pancreatic and colorectal cancer metastases in the liver develop through multiple steps. Local invasion by cancer cells is followed by their intravasation into the tumor vasculature. Cancer cells then enter the portomesenteric venous system as single cells or clusters that might be coated by platelets. CTCs are released into the superior and inferior mesenteric (*green circle*) veins for CRC in the right colon and left colon/rectum, respectively, and in the portal vein (*red circle*) for PDAC. Portal blood flows through the liver and then to other distant organs, after crossing the liver capillaries in portal areas. CTCs follow the same route and might extravasate in the liver parenchyma to start colonization. Portal blood sampling before passage to the liver can improve the CTC recovery rate. The blue arrows show the direction of the blood flow in the veins. CRC, colorectal cancer; *PADC,* pancreatic ductal adenocarcinoma. (From Buscail E, Chiche L, Laurent C, et al. Tumor-proximal liquid biopsy to improve diagnostic and prognostic performances of circulating tumor cells. *Mol Oncol* 2019;13:1811–26.)

forces. The isolated cells are easily accessible and can be extracted individually based on their physical characteristics to deplete any cells nonspecifically bound to beads. The same group has recently developed the magnetic sifter, a miniature microfluidic chip with a dense array of magnetic pores; tumor cells are labeled with magnetic nanoparticles and are captured from whole blood with high efficiency.[35] The use of isolation technologies that take advantage of magnetic fields may lead the way to routine preparation and characterization of liquid biopsies from cancer patients.

Negative selection. This isolation approach is completely independent of the phenotype of CTCs and is based on the depletion of noncancerous peripheral blood cells. A first step is often the lysis of red blood cells (RBCs) and the second step may use specific markers for white blood cells (WBCs) like CD45 or CD61 to magnetically remove them from the sample.[36,37] Another variation of CTC enrichment by negative depletion is the commercially available RosetteSep system (StemCell technologies, Canada): tetrameric antibody complexes target unwanted cells for removal.[38] This approach is independent of the expression of EpCAM on CTCs and has better recoveries than

the conventional density gradient method for the isolation of CTCs from normal leukocytes in blood.

Label-independent circulating tumor cell enrichment systems. Physical properties are another alternative to enrich CTCs from blood samples. During the last decade, numerous marker-independent techniques have been developed for CTC isolation. Label-free enrichment processes based on physical properties, such as density, size, deformability, and electric charges, avoid molecular biases induced by variability of cell biomarker expression associated with tumor heterogeneity. Among physical properties, the size of CTCs is the main characteristic used to enrich them. Indeed, CTCs generally exhibit a larger morphology than leukocytes (8 to 10 μm) and filtration membranes and microfluidic devices using inertial focusing to separate CTCs from blood have been developed.[39–42]

Systems based on density. Density gradient centrifugation using commercially available reagents (e.g., Ficoll, GE Healthcare Life Sciences, Pittsburgh, PA) is one of the most widely used approaches for CTC enrichment.[43] It is based on the lower density of mononuclear cells (including CTCs)

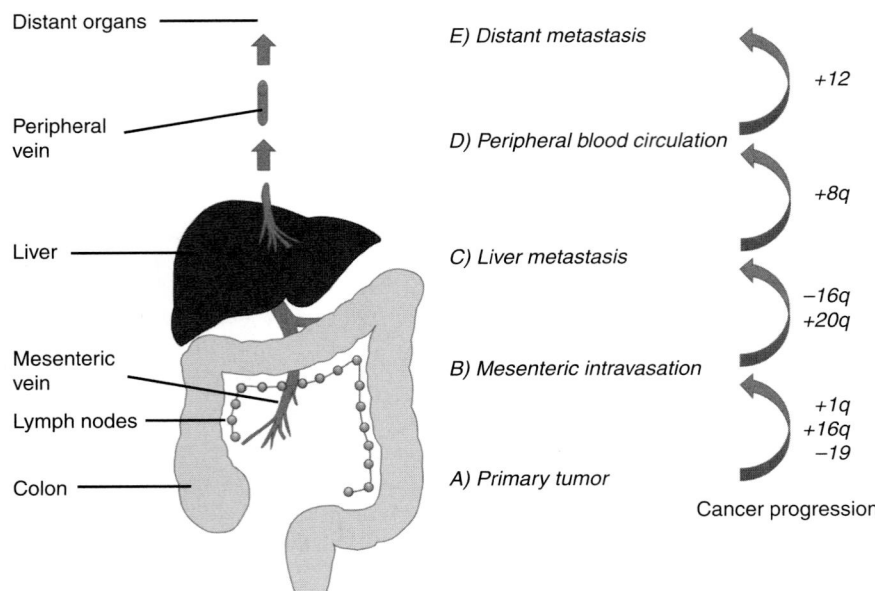

FIGURE 71.8 Chromosomal aberrations are associated with cancer progression. Tumor cells from the primary colorectal cancer disseminate into the mesenteric vein, after which they arrive in the liver and can grow out to become a metastasis. Tumor cells travel further into the peripheral blood circulation, and distant metastasis in organs beyond the liver may finally occur. (From Joosse SA, Souche FR, Babayan A, et al. Chromosomal aberrations associated with sequential steps of the metastatic cascade in colorectal cancer patients. *Clin Chem* 2018;64:1505–12.)

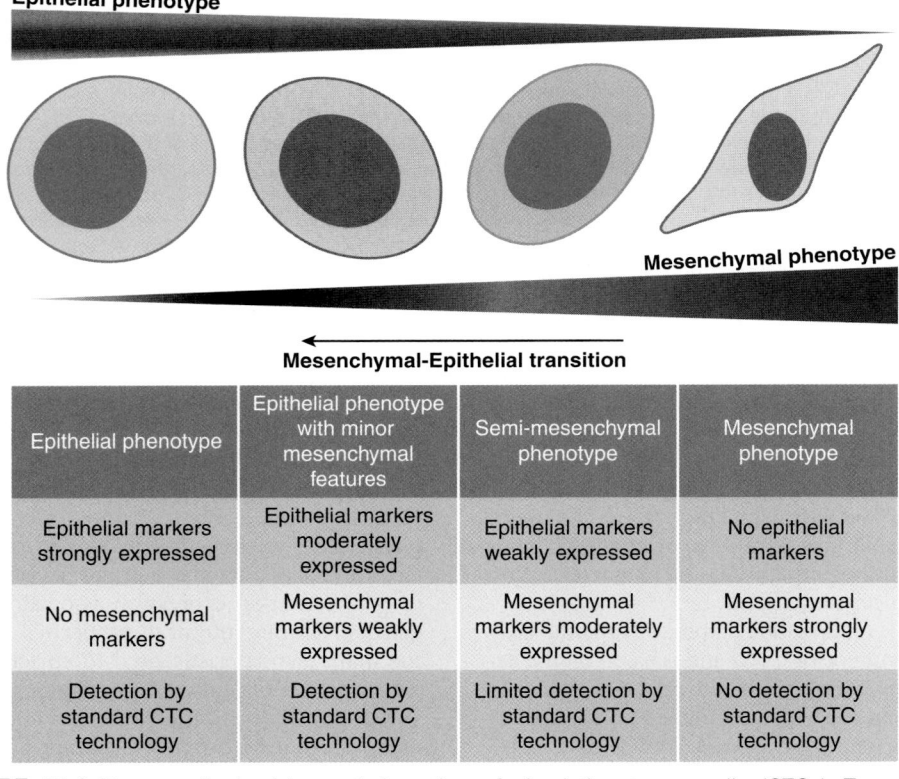

Epithelial phenotype	Epithelial phenotype with minor mesenchymal features	Semi-mesenchymal phenotype	Mesenchymal phenotype
Epithelial markers strongly expressed	Epithelial markers moderately expressed	Epithelial markers weakly expressed	No epithelial markers
No mesenchymal markers	Mesenchymal markers weakly expressed	Mesenchymal markers moderately expressed	Mesenchymal markers strongly expressed
Detection by standard CTC technology	Detection by standard CTC technology	Limited detection by standard CTC technology	No detection by standard CTC technology

FIGURE 71.9 Tumor cell plasticity and detection of circulating tumor cells (CTCs). Tumor cells detected within primary tumors and in the peripheral blood may manifest different continuous phenotypes ranging from epithelial to mesenchymal. These phenotypic changes can influence the yield of CTCs detection by current technologies that are usually based on epithelial markers. (From Bednarz-Knoll, Alix-Panabières, and Pantel, *Cancer Met Rev* 2012.)

compared to RBCs and polymorphonuclear leukocytes.[44] To enrich correctly, the idea is to further combine it to immuno-magnetic enrichment (positive or negative selection). Another alternative is to enrich directly the CTCs with a well-defined Ficoll gradient. The OncoQuick system (Greiner Bio-One, Germany) is an improved version of this approach that uses a porous membrane placed on top of the gradient media to prevent mixing.[45] Experiments performed in cell lines have shown CTC recovery rates of 70 to 90%.[46] Although simple and inexpensive, the OncoQuick system has a relatively low yield and enrichment compared to the Cell-Search system because in the same group of 61 patients, at least one CTC was detected in 23% with OncoQuick and in 54% with CellSearch system.[47]

Systems based on circulating tumor cell size. Size-based isolation systems are independent of tumor markers and separate CTCs (that are usually larger) from smaller leukocytes. Several different size–based systems have been developed and include membrane filters, microfluidic chips, and hydrodynamic methods.[48–50] The first CTC filtration device was described by Vona and colleagues in 2000.[51] Since then, filtration devices have been improved, and many downstream applications have been developed. Filters used for CTC isolation/enrichment are often disposable porous membranes (usually polycarbonate) containing numerous randomly distributed 7- to 8-μm-diameter holes that allow blood constituents to cross but capture the larger CTCs. Specific microfabrication techniques have been applied to build microfilters with controlled pore distribution, size, and geometry[52–54] and different materials like polycarbonate,[51,55,56] parylene C,[57] nickel,[52] and silicon[41] have been used in the fabrication of these membranes.

Polycarbonate membrane filters are usually accompanied by specific syringes or pumps so the pressure on the filter is optimized to keep fragile CTCs intact. Commercially available filtering devices for CTC isolation include the ISET system (isolation by size of epithelial tumor cells, Rarecells, France), ScreenCell (ScreenCell Inc., France), and the CellSieve system (CREATV MicroTech, Potomac, MD).

CTC isolation by size filtration is simple and reliable; filtration and staining are easy to perform, and the method is rapid. CTCs can be identified using classic cytopathologic criteria. No complex instrumentation or specific training is needed. However, false-negative results may be obtained by using filtration devices where small CTCs are missed. Moreover, endothelial cells or rare hematologic cells such as mega-karyocytes may also be present on the filter. For this reason, downstream cytomorphologic, immunocytochemical, and molecular characterization are important to rule out cells that are not CTCs.[58]

Separation based on the electric charge of circulating tumor cells. CTCs are different from peripheral blood mononuclear cells (PBMCs) with respect to morphology and dielectric properties. Dielectrophoresis (DEP) is a technology for CTC isolation based on electrical properties of cancer cells. Dielectric properties (polarizability) of cells are dependent on cell diameter, membrane area, density, conductivity, and volume. Depending on their phenotype and morphology, different cells have different dielectric properties, which is the principle employed for electro-kinetic isolation of CTCs.[59]

Microfluidic systems for circulating tumor cell analyses. The main advantages of microfluidic systems for CTC

isolation/enrichment are their simplicity and the potential to be fully automated, unlike traditional affinity-based CTC isolation techniques. The main disadvantage is the long time needed to run each sample and the low capacity in terms of the volume of peripheral blood that can be processed. These systems are based on a combination of precisely defined topography of microstructures (traps) with laminar flow in microchannels.[16]

With microfluidic-based CTC technology, the chambers are made out of transparent materials that enhance high-resolution imaging, including the use of transmitted light microscopy.[60–62] Most microfluidic devices are reliant on three-dimensional structures that limit the characterization of cells on the chip. This limitation can be overcome by using functionalized graphene oxide nanosheets on a patterned gold surface.[63] In recent years, various sophisticated microfluidic devices have been developed,[64–67] including in situ capture and CTC culture in a three-dimensional co-culture model simulating a tumor microenvironment.[68]

In vivo systems for circulating tumor cell enrichment. The recent development of in vivo systems for CTC isolation from whole blood adds another dimension to the field of CTC isolation. These systems aim to overcome the limitation of small blood sample volumes inherent to the ex vivo CTC isolation techniques previously described.

The first in vivo CTC isolation system used in cancer patients was the CellCollector (CC, Gilupi GmbH, Germany). CellCollector is a nanowire that is coated at its tip (2 cm of length) with pure gold, to which chimeric antibodies directed to EpCAM are covalently attached. The CellCollector is placed into the antecubital vein of a cancer patient for in vivo binding of CTCs.[69] Several studies in patients with lung and prostate cancer have demonstrated technical validity for CTC detection and molecular characterization;[70–73] however, the clinical relevance of CC-detected CTCs is still under investigation. Recently, Dizdar and colleagues evaluated this technology for CTC detection in CRC patients. While CTC detection in M_0 CRC patients was significantly increased with the CC, the clinical relevance of these CTCs appears inferior to the cells identified by the CellSearch system.[74]

Transdermal photoacoustic flow cytometry can also detect CTCs in vivo. A high–pulse repetition rate diode laser shines light through the skin into a vessel that is up to 3 mm deep to detect acoustic vibrations that result from the absorption of laser light by target nanoparticles.[75] By using this technology, circulating melanoma cells were detected in blood.[76] More recently, Galanzha and colleagues reported a completely new Cytophone platform for photoacoustic detection of CTCs in patients with melanoma.[77] The Cytophone could detect individual CTCs at a concentration of $\geq$1 CTC/mL in 20 seconds and could also identify clots and CTC-clot emboli, indicating the potential of in vivo blood testing with the Cytophone in melanoma patients.

Analysis of High Blood Volumes to Increase Circulating Tumor Cell Capture Rate

To analyze a high volume of blood, an alternative to in vivo CTC detection is analysis by leukapheresis. Indeed, leukapheresis is a laboratory procedure in which WBCs or peripheral blood stem cells are separated from blood. During leukapheresis, a patient's blood is passed through a machine that removes the WBCs or peripheral blood stem cells and then returns the balance of the blood back to the patient. Eifler and colleagues first showed that isolation of CTCs via leukapheresis was feasible.[78] Screening leukapheresis products generated from up to 2.5 L of processed blood per patient demonstrated that CTCs can be detected in more than 90% of nonmetastatic breast cancer patients.[79] Label-free enrichment and molecular characterization of viable CTCs can be performed from diagnostic leukapheresis (DLA) products,[80] and DLA has enabled transcriptomic profiling of single CTCs demonstrating intercellular heterogeneity of endocrine resistance in estrogen receptor (ER)-positive breast cancer.[81]

Strategies for Circulating Tumor Cell Detection

After the enrichment step, the samples still contain a substantial number of contaminating leukocytes; thus CTCs need to be specifically identified at the single-cell level by a robust reproducible method that can distinguish them from normal blood cells. CTC detection is achieved by (i) immunofluorescence, (ii) molecular nucleic acid analyses (multiplex RT-qPCR), and (iii) functional assays (EPISPOT and EPIDROP).[8] An outline of the main approaches for CTC detection is presented in Fig. 71.6.

Immunologic Technologies

Immunologic technologies are the most frequent methods employed for CTC detection, and they use a combination of membrane and/or intracytoplasmic anti-epithelial, anti-mesenchymal, and anti–tissue-specific markers and anti–tumor-associated antibodies.[8] Over the past 20 years, keratins as constituents of the cytoskeleton of epithelial cells[82] have been established as detection markers for CTCs in patients with various kinds of carcinomas. Many CTC assays follow principles that are similar to the FDA-cleared CellSearch system, which has been the "gold standard" for many years and will be therefore discussed in more detail. After EpCAM–based immunomagnetic enrichment of CTCs, cells are fluorescently stained for epithelial keratins (CK8, 18, and 19) as markers for CTCs, the common leukocyte antigen CD45 as an exclusion marker, and a nuclear dye (4′,6-diamidino-2-phenylindole [DAPI]) to access cellular integrity (Fig. 71.10), and suspicious events are listed in a photo gallery using automated digital microscopy. The main advantages of the CellSearch system are its high reproducibility and robustness including defined preanalytical steps of blood sampling that ensure stability for 96 hours at room temperature.[83,84] Most importantly, there is a wealth of data from large-scale clinical studies demonstrating the correlation of CellSearch-based CTC counts with clinical outcome in breast cancer and may other solid tumors.[85] However, limitations to this system are that the enrichment and detection steps depend entirely on the expression of the epithelial markers EpCAM and keratins. Thus CTCs that have undergone a complete EMT and do not express EpCAM and keratins (see below) cannot be detected. Therefore there is an ongoing search for additional markers that detect EMT CTCs and are not expressed on contaminating blood cells to ensure both high sensitivity and specificity of CTC detection.

Molecular circulating tumor cell assays. Molecular techniques identify specific tumor DNA or mRNA in lysates of blood cells to indirectly demonstrate the presence of CTCs. Detection involves designing specific primers for transcripts supposedly associated with CTC-specific genes. These genes either code for tissue-, organ-, or tumor-specific proteins or, more specifically, contain known mutations, translocations, or methylation patterns found in cancer cells.[86] RNA-based methods have the highest sensitivity but can lack specificity, owing to the potential of capturing noncancerous cells that generate false-positive signals, thus decreasing the overall accuracy. Considering the heterogeneity of CTCs, multiplex RT-PCR assays could overcome this limitation.[8,87]

Functional Circulating Tumor Cell Assays

Functional assays that exploit aspects of cellular CTC activity can identify "metastasis-competent cells" among the entire pool of CTCs (see Figs. 71.6 and 71.11). The functional epithelial immunospot (EPISPOT, a specific type of ELISPOT or Enzyme-LInked immunoSPOT) assay was introduced for in vitro CTC detection and focuses only on viable CTCs.[88] This technology assesses the presence of CTCs based on secretion, shedding, or release of specific proteins during 24 to 48 hours of short-term culture.[89] This assay has been used in many types of solid cancers, such as breast, colorectal, prostate, and others. The new EPIDROP assay (EPIspot in a DROP) is currently under optimization for the detection of single viable CTCs. It allows the enumeration and characterization of all CTCs, and gives information on their viability and functionality at the single cell level and also on their drug resistance profile in a few hours.[8] More recently, Tang and colleagues described a high-throughput assay for rapid detection of rare metabolically active tumor cells in pleural effusions and the peripheral blood of lung cancer patients.[90]

The establishment of in vitro cultures and permanent lines from CTCs has become a challenging task (Fig. 71.12).[91] Recently, CTC lines have been used to identify key proteins and new pathways involved in cancer stemness and dissemination and to test new drugs to inhibit metastasis-initiator CTCs. Ex vivo CTC cultures have been established for breast,[61,92] prostate,[93] lung,[68] colon,[89] and head and neck cancers.[94] Permanent CTC lines from circulating colon cancer cells have been established both before (CTC-MCC-41)[89,95] and after the initiation of the anticancer treatment.[96] Important information can be obtained by transplantation of patient-derived CTCs into immunodeficient mice; tumors that grow after xenotransplantation of enriched CTCs have the characteristics of metastasis-initiator cells.[97]

Strategies for Circulating Tumor Cell Characterization

Serial CTC measurement can follow the evolution of tumor subclones during treatment and disease progression and hold the key to understand the biology of the metastatic cascade.[91] Improvements in technologies to yield purer CTC populations improve cellular and molecular investigations. Characterization of single CTCs allows better insight into tumor heterogeneity within assays, including immunofluorescence, array comparative genomic hybridization (CGH), massively parallel sequencing (MPS) of both DNA and RNA, and fluorescence in situ hybridization (FISH).

Immunologic detection and characterization allow isolation of stained CTCs for subsequent molecular characterization. While manual isolation by micromanipulation of CTCs is possible,[98] it is rather arduous and time-consuming. An alternative automated single-cell selection device is the DEPArray, which is based on DEP that traps single cells in DEP cages and is designed for single-cell recovery of CTCs.

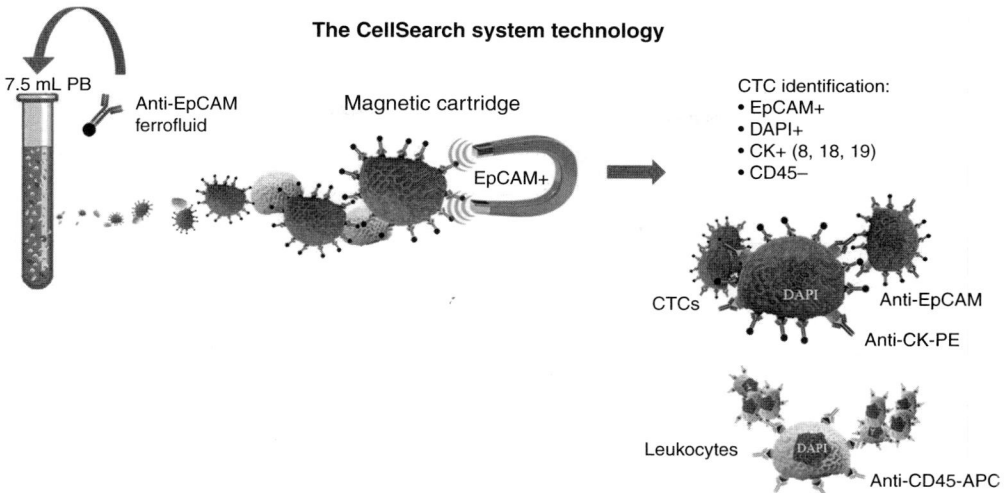

FIGURE 71.10 Positive immunomagnetic isolation and staining of circulating tumor cells (CTCs) on the CellSearch system. Most nucleated cells in the blood are white blood cells (WBC, leukocytes). CTCs are enriched by a magnetic cartridge and are identified by being EpCAM$^+$, CK$^+$, and CD45$^-$. After isolation, they can be enumerated and/or characterized.

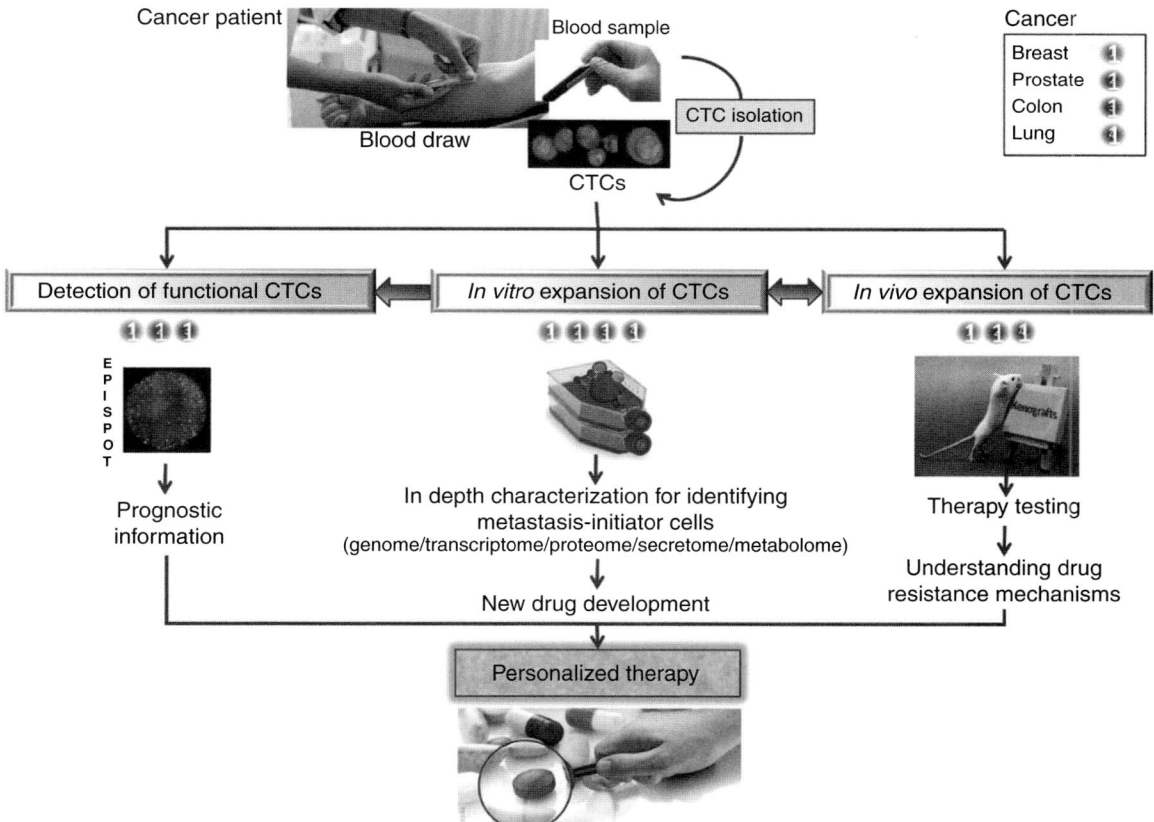

FIGURE 71.11 Functional studies using in vitro and in vivo models for personalized clinical management of cancer patients. After enrichment of circulating tumor cells (CTCs) from blood samples of cancer patients, viable CTCs can be enumerated with a functional assay (EPISPOT) and prognostic information obtained. CTCs can be cultured in vitro, and in-depth characterization of established CTC lines may identify metastasis-initiator cells, a crucial point for new drug development and potential cancer cures. Alternatively, CTCs can be expanded in vivo for therapy testing and to understand drug resistance mechanisms. (From Pantel K, Alix-Panabières C. Functional studies on viable circulating tumor cells. *Clin Chem* 2016;62:328–34)

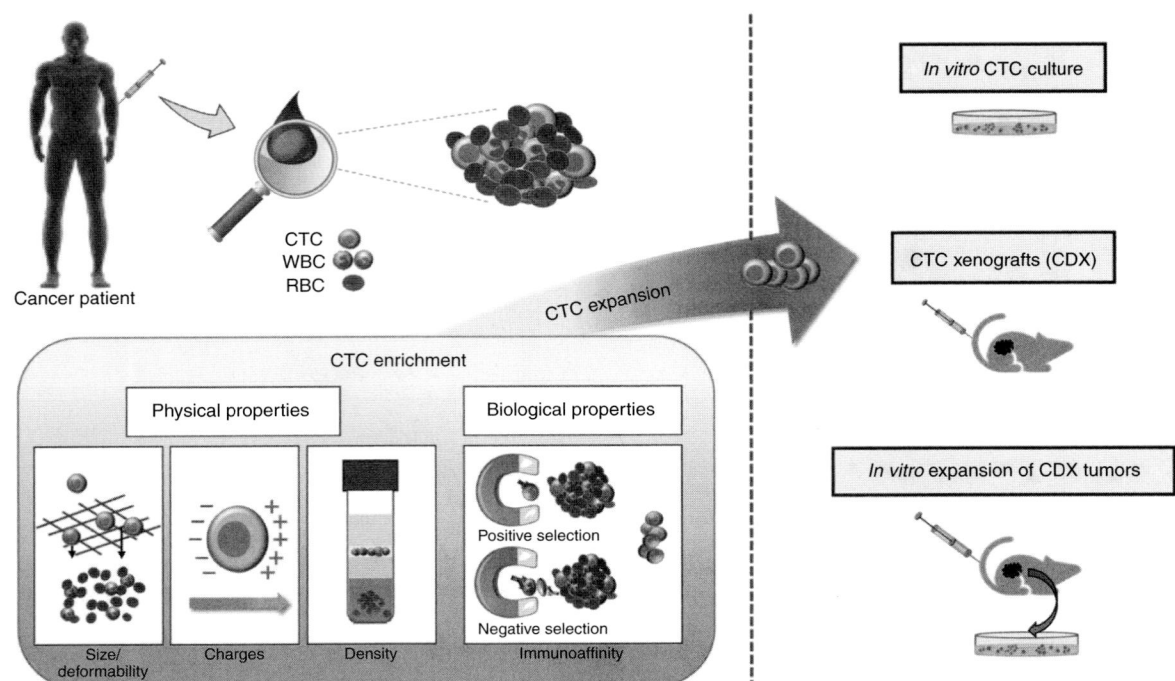

FIGURE 71.12 Circulating tumor cell (CTC) expansion technologies. In vitro CTC cultures are a valuable tool for functional analyses, drug screening, and genome, transcriptome, proteome, secretome, and metabolome studies of metastasis-initiator tumor cells. These analyses bring unique insights that are useful for identifying novel pathways, particularly those implicated in CTC metastatic potential. CTC-derived xenografts (CDX) model the in vivo environment to understand drug resistance mechanisms, identify the properties of metastasis-initiator cells, and assess the capacity of CTCs to induce in vivo tumor growth and metastases. In vitro expansion of CDX tumors (CDX-derived cells) can be used to monitor the sensitivity/response to anti-cancer therapies, identify new biomarkers, and unravel the mechanisms of drug response. (From Cortés-Hernández LE, Eslami-S Z, Alix-Panabières C. Circulating tumor cell as the functional aspect of liquid biopsy to understand the metastatic cascade in solid cancer. *Mol Aspects Med* 2020;72:100816.)

Multiple clinical studies have used this technology to detect and isolate single CTCs for subsequent genetic analyses.[99–102]

Another approach is FISH analysis of single CTCs identified by immunocytochemistry. Recently, padlock probe technology, which enables in situ analysis of AR-V7 in CTCs, showed that 71% (22 of 31) of castration-resistant prostate cancer (CRPC) patients had detectable AR-V7 expression ranging from low to high expression.[103] Patients with AR-V7-positive CTCs respond better to taxane-based chemotherapy than novel hormonal therapies, indicating a treatment-selection biomarker.[104]

Circulating Tumor Cells as a "Window to Metastasis"

In 1889, in the very first issue of *Lancet*, Steve Paget described "the seed and soil hypothesis," in which "metastasis depends on the cross talk between selected cancer cells (the seed) and specific organ microenvironments (the soil)," a hypothesis revisited many years later by Fidler.[105] Detailing the mechanism of metastasis remains a very hot topic in cancer research today (Fig. 71.13).[24,106] Analysis of disease course, tumor growth rates, autopsy studies, clinical trials, and molecular genetic analyses of primary and DTCs all contribute to our understanding of systemic cancer.[13,107] Molecular characterization of CTCs provides a level of detail not previously possible and may be the key to our further understanding of metastatic progression.

CTC biology can be viewed as a "window to metastasis" because CTCs play a critical role in the metastatic spread of carcinomas (see Fig. 71.13).[8,16] If CTCs are effectively targeted or kept in a dormant state, the cancer may be prevented from progressing to metastatic disease. Molecular characterization of CTCs from patients may be the shortest path to determine which and when patients might relapse and to identify specific mechanisms to target these cells. Dormancy gene signatures that identify individuals with dormant disease have also been explored.[108,109] In contrast, CTCs with stemness and EMT features display enhanced malignant and metastatic potential. The role of CTCs in treatment failure and disease progression is likely explained by their biological processes, such as EMT, stemness features, dormancy, and heterogeneity (Fig. 71.14).[110]

Mentioning the evolution of dispersal, it is of utmost interest to evaluate whether similar ecologic and evolutionary principles can be applied to metastasis, and how these processes may shape the spatiotemporal dynamics of CTCs.[111] Indeed, CTCs have themselves been observed to disperse alone and in groups of up to around 100 cells, called clusters or microemboli,[112–114] and cancer cells reproduce asexually, so it is uncertain which of the aforementioned evolutionary outcomes is the most likely to explain a role of kin selection in metastasis (Fig. 71.15).

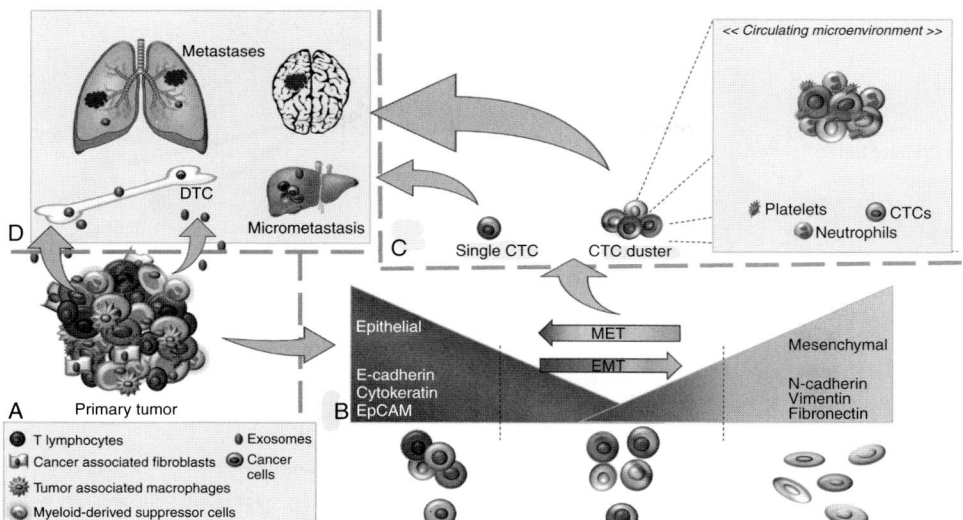

FIGURE 71.13 Metastatic cascade. (A) Primary tumor microenvironment. To keep growing, cancer cells need to interact with several cell types, such as T lymphocytes, cancer-associated fibroblasts, tumor-associated macrophages, myeloid-derived suppressor cells, and also other cancer cells. These interactions are possible due to cell-to-cell communications (i.e., exosomes) that strengthen the epithelial to mesenchymal (EMT) and cancer stem cell (CSC) features to induce the formation of circulating tumor cells (CTCs) and then metastasis-initiator cells (MICs). (B) CTC epithelial-to-mesenchymal plasticity. CTCs can undergo EMT and then mesenchymal to epithelial transition (MET). (C) CTCs may travel in the bloodstream as single cells or in clusters or microemboli. CTC clusters might be made only of CTCs or of CTCs associated with platelets and neutrophils, thus increasing the chance of becoming MICs. (D) Disseminated tumor cells (DTC), micrometastasis, and metastasis. Premetastatic niches are first established by exosomes that originate from the primary tumor. Then, single CTCs or CTC clusters might invade a different body site and remain dormant (in the figure, bone marrow that is a disseminated tumor cell (DTC) reservoir)), form a metastasis (in lung and brain), or a micrometastasis (liver, in the figure). (From Cortés-Hernández LE, Eslami-S Z, Alix-Panabières C. Circulating tumor cell as the functional aspect of liquid biopsy to understand the metastatic cascade in solid cancer. *Mol Aspects Med* 2020;72:100816.)

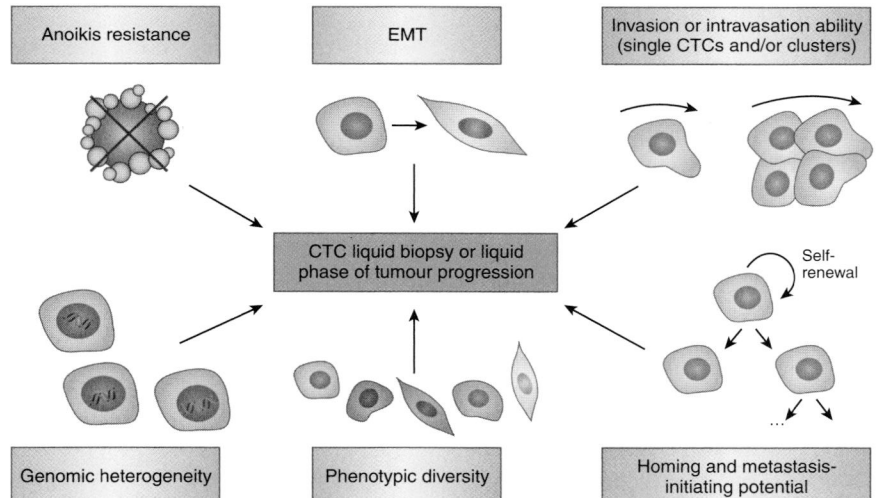

FIGURE 71.14 Current concepts of the cellular and molecular characteristics of circulating tumor cells (CTCs). The scheme summarizes the characteristics of CTCs in cancer patients on the basis of current knowledge. The mechanisms by which viable CTCs avoid cell death in the circulation and the conditions required for the homing and metastasis-initiating potential of CTCs are still under investigation. CTCs may overcome anoikis, a special kind of apoptosis when cells are detached from their basal membrane. Phenotypic plasticity or diversity relates not only to epithelial-to-mesenchymal transition (EMT) but also includes the expression of proteins related to apoptosis, proliferation, invasion, and chemotaxis. Genomic heterogeneity includes HER2, estrogen receptor (ER), androgen receptor (AR), KRAS, and other genes, such as adenomatous polyposis coli (APC), TP53, PIK3CA, neurofibromin 1 (NF1), MLH1, neuron navigator 3 (NAV3), and the gene encoding β-catenin (CTNNB1), as well as copy number variations found in individual CTCs. (From Alix-Panabières C, Pantel K. Challenges in circulating tumour cell research. *Nat Rev Cancer* 2014;14:623–31.)

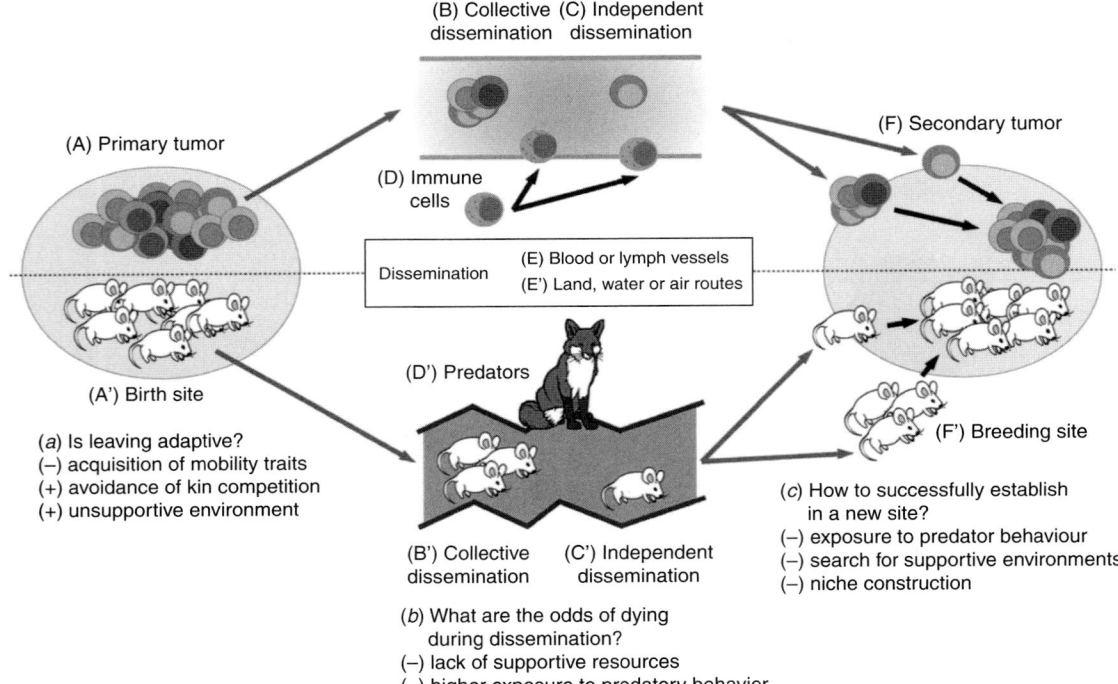

FIGURE 71.15 Comparison between tumor metastasis and mammalian migration. Dispersing cells (*top*) or individuals (*bottom*) have to leave their primary tumor (A) or their birth site (A') to disseminate collectively (B, B') or independently (C, C'). They may be exposed to predatory behavior from immune cells (D) or predators (D') when joining the blood or lymph flow (E) or traveling by land, water, or air (E'), before finally arriving at secondary tumor locations (F) or breeding sites (F'). During all these steps, they are being exposed to beneficial and detrimental factors, which may or may not tip the balance toward dispersal. (From Tissot T, Massol F, Ujvari B, Alix-Panabieres C, Loeuille N, Thomas F. Metastasis and the evolution of dispersal. *Proc Biol Sci* 2019;286:20192186.)

Epithelial and Mesenchymal Transitions of Circulating Tumor Cells

EMT is an essential process in the metastatic cascade.[115–118] This biological process is highly associated with an invasive phenotype and enables detachment of tumor cells from the primary site and migration (Fig. 71.16). The reverse process of mesenchymal epithelial transition (MET) might play a crucial role in the further steps of metastasis when CTCs seed distant organs and establish metastasis. The mechanisms and the interplay of EMT and MET have been intensively studied, and current data suggest the existence of the EMT process in CTCs.[29,87] It is now clear that CTCs from MBC patients exhibit heterogeneous epithelial and mesenchymal phenotypes and display higher frequencies of partial or full-blown mesenchymal phenotype than carcinoma cells within primary tumors. Mesenchymal-like CTCs are also elevated in patients who are refractory to therapy.[115]

Currently, most systems that detect CTCs, including the CellSearch system, are based on the expression of the epithelial marker EpCAM and do not specifically identify CTC subtypes with EMT. Over the past years, several EMT-related markers have been applied in CTC studies. Three EMT markers (*TWIST1*, *AKT2*, and *PI3Kα*) and the stem cell marker *ALDH1* were evaluated in CTCs from 502 primary breast cancer patients by a multiplex RT-PCR assay.[119] A subset of CTCs showed EMT and stem cell characteristics. The expression levels of EMT-inducing transcription factors (*TWIST1*, *SNAIL1*, *SLUG*, *ZEB1*, and *FOXC2*) were also determined in

CTCs from primary breast cancer patients.[120] In another study, rare primary tumor cells simultaneously expressed mesenchymal and epithelial markers, but mesenchymal cells were highly enriched in CTCs, and serial monitoring suggested an association of mesenchymal CTCs with disease progression.[121] Mesenchymal CTCs occurred as both single cells and multicellular clusters, expressed known EMT regulators, including transforming growth factor (TGF)-β pathway components and the *FOXC1* transcription factor. These data support a role for EMT in the blood-borne dissemination of human breast cancer.[121] When the EMT phenotype of CTCs was studied through the expression of two important EMT-connected genes—namely, *VIM* and *SNAIL*—using cytokeratin-negative CTCs from nonmetastatic breast cancer patients, the simultaneous detection of both EGFR and EMT markers may improve prognostic or predictive information.[122] A differential expression pattern of ALDH1 (a stemness marker) and TWIST (an EMT marker) on single CTCs was observed both in early and MBC. CTCs expressing high ALDH1 along with nuclear TWIST were more frequently found in patients with MBC, suggesting that CTCs undergoing EMT may prevail during disease progression.[123]

Counter to expectation, Gorges and colleagues reported low CTC numbers in some patients with late metastatic cancers.[124] These results prompted the search for new markers, including those for mesenchymal-like subpopulations. Plastin-3 is an EMT marker in CTCs in CRC. Aberrant expression of plastin-3 was associated with increased CTCs and poor

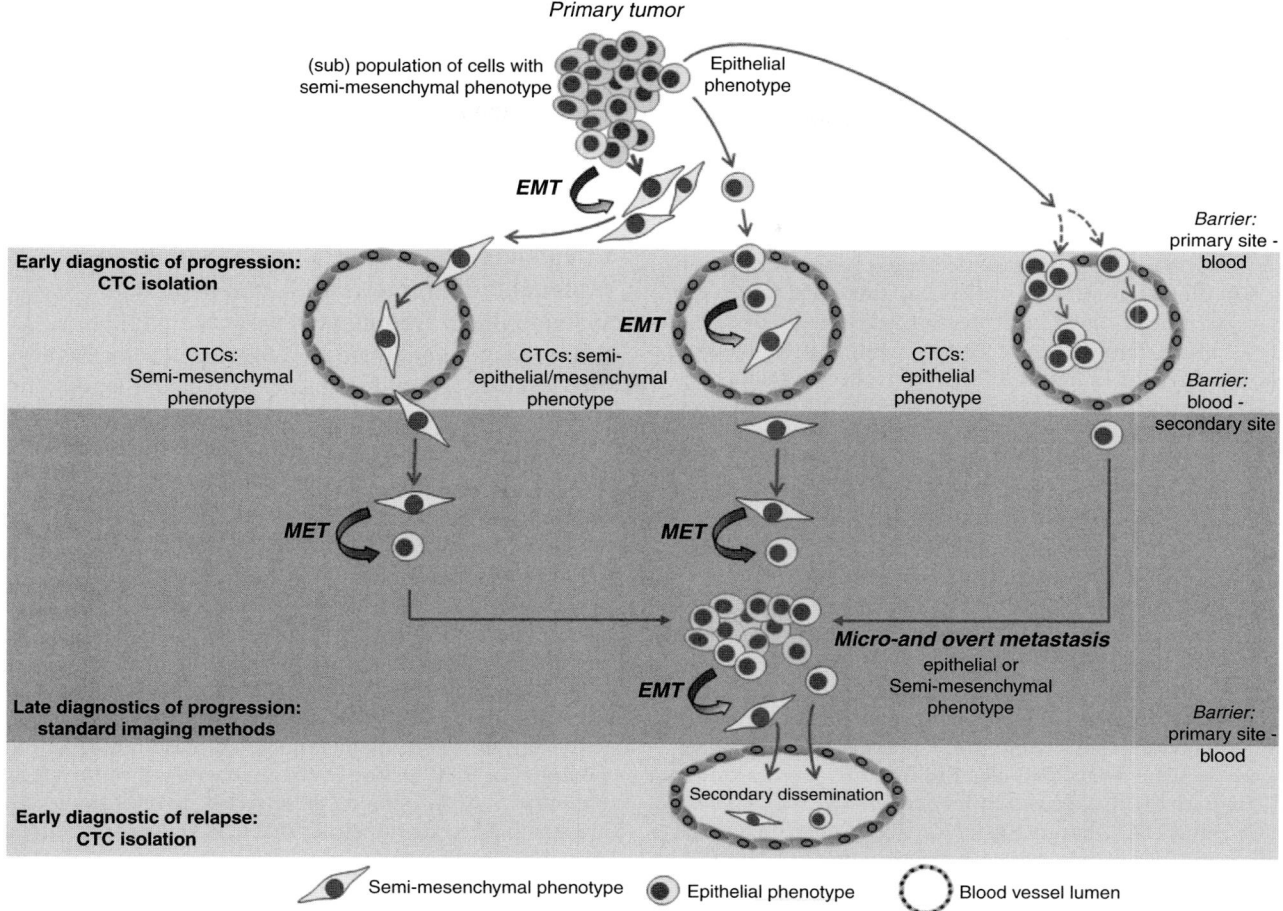

FIGURE 71.16 Models of epithelial-to-mesenchymal transition (EMT)-dependent and -independent tumor cell dissemination. Over time and upon different stimuli, a tumor mass evolves and some cells enter the blood or lymph vessels and disseminate throughout the body. Dissemination is an early phase of tumor progression and may lead to the establishment of micrometastasis, which in the appropriate niche are able to grow out eventually to overt metastasis. Dissemination might take place in two hypothetical ways: EMT dependent or independent. Cancer cells might mechanically infiltrate blood vessels preserving their epithelial phenotype. They might, however, also undergo EMT in the blood stream and hence display a semi-mesenchymal phenotype. Alternatively, a subpopulation of cells localized within the primary tumor might transform into an epithelial phenotype. (From Bednarz-Knoll N, Alix-Panabieres C, Pantel K. Plasticity of disseminating cancer cells in patients with epithelial malignancies. *Cancer Metastasis Rev* 2012;31:673–87.)

prognosis in CRC and may be involved in the regulation of EMT.[125] Cell-surface vimentin is specifically expressed on the surface of CTCs from epithelial cancers undergoing EMT, and the number of CTCs undergoing EMT correlates with disease outcome.

Cytokeratins are widely used for the identification of CTCs by immunocytochemistry, but even these established markers might be modulated during EMT.[82] Breast cancer cells display a complex pattern of cytokeratin expression with potential biological relevance. Individual cytokeratin antibodies may recognize only certain cytokeratins, and important subsets of biologically relevant CTCs in cancer patients may be missed.[126]

EMT and MET transitions are central to the metastatic potential of CTCs; the elucidation of CTC plasticity on the clinical outcome of cancer patients may shed more light on this important topic. Thus far, a large number of prognostic studies in patients with breast cancer and other solid tumors[8]

and recent experimental studies on CTCs[127,128] indicate that CTCs with epithelial attributes are relevant for the onset of metastasis. Thus one might postulate that EMT is important for the release of CTCs from tumor tissues, while MET and the resulting epithelial phenotype of CTCs might allow them to colonize distant organs.[8,87] However, the most important feature might be the plasticity of CTCs to change their phenotype depending on the actual requirements of their changing microenvironments (i.e., blood or diverse organ sites such as bone, liver, or brain). This plasticity is not easily assessable by snapshot analysis but requires longitudinal analysis or experimental models such as cell lines or xenografts established from CTCs.[89,97,129]

Circulating Cancer Stem Cells

Stemness is the ability of cells to self-renew and differentiate into cancer cells.[130] There is substantial evidence that many cancers are driven by a population of cells that display stem cell properties. These cells, called CSCs or tumor initiating cells, not only drive tumor initiation and growth but also mediate tumor metastasis and therapeutic resistance. There is in vitro and clinical evidence that CSCs mediate metastasis and treatment resistance in breast cancer. Novel strategies to isolate CTCs that contain CSCs and the use of patient-derived xenograft models in preclinical breast cancer research have been developed to study the biology of CSCs.[131] Therapeutic resistance, underlying tumor recurrence, and the lack of curative treatments in metastatic disease raise the question as to whether conventional anticancer therapies target the right cells. Indeed, these treatments might miss CSCs that are resistant to many current cancer treatments, including chemotherapy and radiation therapy.[132] Emerging data suggest that the remarkable clinical efficacy of HER-2 targeting agents may be related to their ability to target the breast CSC population. In breast cancers that do not display HER-2 gene amplification, HER-2 is selectively expressed in the CSC population.[133] This expression is regulated by the tumor microenvironment, suggesting that novel and effective adjuvant therapies may need to target the CSC population.[134,135]

EMT induction not only allows for cancer cells to disseminate from the primary tumor but also promotes their self-renewal capability.[136] Breast CSCs have elevated tumorigenicity required for metastatic outgrowth, while EMT may promote CSC character and endows breast cancer cells with enhanced invasive and migratory potential.[137] Emerging evidence indicates that CSCs and EMT cooperate to produce CTCs that are highly competent for metastasis.[138] CTCs with both CSC and EMT characteristics have been identified in the bloodstream of patients with metastatic disease.[119,139] Furthermore, the expression of stemness and EMT markers in CTCs is associated with resistance to conventional anticancer therapies and treatment failure.[136] Some subsets of CTCs have a putative breast CSC phenotype and express EMT markers. The expression of CSC markers such as CD44, CD24, or ALDH1, both by molecular assays and imaging, has also been shown in CTCs.[139–141]

Circulating Tumor Cell Escape From the Immune System

Once in the bloodstream, CTCs face several natural obstacles that hinder the metastatic process. One of the main problems that CTCs face in the circulation is an attack by the immune system (Fig. 71.17). Many studies have been done to understand the mechanisms as to how the immune system could fight cancer. Several biomarkers could be of utmost interest (Fig. 71.18). In CRC, the upregulation of CD47, the "don't eat me signal," protects CTCs from the attack of macrophages and dendritic cells.[142] The most clinically advanced biomarkers are the programmed death-1 (PD-1) and its ligand (PD-L1). Indeed, PD-L1 can be expressed by tumor cells, preventing the immune system from destroying them. The PD-1 receptor is a surface protein expressed on activated T-cells, and its ligand PD-L1 is expressed on the surface of antigen-presenting cells. The formation of the PD-1/PD-L1 complex induces a strong inhibitory signal in the T-cell, which leads to a reduction of cytokine production and a suppression of T-cell proliferation:[143] the immune system is misled by cancer cells expressing PD-L1 and does not destroy them. This crucial point led to the development of immune checkpoint inhibitor therapies (antibodies against PD-1 or PD-L1), and remarkable clinical responses have been observed in several

different malignancies (e.g., melanoma, lung, kidney, and bladder cancers).[143] Immune modulation has also shown promising results in triple negative breast cancer (TNBC) and ERBB2-positive patients.[144] In this context, liquid biopsy in cancer immunotherapy is a very attractive approach as it is minimally invasive, cost-effective, and rapidly gives information to the physician who guides decision-making for therapeutic strategy (Fig. 71.19).[145]

Circulating Tumor Cells: Clinical Significance, Molecular Characterization, and Impact on Individualized Treatment of Cancer Patients

Monitoring of blood samples collected at primary diagnosis and at subsequent time points can enable earlier detection of disease recurrence, months before radiologic detection, and can potentially be translated into a higher chance of cure (see Fig. 71.3).

Breast Cancer

The clinical significance of CTCs has been extensively evaluated in patients with breast cancer. Many clinical studies have shown that CTC detection is associated with OS and PFS both in early and MBC.[8] A comprehensive meta-analysis of published literature on the prognostic relevance of CTC clearly indicates that the detection of CTCs is a reliable prognostic factor in patients both with early-stage and MBC.[146]

At the moment, many clinical studies are evaluating the potential of CTC testing in the management of breast cancer patients.[147] A number of prospective interventional studies are designed to demonstrate that CTC enumeration/characterization may improve the management of breast cancer patients. These include studies to assess CTC-guided hormone therapy versus chemotherapy decisions in M_1 patients, changes in CTC counts during treatment in metastatic patients, and anti–HER-2 treatments in HER-2–negative breast cancer patients selected on the basis of CTCs detection/characterization. The results of these trials will be very important for CTC implementation in the routine management of breast cancer patients.[148]

Clinical significance of circulating tumor cells in metastatic breast cancer. In a seminal paper in 2004, Cristofanilli and colleagues demonstrated that CTCs are an independent prognostic factor for PFS and OS in patients with MBC.[19] The CellSearch system was used with a cutoff of 5 CTCs/7.5 mL of peripheral blood. This paper led to the FDA clearance of the CellSearch assay in MBC. Many clinical studies have since verified the importance of CTC enumeration in MBC.[141,149–153]

It is now clear that MBC patients who present basal counts of 5 CTCs/7.5 mL of blood or greater have a poor prognosis and that enumeration of CTCs during treatment predicts progression of disease earlier than conventional imaging tests.[141] Changing chemotherapy and switching to an alternate cytotoxic therapy was not effective in prolonging OS in patients with persistent increase in CTCs.[154] The independent prognostic effect of CTC count by CellSearch on PFS and OS was further confirmed across 20 studies at 17 European centers that included 1944 eligible patients.[155] CTC analysis may predict the effect of treatment earlier than imaging.[156–158] Correlation between gene expression signatures in CTCs and response to therapy in patients with MBC has also been observed.[159] The prognostic significance of CTC detection is also supported by numerous clinical studies performed on

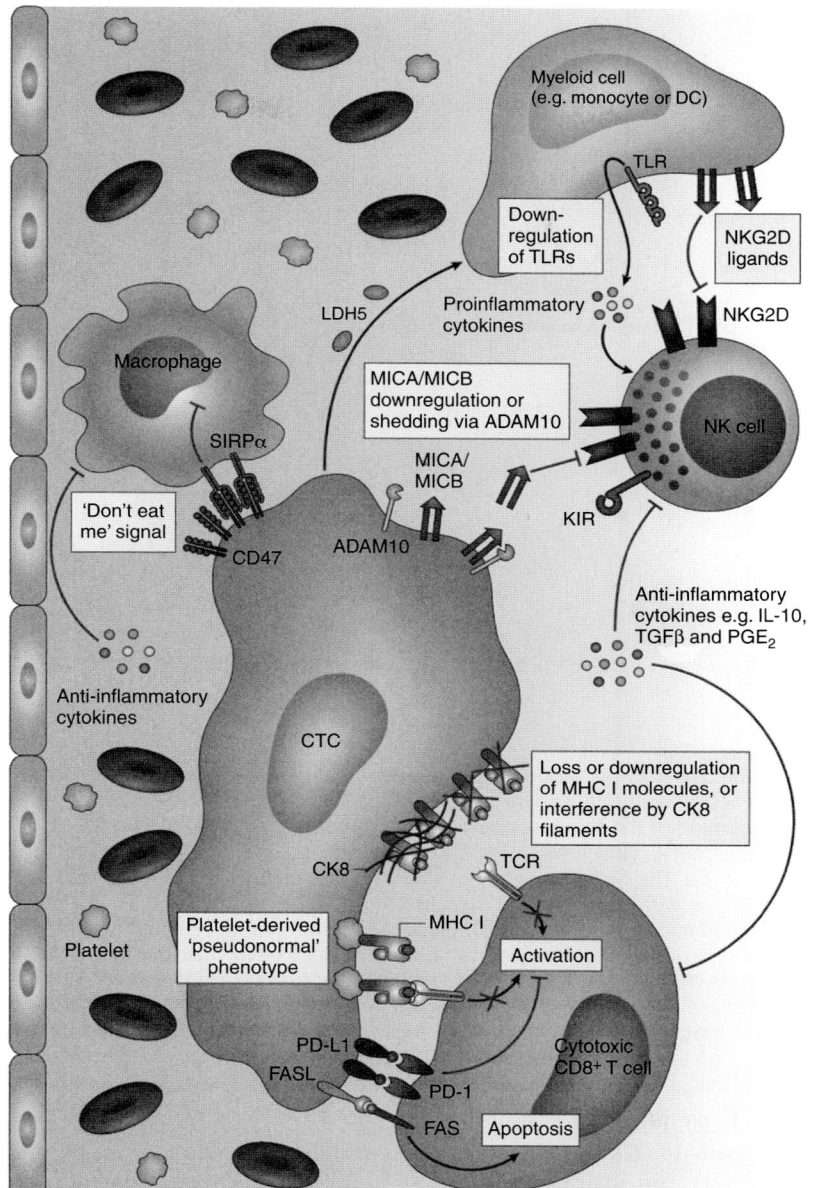

FIGURE 71.17 Immune-escape mechanisms of circulating tumor cells (CTCs) in the peripheral blood. The schematic illustrates mechanisms of immune escape of CTCs, and the interactions between CTCs and immune cells in the peripheral blood. The interplay between CTCs and NK cells is highlighted, with secretion of LDH5 and ADAM10-mediated shedding of the NKG2D ligand MICA/MICB from CTCs preventing recognition and elimination of the cells via NK cell–mediated lysis. LDH5 exerts this effect indirectly by upregulating the expression of NKG2D ligands on circulating monocytes, which results in downregulation of NKG2D expression on NK cells. Three different strategies of CTC escape from MHC I-mediated recognition by NK cells and T cells are depicted: (1) interference with TCR recognition of MHC I molecules by cell-surface-bound cytokeratins (CK8, CD18, and CK19); (2) acquisition of a "pseudonormal" phenotype resulting from membrane transfer from platelets to CTCs; and (3) the downregulation or loss of MHC I expression. Additional mechanisms of immune escape include expression of the inhibitory immune-checkpoint protein PD-L1, presentation of the "don't eat me" signaling receptor CD47, and an altered expression of the apoptotic proteins FAS and/or FASL. *ADAM10,* Disintegrin and metalloproteinase domain-containing protein 10; *CK8,* cytokeratin 8; *CTC,* circulating tumor cell; *DC,* dendritic cell; *FASL,* FAS ligand; *IL-10,* interleukin 10; *KIR,* killer-cell immunoglobulin-like receptor; *LDH5,* lactate dehydrogenase 5; *MHC I,* MHC class I; *MICA,* MHC I polypeptide-related sequence A; *MICB,* MHC I polypeptide-related sequence B; *NK,* natural killer; *NKG2D,* NK-cell receptor D (also known as NKG2-D type II integral membrane protein); *PD-1,* programmed cell-death protein 1; *PD-L1,* programmed cell death 1 ligand 1; *PGE₂,* prostaglandin E2; *SIRPα,* signal-regulatory protein α; *TCR,* T-cell receptor; *TGFβ,* transforming growth factor β; *TLR,* Toll-like receptor. (From Mohme M, Riethdorf S, Pantel K. Circulating and disseminated tumour cells - mechanisms of immune surveillance and escape. *Nat Rev Clin Oncol* 2017;14:155–67.)

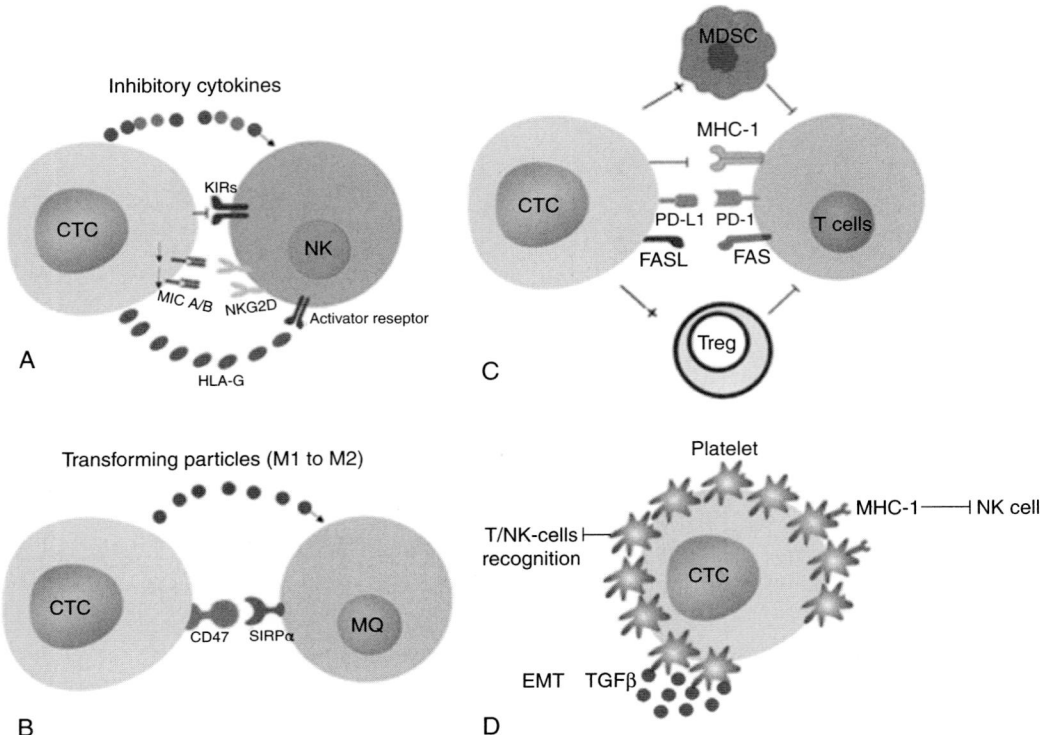

FIGURE 71.18 Circulating tumor cells (CTCs) evade the immune systems in several ways (A–D). (A) CTCs modulate NK cell activity by producing inhibitory cytokines and blocking NK cell activator receptors. (B) CTCs induce production of the tumor-supporting M2 type of macrophage (MQ). (C) PDL-1 and Fas Cell Surface Death Receptor Ligand (FASL): FASL on tumor cells binds to the FAS receptor on T-cells to initiate T-cell apoptosis. The high frequency of FASL[+]/CTCs, Treg cells, FAS[+]/CD8[+]CTLs, and CD4[+] T-helper cells in patients with breast cancer suggests that CTCs mediate immune suppression through the FAS/FASL-induced apoptosis pathway. (D) Platelets interact with CTCs and protect them from antigen recognition by immune cells. Platelets produce MHC-I–positive vesicles, thus sending self-signal to NK cells. Platelets also produce TGF-β, a factor that initiates and maintains EMT, and helps CTCs to evade immune attacks. (From Dianat-Moghadam H, Azizi M, Eslami-S Z, et al. The role of circulating tumor cells in the metastatic cascade: biology, technical challenges, and clinical relevance. *Cancers* 2020;12:867.)

systems other than the CellSearch. RT-PCR assays, especially for the epithelial marker cytokeratin-19 (*CK-19*) alone or in combination with other transcripts, can identify CTCs in MBC.[22] Before the initiation of front-line treatment in patients with MBC, the median PFS and OS were significantly shorter when *CK-19* mRNA-positive CTCs were detected compared with patients who were negative for *CK-19* mRNA.[160] The presence of baseline *CK-19* mRNA-positive CTCs was associated with poor prognosis, and a decrease in mammaglobin mRNA in CTCs may correlate to therapeutic response.[161] The detection of viable CTCs that excrete *CK-19* correlates with OS using the EPISPOT assay.[162]

Clinical significance of circulating tumor cells in early breast cancer. In early breast cancer, CTC numbers are low, and molecular assays are most successful for detection. Nested RT-PCR for *CK-19* expression in the peripheral blood of node-negative breast cancer patients was first shown to be of prognostic value in 2002.[163] Detection of *CK-19* transcripts by using an EpCAM-independent RT-qPCR assay in peripheral blood of early breast cancer patients[164,165] was an independent prognostic factor for disease-free survival (DFS) and OS before,[166] during,[167] and after[168] chemotherapy. Before administration of adjuvant chemotherapy, CTC detection based on

CK-19 positivity by RT-qPCR predicted poor clinical outcome mainly in patients with ER-negative, triple-negative, and HER-2–positive early-stage breast cancer.[169] By using the same EpCAM-independent assay, persistent CTC detection during the first 5 years of follow-up indicated resistance to chemotherapy and hormonal therapy and predicted late relapses in patients with operable breast cancer.[170] Elimination of these *CK-19* mRNA-positive CTCs during adjuvant chemotherapy reflects successful treatment.[171]

CellSearch has also been used in early disease stages, but, to be more sensitive, some groups analyzed up to 20 mL of blood.[172] By using CellSearch, detection of one or more CTCs in the blood sample before neoadjuvant chemotherapy accurately predicted OS.[173] In another CellSearch study, chemonaive patients with nonmetastatic breast cancer at the time of definitive surgery were studied. After a median follow-up of 35 months, the presence of one or more CTCs predicted early recurrence and decreased OS.[174] The REMAGUS02 neoadjuvant study was the first to report the significance of CellSearch CTC detection on distant metastasis-free survival and OS. The detection of CTCs was independently associated with a significantly worse outcome but mainly during the first 3 to 4 years of follow-up.[175] In the German SUCCESS trial, the presence

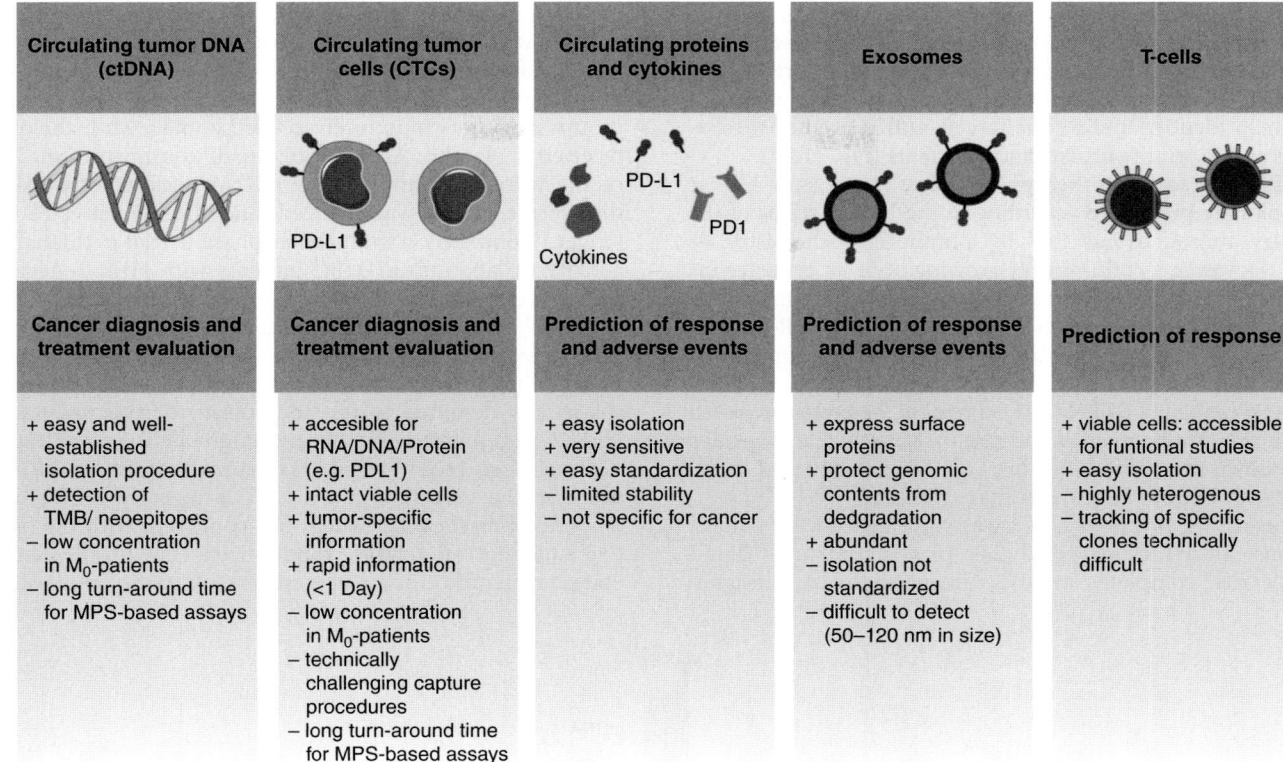

FIGURE 71.19 Suitable targets in liquid biopsy for cancer immunotherapy. All targets used in liquid biopsies share different advantages and disadvantages that favor or disfavor their use in clinical settings as mentioned in the boxes. *TMB,* Tumor mutational burden. (From Hofman P, Heeke S, Alix-Panabières C, Pantel K. Liquid biopsy in the era of immuno-oncology: is it ready for prime-time use for cancer patients? *Ann Oncol* 2019;30:1448–59.

of CTCs was associated with poor DFS, distant DFS, breast cancer–specific survival, and OS, and the prognosis was worse in patients with at least 5 CTCs/30 mL blood. CTCs were confirmed as independent prognostic markers by multivariable analysis for DFS and OS.[176] These findings may change the clinical management of early breast cancer because they clearly indicate the metastatic potential of CTC early in the disease.

Thus reports on thousands of breast cancer patients demonstrate that the CTC counts before neoadjuvant therapy[14,15] and the counts at primary surgery before adjuvant therapy predict the relapse (for review, see Pantel and Alix-Panabières[8]). Encouraging data have also been published for other tumor entities including colorectal[177] and pancreatic cancer.[178] Much less information is available regarding the prognostic relevance of liquid biopsies focusing on the surveillance of MRD through follow-up care studies. Here, we will discuss recent studies indicating that the detection of CTCs months or even years after initial diagnosis predicts metastatic relapse earlier than clinical imaging procedures used to diagnose relapse in breast cancer patients. Trapp and colleagues assessed the CTC counts before and 2 years after chemotherapy in patients with nonmetastatic breast cancer.[179] The multicenter, open-label, phase III SUCCESS A trial compared two adjuvant chemotherapy regimens followed by 2 versus 5 years of zoledronate for early-stage, high-risk breast cancer patients. Two years after chemotherapy, 198 (18.2%) of 1087 patients were CTC positive, and a positive CTC status at this time point predicted a decreased OS and DFS.

Recurrences in hormone receptor-positive breast cancer are characterized by a long latency period ("cancer dormancy") of 5 or more years in at least one-half of all cases.[180] Recently, Sparano and colleagues demonstrated that the presence of CTCs obtained approximately 5 years after diagnosis predicted late recurrence of patients with operable HER2-negative breast cancer.[181] The analysis of 547 women revealed that the recurrence rates per person-year of follow-up in the CTC-positive group was 21.4% (7 recurrences per 32.7 person-years), while being only 2.0% in the CTC-negative group (16 recurrences per 796.3 person-years). Multivariate analysis showed that the detection of CTCs was linked to a 13.1-fold higher risk of recurrence (hazard ratio [HR] point estimate, 13.1; 95% CI, 4.7 to 36.3), thus indicating the clinical validity of CTCs for risk stratification in regard to late breast cancer recurrences.

Recently, Goodman and colleagues evaluated the interaction between radiotherapy, CTC detection, and clinical outcome in patients with early-stage breast cancer.[182] Interestingly, radiotherapy was associated with longer survival in patients with detectable CTCs, suggesting that CTC detection might be a predictive marker for radiotherapy. However, the authors conclude that the study results need to be validated in a prospective interventional trial.

Molecular characterization of circulating tumor cells in breast cancer and its impact on individualized treatment. The main goal of adjuvant therapy is to prevent distant recurrences by targeting residual DTCs. However, many deaths in patients with ER-positive breast cancer occur after 5 years, showing that residual disease can be dormant for very long periods up to 20 years and more.[180] Molecular differences between primary tumors and CTCs could be of crucial importance for therapeutic decisions. Molecular characterization of CTCs may help identify therapeutic targets and resistance mechanisms and to stratify breast cancer patients (Fig. 71.20).[8]

HER-2 for targeted therapy. In breast cancer, anti–HER-2 therapies are prescribed according to the HER-2 status of the primary tumor, as assessed by immunohistochemistry or FISH. However, a continuously growing body of evidence indicates that CTC HER-2 status can be different from that of the corresponding primary tumor. Moreover, CTC HER-2 status can change over time, particularly during disease recurrence or progression.[183–189] By using CellSearch and an automated algorithm to evaluate CTC HER-2 expression, heterogeneity even within the same patient is the rule.[190] Many research groups have shown that HER-2–positive CTCs can be detected in patients with HER-2–negative primary tumors.[183,186,187,191–193]

The HER-2 status of CTCs was correlated to the clinical response of HER-2–targeted therapies in the first "liquid biopsy trial" completed in 2012. Georgoulias and colleagues investigated the effect of trastuzumab in a small number of patients who were HER-2 negative in the primary tumor but were positive for CK[(+)]/HER2[(+)] CTCs as evaluated by immunofluorescence. These patients were randomized into two groups, and one group received trastuzumab, while the other received a placebo. After trastuzumab administration, 75% of the women became *CK-19* mRNA-negative, the risk of disease recurrence was reduced, and the median DFS was longer.[194] Similarly, a multicenter phase II trial evaluated the activity of lapatinib in MBC patients with HER-2–negative primary tumors and HER-2–positive CTCs using the CellSearch.[195] The TREAT-CTC trial, initiated in 2012, is a randomized phase II trial for patients with HER-2 negative primary breast cancer but HER-2–positive CTCs. This trial is specifically designed to test the efficacy of trastuzumab in HER-2–negative early breast cancer. Ignatiadis and colleagues demonstrated recently that trastuzumab treatment did not decrease the detection rate of CTCs in early HER2 non-amplified breast cancer which was consistent with the negative outcome of a large, randomized trial in the United States testing the efficacy of trastuzumab in the same patient

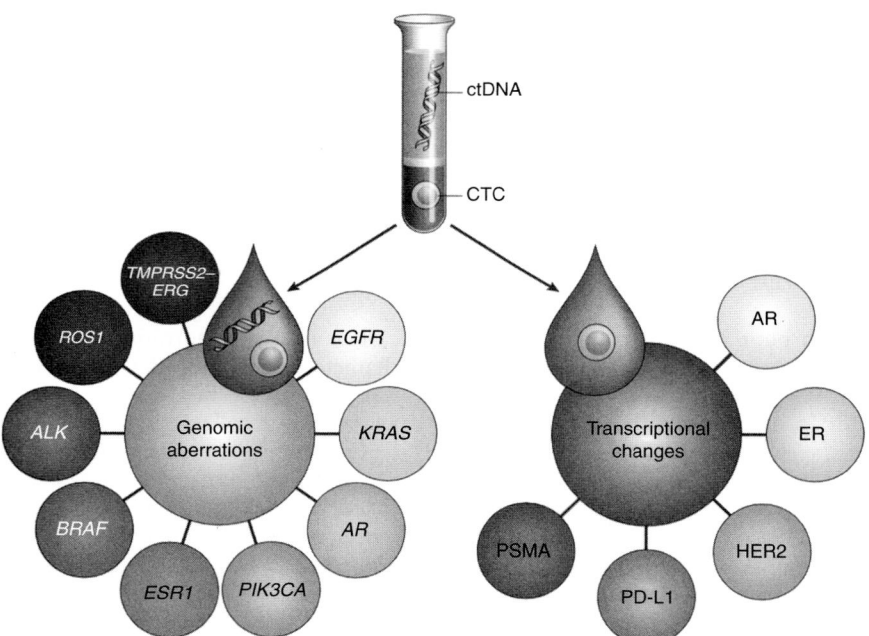

FIGURE 71.20 Therapeutic targets and resistance mechanisms. Analysis of genomic aberrations in circulating tumor cells (CTCs), circulating cell-free tumor DNA (ctDNA) and transcriptional changes in CTCs can be used for the detection of therapeutic vulnerabilities and the real-time monitoring of tumor evolution under the selective pressure of anticancer therapy. This figure provides examples of genes in which aberrations of therapeutic relevance have been defined, predominantly in non–small cell lung cancer (EGFR, ROS1, and ALK), colorectal cancer (KRAS), breast cancer (ESR1 and PIK3CA), prostate cancer (AR and TMPRESS2–ERG fusions), and melanoma (BRAF). Also shown are aberrant transcription of proteins with predominant therapeutic relevance to breast cancer (HER2 and the estrogen receptor [ER]), prostate cancer (androgen receptor [AR], particularly androgen receptor splice variant 7 [AR-V7], and prostate-specific membrane antigen [PSMA]), and for multiple tumor types (programmed cell death 1 ligand 1 [PD-L1]). The majority of ctDNA in plasma is derived from apoptotic cells; however, continuous increases in ctDNA concentrations reflecting particular genetic variants in sequential analyses indicate the evolution of viable tumor cells with resistance to therapy (e.g., ESR1 mutations during endocrine therapy in breast cancer). The capture of CTCs is more cumbersome than the collection of plasma for ctDNA analysis, although CTC analysis enables the detection of changes in gene transcription and protein expression that can be relevant to anticancer therapy, which is not possible with ctDNA. Thus the choice of the most appropriate form of liquid biopsy analysis depends on the drug target, and ctDNA and CTCs can provide complementary information. (From Pantel K, Alix-Panabières C. Liquid biopsy and minimal residual disease – latest advances and implications for cure. *Nat Rev Clin Oncol* 2019;16:409–24.)

population.[196] Thus one could envisage that CTC counts could be developed into an early surrogate endpoint predicting survival in cancer patients.

Estrogen receptor for endocrine treatment. Endocrine treatment is the preferred systemic treatment in MBC patients who have had an ER–positive primary tumor or metastatic lesions. However, 20% of these patients do not benefit from this therapy and demonstrate further metastatic progress. A possible explanation for failure of endocrine therapy might be the heterogeneity of ER expression in CTCs. Similar to the HER-2 story, there is a growing body of evidence that hormone receptor status can change over time, especially during disease recurrence or progression in breast cancer patients.[183–189] In this context, reevaluation of hormone receptor status by molecular characterization of CTCs is a strategy with potential clinical application. Optimal individualized treatment could be selected by characterizing ER status in CTCs and comparing it to the primary tumor.[197] The commercially available AdnaTest Breast Cancer kit (AdnaGen, Qiagen, Germany) can detect EpCAM, MUC-1, and HER-2 transcripts in CTCs; it was found that a major proportion of CTCs in MBC patients showed EMT and tumor stem cell characteristics.[139] Interestingly, when ER and progesterone receptor (PR) CTC expression was assessed by RT-PCR, CTCs were mostly triple-negative regardless of the ER, PR, and HER-2 status of the primary tumor.[189] CTCs frequently lack ER expression in MBC patients with ER-positive primary tumors and show a considerable intrapatient heterogeneity, which may reflect a mechanism to escape endocrine therapy.[198] Single-cell analysis based on whole-genome analysis (WGA) and MPS did not support a role for *ESR1* mutations.[198] In nonmetastatic breast cancer patients, the expression of estrogen, progesterone, and EGFR by immunofluorescence experiments revealed heterogeneous expression of these hormonal receptors in single CTCs in the same patient.[199]

Recently, CK4/6 inhibitors were introduced for the treatment of breast cancer patients resistant to endocrine therapy. Whether CTC counts or molecular analysis of CTCs can predict outcome of this form of therapy is subject of ongoing investigations. In this context, the determination of mutations in the PI3CA gene in CTCs might be a promising approach.[200]

Prostate cancer. In prostate cancer, CTCs have been extensively studied and validated as a prognostic tool.[201] In advanced prostate cancer, CTC enumeration on the Cell-Search system is FDA-cleared as a prognostic test of survival at baseline and post-treatment (for review, see Pantel and colleagues[202]). Integration into routine clinical practice is ongoing. The main CTC studies in advanced and localized prostate cancer highlight the important gains and the challenges posed by various approaches and their implications for advancing prostate cancer management.[202]

Clinical significance of circulating tumor cells in metastatic prostate cancer. In 2008, the FDA cleared the Cell-Search assay for the enumeration of CTCs in CRPC based on data presented by de Bono and colleagues,[203] who showed that CTC enumeration had prognostic value as an independent predictor of OS in CRPC. This study was followed by many others, confirming that CTC enumeration can be used to monitor disease status and therapeutic outcome.[204–207] In patients with metastatic hormone-sensitive prostate cancer, correlation of prostate-specific antigen, Gleason score, and TNM stage with CTC counts showed that CTCs could correctly stage prostate cancer and assess prognosis.[208,209] According to the results of a prospective phase III trial, baseline CTC counts were prognostic and could be used as an early metric to help redirect and optimize therapy.[210]

Clinical trials that evaluate the efficacy of drugs in CRPC need new clinical endpoints that are valid surrogates for survival. In a clinical trial of abiraterone plus prednisone versus prednisone alone for patients with metastatic CRPC, Scher and colleagues evaluated CTC enumeration as a surrogate outcome. They developed a biomarker panel that includes CTC number and LDH concentration as a surrogate for survival at the individual patient level.[211]

Although these findings would require large-scale prospective validation before routine clinical practice, they do show the strong potential of CTC analysis for the management of prostate cancer.

Advances in the understanding of prostate cancer signaling pathways have led to the development and subsequent approval of multiple novel therapies, especially for metastatic CRPC. The androgen receptor (AR) is a key target in prostate cancer, and many current therapies for metastatic CRPC target AR signaling. For example, abiraterone and enzalutamide are novel endocrine treatments that abrogate AR signaling in CRPC, but resistance to these therapies is also common. CRPC therapeutic intervention after clinical progression may be achieved through the characterization of AR activity. Biopsies of bone metastases can also assess AR activity but are highly invasive. On the other hand, the molecular characterization of CTCs offers a minimally invasive approach to study late-stage disease. However, patient benefit is variable with these agents, so development of other predictive biomarkers is very important.

Pretreatment detection of AR splice variant-7 (AR-V7) in CTCs from CRPC patients is associated with resistance to enzalutamide and abiraterone.[212,213] Such androgen ablation therapy induces expression of constitutively active AR splice variants that drive disease progression. Recently, the same group confirmed these results by conducting CTC-based AR-V7 analysis at baseline, during therapy, and at progression.[214] Nuclear AR expression in CTCs of CRPC patients treated with enzalutamide and abiraterone was also evaluated and appeared to predict outcome.[202] However, CTCs exhibit a marked intrapatient heterogeneity in regard to AR and ARv7 expression;[70,103,215] this heterogeneity reflects the high plasticity of tumor cells and might also be an effective way to escape AR-directed or other therapies.

In early-stage, nonmetastatic prostate cancer, the clinical relevance of CTCs is still under investigation.[202] Due to the low CTC counts, there are ongoing efforts to combine different CTC assays that are complementary and based on different approaches to enrich and detect CTCs[71]; for example, the combination of three CTC assays leads to a detection rate of over 80% in high-risk early stage prostate cancer.[72,216] CTCs show a marked intrapatient and interpatient heterogeneity in high-risk early-stage prostate cancer patients.[73] Moreover, CTC analysis has been used to address the question whether prostate biopsies can induce the release of tumor cells into the circulation.[217] However, long-term follow-up studies are now required to assess the clinical relevance of CTC analysis in early prostate cancer.

Colorectal Cancer

A meta-analysis of 12 studies revealed prognostic value of CTCs and DTCs in patients with metastatic CRC.[218] CTC number was an independent predictor of cancer recurrence in six out of nine studies that examined the detection of postoperative CTCs in CRC.[219] The prognostic significance of CTCs in CRC has been reviewed.[220]

Clinical significance of circulating tumor cells in metastatic colorectal cancer. The CellSearch assay was cleared by the FDA for metastatic CRC in 2008.[221] In advanced CRC, CTC enumeration before and during treatment independently predicts PFS and OS and provides additional information beyond CT imaging,[222–224] while surgical resection of metastases immediately decreases CTC levels.[225] CTC numbers are higher in the mesenteric venous blood compartments of patients with CRC, and viable CTCs are trapped in the liver, a finding that may possibly explain the high rates of liver metastasis in this type of cancer.[226] Six CTC markers (tissue specific and EMT transcripts) used in metastatic CRC patients identified therapy-refractory patients not detected by standard image techniques. Patients with increased CTCs numbers, even when classified as responders by computed tomography, showed significantly shorter survival times.[227] The presence of CTCs in stage III colon cancer patients undergoing curative resection followed by mFOLFOX chemotherapy, as determined by telomerase reverse transcriptase, CK-19, CK-20, and CEA transcripts, was an independent predictor of post-chemotherapeutic relapse and strongly correlated with DFS and OS.[228]

Clinical significance of circulating tumor cells in early colorectal cancer. CTC studies in nonmetastatic CRC are more limited compared to metastatic CRC, due to the very low number of CTCs. It was shown that preoperative CTC detection is an independent prognostic marker in nonmetastatic CRC,[229] and the presence of CTCs correlates with reduced DFS in patients with nonmetastatic CRC.[230] CTC detection might help in the selection of high-risk stage II CRC candidates for adjuvant chemotherapy.[231] Previously, plastin-3 mRNA has been suggested as a specific marker for CTCs that helps to distinguish between Duke's stage B patients with low and high risk of recurrences.[177] CEA, CK, and CD133 expression were used to evaluate the clinical significance of CTCs as a prognostic factor for OS and DFS in patients with CRC after curative surgery. In patients with Duke's stage B and C CRC who required adjuvant chemotherapy, detection of CEA/CK/CD133 mRNA in CTCs predicted risk of recurrence and poor prognosis.[232] Interventional studies are now needed to assess whether stage B patients with CTCs will profit from chemotherapy and whether stage C patients without CTCs can be spared from chemotherapy.

Molecular Characterization of Circulating Tumor Cells in Colorectal Cancer: Impact on Individualized Treatment

Patients with benign inflammatory diseases of the colon can harbor viable circulating epithelial cells that are detected as "CTCs" on the CellSearch system because they are of epithelial origin and CD45 negative.[233] Hence, further molecular characterization of CTCs is important in CRC. A considerable portion of viable CTCs are trapped in the liver, as shown by their enumeration in the peripheral and mesenteric blood, using both the CellSearch and EPISPOT assays,[26] potentially explaining the high incidence of liver metastasis in colon cancer. Anti-EGFR therapy in metastatic CRC may select for KRAS and BRAF mutations. However, the occurrence of these mutations in metastatic CRC may vary among primary

tumors, CTCs, and metastatic tumors.[234,235] Using the CellSearch system, the expression of *EGFR*, *EGFR* gene amplification, *KRAS*, *BRAF*, and *PIK3CA* mutations were evaluated in single CTCs of patients with metastatic CRC,[236] and the concordance between *KRAS* mutations in CTCs and primary tumors was 50%.[237] *APC*, *KRAS*, and *PIK3CA* mutations that were found in CTCs were also present at subclonal levels in the primary tumors and metastases from the same patients.[98] When *KRAS* mutations were investigated in CTCs from patients with metastatic CRC throughout the course of the disease and compared to the corresponding primary tumors, CTCs exhibited different *KRAS* mutations during treatment.[238] Plastin-3 is a marker for CTCs undergoing EMT and is associated with CRC prognosis, particularly in patients with Duke's B and C stage tumors.[177] Patients with CTC positivity at baseline had a shorter median PFS compared to patients with no CTCs, and a significant correlation was also found between CTC detection during treatment and radiographic findings at 6 months.[224] CTCs are promising markers for the evaluation and prediction of treatment responses in rectal cancer patients, superior to CEA.[239]

In conclusion, CTC analysis highly correlates to systemic disease spread and disease outcome in CRC patients. Many clinical studies support the potential utility of CTC detection in CRC.

Lung Cancer

CTCs are much more frequent in small cell lung cancer (SCLC) than non–small cell lung cancer (NSCLC). Possible explanations are that current detection methods relying on epithelial markers to identify CTCs are not as effective in NSCLC compared to SCLC, and that CTCs from NSCLC may have a shorter transit time in blood. Even so, there is evidence that in lung cancer CTC numbers are prognostic in both SCLC and NSCLC, and that CTCs counted before and after treatment mirror treatment response. In patients with molecularly defined subtypes of NSCLC, CTCs demonstrate the same molecular changes as the cancer cells of the tumor.[240]

Clinical significance of circulating tumor cells in non–small cell lung cancer. The presence of EpCAM/MUC-1 mRNA-positive CTCs in NSCLC patients preoperatively and postoperatively revealed shortened DFS and OS.[241] In NSCLC patients undergoing surgery, the presence and the number of CTCs were associated with worse survival,[242] and hybrid CTCs with an EMT phenotype were detected.[243] CTCs are detectable in patients with untreated stage III or IV NSCLC and are prognostic.[244]

Clinical significance of circulating tumor cells in small cell lung cancer. SCLC accounts for 15 to 20% of lung cancer cases. It is very aggressive and characterized by early dissemination and dismal prognosis. In most cases, SCLC is not operable, and it is difficult to obtain biopsies to investigate its biology and therapeutic options. In this type of cancer, EpCAM-positive/keratin-positive CTCs circulate in high numbers and are readily accessible through a single blood draw, which can be easily repeated for follow-up over time. Moreover, CTCs in SCLC are tumorigenic in immunocompromised mice; the resultant CTC-derived explants mirror the patient's response to platinum and etoposide chemotherapy and can be used for the selection of appropriate therapies.[245] In patients with SCLC undergoing standard treatment, CTCs and CTC clusters, called circulating tumor microemboli (CTM), can be detected and are independent prognostic factors.[246] Evaluating the presence of CTM also improved diagnostic accuracy in NSCLC patients based on clinical and imaging data.[247] The change in CTC count after the first cycle of chemotherapy, evaluated by using the CellSearch system, provided useful prognostic information in SCLC[248] and was the strongest response predictor for chemotherapy and survival.[246]

Besides CTC enumeration, further molecular downstream analysis can reveal druggable mutations relevant to therapy of NSCLC patients.[249,250] For example, Crizotinib is an effective molecular treatment for *ALK* rearrangement–positive NSCLC. The companion diagnostic test for *ALK* rearrangements in NSCLC for crizotinib treatment is currently done by tumor biopsy or fine-needle aspiration. Pailler and colleagues successfully managed to detect *ALK* rearrangements in CTCs of NSCLC patients, enabling both diagnostic testing and monitoring of crizotinib treatment.[251,252] These results highlight the suitability of CTCs to identify therapeutic resistance mutations in ALK-rearranged patients. Single-CTC sequencing may be a unique tool to assess heterogeneous resistance mechanisms and help clinicians in treatment personalization and resistance options to ALK-targeted therapies.

Cutaneous Melanoma

Cutaneous melanoma is a cancer of the skin derived from transformation of melanocytes. Melanoma is mainly a disease of developed countries, with the highest incidence in Australia, North America, and Europe.[253,254] Unfortunately, melanoma is among the fastest-growing cancers in Western societies. A unique characteristic of primary melanoma is that small lesions can be highly metastatic with very poor prognosis compared to similar-size tumors of other cancers, so early detection of CTCs is very important. Melanoma often metastasizes to regional lymph nodes and to distant organs.[255,256] Melanoma metastasis may occur to almost any organ, but brain, liver, and lung are the most common, so CTCs are particularly interesting due to their aggressive ability to metastasize systemically.[257] Recently, the approval of targeted therapies such as *BRAF* mutation inhibitors (vemurafenib, dabrafenib), the MEK inhibitor trametinib, and immune checkpoint inhibitors PDL-1 (pembrolizumab), PD1 (nivolumab), and ipilimumab alone and in combinations have improved OS and DFS considerably.[258–260]

Clinical significance of circulating tumor cells in cutaneous melanoma. The systemic spread of melanoma as viewed through CTCs is in essence real-time monitoring of metastasis as it occurs.[261,262] The only approved blood biomarker for melanoma is LDH in American Joint Cancer Committee stage III/IV patients. Because melanoma is highly malignant, it is not surprising that studies have found CTC analysis clinically important. CTC analysis of melanoma patients started in the early 1990s and has progressed through the years, along with advancements in molecular assays.[263–265] Circulating melanoma cells have differentiation lineage and tumor-related gene expression patterns that are not found in peripheral blood leukocytes. RT-qPCR can be performed on blood after lysis of RBCs and mononuclear cell preparation. Unlike most other RT-qPCR CTC assays, analysis of melanoma cells does not require antibody capture through cell surface antigens. There are only a few cell-surface melanoma-associated antigens for targeting antibodies.[266–268] Therefore molecular assays that target melanoma transcripts are often

used, including *MART-1, MAGE-A3, PAX3,* and ganglioside *GM2/GD2 glycosyltransferase (GalNAc-T).*[264,269–271]

Melanoma is heterogeneous in genomic aberrations and transcriptome expression. Therefore it is important to use multiple markers to assess CTCs to improve sensitivity.[267,269,272–274] New approaches to detect CTCs include the inertial focusing spiral microfluidics CTChip in the ClearCell FX system (Clearbridge BioMedics, Singapore).[275]

Multiple marker RT-qPCR assays allow monitoring both early- and advanced-stage patients during treatment; several well-annotated studies with long-term follow-up have been published.[270,271,273,276,277] CTC monitoring post- and pretreatment also predicts OS in surgically resected disease-free stage III/IV patients. A recent multicenter international phase III trial demonstrated that CTC analysis predicts the outcome of melanoma patients with positive sentinel lymph nodes after their resection with disease-free status.[277] Multimarker RT-qPCR analysis may be helpful in identifying patients who have high risk of systemic disease progression after surgery or therapy.

Molecular characterization of isolated circulating tumor cells from skin cancer patients. Melanoma CTCs are unique in their associated antigens, mRNA expression patterns, and genomic aberrations.[266,267,272,278–280] Recently, an in-depth genomic analysis was performed on paired primary tumors and CTCs whereby copy number aberrations and loss of heterozygosity were analyzed. CTCs were captured by several antiganglioside cell surface human IgM monoclonal antibodies and then subjected to a genome-wide SNP array.[268] IgM provides better capture of CTCs than IgG. Greater than 90% of SNPs were concordant between the primary tumor and isolated CTCs. Several frequent copy number aberrations were identified and validated in a separate cohort of patients with advanced-stage melanoma. These studies indicate the presence of many unexplored key copy number variants in CTCs that can be used to monitor patients' progression. Other groups have reported known genomic mutations in *BRAF* and *KIT,* using isolated melanoma CTC.[281,282]

Overall CTC analysis is correlated to systemic disease spread and disease outcome in melanoma patients. However, intra-patient heterogeneity poses a challenge to detect circulating melanoma cells, which do not express the epithelial markers used to capture and detect CTC in carcinoma patients.[283] With the current availability of improved therapeutics in melanoma (in particular, antibody-based immune checkpoint inhibition therapy against PDL1 and PD1), the monitoring of CTCs may be important to assess early subclinical recurrence and progression both during and after treatment.

In addition to melanoma, the detection and molecular characterization of CTCs contributes interesting clinical information in Merkel cell carcinomas,[102,284] an aggressive but rare polyomavirus-induced skin cancer which also responded to immune checkpoint inhibition therapy.[257]

Ovarian Cancer

Both molecular and immunocytochemical assays have been used to detect CTCs in ovarian cancer. Molecular assays have been used for the detection and characterization of CTCs in ovarian cancer.[285,286] Aktas and colleagues investigated CTCs in the blood of 122 ovarian cancer patients at primary diagnosis and after platinum-based chemotherapy by using immunomagnetic enrichment and multiplex RT-PCR, and CTCs correlated with shorter OS before surgery and after chemotherapy.[287] When ovarian cancer is studied by the Cell-Search system, some studies show that elevated CTCs impart an unfavorable prognosis,[288] while others find no correlation.[289] Even if CTCs are associated with poor outcomes in ovarian cancer, clinical implementation will require uniform methodology and prospective validation.[290] By using a cell adhesion matrix for functional enrichment and identification, the presence of CTCs was correlated with shorter OS and PFS and had a better positive predictive value than CA-125.[291]

Platinum resistance constitutes one of the most recognized clinical challenges for ovarian cancer. Molecular CTC analysis in ovarian cancer correlates with platinum resistance. Although the immunohistochemistry of ERCC1 protein in primary tumors did not predict platinum resistance, ERCC1[(+)] CTCs did predict platinum resistance at primary diagnosis of ovarian cancer.[292] A meta-analysis of eight studies, including 1184 patients, showed that patients with ERCC1[(+)] CTCs had significantly shorter OS and DFS than patients with ERCC1[(−)] CTCs.[293]

Pancreatic Cancer

Pancreatic cancers frequently spread to the liver, lung, and skeletal system, suggesting that pancreatic tumor cells must be able to intravasate and travel through the circulation to distant organs. The presence of CTCs correlates with an unfavorable outcome in pancreatic cancer.[294,295] However, as stated by Gall and colleagues, CTCs are rare in pancreatic cancer, and it is unclear whether CTCs actually contribute toward tumor invasiveness and spread in such an aggressive cancer.[296] Nevertheless, a recent study shows that CTCs can be used for risk stratification.[178] Moreover, a meta-analysis including nine studies with a total of 623 pancreatic cancer patients showed that 268 CTC-positive patients had poorer PFS and OS compared to 355 CTC-negative patients.[297] Larger studies, as well as characterization of the CTC population, are required to achieve further insight into the clinical implications of CTC analysis in pancreatic cancer.

Head and Neck Cancer

Head and neck squamous cell carcinoma (HNSCC) is the sixth most common cancer and causes high morbidity due to the lack of early detection. A comprehensive review details studies over the past 5 years on the detection of CTCs in HNSCC.[298] When CTCs from locally advanced NHSCC are enriched by the CellSearch system, CTCs are detected in only a low fraction of cases.[299] Recently, the prognostic value of CTCs in advanced HNSCC was confirmed in the prospective CIRCUTEC study.[38] A meta-analysis of eight studies and 433 patients with HNSCC concluded that the presence of CTCs portends a poor prognosis compared to patients without CTCs.[299] In patients with HNSCC undergoing surgical intervention, patients with no detectable CTCs had a higher probability of longer DFS.[300,301] In both of these studies, CTCs were isolated only by negative enrichment that is not dependent on the expression of surface epithelial markers. Another prospective multicentric study evaluated the role of CTC detection in locally advanced head and neck cancer; a decrease in the CTC number or their absence throughout treatment was related to nonprogressive disease.[302] Current staging methods for squamous cell carcinomas of the oral cavity need to be improved to predict the risk to individual patients. This can be achieved by counting bone marrow

DTCs and peripheral blood CTCs that predict relapse with higher sensitivity than routine staging procedures.[303] The persistence of CTCs after upfront tumor surgery may be useful for the identification of patients who benefit from treatment intensification in locally advanced HNSCC.[304]

Hepatocellular Carcinoma

CTC analysis in hepatocellular carcinoma (HCC) is a rather under-investigated field.[305] A large variation of CTCs with epithelial, mesenchymal, liver-specific, and mixed characteristics, including different size ranges, is observed among patient groups and is associated with therapeutic outcome.[306] Frequent EpCAM[+] CTCs in intermediate or advanced HCC are seen,[307] and they predicted clinical outcome after curative liver resection.[307] In HCC patients undergoing curative resection, stem cell-like phenotypes have been observed in EpCAM[+] CTCs. Preoperative CTC numbers predicted tumor recurrence in HCC patients after surgery, especially in patient subgroups with α-fetoprotein concentrations of up to 400 ng/mL.[308]

Bladder Cancer

CTCs may be used as a noninvasive, real-time tool for the stratification of early-stage bladder cancer patients according to individual risk of progression.[309,310] The potential prognostic value of CTCs in patients with advanced nonmetastatic urothelial carcinoma of the bladder was shown in a recent clinical study, where CTC-positive patients had significantly higher risks of disease recurrence, as well as cancer-specific and overall mortality.[309] CellSearch was also used to detect and evaluate prospectively the biological significance of CTCs in patients with nonmetastatic, advanced bladder cancer. According to this study, the presence of CTCs may be predictive for early systemic disease because CTCs were detected in 30% of patients with nonmetastatic disease.[311] The prognosis of T1G3 bladder cancer is highly variable and unpredictable from clinical and pathologic prognostic factors. When survivin-expressing CTCs were evaluated in patients with T1G3 bladder tumors, the presence of CTCs was an independent prognostic factor for DFS.[312] Furthermore, assessment of the phenotype of CTCs with regard to immune checkpoint inhibitors such as PD-L1 used for therapy in bladder cancer is now possible[310] and might be used in future studies for patient stratification and monitoring.

POINTS TO REMEMBER

Circulating Tumor Cells

- CTC enumeration tests in metastatic breast, colorectal, and prostate cancer are cleared by the FDA.
- A plethora of analytical systems are available for CTC isolation, detection, and molecular characterization and are currently under analytical and clinical evaluation.
- CTC molecular characterization may be translated into individualized targeted treatments.
- Single-cell analysis of CTCs holds considerable promise for the identification of therapeutic targets and resistance mechanisms in CTCs, as well as for real-time monitoring of the efficacy of systemic therapies.
- Quality control and standardization of CTC isolation, detection, and molecular characterization are required for the incorporation of CTC analysis into routine clinical laboratory practice.

CIRCULATING TUMOR DNA

As mentioned above, cancers release several components within the circulation including cell-free nucleic acids (see Fig. 71.1) from which the DNA fraction (ctDNA) has attracted much interest. In addition to its non- or minimally invasive nature, analysis of ctDNA released by the patient′s cancer should give a view of both intra- and intertumor heterogeneity (especially compared to single biopsy analysis), and thus provide a pertinent tool to perform serial real-time monitoring of tumor progression and evolution in patients (see Figs. 71.2 and 71.3). Development of new technologies has been key to the progress we have recently seen in ctDNA clinical applications, including more efficient handling and detection that allows a greater understanding of its biology and its use as a potential cancer biomarker. A wide range of comprehensive reviews have been published (see references[3,4,313–316] for recent reviews). Technologies for the analysis of ctDNA have been reviewed in detail elsewhere.[3,313,317–319] Thus in this chapter we only briefly summarize the principles of some of the key technologies and their application in patients with cancer (Fig. 71.21).

ctDNA HISTORICAL BACKGROUND

The presence of cell-free circulating nucleic acids in human plasma was first described in 1948 by Mandel and Métais.[320] Increased levels of circulating cell-free DNA (ccfDNA) were subsequently described in several pathologies compared to healthy subjects.[321,322] Leon and colleagues made similar observations in 1977 in the serum of cancer patients.[323] A decade later, Stroun and colleagues described that some of this ccfDNA was of neoplastic origin.[324] In 1994, Sorenson showed the presence of mutated *KRAS* sequences in the plasma of patients with pancreatic adenocarcinoma presenting with the same mutation of the *KRAS* oncogene.[325] Recent developments in molecular assays such as MPS or ultrasensitive and digital PCR methods have initiated an enormous re-vitalization of the ccfDNA research field with the first applications entering clinical practice. These discoveries and chosen subsequent investigations are summarized in Fig. 71.22 (see references[326,327] for reviews).

Origin and Specific Features of ctDNA

Even if it is still a matter of debate (see Aucamp and colleagues[328] for an extensive review), the main sources of fragmented ccfDNA in healthy individuals, in the absence of inflammation or physical exercise, are apoptotic cells, perhaps predominantly apoptotic WBCs. Necrosis and active transport through the plasma membrane are the other main sources of ccfDNA.[328,329] As other components of cells, such as RNA, lipids, metabolites, and cytosolic and cell-surface proteins, DNA can be contained in EVs, including exosomes.[330]

Increased levels of ccfDNA have been associated with pregnancy, noncancer pathologic processes (including diabetes, autoimmune diseases, inflammation, and infection) and tissue damage (intensive exercise or soft-tissue injury), as well as cancers.[315,331,332] However, due to the non–cancer-specific nature of ccfDNA, most literature refers to analysis of the fraction that originates from the tumor. This analysis is generally performed by the specific detection of tumor-specific genetic or epigenetic alterations (see below).[333]

ctDNA arises from apoptosis or necrosis of primary and metastatic solid tumors and from degradation of CTCs. In addition, active release of ctDNA embodied in EVs such as exosomes has also been reported.[334,335] Increased secretion of exosomes, including genomic DNA containing ones, have been described in several cancer contexts.[334,335] ctDNA may also be derived from CTCs that are disrupted in the bloodstream but their quantitative contribution to total ctDNA is not clear and likely depends on the cancer stage and treatment.

Due to the different cell death mechanisms involved in the liberation of ccfDNA and ctDNA, many reports have described significant size distribution differences between ccfDNA and ctDNA (see below). Although contradictory results have been described concerning the size distribution of ccfDNA and ctDNA,[336,337] recent work tends to demonstrate a high fragmentation of ctDNA.[317] For example, Cristiano and colleagues analyzed the ccfDNA fragmentation patterns of healthy individuals and cancer patients and found that ccfDNA profiles of healthy individuals reflected nucleosomal patterns of WBCs, while patients with cancer had altered fragmentation profiles (see below).[338]

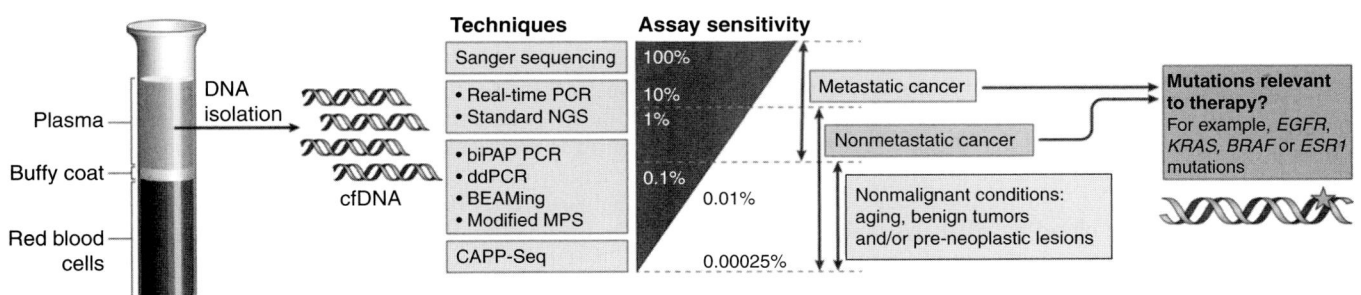

FIGURE 71.21 Methods for ctDNA detection. Tumor-specific genetic or epigenetic alterations can be detected in cfDNA extracted from body fluids including blood using an increasing number of technologies. The scheme summarizes the described sensitivities of several of the technologies that can be used to perform ctDNA detection. Moreover, it indicates the typical ranges of concentrations of tumor-associated mutations that have been reported for patients according to disease stage and healthy subjects. In the latter case, the presence of such mutations has been associated with benign or premalignant lesions or aging (i.e., associated with clonal hematopoiesis of indeterminate potential). *BEAMing,* Beads, emulsification, amplification, and magnetics; *CAPP-Seq,* cancer personalized profiling by deep sequencing; *ddPCR,* droplet-based digital PCR; *MPS,* massively parallel sequencing. (From Pantel K, Alix-Panabières C. Liquid biopsy and minimal residual disease – latest advances and implications for cure. *Nat Rev Clin Oncol* 2019;16:409–24.)

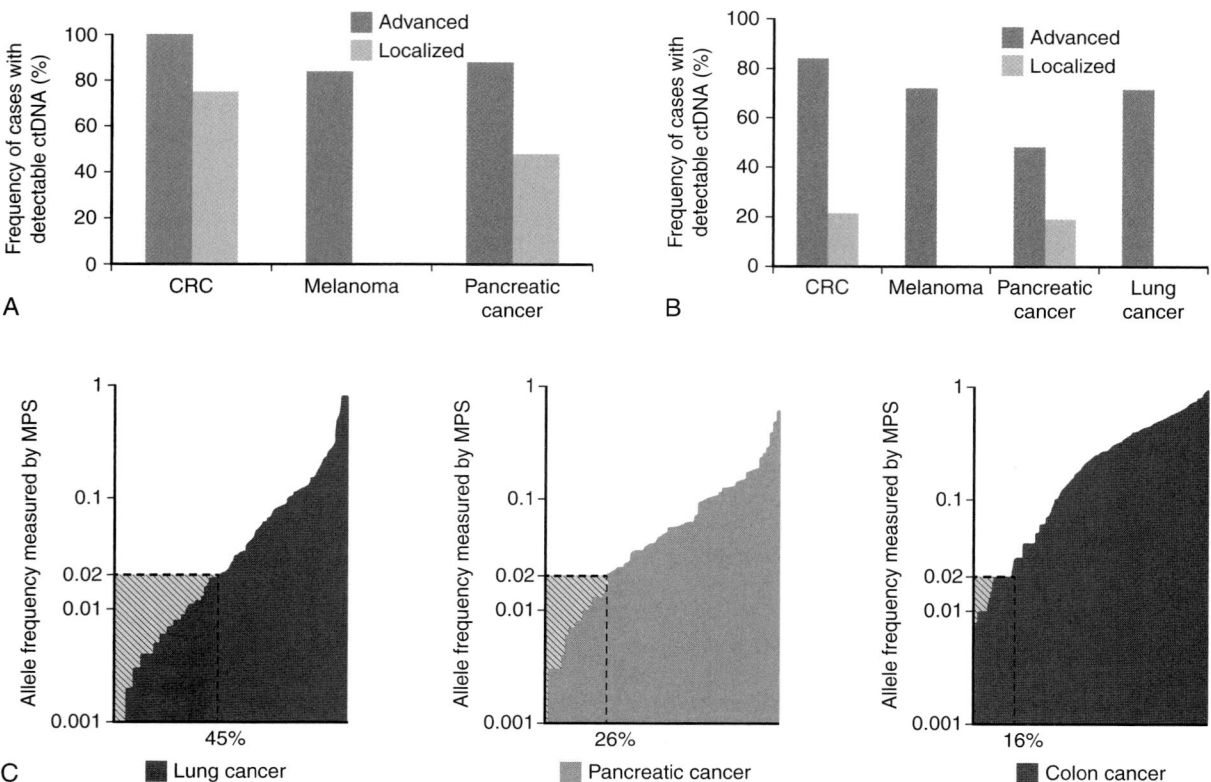

FIGURE 71.22 The percentage of detectable ctDNA and mutant allele frequencies in liquid biopsies of different cancers. (A) Percentage of patients with detectable ctDNA in localized and advanced cancers from one study.[354] CRC (*n* = 24), melanoma (*n* = 18), and pancreatic (*n* = 34) cancers are compared. (B) Similar data summarized from four additional studies.[363,437,503,504] CRC (*n*=50 advanced and *n* = 250 localized cancers), melanoma (*n* = 11 advanced cancers), pancreatic (*n* = 104 advanced and *n* = 31 localized cancers), and lung (*n* = 105 advanced cancer) cancers are shown. (C) Distribution of mutated allele frequencies found in colorectal (*n* = 293), lung (*n* = 273), and pancreatic (*n* = 100) cancers. (From Pécuchet N, Rozenholc Y, Zonta E, Pietrasz D, Didelot A, Combe P, et al. Analysis of baseposition error rate of next-generation sequencing to detect tumor mutations in circulating DNA. *Clin Chem* 2016;62:1492–503. From Postel M, Roosen A, Laurent-Puig P, Taly V, Wang-Renault SF. Droplet-based digital PCR and next generation sequencing for monitoring circulating tumor DNA: a cancer diagnostic perspective. *Expert Rev Mol Diagn* 2018;18:7–17.)

Presence of ctDNA in Body Effluents

CcfDNA can be detected in body effluents including blood, urine, cerebrospinal and pleural fluids, and even stool (see references[316,339,340] for reviews). Most literature, however, refers to ctDNA circulating in the blood stream and more particularly in plasma. We will here briefly review different sources of ctDNA and then focus on plasmatic ctDNA detection (Fig. 71.23).

For studies involving blood-based analysis, plasma is generally described as a more suitable source for ctDNA analysis with a lower background of ccfDNA coming from nontumor cells.[331] Indeed, compared with plasma, a larger proportion of "wild-type" DNA (i.e., not presenting tumor-specific mutations) is indeed generally observed in serum.[341–344] Presence of this DNA will further dilute ctDNA and thus potentially decrease reachable sensitivity. This nontumor DNA could be due to the clotting process of WBCs in the collection tube leading to their lysis.[342,345,346] In a prospective study studying ctDNA for metastatic CRC patient follow-up, Boeckx and colleagues performed a comparative analysis of ctDNA extracted from serum and plasma samples collected at baseline. They observed a significantly higher concentration of cfDNA in serum samples compared to plasma samples (*P* < .001) but the fraction of ctDNA was higher in the plasma samples (measured by detection of tumor-specific mutations and methylation markers, see below, *P* < .001).[347]

Urine is an attractive source of ctDNA since it is truly noninvasive, therefore sample collection is simple and allows for large volume collections. Both high- and low-molecular-weight DNAs (<100 base pairs) can be found in urine, probably originating from genomic DNA of the urinary tract and cfDNA, respectively.[348] Earlier studies have evaluated DNA originating from urinary cells (analyzed from urine sediment) as shown for invasive bladder cancer.[348] However, urine ccfDNA is also present in a nontumor context, originating from renal clearance of blood cfDNA.[316] For patients with urogenital cancers, detected ctDNA fragments might result from shedding of tumor cells or their breakdown products into the urinary tract.[316] Detection of ctDNA in urine is particularly attractive for cancers of the urogenital system,[316,340] but some studies have described its potential in other cancers including non–small cell cancers,[349] and HCC.[350] Degradation of DNA in urine and high fragmentation of urinary ctDNA, however, raises several technical

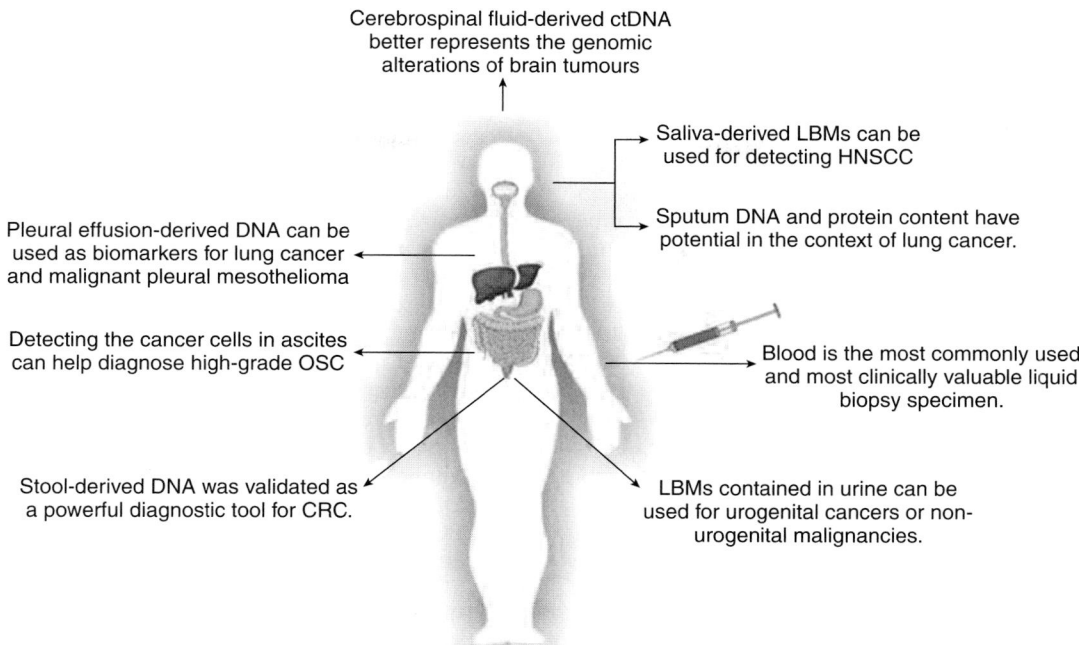

FIGURE 71.23 The body fluids suitable for liquid biopsies and their applications in tumor diagnosis and screening. *CRC,* colorectal cancer; *HNSCC,* head and neck squamous cell carcinoma; *LBMs,* liquid biopsy markers; *OSC,* ovarian serous carcinoma. (From Wu J, Hu S, Zhang L, et al. Tumor circulome in the liquid biopsies for cancer diagnosis and prognosis. *Theranostics* 2020;10:4544–56.)

concerns. Moreover, as for other bodily fluids, several clinical and biological factors are thought to influence the proportion of ctDNA that can be detected in urine and needs to be further evaluated before clinical implementation.[316,351]

CSF is an important source for detection of ctDNA in patients with primary brain tumors (e.g., gliomas) and central nervous system metastases.[316,352,353] Compared to other patients with advanced cancers, plasma ctDNA concentrations are rather low in patients with brain tumors (including high-grade gliomas and medulloblastomas), possibly due to the blood-brain barrier that can block the release of ctDNA into the blood circulation.[316,354] Although obtained through an invasive procedure, CSF is routinely collected in several brain pathologies and could thus represent a pertinent choice for ctDNA analysis of these patients. The CSF in general has less protein, lipids, and cells compared to blood, which allows for easier extraction of ctDNA. De Mattos-Arruda and colleagues showed that, for central nervous system cancers, ctDNA is more abundantly present in CSF than in plasma.[355] MPS applied to CSF here was more comprehensive than plasma, allowing for the identification of putative actionable somatic mutations. For gliomas in particular, detection of ctDNA in CSF is strongly correlated with the stage of disease and leptomeningeal metastasis.

Interest of other bodily effluents for ctDNA analysis have been evaluated in different cancers (see references[316,339] for reviews) including saliva for patients with oral cancers[356] and pleural effusion fluid or bronchial washing samples for patients with NSCLC.[357,358]

In order to achieve optimal sensitivity for ctDNA detection, the choice of pertinent biological fluid should be linked to tumor localization as highlighted by Siravegna and colleagues.[316] Moreover, several studies have described the influence of several biological and clinical factors on ctDNA

concentrations and dynamics. Finally, the biology of the ccfDNA release in healthy individuals is relatively poorly understood. There is thus a need for large and well-designed studies that could investigate the influence of these parameters on the performance of ctDNA analysis. The rest of this review will mainly focus on plasma ctDNA.

Half-Life of ctDNA

The half-life of ctDNA is important in the assessment of cancer patients. Understanding the rapid clearance and/or degradation from the circulation is needed to interpret patient results. The half-life of ctDNA in the bloodstream is estimated to be between 16 minutes and 2.5 hours.[359] For example, thanks to the serial analysis of plasma samples collected after complete tumor resection of a patient, Diehl and colleagues measured a half-life of ctDNA monitored by a specific tumor alteration of around 114 minutes.[360] Such rapid decay upon therapeutic interventions makes it an appealing tool for cancer evolution dynamic monitoring (real-time).

Important factors may include ctDNA degradation by enzymes in blood, binding to blood lipids/proteins, binding to nucleoprotein, uptake by leukocytes in blood and tissues, and clearance by normal physiologic mechanisms in the liver and kidney. Tumors located in highly vascular organs or with active angiogenesis will have higher access and release into the systemic circulation. In addition, ctDNA can be taken up by cells in the surrounding microenvironment, as well as be incorporated into vesicles of cancer cells and released as exosomes.[361,362] Finally, brain cancer patients, even in advanced stages, will present very low blood concentrations of ctDNA compared to other cancers, possibly due to the blood-brain barrier that can block release of ctDNA into peripheral blood (see above).[316,354]

The quantity of ctDNA is linked to the localization of the primary tumor and metastasis.[316] In advanced CRC, Bachet and colleagues showed that low or undetectable concentrations of ctDNA were observed more frequently in patients with primary tumor resection, metachronous metastases, and peritoneal carcinomatosis while the presence of liver metastases was associated with higher ctDNA concentrations.[363] Moreover, in this same study, the presence or absence of ctDNA was also associated with several biological factors such as leukocyte counts and concentrations of LDH, alkaline phosphatase, albumin, CA 19-9, and CEA. High ctDNA concentrations were also associated with the presence of liver metastases in advanced lung cancer.[361] A higher concentration of ctDNA is observed in advanced cancers compared with localized ones,[354,364] and was described as associated with higher tumor burden as evaluated by RECIST criteria.[360,365] In early cancers, the total amount of ctDNA might be less than 0.01% of the total ccfDNA as described in CRC by Diehl and colleagues.[343] These extremely low concentrations occur during the early stages of cancer in patients without overt metastases. Moreover, even in the case of advanced cancers, the proportion of patients with detectable amount of ctDNA can be low. For example, Laurent-Puig and colleagues described that, using BPER optimized MPS (i.e., allowing to reach <0.1% sensitivity), 45% of lung cancer patients, 26% of pancreas patients, and 16% of CRC patients, release less than 2% of the ctDNA.[331,366]

Preanalytical and Analytical Considerations for the Assessment of ctDNA

The ctDNA particularities mentioned above link the quality and reproducibility of results to both the preanalytical handling of samples and the accuracy and sensitivity of the technologies.[367–369] Generalizations on the use of ctDNA are therefore dependent on our ability to establish strong and detailed guidelines largely shared among the cancer community. This also includes, for example, the development of pertinent reference materials and standardized experimental protocols for ctDNA analysis.[370,371] Large consortia such as CANCER-ID (www.cancer-id.eu) or ELBS (www.elbs.eu) (see below) will be instrumental in developing, validating, and implementing standard operating procedures for the efficient analysis of ctDNA.[372]

Several factors can lead to variations in results that compromise ctDNA clinical validation. These factors include the choice of blood collection tubes, timing between sample collection and blood processing (partly resolved with the choice of appropriate tubes for blood collection), choice of DNA extraction methods, and sample storage.[373–379] This has been extensively reviewed elsewhere and will not be discussed in detail here.[3,380–382]

The importance of preanalytical standardization has been highlighted by several groups.[378,383,384] First, inappropriate sample storage conditions and delays in analysis may lead to nuclease cleavage of released DNA and unwanted lysis of nucleated blood cells leading to normal cell DNA release and thus even higher dilution of tumor DNA.[331] According to several reports, ethylenediaminetetraacetic acid (EDTA) collected blood should ideally be processed within 2 hours.[373–375] However, several new tubes have been recently developed, involving nucleated blood cell stabilization, including the Cell-Free DNA BCT blood collection tubes (Streck, La Vista, NE).[383] Such tubes permit better stabilization of ccfDNA (according to the manufacturer, up to 14 days between 6 and 37 °C) and prevent

ccfDNA degradation,[374] but also cost more than conventional EDTA tubes. However, they are especially important for centralized testing centers and large multi-centric clinical studies crucial for further ctDNA developments. In addition, ccfDNA extraction methods are also critical as they can cause analysis discrepancies.[369,379,385,386] CcfDNA isolation procedures not only determine the isolation efficiencies of ccfDNA but also the representation of smaller DNA fragments (potentially enriched in ctDNA),[387] further reinforcing the need to apply standardized preanalytical processes.[369,388]

After extraction, accurate quantification of ccfDNA is also important, especially for future clinical implementation. For example, accurate quantification ensures that input ccfDNA quantity is sufficient to achieve required sequencing depth[388] and thus increases the chance to reach the targeted sensitivity. Methods for ccfDNA quantification include ultraviolet (UV) spectrophotometry, electrophoresis, spectrofluorimetry using fluorogenic binding agents (such as PicoGreen),[389] quantitative PCR (qPCR), and digital PCR. UV spectrophotometry can assess extracted sample purity, but it is typically not sensitive enough for ccfDNA quantification. Moreover, strong correlations are generally observed between fluorogenic assays (e.g., Qubit 3.0 fluorimeter, Thermo Fisher Scientific) and both qPCR and droplet-based digital PCR (ddPCR), but to a lower extent with UV-spectrophotometry (e.g., Nanodrop 2000 spectrophotometer, Thermo Fisher Scientific).[390] Assays based on qPCR are often used for ccfDNA quantification[391] but have increased variability at low DNA quantity, which may lead to the introduction of imprecision and bias.[388] (ddPCR) allows for absolute quantification and does not require standard curves (as qPCR does).[388] Microfluidic electrophoresis platforms, such as the 4200 TapeStation instrument from Agilent, can perform size distribution and concentration measurements of ccfDNA.[392] Newly developed capillary electro-driven DNA concentration and separation systems or specifically designed ddPCR assays can allow for accurate determination of ccfDNA concentrations and size profiles.[393,394] Finally, several strategies have been designed that couple different methods for efficient ccfDNA quantification and/or sizing.[377]

The development and validation of pertinent reference materials can also increase interlaboratory reproducibility by identifying and correcting for preanalytical variables.[370,388] Indeed, the use of quality control assays, reference materials, and standards available from companies and academic initiatives should enable the development of robust and standardized workflows that facilitate the implementation of ctDNA analysis into clinical practice.[391]

Hypothesis on the Potential Function of ctDNA

ctDNA may have physiologic functions that influence normal cells, particularly those adjacent to the tumor. Single- and double-stranded DNA bind to toll-like receptors (TLRs) expressed on the surface of tumor cells and tumor-infiltrating cells.[395] ctDNA can bind to TLRs on leukocytes and activate various specific signal transduction pathways that may alter host-immune responses to tumor cells in the tumor microenvironment. Activation of TLRs can initiate signal transduction pathways that result in cytokine release and other functional changes in the targeted binding cells. The release of ctDNA may have direct effects on tumor microenvironment immune cells, as well as distant organ sites. Experimental studies have indicated that ctDNA may also act through horizontal gene transfection into normal cells in the tumor microenvironment,[396] and cellular transformation and tumorigenesis have been implicated with oncogene-containing DNA transfected in vivo.[396–398] The possibility that metastases might develop after transfection of susceptible cells in distant organs by circulated oncogenes derived from the primary tumor is central to the hypothesis of "genometastasis" proposed by García-Olmo and colleagues.[399–401] At present, it is, however, unclear to what extent these ctDNA-mediated effects may actually influence the pathophysiology of cancer patients.

Detection of ctDNA

Markers for ctDNA Detection

A wide range of genetic and epigenetic alterations has been described and validated for ctDNA detection (Fig. 71.24). On one hand, ctDNA can be used to highlight mutation(s) that predict responses to US Food and Drug Administration

(FDA) – approved targeted therapies. On the other hand, follow-up of single tumor-specific alteration(s) previously highlighted in the primary tumor is commonly performed.[402] Even if most studies use cancer specific mutations (i.e., single-nucleotide variants [SNVs], small insertions or small deletions) for ctDNA detection, several other types of alterations have been described for ctDNA including tumor-agnostic ones. These potential markers includes dysregulation of gene methylation, microsatellite loss of heterozygosity, DNA integrity, gene fusion, copy number variation (CNV), and cancer viral DNA.[402] The first two ctDNA blood-based assays approved by FDA in 2016 were for the detection of EGFR mutations in NSCLC patients (cobas EGFR Mutation Test v2, Roche Molecular Systems) and methylation of the SEPTIN9 gene in colon cancer (Epi proColon, Epigenomics).[370,403] Moreover, the European Medicine Agency (EMA) authorized the use of ctDNA obtained from blood when tumor tissue was not available in patients with locally advanced or metastatic NSCLC

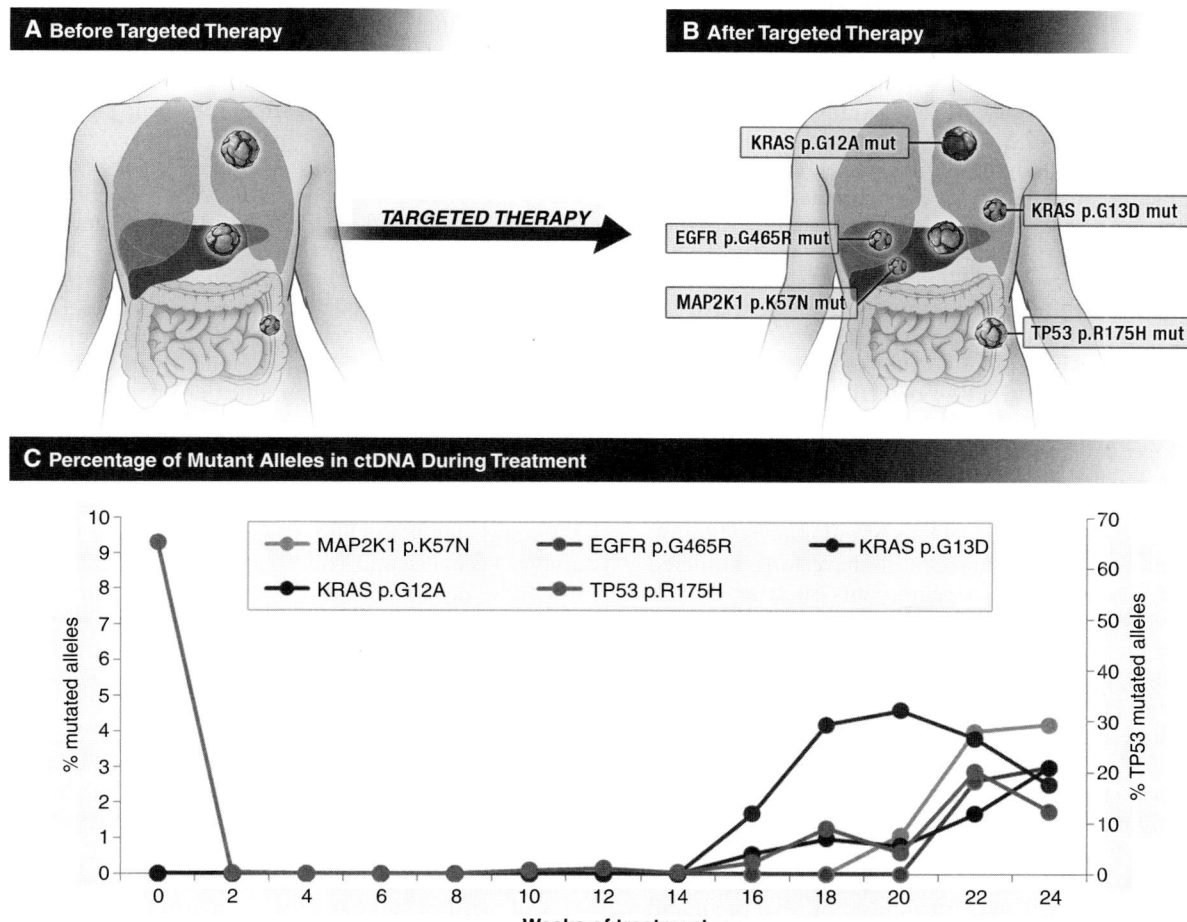

FIGURE 71.24 Liquid biopsies to monitor cancer evolution during targeted therapy. Due to the intrinsic heterogeneity of human tumors, distinct drug resistance mechanisms can evolve within a single patient and even within individual metastatic lesions. Tissue biopsies are inherently unable to capture this heterogeneity while liquid biopsies can profile more comprehensively clonal evolution in space and time. As an example, we describe a patient with metastatic colorectal cancer: upon treatment with anti- epidermal growth factor receptor (EGFR) antibodies, resistant clones progressively emerge carrying resistance mutations. Circulating free DNA allows identification, tracking, and quantification of clones bearing distinct alleles. Monitoring of a stem (truncal) mutation in the TP53 gene tracks tumor burden, while lesion-specific mutations (KRAS, MAPK) provide a measure of clonal evolution during therapy. (From Bardelli A, Pantel K. Liquid biopsies, what we do not know (yet). *Cancer Cell* 2017;31:172–9.)

when considering the use of tyrosine kinase inhibitors (IRESSA). Furthermore, they recommended that EGFR mutation status of ctDNA should be performed using "robust, reliable and sensitive test(s) with demonstrated utility for the determination of EGFR mutations... to avoid false negative or false positive results."[404] Similarly, the NCCN guidelines recommend the use of plasma for detection of variants in ctDNA when it is not feasible to obtain tissue for testing.

The development of universal markers of ctDNA based on methylation dysregulation of specific gene promoter regions or DNA integrity are promising approaches, notably in cancers with multiple molecular alterations of low incidence requiring large molecular screening.[364,405,406] In the blood of cancer patients, dysregulations of CpG methylation can be detected and can be used for early cancer detection, prognosis, and treatment monitoring (see references[316,405,407–411] for reviews). Moreover, analysis of methylation patterns can also determine the tissue of origin of circulating DNA[412] including its tumor fraction when present.[413,414] As mentioned above, ctDNA can also be differentiated from non–cancer-related ccfDNA by its size.[329,415,416] Several methods have been described for DNA integrity determination (see Zonta and colleagues[329] for a review). DNA integrity analysis is a ctDNA biomarker with applications in many cancers,[338,415] although the specific calculations and cutoffs may vary between cancer types. Moreover, as mentioned above, preanalytical sample handling, including collection tubes and ccfDNA extraction procedures, can strongly bias DNA integrity measurements and should thus be carefully standardized to allow for interlaboratory comparison.

Several cancers have an etiology strongly linked to viral DNA integration. In these cancers, ctDNA can be tested for specific cell-free viral DNA. The advantage of assessing viral ctDNA is high specificity and detection sensitivity. Examples include Epstein Barr virus (EBV) detection in nasopharyngeal cancer[417] and human papilloma virus (HPV) for head and neck cancer, anal, and cervical cancer.[418–422]

Technologies for ctDNA Detection

The low concentrations of ctDNA in blood and its dilution by DNA coming from noncancer cells have long hindered its detection. Technological developments such as ddPCR and optimized MPS now provide unprecedented sensitivity and accuracy for the detection of cancer-specific genetic and epigenetic alterations within biological samples including body-effluents. The high sensitivity, specificity, and accuracy offered by these technologies have been key to the massive developments observed recently in the use of ctDNA in cancer patient management (see Fig. 71.21).

The principles of digital PCR have been described elsewhere.[331,423,424] Briefly, limiting dilution, PCR amplification and Poisson statistics are used to accurately quantify a given molecule.[425] The term "dPCR" was introduced by Vogelstein and collaborators in 1999.[426] In 2003, the same team described a new version of the technology, "BEAMing" (*beads, emulsion, amplification and magnetics*), that used aqueous microdroplets and beads for the detection and enumeration of genetic variants.[427] BEAMing has been successfully used in the context of liquid biopsy,[343,428–431] but requires a complex experimental procedure that has limited its broad use in clinics. The coupling of emulsion PCR and microfluidics has improved robustness and facilitated experimental procedures leading to several commercial platforms and its broad adoption.[315,424]

Compared to those that are MPS-based, experiments using dPCR are more sensitive, easier to set-up, faster, and do not require complex informatics support for development and analysis. However, dPCR requires previous knowledge of genetic or epigenetic changes. Single tumor-specific mutations or a limited panel of mutations previously known from prior genomic analysis of resection or biopsy specimens are generally used to detect ctDNA (usually as a measure of MRD). However, multiplexing is often limited[315,331] to 3-4-plexes for precise identification of each single tested sequence when using nanoliter-sized compartments. Other multiplexing strategies have been described that allow screening of a pool of alterations including *RAS/RAF* mutations[432] or EGFR exon 19 deletions.[433]

In contrast, MPS has massive multiplexing capabilities and could thus in theory, identify novel genetic or epigenetic modifications. However, MPS is time consuming and requires powerful informatic support. Strategies based on whole-genome sequencing (WGS) or whole-exome sequencing (WES) can be used for copy-number aberrations, point mutations, and/or other genetic aberrations. However, they usually generate low sequencing coverage leading to low sensitivity for ctDNA analysis.

Targeted MPS-based cancer-specific gene panels are largely used for screening of tumor biopsies. However, analytical sensitivity was initially limited to around 2% (as reported for the use of Ion Torrent AmpliSeq Panels).[366] Low depth of sequencing, high background error noise, and methodological pipelines used for data analysis contribute to relatively low performance.[366] Highly sensitive targeted and optimized MPS procedures have recently been developed to overcome such issues. For example, molecular identifiers such as the Safe-sequencing system (Safe-SeqS),[434] tagged-amplicon deep sequencing (TAm-Seq),[435] and strategies that remove background error noise such as Base-Position Error Rate (BPER) Analysis[366] and cancer personalized profiling by deep sequencing (CAPP-Seq)[436] can reduce detection limits to below 0.01%.[57]

Interestingly, several studies have combined the use of MPS and dPCR for liquid biopsy analysis.[354,437–439] For example, Pécuchet and colleagues combined BPER MPS and dPCR to detect ctDNA from lung and pancreatic cancer patients. They observed high detection sensitivity and specificity for both methods. Moreover, significant consistency between these two methods for *EGFR* and *KRAS* mutations detection was observed (κ 0.90 [0.73 ± 1.06]).[366]

As mentioned above, both targeted MPS and dPCR require detailed prior information on the mutational spectrum of the tumor in the individual patient. The ability to detect subclonal mutations that are under-represented in the primary lesion but are selected during adjuvant therapy or during the natural postoperative course of the disease is a potential advantage of sensitive nontargeted approaches. Recently, Mouliere and colleagues presented a new approach to enrich shorter ccfDNA fragments (90 to 150 bp), which considerably increased assay sensitivity. Selecting fragments between 90 and 150 bp improved detection of tumor DNA, with more than a twofold median enrichment in greater than 95% of cases, and more than fourfold enrichment in greater than 10% of cases.[440] Using low-pass WGS (0.4×) of size-selected ccfDNA identified clinically actionable mutations and copy number alterations that were otherwise not detected. Identification of advanced cancers was improved by predictive models integrating fragment length and copy number analysis of ccfDNA, with AUC greater than 0.99 compared to AUC less than 0.80 without fragmentation features. Increased identification of ccfDNA from patients with glioma, renal, and pancreatic cancer was achieved with area under the curve (AUC) greater than 0.91, compared to AUC less than 0.5 without fragmentation features. Fragment size analysis and selective sequencing of specific fragment sizes can boost ctDNA detection and can complement or provide an alternative to deeper sequencing of cell-free DNA.

CtDNA detection can be also improved by MPS when hundreds to thousands of mutations are identified by tumor genotyping. Recently, Wan and colleagues[441] combined patient-specific mutation lists with both custom error-suppression methods and signal enrichment based on biological features of ctDNA. In this framework, the sensitivity can be estimated independently for each sample based on the number of informative reads, which is the product of the number of mutations analyzed and the average depth of unique sequencing reads. Applying their INVAR approach to deep sequencing data generated by custom hybrid-capture panels showed that when ~10^6 informative reads were obtained, INVAR allowed detection of tumor-derived DNA fractions to parts per million (ppm). The authors further demonstrated that INVAR can be generalized and allows improved detection of ctDNA from whole-exome and low-depth WGS data.

Efficient patient follow-up requires a large panel of sequences since gene mutations and hotspot codons vary widely among cancer patients, thus strongly complicating the detection procedure. "Universal" ctDNA markers such as methylation or DNA integrity can be used.[329,331,364,406] For example, analysis of two methylation markers can successfully screen most, if not all, CRC patients.[364] This can clearly decrease the number of tests required, simplify the detection procedure, and allow the monitoring of tumor DNA dynamics without the need of developing individualized assays for each cancer patient. Furthermore, the combined analysis of different markers such as ctDNA mutations and methylation biomarkers might allow breakthroughs in early-stage cancer diagnosis. Cristiano and colleagues[338] developed the DELFI approach (DNA evaluation of fragments for early interception) to evaluate ccfDNA fragmentation patterns across the genome and applied it to 236 patients with breast, colorectal, lung, ovarian, pancreatic, gastric, or bile duct cancer and 245 healthy individuals. In addition to highlighting interesting features of ccfDNA, the authors demonstrated sensitivities of detection ranging from 57 to greater than 99% among the seven cancer types at 98% specificity, with an overall AUC of 0.94. Combined with mutation analyses, the authors detected 91% of patients with a specificity of 98% and highlighted the possibility of identifying the source of ctDNA. Similarly, Shen and colleagues demonstrated the ability to detect large-scale DNA methylation changes in ccfDNA for the detection and classification of AML, pancreatic, colorectal, breast, lung, bladder, and renal cancers.[442] Targeted methylation analysis of ccfDNA was used to detect and localize multiple cancer types (50 in total) across all stages by the Circulating Cell-free Genome Atlas (CCGA) consortium.[443] In short, for stage I to III cancers when considering a predefined set of 12 cancer types accounting for around 63% of US cancer deaths annually (anus, bladder, colon/rectum, esophagus, head and neck, liver/bile-duct, lung, lymphoma, ovary, pancreas, plasma cell

neoplasm, stomach), a sensitivity of 67.3% (CI: 60.7 to 73.3%) was achieved with 43.9% (CI: 39.4 to 48.5%) across all cancer types. Tissue of origin localization was predicted in 96% of apparent cancer samples and appeared accurate in 93% of samples. Performance, especially for early cancer stages, would probably be further enhanced by combining different markers.

ctDNA Analysis in Clinical Oncology

Evaluation of the potential impact of ctDNA for cancer patient management has been central to a wide range of studies that highlight the pertinence of ctDNA for diagnosis, prognosis, follow-up, and treatment management (see Fig. 71.22). Moreover, the development of highly sensitive and quantitative analysis of ccfDNA allows fine-tuned monitoring of ctDNA levels[444] paving the way for the detection of early cancer recurrence, the tracking of resistant subclones, and the early and cost-effective evaluation of treatment efficacy (see Figs. 71.19 and 71.20). It is now well accepted that the quantity of ctDNA is related to tumor burden[316,354,445] and strong correlations between mutations detected in plasma and in the tumor tissues and/or in metastasis have been reported, leading to strong implications for precision medicine. Variations in the amount of ctDNA correlate better with treatment response than conventionally used serum markers[365,438,439] or conventional imaging.[446,447] Moreover, blood ctDNA analysis allows shorter median turn-around time of testing compared to conventional tissue-based procedures.[448,363] Serial analysis of ctDNA permits the monitoring of clonal evolution during treatment,[316,449] early detection of known treatment resistance mutations,[446] and identifies new resistance mechanisms via sequencing analysis.[450,451]

In the following sections, we provide an overview of key reports that have described the correlation of ctDNA with clinical outcomes in patients with advanced and early-stage cancers, including those with breast, prostate, colorectal, and lung cancer. These tumor types have divergent molecular characteristics, yet all frequently result in MRD after standard curative-intent treatment. Early detection of cancer has been reviewed elsewhere and will not be presented here.[314,331,415,452]

Breast Cancer

The activation of the PI3K signaling pathway by mutations in *PIK3CA* can result in resistance to HER2-targeted therapies in patients with breast cancer.[453] CTC analysis has revealed the presence of *PIK3CA* mutations in 7 (15.9%) of 44 patients with MBC;[454] those with HER2$^+$ CTCs had received anti-HER2 therapy with the tyrosine-kinase inhibitor lapatinib. Striking levels of intrapatient heterogeneity in *PIK3CA* mutational status have also been revealed by the analysis of single CTCs.[200,455–457] *PIK3CA* mutations were also enriched in ctDNA from patients with MBC who developed resistance to endocrine therapy.[458] Moreover, in an analysis of serial plasma samples from patients with advanced-stage breast cancer involved in the phase III PALOMA-3 trial, O'Leary and colleagues[459] found that the relative change in *PIK3CA*-mutant ctDNA after 15 days of treatment with the CDK4/6 inhibitor palbociclib plus fulvestrant was strongly predictive of PFS (change above the median value: HR = 3.94, 95% CI 1.61 to 9.64; log-rank P = .0013). Thus *PIK3CA* mutations might occur in micrometastases and postsurgical MRD surveillance for such mutations in ccfDNA or CTCs could potentially guide future therapeutic strategies to block metastatic relapse. Recently the FDA approved the use of a companion diagnostic test for the detection of PIK3CA mutations in tissue and/or liquid biopsy (ctDNA) from patients with Hormone Receptor-positive, HER2-negative advanced MBC (https://www.fda.gov/news-events/press-announcements/fda-approves-first-pi3k-inhibitor-breast-cancer). If the liquid biopsy is negative, a tumor biopsy should be tested.

Mutations in *ESR1* which encodes the ER, occur in ~20% of patients with ER⁺ MBC who develop resistance to hormone therapy;[460,461,462] these mutations confer resistance to several endocrine agents through constitutive activation of the ER. The findings of a MPS-based study in five patients with MBC suggested that ctDNA profiles reflect the heterogeneous mutational spectrum of multiple individual CTCs.[462] *ESR1* mutations can readily be identified in the ctDNA of patients with MBC who are developing resistance to endocrine therapy,[458,463,464] and in some patients these mutations were not detected through sequencing of tumor DNA from a single metastatic lesion.[464] In another analysis of plasma ctDNA from patients involved in the PALOMA-3 study (*n* = 195), O'Leary and colleagues[465] showed that clonal evolution frequently occurs during treatment, reflecting substantial sub-clonal complexity in breast cancer that has progressed after prior endocrine therapy; new driver mutations emerged in *PIK3CA* and *ESR1* (in particular, *ESR1* Y537S) after treatment with either palbociclib plus fulvestrant or placebo plus fulvestrant.

Initial insights into the utility of ctDNA measurements in monitoring for MRD in patients with high-risk early-stage breast cancer were provided by Garcia-Murillas and colleagues in 2015.[466] In this study, personalized dPCR assays were used to probe ccfDNA samples from 55 patients for the presence of somatic mutations known to be present in their primary tumors. Single or serial blood samples were obtained at different postsurgical time points (all patients had also received neoadjuvant chemotherapy) and the detection of ctDNA was correlated with an increased risk of metastatic relapse.[466] Interestingly, the detection of ctDNA preceded the clinical diagnosis of disease relapse by a median of 7.9 months. In another pilot study, Chen and colleagues[467] used the Oncomine Research Panel consisting of 134 cancer-related genes to assess the suitability of ctDNA as a biomarker of MRD. Among 38 patients who had residual TNBC after neoadjuvant chemotherapy, 33 had at least one mutation identified in their primary tumor, only 4 of whom had mutations detected in ccfDNA samples obtained during adjuvant therapy (a total of three *TP53* mutations, one *AKT1* mutation, and one *CDKN2A* mutation).[467] Nevertheless, the four patients with detectable ctDNA had disease relapse within 9 months,[467] although this cohort is obviously too small to draw firm conclusions.

Serial monitoring of ctDNA in a retrospective pilot study by Olsson and colleagues[468] involved 20 patients with nonmetastatic breast cancer. Low-coverage WGS was used to screen primary tumors for patient-specific chromosomal rearrangements and, subsequently, droplet digital PCR (ddPCR) with rearrangement-specific primers was performed to quantify ctDNA levels in plasma samples. Follow-up analyses revealed that postsurgical ctDNA monitoring enabled accurate discrimination between patients with and those without eventual distant recurrence (sensitivity 93%, specificity 100%).[468] The average lead time between ctDNA detection and the clinical diagnosis of metastatic relapse was 11 months (range 0 to 37 months).[468]

ctDNA was not detected in patients who remained disease-free after surgery; however, this patient subset was very small (*n* = 6) and larger cohorts need to be analyzed.[468]

Another study of 46 patients with nonmetastatic TNBC was conducted by Riva and colleagues[469] with the aim of investigating whether ctDNA detection can monitor the tumor response to neoadjuvant chemotherapy. Serial blood samples were analyzed for ctDNA harboring patient-specific *TP53* mutations using customized ddPCR assays. CtDNA was detected at baseline in 27 (75%) of 36 evaluable patients, with ctDNA levels decreasing during therapy in almost all of these patients.[469] Of potential prognostic relevance, ctDNA detection after one cycle of neoadjuvant chemotherapy was correlated with shorter DFS and OS.[469]

Recently, Garcia-Murillas and colleagues[470] assessed 101 patients with early-stage breast cancer irrespective of hormone receptor and HER2 status who were receiving neoadjuvant chemotherapy followed by surgery or surgery before adjuvant chemotherapy. Detection of ctDNA during follow-up was associated with relapse (HR 25.2; 95% CI, 6.7 to 95.6; *P* < .001) in breast cancer patients. Detection of ctDNA at diagnosis, before any treatment, was also associated with relapse-free survival (HR 5.8; 95% CI, 1.2 to 27.1; *P* = .01). ctDNA detection had a median lead time of 10.7 months (95% CI, 8.1 to 19.1 months) compared with clinical relapse and was associated with relapse in all breast cancer subtypes. Distant extracranial metastatic relapse was detected by ctDNA in 22 of 23 patients (96%). Brain-only metastasis was less commonly detected by ctDNA (one of six patients [17%]), suggesting relapse sites less readily detectable by ctDNA analysis.[470]

Prostate Cancer

Mutations in the androgen receptor gene (*AR*) have been detected in CTCs of patients with CRPC.[471] Many of the mutations were also detected in tumor specimens and were associated with resistance to androgen-deprivation therapy.[471] Similar information can be obtained from the profiling of ctDNA from patients with prostate cancer.[472] Potential implications of these findings for MRD assessment relate to the assumption that these mutations already occur before overt metastases signals castration resistance; therefore their detection might enable earlier intervention to delay or prevent the occurrence of metastasis.

Mayrhofer and colleagues used a combination of targeted and low-pass WGS to perform ccfDNA and matched WBC germline DNA analysis in 364 blood samples from 217 metastatic prostate cancer patients.[473] Detection of ctDNA was successful in 85.9% of the baselines samples, correlated with therapy, and was mirrored by CTC enumeration of synchronous blood samples. Continuous evolution of AR variants was observed during the course of the disease. Interestingly, the authors analyzed not only frequent genetic alterations (for example in DNA repair deficiency genes), but also the microsatellite instability phenotype and biallelic inactivation (by sequencing of nonrepetitive intronic and exonic regions of PTEN, RB1, and TP53). Moreover, concomitant analysis of WBC germline DNA identified patients with false-positive variants (14.6% of patients) due to clonal hematopoiesis. Adalsteinsson and colleagues also applied WGS to ctDNA analysis of advanced prostate cancers.[474]

By studying WES and whole-genome bisulfite sequencing of ccfDNA and matched metastatic tumor biopsies from patients with metastatic prostate adenocarcinoma and castration-resistant neuroendocrine prostate cancer (CRPC-NE), Beltran and colleagues identified genetic and epigenetic features specific to ctDNA of CRPC-NE. In particular, a combined set of genomic (TP53, RB1, CYLD, AR) and epigenomic (hypo- and hypermethylation of 20 differential sites) alterations identified patients with CRPC-NE.[475]

Colorectal Cancer

The effectiveness of anti-EGFR antibody therapy in patients with CRC is negatively affected by mutations in *KRAS*, which encodes a key GTPase that orchestrates signaling downstream of EGFR. An in-depth analysis of individual CTCs from patients with CRC demonstrated the striking levels of intrapatient and interpatient heterogeneity in *KRAS* status.[234,236] A comparative analysis of CTCs from patients with localized primary tumors and those with metastatic disease also revealed mutations in genes with a known driver role in CRC development and progression (such as *APC*, *KRAS*, or *PIK3CA*).[98] Remarkably, CDK8 was amplified in some CTCs, thus pointing to targeting of CDK8 with CDK inhibitors as a potential new therapeutic strategy for some patients with CRC.[22] The presence of these mutations in both primary tumors and metastases indicates that these mutations might be relevant to the development of metastatic disease and could, therefore be applicable to strategies for therapeutic targeting of MRD.

The analysis of ctDNA has also contributed to a better understanding of tumor evolution and response to therapy in patients with CRC. The level of concordance between the mutational status of *KRAS* in tumor tissue and ctDNA is high,[316,354] but ctDNA sometimes harbors KRAS mutations that are not detected in primary tumor specimens.[98] Technical issues notwithstanding, these mutations might reflect minor, overlooked subclones present in the primary tumor or in occult micrometastases. Sequential ctDNA analysis during EGFR inhibition reveals that *KRAS* and *NRAS* mutations can rapidly emerge as a result of the selective pressure exerted by targeted therapy.[476] Interestingly, it has been proposed that the emergent population of *KRAS*-mutant subclones declines upon withdrawal of anti-EGFR therapy,[476] suggesting guided "cyclical therapy" characterized by sequential withdrawal and reintroduction of EGFR inhibitors on the basis of genetic data from ctDNA analyses. However, the clearance of RAS mutations in patients treated by chemotherapy for a RAS mutated mCRC is a rare event and should be investigated using appropriate tools to avoid erroneous interpretation. In particular, Moati and colleagues[476a] demonstrated that monitoring tumor mutations in plasma samples only makes sense in combination with strict control of the presence of ctDNA. In this study, presence of ctDNA was assessed by the use of CRC-specific methylation markers (WIF1 and NPY promoters) and/or mutations in cancer-specific genes using highly sensitive optimized targeted MPS (BPER method). The therapeutic impacts of RAS clearance need to be further explored.[402]

In a study involving 44 patients with CRC,[477] patient-specific somatic mutations were detected through genomic analysis of primary tumor samples, thus enabling the development of personalized ctDNA assays. Using these assays, ctDNA was detected in 11 (73.3%) of 15 patients at or before the time of clinical or radiologic recurrence of CRC.[477] Furthermore, the molecular analyses also assisted in distinguishing recurrent CRC from a second primary cancer.[477]

In a prospective study enrolling 88 metastatic CRC patients treated with first- (82.9%) or second- (17.1%) line chemotherapy, Garlan and colleagues[439] demonstrated the importance of early changes in ctDNA concentration as a marker of therapeutic efficacy. In this work, ctDNA was assessed in plasma collected before the first (C_0), second (C_1), and/or third (C_2) chemotherapy cycle, using ddPCR assays targeting either gene mutations (*KRAS, BRAF, TP53*) or hypermethylation (*WIF1, NPY*). In this work, patients with a high (>10 ng/mL) versus low (≤0.1 ng/mL) ctDNA concentration at inclusion had a shorter OS (6.8 versus 33.4 months: adjusted HR = 5.64; CI$_{95\%}$[2.5 to 12.6], $P <$ .0001). Moreover, by monitoring the ctDNA concentration at inclusion and before the second or third chemotherapy cycle, patients could be clearly classified in "good ctDNA responders" ($n = 58$) and "bad ctDNA responders" ($n = 15$). Patients from the first group had both a better objective response rate ($P < .001$) and a longer median progression-free survival (8.5 versus 2.4 months: HR=0.19, CI$_{95\%}$[0.09 to 0.40], $P < .0001$) and OS (27.1 versus 11.2 months: HR=0.25, CI$_{95\%}$[0.11 to 0.57], $P < .001$).[47]

The analysis of ctDNA in nonmetastatic colon cancer may be of great help for the physician to identify higher-risk patients. In one study involving 96 newly diagnosed stage III colon cancer patients, Tie and colleagues[478] investigated ctDNA detection after surgery as a promising prognostic marker. The ctDNA was assessed using personalized assays based on previous analysis of patients' individual tumors using MPS of 15 genes commonly mutated in CRC. ctDNA was detected after surgery in 20 of 96 (21%) postsurgical samples and was associated with a shorter recurrence-free interval (RFI; HR 3.8; 95% CI, 2.4 to 21.0; $P < .001$). CtDNA status was independently associated with RFI after adjusting for known clinicopathologic risk factors (HR 7.5; 95% CI, 3.5 to 16.1; $P < .001$). CtDNA was detected in 15 of 88 available post-chemotherapy samples (17%). The estimated 3-year RFI was 30% for these patients versus 77% for the patients with ctDNA not detected (HR 6.8; 95% CI, 11.0 to 157.0; $P < .001$). Such data suggests that the analysis of ctDNA after completion of adjuvant chemotherapy may identify patients that remains at high risk of recurrence.[478]

The same group previously demonstrated similar results on the prognostic impact of postsurgical detection of ctDNA for stage II colon cancer patients. In a prospective analysis of 1046 plasma samples from 230 patients with stage II colon cancer using MPS-based assays,[479] ctDNA was detected after surgery in 14 (7.9%) of 178 patients who received no adjuvant chemotherapy. After a median follow-up of 27 months, the recurrence rate was higher in the ctDNA-positive patients than in the ctDNA-negative patients (78.7 versus 9.8%; HR 18.0, 95% CI, 7.9 to 40.0; $P < .001$).[479] ctDNA detection after completion of adjuvant chemotherapy was also associated with shorter RFS (HR 11.0, 95% CI, 1.8 to 68; $P = .001$). Taken together, these results indicate that postoperative ctDNA detection provides evidence of MRD that is relevant to the clinical outcomes of patients with colon cancer.

A proof of principle study by Schøler and colleagues[480] in 45 patients with CRC also suggests that postoperative ctDNA detection provides evidence of MRD that is linked to an increased risk of relapse. In this study,[480] MPS was again used to identify somatic mutations, which were subsequently used as markers to detect ctDNA and thereby quantify MRD during a 3-year follow-up period. Sequential analyses of blood samples from 27 patients revealed the presence of ctDNA postoperatively in all relapsing patients ($n = 14$), with an average lead time of 9.4 months compared with CT-based detection of CRC recurrence; no patient without disease relapse had detectable ctDNA. Among 21 patients with localized disease, 6 (28.6%) had detectable ctDNA within 3 months after surgery and this finding was strongly correlated with the riskof relapse (HR 37.7, 95% CI, 4.2 to 335.5; $P < .001$). The same group recently[481] performed a multicenter cohort study involving 829 plasma samples, from 125 stage I–III patients collected before surgery, after surgery (day 30), and every 3 months for up to 3 years. Using ultra-deep personalized multiplex MPS, the authors demonstrated strong associations between ctDNA detection and risks of relapse before surgery, after surgery, and also shortly after adjuvant chemotherapy. This work shows that analysis of serial ctDNA detects disease recurrence up to 16.5 months before conventional radiologic examination (mean: 8.7 months; range: 0.8 to 16.5 months). Moreover, actionable mutations were identified in 81.8% of the ctDNA-positive relapse samples.

Taieb and colleagues recently showed that ctDNA was highly predictive of recurrence in stage III patients coming from a large phase III prospective trial. They also observed that 3 months of adjuvant FOLFOX seemed insufficient in ctDNA+ patients compared to 6 months treatment, further suggesting that ctDNA could be a highly pertinent tool to guide therapeutic strategy in the adjuvant setting.[482] The same group is now involved in an ongoing trial, CIRCULATE-PRODIGE 70 (national phase III trial, NCT 2019-000935-15, conducted in more than 100 centers in France), aiming to evaluate the efficacy of risk stratification in stage II patients based on postoperative ctDNA detection and the efficacy of adjuvant therapy in patients with ctDNA.[483]

Lung Cancer

Non–small cell lung cancer. Mutations in *EGFR* have been the prime candidates for ctDNA liquid biopsies because these mutations determine the effectiveness of EGFR-targeted therapies in patients with NSCLC. For example, sensitivity to the EGFR tyrosine kinase inhibitors erlotinib and gefitinib is dependent on the presence of activating aberrations, such as the $EGFR^{L858R}$ mutation or exon 19 deletions, whereas the $EGFR^{T790M}$ mutation is associated with resistance to these agents. Assessment of EGFR mutational status in ccfDNA from patients with NSCLC has high specificity but limited sensitivity (that is, the mutation detected in the tumor specimen is not always detectable in ccfDNA samples from the same patient).[88–90] For example, the Cobas EGFR mutation test v2 has a reported specificity and sensitivity of 99.8 and 65.7%, respectively.[91] Nevertheless, this test has been approved by the FDA and the European Medicines Agency with the recommendation that plasma ccfDNA analysis be performed first in order to avoid unnecessary invasive biopsies of the lung (with subsequent tumor biopsy analysis if no *EGFR* mutation is detected in ccfDNA).[92] The potential relevance of such assays for MRD assessment remains under investigation. Even through liquid biopsy for NSCLC patients is a key advantage, the amount of ctDNA in these patients is low (i.e., Pecuchet and colleagues described 45% of patients with less than 2% of ccfDNA in advanced NSCLC).[366]

Using CAPP-seq, Newman and colleagues developed an assay able to identify somatic mutations in more than 95% of NSCLC tumor tissues.[436] CtDNA was detected in 100% of stage II to IV and 50% of stage I NSCLC patients, with 96% specificity for mutant allele fractions down to ~0.02%. Concentrations of ctDNA were correlated with tumor volume and provided earlier response assessment than radiographic approaches. Moreover, their approach was also designed to detect rearrangements of the receptor tyrosine kinases, ALK (anaplastic lymphoma receptor tyrosine kinase), ROS1 (c-ros oncogene 1 tyrosine kinase), and the RET proto-oncogene (harbored in approximately 8% of NSCLC). Interestingly, they also investigated biopsy-free tumor screening and genotyping with CAPP-Seq and found, in a proof of principle experiment, that they correctly classified 100% of plasma samples with ctDNA above a fractional abundance of 0.4% with a false positive rate of 0% and identified 100% of EGFR and KRAS mutations at allelic fractions greater than 0.1% with 99% specificity.

The prognostic value of ctDNA detection at baseline and during early follow up has also been investigated. Using a strategy combining BPER optimized MPS and ddPCR, Pécuchet and colleagues performed a prospective observational study involving 124 newly diagnosed advanced NSCLC patients.[365] In this study, a marker-mutation for ctDNA follow-up was found in 89% patients. ctDNA positivity at baseline was an independent marker of poor prognosis with a median OS of 13.6 versus 21.5 months (adjusted HR 1.82, 95% CI, 1.01 to 3.55, $P < .05$) and a median progression-free survival of 4.9 versus 10.4 months (adjusted HR 2.14, 95% CI, 1.30 to 3.67, $P = .002$). The presence of ctDNA was related to the presence of liver metastasis. After treatment initiation, residual ctDNA at first evaluation was an early measure of treatment benefit and was related to the best radiologic response, progression-free survival, and OS. Negative ctDNA at first evaluation predicted OS independently of RECIST evaluation ($P = .0007$). McCoach and colleagues identified ALK fusions using the Guardant360 MPS test to characterize resistance mechanisms for progression for patients with NSCLC.[484]

Data on postsurgical ctDNA measurements in patients with early-stage NSCLC are more limited.[56] In a landmark study, Abbosh and colleagues[483a] developed MPS-based, patient-specific mutational panel assays (comprising 12 to 30 SNVs) that were used for longitudinal ctDNA profiling in 24 patients enrolled in the TRACERx lung cancer study, with accompanying clinical and radiologic follow-up. Despite the small cohort size, the detection of SNVs in ctDNA seemed to be correlated with clinical evidence of NSCLC relapse. The threshold of ctDNA detection was less than 0.1%, and the median lead time to clinical and radiologic detection of disease recurrence was 70 days with a broad range of 10 to 346 days.

Chaudhuri and colleagues[483b] have shown that ctDNA analysis can be applied without prior knowledge of primary tumor genetics. In 40 patients with stage I to III lung cancer, a panel of 128 genes was targeted using CAPP-Seq and ctDNA was detected in the first post-treatment blood sample within 4 months of primary treatment in 94% of patients with subsequent recurrence. In 72% of patients, ctDNA was detected before radiologic recurrence, with an average lead time of 5.2 months. In one of five patients who received surgery and chemotherapy, ctDNA was detectable at a very low concentration of 0.04% greater than 20 months before radiologic evidence of relapse.

Pritchett and colleagues[485] analyzed the plasma of 264 patients with untreated, advanced NSCLC using a ctDNA

MPS assay to detect genomic alterations in 36 commonly mutated genes. Concordance of plasma analysis with matched tissue profiling was 97.8% with 82.9% positive predictive value, 98.5% negative predictive value, 70.6% sensitivity, and 99.2% specificity. Considering specific alterations in eight genes that most influence patient management, the positive predictive value was 97.8%, with 97.1% negative predictive value, 73.9% sensitivity, and 99.8% specificity. Across the entire study, 48 patients with actionable alterations were identified by ctDNA testing compared with only 38 by tissue testing. Thus the use of plasma-based molecular profiling using MPS detected 26% more actionable alterations compared with standard-of-care tissue testing.[485]

Beyond CTC analyses, the efficacy of immune-checkpoint inhibition could potentially be predicted using ctDNA-based assessments of tumor mutational burden (TMB).[486] Tumor cells with higher TMBs may present greater numbers of neoantigens, which makes them prone to immune recognition by T cells.[487] Despite promising initial results, the technical and clinical validation of TMB assessment using ctDNA is ongoing.[486] Moreover, surveillance of NSCLC long-term responders to PD-(L)1 blockade via ctDNA analysis to differentiate those who will achieve ongoing benefit from those at risk of eventual progression has been recently proposed.[488] In this study, Hellmann and colleagues use CAPP-seq to analyze plasma samples of 31 NSCLC patients with long term benefit to PD-(L)1 blockade (PFS > 12 months), collected at a median surveillance time point of 26.7 months after initiation of therapy (near the end or after treatment). While all patients with baseline plasma samples available ($N = 9$) had detectable ctDNA prior to therapy initiation, only 4/31 were positive for ctDNA detection at the surveillance time point and all eventually progressed. In contrast, among the 27 patients negative for ctDNA detection, 25 (93%) remained progression-free (Fisher's $P < .0001$ with a PPV of 1.00 [95% CI, 0.51 to 1.00], and a NPV of 0.93 [95% CI, 0.80 to 0.99]). The authors suggested that ctDNA surveillance, if validated, could facilitate personalization of the duration of immune checkpoint blockade and enable early intervention in patients at high risk for progression.[488]

Small cell lung cancer. Compared to other tumor types, few studies of ctDNA in SCLC have been published.[489,490] SCLC is an aggressive disease presenting a high mutation burden, intratumoral and intertumoral heterogeneity, and few targets that are readily druggable.[490] Treatment options are limited for these poor-prognosis patients. In this context, ctDNA could help during the course of treatment to understand acquired chemotherapy resistance and, as more novel targeted treatments reach the clinic, to stratify patients with SCLC as has been done with other tumor types including NSCLC (see above).[491] Using targeted MPS, Almodovar and colleagues analyzed ccfDNA from SCLC patients undergoing therapy for the presence of genetic alterations frequently altered in SCLC (i.e., single nucleotide variants, copy number alterations, insertions and deletions in 14 different genes).[491] One-hundred forty plasma samples from 27 patients (59% with extensive stage disease) obtained during 26 months of patient follow-up were examined. Disease associated alterations were observed in 85% of the samples (mutant allele frequencies between 0.1 and 87%). The observed allele frequencies and copy number alterations tracked closely with treatment responses. In several patients, the analysis of cfDNA provided evidence of disease relapse before conventional imaging.

In a randomized phase II study of the Aurora A kinase inhibitor, alisertib, plus paclitaxel as second-line therapy for SCLC patients, Owonikoko and colleagues[492] evaluated the association of genetic alterations in ctDNA with clinical outcome. The presence of genetic alterations in ccfDNA was assessed retrospectively by MPS targeting a custom panel of 80 genes (PlasmaSelect-R, Personal Genome Diagnostics) selected from the literature based on reported recurrent dysregulations in SCLC. The assay targets a read coverage of $20,000\times$ with a sensitivity greater than 0.1% for single nucleotide variants and greater than 0.2% for amplifications. Analysis of 155 baseline plasma samples led to 142 successful sequencing runs among which 140 presented genetic alterations (80%). The genetic mutation profiles revealed from the SCLC plasma ctDNA samples were concordant with the literature. Moreover, the presence of specific alterations was associated with patient outcome and response to treatment.[492]

Mohan and colleagues[493] identified tumor-related changes in 94% of patients with limited stage (LS) SCLC and 100% of patients with extensive-stage SCLC. Both CTC counts and ccfDNA readouts correlated with disease stage and OS. A simple ccfDNA genome-wide copy number approach provided an effective means of monitoring patients through treatment, and targeted ccfDNA sequencing identified potential therapeutic targets in more than 50% of patients.

POINTS TO REMEMBER

ctDNA

- ctDNA can identify DNA changes in the primary tumor, including mutations, loss of microsatellite heterozygosity, methylation of regulatory regions, DNA integrity, amplification, copy number variations, and the presence of viral DNA.
- ctDNA assays can be performed on several body effluents (e.g., blood, urine, CSF) with blood plasma being most widely used at present.
- Recent technological advances including dPCR and optimized MPS have reached high sensitivities and accuracies further expanding ctDNA applications.
- ctDNA mutation analyses can be used as companion diagnostics for targeted therapies (e.g., EGFR mutations in NSCLC treatment).
- ctDNA is a pertinent tool to assess tumor evolution, minimal residual disease, and progression in individual patients.
- ctDNA allows for monitoring of therapy efficiency both in early- and late-stage cancers.
- ctDNA contributes to the discovery of druggable mutations and genomic resistance mechanisms.
- Standardization of both preanalytical and analytical ctDNA procedures are required and would further enhance its impact on cancer patient management.

COMBINED DISCUSSION OF CIRCULATING TUMOR CELLS AND ctDNA

Future Challenges for Liquid Biopsy Analysis

The future of CTC and ctDNA analyses lies in the hands of investigators in academia and the pharmaceutical and biotechnology industry to validate assays for CLIA and FDA approval for clinical diagnostics. Large clinical multicenter studies are now required to ensure the benefit for cancer patients. Moreover, the establishment of international guidelines for CTC and ctDNA analyses is important.

The full potential of CTC and ctDNA analyses for cancer research and clinics is just starting to be explored efficiently. Several clinical studies now involve serial blood collections, which will undoubtedly enhance our understanding on its pertinence for patient follow-up and on its ability to improve patient survival. With continuous technological improvements, an even wider range of applications should appear. Broad and pertinent clinical usage will depend on standardization of both preanalytical and analytical procedures. A large amount of work has already been performed in this area and is central to large initiatives such as Cancer-ID in Europe[464,465] and will be continued by the ELBS (www.elbs.eu).[10] Standard operating procedures should be developed and broadly validated. Development of appropriate reference materials will also contribute to more standardized quality controls, quantification, and reporting among laboratories.

Continued validation of highly sensitive and specific biomarkers is important. A combination of several markers, especially in the case where early cancer diagnosis is desired, seems to be a valid approach. Interestingly, Cohen and colleagues recently combined the highly sensitive detection of mutations within ctDNA and protein markers for the detection of early-stage cancer patients.[494] The same group also identified the likely organ of origin of several nonmetastatic cancers (CancerSEEK blood test).[495]

Moreover, as for other components of liquid biopsy, large clinical validation studies are now mandatory in order to evaluate/demonstrate the efficiency of liquid biopsy monitoring and its benefit on patient outcome.

Comparison Between Circulating Tumor Cells and ctDNA

Both types of liquid biopsy assays need better quality control and standardization to provide more consistent reporting and comparisons. There are many different ways to detect and procure CTCs, as well as different downstream assays, and the same diversity of assays exists for ctDNA. The development of quality controls and reporting standards is needed to allow comparisons between different assays and to determine clinical utility. Quality control issues include blood tube collection, transport to a reference or hospital laboratory, reference standards, isolation, reproducibility, robustness, accuracy, and reporting format. Proficiency testing for standardization and insight into the performance of ctDNA assays is available through the College of American Pathology PT program (https://www.cap.org/laboratory-improvement/proficiency-testing).

Applications for CTCs and ctDNA have greatly advanced in the last decade. Both approaches provide overlapping information and unique information for specific cancers. CTC detection provides real-time information on tumor spread. If CTCs are sampled repetitively over days to weeks and their numbers increase, the tumor is progressing and active metastasis is occurring. Assessing the presence of CTCs in blood may be important before, during, and after therapy because their presence suggests potential metastasis and colonization in distant sites. Continued development of better markers for CTCs that predict survival and establishment of metastasis is important. Moreover, molecular characterization of CTCs in addition to quantification can provide information beyond the genomic level. Transcriptional plasticity can be an important driver for resistance to cancer therapy and CTCs can be interrogated at the RNA and protein level, which provides additional guidance for treatment decisions. Transcriptional analysis of CTCs may also predict which organ site is likely to be colonized; different organ microenvironments can select different types of tumor cells and induce different transcriptional activities as a consequence of the crosstalk between the tumor cells and the surrounding organ. Finally, single cell CTC analysis provides information on intrapatient heterogeneity,[496] which is an important mechanism of resistance to therapy in prostate cancer.[497]

Similar to CTCs, ctDNA is also diluted in a sea of ccfDNA released from normal cells, therefore requiring the use of sensitive molecular assays.[8] The detection of ctDNA indicates there is tumor present in the patient, but unlike CTCs, it does not indicate if it is spreading through the circulation and most ctDNA is derived from dying cancer cells which may or may not represent the pool of living cancer cells in the patient body. However, consistent detection or increasing concentrations over time suggest that the tumor is active (progressing or rapidly renewing cell turnover). Sequential assessments of ctDNA contribute to the detection of MRD after tumor resection and disease progression in advanced cancer patients. Moreover, druggable mutations and genomic resistance mechanisms (e.g., T790M mutations in NSCLC, KRAS mutations in colon cancer or ER gene mutations in breast cancer) can be detected within ctDNA and may empower selection of the best therapy for individual cancer patients.

Capture of ccfDNA from blood plasma is much easier than capture of CTCs, but sophisticated downstream analysis of ctDNA also requires expert skills; thus the concordance between different technologies and laboratories is not high, especially in samples with low ccfDNA concentrations.[383] Another issue for CTCs and ctDNA is the volume of blood needed (>5 mL) to accurately assess CTCs, particularly in early-stage cancer patients. Although ctDNA has in principle a higher dynamic range than CTCs, the number of ctDNA molecules can also become a limiting factor in early cancer detection where the tumor burden is very low. The recent development of assays with high sensitivity and the ability to assess a broad spectrum of mutations on fragments of ctDNA may overcome this limitation.

As better CTC isolation methods develop, downstream CTC analysis has improved and is now more informative.[8] Because CTCs are heterogeneous, not all detected CTCs may be equally relevant in assessing metastatic potential, which points to the relevance of further downstream analysis of CTCs to identify the metastasis-initiating subset in future studies. In this context, the establishment of CTC lines or xenografts as models to study the biology of CTCs in depth is an important research area.

The combination of both CTCs and ctDNA as a liquid biopsy may augment the accurate assessment of cancer patients. Both can be used together to provide informative patient results.[271] In addition, the use of liquid biopsy (CTC and/or ctDNA) may be combined with imaging and blood protein/analyte tumor biomarkers to give a more comprehensive evaluation of the patient status. The real challenge is to combine all the information into an interpretable result for the clinician to enable decisions on treatment: analyses of CTCs and ctDNA have paved new diagnostic avenues and are to date the cornerstones of liquid biopsy diagnostics (Fig. 71.25).

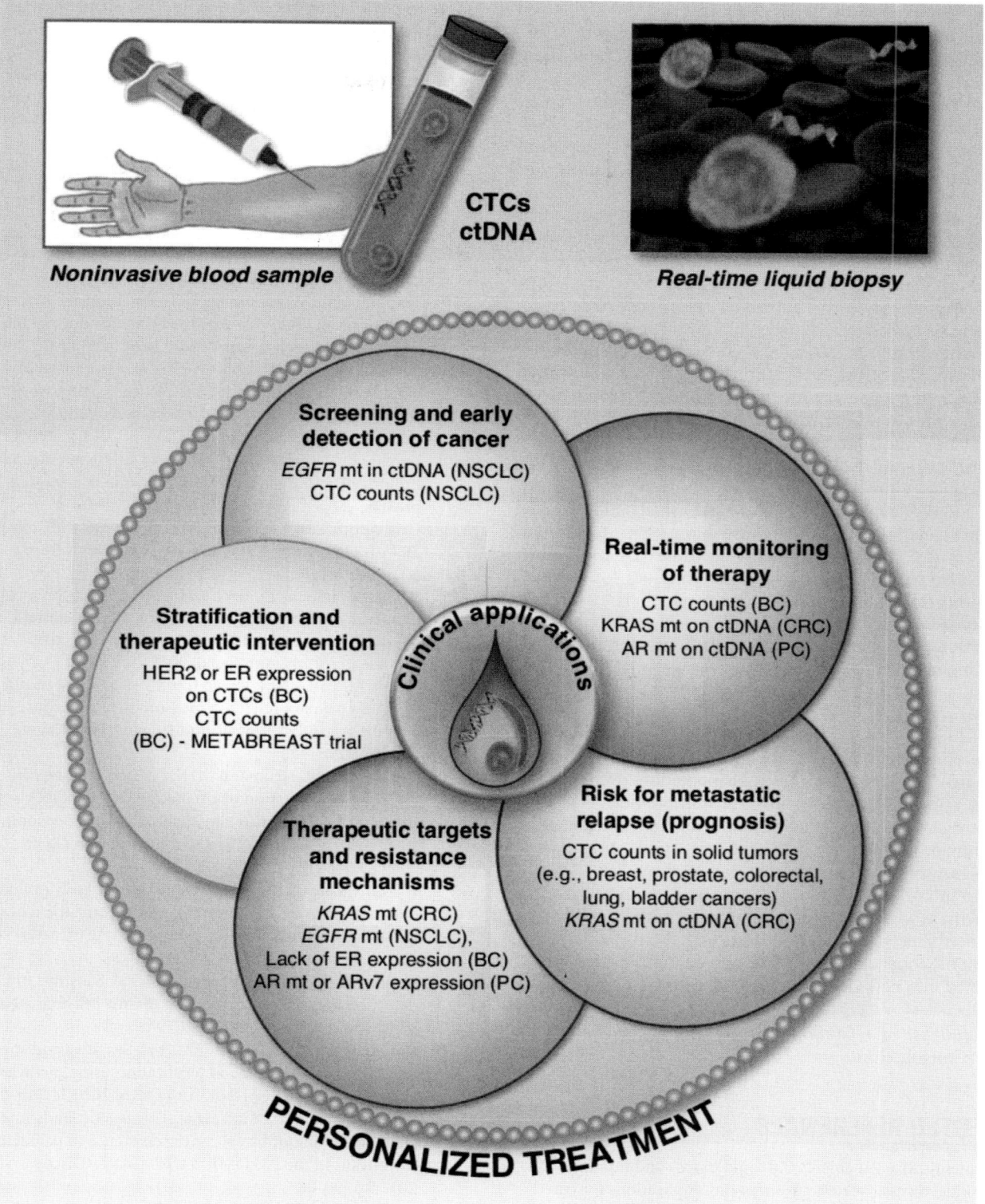

FIGURE 71.25 Clinical applications of circulating tumor cells (CTCs) and ctDNA as liquid biopsies for personalized medicine. Blood samples can be sampled repeatedly to predict relapse in M0 patients or metastatic progression in M1 patients, monitor the efficacy of therapies, and understand potential resistance mechanisms. Before therapy, patients can be stratified to the most effective drugs, whereas after initiation of treatment, persistent increases of CTCs/ctDNA indicates resistance to therapy, and this information may allow an early switch to a more effective regimen before the tumor burden is excessive and incurable. *BC,* Breast cancer; *CRC,* colorectal cancer; *mt,* mutation; *PC,* prostate cancer. (From Alix-Panabières C, Pantel K. Clinical applications of circulating tumor cells and circulating tumor DNA as liquid biopsy. *Cancer Discov* 2016;6:479–91.)

Liquid Biopsy versus Tumor Biopsy

A major objective in the field is to determine whether CTCs and ctDNA analysis can replace tumor biopsies. Liquid biopsies are minimally invasive and can be performed repetitively without the complications of tumor biopsy. Tumor biopsies cannot always be performed because of the tumor site location, and repetitive samples may not be sufficient or representative of the tumor. Repeat ctDNA molecular analysis may be more consistent than tumor biopsies because of tumor sampling error. CTC analysis of genomic aberrations can now be performed with the same potential quality as a tumor biopsy such as a fine-needle aspiration. While initial diagnosis is best performed by tumor biopsy and conventional histopathology, liquid biopsies may in the future be used once validated for targeted therapy stratification and monitoring patients. With the advent of MPS, ctDNA and CTC assays have become more informative and offer better homogeneity than a solid tumor for sequencing analysis. As liquid biopsies become better validated, they may be used in cases where tumor biopsies are difficult or impossible to obtain. CtDNA and CTC analysis may enable rapid decisions for treatment stratification and modification during therapy. The European consortium, CANCER-ID (2015–2019),[372] has established guidelines for clinical validation of liquid biopsy biomarkers to evaluate ctDNA and CTC in breast and lung cancer by multicenter prospective trials aimed to evaluate techniques for assessing CTCs and ctDNA in different laboratories.[498] The objectives of CANCER-ID are continued by the newly established ELBS consortium, which consists of almost 100 partner institutions including non-European participants (www-elbs.eu).

CONCLUSIONS

The development of liquid biopsy (CTCs and ctDNA) provides many new opportunities for implementation over the next 5 years. These assays, upon validation, may provide better clinical management in treatment monitoring and understanding of tumor progression for many different types of cancers. As new biosensors, molecular procedures, and molecular devices develop in both CTC and ctDNA analyses, the sensitivity and specificity, as well as logistics, will improve. With the resource of the cancer gene atlas (TCGA NIH USA[1]), there is a significant amount of sequencing data of multiple cancer types that can be translated into new CTC and ctDNA targets in the future.

For a full list of references for this chapter, please refer to ExpertConsult.com.

SELECTED REFERENCES

8. Pantel K, Alix-Panabières C. Liquid biopsy and minimal residual disease – latest advances and implications for cure. Nat Rev Clin Oncol 2019;16:409–24.

14. Bidard FC, Michiels S, Riethdorf S, et al. Circulating tumor cells in breast cancer patients treated by neoadjuvant chemotherapy: a meta-analysis. J Natl Cancer Inst 2018;110:560–67.

15. Riethdorf S, Müller V, Loibl S, et al. Prognostic impact of circulating tumor cells for breast cancer patients treated in the neoadjuvant 'Geparquattro' trial. Clin Cancer Res 2017;23:5384–93.

17. Müller C, Holtschmidt J, Auer M, et al. Hematogenous dissemination of glioblastoma multiforme. Sci Transl Med 2014;6:247ra101.

28. Joosse SA, Souche FR, Babayan A, et al. Chromosomal aberrations associated with sequential steps of the metastatic cascade in colorectal cancer patients. Clin Chem 2018;64:1505–12.

87. Keller L, Pantel K. Unravelling tumour heterogeneity by single-cell profiling of circulating tumour cells. Nat Rev Cancer 2019;19:553–67.

89. Cayrefourcq L, Mazard T, Joosse S, et al. Establishment and characterization of a cell line from human circulating colon cancer cells. Cancer Res 2015;75:892–901.

179. Trapp E, Janni W, Schindlbeck C, et al. Presence of circulating tumor cells in high-risk early breast cancer during follow-up and prognosis. J Natl Cancer Inst 2019;111:380–7.

181. Sparano J, O'Neill A, Alpaugh K, et al. Association of circulating tumor cells with late recurrence of estrogen receptor-positive breast cancer: a secondary analysis of a randomized clinical trial. JAMA Oncol 2018;4:1700–6.

206. Lorente D, Olmos D, Mateo J, et al. Decline in circulating tumor cell count and treatment outcome in advanced prostate cancer. Eur Urol 2016;70:985–92.

338. Cristiano S, Leal A, Phallen J, et al. Genome-wide cell-free DNA fragmentation in patients with cancer. Nature 2019;570:385–9.

363. Bachet JB, Bouché O, Taieb J, et al. RAS mutation analysis in circulating tumor DNA from patients with metastatic colorectal cancer: the AGEO RASANC prospective multicenter study. Ann Oncol 2018;29:1211–9.

368. Whale AS, Jones GM, Pavšič J, et al. Assessment of digital PCR as a primary reference measurement procedure to support advances in precision medicine. Clin Chem 2018;64:1296–1307.

383. Lampignano R, Neumann MHD, Weber S, Heitzer E. Multicenter evaluation of circulating cell-free DNA Extraction and downstream analyses for the development of standardized (pre)analytical work flows. Clin Chem 2019;65:306837.

439. Garlan F, Laurent-Puig P, Sefrioui D, et al. Early evaluation of circulating tumor DNA as marker of therapeutic efficacy in metastatic colorectal cancer patients (PLACOL study). Clin Cancer Res 2017;23:5416–25.

442. Shen SY, Singhania R, Fehringer G, et al. Sensitive tumour detection and classification using plasma cell-free DNA methylomes. Nature 2018;563:579–83.

443. Liu MC, Oxnard GR, Klein EA, et al. Sensitive and specific multi-cancer detection and localization using methylation signatures in cell-free DNA. Ann Oncol 2020;31:745–59.

465. O'Leary B, Cutts RJ, Liu Y, et al. The genetic landscape and clonal evolution of breast cancer resistance to palbociclib plus fulvestrant in the PALOMA-3 trial. Cancer Discov 2018;8:1390–403.

479. Tie J, Wang Y, Tomasetti C, et al. Circulating tumor DNA analysis detects minimal residual disease and predicts recurrence in patients with stage II colon cancer. Sci Transl Med 2016;8:346ra92.

494. Cohen JD, Li L, Wang Y, et al. Detection and localization of surgically resectable cancers with a multi-analyte blood test. Science 2018;359:926–30.

72

Circulating Nucleic Acids for Prenatal Diagnostics

Rossa W.K. Chiu and Yuk Ming Dennis Lo

ABSTRACT

Background

Prenatal diagnosis is becoming an essential part of prenatal care for a growing number of patients. To make a definitive diagnosis, traditional methods of sampling fetal genetic material, such as chorionic villus sampling and amniocentesis, are invasive and introduce a risk of spontaneous miscarriage. The discovery of cell-free fetal DNA (cffDNA) in the circulation of pregnant women led to the possibility of noninvasive genetic and chromosomal assessment of the fetus through the sampling of maternal peripheral blood. The clinical introduction of cffDNA tests has led to a substantial reduction in the number of invasive procedures performed worldwide.

Content

This chapter describes the biological properties of circulating cffDNA, the applications that have been developed, and their clinical uses. Additionally, analytical characteristics of cffDNA testing are highlighted. Circulating cffDNA is derived from placental cell turnover. This DNA from apoptotic placenta cells is highly fragmented, with the majority of fragments less than 200 bp in length. Circulating cffDNA exists with a substantial background of maternal DNA. Circulating cffDNA can be detected from early pregnancy onward, and it rapidly (about 1 hour half-life) disappears from maternal circulation following delivery of the newborn. The analysis of cffDNA is now clinically used for the assessment of sex-linked diseases, fetal blood group incompatibility, fetal chromosomal aneuploidies, and some single-gene diseases. Analytical protocols are designed to maximize the yield of fetal DNA by minimizing maternal DNA contamination and by preserving the abundance of short DNA molecules. The inclusion of internal positive controls for the presence of fetal DNA or the measurement of fetal DNA fraction is an important quality control parameter.

BRIEF OVERVIEW OF THE EARLY DEVELOPMENTS OF PRENATAL GENETIC DIAGNOSTICS

Prenatal diagnosis is an important part of prenatal care for many women. It encompasses both diagnostic and screening tests that detect or exclude morphologic, structural, functional, chromosomal, and molecular defects in a fetus. Amniocentesis was first introduced in 1952 for the prenatal assessment of fetal hemolytic disease.[1] This was followed by karyotyping of amniotic fluid cells in 1966,[2] and then ultrasonography for fetal structural abnormalities in the 1970s.[3,4] Later, maternal serum biochemistry testing was shown to be of value in the screening of neural tube defects[5,6] and fetal aneuploidies.[7] In the early 1980s, chorionic villus sampling (CVS) became available as an alternative to amniocentesis for prenatal genetic assessment.[8] For many years, amniocentesis and CVS were the key approaches for providing fetal genetic material used in prenatal testing.

The main disadvantage of amniocentesis and CVS is the procedure-related risk of fetal miscarriage. The fetal loss rate associated with the performance of these invasive procedures is between 0.1 and 0.3%.[9] The risk may be small but it is finite. Efforts have therefore been devoted to the development of noninvasive approaches to identify high-risk pregnant women.

STRATEGIES TO MITIGATE RISKS OF INVASIVE PRENATAL DIAGNOSIS

The risk for Down syndrome, with an incidence rate of 1 in 800 pregnancies,[10] is one of the predominant reasons for women seeking prenatal diagnosis. Strategies have been devised to identify high-risk pregnancies by the combined assessment of maternal age, serum biochemical markers, and ultrasonography findings. The purpose of this assessment is to risk stratify pregnancies where the chance of having an affected fetus is higher than the chance of a procedure-related fetal loss. Different combinations of screening strategies have been practiced, with different levels of specificity and sensitivity.[11]

Maternal Age

The probability of giving birth to an infant with Down syndrome increases with advancing maternal age.[12] The risk of giving birth to an affected infant at term is estimated to be less than 1 in 1000 at a maternal age of 29 years and younger, but it increases to 1 in 385 at 35 years of age.[13] Hence, prior to the development of more elaborate prenatal screening strategies, it was customary to offer prenatal diagnosis to women aged 35 years or older. However, because a significant proportion of women become pregnant before 35 years of age, maternal age alone would only identify 51% of Down syndrome–affected pregnancies at a 14% false-positive rate.[14]

Serum Biochemistry Screening

The combination of maternal age assessment with maternal serum screening of various biomarkers between 15 and 22 weeks of gestation was later developed as a second trimester screening protocol to identify high-risk pregnancies. This screening strategy is referred to as the "triple test," and the serum biomarkers include alpha-fetoprotein, human chorionic gonadotropin, and unconjugated estriol. When the analytical cutoff values are set to give a 5% false-positive rate, the detection sensitivity for Down syndrome is 70%.[15] Testing maternal serum inhibin A and the triple test markers during the second trimester, termed the "quadruple test," provided a detection sensitivity of 75% at a false-positive rate of 5%.[14]

First Trimester Screening

While the triple and quadruple tests are used during the second trimester, alternative Down syndrome screening strategies have been developed for testing during the first trimester. One of these strategies for first trimester Down syndrome screening measures free β-human chorionic gonadotropin and pregnancy-associated plasma protein A.[16,17] Down syndrome is associated with an increase in fetal nuchal translucency measured by first trimester ultrasound.[18] Subsequently, the combination of first trimester biochemical markers, fetal nuchal translucency, and maternal age assessments came to be known as the "first trimester combined test." With a false-positive rate of 5%, the test could detect 95% of Down syndrome fetuses.[19]

The approaches described above have been incorporated into many prenatal screening programs. However, the main disadvantage of these tests lies in their high false-positive rates. Most of the test cutoff values used to identify those deemed to be at high risk had false-positive rates of 5%. This meant that 1 in every 20 women would be labeled as high risk and would need to face the decision of whether or not to undergo an invasive diagnostic procedure. Because the average Down syndrome risk is 1 in 800, this meant that a substantial number of women undergoing an invasive diagnostic procedure did not carry an affected fetus. Therefore there was a need to identify or develop more robust screening methods that had lower false-positive rates and improved detection rates.

NONINVASIVE FETAL DNA ANALYSIS

The prenatal screening methods described above are based on the detection of prenatal phenotypic features that tend to be associated with Down syndrome. The rationale was that to improve the sensitivity and specificity of prenatal screening, methods directed at the detection of the fundamental genetic lesion pathognomonic of the condition are required—for example, trisomy 21 for Down syndrome or the fetal mutations for single-gene diseases. To this end, noninvasive methods have been developed to provide access to fetal DNA for analysis.

Fetal Cells in Maternal Blood

More than a century ago, a German pathologist, Schmorl,[20] observed the presence of trophoblasts in the lung tissues of women who died of preeclampsia. The existence of such circulating fetal cells was later confirmed by molecular techniques based on the detection of Y-chromosome DNA sequences in the blood of women pregnant with male fetuses.[21] The idea of noninvasive prenatal diagnosis based on maternal blood sampling began to emerge. It was subsequently realized that intact fetal cells are present in maternal circulation rarely, with about just one cell per milliliter of maternal blood.[22] Protocols have since been developed to isolate and enrich for these rare fetal cells, including fluorescence and magnetic activated cell sorting,[23,24] and more recently by nanofluidics.[25] Though the identification and isolation of intact fetal cells in maternal circulation is somewhat challenging, once isolated, they may be amenable to single-cell whole-genome analysis for the potential identification of fetal genetic and genomic abnormalities.[26] If more robust approaches for fetal cell isolation and identification could be achieved, circulating fetal cell–based noninvasive prenatal diagnostics may be a clinically viable option in the future.

Cell-free Fetal DNA in Maternal Plasma

Instead of intact cells, Lo and colleagues[27] searched for fetal DNA in the cell-free portion of maternal blood—namely, plasma and serum. Y-chromosome DNA was detected in the plasma and serum of women who were pregnant with male fetuses but not in women with female fetuses. Since this first report in 1997, much research investigated the properties and potential utilities of circulating cffDNA. cffDNA analysis is currently used for routine prenatal testing.

THE BIOLOGY OF CIRCULATING CELL-FREE FETAL NUCLEIC ACIDS IN MATERNAL PLASMA

Every milliliter of maternal plasma contains thousands of genome-equivalents of cell-free DNA, with the fetus contributing a minor proportion.[28] In other words, the majority of the cell-free DNA in maternal plasma is derived from the mother. The median amount of cffDNA as a proportion of the total DNA in maternal plasma, termed the "fetal fraction," is around 10% in the first and second trimesters and around 20% during the third trimester.[29] The absolute concentration of cffDNA increases with gestational age, probably as a consequence of the increase in placental tissue mass. Nonetheless, its abundance in the maternal circulation far exceeds that of intact fetal cells.

POINTS TO REMEMBER
Biological Properties of cffDNA

- cffDNA is a by-product of placental cell turnover.
- cffDNA coexists in maternal plasma with a major background of maternal DNA.
- cffDNA is highly fragmented and is generally less than 200 bp long.
- cffDNA fragmentation is a nonrandom process.
- cffDNA has rapid clearance kinetics and an apparent half-life of 1 h.
- cffDNA is detectable in early pregnancy. It is most reliably detected from the late first trimester onward.

Fetal DNA molecules are detectable in maternal plasma quite early in pregnancy. Depending on the analytical platform used, cffDNA is detected from around the 10th week of gestation.[30] cffDNA is cleared from maternal plasma very rapidly after delivery.[31] Using sensitive methods to measure cffDNA serially after delivery, the half-life of cffDNA in the postpartum maternal serum is about an hour.[32] No cffDNA could be detected in maternal plasma 1 day after delivery. These observations reveal that fetal DNA molecules in maternal plasma have a high turnover rate with efficient clearance mechanisms. Renal clearance studies performed by serial monitoring of cffDNA in maternal plasma and maternal urine after delivery show that renal excretion is only a minor component of fetal DNA clearance.[32]

Despite the rapid clearance kinetics, cffDNA amounts to approximately 10 to 20% of the total DNA in maternal plasma; this suggests that substantial amounts of fetal DNA may be released by a tissue source at any point in time. At least two lines of evidence demonstrate the placenta as the predominant tissue that releases fetal DNA into the maternal circulation: first, epigenetic markers specific to the placenta are detectable in maternal plasma[33,34]; second, chromosomal abnormalities confined to the placenta are detectable in maternal plasma.[35] On the other hand, the main contributors of cell-free DNA from the mother are maternal hematologic cells.[34,36]

Cell-free DNA is a metabolic by-product of cell death and is therefore present in the circulation as short fragments in a "cell-free" form. Researchers studied the size profile of maternal plasma DNA in a high-resolution manner (Fig. 72.1).[37,38] Cell-free DNA molecules are generally shorter than 200 bp. The most frequently represented size in plasma is 166 bp in length. 166 bp corresponds to the length of DNA that is wound around a histone core with a linker. This characteristic

size reflected that cell-free DNA is mainly derived from mononucleosomes. Interestingly, cffDNA molecules are somewhat shorter, and the most frequently represented size is 142 bp in length.[37] This shorter length corresponds to the length of DNA wound around a histone core without a linker. This implies that the fetal DNA molecules may have undergone further steps of degradation compared to maternal DNA in maternal plasma. In addition to these dominant peaks, there are smaller amounts of cell-free DNA that are successively shorter in 10-bp increments.

There is now evidence to show that the fragmentation of cell-free DNA, including cffDNA is not a random process. There are locations in the genome which serve more frequently as the fragmentation or ending sites than others.[39] The cffDNA and the cell-free maternal DNA share some preferred fragmentation sites but there are also some genomic locations favored by the fetal DNA rather than the maternal DNA as ending sites and vice versa. The fragmentation process involves a series of enzymatic cutting steps and is partly influenced by chromatin structure.[40] For example, the presence of histones seem to be required to fix DNA in a conformation such that nucleases cut the DNA at the minor grooves of nucleosomes to generate short cell-free DNA molecules that are successively shorter by 10 bp.[40]

DIAGNOSTIC APPLICATIONS OF CIRCULATING cffDNA

Cell-free fetal DNA is a source of fetal genetic material that may be sampled noninvasively by maternal phlebotomy. Its relative high abundance in maternal plasma from early

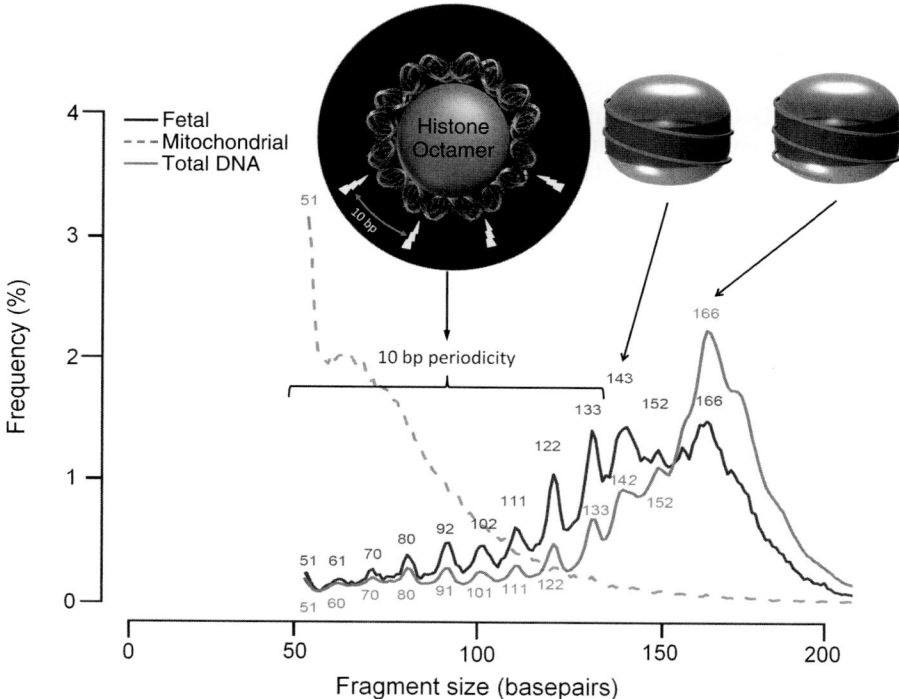

FIGURE 72.1 Size distribution of fetal, mitochondrial, and total DNA. Numbers denote the DNA size in bps at the peaks. Schematic illustrations of the structural organization of a nucleosome are shown above the graph. From left to right, DNA double helix wound around a nucleosomal core unit with the sites for nuclease cleavage shown; a nucleosome core unit with approximately 146 bp of DNA wound around it; and a nucleosomal core unit with an approximately 20-bp linker intact.

pregnancy, with no postpartum persistence, has facilitated the development of a number of applications for noninvasive prenatal assessment.

Fetal Sex Assessment for Sex-associated Disorders

The first report of cffDNA was based on the detection of male fetal DNA sequences in the plasma of women pregnant with male fetuses.[27] This noninvasive test for fetal sex assessment was immediately useful for clinical purposes. The accurate assessment of fetal sex is useful for the prenatal management of diseases with sex-linked patterns of inheritance and conditions such as congenital adrenal hyperplasia, where the disease manifestation differs between male and female offspring. For sex-linked genetic diseases, such as hemophilia and Duchenne muscular dystrophy, invasive prenatal diagnostic procedures could be avoided if the noninvasive fetal sex assessment suggested a female fetus. For congenital adrenal hyperplasia secondary to 21-hydroxylase deficiency, female fetuses are at risk of virilization. Thus steroid therapy and further prenatal genetic assessment may be avoided if the noninvasive fetal sex assessment suggested a male fetus. In general, the specificity for male cffDNA detection approaches 99%.[30] In terms of sensitivity, Devaney and colleagues showed that higher sensitivities could be reached by using later gestational ages, more replicate analyses, and higher-sensitivity analytical approaches.[30] For example, real-time PCR provides higher sensitivity than conventional PCR.

Fetal Rhesus D Status Determination

Rhesus (Rh) D incompatibility occurs when an RhD-negative woman is pregnant with an RhD-positive fetus. RhD-negative blood cells lack the RhD antigen. Therefore when the RhD-negative maternal immune cells are presented with the RhD antigen of the RhD-positive fetal blood, alloimmunization occurs. Upon the next pregnancy with an RhD-positive fetus, the sensitized woman and the anti-RhD antibodies may cause destruction of the fetal tissues, causing hemolytic disease of the newborn. However, such risks do not exist if the woman is pregnant with an RhD-negative fetus. Therefore prenatal RhD genotyping of the fetus is useful in the management of RhD-negative pregnant women. The great majority of RhD-negative individuals lack the RhD gene, *RHD*, due to gene deletion. Therefore one could noninvasively assess the fetal RhD status by detecting the presence of *RHD* in the plasma of RhD-negative pregnant women.[41,42] Unlike conventional methods, such as amniocentesis or CVS, noninvasive methods are free from the risk of inducing fetomaternal

hemorrhage and further sensitization. The analysis of cffDNA for noninvasive fetal RhD genotyping has been globally implemented for clinical use. In addition, the test has also been used as the basis for rationalizing the administration of prophylactic anti-D immunoglobulin only to pregnancies involving an RhD-positive fetus.[43] Such an approach may minimize the unnecessary use of the scarce and expensive anti-D immunoglobulin, as well as reduce the need to unnecessarily expose the pregnant woman to the anti-D blood product. Hemolytic disease of the newborn is further discussed in Chapter 59.

Fetal Chromosomal Aneuploidy Screening

Down syndrome is one of the key reasons for couples to consider prenatal diagnosis. Down syndrome is typically caused by the presence of an additional dose of chromosome 21—namely, trisomy 21—in the genome of affected individuals. Therefore the key to achieving noninvasive prenatal detection of Down syndrome is to provide evidence that increased copies of chromosome 21 are present in maternal plasma. The majority of the DNA in maternal plasma, including DNA from chromosome 21, originates from the mother who is assumed to have a normal amount of chromosome 21. If the fetus has trisomy 21, it would contribute additional amounts of chromosome 21 into maternal plasma. Therefore the additional amount of cell-free chromosome 21 DNA molecules in maternal plasma is dependent on the fetal fraction (i.e., the percent of fetal DNA in the background of maternal DNA in the plasma). The higher the fetal fraction, the easier the identification of trisomy 21–associated changes in maternal plasma DNA analysis.

Methodological Approaches

To precisely quantify and detect this small additional amount of chromosome 21 DNA, most protocols utilize massively parallel sequencing (see Chapter 65). One approach is based on random or shotgun sequencing of maternal plasma DNA.[44] The rationale is that among the cell-free DNA fragments in maternal plasma, if one sequences a random fraction of all the molecules, the relative amount of DNA obtained from each segment across the genome should reflect the relative DNA contribution of that segment in the genome of the tested individual. To determine the relative amount of DNA from each segment—such as, each chromosome—one could determine the number of DNA molecules sequenced from that chromosome as a proportion of all molecules sequenced from the sample. The relative amount, or genomic representation, is then compared with the expected amount for the same chromosome among a control group of samples representing euploid pregnancies (Fig. 72.2). If a sample shows a genomic representation of chromosome 21 that is significantly increased (e.g., more than 3 standard deviations) from the control group, the amount of chromosome 21 is considered elevated and therefore suggestive of trisomy 21.

Because this approach is based on random whole-genome sequencing, it could in principle be applied to other chromosomal aneuploidies, such as trisomy 18 and trisomy 13, and the sex chromosome aneuploidies, such as Turner syndrome, 45 X, and Klinefelter syndrome, 47 XXY.[45] The protocol could be repurposed for the detection of microdeletion and microduplication syndromes.[46,47] Molecular karyotyping at Mb-level of resolution covering most parts of the

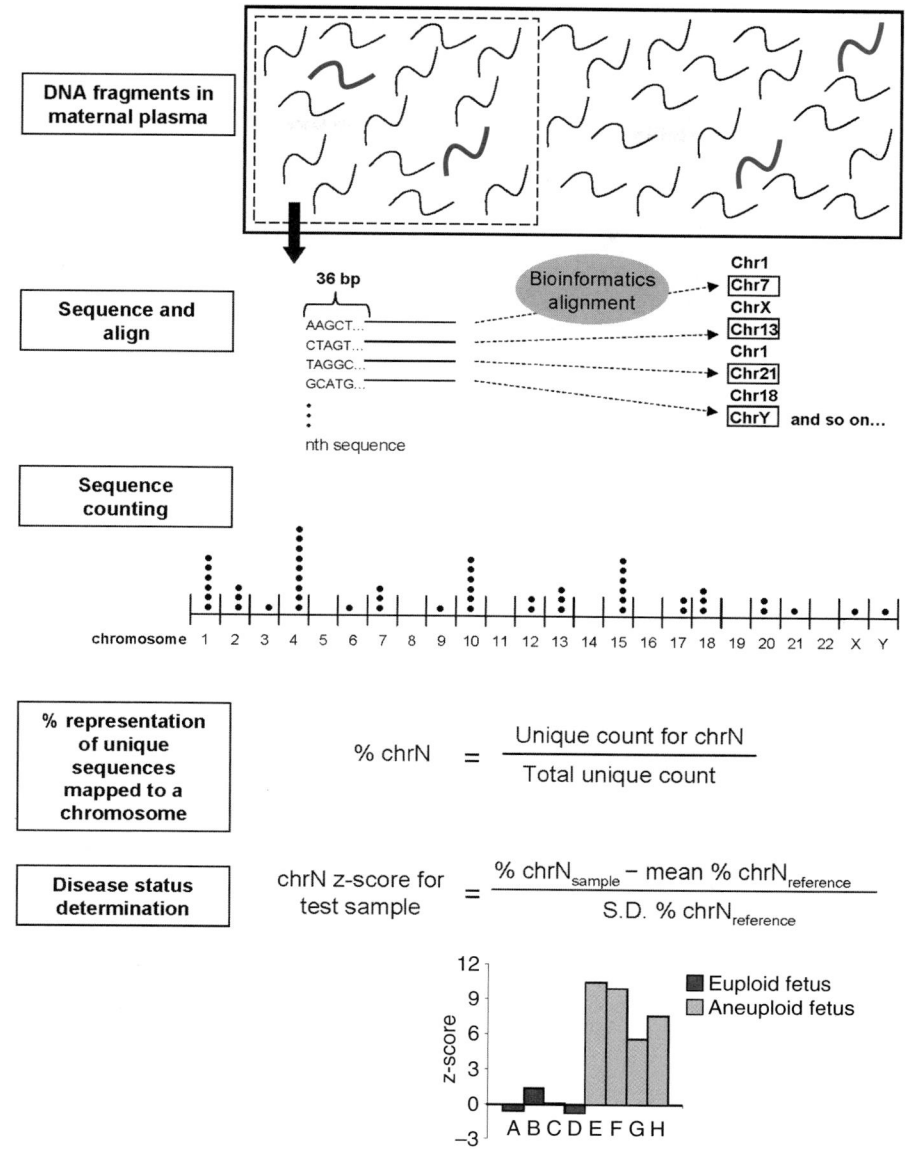

FIGURE 72.2 Schematic illustration of the procedural framework for using massively parallel genomic sequencing for the noninvasive prenatal detection of fetal chromosomal aneuploidy. Fetal DNA *(thick red fragments)* circulates in maternal plasma as a minor population among a high background of maternal DNA *(black fragments)*. A sample containing representative DNA molecules in maternal plasma is obtained. Plasma DNA molecules are sequenced, and the chromosomal origin of each molecule is identified through mapping to the human reference genome by bioinformatics analysis. The number of sequences mapped to each chromosome is counted and then expressed as a percentage of all unique sequences generated for the sample, termed *%chrN* for chromosome N. Z-scores for each chromosome and each test sample are calculated using the formula shown. The z-score of a potentially aneuploid chromosome is expected to be higher for pregnancies with an aneuploid fetus (cases E to H) than those with a euploid fetus (cases A to D). (From Chiu RWK, Chan KCA, Gao Y, et al. Noninvasive prenatal diagnosis of fetal chromosomal aneuploidy by massively parallel genomic sequencing of DNA in maternal plasma. *Proc Natl Acad Sci U S A* 2008;105:20458–63.)

genome appears possible.[46,47] As described in the section on analytical aspects, the successful implementation of these protocols relies on the precise quantification of the genomic segment of interest. For example, the signal-to-noise ratio for relative quantification of a genomic region is partly governed by the sequencing depth.[47,48] Thus the sequencing depth may need to be adjusted if the analysis is intended for the detection of subchromosomal changes instead of whole-chromosome aneuploidies. In addition, target capture of cell-free DNA originating from chromosomal regions of interest followed by targeted analysis could similarly achieve relative genomic representation assessment.[48]

To detect the presence of extra or missing copies of chromosomes, allelic ratio approaches have also been developed.

Such approaches take advantage of polymorphic differences between homologous chromosomes between the mother and the fetus.[49] In principle, such polymorphic loci may include loci where the mother is homozygous and the fetus is heterozygous, or when the mother is heterozygous and the fetus is homozygous. The rationale is that when the fetus has aneuploidy, the ratio between alleles on that chromosome will be skewed. However, the extent of skewing between the alleles is dependent on the configuration of the polymorphic markers between the fetus and the mother and the fetal fraction. To implement this method, the allelic information of each cell-free DNA fragment needs to be compared to relative amounts of the homologous chromosomes.

Clinical Implementation

cffDNA-based noninvasive prenatal screening for fetal chromosomal aneuploidy became clinically available in 2011[50] and is now available worldwide. In general, cffDNA-based noninvasive prenatal screening achieved detection rates of about 99% for Down syndrome with less than 1% false-positive rates.[51,52] Depending on the specific protocol used, the detection rates for trisomy 18 and trisomy 13 are about or greater than 90%, with less than 1% false-positive rates.[51,52] In other words, cffDNA-based prenatal screening achieved better detection sensitivities and specificities than those screening modalities based on maternal serum biochemistry and/or fetal ultrasonography. Consequently, there are a number of professional guidelines and recommendations incorporating the use of cffDNA-based prenatal assessment as one of the options for fetal chromosomal aneuploidy screening.[53,54] However, it is noteworthy that there are false-positive cases (see discussion below). Therefore cffDNA assessment is a screening procedure and not a definitive diagnostic tool. All clinical guidelines recommend that cffDNA tests with positive findings suggestive of chromosomal aneuploidy should be confirmed by tests on fetal genetic material collected by conventional invasive methods such as chorionic villus sampling or amniocentesis.

While the performance profile of the cffDNA-based tests is quite attractive for screening, the direct costs are higher than that of maternal serum biochemistry screening. To balance the overall costs, various modalities for incorporating the cffDNA-based tests into prenatal screening programs have evolved.[51] One option is to recommend cffDNA testing only to pregnant women who are identified as high risk and who would otherwise be recommended for conventional invasive prenatal diagnosis. For example, women who receive a high-risk score upon having undergone the first trimester combined screening test may consider the option of cffDNA testing. In this scenario, the cffDNA assessment is only performed for the 5% of pregnancies with high-risk scores. With their high-specificity profile, the cffDNA tests should be able to further identify 99% of the unaffected pregnancies. As a result, the number of pregnancies recommended for invasive testing would be reduced to only those patients with a positive cffDNA test result. In practice, since the implementation of cffDNA testing in the clinical setting, the reduction in invasive prenatal diagnostic procedures is between 26 and 69%.[55–57]

The two-step screening approach described above has the advantage of reducing the high false-positive rate of the conventional prenatal screening program. However, it does not raise the aneuploidy detection rates that are limited by the detection performance of first-tier screening tests. Consequently, some groups have proposed a "contingent approach" where the threshold to label a pregnancy as "high risk" by the conventional screening tests is relaxed to include a greater proportion of the population (e.g., 10% of all pregnancies).[51] Theoretically, this would increase the detection rates for fetal chromosomal aneuploidies without an increase in the overall false-positive rate in the context of a two-tier screening program where cffDNA analysis serves as the second-tier test.

Recently, evidence has emerged that cffDNA tests for chromosomal aneuploidies have similar detection sensitivities and specificities among high- and average-risk pregnant women.[58–60] This has led to discussions on applying the cffDNA tests as a primary screening test.[53,61] Bianchi and colleagues[61] reported that the positive predictive values of the cffDNA sequencing tests were substantially higher than that of maternal serum biochemistry–based screening. For trisomy 21 detection, the positive predictive value of cffDNA sequencing was 45.5%, while that of conventional screening was 4.2%. For trisomy 18 detection, the positive predictive value of cffDNA sequencing was 40.0% and 8.3% for conventional screening. In this study, the negative predictive values for trisomy 21 and trisomy 18 detection were 100% for both cffDNA sequencing and conventional screening. If the cost of cffDNA testing could be substantially reduced, cost-benefit studies have identified it as the preferred primary screen for aneuploidies.[62]

Discordant Results

While cffDNA tests demonstrate high sensitivities and specificities, there are false-negative and false-positive results. Some of the false-negative cases are a result of low fetal DNA fraction.[63] In these cases, the proportion of fetal DNA in the sample is too low to produce a statistically significant change in the genomic representation, even in the presence of chromosome aneuploidy. Other false-negative cases are due to the mosaic nature of some chromosomal abnormalities. Mosaicism refers to the situation when only a proportion of the fetal cells harbor the chromosomal abnormality. Because the proportion of fetal cells that are contributing the DNA from the affected chromosome is reduced, the ability of the analytical method to detect the abnormality is also reduced.[63] Interestingly, some of the false-negative cases are a result of the absence of the chromosomal aneuploidy in the placental tissue.[64] In other words, the chromosomal aneuploidy is present in the fetus proper but not in the placenta or is present at an exceedingly low proportion of the placental cells. cffDNA in maternal plasma is mainly placental DNA, and this discrepancy between aneuploidy in the placenta and the fetus may result in false-negative test results.

POINTS TO REMEMBER
Reasons for Discordant cffDNA Results

- False-negative results due to low fetal fraction, mosaicism, and absence of the abnormality in the placenta
- False-positive results due to statistical reasons, confined placental mosaicism, and maternal DNA abnormalities
- Incidental findings could be due to occult maternal malignancy or diseases with plasma DNA abnormalities, such as systemic lupus erythematosus.

False-positivity can be statistical. For example, chromosome 21 DNA amount is considered elevated when it is 3 standard deviations above that of a control population. However, 0.01% of the control population falls beyond 3 standard deviations in a one-tailed normal distribution. Therefore the choice of a cut-off value for aneuploidy detection influences the theoretical false-positive rate of the test. A relatively common biological reason for "false-positive" results is confined placental mosaicism.[65] Confined placental mosaicism refers to chromosomal aneuploidy in the placenta but not the fetus proper; one report showed that placental mosaicism occurred in 2% of cases by chorionic villus sampling.[66] Because cffDNA is placental DNA, placental mosaicism may cause false-positive test results reflecting the state of the placenta, not the fetus. In fact, only 13% of mosaic chorionic villus abnormalities are detected in amniocytes.[66] Finally, another reason for "false-positive" fetal aneuploidy detection relates to aneuploidies of the mother. This is especially the case for subclinical mosaic sex chromosome aneuploidies. It has been reported that 8.6% of the sex chromosome aneuploidies detected by cffDNA testing occur when the maternal blood cell DNA showed the same finding.[67] This most commonly occurs with monosomy X (45, X) and triple X (47, XXX). Consequently, some centers offer reflex confirmatory testing for maternal DNA when the cffDNA test suggests the presence of sex chromosome aneuploidy.[67]

Other non–pregnancy-related diseases may confound the use of cffDNA testing. For example, malignant tumors release cell-free DNA (see Chapter 71).[68] Occult malignancies have been suspected in pregnant women after cffDNA testing.[69] Suspicion arises when multiple chromosomal aneuploidies are detected in the same sample, or the cell-free DNA chromosomal copy number aberration shows a magnitude that is substantially larger than that expected for the measured fetal fraction. Other conditions, such as systemic lupus erythematosus, are also associated with abnormalities in the cell-free DNA profile.[70] If these abnormalities preexist in the plasma of a woman, the cffDNA test interpretation may become more challenging during pregnancy.

In summary, cffDNA results for chromosomal aneuploidy screening may, in rare instances, be inaccurate. Positive results require confirmation by definitive invasive testing. The obstetric history, other obstetric findings, and ultrasound features should be taken into account for the interpretation of the cffDNA tests. Each couple considering cffDNA testing for fetal chromosomal aneuploid screening should therefore be provided with pre- and post-test counselling so that informed decisions could be made.[71]

Single-Gene Diseases

Besides fetal chromosomal aneuploidies, many prenatal programs address the screening and diagnosis of single-gene diseases, such as cystic fibrosis, sickle cell anemia, and thalassemias. Noninvasive prenatal diagnosis of autosomal dominant diseases of paternal origin may be achieved in a similar manner to fetal rhesus D genotyping. For example, when a paternal mutation is detected in the plasma of a mother known not to share the same mutation as the father, this may imply that the fetus has inherited the paternal mutation.[72] Maternally inherited mutations, on the other hand, are more challenging to diagnose by cffDNA analysis because cffDNA is surrounded by maternal DNA molecules that harbor the mutation. In view of the maternal DNA interference, the fetal

inheritance of the maternal mutation can be assessed by quantifying the ratio between the variant and the wild-type alleles in the sample—namely, the relative mutation dosage approach (Fig. 72.3).[73] For example, for a person with a heterozygous mutation, there should be equal amounts of variant and wild-type alleles among the cell-free DNA molecules. When the person is pregnant with a heterozygous fetus, the relative amounts between the variant and wild-type alleles remain equal. If the fetus has not inherited the maternal mutation and is homozygous for the wild-type allele, there should be a slight overrepresentation in the wild-type allele compared with the variant allele. Finally, if the fetus is homozygous for the mutation (maternal mutation and the same mutation from the father), there would be a slight overrepresentation of the variant allele when compared with the wild-type allele. On the other hand, to detect compound heterozygous mutations, a combination approach could be used (i.e., direct detection of the paternal mutation combined with the allelic ratio assessment for the maternal mutation in maternal plasma) (see Fig. 72.3).

Protocols based on digital PCR[74] or sequencing have been developed for quantifying amounts of the maternal variant allele and wild-type allele in maternal plasma. Digital PCR protocols for the noninvasive assessment of beta-thalassemia, hemophilia, and sickle cell disease exist.[75,76] Sequencing-based protocols, such as those for beta-thalassemia and congenital adrenal hyperplasia,[77] use targeted capture of the disease locus. To render the protocols even more cost effective, haplotype-based analyses have been developed, termed *relative haplotype dosage analysis* (RHDO).[37,77] In the RHDO method, haplotypes of the variant and wild-type alleles are known. During interpretation of the maternal plasma DNA sequencing results, the number of DNA molecules detected that cover single nucleotide polymorphism (SNP) alleles belonging to the inheritance block that contains the mutation are counted. The counts from each consecutive informative SNP allele are combined. The same analysis is performed for the homologous allele that does not contain the mutation. The total number of DNA molecules that originate from the haplotype block of the allele containing the mutation are compared with the count for the haplotype block of the allele not containing the mutation. Based on a statistical comparison, an interpretation is made regarding which haplotype block the fetus has likely inherited—namely, the variant or the wild-type allele.[37,77] Targeted sequence analysis covering genomic loci of clinical importance may be the approach of choice to deliver noninvasive prenatal diagnosis of single-gene diseases. To realize this, more convenient methods to generate long-range haplotype information are needed.[77]

NONINVASIVE FETAL "OMICS"

Many advances have occurred in cffDNA analysis. Massively parallel sequencing (also known as next generation sequencing) has enabled an approach to determine the fetal genome noninvasively. Studies have demonstrated that the entire fetal genome is represented in maternal plasma.[37,39,78] Therefore fetal genotype determination for any disease loci is theoretically possible. Besides the fetal genome, the transcriptome[79] and the DNA methylome of the placenta[34] may be determined directly from maternal plasma analysis. These developments are particularly important because they offer the

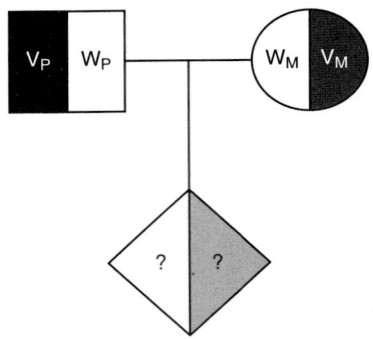

Condition	Approach
Autosomal dominant traits or mutations	
Paternally inherited	Qualitative detection of V_P
Maternally inherited	Quantitative comparison between V_M and W. If V_M = W, fetus has inherited V_M. If V_M < W, fetus has not inherited V_M.
Autosomal recessive conditions or diseases	
When V_P and V_M are identical	Quantitative comparison between V and W. If V = W, fetus is heterozygous. If V > W, fetus is homozygous for the variant. If V < W, fetus has not inherited the variant.
When V_P and V_M are different	Assess which paternal allele has been transmitted to the fetus by qualitative detection of V_P or W_P by a polymorphism that distinguishes W_P from V_P, V_M and W_M. Assess which maternal allele has been transmitted to the fetus by quantitative comparison between V_M and W. If V_M = W, fetus has inherited V_M. If V_M < W, fetus has not inherited V_M.

FIGURE 72.3 Approaches to noninvasive prenatal diagnosis of monogenic diseases by maternal plasma DNA analysis. *V,* Variant allele; V_M, maternally inherited variant allele; V_P, paternally inherited variant allele; *W,* wild-type allele; W_M, maternally inherited wild-type allele; W_P, paternally inherited wild-type allele.

means to monitor placental function. Placental dysfunction occurs or is suspected to occur in some pregnancy-associated diseases, such as preeclampsia, preterm labor, and intrauterine growth retardation. The ability to noninvasively monitor the health of the placenta by molecular means, which was previously not possible, means that the utility of maternal plasma cell-free nucleic acid analysis could be extended beyond the assessment of fetal genetic and chromosomal diseases.

ANALYTICAL ASPECTS

Cell-free nucleic acids exist in plasma in the form of short fragments and are present in low abundance. In addition, the key to successful analysis of cffDNA lies in the preservation and maximization of the fetal fraction in the maternal blood sample. Thus attention to a number of preanalytical and analytical details, as outlined below, is important to ensure the quality of the analysis.

Maternal Blood Sample Collection and Processing

One advantage of cffDNA analysis for prenatal screening is that, unlike maternal serum biochemistry testing, the use of the cffDNA tests is not restricted to a specific gestational period. This is because the cffDNA tests target the detection of the core pathologies of the fetus—for example, inherited mutations or chromosomal aneuploidies. These pathologies exist throughout the pregnancy. However, during the earliest stage of pregnancy, there may not be a sufficient amount of fetal DNA in the maternal circulation. While cffDNA has been detected in maternal plasma in individual pregnant women from as early as 18 days of pregnancy,[80] it becomes quantitatively sufficient for most testing purposes from about the 11th week of pregnancy. Between 9 and 13 weeks of gestation, 2% of pregnancies show fetal DNA fractions that are below 5% and are prone to potential false negativity.[50] Therefore some cffDNA testing programs specify the minimum gestational age for samples that are acceptable.[63]

As will be discussed, maximizing the fetal DNA fraction in the maternal sample is a key factor to many cffDNA tests. With such a consideration, maternal plasma is preferred over maternal serum since clotting of the maternal blood cells results in the release of more maternal DNA into serum as compared to plasma.[28] While the absolute fetal DNA amounts in plasma and serum are similar, the fetal DNA fraction is significantly reduced in serum. Even for plasma, different anticoagulants show varying degrees of efficacy in suppressing the rise in maternal background DNA over time. EDTA is more effective than heparin and citrate in maintaining a relatively stable total plasma DNA concentration and fetal DNA fraction up to about 24 hours after phlebotomy.[81] Some companies manufacture blood collection tubes containing proprietary cell-stabilizing reagents that are effective in maintaining the plasma DNA concentration and fetal fraction for up to 14 days.[82] The availability of these tubes has helped to facilitate the shipping of maternal blood samples across long distances for cffDNA testing.

After the maternal peripheral blood samples are collected, plasma is harvested via centrifugation. The goal of centrifugation is to minimize the residual maternal blood cells in the sample. Furthermore, it is not recommended to use hemolyzed samples for cffDNA analysis. Reduction in maternal DNA contamination results in maximization of the fetal fraction. Therefore two-step centrifugation protocols are recommended.[83] The plasma supernatant is carefully harvested after the first centrifugation with care not to disturb the underlying maternal blood cell layer. With the second centrifugation, the remaining cells in the form of a cell pellet are separated from the final supernatant. The resultant plasma can be stored frozen until further analysis.

Circulating Cell-free Fetal DNA Analysis

A significant amount of cffDNA has a length shorter than 100 bp.[37,38,84] For plasma DNA extraction, a protocol that is efficient in preserving the small DNA molecules is advantageous.[85] For the same reason, PCR assays intended for cffDNA or placental RNA detection should be designed to amplify shorter products, preferably less than 100 bp.[29,84,86] The fact that circulating fetal DNA molecules are generally shorter than maternal DNA can be used to enhance the detection of fetal DNA. Researchers have used size-selection methods to increase the proportional representation of short DNA within the sample or dataset to improve the detection of fetal DNA.[73,87,88] In addition, the detection of short DNA from maternal plasma can be used to detect fetal disorders.[89] The rationale is that when the fetus has an aneuploidy, such as trisomy 21, there should be an additional dose of short DNA from chromosome 21. Therefore the overall size profile of the chromosome 21 DNA molecules would be shorter than that of other nonaneuploid chromosomes. If the fetus has monosomy X, it is then expected that there would be less short DNA from chromosome X, and thus the overall size profile of chromosome X would be longer than the other nonaneuploid chromosomes.

Besides the need for maximizing the fetal DNA fraction, there are circumstances where it may be advantageous to employ measures to minimize the maternal DNA interference. Unless the fetal DNA sequence of interest is absent in the maternal genome—for example, chromosome Y or *RHD* in rhesus-negative women—the need to minimize the

background maternal DNA interference is particularly relevant when one aims to directly detect a fetal-specific sequence in maternal plasma. For example, for the detection of fetal-specific genetic variants in maternal plasma, the large background of wild-type DNA often results in nonspecificity of the assay.[90] Researchers have used a number of different approaches to minimize background maternal DNA. Minisequencing or primer extension assays have been designed that only allow the extension of the fetal DNA sequence but not the maternal DNA sequence.[90] Peptide nucleic acid clamping has been used to suppress the maternal DNA from interacting with the detection reagents of the fetal-specific assay.[91] Restriction enzyme cutting has been used to remove the maternal DNA sequence from the sample.[92] Single-molecule or digital PCR is conducted when the average amount of template DNA per reaction well is less than one molecule. Therefore the fetal DNA sequence is separated from the maternal counterpart sequence in the reaction environment and therefore is less prone to nonspecific amplification of the maternal DNA sequence.[73]

Measuring the Fetal DNA Fraction

Analysis of the fetal DNA fraction is an important quality control parameter for cffDNA analysis. For assays that aim to detect the presence of a fetal-specific DNA sequence, such as the presence of Y-chromosome sequences for determining male fetal sex and the presence of *RHD* to determine a rhesus D positive fetus, the inclusion of an internal fetal DNA control is preferable. The internal fetal DNA control is particularly useful when the assay reveals that the target sequence is negative. For example, when the Y-chromosome assay shows negative results, it may either mean the presence of the female fetus or the lack of fetal DNA in the sample. When the *RHD* assay is negative, it may mean the fetus is rhesus D negative or the sample lacked fetal DNA. The positive detection of an internal fetal DNA control in such situations would exclude the scenario of lack of fetal DNA. Thus the report for the female fetus or rhesus D negative fetus could be issued with confidence.

There are several different methods for detecting the presence of fetal DNA.[93] Some laboratories detect the fetal Y-chromosome sequence as the indicator of the presence of fetal DNA in the case of male fetuses. Some laboratories include the analysis of a panel of polymorphisms with the target sequence analysis. The panel aims to detect alleles that are not present in the maternal DNA or that show a minor contribution as an indicator of the presence of fetal DNA in the sample. Another approach is to detect placental-specific methylation signatures in maternal plasma. These are gene loci where the methylation status is opposite in the placenta as compared to the maternal blood cells. Assays specific for the detection of the placental form of the gene are used for maternal plasma analysis. The assay is designed to only detect the placental and not the maternal form of the DNA sequences. For example, the *RASSF1A* gene was shown to be hypermethylated in the placenta and not the maternal blood cells.[92] The presence of the methylated form of *RASSF1A* in maternal plasma suggests the presence of fetal/placental DNA.

There are a number of cffDNA tests where ensuring the presence of a minimum amount of fetal DNA in the sample—namely, the fetal DNA fraction—is an important quality control parameter.[63] For example, the noninvasive detection of fetal chromosomal aneuploidies by maternal plasma DNA sequencing and the assessment of the fetal inheritance of the maternal allele by relative mutation dosage or relative haplotype dosage all rely on the sample containing a certain minimum amount of fetal DNA.[63,73] The statistics developed to determine the presence or absence of a statistically significant difference in chromosome dosage or allelic ratio is dependent on the sample containing at least a certain amount of fetal DNA. Therefore for the tests based on massively parallel sequencing, the proportion of Y-chromosome sequences is often used as a fetal fraction measurement for chromosome Y–positive samples.[60] A panel of placenta-specific DNA methylation markers has also been developed to quantify the fetal DNA.[94] Recently, the proportion of short DNA in a sample has also been shown as a reasonable measure of the fetal DNA fraction.[89]

Massively Parallel Maternal Plasma DNA Sequencing

The advantage of massively parallel sequencing–based cffDNA assessment is that many maternal plasma DNA molecules can be analyzed per sample, regardless of whether the DNA fragment is originating from the fetus or the mother. For quantitative sequencing applications, such as for fetal chromosomal aneuploidy detection or relative haplotype dosage analysis, the key to success is to maximize the signal-to-noise ratio of the sequencing data covering the genetic abnormality of interest. Trying to maximize the fetal fraction improves the chance of detecting the fetal abnormality. Increasing the sequencing depth either for random or targeted sequencing improves the precision, and thus reduces the noise, for genomic representation or allelic ratio assessments.[50] The size of the genomic locus of interest also matters. At the same sequencing depth, larger loci, such as whole chromosome aneuploidies, are much easier to detect than subchromosomal aneuploidies.[46,47] Thus protocols for the detection of subchromosomal aneuploidies require higher sequencing depths. The current massively parallel sequencing protocols also suffer from a certain extent of GC bias. To reduce the imprecision surrounding the quantitative measurement of cffDNA by sequencing, GC normalization steps are typically included in the bioinformatics analysis of the data. This is especially important for the detection of aneuploidies in GC-rich chromosomes, such as chromosomes 13 and 18.

On the other hand, current massively parallel sequencing protocols have a sequencing error rate that cannot be ignored. This has an impact on the detection of single-nucleotide variants of the fetus. Because cffDNA is the minor species of DNA in maternal plasma, high-depth sequencing is needed to detect fetal single-nucleotide variants. Yet, the higher the total number of bases sequenced, the higher the chance for sequencing errors.[78] Thus extra care is needed in designing protocols for the detection of fetal single-nucleotide variants by sequencing. For example, targeted capture of loci of interest followed by sequencing is one feasible option. Targeted sequencing allows a high depth to be achieved without sequencing a high total number of bases, thereby reducing the number of sequencing errors detected and improving the signal-to-noise ratio.

POINTS TO REMEMBER
Analytical Factors to Be Mindful of

- EDTA plasma is preferred over serum.
- When delayed blood processing is expected, collection of blood into tubes containing cell-stabilizing agents is recommended.
- Avoid hemolysis.
- Harvest the plasma using protocols to remove as much of the maternal blood cells as possible.
- Use protocols that preserve the short cell-free DNA molecules.
- Design assays to maximize the chance of detecting the short cffDNA molecules.
- Consider approaches to further minimize the effect of the maternal DNA interference.
- Include an internal control to indicate the presence of fetal DNA or measure the fetal DNA fraction.
- Maximize the signal-to-noise ratio of the massively parallel sequencing protocols used for cffDNA analysis.

CONCLUSION

Cell-free fetal nucleic acids in the maternal circulation are a reliable and noninvasive source of fetal genetic material. Knowledge about their biological properties has translated into useful information for guiding the design of the preanalytical and analytical approaches relevant for cffDNA analysis. cffDNA analysis is useful for the prenatal assessment of fetal chromosomal aneuploidies and genetic diseases. Its effectiveness in some of these areas has led to a major reduction in the number of amniocenteses performed worldwide. cffDNA analysis has the potential to detail the entire fetal genome noninvasively before the birth of the child. Nonetheless, the vast amount of information that one may be able to access before the birth of the child has raised some potential concerns and spurred research interests in studying the ethical, legal, and social implications of such technologies.[95] It remains to be seen how noninvasive prenatal diagnostics will continue to develop and how it will contribute to improving and maintaining fetal and maternal health.

SELECTED REFERENCES

27. Lo YMD, Corbetta N, Chamberlain PF, et al. Presence of fetal DNA in maternal plasma and serum. Lancet 1997;350:485–7.
28. Lo YMD, Tein MS, Lau TK, et al. Quantitative analysis of fetal DNA in maternal plasma and serum: Implications for noninvasive prenatal diagnosis. Am J Hum Genet 1998;62:768–75.
30. Devaney SA, Palomaki GE, Scott JA, Bianchi DW. Noninvasive fetal sex determination using cell-free fetal DNA: a systematic review and meta-analysis. JAMA 2011;306:627–36.
37. Lo YMD, Chan KCA, Sun H, et al. Maternal plasma DNA sequencing reveals the genome-wide genetic and mutational profile of the fetus. Sci Transl Med 2010;2:61ra91.
40. Han DSC, Ni M, Chan RWY, et al. The biology of cell-free DNA fragmentation and the roles of DNASE1, DNASE1L3, and DFFB. Am J Hum Genet 2020;106:202–14.

43. van der Schoot CE, Hahn S, Chitty LS. Non-invasive prenatal diagnosis and determination of fetal RH status. Semin Fetal Neonatal Med 2008;13:63–8.

44. Chiu RWK, Chan KCA, Gao Y, et al. Noninvasive prenatal diagnosis of fetal chromosomal aneuploidy by massively parallel genomic sequencing of DNA in maternal plasma. Proc Natl Acad Sci U S A 2008;105:20458–63.

46. Srinivasan A, Bianchi DW, Huang H, Sehnert AJ, Rava RP. Noninvasive detection of fetal subchromosome abnormalities via deep sequencing of maternal plasma. Am J Hum Genet 2013;92:167–76.

49. Ryan A, Hunkapiller N, Banjevic M, et al. Validation of an enhanced version of a single-nucleotide polymorphism-based noninvasive prenatal test for detection of fetal aneuploidies. Fetal Diagn Ther 2016;40:219–23.

54. Gregg AR, Skotko BG, Benkendorf JL, et al. Noninvasive prenatal screening for fetal aneuploidy, 2016 update: A position statement of the American College of Medical Genetics and Genomics. Genet Med 2016;18:1056–65.

61. Bianchi DW, Parker RL, Wentworth J, et al. DNA sequencing versus standard prenatal aneuploidy screening. N Engl J Med 2014;370:799–808.

62. Neyt M, Hulstaert F, Gyselaers W. Introducing the non-invasive prenatal test for trisomy 21 in belgium: a cost-consequences analysis. BMJ Open 2014;4:e005922.

63. Hui L, Bianchi DW. Fetal fraction and noninvasive prenatal testing: What clinicians need to know. Prenat Diagn 2020;40:155–63.

65. Bianchi DW, Chiu RWK. Sequencing of circulating cell-free DNA during pregnancy. N Engl J Med 2018;379:464–73.

69. Dharajiya NG, Grosu DS, Farkas DH, et al. Incidental detection of maternal neoplasia in noninvasive prenatal testing. Clin Chem 2018;64:329–35.

71. Sachs A, Blanchard L, Buchanan A, Norwitz E, Bianchi DW. Recommended pre-test counseling points for noninvasive prenatal testing using cell-free DNA: A 2015 perspective. Prenat Diagn 2015;35:968–71.

75. Camunas-Soler J, Lee H, Hudgins L, et al. Noninvasive prenatal diagnosis of single-gene disorders by use of droplet digital PCR. Clin Chem 2018;64:336–45.

77. Hui WWI, Jiang P, Tong YK, et al. Universal haplotype-based noninvasive prenatal testing for single gene diseases. Clin Chem 2017;63:513–24.

89. Yu SCY, Chan KCA, Zheng YW, et al. Size-based molecular diagnostics using plasma DNA for noninvasive prenatal testing. Proc Natl Acad Sci U S A 2014;111:8583–8.

95. Greely HT. Get ready for the flood of fetal gene screening. Nature 2011;469:289–91.

73

Pharmacogenetics*

Gwendolyn Appell McMillin, Mia Wadelius, and Victoria M. Pratt

ABSTRACT

Background

Pharmacogenetics describes how genes influence drug response. Genes can impact either the pharmacokinetics or pharmacodynamics of a drug to influence the dose required and associated therapeutic or toxic effects. Pharmacogenetic testing performed before drug administration may guide the selection of drugs and drug dosing. Post-therapeutic pharmacogenetic testing can explain an adverse drug reaction, including therapeutic failure.

Content

This chapter reviews pharmacokinetics and pharmacodynamics, the two major processes involved in drug response,

and describes how genes that encode for proteins involved in these processes influence drug response. Important nongenetic factors that influence drug response, such as drug formulation differences, drug–drug and food–drug interactions, and clinical status are discussed, along with appropriate specimens and analytical strategies for performing, reporting, and interpreting pharmacogenetic testing results. In addition, specific gene–drug examples are described in detail relative to the nomenclature of genetic variants and allele assignments, genotype-phenotype predictions, clinical applications, and associated guidance for dosing.

---

*The full version of this chapter is available electronically on ExpertConsult.com.

Hematology and Coagulation

Exam questions, case studies, and additional resources are available on ExpertConsult.com.
*Full versions of these chapters are available electronically on www.ExpertConsult.com.

74

Automated Hematology*

Devon S. Chabot-Richards, Qian-Yun Zhang, and Tracy I. George

ABSTRACT

Background

The roots of automated hematology began with manual microscopy and laborious cell counting techniques. Using the Coulter principle and advances in laboratory methodology, automated hematology is now rapid and inexpensive with the complete blood cell count (CBC) being one of the most commonly ordered tests in medicine.

Content

This chapter describes the principles of automated hematology, including how we measure red blood cells (RBCs), white blood cells (WBCs), and platelets from whole blood. Next, the laboratory parameters that are derived from the measurement of RBCs, WBCs, and platelets are discussed. These include standard laboratory measurements of the CBC which help describe anemia, such as the mean corpuscular volume (MCV), to newer measurements which quantitate immature granulocytes (IG), immature platelets (IPF), and immature reticulocytes (IRF). The uses of recently introduced laboratory parameters in automated hematology are also described.

*The full version of this chapter is available electronically on ExpertConsult.com.

Leukocyte Morphology in Blood and Bone Marrow*

Daniel Babu, Tracy I. George, and Devon S. Chabot-Richards

ABSTRACT

Background
Leukocytes comprise a wide variety of cell types, and evaluation of these components is critical in medical and clinical laboratory practice. Although sensitive laboratory methods may offer strong clues about leukocyte abnormalities, accurate morphologic evaluation of these cells is key in confirming suspicion for a pathologic process and in guiding clinical decision making. However, proper assessment of these cells requires understanding of normal quantitative and morphologic parameters and the deviations from these that are seen in neoplastic and non-neoplastic states.

Content
This chapter discusses essential aspects of evaluating of leukocyte components most commonly found in peripheral blood and bone marrow specimens. The clinical value of leukocyte morphologic examination will be discussed with an overview of specimen preparation and normal quantitative ranges. Morphologic features of granulocytes, maturing myelomonocytic cells, lymphocytes, plasma cells, and other special cell types will be detailed. Importantly, this chapter describes cytomorphologic changes of such cells representing a spectrum of neoplastic and non-neoplastic conditions.

---

*The full version of this chapter is available electronically on ExpertConsult.com.

Red Blood Cell Morphology and Indices: The Clinical Chemistry Interface*

Hooman H. Rashidi, Nam K. Tran, and Ralph Green

ABSTRACT

Background

A fundamental understanding of the basis and clinical significance of standard laboratory tests in hematology and associated peripheral blood smear findings is essential for analysis and interpretation of certain chemistry test results. The overlap between hematology and chemistry is also an important aspect in most chemistry and hematology laboratories. Rigorous quality control ensuring accuracy and precision applies to both. These inter-relationships are bidirectional; perturbations of blood chemistry can influence hematologic measurements, and conversely, hematologic abnormalities may affect analyte determinations in the clinical chemistry laboratory.

Content

This chapter describes the basic concepts and definitions in hematology, specifically looking at metric data on red blood cell parameters generated in the automated complete blood count and the most common peripheral blood smear red blood cell findings, with particular focus on the overlap of certain hematology and chemistry tests. Perturbations of numerous blood analytes and substances and abnormal hematologic conditions can introduce spurious results in various output measurements in the clinical laboratory, especially within hematology and chemistry domains. Certain substances and conditions can lead to false increase or false decrease in various test results, and, if not corrected or noticed, they may lead or contribute to misleading information with adverse patient outcomes. An awareness of such substances and conditions in patient management and in the scope of accurate laboratory test usage will ultimately enhance patient care and minimize adverse effects and unnecessary or inappropriate treatments.

Just as the automated chemistry analyzer represents the backbone instrument used in the clinical chemistry laboratory that provides essential information covering a broad swath of clinical decision making, so the automated blood counting instrument is the engine that drives and informs most decisions that emanate from the laboratory hematology section of a modern clinical laboratory.

Although widely diverse in their design and purpose—blood cell counters focus on the formed elements of the blood, whereas chemistry analyzers are concerned largely with the composition of the plasma—the functionality and the integrity of the data generated by both of these two mainstay instruments have important and sometimes critical intersections. Aberrations in blood chemistry composition can substantially affect the results generated by blood counting instruments, and abnormalities that arise in the formed elements of the blood that are the feature of hematologic disorders can be associated with or lead to changes in blood chemistry composition that are reflected in real or spurious abnormalities in clinical chemistry values.

---

*The full version of this chapter is available electronically on ExpertConsult.com.

Hemoglobin and Hemoglobinopathies

Jason C.C. So and Edmond S.K. Ma[a]

ABSTRACT

Background

Disorders of hemoglobin (Hb) are collectively the commonest Mendelian disease found in humans. These disorders encompass both thalassemia and hemoglobinopathies. Thalassemia refers to quantitative deficiencies of one or more globin sub-units of the Hb molecule, with α-thalassemia and β-thalassemia being defined as reduced or absent production of α-globin and β-globin chains, respectively. Hemoglobinopathies are a qualitative defect resulting from globin gene mutations that change the amino acid sequence and lead to the production of Hb variants. Overlaps between the two forms of globin disorders occur. Some forms of β-thalassemia result from structural hemoglobin variants that are not effectively synthesized or are unstable, leading to a functional deficiency of β-globin chains and a thalassemic phenotype. Globin disorders are the first genetic diseases to be characterized at the molecular level and early work in the field opened up the era of molecular medicine. Thalassemia and hemoglobinopathies occur at the highest frequency in countries of the tropics, although they are seen at increasing frequencies among the emigrants from this region to other countries, hence causing significant health care burden worldwide.

Content

This chapter describes the protein structure, biosynthesis, switching, and physiologic function of hemoglobin. Emphasis is placed on the analytical methods, ranging from hematologic investigation and hemoglobin study to molecular methods of detection. Challenges and caveats on the interpretation of laboratory data are discussed. Clinical aspects of thalassemic syndromes and hemoglobinopathies are described to illustrate the significance of the laboratory studies.

BIOCHEMISTRY, GENETICS, AND PHYSIOLOGY OF HEMOGLOBIN

Hemoglobin is a hemoprotein whose primary function is to transport oxygen from the lungs to body tissues. It was first isolated in 1849, and was the first oligomeric protein to be characterized by ultracentrifugation and to have (1) its molecular mass accurately determined, (2) its physiologic function described, and (3) after the 25-year study of Perutz and colleagues in Cambridge, its structure defined by x-ray crystallography.[1] In 1949, Pauling and colleagues[2] showed that Hb from patients with sickle cell disease differed from normal Hb because it has two to four additional net positive charges. Later, the reasons for the charge difference were elucidated by locating the single amino acid difference between Hb from normal individuals and Hb from those with sickle cell disease.[3–6]

Biochemistry

Hemoglobin is a globular protein with a diameter of 6.4 nm and a molecular mass of approximately 64,500 Da. As shown in Fig. 77.1, Hb consists of four globin subunits (two α- and two non–α- [β-, γ-, or δ]-chains), with each looped around itself to form a pocket or cleft in which the heme group nestles. Normally, this heme pocket is formed entirely by nonpolar (hydrophobic) amino acids. The heme moiety (see Fig. 77.1) is suspended within this pocket by an attachment of its Fe atom to the imidazole group of the proximal histidine (position 92 of the β-chain [β92] or position 87 of the α-chain [α87]). The imidazole group of the distal histidine (β63 or α58) is also in contiguity with the Fe of heme, but it appears to swing into and out of this position to permit the passage of oxygen into and out of the Hb molecule. The four Fe atoms are in the divalent state, whether Hb is oxygenated or deoxygenated.

Protein Structure

As with all proteins, the function of Hb is dictated by its primary, secondary, tertiary, and quaternary structures.

Primary structure. The α- and non–α-globin chains of Hb are 141 and 146 amino acid residues in length, respectively. Some sequence homology has been noted, with 64 individual amino acid residues in identical positions in both α- and β-chains. The β-chain differs from the δ- and γ-chains by 39 and 10 residues, respectively. The amino terminal of the β-globin chain is the site of attachment of glucose (HbA_{1c}), urea, and salicylate.[7] The carboxy terminal amino acid of the β-chain is tyrosine and can function as a part of salt bridges. Although no disulfide bonds are present, six SH groups have

[a]The authors gratefully acknowledge the contributions of M. Domenica Cappellini, Stanley F. Lo, and Dorine W. Swinkels, upon which portions of this chapter are based.

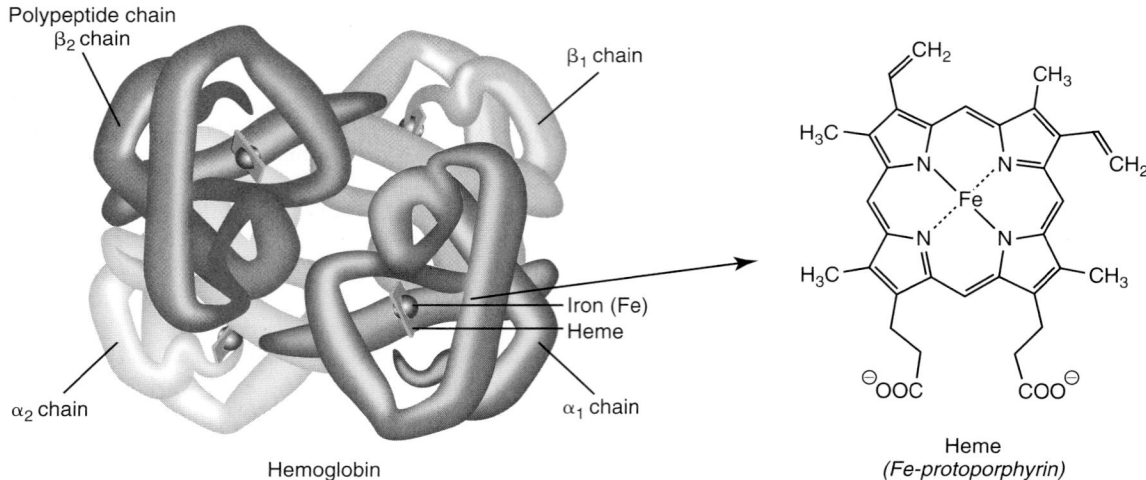

FIGURE 77.1 Model of the hemoglobin tetramer with the α-chain subunits facing the reader. Each subunit contains a molecule of heme attached to an atom of iron.

been noted (from cysteine at positions α104, β93, and β112). The γ-chain has a glycine amino terminal, and the alkali resistance of Hb F is attributed to the presence of threonine and tryptophan at positions 112 and 130 of the γ-chain, respectively. The γ-chain is unique in that it is the only globin chain to be highly susceptible to acetylation, and acetylated Hb F is a prominent feature in cord and neonatal blood, and may form as much as 25% of the total Hb. The N-terminal valine of the β-globin chain of HbA$_{1c}$ can also be acetylated to a smaller degree (<1 to 3%), for example, in alcoholic liver disease.[7]

Secondary structure. Approximately 75 to 80% of polypeptide chains of the α- and non–α-chains are arranged in helices, with the remainder forming nonhelical turns. The β-chain of Hb A is arranged into eight helices identified as A through H. In contrast, the α-chain is missing an equivalent of the D helix and has only seven helices. Nomenclature within the helices identifies the helix and the position within the helix of the amino acid residue (e.g., F3 is the third amino acid residue in the F helix). Amino acid residues in the peptide chains that join adjacent helices are described by the identification of two adjacent helices and the position of residues within the joining peptide. For example, EF3 would be the third residue in the peptide joining the E and F helices.

Tertiary structure. The tertiary structure of Hb refers to the arrangement of helices into a three-dimensional, pretzel-like structure. The heme group, located in a crevice between the E and F helices, is attached to histidine residues in each globin chain. Heme iron is axially hinged to globin proteins by an invariant histidine residue in helix F8, termed the proximal histidine. The opposite axial position binds O$_2$, which is stabilized by interaction with the conserved distal histidine in helix E7. This attachment is essential to maintaining the secondary and tertiary structure of the globin chains.

Quaternary structure. The quaternary structure of Hb results from the attachment of the four globin chains to each other. Within the Hb tetramer, each globin subunit binds the unlike chain through two distinct interfaces, termed the

α1β1 and α1β2. The globin dimers are formed through the extremely high affinity α1β1 interaction. Globin monomers are relatively unstable compared with dimers, which tend to precipitate inside the red cell and cause erythrotoxicity. Thus mutations that impair α1β1 interaction may cause hemolytic anemia. On the other hand, the α1β2 interaction is of lower affinity and mediates tetramerization. Oxygen binding destabilizes the α1β2 interaction that results in the transition of quaternary structure from the T state (tense, deoxygenated) to the R state (relaxed, oxygenated), which facilitates O$_2$ binding to additional subunits. This process causes cooperative O$_2$ binding as illustrated by the characteristic sigmoidal shape of the oxygen dissociation curve. Mutations within the α1β2 interaction region alter the functional property of Hb by disturbing O$_2$ binding characteristics. Cooperativity represents a general phenomenon termed allosteric regulation, in which effector molecules exert effect by binding to regions that are distinct from the active site. In addition to O$_2$, another allosteric regulator H$^+$ binds Hb to promote O$_2$ release in a process termed the Bohr effect.[8] The compound 2,3-biphosphoglycerate (2,3-BPG), formed as a result of glycolysis and present at relatively high concentrations in red blood cells, is another important allosteric regulator.

Modified Hemoglobins

In addition to the Hbs discussed previously, carboxyhemoglobin, methemoglobin, and sulfhemoglobin are other Hbs whose structures have been environmentally or chemically modified.

Each of the modified Hbs has a characteristic spectral pattern, as shown in Fig. 77.2. These spectral characteristics form the basis of analysis in the many co-oximeters and blood gas analyzers (see Chapter 37) that provide, in a single analysis, the simultaneous quantitative measurement of carboxyhemoglobin, methemoglobin, and sulfhemoglobin. The spectral scans are performed using multidiode arrays covering a number of wavelengths, followed by patented calculations that discriminate between normal and modified Hbs.

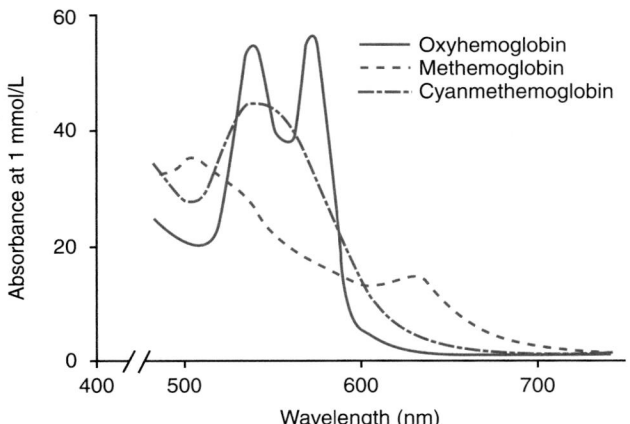

FIGURE 77.2 Spectrophotometric absorption curves for oxyhemoglobin, methemoglobin, and cyanmethemoglobin. Oxyhemoglobin and cyanmethemoglobin are used in measuring the concentration of hemoglobin *(Hb)*. The peak at 630 nm, which is distinctive for methemoglobin, is abolished by addition of cyanide, and the resultant decrease in absorbance is directly proportional to the methemoglobin concentration. All heme proteins exhibit their maximum absorbance in the Soret band region of 400 to 440 nm. Because the absorbance of Hb in the Soret region is approximately 10 times the absorbance at 540 nm, the Soret peaks have been omitted from this diagram. The absorbance curve for methemoglobin is greatly influenced by small changes in pH. The curve given here was obtained at a pH of 6.6.

Carboxyhemoglobin

Carboxyhemoglobin is formed by the preferential attachment of carbon monoxide instead of oxygen to Hb. Carboxyhemoglobin concentrations (usually expressed as a carboxyhemoglobin saturation) have been known to reach 20% in individuals who are exposed to significant workplace concentrations of carbon monoxide. For example, police directing traffic at busy intersections and workers in radiator and welding shops have high carboxyhemoglobin concentrations at the end of the working day. The ability to perform heavy manual work or complex tasks is impaired at carboxyhemoglobin concentrations of 10% or even less for some individuals.[9] Faulty home furnaces and automobile exhaust systems have been known to produce large amounts of carbon monoxide, sometimes with tragic results. Carboxyhemoglobin saturation that varies from 15 to 25% may be associated with dizziness, headaches, and nausea, and greater than 50% saturation is considered life threatening.[10] After removal of the exposed individual from the carbon monoxide source, a slow decline in carboxyhemoglobin saturation occurs, in keeping with the half-life of 4 to 5 hours at sea level.[11]

Methemoglobin

The Fe of heme is normally in the reduced ferrous state (Fe^{2+}). Under alkaline conditions, the Fe is oxidized to the ferric state (Fe^{3+}) by toxic agents, such as nitrates (found in some well waters), aniline dyes, chlorates, drugs (e.g., quinones, phenacetin, and sulfonamides), or local anesthetics (e.g., procaine, benzocaine, and lidocaine). This oxidation converts the heme to hematin[12] and the Hb to methemoglobin. Patients with methemoglobin are cyanotic because ferric hemes of methemoglobin bind oxygen irreversibly. These patients are labeled as pseudocyanotic since the O_2 saturation

of Hb is low despite adequate arterial oxygenation. Low levels of methemoglobin are normally reduced to Hb in the cell by the reduced form of the nicotinamide-adenine dinucleotide–cytochrome reductase system.

Hereditary methemoglobinemia is a rare condition that was first described in Europeans, but was later found in individuals of many racial backgrounds. Familial methemoglobinemia in an autosomal recessive mode of transmission is due to a deficiency in the enzyme nicotinamide-adenine dinucleotide–cytochrome b5 reductase. Hb variants, Hb M Saskatoon, Hb Freiburg, and Hb St. Louis stabilize the ferric Fe state and are associated with an autosomal dominant familial methemoglobinemia. The presence of methemoglobin in unexplained cyanosis can be identified through measurement of its absorption spectrum, either by simple spectroscopy or more definitely by spectrophotometry. Methemoglobinemia is treated by the administration of methylene blue. Ascorbic acid is less effective and may be used where methylene blue cannot be used.

Sulfhemoglobin

Sulfhemoglobin is produced by the reaction of sulfur-containing compounds with heme to form an irreversible chemical alteration and oxidation of Hb by the introduction of sulfur in one or more of the porphyrin rings. The most common cause of sulfhemoglobinemia is exposure to drugs,[13] such as phenacetin and sulfonamides. Sulfhemoglobin cannot transport oxygen, and cyanosis is noted at low concentrations.

Biosynthesis

The biosynthesis of Hb requires the biosynthesis of both heme and the globin polypeptide chains.

Heme Biosynthesis

Heme, ferrous protoporphyrin IX, consists of four pyrrole rings surrounding an iron (Fe) atom with four of the six electron pairs of Fe attached to the nitrogen atoms in the pyrrole rings (see Chapter 40). One of the remaining electron pairs attaches to a histidine residue in a globin chain, and the other pair is available for binding and transporting an oxygen molecule. The latter electron pair is protected from oxidation by the surrounding nonpolar amino acid residues of the globin chain. Hemin results from the relatively easy oxidation of the Fe of heme, from the ferrous to the ferric state.[12] To remain electrically neutral, a halide molecule, usually chloride, becomes attached to hemin. In alkaline solution, hematin is formed by the replacement of the halide atom of hemin by a hydroxyl group.

The biosynthesis of heme, shown schematically in Fig. 77.3, takes place primarily in the bone marrow and the liver, and is an eight-step process, with each step involving a different genetically controlled enzyme. Details of this process are given in Chapter 40.

Heme synthesis is controlled by a regulatory negative feedback loop that relies on post-translational regulation through the interaction of iron-regulatory proteins (IRP) with iron-responsive elements (IRE) on the messenger ribonucleic acid (mRNA) that encodes iron transporters, ferroproteins, and enzymes involved in cellular iron homeostasis. Excess heme inhibits the activity of ferrochelatase and the acquisition of Fe from the transport protein transferrin. The decrease in Fe acquisition leads to a decrease in Fe uptake

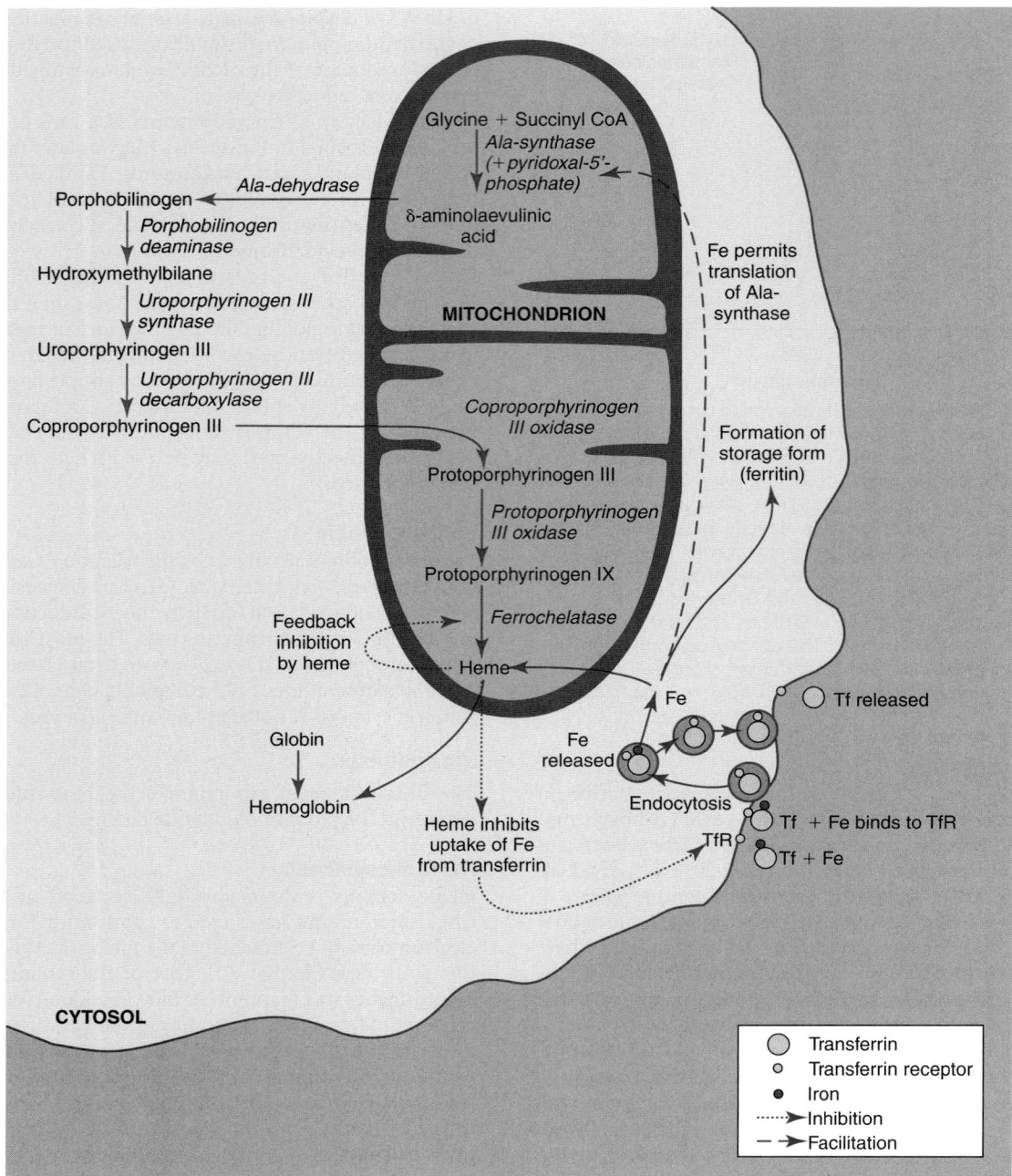

FIGURE 77.3 Heme synthesis. *CoA*, Co-enzyme A; *Fe*, iron; *TfR*, transferrin receptor. (From Bain BJ. *Haemoglobinopathy diagnosis.* London: Blackwell; 2001.)

into the cell, with a subsequent decrease in δ-aminolevulinic acid and heme production. Conversely, Fe deficiency and increased erythropoietin synthesis lead to the combination of the IRP with the IRE in the 3′-end of the transferrin receptor protein mRNA. This combination in turn leads to protection of the mRNA from degradation with subsequent increased uptake of Fe into erythroid cells caused by the increased expression of transferrin receptors on the cell membrane.

Globin Synthesis and Globin Gene Families
The genes that control the α-like and ζ-globin chains are located in a cluster on chromosome 16 at position 16p13.3,

which is near the chromosome 16 telomere (Fig. 77.4). The α-like gene extends more than 28 kb, and contains, reading from the upstream (5′) end to the downstream (3′) end of the DNA segment, an embryonic α-like ζ-globin gene, a hypervariable region, a pseudo(ψ)–ζ-gene, a pair of pseudo (ψ)–α-genes, a pair of functional α-globin genes, an unexpressed α-like θ gene, and finally, another hypervariable region. Approximately 25 to 65 kb upstream of the α-globin genes are four highly conserved noncoding sequences known as multispecies conserved sequences (MCS) and termed MCS-R1 to MCS-R4, which are involved in the regulation of the α-globin genes. Of these elements to date, only MCS-R2,

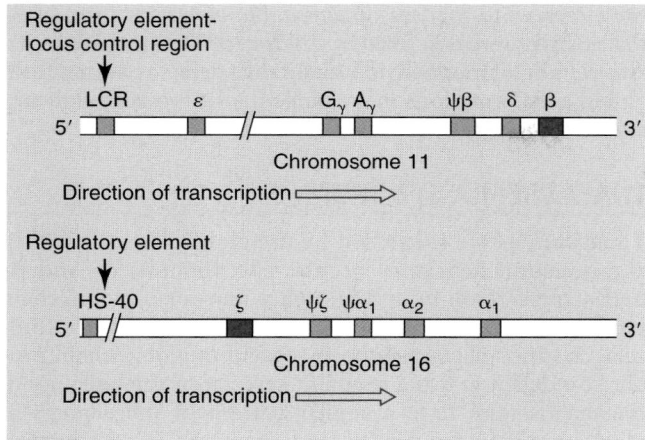

FIGURE 77.4 Globin α- and β-gene clusters. *LCR,* Locus control region. (From Bain BJ. *Haemoglobinopathy diagnosis.* London: Blackwell; 2001.)

TABLE 77.1 Hemoglobins in Embryonic, Fetal, and Adult Life			
	GLOBIN CHAINS		
Stage of Development	**α-Cluster**	**β-Cluster**	**Hemoglobins**
Embryonic	ζ, α	ε	Hb Gower 1 ($\zeta_2\varepsilon_2$)
			Hb Gower 2 ($\alpha_2\varepsilon_2$)
			Hb Portland 1 ($\zeta_2\gamma_2$)
			Hb Portland 2 ($\zeta_2\beta_2$)
Fetal	α	γ	Hb F ($\alpha_2\gamma_2$)
Adult	α	β, γ, δ	Hb A ($\alpha_2\beta_2$)
			Hb F ($\alpha_2\gamma_2$)
			Hb A_2 ($\alpha_2\delta_2$)

also known as HS-40, has been shown to be essential for α-globin gene expression.[14] Alpha-thalassemia arises from the deletion of one or more α-globin genes or point mutations. Deletion of all four genes results in the condition of Hb Bart hydrops fetalis and is typically incompatible with life. Substantial genetic variability is seen between individuals and ethnic groups with respect to the copy number of the ζ-, ψζ-, and α-genes.

The β-, γ-, and δ-globin genes are clustered closely together on chromosome 11. Reading from the 5′ end, the gene sequence is an ε-gene followed by two γ-genes (designated Gγ and Aγ, respectively), a pseudo–ψβ-gene, a δ-gene, and a β-gene. Therefore two genes encode the γ-chain, with one gene each encoding the δ- and β-chains. Upstream to the β-globin locus is the locus control region (LCR), consisting of several DNase I hypersensitive sites that contain binding motifs for transcription activators. The LCR functions as an enhancer to regulate the spatiotemporal transcription of the globin genes. When the globin gene is actively transcribed, the LCR hypersensitive sites are positioned in close proximity to the active gene, forming a chromatin loop.

The globin genes have three exons and two introns with a promoter region (specific for the globin chain) at the 5′ end of each gene. This structure has been highly conserved throughout evolution. The upstream regions flanking the first exon contain a number of sequence motifs that are necessary for specifying correct transcriptional initiation, such as a TATA box found 30 bp upstream of the initiation site, and one or more CCAAT sites at 70 bp upstream. The gene promoters also contain a CACCC or CCGCCC box that binds erythroid Krüppel-like factor 1, and some have binding sites for erythroid transcription factor GATA-1. In model systems, mutations introduced into such sequences lead to reduction in the level of transcription and are known as transcriptional mutants.[15]

Hemoglobin Switching

In normal human adults, Hb A is composed of two normal α- and two normal β-polypeptide chains and is represented symbolically as $\alpha_2\beta_2$ (Table 77.1); it represents at least 96% of the total Hb. Hb A_2 is typically approximately 2.5 to 3.5% of total Hb; it contains two α- and two δ-chains, and is designated as $\alpha_2\delta_2$. HbA2′ is considered a variant of Hb A_2

and is the result of a glycine-to-arginine substitution in the 16th position of the δ-chain; it occurs in 1 to 2% of African Americans. It rarely forms more than 3% of the total Hb and has no clinical implication. Fetal Hb (Hb F) predominates during fetal life but rapidly diminishes during the first year of postnatal life. In normal adults, less than 1% of Hb is Hb F. It consists of two α- and two γ-chains ($\alpha_2\gamma_2$).

In early embryonic life, the yolk sac produces the globin chains ζ and ε (see Table 77.1). These globin chains combine to form the major embryonic Hbs, Hb Gower 1 ($\zeta_2\varepsilon_2$) and 2 ($\alpha_2\varepsilon_2$), and Hb Portland 1 ($\zeta_2\gamma_2$) and 2 ($\zeta_2\beta_2$). Production of the ζ-chain ceases at the gestational age of approximately 4 months.

Production of α- and γ-chains starts at approximately 6 weeks' gestation, with Hb F ($\alpha_2\gamma_2$) increasing in concentration to become the major Hb found in the fetus (Fig. 77.5). Glycine or alanine may be found at position 136 of the γ-chain in the fetus, giving rise to two distinct γ-chains designated Gγ and Aγ, respectively. Formation of Hb A ($\alpha_2\beta_2$)

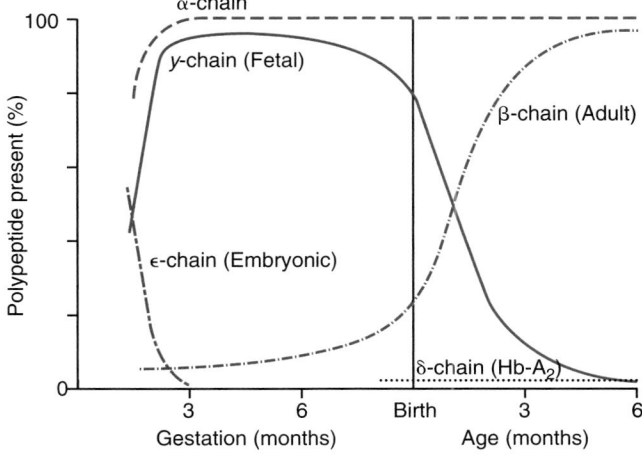

FIGURE 77.5 Changes in relative proportions of globin chains at various stages of embryonic, fetal, and postnatal life. *Hb-A₂,* Glycosylated hemoglobin. (Reprinted from Huehns ER, Dance N, Beaven GH, Hecht F, Motulsky AG. Human embryonic hemoglobins. *Cold Spring Harbor Symp Quant Biol* 1965;29:327–31.)

commences at approximately 28 weeks of gestation, and at birth it can form up to 15% of the total Hb, with the remainder of the Hb consisting mainly of Hb F with a small amount of Hb A_2. Production of the γ-chain declines after birth, and normal adult Hb F concentrations are usually obtained by 1 year of age but may be elevated until 2 years of age.

Physiologic Role

The Fe of heme is in the ferrous state and is able to combine reversibly with oxygen to act as the major oxygen-carrying moiety. The term *cooperativity* is used to describe the interaction of globin chains in such a way that oxygenation of one heme group enhances the probability of oxygenation of the other heme group. The *Bohr effect*[8] refers to reduction of oxygen affinity due to a decrease in pH from the physiologic range (7.35 to 7.45) to 6.0, and is another result of this cooperativity. Because the pH of the tissue decreases as a result of the presence of the end products of anaerobic metabolism, carbon dioxide (CO_2) and carbonic acid, the delivery of oxygen to the exercising tissue is enhanced. The oxygen dissociation curve of normal blood Hb is sigmoidal (Fig. 77.6). Physiologically, the CO_2 reversibly combines with the amino terminal groups of Hb to form carbamated Hb, which facilitates the removal of approximately 10% of the CO_2 that forms because of metabolism in the tissue to the lungs. Removal and transport of CO_2 from the tissue are enhanced by the preference for the attachment of more CO_2 by carbamated Hb.

Clinical Significance of Hemoglobin Disorders

The thalassemia syndromes and hemoglobinopathies are clinical disorders related to Hb. They are collectively the commonest Mendelian or single gene disorders in the world. Although their clinical manifestations may overlap,[15] they form two distinct groups of genetic disorders. Thalassemia refers to quantitative deficiency of one or more globin subunits of the Hb molecule. The name *thalassemia* is derived from the Greek word for "sea," *thalassa*, because early cases of β-thalassemia were described in children of Mediterranean origin. Hemoglobinopathy is a qualitative defect resulting from globin gene mutations that change the amino acid sequence and lead to the production of Hb variants.

THALASSEMIA SYNDROMES

Thalassemias are identified by the globin chain in which a production deficiency occurs. For example, α- and β-thalassemias result from a deficiency in α- or β-globin chain production, respectively (Box 77.1). They are further clinically classified depending on the extent of globin chain production deficit and the resultant severity of the anemia. All the thalassemias have a similar pattern of inheritance: in most cases the gene defects are transmitted in a Mendelian autosomal recessive fashion. Thus the severe symptomatic clinical forms result from the inheritance of homozygous or compound heterozygous genotypes. The inheritance of α-thalassemia is more complicated because it involves the products of the linked pairs of α-globin genes (αα).

α-Thalassemias

The α-thalassemias arise from deficiencies in production of the α-globin chains and are caused by deletions or (less frequently) point mutations in one or more of the four α-globin genes.[16] The conventional nomenclature for the point mutations of an α-gene is "$\alpha^T\alpha$," and for deletion, it is "−α." Deletion of one α-globin gene (−α/) is termed α^+-thalassemia (or α-thal-2) while deletion of two α-globin genes on the same chromosome (− −/) is termed α^0-thalassemia (or α-thal-1). Point mutations are much less frequent. The clinical spectrum of α-thalassemias correlates well with the number of the affected α-genes (i.e., from normal to the loss of all four genes). The inheritance of one or two α-globin gene deletion or mutation in various genotypic configuration results in a "α-thalassemia minor"

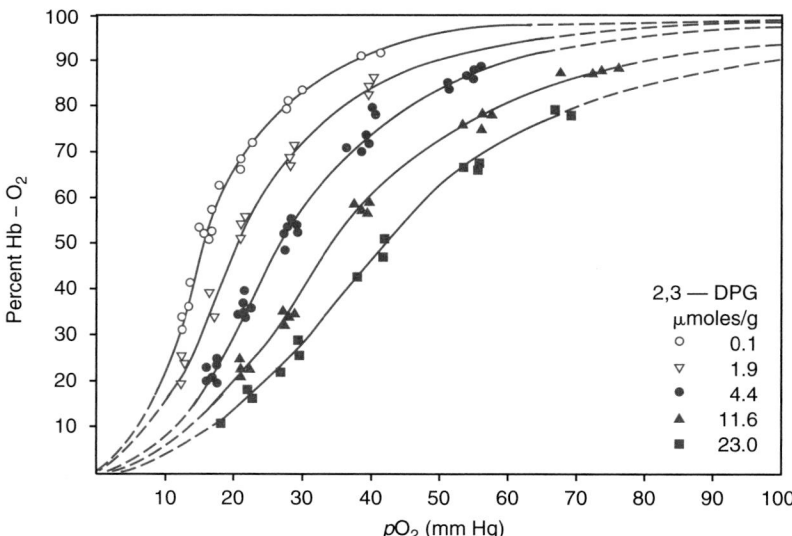

FIGURE 77.6 Normal oxygen dissociation curve of hemoglobin *(Hb)*. Changes in 2,3-diphosphoglycerate *(2,3-DPG)* concentration in the erythrocyte greatly influence the position of the curve. As the concentration of 2,3-DPG increases, the curve shifts to the right. pO_2, Partial pressure of oxygen. (From Duhm J. The effect of 2,3-DPG and other organic phosphates on the Donnan equilibrium and the oxygen affinity of human blood. In: Roth M, Astrup P, eds. *Oxygen affinity of hemoglobin and red cell acid base status [Alfred Benzon Symposium, IV]*. Copenhagen, Denmark: Alfred Benzon Foundation; 1972.)

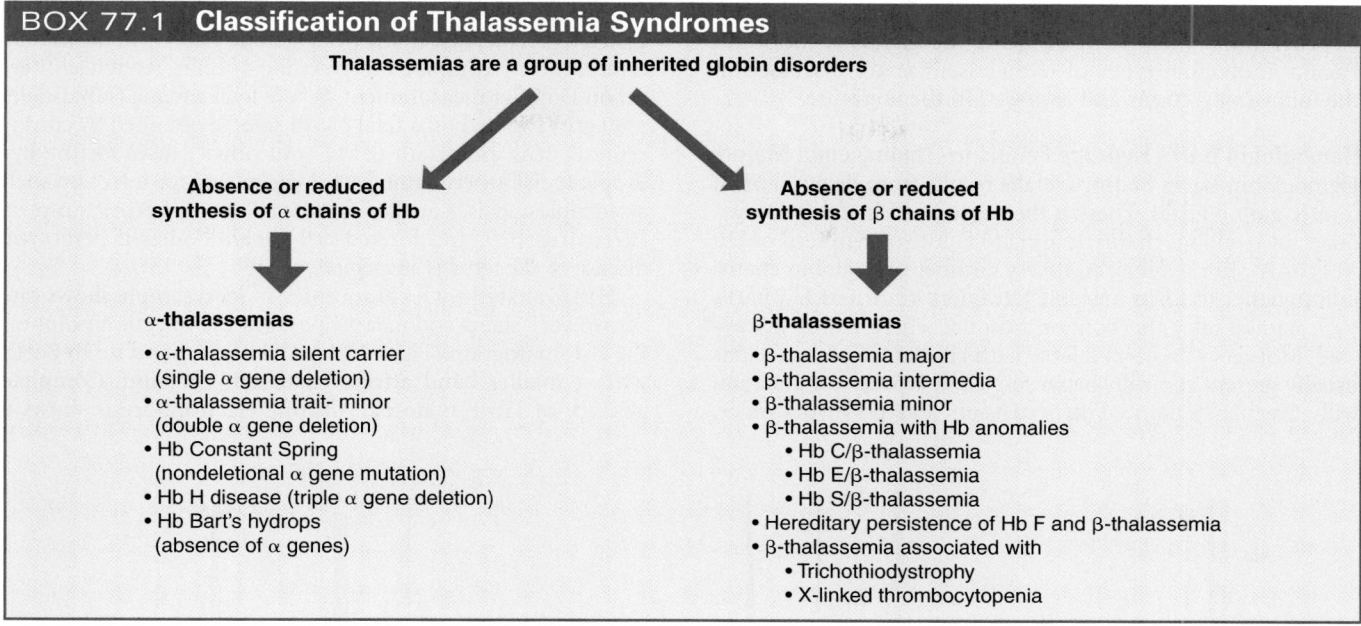

BOX 77.1 **Classification of Thalassemia Syndromes**

Thalassemias are a group of inherited globin disorders

Absence or reduced synthesis of α chains of Hb

Absence or reduced synthesis of β chains of Hb

α-thalassemias
- α-thalassemia silent carrier (single α gene deletion)
- α-thalassemia trait- minor (double α gene deletion)
- Hb Constant Spring (nondeletional α gene mutation)
- Hb H disease (triple α gene deletion)
- Hb Bart's hydrops (absence of α genes)

β-thalassemias
- β-thalassemia major
- β-thalassemia intermedia
- β-thalassemia minor
- β-thalassemia with Hb anomalies
  - Hb C/β-thalassemia
  - Hb E/β-thalassemia
  - Hb S/β-thalassemia
- Hereditary persistence of Hb F and β-thalassemia
- β-thalassemia associated with
  - Trichothiodystrophy
  - X-linked thrombocytopenia

$(-\alpha/\alpha\alpha; \ --/\alpha\alpha; \ -\alpha^T/\alpha\alpha; \ \alpha^T\alpha/-\alpha; \ -\alpha/-\alpha)$. In general, carriers of such genotypes are asymptomatic and may range from hematologically silent to hypochromic microcytic red cell indices in association with a normal Hb level or slight anemia. The peripheral blood smear is quite variable, showing various degrees of hypochromia with some target cells and occasional poikilocytes. In carriers of α^0 thalassemia $(--/\alpha\alpha)$, it is possible to observe a few red cells that contain Hb H inclusions after supravital staining, which are β_4 tetramers that are due to an excess of the β chains. The Hb concentration in adult carriers of α^+ or α°-thalassemia can be indistinguishable from normal, but the percentage of Hb A_2 is slightly lower. Since α-chains bind more readily to β-chains than to the positively charged δ-chains, the HbA_2 level is decreased in limiting levels of α-chains as seen in α-thalassemia. Traces of Hb Bart's (γ_4) in the neonatal period are detectable in a large proportion of neonates with α-thalassemia, and they decline during the first 6 months after birth. The Hb Bart's level in cord blood allows the detection of α^+-thalassemia carrier (<2% Hb Bart's), α°-thalassemia carrier (2–5% Hb Bart's) and Hb H disease (20 to 40% Hb Bart's). In the California Newborn Screening Program, screening for Hb H disease is based on an elevated level (>25%) of a fast-eluting peak on high-performance liquid chromatography (HPLC), which is then subject to confirmation by DNA study.[17] This program shows that α-thalassemia syndromes such as Hb H disease have become the most common nonsickle hemoglobin disorder in California.

Alpha-thalassemias are common in areas where β-thalassemia is also found at a high frequency. Thus the coinheritance of α- and β-thalassemia traits may occur and even ameliorate the hematologic parameters. Depending on the thalassemia status of the partner, subjects who are concurrent α- and β-thalassemia carriers are potentially at risk of being parents to offspring affected by β-thalassemia major, Hb H disease, and Hb Bart's hydrops fetalis. In some cases for genetic counseling in families in whom α- and β-thalassemias are present, genotype diagnosis is essential to fully prevent hydrops fetalis since the α°-thalassemia is masked in carriers of concurrent α- and β-thalassemias.[18,19]

TABLE 77.2 **The Alpha-Thalassemias**

Condition	Affected Number of Alpha-Globin Genes	Phenotype
Silent carrier	One gene affected	Asymptomatic or occasional low red blood cell indexes
Alpha-thalassemia trait	Two genes affected	Mild microcytic and hypochromic anemia
Hb H disease	Three genes affected	Mild-to-moderate anemia, splenomegaly, jaundice
Alpha-thalassemia major/Hb Bart's hydrops	Four genes affected	Most severe form Hb Bart's hydrops Death in utero or at birth

Hb, Hemoglobin.
Data from Vichinsky EP. Alpha thalassemia major—new mutations, intrauterine management, and outcomes. *Hematology Am Soc Hematol Educ Program.* 2009;35–41.

Point mutations of the α-globin gene, although less common than deletions, are important since their coinheritance with α°-thalassemia may result in nondeletional Hb H disease. An example is the chain termination mutation of the α-globin gene, Hb Constant Spring (α142 Gln) or Hb^{CS}. The unstable mutant Hb^{CS} causes not only a reduction in α_2 globin expression from the affected chromosome, but also red cell membrane damage by the partially oxidized α^{CS} chains in addition to the excess β chains; therefore the carriers, but particularly the homozygotes, have a more severe phenotype than α-thalassemia minor, but it is not as severe as most cases of Hb H disease (Table 77.2).

The α-thalassemias occur worldwide and are particularly prevalent in Southeast Asia, Southern China, Mediterranean countries (particularly Greece and the Greek Cypriot part of Cyprus), India, the Middle East, and the islands of the South Pacific. Individual types of α-thalassemias are discussed in the following sections and reviewed in the literature.[20]

Hemoglobin Bart's Hydrops Fetalis (α-Thalassemia Major)

Hemoglobin Bart's hydrops fetalis results from deletion of all four α-globin genes. There is the subsequent inability to produce any α-globin chains, leading to failure of synthesis of Hb A, F, or A_2. In the fetus, an excess number of γ-globin chains join together to form unstable tetramers known as Hb Bart's ($γ_4$), named after the London hospital where it was discovered. Mothers who carry a fetus with Hb Bart's hydrops fetalis usually present clinically between 20 and 26 weeks of gestation with pregnancy-induced hypertension and polyhydramnios.

Ultrasound of the fetus shows hydrops. Fetal anemia is suggested by an increase in the peak systolic velocity in the middle cerebral artery compared to gestation-specific reference interval on Doppler measurement. Severe fetal anemia (Hb usually <80 g/L) is noted on a fetal blood sample obtained by cordocentesis. It is important to rule out other causes for the hydropic fetus by performing serologic testing for infection such as toxoplasmosis, rubella, cytomegalovirus, herpes simplex, Parvovirus B19, and for red cell alloantibodies if hemolytic disease of the fetus is suspected.

HPLC analysis of a cordocentesis blood sample shows one or two very sharp and narrow peaks at the injection point on the chromatogram (Fig. 77.7A). The major band is Hb Bart's with a smaller band attributed to Hb Portland. Complete absence of Hb F is noted. Alkaline electrophoresis shows a

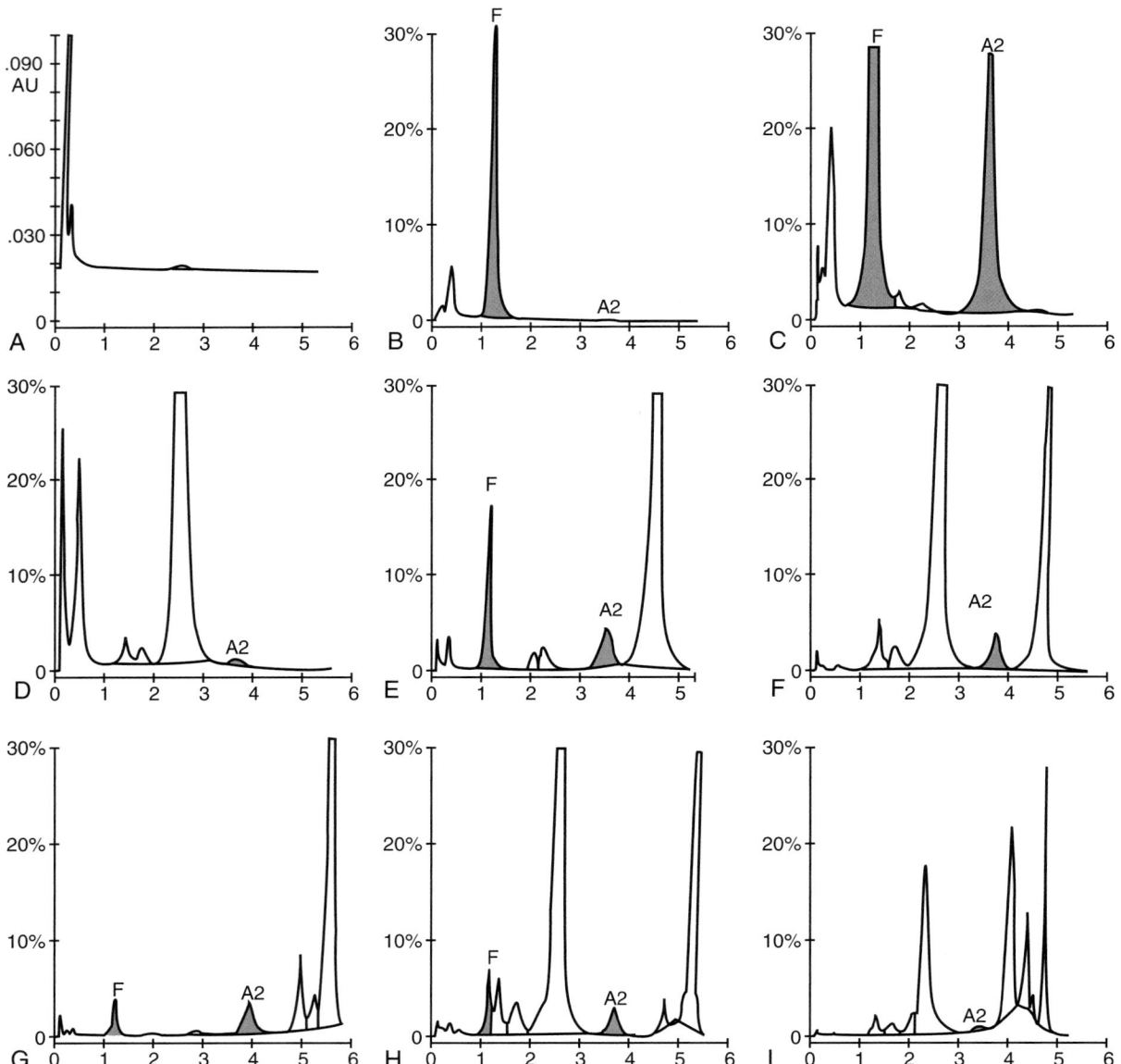

FIGURE 77.7 High-performance liquid chromatography chromatograms obtained on the Bio-Rad Variant β-thal short program for (A) hemoglobin *(Hb)* Bart's; (B) β⁰-thalassemia major; (C) HbE/B⁰-thalassemia; (D) Hb H; (E) homozygous S; (F) S trait; (G) homozygous C; (H) C trait; and (I) Hb S-Hb G Philadelphia. (From Clarke GM, Trefor N, Higgins TN. Laboratory investigation of hemoglobinopathies and thalassemias: review and update. *Clin Chem* 2000;46:1284–90.)

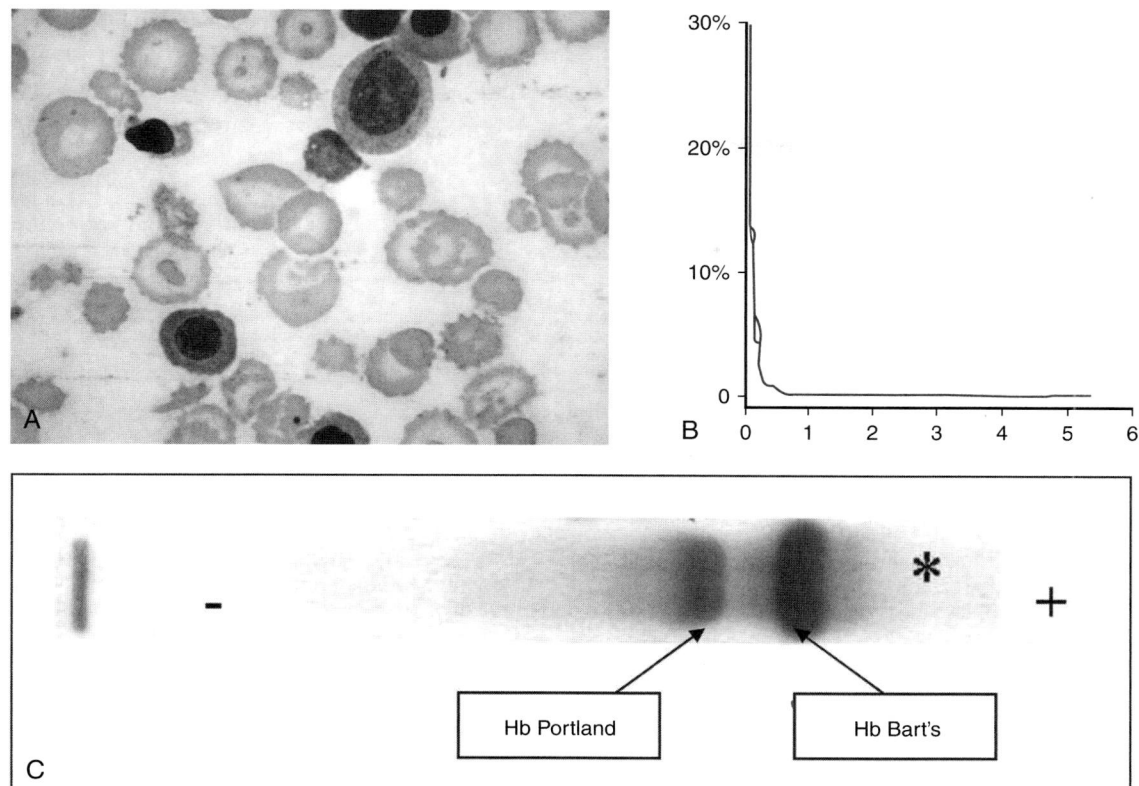

Figure 77.8 Diagnosis of Hb Bart's hydrops fetalis. (A) Peripheral blood smear in a stillbirth showing leukoerythroblastic picture with immature granulocytes and nucleated red cells. Note the hypochromic red cells. (B) HPLC showing predominance of Hb Bart's and absence of α-globin chain–containing hemoglobins. (C) Alkaline electrophoresis showing absence of Hb F, Hb Portland occupying position of Hb A and predominance of the fast-migrating Hb Bart's.

band migrating at the anodal position (Hb Bart's), with another band in the Hb A position (Hb Portland) (Fig. 77.8)

Hb Bart's hydrops fetalis is almost invariably fatal if left untreated,[21] with some fetuses dying in utero, and others surviving a few hours after birth. Treatment using intrauterine transfusion may be able to salvage the fetus, but risks of complications including growth retardation and severe brain damage remain, which may be related to hypoxemia following long-standing intrauterine anemia.

Laboratory investigation of the parents of fetuses with Hb Bart's hydrops fetalis shows a normal HPLC pattern with normal Hb F and A_2 quantification. Parental analysis typically shows a decreased concentration of Hb and decreased MCH and MCV, with the blood smear showing hypochromic, microcytic red cells. The Hb H inclusion body test is usually positive in the parents. A two α-gene *cis*-deletion ($-- /\alpha\alpha$) or a three gene deletion ($-- /-\alpha$) is seen in genetic testing of both parents. This requirement restricts the incidence of Hb Bart's hydrops fetalis to a much smaller population than would be expected based on the worldwide distribution of α-thalassemias because the presence of *trans*-deletions ($-\alpha/-\alpha$) in both parents would not give rise to a four gene deletion in the offspring. Hb Bart's hydrops fetalis is relatively common in Southeast Asia, particularly in Thailand, the Philippines, and Hong Kong, where there is a high prevalence of the $--^{SEA}/(SEA)$ deletion. Deletions that remove the embryonic ζ-globin gene together with both α-globin genes

(e.g. $-^{FIL}$, $-^{THAI}$) can lead to early death of the embryo and usually presents as missed abortions.

Hemoglobin H Disease (α-Thalassemia Intermedia)

This disorder is usually caused by a three α-globin gene deletion ($-- /-\alpha$) and is characterized by a chronic anemia of variable severity.[22] Individuals with nondeletional Hb H disease ($\alpha^T\alpha/--$) are usually more severely affected and are more likely to require transfusion therapy than those with deletional Hb H disease.[23] Significant underproduction of α-globin chains occurs with subsequent joining of free β-globin chains to form the insoluble β-globin chain tetramer Hb H. HPLC analysis of a hemolysate from an individual with Hb H disease shows two bands with short retention times forming a doublet together with a normal Hb A band. Hb F concentration is within the reference interval (see Fig. 77.7D) but the Hb A_2 level is reduced. Electrophoresis at alkaline pH shows a fast-moving band together with a band in the Hb A position that possibly has reduced staining compared with other samples run concurrently. The complete blood count (CBC) shows a moderately reduced concentration of Hb, markedly reduced MCV and MCH, and a markedly increased red cell distribution width (RDW). RBC count is normal or slightly raised. Fe studies are normal, although the ferritin concentration may be elevated. However, the use of automated cell counters may flag adult patients with Hb H disease as iron deficiency, and vigilance should be exercised to

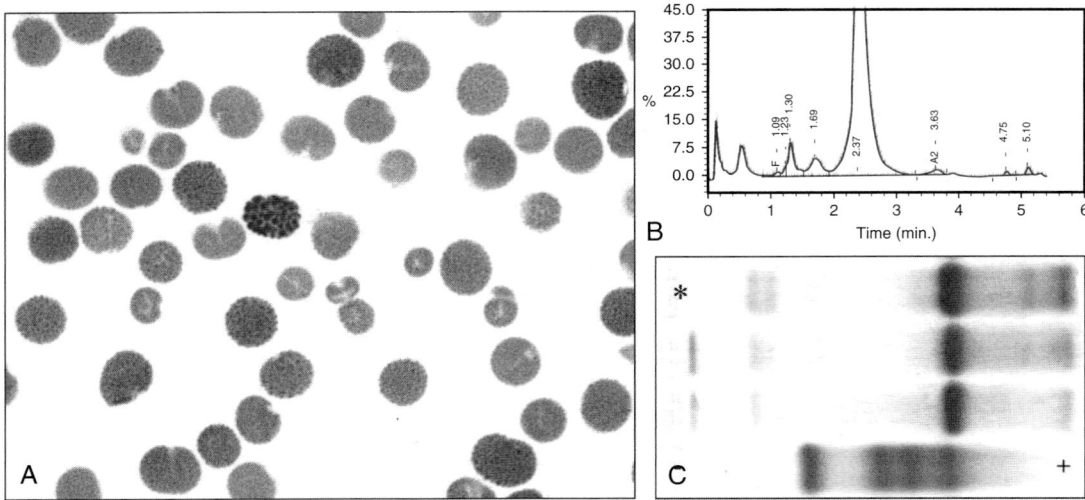

FIGURE 77.9 Diagnosis of nondeletional hemoglobin Constant Spring-H disease by (A) supravital staining showing numerous Hb H inclusion bodies, (B) HPLC showing early eluting peaks compatible with Hb Bart's and Hb H and late-eluting peaks compatible with Hb Constant Spring, and reduced Hb A_2, and (C) alkaline electrophoresis showing in the uppermost lane from cathode to anode Hb Constant Spring (2 bands), Hb A, Hb Bart's, and Hb H.

avoid misdiagnosis. A blood film after staining with brilliant cresyl blue shows many red cells with inclusion bodies (Fig. 77.9A). Hb H disease, according to a recent clinical classification, can be considered a non–transfusion-dependent thalassemia.[24] Fe therapy is not indicated, and transfusion therapy is usually unnecessary except for during an acute illness or in pregnancy. Red cell aplastic crisis is an uncommon complication during an acute Parvovirus B19 infection. Genetic counseling is recommended to prospective parents at risk of having an offspring with Hb H disease.[25]

α-Thalassemia Minor

α-Thalassemia minor is the result of two α-chain gene deletions. These deletions may be seen on the same chromosome ($--/\alpha\alpha$, heterozygous α°-thalassemia or α-thal-1), described as a *cis* deletion, or on different chromosomes ($-\alpha/-\alpha$, homozygous α⁺-thalassemia or α-thal-2), described as a *trans* deletion. The CBC of affected individuals shows a mildly reduced Hb with low MCV and MCH. HPLC analysis shows no abnormal Hb peak, and Hb F and Hb A_2 concentrations are within the reference intervals. Fe studies are normal. The blood film shows occasional red cells with Hb H inclusions on supravital staining in most subjects with heterozygous α°-thalassemia, but they are rarely seen in heterozygous or even homozygous α⁺-thalassemia. Therefore this test is not performed in many parts of the world where α°-thalassemia is not prevalent and the diagnosis of α-thalassemia minor is based on exclusion criteria rather than definitive tests in many routine clinical laboratories. After exclusion of Fe deficiency, the presence of hypochromic microcytic red cell indexes in a patient with normal Hb A_2 and Hb F quantification forms the basis for a presumptive diagnosis of α-thalassemia minor, particularly in the setting of a positive family history. Definitive diagnosis of an α-thalassemia trait (α⁺ or α°-thalassemia) can be achieved by DNA analysis using different methods (gap-polymerase chain reaction [PCR], multiplex ligation-dependent probe amplification [MLPA], allele specific oligonucleotide hybridization [ASO] sequencing).

TABLE 77.3 **Effects of α-Thalassemia on the Percentage of β-Chain Variant Hemoglobin in Heterozygotes**

	AS	AC	AE
αα/αα	41.0 ± 1.8	43.8 ± 1.5	30.0 ± 1.5
αα/α−	35.4 ± 1.6	37.5 ± 1.4	27.0 ± 2.0
α⁻/α⁻ or αα/⁻	28.1 ± 1.4	32.2 ± 0.8	22.0 ± 2.0

AS, Carrier of hemoglobin (Hb) S; *AC*, carrier of Hb C; *AE*, carrier of HbE.
Modified from Bunn HF, Forget BG, eds. *Hemoglobin: molecular genetic and clinical aspects.* Philadelphia: Saunders; 1986.

Molecular diagnosis is required for prenatal diagnosis in couples at risk for Hb Bart's hydrops fetalis.[26]

Silent α-Thalassemia Trait

A silent α-thalassemia trait results from a single α-globin gene deletion or mutation ($-\alpha/\alpha\alpha$; $\alpha^T\alpha/\alpha\alpha$). A single α-globin gene deletion or mutation is frequently clinically and hematologically silent.[27] A CBC of an individual with this trait shows a normal or marginally decreased Hb concentration, MCV, and MCH. Fe studies are normal, and no abnormal Hb peaks are seen on HPLC analysis.

The effects of various α-thalassemias on the percentage of β-chain Hb variants are shown in Table 77.3.[28] In general, the percentage of the Hb variant decreases as a percentage of total Hb as the number of α-globin gene deletions increases. The proportion of β-chain variants is affected by charge. Positively charged β-chain Hb variants such as Hb S, C, D-Los Angeles, and E constitute less than half of the total Hb in the heterozygous state and are reduced further in the presence of α-thalassemia, due to increased competition between normal and mutant β-chain for the limited amounts of α-chain. Conversely, negatively charged β-chain Hb variants such as Hb J-Baltimore and J-Iran, in conjunction with α-thalassemia, show an increased proportion of the mutant Hb since the β-chain variant out-competes normal β-chain for the limited amounts of α-chain in the presence of α-thalassemia.[29]

β-Thalassemias

The β-thalassemias result from a reduction in the synthesis of the β-globin chain[30] and are commonly found in (1) the Mediterranean region, (2) Africa, (3) the Middle East, and (4) Southeast Asia, especially the southern provinces of China, including Hong Kong, the Indian subcontinent, the Malay peninsula, Myanmar (Burma), and Indonesia.[31] The frequency of gene distribution is estimated at 3 to 10% in some populations. The high frequency of β-thalassemia in the tropics is believed to reflect a survival advantage of heterozygotes against *Plasmodium falciparum* malaria. With increasing migration, β-thalassemia, once considered a rare genetic disease in Northern Europe, Australia, and North America, is now becoming more common all over the world. More than 250 β-thalassemia mutations have been described; however, in each ethnic group, a relatively small number of mutations account for most cases (the ratio most often quoted is that ≤20 mutations account for ≥80% of cases). The β-thalassemia alleles can be classified into $β^0$-thalassemia, in which there is no β-globin gene production, and $β^+$ or $β^{++}$-thalassemia, in which there is marked or mild reduction in the production of β-chains, respectively. Most are point mutations, small insertion or deletions within the gene or its immediate flanking sequence. They may affect any level of gene expression and are categorized according to the mechanism by which they affect gene function, namely transcription, RNA processing, and RNA translation.

a. Mutations that affect transcription can either involve the β-globin gene promoter or the stretch of 50 nucleotides in the 5′-untranslated region (5′-UTR). Generally speaking, they result in a minimal to mild deficit in the output of β-globin chains as reflected by the relatively mild $β^+$-thalassemia phenotype of those affected.

b. Mutations that affect RNA processing can involve either of the invariant dinucleotides (GT at 5′ and AG at 3′) at the splice junction in which case normal splicing is abolished in entirety, resulting in the phenotype of $β^0$-thalassemia. Mutations within the consensus sequences that flank the splice junctions reduce efficiency of normal splicing to varying degrees, producing a $β^+$-thalassemia phenotype that ranges from mild to severe. Other splice mutations involve base substitutions within introns or exons. For instance, a cryptic splice site sequence of GT GGT GAG G is found in exon 1 spanning codons 24 to 27. Three mutations within this region activate this cryptic site, causing it to serve as an alternative donor site in RNA processing. The Hb E mutation (β26 GAG→AAG; Glu→Lys) also activates this cryptic splice site causing abnormal RNA processing so that normal splicing which produces Hb E variant is reduced. Other RNA processing mutants affect the polyadenylation signal (AATAAA) and the 3'-UTR. These are usually mild $β^+$-thalassemia alleles.

c. Mutations that affect mRNA translation at either the initiation or extension phases of globin synthesis are associated with a $β^0$-thalassaemia phenotype. Roughly half of the β-thalassemia alleles are characterized by premature termination of β-chain extension. They result from introduction of termination codons due to frameshift or nonsense mutations and nearly all terminate within exons 1 and 2. Terminations early in the sequence are associated with minimal steady state levels of β-mRNA in erythroid cells, due to accelerated decay of the abnormal mRNA referred to as nonsense-mediated decay (NMD). In contrast, exon 3 mutations usually are not subject to NMD and hence result in substantial amounts of mutant mRNA with respect to normal mRNA, which presumably is translated into highly unstable variant β-chains and can lead to severe hemolysis and a dominantly inherited phenotype.[32] Precipitation of unstable β-chains and concurrent excess α-globin chains also overload the intracellular proteolytic mechanisms of erythroblasts in the bone marrow, which aggravates ineffective erythropoiesis.[33]

A few β-thalassemia mutations that segregate independently of the β-globin gene cluster have been described, presumably involving *trans*-acting regulatory factors. An updated list of these mutations is accessible at the Globin Gene Server Website (http://globin.cse.psu.edu).[34,35] Simple deletions of the β-globin gene are rare,[36] ranging in size from 290 bp to more than 100 kb and are necessarily $β^0$-thalassemias. The 619-bp deletion at the 3′ end of the β-globin gene is relatively common among Sindhi and Punjabi populations in India and Pakistan, whereas the 100-kb Chinese $(^Aγδβ)^0$ deletion which includes the δ and β-globin gene are relatively common in Southern Chinese populations. Some deletions are associated with an unusually high level of Hb A_2 or Hb F. Large deletions that affect the entire β-globin gene cluster $(εγγδβ)^0$ are rare and restricted to single families.

The clinical classification of β-thalassemia includes thalassemia major (TM; transfusion-dependent), thalassemia intermedia (TI; of intermediate severity, nontransfusion-dependent), and thalassemia minor (asymptomatic). The severity of the clinical manifestations correlates well with the degree of imbalance of globin chains, depending on the β-globin gene defects and their interaction. The production of β-globin chains is quantitatively reduced to different degrees, whereas the synthesis of α-globin continues as normal, resulting in accumulation of excess unmatched α-globin chains in the erythroid precursors. Clinical manifestations of β-thalassemia range from mild anemia to severe life-threatening disease that requires lifelong transfusions (Fig. 77.10).

β-Thalassemia Major

This is sometimes called Cooley's anemia, after the physician who first described the condition in 1925 in the children of Italian and Greek immigrants in New York.

β-Thalassemia major (TM) results from homozygous or compound heterozygous $β^0$-thalassemia mutations that severely interfere with RNA splicing or translation. Mutations that interfere with translation account for almost 50% of all β-thalassemia mutations.

Clinical presentation usually occurs at younger than 1 year of age, with features such as small size for age, abdominal girth expansion, and failure to thrive. Physical examination of the patient may reveal frontal bossing[37] (an unusually prominent forehead) caused by thickening of the cranial bones, pallor, and prominence of the cheek bones, which in older children obscures the base of the nose and exposes the teeth. These features are a result of marrow expansion (up to a 30-fold increase) caused by ineffective erythropoiesis with production

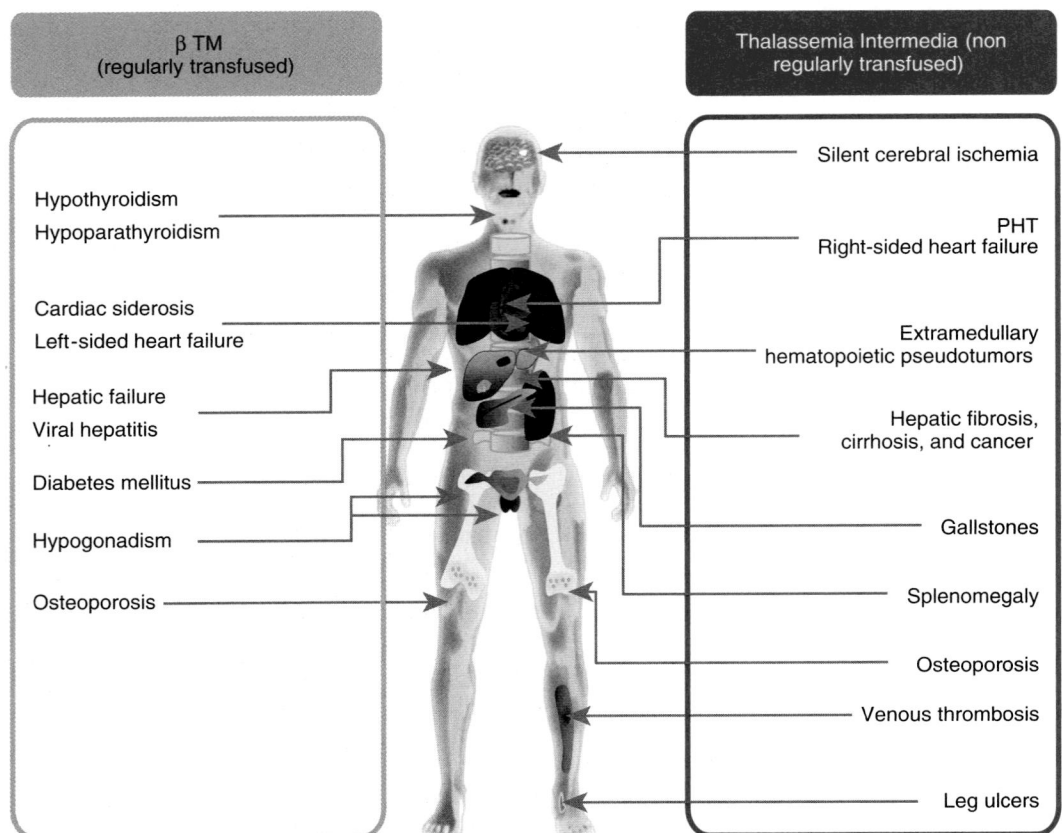

FIGURE 77.10 Clinical complications in thalassemia major and in thalassemia intermedia. *β-TM*, β-thalassemia major; *IOL*, iron overload; *PHT*, pulmonary hypertension. (Modified from Musallam K, Rivella S, Vichinsky E, Rachmilewitz EA. Non-transfusion-dependent thalassemias. *Haematologica* 2013;98:833–44.)

of highly unstable α-globin tetramers, leading to a sequence of events responsible for bone marrow expansion, anemia, hemolysis, splenomegaly, and increased Fe absorption.

Typical CBC results include severe anemia with Hb concentration between 30 and 65 g/L, MCV of 48 to 72 fL, and MCH of 23 to 32 pg. A characteristic markedly abnormal RBC morphology is noted on the peripheral blood smear; this includes a large number of microcytes and/or macrocytes, prominent basophilic stippling, numerous target cells, which may have a bridge joining the central and peripheral pigment zones, polychromasia, and occasional spherocytes, schistocytes, and nucleated red cells. Circulating nucleated red cells often poorly hemoglobinized are rather characteristic of β-thalassemia major or intermedia. Typical peripheral blood on a patient with β° thalassemia major is shown in Fig. 77.11.

White blood cell (WBC) and platelet counts are usually normal. Ferritin is usually within the upper half of the reference interval at the time of diagnosis, and total bilirubin is mildly elevated mainly due to elevation in the unconjugated fraction. Urinalysis frequently shows increased urobilinogen or urobilin concentration, and urine is often dark brown to black because of the presence of dipyroles and mesobilifuscin. The latter features reflect ineffective hematopoiesis with intramedullary red cell destruction. HPLC analysis (see Fig. 77.7B) shows a major Hb F peak with absence of an Hb A peak and variable Hb A₂ (reference interval, 1 to 5.9%; mean, 1.7%) peak. Electrophoresis at alkaline and acid pH shows a dominant band in the F position in both gels.[38]

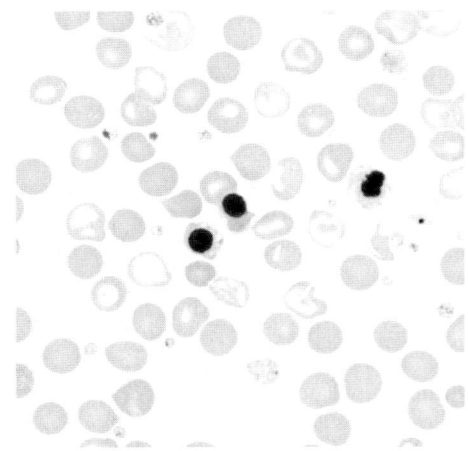

FIGURE 77.11 Peripheral blood smear of an individual with β⁰-thalassemia. (From Rodak BF, Carr JH. *Clinical Hematology Atlas.* 5th ed. Philadelphia: Elsevier; 2017.)

Family studies on both parents and siblings should be performed, and the classical β-thalassemia minor pattern, described later in the chapter, should be found in the parents. Siblings may be normal or may have β-thalassemia minor. A family case history is seen in Fig. 77.12.

The conventional treatment for TM patients includes regular transfusion therapy and Fe chelation. Many patients with TM require splenectomy because of hypersplenism.

TEST/REF	INDEX PAT 7 MO F	MOTHER 33 YRS	FATHER 40 YRS	SIBLING 3 YR F
Hb	↓ 72 G/L	↓ 114	↓ 132	122
REF	105-135	120-160	135-175	115-135
RBC	↓ 3.23 (10¹²/L)	5.19	↑ 6.61	4.42
REF	3.70-5.30	4.10-5.20	4.50-6.00	3.90-5.30
MCV	↓ 69 fL	↓ 68	↓ 63	80
REF	70-86	80-100	80-100	75-87
MCH	↓ 22 pg	↓ 22	↓ 20	28
REF	26-35	26-35	26-35	26-35
HbA	↓ 0.00	0.94	↓ 0.93	0.96
REF	0.94-0.98	0.94-0.98	0.94-0.98	0.94-0.98
HbA2	0.030	↑ 0.054	↑ 0.058	0.030
REF	<0.03	<0.03	<0.03	<0.03
HbF	0.97	<0.01	<0.01	<0.01
REF	<0.10	<0.01	<0.01	<0.01

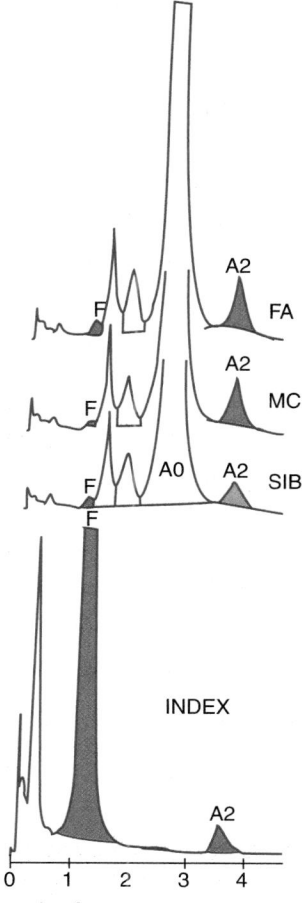

FIGURE 77.12 High-performance liquid chromatograms and complete blood count results from a family study of a child with β⁰-thalassemia. *Hb*, Hemoglobin; *MCH*, mean cell hemoglobin; *MCV*, mean corpuscular volume; *RBC*, red blood cell. (From Berendt HL, Blakney GB, Clarke GM, Higgins TN. A case of β-thalassemia major detected using HPLC in a child of Chinese ancestry. *Clin Biochem* 2000;33:311–13.)

However, optimal clinical management may delay or even obviate the need for splenectomy, which was common in the past. After splenectomy, inclusion bodies consisting of denatured α-chains (also termed Fessas bodies) can be observed in the blood smear after staining with methyl violet. Fe overload is an inevitable and serious complication of long-term blood transfusion therapy that requires adequate treatment to prevent early death mainly from Fe-induced cardiac disease. Puberty is often delayed, incomplete, or completely absent. In boys, active spermatogenesis may occur, and Leydig cell function is normal. The quality and duration of life of TM patients has been transformed over the last 20 years, with life expectancy increasing well into the fourth and fifth decades. Many children who are adequately transfused and are fully compliant with Fe chelation therapy develop normally, enter puberty, and become sexually mature. The availability of oral Fe chelators, such as Deferiprone (ApoPharma, Toronto, Canada) and Deferasirox (Novartis, Basel, Switzerland), has significantly improved the adherence to chelation, which has affected survival.[39] Nevertheless, prolongation of life is accompanied by several complications, partly due to the underlying disorder and partly as a consequence of the treatment with blood transfusions and Fe overload, such as diabetes mellitus, hypothyroidism, hypoparathyroidism, and liver disease.[39]

Allogeneic hemopoietic stem cell transplantation is currently the only method available to cure transfusion-dependent TM; it has been used worldwide.[40] Gene therapy and other innovative therapeutic modalities for the cure of TM are under investigation.[41]

β-Thalassemia Intermedia

β-Thalassemia intermedia (TI) is a clinical term used to describe patients with anemia and splenomegaly, but who do not have the full spectrum of clinical severity found in β-TM.[42] The clinical phenotypes of β-TI lie between those of thalassemia minor and major, encompassing a wide clinical spectrum. Mildly affected patients are almost completely asymptomatic until adult life, experiencing only mild anemia and spontaneously maintaining Hb levels between 7 and 10 g/dL (70 and 100 g/L). Patients with more severe TI generally present between the ages of 2 and 6 years, and although they are able to survive without regular transfusion therapy, growth and development can be retarded. Most β-TI patients are homozygotes or compound heterozygotes for β-gene mutations (β⁺/β⁺; β°/β⁺). Because the clinical severity of the disease is dictated by the different extent of globin chain imbalance, at least three different mechanisms may promote the milder clinical characteristics of TI compared with TM: inheritance of mild or silent β-gene mutations; coinheritance of determinants associated with increased γ-chain production[43] that contributes to neutralizing the large proportion of unbound α-chains; and coinheritance of α-thalassemia that reduces the synthesis of α-chains, thereby reducing the α/non–α-chain imbalance. Increased Hb F production not only improves globin chain imbalance, but also raises the total hemoglobin level. Other molecular mechanisms of β-TI include compound heterozygosity for β-thalassemia and δβ-thalassemia or hereditary persistence of fetal hemoglobin (HPFH), compound heterozygosity for β-thalassemia and Hb E, and simple heterozygosity for β-thalassemia with coexisting amplification of α-globin genes.

β-TI is clinically labeled as non–transfusion-dependent thalassemia (NTDT) because the affected patients do not require lifelong regular transfusions for survival, although they may require occasional or even frequent blood transfusions in particular situations such as pregnancy, surgery, and infections.

HPLC analysis shows a variable Hb F peak with a reduced Hb A peak. Hb A_2 is usually increased. Bands in the A and F positions are seen on electrophoresis at both alkaline and acid pH. Hb is significantly reduced to values between 6 and 10 g/dL (60 and 100 g/L). The peripheral blood smear shows the same features seen in β-TM, including anisocytosis, hypochromia, target cells, basophilic stippling, and nucleated RBCs.

β-Thalassemia Minor (β-Thalassemia Trait)

Subjects with β-thalassemia minor are asymptomatic. The CBC shows low normal or mildly decreased Hb concentration and hematocrit (Hct), decreased MCV (<80 fL) and MCH (<25 pg), and normal to slightly increased RDW. The peripheral blood smear shows microcytic hypochromic RBCs with occasional basophilic stippling and target cells. Note that for patients with liver disease, megaloblastic anemia[44] or myelodysplastic syndrome in association with concomitant underlying β-thalassemia, the MCV value may be spuriously normalized. If these combinations are suspected, careful examination of the blood smear for dimorphic red cell populations is warranted.

The diagnosis of β-thalassemia minor, with appropriate indexes in the CBC, is dependent on the finding of a raised Hb A_2 (≥4%). Even when the quality of measurement is assured, there are subjects in whom Hb A_2 level is borderline raised, typically in the range of 3.1 to 3.9%. Recently, it was found that a significant proportion of these individuals may have underlying heterozygous *KLF1* mutations.[45] However, there are rare β-thalassemia carriers who show normal to borderline raised Hb A_2 level, often due to coinheritance of linked β-globin gene and δ-globin gene mutations.[46] Certain mild to silent β-thalassemia mutations, such as those involving the promoter or 5′ untranslated region, may be associated with normal to mildly reduced MCV and a borderline raised Hb A_2 level. The clinical relevance of these mutations is that, if the partner is having β-thalassemia trait, the couple is at risk of offspring affected by intermediate forms of β-thalassemia. Nevertheless, in routine practice it is difficult, if not impossible, to predict for this risk without resorting to gene sequencing study. There is a long-standing belief that the presence of iron deficiency may spuriously lower the Hb A_2 level in β-thalassemia carriers. Recent data do not support this, but rather show that concomitant iron deficiency does not mask a diagnosis of β-thalassemia trait by Hb A_2 measurement.[47] However, when faced with a patient with hypochromic microcytic anemia, it is always prudent to first exclude iron deficiency and find out its underlying

cause, and consider a Hb pattern study if microcytosis is persistent after adequate iron replacement. The phenotype of normal HbA$_2$ β-thalassemia is also seen in heterozygous εγδβ-thalassemia due to the deletion of the delta-globin gene.

At the other end of the spectrum, an unusually high Hb A_2 level is associated with β-thalassemia trait caused by the uncommon β-globin gene deletions that include the promoter region. Hb A_2 may also be elevated in HIV-positive women without hypochromic microcytic indexes,[48] those with hyperthyroidism or megaloblastic anemia, and individuals with some unstable Hbs.[49] HPLC is the preferred method for this quantification; densitometric scanning of the Hb A_2 band on an alkaline electrophoresis gel is not recommended because of its poor precision and accuracy.[49] In 30 to 40% of all cases of β-thalassemia minor, Hb F could be mildly elevated (1 to 2%). The life span of the RBC may be reduced, and individuals with diabetes may show a lower HbA$_{1c}$ compared with normal individuals with equivalent glycemic control. The β-thalassemia mutations can be identified by direct sequencing or by multiplex PCR-based molecular testing.

δ-β-Thalassemia

The δβ-thalassemias are the result of deletions that affect various parts of the β-globin locus. These deletions are partially compensated by an increased expression of the γ genes that raises the level of Hb F. The length of deletion accounts for different forms of δβ-thalassemia, including both $^Gγ$ and $^Aγ$ genes or only $^Aγ$, and vary from 9 to 100 kb. Hb Lepore is a hybrid of δ- and β-chains that result from a crossover between the two misaligned genes; this Hb is synthesized inefficiently and gives rise to a form of δβ-thalassemia.

Both heterozygous and homozygous conditions have been described. It is found in a variety of ethnic groups, but it is most prevalent in Eastern Mediterranean countries, especially Greece and Italy. CBC analysis of heterozygotes often shows a reduced concentration of Hb (8 to 13.5 g/dL; 80 to 135 g/L) with reduced MCV and MCH, and sometimes an increased RDW. HPLC analysis shows an Hb A peak with a normal or reduced Hb A_2 concentration and a raised Hb F concentration (between 5 and 20%), with the highest Hb F concentration seen in the Sardinian type of δβ-thalassemia.

Hereditary Persistence of Fetal Hemoglobin

The term hereditary persistence of Hb F (HPFH) is used to describe a group of genetic conditions in which the concentration of Hb F is increased above the upper limit of the reference interval because of a reduction in β-globin synthesis and an increase in γ-globin synthesis. As for δβ-thalassemias, deletions of δ and β genes are the molecular basis for many forms of HPFH. However, the level of Hb F production in HPFH is higher than that seen in the δβ-thalassemias. Several deletional variants of HPFH have been described, including Greek, Indian, Italian, Thai, Corfu, and black. In black HPFH, the Hb F is raised to between 10 and 36% of the total Hb with normal Hb A_2 concentrations. Hb, MCV, and MCH are within the reference intervals. This condition is clinically innocuous and asymptomatic. Similarly, no clinical abnormalities are associated with Greek and Thai HPFH, although the concentration of Hb F is in the range of 15 to 25%. By mapping a variety of deletions within the β-globin gene locus that either result in δβ-thalassemia with a modest increase in Hb F and some remaining globin chain imbalance present, or HPFH with a higher Hb F level and balanced globin chain synthesis (hence normochromic normocytic red cell indices), it is found that an approximately 3-kb region upstream of the δ-globin gene is necessary for the silencing of the γ-globin genes. This region harbors binding sites of BCL11A, along with its partners, GATA-1 and HDAC1.[50] Note that some β-thalassemia deletions, such as the Southeast Asian (Vietnamese) deletion, are associated with elevations of both Hb A_2 and Hb F (10 to 20%) in the heterozygous state.

Other HPFHs are due to point mutations in the promoter region upstream from the transcription start site in either the $^G\gamma$ and $^A\gamma$ genes, which alter the binding of one or more transcription factors; these are known as "nondeletional HPFHs."

The increase in Hb F in nondeletional HPFH is distributed heterogeneously among the red cells (heterocellular) in otherwise normal individuals. The Hb F concentration varies between 1 and 13% of total Hb in heterozygotes and between 19 and 21% in homozygotes. No clinical or hematologic abnormalities are noted. The Hb F distribution is also heterocellular in δβ-thalassemia, while it is pancellular in deletional HPFH. Assessment of cellular Hb F distribution and enumeration of F-cells (Hb F-containing red cells) particularly in the very low range is more accurately performed by flow cytometric measurement using an anti–γ-globin chain monoclonal antibody. The quantification of Hb F level and enumeration of F-cells are also useful: (1) as a laboratory endpoint in clinical studies on the augmentation of Hb F production in sickle cell disease and β-thalassemia syndromes; and (2) as a precise hematologic marker for genetic association studies to identify candidate quantitative trait loci that are associated with enhanced γ-globin chain production and amelioration of β-globin disorders.

HEMOGLOBINOPATHIES

If only single point mutations are considered, there are 1695 possible Hb variants of which 733 were identified by mid-2007.[51] Currently, more than 900 hemoglobinopathies have been described, but only a handful show clinical significance. Recent migration from regions with a high frequency of hemoglobinopathies (Southeast Asia or Africa) to regions that had low frequencies (Western Europe, Central and South America, and Canada) has increased the incidence of hemoglobinopathies in these areas to such an extent that some western European countries have introduced neonatal testing for Hb variants. The incidental finding of a hemoglobinopathy during HPLC analysis for HbA$_{1c}$ has increased both the number and the incidence of Hb variants.[52,53] Several Hb variants (e.g., Hb Rambam, Niigata, Camden) interfere with HPLC methods for quantifying HbA$_{1c}$[54] (for a more extensive list, see Elder and colleagues[55]), and Hb variants have also been found as a result of interference in pulse oximetry measurements.[56]

Nomenclature

Hemoglobin variants are named using (1) letters (Hb S, D, E, and so on), (2) the family name of the index case (Hb Lepore), (3) the place of discovery of the variant or place of origin of the propositus (Hb Edmonton), or (4) the name of the river (Hb Saale) flowing through the city in which the propositus lived. In some cases, both a letter and a name are used, as in Hb J-Baltimore, indicating that the Hb is classified as having an electrophoretic mobility similar to that of other

J Hbs, but differs from them in amino acid sequence, and was originally discovered in Baltimore. The term *AS trait* (sometimes abbreviated to *S trait*) is used to describe a heterozygous state in which one of the β-globin chains is S and the other is A. In instances in which no normal β-globin chain is present (e.g., Hb SD), the β-globin chain present in the higher concentration is usually, although not always, placed first. A systematic nomenclature system is now used alongside the variant name to describe the affected chain and location on the chain and the amino acid substitution. For example, Hb Spanish Town [α27(β8)$^{Glu \to Val}$], a Hb variant named after a district in Kingston, Jamaica, and found in Jamaicans of African descent, results from a substitution of valine for glutamic acid in position 27 of the α-globin chain, which is located in position 8 of the B helix of the α-chain.

Classification of Hemoglobin Variants

Hemoglobin variants are classified according to the type of mutation.[28] Single point mutations in α-globin chains give rise to substitution of one amino acid residue. As an example, Hb San Diego [β109(G11)$^{Val \to Met}$] has a methionine residue instead of the normal valine at position 109 of the β-chain. Hb C Harlem [β6(A3)$^{Glu \to Val}$; β73(E17)$^{Asp \to Asn}$] is an example of an Hb variant in which two amino acid residues are substituted, namely, valine replaces glutamic acid at position 6 and asparagine replaces aspartic acid at position 73 of the β-chain. Hb C Harlem is electrophoretically similar to Hb C but behaves like Hb S in every other aspect, including clinical manifestations. Deletional Hb variants arise from the deletion of one to five amino acid residues in the globin chain. Hb Vicksburg [β75(E19)$^{Leu \to 0}$] is an example of this category, having a deletion of leucine in position 75 of the β-chain. Insertion Hbs arise from insertion of one to three amino acid residues into the globin chain. Hb Grady is an example of this category, with an insertion of a three amino acid residue sequence (glutamine-phenylalanine-threonine) between positions 118 and 119 of the α-chain. Deletion–insertion Hbs arise from the deletion of a portion of the normal amino acid residue sequence and the insertion of another sequence, with resultant lengthening or shortening of the globin chain. An example of this type of Hb variant is Hb Montreal, in which the three normal amino acid residues between positions 72 and 76 of the β-globin chain are replaced with a four amino acid residue sequence. Elongation Hbs result from a single bp mutation or frameshift at the 3′ end of exon 3 or the 5′ end of exon 1 of the α$_2$- or the β-globin chain. The elongation Hb, Hb Constant Spring (named after an ethnic Chinese family from the Constant Spring district of Jamaica), has an additional 31 amino acid residues joined at position 142 (the carboxy terminal) of the α-chain. Fusion Hbs result from the fusion of an α- or β-globin chain with a portion of another globin chain. Hb Lepore-Hollandia results from the fusion of the first 22 amino acid residues of the δ-chain with the amino acid sequence from position 50 onward of normal β-globin. For the latter four categories, the systematic name is long and cumbersome, prompting universal use of the variant name rather than the systematic nomenclature.

Apart from the type of mutation and structure, Hb variants can also be classified functionally into the following. (1) Unstable variants. These Hb variants frequently cause congenital Heinz body hemolytic anemia that present with clinical symptoms and are detectable by laboratory testing. Mutations that alter any step in globin processing can destabilize Hb, such as amino acid substitutions within the heme pocket, disruption of secondary structure, substitution in the hydrophobic interior of the subunit, amino acid deletion, and elongation of the subunit. (2) High oxygen affinity variants. These Hb variants commonly result from amino acid substitutions that stabilize the R (high O_2 affinity) state relative to the T (low O_2 affinity) state and/or inhibit responses to environmental allosteric regulators that stimulate O_2 release, including H^+ (Bohr effect) or 2,3 BPG. (3) Low oxygen affinity variants. These Hb variants are caused by amino acid substitutions that shift the quaternary equilibrium of the Hb tetramer from the high-affinity R state to the low-affinity deoxygenated T state. (4) Methemoglobin variants. These Hb variants result from amino acid substitution within the heme pocket that causes stabilization of the heme iron in the oxidized Fe^{3+} form. Affected patients may present with low Hb oxygen saturation despite adequate arterial oxygenation (pseudocyanosis).

Types of Hemoglobin Variants

In α-chain variants, the variant usually forms less than 25% of the total Hb (Hb G Philadelphia and Hb Q Thailand are notable exceptions) because the mutation typically occurs in only one of the four genes that code for the α-globin chain. For β-chain variants in the heterozygous state, the variant forms more than 25% but is usually not at 50% of the total Hb. Based on the mutation of only one of the two β-globin chain genes, the β-chain variant theoretically should form 50% of total Hb. However, when the amino acid substitution results in a net negative charge to the normal β chain, then the variant chain competes more effectively for α-chains and the percent of the Hb variant is greater than Hb A (e.g., Hb N-Baltimore). The converse is true; a decrease in negative charge results in a percent of the variant Hb being less than Hb A (e.g., Hb S).[29] This information can be used to categorize an unknown Hb variant as an α- or β-globin chain variant and in preliminary Hb variant identification.

Hemoglobin S [β6(A3)$^{Glu→Val}$]

Hemoglobin S in the heterozygous or homozygous state is the most widespread of the Hb variants and arises from a substitution of valine for glutamic acid at position 6 in the A helix of the two β-globin chain. Hb S is found frequently in West and North Africa, the Middle East (especially Saudi Arabia), and the Indian subcontinent. Approximately 8% of African Americans are heterozygous for Hb S, and homozygous Hb S is found in 1 in 500 newborns in this group. Four haplotypes originating from different geographic locations have been described. The widespread distribution of the single point gene mutation responsible for the synthesis of Hb S in areas where *P. falciparum* malaria is endemic is due to protection of Hb S heterozygotes from the worst manifestations of this malaria.

Homozygous Hemoglobin S

In homozygous Hb S (Hb SS), a valine for glutamic acid substitution occurs on both β-globin chains because of the inheritance of mutated β-globin chain genes from both parents. This condition is described as "sickle cell anemia" or "sickle cell disease" because of the sickle-shaped RBCs that occur when a sickle cell crisis occurs. It sometimes is written as $β^Sβ^S$.[57]

HPLC analysis (see Fig. 77.7E) of a hemolysate of an individual homozygous for Hb S shows no Hb A peak and a small

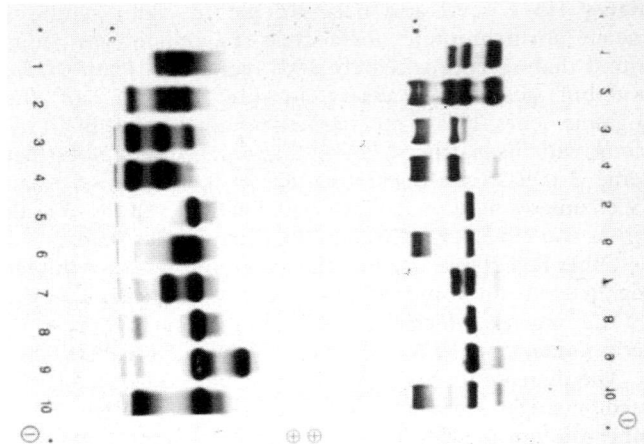

FIGURE 77.13 Alkaline *(left)* and acid *(right)* electrophoresis of various hemoglobinopathies. Lane 1, hemoglobin *(Hb)* S, Hb FA control. Lane 2, HB S, Hb F, HbCA control. Lane 3, transfused SC disease. Lane 4, SC disease. Lane 5, Hb A (normal). Lane 6, Hb Presbyterian. Lane 7, Hb S. Lane 8, raised Hb A2 (β-thalassemia trait). Lane 9, Hb J Baltimore. Lane 10, Hb C.

Hb A_2 peak. The apparent Hb A_2 concentration may be falsely increased because of the presence of carbamylated Hb S. However, note that the Hb A_2 level may also be increased in sickle cell anemia due to an underlying α-thalassemia carrier state, and correlation with the red cell indices is required. Hb S forms 85 to 90% of the total Hb. The Hb F concentration is variable, with females having higher concentrations than males, and is somewhat, although not exclusively, haplotype dependent. The highest Hb F concentrations (10 to 25%) are found in individuals from the Middle East and the Indian subcontinent with the Arab-Indian haplotype. Low Hb F concentrations (5 to 6%) are found in the West African Cameroon (sometimes called Senegal) haplotype. The remaining haplotypes, the Benin and Bantu, have Hb F concentrations in the range of 6 to 7%. Increased concentrations of Hb F mitigate the clinical manifestations of sickle cell anemia to some extent. Electrophoresis (Fig. 77.13) at both alkaline and acid pH shows a single large band in the Hb S position with small bands at the Hb A_2 and Hb F positions. The sickle cell screen test is positive.

CBC analysis of an individual homozygous for Hb S indicates a moderate to a major decrease in Hb concentration (60 to 100 g/L), with normal to increased MCV and MCH. In individuals with a concurrent thalassemia, the Hb is further decreased, and both MCV and MCH are lowered. In the neonate, the peripheral blood smear shows occasional sickle and target cells and Howell-Jolly bodies. As a patient's age increases, these features of hyposplenism become increasingly evident. In the adult, the percentage of sickle cells observed can be as great as 30 to 40%. In the setting of a sickle cell crisis, fewer sickle cells may be present than when individuals are clinically well. Howell-Jolly bodies, target cells, Pappenheimer bodies, boat-shaped cells, and nucleated RBCs are noted. The platelet count and neutrophil counts are elevated. Sometimes blister cells, in which the Hb appears to be present in only one half of the cell, are observed.

Treatment of children with homozygous Hb S includes the use of hydroxyurea, with an increase in the quantity of Hb F, sometimes to 25%. In adults, regular transfusion or exchange transfusion are needed to keep Hb S at less than 40%.

Heterozygous Hemoglobin S (Hemoglobin S Trait)

High-performance liquid chromatography analysis (see Fig. 77.7F) of a hemolysate of a blood sample from an individual who is heterozygous for Hb S shows peaks in the Hb A and S positions, with 40% of the total Hb found in the Hb S peak. Hb S concentrations less than 30% are suggestive of coinheritance of α-thalassemia. Hb F concentration is variable. Electrophoresis (see Fig. 77.13) at both alkaline and acid pH shows bands in the A and S positions.

CBC analysis from an individual who is heterozygous for Hb S shows a slightly decreased concentration of Hb, and sickle cells are not typically seen on the peripheral blood film. Patients are often asymptomatic, and the first time an individual is diagnosed as heterozygous for Hb S (sickle cell trait) is often when an HbA$_{1c}$ analysis is requested for the individual or when a family study is initiated for genetic counseling. In the United States, neonatal screening programs are designed specifically to detect both heterozygous and homozygous Hb S in newborns. Although individuals with the sickle cell trait are clinically asymptomatic, genetic counseling should be considered because coinheritance of two β-globin gene abnormalities from heterozygous parents may contribute to a sickle cell disorder. Alpha- and β-thalassemia can be coinherited with heterozygous Hb S.

Hemoglobin SC (Hemoglobin SC Disease)

Hemoglobin SC disease arises when both β-globin chains are substituted at position 6 with valine (Hb S) or lysine (Hb C). On HPLC and capillary electrophoresis, analysis peaks are noted in the S and C positions, with the S peak forming most of the Hb present.

Electrophoresis (see Fig. 77.13) at both alkaline and acid pH shows bands in the S and C positions, and the sickling test is positive.

Hemoglobin SD

Hemoglobin S may be coinherited with Hb D (SD disease). Individuals with this disease have similar but milder clinical presentation compared with that of sickle cell disease (Hb SS). HPLC analysis shows two peaks—one in the Hb S position that forms approximately 38 to 42% of the total Hb, and the other in the Hb D position that forms 43 to 45% of the total Hb. The Hb F concentration is usually within the reference interval, although concentrations as high as 14% have been observed in some individuals with SD disease. Alkaline electrophoresis shows a band in the S position. Acid electrophoresis shows bands in the S and A positions. The sickling test is positive. CBC analysis shows a greatly decreased concentration of Hb, with normal to slightly elevated MCV. Target, boat-shaped, nucleated red, and sickle cells—together with anisocytosis and poikilocytosis—are noted on the peripheral blood smear (Fig. 77.14).

Hemoglobin S/O Arab

Coinheritance of Hb S and Hb O Arab presents a similar or somewhat milder clinical presentation to sickle cell disease and is found in the Middle East and North Africa.

Hemoglobin S/G Philadelphia

One or more abnormal α-globin chains can combine with Hb S. In African Americans and West Africans, the combination of Hb G Philadelphia [α68(E17)$^{Asn→Lys}$] with Hb S is

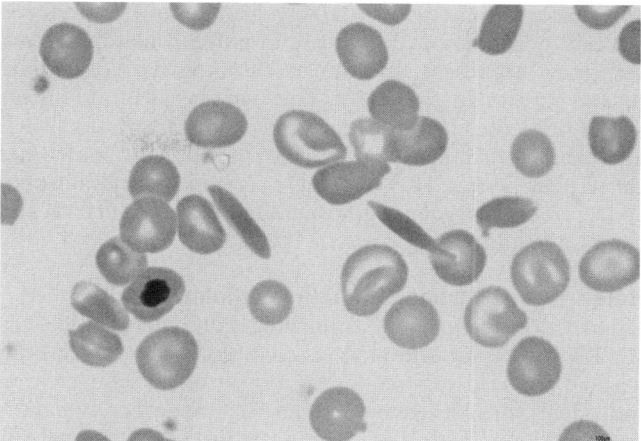

FIGURE 77.14 Peripheral blood smear of Hb SD disease, showing sickle cells and auto-splenectomy changes. Wright-Giemsa ×1000.

prevalent. HPLC analysis (see Fig. 77.7I) of blood samples from these individuals shows at least two major peaks and two smaller peaks. The two major peaks are due to combinations of the normal α-chain with the normal β-chain and the abnormal α-chain with the normal β-chain. The two smaller peaks are due to combinations of the normal α-chain with the abnormal β-chain and the abnormal α-chain with the abnormal β-chain. Electrophoresis at alkaline pH shows major bands in the A and S positions, with a minor band in the C position. At acid pH, bands are seen in the A and S positions. CBC analysis gives a slightly decreased Hb concentration with normal MCV and MCH. α- or β-thalassemia can be coinherited with Hb G Philadelphia and Hb S. In these cases, CBC analysis results in markedly decreased MCV and MCH with reduced Hb concentration.

Double heterozygosity Hb G Philadelphia/Hb S occurs in 1 in 125,500 African Americans. In African Americans, the Hb G Philadelphia mutation commonly occurs with an α-chain deletion, which is *cis* to the mutated allele (-α^G/αα). This results in a change in the amount of mutated α-chain (α^G) from the usual 25% to approximately 30%. No clinical or hematologic manifestations are noted with Hb G Philadelphia/Hb S.

Hemoglobin C [β6(A3)$^{Glu→→Lys}$]

Hemoglobin C arises from a substitution of lysine for glutamic acid at position 6 of the β-globin chain. Hb C may be found in the homozygous (Hb C disease, β^{C}β^C) or heterozygous (Hb C trait) state. Hb C is commonly found in West Africa and the Caribbean. It is the second most commonly studied of all the Hb variants after Hb S.

Homozygous Hemoglobin C (Hemoglobin C Disease)

HPLC analysis (see Fig. 77.7G) of samples from individuals with homozygous Hb C shows a large peak in the C position, with Hb C forming 90 to 95% of the total Hb. Hb F concentrations are variable. Glycated Hb C is found as a small peak eluting before the Hb C peak. The interval of the elution times between glycated Hb C to Hb C is the same as that between HbA$_{1c}$ and Hb A. Electrophoresis at alkaline and acid pH shows a single band in the C position.

Mild to moderate anemia is the most common clinical presentation. CBC analysis shows normal or slightly decreased

Hb concentrations with a normochromic and normocytic red cell morphology. An increase in polychromatophilic red cells may be present, and the reticulocytes may contribute to an increase in the MCV. The peripheral blood smear shows numerous target cells, with occasional nucleated RBCs and characteristic irregular contracted red cells (sometimes called pyknocytes). Hb C crystals may be seen, and bilirubin concentrations may be slightly elevated. Red cell survival and osmotic fragility are decreased.

Heterozygous Hemoglobin C (hemoglobin C trait)

High-performance liquid chromatography analysis (see Fig. 77.7H), capillary electrophoresis, and electrophoresis at both alkaline and acid pH (see Fig. 77.13) on blood samples from individuals who are heterozygous for Hb C reveal bands in the A and C positions, with Hb C forming 38 to 45% of the total Hb. CBC analysis may show target cells and is generally normochromic, with the MCV near the lower limit of the reference interval.

Heterozygous Hb C individuals are usually asymptomatic. Genetic counseling may be useful when prospective parents have abnormalities in the β-globin gene.

Hb C may be coinherited with both α- and β-thalassemias, and the concentration of Hb C is related to the number of functioning α-genes. With only two functioning α-genes, the Hb C concentration can fall to 32% of the total Hb. Coinheritance of Hb C with $β^0$- or $β^+$-thalassemia results in moderately severe anemia with splenomegaly. The Hb F concentration is often increased.

Hemoglobin D Punjab [$β121(GH4)^{Glu \rightarrow \rightarrow \rightarrow Gln}$]

Hemoglobin D Punjab is an Hb variant in which glutamic acid at position 121 of the β-globin chain is replaced with glutamine. The names Hb D Los Angeles and Hb D Punjab are used to describe this variant, with the former name used more often in North America and the latter in the United Kingdom. Hb D Punjab is found in the Punjab region of the Indian subcontinent, especially in Sikhs from the Lycus Valley. Large-scale immigration from this area to the United Kingdom, the United States, and Canada has widened the distribution of Hb D Punjab. Hb D Punjab is also found in Caucasians whose ancestors lived in the Indian subcontinent at the time of the British Raj. Hb D Punjab is found in both heterozygous (Hb D Punjab trait) and homozygous (Hb D Punjab disease, $β^Dβ^D$) states.

HPLC analysis of blood from an individual with homozygous Hb D Punjab shows normal or marginally raised Hb F and Hb A_2 peaks, with a large peak in the Hb D position forming more than 90% of the total Hb. Electrophoresis at alkaline pH shows a band in the S position, which migrates to the A position in acid electrophoresis. CBC analysis shows a mild decrease in Hb concentrations, MCV, and MCH, with target cells observed in the blood smear. Patients present clinically with mild anemia.

HPLC analysis of individuals with the Hb D Punjab trait shows two peaks—one at the A position and the other at the D position—with Hb D forming 30 to 40% of the total Hb. The Hb F and Hb A_2 concentrations are within or slightly above the reference intervals. Electrophoresis at alkaline pH shows two bands—one in the A position and the other in the S position. On electrophoresis at acid pH, a single band in the A position is noted. HPLC is the preferred method for identification of Hb D because a similar electrophoretic pattern, on both alkaline and acid pH, is seen with Hb G. CBC analysis is unremarkable except for the presence of target cells on the blood smear. Individuals with Hb D Punjab trait are clinically asymptomatic.

Hemoglobin D Iran [$b22(B4)^{Glu \rightarrow \rightarrow Gln}$]

Hemoglobin D Iran is a β-globin chain variant in which glutamine replaces glutamic acid at position 22 of the β-globin chain.

On HPLC analysis, peaks are seen in the A and A_2 positions with quantification for Hb A_2 far above what is normally expected. Alkaline electrophoresis shows two bands—one in the A position and the other in the S position. On acid electrophoresis, a single band in the A position is noted. Individuals with Hb D Iran are asymptomatic.

Hemoglobin E [$b26(B8)^{Glu \rightarrow \rightarrow Lys}$]

Hemoglobin E is a β-chain variant with lysine replacing glutamic acid at position 26 of the β-globin chain. It's a common variant in Southeast Asia. Hb E is found in both homozygous and heterozygous states and may be combined with β-thalassemia. It is widespread in the Far East, including Southern China, Cambodia, Thailand, and Laos. Hb E has been increasingly found in the United States and Canada, which is caused by emigration from these areas. It may be believed to be the "thalassemic variant" because some of the features of the CBC resemble thalassemia, especially in the homozygous state.

HPLC analysis of blood from individuals with homozygous Hb E (Hb E disease, $β^Eβ^E$) shows a single peak (>90% of the total Hb) coeluting with Hb A_2. Hb F is within or marginally above the reference interval. On alkaline electrophoresis, a single band is noted in the C position, which migrates to the A position in acid electrophoresis. CBC analysis shows normal to marginally decreased Hb concentrations with low MCV and MCH. Target cells are noted in the peripheral blood smear. Fe studies are normal. Homozygous Hb E individuals are usually asymptomatic, although slight anemia may be present.

HPLC analysis of blood from individuals with heterozygous Hb E reveals two peaks—one in the A position and the other in the A_2 position. Hb E forms approximately 30% of the total Hb. CBC analysis shows normal Hb concentrations and occasionally low MCV. Target cells are noted in the peripheral blood smear. Fe studies are normal. Heterozygous Hb E individuals are usually asymptomatic, although slight anemia may be present.

Coinheritance of heterozygous Hb E with α-thalassemia produces a mild anemia with low Hb, MCV, and MCH. Target cells are noted on the peripheral blood smear, together with microcytosis and hypochromia. Patients who are pregnant may need to be monitored closely, although transfusion is not usually required.

Hb A_2 is higher in patients with Hb E than in patients without a Hb variant or thalassemia because of decreased synthesis of the abnormal β-globin chain, which allows for increased binding between the excess α-globin and δ-globin chains producing Hb A_2.[58,59] Quantification of Hb A_2 provides a challenge to the laboratory, in that Hb E and Hb A_2 coelute. Hb E shows retention time similar to that of Hb A_2 and these hemoglobins cannot be positively separated by this method (see Fig. 77.15C). Capillary zone electrophoresis is capable of separating Hb E from Hb A_2 and hence can give an accurate quantification of Hb A_2 in the presence of Hb E (see Fig. 77.15D).

Hemoglobin O Arab [$b121(GH4)^{Glu \rightarrow \rightarrow \rightarrow Lys}$]

Hemoglobin O Arab is a β-chain variant with lysine replacing glutamic acid at position 121 of the β-globin chain. Hb O

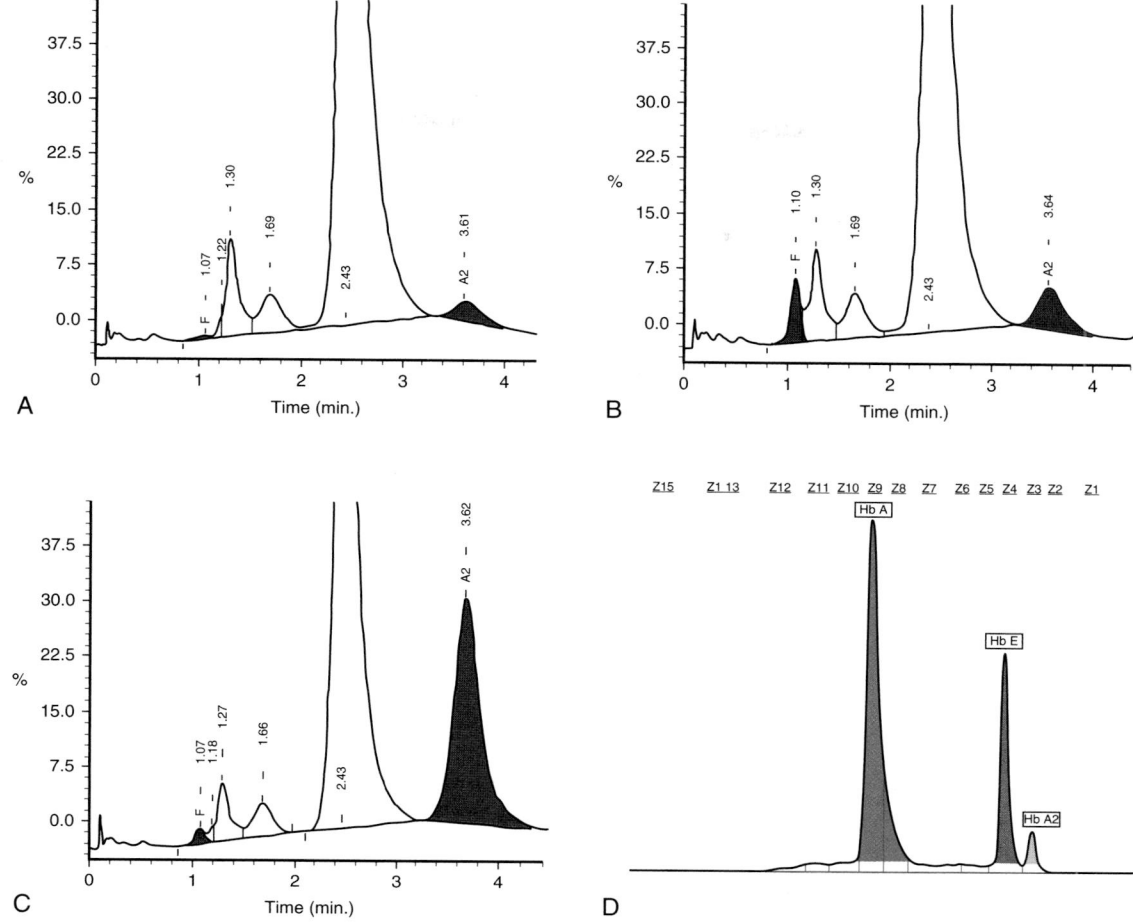

FIGURE 77.15 High-performance liquid chromatography (HPLC) chromatograms in (A) a normal subject, (B) a patient with β-thalassemia trait showing raised Hb A2 level, (C) a patient with heterozygous Hb E showing apparently markedly raised Hb A2 due to co-elution of Hb E with Hb A2, and (D) electropherogram of capillary zone electrophoresis in a patient with heterozygous Hb E showing separation of Hb E and Hb A2 into different zones.

Arab is found in a wide variety of ethnic groups in North Africa and Eastern Europe, and is not confined, nor is it even common, among Arab populations. Hb O Arab has been found in both heterozygous and homozygous states.

HPLC analysis of blood from an individual with homozygous Hb O Arab shows a single band between the S and C positions, with Hb O Arab forming more than 90% of the total Hb. Electrophoresis at alkaline pH shows a band close to the C position. On electrophoresis at acid pH, a band is seen between the A and S positions (but closer to A). CBC analysis shows a normal or marginally low Hb concentration, MCV, and MCH. The peripheral blood smear shows slight microcytosis.

No unusual hematologic features are noted in individuals with heterozygous Hb O Arab. HPLC analysis of blood from these individuals shows two peaks—one in the A position and the other eluting close to the C position and forming 30 to 40% of the total Hb. Electrophoresis at alkaline electrophoresis shows bands in the A position and close to the C position. On acid electrophoresis, two bands are noted—one in the A position and the other in a position between the A and S positions.

Thalassemic Hemoglobinopathies

Amino acid substitutions and other mutations can produce multiple effects on the globin protein. The term thalassemic

hemoglobinopathies is used to refer to a group of Hb variants with features that overlap with thalassemia. For example, Hb E (β26 [B8] Glu > Lys), a common hemoglobinopathy in Southeast Asia, contains an amino acid substitution that renders β chains mildly unstable in vitro with minimal clinical significance. This mutation also creates an alternative splice site in the β-globin mRNA, resulting in reduced synthesis of the productive transcripts and consequently a thalassemic picture. Other examples of thalassemic hemoglobinopathies are hybrid hemoglobins such as Hb Lepore and anti-Lepore, and elongated hemoglobins such as Hb Constant Spring.

Hybrid Hemoglobins

Hybrid Hbs, or crossover Hbs, describe a group of Hb variants in which one of the globin chains is a hybrid of amino acid sequences of two other globin chains. The term crossover Hb is sometimes used because there is a point in the amino acid sequence at which there is crossover from the amino acid sequence of one globin chain to another globin chain. Individuals with these hybrid Hb variants present with clinical features and laboratory findings, particularly in their CBCs, which are similar to those of thalassemia. Production of the hybrid globin chain is reduced. Hb Lepore is the prototypical hybrid Hb.

Hemoglobin Lepore

Hemoglobin Lepore is classified as a δβ-hybrid Hb variant on the basis that the non–α-chain is a hybrid of δ- and β-globin chains. It is unique in that it is the only hemoglobinopathy named after the family name of the index case. δ-/β-Hybrid Hbs arise because there are deletions of the 3′ portion of the δ-globin gene and of the 5′ portion of the β-globin chain, with resultant formation of a δβ-fusion gene. Three distinct variations of Hb Lepore have been described. In Hb Lepore-Hollandia (δβ-hybrid [δ through 22; β from 50]), a variant found in Canada and Papua New Guinea, fusion occurs at the first 22 amino acid residues of the δ-globin chain, with the amino acids from position 50 onward of the β-globin chain. In Hb Lepore-Baltimore (δβ-hybrid (δ through 50: β from 86]), which is found mainly in individuals of Spanish ancestry, the first 50 amino acid residues of the δ-globin chain are fused with amino acid residues from position 86 of the β-globin chain. In Hb Lepore-Boston-Washington (δβ-hybrid [δ through 87; β from 116]), the most common Hb Lepore, the first 87 amino acid residues of the δ-globin chain are fused with amino acid residues from position 116 onward of the β-globin chain. Hb Lepore-Boston-Washington, sometimes called Hb Lepore-Boston, is found mainly in individuals of Italian descent, although it has been found in individuals from Eastern Europe.

HPLC analysis of blood from individuals with Hb Lepore shows greatly elevated Hb A2 concentration with marginally reduced Hb A. The Hb A2 concentration is usually greater than 10% of the total Hb and is falsely increased because of the coelution of Hb A2 and Hb Lepore. Electrophoresis at alkaline pH shows a band in the S position for Hb Lepore-Boston-Washington and in a position between the A and S positions for the other Hb Lepore variants. At acid pH, a single band is present in the A position for all Hb Lepore variants. Hb A2 and Hb Lepore are resolved on capillary electrophoresis.

CBC analysis shows greatly reduced concentrations of Hb, MCV, and MCH in Hb Lepore homozygotes. Hematologic findings are similar to those of β-TM or β-TI. CBC analysis of heterozygotes shows slightly reduced MCV and MCH. Hematologic findings are similar to those of the β-thalassemia trait. Fe studies are normal in both heterozygotes and homozygotes. The similarity of the hematology in Hb Lepore and in β-thalassemia makes careful review of HPLC and electrophoretic analysis essential. A greatly elevated Hb A2 by HPLC analysis and a small band in the S position on electrophoresis at alkaline pH suggest Hb Lepore.

Hemoglobin Anti-Lepore

Hemoglobin anti-Lepore is classified as a βδ-hybrid Hb variant on the basis that the non–α-chain is a hybrid of β-chain like residues at the N-terminal end and δ-chain like residues at the C-terminal end. While the heterozygous state of Hb anti-Lepore is clinically silent, compound heterozygous Hb anti-Lepore and β0-thalassemia may produce a thalassemia intermedia phenotype in the affected patient.[60]

Elongation Hemoglobins

Elongation Hbs, of which there are 13 (7 α-chain and 6 β-chain variants) result from lengthening of the C or N terminus of either globin chain. The most important, from a clinical perspective, are the five C-terminal, α-chain variants in which the terminal codon TAA is changed and an amino acid

sequence is added. The prototypical elongation Hb is Hb Constant Spring. In this variant, the C-terminal TAA codon is changed to CAA in the α2-gene, and a 31-amino-acid sequence is added at the C-terminal end to give an α-globin chain length of 173-amino-acid residues, rather than the normal 142 residue length. This increase in length results in instability of the Hb variant, and synthesis of this elongated globin chain is reduced. Hb Constant Spring is found in Southeast Asia, especially in Vietnam, Cambodia, and Laos, and is found in both the heterozygous and homozygous states.

Patients with heterozygous Hb Constant Spring present with slightly reduced Hb, MCV, and MCH, with hypochromia and microcytosis in the peripheral blood smear. Fe studies are often normal. Homozygous patients have reduced red cell survival and more significant anemia and reduction of MCH, but MCV is normal because of reticulocytosis.

The instability of Hb Constant Spring presents a challenge to the laboratory diagnosis of this variant. The blood used for analytical procedures should be as fresh as possible. Samples older than 24 hours should not be used. HPLC analysis of blood from individuals with Hb Constant Spring demonstrates a small peak in the C position, which forms approximately 4 to 6% of the total Hb in the homozygote and 1 to 3% in the heterozygote. On electrophoresis at alkaline pH, a small band migrating cathodally to the application point may be seen. This alkaline electrophoretic mobility is unique because it is the only Hb variant that moves toward the cathode rather than the anode.

Hb Constant Spring is commonly found in combination with α0-thalassemia, especially the (−SEA) mutation. The clinical presentation of this combination results in a severe form of Hb H disease (see Fig. 77.9).

Database of Hemoglobin Variants

A comprehensive database of hemoglobin variants and thalassemia is found at the Globin Gene Server http://globin.cse.psu. edu/. It contains more than 1800 entries that include more than 1300 hemoglobin variants and more than 500 thalassemia mutations (accessed January 2020).[35,61] Many benign Hb variants are identified incidentally through routine newborn testing, HbA1c testing or through investigation of cyanosis with adequate arterial oxygenation and no cardiopulmonary disease, erythrocytosis with a normal or elevated erythropoietin level, and family history of Hb variant. The importance of referencing the Hb variant database for clinical correlation is to minimize additional diagnostic procedures, hence sparing expense and patient risk. Laboratories should maintain a bank of hematologic and chromatographic data for Hb variants found in their facilities.

Interactions Between α-Thalassemia and β-Thalassemia

β-Thalassemia Heterozygotes With Concurrent SEA Deletion

β-Thalassemia heterozygotes with concurrent SEA deletion are at risk of producing offspring affected by: (1) β-thalassemia major, if the partner is a β-thalassemia carrier, (2) Hb Bart's hydrops fetalis, if the partner is a SEA deletion carrier, and (3) Hb H disease, if the partner is a carrier of single α-globin gene deletion.[18] In terms of phenotype, double heterozygotes for β-thalassemia and α0-thalassemia show higher MCV and MCH values than those who are heterozygous for either trait alone. Hemoglobin pattern study in these subjects shows an increased Hb A_2 only and thus resembles simple β-thalassemia carrier. The Hb H inclusion test is not suitable for the diagnosis of double α- and β-heterozygotes, as it is negative in nearly all cases due to a reduced chain imbalance and fewer free β-globin chains to form Hb H. It follows that if one partner of a couple is a known carrier of $α^0$-thalassemia, it is imperative to screen for $α^0$-thalassemia in the other partner, even though he or she may appear to be a β-thalassemia carrier based on hematologic findings (discordant α/β couples), to predict for the risk of hydrops fetalis.[19] Secondly, the presence of SEA deletion should be determined in couples at risk of conceiving a fetus affected by $β^0/β^+$-thalassemia (i.e., parents who are discordant carriers of $β^0$- and $β^+$-thalassemia mutations), so that the consistent phenotypic amelioration effect may be incorporated into the genetic counselling of such couples.[62] The screening for concurrent ($—^{SEA}$) α-thalassemia mutation in these subjects can be performed by standard gap-PCR.

Hb H Disease and Heterozygous β-Thalassemia

These patients show anemia with markedly hypochromic and microcytic red cells, variable levels of Hb A_2, and significant globin chain imbalance. Hb H inclusion bodies may not be present at all, although in a few cases, a trace amount of Hb Bart's is detected. Genotype analysis therefore serves as an important diagnostic tool to investigate adult patients with unexplained moderate to severe hypochromic microcytic anemia, without which the definitive diagnosis may be considerably delayed and unnecessary investigations for other causes of anemia may be undertaken.[63] A family study is also useful in these cases.

Triplicated α-Globin Genes and Heterozygosity for $β^0$-Thalassemia

The presence of extra copies of α-globin genes in β-thalassemia heterozygotes leads to aggravation of the globin chain imbalance in such individuals and predicts for a thalassemia intermedia phenotype. Triplication of the α-globin gene is formed as a result of mispairing of homologous sequences in the α-globin gene followed by unequal cross-over, which also gives rise to single α-globin gene deletions. Triplication commonly exists in two forms, $ααα^{anti-3.7}$ configuration or $ααα^{anti-4.2}$ configuration. A genotype of triplicated α-globin genes ($ααα/αα$) and heterozygosity for β-thalassemia, with a few exceptions, is associated with thalassemia intermedia of mild severity, and has been recognized in various ethnic groups.[64] Clinical behavior as β-thalassemia trait is also reported and the reason for the phenotypic heterogeneity is uncertain, but there may be progressive anemia associated with increase in age.

Patients with triplicated α-globin gene with heterozygous β-thalassemia are often mistaken as a simple β-thalassemia carrier, because of the superficial resemblance of MCV, MCH, and Hb A_2 results. The hemoglobin level in these patients is lower than expected for simple β-thalassemia minor and, in view of the frequent occurrence of jaundice and splenomegaly, often leads to exhaustive investigations for a presumptive diagnosis of concurrent hemolytic anemia. Several diagnostic clues will help to raise the clinical suspicion of triplicated α-globin gene in heterozygous β-thalassemia. First, the red cell abnormalities, in terms of hypochromasia, anisocytosis, and poikilocytosis, are more marked than that seen in β-thalassemia minor. Second, circulated normoblasts are uniformly

noted in the blood film even in the absence of splenectomy, which is not expected for β-thalassemia minor. Finally, the Hb F level of these patients is significantly higher than in β-thalassemia minor. Although an increase in Hb F level is not specific and may be attributable to other factors, the presence of extra copies of the α-globin gene should be considered in apparent β-thalassemia heterozygotes with a higher Hb F level and a lower hemoglobin level than expected. Higher order amplifications of the α-globin genes are also rarely detected, with a predictable more severe phenotype when co-existing with heterozygous β-thalassemia.

The genotype of triplicated or higher order amplification of α-globin genes in β-thalassemia heterozygotes may explain the inheritance of families with children affected with β-thalassemia intermedia in which only one parent showed abnormalities on hemoglobin analysis.

Interactions Between Thalassemia and Hemoglobinopathy

Most variant hemoglobins are clinically benign. However, coinheritance of a hemoglobin variant with thalassemia may result in significant disease. An example is compound heterozygosity for Hb E and β-thalassemia.[65] Approximately half of the patients with Hb E/β-thalassemia behave as β-thalassemia intermedia and the other half as β-thalassemia major. The determining factors are still not completely understood, but Hb F expression level is one important disease modifying factor. Due to emigration and hence admixture of the world's population, the chance of coinheriting an unusual hemoglobinopathy and thalassemia combination is increased, for example compound heterozygosity for Hb Malay, prevalent in Southeast Asia, and a β-thalassemia mutation in the Chinese.[66] Careful clinical and laboratory correlation is therefore required to determine if additional investigations are indicated to precisely characterize the globin gene mutations.

The coinheritance of Hb H disease genotypes (either three-gene deletion or two-gene deletion and nondeletional α-globin gene mutation such as Hb CS) and heterozygous Hb E result in hemoglobin A + E + Bart's disease. The clinical phenotype is similar to Hb H disease, showing a variable degree of anemia and splenomegaly. Unlike Hb H disease, there are relatively few Hb H inclusion bodies. The hemoglobin comprises Hb A, Hb E (~14%), Hb Bart ($~8\%$), and Hb F (1–2%), and occasionally a small amount of Hb H.[22] In this condition, the $β^A$, $β^E$, and γ chains compete for a limited number of α chains. There is a competitive advantage for $β^A$ to bind with α chains, resulting in an excess of $β^E$ and γ chains. Although the $γ_4$ tetramer is stable, the $β^E_4$ tetramer is most probably not and hence, these patients have Hb Bart's and reduced Hb H level. The same reduction of β-globin variant percentage applies to most β-globin variants with coinheritance of α-thalassemia. Another well-known example is heterozygous Hb S with coinherited α-thalassemia, which leads to reduction of Hb S level to 25 to 30%.

Similarly, when an α-chain hemoglobin variant is coinherited with β-thalassemia, the percentage of the α-chain variant is usually lower in the doubly affected individual than in the simple heterozygote. The normal α-chains bind preferentially to the β (and γ) chains and, if there is a severe degree of globin imbalance, virtually no variant α-chains combine with the limited number of available β (and γ) chains. The excess variant α-chains presumably are precipitated or subject to proteolytic degradation in the red cell precursors.

The percentage of a β-globin variant is increased to 70 to 90% in a patient who has coinherited β-thalassemia. The exact proportion of variant depends on the nature of the β-thalassemia mutation that determines the amount of residual $β^A$-globin chain production. The same applies to coinheritance of α-globin variant and α-thalassemia. An example is Hb Q-Thailand. As this α1-globin gene variant is linked with α2-globin gene deletion, the percentage of the variant in the heterozygous state is around 30%. In the homozygous state or compound heterozygous with SEA deletion (Hb Q-H disease),[67] the percentage of Hb Q-Thailand is over 95% and Hb A is absent.

Rarely, coinheritance of α-thalassemia, β-thalassemia, and a hemoglobin variant is seen. One interesting example is Hb H genotype with homozygous Hb E or Hb E/$β^0$-thalassemia, the hemoglobin E + F + Bart's disease, with the hemoglobin pattern characteristically showing Hb E (70 to 95%), Hb F (1 to 25%), and Hb Bart's (1 to 7%).[22]

Coinheritance of Hb D Punjab with β-thalassemia is common in Southern Asians. CBC analysis of these patients shows decreased concentrations of Hb with markedly decreased MCV and MCH. Target and irregular contracted cells, together with hypochromia and anisocytosis, are seen on the blood smear. Quantification of Hb A_2 in individuals with coinheritance of Hb D Punjab and β-thalassemia presents a challenge to the laboratory, because HPLC analysis underestimates the Hb A_2 concentration due to an unstable rising baseline in these individuals. Capillary zone electrophoresis allows accurate quantification of Hb A_2 in this situation.

Similar to the scenario of interaction between α-thalassemia and β-thalassemia, molecular methods and family studies are needed to resolve complex syndromes resulting from interaction between thalassemia and the hemoglobinopathies.

ANALYTICAL METHODS

The laboratory plays a crucial role in detection and characterization of the hemoglobinopathies and thalassemias, as discussed in the next sections.[68] Several recommendations have been put forth for laboratory investigations of abnormal Hbs and thalassemias.[69–71] For example, in 1978, the International Committee for Standardization in Hematology expert panel on abnormal Hbs published recommendations for the laboratory investigation of these conditions.[72] In its initial investigation, (1) a CBC, (2) electrophoresis at pH 9.2, (3) tests for solubility and sickling, and (4) quantification of Hb A_2 and Hb F were recommended. If an abnormal Hb was found as a result of these initial tests, further tests, including electrophoresis at pH 6.2, globin chain separation, and isoelectric focusing, were recommended by the panel. If the presence of an unstable Hb or Hb with altered oxygen affinity was suspected, then heat and isopropanol stability tests were recommended. Although new techniques have replaced some of these tests, the approach of using multiple assays in the initial investigation of hemoglobinopathies and thalassemias is an accepted practice that is used in many laboratories involved in the investigation of these disorders. In addition to these tests, the Fe status of the patient should be ascertained by measurement of ferritin or by the Fe/total Fe-binding capacity/saturation index. Information on the ethnicity and/or nationality of the patient, when allowed under patient confidentiality rules, may provide useful information

because thalassemias (e.g., β-thalassemia in individuals of Mediterranean origin) and certain hemoglobinopathies (e.g., Hb S trait and homozygous S in African Americans) are associated with particular ethnic and/or national groups.

The 2010 guidelines of the British Committee for Standards in Haematology[73] for the laboratory diagnosis of hemoglobinopathies recommend that qualification for genetic counseling requires identification of Hbs S, C, D Punjab, O Arab, E, Lepore, and H, and the detection of carriers of $α^0$-thalassemia and β-thalassemia traits. To accomplish this, it is recommended that "all ethnic groups" be screened for the β-thalassemia trait when the mean cell (or corpuscular) Hb (MCH) is less than 27 pg. All ethnic groups, except for Northern European Caucasians, should be screened for Hb variants. Selected ethnic groups should be screened for $α^0$-thalassemia trait when the MCH is less than 25 pg. Recommended methods include HPLC and Hb electrophoresis for identification of Hb variants, and HPLC and microcolumn chromatography for quantification of Hb A_2. Electrophoresis is not recommended for the quantification of Hb A_2. In addition, it is recommended that two methods, based on different analytical principles, be used to establish a presumptive identification of the Hb variant. A flowchart (Fig. 77.16) is suggested for identification of $α^0$-, β-, and δβ-thalassemia traits and Hb variants.

Indications for the Investigation of Globin Disorders

The indications for initiating an investigation of thalassemia or hemoglobinopathy are either clinical and laboratory features that raise a suspicion of the disorder, or screening in at-risk subjects.

1. Clinical suspicion of thalassemia or hemoglobinopathy such as unexplained anemia, splenomegaly, jaundice, polycythemia, hemolytic anemia, cyanosis, spurious hypoxemia, or suspected sickle cell crisis.
2. Laboratory evidence of thalassemia or hemoglobinopathy such as hypochromic microcytic red cell indices not due to iron deficiency or chronic disorder, abnormal red cell morphology of unknown cause, and hemoglobin variants incidentally discovered during HbA_{1c} measurement.[54]
3. Family study of an individual diagnosed to have thalassemia or hemoglobinopathy.
4. Premarital, preconception, or antenatal carrier screening in couples from high-prevalence populations for genetic counseling and reproductive decision.
5. Follow up study of patients with severe thalassemia or hemoglobinopathy to determine treatment response, for example, hematopoietic stem cell transplantation or augmentation of Hb F production.
6. Preoperative screening for Hb S in at-risk ethnic populations.

Why Is the Recognition of Globin Disorders Clinically Important?

Correct diagnosis and early recognition of the patients and carriers of hereditary globin disorders is clinically important for several reasons.

1. Planning for appropriate medical treatment strategy such as blood transfusion and chelation regimens in β-thalassemia major.
2. Predicting the prognosis of affected patients through accurate diagnosis and genotype–phenotype correlation.
3. Prevention of fetuses affected by severe thalassemia through carrier detection, genetic counseling, and prenatal diagnosis in high-prevalence populations.

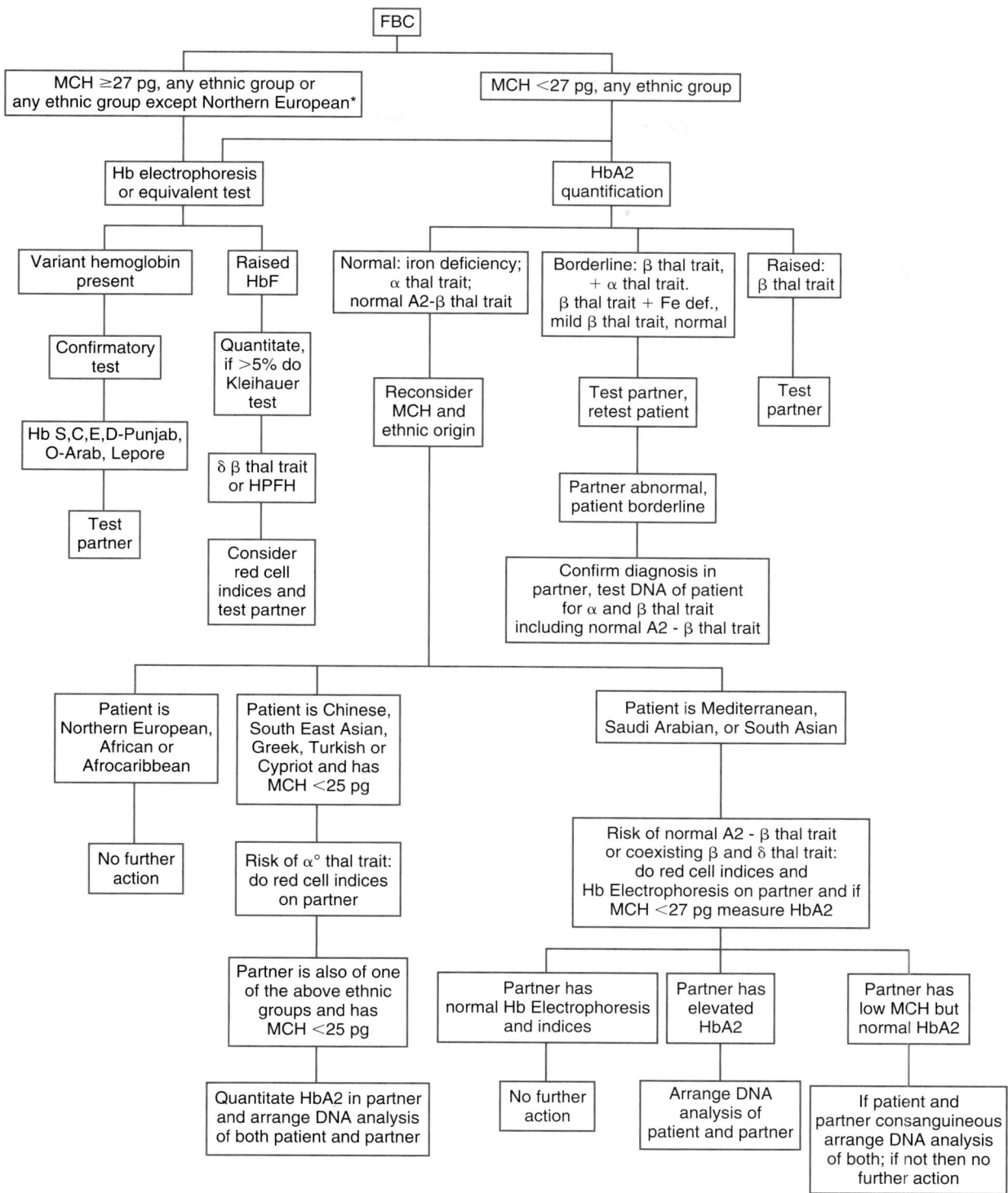

FIGURE 77.16 Flowchart demonstrating procedures for diagnosis of α⁰-, β-, and δβ-thalassemia traits and clinically significant hemoglobin variants in pregnant women ("patients") and their partners. Selective screening is acceptable in low-incidence areas but only if accurate information on ethnic origin is available. *FBC,* Full blood count; *Hb,* hemoglobin; *Hb S, C, E, D-Punjab, O-Arab, Lepore,* various types of hemoglobin; *MCH,* mean cell hemoglobin; *thal,* thalassemia. (Modified from Laboratory diagnosis of haemoglobinopathies. *Br J Haematol* 1998;101:783–92.)

4. Deciphering complex cases of unexplained anemia and elucidating family inheritance.
5. Avoidance of unnecessary invasive procedures such as bone marrow examination or endoscopy and unsuitable treatment such as iron supplement in patients with globin disorders presenting as unexplained anemia, and avoidance of unnecessary invasive procedures such as cardiac catheterization or arterial oxygen saturation studies in patients with hemoglobin variants presenting as spurious hypoxemia.
6. Avoidance of oxidative drugs in unstable hemoglobin variants.
7. Instituting appropriate preventive medical measures such as penicillin prophylaxis and pneumococcal vaccination in infants with sickle cell disease.

Background Patient Information

Although thalassemia and hemoglobinopathies are prevalent in geographical areas where malaria infection is endemic, these globin disorders are now also found in North America, Europe, and all parts of the world because of population migration. Since the spectrum of globin mutations varies with different populations, knowledge of the ethnicity of the patient is always helpful to the laboratory when detection of globin disorder is considered clinically indicated.

The family history should be thoroughly taken. While a positive family history of anemia should alert the clinician to the possibility of inherited globin disorders, the lack of relevant family history does not exclude the possible presence of globin gene mutations since heterozygote carriers are clinically asymptomatic. Importantly, two or more globin gene mutations, for example interaction between α- and β-thalassemia, may be present in the same individual. Appropriate family study is required to characterize these complicated genotypes and to explain the inheritance pattern. It should be noted that nonpaternity and de novo or sporadic mutation are also confounding factors in the correct interpretation of family studies.

Clinical information on the age, gender, marital status, reproductive plan, and concurrent medical illness is necessary for the investigation of globin disorders. When a pregnant woman is referred for a hemoglobin study, there is an urgency to make the correct diagnosis and to screen the partner in a timely manner for genetic counseling and prenatal diagnosis, if needed. Concurrent medical illness, for example chronic inflammatory conditions or renal impairment, may cause anemia or lower the hemoglobin level in thalassemia carriers, and conditions associated with stress erythropoiesis may cause acquired elevation of Hb F level.

Preferred Specimen

The preferred blood sample for use in detection and characterization of thalassemia and hemoglobinopathies is one collected with potassium or sodium salts of ethylenediaminetetraacetic acid as the anticoagulant. To minimize the formation of degradation products, which are especially noticeable as small bands eluting with similar retention time as HbA_{1c} and Hb F on HPLC analysis, testing should be performed within 5 days of collection, and samples should be stored at 4 °C.

Laboratory Techniques of Hemoglobin Study

Analytical techniques used to measure RBCs and their indexes, Hb, and related compounds include (1) determination of CBC, (2) electrophoresis, (3) separation techniques such as HPLC, capillary electrophoresis, and mass spectrometry, (4) DNA analysis, and (5) specific tests for specific variants.

Red Blood Cell Parameters

A complete blood count (CBC) of a whole blood sample consists of (1) numbers of RBCs (erythrocytes), (2) numbers of WBCs, (3) numbers of platelets, (4) a measure of Hb, (5) estimates of red cell volume, and (6) estimation of WBC subtypes. (Note: A CBC is also known as a full blood count, a full blood examination, or a blood panel.) Red cell parameters (or indices) are routinely available on automated hematology cell counters. With exceptions, the hemoglobin (Hb) level, RBCs, and mean cell volume (MCV) are direct or primary measurements by the cell counter, whereas hematocrit (HCT), mean cell hemoglobin (MCH), and mean cell hemoglobin concentration (MCHC) are derived parameters. The red cell distribution width (RDW) is the coefficient variation of red cell volume and some automated cell counters also report the standard deviation. Please see Chapter 74 for more details.

Knowledge of red cell indices[74,75] and the information obtained from microscopic examination of a peripheral blood film is vital to the diagnosis of both α- and β-thalassemias. Hemoglobinopathies often have a lesser impact on red cell indexes, but may present with abnormal red cell morphology on peripheral blood films.

Mean cell volume. In thalassemias, the Hb concentration and the MCV, an index of cell size, are decreased, sometimes markedly, whereas in hemoglobinopathies, both are often normal. The MCV is a reliable measurement that is often used to guide thalassemia screening. There are, however, several catches to note: First, red cells tend to swell up after being stored in EDTA for 2 to 3 days and hence, in the aged sample a spuriously elevated MCV value may result. Analysis of red cell parameters therefore should not be excessively delayed. Second, concurrent thalassemia trait and megaloblastic anemia[44] tend to normalize the MCV value. Examination of other red cell parameters, such as the RDW and blood smear features, will offer hints to these combined conditions. Third, the reference range of MCV in infancy and childhood is significantly different from adults. The MCV value is high at birth, falls to a nadir at around 1 year of age and reaches adult value after 18 years of age (Table 77.4). It is important to bear this point in mind to avoid overzealous investigation of low MCV and MCH values especially in early childhood. Fourth, some mild types of thalassemia mutations may present with a normal MCV,[76] as will most hemoglobin variants.

Mean cell hemoglobin and mean cell hemoglobin concentration. The MCH, despite a calculated value derived from primary cell counter measurements, remains relatively stable over time even when blood sample is stored for 2 to 3 days. Therefore in the United Kingdom the MCH is advocated as a cutoff parameter for the purpose of thalassemia screening. If specimen transport time is short and samples are analyzed without much delay, MCV remains a very reliable screening parameter for thalassemia.

The MCHC theoretically should reflect red cell hemoglobinization. However, in practice the MCHC values generated by automated cell counters usually fall within a narrow range that may not adequately demonstrate the degree of

TABLE 77.4 Reference Intervals of Mean Corpuscular Volume With Respect To Age

Age	MCV (fL)
At birth (term infants)	100–125
2 weeks	88–110
2 months	84–98
6 months	73–84
1 year	70–82
2–6 years	72–87
6–12 years	76–90
12–18 years	77–94
Adult	80–96

MCV, Mean corpuscular volume.
Reference intervals vary depending on test methodology and the reference population.
Data excerpted from Lilleyman JS, Hann IM, Blanchette VS. *Pediatric hematology*. 2nd ed. London: Churchill Livingstone; 1999. pp 2.

hypochromasia that is present. The MCHC is more often used as an internal quality control parameter of automated cell counters for the stability of red cell measurements.

One model of automated cell counter is capable of directly measuring the hemoglobin concentration of individual red cells and their mean value, giving a parameter known as corpuscular hemoglobin concentration mean (CHCM), which is different from and should not be confused with MCHC (see Chapter 74). Direct hemoglobin concentration measurement assists in distinguishing thalassemia trait from iron deficiency through analysis of the erythrogram, which is a plot of red cell volume (*y axis*) versus red cell hemoglobin concentration (*x-axis*) (Fig. 77.17)

MCV and MCH cutoff for thalassemia screening. Since it is not cost effective to perform thalassemia screening on every subject, MCV and MCH cutoff values are usually employed to decide whether hemoglobin pattern study is justified. Needless to say, this strategy may potentially miss carriers of mild to silent thalassemia mutations, but it serves the overall goal of thalassemia screening to prevent fetuses affected by severe thalassemia, namely Hb Bart's hydrops fetalis and β-thalassemia major.

One study recommends that an MCV of less than 72 fL (reference interval 80 to 100 fL; reference intervals vary depending on test methodology and the reference population)[77] is maximally sensitive and specific for the presumptive diagnosis of thalassemia. However, an MCH less than 27 pg (reference interval 26 to 35 pg)[77] has been recommended as the decision point for further investigation for iron deficiency anemia (IDA) and thalassemia. The rationale for the selection of MCH over MCV as the decision point for further investigation is the potential increase of up to 5 fL in MCV in samples older than 24 hours.

Another study from Hong Kong shows that employing MCV < 80 fL or MCH < 27 pg as cutoff value for thalassemia screening detects all heterozygous carriers of (—SEA) α-thalassemia (SEA deletion) and the common β-thalassemia mutations including codons 41 to 42 (-CTTT), IVSII-654 (C→T), nt-28 (A→G), and codon 17 (A→T). Two less common carrier states, namely: (1) compound heterozygosity for (—SEA) α-thalassemia and triplicated α-globin gene (—SEA/ααα) and (2) concurrent (—SEA) α-thalassemia and β-thalassemia carrier, are covered. However using the above cutoff values will not detect: (1) around 50% of carriers of Hb E; (2) around 50% of carriers of single α-globin gene deletion (−α3.7 or −α4.2) and nondeletional α-globin gene mutations (e.g., Hb CS or Hb QS); and (3) the rare silent β-thalassemia carriers.[27]

Investigation of hypochromic microcytic anemia. Anemia associated with hypochromic microcytic red cell indices can be due to IDA, thalassemia, anemia of chronic disorder (ACD), and sideroblastic anemia. Apart from sideroblastic anemia, the three other causes of hypochromic microcytic anemia are commonly encountered in clinical practice. Accurate detection and distinguishing one diagnosis from another is therefore clinically relevant.

The RBC count may be in the upper half of or above the reference interval in thalassemias, but within the reference interval in most hemoglobinopathies without a coinherited thalassemia. In contrast, the RBC count is low in IDA and ACD and is proportionally related to the decrease in Hb concentration. The RDW, a measure of variation in the size of the RBC (anisocytosis), tends to be above the reference interval in IDAs and other microcytic anemias. The RDW in thalassemias is usually within or close to the reference interval, reflecting the uniformity of red cell size. Of note, in Hb H disease and β-thalassemia intermedia and major, the RDW is markedly increased. Some authors have suggested the use of the ratio between the percentage of microcytes and the percentage of hypochromic cells (M/H ratio) in the differentiation between IDA and the β-thalassemia trait. This ratio has been found to be higher for β-thalassemia traits than for IDA.[78]Several other algorithms or discriminant functions, based on conventional and more innovative parameters[79] from the CBC, have been developed and evaluated for the differentiation between Fe deficiency from thalassemia[77,80–83] (Table 77.5).[84]

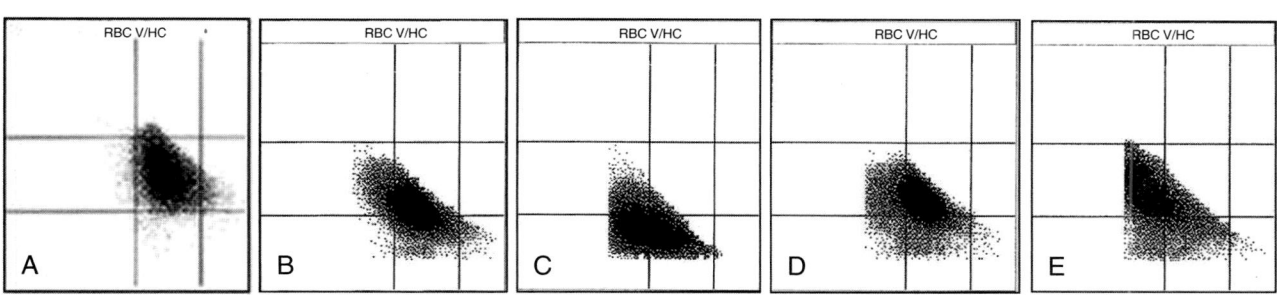

FIGURE 77.17 Erythrograms patterns in: (A) normal, (B) thalassemia trait, (C) iron deficiency anemia, (D) combined thalassemia and iron deficiency anemia, and (E) hemoglobin H disease.

TABLE 77.5 Discriminant Functions for Distinguishing Thalassemia Trait From Iron Deficiency Anemia in Patients With Microcytic Red Blood Cells

Discriminant Index	Calculation	Cutoff Value[a]
England and Fraser	MCV − RBC − (5 Hb) − 3.4	0
RBC	RBC	5.0
Mentzer	MCV/RBC	13
Srivastava	MCH/RBC	3.8
Shine and Lal	$MCV^2 \times MCH$	1.53
Bessman	RDW	15
Ricerca	RDW/RBC	4.4
Green and King	$MCV^2 \times RDW/100\ Hb$	65
Jayabose (RDW index)	MCV/(RBC × RDW)	220
Sirdah	MCV − RBC − (3 Hb)	27.0
M/H ratio	Microcytic RBC %/ hypochromic RBC %	3.7
Ehsani	MCV − (10 RBC)	15

[a]Cutoff values transformed into general used units: Hb in grams per deciliter; RBC in 10^{12}/L; MCV in femtoliter; MCH in picograms; and RDW in percentage.

Hb, Hemoglobin; *MCH*, mean cell Hb; *MCV*, mean cell volume; *RBC*, red blood cell; *RDW*, red cell distribution width.

Data from Hoffmann JJ, Urrechaga E, Aguirre U. Discriminant indices for distinguishing thalassemia and iron deficiency in patients with microcytic anemia: a reply. *Clin Chem Lab Med* 2015;53:1883–94.

TABLE 77.6 Laboratory Differentiation of Hypochromic Microcytic Anemia

Laboratory Parameter	Thalassemia Trait	IDA	ACD	ACD + IDA
RBC count	↑/N	↓	↓	↓
MCV	↓	↓	N/↓	↓
MCH	↓	↓	N/↓	↓
RDW	N	↑	N/↑	↑
Serum iron	N	↓	↓	↓
TIBC/transferrin	N	↑	↓	↓
Transferrin saturation	N	↓	↓	↓
Ferritin	N	↓	↑/N	↑/N
Soluble transferrin receptor (sTfR)	N	↑	N	↑
sTfR/log ferritin ratio	N	↑ (>2)	↓ (<1)	↑ (>2)
CHr or RET-He	↓	↓	N/↓	↓

The typical profile of each clinical scenario is depicted.
ACD, Anemia of chronic disorder; *IDA*, iron deficiency anemia; *N*, normal; ↑, increased; ↓, decreased.

A recent meta-analysis of the most frequently used discriminant functions has demonstrated high variation in the performance of these parameters for distinguishing thalassemia trait from IDA.[84] In general, the newer functions seem to be able to make this distinction better than the more traditional formulas. The M/H ratio was shown to be superior to other discriminant indexes. Notwithstanding its high performance, even the M/H ratio cannot be used for making a final diagnosis of the thalassemia trait. Its value lies in screening of microcytic individuals, to select those in whom additional laboratory investigations are warranted for confirming the presence of thalassemia. An algorithm based on MCV, MCH, Hb A$_2$, and Hb F quantifications has been advocated to better discriminate among β-thalassemia minor, Fe deficiency, δβ-thalassemia, and HPFH.[85] For more information on the clinical usefulness of these CBC parameters and discriminative algorithms, and for conditions leading to microcytic anemia, the reader is referred to the literature.[80–84]

Although the CBC parameters are often the first indication that the patient might have a thalassemia or a hemoglobinopathy, these data are not sufficient to allow the final diagnosis. To investigate hypochromic microcytic anemia, an iron study is often requested together with a hemoglobin pattern study. A biochemical iron profile includes serum iron, total iron binding capacity (TIBC) or transferrin level, serum ferritin, and transferrin saturation (see Chapter 40). Thalassemia carriers show a normal iron study. Typical IDA shows low serum iron, high TIBC and transferrin, low serum ferritin, and low transferrin saturation. Typical iron profile in ACD shows low serum iron, low TIBC and transferrin, high serum ferritin, and low transferrin saturation.

The same patient may have more than one of these causes. For example, a subject with thalassemia trait can have concomitant iron deficiency. Iron replacement therapy is indicated and does not alter the underlying thalassemic condition. ACD superficially mimics iron deficiency based on low serum iron and low transferrin saturation, but the ferritin being an acute phase reactant is elevated. When true iron deficiency coexists with ACD, the former is often masked because of the elevated ferritin level. Since ferritin is no longer a useful marker for the detection of iron deficiency in this setting, newer markers such as soluble transferrin receptor and reticulocyte hemoglobin content have a role to play (Table 77.6). Patients with high soluble transferrin receptor level or high soluble transferrin receptor (in mg/L) to log ferritin (in μg/L) ratio indicates iron deficiency. Low reticulocyte hemoglobin content further strengthens the presence of iron deficiency when the soluble transferrin receptor to log ferritin ratio is high.

Reticulocyte count. A reticulocyte count is helpful in hemoglobin study to reflect hemolysis that may accompany an unstable hemoglobinopathy. The reticulocyte count is often elevated in the intermediate to severe forms of thalassemia, indicating shortened red cell survival as a pathogenic mechanism in these disorders. The reticulocyte count in thalassemia trait is normal while in IDA it is often normal or inadequately elevated for the degree of anemia. Quick and accurate enumeration of reticulocytes is achievable by automated cell counters.

Red cell morphology. Important clues to the diagnosis of hemoglobin disorders are often available through morphologic examination of red blood cells in a well-prepared blood film, which should be an integral part of hemoglobin study.

In thalassemias, the RBCs in the peripheral blood smear are hypochromic and microcytic. The microcytosis and hypochromasia in thalassemia trait is disproportionately low for the hemoglobin level. Red cells usually show minimal anisocytosis. Occasional target cells and basophilic stippling are encountered, the latter mainly in β-thalassemia trait. The degree of microcytosis and hypochromasia in iron deficiency frequently parallels the anemia. There is more anisocytosis and poikilocytosis in iron deficiency. Elliptocytes and pencil-shaped cells are frequently identified. In general, the appearance of red cells on blood film examination is more microcytic in thalassemia trait and more hypochromic in iron deficiency. In intermediate and severe thalassemia, the degree of hypochromasia is much more prominent. Red cells often appear flattened out and larger than what will have been expected from the MCV value. The presence of nucleated red cells is a useful feature to distinguish these cases from severe IDA.

Hemoglobin variants with altered physical properties may show characteristic red cell features. Characteristic sickle- or crescent-shaped RBCs are seen (Fig. 77.18) in the peripheral blood smear of patients who are homozygous for Hb S (sickle cell disease), and targets are seen in blood smears from patients who are homozygous for Hb E (see Fig. 77.18). Other features in a blood film in sickle cell anemia include boat-shaped cells, target cells, polychromatophilic red cells, basophilic stippling, circulating nucleated reds, and Howell-Jolly bodies. Red cells in homozygous Hb C disease are microcytic with numerous target cells, some irregularly contracted cells and rare, but diagnostic, intracellular Hb C crystals. Compound heterozygosity for Hb S and Hb C (SC disease) shows irregularly contracted cells and misshapen red cells

with straight edges and being angulated or branched (SC poikilocytes) (Fig. 77.19).

In unstable hemoglobinopathy (e.g., Hb Koln, Hb Hammersmith), irregularly contracted cells and bite cells are formed due to membrane damage and loss and removal of Heinz bodies after traversing the splenic sinusoids (Fig. 77.20). Differential diagnoses for this feature include oxidative hemolysis in G6PD deficiency, Hb C, and Hb SC disease.

Determining Hemoglobin H and Zeta Chains and Hb Bart

Supravital staining for Hb H inclusion bodies. Hemoglobin H, an insoluble tetramer consisting of four β-globin chains, arises in α-thalassemia, in which decreased production of α-globin chains causes a subsequent excess of β-globin chains. If these tetramers are oxidized, precipitation occurs, which may be viewed microscopically. In the laboratory, this oxidation is achieved by staining unfixed cells with freshly prepared methylene blue or brilliant cresyl blue at 37 °C. Inclusion of positive and negative controls with each batch of Hb H preparations is essential because substantial batch-to-batch variability is seen in the dye.[86] In Hb H disease, typically 30 to 100% of the red cells contain inclusions, which have been described as looking like golf balls. In α^0-thalassemia (two α-gene deletion *in-cis*), as few as 1 cell with inclusions may be seen per 1000 to 10,000 red cells. The presence of Hb H inclusions serves as confirmation of a presumptive diagnosis of α^0-thalassemia or Hb H disease. Note that in homozygous α^+ (α-thal-2) or $-\alpha/-\alpha$

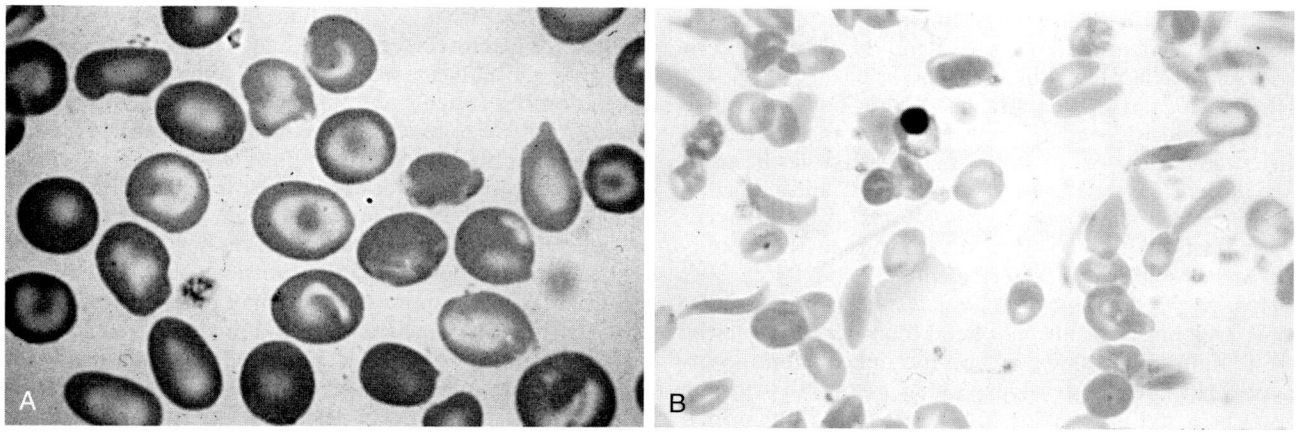

FIGURE 77.18 Peripheral blood smear from patients with (A) homozygous hemoglobin *(Hb)* E and (B) homozygous Hb S.

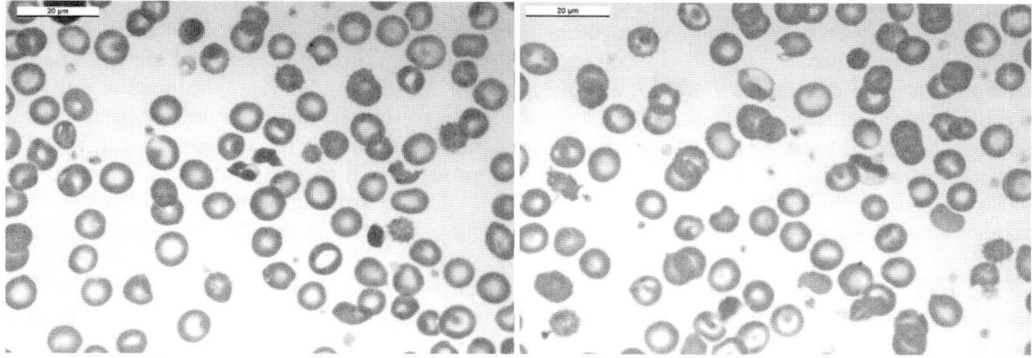

FIGURE 77.19 Peripheral blood smear in compound heterozygous for Hb S and Hb C showing SC poikilocytes containing angulated intracellular crystals. (Courtesy Dr. Alvin Ip.)

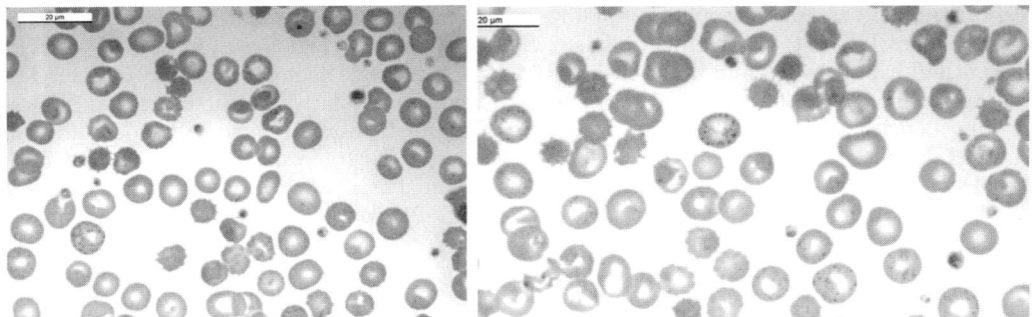

FIGURE 77.20 Peripheral blood smear in heterozygous Hb Hammersmith after splenectomy, showing irregularly contracted red cells, polychromatophilic red cells, basophilic stippling, and Howell-Jolly bodies. Some echinocytes and acanthocytes also seen as a part of post-splenectomy changes. (Images in collaboration with Dr. Alvin Ip.)

genotype, although it also involves deletion of two α-globin genes, Hb H inclusion bodies are not usually detected. Similarly, Hb H inclusion bodies are not regularly detected in nondeletional thalassemia mutations such as in heterozygous Hb Quong Sze and Constant Spring, and in heterozygous α⁺-thalassemia. The diagnosis of silent α-thalassemia or α-thalassemia minor cannot be definitively excluded even in the absence of Hb H inclusions.

Red cell precipitates after supravital staining may arise from staining of reticulin and Howell-Jolly bodies and other protein and nucleic acid entities. However, none of these conditions give an evenly distributed precipitate pattern in a red cell as seen in α-thalassemia. Hb H-like inclusion bodies are found in carriers of Hb New York and should not be confused with *bona fide* Hb H inclusion bodies.[87]

Hb H detection by this method is laborious to perform and is experience dependent. For detection of the two α-gene *cis* deletion (−/αα) or α⁰-thalassemia, the test has been reported to have a clinical sensitivity of only 0.47 and a specificity of 0.99 in a North American laboratory.[88] A much higher test sensitivity of 99% is reported in a Hong Kong study where α-thalassemia is more prevalent.[89]

Detection of embryonic ζ-globin chain. Detection of embryonic ζ-globin chain in peripheral blood erythrocytes by immunofluorescence study or enzyme linked immunosorbent assay (ELISA) was developed to replace the Hb inclusion test especially in the detection of SEA deletion.[90] The principle of the latter assay is based on the increased expression of ζ-globin chains in adult carriers of the SEA deletion. Although the test is shown to be simple and reliable, the limited source of anti-ζ monoclonal antibody and lack of commercialization renders the test hitherto unpopular when compared with other detection methods.

Immunochromatographic strip test for Hb Bart's. A simple, inexpensive, and quick immunochromatographic strip test for Hb Bart's has also been developed to detect α-thalassemia. The sensitivity of α⁰-thalassemia detection is reported to be very high at 97 to 100% in various studies.[91–94] While a negative result almost excludes α⁰-thalassemia, it cannot exclude heterozygous or homozygous α⁺-thalassemia and the non-deletional α-globin gene mutations. False negativity can sometimes be seen in patients double heterozygous for α⁰-thalassemia and β-thalassemia trait. Importantly, a false positive result is seen in patients with an increased Hb F level. Weak positivity can occasionally be seen in β-thalassemia trait and Hb E, and

should not be overcalled. Weak positive reactions should be confirmed by repeating the test. Cases showing repeated weak positivity, or otherwise with unexplained red cell microcytosis, should be further evaluated by molecular studies.

High-Performance Liquid Chromatography

HPLC using a column packed with cation-exchange resin[95–97] provides, in a single analytical protocol, the quantification of Hb F and Hb A₂ (see Chapter 19 for a detailed discussion of HPLC). With it, the initial identification of an Hb variant on the basis of elution time may also be made.

After injection and subsequent adsorption onto the particles of a cation-exchange resin, molecules of Hb are eluted using gradient elution. Detection of eluted Hbs is achieved by monitoring the effluent solvent stream using a dual-wavelength photometer (usually set to measure at wavelengths of 415 and 690 nm). The technique is precise for the quantification of both Hb F and Hb A₂, and presumptive identification of the common Hb variant may be made. These features have made HPLC the method of choice for hemoglobinopathy and thalassemia screening for many laboratories, including those that perform neonatal hemoglobinopathy screening. Fig. 77.7 shows the separation on a commercial system of nine Hb variants.

Several commercial methods have been available for many years, but most of them lack the resolution achieved by noncommercial methods. A noncommercial HPLC method has been described, with the retention time and relative concentration of 40 common Hb variants listed.[97] This system requires a longer time for analysis, provides superior resolution, and overcomes the problem of coelution of several Hb variants that occurs with commercial systems. For example, with one commercial system, Hb E, Hb Osu-Christiansborg, Hb G-Coushatta, Hb Lepore, and Hb G-Copenhagen coelute with Hb A₂, making Hb A₂ quantification and definitive identification of the Hb variants impossible.[98,99] Some newer commercial models have incorporated an optional extended analysis mode with higher resolution to overcome this problem.

Other chromatographic problems, such as rising baseline, have resulted in falsely low Hb A₂ concentration in Hb D patients.[100,101] This may be corrected mathematically to produce a more accurate result. Patients with Hb S have falsely increased Hb A₂ concentrations; this was originally believed to be caused by the coelution of glycated Hb S with Hb A₂.[102] Subsequent studies have shown that the increase in Hb A₂ in patients with Hb S is due to coelution of carbamylated Hb S species.[103] The diagnosis of coinheritance of β-thalassemia with Hb S may be compromised by this false increase in Hb A_2. However, knowledge of the concentration of Hb A_2 is not essential in making the diagnosis of $β^0$- or $β^+$-thalassemia in these patients: in the case of a co-existing $β^0$-thalassemia mutation, no normal β-globin chain is produced, and the electrophoretic pattern and HPLC analysis closely resemble those of a homozygous Hb S patient (large Hb F and Hb S peaks with no Hb A peak); in the case of a co-existing $β^+$-thalassemia mutation, the concentration of Hb S is greater than that of Hb A, a situation that otherwise is seen only in recently transfused patients who have sickle cell disease. Capillary zone electrophoresis and microcolumn methods have been described that eliminate the interference of modified Hb S with Hb A_2 quantification.

The use of relative elution time rather than absolute elution time in the initial identification of an unknown Hb variant is useful and recommended. The reference Hb ideally is one that is found in low concentrations in most individuals. In this regard, Hb A_2 is probably most useful as a reference point despite the number of coeluting Hb variants.

The elution time of the Hb may change slightly with increasing Hb variant concentration. For example, Hb F concentrations obtained by HPLC are often lower than those

POINTS TO REMEMBER

There are some useful clues and caveats when analyzing HPLC chromatograms in the diagnosis of thalassemias and hemoglobinopathies:

a. *"Hb A_2" greater than 10% is not Hb A_2 but a Hb variant co-eluting with the former.* In this situation, the diagnosis of any co-existing β-thalassemia may be suggested by the red cell indices. Use of an alternative method for Hb A_2 quantification or molecular analysis can help to resolve the problem.

b. *Normal HPLC findings do not exclude globin disorders.* A Hb variant can have the same elution time as Hb A. The HPLC chromatogram of α-thalassemia trait is normal. Correlation with other investigation results is needed.

c. *A normal Hb A_2 level does not always exclude β-thalassemia.* A very mild β-thalassemia mutation, β-thalassemia with co-existing delta-thalassemia or an Hb A_2 variant that has a different elution time from Hb A_2 will all result in a normal Hb A_2 level. Always examine the Hb A_2 peak for any abnormal shape and look for any small abnormal peak that may suggest a Hb A_2 variant.

d. *A Hb variant greater than 30% is more likely to be a β-chain variant.* However, rare β-chain variants can show reduced expression to below 30% (e.g., Hb E).

e. *Alpha chain variants are mostly below 30% of total Hb,* unless there is co-existing α-globin gene deletion/thalassemia (e.g., Hb Q-Thailand).

f. *Alpha thalassemia reduces the percentage of most β-chain variants, but increases the percentage of α-chain variants. Beta thalassemia increases the percentage of β-chain variants.*

g. *When Hb A is absent, it is more likely to be due to β-globin gene cluster defects.* Rarely, an α-chain variant plus α-thalassemia can lead to absent Hb A (e.g., Hb Q Thailand-H disease).

h. *Multiple small and variable peaks suggest an unstable Hb.*

obtained from alkaline denaturation and/or spectrophotometric methods that are often quoted in standard hematology texts and used for the diagnosis of juvenile myelomonocytic leukemia and monosomy 7 syndrome. Caution should be used in interchanging Hb F concentrations obtained by HPLC with those obtained by other methods.

It should be noted that hemoglobinopathies may interfere with glycated Hb analysis because results may be falsely increased or decreased, depending on the particular method and the hemoglobinopathy.[7,104,105] Hb variants that cannot be separated from Hb A or HbA_{1c} will produce spuriously increased or decreased results by ion-exchange HPLC[54] (see also Chapter 47 on Diabetes Mellitus).

The higher equipment, reagent, and maintenance costs of HPLC over electrophoresis are offset by the advantages of automation, accurate Hb A_2 and Hb F measurement, and better resolution of hemoglobin variants. Most clinical laboratories favor the use of HPLC as the initial hemoglobin analysis to be supplemented by electrophoresis or other specialized tests for the identification of hemoglobin variants. With increasing experience in HPLC and capillary electrophoresis for hemoglobin variant screening and the wider availability of molecular tests, one can argue that the role of conventional electrophoresis is ever diminishing.

Electrophoresis

Hemoglobin electrophoresis at alkaline and acidic pH. Electrophoresis methods at alkaline and acidic pH are commonly used for hemoglobin separation. The isoelectric point of Hb A molecule, at which it is neutral, is at pH 6.8. Therefore at alkaline pH, it behaves as an anion (bears negative charge) and migrates toward the anode, whereas at acidic pH it behaves as a cation and migrates toward the cathode.

Electrophoresis (see Chapter 18) under alkaline conditions (pH 9.2) is a common initial screening method for the detection and preliminary identification of hemoglobinopathies.[104] Several media, including paper and cellulose acetate, have been used, although agarose[106] is now the medium of choice and the one usually supplied commercially. A pH 9.2 barbital buffer is the most common buffer system. Visualization of separated Hb bands is achieved by using a protein-binding stain, such as Amido Black or Ponceau S. Hb bands stain blue with Amido Black and reddish pink with Ponceau S. After clearing of excess stain, Hb bands on the agarose media are clearly seen against the clear background. The *left panel* of Fig. 77.13 shows an alkaline electrophoresis gel stained with Amido Black. Quantification by densitometry of Hb A_2 and F bands on alkaline electrophoresis, although still performed by laboratories, is not recommended by the College of American Pathologists in the hemoglobinopathy survey critiques,[107] because of high analytical imprecision resulting from limitations of densitometry in quantifying faint bands.

At alkaline pH, Hbs migrate according to electrical charge, with Hb H moving the fastest (closest to the anode). The order of migration (fastest to slowest) is Hb H, Hb N, Hb I, Hb J, Hb A, Hb F, Hb S, and Hb C. Hb D, Hb G, and Hb Lepore comigrate with Hb S, and Hb E, Hb O, and Hb A_2 comigrate with Hb C. Hb Constant Spring migrates slightly toward the cathode. An easy way to remember the sequence is Hb A goes to the anode, whereas Hb C migrates to the cathode. Hb F and Hb S follow after Hb A in alphabetical order.

Electrophoresis at pH 6.4 using a citrate buffer is performed when an abnormal band is noted on alkaline Hb electrophoresis. Agarose is the preferred medium, with acid violet as the preferred stain. The same Hb variants performed on agarose electrophoresis at pH 6.4 and stained with acid violet are shown in the *right panel* of Fig. 77.13. The order of migration (cathode to anode, fastest to slowest) is Hb F, Hb A, Hb S, and Hb C. Hb D, Hb G, Hb I, Hb J, Hb O, Hb A_2, and Hb E comigrates with Hb A.

Based on positions of the bands in acid and alkaline electrophoresis, a presumptive identification of the Hb variant may be made. For example, bands are found on alkaline electrophoresis in both A and C positions. On acid electrophoresis, if bands are found in the A and C positions, then a presumptive identification of the Hb C trait may be made because this pattern is characteristic. However, if a band is found only in the A position on acid electrophoresis, then a presumptive identification of Hb E may be made. If bands are found in the C position on alkaline electrophoresis and between the S and A positions on acid electrophoresis, then a presumptive identification of Hb O may be made. Further testing is required to determine whether the Hb O is Hb O Arab, Hb O Indonesia, or Hb O Padova. Both Hb C and Hb O Arab can be inherited together with Hb S in the African-American population and it is of practical importance to distinguish between compound heterozygosity for Hb S and Hb O Arab from Hb SC disease, since the former combination is clinically more severe. The presence of Hb O Arab facilitates the polymerization of Hb S. Fairbanks[108] described a numbering system for the most common Hb bands on alkaline electrophoresis (Hb H is position 1, Hb A is position 5, Hb S is position 9, and Hb C is position 13) that allowed the position of a band to be described more exactly than the commonly used descriptive term "between S and A positions." However, this system has not found universal acceptance. Laboratories should keep a bank of obtained electrophoretic data to help future identification of unusual Hb variants.

Specific types of electrophoresis that are used for Hb analysis include isoelectric focusing, electrophoresis, and capillary electrophoresis.

Capillary electrophoresis. The introduction of commercial capillary electrophoresis instrumentation for the separation of Hbs has made this technique available to clinical laboratories.[109] Separation in an alkaline buffer at a specific pH using high voltages is based on charge difference, electrolyte pH, and electro-osmotic flow. Capillary electrophoresis in free solution is also known as capillary zone electrophoresis. Hemoglobin molecules migrate through a capillary filled with a salt buffer under alkaline conditions. There is no matrix interaction to introduce complexities or to alter reproducibility. Hb measurement is commonly performed at a wavelength of 415 nm, and identification is based on migration position. All common Hb variants are separated, and quantification of Hb F and Hb A_2 is performed in a single analytical run.[110–112] Cotton and colleagues[110] initially described the application of this technique for the identification of Hb variants and quantification of Hb A_2; others have described the usefulness of the technique in the clinical laboratory.[58,113,114] Advantages of capillary electrophoresis over HPLC include quantification of Hb A_2 in the presence of Hb E (due to incomplete resolution of Hb A_2 from Hb E in HPLC

as shown in Fig. 77.15), quantification of Hb H, and identification of Hb Lepore.

Isoelectric focusing electrophoresis. Isoelectric focusing utilizes an electric current to pass through a supporting medium such as agarose or polyacrylamide gel to generate a stable pH gradient ranging from pH 6.0 at the anode to pH 8.0 at the cathode. Hemolysate is applied to the gel at the cathode end and hemoglobin fractions migrate through the pH gradient until they stop at the pH equivalent to the isoelectric point, where they are focused into sharp and distinct bands. Isoelectric-focusing electrophoresis (IEF)[115] has greater resolving power than conventional electrophoresis, but it is more expensive, time-consuming, and technique-dependent to perform (see Chapter 18). Commercial IEF gels are made of cellulose acetate or polyacrylamide with the pH gradient produced by the inclusion of amphoteric materials of different pHs in bands in the gel. Locations of the Hb bands are identified using stains similar to those used in conventional electrophoresis. The bands or zones produced by IEF (Fig. 77.21) are more clearly defined than with those seen with conventional electrophoresis, and reliable quantification of separated Hbs may be made at high concentrations using densitometry. However, quantification of Hb A_2 and Hb F at low concentrations is imprecise and is not recommended. The Hb elution pattern in IEF is similar to that of alkaline Hb electrophoresis, except that Hb D and Hb G are resolved from each other and from Hb S. Historically, IEF has been used extensively to identify and characterize Hb variants; however, it is currently less frequently used because of the following limitations: (1) A constant temperature of 10 to 15 °C during the procedure is essential to maintain the pH gradient for proper hemoglobin separation; (2) minor and nonspecific bands are often visible due to high resolution of the system that may complicate interpretation; (3) hemoglobin fractions cannot be accurately quantified; and (4) it is more costly than other electrophoretic procedures.

Capillary isoelectric focusing electrophoresis. Capillary IEF[109,110,116–118] combines the detection sensitivity of capillary electrophoresis (see Chapter 18) with the resolution qualities and existing extensive data on Hb variant separation by IEF and the automated sampling and digital data acquisition techniques developed for chromatography. With this approach, the hemolysate is introduced into the capillary chamber using low-pressure injection and then is focused at high voltage (typically $\approx$30 kV and 0.5 to 1.5 μA), during which it is essential to maintain adequate cooling. The separated Hbs are then eluted, using low-pressure and simultaneous voltage, past a single-wavelength spectrophotometric detector set to read at 415 nm or a dual-wavelength detector set at 415 and 450 nm. In routine use, the Hbs are typically separated within 15 minutes, but the elution time may be extended if the presence of an abnormal Hb is suspected. Hb variants[116] are identified by comparison of isoelectric point values and migration times of the unknown, using Hb A as the reference peak, with known controls and published data. Quantification is based on integration of the measured absorbance of the bands, and accurate results have been obtained for Hb A_2 and Hb F concentrations.

Globin chain electrophoresis. Globin chain electrophoresis at acidic and alkaline pH is performed upon dissociation of individual globin chains by dithiothreitol and urea. This method is used to determine whether the hemoglobin variant

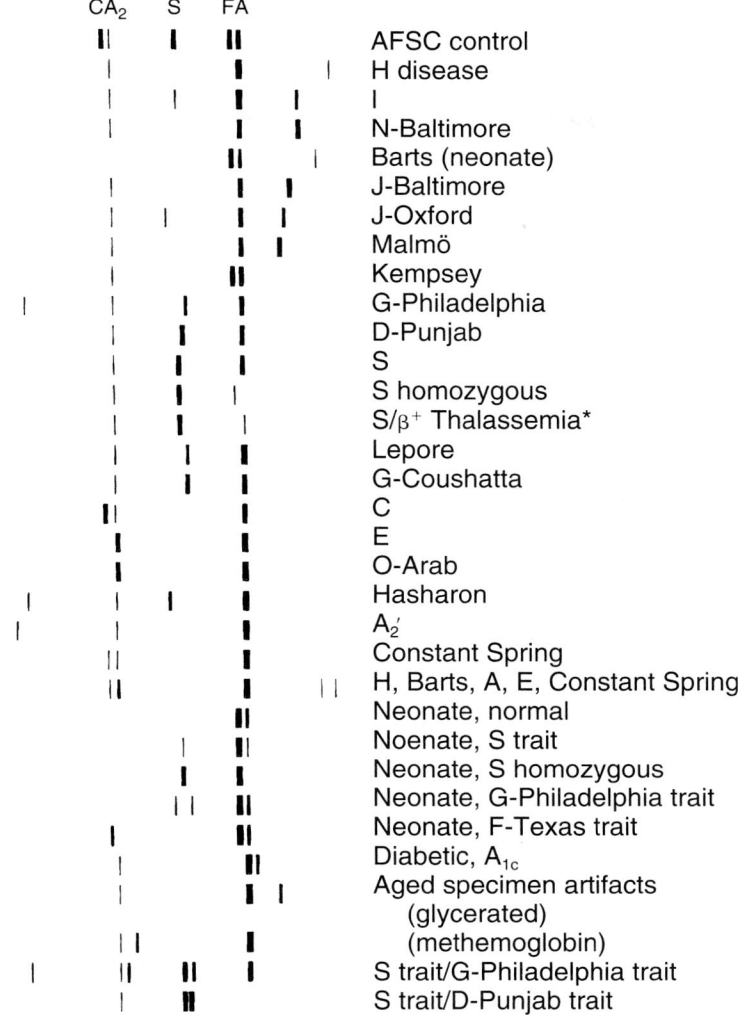

FIGURE 77.21 A diagram of isoelectric focusing patterns for a variety of hemoglobin *(Hb)* variants. The conditions shown represent heterozygotes (traits), unless otherwise indicated. The width of the bars approximates the relative density of the bands observed. The acid anodic (pH 6) side is to the *right*, and the alkaline cathodic (pH 8) side is to the *left*. The same pattern is observed in homozygous patients with Hb S disease who have received Hb A by transfusion.

is a α-chain variant or β-chain variant. In conjunction with hemoglobin electrophoresis at alkaline and acidic pH, globin chain electrophoresis can form an integral part of the systematic identification of hemoglobin variants, especially the rare hemoglobinopathies.

Mass Spectroscopy

Electrospray mass spectrometry (see Chapter 20) is becoming the method of choice[119] for the complete characterization of newly discovered Hb variants.[51–53,99,103,106,120–122] By using this method, the mass of the variant, whether it is an α- or a β-chain variant, as well as the possible location and identity of the amino acid residue substitution and the quantity of variant present, can be derived.

To analyze a sample with this technique, the globin chains first are separated and then are isolated by semipreparative HPLC. The isolated fractions are further concentrated using a variety of techniques, including membrane filtration. The fraction containing the mutant globin chain is digested using

specific endopeptidases that selectively cut at certain amino acid residues of the globin chain. The resultant digested peptide fragments are further separated by preparative HPLC, and the mutant peptide is sequenced using Edman degradation. Another portion of the digested globin chains is entered into the electrospray mass spectrometer, and the resultant mass spectrum provides information on the mass of the mutant globin chain, which can be used to provisionally identify the substituted amino acid. For Hb Rambam,[106] the mass spectrum of the β-globin chain shows the mass of the normal β-chain to be 15,867 Da and the mass of the mutant β-chain to be 15,925 Da. The increase in the mass of 58 in the mutant β-globin chain may be attributed to a change in amino acid residue from glycine (75 Da) to aspartic acid (133 Da).

Another mass spectrometry method of converting molecules into gaseous ions is matrix-assisted laser desorption/ ionization (MALDI). As an accelerating voltage is applied, these particles are separated based on their mass-to-charge ratio. The determination of molecular weight is extremely accurate and can be harnessed to decipher variant hemoglobins. The advanced instrumentation such as tandem mass spectrometry has enabled the determination of variant hemoglobin even in a minute sample of hemolysate without the need for prior separation. Tandem mass spectroscopy has been used for newborn screening for sickle cell disease[123,124] and for the characterization of Hb A_2.[125]

Modern mass spectrometry can undertake amino acid sequencing of proteins and nucleotide sequencing of DNA molecules. In specialized reference laboratories, mass spectrometry is useful in the identification of α-chain variants because direct nucleotide sequencing of the α-globin gene with a high GC content is not simple and straightforward. Highly unstable hemoglobin variants that manifest clinically as hemolytic anemia can be detected by mass spectrometry. These variants often exist in trace amounts and escape detection by other methods. Finally, mass spectrometry provides information on the post-translational modifications, such as oxidation and glycation.

Specific Tests

Sickling and Hemoglobin S Solubility Tests

Sickling tests are useful in confirming the presence of Hb S in a sample after initial electrophoresis at alkaline pH. When Hb S is oxygenated, it is fully soluble. When Hb S is deoxygenated, polymerization occurs, forming deformed red cells with a characteristic rigid sickle shape. In the laboratory, deoxygenation and lysis of RBCs is achieved using a solution of sodium metabisulfite in a phosphate buffer. Addition of the sodium metabisulfite reagent to an Hb S–containing blood sample induces the typical sickle shape of RBCs (which is the basis of the sickling test by microscopic investigation of the blood film preparation), and it also causes turbidity (which is the basis of the solubility test). In the Hb S solubility test, this turbidity is visualized by holding a lined card or a card with writing on it behind the reaction test tube (Fig. 77.22). In positive samples, lines or letters cannot be seen, whereas in negative samples, lines or letters are clearly visible. Both a positive and a negative control should be used with each test. The hematocrit (Hct) of the blood sample to be tested should be measured, and if it is less than 15%, the amount of blood used in the test should be doubled because low Hb concentration is a cause of falsely negative sickling screens. Lipemic samples and samples with a monoclonal protein (M-protein) may give a false-positive result. Hb C Harlem and Hb Memphis [$\alpha 23(B4)^{Glu}\psi Gln$] also give a positive result in this procedure; therefore it is essential to identify the Hb in all positive tests by other techniques. The solubility test cannot distinguish sickle cell trait from sickle cell disease or Hb S/β-thalassemia. It cannot detect the presence of hemoglobin variants, namely Hb C, Hb D-Punjab, and Hb O Arab, which in combination with Hb S may cause a sickling disorder. The solubility test is negative when the concentration of Hb S is less than 15% of the total hemoglobin fraction. It is not applicable to infants with high Hb F level, and also in patients who have recently been transfused. The Hb S solubility test therefore should not be used as a primary diagnostic test, or for the purpose of genetic counseling and assessment of reproductive risk. The test is subjective, and the combination of two identification techniques, such as HPLC and alkaline electrophoresis, may eliminate the necessity to perform this test on a routine basis.

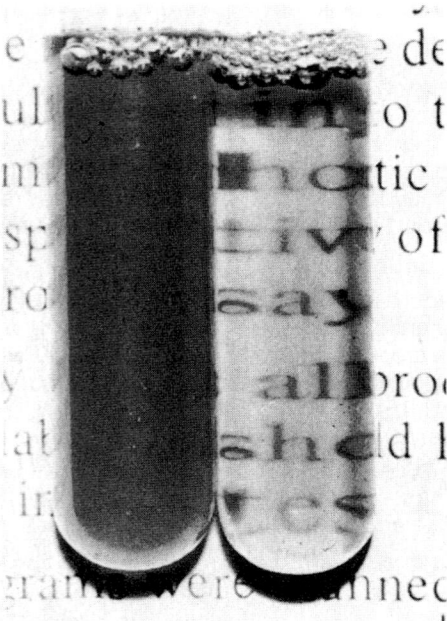

FIGURE 77.22 Solubility test for hemoglobin (*Hb*) S. Deoxyhemoglobin S *(left tube)* is insoluble in 2.3 mol/L phosphate buffer. In contrast, normal hemolysate *(right tube)* is sufficiently transparent that print can easily be read through it.

Tests for Unstable Hemoglobins

These tests use heat or isopropanol to precipitate the unstable Hb and must be performed on fresh blood. More than 100 unstable Hbs are mainly the result of the interchange of nonpolar amino acid residues for polar amino acid residues in positions in the α- or β-globin chain associated with the heme cleft. One notable example is Hb Hasharon [$\alpha 47(CD)^{Asp\psi His}$], an Hb variant found in Ashkenazi Jews, results from substitution of the nonpolar amino acid residue histidine for the polar aspartic acid residue at position 47 of the α-chain.

Nonpolar isopropanol weakens the internal bonds within Hb, decreasing the stability of the Hb molecule. Normal Hb (Hb A) precipitates within 40 minutes at 37°C in the presence of a 17% solution of isopropanol with a pH 7.4 Tris buffer. Unstable Hbs usually precipitate within 5 minutes under these conditions. Both a positive and a negative control should be included with each analysis, although a positive control may not always be readily available. An umbilical cord blood or neonatal sample, not fresh, may be an acceptable alternative as a positive control. At the time of reading, the negative control should be clear, and the positive control should have some flocculation.

Normal Hb is stable when heated to 50°C. However, unstable Hbs precipitate to varying extents when similarly treated. A hemolysate of the sample in a pH 7.4 Tris-phosphate buffer is divided into two aliquots. One is stored at 4 °C, the other is heated at 50 °C for 2 hours. Both samples are centrifuged, and Hb quantification is performed on each supernatant.

Frequently, both heat and isopropanol stability tests are performed when a suspected unstable Hb variant is investigated. Unstable Hb variants may not appear on HPLC or electrophoresis, especially if the variant is unstable enough to precipitate before analysis by these techniques.

The Heinz body preparation to detect oxidized denatured hemoglobin can provide a useful clue to the presence of unstable hemoglobin.

Tests for High-Affinity Hemoglobins

Investigation of hemoglobin function is required in rare instances to detect variant hemoglobins with altered oxygen affinity, by measuring the P_{50} and determining the oxygen dissociation curve. These variants may escape detection if the electrophoretic mobility is similar to that of Hb A. High oxygen affinity hemoglobin variants are associated with erythrocytosis.

Globin Chain Synthesis Study

The α-globin chain and β-globin chain synthesis studies, based on incubating reticulocytes with radioactive leucine, separating globin chains chromatographically and determining the amount of radioactivity incorporated, can help to determine whether a patient may have α-thalassemia or β-thalassemia. However, with the technological advancement in mutation detection methodology, globin chain synthesis studies are very rarely used for clinical purposes.

DNA Analysis

Clinical Indications

DNA-based mutational analysis is now widely employed as a definitive diagnostic test for thalassemia and hemoglobinopathies. Advances in molecular genetics allow rapid and accurate mutation detection testing to be carried out at a manageable cost. At the clinical laboratory, globin genotyping is performed for the following indications:

1. Prenatal diagnosis. Direct detection of globin gene mutation in fetal DNA enables prenatal diagnosis to be performed at early gestation based on small sample obtained from chorionic villous biopsy and amniocentesis. The test result is essential for genetic counseling and reproductive decision-making. Both chorionic villous sampling and amniocentesis are invasive procedures associated with a 1% risk of abortion. Noninvasive methods of prenatal diagnosis such as utilizing fetal cells in the maternal circulation or cell-free fetal DNA in the maternal plasma are feasible. In vitro fertilization and preimplantation genetic testing[126] based on embryo biopsy is an established clinical service in reproductive medicine. There are several advantages of preimplantation genetic testing over conventional

prenatal diagnosis: (a) Obviates the need for abortion of affected fetus; (b) Applicable to infertile couples who are also at risk of fetus affected by severe globin disorder; (c) Enables genotyping to be performed on HLA loci in addition to the globin genes, which facilitates the decision of saving the cord blood of an unaffected fetus for consideration of transplanting an affected sibling.

2. Genotype–phenotype correlation. The ability to predict phenotype from genotype allows anticipation of clinical course and prognosis of the patient, upon which management decisions may be based.[127] The genetic information generated is also valuable for genetic counseling and prenatal diagnosis of couples at risk of conceiving a fetus affected by hemoglobin disorders such as severe β-thalassemia.

3. Diagnosis of complicated cases. DNA diagnosis can give a verdict on complicated cases in which a definite conclusion is difficult or even impossible based on hemoglobin study (Table 77.7). This is particularly relevant in geographical areas where both α-globin gene[128–130] and β-globin gene[131–134] mutations are prevalent. Two examples of complex α/β interactions that require DNA diagnosis are concurrent Hb H disease and heterozygous β-thalassemia[63] and β-thalassemia intermedia due to triplicated α-globin gene and heterozygous β-thalassemia.[64] Genotyping is also needed for an unequivocal diagnosis of hemoglobin variants or molecular characterization of potentially novel hemoglobin variants, applicable to screening at-risk populations for clinically significant Hb variants.[131,135]

Molecular Diagnostic Techniques

Deletions. Large deletions of the α-globin gene locus are the major cause of α-thalassemia. Large deletions of the β-globin gene locus are uncommon, and result in deletional forms of hereditary persistence of fetal hemoglobin (HPFH), $\delta\beta$-thalassemia, and more rarely, deletional forms of β-thalassemia. Although Southern blot analysis is considered the gold standard and mainstay of detecting large deletions, the use of radioactive probes and the long turn-around time limit its clinical utility. Gap-polymerase chain reaction (PCR), performed singly or in multiplex form and followed by gel electrophoresis, is increasingly employed to detect common deletions with known breakpoints. For example, a multiplex gap-PCR that detects ($-^{SEA}$) α-thalassemia deletion, ($-\alpha^{3.7}$) rightward single α-globin gene deletion and

TABLE 77.7 Examples of Atypical Phenotypes in Thalassemia and Possible Causes

Atypical Phenotype	Possible Cause due to Genetic Interaction	Possible Cause due to Unusual Globin Mutation
β-Thalassemia trait with high HbF	Heterozygous β-thalassemia mutation + HPFH	β-Thalassemia due to deletion or promoter mutation
β-Thalassemia trait with near normal MCV	Heterozygous β-thalassemia mutation + masked single or two-α-globin gene deletion	Very mild β-thalassemia mutation
β-Thalassemia trait with significant anemia	Heterozygous β-thalassemia mutation + silent triplicated α-globin gene configuration	Dominant β-thalassemia
Hb E trait with low percentage of Hb variant	Heterozygous Hb E mutation + α-thalassemia	Hemoglobin anti-Lepore Hong Kong ($\beta\delta$-fusion gene)[60]
Thalassemic red cell indices with reduced Hb A_2	Heterozygous β-thalassemia mutation + δ thalassemia mutation or variant such as Hb A_2 Hong Kong[46]	$\delta\beta$-Thalassemia

Modified from Ip H-W, So C-C. Diagnosis and prevention of thalassemia. *Crit Rev Clin Lab Sci* 2013;50(6):125–41.

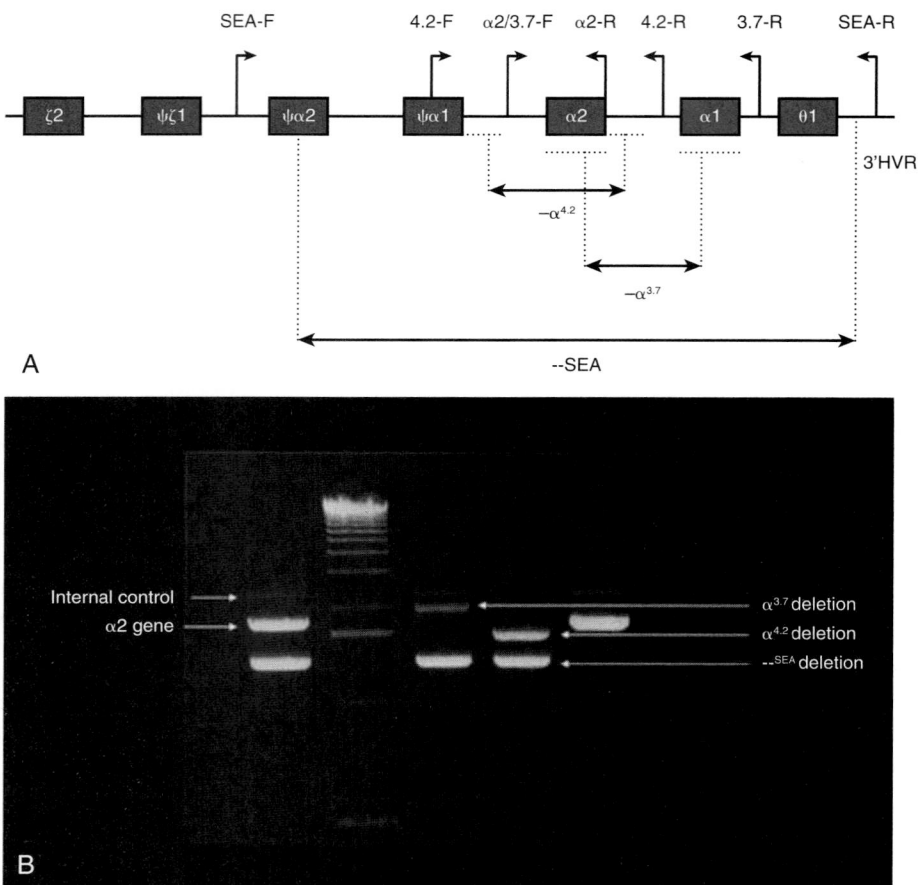

FIGURE 77.23 (A) Primer binding sites in the multiplex gap-polymerase chain reaction (PCR) for detection of the three common α-globin gene deletions in Chinese. (B) Electrophoretic results of multiplex gap-PCR products on 1% agarose gel in Chinese patients with different forms of α-globin gene deletions.

$(-\alpha^{4.2})$ leftward single α-globin gene deletion already detects a majority of all α-thalassemia alleles in the Chinese (Fig. 77.23), the remaining being nondeletional α-globin gene mutations or uncommon deletions.[86,136] One caveat of the gap-PCR approach is that unusual rearrangements such as the HKαα allele,[137] a nondeleterious allele that contains neither deletion or triplication and is found in 0.33% of the Southern Chinese population,[138] may be mistaken as $-\alpha^{3.7}$ without further confirmation.

A useful technique to detect gene deletion is multiplex ligation-dependent probe amplification (MLPA).[36] Multiple probes are designed to bind to target sequences along the α- or β-globin gene cluster. Each probe comprises two oligonucleotides that bind adjacent to its respective target sequence. A ligation reaction takes place and the intact probes are amplified in a PCR using one single set of labeled primers since all probes are constructed to have the same primer recognition ends. Amplification products differ in size, which can be separated by electrophoresis using an automated sequencer. The peak height or area of a probe represents the amount of amplification product, which is in turn proportional to the copy number of the target sequence in the sample. This technique has been applied to diagnose common and uncommon α-thalassemia and β-thalassemia deletions, and obviates the need for Southern blot study. The

thalassemia deletions as detected by MLPA are usually confirmed by gap-PCR followed by direct sequencing of the PCR product (Fig. 77.24), as it can be difficult to determine exact breakpoints by MLPA. This technique can also detect globin gene amplifications.

Point mutations. Dot blotting or reverse dot blotting using allele-specific oligonucleotide probes have been commonly employed to detect point mutations in globin genes. Specific hybridization between a probe and the PCR product reveals a particular point mutation. Although reverse dot blot arrays capable of simultaneously detecting many point mutations are available, automation of the tedious post-PCR manipulation steps is needed. To detect several commonly found mutations in an ethnic population, a multiplex system such as multiplex PCR with allele-specific primers or multiplex amplification refractory mutational system (ARMS) are now widely used. The presence of a PCR product of predicted size in gel electrophoresis indicates the presence of the corresponding mutation (Fig. 77.25). A more sophisticated technique of point mutation detection is mini-sequencing, usually performed as in a multiplex fashion for several common mutations on an automated sequencer.[130] In mini-sequencing, site-specific primers (just one nucleotide 5′ to the point mutation) of different lengths are subjected to multiple rounds of annealing and single nucleotide extension in the

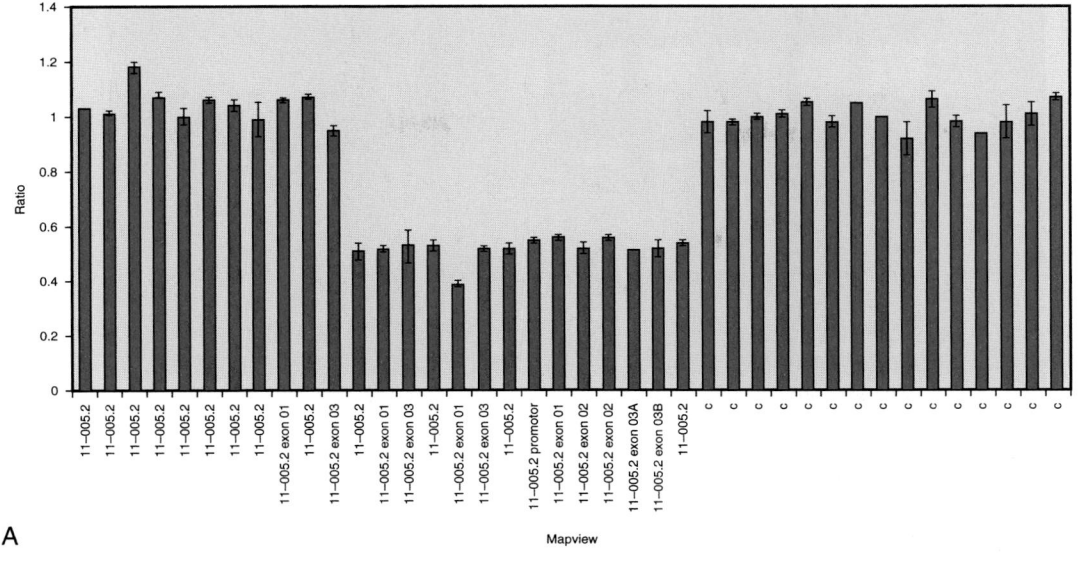

A

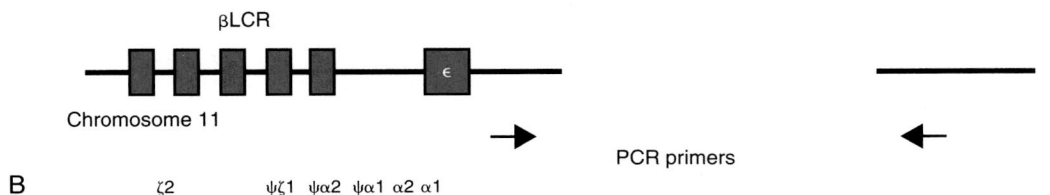

B

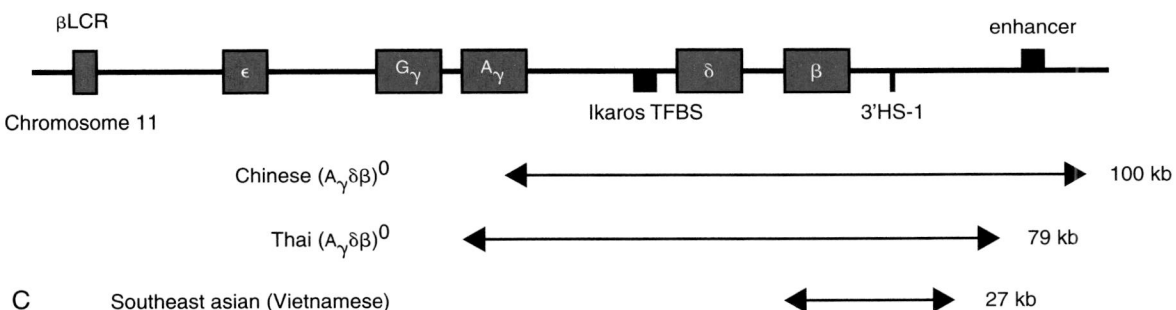

C

FIGURE 77.24 (A) Ratio plot of multiplex ligation-dependent probe amplification (MLPA) probes for β-globin gene cluster showing heterozygous deletion. (B) Gap-polymerase chain reaction *(PCR)* primers designed to map deletion breakpoints based on information from probes deleted. (C) Deletions of β-globin gene cluster in Chinese characterized by MLPA. *LCR,* Locus control region.

presence of thermostable DNA polymerase and the four dideoxynucleotides each labeled with a different fluorophore. The mini-sequencing products are separated and detected by capillary electrophoresis, followed by automated genotyping.

To detect uncommon mutations, direct nucleotide sequencing of the PCR amplified globin gene is usually performed. While straightforward for the β-globin gene, the high GC content of the α-globin gene renders the process more difficult. With the wider availability and reducing cost of DNA sequencing, conventional methods for screening uncommon or unknown mutations including single strand conformation polymorphism, denaturing gradient gel electrophoresis, and restriction endonuclease analysis are less

commonly performed. Nevertheless, two fast mutation scanning methods, namely denaturing high-performance liquid chromatography (D-HPLC) study and high-resolution melting (HRM) curve analysis on real-time quantitative PCR platform, have been explored for globin mutation detection. D-HPLC involves amplification of the globin gene target sequence, formation of homoduplexes and heteroduplexes if a mutation is present, anchoring of the duplexes to a cartridge, followed by D-HPLC study on the DNA fragment analysis system. Homoduplexes and heteroduplexes are eluted off the cartridge by a solution with changing ionic concentration and collected at different times (Fig. 77.26). HRM study subjects amplified globin gene products to increasing temperature and

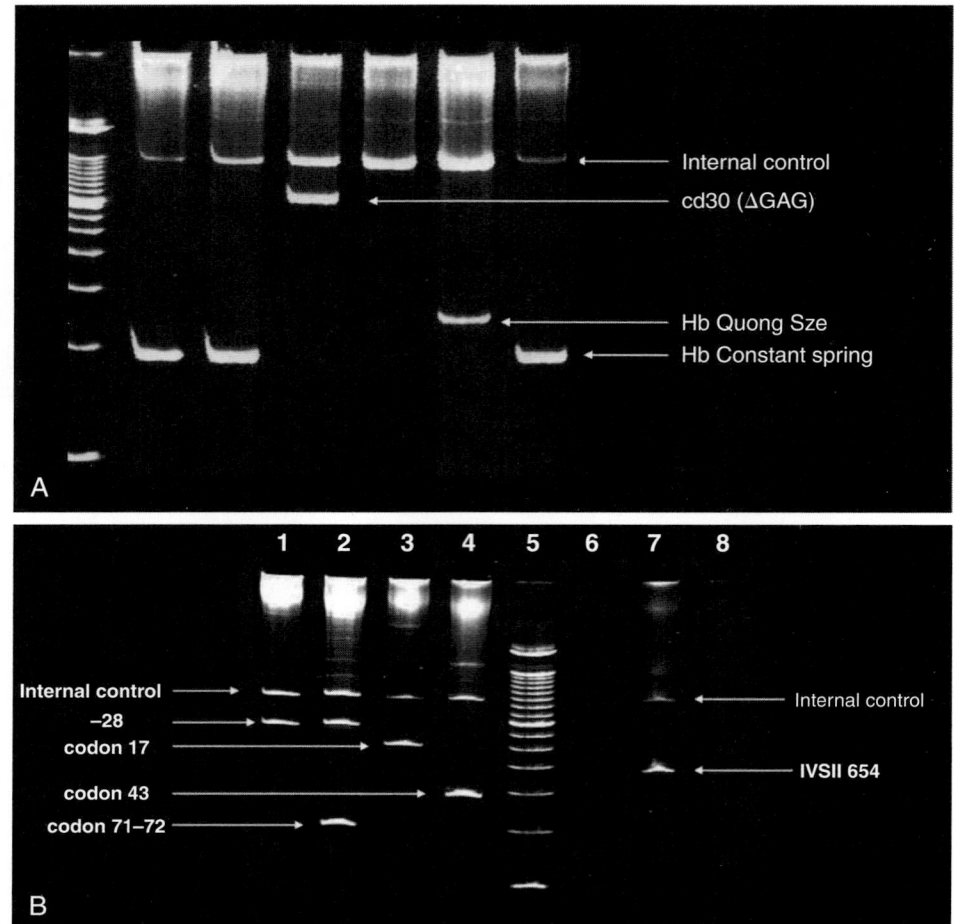

FIGURE 77.25 (A) Electrophoretic results of multiplex amplification refractory mutational system (ARMS) products on aqueous 8% polyacrylamide gel in Chinese patients with the common nondeletional α-thalassemia mutations. (B) Electrophoretic results of multiplex ARMS products on aqueous 8% polyacrylamide gel in Chinese patients with the common β-thalassemia point mutations.

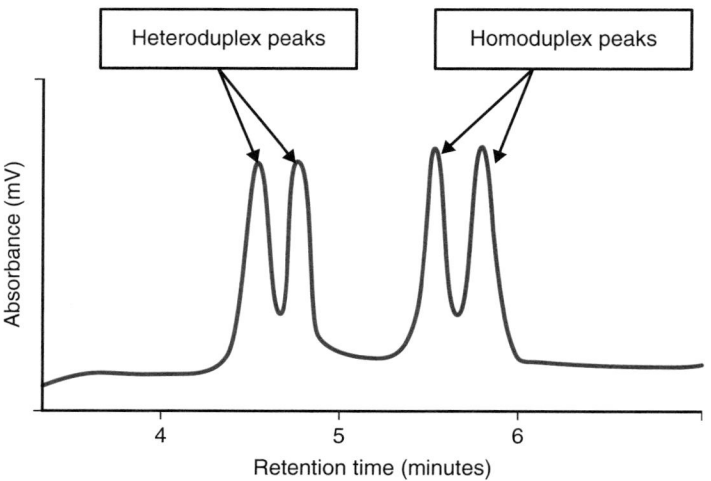

FIGURE 77.26 Chromatogram of denaturing high-performance liquid chromatography (D-HPLC) showing differentiation among heteroduplexes, wide-type homoduplex, and mutant homoduplex based on different elution times.

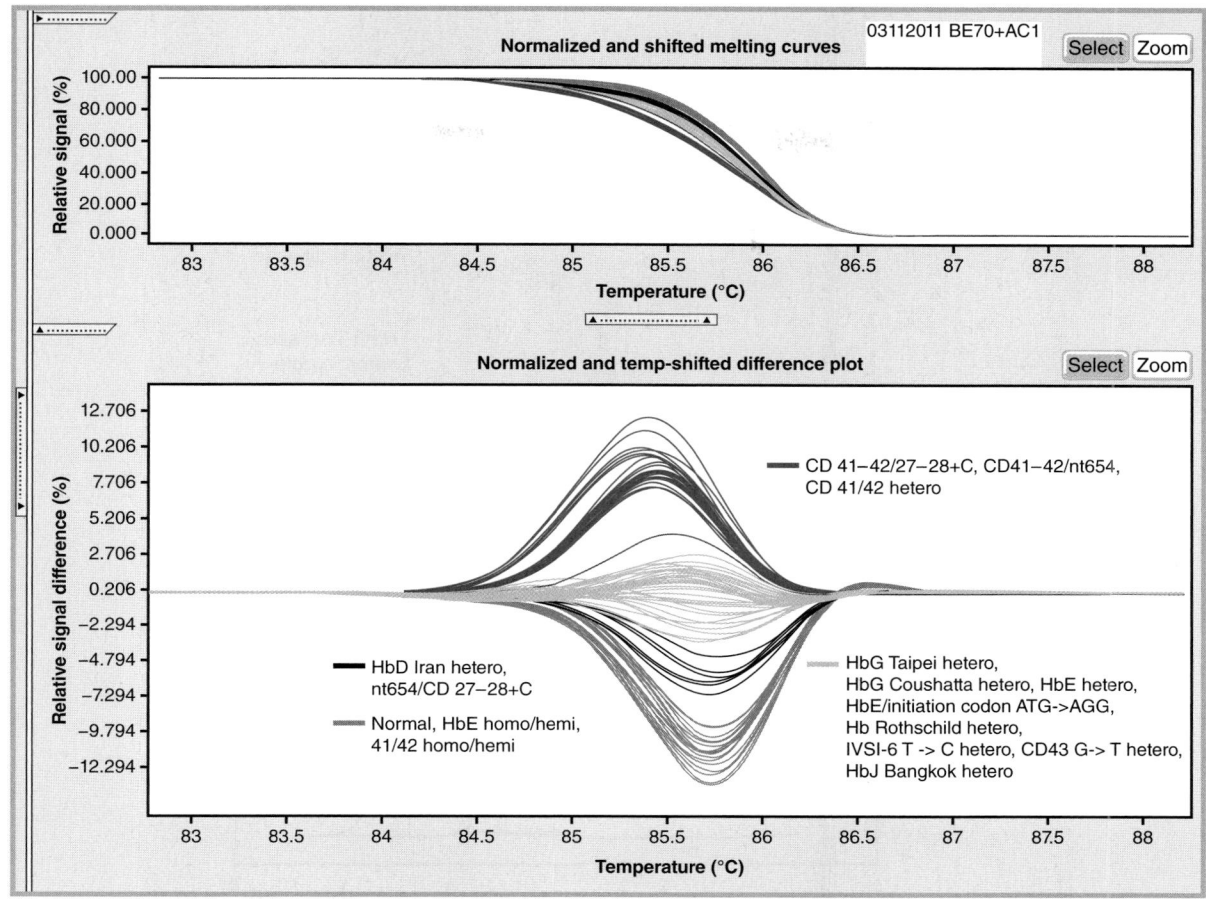

FIGURE 77.27 High-resolution melting (HRM) analysis. *(Upper panel)* Melting curves of different heterozygous and homozygous hemoglobin variants and thalassemia mutants. *(Lower panel)* Relative signal difference plots of various mutants and normal.

records the details of their dissociation from double-stranded DNA (dsDNA) to single-stranded DNA (ssDNA), in the presence of a fluorescent dye that binds only to dsDNA. In a melting experiment, fluorescence is initially high because the sample starts as dsDNA but diminishes as the temperature is raised and DNA dissociates into single strands, and how the DNA melts is entirely sequence dependent, with heteroduplex having a lower melting temperature than homoduplex. Monitoring the shape of the melting curve thus gives information as to the presence and type of any point mutation in the amplicon (Fig 77.27). Array or DNA chip-based thalassemia mutation detection has been described but the popularity is limited by the sophistication of instrumentation.[139]

Hb H disease genotyping. A practical laboratory strategy for genotyping hemoglobin H disease is to employ upfront a combination of multiplex Gap-PCR for the common deletions and multiplex ARMS for the common nondeletional mutations, which covers the vast majority of cases.[86] If indicated, the rare deletions are detected by Southern blot analysis or MLPA, and the rare mutations are detected by direct nucleotide sequencing. One caveat of this approach is that, without reference to the hemoglobin pattern study result, Hb Q-H disease[67] (compound heterozygosity for SEA deletion and Hb Q-Thailand) may masquerade as simple deletional hemoglobin H disease due to compound heterozygosity for

SEA deletion and $-\alpha^{4.2}$, since the Hb Q-Thailand is linked with and always found on $-\alpha^{4.2}$ chromosome. Further sequencing of apparent $-^{SEA}/-\alpha^{4.2}$ will reveal Hb Q-Thailand. However, on cellulose acetate electrophoresis, the characteristic picture of a fasting moving Hb H band, absence of Hb A (due to absence of normal α-globin gene), and a slow-moving band migrating between Hb F and Hb S is unmistakable (Fig. 77.28). This underscores the important of taking all the hematologic and genotype results into account when making a diagnosis of hemoglobin disorder.

Next-generation sequencing. Next-generation sequencing (NGS) is established in clinical molecular diagnostics as a high-throughput, multiplex, and accurate method of variant detection in genetic disorders (see Chapter 65). The challenge of NGS application to thalassemia and hemoglobinopathy is the wide spectrum of globin gene variants, ranging from single nucleotide variants (SNV) and small insertions/deletions (indels) to large genomic rearrangements that in total number over 1800 different mutations. Therefore a comprehensive NGS platform should target the entire coding regions of the globin genes, the key regulatory regions, known pathogenic copy number variation regions, and known SNV and indels in the noncoding regions of the globin genes. The important genetic modifier genes may also be incorporated into the NGS test.[140] Bioinformatic pipelines can be tailored to

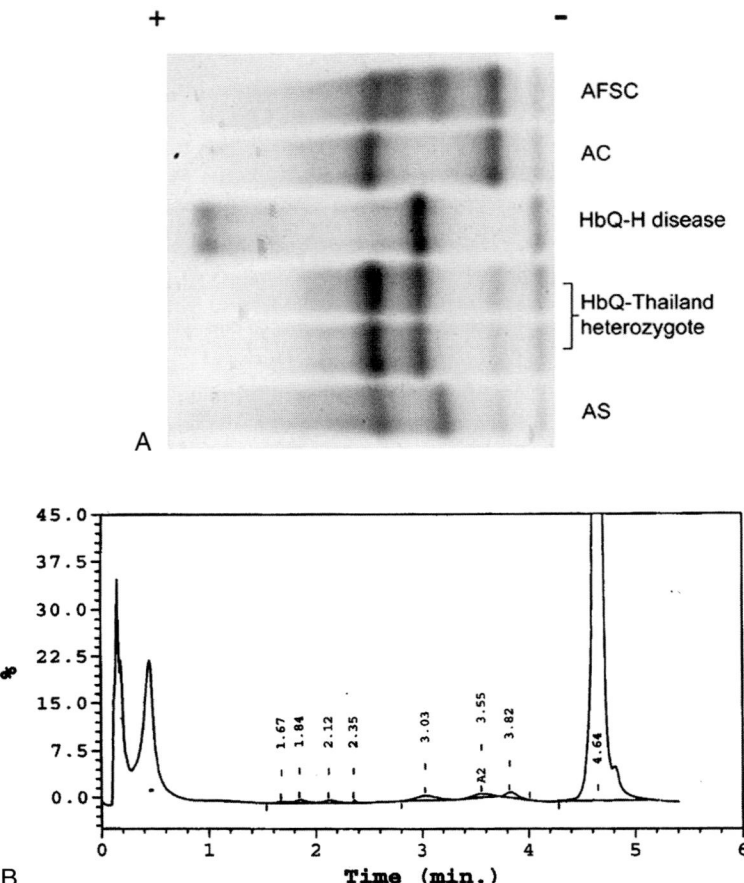

FIGURE 77.28 (A) Cellulose acetate electrophoresis at alkaline pH for HbQ-H disease and HbQ-Thailand heterozygotes. *Lane 1*, HbA, HbF, HbS and HbC control from anode to cathode. *Lane 2*, HbA and HbC from a heterozygote carrier of HbC. *Lane 3*, HbQ-H disease. Note the fasting moving HbH band, absence of HbA and a strong band migrating between HbF and HbS that corresponds to HbQ-Thailand. *Lanes 4* and *5*, Hb Q-Thailand heterozygote showing an extra band migrating between HbF and HbS. *Lane 6*, HbA and HbS from a heterozygote carrier of HbS. (B) HPLC showing a predominant peak in the S-window that corresponds to HbQ-Thailand, which elutes at 4.64 minutes and constitutes 96.9% of the total Hb. The small overlapping peak on the right side of the HbQ peak represents HbQ$_2$ from the a chain variant combined with normal d chain. Note the absence of HbA and fasting eluting Hb fractions compatible with HbH and Hb Barts. The HbA^2 level is reduced to 0.6%. (Images in collaboration with Dr. Alvin Ip.)

characterize structural variants and for breakpoint mapping in rearrangements of the globin gene clusters.[141] The NGS approach is applicable to large-scale thalassemia carrier screening among premarital couples in high-prevalence populations to prevent offspring affected by severe thalassemia.[142]

SELECTED REFERENCES

16. Higgs DR, Gibbons RJ. The molecular basis of alpha-thalassemia: a model for understanding human molecular genetics. Hematol Oncol Clin North Am 2010;24:1033–54.

17. Lorey F, Cunningham G, Vichinsky EP, et al. Universal newborn screening for Hb H disease in California. Genet Test 2001;5:93–100.

20. Piel FB, Weatherall DJ. The alpha-thalassemias. N Engl J Med 2014;371:1908–16.

21. Chui DH, Waye JS. Hydrops fetalis caused by alpha-thalassemia: an emerging health care problem. Blood 1998;91:2213–22.

22. Fucharoen S, Viprakasit V. Hb H disease: clinical course and disease modifiers. Hematology Am Soc Hematol Educ Program 2009;1:26–34.

23. Chen FE, Ooi C, Ha SY, et al. Genetic and clinical features of hemoglobin H disease in Chinese patients. N Engl J Med 2000;343:544–50.

25. Chui DH, Fucharoen S, Chan V. Hemoglobin H disease: not necessarily a benign disorder. Blood 2003;101:791–800.

32. Thein SL, Hesketh C, Taylor P, et al. Molecular basis for dominantly inherited inclusion body beta-thalassemia. Proc Natl Acad Sci U S A 1990;87:3924–8.

34. Hardison RC, Chui DH, Riemer C, et al. Databases of human hemoglobin variants and other resources at the globin gene server. Hemoglobin 2001;25:183–93.

39. Borgna-Pignatti C, Marsella M. Iron chelation in thalassemia major. Clin Ther 2015;37:2866–77.
40. Baronciani D, Angelucci E, Potschger U, et al. Hemopoietic stem cell transplantation in thalassemia: a report from the European Society for Blood and Bone Marrow Transplantation Hemoglobinopathy Registry, 2000–2010. Bone Marrow Transplant 2016;51:536–41.
42. Thein SL. Genetic modifiers of beta-thalassemia. Haematologica 2005;90:649–60.
45. Perseu L, Satta S, Moi P, et al. KLF1 gene mutations cause borderline HbA(2). Blood 2011;118:4454–8.
50. Sankaran VG, Xu J, Byron R, et al. A functional element necessary for fetal hemoglobin silencing. N Engl J Med 2011;365:807–14.
61. Giardine B, Borg J, Viennas E, et al. Updates of the HbVar database of human hemoglobin variants and thalassemia mutations. Nucleic Acids Res 2014;42:D1063–9.
65. Fucharoen S, Weatherall DJ. The hemoglobin E thalassemias. Cold Spring Harb Perspect Med 2012;2:229–43.
81. Schoorl M, Schoorl M, Linssen J, et al. Efficacy of advanced discriminating algorithms for screening on iron-deficiency anemia and beta-thalassemia trait: a multicenter evaluation. Am J Clin Pathol 2012;138:300–4.
127. Ho PJ, Hall GW, Luo LY, Weatherall DJ, Thein SL. Phenotypic prediction in beta-thalassemia. Ann N Y Acad Sci 1998;850:436–41.
141. Clark BE, Shooter C, Smith F, et al. Next-generation sequencing as a tool for breakpoint analysis in rearrangements of the globin gene clusters. Int J Lab Hematol 2017;39(Suppl 1):111–20.
142. He J, Song W, Yang J, et al. Next-generation sequencing improves thalassemia carrier screening among premarital adults in a high prevalence population: the Dai nationality, China. Genet Med 2017;19:1022–31.

Enzymes of the Red Blood Cell

Minke A.E. Rab and Richard van Wijk

ABSTRACT

Background

Red cell metabolism provides the cell with energy to pump ions against electrochemical gradients, maintain its shape, keep iron from hemoglobin in its reduced form, and maintain enzyme and hemoglobin sulfhydryl groups. The main source of metabolic energy comes from glucose. Glucose is metabolized through the Emden-Meyerhof glycolytic pathway and through the hexose monophosphate shunt, producing adenosine triphosphate (ATP) and nicotinamide-adenine dinucleotide (NADH). 2,3-Bisphosphoglycerate, an important regulator of the oxygen affinity of hemoglobin, is also generated during glycolysis. The hexose monophosphate shunt oxidizes glucose-6-phosphate, thereby generating nicotinamide adenine dinucleotide phosphate (NADPH). NADPH mainly serves the red cell to maintain high concentrations of reduced glutathione (GSH). The red cell lacks the capacity for de novo purine synthesis but has a salvage pathway that permits synthesis of purine nucleotides from purine bases.

Content

Hereditary red blood cell (RBC) enzymopathies are genetic disorders affecting genes encoding RBC enzymes involved in red cell metabolism. They cause a specific type of anemia designated hereditary nonspherocytic hemolytic anemia (HNSHA). HNSHA is a normocytic normochromic hemolytic anemia. In contrast to other hereditary red cell disorders, such as membrane disorders or hemoglobinopathies, morphologic abnormalities of the RBC are absent. The diagnosis is based on detection of reduced specific enzyme activity and molecular characterization of the defect on the DNA level. The most common enzyme disorders are deficiencies of glucose-6-phosphate dehydrogenase (G6PD) and pyruvate kinase. However, there are a number of additional enzyme disorders, more rare and often much less known, causing HNSHA.

INTRODUCTION

Red blood cells (RBCs) perform a variety of functions, the most important being the binding, transport, and delivery of oxygen to all tissues. To do so, they must be capable of passage through microcapillaries—a feature that is achieved by modifications of the red cell's biconcave shape. This shape change is possible because, unlike most other cells in the body, the human RBC loses its nucleus and organelles before entering the circulation from the bone marrow. In addition, remaining RNA in the reticulocyte is lost within the first 2 days in circulation, thereby making further protein synthesis in the mature red cell no longer possible.

Normal human red cells survive in circulation for approximately 120 days, using energy to maintain the electrolyte gradient between plasma and red cell cytoplasm and to keep hemoglobin and the sulfhydryl groups of the red cell enzymes and membrane proteins in the reduced state. Because of the absence of a nucleus and mitochondria, the red cell is incapable of generating energy via the (oxidative) Krebs cycle and depends mainly on the anaerobic conversion of glucose by the Embden-Meyerhof pathway (EMP or direct glycolytic pathway) and the oxidative hexose monophosphate pathway (HMP or pentose phosphate shunt) (Fig. 78.1). Numerous red cell enzymes are involved in these pathways, thereby providing the cell with the necessary high-energy phosphates (primarily adenosine triphosphate [ATP]) and reducing power (nicotinamide adenine dinucleotide phosphate [NADPH]).

Deficiencies of any of these red cell enzymes may result in impaired ATP generation or the inability to withstand oxidative stress and, consequently, loss of function of the RBC. By far, the majority of these disorders are hereditary in nature, although acquired deficiencies have been described, mainly in malignant disorders involving the bone marrow.[1] Hereditary enzymatic defects in these pathways are able to (1) disturb the red cell's integrity, (2) shorten its survival, and (3) produce hereditary nonspherocytic hemolytic anemia (HNSHA). In general, deficiencies of enzymes involved in ATP generation lead to chronic hemolytic anemia. Other enzyme deficiencies cause acute episodes of severe hemolysis [e.g., when oxidative stress on the red cell is increased (as in some types of G6PD deficiency)]. Red cell morphology is, in general, unremarkable, except for pyrimidine 5′-nucleotidase deficiency, which is characterized by prominent basophilic stippling (see pyrimidine-5′-nucleotidase-1).

Many RBC enzymes are expressed in other tissues as well but cause notable symptoms predominantly in red cells because of its long life span after loss of protein synthesis; once an enzyme is degraded or otherwise becomes nonfunctional,

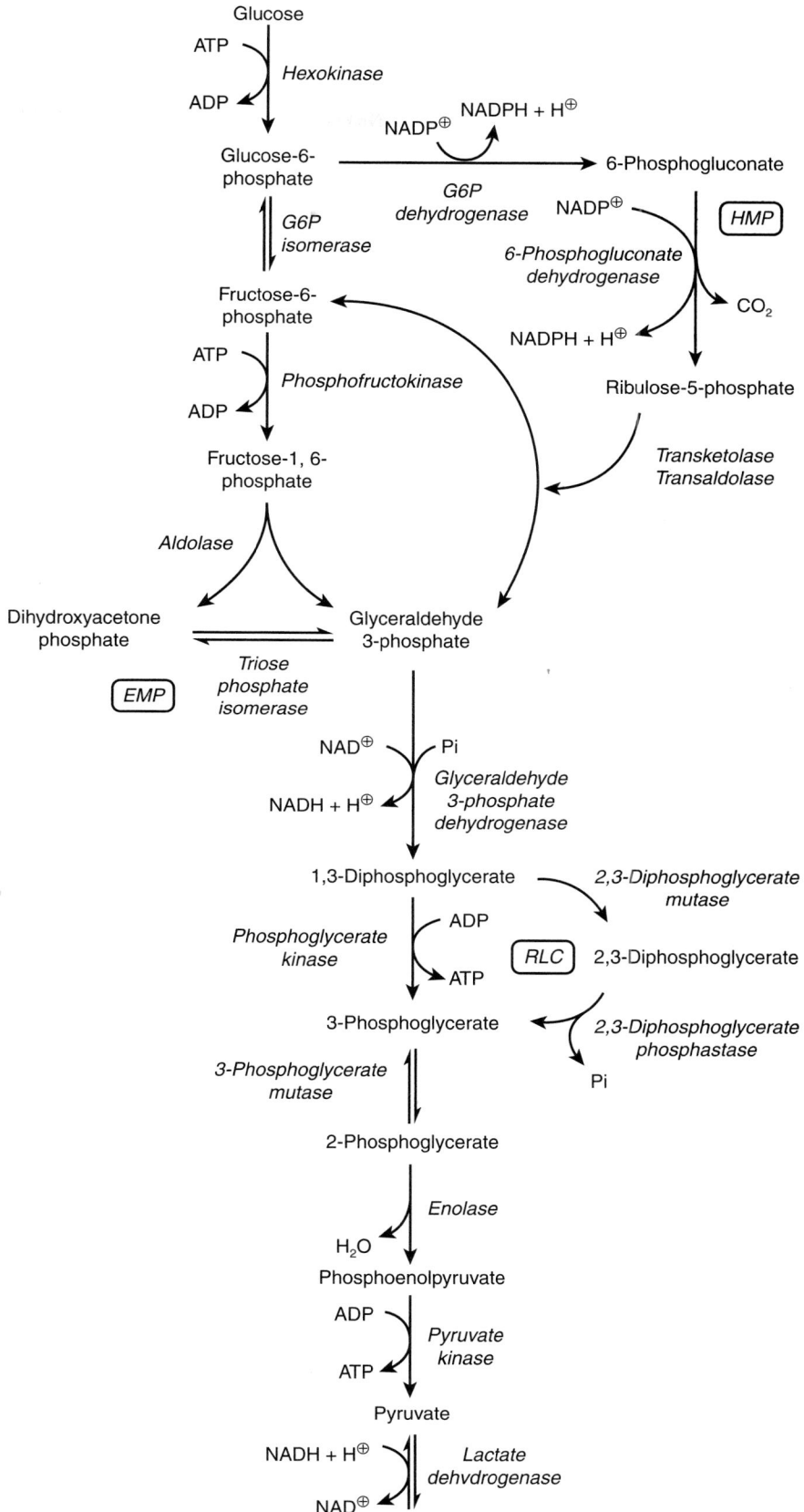

FIGURE 78.1 Major glycolytic pathways of the red blood cell. Substrates are in uppercase type, and enzymes are in parentheses. *ADP*, Adenosine diphosphate; *ATP*, adenosine triphosphate; *EMP*, Embden-Meyerhof pathway; *HMP*, hexose monophosphate pathway or pentose shunt; *NAD+*, nicotinamide-adenine dinucleotide; *NADH*, reduced nicotinamide-adenine dinucleotide; *NADP+*, nicotinamide-adenine dinucleotide phosphate; *NADPH*, reduced nicotinamide-adenine dinucleotide phosphate; *RLC*, Rapoport-Luebering cycle. The step from ribulose 5-phosphate, which is shown as being catalyzed by transketolase and transaldolase, is an abbreviation of this portion of the HMP. Note that diphosphoglycerate and diphosphoglyceric acid are also called bisphosphoglycerate and bisphosphoglyceric acid, respectively.

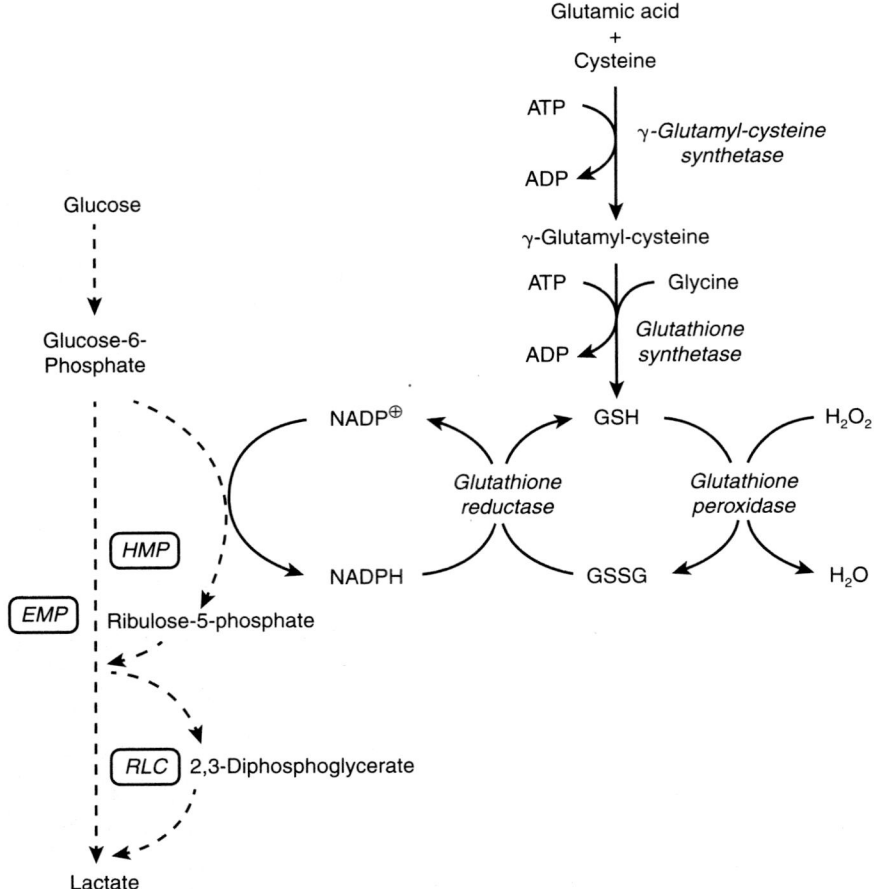

FIGURE 78.2 Interrelationship of hexose monophosphate and glutathione pathways. *ADP,* Adenosine diphosphate; *ATP,* adenosine triphosphate; *EMP;* Embden-Meyerhof pathway; *GSH,* Reduced glutathione; *GSSG,* oxidized glutathione; *HMP,* Hexose monophosphate pathway; *NADP,* nicotinamide-adenine dinucleotide phosphate; *NADPH,* reduced nicotinamide-adenine dinucleotide phosphate; *RLC,* Rapoport-Luebering cycle.

it cannot be replaced by new or other "compensating" proteins because nucleus, mitochondria, ribosomes, and other cell organelles are lacking in mature red cells.

Disorders have been described in the EMP, HMP, the Rapoport-Luebering cycle, the glutathione pathway (Fig. 78.2), purine-pyrimidine metabolism, and methemoglobin reduction. This section describes the clinically important red cell enzymes involved in these metabolic pathways and the disorders associated with defects in these pathways (Table 78.1). In addition, diagnostic strategies and pitfalls of laboratory diagnostics for these enzyme deficiencies are explained. The laboratory methods described have been used for decades and are well documented. During the past few years, however, molecular diagnostics have proven to be an indispensable tool in the diagnosis of hereditary red cell enzyme deficiencies.

THE EMBDEN-MEYERHOF PATHWAY

Glucose is the energy source of the red cell. In a normal situation (without increased "oxidative stress"), 90% of glucose is catabolized anaerobically to pyruvate or lactate by the direct glycolytic pathway, or EMP. Although one mole of ATP is used by hexokinase and an additional mole of ATP by phosphofructokinase, the net gain is 2 moles of ATP per mole of glucose since a total of 4 moles of ATP is formed per mole of glucose by phosphoglycerate kinase and pyruvate kinase. In addition, reducing energy is generated in the form of reduced NADH in the reaction catalyzed by glyceraldehyde-3-phosphate dehydrogenase. This reducing energy can be used to reduce methemoglobin to hemoglobin by NADH-cytochrome b5 reductase. If this reaction takes place, the end product of the glycolysis is pyruvate. However, if NADH is not reoxidized here, it is used in reducing pyruvate to lactate by lactate dehydrogenase (LD) in the last step of glycolysis.

Although the pathway is reasonably straightforward, it is subjected to a complex mechanism of inhibiting and stimulating factors. Some of the enzymes involved are allosterically stimulated by intermediates of the pathway (e.g., stimulation of pyruvate kinase by fructose 1,6-bisphosphate); others serve as strong inhibitors (e.g., glucose 6-phosphate for hexokinase).

Hexokinase

Hexokinase (HK; Enzyme Classification [EC] number 2.7.1.1 [https://www.qmul.ac.uk/sbcs/iubmb]) catalyzes the phosphorylation of glucose to glucose-6-phosphate using ATP as a phosphoryl donor. The activity of HK is significantly higher in reticulocytes compared with mature red cells, where it is

TABLE 78.1 Clinically Relevant Enzyme Disorders of the Red Blood Cell

Enzyme Deficiency	Gene	Chromosome	Frequency	Hematologic Symptoms	Nonhematologic Symptoms	Inheritance	OMIM
Embden-Meyerhof Pathway							
Hexokinase	HK1	10q22	10–100 cases reported	HNSHA	—	AR	235700
Glucose phosphate isomerase	GPI	19q13.1	>100 cases reported	HNSHA	Neurologic abnormalities	AR	172400
Phosphofructokinase	PFKM	12q13.3	10–100 cases reported	HNSHA and/or muscle glycogen storage disease	Myopathy	AR	610681
Aldolase	ALDOA	16p11.2	<10 cases reported	HNSHA	Mild liver glycogen storage; myopathy, mental retardation	AR	611881
Triosephosphate isomerase	TPI1	12p13	10–100 cases reported	HNSHA	Severe neuromuscular disease	AR	190450
Phosphoglycerate kinase	PGK1	Xq13	10–100 cases reported	HNSHA	Myoglobinuria; neuromuscular disorder	SL	311800
Pyruvate kinase	PKLR	1q21	>100 cases reported	HNSHA	—	AR	266200
Hexose Monophosphate Pathway							
Glucose-6-phosphate dehydrogenase	G6PD	Xq28	very common	HNSHA; drug- or infection-induced hemolysis; favism	—	SL	305900
Rapoport-Luebering Shunt							
Bisphosphoglycerate mutase	BPGM	7q31-34	0–10 cases reported	erythrocytosis	—	AR	222800
Glutathione Pathway							
Glutamate cysteine ligase	GCLC	6p12	10–100 cases reported	HNSHA, drug- or infection-induced hemolysis	Neurologic abnormalities	AR	230450
Glutathione synthetase	GSS	20q11.2	10-100 cases reported	HNSHA; drug- or infection-induced hemolysis	5-Oxoprolinuria and neurologic defect	AR	231900
Glutathione reductase	GSR	8p21.1	0-10 cases reported	HNSHA; drug- or infection-induced hemolysis; favism	—	AR	
Purine-Pyrimidine Metabolism							
Pyrimidine 5'-nucleotidase	NT5C3A	7p14.3	>100 cases reported	HNSHA	Mental retardation in some cases	AR	266120
Adenylate kinase	AK1	9q34.1	10-100 cases reported	HNSHA	—	AR	612631
Adenosine deaminase (increased activity)	ADA	20q13.12	0-10 cases reported	HNSHA	—	AD	102730
Methemoglobin Reduction							
Cytochrome b5 reductase	CYB5R3	22q13.2	>100 cases reported	Methemoglobinemia; cyanosis; erythrocytosis	Mental retardation	AR	250800

AR, Autosomal recessive; *AD,* autosomal dominant; *HNSHA,* hemolytic nonspherocytic hemolytic anemia; *SL,* sex-linked.

very low. The HK reaction is one of two rate-limiting steps in this pathway, the other being the phosphofructokinase reaction.

In mammalian tissues, four isozymes of HK with different enzymatic properties exist, HK-I to III with an Mr of 100 kDa, and HK-IV (or glucokinase) with an Mr of 50 kDa. HK-I is the predominant HK isozyme in tissues that depend strongly on glucose use for their physiologic functioning, such as brain, muscle, and red blood cells. HK-I displays unique regulatory properties in its sensitivity to inhibition by physiologic concentrations of the product G6P and relief of this inhibition by inorganic phosphate and by high concentrations of glucose.[2] HK is a homodimer[3,4] and elucidation of the structures of human and rat HK-I has provided substantial insight into ligand-binding sites and subsequent modes of interaction.[4,5]

Apart from HK-I, RBCs contain a specific subtype of HK: HK-R.[6] Both HKs are encoded by the gene *HK1*, localized on chromosome 10q22 and spanning more than 100 kb.[7] The structure of *HK1* is complex: it encompasses 29 exons that, by tissue-specific transcription, generate multiple transcripts through alternative splicing of different 5′ exons.[7,8] Erythroid-specific transcriptional control results in a unique red cell–specific mRNA that differs from HK-I mRNA at the 5′ untranslated region (5′-UTR) and at the first 63 nucleotides of the coding region.[9–11] HK-R is mainly present in erythroblasts, reticulocytes, and young red cells. HK-1 replaces HK-R as the RBC matures[6] and, as a result, mature red cells contain only 2 to 3% of the HK activity of reticulocytes.[12]

HK deficiency (OMIM 235700; see Online Mendelian Inheritance in Man database: www.omim.org/) is a rare, recessively inherited disease with chronic nonspherocytic hemolytic anemia (CNSHA) as the predominant clinical feature. The phenotypic expression of the disease is heterogeneous, as with most glycolytic red cell enzyme deficiencies. The spectrum ranges from severe neonatal hemolysis and death to a fully compensated chronic hemolytic anemia. In general, patients benefit from splenectomy. Since HK activity is strongly dependent on red cell age, reticulocytosis, usually present in HK-deficient patients, may obscure the enzyme deficiency. Other age-dependent red cell enzymes (e.g., pyruvate kinase [PK], G6PD) should be measured simultaneously to assess the influence of reticulocyte enzyme activity.

Approximately 30 patients with HK deficiency have been described to date.[13–19] Most patients are compound heterozygous for missense mutations in *HK1*, some of which have been shown to affect enzyme stability[13,20] or the enzyme's active site.[16] A lethal case of HK deficiency was found to be due to a intragenic deletion of 9.5 kb, causing the deletion of exons 5 to 8 of HK1, resulting in a null allele.[15] In three patients from two unrelated families, HK deficiency was found to be due to a mutation in the erythroid-specific promoter (−193A>G), which downregulates erythroid-specific transcription of *HK1* and, hence, specifically affects HK-R production.[17] These findings underscore the importance of including promoter mutation analysis in the molecular diagnosis of red cell enzyme deficiencies.[21]

Mutations in *HK1* have also been associated with Russe type hereditary motor and sensory neuropathy, retinitis pigmentosa 79, and neurodevelopmental abnormalities with visual impairment. In all these cases, HK enzymatic activity was normal and HNSHA was absent, suggesting a different pathogenic mechanism for the dominant missense variants in *HK1*.[22]

Glucose-6-Phosphate Isomerase

Glucose-6-phosphate (G6P) isomerase (GPI; EC 5.3.1.9) (also known as phosphoglucose isomerase [PGI]), catalyzes the interconversion of G6P and fructose-6-phosphate (F6P)—the second step of the EMP. As a result of this reversible reaction, products of the HMP can be recycled to G6P. Besides being a housekeeping enzyme of glycolysis, GPI also functions as a neuroleukin, an autocrine motility factor, a nerve growth factor, and a mediator of differentiation and maturation.[23,24] These nonerythroid functions have been proposed to account for the nonhematologic features, such as neuromuscular symptoms, that occur in some cases of GPI deficiency.[25] Alternatively, disturbed glycerolipid biosynthesis may also play a role by affecting membrane formation, membrane function, and axonal migration.[26]

The crystal structure of human GPI has been resolved. The enzyme is a homodimer consisting of two subunits of 63 kDa each. The dimeric form of GPI is a prerequisite for catalytic activity because the active site of the enzyme is composed of polypeptide chains from both subunits.[27]

The gene encoding GPI (*GPI*) is located on chromosome 19q13.1 and consists of 18 exons, spanning at least 50 kb, with a cDNA 1.9 kb in length.[28]

GPI deficiency (OMIM 172400) is an autosomal recessive disease and, after G6PD and PK deficiency, considered the third most common red cell enzymopathy. Patients are homozygous or compound heterozygous for mutations in *GPI* and show mild to severe chronic hemolytic anemia. Neonatal death,[29] hydrops fetalis,[30,31] neurologic symptoms, and granulocyte dysfunction[32] have been reported. GPI knockout mice die in the embryonic state.[33]

Usually, a marked reticulocytosis is seen. Unlike HK, GPI activity in reticulocytes is only marginally higher than that in older cells. Splenectomy appears to result in a slight increase in hemoglobin levels but reduces transfusion requirements.[34] As in PK deficiency, there is a tendency for an increase in the number of reticulocytes after splenectomy.[34]

To date, approximately 60 families with GPI deficiency have been characterized worldwide.[34–37] By far, the majority of the 50 identified mutations are missense mutations, some of which are recurrent: c.301G>A p.(Val101Met), c.584C>T p.(Thr195Ile), c.1039C>T p.(Arg347Cys), and c.1040G>A p.(Arg347His).[34,37] Using the three-dimensional model of GPI, many of the missense mutations illustrate just how critical the precise three-dimensional structure is for correct function. Most of the mutations disrupt key interactions that contribute directly or indirectly to the active site architecture.[27,38]

Phosphofructokinase

Phosphofructokinase (PFK; EC 2.7.1.11) catalyzes the irreversible phosphorylation of fructose-6-phosphate by ATP to fructose-1,6-bisphosphate (FBP; also called fructose 1,6-diphosphate, FDP). This conversion is rate limiting. PFK activity is tightly controlled by many metabolic effectors,[39,40] by binding to calmodulin,[41] as well as the association of the enzyme with the red cell membrane.[42]

The enzyme is a homotetramer or heterotetramer with a molecular mass of around 340 kDa. Three distinct isoenzymes have been identified in humans: PFK-M (muscle),

PFK-L (liver), and PFK-P (platelet). In RBCs, the L- and M-isoforms are expressed; consequently, five forms of phosphofructokinase can be identified that differ in composition: M_4, M_3L_1, M_2L_2, ML_3, and L_4.

The genes encoding PFK-L (*PFKL*) and PFK-M (*PFKM*) are located on chromosome 21q22.3 and 12q13.3, respectively. The *PFKM* gene spans 30 kb, containing 27 exons and at least three promoter regions.[43] *PFKL* contains 22 exons and spans more than 28 kb.[44] A preliminary model of the structure of human muscle PFK has been presented.[45]

PFK deficiency is a rare autosomal recessively inherited disorder. Because red cells contain both M and L subunits, mutations affecting either of the genes coding for these subunits will affect PFK activity. Thus when the L-subunit is affected, red cells contain only M_4 PFK homotetramers and are partially PFK deficient. Similarly, when the M subunit is deficient, the partial PFK deficiency in red cells is accompanied by virtually absent PFK activity in muscle. This causes mild to severe myopathy, characterized by exercise intolerance, cramps, and myoglobinuria (Tarui disease or glycogen storage disease VII, OMIM 610681).[46] The accompanying hemolysis is generally mild and may be absent. PFK-deficient red cells display a metabolic block at the PFK step in glycolysis and have decreased concentrations of 2,3-bisphosphoglyceric acid (2,3-BPG, also called 2,3-diphosphoglyceric acid, 2,3-DPG; see Rapoport-Luebering Shunt).

To date, approximately 100 cases with PFK deficiency have been reported and 25 different mutations in *PFKM* associated with PFK deficiency have been identified.[47–52] About 60% of these mutations are missense mutations, with the remaining ones mainly affecting pre-mRNA processing.[46,47] Approximately one-third of identified PFK-deficient patients are of Ashkenazi Jewish origin. In this population, the most frequently encountered mutations are an intronic splice-site mutation in intron 5, c.237+1G>A, causing in-frame skipping of exon 5,[53] and a single base-pair deletion in exon 22, c.2003delC, that disrupts the reading frame creating a premature stop codon (p.(Pro668Glnfs*17)).[54]

To date, there has been only one reported case in which an unstable L subunit was identified. This patient exhibited no signs of myopathy or hemolysis.[55]

The fact that PFK deficiency in dogs is associated with hemolytic crises after strenuous exercise, as well as the exercise intolerance, progressive cardiac hypertrophy, and reduced life span seen in *Pfkm* null mice indicate that Tarui disease is not simply a muscle glycogenosis, but rather a complex systemic disorder.[56,57]

PFK is relatively unstable, and PFK enzyme activity assays should be carried out on fresh blood samples, as activity will decrease rapidly upon prolonged storage.

Aldolase

Aldolase (fructose-bisphosphate aldolase; EC 4.1.2.13) catalyzes the reversible conversion of fructose-1,6-bisphosphate to glyceraldehyde-3-phosphate and dihydroxyacetone phosphate. The enzyme is a 159-kDa tetramer of identical subunits of 40 kDa. Three isoenzymes have been identified to date: aldolases A, B, and C. Aldolase A is the isoenzyme that is expressed in the red cell but is also expressed in muscle.[58] The flexible C-terminal region of aldolase A has been implicated in the catalytic function of the enzyme.[59,60] Red cell aldolase binds to actin, and the N-terminal domain of band 3,[61]

thereby inhibiting the enzyme's activity.[62] Aldolase activity is also influenced by red cell age.

The gene for aldolase A (*ALDOA*) is located on chromosome 16p11.2. It spans 7.5 kb and contains 12 exons. Several transcription-initiation sites were identified that direct tissue-specific splicing.[63]

Aldolase deficiency (OMIM 611881) is a very rare disease; only seven cases have been described. All but one patient displayed chronic hemolytic anemia. In some patients, hemolysis is the sole clinical feature,[64] whereas in other patients, hemolytic anemia is accompanied by myopathy,[60,65] rhabdomyolysis,[66] psychomotor retardation,[65] or mental retardation.[58,65] Intriguingly, the one patient without hemolytic anemia presented with severe fever-induced rhabdomyolysis, possibly due to tissue-specific thermal instability of the mutant aldolase.[67]

Triosephosphate Isomerase

Triosephosphate isomerase (TPI; EC 5.3.1.1) is the enzyme of the anaerobic glycolytic pathway with the highest activity. This ubiquitously expressed enzyme catalyzes the interconversion of glyceraldehyde-3-phosphate and dihydroxyacetone phosphate. TPI is active as a dimer, consisting of two identical 27-kDa subunits of 248 amino acids. The three-dimensional structures of the human enzyme obtained by crystallography[68,69] show that the active site is located at the dimer interface and that several water molecules are an integral part of the dimer interface. No isoenzymes of TPI are known; only three distinct electrophoretic forms attributable to minor post-translational modifications have been identified.[70,71] RBC TPI activity is not related to red cell age.

TPI is transcribed from a single gene (*TPI1*), located on chromosome 12p13. The gene spans 3.5 kb and contains seven exons that encode the 248 amino acids-long TPI subunit. Three processed pseudogenes have been found.[72]

TPI deficiency (OMIM 190450) is a rare autosomal recessive systemic disorder and clinically the most severe disorder of glycolysis. The disease is characterized by hemolytic anemia, severe neuromuscular defects, increased susceptibility to infection, and cardiomyopathy.[73,74] Patients usually die in childhood, although intriguing exceptions have been reported.[75] Because of the metabolic block at the TPI step, a 20- to 60-fold increase in red cell concentration of dihydroxyacetone phosphate occurs. The resulting elevated levels of toxic methylglyoxal, and consequent formation of advanced glycation end products is proposed to be a key factor in the pathophysiology of TPI deficiency-related severe neuromuscular disease. In addition, molecular changes in the TPI dimer interface may cause a functional synaptic defect in TPI deficiency resulting in neurologic dysfunction.[76]

To date, 20 different mutations, mostly missense, have been identified in the gene encoding TPI, and approximately 50 patients have been reported.[77–83] Mutations result in decreased enzymatic activity and/or dissociation of the TPI dimer into inactive monomers.[74] The most common mutation is c.315G>C p.(Glu105Asp), a mutation detected in approximately 80% of patients. While TPI activity itself is not affected, this mutation impairs the formation of active dimers by disrupting the water-protein and water-water interactions that join the two monomers.[69] Haplotype analysis suggest a single origin for this mutation with the common ancestor in Northern Europe.[84]

Phosphoglycerate Kinase

Phosphoglycerate kinase (PGK, EC 2.7.2.3) catalyzes the reversible conversion of 1,3-bisphosphoglycerate (also called 1,2-diphosphoglycerate) to 3-phosphoglycerate, thereby generating one molecule of ATP. The reaction can be bypassed by the Rapoport-Luebering shunt at the expense of one molecule of ATP (see Rapoport-Luebering shunt and Fig. 78.1) This alternative routing of glycolytic intermediates has been called the *energy clutch* of glycolysis.[85]

In humans, two isoenzymes (PGK-1 and PGK-2) exist. PGK-1 is ubiquitously expressed in all somatic cells; PGK-2 is expressed only in spermatozoa.[86] PGK-1 is a 48-kDa monomeric enzyme consisting of 417 amino acids.[87] The gene encoding PGK-1 (*PGK1*) is located on the long arm of the X-chromosome (Xq13). The gene spans 23 kb and is composed of 11 exons.[88] Nonfunctional pseudogenes have been found on the X chromosome and chromosome 19.[86]

PGK deficiency (OMIM 311800) is one of the uncommon causes of HNSHA. Sometimes the deficiency manifests only mild to severe chronic hemolytic anemia, but in many other cases other clinical findings are present, particularly neurologic symptoms and myopathy; these may occur with or without hemolytic anemia.[89] More than 50 patients with PGK deficiency have been characterized.[90–92] Multiorgan involvement in patients with PGK deficiency appears to be associated with lower residual enzyme activity, as compared to patients displaying only myopathy.[93] Most of the 29 mutations reported to date are missense ones, mainly affecting thermal stability of the protein.[94] They are mostly unique mutations except for the c.491A>T (p.Asp164Val) change, which has been encountered three times, each in the context of a different haplotype,[95] suggesting independent origins of this mutation.[89] Review of amino acid substitutions in PGK has gained some insight into the genotype-to-phenotype correlation in PGK deficiency,[96] but the reason for the range of manifestations in PGK deficiency remains unclear, suggesting that other yet unknown environmental, metabolic, genetic, and/or epigenetic factors are involved.[96,97]

Pyruvate Kinase

Pyruvate kinase (PK; EC 2.7.1.40) catalyzes the conversion of phosphoenolpyruvate to pyruvate with the concomitant generation of the second molecule of ATP in glycolysis (see Fig. 78.1). Pyruvate is crucial for several metabolic pathways, and PK represents one of the major regulatory enzymes of glycolysis. PK is allosterically activated by its substrate and by FBP (fructose-1,6-bisphosphate), and its enzymatic activity strongly depends on red cell age. Therefore because the youngest red cells have the highest activity, a deficiency of PK may easily be masked by reticulocytosis.

PK is a homotetrameric enzyme. In mammals, four isozymes are expressed. PK-M1 is expressed in skeletal muscle, heart, and brain. It is the only PK isozyme that is not allosterically regulated. PK-M2 is expressed in early fetal tissues and in adult tissues, including leukocytes and platelets. Both M1 and M2 isozymes are produced from a single gene (*PKM2*) by means of alternative splicing.[98,99] PK-L is predominantly expressed in the liver, whereas the expression of PK-R is confined to the red cell.[100] The PK-L and PK-R subunits are transcribed from a single gene (*PKLR*) located on chromosome 1q21 by the use of tissue-specific promoters.[100,101] The *PKLR* gene consists of 12 exons and is approximately 9.5 kb

in size.[102] Exon 1 is exclusively expressed in erythroid cells, whereas expression of exon 2 is confined to the liver. Hence, the PK-R monomer is composed of 574 amino acids.[103] The PK-L subunit comprises 531 amino acids.[104]

In basophilic erythroblasts, both the PK-M2 and PK-R isozymes are expressed. During further erythroid differentiation and maturation the PK-R isozyme progressively replaces PK-M2.[105–107] In addition, the red cell limited proteolytic degradation of the 63-kDa PK-R subunit renders a subset of PK-R monomers of 57 to 58 kDa.[108] Consequently, in young and mature human red cells two distinct species can be distinguished, PK-R1 and PK-R2, that differ in PK-R and "processed" PK-R subunit composition.[109]

The crystal structure of human red cell PK has been elucidated.[110] Each PK-R subunit is composed of four domains: N, A, B, and C. The active site lies in a cleft between the A-domain and the flexible B-domain. The B-domain is capable of rotating with respect to the A-domain, generating either the "open" or "closed" conformation. The C-domain contains the binding site for FBP. In the PK tetramer, subunit interactions at the interfaces between the A and C domains, as well as A/B and A/C domain interactions, within one subunit are considered to be key determinants of the allosteric response, involving switching from the low-affinity T-state to the high affinity R-state.[110–114]

Pyruvate kinase deficiency (OMIM 266200) is the most common cause of nonspherocytic hemolytic anemia due to defective glycolysis. It is an autosomal recessive disease. In the general white population, the allelic frequency is estimated to be around 2%.[115]

The two major metabolic abnormalities resulting from PK deficiency are ATP depletion and increased levels of 2,3-BPG. The precise mechanisms by which the enzyme deficiency leads to a shortened RBC lifespan are unknown. An important feature, however, is the selective sequestration of PK-deficient reticulocytes by the spleen.[116] It has been suggested that the metabolic disturbances of the enzyme deficiency may affect not only red cell survival, but also the maturation of PK-deficient erythroid progenitors, resulting in ineffective erythropoiesis.[117]

PK-deficient patients display a highly variable degree of chronic hemolysis with variable clinical severity. Clinical symptoms range from severe anemia and death at birth, severe transfusion-dependent chronic hemolysis, or moderate hemolysis with exacerbation during infection, to a well-compensated hemolysis without anemia.[118] Common complications are iron overload and gallstones, and perinatal complications include anemia requiring transfusion, hyperbilirubinemia, hydrops, and prematurity.[119] Splenectomy is, in general, beneficial, as it is associated with an increase in hemoglobin and decreased transfusion burden.[119] PK deficiency has been treated successfully by stem cell transplantation.[120] Gene therapy strategies have been shown to be able to correct the PK-deficient phenotype in mice.[121] Recent evidence indicates that small molecule activation of mutant PK restores glycolysis and normalizes red cell metabolism in PK deficiency,[122] and clinical trials using small molecule allosteric activators of PK have reported an increase in hemoglobin level in half of the PK-deficient patients who were administered the drug.[123]

To date, more than 260 mutations in PKLR have been reported to be associated with pyruvate kinase deficiency.[124]

Two-thirds of these mutations are missense mutations affecting conserved residues in structurally and functionally important domains of PK. The most frequently detected mutations are missense mutants c.1456C>T (p.Arg486Trp), c.1529G>A (p.Arg510Gln), c.994G>A (p.Gly332Ser), and nonsense mutant c.721G>T (p.Glu241*). Evaluating the protein structural context of affected residues using the three-dimensional structure of recombinant human tetrameric PK has provided a rationale for the observed enzyme deficiency.[110,125,126] From a large cohort of PK-deficient patients, a limited genotype-to-phenotype correlation was identified: patients with two missense mutations had a lower likelihood of splenectomy, fewer transfusions, and a lower rate of iron overload, whereas patients with two nonmissense mutations were less likely to have a complete or partial response to splenectomy.[119] It is important to note that because most PK-deficient patients are compound heterozygous for two different (missense) mutations, up to seven different tetrameric forms of PK may be present in such patients, each with distinct structural and kinetic properties. This complicates genotype-to-phenotype correlations as it is difficult to infer which mutation is primarily responsible for deficient enzyme function and the clinical phenotype.[125]

Pyruvate kinase deficiency has been reported to have a protective effect against replication of the malarial parasite in human RBCs,[127,128] and malaria has been found to act as a selective force in the *PKLR* genomic region.[129] This protective effect may be related to the reduced ATP levels in PK-deficient red blood cells.[130]

PK levels are also decreased in patients with red cell disorders caused by mutations in *KLF1*, probably due to altered binding of mutant KLF1 to the erythroid promoter region of *PKLR*.[131]

Lactate Dehydrogenase

LD catalyzes the conversion of pyruvate to lactate, the last step in the EMP. Deficiency of this enzyme is not associated with hematologic disease. LD is described in Chapter 32.

HEXOSE MONOPHOSPHATE PATHWAY

Normally, approximately 10% of glucose is catabolized through the HMP (see Fig. 78.1). The primary function of this pathway is to reduce 2 moles of $NADP^+$ to NADPH, by means of oxidizing G6P. The amount of glucose passing through this pathway is regulated by the amount of $NADP^+$ that has been made available by the oxidation of NADPH. In the red cell, NADPH is required mainly for the regeneration and preservation of the reduced form of glutathione (GSH), which is crucial to the cell to detoxify hydrogen peroxide, thereby protecting against oxidative stress. Because the red cell has no other ways of generating NADPH, it depends strongly on the activity of the prime enzyme of NADPH production: glucose 6-phosphate dehydrogenase.

Glucose-6-Phosphate Dehydrogenase

G6PD (EC 1.1.1.49) is expressed in all cells and catalyzes the first step and rate-limiting step in the HMP—the conversion of glucose 6-phosphate to 6-phosphogluconolactone, which is readily converted to 6-phosphogluconate. In the process, an equivalent number of moles of NADPH is generated. G6PD activity is higher in reticulocytes than in mature red cells.

The active enzyme is predominantly a homodimer that comprises 59-kDa subunits of 515 amino acids each. Lowering the pH causes a shift from the dimeric to the tetrameric form.[132] In the absence of $NADP^+$, G6PD dissociates into inactive subunits. Each G6PD subunit is built up by two domains. The extensive interface between the two monomers is of crucial importance for enzymatic stability and activity. The importance of $NADP^+$ for stability is explained by the structural $NADP^+$ site, distant from the active site but close to the dimer interface.[133]

The gene coding for G6PD is located on the long arm of the X-chromosome (Xq28). It spans 18 kb and consists of 13 exons, of which exon 1 is noncoding.

G6PD deficiency (OMIM 305900) is the most common enzymopathy, affecting an estimated 220 million males worldwide and an estimated 133 million females across all malaria endemic countries.[134] The parallel between the high frequency of G6PD deficiency and the worldwide distribution of malaria implies that G6PD deficiency confers a selective advantage.[135–137] This hypothesis is supported by several lines of evidence,[138,139] indicating that the uniform state of G6PD deficiency in hemizygous males, and probably also homozygous females, confers significant protection against severe, life-threatening malaria.[140–142]

G6PD variants have been grouped into categories (class I to V) according to the level of residual enzyme activity and clinical manifestations (Table 78.2).[143] More than 400 variants and more than 200 different mutations have been reported,

TABLE 78.2 Classes of Severity of Glucose-6-Phosphate Dehydrogenase (G6PD) Deficiency

Class	Description	Clinical Manifestations
Class I	Severe deficiency (<10% residual activity), e.g., G6PD Guadalajara	Chronic nonspherocytic hemolytic anemia, neonatal jaundice, acute exacerbations of hemolysis
Class II	Severe deficiency (<10% residual activity), e.g., G6PD Mediterranean	Acute hemolysis
Class III	Moderate to mild deficiency (10–60% residual activity), e.g., G6PD A−	Acute hemolysis
Class IV	Very mild or no deficiency, 60–150% residual activity, e.g., G6PD A	None
Class V	Increased activity (only one variant known, G6PD Hektoen)	None

G6PD, Glucose-6-phosphate dehydrogenase.
Glucose-6-phosphate dehydrogenase deficiency. Who working group. *Bull World Health Organ* 1989;67:601–11.

most of which encode the substitution of a single amino acid.[144,145] The most common deficient variant in people from African descent is G6PD A−. This variant is characterized by the c.376A>G p.(Asn126Asp) mutation, in most cases with a second mutation *in cis*, c.202G>A p.(Val68Met). G6PD Mediterranean, c.563C>T p.(Ser188Phe), is the most common G6PD variant in people from Mediterranean countries.

Clinically, G6PD deficiency can manifest itself as:
- Drug-induced hemolysis
- Infection-induced hemolysis
- Favism
- Neonatal jaundice (NNJ)
- CNSHA

Most G6PD-deficient individuals are asymptomatic throughout life. They develop acute hemolysis only during periods of increased oxidative stress, elicited by certain drugs (Table 78.3),[146] infections, or the ingestion of fava beans. Clinically, such hemolytic episodes are characterized by anemia accompanied by increased levels of bilirubin and LDH in plasma and reticulocytosis. The exact mechanism by which increased oxidative stress leads to acute hemolysis is unknown, but it

TABLE 78.3 Drugs That May Trigger Hemolysis in Glucose-6-Phosphate Dehydrogenase-deficient Individuals

Category of Drug	Predictable Hemolysis	Possible Hemolysis
Anti-malarials	Dapsone containing combinations	Chloroquine
	Primaquine	Quinine
	Pamaquine	Quinidine
	Methylene blue	Mepacrine
Analgesics/ Antipyretic	Phenazopyridine	Aspirin (Acetylsalicylic acid, high doses)
		Paracetamol (Acetominophen)
Anti-bacterials	Cotrimoxazole	Sulfasalazine
	Niridazole	Sulfadiazine
	Quinolones (including nalidixic acid, ciprofloxacin, ofloxacin, movifloxacin, norfloxacin)	Sulfonylureas
	Nitrofurantoin	
Other	Rasburicase	Chloramphenicol
	Toluidine blue	Isoniazid
		Ascorbic acid
		Glibenclamide
		Vitamin K analogs
		Isosorbide dinitrate
		Sulfonylureas
		Dimercaptosuccinic acid

Adapted from Luzzatto L, Nannelli C, Notaro R. Glucose-6-phosphate dehydrogenase deficiency. *Hematol Oncol Clin North Am* 2016;30: 373–93.

results from the inability of G6PD-deficient red cells to withstand oxidative damage induced by the triggers mentioned previously. This is generally accompanied by the formation of Heinz bodies. Such cells are rapidly eliminated from the circulation by the spleen. Older red cells are more susceptible to destruction than young ones and are selectively removed from the circulation, characterizing a self-limited course of hemolysis. The reticulocytosis that is elicited as a result of hemolysis may obscure the enzyme deficiency as these very young RBCs have the highest enzyme activity. The administration of drugs that are capable of inducing hemolysis in G6PD-deficient individuals is often accompanied by methemoglobin formation.

Notably, as a result of X-chromosome inactivation, heterozygous females are genetic mosaics. As a consequence of (skewed) X-chromosome inactivation, they may display enzymatic activities ranging from normal to as low as hemizygous males. Hence, they may express the same pathophysiologic phenotype as their hemizygous male counterparts.[148–150]

G6PD-deficient neonates who have co-inherited a TA$_{(n)}$ repeat variation mutation in the uridine-diphosphate-glucuronosyl-transferase-1 (*UGT1A1*) promoter, causing downregulated expression of the enzyme,[151] are particularly at risk for developing NNJ and even kernicterus.[152,153]

A small proportion of G6PD-deficient individuals display the phenotype of CNSHA. The hemolytic anemia in these class I G6PD-deficient patients may be severe. Mutations associated with class I G6PD deficiency are generally clustered in exons 10, 11, and 12 designating the subunit interface.[133]

For further reading on the extensive topic of G6PD deficiency we refer to excellent reviews.[154–157]

6-PHOSPHOGLUCONATE DEHYDROGENASE (DECARBOXYLATING) (EC 1.1.1.44)

Even though the oxidation of phosphogluconate to ribulose-5-phosphate by 6-phosphogluconate dehydrogenase generates an equal number of moles of NADPH, the few cases of 6-phosphogluconate dehydrogenase deficiency are usually not associated with hemolysis.[158]

Transketolase

Transketolase (EC 2.2.1.1) is decreased in thiamine deficiency,[159] and its expression was found to be downregulated in patients with pyrimidine-5′-nucleotidase deficiency.[160] Low values of it have also been found in chronic alcoholism (see Chapter 51 for more details).

RAPOPORT-LUEBERING SHUNT

Red cell 2,3-BPG is important in the regulation of the oxygen affinity of hemoglobin.[161–163] 2,3-BPG is synthesized and dephosphorylated in the Rapoport-Luebering shunt. Thus this unique glycolytic bypass represents an important physiologic means for the regulation of the oxygen-affinity. At the same time, the Rapoport-Luebering shunt provides the red cell with flexibility with regard to the generation of ATP. From an oxygen-transport point of view, the EMP serves principally the generation of 2,3-BPG, because in terms of quantity, it is the principal glycolytic intermediate: the concentration of 2,3-BPG is about equal to the sum of all other glycolytic intermediates. In PK deficiency, 2,3-BPG is increased as a result of the metabolic block at the PK step and of retrograde accumulation of glycolytic intermediates. Increased 2,3-BPG levels result in decreased oxygen affinity of hemoglobin, so that oxygen is more readily transferred to tissues.[164] This beneficial circumstance is absent in those glycolytic enzyme defects that cause a decrease in 2,3-BPG levels (e.g., HK and GPI deficiency).

Both reactions in the Rapoport-Luebering shunt are catalyzed by one multifunctional protein: 2,3-BPG mutase (BPGM, EC 5.4.2.4). The mutase activity of this enzyme converts the glycolytic intermediate 1,3-BPG to 2,3-BPG. BPGM also has phosphatase activity (2,3-BPG phosphatase [BPGP]; EC 3.1.3.13), converting 2,3-BPG to 3-phosphoglycerate, which then re-enters the glycolytic pathway (see Fig. 78.1).

BPGM is a homodimer with 30-kDa subunits consisting of 258 amino acids. Elucidation of the crystal structure of human BPGM has provided a structural basis for the different enzymatic activities of this enzyme.[165,166]

The gene for BPGM (*BPGM*) is located on chromosome 7q31-34. It consists of three exons, spanning more than 22 kb.[167] It is expressed only in erythroid tissue, during the late stages of differentiation.[167]

BPGM deficiency (OMIM 222800) is a very rare disorder that results in reduced levels of 2,3-BPG.[168] As a result, the oxygen affinity of hemoglobin is increased, causing a decrease in tissue oxygenation and, consequently, erythrocytosis. Only five families with BPGM deficiency and four mutations in *BPGM* have been described.[169–172] BPGM deficiency appears to be an autosomal recessive disorder, although some heterozygous individuals also display increased hemoglobin concentrations.[169–171]

GLUTATHIONE PATHWAY

The sulfhydryl-containing tripeptide reduced glutathione (GSH) is present in high concentrations in most mammalian cells.[173,174] In RBCs, GSH protects hemoglobin and other critical red cell proteins from peroxidative injury.[175] In this process, which involves the reduction of peroxides or oxidized protein sulfhydryl groups, GSH is converted to GSSH (oxidized glutathione) (see Fig. 78.2). Enzyme deficiencies in this pathway, except for glutathione peroxidase deficiency, lead to mild CNSHA, accompanied by drug- and infection-induced hemolytic episodes. The pathogenesis of hemolysis of such enzyme deficiencies is probably similar to that in G6PD deficiency (180).

Glutamate Cysteine Ligase

Glutamate cysteine ligase (EC 6.3.2.2), also known as gamma-glutamylcysteine synthetase, catalyzes the first step in glutathione biosynthesis. The enzyme mediates the formation of γ-glutamylcysteine, adenosine diphosphate (ADP), and P_i from glutamate, cysteine, and ATP. This amide linking is the rate-limiting step in glutathione synthesis. There is a feedback inhibition by glutathione. Glutamate cysteine ligase is a heterodimer composed of a catalytic heavy chain (GCS$_h$,) of 637 amino acids and 73 kDa and a regulatory light chain (GCS$_l$) of 274 amino acids and 31 kDa.[176,177]

The genes for GCS$_h$ (*GCLC*) and GCS$_l$ (*GCLM*) are localized on chromosome 6p12 and chromosome 1p22.1, respectively.[178,179]

Hereditary glutamate cysteine ligase deficiency (OMIM 230450) is an autosomal recessive disorder that is very rare.

It is generally associated with mild HNSHA. Drug- and infection-induced hemolytic crises may occur. Twelve cases of glutamate cysteine ligase deficiency have been described and a total of six different mutations have been reported, all of which affected the heavy subunit of glutamate cysteine ligase.[180] In about one-third of patients given a diagnosis of glutamate cysteine ligase deficiency, the hemolytic anemia is accompanied by neurologic manifestations.[180] The homology model of the human catalytic subunit, based on the crystal structure of *Saccharomyces cerevisiae*, has been generated to explain the molecular basis of glutamate cysteine ligase deficiency.[181]

Glutathione Synthetase

Glutathione synthetase (EC 6.3.2.3; GS) mediates the second irreversible ATP-dependent step in the synthesis of GSH. The enzyme catalyzes the addition of glycine to the dipeptide γ-glutamylcysteine. Glutathione synthetase is a homodimer of 52 kDa.[182]

The 23 kb spanning gene for glutathione synthetase (*GSS*) is located on chromosome 20q11.2 and contains 13 exons, of which the first is noncoding, that encode 474 amino acids.[183]

Deficiency of glutathione synthetase (OMIM 231900) is rare, but it is the most common abnormality of glutathione metabolism. The disorder is inherited in an autosomal recessive mode. Three distinct clinical forms of GS deficiency can be distinguished on the basis of their severity.[184] The mildest form displays hemolytic anemia as the only clinical manifestation. In moderate and severe forms, the hemolytic anemia is accompanied by metabolic acidosis and 5-oxoprolinuria,[185] which results from accumulation of γ-glutamylcysteine.[175] Patients with the severe type of GS deficiency develop, in addition, progressive central nervous system damage. Approximately one-third of all patients die in childhood, often in the neonatal period.[186] It is important to note that 5-oxoprolinuria (or pyroglutamic aciduria) can also be associated with other disorders,[187,188] including acetaminophen-induced 5-oxoproline metabolic acidosis (see also Chapter 50 and 51 on paracetamol induced metabolic acidosis).[189,190]

More than 75 patients and 40 mutations have been described as associated with GS deficiency.[175,191–198] Most mutations are missense ones, and mapping them onto the structure of GS provides a molecular basis for understanding their effects.[199,200] To some extent, the type of mutation, GS activity, and GSH levels can predict a mild versus a more severe phenotype.[191]

Glutathione Reductase

Glutathione reductase (glutathione-disulfide reductase; EC 1.8.1.7; GSR) links the glutathione pathway to the HMP through reversible oxidation and reduction of NADP. The enzyme maintains high levels of reduced glutathione in the RBC and requires flavin adenine dinucleotide (FAD) as a cofactor. Two GSR isoforms exist: a mitochondrial form and a cytoplasmic form, which may be produced by alternative initiation of translation.[201] The active enzyme is a homodimer, linked by a disulfide bridge. Each subunit (522 amino acids; 56 kDa) is divided into four domains, of which domains 1 and 2 bind FAD and NADPH, respectively. Domain 4 is involved in the dimer interface.[202,203]

The gene encoding GSR (*GSR*) is located on chromosome 8p21.1, spans 50 kb, and contains 13 exons.[204]

Since GSR activity is strongly influenced by diet,[205] acquired GSR deficiency is common in malnourished populations. Except when very severe, the deficiency is not associated with hemolysis. Hereditary glutathione reductase deficiency (OMIM 138300) is a very rare autosomal recessive disease. Only two families have been reported. Red cells of patients contained no detectable GSR enzymatic activity. Patients from one family[206] presented with favism and were found to be homozygous for a large genomic deletion of 2246 bp (c.1286-229_*499del2246 p.(Asp429Alafs*6).[207] The patient from the other family displayed severe NNJ without hemolysis and was found to be compound heterozygous for a c.993G>A p.(Trp331*) nonsense mutation, and a c.1121G>C p.(Gly374Ala) missense mutation.[207]

Similar to other red cell disorders like PK deficiency, GSR deficiency may provide protection against malaria.[208]

Glutathione Peroxidase

Glutathione peroxidase (GPX, EC 1.11.1.9) catalyzes the conversion of hydrogen peroxide to water, thus reducing peroxidative stress to proteins in the cell. It is active as a homotetrameric enzyme consisting of 21-kDa subunits and encoded by the *GPX1* gene on chromosome 3p21.3.[209] Enzyme levels of GPX are regulated by selenium.[210] Because red cells also have high catalase (EC 1.11.1.6) activity to convert H_2O_2 to water and O_2, the activity of GPX may be redundant. In fact, deficiencies of either catalase or GPX are without clinical consequences.[211,212]

Low GPX activities occur commonly in healthy persons in some population groups,[213] and although the association with hemolysis has been reported,[213,214] a clear cause-effect relationship has not been established.

PURINE-PYRIMIDINE METABOLISM

Because RBCs cannot synthesize nucleotides de novo, they have evolved nucleotide salvage pathways to effectively preserve them. This is particularly important to maintain the pool of adenosine phosphates, which comprises about 97% of the total nucleotide content of the red cell. In contrast, pyrimidine ribonucleotides that result from the breakdown of ribosomal RNA during maturation are efficiently lost from the red cell. Deficiencies of some enzymes in these pathways lead to HNSHA, whereas deficiencies of others cause metabolic disease, but are without an apparent effect on the red cell.[215,216]

Pyrimidine-5′-Nucleotidase-1

Pyrimidine-5′-nucleotidases (P5′N) are a group of enzymes dephosphorylating pyrimidine nucleotides to the corresponding nucleosides and inorganic phosphates. These nucleosides are able to freely diffuse across the membrane out of the cell, thereby preventing their accumulation. Two cytoplasmic forms of the enzyme were identified in the red cell: P5′N-1 and P5′N-2. These enzymes are encoded by different genes and have different molecular properties and substrate specificities.[217,218] Because no known disorders are associated with deficiency of P5′N-2, this enzyme will not be further discussed here.

Pyrimidine-5′-nucleotidase-1 (P5′N-1; EC 3.1.3.5) is a monomeric 34 kDa protein consisting of 286 amino acids.[219] The enzyme activity has optimal substrate specificity for uridine 5′-monophosphate and cytidine 5′-monophosphate.[220]

P5′N-1 activity is highly dependent on RBC age. Its activity is highest in reticulocytes, and a rapid decline occurs during the first few days of maturation, followed by further decline throughout the life span of the red cell.[221]

The gene encoding P5′N-1 (*NT5C3A*) maps to chromosome 7p14.3, spans about 50 kb, and consists of 11 exons.[222] Three transcripts are formed by means of alternative splicing of pre-mRNA. The 286 amino acids–long protein from red cells is translated from mRNA lacking exons 2 and R.[222,223]

The three-dimensional model of the crystal structure of mouse P5′N-1 has provided insight into kinetic mechanisms of the human enzyme.[224]

P5′N-1 deficiency (OMIM 266120) is the most frequent disorder of red cell nucleotide metabolism and a relatively common cause of nonspherocytic hemolytic anemia. Its hallmark is the accumulation and precipitation of pyrimidine nucleotides that lead to a shortened RBC life span by yet unknown mechanisms[220,225] The deficiency is inherited in an autosomal recessive manner. It is the only red cell enzyme deficiency in which red cell morphology is helpful: prominent basophilic stippling is visible in blood smears from P5′N-1-deficient patients, representing the accumulation of pyrimidine nucleotides.

More than 100 patients have been diagnosed with P5′N-1 deficiency, but because of the relatively mild phenotypic expression many cases may remain undetected.[226] To date, 30 different mutations have been reported and most patients are homozygous for a given mutation in *NT5C3A*.[220,227–231] One-third are missense mutations, and the other mutations are small deletions and insertions, or affect splicing. Strikingly, none of the missense mutations concern residues directly involved in catalysis. Therefore it is likely that reduced enzymatic activity and/or protein instability in those cases is due to secondary effects related to conformational changes.[224,227]

Notably, lead poisoning causes acquired P5′N-1 deficiency and may be associated with hemolytic anemia and marked basophilic stippling; Pb^{2+} binding to the active site prevents binding of Mg^{2+}, which is a cofactor essential for the enzyme's activity.[224] For more details on lead poisoning, refer to Chapter 44. P5′N1 activity is also inhibited in β-thalassemia.[232]

Adenylate Kinase

Adenylate kinase (AK; EC 2.7.4.3) catalyzes the reversible interconversion of the adenine nucleotides, ATP and AMP, to ADP. The gene for AK (*AK1*) has been localized to chromosome 9q34.1, is 12 kb in size, and consists of 7 exons, of which exon 1 is noncoding. The mRNA codes for a monomeric enzyme of 194 amino acids.[233]

AK deficiency (OMIM 612631) is a rare autosomal recessive disorder. More than 10 patients have been described and 12 different mutations have been identified, two-thirds of which are missense mutations.[234,235] AK-deficient patients display moderate to severe hemolytic anemia. In some patients, hemolysis is accompanied by mental retardation and psychomotor impairment.[234] The study of altered properties of mutant AKs has provided support for the cause-effect relationship between *AK1* mutations and hemolytic anemia.[236]

Adenosine Deaminase

Adenosine deaminase (ADA; EC 3.5.4.4) is the enzyme of purine metabolism that transfers the amine group from adenosine and 2′-deoxyadenosine to inosine and 2′-deoxyinosine, respectively. Deficiency of ADA leads to severe combined immunodeficiency disease (SCID) without hemolysis.

A hereditary increase in red cell ADA activity (OMIM 102730) results in depletion of red cell ATP[237] and causes nonspherocytic hemolytic anemia. It is the only RBC enzymopathy that is inherited as an autosomal dominant disorder. Only a few cases have been described, displaying a 30- to 70-fold increase in ADA activity. The molecular basis of this disorder has not been elucidated. In patients, high levels of normal ADA mRNA were present, suggesting the mutation of an in cis transcriptional regulatory element in close proximity of the gene that results in overproduction of an otherwise normal enzyme.[238–240]

Less pronounced increases of ADA activity, approximately two- to sixfold, are seen in the majority of patients with Diamond-Blackfan anemia, a congenital form of erythroid aplasia.[241,242] The reason for this is not understood.

METHEMOGLOBIN REDUCTION

Hemoglobin can bind oxygen only in the reduced ferrous (Fe^{2+}) state. Thus when hemoglobin is oxidized to the ferric (Fe^{3+}) state, the capacity to bind oxygen is lost. The oxidized state of hemoglobin, called *methemoglobin*, represents less than 1% of total hemoglobin in healthy red cells. To preserve oxygen-binding capacity, the RBC keeps hemoglobin in the reduced state by a process that strongly depends on the NADH-dependent cytochrome b5/cytochrome b5 reductase system.

Cytochrome B5 Reductase

NADH-cytochrome b_5 reductase, or methemoglobin reductase, (Cb5R, EC 1.6.2.2) uses the NADH generated by glyceraldehyde-3-phosphate dehydrogenase in the EMP to reduce the 12-kDa electron transport protein cytochrome b5. In turn, cytochrome b5 reduces methemoglobin to hemoglobin.

The enzyme is present in two different forms. The membrane-bound form is a 35-kDa protein of 301 amino acids that is anchored to the endoplasmic reticulum and outer mitochondrial membrane where it is involved in a number of physiologic processes, such as fatty acid desaturation and cholesterol biosynthesis.[243] The membrane-bound form is present in all cell types except red cells. The second, soluble, form of Cb5R is a red cell specific protein of 278 amino acids.[244] The two isoforms share an identical hydrophilic C-terminal domain, but the N terminus of the cytoplasmic form lacks the 25 hydrophobic amino acids that constitute the membrane binding domain.[245]

Both forms of Cb5R are transcribed from the *CYB5R3* gene (previously known as *DIA1*) on chromosome 22q13.2. The gene is 32 kb in length and contains nine exons.[246] Exon 1 is lacking from the red cell-specific mRNA.

Several three-dimensional structures, including human red cell cytochrome b_5 reductase,[247] have been solved by crystallography. This revealed two distinct, highly conserved regions called the FAD domain, containing the FAD prosthetic group, and NADH domains. The two domains are connected by a "hinge" region.[248]

NADH-cytochrome b5 reductase deficiency (OMIM 250800) is a rare autosomal recessive disorder, causing hereditary methemoglobinemia. The methemoglobinemia may be accompanied by compensatory secondary erythrocytosis,

due to a leftward shift in the oxyhemoglobin dissociation curve.[249] CB5R-deficiency was the first identified hereditary enzymopathy.[250] Two distinct clinical forms (types I and II) can be distinguished.[251] The typically blue color of the skin—cyanosis—due to lack of oxygen in the blood, is a prominent feature of both types. In patients with type I methemoglobinemia, the enzyme deficiency is confined to the red cells. Patients with type II deficiency are more severely affected due to the loss of both membrane-bound and soluble enzyme function in tissues. Patients seldom reach adulthood because of a myriad of severe clinical symptoms, such as progressive encephalopathy.[243,252]

Importantly, acquired acute methemoglobinemia is more frequent and may occur as a result of the intake of oxidizing medications or drugs.

Approximately 80 different mutations in *CYB5R3* have been identified that are associated with hereditary methemoglobinemia.[253,254] Most are missense mutations, but nonsense, splice site mutations and small deletions have also been reported. There are no mutational hotspots, and only very few of the mutations are common to both types of methemoglobinemia.[251,253] Interestingly, there are examples of different mutations of the same amino acid leading to different forms of the disease, raising the hypothesis that the phenotype is related to residual enzymatic activity, as determined by the different combinations of mutations.[253]

DETECTION OF HEREDITARY RED CELL ENZYME DEFICIENCIES

Other than deficiencies of G6PD and PK, red blood cell enzymopathies are rare to very rare. Therefore testing should be done in specialized laboratories with experience with these assays. Specimens should be shipped by mail or courier service to reference laboratories that specialize in performance of these assays. As a rule, whole-blood specimens anticoagulated with EDTA are suitable, and specimens should be shipped at 4 °C.[255] Exceptions are assays for phosphorylated sugar intermediates, 2,3-BPG, and nucleotide intermediates, which are unstable in freshly drawn blood and require immediate deproteinization in perchloric acid.[255]

Care should be taken for proper removal of leukocytes and platelets before testing, because these cells also contain enzymatic activity, thereby potentially obscuring a deficiency of the red cell enzyme.[255]

Other pitfalls in the correct diagnosis of glycolytic enzyme deficiencies include the RBC age-dependent behavior of a number of enzymes (in particular, PK, HK, P5′N1, and G6PD). For proper evaluation of a single enzyme measurement, its activity should be compared with simultaneous measurement of the activity of a reference enzyme (e.g., HK), for instance, by calculating the ratio between the two enzymes.[256]

Many patients suffering from severe hemolysis may have already received blood transfusions. In this case, results from red cell enzyme assays must be interpreted with great care, because the presence of donor red cells may obscure an enzyme deficiency. In addition, some mutant enzymes display normal activity in vitro, whereas severe impairment of enzymatic activity may occur in vivo. More sophisticated assays, for example, heat instability tests and enzyme kinetics, are required to identify an enzyme deficiency in those cases.[257]

Over the past few years, most of the genes coding for the red cell enzymes have been localized and characterized. This has made molecular diagnostics possible, and many causative mutations have been identified. Molecular diagnostics at the DNA level are very attractive in situations in which the diagnosis of enzyme deficiency is difficult or impossible by activity measurements, as may occur in transfused patients, as explained previously. Nowadays, many of the genes encoding RBC enzymes are included in NGS panels.[258,259] DNA diagnostics also offer the possibility of prenatal diagnosis. The ability to study the effects of mutations in three-dimensional models of the enzymes and the possibility of expressing recombinant mutant enzymes will lead to a better understanding of the genotype-to-phenotype correlation noted in RBC enzymopathies.

METHODS

In this section, methodologic principles and reference values are given for the methods used to measure red cell G6PD and PK enzyme activities.[255] Deficiencies of G6PD and PK are the most frequently occurring red cell enzymopathies and guidelines/recommendations on the laboratory diagnosis have been published.[256,260] In addition, the method to measure HK activity is described, which serves as a reference enzyme to evaluate results compared to the mean RBC age.

Method Summary for Determination of Glucose-6-Phosphate Dehydrogenase

Principle

G6PD catalyzes the oxidation of glucose-6-phosphate (Glucose-6-P) to 6-phosphogluconate (6-PGA) with concurrent conversion of $NADP^+$ to NADPH. The activity of G6PD is determined by measurement of the rate of increase in NADPH concentration. Unlike $NADP^+$, NADPH strongly absorbs ultraviolet (UV) light. Therefore the rate of increase in absorbance at 340 nm is a measure of G6PD enzyme activity.

$$\text{Glucose-6-P} + NADP^+ \xrightarrow{\text{G-6-PD}} \text{6-PGA} + NADPH + H^+$$

Reference Intervals

The reference interval for G6PD in red blood cells is 6 to 11 U/g Hb. Values greater than 11 U/g Hb are often encountered in any condition associated with younger than normal RBCs (as in hemolytic anemia not due to G6PD deficiency).

Method Summary for Determination of Pyruvate Kinase Activity

Principle

Pyruvate kinase catalyzes the phosphorylation of ADP to ATP by phosphoenol pyruvate (PEP). The rate of formation of pyruvate is measured by linking the PK reaction with the lactic dehydrogenase (LDH) reaction, in which NADH is oxidized to NAD^+. Because LD is present in excess, the rate of NADH oxidation is limited by the activity of PK. The reaction rate is measured by the rate of decrease in absorbance at 340 nm.

1. $PEP + ADP \xrightarrow[Mg^{2+}, K^+]{PK} \text{Pyruvate} + ATP$

2. $\text{Pyruvate} + NADH + H^+ \xrightleftharpoons{LDH} \text{Lactate} + NAD^+$

Reference Intervals

Reference interval for pyruvate kinase enzyme activity is 6 to 12 U/gHb. Values greater than 12 U/g Hb are often encountered in any condition associated with younger than normal RBCs (as in hemolytic anemia not due to PK deficiency).

Method Summary for Determination of Hexokinase Activity

Principle

Hexokinase catalyzes the phosphoryl transfer from ATP to glucose, whereby glucose-6-phosphate and ADP are formed. The formation of glucose-6-P is measured by linking its further oxidation to 6-phosphogluconate to the reduction of $NADP^+$ through the G6PD reaction. The rate of increase in absorbance at 340 nm is a measure of HK enzyme activity:

1. $ATP + \text{glucose} \xrightarrow[Mg^{2+}]{HK} \text{Glucose-6-P} + ADP$

2. $\text{Glucose-6-P} + NADP^+ \xrightarrow{\text{G-6-9}} \text{6-Phosphogluconate} + NADPH + H^+$

Reference Intervals

Hexokinase is the red cell enzyme with the lowest enzymatic activity. Reference interval for hexokinase enzyme activity is 0.8 to 1.5 U/gHb. Because enzymatic activity is strongly dependent on red cell age, values greater than 1.5 U/g Hb are often encountered in any condition associated with younger than normal RBCs (as in hemolytic anemia not due to hexokinase deficiency).

POINTS TO REMEMBER

- Red blood cell (RBC) enzyme disorders cause a variable degree of hereditary nonspherocytic hemolytic anemia.
- Deficiencies of bisphosphoglycerate mutase and cytochrome b_5 reductase cause congenital erythrocytosis and methemoglobinemia, respectively.
- Glucose-6-phosphate dehydrogenase deficiency and pyruvate kinase deficiency are the most common red cell enzyme deficiencies.
- A number of enzyme deficiencies affect tissues other than the RBC.
- The red cell age-dependent activity of several enzymes represents an important diagnostic pitfall.

SELECTED REFERENCES

14. Kanno H. Hexokinase: Gene structure and mutations. Bailliere's best practice & research 2000;13:83–8.

34. Fermo E, Vercellati C, Marcello AP, Zaninoni A, Aytac S, Cetin M, et al. Clinical and molecular spectrum of glucose-6-phosphate isomerase deficiency. Report of 12 new cases. Front Physiol 2019;10:467.

47. Fujii H, Miwa S. Other erythrocyte enzyme deficiencies associated with non-haematological symptoms: Phosphoglycerate kinase and phosphofructokinase deficiency. Bailliere's best practice & research 2000;13:141–8.

66. Yao DC, Tolan DR, Murray MF, Harris DJ, Darras BT, Geva A, Neufeld EJ. Hemolytic anemia and severe rhabdomyolysis caused by compound heterozygous mutations of the gene for erythrocyte/muscle isozyme of aldolase, aldoa[arg303x/cys338tyr]. Blood 2004;103:2401–3.

74. Orosz F, Olah J, Ovadi J. Triosephosphate isomerase deficiency: New insights into an enigmatic disease. Biochim Biophys Acta 2009

89. Beutler E. Pgk deficiency. Br J Haematol 2007;136:3–11.

109. van Wijk R, van Solinge WW. The energy-less red blood cell is lost: Erythrocyte enzyme abnormalities of glycolysis. Blood 2005;106:4034–42.

119. Grace RF, Bianchi P, van Beers EJ, Eber SW, Glader B, Yaish HM, et al. Clinical spectrum of pyruvate kinase deficiency: Data from the pyruvate kinase deficiency natural history study. Blood 2018;131:2183–92.

146. Luzzatto L, Seneca E. G6pd deficiency: A classic example of pharmacogenetics with on-going clinical implications. British journal of haematology 2014;164:469–80.

156. Luzzatto L, Arese P. Favism and glucose-6-phosphate dehydrogenase deficiency. N Engl J Med 2018;378:60–71.

170. Petousi N, Copley RR, Lappin TR, Haggan SE, Bento CM, Cario H, et al. Erythrocytosis associated with a novel missense mutation in the bpgm gene. Haematologica 2014;99:e201–4.

174. Ristoff E. Inborn errors of gsh metabolism. In: Masella R, Mazza G, editors. Glutathione and sulfur amino acids in human health and disease: John Wiley & Sons, Inc; 2009. p. 343–62.

219. Zanella A, Bianchi P, Fermo E, Valentini G. Hereditary pyrimidine 5'-nucleotidase deficiency: From genetics to clinical manifestations. Br J Haematol 2006;133:113–23.

235. Abrusci P, Chiarelli LR, Galizzi A, Fermo E, Bianchi P, Zanella A, Valentini G. Erythrocyte adenylate kinase deficiency: Characterization of recombinant mutant forms and relationship with nonspherocytic hemolytic anemia. Exp Hematol 2007;35:1182–9.

250. Percy MJ, Lappin TR. Recessive congenital methaemoglobinaemia: Cytochrome b(5) reductase deficiency. Br J Haematol 2008; 141:298–308.

255. Bianchi P, Fermo E, Glader B, Kanno H, Agarwal A, Barcellini W, et al. Addressing the diagnostic gaps in pyruvate kinase deficiency: Consensus recommendations on the diagnosis of pyruvate kinase deficiency. American journal of hematology 2019;94:149–61.

Physiology of Hemostasis*

Russell A. Higgins, Steve Kitchen, Dong Chen, and Marco Cattaneo

ABSTRACT

Background

Hemostasis is a physiologic process involving platelets, coagulation and fibrinolysis proteins, and blood vessels that maintain blood in the fluid state under normal conditions but rapidly form a blood clot at sites of injury. Intact endothelial cells lining the blood vessels prevent activation of platelets and coagulation factors. When an injury occurs, platelets and coagulation factors form a blood clot to prevent hemorrhage. Blood clots must be limited to the site of injury to prevent intravascular clotting; therefore coagulation and platelet activation is highly regulated. This chapter sets the stage for discussions of pathophysiology and laboratory testing in subsequent chapters.

Content

This chapter describes the basic roles and interactions of platelets, coagulation factors, and blood vessels/endothelium in hemostasis. Blood vessels contract to slow down bleeding, and the subendothelial matrix provides stimuli for platelet adhesion and coagulation. Primary hemostasis refers to the platelets' response at the site of injury that results in a platelet plug. The plasma coagulation cascade is initiated by tissue factor exposed at the injury site and is propagated by a complex cascade of reactions resulting in a fibrin clot on top of the platelet plug. Fibrinolysis cleaves the fibrin clot into soluble fragments and begins the healing process. Endothelial cells participate in the regulation of hemostasis through secretion of molecules and complex interactions on the endothelial surface. Basic molecular mechanisms and cell interactions involved in the regulation of primary hemostasis, plasma coagulation, and fibrinolysis are described below.

---

*The full version of this chapter is available electronically on ExpertConsult.com.

Platelets and von Willebrand Factor

Russell A. Higgins, Steve Kitchen, and Dong Chen

ABSTRACT

Primary hemostasis is characterized by vascular contraction, platelet adhesion, and formation of a platelet thrombus. It begins immediately after endothelial disruption with platelets and von Willebrand factor (VWF) being the key components in the initiation of hemostatic process. This chapter describes the laboratory testing of platelets and VWF and provides an overview of pathologic disorders.

TEST METHODS FOR EVALUATION OF PLATELETS

Laboratory testing can assess many of the platelet activities such as adhesion, aggregation, secretion, clot retraction, and those related to plasma coagulation and damaged endothelium. In addition to functional tests, platelet morphology, ultrastructure, and quantity can be evaluated by a variety of methods.

Platelet Light Microscopy and Platelet Indices

Automated and manual platelet counting are covered in Chapter 74. Alternatively, the proportion of platelets to red blood cells on a Giemsa-Wright stained blood film can be used along with the red blood cells counted on an automated hematology analyzer to calculate the platelet count.[1,2] Besides a platelet count, an automated hematology analyzer can provide other indices such as mean platelet volume (MPV), plateletcrit (PCT), platelet distribution width (PDW), platelet large cell ratio (P-LCR), and immature platelet fraction (IPF). MPV, PDW, and IPF increase with peripheral platelet destruction because young platelets released from the bone marrow are larger and can be a helpful indication of bone marrow response. The MPV is an important laboratory variable since it can help to categorize different inherited platelet disorders (IPDs). For instance, small platelets (microcytic platelets) are characteristic of Wiskott–Aldrich syndrome (WAS)[3]; conversely, large platelets (macrocytosis) are characteristic of Bernard-Soulier syndrome (BSS)[4] and *MYH9* mutation-associated platelet diseases.[5] Under the light microscope, a platelet should be less than one-third the size of a red blood cell and contain purple cytoplasmic granules, which are alpha granules (Fig. 80.1A). An absence of these purple granules is characteristic for gray platelet syndrome (GPS) (see Fig. 80.1B). White cells should also be examined since the presence of Döhle body-like pale blue cytoplasmic inclusions in neutrophils, in conjunction with large platelets, is characteristic for May-Hegglin anomaly or other *MYH9*-mutation associated platelet disorders (see Fig. 80.1C).[5–7]

Platelet Structure by Platelet Transmission Electron Microscopy

Platelet transmission electron microscopy (PTEM) is a valuable tool for the laboratory diagnosis of various hereditary platelet disorders since it was first used to visualize fibrin-platelet clot formation in the 1950s.[8,9] PTEM employs two main methods to visualize platelet ultrastructure, whole mount (WM) TEM and thin section (TS) TEM.[10,11] WMTEM is a quick and simple way to examine platelet electron opaque inclusions and dense granules (DG), also known as delta granules, by laying platelet-rich plasma (PRP) on a TEM grid. The high calcium content in DG blocks the electron beam of TEM and creates a sharp dark shadow (Fig. 80.2).[12] WMTEM is considered the gold standard test for diagnosing DG deficiencies in Hermansky-Pudlak syndrome (HPS),[13–15] combined alpha-delta platelet storage pool deficiency,[16,17] Paris-Trousseau-Jacobsen syndrome,[18] WAS,[19] thrombocytopenia with absent radii syndrome (TAR),[20] Chediak-Higashi syndrome,[10] and other platelet DG deficiencies. TSTEM is a preferred method to visualize platelet alpha granules, other organelles, and inclusions (Fig. 80.3). Distinct and sometimes pathognomonic ultrastructural abnormalities are found in GPS with virtually absent alpha granules,[16,17] White platelet syndrome,[21] Medich giant platelet disorder,[22] X-linked GATA-1 macrothrombocytopenia,[18,23,24] and the recently described York platelet syndrome.[25,26]

Bleeding Time

To assess the platelet functions as summarized in Table 80.1, over the past century, many iterations of the bleeding time were employed.[27,28] The test is performed on the volar aspect (the surface of the arm on the same side as the palm) of the forearm. A blood pressure cuff is applied at 40 mm Hg to provide uniform intravascular pressure at the site of the incision. A small incision (1 cm long and 1 mm deep) is made using a disposable template that provides a uniform incision from test to test. The result is influenced by the direction of

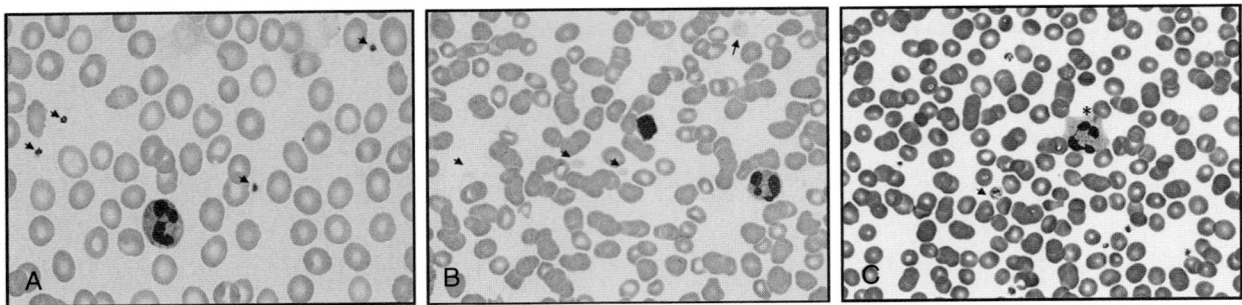

FIGURE 80.1 Platelet light microscopy. (A) Giemsa-Wright-stained peripheral blood smear shows normal platelets (*arrows*). (B) Giemsa-Wright stain of peripheral blood from a patient with gray platelet syndrome. *Arrows* point to the hypogranular platelets. (C) Giemsa-Wright stain of peripheral blood from a patient with *MYH9*-associated platelet disease. The *arrow* points to a large platelet. *Cytoplasmic inclusion in a neutrophil.

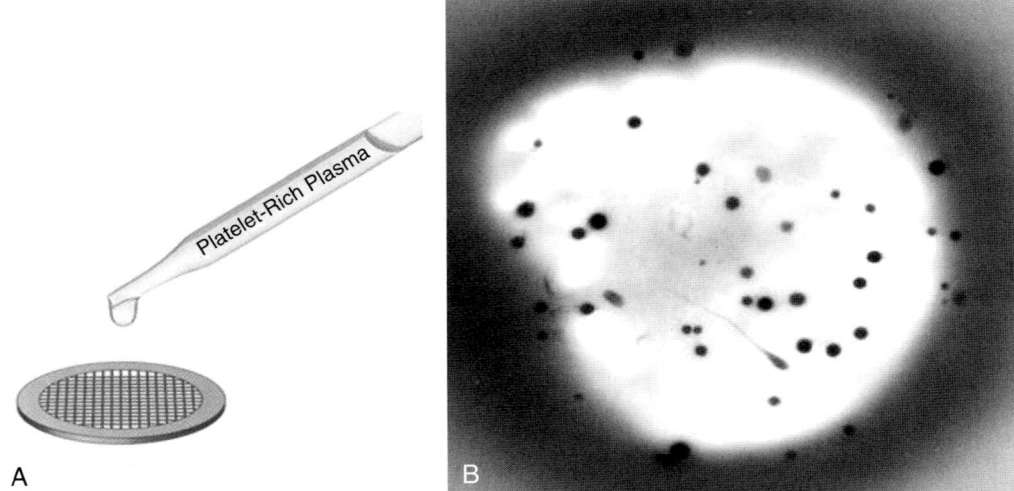

FIGURE 80.2 Platelet whole mount transmission electron microscopy. (A) Whole blood samples collected in ACD tubes are first centrifuged to prepare platelet-rich plasma, which is then dropped onto a coated copper grid. After being air-dried, the grid is then directly examined by transmission electron microscopy. (B) A micrograph of the whole mount image of a platelet. Calcium in the dense granules can block the electron beam and causes an ink-dot-like shadow. While most are round, rare dense granules have tails.

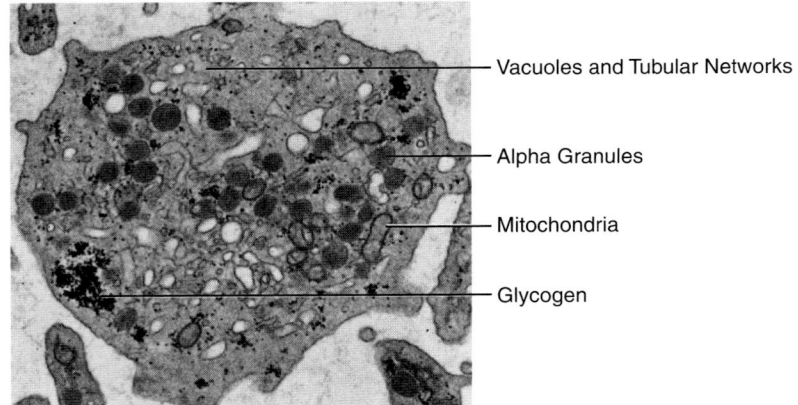

FIGURE 80.3 Ultrastructure of platelet by thin section transmission electron microscopy. Platelet size, shape, alpha-granules, canalicular systems, Golgi complex, and aberrant inclusions can be assessed.

TABLE 80.1   Summary of Platelet Functions

Function	Description
Adhesion	Upon activation, the platelet recognizes surfaces other than normal endothelium and adheres to those surfaces.
Aggregation	Upon activation, the platelet recognizes and attaches (aggregates) to other platelets.
Secretion	Upon activation, the platelet secretes the contents of the alpha granules and dense granules.
Support of plasma coagulation	At the site of injury, the platelet serves as a surface upon which macromolecular enzyme complexes form, and plasma coagulation is accelerated.
Clot retraction	Following clot formation, the filipodia of platelets attach to the fibrin strands and, through contraction, reduce clot size and express serum in vitro and juxtapose edges of the injury in vivo.
Support of damaged endothelium	Platelets adhere to damaged endothelium, fuse with the membrane, and become incorporated with the endothelial cytoplasm.

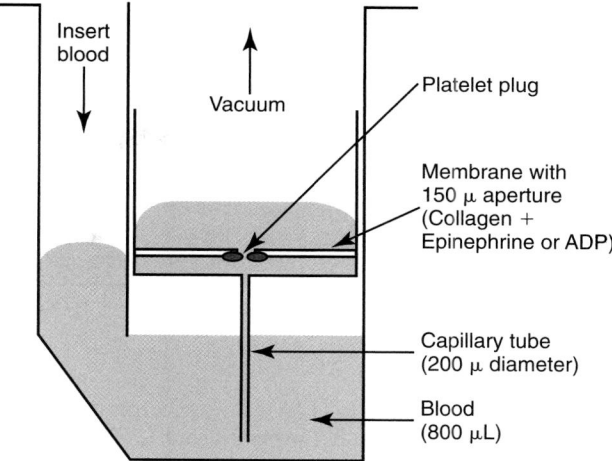

FIGURE 80.4 Schematic of the PFA-100 Analyzer. The PFA-100 analyzer provides a global measure of platelet function in a whole blood specimen. Blood anticoagulated with citrate is pipetted into the cuvette with a reaction membrane with collagen/epinephrine or collagen/adenosine diphosphate (*ADP*). Using a vacuum (syringe suction), blood is aspirated through the capillary tube at a rate sufficient to produce a wall shear rate of 1000 seconds^{-1}. Blood containing shear stress–activated platelets enters a small chamber and passes through the aperture of the membrane. At the aperture, the platelets adhere and aggregate until the aperture is closed and flow is obstructed. The time to achieve closure is referred to as *closure time.*

TABLE 80.2   Expected Results of the PFA-100 Analyzer

Condition	Collagen/Epinephrine Cartridge Closure Time	Collagen/ADP Cartridge Closure Time
Normal	Normal	Normal
Medication (aspirin effect)	Prolonged	Normal
Platelet function defect and von Willebrand disease	Prolonged	Prolonged

PFA-100, Platelet Function Analyzer, Siemens Healthcare Diagnostics, Deerfield, Ill. *ADP,* Adenosine diphosphate.

incision, with a shorter time obtained if the incision is parallel to the sides of the forearm compared with a perpendicular incision. Blood at the site of injury is gently blotted with a filter paper every 30 seconds until no blood is detectable on the paper (time required, 4 to 8 minutes). Because the test lacks sensitivity and specificity for diagnosing bleeding diatheses and exhibits high intertechnologist imprecision, it is no longer routinely used.

Platelet Function Analyzer (PFA-100 and PFA-200)

The PFA-100 analyzer (Fig. 80.4) is a global test of platelet and VWF function under high shear flow.[29,30] The analyzer utilizes whole blood specimens collected in a 3.2% buffered citrate tube (109 mmol/L trisodium citrate). When platelets pass through a small perforation in a membrane with embedded activators (collagen/epinephrine and collagen/adenosine diphosphate [ADP]), they are activated and interact with VWF. The time required for adhering and aggregating platelets to close the perforation is measured, known as the closure time. Prolonged collagen/epinephrine closure time (PFA-CEPI) and normal collagen/ADP closure time (PFA–CADP) are likely related to aspirin effect (Table 80.2).[31] Prolonged PFA–CEPI and–CADP can be seen in inherited or acquired platelet disorders and von Willebrand disease (VWD; see Table 80.2).[32] PFA-100 is not affected by coagulation factor deficiencies such as hemophilia A or B. Although PFA-100 is simple to operate, it has several limitations. The closure times can be affected by anemia or thrombocytopenia, and it is insensitive to some platelet disorders such as storage-pool deficiency[33] and the antiplatelet effect of thienopyridine drugs.[34] To overcome the latter, a new INNOVANCE PFA-200 System

(Siemens Healthcare Diagnostics, Deerfield, IL) was developed[35] and has shown promising results,[36] though its laboratory performance remains to be independently evaluated in both clinical and laboratory studies.

Platelet Aggregation Tests

The original platelet aggregation method and the first aggregometer were described by Dr. Gustav Born in 1962,[37] which laid the foundation for understanding platelet biology and clinical laboratory testing for platelet dysfunction. After this invention, various platelet aggregation tests using an array of agonists (Table 80.3) were established.[38–40] Platelet aggregation can be detected by either light transmission or electrical impedance methods. Both methods have become preferred platelet function tests. Of the two methods, light

TABLE 80.3 Commonly Used Platelet Aggregation Agonists

Collagen	Activates receptor GP VI, GPIa/IIa
ADP	Activates receptors P_2Y_1 and P_2Y_{12}
TRAP	Activates the thrombin receptors PAR_1 and PAR_4
Epinephrine	Activates the alpha 2 receptor
Arachidonic acid	Activates the cyclooxygenase pathway
Ristocetin	Activates VWF binding to GP Ib/V/IX

ADP, Adenosine diphosphate; *GP,* glycoprotein; *TRAP,* thrombin receptor activation peptide.

transmission aggregometry (LTA) is more commonly used.[41] It employs PRP and platelet-poor plasma (PPP) harvested from whole blood collected into 109 mmol/L trisodium citrate. Since the platelet count can affect results, PRP is then adjusted to approximately 250×10^9/L to assure reliable results. After adjusting the maximum light transmission by PPP, the patient's PRP is placed in the testing chamber in the light path and warmed to 37 °C with continuous stirring and continuous measurement of light transmittance. After an agonist is added, increased transmission of light is recorded over time as the platelets aggregate (see Fig. 80.5). The tracing of platelet aggregation with epinephrine or ADP usually shows two waves. Right before the first wave of aggregation, there is an initial increase of turbidity immediately after the addition of an agonist. This is caused by an initial platelet shape change. During the first wave of aggregation, platelet granule and cytoplasmic contents are released. The released ADP and thromboxane A2 (TXA2) cause further activation of platelets, which triggers the second wave of aggregation. Sometimes, the first wave of aggregation is reversible when a low dose agonist (e.g., 2μM ADP) is used, and the secondary wave does not occur. Other agonists, like collagen and arachidonic acid, do not demonstrate separate primary and secondary waves because aggregation and secretion are coinciding. The maximum percentage of aggregation is frequently used as the final result to assess platelet function. An alternative method was developed using anticoagulated whole blood. In this case, an electric probe is placed in the specimen, and an alternating current is passed through the blood. Upon activation, platelets are attracted to the electrodes. As more platelets attach to the electrodes, the flow of current is impeded and plotted over time. Although LTA remains the "gold standard" for platelet aggregation, the impedance method has several advantages, such as no preanalytical sample preparation and a smaller sample size requirement. The patterns of responses to different agonists can be used to diagnose platelet disorders (Table 80.4).

Platelet Secretion Studies

Upon initial activation, platelets secrete a wide variety of mediators into the microenvironment. These mediators are stored in the platelet dense and alpha granules, as summarized in Table 80.5. DG secretion was initially evaluated by exploiting the ability of platelets to take up radioactively labeled serotonin and then release of the label following platelet activation.[42] This serotonin release assay (SRA) is very labor-intensive and requires the use of radioisotopes. An alternative method is adenosine triphosphate (ATP) release using a lumi-aggregometer, in which luciferin and luciferase are added to the patient specimen before an agonist is added.[43] Conversion of luciferin to its product by luciferase is dependent on ATP, the only source of which is released from the platelet DG. In the conversion of luciferin to its product, photons are emitted and are detected by a fluorometer in a quantity that correlates with the ATP released. This method allows for the simultaneous assessment of aggregation and secretion in the same reaction by using either LTA or impedance aggregometry.

Platelet Support of Plasma Coagulation

Platelets contribute to the coagulation cascade by providing phospholipids, such as phosphatidylserine,[44] which is required by the coagulation factors' activation. They also secret coagulation factors V,[45] XIII,[46] VIII, and VWF[47] from alpha granules to facilitate local clot formation. Platelet support of plasma coagulation can be evaluated by measuring the amount of residual prothrombin in a serum specimen after coagulation in the test tube is complete.[48] However, this test is not routinely performed in clinical laboratories.

Platelet Contractile Function

Platelet contractile function can be evaluated by measuring clot retraction. Upon activation, platelets form filopodia, slender

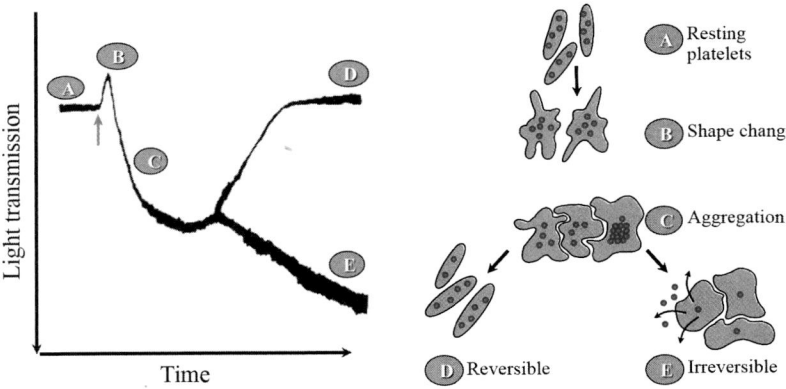

FIGURE 80.5 An exemplar tracing of a platelet aggregation study. Platelet aggregation tracing includes an initial baseline (A), a spike of increased turbidity due to platelet shape change (B), the first wave of platelet aggregation (C), and second wave of aggregation (E). Sometimes the first wave of aggregation is reversible (D), while the second wave of aggregation is usually irreversible.

TABLE 80.4 The Patterns of Responses to Different Agonists of Platelet Disorders

Normal/Disease	ARACHIDONIC		ADP		Epinephrine	COLLAGEN		Ristocetin
	Acid	U$_{46619}$	5 μM	20 μM		Low	High	
Normal	N	N	N	N	N/↓	N	N	N
Storage pool defect	N/↓	N	N	N	N/↓	N/↓	N	N
Bernard-Soulier syndrome	N	N	N	N	N	N	N	↓↓
Glanzmann thrombasthenia	↓↓	↓↓	↓↓	↓↓	↓↓	↓↓	↓↓	N/↓
P2Y12/P2Y1 defect	V	V	↓↓	↓↓	V	V	V	N/V
GPIa/IIa defect	N	N	N	N	N	↓	N/↓	N
GPVI defect	N	N	N	N	N	↓↓	N/↓	N
TXA2 synthesis defect	↓↓	N	N	N	N	N	N	N
TXA2 receptor defect	↓↓	↓↓	N	N	N	N	N	N

TABLE 80.5 Representative Contents of Alpha and Dense Granules in Platelets

Representative alpha granule contents	Adhesion proteins
	Chemokines
	Coagulation factors
	Growth factors
	Immunoglobulins
Representative dense granule contents	Amines
	Nucleotides
	Ions
	Transmitters

TABLE 80.6 Platelet Glycoproteins and Associated Diseases

Glycoprotein	Alternative Name	Disease if Deficient
GP IIb	CD41	Glanzmann thrombasthenia
GP IIIa	CD61	
GP Ib-a	CD42b	Bernard Soulier syndrome
GP IX	CD42a	
GP Ia/IIa	CD49b	Collagen receptor deficiency
GP VI	GP6	

projections from the surface of the platelets that attach to fibrin(ogen) strands via their surface receptors glycoprotein (GP) IIb/IIIa. Platelet actin tethers to membrane receptors and organizes with cytoplasmic myosin within these filipodia, forming a rudimentary muscle that contracts at the conclusion of the hemostatic process.[49] This has been described as the in vivo suture, drawing the edges of the injury closer together as healing is initiated. This clot retraction is dependent on the contractile proteins in platelets and can be qualitatively measured in a test tube.[50] Clot retraction is abnormal in Glazmann thrombasthenia and some acquired disorders, most notably with monoclonal gammopathy; nevertheless, platelet contractile function is not routinely tested in clinical laboratories.

Platelet Receptors and Function Using Flow Cytometry

Flow cytometry is a useful adjunct in evaluating platelet function in selected situations.[51] Flow cytometry can be used to evaluate the platelet surface antigen expression and activation state. Platelet surface antigens include the VWF binding receptor glycoprotein (GP) complex Ibα/β-IX-V (CD42a–d), fibrinogen receptor GPIIb/IIIa (CD41/CD61), and collagen binding receptors GPIa (CD49b) and GPVI. GP surface expressions can be measured with the use of fluorescent-conjugated GP-specific antibodies. The fluorescent intensities correlate with GP expressions. Flow cytometry can be used to measure platelet surface glycoprotein deficiencies in BSS, Glanzmann thrombasthenia (GT), and collagen receptor deficiencies (Table 80.6).

Flow cytometry can be used to evaluate platelet function by measuring activation markers upon platelet activation. The most commonly used platelet activation markers are P-selectin

(CD62P),[52] activated GPIIb/IIIa complex,[53] and lysosomal-associated membrane protein (CD63).[54] CD62P is located on the alpha granule membrane, while CD63 is on the membrane of DG and lysosomes. Both CD62P and CD63 translocate to the surface of plasma membrane after platelet activation with ensued granule release. Decreased expression of CD62P and CD63 upon platelet activation can be seen in AG or DG deficiencies, respectively. PAC-1 is a mouse monoclonal antibody that detects the neoepitope of GPIIb/IIIa conformation changes upon platelet activation. PAC-1 binding on the platelet surface is indicative of platelet activation. A lack of PAC-1 binding by activated platelets suggests GT or other platelet disorders. Currently, the flow cytometric method of platelet function testing remains largely a research tool and has not been widely used in clinical laboratories.[55]

Molecular Genetic Testing

Genotyping has a confirmatory role in the diagnosis of IPD. Molecular genetic analysis by Sanger sequencing was first employed in the early 1990s to identify the causal mutations in the genes coding for GPIIb/IIIa[56] and GPIbα/β−IX-V[57] in GT and BSS, respectively. With the advent of next-generation sequencing (NGS), several novel platelet disorder-associated gene mutations have been identified, for example, *NBEAL2*, *GFI1B* and *VPS33b* for GPS, *ACTN1* for autosomal dominant thrombocytopenia, *RBM8A* for thrombocytopenia absent radii, *STIM1* for York platelet syndrome, and *ANKRD26*, *ETV6*, *GATA-1*, *GATA-2* and *RUNX1* for thrombocytopenia with a predisposition to hematologic malignancy. For further discussion on these molecular techniques, refer to Chapter 64. Although NGS-based approaches may potentially revolutionize the diagnosis of IPD, preliminary clinical and laboratory phenotypic characterization remain crucial and indispensable.[58] Due to the growing list of heritable thrombocytopenias and their disease associations, a new, evolving classification has been proposed.[59,60]

AT A GLANCE

Molecular Classification of Hereditary Platelet Disorders

- Inherited platelet disorders affecting only platelets
  Examples: Glanzmann thrombasthenia, Bernard-Soulier disease, Gray platelet syndrome
- Inherited platelet disorders with a syndromic phenotype
  Examples: *MYH9*—*MYH9* mutation-related disorders, *STIM1*—New York Platelet syndrome, *RBM8A*—thrombocytopenia with absent radii
- Inherited platelet disorders associated with increased risk of hematologic malignancies
  Examples: ANKRD26, ETV6, RUNX1, GATA-1, GATA-2

Evaluation of Antiplatelet Medication

Antiplatelet medications are commonly used in patients with cardiovascular conditions (see Table 80.7). Evaluation of the effects of antiplatelet medication has two main clinical indications. First, it is crucial to know whether the medication is effectively inhibiting the platelet functions as intended for the patient to receive the desired reduced risk of thrombosis. Second, many patients who are taking antiplatelet medications need emergency or elective procedures and may be at increased risk for hemorrhage during those procedures. Increased risk of hemorrhage in patients taking antiplatelet medications has been demonstrated but is widely variable among patients. Unfortunately, whether laboratory tests of the medication effects on platelet function indeed can accurately predict hemorrhagic or thrombotic outcome is still controversial.[61–66] Several techniques are used to measure the effects that medications have on platelet function. They include the PFA-100 and -200 analyzers, Verify-Now, PlateletWorks, Multiplate, Thromboelastography (TEG), Platelet Mapping, and platelet aggregation assays.

TABLE 80.7   Examples of Medications Affecting Platelet Function

Class of Medication	Examples
Nonsteroidal anti-inflamatory	Aspirin, naproxen, ibuprofen, indomethacin
GP IIb/IIIa antagonists (antibodies)	Abciximab, eptifibatide, tirofiban
Thienopyridines	Clopidogrel, ticlopidine
Increase cAMP and/or cGMP	Iloprost, dipyridamole, prostacyclin
Cardiovascular medications	Many
Volume expanders	Dextran, hydroxyethyl starch
Chemotherapeutic agents	Mitomycin, daunorubicin, carmustine
Psychotropic medications	Many
Others	Antihistamines, clofibrate, rad contrast agents

cAMP, Adenosine 3′,5′-cyclic monophosphate; *cGMP*, guanosine 3,5-cyclic monophosphate; *GP*, glycoprotein.

Since some of these tests are still being clinically validated and are beyond the general scope of this chapter, only selected methods are discussed.

Platelet Aggregation

The "gold standard" for medication effect on platelet function is platelet aggregation using LTA or impedance with the appropriate agonist for the medication (ADP for the thienopyridines; arachidonic acid or collagen for aspirin). Other methods can be compared against this reference method.[67] Both LTA and impedance assays are labor-intensive and infeasible for urgent or routine testing.

PFA-100

The PFA-100 was described earlier in the chapter. The prolongation of epinephrine cartridge closure time is indicative of aspirin effect. It can be used to assess the antiplatelet effect of aspirin. PFA-100 CADP is insensitive for thienopyridine drugs, which could be overcome by the new PFA-200 method. Both cartridges are very sensitive in detecting GP IIb/IIIa antagonists such as abciximab, eptifibatide, and tirofiban.[35,68]

Verify-Now

Verify-Now (Accumetrics, San Diego, CA) is a rapid turbidimetric assay that exploits the affinity of activated platelets for fibrinogen. A tube of the patient's whole blood, containing 109 mmol/L trisodium citrate as an anticoagulant, is inserted into a disposable cartridge on the instrument. The blood is drawn from the citrate tube into cartridge chambers containing a platelet agonist and fibrinogen-coated microparticles. Chambers contain different agonists, including thrombin receptor activation peptide (TRAP), as a control agonist for the capacity of platelet function, and ADP or arachidonic acid, depending on the cartridge type, to assess medication effect. "Aggregation" of the fibrinogen-coated beads by platelets in the chambers is measured, and the effect of antiplatelet medication is reported in arbitrary units, such as aspirin reactivity units (ARU) or platelet reactivity units (PRU).[69–71] Separate cartridges have been used to assess aspirin or thienopyridine (e.g., clopidogrel). The clinical efficacy of using Verify-Now to guide the dosing of antiplatelet therapy is still controversial in the literature, though it offers an option to assess platelet function in the corresponding patient population.[72]

CLINICAL APPLICATION OF TESTS FOR PLATELET DISORDERS

The assays and devices discussed earlier are used to detect both inherited and acquired platelet disorders.

Inherited Platelet Disorders

Although there have been no large population studies, the prevalence of hereditary platelet disorders is estimated to be close to 0.1–1%.[73,74] These disorders can be roughly classified into four categories: (1) platelet generation deficiency, which can cause congenital thrombocytopenia, (2) surface receptor deficiency, (3) signal transduction deficiency, and (4) storage-pool deficiency. This is a simplified categorization of the growing list of IPDs. Some of the diseases may have a combination of any of the four defects. Examples of IPDs are summarized in Table 80.8.

TABLE 80.8 Examples of Platelet Disorders

	Inheri-tance	Platelet Count	Peripheral Blood Smear	Platelet Aggregation	Platelet ATP Secretion	Flow Cytometry	Diagnostic EM Features	Gene Mutation
Congenital Thrombocytopenias								
Wiskott-Aldrich syndrome	XR	Mod. to severe ↓	Small platelets	AA ↓/NL ADP NL Epi ↓/NL Col NL Risto NL	↓	↓CD63 upon stimulation	Dense granule deficiency	WAS
MYH9-related disorders	AD	Mild to mod. ↓	Large platelets, leukocyte inclusions	NL	NL	NL	Inclusions in white cells	MYH9
Congenital amegakaryocytic thrombocytopenia	AR	Severe ↓	Rare to absent platelets	NA	NA	↓c-Mpl expression	NL	MPL
X-linked thrombocytopenia with dyserythropoiesis	XR	Mod. ↓	Small platelets	NA	NA	NL	Decreased dense granules	GATA-1
Surface Receptor Defects								
Glanzmann thrombasthenia	AR	NL or mild to mod. ↓	Normal platelets	AA ↓ ADP ↓ Epi ↓ Col ↓ Risto NL	NL	Absent GPIIb, GPIIIa	NL	ITGA2B, ITGB3
Bernard-Soulier syndrome	AR	Mod. to severe ↓	Giant platelets	AA NL ADP NL Epi NL Col NL Risto ↓	NL	Absent GPIbα, GPIbβ, GPIX	Giant platelets	GP1BA GP1BB GP9
Collagen receptor GPVI deficiency	AR	Mild ↓ or NL	NL	AA NL ADP NL Epi NL Col ↓ Risto NL	↓/NL	↓GPVI	NL	GP6
ADP receptor defect	AR	NL	NL	AA ↓2nd W ADP ↓ Epi ↓2nd W Col NL Risto NL	↓/NL	NL	NL	P2RY12
Thromboxane A2 receptor deficiency	AR	NL	NL	AA ↓ or delayed ADP NL Epi ↓2nd W Col NL Risto NL U46619 ↓	↓/NL	NL	NL	TBXA2R
Storage Pool Disorders								
Gray platelet syndrome	AD or AR	Mild ↓	Large and pale platelets	AA NL ADP NL Epi NL Col NL Risto NL	NL	↓P-selectin upon sTRAP, ADP or convulxin stimulation	Lack alpha granules	NBEAL2

Continued

TABLE 80.8 **Examples of Platelet Disorders—cont'd**

	Inheritance	Platelet Count	Peripheral Blood Smear	Platelet Aggregation	Platelet ATP Secretion	Flow Cytometry	Diagnostic EM Features	Gene Mutation
Paris-Trousseau Jacobsen syndrome	AD	Mod. to severe ↓	NL or large platelets	AA NL ADP NL Epi NL Col NL Risto NL	↓	N/A	Dense granule deficiency Giant α-granules	Del11q23 (*FLI1*)
Hermansky-Pudlak syndrome	AR	NL	NL	AA ↓/NL ADP NL Epi ↓2nd W Col NL Risto NL	↓	↓ CD63 after stimulation	Absent platelet dense body by whole mount	*HPS1-7* *AP3B1,* *AP3D1* *DTNBP1,* *BLOC1S3,* *BLOC1S6* *PLDN*
Chediak-Higashi syndrome	AR	NL	Leukocyte inclusions	AA ↓/NL ADP ↓ Epi ↓ 2ndW Col NL Risto NL	↓	↓CD63 upon stimulation	Leukocyte lysosomal inclusions Decreased platelet dense granule deficiency	*LYST*
Combined αδ granule deficiency	AR/AD	NL	NL	AA NL/↓ ADP NL/↓ Epi NL/↓ Col NL/↓ Risto NL/↓	↓	↓P-selectin ↓CD63 upon stimulation	Platelet alpha and dense granule deficiency	*GFI1B*
Signal Transduction Defects								
G-protein activation defect	AD	NL	NL	AA NL/↓ ADP ↓ Epi ↓ Col ↓ Risto NL/↓	↓/NL	↓ activation with PAC-1	NL	*GNAS*
Thromboxane synthase deficiency	AD	NL	NL	AA absent ADP NL Epi ↓ Col ↓/NL Risto NL	↓/NL	NL	NL	*TBXAS1*
Cyclooxygenase deficiency	AD	NL	NL	AA absent ADP NL Epi ↓ Col ↓/NL Risto NL	↓/NL	NL	NL	*PTGS1*
Calcium mobilization defects	unknown	NL	NL	AA NL ADP NL Epi ↓ Col NL Risto NL	↓	↓ CD63 after stimulation	NL	*STIM1*

↓, Decrease; *AA*, arachidonic acid; *Col*, collagen; *Epi*, epinephrine; *Mod.*, moderate; *NL*, normal; *Risto*, ristocetin

Congenital Thrombocytopenia

Congenital thrombocytopenia is frequently an incidental finding. Depending on the platelet count and other comorbidities, the patient may have various bleeding diatheses. A group of diseases have large platelets and are thus called macrothrombocytopenia. The advent of NGS has uncovered many genetic abnormalities behind these disorders.[75] Platelet function analysis may be normal or abnormal. However, platelet function testing is frequently hindered by thrombocytopenia. Therefore PTEM and flow cytometry tests could be useful in this setting.

AT A GLANCE
Inherited Platelet Disorders

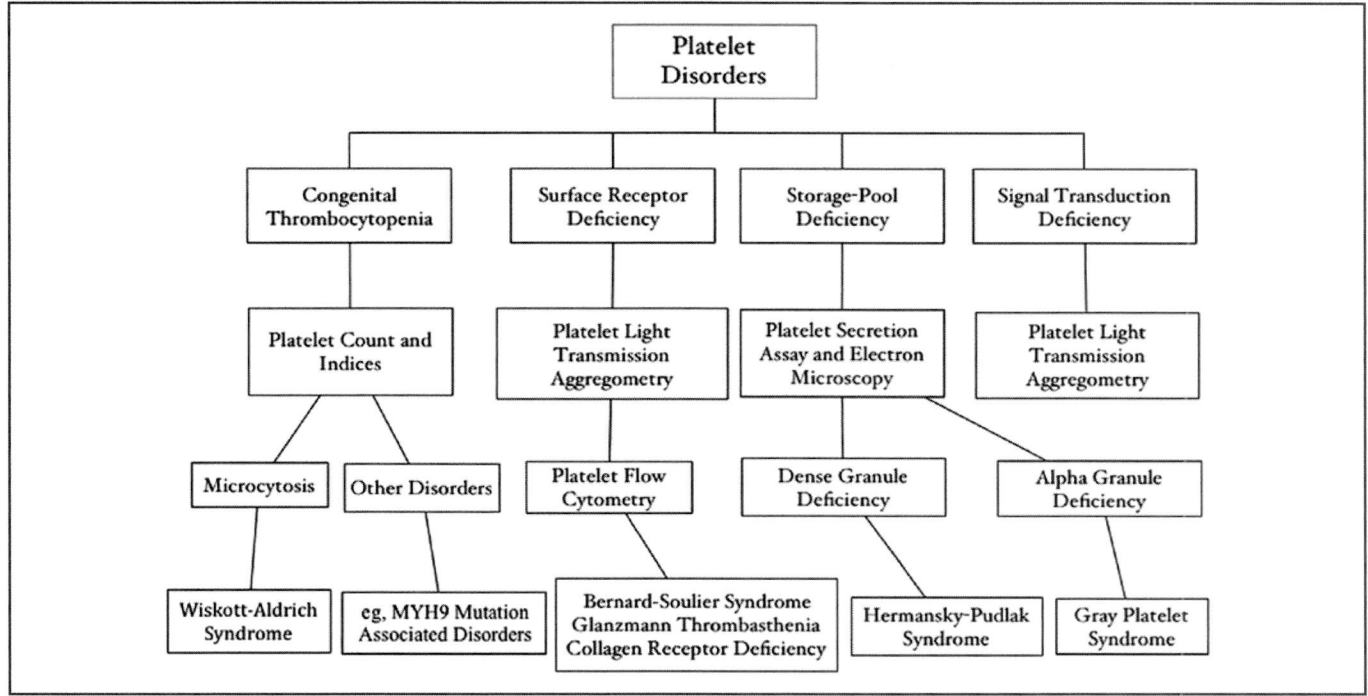

Surface Receptor Deficiency

Prototypical surface protein deficiencies are BSS and Glanzmann thrombasthenia.

Bernard-Soulier syndrome (BSS) is a disorder of platelet function that is caused by the defect of VWF receptor (GP Ib/V/IX) with a prevalence of less than 1:1,000,000 in the general population.[76,77] It is one of the giant platelet syndromes with concurrent thrombocytopenia and is associated with moderate to severe bleeding. Mutations have been reported in the genes coding for GPIb alpha (gene symbol *GP1BA*) and GPIX (*GP9*), but not GPV (*GP5*). BSS is inherited as mainly an autosomal recessive trait with bleeding seen only in homozygotes, and it is seen most frequently in consanguineous relations. However, there are autosomal dominant variants due to distinct mutations of *GP1BA*.[78,79] Platelet macrocytosis and a distinct platelet aggregation pattern of absent or markedly decreased ristocetin-induced platelet aggregation (RIPA; see Table 80.4) usually are sufficient to render the diagnosis. BSS can be further verified by either platelet GPIb and IX assessment by flow cytometry or genetic testing.

Glanzmann thrombasthenia (GT) is caused by the absence or abnormality of the platelet integrin, GP IIb/IIIa, the receptor for fibrinogen in aggregation.[80] Mutations (deletions or other mutations) in the genes for GP IIb or GP IIIa membrane proteins have been identified.[81] The disorder is inherited as an autosomal recessive trait that leads to a mild to moderate bleeding diathesis. It is a rare disorder, affecting approximately 1:1,000,000 in the general population; however, it is more prevalent in populations with consanguineous relations. The platelet count is normal; however, platelet aggregation with all agonists except ristocetin is abnormal (see Table 80.4). In addition, the bleeding time is prolonged,

the PFA-100 value is prolonged, and clot retraction is abnormal. The diagnosis can be further confirmed by either assessment of GP IIb and IIIa by flow cytometry or genetic testing.

Collagen receptor deficiencies are caused by defective collagen receptors on the surface of platelets, GPIa, or GPVI. Patients with severe collagen receptor deficiencies usually present with a lifelong bleeding diathesis and an absence of platelet aggregation response to collagen. GPIa is the minor platelet collagen receptor, and its expression levels can vary with different genetic variants of the α2 subunit gene *ITGA2*.[82] GPVI is the primary platelet collagen receptor, and its deficiency is frequently associated with decreased collagen-induced platelet aggregation.[83]

Signal Transduction Deficiency

Signal transduction deficiency most commonly includes protein Gi signal pathway defects caused by either ADP or epinephrine receptor deficiencies or defects in their signal transduction.[84] In rare cases, platelet signal transduction of the TXA2 pathway is defective.[85] When platelet aggregation studies are performed, the pattern is similar to those of patients who are taking aspirin. The arachidonate induced platelet aggregation is abolished, and there is no epinephrine induced secondary wave of platelet aggregation. The potential defects include arachidonate-release enzyme deficiency, prostaglandin synthase (also known as cyclooxygenase 1, COX1) deficiency, TXA2 synthase deficiency, or TXA2 receptor deficiency. These patients frequently also have decreased serum and urine thromboxane B2, a metabolite of TXA2.

Storage-Pool Deficiency

Platelet storage-pool deficiencies are caused by abnormal dense or alpha granules. The prototypic disease of DG deficiency is

HPS.[13,86] Patients with HPS usually have virtually no DG in platelets. Mild DG deficiency exists; however, their diagnosis is hindered by a lack of reference interval of DG.[14] DG deficiency can be detected by abnormal platelet serotonin or ATP release test or WMPTEM. GPS is caused by severe alpha granule deficiency.[16,17] It can be easily detected by peripheral blood film review (see Fig. 80.1B) since the platelets appear gray due to a lack of purple granules. GPS can be definitively diagnosed by TSPTEM. Neither PFA-100[33] nor platelet aggregation testing has sufficient sensitivity for detecting storage-pool deficiencies. Therefore if a platelet defect is suspected, and routine platelet testing is normal, PTEM or serotonin/ATP secretion tests should be considered.

Acquired Platelet Disorders

Acquired platelet disorders are the more common IPD. Potential contributing factors include medications, renal failure, paraproteinemia, and primary bone marrow disorders.

Medication Effects

Many medications affect platelet function. Drugs such as aspirin, thienopyridines, and monoclonal inhibitors of GP IIb/IIIa are explicitly used to reduce platelet function and consequently prevent thrombosis, particularly arterial thrombosis. In other cases, the effects on platelet function are adverse complications of the medication. These effects generally are not enough to lead to a bleeding complication; however, if the medication is used in patients with inherited or acquired platelet disorders or other disorders of hemostasis, the effect may increase bleeding. Examples of medications that affect platelet function are listed in Table 80.7.

Renal Failure

In patients with renal failure, platelet functions tend to be inhibited at urea nitrogen of 60 mg/dL (21 mmol/L) or greater and creatinine of 3 to 4 mg/dL (265–354 μmol/L) or greater.[87–89] In vitro studies have confirmed the deleterious effects of organic acids and the rapid rate at which normal platelets demonstrate loss of function.[90,91] For this reason, the use of platelet transfusion in managing bleeding in uremic patients is ineffective. Management is difficult; however, treatment with dialysis to reduce retained acids is often effective. In addition, the use of DDAVP (Desmopressin) to increase the platelet adhesion protein VWF has proven effective in some patients.[92]

Paraproteinemia

Patients with multiple myeloma or Waldenström macroglobulinemia often have remarkably increased concentrations of immunoglobulins, which can interfere with platelet functions by masking the surface receptors.[93] Similar acquired platelet dysfunction is also observed in other lymphomas.[94] Besides possible secondary thrombocytopenia, patients may have prolonged PFA-100 closure times and abnormal results of platelet aggregation studies. These problems are managed by treating the underlying disease. In acute situations, plasmapheresis is effective in reducing paraprotein concentrations, but only for short-term management.

Primary Bone Marrow Disorders

Production and function of platelets can be affected in various myeloid neoplasms or acquired bone marrow disorders.

These effects may include, but are not limited to, increased or decreased platelet counts, reduced granules, reduced or abnormal membrane receptors, adsorption of high-molecular-weight VWF multimers causing an acquired type 2 VWD syndrome in patients with marked thrombocytosis (see von Willebrand Disease and Acquired von Willebrand Syndrome section below),[95] or abnormal signal transduction mechanisms. As a result of these variable effects, patients may manifest abnormal bleeding, or paradoxically, thrombosis. Bleeding episodes may be managed with platelet transfusion; patients at thrombotic risk may benefit from antiplatelet medication.

POINTS TO REMEMBER

Platelet Disorders

- Platelets and von Willebrand factor have essential roles in primary hemostasis.
- Platelet laboratory testing includes platelet count, indices, platelet function tests, platelet flow cytometry, platelet transmission electron microscopy, and genotyping studies.
- Platelet disorders can be congenital or acquired.
- Inherited platelet disorders can be divided into (1) platelet generation disorders, (2) surface receptor deficiency, (3) signal transduction deficiency, and (4) storage-pool deficiency
- Acquired platelet disorders include medication effect, renal failure, paraproteinemia, and primary bone marrow disorders (e.g., myeloproliferative disorders)

TEST METHODS FOR EVALUATION OF VON WILLEBRAND FACTOR

VWF plays an essential role in platelet adhesion to collagen at the site of injury. In addition to the adhesion function, VWF is the carrier of factor VIII in circulation, protecting it from early clearance. Various assays have been designed to diagnose, characterize, and monitor VWD. VWF antigen assays measure the quantity of VWF. Methods assessing VWF functional activity include RIPA, VWF–ristocetin cofactor activity, VWF–collagen binding activity, VWF-glycoprotein Ib binding (immunoactivity) activity, and von Willebrand factor-factor VIII binding activity. All functional assays are most sensitive to loss of high-molecular-weight VWF multimers, which contain the most functional epitopes. The VWF multimer assay allows visualization of multimers and confirms the presence or absence of high-molecular-weight VWF multimers.

Ristocetin-induced Platelet Aggregation Assay

Ristocetin is an antibiotic that was initially derived from the cultures of *Norcardia lurida*. It was found to cause in vivo and in vitro aggregation of platelets by inducing a conformational change in VWF and allowing binding to the platelet receptor. RIPA is mediated by VWF. When aggregation is induced by ristocetin in the patient's PRP, the test will reflect both the activity of VWF in the plasma and function of the receptor for VWF in the platelet membrane (GP Ib-V-IX complex).[96] The methods used to detect aggregation of the platelets are the same as those described in the section on platelet aggregation (see earlier section). Testing is done at a high concentration of ristocetin to detect VWF ristocetin cofactor (VWF:RCo) activity, and at low concentration to detect abnormally increased affinity of VWF:RCo for its receptor on the platelet. Notably, RIPA differs from the other VWF activity methodologies below in that it incorporates the patient's platelets; consequently, increased VWF-platelet binding activity can be detected when abnormal VWF (e.g., type 2B VWD) is absorbed onto the platelet surface. The tests below use PPP rather than PRP.

von Willebrand Factor–Ristocetin Cofactor Assay (VWF:RCo)

The most common of the assays for VWF activity, VWF:RCo, exploits the binding of VWF to platelets in the presence of ristocetin.[97] Platelets are prepared free of VWF using gel filtration or washing. Platelets are used fresh for the assay or, as is done for commercial assays, are lyophilized for longer storage. Platelets are used in an agglutination reaction with ristocetin as the agonist. The specimen used is PPP harvested from whole blood anticoagulated with 109 mmol/L trisodium citrate. Using dilutions of normal pooled plasma, a calibration curve is developed based on the rate or extent of agglutination. The rate or extent of agglutination of the patient's specimen is then compared with the calibration curve, and the value is extrapolated. This original method for determining the activity of VWF is very labor intense, but despite difficulty with imprecision, it remains the gold standard for the development and validation of other methods.

von Willebrand Factor GPIb Binding Assays (VWF:Ab, VWF:GPIbR, VWF:GPIbM)

The VWF:RCo is the gold standard for measuring the ability of VWF to bind platelets, but it is laborious, and other types of assays for the evaluation of VWF-platelet binding have emerged. Three types of methods assess the ability of the VWF molecule to bind the platelet receptor, GPIb, without the use of platelets.[98] The first method (VWF:Ab) takes advantage of monoclonal antibodies to platelet binding functional GPIb-binding epitopes in the VWF (e.g., GPIb-binding site). An automated homogeneous immunoturbidimetric assay with antibody-coated latex beads shows a direct correlation between the degree of agglutination and VWF activity in the plasma.[99] The second type of method (VWF:GPIbR) has similarities to the ristocetin cofactor assay, using ristocetin to expose GPIb binding sites in VWF. Rather than platelet agglutination, as occurs in the ristocetin cofactor assay, recombinant GPIb fragments are captured onto a solid surface by monoclonal antibodies, and then VWF from test plasma recognizes the GPIb in the presence of ristocetin. Both automated latex particle and solid-phase capture methods have been described. In the third type of method (VWF:GPIbM), GPIb with a gain-of-function mutations can bind VWF without the addition of ristocetin.[100] The mutant GPIb fragments are captured onto a solid surface, and then VWF from test plasma binds spontaneously (without ristocetin). Both solid phase capture and automated latex methods have been developed. VWF:Ab, VWF:GPIbR, and VWF:GPIbM methods have been automated on coagulation analyzers, and most demonstrate improved performance characteristics, especially at activity values lower than 30 U/dL, compared to VWF:RCo by aggregometry.[101] Automated methods described correlate well with VWF:RCo by aggregometry for diagnosis and subclassification of VWD; however, all studies demonstrate examples of discrepancies. Therefore more than one type of VWF activity assays may be necessary to diagnose or subclassify VWD.

POINTS TO REMEMBER

VWF Platelet/GPIb Binding Activity

- VWF:RCo by aggregometry is the "gold standard" activity assay.
- VWF:RCo measures agglutination/aggregation of **platelets** in the presence of patient VWF.
- Alternative methods VWF:Ab, VWF:GPIbR, and VWF:GPIbM do not require platelets.
- VWF:Ab measures agglutination of latex beads coated with a monoclonal antibody against the GPIb-binding domain of VWF and **does not require ristocetin**.
- VWF:GPIbR measures the binding of patient VWF to recombinant GPIb in the presence of ristocetin.
- VWF:GPIbM measures the binding of patient VWF to mutated, gain-of-function GPIb, and **does not require ristocetin**.

---

von Willebrand Factor–Collagen-Binding Assay (VWF:CB)

The binding of VWF to the collagen matrix initiates the process of platelet adhesion and the hemostatic process. This VWF activity can be quantified using the collagen-binding function (VWF:CB).[102] The specimen used is PPP harvested from whole blood containing 109 mmol/L trisodium citrate as an anticoagulant. The methods available are primarily enzyme-linked immunosorbent assay (ELISA)-type assays in which VWF binds to stationary phase collagen (collagen types I and III—alone or in combination—derived from human, equine, or bovine tendon), followed by quantification of the bound VWF. The concentration of VWF:CB tends to parallel that of VWF:RCo in most settings. Some assays of VWF:CB are more sensitive to high-molecular-weight VWF multimers and may detect type 2 VWD (see later) more readily.

von Willebrand Factor-Factor VIII Binding Activity

The VWF-factor VIII binding activity evaluates the factor VIII binding domains of VWF rather than the platelet or collagen binding domains.[103] The VWF-factor VIII binding assay is an ELISA method that uses monoclonal anti-VWF to capture patient VWF onto the solid surface, followed by exposure of the patient's captured VWF to recombinant factor VIII. Separate determinations of VWF quantitation and VWF bound-factor VIII activity are made by a VWF detection antibody and chromogenic factor VIII, respectively. The results are expressed as a ratio of factor VIII activity to VWF.

von Willebrand Factor Antigen Assays (VWF:Ag)

The original assay for VWF:Ag was the immunoelectrophoretic method of Laurell (referred to as the Laurell rocket assay).[104] With this method, polyclonal monospecific antibody to VWF is uniformly distributed in a porous agarose gel. Controls and patient specimens are electrophoresed into the gel, and the distance of a precipitin "rocket" from the sample well is proportional to the quantity of VWF protein. This method is labor-intensive and time-consuming and has been replaced by classic ELISA assays. To simplify the assay and allow for easier automation, popular microparticle agglutination assays were developed and are most commonly used. Monoclonal antibody to VWF is coated on microparticles (latex immunoassay [LIA]). VWF directly agglutinates the microparticles with the endpoint measured by turbidometric or nephelometric methods. The specimen used is PPP harvested from whole blood anticoagulated with 109 mmol/L trisodium citrate. An acceptable correlation of the classic ELISA with the LIA has been noted. Although LIA assays may give higher results than the ELISA, a good agreement among results is currently obtained with different methods in proficiency testing exercises.[105]

von Willebrand Factor Multimer Analysis

In megakaryocytes and endothelial cells, the *VWF* gene codes for a subunit protein of approximately 220 kDa. Postribosomally, carbohydrate is added to the subunit, dimers of the subunits are formed, and the dimers undergo polymerization. The VWF secreted is a population of multimeric molecules varying in size from 500 kDa to as large as 20,000 kDa or more. The size of these VWF multimers is controlled in the plasma by a metalloprotease, ADAMTS13 (see later), the size of the multimers being related to the function of the molecule. VWF multimers are qualitatively detected in the plasma using electrophoresis in a porous gel, followed by visualization with a radiolabeled or enzymatically labeled antibody to VWF.[106,107] Analysis of the multimer patterns is subjective. The specimen used is PPP harvested from whole blood containing 109 mmol/L trisodium citrate as an anticoagulant. Loss of the high-molecular-weight multimers (HMWM) is associated with a reduced function (type 2A or 2B VWD), as described later (see Fig. 80.6).

Genetic Testing for von Willebrand Disease

Genetic testing at this moment is not required for the laboratory diagnosis of VWD. Approximately 50% of type I VWD patients may not have identifiable mutations. Mutations are highly relevant in types 2 and 3 VWD.[108] Genetic testing

for VWD is usually not required, but it may be helpful to confirm a VWD diagnosis or differentiate the various types of VWD.

CLINICAL APPLICATION OF TESTS FOR VON WILLEBRAND DISEASE AND ACQUIRED VON WILLEBRAND SYNDROME

VWD is an autosomal inherited bleeding diathesis, caused by the deficiency of VWF, which participates in the initial hemostasis by interacting with platelets. The prevalence of VWD is about 1% of the general population, but only approximately 1/10th of individuals are clinically symptomatic.[109–111] Acquired von Willebrand syndrome (AVWS) is caused by abnormal VWF secondary to various medical conditions.[112] Etiologies of AVWS include immunologic disorders with monoclonal proteins, severe hypothyroidism, cardiovascular abnormalities associated with nonlamellar flow, myeloproliferative disorders with a high platelet count, and some neoplasms associated with absorption of VWF (e.g., Wilms tumor).[112] Accurate diagnosis and classification of VWD and AVWS rely on a correlation between clinical observation and laboratory testing results.

VWD is classified as a quantitative or qualitative deficiency of plasma VWF, often accompanied by secondary deficiency of coagulation factor VIII activity (FVIII:C). There are three major types of VWD[113,114] as illustrated in Table 80.9. Type 1 VWD, the most common type, reflects a quantitative deficiency of normally functioning VWF. Type 3 VWD, a recessively inherited rare disorder, denotes a virtual absence of VWF. Type 2 VWD represents qualitative VWF abnormalities that are categorized into four variant groups. Type 2A VWD is characterized by the absence of the most hemostatically-effective VWF HMWM, due either to defective multimer assembly or to accelerated proteolysis. Type 2B VWD is caused by secondary clearance of the HMWM due to their abnormally high binding affinity to the platelet surface

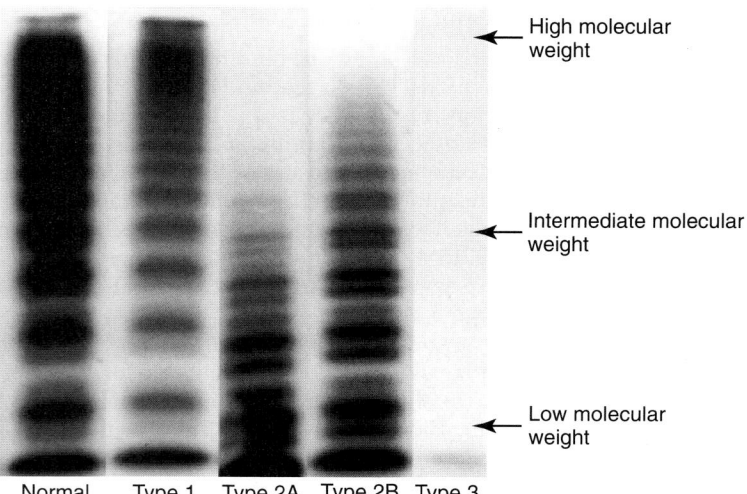

FIGURE 80.6 Multimeric analysis of VWF-Ag. Plasma is electrophoresed into a porous gel of agarose or agarose and acrylamide, the multimers are separated, and the VWF:Ag multimers are radiolabeled with antibody to VWF:Ag. Typical patterns of normal and VWD types 1, 2A, 2B, and 3 are shown in the autoradiograph. The pattern seen in type 2M is like that of type 1.

TABLE 80.9   Classification and Laboratory Features of von Willebrand Diseases

	Normal	VWD VARIANTS					
		1	2A	2B	2M	2N	3
Prevalence in VWD (%)		70–80	10–15	5	<1	<1	<1
Screening Tests							
Platelet count	NL	NL	NL	NL or ↓	NL	NL	NL
FVIII:C	NL	NL or ↓	NL or ↓	NL or ↓	NL	↓↓	↓↓↓
VWF:Ag	NL	↓ or ↓↓	NL or ↓/↓↓	NL or ↓/↓↓	NL or ↓/↓↓	NL or ↓	Absent
VWF:RCo or other tests	NL	↓ or ↓↓	↓/↓↓	NL or ↓/↓↓	NL or ↓/↓↓	NL or ↓	Absent
VWF:RCo/VWF:Ag	>0.5–0.7	>0.5–0.7	<0.5–0.7	<0.5–0.7	<0.5–0.7	>0.5–0.7	NA
VWF:CB/VWF:Ag	>0.5–0.7	>0.5–0.7	<0.5–0.7	<0.5–0.7	<0.5–0.7[a]	>0.5–0.7	NA
Supplemental Tests							
VWF multimer analysis patterns	Normal multimer distribution	Normal multimer distribution	Decreased HMWM Abnormal satellite bands	Decreased HMWM Abnormal satellite bands	Normal (ultra large and/or smeary multimers in some variants)	Normal multimer distribution	Absent
RIPA (low-dose ristocetin)	NL	NL	NL	↑	NL	NL	NL
VWF:FVIIIB	NL	NL	NL	NL	NL	↓↓↓	Absent

[a]May be insensitive in certain assays.
↓, Decrease; ↑, increase; *Ag*, antigen; *CB*, collagen binding activity; *FVIII:C*, factor VIII activity; *HMWM*, high-molecular-weight multimers; *NL*, normal; *RCo*, ristocetin cofactor activity; *VWD*, von Willebrand disease; *VWF*, von Willebrand factor.

glycoprotein GP Ib-V-IX. Type 2M (with M representing multimer) VWD exhibits decreased VWF platelet-binding activity without substantive deficiency of VWF HMWM. It is important to be aware that *VWF* exon 28 single nucleotide polymorphisms (SNPs), I1380V, N1435S, and D1472H, are associated with a significantly lower VWF:RCo/VWF:Ag ratio, which should not be misdiagnosed as type 2M VWD.[115] Finally, type 2N (Normandy) VWD has a laboratory phenotype of plasma FVIII deficiency that is secondary to defective VWF binding of FVIII.

AVWS may be under-recognized and could be suspected in adults without a history of life-long or family history of bleeding; however, AVWS also occurs in the pediatric setting, particularly with congenital heart defects that cause turbulent blood flow. AVWS has several mechanisms and associated disease processes. Patients with lymphoproliferative disorders and monoclonal proteins (e.g., multiple myeloma or monoclonal gammopathy of undetermined significance) or autoimmune disease may produce antibodies that recognize VWF.[116,117] Increased turbulent blood flow associated with congenital heart defects, such as aortic stenosis or ventricular septal defects, can cause AVWS. In adults, aortic stenosis and, especially, ventricular assist devices are associated with AWVS and bleeding. The shear stress causes VWF to unfold from its globular tertiary structure, exposing sites for proteolysis into smaller multimer forms.[108] Patients with myeloproliferative disorders may develop AVWS, which may be due to the adsorption of VWF HMWM onto the surface of platelets. Similarly, some neoplasms, such as Wilms tumor or lymphoproliferative disorders, may express GPIb and adsorb high-molecular-weight VWF

multimer. Patients with hypothyroidism may develop AVWS, probably through reduced synthesis and secretion.[118] AVWS may mimic any type of VWD,[119] or it may not demonstrate the abnormality of VWF:Ag, VWF:RCo, or factor VIII. In the latter cases, a VWF mulitmer analysis may be needed to demonstrate acquired loss of HMWM, particularly in patients with underlying cardiovascular diseases.

Initial von Willebrand Disease Laboratory Testing

Recommended initial laboratory tests include measurements of plasma VWF antigen (VWF:Ag), VWF-platelet GPIb complex binding activity such as ristocetin cofactor activity (VWF:RCo), and factor VIII coagulant activity (FVIII:C).[113] Both National Heart, Lung, and Blood Institute (NHLBI) of the National Institutes of Health (NIH)[113] and International Society on Thrombosis and Haemostasis (ISTH)[113] recommended supplemental tests, assays of VWF platelet-binding activity (RIPA: ristocetin-induced platelet aggregometry) and derived VWF activity/antigen ratios, in conjunction with plasma VWF multimer analysis, for VWD classification. VWF:RCo assay is considered the gold standard method for assessing VWF function. It measures ristocetin-dependent VWF-mediated agglutination of washed or fixed platelets. This method was initially developed from observations of ristocetin-induced VWF-dependent platelet agglutination, measured either by LTA or by macroscopic agglutination of washed formalin-fixed platelets.[120,121] VWF:RCo by LTA (VWF:RCo-LTA) is considered the reference method. Except for type 2N VWD, the derived VWF:RCo/VWF:Ag ratio cut off at 0.5 to 0.7 has been suggested to help distinguish type 2 from type 1 VWD (see Table 80.9). Various alternative methods have been explored to supplement and ultimately replace the VWF:RCo-LTA assay. These assays include the following: (1) VWF collagen-binding methods by ELISA[122]; (2) an automated ristocetin cofactor activity assay using lyophilized normal donor platelets and photo-optical coagulation analyzers[123]; (3) a latex particle–enhanced immunoturbidimetric VWF activity assay using an optical coagulation analyzer (VWF:Ab)[99]; (4) recombinant platelet wild-type (VWF:GPIbR) or gain-of-function (VWF:GPIbM) recombinant GPIb-based enzyme-linked immunosorbent assays[100]; and (5) flow cytometric methods.[124]

POINTS TO REMEMBER

von Willebrand Disease
- Prevalence of VWD is about 0.1–1% in general population.
- The variants of VWD include types 1, 2A, 2B, 2M, 2N and 3.
- VWD type 1 and 3 are quantitative VWF deficiencies.
- VWD type 2A, 2B, and 2M are qualitative VWF deficiencies.
- VWF antigen, activity and factor VIII activity testing are recommended initial tests for laboratory diagnosis of a VWD.
- Three major supplementary tests for classifying type 2 VWD: VWF multimer analysis, VWF-FVIII binding activity assays and ristocetin-induced platelet aggregation.

Acquired von Willebrand Syndrome
- Lack of a personal life-long bleeding (adults) or family history of bleeding.

- Can mimic laboratory phenotype of VWD type 1, 2, or 3.
- Some cases display only a loss of the highest molecular weight multimers with normal VWF:Ag, VWF:RCo, and factor VIII.
  1. Autoantibodies—lymphoproliferative disorders, multiple myeloma; monoclonal gammopathy of unknown significance.
  2. Adsorption onto cells—Wilms tumor expressing GPIb; myeloproliferative disorders, typically with high platelet count.
  3. Increased proteolysis—increased shear forces due to congenital and acquired heart disease, aortic stenosis, ventricular assist devices.
  4. Hypothyroidism—decreased synthesis or secretion of VWF.

Supplementary Testing

There are three major supplementary tests for classifying type 2 VWD (see Table 80.9). VWF multimer analysis is usually required to confirm the diagnosis of types 2A, 2B and 2M VWD. There are various VWF multimer electrophoresis and imaging methods,[125,126] and examples of common type 2 VWD variants are available on the ISTH-related web site, von Willebrand factor Variant Database (http://www.vwf.group.shef.ac.uk/). VWF-FVIII binding activity assays are used for diagnosing type 2N VWD, in which an aberrantly low VWF-FVIII binding capacity is indicative of type 2N VWD.[127] Finally, an abnormal RIPA with low dose ristocetin (approximately 0.5 mg/mL) is diagnostic for type 2B VWD.[128] Most known disorders of adhesion are due to defects in VWF rather than the intrinsic platelet defects. A rare exception is platelet type VWD caused by a defect in GP Ib. Platelet type VWD mimics the laboratory pattern, including increased RIPA (low dose), of VWD type 2B, so specialized ELISA

AT A GLANCE
von Willebrand Disease Classification

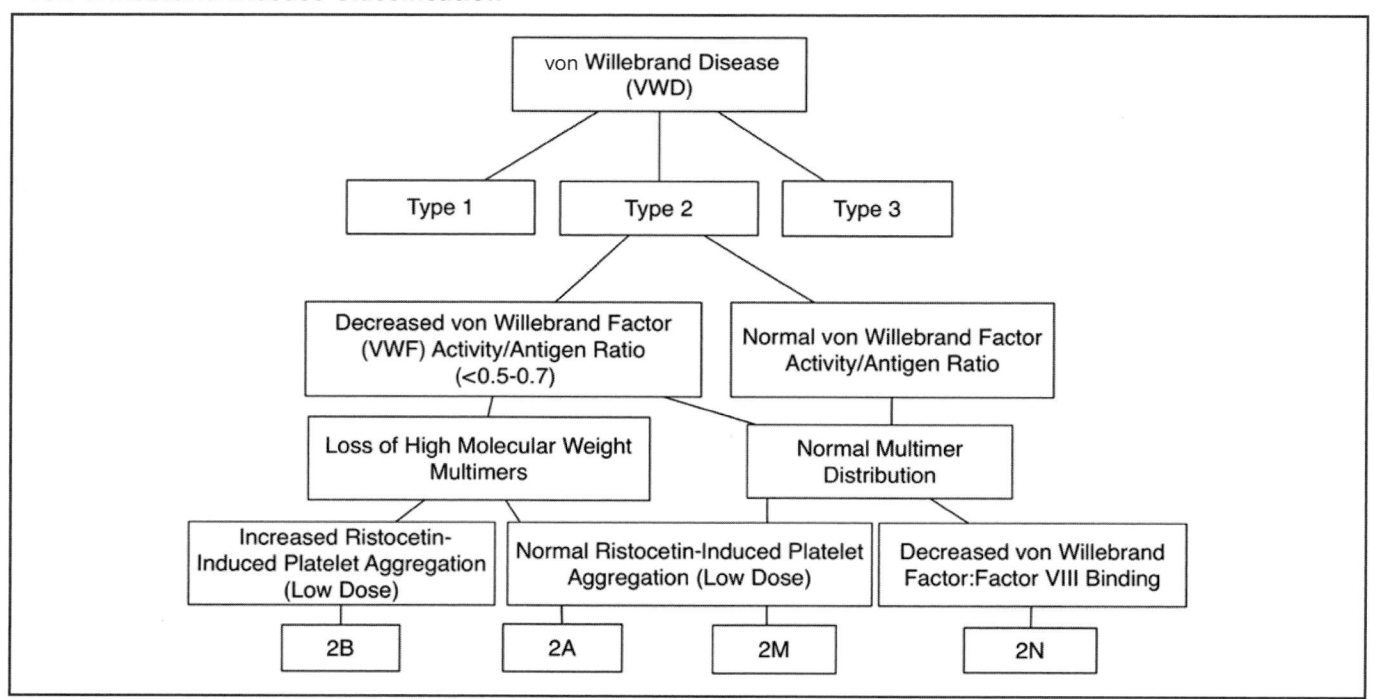

based VWF:platelet binding assays (decreased in VWD type 2B and normal in platelet type VWD), or genetic testing, may be needed. The distinction between type 2B VWD and platelet type VWD is important because the latter requires platelet transfusion rather than VWF concentrates for therapy.

THROMBOTIC DISORDERS DUE TO PLATELET ACTIVATION

Although they are predominantly clinical diagnoses, heparin-induced thrombocytopenia (HIT) and thrombotic thrombocytopenic purpura (TTP) may be confirmed with the HIT assays and ADAMTS13 assays, respectively.

Heparin-induced Thrombocytopenia

Heparin-induced thrombocytopenia (HIT) is a serious complication of heparin therapy because patients with HIT have a substantially increased thrombotic risk. HIT is thought to be caused by the development of antibodies that recognize neoantigens formed from complexes of platelet factor 4 in the presence of heparin. HIT antibodies can activate platelets, presumably contributing to thrombocytopenia and thrombosis. Thrombocytopenia or thrombosis without the presence of heparin-dependent antibodies is not HIT, nor is the isolated presence of such antibodies without thrombocytopenia or thrombosis. The diagnosis of HIT is therefore based on both clinical and laboratory features. The frequency of HIT is greater in surgical than in medical patients and is greater with unfractionated heparin (UFH) than low-molecular-weight heparin (LMWH). In orthopedic patients given prophylactic subcutaneous heparin, the incidence is around 5%, which is approximately 10-fold higher than the incidence with LMWH in this group. For medical patients on therapeutic UFH, the incidence is around 0.5 to 1%. When HIT develops, the platelet count typically decreases 5 to 14 days following initiation of therapy in patients who were not previously exposed to heparin therapy. If patients have had heparin in the previous 3 months, preexisting antibodies may appear as soon as heparin is used. The platelet count must be checked regularly in patients treated with UFH, and a decreased platelet count by more than 50% is an important warning sign of HIT. Severe thrombocytopenia ($<15 \times 10^9$ cells/L) is rare. Approximately half of patients who develop HIT will have associated thrombosis if not promptly diagnosed and treated. The initial assessment is clinical and is based on a system that has been termed the 4 Ts system (**t**hrombocytopenia; **t**iming of fall in platelets; **t**hrombosis; o**t**her causes of thrombocytopenia not evident). This system generates a pretest probability score (summarized in Table 80.10) that guides testing and treatment decisions. If the score is moderate or high, then HIT testing is indicated, and heparin therapy must be terminated and alternative anticoagulants used. If the score is low, then HIT testing is not indicated, and the clinical team can continue heparin. Since fewer than 2% of patients with low pretest probability scores have laboratory evidence of HIT, preventing HIT testing in these patients can help prevent unnecessary testing and therapy.[129]

It is important to remember that the diagnosis and management of HIT are clinical, with the laboratory used only for confirmatory purposes. Several laboratory tests available for these purposes are based on platelet activation (functional) or immunologic assays using PF4-heparin complexes as an antigen. Functional assays (e.g., SRA or aggregometry based heparin-induced platelet activation assays [HIPA]) require a healthy subject as a source of donor platelets, and not all subjects are suitable because responsiveness to HIT antibodies varies. In functional assays, patient serum is incubated with donor platelets, and then platelet activation is assessed. These tests are performed at low (,0.1 to 0.3 IU/mL) and high (100 IU/mL) heparin concentrations to evaluate the heparin-

TABLE 80.10	The Four Ts of Pretest Probability for Heparin-induced Thrombocytopenia			
		SCORE		
		2	**1**	**0**
Thrombocytopenia		PLT count drop >50% from baseline and nadir PLT count ≥20 × 10⁹/L	PLT count drop 30–50% or nadir PLT count 10–19 × 10⁹/L	PLT count drop <30% or PLT count nadir <10 × 10⁹/L
Timing of PLT fall with heparin	No prior exposure	5–10 days or	5–10 days (unclear data) or >10 days	<4 days
	Prior exposure	≤1 day with heparin exposure in prior 30 days	≤1 day with heparin exposure in prior 30–100 days	
Thrombosis	Thrombosis	New confirmed thrombosis	Progressive or recurrent or unproven thrombosis	No thrombosis
	Other presentations	Skin necrosis at the injection site or acute systemic reaction (unfractionated heparin)	Non-necrotizing skin lesions at the injection site	
Other causes of thrombocytopenia		None	Possible	Definite

Interpretation:
Total score 6 to 8 = high pretest probability → Testing indicated
Total score 4 to 5 = intermediate probability → Testing may be indicated
Total score ≤3 = low pretest probability → Testing not indicated
PLT, Platelet; *UFH,* unfractionated heparin.
Modified from Lo GK, Juhl D, Warkentin TE, et al. Evaluation of pretest clinical score (4 T's) for the diagnosis of heparin-induced thrombocytopenia in two clinical settings. *J Thromb Haemost* 2006;4:759–65.

dependent platelet release/activation. The presence of HIT antibodies causes platelet release at low heparin concentrations, but high heparin concentrations neutralize the antibody. Platelet activation in the presence of the high concentration of heparin is considered nonspecific. SRA are both sensitive (100%) and specific (95.1%) for clinical HIT[130] and are considered the gold standard laboratory method. SRA may require radioactive material and are technically difficult; hence, these tests are typically limited to large reference laboratories. HIPA was originally read visually with indirect light, but many methods have been adapted, including LTA, lumi-aggregometry, whole blood aggregometry, or even flow cytometric methods to assess platelet activation. In general, the sensitivity of HIPA is lower than SRA, even if platelets are washed. SRA and HIPA are typically found in reference laboratories.

Because SRA or HIPA are time-intensive and laborious, ELISA or EIA assays are most often performed as a first-line test. In these assays, PF4 along with a heparin (or other negatively charge polyanion like PF4-polyvinyl sulfonate) is coated on the solid phase. When test serum contains HIT antibodies, the labeled detection antibody creates a color change that is read as optical density (OD). The degree of positivity is important in that strong positivity is associated with thrombosis. Positive results can be followed up with an inhibition step that involves the use of high dose heparin (100 IU/dL) to neutralize HIT antibodies; a large decrease in OD compared to the OD without heparin indicates a heparin dependent antibody, as opposed to a nonspecific antibody. Antibody assays have a clinical sensitivity close to 100% but have lower specificity for the syndrome (74% for polyspecific assays detecting IgG, IgA, and IgG assays or 89% of IgG specific assays) than SRA or HIPA.[130] False positives are common due to the use of these ELISAs, so the application of pretest probability is necessary. Some experts believe that only immunoglobulin (Ig) G antibodies cause the clinical disorder.[131] Many commercial antigen assays detect IgM and IgA antibodies, as well as IgG. Without patient selection with pretest probability, the false-positive rate of ELISAs detecting IgG, IgA, and IgM may be close to 50%.[129] For full reviews and guidance, see Linkins and coworkers.[132,133]

Thrombotic Thrombocytopenic Purpura and ADAMTS13

TTP is a medical emergent disease that carries 80% mortality if not recognized promptly and treated with plasma exchange.[134] The classic clinical symptoms include (1) microangiopathic hemolytic anemia, (2) thrombocytopenia, (3) fever, (4) renal failure, and (5) central nervous system abnormalities, also known as "pentad" clinical features. The differential diagnosis includes disseminated intravascular coagulation (DIC) and atypical hemolytic uremic syndrome. TTP is caused by congenital or acquired ADAMTS13 deficiency. ADAMTS13 a VWF-cleaving protease, which depolymerizes VWF after secretion from the endothelial cell. When ADAMTS13 activity is markedly decreased (typically <10%), platelets bind to ultra-high-molecular-weight multimer and cause spontaneous platelet thrombi in the microvasculature, such as in the kidney and brain. ADAMTS13 deficiency is most often acquired due to an autoantibody that either inhibits ADAMTS13 function or clears ADAMTS13 from circulation, with the former being the most common. Other secondary mechanisms of ADAMTS13 deficiency include medications, pregnancy, infections, malignancy, and hematopoietic stem cell transplantation. Rare congenital ADAMTS13 deficiency, also known as Upshaw Schulman syndrome, also occurs in children and young adults. TTP is treated with plasma exchange with fresh frozen plasma. This therapy presumably removes inhibitors and ultra-high-molecular-weight VWF and replaces ADAMTS13.

ADAMTS13 activity test is required for the definitive diagnosis of TTP. The older functional assay for this molecule is based on the ability of the patient's plasma to cleave the HMWMs of VWF. It requires lengthy incubation followed by VWF multimer analysis, taking up to 2 days; thus it is no longer routinely used in clinical laboratories. New assays have become available, including the fluorescence resonance energy transfer (FRET) assay[135] and ELISA,[136] which are proving to be of greater diagnostic usefulness. An additional mixing step with plasma evaluates for the presence of an inhibitor, and some laboratories report an inhibitor titer, using similar steps as those in the factor VIII Bethesda assay. To accurately measure patients' own ADAMTS13 activities, samples must be collected before therapy to avoid false elevation of ADAMTS13 from plasma products.

POINTS TO REMEMBER
Heparin-Induced Thrombocytopenia

- HIT is predominantly a clinical diagnosis, but laboratory testing may confirm the diagnosis.
- Serotonin release assays detect the release of radiolabeled serotonin from donor platelets stimulated by HIT antibodies in the presence of heparin (low dose).
- Serotonin release assays are sensitive and specific but are not widely available.
- ELISAs detect antibodies to the PF4-heparin complex (or PF4-polyanion).
- ELISAs are widely used and have high sensitivity but suffer from low specificity, resulting in false positives.
- Pretest probability decreases unnecessary testing and decreases false-positive test results.
- Pretest probability is based on the 4 Ts:
  - Thrombosis
  - Thrombocytopenia
  - Timing
  - Other causes of thrombocytopenia

POINTS TO REMEMBER
Thrombotic Thrombocytopenic Purpura

- High mortality if not diagnosed promptly.
- The pentad clinical features include (1) microangiopathic hemolytic anemia, (2) thrombocytopenia, (3) fever, (4) renal failure, and (5) central nervous system abnormalities.
- It is caused by congenital or acquired severe ADAMTS13 deficiency (<10%).
- Acquired ADAMTS13 is caused by specific inhibitors that can be measured by a Bethesda assay or ELISA.

SLECTED REFERENCES

1. Zeigler Z, Murphy S, Gardner FH. Microscopic platelet size and morphology in various hematologic disorders. Blood 1978;51:479–86.
3. Murphy S, Oski FA, Naiman JL, et al. Platelet size and kinetics in hereditary and acquired thrombocytopenia. N Engl J Med 1972;286:499–504.
14. White JG. Platelet granule disorders. Crit Rev Oncol Hematol 1986;4:337–77.
37. Born GV. Aggregation of blood platelets by adenosine diphosphate and its reversal. Nature 1962;194:927–9.
38. Hayward CP, Moffat KA, Raby A, et al. Development of North American consensus guidelines for medical laboratories that perform and interpret platelet function testing using light transmission aggregometry. Am J Clin Pathol 2010;134:955–63.
39. Harrison P, Mackie I, Mumford A, et al. Guidelines for the laboratory investigation of heritable disorders of platelet function. Br J Haematol 2011;155:30–44.
41. Cattaneo M, Hayward CP, Moffat KA, et al. Results of a worldwide survey on the assessment of platelet function by light transmission aggregometry: a report from the platelet physiology subcommittee of the SSC of the ISTH. J Thromb Haemost 2009;7:1029.
51. Michelson AD, Barnard MR, Krueger LA, et al. Evaluation of platelet function by flow cytometry. Methods 2000;21:259–70.
58. Blaauwgeers MW, van Asten I, Kruip M, et al. The limitation of genetic testing in diagnosing patients suspected for congenital platelet defects. Am J Hematol 2020;95:E26–8.
59. Noris P, Pecci A. Hereditary thrombocytopenias: a growing list of disorders. Hematology Am Soc Hematol Educ Program 2017;2017:385–99.
64. Shore-Lesserson L. Platelet inhibitors and monitoring platelet function: implications for bleeding. Hematol Oncol Clin North Am 2007;21:51–63.

70. Fontana P, Reber G, de Moerloose P. Assessing aspirin responsiveness using the Verify Now Aspirin assay. Thromb Res 2008;121:581–2.
75. Bunimov N, Fuller N, Hayward CP. Genetic loci associated with platelet traits and platelet disorders. Semin Thromb Hemost 2013;39:291–305.
95. Budde U, van Genderen PJ. Acquired von Willebrand disease in patients with high platelet counts. Semin Thromb Hemost 1997;23:425–31.
113. Nichols WL, Hultin MB, James AH, et al. von Willebrand disease (VWD): evidence-based diagnosis and management guidelines, the National Heart, Lung, and Blood Institute (NHLBI) Expert Panel report (USA). Haemophilia 2008;14:171–232.
114. Sadler JE, Budde U, Eikenboom JC, et al. Update on the pathophysiology and classification of von Willebrand disease: a report of the Subcommittee on von Willebrand Factor. J Thromb Haemost 2006;4:2103–14.
117. Federici AB, Rand JH, Mannucci PM. Acquired von Willebrand syndrome: an important bleeding complication to be considered in patients with lymphoproliferative and myeloproliferative disorders. Hematol J 2001;2:358–62.
130. Warkentin TE, Sheppard JA, Moore JC, et al. Laboratory testing for the antibodies that cause heparin-induced thrombocytopenia: how much class do we need? J Lab Clin Med 2005;146:341–6.
132. Linkins LA, Dans AL, Moores LK, et al. Treatment and prevention of heparin-induced thrombocytopenia: Antithrombotic Therapy and Prevention of Thrombosis, 9th ed: American College of Chest Physicians Evidence-Based Clinical Practice Guidelines. Chest 2012;141:e495S–530S.
135. Kokame K, Nobe Y, Kokubo Y, et al. FRETS-VWF73, a first fluorogenic substrate for ADAMTS13 assay. Br J Haematol 2005;129:93–100.

81

Coagulation, Anticoagulation, and Fibrinolysis

Russell A. Higgins, Steve Kitchen, and Dong Chen

ABSTRACT

Background

A subset of hemostatic disorders are due to an imbalance in coagulation or fibrinolysis. Disorders of coagulation or fibrinolysis can be either inherited (e.g., hemophilia A) or acquired (e.g., liver disease), and the clinical presentation is typically either bleeding or thrombosis. Laboratory testing is used to diagnose and to monitor the therapy of patients with these disorders. Additionally, a growing list of anticoagulant medications need laboratory testing to adjust the dose or to assess the risk for bleeding or thrombosis.

Content

This chapter describes laboratory testing for disorders of coagulation and fibrinolysis. Prothrombin time (PT), activated partial thromboplastin time (aPTT), thrombin time, and fibrinogen are routine tests in coagulation laboratories and are used in the initial evaluation of bleeding or thrombosis. Mixing studies and specialized testing of the coagulation and fibrinolytic pathways are used in an algorithmic fashion to complete the diagnostic workup. D-Dimer testing is a marker of fibrinolysis used to assess disseminated intravascular coagulation or to exclude venous thromboembolism (VTE). Thrombotic disorders may be investigated with protein C, protein S, antithrombin, factor V Leiden (FVL) mutation, prothrombin *G20210A* mutation, and lupus anticoagulant (LAC) tests. Laboratory testing of patients on a variety of anticoagulant medications are also described.

GENERAL CONSIDERATIONS FOR COAGULATION TESTING

Coagulation tests have unique preanalytic and analytic issues that require discussion before the specific tests are addressed. The basic principles of clotting tests and chromogenic tests as they apply to coagulation are outlined.

Preanalytic Variables for Coagulation-based Assays

Control of preanalytical issues in coagulation testing is paramount for good laboratory performance (see also "Hemostasis Testing" section in Chapter 5). In addition to the common issues of hemolyzed, icteric, or lipemic samples, some preanalytical factors of particular importance in coagulation testing include (1) clotted specimens, (2) improper blood-to-anticoagulant ratio, and (3) contamination with saline, heparin, or other anticoagulants. Traumatic venipuncture, activation of coagulation within the collection device, or improper mixing of the anticoagulant with blood may result in clotting, which consumes coagulation factors, making testing unreliable. Blood for coagulation testing should be collected by standard venipuncture techniques into 109 mmol/L (3.2%) trisodium citrate, such that the final proportion of blood to anticoagulant is 9 : 1. Blood is commonly collected into commercially available tubes with prealiquoted trisodium citrate and a line indicating the appropriate volume of blood to be drawn. Collection of a volume of blood less than the recommended volume ("a short draw") will result in excess anticoagulant compared to plasma and prolonged clotting times. Likewise, samples with a high hematocrit (>55%) will require a decreased volume of anticoagulant because of a lower plasma volume (Box 81.1).

Some coagulation testing, such as activated clotting time (ACT), may be performed on whole blood; however, most routine clot-based assays are performed on plasma, separated from the cellular components by centrifugation. Plasma prepared from citrate tubes is referred to as citrated plasma. Lipemia, hemolysis, and icterus are interferences in serum and plasma, affecting both chemistry and coagulation tests[1]; however, clot-based tests are sensitive to additional preanalytic factors (see Points to Remember box). To avoid interference from phospholipid, platelet poor plasma (PPP) with a platelet count less than 10×10^9/L is prepared by centrifugation, typically at $1500 \times g$ for at least 15 minutes.[2] Higher speeds and shorter times have been used to prepare plasma for PT, aPTT, and thrombin time (TT), because these tests may not be affected by platelet counts up to 200×10^9/L; this rapid processing is not suitable for heparin assays or LAC testing. If this rapid centrifugation approach is used, the coagulation tests should be performed immediately to prevent release of platelet phospholipid from activated platelets into the plasma. Ultimately, the laboratory should confirm that PPP is produced or that their method of plasma preparation does not affect coagulation results. Reagent phospholipids are important for the spatial orientation of coagulation molecules, so exogenous phospholipid may have a significant impact on the aPTT. Centrifugation and testing of the derived plasma should occur as soon as possible, usually within

BOX 81.1 Adjusting Citrate Volume for Hematocrit > 55%

$$C = (1.85 \times 10^{-3}) (100\text{-hct})(V_{blood})$$
- C; appropriate volume of citrate
- hct; hematocrit of patient
- V; volume of blood in tube
- 1.85×10^{-3}, constant

24 hours for PT, or within 4 hours for aPTT or other clot-based tests.[2] Plasma should be stored at room temperature for PT but may be stored at either room or refrigerated temperatures (2 to 8 °C) for aPTT. Whole-blood samples should be stored at 18 to 24 °C, whereas refrigerated temperatures should be avoided because of possible "cold activation" of factor VII.[3] Refrigeration of whole blood also decreases factor VIII and VWF and may cause the misdiagnosis of hemophilia A or VWD. If the sample is centrifuged and the plasma aliquoted, cold storage may be acceptable for tests other than PT. Samples for monitoring unfractionated heparin (UFH) therapy should be centrifuged within 1 hour to avoid neutralization of heparin by platelet factor 4 (PF4) released from platelets. When coagulation testing is delayed beyond 24 hours, the plasma should be separated from the cells and kept below −20 or at −70 °C for longer storage.[2] The freeze–thaw cycles disrupt platelet membranes, so PPP is especially important for frozen plasma. Therefore double centrifugation is the best practice to avoid this phospholipid contamination when freezing plasma. Household-grade freezers with auto-defrost cycles are not suitable. Frozen samples should be rapidly defrosted at 37 °C and then mixed to resuspend any precipitate that may contain coagulation proteins.

POINTS TO REMEMBER

Preanalytic Issues and Interferences

- Underfilled citrate tubes cause prolongation of clotting tests.
- Overfilled citrate tubes cause shortening of clotting tests.
- Activated factors from clotted samples, traumatic draws, or therapy with activated factors shorten clotting times.
- High hematocrit (>55%) decreases the plasma-to-citrate ratio and prolongs clotting times.
- Loss of labile factors VIII and V secondary to increased storage time (>4 h) prolongs clotting times.
- Cold activation of whole blood stored at 2–4 °C for 4 h decreases factor VIII and VWF.
- Prolonged cold storage (overnight) of whole blood may shorten PT.
- Lipemia, icterus, and hemolysis interfere with optical and in some cases mechanical clot detection.
- LACs prolong phospholipid-dependent (Russell's viper venom time [DRVVT], PTT > PT) clotting times.
- Frozen plasma specimens must be platelet poor to prevent prolongation of clotting times from platelet-derived phospholipids.
- Contamination from heparin or saline drips may prolong clotting times.

Optical versus Mechanical End Point Detection

Clot-based tests (e.g., PT/INR, aPTT, and TT) detect the time interval from initiation of coagulation to clot formation. Detection of clot formation as an end point has been accomplished in a number of ways. Early methods used a tilt-tube technique that depended on visually identifying clot formation in plasma samples. A water bath was necessary to keep the temperature at 37 °C. Currently, this time-intensive manual method is used only with international reference thromboplastins.

As a result of high-volume testing, most coagulation testing is now performed on automated instruments that control the temperature of the reaction and detect end points by use of any one of several methods. Most methods detect either a change in physical/mechanical properties or a change in the light transmission produced by polymerized fibrin. Numerous approaches for mechanical end point detection have been developed. One mechanical method consists of a metal ball at the bottom of a sample cuvette that is sent into a back-and-forth motion by a magnet; the end point is detected when fibrin monomers polymerize into fibrin strands and impede the motion of the ball. Another mechanical detection system uses a magnet to hold a ball to the side of a rotating cuvette until fibrin strands physically displace the ball. Optical methods (usually nephelometric but occasionally turbidimetric; see Chapter 16) use the decrease in light transmission or increased light scatter as fibrin monomers are polymerized into fibrin strands.[4] Optical end points may occur at preset thresholds or use the kinetics, such as maximum acceleration of fibrin polymerization, to define end points. Light sources have traditionally been halogen lamps or lasers, but newer instruments may use light-emitting diodes (LEDs) that increase longevity and allow measurement at wavelengths that have less overlap with interfering substances. A potential advantage of mechanical over optical end point detection is less interference from substances, such as hemoglobin, bilirubin, or lipid that interfere with optical methods. When an end point cannot be detected with an instrument using an optical end point method, laboratories should have a protocol, such as a backup mechanical method or a send-out laboratory, to obtain a result.

Chromogenic Assays

Chromogenic assays have been used to bypass the complexity of the clotting cascade, including the effects of elevated coagulation factors, anticoagulant medications, and LACs (discussed later). In these assays, serine proteases (such as thrombin, factor Xa, factor IXa, factor XIa, and factor XIIa) of the clotting cascade cleave oligopeptide substrates, releasing chromogens that are then detected optically, most commonly at a wavelength of 405 nm:

Serine protease + Chromogenic substrate → p-Nitroaniline (detected at 405 nm)

The chromogenic method is commonly applied to assays that measure (1) factor VIII, (2) factor IX, (3) antithrombin, (4) protein C, (5) factor X, and (6) heparin concentration (anti-Xa method). However, numerous other applications are possible.

TEST METHODS FOR COAGULATION

The coagulation cascade culminates in the formation of a fibrin meshwork. Tests commonly used in the initial evaluation of bleeding include (1) PT and INR, (2) aPTT, (3) fibrinogen assays (Clauss and derived), and (4) TT, whereas (4) mixing studies, (5) factor assays, (6) inhibitor assays, and (7) factor XIII assays are used in an algorithmic fashion to finalize the diagnosis. Many of these tests are also used to monitor therapy or to measure anticoagulant effect.

The coagulation assays measured in seconds, like PT, aPTT, and TT, are not standardized, and intermethod comparison can be high. The PT has been harmonized globally by calculating and reporting the INR, specifically for patients on stable therapeutic warfarin (see "Therapy With Vitamin K Antagonists"). On the other hand, most coagulation factor assays are now traceable to a plasma international standard and are measured in % activity or international units of activity (e.g., IU/mL).[5] Calibrators, reagents, and instruments are all known to cause differences between methods in factor assays. Even fibrinogen, with an international standard potency assignment in milligrams (e.g., mg/dL), has substantial interlaboratory variability, in part due to differences in methodology (See Fibrinogen). Moreover, population differences in factor levels, particularly with factor VIII, have contributed to the complexity of standardizing coagulation factor assays. The methodology, reagent, and population variables underscore the need for locally verified or established reference ranges for all coagulation assays.

Prothrombin Time

The PT is a clot-based assay that reflects the activity of *extrinsic* and *common pathway* factors of the coagulation cascade. The PT cannot be compared across different laboratories because the specific thromboplastin/instrument combination determines the responsiveness of the test. The INR, which is derived mathematically from the PT, allows harmonization of the PT across laboratories for the purpose of monitoring vitamin K antagonists (VKAs) (see "Therapy With Vitamin K Antagonist").

The PT is performed on PPP at 37 °C. It is initiated by the addition of a thromboplastin reagent containing TF, calcium, and phospholipid. The TF in the reagent initiates the extrinsic pathway of the coagulation cascade (see Fig. 81.1), the phospholipids provide a surface for assembly of coagulation factors, and the calcium chloride counteracts the binding of plasma calcium by citrate, making calcium available for the coagulation process. The timer is started when reagent is added, and the end point occurs when fibrin monomer polymerization is detected.

Patient plasma + Thromboplastin (tissue factor and phospholipid) + $CaCl_2$ → Fibrin clot

The addition of TF activates the extrinsic pathway much like the natural process; however, clotting occurs before the intrinsic pathway is significantly propagated, as occurs with in vivo coagulation. Consequently, the PT is not sensitive to factor VIII or other intrinsic coagulation factors, and PT could be considered a test of the initiation phase of coagulation.

The PT is used to identify deficiencies or inhibitors of factors VII, X, V, and II and fibrinogen. Expected results of clotting assays, including PT, are shown in Table 81.1 for key inherited and acquired disorders. The sensitivity of PT reagents to the deficiency of coagulation factors varies with the specific reagent and instrument combination. Therefore it is useful for laboratories to determine the sensitivity of a given PT system to factors VII, X, V, and II (see Fig. 81.2 for illustration of the principle, although this example uses the aPTT test rather than PT). Alternatively, manufacturers may provide data regarding responsiveness to coagulation factors. If a reagent is overly sensitive to decreases in a factor (e.g., 0.5 IU/mL factor VII), the laboratory may detect clinically insignificant prolongations of the PT. Needless laboratory evaluations and delays in surgical interventions may be avoided if reagents are selected carefully.

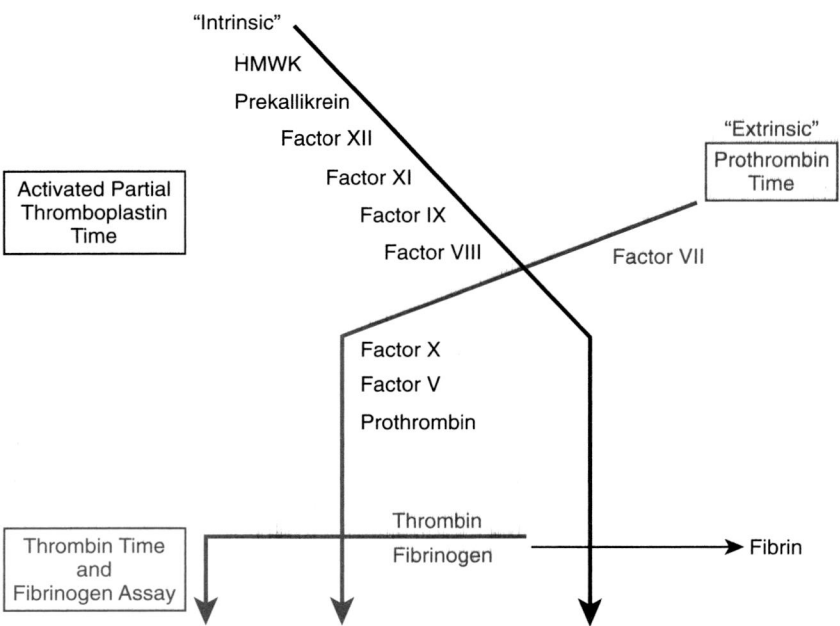

FIGURE 81.1 Model of the in vitro coagulation cascade. Extrinsic, intrinsic, and common pathways of coagulation are shown. In vivo coagulation occurs in phases and does not require contact factor activation of factor XII, prekallikrein, and high-molecular-weight kininogen *(HMWK)* for clot formation.

TABLE 81.1 Clinical Settings and Coagulation Tests

	Presentation	aPTT	PT	TT	Fibrinogen
Inherited Disorders					
Contact factor deficiencies (HMWK, prekallikrein, and factor XII)	None	↑	NI	NI	NI
Intrinsic pathway procoagulant deficiencies (factor XI, IX, and VIII)	Bleeding	↑	NI	NI	NI
Extrinsic pathway procoagulant deficiencies (factor VII)	Bleeding	NI	↑	NI	NI
Common pathway deficiencies (factor X, V, and II)	Bleeding	↑	↑	NI	NI
Congenital hypofibrinogenemia	Bleeding	↑	↑	↑	↓
Congenital dysfibrinogenemia	Bleeding/thrombosis	NI or ↑	NI or ↑	↑	↓activity
Natural anticoagulant deficiencies (protein C, protein S, and antithrombin)	Thrombosis	NI	NI	NI	NI
von Willebrand disease	Bleeding	NI or ↑	NI	NI	NI
Glanzmann thrombasthenia	Bleeding	NI	NI	NI	NI
Bernard-Soulier syndrome	Bleeding	NI	NI	NI	NI
Acquired Disorders					
Liver disease	Bleeding/thrombosis	NI or ↑[a]	↑	↑	NI or ↓
Disseminated intravascular coagulation	Bleeding/thrombosis	NI or ↑[a]	↑	↑	↓
Vitamin K deficiency	Bleeding	NI or ↑[a]	↑	NI	NI
Lupus anticoagulant	Thrombosis or asymptomatic	↑	NI[b]	NI	NI
Specific intrinsic pathway factor inhibitors (factor XI, IX, and VIII)	Bleeding	NI	↑	NI	NI
Specific common pathway factor inhibitors (factor X, V, and II)	Bleeding	↑	↑	NI	NI
Medications					
Unfractionated heparin		↑	NI or ↑[c]	↑	NI
Low-molecular-weight heparin		↑[d]	NI	↑	NI
Fondaparinux		↑	↑	NI	NI
Direct thrombin inhibitors (oral and intravenous)		See Table 81.7	See Table 81.7	↑	↓[e]
Direct oral Xa inhibitors		See Table 81.7	See Table 81.7	NI	NI
Anti–vitamin K (warfarin)		NI or ↑[a]	↑	NI	NI

[a]Prolongation of aPTT depends on the sensitivity of the reagents and the degree of factor deficiency.
[b]Strong lupus anticoagulants prolong PT in addition to aPTT.
[c]PT reagents may contain heparin-neutralizing reagents (usually up to 1–2 U/mL).
[d]aPTT is not predictably prolonged by low molecular weight heparin.
[e]Direct thrombin inhibitors (e.g., argatroban) may cause underestimation of fibrinogen by the Clauss method (depending on thrombin concentration in reagent).
NI, Normal.

The PT/INR has been used to monitor VKA therapy because it is sensitive to vitamin K–dependent factors, II, VII, and X. Monitoring during bridging or conversion of patients from heparin therapy to therapy with VKAs is made possible by the addition of heparin-neutralizing substances. VKA therapy and its monitoring are addressed in greater detail later.

Activated Partial Thromboplastin Time

The aPTT is a clot-based assay initiated by activation of contact factors and reflects the activity of the intrinsic and common coagulation pathways (see Fig. 81.1). Activation of contact factors (high molecular weight kininogen [HMWK], prekallikrein, and factors XII and XI) is achieved by the addition of one of a wide variety of activators. With the exception of ellagic acid, these substances have negatively charged surface responsible for contact factor activation. Activators including kaolin, celite, and micronized silica have been used extensively when mechanical end points are determined by coagulometers (see earlier); however, if optical detection is used, micronized silica or the soluble chemical

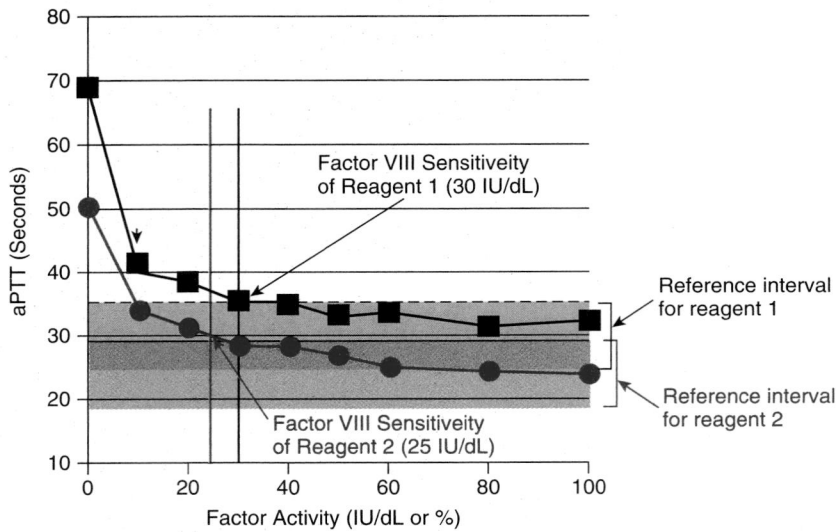

FIGURE 81.2 Relationship of activated partial thromboplastin time *(aPTT)* to factor VIII activity. The graph demonstrates typical relationships of factor activity to clotting time. Response curves are shown for two aPTT reagents. Reference intervals for the reagents are represented as *gray* and *red* shaded areas for reagent 1 and reagent 2, respectively. Determining reagent responsiveness is accomplished by measuring the aPTT in a dilutional series of factor-deficient plasma with normal pooled plasma. The factor activity at which aPTT prolongs above the reference interval is the limit of detection of the reagent (shown as *black* or *red arrows*). The graph demonstrates that aPTT reagents vary in their response to coagulation factors. Reagent 2 has a lower sensitivity than reagent 1 for factor VIII and may be less useful in detecting mild hemophilia A. Prothrombin time (PT) reagents (and instrument combinations) also vary in their responses to extrinsic and common pathway factors and are assessed in a similar manner. The *arrowhead* indicates the effect of a 10-fold dilution used for the factor VIII activity assay. The dilution takes advantage of the dynamic part of the curve, in which larger changes in aPTT indicate smaller changes in factor VIII activity.

activator ellagic acid is used because they do not interfere with light transmission.

The aPTT is carried out in two stages. First, reagent containing a contact activator and phospholipids is added and incubated with the citrated plasma at 37 °C for several minutes (varies with the method). Second, the plasma is recalcified with calcium chloride, which is required for subsequent activation of downstream coagulation factors and the timer is started. The timer is stopped when the end point is detected.

(Stage 1) Patient plasma + Activator + Phospholipid
→ Factor XIIa + Factor XIa

(Stage 2) CaCl₂ + Factor XIIa + Factor XIa
+ Other coagulation factors → Fibrin clot

Although aPTT, activated partial thromboplastic time, implies the addition of thromboplastin, this is not the case. This ambiguity is a result of use of the term *partial* thromboplastin by Langdell and associates[6] to describe a group of reagents that produced clotting that was less rapid in hemophiliac plasma than in normal plasma. This was contrasted with "complete" thromboplastin reagents used in the PT assay, which did not discriminate normal and hemophiliac plasmas. Partial thromboplastin activity was achieved by replacing thromboplastin with phospholipid preparations, sometimes called cephalin; however, the overall effect was to dilute the thromboplastin activity, making the contribution of the intrinsic pathway measurable. Subsequently, the addition of activators led to the aPTT that we recognize today.

The aPTT is sensitive to activities of the intrinsic and common pathway factors (1) HMWK, (2) prekallikrein, (3) XII, (4) XI, (5) IX, (6) VIII, (7) X, (8) V, (9) II, and (10) fibrinogen.[7] Common uses of the aPTT include monitoring of heparin therapy and screening for deficiencies or inhibitors of intrinsic and common pathway factors. The use of aPTT for monitoring heparin therapy is discussed later. The response of aPTT reagents to heparin,[8] factor deficiency, specific factor inhibitors, and LACs[9] varies widely. If a clinical laboratory intends to use aPTT to detect factor deficiencies, it is important to know the threshold of factor deficiency that prolongs the aPTT (see Fig. 81.2). The response of aPTT to factors VIII, IX, and XI is particularly important because of the prevalence of hemophilias and their clinically significant bleeding risk. In general, the desired response threshold (i.e., the level of factor deficiency associated with prolongation of aPTT) to factors VIII, IX, and XI should be approximately 30 to 40 IU/dL. Alternatively, manufacturers may provide data regarding responsiveness to coagulation factors. Very sensitive reagents may create unnecessary laboratory follow-up or treatment delay, whereas insensitive reagents may not detect mild factor deficiency.

The aPTT is prolonged in a variety of clinically significant and insignificant scenarios. Table 81.1 summarizes some causes of prolonged aPTT and/or PT. Six potential causes of isolated prolongation of aPTT include (1) a procoagulant deficiency or deficiencies that may be associated with a bleeding history, (2) a contact factor deficiency without bleeding risk (XII, prekallikrein, HMWK), (3) a specific inhibitor acquired as an alloimmune or autoimmune phenomenon (e.g., factor VIII inhibitor), (4) a nonspecific inhibitor such as a LAC, (5) a medication effect or contamination (e.g., heparin, direct thrombin inhibitor), and (6) a spurious result. A prolonged aPTT reflects clinically significant deficiencies of coagulation factors (factors XI, IX, and VIII) and is an important test for identifying these deficiencies. However, deficiencies of several intrinsic coagulation factors, HMWK, prekallikrein, and factor XII, prolong the aPTT but are not associated with bleeding.

Fibrinogen (Clauss and Derived Method)

Coagulation ultimately depends on the conversion of fibrinogen to fibrin monomer by thrombin (see Fig. 81.1). The Clauss method[10] is the most commonly used method to measure fibrinogen concentration. Initial dilution of plasma (usually 1:10) serves to dilute fibrinogen, and then excess thrombin (final concentration 30 to 100 U/mL) is added to the diluted plasma. With the enzyme (thrombin) at saturating concentrations and the substrate (fibrinogen) at limiting concentration, the rate of fibrin formation depends on the concentration of fibrinogen:

Patient plasma (diluted) + Thrombin (high concentration)
→ Fibrin clot

The fibrin end point is used to determine fibrinogen concentration from a calibration curve. Five dilutions of the fibrinogen calibrator are made, and a calibration curve is generated by plotting fibrinogen concentration against the rate of fibrin clot formation.

Another method of fibrinogen determination is PT-derived fibrinogen, also known as PT-fibrinogen. The fibrinogen concentration is proportional to the maximal change in absorbance in an optical PT measurement. A calibrator is used to create a calibration curve relating the change of absorbance of PT to the fibrinogen concentration. The PT-fibrinogen assay may overestimate fibrinogen concentration in patients with DIC, patients on fibrinolytic therapy, and many patients with dysfibrinogenemia. In addition, some fibrinogen calibrators contribute more turbidity and may not be optimal for PT-fibrinogen measurements. The Clauss method is considered by many to provide a more meaningful fibrinogen measurement because fibrinogen degradation products are not detected, whereas PT-fibrinogen methods are more sensitive to fibrinogen degradation products. FDPs prolong some clot-based tests by interfering with fibrin monomer polymerization, but they may also act as anticoagulants and contribute to hemorrhage in DIC.[11]

Mixing Studies

Mixing studies are performed on abnormally prolonged clot-based assays such as aPTT and PT. The purpose of mixing studies is to determine whether prolonged clotting times are due to factor deficiency or inhibitor activity. Mixing studies are useful for guiding the coagulation work-up, but they lack clinical sensitivity and specificity. Hence, the results of mixing studies are followed with LAC tests, factor assays, and possibly specific functional inhibitor studies for confirmation. Inhibitors are categorized as nonspecific or specific types. Nonspecific inhibitors (e.g., heparin, LAC) have activity against multiple procoagulants, whereas specific inhibitors are directed at a single factor. LACs are a heterogeneous

group of immunoglobulins with phospholipid-dependent activity against coagulation factors; they are discussed in greater detail later. Specific factor VIII inhibitors are usually seen as alloantibodies in the setting of hemophilia A treated with factor VIII concentrates, but they may be seen in nonhemophiliac patients as an autoantibody. Although rare, specific inhibitors may occur against any factor, and a high degree of clinical suspicion is needed when bleeding is otherwise unexplained.

Mixing studies are useful when clotting time (e.g., aPTT, PT) is unexpectedly prolonged outside the reference interval. They are also recommended for LAC testing (see section on DRVVT and LAC studies later) to confirm the inhibitor effect. Patient plasma is mixed in a 1 : 1 ratio with NPP using the same anticoagulant, and then the clotting assay is repeated *immediately*. NPP should contain 100 (±20 IU/dL) of all factors. If a factor deficiency in the patient plasma exists, the NPP supplies the factors needed to correct the clotting time back into the reference interval. If an inhibitor is present, the mixed specimen will not correct the clotting time into the reference interval.

The utility of mixing studies largely depends on the patient population and the clinical setting. For example, aPTT mixing studies are performed more frequently than PT mixing studies because LACs, which are common, affect aPTT to a much greater extent than PT. When aPTT is prolonged and mixing studies fail to adequately correct into the reference interval, an inhibitor is suspected. If the patient is asymptomatic or has a history of thrombosis, the next step should be to look for LAC rather than measure factor VIII, IX, and XI concentrations. Conversely, if the patient has a bleeding presentation, a specific inhibitor may be suspected and factor activities should be measured. PT mixing studies may be less helpful because the differential diagnosis of an isolated prolongation of PT is limited.

Immediate aPTT mixing studies that correct to the reference interval require incubated mixing to assess for time-dependent inhibitors. In such studies, the patient's plasma is mixed with NPP and they are incubated together for 1 or 2 hours at 37 °C. The aPTT is then repeated and compared with a control. The control consists of patient plasma and NPP incubated at 37 °C separately, followed by mixing and aPTT measurement. This control step is important because it controls for loss of labile factors during the incubation process (Fig. 81.3). One approach to interpretation is to consider a 10% difference between the test and the control to indicate a time-dependent inhibitor. Acquired alloantibodies to factor VIII are frequently time dependent; however, up to 15% of LAC measurements are also time dependent.[12] Considering the high prevalence of LAC relative to the low prevalence of acquired factor VIII inhibitors in hemophilia patients (1 to 2 per million of population per year), laboratories are more likely to encounter time-dependent LACs than time-dependent acquired factor VIII inhibitors (Table 81.2).

The performance characteristics of mixing studies depend on the factor and phospholipid content of NPP, titer and strength of inhibitor, presence of multiple factor deficiencies, heparin contamination, and criteria for interpretation. Weak inhibitors or very sensitive aPTT reagents may cause substantial difficulties. Phospholipid-poor assay reagents are more sensitive to LACs, so perhaps weaker LACs are detected before mixing, but they are rapidly diluted out by 1 : 1 mixing. *If the aPTT*

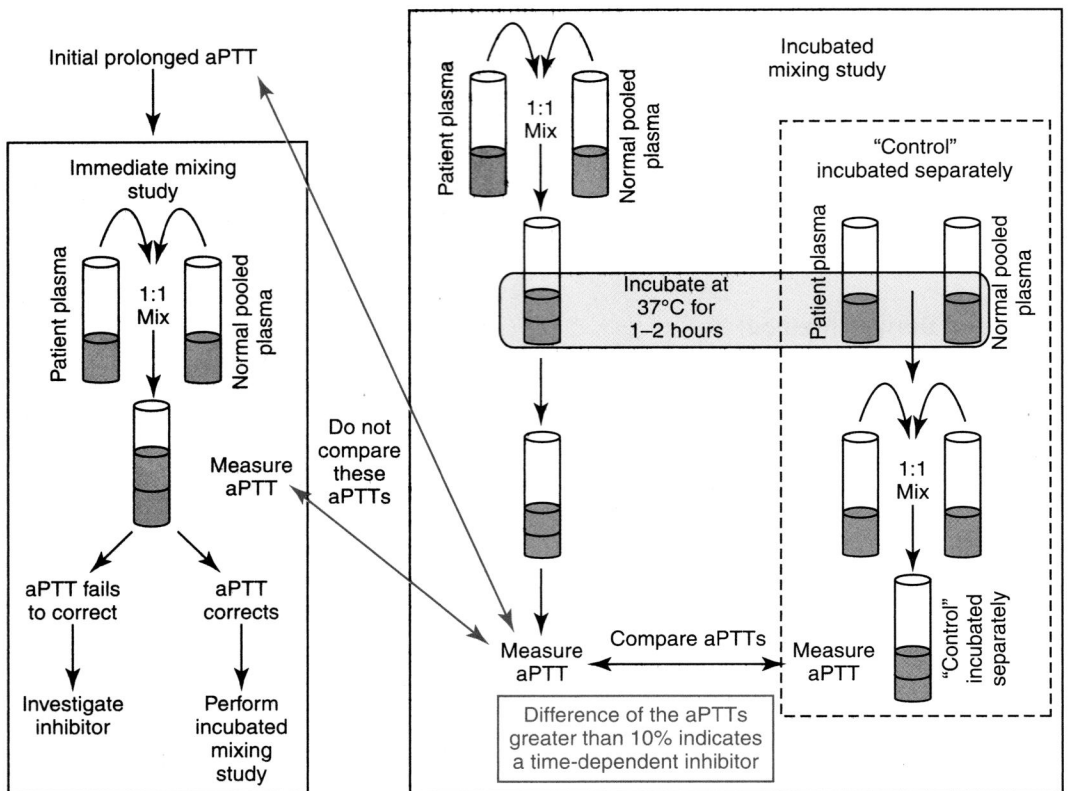

FIGURE 81.3 Sequence for the performance of mixing studies. In this example, a 1 : 1 mixing study is used. An immediate mixing study is shown on the *left*. Equal volumes of patient plasma and normal pooled plasma are mixed, and then the activated partial thromboplastin time *(aPTT)* is measured. If aPTT fails to correct (e.g., into the reference interval), there is evidence of an inhibitor and the mixing study is complete. If the immediate mixing study corrects, an incubated mixing study is needed to exclude a time-dependent inhibitor. The incubated mixing study starts with mixing equal volumes of patient plasma and normal pooled plasma. The 1 : 1 mix is incubated for 37 °C for 1 to 2 hours, and then an aPTT is performed. Interpretation of the incubated mixing study relies on the control shown in the *dashed black box,* in which patient plasma and normal pooled plasma are incubated separately (i.e., mixed after incubation) to control for loss of labile factors. The control aPTT is used for comparison with the incubated mixing study; neither the initial aPTT nor the aPTT of the immediate mix should be used for comparison.

TABLE 81.2 Prevalence of Time-Dependent Inhibitors in a Population of 300 Million

Inhibitor Type	Population Affected by Disorder	Prevalence of Inhibitor in Affected Population (%)	% Time Dependence	Number of Time-Dependent Inhibitors
Lupus anticoagulants	9×10^6	3	10	900,000
Factor VIII inhibitor in hemophilia A	30,000	15	90	4050[a]
Acquired hemophilia A	300	100	~100 (most)	~300

[a]Time-dependent inhibitors are 222 times more likely to be due to lupus anticoagulant than to specific factor VIII inhibitor.

is only minimally elevated (e.g., <5 seconds above the reference interval), 1 : 1 mixing studies are not useful, because the clotting times may correct despite the presence of an inhibitor. Some laboratories use an alternative mixing study with four parts patient plasma and one part NPP to improve sensitivity for these weak inhibitors.[13] Mixing studies certainly are not quantitative, and the clinical significance of these "weak" inhibitors is not known. NPP should be prepared from at least 20 apparently healthy individuals to ensure 100 (±20 IU/dL) of all factors. It is also important that NPP be platelet poor because contamination,

especially in frozen aliquots, may contribute to phospholipid content that will neutralize LACs. In some instances, 1 : 1 mixing may not correct when multiple factors are deficient, as may be seen in samples from patients who are supratherapeutic on VKAs. Heparin, direct thrombin inhibitors, or direct anti-Xa inhibitors also may behave like inhibitors in mixing studies. Additional clinical correlation and laboratory investigations may be needed to exclude these medications.

Interpretation of mixing studies is not always straightforward, and criteria for interpretation may vary somewhat across laboratories. Although laboratories have commonly considered correction of the immediate 1 : 1 mix to be within the reference interval (+2 standard deviations), many variations are used (e.g., +3 standard deviations of the mean aPTT). Because addition of NPP substantially dilutes weak LACs in test plasma, the requirement for correction into the reference interval may be too stringent and may result in false-negative interpretations.[14] Rosner and colleagues[15] suggested an index, and Chang and coworkers demonstrated improved performance when using a percent correction and a 4 : 1 mix.[13] The performance of the percent correction and Rosner index has been verified for LAC-sensitive aPTT 1 : 1 mixing studies in a single laboratory.[16] Currently, there is no uniformity in the performance of mixing studies, nor are there uniform criteria for interpretation; ultimately, the laboratory director must decide the appropriate approach and each result should be accompanied with an interpretation.[17]

Factor Assays

The most commonly performed factor assay is the one-stage factor assay. One-stage assays are based on the aPTT or the PT, depending on which factor is being measured. The assay is performed on dilutions of patient plasma that are then mixed 1 : 1 with factor-deficient plasma. Factor-deficient plasma is deficient in a single factor but contains essentially 100 IU/dL of all other factors. Plasma from patients with severe hemophilia has been used historically; factor-deficient plasmas manufactured by immunodepletion methods are now commercially available. Mixing of patient plasma with deficient plasma ensures that clotting times are dependent on the factor being measured. aPTT-based one-stage assays are used to measure factor activity of intrinsic factors, while PT-based assays are mostly used to measure factor VII and factors of the common pathway. Factor activity is then determined from a calibration curve created by plotting the clotting time (PT or aPTT) in seconds versus the concentration of factor (Fig. 81.4).

The aPTT-based one-stage factor VIII assay consists of a dilutional series of patient plasma samples that are then mixed with factor VIII–deficient plasma. The aPTT changes minimally when factor concentration is near 100 IU/dL; thus the initial dilution (typically 1 : 10) prolongs the aPTT into a

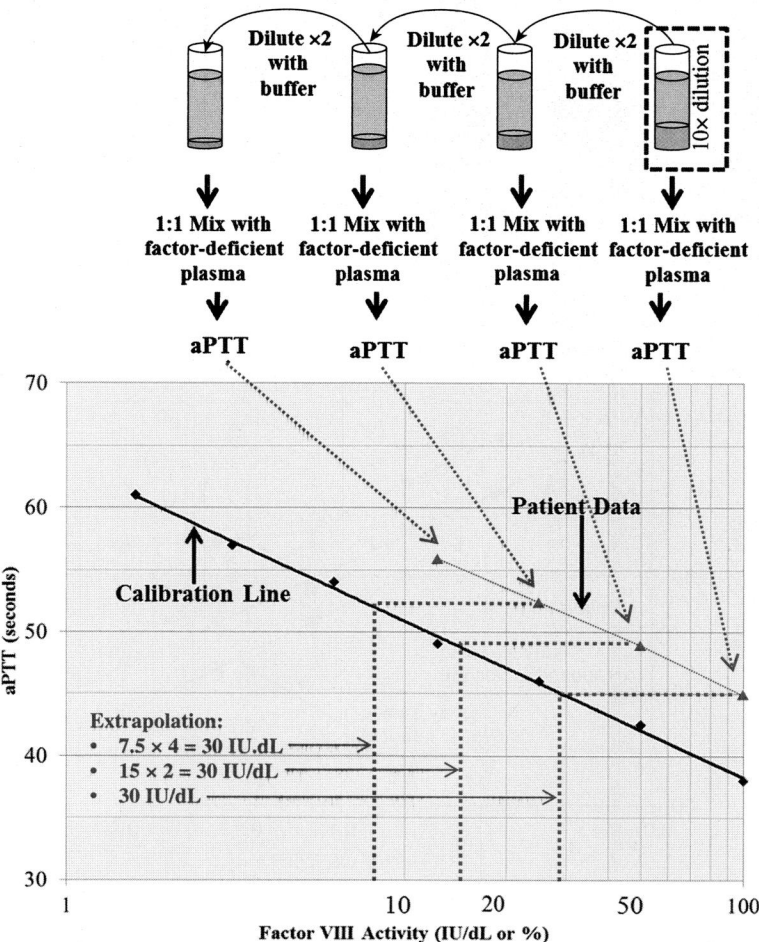

FIGURE 81.4 Activated partial thromboplastin time *(aPTT)*-based one-stage factor VIII assay. Dilutions of patient plasma into factor VIII–deficient plasma are made by starting with a 1:10 dilution. The aPTT of diluted plasmas is used to extrapolate factor VIII activity from the calibration curve. The 1:10 dilution is considered the starting point for comparison with the calibration line, which also starts with a 1:10 dilution. Each subsequent dilution in the series needs to be multiplied by a dilution factor to achieve the equivalent of the 1:10 dilution.

steeper part of the relationship between clotting time and factor activity (see Fig. 81.2). At least three dilutions are needed because clot-based tests are subject to interference from inhibitors. The aPTTs of the dilutional series are used to extrapolate factor VIII activity from the calibration line. The 1 : 10 dilution is considered the starting point for comparison with the calibration line, which also starts with a 1 : 10 dilution. Historically, calibrators were created locally by pooling large numbers of donor plasmas, and factor VIII was assumed to be 100%. However, studies demonstrated differences in factor VIII between populations. Currently, calibrators are assigned values in international units (IU) traceable to the international standard plasma established by the World Health Organization (WHO). The amount of factor VIII in 1 mL of fresh pooled plasma collected from a large number of donors was defined as 1 international unit when this unitage and the 1st WHO International Standard for FVIII was established. A calibration line is created by diluting the calibrator in a manner similar to the patient samples. Various mathematical transformations, most commonly log transformation, are employed to create a straight calibration line.

Various inhibitors such as lupus anticoagulant, anticoagulant medication, or specific factor inhibitor (e.g., factor VIII inhibitor), cause interference with the one-stage factor assay. Factor activity should be determined with at least three dilutions (e.g., 1:10, 1:20, and 1:40) to enhance accuracy and allow for detection of inhibitors by assessing parallelism between patient data and the calibration curve (Fig. 81.5). Serial dilutions, when parallel, should return the same activities after multiplying by the dilution factors. If increasing activities are obtained as dilutions increase, the patient's curve will be nonparallel to the calibration curve, and an inhibitor is suspected. Additional higher dilutions can be used in an attempt to dilute an inhibitor. When at least two consecutive dilutions produce similar activities, the inhibitor effect has been diluted out; the activity is then reported using the average of these activities, after correction for dilution. It may not be possible to dilute out strong or high titer inhibitors. The one-stage factor assay depicting elevated, reduced, and inhibited assays is shown in Fig. 81.5.

The two-stage assay is only used by specialized laboratories as an alternative method to measure factor VIII activity. The first stage involves the production of factor Xa, and the second stage determines the amount of factor Xa produced. The first stage contributes exogenous coagulation factors needed for formation of the prothrombinase complex, except for factor VIII. In this first stage, the formation of Xa depends on the amount of factor VIII in the patient's plasma. In the second stage, NPP is added to the reaction as a source of prothrombin and fibrinogen so that fibrin clotting will occur. The clotting time will be dependent on factor Xa generated in the first stage, which is dependent on factor VIII concentration; thus the clotting time in the second step is proportional to the amount of factor VIII in the patient sample. A calibration curve is then used to determine the factor VIII activity.[18]

Chromogenic factor VIII assays are based on the two-stage assay (Fig. 81.6). Similar to the two-stage assay, the first stage allows for the generation of factor Xa by the addition of reagents needed to the form intrinsic tenase complex. Calcium, phospholipid, excess purified factor IXa, and excess factor X are added such that the amount of factor Xa generated during this first stage depends on the amount of factor VIII in the patient sample. The second stage measures the absorbance developed from the enzymatic release of *p*-nitroaniline from a

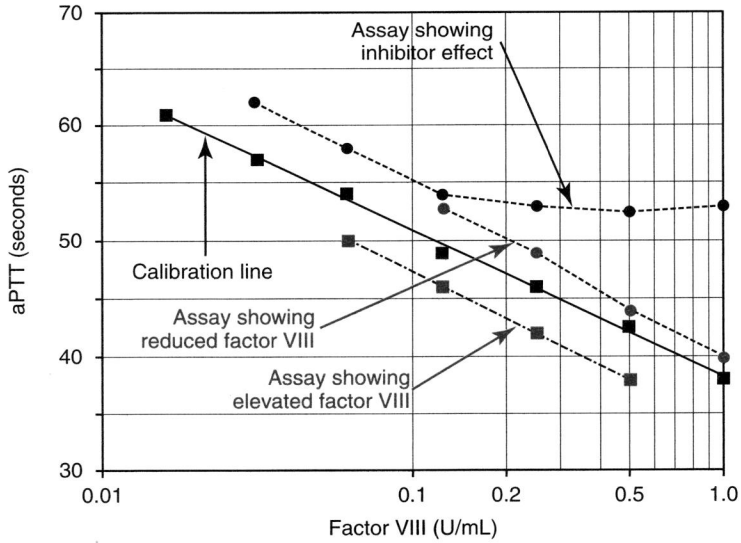

FIGURE 81.5 Factor VIII assay demonstrating the effect of an inhibitor. Parallelism should be demonstrated to ensure accurate measurement of factor activity. The dilutional series of three separate patient plasmas are shown. Parallelism between the calibration curve and the patient plasma dilutions is seen in two of the factor VIII assays *(red boxes* and *red circles)*. A third patient plasma containing lupus anticoagulant shows a nonparallel series *(black circles)*. The first three dilutions of the nonparallel series recover increasing amounts of factor activity (after correction for dilution). However, the last three dilutions show that the line becomes parallel to the calibration curve as the lupus anticoagulant is diluted out. The first two dilutions that become parallel are used to acquire an accurate factor VIII activity, by averaging factor activity after correction for dilution. *aPTT,* Activated partial thromboplastin time.

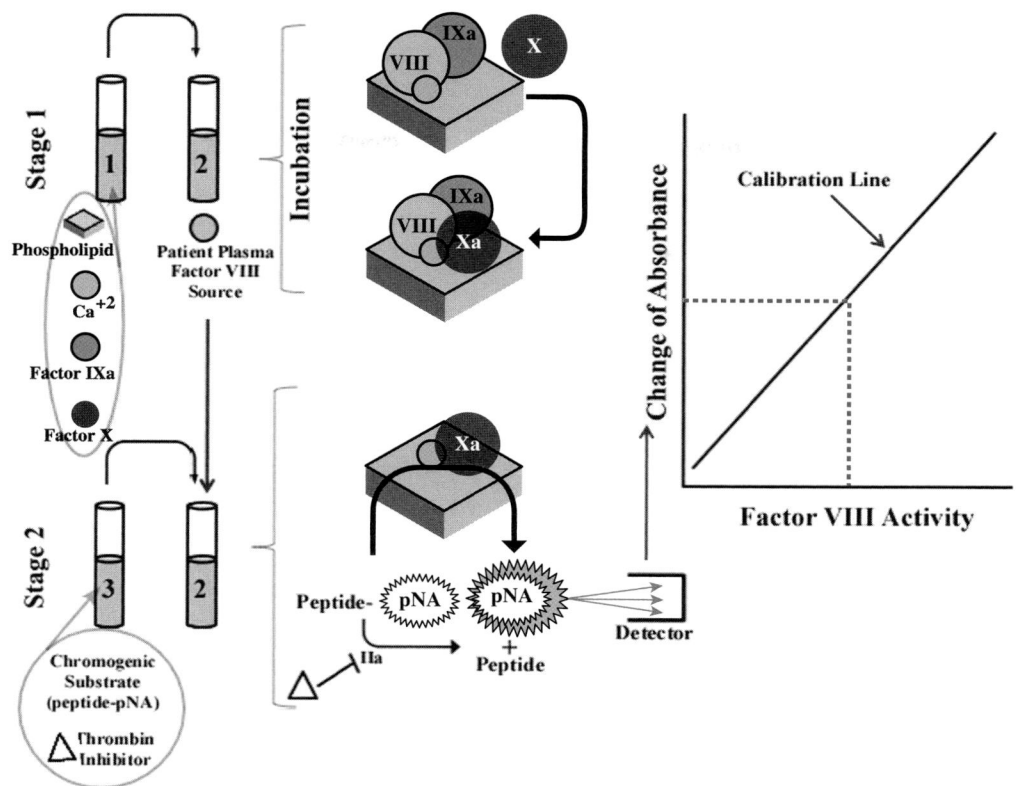

FIGURE 81.6 Schematic of the chromogenic assay for factor VIII. The chromogenic factor VIII assay is modeled after the classic two-stage factor VIII assay. The patient sample *(tube 2)* is highly diluted with buffer, allowing measurement in the presence of lupus anticoagulant. During the first stage, substrates *(tube 1)* are added to the diluted patient plasma to allow formation of the tenase complex and subsequent conversion of factor X to factor Xa. Conversion of factor X to factor Xa is dependent on factor VIII activity supplied by patient plasma. The second stage starts when chromogenic substrate is added to tube 2. Factor Xa generated during the first stage hydrolyzes the chromogenic peptide substrate and releases *p*-nitroaniline *(pNA)*. A thrombin inhibitor prevents nonspecific hydrolysis of the chromogenic substrate by thrombin. Absorbance resulting from the release of pNA is detected at 405 nm and is used to extrapolate factor VIII activity from the calibration curve.

chromogenic substrate by Xa. A direct thrombin inhibitor is often added to the second stage to decrease cleavage of the chromogenic substrate by thrombin (factor IIa). A calibration curve relates the change in absorbance at 405 nm to factor VIII activity in the specimen.[19]

(Patient plasma [source of Factor VIII] + Buffer [1:50]) + (IXa and X [excess]) + $CaCl_2$ + Phospholipid → Xa

Xa + Substrate + Direct thrombin inhibitor → p - Nitroaniline [detected at 405 nm]

Important differences have been observed in factor VIII activity depending on the method used. Two-stage assays and chromogenic assays are less sensitive to LACs[20] because of the higher initial plasma dilutions employed. Some chromogenic assays include thrombin to fully activate factor VIII to VIIIa; others rely on feedback activation of factor VIII by thrombin generation analogous to the in vivo propagation phase of coagulation. One-stage assays sometimes will overestimate factor VIII activity compared with two-stage or chromogenic assays.[21,22] It is important to keep this in mind because a one-stage assay may not exclude a mild hemophilia A, and clinical correlation with bleeding symptoms and family history may

be needed. The incubation times in the first stage of chromogenic assays are not uniform across different commercially available assays, and longer incubation times allow for the detection of some types of mild hemophilia A.[23] Less frequently, two-stage assays will recover more factor VIII activity than one-stage assays.

Factor Inhibitor Assays

Inhibitors are quantified with a functional inhibitor assay. The Bethesda assay established the framework for functional inhibitor assays and defined the Bethesda unit (BU).[24] The primary focus of this assay and unit was to create uniformity in the measurement of factor VIII inhibitors in patients with hemophilia A. This is accomplished by creating an incubated mix of patient plasma (containing the inhibitor) with NPP (containing ∼100 IU/dL factor VIII activity), and then measuring the remaining factor VIII activity. Strong inhibitors reduce the resultant factor VIII activity more than weak inhibitors do. Titration of this effect is possible using serial dilutions of patient plasma before mixing.

The Bethesda assay begins with undiluted patient plasma or dilutions of patient plasma with imidazole buffer. The patient sample is then mixed with NPP. The mixed sample is incubated for 2 hours at 37 °C, and then factor VIII is assayed. A reference mix, consisting of a 1 : 1 incubated mix of imidazole buffer and NPP, is crucial to control for loss of labile factors during incubation. The residual factor activity is calculated as follows:

Residual factor activity (%) = Factor activity (IU/mL) of patient mix/factor activity of control mix (IU/mL)

Finally, the residual factor activity is translated into Bethesda units. One BU per milliliter is defined as the inhibitor activity producing a residual factor activity of 50% of the starting concentration of factor VIII in the reference mix. A value of 2 BU/mL is then the inhibitor activity producing a residual factor activity of 25%. A log-linear graph of factor activity and BU/mL is drawn according to this definition. For ease of use, a chart relating residual factor to Bethesda unit per milliliter is constructed. Parallelism of dilutions should be expected to confirm the precision of the result.

Nijmegen modifications of the Bethesda assay improve specificity near the low analytical limit of detection (Fig. 81.7).[25] The Nijmegen modifications include replacing imidazole buffer with factor-deficient plasma for dilutions and buffering the NPP at pH 7.4. Both of these changes reduce loss of factor VIII during incubation. Buffering the NPP prevents increasing pH, and diluting with factor deficient plasma normalizes protein concentrations in the reference plasma. An additional

modification has included heating patient plasma to denature residual factor activities. Many laboratories in the North American Specialized Coagulation Laboratory (NASCOLA) survey were found to be using a hybrid of the classic Bethesda and Nijmegen procedures in which a commercially available buffered NPP was used, but imidazole buffer was used for dilutions of patient plasma. The high coefficient of variation (CV) and the variation in laboratory procedures make standard treatment guidelines based on BU/mL difficult.[26] To assay other factor inhibitors, the factor VIII deficient plasma used in the assay is replaced with the corresponding factor deficient plasma.

The behaviors of inhibitors in laboratory tests are not uniform. Although most inhibitors demonstrate an expected increase in residual factor VIII activity with increasing dilutions (type I inhibitor), some inhibitors (type II inhibitors) lack this relationship. Type II inhibitors lack parallelism to the calibration curve and may be difficult to titer. In these cases, dilutions of patient plasma corresponding to approximately 50% residual activity are used to estimate BU/mL.[27] In addition, some factor VIII inhibitors increase factor VIII clearance but do not affect factor VIII activity. These non-neutralizing factor VIII inhibitors cannot be detected with a mixing study, nor can they be titered with a functional inhibitor assay. ELISA assays for detecting factor VIII antibodies can be used to detect non-neutralizing types of inhibitors.[28]

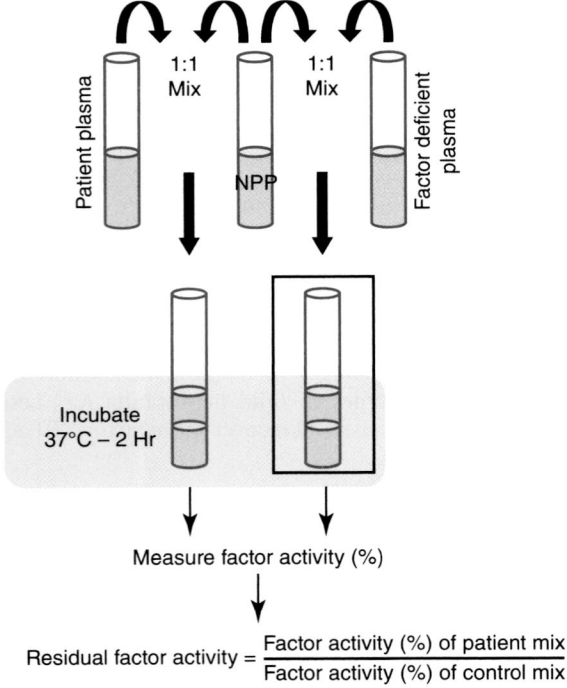

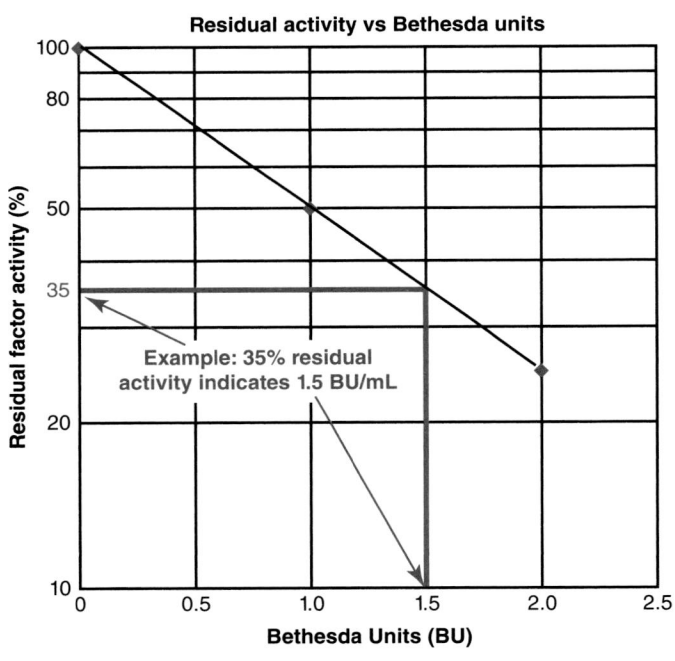

FIGURE 81.7 Schematic of the functional inhibitor assay. Patient plasma is the source of inhibitor, and buffered normal pooled plasma (NPP) is the source of coagulation factors. Patient plasma is mixed with an equal volume of buffered NPP. The mix is then incubated for 1 to 2 hours at 37 °C, allowing time-dependent inhibitors to work. A control mix consists of an incubated mix of equal volumes of factor (e.g., factor VIII)-deficient plasma (without inhibitor) and buffered NPP. One-stage factor assays are used to determine the factor activities of the patient mix and the control mix. Residual factor activity is then calculated. The definition of a Bethesda unit provides a calibration line, and residual factor activity is used to extrapolate the titer in Bethesda units/mL. When high titers of inhibitor are present, initial dilutions of the patient plasma into factor-deficient plasma are required *(not shown)*.

Factor XIII Assays

Plasma factor XIII is a zymogen that is activated by thrombin in a calcium-dependent reaction. The active enzyme catalyzes the covalent cross-linking of fibrin molecules and polymers, producing a stable clot. Factor XIIIa is a transglutaminase that links glutamine residues to lysine residues via the transfer of an acyl group and the release of ammonia. Because noncovalently linked fibrin polymer is sufficiently stable to support the end point in these tests, factor XIIIa activity is not reflected in clot-based assays such as aPTT and PT.

The urea solubility screen, or a variation thereof, is a common screening method for factor XIII deficiency. Before the actions of factor XIIIa take place, fibrin polymer structure is held together by hydrogen bonds and is soluble when subjected to weak alkalis and acids[29] or to high concentrations of solute such as urea. This is the basis of factor XIII screening methods. In the urea solubility screen, fibrin clot is formed from citrated patient plasma and then is suspended in 6 mol/L urea. The clot is visually observed at intervals for dissolution. Covalently linked fibrin clots do not dissolve. Noncovalently linked fibrin clots are dissolved after 1 to 3 hours in severe factor XIII–deficient plasmas. A fibrin clot prepared from NPP serves as the control. This method detects only very severe factor deficiency, as very little factor XIIIa activity is required to stabilize a fibrin clot.

Data from UK National External Quality Assessment Scheme (NEQAS) Surveys demonstrated variability in screening methods.[30] Fibrin clots were achieved with calcium alone, calcium and thrombin, or thrombin alone; moreover, when thrombin was used, the concentration was not uniform. Acetic acid, urea, and monochloroacetic acid were used as solvents. Altogether, 15 different combinations of solvents and clot preparations were used, contributing to variable responses. Further evaluation of plasmas spiked with factor XIII confirmed that a combination of thrombin and acetic acid provided the best sensitivity, which was in the interval of 1 IU/dL to 5 IU/dL factor XIII. Positive solubility screens for factor XIII need confirmation by quantitative methods that may be factor XIII antigen assays or factor XIII activity assays.[31]

Thrombin Time

TT is a clot-based assay reflecting two steps: conversion of fibrinogen to fibrin monomer by thrombin and polymerization of fibrin monomers. A low concentration of thrombin (final concentration of 0.1 to 0.3 U/mL depending on source of thrombin) is added to citrated plasma, fibrin is generated, and the time it takes to form the clot is measured.

Patient plasma (undiluted) + Thrombin (low concentration) → Fibrin clot

Note that TT is different from the Clauss fibrinogen measurement: in the Clauss fibrinogen method, patient plasma is diluted, and a higher concentration of thrombin is used. Although TT is still sensitive to low fibrinogen concentrations, TT is more sensitive to thrombin inhibitors, abnormal fibrinogen (dysfibrinogen), and substances that interfere with fibrin polymerization compared with the Clauss fibrinogen assay. Thrombin inhibitors prolong TT and are commonly encountered as therapeutic anticoagulants, including heparin and direct thrombin inhibitors. Because these inhibitors may interfere with other clot-based tests, many laboratories use TT as a tool to detect the

unexpected presence of these therapeutic agents. If TT is used for this purpose, the laboratory should determine the responsiveness of its TT assay to direct thrombin inhibitors and heparin. TT assays with low concentrations of thrombin (0.1 U/mL) are exquisitely sensitive to subtherapeutic levels of unfractionated heparin (0.2 IU/mL), resulting in TT greater than 120 seconds. TT is also very sensitive to direct thrombin inhibitors like argatroban or dabigatran. TT is less responsive to low molecular weight heparin (LMWH), which produces mild to moderate elevations in TT.

Inhibitors to bovine thrombin and/or factor V occur in some individuals exposed to topical bovine thrombin during surgical procedures. Bovine thrombin combined with a source of fibrinogen, such as cryoprecipitate, is an effective hemostatic agent. However, topical bovine thrombin preparations also contain bovine factor V, so inhibitors to both bovine factors II and V can be produced. Bovine factor V inhibitors may cross-react with human factor V to produce bleeding, but cross-reactivity of bovine thrombin inhibitors with human thrombin is rare. There is, however, prolongation of the TT if bovine thrombin is used for TT assays instead of human thrombin; this will be confirmed by a normal TT using human thrombin.

TT may be prolonged in the presence of structurally abnormal fibrinogens, called dysfibrinogens. Congenital dysfibrinogenemia occurs only rarely, and it is much more common to see acquired dysfibrinogenemia. Individuals with dysfibrinogenemia are typically asymptomatic, but some may be at risk for bleeding or thrombosis. Both bleeding and thrombosis may occur in the same patient. Liver and biliary diseases are common causes of acquired dysfibrinogenemia and produce fibrinogen molecules with increased sialylation of carbohydrate moieties. As a result, an increase in negative charge retards fibrin polymerization[32] and prolongs the TT. TT and the closely related reptilase time are considered initial screening tests for dysfibrinogenemia. The laboratory diagnosis of dysfibrinogenemia is confirmed by finding a discrepancy in the ratio of fibrinogen clotting activity to the fibrinogen antigen concentration.[33]

Prolonged TTs occur in a wide variety of settings and are not specific for dysfibrinogenemia (Table 81.3). For example, substances that prolong TT include paraproteins, fibrinogen degradation products, and high fibrinogen concentrations. Paraproteins affecting TTs may be of any heavy chain and are seen in the clinical setting of Waldenström macroglobulinemia or multiple myeloma. Paraproteins may affect other tests of hemostasis, including aPTT and bleeding time.[34] These patients may even have clinical symptoms of bleeding, but it is not possible to predict bleeding based on any laboratory test. Increased FDPs and increased fibrinogen, by virtue of their structural similarities to fibrin, may prolong the TT by competing with normal fibrin monomers in the polymerization process. High concentrations of FDPs are seen in DIC and after fibrinolytic therapy. High concentrations of fibrinogen are commonly encountered as part of an acute-phase reaction in hospitalized patients. Thus fibrinogen assays are useful in the evaluation of prolonged TT.

CLINICAL APPLICATION OF LABORATORY TESTS FOR COAGULATION DISORDERS

Laboratory tests described earlier are used in the diagnosis and evaluation of inherited and acquired disorders of coagulation.

TABLE 81.3 Thrombin Time in Various Clinical Settings

Clinical Settings	Thrombin Time	Mechanism
Inherited dysfibrinogenemia	Prolonged	Inhibition of fibrinopeptide A and B Inhibition of fibrin monomer polymerization
Acquired dysfibrinogenemia	Prolonged[a]	Inhibition of fibrin monomer polymerization
AL amyloidosis	Prolonged	Unknown
Monoclonal immunoglobulins	Prolonged	Inhibition of thrombin Inhibition of fibrin monomer polymerization
Fibrin degradation products	Prolonged	Inhibition of fibrin monomer polymerization
Low fibrinogen	Prolonged	Decreased fibrinogen substrate
Elevated fibrinogen	Prolonged	Interference with fibrin-monomer polymerization
Medications/Iatrogenic Settings		
Argatroban	Prolonged	Inhibition of thrombin
Hirudin and related medications	Prolonged	Inhibition of thrombin
Unfractionated heparin	Prolonged	Inhibition of thrombin
Fractionated heparin	Prolonged	Inhibition of thrombin
Bovine thrombin, topical	Prolonged	Development of alloantibodies to thrombin[a]
Dextran	Shortened	Increased rate of fibrin monomer polymerization
Hydroxyethyl starch	Shortened	Unknown
Thrombolytics (urokinase, tissue plasminogen activator)	Prolonged	Inhibition of fibrin monomer polymerization secondary fibrin degradation products Decreased fibrinogen substrate
Radiocontrast agents	Prolonged	Inhibition of fibrin monomer generation and polymerization

[a]Thrombin time is most commonly affected when bovine thrombin is used as a reagent.
Modified from Cunningham MT, Brandt JT, Laposata M, Olson JD. Laboratory diagnosis of dysfibrinogenemia. *Arch Pathol Lab Med* 2002;126:499–505.

Inherited Coagulation Disorders

The most common inheritable bleeding disorders resulting from coagulation factor deficiencies include (1) hemophilia A (factor VIII deficiency), (2) hemophilia B (factor IX deficiency), and (3) factor XI deficiency (historically referred to as hemophilia C). In the laboratory, deficiencies of the intrinsic pathway produce isolated prolongation of aPTT. Factor XII, prekallikrein, or HMWK deficiency are in the differential diagnosis of isolated prolongation of aPTT, but these contact factor deficiencies do not cause clinical bleeding. LACs prolong the aPTT, but are paradoxically associated with thrombosis. Only rare cases of LAC hypoprothrombinemia syndrome are associated with bleeding.[35]

Inherited factor VII deficiency, or less likely mild factor X, V, or II deficiency, causes isolated prolongation of the PT without prolongation of the aPTT. Factor VII deficiency is the most common of these inherited deficiencies, with factor activities typically in the range of 0 to 20 IU/dL. Factor VII Padua, a factor VII variant, causes variable responsiveness to thromboplastins derived from rabbits, humans, and oxen. Factor VII Padua is probably not associated with a risk for hemorrhage, but it produces interlaboratory discrepancy in PT/INR and factor VII results.[36] Consequently, laboratories using rabbit thromboplastin will find decreased factor VII activity, laboratories using ox thromboplastin will find normal factor VII, and laboratories using human thromboplastin will find intermediate factor VII activity. Factor VII Padua is considered a type 2 deficiency because factor VII activity is decreased (using rabbit reagent), but factor VII antigen is normal. Recognizing factor VII Padua is valuable to explain discrepant laboratory values and to avoid unnecessary treatment or procedure delays.

Clinically significant single deficiencies of factors X, V, II, or fibrinogen prolong both PT and aPTT. aPTT mixing studies show a factor deficiency, and factor activity is markedly decreased. Inherited afibrinogenemia or hypofibrinogenemia also causes prolongation of PT and aPTT, and mixing studies of patient plasma and normal pooled plasma demonstrates a factor deficiency. A functional fibrinogen assay shows markedly decreased fibrinogen. In all cases of inherited deficiency, clinical correlation with a bleeding and family history is needed to make a diagnosis.

Two rare inherited deficiencies of multiple factors are combined factor V and factor VIII deficiency (F5F8D) and vitamin K–dependent clotting factor deficiency (VKCFD).[37] In F5F8D, *LMAN1* or *MCFD2* mutations disrupt the transport of coagulation cofactors from the endoplasmic reticulum to the Golgi apparatus.[38] F5F8D is inherited in an autosomal recessive pattern and reduces cofactors to a range of 5 to 30 IU/dL. F5F8D causes epistaxis, menorrhagia, and bleeding associated with injury or surgery, but other phenotypic consequences have not been described in humans. VKCFD is caused by mutations in γ-carboxylase or vitamin K epoxide reductase that interfere with the vitamin K cycle. Vitamin K–dependent factors are not γ-carboxylated and do not obtain full activity. Intracranial hemorrhage in neonates has been described that is partially responsive to replacement of vitamin K. Antibiotics that decrease vitamin K–producing gut flora also can exacerbate deficiency and have been associated with reports of hemarthrosis and mucocutaneous hemorrhage. Skeletal abnormalities also have been described, presumably because of lack of γ-carboxylation of proteins involved in bone metabolism.[39]

AT A GLANCE
Isolated Prolongation of Activated Partial Thromboplastic Time

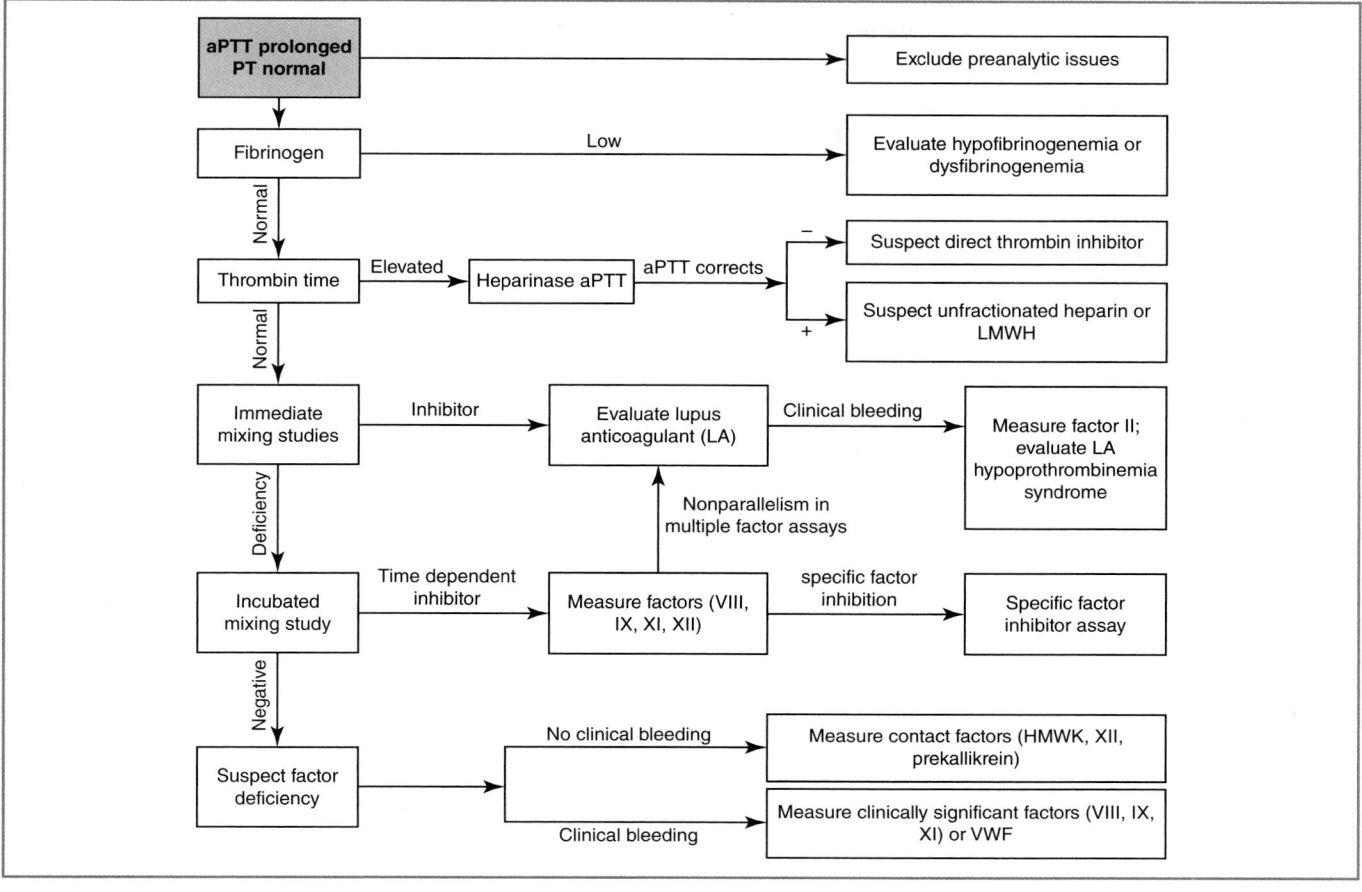

Factor XIII deficiency is a rare disorder of secondary hemostasis with a bleeding phenotype and normal PT, aPTT, TT, and fibrinogen.[31] A urea solubility test demonstrates dissolution of fibrin clot in 1 to 2 hours. Low factor XIII can be confirmed with antigen or activity assays. Platelet function and studies of fibrinolysis are normal.

POINTS TO REMEMBER
Inherited Factor Deficiencies

- Contact factor deficiencies (i.e., prekallikrein, factor XII, and HMWK) are not associated with clinical bleeding.
- Factor VIII, IX, and XI deficiency causes hemophilia A, B, and C, respectively.
- Factor VII deficiency can be associated with clinical bleeding.
- Common pathway factor deficiency (i.e., factor X, factor V, prothrombin, or fibrinogen) is associated with bleeding.
- Factor XIII deficiency is associated with bleeding.
- Combined factor deficiency of factor V and factor VIII result from mutations in the LMAN1/MCFD2-dependent secretory pathway.
- Combined deficiency of vitamin K–dependent clotting factors is caused by mutations in γ-glutamyl carboxylase or vitamin K 2,3-epoxide reductase (VKOR)

Factor VIII Deficiency (Hemophilia A)

Factor VIII deficiency is an X-linked recessive genetic disorder with an incidence of 1 in 5000 live male births. Because one third of mutations occur spontaneously, a family history is not always present. Severity of bleeding correlates with the amount of factor VIII with activities of (1) less than 1 IU/dL, (2) 1 to 5 IU/dL, and (3) greater than 5 to 40 IU/dL associated with severe, moderate, and mild hemophilia A, respectively.[40]

Laboratory studies of individuals with factor VIII deficiency show isolated prolongation of aPTT and normal PT. A normal TT is helpful to exclude heparin contamination as a cause for prolonged aPTT. Mixing studies should help identify a factor deficiency. Factor activities of the intrinsic pathway should be measured to confirm suspicion of an intrinsic pathway deficiency. In a male patient, factor VIII, IX, and XI activity should be measured. Female carriers may have mildly reduced factor VIII activity and mild bleeding symptoms, but investigation of factor XI deficiency and VWD is probably best considered first in females. Because factor VIII is elevated in response to stress and exercise, confirmation of carrier status is best confirmed with molecular studies. Decreased factor VIII activity with normal activity of factors IX and XI is expected in hemophilia A. Patients with normal factor VIII with a one-stage assay, but significantly lower values with a two-stage assay or chromogenic assay, most

AT A GLANCE

Isolated Prolongation of Prothrombin Time

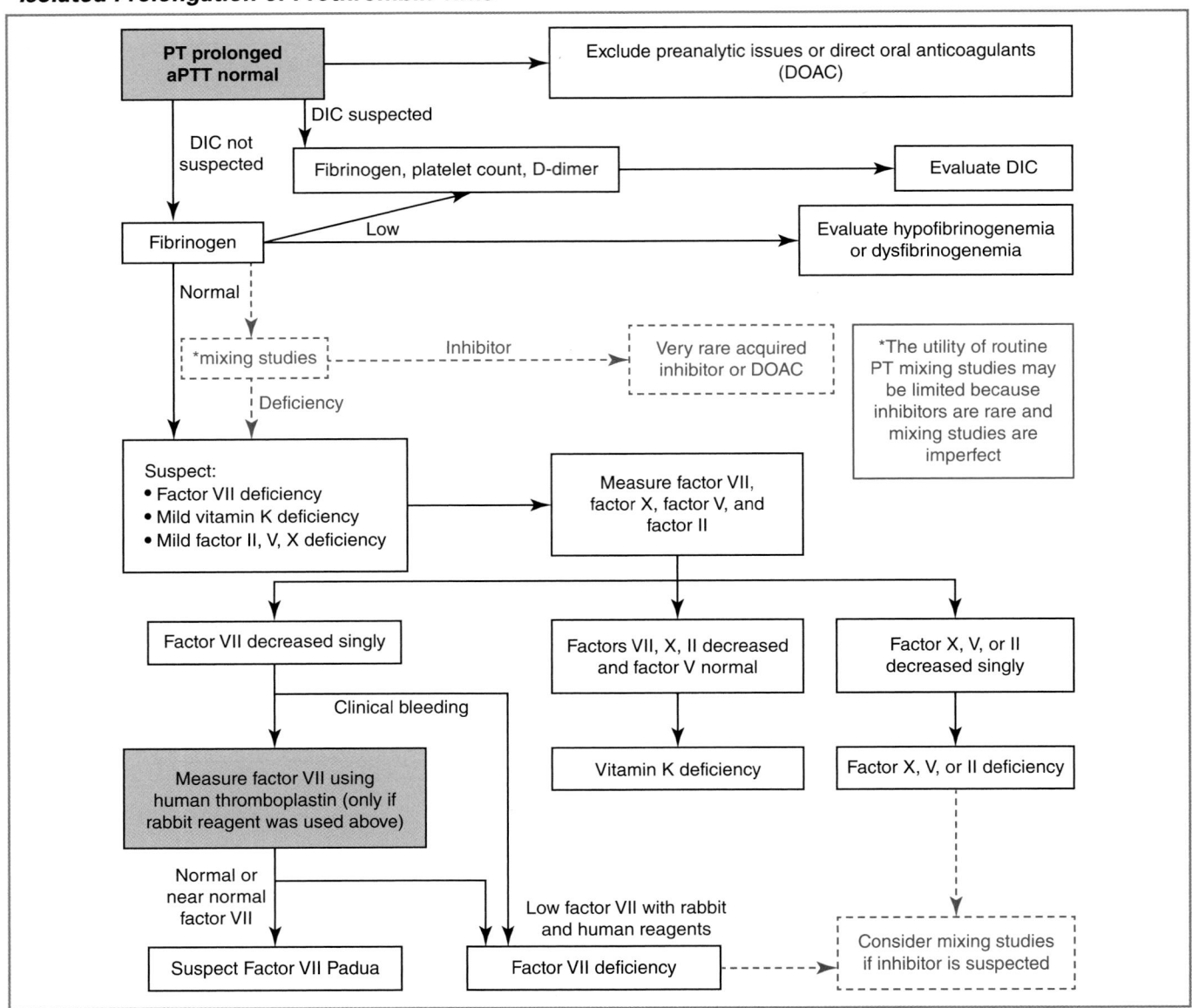

frequently present clinically like a mild hemophilia and have been referred to as mild discrepant hemophilia A. Up to 40% of mild hemophilia A patients may have discrepant results.[21,22] Patients with lower factor VIII with the one-stage assay generally have absent or mild bleeding; however, rare patients with a "reverse" discrepancy do have significant bleeding tendency.[41] For these reasons, the World Federation of Hemophilia has recommended performing both the one-stage and chromogenic (or two-stage) assays at diagnosis.[42]

Patients with other inherited bleeding disorders also present with a low factor VIII. Most VWD patients present with an isolated prolongation of aPTT and low factor VIII activity, so evaluation of VWD is warranted in some cases before a diagnosis is rendered. The distinction of hemophilia A from type 2N VWD is particularly difficult. Type 2N VWD is caused by decreased affinity of VWF for factor VIII, so patients have

decreased factor VIII because it is not protected by binding to VWF. The distinction of type 2N VWD and hemophilia A can be accomplished with a careful family history, a VWF:VIII binding assay (which is performed only at very specialized laboratories), or genetic testing. VWD type 2N is inherited in an autosomal recessive pattern, rather than an X-linked inheritance pattern such as in hemophilia A. A family history of hemophilia may be absent in up to 30% of infant males with hemophilia A, because of spontaneous mutations. Genetic testing to identify a specific factor VIII mutation may be useful in prenatal testing of carrier females. Ultimately the family and clinical history is needed to make a confident diagnosis of an inherited bleeding disorder.

Factor VIII activity is used to monitor factor VIII replacement therapy—the mainstay of prophylaxis and of management of an acute bleeding event. When postinfusion recovery of factor VIII activity is lower than anticipated or the patient fails to respond clinically, a factor VIII inhibitor is suspected. The aPTT is prolonged, but in this case, mixing studies suggest an inhibitor. **Most factor VIII inhibitors are time dependent**; thus an immediate aPTT mixing study may correct the prolonged aPTT. However, an incubated aPTT mixing study reveals prolongation compared with the appropriate control. Factor VIII inhibitor is quantified with a Bethesda assay, and the titer is used to guide therapeutic decisions. Patients with an inhibitor titer of less than 5 BU/mL may respond to high doses of factor replacement; conversely, patients with higher titers are not likely to respond and require alternative treatment. Anamnestic responses may occur, in which low or undetectable inhibitor titers rise 4 to 7 days after re-exposure to factor VIII. Inhibitors have been reported in 10 to 25% of patients and are associated with certain molecular defects in the *F8* (for factor VIII) gene. Most inhibitors occur in severe factor VIII deficiency, but inhibitors may occur in mild disease. Alternative treatments for patients with inhibitors have included replacement with porcine factor VIII or products with factor VIII–bypassing activity, such as recombinant activated factor VIIa concentrate or activated prothrombin complex concentrates.[43] These latter two products activate factor X without factor VIII or IX.

Factor IX Deficiency (Hemophilia B)

Factor IX deficiency, also known as hemophilia B or Christmas disease, is a heritable X-linked recessive bleeding disorder. The incidence is approximately 1 in 30,000 males. Similar to that of hemophilia A, the bleeding manifestations correspond closely to the amount of factor IX activity. Compared to hemophilia A, a lower proportion of these patients inherit severe deficiency.

The laboratory approach to diagnosis is similar to that for hemophilia A. When an isolated prolonged aPTT is present, investigation with mixing studies helps identify a factor deficiency. Measured factor IX activity is low with normal factor VIII and XI activity.

The mainstay of treatment for bleeding episodes with these patients is infusion of factor IX concentrates. The amount infused depends on the severity of bleeding, site of the bleeding, and size of the patient. In susceptible individuals, infusion may induce the development of alloantibodies to factor IX. The incidence of inhibitor formation in hemophilia B is approximately 1 to 3% — much lower than that in hemophilia A. The development of inhibitors can be preceded or accompanied by an allergic or anaphylactic reaction. Bleeding episodes with a factor IX inhibitor titer less than 5 BU/mL in patients who do not produce a significant anamnestic reaction are treated with factor IX concentrates. Higher inhibitor titers (≥5 BU/mL) and high responders

require infusion of products that bypass factor IX (e.g., recombinant factor VIIa).

Monitoring Factor Concentrate Therapy (Hemophilia A and B)

Factor replacement is used in the immediate setting to treat bleeding episodes and prevent surgical bleeding. Target factor concentration is designated according to the risk for bleeding. High-risk sites of bleeding, such as the central nervous system, deep muscle, neck, and gastrointestinal tract, often require a high target factor VIII (e.g., 80 to 100 IU/dL), whereas lower-risk sites of bleeding call for a lower target factor VIII (e.g., 40 to 60 IU/dL for joint and superficial muscle bleeds without neurovascular compromise). Similarly, initial prophylaxis before major surgery requires an 80 to 100 IU/dL target and minor surgery requires a lower target of 40 to 80 IU/dL. Postoperative targets, postbleed maintenance targets, and duration of therapy are also outlined in guidelines from the World Federation of Hemophilia.[42] Monitoring in these settings involves a preinfusion and 15-minute postinfusion sample. Although imperfect, a rule of thumb is 1 unit of factor VIII per kilogram of body weight generally increases the plasma factor VIII by 2 IU/dL. Preinfusion factor VIII results, along with the target concentration, are used to calculate the initial dose (Table 81.4). The 15-minute postinfusion dose is used to assess recovery. Recovery varies among individuals, and subsequent doses are based on recovery of the specific product and the half-life of factor VIII. Low recovery can be an indication of a factor VIII inhibitor.

Early prophylactic factor VIII therapy in children with severe hemophilia A can decrease bleeding episodes and prevent joint damage. This approach is well accepted, but the dose regimen is not uniform and often may be individualized for patients. A commonly used protocol is 25 to 40 IU/kg given 3 days/wk.[42] Another rule of thumb is the plasma factor VIII trough should be kept greater than 1 IU/dL to prevent joint disease, but some studies have shown that this may not necessarily be the case. Because factor concentrates are expensive, it is desirable to give the least amount of factor necessary to treat patients. Some hemophilia centers have used pharmacokinetic studies to calculate the minimum dose needed to achieve a trough greater than 1 IU/dL, whereas others have relied more heavily on the clinical bleeding pattern to individualize doses.[44,45] However, trough levels are not routinely measured because 1 IU/dL is too close to the lower limit of the analytical measurement range.

The approach to replacement therapy for hemophilia B is similar to that of hemophilia A with a few differences. Plasma-derived factor IX concentrates, recombinant factor IX, or activated prothrombin complex concentrate are used

TABLE 81.4 Estimating Initial Factor Concentrate Dose Using Target Factor Concentration and Preinfusion Plasma Factor Level

Factor Concentrate	Formula	
Plasma-derived factor VIII	Body weight in kilograms × Target concentration × 0.5 = Dose of factor in units.	
Plasma-derived factor IX	Body weight in kilograms × Target concentration = Dose of factor in units.	
Recombinant factor IX	Adults	Body weight in kilograms × Target concentration = Dose of factor in units ÷ 0.8
	Children	Body weight in kilograms × Target concentration = Dose of factor in units ÷ 0.7

for replacement. The in vivo recovery is different from that of factor VIII replacement. Factor IX concentrates typically raise the plasma factor IX activity by 1 IU/dL, but recombinant products have less recovery. Initial dose is estimated based on these relationships (see Table 81.4). Because factor IX has a longer half-life, long-term prophylaxis is commonly dosed 2 days per week instead of 3.[42]

Both chromogenic and one-stage factor assays are calibrated to WHO international plasma standards; however, major discrepancies arise when monitoring response to recombinant or modified factor VIII and IX concentrates.[46] Some full-length recombinant factor VIII concentrates produce 30 to 50% more factor VIII activity using chromogenic assays compared to one-stage factor assays when all methods are calibrated with a plasma standard. This is also the case for some recombinant B-domain deleted factor concentrates in which chromogenic assay produces results approximately 50% higher than those obtained by one-stage assays when both methods are calibrated using a plasma standard.[47] Additionally, large discrepancies occur among various one-stage assays in these post-treatment plasma samples. In many instances, calibration of one-stage factor assays with product-specific reference material significantly reduces discrepancies; however, this approach has not yet been widely applied to clinical practice.[47,48] Recombinant factor IX concentrates have also produced discrepancies between chromogenic and one-stage assays.

The engineered extended half-life factor VIII and factor IX concentrates entering the market produce even larger discrepancies, so manufacturers and laboratories will need to define appropriate methodologies for monitoring these products. These products are recombinant factors modified by mechanisms such as covalent binding of factor subunits,

glycopegylation, or fusion with albumin or the Fc portion of immunoglobulin. Although many aPTT based one-stage factor assays can be used to monitor most of the extended half-life factor, some commonly used one-stage factor reagents (i.e., aPTT reagents) should not be used because they significantly over- or underestimate the factor activity.[49–54] Most extended half-life products can be monitored with chromogenic assays, but these methods may not be offered by local laboratories. Table 81.5 and Table 81.6 summarize the monitoring methods for extended half-life factor VIII and factor IX products, respectively.

A new therapeutic product, emicizumab, is now widely used to treat hemophilia A. Emicizumab, or Hemlibra®, is a humanized bispecific monoclonal antibody that simulates factor VIIIa activity by engaging factor IXa and factor X. Emicizumab is advantageous because it is dosed once per week (with monthly injections likely in the future) as a subcutaneous injection, improving the quality of life of patients with hemophilia A with or without factor VIII inhibitors. Emicizumab has created significant challenges for laboratories because it prohibits monitoring of patient endogenous factor activity with routine aPTT-based coagulation tests. Emicizumab shortens the aPTT into or below the reference interval due to its ability to mimic VIIIa, hence the aPTT-based one-stage factor assays, including factor VIII, yield falsely elevated results. Any tests based on aPTT, including lupus anticoagulant tests, activated protein C resistance, some protein C assays, and some protein S assays, are also affected. PT is affected minimally but is not considered clinically significant. PT-based factor assays, thrombin time, Clauss fibrinogen, and immunoassays are not affected.[55,56]

Patients on emicizumab with breakthrough bleeding are treated with recombinant factor VIIa, factor VIII, or activated prothrombin complex concentrates. Although experience is

TABLE 81.5 Factor VIII Extended Half-Life Products

Factor VIII Product	Modification	Monitoring Method
Eloctate®; rFVIIIFc	Fc fusion BDD rFVIII	Most one-stage assays are adequate Chromogenic is adequate
Adynovate®; BAX855	Pegylated rFVIII	Most one-stage assays are adequate Chromogenic is adequate
Afstyla®; rFVIII-Single Chain	Single chain BD truncated rFVIII	Most one-stage assays are adequate but must be multiplied by 2 Chromogenic is adequate
Esperoct®; N8 GP	glycopegylated rFVIII	Avoid one-stage assays with APTT-SP and Synthasil/Siemens Instrument Chromogenic is adequate
Jivi®; Bay 94 9027	pegylated BDD rFVIII	Avoid APTT-SP and APTT-A Chromogenic is adequate

TABLE 81.6 Factor IX Extended Half-Life Products

Factor IX Product	Modification	Monitoring Method
Rebinyn®; N9 GP	glycopegylated rFIX	Avoid STA-PTTA, STA-C.K., Actin, Actin FS, Actin FSL, Pathromtin SL, Synthasil, APTT-SP Chromogenic is adequate
Alprolix®; rFIXFc	Fc fusion rFIX	Avoid STA-C.K. Prest Chromogenic is adequate
Idelvion®; FIX-albumin	Albumin fusion rFIX	Avoid STA-C.K., Actin FS, Actin FSL, and SynthAFax Chromogenic may not be suitable

still limited, guidelines for management of bleeding and laboratory coagulation testing are available.[57,58] In bleeding patients on emicizumab being treated with factor VIII concentrates, factor VIII activity should be measured with a chromogenic assay using *bovine factor IXa and factor X* reagents. Because factor VIII therapy may be used in bleeding patients with factor VIII inhibitor titers less than 5 BU/mL, an accurate factor VIII inhibitor titer is important. Factor VIII inhibitor assays based on one-stage assays cause false negative results, so inhibitor assays must be performed using bovine chromogenic reagents. Factor VIII inhibitor levels should be measured with the bovine chromogenic assay before and after initiation of emicizumab to verify assay performance. Assays calibrated with emicizumab can be used to provide evidence of emicizumab neutralizing antibodies, which were seen in less than 1% of patients in the clinical trials.[59] One-stage factor VIII assays, or chromogenic factor VIII assays using *human-derived* reagents, that are calibrated with emicizumab, can be used to assess emicizumab activity levels. Since the half-life of emicizumab is approximately 30 days, a low emicizumab level indicates the potential presence of an anti-emicizumab antibody.

POINTS TO REMEMBER
Emicizumab and Laboratory Testing

- Emicizumab is a humanized bispecific monoclonal antibody that mimics factor VIIIa activity by binding factor IXa and factor X.
- Emicizumab is indicated for prophylaxic therapy in hemophilia A with or without inhibitors.
- Emicizumab shortens aPTT clotting times into or below the reference interval.
- Emicizumab interferes with aPTT-based assays.
- Emicizumab falsely elevates aPTT-based one-stage factor assays, including factor VIII.
- Emicizumab produces false negative factor VIII inhibitor levels.
- Factor VIII activity and factor VIII inhibitor levels can be measured with chromogenic factor VIII using *bovine-derived* reagents.
- Emicizumab levels may be used to confirm suspicion of a neutralizing antibody against emicizumab.

Factor XI Deficiency (Hemophilia C)

Factor XI deficiency is a rare autosomal recessive disorder with a high incidence in the Ashkenazi Jewish population.[60,61] Terms for this disorder include plasma thromboplastin antecedent deficiency, Rosenthal syndrome, and hemophilia C. More recently, autosomal dominant forms have been described. The bleeding symptoms are heterogeneous, and, in contrast to factor VIII or IX deficiency, bleeding severity does not correlate well with plasma factor activity. Bleeding at mucosal sites or after surgical challenges is common, so deficiency is not discovered until adulthood in some cases.

aPTT is typically prolonged and factor XI activity is decreased. Patients with normal aPTT results have also been reported, so testing factor XI activity may be indicated in individuals with a convincing bleeding history.[62] Two mutations are responsible for most (88%) of the classic autosomal recessive disease in the Ashkenazi Jewish population;

combinations of these mutations produce factor XI activities in the 1 to 10 IU/dL interval.[60,61] Heterozygotes for factor XI present with moderately reduced factor XI activity. The relationship between factor activity and bleeding risk is not always predictable, and bleeding may occur with surgical procedures when factor XI activities are above 50 IU/dL.[63] Mixing studies of aPTT suggest a deficiency. Inhibitors may occur after treatment with plasma and may be titered with functional inhibitor assays. Inhibitors occur frequently in patients with low factor XI concentrations when exposed to plasma as replacement therapy.[64] Plasma concentrates are not available in all regions and recombinant products are not available.

Factor XIII Deficiency

Inherited deficiency of factor XIII is rare, with an estimated prevalence of 1 to 2 per million.[65] The classic presentation of umbilical stump bleeding, excessive bleeding after trauma, and abnormal scar formation was described in 1960.[66] Severe factor XIII deficiency is associated with recurrent spontaneous abortion.[67] Bleeding risk is expected when factor XIII activity falls below 3 IU/dL. Severe factor XIII deficiency is treated with fresh frozen plasma (FFP) or cryoprecipitate.

A limited number of clinical settings may warrant detection of factor XIII above 5 to 10 IU/dL.[68] Monitoring with quantitative assays may be helpful in demonstrating recovery and in timing doses. Monitoring also may be helpful during pregnancy in women with factor XIII deficiency, because a factor XIII concentration above 10 IU/mL has been suggested to support pregnancy.[65,67] Rarely, acquired deficiencies or inhibitors of factor XIII have been encountered that may be associated with greater factor XIII activity than that of classic factor XIII deficiency. Some less sensitive solubility-based screening methods may not detect these mild to moderate factor XIII deficiencies, so quantitative methods may be desirable when these clinical scenarios are evaluated.

Acquired Coagulation Disorders

Many conditions cause acquired disorders of coagulation that manifest as hemorrhage (see Table 81.1). LACs are acquired inhibitors associated with prolongation of aPTT; however, LACs are associated with thrombophilia, rather than hemorrhage. LACs will be discussed later. Specific factor inhibitors, except for factor XII inhibitor, cause a bleeding phenotype. Specific factor inhibitors prolong PT, aPTT, or both, depending on the targeted factor. The work-up for specific factor inhibitors includes demonstration of an inhibitor with mixing studies, demonstration of decreased factor activity, measurement of the inhibitor titer, and clinical correlation with a bleeding phenotype.

Anticoagulant medications including UFH, LMWH, direct thrombin inhibitors, and direct factor Xa inhibitors are examples of pharmacologic inhibitors that prolong PT and/or aPTT. Mixing studies typically demonstrate an inhibitor. Because anticoagulant medication may interfere with testing or cause unnecessary laboratory , several tests are used to evaluate these in the laboratory. TT is useful to evaluate for the presence of heparin or direct thrombin inhibitor, and anti-Xa assays may be used to evaluate for direct factor Xa inhibitor medications that are becoming widely used.

Acquired factor deficiencies often involve deficiency of multiple coagulation factors. A notable exception is the rare association of AL amyloidosis with factor X deficiency. Vitamin K deficiency or VKA therapy (discussed earlier) decreases activities of factors II, VII, IX, and X. DIC (discussed in greater detail later under "Fibrinolysis") is a pathologic disorder that consumes fibrinogen and multiple coagulation factors. Because many coagulation factors are synthesized in the hepatocytes, liver disease is associated with multiple factor deficiencies. Dilutional coagulopathy in patients receiving aggressive fluid replacement or massive transfusions of cellular components without sufficient plasma replacement is another example of acquired deficiency of multiple coagulation factors. These acquired deficiencies of multiple coagulation factors can cause isolated prolongation of PT or prolongation of both PT and aPTT. Mixing studies for aPTT can be challenging to interpret in multiple factor deficiency because a 1:1 mix may not correct the aPTT to the reference interval. In these cases, clinical correlation and additional laboratory tests, including TT and measurements of D-dimer, fibrinogen, and specific factors, are often helpful.

Liver Disease

Traditionally, severe chronic liver disease was thought to be associated with impairment of secondary hemostasis resulting in a bleeding phenotype. Hepatocytes synthesize most of the procoagulant factors; therefore cirrhosis is associated with multiple factor deficiencies and prolongation of clotting tests. Factor VIII is made by endothelial cells and is often elevated with liver disease, as part of an acute-phase reaction. PT and aPTT are usually prolonged in cirrhosis, and PT, in particular, has been used to assess bleeding risk and to guide therapy with FFP before procedures are undertaken. Unfortunately, PT does not reliably predict bleeding risk in severe liver disease.

It has been suggested that bleeding risk in cirrhosis may be partially attributed to hyperfibrinolysis due to deficiencies of naturally occurring fibrinolysis inhibitors that are produced in the liver, such as thrombin-activatable fibrinolysis inhibitor (TAFI), α_2-antiplasmin, and PAI-1. Similarly, thrombotic complications (e.g., portal vein thrombosis) in cirrhosis have been attributed to deficiencies of natural anticoagulants (e.g., PC, PS) or plasminogen, all of which are produced by the liver. Clotting assays do not reflect the contributions of these liver-derived molecules to in vivo hemostasis. Likewise, measurement of individual components of fibrinolysis or secondary hemostasis may not be informative in isolation. Modern models of hemostasis in severe liver disease suggest that it is the summative balance of secondary hemostasis and fibrinolysis that determines risk.[69] Moderate to severe thrombocytopenia associated with cirrhosis also may contribute to bleeding risk. Following platelet count is an important part of assessing bleeding risk in cirrhotic patients.

INR is used in the model for the end-stage liver disease (MELD) score, an index of severity of liver disease used to prioritize liver transplantation.[70] The current INR system was designed to monitor patients on VKA therapy. As a consequence, the international sensitivity index (ISI) does not harmonize INRs across laboratories for the purpose of monitoring liver disease. Interlaboratory variation in INR systems contributes to variation in MELD scores. Harmonizing results with a liver-specific ISI is effective,[71,72] but currently laboratories are poorly equipped to handle two INR systems and commercial thromboplastins do not have an assigned ISI for liver disease. Recent studies have shown that when the VKA ISI is close to 1, liver-specific ISI is also close to 1, which may provide some unification of liver-specific INR assessment.[73]

Vitamin K Deficiency

Vitamin K deficiency may manifest with bleeding or may be identified incidentally with an isolated prolongation of PT or combined prolongation of PT and aPTT. TT and fibrinogen are normal. Vitamin K deficiency is typically investigated clinically by treating with vitamin K in a patient with a clinical risk factor for vitamin K deficiency. Mixing studies can potentially be useful, but multiple-factor deficiency may not correct after mixing. Measuring vitamin K–dependent factors can help confirm the diagnosis. Measuring several vitamin K–dependent factors, along with at least one non–vitamin K–dependent factor for comparison, is a reasonable approach. If administration of vitamin K fails to correct the PT/INR, serum vitamin K_1 or proteins induced by VKA or absence (PIVKA-II) can be measured. PIVKA-II represents the under-carboxylated, nonfunctional form of prothrombin produced during vitamin K deficiency or during therapy with VKAs. Hence, in a vitamin K–deficient state, vitamin K will be decreased and PIVKA-II elevated. Because it has a half-life of approximately 60 hours, elevated PIVKA-II may be used to confirm vitamin K deficiency even several days after vitamin K replacement has started.[74]

Without vitamin K prophylaxis, neonates are at risk for vitamin K deficiency. The classic hemorrhagic disease of the newborn, now called vitamin K deficiency bleeding, occurs in the first week of life. Neonatal risk for vitamin K deficiency is due to a combination of low vitamin K stores at birth, inadequate vitamin K intake, and lack of intestinal flora—an important source of vitamin K. Bleeding from neonatal vitamin K deficiency is avoided by treating neonates with vitamin K, but vitamin K deficiency bleeding may still be seen in countries where access to health care is limited. Late vitamin K deficiency bleeding occurs from 2 to 24 weeks and has been most frequently attributed to inadequate or absent vitamin K prophylaxis. Formula-fed infants rarely develop vitamin K deficiency because formula is supplemented, but breastfed infants are at increased risk because of low levels of vitamin K in breast milk. Cholestasis secondary to undiagnosed hepatobiliary disease is another risk factor for late vitamin K deficiency bleeding.[75] Even in countries with prophylaxis programs, late vitamin K deficiency bleeding has occurred because of refusal of vitamin K prophylaxis.

Adult vitamin K deficiency may be due to drugs that affect vitamin K metabolism, inadequate intake, liver or biliary disease, or inadequate intestinal adsorption. Postsurgical patients receiving parenteral nutrition are at risk for acquired deficiency because the vitamin K stored in the liver can be depleted in a short time. Antibiotic therapy that alters the intestinal flora may contribute to deficiency of vitamin K.

Disseminated Intravascular Coagulation

Overt, or acute, DIC is an excessive uncontrolled thrombin generation and fibrinolysis, exceeding the regulatory capacity of the endothelium and plasma inhibitors. Fibrin thrombi are formed in the microvasculature, trapping platelets and shearing RBCs into schistocytes as they pass through the fibrin strands. Ultimately, DIC consumes coagulation factors, inhibitors, platelets, and red blood cells. Clinically, patients with DIC present with bleeding and thrombosis, although thrombosis may not be as readily apparent because these clots primarily occur in the microvasculature. Ecchymoses, petechiae, and oozing from intravenous access sites or surgical incisions are frequent hemorrhagic presentations. Occlusion of small vessels leads to end-organ damage. DIC is not a disease, but rather a manifestation of a wide variety of possible underlying disorders (see At a Glance). The clinical diagnosis begins with recognizing the thrombohemorrhagic picture, which should then trigger a search for the underlying disease process. While severe DIC often leads to a hemorrhagic clinical picture due to consumption of coagulation factors and platelets, nonovert DIC caused by a more chronic disease process may present with thrombosis or hemorrhage. In nonovert/chronic DIC, the regulatory mechanisms are not completely overwhelmed, and consumption of RBCs, platelets, and hemostatic factors is mitigated.

Because the clinical presentations and therapies for DIC vary with the underlying disease process, many forms of DIC have been studied in the context of a specific clinical scenario. Sepsis is the most common cause of DIC and is managed by treating the infection with antibiotic therapy or surgical drainage of an abscess. Nonovert, or chronic, DIC due to cancer is often associated with prothrombotic manifestations and may be treated with prophylactic anticoagulant medications, such as LMWH. Trauma-induced coagulopathy refers to DIC due to traumatic injury itself and manifests with a fibrinolytic phenotype; hence, there is interest in treating trauma-induced coagulopathy with antifibrinolytic agents. DIC caused by acute promyelocytic leukemia with t(15;17) also manifests with prominent fibrinolysis, but early therapy with all-*trans*-retinoic acid targets the underlying neoplasm and mitigates the risk of hemorrhage and thrombosis. Treatment of DIC may be supported by transfusion of blood components, anticoagulants (e.g., heparin), and/or antifibrinolytics, but definitive therapy relies predominantly on clinical management of the underlying disease process.

Stereotypical laboratory data for overt DIC include: (1) prolonged clotting times (aPTT, PT, and TT), (2) low fibrinogen, (3) elevated fibrin/FDP, (4) elevated D-dimer, (5) thrombocytopenia, and (6) anemia, often with schistocytes on a peripheral smear. Clotting times are prolonged because of hypofibrinogenemia, interference from FDPs, or consumption of coagulation factors. Prolongation of clotting assays, however, is not always present in DIC because circulating activated factors accelerate/shorten clotting times; in fact, aPTT below the reference interval can be an indicator of early DIC. Fibrinogen concentration may be low from consumption, but it is not low in every case. Likewise, platelet count varies significantly in patients with DIC, and schistocytes are not always present. Nonetheless, clotting assays, fibrinogen assays, platelet counts, and reviews of peripheral smears are important tests for evaluating DIC.

The International Society on Thrombosis and Haemostasis (ISTH) published a scoring system for the diagnosis of overt DIC (see At a Glance).[76] Since the original description, new D-dimer cut-offs and overall DIC score cut-off have been proposed.[77] Scoring systems for DIC have primarily been used as research tools but may be clinically useful to educate physicians and standardize the approach. The ISTH has also provided an approach to nonovert DIC. The diagnosis of nonovert DIC is more difficult, relying on the daily trend of laboratory test results rather than on a single set of laboratory data.

AT A GLANCE

International Society of Thrombosis and Hemostasis Criteria for Diagnosis of Overt Disseminated Intravascular Coagulation

Clinical Conditions Associated With DIC
- Sepsis, severe infection
- Trauma, burns, surgery
- Organ destruction
- Malignancy
- Obstetric calamities
- Vascular abnormalities
- Severe hepatic failure
- Severe toxic or immunologic reactions

Diagnostic Algorithm for the Diagnosis of Overt DIC
1. Risk assessment: Does the patient have an underlying disorder known to be associated with overt DIC (from list above)?
   If yes: Proceed to step 2.
   If no: Do not use this algorithm.
2. Order global coagulation tests (platelet count, prothrombin time [PT], fibrinogen, and D-dimer).
3. Score global coagulation test results.
   Platelet count (K/µL)
   ($>100 = 0$; $<100 = 1$; $<50 = 2$)
   Elevated D-dimer (µg/mL FEU)
   (D-dimer $<3 = 0$; D-dimer ≥ 3 but $< 7 = 2$; D-dimer $\geq 7 = 3$)
   Prolonged PT (seconds above reference interval)
   (<3 s $= 0$; >3 s but <6 s $= 1$; >6 s $= 2$)
   Fibrinogen level (g/L)
   ($>1 = 0$; $<1 = 1$)
4. Calculate score.
5. If ≥ 5: Compatible with overt DIC (cutoff ≥ 4 has been proposed with the D-dimer thresholds listed above).
   If < 5: Suggestive (not affirmative) for nonovert DIC; repeat score next 1 to 2 days.

TEST METHODS AND THEIR CLINICAL APPLICATION FOR FIBRINOLYSIS

Fibrinolysis is the process of converting insoluble fibrin to soluble products that are then cleared from the circulation by the liver. Fibrinolysis serves to balance the activity of coagulation. Perturbations in fibrinolysis disrupt the balance and may create risk for thrombosis or hemorrhage.

Various tests are used to evaluate fibrinolytic activity, including: (1) TT, (2) FDP assays, (3) D-dimer assays, (4) PAI-1 assays, (5) α_2-antiplasmin assays, and (6) plasminogen assays. Inherited disorders of PAI-1, α_2-antiplasmin, and plasminogen are rare and are discussed briefly with the specific tests described in the following section. Acquired fibrinolysis is most frequently encountered as DIC, a disorder of both coagulation and fibrinolysis (See previous "Disseminated Intravascular Coagulation" section).

Thrombin Time

TT was discussed in detail earlier in relation to coagulation testing. However, TT also is used in evaluation of fibrinolytic activity. Increased FDPs in settings of increased fibrinolysis such as DIC and thrombolytic therapy interfere with fibrin polymerization, prolonging the TT.

Fibrin and Fibrinogen Degradation Product Assays

Under physiologic conditions, plasmin cleaves cross-linked fibrin into soluble FDPs of various molecular weights and compositions (Fig. 81.8). If plasmin activity exceeds the capacity of antiplasmin activity in the circulation, fibrinogen may be cleaved into fibrinogen degradation products. Fibrinogen is cleaved into high molecular weight fragments, known as X and Y fragments. Further enzymatic degradation yields lower molecular weight D and E fragments.[78] Collectively, fibrin and fibrinogen products are referred to as FDP. FDP titers are determined by immunoassays, usually manual semiquantitative latex-agglutination immunoassays using monoclonal antibodies raised against FDP. Serum is tested in assays that employ antibodies that are reactive against fibrinogen; plasma or serum may be used in assays employing antibodies without fibrinogen reactivity.

Primary fibrinolysis is part of the normal hemostatic process. When increased plasmin activity (e.g., from increased urokinase after prostate surgery) is the prevailing pathologic issue, the process is referred to as secondary fibrinolysis and may be associated with bleeding. The clinical utility of FDP assays is limited because of poor low-end sensitivity compared to that of many current quantitative D-dimer assays.

D-Dimer Assays

D-Dimer moieties are formed specifically by the cross-linkage of D-domain subunits of fibrin strands by factor XIIIa. D-Dimers are detected in plasma after plasmin has enzymatically cleaved cross-linked fibrin clot (see Fig. 81.8). Therefore detection of D-dimer in plasma signifies cleavage of cross-linked fibrin, but not

cleavage of fibrinogen, fibrin monomers, or non–cross-linked fibrin strands. Quantitative D-Dimer assays are useful for the evaluation of DIC and, if the assay has sufficient negative predictive value, for the evaluation of patients with DVT or pulmonary embolism.[79]

Immunoassays used to measure concentrations of D-dimer include ELISA, immunoturbidimetric assay, LIA techniques, and luminescence immunoassay. Semiquantitative tests by latex agglutination generally lack sensitivity and are inappropriate for exclusion of thromboembolism. FDP containing D-dimer moieties are not uniform, and various dimer, trimer, and tetramer species of fragments occur. Also, monoclonal antibodies vary in their ability to recognize the wide variety of D-dimer species, and calibrators vary in their content of these D-dimer species. This variability has led to considerable difficulty in standardizing D-dimer assays. Therefore rather than standardization, international efforts have focused on harmonization of D-dimer testing. Further difficulty has arisen from inconsistency in reported D-dimer units. It is imperative that both the unit type and the unit of concentration are reported correctly. D-Dimer units may be D-dimer units (D-DU) or fibrinogen equivalent units (FEU). D-DU (185 kDa) is approximately half the weight of FEU (340 kDa). The appropriate unit type (D-DU vs. FEU) and unit of concentration (e.g., nanogram per milliliter, microgram per liter) are determined by the calibrator used in the assay and should be available in the package insert. Using the wrong units may result in poor interlaboratory agreement (failed proficiency testing) and, more importantly, improper laboratory thresholds for excluding DVT and pulmonary embolism (PE).[80,81] The clinical utility of D-dimer is discussed in the previous section "Disseminated Intravascular Coagulation" and following section "D-Dimer for Exclusion of Venous Thromboembolism."

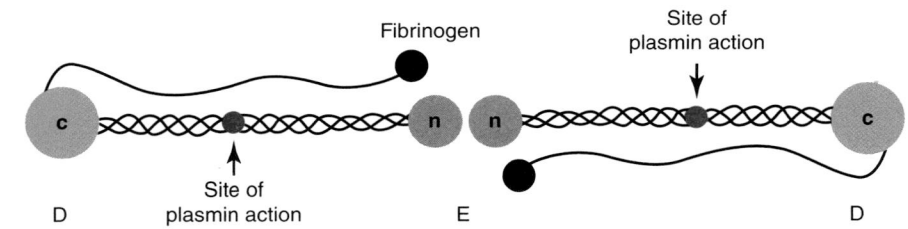

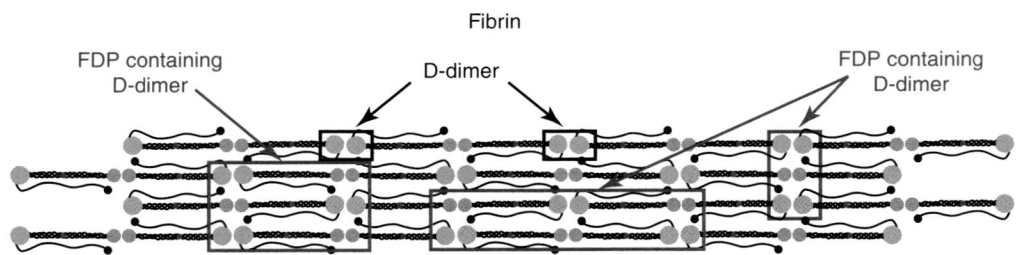

FIGURE 81.8 Fibrinogen, fibrin, and the formation of D-dimer. Fibrinogen (340 kDa) is cleaved by thrombin into fibrin monomer. Fibrin monomers polymerize end to end and side to side forming a fiber, fibrin, in a process that is not enzymatically driven. As depicted, the polymerization of fibrin monomer occurs with the association of the D domains of two fibrin monomers with the E domain of a third. Cross-linking of D domains occurs with the action of a transamidase, factor XIIIa, forming D-dimer epitopes. Plasmin, the key enzyme for fibrinolysis, cleaves the fibrin molecule between the D and E domains. Soluble fragments of fibrin (fibrin degradation products [FDPs]) that contain variable numbers of the D-D epitopes (d-dimer) are produced.

Plasminogen Activator Inhibitor Type 1 Assays

PAI-1 deficiency has been reported as a congenital defect but may be acquired as well. Congenital PAI-1 deficiency is associated with bleeding risk, but experience is limited and the prevalence is unknown. High concentrations of PAI-1 have been associated with a risk for arterial thrombosis; however, PAI-1 is not commonly measured for this purpose. PAI-1 assays are not widely performed in clinical laboratories but testing at reference laboratories may be useful after common causes of bleeding have been excluded. As with other enzymes of coagulation and fibrinolysis, qualitative and quantitative defects of PAI-1 have been reported, and a functional assay for screening purposes is desirable.

A specific chromogenic substrate for plasmin simplifies functional assays for PAI-1, plasminogen, and α_2-antiplasmin. A general scheme for PAI-1 functional assays is to add a known amount of plasminogen activator (tPA or urokinase) to citrated patient plasma, followed by excess plasminogen. Plasmin activity is measured by its cleavage of a chromogenic substrate. Residual plasmin activity is inversely proportional to the PAI-1 of the subject plasma. Inhibitors of α_2-antiplasmin and other plasmin inhibitors are added to prevent interference.[82]

PAI-1 activity assays were developed to detect increased PAI-1, and the available assays do not perform acceptably at low concentrations. Zero activity has been included in the reference interval with this strategy. Agren and associates[83] modified a PAI-1 activity assay by adding calibration points to the low end of the calibration curve. The same group has established that PAI-1 activity below 1 U/mL is associated with increased plasminogen activation and clinical bleeding.

PAI-1 deficiency is an important consideration in patients with convincing bleeding histories, but without overt factor deficiency, because antifibrinolytic therapies may be beneficial. PAI-1 deficiency is a difficult diagnosis to make and requires exclusion of more common hemorrhagic diatheses. Data on PAI-1 are difficult to interpret because of their diurnal variation and its elevation as an acute-phase reactant; in addition, PAI-1 is sensitive to poor phlebotomy technique. If the tourniquet is left on too long, tPA is secreted by endothelial cells and degrades PAI-1. PAI-1 activity should be combined with PAI-1 antigen and tPA assays to assist interpretation of results. Testing for PAI-1 is often performed at the same time as α_2-antiplasmin deficiency as part of an investigation of a fibrinolytic disorder. Strict clinical correlation and sometimes studies of family members are needed to make a diagnosis.

α_2-Antiplasmin

Congenital α_2-antiplasmin deficiency is a rare disorder associated with bleeding. Bleeding symptoms may be delayed, reminiscent of other deficiencies affecting clot stability, such as factor XIII deficiency or PAI-1 deficiency. Acquired deficiencies also occur with liver disease. Similar to other rare disorders of fibrinolysis, careful clinical and laboratory exclusion of more common bleeding disorders is required before a diagnosis of α_2-antiplasmin deficiency is pursued. Quantitative and qualitative types of α_2-antiplasmin deficiency have been reported.[84]

For functional α_2-antiplasmin assays, excess plasmin is added to citrated patient plasma. α_2-Antiplasmin from the patient sample will form inactive plasmin-antiplasmin complexes. Residual plasmin activity is measured by the addition of a chromogenic substrate. Residual plasmin is inversely

proportional to antiplasmin in the patient plasma. A calibration curve relates the absorbance change resulting from plasmin activity to α_2-antiplasmin activity of the test plasma. Antigen assays may be considered in individuals with decreased functional activity to substantiate findings or to define qualitative deficiency.

Plasminogen

Plasminogen deficiency is a rare congenital disorder. Originally, plasminogen deficiency was reported to be associated with thrombosis, but other reports challenge its importance as an independent risk factor. More importantly, severe congenital plasminogen deficiency results in the unusual clinical finding of fibrin pseudomembranes at various mucosal surfaces. The most common site of pseudomembrane deposition is the eye, referred to as ligneous conjunctivitis. Quantitative and qualitative deficiencies have been identified, but pseudomembrane deposition is thought to be associated with quantitative deficiencies. Acquired plasminogen deficiency (e.g., in liver disease) may occur, but the clinical importance is not clear.[85]

When testing plasminogen, excess tPA is added to citrated patient plasma. Plasmin activity is then measured chromogenically, and the plasminogen is extrapolated from a calibration curve. Antigenic assays are also available.

POINTS TO REMEMBER
Inherited Deficiency of Fibrinolysis

- Common coagulation factor deficiency, von Willebrand disease, and platelet disorders should be excluded before evaluating for PAI-1 or α_2-antiplasmin deficiency.
- PAI-1 deficiency typically presents with delayed bleeding.
- α_2-antiplasmin deficiency typically presents with delayed bleeding.
- PAI-1 activity, PAI-1 antigen, and tPA are needed together for interpretation.
- Plasminogen deficiency is **not** associated with bleeding or thrombosis.
- Plasminogen deficiency is associated with deposition of fibrin on mucous membranes, or pseudomembranes.
- Pseudomembranes deposition on the conjunctiva due to plasminogen deficiency is called ligneous conjunctivitis.

THROMBOSIS

Thrombosis is the formation or presence of a blood clot in a blood vessel. The vessel may be any vein or artery as, for example, in DVT or coronary (artery) thrombosis. The clot itself is termed a *thrombus*. If the clot breaks loose and travels through the bloodstream, it is a thromboembolism.

Regulation of hemostasis was discussed in Chapter 79. Thrombophilia refers to an elevated risk for thrombosis and can be further categorized into acquired or inherited thrombophilia. Deficiencies (e.g., AT deficiency) or abnormalities (e.g., Factor V Leiden (FVL)) of natural anticoagulants may produce elevated risk for thrombosis. Assays used to measure anticoagulant function include aPC resistance, FVL mutation detection, PC, PS, and AT assays. In addition to natural anticoagulant deficiency and dysfunction, elevated levels of some procoagulants increase thrombotic risk.

Assays that address elevated procoagulants include (1) prothrombin *G20210A* mutation detection, (2) fibrinogen, and (3) factor VIII activity. The above tests are most often employed to detect inherited thrombophilia; however, some of these tests are used to detect acquired thrombophilia (e.g., PC deficiency related to trauma) or, in the case of AT, to ensure adequate response to heparin therapy. LACs and heparin-induced thrombocytopenia (HIT) can impart an acquired thrombotic risk and are discussed in the following section (see "Clinicopathologic Diagnosis of Other Thrombotic Disorders").

Venous Thromboembolism (VTE) is a major cause of morbidity and mortality, and rapid diagnosis is necessary for timely therapeutic interventions. Unfortunately, no laboratory test has sufficient positive predictive value to be useful to predict the presence of thromboembolism, but quantitative D-dimer tests (see previous discussion of D-dimer in "Test Methods for Fibrinolysis") have excellent negative predictive value and are used to exclude proximal VTE.

D-Dimer for Exclusion of Venous Thromboembolism

Quantitative D-dimer is widely used to exclude DVT and PE. An exclusionary approach uses the D-dimer concentration combined with the degree of clinical suspicion of DVT for PE (low, moderate, or high pretest probability) to decide whether diagnostic imaging is indicated. The value of the D-dimer assay for this purpose derives from its high negative predictive value. A D-dimer concentration below the established threshold, in a patient with low or moderate pretest probability, strongly suggests that DVT or PE is not present, and imaging studies are not pursued. Patients with high pretest probability require diagnostic imaging, and D-dimer should not be measured. Only quantitative D-dimer assays meeting criteria for negative predictive value, established in large clinical studies for evaluation of DVT and PE, should be used to exclude thromboembolism. The minimum performance criteria at the threshold D-dimer value

for excluding thromboembolism are a 98% negative predictive value with the lower confidence interval at 95% and a 98% sensitivity with the lower confidence interval at 90%. Because hundreds of patients are needed to establish a statistically meaningful threshold, laboratories often rely on clinical studies performed by manufacturers of commercial D-dimer kits. Moreover, the performance characteristics and threshold for exclusion should be carefully defined in terms of low and/or moderate pretest probability. Semiquantitative tests by latex agglutination generally lack sensitivity and are inappropriate for exclusion of thromboembolism. D-Dimer assay methodology is discussed previously in the "Test Methods for Fibrinolysis" section.

TEST METHODS AND THEIR CLINICAL APPLICATION FOR THROMBOTIC RISK

Expert groups have recommended that thrombophilia testing must be supervised by experienced laboratory staff and that the clinical significance of results must be interpreted by an experienced clinician who is aware of all the relevant factors that may influence individual test results in each case.[86] Heritable thrombophilia testing is most often performed as a panel of AT, PC, PS, FVL (or aPC reflexed to FVL), and prothrombin *G20210A*. A thrombotic event is typically the impetus for ordering thrombophilia testing. Because the relative risk for re-thrombosis with most inherited thrombophilia is marginal, patient selection for testing is predominantly based on the presence of transient risks at the time of thrombosis. Events close to major transient risks including surgery, trauma, or prolonged immobility are classified as provoked VTE and inherited thrombophilia testing is not indicated. Other minor transient risks such as pregnancy, oral contraceptives, and travel-associated immobility are more complicated; however, in most cases the presence of an inherited thrombophilia would not alter patient management. A strong family history

---

AT A GLANCE

Exclusion of Venous Thromboembolism

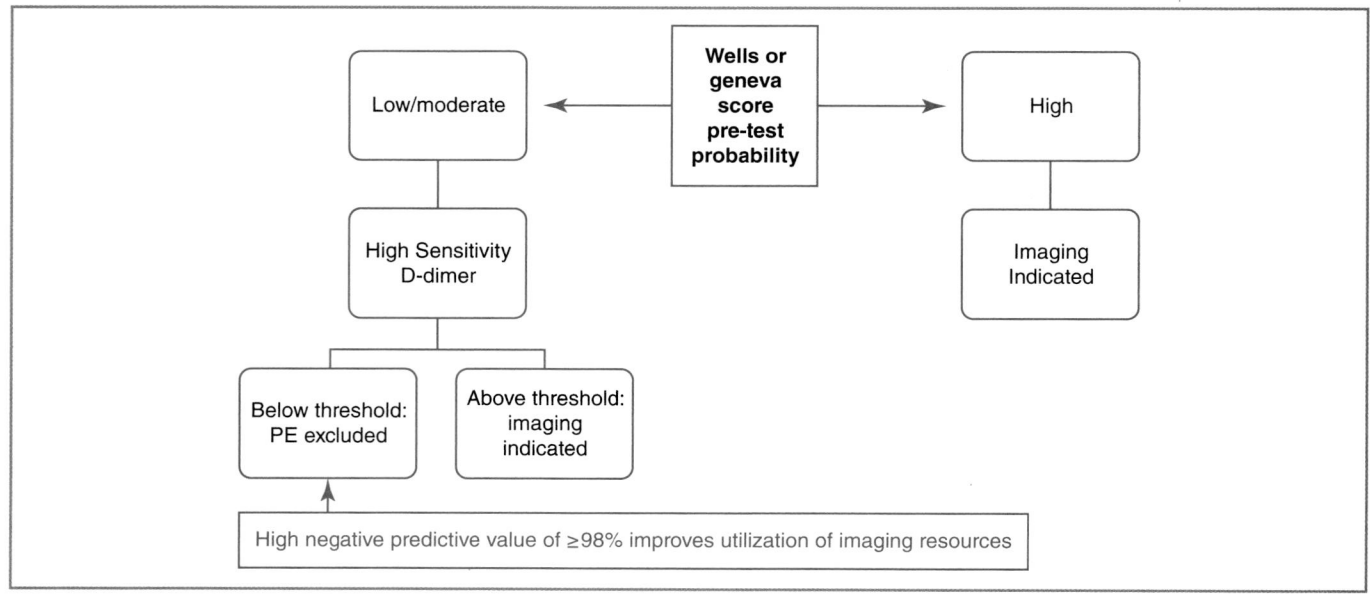

High negative predictive value of ≥98% improves utilization of imaging resources

of unprovoked VTE may be an indication if clinical management would be affected by the result. Other information considered when deciding which patients to test includes age, unusual sites of thrombosis, and bleeding risk while on anticoagulant medication. Guidelines have addressed thrombophilia testing.[86]

Antiphospholipid antibody syndrome (APS) is addressed later in the "Clinicopathologic Diagnosis of other Thrombotic Disorders" section. APS is an acquired disorder with a risk for recurrent thrombosis; therefore testing for APS can have an impact on clinical management, such as the decision to stop anticoagulant therapy.

THROMBOPHILIA TESTING

Activated Protein C Resistance Assays

Addition of aPC to plasma leads to an anticoagulant effect, because aPC degrades the activated forms of factor V (FVa) and factor VIII (FVIIIa), thus slowing the clotting process. Activated protein C resistance (aPCR), which was first described by Dahlback and coworkers,[87] is defined as impairment of this anticoagulant response to aPC. These authors reported that aPCR was associated with a predisposition to thrombosis. aPC cleaves factor Va, and a vast majority of patients with familial aPCR have a point mutation at the cleavage site on factor V.[88] This abnormal factor V protein, in which the arginine at position 506 is replaced with a glutamine (Arg506Gln or R506Q), has been named FVL.[88]

The first assay established for determination of aPCR measured aPTT with and without purified human aPC in the calcium chloride reagent. The aPTT with aPC is divided by the baseline aPTT, and the quotient is called the aPCR ratio. A low ratio indicates the presence of aPCR. A number of tests are now available to detect the abnormal phenotype or the presence of the genetic defect.[88]

Because phenotypic aPCR tests may be influenced by in vitro platelet activation and platelet contamination, plasma should be double-centrifuged at 2000 × g for 15 minutes to reduce the residual platelet count to a minimum. Other factors that affect the test include reduced concentrations of clotting factor II or factor X (decreased ratio) and increased quantities of factor VIII (increased ratio). The presence of LAC has been known to increase aPCR. The original aPCR test[89] should not be used during VKA anticoagulant therapy and is unreliable if the patient has a prolonged PT/INR or aPTT for other reasons. Increased aPCR has been observed to occur in the absence of FVL and has been reported to increase the risk for thrombosis.[90] The original test detects both FVL- and non–FVL-related causes of aPCR, but many centers use a modified version that is more sensitive and more specific for the presence of FVL. This involves a 1:5 or 1:10 dilution of patient plasma in factor V–depleted plasma before analysis. A normal result in this modified aPCR test result excludes the presence of FVL and is not affected by test plasma clotting factor concentrations. Direct oral anticoagulants (DOACs), including FXa inhibitors such as rivaroxaban[91] and FIIa inhibitors such as dabigatran,[92,93] can falsely elevate the aPC ratio depending on the concentration of drug and the laboratory method used for testing.

Good separations of aPCR results are often noted in (1) normal subjects, (2) patients with heterozygous deficiency of FVL, and (3) homozygous individuals. Thus a very low aPCR test (with or without plasma dilution in factor V–depleted plasma) result may be suggestive of homozygous FVL or compound heterozygosity for FVL and factor V deficiency. In the latter case, only FVL is present in plasma, and such patients are described as pseudo-homozygous for FVL. Misdiagnosis of homozygous FVL could have serious consequences in terms of genetic counseling, so suspicion for FVL based on phenotypic tests is best confirmed by genetic analysis.

Several so-called global screening tests are variations of the original aPCR test and may detect deficiencies of PC and PS, as well as aPCR and FVL. Several of these tests use a PC activator from the venom of the southern copperhead viper (*Agkistrodon contortrix contortrix*).[94] The venom contains an enzyme that converts PC to aPC in the sample. The aPC, catalyzed by PS, greatly prolongs the clotting time, unless FVL and/or aPCR are present. Results of currently available global screening tests may be normal in the presence of mild deficiency of PC and PS[95]; thus a normal result cannot be used to exclude a deficiency of these factors.

Factor V Leiden Mutation Detection

Heterozygous FVL has a prevalence of approximately 3% in whites, but it is more prevalent in Sweden, where the defect was first identified. It is practically absent from some Eastern populations and the black populations of Africa.

FVL was originally detected using amplification of the *F5* gene DNA by use of the polymerase chain reaction, with which DNA fragments were amplified before digestion with a restriction enzyme.[88] Such assays using restriction enzyme digestion of DNA are labor-intensive compared with other methods and may include hazardous components. Alternative methods include the allele-refractory mutation system (ARMS) and real-time polymerase chain reaction with melting analysis of the products. Details of molecular methods are found in Chapter 64.

External quality assurance (QA) is available for FVL and prothrombin *G20210A* analysis with an error rate of 3 to 6% among approximately 50 centers performing such tests.[96] Errors identified include sample mismatching, equipment malfunction, and transcription errors. Similar results have been reported in other programs. Genetic tests are generally considered to be definitive, and mistakes are serious errors. For a review of quality issues related to genetic testing in inherited thrombophilia disorders, see the 2012 report by Cooper and associates.[97]

Protein C Assays

Heritable PC deficiency has a prevalence of approximately 1 in 700 in the general population and 2 to 4% in selected subjects with a personal history of venous thrombosis. PC deficiency is associated with a 5-fold to 10-fold increased risk for VTE, although some kindreds appear to have no such increased risk. Combined defects with coinheritance of PC deficiency and FVL markedly increase thrombotic risk, beyond that caused by inheritance of either defect alone.[98]

PC concentration is very low in the newborn. PC concentrations may only reach adult values at 16 years of age, with further increases occurring up until approximately 30 years of age.[88] PC concentrations may be reduced in patients with liver disease and vitamin K deficiency and by VKAs such as warfarin. In vitamin K deficiency, the PC assay result depends on the measurement system. When a low concentration of

PC is detected, physiologic, clinical, and pharmacologic causes should be excluded. PT/INR should be performed as an indication of normal liver function. Not all cases with genetic defects of PC have reduced activity by PC assay. Some carriers have PC concentrations within the normal reference interval.

On initiation of warfarin therapy, PC concentrations fall with a half-life of approximately 4 to 6 hours, similar to factor VII, but much shorter than other vitamin K–dependent clotting factors such as IX, X, II, and PS. It should be noted that it is not possible to diagnose PC deficiency in patients who are in the induction phase of warfarin therapy, and testing is not recommended in patients on stable VKA therapy. PC deficiency is the prototypical thrombophilia associated with warfarin-induced skin necrosis,[99] although it also occurs with other thrombophilias or even in the absence of recognized thrombophilia. The additional decrease in PC caused by warfarin puts patients with inherited PC deficiency at additional risk for thrombosis. The predilection for skin reflects the importance of the PC and PS system to protect cutaneous vessels from thrombosis. Warfarin-induced skin necrosis is rare, but its recognition and discontinuation of warfarin can prevent loss of limbs or death. Screening for PC deficiency to prevent warfarin-induced skin necrosis is not practical because most patients with PC deficiency who are treated with warfarin do not develop skin necrosis.

Clotting, chromogenic, and antigenic assays are available for measuring PC concentrations. Clotting-based PC assays require the addition of test sample to PC-depleted plasma, then southern copperhead viper activator converts PC to aPC, which prolongs clotting time through destruction of factors Va and VIIIa. The clotting end point is based on aPTT, PT, or the addition of snake venoms. Assays based on aPTT may be influenced by the phospholipid composition of the reagent and concentration of factor VIII.

PC assays based on aPTT may underestimate PC in samples with high concentrations of factor VIII. The presence of FVL, particularly homozygous FVL, may falsely reduce concentrations of PC reported by clotting-based assays because FVL is resistant to destruction by aPC, and clotting time does not fully reflect aPC activity. Predilution of patient plasma in PC-depleted plasma may reduce or remove the influence of FVL.[100] PC can be overestimated through the anticoagulant influence of LAC. DOACs such as dabigatran and rivaroxaban may cause overestimation of PC activity in clot-based PC assays (see Table 81.7) with the potential for a false normal result in patients with PC deficiency.[93,101] Because they are less subject to interferences, UK guidelines suggest that chromogenic PC assays may be preferable to clot-based techniques.[86] The advantage of clotting-based assays is that they may detect rare heritable functional defects that remain undetected by other techniques.

Chromogenic assays of PC generally use southern copperhead viper activator conversion of PC to aPC. However, currently available chromogenic substrates for aPC measurement lack complete specificity and are cleaved by a variety of proteases. Partially clotted samples and serum may give falsely high chromogenic PC activity results because of background protease activity. Some southern copperhead viper activator–based chromogenic assays are unable to detect all patients with type II PC deficiency, in the case of disparity between antigen and functional activity.

PC antigen is now typically determined by automated latex-based immunoassay or by ELISA-based methods, which are relatively precise and very sensitive to low concentrations of PC. These have been used to differentiate types I and II deficiency. Approximately three-quarters of patients recorded as having PC deficiency have type I deficiency (low antigen and function), with most of the rest having type II deficiency, which is characterized by normal concentrations of protein but low PC as measured by both clotting and chromogenic assays.

Protein S

PS is a glycoprotein whose amino acid sequence is coded by the *PROS1* gene. As stated earlier, approximately 60 to 70% of plasma PS is bound to C4b-binding protein and has no significant role in hemostasis. The remainder is termed free PS and functions as a cofactor for the degradation of factors Va and VIIIa by aPC. Deficiency of PS is associated with a fivefold increased risk for venous thrombosis, and the combination of the FVL mutation and the PS deficiency is associated with a high risk for thrombosis.[102] The incidence of familial PS deficiency is approximately 1 in 700 to 1 in 3000 of the general population in the United Kingdom.[103]

TABLE 81.7   Effect of Direct Oral Anticoagulants at Usual Peak Concentration

	Rivaroxaban	Apixaban	Dabigatran
PT/INR	Prolonged + or + +	Normal or prolonged	Prolonged +
aPTT	Prolonged +	Normal or prolonged +/–	Prolonged + +
Thrombin time	No effect	No effect	Grossly prolonged at trough (low) levels
Clauss fibrinogen	No effect	No effect	Unaffected or reduced
PT-based factors II, V, VII, X assays	Reduced activity at low plasma dilutions		
aPTT-based factors VIII, IX, XI, XII assays	Reduced activity at low plasma dilutions		
Clot-based PC or PS	Potential for overestimation		
Antithrombin: Xa based	Potential for overestimation		No effect
Antithrombin: IIa based	No effect		Potential for overestimation
DRVVT/LAC testing	Potential to misclassify normal as LAC present		
aPCR	Increased ratios for some methods		

aPCR, Activated protein C resistance; *aPTT,* activated partial thromboplastin time; *DRVVT,* dilute Russell viper venom time; *INR,* international normalized ratio; *LAC,* lupus anticoagulant; *PC,* protein C; *PS,* protein S; *PT,* prothrombin time.

Heritable PS deficiency is classified as type I, II, or III. Type I is defined by reduced concentrations of total PS antigen (total PS) and free PS antigen (free PS) and reduced PS activity. Type II deficiency is characterized by isolated deficiency of PS activity. Type III deficiency displays normal concentrations of total PS, but a reduced concentration of free PS and reduced activity of PS. Type III PS deficiency, however, may not be a separate disorder because it has occurred with some of the same gene mutations that cause type I deficiency in other family members. PS concentrations are lower in women than in men and may be further decreased by certain oral contraceptives; its quantities are particularly low in the newborn. Gender-specific reference intervals are therefore useful. Low total PS with normal concentrations of free PS occur in patients with low concentrations of C4bBP. Pregnancy, acute-phase reactions, oral contraceptives, and hormone replacement therapy may reduce concentrations of free PS, but not total PS. Again similar to PC, PS concentrations are reduced in liver disease, vitamin K deficiency, and VKA therapy. Testing of patients while they are anticoagulated is problematic. Measurement of total PS antigen probably is not helpful in most cases, and an assay that measures the concentration of free PS antigen is preferred. In normal subjects, the free PS antigen concentration reflects the functional PS activity in plasma. Free PS has been measured by ELISA but is increasingly measured using latex-based assays in automated analyzers. Many of these methods have removed the need to first separate free PS from that bound to C4bBP, usually by precipitation of bound PS using polyethylene glycol. Measurement of free PS antigen has been shown to be more reliable at detecting PS deficiency in subjects with *PROS1* gene defects than measurement of total PS.[104]

Functional assays of PS are based on the ability of PS to act as cofactor in aPC-mediated destruction of activated V and/or VIII. This anticoagulant activity may be detected through PT, aPTT, or venom-based clotting time. Functional assays of PS may be sensitive to type II defects, which are missed by antigenic assay. However, problems arise when many functional assays are used. Some patients were incorrectly diagnosed as having type II PS deficiency when aPC resistance resulted in underestimation of PS by functional assay.[105] Results obtained in proficiency testing surveys indicate that even in normal subjects, activity results determined by different assays are not interchangeable. As with PC, PS can be overestimated through the additive anticoagulant influence of LAC. DOACs such as dabigatran and rivaroxaban may cause overestimation of PS activity in clot-based assays (see Table 81.7) with the potential for a false normal result in patients with PS deficiency.[93,101] Consequently, many laboratories currently avoid use of functional assays because of these problems. Furthermore, the British Committee for Standards in Haematology state that immunoreactive assays of free PS antigen are preferable to functional assays, and if a functional assay is performed in the initial screen, low results should be investigated further using an immunoreactive free PS antigen assay.[86]

Antithrombin Assays

AT, previously known as antithrombin III, deficiency may be inherited as the result of a molecular defect, but it may also be acquired (1) through decreased production (e.g., liver disease), (2) through increased turnover (e.g., consumption, heparin therapy), or (3) by renal loss in nephrotic syndrome.

The in vivo half-life of plasma AT is approximately 65 hours, although it may be shorter for AT infused as replacement therapy.

Two main categories of AT deficiency are known: type I, which is characterized by parallel reduction in activity and antigen concentration, and type II, in which activity and antigen concentration are discordant. Three types of qualitative functional defects have been identified, including those in the heparin-binding site, those in the reactive site, and pleiotropic/multiple effects. Heritable AT deficiency has a prevalence of approximately 1 in 3000 of the population and is associated with a 10- to 50-fold increased risk for venous thrombosis. Not all defects are equally thrombotic, and individuals with heterozygous heparin-binding site defects may have no increased risk.

Because antigen concentrations are normal in many type 2 defects, a functional AT assay is essential. Most experts prefer an assay sensitive to all type 2 defects. The reference interval for AT concentration is narrow, and accurate assays are required to distinguish normal from abnormal. Suitable chromogenic assays are available based on the ability of the sample to inhibit generation of color by the action of either thrombin or factor Xa (in the reagent) on a chromogenic substrate specific for the protease (thrombin or Xa).

AT variants may react poorly with one enzyme (thrombin or Xa) and normally with another; this pattern may vary in the presence and absence of heparin. Heparin cofactor II (HC II), whose activity is enhanced by heparin, is an additional protein that neutralizes human thrombin. The presence of HC II in plasma may reduce the specificity of AT assays, particularly those using human thrombin, where there is an assay incubation time with thrombin of longer than 30 seconds.[106] This problem is partially solved by using bovine thrombin or factor Xa. Thrombin-based AT assays should not be used in patients receiving direct thrombin inhibitors because concentrations can be substantially overestimated.[92] Similarly, factor Xa–based assays should not be used in patients receiving anti–Xa inhibitors such as rivaroxaban; the same problem of overestimation may occur.[91]

Results obtained with different assays vary, so that in some defects normal results occur in one assay type whereas activity is low in another. Many variant AT defects have been described when these problems occur, so results should be interpreted only with knowledge about the assay characteristics.

Chromogenic substrate assays are preferred for measurement of AT concentration. These generally involve the incubation of enzyme (thrombin or factor Xa) with diluted plasma in the presence of heparin before a chromogenic substrate is added; *p*-nitroaniline (pNA) release from the substrate is monitored at 405 nm. AT inhibits the enzyme, and the decrease in absorbance at 405 nm with sample compared with no sample is proportional to the AT concentration. Precision varies across assays. For example, bovine-thrombin–based assays typically show a CV of approximately 1.5%, whereas factor Xa–based assays tend to have a CV of approximately 2.5%. The determination of the reference interval (to include the 2.5 to 97.5 percentile) for AT should use nonparametric methods because the distribution of results is not Gaussian. Factors such as age, sex, oral contraceptive use, and circadian rhythm influence AT concentrations to varying degrees.[107] However, for practical purposes, it is acceptable to use a single (adult) reference interval that includes similar numbers of men and women. AT concentrations are low in neonates. AT is consumed during clotting, and artificially low concentrations are found in clotted samples, whereas genuinely low concentrations may occur as a consequence of recent massive thrombosis. Because liver disease and heparin therapy will reduce AT concentrations, a PT/INR should be performed on specimens with low AT concentration to assess whether the sample is clotted or the patient has liver disease.

When a congenital deficiency is suspected, AT antigen is measured to differentiate type I from type II AT deficiency. AT antigen is measured by immunoassays such as ELISA, immunoelectrophoresis, radial immunodiffusion, and immunoturbidimetry. Genetic analysis is useful to identify the defect at a molecular level because different defects are associated with different thrombotic risk.

Prothrombin *G20210A* Detection

The prothrombin *G20210A* mutation is a genetic defect that leads to an increase in the concentration of factor II in plasma and confers an increased risk for venous thrombosis. This defect *(PT G20210A)* occurs in approximately 2 to 3% of Caucasians and leads to a twofold to threefold increased risk for VTE.[108] Increased prothrombin concentration alone will not reliably identify carriers of the genetic defect.

Factor VIII and von Willebrand Factor

It has been reported that elevated activity of factor VIII is an independent risk factor for venous thrombosis.[109] For example, elevated activities of factor VIII are found in approximately 20% of subjects with VTE. The elevation is independent of the acute-phase response (which causes transient but marked increases in factor VIII). The risk increases as factor VIII rises above 150 IU/dL, with an eightfold increase in risk above 270 IU/dL. Elevated activities of factor VIII, however, do occur in a number of other situations, and activities above 150 IU/dL are found in 10 to 30% of apparently healthy subjects. For this reason, many laboratories do not routinely include factor VIII determination in the standard panel of tests used to investigate patients for heritable thrombophilia, and it is not recommended in some countries, such as the United Kingdom.[86]

It has been reported that risk for VTE is increased as the activity of VWF is increased.[110] One function of VWF is to transport factor VIII in plasma, forming a relationship between the two molecules. Higher quantities of VWF lead to greater quantities of factor VIII, and when multivariate analysis is performed, factor VIII is shown to be an independent risk factor, whereas VWF is not; increased risk for thrombosis is a consequence of the increased quantities of factor VIII.[109]

Fibrinogen

Numerous studies have shown that the concentration of fibrinogen is associated with risk for coronary heart disease and stroke, and a meta-analysis of 31 such studies has confirmed this.[111] Although this finding is independent of other markers of the acute-phase response such as C-reactive protein, it remains unclear whether higher fibrinogen causes coronary heart disease, and no consensus has been reached on whether measurement of the concentration of fibrinogen is clinically useful for assessing risk in individual patients. Currently, it seems likely that the independent effect of fibrinogen is small. At present, most experts would suggest that it is not cost-effective to consider population-wide screening of fibrinogen concentrations.

Antiphospholipid Antibodies and Lupus Anticoagulant

APAs, including LAC antibodies, anticardiolipin antibodies, and β_2-glycoprotein I (GPI) antibodies, occur in antiphospholipid antibody syndrome (APS).[112] APS is an acquired disorder of the immune system characterized by excessive clotting of blood and/or certain complications of pregnancy. APS is diagnosed when particular clinical symptoms coincide with the presence of APA in laboratory tests. Some antibodies are transient; thus a diagnosis of APS requires repeat testing for confirmation after 12 weeks. The most common thrombotic symptoms are VTE and ischemic stroke, with some patients having thrombocytopenia. Types of pregnancy failure that are consistent with APS include: (1) three or more unexplained consecutive abortions before 10 weeks, (2) unexplained death of a morphologically normal fetus at or after 10 weeks, and (3) premature birth before 34 weeks as a result of severe preeclampsia or placental insufficiency. Internationally, classification criteria have been published.[113]

At present, the degree of standardization of tests for APA is poor, and the limitations of such tests must be kept in mind when patients are assessed for possible APS. Several types of APA are undoubtedly linked to thrombosis and pregnancy loss. These include anti–β_2-GPI (anti–β_2-GP-1), LAC, and anticardiolipin antibodies. Other types of APA, such as prothrombin antibodies, have been reported to be linked to APS, but currently no consensus has been reached on their clinical relevance.

It has long been recognized that some individuals with systemic lupus erythematosus (SLE) have prolonged aPTTs. This was shown to be due to the presence of an in vitro inhibitor called LAC. These inhibitors previously were thought to work against phospholipid, but these antibodies were found to be active against proteins that bind to lipids; these proteins include β_2-GP1, prothrombin, annexin V, and others.[114–116] Antibodies that prolong phospholipid-dependent clotting tests are collectively termed LAC. This group is very heterogeneous in relation to clinical picture and laboratory features. It should be noted that although some SLE individuals are positive for LAC, most cases of LAC are not associated with SLE, even though the term *lupus anticoagulant* has continued to be used. In addition, it should be noted that not all APAs prolong these clotting tests. Some cases with detectable LAC do not have clinical features and therefore are not classified as APS. The aPTT, however, is not prolonged in all cases in which LAC is present, and most cases with LAC and prolonged aPTT have no bleeding symptoms but may have thrombosis as described previously. Only rarely is LAC associated with bleeding, usually when acquired prothrombin deficiency is a consequence of high concentrations of anti-prothrombin antibody.[35]

Criteria and guidelines for LAC detection have been published by the Scientific and Standardization Committee (SSC) of the ISTH, British Committee for Standards in Haematology (BCSH), and Clinical and Laboratory Standards Institute (CLSI).[117–121] The ISTH criteria from 1995 (see At a Glance) have been updated, especially with regard to the application of mixing studies and patients on vitamin K antagonists. The ISTH 2009 update addresses a number of important aspects of standardization. For example, the quality of the sample affects results of LAC tests, and if there are residual platelets, they can rupture during the testing, leading to loss of antibody and false-negative results. This is a particular problem if plasmas are frozen before testing; therefore double centrifugation is required before deep freezing. Filtering to remove residual platelets, however, is not recommended. The guidelines also recommend that the DRVVT should be the first test performed and the second test should be a LAC sensitive aPTT-based test; however, the BCHS and CLSI guidelines allow other test systems. The DRVVT is a clot-based test that is initiated by the addition of a Russell viper venom that directly activates factor X, thereby bypassing effects of extrinsic and intrinsic pathways. Only the DRVVT or the aPTT test needs to be positive to be considered evidence of LAC, although in most cases, both will be positive. For a screening test (e.g., aPTT or DRVVT) to be sensitive to the presence of LAC, the reagent should have a low phospholipid concentration. A confirmatory step is required for each individual LAC test to confirm the phospholipid-dependent nature of the inhibitor. This confirmation is achieved by repeating the test with a higher phospholipid concentration to neutralize the phospholipid-dependent inhibitors. There is also a role for performing a mixing study of LAC tests to help differentiate between a clotting factor deficiency (e.g., warfarin therapy) and a lupus inhibitor. Mild prolongation of screening aPTT or DRVVT may correct with mixing studies due to dilution effect, causing false negative LAC; therefore the subsequent guidelines have adopted alternative approaches.[122] The 2009 ISTH update upholds the traditional screen, mix, and then confirm approach, but it introduces the concept that mixing studies for integrated test systems (e.g., DRVVT screen and DRVVT confirm performed in parallel) utilizing a screen/confirm ratio may not always require mixing studies. CLSI reorders the approach (i.e., screen, confirm, mix) and recommends performing mixing studies to clarify positive screen/confirm ratios (or positive percent corrections) when the undiluted confirm test or a LAC-unresponsive aPTT is above the reference interval, suggesting a non-LAC prolongation of clotting tests. Specific factor inhibitors, such as factor VIII inhibitors, are associated with bleeding and should be excluded clinically.

As a consequence of thrombosis, many patients with LAC require oral anticoagulant therapy. Interpretation of LAC tests is difficult during VKA therapy because reductions in the quantities of various coagulation factors during VKA therapy will affect the DRVVT and aPTT tests. The SSC LAC guideline recommends that such testing should be done 1 to 2 weeks after discontinuation of VKA therapy.[118] If testing is necessary at the time of VKA therapy, it is recommended that the DRVVT should be performed when the INR is less than 1.5, testing should not be done when the INR is greater than 3.5,

and a mix of test and normal plasma should be considered when the INR is between these limits. In addition, the SSC guideline does not recommend use of dilute PT, assays based on snake venoms, or kaolin-clotting time for LAC detection.

Various solid-phase ELISA tests are available for the detection of APA. These include tests for ACA for which commercial kits have been available for many years. Standardization of such kits, however, is rather poor, and comparisons consistently demonstrate that even concordance as to whether a sample is positive or negative is frequently absent when testing is done with two or more different kits.[123] Both IgG and IgM forms of ACA occur. Evidence that the IgM isotype is of clinical relevance is weak, and many laboratories test only for IgG. Some but not all ACA assays incorporate β_2-GP-1 in the reagents so that cardiolipin bound to the surface of a microtiter plate will be associated with β_2-GP-1. Some ACA kits detect only β_2-GP-1–dependent antibodies, whereas others detect non–β_2-GP-1–dependent antibodies. Evidence suggests that it is the β_2-GP-1–dependent antibodies that have the greatest clinical significance in APS, so β_2-GP-1–dependent ACA is recommended by the SSC of ISTH.[124–126] As for ACA kits, standardization of APS kits is poor, and there will be patients with APS who are negative by one kit and positive by another.[123]

MONITORING ANTICOAGULANT THERAPY

Several guidelines are available from the American College of Chest Physicians on the monitoring of anticoagulant therapy. They address anticoagulants such as argatroban, bivalirudin, fondaparinux, hirudin, LMWH, UFH,[127,128] and VKAs, and DOACs.[129,130] Details of several of these substances are discussed in the following sections.

Unfractionated Heparin

Heparin is a highly sulfated polysaccharide used as an anticoagulant for the treatment and prevention of thromboembolic disease. For many years, clinical preparations were unfractionated, containing mixtures of polysaccharide chains of different lengths. Such unfractionated materials typically have average molecular weights of 12,000 to 15,000 Da.

Diagnosis of Antiphospholipid Antibody Syndrome (APS)

- The diagnosis of APS requires **both** clinical and laboratory criteria.
- Clinical criteria (any one of the following)
  - Thrombosis
  - Pregnancy complication
- Three or more unexplained consecutive abortions before 10 weeks
- Unexplained death of a morphologically normal fetus at or after 10 weeks
- Premature birth <34 weeks due to severe preeclampsia or placental insufficiency
AND
- Laboratory criteria (any positive test present on 2 or more occasions at least 12 weeks apart)
- Anticardiolipin (IgG or IgM)
- Anti–β_2 glycoprotein I (IgG or IgM)
- Lupus anticoagulant

The anticoagulant effect of UFH is exerted by potentiating the action of AT. After binding to heparin, the AT undergoes a conformational change, facilitating very rapid inactivation of thrombin and several other activated clotting factors, which, like thrombin, have serine in their active site (so-called serine proteases). These include factor Xa, factor IXa, factor XIa, and factor XIIa. The number of saccharide units in the polysaccharide chain of heparin influences these reactions. At least five saccharide units are required for some anticoagulant activity. Polymers measuring less than five saccharide units in length have no anticoagulant activity. For inhibition of thrombin, heparin chains must bind to both AT and thrombin and thus need to be 18 or more units in length. Simultaneous binding is not required for neutralization of factor Xa, and chains between 5 and 17 units long catalyze neutralization of Xa without affecting thrombin directly. So-called LMWHs, containing a more uniform population of these shorter polysaccharides, are manufactured from UFH by controlled depolymerization. LMWH is discussed later. Guidance on use of UFH in several settings has been published.[131]

aPTT for Monitoring Unfractionated Heparin

There is no strong evidence that monitoring of UFH therapy improves clinical outcomes.[132] Nevertheless laboratory monitoring is standard practice because the dose needed for protection from thrombosis varies across subjects, and overdose is associated with hemorrhagic risk. The most widely used test for monitoring UFH is the aPTT (discussed previously). In an early study, it was demonstrated that the risk for VTE was reduced when the aPTT ratio (patient to control value) was greater than 1.5, and a therapeutic range of 1.5 to 2.5 was suggested.[133] However, several subsequent studies have shown marked differences among aPTT reagents and methods in terms of heparin responsiveness.[134] Thus a specific reference interval of 1.5 to 2.5 is not appropriate for all reagents. For each aPTT method, it is necessary to establish a therapeutic range by measurement of aPTT and heparin concentration by protamine sulfate titration or anti-Xa assay. For example, for the early studies,[133] an aPTT

reference interval of 1.5 to 2.5 was found to be equivalent to 0.2 to 0.4 IU of heparin/mL by protamine sulfate titration assay or 0.3 to 0.7 IU/mL by anti-Xa assay.[127] Laboratories using aPTT to monitor heparin must determine the therapeutic interval for its specific aPTT/instrument combination using samples from patients on heparin. (Note that these samples have been referred to as ex vivo samples in some literature.) Regression analysis is used to establish the interval of aPTT (or aPTT ratios) corresponding to heparin concentrations between 0.3 and 0.7 IU/mL determined by anti-Xa methodology (Fig. 81.9).[134] This should not be done using plasmas spiked with heparin in vitro, because the therapeutic interval established may be different from that determined using samples from patients on heparin. The therapeutic interval should be established using between 30 and 60 samples, although some have suggested that several hundred specimens may be needed.

If the aPTT ratio is used, it should be calculated using the midpoint of the normal reference interval as the denominator. It should be noted that there is a poor correlation between aPTT and heparin concentration, possibly reflecting the poor specificity of aPTT for heparin effect. The aPTT is influenced by the concentrations of other clotting factors, including those affected by warfarin (see later), by factor XII, or especially by the quantity of factor VIII, which will change dramatically as a patient with acute thrombosis recovers, that is, as the acute-phase response changes. Because of variability in the process, the therapeutic range should be checked for all new lot numbers of aPTT reagent. In practice, laboratories often sequester large amounts of a single reagent lot to avoid the labor-intensive process of calibrating the aPTT assay for new lots. Preanalytic variables dramatically affect the results of aPTT in samples containing UFH. For example, when citrate is used as an anticoagulant, platelets in the blood sample are activated, leading to release of a granule constituent, PF4, which neutralizes heparin. CLSI states that citrated samples for monitoring heparin therapy should be tested within 1 hour of collection or centrifuged and tested within 4 hours[2]; however, this is logistically challenging for many laboratories. Citrate samples for monitoring heparin should be analyzed as soon as possible because aPTT increases and heparin activity (anti-Xa) decreases progressively; shortening of aPTT and loss of heparin activity over time is variable, but significant change occurs rapidly over 4 hours in some individuals.[135] The problem with citrated samples is particularly marked if a blood sample has a large air space within the tube, with much more rapid and marked loss of heparin.[136] The problem is avoided if blood samples are collected into an anticoagulant cocktail comprising citrate, theophylline, adenosine, and dipyridamole that is commercially available and that inhibits platelets, thereby avoiding this problem. Such samples are stable with respect to aPTT for much longer than 4 hours, but this tube type must be validated by the laboratory.

If UFH is given by intravenous infusion or subcutaneous injection, the sample should be collected 4 to 6 hours after initiation of therapy or after any dose adjustment, to allow steady state to be reached.

On various occasions, aPTT is inappropriate for monitoring UFH because of lack of specificity. Thus the aPTT may be within the therapeutic range despite suboptimal heparin concentrations because of: (1) the presence of LAC, (2) combined UFH and VKA, (3) combined UFH and thrombolytic therapy, and (4) congenital or acquired factor deficiency. On the other

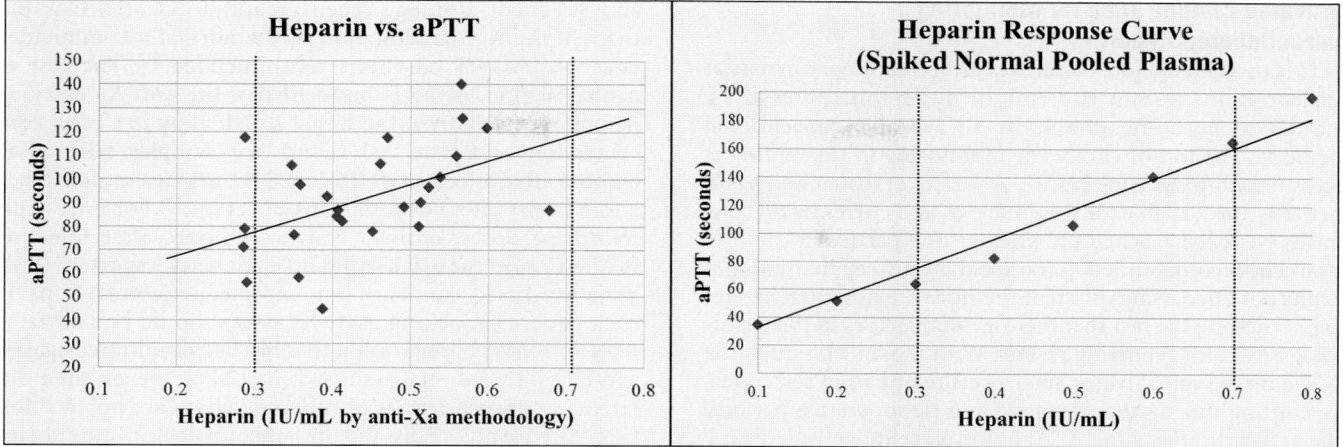

FIGURE 81.9 Establishing an activated partial thromboplastin time *(aPTT)* therapeutic range for monitoring unfractionated heparin (UFH). On the *left,* the graph displays the relationship of aPTT in samples from heparin treated patients to UFH measured by an anti-Xa method. Although the response to one individual patient may be linear, there is extensive interpatient variability in UFH responsiveness. Despite this loose relationship, one popular approach to establishing an aPTT therapeutic range is to fit a line through the points; the intersections of the regression line with the widely accepted UFH therapeutic range of 0.3 to 0.7 IU/mL establishes the laboratory-specific aPTT therapeutic range. Using the method on the *left,* the therapeutic aPTT interval is 75 to 120 seconds. With some reagents, the linear regression (e.g., lacking a positive correlation) does not adequately estimate the aPTT range. On the *right,* the graph displays the relationship of the same aPTT reagent to normal pooled plasma spiked with increasing concentrations of UFH. Here the same aPTT reagent would have a therapeutic range of 75 to 160 seconds. This method consistently overestimates the aPTT therapeutic range and is not recommended.

hand, heparin resistance, with subtherapeutic aPTT despite large doses of heparin, is caused by antithrombin deficiency. When monitoring with aPTT, apparent "heparin resistance" also occurs with markedly elevated factor VIII, as occurs with an acute phase response, due to shortening of the aPTT. In these cases, measurement of unfractionated heparin by anti-Xa method (see below), which is not sensitive to factor VIII, may prevent escalation of heparin.[137] The effect of UFH is rapidly reversed by infusion of protamine sulfate; however, excessive protamine sulfate administration can cause prolongation of the aPTT and other clotting tests, including the activated clotting time.

Heparin Assays for Monitoring Unfractionated Heparin

Historically, a heparin assay based on protamine sulfate titration was used in North America to establish the therapeutic range for UFH therapy (see earlier section on aPTT). However, this assay was poorly standardized, not commercially available, not well suited to automation, and is practically obsolete in terms of current usage. Currently, the most popular assays used to measure heparin activity are based on the ability of heparin to neutralize factor Xa that has been added to the test sample. They are known as anti-Xa assays and measure the ability of heparin-accelerated AT to inhibit Xa, with residual Xa activity measured through its ability to clot plasma or more often by the amidolytic cleavage of a small chromogenic substrate. In the latter assay, a peptide substrate is cleaved to release pNA, with the change in absorbance being inversely proportional to heparin concentration. Some anti-Xa assays include the addition of exogenous AT to the test sample, ensuring an excess of AT. Other heparin assays do not

add exogenous AT, the rationale being that the assay should reflect the ability of heparin to exert an anticoagulant effect, dependent on the quantity of AT present in the patient's plasma. Therefore these assays may be more likely to correlate with clinical efficacy. This is especially important in that infusion of UFH could lead to a reduction in the quantity of patient AT through increased clearance and a shorter half-life. Similar available assays employ thrombin (FIIa) in place of factor Xa; they are therefore anti-IIa assays. Both anti-Xa and anti-IIa assays for UFH need to be calibrated with a heparin that has been calibrated against a WHO international standard. If anti-Xa is used to monitor UFH, the therapeutic range is 0.3 to 0.7 IU/mL.[138]

Thrombin Time for Monitoring Unfractionated Heparin

Thrombin clotting time (TCT) is prolonged by UFH, the magnitude of which depends on the reagents, the method, and the concentration of heparin. Although it has been proposed as suitable for monitoring therapy, the test is rarely selected for this purpose. One problem is that for many methods, the TCT becomes difficult to measure at doses of heparin within or just above the upper limit of the therapeutic range. This problem is removed by the use of higher concentrations of thrombin, or by the inclusion of calcium in the TT reagent, which may improve the correlation between TCT and concentration of UFH. However, some versions of TCT methods are useful even at low concentrations of heparin. Such methods are useful in the detection and exclusion of heparin as a cause of prolonged aPTT, where clinical information is lacking, or where contamination of heparin in a sample is suspected.

Activated Clotting Time for Monitoring Unfractionated Heparin

UFH is used in high doses during cardiopulmonary bypass at concentrations of 3 to 10 U/mL or more; this causes aPTT and TT to be unmeasurable by all available conventional methods. The test of choice for monitoring in this setting is Activated Clotting Time (ACT). A variety of instruments and methods are available for this purpose, and currently no consensus has been reached on whether one particular method should be recommended. It is important to keep in mind that results obtained using different methods are not interchangeable,[139] despite the fact that there are similarities in the terminology used for reporting results. With most techniques, the ACT employs an activator such as celite or kaolin to accelerate clotting during the operative and perioperative periods. The activator affects the ACT; however, celite-activated ACT is prolonged relative to an ACT determined using kaolin. In addition, ACT may be prolonged by the hypothermia and hemodilution that may accompany cardiopulmonary bypass procedures. Thus a poor correlation has been noted between heparin concentration as measured in specific assays and results obtained by ACT. Aprotinin prolongs celite-activated ACT in a dose-dependent way independently of heparin, and if aprotinin is used, ACT should be maintained at a higher result to ensure adequate heparinization, perhaps with twofold higher ACT results. When all factors are taken into account, management protocols often need to be device and anticoagulant specific.

ACT results are affected by the quantities of several clotting factors. For example, if the patient has severe deficiency of factor XII, HMWK, or prekallikrein, the contact phase is compromised and the baseline value is grossly prolonged to values similar to those achieved by the high-dose heparin used for anticoagulation during cardiopulmonary bypass and other procedures. In these cases, the test cannot be used safely, so tests specific for the action of heparin such as anti-Xa assay must be considered. Therefore a preheparinization baseline ACT is needed to exclude the presence of such an abnormality.

Low-Molecular-Weight Heparin

Updated evidence-based practice guidelines for anticoagulant therapy were published in 2012,[127,132] including use for prevention of VTE in nonsurgical[140] and surgical[141] patients. As mentioned previously, LMWHs are derived from UFH by depolymerization of the polysaccharide chains. The ratio of activity against factor Xa to activity against thrombin is high but varies across different preparations. LMWHs are favored over UFH as the treatment of choice in a number of clinical situations for several reasons, including a better benefit-to-risk ratio, more predictable dose response with reduced requirement for monitoring, and a lower incidence of heparin-induced thrombocytopenia. Most LMWHs have an average molecular weight below 5000 Da, and their bioavailability is approximately 90% after subcutaneous injection, with a half-life of between 3 and 6 hours. Prophylactic doses are given as fixed doses or weight-adjusted doses; therapeutic doses are weight-based. For most patients, monitoring is not necessary, but some experts recommend monitoring in special populations, including obese patients (less reliable dose-response relationship), pediatric patients, patients with renal insufficiency (LMWHs are cleared by the kidney),

and pregnant women. When creatinine clearance is less than 30 mL/min, a reduction of the normal recommended dose of LMWH has been recommended.[132] The test of choice if monitoring is performed is the anti-Xa assay. In neonates or children, the target for therapy is a peak concentration of 0.5 to 1.0 IU/mL for samples taken 4 to 6 hours after injection or 0.5 to 0.8 IU/mL in a sample taken 2 to 6 hours after subcutaneous injection.[131] For once-daily treatment doses, anti-Xa activity 4 hours after injection is often more than 1 U/mL and may be closer to 2 U/mL. Evidence-based guidance on expected concentrations in such patients is lacking. Anti-Xa assays should be calibrated with an LMWH preparation that has been calibrated against a WHO international standard for LMWH; even then differences between results of different assays are noted. Clotting-based anti-Xa assays are unsuitable for monitoring LMWH. The anti-Xa activity of LMWH is poorly reversed by protamine sulfate.

Fondaparinux

Fondaparinux (trade name Arixtra) is a synthetic pentasaccharide with a molecular weight of ≈1700 Da that binds AT with higher affinity than does heparin. It has a half-life of 17 hours after subcutaneous injection. A predictable anticoagulant response allows once-daily subcutaneous injection in fixed doses without the need for laboratory monitoring. It is contraindicated in renal insufficiency. In circumstances in which it may be useful to determine the activity of fondaparinux, the assay of choice is anti-Xa, but in this case, the assay must be calibrated using fondaparinux in the standard plasma—not LMWH.[138] Expected mean 3-hour peak concentrations after 2.5 and 7.5 mg daily doses are 0.39 to 0.5 mg/L and 1.20 to 1.26 mg/L, respectively, although the therapeutic range has not been established.[127] Fondaparinux is not reversed by protamine sulfate.

Parenteral Direct Thrombin Inhibitors

The most widely used parenteral anticoagulants, including UFH and LMWH, have a number of limitations that have led to the development of newer alternatives. Several direct thrombin inhibitors have now been licensed for use in particular clinical settings. For example, recombinant hirudin is licensed for treatment of arterial or venous thrombosis in which HIT is present (see later discussion of HIT), and for use in cardiopulmonary bypass. In most studies, increased bleeding compared with alternatives has restricted its use somewhat. Argatroban is a parenteral direct thrombin inhibitor used for prophylaxis or treatment of thrombosis in patients with HIT. A synthetic hirudin analog named bivalirudin is also available and may be useful in certain settings.

Direct Oral Anticoagulants

Several new direct oral anticoagulants have been licensed in the last few years in a number of countries. Several different terms have been used to describe this category of drugs, including new or novel oral anticoagulants (NOACs), non–vitamin K oral anticoagulants (NOACs), and target-specific oral anticoagulants (TSOACs). Recently the term *direct oral anticoagulants* (DOACs) has been recommended by ISTH and SSC based on a survey of a number of societies in the area of thrombosis.[142]

DOACs recently licensed in the United States and Europe include dabigatran etexilate (Pradaxa, Boehringer Ingelheim,

Ingelheim, Germany), rivaroxaban (Xarelto, Bayer Pharma AG, Berlin, Germany), apixaban (Eliquis, Bristol-Myers Squibb, New York, NY), edoxaban (Savaysa, Daiichi Sankyo, Tokyo, Japan), and betrixaban (BEVYXXA, Portola, San Francisco, CA). Dabigatran etexilate is a direct thrombin inhibitor, and rivaroxaban, apixaban, edoxaban, and betrixaban are direct Xa inhibitors. Their use is increasing for stroke prevention in nonvalvular atrial fibrillation and thromboprophylaxis after knee or hip replacement. These DOACs share some common features of rapid action and the ability to bind both free and surface-bound forms of their target activated serine protease. Randomized clinical trials have established that pharmacokinetic and pharmacodynamic responses in different individuals are sufficiently similar to ensure that these drugs are safe and efficacious at fixed doses without monitoring in the majority of patients. On the other hand, many clinical trials exclude patients with renal impairment, children, the very elderly, those with increased bleeding risk, and those at the extremes of body weight and therefore there are circumstances in which it may be useful to determine the concentration of anticoagulant in particular patients. Circumstances in which measuring DOAC may be helpful are summarized in Box 81.2.

Both direct IIa and direct Xa inhibitors interfere in many clot-based coagulation tests and assays and some chromogenic assays, some of which were described previously in relation to PC, PS, AT, and aPCR testing.[138] For a review of DOACs in the laboratory, see a report by Adcock and Gosselin.[143,144] The effects of DOAC on screening tests is very much dependent on the reagents used for testing, so laboratories should be aware of the sensitivity of the reagents in local use. Safe interpretation of clotting test results in the presence of DOACs must take the laboratory method and reagent sensitivity into account. Drugs in the same class have different effects on clotting tests; for example, for most reagents, rivaroxaban has more impact on PT and aPTT than apixaban for any particular plasma concentration of drug. A summary of these effects is shown in Table 81.7. Data obtained by study of one drug should not be used to predict actions of another from the same class.

BOX 81.2 Circumstances When Measurement of Direct Oral Anticoagulants May Be Useful

- When there is spontaneous or traumatic bleeding
- If overdose is suspected
- When patients are taking other drugs known to interact
- In patients with new thrombosis while taking the drug
- If emergency surgery is needed
- If thrombolysis is being considered
- Before elective surgery in which drug may still be present
- In patients requiring neuraxial anesthesia before surgery
- In patients with renal impairment
- During bridging between anticoagulants
- To assess compliance
- Extremes of body weight
- To assess possible accumulation in very old patients
- In patients in whom absorption may be affected by intestinal surgery
If reversal agents are being used

Direct Xa Inhibitor Assays

The concentration of direct factor Xa inhibitors can be determined in plasma using liquid chromatography–mass spectrometry, but this technique is not suitable for rapid assays and is not widely available. The most frequently used methods for measurement of direct factor Xa inhibitors are anti-Xa activity assays. A number of studies have shown these to be more sensitive and more specific than routine clot-based tests.[138] There is excellent correlation between levels determined by anti-Xa and by liquid chromatography/mass spectrometry methods, which is not the case for levels estimated by PT.[130] The anti-Xa assay reagents and method should be optimized for use with DOACs because some methods developed for use with LMWH are unsuitable for assay of samples containing rivaroxaban or apixaban. It is recommended that product-specific calibrators are used,[138] and it may be necessary to establish different calibrations for samples with high and low levels in some cases.[145] PT and aPTT should not be used to determine drug concentrations because these tests are sensitive to many other effects in addition to the presence of DOACs.

Direct IIa Inhibitor Assays

As for direct Xa inhibitors, the concentration of direct factor IIa inhibitors can be determined in plasma using liquid chromatography–mass spectrometry, but this technique is not suitable for rapid assays and is not widely available. A number of types of assay are available. Specific chromogenic anti-IIa assays can be used to determine concentrations of dabigatran, argatroban, or lepirudin in plasma. Thrombin-based clotting assays also can be used with product-specific calibrators. One particular commercial thrombin-based assay has been more widely used and shows good linearity between dabigatran concentration and clotting time up to 300 ng/mL or higher.[146] Because the test plasma is diluted between 1 in 8 and 1 in 20, the clotting time and assay results are largely independent of the test plasma fibrinogen, rendering the test highly specific for presence of thrombin inhibitors. Supratherapeutic concentrations of UFH can prolong the clotting time in this assay. Other options for assay of direct thrombin inhibitors include ecarin clotting and chromogenic assays or prothrombinase-induced clotting time.[147]

Therapy With Vitamin K Antagonists

VKAs such as warfarin are used as oral drugs for the treatment of VTE and as prophylaxis in patients with atrial fibrillation, artificial heart valves, or various thrombophilic states. The number of patients requiring long-term VKA therapy continues to grow and is estimated at 750,000 to 1 million at present in the United Kingdom, with a similar prevalence in many developed Western populations. This number is expected to continue to rise, even though possible new anticoagulant drugs are being investigated in clinical trials.

VKAs function as anticoagulants by interfering with the vitamin K cycle, which is needed for the postribosmal modification of clotting factors II, VII, IX, and X, as well as the anticoagulant proteins PC and PS. A consequence of VKA therapy is that these factors are no longer fully functional. Typically in the clotting process, multiple amino acids in these clotting factors are carboxylated in a way that facilitates binding of the factors to calcium and phospholipid surfaces. Without these modifications, binding is reduced and clotting proceeds much more slowly. The problem is that the dose

POINTS TO REMEMBER
Laboratory Issues With Direct Oral Anticoagulants

- DOACs are safe and effective, without routine laboratory monitoring of drug levels in the majority of patients.
- Measurement of plasma drug concentration may be useful in selected cases, including renal impairment, before surgery, at extremes of body weight, and when bleeding or thrombosis occurs during therapy.
- The method of choice for rapid determination of plasma concentrations of direct oral factor Xa inhibitors is an anti-Xa method validated for use with DOAC and calibrated with drug-specific calibrators.
- The method of choice for rapid determination of plasma concentrations of direct oral thrombin inhibitors is dilute TT, ecarin time, or chromogenic assay, all of which should be calibrated using drug specific calibrators.
- Prolongation of PT and aPTT by DOACs varies across different drugs (even between drugs with the same target).
- The prolongation of PT and aPTT by DOAC varies markedly according to which reagents are used for testing (see also Table 81.6).
- Normal PT and aPTT do not always exclude presence of peak levels of DOACs
- DOACs may interfere in a range of clot-based coagulation tests and some chromogenic assays (see also Table 81.7).

response is variable, so dosage must be very closely monitored to avoid over-anticoagulation or under-anticoagulation.

Many different types of VKA are used; warfarin (also known as Coumadin, Jantoven, Marevan, Lawarin, and Waran) is most common in North America and the United Kingdom. Numerous drugs affect the action of VKA in an unpredictable fashion, making monitoring necessary. Indeed, optimal oral anticoagulant therapy requires regular monitoring to ensure an appropriate balance between antithrombotic effects and unwanted hemorrhagic side effects. As discussed earlier, the test of choice for this monitoring in most countries is measurement of PT. Because of variability in different lots of thromboplastins, a normalization model has been developed that is based on expression of results using the INR.

As discussed in greater detail earlier in this chapter, the INR is based on the source of thromboplastins, and series of international standard thromboplastins are available from the WHO. Commercial thromboplastins are calibrated against the WHO reference thromboplastin by determination of paired PTs performed with the reference and commercial thromboplastin on a series of plasma specimens from healthy normal subjects and plasmas from patients stabilized on VKA therapy. The $\log_{10}$ of paired PTs is plotted, and a regression line fitted through the data. The slope of the line indicates the responsiveness of the commercial thromboplastin relative to the WHO international standard. This is used to derive the ISI. The ISI is then used to convert PT into INR using the equation:

$$INR = [PT\ (patient)/PT\ (geometric\ mean\ of\ normal\ patients)]^{ISI}$$

The ISI is influenced by the analyzer used to perform testing; thus a single thromboplastin may have different ISIs when used with different analyzers. The reagent manufacturer, therefore, provides specific ISI values for reagent/instrument combinations.

It has been reported that some analyzers of the same model type vary to the extent that local calibration of the ISI may be needed. For a full review, see Tripodi.[148] When the INR system is used, the same result should be obtained, irrespective of the methods that have been used to derive the value, but on some occasions, this does not occur. For example, this is a particular problem when INRs are elevated substantially above the therapeutic range. It also may occur when patients have LAC in which prolongation of PT/INR is a combination of VKA therapy and interference with the test by LAC. Some reagents and certain patients are particularly prone to this problem. To monitor VKA therapy when the PT/INR is affected by LAC, it is necessary to select a PT/INR system (perhaps by sending samples to other laboratories) that is not responsive to the LAC effect in that patient (as evidenced by a normal PT/INR before commencement of VKA therapy) or use of alternative assays such as chromogenic factor X or chromogenic factor II activity.[149] For clinical recommendations on targets for INR in VKA therapy, see the report by Ansell and associates.[150]

Point of Care for Monitoring Vitamin K Antagonist Therapy
Much of the testing for monitoring anticoagulant therapy continues to be performed in core or reference clinical laboratories, but there is a trend toward performing such measurements near the patient.[151] This type of testing is known as point-of-care (POC) testing (see Chapter 30),[152] and POC devices are now available that allow the patient to measure INR at home.[153] Consequently, the patient is able to adjust his or her VKA dose, and guidelines and recommendations have been established for self-testing and self-management of oral anticoagulation.[154,155] However, it should be noted that results from a 2010 study did not support the superiority of self-testing over clinic testing in reducing the risk for stroke, major bleeding episodes, and death among patients taking warfarin therapy.[153]

Determination of INR with POC instruments involves insertion of an individual test strip or cartridge into the monitor, followed by addition of the patient's blood sample. The blood reconstitutes dried thromboplastin reagent and initiates clotting reactions in the presence of calcium, leading to thrombin generation or clot formation. Within POC-INR devices are many types of end-point detection systems. For some systems, electronic quality control (QC) is available, in which an electronic device is inserted into the monitor in place of the test strip and an electronic signal is produced that tests the electronic system within the POC monitor. Table 81.8 provides a list of currently used POC-INR systems.

Some manufacturers of POC-INR systems produce test strips for INR determination with built-in QC. For example, the CoaguChek XS and CoaguChek XS Plus devices (Roche Diagnostics, Indianapolis, Indiana) have a test strip integrity check. With these devices, a test strip containing a compound (Resazurin) that is sensitive to factors such as light, humidity, and temperature is analyzed. Chemical changes that occur are measured electrochemically, and the patient INR is displayed only if the test strip integrity check is acceptable. In addition to internal QC checks, external QA (EQA) is available for POC-INR testing in the United States and Europe.[156]

Participation in EQA/proficiency testing is recommended in some countries for health care professionals performing POC INR tests.[154] Proficiency testing programs typically compare the local result to a target range derived from results returned by other users of the same device. The most commonly

TABLE 81.8 Some Prothrombin Time and International Normalized Ratio Point-of-Care Devices

Device	End-Point Detection	Memory Storage	Sample Volume (µL)	Quality Control Available	Sample Type	Tests Other Than INR
CoaguChek S (Roche)	Iron oxide particles	60	10	Liquid QC	Capillary/venous native whole blood	No
CoaguChek XS (Roche)	Electrochemical cleavage	100	10	Built-in QC	Capillary/venous native whole blood	No
CoaguChek XS Plus (Roche)	Electrochemical cleavage	500	10	Liquid and built-in QC	Capillary/venous native whole blood	No
Hemochron Signature Series (ITC/Thoratec Corporation)	Blood flow through a restriction channel	200+ basic model 600+ top model	50	Liquid QC	Native or citrated capillary/venous whole blood	Yes
i-STAT (Abbott Diagnostics)	Electrochemical cleavage	5000	20	Liquid QC	Native whole blood	Yes
INRatio (Hemo-Sense/Inverness Medical)	Electric impedance	60	15	Built-in QC	Native capillary whole blood	No
ProTime (ITC/Thoratec Corporation)	Photoptic detection of decreased blood flow	50	27	Liquid and built-in QC	Capillary/venous native whole blood	No

QC, Quality control.

used target is a range spanning 15% above the peer group median to 15% below the median although a number of other ranges have been used.[157]

It should be noted that POC-INR results may not agree with those generated in local clinical laboratories, particularly when values are beyond the therapeutic interval. As part of the QC process, a venous sample is collected at the same time as the POC test and is analyzed in an appropriate laboratory. Some patients show discrepancies between INRs determined by two different techniques, despite being stabilized on oral anticoagulant therapy. One cause of this is the presence of LAC, although discrepancies also occur without LAC. POC instruments with an electrochemical end-point detection are insensitive to low fibrinogen levels.[158,159]

In a 2008 study, Murray and colleagues[160] concluded that patients could successfully participate in a formal EQA program using the same freeze-dried test samples as are used in conventional laboratory EQA programs. The same study demonstrated that comparing the patient POC device with a reference device was an effective form of EQA. Recommendations in relation to QC and QA related to patients who self-test or self-manage their VKA therapy are available.[161]

SELECTED REFERENCES

2. CLSI. Collection, transport and processing of blood specimens for testing plasma-based coagulation assays and molecular assays; approved guideline—fifth edition. CLSI document H21-A5. Wayne, PA: Clinical and Laboratory Standards Institute; 2008.
6. Langdell RD, Wagner RH, Brinkhous KM. Effect of antihemophilic factor on one-stage clotting tests; a presumptive test for hemophilia and a simple one-stage antihemophilic factor assy procedure. J Lab Clin Med 1953;41:637–47.
17. One-stage prothrombin time (PT) and activated partial thromboplastin time (APTT) test. H47-A2. 2nd ed. Wayne, PA: CLSI; 2008.
25. Verbruggen B, Novakova I, Wessels H, Boezeman J, van den Berg M, Mauser-Bunschoten E. The Nijmegen modification of the Bethesda assay for factor VIII:C inhibitors: improved specificity and reliability. Thromb Haemost 1995;73:247–51.
40. White GC II, Rosendaal F, Aledort LM, Lusher JM, Rothschild C, Ingerslev J. Definitions in hemophilia. Recommendation of the scientific subcommittee on factor VIII and factor IX of the scientific and standardization committee of the International Society on Thrombosis and Haemostasis. Thromb Haemost 2001;85:560.
58. Jenkins PV, Bowyer A, Burgess C, et al. Laboratory coagulation tests and emicizumab treatment A United Kingdom Haemophilia Centre Doctors' Organisation guideline. Haemophilia 2020;26:151–5.
76. Taylor FB, Jr., Toh CH, Hoots WK, Wada H, Levi M. Towards definition, clinical and laboratory criteria, and a scoring system for disseminated intravascular coagulation. Thromb Haemost 2001;86:1327–30.
79. Quantitative D-dimer for the exclusion of venous thromboembolic disease. H59-A. Wayne, PA: Clinical and Laboratory Standards Institute; 2012.
86. Baglin T, Gray E, Greaves M, et al. Clinical guidelines for testing for heritable thrombophilia. Br J Haematol 2010;149:209–20.
91. Hillarp A, Baghaei F, Fagerberg Blixter I, et al. Effects of the oral, direct factor Xa inhibitor rivaroxaban on commonly used coagulation assays. J Thromb Haemost 2011;9:133–9.
93. Adcock DM, Gosselin R, Kitchen S, Dwyre DM. The effect of dabigatran on select specialty coagulation assays. Am J Clin Pathol 2013;139:102–9.
112. Giannakopoulos B, Krilis SA. The pathogenesis of the antiphospholipid syndrome. N Engl J Med 2013;368:1033–44.

113. Miyakis S, Lockshin MD, Atsumi T, et al. International consensus statement on an update of the classification criteria for definite antiphospholipid syndrome (APS). J Thromb Haemost 2006;4:295–306.

118. Pengo V, Tripodi A, Reber G, et al. Update of the guidelines for lupus anticoagulant detection. Subcommittee on Lupus Anticoagulant/Antiphospholipid Antibody of the Scientific and Standardisation Committee of the International Society on Thrombosis and Haemostasis. J Thromb Haemost 2009;7:1737–40.

119. Keeling D, Mackie I, Moore GW, Greer IA, Greaves M, British Committee for Standards in H. Guidelines on the investigation and management of antiphospholipid syndrome. Br J Haematol 2012;157:47–58.

121. Laboratory Testing for lupus anticoagulant. H60-A. 1st ed. Wayne, PA: Clinical and Laboratory Standards Institute; 2014.

134. Brill-Edwards P, Ginsberg JS, Johnston M, Hirsh J. Establishing a therapeutic range for heparin therapy. Ann Intern Med 1993;119:104–9.

144. Gosselin RC, Adcock DM, Douxfils J. An update on laboratory assessment for direct oral anticoagulants (DOACs). Int J Lab Hematol 2019;41(Suppl 1):33–9.

148. Tripodi A. Monitoring oral anticoagulant therapy. In: Kitchen S, Olson JD, Preston FE, eds. Quality in laboratory hemostasis and thrombosis. Hoboken, NJ: Wiley-Blackwell; 2009.

Microbiology

Exam questions, case studies, and additional resources are available on ExpertConsult.com.
*Full versions of these chapters are available electronically on www.ExpertConsult.com.

82

Introduction to Infectious Diseases

Michael TeKippe and Erin McElvania

ABSTRACT

Almost every portion of the human body can be infected in some manner by bacteria, viruses, fungi, or parasites. Symptoms of infection range widely from a mild or asymptomatic upper respiratory virus to severe and life-threatening infections such as meningitis. The variation in symptoms and disease severity is due to both differences in the pathogenic potential of the infecting organism and the response of the host. The pathogens that infect our bodies vary by geographic location and the time of year. Some pathogens are externally introduced into the body while others are members of our commensal microbiota that have gained access to normally sterile sites allowing them to proliferate and cause infection. The host immune system is responsible for eradicating pathogens when they invade, but it varies in efficacy due to age, genetic defects of the immune system, or immunosuppressive therapies such as chemotherapy and biologic treatments. This chapter is divided into sections mostly by organ system: bloodstream and endovascular, central nervous system (CNS), upper respiratory, lower respiratory, gastrointestinal, genitourinary, bone and joint, skin and soft tissue, multi-system, and congenital infections. In each section, we describe the most common types of infection, the most common pathogens responsible for these infections, the mechanisms of infection, and special considerations for pediatric and immunocompromised individuals. This chapter is a launching point from which the pathogens covered in subsequent chapters can be placed into clinical context.

INTRODUCTION

Almost every portion of the human body can be infected in some manner by bacteria, viruses, fungi, or parasites (see At a Glance: Overview of body systems and associated major human pathogens). Symptoms of infection range widely from a mild or asymptomatic upper respiratory virus to severe and life-threatening infections such as meningitis. The variation in symptoms and disease severity is due to both differences in the pathogenic potential of the infecting organism and the response of the host. The pathogens that infect our bodies vary by geographic location and the time of year. Some pathogens are externally introduced into the body while others are members of our commensal microbiota that have gained access to normally sterile sites allowing them to proliferate and cause infection (see At a Glance: Overview of major human pathogens and associated infections). The host immune system is responsible for eradicating pathogens when they invade, but it varies in efficacy due to age, genetic defects of the immune system, or immunosuppressive therapies such as chemotherapy and biologic treatments. This chapter is divided into sections mostly by organ system: bloodstream and endovascular, CNS, upper respiratory, lower respiratory, eye, gastrointestinal (GI), genitourinary (GU), bone and joint, skin and soft tissue, multi-system, and congenital infections. In each section, we describe the most common types of infection, the most common pathogens responsible for these infections, the mechanisms of infection, and special considerations for pediatric and immunocompromised individuals. This chapter is a launching point from which the pathogens covered in subsequent chapters can be placed into clinical context.

POINTS TO REMEMBER

- Human infections can be caused by bacteria, viruses, fungi, and parasites.
- Common pathogens at a specific body site vary and are a result of the route of infection.
- Infection severity is influenced by the pathogenic potential of a microorganism, host immune status, and the organ system infected.

AT A GLANCE

Overview of Body Systems and Associated Major Human Pathogens

Bloodstream
- *Staphylococcus aureus*, Enterobacterales
- *Candida* spp.
- *Plasmodium* spp.

Central Nervous System
- *Streptococcus pneumoniae, Haemophilus influenzae, Neisseria meningitidis*
- *Cryptococcus neoformans*
- Herpes simplex virus, Enterovirus, West Nile virus

Respiratory
- *S. pneumoniae, S. aureus, Pseudomonas aeruginosa*
- *H. influenzae, Klebsiella* spp., *Mycobacterium tuberculosis, Mycoplasma pneumoniae, Legionella* spp.
- *C. neoformans, Aspergillus* spp., *Pneumocystis jirovecii*
- *Coccidioides* spp., *Blastomyces dermatitidis, Histoplasma capsulatum*
- Influenza virus, Respiratory syncytial virus, Rhinovirus, Coronavirus

Gastrointestinal
- *Salmonella, Campylobacter, Shigella, Escherichia coli* O157
- Norovirus, Rotavirus, Hepatitis A
- *Giardia lamblia, Cryptosporidium, Entamoeba histolytica*

Urogenital
- Urinary tract
  - *E. coli, Klebsiella* spp., *P. aeruginosa, Staphylococcus saprophyticus*
  - *Schistosoma haematobium*
- Genital Tract
  - *Chlamydia trachomatis, Neisseria gonorrhoeae, Mycoplasma genitalium, Treponema pallidum*
  - *Candida* spp.
  - Herpes simplex virus, human papillomavirus
  - *Trichomonas vaginalis*

Bone and Joint
- *S. aureus*, coagulase-negative *Staphylococcus, Cutibacterium acnes, N. gonorrhoeae, Borrelia burgdorferi*
- Chikungunya virus

Skin and Soft Tissue
- *S. aureus, Streptococcus pyogenes, Pasteurella multocida, Clostridium perfringens*
- *Trichophyton* spp., *Microsporum* spp., *Epidermophyton* spp.
- Varicella zoster virus (VZV), molluscum contagiosum, Herpes simplex virus (HSV)
- *Sarcoptes scabiei* (scabies) and *Pediculus* spp. (lice)

BLOODSTREAM AND ENDOVASCULAR INFECTIONS

Bacteremia and fungemia are the presence of bacteria or fungi in the bloodstream. This can occur transiently, intermittently, or continuously. The most common type of bacteremia is transient, in which small amounts of bacteria breach the mucus membranes to enter the blood, such as occurs when one brushes their teeth. The microorganisms are cleared rapidly by the host immune system and for the most part do not cause further complications for the host. However, a number of infections at other body sites (e.g., osteomyelitis, urinary tract infection [UTI], pneumonia, intraabdominal infection) can lead to intermittent seeding of the bloodstream with microorganisms. Blood cultures are used to capture this seeding. Under certain circumstances the endovascular system itself can become directly infected, causing continuous infection. These situations include suppurative thrombophlebitis and infective endocarditis. In this section, we discuss the pathogenesis responsible for bloodstream and endovascular infections. A table of common microorganisms causing these infections can be found in Table 82.1.

Suppurative Thrombophlebitis

Suppurative thrombophlebitis, also known as septic thrombophlebitis, refers to the development of venous thrombosis in the presence of bacteremia. In this setting, the thrombus provides a nidus of infection for colonization and growth of the bacteria. In the peripheral veins, the presence of an intravenous

catheter is the most common precipitating factor although burns and intravenously injected drugs are also predisposing factors.[1-3] Suppurative thrombophlebitis of the vena cava largely occurs in the presence of central venous catheters (CVCs). *Staphylococcus aureus* is the most common pathogen responsible but other bacteria including *Streptococcus pyogenes* (also known as group A *Streptococcus* or GAS) and enteric gram-negative bacilli have been described.[4] *Candida* species are the most common fungal cause of infection.[4]

Suppurative thrombophlebitis may also develop secondary to other ongoing infections. Osteomyelitis, particularly in children with subperiosteal abscesses secondary to *S. aureus*, can induce thrombophlebitis in nearby veins. Pylephlebitis, suppurative thrombosis of the portal vein, can occur secondary to any intra-abdominal infection with drainage through the portal vein and septic dural sinus thrombosis can occur following head and neck infections.[3,5] *Escherichia coli* and *Bacteroides* species are most commonly associated with pylephlebitis but other enteric bacteria can also be present.[5] *S. aureus* remains the most common cause of septic dural sinus thrombosis, but streptococci and anaerobes such as *Bacteroides* and *Fusobacterium* are also noted.[6,7]

Suppurative thrombophlebitis of the jugular vein is known by a variety of names including Lemierre syndrome, postanginal sepsis, and necrobacillosis. It is primarily associated with a preceding episode of pharyngitis. Septic emboli to the lungs are common, and lung abscesses and empyema can result. The most common etiologic agent is the anaerobe *Fusobacterium necrophorum*, but other oral microbiota

TABLE 82.1	Common Pathogens Causing Bloodstream and Endovascular Infections		
	Bacteria	**Fungi**	**Parasites**
Suppurative thrombophlebitis	Staphylococcus aureus Streptococcus pyogenes Escherichia coli and other Enterobacterales Fusobacterium necrophorum	Candida spp.	
Infective endocarditis	S. aureus Streptococcus spp., primarily viridans group streptococci and Streptococcus bovis Enterococcus spp. Coagulase-negative staphylococcus spp. HACEK gram-negative bacteria	Candida spp.	
Catheter-related infections	S. aureus Staphylococcus lugdunensis Coagulase-negative staphylococcus spp. Enterobacterales Enterococcus spp. Pseudomonas aeruginosa	Candida spp.	
Asplenic patients	Streptococcus pneumoniae Neisseria meningitidis Haemophilus influenzae		Plasmodium spp. Babesia spp.
Parasites			Plasmodium spp. Babesia spp. Trypanosoma spp.
Immunocompromised host	Viridans group streptococci	Cryptococcus neoformans Fusarium spp.	
Pediatrics	Streptococcus agalactiae E. coli Listeria monocytogenes		

including streptococcal species (particularly *S. pyogenes*), *Eikenella corrodens*, and other *Fusobacterium* species can be responsible.[5]

Infective Endocarditis

Infective endocarditis is infection of the endovascular surfaces of the heart. The infection is most frequently established on the heart valves, but it can also develop directly on the wall of the chamber, often in locations where septal defects create turbulent flow. Although technically not part of the endocardium and hence not true endocarditis, infections of cardiac shunts or those related to coarctation of the aorta are considered in this group of infections due to their similar clinical manifestations, microbiologic causes, and treatments.

The clinical manifestations of infective endocarditis typically include fever along with nonspecific findings such as malaise, headache, myalgias, night sweats, vomiting, and abdominal pain. Signs of emboli including splinter hemorrhages, Janeway lesions (nodular erythematous macules of the palms and soles), kidney and splenic infarcts, lung abscess/empyema, osteomyelitis, septic arthritis, embolic stroke, and intracranial hemorrhage. Systemic immune reactions such as glomerulonephritis, Osler's nodes (tender subcutaneous nodules on the fingers and toes), and Roth spots (hemorrhagic lesions of the retina) may also be present. Diagnosis is made using the modified Duke criteria to stratify patients into definite or possible infective endocarditis or to reject that diagnosis outright. Major criteria include two or more blood cultures with microorganisms associated with infective

endocarditis or echographic evidence of endocarditis. Minor criteria include a predisposing condition, fever, evidence of emboli, immunologic phenomena, and a positive blood culture that does not meet major criteria.[8]

The vast majority of infective endocarditis cases are secondary to gram-positive organisms. *S. aureus* is the leading cause worldwide and was responsible for 31% of cases in a large cohort of ~2800 cases.[9] Streptococci were responsible for 29% of cases with viridans group streptococci causing 17% and *Streptococcus bovis* leading to 6% of total cases respectively. Enterococci were responsible for 10% of cases as well. Although not considered an endocarditis-associated organism by the modified Duke criteria, coagulase-negative staphylococci are a relatively common cause of infective endocarditis at 11% of cases.[9]

Gram-negative organisms are much less commonly associated with infective endocarditis than gram-positive organisms and only comprised 4% of cases in the same study.[9] The most common organisms are a collection of gram-negative bacteria that colonize the oral-pharyngeal cavity called the HACEK organisms. Members of this group include *Haemophilus* spp., *Aggregatibacter* spp. (primarily *A. aphrophilus*, *A. paraphrophilus*, and *A. actinomycetemcomitans*), *Cardiobacterium hominis* and *C. valvarum*, *E. corrodens*, and *Kingella kingae*. Historically, the fastidious nature of these organisms may have prevented them from growing in blood culture broth within a 5-day period, but with modern automated blood culture systems, the HACEK organisms are reliably isolated within the 5-day window, generally in 2 to 3 days.[10]

Fungal endocarditis is even less prevalent than gram-negative cases and is usually secondary to *Candida* species. Cases of *Aspergillus* endocarditis, which is likely the second leading cause of fungal endocarditis, have also been reported.[11]

Immunocompromised Patients and Health Care–Associated Bloodstream and Endovascular Infections

The rate of endovascular infection rises dramatically in the health care setting. One of the leading causes for this is the presence of CVCs. Although these lines provide a location for the development of suppurative thrombophlebitis as discussed earlier, CVCs can also lead to infection in the absence of clots. CVCs both serve as a portal for direct access to the bloodstream and as a nidus of biofilm formation and ongoing infection. Central line-associated bloodstream infections (CLABSIs) are largely introduced in one of three ways: skin colonization leading to migration of organisms along the intracutaneous tract and through the fibrin sheath surrounding the catheter, intraluminal colonization of the catheter or hub, and hematogenous seeding from another location. The organisms associated with CLABSIs reflect those routes of infection. *S. aureus* and coagulase-negative staphylococci, which are key components of the skin microbiota, are leading causes of CLABSIs.[12] However, considerable effort has been placed on infection prevention methods, including skin cleansing and catheter care.[13] There is evidence that these preventive methods have been effective at reducing rates of CLABSI.[14] Enterobacterales (particularly *Klebsiella, E. coli,* and *Enterobacter*) and *Candida* species are now the leading groups of organisms responsible for CLABSIs in the United States based on reporting to the National Healthcare Safety Network.[12] *Enterococcus* species and *Pseudomonas aeruginosa* are also key causes of CLABSIs.

The rate of infective endocarditis is increased dramatically in the presence of indwelling foreign material, which lacks many of the protective barriers of normal tissue and can thus better serve as a nidus for infection. Prosthetic valves in particular have high rates of infection, with older studies suggesting rates ranging from 1 to 6%.[15–18] A more recent study still shows similar rates of 1.9%.[19] Causative organisms are similar to those with native valve endocarditis.[9]

Immunocompromised oncology and transplant patients demonstrate endovascular infections at much higher rates than immunocompetent individuals due to high rates of CVC usage and loss of intestinal mucosal barrier function, in addition to loss of immune function. Immunocompromised patients are also at increased risk of bone marrow infections caused by hematogenous seeding. Viridans group streptococci are a major concern in this population,[12] but a wide variety of bacteria and fungi can lead to endovascular infection in these patients.

One set of immunocompromised patients worth noting here are asplenic and functionally asplenic patients. The spleen plays a critical role in the prevention of bacteremia from a number of encapsulated bacteria (*Streptococcus pneumoniae, Neisseria meningitidis,* and *Haemophilus influenzae* most prominently), and the absence of a functional spleen greatly increases the risk of bacteremia and subsequent complications from these organisms. Management of that risk includes vaccinations against these organisms and antibiotic prophylaxis in high-risk asplenic patients. Of note, the spleen is also important in helping to control the parasitic infections of malaria and babesiosis discussed later in this section; asplenic patients with those infections exhibit more severe symptoms.[20]

Pediatric Considerations

For the most part, pediatric endovascular infections are caused by similar organisms as adult infections. However, otherwise healthy neonates are particularly prone to higher rates of bacteremia and may present with fever or a period of hypothermia as the only symptom. Bacteremia and corresponding sepsis in these neonates is divided into early-onset (less than 7 days of age) and late-onset (greater than 7 days of age).[21] Historically, *Streptococcus agalactiae* (also known as group B *Streptococcus* or GBS) was the leading cause of neonatal sepsis. Maternal screening and antibiotic prophylaxis have dramatically decreased the rate of early-onset GBS sepsis but has not changed the rate of late-onset sepsis.[22] *E. coli* is the second leading cause of sepsis in the neonatal period and now has similar rates to GBS.[21] *Listeria monocytogenes* is also well known to cause early-onset infection, but today only causes rare sporadic cases.[23]

Parasitemia

Although the number of cases of bacteria and fungi causing isolated bloodstream infections in otherwise healthy individuals is low, there are a number of significant parasites that do cause such infections. The most significant of these infections is malaria, which is caused by parasites of the genus *Plasmodium*. In 2018, there were an estimated 228 million cases of malaria worldwide resulting in 405,000 deaths with two-thirds in children under 5 years of age.[24] Malaria is spread to humans via the bite of female mosquitoes of the genus *Anopheles*. Infections are found throughout most of the tropics with ongoing transmission in 89 countries. The vast majority of cases (92%) occur in Africa with six countries (Nigeria, Democratic Republic of the Congo, Uganda, Côte d'Ivoire, Mozambique, and Niger) being responsible for more than half of all infections worldwide.[24]

Malaria is caused by four *Plasmodium* species that primarily infect humans: *P. falciparum, P. vivax, P. ovale,* and *P. malariae*. Two other species that are simian parasites have been shown to infect humans, although it is unclear if natural human-to-mosquito-to-human transmission occurs: *P. knowlesi* and *P. simium*. *P. falciparum* is responsible for the vast majority of cases and tends to have the most severe presentation. Over 99% of cases in Africa and a majority of cases in the Eastern hemisphere are caused by *P. falciparum*.[24] *P. vivax* is the second most common cause of malaria worldwide causing 3.3% of cases, including almost half of the cases in India. *P. vivax* is also the leading cause of malaria in the Americas causing 75% of cases.[24] *P. ovale* is endemic to tropical western Africa and can also be found in Southeast Asia and Oceania although at much lower levels than either *P. falciparum* or *P. vivax. P. malariae* is a relatively rare cause of malaria that is distributed throughout a similar area as *P. falciparum*.[25] *P. knowlesi* is similar in morphology to *P. malariae*, sometimes resembling a mixed *P. malariae* and *P. falciparum* infection, and has been shown to cause malaria, including severe malaria, in Southeast Asia.[26] Likewise, *P. simium* is similar in form to *P. vivax* and was recently discovered in patients in Brazil.[27] Both *P. vivax* and *P. ovale* have life cycle stages as hypnozoites, which are dormant stages that reside in the liver. These *Plasmodium* species require additional treatment to clear the hypnozoite stage, without which patients are at risk for recrudescence of disease.

The clinical manifestations of malaria are usually nonspecific such that malaria should be suspected in any febrile patient with exposure to a malaria endemic region. Initial symptoms of uncomplicated malaria include fever, headache, fatigue, nausea, vomiting, diarrhea, arthralgias, and myalgias. Severe malaria can lead to severe anemia, hypoglycemia, metabolic acidosis, acute respiratory distress syndrome, liver failure, renal failure, disseminated intravascular coagulation, and circulatory collapse. An encephalopathy with impaired consciousness, delirium, or seizures known as cerebral malaria can also be present.

Babesiosis is another parasitic disease that affects the circulatory system. Parasites from the genus *Babesia* invade and infect red blood cells similarly to *Plasmodium* species. Humans are infected primarily through *Ixodes scapularis* tick bite and are dead-end hosts. A variety of other mammals serve as a reservoir for the parasite. *Babesia microti* is the main agent of babesiosis in the United States, primarily located in the northeastern and upper Midwestern areas of the country. Cases in Europe have been associated with *B. divergens,* while *B. venatorum* is endemic in northeastern China. Symptoms range from asymptomatic to mild disease with fever, fatigue, and myalgias to severe disease. Severe disease is largely limited to elderly or immunocompromised patients, particularly asplenic patients. Acute respiratory distress syndrome and disseminated intravascular coagulopathy are the most common presentation of severe babesiosis. Infection often resolves without treatment in immunocompetent individuals, but treatment is recommended for all symptomatic patients.[28]

African trypanosomiasis, also known as sleeping sickness, is caused by parasites that are transmitted by the tsetse fly. These parasites then infect the bloodstream, enter the lymphatics and distribute widely throughout the body, ultimately entering the cerebral spinal fluid (CSF) and brain. There are two forms of trypanosomiasis: *Trypanosoma brucei gambiense* and *Trypanosoma brucei rhodesiense. T.b. gambiense* is found in 24 countries in western and central Africa and is the cause of 97% of all trypanosomiasis. This species causes a chronic infection where symptoms do not develop until months or years after infection. *T.b. rhodesiense* is found in 13 countries of eastern and southern Africa. Infection results in clinical presentation weeks to months after initial infection. Early symptoms of African trypanosomiasis include intermittent headache, fever, fatigue, myalgias, and arthralgias. A painless skin lesion (chancre) may also develop at the site of the infected bite, which is more common with *T. b. rhodesiense* than with *T. b. gambiense.* Lymphadenitis can also occur. Late-stage disease is classified as involvement of the CNS. A diffuse meningoencephalitis develops leading to encephalopathy with psychosis, seizures, delirium, and increasing somnolence, hence the sleeping sickness name.[29] Fatality of late-stage disease is nearly 100% if untreated.[30] Due to sustained efforts including surveillance, vector control, and case treatments, reported cases of African trypanosomiasis continue to drop with fewer than 3000 cases reported in 2015.[31,32]

The related parasite *Trypanosoma cruzi* causes a different infection known as American trypanosomiasis or Chagas disease. These parasites are spread by insects of the Triatominae subfamily (kissing bugs). The disease is found throughout the Americas from the southern United States to northern Argentina and Chile. Acute infection consists of a phase typically lasting 8 to 12 weeks after infection characterized by circulating parasites. Most patients are asymptomatic or have mild nonspecific symptoms during this phase and do not present for medical attention. A very small percentage may develop severe acute symptoms, most prominently acute myocarditis. After the acute phase, parasitemia will drop to an undetectable level, and infection will only be identifiable by serology. Patients can remain in an asymptomatic phase called the indeterminate form for decades. However, 30% to 40% of chronically infected patients will develop additional complications. The most common are cardiac issues where conduction system abnormalities occur and lead to development of heart failure. Involvement of the GI system is the other major complication of chronic Chagas disease occurring in 10% to 15% of patients infected. These complications include megaesophagus (with dysphagia, regurgitation, epigastric pain, and malnutrition) and megacolon (with constipation, abdominal distension, and sometimes large bowel obstruction).[33]

POINTS TO REMEMBER

- Bacteremia and fungemia are the presence of bacteria or fungi in the bloodstream, which can occur transiently, intermittently, or continuously.
- Gram-positive bacteria are the most common cause of bacteremia, including *Staphylococcus aureus,* streptococci, and enterococci.
- *Plasmodium* spp. are the most common cause of bloodstream infection in immunocompetent hosts.

CENTRAL NERVOUS SYSTEM INFECTIONS

Infections of the CNS include meningitis, encephalitis, and brain abscesses. Pathogens enter the CNS by crossing the blood brain barrier, trauma, the introduction of hardware such as shunts, or by direct extension from the sinuses. Infected patients can be asymptomatic, have mild, nonspecific symptoms, or develop fever, headache, and altered mental status. Depending on the infectious agent and the patient immune status infection can range from asymptomatic to deadly. CNS infections are most common in the first month of life and they are most severe and have the highest risk of morbidity and mortality in the very young and very old.[22,34,35]

Diagnosis of CNS infections relies on the collection of CSF. During the lumbar puncture the opening pressure is measured. High opening pressures are a signal that there is pressure in the CNS space that raises the suspicion for infection. The fluid is then examined for the presence of different types of white blood cells, along with levels of protein and glucose, to get a measure of overall inflammation.[34,35] Radiologic imaging is used to support the diagnosis of CNS infection. In this section we discuss the pathogenesis responsible for CNS infections. A diagram of CSF flow through the brain can be viewed in Fig. 82.1 and the most common microorganisms causing CNS infections are listed in Table 82.2.

Meningitis

Meningitis is inflammation of the meninges, the membranes that cover the brain and spinal cord. They contain the CSF, which bathes the brain. To enter this space, pathogens must cross the blood-brain barrier, entering either by direct extension from the sinuses—a situation which occurs most frequently in the presence of anatomical defects—or by way of trauma. Once in the CNS, pathogens multiply and are recognized by circulating immune cells causing the recruitment of additional immune cells to the CSF and the release of large amounts of proinflammatory cytokines. This inflammation causes increased pressure in the CNS, resulting in the symptoms of meningitis.

Viruses are the most frequent cause of acute meningitis with enteroviruses, arboviruses such as West Nile virus, and herpesviruses being the most common etiologies. Patients with acute meningitis present with fever, headache, neck stiffness, and/or altered mental status. Viral infections cause mild to moderate symptoms and self-resolve in otherwise healthy individuals. Symptoms are much more severe in acute bacterial meningitis, such that most patients seek medical attention within hours to a day of onset. The most common causes of bacterial meningitis in the community setting are *S. pneumoniae*, *N. meningitidis*, and *H. influenzae*, although the use of vaccines for these organisms over the last 20+ years has led to marked decrease in the rates of meningitis due to these organisms.[36] *L. monocytogenes* is another important cause of acute meningitis, primarily infecting the very young and old. *S. aureus* very rarely leads to isolated meningitis but is an important cause of acute meningitis in patients with endocarditis or paraspinal abscess. Parasitic causes of acute meningitis are rare in the United States but the free-living amoeba *Naegleria fowleri* is the most common in immunocompetent patients. Worldwide, the roundworm *Angiostrongylus cantonensis* is an important cause of eosinophilic meningitis.[34,35]

The presence of CSF hardware such as ventriculoperitoneal shunts increases the risk of infection and dramatically changes the types of pathogens responsible for infection. Gram-positive skin microbiota such as coagulase-negative staphylococci and *Cutibacterium acnes* (formerly *Propionibacterium acnes*) are much more prevalent. Gram-negative infections, particularly with enteric gram-negative bacteria such as *E. coli* and *Klebsiella* species also happen more frequently in the presence of CSF hardware, albeit at lower rates than with gram-positive skin microbiota.

Chronic meningitis shares many of the symptoms seen with acute meningitis, but symptom onset is gradual over weeks to months. Often patients will present with low-grade fevers and lethargy in addition to headache and altered mental status. Chronic meningitis is most often caused by mycobacteria, spirochetes, and fungi. *Mycobacterium tuberculosis* meningitis is the most common form of chronic meningitis, although it can

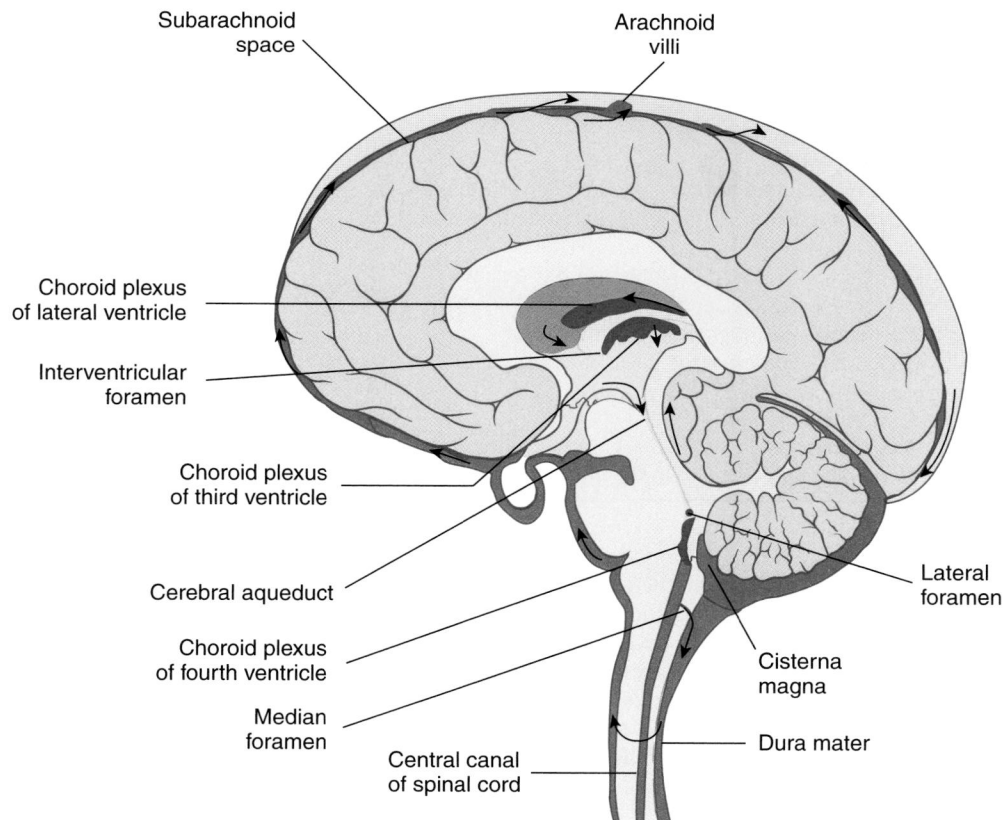

FIGURE 82.1 Flow of cerebral spinal fluid (CSF) through the brain. CSF originates in the choroid plexus and flows through the ventricles and subarachnoid space and into the bloodstream. (Reproduced with permission from Tille P, editor. *Bailey and Scott's diagnostic microbiology.* 14th ed. St. Louis: Elsevier; 2017.)

	Bacteria	Viruses	Fungi	Parasites
Acute meningitis	*Streptococcus pneumoniae* *Haemophilus influenzae* *Neisseria meningitidis* *Listeria monocytogenes* *Staphylococcus aureus*			*Naegleria fowleri* *Angiostrongylus* *cantonensis*

Chronic meningitis	*Mycobacterium tuberculosis*
	Treponema pallidum
	    (syphilis)
	Borrelia burgdorferi
	    (Lyme disease)
			Cryptococcus gattii
			Coccidioides spp.
			Histoplasma
			    capsulatum
				Acanthamoeba spp.
				Balamuthia mandrillaris

Encephalitis	*Mycoplasma pneumoniae* *Bartonella henselae* *Rickettsia rickettsii* *Ehrlichia chaffeensis*	Arboviruses (West Nile, eastern equine encephalitis, western equine encephalitis, St. Louis encephalitis, La Crosse encephalitis, Venezuelan equine encephalitis, and Japanese encephalitis viruses) Chikungunya virus Herpes viruses, primarily HSV-1 Enterovirus Influenza and other respiratory viruses		
Brain abscess	*Streptococcus anginosus* group *S. aureus* *H. influenzae* *Nocardia* spp. Anaerobic oral microbiota (*Fusobacterium* spp., *Bacteroides* spp., and *Prevotella* spp.)		*Cladophialophora bantiana* *Rhinocladiella mackenziei*	*Taenia solium* (Cysticercosis) *Entamoeba histolytica* *Schistosoma japonicum* *Paragonimus* spp.
Immunocompromised host	Skin microbiota entering through shunts	Cytomegalovirus (CMV) Human herpesvirus 6 (HHV-6) JC polyomavirus	*Cryptococcus neoformans* Candida spp.	*Toxoplasma gondii*
Pediatrics	*Streptococcus agalactiae* *Escherichia coli, Klebsiella* spp., and *Enterobacter* spp. *L. monocytogenes* *S. pneumoniae* *N. meningitidis*	Herpes simplex virus (HSV) Enterovirus Parechovirus		

TABLE 82.2 Common Pathogens Causing Central Nervous System Infections

present in an acute manner in children. For spirochetes, *Treponema pallidum* and *Borrelia burgdorferi,* the etiologic agents responsible for syphilis and Lyme disease, respectively, cause chronic meningitis although their most common presentation is encephalitis. Fungal causes of chronic meningitis include *Cryptococcus* species and endemic fungi such as *Coccidioides* and *Histoplasma.* The parasites *Acanthamoeba* and *Balamuthia* are rare causes of chronic parasitic meningitis.[34]

Encephalitis
Encephalitis is irritation, inflammation, or swelling of the brain. It differs from meningitis in that the brain parenchyma

is directly affected. As such, altered mental status including speech disturbances, confusion, agitation, hallucinations, and decreased levels of consciousness are strongly indicative of encephalitis. It can also cause seizures and partial paralysis. In reality, the distinction between meningitis and encephalitis is blurred with many patients often having both features, a condition referred to as meningoencephalitis. However, it is important to note the difference in presentation as the differential for the conditions are quite different. In terms of infectious encephalitis, viral infections are overwhelmingly the most common cause. In the United States, West Nile virus is the most common proven cause of infectious encephalitis. Other arboviruses such as St. Louis encephalitis, La Crosse encephalitis, Eastern equine encephalitis, and Western equine encephalitis play roles in the US while Chikungunya, Japanese encephalitis, and Venezuelan equine encephalitis are among the many important arboviral agents of encephalitis worldwide.[34] The herpesviruses, especially herpes simplex virus-1 (HSV-1) are also significant causes of encephalitis. Enteroviruses and other respiratory viruses, particularly influenza, are also known causes of encephalitis. Most bacterial causes of CNS infection lead to a meningitic rather than encephalitic presentation, but *Mycoplasma pneumoniae*, *Bartonella henselae*, *Rickettsia rickettsii*, and *Ehrlichia chaffeensis* are bacteria that can lead to a presentation of encephalitis.[34]

Brain Abscesses

Pathogens causing brain abscesses gain access to the brain by hematogenous spread through the blood-brain barrier, trauma to the brain, or contiguous spread to the brain from infections such as sinusitis, otitis media, or mastoiditis. Individuals present with symptoms of headache, nausea, vomiting, and neurologic findings such as seizure. Fever is present in less than 50% of patients with brain abscesses, much lower than for patients with meningitis and encephalitis. Bacteria are the most common cause of brain abscesses. Infections resulting from direct spread are usually polymicrobial including both facultative anaerobic bacteria such as streptococcal species (particularly *Streptococcus anginosus* group), *S. aureus*, and *H. influenzae* and obligate anaerobic bacteria such as *Bacteroides*, *Fusobacterium*, and *Prevotella* species. Neurotropic fungi causing brain abscesses include *Cladophialophora bantiana* and *Rhinocladiella mackenziei*.[37,38] Infections from hematogenous spread are more likely to be monomicrobial and secondary to other infections such as endocarditis. Parasitic infections are common in the developing world, but very rare in the United States, with cysticercosis due to the tapeworm *Taenia solium* being the most common. *Entamoeba histolytica*, *Schistosoma japonicum*, and *Paragonimus* species are also associated with brain abscesses.[34]

Immunocompromised Patients

Immunocompromised patients are susceptible to a broad differential of pathogens causing CNS disease. Human immunodeficiency virus (HIV) can directly affect the CNS leading to HIV encephalitis. Additionally, HIV-infected patients with severe immunosuppression are very susceptible to CNS infection with the fungal pathogen *Cryptococcus neoformans* and the parasite *Toxoplasma gondii*, both of which cause chronic meningitis or encephalitis. Immunocompromised patients are also at risk for encephalitis due to herpesviruses, particularly cytomegalovirus (CMV) and human herpesvirus-6 (HHV-6). Other types of fungal meningitis that are very rare in immunocompetent individuals such as *Candida* meningitis and *Scedosporium* meningitis, which is associated with near-death drowning,[39] are seen at higher rates in immunocompromised patients. The JC polyomavirus, a very common virus with few effects in immunocompetent individuals, is associated with progressive multifocal leukoencephalopathy (PML), a demyelinating disorder that leads to rapidly progressive focal neurologic deficits.

Pediatric Considerations

The first month of life has a greater risk for CNS infection than at any other point in an individual's life, as the blood-brain barrier is inadequately developed at that time. Classically, *S. agalactiae* (GBS) was the leading cause of bacterial meningitis in these infants, but maternal screening and intrapartum antibiotic prophylaxis has decreased this rate. Today, the rate of GBS meningitis in neonates is similar to that due to *E. coli*. Combined, GBS and *E. coli* meningitis account for more than 80% of neonatal bacterial meningitis. Other gram-negative organisms, including *Klebsiella* and *Enterobacter* species, are the next most common with gram-positive organisms such as *Listeria* comprising a small number of cases. The more common causes of bacterial meningitis in elderly patients, *S. pneumoniae*, *N. meningitidis*, and *H. influenzae*, are also the most common causes of meningitis between 1 month and 1 year of age.

Viral encephalitis and meningitis are also more common in young infants than older individuals, with enterovirus being particularly frequent. Parechovirus, which is closely related to the enteroviruses, is a cause of meningitis and encephalitis that is largely isolated to infants. Finally, a special note should be made of neonatal HSV meningoencephalitis. This infection, most commonly seen in the first 3 weeks of life but possibly as late as 6 weeks, can be caused by either HSV-1 or HSV-2 but is more commonly associated with HSV-2. With this infection, HSV enters the CNS either from retrograde spread from the nasopharynx and olfactory nerves or through hematogenous spread. Once present, it causes a profound meningoencephalitis often associated with lifelong neurologic impairment or death.

POINTS TO REMEMBER

- Central nervous system (CNS) infections include meningitis, encephalitis, and brain abscesses.
- Infections occur when pathogens cross the blood brain barrier, are introduced through trauma or surgery, form biofilms on hardware such as shunts, or gain access to the CNS space by direct extension from the sinuses.
- Individuals are at greater risk for CNS infection during the first month of life.

EYE INFECTIONS

The eye is a complex organ consisting of many different portions, each of which is susceptible to different microbial pathogens. Conjunctivitis, keratitis, endophthalmitis, and uveitis are all inflammatory reactions in different components of the eye, and all can be caused by infectious etiologies. These infections range from being very common but mostly benign, such as viral conjunctivitis, to being less frequent but potential causes of blindness. Diagnosis and management of many of these infections requires involvement of ophthalmologists. A diagram of the eye can be found in Fig. 82.2 and the most common causes of eye infection are found in Table 82.3.

Conjunctivitis

The conjunctiva is the mucous membrane that covers the inner surface of the eyelid and the globe of the eye up to the junction of the sclera and cornea. Inflammation of this

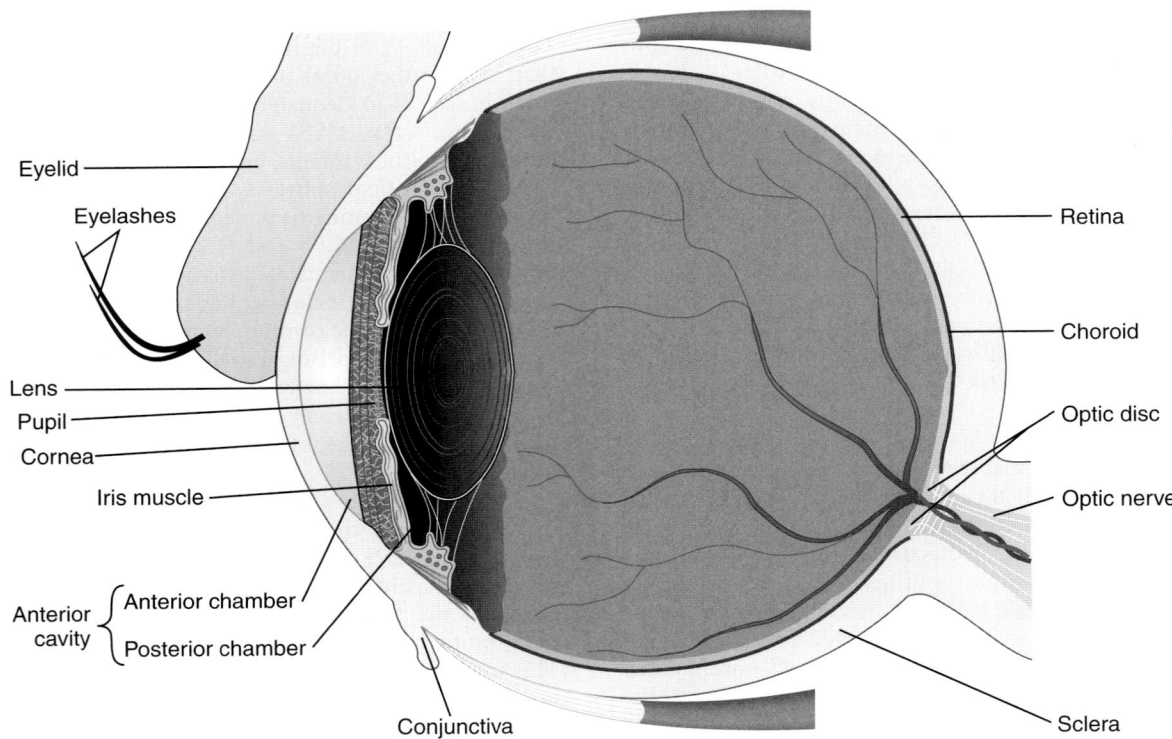

Eyelid

Eyelashes

Lens

Pupil

Cornea

Iris muscle

Anterior cavity { Anterior chamber

Posterior chamber

Conjunctiva

Retina

Choroid

Optic disc

Optic nerve

Sclera

FIGURE 82.2 Basic anatomy of the eye. (Reproduced with permission from Tille P, editor. *Bailey and Scott's diagnostic microbiology.* 14th ed. St. Louis: Elsevier; 2017.)

mucous membrane is termed conjunctivitis, and infectious conjunctivitis is the most common type of eye infection. Both viral and bacterial etiologies of conjunctivitis are common while fungal or parasitic causes are quite rare.

Viral causes are thought to be the most frequent infectious causes of conjunctivitis, which is often called "pink eye" and classically presents with copious watery discharge and conjunctival erythema. It can be unilateral at presentation but usually spreads to become bilateral. Fever, rhinorrhea, and pharyngitis may be present. Adenoviruses are the most common etiologic agents, as they are highly contagious. Symptoms typically resolve spontaneously within 2 weeks, but some adenovirus serotypes can lead to epidemic keratoconjunctivitis, which includes involvement of the cornea and where symptoms can last weeks to months. HSV and varicella zoster virus (VZV) can also lead to conjunctivitis, with few clinical complications when these infections are limited to the conjunctiva. Both HSV and VZV can extend to other parts of the eye, however, and these infections will be discussed further later in this section. Other rare viral causes of conjunctivitis are self-limited and include influenza, Epstein-Barr virus (EBV), measles, mumps, rubella, papillomavirus, and molluscum contagiosum.[34]

Determining the incidence of acute bacterial conjunctivitis is difficult, as many cases of viral conjunctivitis are treated as bacterial in origin. Classically, unilateral presentation is thought to be more common, but bilateral bacterial conjunctivitis also occurs. *S. aureus, S. pneumoniae, H. influenzae,* and *Moraxella catarrhalis* are the most common bacteria associated with conjunctivitis.[40] In adults, *S. aureus* predominate while other organisms have historically been more common in children.[40] Bacterial conjunctivitis from these organisms is

largely self-limited as with viral conjunctivitis and the benefit of antibiotic therapy is unclear.[41] Topical antibiotics are typically prescribed when therapy is given. *Neisseria gonorrhoeae* and to a lesser extent *N. meningitidis* can cause hyperacute bacterial conjunctivitis.[34] Infection is marked by copious, thick, yellowish-green discharge and requires systemic antibiotics for successful therapy.

Chlamydia trachomatis is another critically important cause of conjunctivitis. Infection is typically sexually acquired and inoculation into the eye results in redness and mucopurulent discharge.[34] *C. trachomatis* serotypes A, B, Ba, and C are associated with trachoma, which is the leading infectious cause of blindness worldwide. Blindness occurs following repeated bouts of infection, leading to eyelid scarring and ultimately corneal scarring. *C. trachomatis* is highly contagious and spread rapidly among families through secretions on fingers and fomites. In 1998, the World Health Organization launched a global initiative to eliminate trachoma using a combined strategy abbreviated "SAFE": surgery for trichiasis (in turned eyelashes), antibiotics for active infection, facial cleanliness, and environmental improvement. These efforts have made a significant global impact, bringing the population at risk of blindness down to 142 million in 2019 (from 1.5 billion in 2002) and decreased the number of people requiring surgery from 7.6 million to 2.5 million over that same time frame.[42]

Keratitis

Keratitis is inflammation of the cornea, which can have an infectious or noninfectious source. Infectious keratitis can be caused by bacteria, viruses, fungi, or parasites. The most common risk factor for the development of microbial

TABLE 82.3 Common Pathogens of Eye Infections

	Bacteria	Viruses	Fungi	Parasites
Conjunctivitis	Staphylococcus aureus Streptococcus pneumoniae Haemophilus influenzae Moraxella catarrhalis Neisseria gonorrhoeae Neisseria meningitidis Chlamydia trachomatis	Adenoviruses Herpes simplex virus (HSV) Varicella zoster virus (VZV) Influenza Epstein-Barr virus (EBV) Measles Mumps Rubella Papillomavirus Molluscum contagiosum		
Keratitis	Pseudomonas aeruginosa S. aureus S. pneumoniae Other Streptococcus spp. Haemophilus spp. Moraxella spp. Proteus spp. Klebsiella spp. Enterobacter spp. Citrobacter spp. Serratia marcescens Mycobacterium tuberculosis Rapidly growing Mycobacterium spp.	Herpes simplex virus (HSV) Varicella zoster virus (VZV)	Fusarium spp. Aspergillus spp. Candida spp. Paecilomyces spp. Phialophora spp. Curvularia spp. Alternaria spp. Sporothrix spp. Blastomyces spp. Scedosporium spp.	Acanthamoeba spp. Leishmania spp. Microsporidia Onchocerca volvulus
Endophthalmitis	Coagulase-negative staphylococci S. aureus S. pneumoniae Other Streptococcus spp. Enterococcus spp. H. influenzae Bacillus cereus Escherichia coli Klebsiella pneumoniae Hypermucoid K. pneumoniae		Candida spp. Cryptococcus spp. Fusarium spp. Aspergillus spp.	
Uveitis	Treponema pallidum (syphilis) M. tuberculosis Borrelia burgdorferi Bartonella henselae Leptospira spp. Brucella spp. Mycobacterium leprae	Herpes simplex virus (HSV) Varicella zoster virus (VZV) Cytomegalovirus (CMV) West Nile virus Chikungunya virus Ebola virus		Toxoplasma gondii
Pediatrics	N. gonorrhoeae C. trachomatis T. pallidum (syphilis)	Adenoviruses Herpes simplex virus (HSV) Cytomegalovirus (CMV)		T. gondii

keratitis is contact lens use. Other risk factors include other disruptions of the cornea including surgical and nonsurgical trauma, dysfunctional tearing such as secondary to Sjögren syndrome, diabetes mellitus, and systemic immunodeficiency.

Bacterial keratitis is thought to cause approximately 90% of microbial keratitis with *P. aeruginosa* being the most common causative agent.[43] *S. aureus, S. pneumoniae,* and *Serratia marcescens* are also common causes of keratitis.[43] A variety of other species are found at lower rates including other *Streptococcus, Haemophilus, Moraxella, Proteus, Klebsiella, Enterobacter,* and *Citrobacter* species.[34] Patients typically

present with severe eye pain that is often accompanied by significant conjunctival infection and tearing. Edema and infiltration of inflammatory cells result in a loss of corneal transparency resulting in reduced vision.

Mycobacterial keratitis can also occur, although it is rare. This includes infections both from *M. tuberculosis* and other nontuberculous mycobacteria (NTM).[34] Rapid growing NTM such as *Mycobacterium fortuitum, Mycobacterium chelonae,* and *Mycobacterium abscessus* make up the majority of cases with trauma, particularly laser-assisted in situ keratomileusis (LASIK), almost always serving as a risk factor.[44] Outbreaks of NTM keratitis have occurred worldwide following LASIK secondary to improper sterilization techniques.[44] Diagnosis is difficult due to the chronic and indolent nature of these infections compared to more common bacterial keratitis.

Fungal causes of keratitis are much less frequent than bacterial causes but can be quite severe and difficult to treat. Furthermore, as with NTM keratitis, the presentation can be indolent and chronic. A huge spectrum of fungi can lead to cases of fungal keratitis including *Fusarium, Candida, Aspergillus, Paecilomyces, Phialophora, Curvularia, Alternaria, Sporothrix, Blastomyces,* and *Scedosporium* among others.[34] *Fusarium* and *Aspergillus* though seem to be the most common causes worldwide.[45] A multi-state outbreak of *Fusarium* keratitis associated with contaminated contact lens solution occurred in the United States in 2006.[46] Outbreaks have also been noted in Singapore,[47] France,[48] and Spain.[49]

Parasitic keratitis can also be associated with contact lens use. *Acanthamoeba* are free-living amoeba found commonly in water and soil. They are resistant to desiccation, freezing, and standard chlorination techniques.[50] There have been outbreaks associated with contaminated contact lens solution, but sporadic cases continue as *Acanthamoeba* can be found in tap water. Presentation typically involves photophobia and eye pain.[34]

Other parasites including *Leishmania* and the obligate intracellular parasites known as Microsporidia have been found to induce keratitis in patients infected with HIV.[34] Historically, the most important parasitic cause of keratitis is the microfilariae *Onchocerca volvulus*. This parasite leads to the disease onchocerciasis, or river blindness, which is transmitted by the black fly. The name river blindness refers to the fact that the black fly lays their eggs on rocks and vegetation in rivers and streams. The vast majority of onchocerciasis is found in Africa, but it is also endemic within small areas of Brazil, Venezuela, and Yemen. Although WHO efforts including insecticide treatment against the black fly vector and anti-helminth treatments directed against *O. volvulus* have reduced transmission, there remained a reported 1.15 million cases of vision loss in 2017.[51]

Viral keratitis is overwhelmingly the result of infection with HSV and to a lesser extent VZV. Approximately 500,000 people in the United States and 1.5 million globally are affected by HSV keratitis.[52] Infection can be due to primary infection with either HSV or VZV, but in both instances infections are more common with recurrences of these viruses in the form of reactivation of latent virus.[34] Both viruses can lead to a variety of corneal lesions along with causing decreased corneal sensation. Unlike most other kinds of keratitis, the latent nature of these viral infections can lead to chronic and recurrent infections.[52]

Endophthalmitis

Infection of the vitreous or aqueous humors is known as endophthalmitis. It is exclusively caused by bacteria and fungi, as viral and parasitic infections that may involve the vitreous or aqueous humors are classified under uveitis. Patients present with decreased vision and eye pain can also be present.

Most bacterial cases of endophthalmitis are associated with eye trauma caused by surgical or medical treatment for cataracts, glaucoma, or macular degeneration. Depending on the type of surgery, the microbial causes of infection change. Infection occurs most frequently following cataract surgery and coagulase-negative staphylococci comprises about 70%

of infections. *S. aureus, S. pneumoniae,* other *Streptococcus* species, *Enterococcus* species, and *H. influenzae* can all also play a role in postsurgical endophthalmitis. Nonsurgical trauma can also lead to endophthalmitis; these infections have a much wider variety of microbial causes with *Bacillus cereus* as the leading cause of significant infection.[53]

Besides trauma, the other route of developing bacterial endophthalmitis is secondary to bacteremia and seeding of the eye. Endocarditis and urosepsis are often the source of bacteremia. In North America, *S. aureus* is the most common pathogen but viridans group streptococci, *S. pneumoniae, S. pyogenes, E. coli,* and *K. pneumoniae* can also be causes. In East Asia, hypermucoid *K. pneumoniae* associated with liver abscess is the leading cause of endogenous bacterial endophthalmitis.[53]

Fungal endophthalmitis is divided into infections caused by yeasts and filamentous fungi. Endophthalmitis secondary to yeast is almost exclusively due to *Candida* species, although *Cryptococcus* and other yeasts have caused rare infections. *Candida* endophthalmitis is primarily acquired through endogenous infection secondary to active fungemia. It is the most common cause of fungal endophthalmitis in North America and Europe. Risk factors are the same as those for candidemia including neutropenia, receiving total parental nutrition, having indwelling catheters, and receiving broad-spectrum antibiotics. Endophthalmitis caused by filamentous fungi is more common in tropical regions, where it exceeds *Candida* endophthalmitis in frequency. Although endophthalmitis caused by filamentous fungi can be acquired endogenously through fungemia, it is more commonly acquired through exogenous methods either by direct extension from fungal keratitis or secondary to penetrating trauma to the globe. *Fusarium* species, the most common cause of fungal keratitis, is the leading cause of filamentous fungal endophthalmitis. *Aspergillus* species also are a major cause of endophthalmitis.[54]

Uveitis

Inflammation of the uvea, the pigmented, vascular middle layer of the eye between the cornea and the retina, is known as uveitis. The uvea consists of the iris, the ciliary body, and the choroid which supplies oxygen and nutrients to the retina. Although the retina is structurally distinct from the uvea, retinitis is considered part of uveitis as it commonly occurs in conjunction with involvement of the choroid. Most causes of uveitis are idiopathic or autoimmune, but a number of infectious etiologies can lead to uveitis.[34]

The most common cause of infectious uveitis worldwide is the parasite *T. gondii*. In contrast with CNS *T. gondii* infection, most patients with ocular *T. gondii* infection are immunocompetent. Infection typically begins in the retina and spreads to the choroid. Patients usually present with floaters and vision loss.[55]

The herpesviruses HSV, VZV, and CMV are all causes of infectious uveitis. HSV can induce an anterior uveitis, most commonly affecting the iris. These patients often also have complications of HSV keratitis. HSV and VZV can both induce a rapidly progressive necrotizing retinitis known as acute retinal necrosis. This condition typically starts with anterior uveitis before spreading posteriorly. Patients usually have mild eye pain or photophobia, followed by decreasing vision in the affected eye. CMV is classically associated with

CMV retinitis, which presents as painless vision loss. CMV retinitis occurs in immunocompromised patients, most commonly those with advanced HIV infection. Fortunately, increases in the use of highly active antiretroviral therapy for HIV has led to decreased rates of CMV retinitis. Other rare viral causes of uveitis include West Nile virus, chikungunya virus, and Ebola virus.[34]

Bacterial causes of uveitis are relatively rare. Syphilis is the most common, and it can be the presenting feature of syphilis infection. Ocular syphilis can also lead to keratitis, but uveitis involving any portion of the uvea is more common. Other rare bacterial causes of uveitis include *M. tuberculosis* (tuberculosis), *B. burgdorferi* (Lyme disease), *B. henselae* (cat scratch disease), *Leptospira* species (leptospirosis), *Brucella* species (brucellosis), and *Mycobacterium leprae* (leprosy).[56]

Pediatric Considerations

For the most part, children suffer from similar eye infections as adults. Conjunctivitis is an incredibly common issue with adenovirus being the most common causative agent. However, in the neonatal period, infants are prone to ocular infections of sexually transmitted organisms. Specifically, neonatal conjunctivitis secondary to *N. gonorrhoeae* and *C. trachomatis* requires prompt recognition. HSV can lead to ocular infection both in the form of conjunctivitis and keratitis in the neonatal period. However, unlike in adults, where 80% of ocular HSV infections are secondary to HSV-1, HSV-2 is the more frequent cause of ocular infection in the pediatric time period.[34] Some congenital infections, specifically CMV, toxoplasmosis, and syphilis can have ocular involvement, primarily in the form of uveitis/retinitis.

POINTS TO REMEMBER

- Conjunctivitis, keratitis, endophthalmitis, and uveitis are caused by inflammation of the eye secondary to infectious and noninfectious etiologies.
- Viral conjunctivitis is the most common type of eye infection.
- Ninety percent of keratitis is caused by bacteria, with *Pseudomonas aeruginosa* being the most common organism.
- *Onchocerca volvulus*, the cause of river blindness, and *Acanthamoeba* are notable parasitic causes of keratitis.

UPPER RESPIRATORY TRACT INFECTIONS

Upper respiratory tract infections (URTIs) include infections of the nose, nasal passages, paranasal sinuses, pharynx, and the larynx above the vocal cords. The middle ear is also connected to these passages through the eustachian tube, and ear infections will be discussed here as well. This area is colonized by bacteria and exposed to circulating viruses. Most URTIs are caused by viruses which cause damage to the mucosal lining of the upper respiratory tract and can be an entry point for bacterial infections. Although most infections are self-limited, occasionally URTIs can be chronic or life-threatening, and these infections can develop into lower respiratory tract infections (LRTIs) with more severe consequences. A diagram of the respiratory tract can be found in Fig. 82.3 and the most common causes of URTIs are found in Table 82.4.

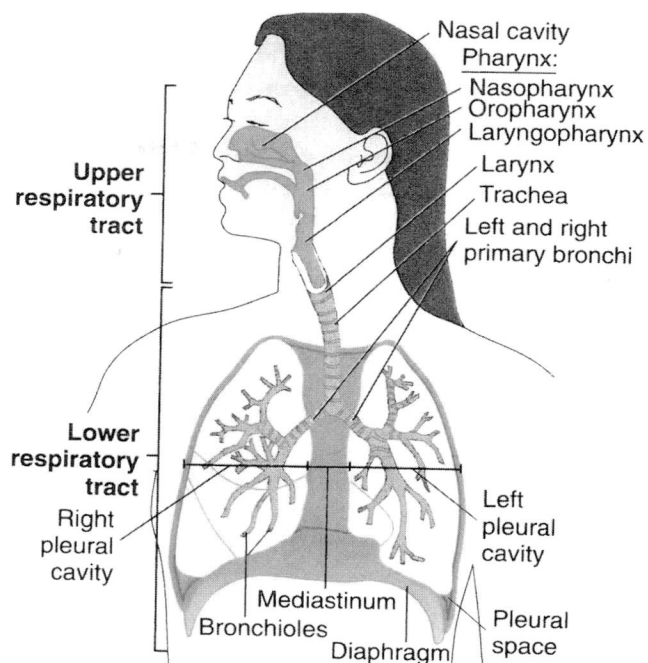

FIGURE 82.3 Basic anatomy of the respiratory tract, including the upper and lower respiratory tract regions. (Reproduced with permission from Tille P, editor. *Bailey and Scott's diagnostic microbiology.* 14th ed. St. Louis: Elsevier; 2017.)

Viral Upper Respiratory Tract Infections

Among the most common causes of infection are viral URTIs. In otherwise healthy individuals these infections cause mild disease, but infections can be serious and even deadly in young children, the elderly, and those with immunocompromising conditions. The classic presentation of viral URTIs are the symptoms of the "common cold": nasal congestion, rhinorrhea, sneezing, cough, and fatigue. Fever is often but not always present. Among the viral causes of URTI, the most frequent cause of severe symptoms is influenza virus, a segmented RNA virus that causes yearly seasonal infection and occasional pandemics, most recently the H1N1 pandemic of 2009 to 2010. The virus undergoes antigenic drift (point mutations) and antigenic shift (segment reassortment) which allow it to evade the immune system year after year.[57] Development of influenza pneumonia and secondary bacterial pneumonia causes high morbidity and mortality. There is a vaccine against this viral infection, but due to antigenic drift and shift, vaccine effectiveness varies from year to year.[57] Antivirals with some efficacy against influenza exist but the benefits of those treatments are limited. Respiratory syncytial virus (RSV) causes mild URTI in otherwise healthy adults but can cause serious LRTI in very young children and the immunocompromised. Other viral causes of URTI are rhinoviruses (the most frequent infection), parainfluenza viruses 1 to 4, adenoviruses, human metapneumovirus, enteroviruses, bocavirus, and coronaviruses.

Pharyngitis

Pharyngitis, characterized as sore throat, fever, and inflammation of the pharynx, often including inflammation of the tonsils, is also a very common infection. Although pharyngitis

TABLE 82.4 Common Pathogens of Upper Respiratory Tract Infections

	Bacteria	Viruses	Fungi
Viral upper respiratory tract infections		Influenza Respiratory syncytial virus (RSV) Parainfluenza viruses 1–4 Adenoviruses Human metapneumovirus Coronaviruses Human rhinoviruses/enteroviruses Bocavirus	
Pharyngitis	*Streptococcus pyogenes* (Group A) Group C/G large, β-hemolytic streptococci *Arcanobacterium haemolyticum* *Fusobacterium necrophorum* *Corynebacterium diphtheriae* *Neisseria gonorrhoeae*		
Epiglottitis	*Haemophilus influenzae* type b *Streptococcus pneumoniae*		
Acute sinusitis	*S. pneumoniae* *H. influenzae* (nontypeable) *Moraxella catarrhalis* *S. pyogenes* (Group A) *Staphylococcus aureus*		
Chronic sinusitis	Enterobacterales *Pseudomonas aeruginosa* Oral anaerobic bacteria		*Aspergillus* spp. *Bipolaris* spp. and other dematiaceous fungi
Ear infections	*S. pneumoniae* *H. influenzae* (nontypeable) *Moraxella catarrhalis* *P. aeruginosa* *S. aureus*		*Aspergillus* spp., especially *A. niger* *Candida* spp.
Immunocompromised host			*Aspergillus* spp. *Bipolaris* spp. and other dematiaceous fungi *Fusarium* spp. Mucorales *Scedosporium* spp.
Pediatrics		Respiratory syncytial virus (RSV) Parainfluenza viruses (croup)	

can be an isolated infection, more frequently it is associated with a more widespread infection, either of the entire upper respiratory tract or the body at large. Approximately 85% of pharyngitis is caused by viruses such as rhinovirus, enterovirus, adenovirus, EBV, CMV, HSV-1, HSV-2, influenza, and acute HIV infection.[58]

The most common bacterial cause of pharyngitis is *S. pyogenes* (GAS), which presents with symptoms of fever, headache, lymphadenitis, and vomiting but lacks the rhinorrhea, cough, and congestion present with most viral causes of pharyngitis. A diffuse erythematous rash, typically beginning in the axilla and groin, that usually subsequently peels can also be present with *S. pyogenes* pharyngitis; the bright redness of the rash has given this presentation the name scarlet fever. Serious complications of *S. pyogenes* pharyngitis include acute rheumatic fever (ARF) and poststreptococcal glomerulonephritis (PSGN). ARF presents with a fever and a

combination of the major manifestations: carditis/valvulitis, arthritis, subcutaneous nodules, a rash known as erythema marginatum, and CNS involvement in the form of Sydenham chorea.[59] These symptoms develop within weeks of the original episode of pharyngitis. PSGN also occurs within weeks of the initial infection and ranges in severity from asymptomatic microscopic hematuria to severe nephritic syndrome with gross hematuria, edema, and hypertension.[60] Antibiotic treatment of the initial episode of GAS pharyngitis reduces the rate of ARF and likely the rate of PSGN as well although evidence of this is less conclusive.[61]

Other bacterial causes of pharyngitis include Group C and G streptococci, *Arcanobacterium haemolyticum*, and *F. necrophorum*. In sexually active individuals, *N. gonorrhoeae* is another cause. *Corynebacterium diphtheriae* causes severe, toxin-mediated infection and is characterized by the formation of a pseudomembrane covering the tonsils and throat.

This membrane may spread into the tracheobronchial tree, and the resulting inflammation can lead to respiratory failure, particularly in young children with smaller airways. Diphtheria antitoxin was developed in the late 19th century and was shown to decrease mortality; antibiotics also help with treatment by killing bacteria and preventing additional toxin formation.[22] Cases are now exceedingly rare in the United States due to vaccination, but outbreaks occur worldwide, particularly when breakdowns in health care and vaccinations occur. The WHO reported 15,000 cases of diphtheria in 2018.[62]

Epiglottitis

Epiglottitis is inflammation of the epiglottis and surrounding structures. Patients present with fever, difficulty swallowing, and throat pain and will often have stridor and upper airway obstruction that can lead to respiratory failure and death. The infectious causes of this condition in adults are widely varied, but overall the frequency of this infection is very low. In the past, epiglottitis primarily affected children 1 to 4 years of age due to infection with *H. influenzae* type b. Because of the smaller airways of children, epiglottitis can cause airway obstruction leading to suffocation and death. Now that vaccination for *H. influenzae* is widespread, the incidence of epiglottitis in children has been drastically reduced. Other known causes of epiglottitis are other serotypes of *H. influenzae* (types A, F, and nontypable), *S. pneumoniae,* and rarely *S. aureus.*[63,64]

Sinusitis

Sinusitis is caused by inflammation of the paranasal sinuses, and it can be either acute or chronic in presentation. Acute sinusitis is caused by obstruction of the ostia due to edema and damaged ciliated cells, resulting in high amounts of thick, mucus secretions. Most infections are viral and self-limited. Bacterial infection is often preceded by damage to the cellular mucosa caused by viral infection, allergy, cigarette smoking, or swimming. Bacterial causes of sinusitis are primarily *H. influenzae* (predominantly nontypable strains) and *S. pneumoniae.* Less common causes are *S. pyogenes,* *S. aureus,* and *M. catarrhalis.* Acute bacterial sinusitis presents with similar symptoms to viral URTIs (congestion, nasal discharge, headache, and cough) making it difficult to distinguish the infections. Symptoms lasting longer than 10 days, worsening of symptoms following an initial improvement, and severe onset of symptoms with purulent discharge for at least 3 days are suggestions of bacterial involvement that may warrant antibiotic treatment.[65] Complications of acute bacterial sinusitis are caused by direct spread of the infection from the sinuses into the adjoining structures of the head. Extracranial spread can lead to orbital cellulitis (infection of the orbital fat and ocular muscles), orbital abscess, or subperiosteal abscesses of the facial bones; Pott puffy tumor is a swelling of the forehead secondary to a subperiosteal abscess of the frontal bone. Spread into the intracranial cavity can also occur leading to epidural abscess, subdural empyema, meningitis, and intraparenchymal brain abscess.[66]

Chronic sinusitis is a complex process leading to ongoing inflammation of the paranasal sinuses for at least 12 weeks. Although this can be secondary to untreated acute sinusitis, this condition has multifactorial causes and antimicrobial therapy alone is typically inadequate for resolution of symptoms. The microbiology of these inflamed sinuses both includes agents similar to the causes of acute sinusitis (*H. influenzae, S. pneumoniae, M. catarrhalis,* and *S. aureus*) and additional enteric gram-negative bacteria (*Klebsiella, Pseudomonas, Enterobacter,* and *E. coli*) and oral anaerobes (*Prevotella, Peptostreptococcus,* and *Fusobacterium*). Colonization (not infection) of the sinuses with fungal species can lead to an eosinophilic inflammatory response to these fungi known as allergic fungal rhinosinusitis. The most common fungi involved are *Aspergillus* spp. and dematiaceous fungi such as *Bipolaris.*[67]

Otitis Media, Mastoiditis, and Otitis Externa

Acute otitis media (AOM) consists of infection of the middle ear (Fig. 82.4). This infection begins with eustachian tube dysfunction, typically caused by a viral URTI, which induces inflammatory edema. This edema prevents drainage of middle ear fluid. This fluid accumulates and can become infected, which leads to the clinical symptoms of AOM: fever and ear pain. Rupture of the tympanic membrane or placement of myringotomy tubes may lead to presentation with ear drainage. Classically, *S. pneumoniae* has been the most common causative agent followed by *H. influenzae* and *M. catarrhalis;* however, ongoing vaccination efforts against *S. pneumoniae* seem to have reduced the frequency of pneumococcal infection, making *H. influenzae* the most common cause.[68]

Complications from AOM are rare but can occur. The most common is mastoiditis. The mastoid portion of the temporal bone lies adjacent to the middle ear and is filled with interconnected air cells that also connect to the middle ear. Infected fluid can back up from the middle ear and establish an infection in the mastoid, including formation of an abscess that may require surgical drainage for successful treatment.

The external auditory canal is separated from the middle ear and the sinuses by the tympanic membrane and is lined with squamous epithelium rather than respiratory mucosa. Given these features, infection of the external auditory canal known as otitis externa is not caused by the same pathogens responsible for AOM or acute sinusitis. Instead, *P. aeruginosa* is the most common pathogen followed by *S. aureus. Staphylococcus epidermidis* is a colonizer of the ear canal but may also play a role in infection in certain cases.[69] Acute otitis externa typically presents with ear pain and ear drainage; water exposure (particularly swimming) and localized trauma of the canal are risk factors that reduce cerumen (ear wax) and create an environment for the establishment of infection. Fungal species, particularly *Aspergillus niger,* but also other *Aspergillus* and *Candida* species can lead to a chronic otitis externa, predominantly presenting as chronic ear itching in immunocompetent individuals.[70]

Immunocompromised Patients

Immunocompromised individuals are more likely to develop severe symptoms and experience complications following URTIs compared to immunocompetent individuals. In particular, viral URTIs are more likely to lead to LRTIs (both viral and secondary bacterial infections) with corresponding complications including respiratory failure and death.

One type of infection limited almost exclusively to immunocompromised patients is invasive fungal sinusitis. This

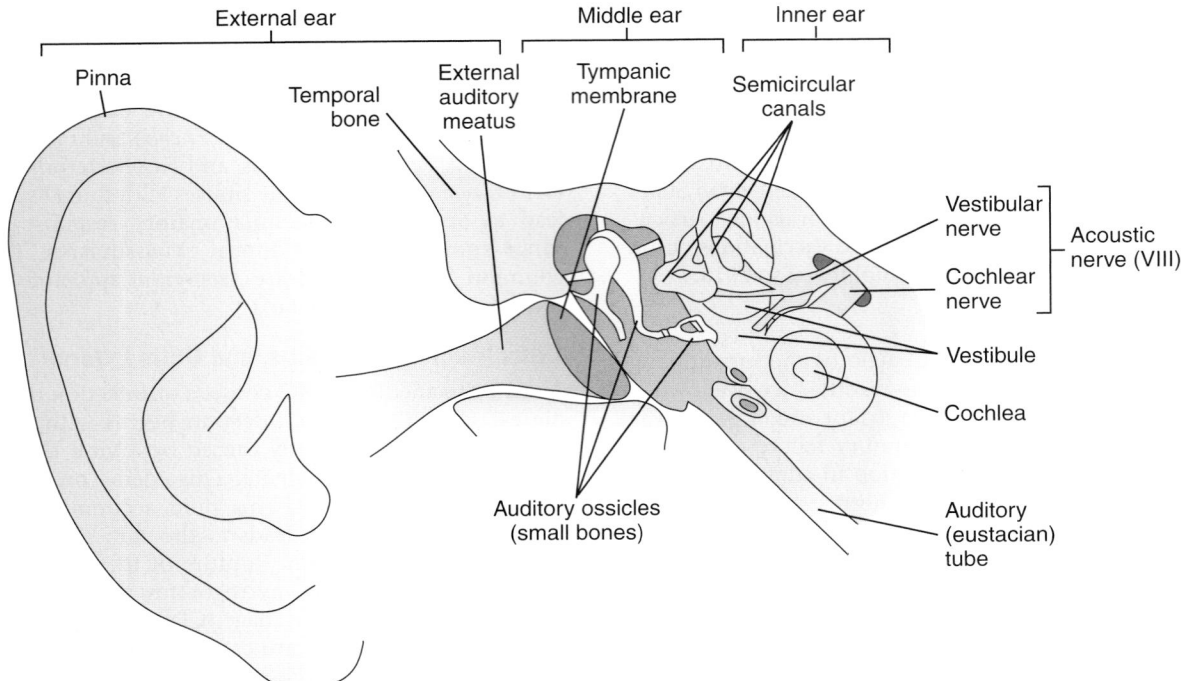

FIGURE 82.4 Basic anatomy of the ear. (Reproduced with permission from Tille P, editor. *Bailey and Scott's diagnostic microbiology.* 14th ed. St. Louis: Elsevier; 2017.)

condition arises from direct fungal invasion and spread through the tissues of the sinuses and adjoining structures. Computerized tomography (CT) and magnetic resonance imaging (MRI) can demonstrate erosions suggestive of the diagnosis, but endoscopic evaluation with biopsy is necessary to confirm the diagnosis. A more acute and severe presentation usually with fever can occur due to infection with *Aspergillus* species, *Fusarium* species, and molds of the order Mucorales. Dematiaceous molds (particularly *Bipolaris, Curvularia,* and *Alternaria*) and *Scedosporium* are more apt to lead to chronic sinusitis with fewer systematic symptoms including fever and metastatic spread. Treatment requires both aggressive surgical debridement and antifungal therapy.[71]

Pediatric Considerations

The infections mentioned in this section occur at much higher rates in pediatric patients than adults, and they are the leading causes for acute care pediatric visits. One cohort study from Germany suggests the annual incidence of URTI was 3.4 episodes per year for the first 2 years of life followed by 2.3 episodes per year through preschool age.[72] AOM occurs in 60% of children by age 7 with 40% of patients having at least 4 episodes.[73] Respiratory viral infections are also more prone to lead to LRTI in younger children as well.

Pediatric patients are also susceptible to the condition known as croup. Croup is characterized by a barking cough and inspiratory stridor secondary to inflammation of the larynx and subglottic airway, which when severe can lead to obstruction of the airway and respiratory distress and failure. The parainfluenza viruses are the most common causes of croup with parainfluenza-3 tending to be the most severe.[74,75] Other viruses including RSV and influenza can also induce croup.

POINTS TO REMEMBER

- Upper respiratory tract infections (URTIs) include infections of the nose, nasal passages, paranasal sinuses, pharynx, and the larynx above the vocal cords.
- Most infections are caused by viruses that damage the mucosal lining of the upper respiratory tract, which can be an entry point for bacterial infections.
- The middle ear is connected to the upper respiratory tract through the eustachian tube, and ear infections are often caused by viruses and bacteria circulating in the upper respiratory tract.
- Although most URTIs are self-limited, occasionally they progress to lower respiratory tract infections with more severe symptoms.

LOWER RESPIRATORY TRACT INFECTIONS

Infection of the lower respiratory tract includes the larynx below the vocal folds, the trachea, bronchi, and bronchioles. Infections are most commonly caused by viruses, but damaged mucosa can lead to secondary bacterial superinfections which can be very severe. These infections are an enormous burden on global health being the most common infectious cause of death with 3 million deaths in 2016 according to the WHO.[76] Tuberculosis, another specific LRTI, was responsible for another 1.3 million deaths. A diagram of the respiratory tract can be found in Fig. 82.3 and the most common causes of LRTI are found in Table 82.5.

Bronchitis

Bronchitis is inflammation of the large and mid-sized airways or bronchi without progression to pneumonia. Symptoms

TABLE 82.5   Common Pathogens of Lower Respiratory Infections

	Bacteria	Viruses	Fungi	Parasites

Bronchitis	*Mycoplasma pneumoniae*
	Chlamydia pneumoniae
	Bordetella pertussis
	Streptococcus pneumoniae
	Haemophilus influenzae
	Moraxella catarrhalis
	Pseudomonas aeruginosa
		Respiratory viruses
		  (see upper respiratory
		  infections)		

Pneumonia	*H. influenzae*
	S. pneumoniae
	Staphylococcus aureus
	Streptococcus pyogenes
	Klebsiella pneumoniae
	P. aeruginosa
	M. catarrhalis
		Respiratory viruses
		  (see upper respiratory
		  infections)
		Novel coronaviruses
		  (SARS, MERS, and
		  SARS-CoV-2)		

Atypical pneumonia	*Legionella* spp. *M. pneumoniae* *C. pneumoniae*			
Aspiration pneumonia	Aerobic and anaerobic oral microbiota			

Ventilator-associated
  pneumonia
	Escherichia coli
	Klebsiella spp.
	Enterobacter spp.
	Acinetobacter baumannii
	P. aeruginosa
	S. aureus
	Stenotrophomonas
	  maltophilia			

Chronic pneumonia	*Mycobacterium tuberculosis*		*Histoplasma capsulatum* *Blastomyces dermatitidis* *Coccidioides* spp. *Aspergillus* spp.	*Paragonimus* spp.
Pleural infections	*Streptococcus anginosus* group *S. aureus* *S. pneumoniae* *H. influenzae*			

Immunocompromised
  host
	Mycobacterium abscessus
	Mycobacterium avium
	  complex
	Mycobacterium kansasii
	Actinomyces spp.
	Nocardia spp.
		Cytomegalovirus (CMV)	*Cryptococcus*
			  neoformans
			Pneumocystis jirovecii
			Aspergillus
			Fusarium spp.
			Scedosporium spp.
			Mucorales	

Cystic fibrosis	*P. aeruginosa* *S. aureus* *H. influenzae* *Burkholderia cepacia* *M. abscessus* *M. avium* complex			
Pediatrics		Respiratory syncytial virus (RSV) Human metapneumovirus Influenza Parainfluenza viruses 1-4 Adenoviruses Coronaviruses Bocavirus		

include nasal congestion, rhinitis, sore throat, malaise, and cough with or without wheezing. The frequency and severity of cough separates bronchitis from an isolated URTI. Viruses are the most common cause of acute bronchitis and infection is generally brief and self-limited.[77] *M. pneumoniae* and *Chlamydia pneumoniae* are the most common bacterial causes.[77] *Bordetella pertussis*, the causative agent of whooping cough, causes bronchitis with a paroxysmal cough and an inspiratory whoop which gives the disease its name. Due to vaccination, rates are relatively low in the United States, but the Centers for Disease Control and Prevention (CDC) reported greater than 15,000 cases in 2018.[78]

Chronic bronchitis is a more serious condition leading to significant morbidity and mortality. It is most commonly seen in patients with chronic lung disease such as chronic obstructive lung disease (COPD). Chronic bronchitis can be caused by common respiratory viruses or by bacteria such as *S. pneumoniae, H. influenzae*, and *M. catarrhalis. P. aeruginosa* is also an important etiologic agent in individuals with severe COPD.[34]

Pneumonia

Infection of the lung air sacs, or pneumonia, is a common infection with over 3 million cases annually in the United States, resulting in significant mortality. Infection presents with symptoms of cough, sputum production, fever, and dyspnea but can also include systemic features such as fatigue.[79] Radiologic imaging is used to support clinical symptoms in the diagnosis of pneumonia. Although pneumonia can occur in patients of any age, the elderly and those with chronic lung disease such as COPD are at highest risk for contracting pneumonia and for those patients, the mortality rate is increased when infection occurs.[76]

Community-acquired pneumonia (CAP) is the most common type of pneumonia and is most frequently due to infection with *H. influenzae* or *S. pneumoniae. S. aureus* and *S. pyogenes* can both cause pneumonia as well and are much more common following an antecedent viral infection, particularly influenza. Infection with these agents is often severe and complicated by a necrotizing component. *P. aeruginosa* pneumonia is associated almost exclusively with patients who have chronic lung disease. A subset of cases of community-acquired pneumonia have been classified as atypical pneumonia. Originally, the term was meant to signify a case with reduced sputum production and a milder and more protracted course. Today though, atypical pneumonia has come to refer to pneumonia caused by an organism that is often not recoverable in sputum culture: most commonly, *M. pneumoniae*, but also *C. pneumoniae* and *Legionella* species. Although *M. pneumoniae* and *C. pneumoniae* often may produce fewer symptoms than seen with typical CAP, there is considerable overlap in clinical courses between typical and atypical cases. Viral causes of CAP are also abundant. Influenza is a leading cause of viral pneumonia, but novel coronaviruses including severe acute respiratory syndrome coronavirus 2 (SARS-CoV-2), severe acute respiratory syndrome (SARS), and Middle East Respiratory Syndrome (MERS) demonstrate the large-scale morbidity and mortality that can be caused by viral pneumonia.[34,35,80,81]

Aspiration pneumonia is caused by aspiration of food or saliva into the lungs. This can occur in a single aspiration event or through repeated undetectable micro-aspirations.

Persons that are elderly and those with esophageal disorders are at higher risk for aspiration events leading to pneumonia. The initial damage from aspiration is mostly caused by a chemical pneumonitis due to the presence of acidic stomach contents. However, a bacterial pneumonia can also be established which can lead to ongoing lung damage. Oral anaerobes including *Peptostreptococcus, Prevotella, Fusobacterium*, and *Bacteroides* play a key role in these infections while the most common aerobic bacteria recovered are gram-negatives and *S. aureus*. Aspiration can also lead to areas of lung necrosis and the development of lung abscess.[56]

Patients in hospital settings and on ventilators are at risk for the development of pneumonia due to a number of factors including depressed consciousness, chronic lung disease, trauma secondary to mechanical ventilation, and aspiration among others. Patients who acquire pneumonia in the hospital are most often infected with aerobic gram-negative bacteria including *P. aeruginosa, Klebsiella* species, *E. coli, Acinetobacter* species, *Enterobacter* species, and *Stenotrophomonas maltophilia* along with the gram-positive bacterium *S. aureus*.[82] Given the acquisition of these organisms in the health care setting, they are frequently resistant to multiple antibiotics; this increasing resistance, particularly among the gram-negative organisms, is a growing issue in infectious diseases today.

Fungal pneumonia in immunocompetent individuals is largely limited to *Cryptococcus gattii* and dimorphic fungi. The common dimorphic mycoses are due to *Histoplasma capsulatum* (located mostly throughout the United States in the Ohio and Mississippi river valleys), *Blastomyces dermatitidis* (located throughout much of the eastern and midwestern United States and Canada), *Coccidioides immitis* and *Coccidioides posadasii* (found in hot and arid areas of the southwestern United States and northern Mexico), and *Paracoccidioides brasiliensis* (located across much of South and Central America). An additional species of *Histoplasma*, *H. duboisii* is found in much of Africa. All of these fungi are dimorphic meaning they manifest as yeast while in a human host, or spherules with endospores in the case of *Coccidioides* spp. and grow in a mold form in environmental conditions. These pathogens enter the body through inhalation of conidia. In the majority of all of these cases, infection is asymptomatic. However, all types can cause an acute or chronic pneumonia along with mediastinal lymphadenopathy. Dissemination to other distal sites including the skin, bones, joints, intra-abdominal organs, and CNS can all occur and happen with different frequencies depending on the specific endemic mycosis.[34,83–86]

Parasitic pneumonia is relatively uncommon, but otherwise healthy individuals who have a history of eating raw or undercooked crab or crayfish may become infected with the parasitic lung fluke *Paragonimus*. Symptoms are initially abdominal pain and diarrhea, but later these patients develop fever, chest pain, and fatigue when the adult worms establish a chronic infection encapsulated into cysts. Infected individuals have a dry cough initially but over time they can produce rusty-colored sputum due to blood. An estimated 20 million people worldwide may be infected with *Paragonimus*.[87]

Pulmonary Tuberculosis

Tuberculosis remains one of the most significant infectious diseases on a global scale; in 2016, it was the leading cause of death worldwide.[76] The causative agent, *M. tuberculosis* (TB), is extremely contagious and spread from person to person by respiratory droplets from individuals with active TB. The bacteria reside within pulmonary macrophages deep in the alveolar spaces of the lung. The vast majority of infected individuals contain the infection and may be asymptomatic for long periods of time, even decades, resulting in a chronic TB infection known as latent TB. In response to TB infection, the host produces an inflammatory reaction that results in granuloma formation with central necrosis; the TB bacteria are contained in these granulomas but cannot be fully eliminated. As a result of the highly infectious nature combined with the prolonged asymptomatic duration of infection, the WHO estimates that approximately a third of the world's population is infected with tuberculosis. The primary risk of latent TB is reactivation to active TB infection, and someone infected with latent TB has a 5 to 10% chance of reactivation during their lifetime. Upon reactivation, most people develop a chronic pneumonia, which can be complicated by pleural effusion. Symptoms consist of persistent cough, intermittent fever, night sweats, and weight loss. The right middle lobe is the most commonly involved, but reactivation can occur anywhere in the lung. Dissemination from the lungs to other sites including skin, bones, joints, and the CNS can also occur. Both dissemination and reactivation are more common in immunocompromised patients. The immune systems of young children can have a difficult time containing the initial infection. They are prone to developing progressive primary tuberculosis that disseminates, especially in the form of TB meningitis.[88]

Pleural Infections

The pleura are thin membranes between the lungs and the chest cavity that act as lubrication to reduce friction and facilitate breathing. Pleural infections are caused by the buildup of fluid in the pleura, outside of the lungs, which makes breathing very difficult and painful. Commonly, these infections take the form of empyemas, which are collections of pus in a body cavity. Pleural fluid is sampled and cultured to determine the source of the fluid. Pleural effusions are separated into exudates, including empyema, and transudates (which result from oncotic pressures in the chest) on the basis of cell count, protein levels, and lactate dehydrogenase (LDH) using a set of criteria known as Light's criteria. Empyema and pleural infection occur due to spread from adjacent bacterial pneumonia. Given that fact, historically the most prevalent causes of pleural infections were *S. pneumoniae* and *H. influenzae*. Vaccinations have reduced the rates of the more virulent strains of these organisms and today the most common bacterial cause is *S. anginosus* group followed by *S. aureus*.[89]

Immunocompromised Patients

Immunocompromised patients are more prone to severe complications from all of the infections described in this section. This includes increased rates of respiratory failure due to viral pneumonia and increased dissemination out of the lungs for tuberculosis and the endemic fungi. However, there are also numerous pathogens which infect the lower respiratory tract of immunocompromised patients that are largely not found in immunocompetent individuals. One such pathogen is *Pneumocystis jirovecii*, a ubiquitous fungus found worldwide. The complete life cycle of *Pneumocystis* is unknown, but it seems to commonly cause asymptomatic infection in immunocompetent individuals. In the immunocompromised though, it can lead to a pneumonia that presents with fever, cough, and dyspnea. Progression to hypoxia and progression to respiratory failure is not uncommon. Prophylaxis of high-risk patients is standard to prevent the development of infection.[34,35]

Immunocompromised individuals are at risk of pneumonia due to a number of other fungal pathogens as well. Pneumonia due to *Aspergillus* is the most common fungal pneumonia in these patients, but other molds including Mucorales, *Fusarium* species, and *Scedosporium* can also cause invasive pulmonary disease in the immunocompromised. The yeast *C. neoformans* initially infects the lungs upon inhalation of aerosolized spores. This can result in pneumonia in immunocompromised individuals and can disseminate to the CNS leading to meningitis.

In addition to fungal pathogens, immunocompromised patients are also more susceptible to unique viral, bacterial, and parasitic pulmonary infections. CMV pneumonitis can be a complication of stem cell or solid organ transplantation. Nontuberculous mycobacteria, particularly those of the *Mycobacterium avium-intracellulare complex* (MAIC) can lead to pneumonia in patients with severe immunosuppression from advanced HIV infection, lung transplantation, or other chronic lung disease.[35]

The helminth *Strongyloides stercoralis* can also cause pulmonary manifestations in the immunocompromised. Infection begins with contact of skin with contaminated soil; the filariform larvae penetrate the skin, travel to the lungs, puncture the alveoli, and ascend the tracheobronchial tree and are swallowed. In the intestine, the larvae develop into adult worms. Some of the larva produced by these adult worms can lead to autoinfection, and thus *S. stercoralis* can complete its entire life cycle in the same host. An intact immune system limits autoinfection, and infected individuals can remain asymptomatic for decades. Immunosuppression can lead to a rapid increase in autoinfection causing the state known as hyperinfection. *Strongyloides* hyperinfection causes increasing respiratory symptoms and even acute respiratory distress syndrome due to inflammation from larval migration through the lungs. Gastrointestinal and dermatologic manifestations are also possible and traversal through the intestinal wall can lead to polymicrobial bacteremia and CNS infection when the worm inoculates GI bacteria into the bloodstream or CNS.[90]

Pediatric Considerations

Pediatric patients are prone to the development of bronchiolitis, an LRTI of the epithelium of the small bronchioles; this leads to inflammation and obstruction. Clinical manifestations include symptoms of a viral URTI (fever, nasal congestion/discharge) coupled with wheezing, crackles, or respiratory distress. RSV is the most common cause, and RSV bronchiolitis is a leading cause of pediatric hospitalization, with a significant global health impact and an estimated 1.4 million hospitalizations and 118,000 deaths annually.[91] Other viral causes include human metapneumovirus and less frequently influenza, parainfluenza, adenovirus, coronavirus, and bocavirus.

Cystic fibrosis (CF) is a relatively common autosomal recessive disorder affecting approximately 1 out of 3000 live births in people of northern European descent.[92] It is caused by mutations to the chloride channel cystic fibrosis transmembrane conductance regulator (CFTR). One of the effects of these mutations is the production of thick mucus secretions and chronic airway obstruction. This allows for the establishment of chronic infection with bacteria including *H. influenzae, S. aureus, P. aeruginosa*, and members of the *Burkholderia cepacia* complex. Nontuberculous mycobacteria including *M. abscessus* and MAIC can also colonize and lead to ongoing infection. Chronic pneumonia in these patients leads to ongoing inflammatory lung damage. Acute episodes of bronchopneumonia also occur and are treated with antibiotics and aggressive chest physiotherapy. Advances in care for patients with cystic fibrosis, including the development of CFTR modulators, has extended the lifespan of these patients greatly, and according to the North American Cystic Fibrosis Foundation, the life expectancy of people with CF is now 44 years. These changes have pushed CF out of being a primarily pediatric disease as now over half of all individuals with CF are over the age of 18 years.[93]

POINTS TO REMEMBER

- Infection of the lower respiratory tract includes the larynx below the vocal folds, the trachea, bronchi, and bronchioles.
- Most infections are caused by viruses, but damaged mucosa can lead to secondary bacterial superinfections which cause high morbidity and mortality.
- Lower respiratory tract infections are the most common infectious cause of death worldwide, accounting for 3 million deaths in 2017 with an additional 1.3 million global deaths caused by *Mycobacterium tuberculosis* alone.

GASTROINTESTINAL AND INTRA-ABDOMINAL INFECTIONS

Gastroenteritis

Infections of the GI tract are the second highest cause of death due to infection worldwide with 1.4 million deaths in 2016.[76] They are spread by fecal-oral transmission or from person to person. Persons at elevated risk of contracting GI illness are young children, children attending or adults working at daycare centers, those living in crowded living conditions, and persons without access to sources of clean water. Infection is generally self-limited and does not require treatment, but young children, the elderly, immunocompromised, and malnourished populations are at higher risk of developing severe symptoms, mostly due to dehydration, and may need antimicrobial or supportive care to overcome their GI infection. These populations are also at increased risk for morbidity and mortality due to GI illness. A diagram of the GI tract can be found in Fig. 82.5, and the most common causes of GI infection are found in Table 82.6.

Acute gastroenteritis is inflammation of the stomach and the small and large intestines. Acute gastroenteritis presents as vomiting and/or diarrhea and lasts less than 2 weeks; it may be accompanied by fever and abdominal pain. Viral gastroenteritis is the most prevalent cause of infectious GI illness and presents as a form of acute gastroenteritis. Viral gastroenteritis is seasonal and peaks in the winter and spring. Norovirus is the most common cause of gastroenteritis in the United States. It is highly contagious and can present both in endemic forms and epidemic. About half of all foodborne outbreaks in the United States are associated with norovirus.[94,95] Symptoms range from asymptomatic infection to sustained fever, vomiting, and diarrhea for 48 to 72 hours with vomiting occurring more frequently than typically seen with other forms of viral gastroenteritis. Rotavirus historically was the most common cause of severe gastroenteritis, but the development of effective rotavirus vaccines has reduced the rate of infection dramatically in countries where vaccine use is prevalent. Other viral causes of acute gastroenteritis include astroviruses, adenoviruses, sapoviruses, and enteroviruses. All of these viruses can lead to self-limited diarrheal disease.[35]

Bacterial gastroenteritis in adults is generally acute in nature and often presents along with other clinical findings including bloody stool, fever, abdominal pain, nausea, and/or vomiting. It comes in two primary forms: direct ingestion of toxins produced by the bacteria prior to ingestion versus direct infection of the GI tract. Examples of toxin-mediated food poisoning include ingestion of toxin produced by *S. aureus, Clostridium perfringens*, and *B. cereus*. These illnesses typically have a rapid onset (within 8 to 16 hours of ingestion) and largely resolve within 24 hours. Direct bacterial infection of the GI tract can lead to a more prolonged infection than would usually be seen with acute viral gastroenteritis. Many of these bacteria produce toxins which cause massive host cell destruction with only small amounts of bacteria being present. Even so, in otherwise healthy individuals these infections are self-limiting and most individuals do not require antibiotic treatment. Immunocompromised persons, young children, and elderly persons greater than 65 years of age are more likely to suffer from severe dehydration due to GI infections or spread of pathogens outside of the GI tract and may need both antibiotic and supportive treatment to overcome infection.[34,35]

Bacterial causes of gastroenteritis vary from region to region, but in the US, the most common causes of bacterial gastroenteritis are *Campylobacter* and *Salmonella*.[96] Both of these bacteria are acquired through consumption of undercooked poultry although *Salmonella* is also associated with eggs, milk products, and less commonly other foods including fresh produce and meats. The next most common bacterial causes of gastroenteritis are *Shigella* species and Shiga-toxin producing *E. coli* (STEC; also known as enterohemorrhagic *E. coli* or EHEC). Both of these infections occur at rates about one-quarter to one-third as frequent as *Salmonella* or *Campylobacter*, but both are more commonly associated with bloody diarrhea. EHEC is significant due to its connection to hemolytic-uremic syndrome (HUS), a combination of hemolytic anemia, thrombocytopenia, and acute kidney injury.[96] HUS is more frequent in children, where it is one of the leading causes of acute kidney injury, but it can occur in adults as well. Infection with *Shigella* can also lead to HUS, but at lower frequency than EHEC infection. *Vibrio cholerae* remains an important cause of bacterial gastroenteritis worldwide being classified as endemic in approximately 50 countries, mostly in Africa and Asia,[97] and leads to outbreaks in other parts of the world as well. Non-cholera *Vibrio* species, particularly *Vibrio parahaemolyticus* (associated with shellfish consumption) also

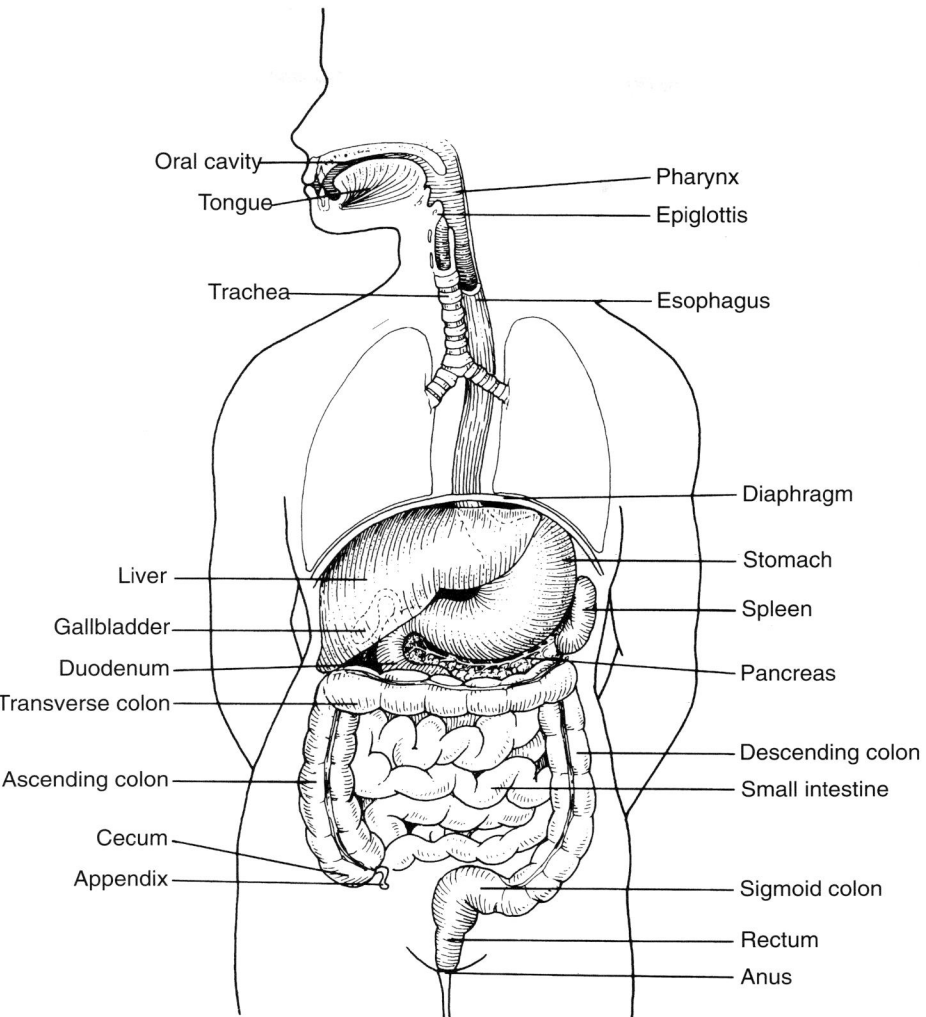

FIGURE 82.5 Basic anatomy of the gastrointestinal tract. (Reproduced with permission from Tille P, editor. *Bailey and Scott's diagnostic microbiology.* 14th ed. St. Louis: Elsevier; 2017.)

TABLE 82.6	**Common Pathogens Causing Gastrointestinal Infections**			
	Bacteria	**Viruses**	**Fungi**	**Parasites**
Gastroenteritis	*Campylobacter*	Norovirus		*Giardia lamblia*
	Salmonella	Astrovirus		*Cryptosporidium parvum*
	Shigella	Adenoviruses 40/41		*Cyclospora cayetanensis*
	Vibrio parahaemolyticus	Sapoviruses		*Entamoeba histolytica*
	Vibrio cholerae	Enteroviruses		
	Listeria monocytogenes			
	Aeromonas spp.			
	Plesiomonas shigelloides			
Toxin-mediated gastroenteritis	*Staphylococcus aureus*			
	Bacillus cereus			
	Clostridium perfringens			
	Clostridioides difficile			
	Shiga-toxin producing *Escherichia coli* (STEC; also known as enterohemorrhagic *E. coli* or EHEC)			

Continued

TABLE 82.6　Common Pathogens Causing Gastrointestinal Infections—cont'd

	Bacteria	Viruses	Fungi	Parasites
Intestinal helminths				*Ascaris lumbricoides* (roundworm) *Trichuris trichiura* (whipworm) *Ancylostoma duodenale* (hookworm) *Necator americanus* (hookworm) *Strongyloides stercoralis* Enterobius vermicularis (pinworm) *Taenia saginata* (beef tapeworm) *Taenia solium* (pork tapeworm) *Dibothriocephalus latus* (fish tapeworm) *Hymenolepis nana* (dwarf tapeworm) *Echinococcus* spp. *Fasciolopsis buski* *Heterophyes heterophyes* *Metagonimus yokogawai*
Esophagitis		Cytomegalovirus (CMV) Herpes simplex virus (HSV)	*Candida* spp.	
Gastritis	*Helicobacter pylori*			
Hepatitis and biliary tree infections		Hepatitis A-E Epstein–Barr virus (EBV) Cytomegalovirus (CMV) Herpes simplex virus (HSV) Adenoviruses Enteroviruses		
Liver abscesses	*Streptococcus anginosus* group Enteric gram-positive and gram-negative microbiota (aerobic and anaerobic) Hypermucoid *Klebsiella pneumoniae* S. aureus Streptococcus pyogenes			*E. histolytica* *Echinococcus* spp.
Peritoneal infections	Enteric gram-positive and gram-negative microbiota (aerobic and anaerobic) *Streptococcus pneumoniae*			
Immunocompro-mised host	*Mycobacterium avium-intracellulare* complex Cutaneous microbiota including coagulase-negative staphylococci and *S. aureus* (peritoneal catheter) *Pseudomonas aeruginosa* and other environmental bacteria (peritoneal catheter)	Cytomegalovirus (CMV)	Microsporidia *Candida* spp. (peritoneal catheter) *Aspergillus, Fusarium,* and other filamen-tous molds (peritoneal catheter)	
Pediatrics	*Yersinia enterocolitica*	Rotavirus		

cause gastroenteritis. Other rare but recognized causes of bacterial gastroenteritis in the United States include *L. monocytogenes* along with *Yersinia enterocolitica* and *Yersinia pseudotuberculosis*, which are most commonly associated with pork consumption, particularly consumption of chitterlings (prepared intestines).[95]

In general, bacterial causes of gastroenteritis rarely lead to chronic infection in immunocompetent individuals. However, *Clostridioides difficile* (formerly *Clostridium difficile*) can cause both an acute gastroenteritis along with a chronic or recurrent gastroenteritis. *C. difficile* asymptomatically colonizes the GI tract in an estimated 5 to 10% of adults. While the organism has the ability to produce toxins that cause diarrheal disease, in asymptomatic patients potential effects of these toxins are kept in check through a homeostatic balance between the host and intestinal microbiota. Disruption of this homeostasis in the form of antibiotic therapy increases the risk of increased toxin production and the development of gastroenteritis caused by *C. difficile*. Unlike other causes of bacterial GI disease, which are rare to contract while hospitalized, *C. difficile* can spread from patient to patient and the high levels of antibiotic use in the health care setting put colonized patients at risk for developing *C. difficile* diarrheal disease. Infection can be severe, especially in immunocompromised and elderly patients, causing pseudomembranous colitis and death.[95,98]

Parasitic GI infections generally have longer incubation periods than bacterial, viral, or toxin mediated infections. Parasitic GI infections are acquired through ingestion of contaminated food or water sources or through fecal-oral spread from human to human. Individuals present with intermittent or persistent diarrhea lasting greater than 1 week and often have diarrhea that persists despite antibiotic treatment. Autoinfection due to poor hand hygiene can be a source of ongoing infection. Anti-parasitic treatment may be required, especially for ongoing infections, young children, elderly, and immunocompromised populations. The most common causes of parasitic gastroenteritis in the United States are *Giardia lamblia*, *Cryptosporidium parvum*, and *Cyclospora cayetanensis*. *Giardia* provides examples of all primary methods of transmission of parasitic diarrhea. Consumption of contaminated water is a leading cause of acquisition; this is a particularly common source of infection for hikers who drink improperly treated water or swimmers in natural bodies of water. Acquisition can also occur via consumption of contaminated foods, particularly raw or undercooked food such as fresh produce, and outbreaks—particularly at childcare centers—can occur via fecal-oral transmission. International travel also serves as a risk factor for acquisition. Similar routes of transmission occur for *Cryptosporidium*. Although daycare transmission is rare, outbreaks associated with swimming pools are more common due to the fact that *Cryptosporidium* oocytes are resistant to many disinfectants including chlorine. *Cyclospora* is more commonly associated with food outbreaks, often with fresh produce. Intestinal amebiasis caused by *E. histolytica* is another important cause of infectious diarrhea globally. *E. histolytica* can also cause extra-intestinal symptoms, most commonly amebic liver abscess, but infrequently pleuropulmonary abscess, pericardial abscess, and brain abscess. Cutaneous infection is also possible, most likely from direct inoculation as it is most common in infants wearing diapers.[34,35,99]

Intestinal Helminths

Helminths, or free-living and parasitic worms, are the most common human parasites with an estimated 1 billion people infected worldwide. Infection is most prevalent in tropical areas with high humidity along with poor sanitation and lack of access to clean drinking water. Humans can be infected by both worms of the phylum Nematoda (roundworms) and two classes from the phylum Platyhelminthes: Cestoda (tapeworms) and Trematoda (flukes). Intestinal nematodes include *Ascaris lumbricoides* (roundworm), *Trichuris trichiura* (whipworm), *Ancylostoma duodenale* (Old world hookworm), *Necator americanus* (New World hookworm), *S. stercoralis*, and *Enterobius vermicularis* (pinworm). They are spread through ingestion of eggs in contaminated food and water or skin penetration by filariform larvae (*S. stercoralis*). Humans are the definitive host for a variety of tapeworms including *Taenia saginata* (beef tapeworm), *T. solium* (pork tapeworm), *Dibothriocephalus latus* (fish tapeworm), and *Hymenolepis nana* (dwarf tapeworm). Cestodes of the genus *Echinococcus*, whose definitive hosts are dogs and other canids, also infect humans where they lead to extra-intestinal cyst formation. Over 70 species of trematodes can infect the human intestine with some of the more common species including *Fasciolopsis buski*, *Heterophyes heterophyes*, and *Metagonimus yokogawai*. Typically, intestinal helminths can range in clinical presentation from asymptomatic to diarrhea and vague abdominal pain. Blood loss associated with their infection can lead to anemia, and infection is also associated with the loss of micronutrients and with cognitive impairment and developmental delay. A person can be infected with multiple intestinal helminths at one time and they can be infected intermittently throughout their lifetime.[99,100]

Esophagitis

Esophagitis is inflammation or irritation of the esophagus. Symptoms include difficult or painful swallowing and chest pain that occurs during eating. Esophagitis is most often caused by stomach acid entering the esophagus, but it can also be infectious. Infection is largely limited to immunocompromised patients with conditions such as advanced HIV, cancer, or use of steroids or other immunomodulating therapy. The primary pathogens responsible for infectious esophagitis are *Candida* spp. along with the viruses CMV and HSV.[34]

Gastritis

Gastritis is inflammation of the protective layer of the stomach. The most common cause of gastritis is *Helicobacter pylori*. It is spread via the fecal-oral route and the prevalence of *H. pylori* is highest in developing countries where people live in crowded conditions with poor sanitation. Approximately half of the world is colonized with *H. pylori*. Those infected are generally asymptomatic, but a subset can develop peptic ulcers and those infected with *H. pylori* have increased risk of developing gastric adenocarcinoma and gastric mucosa-associated lymphoid tissue lymphoma.[101]

Hepatitis and Biliary Tree Infections

Hepatitis is inflammation of the liver. Acute infections cause nonspecific symptoms such as fatigue, nausea, anorexia, and abdominal pain. Chronic infections are those persisting more than 6 months following transmission and cause cirrhosis, abdominal swelling, peritonitis, edema, GI bleeding, and hepatic encephalopathy and extrahepatic conditions. The most common infectious causes of hepatitis are viruses; five unrelated viruses whose primary clinical manifestation is hepatitis have been designated hepatitis A through E.

Hepatitis A and E are spread by fecal-oral and person-person routes of infection, usually through contaminated food and water, daycare exposure, or food handlers. Hepatitis E is endemic in swine and causes zoonotic transmission. Both hepatitis A and E cause self-limiting disease in otherwise healthy individuals. They cannot be transmitted from mother to child and those infected rarely develop chronic disease. Infection can be severe in elderly and pregnant adults, immunocompromised populations, and those co-infected with HIV and Hepatitis B. Vaccination for hepatitis A is available worldwide while a hepatitis E vaccine is available in China.[102,103]

Hepatitis B is a bloodborne pathogen acquired through IV drug use, blood transfusions, sexual contact, and perinatally. Hepatitis B is highly infectious, and the virus can survive for at least 7 days outside of the body. Chronic infection is common and is inversely proportional to the age at which an individual was infected; 90% of neonates infected will develop chronic infection compared to less than 5% of those infected as adults. Chronic infection leads to cirrhosis, hepatocellular carcinoma, as well as extrahepatic manifestations such as progressive liver disease, polyarteritis nodosa, and renal disease. In the United States, vaccination is routinely given at birth to prevent transmission. Hepatitis D is a bloodborne pathogen that requires co-infection with hepatitis B. Infection is spread by IV drug use and hepatitis D can accelerate symptoms seen with hepatitis B infection. There is no vaccine and the only treatment is to eradicate the patient's hepatitis B infection.[104,105]

Hepatitis C is a bloodborne pathogen acquired through IV drug use, transfusions, perinatally, and rarely through sexual contact. Patients are usually asymptomatic during acute infection, but 50 to 80% of adults will develop chronic infection, leading to cirrhosis, risk of developing hepatocellular carcinoma, and extrahepatic diseases such as autoimmune thyroiditis, B-cell non-Hodgkin lymphoma, and glomerulonephritis. New antiviral therapy for hepatitis C has emerged in recent years, but treatment is very expensive and requires 12 weeks or more of medication. There is no vaccine for hepatitis C at this time.[34,106]

In addition to the "hepatitis" viruses, a number of other viruses can also lead to hepatitis. EBV, in the form of infectious mononucleosis, is typically associated with hepatitis, which can also be seen with CMV. Different adenoviruses and enteroviruses have also been associated with hepatitis. Typically, the hepatitis associated with these infections is mild and asymptomatic but in immunocompromised patients and in infants, these infections can be severe and lead to fulminant liver failure and death. In neonates, HSV-1 and HSV-2—viruses that do not cause hepatitis in older individuals—can lead to severe hepatitis resulting in liver failure and death.[34]

Liver Abscesses

The liver can also become the site of abscess formation.[107] Typically, infection occurs due to spread from the biliary tree, hepatic artery, portal vein, direct extension from cholecystitis, subphrenic abscess, perinephric abscess, or through trauma.

These infections are primarily bacterial and are related to the method of spread. Extension from the GI tract is more likely to be caused by gram-negative bacteria such as *E. coli* and *Klebsiella* along with anaerobes such as *Bacteroides* species. Studies have suggested that species of the *S. anginosus* group are a leading cause of liver abscess in the United States.[108] *S. aureus* and *S. pyogenes* have also been associated with liver abscess in select circumstances, largely associated with ongoing bacteremia. Worldwide, the amoeba *E. histolytica* is a common cause of liver abscesses,[109] and since the 1980s, pyogenic liver abscesses from eastern Asia have been associated with hypermucoid strains of *K. pneumoniae*.[110]

Biliary Tract Infection

The biliary tract can also be a site of infection. Cholecystitis is inflammation of the gallbladder, which can be sterile, but is associated with infection in 20 to 50% of cases. Cholangitis is inflammation of the common bile duct and is more commonly associated with infection (greater than 90% of cases). In both cases, infection is due to bacterial traversal from the intestine. This requires some level of dysfunction in the biliary system to allow spread, with gallstones being the most common cause. The classic presentation includes fever and abdominal pain. Jaundice is also classically present with cholangitis in a trio of symptoms known as Charcot's triad. Enteric gram-negative bacteria such as *E. coli, Klebsiella,* and *Enterobacter* along with anaerobes such as *Bacteroides* are the most common causes of infection. *Enterococcus* species are the most common gram-positive organism associated with these infections.[34]

Peritoneal Infections

Peritoneal infections occur in the space between the parietal peritoneum (which surrounds the abdominal wall) and the visceral peritoneum (which surrounds the intestinal organs such as the intestines). Infection of this space happens in three ways. The first is spontaneous bacterial peritonitis. This infection is limited to patients with ascites, which is the accumulation of fluid in the peritoneal space. This is most commonly associated with cirrhosis of the liver, but other causes include cancer, heart failure, and nephrotic syndrome. These infections are typically monomicrobial bacterial infections and occur primarily when bacteria translocate across the gut into the peritoneal space. Other causes of infection including UTIs and bacteremia can also lead to the seeding of the peritoneal cavity. Enteric gram-negative bacteria are the leading cause of infection but *S. pneumoniae* also plays a key role.[91]

The second form of peritonitis is secondary bacterial peritonitis.[111] This occurs when there is a loss of integrity in the GI tract. This type of infection leads to polymicrobial infection primarily with enteric gram-negative and anaerobic bacteria as millions of bacteria enter the peritoneal space. This often leads to the formation of intra-abdominal abscesses, and typically requires surgical management both for drainage of the abscesses and repair of the initial perforation. Causes of these perforations include appendicitis, diverticulitis, and gastric ulceration.

Finally, the peritoneal space can become infected due to peritoneal dialysis and the presence of a dialysis catheter in the peritoneal space. These are primarily gram-positive bacterial infections caused by cutaneous microbiota with coagulase-negative staphylococci alone responsible for 40% of cases.[112] *S. aureus* and *Enterococcus* species are also important causes of these infections while *E. coli, Klebsiella,* and *P. aeruginosa* are the most common gram-negative bacterial causes. Fungal peritonitis is much less common than bacterial but can be incredibly difficult to treat. *Candida* species are the predominant cause of fungal peritonitis, but cases of *Aspergillus, Fusarium,* and other molds have also been reported.[34]

Immunocompromised Patients

Immunocompromised individuals are at risk of contracting the same GI pathogens acquired by otherwise healthy adults, but they are at higher risk for developing severe symptoms, spread to extraintestinal sites, and death. Furthermore, GI infections that typically only cause acute gastroenteritis can lead to chronic gastroenteritis with symptoms persisting for weeks to months or even longer; *Cryptosporidium* and norovirus are agents that can be particularly challenging for immunocompromised patients to overcome. In addition, patients that are severely immunosuppressed, such as those with advanced HIV or AIDS, can also develop diarrhea due to MAIC, CMV, and Microsporidia, which rarely cause symptomatic infection in immunocompetent adults. CMV is of particular significance given its frequency, severity, and its ability to affect all components of the GI tract in immunocompromised patients leading to esophagitis, gastritis, gastroenteritis/colitis, and hepatitis.[113]

Neutropenic patients are also at risk for the development of neutropenic enterocolitis, known as typhlitis, for its most common location of occurrence in the ileocecal region ("typhlon" is the Greek word for cecum). Pathogenesis of this condition is not completely understood but is thought to include dysregulation of the intestinal microbiota leading to invasion of the intestinal walls, which can then progress to necrosis. Treatment involves broad-spectrum antibiotics covering enteric gram-negative bacteria and intestinal anaerobes, restoration of neutrophils, and bowel rest along with additional supportive therapy.

Immunocompromised patients infected with hepatitis often have more severe symptoms and duration of illness compared to otherwise healthy adults. The rate of hepatitis and HIV co-infection is very high in the United States, with 10% of HIV positive individuals co-infected with hepatitis B and 25% co-infected with hepatitis C virus. Due to IV drug use being the route of transmission for both viruses, 75% of IV drug users who are infected with HIV are co-infected with Hepatitis C. This has severe clinical impact as co-infection of HIV and HCV triples risk for liver disease.[114]

Pediatric Considerations

Children are also susceptible to the same GI pathogens as adults; however, their presentation may be more severe. Because children are generally in good health and lack comorbidities, they have very low rates of other infections discussed in this section. Peritonitis occurs much less frequently in children; when it does occur, perforated appendicitis is overwhelmingly the leading cause. Biliary tree infections are also much less common given the much lower rate of gallstones. When biliary tree infections do arise, congenital conditions such as biliary atresia are often responsible.

Preterm infants are vulnerable to the development of necrotizing enterocolitis. This condition involves severe intestinal inflammation ranging from mucosal injury to complete necrosis and bowel perforation. It happens in 2% to 7% of neonates born prior to 32 weeks gestational age but that rate rises to as high as 14% in infants with birth weights less than 1000 g.[115,116] Pathogenesis remains incompletely understood, but it is thought that the immature intestinal tract and immune system leads to dysregulation of the intestinal microbiota and an inappropriate inflammatory response leading to intestinal injury. Treatment involves bowel rest and broad-spectrum antibiotics with surgical removal of necrotic or perforated bowel required at times.

POINTS TO REMEMBER

- Gastrointestinal (GI) tract infections are spread by fecal-oral and person-to-person transmission.
- GI infections primarily affect children and those caring for them, people living in crowded living conditions, and those who lack access to clean drinking water.
- GI tract infections cause the highest number of infectious deaths worldwide after lower respiratory tract infections.
- Infection is generally self-limited and does not require treatment, but young children, the elderly, immunocompromised, and malnourished populations are at higher risk of developing severe symptoms, mostly due to dehydration, and may need antimicrobial or supportive care to overcome infection.

GENITOURINARY TRACT INFECTIONS

Infections of the GU tract include those occurring in organs involved in the production and excretion of urine and organs involved in reproduction. These involve some of the most common infections acquired such as UTIs and sexually transmitted infections (STIs). The most common causes of GU infection are found in Table 82.7 and a diagram of the urinary tract is located in Fig. 82.6.

Urinary Tract Infections

Most UTIs occur when bacteria gain access to the bladder by way of the urethra. Symptoms include burning during urination, an urge to frequently urinate despite an empty bladder, and occasionally pelvic pain. Women are much more likely to develop UTIs than men with a lifetime incidence of greater than 50%.[117] UTIs frequently recur; for women experiencing their first UTI, 27% will have a recurrence within 6 months and 44 to 70% will have recurrence within a year.[118,119] The majority of UTIs remain localized to the lower urinary tract, but in a small percentage of patients bacteria will ascend up the ureters and cause kidney infection. For some patients, bacteria will gain access to the bloodstream causing bacteremia deemed "urosepsis" due to the urinary tract source of infection. The flow of urine is generally sufficient to flush invading bacteria out of the urinary tract, but conditions that cause obstruction of urine flow such as kidney or bladder stones, structural abnormalities of the urinary tract, and use of a urinary catheter put patients at increased risk for the development of a UTI. Enteric gram-negative bacteria such as *E. coli, K. pneumoniae,* and *Proteus* spp. are the most

TABLE 82.7   Common Pathogens of Urogenital Tract Infections

	Bacteria	Viruses	Fungi	Parasites
Urinary tract infections	*Escherichia coli* *Klebsiella* spp. *Proteus* spp. *Enterobacter* spp. *Pseudomonas* spp. *Staphylococcus saprophyticus* *Staphylococcus aureus* Coagulase-negative staphylococci *Enterococcus* spp. *Corynebacterium urealyticum*		*Candida* spp.	*Schistosoma haematobium*
Genital tract infections	*Chlamydia trachomatis* Neisseria gonorrhoeae Mycoplasma genitalium			
Vaginosis	Vaginal microbiota dysbiosis (bacterial vaginosis)		*Candida* spp.	*Trichomonas vaginalis*
Orchitis and epididymitis	*C. trachomatis* *N. gonorrhoeae* *Brucella* spp.	Mumps virus		
Genital ulcers	*Treponema pallidum* (syphilis) *Haemophilus ducreyi*	Herpes simplex virus (HSV) Human papillomavirus (HPV)		
Immunocompromised host	*Mycobacterium bovis* Bacillus Calmette-Guérin (BCG)	BK polyomavirus (BKV) Adenovirus		

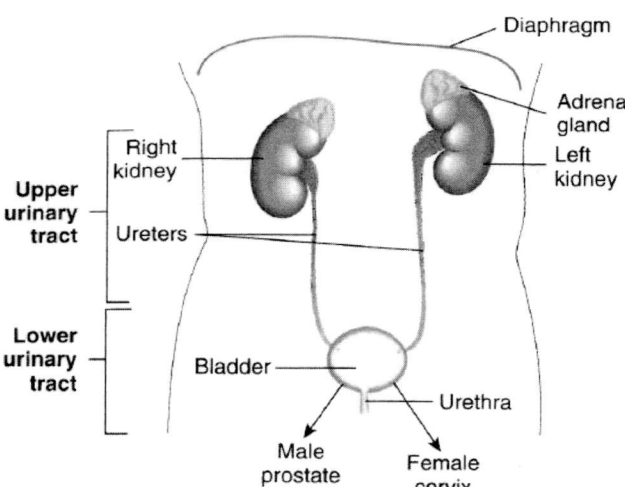

FIGURE 82.6 Basic anatomy of the urinary tract. (Reproduced with permission from Tille P, editor. *Bailey and Scott's diagnostic microbiology.* 14th ed. St. Louis: Elsevier; 2017.)

common causes of lower UTIs, subsequent kidney infections, and urosepsis. Although UTIs caused by gram-positive bacteria are much less prevalent than gram-negative bacteria, the most common causes are *Staphylococcus saprophyticus, Enterococcus* spp., and *Corynebacterium urealyticum.* Asymptomatic bacteriuria is very common, especially in the elderly, and should not be treated in the absence of symptoms. A small percentage of UTIs are caused by hematogenous spread of bacteria from the bloodstream to the kidneys; the most common organisms causing descending UTIs are *S. aureus* and *Candida* species.[34,35]

Schistosoma haematobium is a parasitic cause of chronic UTI. This blood fluke is endemic in Africa, the Middle East, and Corsica and infection is associated with rural, poor areas.[120] *S. haematobium* infection occurs when free swimming cercariae penetrate the skin of individuals using infested water for agricultural, occupational, domestic, or recreational purposes. The parasite enters the circulatory system where it matures into an adult and resides in the vesical and pelvic venous plexus of the bladder. The adult female releases eggs that are excreted in the urine. Symptoms of *S. haematobium* include hematuria, scarring, and calcification, and infection puts an individual at increased risk of developing squamous cell carcinoma of the bladder.[120]

Genital Tract Infections

Genital tract infections involve the urethra, cervix, vagina, epididymis, testicles, and rectum. Infection at these sites is primarily due to sexual transmission but vaginal irritation can also be due to dysbiosis of the normal vaginal microbiome.

Urethritis is inflammation of the urethra. Symptoms include dysuria, urethral itching, or purulent discharge. Cervicitis is inflammation of the cervix. Symptoms include vaginal discharge or bleeding (outside of menses), pain and inflammation, pain during sexual intercourse, and pelvic pressure that can be painful. The main causes of both urethritis and cervicitis are the sexually transmitted bacteria *C. trachomatis* and *N. gonorrhoeae.* Less is known about the clinical significance of the emerging pathogen *Mycoplasma genitalium,*[121] but it may be responsible for up to 30% of cases of recurrent urethritis in males. It is found in 10 to 30% of females with cervicitis, but the clinical significance, especially in females, is an area of ongoing research.

C. trachomatis and *N. gonorrhoeae* infections are often asymptomatic or cause mild symptoms. A study from Uganda found that of patients infected with *C. trachomatis*, only 11% of males and 6% of females had symptoms while 45% of males and 14% of females with *N. gonorrhoeae* had signs of infection.[122] Routine screening for STIs is recommended for any sexually active person and these screens are essential for detection of asymptomatic infections, prevention of long-term sequelae, and prevention of spread to additional partners. For high-risk individuals and men who have sex with men (MSM), throat swab and rectal swab should be tested in addition to urine/vaginal swabs for increased detection of STIs. Undiagnosed *C. trachomatis* and *N. gonorrhoeae* infection in females can lead to pelvic inflammatory disease and infertility. *N. gonorrhoeae* can disseminate to other areas of the body; the most common symptoms of disseminated gonococcal infection are large joint arthritis (knees most often) and skin findings, where it most commonly presents as fever, septic arthritis, tenosynovitis, and nodular/vesicular skin lesions.[123]

Proctitis is inflammation of the rectum. Symptoms include blood and pus present in stool or when wiping and anorectal pain. Proctocolitis is inflammation of the colonic mucosa extending 12 cm distal to the anus. The source of infection for both proctitis and proctocolitis is most often anoreceptive sex. Infectious agents include *C. trachomatis, N. gonorrhoeae,* and *Trichomonas vaginalis.* Lymphogranuloma venereum (LGV) is an invasive disease caused by *C. trachomatis* serovars L1-3. It is spread primarily among MSM and it causes proctitis and proctocolitis which mimics inflammatory bowel disease. Although uncommon in the United States, it is endemic in certain areas of Africa, Southeast Asia, India, the Caribbean, and South America.[123]

Vaginosis is defined by irritation of the vagina resulting in vaginal itching, discharge, discomfort, odor, and often pain with intercourse. There are three main causes: bacterial vaginosis, candidiasis, and trichomoniasis. Bacterial vaginosis is caused by dysbiosis of the vaginal microbiota, resulting in a reduction of *Lactobacillus* spp., which make up the majority of healthy vaginal bacterial microbiota, and an increase in *Gardnerella vaginalis, Prevotella* spp., *Mobiluncus* spp., and other anaerobic bacteria. Vulvovaginal candidiasis is caused by overgrowth of *Candida* spp., usually *Candida albicans.* Trichomoniasis is caused by the sexually transmitted protozoan parasite *T. vaginalis,* which is the most prevalent non-viral STI in the United States infecting an estimated 3.7 million people.[123] Only 30% of infected individuals will develop symptoms. *T. vaginalis* is associated with premature rupture of membranes and preterm delivery for pregnant women, so detection and treatment in pregnant women is of utmost importance.

Orchitis is inflammation of one or both testicles. Epididymitis is inflammation of the tube located at the back of the testicles that stores and carries sperm. Infection occurs when bacteria or viruses ascend the urethra or bladder to the epididymis and testicles. Symptoms include pain and inflammation of the testicles, fever, nausea, vomiting, and malaise. Bacterial causes of orchitis and epididymitis include *C. trachomatis* and *N. gonorrhoeae.* The zoonosis brucellosis, caused by species in the *Brucella* genus, can also lead to orchitis.[124] Mumps virus is another cause of orchitis.[125] Serious complications of infection include shrinking of the testicles, scrotal abscess, and male infertility.

Genital Ulcers

Genital ulcers are skin defects which can present as deep ulceration or superficial erosion. These erosions are located on the genitals, perineum, anus, or perianal skin. Infections that cause genital ulcers often also cause inguinal lymphadenopathy and infected individuals may also have constitutional symptoms. The most common infections causing genital ulcers are syphilis, HSV-1 and HSV-2, and human papillomaviruses (HPV). *Haemophilus ducreyi* causes a painful ulcer-forming STI also known as chancroid. Although prevalent in the past, it is declining and now extremely rare in the United States.[123]

Syphilis is called by the bacterium *T. pallidum* and transmission is caused by direct contact with a genital lesion during sexual contact. There are three stages of syphilis disease. During primary syphilis a chancre that is painless and firm with round borders forms at the site of infection (in or around the penis, vagina, anus, or mouth). Without treatment these lesions last 3 to 6 weeks before resolving. Secondary syphilis is characterized by a painless, macular rash on the palms of the hands and the soles of the feet. Systemic sequelae of secondary syphilis include fever, lymphadenopathy, hepatosplenomegaly, hepatitis, and nephrotic syndrome. After resolution of the symptoms of secondary syphilis, individuals enter the latent phase. In this phase, patients are asymptomatic but continue to harbor *T. pallidum.* The latent phase can last years, but eventually one third of patients with untreated syphilis will go on to develop tertiary syphilis or severe manifestations of *T. pallidum* infection including neurosyphilis, cardiovascular syphilis, or gummatous syphilis.[123]

Herpes simplex viruses (HSV-1 and HSV-2 also called herpes) are very common STIs in the United States with over 10% of sexually active persons infected. Symptoms of herpes infection include vesicular lesions in or around the penis, vulva, rectum, or mouth which rupture and result in painful ulcers that take 2 to 4 weeks to heal. These lesions contain high levels of virus and HSV is transmitted to others through close contact with these infected lesions. Infected individuals can also transmit the virus while asymptomatic and without visible lesions through viral shedding from mucosal surfaces, genital secretions, or oral secretions. HSV infects epithelial cells of the skin after which it travels to the sensory nerve ending and resides in a latent state within the nerve sensory root ganglion nucleus allowing for periodic reactivation of infection. During the initial outbreak, individuals may experience constitutional symptoms such as fever, swollen lymph nodes, body aches, or headaches in addition to genital or oral lesions. Subsequent outbreaks tend to be less severe than the initial outbreak. In the United States, HSV-2 is more commonly associated with genital infections while HSV-1 is typically associated with nonsexual acquisition of the virus through saliva causing oral lesions; however, either virus can become established at whichever mucosal surface first encounters the virus, leading to some individuals with oral HSV-2 lesions and others with genital HSV-1 lesions.[123]

HPV is the most common STI in the United States in both men and women. Transmission occurs through sexual contact with an infected individual at which time HPV infects the basal layer of the skin or mucous membranes. HPV consists of over 200 strain types with about 40 types being sexually transmitted. Clinical presentation depends on which strain type is contracted. The majority of HPV types cause asymptomatic infection which self-resolves in 8 months to 2 years. Types 6 and 11 are responsible for the majority of anogenital warts. Viral proteins of high-risk HPV types act as oncoproteins causing the epithelial cells to continue to divide when they would normally fall into cell cycle arrest, which induces chromosomal abnormalities in the epithelial cells and blocks apoptosis. HPV primarily causes cervical cancer but can also cause cancer of the vagina, vulva, anus, and oropharynx. HPV types 16 and 18 are the cause of most HPV-associated cancers, followed by types 31, 33, 45, 52, and 58. In 2006, an HPV vaccine was released for use in adolescents and young adults. The current 9-valent vaccine covers all HPV types listed above that are known to cause genital warts and cancer.[126] Vaccination uptake has been slow due to the stigma of vaccinating adolescents against an STI. In 2018, around 50% of females and males aged 13 to 17 living in the United States were fully vaccinated against HPV.[126] While HPV-associated cancer primarily affects females, vaccination of both males and females prior to becoming sexually active is important to break the cycle of HPV transmission.[123]

Immunocompromised Patients

Renal transplant patients are at risk of developing several viral infections. Adenovirus acquired through viremia has been shown to cause hemorrhagic cystitis and renal allograft nephropathy in renal transplant patients. Primary BK polyomavirus infection occurs within the first few years of life as an asymptomatic infection after which the virus becomes latent in uroepithelial and renal cells. Ten percent of patients that have received kidney transplants experience BK virus reactivation, usually in the first year following transplant. This process is generally asymptomatic but can be identified by a rise in the patient's serum creatinine. Histopathology is the gold standard for diagnosis of BK neuropathy, but lack of detection of BK virus in urine has a high negative predictive value. A third of patients with detectable BK virus in their urine progress to viremia and neuropathy.[127]

Mycobacterium bovis Bacillus Calmette-Guérin (BCG) is used as a vaccine strain to protect against *M. tuberculosis* outside of the United States. This organism is also used for intravesical immunotherapy for superficial bladder cancer. The mechanism of action for *M. bovis* BCG eradication of bladder cancer is unknown, but it is quite effective and well tolerated. One major side effect is that an estimated 4 to 5% of patients develop disseminated *M. bovis* BCG infections following treatment.[128]

POINTS TO REMEMBER

- Genitourinary tract infections include those occurring in the production and excretion of urine and organs involved in reproduction.
- Most urinary tract infections are caused by bacteria with *Escherichia coli* being the most common.
- *Chlamydia trachomatis, Neisseria gonorrhoeae,* and *Trichomonas vaginalis* are common causes of sexually transmitted infection
- Genital ulcers are most commonly caused by herpes simplex virus and human papillomavirus.

BONE AND JOINT INFECTIONS

Infections of the bones and joints are relatively rare as fully developed bone, in particular, is highly resistant to infection. However, numerous predisposing conditions markedly increase the likelihood of these infections. The severity and difficulty of diagnosis, treatment, and management of these infections makes them of critical importance in the realm of infectious diseases. The most common causes of bone and joint infection are found in Table 82.8.

Bone Infections

Osteomyelitis is infection of the bone, which can be caused by hematogenous seeding, contiguous spread from the joint or surrounding soft tissue, or direct inoculation due to trauma or surgery. Bacteria that seed the bone multiply, causing inflammation at the site of infection and bone necrosis. Symptoms of osteomyelitis are nonspecific, subacute or chronic, and generally localized to the site of infection rather than being systemic. The diagnosis of osteomyelitis is supported by imaging studies (primarily MRI), elevation of the inflammatory markers erythrocyte sedimentation rate (ESR) and C-reactive protein (CRP), and recovery of microorganism in culture. Surgical debridement and long courses of antibiotics are typically required to eliminate infection. Hematogenous osteomyelitis is typically monomicrobial, and *S. aureus* is the primary cause. In vitro models have shown that *S. aureus* can persist in a dormant state within osteoclasts for long periods of time, which may explain the high relapse rate seen clinically when using short courses of antibiotics.[34]

For patients with indwelling hardware or prosthetic joints, coagulase-negative staphylococci are the leading cause of infection. Almost any bacteria including *S. aureus*, groups A, B, C, and G streptococci, *Enterococcus*, enteric gram-negative bacteria, anaerobes, and nonpathogenic skin microbiota such as *C. acnes* and *Corynebacterium* spp. have been associated with prosthetic bone and joint infections. Between 1 and 2% of prosthetic joints become infected.[129] These infections can be acquired hematogenously or through local introduction either from wound infection or surgical contamination.[129] Infection typically involves the osseous structures adjacent to the foreign material and happen early in the postimplantation period. Treatment of these infections is complicated by the foreign material, which provides a local environment for the establishment of biofilms leading to an inability to clear the infection. Thus successful treatment of these infections generally requires removal of the foreign material in addition to antibiotic therapy. In cases where the material cannot be removed, indefinite suppressive antibiotic therapy has been used to mitigate the infection.[130]

Patients with open fractures and penetrating wounds are at risk for *S. aureus* but can develop osteomyelitis with a broad range of environmental and cutaneous microorganisms including aerobic gram-negative rods, fungi, and nontuberculosis *Mycobacterium* spp. These infections reflect the nature of the contaminating process with dirty wounds being more likely to develop polymicrobial infections caused by environmental organisms. Patients with diabetes mellitus are prone to the development of nonhealing chronic ulcers secondary to vascular insufficiency and neuropathy; approximately 15% of diabetic patients will develop a foot

TABLE 82.8 Common Pathogens Causing Bone and Joint Infections

	Bacteria	Viruses	Fungi
Osteomyelitis	*Staphylococcus aureus*		
Open fractures and penetrating wounds	*S. aureus* Non-tuberculosis *Mycobacterium* spp. Environmental gram-negative bacilli		Environmental molds
Prosthetic bone and joint infections	Coagulase-negative staphylococci *Cutibacterium acnes* *Corynebacterium* spp. *S. aureus* β-hemolytic streptococci *Enterococcus* spp. Enteric gram-negative bacteria Anaerobic bacteria		
Septic arthritis	*S. aureus* β-Hemolytic streptococci *Pseudomonas aeruginosa* *Neisseria gonorrhoeae* *Borrelia burgdorferi* (Lyme disease)	Parvovirus B19 Rubella Chikungunya, Zika, and dengue virus Human T-cell lymphotropic virus type 1 (HTLV-1) Human immunodeficiency virus (HIV) Acute hepatitis B virus (HBV) Acute hepatitis C virus (HCV)	
Chronic septic arthritis	*Tropheryma whipplei* (Whipple disease)		*Candida* spp. *Coccidioides* spp. *Blastomyces dermatitidis* *Histoplasma capsulatum* *Sporothrix schenckii*
Pediatrics	*Kingella kingae* *S. aureus* *Haemophilus influenzae* type b *Streptococcus pyogenes* (Group A)		

ulcer in their lifetime.[34] These ulcers are apt to develop into polymicrobial osteomyelitis through direct spread. Diagnosis of the causative agents requires deep tissue culture or surgical bone biopsy because superficial necrotic tissue is contaminated with cutaneous and environmental bacteria which are not indicative of the causative agent of the osteomyelitis. Treatment, as with most other forms of osteomyelitis, requires a combination of surgical debridement and prolonged use of antibiotics.

Joint Infections

Joint infections occur at a higher rate than bone infections due to the structure of the joint. Acute bacterial arthritis, also known as septic arthritis, is the most common joint infection and can cause permanent joint destruction and morbidity despite proper treatment. In most cases, joint infection is acquired through occult bacteremia. The synovial space has extensive vasculature. Bacteria entering through the vasculature adhere to the synovial membrane, proliferate in the synovial fluid, and incite a massive host inflammatory response that causes joint destruction. Bacterial infection is typically monomicrobial and affects a single joint. Infection can occur in patients with native joints, but infection is more likely in a joint with preexisting arthritis such as rheumatoid arthritis, osteoarthritis, gout, or pseudogout. Immunocompromised patients, including those patients with diabetes, are at higher risk of infection. Patients with rheumatoid arthritis are at particular risk as they already have underlying changes to the joint that increase the risk of infection and are also often on immunosuppressive medication. Besides hematogenous spread, septic arthritis can be acquired through trauma to the joint space, surgery, or contiguous spread from bone or soft tissue. Diagnosis of septic arthritis depends on acquisition of synovial fluid for cell count analysis and culture; sensitivity of culture can be relatively low (60 to 70%), and molecular testing is used at times to increase detection of causative agents.[34]

Although the bacterial differential for joint infections is large depending on the source of infection and host factors, bacteria such as *S. aureus* (35 to 65% of all cases) and β-hemolytic streptococci contain virulence factors that predispose these organisms for infections of the joint space. *S. agalactiae* has become a more frequently recognized cause of septic arthritis, particularly in patients with diabetes mellitus.[34] Enteric gram-negative organisms rarely cause joint infections except in the very young, elderly, and immunocompromised patients. Patients using intravenous drugs demonstrate higher rates of *P. aeruginosa* septic arthritis. Sexually active adults are susceptible to gonococcal joint infections; for young adults, this is among the leading causes of septic arthritis. Patients with the appropriate exposures can develop acute septic arthritis secondary to *B. burgdorferi*, the causative agent of Lyme disease; this presentation typically occurs months after the initial infection and requires a combination of clinical suspicion, serologic testing, and PCR testing of synovial fluid for diagnosis. Direct inoculation of bacteria into the joint space leads to a different variety of infectious organisms depending on the environment of the trauma. Bite wounds, particularly in the hand, can lead to septic arthritis. *Pasteurella multocida* and *Capnocytophaga* species are commonly associated with dog and cat bites while *E. corrodens* is a leading cause associated with human bites.

Chronic septic arthritis is rare and characterized by slow onset with few symptoms, but it can result in joint destruction and loss of function. Due to the presentation, diagnosis is often delayed, and it is difficult to identify a pathogenic cause in many cases. Tuberculosis is a leading cause of chronic septic arthritis, but other slowly growing mycobacteria, fungi, or atypical bacteria have been associated with chronic infections, including noncultivable *Tropheryma whipplei* (Whipple disease). Fungal arthritis is most commonly associated with *Candida* species, although the dimorphic fungi *Coccidioides*, *Blastomyces*, *Histoplasma*, and *Sporothrix* also are associated with joint infections. The incidence of chronic arthritis is highest in immunocompromised patients.[34]

Viral joint infections are usually associated with systemic viral infection and are often accompanied by fever and other systemic sequalae. Causes of viral arthritis are parvovirus B19, rubella, acute hepatitis B and C, retroviruses HIV and HTLV-1, and arboviruses such as chikungunya, dengue, and Zika. Viruses can infect the synovium or symptoms can be due to immune-mediated inflammation in the joint. Viral arthritis generally involves multiple joints and inflammation typically lasts for a few weeks before resolving without long-term joint damage. Chikungunya virus, however, has been associated with debilitating polyarthritis that recurs and can last for months up to years.

Infections can also be associated with reactive arthritis, which is an acute arthritis, typically mono- or oligoarticular and more commonly in the lower extremities, following an antecedent infection. The infection usually precedes the arthritis by days to weeks and has been most commonly associated with GI infection (*Salmonella*, *Shigella*, *Yersinia*, *Campylobacter*, and *C. difficile*) or GU tract infection (*C. trachomatis* classically but *Ureaplasma urealyticum* and *M. genitalium* have also been reported as well). *S. pyogenes* has also been associated with postinfectious arthritis both in the form of rheumatic fever and poststreptococcal reactive arthritis.

Pediatric Considerations

Prepubescent bones are radically different in structure than adult bones and feature a rich vascular supply. This makes them far more prone to infection, particularly at the metaphysis of the long bones with the femur and tibia being the two most commonly infected bones.[131] Infection is acquired through acute hematogenous spread and is relatively common with rates as high as 1 in 10,000 in the developed world and 1 in 500 in developing countries.[131] Septic arthritis can also be acquired hematogenously, but in children, it often occurs as the product of direct invasion of the joint from adjoining osteomyelitis. Pediatric patients often present with fever and systemic symptoms in addition to localized pain. Treatment often does not require surgery unless large abscesses are present (although sampling for culture can be

useful) and short courses of IV therapy followed by a few weeks of oral antibiotics is typically sufficient.[132]

S. aureus is overwhelmingly the most common cause of these infections.[132] *H. influenzae* type B used to be a much more significant cause as well, but rates have dropped precipitously in the setting of vaccination. Today, *S. pyogenes* is the second leading cause of pediatric acute osteomyelitis.[131] *K. kingae*, a gram-negative organism which is part of the oral microbiota, is increasingly identified as a cause of osteomyelitis and septic arthritis in children under 4 years of age.[133] Neonates are particularly susceptible to osteomyelitis from *S. agalactiae* and *E. coli*, which are the leading causes of bacteremia at that age. Patients with sickle cell disease are at increased risk for osteomyelitis at any age, but coupled with the structure of pediatric bones, they are at highest risk during childhood. *S. aureus* remains an important cause of osteomyelitis in patients with sickle cell disease but gram-negative organisms, particularly *Salmonella* and *E. coli*, along with encapsulated organisms such as *S. pneumoniae*, *N. meningitidis*, and *H. influenzae* (secondary to decreased splenic function) cause much higher rates of bone and joint infection in individuals with sickle cell disease than in the population at large.

POINTS TO REMEMBER

- Osteomyelitis and joint infections are caused by hematogenous seeding, contiguous spread from the joint or surrounding soft tissue, or direct inoculation due to trauma or surgery.
- Osteomyelitis is more prevalent in prepubescent children than adults due to the rich vascular supply in developing bones.
- Bacteria cause the majority of bone and joint infections in children and adults.

SKIN AND SOFT TISSUE INFECTIONS

Skin separates the body from the outside world and serves as a barrier to invasion and infection by pathogens. The skin uses multiple mechanisms to prevent infection including an overlapping layer of skin cells known as corneocytes, which produce antimicrobial peptides and are embedded in a lipid matrix that is acidic thereby reducing microbial growth. Despite this protection, skin infections are still frequent and are caused by all categories of pathogens: viruses, bacteria, fungi, and parasites. Skin infections can be the primary location of infection and numerous other infections throughout the body can produce dermatologic findings. The most common causes of skin and soft tissue infection are found in Table 82.9.

Bacterial Skin and Soft Tissue Infections

Bacterial infection of the skin is quite varied in appearance depending on the portion of the skin that is infected. The vast majority of these infections are secondary to *S. pyogenes* and *S. aureus* but other organisms can be involved under select circumstances.

Impetigo

Impetigo is a superficial bacterial infection that comes in two forms: nonbullous and bullous. Nonbullous impetigo is the

TABLE 82.9	**Common Pathogens Causing Skin and Soft Tissue Infections**			
	Bacteria	**Viruses**	**Fungi**	**Parasites**
Impetigo and ecthyma	*Staphylococcus aureus* *Streptococcus pyogenes* (Group A)			
Folliculitis	*S. aureus* *Pseudomonas aeruginosa*			
Cellulitis	β-Hemolytic streptococci *S. aureus* *Pasteurella multocida* (animal bite) *Capnocytophaga canimorsus* (animal bite) *Eikenella corrodens* (human bite) *Erysipelothrix rhusiopathiae* (animal exposure, particularly swine) *Streptococcus pneumoniae* (periorbital/orbital cellulitis) *Haemophilus influenzae* (periorbital/ orbital cellulitis) *Aeromonas hydrophila* (freshwater exposure) *Vibrio* spp. (saltwater exposure)			
Fasciitis and myositis	β-Hemolytic streptococci, primarily *S. pyogenes* (Group A) *Clostridium* spp., primarily *C. perfringens* Anaerobic bacteria			
Toxic shock syndromes	*S. aureus* *S. pyogenes* (Group A)			
Other skin infections	*Borrelia burgdorferi* (Lyme disease) *Bacillus anthracis* (anthrax) *Mycobacterium leprae* (leprosy)	Varicella zoster virus (VZV) Molluscum contagiosum Herpes simplex virus (HSV) Human papillomavirus (HPV)	*Trichophyton* spp. *Microsporum* spp. *Epidermophyton* spp. *Malassezia* spp. *Candida* spp. *Sporothrix schenckii*	*Leishmania* spp. *Sarcoptes scabiei* (scabies) *Pediculus* spp. (lice) *Dermatobia hominis* (human botfly) *Cordylobia anthropophaga* (tumbu fly) *Ancylostoma braziliense* and *Ancylostoma caninum* (hookworms)

more common form. It begins as papules that progress to pustules and break apart to form a classic honey-colored crust; these lesions are usually secondary to *S. pyogenes* infection. The bullous form of impetigo is secondary to strains of *S. aureus* that produce exfoliative toxin A. This toxin leads to the loss of cell adhesion in the epidermis, causing the formation of bullae filled with a translucent yellowish fluid. The bullae ultimately rupture leaving a thin brown crust. Systemic symptoms are rare with impetigo.[22]

Ecthyma

Ecthyma is an infection where ulcerative lesions extend from the epidermis into the dermis; the lesions evolve into a crusted ulcer surrounded by a raised rim. These lesions are secondary to *S. pyogenes* infection and are typically associated with another pruritic skin condition such as scabies or an insect bite. Ecthyma gangrenosum is a necrotizing ulcer covered with a black eschar that is characteristic of *P. aeruginosa* infection. This infection usually occurs in the setting of neutropenia or neutrophil dysfunction and is indicative of hematogenous spread, often coupled with ongoing bacteremia.

Folliculitis

Folliculitis is a superficial infection that does not extend into the dermis. It is most frequently caused by *S. aureus*. Immersion in contaminated water can lead to a diffuse "hot-tub folliculitis" which is secondary to *P. aeruginosa*. Deeper extension of infection along the hair follicle into the dermis with development of a surrounding nodule is a furuncle (also called a boil). Furuncles often serve as the nidus of the formation of a skin abscess, which are collections of pus in the dermis and deep skin tissues. Carbuncles are collections of several furuncles that have coalesced into one mass. Furuncles, carbuncles, and skin abscesses are overwhelmingly caused by *S. aureus* although injections into the skin (as with IV drug use) can lead to a wider variety of causative organisms. Perianal abscesses are frequently polymicrobial secondary to enteric gram-negative bacteria and may contain an anaerobic component.

Cellulitis

Cellulitis is an acute infection of the dermis and subcutaneous tissues. A subset of cellulitis is erysipelas, which is characterized by a bright red plaque with well-demarcated borders. Erysipelas differs from other cellulitides in that manner as cellulitis may have a more varied intensity and ill-defined borders. Erysipelas is most commonly due to *S. pyogenes* but can also occur secondary to the other large, β-hemolytic streptococci (groups B, C, and G). Cellulitis has a more diverse set of infectious causes, but *S. pyogenes* remains the most common. *S. aureus* is another major cause of cellulitis, particularly for cellulitis associated with abscess formation where it is the predominant cause of infection. A number of other bacteria can induce cellulitis particularly under the correct circumstances; these include but are not limited to the following: *P. multocida* (animal bite), *Capnocytophaga canimorsus* (animal bite), *E. corrodens* (human bite), *Erysipelothrix rhusiopathiae* (animal exposure particularly swine), *S. pneumoniae* (periorbital/orbital cellulitis), *H. influenzae* (periorbital/orbital cellulitis), *Aeromonas hydrophila* (freshwater exposure), and *Vibrio* species (saltwater exposure).

Fasciitis and Myositis

The soft tissues underlying the skin can also become infected with bacteria. This includes fasciitis (infection of the muscle fascia and overlying subcutaneous fat) and myositis (infection of the skeletal muscle). The most common form of myositis is pyomyositis, which is secondary to hematogenous seeding. *S. aureus* causes the vast majority of cases followed by *S. pyogenes*. Trauma can also lead to the development of myositis with a much broader differential of organisms. This includes *Clostridium* species, which can induce a rapidly progressive infection known as clostridial myonecrosis or gas gangrene. The trauma both introduces the bacteria and creates a devascularized zone of tissue which allows the organisms to proliferate. The majority of cases are secondary to *C. perfringens* with the remaining cases due to other *Clostridium* species, most notably *Clostridium septicum*. Modern trauma care has reduced rates of these infections, and treatment requires a combination of surgery and antibiotics.[134]

The most concerning form of fasciitis is necrotizing fasciitis. This rare infection can spread rapidly along the fascial plane due to its poor blood supply, and it is a surgical emergency, as effective treatment requires surgical debridement in addition to antibiotics. Diagnosis can be complicated by the fact that the overlying skin can retain a normal appearance as skin involvement need not be present. Clinical manifestations suggestive of necrotizing fasciitis include fever, crepitus, and severe pain (out of proportion to exam).[135] Necrotizing fasciitis comes in two major forms. Type I infection is a polymicrobial infection involving both anaerobes (usually *Bacteroides*, *Clostridium*, or *Peptostreptococcus*) and aerobic gram-negative bacteria. This type of necrotizing fasciitis is largely limited to older individuals with underlying medical conditions, most commonly diabetes mellitus with associated peripheral vascular disease. Type II infection can occur at any age and without any medical comorbidities. It is monomicrobial in nature, usually secondary to *S. pyogenes*, although other β-hemolytic streptococci and *S. aureus* are other rare causes. Infection can occur from direct seeding (either from penetrating trauma or overlying cutaneous lesions) or from hematogenous seeding often to the site of minor, nonpenetrating trauma.[134,135]

Toxic Shock Syndromes

Another pair of conditions that have skin involvement with bacterial infection are staphylococcal toxic shock syndrome and streptococcal toxic shock syndrome. Both are secondary to the production of toxins by the respective bacteria that act as superantigens, resulting in massive cytokine production. Both conditions feature erythematous rashes that resemble sunburns that can be confused for cellulitis; the rashes ultimately lead to desquamation. Hypotension and shock are key features of the conditions, and end organ dysfunction in the form of diarrhea, acute kidney injury, and altered mental status can occur. Tampon use was initially described as the major risk factor for staphylococcal toxic shock, but now nonmenstrual causes are more common.[136] Streptococcal toxic shock is associated with any invasive *S. pyogenes* infection including necrotizing soft tissue infections, myositis, bacteremia, and pneumonia.

Other Bacterial Skin Infections

A variety of other bacteria can also cause skin infections. Early Lyme disease leads to the development of a circular rash known as erythema migrans at the site of the tick bite.[137] Cutaneous anthrax occurs after subcutaneous entry of spores and causes a lesion which develops from a vesicle or bulla into a painless necrotic ulcer with black eschar.[138] Leprosy, caused by the bacteria *M. leprae*, remains an ongoing issue worldwide with 208,000 new cases in 2018 according to the WHO.[139] Leprosy is marked by hypopigmented or reddish patches with decreased or absent sensation. Multi-drug therapy exists and can eliminate the disease and prevent the development of disability.[140]

Viral Skin and Soft Tissue Infections
Systemic Viral Infections

HSV and HPV are two viral infections discussed previously that can also cause skin infections. HSV can lead to the development of painful vesicles that are erythematous and tender. This happens more frequently in areas of skin trauma such as eczema (eczema herpeticum), finger chewing (herpetic whitlow), or wrestling (herpes gladiatorum). These lesions resolve on their own, but treatment with acyclovir or valacyclovir may speed the process. Relapses occur as well. Some of the more than 200 strain types of HPV have a predilection for infection of skin rather than the GU mucosa. These isolates lead to the development of warts, an exceedingly common infection affecting up to 10% of all children.[141]

Molluscum contagiosum is another common viral skin disease of childhood. It is caused by a poxvirus known as molluscum contagiosum virus. It leads to the development of firm, dome-shaped papules. The lesions are painless but may be pruritic and can become inflamed and secondarily infected (at which time they become painful).[22] The frequency of infection in adults is less than children, but molluscum can occur and is often sexually transmitted. Immunocompromised patients, particularly those with advanced HIV can have profound spread and involvement.

A number of multi-system viral infections have prominent skin findings. One of the most notable such infections is caused by VZV. Primary infection with VZV leads to the development of varicella, also known as chicken pox. Infection occurs after inhalation of infected droplets or through direct contact of an infected vesicle. During the incubation period, the virus enters the bloodstream and spreads throughout the body. A prodrome of fever and malaise develops followed 24 hours later by the appearance of a diffuse vesicular rash, frequently described as "dew drops on a rose petal." The rash is found in different stages and is usually pruritic. The rash can become secondarily infected, most commonly with *S. pyogenes*, and sepsis can result. Other complications of primary VZV infection include encephalitis (most commonly in the form of acute cerebellar ataxia but also with a diffuse encephalitis), pneumonia, and hepatitis. After resolution of the initial infection, the virus establishes a latent phase in the sensory neurons. At a later date, the virus can reactivate leading to the development of herpes zoster, also known as shingles. Herpes zoster presents as a painful vesicular rash following a dermatomal distribution. Reactivation is more common in immunocompromised patients but also occurs in immunocompetent individuals.[22] Other multi-system viruses with skin manifestations include measles, rubella, enterovirus, and parvovirus among others.

Fungal Skin and Soft Tissue Infections

Fungal infections of the skin are very common. The most common of these are superficial infections caused by dermatophytes, which are mold species that live off the keratin produced by skin. These infections are caused primarily by fungi of the genera *Trichophyton, Microsporum,* and *Epidermophyton*. Rather than being named for the causative agent, these infections are named for the portion of the body affected: tinea capitis (infection of the scalp hair), tinea pedis (infection of the foot commonly known as athlete's foot), tinea cruris (infection of the groin commonly known as jock itch), and tinea corporis (infection of the rest of the body commonly known as ringworm). Topical treatment is largely effective except for tinea capitis, which requires systemic oral therapy.[142,143]

Fungi of the genus *Malassezia* are normal skin colonizers but overgrowth and transition from yeast to the mycelial form can lead to the development of macules of differing pigmentation known as tinea versicolor.[143]

Candida can also lead to skin infections. This is most common in young, diapered children who often develop candidal dermatitis in the diapered region. Older individuals with comorbidities or immunosuppression can also develop candidal skin infections.[143]

The dimorphic fungus *Sporothrix schenckii* can cause infection of the skin and underlying tissues known as sporotrichosis. Infection typically begins as an erythematous papule, which may then ulcerate. Spread occurs down the lymphatic tract with development of similar lesions along the drainage course. Primary risk factors for the infection include working with soil, landscaping, and gardening; hence, it also has the name rose gardener's disease.[142,143]

Parasitic Skin and Soft Tissue Infections

One of the most significant parasitic diseases of the skin is leishmaniasis. This is caused by protozoa from the genus *Leishmania*, which are transmitted by the bite of sand flies. Geographical locations contain distinct species of *Leishmania* which cause New World and Old World disease. The most common presentation for all species is cutaneous leishmaniasis, which begins as an erythematous papule that

enlarges into a nodule and ultimately ulcerates, creating a lesion with an indurated border. The ulcer winds up being covered, often with a hyperkeratotic eschar for Old World disease or a thick fibrinous material for New World disease. Some species of *Leishmania* can also cause visceral leishmaniasis, also known as kala-azar. In this condition, heavy loads of parasites accumulate in the spleen, liver, and bone marrow leading to severe anemia, thrombocytopenia, immunosuppression, and liver failure. Untreated cases are almost universally fatal.[144]

Scabies is caused by infestations of the mite *Sarcoptes scabiei*, which causes very pruritic eruptions. Classically, the site of infection is the interdigital spaces of the hands, but it can spread across the body. In infants, heavy involvement is often noted with spread across the entire body and reactions can be robust, appearing vesicular or bullous in nature. Immunocompromised patients can develop crusted scabies where scaly patches form featuring high numbers of mites; pruritus can be minimal in these patients.[22]

Three species of lice infect humans: *Pediculus humanus capitis* (the head louse), *Pediculus humanus humanus* (the body louse), and *Pthirus pubis* (the crab louse, responsible for pediculosis pubis). All three species cause pruritus and skin irritation. *P. h. humanus* is a key vector for the transmission of *Bartonella quintana* (the causative agent of trench fever and a cause of endocarditis), *Rickettsia prowazekii* (the agent of epidemic typhus), and *Borrelia recurrentis* (the agent of relapsing fever).[145]

Two species of flies have also been known to cause larval infestation of the skin known as myiasis. In these cases, the larvae infest the skin where they remain and develop. This causes local irritation and pain. The human botfly, *Dermatobia hominis*, is found throughout much of the Americas; the female fly hijacks mosquitos and lays eggs on them, and subsequently the mosquitos bring the eggs and hatched larva to the host. Another cause of myiasis is the tumbu fly, *Cordylobia anthropophaga*, which is found in east and central Africa. Treatment for the condition is removal of the larva.[146]

Cutaneous larva migrans occurs when humans are infected by hookworms that are not natural human parasites. Most commonly this is associated with the dog and cat hookworms, *Ancylostoma braziliense* or *Ancylostoma caninum*. One study from France revealed that cutaneous larva migrans was the most common dermatologic issue in returning travelers.[147] As these worms lack the collagenase necessary to break through the basement membrane of the skin, they continue to track through skin and produce an inflammatory reaction along their path.[148]

POINTS TO REMEMBER

- Skin and soft tissue infections include impetigo and ecthyma, folliculitis, cellulitis, fasciitis and myositis, and infections caused by toxin production and range in severity from mild to life-threatening.
- Bacteria cause the majority of skin and soft tissue infections with *Staphylococcus aureus* and *Streptococcus pyogenes* being the most common.
- Systemic viral infections often cause rashes or lesions as part of their sequelae.
- *Leishmania* spp., mites, and lice are important parasitic causes of skin and soft tissue infection.

MULTI-SYSTEMIC INFECTIONS

A number of infections do not have a single primary site of infection but instead quickly spread throughout multiple systems in the body. Many of these infections are viruses and are often transmitted through respiratory secretions. Some of the noteworthy infections are covered in this section and are summarized in Table 82.10.

Multi-System Viral Infections

Measles is a prototypical example of such an infection.[22] The infection is initially established with viral entry through the respiratory mucosa or conjunctiva. Viral replication occurs locally before disseminating into the bloodstream producing viremia. Once the incubation period completes, the prodrome begins with fever and malaise developing into conjunctivitis, cough, and coryza. Koplik spots, which are 1- to 3-mm whitish spots located primarily on the buccal mucosa may also develop during this time. These symptoms persist for 2 to 4 days prior to the development of the classic measles rash, which is a diffuse, erythematous, blanching, maculopapular rash which usually progresses cranially to caudally across the body. Typically, the fever breaks 2 to 3 days after the development of the rash with the remaining symptoms resolving in 1 to 2 weeks. Complications of measles include pneumonia (which is the most common cause of measles-associated death), gastroenteritis, and encephalitis. Subacute sclerosing panencephalitis (SSPE) is a fatal, progressive degenerative disease that typically occurs 7 to 10 years after the initial measles infection. The greatest risk factor for the development of SSPE is infection at an early age. A review of cases from California suggests the rate of SSPE may be 1:1367 for children with measles infection before the age of 5 years and 1:609 for children infected prior to the age of 1 year.[149] Measles also serves to lower overall immunity for an extended time after initial infection; evidence links this loss of immunity to increased mortality for 2 to 3 years following infection.[150]

Mumps is another multi-system virus spread through contact with respiratory droplets, direct contact, and contaminated fomites. The typical presentation involves fever, fatigue, myalgias, and headache followed by inflammation of one or both parotid glands. The most common complications include orchitis (15 to 30% of postpubescent males) and inflammation of the ovaries (5% of postpubescent females).[125] CNS complications also occur including meningitis and encephalitis and sensorineural hearing loss.

Adenoviruses consist of greater than 60 serotypes that cause a wide range of infectious presentations in humans including pharyngitis, bronchiolitis, otitis media, and pneumonia. Adenovirus is a common cause of conjunctivitis, and gastroenteritis and hepatitis are also known to be associated with certain serotypes of adenovirus. In children, adenovirus can lead to a combination of fever, rash, and conjunctivitis that resembles the autoinflammatory vasculitis Kawasaki disease. In neonates and immunocompromised patients, adenovirus can lead to a severe disseminated disease and death.

A number of the herpesviruses can produce multi-systemic infection. Primary VZV infection leads to a multi-system infection that was discussed in the section on skin and soft tissue infections. HHV-6 is the most frequent cause of roseola in children. Roseola involves 3 to 5 days of high fever, followed by abrupt resolution and development of a rash, and it occurs in approximately one quarter of patients with primary HHV-6 infection.[151] It is unclear exactly what percentage of HHV-6 infections are symptomatic, but fever and fussiness are thought to be common with infection and cases of encephalitis and febrile seizures also reported.[151] EBV can also cause multi-system infection. Although often asymptomatic upon initial infection, primary EBV infection can lead to infectious mononucleosis characterized by pharyngitis, fever, lymphadenopathy, fatigue, hepatitis, and splenomegaly. Latent EBV infection is also associated with lymphoproliferative disorders, including hemophagocytic lymphohistiocytosis (HLH), lymphomatoid granulomatosis, and post-transplant lymphoproliferative disease (PTLD). Due to the latent infection and transformative properties of EBV, a number of malignancies are also associated with EBV in certain populations including Burkitt lymphoma, Hodgkin lymphoma, non-Hodgkin lymphoma, T-cell lymphoma, nasopharyngeal carcinomas, and smooth muscle tumors. CMV is yet another herpes virus with multi-system involvement. Although it can lead to infectious mononucleosis with primary infection, it is of much greater significance in the immunocompromised population where it can cause retinitis, pneumonitis, hepatitis, colitis, encephalitis, and graft loss.

Acute HIV infection, although localized to components of the immune system, behaves as a generalized infection in the acute phase. It is not clear exactly what percentage of patients develop symptoms during the acute infection. One study indicated that most patients develop some symptoms, but they are typically mild and nonspecific.[152] Patients who do present with symptoms typically complain of fever, pharyngitis, lymphadenopathy, fatigue, and rash not dissimilarly to patients with infectious mononucleosis. Headache and aseptic meningitis also have been found to occur. Opportunistic infections are rare in the acute phase with oral and esophageal candidiasis being the most frequent. Left untreated, HIV infection ultimately leads to the loss of CD4 T cells and opportunistic infections.

TABLE 82.10	Common Pathogens Causing Multi-System Infections	
	Bacteria	**Viruses**
Pathogens causing multi-system infections	*Rickettsia* spp. *Orientia tsutsugamushi* *Ehrlichia* spp. *Anaplasma* spp.	Measles virus Mumps virus Adenoviruses Cytomegalovirus (CMV) Epstein–Barr virus (EBV) Varicella zoster virus (VZV) Human herpesvirus 6 (HHV-6) Acute human immunodeficiency virus (HIV)

Rickettsiales

Bacteria of the order Rickettsiales cause a variety of related diseases across all of the inhabited continents.[153] Members of this family are obligate intracellular bacteria, and they are transmitted from host to host via arthropods. The best studied of these infections is Rocky Mountain spotted fever (RMSF) caused by *R. rickettsii*, which is the most prevalent rickettsial infection in the United States. In the case of *R. rickettsii*, the principal vector is the American dog tick, *Dermacentor variabilis*. Patients with RMSF initially present with features common to rickettsial infections: fever, headache, arthralgias, and myalgias. Rash develops in most patients but typically not until day 3 to 5 of symptoms and thus is often not present at the initial presentation to health care. Classically, the rash begins with blanching erythematous macules on the wrists and ankles that spreads and becomes petechial. Rash in the palms and soles is often suggestive of RMSF, but this aspect develops later in the course. Eschar, which is common with other spotted fever rickettsia, is rare. Patients develop thrombocytopenia and often present with hyponatremia. Complications include acute respiratory distress syndrome, encephalitis, and sepsis. Most cases respond quickly to treatment with doxycycline but failure to recognize the disease and treat appropriately can lead to death.

Besides *R. rickettsii*, the other members of the order Rickettsiales cause similar symptoms including fever, myalgias, and rash/eschar. The family Rickettsiaceae consists of two genera: *Orientia* and *Rickettsia*, with *Rickettsia* subdivided into the spotted fever group (including *R. rickettsii*) and the typhus group. Diseases caused by the spotted fever group include but are not limited to African tick bite fever (*R. africae*), rickettsialpox (*R. akari*), Queensland tick typhus (*R. australis*), Mediterranean spotted fever (*R. conorii*), Flinders Island spotted fever (*R. honei*), Japanese spotted fever (*R. japonica*), and Siberian tick typhus (*R. sibirica*).[154] The typhus group of *Rickettsia* includes the agents of murine typhus (*R. typhi*) and epidemic typhus (*R. prowazekii*). The genus *Orientia* does include one pathogen of note: *O. tsutsugamushi* is responsible for the mite-borne disease known as scrub typhus.

Members of Anaplasmataceae, the other major family in the order Rickettsiales that are responsible for human disease, include species in the genera *Ehrlichia* and *Anaplasma*. *E. chaffeensis*, the agent of human monocytic ehrlichiosis (HME) and *A. phagocytophilum*, the agent of human granulocytic anaplasmosis (HGA) are the two most commonly recognized pathogenic species. Patients with these infections also present with fever, headache, and myalgias; severity can range from asymptomatic to severe, but symptoms tend toward less severe disease than RMSF. Rash is rare with HGA and occurs in about one-third of cases of HME.[155,156]

POINTS TO REMEMBER

- Several bacteria and viruses do not have a primary site of infection but spread rapidly throughout the body causing sequelae in multiple organ systems.
- Viruses causing multi-system infection include respiratory-transmitted viruses such as measles, mumps, adenoviruses, and herpes viruses and human immunodeficiency virus.
- Bacteria causing multi-system infections include *Orientia tsutsugamushi*, *Rickettsia*, *Ehrlichia*, and *Anaplasma* species.

CONGENITAL INFECTIONS

Congenital infections are a significant cause of fetal demise and the combination of prenatally and perinatally acquired infections leads to morbidity and mortality in the neonatal period and beyond. Rates of these infections vary wildly across the globe with lower- to middle-income countries experiencing a much higher burden of disease. The most common causes of congenital infection are found in Table 82.11. For many of these infections, prevention and treatment strategies exist making them potential areas to improve global health.

The acronym TORCH was initially coined in the early 1970s to describe a collection of four prenatally acquired infections that featured overlapping presentations including skin lesions, ocular disease, and CNS involvement: *T. gondii*, **r**ubella virus, **C**MV, and **H**SV.[157] Since that time, TORCH infection has become a general catch-all term for congenital infection with the "O" coming to stand for "other" and including additional infections that cause fetal abnormalities including syphilis, VZV, parvovirus, and most recently Zika virus. At times, HIV, hepatitis B, and hepatitis C, which are far more commonly acquired perinatally than prenatally are also considered part of the TORCH infection group.

In the United States, CMV is the most common congenital infection with 0.5 to 1% of all infants—approximately 40,000 per year—being infected.[158] However, approximately 90% of infections will be asymptomatic. Congenital CMV

TABLE 82.11 Common Pathogens Causing Congenital and Perinatally Acquired Infections

	Bacteria	Viruses	Parasites
Congenital infections	*Treponema pallidum* (syphilis)	Rubella virus Cytomegalovirus (CMV) Herpes simplex virus (HSV) Varicella zoster virus (VZV) Zika virus Parvovirus	*Toxoplasma gondii*
Perinatally acquired infections		Human immunodeficiency virus (HIV) Hepatitis B virus (HBV) Hepatitis C virus (HCV)	

manifestations include small size for gestational age, petechiae, purpura, thrombocytopenia, jaundice, hepatitis, chorioretinitis, microcephaly, intracranial calcifications, and sensorineural hearing loss. Hearing loss can be present at birth or can develop later, requiring these children to have frequent hearing screens. Studies over the last two decades have indicated that treatment with the antiviral valganciclovir has been associated with reduced rates of hearing loss and higher scores on neurodevelopmental tests.[22,159] Infection can occur either from primary CMV infection or recurrent/reactive infection, but the risk of vertical transmission is much higher with primary CMV infection.

Congenital toxoplasmosis occurs most commonly from transplacental migration of the parasite during maternal primary infection. It occurs at about 1/10 the rate of congenital CMV infection (0.01 to 0.1% of live births), and 70 to 90% of infected infants are asymptomatic at birth. The classic triad of congenital toxoplasmosis is chorioretinitis, hydrocephalus, and intracranial calcifications. This complete combination is rare and other manifestations include anemia, thrombocytopenia, jaundice, hepatosplenomegaly, and seizures. Treatment of symptomatic congenital toxoplasmosis is typically done with pyrimethamine, sulfadiazine, and folinic acid, but there is considerable variation in treatments as optimal doses, durations, and effectiveness are unknown.[22]

Congenital rubella syndrome (CRS) has the classic manifestations of sensorineural hearing loss, cataracts, and cardiac defects in a small for gestational age infant. Other findings that may be present include other ocular findings (microphthalmia, chorioretinitis), petechiae/purpura (blueberry muffin rash), thrombocytopenia, and hepatosplenomegaly. Vaccination against rubella has dramatically cut rates of CRS. In the United States, rubella transmission and CRS were declared eliminated in 2004.[22] Worldwide, though, it is estimated that more than 100,000 infants per year are born with congenital rubella.[160] With the spread of rubella vaccination programs throughout the 2010s, this number should continue to drop.

Historically, HSV was the fourth TORCH infection. Although HSV can lead to congenital infection with skin lesions including petechiae/purpura, chorioretinitis, and hearing loss, congenital infection is quite rare. Of more significance is perinatal acquisition of HSV. This can lead to infection of the skin, eyes, and mucous membranes (so called SEM disease) with visible vesicular lesions. However, more serious involvement in the form of CNS disease or disseminated HSV (with the liver and lungs most commonly involved) is also possible. These infections have high rates of morbidity and mortality and require aggressive treatment with IV acyclovir to limit complications such as neurologic deficits.

Syphilis was not included in the original TORCH acronym due to the fact that congenital syphilis lacks some of the common features of the other TORCH infections. Its importance as a congenital infection though has led to different attempts to rebrand the TORCH acronym (as STORCH or TORCHES). Although these rebrands have largely not stuck, syphilis remains the first infection considered in the "other" category. Symptoms of congenital syphilis may be present early including snuffles (nasal secretions), mucous membrane lesions, hepatosplenomegaly, anemia, thrombocytopenia, maculopapular rash, and osteochondritis. However, many symptoms will not present for months or even years including musculoskeletal lesions,

teeth changes, ocular involvement, and meningitis/CNS changes. Maternal screening and treatment with penicillin is the mainstay of prevention and treatment.[22]

Zika virus is a recently recognized pathogen that causes significant congenital infection. Initially recognized in 2015 in association with the Zika outbreak in Brazil, congenital Zika syndrome described infants with microcephaly, hypertonia, ocular abnormalities, hearing loss, and seizures. However, the full clinical picture of this syndrome is still being determined at this time. No treatment exists. Screening protocols vary but largely involve testing neonates whose mothers had evidence of Zika infection during pregnancy or symptomatic infants with an appropriate potential exposure.[22,161]

Although typically acquired perinatally rather than congenitally, HIV, HBV, and HCV are worth mentioning. These infections affect millions of people worldwide: 38 million for HIV,[162] 71 million for HCV,[163] and 360 million for HBV.[164] Typically, infants born with these infections are initially asymptomatic before progressing to develop the chronic manifestations. For HIV and HBV, perinatal transmission is high in an untreated state, but screening and treatment programs can reduce transmission markedly. For HIV, maternal screening along with maternal antiretroviral treatment and postnatal antiretroviral treatment of infants has reduced global rates of new infant HIV infection to ~150,000 cases per year down from around 280,000 infants per year in 2010.[162] For HBV, maternal screening allows for administration of hepatitis B immunoglobulin and initiation of HBV vaccination within 12 hours of birth, thereby reducing rates of transmission.[22] Perinatal transmission rates of HCV are lower than untreated HIV or HBV, but still lead to a significant burden of disease. Currently, no systematic treatment strategies for the reduction of perinatal HCV transmission have been developed, but the recent development of highly effective antivirals to eliminate chronic HCV infection may ultimately lead to reduced perinatal transmission.

POINTS TO REMEMBER

- Congenital and perinatally acquired infections are primarily caused by viruses acquired during pregnancy or around the time of birth.
- Cytomegalovirus is the most common congenitally acquired infection in the United States
- *Treponema pallidum*, causing syphilis, and *Toxoplasma gondii* are important bacterial and parasitic causes of congenital disease, respectively.
- Congenital and perinatally acquired infections can cause fetal demise and significant morbidity in the neonatal period and beyond.

SELECTED REFERENCES

8. Baddour LM, Wilson WR, Bayer AS, et al. Infective endocarditis in adults: diagnosis, antimicrobial therapy, and management of complications: a scientific statement for healthcare professionals from the American Heart Association. Circulation 2015:1435–86.
22. Kimberlin DW. Red Book: 2018-2021 report of the committee on infectious diseases. Red B. 2018-2021 Report of the

Committee on Infectious Disease. American Academy of Pediatrics; 2018.

24. World malaria report 2019. Geneva: World Health Organization; 2019.

34. Bennett J, Dolin R, Blaser MJ, editors. Mandell, Douglas, and Bennett's principles and practice of infectious diseases. 9th ed. Philadelphia, Elsevier; 2019.

35. Spec A, Escota G, Chrisler C, et al., editors. Comprehensive review of infectious diseases. 1st ed. Edinburgh, Elsevier; 2020.

76. The top 10 causes of death. [cited 2020 Feb 29]. Available from: https://www.who.int/news-room/fact-sheets/detail/the-top-10-causes-of-death.

80. Metlay JP, Waterer GW, Long AC, et al. Diagnosis and treatment of adults with community-acquired pneumonia. Am J Respir Crit Care Med 2019;200:E45–67.

82. Jones RN. Microbial etiologies of hospital-acquired bacterial pneumonia and ventilator-associated bacterial pneumonia. Clin Infect Dis 2010;51(Suppl 1):S81–7.

92. O'Sullivan BP, Freedman SD. Cystic fibrosis. Lancet 2009;373: 1891–904.

95. DuPont HL. Acute infectious diarrhea in immunocompetent adults. N Engl J Med 2014;370:1532–40.

109. Haque R, Huston CD, Hughes M, et al. Amebiasis. N Engl J Med 2003;348:1565–73.

123. Workowski KA, Bolan GA. Sexually Transmitted Diseases Treatment Guidelines, 2015. MMWR Recomm Rep 2015;64(3).

134. Burnham JP, Kollef MH. Treatment of severe skin and soft tissue infections: a review. Curr Opin Infect Dis 2018;31:113–9.

146. Francesconi F, Lupi O. Myiasis. Clin Microbiol Rev 2012;25:79–105.

153. Parola P, Paddock CD, Socolovschi C, et al. Update on tick-borne rickettsioses around the world: a geographic approach. Clin Microbiol Rev 2013;26:657–702.

157. Epps RE, Pittelkow MR, Su WP. TORCH syndrome. Semin Dermatol 1995;14:179–86.

83

The Role of the Clinical Laboratory in Infection Prevention and Antimicrobial Stewardship

Catherine A. Hogan, Niaz Banaei, Matthew M. Hitchcock, and Stanley C. Deresinsky

ABSTRACT

Background

The clinical laboratory occupies an important role in enabling effective infection prevention and control (IPC) and antimicrobial stewardship program (ASP) interventions. Indeed, the clinical laboratory generates the microbiologic data to guide clinical practice and recognize new trends that may signal nascent outbreaks and provides timely and accurate testing results that have the potential to impact patient care. In addition, the IPC and ASP groups offer key expertise in clinical care and facility operations that help the laboratory prioritize implementation of clinically relevant technologies. These groups serve as important liaisons between the laboratory and frontline clinicians, ensuring that results are interpreted correctly and translated into meaningful changes in health care delivery.

Content

In this chapter, we present key areas of opportunity within the clinical laboratory to produce high-quality testing results that will guide IPC and ASP decision-making. Data are briefly summarized for each category, with a focus on rapid diagnostic methods, detection of resistant organisms, and biomarker-based management. Recent developments in rapid diagnostic platforms and other diagnostic areas are described and are expected to continue to expand in the near future. Strategies on outcome-based assessment are also addressed. Finally, a framework for effective collaboration between the three respective groups is presented with the goal of enhancing patient care and clinical outcomes.

INTRODUCTION

Beyond its direct clinical care role, the clinical laboratory resides at the strategic interface between microbiological testing and actionable results used by infection prevention and control (IPC) and the antimicrobial stewardship program (ASP) within an institution. Indeed, the clinical laboratory generates key microbiological data that allow the IPC department and ASP to function effectively and leads the selection and validation of assays that hold potential to impact patient care. Lack of local data would severely impair the ability of IPC and ASP to plan and optimize detailed interventions that are tailored to local epidemiologic trends. This is not a one-way relationship, however, as IPC and ASP provide the laboratory with essential input regarding the need and implementation of new tests and result reporting and interpretation that enable the laboratory to produce clinically actionable results that translate to real impact on antimicrobial prescribing, institutional costs, and patient outcomes. These three separate but interdependent entities work best with open collaboration, communication, and shared goals.[1–4] This chapter will serve as an introduction to the roles and objectives of these key programs and present specific areas of opportunity for the clinical laboratory to enhance clinical impact and successfully collaborate with the IPC and ASP groups.

ROLES AND OBJECTIVES OF KEY STAKEHOLDERS

Clinical Laboratory

The clinical microbiology and virology laboratories are at the forefront of optimal patient care given their capacity for early identification of organisms including unusual or unsuspected pathogens, timely detection of antimicrobial resistance, emergence of potential outbreaks, and recognition of potential bioterrorism organisms.[5] To do so, they require the appropriate tools, staffing, and resources to fill their mandate to provide highly accurate and reproducible results. In many settings, the current context of the clinical laboratory practice has been challenged by diversion of financial resources resulting from payment restructuring, increasingly complex and expensive assays, gradual loss of conventional microbiology and virology expertise, and large-scale laboratory consolidation.[6,7] However, this is also a world of tremendous opportunity with the recent revolutionary introduction of matrix-assisted laser desorption/ionization time-of-flight mass spectrometry (MALDI-TOF MS) for organism identification, greater importance of molecular testing, and implementation of laboratory automation.[8,9] Clinical laboratories must carefully decide which assays to adopt, implement cost-effective workflows, and efficiently collaborate with key clinical groups. Among these, the IPC and ASP groups are two key partners with whom the clinical laboratory has the potential to establish mutually beneficial relationships to enhance patient care (At a Glance 83.1).[10–12]

AT A GLANCE
Shared Activities

Shared activities between the clinical microbiology laboratory, antimicrobial stewardship program (ASP), and infection prevention and control (IPC)

In North America, clinical laboratories are led by MD- or PhD-trained microbiologists and are staffed by clinical laboratory scientists and laboratory assistants.[13] This model may vary in other settings.[14] The clinical laboratory serves many roles that span the full spectrum of testing, from the preanalytical to the postanalytical components.

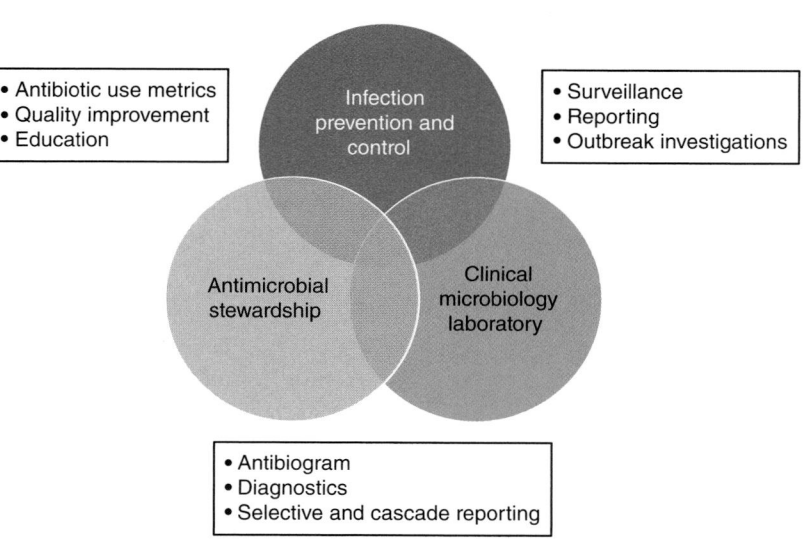

- Antibiotic use metrics
- Quality improvement
- Education

Infection prevention and control

- Surveillance
- Reporting
- Outbreak investigations

Antimicrobial stewardship

Clinical microbiology laboratory

- Antibiogram
- Diagnostics
- Selective and cascade reporting

Preanalytical

Despite significant technological improvements in microbiology, there is still no substitute for high-quality specimen submission. Indeed, the quality of test results and interpretation directly depend on the quality of the sample received in the laboratory. As such, all individuals involved should strive to maintain optimal quality along the spectrum of testing.[15] The laboratory can optimize this process by providing guidance on optimal test selection, test ordering, sample collection, sample transport, and sample processing.[16] The preanalytical phase is also important as it is the most error-prone, with approximately 70% of laboratory errors occurring in this phase.[17] These preanalytical components need to be considered when discussing testing strategy between the clinical laboratory, IPC, and ASP. For example, the accuracy of ruling out tuberculosis from respiratory samples depends on the quality of the sample submitted.[18] As such, the clinical laboratory and the IPC group can work together to ensure optimal sample collection takes place, and that criteria and procedures are followed at the laboratory to optimize organism recovery.

Analytical

For the analytical phase, the clinical laboratory is involved in many aspects to ensure the testing performed is of high quality. The clinical laboratory oversees quality management procedures that include quality control (QC), or the initial step of controlling a procedure, and quality assurance (QA), which is a broader component that includes proficiency testing, personnel competency testing, monitoring of inventory, and calibration and maintenance of equipment. Importantly, the clinical laboratory actively monitors key QA metrics including test result positivity rates (e.g., proportion of positive blood cultures and molecular assays, blood culture contamination rates), turnaround time of critical test results, and test accuracy.[19] Regular review of these metrics allows identification of irregularities that may require further investigation to address the root cause of the issue and/or communication to other stakeholders including higher levels of management.

Postanalytical

The clinical laboratory also reviews postanalytical performance, including review and approval of test results, proper communication of results, and sample storage conditions. Furthermore, microbiology laboratories take on the task of generating a cumulative antibiogram annually and selecting antimicrobials for susceptibility testing and reporting in collaboration with ASP and other clinical colleagues. Standardized methods for production of a facility-specific antibiogram have been published by the Clinical and Laboratory Standards Institute (CLSI).[20] If a sufficient number of isolates are available, unit-specific antibiograms can be produced in cases where a facility may have a specific unit with unique resistance patterns such as in the intensive care unit(s), and empiric therapy choices may differ based on the location of the patient.[21] These steps require close collaboration with ASP to ensure relevance to local practice and increase their uptake. The clinical laboratory is actively involved as all of the steps outlined require continual review and improvements to achieve consistent quality testing results.

CLINICAL LABORATORY ROLE FOR ASP

For the purpose of ASP, distinct microbiology laboratory roles, of which some may occur in collaboration with other

BOX 83.1 Microbiology Laboratory Roles in Antimicrobial Stewardship Programs

1. Stratified cumulative antibiogram susceptibility reporting
2. Selective or cascade reporting of antimicrobial susceptibility testing
3. Rapid viral testing for respiratory pathogens
4. Rapid diagnostic assays for positive blood culture broth
5. Use of procalcitonin (PCT) testing and algorithms for ICU patients
6. Use of non–culture-based fungal markers for patients with hematologic malignancies

BOX 83.2 Roles of Clinical Microbiology in Infection Prevention and Control

1. Surveillance and early warning system
   a. Notify infection control staff of infection clusters, unusual resistance patterns, possible patient-to-patient transmission
2. Assist and advise regarding inclusion of laboratory diagnosis in case definition
3. Perform laboratory confirmation of diagnosis
   a. Characterize isolates with high accuracy
   b. Store clinically important isolates (e.g., unusual, resistant, and/or outbreak-related)
   c. Search the laboratory information system (LIS) for cases
4. Provide data for use in ongoing surveillance
5. Perform molecular typing of strains (or send out if testing not offered in-house)
6. Assess laboratory procedures and adjust as necessary
7. Maintain surveillance and early warning system

TABLE 83.1 Infection Prevention and Control Areas of Involvement to Mitigate Infectious Risk

Hospital building	Water distribution
	Heating, ventilation, air conditioning (HVAC)
	Renovation and construction projects
	Monitoring of surveillance cultures from air, water, and surfaces, especially in high-risk areas
Hospital services	Food services
	In-facility laundry
	Environmental Cleaning
Disinfection	Disinfection and sterilization of reusable medical equipment
Surveillance	Active surveillance for hospital- and health care–associated infections
Best clinical practice	Contact and isolation precautions
	Hand hygiene
	Infection prevention processes for surgical procedures
	Risk reduction for infection with use of medical devices

clinical laboratories, have been identified from the Infectious Diseases Society of America (IDSA) ASP guidelines and are presented in Box 83.1.[22]

These examples showcase the potential for clinical laboratory involvement with ASP. However, in practice, this often proves to be a challenge as laboratory input to stewardship programs may be limited. Indeed, surveys from multiple countries have shown varied microbiologist representation in ASP activities ranging from 26% to 89%.[2] It is thus crucial to better understand the respective role of each of these groups and how best to integrate them.

CLINICAL LABORATORY ROLE FOR IPC

For the purpose of infection control (IC), similar roles specific to the microbiology laboratory have been outlined by expert opinion and are included in Box 83.2.[3] Thus there are multiple areas of opportunity for collaboration between the clinical laboratory, ASP, and IPC, which will be described in further detail in this chapter.

Infection Prevention and Control

Infection Control and Prevention (IPC; sometimes referred to as IPAC), also known in some locations as Hospital Epidemiology and Infection Control (HEIC) or IC, is a hospital department primarily focused on the prevention of hospital-acquired

infections. To this end, IPC is involved in the mitigation of the risk of infection to patients and staff in all aspects of the hospital environment and during the provision of health care.[23,24] It is led by an IC professional, often a physician hospital epidemiologist or a nurse with IC training, and staffed by infection preventionists, who generally have a background in nursing, though programs in smaller facilities may be structured differently.[23,25]

The mitigation of infectious risks is achieved through multiple avenues and activities. This includes compliance with industry standards and regulations regarding the built environment of the hospital, which involves oversight of diverse systems and processes, as well as surveillance of clinical care to ensure best practices for infection prevention are implemented (Table 83.1).[26–32] IPC is also tasked with the critical task of active surveillance for classical hospital- or health care–acquired infections, including surgical site infections (SSIs), device-associated infections such as catheter-associated urinary tract infections (CAUTIs) and central line-associated bloodstream infections (CLABSIs), ventilator-associated pneumonias (VAPs), and *Clostridioides difficile* infection (CDI).[23,24] The results of longitudinal surveillance for these infections are publicly reported as quality measures and form the basis for ongoing quality improvement projects within IC.[23] IPC also identifies and investigates clusters of infections that may be transmitted through the health care environment, oversees data-driven interventions to prevent further transmission or occurrence of infection, and plays a key role in emergency preparedness for management of outbreaks of novel pathogens and bioterrorism events.[23,24]

Especially in the surveillance aspect, IPC is heavily dependent on the clinical laboratory for the identification of individual hospital-acquired infections, as well as clusters or changes in the rates over time, in order to evaluate for lapses in IC procedures or areas where practice improvement is needed.[3] In outbreak settings where epidemiologic links can be identified between infections caused by the same species of organism, the clinical laboratory may also be needed to provide additional information on the relatedness of the causative organisms in each infection. This can be performed by molecular typing methods including next-generation sequencing (NGS) to determine if the outbreak is associated with general lapses in IC procedures, which would be suggested by the presence of unrelated organisms, or is more specific in origin, emanating from a single source or through cross-transmission. Such testing can guide the eventual recommendations to general reinforcement of proper IC procedures or more directed interventions to interrupt transmission channels.[24,33–35]

Antimicrobial Stewardship

Antimicrobial stewardship can be defined by both goals and practices. As a general concept, antimicrobial stewardship is "a coherent set of actions which promote using antimicrobials responsibly [to ensure] sustainable access to all who need them," as antimicrobials are a class of drugs with potential clinical impact on both the treated individual and the community.[36] In practice, antimicrobial stewardship can be defined as "coordinated interventions designed to improve and measure the appropriate use of antimicrobial agents by promoting the selection of the optimal antimicrobial drug regimen including dose, duration of therapy, and route of administration,"[12] or, more simply, as optimization of the use of antimicrobial agents in the treatment of patients with infections.[37] This involves more than ensuring that patients are receiving appropriate antibiotics for identified infections and also encompasses concordance with published guidelines for empiric therapy,[38] optimization of antibiotic choice and dosing for identified infections,[39,40] treatment of infection for the shortest effective duration,[41,42] preferential use of antibiotics with lower risks of CDI or other serious side effects,[43–45] proper choice and duration of surgical antimicrobial prophylaxis,[28,46] and avoidance of antibiotic use in conditions where they are not indicated, such as viral upper respiratory syndromes and asymptomatic bacteriuria.[47,48]

In the United States, ASPs are organized around seven core elements as defined by the Centers for Disease Control and Prevention (CDC).[49] Similar core elements for antimicrobial stewardship in other regions have been described elsewhere.[10] The CDC core elements are presented in Box 83.3.

Implementation of the core elements can vary from facility to facility based on size and complexity of operations. In general, the ASP is run by a physician and pharmacist, ideally with subspecialty training in infectious diseases and antimicrobial stewardship.[11,50] Recommendations for staffing requirements based on facility size and acuity have been published.[50,51] While the CDC core elements emphasize the centrality of pharmacy expertise in an ASP, other publications recommend expertise in "infection management" more generally.[10] This more holistic approach recognizes that proper treatment of infections involves much more than simply the correct choice (empiric or directed) of antimicrobial agent. For example, intra-abdominal infections can be treated with antibiotic courses as short as 4 days following achievement of source control via surgical or interventional procedures,[52] which highlights the importance of source control compared to antibiotic therapy in management of these and related types of infections.

The activities performed by a specific ASP will depend on the staffing, with proportionally larger programs often being

---

> ### BOX 83.3 CDC Core Elements of Antimicrobial Stewardship
>
> 1. **Hospital leadership commitment:** dedication of necessary human, financial, and information technology resources to antimicrobial stewardship
> 2. **Accountability:** appoint a leader or co-leaders responsible for program management
> 3. **Pharmacy experience:** pharmacist with expertise in the pharmacology of antibiotics, ideally as a co-leader of the antimicrobial stewardship program, leads implementation efforts to improve antibiotic use
> 4. **Action:** implement interventions to improve antibiotic use
> 5. **Tracking:** monitor antibiotic prescribing, the impact of interventions, and important outcomes such as *Clostridioides difficile* infection rates and changes in resistance patterns
> 6. **Reporting:** regularly report antibiotic use and resistance patterns to prescribers, pharmacists, nurses, and hospital leadership
> 7. **Education:** educate prescribers, pharmacists, and nurses about adverse reactions from antibiotics, antibiotic resistance, and optimal prescribing

---

capable of more intensive interventions. Typical ASP activities range from distribution of national guidelines for the antibiotic course and duration for the treatment of identified infections, development of local guidelines based on local/regional resistance data (i.e., the cumulative antibiogram) and preferential use of antibiotics with fewer side effects or lower risk of CDI, pre-authorization for use of restricted antibiotics, prospective audit and feedback, either for targeted antimicrobials or a more intensive form known as "handshake stewardship" due to the focus on face-to-face feedback and discussion, enforcement of antibiotic timeouts for reappraisal of current antibiotic necessity, pharmacokinetic monitoring for aminoglycosides and vancomycin, and educational interventions.[10,38,43–45,53,54] There are many opportunities to utilize information technology for stewardship purposes, either through electronic medical record (EMR) platforms or third-party software, and these may include the construction of order sets and other decision-support tools at the point of ordering, monitoring for appropriateness of target antibiotic usage and bug-drug mismatches, opportunities for conversion from intravenous to oral formulations, and real-time alerts for critical microbiological results.[55–59] The major outcomes tracked by ASPs include antibiotic utilization, usually normalized as days of therapy per bed-days of care for in-patient units, patient outcomes such as mortality and hospital length-of-stay (LOS), process measures such as the appropriateness of antibiotic prescriptions, as well as key complications of antibiotic use such as CDI.[22,60–62] Reporting to leadership may be done within the facility IC committee as a way to formally link the ASP and IPC, and stewardship guidelines also suggest that the hospital epidemiologist be part of the stewardship team.[11,23,63]

As with IPC, ASPs are heavily dependent on data generated by the clinical laboratory to direct their interventions, and close collaboration between ASP and the laboratory is critical.[10–12] Essentially any intervention aside from general education or dissemination of national guideline recommendations, even pre-authorization of the use of restricted antimicrobial agents, requires knowledge of local resistance patterns or specific culture results for an individual patient. As presented above, one of the most common collaborations between ASP and the clinical microbiology laboratory is the production and dissemination of the cumulative antibiogram, which is a cumulative assessment of antimicrobial susceptibility profiles within the facility that can be used to monitor for changes in resistance patterns, optimize decisions on empiric antimicrobial therapy for specific syndromes based on these patterns, and may also help direct IC measures.[64]

ASPs may also work with the clinical microbiology laboratory on the implementation of selective antibiotic susceptibility reporting, or the subset known as cascade reporting, in order to nudge providers to the use of optimal first-line therapies or narrower-spectrum antibiotics and avoid use of formulary-restricted antibiotics or other agents associated with higher rates of toxicities or other complications in the treatment of uncomplicated infections.[65–69] ASPs can also collaborate with the clinical microbiology laboratory on the implementation of rapid diagnostic platforms, which may allow for earlier switch from empiric to targeted therapy, and studies have shown that diagnostic test or antibiotic susceptibility results, rapid or otherwise, may have a higher effect on management by frontline providers when integrated into clinical care in the context of a stewardship intervention.[4,22,70–73]

POINTS TO REMEMBER

- Infection prevention and control (IPC) is dedicated to the prevention of infections in the health care setting.
- The core function of the antimicrobial stewardship program (ASP) is to promote the responsible use of antimicrobial agents.
- ASPs are organized around seven core elements.
- IPC and ASP activities are broad in scope and nature.
- Collaboration with the clinical laboratory is essential for IPC and ASP programs.

WORKFLOW AND COMMUNICATION BETWEEN THE LABORATORY, INFECTION PREVENTION AND CONTROL, AND ANTIMICROBIAL STEWARDSHIP PROGRAM

Communication is the bedrock of collaboration between the clinical laboratory, IPC, and ASP and should occur at many levels within the hospital or health care system. More formal areas for communication and collaboration between services include the IC committee, which is generally chaired by the hospital epidemiologist and should include representation from the clinical laboratory in addition to other clinical and ancillary services and is tasked with review of surveillance data, including outbreaks and necessary responses, and approval of IC policies and procedures.[24] Antimicrobial stewardship guidelines recommend that the clinical microbiologist and hospital epidemiologist be included as key members of the stewardship team, which may be structured as a formal committee or a more informal working group.[10–12] Information must also flow freely from the clinical microbiology laboratory to both IPC and ASP, as the function of each is deeply dependent on data generated in the laboratory.

Results of active surveillance cultures or molecular tests for multidrug-resistant organisms (MDROs) must be rapidly communicated from the laboratory to IC to ensure that the appropriate isolation and contact precautions are used during clinical care to limit transmission within the hospital environment and ensure that any necessary enhanced cleaning procedures are followed.[29,74] As clinical care, especially in large centers, is fragmented between many teams and services, clinical laboratory personnel may be the first to notice clusters or outbreaks and can alert IC of these concerns.[75]

Collaboration with the clinical laboratory is also essential to the practices of antimicrobial stewardship, as the core functions of ASP depend on knowledge of culture and susceptibility results for individual patients. Antibiograms or local treatment guidelines are updated periodically and are not time-critical products. In contrast, most ASP interventions performed on a daily basis such as prospective audit and feedback, are dependent on culture and susceptibility results,[11] and this is an area where rapid communication of laboratory results to ASPs can make a significant impact on antimicrobial use and patient care. As rapid molecular diagnostic tests for organism identification and antimicrobial susceptibility become more common, these provide new opportunities to shorten the time to appropriate, targeted antimicrobial therapy,[76] which is facilitated by integrated communication from the clinical laboratory to ASP and the primary team.[71–73,77–83]

LABORATORY DIAGNOSTIC METHODS TO SUPPORT INFECTION PREVENTION AND CONTROL AND ANTIMICROBIAL STEWARDSHIP PROGRAM

Rapid Identification of Bloodstream Infections

Bloodstream infections continue to be associated with significant morbidity and mortality, particularly in septic shock.[84] Early initiation of appropriate antimicrobial therapy in this setting is crucial to achieve favorable clinical outcomes[85–89] but may be challenging to achieve with current microbiological methods given the lengthy turnaround time required for testing. This is especially important in cases of resistant or unusual microorganisms, where standard empiric therapy may not be active. Thus given the crucial role of the microbiology laboratory in these settings, there has been major interest in technology development to reduce time to organism identification and antimicrobial susceptibility testing (AST). Methods for the rapid identification and AST of organisms causing bloodstream infections have the potential to improve many ASP targets, including shortened time to initiation of appropriate therapy (either antibiotic de-escalation or escalation) and reductions in hospital LOS, mortality, antimicrobial-related side effects, and antibiotic selection pressure. Rapid identification of genetic markers of resistance such as for methicillin-resistant *Staphylococcus aureus* (MRSA) (gene: *mecA*) and vancomycin-resistant enterococcus (VRE) (genes: *vanA*, *vanB*, and others) may also quickly guide the implementation of appropriate IC measures including contact precautions and use of single-patient rooms. However, in real-world practice, factors other than timing of organism identification that influence clinical outcomes should also be considered. These include severity of clinical presentation, host factors such as immune compromise, availability of expert ASP advice, baseline clinical education level of providing teams, and effectiveness of communication of results to providers. Moreover, given that new technologies are often significantly more costly than previous traditional methods, thoughtful design and implementation of workflows that optimize communication of actionable results between the microbiology laboratory, ASP, and IPC is necessary to optimize cost-effective practices and maximize the benefits of the resources that are used. Direct communication of results from the clinical laboratory to the ASP and/or treating team have been shown to be effective.[81,90,91] Furthermore, as a general principle, the clinical laboratory should be involved in all aspects of result communication implementation.[92]

MALDI-based Methods

Matrix-assisted laser desorption/ionization–time of flight mass spectrometry (MALDI-TOF MS) technology has completely revolutionized microbial identification in the clinical microbiology laboratory by enabling faster, simpler, and more accurate results in a cost-effective way.[93,94] This technology was initially developed for use on fresh (16- to 24-hour growth), isolated bacterial colonies. It was subsequently adapted for use from rapid (2- to 6-hour) organism subculture, and from positive blood culture broth after short processing. The direct processing approach accuracy rate is lower than for subculture but allows more rapid organism identification.[95] Different MALDI-TOF MS approaches directly from positive blood culture broth are available: a commercial kit that is CE-marked but not cleared by the US Food and Drug Administration (FDA) (Sepsityper by Bruker Daltonics, Inc., Billerica, MA) and in-house developed protocols.[95–97]

MALDI-TOF MS-based identification has shown value beyond that of the Gram stain result alone, particularly to guide empiric therapy with identification of organisms with an increased risk of resistance such as AmpC-producing *Enterobacterales*.[98] In addition, rapid MALDI-TOF MS procedures (either through rapid subculture or direct processing) have been shown to significantly reduce the time to organism identification compared to standard subculture, with a time benefit ranging from 11.7 to 30 hours depending on the protocol and comparator method used.[99–103] In adults, rapid MALDI-TOF MS identification has been associated with reduced LOS, hospital costs, and mortality,[101,103,104] though these studies were implemented as a bundle including rapid AST and/or ASP intervention which may partly explain the observed benefit. In children, the clinical impact of rapid MALDI-TOF MS identification has been associated with reduced time to appropriate antimicrobial treatment in inpatients, reduced infection-related LOS, but not with a mortality benefit.[99,105] Similarly, these pediatric studies have included an ASP component to their diagnostic intervention, again highlighting the importance of a strong partnership between the laboratory and ASP.

Molecular Methods

Multiplexed syndromic panels have emerged over the last few years for organism detection and identification of antimicrobial resistance genes and have been widely adopted in microbiology laboratories across the United States. At the time of chapter preparation, eight FDA-cleared multiplex panels from positive blood culture broth are available based on different technologies: FilmArray BCID (BioFire Diagnostics, LLC, Salt Lake City, UT), Verigene BC-GP and BC-GN (Luminex Corp,

Austin, TX), ePlex BCID-GP, BCID-GN, and BCID-FP (GenMark Diagnostics, Carlsbad, CA), and iC-GPC and iC-GNR (iCubate, Huntsville, AL).

These panels include 8 to 29 bacterial and/or fungal targets, and three to nine antimicrobial resistance genes. Detection of antimicrobial resistance genes is of limited utility in settings with low prevalence of resistant organisms. Turnaround time ranges from 1 to 4.5 hours, and studies have demonstrated robust test performance characteristics with sensitivity and specificity greater than 90% for most organisms tested across platforms.[106–114] However, as with the other multiplexed syndromic molecular assays, false positive results due to contamination may occur, including from the matrix used for testing such as blood culture broth and stool transport media such as Cary-Blair medium.[106,115]

Of the syndromic multiplex panels for positive blood cultures, the FilmArray BCID and the Verigene BC-GP and BC-GN panels have been available commercially for the longest, with FDA approval in 2013, 2012, and 2014, respectively. These assays have been the most extensively studied so far for their test performance and impact on clinical and economic outcomes.[116] The FilmArray BCID panel in combination with ASP intervention was shown to be associated with reduced turnaround time to organism identification and time to effective or optimal antimicrobial therapy.[82,91,117,118] However, its impact on LOS was mixed, with a beneficial impact seen in one study for coagulase-negative staphylococci,[117] and no effect in others.[82,91] One of these studies also demonstrated cost-effectiveness of BCID implementation when coupled with ASP intervention for the rapid identification of coagulase-negative staphylococci contaminants.[117] Similarly, the Verigene BC-GP and BC-GN panels have demonstrated favorable impact on turnaround time, but mixed results on LOS and mortality.[119–123]

These results are promising and support the role of rapid molecular diagnostics for positive blood cultures. However, as for rapid MALDI-TOF MS identification, the findings must be considered carefully as rapid diagnostic methods are often implemented in a bundled fashion with heterogeneous ASP interventions such that it may be difficult to discern the benefit of the diagnostic method alone.[124] Moreover, timely and effective communication of the rapid results to the clinician is critical to produce a favorable clinical impact.[91] The main limitations of the blood culture multiplex panels, high cost and low throughput, may be of greater importance in high-volume laboratories and should be considered.

Other Methods

Accelerate Pheno system. The first rapid commercial identification and phenotypic AST platform to receive FDA clearance was the Accelerate Pheno system (Accelerate Diagnostics, Inc., Tucson, AZ) in 2017. Automated gel electrofiltration and fluorescence in-situ hybridization (FISH) enables the identification of 16 targets (6 gram-positive, 8 gram-negative, and 2 fungal) with turnaround time of 2 hours. This is followed by phenotypic AST by morphokinetic cellular analysis, which measures the response of individual cells and colonies to antibiotics over time. Testing turnaround time is approximately 7 hours. The Accelerate Pheno system has shown high test performance characteristics with greater than 90% overall sensitivity and specificity for organism identification, and similarly high performance for susceptibility testing in bloodstream infection.[125,126] However, similar to the multiplexed molecular panels, organism identification is limited to on-panel targets, instrument acquisition and cartridge costs are high, and suboptimal performance in cases of polymicrobial infection remains a limitation.[127] Clinical studies have now been published showing improved time to optimal antimicrobial therapy, but no change in clinical outcome or antibiotic usage with the Accelerate Pheno system combined with ASP intervention.[128–130] In addition, two studies exploring its hypothetical impact have projected it to be beneficial in generating more rapid results.[131,132]

T2Bacteria panel. The T2Bacteria Panel (T2 Biosystems, Lexington, MA) was CE-marked in 2017 and FDA-cleared in 2018 for the detection of bacterial organisms directly from whole blood, thus enabling more rapid diagnosis of sepsis etiology. The panel includes five targets: *S. aureus, E. faecium, Klebsiella pneumoniae, Escherichia coli,* and *Pseudomonas aeruginosa.* The platform detects organisms based on polymerase chain reaction (PCR) and miniaturized magnetic resonance, provides results within 3 to 5 hours, and does not include the capacity for resistance testing at this time. The largest study performed to date on its diagnostic accuracy has shown per-patient sensitivity and specificity of 90% for proven bloodstream infection for the five targets on the panel.[133] There are no data supporting beneficial clinical impact at this point, and the risk of putative false-positive results (defined as discordant T2Bacteria positive, blood culture negative) reached 40% in the previous study, raising concern for increased inappropriate antibiotic use.[134]

T2Candida panel. The T2Candida Panel (T2 Biosystems) was the first FDA-cleared assay for the detection of *Candida* spp. directly from whole blood in 2014. This panel includes 5 *Candida* targets: *C. albicans* and/or *C. tropicalis, C. krusei* and/or *C. glabrata,* and *C. parapsilosis.* Organism detection technology and turnaround time are the same as for the T2Bacteria panel. A recent meta-analysis on the diagnostic accuracy of the T2Candida panel showed the pooled sensitivity and specificity to be 91% and 94%, respectively.[135] Limited data have been published in support of a clinical benefit; however, patient population and expected pretest probability are important factors to consider prior to implementing this technology for clinical use.

KARIUS TEST

The Karius test (Karius Dx, Redwood City, CA) is based on metagenomic NGS of microbial cell-free DNA from plasma and permits the identification of over 1000 organisms including bacteria, fungi, parasites, and DNA viruses. This non–FDA-cleared test is performed at the CLIA-certified Karius laboratory, with turnaround time of 48 hours or less from sample receipt. Although promising in nature given its broad-range pathogen detection, this diagnostic technology has shown limited positive and negative percent agreement of 93.7% and 40.0%, respectively, compared to patients with positive and negative initial blood cultures. In addition, it has shown potential for earlier detection of bloodstream infection in immunocompromised hosts,[136] though its clinical impact has been variable.[137,138]

SEPTIFAST

The SeptiFast test (Roche Diagnostics, Basel, Switzerland) is a CE-marked, non–FDA-cleared multiplexed assay that has been extensively studied in Europe for the rapid molecular diagnosis of sepsis from whole blood and for prediction of complicated bloodstream infection.[139–142] This method can identify 25 pathogens (19 bacteria, 5 *Candida* spp., and *Aspergillus fumigatus*) and *mecA* in *S. aureus* positive samples based on multiplexed real-time PCR. Test performance characteristics have shown favorable results especially as an adjuvant test, but increased contamination rates relative to conventional blood cultures remain an issue.[139,140,142,143]

SUMMARY OF RAPID BLOODSTREAM INFECTION IDENTIFICATION

In summary, the clinical microbiology laboratory plays a critical role in identifying bloodstream infections in a timely manner, and effectively communicating these results with the treating medical team and the ASP group to achieve timely therapeutic decision-making. In addition, prompt communication to the IPC team may be required after identification of organisms of importance (MRSA, VRE, carbapenemase-producing *Enterobacterales, Candida auris,* etc.) and other unusual, resistant, or bioterrorism organisms as required by institutional policy. Many new microbiology technologies have reached the market in recent years to support this effort by rapidly identifying organisms from positive blood cultures or whole blood, and rapid molecular or phenotypic resistance testing to guide patient care (Table 83.2). The evidence base to support favorable clinical impact with these new assays is currently more robust for the multiplex assays in contrast to the newer phenotypic and magnetic resonance-based methods. Real-world challenges in the interpretation of results and dealing with polymicrobial samples will require improvements in the future, especially given the significantly higher costs of these assays compared to conventional testing.

POINTS TO REMEMBER

- Many rapid technologies are available for the diagnosis of bloodstream infections.
- New technologies continue to emerge for rapid antimicrobial susceptibility testing.
- Prompt communication of important laboratory results to ASP and IPC is key to enable effective intervention.
- Additional data are needed to fully leverage these rapid tests and to balance their increased cost.

Other Multiplex Syndromic Panels

Other multiplex syndromic panels were implemented for clinical testing in the last few years and have significantly modified the diagnostic testing approach for the clinical syndromes of upper and lower respiratory infections, gastrointestinal (GI) infections, and meningitis/encephalitis. Indeed, instead of the clinician having to choose target-specific testing in a stepwise fashion, one can now order a single test to detect up to 27 organisms.[116] Their availability has generated significant enthusiasm in the clinical world given the comprehensive nature of testing and potential to accelerate turnaround time of actionable results. Potential advantages mirror those presented with the bloodstream infection panels, with reduced time to appropriate antimicrobial therapy, reduced LOS, and improvement of

TABLE 83.2 Summary of Rapid Bloodstream Infection Organism Identification and Antimicrobial Susceptibility Testing

Level of Identification	Method	Selected Examples
Organism identification	MALDI-TOF MS	Sepsityper (Bruker) Laboratory-developed protocols
	PCR and miniaturized magnetic resonance	T2Bacteria Panel (T2 Biosystems) T2Candida Panel (T2 Biosystems)
	Cell-free DNA next-generation sequencing	Karius test (Karius)
Organism identification and detection of antimicrobial resistance genes	Multiplex molecular methods	FilmArray BCID (BioFire) Verigene BC-GP and BC-GN (Luminex) ePlex BCID-GP BCID-GN and BCID-FP (GenMark) iC-GPC and iC-GNR (iCubate) SeptiFast test (Roche)
Organism identification and phenotypic antimicrobial susceptibility testing	FISH and morphokinetic cellular analysis	Pheno system (Accelerate)
	Direct or rapid MALDI-TOF MS followed by various phenotypic methods (e.g., lysis and centrifugation followed by rapid automated AST)	Laboratory-developed protocols

AST, Antimicrobial susceptibility testing; *DNA*, deoxyribonucleic acid; *FISH*, fluorescence in situ hybridization; *MALDI-TOF MS*, matrix-assisted laser desorption/ionization-time of flight mass spectrometry; *PCR*, polymerase chain reaction.

antimicrobial stewardship targets. However, these also share the challenge of contamination risk, risk of false-positive results, limited experience with rare targets, over-treatment from physician unfamiliarity with the significance of all panel targets, and significant associated expense.[115,116] Thus the microbiology and infectious diseases fields have started to interrogate the appropriate utilization of these syndromic tests, and how best to integrate them into diagnostic algorithms. Indeed, laboratories should carefully consider their local epidemiology and the potential for syndromic tests to impact clinical practice in their settings prior to implementing these assays. Here, we will briefly discuss the evidence and considerations specific to commercially available panels for the diagnosis of respiratory infections, GI infections, and meningitis and/or encephalitis. Multiplex syndromic panel testing has largely remained in centralized laboratories for the moment, although their use is expected to expand in the future, leading to additional considerations for implementation of testing.

Respiratory Infections

There are currently several FDA-cleared multiplex syndromic assays that include more than three targets for the diagnosis of respiratory infections including the FilmArray RP and RP2 (BioFire Diagnostics LLC), NxTAG-RPP and Verigene RP *Flex* (Luminex Corp), and ePlex and eSensor RVP (GenMark Diagnostics). In addition, the FilmArray RP2.1 panel received FDA emergency use authorization in May 2020 and includes detection of severe acute respiratory syndrome coronavirus 2 (SARS-CoV-2).[144] Other FDA-cleared molecular assays with 2 to 3 viral targets are available and may be advantageous for cost and turnaround time when positive. The syndromic assays include 8 to 21 viral and bacterial targets, and turnaround time ranges from 1 to 8 hours. Test performance characteristics are good with overall sensitivity greater than 84% and specificity greater than 99%.[116]

Several quasi-experimental (pre- and post-implementation) studies have examined the clinical impact of respiratory multiplex assay use and found them to be associated with positive outcomes including faster time to virus identification, decreased antimicrobial use, and decreased LOS in adults and pediatrics.[145–147] Impact was further supported in a randomized controlled trial (RCT) of point-of-care testing respiratory assay versus laboratory PCR assays with reduced LOS; however, there was no difference in proportion treated with antibiotics or mean duration of therapy.[148] Similarly, a recent RCT comparing communication of multiplex PCR results within 24 hours of testing versus after a 7-day hold period showed no difference in antibiotic use or LOS.[149] Thus clinical impact needs to be considered through the testing platform used, testing setting, and how results will be integrated into clinical decision-making.

Gastroenteritis

There are currently several FDA-cleared multiplex syndromic assays for the diagnosis of GI infections including the FilmArray GIP (BioFire Diagnostics LLC), Verigene EP (Luminex Corp.), and Luminex x-TAG-GPP (Luminex Corp.). These assays include a total of 9 to 22 viral, bacterial, toxin, and parasitic targets, and turnaround time ranges from 1 to 5 hours. Test performance has been mostly studied for the FilmArray and Verigene panels, although all panels have shown high sensitivity and specificity greater than 95%, with exceptions for the rarer targets.[116,150] Overall positivity of these panels ranges from 15% to 50%, which is significantly higher than that previously seen with conventional methods and may reflect colonization rather than infection with some targets on the assays.[116]

Mounting evidence has been published assessing the clinical impact of multiplex syndromic panels for the diagnosis of GI infections. Although performing the assay is more costly than conventional testing, it was nonetheless cost-effective by improving IC measures for patient isolation.[151,152]

Moreover, recent data support the beneficial impact of such assays on reducing need for endoscopy, abdominal imaging, and antibiotic use, likely as a result of the improved test performance characteristics of these assays.[153,154] Given the frequent self-resolving nature of GI infections, these data are particularly important to justify implementation of syndromic multiplex panels in clinical laboratories.

Meningitis/Encephalitis

There is currently only 1 FDA-cleared multiplex syndromic assay for the diagnosis of meningitis and/or encephalitis, the FilmArray ME panel (BioFire Diagnostics LLC) that was FDA-cleared in 2015. This panel includes a total of 14 targets (bacterial, viral, and fungal) with a turnaround time of 1 hour. This panel was shown to have excellent performance with overall sensitivity around 90% and specificity greater than 95%.[155] However, inclusion of very few specimens positive for *E. coli*, *Haemophilus influenzae*, *Neisseria meningitidis*, *Streptococcus agalactiae*, and *Cryptococcus neoformans/gattii* made it difficult to extrapolate test performance for these organisms.[156] As such, one must stay attuned to the risk of false-positive (especially *Streptococcus pneumoniae* and *S. agalactiae*) and false-negative results (herpes simplex virus [HSV-1 and HSV-2], enterovirus, and *C. neoformans/gattii*) which may have important potential negative consequences.[155,157,158] Moreover, there is ongoing concern regarding the decreased analytical sensitivity of the ME panel compared to targeted HSV PCR, and the risk of missing low-burden HSV CNS infection.[157]

A number of studies have been recently published on the favorable clinical impact of the ME panel.[158] This assay has shown potential to identify the etiology of culture-negative meningitis allowing specific targeted therapy,[159] decreased time to appropriate therapy, timely appropriate antibiotic cessation, and/or a trend toward lower LOS.[158,160,161]

SUMMARY FOR OTHER MULTIPLEX SYNDROMIC PANELS

Multiplex syndromic panels demonstrate significant potential to improve clinical care and have unleashed a paradigm change within clinical laboratory testing. However, their cost is high and certain limitations to test performance remain. The microbiology laboratory plays an important role in selecting which patients to test with these assays and under what circumstances.[162] Indeed, preanalytical selection criteria for testing should be considered to optimize pretest probability and use of the tests.[163,164] Furthermore, given the ASP and IPC implications, workflows should be established that allow effective communication of results to clinicians and health care providers for timely decision making.

Antimicrobial Susceptibility Testing
Genotypic Markers of Antimicrobial Resistance

As highlighted earlier, timely selection of appropriate antibiotic therapy requires the capacity to rapidly identify organism resistance. Ideally, methodologies for rapid phenotypic AST would be used, providing full information on susceptibility and resistance results. However, conventional phenotypic AST method turnaround time remains in the range of around 1 to 2 days. Molecular testing provides a more rapid alternative to accurately detect genes associated with antimicrobial resistance.[165]

This approach has proven more straightforward for gram-positive pathogens such as *Staphylococcus* spp. and *Enterococcus* species which encode a monogenic resistance mechanism for beta-lactams and vancomycin, respectively. Such an approach may also be considered for *Candida* spp. resistance to echinocandin antifungal agents via FKS mutations.[166] In contrast, gram-negative rods have many resistance mechanisms which are not as amenable to rapid, on-demand nucleic acid amplification testing (NAAT) for clinical use except for specific indications such as identification of carbapenemase-producing carbapenem-resistant Enterobacterales (CP-CRE).

mecA, vanA, and *vanB*

Many options are currently available for detection of *mecA* (encoding beta-lactam resistance in staphylococci), as well as *vanA* and *vanB* (encoding vancomycin resistance in *Enterococcus*), including single-target commercial NAATs,[167] in-house laboratory-developed tests,[168] penicillin-binding protein 2a (PBP2a) lateral flow assays,[169] and multiplexed panels as presented earlier. Although molecular resistance testing is more expensive than conventional phenotypic testing, this may be offset by its clinical benefit. For example, vancomycin is typically used for the empiric coverage of possible infection with gram-positive pathogens. However, this therapy is inferior to beta-lactams (nafcillin, cloxacillin, flucloxacillin, or cefazolin) for the treatment of methicillin-susceptible *S. aureus* (MSSA) bacteremia, and has been associated with poorer clinical outcomes and increased mortality.[170,171] Molecular testing of *mecA*, which is used for the rapid detection of MRSA, thus provides the opportunity to confidently and rapidly guide the choice of optimal therapy and influence clinical outcome.

The impact of such testing has been studied in adults and children with the use of real-time PCR for *mecA* detection from blood and other sterile body sites which showed reduced vancomycin usage, reduced time to optimal therapy, and reduced LOS.[168,172,173] Additional studies have evaluated the use of MRSA nasal PCR screening as a formal tool for antimicrobial stewardship-driven de-escalation in the management of patients with pneumonia and have consistently shown that vancomycin can be stopped an average of 2 days earlier when use is guided by MRSA nasal PCR results compared to standard management with no increase in adverse outcomes.[174–176] Use of MRSA nasal screening to guide antibiotic coverage in this way was mentioned as a strategy for management of community-acquired pneumonia (CAP) in the 2019 ATS/IDSA guidelines.[177] In addition, molecular detection of *vanA/vanB* has also been shown to save isolation days and transmission risk days when performed directly on rectal screening.[178]

CARBAPENEMASE GENES

The most common carbapenemases in the United States are *K. pneumoniae* carbapenemase (KPC), New Delhi Metallo-beta-lactamase (NDM), Verona Integron-Encoded Metallo-beta-lactamase (VIM), imipenemase (IMP), and oxacillinase-48-like (OXA-48-like).[179] KPC, VIM, and IMP have been reported worldwide, whereas OXA-48 has been mostly identified in Europe and India.[180] Similarly, although NDM emerged in the Indian subcontinent, it has now been identified globally with multiple variants.[181] Prompt identification of these resistance mechanisms in cultured isolates and screening samples are important to enact appropriate IC measures, inform appropriate therapy, and plan additional antibiotic testing as appropriate.[182] Indeed, these organisms can readily spread in hospitalized patients and lead to outbreaks that may be very difficult to control. One of the first steps to enable recognition of CP-CRE is accurate susceptibility testing to prevent reports of false susceptibility to carbapenems and missed identification of carbapenemase-producers. Clinical laboratories can facilitate recognition and subsequent IC efforts by ensuring they are using current breakpoints for antimicrobial susceptibility interpretation. Indeed, studies have demonstrated the potential for missed CP-CRE detection with outdated breakpoint usage.[183,184] Further discussion on screening for these organisms is discussed in the IPC screening tests section below.

Multiplex PCRs to detect the most common carbapenemase enzymes with high accuracy have been developed as laboratory-developed tests[185,186] and commercially.[187,188] Recently, multiplexed lateral flow assays have also been developed to detect either the three or five most common carbapenemase enzymes with high test performance, enabling a rapid and simple testing method.[189,190] Such testing can be performed from positive blood culture broth after simple processing and from pure colonies, and is available commercially (NG-Test Carba 5, Hardy Diagnostics, Santa Maria, CA).[191–193] In addition, several phenotypic methods for carbapenemase identification are also available (Carba-NP, modified Hodge test, modified carbapenemase inactivation method [mCIM]) as lower-cost alternatives to molecular methods, though these do not detect the specific resistance mechanism and turnaround time is longer.[194] Strategies on how to integrate such assays into IPC algorithms for screening and diagnosis of CPE clinical isolates is discussed in more detail below.

Rapid Phenotypic Susceptibility Testing
Rapid Disk Diffusion Testing
Disk diffusion testing from fresh, isolated colonies has been used for decades as a reference method for AST. Given this method requires overnight incubation after a fresh subculture, results are available after a total of approximately 48 hours. Recently, rapid disk diffusion methods that produce results in as few as 4 hours have been validated from positive blood cultures for Enterobacterales and *Acinetobacter*, providing a low-cost manual alternative to the rapid testing methods presented above.[195,196] Further work is expected in this area for additional sample types.

Other Rapid Phenotypic Antimicrobial Susceptibility Testing Methods
The Accelerate Pheno system, discussed earlier in this chapter, is currently the only commercial platform FDA-cleared for rapid phenotypic AST. In addition, a number of laboratory-developed protocols have been validated successfully as method adaptations to longstanding commercially available automated AST platforms such as VITEK2 (bioMérieux, Marcy l'Étoile, France), Phoenix (Becton, Dickinson and Company, Franklin Lakes, NJ), and Micro-Scan Walkaway (Beckman Coulter, Brea, CA).[197–202] These approaches produce rapid, highly accurate results with relatively simple sample processing and inexpensive reagent costs.

Other Pathogens of Infection Prevention and Control Importance
Mycobacterium Tuberculosis Polymerase Chain Reaction
Mycobacterium tuberculosis (TB) represents a pathogen of importance given its potential for transmission in health care settings, particularly when it is unsuspected and the diagnosis is delayed. Active respiratory disease with TB (pulmonary or laryngeal involvement) is contagious and can be transmitted through coughing or sneezing, and through aerosolization from procedures such as bronchoscopy and autopsy. Risk of TB transmission depends on a number of factors including organismal load as assessed by acid-fast bacilli (AFB) smear status (i.e., smear positive versus negative), location of TB disease, HIV status, endoscopic or surgical procedure, lack of active TB therapy, and inadequate ventilation and isolation precaution measures.[203] When a case is suspected, IPC should be informed and airborne precautions should be instituted promptly to reduce risk of transmission until TB disease is until TB disease is confirmed, ruled out, or an alternative diagnosis is made. As such, test performance characteristics and turnaround time of diagnostic methods to evaluate for TB are important factors to consider and directly link the clinical laboratory to IC implications.

TB detection from direct specimens has historically been performed by conventional AFB smear (Ziehl-Neelsen or Kinyoun) or fluorescent smear (auramine or auramine/rhodamine). Although inexpensive, these methods are hampered by low sensitivity and low specificity from cross-reactivity with other non-tuberculous mycobacteria.[204,205] TB NAATs have emerged as a beneficial alternative to AFB smear for more rapid turnaround, greater sensitivity (>95% for smear-positive; between 50% and 75% for smear-negative), and greater specificity (>99%), prompting many laboratories and health settings in the US and globally to incorporate these into the diagnostic evaluation for TB.[206,207] In 2015, the FDA approved the modification of the Xpert MTB/Rif assay to allow it to replace smear results to guide discontinuation of airborne precautions.[208] Indeed, a single NAAT has shown a negative predictive value (NPV) of 99.7% for predicting absence of AFB-smear-positive/culture-positive TB, and two NAATs demonstrated a NPV of 100%.[209] Since then, multiple IC protocols based on two negative TB NAAT results have demonstrated the safety and advantages of NAAT over smear microscopy including decreased duration of isolation, decreased LOS, and cost-effectiveness.[210,211] Furthermore, the Association of Public Health Laboratories (APHL) and the National Tuberculosis Controllers Association (NTCA) have integrated NAAT-based testing in their recommended algorithms.[212,213] TB culture must nonetheless continue to be performed for susceptibility testing and for diagnosis in NAAT-negative, culture-positive TB cases. Several public health laboratories have already incorporated NGS testing of TB isolates, which has shown good test performance and reduced turnaround time for characterizing drug resistance and may eventually be adopted in clinical laboratories.[214,215]

Implementation of rapid and effective TB evaluation protocols thus requires close collaboration between the clinical laboratory, IPC, and other clinical providers such as respiratory therapists and nurses.[216] Rapid access to induced sputum production, prompt sample transport to the laboratory, and timely sample processing and reporting of results allows safe discontinuation of airborne precautions. However, given the labor-intensive nature of respiratory sample processing, planning is required to optimize laboratory workflows and impact of results including if, when, and how to batch specimen processing, processing on weekends or not, performing NAAT on all AFB samples or only on demand, in addition to other concerns.

C. difficile Nucleic Acid Amplification Testing and Other Diagnostics

Clostridioides (previously *Clostridium*) *difficile* infection (CDI) is the most common infectious cause of nosocomial diarrhea, with an estimated 450,000 cases and 15,000 CDI-associated deaths annually in the United States.[217,218] In addition to the clinical impact, CDI rates are of particular importance to IC and hospital leadership, as these are publicly reported data with associated financial penalties.[219,220] The incidence of CDI rose dramatically in the previous two decades, driven by both the emergence of the epidemic BI/NAP1/027 strain and the shift toward more analytically sensitive testing for the presence of toxigenic *C. difficile* organisms.[221,222] The transition from the widespread use of toxin assays, which detect the presence of *C. difficile* toxins A and/or B, typically using ELISA or EIA technology, to the use of NAATs that detect toxin genes, was associated with a 43% to 97% increase in the CDI incidence in facilities that directly switched, despite no evidence of increased transmission events or antibiotic use, suggesting that NAATs were identifying not only patients with CDI but also those with subclinical disease or who may simply have been colonized with *C. difficile* and had diarrhea from another cause.[223–228] Indeed, many studies have shown *C. difficile* colonization rates range anywhere from 5% to greater than 25% depending on the patient population tested, which underscores the risk of CDI overdiagnosis posed by highly sensitive NAATs, especially if strict testing criteria are not enforced.[229–237]

Because CDI is a toxin-mediated disease state and identification of the organism is insufficient to establish the diagnosis, the optimal diagnostic testing strategy for CDI remains undefined. As alluded to above, direct toxin assays fell out of favor due to insufficient analytic sensitivity as a single test.[238–240] These were initially replaced by NAATs, which have sensitivity comparable to toxigenic culture, the gold standard for isolation of toxigenic *C. difficile* organisms,[241] but a positive NAAT result by itself cannot differentiate between colonization and toxin-mediated disease, especially when clinical symptoms are not considered.[242] Indeed, multiple recent studies have shown that when different testing modalities are used, patients who are positive by both NAAT and direct toxin assays have longer duration of diarrhea, longer hospital stays, and higher mortality rates compared to those positive only by NAAT, and outcomes are similar between patients positive only by NAAT and those who test negative for *C. difficile* by all methods.[243–248] As studies have shown that the difference in sensitivity between NAATs and toxin tests is mediated, at least in part, by organismal burden, with samples positive by toxin assays having significantly higher organismal loads than those positive only by NAAT, and the PCR cycle threshold (CT) is inversely correlated with organismal load,[249–251] some have used the PCR CT value to predict direct toxin assay positivity.[252,253] Similar to direct toxin assay results, multiple studies have shown that lower CT values, corresponding to higher bacterial loads and predicted positive toxin assay results, are associated with more severe disease and risk of recurrence compared to predicted toxin-negative

results.[254–261] While this methodology is attractive as it maintains the high sensitivity of NAATs while providing an additional level of information from the qualitative PCR result without a second test, it remains in limited use, and some studies have shown significant overlap of CT values between toxin-positive and toxin-negative results, leading to lower specificity for the diagnosis of CDI.[259,262] Given the downsides of current direct toxin assays and NAATs, new diagnostics are in development. The most promising tests are ultrasensitive toxin assays, which have superior sensitivity to current toxin assays and may be less prone to overdiagnosis than NAATs, but none are yet available for commercial use.[263–267]

Given the complexities of diagnostic testing and contrasting strengths and weaknesses of the available assays, current guidelines from the United States and Europe recommend the use of multi-step algorithms rather than use of NAATs alone and to enact institutional testing criteria to avoid testing in patients without clinically significant diarrhea or who have a readily identifiable alternative cause.[268–271] Strict testing criteria have been shown to reduce inappropriate testing rates.[237] Multi-step algorithms can add additional information regarding the likelihood of true, toxin-mediated CDI rather than colonization, and allow identification of patients, especially those who have milder or atypical symptoms, who can be safely monitored without antimicrobial therapy.[254] In addition, while any patient diagnosed with CDI may be an appropriate target for antimicrobial stewardship interventions,[272] patients ultimately deemed to be carriers may be the most important stewardship targets as avoidance of additional antibiotic exposure could potentially reduce the significant risk these patients carry of later conversion to true, toxin-mediated infection.[234,235,273]

When choosing a diagnostic testing algorithm, it is beneficial for the laboratory to work collaboratively with IPC and ASP during development, as factors beyond the analytical will need to be considered. As the surveillance definition for public reporting of hospital-onset CDI (HO-CDI) cases transitioned from a clinical case definition to a laboratory-identified (LabID) event, with a new, positive result on hospital day 4 or later classified as a hospital-onset case regardless of degree of symptoms or when they began, overdiagnosis is common when testing criteria are lax or testing is not done promptly for diarrheal symptoms present on admission.[274] This may lead to an inflated HO-CDI rate and a risk of undue public scrutiny or a potential financial penalty.[219,275,276] In addition, in multi-step algorithms, the specific order of tests used may have significant effects on CDI surveillance and publicly reported rates.[277] Beyond the issue of surveillance, admitted patients with active CDI or who are merely carriers of *C. difficile* are significant sources of transmission to other patients, either directly through contact or indirectly through the hospital environment.[278–281] Therefore positive *C. difficile* results must be promptly conveyed to IPC so proper isolation and enhanced environmental cleaning procedures can be put into place.[29,282–284] ASP involvement in the management of CDI cases has been associated with higher rates of concordance with guidelines and optimization of treatment.[285–287]

New and Emerging Technologies

Many new and/or emerging technologies have been presented earlier in this chapter. In clinical microbiology, further advances are expected in diagnostics that facilitate a more rapid diagnosis of bloodstream infections such as assays that can be performed directly from whole blood with high test performance. Significant progress is expected in molecular methods, including the upgrade of multiplexed syndromic panels to include more targets and clinical applications (e.g., rapid diagnosis of the etiology of septic arthritis), broadening of NAAT-based resistance testing (e.g., including *mecC* testing for *S. aureus* methicillin resistance), expansion of testing by cell-free DNA (e.g., noninvasive diagnosis of TB), and improvements in metagenomic NGS (e.g., increasing analytical sensitivity through improved host depletion methods, reducing turnaround time and cost).[288] Furthermore, technologies that complement our current diagnostic arsenal such as flow cytometry offer the promise of rapidly ruling out infections (e.g. rapid and simple rule-out of urinary tract infection).[289,290]

Artificial intelligence including machine learning algorithms are also expected to take on an increasingly prominent role in microbiology diagnostics and in guiding clinical decision-making. For example, machine learning approaches have shown great promise in prediction of organism resistance compared to standard antibiograms by incorporating a high number of patient-specific and institution-specific factors.[291-294]

In addition, whole-genome sequencing is becoming increasingly used in research and clinical practice, particularly for nosocomial outbreak investigation and IC purposes.[35] Application of this technology was indispensable in the investigation and eventual mitigation of carbapenem-resistant *K. pneumoniae* outbreak in a nosocomial setting.[295] This area is expected to develop further in the near future, becoming increasingly cheaper, portable, more rapid, and used in real-time investigations.

POINTS TO REMEMBER

- The diagnostic arsenal continues to expand for the clinical laboratory, spanning multiple technologies.
- Cost versus added utility need to be balanced.
- Artificial intelligence has already started to be used in the clinical laboratory, and is expected to become increasingly useful.

ANTIMICROBIAL SUSCEPTIBILITY TESTING CONSIDERATIONS

Selective and Cascade Reporting

One of the most important roles of the clinical laboratory is to perform AST, and convey interpretation and/or minimal inhibitory concentrations (MICs) to clinicians. Although this may appear as a passive process at face value, meticulous care must be taken to design and implement an algorithm by which these results are released to optimize uptake of these results. This can be achieved by establishing a set of built-in rules integrated within the LIS for tailored reporting per institutional guidelines.

Selective testing is an important component of laboratory-based antimicrobial stewardship, and refers to including only a selected number of first-line agents for testing and reporting, instead of reporting results for all available drugs

up front. Examples of selective reporting include specific bug-drug combinations for which testing is inappropriate (e.g., avoid testing daptomycin for respiratory isolates), reporting is inappropriate (e.g., avoid reporting certain antibiotics contra-indicated in pediatrics), or for which the literature supports worse outcomes despite in vitro susceptibility (e.g., avoid reporting piperacillin-tazobactam result for ceftriaxone-nonsusceptible *E. coli* and *K. pneumoniae* regardless of MIC).[22,296] In its M100 document, the document that details the performance standards for interpretation of AST, CLSI has outlined an approach based on groups for testing and reporting and divided into five categories: group A agents (routinely test and report), group B (antimicrobial agents that may warrant testing but may be reported selectively), group C (alternative or supplemental agents, or for reporting to IPC group), group U (antimicrobial agents used only or primarily to treat urinary tract infections), and group O/other (antimicrobial agents that have a clinical indication but are not used for routine testing and reporting in the United States).[297] This document provides a useful general approach, but ultimately each institution must determine which step-wise test/report sequence best suits their needs. This is ideally decided with multiple stakeholders in a group setting such as an antibiotic subcommittee meeting that includes the clinical laboratory, infectious disease clinicians, pharmacists, emergency physicians, and others, and must be reassessed at regular intervals. For example, in an institution with previous universal reporting of ciprofloxacin for *Enterobacterales*, suppression of ciprofloxacin AST when other agents were susceptible led to a sustained decrease in ciprofloxacin use.[65] Similarly, selective reporting of AST results from urine cultures led to increased adherence to first-line treatment guidelines, and high level of provider acceptability in general practice.[298] Such anticipated impact can help motivate meaningful partnership between the clinical laboratory, ASP, and IPC groups to achieve important targets.

In the future, it is anticipated that more advanced antimicrobial reporting software will allow incorporation of individual-level data (weight, creatinine clearance, albumin level, concomitant drugs) in addition to organism identification and MIC data to provide personalized reporting that will eventually replace breakpoints.

Cascade reporting refers to the practice of reporting AST results to optimize use of first-line therapies and narrower-spectrum antibiotics, and to avoid use of formulary-restricted, broad-spectrum, and/or more expensive antimicrobials when first-line agents are susceptible.[20,65-69] As such, it can be considered as a component of selective reporting.[20] Examples of cascade reporting strategies include suppression of cefepime and carbapenem susceptibilities when Enterobacterales isolates are susceptible to ceftriaxone,[299] and nonreporting of ciprofloxacin susceptibility when an Enterobacterales isolate is susceptible to narrower agents such as ampicillin, cefazolin, and trimethoprim-sulfamethoxazole.[65] Although there are limitations to this approach, including challenges to capture the true cost of drug and imbalances in emergence of resistance among members of an antimicrobial class, this nonetheless presents a means by which to optimize cost-effective drug selection by nudging the clinician upstream. Similar to selective reporting, decisions regarding the algorithmic rules of cascade reporting should be made jointly by the clinical laboratory and ASP.

Cumulative Antibiogram

One of the most helpful contributions of the clinical laboratory is to generate a yearly cumulative antibiogram of susceptibility results across isolates and patient populations for its institution. These data provide the most useful information to guide empiric antibiotic therapy selection while awaiting confirmatory microbiological results. Given the complexity of producing this report, recommendations on how to proceed with the different phases of AST data collection, analysis, presentation, and dissemination of results can be found in the CLSI M39 document.[20] This guideline covers the basics on how to generate a cumulative antibiogram and includes the principles listed in Box 83.4.[20]

Given the design, the cumulative antibiogram is not well suited to detect the emergence of resistance, which may require follow-up of multiple isolates from a patient over time. For this purpose, ongoing data verification as a part of a Quality Management System is more appropriate. If sufficient isolates are available, an enhanced antibiogram can be produced which stratify the data by different parameters including hospital unit (e.g., ICU), by an organism's resistance profile (e.g., VRE), by specimen type (e.g., blood isolates only), or by patient population (e.g., cystic fibrosis patients).[20] ICU-specific data may be particularly useful given empiric therapy choices may differ based on the location of the patient.[21]

Challenging Situations

Challenging situations arise in the clinical laboratory when requests are received for specialized testing for which there is

POINTS TO REMEMBER

- Selective testing refers to including only a selected number of first-line agents for testing and reporting and is an important strategy to improve antimicrobial use.
- Cascade reporting refers to the practice of reporting antimicrobial susceptibility testing results to optimize use of first-line therapies and narrower-spectrum antibiotics when first-line agents are susceptible.
- The clinical laboratory should produce a yearly cumulative antibiogram to be used to guide empiric therapy.

BOX 83.4 Principles of a Cumulative Antibiogram

- Produce an annual antibiogram.
- Include only species for which there are >30 isolates (or use a disclaimer when there are less).
- Report data as % susceptible.
- Only include the first isolate of a given species per patient per analysis period.
- Only include antimicrobial agents that are routinely tested including those that may be suppressed per selective reporting.
- Only include isolates collected for diagnostic purposes, not those collected for surveillance.
- Include meningitis and non-meningitis breakpoints for *Streptococcus pneumoniae*.
- Separate methicillin-resistant (MRSA) and methicillin-susceptible (MSSA) *S. aureus*.

lack of proper guidance on the significance of testing to inform clinical outcomes. These include requests for susceptibility testing of new antimicrobial agents, MDROs, and situations for which there are no breakpoints available for the organism-drug combination of interest. A full discussion of these topics is beyond the scope of this chapter but can be explored further in other references.[300,301]

BIOMARKERS

C-reactive Protein

C-reactive protein (CRP) is one of the most commonly used biomarkers of the inflammatory state.[302] It was first isolated in the sera of patients with pneumonia in 1930 as a protein capable of precipitating polysaccharide fractions from *S. pneumoniae*.[303] It is an acute phase reactant produced by the liver in response to inflammatory cytokines, most prominently interleukin-6.[302,304,305] It is involved in the induction of additional inflammatory cytokines and can also activate the complement system and bind to phagocytic cells.[305] It rises proportionally to the degree of inflammation, as the serum levels are determined only by the rate of production, begins to rise within 6 to 12 hours of the initial insult, and peaks in 2 to 3 days, though levels may be affected by underlying liver dysfunction given the single-organ origin.[302-304,306] CRP levels are correlated with severity of inflammation, improve in response to appropriate antibiotic therapy when elevated due to infection, and poor patient outcomes are associated with persistently elevated levels.[302,303,307-310] In a systematic review and meta-analysis, CRP had an estimated pooled sensitivity of 75% and specificity of 67% for differentiating bacterial infection from noninfectious causes of inflammation,[304] though extremely elevated levels may be more useful, as one study showed that infection was present in 88% of cases with a CRP value greater than 500 mg/L.[311] One study of pediatric patients with a systemic inflammatory response found that use of a panel of eight biomarkers that included both CRP and procalcitonin (PCT) had a 90% NPV in identifying patients without a bacterial infection.[312] CRP is often used in the diagnosis of bone and joint infections, both in children and adults,[313-315] and serial CRP measurements have been shown to correlate with resolution of these infections, as well as SSIs, soft tissue infections such as cellulitis, VAP, bloodstream infections, and sepsis,[308,309,316-319] and have been used as a marker for timing of stepdown to oral antibiotic therapy in the management of bone and joint infections in children.[320,321] One recent RCT compared CRP-guided antibiotic therapy in which antibiotic discontinuation was recommended upon 75% reduction from peak CRP value to fixed durations of 7 and 14 days in the treatment of uncomplicated gram-negative bacteremia. The study showed that patients who received the CRP-guided course had a median duration of 7 days of antibiotic therapy with no difference in the composite primary outcome of relapse, suppurative or distant infectious complications, and all-cause mortality at 30 days between the treatment arms.[322]

One major area in which CRP has been used to affect antibiotic therapy decisions is in acute exacerbations of chronic obstructive pulmonary disease (COPD). The Global Initiative for Chronic Obstructive Lung Disease (GOLD) recommendations for management of acute COPD exacerbations recommends antibiotics for acute exacerbations when there is an increase in the three cardinal symptoms of dyspnea, sputum purulence, and sputum volume, if two cardinal symptoms are present but one is sputum purulence, or for severe exacerbations requiring mechanical ventilation.[323] Current GOLD guidelines discuss biomarkers to direct antibiotic use but do not formally recommend incorporation into management or use to guide antibiotic usage.[323] The most recent Cochrane review on the use of antibiotics in this setting found inconsistent effects on treatment outcomes aside from patients with severe exacerbations requiring ICU-level care, who had a strong beneficial effect from antibiotic therapy.[324] Prior studies in COPD exacerbations have shown that CRP is more elevated in COPD exacerbations brought on by bacterial respiratory infections,[325,326] and thus could be used to help differentiate patients who may benefit from antibiotics in addition to standard therapies from those who may not. Two trials of CRP-guided acute COPD therapy management were recently published. Butler et al. randomized patients to COPD management guided by point-of-care CRP measurement at presentation compared to usual care and found that fewer patients in the CRP arm received antibiotics at the initial visit compared to usual care (47.7% versus 69.7%) and in 4 weeks of follow-up (59.1% versus 79.7%), and there was no difference in adverse outcomes in 6 months of follow-up.[327] Prins et al. randomized patients to a CRP-guided strategy versus a GOLD-guided strategy with regard to the use of antibiotics as part of acute COPD exacerbation and found that fewer patients in the CRP-guided arm received antibiotics in the first 24 hours compared to the GOLD-guided arm, despite treatment cross-over.[328] There was no difference in treatment failure rate, time to next exacerbation, hospital LOS, or mortality, both 30-day and 1-year.[328] These authors concluded that CRP could be used to safely guide and reduce antibiotic use in the treatment of acute COPD exacerbation,[327,328] though these results have not yet been translated into clinical practice outside of these trial settings. If further studies support the use of CRP to guide antibiotic therapy in the management of acute COPD exacerbations, ASPs could incorporate this into treatment algorithms to reduce inappropriate antibiotic therapy at a local level.

Procalcitonin

Procalcitonin (PCT) is a precursor of the hormone calcitonin that is secreted by nonendocrine, parenchymal cells in numerous tissues at high concentrations in response to inflammatory cytokines such as TNF-α and IL-1β, as well bacterial toxins such as lipopolysaccharide, and thus can function as a marker of inflammatory states.[329–331] PCT release in response to inflammatory cytokines is attenuated by interferon-γ, which is hypothesized to produce lower levels of PCT in response to viral compared to bacterial infections.[330] While severe infection is one of the most common causes of an elevated serum PCT, it is also released in noninfectious inflammatory states such as pancreatitis, severe ischemia, inhalational injury, major burns, heatstroke, massive trauma, and following extensive surgical procedures and can also be chronically elevated in patients with advanced kidney disease.[331,332] Despite the lack of complete specificity for infection, there is widespread interest in the use of PCT in the diagnosis and management of infection.

Multiple studies have shown that, in the context of infection, PCT levels begin to rise within 4 to 6 hours of the onset of the inflammatory state, though can have a delayed peak, and tend to be most elevated in severe, systemic bacterial infection compared to viral or localized bacterial infections.[331,333–335] Levels fall rapidly in response to appropriate antimicrobial therapy and infection management and the kinetics, especially over the first 72 hours of hospitalization, are associated with patient outcomes.[333,336,337]

These broad characteristics have led to attempts to use PCT levels to discriminate between infectious and noninfectious states, bacterial and viral infections, especially in syndromes such as CAP, and also to use serial PCT levels to determine when antibiotics can be stopped. While it is sometimes used in such a way in clinical care, multiple studies have concluded that, while PCT levels are positively correlated with presence of invasive bacterial infection, a single PCT value is insufficient to determine if an individual patient has an infection and should receive antibiotics and must be used as a complement to clinical evaluation.[335,338–342] While there is heterogeneity in the literature due a diversity of specific PCT assays used, one systemic review and meta-analysis estimated that, at the most common threshold value of 0.5 ng/mL, PCT had a pooled sensitivity of 76% and specificity of 69% for presence of bacteremia, with an area under the receiver-operator curve of 0.79.[343] Another systematic review that included only studies that evaluated CAP showed much more dismal results, with a pooled sensitivity of 55% and specificity of 76% to distinguish bacterial from viral pneumonia,[341] although the most recently completed multicenter study included in this meta-analysis showed an 81% sensitivity and 52% specificity at a cut-off of 0.1 ng/mL.[335]

There are much more promising results in studies that have used a PCT-guided algorithm to direct antibiotic use, and specifically cessation, in critically ill patients or those with confirmed infections. Although there is considerable heterogeneity in these data, a recent meta-analysis evaluating pooled data from 11 trials with 4482 patients showed similar results, with a shorter duration of antibiotic therapy for patients receiving PCT-guided care (9.3 versus 10.4 days), as well as lower 30-day mortality (21.1% versus 23.7%) compared to those who did not.[344] A separate meta-analysis showed similar results, though concluded that there were methodological concerns across many trials.[345]

Many other studies have specifically evaluated the use of PCT to guide therapy in lower respiratory tract infections (LRTIs) given the common inability to distinguish viral and bacterial etiologies on clinical grounds alone, and PCT levels tend to be higher in patients with bacterial pneumonia compared to viral infections or acute exacerbations of COPD.[341,346] On the whole, these have shown similar results to the trials in sepsis patients, with lower antibiotic use and similar outcomes with PCT-guided therapy compared to standard care.[347–349] A patient-level meta-analysis of PCT-guided therapy in acute respiratory infections included 6708 patients and found that use of an algorithm reduced antibiotic exposure by 2.4 days (5.7 versus 8.1) with a slight reduction in 30-day mortality (9% versus 10%) and a 30% reduction in antibiotic-associated side effects.[350] These results were consistent with prior meta-analyses on this subject.[351,352]

PCT-based algorithms have also been used specifically in the management of acute COPD exacerbations, though many of these have been folded into larger LRTI trials and not studied separately. Older studies have shown conflicting benefits of PCT to guide antibiotic usage in acute COPD exacerbations.[325,326] Some more recent data demonstrated PCT could be used to reduce antibiotic usage without worsening 30-day hospital re-admission rate,[353–355] but another study demonstrated no change in antibiotic usage and higher 3-month mortality in intensive care patients in the PCT arm.[356] A recent meta-analysis including 1376 patients from eight trials concluded that PCT use was associated with fewer antibiotic prescriptions at the beginning of care, but did not affect overall antibiotic exposure when those received in follow-up were considered, though there was no difference in mortality or readmission.[357] Interestingly, PCT for antibiotic guidance in acute COPD exacerbations has had low uptake in the United States, with levels obtained in only 5% of greater than 200,000 hospitalizations for acute COPD exacerbations,[358] which may reflect providers' assessment of the uncertain utility in this area.

Ultimately, PCT appears to be most useful when applied as a stewardship intervention with particular focus on stopping antibiotics when no longer necessary rather than being strictly used as a test to prevent them from being started.[342] It should be utilized in a systematic approach with a clearly defined algorithm.[359]

Fungal Infections
1,3-β-D-Glucan
Polysaccharides are the main structural component of fungal cell walls, and include glucan (most important and abundant), chitin, and mannan. β-D-glucan (here, specifically (1,3)-β-D-glucan) is a component present in most fungi except for low or absent levels in members of the *Mucorales* family and *Cryptococcus* spp.[360,361] The Fungitell assay (Associates of Cape Cod, Inc., East Falmouth, MA) was FDA-approved in 2004 for use as an aid for the diagnosis of invasive fungal infection (IFI) from serum. Its use was subsequently studied from cerebrospinal fluid (CSF) and bronchoalveolar lavage (BAL), alone and in combination with serum, as a biomarker for the diagnosis of fungal disease.[362–364] This assay is based on the measurement of activated Factor G detection by a spectrophotometric reader which converts optical density to β-D-glucan concentration. Result interpretation is categorized as follows: negative (<60 pg/mL), indeterminate (60 to 79 pg/mL), and positive (≥80 pg/mL).[365] False-positive results have been reported from many sources including from hemodialysis with cellulose membranes, albumin, and certain antibiotics including older formulations of piperacillin-tazobactam.[366,367] The use of intravenous immunoglobulin is also an important source of false positives that can persist over 2 weeks after administration of the infusion.[368]

β-D-glucan has generated interest as a potential adjunct for the diagnosis of IFI given it is found in a broad range of fungi and uses a readily available and noninvasive sample source, serum, that can also be used for serial testing.[369] Indeed, invasive sampling may be unavailable or contraindicated in many instances of suspected IFI, and patients may already be treated with broad-spectrum antifungal agents, reducing the sensitivity of fungal culture. Many studies have evaluated performance of this assay, with a meta-analysis including heterogeneous patient populations (hematologic, cancer, ICU, and immunocompromised patients but excluding *Pneumocystis jirovecii* pneumonia

[PCP]) showing a pooled sensitivity of 76.8% and specificity of 85.3% for patients with proven or probable IFI.[370] A subsequent meta-analysis showed that two consecutive tests performed better than a single one, with sensitivity of 49.6% and specificity of 98.8% for the diagnosis of IFI.[371] When restricting the indication to ruling out PCP, test performance improved to a sensitivity of 94.8% and specificity of 86.3%.[372] β-D-glucan may thus serve as a useful diagnostic adjunct when PCP is suspected but invasive testing cannot be performed.[373] Furthermore, limited evidence suggests (1,3)-β-D-glucan may be more sensitive than galactomannan (GM) for the detection of invasive aspergillosis (IA),[367] and that combining it with GM may be useful to rule out false-positive results from either test.[374] Current recommendations from the IDSA are to perform serum testing for (1,3)-β-D-glucan for the diagnosis of IA for high-risk patients (hematologic malignancy and allogeneic hematopoietic stem-cell transplant), and to consider its use from serum and/or BAL in support of a preemptive approach to antifungal therapy in these patients.[375] This contrasts slightly with the European Society of Clinical Microbiology and Infectious Diseases (ESCMID) assessment that (1,3)-β-D-glucan testing alone shows limited utility, and that combining it with GM is recommended.[376]

Testing with the (1,3)-β-D-glucan assay is an interesting area of opportunity between the clinical laboratory and ASP given the potential for negative results to facilitate the appropriate de-escalation of empiric antifungal therapy as recommended by guidelines.[22] Some institutions have adopted ASP algorithms based on the NPV of (1,3)-β-D-glucan testing; however, prospective data assessing the impact of testing alone are currently lacking.[377,378] Furthermore, interpretation of negative results should consider the clinical possibility of *Cryptococcus* or *Mucorales* infection given these organisms do not produce (1,3)-β-D-glucan. Turnaround time should also be considered in such decision-making given testing in most US settings is performed as send out.

In summary, given the lack of robust fungal diagnostics with high test performance across fungal organisms, patient populations, and clinical syndromes, (1,3)-β-D-glucan continues to be used as an aid for the diagnosis of IFI. Proper consideration should be given to selecting the right patient population to test, incorporating testing into institution-specific diagnostic workflows that favor test performance and cost-effectiveness, and ensuring clinicians understand the sensitivity and specificity limitations of testing given the important clinical implications.

Galactomannan
GM is a polysaccharide that is an important component of the *Aspergillus* spp. cell wall, and is largely absent from other fungi.[379] The Platelia Aspergillus Ag assay (Bio-Rad Laboratories, Hercules, CA) is an immunoenzymatic sandwich microplate assay for detection from serum and BAL that was FDA-approved in 2003 as an aid in the diagnosis of IA. The result is reported as an optical density index, with thresholds for positivity that vary by sample type. The FDA approved a threshold of ≥0.5 as positive, but higher values have shown improved specificity.[380,381] The performance of the GM detection for diagnosis of IA from serum in a heterogeneous immunocompromised patient population was assessed in a large meta-analysis that showed a sensitivity of 82% and specificity of 81% using a cut-off threshold of 0.5.[381]

TABLE 83.3 Synopsis of the Clinical Use of the Various Biomarkers Discussed in This Chapter

Inflammatory Marker	Utility
C-reactive protein	• Diagnosis of infection • Antibiotics for COPD exacerbation • Stepdown to oral antibiotic therapy • Discontinuation of antibiotic therapy
Procalcitonin	• Diagnosis of infection • Discontinuation of antibiotic therapy
Fungal Diagnostics	**Utility**
Galactomannan (1,3)-β-D-glucan	• Invasive aspergillosis • Invasive fungal infection, with the exception of *Cryptococcus*, *Mucorales* agents and *Fusarium* • *Pneumocystis* pneumonia

The role of GM is predominantly for screening in high-risk patient populations to facilitate appropriate initiation of *Aspergillus* therapy, and can be considered as a surrogate marker for poor clinical outcomes when elevated.[382] Serum and BAL GM testing is recommended for the diagnosis of IA in high-risk adult and pediatric patients by IDSA.[375] The usefulness of GM screening has been established for high-risk patient groups only, and serum testing of solid organ transplant (SOT) recipients and individuals with chronic granulomatous diseases (CGD) is not recommended.[375] Similarly, serum-based GM testing for patients already on mold-active therapy or prophylaxis is not recommended.[375] Thus GM represents an important diagnostic tool to aid in the diagnosis of IA and is more specific than (1,3)-β-D-glucan for this purpose. Several studies have explored the use of serial GM alone or in combination with *Aspergillus* PCR in a preemptive approach to avert unnecessary initiation of antifungal therapy with varying results.[383–385] Further data in this area would be helpful to inform practical strategies on how to integrate GM testing in antifungal stewardship efforts, especially in the current context of widespread use of mold-active prophylaxis. A summary of the utility of biomarkers for infectious disease diagnosis is included in Table 83.3.

SCREENING TESTS FOR INFECTION PREVENTION AND CONTROL

Both culture-based and molecular diagnostics have applications outside of direct clinical care of patients and can be used for both IC and antimicrobial stewardship purposes. The most common use of these tests from an IC standpoint is for identification of patients who harbor multi-drug-resistant organisms (MDROs) such as MRSA, VRE, CP-CRE, and *C. difficile*, as these organisms can be transmitted within a health care environment through patient care activities, and thus transmission from carriers may be reduced by application of enhanced IC measures such as use of isolation and contact precautions.[29,74,386,387] Active surveillance, the screening of patients for asymptomatic colonization with MDROs, especially MRSA, is a common practice in IC,[74] though the breadth and intensity of screening at a given facility will differ and may be dependent on such factors as legislative mandate,

health system standards, and local epidemiologic trends. Screening can be universal or targeted in nature, including all patients within a facility or only those in high-risk areas such as the ICU.[388–391] The choice between culture and molecular diagnostics for surveillance should be made in consultation between IC and the clinical laboratory in order to determine the most efficient screening method based on analytic sensitivity, turnaround time, and cost.[391] While molecular diagnostics such as PCR are more expensive compared to culture-based methods, they are quicker and more sensitive, and the rapid turnaround time may help avoid universal use or overly delayed application of isolation and enhanced precautions pending screening results, though surveillance with molecular assays has not been shown to significantly reduce MRSA or ESBL transmission compared to culture-based methods.[391–393] Active surveillance is less commonly performed for VRE and CRE as these organisms are not as widely prevalent as MRSA, though surveillance of high-prevalence facilities or high-risk locations within a facility may be appropriate based on local epidemiology,[394,395] and some studies have associated active VRE surveillance with decreased risk of hospital-acquired VRE infections.[396,397] CRE screening is on the rise as these organisms become more common,[398–400] and active CRE surveillance may become more necessary over time as monitoring of clinical cultures underestimates the prevalence of CRE.[401] While molecular assays are appropriate for surveillance for MRSA and VRE due to the limited number of genetic mechanisms that produce the resistant phenotype, molecular diagnostics have significant limitations in the detection of CRE due to the numerous mechanisms, both enzymatic (carbapenemase-producing) and nonenzymatic, that can produce a CRE phenotype, so culture-based surveillance may be preferred, at least for initial testing.[392,400] Active surveillance for *C. difficile* carriage in asymptomatic patients is uncommon outside of study or outbreak settings or in high-risk populations such as patients on hematopoietic stem cell transplant wards.[234,402–405]

While isolation and use of contact precautions remain common in the management of hospitalized patients colonized with MDROs, their efficacy has been questioned,[406] especially in light of the association of contact precautions with noninfectious adverse effects and reduced patient well-being during hospitalization.[407–410] Multiple studies have evaluated the effect of discontinuation of routine contact precautions, often in a pre- and postintervention analysis and have consistently demonstrated no increase in MRSA and VRE infection rates following discontinuation of contact precautions for patients colonized with these MDROs.[411–415] A follow-up study after routine precaution discontinuation showed the rate of noninfectious adverse events was reduced, with a particularly profound reduction in patients colonized with MDROs.[416] While this evidence is still emerging, CDC guidelines continue to recommend the use of isolation and contact precautions for patients with a history of infection or colonization with MDROs such as MRSA and VRE, with possible criteria for discontinuation including: repeatedly negative surveillance cultures; a duration free of infection, hospitalization, or receipt of broad-spectrum antimicrobials such as 6 or 12 months; or completion of an effective decolonization protocol (applicable only to MRSA).[29,74] The duration of contact precautions for patients known to carry *C. difficile* remains controversial. Contact precautions are recommended to continue for at least 48 hours after cessation of diarrhea, though may be extended for the duration of acute care hospitalization even after diarrhea resolution due to the risk of continued shedding of spores into the environment.[268,284] In contrast to these recommendations, though, one single-center study from Switzerland evaluated transmission after routine contact precautions were discontinued for patients with CDI and found that over a 10-year period only 6% ($n = 451$) of close contacts of a CDI patient had detectable toxigenic *C. difficile* on surveillance rectal swabs, 1.3% had a similar ribotype as the index patient, and only two pairs (0.4%) had transmission confirmed via NGS.[417]

While isolation and contact precautions are used to prevent transmission of MDROs from patients to other patients or the environment,[74] other interventions can be done to reduce the prevalence of MDROs. One of the most common approaches is decolonization, which is most established in patients with MRSA.[418,419] Protocols for MRSA decolonization can be varied, often involving a combination of a nasal treatment, typically mupirocin or a non-antibiotic treatment such as an alcohol-based antiseptic or povidone iodine, as well as a topical agent such as chlorhexidine gluconate. Decolonization may be targeted to known carriers of MRSA or applied universally, especially in high-risk locations such as the ICU and has been associated with lower rates of MRSA infection.[418,420–426] An extended decolonization protocol with bi-monthly nasal mupirocin and chlorhexidine gluconate wash for 6 months beyond the index inpatient admission has also been associated with a lower rate of future MRSA infection.[427] Multiple modeling studies estimate that decolonization protocols can be cost saving due to the prevention of future infections.[428,429] Decolonization strategies are less established for management of patients who are carriers of VRE or CRE given the inherent difficulties with eradication of highly resistant organisms in the gut, and currently exist only in case reports or small series with various methods used.[430–433]

Surveillance cultures and molecular diagnostics also inform antimicrobial stewardship practices. Knowledge of local MDRO prevalence and colonization status of individual patients can help guide empiric antimicrobial choice, especially in critically ill patients, and inform local treatment guidelines produced by ASPs.[10,22,434,435] One example of a more specific way that methods originally developed for active surveillance can be co-opted into stewardship interventions is with the use of MRSA nasal screening to de-escalate empiric antibiotic regimens in the treatment of pneumonia. Multiple studies have shown that the MRSA nasal PCR has a NPV of greater than 98% for presence of MRSA pneumonia when obtained at or near the time of clinical diagnosis, especially in patients admitted from the community, which could allow for early discontinuation of MRSA-directed antibiotics, primarily vancomycin, and lead to favorable clinical outcomes.[174–176,436–443]

TRANSLATING MICROBIOLOGICAL RESULTS INTO CLINICAL IMPACT

Building the Case for Clinical Impact of Microbiological Results

Beyond a strong partnership between the clinical laboratory and the ASP and IPC groups, it is essential to secure adequate support and resources from the hospital administration to enable the laboratory to develop and pursue its activities. Requesting additional resources for test development, assay, or implementation alone may be a challenge. However, presenting a well-described and researched case for how these laboratory interventions will impact patient care for tangible patient outcomes (e.g., length of stay, ED isolation time) may increase likelihood of success. To this end, some institutions are now incorporating cost-savings programs, whereby the clinical laboratory can submit projects that will achieve cost-savings for the hospital and in exchange receive a portion of the cost-savings in return. Other similar projects have also been explored. Nonetheless, such discussion and negotiations may be challenging, and a strong advocate for the clinical laboratory is essential and may come from the ASP and IPC groups themselves given the strong interdependence of their practice with the laboratory.

Assessment of Effectiveness of Interventions

Performance metrics are an important component to include in the practice of the clinical laboratory, ASP, and IPC, both to assess their own work and to liaise more effectively with higher management.[6] For the clinical laboratory, metrics to monitor performance are well established and need to be appropriately followed, such as to establish and maintain College of American Pathologists (CAP) accreditation.[444] However, additional tailored metrics should be defined and followed for a more detailed assessment of performance for specific procedures of interest for each laboratory. Evaluation of the efficacy of interventions is also a critical aspect of ASP practice, to assess overall performance and to adjust interventions when they fail to achieve expected outcomes.[22] Prior demonstration of increased impact of rapid diagnostics tests on clinical care when implemented as part of a stewardship intervention supports that collaboration between the laboratory and ASP should be pursued whenever possible, and thus certain metrics may be assessed collaboratively.[4,22,71] From a financial standpoint, rapid diagnostic tests introduced by the clinical laboratory are expected to reduce facility costs or patient length of stay, or significantly improve quality of care or patient outcomes in order to justify the additional costs of the rapid tests.[92] Prior to implementing an ASP intervention, key baseline data should be reviewed and specific metrics of interest and expected outcomes should be defined. The laboratory and ASP can each provide critical pieces of these data.[76] Furthermore, clear roles and objectives for each group should be agreed upon, and clear objectives for which each group is accountable with a predefined timeline should be set.

Stewardship interventions that incorporate rapid diagnostic tests should assess antibiotic usage (both overall and targeted agents), time to effective or optimal antibiotic therapy, time to appropriate de-escalation or escalation, use of broad-spectrum therapy, and patient-level outcomes such as length of stay, re-admission rate, and mortality, and rates of adverse drug events and CDI.[11,22,76] Further stewardship-specific metrics may include the proportion of cases ASP directly intervened in, time to ASP intervention, rate of uptake of ASP recommendations, and reasons for refusal to follow ASP recommendations. Similarly, in addition to its surveillance for classical hospital- or health care–acquired infections, IPC should define and follow its own metrics of performance including hospital-wide and emergency department isolation days, frequency of unusual or possible nosocomially spread pathogens, and others. Regular assessment of performance through review of these metrics enables the clinical laboratory, ASP, and IPC to identify areas of strength and weakness to more effectively pursue their work and collaboration.

DIAGNOSTIC STEWARDSHIP

Diagnostic stewardship is an emerging term for the judicious use of diagnostic testing to avoid use in low-probability settings, ensuring that results are clinically meaningful and increase the likelihood of a correct diagnosis.[70,445] It can involve educational initiatives on appropriate testing criteria, as well as modification to all facets of the testing process, including ordering, sample collection, laboratory processes during test performance, and reporting of the results.[445,446] Diagnostic stewardship principles have become more salient with the advent of molecular diagnostics, especially the development of multiplex, syndromic assays and will likely be even more critical in the future as the use of NGS becomes more widespread.[70] Diagnostic stewardship principles complement ASP measures and may be implemented as part of holistic stewardship interventions.[446]

While the principles can be applied to any diagnostic test, one of the illustrative areas of the current literature regarding the application of diagnostic stewardship involves *C. difficile* testing, and includes interventions as varied as sample rejection in the lab based on stool characteristics or clinical criteria,[237,268,271] clinical decision support tools embedded in the electronic order entry system,[447–452] postordering review and/or pre-authorization of in-patient *C. difficile* testing,[453–455] educational initiatives,[456,457] implementation of multi-step algorithms,[254,268,270,458,459] or combinations of the above. Other examples of implementation of stewardship principles into diagnostic testing for infectious diseases include changes to urine culture ordering, such as "reflex culture" only when the screening urinalysis is abnormal, or altered reporting of urine culture results in order to reduce identification, and thus treatment, of asymptomatic bacteriuria,[460–462] only obtaining respiratory cultures in intubated patients with a high probability of VAP based on clinical and imaging factors,[463] and restricting the use of multiplex PCR panels for gastroenteritis in the in-patient setting where results are unlikely to be positive.[164,464]

SUMMARY

In summary, the clinical laboratory is a vital partner for IPC and ASP by providing the underlying data necessary for these groups to fulfill their institutional roles. At the same time, these groups offer important expertise in clinical care and facility operations that help the laboratory implement key technologies to produce more rapid and useful microbiological results that positively affect patient care and can serve as important liaisons between the laboratory and frontline clinicians, ensuring that results are interpreted correctly and translated into meaningful changes in health care delivery. There are numerous opportunities for collaboration as rapid diagnostic platforms expand and molecular and other diagnostics increase in complexity and availability. A close, respectful partnership with open communication between these groups is vital to maximize the benefit of existing interventions and evaluate their impact, monitor for areas of improvement, and strategically plan for the future.

SELECTED REFERENCES

2. Morency-Potvin P, Schwartz DN, Weinstein RA. Antimicrobial stewardship: how the microbiology laboratory can right the ship. Clin Microbiol Rev 2017;30(1):381–407.

3. Diekema DJ, Saboulle MA. Clinical microbiology and infection prevention. J Clin Microbiol 2011;49(Suppl 9): S57–60.

22. Barlam TF, Cosgrove SE, Abbo LM, et al. Implementing an antibiotic stewardship program: guidelines by the Infectious Diseases Society of America and the Society for Healthcare Epidemiology of America. Clin Infect Dis 2016;62(10): e51–77.

23. Bryant KA, Harris AD, Gould CV, et al. Necessary infrastructure of infection prevention and healthcare epidemiology programs: a review. Infect Control Hosp Epidemiol 2016;37(4):371–80.

38. Schuts EC, Hulscher M, Mouton JW, et al. Current evidence on hospital antimicrobial stewardship objectives: a systematic review and meta-analysis. Lancet Infect Dis 2016;16(7): 847–56.

44. Dingle KE, Didelot X, Quan TP, et al. Effects of control interventions on Clostridium difficile infection in England: an observational study. Lancet Infect Dis 2017;17(4): 411–21.

49. Centers for Disease Control and Prevention. The core elements of hospital antibiotic stewardship programs: 2019. 2019.

70. Patel R, Fang FC. Diagnostic stewardship: opportunity for a laboratory-infectious diseases partnership. Clin Infect Dis 2018;67(5):799–801.

77. Timbrook TT, Morton JB, McConeghy KW, et al. The effect of molecular rapid diagnostic testing on clinical outcomes in bloodstream infections: a systematic review and meta-analysis. Clin Infect Dis 2017;64(1):15–23.

91. Banerjee R, Teng CB, Cunningham SA, et al. Randomized trial of rapid multiplex polymerase chain reaction-based blood culture identification and susceptibility testing. Clin Infect Dis 2015;61(7):1071–80.

116. Ramanan P, Bryson AL, Binnicker MJ, et al. Syndromic panel-based testing in clinical microbiology. Clin Microbiol Rev 2018;31(1):e00024–17.

243. Polage CR, Gyorke CE, Kennedy MA, et al. Overdiagnosis of Clostridium difficile infection in the molecular test era. JAMA Intern Med 2015;175(11):1792–801.

288. Mitchell SL, Simner PJ. Next-generation sequencing in clinical microbiology: Are we there yet? Clin Lab Med 2019;39(3): 405–18.

297. Clinical and Laboratory Standards Institute (CLSI). Performance standards for antimicrobial susceptibility testing. 30th ed. CLSI Supplement M100. Wayne, PA: 2020.

350. Schuetz P, Wirz Y, Sager R, et al. Effect of procalcitonin-guided antibiotic treatment on mortality in acute respiratory infections: a patient level meta-analysis. Lancet Infect Dis 2018;18(1):95–107.

370. Karageorgopoulos DE, Vouloumanou EK, Ntziora F, et al. beta-D-glucan assay for the diagnosis of invasive fungal infections: a meta-analysis. Clin Infect Dis 2011;52(6): 750–70.

413. Bearman G, Abbas S, Masroor N, et al. Impact of discontinuing contact precautions for methicillin-resistant staphylococcus aureus and vancomycin-resistant enterococcus: an interrupted time series analysis. Infect Control Hosp Epidemiol 2018;39(6):676–82.

443. Parente DM, Cunha CB, Mylonakis E, et al. The clinical utility of Methicillin-Resistant Staphylococcus aureus (MRSA) nasal screening to rule out MRSA pneumonia: a diagnostic meta-analysis with antimicrobial stewardship implications. Clin Infect Dis 2018;67(1):1–7.

446. Messacar K, Parker SK, Todd JK, et al. Implementation of rapid molecular infectious disease diagnostics: the role of diagnostic and antimicrobial stewardship. J Clin Microbiol 2017;55(3): 715–23.

453. Christensen AB, Barr VO, Martin DW, et al. Diagnostic stewardship of C. difficile testing: a quasi-experimental antimicrobial stewardship study. Infect Control Hosp Epidemiol 2019;40(3):269–75.

Bacteriology*

William D. Lainhart, A. Brian Mochon, Morgan A. Pence, and Christopher D. Doern

ABSTRACT

The diagnosis of bacterial infection is one of the many important services provided by the clinical microbiology laboratory. The past decade has resulted in a dramatic shift in the manner in which clinical microbiologists identify bacteria. With the widespread adoption of matrix-assisted laser desorption/ionization time-of-flight mass spectrometry (MALDI-TOF MS) and molecular methods such as 16S rDNA sequencing, clinical microbiologists are increasingly less reliant on traditional, growth-based, biochemical and metabolic methods.

This chapter describes bacteriology in its current state and as it will likely be practiced going forward rather than reiterating how it was traditionally practiced. By way of introduction, important preanalytical considerations, including specimen collection and submission, are discussed. Identification of bacteria is then detailed in addition to key principles in biochemical identification. Of note, organism categorization will be discussed in the context of modern diagnostic methods such as MALDI-TOF MS and sequence-based identification. In addition, this chapter includes a comprehensive discussion of bacterial infections with a focus on the laboratory methods required to diagnose them.

---

*The full version of this chapter is available electronically on ExpertConsult.com.

Antimicrobial Susceptibility Testing*

Romney M. Humphries and April N. Abbott

ABSTRACT

Background

Antimicrobial susceptibility testing is one of the most important tasks of the clinical microbiology laboratory. Antimicrobial resistance is common, and early recognition of patients with resistant pathogens and appropriate optimization of their antimicrobial therapy significantly improves outcomes.

Content

This chapter reviews the key aspects of antimicrobial susceptibility testing (AST) of bacteria, mycobacteria, and yeast. In most circumstances, AST is performed by evaluating the effect of antimicrobial agents on the growth of an organism, in culture. The relative effect (measured as either a zone of inhibition surrounding a disk containing the antimicrobial, or a minimum inhibitory concentration [MIC] for dilution methods) is interpreted using clinical breakpoints set by international standards organizations. Standardization of AST is achieved through use of consistent inoculum concentrations, test media, and incubation conditions. The concepts of surrogate agent testing, detection of resistance mechanisms, use of commercial systems, and molecular methods for susceptibility testing are discussed. In some instances, additional testing is required to detect important resistance, including methicillin-resistant *Staphylococcus aureus* (MRSA) and vancomycin-resistant *Enterococcus* (VRE). Key concepts for testing bacteria, fungi, and mycobacteria are presented. Common antimicrobials used in clinical practice are also discussed.

*The full version of this chapter is available electronically on ExpertConsult.com.

Mycobacteriology*

Adam J. Caulfield, Rachael M. Liesman, Derrick J. Chen, and Nancy L. Wengenack[a]

ABSTRACT

Background

There are currently approximately 200 recognized species of mycobacteria. Although some species are strictly environmental organisms, several are significant human pathogens, including *Mycobacterium tuberculosis*. *M. tuberculosis* is responsible for nearly 1.5 million deaths each year, and nontuberculous mycobacteria (NTM), such as *Mycobacterium avium* complex (MAC), are also responsible for significant morbidity and mortality.

Content

This chapter describes the laboratory methods used for the detection and identification of *Mycobacterium* species. Methods used for mycobacteria detection and identification are continually evolving to achieve more rapid, cost-effective, and accurate results. Traditional microbiologic methods such as morphology and biochemical profiling have given way to molecular detection and identification methods; however, acid-fast staining and culture for mycobacteria remain at the core of any diagnostic algorithm. After growth in culture, molecular technologies such as nucleic acid hybridization probes, matrix-assisted laser desorption/ionization time-of-flight mass spectrometry (MALDI-TOF MS), and DNA sequencing are used for definitive species identification. Nucleic acid amplification methods allow for culture-independent, direct detection of the *M. tuberculosis* complex (MTBC) and MAC within respiratory specimens and predict susceptibility to anti-infective therapy, which leads to more rapid diagnoses of appropriate patient care.

---

*The full version of this chapter is available electronically on ExpertConsult.com.

[a]This chapter is adapted in part with permission from Caulfield AJ, Wengenack NL. Diagnosis of active tuberculosis disease: from microscopy to molecular techniques. *J Clin Tuberc Other Mycobact Dis* 2016;4:33–43.

Mycology*

Ingibjörg Hilmarsdóttir, Sarah E. Kidd, and Anna F. Lau[a]

ABSTRACT

Background

Ubiquitous in nature, fungi may be opportunistic organisms in compromised hosts or primary pathogens in immunocompetent individuals. Commensal fungi reside in the human body as part of the resident microbiota and cause opportunistic infections. Diagnosis of fungal infections relies on assessment of several factors, including geographical exposure, underlying host condition, clinical manifestations, and diagnostic accuracy of laboratory tests such as culture, anatomic pathology tests, immunologic assays, and molecular tests.

Content

A perspective on the importance of fungi in their natural environment is provided, and their differences in relation to other microorganisms are highlighted. Prevalent and emerging fungal infections are discussed, and a review of

nomenclature changes in medical mycology is listed with the understanding of continued uncertainty regarding phylogenetic relationships between fungal taxa. Preanalytical, analytical, and postanalytical procedures for the laboratory diagnosis of fungal infections are reviewed, with emphasis on fungal morphology and issues that require close communication with the clinical team. Common histopathologic and cytologic features related to anatomic pathology are discussed. Given the suboptimal sensitivity, specificity, and relatively long turnaround time for culture-based detection and identification of fungi, a review of nonphenotypic methods such as mass spectrometry, immunologic assays, and molecular tests is provided. Finally, the principal features of fungal infections are summarized, including patient populations affected, clinical manifestations, relevant diagnostic approaches and tests, and therapeutic issues related to antifungal resistance.

*The full version of this chapter is available electronically on ExpertConsult.com.

[a]We are grateful to Gabriel Lecso of the Service de Parasitologie-Mycologie, Hôpital Universitaire Pitié-Salpêtrière, Paris, France, and to the Kaminski Digital Image Library of Medical Mycology by David H. Ellis, University of Adelaide, Australia, for their collection of photographs that greatly enhanced the value of our chapter.

Parasitology*

Blaine A. Mathison and Bobbi S. Pritt ª

ABSTRACT

Background

Parasites are an important cause of human morbidity and mortality worldwide. They include a diverse array of single-celled eukaryotic organisms (protozoans), multicellular worms (helminths), and arthropods that live in or on the human body and can cause mild to severe life-threatening disease. While many parasites primarily infect impoverished individuals in tropical and subtropical regions of the world, others cause infection in the world's temperate regions including those living in resource-rich, affluent countries. The study of parasitology has gained a renewed importance in recent decades due to the ease in which humans, animals, and food can move rapidly and widely across the globe and the increased number of individuals who are immunocompromised and at risk for severe disease.

Content

This chapter provides an overview of human parasitology and the general laboratory approaches for identifying important parasites in various specimens. Both conventional and state-of-the-art diagnostic methods are covered, including light microscopy, serology, antigen detection, and nucleic acid amplification. Particular attention is paid to testing in blood and fecal specimens, as these are the most common specimens received in the clinical laboratory for detection of parasites. The most important human parasites are discussed individually, with an emphasis on the fundamental clinical and biologic information needed for accurate diagnosis and management of infection. The categories of parasites covered include the blood and tissue protozoa, intestinal protozoa, intestinal helminths, tissue helminths, and medically important arthropods.

*The full version of this chapter is available electronically on ExpertConsult.com.
ªThe authors would like to thank Dr. Esther Babady for her previous contribution to this chapter. Henry Bishop and Sarah Sapp of the DPDx Team (Centers for Disease Control and Prevention, Atlanta, GA) kindly provided updated life cycles.

Virology

Blake W. Buchan and Neil W. Anderson

ABSTRACT

Background

Viral illness has a wide variety of clinical manifestations ranging from focal to systemic and affecting nearly every organ system. Infections may be asymptomatic, acute, or chronic in nature. The viruses causing these syndromes are diverse; however, unrelated viruses may cause clinically indistinguishable disease. Combined, these factors drive the importance of rapid and accurate laboratory diagnosis to enable effective patient management.

Content

In this chapter we discuss the use of qualitative and quantitative nucleic acid amplification and detection methods to diagnose and monitor viral infections. We also provide alternative diagnostic methods for those syndromes not optimally diagnosed by molecular techniques. Specific topics covered in this chapter include viral infections of the respiratory tract, viral illness in immunocompromised populations, infections of the central nervous system (CNS), sexually transmitted viral illness, viral hepatitis, viral hemorrhagic fever (VHF), and diagnosis of vaccine preventable viral infections. Epidemiology of key organisms responsible for each of the clinical syndromes are highlighted and factors impacting laboratory diagnosis and interpretation of results are discussed. Examples include optimal specimen type, availability of standardized assays, utility of qualitative versus quantitative results, multiplexed detection strategies, and potential shortcomings of current diagnostic approaches.

INTRODUCTION AND HISTORICAL PERSPECTIVE

Viruses are among the most common and potentially devastating infectious agents associated with human illness. Non-specific symptoms, asymptomatic carriage, and ease of dissemination via aerosol or contact with bodily fluids enable viruses to infect millions of people during endemic exposure or epidemic outbreaks. Global pandemics such as the 1918 to 1919 influenza claimed 50 to 100 million lives and seasonal influenza epidemics continue to burden health care systems with thousands of hospitalizations annually.[1,2] More recently, the SARS-CoV-2 pandemic, which began in China in December of 2019, has poignantly demonstrated the ability of a novel viral pathogen to rapidly spread, cause over 1 million deaths, and upset the global economy and everyday lives of people on every continent. All this despite fantastic advances in modern medicine including antiviral and vaccine development since the 1918 pandemic. Other viral pandemics, such as human immunodeficiency virus (HIV), have persisted for decades without a vaccine or cure and continue to be a leading cause of mortality in the developing world and requiring costly lifelong suppressive therapies. Chronic viral infection with hepatitis B, hepatitis C, or human papillomavirus (HPV) affects millions of individuals globally and all are strongly associated with human carcinogenesis. Among the most insidious of viral pathogens are those that establish a lifelong latency within the human host including the herpesviruses and polyomaviruses. These latent infections remain largely asymptomatic but may reactivate to cause acute life-threatening disease in the immunocompromised host.

Traditionally, viral culture methods were used to diagnose acute and chronic viral infections. These methods were insensitive, required technical expertise, and results were of limited utility in guiding early therapy because of extended time to result. Additionally, many important viral pathogens lack in vitro models and cannot be efficiently cultured using standard methods. Prime examples of this include norovirus, a leading cause of community acquired and health care–associated gastroenteritis, and hepatitis A and E viruses, which are common causes of acute hepatitis in developing countries. Despite these limitations, maintenance of viral culture capabilities is still of value for phenotypic evaluation of antiviral resistance and for the detection of novel viral pathogens; however, this expertise is largely centralized in regional reference, public health, or government laboratories. Direct antigen detection methods have emerged as a tool to provide more rapid results and in situ detection of noncultivable viruses, but these methods often lack sensitivity and are not available for the majority of viral infections.

Over the past decade, clinical virology has experienced a dramatic shift toward the use of molecular diagnostics. This shift has been driven equally by the benefits to patient care and, in the United States, by the increasing availability of Food and Drug Administration (FDA)-cleared molecular assays. These assays increase precision, accuracy, and commutability of molecular results through automation and standardization of test parameters including specimen type, extraction method, and thermal cycling conditions. Additionally, quantitative assays often include internal and external standards for calibration or conversion of results to an international standard for quantification. This is especially important for management of some chronic viral infections such as HIV or cytomegalovirus (CMV).

In the United States, increased availability of easy-to-use assays designated as "waived" and/or "moderate complexity" by the Clinical Laboratory Improvement Amendments (CLIA) has further expanded molecular diagnostics into nonspecialized or near point of care (POC) laboratories. These tests do not require technical expertise or interpretation of results and have a turn-around time (TAT) of 15 minutes to 3 hours, which enables early patient management decisions. More recently, the development of large multiplexed "syndromic panels" (i.e., molecular assays that simultaneously detect many pathogens associated with a particular disease syndrome) have enabled the detection of multiple viral pathogens (and bacterial, parasitic, and fungal pathogens) associated with a specific clinical syndrome such as respiratory and gastrointestinal tract infections. While these tests simplify ordering for physicians and consolidate testing platforms for the laboratory, they often come at an increased pretest cost per test; further, clinical interpretation of results may be complicated when an unexpected virus is detected or when multiple pathogens are detected in a specimen.[3]

Herein, we discuss the use of currently available qualitative and quantitative nucleic acid amplification and detection methods utilized for the diagnosis and management of patients with viral illnesses (see At a Glance). We also discuss alternative diagnostic methods for infections that are not amenable to diagnosis using molecular methods or those where molecular methods are not well established, standardized, or available to highlight the continued challenges facing laboratory diagnosis of these conditions.

VIRAL INFECTIONS OF THE RESPIRATORY TRACT

Introduction

Respiratory viruses are a taxonomically diverse group of pathogens capable of causing disease within the upper or lower respiratory tract. This group includes influenza, parainfluenza, respiratory syncytial virus (RSV), human metapneumovirus (hMPV), adenovirus, coronavirus, rhinovirus,

---

AT A GLANCE

Considerations for Diagnosis and Monitoring of Select Viral Pathogens

Human Immunodeficiency Virus (HIV)
HIV Fourth-Generation Diagnostic Algorithm:
- Initial diagnostic screening is by the fourth-generation antigen-antibody immunoassay.
- Reactive screens are confirmed by a HIV1/HIV2 antibody differentiation immunoassay.
- Patients with reactive antigen-antibody assays and nonreactive differentiation assays are confirmed by molecular testing.

Influenza
- Most rapid antigen tests for influenza lack sensitivity, particularly in adults.
- Viral culture for influenza is sensitive and specific, though time consuming and technically demanding.
- Molecular testing for influenza is highly sensitive and specific.
- Uniplex or limited multiplex molecular assays (i.e., detect 2–3 targets) may exhibit higher sensitivity for influenza than multiplex syndromic panels.

Hepatitis C Virus (HCV)
- Patients should initially be screened for HCV using serology.
- Negative serologic results should be confirmed with follow-up RNA testing if immunocompromised or acute infection suspected.
- Positive serologic results should be confirmed with follow-up RNA testing.
- If positive serology results do not confirm by RNA testing and HCV infection is still suspected, testing with a different HCV antibody test or repeat molecular testing within 6 months should be considered.

Herpes Simplex Virus (HSV)
HSV meningitis and cerebritis
- HSV is a leading cause of recurrent aseptic meningitis in young adults and can be life threatening in immunocompromised individuals.

- Culture of HSV from cerebrospinal fluid (CSF) in symptomatic patients is 4–20% sensitive and should not be used to rule out HSV involvement.
- Serologic assessment of CSF is of limited utility because of the extended time to detection (1–4 weeks) and propensity for IgM detection during periods of asymptomatic reactivation.
- Qualitative assessment of CSF for HSV is preferred for diagnosis; detection of any viral DNA is abnormal.

Cytomegalovirus (CMV)
Considerations for viral load monitoring:
- A significant change (>0.5–1.0 $\log_{10}$ copies or IU/mL) in consecutive viral load measurements is a better prognostic indicator than a single viral load value.
- Serial viral load measurements should not be conducted more often than once per 5–7 days, viral DNA half-life in blood is 3–8 days.
- When following viral load trends, be sure results were obtained using the same assay and sample type. Interassay variability can range from 0.5 to 1.5 $\log_{10}$ copies/mL.
- Whole blood viral load values are approximately 0.8–1.2 $\log_{10}$ higher than in matched plasma specimens.

Mumps
- In unvaccinated persons, serologic detection of anti-mumps IgM is 80–90% sensitive if specimen is collected greater than 3–5 days from symptom onset.
- In persons who have received the mumps vaccine, serologic detection of anti-mumps IgM is as little as 9–47% sensitive.
- Detection of mumps DNA by nucleic acid amplification test (NAAT) in saliva is greater than 90% sensitive if specimen is collected ≤2 days from symptom onset.
- Collection of blood (serology) and buccal swab (NAAT) is recommended to confirm diagnosis in all patients with compatible signs and symptoms.

enterovirus, and other less common viruses (e.g., human bocavirus). Infections involving the upper respiratory system are often manifested by rhinitis, sinusitis, or pharyngitis, whereas infections involving the lower respiratory tract often result in bronchitis and pneumonia. In North America, the prevalence of both influenza and RSV is the highest during the winter months, including late fall and early spring.[4–7] In contrast, infections with enterovirus exhibit an opposite seasonality, occurring mainly during the summer months.[8] Parainfluenza occurs predominantly in the fall months, with the exception of parainfluenza virus (PIV) 3, which occurs in the summer.[9] Adenovirus and rhinovirus are common causes of respiratory infections throughout the year.[10]

Infections with respiratory viruses are relatively common, even among immunocompetent patients. Influenza often causes fever, upper respiratory symptoms, and occasionally lower respiratory symptoms in immunocompetent hosts. In 2017, influenza was responsible for 55.0 hospitalizations per 100,000 people in the United States and 123.8 per 100,000 globally, with a disproportional preference for elderly patients.[11,12] Influenza is also attributed to an estimated 6% of all outpatient physician visits with the highest incidence among children aged 2 to 17 years.[13] RSV classically causes bronchiolitis, a lower respiratory infection associated with fever, cough, and wheezing most commonly in the pediatric population. Severe infections requiring hospitalization affect an estimated 57,000 to 100,000 children annually in the United States, with an estimated cost of up to $300 million.[6,14] Related mortality rates in children less than 5 years of age surpass those of influenza.[15] PIV is another important respiratory virus in this patient population. Bronchiolitis, croup, and pneumonia resulting from PIV is responsible for approximately 1.1 hospitalizations per 1000 children under the age of 5 annually.[16] Finally, while not as severe as influenza and RSV, mild upper respiratory infections caused by rhinovirus, coronavirus, and enterovirus have a significant impact on immunocompetent populations. The economic burden of these infections is staggering, estimated at approximately $40 billion annually.[17] More than half of these seemingly mild infections are due to rhinovirus, which has been associated with asthma exacerbations, cystic fibrosis exacerbations, chronic obstructive pulmonary disease, and other respiratory complications.[18]

In immunosuppressed patients, illnesses due to respiratory viruses are typically more severe. For example, influenza was more likely to cause severe disease, secondary complications, and prolonged viral shedding in this population.[19] Immunosuppressed patients also exhibited fewer clinical signs of infection, making diagnosis challenging. RSV has been reported to cause severe pneumonia in solid organ and bone marrow transplant (BMT) patients with mortality rates as high as 70%.[20,21] hMPV also appears to disproportionally affect immunosuppressed patients. Specifically, hMPV was found to be the most prevalent respiratory virus causing symptoms in lung transplant recipients.[22] More recent data suggest that this virus is also an important pathogen in children and critically ill adult populations.[23,24] Similarly, adenovirus infections in immunosuppressed hosts can be of high severity resulting in pneumonia, acute respiratory distress syndrome, and occasionally death. Adenovirus has been found to infect 4.9 to 29% of patients following stem cell transplant, often resulting in severe lower respiratory

infections.[25] In lung transplant patients, adenovirus has been associated with significantly higher rejection rates, bronchiolitis obliterans, and increased overall mortality.[26,27]

Influenza Virus

Culture and Antigen Tests for Influenza Virus

Historically, viral culture was commonly utilized for the diagnosis of influenza infection. This approach had moderate sensitivity with the advantage of enabling simultaneous detection of other respiratory viruses. A significant disadvantage of this approach is the need for examination by technologists trained in identifying cytopathic effect (CPE), which is the change induced by viral infection in a cultured cell line. This change can be subtle and difficult to perceive to the untrained eye. When present, CPE typically signifies a positive result and specific morphologic features can suggest a specific viral pathogen. Positive results require 4 days to obtain on average, and additional steps such as hemagglutination or immunostaining are necessary for confirmation and definitive identification of the virus. Rapid cell culture methods utilizing shell vials have been described which enable viral identification in 1 to 3 days; however, these methods remain laborious and require technical expertise.

Antigen-based influenza detection assays address many of the disadvantages associated with viral culture. These assays are available in a variety of formats, ranging from micro-well–based enzyme-linked immunosorbent assays (ELISAs) to lateral flow immunoassays (IAs). Recently developed versions of these tests provide answers within minutes and are commonly referred to as rapid influenza diagnostic tests (RIDTs). The ease of performance has resulted in CLIA "waived" designation for many of these tests, allowing for POC use. Given the rapidity and simplicity of RIDTs, they are commonly used throughout the United States. Following the 2009 H1N1 outbreak, a survey of community hospital laboratories revealed that approximately 84% utilized RIDTs.[28] Despite widespread use, RIDTs have important limitations. Most notable is the low sensitivity, which is dependent on influenza strain but may be only 50 to 80% compared with nucleic acid amplification tests assays (NAATs).[29,30]

Several factors contribute to the comparatively poor sensitivity of RIDTs. First, these tests are highly dependent on the presence of an adequate amount of viral antigen for detection. As such, they perform better in individuals with higher levels of viral replication during infection (i.e., children) than in those with a lower viral burden (i.e., adults).[31] The need for adequate antigen also necessitates proper specimen collection. Nasopharyngeal swabs allow for adequate sampling of infected cells and therefore have a significantly greater sensitivity compared to specimens such as nasal swabs. The efficacy of these assays is also highly dependent upon the antigenic make-up of the influenza virus in circulation in a given year. During the 2009 H1N1 influenza epidemic, RIDTs were found to have estimated sensitivities as low as 40%.[32] Despite variable sensitivity, RIDTs are routinely used to make decisions regarding whether or not to provide treatment for patients with influenza-like illness. During the 2009 H1N1 epidemic it was estimated that approximately 88% of patients with negative RIDTs and symptoms suggesting influenza did not receive treatment.[33] This prompted intervention from the FDA in the form of mandated minimal performance criteria for RIDTs prior to marketing and a reclassification from Class I in vitro devices (IVDs) to Class II IVDs with special controls.[34] During clinical trials, the analytical performance characteristics of RIDTs must now be compared to either culture or molecular methods. The sensitivity when compared to culture must be at least 90% for influenza A and 80% for influenza B. When compared to molecular methods, the sensitivity for both influenza A and influenza B should be a minimum of 80%. Additionally, assay performance must be reassessed annually by the device manufacturer to assess the ability to detect currently circulating strains.

NAATs for Influenza and RSV

The adoption of molecular testing represents a significant breakthrough for influenza diagnostics (see Chapter 67 for additional discussion). Many available molecular tests have sensitivities comparable to culture with the added advantage of providing same-day results.[35] The dominant technology employed by molecular influenza diagnostics is real-time polymerase chain reaction (PCR) (RT-PCR) (for additional discussion on this technique, refer to Chapter 64). Since the virus has a segmented RNA genome, each RT-PCR assay must include a reverse transcription step to generate a complementary DNA (cDNA) template prior to target amplification and detection. A comprehensive list of FDA-cleared molecular influenza diagnostics is available at https://www.fda.gov/medical-devices/vitro-diagnostics/nucleic-acid-based-tests.[36] At the time of preparation of this chapter, 28 molecular tests for influenza have attained FDA-cleared status. These assays are available in different formats, which impact laboratory workflow and utility. Uniplex assays designed to detect influenza without differentiating type A from B impede selection of appropriate antiviral therapy since influenza B is universally resistant to the antivirals amantadine and rimantadine.[37,38] The inability to subtype influenza A may also limit the utility of these assays. This was best illustrated during the 2009 H1N1 influenza epidemic when it was revealed that a significant portion of the seasonal H1N1 viruses were oseltamivir resistant, while the 2009 H1N1 strain retained greater than 99% susceptibility.[39] Multiplexed PCR assays such as the Cepheid Xpert Flu and Prodesse ProFLU + assay are capable of differentiating influenza A and influenza B, as well as performing limited subtyping of influenza A.[40]

An important enhancement to recently developed influenza molecular assays is the simultaneous testing of RSV, which has a similar seasonal and symptomatic pattern to influenza. Although RSV has historically been associated primarily with disease in young children, the virus is now recognized as an important cause of respiratory disease in older adults (177,000 hospitalizations, 14,000 deaths annually in the United States).[6] The Simplexa Flu A/B & RSV Direct assay (DiaSorin) and the Xpert Flu/RSV assay (Cepheid) both detect and differentiate influenza A and B and RSV simultaneously using multiplex PCR while maintaining high sensitivity for each target.[41–43] Recently, simplification of diagnostic platforms has resulted in the development of CLIA-waived molecular influenza assays such as the Roche Cobas Liat Influenza A/B and Abbott ID NOW Influenza A & B 2 assays. The Liat Influenza A/B is performed in a closed system, provides results within 20 minutes, and demonstrates a 99.2% sensitivity compared to previously existing molecular methods.[44] The Abbott ID NOW Influenza A & B 2 is a similar molecular test designed for near POC use with sensitivity and

specificity of greater than 95 and 100%, respectively, when compared to currently available molecular tests.[45] The appeal of these assays is the combination of the speed and ease of use of RIDTs with the sensitivity of molecular methods.

The positive impact of these waived molecular tests on patient care has been well documented. Martinot and colleagues demonstrated reduced time to antiviral administration, a decrease in antibacterial utilization, and a shortened length of stay in the emergency department following implementation of the Abbott ID NOW test,[46] while Benirschke and colleagues demonstrated a similar positive impact to clinical care following implementation of the Roche LIAT Influenza A/B assay in an urgent care setting.[47] Despite the advantages of POC molecular testing, introduction of molecular testing into the POC environment necessitates careful consideration. Molecular methodologies are attractive due to their high analytical sensitivity, an attribute that also makes them more susceptible to environmental contamination than less sensitive antigen tests. Moving molecular testing from controlled laboratory environments into relatively chaotic settings, such as primary care offices or emergency departments, requires careful education regarding molecular techniques and the adoption of practices to detect and prevent environmental contamination. These risks were addressed in 2019 by the College of American Pathologists (CAP) when the adoption of specific mitigation and monitoring strategies became a formal requirement for CAP-accredited laboratories that employ CLIA-waived testing methods.

Diagnostic Tests for Other Common Respiratory Viruses

Culture has historically been considered the gold standard for the diagnosis of other respiratory viruses and shares many of the same advantages and disadvantages previously discussed for influenza culture.[48–50]

Similar to influenza and RSV, molecular methods are being used more frequently to identify other respiratory viruses due to their decreased TAT and high sensitivity. In contrast to influenza and RSV, commercially available assays for the detection of other respiratory viruses are more limited.[51] As a result, many laboratory-developed tests (LDTs) that detect one or several of these pathogens have been described. These tests are often multiplexed to simultaneously detect rhinovirus, PIV, hMPV, and various other respiratory viruses.[52–54] The development and maintenance of such assays can be challenging. Differences in primer and probe design, as well as nucleic acid extraction techniques can drastically affect assay sensitivity.[51] Additionally, while many FDA-cleared assays are designed to be "moderate complexity" sample-to-answer tests, LDTs are highly complex and require separate extraction, amplification, and detection steps. The implementation and use of laboratory-developed molecular assays also requires a degree of technical expertise which may not be present in every clinical laboratory.

The introduction of highly multiplexed FDA-cleared molecular assays has made testing for common and uncommon respiratory pathogens more accessible to clinical laboratories. Currently, four test platforms (and their later iterations) are FDA-cleared for the detection and differentiation of greater than 10 respiratory viral pathogens.[36] These assays come in various formats requiring different workflows. The Luminex xTAG RVP multiplex assay (Luminex, Austin, TX) uses an initial multiplex PCR to amplify numerous viral targets followed by target identification using a fluorescent-labeled bead array sorted by flow cytometry.[55–57] A later version of the test, the Luminex xTAG RVP Fast, boasts a more rapid TAT but does not detect PIV or differentiate RSV A and B.[56] The GenMark eSensor RVP (GenMark, Carlsbad, CA) is similar to the Luminex xTAG RVP in that it initially employs a multiplex PCR to amplify numerous viral targets. Targets are then sorted and identified using capture and signal probes coupled to ferrocene labels and gold electrodes arranged in a microarray. Target binding is detected using voltammetry as a current is applied to each electrode.[58–60] A potential disadvantage of both of these assays is the need for an initial "off-line" end-point PCR step followed by a manual transfer of the amplified product to a second analyzer for target detection. This approach increases the total hands-on time, time to result, and creates the potential for amplicon contamination. These weaknesses have been addressed by more recent iterations of these assays. An updated version of the Luminex platform, the NxTAG RVP, enables streamlined processing of previously extracted nucleic acid without the need for amplified DNA handling. This assay was cleared by the FDA for nasopharyngeal swab testing in 2015. Initial evaluation of this assay demonstrated overall robust performance and simplified workflow; however, the authors noted a sensitivity of 66% for select Coronavirus types OC43 and NL63.[61]

The BioFire FilmArray (BioFire Diagnostics, Salt Lake City, UT) and Luminex Verigene systems are also highly multiplexed but are designed to be sample-to-answer assays, eliminating the need to manipulate extracted or amplified DNA products. The FilmArray incorporates nucleic acid extraction, nested PCR, and target detection using SYBR Green fluorescence into a single-use enclosed test pouch.[41,59,62] Target-specific primers are separated into an array of microwells allowing for the discernment of specific targets. Similarly, the Verigene system employs multiplex PCR for target amplification but uses a standard microarray-based approach involving immobilized capture probes for detection of target amplicon. Sensitivity is maximized through signal amplification using gold nanoparticle-conjugated detection probes thus allowing for visualization by a separate automated array reader.[63,64] Several studies comparing the accuracy and efficacy of all four of these systems have been conducted.[59,64,65] A large comparative study of the eSensor, FilmArray, and xTAG systems revealed differences in sensitivities for individual targets, most notably for influenza A/B and adenovirus.[66]

A significant advantage of large, multiplexed panels is the ability to test for many different viruses with overlapping symptomatology. This allows for providers to order a single test for patients who present with respiratory symptoms, a process referred to as "syndromic testing." Since providers do not have to individually order testing for each specific pathogen, they are more likely to detect pathogens they did not previously suspect. This can be useful in patient populations such as the immunosuppressed who are at high risk for serious respiratory infections from a wide range of pathogens. The detection of unexpected pathogens can also be a double-edged sword. If there is a low pretest probability for a particular diagnosis, false positive results will contribute to a poor positive predictive value (PPV) and may be a distractor from the patient's more acute pathologic process. Additionally, many of the targets present on multiplex panels are not

clinically actionable since pharmacologic therapy is only available for a minority of respiratory viruses. Given the added price of multiplex tests, patients not at risk for severe disease may be better served by symptom management/supportive care rather than an expensive diagnostic test. One potential approach is to reserve syndromic testing for immunosuppressed patients who are at a higher risk for severe infection by several respiratory viruses or immunocompetent patients presenting in acute respiratory distress. This approach requires flexibility in testing that is currently being integrated into some of the existing multiplex tests. The most updated version of the Verigene assay, the FDA cleared Verigene RP *Flex* assay, allows for selective ordering and reporting of a panel of 16 respiratory pathogens. At the time of this writing, data regarding the performance of this assay are unavailable.[65]

Diagnostic Tests for Emerging Respiratory Viruses

Over the past decade, several respiratory viruses have been identified as important public health concerns due to their disease severity and their potential for epidemic and pandemic spread. Extreme caution should be used when manipulating specimens from patients with suspected highly pathogenic respiratory viruses. In general, culture of these viruses should not be attempted, and testing should be deferred to specialized laboratories with the appropriate biocontainment facilities. As such, local and national reference laboratories should always be consulted when testing for any of the following pathogens is warranted.

Avian influenza A (H5N1) first emerged in 1997 as a potentially fatal human pathogen.[67] At this time, virus transmission from poultry was responsible for 18 human infections in Hong Kong leading to 6 deaths.[37] Since then, sporadic human infections have been reported in Africa, Asia, Europe, and the Middle East, often in association with zoonotic transmission from birds.[68,69] In 2013 another avian influenza type A strain (H7N9) was observed to be a cause of human infection in China.[70] Since these initial reports, there have been greater than 600 cases predominantly in Eastern China.[71–73] Preferred specimens for testing are nasopharyngeal swabs or aspirates.[73] The analytical sensitivity of RIDTs for the detection of avian influenza A (H5N1) and (H7N9) has been shown to be very low by several studies, requiring at least a 10^4 median tissue culture infective dose ($TCID_{50}$) for positivity.[74,75] Conventionally used FDA approved molecular diagnostics for influenza have not been thoroughly evaluated for the detection of either avian influenza A (H5N1) or (H7N9). While some of these molecular tests may fail to detect virus, others may identify these viruses as influenza A (nontypeable).[72]

In 2014, enterovirus D68 (EV-D68) was identified as the cause of severe respiratory symptoms including wheezing and shortness of breath in a cohort of children from the Midwestern United States.[76] This virus was initially described in 1962 and had previously been associated with sporadic outbreaks of respiratory illnesses throughout the world.[77,78] The 2014 outbreak in the United States lasted 4 months and affected approximately 1152 people in 49 states.[79] In addition to severe respiratory symptoms, neurologic sequelae such as flaccid paralysis similar to that seen in polio were later described in a small proportion of the affected patients.[80] Subsequently, outbreaks of acute flaccid paralysis associated with EV-D68 have been identified in late summer to fall in a biannual pattern (e.g., 2014, 2016, and 2018). While EV-D68 is not identified to subtype by any commercial assay, affected patients notably tested positive for "Rhinovirus/Enterovirus" using the BioFire FilmArray Respiratory Panel.[81] The preferred specimens for testing are nasopharyngeal, oropharyngeal, or other upper respiratory specimens.[82]

Finally, members of the coronavirus family have also emerged from zoonotic reservoirs to become highly pathogenic human viruses. In 2003 a coronavirus was found to be responsible for an international outbreak of patients afflicted with severe acute respiratory syndrome (SARS).[83] The implicated virus, now referred to as SARS-CoV (SARS associated coronavirus), was acquired by humans from horseshoe bats.[84] A second coronavirus, MERs-CoV (Middle Eastern Respiratory Syndrome associated coronavirus), emerged in Saudi Arabia in 2012.[75] Both viruses cause severe respiratory illness with associated mortality of 30 to 40%.[75] Multiple specimens should be submitted from upper and lower respiratory sites in order to enhance diagnostic sensitivity. A RT-PCR assay has been developed by the CDC and is currently available at most state laboratories.[75,82] In 2019, a third highly pathogenic coronavirus emerged in Wuhan, China. Although initial data regarding this virus suggest a mortality of approximately 4%, these data also suggest this virus results in an increased need for ICU care and is readily transmissible in health care settings.[85] Unlike the previous two zoonotic coronaviruses (SARS-CoV and MERS-CoV), efficient human-to-human transmission of SARS-CoV-2 has resulted in a global pandemic. Epidemiology and diagnostic approaches for SARS-CoV-2 are discussed in detail in the following section.

Severe Acute Respiratory Syndrome-related Coronavirus-2 (SARS-CoV-2)
Epidemiology of SARS-CoV-2
Severe acute respiratory syndrome coronavirus-2 (SARS-CoV-2) is a member of the *Coronaviridae* family of enveloped RNA viruses, further classified as genus *Betacoronavirus* and subgenus Sarbecovirus. Taxonomically it shares greater than 96% genome sequence identity with a coronavirus of bat origin and while not a direct descendant, also clusters closely with 2003 SARS-CoV.[86,87] Human infections with SARS-CoV-2 were initially identified in Wuhan, China in December 2019 and rapidly spread via human-to-human transmission to every continent except Antarctica, accounting for greater than 30 million infections and over one million deaths in the ensuing months (https://coronavirus.jhu.edu/map.html, accessed October 2020). The clinical presentation of patients infected with SARS-CoV-2 can range from asymptomatic to severe acute respiratory distress with multi-organ failure. Patient-specific factors including age greater than 60, underlying cardiovascular disease, and diabetes have been associated with increased risk of severe disease and mortality; however, severe symptoms requiring hospitalization, respiratory support, and mortality have been reported in immunocompetent individuals of all ages. The primary route of transmission is via respiratory droplets or aerosols. SARS-CoV-2 RNA is rarely detected in blood or urine of acutely ill individuals but can be present at a high concentration in stool, though there is little evidence to support transmission via fecal-oral route.[88,89]

Diagnostic Approaches for SARS-CoV-2
There are multiple diagnostic approaches to identify patients with acute symptomatic or asymptomatic infection including viral culture, NAATs including reverse transcriptase PCR (RT-PCR), and rapid antigen detection tests (RADTs). These methods have been applied to various upper and lower respiratory specimen types including nasopharyngeal swab, nasal swab, throat swab, saliva, sputum, and bronchioalveolar lavage (BAL) fluid. In addition, serologic tests capable of detecting SARS-CoV-2 specific IgG, IgM, IgA, and total antibody have been developed to assess prior exposure to the virus. It is critical to recognize the differences in performance and optimal utility to correctly interpret test results.

Direct detection methods. SARS-CoV-2 can be cultured from clinical specimens using routine methods and forms visible plaques in VeroE6 and Vero CCL81 cells within 2 to 3 days of inoculation.[90] While useful in studying the basic biology of the virus, viral culture requires biosafety level-3 (BSL-3) safety precautions and is not recommended for routine diagnosis. Further, the sensitivity of culture methods may be inferior to NAATs as indicated by an inability to recover virus from respiratory specimens with less than 10^4 RNA copies/mL.[88]

RADTs are an inexpensive and direct method to detect the presence of SARS-CoV-2 in clinical specimens. These tests are simple-to-use lateral flow assays that can be read either visually, based on the appearance of colored indicator lines, or automatically, using a simple device to detect a fluorescent signal. At the time of writing, five such assays have received emergency use authorization (EUA) by the FDA. A major benefit of these tests is the ability to deploy them outside of a high-complexity laboratory, at or near the POC to rapidly identify persons with SARS-CoV-2 infection. Importantly, these tests have generally been approved for use in symptomatic patients within 1 week of symptom onset when viral load (VL) is the highest to maximize sensitivity. An independent clinical evaluation of two RADTs (BD Veritor, Becton, Dickinson and Co., Sparks, MD and Sofia 2, Quidel Corp., San Diego, CA) demonstrated approximately 80 to 85% sensitivity compared to a PCR-based test for SARS-CoV-2 in nasal specimens collected from patients less than 7 days from symptom onset.[91] Importantly, the performance of these tests has not been evaluated when used as a screening test in asymptomatic populations where VL (and thus sensitivity) may be lower. A commercially available RADT without EUA designation found the test to be 3 $\log_{10}$ less sensitive than viral culture and 5 $\log_{10}$ less sensitive than PCR in analytic limit of detection (LoD) analysis.[92] Because of potential shortcomings in sensitivity, the CDC and WHO recommend that negative results in symptomatic patients be considered presumptive and confirmed by a PCR-based test to rule out infection.[93,94] Conversely, if used to screen asymptomatic individuals (an off-label application), positive results may require PCR confirmation in low-incidence populations.

NAATs provide the most sensitive method for direct detection of SARS-CoV-2 in clinical specimens and are considered the "gold standard" method for detection of SARS-CoV-2 and diagnosis of Coronavirus Infectious Disease 2019 (COVID-19). Approximately 6 months following the first reported transmission in the United States, greater than 200 different NAATs were made commercially available through the FDA EUA regulatory pathway. This includes high-complexity batched testing platforms, moderate complexity sample-to-answer platforms, and "rapid" POC tests. The absolute sensitivity of these NAATs is difficult to ascertain due to lack of true "gold standard" and is likely influenced by multiple factors including specimen type, collection method, and test design (e.g., genomic target, detection chemistry, etc.). The majority of available tests are designed to detect two or three distinct genomic targets specific to SARS-CoV-2 and/or are conserved among the subgenus *Sarbecovirus* which includes 2003 SARS-CoV and other nonhuman SARS-CoVs. The goal of utilizing multiple assay targets is to increase sensitivity and provide redundancy to insulate against the impact of potential viral mutation events on test performance. However, in instances for which solely pan-*Sarbecovirus* targets are detected, results are typically considered preliminarily positive given the possibility of cross-reactivity with other viruses in the family. Multiple split-sample studies have compared the performance of available laboratory-based RT-PCR tests and report 96 to 100% positive agreement (i.e., sensitivity) among these tests based on consensus result.[95–98] A rapid isothermal amplification test has been designed for use at the POC and delivers a result in as little as 5 minutes; however, reduced sensitivity of 75 to 90% has been reported compared to "traditional" laboratory-based RT-PCR assays.[96,99,100] This difference in sensitivity is likely due to a difference in the LoD between laboratory-based RT-PCR tests (39 to 779 copies/mL) and the POC test (3000 to 20,000 copies/mL).[96,98,100]

The sensitivity of NAATs can also be influenced by the type of specimen analyzed and when in the course of infection the specimen is collected. Among upper respiratory specimens, nasopharyngeal, throat, saliva, and anterior nares have all been evaluated. A limited number of studies have directly compared the sensitivity of viral detection in each specimen type. Results appear to support similar statistical performance among most specimen types with slightly higher sensitivity observed in NP than throat.[89,101,102] Viral RNA may be detected as early as 1 week prior to symptom onset, but typically peaks at or near the time of recognized symptoms. Following symptom onset, the VL begins to decrease in all respiratory specimens but remains detectable in lower respiratory specimens such as sputum or BAL significantly longer than upper respiratory specimens such as nasal or nasopharyngeal swabs.[88,103] In addition, positive BAL specimens have been reported in symptomatic and immunocompromised patients with negative NP or throat results.[104] Therefore consideration may be given to testing a lower respiratory specimen in patients with compatible symptoms and a negative NP or nares result. Importantly, persistence in the lower respiratory tract is frequently at less than 10^4 copies/mL, which as mentioned above correlates with a failure to recover virus in culture. The significance of long-term, low-level persistence as it related to risk of relapse or transmission is currently unclear.

Indirect detection methods. The use of serologic methods to indirectly detect individuals who are currently infected or have been exposed to SARS-CoV-2 has been widely explored. Multiple technologies including highly automated laboratory-based IAs and POC "rapid" lateral flow tests are commercially available and have obtained EUA status from the US FDA (https://www.fda.gov/medical-devices/emergency-situations-medical-devices/eua-authorized-serology-test-performance, accessed June 29, 2020). These assays most commonly utilize purified viral nucleocapsid or spike proteins to detect the presence of one or more antibody classes (e.g., IgG, IgM, IgA, total antibody). The sensitivity of these assays ranges from approximately 75% to greater than 99%, with reported specificities of approximately 90% to greater than 99%. The sensitivity of serologic tests is dependent on the time from exposure to the virus, known as the "diagnostic window." For SARS-CoV-2, the development of specific IgM and IgG class antibodies appears to occur nearly simultaneously, with 95% of individuals generating a detectable antibody response by 14 days postexposure, and essentially 100% by 21 days postexposure.[103,105,106] This response reaches a plateau within 1 week of detection and then both IgG and IgM titers begin to decline. The decline in IgG titer is less abrupt than IgM; however, at this point it is not clear how long antibody remains detectable after initial exposure. Cross-reactivity with the four "human coronaviruses" appears to be negligible for most commercially available assays, though this may vary based on assay design.[106]

The utility and interpretation of serologic results remains in question. As of time of writing, the seroprevalence in much of the world is likely 1 to 5%. This low prevalence renders even the most specific serologic assays a PPV as low as 80%. Further, the extent and duration of protective immunity correlated with a positive serologic result has not been established. Therefore the current utility of serologic assays lies primarily in the epidemiologic assessment of exposure to SARS-CoV-2 in various populations, which may be used to guide RT-PCR based screening strategies, and in retrospective diagnosis of late-stage infections (>2 weeks after symptom onset) when direct detection tests including RT-PCR may have converted to negative.

POINTS TO REMEMBER
Respiratory Viruses

- Influenza and RSV are the most common causes of severe respiratory disease in healthy populations.
- Respiratory viral culture is time consuming, technically demanding, and no longer commonly used.
- Influenza rapid antigen tests have poor sensitivity and should not be used to rule out infection.
- Molecular assays are the primary method used for the diagnosis of respiratory pathogens and range from uniplex to massively multiplexed (>20 targets).
- Testing for highly pathogenic emerging respiratory viruses, including MERS-CoV and pandemic influenza, should be coordinated with local and national reference laboratories.

VIRAL INFECTIONS IN IMMUNOCOMPROMISED POPULATIONS

Introduction

Viruses are the most common cause of infectious disease in humans. The vast majority of viral infections are self-limited or asymptomatic in persons with normal immune function and do not require medical intervention. In contrast, these same agents can cause devastating disease in persons with impaired immune function resulting from genetic disorders, infectious agents such as HIV, hematologic malignancies, or iatrogenic immunosuppression following hematopoietic or SOT. Severe viral syndromes in these populations can result from primary infection or reactivation of viruses that have established lifelong latency following initial infection, notably the herpesviruses and polyomaviruses. Reactivation of these latent viruses may include intermittent and asymptomatic shedding of virus in bodily fluids, or symptomatic illness ranging from mild fever and rash to superficial lesions to fulminant multiorgan or systemic disease. Presentation and course can be impacted by the immune status of the host and site of viral latency. Therefore several diagnostic approaches are necessary to aid in differentiating active versus latent infection status, to monitor disease progression, identify potential antiviral resistance, and to stratify risk of severe disease when considering immunosuppressive therapy or evaluating potential transplant candidates.

Herpesviruses

Cytomegalovirus

CMV, also known as human herpes virus 5 (HHV-5), is an obligate human pathogen and member of the *Betaherpesviridae* subfamily. Seroprevalence of CMV increases with age and is reported to be 50 to 80% by midlife; however, this can approach 100% in specific populations.[107,108] CMV is capable of infecting and replicating within a broad range of human tissues and cell types including differentiated epithelial, endothelial, parenchymal, smooth muscle, lymphoid, and myeloid cells.[109,110] Following primary infection, CMV establishes a lifelong association with its host, existing as an episomal circularized genome within undifferentiated cells primarily of myeloid lineage.[110,111] In healthy individuals, latent, non-replicating CMV can be found in $1:10^4$ to $1:10^5$ circulating monocytes. Normal physiologic processes including cellular differentiation and immune response to infections can trigger asymptomatic viral reactivation and shedding of infective virions in nearly all bodily fluids (e.g., blood, urine, saliva, stool, semen, breast milk).[109,110] Specifically, intermittent shedding of CMV in saliva has been reported in 1 to 2% of asymptomatic immunocompetent adults and in up to 46% of asymptomatic HIV-positive patients.[112,113] Additionally, CMV can be transmitted in utero resulting in congenital CMV disease which can result in mortality or cause immediate or progressive hearing, visual, and mental deficits.[114,115]

The majority of CMV infections in the immunocompetent host are mild and self-resolving and go unnoticed or unreported.[116] In contrast, primary infection or reactivation of latent virus can cause devastating illness in an immunocompromised host. Specific syndromes include pneumonitis, colitis, retinitis, meningitis, and systemic viral sepsis. The risk of CMV disease is highest in individuals with advanced HIV/AIDS and in patients undergoing immunosuppressive therapies following SOT or hematopoietic stem cell transplant (HSCT). Rates can be 8 to 41% following SOT or HSCT, with the highest incidence seen in heart and lung transplant patients.[117–119] Among opportunistic infections, the presence or absence of CMV disease is a leading factor in successful transplantation and survival.[120]

Laboratory approaches for the diagnosis and monitoring of CMV disease include serologic, nucleic acid-based, and antigen-based approaches. Serologic tests provide indirect evidence of exposure to CMV but are not used for diagnosis or monitoring of active disease. In contrast, direct detection methods such as PCR or viral antigen tests provide methods to detect and monitor active disease. Measurement of CMV antigenemia based on the quantification of CMV structural protein pp65 was an early approach to quantify the amount of actively replicating virus in circulation.[121,122] This approach was beneficial in monitoring patients for viral relapse, but quantification lacked standardization and assays were technically demanding to conduct. Subsequently, quantitative NAATs have been developed that offer a comparatively simplified workflow, standardization to an international scale, and increased sensitivity.

Serologic tests for CMV. Serologic tests hold no utility for the diagnosis or monitoring of CMV disease. The titer of anti-CMV IgG is not correlated with active disease, and anti-CMV IgM is commonly associated with episodes of asymptomatic viral reactivation.[107] The chief utility of CMV serology is to establish the serostatus of two specific populations: women, as part of a prenatal or perinatal screen, and potential donors and recipients prior to SOT or HSCT. The presence of CMV-specific IgG and IgM is determined using enzyme immunoassays (EIAs), chemiluminescent immunoassays (CIA), or indirect immunofluorescence assays (IFAs). For transplant patients determination of serostatus aids in stratifying risk and severity of potential CMV disease, and also guides dose and duration of antiviral therapy following transplant.[123] In one study, donor positive/recipient negative (D+/R−) transplant carried a 19 to 31% risk of subsequent CMV disease compared with only 2 to 3% risk in D-/R− transplants.[124] Extension of antiviral prophylaxis in D+/R− organ recipients may reduce the incidence of late onset CMV disease.[125]

Beyond establishment of serostatus, differentiation between primary and past infection holds prognostic implications for the risk of congenital CMV disease. The presence of anti-CMV IgM should not be independently interpreted as evidence of primary infection due to long-term persistence (6 to 9 months) following primary infection, presence during episodes of viral reactivation, and cross-reactivity with other *Herpesviridae*[126]; however, absence of IgM effectively rules out recent infection.[126,127] Anti-CMV IgG avidity testing can be used to distinguish primary from past infection in women with dual positive IgG and IgM results. The presence of high avidity IgG is an indication that primary infection occurred 18 to 20 weeks prior to testing, that is, past infection[127] and is associated with a 1 to 2% risk of congenital CMV infection compared with a risk of 12 to 75% in women with low avidity IgG.[127,128] Despite these prognostic implications, routine serologic screening of pregnant women for CMV is not currently recommended due to the remaining potential for congenital infection, regardless of maternal immune status, and lack of therapeutic intervention to prevent congenital transmission.[129] IgG avidity testing has also been used as a prognostic tool in post-transplant patients. In this group, failure to develop high avidity antibodies following primary infection may be associated with increased risk for severe CMV infection or organ rejection.[130,131] Several ELISA-based CMV IgG avidity tests are commercially available; however, none have received FDA clearance to date.[132] Laboratories that offer testing must conduct internal assay validation studies and may establish different thresholds to define high and low avidity results which contributes to variability in analytic and prognostic performance of these assays. Therefore results must be interpreted in the context of other laboratory and clinical findings.

Qualitative NAATs for CMV. Qualitative NAATs are used to aid in diagnosis of localized infections such as pneumonia, retinitis, meningitis, gastrointestinal, or other "end organ disease." Potential specimens include tissue biopsy, bronchoalveolar lavage (BAL), cerebrospinal fluid (CSF), and vitreous fluid. Direct detection of CMV in these specimens is important because 50 and 70% of patients with end organ disease have undetectable CMV in whole blood (WB) or plasma specimens.[133–136] The high sensitivity and negative predictive value (NPV) of qualitative NAATs can be used to essentially rule out active CMV infection in cases of presumed CMV pneumonitis, retinitis, or gastrointestinal disease.[136–138] Conversely, a positive result should not be used to define "proven infection" due to an inability to differentiate asymptomatic shedding from end organ disease.[139] While higher VLs have been associated with increased specificity for disease, specimen heterogeneity and a lack of assay standardization has precluded the development of reliable quantitative thresholds to define active infection. Therefore all positive results obtained from fluids and tissues should be confirmed by a more specific method such as histologic examination and must be correlated with clinical symptoms to support a probable diagnosis of CMV disease.[137–139]

There are currently no FDA-approved qualitative CMV NAATs, but several tests are commercially available as analyte specific reagents (ASRs) or have received CE marking for use in the European Union (Table 89.1). An evaluation of five of these NAATs, as well as an LDT, was conducted using 200 prospectively collected clinical samples representing respiratory, urine, CSF, biopsy tissue, and other clinical specimens.[140] The analytic LoD ranged from 10^2 to 10^3 copies/mL for all six tests. The clinical sensitivity of 5 of 6 assays was 100%, with one of the assays demonstrating only 89% (41/46) sensitivity for detection of CMV in the clinical specimens. These data support the utility of qualitative NAATs as a high-sensitivity screen for the presence of CMV in various specimen types and an effective method to rule out CMV as the etiologic agent in these cases.

Quantitative NAATs for CMV. An important factor in predicting and monitoring CMV disease is the change in blood or plasma VL. Rapid changes in VL are prognostic for stratifying risk of disease and severity of symptoms.[146,147] Results of VL tests also impact decisions to initiate or discontinue therapy and aid in early recognition of antiviral resistance.[148–150] Therefore the use of quantitative NAAT is recommended by several national and international guidelines as an important component in patient management.[120,149]

The type of specimen tested impacts test sensitivity and the quantitative CMV VL value obtained, which in turn affects the interpretation of results. Assays using WB quantify latent, cell-associated virus in addition to infective extracellular virions. Therefore WB-based assays are more sensitive for the qualitative detection of CMV, and quantitative VL values are approximately 0.8 to 1.2 log higher than matched plasma specimens, albeit with a poor correlation coefficient (r^2 value, 0.19 to 0.79).[151–153] Importantly, the increased sensitivity of WB assays has not demonstrated a prognostic advantage for determination of CMV disease compared to plasma-based tests.[145,152] The rate of virologic recurrence was similar in patients with undetectable VL in matched WB and plasma (23.6%) as it was in patients with a quantifiable VL in WB and CMV negative plasma (23.1%), owing to the detection of latent inactive virus in WB specimens.[152]

Increasing analytical sensitivity of quantitative NAATs has lowered the threshold of detection to as few as 6 to 150 copies/mL in WB or plasma specimens.[151,154] At these low levels of detection, the presence of cell-associated virus or free viral DNA may contribute to a detectable VL, even following effective antiviral treatment. This is supported by the finding of detectable VL in both WB (~70%) and plasma (~48 to 59%) specimens in asymptomatic patients.[152,155] These data suggest that even when using plasma, a low VL does not indicate a risk of CMV disease. Further, the inability to achieve an undetectable VL can result in unnecessary antiviral therapy and increase the risk of resistance if a "treat to negative" paradigm is used.[120,156]

Absolute quantitative VL thresholds ranging from 1000 to 10,000 CMV copies/mL have been evaluated as clinical decision points to define active infection and drive initiation or discontinuation of antiviral therapy.[145,147,157] Unfortunately, the establishment of a single reliable threshold to predict disease has been hindered by a lack of standardization among commercially available and laboratory developed tests, including the use of different calibration materials, which causes interassay variability of 0.5 to 2.0 $\log_{10}$ copies/mL.[158]

A significant step toward standardization of CMV VL testing was made with the introduction of an international standard by the World Health Organization (WHO) in 2010. This allows laboratories to calibrate VL results to a single international unit (IU) standard regardless of which test is being used, thereby enabling a more accurate comparison of viremia values across institutions. Standardized IVD assays can

TABLE 89.1 Characteristics of Cytomegalovirus Direct Detection Assays

	Target	TAT	Test Platforms	Sensitivity (%)	Specificity (%)	Reference
Culture	CMV		Routine, Shell vials	8–48	99–100	135, 141
Antigenemia	pp65 tegument protein	2–6 h	None	38–100	55–99	135, 142–145
Qualitative NAAT						
Leukocytes			LDT	94	50	144
CSF, urine, tissue, BAL, throat swab	Varies by assay	1–3 h	ASR or CE-Mark; EraGen Multicode, Liaison MDX, Elitech MGB Alert, Roche CMV ASRs, Abbott CMV	89–100	97–100	140

ASRs, Analyte-specific reagents; *BAL,* bronchioalveolar lavage; *CMV,* cytomegalovirus; *CSF,* cerebrospinal fluid; *LDT,* laboratory-developed test; *NAAT,* nucleic acid amplification test; *TAT,* turn-around time.

achieve precision within as little as 0.1 $\log_{10}$ copies/mL, which may be less variation than what is observed biologically during chronic infection.[155] Specifically, a multicenter study of an FDA-cleared plasma-based NAAT calibrated to the IU standard demonstrated a narrow 95% confidence interval (CI) of 0.14 to 0.17 $\log_{10}$ copies/mL for specimens tested across five different laboratories.[158] However, a comparison of ten different CMV NAATs, all calibrated to IU, demonstrated a variance of up to 2.8 $\log_{10}$ IU/mL among clinical specimens analyzed by each assay, with over 40% of specimens giving values greater than 0.5 $\log_{10}$ IU/mL from the mean.[154] Further, the use of IU will not allow for interchangeable comparison of values obtained from different specimen types such WB and plasma. These data demonstrate that even when using a standardized calibrator and reporting results as IU/mL, assay-specific factors including the use of different specimen types, CMV gene targets, cycling conditions, and nucleic acid extraction methods can cause significant inter-assay variability. Taken together, these data underscore the difficulty in obtaining commutable VL results across different laboratories and the barriers to development of a "global" CMV VL threshold for use as a clinical decision point. Until these variables can be addressed, serial VL monitoring for preemptive therapy or identification of therapy failure should be conducted by the same laboratory to avoid potentially misleading results.[159]

An alternative approach to absolute VL thresholds is the observation of change in VL values over time. Several studies have demonstrated that a significant or rapid change in VL is a better prognostic indicator than a single value, especially when the VL is relatively low (10^2 to 10^3 copies/mL) where higher variability in assay results are expected.[135,146,147] CMV replication kinetics or "doubling time" (T_d) has been used to stratify the risk of disease and necessity of antiviral therapy following transplant.[146,160] No definitive T_d threshold exists; however, one study found that use of a T_d less than 2 days as criteria for initiation of therapy was associated with significantly fewer days of viremia and antiviral therapy compared with the use of a VL threshold of 1000 copies/mL.[160] While effective, this approach requires frequent (2- to 3-day interval) collection of specimens which may be inconvenient or impractical for outpatients. Importantly, once antiviral therapy has been initiated serial CMV VL tests should be conducted no more frequently than once per 5 to 7 days since the half-life of CMV DNA in blood is 3 to 8 days.[161] Further, an increase in VL can be expected within 72 h of initiation of antiviral therapy in some patients and is not indicative of therapy failure.[162]

Current assays that have attained FDA and CE regulatory status for IVD use include the Qiagen artus CMV RGQ MDx, the Roche COBAS AmpliPrep/COBAS TaqMan CMV test, and the Roche COBAS CMV test (run on cobas 6800 or 8800 systems). These assays all contain internal quantitative controls calibrated to the IU standard and are indicated for use only with plasma specimens. Each system includes automated nucleic acid extraction followed by RT-PCR amplification and detection of target DNA. The assays have an LoD of 34 to 91 IU/mL and a linear range of ~10^2 to 10^7 IU/mL. Additional quantitative CMV assays that have attained CE Mark or are commercially available as ASRs for the development of LDTs are available for use on various real-time PCR platforms and demonstrate similar limits of detection and quantification to

FDA-cleared tests.[154] However, the use of different extraction methods, thermocyclers, and calibration materials can contribute to variability of VL results. Therefore regardless of assay, it is important to establish a baseline VL for patients entering a health care system or for those with VL results received from a different laboratory.

Antiviral resistance testing in CMV. Antiviral treatment or prophylaxis plays an integral role in the management of patients at risk for CMV infection and disease. The gold standard method to assess antiviral susceptibility involves observation of viral plaques or CPE in cultured cell lines in the presence of increasing concentration of an antiviral agent. This phenotypic method has the advantage of determining a specific inhibitory concentration for an antiviral and is independent of specific resistance mechanisms.[163] The major drawbacks to this approach are the technical expertise required to carry out viral culture, the requirement for isolated virus, and the incubation time necessary to observe CPE, which can be as long as 4 weeks. In contrast, genotypic methods rely on the detection of specific mutations in the viral genome that are associated with antiviral resistance. These methods directly analyze virus present in clinical specimens (i.e., do not require isolation of the virus) and can be completed in as little as 1 to 2 days; however, the accuracy and reliability of results is dependent on knowledge of specific mutations leading to resistance.[163] To date, the majority of mutations resulting in resistance to commonly used antiviral agents ganciclovir, cidofovir, and foscarnet map to specific regions of two CMV genes: UL97, encoding a tyrosine kinase required for activation of ganciclovir, and UL54, the viral DNA polymerase.[164] Molecular assays using PCR to amplify selected regions of the UL97 and UL54 genes, followed by Sanger sequence analysis, have been developed by clinical and reference laboratories and are widely used to identify resistant CMV in clinical specimens. While mutations in UL97 are most common and result in resistance to ganciclovir only, CMV may also develop mutations in UL54 that result in resistance to one or more antiviral agents. Therefore analysis of both UL97 and UL54 should be conducted when patients fail therapy.[164,165]

Varicella-Zoster Virus

Primary infection with varicella-zoster virus (VZV) manifests as a disseminated syndrome involving viral replication within lymphoid and cutaneous tissue. This gives rise to the classic symptoms of fever and vesicular rash associated with chicken pox. Following primary infection VZV achieves latency primarily within trigeminal and dorsal root sensory nerve ganglia.[166] Reactivation of latent virus results in secondary varicella disease known as herpes zoster (HZ), which often presents as a vesicular rash in related dermatomes. VZV is highly contagious and can be transmitted through aerosolization of respiratory secretions or direct contact with vesicular lesions. Seroprevalence of VZV was reported to be 90 to 100% by adolescence even prior to the availability and use of VZV vaccine in 1995.[167,168]

In the compromised host, primary infection or reactivation of varicella can cause severe illness including high fever, meningitis, encephalitis, pneumonia, hepatitis, retinal necrosis, or disseminated visceral disease.[166,169–171] Retinal necrosis is common in individuals with advanced or uncontrolled AIDS, and is accompanied by CNS involvement in up to 75%

of cases.[172,173] Visceral HZ in compromised individuals is an immediate life-threatening condition associated with fever, multiple organ involvement, and disseminated intravascular coagulation (DIC) that can be associated with mortality rates of greater than 50%.[171,174] Importantly, these symptoms may be present in the absence of the characteristic vesicular rash associated with HZ (zoster sine herpete) that can impede clinical diagnosis.[170,171] Populations at the highest risk for HZ are individuals with hematopoietic malignancies, advanced HIV/AIDS, or those undergoing immunosuppressive therapy following SOT or BMT.[166,169,172] The risk of HZ within 4 years of SOT has been estimated at 8 to 11% overall, but is significantly higher in patients greater than 60 years of age.[169] Additionally, the risk of post-transplant HZ was 3.4 times higher in patients who were seronegative at the time of transplant.[169] Therefore establishment of serostatus is important for stratifying risk and identifying patients who would benefit from HZ vaccination prior to transplant.[175]

Serologic tests for VZV. Serologic diagnosis of primary varicella is not routinely performed because it requires comparison of acute and convalescent sera, which delays diagnosis by 10 to 14 days. The establishment of varicella serostatus is however beneficial for screening of health care workers and pretransplant assessment of individuals with no record of vaccination or natural varicella infection. Common methods to assess serostatus include latex agglutination (LA), ELISA, fluorescent antibody to membrane antigen (FAMA), and CIA (Table 89.2).

The FAMA test is based on detection of varicella envelope-specific antibodies in cultured virus.[181] FAMA has been considered the gold standard for the establishment of serostatus because of its high sensitivity and correlation with protective immunity; however, the assay is technically demanding and time consuming. These factors have prevented widespread use of this method in clinical laboratories. LA tests are inexpensive, require no additional equipment, are simple to perform, and can be completed within 10 to 15 minutes. The sensitivity of LA tests (89 to 98%) is similar to FAMA and equivalent or superior to that of traditional ELISA but specificity is low when compared to FAMA.[176,177,182] This may be due to the subjective interpretation of agglutination reactions. Newer

ELISA and CIA tests based on purified envelope glycoprotein (gpELISA) have demonstrated better sensitivity (87 to 100%) than traditional ELISA tests (72 to 98%).[179,180] Additional benefits of ELISA and CIA tests include an objective result and the ability to automate testing, which enables high-throughput screening of sera.

Establishment of serostatus in immunized persons can be difficult because the antibody response to the vOka vaccine is 10-fold lower than the response to natural infection. Additionally, vaccine induced antibodies begin to decline and may become undetectable in 5 to 30% of individuals within 5 to 15 years post vaccination, resulting in 61 to 85% sensitivity of FAMA and LA in immunized populations.[178,181,182] New gpELISA tests demonstrate better performance in detecting seroconversion following immunization (87 to 99% sensitive). However, long-term follow-up studies have not been conducted to determine if sensitivity remains high despite declining antibody concentration.[179-181]

Qualitative NAATs for VZV. NAATs are the preferred method for laboratory diagnosis of acute primary varicella and secondary HZ disease because of the increased speed and sensitivity compared with culture or direct detection (e.g., direct fluorescent antibody [DFA]) methods. In patients with rash consistent with HZ, culture was found to be 20 to 53% sensitive and DFA was found to be 82% sensitive when compared to NAAT.[183,184] VZV NAATs may also be multiplexed to include HSV-1 and HSV-2. This can be valuable in the assessment of cutaneous and mucocutaneous lesions given the similarity in appearance.[183,184] Specifically, one study using a multiplexed VZV and HSV NAAT reported 11% of all positive VZV detections to be from male or female genital sites.[185] In these cases, a VZV-specific test may not have been ordered based on clinical presentation and location of the lesion, supporting the value of combined target NAATs.

Qualitative NAATs also provide a sensitive method to detect VZV in sterile specimens such as CSF, BAL, or vitreous fluid where the presence of any amount of virus is likely causal. Pulmonary varicella or HZ can be severe in adults and if untreated carries up to 30% mortality. Supportive therapy and early treatment with acyclovir can greatly reduce mortality,[186-188] however the clinical diagnosis of VZV pneumonitis is difficult because physical and radiographic findings are nonspecific.[186,188,189] Direct analysis of BAL specimens using NAATs has enabled rapid and definitive detection of VZV in cases of pneumonitis, resulting in early appropriate therapy to improve patient outcome.[189,190] Similarly, clinical symptoms of necrotizing retinitis are nonspecific among the various herpesviruses commonly associated with this condition (VZV, CMV, HSV).[191,192] VZV NAATs have been successfully used to analyze vitreous specimens and provide a rapid and definitive diagnosis.[192-195] The use of aqueous humor rather than vitreous is less invasive, requires as little as 10 to 20 μL fluid, and also appears to be acceptable for laboratory diagnosis of viral retinitis.[192]

Several FDA or CE-Mark qualitative VZV NAATs are commercially available in addition to analyte-specific reagents and published primer sequences (Table 89.3). FDA and CE-Mark assays are often cleared for specific specimen types, typically cutaneous lesions, and require additional verification studies to enable reporting of results on alternative specimen types.

Importantly, up to 5% of individuals receiving the vOka vaccine may develop a characteristic rash.[200,201] Discrimination

TABLE 89.2 Serologic Assays for Determination of Varicella-Zoster Serostatus

Type/Name	Sensitivity (%)	Specificity (%)	Reference
Latex Agglutination			
	97.6–98.0[a]	90.0–97.2[a]	176, 177
	89.1–90.9[b]	76.4–97.5[b]	178
ELISA			
Whole antigen	75.0–98.5[c]	87.6–100[c]	177, 178
	72.7–83.0[b]	94.1–100[b]	178, 179
Glycoprotein	86.9–100[b]	89.4–100[b]	179, 180

[a]Compared to ELISA.
[b]Compared to FAMA.
[c]Compared to LA.
ELISA, Enzyme-linked immunosorbent assay; *FAMA,* fluorescent antibody to membrane antigen; *LA,* latex agglutination.

TABLE 89.3 Molecular Tests for Detection of Varicella-Zoster Virus

Manufacturer	Regulatory Status	Target	Specimen	Instrument	Quantitative (AMR) or Qualitative (LoD)	Reference
Quidel Lyra Direct HSV + VZV	FDA-IVD, CE-IVD	Not available	Vesicular lesion, swab	ABI7500Fast DX	Qualitative	Manufacturer product insert
Roche	CE-IVD	Not available	CSF, vesicular exudate (extracted nucleic acid)	LightCycler 2.0	Qualitative	Manufacturer product insert
Cepheid Benelux (Affigene VZV)	CE-IVD	ORF 62	CSF, vesicular swabs, blood/plasma, respiratory, eye swab, tissue (extracted nucleic acid)	Roter-Gene, ABI, iCycler	Qualitative; LoD 9.3 copies/mL	196
BioFire FilmArray ME	FDA-IVD, CE-IVD	Not available	CSF	FilmArray	Qualitative; LoD ~10^3 copies/mL	197
DiaSorin Simplexa VZV Direct	FDA-IVD, CE-IVD	Not available	CSV, Vesicular swabs	Liaison MDX	Qualitative, ~10^3 copies/mL	Manufacturer product insert
Quidel Solana HSV 1+2/ VZV	FDA-IVD, CE-IVD	Not available	Vesicular swabs	Solana	Qualitative	Manufacturer product insert
LDT	n/a	ORF 28, ORF 29	CSF, Vesicular swabs, Blood/plasma, respiratory, eye swab, tissue (extracted nucleic acid)	Open system	Qualitative; LoD 16 copies/mL	184, 196
LDT	n/a	ORF 62	Vesicular lesions or crusts	ABI Prism 7700	Qualitative; LoD 13 copies/mL	183, 184
LDT	n/a	ORF 29	Whole blood, Plasma, Serum	Perkin-Elmer 9600	Quantitative; Whole blood 80–10^6 copies/mL, Plasma 20–10^6 copies/mL	198, 199

AMR, Analytic measurement range for quantitative tests; *CSF*, cerebrospinal fluid; *FDA*, Food and Drug Administration; *HSV*, herpes simplex virus; *IVD*, in vitro diagnostic, obtained either FDA or CE clearance; *LDT*, laboratory developed test, independently verified without regulatory clearance; *LoD*, limit of detection for qualitative tests; *VZV*, varicella-zoster virus.

between vaccine-induced lesions and acute infection with wild-type VZV in these patients may impact prognosis and infection prevention strategies.[201] Importantly, none of the currently marketed assays differentiate wild-type VZV from vOka. Differentiation has been reliably achieved using additional primers that target a specific polymorphism in ORF 62 and other vaccine-specific SNPs.[183] Currently, this testing is available through the US CDC and other specialized reference laboratories.[201]

It is difficult to assess the absolute sensitivity of NAATs for detection of VZV in various specimens because "gold standard" reference methods including culture are significantly less sensitive than NAAT.[184] Analytic studies typically report a lower LoD of 10 to 200 copies/mL; however, a lack of standardization of methods among LDTs makes the clinical comparison of assays difficult. For example, the initial description of a VZV LDT reported 94% sensitivity when compared to a composite method of culture, DFA, and serology.[184] A subsequent study reported the LDT to be only ~60% sensitive compared to a commercially available VZV NAAT.[196] This

highlights the importance of standardized test methods and the impact of the chosen gold standard comparator when reviewing the performance or comparative performance of a molecular assay(s).

Quantitative NAATs. Quantitative NAATs enable the enumeration of VZV copies/mL in WB, plasma, or other bodily fluids. These assays can have a broad dynamic range of less than 100 copies/mL to greater than 10^7 copies/mL providing both sensitive and accurate determination of VZV VL.[202–204] Using these sensitive NAATs, a low level of VZV DNA has been detected in peripheral blood monocytes (PBMCs) isolated from 0 to 3% of asymptomatic individuals, though it is not clear if this represents differences in test sensitivity, subclinical reactivation, or latent cell-associated virus.[202,204] In patients presenting with characteristic rash, a VL threshold of 20 to 80 copies/mL was found to be 81 to 86% sensitive within 2 days following rash onset and increased to 100% for primary varicella and 80 to 89% for HZ within 1 week of rash onset.[198] A more important role for quantitative VZV NAAT is the evaluation of compromised patients with disseminated disease or visceral HZ sine herpete. Plasma VL can reach levels of 10^3 to 10^6 copies/mL in these patients.[203] Higher VLs were frequently correlated with more severe disease, and in all cases a rapid decrease in VL was observed following antiviral therapy.[198,203,205] Importantly, the detection of VZV in plasma precedes clinical symptoms in some but not all patients, thereby limiting the utility of serial monitoring to predict disease recurrence or initiate antiviral therapy prior to symptom onset.[199,205] These data support a diagnostic and prognostic role for quantitative NAAT in the assessment of VZV in immunocompromised patients; however, it must also be noted that these studies were conducted using nonstandardized LDTs. Therefore specific VL thresholds correlated with infection, disease state, or response to therapy are not universally applicable. Serial VL testing should be conducted at a single laboratory and specific VL thresholds for clinical decision points must be established by individual laboratories or institutions.

Quantitative analysis of VZV in saliva specimens has also been proposed as a noninvasive method to aid in diagnosis of disseminated HZ, HZ with CNS involvement, and in cases of facial palsy without rash. Detection of VZV in saliva was 72 to 100% sensitive in patients with rash and clinically diagnosed HZ.[206,207] VL ranged from 10^1 to 10^7 copies/mL and correlated with subjective pain scores.[207] Importantly, the detection of VZV in saliva is not necessarily indicative of acute HZ. Environmental or medical stress can induce subclinical reactivation and shedding of VZV in saliva in the absence of detectable blood VL or acute disease.[208,209] Given these data, the use of saliva as a specimen may have merit as a noninvasive specimen type when confirming VZV in persons with rash or when investigating atypical presentations of HZ. However, results should be interpreted in the context of other clinical findings.

Human Herpesvirus 6

Human herpesvirus 6 (HHV-6) is part of the *Betaherpesvirus* subfamily and encompasses variants HHV-6A and HHV-6B. These variants are serologically indistinguishable; however, nucleic acid analysis has demonstrated that greater than 95% of symptomatic infections are due to HHV-6B.[210,211] The primary syndrome associated with HHV-6 infection is roseola (sixth disease). This is almost exclusively a childhood illness and accounts for 10 to 30% of emergency department visits in children less than 2 years of age.[212] Like all herpesviruses, HHV-6 is capable of establishing lifelong latency following initial infection which is presumed to be primarily within mononuclear cells.[213] Latency is maintained through integration of the viral genome into the host chromosome, a characteristic unique to HHV-6 among the herpesviruses.[214,215] Seroprevalence of HHV-6 can be variable regionally and in different populations, but is typically greater than 90% by adulthood.[211,213]

In the immunocompromised host, latent virus can reactivate to cause severe illness including pneumonitis, CNS disease, and delayed bone marrow engraftment or graft versus host disease (GVHD).[213,216,217] The incidence of HHV-6 reactivation ranges from ~0 to 80% (average 30 to 50%) in SOT or BMT patients with a slight preference for BMT.[213,218] In contrast to VZV, reactivation of HHV-6 typically occurs in the first month following transplant.[216,218]

Serologic methods are available to identify individuals with antibodies to the HHV-6; however, due to the high seroprevalence of this virus and requirement for comparing acute and convalescent titers they play no practical role in diagnosis of acute to active HHV-6 infection.

NAATs for HHV-6. Both qualitative and quantitative NAATs have been employed for the detection of HHV-6 in clinical specimens using various targets and methodologies. There are currently no FDA-cleared NAATs for detection of HHV-6 in serum, but CE-Marked assays are commercially available and several reference laboratories offer quantitative or qualitative testing (Table 89.4).

A multiplexed panel for qualitative detection of HHV-6 in CSF has recently been cleared by the FDA for IVD use (see meningitis section of this chapter). The specific syndrome or site of infection dictates the specimen most appropriate for analysis by NAAT. These include CSF, BAL fluid, and blood/serum (when disseminated disease suspected).

Quantitative NAATs are the preferred method for laboratory diagnosis of HHV-6 reactivation disease in post-transplant or other at-risk populations. Whole blood, isolated PBMCs, or serum can be used to monitor HHV-6 VL. HHV-6 DNA has been detected in 30 to 90% of peripheral blood or PBMC

TABLE 89.4 Nucleic Acid Amplification Tests for Detection of Human Herpes Virus-6 in Plasma

Amplification Method	Detection Method	Target	Specimen	Quantitative or Qualitative	LoD or AMR	Reference
Nested PCR	Gel electrophoresis	*orf57*	Plasma	Qualitative	10^0–10^1 copies/mL	219, 220
LAMP	Reaction turbidity	*orf31*	Plasma	Qualitative	10^1–10^3 copies/mL	219, 221
Endpoint PCR	Capture EIA	*orf89*	Plasma	Qualitative	10^0 copies/mL	219
Real-time PCR	Fluorescent probe	*orf67*	Plasma, tissue	Quantitative	LoD 10^0–10^1 copies/mL; AMR 10^2–10^6	222
Real-time PCR	Fluorescent probe	*orf67*	Plasma, serum, CSF	Quantitative	LoD 10^0–10^1 copies/mL; AMR 10^3–10^7	223
Real-time PCR	Fluorescent probe	*orf31*	Plasma, whole blood	Quantitative	LoD 10^1–10^2 copies/mL; AMR NR	224
Real-time PCR	Fluorescent probe	NR	Plasma	Quantitative	LoD 10^2–10^3 copies/mL; AMR NR	219

AMR, Analytic measurement range for quantitative tests; *CSF,* cerebrospinal fluid; *EIA,* enzyme immunoassay; *LAMP,* loop-mediated amplification; *LoD,* limit of detection for qualitative tests; *NR,* not reported.

samples obtained from asymptomatic individuals, frequently at levels of 10^3 copies/mL or higher.[202,225] This complicates interpretation of a single VL result in a patient with compatible symptoms. A rapid increase of 3 to 4 $\log_{10}$ in HHV-6 VL, reaching 10^5 to 10^6 copies/10^6 PBMC, has been observed between 0 and 14 days following onset of symptoms.[218,226] The delayed rise in VL precludes the use of post-transplant serial monitoring to predict HHV-6 reactivation disease; however, a rise in HHV-6 VL can be useful in confirming the involvement of HHV-6 when other viral etiologies (CMV, VZV) may also be in the differential. Additionally, VL is a useful prognostic marker since high VL is correlated with delayed tissue engraftment, and VL decreases following antiviral therapy.[218] In contrast to peripheral blood or PBMCs, HHV-6 DNA is only rarely detected in sera of asymptomatic individuals and likely represents viral DNA released from lysed PBMCs rather than active viral replication.[225,227] This suggests the detection of HHV-6 DNA in serum may be more specific for active disease compared to peripheral blood, though sensitivity may be reduced.[227]

The lack of assay standardization and an international calibrator complicate interpretation of quantitative VL results and impede the establishment of a universal threshold for clinical significance. A greater than 15-fold variability between HHV-6 assays at the upper end of quantitation and greater than 200-fold variability in VL results for reference specimens containing ~3 $\log_{10}$ copies/mL has been reported.[219] Recent development of the first WHO International Standard for HHV-6 has the potential to reduce interlaboratory and interassay variation in reported VL values; however, differences in assay target, extraction method, and PCR instrumentation still contribute to variation in VL values obtained from different tests.[228] Therefore it is recommended to use the same test and laboratory when monitoring HHV-6 VL with importance being placed on the change in VL rather than the absolute value.

Chromosomally integrated HHV-6. A particular challenge for molecular diagnostics arises from the chromosomal integration of HHV-6 during latency. Latent infection of germinal cells provides the possibility of hereditary transmission of HHV-6, which in turn results in individuals who carry the full HHV-6 genome in every cell of their body.[229] Inherited chromosomally integrated HHV-6 (iciHHV-6) is present in approximately 1% of the human population.[214,229] Blood or other tissue specimens taken from these individuals frequently have extremely high VL (>5 $\log_{10}$ in plasma, >7 $\log_{10}$ in WB) independent of HHV-6 disease.[230] This may result in misdiagnosis in patients suffering from an illness mediated by other infectious or noninfectious causes. Therefore patients with HHV-6 VL of greater than 5.5 $\log_{10}$ copies/mL in WB should be further evaluated to determine the presence of iciHHV-6 prior to making a diagnosis of acute HHV-6 infection.[231]

Historically, identification of iciHHV-6 was based on detection of HHV-6 DNA in hair follicles or nails obtained from a suspected individual. More recently, digital PCR (dPCR) has been used to accurately quantify and compare HHV-6 copy number to that of a host cell target in WB samples. Since the iciHHV-6 genome is integrated in single copy into every nucleated cell, a ratio of 1 would indicate iciHHV-6 while a ratio higher or lower than one would indicate the presence of nonintegrated, actively replicating HHV-6. This theory has been tested and a ratio of 0.96 to 1.02 was

observed in patients with iciHHV-6 with a coefficient of variation (CV) of 3%.[232]

Definitive identification of iciHHV-6 does not rule out active viral replication and disease; however, it does render both WB and plasma HHV-6 DNA VL values uninterpretable. In patients with iciHHV-6, active viral replication contributes only minimally to the total VL in WB, and latent virus is shed variably and at high levels into plasma during natural cell lysis, both of which minimize or mask clinically significant changes in VL.[231] An alternative approach to diagnosis of active disease in these patients is to monitor HHV-6 mRNA as a proxy for active replication. Caserta et al. reported the detection of HHV-6 DNA in 100% of plasma specimens obtained from individuals with iciHHV-6 compared to only 5% positivity when using reverse-transcriptase PCR to target HHV-6 mRNA.[227] Compared to viral culture, the specificity of a DNA-based test was 84% while the specificity of an mRNA-based test was 98% with no difference in sensitivity for detection of active viral replication. While promising, quantitative mRNA-based tests for HHV-6 lack standardization and are only available for research. Until these assays are verified for clinical use and more widely available, the diagnosis of active HHV-6 infection in a patient with iciHHV-6 is based on clinical assessment and exclusion of other potential etiologies.

Human Herpesvirus 8

Human herpesvirus-8 (HHV-8) can cause acute, reactivation, or asymptomatic latent infection.[233] The seroprevalence of HHV-8 is typically low, ranging from 1 to 15% in the United States, Europe, and Asia but may be as high as 36 to 90% in sub-Saharan Africa.[233] Transmission of HHV-8 likely occurs during intermittent periods of viral shedding in various bodily fluids including saliva.[234,235] Specific risk factors for acquisition of HHV-8 include maternal seropositivity, injection drug use, and high-risk sexual practices.[233,236–238]

Primary infection with HHV-8 is asymptomatic or associated with mild symptoms including rash, diarrhea, and fatigue in healthy adults.[239] Viral reactivation following infectious or iatrogenic immunosuppression results in the clinical syndromes commonly attributed to HHV-8. These include Kaposi sarcoma (KS), primary effusion lymphoma (PEL), and multicentric Castleman disease (MCD). Expression of HHV-8 latency-associated nuclear antigen (LANA) inhibits tumor suppression through interactions with p53 and E2F, resulting in abnormal proliferation of blood vessels (tumor spindle cells).[240] This gives rise to the characteristic brown to red plaques or nodules which are localized to epithelial sites in mild disease, but also occur in the oral cavity, lymph nodes, or internal organs in severe or disseminated disease.

HIV infection is the greatest risk factor for development of KS, with rates in HIV-infected individuals 5000 to 20,000 times greater than in the general population.[241,242] Patients who are positive for both HIV and HHV-8 have a 50% chance of developing KS within 10 years.[237] Symptoms may be mild and limited to cutaneous involvement; however, severe complications including pancytopenia, hepatitis, and visceral involvement leading to patient demise have also been reported.[243,244] Importantly, KS-associated symptoms can diminish if immunosuppression is reduced through effective antiretroviral therapy or reduction in immunosuppressive agents.[240] Therefore accurate laboratory diagnosis of HHV-8 can aid in patient management.

Serologic tests for HHV-8. Among available test modalities for HHV-8, ELISA and EIAs and IFAs are relatively simple and well adapted for routine use in clinical laboratories. These tests can be composed of a single purified antigen (K8.1, *orf73*, *orf65*) or use whole HHV-8 culture lysate. Sensitivity ranges from 70 to 97% depending on antigen target and threshold used, but specificity is typically greater than 95%.[245,246] The sensitivity of these tests is highest in patients with classic KS (80 to 100%) or AIDS-related KS (67 to 97%) but is lower in healthy, asymptomatic controls (16 to 56%). Comparison of HHV-8 serologic results obtained using different tests and algorithms demonstrated 92 to 100% agreement among KS patients but only 80 to 89% agreement among samples from healthy blood donors.[246,247] This makes the use of serologic tests sub-optimal when assessing seropositivity to stratify risk of HHV-8 reactivation disease in pretransplant patients. Further, negative results should be interpreted with caution in patients with clinical signs and symptoms consistent with KS due to low and variable sensitivity of serologic assays during active infection.

Direct antigen and NAATs for HHV-8. Immunostaining for HHV-8 in lesion biopsies is based on detection of LANA (*orf73*), which is expressed in all cells latently infected with HHV-8.[248] Approximately 10% of cells in early KS plaque lesions stain positive for LANA; however this increases to greater than 90% positivity in nodular lesions.[249] Manual microscopic examination of stained tissue sections can be subjective and may contribute to variability in sensitivity, especially in cases where a small percentage of cells in the biopsy is positive for a given marker. Additionally, biopsy is by nature invasive and preparation, staining, and reading of tissue sections are both labor intensive and time consuming. Therefore while tissue biopsy remains the gold standard for diagnosis of localized infection, simpler and less subjective methods for laboratory diagnosis of HHV-8 are of interest.

Available NAATs for the detection of HHV-8 include primarily LDTs that rely on lytic and latent phase genetic targets.[250] Qualitative NAATs have been used to confirm the presence of HHV-8 in tissue biopsy and have demonstrated greater than 90% sensitivity.[234,251] Visceral KS, PEL, or MCD are difficult to diagnose and monitor because of their internal and sometimes diffuse or multifocal locations. HHV-8 DNA is not detected in healthy, immunocompetent individuals; however, up to 10% of HIV-positive patients without KS may have detectable HHV-8 in isolated PBMCs.[202,246] Further, the sensitivity of NAAT in symptomatic patients ranges from 33 to 91% depending on the LoD of the specific test used.[246] Combined, this limits the positive and NPV of qualitative NAAT results in at-risk populations. Quantitative analysis of DNA extracted from PBMCs or serum has shown a 2 to 3 log_{10} increase in VL during clinical exacerbations including a spike in temperature, C-reactive protein, and acute increase of liver enzymes.[252,253] Additionally, higher VL values were associated with a greater number of lesions.[254] While intriguing, quantitative analysis of blood components is not widely used for the diagnosis of HHV-8 related infections and requires further investigation to establish clinical decision points. Further, laboratory-developed qualitative and quantitative NAAT methods lack standardization, a problem that complicates the comparison of results across laboratories.

Polyomaviruses

Polyomaviruses are genetically diverse, nonenveloped DNA viruses that have been identified in humans and other non-human primates. Infection with these viruses is largely asymptomatic which has contributed to their relatively recent discovery and association with clinical disease. The earliest human polyomaviruses, JC and BK, were identified in the early 1970s. These two viruses share ~75% genome homology and are linked to progressive and serious clinical syndromes in compromised patients.[255] Since 2007, nine additional human polyomaviruses have been identified in clinical specimens including nasopharyngeal tissue, skin, urine, stool, and blood. The apparent ubiquity of polyomaviruses in human populations, coupled with the propensity for asymptomatic shedding of virus and environmental stability of virions all likely contribute to a seroprevalence 25 to 92% among these viruses.[256]

BK virus

Exposure to BK virus likely occurs early in life and primary infection is largely asymptomatic. Epidemiologic studies report worldwide seroprevalence of 60 to 100% by early adolescence.[257] BK virus has been isolated from many anatomic sites including lungs, tonsils, spleen, and lymph nodes, but the primary site of latency is epithelial cells of the urinary tract including renal tubules.[257,258] Sporadic asymptomatic shedding of the virus in urine is common with the frequency of viral urinary shedding increasing from ~15% in 20- to 30-year-olds to greater than 40% in 80- to 89-year-olds.[259]

Severe syndromes most commonly associated with BK virus include polyomavirus associated nephropathy (PVAN) and hemorrhagic cystitis (HC).[257,260] These syndromes are observed exclusively in immunocompromised patients. The specific patients at highest risk for PVAN are those who have undergone renal transplant, in which 1 to 10% will develop disease. HC is more commonly observed in patients following HSCT and may affect 5 to 15% of patients. In either case, onset is typically late and is preceded by viruria and viremia. Successful treatment for PVAN or HC relies heavily on the reduction of immunosuppression, which is more effective if implemented early in disease.[257,260] Therefore sensitive, accurate, and early detection of BK virus in at-risk patients is central to improving outcomes.

Diagnostic methods for presumed BK virus infections. Histologic assessment of tissue biopsy is considered the gold standard for diagnosis of BK virus associated nephropathy; however, sensitivity of biopsy may be only 63 to 75% if a single specimen is collected due to the focal nature of renal pathology.[261]

Nucleic acid amplification and detection methods are the most widely used approach to diagnosing BK virus associated nephropathy and cystitis and require minimally or noninvasive specimen types (Table 89.5).

Analysis of urine has the advantage of being noninvasive. Additionally, BK virus DNA may be detected several weeks earlier in urine and reaches a significantly higher VL (2 to 10 log_{10} copies/mL) than that observed in plasma.[262,263] Combined, these factors make NAAT testing of urine a practical method to screen at-risk patients for early signs of BK virus reactivation. Importantly, while sensitive, qualitative detection of BK virus DNA in urine lacks specificity as an indicator of renal disease due to the high frequency of viral shedding

TABLE 89.5 Characteristics of Nucleic Acid Amplification Tests for Detection of Polyomaviruses

Virus	Genetic Targets	Specimens	Viral Load Associated With Clinical Disease	Comment
BK virus	Viral capsid protein (VP1), Large T antigen (LT)	Urine	A threshold of $\geq 10^6$–10^7 copies/mL is 78–85% specific for PVAN	Asymptomatic shedding of BK virus in urine is observed in 7–40% of individuals at viral load of 10^3–10^4 copies/mL
		Plasma	A threshold of $\geq 10^4$ copies/mL is 92–94% specific for PVAN	Asymptomatic shedding of BK virus in plasma is observed in <1% of individuals
JC virus	Small T antigen, noncodiing regulatory region	CSF	Detection of JC virus at any VL in CSF should be considered clinically significant. Sustained CSF VLs >10^3–10^4 copies/mL are correlated with rapid progression of PML.	Detection of JC virus in urine (common) or plasma (rare) does not correlate with PML

CSF, Cerebrospinal fluid; *PML,* progressive multifocal leukoencephalopathy; *PVAN,* polyomavirus associated nephropathy, *VL,* viral load.

(7 to 27% of asymptomatic patients), which can routinely reach 3 to 4 $\log_{10}$ copies/mL urine.[264] Studies using quantitative NAAT have demonstrated a viruria threshold of greater than 7 $\log_{10}$ copies/mL to be 100% sensitive and 78 to 85% specific for biopsy-confirmed PVAN.[263,265]

Plasma provides a minimally invasive specimen that has the potential for more specific diagnosis of PVAN. In contrast to urine, asymptomatic reactivation and shedding in the bloodstream is rare.[259,264] When present, BK VL in plasma also tends to be lower and within a narrower range than that observed in urine, ranging from 3 to 7 $\log_{10}$ copies/mL.[263,265] Clinical correlation studies have demonstrated a plasma threshold of greater than 4 $\log_{10}$ copies/mL to be 100% sensitive and 87 to 96% specific for predicting biopsy proven PVAN.[263,265] While more specific than viruria, no single threshold for viremia is both 100% sensitive and specific in predicting PVAN in at risk patients. Therefore monitoring of viremia for significant changes over time or demonstrating persistent high viremia is likely a better predictor of PVAN than a single specimen value in either urine or plasma.[262]

The American Society of Transplantation guidelines recommend routine viruria monitoring until a threshold of 7 $\log_{10}$ copies/mL is detected, at which point serum viremia should be monitored with a sustained threshold of 4 $\log_{10}$ indicating PVAN.[260] Others have suggested a more conservative viruria threshold of 4 to 6 $\log_{10}$ as an indication to initiate serum testing or adjust immunosuppressive therapy.[263] This is supported by data demonstrating that viruria of greater than 6 $\log_{10}$/mL is 100% sensitive and 92 to 94% specific for predicting patients with viremia above 4 $\log_{10}$ copies/mL (the plasma threshold for clinical significance).[262,265] Importantly, the level of viruria or viremia does not correlate well with the extent of tissue involvement and, therefore renal biopsy must be conducted to accurately determine the extent of organ involvement present.[266]

Interpretation of quantitative BK virus NAATs. Establishment of absolute viruria or viremia VL thresholds that are highly specific and sensitive for PVAN is complicated by both analytical (assay specific) and biological (virus subtype) factors that impact assay variability. Commercial and laboratory-developed BK NAATs target disparate genetic sequences including a 287 bp typing region; the viral capsid encoding VP1, VP2, or VP3 genes; and the large T antigen gene.[259,262,263,267,268] Further, considerable genetic diversity is present among BK virus subtypes and single nucleotide polymorphisms (SNPs) within assay targets are present in up to 27 to 82% of sequenced strains. Each of these factors has been noted to contribute to variability in VL values reported by different laboratories.[269,270] Split sample studies have found that fewer than 70% of reported VL values are within 0.5 $\log_{10}$ when tested by different laboratories, with a range of values spanning up to 7 $\log_{10}$ copies/mL for some specimens.[267,268,270] Additionally, recent discovery of novel polyomaviruses poses the possibility of previously unrecognized cross-reactivity of assay target sequences.

There are currently no FDA-cleared NAATs for BK virus; clinical laboratories have to verify the performance of commercially available tests with CE-Mark designation or independently develop and validate in-house quantitative NAATs. This results in a lack of standardization of preanalytic specimen processing, extraction methods, primer/probe targets, and calibration standards. In 2016 the first international standard for BK virus was introduced by the WHO.[269] Use of the IU standard effectively reduced the variability in VL values by greater than 0.6 $\log_{10}$ copies/mL between a commercially available NAAT and a laboratory developed test for BK virus.[271] Importantly, IU are not equivalent to copies. Therefore results obtained in IU/mL must be converted back to copies/mL based on laboratory and NAAT-specific comparison studies to enable interpretation by clinicians using VL thresholds (stated in copies/mL) and current guidance documents. While standardization to IU accounts for a major source of VL variability, differences in reported VL of up to 2 $\log_{10}$ can be observed between NAATs even when targeting the same viral sequence.[270] This likely results from differences in preanalytical steps such as specimen input volume and nucleic acid extraction method. Therefore serial monitoring of at-risk patients should be conducted by a single laboratory using a single test to ensure reliability of results in guiding patient management.

JC Virus

JC virus has a global distribution with an average seroprevalence in humans of 60 to 80%.[264,272] Primary infection is asymptomatic and is followed by viral latency in tissues of the kidney, bone, lymph node, spleen, and brain.[273] The frequency of asymptomatic viral shedding in urine is higher than that observed for BK virus, reaching a point prevalence of 58 to 72% in persons over the age of 40.[259] The absolute VL measured in urine is also high, ranging from 5 to 6 $\log_{10}$ copies/mL.[264] Despite these findings, severe disease is almost exclusively associated with CNS manifestations and is not correlated with the detection of JC virus in urine. High urinary shedding does however provide a plausible mechanism for transmission of the virus to naïve hosts.

The most severe syndrome attributed to JC virus is progressive multifocal leukoencephalopathy (PML). This syndrome is seen in patients with underlying immunosuppression including hematologic malignancies, AIDS, or those undergoing monoclonal antibody therapy for multiple sclerosis (MS) or other autoimmune disease.[255] Destructive viral replication causes demyelination of white matter in the brain which manifests as progressive confusion, ataxia, paresis, and death if untreated. Primary therapy for PML is reduction of immunosuppression either through modification of immunomodulatory therapy or adherence to antiretroviral regimens, which can improve the 1-year survival rate by 5-fold.[255]

Diagnostic methods for presumed JC virus CNS infections.
Virus-specific serologic tests play no role in diagnosing active infection; however, determination of serostatus aids in identifying patients at risk for developing PML. Specifically, candidates for treatment with natalizumab may benefit from a serologic assessment because of the increased risk of PML associated with this therapy.[274] In patients testing seropositive for JC virus the rate of PML can vary from 0.56 cases/1000 to 11.1 cases/1000 depending on the duration of natalizumab exposure and prior use of other immunosuppressants.[275] PML has been associated with other immunomodulatory therapies including fingolimod and dimethyl fumarate as well, albeit at a far lower incidence of less than 1/20,000 patients.[276] The STRATIFY JCV assay (Focus Diagnostics) is a commercially available ELISA test which uses immobilized VP1 capsid protein as target for serum antibodies. This assay has a reported sensitivity of greater than 97% and specificity greater than 90% for identification of seropositive patients.[277] Plavina et al. have evaluated this assay and refined risk stratification based on assay index value, noting a tenfold increased risk of developing PML for values greater than 1.5.[278] Based on these results, serologic screening for JC virus may aid in selection of therapy (e.g., shortened duration or alternative immunomodulatory agents) for patients suffering from MS or Crohn disease.

The diagnosis of PML requires a combination of clinical presentation, imaging, and direct detection of JC virus in an appropriate specimen. Viral detection can be accomplished using NAAT or targeting viral proteins through immunostaining. Detection of JC virus DNA in brain or other tissues using NAATs lacks both sensitivity and specificity due to the presence of latent virus in brain tissue of healthy individuals and localized focal nature of infection.[273] Immunostaining for capsid protein (VP1) or large T antigen (LT) which are expressed during viral replication may provide a more accurate assessment of active disease. The presence of either or

both markers was detected in 83 to 96% of patients with PML compared with only 0 to 6% of patients without PML regardless of HIV status.[273] While more accurate, this method relies on invasive sampling of brain tissue in patients with suspected disease. Further, antibodies are cross-reactive among polyomaviruses including BK.

Laboratory diagnosis of acute PML is most commonly achieved by NAAT (see Table 89.5). Potential non- or minimally invasive specimens include urine, blood, or CSF. As discussed above, JC virus is frequently detected in urine; however, urinary shedding is not correlated with viremia or the development of PML.[264,279] JC virus DNA was not detected in plasma samples obtained from healthy blood donors and was found in only 0.3% of patients taking natalizumab for MS, none of which developed PML.[264,279] While point prevalence of JC virus viremia may reach 17% in high-risk patients with HIV infection, longitudinal monitoring of serum for JC virus DNA in these patients indicates no correlation of JC viremia with PML.[280] Given these findings, neither plasma nor urine appear to be adequate surrogate specimens for accurate laboratory diagnosis of PML. Therefore the specimen of choice for diagnosis of presumed cases of PML is CSF.

Unlike molecular assays for BK virus which require accurate quantitation and high precision for monitoring of VL, these factors are less critical when assessing clinical specimens for JC virus. A study of 61 HIV patients with histologically confirmed PML found CSF VL ranging from undetectable to greater than 7 $\log_{10}$ copies/mL at the time of onset of neurologic symptoms.[281] Detection of JC virus in the CSF was 100% specific for PML, indicating that the presence of any amount of virus in a CSF specimen should be considered clinically significant. While unnecessary for diagnosis, quantitative NAAT may be prognostically useful for patients with PML. JC virus CSF VL appears to be significantly higher in patients who do not receive therapy or succumbed to infection within 1 year of diagnosis compared to those whose clinical status improved following therapy.[281,282]

Diagnostic methods for JC virus infections outside the CNS.
JC virus infections outside the CNS appear to be exceedingly rare and difficult to definitively attribute to the virus. JC virus nephropathy in kidney transplant recipients is the most frequently reported of extra-CNS infections; however, there continues to be a vigorous debate surrounding the causal versus correlative role of JC virus in these infections, and if causal, how best to diagnose and monitor for disease.[283–286] JC virus is detected in the urine of up to 50% of renal transplant patients without pathologic signs of disease at a wide range of 10^3 to 10^7 copies/mL which renders testing of urine a poor surrogate for diagnosis of JC nephropathy.[283] JC virus DNA is also detected in serum or blood in up to 25% of renal transplant patients, albeit at lower levels of $\leq 10^3$ copies/mL, in absence of pathologic evidence of renal infection. Further, a recent cases series reported JC viremia in only 4/9 (44%) of patients with histologically observed viral inclusions.[284] Based on these findings, the role of quantitative assessment of JC VL in urine, blood, or serum specimens in renal transplant patients remains controversial and unresolved. Immunostaining for polyomavirus combined with PCR confirmation of species in biopsy specimens provides the best evidence of JC nephropathy.

Interpretation of quantitative JC virus NAATs.
There are currently no FDA-cleared assays for detection of JC virus;

however NAATs developed by commercial laboratories such as Viracor Laboratories and the National Institutes of Health (NIH) have reported an LoD of ~1 to 2 $\log_{10}$ copies/mL.[279,287] Both are approximately 95% sensitive for the detection of JC virus in CSF specimens.[287] By comparison, assays with a reported LoD of 2 to 3 $\log_{10}$ copies/mL exhibit a sensitivity of 76% in biopsy-proven cases of PML.[281] Therefore a low LoD is essential for accurate laboratory diagnosis of PML.

The establishment of accurate quantitative VL values for JC virus is complicated by many of the same factors impacting BK virus quantitation including lack of standardized preanalytical and analytical methods (discussed above). Similar to BK, an international quantitative JC virus standard was developed by the WHO in 2016. However, a genetic analysis of the WHO standard found significant heterogeneity in the copy number of different loci frequently targeted by JC virus NAATs including VP1, large, and small T antigen.[288] This may be due to genetic rearrangements incurred during culture of the virus for preparation of the standard material and is also observed in other commercially available standards. The net effect of these copy number derangements is up to eightfold variation in VL value depending on the specific viral sequence targeted by the assay and the standard used for calibration.[288] Based on these data quantitative VL values are likely not commutable across different laboratories and NAATs, which continues to be a barrier to the establishment of clinically useful VL thresholds to aid in monitoring and prognosis of patients with JC virus infection.

Adenovirus

Human adenoviruses (AdVs) are a genetically and serologically diverse group of nonenveloped DNA viruses. Seven species (A-G) comprise at least 67 known serotypes or genotypes, each with specific tissue tropism and disease association.[289,290] Transmission can occur through direct exposure to respiratory droplets or other bodily fluids (urine, stool), or through contact with fomites where AdVs may persist for days to weeks. Therefore those at greatest risk for transmission include persons in close quarters such as military barracks, childcare facilities, dormitories, and within the health care setting.

In the immunocompetent host AdV infection causes respiratory, gastrointestinal, or conjunctival symptoms depending on the virus serotype and route of infection.[289] These infections are often self-limiting or asymptomatic and may not require medical intervention. In contrast, primary infection in an immunocompromised host can result in severe or protracted lower respiratory or gastrointestinal symptoms and is associated with an increased mortality rate (see respiratory and viral gastroenteritis sections of this chapter). Following primary infection, some AdV species (most notably species-C, AdV-C) establish latency within T-lymphocytes in adenoid and other lymphoid tissues.[291] The specific site of viral latency for other AdV species and serotypes is ill defined.[290,292]

Persons at highest risk for serious AdV disease include both SOT and HSCT recipients. Incidence in these groups varies from 3 to 47% but is highest following allogenic HSCT with peak incidence in children, and usually occurs within 100 days of transplant.[293] Reactivation of latent virus often initiates as focal disease resulting in pneumonia, hepatitis, gastroenteritis, and urinary symptoms including nephritis

and HC.[289,293] Disseminated disease characterized by multi-organ involvement and viremia occurs in 10 to 30% of patients and mortality may exceed 70 to 80%.[289,294] In both SOT and HSCT recipients, AdV species C (AdV-C) appears to be the predominant subgroup causing systemic disease, though serious infections with subgroups A and B are not uncommon.[289,293] Specifically, species B serotypes 7, 11, 34, 35 are strongly associated with HC.[289,291] In addition to serving as an important reservoir for reactivation disease, viral latency is also associated with intermittent asymptomatic viral shedding which can complicate interpretation of positive results in nonsterile specimens such as stool or respiratory secretions. Of specific note, AdV species F serotypes 40 and 41 are most frequently associated with gastroenteritis in both immunocompetent and immunocompromised individuals. For a specific discussion of these AdVs the reader is referred to the chapter section on viruses associated with gastroenteritis.

Diagnostic approaches for patients with presumed AdV disease. Direct detection of AdV in clinical specimens based on viral culture or direct fluorescent antigen (DFA) assays are applicable to various specimen types including respiratory, urine, and stool; however, they lack sensitivity when compared to NAAT.[295] Quantitative NAAT is the current best practice for detection and monitoring AdV replication in post-transplant populations.[296] NAATs are typically designed to target the AdV E1A or hexon gene which is conserved across subgroups and serotypes. Importantly, "universal" primer sets used to detect all AdV subgroups and serotypes should be periodically evaluated *in silico* to assure that they are suitable for newly described AdVs. Though there are no currently FDA-cleared assays, testing is readily available through reference laboratories. These laboratories may have different specimen, transport, and acceptability criteria based on their independent assay validations.

Role of NAAT in screening for AdV infection. Determination of AdV VL in specimens including urine, stool, and serum has been investigated as both a diagnostic and prognostic marker of severe and/or disseminated disease. AdV can be detected by sensitive NAAT in stool specimens from healthy individuals, which has been proposed as a noninvasive specimen to screen for and predict disseminated disease in the immunocompromised host.[295,297] In a study of 182 HSCT patients, AdV was detected in stool specimens (mean VL 5 $\log_{10}$ copies/g; range 4 to 12 $\log_{10}$ copies/g) from 16/18 (88.9%) patients with disseminated AdV infection a median 42 days prior to detection in WB samples.[295] Importantly, 5 (24%) of these patients remained negative using stool antigen detection methods, indicating a diminished role for antigen tests as a screening method. These data are in agreement with Lion et al. who proposed a stool VL threshold of 6 $\log_{10}$ copies/g as a prognostic indicator of invasive disease with approximately 70% PPV.[297] In contrast, others have found stool screening to be less effective, detecting AdV in stool from only 10/26 (38%) patients prior to AdV viremia.[298] Similarly, detection of AdV in throat or urine specimens is not independently correlated with disseminated disease; however, detection of AdV in greater than 2 different specimen types (e.g., stool, throat, and urine) is strongly suggestive of disseminated disease and is correlated with peripheral blood VL of greater than 10^2 copies/mL.[294] Given these data, quantitative NAAT analysis of WB or serum should be conducted on all symptomatic patients with suspicion of AdV disease regardless of findings in other specimen types.

Role of NAAT for diagnosis of AdV infection. Disease caused by AdV can remain localized to a specific body site or organ or can disseminate. In both cases, a rapid diagnosis may be used to initiate antiviral treatment and/or modify immunosuppressive regimens. Focal disease is more common following SOT, and often initiates within the transplanted organ.[290] Patients receiving a kidney transplant are at the highest risk for HC but renal involvement also occurs following HSCT.[291,293,299] For these cases, detection of AdV in urine specimens is highly specific for HC and may precede viremia by 14 days.[299,300] In one study, AdV was detected in urine collected from all 17 (100%) symptomatic kidney transplant patients compared with detection of AdV viremia in only 9 of 21 (43%) cases.[299]

Disseminated AdV disease can carry a mortality rate of up to 80%.[294] Quantitative VL values and changes in VL have been correlated with disease severity and response to therapy.[299,301] Therefore analysis of WB specimens is critical in the diagnosis and management of patients at risk for AdV disease. While over 70% of patients with a high WB or plasma VL (>6 $\log_{10}$ copies/mL) progress to disseminated disease, transient low-level viremia (2 to 3 $\log_{10}$ copies/mL) has been detected in post-transplant patients who do not develop AdV disease.[294,298] This low-level asymptomatic viremia is common in adults, affecting 6 to 8% of SOT recipients.[302] In contrast, low-level asymptomatic viremia is uncommon in pediatric patients and resulting disseminated disease carries a high mortality rate.[301] Based on these findings, a clinical threshold for WB VL that correlates with or is prognostic of disseminated disease would be desirable.

Routine monitoring of blood VL following HSCT has shown some utility in predicting disseminated disease and stratifying risk of severe complications. Several studies have shown that a detectable VL in WB or plasma precedes invasive or disseminated disease by 15 to 21 days.[294,298] In these cases, a VL threshold of ≥ 3 $\log_{10}$ copies/mL was approximately 90% sensitive and specific for predicting invasive disease but

---

POINTS TO REMEMBER

Viral Infections in Immunocompromised Populations

- Most viral illness affecting immunocompromised individuals is attributable to reactivation of latent viral infections rather than primary infection.
- High seroprevalence of herpesviruses and polyomaviruses prevents the use of serologic tests to diagnose active disease; serologic assessment can be important in assessing risk of subsequent disease in at-risk populations.
- Qualitative detection of a virus may not indicate active infection due to asymptomatic reactivation and viral shedding or the presence of latent nonreplicating virus in host cells within the sample.
- Interpretation of quantitative viral load results is dependent on specimen type and assay utilized. Conversion of results using an international standard aids in standardization of results.
- Quantitative viral load results can be used to monitor therapy and suggest the emergence of resistance to antiviral regimens.

---

maximum VL in these patients ranged from 3 to 9 $\log_{10}$ copies/mL. Of note, patients with maximal VL greater than 6 $\log_{10}$ or rapid rise of greater than 1 $\log_{10}$ over 7 to 21 days are at increased risk of severe complications including death.[294,298,303] These data support the practice of monitoring of WB or plasma VL in high-risk patients or to confirm the diagnosis of AdV in patients with compatible symptoms. However, routine monitoring of AdV VL in low-risk or asymptomatic patients should be avoided because of difficulty in interpretation and poor PPV of low-level viremia for predicting invasive disease.[296]

SEXUALLY TRANSMITTED INFECTIONS

Herpes Simplex Virus

HSV is a common cause of sexually transmitted infections (STIs). Within the United States, the estimated seroprevalence of HSV-2 among 14- to 49-year-olds is 15.7%, whereas the estimated seroprevalence of HSV-1 among this group is 53.9%.[304] Both viruses are capable of causing genital herpes, a disease characterized by episodes of painful vesicles and ulcerations affecting the mucocutaneous surfaces of the genitalia. The ability of the virus to lie dormant within the sensory neuronal ganglia prevents eradication of infection and allows for recurrent episodes of symptomatology.[305] Conventionally, HSV-1 has been associated with oral-labial infections whereas HSV-2 has been associated with genital infection. However, an increase in genital infection with HSV-1 has been noted over recent years.[306] This shift in prevalence has been so pronounced that a large-scale 2013 study actually found a higher rate of HSV-1 genital infection among young women than HSV-2.[307] The clinical manifestations of HSV-1 and HSV-2 genital infections are similar so differentiation between the two cannot be achieved using clinical features alone.[305,307] Both are also capable of causing one of the more severe complications of genital HSV infection, neonatal infection. Neonatal HSV infection typically is acquired during a vaginal delivery when the neonate is exposed to virus within the birth canal, resulting in symptomatology ranging from localized skin lesions to severe fully disseminated disease. Evidence suggests that transmission of neonatal infection is more common with HSV-1 than HSV-2.[308,309]

Serologic Methods for Diagnosis of HSV

Serologic assessment is not useful for diagnosis of patients presenting with genital lesions and is reserved primarily for prenatal screening or to determine serostatus in potentially serodiscordant couples. The earliest serologic tests were Western blot assays designed to detect serum antibodies against whole antigen preparations separated by electrophoresis.[310] Differentiation of HSV-1 and HSV-2 was based on unique banding patterns. These assays have since evolved into modern ELISAs that are more rapid, easier to perform, and less expensive.

ELISAs utilized crude HSV antigen preparations and were not capable of HSV typing.[311,312] Given the crude nature of the antigen preparation, assay sensitivity and specificity were low. Current HSV serologic assays utilize purified preparations of HSV-1 and HSV-2 glycoprotein G (gG-1 and gG-2).[313,314] This antigen differs significantly between HSV-1 and HSV-2, allowing for type-specific IgG serology results. Rapid variations of type-specific ELISA and CIA are now available which allow for POC antibody detection with sensitivity and specificity comparable to lab-based testing.[315–317] An important consideration for the serologic detection of HSV is the high background seropositivity. For HSV-1 this can range from 70% in developed countries to nearly 100% in developing countries.[318,319] This fact negatively affects the PPV of serology, making results difficult to interpret. A potential solution is the use of IgM-based serology as a marker of active infection. However, positive results for IgM are also difficult to interpret since IgM has been shown to persist following an acute infection, can reappear upon reactivation, and exhibits cross-reactivity with other Herpesviridae (including CMV and VZV). HSV IgM testing also has a relatively low sensitivity for the diagnosis of genital herpes, estimated at approximately 73.9%.[320] Overall, given the limitations of HSV serologic testing, results should always be interpreted within the context of other testing and patient history.

Direct Detection Methods for Diagnosis of HSV

Traditional culture techniques involved inoculating a patient specimen onto a permissive cell line and observing for CPE. Subsequent typing of HSV is accomplished using monoclonal antibodies.[321,322] An advantage of culture is the ability to simultaneously test for other viruses including VZV, which may resemble HSV clinically. A significant disadvantage of culture is the extended TAT and technical expertise required. While HSV has a rapid growth rate, the appearance of CPE may still take 2 to 5 days to develop.[323] Shell vial culture is a rapid culture methodology that employs centrifugation to concentrate the virus onto a coverslip containing permissive cells. This coverslip is then stained with fluorescently labeled monoclonal antibodies and microscopically examined after 24- to 48-hour incubation.[324–326] A similar methodology, the enzyme linked virus inducible system (ELVIS), allows detection after 24 hours using cell lines designed to express β-galactosidase in HSV-infected cells.[324,327] Of note, the sensitivity of all culture-based approaches is affected by the age of the lesion, with the highest sensitivity being achieved from vesicular stage lesions.[328]

Molecular methods have emerged as the preferred approach for the diagnosis of primary or recurrent lesions due to HSV. Early LDTs targeted highly conserved regions of HSV to amplify both HSV-1 and HSV-2 without differentiation.[329] Newer assays have taken advantage of genetic polymorphisms between HSV-1 and HSV-2 allowing for methods such as melting curve analysis for type differentiation.[330–332] For additional information on melting curve analysis, refer to Chapter 64. A commonality shared by nearly all NAATs for the detection of HSV is a high sensitivity, often greater than that of culture.[330,332,333] The added sensitivity of NAAT and lack of necessity for viable virus or accurate quantitation diminish the impact of specimen collection and transport on assay performance. However, maximum sensitivity is obtained by swabbing unroofed vesicular lesions.[334]

Multiplexed molecular assays have also been designed to simultaneously detect additional pathogens that may resemble HSV lesions clinically such as *Treponema pallidum* and VZV.[335,336] The availability of these assays has highlighted previously underappreciated epidemiologic aspects of STIs. A study analyzing 2113 swab specimens collected from genital lesions using a multiplexed molecular assay designed to detect HSV-1, HSV-2, and VZV revealed 14 instances of VZV

positivity.[185] This suggests that VZV can mimic genital herpes and may be more common than traditionally believed.

The requirement for technical expertise in molecular methods has been addressed by the recent availability of FDA-cleared "moderately complex" molecular HSV tests. These assays have sensitivities and specificities comparable or superior to their LDT counterparts. Current versions of these tests are FDA-cleared for the detection of HSV-1 and HSV-2 from cutaneous and mucocutaneous lesions only, with the exception of the Focus Simplexa HSV 1/2 Direct and FilmArray ME assays, which have an indication for detection of HSV in CSF (see meningitis section of this chapter). While the Simplexa, Lyra Direct HSV 1+2/VZV (Quidel), and many other FDA-cleared HSV molecular tests utilize RT-PCR, others employ helicase dependent amplification (HDA) and loop mediated amplification (LAMP) methods.[337,338] These processes allow for the isothermal amplification of a molecular target, which eliminates the need for thermocycling, making them both rapid and easy to perform.

Human Papillomavirus

HPV has a circular double-stranded DNA genome and is taxonomically divided into greater than 200 different genotypes based on sequence variations. HPV is common among human populations throughout the world and is typically acquired through sexual contact. A prospective study of 2011 sexually active women estimated a cumulative risk of 44% for acquiring HPV.[339] Introduction of a vaccine against the most common genotypes has resulted in a 5 to 10% drop in prevalence of HPV 16 and HPV 18 in two recent studies.[340,341] Among at-risk groups without vaccination, the incidence remains high and far exceeds that seen for other STIs.[342,343]

HPV causes hyperproliferation of infected basal epithelial cells of the skin and mucosal surfaces resulting in the formation of condyloma acuminata (genital warts). These lesions are noninflammatory and typically regress without intervention. However, they can be disfiguring and cause significant emotional distress.[344,345] In contrast to skin lesions, lesions that occur within the cervical or anal mucosa are often asymptomatic. This makes identification of infected individuals difficult, which greatly contributes to the spread of infection. Following regression of epithelial lesions, the virus enters a period of latency and is capable of causing additional episodes of condyloma acuminata throughout the life of the patient. The most severe consequence of persistent infection is the development of cervical carcinoma, which is associated with so-called "oncogenic" or "high-risk" genotypes.[346] Among these, HPV types 16 and 18 are associated with the greatest risk of cervical cancer which is estimated to be 15 to 20% within 10 years of infection.[346,347]

HPV oncogenesis is most frequently associated with squamous cell carcinoma of the cervix; however, the virus is also strongly associated with adenocarcinoma of the cervix and squamous cell carcinomas of the rectum, head, and neck.[348–350] The significant role of HPV in these other malignancy types has been well characterized over the past decade. From 2008 to 2012 the CDC estimates that approximately 79% (n = 30,700) of cases of newly diagnosed head and neck cancer are HPV-related, with the vast majority being secondary to HPV 16.[351] The prevalence of HPV-related anal cancer is estimated at 5.1 per 100,000 individuals, though is much higher in HIV-positive men at 45.9 per 100,000 individuals.[352] The highest

TABLE 89.6   **FDA-Cleared Molecular Tests for Detection of Human Papillomavirus**

Assay	Genetic Target	Genotyping	Approved Indication for Primary Screen	Approved Collection Medium
Cervista HPV 16/18 and HR (Hologic)	DNA	Cervista HPV HR detects 14 high-risk genotypes without differentiation Cervista HPV 16/18 reports genotype for 16, 18 if present	No	ThinPrep
Digene HC2 HPV DNA Test (Qiagen)	DNA	Detects 18 high-risk genotypes, without differentiation	No	SurePath and ThinPrep
Cobas HPV test (Roche)	DNA	Detects 14 high-risk genotypes, specifically differentiates 16, 18 (others reported as "High risk HPV detected")	Yes	SurePath and ThinPrep
Aptima HPV assay (Hologic)	mRNA	Detects 14 high-risk genotypes, without differentiation	No	ThinPrep
Aptima HPV 16, 18/45 genotype assay (Hologic)	mRNA	Specifically detects and differentiates genotypes 16, 18/45	No	ThinPrep
Onclarity HPV assay (BD)	DNA	Detects 17 high-risk genotypes, specifically differentiates 16, 18, 45	Yes	SurePath

HPV, Human papillomavirus.

risk factor for both HPV-related head and neck carcinomas and anal carcinomas appear to be sexual contact with infected individuals, suggesting possible mitigation through effective screening and vaccination approaches.

Diagnostic Cytology Methods for HPV

The goal of testing for HPV is early detection to aid in prevention of HPV-related malignancies. Since its introduction in 1941, cervical cytology has remained the mainstay for HPV screening. During cervical cytology, the transitional zone of the cervix is sampled using a brush and exfoliated cells are examined for cytologic abnormalities. Sensitivity of this method is highly dependent on collection of brushings from the region of the cervix most commonly affected by HPV.[353] Cytology results are interpreted using the Bethesda classification system in which atypical cells are classified as "low-grade squamous intraepithelial lesions" (LSIL) and "high-grade squamous intraepithelial lesion" (HSIL).[354–356] Atypical cells that lack all necessary features to be classified as LSIL or HSIL may be classified as atypical squamous cells of undetermined significance (ASC-US) or atypical squamous cells—cannot exclude HSIL (ASC-H). If a high-grade lesion is suspected based on cytology, a cervical biopsy is often performed. Atypia observed on a cervical biopsy is classified using a different standardized classification system, cervical intraepithelial neoplasia (CIN) 1 to 3. A diagnosis of CIN 1 is rendered when typical viral CPE is present, a finding correlating to LSIL. CIN 2 corresponds to dysplasia confined to the basal two thirds of the epithelium whereas in CIN 3 the dysplasia is full thickness (carcinoma in situ). If deep invasion of atypical cells is observed, a diagnosis of invasive carcinoma is rendered. The American Society for Colposcopy and Cervical Pathology (ASCCP) published updated guidelines in 2019 regarding the further management of patients with different cytology and biopsy results.[357]

Molecular Tests for Screening and Diagnosis of Invasive HPV

Molecular detection of HPV has emerged as a method to augment cytologic screening of patients for the risk of HPV-related malignancy. Molecular assays vary substantially based on the type of nucleic acid they detect (DNA vs. RNA) and the specific HPV genotypes they detect and differentiate (Table 89.6). Current FDA-approved HPV assays that detect DNA include the Cervista HPV 16/18 and high-risk (HR) tests (Hologic), the Digene HC2 HPV DNA Test (Qiagen), and the Cobas HPV test (Roche). Studies comparing these tests have shown comparable performance between these tests with slightly lower sensitivity exhibited for the HC2 assay.[358–361] This is likely multifactorial, resulting from the underlying chemistry of the HC2 (probe-based rather than PCR-based) and the lack of internal specimen adequacy control which can lead to an interpretation of "negative" for specimens that would be considered inadequate by other systems.

The Aptima HPV assay (Hologic) differs from the previously discussed tests in that it targets RNA rather than DNA. Specifically, Aptima HPV detects HPV E6 and E7 oncogene mRNA transcripts present in infected host cells. It is capable of detecting 14 different high-risk HPV types, including 16 and 18, though it does not differentiate them. A second, the Aptima HPV 16 18/45 Genotype Assay, can be performed on positive samples to specifically identify HPV 16 and HPV 18/45. By detecting mRNA rather than DNA, the APTIMA assay has the potential to more specifically identify active infection since large amounts of RNA are not present during viral latency. Several recent comparisons of the Aptima assay to other commercially available DNA-based assays support this hypothesis.[362,363] In 2018, a fifth HPV assay was approved by the FDA, the BD Onclarity HPV Assay. The Onclarity assay targets the E6 and E7 genes, similar to the Aptima HPV assay; however, the Onclarity assay uses real-time PCR and specifically differentiates HPV 16, 18, and 45. Initial evaluations of the BD Onclarity assay have supported good overall concordance with its predecessors.[364] When considering which assay to implement it is important to recognize the specific specimen types approved for each assay. The Digene HC 2 assay and the COBAS 4800 HPV assay are FDA approved for both SurePath and ThinPrep cervical cytology collection devices. The Aptima and Cervista assays are approved for ThinPrep specimens only, whereas the BD Onclarity assay is approved for SurePath only.[365]

Diagnostic Algorithms for HPV

The use of cytology, biopsy, and molecular testing for HPV has evolved much over recent years. The ASCCP provides formal guidance regarding how these tests should be used in different age groups. Initial guidelines released in 2012 addressed how commonly utilized molecular tests should be integrated into the cervical cancer screening algorithm.[366] These guidelines recommended screening by cytology every 3 years from the ages of 21 to 65 years as acceptable practice. However, for women ages 30 to 65 years the preferable screening method was "co-testing," which includes the use of both cytology and molecular methods simultaneously. If this strategy was applied, screening could be reduced to every 5 years. This recommendation was based on meta-analysis data supporting the high sensitivity of HPV molecular testing for the early detection of cervical carcinoma.[367]

A consequence of "co-testing" has been an increased number of patients reported as positive for high-risk HPV by molecular methods though negative by cytology. While the ASCCP guidelines state these women can be retested 1 year later, investigators have shown it is possible to further risk stratify these patients based on HPV genotyping. The ATHENA (Addressing the Need for Advanced HPV Diagnostics) study demonstrated that positivity for HPV 16 and/or HPV 18 carries nearly double the risk for CIN 2 lesions or greater compared to other high-risk HPV types (11.4% versus 6.1%).[368,369] This and other similar studies clearly demonstrate the added value of specific genotyping among high-risk HPV types. This increased risk is reflected in the current guidelines, which recommend that patients between ages 30 and 65 with molecular positivity for HPV 16 or HPV 18 be managed more aggressively than patients with positivity for other HPV types, necessitating immediate colposcopy rather than rescreening 1 year later. A second important insight from this trial was the considerable laboratory-to-laboratory variation in cytologic abnormality rates, suggesting the subjectivity of this approach may have a significant effect on patient results.[370] In contrast, molecular positivity rates did not vary significantly among sites, suggesting molecular methods are less subject to bias and perhaps better suited as the initial screening methodology.

In 2014, the Cobas HPV test (Roche) became the first FDA-approved molecular assay indicated for primary HPV screening of ThinPrep specimens obtained from women age 25 and older. In 2018 it was joined by the BD Onclarity, which obtained approval for primary screen utilizing Sure-Path specimens.[365] Initial studies examining this approach suggest molecular screening has higher sensitivity and accuracy compared to cytology.[371] In 2018, the American Academy of Obstetrics and Gynecology endorsed primary HPV screening as an acceptable approach to HPV management in women 30 to 65 years of age.[372] Updated patient management guidelines published by the ASCCP in 2019 also support the acceptability of primary screening.[357] These guidelines state that either co-testing or primary screening can be used interchangeably, provided the assay in use has attained FDA approval for primary screening. These updated guidelines also state that cytology alone is only acceptable as a screening approach when concurrent molecular testing is not feasible.

Human Immunodeficiency Virus

HIV is the causative agent of acquired immunodeficiency syndrome (AIDS). There are two different species of HIV, HIV-1 and HIV-2, as well as several subtypes. HIV-2 is uncommon in most regions of the world and is primarily limited to the African continent. In contrast, HIV-1 is found throughout the world and is responsible for the current AIDS pandemic. Both viruses are sexually transmitted, though can also be transmitted through bodily fluids such as blood. Though severity of disease and overall mortality is significantly lower in patients infected with HIV-2, both viruses are capable of causing a prolonged infection leading to profound immunosuppression, opportunistic infections, and ultimately death.[373,374] Acute infection with HIV is marked by symptoms in approximately 40 to 90% of patients, including fever, malaise, rash, headache, and lymphadenopathy.[375] These symptoms are nonspecific, transient, and often cause the initial infection to be overlooked or misdiagnosed. During infection the virus replicates in CD4+ T lymphocytes, exhibiting an initial replicative peak within days after infection followed by a plateau of steady state replication that can persist for years. During this time CD4+ T lymphocytes gradually decline in number, eventually putting the patient at risk for life threatening opportunistic infections. Patients are contagious during the entire time course of infection but are particularly contagious during the acute stage when VL can be greater than 6 $\log_{10}$ copies/mL. Therefore early diagnosis of acute HIV infection is critical in reducing the spread of disease. Current CDC estimates suggest an average 1.2 million people are living with HIV in the United States and approximately 12.8% have not been diagnosed.[376] Worldwide there are approximately 38 million people living with HIV, with sub-Saharan Africa accounting for approximately two thirds of infected individuals.[377]

Serologic and Molecular Methods for Diagnosis of HIV

Laboratory diagnosis of HIV is typically achieved through serologic testing. Serologic tests have substantially evolved throughout the years and are referred to as first to fifth generation tests. These tests are all ELISA based, though with key differences. First-generation EIAs detect IgG antibody against crude preparations of HIV antigen derived from viral lysates. As such, they lacked both sensitivity and specificity and were only in use for a brief period of time.[378,379] Second-generation EIAs substituted viral lysates for purified viral proteins, a change that reduced the window of detection from approximately 56 to 42 days following infection.[379,380] Third-generation assays allowed for the detection of both IgG and IgM, further shortening the detection window to 3 to 4 weeks. Since their release in the early 1990s, third-generation HIV assays have been the predominant assays in use throughout the world. A subset of third-generation assays has been adapted into lateral flow formats allowing for rapid POC testing. These rapid HIV tests have greatly extended screening capabilities by allowing testing to be performed in emergent situations and in low-income locations with limited testing capabilities.[381] A more recent improvement in HIV testing is the introduction of fourth-generation ELISAs, which improve upon their predecessors by adding the ability to detect p24 antigen in addition to IgG and IgM. Since p24 antigen appears prior to HIV-specific antibodies, these assays have the shortest window of detection among available EIAs, allowing detection of HIV within approximately 2 to 3 weeks of infection onset.[382,383] Most recently, the BioPlex 2200 HIV Ag-AB assay (Bio-Rad) was developed as a "fifth-generation" test. This test is capable of detecting p24 antigen in addition to antibodies to HIV-1 and HIV-2 like its fourth-generation predecessors while simultaneously differentiating between the three analytes. Evaluation of the BioPlex assay has shown similar performance to other commercially available fourth-generation assays.[384]

Diagnostic Algorithms for HIV

Since none of the currently available EIAs are 100% specific, confirmatory testing is required prior to rendering a diagnosis of HIV. Traditionally, confirmation was performed using the HIV Western Blot (WB) to detect the presence or absence of patient antibodies to specific HIV proteins. Based on the pattern of reactivity, patients were classified as negative, positive, or indeterminate. The window period for WB positivity is extremely variable, typically taking several weeks to months following exposure. An indeterminate WB result may indicate cross-reactive antibodies in the EIA screen or a true infection which may be revealed with repeat testing up to 6 months later.[385] This long period of diagnostic uncertainty can cause a significant amount of emotional distress in patients.

In 2014 the CDC recommended a new algorithm for HIV diagnosis, commonly referred to as the "fourth-generation algorithm."[383] Rather than screening with third-generation ELISAs, this algorithm incorporates screening with the more sensitive fourth-generation EIAs, allowing for the earlier detection of acute HIV infection. Another improvement is the elimination of WB as the primary confirmatory test. In its place, an EIA capable of differentiating antibodies against HIV-1 and HIV-2 is employed. There are several advantages to this approach. The use of a differentiation assay allows for a better detection and identification of HIV-2 infections that may be under diagnosed by the WB.[386] Additionally, an EIA is easier to interpret and quicker to perform than WB that enables confirmatory results within 24 hours of the initial screening result.[387] Importantly, the confirmatory HIV-1/HIV-2 differentiation assay is a second-generation immunoassay whereas the antigen/antibody screen is a fourth-generation assay. Therefore in the setting of acute HIV infection, patients may test positive with the screening assay but negative with the confirmatory test. As such, patients with this testing pattern require additional confirmatory testing using an FDA-approved HIV NAAT.[383] In the setting of acute HIV-1 infection, nucleic acid will be detectable prior to fourth-generation antigen/antibody screening assays and can be used to make a definitive diagnosis. Since none of the FDA-approved NAATs currently detect HIV-2, patients with risk factors for HIV-2 (i.e., residence in or travel to an endemic area) require either demonstration of seroconversion over time or confirmation with an HIV-2 specific NAAT. Studies examining the performance of the fourth-generation algorithm demonstrated nearly 100% sensitivity and specificity for the diagnosis of HIV-1 in various populations.[388,389]

There are currently five commercially available fourth-generation platforms and a sixth fifth-generation platform that are considered acceptable screening assays for the fourth-generation algorithm (https://www.cdc.gov/hiv/pdf/testing/hiv-tests-laboratory-use.pdf). Head-to-head comparisons of these assays suggest similar performance.[390] The options for HIV-1/2 differentiation assays (second step of the algorithm) are less diverse. Until 2017 the Multispot HIV-1/HIV-2 rapid test (Bio-Rad) was the only assay recommended by the CDC

and the Association of Public Health Laboratories (APHL) as an acceptable supplemental assay in the fourth-generation algorithm. When used in the context of the fourth-generation algorithm, the Multispot exhibits superior performance when compared to the Western Blot, in particular due to its ability to accurately identify HIV-2 infections.[386] In 2017, the Multispot was discontinued and replaced by its successor, the Geenius HIV 1/2 Supplemental system (Bio-Rad). Functionally, the Geenius is very similar to the Multispot with the ability to detect and differentiate antibodies to HIV-1 and HIV-2. However, whereas the Multispot used two antigen targets for the detection of HIV-1 and one target for HIV-2, the Geenius uses four targets for HIV-1 and two targets for HIV-2. This redesign has resulted in some differences in performance and interpretation compared to its predecessor. The Geenius demonstrates better detection of acute HIV infections[391] but also suffers increased occurrence of cross-reactivity between HIV-1 and HIV-2 (i.e., HIV-1 reactive with HIV-2 cross-reactivity).

Currently the only FDA-cleared molecular test for the diagnosis of HIV is the Aptima HIV-1 Qualitative Assay. This assay shows high sensitivity for the detection of acute HIV-1.[392] Of note, patients with acute HIV-1 rapidly develop high VLs. If acute HIV is suspected and a low VL less than 1000 copies/mL is obtained, laboratories should investigate further for the possibility of preanalytical error. There are, however, a cohort of patients who may have low or undetectable VL at the time of diagnosis. These patients are able to control the virus with their own immune systems through a variety of mechanisms and are known as "elite controllers" or "long-term nonprogressors."[393] Though these patients constitute a minority of those infected with HIV, identification of them is important because a proportion will eventually lose their ability to control the virus and progress to AIDS. While these patients may have an undetectable VL, they still exhibit the appropriate seroconversion and will be diagnosed appropriately if the fourth-generation algorithm is used.

Another unique population that must be considered when establishing a diagnosis of HIV is neonates. Since IgG antibodies cross the placenta, serologic testing in neonates reflects the serologic status of the mother and as such cannot be used. This necessitates a molecular approach. Guidelines regarding how often to test a child following birth exist and are dependent on the mother's HIV status and overall risk of transmission to the child.[394] In this setting, diagnosis is initially established using molecular testing. Therefore it is recommended that all positive molecular results be confirmed by eventual demonstration of seroconversion. Another complication of testing in this population is that at-risk infants are also being treated with antiretroviral prophylaxis or empiric therapy. As such, testing with an RNA-based test may in theory be a suboptimal approach given the potential for viral suppression. For this reason, testing using either DNA-based or RNA/DNA combination-based assays has been recommended in infants since proviral DNA should not be affected by therapy. While this may be intuitive, some investigators have suggested that this may not be needed, and that RNA-based assays are equally effective for diagnosis in this setting.[395] Regardless, there are currently no FDA-approved assays that detect HIV DNA. Given the current availability of only a single HIV qualitative test that detects RNA only, there is an overall need for additional options.

Several CE-marked assays have been described, though they are currently unavailable in the United States.[396,397] A better availability of qualitative molecular tests will be of particular benefit to perinatal management.

Challenges to Implementation of HIV Algorithm-based Testing

Adherence to the fourth-generation algorithm for diagnosis of acute HIV may necessitate up to three different tests using two different methodologies (serologic and molecular), creating a challenge for specimen management. Molecular tests are exquisitely sensitive, and many serologic tests are performed in laboratories with techniques that may not be adequate to prevent contamination. Viral contamination of automated and manual processes in clinical chemistry laboratories has been well documented.[398,399] This creates a potential for specimen contamination and false positivity if a single patient specimen is used to perform all patient testing for HIV diagnosis. Laboratories have addressed this by requiring separate patient specimens for serologic and molecular testing, though the patient may no longer be available when it becomes known that a second specimen is needed for confirmation. Another strategy is to adopt processes to prevent contamination, yet still allow testing on a single specimen (i.e., aliquoting all received specimens for potential molecular testing prior to placement on an automated line for serologic testing). The degree to which specimen contamination is a risk differs from laboratory to laboratory; it is the responsibility of each laboratory to evaluate this risk.

Despite the strong diagnostic performance of the current fourth-generation algorithm there are situations in which patients may be tested using alternative approaches. HIV rapid tests are simple-to-perform screening assays that are designed to be implemented as POC devices. The majority of these are third-generation immunoassays that utilize lateral flow chemistry. An advantage to these tests is their rapidity, allowing screening results to be communicated with a patient often during a single encounter. This rapidity is also helpful in settings in which urgent decisions are required (i.e., the decision to give antivirals during an emergent delivery). Their ease of use also allows implementation in settings outside of the clinical laboratory, creating a greater availability of HIV diagnostics. A significant disadvantage of these assays is their generally inferior performance when compared to antigen/antibody screening assays in terms of both sensitivity and specificity.[400,401] As such, the CDC has historically recommended that all positive rapid antibody tests be confirmed using an antigen/antibody assay. If positive, further testing should be performed according to the fourth-generation algorithm. If negative by a fourth-generation immunoassay, additional testing is not needed.[383] In 2018 the CDC acknowledged an exception to this rule. If the Determine HIV 1/2 Ag/Ab rapid test (currently the sole fourth-generation rapid assay) is utilized on serum or plasma it can serve as an acceptable first step in the fourth-generation algorithm. Importantly, if this approach is taken, laboratories must adopt reporting language that acknowledges the resultant decreased sensitivity for acute HIV.

Molecular Methods for Monitoring and Management of Patients With HIV

During the period of clinical latency, CD4+ T cell count gradually decreases along with an increasing VL. Early studies examined the utility of these targets as markers of disease progression. The measurement of CD4+ T cell count is a good indicator of immune status at diagnosis and conveys the urgency of starting treatment, whereas VL is prognostic of disease progression and serves as a marker to monitor response to antiviral therapy.[402–404] As such, patients with HIV are now routinely tested for VL and guidelines for utilization of these data are available from the US Department of Health and Human Services (DHHS).[402] The main goal is to achieve and maintain an undetectable VL by 24 weeks of therapy. This endpoint differs depending on the assay used.

Assays that detect and quantify viral RNA use a variety of chemistries. Early assays included the Cobas Amplicor assay (Roche) that utilized endpoint PCR, the Versant HIV-1 RNA assay (Bayer) which utilized branch DNA for target capture and signal amplification, and the Nuclisens HIV-QT assay that utilized a chemistry similar to transcription mediated amplification (TMA). Original versions of these assays had analytical sensitivities ranging from 75 to 400 copies/mL. Variation in chemistry and design prevented interassay comparison of VL and resulted in variable sensitivity for specific HIV subtypes.[405] These limitations prompted a second generation of HIV VL assays with improved analytical sensitivity. Currently two of these assays are FDA-approved, the Cobas AmpliPrep/Cobas TaqMan HIV-1 Assay (Roche) and the Real-Time TaqMan HIV-1 assay (Abbott). Both utilize RT-PCR and target conserved genetic regions unaffected by mutations conferring resistance to antiviral drugs. These assays are capable of detecting and quantifying extremely low VLs (20 to 40 copies/mL) and demonstrate better interassay correlation than their earlier counterparts.[406,407] The acceptable interassay variation in VL is ~0.5 $\log_{10}$ copies/mL.[402] An unintended consequence of increased analytical sensitivity was the detection of HIV in patients with previously undetectable VL and the resulting unnecessary modifications to therapy, additional cost, and added confusion.[408,409] Low and intermittent VL values likely represent "viral load blips" which are now addressed in the DHHS VL monitoring guidelines.[402] VL blips are defined as transiently detectable VLs less than 400 copies/mL and should be regarded as clinically insignificant. At this time, data are conflicting regarding the clinical significance of persistent low-level VL.[410,411]

Resistance to antiviral therapy is mediated by mutations in specific drug targets. Testing for these mutations is commonly referred to as HIV genotyping. The majority of resistance mutations occur in genes encoding the viral protease and reverse transcriptase enzymes, since these are the most common targets of antiviral therapy. There is currently one FDA-approved genotyping kit available, the ViroSeq HIV-1 Genotyping System (Abbott).[412,413] This assay amplifies the protease and reverse transcriptase genes which are then sequenced using traditional Sanger sequencing methods. Resulting sequence data are compared to a reference library of characterized antiviral resistance mutations. While several libraries exist, the Stanford University HIV Drug Resistance Database is the most complete and commonly utilized. An important limitation to this methodology is that it only detects resistance to antivirals that target the protease and reverse transcriptase genes. The introduction of new drug classes, such as integrase inhibitors, has created a need for detecting mutations in alternative genes. Several integrase inhibitor genotype assays have been developed for this purpose, though none are FDA-approved.[414,415] A second limitation of HIV genotyping is an inability to detect low-level mutations present in mixed viral populations. Sanger sequencing requires a mutation to comprise of at least 25 to 30% of a mixture in order to be detected.[416] Next-generation sequencing technologies are highly suited to address this challenge (for additional discussion on next-generation sequencing, refer to Chapter 64). This technology has been applied to detect mutational frequencies as low as 1% in mixed populations.[417,418] The clinical significance of low-frequency mutations detected by next-generation sequencing but not by Sanger-based methods remains uncertain. A recent study suggested limited utility of the next-generation sequencing approach beyond the routine Sanger result.[419] In this study, additional low-frequency mutations identified by next-generation sequencing did not appear to predict antiviral treatment failure or correlate with disease relapse or prognosis.

Phenotypic resistance testing may be used when genotyping fails to identify a genetic basis for observed resistance or for the determination of viral tropism. Phenotyping is a complicated process of isolating and amplifying viral RNA followed by cloning the product into an HIV vector containing a reporter gene (e.g., luciferase). Growth of the virus in vitro is then quantified in the presence of various antivirals. Results are compared to those obtained from wild-type virus and antiviral concentrations that inhibit 50 and 90% of viral growth are reported. In the United States, these tests are only available at two reference laboratories, Virco Lab, Inc (Bridgewater, NJ) and Monogram Biosciences (San Francisco, CA). Co-receptor tropism assays share much of the same methodology.[420] These methods test whether the patient's virus is CXCR4 tropic or CCR5 tropic by examining the ability of cloned virus to infect cells with either co-receptor. Maraviroc, a CCR5 antagonist, will only be effective in patients with CCR5 tropic virions.

An important limitation to both phenotypic and genotypic methodologies for the assessment of resistance is the need for a threshold amount of virus (typically 500 to 2000 copies/mL) for successful sequencing or cloning. Newer assays utilizing proviral DNA rather than RNA have been developed to address this challenge; however, results obtained using proviral DNA may not correlate well with results based on RNA.[421,422]

POINTS TO REMEMBER
Sexually Transmitted Viruses

- HSV serology can be difficult to interpret given high seroprevalence for HSV-1 and HSV-2.
- Diagnosis of HSV is best accomplished through highly sensitive and specific molecular detection techniques.
- Molecular methods that target HPV high-risk types and specific identification of genotypes 16 and 18 allows for identification of patients at high risk for carcinoma.
- HIV is typically diagnosed with serology and occasionally molecular methods, whereas HIV progression is monitored by quantitative viral load assays.
- The currently recommended fourth-generation screening algorithm for HIV entails use of a screening test that includes p24 antigen.

VIRAL INFECTIONS OF THE CENTRAL NERVOUS SYSTEM

Introduction

Infections of the CNS can be attributed to bacterial, fungal, viral, and protozoan pathogens. Symptoms can range from mild fever and headache to severe debilitating headache, photophobia, nuchal rigidity, fever, altered mental status, and death. Viral etiologies are the most common cause of infectious meningitis and as a whole these infections are less severe than bacterial or fungal meningitis. The majority of viral meningitis infections are mild, transient, and self-resolving within 7 to 10 days. Medical attention may not be sought for mild cases and a specific pathogen is often not identified. Even among severe meningitis-related deaths, a definitive pathogen is identified in only 30% of cases.[423] Collectively, these infections of unknown etiology are referred to as "aseptic meningitis" and are believed to be largely viral. Viral meningitis is classically characterized by CSF parameters including normal glucose (2.2 to 4.7 mmol/L), moderately increased protein (500 to 1500 mg/L), and mild leukocytosis (50 to 250 × 10^6 cells/L) with a lymphocytic predominance.[424,425] Importantly, transient neutrophilic predominance is common early in viral meningitis and does not exclude a viral etiology.[425]

Three groups of viruses are responsible for the majority of cases of viral meningitis and encephalitis: herpesviruses, arboviruses, and enteroviruses (EVs; Table 89.7). Epidemiology, transmission, and risk factors for viral meningitis among these groups of viruses differ, but all are capable of causing symptomatic illness in immune competent hosts. Culture, serologic, and NAAT-based methods have all been employed for the identification of viral agents associated with meningitis and encephalitis.

Enteroviruses

Infections with non-polio EVs including enterovirus, coxsackie virus, and echovirus and the closely related human parechoviruses (HPeVs) are extremely common, affecting greater than 10 million people annually in the United States.[426] Infections are largely asymptomatic, but may also manifest as fever, rash, respiratory illness, vesicular lesions, or CNS disease (e.g., meningitis, acute flaccid myelitis [AFM], encephalitis). Enteroviral infections are the leading cause of meningitis in children, with 50 to 90% of infections affecting children less than 5 years of age.[426,427] Of note, increased incidence of AFM in children has been observed throughout the United States in late summer to fall on a biannual basis since 2014. These peaks have occurred during outbreaks of enterovirus D68 and A71; however, a causal relationship has been difficult to establish.[428,429] HPeVs are the second leading cause of meningitis in children, accounting for 20 to 30% as many infections as EVs[430]; however, this may be an underestimation since specific diagnostic tests for HPeV are not widely available.

Laboratory diagnostics can play an important role in the management of patients with suspected viral meningitis. Rapid and accurate identification of EV and HPeV in CSF specimens, particularly in children, can reduce hospitalization time and prevent unnecessary antibiotic therapy.[431-433] Specifically, unnecessary antibiotic usage was decreased by an average of 20 hours and total cost of care was reduced by nearly $3000 per patient when the results of EV NAAT were available within 24 hours. These savings can account for a

TABLE 89.7 Characteristics and Approaches to Diagnosis of Central Nervous System Infections due to Select Herpesviruses and Enteroviruses

Virus	CSF Characteristics	Culture	Serology	Molecular
Herpesviruses				
Herpes simplex virus-1 and -2 (HSV-1, HSV-2)	Protein concentration 700–1500 mg/L; leukocyte count 200–500 × 10⁶ cells/L	Limited utility due to poor sensitivity (<20%) and extended time to result (2–14 days).	Limited utility for diagnosis of acute HSV CNS disease. Requires 1–4 weeks to reach diagnostic levels in CSF.	Preferred method. Laboratory developed and FDA-cleared tests available. Sensitivity 75–100%, limit of detection 10^3–10^4 viral copies/mL. Viral DNA may be undetectable 1–3 days following onset of symptoms.
Varicella zoster virus (VZV)	Protein concentration 600–2600 mg/L; leukocyte count 5–450 × 10⁶ cells/L	Limited utility due to poor sensitivity and extended time to result (2–14 days).	Detection of IgG in blood has no utility due to >90% seroprevalence. Detection of IgM in blood may indicate acute infection or viral reactivation. Detection of either IgG or IgM in CSF is consistent with VZV meningitis but may also result from asymptomatic reactivation or transmigration across blood brain barrier. A comparison of antibody titer (CSF vs. serum) can be useful.	Preferred method. Laboratory developed and FDA-cleared tests available. Sensitivity 95–100%, limit of detection 10^0–10^1 viral copies/reaction. Quantitative assays may be used to predict more severe disease in specimens with viral load >10^4 copies/mL.
Epstein-Barr virus (EBV)		Not cultivable using routine methods	Limited utility due to high seroprevalence	Qualitative and quantitative NAATs evaluated. Qualitative NAATs demonstrate 75–100% sensitivity but 66–80% specificity due to latent virus in lymphocytic CSF infiltrates. Quantitative NAATs may be used to increase specificity to >95% if based on threshold of 10^4 copies/mL
Enteroviruses				
	Protein concentration 100–875 mg/L; leukocyte count 0–1300 × 10⁶ cells/L	Limited utility due to poor sensitivity (35–75%) and extended time to result (5–14 days).	Limited utility due to high seroprevalence and potential for positivity during asymptomatic reactivation	Preferred method. Laboratory developed and FDA-cleared tests available. Target conserved 5′UTR of EV genome to detect majority of serotypes (coxsackievirus, enterovirus, echovirus). Sensitivity >95%, limit of detection <50 copies/mL, time to result 2–6 h. May cross-react with rhinovirus. Undetectable VL in serum does not rule out CNS involvement.

CNS, Central nervous system; *CSF,* cerebrospinal fluid; *EV,* enterovirus; *FDA,* Food and Drug Administration; *HPV,* human papillomavirus; *NAATs,* nucleic acid amplification tests; *VL,* viral load; *VZV,* varicella-zoster virus.

10 to 20% reduction in total hospital cost of care if EV NAAT is used for all symptomatic infants.

Diagnostic Methods for Presumed EV or HPeV CNS Infections

Enterovirus can be recovered from various specimen types using viral culture methods; however, these methods are technically demanding, have sensitivity as low as 35%, and require 4 to 14 days for results.[434–436] NAATs targeting the 5′ untranslated region (5′UTR) of the EV genome have been the preferred method for detection of EVs since the early 1990s.[437] The 5′UTR sequence is well conserved across EV species and enables pan-detection of the majority of clinically relevant EVs including EV-D68 and EV-A71.[438] EV and HPeV are present in the CSF during symptomatic infection, and CSF is the specimen of choice for laboratory diagnosis of EV or HPeV meningitis. Importantly, only 55% of patients with EV meningitis had detectable EV RNA in matched serum specimens.[439] Therefore analysis of serum cannot be used to rule out CNS involvement. Conversely, EV is frequently detected at low levels in the CSF of children suffering from EV sepsis in absence of clinical or radiographic evidence of CNS involvement. This may be the result of leakage of a small amount of viral RNA into the CNS compartment from the bloodstream, in which the VL may be as high as 10^5 to 10^6 copies/mL during viral sepsis. In these cases, CSF lymphocytosis may aid in supporting or refuting CNS involvement.[439]

A specific advantage of NAATs is the increased analytical sensitivity (100 to 500 copies/mL) compared with culture.[440,441] This is a critical characteristic given the relatively low VL associated with CNS infection (10^2 to 10^3 copies/mL) and small specimen volume typically submitted for analysis.[439] Qualitative NAATs based on either end-point detection or RT-PCR demonstrate sensitivity of 94 to 100% compared with viral culture, and identify EVs in an additional 8 to 29% of culture negative specimens.[434,435,441] Real-time quantitative PCR (qPCR) assays have also been published with an analytic measurement range spanning 5 $\log_{10}$ copies/mL.[440,442] The clinical sensitivity of qPCR is superior to viral culture, detecting EV in an additional 12% of symptomatic patients.[442] Importantly, EV was not detected in the CSF of asymptomatic controls, which supports the clinical relevance of these additional positive specimens.

Molecular testing for EVs and HPeVs in CSF is still largely conducted using high-complexity LDTs which are independently developed and validated. Two molecular tests for the detection of EVs in CSF have gained FDA-cleared status with a "moderate complexity" designation: Xpert EV (Cepheid, Sunnyvale, CA) and FilmArray ME (BioFire). These tests are fully automated, sample-to-answer, and require as little as 1 to 2.5 hours for results. The Xpert EV assay is designed to detect greater than 60 EV serotypes with a LoD of 10^{-3} to 10^2 TCID$_{50}$/mL[443] and demonstrates greater than 95% sensitivity and 100% specificity when compared to a composite gold standard.[436,443,444] The FilmArray ME is a largely multiplexed assay capable of detecting seven viruses (in addition to six bacteria and one yeast) associated with CNS infection from CSF specimens.[197] An independent clinical evaluation of the FilmArray ME using archived CSF specimens demonstrated 57 to 100% sensitivity and 84 to 100% specificity for detection of viral targets on the multiplex panel as compared to individual uniplex laboratory-developed NAATs. This included 97.4% (37/38) sensitivity for the detection of EVs.[197]

A potential drawback to EV NAATs targeting the 5′UTR sequence is the reported cross-reactivity with rhinovirus[438,443]; however, this may not be a major confounding factor when analyzing CSF since rhinovirus is not associated with meningitis. Further, not all rhinovirus serotypes are cross-reactive as indicated by the analytic specificity studies conducted in evaluations of EV NAATs.[441,442,444] Cross-reactivity is likely multifactorial, depending on specific target sequence, limit or threshold of detection utilized, and the specific rhinovirus serotype present in the specimen. Likewise, use of the 5′UTR target does not allow differentiation of EV serotypes of specific interest such as D68 or A71, which have been associated with acute respiratory symptoms and AFM. LDTs based on EV capsid protein VP1 gene sequences can specifically identify EV-D68[429,445] and are used to confirm the presence of EV-D68 in specimens that test positive using "traditional" 5′UTR-based "pan-EV" tests. Importantly, EV RNA is only

rarely detected in CSF specimens obtained from patients meeting the clinical criteria for AFM diagnosis.[428,429] In contrast, EV-D68 has been detected by NAAT in up to 50% of respiratory specimens and serologically in up to 80% of CSF specimens in these patients. Taken together, these data demonstrate the limitations of standard EV NAATs for diagnosis of EV CNS infections beyond classic meningitis.

Herpesviruses

Several of the human herpesviruses have been associated with CNS manifestations following either primary infection or viral reactivation. Clinical symptoms are nonspecific among the herpesviruses and share common symptoms with other viral CNS infections; however, prognosis and approach to treatment may vary among herpesviruses and other viral agents causing CNS infection. Therefore the laboratory plays an important role in identification and differentiation of these agents.

Herpes Simplex Virus

HSV is the second most commonly identified viral agent associated with CNS infection and is a leading cause of death among CNS infections with known etiology.[423] Important differences in epidemiology, prognosis, and mortality are observed between CNS infections with HSV-1 and HSV-2, making specific identification of these viruses a critical component to patient management. Recurrent aseptic meningitis (Mollaret syndrome) is the most common CNS complication associated with HSV-2. It primarily affects young immunocompetent adults, and has an approximately 1.7:1 predominance in females.[446–449] This is typically a self-limiting meningitis and the specific benefit of antiviral therapy and optimal treatment regimen have not been established.[449] Genital lesions associated with HSV may or may not be present at the time of CNS symptoms.[450,451] HSV-1 accounts for 80% of HSV encephalitis and is the most common cause of sporadic encephalitis in immunocompetent individuals and those with underlying immune suppression or uncontrolled HIV.[452–454] HSV encephalitis is a severe and life-threatening condition requiring immediate medical intervention. Even with effective treatment, the mortality rate for HSV encephalitis can approach 20% and greater than 95% of patients will suffer long-term neurologic defects.[453,454]

Culture of HSV from CSF in symptomatic patients is low yield (4 to 20% sensitive) and should not be used to rule out HSV involvement.[450,455] Serologic assessment of the CSF is also of limited utility in diagnosing acute HSV meningitis or encephalitis. Antibody levels may take 1 to 4 weeks to become detectable in CSF following primary infection and persist at low levels in CSF even in individuals with no history of CNS involvement.[450,455]

NAATs for the detection of HSV in CSF are preferred because of both increased sensitivity and reduced time to result. The VL of HSV in symptomatic CNS infections is variable, but commonly ranges from 10^2 to 10^4 viral copies/mL.[456,457] There is no statistical difference in VL between CNS infections caused by HSV-1 or HSV-2, and VL in HSV meningitis is similar to that observed in encephalitis.[456,458] The impact of CSF VL determination remains an open area for further research. Some studies have demonstrated a correlation of VL with severity of symptoms and prognosis, while others failed to identify a significant association.[453,459] Importantly, viral DNA may not be detected in CSF for 1 to 3 days following acute onset of symptoms so a second test may be considered for patients with compatible symptoms 3 to 7 days after onset.[452]

Several laboratory-developed and FDA-cleared or CE-Marked assays are available for the identification of HSV-1 and -2 in CSF specimens. Published LDTs using various viral targets, primer and probe chemistries, and PCR platforms have demonstrated an LoD of 10^3 to 10^4 copies/mL and sensitivity 70 to 100% for detection of HSV in CSF specimens.[329,452,457] The Aries HSV 1&2 assay (Luminex) has gained FDA clearance for cutaneous lesions but is CE-marked for use with both cutaneous lesions and CSF specimens. A single analytical (spiked specimen) study determined the LoD of this assay to be approximately 1000 copies/mL in CSF for both HSV-1 and -2.[460] One HSV-specific NAAT (Simplexa HSV-1/2 Direct, Focus Diagnostics, Cypress, CA) and one multiplex NAAT (FilmArray ME panel, BioFire Diagnostics), have received FDA clearance with an indication for CSF specimens. The Simplexa assay requires 50 μL of CSF and is fully automated which simplifies workflow and may provide superior reproducibility than the previously discussed LDTs. An initial evaluation of the Simplexa assay demonstrated 97.9% sensitivity and 96.2% specificity for detection of HSV in CSF.[461] The FilmArray ME is a highly multiplexed sample-to-answer test for multiple bacterial and viral pathogens associated with meningitis. This assay requires 200 μL of CSF and demonstrated 93 to 100% sensitivity and greater than 98% specificity for the identification of HSV-1 and -2 in two initial studies.[197,462] Subsequent comparative studies have demonstrated reduced sensitivity of the FilmArray ME, ranging from 50 to 87%, for HSV-1 and 2 when compared to uniplex FDA-cleared or laboratory developed tests.[463,464] In all cases, the discordance occurred in specimens with high cycle threshold values, indicating a very low target concentration. Upon adjudication using clinical chart review and alternative molecular tests, 63% of results initially deemed to be false negative by FilmArray were determined to be truly negative.[464,465] These data suggest that uniplex HSV tests may have a lower absolute LoD; however, the clinical relevance of these additional detections remains unresolved.

Varicella Zoster Virus

Following primary infection, VZV achieves latency within trigeminal and dorsal root sensory ganglia.[166] Primary infection or reactivation of latent virus during periods of immune suppression can manifest as cerebellar ataxia, moderate to severe meningitis, or encephalitis.[466] These CNS complications occur at a rate of approximately 1 in 4000 to 10,000 cases.[187] Cutaneous rash is present in only 42% of patients with confirmed VZV CNS disease.[466] Introduction of the VZV vaccine has dramatically reduced the number of severe VZV infections. However, VZV remains the most common herpesvirus associated with CNS disease in some regions.[467] Further, vaccine coverage is not universal and 15 to 20% of individuals may not have an adequate immune response to a single dose of vaccine. While rare, vaccine-associated diseases including CNS manifestations have been reported.[466]

NAATs have become the preferred method for diagnosing VZV CNS infections. In addition to increased sensitivity and decreased TAT, the decreasing cost and commercial availability of ASRs and test kits with FDA clearance or CE marking have made molecular tests equivalent or less expensive than viral culture.[187]

The majority of VZV NAATs are developed and validated by individual laboratories and include both qualitative and quantitative assays. These tests require nucleic acid extraction or other treatment to inactivate or remove inhibitory substances present in CSF prior to PCR for optimal sensitivity.[468] The sensitivity of LDT uniplex VZV NAATs for CSF is reported to be 96 to 100% with an LoD of 10^0 to 10^1 copies/reaction.[184,196,469] Multiplexed LDTs have also been developed for the simultaneous detection of five herpesviruses associated with CNS infection in a single reaction. Despite a more complex design, the LoD for VZV in CSF was approximately 50 genomes/reaction, which is comparable to that of uniplex tests.[470] Recently, two tests have attained FDA-cleared status for the identification of VZV in CSF specimens. The Simplexa VZV Direct assay (DiaSorin) is a sample-to-answer uniplex test that requires just 50 μL of CSF and returns a result in approximately 60 min. The LoD was determined to be approximately 10^3 copies/mL in analytical studies.[471] This is somewhat higher than the LoD reported for several LDTs; however, there are currently no available studies evaluating the clinical performance of this test. The multiplexed FilmArray ME test has a reported sensitivity of 100% for detection of VZV when compared with uniplex PCR and sequence analysis.[197,462] The qualitative finding of VZV in a CSF specimen is typically associated with causality in the context of compatible symptoms. However, in an immunocompromised patient, low levels of VZV DNA may be present in CSF due to asymptomatic viral reactivation or infiltration from VZV viremia.

Quantitative PCR analysis of the CSF has been explored as a method to differentiate between clinical CNS syndromes and to predict severity of disease. Two independent studies found significantly higher mean CSF VL (~1 log 10) in patients with encephalitis compared to patients with meningitis.[472,473] Importantly, the absolute VL values associated with each syndrome were different between the studies, likely due to nonstandardiziation between the specific assays used. A contrasting study found no significant difference between patients having encephalitis or meningitis; however, both syndromes were associated with higher VL than patients with cranial nerve affection, encephalopathy, or cerebrovascular disease.[467] All studies found VZV VL in CSF to be highly variable ranging from 10^2 to 10^8 copies/mL.[467,472,473] Given these data, it may be difficult to assign a definitive VL threshold to differentiate specific CNS syndromes. Rather, the detection of VZV in CSF should be correlated with clinical investigation, imaging studies, and/or histologic analysis. As a prognostic tool, CSF VL may be useful given the finding that patients with $\leq 10^4$ copies/mL were more likely to survive and less likely to require intensive care.[472,473]

Epstein-Barr Virus

Epstein-Barr virus (EBV) is associated with 20 to 100% of Burkitt lymphoma variants, 40% of Hodgkin lymphoma, and 10% of diffuse large B-cell lymphomas in immune competent individuals.[474] The risk of developing these malignancies is increased in immunocompromised patients including those receiving immunosuppressive drug regimens following allogeneic transplant or in individuals with uncontrolled HIV infection.[474,475] Specifically, nearly 100% of primary CNS lymphomas (PCNSLs) are positive for EBV.[474] Definitive diagnosis often requires histologic exam of CNS tissues, which is invasive and may not be feasible in all cases.

Molecular analysis of CSF specimens using NAAT has been proposed as a direct method to diagnose CNS lymphomas caused by EBV. Studies have demonstrated NAAT to be 75 to 100% sensitive for detection of EBV in HIV-positive patients with histologically confirmed CNS lymphomas.[476–480] However, EBV was also detected in 12 to 22% of patients without CNS lymphoma resulting in a PPV of 29%.[476,478,479,481] Additionally, the presence of EBV in CSF was not correlated with an increased risk of developing CNS lymphomas when compared to patients with undetectable EBV in CSF.[479] The "false positive" EBV results may be attributable to detection of latent virus in lymphocytic infiltrates resulting from the primary cause of meningitis in these patients (e.g., toxoplasmosis, HIV encephalitis, cryptococcal meningitis).[481] Therefore qualitative detection of EBV in CSF must be interpreted with caution because it lacks both specificity for current CNS lymphoma and prognostic value for development of future disease.

Quantitative NAATs to determine EBV VL in both CSF and plasma have addressed the shortcomings of qualitative tests. EBV DNA can be detected in a similar proportion (27 to 31%) of plasma samples obtained from HIV patients with PCNSL and controls.[476] However, a high CSF VL of 10^4 to 10^6 copies/mL or increased CSF:plasma VL ratio is strongly correlated with PCNSL.[476,482] The use of a CSF VL threshold of 10^4 copies/mL increased the specificity of NAAT to 96% compared with 66% specificity when using a qualitative NAAT.[483] Conversely, a CSF threshold of 10^3 copies/mL provided a specificity of 100% but sensitivity of only 50%.[484] While promising, the reliability and widespread utilization of a single VL threshold to define disease is dependent on reproducible, accurate, and consistent quantification of VL.

Currently, there are no available FDA-cleared tests for qualitative or quantitative detection of EBV in CSF or other specimens. Several CE-marked assays or LDTs using commercially available ASRs (Cepheid; Qiagen, Hilden, Germany; Roche Diagnostics GmbH, Germany; Analitica, Padova, Italy) have been described. These assays target conserved regions of the EBV genome and demonstrate an LoD near 10^2 copies/mL with quantitative ranges of 10^2 to 10^7 copies/mL.[485–487] Importantly, absolute VL values reported by each test are variable. One multicenter study comparing 30 LDT and commercially available EBV NAATs noted variability of 2.3 to 4.1 $\log_{10}$ copies/mL for the same specimen, with less than 50% of NAATs reporting VL within 0.5 $\log_{10}$ of the expected value.[488] The first WHO standard for EBV was introduced in 2011 to provide a single calibration standard and reduce intra-assay variability. Subsequent studies have found that use of this standard reduces variability in VL result, though a variation of greater than 1 $\log_{10}$ between assays is not uncommon.[489] The use of commercial assays or ASRs ensures quality of reagents; however, other variables including nucleic acid extraction method, sample collection and input, and assay calibrators are still laboratory dependent and can be significant sources of variability in reported VL.[487] This lack of commutability of results between laboratories has historically prevented the adoption of a universal VL threshold to definitively diagnose EBV-related CNS pathologies.

Human Herpesvirus 6

Greater than 90% of adults are seropositive for HHV-6. Symptomatic HHV-6 infections of the CNS are primarily observed in two populations: children under the age of 2 following primary HHV-6 infection and adult immunocompromised patients as a result of viral reactivation. HHV-6 has been implicated in up to 30% of children with febrile status

epilepticus.[490] The incidence of HHV-6 encephalitis in post-transplant patients can be as high as 12% depending on type of transplant and immunosuppressive regimen and can carry a 40% mortality rate.[491,492] The relationship between serologic assessment of the CSF and detection of viral DNA using NAAT is variable; correlation between NAAT and IgG results was found to be statistically significant ($P = .03$) while correlation between NAAT and IgM was not ($P = .69$).[493] This may be due to (i) detection of latent HHV-6 DNA present in lymphocytic infiltrates during episodes of viral meningitis caused by other viral pathogens, (ii) earlier detection of viral DNA by NAAT, (iii) differences in sensitivity between the two methods, or iv) nonspecific cross-reactivity of serologic assays. Regardless, these data suggest a limited role of serologic analysis for the diagnosis of acute CNS infection.

Highly sensitive qualitative NAATs are well suited for analysis of CSF because active CNS disease can occur at very low viral concentrations and the presence of any HHV-6 in CSF is often indicative of disease.[217,492,493] NAATs based on nested PCR or a combined PCR-EIA method are extremely sensitive, detecting HHV-6 in specimens containing as few as 4 genome equivalents/mL.[219] The multiplexed FilmArray ME panel detects but does not differentiate HHV-6 variants A and B (HHV-6A, HHV-6B) and has demonstrated a 94.7% sensitivity and 100% specificity in clinical specimens.[197] Both HHV-6A and HHV-6B have been detected in CSF specimens; however, HHV-6B is implicated in greater than 99% of primary HHV-6 meningitis cases.[210,494] A significant proportion (~40%) of these patients also have detectable HHV-6B in PBMCs and saliva.[210] HHV-6A has demonstrated neurotropism, can persist in the CSF of asymptomatic patients, and is rarely associated with disease.[210,493] Therefore NAATs that differentiate HHV-6A and B can be beneficial when interpreting positive CSF results.

Interpretation of qualitative HHV-6 detection in CSF is further complicated by asymptomatic viral reactivation and the presence of inherited chromosomally integrated HHV-6 (iciHHV-6, discussed in "Viral Infections in Immunocompromised Populations" section).[210,494] A recent study found HHV-6 to be the most frequent target detected by the FilmArray ME panel; however, neurologic symptoms were attributed to HHV-6 in just 20% of these cases.[495] In these instances, quantitative comparison of VL in serum versus CSF may aid in differentiating latent or iciHHV-6 from active viral replication indicative of CNS disease, though no definitive threshold has been established.[494] Because of these limitations, diagnosis of HHV-6 encephalitis should not be made based on a positive NAAT results alone. Clinical criteria including altered mental status, seizure, and exclusion of other infectious etiologies should be used to support the diagnosis in patients with a positive NAAT result.[492]

Arboviruses

The term "arboviruses" refers to a large and diverse group of viral pathogens belonging primarily to the *Togaviridae, Bunyaviridae,* and *Flaviviridae* families that cause arthropod-borne illness. A number of species within the arbovirus group are notable agents of endemic or epidemic acute CNS disease. The epidemiology of specific species within arboviruses is driven by the geographic and seasonal distribution of the natural host and vector.[496,497] Key characteristics of arboviruses associated with neuroinvasive disease are presented in Table 89.8. Accurate diagnosis is important to rule out other

TABLE 89.8 Characteristics of Arboviruses Associated With Central Nervous System Infection

Taxonomy	Reported CNS Infections/Year	Reservoir	Primary Vector	Range	Manifestation	Diagnostic Approach
Flaviviridae						
West Nile	1200–1500 (USA)	Several types of birds including jays, ducks, crows	*Culex* spp. mosquitoes	North America, Europe, Africa, Asia	Asymptomatic in 80% of infections. Meningitis and encephalitis in <1% of infections, severe disease in adults and elderly with 5–10% mortality.	IgM in CSF. May be cross-reactive with other *Flaviviridae*.
St. Louis encephalitis	10–15 (USA)	Several types of birds including sparrows, jays, pigeons.	*Culex* spp. mosquitoes	North and South America	Encephalitis in adults. Rarely fatal.	IgM in CSF. May be cross-reactive with other *Flaviviridae*, especially Japanese encephalitis and West Nile.
Japanese encephalitis	Rare; <1 case/1 million travelers to endemic region	Pigs, aquatic birds (heron, egret)	*Culex* spp. mosquitoes	Southeast Asia	Asymptomatic infection common, 70% seropositivity in endemic regions. Symptomatic infection (encephalitis) in <1% of cases but may be severe with up to 30% mortality in children. Vaccine available.	IgM in CSF detectable 4 days post infection, detectable in serum 7 days post infection. IgM may cross-react with West Nile, dengue, or other *Flaviviridae* in endemic area. Plaque reduction neutralizing antibody test to confirm etiology.
Murray Valley	0–15 cases/year (Australia)	Aquatic birds	*Culex* spp. mosquitos	Australia, Papua New Guinea	Symptomatic in 1:150–1:1000 infections. Mortality rate 15–30% in symptomatic CNS infections.	IgM in CSF. Neutralizing antibodies cross-neutralize Japanese encephalitis virus.
Powassan	10–15 (USA)	Woodchucks, Squirrels, and white-footed mouse	*Ixodes* spp. ticks	Northeastern and North central United States	Infections are predominantly asymptomatic. Cases progressing to severe encephalitis carry 10% mortality.	IgM in CSF to diagnose acute infection. A fourfold rise in serum IgG can retrospectively confirm diagnosis.
Tick-borne encephalitis	~1000 cases/year (global)	Small rodents including mice and ground squirrels	*Ixodes* spp. ticks	Europe, Russia, Asia, North America	Asymptomatic or mild febrile illness in 70–80% of infections. Severe/invasion CNS disease in 20–30% of infections resulting in 1–20% mortality.	IgM in CSF to diagnose acute infection. A fourfold rise in serum IgG can retrospectively confirm diagnosis. Cross-reactivity exists with other *Flaviviridae*.
Bunyaviridae						
La Crosse	70–100 (USA)	Chipmunks, ground squirrels	*Aedes triseriatus* (woodland mosquito)	Southeastern and Great lakes region (USA), South and central region (Canada)	Severe encephalitis. Majority of cases (>90%) in children. Approximately 0.5–5% case fatality.	IgM in CSF to diagnose acute infection. A fourfold rise in serum IgG can retrospectively confirm diagnosis.

TABLE 89.8 Characteristics of Arboviruses Associated With Central Nervous System Infection—cont'd

Taxonomy	Reported CNS Infections/Year	Reservoir	Primary Vector	Range	Manifestation	Diagnostic Approach
Jamestown Canyon	5–10 (USA)	Deer	Various mosquito genera including *Aedes, Culex, Coquillettidia*	Temperate climates including Northeastern and North central USA, Canada	Encephalitis and meningitis. Bimodal distribution affecting young and elderly. Rarely fatal	IgM in CSF to diagnose acute infection. May cross-react with other Bunyaviridae.
California encephalitis	10–20 (USA)	Chipmunks, ground squirrels	*Aedes triseriatus* (woodland mosquito)	Southeastern and Great lakes region (USA), South and central region (Canada)	Asymptomatic or mild symptoms in 80% of infections. Severe CNS infection resulting in meningitis and seizure in 20% with a mortality rate of <1%.	IgM in CSF to diagnose acute infection. May cross-react with other Bunyaviridae.
Togaviridae						
Eastern equine encephalitis	5–10 (USA)	Passerine birds	*Culiseta melanura*	North, Central, and South America	Encephalitis and meningitis affecting all ages. Mortality rate of 25% or higher.	IgM in CSF to diagnose acute infection. Antigen detection in brain biopsy. A fourfold rise in serum IgG can retrospectively confirm diagnosis.
Western equine encephalitis	5–10 (USA)	Passerine birds	*Culex tarsalis*	Primarily North America. Rare human cases reported in South America	Encephalitis and meningitis. Severe disease seen in elderly and infants. Mortality rate of <5%.	IgM in CSF to diagnose acute infection. Antigen detection in brain biopsy.
Venezuelan equine encephalitis	Very rare in United States; outbreak associated; may affect up to 100,000 people per epidemic.	Horses	Various mosquito genera including *Aedes* and *Psorophora*. Possible transmission via contact or aerosol exposure to equine urine and other body fluids	Primarily Central and South America. Outbreak associated.	Encephalitis and meningitis. Severe disease more common in children than adults. Mortality rate of 20–35% in children.	IgM in CSF to diagnose acute infection. Antigen detection in brain biopsy. A fourfold rise in serum IgG can retrospectively confirm diagnosis.

CNS, Central nervous system; CSF, cerebrospinal fluid.

potential bacterial or viral pathogens for which there may be specific treatment and also for epidemiologic purposes.

The *Flaviviridae* family members most commonly associated with meningitis or encephalitis include West Nile (WNV), St. Louis encephalitis (SLE), Japanese encephalitis (JEV), Powassan (POW), tickborne encephalitis (TBE), and Murray Valley (MVE) viruses.[498] WNV has a global distribution and is the leading cause of arboviral infection in the United States. Approximately 80% of infections are asymptomatic and less than 1% result in neuroinvasive disease; however, because of the ubiquity of the reservoir and vector, WNV is implicated in 1200 to 1500 cases of meningitis and encephalitis per year.[496] Adults and elderly suffer greater than 95% of severe infections, which carry a 5 to 10% mortality rate.[496,499] JEV is a leading cause of arboviral encephalitis in Southeast Asia, where adult seroprevalence is greater than 70%.[500] The majority of infections are asymptomatic, but the attack rate can be 5 to 50 cases per 100,000 in children and up to 30% of cases are fatal.

Bunyaviridae commonly associated with neuroinvasive disease include La Crosse (LCV), Jamestown Canyon (JCV), and California encephalitis virus. LCV has been implicated in greater than 1000 cases of neuroinvasive disease in the United States since its initial discovery in 1960 and accounted for 76 cases in 2014.[496,501] The majority of these cases (79%) were associated with severe encephalitis in children and greater than 95% required hospitalization.[496] JCV is increasingly recognized as a cause of neuroinvasive illness since its initial reporting in 2001, and now accounts for approximately 15 to 20 reported cases per year in the United States.[496,497] Symptoms tend to be less severe than LCV, requiring hospitalization in 48 to 64% of cases with no reported fatalities.[496,497]

Togaviridae associated with neuroinvasive disease include Eastern equine (EEEV), Western equine (WEEV), and Venezuelan equine (VEEV) encephalitis viruses.[498,499] EEEV and WEEV are maintained in passerine birds and are transmitted to humans by mosquitoes. The endemic region for EEEV includes North and South America, where sporadic outbreaks have been reported.[499] Human exposure is likely common, however 2 to 10 cases of neuroinvasive EEEV disease are reported annually in United States with a reported mortality rate of ≥25%.[496,499] WEEV is primarily reported on the North American continent. Infection is less severe than EEEV, with a reported mortality rate of less than 5%.[499] Unlike WEEV and EEEV, VEEV is maintained in horses as a natural reservoir and equine infections typically remain asymptomatic despite high VL.[499,502] Human infection is common based on serologic evidence from residents of southern Florida. However, severe symptomatic infection is rare and carries a mortality of less than 1%.[502,503]

Diagnostic Methods for Presumed Arboviral CNS Infections

The diagnostic approach to patients with suspected arboviral meningitis or encephalitis largely relies on serologic tests. Following infection, viral replication occurs in the bloodstream to produce a low-level viremia. This period precedes the development of CNS symptoms by 5 to 8 days and may be asymptomatic or accompanied by generalized symptoms of fever or rash. During this time the patient will test negative for serum IgM and IgG antibodies. However, viral nucleic acid may be detected in blood samples using PCR.[504,505] By the time of CNS symptom onset, the initial viremia has been neutralized by rising IgM concentrations; therefore PCR analysis of blood specimens is not recommended for the diagnosis of arboviral neuroinvasive disease.[452,504]

Serologic tests for different arboviruses including ELISA, immunofluorescent assay (IFA), and antibody neutralization tests are commonly used to make a serologic diagnosis. Antiviral IgM and IgG are detectable by ELISA in the serum approximately 7 and 11 days postinfection, respectively, and can be used to aid in specific diagnosis.[504] Importantly, IgG antibodies persist at sustained levels for many years and IgM has been found to persist for greater than 1 year in 17 to 58% of persons following primary WNV infection.[506–508] Therefore serologic analysis of CSF to detect intrathecal IgM production provides the most accurate assessment of acute arboviral meningitis.

A drawback to the reliance on serologic diagnostics is the potential for cross-reactivity between species within a viral family or genus. This is especially problematic in regions where multiple viruses causing a similar clinical presentation co-circulate. Evaluations of commercially available IgM ELISAs for detection of JEV have demonstrated greater than 90% sensitivity but variable specificity of 56 to 99% due to cross-reactivity with dengue virus positive sera.[509] Similarly, ELISA assays for *Bunyaviridae* have demonstrated IgM cross-reactivity within the California serogroup (La Crosse, Jamestown Canyon, California encephalitis).[497,510] An international quality assurance study involving a panel of 10 samples containing antisera positive for WNV, other flaviviruses, or negative for arboviral antibodies demonstrated only 73% correct classification of IgM and 95% classification of IgG among 19 laboratories.[511] Definitive identification can be accomplished by demonstrating a fourfold rise in antiviral IgG between acute and convalescent sera or by in vitro plaque reduction neutralization testing (PRNT).[452] Though cross-reactivity may also be observed among neutralizing antibodies (NAb), the true etiologic agent should demonstrate a significantly higher NAb titer than other potentially cross-reactive viruses.[497,510]

Detection of viral nucleic acid in CSF using NAAT has also been explored but demonstrates poor sensitivity compared with serologic detection of virus-specific IgM.[504] Specifically, PCR-based detection of WNV in CSF is positive in less than

---

POINTS TO REMEMBER
Viral Infections of the Central Nervous System

- Most common causes of CNS viral infections belong to the herpesvirus, enterovirus, and arbovirus groups.
- Viral culture of cerebrospinal fluid is low yield and should not be routinely conducted for diagnosis of CNS infections.
- Nucleic acid amplification assays are sensitive methods for detection of CNS infections due to enteroviruses or herpesviruses but have poor clinical sensitivity for detection of arboviral infections.
- Quantitative viral load determination in CSF specimens is not essential for patient management. The presence of any amount of detectable virus is generally indicative of active disease.
- Serologic methods are preferred for the diagnosis of arboviral CNS infections; however, definitive identification of the specific virus is hampered by antibody cross-reactivity.

60% of cases.[452] A specific exception is in the immunocompromised host, where humoral immunity may be compromised. In these patients, direct detection of viral nucleic acid in the CSF may provide a superior diagnostic approach.[512] A particular advantage of NAAT is the high degree of specificity for identification and differentiation of individual viruses, which is somewhat lacking in serologic tests. For these reasons, NAAT is frequently used in the epidemiologic investigation of specimens obtained from host or reservoir species and screening of donor blood units during epidemics.[505]

ARTHROPOD BORNE VIRUSES ASSOCIATED WITH FEVER AND RASH

Introduction

A wide range of viruses can be transmitted from infected humans or from zoonotic reservoirs via arthropod vectors such as mosquitos or ticks. Infection with these viruses can range from asymptomatic to mild self-resolving to life-threatening and include an array of symptoms such as fatigue, arthralgia, fever, rash, neurologic manifestations, and hemorrhage. Three of the most commonly encountered arboviruses associated with nonspecific symptoms of fever and rash are Zika, chikungunya, and dengue. Both Zika and dengue are members of the Flaviviridae family, while chikungunya belongs to the Togaviridae family. In addition to sharing similar clinical presentations all three viruses share the same arthropod vector, the *Aedes* spp. mosquito, and overlapping geographical range consisting of primarily tropical or sub-tropical regions of Southeast Asia, India, China, Central and South America, and Africa. Notably, this range has recently expanded to include autochthonous infections in Southern Europe and the United States, likely to due to expanding range of the *Aedes* mosquito and climate change. The clinical, epidemiologic, and taxonomic similarities between these three viruses complicate specific diagnosis of these infections. While early symptoms are similar and the majority of infections are mild, accurate diagnosis is important since each virus carries unique secondary manifestations or risk factors.

Dengue virus accounts for up to 390 million human infections/year globally. Among these, approximately 25% develop mild symptoms of fever, rash, and headache; however 0.1 to 0.5% result in severe disease including dengue hemorrhagic fever (DHF) that can carry a mortality rate of up to 20% without supportive treatment.[513,514] Chikungunya virus has been recognized as the cause of large outbreaks of human infection since its initial identification in the 1950s.[515] Chikungunya is highly transmissible as indicated by post-outbreak seroprevalence studies and is associated with acute symptoms consisting of fever, arthralgia, and rash in approximately 20% of cases.[515,516] While mortality is rare, up to 50% of infected individuals may suffer long-term post-infection chronic inflammatory rheumatism resulting in significant morbidity and lost productivity.[516] Zika virus was also first identified in humans in the 1950s and until recently received little consideration since symptoms of fever, rash, and arthralgia are mild, nonspecific, and self-resolving.[517] During more recent outbreaks in French Polynesia (2011) and Brazil (2015), more severe postinfectious complications were recognized including Guillain-Barre syndrome (GBS)

and congenital neonatal microcephaly.[517] Post-Zika GBS impacts less than 0.1% of cases and is self-resolving without lasting effect. In contrast, congenital microcephaly or other birth defect impacts up to 10% of all fetuses whose mothers had confirmed Zika infection during their pregnancy and results in life-long disability.[518]

Serologic and Antigen Tests for Arboviral Viruses Associated With Fever and Rash

A major consideration when using serologic methods is the differentiation between primary and past infection in symptomatic individuals residing in endemic areas. This is most pronounced in the diagnosis of dengue, which infects millions annually and reaches seroprevalence of 35% or higher in endemic regions.[519,520] Commercially available IgM capture ELISA (MAC-ELISA) are 96 to 99% sensitive when used ≥5 days after symptom onset and detect all four dengue virus serotypes.[521,522] These tests serve as an important initial screen in symptomatic patients. However, IgM persists for up to 3 months following primary infection and is cross-reactive with other members of the *Flaviviridae* family.[523] Therefore in residents or long-term visitors to endemic areas, a more specific test would be preferred. Antigen-based detection assays targeting the nonstructural protein 1 (NS1) of dengue virus have shown potential in filling this role; NS1 is specific to dengue virus, is detectable in blood earlier than IgM, and is only present in acute and postacute phases of infection (1 to 10 days post onset of symptoms). Commercially available ELISAs targeting NS1 demonstrate 60 to 96% sensitivity during acute phase and little to no cross-reactivity with other flaviviruses, thereby providing an earlier and more specific diagnosis.[521,524] Importantly, the presence of rheumatoid factor may be a significant cause of false positive results in naïve patients.

Zika virus infections have rapidly expanded over the last decade to reach endemic and epidemic status in 75 countries in Africa, Southeast Asia, the Pacific, and the Americas.[525] The geographic distribution and symptoms of Zika infection (fever, rash, conjunctivitis) mirror early symptoms of other arboviral rash viruses, and serologic tests for Zika virus are cross-reactive with dengue virus and other *Flaviviridae*.[526] These factors complicate early serologic diagnosis of Zika infections. Current CDC recommendations updated in 2019 include serologic (IgM) testing for both Zika and dengue virus in patients with compatible symptoms and recent travel to endemic regions, or sexual contact with an individual from an endemic region.[526] Patients with symptom onset of less than 7 days may be in the window period for serologic response, so serum IgM testing is only recommended if NAAT testing is negative. Serum VL testing 1 to 12 weeks after symptom onset may be undetectable and serum IgM analysis is the initial test of choice. Due to significant cross-reactivity among *Flaviviridae*, all positive IgM results must be confirmed using PRNT. Serologic testing is not recommended for diagnosis of acute infection in symptomatic or asymptomatic pregnant women due to persistence of anti-Zika IgM for months to years. For these patients, both serum and urine specimens should be tested by NAAT to aid in assessment of recent infection due to persistence of Zika virus in urine.[526]

Serologic diagnosis of acute chikungunya infection shares similar limitations with dengue and Zika viruses. Antibodies are not detectable until 5 to 7 days after symptom onset, and the majority of cases are in patients living in endemic regions who may have had previous exposure to the virus.[527] Therefore a serologic approach to diagnosis relies on the detection of anti-chikungunya IgM rather than IgG or total antibody, and negative results do not rule out very recent infection. Several serologic tests have been developed and are commercially available for the detection of anti-chikungunya IgM antibodies, including traditional ELISA, capture ELISA (MAC-ELISA), IFA, and rapid lateral flow immunoassays. A multicenter performance evaluation using characterized clinical specimens demonstrated significant performance differences between these tests. In general, laboratory-based ELISA, MAC-ELISA, and IFA tests demonstrated sensitivity of 92 to 100% while rapid test sensitivity ranged from 0 to 13%.[528] No cross-reactivity with dengue or other *Flaviviridae* was observed; however, some nonspecific reactivity occurred in sera positive for other members of the *Togaviridae* family, including o'nyong-nyong and Mayaro viruses. Given these limitations, the CDC currently recommends serologic assessment (IgM ELISA) for individuals ≥6 days from symptom onset, followed by confirmation of positive results with PRNT.[527]

NAATs for Arboviral Viruses Associated With Fever and Rash

Direct detection of viral RNA using NAATs provides definitive evidence of active disease and is the preferred approach for diagnosing acute dengue, Zika, and chikungunya virus infection. The majority of NAATs designed for detection of Zika, chikungunya, and dengue viruses are LDTs and are designed for the qualitative detection of a single target; however, due to the overlapping geographic range and symptomology among these viruses, multiplex tests have also been developed. All three viruses can be detected in blood or serum samples at the time of symptom onset, though the viremia is short-lived and is frequently undetectable by 5 to 7 days post symptom onset.[527,529–531] Therefore an accurate patient history is important in selecting the appropriate testing approach (NAAT versus serology), and most testing algorithms recommend serologic assessment for patients with a negative NAAT result.[526,527,532] In addition to detection of viral RNA in blood during the acute phase, viral RNA may also be detected in other bodily fluids including urine and semen well beyond the acute phase. The clinical and epidemiologic significance of this finding is briefly discussed for each virus below.

Dengue virus is comprised of four serotypes (dengue virus 1 to 4) that are capable of causing clinically indistinguishable disease. Severe forms of dengue including DHF and dengue shock syndrome (DSS) are more frequent in individuals with history of infection with a different dengue virus genotype[530]; therefore discrimination of genotype may be of prognostic utility. The CDC DENV-1-4 RT-PCR Assay is the only test currently FDA-approved for the diagnosis of dengue in blood or serum. The LoD is approximately 10^3 viral copies/mL in serum for each genotype, and the clinical sensitivity ranges from 79 to 97% within the first 3 days of illness.[532,533] Other commercially available research use only (RUO) or LDTs have demonstrated similar performance with stated LoD of 50 copies/mL (Dengue Real-time PCR, CTK Biotech, San Diego, CA) or 1 to 1000 PFU/mL, depending on serotype.[534–536] Importantly, because of the rapid decrease in serum VL following symptom onset, the use of NAAT alone

may not detect up to 40% of infections between days 3 and 5 of symptomatic infection. The highest diagnostic accuracy for dengue is achieved through co-testing with a NAAT and either IgM ELISA or NS1 antigen test.[532]

Following the large Zika virus outbreak in Central and South America in 2015 many commercial assay manufacturers and independent laboratories submitted applications to the FDA for EUA of their tests. These NAATs range in design from simple RT-PCR reagents for use with extracted nucleic acid on a standard thermocycler to highly automated sample-to-answer assays for use on existing high throughput platforms. All assays have an authorized indication for testing serum but many have additional claims for whole blood, plasma, and urine. The limits of detection range from approximately 10 to 500 viral genomic copies/mL of specimen and reported sensitivities are greater than 95% for the majority of assays. Zika virus RNA can be detected in various bodily fluids including serum, urine, saliva, vaginal secretions, breast milk, and semen following primary infection; however, prevalence and persistence in these fluids is variable.[531] Viral RNA in present in greater than 90% of symptomatic patients and ranges from 10^6 to 10^8 copies/mL in the first 3 days of infection. The serum VL then quickly declines resulting in only 50% of patients being detectable by post symptom onset.[531] Similarly, viral RNA is detectable in urine of up to 60% of patients early in infection but rapidly declines. Long-term persistence of Zika virus RNA has been observed in semen, exceeding 120 days in some patients and provides a mechanism for person-to-person spread.[517,531] The frequency of detection in other specimens is low and testing of these specimens does not serve a role in routine diagnosis of symptomatic patients.[531] Specific recommendations for Zika virus testing differ based on patient (pregnancy, symptomatic vs. asymptomatic) and epidemiologic (travel history, time since exposure, current outbreak status) factors. In general, symptomatic patients with potential exposure through travel to an endemic region or sexual contact with someone with recent travel to an endemic region should be tested by NAAT if within 7 days of symptom onset, and serology (IgM) should be added if NAAT is negative or symptoms have been present for greater than 7 days.[526]

There are currently no FDA-cleared NAATs for the detection of chikungunya virus. Commercially available tests such as the RealStar Chikungunya (Altona Diagnostics, Germany) and Genesig Chikungunya (Primerdesign, UK) have received CE marking or are available for RUO in the United States. Alternatively, several reference laboratories offer LDTs, and the CDC has published the primer and probe sequences used in their assay.[527] There are limited published clinical or analytical evaluations of these tests, but data from the manufacturer package inserts indicate LoDs of approximately 100 viral copies or 10 PFU/mL.[527,529] These LoDs should be adequate to provide high sensitivity for the detection of chikungunya in blood samples during acute infection, which ranges from 10^4 to 10^7 PFU/mL in the first week following symptom onset.[529] Chikungunya RNA has also been detected in urine and semen for greater than 30 days post symptom onset and following complete resolution of symptoms.[537] However, the clinical significance of this finding, including implications for transmission, remain unknown, and there are no specific recommendations for testing specimens other than blood or serum. Notably, the sensitivity of NAATs for chikungunya may be impacted by the specific virus genotype. For instance, the CDC has developed two sets of primers and probes: one specific for East Central South African genotypes and one for the Asian genotype that is also the predominant genotype in the Caribbean.[527] While these primer/probe sets are largely cross-reactive, slight differences in sensitivity are observed when detecting viruses of the opposite genotype.[529]

VIRAL GASTROENTERITIS

Introduction

Within the United States, an estimated 179 million cases of acute gastroenteritis (AGE) occur annually, of which a major pathogen is identified in approximately 9.4 million (5.3%) cases.[538,539] Viral pathogens including norovirus, adenovirus, rotavirus, astrovirus, and sapovirus are among the most common etiologies of AGE and cause infections ranging from asymptomatic to severe.

Norovirus is the most common cause of diarrhea in healthy adults, responsible for an estimated 50% of diarrheal outbreaks.[540] Norovirus outbreaks often occur in crowded locations, such as cruise ships, college dormitories, or military barracks and are characterized by vomiting and diarrhea, typically resolving in 1 to 2 days.[541] Thereafter, patients will often asymptomatically shed the virus for several weeks.[542] Coupled with the low infectious dose of Norovirus and high environmental stability, management of institutional outbreaks can be challenging.[543]

Rotavirus is the leading cause of viral gastroenteritis in healthy children, accounting for approximately 2 million child hospital admissions globally every year.[544] Children aged 4 to 23 months are at the greatest risk of severe disease, manifested by severe dehydration, shock, and occasionally death. Vaccination has dramatically reduced the incidence of infection[545]; however, this virus is still an important cause of infant disease and mortality throughout the world, accounting for approximately 197,000 deaths per year.

Finally, the enteric AdVs (serotype 40 and 41) are associated with self-limiting diarrhea in immunocompetent patients throughout the world.[546,547] Importantly, infections with these viruses in the immunosuppressed population are more severe with protracted time course and have been associated with fatal cases of enterocolitis.[548]

Culture and Antigen-based Diagnostic Approaches

The use of culture for the diagnosis of viral gastroenteritis has been largely abandoned because of the extended TAT and poor sensitivity of this method. In many cases, symptomatic patients will have resolved their infection by the time results are available. Furthermore, many of the important viral pathogens are difficult to cultivate. Specifically, norovirus, the most common cause of viral gastroenteritis in adults, is not cultivable in routinely used cell lines.[549,550]

Antigen-based methodologies have been described for several of the agents of viral gastroenteritis. These tests are available as semi-automated EIAs for high-throughput laboratory-based testing and as on-demand immunochromatographic assays designed for rapidity. A 2015 study comparing seven available rotavirus immunochromatographic assays to PCR found that all had suitable diagnostic accuracy in symptomatic patients, though results were often negative in patients with asymptomatic viral shedding.[551] Antigen testing is also commonly utilized for the detection of adenovirus 40 and 41 in stool specimens and demonstrates similar performance to rotavirus antigen testing. The performance of antigen testing for norovirus, astrovirus, and sapovirus is too poor to allow routine diagnostic use.

Molecular Approaches for Laboratory Diagnosis of Viral Gastroenteritis

Given the limitations of culture and antigen testing, viral gastroenteritis is increasingly being diagnosed using molecular methods that demonstrate increased sensitivity compared with culture or antigen detection and often allow for laboratory diagnosis within the same day. Several uni- and multiplex LDTs have been described for the detection of the most common viral pathogens. These assays rely largely on nucleic acid amplification followed by endpoint detection of amplified products using techniques such as gel electrophoresis or immunoassays and have been applied to the detection of norovirus and rotavirus in fresh stool specimens.[552–555] As molecular assays have evolved, there has been a trend toward multiplexing to enable simultaneous detection of multiple agents of viral gastroenteritis. Laboratory developed multiplexed assays designed for simultaneous detection of norovirus, sapovirus, astrovirus, and adenovirus have demonstrated sensitivities superior to antigen detection.[556,557]

Several FDA-cleared multiplexed gastrointestinal assays have become commercially available in recent years allowing for simplified implementation of multiplex testing on stool specimens. These assays utilize different multiplexing technologies to detect and differentiate anywhere from four to greater than 20 viral, bacterial, and parasitic pathogens associated with AGE.[558] The Luminex xTAG Gastrointestinal Pathogen Panel detects 15 bacterial, parasitic, and viral gastrointestinal pathogens, including adenovirus 40/41, norovirus, and rotavirus. The assay employs multiplex PCR for amplification of pathogen-specific targets followed by detection of amplicon using liquid array flow cytometry. This assay demonstrates a greater sensitivity than antigen-based approaches for adenovirus, rotavirus, and norovirus, and comparable sensitivity to other molecular tests designed for these pathogens.[559–561] A limitation of this assay is the need for the transfer of amplified nucleic acid to the flow cytometer for subsequent sorting, thus creating an extra step and potential for amplicon contamination. The BioFire FilmArray gastrointestinal panel detects greater than 20 pathogens, including adenovirus 40/41, norovirus, rotavirus, sapovirus, and astrovirus. This assay is a sample-to-answer assay with a "moderate complexity" classification that includes extraction, two-stage nested PCR, and amplicon detection using SYBR Green fluorescence. Second stage PCR is conducted in an array of individual microwells containing target-specific primers, thereby allowing the differentiation of positive targets. Similar to the Luminex xTAG, the FilmArray gastrointestinal panel demonstrates sensitivities for viral targets comparable to other molecular methods.[562] A third multiplex gastrointestinal panel, the Verigene EP, detects nine enteric pathogens including norovirus and rotavirus. The Verigene EP also relies on multiplex PCR for amplification of pathogen-specific target sequences, but detection is accomplished using an array of capture probes immobilized to the surface of a glass slide. Like the FilmArray, Verigene is a sample-to-answer, moderate complexity molecular assay with a TAT of less than 2 hours.

A significant advantage of testing with large multiplex panels is the ability to perform a single test in patients with a specific syndrome (gastroenteritis), a concept referred to as "syndromic testing." This allows for the detection of pathogens that may have otherwise not been tested for and can be extremely beneficial in patients with severe disease and broad clinical differentials, such as the immunosuppressed or critically ill. However, this approach may not be as beneficial in relatively healthy patients with uncomplicated AGE. Viral gastroenteritis in these populations is typically self-limiting and not clinically actionable, calling into question the utility of a costly multiplex PCR. Further, asymptomatic carriage of enteric pathogens by healthy individuals may lead to diagnostic confusion. A 2014 study comparing two commercially available gastrointestinal multiplex panels revealed a staggering 21.1% of specimens containing multiple potential pathogens among stool specimens submitted for the diagnosis of gastroenteritis.[563] While potentially beneficial, mixed detections may also lead to diagnostic confusion. As these results become more common with a wider utilization of multiplexed testing, further studies are needed to better characterize the clinical significance of these findings.

A recent advance in the realm of gastrointestinal pathogen testing is the adoption of rectal swabs as a suitable specimen type for some molecular testing. This has been shown to be true in both adult and child patient cohorts with a variety of different stool pathogens.[564,565] Collection of rectal swabs rather than stool greatly improves the ease of collection, allowing for more rapid collection of diagnostic specimens. This can have dramatic positive effects, particularly in the setting of outbreak investigation or when managing critically ill children who may be unable to produce a stool specimen on demand.

POINTS TO REMEMBER
Viral Gastroenteritis

- Norovirus is the most common cause of diarrhea in healthy adults.
- Antigen-based tests are commonly used for diagnosis of rotavirus and adenovirus, though perform poorly for diagnosis of norovirus.
- Molecular assays have emerged as the dominant diagnostic method for most gastrointestinal viruses and range from uniplex to massively multiplexed (>20 targets).

VIRAL HEPATITIS
Hepatitis B Virus

Hepatitis B virus (HBV), a member of the *Hepadnaviridae* family, is a causative agent of acute and chronic hepatitis (for additional discussion on hepatitis, refer to Chapter 51). The virus is spread through contact with blood, semen, or other bodily fluids. Patients infected with the virus at a young age (typically acquired during birth) tend to develop chronic hepatitis. This commonly occurs in areas where the virus is highly endemic, such as Southeast Asia and parts of Africa where prevalence can exceed 8% of the general population.[566] Acquisition of the virus during adulthood tends to cause acute hepatitis with infection resolution. Acute hepatitis is manifested clinically by nausea and abdominal pain occasionally coupled with signs of acute hepatic failure, including jaundice and coagulopathy. Patients who progress to chronic hepatitis develop extensive fibrosis of the liver and resultant signs of hepatic cirrhosis. An estimated total of 19,764 new cases of HBV were acquired in the United States in 2013.[295] The most common means of transmission appear to be injection drug use followed by sexual contact.[295]

Serologic Antibody and Antigen Detection for Diagnosis of HBV Infection

Detection of HBV surface antigen (HBsAg) is a sensitive tool for the diagnosis of active infection. High sensitivity results from the presence of HBsAg on infective virions and subviral particles released during infection. Commercially available HBsAg detection assays rely on some form of antibody capture and are designed for high-throughput testing on automated platforms. Analytical sensitivities for wild-type virus are comparable for these assays, ranging from 0.011 to 0.095 IU/mL.[567] Mutations in the antigenic determinant of HBsAg can dramatically affect assay sensitivity and cause false negative results (prevalence ranging from 0.7 to 1%).[567–569] These assays may also occasionally yield false positive results due to nonspecific cross-reactivity. To increase specificity, testing algorithms typically require positivity in duplicate and confirmation by antibody neutralization before a positive result is reported. A development in HBsAg testing over recent years has been the availability of immunochromatographic devices designed for POC testing. While these assays make HBV testing more available to at-risk populations, a recent meta-analysis of available POC HBsAg devices revealed a wide variation in sensitivity among different commercially available tests, ranging from 43.5 to 99.8%.[570]

Serologic assays to detect the presence of antibodies to various components of HBV play an important role in differentiating acute and past infection, as well as determining immune status. Detection of hepatitis B surface antibody (anti-HBsAg) indicates past exposure to wild-type virus or the HBV vaccine. Whether obtained through natural infection or vaccination, anti-HBsAg will be protective against future infection if present in adequate amount. Assays for the detection of anti-HBsAg use similar chemistries as those in use for HBsAg detection and are available in qualitative and quantitative formats. The ability to quantify anti-HBsAg allows for the determination of immunity and can be used to guide subsequent revaccination if necessary. A level of 10 IU/mL is the accepted level needed for immunity by both the CDC and the WHO. Hepatitis B core antibody (anti-HBc) is only acquired during infection and will not be present in vaccinated individuals. Commercial assays are capable of detecting either anti-HBc IgM or total anti-HBc antibody, with estimated false positive rates of approximately 3 to 9%.[571] The combined results of HBsAg, anti-HBsAg, anti-HBc total antibody, and anti-HBc IgM can be used to determine the infection status of an individual (Table 89.9). In acute infections that progress to chronic infections HBsAg and total anti-HBc remain positive. In resolved cases of HBV, the total anti-HBc remains positive and HBsAg will become undetectable as anti-HBsAg appears. The period between this switch is known as the window period and is marked by the absence of both HBsAg and anti-HBsAg. During this window, anti-HBc IgM is the only serologic marker of infection.

Serologic and NAAT Tests for Monitoring Patients With HBV Infection

In addition to diagnosis, serologic markers are also important components of the management of chronic HBV. The NIH consensus guidelines recognize three major phases of chronic HBV infection: immune tolerant, immune active, and inactive carrier phase.[572] A summary of these phases is provided in Table 89.10.

The immune tolerant phase is marked by high viral replication with minimal host response. In the immune active phase, the host mounts a robust immune response, causing hepatic inflammation and scarring which, if chronic and untreated, puts the patient at risk for hepatocellular carcinoma. The inactive carrier phase is characterized by a great reduction in VL, liver damage, and risk for hepatocellular carcinoma. This transition is a positive prognostic indicator for the patient and typically results in the cessation of treatment. Patients can be monitored for this transition by testing for hepatitis B E antigen (HBeAg) and anti-HBeAg antibody. Patients in the immune active phase are typically HBeAg positive and anti-HBeAg negative whereas the reverse is true when the patients progress to the inactive carrier phase.

Another method to monitor the progression of HBV infection is to monitor VL. VLs greater than 1000 copies/mL

(2000 IU/mL) are strong predictors of progression to hepatocellular carcinoma.[573] This risk has been shown to be independent of HBeAg status, with a relative risk of 6.5 for progression to cancer in patients with VL greater than 6 $\log_{10}$ copies/mL.[574] The Hybrid Capture 2 assay (Qiagen) and the Versant HBV DNA 3.0 assay (Siemens) utilize signal amplification strategies (hybrid capture and bDNA, respectively) rather than PCR to determine VL. These two assays have demonstrated strong correlation of results with one another, though both suffer low detection rates in patients who are HBeAg negative.[575] Recently developed assays that utilize RT-PCR have enabled lower limits of detection. These include the Cobas TaqMan HBV v2.0 (Roche), Real-Time HBV PCR (Abbott), and the Artus HBV PCR (Qiagen). Each of these assays' report results in IU/mL rather than copies/mL, which allows results to be indexed to the WHO international standard. All are highly sensitive, with limits of detection ranging from 9 to 54 IU/mL, and demonstrate good interassay agreement.[576–578]

In 2015 the WHO issued guidelines for the management and treatment of HBV. These guidelines recommend that patients should be monitored annually using HBsAg, HBeAg, and HBV VL.[579] Patients with cirrhosis should be treated for HBV and patients greater than 30 years old with abnormal alanine aminotransferase (ALT) values and HBV VLs of greater than 20,000 IU/mL. This latter patient population should receive treatment regardless of HBeAg status. Treatment can be discontinued in patients without cirrhosis, who have demonstrated HBeAg loss, have persistently normal ALT, and have persistently undetectable HBV DNA levels. These patients still require long-term monitoring for disease relapse. Any consistent sign of reactivation, including HBeAg positivity, HBsAg positivity, ALT value increase, or appearance of detectable HBV DNA warrants retreatment.

Special Diagnostic Considerations and HBV Genotyping

There are several situations that may arise during HBV testing which warrant special consideration. The first is the occurrence of surface escape mutations. These occur when the

TABLE 89.9 Interpretation of Typical Hepatitis B Serologic Results

Clinical Status	HBsAg	Anti-HBsAg	Anti-HBcAg Total	Anti-HBcAg IgM	HBeAg	Anti-HBeAg
Vaccinated	−	+	−	−	−	−
Acute infection	+	−	+/−	+/−	+/−	+/−
Resolving acute infection (window period)	−	−	+	+	−	+
Resolved infection	−	+	+	−	−	+
Chronic infection	+	−	+	−	+/−	+/−

Anti-HBcAg, Hepatitis B core antigen antibodies; *Anti-HBeAg,* hepatitis B E antigen antibodies; *Anti-HBsAg,* hepatitis B surface antigen antibodies; *HBeAg,* hepatitis B E antigen; *HBsAg,* hepatitis B surface antigen.

TABLE 89.10 Phases of Chronic Hepatitis B Virus: Clinical and Laboratory Features

Phase of Chronic HBV	Viral Load	HBeAg	Anti-HBeAg	Inflammation	Risk of Carcinoma
Immune tolerant	High	+	−	Low	Low
Immune active	Moderate	+	−	High	High
Inactive carrier	Low/undetectable	−	+	Low	Low

Anti-HBeAg, Hepatitis B E antigen antibodies; *HBeAg,* hepatitis B E antigen; *HBV,* hepatitis B virus.

virus develops mutations in the surface antigen protein allowing it to go unrecognized by the immune system.[580] This can result in vaccine failure and false negative results on commercially available HBsAg assays.[581] Specific mutations in the surface antigen protein have also been associated with a high risk of hepatocellular carcinoma. Surface antigen escape mutations should be suspected in patients with negative HBsAg and high HBV VLs. Another challenge to HBV test interpretation is the presence of core and precore mutants. These mutations cause a loss or significant decrease in the expression of HBeAg. As such, patients who develop these mutations may mistakenly be categorized as having entered the inactive carrier phase. Similar to HBsAg escape mutations, certain precore and core mutations have also been associated with a higher risk of hepatocellular carcinoma.[582] The identification of surface escape mutants, precore mutants, and core mutants is possible through the use of various commercially available assays and LDTs. The detection of these mutations is often considered an integral part of hepatitis B genotyping.

HBV genotyping is performed using a wide variety of technologies. They range from the INNO-LiPA assay (Innogenetics) which utilizes endpoint PCR with amplicon detection via oligonucleotide hybridization on nitrocellulose strips to the Trugene HBV genotyping assay (Siemens) which uses a traditional sequencing approach. Other utilized technologies include multiplex PCR, serotyping, oligonucleotide microarray chips, invader assays, and RT-PCR.[583] While these assays vary in their capabilities, most can be used to identify the previously described HBV variants. They can also be applied to determine the phylogenetic genotype and mutations leading to drug resistance. Phylogenetic genotyping can be used to predict disease outcome. Evidence suggests higher rates of cirrhosis in patients with genotype C and D infections and better response to interferon in genotypes A and B.[584] However, data regarding genotypic dependent treatment response to available nucleoside/nucleotide analogs suggest that genotype plays a limited role in response to these drugs.[585]

Hepatitis Delta Virus

Hepatitis delta virus (HDV) is a replication deficient subviral particle first described in 1977 from patients infected with HBV expressing a new "delta antigen."[586] The expression of this antigen was strongly associated with chronic HBV infected individuals experiencing active liver damage. Three years later animal studies were able to elucidate the infectious nature of HDV and the reliance of this agent on prior HBV infection to initiate disease.[587] Today, HDV is a well-established cause of significant morbidity and mortality among patients with chronic HBV infection.

While HDV has a worldwide prevalence of approximately 4.5% among HBsAg positive individuals, there is a clear geographical stratification of disease.[588] Prevalence is highest in China, Russia, Eastern Europe, Africa, and South America. Cases in the United States typically occur in patients with a history of travel to these regions. Other risk factors for HDV infection include intravenous drug use or concurrent infection with HIV and/or hepatitis C virus (HCV).

Infection with HDV usually follows one of two clinical courses. Situations in which HBV naive patients are simultaneously infected with HBV and HDV are known as "coinfections"

or situations where a person with established HBV infection is infected with HDV, known as "superinfection." In coinfections patients typically experience acute liver damage, often of greater severity than the damage seen in traditional acute HBV infections. Approximately 2 to 8% of HBV-infected individuals progress to chronic infection.[589] HDV superinfection occurs when a patient with chronic HBV infection newly acquires HDV. The hallmark of HDV superinfection is a dramatic worsening in the severity and progression of liver damage. Approximately 90 to 100% of patients will develop chronic HDV infection, with approximately 80% progressing to cirrhosis within 5 to 10 years.[589]

Testing for HDV should be pursued in patients with newly diagnosed or worsening HBV infection and risk factors for HDV infection (including travel to a location of endemicity). Serologic testing is the mainstay for diagnosis. Patients initially infected with HDV will produce anti-HDV IgM, which can be utilized for the diagnosis of acute infection. Chronic infections can be diagnosed by the presence of HDV IgG in the absence of HDV IgM. Although HDV IgG is initially produced in patients who clear the virus, IgG is typically undetectable approximately 32 weeks following exposure.[590] The prolonged presence of HDV IgG should prompt suspicion of chronic infection.

Molecular testing for HDV has also been described, though commercial options are limited, and performance is variable. There is evidence to suggest currently available assays may lack the sensitivity of HDV serologic testing.[591] Although quantitative VL assays may play a role in the monitoring of disease progression, there is still significant assay-to-assay variability and a universal standard does not currently exist.

Hepatitis C Virus

HCV is a member of the *Flaviviridae* family and is a common cause of chronic liver disease worldwide (for additional information on liver disease, refer to Chapter 51). The virus is spread most often through exposure to blood (e.g., intravenous drug use) or through sexual contact. Patients infected with HCV may have initial symptoms consistent with acute hepatitis such as jaundice or abdominal pain, though the majority of acute infections are asymptomatic. Approximately 75% of acutely infected individuals fail to clear the virus and develop a chronic infection. Most patients with chronic infections will remain asymptomatic, though potential complications include cirrhosis and hepatocellular carcinoma. Within the United States, it is estimated that approximately 4.6 million people have been infected with HCV, of which 3.5 million are actively infected.[592] Of those with active infections, it is estimated that 17% developed cirrhosis.[593] This creates a large national burden of disease and has staggering societal consequences. A study of 407,786 patients diagnosed in 2009 estimated a total cost of $2.7 billion dollars paid by Medicare for the management of these patients alone.[594]

Serologic Tests for Diagnosis of HCV Infection

Given the commonality of symptomatic and asymptomatic disease, effective HCV screening approaches are essential. Serologic approaches to detection of anti-HCV IgG antibodies have greatly evolved since their first implementation. First-generation EIA assays utilized nonstructural antigen

(NS4) and took an average of 22 weeks to become positive following infection.[595] Second-generation assays added additional antigens (core and NS3 regions) allowing for detection at approximately 10 weeks following infection.[596] Third-generation assays introduced reconfigured core and NS3 antigens and the NS5 antigen, allowing for detection 2 to 3 weeks earlier than second-generation assays with an increase in overall sensitivity.[597] The majority of currently used third-generation EIAs are performed on automated immune-analyzers allowing high-throughput testing with minimal handling.[598–600] A more recent development is the availability of rapid immunoassays which can be used as POC devices. The sensitivities of these assays are high (approximately 86.8 to 99.3%) and some, such as the Combiquic HIV/HCV test (Qualpro Diagnostics) and the Multiplo Rapid HIV/HCV Antibody Tests (MedMira Laboratories), allow for the simultaneous detection of HIV.[601,602]

An important consideration regarding HCV serologic assays is that they have been designed as screening assays and as such require confirmatory testing. This is true despite the increased specificity observed in third-generation assays (>99%) compared to first- and second-generation tests.[603] While these assays function well in high-prevalence populations, they can have low PPVs in low-prevalence populations.[604] Confirmatory testing was traditionally performed using a recombinant immunoblot assay known as the RIBA. This assay determined the presence or absence of antibodies to specific HCV antigens and is interpreted as negative, positive, or indeterminate. Although initially recommended by the CDC for confirmation of positive serologic results, the RIBA is no longer commercially available.[605] Repeat testing of serologically positive specimens with low signal-to-cutoff ratios using a second serologic assay is one strategy to discern true positives from false positives. Regardless, current CDC guidelines recommend that all patients with positive HCV serologic tests be followed by a molecular test to determine true infection.[605]

NAATs for Monitoring Patients With HCV Infection

Molecular tests for HCV are available in qualitative and quantitative formats. Qualitative assays use either PCR or TMA technologies. The specificity of these tests makes them suitable for the confirmation of infection in seropositive patients. These assays have also been designed to have high analytical sensitivity, with LoDs no greater than 50 IU/mL.[606] This makes them suitable for the diagnosis of acute infection, during which HCV RNA may become detectable 1 month prior to the appearance of antibodies.[607] In some patients, extremely low-level viremia may persist following natural resolution of infection or treatment. Therefore negative molecular test results should be repeated 6 to 12 months later before ruling out infection. Qualitative molecular assays are also useful in cases in which immunodeficiency may cause falsely negative serology or in perinatal cases in which serologic testing is unreliable due to maternal antibodies.

Once a diagnosis of HCV has been established, quantitative molecular tests play an important role in patient management. VL is measured at the initiation of antiviral therapy and is repeated at different intervals throughout therapy. Rapid virologic response (RVR) is defined as undetectable VL within 4 weeks of starting therapy. Early virologic response (EVR) is defined as a VL that decreases by 2 $\log_{10}$

within 12 weeks. Sustained virologic response (SVR) is the goal of treatment and is defined as the lack of detectable virus 6 months following the end of treatment. The ability to accurately assess patients at each of these timepoints is dependent on the technology used. Commercially available quantitative HCV assays use bDNA or real-time RT-PCR technology. Signal amplification using bDNA has a broad dynamic range and is easy to perform; however, with an LoD of 615 IU/mL it has less analytical sensitivity than nucleic acid amplification methods. Real-time RT-PCR based assays have LoDs similar to commercially available qualitative assays (12 to 15 IU/mL), eliminating the need for multiple assays to diagnose and monitor infected patients.[608,609] The two FDA-cleared real-time RT-PCR assays currently available are the Real-Time HCV (Abbott) and the Cobas AmpliPrep/Cobas TaqMan (Roche). Comparisons of these platforms have shown similar performance across the dynamic range of each test. Compared to standard RT-PCR assays, both real-time tests are significantly more effective at predicting SVR when used throughout treatment.[609]

HCV Genotyping

An integral part of HCV management is genotyping, which assigns a phylogenetic genotype (1 to 6) to the patient's virus. The traditional gold standard has been bidirectional sequencing, often of the 5′UTR of the viral genome. Despite high accuracy, sequencing approaches are only able to identify viral variants comprising at least 20 to 25% of the total viral population.[610] A different assay, the Versant HCV genotype assay (LiPA) 2.0, uses reverse hybridization of amplified DNA to oligonucleotide probes immobilized on a nitrocellulose strip to identify HCV genotypes. Compared to sequencing, this methodology is capable of detecting lower quantities of variants within mixed viral populations. HCV genotyping is also available using RT-PCR based approaches including the Abbott Real-Time HCV Genotype II assay. This test is FDA-cleared for the qualitative identification of genotypes 1 to 5 and differentiates subtypes 1a/1b. A direct comparison of the Versant LiPA 2.0 line probe assay and the Abbott Real-Time HCV Genotype (GT) II assay revealed a concordance rate of 99.2% among 225 samples.[611]

Genotyping should be performed at diagnosis and whenever there is a possibility for a new infection. The viral genotype, combined with VL kinetics, helps determine the duration of treatment needed and the likelihood of obtaining SVR. The majority (71.5%) of HCV infections in the United States are due to genotype 1A.[612] Infections with genotype 1 have traditionally been important to recognize since they respond less well to ribavirin and peginterferon α-2a treatment and therefore require longer treatment courses than genotypes 2 or 3.[613,614]

The introduction of direct-acting antivirals (DAAs) has changed the clinical impact associated with genotype 1. These drugs act directly on HCV-associated proteins and include RNA-polymerase inhibitors, protease inhibitors, nonstructural protein inhibitors, and NS5A inhibitors. Interferon-free courses of treatment with the nucleotide polymerase inhibitor sofosbuvir and the HCV NS5A inhibitor ledipasvir have cure rates greater than 90% in patients with genotype 1.[615] While variations in response persist among different genotypes, the use of DAAs has also created the need for targeted antiviral resistance testing to identify specific mutations that reduce the efficacy of these drugs. Specifically, the presence of a Q80K mutation results in resistance to simeprevir (an NS3/4a protease inhibitor) and is more commonly found in genotype 1a infections.[616] The HCV GenoSure NS3/4A (Monogram Biosciences) assay is a commercially available assay for the identification of Q80K mutations and others within the NS3/NS4A region. Similar assays have been developed for the detection of mutations within the NS5B and NS5A regions. The role of genotypic HCV resistance testing is currently unclear; however, as treatment modalities evolve it is likely that the need for genotyping will become less important. Since 2017 several "pangenotypic" treatment regimens have been described with high rates of SVR across all genotypes.[617] The increasing popularity of these regimens as first-line treatment suggest a limited role for HCV genotyping in the future.

Hepatitis A and E

Hepatitis A virus (HAV) and hepatitis E virus (HEV) are both agents of acute hepatitis transmitted primarily through fecal-oral routes (for additional discussion on hepatitis, refer to Chapter 51). Disease with either virus typically causes fever accompanied by abdominal pain and anorexia. Patients often have laboratory signs of acute hepatitis, including increased bilirubin, ALT, and aspartate aminotransferase (AST). While generally self-limiting, in certain at-risk populations these viruses can cause more severe, life-threatening disease. Though the actual incidence of HAV infections in the United States has declined throughout the years (6.0 cases/100,000 to 0.4 cases/100,000), the hospitalization rate due to infection has risen from 7.3 to 24.5%.[618] This increase is largely attributed to the proportion of infected patients with concurrent chronic liver disease (including HBV and HCV), in whom disease is much more severe. The seroprevalence of HEV varies globally, ranging from approximately 6.0% in the United States to 67.7% in Egypt.[619–621] Similar to HAV, HEV has the potential to cause severe disease in patients with underlying liver disease.[622] HEV also has been strongly linked to severe disease in pregnant women. A recent study demonstrated that HEV was responsible for nearly 10% of all pregnancy-related deaths in Bangladesh over a 7-year period.[623]

Diagnostic Approaches for Diagnosis of HAV and HEV

Serology plays an important role in HAV diagnosis. HAV IgG is of limited diagnostic utility though can be used to establish immunity following vaccination. Infections with HAV are typically diagnosed through the detection of HAV IgM, a marker of recent infection. Detection methods range from high-throughput automated immunoassays designed for large clinical laboratories to ELISA-based devices designed for the rapid testing of smaller numbers of samples. Direct comparisons of these assays have demonstrated similar performances and strong overall agreement.[624–626] An important consideration when using these tests is the pretest probability of the patient to be tested. When these tests are performed on patients without symptoms consistent with HAV, results may be difficult to interpret. False positive results have been reported in patients with autoimmune diseases and other viral infections.[627] Since HAV IgM has been shown to remain in the serum for as many as 420 days after infection, a positive result may also represent a past infection and not explain a patient's acute disease.[628] As such, a positive HAV IgM should

always be interpreted in context of a patient's entire clinical presentation. A 2013 study demonstrated that after performing 10,735 tests, 10 of the 35 patients with positive HAV IgM had different established causes of liver disease.[629]

Testing for HEV is now recommended as part of the diagnosis of "drug induced liver injury" and as a result is becoming more common. Similar to HAV, HEV diagnosis is typically established through serology. In contrast to HAV, assays for the detection of HEV antibodies have far less comparable performances. A Swedish study demonstrated concordant IgG and IgM results in only 70% of tested patients.[630] The overall specificity of HEV IgM based assays has been shown to be low, with significant cross-reactivity with other viruses (including EBV and CMV).[631] Strategies have been described to increase diagnostic performance. One approach is to always test HEV IgG and IgM simultaneously. This approach adds specificity since the two immunoglobulins are often present together in true acute infections.[632] A second approach is the adoption of HEV molecular testing for the confirmation of acute cases. Though no assays are currently commercially available, several LDTs have been described for the sensitive and specific identification of HEV.[633] An advantage to this approach is added sensitivity in immunocompromised patients who may be unable to mount detectable immune responses.

POINTS TO REMEMBER
Viral Hepatitis

- Diagnosis and staging (acute, chronic, or resolved) of HBV infection is accomplished through a combination of antigen and antibody testing.
- Progression of hepatitis B infection is monitored by both viral load and a combination of HBeAg and HBeAb detection.
- HCV infection is typically diagnosed using an antibody screen with confirmation by a molecular test.
- Progression of HCV infection is monitored using quantitative viral load testing performed at specific times during treatment to assess for treatment-related milestones, including RVR (response at 4 weeks) and EVR (response at 12 weeks).
- Molecular assays are available for the detection of resistance to HCV antivirals.

VIRAL HEMORRHAGIC FEVERS

Introduction

The syndrome of VHF is often preceded by a nonspecific prodromal period characterized by fever, headache, and malaise. A proportion of infected individuals progresses to symptoms such as severe vomiting, diarrhea, and characteristic hemorrhage from the mouth, eyes, nose, gastrointestinal tract, or vagina. This is often accompanied by thrombocytopenia and hypotension, which ultimately leads to multiorgan failure and death. Despite significant overlap in clinical presentation, VHF syndrome can be caused by a number of unrelated viral families and species. Most notable among these are members of the *Arenaviridae* (Lassa virus), *Flaviviridae* (Yellow fever virus, dengue virus), *Filoviridae* (Ebola and Marburg virus), and *Bunyaviridae* (Congo-Crimean hemorrhagic fever virus, Rift Valley fever virus, hantaviruses) families (Table 89.11).

TABLE 89.11   Viruses Associated With Viral Hemorrhagic Fever

Taxonomy	Global Burden	Reservoir	Transmission	Range, Endemic Areas	Manifestation and Incidence of Severe Disease
Arenaviridae Lassa virus	Endemic spread accounting for 600–1000 deaths/year in Western Africa. Rare imported cases in Europe and USA.	Rodents including *Mastomys* spp. are asymptomatic carriers. Virus shed in urine and feces.	Ingestion of food or water contaminated rodent excrement. Direct contact with blood or bodily fluids from infected human. Airborne transmission unlikely.	West Africa	Symptomatic infection in ~20% of cases with ~15% mortality in this group.
Flaviviridae Yellow fever virus	Estimated 80,00–200,000 symptomatic infections/year globally	Humans and nonhuman primates	Transmitted by mosquitoes of the *Aedes* or *Haemagogus* genus	Tropical and subtropical regions of Africa and South America	Acute mild symptomatic phase progresses to severe phase including high fever, jaundice, and hemorrhage in 15% of infections. Up to 50% fatal in patients with severe symptoms if untreated.
Filoviridae Ebola virus	Outbreak associated. Typically involving <100 individuals but has the potential to cause large outbreaks involving >10,000 individuals	Fruit bats are likely natural reservoir, asymptomatic carriers. Humans serve as primary reservoir for transmission during epidemics	Direct contact with blood or bodily fluids from infected animal or human. Airborne transmission unlikely.	Tropical regions of central and Western Africa	Symptoms in nearly 100% of infections. Fever, severe diarrhea, hemorrhage, and multi-organ failure. Case fatality rate of 25–90% reported for individual epidemic outbreaks.
Marburg virus	Outbreak associated. Typically involving <50 individuals. No large outbreaks reported to date.	Fruit bats are likely natural reservoir, asymptomatic carriers. Humans serve as primary reservoir for transmission during outbreaks	Direct contact with blood or bodily fluids from infected animal or human. Airborne transmission unlikely.	Tropical regions of central and Western Africa.	Symptoms in nearly 100% of infections. Fever, severe diarrhea, hemorrhage, and multi-organ failure. Case fatality rate of 25–90% reported for individual outbreaks.

Bunyaviridae

Crimean-Congo hemorrhagic fever virus (genus *Nairovirus*)	Estimated 500–1000 severe infections/year	Natural reservoirs include cattle, sheep, and goats which are asymptomatic carriers. Humans may also serve as a reservoir during outbreaks	May be transmitted by tick (genus *Hyalomma*) vector or contact with blood of body fluids of infected livestock or humans	Countries in the Middle East, Balkan peninsula, Eastern Asia, Africa, and India	Symptomatic infection in ~20% of cases. Nonspecific febrile illness progresses to altered mental state, photophobia, hepatitis, and hemorrhage. Mortality rate is 30–40%
Rift Valley fever virus (genus *Phlebovirus*)	Outbreak associated. Typically involves 10–100 cases but larger outbreaks have been reported.	Natural reservoirs include cattle, sheep, and goats which are susceptible to infection and suffer 10–90% mortality rates. Humans do not serve as reservoir.	May be transmitted by mosquito (genus *Aedes*) vector or contact with blood or body fluids of infected livestock. Human-to-human transmission has not been documented.	Sub-Saharan Africa and Middle Eastern countries	Majority of human infections are asymptomatic or associated with mild symptoms of fever and myalgia. Severe symptoms including meningoencephalitis and hemorrhagic fever are rare. Overall mortality rate is <1% but may be >50% in patients who develop severe disease.
Hantaan, Seoul, Puumala, and Dobrava viruses (Genus *Hantavirus*)	Estimated 150,000 infections with hantaviruses resulting in hemorrhagic fever per year globally	Small mammals including field mice, rats, and voles serve as the natural reservoir and are asymptomatic carriers.	Inhalation of aerosolized urine or feces from infected rodents or direct contact between these materials and open wounds.	Eastern Asia including China, Korea, and Russia	Primary symptoms include headache and visual impairment. Severe disease includes hypotension, renal failure, and hemorrhage. Mortality rate is 5–15%. Other types of hantaviruses cause severe pulmonary syndrome in North America.

The severity of symptoms and mortality rate associated with infection varies widely with each specific virus, with the development of severe symptoms, including VHF, ranging from 20 to 95% and overall case fatality rates of less than 1 to greater than 90%.[523,634,635] The epidemiology of VHF also varies with each agent and is dictated largely by the geographic range of the natural host or vector for each specific virus and the route of infection. Combined, these factors can result in either endemic transmission or epidemic outbreaks. Given the broad differential for patients presenting with early symptoms of fever and malaise, it is of critical importance to rule out an agent of VHF in patients residing in or returning from an endemic region or with a history of close contact with an individual infected with a VHF virus. Early recognition and specific or supportive care can reduce the mortality rate associated with these infections. Additionally, early recognition enables appropriate infection control and epidemiologic studies to reduce the impact of potential epidemics.

Laboratory Diagnosis of Viral Hemorrhagic Fever

The approach to diagnosis of agents associated with VHF must consider the safety of laboratorians and health care workers. Viral culture of specimens including blood, urine, and stool may be high yield; however, propagation of virus to a high titer and excessive manipulation of cultures present an increased risk of laboratory-acquired infection. Many viruses associated with VHF including Ebola, Marburg, Lassa fever, Crimean-Congo, Rift Valley, and others are designated as category A select agents by the CDC and should not be handled outside of a BSL-4 laboratory. Additionally, viral culture can significantly delay time to definitive diagnosis. For these reasons, viral culture is not widely utilized in the diagnosis of VHF and is discouraged. The most common methods for laboratory diagnosis of VHF include RT-PCR, serologic, and antigen detection assays.

Serologic and Antigen Tests for VHF

Serologic methods are the most widely used approach for assessment of patients with symptoms or exposure consistent with VHF. These include ELISAs or IFAs designed to detect virus-specific IgG and/or IgM antibodies. When using serologic methods as a primary method of diagnosis it is important to consider the window period (the time between exposure and development of detectable antibodies) and specificity of the assay for a given virus. For example, serologic diagnosis of hantaviruses associated with hemorrhagic fever and renal syndrome (HFRS) are available for detection of either IgM or IgG class antibodies and typically target the nucleocapsid protein. Both classes of antibodies may be detectable by 2 to 8 days following onset of symptoms; however, IgM demonstrates 23 to 64% cross-reactivity among hantavirus species whereas IgG may be as little as 6 to 11% cross-reactive at early time points.[636] Conversely, detection of IgM wanes significantly by 2 to 5 months following infection at which point the cross-reactivity of IgG increases to greater than 68% among hantaviruses. Similar cross-reactivity is common within other families of viruses causing VHF (e.g., filoviruses, bunyaviruses), and includes species not associated with VHF such as those primarily associated with aseptic meningitis (see meningitis section). Therefore it is important to consider the patient history with respect to travel or residence in an endemic area when interpreting serologic results.

NAATs for VHF

Molecular methods including RT-PCR and reverse-transcriptase PCR have the potential to provide early, sensitive, and more specific species identification in patients with acute illness. Following infection, active viral replication resulting in viremia coincides with onset of symptoms and often precedes the development of an antibody response. Therefore sensitive NAATs can frequently detect viral nucleic acid 1 to 5 days prior to serologic positivity.[534,637] In addition to earlier detection, NAATs also provide a rapid result. This enables the implementation of appropriate infection control measures for highly infectious and pathogenic viruses such as Ebola and Marburg viruses.[638,639] Use of a RT-PCR assay for Ebola virus demonstrated 98.4% sensitivity and 99.7% specificity in analysis of over 1000 blood specimens obtained during a large outbreak in Uganda.[638] This included a positive result for 50/246 (20.3%) samples which were negative by an antigen test. These data represented both early infections in which subsequent antigen tests were positive, and convalescent phase samples, which were positive for IgM and/or IgG. NAATs are also useful in the diagnosis of acute infection with dengue, hantaviruses, Lassa virus, Rift Valley fever virus and Crimean-Congo hemorrhagic fever virus with reported 90 to 100% sensitivity and 99 to 100% specificity in acute phase samples.[534,536,637,639–641] Importantly, sensitivity can decrease rapidly from near 100% within 3 days of symptom onset to as little as 20 to 50% $\geq$5 days after onset of symptoms.[534,637] Because serum VL drops dramatically upon convalescence, NAATs have been used as a test of cure and to identify sites of viral persistence with potential for transmission. In the cases of Ebola, NAAT has been used to identify potentially infectious virus in bodily excretions including semen, which may persist for up to a year following resolution of symptoms.[642,643]

The majority of NAATs developed for the detection of agents of VHF are LDT uniplex assays. Due to the highly infectious nature of viruses causing VHF, much of the performance data have been based on analytic "spiked" samples containing attenuated virus or viral sequences, or a limited number of retrospective frozen clinical specimens. A multicenter quality assurance study involving 24 laboratories demonstrated variable performance in detecting prepared samples containing Ebola, Marburg, or Lassa virus.[511] Approximately 78 to 93% of laboratories detected these viruses in samples containing $\geq$4 $\log_{10}$ copies/mL. This dropped to as low as 50% of laboratories for specimens containing less than 4 $\log_{10}$ copies/mL. These data reinforce the importance of conducting both NAAT and serologic assessment of patients suspected of VHF and correlating with travel or exposure history when ruling out these etiologies.

A number of NAATs have been developed and have gained FDA EUA status. Among these are the Xpert Ebola Assay (Cepheid), designed to detect Ebola Zaire, and the FilmArray BT test (BioFire Defense, Salt Lake City, UT), a multiplex NAAT designed to detect 16 biothreat agents including Ebola and Marburg viruses. Both are sample-to-answer tests with an indication for whole blood or serum specimens and provide a result in less than 2 hours. The Xpert Ebola test has an estimated LoD of 73 copies/mL based on analytic studies using inactivated virus and has been successfully implemented in low-resource and mobile lab settings to aid in rapid testing and identification for infected patients.[644,645] The FilmArray BT assay was compared to a RT-PCR assay developed by the

CDC using blood samples spiked with inactivated virus and archived clinical specimens. Results demonstrated similar performance between the two assays with an LoD near 2 $\log_{10}$ $TCID_{50}$/mL.[646] In 2019 the FDA extended the EUA authorization of this test and expanded the initial indication for blood specimens to include undiluted urine specimens as well. While both assays provide a rapid solution for initial testing of suspected cases, all results are considered preliminary and must be confirmed by state public health laboratories or the CDC.

POINTS TO REMEMBER

Viral Hemorrhagic Fever

- Viral hemorrhagic fever (VHF) is caused by members of the *Filoviridae, Flaviviridae, Bunyaviridae,* and *Arenaviridae* families.
- Agents of VHF should not routinely be cultured because of the risk of laboratory-acquired infection. Many are considered potential biothreat agents.
- Serologic tests are cross-reactive between species associated with VHF and those in the same viral family which are not associated with VHF.
- NAATs provide the most sensitive and specific method for laboratory diagnosis of viruses associated with VHF but are not widely available.

RE-EMERGING VACCINE-PREVENTABLE VIRAL ILLNESS

Introduction

Vaccines have played an important role in reducing the morbidity and mortality associated with many viral illnesses. Examples include the eradication of variola virus in 1980 and the near eradication of poliovirus, which was responsible for greater than 40,000 US cases/yr in the 1940s and now causes less than 70 reported cases/year globally.[647] Other vaccine-preventable illnesses such as measles and mumps have received renewed interest as sporadic outbreaks in countries thought to be free of disease appear to be increasing in prevalence.[648] The cause of these outbreaks may be a combination of incomplete protective immunity conferred by the vaccine and a recent decrease in the childhood vaccination rate due to unfounded reports linking immunization to autism.[648,649]

Measles (Rubeola Virus)

Rubeola virus, the cause of measles, is an RNA virus belonging to the *Paramyxoviridae* family, genus *Morbillivirus*. Widespread childhood vaccination efforts in developed countries have reduced measles infections by greater than 99.99% since the early 1960s; however, measles remains a large global burden, infecting 20 million people annually.[647,648] International travel to and from endemic regions serves as an important route for continued introduction of the virus into nonendemic regions. This most often results in sporadic outbreaks of measles cases affecting 10 to 100 exposed individuals.[648,650,651] The majority of individuals infected during these outbreaks are of unvaccinated or unknown vaccination status; however, instances of vaccine failure have been reported.[648,652,653] Rubeola virus is highly contagious via aerosol transmission with attack rates of greater than 99% in unvaccinated individuals having close

contact with infected patients. The nonspecific symptoms of fever, cough, coryza, and conjunctivitis combined with the paucity of cases in developed countries may result in delayed recognition of measles virus cases. Therefore rapid and accurate laboratory diagnostics are central to both the management of the individual and infection control efforts.

The detection of anti-rubeola virus IgM in serum using direct or indirect ELISA from a patient with compatible clinical symptoms is currently considered the "gold standard" for laboratory diagnosis of acute measles infection. A comparison of five commercially available assays demonstrated overall sensitivity of 82.8 to 92.2%; however, time of serum collection had a dramatic impact on performance.[654] For specimens collected during early acute phase (0 to 3 days from onset of symptoms), the sensitivity of IgM assays was only 57 to 80%, whereas sensitivity was 92 to 100% for specimens collected during convalescent phase (6 to 14 days from onset of symptoms). The specificity of each assay was variable, ranging from 86 to 99%, and cross-reactivity was most commonly observed in serum specimens reactive for parvovirus, rubella virus, and EBV.[654]

NAATs may be of utility in patients who were recently immunized (i.e., IgM positive, IgG negative) or for those with recent exposure who may be in early acute phase with negative serologic results. Both respiratory (pharyngeal) and urine specimens have been evaluated for use as noninvasive specimens for rubeola virus NAATs. In a study of 165 confirmed cases, 136 (82.4%) were positive by both IgM serology and PCR while an additional 27 (16.4%) cases were positive by PCR only. The majority of PCR positive/IgM negative cases (19/27, 70.4%) were tested ≤3 days from onset of rash. Sensitivity of PCR was greater for pharyngeal specimens (96.2%) than urine (77.7%).[655] Importantly, the sensitivity of PCR on both urine and pharyngeal specimens decreases following onset of rash and is not useful if symptom onset was greater than 7 to 14 days prior to testing.[656] There are currently no FDA-cleared molecular assays for the detection of measles and few clinical laboratories have developed tests. In the United States, if measles infection is suspected, local departments of public health should be notified immediately and specimens should be sent to state or regional laboratories for definitive identification and typing.[648]

Mumps

Mumps virus belongs to the *Paramyxoviridae* family, within the subfamily *Rubulavirinae* and is closely related to PIV. Following a primary infection, nonspecific upper respiratory symptoms or mild fever are present in ~50 to 70% of infections; however, the hallmark of mumps infection is enlargement of one or both parotid glands which is observed in 60 to 70% of cases.[657] While not pathognomonic, mumps is often diagnosed clinically on the basis of these symptoms and should be considered in a patient with a travel history to an endemic area or in close contact with persons showing similar symptomology. Serious complications including pancreatitis, meningitis/encephalitis, orchitis, or oophoritis occur in 1 to 25% of symptomatic infections.[657,658] Although these complications can result in a considerable morbidity, the overall mortality rate for mumps virus infection is less than 0.1%.[647,657] Mumps is highly contagious via exposure to respiratory secretions on fomites or aerosolized droplets and carries an attack rate of 80 to 90% in nonimmune individuals.

An average of 160,000 cases of mumps were reported annually in the United States prior to introduction of the mumps vaccine in 1968. Childhood immunization efforts (two-dose schedule) have reduced the number of mumps infections by 96 to 99% in developed countries.[647,657] Humans are the only host and reservoir for mumps virus, so the source for sporadic outbreak is unvaccinated individuals or vaccine failure.[659,660] Reported vaccine efficacy ranges from 79 to 95% for the recommended two-dose regimen, and it has been speculated that this variability is due to poor efficacy against non–genotype A (vaccine) strains.[658,659]

In nonvaccinated individuals, the serologic diagnosis of mumps is relatively straightforward, indicated by a positive anti-mumps IgM result in absence of detectable IgG. In primary, nonimmune infections, IgM is reliably detected 3 days following clinical symptoms using standard ELISA and persists to 1 to 2 months thereafter.[661] The sensitivity of IgM ELISAs or IFAs is 80 to 90% overall, but decreases to 40 to 50% if blood is collected less than 3 days from symptom onset.[662] In highly vaccinated populations, the diagnosis of acute infection is more complicated. The IgM response to infection in vaccinated individuals may be weak or absent. This is reflected by the reduced sensitivity (9 to 47%) of commercially available IgM ELISAs when used in this group.[662] An IgM capture assay developed by the CDC demonstrated a somewhat higher sensitivity of 46 to 71% in vaccinated individuals; however, this is still too low to adequately rule out acute infection. Additionally, care must be taken in interpreting a positive IgM result in young children who have been recently vaccinated. A vaccine-induced IgM result may be positive in 70% or greater of vaccines and can persist for up to 1 year resulting in potential false positive results.[663] Culture of saliva specimens is a direct method to definitively diagnose mumps in vaccinated or unvaccinated persons and is less susceptible to false positive results, but maximal sensitivity is achieved when specimens are collected 2 days prior to parotitis.[664] By the time symptoms are observed, culture sensitivity may be only 50 to 80%.

Molecular methods have been evaluated as a more direct method to diagnose acute mumps infection. These assays have demonstrated equivalent performance in the detection of mumps regardless of vaccination status of the patient.[662] The specimen of choice for PCR analysis is saliva collected by buccal swab. Viral shedding in saliva occurs 3 days prior to symptoms and lasts for 3 days after onset of parotitis with VL peaking at 1 to 2 days postonset.[664] When collected within 2 days of parotitis, PCR can be up to 90% sensitive but rapidly decreases to as little as 20 to 50% by day 3 of symptoms[662]; therefore prompt collection of the specimen is critical for optimal sensitivity. An additional benefit of molecular detection of mumps is similar performance in both vaccinated and nonvaccinated persons. In one study, RT-PCR was greater than 90% sensitive in nonvaccinated and persons who had received one or two doses of vaccine. The collection of both blood and buccal swab specimens is recommended by the CDC for the diagnosis of mumps. There are no FDA-cleared molecular assays for the detection of mumps virus and few hospital laboratories have developed or validated laboratory-developed PCR assays. If mumps infection is suspected, local departments of public health should be notified immediately and specimens should be sent to state or regional laboratories for identification.

POINTS TO REMEMBER

Re-emerging Vaccine Preventable Viral Illness

- Increasing globalization provides continued opportunity for the introduction of vaccine-preventable illness into low-endemicity regions resulting in misdiagnosis.
- High vaccination rate in developed countries complicates the interpretation of serologic results.
- Nucleic acid amplification tests for measles and mumps are useful for diagnosis of acute infection in immunized individuals but rapidly loses sensitivity upon convalescence.

SUMMARY AND CONCLUSION

Viral illness continues to be a major cause of morbidity and mortality in both industrialized and developing countries. While some historically significant causes of viral disease such as polio, smallpox, measles, and mumps have been reduced through local or global vaccination programs, others persist in under-vaccinated regions or recur in annual epidemics such as influenza. The increased utilization of more advanced immunomodulatory therapies for patients with malignancies undergoing HSCT and in SOT recipients has increased the prevalence of previously uncommon and severe systemic illness resulting from reactivation of latent illness due to herpesviruses and polyomaviruses. These same therapies also result in more severe primary infections by common viruses causing respiratory and gastrointestinal symptoms. As more specific therapies become available for treatment of these pathogens, timely and accurate diagnostic assays are increasingly important for appropriate patient management.

Increasing availability and standardization of molecular diagnostics have made an astounding impact in viral diagnostics over the past two decades through increased sensitivity, specificity, and accurate quantitation of viral pathogens in clinical specimens; however, newer technologies appear poised to expand on current capabilities. Rapid, POC molecular diagnostics are beginning to change workflow for the diagnosis and treatment of influenza with sensitivity rivaling laboratory-based traditional RT-PCR methods and TAT of less than 20 min. These platforms may effectively remove centralized testing from the clinical and molecular laboratories closer to the patient. A decrease in test volume for these relatively simple assays may aid in freeing resources for the development of more complex quantitative or multiplexed testing which will be the cornerstone of laboratory molecular diagnostics.

The introduction of easy-to-use multiplex "syndromic panel" assays has simplified test ordering for physicians when presented with patients suffering respiratory, GI, or CNS symptoms by enabling simultaneous detection of multiple viruses, bacteria, fungi, and parasites associated with a particular symptomology. However, results may be challenging to interpret or even misleading when an unexpected finding is encountered. Additionally, syndromic testing may not be appropriate or cost effective as a first-line approach for all patients. Specifically, otherwise healthy patients presenting to outpatient clinics with upper respiratory illness may gain more benefit from a rapid influenza test. Conversely, a multiplexed syndromic panel may be more appropriate for acutely ill, compromised, or pediatric patients to reach a rapid diagnosis when presenting with nonspecific symptoms.

As complexity of testing modalities, test menus, and interpretation of results continue to grow the laboratory will play a central role offering both technical and clinical expertise to primary patient care providers. A strong relationship between the laboratory, providers, and pharmacy will be critical in the selection of the appropriate test to provide the greatest clinical utility, cost control, and the highest level of patient care.

SELECTED REFERENCES

66. Popowitch EB, O'Neill SS, Miller MB. Comparison of the Biofire FilmArray RP, Genmark eSensor RVP, Luminex xTAG RVPv1, and Luminex xTAG RVP fast multiplex assays for detection of respiratory viruses. J Clin Microbiol 2013;51:1528–33.

88. Wolfel R, Corman VM, Guggemos W, et al. Virological assessment of hospitalized patients with COVID-2019. Nature 2020;581:465–9.

104. Ramos KJ, Kapnadak SG, Collins BF, et al. Detection of SARS-CoV-2 by bronchoscopy after negative nasopharyngeal testing: Stay vigilant for COVID-19. Respir Med Case Rep 2020;30:101120.

110. Sinclair J. Human cytomegalovirus: Latency and reactivation in the myeloid lineage. J Clin Virol 2008;41:180–5.

151. Babady NE, Cheng C, Cumberbatch E, et al. Monitoring of cytomegalovirus viral loads by two molecular assays in whole-blood and plasma samples from hematopoietic stem cell transplant recipients. J Clin Microbiol 2015;53:1252–7.

154. Preiksaitis JK, Hayden RT, Tong Y, et al. Are we there yet? Impact of the first international standard for cytomegalovirus DNA on the harmonization of results reported on plasma samples. Clin Infect Dis 2016;63:583–9.

228. Govind S, Hockley J, Morris C. Collaborative study to establish the 1st who international standard for human herpes virus 6b (HHV-6b) DNA for nucleic acid amplification technique (NAT)-based assays. World Health Organization. 2017. https://apps.who.int/iris/handle/10665/260259.

260. Hirsch HH, Randhawa P, Practice ASTIDCo. BK virus in solid organ transplant recipients. American Journal of Transplantation. 2009;9(Suppl 4):S136–46.

357. Perkins RB, Guido RS, Castle PE, et al. 2019 ASCCP Risk-Based Management Consensus Guidelines for Abnormal Cervical Cancer Screening Tests and Cancer Precursors. J Low Genit Tract Dis 2020;24:102–31.

463. Graf EH, Farquharson MV, Cardenas AM. Comparative evaluation of the Filmarray meningitis/encephalitis molecular panel in a pediatric population. Diagn Microbiol Infect Dis 2017;87:92–4.

499. Go YY, Balasuriya UB, Lee CK. Zoonotic encephalitides caused by arboviruses: Transmission and epidemiology of alphaviruses and flaviviruses. Clin Exp Vaccine Res 2014;3:58–77.

514. Bhatt S, Gething PW, Brady OJ, et al. The global distribution and burden of dengue. Nature 2013;496:504–7.

515. Silva LA, Dermody TS. Chikungunya virus: Epidemiology, replication, disease mechanisms, and prospective intervention strategies. J Clin Invest 2017;127:737–49.

520. Rahman MT, Tahmin HA, Mannan T, Sultana R. Seropositivity and pattern of dengue infection in Dhaka City. Mymensingh Med J 2007;16:204–8.

566. Hou J, Liu Z, Gu F. Epidemiology and prevention of hepatitis B virus infection. Int J Med Sci 2005;2:50–7.

567. Servant-Delmas A, Mercier-Darty M, Ly TD, et al. Variable capacity of 13 hepatitis B virus surface antigen assays for the detection of HBsAg mutants in blood samples. J Clin Virol 2012;53:338–45.

597. Barrera JM, Francis B, Ercilla G, et al. Improved detection of anti-HCV in post-transfusion hepatitis by a third-generation ELISA. Vox Sang 1995;68:15–8.

628. Kao HW, Ashcavai M, Redeker AG. The persistence of hepatitis A IgM antibody after acute clinical hepatitis A. Hepatology 1984;4:933–6.

641. Wolfel R, Paweska JT, Petersen N, et al. Low-density macroarray for rapid detection and identification of Crimean-Congo hemorrhagic fever virus. J Clin Microbiol 2009;47:1025–30.

658. Latner DR, Hickman CJ. Remembering mumps. PLoS Pathog 2015;11:e1004791.

SECTION IX

Transfusion Medicine

Exam questions, case studies, and additional resources are available on ExpertConsult.com.
*Full versions of these chapters are available electronically on www.ExpertConsult.com.

Blood Group Systems and Pretransfusion Testing*

Anh P. Dinh and Edward J. Yoon

ABSTRACT

Background
Specific knowledge of relevant blood group systems is essential for a thorough understanding of blood bank pretransfusion testing methodology and the potential practical applications of that information to clinical practice. In any given patient care setting, the blood bank and transfusion medicine service are tasked with integrating this information to improve the safety of blood transfusion and related activities.

Content
The first portion of this chapter (Blood Group Systems) introduces the commonly assessed carbohydrate and protein blood group systems relevant to clinical and transfusion service practices, including ABO, Lewis, Ii, P1PK, Rh, MNS, Kell, Duffy, and Kidd blood group systems. Salient laboratory details and/or clinical associations are also provided. The second portion of this chapter (Pretransfusion Testing) introduces basic tenets and methods of blood bank laboratory serologic testing and describes the usual stepwise approach for routine pretransfusion testing, including ABO and Rh type, antibody screen and identification, and crossmatch. Direct antiglobulin testing is also briefly discussed, as are situations involving emergency release of blood products.

---

*The full version of this chapter is available electronically on ExpertConsult.com.

Blood Components, Product Modifications, and Blood Donor Screening*

John P. Manis

ABSTRACT

Background

Transfusion of blood requires multiple steps, including blood donation from nonremunerated healthy volunteers, manufacture, testing, and modifications of blood components, and finally administration of the product to a patient. While blood donation and transfusions have steadily decreased in the United States over the past decade, 16 million blood products were generated by collection and about 15 million transfused in 2019.[1] Red cells, platelets, plasma, and cryoprecipitate are manufactured using relatively simple and widely available methods to supply the demand for blood. The safety of the blood supply is ensured using donor history questionnaires, laboratory testing, and quality measures to keep these biologic products derived from millions of donors therapeutically consistent.

Content

The first half of the chapter describes the blood manufacturing process, beginning with the collection of whole blood or apheresis products from a healthy donor to the point where the product is ready to be transfused into a patient. The steps taken to reduce both infectious and noninfectious threats to the blood supply will be discussed. Donor adverse events resulting from both methods of collection will be detailed. Autologous and directed donation will be briefly discussed. The second half of the chapter details the methods of processing whole blood into components. Modifications, such as irradiation, leukocyte reduction, washing, and volume reduction will also be discussed. Understanding the process of obtaining, manufacturing, and transfusing blood is critical to interpreting clinical outcomes of blood administration.

---

*The full version of this chapter is available electronically on ExpertConsult.com.

Indications for Transfusion: RBCs, Platelets, Plasma, and Cryoprecipitate

Edward J. Yoon and Anh P. Dinh

ABSTRACT

Background

Blood transfusion practices should ultimately be driven by evidence-based decisions that integrate clinical observations, laboratory data, and a sound understanding of how patients can realistically benefit from blood products. In addition to acting as stewards of the local blood supply, the blood bank and transfusion medicine service are necessarily involved in ensuring that these concepts are understood and, consequently, that blood transfusions are appropriately conducted.

Content

The focus of this chapter is adult transfusion medicine, as pediatric transfusion medicine is beyond the scope of this material. Following a brief clinical practice foreword regarding

informed consent, this chapter introduces the four commonly encountered blood component products in modern transfusion medicine: packed red blood cells, platelets, plasma, and cryoprecipitated antihemophilic factor. Highlights of evidence-based practices supported by current scientific medical literature at the time of writing are discussed, including clinical and laboratory parameter-related indications for transfusion, appropriate dosing, and expected responses. When applicable, special transfusion considerations for specific clinical situations are also described. In addition, there is a brief discussion of the clinical and logistical aspects of massive transfusion. The chapter concludes with a review of infrequently encountered blood products such as granulocytes and whole blood.

BLOOD TRANSFUSION PRACTICES

Introduction

Blood transfusion is one of the most common medical interventions in modern health care. While the practice at its inception was crudely conceived of and fraught with misguided assumptions, allogeneic blood transfusion (transfusing blood from one source, i.e., donor, to another, i.e., recipient) has since been recognized as having tremendous potential for reducing morbidity and mortality, especially in certain chronically and critically ill patient populations. Furthermore, transfusion practices have evolved considerably since then and continue to be refined with advances in medical and scientific evidence-based research. Although risk is certainly involved and several adverse effects of transfusions have been well described, understanding the contexts whereby transfusions may be beneficial has an integral place in the practice of medicine. This chapter will mainly focus on key aspects of red blood cell, platelet, plasma, and cryoprecipitate transfusion. It is important to note that this discussion will be limited to adults, as pediatric transfusion medicine is a complex, nuanced topic beyond the scope of this material.

Consent for Blood Products

As with all medical interventions or invasive procedures, transfusion requires prior informed consent from the recipient. Documentation of consent (paper or electronic forms) demonstrates that the prospective recipient has been informed of

the relevant benefits and risks, as well as given the opportunity to have any questions addressed. Engagement and mutual understanding are critical for proper medical care while maintaining a patient's rights and autonomy. Blood transfusions should never be forced upon an individual who may otherwise refuse such treatment.

If an individual is deemed to be incompetent and therefore unable to properly make informed health care decisions, a surrogate decision-making individual or party may be authorized to consent on the recipient's behalf. Similarly, parents may have medical decision-making authority for their underage minor children. For critically ill patients who are unable to provide consent (i.e., unconscious trauma patients), hospitals may have emergency provisions that permit physician-prescribed transfusions. In any case, specific local laws and regulations may take precedence and dictate the terms and boundaries of medical decision-making, which includes transfusions. For ambiguous situations involving potential morbidity and mortality, prompt consultation with a hospital ethics board or local authorities is recommended.

Red Blood Cells

Packed red blood cells (pRBCs) were historically believed to provide a panacea-like spectrum of health benefits, including reinforced wound healing and nutritional supplementation. However, current evidence suggests that the sole purpose of pRBC transfusion should be to increase a patient's oxygen-carrying capacity and consequently improve tissue oxygenation. The need to improve oxygenation may be encountered in a wide variety of clinical situations such as hypoproliferative marrow disorders, acute or chronic hemolysis (i.e., sickle cell disease [SCD]), and active blood loss due to bleeding. Decisions of whether to transfuse pRBCs may be complex and must account for multiple concurrent factors. Considerations may include a patient's overall clinical status, the specific diagnosis leading to the oxygenation deficit, medical and surgical comorbidities, physiologic compensatory mechanisms that may prevent the need for transfusion, the availability of alternative therapies, and relevant laboratory values. Of the laboratory values used to guide pRBC transfusion, the hemoglobin (Hb) measurement component of routine complete blood counts (CBC) is typically the most relevant and informative.

Normal reference ranges for Hb are approximately 12 to 16 g/dL for females and 13.5 to 18 g/dL for males.[1] In the absence of exacerbating factors, a certain degree of anemia, as evidenced by a lower Hb measurement, is physiologically tolerable and may be adequately compensated for through increased cardiac output and altered tissue metabolism. Prior studies in healthy volunteers demonstrated tolerance of short-term hemodilution-induced anemia down to 5.1 g/dL.[2] The critical Hb levels tend to be higher for most patient populations that may require pRBC transfusion, although evidence-based thresholds for these values were not established until relatively recently. The Transfusion Requirements in Critical Care (TRICC) trial was the seminal investigation for modern evidence-based pRBC transfusion practices, demonstrating that restrictive thresholds to maintain Hb > 7 g/dL were not inferior to historically higher liberal thresholds to maintain Hb > 10 g/dL, and that restrictive thresholds were associated with improved survival in specific patient groups.[3] Subsequent randomized control trials posed similar questions for various medical and surgical disciplines, including obstetrics, gastroenterology, cardiac surgery, and orthopedic surgery.[4–7] With relatively few exceptions, these studies concluded that there was no apparent clinical benefit to a liberal transfusion strategy. Therefore the consensus of evidence at the time of this writing favors restrictive pRBC transfusion strategies in most situations with Hb thresholds of >7 to 8 g/dL, which is recommended by several published clinical practice guidelines.[7a] It should be noted, however, that there is insufficient high-quality evidence at this time for some critical situations where more liberal transfusion may be warranted, including acute coronary syndromes and acute brain injury.[9] Furthermore, as Hb measurements may be of limited utility in actively bleeding patients, they should not be the sole determinant of transfusion decisions in such cases.

A single unit of pRBCs increases an adult patient's post-transfusion Hb by approximately 1 g/dL and the hematocrit by approximately 3%, although the actual response may depend on certain factors such as blood volume. Patients with smaller or larger total blood volumes may experience a greater or lesser response, respectively, for the same amount transfused. Similarly, there may be suboptimal responses in patients with effectively larger-than-expected circulating volumes due to splenomegaly or treatment with continuous extracorporeal circuits (i.e., continuous venovenous hemodialysis (CVVHD) or extracorporeal membrane oxygenation [ECMO]). Finally, lesser responses would be expected in patients actively losing RBC mass, as observed with active

bleeding and continuous destruction due to immunologic or mechanical etiologies. Therefore while the expectation of 1 g/dL per pRBC unit may be a reasonable starting point, patients may require fewer or more transfusions than initially predicted. Furthermore, with the exceptions of active bleeding and hemodynamic instability, pRBCs should be prescribed and transfused one unit at a time, and the decision to transfuse further should be supported by post-transfusion clinical and laboratory data.

Transfusion-dependent Anemia

There are some special considerations for patients receiving long-term treatment with chronic pRBC transfusion, including those with SCD and transfusion-dependent thalassemia. While chronically transfused patients often benefit from individualized, evidence-based therapy plans that account for their specific diseases and their relative normal laboratory parameters, some generalized advice is presented here. First, the baseline Hb levels in this patient population may be significantly lower than the established reference ranges. Consequently, providers should interpret the anemia with caution and avoid excessive transfusion as evidence suggests that increased RBC mass in these patients may lead to deleterious hyperviscosity effects beyond a certain threshold.[10,11] Second, these patients have a relatively high risk of RBC antigen alloimmunization.[12–19] This risk may be mitigated by selecting pRBCs that express (or do not express) antigens and most closely approximate a patient's native RBCs. This process of RBC phenotype matching typically involves the most common Rh system antigens (i.e., D, C, c, E, and e antigens) and Kell system antigens (i.e., K antigen) at a minimum due to the historical prevalence of their corresponding alloantibodies in chronically transfused patients,[20] although other immunogenic blood group systems may also be accounted for if feasible. Finally, patients with SCD may strongly benefit from receiving pRBCs confirmed to have been collected from hemoglobin S (HbS) negative donors, although this approach is not universally practiced.[21] More drastic situations such as large volume transfusions or RBC exchange transfusions for SCD-related indications may warrant stronger consideration of exclusively transfusing HbS negative products.

Hyperhemolysis Syndrome

Hyperhemolysis syndrome should be recognized as a potential rare complication of and relative contraindication for pRBC transfusion, frequently described in patients with transfusion-dependent hemoglobinopathies, though not exclusively.[22] Hyperhemolysis syndrome presents with clinical and laboratory findings indicative of active hemolysis, along with reticulocytopenia and post-transfusion Hb levels falling even below pretransfusion levels. These distinct findings suggest hemolysis of both recently transfused RBCs and autologous RBCs and therefore represent a paradoxical net loss of circulating RBC mass post-transfusion. The pathophysiology of hyperhemolysis is still incompletely understood and may involve some combination of a cryptic immunologic bystander effect, macrophage activation, complement activation, and erythropoietic suppression.[23,24] While the etiology remains unclear at this time, further pRBC transfusion allogeneic or otherwise should generally be avoided due to the risk of exacerbating the degree of hemolysis. Understandably, this situation can be quite unsettling for clinicians advised to limit pRBC transfusion in the face of sometimes precipitously declining Hb levels. Perhaps more than any other situation involving pRBC transfusion, clear communication of goals and possible non-transfusion treatment modalities is critical.

POINTS TO REMEMBER

- Packed RBC transfusions serve solely to increase oxygen-carrying capacity and improve tissue oxygenation.
- Restrictive pRBC transfusion strategies are generally favored for many common clinical and surgical situations.
- Patients with chronic transfusion-dependent anemias warrant special considerations prior to considering pRBC transfusions.

Platelets

Platelets play a critical role in the initial response to tissue injury for primary hemostasis. As a result, thrombocytopenia, as evidenced by decreased platelets enumerated by routine CBCs, may represent a significant risk for persistent bleeding. Platelet transfusions mitigate this risk by bolstering the quantity of circulating functional platelets. As many clinical bleeding situations are complex and may involve deficiencies of physiologic procoagulant constituents besides platelets, it is essential to remember that platelet transfusion only addresses one specific aspect of the global hemostatic process.

The expected response to platelet transfusion varies by the specific product. Platelets may be separated from whole blood donations or collected using apheresis technology, and these products may be used interchangeably for transfusion support purposes. While a single unit of apheresis-derived platelets elicits an expected post-transfusion increase in the range of 30,000 to 60,000/μL, the increase from a single unit of whole blood-derived platelets is approximately six times less (5000 to 10,000/μL). Consequently, whole blood-derived (WBD) platelets are often pooled from five to six individual units, which in aggregate approximates the post-transfusion response to a single apheresis-derived unit. These distinctions should be clear when discussing transfusion goals to avoid confusion. Additionally, platelet transfusions should be prescribed and transfused one at a time, which typically entails a single apheresis-derived unit or an equivalent pool of five to six WBD units. Post-transfusion clinical and laboratory data should support the decision to transfuse further, if deemed necessary.

Prophylaxis

The normal reference range for platelets is approximately 150,000 to 450,000/μL.[1] However, platelet counts may be significantly lower without any apparent bleeding risk from thrombocytopenia alone. An early study posited a relationship between the platelet count and the frequency and severity of hemorrhage in thrombocytopenic patients undergoing chemotherapy for acute leukemia, suggesting that prophylactic platelet transfusions to maintain platelets $\geq$ 20,000/μL would mitigate the risk of spontaneous bleeding.[25] Subsequent clinical trials lowered this threshold to $\geq$ 10,000/μL, with some reports suggesting that even lower platelet counts may be sufficient to prevent spontaneous hemorrhage.[26-29] Most evidence-based clinical practice guidelines recommend a threshold of $\geq$ 10,000/μL for prophylactic transfusions.[8,30,31] Of note, despite advances in modern chemotherapy and

bone marrow transplantation, patients with hypoproliferative thrombocytopenia secondary to chemotherapy for hematologic disorders continue to constitute a significant portion of patients receiving platelet transfusions in this manner.[32,33]

Active Bleeding

Compared to prophylaxis, platelet transfusion thresholds to address significant bleeding or the risk thereof are more contentious. Most guidelines recommend maintaining platelets $\geq$ 50,000/μL for active bleeding and in preparation for major non-neuraxial surgical procedures, although unanimous recommendations for minor invasive procedures are conspicuously absent. Commonly performed minor procedures for which recommendations exist include central venous catheter placement with platelets $\geq$ 20,000/μL and lumbar puncture with platelets $\geq$ 50,000/μL, for instance, although the quality of supporting evidence for such practices is poor and specific thresholds may vary slightly depending on the source.[8,31] The availability of disparate recommendations for such poorly defined situations necessitates a thorough appraisal of a given patient's situation and bleeding risk, setting realistic goals, as well as clear communication between the clinical and transfusion medicine services. For neurosurgery, posterior-orbit ophthalmic surgical procedures, and related neuraxial bleeding, platelets $\geq$ 100,000/μL is recommended based on expert opinion, low-quality evidence, and the perceived critical nature of achieving hemostasis in these sites.[34]

Finally, it is worth noting that excluding situations of life-threatening hemorrhage secondary to thrombocytopenia, established evidence-based practice guidelines generally advise against platelet transfusions in the settings of immune thrombocytopenia (ITP), heparin-induced thrombocytopenia (HIT), and thrombotic thrombocytopenic purpura (TTP).[35-39] These relative contraindications historically originated from concerns that transfusion is either ineffective in increasing circulating platelet counts due to the immune pathophysiology as in ITP, or that it may precipitate thrombotic exacerbation as in HIT or TTP. However, more recent evidence has challenged the validity of these claims for all three situations and has posited that platelet transfusion may not be as deleterious as once believed.[40,41] Therefore any attempts at platelet transfusion in these cases should be thoroughly justified and approached cautiously.

Thrombocytopathy

The utility of platelet transfusions to address functional thrombocytopenia secondary to platelet dysfunction has also been explored. Acquired platelet dysfunction may occur in the setting of antiplatelet agent use (i.e., aspirin), cardiopulmonary bypass (CPB), and uremia, for example. For antiplatelet agent use and CPB specifically, evidence-based clinical practice guidelines have conceded that platelet transfusion may provide some degree of benefit in bleeding patients, albeit based on weak evidence.[8,42] On the other hand, bleeds stemming from uremia should not be addressed with platelet transfusions. The pathophysiology of the coagulopathy associated with uremia is more complex than pure platelet dysfunction and consequently does not clearly benefit from transfusion.[43] Common alternative therapies include desmopressin (DDAVP), as well as dialysis to remove causative uremic metabolites.[44]

Platelet Refractoriness

Platelet refractoriness is broadly defined as an undesirably poor response to platelet transfusion, as evidenced by a lower-than-expected platelet increment on a post-transfusion CBC. This observation may be relatively frequent, complicating up to 34% of transfusions in certain populations, especially those who are multiply transfused.[45] Causes for suboptimal responses are classified as antibody-mediated (immune causes) versus those that are not (nonimmune causes) (Table 92.1), and this distinction is the crucial first step toward appropriate treatment of a platelet refractory patient.[46] While the incidence may vary by specific patient population, nonimmune causes tend to predominate due to their ubiquity, especially among hospitalized and transfusion-dependent patients. Among the immune causes, refractoriness mediated by alloantibodies formed against human leukocyte antigens (HLA) is commonly encountered and will be the focus of the discussion below, although antibodies against other non-HLA antigens such as human platelet antigens (HPA) may occasionally be implicated in immune refractoriness.

Compared to cases of nonimmune refractoriness, one often distinguishing feature of immune refractoriness is the pattern of platelet increment response observed within one hour post-transfusion. Due to the presence of relevant antibodies immediately interacting with transfused platelets, a relatively minimal increase in platelet count may be detected, if any. By contrast, in cases of nonimmune refractoriness, a considerable increase in platelet count may be observed initially; however, this increment is later diminished by an underlying consumptive process. In either case, if the response pattern assessment is not performed within one hour post-transfusion, potential immune versus nonimmune causes may be indistinguishable (Fig. 92.1). As such, the criteria for defining platelet refractoriness includes this timed assessment. Additionally, patient size may influence the post-transfusion platelet count increment. More rigorous calculations, such as the corrected count increment or percentage platelet recovery, can be used to account for this variable, provided certain patient and laboratory parameters are available (Table 92.2).[47,48] Once an immune etiology is suspected, laboratory investigation is required to identify which platelet-relevant antibodies, if any, are present in the patient. In the case of anti-HLA alloantibodies, those directed against HLA class I antigens (specifically HLA-A and HLA-B antigens) must be detected due to their expression on platelet membranes.[49] It should be noted, however, that patients may have preexisting anti-HLA antibodies due to prior exposure through transfusion or pregnancies. Therefore the mere presence of these antibodies does not necessarily establish causality for platelet refractoriness without other clinical or laboratory evidence of it.

There are several options for transfusion strategies if anti-HLA antibodies are implicated in platelet refractoriness, all of which require close communication with the patient's clinical service, the immunogenetics/HLA laboratory that performs testing, and the donor blood center tasked with procuring

TABLE 92.1	Potential Causes of Platelet Refractoriness
Immune Causes	**Nonimmune Causes**
Human leukocyte antigen (HLA) alloantibodies	Infection
Human platelet antigen (HPA) alloantibodies	High fevers
ABO isohemagglutinins	Antibiotic medications
Platelet autoantibodies	Antifungal medications
Drug-dependent platelet antibodies	Heparin
Immune complexes	Disseminated intravascular coagulation (DIC)
	Bleeding
	Graft-versus-host disease (GVHD)
	Veno-occlusive disorders
	Splenomegaly
	Increasing weight
	Multiple pregnancies

Data from Stanworth SJ, Navarrete C, Estcourt L, Marsh J. Platelet refractoriness—practical approaches and ongoing dilemmas in patient management. *Br J Haematol.* 2015;171(3):297–305. doi:10.1111/bjh.13597.

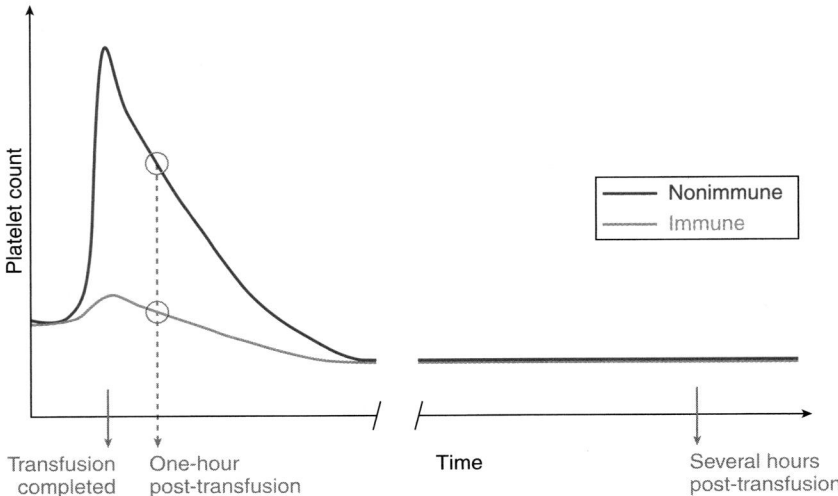

FIGURE 92.1 Schematic example of post-transfusion response patterns for immune and nonimmune platelet refractoriness.

TABLE 92.2 Calculations Used to Assess Platelet Transfusion Response

Calculation Method	Formula	Results Suspicious for Platelet Refractoriness[a]
Post-transfusion platelet increment (PPI)	Post-transfusion platelets (/L) – Pretransfusion platelets (/L)	$<5 \times 10^9$
Corrected count increment (CCI)	$\dfrac{\text{PPI (/L)} \times \text{Body surface area } (m^2)}{\text{Platelets transfused } (10^{11})}$	$<5 \times 10^9$
Percentage platelet recovery (PPR)	$\dfrac{\text{PPI (/L)} \times \text{Total blood volume (L)} \times 100\%}{\text{Platelets transfused } (10^{11})}$	$<20\%$

[a]Based on two sequential transfusion events. Calculations are performed within 1 hour post-transfusion.
Data from Tinmouth AT, Semple E, Shehata N, Branch DR. Platelet immunopathology and therapy: a Canadian Blood Services Research and Development Symposium. *Transfus Med Rev.* 2006;20(4):294–314. doi:10.1016/j.tmrv.2006.05.008.

TABLE 92.3 Comparison of Strategies for Identifying Human Leukocyte Antigens–Compatible Platelets

Method	Necessary Patient Information	Necessary Donor Information	Advantages	Disadvantages
HLA matching	HLA antigen phenotype	HLA antigen phenotype	Potential for the highest-compatibility donor(s)[a] Low or no risk of further HLA antigen alloimmunization[a]	Limited potential donor pool[a] Time necessary for patient phenotyping
HLA antigen avoidance	Anti-HLA antibody specificities	HLA antigen phenotype	Large potential donor pool Relatively rapid turnaround times	Risk of further HLA antigen alloimmunization
Platelet crossmatching	None specific	None specific	No specific patient or donor information required Most rapid turnaround times	Highly technical process that may not always be available New patient samples required periodically Risk of further HLA antigen alloimmunization

[a]Dependent on HLA match grade.
HLA, Human leukocyte antigens.

products (Table 92.3). HLA matching is the most comprehensive strategy, in which platelet donors are selected based on their HLA-A and HLA-B antigen expression to best approximate that of the patient. Conceptually analogous to phenotype matching for RBCs, the best HLA-matched platelets would come from a donor with the same HLA-A and HLA-B antigen phenotype as the patient, which are therefore not affected by anti-HLA alloantibodies. Additionally, there would be no risk of further alloantibody formation since antigens would not be perceived as foreign. Notably, however, not all platelets classified as HLA-matched are necessarily matched to the same degree. Grades A and BU (B1U and B2U) are the highest grades (recipient will not perceive donor antigens as foreign), while grade D is the lowest (at least two antigen mismatches). Lower-grade matches may confer little to no benefit over random, nonmatched platelets depending on the patient's sensitization history, so the various match grades should be considered when selecting platelets for transfusion (Table 92.4).[50] Given the stringent requirements for favorable high-grade matching, the potential donor pool at any given time may be very limited. Furthermore, HLA matching also requires knowledge of the patient's HLA antigen phenotype, which may require additional time to obtain.

A popular alternative for HLA-compatible platelets, antigen avoidance, uses the patient's anti-HLA antibody profile to avoid selecting platelet donors who possess the corresponding HLA antigen specificities. Instead, platelet donors who lack these specificities are selected. This approach is conceptually analogous to transfusing antigen-negative pRBCs to a patient with specific RBC alloantibodies to ensure compatibility. Antigen avoidance has the inherent advantage of a vastly larger potential donor pool compared to HLA matching, in addition to relatively rapid turnaround times since HLA phenotyping of the patient is not required. However, the avoidance of specific antigens does not preclude the formation of new anti-HLA antibodies against other antigens unaccounted for, which may further complicate future transfusion support.

Lastly, platelet crossmatching serves as a final recourse in cases where immune refractoriness is strongly suspected, no patient information is available, and rapid turnaround times are paramount, although it does not necessarily have to be confined to such dire situations. In brief, representative samples from available donor platelets are reacted with a patient's serum using the solid phase red cell adherence (SPRCA) method. A positive serologic response is elicited, presumably

TABLE 92.4 Match Grades for Human Leukocyte Antigens–matched Platelet Products

Match Grade	Description
A	4 of 4 (4/4) identical antigens
B1U	3 of 4 (3/4) identical antigens, one (1/4) unknown antigen (possible homozygosity)
B2U	2 of 4 (2/4) identical antigens, two (2/4) unknown antigens (possible homozygosity)
B1X	3 of 4 (3/4) identical antigens, one (1/4) cross-reactive antigen
B2X	2 of 4 (2/4) identical antigens, two (2/4) cross-reactive antigens
B2UX	2 of 4 (2/4) identical antigens, one (1/4) unknown antigen, and one (1/4) cross-reactive antigen
C	3 of 4 (3/4) identical antigens, one (1/4) mismatched antigen
D	2 or more (≥2/4) mismatched antigens.
R	Random donor. Antigen and mismatch status unknown

Note: Four (4) total Class I antigens (two HLA-A antigens and two HLA-B antigens)

HLA, Human leukocyte antigens.
From Moroff G, Garratty G, Heal JM, et al. Selection of platelets for refractory patients by HLA matching and prospective crossmatching. *Transfusion.* 1992;32(7):633–640. doi:10.1046/j.1537-2995.1992. 32792391036.x.

if the patient has antibodies against a specific donor's platelet antigens. Theoretically, then, all nonreactive donor units are compatible for transfusion. When feasible, platelet cross-matching has the advantages of the most rapid potential turnaround times without the need for any specific patient or donor HLA-related information. However, the process is technically complicated, may not always be available, and periodically requires new patient samples for testing if continued transfusion support is necessary. Furthermore, like antigen avoidance, there is the additional risk of further alloimmunization.

POINTS TO REMEMBER

- Platelet transfusion for thrombocytopenia addresses a potential defect in primary hemostasis.
- Accepted platelet transfusion thresholds vary based on the clinical situations of prophylaxis (10,000/μL), active bleeding or major surgery (50,000/μL), or neuraxial surgery (100,000/μL).
- Platelet refractoriness may be due to immune or non-immune etiologies, and refractoriness caused by anti-HLA antibodies is an important immune-mediated cause.

Plasma

Plasma contains the coagulation-related proteins necessary for secondary hemostasis. A unit of fresh frozen plasma collected from a normal, non-coagulopathic donor is approximately

200 to 250 mL and contains 1 IU/mL of all plasma coagulation factors, anticoagulation factors, and approximately 2 to 4 mg/mL of fibrinogen.[51] Despite this relatively straightforward fact, reports indicate that plasma transfusions often occur for non–evidence-based indications or outside of existing practice guidelines.[52,53]

Clinical indications for plasma transfusion include bleeding associated with deficiencies of multiple coagulation factors (i.e., disseminated intravascular coagulation (DIC), massive hemorrhage) and deficiencies of individual factors if an alternative pharmacologic concentrate is unavailable.[54] While the procoagulant factors are routinely considered for this purpose, plasma also contains natural direct and indirect anticoagulant proteins such as protein C, protein S, and antithrombin (AT) that balance these complex processes.

While coagulation factor activity levels could theoretically inform plasma transfusion support decisions, such assays are not widely available and usually entail lengthy turnaround times. Consequently, the more quickly and readily available laboratory tests that are often utilized for this purpose include the prothrombin time (PT), international normalized ratio (INR), and activated partial thromboplastin time (aPTT). While the intended use of these values is to provide information regarding the functional status of the historically defined extrinsic/common and intrinsic/common arms of the coagulation cascade, respectively, results above the normal reference ranges do not necessarily correlate with a physiologic hemostatic defect. This limitation occurs because truly irrelevant decreases in coagulation factor activity from a hemostasis perspective can exert disproportionately drastic effects on these assays, leading to overestimates of a patient's bleeding risk. Bleeding risks have only been reported to increase when most coagulation factors fall approximately below 30%.[55] Consequently, for situations in which plasma is indicated, the post-transfusion goal should be thought of as the therapeutic repletion of coagulation factors past the hemostatic threshold rather than full replacement toward an arbitrary reference value.

Prophylactic plasma transfusions in nonbleeding patients occur frequently, often motivated by abnormal coagulation testing, typically involving mildly elevated results less than 1.5 times the upper limit of normal reference ranges, and an imminent invasive procedure that represents a potential hemostatic challenge. As previously mentioned, the PT, aPTT, and INR are poor predictors of bleeding in nonbleeding patients and are consequently poor risk-assessment tools for this purpose. Mild to moderate elevations, in particular, are commonly encountered in clinical practice and may not represent any actual hemostatic deficiencies. Additionally, several clinical trials and observational data have demonstrated no benefit of prophylactic plasma transfusions toward bleeding outcomes, further delegitimizing this practice.[56] There is even evidence to support withholding prophylactic plasma transfusion in nonbleeding patients with advanced liver disease, whose often significantly abnormal coagulation test results may signify an offset but rebalanced hemostasis rather than a bleeding diathesis.[57–59]

Proper dosing of plasma transfusions is based on the intended recipient's weight rather than a fixed number of units per dose. While a unanimous recommendation that applies to all scenarios does not exist, prescribing plasma at 10 to 20 mL/kg is generally accepted as a reasonable dose intended to simultaneously increase all coagulation-related proteins by approximately 25% to 30% activity. This strategy reflects the notion of treating a hemostatic threshold rather than scaling with the magnitude of a test abnormality. That said, laboratory assessment of response can be difficult since routine coagulation tests tend not to vary linearly with the amount of plasma transfused. Larger post-transfusion decreases for PT, INR, and aPTT are observed with greater initial derangements, while the same plasma transfusion dose yields diminishing results as the initial derangement approaches normal reference ranges. In other words, attempts to correct only mildly elevated coagulation abnormalities even with high doses of plasma may prove to be futile and result in only minor normalization of test results, if any.[60]

The terminology for different plasma products stems from regulatory requirements, but these products can be considered interchangeable for almost all indications. Strictly speaking, fresh frozen plasma (FFP) is placed in a freezer within 8 hours of collection, which may be logistically challenging for blood collection and processing operations to accomplish regularly. Compared to FFP, the common alternative plasma frozen within 24 hours of collection (PF24) has a slightly lower level of Factor VIII, but both products have adequate factor activities to maintain hemostasis and are interchangeable for all practical purposes.[61] After thawing, both FFP and PF24 may be kept refrigerated for up to 24 hours, although subsequent relabeling of the product to "thawed plasma" extends its allowable refrigeration up to 120 hours post-thaw.

Warfarin Reversal

Therapeutic anticoagulation is used to prevent and treat many conditions that may otherwise predispose a patient to thromboembolic complications. Warfarin is among the most frequently prescribed anticoagulants for this purpose, especially in the outpatient setting, due to its relatively straightforward dosing, simple oral administration, and ease of therapeutic monitoring using INR measurements. Due to its structural similarity to vitamin K (VITK), warfarin competitively inhibits the ability of certain epoxide reductase enzymes to convert oxidized VITK into a reduced form. Reduced VITK is necessary for the terminal carboxylation and proper hemostatic function of otherwise inactive VITK-dependent coagulation factors (protein C, protein S, and factors II, VII, IX, and X); Warfarin, therefore exerts its therapeutic effect by inhibiting the final activation of nearly functional proteins. This intended effect becomes problematic, however, when an actively anticoagulated patient encounters an unexpected bleeding challenge such as a life-threatening bleed or a sudden need for a major invasive procedure. Depending on the specific situation, urgent warfarin reversal may be indicated to address its then undesired anticoagulant effect immediately.

In the past, cessation of warfarin alongside exogenous VITK administration and plasma transfusion was the preferred approach for urgent warfarin reversal. In some hospital settings, attempted warfarin reversal was cited as being the most common indication for plasma transfusion.[62] In theory, because plasma contains all relevant coagulation proteins, including the VITK-dependent factors and VITK epoxide reductase, it can nonspecifically counteract the effect of warfarin provided the concomitant addition of VITK. The theoretical requisite plasma dose to accomplish this reversal may

be considerable, up to 30 mL/kg. However, due to the impracticalities of such large dosing for urgent situations, realistic dosing would likely be closer to more routine calculations of 10 to 20 mL/kg, which has been used in prior studies assessing the efficacy of plasma in this role.[63] Regardless, several logistical difficulties must be considered for urgent plasma transfusion. First, plasma must be ABO compatible with the intended recipient. This requirement, combined with the fact that compatible thawed plasma may not always be available, may result in considerable delays while plasma is thawed and prepared by the blood bank. Second, even using the most conservative therapeutic dose of 10 mL/kg, the resultant volume of plasma is likely to be several hundreds of milliliters or more for an adult patient, which will be nearly impossible to transfuse-rapidly without risking complications of transfusion associated circulatory overload (TACO). This delicate situation may also be exacerbated if the patient is unable to tolerate large fluid burdens at baseline or is hemodynamically unstable.

Prothrombin complex concentrates (PCC) have emerged as an alternative pharmacologic means of urgent warfarin reversal in recent years. Contemporary four-factor concentrate (4F-PCC) preparations are derived from donor plasma, but deliver nonactivated VITK-dependent factors II, VII, IX, and X in much higher concentrations than can be physiologically found in equivalent volumes of plasma. Consequently, they can be reconstituted in much smaller volumes regardless of dose (less than 100 mL), can be safely rapidly infused, and do not require ABO group compatibility, although the cessation of warfarin and exogenous VITK administration are still required. Recent evidence demonstrated that 4F-PCCs were at least as effective as plasma in achieving hemostasis for patients experiencing major acute bleeding while anticoagulated with warfarin.[63,64] In addition, patients treated with 4F-PCCs achieved significantly faster corrections of deranged INR values and were found to have higher levels of relevant coagulation factors postinfusion than those treated with plasma. Furthermore, given that no significant differences in adverse events were detected, including thromboembolic complications, the conclusion was that 4F-PCC treatment had supplanted plasma transfusion as the definitive modality of urgent warfarin reversal. Similarly, the American College of Cardiology recently published its position that patients who are anticoagulated with warfarin with life-threatening bleeding or major bleeding at critical sites should be appropriately treated with 4F-PCC. Plasma transfusion should be reserved for situations where 4F-PCCs are unavailable or otherwise contraindicated.[65] The evidence and guidelines for warfarin reversal agents are relatively new. Given the long-standing historical role of plasma prior to PCCs as the definitive warfarin reversal agent, physicians may be reluctant to abandon this practice or insist on transfusing plasma even when it is strictly not indicated. Clear communication will be required in such cases, which should necessarily aim to understand the motivation for requesting plasma transfusion, whether therapeutic intervention is warranted at all, and if so, what evidence-based approaches are in the best interest of the patient.

It should be noted that anti-inhibitor coagulant complexes (AICC), which also contain VITK-dependent coagulation factors, are available in many institutions. In contrast to 4F-PCCs, however, these AICCs are indicated for the management of patients with hemophilia A or B and concomitant inhibitor antibodies that blunt the hemostatic response to routine factor-replacement therapy.[66] They are not specifically indicated for the urgent reversal of anticoagulant medications, including warfarin. Available formulations (i.e., Factor VIII Inhibitor Bypassing Activity [FEIBA]) supply activated factor VII as the primary driver of inhibitor-bypassing activity, along with nonactivated factors II, IX, and X, as well as some amount of factor VIII.[67]

POINTS TO REMEMBER

- Plasma transfusion addresses bleeding associated with the simultaneous deficiency of multiple coagulation factors.
- Even for adult patients, the proper dosing of plasma for transfusion is weight-based rather than a fixed dose.
- Urgent reversal of warfarin is ideally addressed with four-factor prothrombin complex concentrates (4F-PCC), and plasma transfusion should only be considered if a 4F-PCC is unavailable or otherwise contraindicated.

Cryoprecipitate

Cryoprecipitate (cryoprecipitated antihemophilic factor) is derived from the insoluble portion of plasma that precipitates out of solution as a unit of frozen plasma is thawed in refrigerated conditions. The resulting single unit of cryoprecipitate is relatively enriched for some, but not all, procoagulant proteins: fibrinogen (factor I), von Willebrand factor (vWF), factor VIII, factor XIII, and fibronectin. These substances are found in higher concentrations than in the same volume of normal plasma, which makes cryoprecipitate the more efficient transfusion option over plasma if the repletion of these substances is necessary. However, all other relevant coagulation-related proteins typically present in normal plasma are absent in cryoprecipitate in appreciable therapeutic quantities. As such, cryoprecipitate and plasma should not be considered interchangeable.

Cryoprecipitate is indicated for fibrinogen repletion in cases of acquired hypofibrinogenemia as evidenced by laboratory measurements (normal reference range of 200 to 450 mg/dL for nonpregnant adults) and is transfused almost exclusively for this purpose. Given that the conversion of fibrinogen into fibrin is critical for proper secondary hemostasis, hypofibrinogenemia represents a bleeding risk. Common scenarios resulting in acquired hypofibrinogenemia include obstetrical hemorrhage, cardiac surgery with CPB or use of ECMO circuits due to active consumption, and liver disease due to underproduction. Of note, baseline fibrinogen levels as high as 600 mg/dL are often seen during pregnancy and the immediate postpartum state.[68] Consequently, for obstetric patients, fibrinogen results that are apparently within reference ranges can be misleading and may represent hypofibrinogenemia.

Pharmacologic factor concentrates have become much more readily available for vWF, factor VIII, and factor XIII. As these are currently the superior alternatives, cryoprecipitate transfusion is no longer indicated to address isolated deficiencies of these substances.[69] While fibrinogen concentrates also exist in the United States, they are only specifically indicated for acute bleeding in patients with congenital fibrinogen deficiencies and should not be used interchangeably with cryoprecipitate. Stated indications for fibrinogen concentrates remain similar for European formulations; however, their utility in cases of acquired perioperative hypofibrinogenemia has been investigated.[70]

For adults, cryoprecipitate pools of up to 10 units are typically transfused as a therapeutic dose. The expected post-transfusion response to this dose is an approximate increase in measurable fibrinogen by 50 to 70 mg/dL; however, this response is highly variable and may be blunted by factors such as ongoing bleeding, consumption, or a large total blood volume. In situations where more precise dosing based on a target fibrinogen level is required, the number of individual cryoprecipitate units to be pooled pretransfusion can be calculated based on the assumption that each unit likely contains $\geq$ 250 mg of fibrinogen (although the minimum requirement per regulation is a more conservative 150 mg/unit) (Fig. 92.2). Pools often combine units of the same donor ABO group, although mixed ABO pools may also be available. Though there is a theoretical risk of minor incompatibility between donor isohemagglutinins and recipient RBCs, ABO group compatibility is not strictly required for adult cryoprecipitate transfusion.

POINTS TO REMEMBER

- Cryoprecipitate is enriched for certain procoagulant proteins and is typically transfused to address hypofibrinogenemia.
- Cryoprecipitate should not be thought of as therapeutically interchangeable with plasma or specific pharmacologic factor concentrates.
- A typical adult dose of cryoprecipitate is a single pool that combines up to 10 individual units.

Massive Transfusion

A common definition for massive transfusion is the transfusion of at least one circulating patient blood volume within 24 hours. An approximate alternative definition for an average-sized adult patient may be the transfusion of 10 or more pRBC units within 24 hours.[54] Regardless of these definitions, situations requiring massive transfusion are often recognized well in advance of such substantial blood loss and replacement

$$\frac{\left[(\text{Desired fibrinogen} - \text{Initial fibrinogen}) \times (\text{Patient plasma volume}) \times \left(\frac{1\ dL}{100\ mL}\right)\right]}{250\ mg/unit}$$

NOTES: Fibrinogen expressed in *mg/dL*; plasma volume expressed in *mL*; assumes 250 mg fibrinogen per unit

FIGURE 92.2 Calculation of cryoprecipitate dosing.[71] (Petrides M, AuBuchon J. To transfuse or not to transfuse: an assessment of risks and benefits. In: Mintz P, ed. *Transfusion therapy: clinical principles and practice.* 3rd ed. Bethesda: AABB; 2011:887.)

and are therefore highly dependent on the experience and clinical acumen of the requesting physicians. While situations such as a trauma with significant hemorrhage may be relatively straightforward for expecting massive transfusion, others such as gastrointestinal bleeding or postpartum hemorrhage may be more subtle. Whatever the indication, prompt recognition of a massive transfusion need is critical for the patient's well-being and maximized efficiency from the blood bank working to supply that patient.

While it may seem obvious, it is important to remember that patients undergoing significant blood loss are actively losing whole blood rather than selectively losing specific blood constituents such as RBCs or coagulation factors. However, the mainstay of modern transfusion medicine is blood component therapy, which is typically prescribed as individual blood product units to address a specific patient need. While usually not an issue for hemodynamically stable patients, this approach is problematic for one who is hemorrhaging since various components are needed, and the intervals between individual transfusions may be prolonged. This approach also poses a problem for the ordering physician, as they are responsible for actively managing which components are needed and when they are given, all while predicting future transfusion requirements. The blood bank is also adversely affected as blood bank personnel receive new orders on a continuous but altogether unpredictable basis with no clear direction of which components may be needed next. Consequently, many institutions have adopted a massive transfusion protocol (MTP) to streamline this potentially chaotic process as soon as a need is recognized.

The goal of an MTP is to efficiently provide multiple blood components in quantities and approximate physiologic ratios that recapitulate the whole blood being lost by a patient. While there is no universally accepted standard for an MTP, most practicing institutions have a predetermined amount of pRBC, plasma, and platelet units that are prepared by the blood bank and subsequently issued as a single "MTP pack." For example, a single MTP pack may contain six pRBC units, six plasma units, and one unit of apheresis platelets (the equivalent of 6 whole blood-derived platelet units). This pack exemplifies a typical 1:1:1 unit-ratio of plasma, whole blood-derived platelets, and pRBCs, respectively, although there is some evidence to suggest that a 1:1:2 strategy favoring pRBC units may be just as efficacious in relevant patient populations.[72] Ultimately, the specific amounts and ratios of these components in an MTP pack and whether other products such as cryoprecipitate or factor concentrates are incorporated should be agreed upon by an institution's blood bank and key stakeholder clinical services.

Once the first pack is issued, the blood bank immediately assembles the next pack and continues assembling subsequent packs until informed otherwise by the ordering physician (i.e., patient stabilization or patient death). Given the disproportionate amount of time and resources spent for a single patient requiring MTP, clear communication is critical between the blood bank and clinical services to ensure the smooth provision of blood products without unduly compromising the other operations of the blood bank. Additionally, the MTP process benefits tremendously from the thoughtful incorporation of other core laboratory services such as chemistry, hematology, and coagulation testing for evaluating the potential need for blood products or other

interventions in as close to real time as possible. If incorporated, processes should be clearly defined, including prompt notification of the laboratory and the necessary prioritization of MTP-related patient samples for testing.

POINTS TO REMEMBER

- A common definition of massive transfusion is the transfusion of at least one circulating patient blood volume within 24 hours, although alternative definitions exist.
- Massive transfusion protocols aim to efficiently provide multiple blood components in quantities and approximate physiologic ratios that recapitulate whole blood being lost from active bleeding.
- Clear communication between the blood bank and requesting clinical service is crucial to ensure the smooth execution of a massive transfusion protocol.

Granulocytes

While nowhere near as common of a practice today as the transfusion of more conventional blood components, granulocyte components may still be requested for transfusion. The historical rationale behind granulocyte transfusion was to provide allogeneic neutrophil support to patients with severe, prolonged neutropenia suffering from bacterial and fungal infections. However, the perceived need for this niche component became somewhat obviated over time due to advances in preferable antimicrobial therapy, increasing reports of pulmonary toxicity and CMV-related adverse events, and the significant potential for alloimmunization that could complicate future transfusion support.[73,74] Even with advances in cellular mobilization and modern apheresis granulocyte collection technology to increase potency, the general interest in granulocyte transfusion remains relatively low, likely due to a combination of its perceived limited utility and procurement difficulty.

In perhaps the highest-profile randomized study of efficacy, the Resolving Infection in Neutropenia with Granulocytes (RING) trial demonstrated no overall effect of granulocyte transfusion on its primary endpoint of clinical success of treatment, a composite of patient survival plus microbial response.[75] However, due to lower-than-expected accrual, this study was ultimately underpowered to appropriately detect beneficial outcomes, although other similarly underpowered studies have suggested the same.[74] Therefore the overall efficacy of granulocyte transfusion remains unproven and controversial.

Should granulocyte transfusion be considered, some objective indication criteria have been proposed, including severe neutropenia (absolute neutrophil count $< 0.5 \times 10^9$/L), ongoing active treatment (i.e., antimicrobial therapy), evidence of fungal or bacterial infection that is unresponsive to antimicrobial therapy, and a reasonable expectation of the resolution of neutropenia with treatment.[76] Assuming a prospective recipient meets these criteria, the understanding is that granulocyte transfusions should serve only as a temporizing measure until the patient's marrow elicits a durable response to resolve the infection. The frequency of granulocyte transfusions and the ultimate expectations of therapy should be thoroughly discussed with the requesting clinical service and the collecting blood donor center before initiation.

Whole Blood

Before individual component therapy in the early twentieth century, non-componentized whole blood transfusion was utilized to varying degrees of success. These transfusions were especially performed in combat settings to mitigate injury-related hemorrhagic shock and largely due to a lack of alternative treatments. These nonideal circumstances were exacerbated by limited blood collection, storage, and infusion technologies, as well as a yet incomplete understanding of certain serologic principles. Individual blood component therapy subsequently became available and has remained the mainstay of modern blood transfusion practices. Such practices have been reinforced over time due to advances in blood component collection techniques, improved storage conditions, and the consensus among the medical community favoring targeted, precise therapy for specific patient needs. For instance, isolated anemia may be addressed with pRBC transfusion, and isolated thrombocytopenia may be addressed with platelet transfusion. Recently, however, whole blood transfusion has resurfaced as a potentially desirable practice for patients who would otherwise require extensive transfusion with multiple components. This renewed interest was once again prominently driven by recent military experiences, and to date, has pervaded certain noncombat civilian settings such as trauma surgery and obstetrics.[77,78]

The rationale behind whole blood transfusion over component therapy in high-acuity settings stems from the fact that, compared to components, whole blood contains all of the relevant physiologic contributors to oxygen-carrying capacity and hemostasis in relatively undiluted, near-physiologic ratios which can be administered as a single infusion. In addition, the collection and storage of a single whole blood product are logistically simpler than for multiple components with varying requirements, which carries implications for potentially wider availability.[79] Presently, however, relatively few hospitals stock and transfuse whole blood, and collections are limited to group O blood donors to ensure major compatibility of RBCs with recipients of all blood groups. These donors must also have demonstrable low titers of plasma isohemagglutinins by laboratory testing due to the potential for hemolysis secondary to minor incompatibility for non–group O recipients, which is an unavoidable consequence of ensuring major compatibility.[77] Among institutions that transfuse low-titer group O whole blood (LTOWB), there is little to no consensus of the parameters of transfusion, what acceptable upper limits of transfusion are, which patient groups qualify, or even what isohemagglutinin titer constitutes a low titer.[80] Despite an increasing body of evidence for its utility, the role of LTOWB in modern transfusion practices remains a controversial subject at this time, and whether it garners more widespread adoption is yet to be seen.

SELECTED REFERENCES

3. Hébert PC, Wells G, Blajchman MA, et al. A Multicenter, Randomized, Controlled Clinical Trial of Transfusion Requirements in Critical Care. N Engl J Med 1999;340(6):409–17. doi:10.1056/NEJM199902113400601.
7. Carson JL, Terrin ML, Noveck H, et al. Liberal or Restrictive Transfusion in High-Risk Patients after Hip Surgery. N Engl J Med 2011;365(26):2453–62. doi:10.1056/NEJMoa1012452.
7a. Carson JL, Guyatt G, Heddle NM, et al. Clinical practice guidelines from the AABB: Red blood cell transfusion thresholds and storage. JAMA - J Am Med Assoc. 2016;316(19):2025–35. doi:10.1001/jama.2016.9185.
8. Kaufman RM, Djulbegovic B, Gernsheimer T, et al. Platelet transfusion: a clinical practice guideline from the AABB. Ann Intern Med 2015;162(3):205–13. doi:10.7326/M14-1589.
16. Yazdanbakhsh K, Ware RE, Noizat-Pirenne F. Red blood cell alloimmunization in sickle cell disease: pathophysiology, risk factors, and transfusion management. Blood 2012;120(3):528–37. doi:10.1182/blood-2011-11-327361.
20. Vichinsky EP, Luban NL, Wright E, et al. Prospective RBC phenotype matching in a stroke-prevention trial in sickle cell anemia: a multicenter transfusion trial. Transfusion 2001;41(9):1086–92. doi:10.1046/j.1537-2995.2001.41091086.x.
28. Slichter SJ, Kaufman RM, Assmann SF, et al. Dose of prophylactic platelet transfusions and prevention of hemorrhage. N Engl J Med 2010;362(7):600–13. doi:10.1056/NEJMoa0904084.
47. Leukocyte reduction and ultraviolet B irradiation of platelets to prevent alloimmunization and refractoriness to platelet transfusions. N Engl J Med 1997;337(26):1861–69. doi:10.1056/NEJM199712253372601.
56. Yang L, Stanworth S, Hopewell S, Doree C, Murphy M. Is fresh-frozen plasma clinically effective? An update of a systematic review of randomized controlled trials (CME). Transfusion 2012;52(8):1673–86. doi:10.1111/j.1537-2995.2011.03515.x.
64. Goldstein JN, Refaai MA, Milling TJ, et al. Four-factor prothrombin complex concentrate versus plasma for rapid vitamin K antagonist reversal in patients needing urgent surgical or invasive interventions: a phase 3b, open-label, non-inferiority, randomised trial. Lancet 2015;385(9982):2077–87. doi:10.1016/S0140-6736(14)61685-8.
72. Holcomb JB, Tilley BC, Baraniuk S, et al. Transfusion of plasma, platelets, and red blood cells in a 1:1:1 vs a 1:1:2 ratio and mortality in patients with severe trauma: the PROPPR randomized clinical trial. JAMA 2015;313(5):471–82. doi:10.1001/jama.2015.12.
75. Price TH, Boeckh M, Harrison RW, et al. Efficacy of transfusion with granulocytes from G-CSF/dexamethasone-treated donors in neutropenic patients with infection. Blood 2015;126(18):2153-2161. doi:10.1182/blood-2015-05-645986.

93

Transfusion Reactions and Adverse Events Associated With Transfusion

Jacqueline N. Poston and Monica B. Pagano

ABSTRACT

Transfusion reactions remain a major issue particularly for patients with chronic transfusion requirements. The majority of reactions are mild, but some are severe and rarely fatal. In 2017, 44 fatal transfusion reactions occurred in the United States.[1] Transfusion reactions and adverse events from transfusion can be divided between events that occur during or within several hours of the transfusion (acute) or events that occur over 24 hours after the end of the transfusion (delayed). While patients do not always meet the standard definition of a particular transfusion reaction, it is essential to categorize reactions to accurately track, manage, and prevent future reactions. This chapter will focus on the presentation, physiology, management, and prevention strategies of the major types of transfusion reactions.

CLASSIFICATION AND TRACKING TRANSFUSION REACTIONS

The first known human blood transfusions were associated with high rates of fatality likely due to incompatible transfusions.[2,3] Following Karl Landsteiner's discovery of the ABO blood group system, blood transfusions have become an increasingly safe cornerstone of medical therapy.[4] While the rates of transfusions are declining in the United States, millions of transfusions are still given each year.[5] Hemovigilance systems have been implemented throughout the world to monitor and improve the safety of blood transfusions.[6] In the United States, the Centers for Disease Control (CDC) started a voluntary hemovigilance database in 2010 called the National Healthcare Safety Network (NHSN) Hemovigilance Module (HM).[7,8] The NHSN HM provides valuable safety data for transfusions in the United States; however, the voluntary, passive reporting system likely leads to underreporting.[9] Adverse events are tracked across the entire transfusion process from donor collection to transfusions to patients. To standardize reporting, the NHSN HM uses a classification system for different transfusion reactions (Tables 93.1 and 93.2).

ACUTE TRANSFUSION REACTIONS

Acute reactions occur during or within several hours of a blood transfusion. Allergic transfusion reactions accounted for almost half (46.8%) of adverse transfusion reactions reported to the NHSN HM between 2010 and 2012.[10] The majority of acute reactions are mild and occur more frequently with platelet transfusions (421.7/100,000) compared to other blood products.[11,10]

ACUTE HEMOLYTIC TRANSFUSION REACTION

Physiology

An acute hemolytic transfusion reaction (AHTR) occurs when the recipient's immune system hemolyzes or rapidly clears the donor's red blood cells. This typically occurs in cases of major incompatible transfusions, when the recipient has pre-formed preformed antibodies against antigens expressed on donor red blood cells. Whether a recipient develops intravascular or extravascular hemolysis depends on the capacity of the recipient's alloantibody to activate complement. The onset of symptoms is likely due to the titer and capacities of the alloantibody, as well as the density of the donor's antigen, with immediate reactions occurring with high titer alloantibodies that have high affinity for a donor antigen present at higher levels on donor red blood cells.[12,13] The most severe AHTRs are associated with ABO incompatibility due to the presence of circulating naturally occurring isoagglutinins. Recipient isoagglutinins directed against the A and B antigens are IgM and can bind the donor's red blood cells leading to complement activation and rapid intravascular hemolysis. The most common cause of major ABO incompatible transfusions are clerical errors (patient identification at the time of sample collection or at the time of blood administration).[14] Non-ABO antigen incompatible hemolytic reactions are more frequent but less severe.[13] Extravascular hemolysis can typically occur with non-ABO red blood cell antigens, is IgG mediated, and donor cells are removed from circulation by the recipient's reticuloendothelial system.

Minor ABO incompatible hemolytic reactions occur when donor isoagglutinins react against the recipient's red blood cells. This can occur from products with high content of donor plasma such as plasma units and platelets. There are a

TABLE 93.1 Summary of Acute Transfusion Reactions[8]

ACUTE TRANSFUSION REACTIONS

Reaction	Diagnosis		Management
Acute hemolytic transfusion reaction (AHTR)	1. Any key symptom during or ≤24 h post-transfusion 2. ≥ 2 hemolysis laboratory findings 3. Either positive direct anti-globulin test (DAT) and positive elution OR negative serologic testing and confirmed physical cause	Key symptoms Back/flank pain; chills/rigors; DIC; epistaxis; fever; hematuria; hypotension; oliguria/anuria; pain and/or oozing at IV site; renal failure Hemolysis labs Fibrinogen; haptoglobin; bilirubin; LDH; hemoglobinemia; hemoglobinuria; plasma discoloration c/w hemolysis; spherocytes on smear	Stop transfusion and avoid additional incompatible transfusions; Supportive care. Consider exchange transfusion with antigen-negative blood depending on clinical severity. IVIG may be useful particularly for patients with sickle cell anemia and AHTR
Febrile nonhemolytic transfusion reaction (FNHTR)	Occurs during or ≤4 h with either fever (≥38 °C and ≥1 °C change from pretransfusion value) OR chills/rigors with no other clear cause of fever		Stop transfusion and rule out hemolytic transfusion reaction; Consider giving antipyretic and restarting transfusion depending on severity of reaction. Consider culturing blood product unit and patient.
Allergic	≥2 allergic symptoms during or ≤4 h post-transfusion	Allergic symptoms Conjunctival edema; edema of lips, tongue or uvula; erythema/edema or periorbital area; Flushing; hypotension; localized angioedema; maculopapular rash; pruritus; respiratory distress/bronchospasm; urticaria	Stop transfusion and administer an antihistamine. Consider restarting transfusion at slower rate when symptoms improve (depending on severity).
Anaphylactic/Severe Allergic	Severe presentation of allergic transfusion reaction. May involve circulatory shock and/or airway obstruction (upper or lower)		Stop transfusion and administer epinephrine, antihistamine. Consider hydrocortisone if prolonged or severe symptoms
Transfusion-related acute lung injury (TRALI)	1. No evidence of acute lung injury before transfusion 2. Acute lung injury ≤6 h post-transfusion 3. Hypoxemia 4. Bilateral infiltrates on imaging 5. No left atrial hypertension (i.e., circulatory overload)		Supportive care. Glucocorticoids unlikely to be helpful.
Transfusion-associated circulatory overload (TACO)	New or exacerbation of ≥3 TACO symptoms within 6 h post-transfusion	TACO symptoms Acute respiratory distress; BNP; CVP; left heart failure; positive fluid balance; Imaging evidence of pulmonary edema	Stop transfusion; Supportive care with focus on diuresis and respiratory support.
Septic	Laboratory evidence of pathogen in transfusion recipient with evidence of pathogen in transfusion component and/or donor and/or same pathogen in different recipient of component from same donor		Stop transfusion; supportive care and anti-microbial coverage
Hypotensive	Hypotension within 1 hr after transfusion and no other known cause		Stop transfusion (usually rapid improvement within 10 min; if not, evaluate for other causes); Supportive care

CDC. *National Healthcare Safety Network biovigilance component hemovigilance module surveillance protocol* [monograph on the internet]. Available from: https://www.cdc.gov/nhsn/pdfs/biovigilance/bv-hv-protocol-current.pdf.

TABLE 93.2	Summary of Delayed Transfusion Reactions[8]	
DELAYED TRANSFUSION REACTIONS		
Reaction	**Diagnosis**	**Management**
Delayed hemolytic transfusion reaction (DHTR)	1. Positive DAT between 24 h and 28 days after transfusion 2. Positive elution OR new RBC alloantibody in recipient serum 3. Inadequate rise of post-transfusion Hb level OR spherocytes of no other known cause	Supportive care. Consider exchange transfusion with antigen-negative blood depending on clinical severity. IVIG may be useful particularly for patients with sickle cell anemia and DHTR
Delayed serologic transfusion reaction (DSTR)	1. No clinical signs of hemolysis 2. New clinically significant antibodies against RBCs (+DAT or +antibody screen with new RBC alloantibody)	Avoid future incompatible blood transfusions.
Transfusion-associated graft-versus-host disease (TA-GVHD)	1. Symptoms 2 days to 6 wk after transfusion 2. Characteristic findings on skin or liver biopsy — TA-GVHD symptoms Rash (erythematous, maculopapular eruption spread centrally to extremities; can progress to erythroderma and hemorrhagic bullous); diarrhea; fever; hepatomegaly; liver dysfunction; marrow aplasia; pancytopenia	Immunosuppression; consider stem cell transplantation
Post-transfusion purpura (PTP)	1. Recipient antibody against human platelet antigen (HPA) or other platelet-specific antigen detected at or after onset of thrombocytopenia 2. Thrombocytopenia (post-transfusion platelet count < 20% of pretransfusion count). Onset typically 5–12 days post-transfusion with no other causes of thrombocytopenia	IVIG; consider glucocorticoids (unclear efficacy); Depending on clinical severity, consider whole blood exchange or plasma exchange; Transfuse antigen-negative platelets if patient has active bleeding
Iron overload	Evidence of iron overload based on iron stores. Confirm iron overload with T2*MRI and/or tissue biopsy.	Consider evaluating for hereditary hemochromatosis depending on patient's risk factors for transfusion related iron overload; Phlebotomy and/or iron chelation.

CDC. *National Healthcare Safety Network biovigilance component hemovigilance module surveillance protocol* [monograph on the internet]. Available from: https://www.cdc.gov/nhsn/pdfs/biovigilance/bv-hv-protocol-current.pdf.

number of cases reported in the literature describing hemolytic transfusion reactions associated with passive transfer of anti-A or anti-B isoagglutinins through platelet transfusions.[15] Isoagglutinin titers may determine the risk for hemolysis, but whether there is a critical titer is still controversial.[16] Isoagglutinin titers can be reduced in platelet products with plasma additive solutions, which replace ~70% of the plasma content.[17]

Incidence

AHTRs are an uncommon event. The rate of a hemolytic transfusion reaction is 1 in 367,393 red blood cell units per year, based on the SHOT hemovigilance database from the United Kingdom.[18] In 2017, only seven fatal hemolytic transfusion reactions were reported to the FDA; the majority (six of seven) were from non-ABO incompatible transfusions.[1]

Presentation and Differential Diagnosis

The classic description of an AHTR with intravascular hemolysis consists of fever, flank pain, and red urine from hemoglobinuria. However, symptoms are often subtle and nonspecific. Of the symptoms seen in other forms of transfusion reactions, only hives has not been described in an AHTR. A high index of suspicion is necessary particularly for patients who are not interactive such as during anesthesia. In these cases, the only sign of an AHTR may be disseminated intravascular coagulopathy (DIC). If unrecognized, patients may continue to receive incompatible transfusions. In one series of 35 patients who developed an AHTR during anesthesia, 25% received up to 6 additional units due to ongoing bleeding.[19]

Alternative etiologies of hemolysis should be considered such as autoimmune hemolytic anemia, artificial heart valve dysfunction, drug-induced hemolysis, microangiopathic hemolytic anemias, and infections associated with hemolysis such as malaria.

NHSN Hemovigilance Diagnostic Criteria[8]

1. Any key symptom during or <24 hours post-transfusion
   a. Back/flank pain; chills/rigors; DIC; epistaxis; fever; hematuria; hypotension; oliguria/anuria; pain and/or oozing at IV site; renal failure
2. Greater than two laboratory findings consistent with hemolysis:
   a. Decreased fibrinogen; decreased haptoglobin; increased bilirubin; increased LDH; hemoglobinemia; hemoglobinuria; plasma discoloration consistent with hemolysis; spherocytes on smear
   i. Note that hemolysis may be intravascular, extravascular, or both.
3. Positive direct antiglobulin test (DAT) and positive elution (immune-mediated hemolysis) or negative serologic testing and confirmed physical cause (non–immune-mediated hemolysis)

Management. If an AHTR is suspected during a transfusion, the transfusion should be immediately stopped and work up should be done to confirm hemolysis with visual examination and DAT. It is critical to avoid additional incompatible transfusions and to provide supportive care including intravenous hydration to prevent renal damage. If the patient needs to continue transfusion support during the transfusion reaction investigation, transfusing with group O red blood cell units minimizes the risk of ABO incompatibility. Depending on timing and clinical severity, an exchange transfusion with antigen negative blood can be considered.[20] For non-ABO and IgG-mediated acute hemolytic reactions, intravenous immunoglobulin (IVIG) may be useful, particularly for patients with sickle cell anemia.[21,22]

Prevention. Prevention of AHTRs should focus on reducing the risk of an incompatible transfusion. This means providing appropriate ABO compatible transfusions, but also focusing on antigen appropriate units for patients with alloantibodies. Notably, the majority of fatalities from hemolytic transfusion reactions in the US in 2017 were from non-ABO antigen incompatible transfusions.[1] To prevent incompatible transfusions, clinical providers and transfusion services must focus on limiting the rate of "wrong blood in tube" (WBIT) events, or mislabeled pretransfusion samples, as well as reducing the rate of providing incorrect products to patients.[23]

FEBRILE NONHEMOLYTIC TRANSFUSION REACTION

Physiology

The pathophysiology of febrile nonhemolytic transfusion reactions (FNHTRs) is not fully defined. Some correlative studies suggest that donor derived antibodies directed against the recipient's HLA or granulocyte antigens drives the recipient's inflammatory response.[24] Another hypothesis is that donor cytokines accumulated during storage are the main cause of febrile reactions.[25]

Incidence

FNHTRs are the second most common adverse transfusion reaction after allergic reactions.[10] FNHTRs accounted for 36.1% of adverse reactions reported to the NHSN HM between 2010 and 2012. Any blood product can cause a FNHTR, and children appear to be more likely to develop FNHTRs than adults.[26]

Presentation and Differential Diagnosis

FNHTR is a diagnosis of exclusion. The classic presentation is a new fever and/or chills during or within 4 hours of the transfusion. These clinical signs are indistinguishable from numerous causes of fever and/or chills including AHTR, septic transfusion reaction, or another underlying cause of fever such as a preexisting infection.

NHSN Hemovigilance Diagnostic Criteria[8]
1. Occurs during or <4 hours after transfusion
2. Fever (>38 °C and ≥1 °C change from pretransfusion value) **OR** chills/rigors with no other clear cause of fever

Management. If the patient develops signs of a FNHTR during the transfusion, the transfusion should be immediately stopped. Given the signs and symptoms are indistinguishable

from an AHTR, hemolysis should be ruled out before classifying the reaction as a FNHTR. Additionally, a septic transfusion reaction must also be considered; however, practices differ on which clinical situations warrant further culturing of the blood product. Depending on the severity of the reaction, antipyretics may be beneficial.

Prevention.

Patient specific factors. Approximately 40% of recipients with a history of a FNHTR will experience another FNHTR.[27,28] Many providers prescribe premedication with acetaminophen and/or an antihistamine for patients with a history of FNHTR. Patients should not receive premedication if they have never had a FNHTR, as this practice does not reduce the rate of FNHTR in patients with no prior history of transfusion reactions.[29] A single center prospective study found that premedication reduces the rate of fever, but does not mitigate other symptoms such as chills.[30] Notably, premedication can mask a fever potentially preventing early recognition of an AHTR or another cause of fever. This is particularly important in patient populations at higher risk of infection such as patients with severe neutropenia.

Product specific factors The incidence of FNHTRs has decreased since the implementation of prestorage leukoreduction supporting the contributing role of donor leukocytes in FNHTRs.[31–33] Platelet products have higher rates of FNHTRs compared to red blood cells, which may be due to the higher concentration of donor plasma in conventional platelet products.[34] Platelet products appear to have similar rates of FNHTR regardless of whether the product is an apheresis unit or derived from pooled whole blood donation.[35,36] Reducing donor plasma with platelet additive solutions (PAS) reduces the incidence of FNHTRs compared to conventional platelets.[37] Prestorage leukoreduction may also decrease the incidence of FNHTR with platelet products compared to leukoreduction after storage.[38]

ALLERGIC AND ANAPHYLACTIC TRANSFUSION REACTIONS

Physiology

The underlying physiology of allergic transfusion reactions is unknown but appears to be a combination of recipient and product factors.[39] Platelet products, followed by plasma products, have the highest rates of allergic transfusion reactions. This combined with the fact that reducing donor plasma in products reduces the incidence of allergic transfusion reactions, suggests that something in donor plasma contributes to an allergic reaction. However, donor plasma alone does not explain the majority of reactions as recipients of split apheresis platelets from the same donor rarely have similar rates of allergic reactions.[40] Recipient factors also contribute to allergic reactions. Recipients with higher levels of IgE and atopic predisposition have an increased risk of allergic reactions.[41,42]

In rare cases, allergic transfusion reactions are due to antibodies in individuals with protein deficiencies, such as IgA, haptoglobin, and C4, but the pathophysiologic role of these antibodies remains uncertain.[43–46] Some allergic reactions may be from passive transfer of donor antibodies to food antigens such as peanuts.[47] However, these particular scenarios are too rare to account for the majority of allergic reactions.[39]

Incidence

Allergic transfusion reactions occur in 1 to 4% of transfusions.[48] Anaphylaxis, a severe form of an allergic reaction, is rare, occurring in less than 10% of all allergic transfusion reactions.[49] Fatalities are exceedingly uncommon; in 2017, three probable fatal allergic transfusion reactions were reported to the FDA.[1]

Presentation and Differential Diagnosis

Pruritus and urticaria are the most common symptoms in allergic transfusion reactions; however, multiple organ systems can be involved. Other etiologies of an allergic reaction should be considered particularly if the onset of the allergic reaction correlates more with exposure to another therapy.

NHSN Hemovigilance Diagnostic Criteria[8]

1. ≥2 allergic symptoms during or ≤4 hours after transfusion.
   a. Allergic symptoms: conjunctival edema; edema of lips, tongue, or uvula; erythema/edema or periorbital area; flushing; hypotension; localized angioedema; maculopapular rash; pruritus; respiratory distress/bronchospasm; urticaria

An anaphylactic or severe allergic reaction is a more severe presentation that may involve circulatory shock and/or airway obstruction.

Management. If a patient develops allergic symptoms during a transfusion, the transfusion should be immediately stopped and the patient should be treated supportively based on symptoms. H1 receptor antagonists, such as diphenhydramine, can relieve symptoms. The transfusion may be restarted depending on the severity of the reaction and the recipient should be reassured that additional allergic transfusion reactions are unlikely with subsequent transfusions. Common practice includes transfusing at a slower rate; however, both transfusion volume and rate do not appear to influence the incidence of allergic reactions.[49]

If the recipient has signs of anaphylaxis, the transfusion should be immediately stopped and epinephrine should be given. If possible, epinephrine should be administered intramuscularly; subcutaneous administration results in slower onset of effect due to vasoconstriction.[50] Intravenous epinephrine should be avoided unless no other route is feasible to limit the inotropic and chronotropic side effects. Glucocorticoids have been used for prolonged allergic symptoms for patients with severe anaphylaxis but lack randomized data and have not been studied in the transfusion setting.[51]

Prevention.

Patient-specific factors. Premedication with acetaminophen and/or antihistamines does not reduce the incidence of allergic transfusion reactions and should not be used to prevent allergic reactions in patients who have not had recurrent allergic transfusion reactions.[52] The majority of recipients who experience an allergic transfusion reaction will not have recurrent reactions; subsequent transfusions may instead desensitize recipients and prevent future allergic reactions.[39]

For patients with recurrent allergic reactions and/or anaphylaxis, the indication and need for the transfusion should be evaluated. If transfusion is required, premedication can be offered. The majority of providers prefer H1 antihistamines for premedication; however, nonsedating H2 histamine receptor blockers can also be considered. However, neither H1 nor H2 antihistamines have high-quality evidence for the treatment of anaphylaxis.[53]

Product Specific Factors

Platelets. Reducing the amount of donor plasma in platelet products reduces the incidence of allergic transfusion reactions. This can be done through volume reduction or washing, both of which will reduce the function of the platelet unit and thus should be reserved only for recipients with persistent allergic reactions despite premedication.[54,55] Platelets can be stored in platelet additive solutions (PAS), which replaces two thirds of the plasma content of the unit. PAS decreases the incidence of allergic transfusion reactions.[17] Although some reports demonstrate conflicting data, a meta-analysis suggests there is no difference in allergic transfusion reactions with pooled versus apheresis platelets.[35] Similarly, ABO-matched and ABO-mismatched apheresis platelets have equivalent rates of allergic transfusion reactions.[41]

Plasma. Plasma products are the second most likely product to cause allergic transfusion reactions. Solvent detergent treated plasma products may reduce the risk of allergic reactions.[56]

Red blood cells. Allergic reactions rarely occur with red blood cell transfusions.[39] However, if a recipient has severe allergic reactions to red blood cells, washing could be considered as it also decreases the rate of allergic transfusion reactions from red blood cells.

IgA deficiency. IgA-deficient blood products may be required for patients with IgA deficiency who have proven anti-IgA antibodies and a history of an allergic or anaphylactic transfusion reaction; however, there is conflicting data to suggest IgA is implicated in allergic transfusion reactions.[46] Additionally, blood products from donors with IgA deficiency do not increase the rate of allergic transfusion reactions, despite the fact that some of these donors have anti-IgA in their plasma.[57]

Donor-specific factors. A minority of allergic reactions are due to products from a particular donor. This may be due to donor antibodies, but additional investigation is required before screening tests can be implemented to identify which donors are most likely to cause an allergic reaction in most recipients.[58]

TRANSFUSION-RELATED ACUTE LUNG INJURY

Physiology

Transfusion-related acute lung injury (TRALI) is hypothesized to be a two-hit phenomenon.[59] First, the recipient's neutrophils are primed and sequester in the lung microenvironment as a response to an underlying risk factor or endothelial injury. Second, the transfused blood product activates the recipient's primed neutrophils resulting in lung damage from inflammation and capillary leak. Antibodies directed against white blood cells (human leukocyte antigens class I and II, as well as anti-neutrophil antibodies) in the donor plasma are thought to be a primary activator of recipient neutrophils.

Incidence

Historically, TRALI occurred in 1 in 5 to 10,000 of plasma containing products.[60] After implementation of policies to avoid plasma products from female donors, the incidence of

TRALI has decreased and fatalities from TRALI now are less common than from transfusion related circulatory overload (TACO).[1] In 2017, five possible and likely fatalities due to TRALI were reported to the FDA.[1] In 2009, TRALI occurred in 0.81 per 10,000 units at two academic centers.[61] The true incidence of TRALI is likely underestimated both due to underreporting and the difficulty to delineate TRALI from other common forms of respiratory distress in hospitalized patients. This is particularly notable as TRALI is more likely in critically ill patients.[62]

Presentation and Differential Diagnosis

Patients with TRALI usually develop acute respiratory distress during or immediately after transfusion, but by definition, it can occur up to 6 hours afterward. All patients must have hypoxemia and pulmonary infiltrates. Other signs and symptoms may include fever (33% of cases), hypotension (32% of cases), and cyanosis (25% cases). Alternative etiologies of acute respiratory distress such as acute respiratory distress syndrome (ARDS) should be considered.

NHSN Hemovigilance Diagnostic Criteria[8]

1. No evidence of acute lung injury before transfusion
2. Acute lung injury ≤6 hours post-transfusion
3. Hypoxemia
4. Bilateral infiltrates on imaging
5. No left atrial hypertension (i.e., circulatory overload)

Notably, an international expert panel in 2019 proposed two updated TRALI definitions and recommended removing the term "possible TRALI."[63] TRALI type I occurs when patients develop TRALI without any risk factors for ARDS, which is consistent with the NHSN HM criteria listed above. TRALI type II is the term suggested for patients with preexisting mild ARDS prior to the transfusion event and/or risk factors for ARDS.

Management
Clinical Support of the Patient

If TRALI is suspected during a transfusion, the transfusion should be discontinued immediately and clinical providers should focus on providing respiratory support. There are no prospective trials on how to manage TRALI if patients require intubation. Most providers extrapolate ventilator support strategies from the ARDS guidelines. Extracorporeal membrane oxygenation (ECMO) has been used to manage severe TRALI, but there is limited evidence to support this practice.[64] Given the potential for hypotension with TRALI, diuresis should be used cautiously and fluid resuscitation should be considered to maintain adequate end-organ perfusion. It is unclear if glucocorticoids are beneficial in TRALI, but most providers avoid giving glucocorticoids if the lung injury occurred more than 14 days ago; this is based on the risk of increased lung damage with late glucocorticoid administration in patients with ARDS.[65]

Laboratory Investigation

If there is high suspicion for TRALI, the blood collection facility must quarantine all existing products related to that donor. If the donor donated multiple blood products, these products should be evaluated to see if other recipients also had reactions consistent with TRALI. The donor(s) should be tested for the presence of anti-human leukocyte antigens (HLA) and potentially anti-human neutrophil antigen (HNA) antibodies.[66] Anti-HNA3a antibodies in particular are associated with an increased risk of TRALI. If the donor has anti-leukocyte antibodies against the recipient's leukocyte antigens, then the donor should be deferred from future blood donations. Note that TRALI is a clinical diagnosis, and the absence of antibodies in the donor does not rule out the diagnosis. Blood collection facilities should evaluate these donors for eligibility criteria to continue donating high plasma blood products even in the absence of HLA antibodies.

Prevention
Patient-specific Prevention Strategies

Patients with a history of TRALI may receive additional transfusions. There does not appear to be an increased risk for a second episode of TRALI provided these patients do not receive additional products from the donor implicated in the prior episode of TRALI.[67] Recipients at higher risk for TRALI include patients with preexisting lung diseases, concurrent sepsis, and recipients of massive transfusion resuscitation.[68] TRALI may be related to other physiologies besides donor anti-HLA antibodies as the rate of postsurgical TRALI has not improved with the advent of donor risk mitigation strategies.[69] Further, TRALI has been described in a recipient of autologous units.[70]

Product-specific Factors

Donations from donors with known anti-HLA antibodies and donors at higher risk for anti-HLA antibodies should not be used to make products with higher proportions of plasma, such as apheresis platelets, plasma, and whole blood. Blood centers are required to test donor populations at risk for HLA alloimmunization (i.e., females with pregnancy history, females in childbearing age) for the presence of anti-HLA antibodies. If identified, these donors are deferred from donating products with higher volumes of plasma. Pregnancy can cause the development of anti-HLA antibodies that can persist years after the pregnancy. Multiparity is further associated with an increased rate of anti-HLA antibodies compared to women with a history of a single pregnancy.[71] Women without a history of pregnancy have similar rates of anti-HLA antibodies compared to men.[71]

In the United States and in parts of Europe, the majority of plasma products are from male donors. Since implementing this strategy, there has been a reduction in the rate of TRALI in Germany, the United Kingdom, and in the United States.[72–74] At two centers in the United States, the rates of TRALI decreased from 2.57 per 10,000 transfused units to 0.81 per 10,000 transfused units after deferring female donors for plasma donation.[61] This has been the single most effective strategy to prevent TRALI.

Additionally, solvent/detergent treated plasma may have a reduced rate of TRALI compared to nonsolvent/detergent plasma based on the lack of detectable anti-HLA antibodies in solvent/detergent treated plasma. This is likely from dilution of any one particular donor's anti-HLA antibodies.[75] Soluble HLA antigens may also be binding any anti-HLA antibodies in the product.

Risk strategies for reducing the rate of TRALI from platelet products have focused on plasma reduction particularly since using all male donors for platelet products would not be feasible due to the higher demands for platelet products compared to plasma. Platelet additive solutions (PAS) have been used to reduce the quantity of plasma levels. Data from the French Hemovigilance database suggests PAS reduces the rate of TRALI from whole blood buffy coat derived platelets, but not from apheresis platelets.[76]

Since the advent of donor deferral policies and leukoreduction, red blood cell transfusions have become the number one cause of TRALI. This speaks to another mechanism driving TRALI from red blood cell transfusions besides donor anti-HLA antibodies as there are some studies demonstrating that multiparous female donors do not increase the risk of TRALI from red blood cell transfusions.[77,78]

TRANSFUSION-ASSOCIATED CIRCULATORY OVERLOAD

Physiology

TACO occurs when a recipient develops hypervolemia from a transfusion with resultant cardiogenic pulmonary edema. Inflammation and altered endothelial activation may contribute to TACO in addition to the volume load of the transfusion.[79] Recipients who develop TACO often have risk factors for hypervolemia such as preexisting renal and/or cardiovascular disease.

Incidence

TACO occurs in 1 to 6% of transfused recipients with higher rates occurring in patients with increased risk factors for hypervolemia.[80] TACO is the leading cause of transfusion related mortality in the US. In 2017, 11 fatalities were reported that were at least possibly due to TACO.[1] The increasing mortality rate of TACO is likely due to improved reporting since the AABB introduced in their standards strategies to reduce the rate of TACO in patients at higher risk for hypervolemia.

Presentation and Differential Diagnosis

Patients with TACO present with signs of hypervolemia and cardiogenic pulmonary edema within 6 hours of transfusion. Noncardiogenic pulmonary edema should be ruled out to confirm the patient is not experiencing TRALI. Additionally, other etiologies or contributing risk factors for hypervolemia should be considered and managed.

NHSN Hemovigilance Diagnostic Criteria[8]

1. New or exacerbation of ≥3 TACO symptoms within 6 hours of the transfusion
   a. Acute respiratory distress; increased brain natriuretic peptide (BNP); increased central venous pressure (CVP); left heart failure; positive fluid balance; imaging evidence of pulmonary edema

Management

If the recipient develops signs of respiratory distress or hypervolemia during the transfusion, it should be immediately discontinued. The primary treatment of TACO is supportive with focus on diuresis and respiratory support.

Prevention

Patient-specific factors. The main focus for preventing TACO is reducing unnecessary transfusions. The risk of TACO increases with the number of units and the rate of transfusion.[81,82] Patients at higher risk for TACO should be identified prior to transfusion. The risk of TACO increases with

preexisting hypervolemia, as well as heart and/or renal disease. Additional risk factors include increasing age, female sex, Caucasian race, and underlying chronic lung disease.[81] Patients transfused in the intensive care unit have higher rates of TACO likely due to multiple preexisting risk factors for hypervolemia. Patients with risk factors for TACO should be optimized from a volume standpoint prior to transfusion.

Product-specific factors. For patients at particularly high risk for TACO who still require transfusion, providers can consider reducing the transfusion rate, as well as decreasing the plasma content of platelet units.

TRANSFUSION-ASSOCIATED SEPSIS

Physiology

Transfusion-associated sepsis or septic transfusion reactions occur when pathogens contaminate blood products and cause sepsis in the recipient. The majority of transfusion-associated sepsis occurs from bacterial contaminated platelet products as platelet products are more conducive to bacterial growth due to room temperature storage conditions, whereas other blood products are stored in cold temperatures.[83,84] Common bacteria implicated are skin flora (derived from the donor's and/or phlebotomist's skin during collection), as well as environmental organisms. Enteric bacteria can contaminate blood products if the donor has asymptomatic bacteremia from gut translocation of enteric bacteria. Tick-borne infections such as Babesiosis have also been transmitted to recipients through transfusions.[85] The risk of acquiring blood borne parasitic infections, such as malaria, increases in endemic areas. Viral infections can also be transmitted through transfusion but are less likely to cause septic transfusion reactions.

Incidence

Platelets are the most common blood products implicated in transfusion-associated sepsis. A US-based surveillance study found that septic reactions occur in 10 per million single donor platelet units, 10.6 per million pooled platelet units and 0.2 per million red blood cell units.[84] In fiscal year 2017, five fatalities from bacterial contamination and two fatalities from viral contamination were reported to the FDA.[1] The cases involving bacteria involved contaminated apheresis platelets, except for one case of *Anaplasma phagocytophilum* from a contaminated red blood cell unit. Both viral cases were due to West Nile Virus; one from thawed plasma and the other an apheresis platelet unit.

Presentation and Differential Diagnosis

Patients with transfusion-associated sepsis classically present with clinical signs of sepsis including fever, hypotension, tachycardia, rigors, and/or chills. However, patients may have nonspecific symptoms such as nausea, vomiting, abdominal pain, and back pain. The timing and severity of symptoms varies based on the recipient's immune response, as well as the bacterial load in the blood product and the type of bacteria implicated. The majority of recipients develop symptoms 30 minutes after receiving the transfusion.[83] A higher index of suspicion is required in patients with therapy or disease-related neutropenia who may not present with classic signs of sepsis.

Symptoms from a transfusion transmitted infection may be indistinguishable from sepsis from sources unrelated to the transfusion; transfusion-associated sepsis can be differentiated with clinical history, as well as through blood cultures from both the recipient and the blood product. Other transfusion reactions with similar symptoms should be ruled out including hemolytic transfusion reactions, FNHTRs, and allergic reactions.

NHSN Hemovigilance Diagnostic Criteria[8]

1. Lab evidence of pathogen in transfusion recipient with evidence of pathogen in transfusion component and/or donor and/or same pathogen in different recipient of component from same donor

Management

The transfusion should be discontinued if a recipient develops high-grade fevers, rigors, chills, abdominal discomfort, nausea, vomiting, or any other signs and symptoms concerning for sepsis during transfusion. Supportive care including fluid resuscitation and empiric antibiotics should be administered when clinically appropriate. Antimicrobial therapy can be tailored to the particular bacteria once it has been identified from blood cultures. When the clinical suspicion for a septic reaction is high, the blood supplier should be alerted as the implicated pathogen may be identified in other blood products from the same donation ("co-components"). These co-components should be cultured and/or quarantined from distribution depending on the index of suspicion that a transfusion transmitted infection occurred. The blood supplier will perform a market withdrawal by recommending that other hospitals quarantine co-components to prevent exposing additional recipients.

Prevention

The low rates of transfusion-associated sepsis are likely due to multiple factors including volunteer donation, donor screening, and testing of platelet products for bacterial contaminants. Additionally, recipients may have transient asymptomatic bacteremia that does not result in fulminant sepsis due to low bacterial burden in the blood product that was below the limit of detection with pretransfusion bacterial testing. Some chronically transfused patient populations, such as patients with acute myelogenous leukemia, are frequently on prophylactic antibiotics, which may also prevent transfusion-associated sepsis.

Product-specific factors. There are several approaches to mitigate the risk of bacterial contamination, including sample diversion at the time of the collection, testing for presence of bacteria in the collected unit through culture or rapid testing, and pathogen inactivation.[86–88] The FDA issued an updated guidance in 2019 for preventing bacterial contamination of platelet products.[89] Under this guidance, all platelet products require some form of testing for bacterial contamination except for pathogen reduction technology (PRT) treated apheresis platelets. The guidance allows storage of apheresis platelets to be extended from 5 to 7 days with either large volume delayed sampling or secondary culture.

HYPOTENSIVE TRANSFUSION REACTIONS

Physiology

Hypotensive transfusion reactions are thought to be due to vasodilation from substances such as bradykinin.[90] This has

been described in situations associated with increased production or abnormal bradykinin metabolism: extracorporeal circulation (including dialysis and apheresis), as well as the use of angiotensin converting enzyme (ACE) inhibitors. Typically, when the transfusion is stopped, the blood pressure returns quickly to baseline without additional interventions.[91]

Incidence

Hypotensive transfusion reactions are rare. One retrospective study from the US reported hypotensive reactions in 1.33 per 10,000 transfusions with a rate of 0.019% for platelet transfusions, 0.015% for red blood cell transfusions, and 0.006% for plasma.[91]

Presentation and Differential Diagnosis

Hypotensive reactions are a diagnosis of exclusion. Alternative causes of hypotension should be ruled out, as well acute transfusion reactions also associated with hypotension including AHTRs, TRALI, anaphylaxis, and transfusion-associated sepsis.

NHSN Hemovigilance Diagnostic Criteria[8]

1. Hypotension within 1 hour after transfusion and no other known cause

Management

The transfusion should be stopped. Hypotensive transfusion reactions rapidly resolve without intervention.

Prevention

Hypotensive transfusion reactions have been reported in patients taking ACE inhibitors who received transfused blood products with negatively charged bedside filters.[92] This practice is no longer common and should be avoided particularly in patients on ACE inhibitors. Patients on ACE inhibitors who receive a transfusion while undergoing cardiopulmonary bypass also appear to be at risk for hypotensive transfusion reactions.[93] Even without exposure to ACE inhibitors, patients can develop hypotensive transfusion reactions if they receive transfusions while on an extracorporeal circuit.[91]

POINTS TO REMEMBER

Acute Transfusion Reactions

- The most frequent cause of fatal ABO incompatible transfusion is patient misidentification at the bedside.
- Transfusion-associated circulatory overload (TACO) is a leading cause of transfusion-associated mortality and can be prevented by avoiding unnecessary transfusions.
- Red blood cells are the most frequent product associated with transfusion-related acute lung injury.

DELAYED TRANSFUSION REACTIONS

Delayed Hemolytic and Serologic Transfusion Reactions

Terminology

The term "alloimmunization" refers to a recipient developing an antibody against an alloantigen. Alloimmunization can occur with any transfused blood product. The terms "delayed hemolytic transfusion reaction" (DHTR) and "delayed serologic transfusion reaction" (DSTR) both refer specifically to developing an alloantibody to a red blood cell antigen. The difference between the two denominations is the presence of hemolysis in DHTR, and the absence of hemolysis in DSTR. However, recipients can also develop alloantibodies against human leukocyte antigens (HLA) after platelet transfusions, which can be a cause of inadequate response to platelet transfusion.

Physiology

Delayed hemolytic and serologic transfusion reactions both consist of developing a previously undetectable alloantibody against a red blood cell antigen days to months after an antigen positive red blood cell transfusion. In a DHTR, the alloantibody hemolyzes the remaining donor red blood cells, whereas there is no evidence of hemolysis in a DSTR.

In DHTR, the hemolysis is usually the result of an anamnestic antibody response, where the recipient had prior exposure to the alloantigen and subsequent evanescence of the alloantibody before re-exposure during transfusion. A DHTR can also occur with de novo generation of an alloantibody.[94] The hemolysis is typically extravascular due to phagocytosis of IgG-opsonized donor red blood cells by the reticuloendothelial system. However, evidence of complement binding has been noted in some cases of DHTR, particularly in patients with sickle cell anemia.[95,96]

Incidence

DHTRs and DSTRs are estimated to occur in 1 in 2500 red blood cell transfusions. DSTRs occur twice as frequently as DHTRs.[97] The incidence is likely underestimated, as many recipients do not have additional antibody screening after transfusion.

Presentation and Differential Diagnosis

It can be difficult to differentiate a DHTR from a DSTR in patients with other concurrent etiologies for hemolysis (such as a hemoglobinopathies). The majority of DHTRs are clinically silent except for laboratory evidence of hemolysis as the extravascular hemolysis of the remaining donor red blood cells causes a minor fluctuation in hemoglobin/hematocrit.

Some populations are more likely to be symptomatic from a DHTR especially if there is a component of intravascular hemolysis as seen in patients with sickle cell anemia. Patients with sickle cell anemia are also at risk for hyperhemolysis following a DHTR, which can result in profound anemia due to destruction of both donor and recipient red blood cells.[96] These cases represent a diagnostic and therapeutic challenge and can be fatal.[98]

NHSN Hemovigilance Diagnostic Criteria: Delayed Hemolytic Transfusion Reaction[8]

1. Positive DAT between 24 hours and 28 days after transfusion
2. Positive elution OR new red blood cell alloantibody in recipient serum
3. Inadequate rise of post-transfusion hemoglobin level OR spherocytes of no other known cause

NHSN Hemovigilance Diagnostic Criteria: Delayed Serologic Diagnostic Criteria[8]

1. No clinical signs of hemolysis
2. New clinically significant antibodies against red blood cells: positive DAT OR positive antibody screen with new red blood cell alloantibody

Management. If patients are symptomatic from a DHTR, they should be treated with supportive care. If additional transfusions are required, patients should receive red blood cell units that do not express the antigen that the patient has developed an alloantibody against. Depending on the severity of the hemolysis, patients with sickle cell anemia and a DHTR may require an exchange transfusion with antigen-negative red blood cells.

Prevention.

Recipient-specific factors. The risk of alloimmunization with red blood cell transfusions correlates with increased transfusion; however, some patient populations are at higher risk of alloimmunization than others.

Sickle cell anemia and red blood cell alloimmunization. Patients with sickle cell anemia are at higher risk for alloantibodies with red blood cell transfusions. The cause seems to be multifactorial. Chronic transfusion, an underlying inflammatory state, and antigen expression discrepancies between mainly Caucasian donor population and recipients of African descent have been postulated to contribute to the increased risk of alloimmunization.[99] To mitigate this risk, patients with sickle cell anemia are often transfused red blood cells that are antigen matched for highly immunogenic antigens (the Rh antigens: D, C/c, E/e, and the K antigen in the Kell blood group system). Although this strategy is considered standard practice, patients with sickle cell anemia continue to be at risk of red blood cell alloimmunization.[100]

Other chronically transfused populations. Patients with myelodysplastic syndrome (MDS) and chronic myelomonocytic leukemia (CMML) have a higher rate of alloimmunization: in one retrospective study, 15% of chronically transfused patients with MDS and CMML developed red blood cell alloantibodies.[101] Prophylactic extended antigen matching has not been widely implemented in this population and it is unknown if the benefits would outweigh the costs. The rate of alloimmunization is considerably lower at 2.3% in chronically transfused patients with bone marrow failure syndromes, suggesting that the underlying disease affects the risk of alloimmunization.[102]

Impact of pregnancy and female sex. Women with a history of pregnancy are at higher risk of HLA alloimmunization with platelet transfusions compared to men and women with no known history of pregnancy.[103] This is likely due to in utero exposure to fetal HLA antigens, but the underlying mechanisms of this physiology are poorly understood. Female sex does not increase the risk of red blood cell alloimmunization except in women with a history of sickle cell anemia.[104]

Impact of massive transfusions. Patients who receive several units in a short time period (such as during a massive transfusion) do not appear to have an increased risk of red blood cell alloimmunization compared to patients that required transfusion but did not require the same initial intensity.[105]

Product-specific factors.

Impact of leukoreduction. Leukoreduction reduces the risk of HLA alloimmunization and refractoriness for platelet transfusions. However, leukoreduction of red blood cell units does not reduce the rate of alloimmunization to red blood cell antigens.[103,106]

Impact of irradiation. Irradiation of red blood cell components does not seem to increase the risk of red blood cell alloimmunization.[107]

Impact of pathogen reduction technology. PRT is under investigation for red blood cell products and there is limited data on the impact of PRT on red blood cell alloimmunization. PRT is available for platelet and plasma products and is widely used in multiple European countries. There is conflicting data on the impact of PRT on alloimmunization with platelet transfusions: some studies suggest that PRT treated platelet products have at least equivalent rates of HLA alloimmunization compared to standard platelets, while another study showed higher rates of alloimmunization with PRT treated platelets.[108–110] Additional randomized controlled trials currently underway may clarify the impact of PRT treated platelets on HLA alloimmunization.[111]

TRANSFUSION-ASSOCIATED GRAFT-VERSUS-HOST DISEASE

Physiology

Transfusion-associated graft-versus-host disease (TA-GVHD) occurs when donor T lymphocytes present in a cellular blood product recognize and attack the recipient's tissues. Viable donor T lymphocytes present in the unit are transfused as part of the blood product and subsequently engraft in the recipient's bone marrow. The donor T lymphocytes recognize and attack the recipient's tissues via the T cell's major histocompatibility complex (MHC; also known as HLA). MHC class II presentation is most commonly implicated, although other donor lymphocytes may also attack the recipient's cells and tissues via MHC class I presentation.[112] Donor T lymphocytes are more likely to recognize and attack the recipient as a pathogen when the donor and recipient have similar or partially matched MHC haplotypes. Recipients who are immunocompromised are at higher risk for TA-GVHD as their immune systems are unable to prevent engraftment and proliferation of donor lymphocytes.

Incidence

TA-GVHD is an extremely rare complication of transfusion. Prior to the implementation of γ-irradiation, the risk of TA-GVHD was estimated to be 0.1 to 1% for higher risk groups such as immunocompromised populations, as well as recipients with similar HLA as the donor of the blood product.[113] Since the advent of γ-irradiation, the true incidence of TA-GVHD is unknown and the literature consists primarily of case reports.

Presentation and Differential Diagnosis

Recipients with TA-GVHD typically develop symptoms between 8 and 10 days after transfusion. Symptoms are similar to acute graft versus host disease in allogeneic hematopoietic stem cell transplantation with multi-organ system involvement except TA-GVHD also causes bone marrow aplasia and pancytopenia. Rash, diarrhea, and liver dysfunction are common. Hemophagocytic lymphohistiocytosis, as well as some drug reactions and viral infections, can cause similar symptoms and should be considered as part of the differential diagnosis.

NHSN Hemovigilance Diagnostic Criteria[8]

1. TA-GVHD symptoms 2 days to 6 weeks after transfusion:
   a. Rash (erythematous, maculopapular eruption spread centrally to extremities; can progress to erythroderma and hemorrhagic bullous); diarrhea; fever; hepatomegaly; liver dysfunction; marrow aplasia; pancytopenia
2. Characteristic findings on skin or liver biopsy

TA-GVHD is definitively diagnosed by the presence of donor-recipient white blood cell chimerism and no alternative diagnosis.

Management

The majority of cases of TA-GVHD have been fatal despite treatment. Immunosuppression and allogeneic stem cell transplantation have been used with limited success.[113]

Prevention

Product-specific factors. Inactivating donor T lymphocytes prevents TA-GVHD. γ-Irradiation of cellular blood components is the gold standard for preventing TA-GVHD. Sufficient irradiation requires a minimum dose of 25 Gy to the central portion of the blood product container and a minimum of 15 Gy to the remainder of the bag. Pathogen reduction technologies also inactivate donor T lymphocytes and are being used instead of γ-irradiation to reduce the risk of TA-GVHD.[114] Leukoreduction alone without γ-irradiation does not prevent TA-GVHD.

Donor-specific factors. The AABB *Standards* requires γ-irradiation of cellular blood products for patient populations and forms of transfusion that are higher risk for TA-GVHD:

- Intrauterine transfusions
- Newborns that are premature, low birth weight, and/or have erythroblastosis fetalis
- Congenital immunodeficiencies
- Hematologic malignancies or solid tumors (Hodgkin lymphoma, sarcoma, neuroblastoma)
- Hematopoietic stem cell transplantation
- Blood product components that are crossmatched, HLA matched, or from directed donations (from family members or related donors)
- Patients receiving fludarabine chemotherapy
- Granulocyte transfusions

Other potential indications for γ-irradiation include patients with other malignancies particularly if these patients are receiving cytotoxic therapies, as well as donor-recipient pairs from a genetically homogenous population. In Japan, all recipients receive γ-irradiated blood products due to HLA homogeneity in the population that previously resulted in higher rates of TA-GVHD.

Typically, γ-irradiation is not routinely used for all patients in the United States. In addition to increased cost and potential for irradiation exposure to blood bank personnel, γ-irradiation reduces the shelf life and increases the amount of potassium in the supernatant of red blood cell units. Irradiated platelet products can have lower recovery and may increase the risk of alloimmunization.[115,116]

POST-TRANSFUSION PURPURA

Physiology

Post transfusion purpura (PTP) is destruction of donor platelets and often the recipient's platelets after a platelet transfusion. This destruction is typically from the recipient's preexisting alloantibody directed against a platelet-specific antigen(s) expressed on the donor's platelets. The majority of alloantibodies are against human platelet antigen-1a (HPA-1a) in recipients who are HPA-1a negative.[117] Multiparous women are at higher risk of PTP suggesting that the alloantibody first develops from exposure to alloantigens on fetal platelets during pregnancy. The alloantibody is thought to be amnestic as the majority of cases present with delayed thrombocytopenia 5 to 12 days after the platelet transfusion.

Passive transfer of donor antibodies against platelet specific antigens in transfusions has been implicated as an etiology of PTP.[118] In this setting, the onset of thrombocytopenia occurs within hours of the transfusion.

Patients with PTP have profound thrombocytopenia with proven destruction of both donor and the recipient's own circulating platelets. The pathophysiology driving autologous platelet destruction is poorly understood, but possible explanations include the presence of polyclonal, pan-reactive IgM and IgG platelet antibodies that bind to donor and recipient platelets, and the presence of soluble HPA-1a in the transfused donor blood that could coat recipient's platelets allowing the alloantibody to bind.[117]

Incidence

Platelet units are the most frequently implicated product in PTP, but it can occur with other platelet containing products such as red blood cells and plasma. The incidence of PTP is unknown and the majority of data comes from case reports. In a retrospective study of Medicare claims data between 2011 and 2012, 78 cases of PTP were identified in hospitalized older patients (ages ≥65); the rate of PTP was estimated to be 1.8 per 100,000 hospitalizations involving transfusions.[119] Multiparous women are most likely to develop PTP, although the risk appears to decrease with age. Older patients who develop PTP are more likely to have a hematologic malignancy or coagulopathy, as well as prolonged hospitalizations and higher platelet transfusion requirements.

Presentation and Differential Diagnosis

Patients with PTP typically present 5 to 12 days after transfusion with thrombocytopenia with rapidly declining platelet counts that may drop to below 10×10^9/L within 24 hours of the onset of thrombocytopenia. Unlike patients with immune thrombocytopenia (ITP), patients with PTP often have diffuse mucocutaneous bleeding and purpura. If there is concern for PTP, the recipient should be screened for antibodies against platelet specific antigens. Given the rarity of PTP, other etiologies of thrombocytopenia such as drug induced thrombocytopenia and ITP should be considered.

NHSN Hemovigilance Diagnostic Criteria[8]

1. Recipient alloantibody against HPA or other platelet specific antigen detected at or after onset of thrombocytopenia
2. Thrombocytopenia (post transfusion platelet count <20% of pretransfusion count). Onset typically 5 to 12 days post-transfusion with no other causes of thrombocytopenia
Management. PTP should be treated with high-dose IVIG. In a retrospective case series of patients with PTP, the majority (16 out of 17) responded to high dose IVIG.[120] Glucocorticoids and plasma exchange have also been used with success in some case reports.[121,122] Platelet transfusions may be used if the recipient has active bleeding, although not all recipients with PTP will respond to platelet transfusion. Preferably, the platelet unit should be from a donor who does not express

the platelet antigen that matches the specificity of the recipient's alloantibody.[123]

Prevention. Recipients with a history of PTP who require platelet transfusions in the future should be transfused with platelets that do not express the antigen(s) that the recipient has alloantibodies against.

POINTS TO REMEMBER
Delayed Transfusion Reactions

1. Delayed hemolytic reactions can result in varied severity of hemolysis ranging from asymptomatic to devastating.
2. Alloimmunization to red blood cell antigens through red blood cell transfusion, transplantation, or pregnancy, and HLA antigens through platelet transfusion (or pregnancy) can result in delayed hemolytic reactions and platelet transfusion refractoriness, respectively.
3. Pathogen inactivation and γ-irradiation are effective strategies to prevent transfusion-associated graft-versus-host disease.

OTHER TRANSFUSION RELATED ADVERSE EVENTS

Transfusion-Related Iron Overload
Physiology

Iron overload causes end organ damage from reactive oxygen species that form when plasma iron levels exceed the iron binding capacity of transferrin. Iron homeostasis is primarily regulated by absorption; beyond excreting approximately 1 mg of iron per day (via stool loss), the human body is unable to remove iron outside the setting of bleeding. Excessive iron intake through red blood cell transfusions can lead to iron overload. A single unit of red blood cells contains approximately 250 mg of iron. In recipients without preexisting iron deficiency, clinically significant iron overload can develop after 50 to 100 units. The risk of free iron increases after 15 to 20 units of red blood cells, at which point the iron carrying capacity of transferrin is saturated. Some recipients develop iron overload with fewer transfusions due to preexisting, ongoing iron deposition from ineffective erythropoiesis.[124] Other higher-risk populations include recipients with hereditary hemochromatosis, as well as recipients with underlying liver disease.[125]

Incidence

Transfusion related iron overload occurs at higher rates in frequently transfused patient populations. Patients with transfusion-dependent thalassemia, sickle cell anemia, aplastic anemia, and some hematologic malignancies associated with ineffective hematopoiesis are at risk for iron overload.[126] After hematopoietic stem cell transplantation, approximately 32 to 58% of patients have elevated ferritin, an estimate of iron stores.[127] An autopsy study of patients who died after hematopoietic stem cell transplantation found iron overload in 40% of patients based on high liver iron content (LIC) 5.6 mg/g.[128]

Presentation and Differential Diagnosis

Patients with end organ damage from iron overload can present with a variety of symptoms depending on which organs have been damaged. Organs particularly susceptible to end organ damage from iron overload include the liver, heart, endocrine organs, skin, and joints. The organs affected can vary based on the underlying disease and the etiology of the iron overload. Other drivers of iron overload, such as hemochromatosis, should be considered particularly when iron overload is out of proportion with the number of red blood cell transfusions and the patient's underlying disease.

Diagnostic criteria. Laboratory testing with ferritin and transferrin saturation can be used to screen for iron overload, but are not specific enough to definitely diagnose iron overload. Ferritin levels consistently over 1000 ng/mL are concerning for iron overload. However, ferritin does not consistently correlate with iron overload; some patients may have iron overload out of proportion of ferritin levels as seen in patients with hemoglobin H Constant Spring disease.[129] Even if ferritin is not above 1000 ng/mL, iron overload should be considered if patients have a significant lifetime history of red blood cell transfusions and/or clinical signs concerning for end organ damage from iron overload.

Traditionally, iron overload has been diagnosed with tissue biopsy (such as liver or bone marrow). Iron overload can also be diagnosed using magnetic resonance imaging (MRI) using T2* and R2.[130,131]

Management. Patients with iron overload can be treated with phlebotomy and/or iron chelation depending on their clinical condition and preferences.[126] The duration and goals of therapy will depend on the patient's ongoing transfusion requirements and underlying disease. Some patient populations continue to be at risk of iron overload outside of ongoing transfusion requirements, such as patients with ineffective erythropoiesis, as well as patients with hereditary hemochromatosis.[126]

Prevention. The primary focus on preventing transfusion related iron overload should be to reduce unnecessary red blood cell transfusions. If patients require chronic red blood cell transfusions, laboratory screening with transferrin saturation and ferritin can be used as a surrogate for iron stores with the caveat that ferritin can be elevated from multiple etiologies besides iron overload.[126] Imaging with liver and/or cardiac MRI can also be used as part of a screening protocol in chronically transfused populations.[126]

DONOR CONSIDERATIONS

Donor Reactions and Fatality

Donors can develop syncope or presyncope with donation. This is most common after the first whole blood donation. Donors who experience syncope after their first donation are less likely to donate blood in the future.[132]

Serious adverse reactions are more common in donors undergoing apheresis compared to whole blood donation.[133] Although rare, donors can die as complications of donation likely due to preexisting conditions that make the donor particularly susceptible to fluid loss from donation. In 2017, 14 donor fatalities were reported to the FDA; only 2 of these fatalities were deemed probable or likely due to the donation process and none were definitively attributable to the donation.[1]

Iron Deficiency

Iron depletion occurs in approximately 33% of donors in the United States. The risk increases with frequent donations and in female donors.[134] Teenage donors (ages 16 to 18 years) are at higher risk for iron depletion and have a higher rate of deferral due to insufficient hemoglobin levels at subsequent donations compared to 19- to 49-year-old women.[135] Daily supplemental oral iron can replace iron stores (compared to no supplementation) and is particularly beneficial in the first 8 weeks after donation.[136] Increasing the interval between donations can also mitigate the risk of iron deficiency.[137]

SELECTED REFERENCES

6. Edens C, Haass KA, Cumming M, et al. Evaluation of the National Healthcare Safety Network Hemovigilance Module for transfusion-related adverse reactions in the United States. Transfusion 2019;59:524–33.

12. Bolton-Maggs PH. SHOT conference report 2016: serious hazards of transfusion - human factors continue to cause most transfusion-related incidents. Transfus Med 2016;26:401–5.

14. Karafin MS, Blagg L, Tobian AA, et al. ABO antibody titers are not predictive of hemolytic reactions due to plasma-incompatible platelet transfusions. Transfusion 2012;52:2087–93.

32. King KE, Shirey RS, Thoman SK, et al. Universal leukoreduction decreases the incidence of febrile nonhemolytic transfusion reactions to RBCs. Transfusion 2004;44:25–9.

38. Savage WJ, Tobian AA, Savage JH, et al. Scratching the surface of allergic transfusion reactions. Transfusion 2013;53:1361–71.

45. Sandler SG, Eder AF, Goldman M, et al. The entity of immunoglobulin A-related anaphylactic transfusion reactions is not evidence based. Transfusion 2015;55:199–204.

47. Heddle NM, Blajchman MA, Meyer RM, et al. A randomized controlled trial comparing the frequency of acute reactions to plasma-removed platelets and prestorage WBC-reduced platelets. Transfusion 2002;42:556–66.

62. Vlaar APJ, Toy P, Fung M, et al. A consensus redefinition of transfusion-related acute lung injury. Transfusion 2019;59:2465–76.

70. Triulzi DJ, Kleinman S, Kakaiya RM, et al. The effect of previous pregnancy and transfusion on HLA alloimmunization in blood donors: implications for a transfusion-related acute lung injury risk reduction strategy. Transfusion 2009;49:1825–35.

73. Eder AF, Herron Jr RM, Strupp A, et al. Effective reduction of transfusion-related acute lung injury risk with male-predominant plasma strategy in the American Red Cross (2006-2008). Transfusion 2010;50:1732–42.

78. Roubinian NH, Hendrickson JE, Triulzi DJ, et al. Incidence and clinical characteristics of transfusion-associated circulatory overload using an active surveillance algorithm. Vox Sang 2017;112:56–63.

84. Benjamin RJ, Kline L, Dy BA, et al. Bacterial contamination of whole-blood-derived platelets: the introduction of sample diversion and prestorage pooling with culture testing in the American Red Cross. Transfusion 2008;48:2348–55.

86. Benjamin RJ, Braschler T, Weingand T, et al. Hemovigilance monitoring of platelet septic reactions with effective bacterial protection systems. Transfusion 2017;57:2946–57.

89. Pagano MB, Ness PM, Chajewski OS, et al. Hypotensive transfusion reactions in the era of prestorage leukoreduction. Transfusion 2015;55:1668–74.

95. Vamvakas EC, Pineda AA, Reisner R, et al. The differentiation of delayed hemolytic and delayed serologic transfusion reactions: incidence and predictors of hemolysis. Transfusion 1995;35:26–32.

96. Dean CL, Maier CL, Chonat S, et al. Challenges in the treatment and prevention of delayed hemolytic transfusion reactions with hyperhemolysis in sickle cell disease patients. Transfusion 2019;59:1698–705.

97. Chou ST, Jackson T, Vege S, et al. High prevalence of red blood cell alloimmunization in sickle cell disease despite transfusion from Rh-matched minority donors. Blood 2013;122:1062–71.

101. Trial to Reduce Alloimmunization to Platelets Study Group. Leukocyte reduction and ultraviolet B irradiation of platelets to prevent alloimmunization and refractoriness to platelet transfusions. N Engl J Med 1997;337:1861–9.

110. Kopolovic I, Ostro J, Tsubota H, et al. A systematic review of transfusion-associated graft-versus-host disease. Blood 2015;126:406–14.

116. Menis M, Forshee RA, Anderson SA, et al. Posttransfusion purpura occurrence and potential risk factors among the inpatient US elderly, as recorded in large Medicare databases during 2011 through 2012. Transfusion 2015;55:284–95.

SECTION X

Clinical Immunology

Exam questions, case studies, and additional resources are available on ExpertConsult.com.
*Full versions of these chapters are available electronically on www.expertconsult.com.

94

Systemic Autoimmune Disease

Melissa R. Snyder, Anne E. Tebo, Aaruni Khanolkar, and Xavier Bossuyt

ABSTRACT

Background

The systemic autoimmune diseases are a broad category of conditions characterized by chronic inflammation with a proven or suspected autoimmune etiology. Autoimmunity results from loss of immune system tolerance, leading to reactions against self-proteins. In many cases, autoantibodies are produced as part of this process. In some cases, these autoantibodies have well-defined antigen specificities and are clearly pathogenic, playing a major role in the disease process. In some diseases, the production of autoantibodies is hypothesized to be more a consequence of the disease. Lastly, for some conditions, a disease-associated autoantibody has yet to be identified.

Across various autoimmune diseases, studies have consistently demonstrated that autoantibody production can occur years before development of clinical symptoms. This has led to new models in which a combination of environmental and genetic "hits" leads to loss of tolerance, resulting in a stage of "preclinical" autoimmunity. Although initially asymptomatic, the ongoing inflammation process, driven by constant autoantigen exposure, will eventually lead to tissue damage and manifestations of clinical symptoms associated with a specific disease process.

Content

The central role of the clinical laboratory in the diagnosis of the systemic autoimmune diseases is antigen-specific autoantibody serology. This chapter will begin with a discussion of autoimmune processes and autoantibody methodologies, with a focus on challenges related to this type of testing. This will be followed by presentation of the most current information on the diagnosis, epidemiology, and laboratory testing for the antinuclear antibody-associated rheumatic diseases, rheumatoid arthritis, antiphospholipid syndrome, and the systemic vasculitides.

INTRODUCTION TO SYSTEMIC AUTOIMMUNITY

Mechanisms of Autoimmunity

Since most patients with autoimmune disease develop symptoms well after the abnormal immune reactions begin, it is often difficult to pinpoint the factors responsible for the initiation of disease. The use of animal models has greatly influenced our understanding of some immunologic mechanisms; however, there are in fact few models of spontaneous autoimmunity that reliably mimic the human disorders. Nevertheless, studies using existing models, as well as genetic and other analyses, are beginning to reveal some of the abnormalities that account for the early steps in the autoimmune reactions. Systemic autoimmune diseases, like many other complex disorders, are believed to arise from a combination of immunologic, genetic, and environmental factors.

Immune Tolerance

Autoimmune reactions reflect disproportionate responses between effector and regulatory arms of the immune system which typically develop through stages of initiation and propagation, and often show phases of resolution (indicated by clinical remissions) and exacerbations (indicated by symptomatic flares). The fundamental underlying mechanism of autoimmunity is defective elimination and/or control of self-reactive lymphocytes, a phenomenon referred to as immune tolerance. The immune system has evolved to discriminate between "foreign" and "self."[1] This property enables the immune system to confront "foreign" entities, such as pathogens, and maintain tolerance toward one's own tissues ("self"). Foreign entities perceived as being dangerous to the host evoke a well-orchestrated series of immunologic events that enable the immune response to effectively purge or contain the foreign entity in an effort to try and minimize morbidity in the host. In healthy, immunocompetent individuals, the immune response operates within a well-defined framework of checks and balances and when this system of checks and balances goes amiss, the result is immunologic anarchy that can include a breakdown of immune tolerance to "self," which then allows the immune response to attack the host's own tissues (autoimmunity).

The concept of immune tolerance was first proposed by Burnet and Fenner in 1949, and experimentally demonstrated by Peter Medawar in 1953.[2,3] The pivotal role that this concept and original experimental proof played in enhancing our fundamental understanding of the immune system is evident by the fact that Burnet and Medawar were awarded the Nobel Prize in 1960.[1]

The major players in the realm of immune tolerance are the T cells and the B cells and the two main tenets that underpin the concept of immune tolerance are "central tolerance" (which is established in the bone marrow for the B cells and in the thymus for the T cells) and "peripheral tolerance," which as the name suggests is enforced in the peripheral tissues.[1] Central tolerance can be characterized as a phase of immunologic instruction that all immature B cells and T cells have to undergo as part of their developmental program, where they are trained to distinguish "foreign" from "self" before they mature and are subsequently released into the peripheral tissues to execute their immune-surveillance functions. Peripheral tolerance represents an extra layer of checks and balances in the peripheral tissues that prevents errant T cells and B cells that might have escaped central tolerance, from behaving abnormally and attacking "self" tissues.

T-Cell Tolerance

A significant number of self-reactive thymus-derived (T-)lymphocytes requiring defined avidity for antigen are purged in the thymus. Thymic deletion of self-reactive T cells for ubiquitously expressed self-antigens as a concept is very easy to understand. However, this has not been the case for deletion of T cells bearing receptors directed to antigens restricted to particular tissues.

Central Tolerance

Immature T cells migrate from the bone marrow to the thymus where they undergo thymic education as part of their developmental program.[4] The thymus is an encapsulated, lobular organ that lies in the anterior mediastinum behind the sternum and is histologically comprised of an outer cortex and an inner medulla.[5]

The cortex is populated with cortical thymic epithelial cells that are ectodermal in origin, as well as some bone marrow–derived macrophages along with the immature T cells. It is in the cortex where immature T cells undergo "positive selection," wherein only the T cells that recognize self-peptides presented by human leukocyte antigen (HLA) molecules expressed on the surface of cortical antigen presenting cells (APCs) with moderate to high avidity are selected to move forward into the medulla.[6–9] The T cells that display weak interactions with the self-peptide/HLA complexes in the cortex are eliminated at this stage as they are deemed unfit for immune surveillance which requires optimal recognition of foreign peptides expressed in the context of self-HLA molecules in the peripheral tissues.

The medulla is comprised of medullary thymic epithelial cells that are endodermal in origin, bone marrow–derived macrophages and dendritic cells, as well as specialized structures called "Hassall's corpuscles" that are sites of cellular destruction.[5] The positively selected immature T cells that enter the medulla from the cortex then undergo "negative selection." Negative selection serves to weed out potentially autoreactive T cells by culling immature T cells that display high avidity for self-peptide/HLA complexes expressed on the surface of medullary APC.[6,10,11] A notable exception to this rule is the thymic selection of regulatory T cells (Tregs) that go on to help enforce peripheral tolerance after their egress from the thymus. Treg development in the thymus requires high-avidity interactions with self-peptide-HLA complexes on the surface of medullary thymic epithelia cells and the presence of IL-2.[12–15]

For many years a dilemma in the field of tolerance centered on how negative selection was able to ensure the elimination of T cells that might react against the multitude of tissue-specific antigens present in the body. The discovery of

AIRE (AutoImmune REgulator), a transcription factor that induces ectopic expression of tissue-specific antigens within the thymic medulla has helped to resolve part of this puzzle.[16,17] Patients who are deficient in AIRE suffer from a syndrome characterized by autoimmune polyendocrinopathy, candidiasis, and ectodermal dysplasia, thus providing proof-of-principle regarding the critical role it plays in tolerance.[16] Recent discoveries have also highlighted the role of FezF2 that can also regulate thymic medullary expression of tissue-specific antigens independently of AIRE.[18] Furthermore, the identification of patients with combined hypomorphic and activating mutations in the T-cell signaling protein ZAP70, who display prominent autoimmune features, also suggest that alterations in T-cell signaling thresholds may disrupt the integrity of the negative-selection process in the thymus thereby potentially predisposing the host to autoimmunity.[19]

Finally, immunologic evidence obtained from patients who have undergone thymic transplantation, where HLA matching between donor and recipient is not routinely performed, suggest that the processes of positive and negative selection may be more nuanced than prevailing dogma might suggest.[6]

Peripheral Tolerance

Silencing autoreactive T cells in the periphery is required as a back-up mechanism to regulate autoreactive T cells that escape central tolerance. This can involve T-cell intrinsic adaptive features that recalibrate signaling cascades within T cells in the face of chronic stimulation with self-antigens. Examples of such adaptive tolerance include reduced ability to mobilize intracellular calcium and transcription factors downstream of T-cell receptor (TCR) engagement, and re-setting the balance between kinases and phosphatases to perturb the positive signaling machinery.[20–22] Additionally, potentially autoreactive T cells can also upregulate inhibitory co-receptors such as cytotoxic T-lymphocyte associated protein 4 (CTLA-4), programmed cell death 1 (PD-1), and the T-cell immunoglobulin mucin (TIM) family which elevates their activation threshold.[23] Indeed, polymorphisms in the *CTLA-4* locus have been associated with autoimmune endocrine disorders.[24] In addition to these T-cell intrinsic mechanisms, the presence of Tregs provides an additional layer of control. As indicated above, natural Tregs are generated in the thymus and co-express CD4, CD25, and the transcription factor, Forkhead box P3 (FoxP3).[12–15] Tregs can also be induced to develop from conventional naïve CD4 T cells in the periphery in the presence of certain cytokines such as transforming growth factor β (TGFβ).[20] The importance of Tregs in suppressing autoimmune responses is highlighted in patients who harbor mutations in the *FOXP3* locus as they suffer from an X-linked disorder featuring immunodeficiency, polyendocrinopathy, and enteropathy.[25] The mechanisms that Tregs employ to dampen responses of autoreactive T cells can include CTLA-4 mediated trans-endocytosis or trogocytosis of co-stimulatory B7 molecules from the surface of professional APCs which impedes the B7-induced co-stimulatory activation signals directed to CD28 on the surface of effector T cells.[26] There is also evidence that Tregs can limit the availability of IL-2 to other effector T cells, as well as elaborate immunosuppressive cytokines, such as TGFβ and IL-10, that bind to their cognate receptors expressed on the surface of effector T cells to attenuate effector T-cell responses.[27,28] Other cellular subsets that may display regulatory potential, such as natural killer T (NKT) cells and γδ T cells, have also been reported to curb disease progression in type I diabetes (T1D), rheumatoid arthritis (RA), and systemic lupus erythematosus (SLE).[20,29]

B-Cell Tolerance

Autoreactive B cells generate antibodies that can directly affect the function of their target molecules or form immune complexes (ICs) with their targets which can deposit in various organs and stimulate complement and tissue-damaging inflammatory myeloid cells via Fc-receptors (FcRs) and/or Toll-like receptors (TLRs) such as TLR-7/8/9, that can recognize nucleic acids bound to autoreactive antibodies.[30–33] Serologic evidence of autoimmune responses often precedes the development of clinically evident disease by many years suggesting that tolerance checkpoints may be compromised early in the pathology of the disease.[34,35]

Central Tolerance

The first phase of instruction that is imparted to immature, developing B cells to help them discriminate "self" from "foreign" occurs in the bone marrow. B-cell intrinsic defects in the genes that encode for molecules associated with the B-cell receptor (BCR) and TLR pathways such as Bruton's tyrosine kinase (BTK), adenosine deaminase (ADA), Wiskott-Aldrich syndrome protein (WASP), myeloid differentiation primary response gene 88(MyD88), interleukin 1 receptor-associated kinase 4 (IRAK-4), transmembrane activator and CAML interactor (TACI), and activation-induced cytidine deaminase (AID) impair central tolerance.[36–41] Under normal circumstances, potentially autoreactive B-cell clones experience one of three different fates: clonal deletion/death, functional silencing/anergy, and "receptor editing."[42–45] Receptor editing involves an additional round of V(D)J gene segment recombination mediated by recombinase-activating genes (RAG) to replace the potentially autoreactive BCR.[45] Recent studies involving a subset of RA patients have revealed that newly generated, circulating, naïve B cells display defects in such secondary recombination events due to aberrant activity of ataxia-telangiectasia mutated (ATM) protein that promotes repair of double-stranded DNA (dsDNA) breaks mediated by the RAG proteins.[46] Moreover, in contrast to healthy control donors, patients with certain autoimmune disorders display marked diversity in their immunoglobulin (Ig) heavy chain variable region gene usage indicating dysregulated B-cell development.[47,48] Data from other carefully executed studies that have also evaluated circulating new emigrant/transitional B cells for the expression

of autoreactive and/or polyreactive antibodies suggest that central tolerance checkpoints may not function optimally in untreated patients suffering from SLE, RA, T1D, Sjögren syndrome (SjS), myasthenia gravis (MG), and neuromyelitis optica spectrum disease (NMOSD).[49–55] Entry of these autoreactive naïve B cells into the circulation can contribute to an environment that is permissive to the development of autoimmunity following presentation of self-antigens to circulating, autoreactive T cells as a result of ensuing somatic hypermutation of the BCR induced by this crosstalk. Multiple lines of evidence indicate that CD19hiCD27−CD21−/lo B cells are present at high frequencies in the blood of patients with several autoimmune diseases.[56–59] The presence of this subset of B cells in the circulation of RA patients correlates with an increased prevalence of erosive joint disease, and similar elevations of this B-cell subset in SLE patients are often associated with more severe autoimmune manifestations.[46,60] Genome wide association studies (GWAS) have also identified the 1858T polymorphism in the *PTPN22* gene as a prominent genetic risk factor for the development of RA, T1D, and SLE.[40,61] This polymorphism can operate in a dominant-negative fashion and is associated with disruptions in BCR and TLR signaling pathways and tolerance checkpoints.[40] Indeed, preliminary data suggest that decreased TLR9 function in SLE-associated B cells may prevent deletion of autoreactive B cells that normally occurs following cross-linking of the BCR and TLR9 with dsDNA.[62,63]

Peripheral Tolerance

The majority of the naïve mature B cells that enter the circulation from the bone marrow require CD4 T-cell help in order to generate isotype-switched antibodies.[20] In the absence of such help, the activation process induced following antigen exposure is often short lived and abortive, resulting in premature death of the B cell.[20] This property of reliance on T-cell help serves to limit autoreactive B-cell activation, as it requires the presence of both the B cell and a CD4 T-cell clone that recognize the appropriate antigenic determinants derived from the same self-antigen; the likelihood that a given autoreactive B-cell clone and its companion autoreactive CD4 T-cell clone have both escaped established tolerance checkpoints is generally low.[20] Experimental evidence also supports the notion of clonal anergy (functional silencing) of autoreactive B cells in the face of high doses of soluble antigens administered intravenously.[64] As previously discussed with T-cell tolerance, functional silencing can involve upregulation of B-cell associated inhibitory receptors such as CD22 and FcγRIIb (CD32b) and rebalancing of positive and negative signaling cascades in the face of chronic antigen exposure and additional adaptations such as impaired migration to follicular zones within secondary lymphoid tissues that facilitate B cell and T helper cell interactions.[65–67] Finally, Tregs can also suppress autoreactive B-cell activation quite likely through the same mechanism they exert toward other professional APCs as described earlier. This notion is clearly supported by the detection of circulating, autoreactive B-cell clones in patients with conditions that impair Treg numbers and/or function, such as ADA-, CD40L-, dedicator of cytokinesis 8 (DOCK8)-, HLA class II-, and WASP deficiency.[36,37,68–70]

Altered Self-Antigens

Autoimmune disease occurs when a specific adaptive immune response is directed against self-antigens. In immune

TABLE 94.1	Effective Control of Immune Response
Characteristics	**Specifics of Immune Response**
Specific	Recognize self from non-self
	Non-self recognized as foreign
	Distinguish between intracellular and extracellular pathogens
Intensity	Must be sufficient and appropriate to eliminate pathogen and confer protection
	Optimal downregulation (homeostasis) to minimize deleterious effects
Duration	Long enough to generate protection
	Should persist after resolution of challenge
	Develop memory to confer protection upon re-challenge

competent individuals, immune response to a foreign agent such as a virus is followed by its clearance from the body and return to homeostasis (Table 94.1). Failure to clear dying cells can lead to antigen modification, immune dysfunction, and tissue damage.[71] Studies from a number of investigations have demonstrated that alterations of autoantigen structure and the distribution in apoptotic cells may play a significant role in the pathogenesis of SLE.[72] Rapid clearance of apoptotic cells is associated with anti-inflammatory consequences. It is therefore likely that delayed apoptotic clearance may enhance the immune recognition of post-translationally modified antigens leading to autoimmunity. While post-translational modifications (e.g., methylation, phosphorylation, acetylation, lipidation, or glycosylation) of proteins play important biological functions under normal conditions, some of these changes can create novel self-antigens or mask antigens that are recognized by the host immune system. Modification of host antigens can greatly influence recognition by immune cells and their effector functions resulting in autoimmune reactions. In patients with RA, recognition of modified proteins has been described, with anti-citrullinated protein antibodies (ACPAs) being the best characterized (Fig. 94.1).[66,71,73,74]

Autoantibodies: Natural and Pathogenic

A key feature of an autoimmune disease is the unfolding of an excessive self-reactive, antigen-driven immune response. While

T cells play a critical role in initiating autoimmune diseases, production of autoantibodies mediated by B cells are useful for serologic diagnosis, disease prediction and, in some cases, can yield insight into pathogenesis. Autoantibodies may also be harmless footprints of an etiologic agent. Thus two main types of autoantibodies have been recognized, natural and pathogenic.

Antibodies that react with self-molecules occur in healthy individuals and are referred to as natural antibodies or natural autoantibodies. These natural autoantibodies are mainly IgM, are encoded by unmutated V(D)J genes, and display a moderate affinity for self-antigens.[75] Natural autoantibodies form a network that serves as first-line defense against self and external (foreign) signals, probably serve housekeeping functions, and contribute to the homeostasis of the immune system. In a minority of individuals, natural autoantibodies can lead to manifestations of autoimmune diseases.

High-affinity, somatically mutated IgG autoantibodies reflect a pathologic process whereby homeostatic pathways related to cell clearance, antigen-receptor signaling, or cell effector functions are disturbed.[75] In some autoimmune disorders, autoantibodies might be present prior to disease onset or the preclinical phase of disease. The mechanisms responsible for autoantibody-induced pathology significantly differ in autoimmune diseases. Autoantibodies directed against the same antigen, depending on the targeted epitope, can result in a range of effects. The location of the likely target antigen most critically influences the pathogenic potential of autoantibodies. Autoantibodies directed against cell surface antigens are clearly pathogenic while those directed against intracellular targets are usually not pathogenic and/or contribute to disease progression. A number of criteria have been used to classify autoantibodies as pathogenic. Three suggested criteria include (1) demonstration that autoantibody titers correlate with disease activity; (2) the specific autoantibody is strongly associated with the relevant disease pathology, being present with the disease or disease subset and absent in healthy individuals and those with other diseases; and (3) the antibody and antigen are localized to the site of tissue damage. In addition, animal models can provide evidence that the autoantibodies against specific autoantigens are pathogenic, where the passive transfer of autoantibodies or antigen-induced immunization can recapitulate clinical features of the disease.[76]

The functional or pathogenic role of autoantibodies in antinuclear antibody (ANA)–associated rheumatic diseases (SLE, SjS, systemic sclerosis [SSc], idiopathic inflammatory myopathies [IIM]) has a long history of intrigue. How autoantibodies

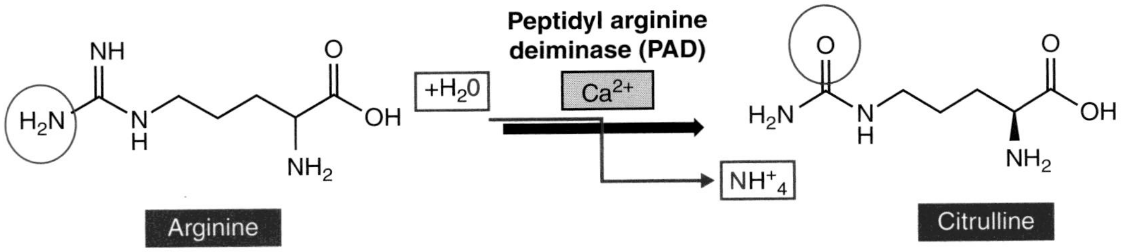

FIGURE 94.1 Citrullination, the conversion of the amino acid arginine in a protein into the amino acid citrulline by the enzyme peptidyl arginine deiminase *(PAD)*. Dysregulated citrullination is a key mechanism that drives the production and maintenance of antibodies to citrullinated proteins, a hallmark in rheumatoid arthritis.

directed to intracellular targets such as topoisomerase I (Scl-70) and RNA polymerase III could translate to the pathophysiology of SSc, however, remain an enigma.[77] Intracellular antigens may be implicated in the induction of disease via three possible mechanisms. First, the antigen is released from inside the cell and binds onto a cell-surface receptor or other extracellular location, such as proteinase 3 (PR3) associated with the anti–neutrophil cytoplasmic antibodies (ANCAs) in patients with granulomatosis with polyangiitis (GPA). Second, the antigen moves to an aberrant site on the cell surface, such as, perhaps, the small ribonucleoprotein antigen Ro. Lastly, the target antigen is cross-reactive and is at an accessible location, such as the membrane ribosomal P-like protein in patients with SLE.

Autoantibodies may induce pathology via a number of mechanisms. These include mimicking receptor stimulation, blocking neural transmission, induction of altered signaling and uncontrolled triggering, cell lysis, activation of neutrophils, induction of inflammation, and microthrombosis.[78] In systemic autoimmune diseases, autoantibodies react with free molecules, such as phospholipids (PL), as well as cell surface and nucleoprotein antigens, forming pathogenic antigen–antibody (immune) complexes. These autoantibodies injure tissues and organs through engagement of FcγR activation of complement and internalization and activation of TLRs. Activation of intracellular TLRs in plasmacytoid dendritic cells leads to the production of type I interferon (IFN), whereas engagement of intracellular TLRs on APCs stimulates cell activation and the production of other inflammatory cytokines. Thus ICs might perpetuate a positive feedback loop amplifying inflammatory responses.[75]

Genetics and Autoimmunity

Autoimmune diseases are characterized by diverse etiologies with complex interactions in which diverse genetic factors are associated not only with disease susceptibility but also with specific autoantibodies and disease phenotypes. Genetic involvement in autoimmunity can be inferred from the possibility of predicting disease through at least three levels of evidence (Table 94.2).[79] First is the idea that more than one autoimmune disease may co-exist in a single patient as seen in a number of systemic autoimmune diseases, a phenomenon referred to as poly-autoimmunity. The second evidence refers to the pathophysiologic mechanisms shared between autoimmune diseases. Lastly, familial clustering of autoimmune diseases has been long recognized and supports a role for shared genetic predisposition. A number of investigations have identified different genetic loci suspected to be involved in systemic autoimmune disease pathogenesis. Of interest, these share several risk loci suggesting that common pathways in immune loss of tolerance may be involved in induction, propagation, and maintenance of these diseases.

Early genetic susceptibility studies focused on genes within the HLA region (also referred to as the major histocompatibility complex [MHC] family); however, there is support for genetic loci that are shared across autoimmune diseases outside the HLA region.[79–81] Many of the identified genetic loci in autoimmunity involve pathways related to B-cell or T-cell activation and differentiation, innate immunity, and regulation of cytokine signaling. In the context of susceptibility genes relating to lymphocytic activation, the role of the HLA region is prominent. Polymorphisms affecting HLA sequences responsible for binding antigens significantly contribute to the pathophysiology of RA and SLE.[81–83] In RA, massive genetic interactions between the *HLA-DRB1* shared epitope (SE) alleles and non-HLA genetic variants in ACPA-positive RA patients have been reported at genome-wide level for two independent cohorts.[82] The primary SLE association signal in the entire MHC region is located at *HLA-DRB1*-associated long-range HLA-gene haplotypes in multiple ancestral populations.[83]

The non-HLA genes encode proteins that have immune-mediating functions, including CTLA-4 (CD152). The CTLA-4 is a type I transmembrane protein of the Ig superfamily and homologue of the co-stimulatory molecule CD28. CTLA-4 serves a critical role in negative regulation of the T-cell immune response.[24,79,80] Another non-HLA susceptibility gene related with the innate immune response is interferon regulatory factor 5 (IRF5). This gene is involved in IFN-mediated signaling, featuring many polymorphisms that are associated with RA, SLE, and SSc.[81–83] While RA, SLE, and SSc are characterized by activation of innate immune system and associated impaired downstream pathway of type 1 IFN responding genes (IFN signatures), there is emerging evidence of diversity and abundance of these in RA when compared to SLE and SSc.[84] Other variants implicated in RA susceptibility include PTPN22, TRAF1-C5, PADI4, and STAT4 genes. These genetic factors seem to contribute to the erosive damage seen in RA. There is also additional evidence that suggests an association between radiographic damage and polymorphisms of genes encoding TNF, IL-1, IL-6, IL-4, IL-5, OPN, and PRF1 in RA.[79,80,82] The heterogeneous etiology of SLE is supported by a wide variety of disease-associated loci that have modest effect sizes but surpass the genome-wide significance threshold for the genetic association with this disease.[83] To date, more than a hundred non-HLA loci with SLE susceptibility have been described. These genes are usually mapped at the noncoding variants suggesting that they may be involved in a regulatory role in the expression of genes that could drive the development of specific phenotypes in SLE. Notable SLE susceptibility non-HLA risk loci include STAT4, PTPN22, IFIH1, and TRAF3IP2. Given the protean clinical picture of this autoimmune disease, there is limited evidence that genetic variants are associated with the development of different SLE phenotypes.[79,83]

Significant discoveries in genetic studies have shifted the dynamics toward gene interplay with environmental and

TABLE 94.2	Evidence for Genetic Involvement in Systemic Autoimmune Diseases	
Evidence	**Description**
Poly-autoimmunity	Co-existence of multiple systemic autoimmune diseases in a single patient
Pathophysiologic mechanisms	Most systemic autoimmune diseases share common mechanisms of disease initiation, propagation, and maintenance
Familial clustering	Shared genetic predisposition

host-specific factors. Understanding the interplay between these elements may enable us to better understand not only the pathogenic mechanisms of these diseases but also decipher clues for more tailored treatments and disease management.

Triggers of Autoimmunity

Despite their heterogeneity, systemic autoimmune diseases share epidemiologic, pathogenic, and clinical features. Exogenous triggers have been reported in a number of systemic autoimmune diseases notably SLE, SSc, RA, and certain inflammatory myopathies such as the statin-induced necrotizing autoimmune myopathy (NAM). These triggers can generally be categorized as noninfectious or infectious. Molecular mimicry is one of the main mechanisms by which infectious or noninfectious agents may induce autoimmunity. Table 94.3 shows a few documented infectious agents implicated in molecular mimicry in the indicated systemic autoimmune diseases. Molecular mimicry is thought to occur when similarities between foreign and self-antigens favor the activation of autoreactive T or B cells by a foreign-derived antigen in a genetically susceptible individual. In addition to molecular mimicry, other mechanisms such as loss of tolerance, nonspecific bystander activation, or persistent antigenic stimuli (among others) may also contribute to the development of autoimmune diseases. Understanding the interplay between genetics, the host microbiome, and environmental factors will contribute significantly to our understanding of the concept of molecular mimicry and the role of the diverse immunologic players.

Noninfectious Triggers

The noninfectious triggers of systemic autoimmunity are very diverse. Most systemic autoimmune diseases affect more women, frequently of reproductive age, than men. This observation draws attention to the environmental etiology, especially the role of sex hormones and X-chromosome genes in autoimmune disorders. A number of studies have investigated exogenous sex hormones, silica, silicone, solvents,

smoking, pesticides, mercuric chloride, and hair dyes as putative risk factors for the development of these diseases.[85–90] Exposure to these agents in the environment may alter posttranslational modifications, affecting immunogenicity of self-proteins and triggering an autoimmune response.[85] For example, citrullination is linked to smoking in RA.[86] In this study by Klareskog and colleagues, a correlation between smoking and HLA-DR SE genes was evident for ACPA-positive RA, but not for ACPA-negative RA. The combination of a history for smoking and the presence of double copies of HLA-DR SE genes increased the risk for RA by 21-fold compared with the risk among nonsmokers carrying no SE genes. In SLE, the strongest epidemiologic evidence exists for increased risk associated with exposure to crystalline silica, cigarette smoking, use of oral contraceptives, and postmenopausal hormone replacement therapy, while there is an inverse association with alcohol use.[87,88] Limited research evidence points to exposure to solvents, residential and agricultural pesticides, heavy metals, and air pollution to risk of SLE too. Mechanisms linking environmental exposures and SLE include epigenetic modifications resulting from exposures, increased oxidative stress, systemic inflammation and inflammatory cytokine upregulation, and hormonal effects.[87–90] In other studies, estrogen replacement therapy in postmenopausal women demonstrates an increased but relatively modest risk for SSc and Raynaud disease.[85] Environmental endocrine modulators, in the form of pesticides, may represent another opportunity for estrogen-like effects to occur, but there is scant evidence that these agents play a role in human systemic autoimmune disease.

Infectious Triggers

It has long been recognized that infections may act as triggers and persistent drivers of various autoimmune diseases. A variety of different and often interrelated mechanisms by which infections trigger and perpetuate autoimmune disease in predisposed patients have been proposed. Experimental evidence suggesting that the joint may become targeted secondarily after the ACPA immune response has been initiated at another site as a consequence of an inflammatory event triggered by a common environmental exposure (periodontal infection/inflammation and/or smoking) have been reported.[86,91] Furthermore, ACPA-positive sera from a subset of RA patients demonstrate cross-reactivity with in vitro citrullinated peptides from Epstein-Barr virus (EBV) and human papilloma virus (HPV).[92,93] Prospective studies defining the kinetics of these antibody responses during natural infection will be important in assessing their role in disease pathogenesis.

In antiphospholipid syndrome (APS), studies in animal models have demonstrated the production of antibodies to β_2-glycloprotein I (β_2GPI) in response to immunization with *Haemophilus influenzae, Neisseria gonorrhoeae*, and tetanus toxoid.[94–96] In addition, studies using peptides from microorganisms with structural similarity to β_2GPI demonstrate induction of β_2GPI antibodies, thrombosis, fetal loss, and inflammation.[94,95] It remains to be determined whether molecular mimicry of viral or bacterial antigens leads to the production of pathogenic antiphospholipid antibodies (aPL) or if epitope spreading to other autoantigens is required for pathogenicity.[96] In ANCA-associated vasculitides, an indirect mechanism of molecular mimicry leading to typical PR3-ANCA has been proposed by Pendergraft and colleagues.[97] In selected ANCA-positive patients, antibodies

TABLE 94.3 Infections, Systemic Autoimmune Diseases, and Molecular Mimicry

Systemic Autoimmune Disease	Infectious Agent
ANCA-associated vasculitides	*Staphylococcus aureus*
Antiphospholipid syndrome	CMV, *H. influenzae, N. gonorrhoeae, C. tetani*
Rheumatoid arthritis	*P. gingivalis, P. mirabilis, E. coli*, EBV, HPV
Systemic lupus erythematosus	EBV
Sjögren syndrome	EBV, HTLV-1, HCV, and HBV
Systemic sclerosis	CMV

ANCA, Anti–neutrophil cytoplasmic antibodies; *C. tetani, Clostridium tetani; CMV*, cytomegalovirus; *E. coli, Escherichia coli; EBV*, Epstein-Barr virus; *H. influenza, Hemophilus influenzae; HBV*, hepatitis B virus; *HCV*, hepatitis C virus; *HPV*, human papilloma virus; *HTLV-1*: human T- cell leukemia virus, type 1; *N. gonorrhoeae, Neisseria gonorrhoeae; P. gingivalis, Porphyromonas gingivalis; P. mirabilis, Proteus mirabilis; S. aureus; Staphylococcus aureus.*

against complementary peptides (antisense peptide sequence) to PR3 (cPR3) were recognized. The cPR3 peptides, which may represent mimics of microbial peptide sequences, were found to share homologies with *Staphylococcus aureus* sequences.

Interactions between host-specific factors (immunologic, genetics, and microbiome) and the environment play significant roles in the pathogenesis and development of autoimmune disease. Of the systemic autoimmune diseases, significant progress has been made in understanding these interactions in SLE and RA. There is evidence that other diseases such as SSc, APS, and SjS also share these attributes. Elucidating the interplay between elements involved in the diverse mechanisms associated with autoimmunity is likely to unravel optimal tools for diagnosis, prognosis, and treatment of these diseases.

Methodologies

The primary role of the clinical immunology laboratory in supporting the diagnostic evaluation of suspected systemic autoimmune disease is through detection of disease-associated, antigen-specific autoantibodies. Testing for autoantibodies, in one form or another, has been around for well over half a century.[98,99] All methods are based on the antigen/antibody interaction, in which a source of relevant antigen is used to "capture" the autoantibody of interest. These various methods can be classified according to the technique used to detect this interaction (Table 94.4). IC-based methods use precipitation or light scatter to directly assess for the presence of the antigen/antibody complex, while immunoassays use a labeled form of an anti-human Ig antibody or antibody fragment as the detection reagent. This difference in detection methods between the two categories has implications for the autoantibody isotypes that are identifiable. The IC-based methods tend to identify autoantibodies of the IgM isotypes more efficiently, although the IgG isotype may also be detected. In addition, using the IC-based methods does not allow for determination of the autoantibody isotype. In comparison, use of detection antibodies in immunoassays allows for specific detection and identification of IgG, IgM, and IgA isotypes. Over the years, methods for identification and characterization of autoantibodies have evolved, generally moving from manual assays to more automated platforms. However, even historic methods may still be employed within the clinical laboratory. In this next section, the general principles of the various methods for detection of antigen-specific autoantibodies will be discussed. For additional information on immunoassays as applied to a wider range of analytes, see Chapter 26 "Immunochemical Techniques."

Immune Complex–based Methods

Gel-based Methods

Gel-based methods are based on formation of an IC between the antigen and autoantibodies that occurs within a solid phase, usually an agarose gel. There are multiple variations of this method.[100] Radial immunodiffusion uses a gel impregnated with the relevant antigen. A well is formed in the gel, into which the patient sample is added. The proteins from the sample will diffuse in a circle into the gel, forming a concentration gradient. Optimal IC formation occurs at the zone of equivalence between the antigen and the autoantibody. If the concentration of autoantibody is sufficient, a precipitin line will be observed; a nonspecific protein stain can also be employed to improve visualization of the precipitin. Rocket immunoelectrophoresis is a

variation of radial immunodiffusion. In this method, instead of allowing circular diffusion to occur, an electric field is applied to the gel, causing the proteins to migrate in a single direction from the well. This allows for improved sensitivity as the effective concentration of the autoantibody migrating into the gel is increased.

Another variation of the gel-based methods is double-immunodiffusion. In this format, the antigen of interest and the patient's sample are placed in two adjoining wells, both of which will diffuse into the gel in a radial pattern. As the antigen and antibody migrate toward each other, ICs will form. At the point of maximal IC formation, a precipitin line may be observed. One advantage of the double immunodiffusion technique is that a patient's sample may be assessed for multiple autoantibodies by surrounding the patient's sample well with multiple wells, each containing a unique antigen. Counterimmunoelectrophoresis is a variation of double immunodiffusion in which an electric current is applied such that the antibody and patient's sample are directed to migrate toward each other, rather than to diffuse radially from the well. As with rocket immunoelectrophoresis, this raises the concentration of antigen and autoantibody that will interact, thereby improving the sensitivity of the method.

Solution Phase Methods

Other methods based on formation of IC are immunoprecipitation and nephelometric/turbidimetric assays. For each of these methods, the IC forms between the antigen and autoantibody in the solution phase. In an immunoprecipitation assay, an IC forms between the autoantibody and a labeled form of the antigen of interest. The IC is then precipitated out of solution by altering the ionic strength of the solution by adding a salt, such as ammonium sulfate. The precipitate is collected and washed; the amount of precipitated antigen, which is proportional to the amount of autoantibody present in the sample, is measured based on the label used. This measurement is compared to a standard curve, which allows for calculation of a semi-quantitative value. A classic example of the immunoprecipitation method is the Farr assay, in which a radiolabeled form of double-stranded DNA (dsDNA) is precipitated by the presence of anti-dsDNA antibodies.[101]

Nephelometric and turbidimetric assays are also based on the principle of IC formation, with the formation of the IC detected by light scatter.[102] In nephelometry, the amount of light scattered is measured at a 90° angle from the incident light; the amount of scattered light detected is directly proportional to the amount of autoantibody in the patient's sample. In turbidimetry, the light that passes through the sample (transmittance) is measured, which is indirectly proportional to the autoantibody concentration. For each of these methods, the signal is compared to a standard curve, which allows for calculation of a numeric value that is a reflection of how much autoantibody the patient has in circulation.

Immunoassay Methods

Indirect Immunofluorescence Methods

Historically, the first type of immunoassay used routinely for detection of antigen-specific autoantibodies was the indirect immunofluorescence (IIF) assay.[103] In this assay, the source of the antigen is an intact cell or tissue which has been adhered onto a slide. Detection of autoantibody binding to the cellular substrate is accomplished through an anti-human Ig labeled

TABLE 94.4 **Characteristics of Various Methodologies Used for Detection of Antigen-specific Autoantibodies**

Category	Methodology	Able to Differentiate Autoantibody Isotype?	General Principle of Method	Detection Method	Examples of Commonly Tested Autoantibodies
Immune complex-based	Gel-based	No	Diffusion or directed migration of antibody and/or antigen in solid-phase gel	Visualization of precipitin line	Anti-Sm/RNP antibodies
	Solution-phase	No	Formation of IC between antibody and labeled antigen in solution, followed by precipitation of complex	Immunoprecipitation: Measurement of precipitate	Farr assay for measurement of anti-dsDNA antibody
			Formation of IC between antibody and antigen in solution, followed by passage of light signal through sample	Nephelometry: Light scatter Turbidimetry: Light transmittance	Rheumatoid factor
Immunoassay	IIF	Yes	Use of intact tissue or cellular substrate to detect antibodies with various antigen specificities	Fluorescently labeled anti-hIg	ANA using Hp-2 cells
	Line/dot blot	Yes	Use of antigens immobilized on nitrocellulose membrane to detect antigen-specific antibody	Enzyme-labeled anti-hIg and visual detection	Myositis-associated autoantibodies
	ELISA	Yes	Use of plate-bound immobilized antigen (purified or recombinant) to detect antigen-specific antibody	Enzyme-labeled anti-hIg and absorbance detection	Anti-CCP antibody
	FEIA	Yes	Use of immobilized antigen (purified or recombinant) to detect antigen-specific antibody	Enzyme-labeled anti-hIg and fluorescence detection	Anti-CCP antibody
	CLIA	Yes	Use of antigen (purified or recombinant) bound to paramagnetic beads to detect antigen-specific antibody	Isoluminol-labeled anti-hIg and chemiluminescence detection	Antibodies to ENAs
	ALBIA	Yes	Use of multiplex antigen array (bead or chip-based) to simultaneously detect antibodies with different antigen specificities	Fluorescently labeled anti-hIg	Antibodies to ENAs

ALBIA, Addressable laser bead immunoassay; *ANA*, antinuclear antibody; *CCP*, cyclic citrullinated peptide; *CLIA*, chemiluminescence immunoassay; *ELISA*, enzyme-linked immunosorbent assay; *ENA*, extractable nuclear antigen; *FEIA*, fluoroenzyme immunoassay; *IIF*, indirect immunofluorescence assay.

with a fluorescent molecule, often fluorescein-5-isothiocyanate (FITC). The presence of an autoantibody would be identified by fluorescence of the target cell or tissue. In some cases, the autoantibody may be associated with visualization of a specific fluorescence pattern, which is related to the localization of the antigen within the cell or tissue. For some IIFs, the fluorescence pattern is reported to the patient's medical record, depending on diagnostic relevance and antigen association. In addition,

IIFs may be reported with a titer, based on analysis of serial dilutions, which reflects the amount of autoantibody present in the sample.

Line/Dot Blot Immunoassay

In comparison to IIF, all other immunoassays use some form of purified or recombinant antigen as the capture reagent. In the line or dot blot immunoassay, the antigen is applied as

METHODOLOGIES

Challenges of Autoantibody Testing

Antibody Heterogeneity

- Autoantibody repertoire for an individual composed of multiple antibodies with differing epitope specificities and binding avidities
- Autoantibody repertoire can change over time due to epitope spreading
- Selection of antigen for diagnostic testing has significant implications related to clinical sensitivity and specificity

Quantitation

- Autoantibody assays should be interpreted as "semi-quantitative" methods
- Numeric result determined by both amount of antibody present and avidity of antibody/antigen interaction
- Autoantibody assays report in arbitrary units which are manufacturer-specific

Standardization

- Qualitative standardization relates to positive/negative agreement between methods
- Differences in antigen and calibration may lead to qualitative discordance between methods
- Quantitative standardization requires use of certified reference material for traceable calibration
- Due to autoantibody heterogeneity, even use of a certified reference material does not guarantee quantitative standardization

either a line or dot on a membrane.[104] This technique is analogous to a Western blot, although, in this case, the antigen is directly applied to the membrane without transfer from an electrophoretic gel. The diluted patient sample is applied to the membrane, during which time the antigen-specific antibody would be captured. After washing, an enzyme-labeled anti-human Ig antibody is added. After a second wash step, a substrate is added which is converted to a colored product on the membrane by the enzyme label. The presence of the patient's antibody is determined by visualization of the membrane or through use of an automated reader. Although the intensity of the band or dot is related to the amount of antibody present in the patient sample, line/dot blots are often reported qualitatively. One advantage of the line/dot blot is the ability to multiplex, by including multiple antigens on a single membrane.

Sandwich Immunoassay

Sandwich immunoassays refer to assays in which the patient autoantibody is "sandwiched" between an immobilized capture antigen (purified or recombinant) and a labeled anti-human Ig antibody. There are several variations of the sandwich immunoassay. In the enzyme immunoassay (EIA) or enzyme-linked immunosorbent assay (ELISA), the antigen is adhered to the bottom of a 96-well plate.[105] Detection of the antigen-specific autoantibody binding to the antigen is performed using an enzyme-labeled anti-human Ig antibody; the enzyme label converts a colorless substrate to a colored product, the intensity of which is measured through light absorbance at the appropriate wavelength. Another format of

the sandwich immunoassay is the fluoroenzyme immunoassay (FEIA). For FEIA, the antigen may be immobilized on a number of supports, including a 96-well plate. The detection antibody is also labeled with an enzyme, which converts the substrate to a fluorescent product. In the third variation of the sandwich immunoassay, the chemiluminescent immunoassay (CLIA), antigen is immobilized on paramagnetic beads.[106] The detection antibody is labeled with a luminescent molecule, commonly isoluminol. Under appropriate conditions, the isoluminol will undergo a chemical reaction. The chemical reaction provides energy to move electrons from the ground to excited state; when the electrons return from the excited state, light is released. In all variations of the sandwich immunoassay, the signal generated from the detection antibody (absorbance, fluorescence, luminescence) is directly proportional to the amount of autoantibody that has bound to the antigen.

Multiplex Immunoassays

Another type of immunoassay routinely used for autoantibody serology is generically referred to as the multiplex immunoassay (MIA).[107–109] There are various formats of MIA testing; however, the most commonly used in the clinical laboratory is the addressable laser bead immunoassay (ALBIA) platform. In this type of assay, individual bead sets, each with a unique fluorescent signal, are coupled to various antigens of interest. The bead sets are then combined into a bead mixture. Autoantibody binding to the beads is detected through use of an anti-human Ig antibody labeled with a fluorescent marker, such as FITC. Measurement of the mean fluorescent intensity (MFI) for each bead, and identification of the individual bead, is accomplished by using a fluidics and laser system analogous to a flow cytometer. Identification of the bead set allows for determination of the antigen specificity of the autoantibody, while measurement of the MFI is directly proportional to the amount of autoantibody that has bound to each bead set.

Challenges

Autoantibody detection and measurement face challenges not generally encountered for other protein analytes.[110–114] Antibodies are heterogeneous molecules, which is necessary in their physiologic role in the adaptive immune response. In addition, antigen-specific autoantibodies must be differentiated from all the other Igs that make up the patient's antibody repertoire. These issues of heterogeneity and specificity require careful selection of the antigen when designing an assay for detection of an autoantibody. Another issue is quantitation; most immunoassays for detection of autoantibodies are semi-quantitative, rather than being truly quantitative, for reasons that will be highlighted in the following section. Lastly, standardization across methods, platforms, and assays remains a challenge. This is an area that deserves increased attention, particularly for autoantibodies that are included as part of the classification criteria for some systemic autoimmune diseases.

Heterogeneity and Antigen Selection

In contrast to most protein analytes for which testing is performed in the clinical laboratory, variation between autoantibodies, both within an individual and between individuals, is significant. Within an individual, the autoantibody response is polyclonal, with production of multiple antibodies that may have different epitope specificities and binding avidities.[115] This would be referred to as the individual's autoantibody repertoire. To add further complexity, an individual's autoantibody repertoire will likely change over time, due in part to epitope spreading. Epitope spreading occurs when the immune response, which was initiated against a single antigenic epitope, expands to include recognition of additional epitopes which may be from the same or different protein molecules. Between individuals, the same heterogeneity is observed. Each individual's autoantibody repertoire will be unique. For example, consider two patients with RA. Each patient might have an immune response which leads to production of autoantibodies that bind to citrullinated peptides. However, the autoantibody repertoire from each individual will probably recognize different citrullinated peptides, possibly originating from different protein molecules. It is also probable that there will be differences in avidity with which the various autoantibodies bind to these different citrullinated peptides. Because of this complexity, designing an assay that will detect autoantibodies from both individuals can be very challenging.[116] In addition, an assay must be able to "pick out" the relevant autoantibody from the other Igs that constitute the individual's complete antibody repertoire. These two challenges combine to have significant impacts on the performance characteristics of an assay, specifically related to clinical sensitivity and specificity. Overcoming these challenges requires careful selection of the capture antigen. The antigen used in the assay must be broad enough to detect relevant autoantibodies that have different epitope specificities, while not including epitopes that might detect diagnostically irrelevant antibodies. Using an epitope-restricted antigen could lead to an assay with decreased sensitivity, although using a broad mixture of antigens could result in decreased specificity. Recombinant antigens may be used, although it is critical to understand the similarities and differences of the epitopes compared to the native antigen. Native antigen may be a viable option, although impurities resulting from other co-purified proteins could affect the specificity of the assay.[117]

Characteristics of Quantitation

Most immunoassays for antigen-specific autoantibodies are reported with a numeric value. The numeric value is compared to a "cutoff," or reference interval, a result above which would be considered "positive" for the presence of the autoantibody. This numeric value is presumed to be a reflection of the concentration of the autoantibody in the patient sample.[98,118] However, this relationship is more complicated. In reality, most immunoassays for autoantibodies should be viewed as "semi-quantitative" methods. While the result generated from an immunoassay is determined, in part, by the amount of autoantibody, avidity of the autoantibody/antigen interaction also affects the observed signal. This "semi-quantitative" character is also evidenced in the reported result units. Virtually all immunoassays for autoantibodies report in arbitrary units, "U" or "U/mL," rather than mass-based units. These units are generally defined by each manufacturer for their specific assay based on their calibrator material. Because of this, the patient result is only a relative comparison to the assay-specific calibrator, rather than a mass-based quantitative value.

With all these limitations, numeric autoantibody results have some diagnostic implications. For many autoantibodies, significantly elevated values are more predictive for the presence of an autoimmune disease compared to results that might be only slightly above the cutoff. In addition, in some conditions, "strongly positive" autoantibody results are linked to more aggressive disease. However, it is important to realize that most autoantibody assays are not truly "quantitative" due to complexities of the antibody avidity, antibody repertoire, and assay-specific calibration schemes.

Standardization

Standardization refers to comparability of results between different assays. For autoantibody assays, standardization can be thought of as "qualitative" or "quantitative."[119] Qualitative standardization requires having positive/negative agreement between assays, while quantitative standardization requires comparability of numeric values. Lack of qualitative standardization can result from differences in antigenic epitopes or assay calibration. Differences in antigens between two assays could lead to a patient sample demonstrating a relatively high positive result on one assay and a low positive or even negative result on another. This pattern of results could suggest that the patient's autoantibody is binding to an epitope present in the antigen used in the first assay, which is not present in the antigen used for the second assay. Assay calibration can also lead to qualitative discrepancies between assays, usually around the cutoff. In other words, if one assay has a cutoff set lower to maximize sensitivity and a second assay has a cutoff set higher to improve specificity, some patient samples may have a weak positive result on one assay and a negative result on the other.[120]

Quantitative comparability adds even further challenges to autoantibody standardization. The only way to achieve quantitative standardization is through the use of certified reference materials (CRMs).[121] CRMs are available for only a handful of autoantibodies, and those that are available have not been routinely used as traceable calibration materials.[122] However, it is critical to point out that the availability and use of a CRM does not guarantee quantitative standardization.[123] This can be attributed again to autoantibody heterogeneity. Even if two assays are calibrated with traceability to the same CRM, but are detecting different subsets of autoantibodies, the quantitative results between the two methods will not be equivalent. Standardization of autoantibody assays faces significant difficulties, some of which are inherent to the autoantibody itself. Qualitative and quantitative comparability should both be considered as goals for future assay development, with the understanding that complete standardization may not be possible. For more detailed information regarding clinical laboratory test standardization, see Chapter 7 "Standardization and Harmonization."

ANTINUCLEAR ANTIBODY-ASSOCIATED RHEUMATIC DISEASES

SjS, SLE, SSc, mixed connective tissue disease (MCTD), and IIMs are classically considered ANA-associated rheumatic diseases. In the first part, an overview of these diseases and the specific ANAs associated with these diseases will be provided. A historical overview of a selection of specific antibodies found in patients with an ANA-associated disease is given in Table 94.5.[124–149] In the second part the assays and methods used for detection of these antibodies will be described in additional detail.

Sjögren Syndrome

Epidemiology, Clinical Features, and Classification Criteria

Primary SjS is a systemic autoimmune disease typified by focal lymphocytic infiltration of the exocrine glands causing

TABLE 94.5 **Historical Overview of Descriptions of Selected Autoantibodies in Antinuclear Antibody–associated Rheumatic Diseases**

Year	Antibody	Year	Antibody
1958		1986	Anti-PL-12[138]/anti-SRP[139]
1959	Anti-nucleoprotein/anti-DNA[124]	1987	
1960		1988	
1961		1989	
1962		1990	Anti-OJ/anti-EJ[140]
1963		1991	
1964		1992	
1965		1993	Anti-RNA pol III[141]
1966	Anti-Sm[125]	1994	
1967		1995	
1968		1996	
1969	Anti-Ro[126]	1997	
1970		1998	
1971	Anti-RNP[127]	1999	Anti-KS[142]
1972		2000	
1973		2001	
1974	Anti-La[128]	2002	
1975		2003	
1976	Anti-Mi2[129]	2004	
1977		2005	Anti-MDA5[143]
1978		2006	Anti-TIF-1γ[144]
1979	Anti-Scl-70[130] Ro=SSA/La=SSB[131]	2007	Anti-NXP-2[149]/anti-SAE[145]/anti-Zo[146]
1980	Anti-centromere[132]/Jo-1[133]	2008	
1981	Anti-Ku[134]	2009	
1982	Anti-Th/To[135]	2010	
1983		2011	Anti-HMGCR[147]
1984	Anti-PL-7[136]	2012	
1985	Anti-fibrillarin[137]	2013	Anti-cN1A[148]

dry eyes and dry mouth.[150] Secondary SjS is the condition in which focal lymphocytic infiltration of the exocrine glands occurs as a late complication in patients with another rheumatic disease such as RA, SLE, or SSc.[150]

Primary SjS occurs in 0.1 to 0.6% of the general adult population with a female:male ratio of at least 9:1 and a mean age of diagnosis at around 50 years.[150] In addition to dry eyes and dry mouth, patients may also present with symptoms of arthralgia, fatigue, and malaise.[151] In some patients, systemic features such as inflammatory arthritis, Raynaud phenomenon, fever, and photosensitivity can be present as well.[152]

The 2016 American College of Rheumatology (ACR) and the European League Against Rheumatism (EULAR) classification criteria for SjS[153] are summarized in Table 94.6. Although such criteria are aimed for research, they can also be useful in clinical practice.

Autoantibodies

In a majority (>70%) of patients with SjS, antibodies to SSA/Ro and SSB/La are found. In SjS, the presence of anti-SSA alone is less common than the presence of both anti-SSA and anti-SSB antibodies. Anti-SSB alone is uncommon, and the Sjögren's International Collaborative Clinical Alliance (SICCA)

Research Groups reported that the presence of anti-SSB, without anti-SSA antibodies, had no significant association with SjS phenotypic features, relative to seronegative participants.[154] Therefore SSB was not included in the 2016 classification criteria.

In patients with primary SjS, hypergammaglobulinemia, low C4 levels, and rheumatoid factor (RF) can be found.[155] Thus in a patient with RF (without ACPAs), arthritis, and dryness, a diagnosis of primary SjS should be considered.[150]

Anti-SSA-60 and anti-TRIM21. It is important to distinguish anti-SSA-60 antibodies from anti-SSA-52 antibodies as the target antigens and their immunologic functions are different. Ro60 is a protein component of small cytoplasmic ribonucleoprotein complexes (hY-RNA complexes) that can bind misfolded noncoding RNA. Ro60 likely is involved in the targeted degradation of noncoding RNA.[156] In mice and certain bacteria, Ro60 is important for cell survival after ultraviolet irradiation.[156] The antigenic target of anti-SSA-52 (Ro52) antibodies is Tripartite Motif 21 (TRIM21), a cytosolic Fc receptor. TRIM21 links Fc-mediated antibody recognition to the ubiquitin proteasome system[157] and is involved in innate immune signaling and antigen degradation.[157] TRIM21 has also been linked to initiation of autophagy.[157]

TABLE 94.6   American College of Rheumatology/European League Against Rheumatism 2016 Classification Criteria for Sjögren Syndrome

Classification Item	Score
Anti-SSA/Ro antibody positivity	3
Focal lymphocytic sialadenitis with a focus score[a] of ≥1 foci/4 mm²	3
Abnormal Ocular Staining Score of ≥5 (or van Bijsterveld score of ≥4)	1
Schirmer's test[b] result of ≤5 mm/5 min	1
Unstimulated salivary flow rate of ≤0.1 mL/min	1
Individuals with signs and/or symptoms suggestive of SjS (ocular or oral dryness) who have a total score of ≥4 meet the criteria	

[a]Focus score (histology): 50 or more lymphocytes per high power field around a salivary duct
[b]The Schirmer test uses standardized blotting paper strips to measure tear flow over a 5-minute period: 5 mm or less of wetting is considered dry
Protocols for ocular staining score (estimation of ocular surface epithelial damage) and salivary flow rate are referred to in Shilbosk et al.[153]
From Shiboski CH, Shiboski SC, Seror R, et al. 2016 American College of Rheumatology/European League Against Rheumatism classification criteria for primary Sjogren's syndrome: a consensus and data-driven methodology involving three international patient cohorts. *Ann Rheum Dis* 2017;76:9–16.

Antibodies to Ro60 are found in patients with SjS, SLE, subacute cutaneous lupus erythematosus, and neonatal lupus erythematosus. Antibodies to Ro52 are associated with a broad range of conditions. They have been associated with myositis and with interstitial lung disease in connective tissue diseases (CTDs).[158,159] A recent French retrospective, observational study found that in patients with antibodies to both TRIM21 (Ro52) and Ro60, primary SjS was the most likely associated disease, especially if combined with antibodies to SSB.[160] In patients negative for antibodies to TRIM21 (Ro52) but positive for antibodies to Ro60, SLE was the most frequent diagnosis (48.5%).[160] Finally, patients with isolated anti-TRIM21 (Ro52) had a wide variety of diseases associated (autoimmune and nonautoimmune). Among autoimmune diseases there was an association with inflammatory myositis.[160] Similar findings were reported by Murng and Thomas.[161]

Neonatal "Lupus" Syndrome
Neonatal "lupus" syndrome can occur in infants born to mothers who carry anti-Sjögren syndrome A (anti-SSA/Ro) and anti-Sjögren syndrome B (anti-SSB/La) antibodies (primary SjS patient or patient with SLE) and is caused by maternal-fetal transmission of these antibodies. The neonates have a rash resembling discoid lupus erythematosus and occasionally also other abnormalities such as hepatosplenomegaly or heart block. Anti-SSA/Ro antibodies can bind to fetal heart conduction tissue and can inhibit cardiac repolarization, resulting in atrioventricular block.[162]

Systemic Lupus Erythematosus
Epidemiology, Clinical Features, and Classification Criteria
SLE typically affects women of childbearing age.[163] The female:male ratio is 13:1 in the age group 15 to 44 years old and 2:1 in children and the elderly.[163] SLE occurs in all ethnicities with a higher prevalence in non-Caucasians than in Caucasians. Although the disease is considered rare in Africa, the prevalence of SLE in Europe and the United States is higher in people from African descent than in Caucasians.[163]

SLE is a prototype systemic autoimmune disease. The disease has a heterogeneous clinical picture and patients may present with different manifestations during their disease course, which typically presents with flares and remissions.[164]

The 2012 Systemic Lupus International Collaborating Clinics (SLICC) classification criteria have not only been used for research but also for diagnosis, as they are sensitive and wide-ranging. According to the SLICC criteria[165] the patient must satisfy at least four criteria, including at least one clinical criterion and one immunologic criterion OR the patient must have biopsy-proven lupus nephritis in the presence of ANAs or anti–double-stranded DNA (dsDNA) antibodies.
- The clinical criteria include acute cutaneous lupus, chronic cutaneous lupus, oral or nasal ulcers, synovitis, serositis, proteinuria or red blood cell casts, neurologic manifestations, hemolytic anemia, leukopenia or lymphopenia, and thrombocytopenia.
- The immunologic criteria include ANA, anti-dsDNA, anti-Smith, antiphospholipid antibodies (aPL), hypocomplementemia, and direct Coombs test.
- In 2018, the ACR and EULAR developed classification criteria for SLE. In these criteria, an ANA of 1:80 or higher by IIF or an equivalent positive test (ever) is an entry criterion.[166] If ANA is absent, one cannot classify as SLE. To fulfill the criteria one must have at least 10 points and at least one clinical criterion. The domains and criteria are summarized in Table 94.7.

Skin involvement occurs in almost 90% of SLE patients (acute cutaneous lupus, subacute cutaneous lupus, chronic cutaneous lupus). A biopsy is important to diagnose cutaneous lupus. An important feature of cutaneous lupus erythematosus is the photosensitivity. The photosensitive rash typically occurs days after ultraviolet light exposure, lasts for over 3 weeks, and may be associated with systemic symptoms such as arthralgia or fatigue.[163]

Musculoskeletal involvement in SLE is common with arthralgia and synovitis occurring in almost 90% of the patients.[165] It typically concerns a symmetric polyarthritis involving metacarpophalangeal, proximal interphalangeal, and knee joints.[163]

Renal involvement is present in 50% of patients (70% in African Americans) and is a major cause of morbidity and mortality in SLE. SLE patients should be checked for proteinuria (e.g., protein/creatinine ratio or 24-hour proteinuria). In addition to proteinuria, lupus nephritis might be further suggested by hypocomplementemia and by increased anti-dsDNA antibody concentrations. The diagnosis is made by a renal biopsy.

TABLE 94.7 American College of Rheumatology/European League Against Rheumatism 2018 Classification Criteria for Systemic Lupus Erythematosus

EULAR and ACR 2019 SLE Classification criteria[166]

Entry criterion: ANA titer of ≥1:80 on HEp-2 cells or an equivalent positive test (ever)

Additive criteria
- Clinical domains and criteria (points are given in parentheses):
  - constitutional [fever (2)]
  - hematologic [neutropenia (3), thrombocytopenia (4), autoimmune hemolysis (4)]
  - neuropsychiatric [delirium (2), psychosis (3), seizure (5)]
  - mucocutaneous [nonscarring alopecia (2), oral ulcers (2), subacute cutaneous or discoid lupus (4), acute cutaneous lupus (6)]
  - serosal [pleural or pericardial effusion (5), acute pericarditis (6)]
  - musculoskeletal [joint involvement (6)]
  - renal [proteinuria >0.5 g/24 h (4), biopsy class II or V lupus nephritis (8), class III or IV lupus nephritis (10)]
- Immunology domains and criteria (points are given in parentheses):
  - antiphospholipid antibodies [anti-cardiolipin (aCL) OR anti-β_2-glycloprotein I (anti-β2G1) OR lupus anticoagulant (LA) (2)]
  - complement [low C3 or C4 (3), low C3 and C4 (4)]
  - SLE-specific antibodies [anti-dsDNA or anti-Sm (6)].

SLE classification requires at least one clinical criterion and ≥10 points

Within each domain, only the highest weighted criterion is counted toward the total score.[166]

Criteria need not occur simultaneously and occurrence of a criterion on at least 1 occasion is sufficient.[166]

From Aringer M, Costenbader K, Kaikh D, et al. 2019 European League Against Rheumatism/American College of Rheumatology classification criteria for systemic lupus erythematosus. *Ann Rheum Dis* 2019;78:1151–9.

In SLE, central nervous disease can be present with neuropsychiatric manifestations and cognitive impairment (depression).

Autoantibodies

Antinuclear antibodies. The presence of serum ANAs detected by IIF is an important serologic marker for SLE. The majority of the SLE patients are positive for ANA by IIF at some point in the disease course.

The sensitivity of ANA by IIF for SLE is considered high (>95%). In a recent SLICC study that included 1137 recent onset SLE patients, 92.3% of the patients were ANA positive, 6.2% were anti-cellular antibody negative, and 1.5% had isolated cytoplasmic and/or mitotic cell patterns.[167]

The two most prevalent ANA patterns in SLE patients are the homogeneous pattern and the speckled pattern.[168] Some patients may switch patterns over time.[168] Recent evidence shows that a portion of SLE patients (13% in a recent Swedish study) loses ANA positivity over time.[168] Thus patients with established disease may be seronegative, but differences between different commercial assays have been noted.[169]

The specific antibodies found in SLE (and their prevalence, as reported in two studies performed in Sweden and Belgium, respectively)[168,170] are dsDNA (44 to 45%), Ro52 (41 to 38%), Ro60 (41 to 48%), SSB/La (20.4 to 19%), Sm (11 to 6%), U1RNP (28 to 16%), and ribosomal P (11 to 9%).

A large study using the US military cohort found that formation of ANAs can precede the clinical onset of SLE by many years.[34] This was shown for anti-dsDNA antibodies (in 55% of patients), anti-SSA/Ro antibodies (in 47%), anti-SSB/La antibodies (in 34%), anti-Sm (in 32%), anti-RNP (in 26%), and aPL antibodies (in 18%).

Anti-dsDNA antibodies. Anti-dsDNA antibodies are not only used to diagnose and to classify SLE, but they are also a marker for renal involvement and disease activity (flares).[171] Especially increased anti-dsDNA levels in combination with low complement are associated with renal involvement.[168,171]

It is important that the assay used for anti-dsDNA measurement specifically detects antibodies to dsDNA because antibodies to single-stranded DNA (ssDNA) are found in a whole range of diseases and are not specific for SLE. Among the antibodies to dsDNA some have a high avidity whereas others have a low avidity. It is mainly the high avidity antibodies that have been advocated to be SLE-specific, to reflect disease activity, and to be associated with lupus nephritis.[123]

There are different methods available for measurement of anti-dsDNA antibodies and each method has its merits and disadvantages. The Farr radioimmunoassay (RIA) is based on precipitation of radiolabeled dsDNA complexed with anti-dsDNA antibodies using high ammonium sulfate concentrations. Antibodies are detected by measurement of the radioactivity in the precipitated pellet. This method is considered a reference method because high-avidity antibodies are precipitated. The disadvantage is the use of radioactivity and that all isotypes (IgG, IgA, and IgM) are precipitated. The *Crithidia luciliae* immunofluorescence test (CLIFT) detects antibodies that bind to the kinetoplast (a modified mitochondrion that contains dsDNA) of the *Crithidia luciliae* hemoflagellate adhered to a glass slide. Antibodies are detected by IIF using a fluorescent-dye coupled secondary anti-human IgG (or IgM, IgA) antibody. This method has a high specificity, but the sensitivity is low (typically 20 to 35%).[123] The ELISA detects antibodies to dsDNA coated (e.g., through poly-lysine) onto 96-well polystyrene plates. Antibodies are detected by using an enzyme-coupled secondary anti-human IgG (or IgM, IgA) antibody. Generally, ELISAs detect high-avidity and low-avidity antibodies, and hence have a high sensitivity but a low specificity. ELISA systems are increasingly replaced by fully automated solid-phase assays such as FEIA, chemiluminescence immunoassay (CLIA), and ALBIA (see Table 94.4).

Even though an international standard has been available (W0/80) and has been widely applied by the manufacturers, results of anti-dsDNA antibodies may differ between the different assays/manufacturers. This might be related to differences in methodology, antigen source, buffer composition, conjugate used.[123] The W0/W80 reference material is depleted and a new candidate preparation has been proposed.[172]

Anti-SSA antibodies. Anti-SSA antibodies have been associated with neonatal lupus, skin involvement (photosensitivity), and sicca symptoms. The antibodies do not seem to fluctuate over time.[168] For more information, see section on SjS.

Anti-U1RNP antibodies. High titers of anti-U1-RNP antibodies are diagnostic for MCTD. In SLE, the prevalence of anti-U1-RNP is 25 to 47%.[172] Anti-U1RNP antibodies (in SLE) have been associated with Raynaud phenomenon.[168,173]

The antigens to which anti-RNP antibodies react reside in 3 proteins (68/70 kDa, protein A, and protein C) complexed with small nuclear U1-RNA. This complex is called small nuclear U1 ribonucleoprotein (snU1-RNP). snU1-RNP is involved in the splicing of precursor messenger RNA. Most anti-U1-RNP antibodies react to the proteins. However, a small fraction of sera recognize the complex of U1-RNA with the protein and not the protein alone.[174]

Anti-Sm antibodies. The prevalence of anti-Sm antibodies (5 to 30%) depends on racial background (more prevalent in individuals of African descent) and the antibody detection system.[175] Anti-Sm antibodies are frequently associated with anti-RNP antibodies.[174] Frodlund reported that anti-Sm antibodies can fluctuate over time in SLE patients, but the clinical relevance needs to be determined.[168]

The antigen to which anti-Sm antibodies bind is composed of a complex of core proteins (B/B′, D1, D2, D3, E, F, and G) (which form a heptamer ring) and uracil-rich snRNAs (U1, U2, U4–U6, and U5). The Sm autoantigen is part of the spliceosome complex involved in the splicing of precursor messenger RNA.

The B/B′ and D polypeptides are the polypeptides that are most frequently involved in the anti-Sm antibody response. The B/B′ proteins share cross-reactive proline-rich octapeptide epitopes (with homology to EBV nuclear antigen) with RNP-A and RNP-C.[176,175] These epitopes are frequently targeted by antibodies present in patients with MCTD.[175] A gly-arg-gly motif including a symmetrical dimethylarginine post-translational modification in the B/B′, D1, and D3 proteins are also major Sm epitopes. The SmD peptides (with the dimethylated arginine residues) are the Sm autoantigens that are most specific for SLE.[175] It is important to know the exact nature of the antigen used in anti-Sm antibody assays in order to better understand its clinical performance.

Anti-ribosomal P antibodies. The reported prevalence of anti-ribosomal P antibodies in SLE ranges from 10 to 47%.[177] The variability in prevalence probably depends on the assay used, ethnicity, the cohort studied, and the age of the patients.[177]

The ribosomal proteins include P0, P1, and P2 with molecular weights of 38, 19, and 17 kDa, respectively. These cytoplasmic phosphoproteins comprise a multi-molecular complex that is a component of the 60S ribosomal subunit (important for the elongation step of protein synthesis).

A recent systematic review and meta-analysis concluded that anti-ribosomal P antibodies are associated with severe manifestations of SLE, mainly lupoid hepatitis and neuropsychiatric lupus, but also lupus nephritis and higher disease activity scores.[177] There is variability between studies, which might be related to differences in assays used and target antigens. Immu-

noassays for detection of anti-ribosomal P antibodies generally use (combinations of) P0, P1, or P2 as autoantigen or a C-terminal 22 amino acid peptide, which is a conserved epitope on all three RibP (P0, P1, P2) proteins.[177]

Anti-nucleosome antibodies. The nucleosome is composed of a histone octamer ([H2A–H2B–H3–H4]2) around which approximately 200 bp dsDNA is wrapped twice and to which histone H1 is bound on the outside.[178] Anti-nucleosome antibodies can be directed to conformational epitopes of the nucleosome or to histone or dsDNA epitopes.[178]

In a comparative analysis based on 26 studies in which the performance of anti-nucleosome and anti-dsDNA antibodies was studied, Bizzaro et al.[178] found that anti-nucleosome antibodies had a higher diagnostic sensitivity than anti-dsDNA antibodies (59.9 versus 52.4%) and a comparable specificity (94.9% versus 94.2%). The specificity of the anti-nucleosome assay was higher for assays that used H1-stripped nucleosomes compared to assays that used intact nucleosomal antigen (95.7 versus 87.5%).[178] Anti-nucleosome antibodies were associated with disease activity.[178] In order to be used in clinical practice, anti-nucleosome antibody measurement should be standardized and there should be consensus on how nucleosomes should be prepared.[179]

Anti-histone antibodies. The target antigens of anti-histone antibodies are the histones H1, H2A, H2B, H3, and H4. Anti-histone antibodies (anti-H2A-H2b antibodies) are found in a majority (>95%) of patients with SLE induced by procainamide, penicillamine, isoniazid, and methyldopa.[180] However, anti-histone antibodies are also found in a variety of other disorders including not only idiopathic SLE but also RA, Felty syndrome, SjS, SSc, primary biliary cirrhosis (PBC), infectious diseases, and neurologic diseases.[180] Thus anti-histone antibodies have a low specificity for drug-induced SLE.

MIXED CONNECTIVE TISSUE DISEASE

For MCTD, the classification criteria of Alarcon-Segovia are frequently used.[181] These criteria include the presence of anti-RNP antibodies in high titer (≥1:1600) and the following clinical features: synovitis, Raynaud phenomenon, hand edema, myositis, and acrosclerosis.

For a description of anti-U1-RNP antibodies, see the section on SLE.

Systemic Sclerosis

Epidemiology, Clinical Features, and Classification Criteria

SSc is a rare CTD. In the United States, the prevalence was estimated to be 275 cases per million with an annual incidence of 19 new cases per million.[182] Women are more affected than men, and disease is more severe in African Americans than in Caucasians.[183]

SSc is characterized by autoantibody production, microvascular dysfunction (small-vessel vasculopathy), and fibrosis of skin and other organs (with varying involvement of internal organs).

SSc is subdivided into limited (skin lesion limited to areas distal to elbows and knees with or without facial involvement) and diffuse cutaneous disease (skin lesions involve proximal extremities and/or trunk).[184] Extra-cutaneous findings include interstitial lung disease, pulmonary hypertension, arthritis, gastrointestinal dysmotility, renal disease (renal crisis), myositis, and cardiac disease.[184] In 2013, a joint committee of the ACR and EULAR published the most recent classification criteria for SSc (Table 94.8).[185]

Autoantibodies

Antinuclear antibodies. ANAs are present in ±94% of the patients with SSc.[186] The most established autoantibodies in SSc are directed to topoisomerase I (Scl-70), centromere proteins, and RNA polymerase III. These antibodies are included in the latest SSc classification criteria[185] and are mostly mutually exclusive. Besides, a number of other autoantibodies have been reported in SSc, including autoantibodies directed to the PM/Scl complex (also known as the exosome), U3RNP/fibrillarin, U11/U12 snRNA, Th/To autoantigens, and Ku.

Anti-centromere antibodies yield the typical centromere staining. Anti-topoisomerase I antibodies yield a specific ANA pattern and anti-polymerase III antibodies a speckled nuclear pattern. When anti-polymerase I antibodies co-exist, a nucleolar pattern is observed as well. Anti-U3 RNP/fibrillarin, anti-Th/To, and anti-PM-Scl antibodies yield a nucleolar pattern, which is fairly characteristic for SSc.

Anti-centromere antibodies. Anti-centromere antibodies have been associated with SSc with limited skin involvement. Anti-centromere antibodies were previously associated with CREST syndrome (calcinosis, Raynaud phenomenon, esophageal dysmotility, sclerodactyly, telangiectasia). Patients with anti-centromere antibodies are less prone to interstitial lung disease (e.g., compared to patients with anti-Scl-70 antibodies)[187] but could be more prone to pulmonary hypertension,[184,188] which is a major cause of death in the subgroup of anti-centromere-positive patients.[184] The main target antigen is centromere protein B, but other centromere proteins can also be the target, such as centromere protein A and C.

Anti-topoisomerase I (Scl-70) antibodies. Anti-topoisomerase I antibodies are found in 15 to 42% of patients with SSc (across all ethnic groups) and are associated with diffuse cutaneous disease (present in 2/3 of patients with anti-topoisomerase I antibodies) and interstitial lung disease.[184,189,190] As interstitial lung disease is now a major cause of mortality in SSc, anti-topoisomerase I antibodies are associated with a poor prognosis.[186]

Anti-RNA polymerase III antibodies. Antibodies to RNA polymerase III commonly co-exist with antibodies to RNA polymerase I. Anti-RNA polymerase III antibodies are associated with a higher risk for renal crisis[191] and a higher risk for malignancy (coincident at diagnosis).[192–194] Patients with anti-RNA polymerase III antibodies should be monitored for scleroderma renal crisis and appropriately treated if needed.

Anti-U3 RNP (fibrillarin) antibodies. Anti-U3 RNP (fibrillarin) antibodies precipitate the U3 ribonucleoprotein (U3 RNA and 34-kDa fibrillarin). Anti-U3 RNP antibodies are detected in 4 to 10% of SSc-patients and are particularly common in patients of African American descent: 27 versus 5% of a Caucasian descent.[195] Anti-U3 RNP-positive patients have more frequent skeletal muscle involvement (which is distinct from myositis overlap) and pulmonary arterial hypertension (a common cause of death).[195,196]

Anti-Th/To antibodies. Anti-Th/To antibodies have been associated with the limited form of cutaneous SSc. The reported prevalence of anti-Th/To in SSc ranged from 1 to 13%. Mitri et al. reported that survival among anti-Th/To-positive patients was reduced compared to survival among anti-centromere-positive patients.[197] The antibody is associated with interstitial lung disease and pulmonary arterial hypertension.[197]

The Th/To autoantigens are a macromolecular protein–RNA complex (human RNase mitochondrial RNA processing [MRP] complex and the related RNase P complex) consisting of a catalytic RNA and at least 9 proteins including Rpp14, Rpp20, Rpp21, Rpp29 (hPop4), Rpp25, Rpp30, Rpp38/40, hPop1, and hPop5.[198,199] RNase MRP is an endoribonuclease that cleaves ribosomal, messenger, and mitochondrial RNAs.[198] Rpp25, Rpp38, and hPop1 have been described as the main autoantigens.[199,200]

Anti-PM/Scl antibodies. Anti-PM/Scl antibodies are mainly found in patients with overlap syndromes of SSc with polymyositis (PM)/dermatomyositis (DM) and more rarely in

TABLE 94.8 Classification Criteria for Systemic Sclerosis

2013 Classification Criteria[a]

Item	Subitem	Weight/Score
Skin thickening proximal to metacarpal phalangeal joints		9
Skin thickening of the fingers	Puffy fingers	2
	Sclerodactyly	4
Fingertip lesions	Ulcers	2
	Pitting scars	3
Telangiectasia		2
Abnormal nail fold capillaries		2
Pulmonary arterial hypertension and/or interstitial lung disease	PAH	2
	interstitial lung disease	2
Raynaud phenomenon		3
SSc-related autoantibodies	Anti-centromere	3
	Anti-topoisomerase I	
	Anti-RNA polymerase III	

[a]If skin thickening proximal to metacarpal phalangeal joints not present, score ≥9 classified as having SSc.
From van den Hoogen F, Khanna D, Fransen J, *et al.* 2013 classification criteria for systemic sclerosis: An American College of Rheumatology/European League Against Rheumatism collaborative initiative. *Arthritis Rheum* 2013;65:2737–47.

patients with PM, DM, or SSc. Depending on the cohort and method of detection used, these antibodies have been found in 2 to 12% of patients with SSc and 21 to 24% of patients with PM/SSc overlap disease.[201,202]

The PM/Scl complex consists of up to 16 proteins and is located primarily in the nucleolus of the cell. It is homologous to the yeast exosome and has a role in RNA degradation and processing (including ribosome assembly). The major antibody targets of the PM/Scl complex are PM/Scl-100 and PM/Scl-75 (the numbers indicate the molecular weight).[203] Epitope mapping of PM/Scl-100 revealed that the antibody response is mainly directed against 15 amino acids at position 231 to 245 of the N-terminal part of the protein.[201] Some assays incorporate this major epitope of PM/Scl-100 as a synthetic peptide, labeled PM-1α. In a large study that measured antibodies to PM-1α, antibodies were present in 7.2% of SSc patients of whom almost 50% had no other SSc-specific antibodies (anti-centromere, anti-topoisomerase I, and anti–RNA polymerase III). Features positively associated with the presence of monospecific anti-PM-1α antibodies included younger age at disease onset, skeletal muscle involvement, calcinosis, inflammatory arthritis, and overlap disease.[201]

Anti-U11/U12 RNP antibodies. Anti-U11/U12 RNP antibodies target small nuclear ribonucleoproteins that are components of the spliceosome that catalyze pre–messenger RNA splicing.[204] These autoantibodies were initially found to react to U11 RNA and U12 RNA by RNA immunoprecipitation.[205] Anti-U11/U12 RNP antibodies are found in 3% of SSc patients.[205] They are found in limited and in diffuse SSc and are associated with severe (and rapidly progressing) pulmonary fibrosis.[205] Anti-U11/U12 RNP antibodies yield a speckled nuclear staining pattern on immunofluorescence.[205]

Anti-NOR90 antibodies. Anti-NOR90 antibodies are directed to the nucleolus-organizing region. The target antigen is human upstream binding factor (hUBF), two polypeptides (93 and 89 kDa) involved in RNA polymerase I transcription.[206] In a study using a line immunoassay, anti-NOR90 antibodies were found in 4.8% of patients with SSc.[207] The antibodies have also been reported in RA, SLE, SjS, and hepatocellular carcinoma.[208,209] Anti-NOR90 antibodies yield a nucleolar staining pattern on immunofluorescence.[210]

Anti-Ku antibodies. Anti-Ku antibodies have been described (in low frequency) in myositis, SSc, SLE, MCTD, SjS, and RA.[211] Anti-Ku patients often have an overlap (connective tissue) syndrome, for example SSc with inflammatory myopathy or with features of SLE.[186,211]

A recent study showed that in anti-Ku patients, distinct phenotypes can be distinguished: in patients with anti-Ku and anti-dsDNA antibodies, glomerulonephritis frequently occurs (and may result in terminal renal failure) whereas in anti-Ku patients with elevated CK levels interstitial lung disease frequently developed.[212]

The antibodies target a heterodimer that binds to the ends of dsDNA-binding fragments. It is involved in DNA repair and the regulation of phosphorylation of nuclear proteins.[213]

Anti-U1-RNP antibodies. Anti-U1RNP antibodies are a marker for MCTD, but can also be found in SLE, SSc, PM/DM, and primary SjS. SSc patients with this antibody usually present with inflammatory symptoms, such as myositis and arthritis. Most of them have limited cutaneous SSc, although approximately 20% develop diffuse cutaneous SSc.[186]

Inflammatory Myopathies

Epidemiology, Clinical Features, and Classification Criteria

IIMs (myositis) are a heterogeneous group of disorders characterized by muscle weakness, inflammation, and immune-mediated lesions[214] that can be associated with systemic inflammation including joints, skin, lungs, and heart. The clinical spectrum of IIM is broad. It includes not only muscle weakness or muscle pain, but also extra-muscular manifestations such as skin symptoms (e.g., heliotrope rash, mechanic hands, or Raynaud phenomenon), respiratory symptoms (dyspnea, cough), articular symptoms (arthralgia or arthritis), and constitutional symptoms. Table 94.9 gives an overview of the most recent EULAR/ACR classification criteria for IIM.[214]

Classically, IIM have been classified into two categories: DM (myositis with characteristic skin changes) and PM (muscle weakness, elevated muscle enzymes, inflammatory alterations on muscle biopsy, and myopathic features on electromyography, without DM skin rash).[215] Currently, four main IIM groups have been proposed: DM, overlap myositis including mainly

---

TABLE 94.9 **2017 EULAR/ACR Classification Criteria for Inflammatory Myopathy—Without Biopsy**

Criteria		Points
Age of onset	>18 and <40 years	1.3
	≥40 years	2.1
Muscle weakness	Objective symmetric weakness of the proximal upper extremities	0.7
	Objective symmetric weakness of the proximal lower extremities	0.8
	Neck flexors are relatively weaker than neck extensors	1.9
	In the legs proximal muscles are relatively weaker than distal muscles	0.9
Skin manifestations	Heliotrope rash	3.1
	Gottron papules	2.1
	Gottron sign	3.3
Other clinical manifestations	Dysphagia or esophageal dysmotility	0.7
Laboratory measurements	Anti-Jo-1 (anti-histidyl-tRNA synthetase)	3.9
	Elevated serum levels of CK or LDH or ASAT/AST/SGOT or ALAT/ALT/SGPT	1.3

From Lundberg IE, Tjarnlund A, Bottai M, et al. 2017 European League Against Rheumatism/American College of Rheumatology classification criteria for adult and juvenile idiopathic inflammatory myopathies and their major subgroups. *Ann Rheum Dis* 2017;76:1955–64.

anti-synthetase syndrome, immune-mediated necrotizing myopathy (IMNM), and inclusion body myositis (IBM).[216-220]

Dermatomyositis: skin rash (Gottron sign or papules, heliotrope rash [liliaceous eyelid edema]) with or without (clinically amyopathic DM) muscle involvement. A third of DM patients have normal creatine kinase concentrations. Some patients have polyarthritis, rapidly progressive interstitial lung disease, or malignancy. These DM subtypes are associated with specific antibodies.

Anti-synthetase syndrome: triad of myositis, interstitial lung disease, and (symmetrical polyarticular) arthritis, which can be accompanied with Raynaud phenomenon, mechanic's hands, and fever. The anti-synthetase syndrome is linked to the presence of anti-synthetase antibodies.

Immune-mediated necrotizing myopathy: severe muscle weakness with typical myofiber necrosis (and only minimal inflammation) on biopsy. Patients often present with high creatine kinase levels resistant to immunosuppressant strategies.[221-223] This subtype is associated with specific antibodies.

Inclusion body myositis: characteristic muscle biopsy with inflammation and signs of muscle degeneration (rimmed vacuoles). This type occurs only after the age of 40 years, has a slow course, and does not respond to immunosuppressive drugs.

Taken together, IIM is a complex group of disorders and myositis-specific antibodies can help in the diagnosis, classification, and estimation of prognosis.

Autoantibodies

The autoantibodies associated with IIM are divided into myositis-specific antibodies and myositis-associated autoantibodies. Myositis-specific antibodies are specific for IIM and are generally mutually exclusive. They are found in up to ± 50% of IIM patients and most of them are associated with specific clinical features of IIM. Myositis-associated antibodies are found in IIM, but also in other systemic rheumatic diseases and in patients with overlap disease.

Antibodies Related to Dermatomyositis

Anti-Mi-2 antibodies. Anti-Mi-2 antibodies are associated with DM (up to 31%) with relatively mild disease and typical cutaneous lesions.[129,224] The antibodies target a component of the nucleosome remodeling-deacetylase (NuRD) complex, involved in transcription regulation.

Anti-MDA-5 antibodies. Anti-MDA-5 antibodies are associated with clinically amyopathic DM (DM rashes but no myositis).[143] This disease can be complicated with rapidly progressive, therapy-resistant, and fatal interstitial lung disease.[225-227] The antibodies were initially reported in an East-Asian population, but they are also reported in other populations with reports of an expanded clinical phenotype (e.g., inflammatory arthritis).[228-230] The antibodies target RNA helicase encoded by melanoma differentiation associated gene 5 (MDA-5). RNA helicase is involved in the innate immune defense against viruses.

Anti-TIF-1γ antibodies. Anti-TIF-1γ (p155/140) antibodies are associated with aggressive skin lesions. They are found in adult and juvenile DM.[144] In adults (>40 years), anti-TIF-1γ antibodies are associated with malignancy (in up to 75% of anti-TIF-1γ positive patients).[231,232] The antibodies target transcriptional intermediary factor 1γ (TIF-1γ), a nuclear transcription factor overexpressed in solid tumors.

Anti-NXP-2 antibodies. Anti-NXP-2 antibodies are associated with severe cutaneous lesions, including calcinosis. They are found in juvenile and adult DM. In adults, an association with malignancy has been suggested, but difficult to prove.[233] The antibodies target nuclear matrix protein 2 (NXP-2),[149] which plays roles in diverse nuclear functions, including RNA metabolism, maintenance of nuclear architecture, and regulation of activation of tumor suppressor gene p53.

Anti-SAE antibodies. Anti-SAE antibodies are associated with DM.[146] Characteristic features have not yet been identified. The antibodies target small ubiquitin-like modifier activating enzyme (SAE), which is involved in post-translational modification of numerous target proteins ("protein SUMOylation").[234]

Anti-aminoacyl-tRNA synthetase antibodies. The anti-synthetase syndrome is associated with anti-aminoacyl-tRNA synthetase autoantibodies. Aminoacyl tRNA synthetases attach dedicated amino acids to their cognate tRNA. Eight anti-synthetase antibodies are known: anti-Jo: Histidyl tRNA synthetase, anti-PL12: Alanine tRNA synthetase, anti-PL7: Threonyl tRNA synthetase, anti-EJ: Glycyl tRNA synthetase, anti-OJ: Isoleucyl tRNA synthetase, anti-Zo: Phenylalanyl tRNA synthetase, anti-Ha: Tyrosyl tRNA synthetase, anti-KS: Asparaginyl tRNA synthetase.[a] The most frequently found anti-synthetase antibody is anti-Jo-1 antibody. Correlations between the type of antibody and clinical features have been proposed. For example, myositis and joint involvement was more common and interstitial lung disease less frequent in patients with anti-Jo-1 antibodies than in patients with anti-PL7 or anti-PL-12 antibodies.[133,234,235] Survival was lower in patients with non–anti-Jo-1 than in patients with anti-Jo-1 antibodies.[236,237] Interstitial lung disease can be the only clinical feature of the anti-synthetase syndrome. As the prognosis of interstitial lung disease associated with anti-synthetase antibodies is better than the prognosis of idiopathic interstitial lung disease, it is valuable to detect these antibodies in patients with interstitial lung disease.[238]

Antibodies Related to Immune-mediated Necrotizing Myopathy

IMNM is associated with antibodies to signal recognition particle (SRP) and 3-hydroxy-3-methylglutaryl CoA reductase (HMGCR).[139,147,221,239] A characteristic feature is the diffuse necrotizing myopathy on muscle biopsy.

Anti-SRP antibodies are associated with severe symmetric proximal muscle disease, and with dysphagia and interstitial lung disease.[240]

Anti-HMGCR antibodies are associated with statin use, but the antibodies have also been found in patients who did not take statins.[147,241,242] Disease course is worse in younger and juvenile anti-HMGCR–positive patients.[243]

Antibodies Related to Inclusion Body Myositis

Anti-cytosolic 5′-nucleotidase 1A autoantibodies (anti-cN1A; previously anti-Mup44) are the only known autoantibodies associated with IBM.[148] Anti-cN1A autoantibodies are present in 30 to 50% of patients with IBM but have also been found in patients with juvenile DM, SjS, and SLE.[148,244]

---

[a]References 133, 136, 138, 140, 142, and 146.

Common Myositis-associated Autoantibodies

Patients with anti-PM/Scl antibodies classically have an overlap disease of myositis and SSc.[151] Patients with anti-U1RNP antibodies classically have an overlap with MCTD. Anti-Ro52 co-occurs frequently with anti-Jo-1 antibodies and potentially identifies patients with more severe interstitial lung disease.[245,246] For anti-Ku, see above.

ANTINUCLEAR ANTIBODY-ASSOCIATED RHEUMATIC DISEASES

Detection of Antinuclear Antibodies

Screening for antinuclear antibodies by indirect immunofluorescence
- Has a high sensitivity but a low specificity when a low cutoff titer is used
- Titer and pattern are important to report
- Should be followed by assays that measure specific antibodies
- It is useful to correlate the pattern with the results of specific antibody testing

Screening for antinuclear antibodies by solid phase assays
- It is important to know what antibodies are screened for
- It is important to know the advantages and limitations of the assay (e.g., may not detect all antibodies)

Autoantibodies
- Can have a diagnostic and prognostic value
- Should be interpreted in the clinical context

Detection of Antinuclear Antibodies

Screening Assays

Detection of ANA is classically performed by IIF assay on HEp-2 cells, which is considered a convenient screening assay for autoantibodies in patients suspected to suffer from an ANA-associated rheumatic disease. With IIF, the autoantibodies that bind to the HEp-2 cell substrate are visualized by a fluorescence microscope after staining with fluorescein-labeled anti-human antibodies. The titer of the antibody and the pattern is reported.

Usually a cutoff is suggested for interpretation of the results. The international recommendations by European Autoimmunity Standardization Initiative (EASI) and International Union Immunology Societies (IUIS) propose to use as cutoff the titer that corresponds to the 95th percentile of local age- and gender-matched healthy subjects.[247] Tan et al.[248] reported that such a cutoff corresponds to a titer of 1:160. However, as recognized by the international recommendations, the sensitivity at a 1:160 cutoff is not optimal and a negative result does not exclude an ANA-associated rheumatic disease.[247] The recent SLE classification criteria include ANA with a 1:80 cutoff as an entry criterion.[166] ANA with a 1:80 cutoff has a high sensitivity (98.4%); however, the specificity is low (66.9%).[249] The higher the titer of the ANAs, the higher the chance for a systemic rheumatic disease.[250] In order to circumvent the disadvantage of using a single cutoff (dichotomous interpretation), it has been suggested to report test result specific likelihood ratios.[251]

In addition to the titer, a pattern is reported. The main ANA staining patterns are homogeneous, speckled, nucleolar, and centromere. A consensus on nomenclature and description of the patterns has been proposed by the International Consensus on ANA Patterns (ICAP) initiative (www.ANApatterns.

org).[252–254] Tables 94.10 and 94.11 give an overview of the various nuclear and cytoplasmic patterns that can be distinguished by IIF and Fig. 94.2 shows examples of various patterns. Except for anti-centromere, a pattern does not allow for identification of the target of the antibodies. However, it might give an indication of the underlying specific antibody. As such it can guide follow-up testing for antibodies to dsDNA or antibodies to extractable nuclear antigens (see Tables 94.10 and 94.11).

The nuclear patterns associated with SLE are the homogeneous (anti-dsDNA antibodies), fine speckled (anti-SSA/Ro), and coarse speckled (anti-Sm, anti-RNP) patterns. The nuclear pattern associated with SjS is the fine speckled pattern (anti-SSA/Ro, anti-SSB/La). The nuclear pattern associated with MCTD is the coarse speckled pattern (anti-U11RNP). The nuclear patterns associated with SSc are the centromere (anti-centromere antibodies), nucleolar (anti-PM-Scl, anti-fibrillarin, anti-NOR90 and anti-Ku), TOPO-I and nuclear speckled patterns (anti-polymerase III, anti-Ku). The nuclear patterns associated with the myositis-specific antibodies include the fine speckled patterns for anti-Mi-2 and anti-TIF-1γ autoantibodies, and the multiple nuclear dots patterns for anti-NXP-2 autoantibodies. Anti-Jo-1 antibodies are associated with a fine speckled cytoplasmic pattern and anti-SRP and antibodies to anti-synthetases other than Jo-1 give a dense fine speckled (DFS) cytoplasmic pattern. It has been suggested that anti-HMGCR antibodies are associated with cytoplasmic staining.[255] However, this is not consistently found and may be substrate dependent. Important to mention is the recent interest in the nuclear DFS pattern on HEp-2 cells. The target antigen is lens epithelium-derived growth factor (LEDGF). This pattern can be found (in high titer) in 1 to 8% of healthy blood donors (mainly young females)[256] and in individuals with a wide variety of diseases.[257,258] As microscopic evaluation can be difficult, it is advised that the antibody is confirmed by a specific test for anti-DFS-70 (LEDGF having a molecular weight of approximately 70 kDa). Anti-DFS-70 antibodies can be found in patients with a systemic rheumatic disease, but mono-specificity for anti-DFS-70 (i.e., no other antibodies are present) is considered rare in systemic rheumatic diseases.[257]

IIF might miss anti-SSA antibodies. Thus in case of a high clinical suspicion of the presence of anti-SSA antibodies (e.g., SjS or neonatal lupus) with negative IIF analysis, a specific assay for anti-SSA should be performed. IIF might also miss myositis-specific antibodies, such as for example the anti-synthetase antibody Jo-1.[247] Therefore in case of a clinical suspicion of IIM, a multispecific assay for the whole spectrum of myositis-specific antibodies should be performed.

IIF on HEp2 cells is not only useful to screen for ANA-associated rheumatic diseases, but also for autoimmune hepatitis, PBC, and juvenile idiopathic arthritis. In all these diseases, ANA are part of the diagnostic/classification criteria.[259–262]

Alternative, automated solid-phase assays have gradually been introduced in clinical laboratories to screen for systemic rheumatic diseases.[263] In these assays, the solid phase is coated with a blend of clinically important specific autoantigens. In the more recently developed and comprehensive assays (e.g., from Inova diagnostics and Thermo Fisher), such antigen blends typically include SSA, SSB, dsDNA, Sm, RNP, topoisomerase I, centromere protein B, RNA polymerase III, PM-Scl, Jo-1, Mi-1, PCNA, and, depending on the manufacturer fibrillarin or Ku and Th/To. The exact composition, however, depends on the assay and the manufacturer. These assays are referred to as CTD

TABLE 94.10 Antinuclear Antibody Nuclear Patterns, Associated Clinical Suspicions, and Proposed Follow-up Tests

Nuclear Pattern	AARD		AUTOIMMUNE LIVER DISEASE	
	Clinical Suspicion	Follow-up Test	Clinical Suspicion	Follow-up Test
Homogeneous	SLE	dsDNA	AIH	
		Nucleosome/chromatin		
	JIA			
Dense fine speckled	No AARD (if no ENA)	DFS70		
Centromere	Limited SSc (SjS with SSc)	CENP-B	PBC (with SSc)	
Fine speckled	SjS, SLE, SCLE, NLE, CHB	SSA, SSB		
	IIM	Mi-2, TIF1γ		
	SSc-IIM-SLE overlap	Ku		
Large speckled	SLE	Sm, U1-RNP		
	SSc	RNApol III		
	MCTD	U1-RNP		
Homogenous nucleolar	SSc	Th/To		
	SSc-IIM overlap	PM/Scl		
Clumpy nucleolar	SSc	Fibrillarin		
Punctate nucleolar	SSc, Raynaud, SjS	NOR90		
TOPO-like	SSc	Topoisomerase-1 (Scl-70)		
Multiple nuclear dots	IIM	NXP-2	PBC	Sp100
Few nuclear dots				
Punctate nuclear envelope			PBC	gp210
PCNA-like	SLE	PCNA		

TOPO-like pattern: (1) nuclear compact fine speckled pattern in interphase cells; (2) fine speckled staining of condensed chromatin in mitotic cells; (3) staining of nucleolar organizing region (NOR) (may be obscured); (4) delicate and weak cytoplasmic web-like staining; and (5) inconsistent staining of the nucleoli.[254]

AARD, ANA-associated rheumatic disease; *AIH,* autoimmune hepatitis; *CHB,* congenital heart block; *ENA,* extractable nuclear antigens; *IIM,* idiopathic inflammatory myopathy; *JIA,* juvenile idiopathic arthritis; *MCTD,* mixed connective tissue disease; *NLE,* neonatal lupus erythematosus; *PBC,* primary biliary cholangitis; *PCNA,* proliferating cell nuclear antigen; *SCLE,* subacute cutaneous lupus; *SjS,* Sjögren syndrome; *SLE,* systemic lupus erythematosus; *SSc,* systemic sclerosis.

Table is based on Damoiseaux J, Andrade LEC, Carballo OG, et al. Clinical relevance of HEp-2 indirect immunofluorescent patterns: The international consensus on ANA patterns (ICAP) perspective. *Ann Rheum Dis* 2019;78:879–89.

TABLE 94.11 Anti-Cytoplasmic Antibody Patterns, Associated Clinical Suspicions, and Proposed Follow-up Tests

CYTOPLASMIC PATTERN	AARD		AUTOIMMUNE LIVER DISEASE	
Pattern	Clinical Suspicion	Follow-up Test	Clinical Suspicion	Follow-up Test
Fibrillar linear			AIH type 1	Smooth muscle (F-Actin)
Fibrillar filamentous				
Fibrillar segmental				
Discrete dots				
Dense fine speckled	SLE	Rib-P		
	IIM—necrotizing	SRP		
	IIM—Anti-synthetase syndrome	Anti-synthetases		
Fine speckled	IIM—Anti-synthetase syndrome	Jo-1		
Reticular / AMA	SSc-PBC overlap		PBC	AMA
Golgi-like				

AARD, ANA-associated rheumatic disease; *AIH,* autoimmune hepatitis; *AMA,* anti-mitochondrial antibodies; *IIM,* idiopathic inflammatory myopathy; *PBC,* primary biliary cholangitis; *SLE,* systemic lupus erythematosus; *SSc,* systemic sclerosis.

Table is based on Damoiseaux J, Andrade LEC, Carballo OG, et al. Clinical relevance of HEp-2 indirect immunofluorescent patterns: The international consensus on ana patterns (ICAP) perspective. *Ann Rheum Dis* 2019;78:879–89.

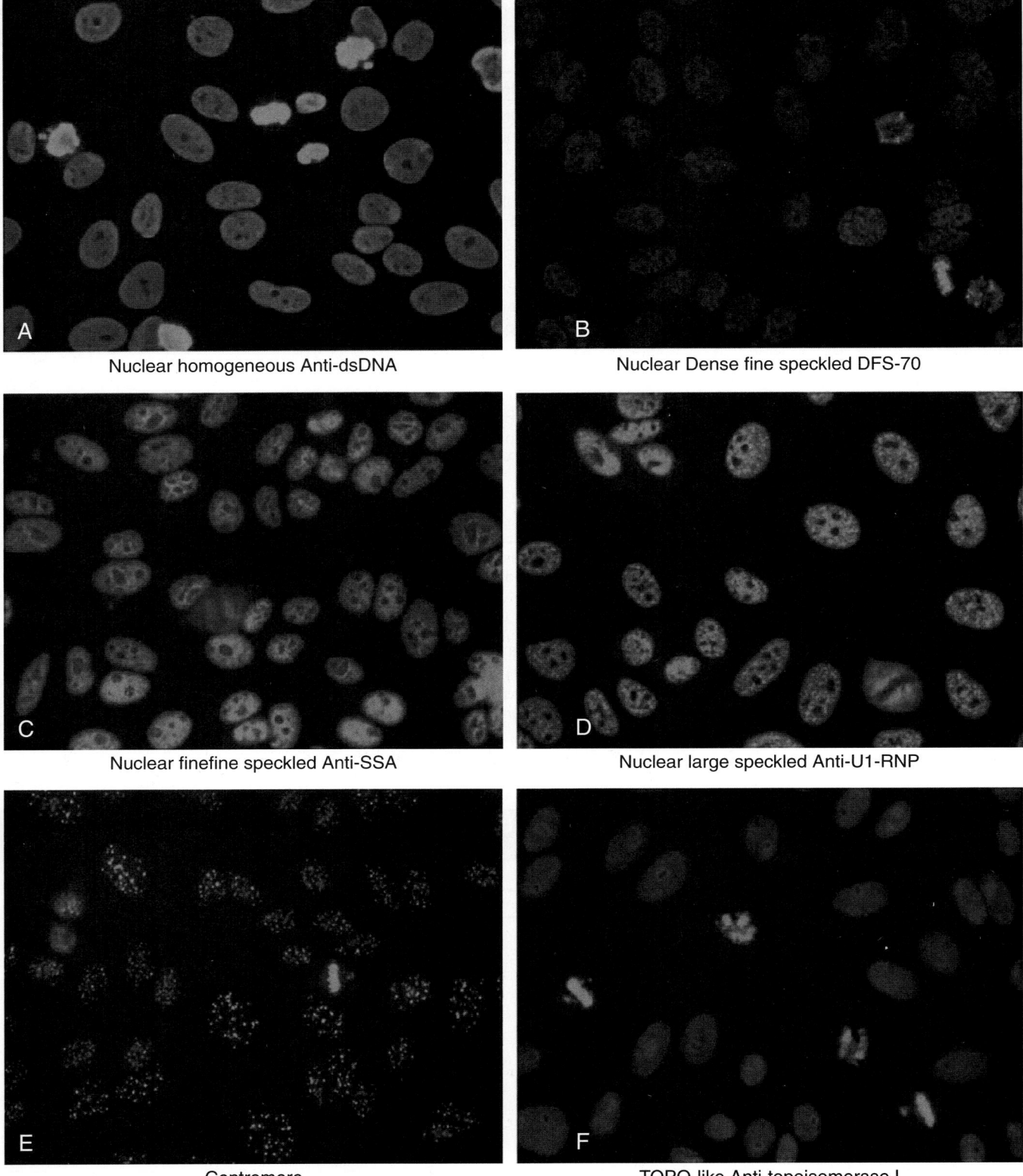

Nuclear homogeneous Anti-dsDNA

Nuclear Dense fine speckled DFS-70

Nuclear finefine speckled Anti-SSA

Nuclear large speckled Anti-U1-RNP

Centromere

TOPO-like Anti-topoisomerase I

FIGURE 94.2 Antinuclear antibody (ANA) indirect immunofluorescence (IIF) on HEp-2 cells. ANAs can produce a variety of nuclear staining patterns on HEp-2 cells, including homogeneous (A), dense fine speckled (B), fine speckled (C), large speckled (D), centromere (E), TOPO-like (F),

Continued

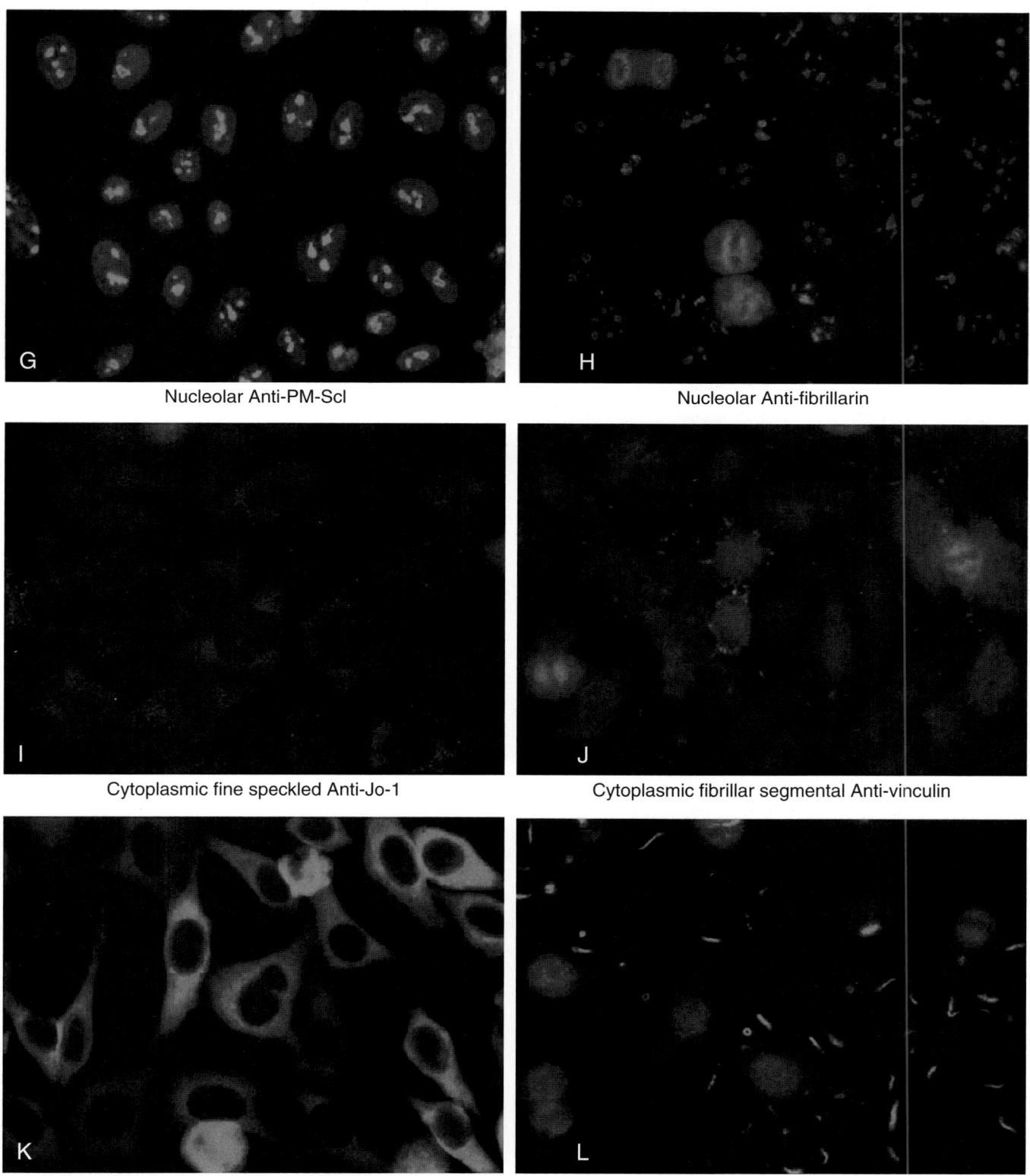

Nucleolar Anti-PM-Scl

Nucleolar Anti-fibrillarin

Cytoplasmic fine speckled Anti-Jo-1

Cytoplasmic fibrillar segmental Anti-vinculin

Cytoplasmic dense fine speckled Anti-PL-12

Cytoplasmic rods and rings

FIGURE 94.2, cont'd and nucleolar (G and H). Each of these patterns can be associated with certain antigen specificities, although follow up testing is generally required for confirmation. Some antibodies produce cytoplasmic patterns, including fine speckled (I), fibrillary segmental (J), dense fine speckled (K), rods and rings (L),

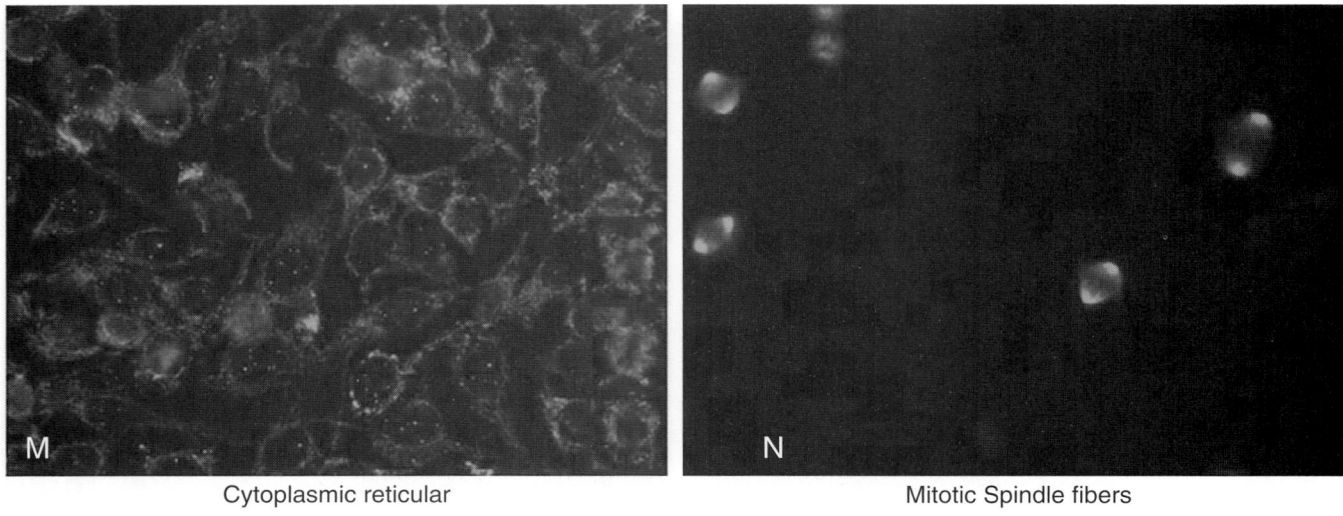

Cytoplasmic reticular

Mitotic Spindle fibers

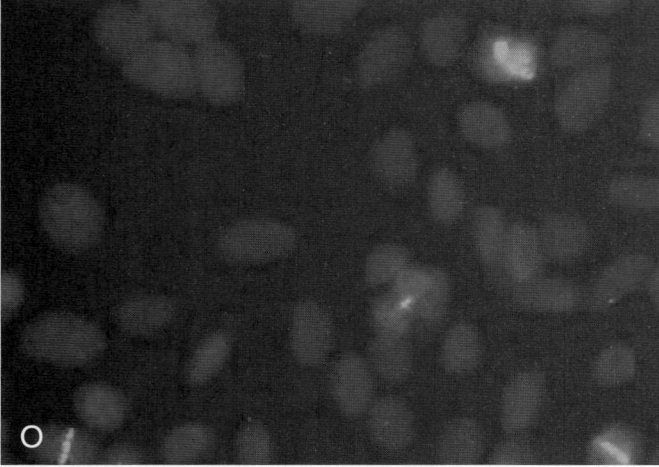

Mitotic Intercellular bridge

FIGURE 94.2, cont'd   and reticular (M). Occasionally, mitotic patterns will be observed, characterized by staining of the dividing cells only, such as spindle fibers (N) and intercellular bridge (O).

screening assays, indicating that they are designed to screen for relevant antibodies in ANA-associated rheumatic diseases. In some assays, such blends of isolated antigens can be supplemented with a cell extract. Autoantibodies that react with the antigens are detected with a detection antibody. Different assay platforms exist: ELISA, FEIA, CLIA, and ALBIA (see Table 94.4).

Most data on the performance of the CTD screen assays is available for the EliA CTD screen assay from Thermo Fisher. Compared to IIF, the major advantages of the solid-phase assays are higher specificity, automation, and reproducibility. A disadvantage of the solid-phase assays, however, is somewhat lower sensitivity compared to IIF. This is mainly the case for SLE and SSc. For SjS, solid phase assays are at least as sensitive as IIF. Combining solid phase assays with IIF yields the most clinically useful information.[264–270]

Specific Assays

In case of a positive screening test (either by IIF or solid-phase assay) follow-up testing is performed in order to identify the target antigen. Direct testing for specific antibodies can also be done in case of a clinical suspicion for a particular disease or a particular antibody.

Several antibodies have initially been identified by immunoprecipitation and immunoprecipitation is still considered a reference technique. However, as it is a manual technique that relies on the use of radiolabeled substances it is not widely available. Alternative (automated) techniques are on hand to test for specific antibodies, including ELISA, FEIA, or CLIA. Also multiplexed assays such as ALBIA, CytoBead, and line/dot blots are frequently used.

It is important to evaluate the technical and clinical performance characteristic of the assays used for identification of specific antibodies. For example, dot blot assays are not standardized and might give different results depending on the assay used.[271] This was most pronounced for antibodies to TIF-1γ antibodies,[271] but differences between assays were also observed for anti-Jo-1 antibodies, which are included in the classification criteria.

It might also be useful to check whether results obtained by assays that detect specific antibodies fit with the results obtained by IIF on HEp-cells. For example, in the majority of cases, anti-dsDNA antibodies should have a homogeneous pattern on IIF analysis and anti-Sm antibodies a coarse speckled pattern. As some line/dot blot systems are prone to weak false-positive results, checking with IIF can have added value. This has for example been shown for anti-SRP antibodies. Ninety-one percent of patients that tested positive for anti-SRP by line/dot immunoassay with the presence of the typical anti-SRP patterns on IIF analysis suffered from IIM compared to only 22% of patients that tested positive with line/dot immunoassay without the typical IIF staining.[272]

RHEUMATOID ARTHRITIS

RA is a chronic disease which is characterized by inflammation of the synovial joints.[273] Although joint damage is one of the hallmarks of RA, many other organ systems may become involved, which is why most physicians and scientists view RA as a systemic condition.[274] Although the pathogenesis is not completely understood, RA is classified as an autoimmune disease based on several characteristics, including production of autoantibodies. In the United States and in Europe, the estimated prevalence is 0.5 to 1.0%. Although RA can be diagnosed at any age, the peak age for onset is 50 years. RA is more prevalent in females, with a female:male ratio of 2:1.[275]

Clinical Symptoms and Complications
Articular Symptoms
The articular manifestations of RA affect, almost exclusively, the synovial diarthrodial joints. The synovial joints are classified based on shape, and include hinge (interphalangeal), saddle (first carpometacarpal), plane (patellofemoral), and ball-and-socket (hip) joints. In RA, it is the interphalangeal joints that are most commonly affected. In the normal synovial joint, the ends of the bone are covered with articular cartilage and are separated by the joint cavity, which is filled with synovial fluid.[276] The synovial fluid is produced by the synovial membrane, which constitutes the inner lining of the joint capsule. The synovial membrane is composed of the subintima (outer layer) and the intima (inner layer). The subintima is acellular, being composed of connective tissue, and is where the synovial blood vessels are located. The intima contains mostly fibroblasts and macrophage-like synovial cells and is normally only a few cells in thickness. In the RA joint, there is intimal hyperplasia, increasing to 8 to 10 cells thick. The subintimal layer becomes infiltrated with a variety of inflammatory cells, along with growth of new blood vessels. This hypertrophied synovium is known as the pannus, which will ultimately invade and erode the joint cartilage and bone if the underlying disease is not treated. Clinical symptoms associated with synovitis are joint stiffness (usually most apparent in the morning), swelling/edema, painful to pressure, and warmth to the touch.[277]

Extra-Articular Complications
In addition to the joint involvement that characterizes RA, other organ systems may become affected, leading to the classification of RA as a systemic autoimmune disease.[278] Although there is no set definition, these manifestations can be classified as extra-articular manifestations of RA or complications/comorbid conditions.[279] Some of the more common extra-articular manifestations are nodules (firm lumps of inflammatory tissue that occur under the skin), Raynaud phenomenon (discoloration of skin in the fingers or toes upon exposure to cold temperatures), and secondary SjS. Other extra-articular manifestations are rarer, but can have a significant impact on mortality; these manifestations include interstitial lung disease, pericarditis/pleuritis, Felty syndrome, and various forms of neuropathy. In addition, there is an increased risk of mortality with other manifestations classified as complications or comorbid conditions. As with many autoimmune diseases, non-Hodgkin lymphoma is more common in RA compared with the general population and is one of the primary causes of accelerated mortality.[280] In addition, there is an increased risk for ischemic heart disease in patients with RA.[281–283]

Disease Pathogenesis
Genetic Risk Factors
RA as a disease develops through a complex process involving genetic and environmental factors.[284] Current models for RA progression hypothesize that a combination of multiple genetic and environmental risk factors work together to break self-tolerance; this is the point when autoimmunity is initiated. As the autoimmune process develops and progresses, the person will eventually reach a point of "preclinical RA." This individual, while still asymptomatic, will have evidence of autoimmunity, including the presence of autoreactive lymphocytes and the production of autoantibodies.[285] After a period of time, which could range from months to years to decades, the patient will develop clinical symptoms of the disease, and ultimately be diagnosed or classified as having RA.

Much of the known genetic risk for developing RA is attributed to a set of MHC alleles referred to as the "shared epitope" (SE).[286] These MHC alleles share certain sequence similarities, specifically at positions 70 to 74 in the third hypervariable region of the DRB chain. A recent classification of the HLA-DRB1 alleles has demonstrated that all the SE alleles have RAA at positions 72 to 74, with variations at positions 70 and 71, which affect the odds ratio (OR) for developing RA.[287,288] Because the SE is near the peptide-binding cleft of the MHC molecule, it has been hypothesized that the associated MHC molecules preferentially present certain self-peptides, which would lead to autoreactive T-cell activation and autoantibody production. Although some studies have data to support this mechanism, other hypotheses have been proposed as well, including effects on the development of the T-cell repertoire in the thymus or having the SE function as an autoantigen.

In addition to the contribution of the MHC alleles, over 100 other genes have been identified as potential risk factors for RA.[289] Some genes, such as *PTPN22*, are involved in the regulation of the immune response. The allele of *PTPN22* associated with RA is a gain-of-function polymorphism, which is purported to lower the threshold for activation of T cells.[290] Another gene identified as a potential risk factor is peptidyl arginine deiminase (PAD).[291] PAD enzymatically deiminates arginine residues in a process known as citrullination (see Fig. 94.1).[292] It is hypothesized that enhanced citrullination could contribute to the breakdown in tolerance, possibly through production of novel self-antigens.

Environmental Risk Factors
The environmental risk factors linked to RA are equally, or even more, complex than the genetic susceptibility. One of the strongest environmental risk factors, which is consistent across multiple studies, is exposure to tobacco smoke.[293] Interestingly, the mechanism by which smoking is thought to

contribute to the development of RA is linked to several of the genetic risk factors, specifically PAD and the SE.[294] Smoking has been shown to lead to increased protein citrullination as mediated by PAD.[295] The gain-of-function mutation in PAD may combine additively or synergistically with smoking to enhance citrullination of certain peptides. This is subsequently linked to the MHC alleles[296]; some studies have demonstrated that citrullinated peptides bind more efficiently to the SE alleles in comparison to the native peptides.[297] This could contribute to the breakdown of tolerance to self-antigens and explain why the effects of smoking are enhanced in individuals who possess the SE.

Other environmental factors have been associated with increased risk for development of RA, although the effects appear to be weaker and with less obvious mechanistic explanations. Female sex is a risk factor for RA, although the exact link is unclear.[298] Increased risk for RA has been associated with early menopause and polycystic ovary syndrome. Hormonal variations are thought to play a role, although the exact etiology is still undefined. Exposure to certain microbes, particularly at the mucosal surfaces, is postulated to contribute to the loss of tolerance, possibly through molecular mimicry. However, a specific organism has yet to be identified. Lastly, a healthy lifestyle characterized by regular physical activity, healthy diet, and low body mass index (BMI) seems to be protective against RA.[298] Why this is the case is not exactly clear, but these are modifiable risk factors that could be important for individuals who are high risk for developing RA.

RHEUMATOID ARTHRITIS-ASSOCIATED AUTOANTIBODIES

The first autoantibody shown to be associated with RA was RF.[299] RF is an autoantibody that specifically binds to the constant region (Fc) of human IgG. RFs themselves can be of the IgM, IgG, or IgA isotype. RFs are detectable in 60 to 80% of patients with RA. Although reasonably sensitive, the specificity of this testing is an issue. RF can be found in other CTDs, including SjS (up to 70%), SLE (up to 30%), and MCTD (up to 25%).[274] RFs are also detected frequently in patients with cryoglobulinemia, up to 70%. The presence of RFs is also associated with a variety of bacterial and viral infections, although these antibodies are often lower in concentration and transient in nature. RF is routinely measured in the clinical laboratory by a variety of methods. Nephelometric assays using IgG-coated latex particles are available; turbidimetric methods are also available on various automated systems. Nephelometry and turbidimetry detect RF of the IgG and IgM isotypes, although it is not possible to distinguish between the two isotypes using these methods. In contrast, immunoassays are able to specifically detect and differentiate between the presence of IgM, IgG, and IgA RFs.

Because RF has limited clinical specificity, physicians and scientists were always on the lookout for improved serology markers for RA.[300] This work led to the discovery of anti-keratin and anti-perinuclear factor autoantibodies.[301,302] Ultimately, it was determined that these autoantibodies were targeting peptides containing citrullinated residues.[73] Collectively, these autoantibodies are referred to as anti-citrullinated peptide antibodies (ACPAs).[303] As described in previous sections, citrullination is an enzymatically mediated post-translational modification resulting from deimination of arginine (see Fig. 94.1). Citrullination can

be found in many different proteins, any of which could be the target of ACPAs.[304] Most studies have shown that ACPAs have a sensitivity of approximately 90% for RA, and a similar specificity. Most testing for ACPAs is done by EIA or MIA.[305] The capture antigens used in these assays are citrullinated peptides that originate from a variety of proteins, including collagen, vimentin, and fibronectin, and the artificial cyclic citrullinated peptide (CCP).[306–308] CCPs are not found in nature, but are useful as in vitro reagents for detection of ACPAs.[309] Variations in sensitivity and specificity can be observed between assays, depending on the included antigen and the repertoire of ACPAs that are detectable.[310–314]

Both RF and ACPAs are associated with the genetic risk factors for RA, being detected at higher frequencies in patients who possess the SE.[315] As stated previously, this suggests that MHC molecules with the SE could preferentially be presenting certain peptides, possibly citrullinated peptides, which lead to autoantibody production. RF and ACPAs are also detectable in individuals prior to development of clinical symptoms.[316] Asymptomatic individuals who are RF or ACPA positive are at increased risk for developing RA.[317] This population is the target of a number of RA prevention trials, the goal of which is to use mild treatment strategies to prevent or delay RA development/progression in high-risk individuals.[318] Individuals diagnosed with RA and who are RF or ACPA positive tend to have more severe disease, have poorer outcomes, and require more aggressive treatment compared to patients who are negative for these autoantibodies.[319–321] This is especially true for individuals who are positive for both RF and ACPA.[322]

Classification Criteria

The diagnosis of RA is based largely on clinical evaluation, with supporting information supplied by laboratory testing. Although diagnostic criteria for RA have yet to be established, the evolution of the diagnostic evaluation, specifically focusing on detection of early RA, can be seen in the change between previous and current classification criteria.[323,324] In 1987, the ACR released classification criteria for RA, which was a revision of criteria from 1958.[325] The 1987 criteria was dominated by clinical evaluation, and included presence of joint morning stiffness of at least 1 hour, arthritis in 3 or more joints, arthritis of the hand joints, symmetrical arthritis, rheumatoid nodules, and evidence of erosions on radiographic evaluation. The only laboratory parameter in the 1987 criteria was positivity for RF. In order to be classified as RA, 4 criteria had to be present. One significant drawback of these criteria is that some of the parameters, including erosions and nodules, are more associated with late disease processes. In 2010, new classification criteria were agreed upon by the ACR and the EULAR.[326] These criteria were simplified in comparison to the 1987 version, as well as targeting individuals with earlier disease and expanding the laboratory parameters (Table 94.12).[327,328] To begin, the 2010 criteria defined an entry criterion, specifically that patients must have at least one joint with definite synovitis for which there is no other pathogenic explanation. These patients are then evaluated for joint involvement (up to five points based on number and size of involved joints), positivity for RF or ACPAs (up to three points), elevated acute phase reactants erythrocyte sedimentation rate (ESR) or C-reactive protein (CRP) (up to one point), and duration of clinical symptoms (up to one point). An individual with six or more points would

TABLE 94.12 2010 EULAR/ACR Classification Criteria for Rheumatoid Arthritis

Criteria Classification	Specific Criteria	Points
Joint involvement	1 large joint	0
	2–10 large joints	1
	1–3 small joints	2
	4–10 small joints	3
	>10 joints (at least 1 small joint)	5
Serology	Negative RF and ACPA	0
	Low-positive RF or ACPA	2
	High-positive RF or ACPA	3
Acute-phase reactants	Normal ESR and CRP	0
	Abnormal ESR or CRP	1
Duration of symptoms	<6 weeks	0
	≥6 weeks	1

ACPA, Anti-citrullinated peptide antibody; *CRP*, C-reactive protein; *ESR*, erythrocyte sedimentation rate; *RF*, rheumatoid factor. Table is based on Aletaha D, Neogi T, Silman AJ, et al. 2010 rheumatoid arthritis classification criteria: An American College of Rheumatology/European League Against Rheumatism collaborative initiative. *Annals Rheum Dis* 2010;69:1580–8.

be classified as having RA. It is interesting to note that the criteria are still dominated by clinical symptoms, as a patient with extensive joint involvement for more than 6 weeks could be classified as RA in the absence of any abnormal laboratory tests. However, positivity for RA and ACPA, even in the context of elevated CRP and ESR, is not sufficient to fulfill the classification criteria. As increasing evidence demonstrates the importance of early intervention in patients with RA, in an attempt to prevent joint damage and other organ involvement, the question of including "preclinical" individuals who are positive for ACPA in the classification criteria will need further discussion.

ANTIPHOSPHOLIPID SYNDROME

Historic Background to Antiphospholipid Antibodies

Antiphospholipid antibodies were first reported in 1906 by Wasserman and colleagues based on the association between syphilis and serum reactivity to PL.[329] This observation led to the development of the Venereal Disease Research Laboratory (VDRL) test for syphilis that is still in use. In 1941, Pangborn identified the PL responsible for the reactivity from bovine heart and called it cardiolipin (CL).[330] Screening of large numbers of patients for syphilis revealed a population of patients with false-positive results. These false-positive results were found to be associated with other infectious diseases and with an increased risk of developing SLE.[331,332] Concurrently, Conley and Hartmann detected a plasma factor that prolonged coagulation time in patients with SLE.[333] Loelinger reported similar findings even when normal pooled plasma was added to the reaction.[334] However, it wasn't until 1963 that this anticoagulant was shown to be associated with thrombosis instead of bleeding.[335] The anticoagulant activity was subsequently shown to also be associated with fetal loss.[336] In 1972, Feinstein and Rappaport called the factor "lupus anticoagulant" (LA),[337] a term that is clearly a misnomer, since not all patients positive for LA have SLE, and LA has anticoagulant effects in vitro and prothrombotic effects in vivo.

A significant milestone in the detection of antibodies to PL (aPL) was the development of a RIA to detect anti-cardiolipin autoantibodies (aCL) in 1983 by Harris and colleagues.[338] The RIA was subsequently replaced with a semi-quantitative ELISA method in 1985.[339] The ELISA was recognized to be significantly more sensitive than the VDRL test for the detection of aCL in patients with SLE, and the antibodies detected demonstrated a strong association with false-positive VDRL results, LA, and thrombosis.[338] Using the aCL ELISA to screen a large population of SLE patients, the authors identified a subset of patients with increased aCL and a high incidence of fetal loss or thrombosis.[340] This condition was initially referred to as the "anticardiolipin syndrome" but was subsequently changed to "antiphospholipid syndrome" (APS) to incorporate the association with LA (Table 94.13).[341]

Antiphospholipid Antibodies and the Pathophysiology of Antiphospholipid Syndrome

The pathogenic mechanisms responsible for thrombosis and obstetric complications in APS are unclear but most likely involve a combination of factors, including aPL antibody activation of cellular elements (endothelial cells, monocytes, and/or platelets), hemostatic reactions, and inflammation, particularly complement activation. In addition, genetic associations between the

TABLE 94.13 Historic Events in the Serologic Evaluation of Antiphospholipid Syndrome

Year	Main Events
1906	Development of the VDRL test for syphilis
1941	Identification of syphilis as a major antigen in the VDRL test
1952	Observation of "false-positive" syphilis test in patients without syphilis reported
1952	Discovery of an inhibitor that prolonged coagulation time in vitro
1954	Initial report correlating prolonged clotting in vitro and pregnancy loss
1963	Initial report of prolonged clotting time and thrombosis
1983	Development of an ELISA for detecting anticardiolipin antibodies
1990	Recognition of beta$_2$ glycoprotein I as a phospholipid binding protein
1991	Discovery of prothrombin a major autoantibody target in antiphospholipid syndrome
1999	Preliminary Sapporo classification criteria for antiphospholipid syndrome
1999	Clinical significance of prothrombin antibodies is dependent of assay principle
2006	Revised 1999 Sapporo classification criteria for antiphospholipid syndrome

ELISA, Enzyme-linked immunosorbent assay; *VDRL*, Venereal Disease Research Laboratory.

production of aPL and predisposition to APS and HLA-DR and HLA-DQ alleles, proinflammatory signaling pathways, genes encoding platelet glycoproteins, and genetic defects in IgA or complement, as well as β₂GPI polymorphisms have been reported.[342–345] The fact that not all patients positive for aPL develop thrombosis or obstetric complications and those that do have varied presentation indicates that aPL are not sufficient to trigger APS in isolation but may instead function to promote or sustain the pathologic response.[346] Thus it has been suggested that two types of aPL exist, functional antibodies with LA activity in vitro contributing to APS disease pathogenesis, and nonfunctional ones which do not seem to play a role in disease.[347,348] This dichotomy in functionality begs the question as to whether aPL are a cause or consequence of APS, which may differ based on the specificity of individual aPL and associated clinical manifestation(s).

A two-hit hypothesis has been suggested for APS-associated thrombosis in which an initial hypercoagulant/proinflammatory environment induced by aPL results in thrombosis after an inciting factor like trauma or infection. Proposed mechanisms by which aPL create a hypercoagulable environment include interference with or inhibition of coagulation factors, impairment of fibrinolytic activity, activation of complement, and direct effects on cell signaling, cytokine, and chemokine production.[349–353]

Although the same aPL are associated with fetal loss and thrombosis in APS, they are believed to cause obstetric disease through different pathogenic mechanisms since the clinical and biological manifestations differ considerably. The pathogenic effects of aPL in obstetric complications are proposed to involve inflammation in the placenta, and inappropriate cytokine/chemokine production which could compromise invasiveness, migration, and/or survival of trophoblasts.[351,352] There are different categories of pregnancy complications and/or morbidity in APS, with various pathogenic mechanisms likely to be of varying importance in different categories. For loss of the conceptus before 10 weeks, issues with placentation and trophoblast migration rather than thrombosis are likely important, while thrombosis may be an important component of premature deliveries due to placental insufficiency.[353] While it is possible that an additional hit is required to induce fetal loss in aPL-positive patients based on differences in presentation and prevalence, whether it is a requirement is less clear since passive transfer of aPL into pregnant mice induces fetal loss.[352]

The heterogeneous nature of aPL poses diagnostic challenges in the context of a number of diseases not necessarily associated with thrombosis or obstetric complications.[353,354] This heterogeneity and lack of specificity also extends to functional and nonfunctional aPL since both types of antibodies may be detected using the same assay(s). Thus it remains to be determined whether different manifestations are caused by subpopulations of autoantibodies against different epitope specificities that are currently detected using the same test(s). Heterogeneity for aPL criteria immunoassays is best described for antibodies to β₂GPI. Antibodies against β₂GPI have been shown to vary in affinity, pathogenicity, and phospholipid dependence.[354] Although β₂GPI-dependent CL testing has been shown to decrease false-positive aCL results associated with certain infectious diseases, animal models have demonstrated production of antibodies to β₂GPI in response to immunization with *H. influenzae*, *N. gonorrhoeae*, and tetanus toxoid.[94] In addition, studies using peptides from

microorganisms with structural similarity to β₂GPI demonstrate induction of β₂GPI antibodies, thrombosis, fetal loss, and inflammation in animal models.[96] Thus the delineation between infectious and noninfectious aPL does not necessarily translate to nonpathogenic and pathogenic (i.e., false versus true positive). It remains to be determined whether molecular mimicry of viral or bacterial antigens leads to the production of pathogenic aPL or if epitope spreading to other autoantigens is required for pathogenicity.[95,96,355] Despite the fact that their exact mechanism(s) of action remains to be determined, there is little doubt that a correlation between the specificity of aPL and the clinical manifestations exists.

APS is also significantly associated with the presence of established cardiovascular diseases, inherited thrombophilia, trauma, age, immobilization, surgery, malignancy, nephrotic syndrome, and the use of oral contraceptives.[356] However, the interplay between these risk factors and APS pathogenesis remains to be clarified. Further knowledge about the role of specific aPL in the pathogenesis of APS should improve both the diagnosis and management of individuals with APS.

Classification of Antiphospholipid Syndrome

In the early 1990s, it was discovered that the antibodies associated with APS did not react solely with PL, but also with their binding proteins either independently or in protein-PL complexes. Some of the antibodies detected in the aCL assay were found to bind β₂GPI in complex with CL,[357,358] and tests utilizing complexes of the two as the antigenic targets were shown to decrease the false-positive rate associated with certain infectious diseases.[357–359] Similarly, LA activity was shown to be dependent on both β₂GPI and prothrombin (PT),[357,359–363] and a number of studies showed that single positivity for anti-β₂GPI was implicated in thrombotic events in the absence of LA or aCL and/or contributed to the better characterization of APS patients.[364–367] Subsequently, testing for IgG and IgM antibodies to β₂GPI was added to the 2006 Sydney revised Sapporo consensus guidelines for the diagnosis of APS.[368]

These criteria presented a significant step in improving the diagnosis and management of patients with APS. The major changes compared with the original Sapporo classification criteria published in 1999[369] were inclusion of medium- or high-titer IgG and IgM anti-β₂GPI antibodies among the laboratory classification criteria, addition of pregnancy morbidity symptoms, and a change in the definition of the interval for persistent aPL positivity from 6 to 12 weeks (Fig. 94.3).[356,368]

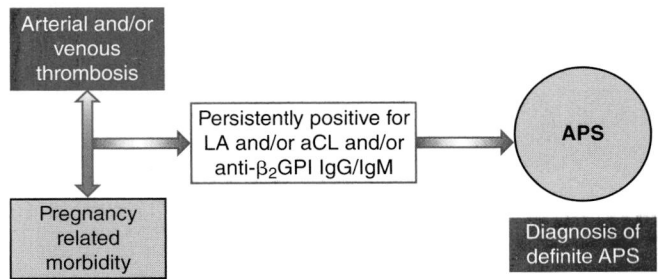

FIGURE 94.3 Current recommendations for the diagnosis of antiphospholipid syndrome. The chart shows the clinical and laboratory criteria for the diagnosis of definite antiphospholipid syndrome *(APS)*. Persistence is defined by positivity separated by at least 12 weeks.

Other significant improvements included two suggestions to categorize patients with APS according to the presence or absence of other acquired or inherited risk factors that may contribute to thrombosis and to sub-classify patients with APS into four different categories according to the extent or type of aPL positivity. The latter is based on evidence suggesting that multiple aPL positivity is associated with a more severe course of the disease.[370] The expert committee also attempted to clarify the definition of medium and high antibody titers and introduced a statement that the threshold for medium antibody titers should be greater than 40 IgG phospholipid units (GPL) or IgM phospholipid units (MPL) (for aCL assays) that can be traced to the Harris standard[2] or greater than the 99th percentile of the reference population (for both aCL and anti-β_2GPI assays).

The main purpose of the original and revised classification criteria was to create common ground for conducting clinical research, exchanging and comparing results, and analyzing data originating from different cohorts, and not for use as diagnostic criteria. Therefore in reality, the diagnosis of APS may still be made by the physician in patients who do not fulfill the requirement of one laboratory or one clinical classification criterion. A main challenge of the laboratory criteria is the definition of the cutoff for medium-positive antibody titers or levels. The suggested threshold of 40 GPL or MPL units for aCL assays is frequently significantly different from the 99th percentile value derived from the reference population.[371,372] In fact, the definition of medium-positive antibody titers depends on the performance characteristics of the particular assay, the calculation method used to determine the cutoff values, and the reference population that is being tested. The revised classification criteria guidance mentioned the lack of suitable evidence and specifically commented that these values are to be used "*until an international consensus is reached.*" The publication also mentioned that the measurement of aCL and anti-β_2GPI antibodies should be performed by "standardized ELISA" methods. In reality, the standardization of these assays is still far from complete.[356] Moreover, some of the widely used tests existed prior to the publication of this guidance, and other newly developed immunoassays may have superior analytical performance compared with the traditional ELISA methodology. Overall, while the 2006 revised Sapporo classification criteria was a major milestone in the diagnosis and management of APS, as new evidence emerges, the classification criteria will require further revision and validation.

Clinical Manifestations and Epidemiology of Antiphospholipid Syndrome

The main clinical features of APS includes thrombosis which could be arterial and/or venous and specific pregnancy-related morbidities as outlined in the 2006 revised Sapporo classification criteria.[368] Neurologic events (chorea, myelitis, and migraine), hematologic abnormalities (thrombocytopenia and hemolytic anemia), livedo reticularis, nephropathy, and valvular heart disease are clinical manifestations not included in the classification criteria but have been reported in a number of APS epidemiologic studies.[368,373–377] In one such report of 1000 APS patients, 53.1% with APS only (primary) and 36.2% affected by SLE and APS (secondary), the most common manifestations were deep vein thrombosis (DVT), thrombocytopenia, livedo reticularis, stroke, and pulmonary embolism (PE).[374] Less frequent features included superficial thrombophlebitis, transient ischemic attacks, hemolytic anemia, and epilepsy. In this series of patients, pregnancy-related morbidities accounted for 14% of the predominant manifestations in female subjects. In rare cases, catastrophic APS (CAPS) associated with the development of excessive thrombosis at multiple sites usually affecting small vessels and leading to multi-organ dysfunction and organ failure have been described.

The true prevalence of APS remains uncertain with wide variabilities reported in different studies. These variations may be due to methodological differences in the diagnostic assays and/or the characteristics of the population evaluated. Some estimates indicate that the incidence of APS is around 5 new cases per 100,000 persons per year and the prevalence around 40 to 50 cases per 100,000 persons. Furthermore, aPL antibodies were found in approximately 13% of patients with stroke, 11% with myocardial infarction, 9.5% of patients with DVT, and 6% of patients with pregnancy-related morbidity.[376] In one healthy population, the incidence of aPL ranged from 1 to 5% and was shown to increase with age and the coexistence of chronic diseases.[373] In this study, the clinical suspicion of APS was significantly increased in young patients who have additional features to the syndrome. It should be noted that aPL antibodies are also found in patients with a variety of clinical conditions such as infections, cancer, and the use of certain drugs including vaccinations. In these conditions, the aPL antibodies are usually transient, demonstrate low-positive reactivity, and are independent of the presence of β_2GPI. The prevalence of aPL antibodies in healthy women of child-bearing age is poorly documented since these antibodies are implicated in pregnancy-related morbidity.

Antiphospholipid Antibody Tests
Anticardiolipin Antibodies

Testing for aCL antibodies can be traced to the development of the RIA by Harris et al. that was subsequently replaced with a semi-quantitative ELISA method.[338,339] The aCL ELISA is sensitive but not specific for APS particularly at low positive levels and certain infections. Despite these limitations, testing for aCL antibodies continues to play a significant role in the diagnosis and management of APS due to its high sensitivity, absence of interference with anticoagulants, ability to test in serum and plasma, as well as ease of testing. With respect to anti-β_2GPI IgG and IgM testing, three groups in 1990 independently reported the identification of β_2GPI (also termed apolipoprotein H) as a critical plasma protein required for the binding of aCL antibodies to CL.[357–359] These studies demonstrated that purified aCL antibodies from patients with APS could bind to CL only in the presence of β_2GPI (β_2GPI-dependent aCL). In contrast, aCL found in patients with syphilis bound to CL in the absence of β_2GPI (β_2GPI-independent aCL). Therefore aCL associated with autoimmune disease (and an increased thrombotic risk) could be distinguished from aCL found in syphilis and other infectious diseases that generally were not associated with an increased thrombotic risk.[357,378] An early study of anti-β_2GPI IgG and IgM tests in patients with APS, SLE, and other CTDs demonstrated that these antibodies were generally not as sensitive (i.e., some aCL-positive patients with definite APS were negative by these assays) as aCL or LA but are more specific for APS.[357]

Anti-Beta2 Glycoprotein I Antibodies

A number of epidemiologic studies and a systematic review of the literature show that anti-β_2GPI antibodies are heterogeneous and the IgG isotype is more strongly associated with thrombosis than IgM and tends to coexist with aCL autoantibodies and/or LAC activity.[357,379-382] In a systematic review, Galli et al. reported that aCL antibodies were not such strong risk factors for thrombosis as LA and were associated with cerebral stroke and myocardial infarction and not DVT.[381] In a 2016 review, Kelchtermans and colleagues found significantly more correlations with thrombosis for aCL IgG and anti-β_2GPI IgG than for their IgM isotype counterparts.[382] Based on this review, unavailability of paired IgG and IgM results for aCL and anti-β_2GPI hampers evaluating the added value of IgM positivity. Thus the role of IgM isotype testing in the evaluation of APS remains controversial.

Lack of Harmonization or "Seronegative" Antiphospholipid Syndrome

Interpretation of aPL antibodies is challenging as antibodies are heterogeneous targeting PLs, PL-binding plasma proteins, and PL-protein complexes (Fig. 94.4). Available immunoassays for the detection of aPL antibodies demonstrate variable performance characteristics likely due to the absence of reference materials necessary for harmonization.[354,356,383] Despite years of use and attempts at standardizing and/or harmonizing the current criteria aPL immunoassays, there is still considerable variability in both the analytical and diagnostic performance characteristics of these tests. Sources of analytical variation in the immunoassays include the types of solid support and methods of immobilization of antigen, the nature and purity of the antigens, composition of diluent, type and composition of reference materials and/or calibrators, difference in reference interval determination, types of calibration, and the methods of detection.[b]

The recognition that aPL represent a heterogeneous group of autoantibodies and that their specificity is poor with respect to certain infectious, autoimmune, or malignant diseases has fueled investigation to identify more specific and reliable markers

---

[b]References 354, 356, 357, 359, 371, 372, and 378.

with better predictive value for the evaluation and management of APS.[377,384,385] Furthermore, reports of patients strongly suspected to have APS, but negative for all three of the current criteria aPL ("seronegative APS") highlights the need for improvement of existing tests and/or the development of additional assays for diagnosis and management. All these factors have led to a persistent search for alternative and more robust biomarkers to effectively diagnose and predict specific clinical manifestations and guide therapeutic management in APS.

"Noncriteria" Antiphospholipid Antibody Tests

Several autoantibodies directed against plasma proteins (β_2GPI, PT, protein C, protein S, and annexin V) or certain PLs and/or their complexes (antiphosphatidic acid [aPA]; anti-phosphatidylinositol (aPI); anti-phosphatidylserine (aPS); anti-phosphatidylethanolamine (aPE); a proprietary mixture of phospholipid antigens (aPhL); antiprothrombin/phosphatidylserine (aPS/PT)] have been recognized and suggested to have diagnostic and/or prognostic relevance for APS.[384-388] The different noncriteria aPL antibodies based on their characteristic are shown in Table 94.14. In addition to aCL and anti-β_2GPI antibodies of IgG and IgM isotypes, aCL IgA and anti-β_2GPI IgA specificities have also been reported to be of diagnostic utility in some patients at risk for APS.[386,387] Studies on the use on negatively charged PL assays such as aPS, aPI, and aPA do not demonstrate significant improvement in the diagnosis of APS except for possibly aPS in patients with pregnancy-related morbidities associated with disease.[388-390] Increased understanding of specific immune targets such as PS/PT and domain I of β_2GPI protein in APS and their potential role(s) in the pathophysiology of disease suggest that these molecules may provide diagnostic, prognostic, and/or therapeutic clues.[385]

Recent efforts to better diagnose, estimate, or stratify patients with APS or at risk for specific clinical manifestations have focused on understanding the performance characteristics of aPS/PT IgG/IgM and anti-domain I IgG antibodies. To address these needs, markers have been evaluated alone or together with respect to current criteria aPL using diverse strategies; alternative to current diagnostic paradigms, additional benefits to current tests ("seronegative" gaps), markers of disease stratification, as well as risk assessment in case of aPL carriers.[391-405]

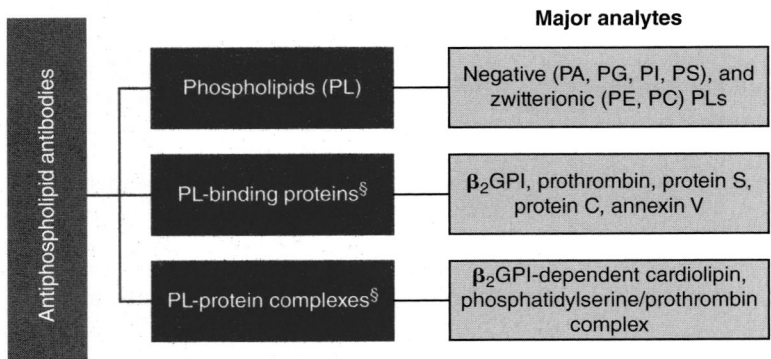

Major analytes

Antiphospholipid antibodies
- Phospholipids (PL) → Negative (PA, PG, PI, PS), and zwitterionic (PE, PC) PLs
- PL-binding proteins[§] → β_2GPI, prothrombin, protein S, protein C, annexin V
- PL-protein complexes[§] → β_2GPI-dependent cardiolipin, phosphatidylserine/prothrombin complex

FIGURE 94.4 Antiphospholipid antibodies have diverse targets with varying clinical implications. The presence of these targets is thought to have pathologic roles in antiphospholipid syndrome (APS), have the potential to more accurately diagnose disease, and influence the design of targeted therapies. The major analytes for each group are shown. *PA,* Phosphatidic acid; *PC,* phosphatidylcholine; *PE,* phosphatidylethanolamine; *PG,* phosphatidylglycerol; *PI,* phosphatidylinositol; *PS,* phosphatidylserine.

TABLE 94.14   Noncriteria Antiphospholipid Antibodies of Interest

Analyte	Isotype(s)
Cardiolipin, aCL	IgA
Beta$_2$ glycoprotein I, anti-β$_2$GPI	IgA
Prothrombin, aPT	IgG and IgM
Phosphatidylserine/Prothrombin complex (aPS/PT)	IgG and IgM
Domain 1 beta$_2$ glycoprotein I domain 1 (aDI)	IgG
APhL[a]	IgG and IgM
Annexin V	IgG and IgM
Negatively (anionic charge) phospholipids[b]	IgG and IgM
Zwitterionic (no net charge) phospholipids[c]	IgG and IgM

[a]APhL, Proprietary mixture of phospholipids (PLs) and PL-binding protein.
[b]Negatively charged PLs (PG, phosphatidylglycerol; PS, phosphatidylserine; PI, phosphatidylinositol).
[c]Zwitterionic PL (PE, phosphatidylethanolamine; PC, phosphatidylcholine.)

Anti-Prothrombin/Phosphatidylserine Antibodies

Antibodies targeting human prothrombin alone (aPT) by ELISA was first reported in 1995.[406] Subsequent studies demonstrated that aPT antibodies were heterogeneous and bind not only to PT coated on gamma-irradiated or activated polyvinyl chloride ELISA plates but also to PT exposed to immobilized phosphatidylserine (PS/PT).[407,408] Funke and colleagues reported that aPS/PT antibodies conferred an OR of 2.8 for venous thrombosis and 4.1 for arterial thrombosis in patients with SLE.[409] In a Japanese cohort, the presence of aPS/PT antibodies conferred an OR of 3.6 for APS in patients with systemic autoimmune diseases.[410] A subsequent study by Bertolaccini and colleagues confirmed the association between aPS/PT IgG and/or IgM isotype with arterial and/or venous thrombosis.[408] In this study, the sensitivity and specificity of aPS/PT for the diagnosis of APS were higher to that of aCL and their presence was not attributable to cross-reactivity with aCL or anti-β$_2$GPI. In addition, aPS/PT antibodies strongly correlated with the presence of LA suggesting that aPS/PT marker may be used as a "screening" or "confirming" assay for APS-associated LA.[408,410] Early recognition of the relative increased sensitivities and correlations with LA of aPS/PT compared to aPT antibodies has prompted a number of recent studies that have examined the relationships between APS-related clinical features, current criterial aPL tests, and the presence of aPS/PT.[391-400] Some of these studies have confirmed an incremental diagnostic role for aPS/PT antibodies for APS,[388,390-392] the positive correlation between aPS/PT IgG and LA,[392,394,395] as well as the relevance of aPS/PT IgG in stratification of patients with thrombosis[393-397] and intrauterine growth retardation in APS.[398] In one recent study, type I and II novel subpopulations of aPS/PT IgG antibodies had different mechanisms of PT recognition and function indicating the possibility of further stratifying patients with thrombosis if independently confirmed.[411] With respect to aPL carriers or persistence of aPL antibodies,[410] there is emerging data for the role of aPS/PT antibodies in risk stratification and diagnosis as these antibodies appear to be stable over the period of investigation.[396,399,412]

Anti-Domain I IgG Antibodies

β$_2$GPI is recognized as one of the most important antigens implicated in the pathophysiology of APS.[413] The protein consists of 326 amino acids organized in five complement control protein domains with the first four comprised of 60 amino acids except for domain five with 82 amino acids. Autoantibodies targeting β$_2$GPI are recognized to be diverse and may target different epitopes in the different domains. The first study to show that the presence of anti-domain I antibodies was found to be better associated with predominantly venous thrombosis, compared to reactivities against the whole protein or other domains.[414] This observation was confirmed in a double-blinded multicenter study including 442 patients all positive for anti-β$_2$GPI antibodies.[415] Anti-domain I antibodies were shown to be present in the plasma in 55% of patients, the majority of whom had a history of thrombosis, resulting in an OR of 3.5 (2.3 to 5.4, 95% confidence interval). Interestingly, the presence of these antibodies was also associated with pregnancy-related morbidity. Another early study by Banzato and colleagues showed that APS patients with triple aPL antibody positivity (i.e., positive for LA, aCL IgG, and anti-β$_2$GPI IgG) had the highest risk for thrombosis and that this population of patients had a significantly higher prevalence of anti-domain I antibodies when compared to those with single or double aPL positivity.[416] There is considerable evidence for a central role for domain I of β$_2$GPI in APS disease stratification based on several recent reports in patients with APS and aPL antibody carriers.[401-405]

ANTIPHOSPHOLIPID SYNDROME

Revised 1999 Sapporo Classification Criteria for the Diagnosis of Antiphospholipid Syndrome

Laboratory Criteria
- Presence of lupus anticoagulant
- IgG or IgM aCL antibodies
  - Moderate or high titer (>40 GPL or MPL units or >99th percentile for the testing laboratory
- IgG or IgM anti-β$_2$GPI antibodies
  - >99th percentile for the testing laboratory according to recommended procedures
- Documentation of persistent positivity on two or more occasions at least 12 weeks apart

Clinical Criteria
- Vascular thrombosis
  - Arterial and/or venous thrombosis
  - Confirmed by imaging or histopathology
  - Histopathology: thrombosis without significant evidence of inflammation
- Pregnancy-related morbidity
  - ≥1 unexplained fetal death at or beyond 10 weeks of gestation
  - ≥1 premature birth before 34 weeks
- Eclampsia or severe preeclampsia or feature of placental insufficiency
  - ≥3 unexplained consecutive spontaneous abortions before 10 weeks

At least one criterion of laboratory and clinical criteria must be met for a diagnosis of APS to be made.

Immunoassays Detecting Antiphospholipid Antibodies

Immunoassays to detect aPL antibodies provide clinicians with additional information that is not obtainable with the LA tests. This information includes detection of specific aPL analytes, their isotype class (IgG or IgM), and their relative concentrations (levels) important for risk estimation and stratification. More important, the solid-phase immunoassays are not significantly affected by analytical variables like the functional-based LA assays. For example, the use of anticoagulation (oral or subcutaneous) or anti-platelet therapy may interfere with LA testing.

Since the development of the initial ELISA to detect aCL antibodies, a number of immunoassays of similar principles as those of the ELISA have been developed and implemented in the clinical laboratories as shown in Table 94.15. These non-ELISA methods include tests to detect single or multiple antibody specificities such as line immunoassays (LIAs) and ALBIAs, or CLIAs and the FEIAs for single aPL measurements.[356,383,386,387,417–422] Except for LIA, which is not widely used, criteria aPL are routinely tested by ELISA, ALBIA, CIA, and FEIA in clinical diagnostic laboratories. Testing for aPS/PT antibodies is currently limited to the ELISA method,[411] and the anti-domain 1 to the CIA and ELISA methodologies.[421] The immunoassays for the detection of all aPL tests have been developed in the absence of internationally acceptable standards; as such their performance characteristics are largely dependent on conditions established by the respective manufacturers.[354,356] These include the assay plates and other types of solid phases, buffers (blocking, sample diluents, and washing), standards and reference preparations for quality control and assurance, as well as units of measurements. Recent studies comparing the detection of aCL and anti-β_2GPII antibodies across platforms indicate that there appears to be differences between methods without significant influence on the diagnostic outcome for APS.[419,420] However, correlations between triple aPL antibody positivity have been reported to depend on the types of immunoassays used.[422]

Currently, aPS/PT and anti-domain I antibodies are tested using a limited number of immunoassays. Thus very few groups have examined the relative performance of available aPS/PT tests[412,423–425] and anti-domain 1 antibodies.[426] However, investigations from independent studies have demonstrated similar diagnostic performance characteristics in APS for the most part. For aPS/PT assays, these investigations report acceptable agreements (Cohen Kappa) and/or positive correlations and predictions for clinical manifestations for APS with the aPS/PT IgG assays.[423–425] The correlations between the aPS/PT IgM kits range from weak to moderate, and

TABLE 94.15 Characteristics of Common Immunoassays for Antiphospholipid Antibodies

Characteristics	ELISAs	Other Solid-Phase Immunoassays[a]	Multiplexed Bead Immunoassays
Type of solid phase	Usually 96-well microtiter plate	Uniformly sized paramagnetic microparticles or individual wells	Uniformly sized paramagnetic microparticles
aCL/β_2GPI attachment/wash buffer	Adsorption/detergent in aCL wash buffer may not be allowed	Passive absorption or covalent coupling/detergent in aCL wash buffer may not be allowed	Covalent coupling/detergent in aCL wash buffer allowed
Anti-human Ig	Enzyme-conjugated anti-human immunoglobulin	Enzyme-, isoluminol-, or acridinium-conjugated anti-human Ig	Fluorochrome-conjugated anti-human Ig
Detection method/readout	Colorimetric/absorbance	Light detection/chemiluminescence, fluorescence	Fluorescence
Automated vs. manual	Manual or semiautomated	Fully automated	Fully automated
Internal controls	Internal controls not included	Internal controls included	Internal controls included
Equipment type	Microplate reader with filters. Manual or semiautomated processing instruments	Specialized equipment, closed system	Specialized equipment, closed system
Economic use	Samples may or may not be batched	Generally continuous random access, with no batching required	Continuous random access, no batching required, multiplexed results
Sensitivity to environmental factors	Sensitive	Not sensitive; controlled reaction conditions	Not sensitive; controlled reaction conditions
Time to first result	1.5–2 h	<1 h	<1 h
Random access	No	Yes	Yes
Calibration	Calibrators have to be assayed with every run	Stored calibration curves	Stored calibration curves
Analytical sensitivity	Medium to high	High to very high	Very high
AMR	Narrow	Potentially wide	Potentially wide
Precision	Medium to high (10–15%)	Very high (<10%)	Very high (<10%)
Calculation of results	Manual (plotting) or with special software	Automatic (stored curve)	Automated (stored curve)

[a]Assays except multiplex immunoassays. *aCL*, Anticardiolipin; *AMR*, analytical measurement range; *β2GPI*, $\beta_2$glycoprotein I; *ELISA*, enzyme-linked immunosorbent assay; *Ig*, immunoglobulin.

TABLE 94.16 Characteristics of Antiphospholipid Antibodies in Antiphospholipid Syndrome

	Description
1	Risk for antiphospholipid syndrome (APS) is dependent on antiphospholipid (aPL) antibody characteristics
2	Of the criteria aPL, lupus anticoagulant has the best predictive value for APS
3	Triple aPL positivity is associated with high risk for a first thrombotic event and recurrence
4	Correlation between anti-domain I IgG and triple aPL positivity is dependent on characteristics of immunoassays used
5	IgG aPL not IgM antibodies confer higher risk.
6	"Medium-to-high" IgG anti-cardiolipin (aCL) antibodies associated with increased risk for thrombosis
7	Anti-beta$_2$ glycoprotein IgG is least sensitive but most specific of criteria aPL tests
8	Antibody "levels" and units are not commutable between different assays
9	Low-positive (95th–99th percentile) aPL antibodies *may* have limited clinical significance
10	Role of isolated IgM aPL antibodies in APS remains uncertain

do not consistently associate with the APS manifestations and LA activity. With respect to anti-domain 1 IgG antibodies, a recent report by Yin et al suggested that optimal exposure of the highly cryptic epitope containing Glycine40-Arginine43 (G40-R43) is critical and may be responsible for inconsistent results in the correlations between assays and for clinical symptoms.[426]

With respect to the units and reference intervals for reporting and interpreting aPL antibody test results, recent studies reporting on aPS/PT and anti-domain 1 assays have not adhered to the revised Sapporo guidance. Reference intervals established based on 97th and 99th percentiles with varying number of normal controls,[427,428] as well as the mean plus 10 standard deviations[429] have been employed. While most studies on anti-domain 1 antibodies have been performed using the in-house ELISA and commercial CIA methods, no formal direct comparisons have been published. Thus the same challenges experienced with other aPL tests are likely to apply. Overall, the interpretation of aPL antibodies in APS is dependent on a number of variables attributable to analytical and clinical characteristics (Table 94.16).

Laboratory Approaches For Antiphospholipid Antibody Testing

Testing for LA and IgG and IgM antibodies for aCL and anti-β$_2$GPI is currently recommended for the evaluation of APS. A number of studies have examined the use of aPS/PT antibodies and/or anti-domain IgG in various combinations with current criteria aPL tests to determine the optimal diagnostic approach for evaluating patients at-risk for disease.[c] Given the heterogeneity of the APS disease cohorts, the variability of the analytes (aPL), diversity of platforms and the way patients are diagnosed with APS, no consensus has emerged. Comparisons between criterion and noncriterion aPL biomarkers are limited by the lack of acceptable standards. Thus the estimates of the diagnostic performance of criterion markers are likely to be biased due to the fact that these tests are part of the laboratory criteria for APS. In contrast, estimates for the noncriterion makers do not suffer from incorporation bias. Because of this, it is difficult to make a direct comparison of the diagnostic performance of

criterion and noncriterion markers. This type of bias is known as incorporation bias. Studies with incorporation bias will overestimate diagnostic performance.[430] The impact of incorporation bias should be considered when making such comparisons as the incremental value of new biomarkers for APS will depend on the criteria used to identify cases. A new biomarker that is highly correlated with criterion biomarkers may offer some operational advantages but would provide little or no additional diagnostic information. Thus studies on the utility of novel biomarkers are subject to potential selection bias depending on the distribution of criterion biomarkers that were used in the initial diagnosis.[400] De Craemer et al. (2016) investigated the role of anti-domain 1 antibodies in the diagnosis and risk stratification of APS and showed their relevance in predicting thrombosis and triple aPL positivity.[402] A subsequent study by Chayou and colleagues showed that identification of APS patients with high risk for thrombosis associated with triple aPL positivity is dependent on the assays used to detect aCL and anti-β$_2$GPI antibodies.[422] This observation implies careful examination of existing tests for APS and their correlations with anti-domain 1 antibodies by clinical laboratories prior to their adoption. Compared to anti-domain 1 antibodies, the evaluation of aPS/PT as a diagnostic marker has focused on its correlations with LA and alternative to aCL testing given its high sensitivity.[334,336,337,362,363] In a recent investigation, the use of aPS/PT antibodies and anti-domain I antibodies were proposed as first-line noncriteria aPL tests.[395] Given the consistent characterizations and availability of commercial tests with comparable analytical performance characteristics to current criteria aPL antibody assays, it appears logical to integrate aPS/PT antibodies and anti-domain I testing in patients at risk for APS who are "seronegative" in criteria tests. In addition, both markers may be useful when current tests are equivocal for APS or in the case of aPL carriers.

In conclusion, the clinical laboratory plays a significant role in the evaluation of APS. A definite diagnosis of APS is difficult as there are numerous nonautoimmune causes of thrombosis and pregnancy-related morbidity. Misdiagnosis of APS can have significant adverse consequences. Thus the goal is to develop and standardize the most comprehensive, sensitive, specific, reliable, robust, and cost-effective panel of aPL tests that ideally will only detect clinically relevant antibodies.

[c]References 391–398, 401–404, 416, 425, 427, and 428.

VASCULITIS

Vasculitis is defined as an inflammation of the blood vessel wall. This inflammation can occur in arteries or veins of any size. Because of the breadth of potentially affected vessels, the clinical features of the systemic vasculitides can vary significantly. The vasculitides are categorized according to size of the involved vessels, specifically large-, medium-, and small-vessel disease.[431] The large-vessel vasculitides affect the aorta and its major branches, and the corresponding veins. The medium-vessel vasculitides primarily show involvement of the main and initial branches of the visceral arteries and veins, while the small-vessel diseases impact the intraparenchymal arteries, arterioles, capillaries, venules, and veins. Despite the commonality of an inflammatory process within the vessel walls, there is significant variation in the pathologic mechanisms that lead to development of the different vasculitides. In addition, the manner in which a specific diagnosis is established is dependent upon the category of disease, with the clinical laboratory playing a role primarily in the diagnosis of small-vessel vasculitides.[432] This section will provide an overview of the large-, medium-, and small-vessel categories, although particular attention will be given to the vasculitides for which the laboratory makes a substantial contribution to the diagnostic evaluation (Table 94.17).

Large-Vessel Vasculitides

Takayasu arteritis (TAK) and giant cell arteritis (GCA) are large-vessel vasculitides which primarily affect the aorta and its major branches.[433,434] The pathology of both diseases shows

TABLE 94.17   Characteristics of Large-, Medium-, and Small-Vessel Vasculitides

Category	Subcategory	Diseases	Description	Role of the Laboratory in Diagnostic Evaluation
Large-vessel	NA	Takayasu arteritis	Granulomatosus arteritis affecting the aorta and its major branches	Limited to assessment for inflammatory response (CRP and ESR)
		Giant cell arteritis	Granulomatosus arteritis affecting the aorta and its major branches, with particular involvement of the extracranial branches of the carotid artery	
Medium-vessel	NA	Polyarteritis nodosa	Necrotizing arteritis that is acute in presentation and sometimes associated with HBV infection	Assessment for HBV status, based on evidence as risk factor
		Kawasaki disease	Necrotizing arteritis that is characterized by mucocutaneous lymph node syndrome and occurs almost exclusively in children	None
Small-vessel	Immune complex-mediated	Anti-GBM disease	Caused by antibody specific for type IV collagen, leading to immunoglobulin deposits in renal and pulmonary basement membranes	Detection of anti-GBM antibodies
		Cryoglobu-linemic vasculitis	Caused by immunoglobulins which precipitate at temperatures lower than 37 °C, leading to deposition in the capillaries, venules, and arterioles	Quantitation and characterization of cryoglobulins
		IgA vasculitis	Characterized by deposition of ICs in capillaries, venules, and arterioles which are predominantly composed of IgA1	None
	ANCA-associated	Granulomatosus with polyangiitis	Necrotizing, pauci-immune vasculitis characterized by presence of granulomas and involvement of upper respiratory system, lungs, and kidneys	Detection of ANCAs by IIF and anti-PR3/anti-MPO antibodies by immunoassay
		Microscopic polyangiitis	Necrotizing, pauci-immune vasculitis without granuloma formation that primarily targets the kidneys and lungs	
		Eosinophilic granulomatosus with polyangiitis	Necrotizing, pauci-immune vasculitis characterized by presence of granulomas and extravascular eosinophils, often associated with asthma, nasal polyps, and eosinophilia	

ANCA, Anti–neutrophil cytoplasmic antibody; *Anti-GBM*, anti-glomerular basement membrane; *CRP*, C-reactive protein; *ESR*, erythrocyte sedimentation rate; *HBV*, hepatitis B virus; *ICs*, immune complexes; *IIF*, indirect immunofluorescence; *MPO*, myeloperoxidase; *PR3*, proteinase 3.

granulomatous inflammation.[435] A granuloma is a tightly organized collection of macrophages, some of which may fuse together to form multinucleated giant cells. Interestingly, the epidemiology of the twp diseases is very different. The incidence of TAK is very low, only 1 to 2 cases/1 million population/year, making epidemiologic studies very difficult. However, it appears that the incidence rates are highest in Asia and South America, while GCA is most frequently found in northern Europe and in North American individuals of Scandinavian descent. The peak age of incidence is an important diagnostic clue. TAK occurs prior to the age of 50 years, with GCA being diagnosed almost exclusively in patients above the age of 50.[431] One commonality between the two diseases is a female predominance.

GCA primarily affects the aorta and extracranial branches of the carotid artery, which leads to the classic clinical symptoms of severe headache and scalp tenderness.[436] Patients with GCA are at risk for blindness, stroke, and aortic aneurysm. Patients with TAK commonly have bruit, reflecting turbulent blood flow due to narrowing of the artery, and claudication, particularly in the arms or legs. Some patients may have reduced or absent pulse, or asymmetrical blood pressure. In both conditions, a systemic acute phase response may be observed, with significant elevation in ESR or CRP. However, this has limited diagnostic utility as neither marker is specific for the large-vessel vasculitides. In addition, some patients, despite significant inflammation in the blood vessel, may have relatively normal ESR and CRP results. Laboratory testing is generally not useful for the diagnosis of the large-vessel vasculitides. TAK is usually diagnosed by angiogram or magnetic resonance imaging, while GCA generally relies on biopsy of the temporal artery.

Medium-Vessel Vasculitides

The medium-vessel diseases are unique within the vasculitides. Polyarteritis nodosa (PAN) and Kawasaki disease (KD) are both characterized by necrotic inflammation of medium-sized vessels.[435] Both are acute conditions that generally do not recur, in comparison to the chronic, relapsing inflammation of other vasculitides.[437] There have been no genetic risk factors identified for either PAN or KD. A strong environmental risk factor for PAN is infection with hepatitis B virus (HBV), although the exact etiology of how this leads to vessel inflammation is not known.[438] An infectious cause for KD is also suspected although the specific organism has not been identified.[439] The likelihood of an infectious trigger is high, given that the condition primarily affects children less than 2 years of age. The clinical features of KD are defined by mucocutaneous lymph node syndrome, which is characterized by oral mucosal changes ("strawberry" tongue, dry lips), skin lesions, bilateral conjunctivitis, and lymphadenopathy. The clinical features of PAN include erythematous nodules/ulcers of the skin, peripheral neuropathy, myalgias which may be accompanied by elevated muscle enzymes, and visceral pain and dysfunction. The diagnosis of PAN is usually based on biopsy which shows necrotizing vasculitis and imaging studies which could show evidence of pseudoaneurysm, visceral infarcts, or gut perforation.[440] Interestingly, while PAN shows no evidence of an autoimmune etiology, KD has been associated with the presence of anti-endothelial cell antibodies (AECA).[441] Although the autoantigen has not been conclusively identified, tropomyosin has been postulated as a potential target of the autoimmune response. Detection of AECA is not used routinely for diagnosis of KD, which still requires biopsy or imaging evaluation.

In the spring of 2020, cases of a Kawasaki-like disease associated with SARS-CoV-2 infection were reported.[442,443] This condition was ultimately given the designation "multisystem inflammatory syndrome in children" (MIS-C). Patients with MIS-C can present with symptoms similar to KD, including fever, rash, oral mucosal redness, and dilation of conjunctival blood vessels.[444] However, these are relatively nonspecific findings, and the epidemiology of MIS-C and KD are substantially different, including the age and ethnicity of affected children. The US Centers for Disease Control and Prevention (CDC) has developed a case definition for MIS-C.[445] This case definition includes fever of $\geq$38.0 °C and laboratory evidence of an inflammatory response in an individual less than 21 years of age who demonstrates evidence of severe illness requiring hospitalization with more than two organ systems involved AND for which there is no other reasonable diagnosis AND a positive molecular, serologic, or antigen test for SARS-CoV-2 (current or recent) or exposure to a confirmed case during 4 weeks prior to symptom onset. There is currently no specific treatment for MIS-C, and care focuses on anti-inflammatory agents, fluid resuscitation, and respiratory support.

Small-Vessel Vasculitides

Small-vessel vasculitides are characterized, pathologically, by necrotizing vasculitis of intraparenchymal arteries, arterioles, capillaries, and venules.[435] There are two subclasses of small-vessel vasculitides—IC-mediated and ANCA-associated.[431] The IC-mediated diseases include anti-glomerular basement membrane (GBM) disease, cryoglobulinemic vasculitis, IgA vasculitis, and hypocomplementemic urticarial vasculitis (HUV). The ANCA-associated small-vessel vasculitides are microscopic polyangiitis (MPA), granulomatosus with polyangiitis (GPA), and eosinophilic granulomatosus with polyangiitis (EGPA). These two subclasses are distinguished from one another by an interesting pathologic finding: IC-mediated small-vessel vasculitides are characterized by significant IC and complement deposition in the vessel wall, while ANCA-associated diseases have little to no Ig detectable in the vessel wall. In addition, the ANCA-associated vasculitides are defined by their association with various ANCAs.[446] ANCAs are so named because they bind to antigens in the neutrophilic granules and produce cytoplasmic staining patterns.

Immune Complex–Mediated Small-Vessel Vasculitides

Anti–glomerular basement membrane disease. Anti-GBM disease is a classic autoantibody-mediated autoimmune disease.[447] In this small-vessel vasculitis, anti-GBM autoantibodies, which are specific for the α3 chain of type IV collagen, deposit in the basement membranes of capillaries in the kidney and lungs.[448] Formation of in situ ICs in the kidneys can lead to acute glomerulonephritis, while deposits in the lungs can result in alveolar hemorrhage. The combination of pulmonary and renal involvement is referred to as Goodpasture syndrome.

Detection of anti-GBM antibodies is an important part of the diagnosis of this condition. This is generally accomplished using an immunoassay with type IV collagen as the capture antigen. Because the glomerulonephritis can be rapidly progressive, and with the risk of pulmonary hemorrhage, treatment for anti-GBM disease must be initiated quickly. As anti-GBM antibodies are clearly pathologic, initial treatment usually involves removal of the autoantibodies from circulation. This is accomplished by either plasmapheresis or plasma exchange. In order to gauge the success of this treatment strategy, clinicians will frequently monitor serial measurements of the anti-GBM antibody.

Cryoglobulinemic vasculitis. Cryoglobulinemic vasculitis is caused by deposition of cryoglobulins in the capillaries, venules, or arterioles.[449] Cryoglobulins are Igs that precipitate out of solution at temperatures lower than 37 °C. Precipitation and deposition of the cryoglobulin leads to activation of complement and occlusion of the small vessels. The most common clinical symptoms associated with cryoglobulinemic vasculitis are skin lesions, arthralgias, and peripheral neuropathy.[450] There are three types of cryoglobulins.[451] Type I cryoglobulins consist of a monoclonal Ig and are generally associated with a B-cell lymphoproliferative disorder such as multiple myeloma or Waldenstrom macroglobulinemia. Type II and type III cryoglobulins are referred to as mixed cryoglobulins. Type II cryoglobulins are composed of a monoclonal Ig with polyclonal Ig, while a type III cryoglobulin is composed only of polyclonal Ig. Type II and type III cryoglobulins are usually characterized by RF activity of the monoclonal Ig or one of the polyclonal Igs, respectively. Type II and type III cryoglobulins are most strongly associated with HCV infection; however, these types of cryoglobulins can also be detected in individuals with other infections or with various autoimmune diseases.

Laboratory testing for cryoglobulins involves measuring the amount of protein that precipitates at cold temperatures and characterizing the precipitated Igs.[452,453] Serum is chilled up to 24 hours and then visually inspected for the presence of precipitate. If precipitate is present, the sample is centrifuged and the amount of precipitate is measured and reported as a percentage of the total volume. The isolated precipitate is washed and re-dissolved at increased temperature. These proteins are then characterized by immunofixation electrophoresis to detect the isotype and clonality of the Ig(s). Correct preanalytical procedures are key to this testing. Samples should be collected in warmed red-top serum tubes, and maintained at 37 °C through the clotting and centrifugation processes. If samples are not kept at 37 °C, there is a risk that the cryoglobulin could precipitate and be centrifuged out of the serum with the cellular blood components, resulting in a false-negative result.

IgA vasculitis. IgA vasculitis is characterized by deposition of IgA-containing ICs in the small vessels. Among the small-vessel vasculitides, the epidemiology of this disease is unique, with at least 75% of cases being diagnosed in children mostly under 10 years of age.[454] The incidence of IgA vasculitis also demonstrates seasonal variation, with more cases identified in fall and winter. This suggests a link to an environmental risk factor, likely infection. Data from several studies support this hypothesis, specifically the identification of a temporal relation between the incidences of IgA vasculitis and respiratory syncytial virus (RSV), influenza, and norovirus. The role of infection is also attractive, given that IgA is expressed at the mucosal surface.

The pathophysiology of IgA vasculitis has been linked to abnormal forms of the Ig, manifested as deficient glycosylation.[455] Increased concentrations of galactose-deficient IgA1 have been detected in patients with IgA vasculitis. It is hypothesized that abnormal glycosylation leads to formation of neoepitopes, resulting in production of IgG antibodies against the IgA. This ultimately results in the ICs that deposit in the small vessels.

More than 95% of patients with IgA vasculitis present with a purpuric rash that almost always involves the legs and buttocks. In addition to the skin involvement, many patients also present with gastrointestinal, musculoskeletal, and renal manifestations. The diagnosis of IgA vasculitis is largely based on clinical evaluation. Current classification criteria as proposed by EULAR include the requirement of purpura of the lower limbs and at least one of the following: acute onset abdominal pain, leukocytoclastic vasculitis or proliferative glomerulonephritis with IgA deposits, acute onset arthralgias, or proteinuria/hematuria.[456]

ANCA Anti–Neutrophil Cytoplasmic Antibody–associated Vasculitides

Granulomatosis with polyangiitis. GPA is characterized clinically by involvement of the upper respiratory tract, lungs, and kidneys.[457,458] Nasal symptoms are the most common, being found in more than 90% of patients. Nasal symptoms may include bleeding, crusting, and obstruction. In some patients, inflammation damages the cartilage, which could lead to a manifestation known as the saddle-nose deformity. The most common pulmonary manifestations are nodules and cavitary lesions. Radiographic findings in the lung of a patient with GPA might be confused with pneumonia. In the kidney, the classic finding in GPA is a rapidly progressive glomerulonephritis.

A biopsy is generally performed to confirm the diagnosis. The most common sites for biopsy are pulmonary nodules and the kidney. A lung biopsy might show evidence of both vasculitis and necrotizing granulomas, with granulomas being one of the pathologic hallmarks of this condition. In the kidney, classic histopathology is a necrotizing crescentic glomerulonephritis.

Microscopic polyangiitis (MPA). MPA is similar to GPA in terms of renal involvement, with patients also at risk for glomerulonephritis.[457,459] Patients with MPA also can present with lung involvement, although these patients are at risk for pulmonary hemorrhage due to inflammation of the pulmonary capillaries. In contrast, one clinical feature that distinguishes MPA from GPA is the absence of nasal involvement.

Pathologically, the kidney biopsy will show evidence of necrotizing crescentic glomerulonephritis, similar to GPA. However, an important distinguishing feature of MPA is the absence of granulomas in the setting of a pauci-immune necrotizing vasculitis. The lack of granulomas in MPA is unique among the ANCA-associated vasculitides.

Eosinophilic granulomatosis with polyangiitis. EGPA also presents frequently with lung and upper respiratory tract involvement.[460] Lung disease may initially manifest as asthma, which may be chronic and occur prior to other evidence of vasculitis. Individuals with EGPA may also have a history of nasal polyps. One clinical feature that may occur in up to 70% of patients with EGPA is mononeuritis or polyneuritis, which is unique among the ANCA-associated vasculitides. Another hallmark of EGPA is peripheral blood eosinophilia, in which eosinophils may account for up to 50% of the white blood cell count. Pathologically, biopsy specimens may be quite similar to GPA, showing the necrotizing vasculitis with limited Ig deposition and granulomas. However, the presence of extravascular eosinophils is a specific characteristic of EGPA.

Anti–neutrophil cytoplasmic antibodies. ANCAs are defined by their antigen specificity and IIF staining pattern.[461] The two most well-characterized antigen specificities are PR3 and myeloperoxidase (MPO).[462] Both of these proteins are found in the cytoplasmic granules of neutrophils. If neutrophils are fixed with formalin, anti-MPO and anti-PR3 antibodies both will produce granular cytoplasmic staining. In contrast, if ethanol-fixed neutrophils are used, two different staining patterns are observed. Anti-PR3 antibodies will produce the same cytoplasmic staining patterns as visualized on formalin-fixed neutrophils. In contrast, anti-MPO antibodies will lead to a perinuclear staining pattern on ethanol-fixed neutrophils. This is an artificial phenomenon and is caused by disruption of the cellular membranes. MPO is highly positively charged and, with alteration in the membranes, migrates to the nucleus through electrostatic interaction with the dsDNA. This results in production of a perinuclear staining pattern referred to as pANCA. This is differentiated from the cytoplasmic, or cANCA, pattern associated with the presence of anti-PR3 antibodies (Fig. 94.5).[463]

The cANCA pattern and anti-PR3 antibody are highly correlated with one another, and this combination is associated with GPA. The pANCA pattern in the presence of an anti-MPO antibody is consistent with MPA. In addition, some patients with EGPA (up to 50%), primarily those with renal disease, are positive for a pANCA pattern. However, the pANCA pattern is not strictly correlated with the MPO antigen, and other antigen specificities have been associated with the IIF pattern in this clinical scenario.[464] It is not uncommon for a laboratory to identify a pANCA pattern in the absence of a detectable anti-MPO antibody. In some cases, this reflects the presence of a true pANCA-associated antigen specificity other than MPO. In other situations, it may be due to the presence of an interfering antibody. One relatively common autoantibody, the ANA, can interfere with ANCA testing. On ethanol-fixed neutrophils, some ANAs, particularly the homogenous pattern, produce a staining pattern that could be misinterpreted as a pANCA. The ANA and pANCA can be differentiated from one another by using formalin-fixed neutrophils, on which the ANA should show no detectable fluorescence, and by incorporating HEp-2 cell IIF on which a true pANCA will be negative.

ANCA testing is performed by IIF using ethanol-fixed neutrophils, either alone or in combination with formalin-fixed neutrophils. Specific detection of anti-PR3 or anti-MPO antigens is accomplished by immunoassay such as EIA or ALBIA. These are the only two antigen specificities that are

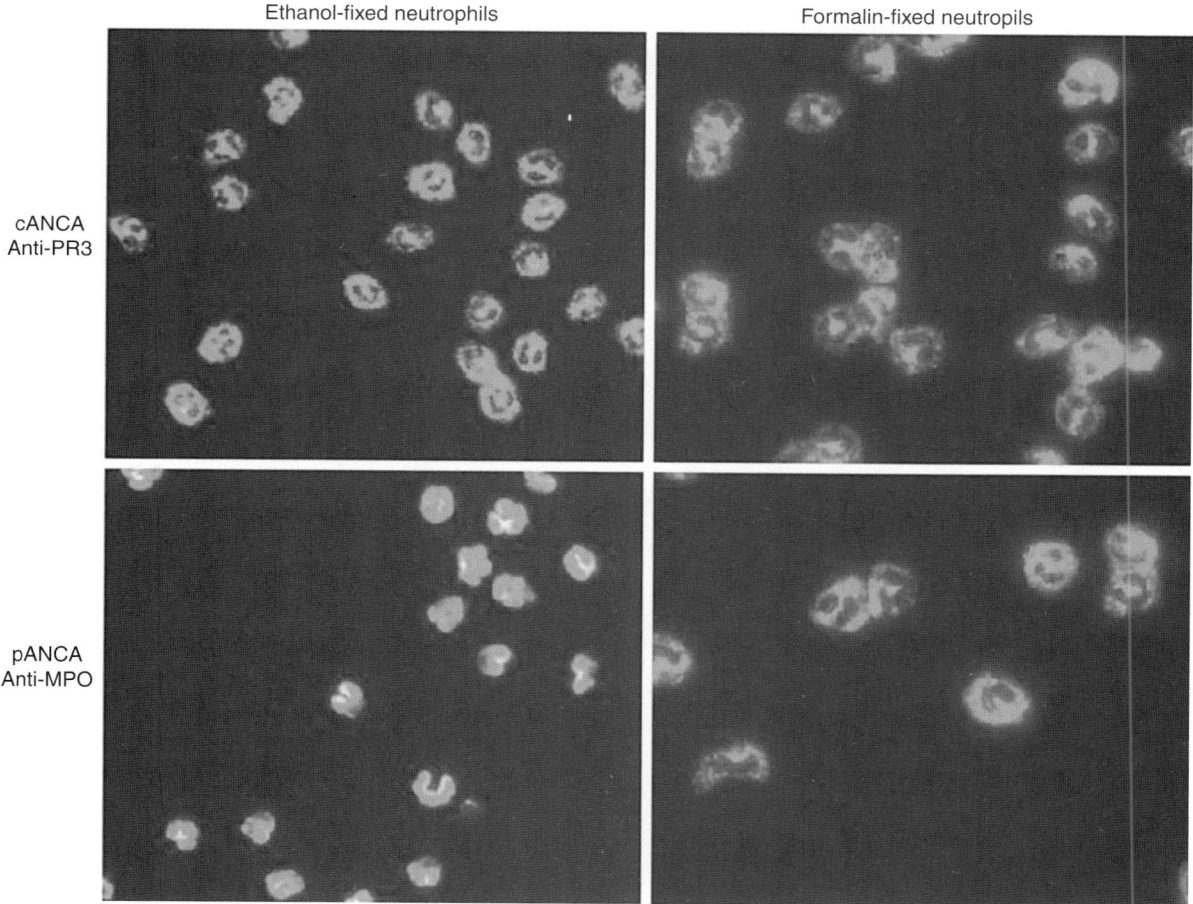

FIGURE 94.5 Anti–neutrophil cytoplasmic antibody (ANCA) indirect immunofluorescence (IIF). Both anti-PR3 and anti-MPO antibodies display cytoplasmic staining on formalin-fixed neutrophils. However, only anti-PR3 antibodies also have a cytoplasmic staining pattern on ethanol-fixed neutrophils, which is interpreted as a cANCA pattern. Anti-MPO antibodies result in a perinuclear pattern on ethanol-fixed neutrophils, which results in a pANCA interpretation.

available for routine laboratory testing. Previous guidelines had suggested that laboratories screen all patient samples using ANCA IIF. It was believed that ANCA was a more sensitive test; any positive or indeterminate samples would then be tested for anti-PR3 and anti-MPO antibodies. However, current guidelines now suggest that the anti-PR3 and anti-MPO immunoassays should be the initial screening test, with ANCA IIF testing recommended in situations where there is a high index of suspicion for an ANCA-associated vasculitis but where the anti-PR3 and anti-MPO testing is negative.[465] The authors cite improvements, particularly in clinical sensitivity, of the anti-PR3 and anti-MPO immunoassays[466,467]and issues with reproducibility of ANCA tests due to the subjective nature of the IIF method,[468,469] in making these new recommendations.

SUMMARY

The systemic autoimmune diseases are a heterogeneous group of diseases, each of which arises from a complex interaction between genetics and the environment. Although the diagnosis of these conditions is largely based on clinical and pathologic evaluation, the clinical laboratory still plays a significant role through autoantibody serology testing. This type of testing poses a number of unique challenges to the clinical laboratory, including varying analytical methodologies, assay standardization, and test interpretation. There are many opportunities for improvements in this testing, which will be key to enhancing the diagnostic approaches to the patient with a suspected systemic autoimmune disease.

SELECTED REFERENCES

20. Singh NJ, Schwartz RH. Primer: mechanisms of immunologic tolerance. Nat Clin Pract Rheumatol 2006;2:44–52.
61. Cho JH, Gregersen PK. Genomics and the multifactorial nature of human autoimmune disease. N Eng J Med 2011;365:1612–23.
71. Rosen A, Casciola-Rosen L. Autoantigens in systemic autoimmunity: critical partner in pathogenesis. J Intern Med 2009;265:625–31.
75. Elkon K, Casali P. Nature and functions of autoantibodies. Nat Clin Pract Rheumatol 2008;4:491–8.
118. Bossuyt X, Coenen D, Fieuws S, et al. Likelihood ratios as a function of antibody concentration for anti-cyclic citrullinated peptide antibodies and rheumatoid factor. Ann Rheum Dis 2009;68:287–9.
123. Mummert E, Fritzler MJ, Sjowall C, et al. The clinical utility of anti-double-stranded DNA antibodies and the challenges of their determination. J Immunol Methods 2018;459:11–9.
166. Aringer M, Costenbader K, Daikh D, et al. 2019 European League Against Rheumatism/American College of Rheumatology classification criteria for systemic lupus erythematosus. Ann Rheum Dis 2019;78:1151–9.
167. Choi MY, Clarke AE, St Pierre Y, et al. Antinuclear antibody-negative systemic lupus erythematosus in an international inception cohort. Arthritis Care Res (Hoboken) 2019;71:893–902.
247. Agmon-Levin N, Damoiseaux J, Kallenberg C, et al. International recommendations for the assessment of autoantibodies to cellular antigens referred to as anti-nuclear antibodies. Ann Rheum Dis 2014;73:17–23.
252. Chan EK, Damoiseaux J, Carballo OG, et al. Report of the first international consensus on standardized nomenclature of antinuclear antibody HEp-2 cell patterns 2014-2015. Front Immunol 2015;6:412.
294. Willemze A, van der Woude D, Ghidey W, et al. The interaction between HLA shared epitope alleles and smoking and its contribution to autoimmunity against several citrullinated antigens. Arthritis Rheum 2011;63:1823–32.
318. Deane KD. Preclinical rheumatoid arthritis and rheumatoid arthritis prevention. Curr Rheumatol Rep 2018;20:50.
326. Aletaha D, Neogi T, Silman AJ, et al. 2010 rheumatoid arthritis classification criteria: an American College of Rheumatology/European League Against Rheumatism collaborative initiative. Ann Rheum Dis 2010;69:1580–8.
356. Lakos G, Favaloro EJ, Harris EN, et al. International consensus guidelines on anticardiolipin and anti-beta2-glycoprotein I testing: report from the 13th International Congress on Antiphospholipid Antibodies. Arthritis Rheum 2012;64:1–10.
368. Miyakis S, Lockshin MD, Atsumi T, et al. International consensus statement on an update of the classification criteria for definite antiphospholipid syndrome (APS). J Thromb Haemost 2006;4:295–306.
370. Pengo V, Biasiolo A, Pegoraro C, et al. Antibody profiles for the diagnosis of antiphospholipid syndrome. Thromb Haemost 2005;93:1147–52.
386. Bertolaccini ML, Amengual O, Atsumi T, et al. 'Non-criteria' APL tests: report of a task force and preconference workshop at the 13th International Congress on Antiphospholipid Antibodies, Galveston, TX, USA, April 2010. Lupus 2011;20:191–205.
431. Jennette JC, Falk RJ, Bacon PA, et al. 2012 revised International Chapel Hill Consensus Conference nomenclature of vasculitides. Arthritis Rheum 2013;65:1–11.
465. Bossuyt X, Cohen Tervaert JW, et al. Position paper: revised 2017 international consensus on testing of ANCAs in granulomatosis with polyangiitis and microscopic polyangiitis. Nat Rev Rheumatol 2017;13:683–92.
466. Damoiseaux J, Csernok E, Rasmussen N, et al. Detection of antineutrophil cytoplasmic antibodies (ANCAs): a multicentre european vasculitis study group (EUVAS) evaluation of the value of indirect immunofluorescence (IIF) versus antigen-specific immunoassays. Ann Rheum Dis 2017;76:647–53.

Transplant, Solid Organ*

Andrew J. Bentall and Mariam Priya Alexander

ABSTRACT

Background

The development of transplantation for organ failure constituted a significant advance in the management of humans with solid organ failure, which progressed rapidly over the second half of the 20th century. The development of successful outcomes in different disciplines to achieve improved clinical and patient-centered outcomes has been a testament to dedicated clinicians and scientists worldwide. The changes in immunosuppression have improved outcomes but have also brought with them complications. Improving longer-term outcomes of transplant recipients continues to be a significant hurdle throughout all solid organ transplantation, and interventions at each point in the transplant management process are being investigated.

Content

This chapter describes the background to solid organ transplantation and the critical immunologic steps to achieve significant outcomes at the time of the transplant and in the ongoing management. The different immunosuppression currently in use is described with associated benefits and side effects with the outcomes of different organ transplants. The complications associated with transplantation, monitoring organ function, future direction, and nontransplant management of organ failure are discussed.

---

*The full version of this chapter is available electronically on ExpertConsult.com.

Hematopoietic Cell Transplantation*

David Buchbinder and Shanmuganathan Chandrakasan

ABSTRACT

Background
Since the first successful application of hematopoietic cell transplantation (HCT) in the 1950s there has been a consistent evolution in the practice of HCT, which has supported an increasing number of HCT survivors worldwide. HCT is a complex procedure which offers a curative option for many malignant and nonmalignant disorders.

Content
High-dose chemotherapy followed by autologous HCT is used as a therapeutic strategy for specific malignant disorders and autoimmune disorders. Chemotherapy sometimes in combination with radiation followed by allogeneic HCT is also used as a therapeutic strategy for malignant disorders and various nonmalignant disorders. In the case of a malignant disorder, immune effector cells from the donor may provide a graft versus malignancy effect. The infused donor hematopoietic stem cells (HSCs) can repopulate the ablated marrow of the recipient. Immune tolerance eventually develops which prevents rejection of the donor HSCs. A greater understanding has evolved pertaining to critical aspects of HCT including conditioning regimen choice, tailoring of conditioning regimen intensity to the unique needs of individual patients and disorders and donor and graft source choice. The importance of supportive care measures has also been underscored ensuring judicious use of antifungal, antiviral, and antibacterial agents. Although the risk of morbidity and mortality associated with infectious complications, and devastating complications of HCT including graft-versus-host disease have been ameliorated to an extent, there is still a vital need to continue to prevent HCT-related complications that are associated with increased morbidity and mortality.

---

*The full version of this chapter is available electronically on ExpertConsult.com.

Transplant Compatibility Testing

Justin D. Kreuter and Manish J. Gandhi

ABSTRACT

Background

Transplant compatibility testing is focused on developing an immune risk profile, which consists of three types of testing—human leukocyte antigen (HLA) typing, HLA antibody screening, and compatibility crossmatch. This immune risk profile is then put into clinical context by the transplant team to make clinical decisions.

Content

This chapter will begin by explaining the structure and clinically relevant properties of HLA. Typing methods for HLA will be described with focus on the evolution of specificity.

The evolution of compatibility testing will elucidate how methods have developed increasing sensitivity and what this means for transplant decisions. Similarly, the evolution of increasingly sensitive methods for detecting HLA antibodies will be described. Beyond transplant-specific testing, this chapter will explain how HLA testing is used to support transfusion medicine. Specifically, selection of platelets for the platelet transfusion refractory patient and transfusion-related acute lung injury (TRALI) testing will be discussed. This chapter will finish by explaining how these HLA tests are used for disease association testing and pharmacotherapy decisions.

INTRODUCTION

The laboratory that performs transplant compatibility testing may go by several names—human leukocyte antigen (HLA) laboratory, tissue typing laboratory, histocompatibility laboratory, or transplant immunology laboratory. Regardless of name, the testing performed in this laboratory supports multiple aspects of clinical practice. First, the primary focus of this laboratory is to provide an immunologic risk profile for the transplant team. Second, transfusion medicine relies on testing and expertise from this laboratory to select compatible platelet units for patients who are refractory to platelet transfusion and investigation of suspected transfusion-related acute lung injury (TRALI) cases. Third, physicians may order HLA typing to assess the risk of certain genetic diseases that have strong HLA associations. Fourth, the field of pharmacogenomics is developing a place in this laboratory to avoid certain adverse drug effects. The diversity of these clinical activities speaks to the important biologic roles of HLA.

HUMAN LEUKOCYTE ANTIGEN STRUCTURE AND PROPERTIES

The major histocompatibility complex (MHC) on the short arm of chromosome 6 is the genetic location of the HLA genes. HLA genes are inherited as a haplotype, co-dominantly expressed, extremely polymorphic, and highly immunogenic. When expressed, HLA proteins are "loaded" with peptides and trafficked to the cell surface, where the immune system is able to monitor the peptides displayed. There are several genes in this MHC region of the human genome; however, this chapter will focus on class I and class II HLA.

POINTS TO REMEMBER ABOUT HUMAN LEUKOCYTE ANTIGEN

- Multiple proteins divided into class I (HLA-A, B, and C) and class II (HLA-DR, DQ, DP)
- Present antigens to T cells, which determine if it is a self-peptide
- Most polymorphic and immunogenic system in humans

Classical class I genes includes the following HLA: A, B, and C. Classical class II genes includes the following HLA: DR, DQ, and DP.[1] The structure of class I HLA consists of an α chain that is covalently bound to a β-2-microglobulin (Fig. 97.1A). In contrast, class II HLA is a haplo-dimer that consists of an α and β chain (Fig. 97.1B). Because the function of HLA is to present peptides to the immune system for surveillance, the most critical aspect of these structures is their peptide-binding groove. In HLA class I the peptide-binding groove is formed by two domains on the α chain. In HLA class II the peptide-binding groove is formed by the combination of domains on the α and β chains. The physical proximity of the HLA genes means that they are inherited together from each parent as a haplotype. This means that HLA genes occur in particular combinations far more frequently than would have been predicted (i.e., linkage disequilibrium). The experienced individual can use this linkage disequilibrium information to check for a potential error in typing. Inheriting HLA as a haplotype means that each child will inherit one full haplotype from each parent (Fig. 97.2). Furthermore, any two full siblings have a 25% chance inheriting the same two HLA haplotypes (i.e., HLA identical match), 50% chance of inheriting one identical

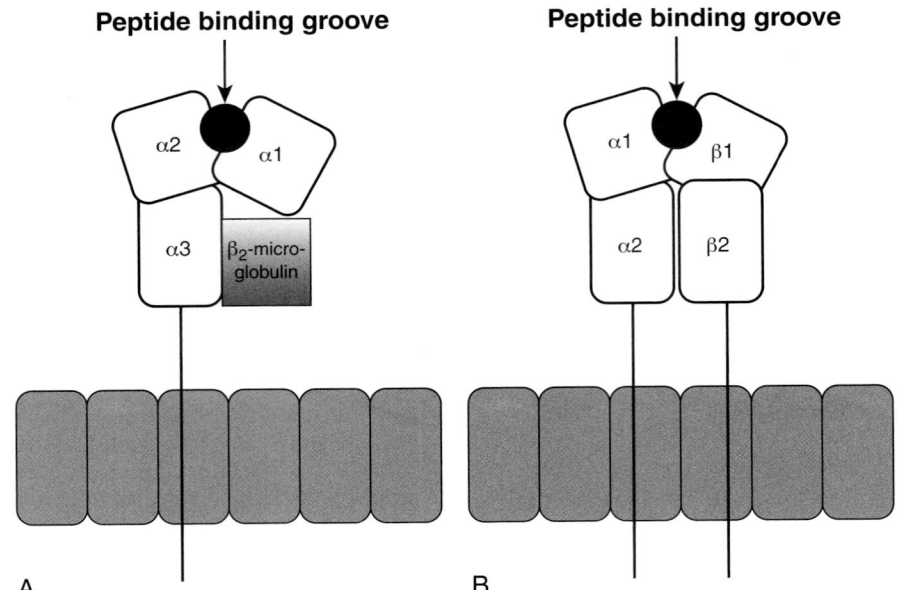

FIGURE 97.1 (A) Structure of human leukocyte antigen (HLA) class I. (B) Structure of HLA class II.

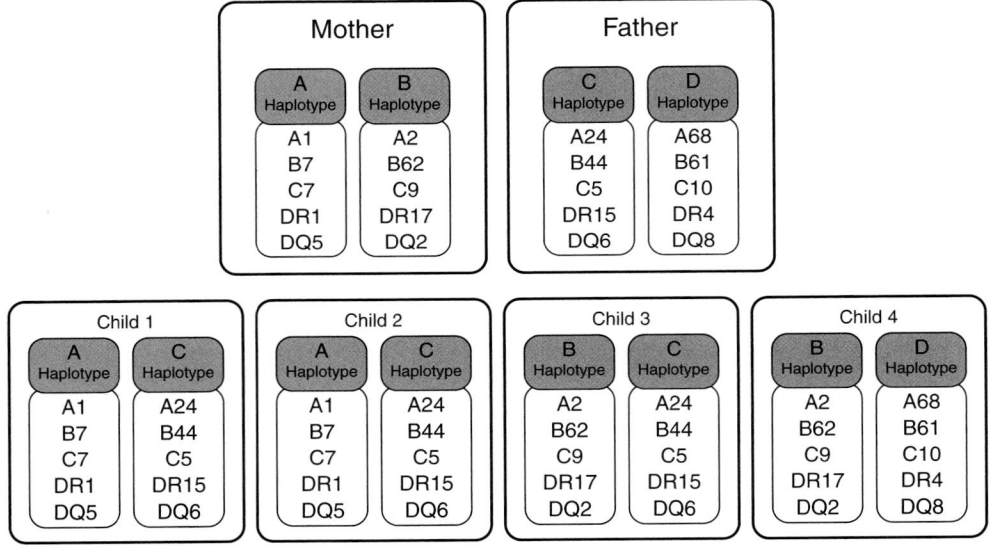

FIGURE 97.2 Haplotype inheritance. Every child inherits one haplotype from each parent. Children 1 and 2 are human leukocyte antigen (HLA) identical, because they inherited the same haplotypes from each parent. Children 3 and 4 are haploidentical, because they have one haplotype in common. Children 1 and 4 inherited completely different haplotypes from each parent.

HLA haplotype (i.e., haploidentical), and 25% chance of inheriting two different HLA haplotypes (i.e., HLA mismatch). Beyond the immediate family, it is rare to identify HLA matches (unless consanguineous marriage is practiced in the community).

Any given HLA protein is able to bind and present a subset of potential peptides in its peptide-binding groove. Presumably for this evolutionary reason, HLA proteins demonstrate co-dominant expression to maximize the number of potential antigens that the immune system is able to present on HLA proteins. HLA genes are co-dominantly expressed, which equips the individual with the greatest number of HLA proteins for immune surveillance. HLA class I and class II

proteins have different patterns of expression, based on cell type. Class I proteins are expressed on all nucleated cells (which includes platelets, since they are fragments of the nucleated megakaryocyte); whereas class II proteins are typically restricted to antigen presenting cells (APCs) such as: B lymphocytes, monocytes/macrophages, and dendritic cells. However, in the presence of inflammation, most cells can be induced to express these class II HLA proteins.[2] Differential expression is important for understanding why support of the platelet refractory patient is focused on class I HLA and why solid organ transplant rejection can be mediated by antibodies to both class I and class II HLA. There are also differences in expression of the amount of HLA proteins on the cell surface by locus. The higher expressed HLA loci are HLA-A, HLA-B, and HLA-DRB1. The lesser expressed HLA loci are HLA-C, HLA-DRB3/4/5, HLA-DQB1, and HLA-DPB1.[3] Understanding expression levels help to appreciate why HLA testing practices evolved as they did—beginning with the higher expressed proteins.

The highly polymorphic nature of HLA cannot be overstated. Because of its role in discriminating self from nonself, the HLA proteins function like a combination lock. This makes it nearly impossible for infectious organisms to perfectly mimic an individual's HLA, maintaining the integrity of immune surveillance. While the complexity inherent in the HLA protein is beneficial for immune surveillance, this creates compatibility challenges for organ transplantation.

HLA molecules are highly immunogenic. During immune surveillance, HLA has the critical role of presenting antigens to T cells. In the case of HLA class I, the intracellular environment is continuously sampled and presented to CD8+ T cells. If the cell presents a fragment of virus in the peptide-binding groove, then the CD8+ T cell becomes activated and promotes a cell-mediated cytotoxic immune response. In the case of HLA class II, the intercellular environment is continuously sampled and presented to CD4+ T cells. If the cell presents a fragment of bacteria in the peptide-binding groove, then the CD4+ T cell becomes activated, releasing cytokines and differentiating into different cells to promote a humoral immune response.

Significance of Human Leukocyte Antigen for Transplant

The highly polymorphic and immunogenic natures of HLA are a hindrance for successful transplantation. When allorecognition occurs, it can result in rejection of the transplanted organ.[4] Allorecognition most often occurs when the donor's APCs displaying donor antigens are recognized directly by the recipients T cells (which is unique to transplantation only). The subsequent inflammatory response in the transplanted organ precipitates upregulation of HLA.[2] This normally helpful response establishes a positive feedback loop for rejection of the donor organ. This highlights the important role of the laboratory to continue to monitor for new and increased donor-specific antibodies after the transplant process.

A second immune reaction associated with HLA is graft-versus-host disease (GvHD). In this situation, it is the donor's T cells that recognize host (i.e., recipient) HLA expressed on other tissues. The risk of GvHD is proportional to the number of lymphocytes in the donor organ. The highest risk of GvHD occurs in hematopoietic stem cell transplantation due to the donor-derived immune system proliferating and recognizing any differences in the host tissues. GvHD is also seen in solid organ transplant, due to "passenger" lymphocytes contained in the donated organ.[5]

Role of the Laboratory

The role of the laboratory is to determine the immune risk profile for each and every transplant. To create this profile, the laboratory must perform a battery of tests: HLA typing both the recipient and donors, screening for anti-HLA antibodies in the recipient, and performing compatibility testing. Over time, both the methods for HLA typing and detecting HLA antibodies have improved, but every test has

limitations. False-positive and false-negative results do occur. Therefore any assessment of immune risk needs to be interpreted in the particular clinical context. A collaborative laboratory-clinical partnership is crucial for optimizing transplant decisions.

Human Leukocyte Antigen Typing

A hierarchical naming convention for HLA has been developed to facilitate clear communication despite the highly polymorphic nature of HLA. For example, when naming a particular HLA-A allele, the prefix HLA, followed by a hyphen, and the specific gene is used (i.e., HLA-A). An asterisk is inserted as a separator between the gene and field 1, which designates the allele group (i.e., HLA-A*02). Successive fields are separated by a colon. Field 2 designates a specific HLA protein (i.e., HLA-A*02:01). Field 3 designates synonymous DNA substitution within the coding region (i.e., HLA-A*02:01:01). Field 4 designates differences in a noncoding region (i.e., HLA-A*02:01:01:02). And finally, a suffix is used to indicate changes in expression (i.e., HLA-A*02:01:01:02N, where "N" indicates that the allele is "null"/not expressed). Later in this chapter, the evolution of HLA typing methodologies will describe how serology was limited to the first field and massively parallel sequencing (MPS) is able to achieve a typing result to the fourth field.[6–8]

A few commonly used HLA typing terms used in clinical practice should be defined.[9] Low resolution typing is just a result for field 1 in the naming convention above. In contrast, higher resolution refers to results from the second field onward. Transplant agreements between a laboratory and the transplant service should specify what fields are required per clinical context. Verification typing is when a different sample is used to verify concordance with an initial HLA typing result. In contrast, extended typing is when further testing is performed on a sample (i.e., additional loci or higher resolution).

POINTS TO REMEMBER ABOUT RESOLUTION OF HUMAN LEUKOCYTE ANTIGEN TYPING

- Low resolution, also called antigen-level typing, refers to results that are limited to the first field in the HLA nomenclature.
- Higher resolution includes results from the second field onward.

HLA was initially typed using a serologic method—complement dependent cytotoxicity (CDC). In this method, lymphocytes are harvested from blood using density gradient centrifugation, and then added to a microtiter plate. Each well of this microtiter plate contains a different typing serum. Typing sera with apparent mono-specific antibodies were sourced from alloimmunized patients. If the antibody in the well recognizes the antigen on the individual's cells during incubation, then after a source of complement is added, cell death can be identified. Availability of quality reagents, reagents for typing nonwhite individuals, and need for reproducible class II typing were primary drivers for developing molecular methods.

The sequence-specific oligonucleotide (SSO) method begins with a polymerase chain reaction (PCR) to amplify selected areas in the MHC. The oligonucleotide primers are designed to hybridize in the conserved HLA region to amplify complete exons initially (exons 2, 3, and 4 of class I genes and exons 2 and 3 of the class II β chain genes). Once amplified, the DNA is then hybridized to labeled probes. Specific polymorphisms in the exons are identified by hybridization to the probes. Specificity of SSO comes from the particular probes used and stringency used during the hybridization step. This method is relatively fast and reliably provides accurate results in most cases to the first field. However, when additional probes are used, second field typing can sometimes be obtained.

The sequence-specific primer (SSP) method begins with hybridization of oligonucleotide primers that are specific for a given HLA allele. After PCR amplification, amplicons are separated by gel electrophoresis. HLA type is determined by looking at the pattern of which primers had a target to bind and amplify. This method is fairly labor- and time-intensive, needing multiple PCR amplifications per HLA loci. However, SSP is able to provide more specific results, consistently up to second field resolution.

Sequence-based typing follows this pattern of progressively more specific or higher resolution HLA typing. Depending on the laboratory's needs, either Sanger sequencing or MPS may be used to achieve third or fourth field resolution, respectively. In Sanger sequencing a terminating labeled nucleotide is randomly added, capillary electrophoresis separates the sequences by length, then information from the nucleotide labels can be integrated with length information to determine the sequence. The international immunogenetics information system (http://www.imgt.org) is queried to help determine clinical HLA typing results.

Methods described so far interrogate only a small portion of the HLA gene and a major limitation of this is that it may yield an ambiguous result (i.e., multiple HLA types are possible). It is important to appreciate that it is the specific combination of many polymorphisms that define each specific HLA allele. Ambiguities may occur for two reasons. First, if two or more alleles differ by a nucleotide polymorphism outside of the DNA regions interrogated, then the true HLA type is ambiguous. Second, ambiguities can also result from an inability to phase the data. All the distinguishing polymorphisms can be known; however, the ambiguity occurs because there is a combination of maternal and paternal alleles mixed together in every patient. Since each HLA type is based on the specific combination of polymorphisms, the maternal and paternal alleles need to be distinguished (Fig. 97.3). Depending on the type of the ambiguity and the level of typing, in most cases, this needs additional testing by alternate methods and/or interrogation of additional regions of the HLA gene. This helps resolve the most common ambiguities that are reported.

For HLA typing, MPS has been used in two ways. The first way is to interrogate exons, similar to previous typing strategies. The advantage of MPS is the increased throughput that comes with the ability to pool multiple patient samples on a single run,[10,11] resulting in decreased cost of the test. The second way is to sequence the complete or major portions of the HLA-gene, including the exons and introns and, in some cases, also the 3′ and 5′ UTR. This helps in resolving most of the ambiguities seen by targeted exonic sequencing only. In addition, accurate fourth field typing can be achieved. Limitations include multiple steps in sample preparation, including library preparation, need for multiple samples to be cost effective, longer turnaround times, computing power requirements, robust software for data analysis, and space for data storage. Moreover, MPS comes with challenges that require significant investment from the laboratory. First, the library preparation is extensive but necessary for being able to organize sequence fragments. Second, the amount of information generated by the massive parallel sequencing requires significant computing power.[12] All of the early reports on HLA MPS were performed using the 454 technology, but Roche ended production of this first generation technology in 2016.[13] Current commercial HLA kits are predominantly available on the second generation NGS platforms using the Ion-Torrent (Thermo-Fisher, Waltham, MA) or Ilumina sequencers (Ilumina, San Diego, CA).[10] These are short read sequencing technologies requiring extensive library preparation and complex bioinformatics for data interpretation. As these methods have been in use for a long time, they provide accurate typing information up to the fourth field in most cases. Third-generation sequencers on the other hand provide longer read lengths and minimal library preparation, thus decreasing the turnaround time. These include sequencers from Pacific Biosciences (Menlo Park, CA) and Oxford Nanopore Technologies (Oxford, UK). Commercial kits using these technologies are in development.

Preferential amplification remains a concern whenever a patient appears to be homozygous or there is an allelic imbalance. This could have devastating consequences in a transplant situation, if a truly heterozygous patient was typed homozygous at a particular locus. This is a reminder that understanding linkage disequilibrium and monitoring of quality metrics from the MPS run (e.g., probability of an incorrect call, read depth, and uniformity of coverage) may be helpful for recognizing the error. In addition, loss of heterozygosity has been described in hematologic malignancies.[14]

Compatibility

The original test for organ compatibility was CDC. Dr. Terasaki's seminal 1969 paper demonstrated the clinical utility for his crossmatch test to improve kidney transplant decisions.[15] In his study, patients with a negative crossmatch experienced a 4% rate of rejection, whereas those with a positive crossmatch experienced an 80% rate of rejection. The original

A*01:01:01:01	A	T	G	A	A	G	G	C	C	A	C	T	C	A	C	A	G	A	C	T	G	A	C	C	G	A	G	C	G
A*01:17	A										G																	C	
A*11:01:01	G										G																	T	
A*11:19	G										C																	T	

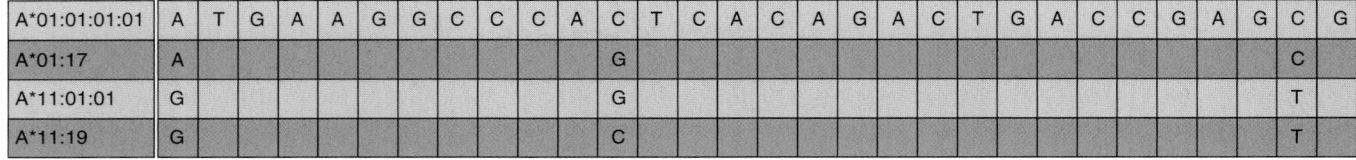

FIGURE 97.3 Human leukocyte antigen (HLA) typing ambiguity. Given this sequencing data with three points of heterozygosity, it is ambiguous which two of the four possibilities are the correct HLA type.

crossmatch was a CDC assay. Cells from the potential donor and serum from the potential recipient would be incubated with complement, and then cell death was visualized to determine if the crossmatch was positive or negative.

This assay was designed to detect anti-HLA IgG antibodies; however, there are additional causes for a positive CDC crossmatch.[16] Autoimmune disease, therapeutic monoclonal antibodies, or anticoagulants in the recipient's sample are a few of the common interfering factors. Because anti-HLA antibodies tend to be IgG, while other autoantibodies tend to be IgM, pretreatment with dithiothreitol or heat inactivation may be used to inactivate IgM present in the sample. Some therapeutic monoclonal antibodies may be absorbed out (see Chapter 98 on therapeutic monoclonal antibodies). Using a serum sample is preferred from the potential recipient, as this avoids additional anticoagulants in the test. Because of these potential interferences, any unexpected positive result should prompt a review of the patient's medical record for sources of interference.

After implementation, the false-negative rate was a driver for systematically improving the sensitivity of this assay. At first, the incubation times were increased, and wash steps were added. The addition of anti-human globulin (AHG) improved sensitivity 10-fold;[17] however, this didn't work for class II donor specific antibodies. Since B cells express surface immunoglobulin, adding AHG gave many false-positive B-cell crossmatches.

Flow cytometry improves both the sensitivity and specificity of crossmatch testing relative to the CDC assay with AHG enhancement.[18,19] In a flow cytometric crossmatch, the recipient serum is incubated with donor cells. Viable cells from the organ donor are needed to perform a flow cytometric crossmatch. The histocompatibility laboratory will receive peripheral blood, lymph node, or a spleen sample to isolate donor cells. This step should be performed to achieve the optimal cell to serum ratio as determined locally. One of the key challenges of the flow cytometric crossmatch is its sensitivity. It is very sensitive for rejection-causing HLA antibodies; however, nonspecific immunoglobulins, autoantibodies, and therapeutic antibodies (e.g., rituximab, daclizumab, alemtuzumab, anti-thymocyte globulin) may also cause a positive result. One way to mitigate nonspecific binding is to pretreat donor cells with pronase, a blend of proteolytic enzymes. Pronase cleaves Fc receptors on B cells, which removes nonspecific antibody binding. However, this is a balancing act as pronase can also destroy HLA epitopes (giving a false-negative result) and even expose cryptic epitopes (giving a false-positive result).[20] Considering treated and nontreated results in parallel may mitigate errors. With appropriate controls, the results of a flow crossmatch are usually reported as mean channel shift with an interpretation based on lab-derived cut-offs. A negative or positive flow crossmatch has important predictive value for transplant patients,[20–22] yet the overall decision should be based on putting all the laboratory data into clinical context.

POINT TO REMEMBER

Crossmatch Testing
- Compatibility testing is currently done by flow crossmatch.
- Donor T and B lymphocytes are reacted with recipient serum.

Detection of Human Leukocyte Antigen Antibodies

Anti-HLA antibodies are a major barrier to successful transplantation. The previous section described the evolution of compatibility testing. As soon as that first crossmatch demonstrated clinical value, it started a search for testing that could assess immunologic risk without a crossmatch. If the flow crossmatch is falsely negative, then an incompatible kidney may be transplanted into the "wrong" patient. On the other hand, if the flow crossmatch is falsely positive, then a "good" recipient may be denied a compatible transplant. Characterizing the antibody profile of a patient is an important piece of additional information to assess the immunologic risk of a particular transplant.

Anti-HLA antibody testing began as a CDC assay, which used leukocytes from a different community blood donor in each well. The patient serum could then be incubated with the whole tray, and then the percent of wells showing cell death could be counted. In this way, it could be extrapolated what percentage of the general population would be incompatible with the patient. This percentage is known as the panel reactive antibody (PRA). Although informative if the ethnicity of the panel is reflective of the donor population, the PRA is not specific to a given donor.

In an effort to achieve greater specificity, anti-HLA antibody detection evolved to solid phase ELISA using AHG, then flow cytometry using latex beads, and current practice depends on polystyrene beads in an array.[17]

Different sets of beads can be utilized, depending on the particular context. For example, mixed beads are used to broadly screen for anti-HLA antibodies. Each bead has HLA from multiple cell lines fixed onto its surface (e.g., LABScreen, One Lambda, Los Angeles, CA). PRA beads are more specific with each bead coated with HLA from one cell line fixed onto its surface. Finally, single antigen beads detect specific anti-HLA antibodies present in the patient sample. Recombinant HLA are produced, purified, and coated onto each bead. By having only a single HLA antigen on each bead, the relative amount of each specific anti-HLA antibody can be determined. Despite being approved as a qualitative assay, many transplant centers integrate a range of numerical mean fluorescence intensities into their mental calculus when assessing the immunologic risk for transplant. The goal of developing anti-HLA antibody testing is to predict crossmatch results and the current iteration of antibody testing is more sensitive than the flow crossmatch.

Luminex based assays are commonly used to assess donor-specific antibodies before transplant to facilitate allocation decisions and after transplant monitoring for acute rejection.[23–25] Post-transplant monitoring should consider immunoassay results in the context of current histopathology and clinical organ function. This is because the immunoassay for HLA antibodies does not include all the elements that may precipitate rejection (i.e., false negatives) and the presence of antibodies does not always indicate the damage potential (i.e., false positives). Detection of antibodies in the absence of clinical rejection may be repeated to understand if the antibodies detected are persistent or transient. Regardless of when this testing is performed, relative to a transplant, the presence of and rate of change in detectable antibodies informs the frequency of future antibody testing.

Luminex based assays in the histocompatibility laboratory use a combination of beads with different antigens—phenotypic beads, multiple antigen beads, and single antigen beads. There are various approaches to Luminex screening (i.e., which of these beads to use when, and in what combination). Approved as a qualitative assay, this test measures the amount of antibody that binds to the target antigen on a particular bead. This flow-based system uses two lasers. The first laser determines the bead (antigen) identity, and the second laser assesses the amount of antibody bound to that bead.

POINTS TO REMEMBER

Antibody Detection

- Antibody detection is currently assessed by solid phase bead-based assays that screen for the presence of anti-HLA antibodies and are also able to identify the specificity of the antibody.
- Mixed beads have HLA from multiple cell lines fixed onto each bead surface.
- PRA beads have HLA from a single cell line fixed onto each bead surface.
- Single antigen beads have a single purified recombinant HLA fixed onto each bead surface.

Bead-based assays are marketed as qualitative assays; however, they provide a fluorescence signal that is clinically used in a semi-quantitative manner. Thus three key challenges come into play with these bead-based assays: determining a positive cutoff, understanding the day-to-day variability, and identifying both false-positive and false-negative results. First, determining a positive cutoff based on the fluorescent signal can be challenging because of the variable HLA expression on different organs and also given the different risk tolerance for the transplant program in clinical context.[26] Cutoffs are thus determined locally based on the organ (e.g., there can be different cutoffs for kidneys versus hearts) with respect to the clinical situation (e.g., an alloimmunized recipient who will be subject to a desensitization protocol may have a different cutoff compared to a patient with no alloimmunization). These assays have high coefficients of day-to-day variability and this needs to be factored in when assays are used to monitor for changes in antibody levels both prior to and after transplantation.[27] Lastly, there are a few causes of false-positive reactivity (e.g., auto-antibodies, anti-CD20 treatment, antibodies to denatured antibodies)[26] and false-negative results due to the prozone effect (also described as serum interference).[27,28] Pretreatment with EDTA is one way to circumvent complement-mediated prozone; however, there are additional causes and laboratory strategies for navigating this interference.[28–30] Despite these challenges, bead-based assays have a central role in the transplant laboratory and are continuing to expand with an increased repertoire of antigen beads.[26,28–30]

Interest in performing virtual crossmatches has grown in recent years.[31] This is not a test, per se, but a review of available testing performed on a potential recipient and making a judgement about likelihood of organ compatibility. While certainly a quick process compared with other compatibility tests, there are limitations. First, patients who are highly al-loimmunized are probably best served with a traditional test for compatibility, such as a flow cytometric crossmatch. Second, one should be cautious if a donor's mismatched antigen is not present on previously tested assays. The absence of information is not the same as a negative result. Third, the antibody testing available for review should be reflective of the patient's current immune status. If the patient hasn't had any recent immunizing events, then an older sample may be appropriate. On the other hand, if the patient has had an immunizing event since their last assessment of immune status, then a virtual crossmatch may not accurately predict compatibility. Because of these limitations, each transplant program is wise to determine local practice about criteria for who is eligible for a virtual crossmatch.

Transfusion Support: Platelet Selection for the Refractory Patient

When patients develop critical thrombocytopenia, increasing the platelet count is important to raise the patient above the minimum threshold needed to mitigate catastrophic bleeding risk; however, some patients fail to increment their platelet count after a platelet transfusion. Repeated failure to increment defines the platelet refractory state. Most patients are refractory because of a nonimmune cause. However, when it is due to an immune cause, refractoriness is most likely due to HLA-antibodies.

Laboratory evaluation to determine the cause of the platelet refractory patient may involve a battery of tests.[32,33] Some of the relevant tests have been mentioned previously—low-to-intermediate resolution class I HLA typing, performed on both the platelet donor and refractory patient and the Luminex assay to detect HLA antibodies, performed on the refractory patient. Most blood providers (e.g., the American Red Cross, Washington DC) will already have performed class I HLA typing on the majority of their platelet donors. This practice speeds the identification of compatible platelets. There are two additional tests that have not yet been discussed and are relevant to supporting platelet refractory patients—platelet crossmatch and human platelet antigen (HPA)-antibody testing.

A platelet crossmatch is only performed in platelet refractory situations. It is a solid phase test system with wells coated with a platelet binding agent. A fresh sample is taken from a platelet unit, ideally from a fresh segment that is heat sealed-off and incubated in the test well to allow binding of donor platelets. Fluid is removed from the well. Next, serum from the refractory patient is added and incubated. Finally, red blood cells coated with anti-IgG are added and the test wells are centrifuged. The bottom of the wells has a slight cone shape. If the patient has an antibody that has bound to the donor platelets, then the coated red blood cells bind like a secondary antibody creating an even red carpet over the bottom of the well. If the patient does not have an antibody that binds to the donor platelets, then the coated red blood cells form a dense pellet in the middle of the well after being centrifuged. In this way, a crisp red dot is a negative reaction and should be interpreted as a compatible platelet crossmatch. Anything other than a crisp red dot is some degree of a positive crossmatch and should be interpreted as an incompatible platelet crossmatch. A variation of the platelet crossmatch uses wells that are preloaded with platelets from different donors. Although this does not identify compatible platelets currently in inventory, it is helpful for many centers that do not maintain a large platelet inventory and would still like to screen refractory patients for antibodies.

Approximately 2 to 3% of patients who are platelet refractory will have antibodies directed toward HPA.[34] These are antigenic epitopes on surface glycoproteins. There are two test systems for detecting these antibodies. The first is a solid phase ELISA that has test wells that contain a particular combination of glycoproteins (i.e., IIb/IIIa, Ib/IX, Ia/IIa, and IV). In addition, there is a well that contains a combination of HLA class I antigens. This enables screening for a diverse number of antibodies known to cause a platelet refractory state. The second test system for anti-HPA antibodies is a Luminex bead assay. This uses the same methodology as previously discussed. In the Luminex assay, the epitopes of HPA-1a/b, HPA-2a/b, HPA-3a/b, HPA-4a/b, HPA-5a/b, GPIV, and a mixture of HLA class I are fixed on different colored beads. This allows a flow platform to screen for and discriminate among IgG antibodies to these epitopes.

There are a few different strategies to select platelets for the platelet refractory patient. First, one could select platelet units that are negative for certain antigens, based on the patient's antibody profile. This strategy depends on availability of current information about the patient's antibodies. A second strategy is providing cross-matched platelets. This strategy depends on a sufficient platelet inventory, given the patient's degree of alloimmunization, for identifying compatible units in inventory. A third strategy is to order/select HLA-identical platelet units. Because actually finding an HLA-identical platelet in inventory may be challenging, this strategy depends on critical review of any HLA mismatch and a current patient antibody profile. A fourth strategy is to select platelet units based on epitope analysis. This strategy depends on use of a publicly available website (http://www.epitopes.net/) and at least inferred high resolution HLA typing. Regardless of which strategy is used, the evaluation should be methodical and individualized for patient need and local resources.

Transfusion Related Acute Lung Injury

TRALI was first described in the mid-1980s and was rapidly recognized to be the most common cause of transfusion-related fatality by the mid-2000s.[35,36] The majority of TRALI reactions occur when HLA antibodies in the donated blood product are transfused into patients that express the cognate HLA antigen. The donor's antibody binds to the cognate antigen on recipient granulocytes, which are prominent in the pulmonary vasculature, causing degranulation and subsequent tissue damage. TRALI is characterized by dramatic, noncardiac, pulmonary compromise during or within 6 hours of transfusion. The Centers for Disease Control criteria, first released in 2009 and most recently updated in 2018, lists the diagnostic criteria and case definitions for TRALI.[37] Clinical experts have recently divided TRALI into type I and type II cases depending on the absence or presence of acute respiratory distress syndrome before transfusion, respectively.[38] This practice update highlights that TRALI remains a valid clinical diagnosis for a patient with preexisting acute respiratory distress syndrome.

In an effort to attenuate the rate of TRALI, female blood donors who have been pregnant are now screened for HLA antibodies.[39] Blood donors who screen positive for HLA antibodies are not permitted to donate plasma-rich blood products. This and other mitigation efforts have reduced the risk of TRALI, which continues to be closely monitored.[40]

TABLE 97.1 Common Human Leukocyte Antigen Disease Associations

Disease	Associated HLA
Ankylosing spondylitis	B27
Celiac disease	DQ2
	DQ8
Narcolepsy	DQB1*06:02
Bechet's disease	B51
Type 1 diabetes	DR17-DQ2

HLA, Human leukocyte antigen.

TABLE 97.2 HLA Alleles Associated With Adverse Drug Reactions in Which Human Leukocyte Antigen Testing Is Required According to the FDA-Approved Package Insert

Drug	HLA Allele
Abacavir	B*57:01
Allopurinol	B*58:01
Carbamazepine	B*15:02
	A*31:01

HLA, Human leukocyte antigen.

Disease Association Testing

In addition to transplant work, many HLA laboratories also perform disease association testing. Several autoimmune diseases have a very strong HLA-association (Table 97.1).[41] It is important to appreciate that having the associated HLA allele is just a risk factor and does not, in fact, diagnose any disease. The value of disease association testing is its negative predictive value. For example, an individual with symptoms suggestive of celiac disease who tests negative for DQ2 and DQ8 most likely has some other inflammatory bowel disease.[42]

Due to the diversity and developing understanding of disease associated HLA types, many labs will perform an intermediate-to-high resolution class I and class II HLA typing (as described above). This serves two purposes. First, it maintains simplicity to have just one orderable test that can be used for an expanding number of HLA disease associations. Second, the HLA typing result continues to provide value if newer information is published.

Pharmacotherapy

In recent years, rare drug reactions have become associated with specific HLA alleles.[43] Certain drugs now require HLA typing before prescribing the medication (Table 97.2). Depending on the situation, intermediate-to-high resolution HLA typing is required to identify which patients are at risk for developing a specific drug reaction. If the patient does have an at-risk HLA allele, then a different medication is selected to avoid the adverse drug reaction.

LOOKING TO THE FUTURE OF HUMAN LEUKOCYTE ANTIGEN TESTING

The future of HLA testing will both stay focused on improving transplant outcomes and expand with the development of personalized medicine. The recent advancements in MPS testing has made HLA typing to the fourth field possible for routine clinical practice. A recent publication demonstrates that a donor matched to the fourth HLA field is associated with superior survival,[44] although additional studies are needed to confirm these findings. As efforts for personalized medicine continue, the role of HLA testing as a companion diagnostic will expand. With newer personalized drugs, HLA type may predict therapeutic effect or risk for an adverse event before initiating treatment. Analogous to the role of HLA-C expression in the control of HIV-1 infection,[45] future research will likely expand the interaction between HLA and infectious agents, including Covid-19.[46,47] With better understanding of drug metabolism, one can also envision a broadening role of HLA typing and pharmacogenomics. Lastly, HLA testing will likely evolve into prognostic testing with loss of heterozygosity testing in tumors. Transplantation, companion diagnostics, infectious disease, and solid cancers all suggest a diverse and interesting future for HLA testing.

POINT TO REMEMBER

Human Leukocyte Antigen Testing Is Indicated for
- Transplantation
- Disease association
- Pharmacogenomics
- Transfusion support

SELECTED REFERENCES

1. Robinson J, Halliwell JA, Hayhurst JD, et al. The IPD and IMGT/HLA Database: Allele Variant Databases. Nucleic Acids Res 2015;43:D423–31.
6. McCluskey J, Kanaan C, Diviney M. Nomenclature and serology of HLA class I and class II alleles. Curr Protoc Immunol 2017;118:A.1S.1–6.
7. Marsh SG, Albert ED, Bodmer WF, et al. Nomenclature for factors of the HLA system, 2010. Tissue Antigens 2010;75:291–455.
9. Nunes E, Heslop H, Fernandez-Vina M, et al. Definitions of histocompatibility typing terms. Blood 2011;118:e180–3.
11. Yohe S, Thyagarajan B. Review of clinical next-generation sequencing. Arch Pathol Lab Med 2017;141:1544–57.
13. Gabriel C, Furst D, Fae I, et al. HLA typing by next-generation sequencing—getting closer to reality. Tissue Antigens 2014;83:65–75.
15. Patel R, Terasaki PI. Significance of the positive crossmatch test in kidney transplantation. N Engl J Med 1969;280:735–9.
17. Gebel HM, Bray RA. Laboratory assessment of HLA antibodies circa 2006: making sense of sensitivity. Transplant Rev 2006;20:189–94.
18. Gebel HM, Bray RA, Nickerson P. Pre-transplant assessment of donor-reactive, HLA-specific antibodies in renal transplantation: contraindication vs. risk. Am J Transplant 2003;3:1488–500.
20. Jaramillo A, Ramon DS, Stoll ST. Technical aspects of crossmatching in transplantation. Clin Lab Med 2018;38:579–93.
26. Schinstock CA, Gandhi MJ, Stegall MD. Interpreting anti-HLA antibody testing data: a practical guide for physicians. Transplantation 2016;100:1619–28.
27. Reed EF, Rao P, Zhang Z, et al. Comprehensive assessment and standardization of solid phase multiplex-bead arrays for the detection of antibodies to HLA. Am J Transplant 2013;13:1859–70.
28. Greenshields AL, Liwski RS. The ABCs (DRDQDPs) of the prozone effect in single antigen bead hla antibody testing: lessons from our highly sensitized patients. Hum Immunol 2019;80:478–86.
33. Juskewitch JE, Norgan AP, De Goey SR, et al. How do I manage the platelet transfusion-refractory patient? Transfusion 2017;57:2828–35.
34. Vassallo RR. Recognition and management of antibodies to human platelet antigens in platelet transfusion-refractory patients. Immunohematology 2009;25:119–24.
36. Toy P, Gajic O, Bacchetti P, et al. Transfusion-related acute lung injury: incidence and risk factors. Blood 2012;119:1757–67.
40. Vossoughi S, Gorlin J, Kessler DA, et al. Ten years of TRALI mitigation: measuring our progress. Transfusion 2019;59:2567–74.
41. Caillat-Zucman S. Molecular mechanisms of HLA association with autoimmune diseases. Tissue Antigens 2009;73:1–8.
43. Fan WL, Shiao MS, Hui RC, et al. HLA association with drug-induced adverse reactions. J Immunol Res 2017;2017:3186328.
45. Parolini F, Biswas P, Serena M, et al. Stability and expression levels of HLA-C on the cell membrane modulate HIV-1 infectivity. J Virol 2017;92:e01711–7.

Monoclonal Antibody Therapeutics and Immunogenicity

Eszter Lázár-Molnár, Maria Alice Vieira Willrich, and Julio C. Delgado[a]

ABSTRACT

Background
The introduction of monoclonal antibody drugs has had major impact in medicine, leading to extraordinary progress in the treatment of a wide variety of diseases, particularly malignancies and chronic inflammatory and autoimmune diseases.

Content
This chapter provides a general overview of monoclonal antibody drugs approved for clinical use, including the basic biology of antibodies, production, pharmacologic characteristics, nomenclature, and various clinical indications. Because of the widespread use of tumor necrosis factor (TNF) antagonists in clinical medicine, we focus on the clinical use of this class of monoclonal antibody drugs to explain the mechanisms that elicit immunogenicity and to describe methodologies for drug monitoring and immunogenicity testing in the clinical laboratory. Finally, interference of monoclonal antibodies with clinical laboratory testing is reviewed since this is an emerging issue increasingly faced by laboratories as the number of patients treated with these drugs is on the rise.

Monoclonal antibody therapeutics (MAT) were initially introduced in transplantation medicine[1,2] following the approval of the first monoclonal antibody drug, muromonab-CD3, by the United States Food and Drug Administration (FDA) in 1985 as an antirejection agent in renal transplant patients.[3] Subsequently in the 1990s several other monoclonal antibodies were approved for clinical use such as rituximab in 1997, followed by trastuzumab and infliximab a year later. All three of these MAT achieved remarkable success, ranking among the top best-selling drugs ever since. The implementation of MAT led to unprecedented progress in the treatment of a wide variety of diseases, including malignancies and chronic inflammatory and autoimmune diseases. MAT are used in oncology, rheumatology, gastroenterology, neurology, and many other areas of medicine. In recent years there have been dramatic advancements in cancer immunotherapy with the introduction of antibody drugs targeting checkpoint inhibitors cytotoxic T lymphocyte-associated 4 (CTLA-4) and programmed cell death-1 (PD-1).[4]

As of the end of 2019, there were 100 unique monoclonal antibody, antibody fragment, or Fc fusion-based drugs, and 20 biosimilars approved by the FDA for the treatment of various diseases. These numbers are expected to increase dramatically in coming years since many more are currently in development.

BIOLOGY OF ANTIBODIES

Antibodies, also known as immunoglobulins (Ig), are naturally occurring large glycoprotein molecules that can be found membrane-bound on the surface of B cells, or in secreted form produced by B cell-derived plasma cells. In addition to recognizing and binding specific antigens, they can induce effector functions such as complement binding and activation of the complement cascade, or induce antibody-dependent cellular cytotoxicity (ADCC). Both of these mechanisms are aimed at eliminating the antigen source by inducing cell killing. Diversity and specificity are essential features of antibodies: the immune system is genetically capable of producing antibodies to virtually any antigen that it encounters, and the antibodies produced are highly specific to that antigen. Antibody-mediated responses constitute crucial mechanisms of the adaptive immune system to provide protection against viruses, bacteria, parasites, and other pathogens.

Ig are large Y-shaped molecules.[5] Each Ig consists of two identical heavy chains (H, 55 kD) and two light chains (L, 22 kD) (Fig. 98.1A). Light chains can be of either lambda (λ) or kappa (κ) isotype, which are functionally identical (for additional information, refer to Chapter 31). Ig heavy chains belong to five different isotypes, which are functionally and structurally different and define the five major Ig classes in humans: IgM, IgD, IgA, IgE, and IgG. IgG is the major type of Ig in normal human serum. It functions predominantly in the secondary phase of the immune response, since it takes at least 2 to 3 weeks for it to appear in the serum following antigenic encounter. IgG can be further subdivided into IgG1, IgG2, IgG3, and IgG4 subclasses in humans, which vary in abundance, the type of antigen they bind to, and in their ability to induce effector functions.[5] Antibody subclass isotype determines the type of effector function induced; IgG3 and IgG1 are the most potent activators of the complement pathway by interacting with C1q and induce complement-dependent cytotoxicity (CDC). IgG3 and IgG1 also bind to Fc receptors on effector cells activating cellular responses such as ADCC. IgG1 is most abundant in serum, followed by IgG2, IgG3, and IgG4. Except for IgG3,

[a]The authors would like to thank Ms. Mary Paul and Ms. Natalya Wilkins-Tyler for their assistance in preparing the figures.

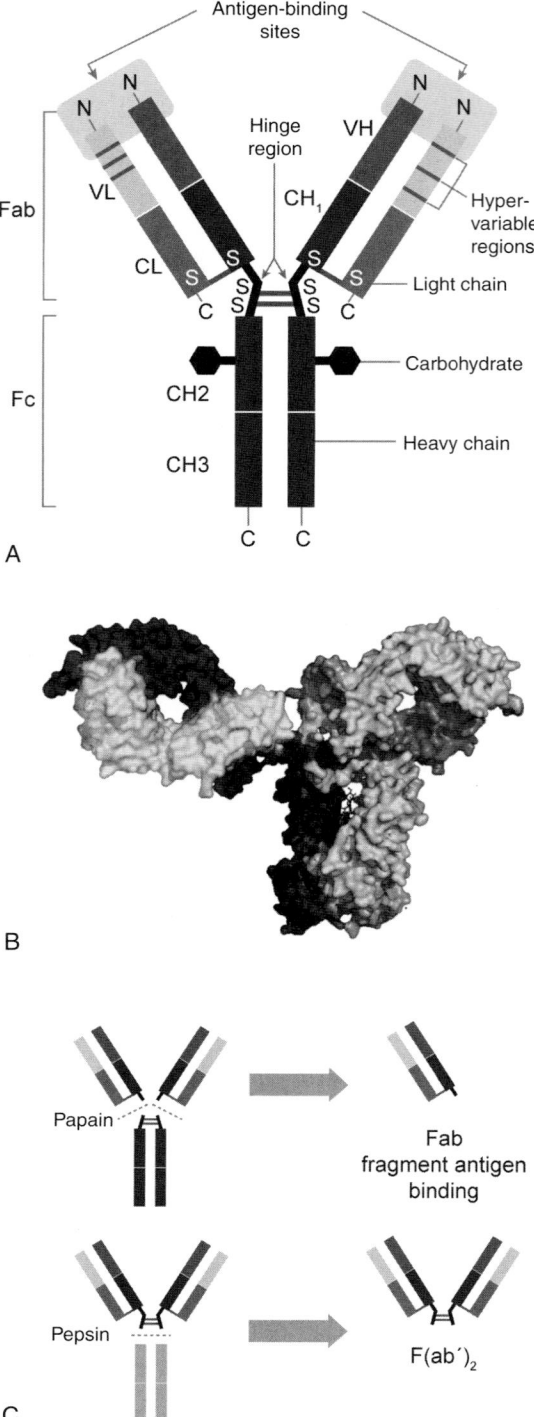

FIGURE 98.1 Structure of the IgG Immunoglobulin Molecule. (A) The IgG molecule consists of two copies of heavy (H) and light (L) polypeptide chains. The L chain has one variable (VL) and one constant (CL) domain, while the H chain has one variable (VH) and three constant (CH1, CH2, CH3) domains. The four chains are connected by disulfide bridges (S). The antigen binding sites are at the N terminal end of the variable domains and are organized into three hypervariable or complementarity determining regions. Glycosylation by carbohydrate molecules are indicated on the heavy chains. (B) Crystal structure of a human IgG1 determined at 2.7Å resolution indicates an asymmetric conformation (protein data bank [PDB] ID: 1HZH). The two IgG1 heavy chains are shown in red and pink; light chains are shown in gray. Carbohydrate chains forming the contact between the CH2 domains are shown in ball-and-stick. The figure was prepared using PyMOL. (C) Enzymatic cleavage of monoclonal antibodies results in fragments that are also targets for therapeutic drug design. Papain digestion yields two Fab fragments with one antigen binding site for each. Pepsin cleaves off the Fc portion below the interchain disulfide bond, leaving a single fragment F(ab')2 that preserves the two antigen binding sites.

which has a serum half-life of about 7 days, the rest of the IgG subclasses have half-lives of ~21 days. When effector functions such as ADCC are desired, IgG1 is the isotype of choice for MAT development (such as in oncology). When blockade rather than engaging immune effector functions is required, IgG2 and IgG4 have been used. Overall, IgG1 is the most frequently used isotype in MAT.

Structurally the IgG heavy and light chains are held together by interchain disulfide bonds in the hinge region (see Fig. 98.1A). Although the structures are diverse, they contain well-defined domains such as the Ig variable (V) and constant (C) domains.[5] These domains are composed of ~100 amino acid residues that share a common two-layered structure composed of two antiparallel β-sheets. The L chain folds into two domains, VL and CL, while the larger H chain consists of four domains, VH, CH1, CH2, and CH3. The antigen binding sites are located at the amino terminal variable region of both the H and the L chain, also called hypervariable regions or complementarity determining regions (CDR), which form a unique antigen binding site known as idiotype. Each variable domain contains three CDR regions, CDR1, CDR2, and CDR3, which show very high degree of sequence variability, and determine antibody specificity. Antibody diversity is generated by complex genetic mechanisms such as somatic hypermutation and affinity maturation. Despite sequence diversity, all Ig domains have highly similar three-dimensional structures. The available highest-resolution crystal structure of a typical full-length human IgG1 determined by x-ray crystallography is shown on Fig. 98.1B. The structure indicates a highly asymmetric conformation ranging from Y shape to T shape, due to high molecular flexibility in the hinge region, which makes structure determination of complete IgG molecules difficult. However, mild enzymatic cleavage with proteolytic enzymes papain or pepsin results in fragments that are easier to crystallize (Fig. 98.1C). Cleavage of an intact antibody molecule with papain results in two monovalent Fab fragments and one dimeric crystallizable fragment (Fc). Cleavage with pepsin results in a bivalent, single F(ab') fragment. In addition to intact Ig, these well-defined Ig fragments have medical and therapeutic applications themselves. The Ig domain structure is conserved in nature; its variants are commonly found as part of other proteins, including Fc receptors, adhesion molecules, costimulatory receptors and ligands, and many others.

THERAPEUTIC ANTIBODIES

The concept of using serum therapy for treatment of disease dates back to the discovery of diphtheria antitoxin by Emil Adolf von Behring (1890), who was awarded a shared Nobel prize in 1901 for the development of serum therapies against diphtheria and tetanus.[6] Serum polyclonal antibody preparations and pooled IgG from healthy individuals have been used for prevention of several infectious diseases (e.g., hepatitis A), or for replacement therapy in patients with Ig deficiencies. Intravenous Ig, approved in 1980, and subcutaneous Ig, approved in 2006, are widely used as replacement therapy, or for the treatment of various autoimmune diseases or as part of desensitization protocols or treatment of rejection in transplantation.

Polyclonal antibodies used for therapeutic interventions include Rh (D) Ig, an enriched fraction of antibodies directed to the D blood group antigen for the prevention of rhesus D alloimmunization in pregnancy. Anti-thymocyte globulin (ATG) is another example of a widely used polyclonal

antibody therapeutic prepared by immunizing mammals (commonly rabbit or horse) with human thymic lymphocytes. ATG administered to patients binds to lymphocytes and depletes them, leading to a profound suppression of the cellular immune response. ATG is used for the treatment of aplastic anemia and organ rejection.

Generation of Monoclonal Antibody Therapeutics

Development of the hybridoma technology in 1975 allowed for production of monoclonal antibodies in vitro, using a hybridoma cell obtained by fusing an immortal myeloma cell (plasma cell-derived tumor cell) and a splenic normal B-cell derived plasma cell.[7] This technology allowed for in vitro production of large amounts of MAT against a wide range of targets, including soluble and cell surface proteins. Early MAT products contained large amounts of nonhuman (i.e., mouse) proteins due to the use of mouse spleen derived plasma cells, which was responsible for the development of adverse effects due to the generation of human anti-mouse antibodies. Clinical experience with the first MAT, murine anti-CD3 muromonab, indicated poor pharmacokinetics and high immunogenicity, making treatment ineffective, which eventually resulted in withdrawal of the drug.[8]

Using recombinant DNA technologies and better understanding of antibody structure-function correlation allowed for the development of chimeric (>65% human on average), humanized (>80% human), and fully human (>95% human) antibodies.[9] Chimeric antibodies contain murine sequences in the variable region since they are initially developed as mouse antibodies. The rest of the molecule is replaced with human sequences, which reduces, but does not eliminate immunogenicity, and improves effector functions due to the presence of the human Fc part. The first chimeric antibody, abciximab, a human-mouse Fab fragment, was approved in the US in 1994, followed by rituximab in 1997, the first chimeric full-length antibody. The next phase of technology development allowed for the exchange of rodent sequences almost entirely to human sequences throughout the molecule, by grafting of the rodent CDR onto human IgG. The first humanized antibody, daclizumab, an antibody to IL-2 receptor α subunit, was approved in the United States in 1997 for the treatment of transplant rejection (withdrawn in 2009). Generation of fully human antibodies became possible with the development of phage-display technology, and transgenic mouse platforms. Phage display platform has become a commodity since the technology patents expired recently.[10] It allows for designing and manipulating the repertoire of antibody genes used as antibody sources, followed by in vitro selection. The first antibody to reach the US market developed by this technology was the tumor necrosis factor (TNF) antagonist adalimumab, approved in 2002.[11] In contrast to phage display platform, transgenic animal technology allows for in vivo selection process and requires less optimization and shorter timelines to reach clinical development.[12] Antibody-producing plasma cells isolated from the spleen of immunized, genetically modified mice that express fully human monoclonal antibodies but are unable to produce mouse antibodies, are used to create hybridomas, which are used for subsequent large-scale production. MAT produced by transgenic technologies include panitumumab, approved in 2006 for oncology, and golimumab, a TNF antagonist approved in 2009.

As of the end of 2019, there were 100 unique monoclonal antibody-based drugs approved in the United States (Table 98.1). Eighty-six of these are monoclonal antibodies or

TABLE 98.1 **Monoclonal Antibody Therapeutics Approved by the US Food and Drug Administration as of December 2019**

Product (Proper) Name	Proprietary Name	Date of Licensure (month/day/year)	Molecular Target	Protein Format	Source	Major Indication
Oncology						
Capromab pendetide	ProstaScint	10/28/1996	Prostate specific membrane antigen (PSMA), or glutamate carboxypep-tidase 2	Murine IgG1, conjugated to Indium-111-pendetide	Mouse hybridoma	Imaging of prostate cancer
Rituximab	Rituxan	11/26/1997	CD20	Chimeric human-murine IgG1κ	CHO cells	NHL, CLL, RA
Trastuzumab	Herceptin	09/25/1998	EGFR (HER2)	Humanized IgG1κ	CHO cells	HER2-positive breast cancer
Alemtuzumab	Campath, Lemtrada	05/07/2001	CD52	Humanized rat IgG1κ	CHO cells	B-cell CLL
Ibritumomab tiuxetan	Zevalin	02/19/2002	CD20	Murine IgG1 conjugated to Indium or yttrium	CHO cells	NH lymphoma
Cetuximab	Erbitux	02/12/2004	EGFR	Chimeric murine-human mAb Fab	SP2/0 murine myeloma	Metastatic colorectal carcinoma (EGFR+)
Bevacizumab	Avastin	02/26/2004	VEGF	Humanized IgG1	CHO	Metastatic colorectal cancer, Her2 negative metastatic breast cancer
Panitumumab	Vectibix	09/27/2006	EGFR	Human IgG2	Transgenic technology/ Hybridoma cells	Metastatic colorectal carcinoma
Ofatumumab	Arzerra	10/26/2009	CD20	Human IgG1κ	Mouse hybridoma	CLL
Ipilimumab	Yervoy	03/25/2011	CTLA-4	Human IgG1κ	CHO cells	Metastatic melanoma
Brentuximab vedotin	Adcetris	08/19/2011	CD30	Chimeric human-murine IgG1 coupled with monomethyl auristatin E (MMAE), a microtubule disrupting agent, through a protease-cleavable linker	CHO cells for the mAb	HL, anaplastic LCL
Pertuzumab	Perjeta	06/08/2012	EGFR (HER2)	Humanized IgG1	CHO cells	HER2-positive breast cancer
Ziv-aflibercept	Zaltrap	08/03/2012	VEGF	VEGFR fused to human IgG1 Fc	CHO cells	Metastatic colorectal cancer
Ado-trastuzumab emtansine	Kadcyla	02/22/2013	EGFR (HER2)	Humanized IgG1k linked to anti-microtubule agent DM1	CHO cells for the mAb	HER2-positive breast cancer
Obinutuzumab	Gazyva	11/01/2013	CD20	Humanized IgG1	CHO cells	CLL
Ramucirumab	Cyramza	04/21/2014	VEGFR2	Human IgG1	Hybridoma cells	Gastric adenocarcinoma
Pembrolizumab	Keytruda	09/04/2014	PD-1 (CD279)	Humanized IgG4κ	Hybridoma	Melanoma, NSCLC, Head and Neck cancer
Blinatumomab	Blincyto	12/03/2014	CD19, CD3d	Murine antibody, constructed BiTE (bi-specific T-cell engager)	CHO cells	B-cell ALL

TABLE 98.1 Monoclonal Antibody Therapeutics Approved by the US Food and Drug Administration as of December 2019—cont'd

Product (Proper) Name	Proprietary Name	Date of Licensure (month/day/year)	Molecular Target	Protein Format	Source	Major Indication
Nivolumab	Opdivo	12/22/2014	PD-1 (CD279)	Human IgG4	Transgenic mouse technology	Metastatic melanoma
Dinutuximab	Unituxin	03/10/2015	GD2, disialoganglioside	Chimeric IgG1κ	Murine hybridoma	Neuroblastoma
Daratumumab	Darzalex	11/16/2015	CD38	Human IgG1κ	CHO cells	Multiple myeloma
Necitumumab	Portrazza	11/24/2015	EGFR	Human IgG1κ	NSO Myeloma cells	NSCLC
Elotuzumab	Empliciti	11/30/2015	SLAMF7	Humanized IgG1κ	NSO Myeloma cells	Multiple myeloma
Atezolizumab	Tecentriq	05/18/2016	PD-L1 (CD274)	Humanized IgG1, Fc engineered (nonglycosylated)	Mouse hybridoma	Urothelial carcinoma
Olaratumab	Lartruvo	10/19/2016	PDGFRa	Human IgG1	NSO Myeloma cells	Soft tissue sarcoma (STS)
Avelumab	Bavencio	03/23/2017	PD-L1 (CD274)	Human IgG1λ	CHO cells	Metastatic Merkel cell carcinoma
Durvalumab	Imfinzi	05/01/2017	PD-L1 (CD274)	Human IgG1κ	CHO cells	Urothelial carcinoma
Rituximab and Hyaluronidase human	Rituxan Hycela	06/22/2017	CD20	Chimeric human-murine IgG1κ	CHO cells	Follicular lymphoma, diffuse large B-cell lymphoma, CLL
Inotuzumab Ozogamicin	Besponsa	08/17/2017	CD22	Humanized IgG4κ attached to N-acetyl-γ-calicheamicin dimethylhydrazide	CHO cells	ALL
Tisagenle-cleucel	Kymriah	08/30/2017	CD19	Chimeric antigen receptor (CAR)	Expressed by patient's own cells by in vitro molecular engineering	ALL
Gemtuzumab ozogamicin	Mylotarg	09/01/2017	CD33	Humanized IgG4κ attached to calicheamicin	NSO Myeloma cells	CD33 positive AML
Axicabtagene ciloleucel	Yescarta	10/18/2017	CD19	Chimeric antigen receptor (CAR)	Expressed by patient's own cells by in vitro molecular engineering	Large B-cell lymphoma
Mogamulizumab-kpkc	Poteligeo	08/08/2018	CCR4	Humanized IgG1κ	CHO cells	T-cell malignancies: mycosis fungoides or Sézary syndrome
Moxetumomab pasudotox-tdfk	Lumoxiti	09/13/2018	CD22	Murine IgV fused to Pseudomonas exotoxin PE38	*Escherichia coli*	Hairy cell leukemia
Cemiplimab-rwlc	Libtayo	09/28/2018	PD-1 (CD279)	Human IgG4	CHO cells	Cutaneous squamous cell carcinoma (CSCC)
Trastuzumab and Hyaluronidase-oysk	Herceptin Hylecta	02/28/2019	EGFR (HER2)	Humanized IgG1κ	CHO cells	HER2-positive breast cancer
Polatuzumab vedotin-piiq	Polivy	06/10/2019	CD79b	Humanized IgG1 fused to anti-mitotic agent MMAE through protease-cleavable linker	CHO cells	Diffuse large B-cell lymphoma

Continued

TABLE 98.1   Monoclonal Antibody Therapeutics Approved by the US Food and Drug Administration as of December 2019—cont'd

Product (Proper) Name	Proprietary Name	Date of Licensure (month/day/year)	Molecular Target	Protein Format	Source	Major Indication
Enfortumab vedotin-ejfv	Padcev	12/18/2019	Nectin 4	Human IgG1κ conjugated to ani-mitotic agent monomethyl auristatin E (MMAE) through protease-cleavable linker	CHO cells	Advanced or metastatic urothelial cancer
Fam-trastuzumab deruxtecan-nxki	Enhertu	12/20/2019	Her2	Humanized IgG1 linked to topoisomerase inhibitor DXd through protease cleavable linker	CHO cells	Metastatic breast cancer
Rheumatology						
Infliximab	Remicade	08/24/1998	TNF	Chimeric human-murine IgG1κ	Mouse hybridoma	RA, PsA, AS, Crohn disease, PsO
Etanercept	Enbrel	11/02/1998	TNF	p75 TNFR2—huIgG1 Fc fusion	CHO cells	RA, PsO, AS, JIA, plaque psoriasis
Adalimumab	Humira	12/31/2002	TNF	Human IgG1κ	CHO cells	RA, PsA, AS, JIA, Crohn disease, plaque psoriasis, hidradenitis suppurativa, uveitis
Abatacept	Orencia	12/23/2005	CTLA-4 ligands CD80 (B7-1), CD86 (B7-2)	CTLA-4 fused to IgG1 Fc	CHO cells	RA, PsA, JIA
Certolizumab pegol	Cimzia	04/22/2008	TNF	Humanized IgG4 Fab	E. coli	RA, PsA, AS, Crohn disease
Golimumab	Simponi	04/24/2009	TNF	Human IgG1κ	Mouse SP2/0 hybridoma	RA, PsA, AS, Spondyloarthritis, UC
Tocilizumab	Actemra	01/08/2010 10/21/2013	IL-6R (CD126)	Humanized IgG1κ	Hybridoma	RA, JIA, Giant cell arteritis, Cytokine release syndrome
Golimumab	Simponi Aria	07/18/2013	TNF	Human IgG1κ	Transgenic mouse technology	RA, PsA, AS
Sarilumab	Kevzara	05/22/2017	IL-6R (CD126)	Human IgG1	CHO cells	RA
Secukinumab	Cosentyx	01/21/2015	IL-17A	Human IgG1κ	CHO cells	Psoriasis, AS
Ustekinumab	Stelara	09/25/2009 09/23/2016	p40 subunit of IL-12 and Il-23	Human IgG1κ	SP2/0 murine myeloma	Plaque psoriasis, PsA, Crohn disease
Canakinumab	Ilaris	06/17/2009	IL-1β	Human IgG1κ	Mouse Sp2/0-Ag14 cell line	Cryopyrin-associated periodic syndromes: Familial cold autoinflammatory syndrome and Muckle-Wells syndrome; JIA
Dermatology						
Guselkumab	Tremfya	07/13/2017	IL-23 p19	Human IgG1λ	Mammalian cell line	Plaque psoriasis
Tildrakizumab-asmn	Ilumya	03/20/2018	IL-23 p19	Humanized IgG1κ	CHO cells	Plaque psoriasis
Risankizumab-rzaa	Skyrizi	04/23/2019	IL-23 p19	Humanized IgG1	Mammalian cell line	Plaque psoriasis
Ustekinumab	Stelara	09/25/2009 9/23/2016	p40 subunit of IL-12 and Il-23	Human IgG1κ	SP2/0 murine myeloma	Plaque psoriasis, PsA, Crohn disease

TABLE 98.1 Monoclonal Antibody Therapeutics Approved by the US Food and Drug Administration as of December 2019—cont'd

Product (Proper) Name	Proprietary Name	Date of Licensure (month/day/year)	Molecular Target	Protein Format	Source	Major Indication
Secukinumab	Cosentyx	01/21/2015	IL-17A	Human IgG1κ	CHO cells	Psoriasis, AS
Ixekizumab	Taltz	03/22/2016	IL-17A	Humanized IgG4κ	Mouse hybridoma	Plaque psoriasis
Brodalumab	Siliq	02/15/2017	IL-17RA	Human IgG2	CHO cells	Plaque psoriasis
Dupilumab	Dupixent	03/28/2017	IL-4Ra, IL-4 and IL-13 receptor	Human IgG4	CHO cells	Eczema, atopic dermatitis
Blood Disease						
Emicizumab-kxwh	Hemlibra	11/16/2017	Factor Ixa and Factor X	Humanized IgG4, bispecific	CHO cells	Hemophilia
Caplacizumab-yhdp	Cablivi	02/06/2019	von Willebrand factor	Humanized bivalent antibody fragment (Nanobody, heavy chain fragment from Camelidae)	E. coli	Acquired thrombotic thrombocytopenic purpura (aTTP)
Efmoroctocog alfa	Eloctate	06/06/2014	Factor VIII substitute	Factor VII fused to human IgG1 Fc	HEK cell line	Hemophilia A
Luspatercept-aamt	Reblozyl	11/08/2019	TGF-β superfamily ligands	Activin receptor type IIB linked to human IgG1 Fc domain	CHO cells	Erythroid maturation agent
Crizanlizumab-tmca	Adakveo	11/15/2019	P-selectin	Humanized IgG2κ	CHO cells	Sickle cell disease
Romiplostim	Nplate	08/22/2008	Thrombopoietin receptor c-Mpl	Peptibody, fused to IgG1 Fc	E. coli	chronic immune thrombocytopenic purpura
Eftrenonacog alfa	Alprolix	03/28/2014	Factor IX substitute	Factor IX fused to human IgG1 Fc	HEK293H cell line	Hemophilia B
Idarucizumab	Praxbind	10/16/2015	Dabigatran, thrombin inhibitor drug	Humanized IgG1 Fab	CHO cells	Anticoagulant reversal
Gastroenterology						
Infliximab	Remicade	08/24/1998	TNF	Chimeric human-murine IgG1κ	Mouse hybridoma	RA, PsA, AS, Crohn disease, plaque psoriasis
Adalimumab	Humira	12/31/2002	TNF	Human IgG1κ	CHO cells	RA, PsA, AS, JIA, Crohn disease, plaque psoriasis, hidradenitis suppurativa, uveitis
Certolizumab pegol	Cimzia	04/22/2008	TNF	Humanized IgG4 Fab	E. coli	RA, PsA, AS, Crohn disease
Golimumab	Simponi	04/24/2009	TNF	Human IgG1κ	Mouse SP2/0 hybridoma	RA, PsA, AS, Spondyloarthritis, UC
Ustekinumab	Stelara	09/25/2009 09/23/2016	p40 subunit of IL-12 and Il-23	Human IgG1κ	SP2/0 murine myeloma	Plaque psoriasis, PsA, Crohn disease
Natalizumab	Tysabri	11/23/2004	α4-integrin	Humanized IgG4κ	Murine myeloma	MS, Crohn disease
Vedolizumab	Entyvio	05/20/2014	a4b7 integrin	Humanized IgG1	CHO cells	UC, Crohn disease
Autoinflammatory and Other Immunologic Disease						
Lanadelumab-flyo	Takhzyro	08/23/2018	Plasma kallikrein	Human IgG1κ	CHO cells	Hereditary angioedema (HAE)
Emapalumab-lzsg	Gamifant	11/20/2018	Interferon-γ	Human IgG1	CHO cells	Hemophagocytic lymphohistiocytosis (HLH)
Ravulizumab-cwvz	Ultomiris	12/21/2018	Complement C5	Humanized IgG2/4κ	CHO cells	Paroxysmal nocturnal hemoglobinuria (PNH)

Continued

TABLE 98.1 Monoclonal Antibody Therapeutics Approved by the US Food and Drug Administration as of December 2019—cont'd

Product (Proper) Name	Proprietary Name	Date of Licensure (month/day/year)	Molecular Target	Protein Format	Source	Major Indication
Eculizumab	Soliris	03/16/2007	C5	Humanized IgG2/4κ	Murine hybridoma	PNH
Canakinumab	Ilaris	06/17/2009	IL-1β	Human IgG1κ	Mouse Sp2/0-Ag14 cell line	Cryopyrin-associated periodic syndromes: Familial cold autoinflammatory syndrome and Muckle-Wells syndrome; JIA
Siltuximab	Sylvant	04/23/2014	IL-6	Chimeric IgG1	CHO cells	multicentric Castleman's disease
Rilonacept	Arcalyst	02/27/2008	IL-1	IL-1R and IL-1R accessory protein linked to hu IgG1 Fc	CHO cells	Cryopyrin-associated periodic syndromes: Familial cold autoinflammatory syndrome and Muckle-Wells syndrome
Neurologic Disease						
Ocrelizumab	Ocrevus	03/28/2017	CD20	Humanized IgG1	CHO cells	Progressive MS
Natalizumab	Tysabri	11/23/2004	α4-integrin	Humanized IgG4κ	Murine myeloma	MS, Crohn disease
Erenumab-aooe	Aimovig	05/17/2018	Calcitonin gene-related peptide receptor (CGRP)	Human IgG2λ	CHO cells	Migraine
Fremanezumab-vfrm	Ajovy	09/14/2018	Calcitonin gene-related peptide (CGRP) ligand	Humanized IgG2Δa/κ	CHO cells	Migraine
Galcanezumab-gnlm	Emgality	09/27/2018	Calcitonin gene-related peptide (CGRP) ligand	Humanized IgG4κ	CHO cells	Migraine
Allergy and Asthma						
Reslizumab	Cinqair	03/23/2016	IL-5	Humanized IgG4κ	NSO Myeloma cells	Severe eosinophilic asthma
Omalizumab	Xolair	06/20/2003	IgE	Humanized IgG1κ	CHO cells	Asthma caused by allergies
Benralizumab	Fasenra	11/14/2017	IL-5Ra	Humanized IgG1κ, Fc engineered (afucosylated)	CHO cells	Severe eosinophilic asthma
Mepolizumab	Nucala	11/04/2015	IL-5	Humanized IgG1κ	CHO cells	Severe eosinophilic asthma; Eosinophilic granulomatosis with polyangiitis (EGPA), appr 6/6/19
Dupilumab	Dupixent	03/28/2017	IL-4Ra, IL-4 and IL-13 receptor	Human IgG4	CHO cells	Eczema, atopic dermatitis
Infectious Disease						
Palivizumab	Synagis	06/19/1998	RSV F protein, A antigenic site	Humanized IgG1κ	Mouse hybridoma	RSV infection
Raxibacumab	Raxibacumab	12/14/2012	*Bacillus anthracis* PA toxin	Human IgG1λ	Murine hybridoma	Anthrax
Ibalizumab-uiyk	Trogarzo	03/06/2018	CD4	Humanized IgG4	NSO Myeloma cells	HIV infection

TABLE 98.1 Monoclonal Antibody Therapeutics Approved by the US Food and Drug Administration as of December 2019—cont'd

Product (Proper) Name	Proprietary Name	Date of Licensure (month/day/year)	Molecular Target	Protein Format	Source	Major Indication
Obiltoxaximab	Anthim	03/18/2016	*B. anthracis* PA toxin	Chimeric IgG1κ, affinity enhanced	Mouse hybridoma	Anthrax—Biodefense
Bezlotoxumab	Zinplava	10/21/2016	*Clostridium difficile* toxin B	Human IgG1	CHO cells	*C. difficile* infection
Bone Disease						
Burosumab-twza	Crysvita	04/17/2018	Fibroblast Growth Factor (FGF23)	Human IgG1κ	CHO cells	X-linked hypophosphatemia (XLH), a form of rickets
Romosozumab-aqqg	Evenity	04/09/2019	Sclerostin	Humanized IgG2	CHO cells	Osteoporosis in postmenopausal women
Denosumab	Prolia, Xgeva	06/01/2010	RANKL, NF-κB ligand	Human IgG2	CHO cells	Osteoporosis, bone metastasis from solid tumors
Asfotase alfa	Strensiq	10/23/2015	TNSALP enzyme replacement	Catalytic domain of human tissue nonspecific alkaline phosphatase (TNSALP), fused to human IgG1 Fc, and a deca-aspartate peptide as bone targeting domain	CHO cells	Hypophosphatasia
Cardiovascular Disease						
Abciximab	ReoPro	12/22/1994	GP IIb/IIIa platelet receptor	Chimeric human-murine mAb Fab	Mouse hybridoma	CVD
Alirocumab	Praluent	07/24/2015	PCSK9, paraprotein convertase subtilisin/kexin type 9	Human IgG1	CHO cells	Familial hypercholesterolemia, CVD
Evolocumab	Repatha	08/27/2015	PCSK9, paraprotein convertase subtilisin/kexin type 10	Human IgG2	CHO cells	Familial hypercholesterolemia, CVD
Ophthalmology						
Brolucizumab-dbll	Beovu	10/07/2019	VEGF	Humanized single-chain Fv (scFv) antibody fragment	*E. coli*	Neovascular (Wet) age-related macular degeneration (AMD)
Ranibizumab	Lucentis	06/30/2006	VEGF-A	Humanized IgG1κ mAb fragment	*E. coli*	Macular edema, age-related macular degeneration
Aflibercept	Eylea	11/18/2011	VEGF	VEGFR fused to human IgG1 Fc	CHO cells	Macular edema
Transplant						
Basiliximab	Simulect	05/12/1998	CD25, IL-2Rα	Chimeric human-murine IgG1κ	Mouse hybridoma	Transplant rejection
Belatacept	Nulojix	06/15/2011	CTLA-4 ligands CD80 (B7-1), CD86 (B7-2)	CTLA-4 (2 amino acid mutant) fused to IgG1 Fc	CHO cells	Transplant rejection

Continued

TABLE 98.1 **Monoclonal Antibody Therapeutics Approved by the US Food and Drug Administration as of December 2019—cont'd**

Product (Proper) Name	Proprietary Name	Date of Licensure (month/day/year)	Molecular Target	Protein Format	Source	Major Indication
Systemic Autoimmune						
Belimumab	Benlysta	03/09/2011 iv 07/20/2017 sc	B lymphocyte stimulator protein (BLyS)/ TNFSF13B/BAFF	Human IgG1λ	NSO Myeloma cells	SLE
Mepolizumab	Nucala	11/04/2015	IL-5	Humanized IgG1κ	CHO cells	Severe eosinophilic asthma; Eosinophilic granulomatosis with polyangiitis (EGPA), appr 6/6/19
Metabolic Disease						
Dulaglutide	Trulicity	09/18/2014	GLP-1R	Glucagon-like peptide-1 agonist (GLP-1) fused to human IgG4 Fc	HEK293H cell line	Type II diabetes

ALL, Acute lymphocytic leukemia; *AML,* acute myeloid leukemia; *AS,* ankylosing spondylitis; *CHO,* Chinese hamster ovary; *CLL,* chronic lymphocytic leukemia; *CTLA4,* cytotoxic T lymphocyte-associated 4; *CVD,* cardiovascular disease; *EGFR,* epidermal growth factor receptor; *GD2,* disialoganglioside-2; *GLP-1,* glucagon-like peptide-1; *GP,* glycoprotein; *HEK,* human embryonic kidney; *HL,* Hodgkin's lymphoma; *hu,* human; *Ig,* immunoglobulin; *IL,* interleukin; *JIA,* juvenile idiopathic arthritis; *LCL,* large cell lymphoma; *Mpl,* myeloproliferative leukemia virus oncogene; *MS,* multiple sclerosis; *NHL,* non-Hodgkin's lymphoma; *NSCLC,* non–small cell lung cancer; *PCSK9,* Proprotein convertase subtilisin/kexin type 9; *PD-1,* programmed cell death-1; *PDGFR,* platelet-derived growth factor receptor; *PD-L1,* programmed cell death-1 ligand-1; *PNH,* paroxysmal nocturnal hemoglobinuria; *PsA,* psoriatic arthritis; *PsO,* plaque psoriasis; *RA,* rheumatoid arthritis; *RANKL,* receptor activator of nuclear factor κ-B ligand; *RSV,* respiratory syncytial virus; *SLAMF7,* signaling lymphocytic activation molecule family member 7; *SLE,* systemic lupus erythematosus; *TNF,* tumor necrosis factor; *TNFR,* tumor necrosis factor receptor; *TNFSF,* tumor necrosis factor ligand superfamily; *TNSALP,* tissue nonspecific alkaline phosphatase; *VEGF,* vascular endothelial growth factor.
Data obtained from FDA Center for Drug Evaluation and Research (CDER) list of licensed biological products; from FDA news releases; and from FDA-approved package inserts.

antibody fragments, 12 are Fc fusion proteins or peptides, and 2 are engineered chimeric antigen receptor T-cell (CAR T) therapies. Of the 86 monoclonal antibody drugs 4 are murine, 10 are chimeric, 40 humanized (human-murine, human-rat, human-camelid), and 32 are fully human. Most of these drugs are full-length antibodies, the most common isotype being IgG1, which occurs in 61 (71%) of approved antibodies; 8 are IgG2 (9%), 2 are IgG2/IgG4 hybrid (2%), and 13 are IgG4 (15%). Additional structures include camelid, and single chain Fv fragments. 11 out of the 12 approved Fc fusion drugs contain IgG1, and one is fused to IgG4 Fc. Engineering the Fc part is becoming more common in order to modulate effector functions, such as using glycoengineering to enhance effector function. As an example, afucosylation of IgG1 Fc in benralizumab facilitates binding to FcγRIII on natural killer (NK) cells, enhancing ADCC-mediated apoptosis of eosinophils and basophils, which is beneficial for the treatment of severe eosinophilic asthma. The Fc part can also be modified to silence effector functions such as in abatacept or eculizumab.[13] Another approach for improving pharmacokinetics is to incorporate mutations to increase neonatal Fc receptor (FcRn) binding, such as the YTE mutation in some antibodies in development.[14] Fusing IgG Fc with other proteins or peptides improves their stability and half-life. This approach is used in 12 currently approved MAT including TNF receptor, enzymes (phosphatase), peptides (glucagon-like), and clotting factors (VIII, IX).

In addition to the full-length antibodies, five of the MAT are Fab antibody fragments. Some Fabs are fused to stabilizer molecules to improve pharmacokinetics in the absence of the Fc part, such as certolizumab pegol, which is PEGylated. Another innovative approach takes advantage of bispecific monoclonal antibodies designed as single-chain variable fragments of two different antibodies combined, such as in blinatumomab (approved in 2014 for acute leukemia), which is a bi-specific T-cell engager, connecting T cells via CD3 with tumor cells expressing CD19, facilitating immunologic synapse formation and tumor cell killing. Most of the approved MAT are nonconjugated intact IgG. However, ten of the MAT used in oncology are conjugated with drug molecules such as antimitotic agents, enzymes, or radioisotopes, which provide additional therapeutic benefits aimed at killing the tumor cell.

As a major breakthrough for cancer immunotherapy, two CAR T-cell therapy agents were approved in 2017: tisagenlecleucel for advanced leukemia and axicabtagene ciloleucel for lymphoma. Chimeric antigen receptor (CAR) is engineered as a single-chain variable fragment molecule fused to signaling domains, which is then expressed on host T cells, grafting monoclonal antibody specificity to the T cells. When injected back to the body, engineered host T cells expressing CAR receptors will recognize the target antigen on the cancer cells, such as CD19 on leukemic or lymphoma cells, and will induce tumor cell killing.[15]

Pharmacokinetic/Pharmacodynamic Properties

MAT are administered parenterally by intravenous, subcutaneous, or intramuscular routes.[16] The intravenous route has the advantage of offering systemic delivery, the ability to deliver high volumes, and most importantly, assures complete bioavailability. However, limitations include inconvenience and adverse effects due to infusion reactions. Subcutaneous and intramuscular delivery offers lower bioavailability (24 to 95%) but allows self-administration and decreased rate of infusion-related adverse events.[17] Although MAT distribute to most tissues to varying degrees, due to their large molecular weight (typically ~150 kDa) they are not able to cross the blood brain barrier and cannot enter the central nervous system.[18]

MAT are eliminated from circulation through various mechanisms: antigen-specific target-mediated disposition and elimination through endothelial cells of the reticuloendothelial system.[18] Target-mediated disposition involves antigen recognition and binding, typically to a membrane bound target, and subsequent clearance by endocytosis and lysosomal degradation. Since the number of antigenic targets is limited, this process is saturable and nonlinear. Elimination through the reticuloendothelial system, however, is nonsaturable and linear, and it involves both free and bound drug. These two processes typically occur in parallel, for MAT targeting a membrane-bound antigen.[18] In contrast to small molecule drugs, the liver and kidneys are not considered essential in the elimination of MAT under normal physiologic conditions, but clearance may be affected in the context of kidney injury leading to disruption of endothelial lining of the glomeruli (such as glomerulonephritis). Other routes affecting MAT clearance include loss of the drug through the gastrointestinal tract in protein losing enteropathy in patients with inflammatory bowel disease (IBD).

Since MAT are typically IgG molecules, their expected half-lives are quite long. This is explained by FcRn mediated uptake and endosomal recycling, a process that substantially extends the half-life of IgG (Fig. 98.2). The binding affinity of FcRn for IgG is negligible at physiologic pH, but when IgG is internalized and enters the endosomes, in the acidic environment of endocytic vacuoles (pH 6.5) it binds to FcRn with high affinity, which rescues IgG from degradation, recycling it through transcytosis.[19,20] The poor pharmacokinetics of mouse antibody-based drugs observed in earlier trials can be explained by their low affinity to human FcRn, which makes the recycling process less efficient.[16]

Of interest, high interindividual variability has been observed in pharmacokinetics of several MAT drugs. Based on multiple clinical trials, the most commonly identified

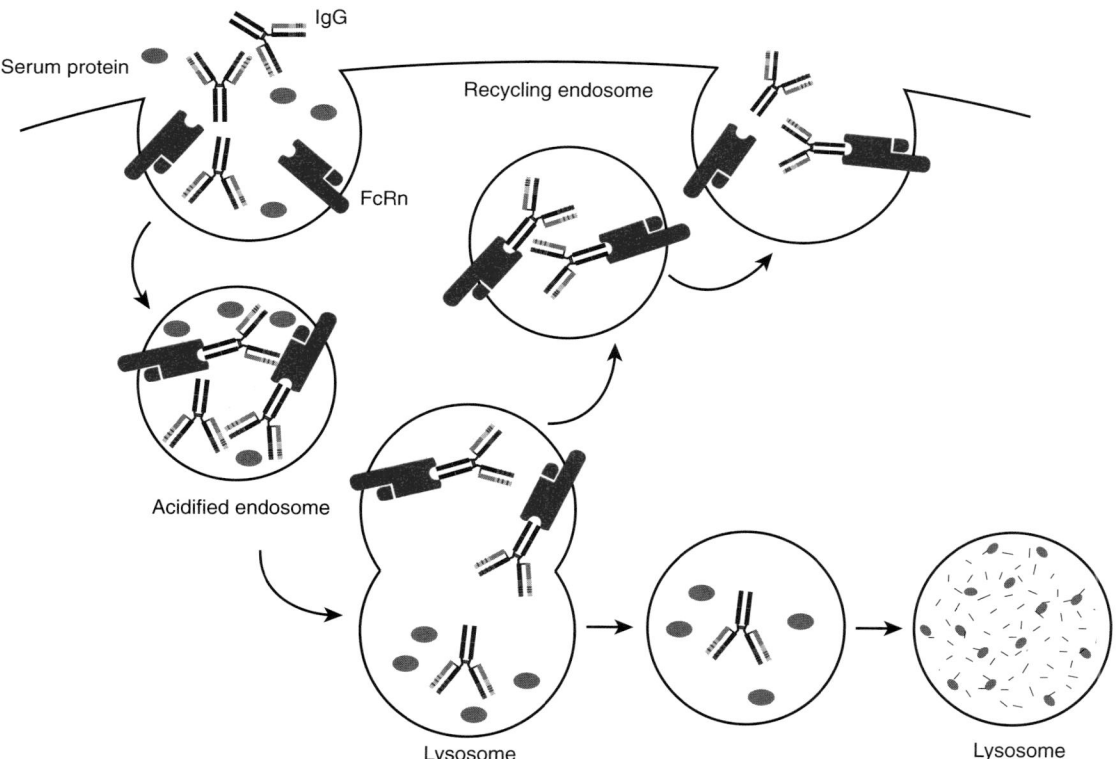

FIGURE 98.2 IgG Plasma Half-Life is Extended by Neonatal Fc Receptor (FcRn) Mediated Cellular Transcytosis and Recycling. The broadly expressed FcRn, a heterodimer consisting of major histocompatibility complex (MHC) class I-like α-domain and β2-microglobulin subunit, interacts with IgG in a pH-dependent manner and maintains IgG homeostasis by rescuing it from lysosomal degradation. IgG does not bind to FcRn at physiologic pH (pH ~7), but when internalized through pinocytosis, it will bind to FcRn with high affinity in the acidified compartments of the endocytic pathway (pH < 6.5). The IgG-FcRn interaction salvages IgG from lysosomal degradation and recycles it to the cell surface, releasing it back to circulation upon exposure to physiologic pH. Excess unbound IgG and other proteins entering the lysosome are degraded. This recycling mechanism occurring primarily in the vascular endothelium is responsible for the relatively long half-life of IgG.

covariates on MAT pharmacokinetics include body weight/ surface area, gender, antidrug antibodies (ADA), creatinine clearance, age, disease severity, and inflammation markers such as C-reactive protein.[21] Other factors influencing inter-individual variability include influence of disease elements such as proteinuria and protein losing enteropathy as mentioned above, or injury to blood-brain barrier, and influence of co-administered drugs.[21] Better understanding of pharmacokinetics and patient-specific covariates paves the way toward personalized MAT therapy, with the goal of increasing efficacy in a cost-effective way, while decreasing toxicity.

Nomenclature

Nomenclature of MAT is currently standardized by international guidelines adopted by the American Medical Association's United States Adopted Names Council. All monoclonal antibody product names end in the suffix –mab (Fig. 98.3). The nomenclature includes a distinct starting prefix to create a unique name, which is followed by an infix representing the target or disease. Infixes indicating the target class, or disease the antibody is used to treat for include tu-/t- for tumor, li-/l- for immunomodulator, vi- for viral, ba- for bacterial, etc. Since the source of the antibody has important safety consideration in that it may induce immunogenicity in patients, a second infix included indicates the source of the antibody (the species on which the Ig sequence of the antibody is based): o for mouse, a for rat, u for human, i for primate. In addition, the degree of presence and origin of nonhuman sequences is further indicated by additional letters in the source infix such as –xi- indicating chimeric (~65% human), –zu- indicating humanized (~80% human), and -u- indicating fully human (>95% human) antibody. For engineered fusion proteins, suffix –cept indicates the presence of receptor molecules as part of the recombinant Fc fusion (such as etanercept for TNF receptor Ig fusion).

Antigens and Diseases Targeted by Monoclonal Antibody Therapeutics

MAT were developed against a number of unique antigen targets. Some antigens show overlap between clinical areas, for example, TNF antagonists are used in rheumatology, as well as gastroenterology for the treatment of Crohn disease (CD). Some antigens are more frequently targeted than others (100 drugs for 61 targets), with TNF and CD20 being the most popular with 6 drugs approved for each, followed by HER2 and VEGF with 5 drugs, and CD19, EGFR, IL-17RA, IL-23 p19, PD-1, and PD-L1 with three antibodies for each. The majority of approved MAT are directed against targets in oncology (35%). Other areas include rheumatology (11%), dermatology (7%), blood disorders (7%), gastroenterology (6%), autoinflammatory and other immunologic disease (6%), allergy and asthma (4%), infectious disease (4%), neurologic disease including multiple sclerosis (4%), bone disorders (4%), cardiovascular disease (3%), ophthalmology (3%), transplant and systemic autoimmune disease (2% each), and type II diabetes (1%).

Antigenic targets for MAT are frequently cell membrane bound receptors such as GPIIb/IIIa, integrins, EGFR, CD20, CD52, CTLA-4, PD-1, PD-L1, or soluble targets including growth factors (VEGF), cytokines (TNF, IL-6, IL-17, IL-12/23), complement (C5), or IgE. While most MAT are designed to recognize human targets, a few of them that are used to treat or prevent infectious diseases bind to microbial protein targets (RSV-F protein, *Bacillus anthracis* PA toxin, *Clostridium difficile* toxin).

MAT targets for oncology can be classified into three different categories. The first category includes tumor-specific

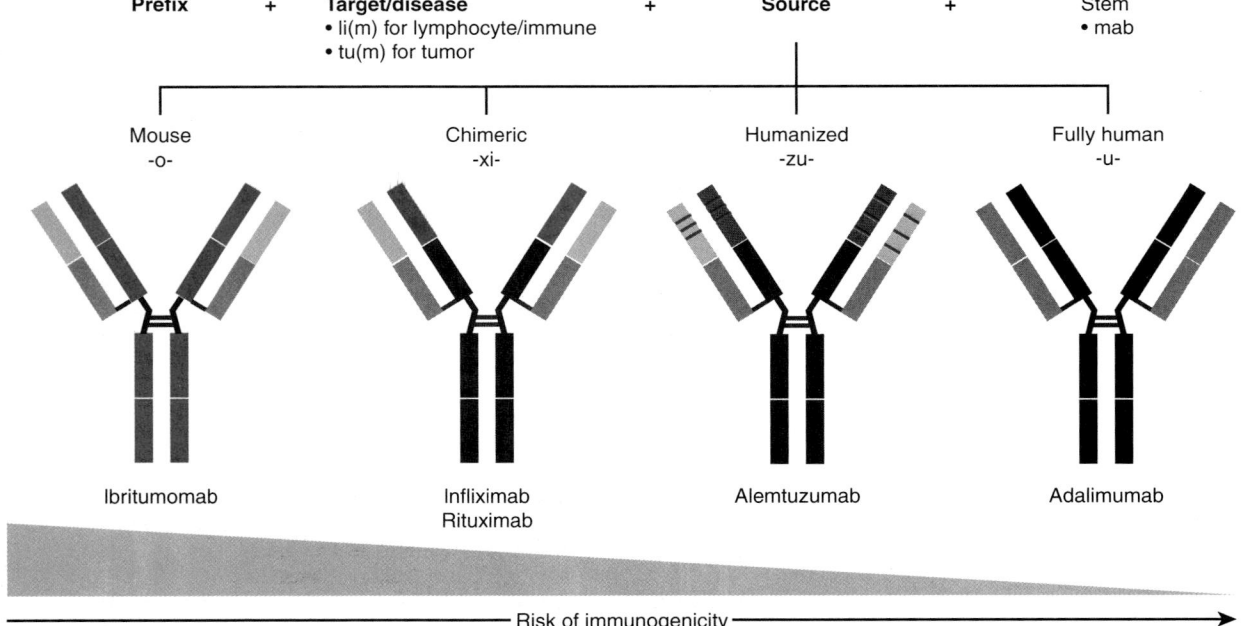

FIGURE 98.3 Standardized Nomenclature for Therapeutic Monoclonal Antibodies. Monoclonal antibody nomenclature includes a unique starting prefix, followed by an infix representing the target or disease, another infix indicating the source, and the stem –mab used as a suffix. Human sequences are shown in grey, mouse sequences in red. Risk of immunogenicity in function of the foreign sequence content is indicated under the figure.

antigens, adhesion molecules serving as "postal addresses" for which killing mechanisms can be targeted.[13] Tumor cell killing can be achieved by activation of immunologic mechanisms following antibody binding to tumor cells (e.g., ADCC or CDC), or by conjugating the antibody to another molecule mediating the killing such as toxins or radioactive isotopes. The second target category overlaps with the first, since it includes tumor cell receptors, which are targeted by MAT with the goal to block ligand binding and signal transduction, for example Her2. The third category includes immunotherapy agents such as checkpoint inhibitors designed to block co-inhibitory signals and thus directly stimulate tumor-specific T-cell responses, or CAR-T cells that express single chain chimeric antigen receptors specific to tumor antigen and are used to induce tumor cell killing.

MAT targeting cytokines include antibodies to pro-inflammatory cytokines IL-1, IL-6, IL-17, and TNF, which play crucial roles in the pathogenesis of numerous chronic inflammatory and autoimmune diseases. These MAT typically block the biological effect by either neutralizing the cytokine or blocking the cytokine receptor that mediates signaling. Due to their pleiotropic biological effects, which include playing a crucial role in host defense against pathogens, systemic pro-inflammatory cytokine blockade may interfere with host defense against infections, which is an unwanted adverse effect.

POINTS TO REMEMBER

- Immunoassays, cell-based assays, and mass spectrometry approaches are available to measure monoclonal antibody therapeutics (MAT) concentrations in the clinical lab.
- It is important to interpret MAT concentration and antidrug antibodies results in the context of the assay used, and timing of blood samples.
- Therapeutic drug monitoring of MAT is relevant in the setting of loss of response to therapy (reactive monitoring) and newer evidence suggests a role for proactive continuous monitoring during different time-points in the course of treatment to adjust therapy before loss of response occurs.
- Interference of MAT with clinical laboratory tests is an emerging concern that can trigger unnecessary additional testing and may delay important therapeutic decisions.
- MAT are mostly of the IgG κ isotype and some of them are given in high enough doses that they show up as monoclonal bands in protein electrophoresis and IgG κ bands upon immunofixation testing. Approaches to differentiate the MAT from an endogenous monoclonal protein have been developed.

THE USE OF TUMOR NECROSIS FACTOR ANTAGONISTS IN CLINICAL MEDICINE

Due to the central role of TNF in inflammation and the pathogenesis of autoimmune and chronic inflammatory diseases, TNF antagonists have revolutionized the treatment of rheumatoid arthritis (RA), ankylosing spondylitis, psoriasis, and IBD including CD and ulcerative colitis.[22,23] The therapeutic benefits have been so dramatic that TNF antagonists are still among the best-selling, most prescribed pharmaceuticals. In recent decades several monoclonal antibody-based TNF antagonists have been developed (Fig. 98.4, Table 98.2). Infliximab is a chimeric mouse/human antibody in which the mouse variable region is preserved, but the rest of the molecule is replaced by human sequences. Adalimumab and golimumab are fully human IgG1 antibodies, produced by phage display or transgenic mouse technology, respectively. Despite containing predominantly human sequences, these molecules may show structural features that are different from the endogenous proteins, such as glycosylation patterns that are characteristic of the producing cells (Chinese Hamster Ovary cells [CHO] or mouse myeloma cells), not necessarily identical to the human glycosylation pattern, which may contribute to immunogenicity.[24] Certolizumab pegol is a humanized antibody Fab fragment, designed by engrafting the mouse CDR into a human IgG4 κ Fab framework, and it has a polyethylene glycol (PEG) molecule attached that prolongs the half-life in the circulation. Etanercept is a fusion protein composed of the extracellular part of human TNF type 2 receptor (TNF-R2, p75) fused to dimeric human IgG1 Fc. Unlike the antibody drugs targeting TNF, etanercept is able to neutralize both TNF receptor ligands, TNF and Lymphotoxin-α.

Biosimilars

Patent expiration of biological drugs created the opportunity for manufacturers to develop biosimilar products, which are highly similar to and have no clinically meaningful differences from existing FDA-approved reference products.[25] An abbreviated pathway for approval was created by Congress through the Biologics Price Competition and Innovation Act of 2009, assuring a shorter and less costly development program with the goal of providing more treatment options, lowering cost through competition, and increasing patient access to treatment. Similarity is determined by extensive structural and functional analysis, comparison of purity, chemical identity, and bioactivity; minor differences are however acceptable (e.g., stabilizer, buffer). For approval of a biosimilar, the manufacturer must demonstrate that there are no clinically meaningful differences compared to the reference product in pharmacokinetics, clinical efficacy, and safety. Assessment of clinical immunogenicity is important during biosimilar development. Due to the complexity of the manufacturing processes for MAT, involving recombinant DNA technology and production by living cells, it cannot be assumed that biosimilars are completely identical to the reference drug (in contrast to small molecule generic drugs, which have chemically identical structure to the reference drug).

Since 2015, 20 biosimilars to MAT have been approved in the US, 18 of which are monoclonal antibodies, along with 2 Fc fusions (Table 98.3). The majority of them are TNF antagonists: four are biosimilars for infliximab, five for adalimumab, and two for etanercept. Biosimilars are expected to show similar immunogenicity profile compared to the reference drug, which is verified during clinical trials.[26] However, due to the variety of assay platforms used across clinical laboratories, internal validation to verify assay performance for the biosimilar compared to the reference drug should be performed before implementing testing for biosimilar drug or ADA to biosimilars.

Treatment Failure to Tumor Necrosis Factor Antagonist Therapy

While administration of TNF antagonists lowers disease activity, inducing clinical remission in the majority of patients,

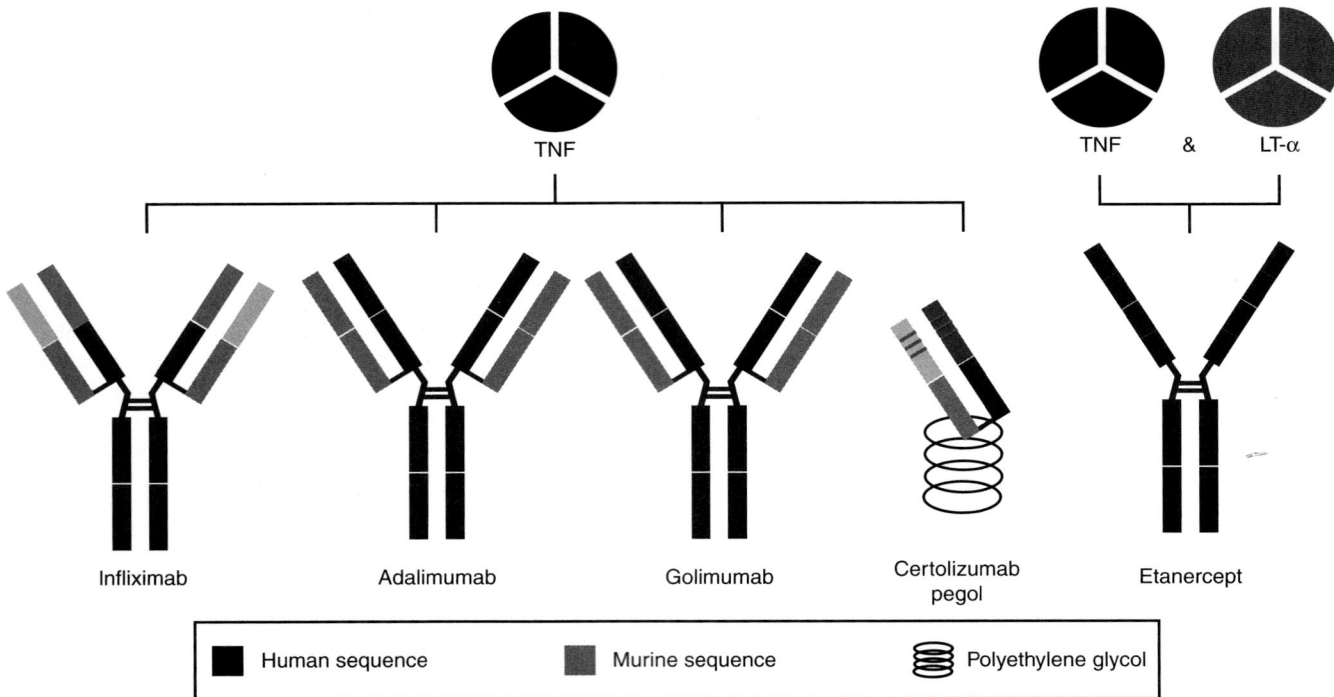

FIGURE 98.4 Tumor Necrosis Factor (TNF) Antagonists Approved for Clinical Use. Infliximab is a chimeric antibody having mouse IgV and human IgG1 constant region. Adalimumab and golimumab are fully human IgG1 antibodies. Certolizumab is a PEGylated humanized antibody Fab fragment with mouse complementarity determining regions. Etanercept is a chimeric fusion protein of TNFR2 and IgG1 Fc. The binding targets for the drugs are indicated. *LT-α*, Lymphotoxin-alpha.

TABLE 98.2	**Tumor Necrosis Factor Antagonists Currently in Clinical Use and Their Structural and Pharmacologic Properties**				

TNF Inhibitors	Etanercept	Infliximab	Adalimumab	Certolizumab Pegol	Golimumab
Molecule	hTNF receptor Fc fusion protein	Chimeric TNF antibody	Human TNF antibody	Humanized antibody Fab, PEGylated	Human TNF antibody
Protein Format	Dimeric hIgG1 Fc fused to hTNF-R2 (p75)	hIgG1κ, murine variable region	hIgG1κ, selected by phage display	hIgG4 Fab, murine CDR, conjugated to 40 kDa PEG	hIgG1κ, produced by transgenic mouse technology
Source	CHO cells	Sp2/0 hybridoma	CHO cells	*Escherichia coli*	SP2/0 hybridoma
Sequence origin	Human	~75% human	Human	~80% human	Human
Method of administration	sc 50 mg once weekly	iv 5 mg/kg at 0, 2, 6, and then every 8 weeks	40 mg every 2 weeks	sc 400 mg at 0, 2, 4, and then every 4 weeks	sc 50 mg once a month; iv 2 mg/kg at 0 and 4, then every 8 weeks
Half-life (days)	3–5	8–10	10–20	14	14
Year of first FDA approval	1998	1998	2002	2008	2009
Indications	RA, JIA, PsA, AS, PsO	CD, UC, RA, AS, PsA, PsO	RA, JIA, PsA, AS, CD, PsO	CD, RA, PsA, AS,	RA, PsA, AS

AS, Ankylosing spondylitis; *CD,* Crohn disease; *CDR,* complementarity determining region; *CHO,* Chinese hamster ovary; *FDA,* Food and Drug Administration; *h,* human; *iv,* intravenous infusion; *PsA,* psoriatic arthritis; *PsO,* plaque psoriasis; *RA,* rheumatoid arthritis; *sc,* subcutaneous injection; *UC,* ulcerative colitis.

therapeutic challenges with TNF antagonists are substantial and may result in inadequate responses in some patients. Some do not respond at all, and others lose response over time, despite increased doses or more frequent administration of the drug.[27,28] The mechanisms of treatment failure can be attributed to many factors, including drug-related immunogenicity; treatment-related factors including dosing and bioavailability

issues and pharmacokinetics and pharmacodynamics of the drug; individual patient-related factors; and disease-specific differences in the pathogenic role of TNF.[29]

Primary Treatment Failure

Primary treatment failure is clinically defined as lack of improvement of clinical signs and symptoms during the induction

TABLE 98.3　US Food and Drug Administration-approved Biosimilars to Monoclonal Antibody Therapeutics

	Product Name	Proprietary Name	Date of Licensure (month/day/year)	Molecular Target	Protein Format	Source	Major Indication	Reference Drug	Reference Drug Proprietary Name	Reference Drug Date of Licensure (month/day/year)
1	Infliximab-dyyb	Inflectra	04/05/2016	TNF	Chimeric IgG1κ	Murine hybridoma	RA, PsA, AS, Crohn disease, UC, PsO	Infliximab	Remicade	08/24/1998
2	Etanercept-szzs	Erelzi	08/30/2016	TNF	Fc fusion, p75 TNFR2—huIgG1 Fc	CHO cells	RA, PsA, AS, JIA, PsO	Etanercept	Enbrel	11/02/1998
3	Adalimumab-atto	Amjevita	09/23/2016	TNF	Human IgG1κ	CHO cells	RA, PsA, AS, JIA, Crohn disease, UC, PsO	Adalimumab	Humira	12/31/2002
4	Infliximab-abda	Renflexis	04/21/2017	TNF	Chimeric IgG1κ	Murine hybridoma	RA, PsA, AS, Crohn disease, UC, PsO	Infliximab	Remicade	08/24/1998
5	Adalimumab-adbm	Cyltezo	08/25/2017	TNF	Human IgG1κ	CHO cells	RA, PsA, AS, JIA, Crohn disease, UC, PsO	Adalimumab	Humira	12/31/2002
6	Bevacizumab-awwb	Mvasi	09/14/2017	VEGF	Humanized IgG1	CHO	Metastatic colorectal cancer, Her2 negative metastatic breast cancer	Bevacizumab	Avastin	02/26/2004
7	Trastuzumab-dkst	Ogivri	12/01/2017	EGFR (HER2)	Humanized IgG1κ	CHO cells	HER2-positive breast cancer	Trastuzumab	Herceptin	09/25/1998
8	Infliximab-qbtx	Ixifi	12/13/2017	TNF	Chimeric IgG1κ	Murine hybridoma	RA, PsA, AS, Crohn disease, UC, PsO	Infliximab	Remicade	08/24/1998
9	Adalimumab-adaz	Hyrimoz	10/30/2018	TNF	Human IgG1κ	CHO cells	RA, PsA, AS, JIA, Crohn disease, UC, plaque psoriasis	Adalimumab	Humira	12/31/2002
10	Rituximab-abbs	Truxima	11/28/2018	CD20	Chimeric IgG1k	CHO cells	NHL	Rituximab	Rituxan	11/26/1997
11	Trastuzumab-pkrb	Herzuma	12/14/2018	EGFR (HER2)	Humanized IgG1κ	CHO cells	HER2-positive breast cancer	Trastuzumab	Herceptin	09/25/1998
12	Trastuzumab-dttb	Ontruzant	01/18/2019	EGFR (HER2)	Humanized IgG1κ	CHO cells	HER2-positive breast cancer, and gastric adenocarcinoma	Trastuzumab	Herceptin	09/25/1998
13	Trastuzumab-qyyp	Trazimera	03/11/2019	EGFR (HER2)	Humanized IgG1κ	CHO cells	HER2-positive breast cancer, and gastric adenocarcinoma	Trastuzumab	Herceptin	09/25/1998
14	Etanercept-ykro	Eticovo	04/26/2019	TNF	Fc fusion, p75 TNFR2—huIgG1 Fc	CHO cells	RA, PsA, AS, JIA, PsO	Etanercept	Enbrel	11/02/1998
15	Trastuzumab-anns	Kanjinti	06/13/2019	EGFR (HER2)	Humanized IgG1κ	CHO cells	HER2-positive breast cancer, and gastric adenocarcinoma	Trastuzumab	Herceptin	09/25/1998
16	Bevacizumab-bvzr	Zirabev	06/28/2019	VEGF	Humanized IgG1	CHO	Metastatic colorectal cancer, NSCLC, recurrent glioblastoma, RCC, cervical cancer	Bevacizumab	Avastin	02/26/2004

Continued

TABLE 98.3 US Food and Drug Administration-approved Biosimilars to Monoclonal Antibody Therapeutics—cont'd

Product Name	Proprietary Name	Date of Licensure (month/day/year)	Molecular Target	Protein Format	Source	Major Indication	Reference Drug	Reference Drug Proprietary Name	Reference Drug Date of Licensure (month/day/year)
17 Rituximab-pvvr	Ruxience	07/23/2019	CD20	Chimeric IgG1κ	CHO cells	NHL, CLL, GPA, MPA	Rituximab	Rituxan	11/26/1997
18 Adalimumab-bwwd	Hadlima	07/25/2019	TNF	Human IgG1κ	Mammalian cells	RA, JIA, PsA, AS, Crohn disease, UC, PsO	Adalimumab	Humira	12/31/2002
19 Adalimumab-afzb	Abrilada	11/18/2019	TNF	Human IgG1κ	CHO cells	RA, JIA, PsA, AS, Crohn disease, UC, PsO	Adalimumab	Humira	12/31/2002
20 Infliximab-axxq	Avsola	12/06/2019	TNF	Chimeric IgG1κ	CHO cells	Crohn disease, UC, RA, AS, PsA, PsO	Infliximab	Remicade	08/24/1998

AS, Ankylosing spondylitis; *CHO,* Chinese hamster ovary; *EGFR,* epidermal growth factor receptor; *GPA,* granulomatosis with polyangiitis; *hu,* human; *Ig,* immunoglobulin; *JIA,* juvenile idiopathic arthritis; *MPA,* microscopic polyangiitis; *NHL,* Non-Hodgkin's Lymphoma; *NSCLC,* non-small cell lung cancer; *PsA,* psoriatic arthritis; *PsO,* plaque psoriasis; *RA,* rheumatoid arthritis; *RCC,* renal cell carcinoma; *TNF,* tumor necrosis factor; *TNFSF,* tumor necrosis factor ligand superfamily; *TNFR,* tumor necrosis factor receptor; *TNSALP,* tissue nonspecific alkaline phosphatase; *UC,* ulcerative colitis; *VEGF,* vascular endothelial growth factor.

Data obtained from FDA Therapeutic Biologic Applications, Biosimilar product information, and from FDA package inserts.

therapy, and has been reported to occur in about one third of patients treated with TNF antagonists, including both RA and CD.[27] The underlying reason for primary failure is not always clear, but may involve rapid clearance of the drug, or may involve bioavailability issues such as inadequate dosing or patient compliance. Beyond altered pharmacokinetics, other causes of primary treatment failure include pharmacodynamics, such as non–TNF-driven disease mechanisms. Immunogenicity is usually not a contributing factor for primary treatment failure since the development of antibodies takes time (several weeks to months).

Secondary Treatment Failure

Secondary treatment failure occurs when patients who had shown improvement of clinical symptoms during the induction therapy lose response over time and show relapses, despite increased or more frequent dosing. It has been shown that as many as 50% of patients with RA and CD develop secondary nonresponse due to loss of effectiveness of the drug over time.[28] The mechanisms of secondary treatment failure can be diverse, but the most common cause is immunogenicity resulting in the development of ADA to the TNF antagonist.[30] ADA will neutralize the drug rendering it noneffective, or induce its rapid clearance through immune complex formation.

In addition to immunogenicity, other factors may also contribute to secondary nonresponse, such as inadequate drug concentrations in the circulation and subsequently in target tissues, which can be due to accelerated drug clearance, or increased consumption in periods of high disease activity. Pharmacodynamic issues that affect the pathologic mechanisms driving inflammation include infections, which can markedly alter the inflammatory process and cytokine balance; concomitant treatment with other drugs may also result in secondary response failure and recurrence of the symptoms.[24]

Immunogenicity to Tumor Necrosis Factor Antagonists

Repeated injections of exogenous proteins have been shown to trigger the immune response and the development of antibodies against the protein, which is commonly associated with a decrease in the effectiveness of the treatment.[31,32] The ability of a therapeutic protein to trigger the immune system is related to its "foreignness": the more it differs from the endogenous counterpart, the higher the chance that it elicits immunogenicity.[32] Immunogenicity of therapeutic proteins is an important factor that affects treatment efficacy and safety. Decreasing or eliminating rodent sequences from MAT decreases the intensity of the immune response against MAT but does not completely eliminate immunogenicity. Fully human antibody drugs produced by phage display technology, or by using humanized mouse models, may still elicit ADA formation. Immunogenicity of fully human antibodies may be related to differences in Ig allotypes between populations and individuals created by genetic diversity.[33] Formation of natural anti-idiotype antibodies has been detected, and the presence of natural anti-idiotype antibodies in polyclonal Ig preparations such as intravenous Ig are thought to contribute to the therapeutic effect of the product.[34]

The mechanism of immunogenicity involves the uptake of these drugs by antigen presenting cells, followed by cleavage into peptides that can be presented by human leukocyte antigen (HLA) molecules. These peptide-HLA complexes are then recognized by specific T-cell receptors, followed by proliferation and expansion of the specific T-cell clone. This alloantigen presentation process is driven by the immunogenic T-cell epitopes that can be found in the therapeutic protein and their ability to trigger an immune response.[35] Development of immunogenicity is influenced by the patient's genetic background,[36] including HLA haplotype,[37–39] and genetic variations in other immune regulatory genes such as IL-10.[40] Importantly, the microenvironment in which the antigen-specific CD4$^+$ T cells encounter antigen affects immunogenicity, as inflammatory cytokines may skew T-cell differentiation into certain lineages, which may then promote antibody formation.[41] This is of interest given the autoimmune or chronic inflammatory status of the patient population treated with TNF antagonists, which may impact the overall immune response to these drugs. Interestingly, patients who develop antibodies against one type of TNF antagonist drug are at higher risk for developing antibodies against another type of drug when switching therapy. IBD patients with previous anti-infliximab antibodies were significantly more prone to develop anti-adalimumab antibodies (33%) when switched to adalimumab, compared to patients without previous anti-infliximab antibodies.[42] Further investigation of patient-related immunogenicity factors could potentially result in predicting which patients are at increased risk for developing ADA, which would allow for risk stratification and individual treatment optimization. Of interest, a recent genome-wide association study has shown that CD patients carrying HLA-DQA1*05 alleles developed antibodies to infliximab and adalimumab at a higher rate, compared to noncarriers (hazard ratio 1.9).[43] This finding has clinical implications as testing patients for the presence of HLA-DQA1*05 before treatment may help personalize the choice of TNF inhibitor and the need for combination therapy with an immunomodulator.

Treatment-related factors such as the mode of administration also play an important role in immunogenicity. Use of high doses of a protein drug may reduce its immunogenicity by inducing immunologic tolerance.[44] Repeated doses over months, or years of treatment increase the risk of developing ADA. Intravenous administration is generally thought to be less immunogenic than subcutaneous or intramuscular administration.[45] Most TNF antagonists are administered through repeated subcutaneous injections (with the exception of infliximab given intravenously), which is similar to the delivery of immunogenic vaccines. Of interest, combination therapy using TNF antagonists and immunosuppressive drugs such as methotrexate often decreases the incidence of antibody formation, enhancing clinical efficacy.[46,47] However, an individualized approach is preferred based on risk-benefit evaluation due to risks commonly associated with long-term immunosuppressive therapy.[48]

Immunogenicity testing is required by regulatory agencies including FDA and European Medicines Agency for submission of the drug for approval.[49] It also has important implications following drug approval, when the drug enters the market. According to a recent comprehensive review, 25.3% of all patients treated with infliximab developed ADA.[47] Adalimumab, a fully human antibody, was shown to elicit antibody response in 14.1% of patients in a combined cohort of RA, spondyloarthritis, and IBD.[47]

Neutralizing ADA have the ability to directly interfere with the biological effect of the drug by decreasing or eliminating its ability to inhibit TNF mediated signaling through cell surface TNF receptors. These antibodies may directly bind to the idiotype of the drug, or to other sites in its proximity, eliciting steric hindrance that in turn prevents binding of the drug to TNF. Non-neutralizing antibodies do not directly interfere with TNF binding but may compromise therapeutic efficacy by contributing to enhanced clearance of the drug from the circulation through immune complex formation and binding to Fc receptors on phagocytic cells.[24] In case of subcutaneous administration, immune complexes may form around the injection site, which will prevent absorption of the drug into the circulation, reducing bioavailability.[50]

In addition to the neutralizing versus non-neutralizing effect, the isotype of the ADA has additional relevance in influencing the pharmacokinetics and the types of adverse effects. Infliximab-specific antibodies are primarily IgG isotypes, although other isotypes such as IgA, IgM, and rarely IgE have been reported.[51,52] Of the IgG type antibodies, IgG1 and IgG4 are most common for both infliximab[51] and adalimumab.[29,53] The presence of IgG4 types of antibodies is consistent with previous observations showing that this subtype is induced by repeated antigen exposure.[54]

Overall, ADA are associated with low serum drug concentration, reduced clinical response or remission of clinical disease, and adverse effects such as hypersensitivity reactions and immune complex disease.[55] Drug bioactivity has been shown to disappear from circulation as soon as ADA appear.[56]

CLINICAL LABORATORY TESTING FOR TUMOR NECROSIS FACTOR ANTAGONISTS

As the number of approved TNF antagonists and biosimilars is increasing, so is the need for optimizing the use of these drugs to achieve the best outcome at an affordable cost. An emerging strategy is to use laboratory-based testing for measuring serum drug concentrations and detection of ADA, which may be responsible for loss of response to treatment or for the development of side effects.[57] This personalized medicine approach provides opportunities for optimizing therapy at the level of the individual patient. For many TNF antagonists, substantial interindividual variability exists in serum drug concentrations. Such variabilities have been reported for other MAT including alemtuzumab, rituximab, eculizumab, and others.[58] Variations of drug concentrations depend on how patients metabolize the drug, but are also affected by target variations, such as increased concentrations of TNF or IL-6 during exacerbation of a chronic inflammatory disease, which have been shown to also correlate with inflammatory markers such as C-reactive protein.[59]

The benefits of laboratory testing for serum drug concentrations and detection of ADA have been recognized for TNF antagonists such as infliximab and adalimumab. Although the majority of patients respond well to these drugs, about 30% of them show lack of response to induction therapy, and 50 to 60% of those previously responding will develop secondary treatment failure, in part due to immunogenicity and the appearance of ADA. Studies have proven that the presence of ADA is associated with significantly higher risk of secondary treatment failure.[60,61] In a cohort of RA patients treated with infliximab, the appearance of ADA correlated

with decreasing serum drug concentrations.[56] Laboratory testing to measure drug concentration and detect ADA allows for adjusting treatment based on the most likely mechanism responsible for treatment failure, according to the patient's individual needs.

In response to clinical need, testing for TNF antagonists and ADA is increasingly adopted in many clinical laboratories. The methodologies used for clinical testing vary between laboratories and show variations in their analytical sensitivities and specificities. Details of the different technologies are provided below; assays that are only used in research laboratories are not presented in this chapter. With some exceptions, the same analytical platforms are used to measure serum drug concentrations and detect ADA. Most of the assays currently in clinical use are binding-based methods including solid phase binding platforms such as enzyme-linked immunosorbent assay (ELISA), and liquid phase binding such as the high-performance liquid chromatography- or HPLC-based homogenous mobility-shift assay (for additional information on chromatography and HPLC, refer to Chapter 19).[62] Liquid chromatography tandem mass spectrometry (LC-MS/MS) is also used by clinical laboratories to measure TNF antagonist drug concentrations (for additional information on mass spectrometry, refer to Chapter 20).[63] Functional assays that are used clinically include a cell-based reporter gene assay (RGA), which measures active drug concentrations based on inhibition of TNF receptor induced signaling activity in live cells.[64]

Expectations for clinical assay development include the requirement to accurately and reliably measure concentrations of functionally active drug and ADA. Challenges of assay development for measuring serum drug concentrations include high concentrations of endogenous Ig in the serum, including occasional interference by rheumatoid factor, heterophilic, or anti-allotype antibodies.[65] Developing assays for detection of ADA poses additional analytical challenges, since both the drug and the ADA are Ig themselves. In addition, there is variation between assays in whether or not they detect binding, and/or neutralizing antibodies, since not all ADA may be neutralizing or contribute to treatment failure equally.

Another challenge for ADA assay development is drug interference caused by the presence of varying concentrations of TNF antagonists in the sera during long-term therapy. Most assays predominantly detect free ADA (not bound to drug) in circulation, when they are present at concentrations that stoichiometrically exceed drug concentrations (Fig. 98.5). During continuous treatment, drug interference may lead to lower analytical sensitivity for antibody detection, which could result in underestimation of the total amount of ADA present, or a false negative result. Drug interference affects most ADA assays, although some are less prone to interference than others due to using an acid dissociation step prior to detection of ADA.[62,66] Second-generation assays that are using the preanalytical acid dissociation step are also referred to as drug tolerant, or total antibody assays, currently available in various formats such as ELISA, electrochemiluminescence immunoassay (ECLIA), and homogeneous mobility-shift assay (HMSA).[67] Using acid to lower the pH of the sample to pH 2.5 to 3 allows for dissociating the endogenous drug from ADA, which can subsequently be captured by the drug in the assay. However, ADA may not be fully recovered even after acid dissociation, as most assays fall short of being 100% drug resistant. To

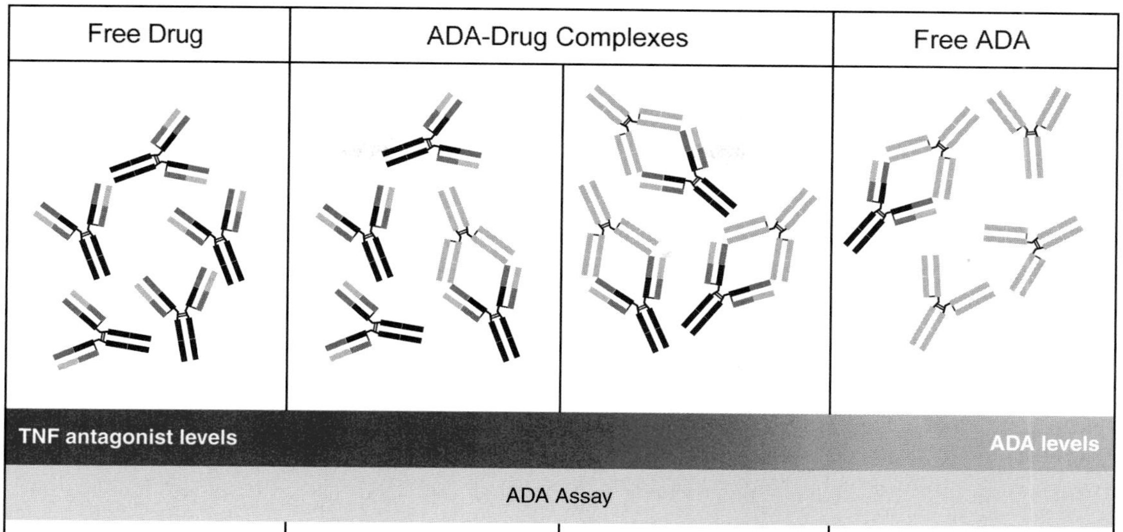

FIGURE 98.5 Detection of Antidrug Antibodies (ADA) in the Presence of Tumor Necrosis Factor (TNF) Antagonists. Detection of ADA varies depending on the assay used and the amount of drug in the serum, which may form immune complexes, decreasing the availability of free ADA detected by most assays. Assays that use acid pretreatment of the serum to dissociate immune complexes, such as HMSA or certain solid phase methods (total ELISA, ECLIA) are less sensitive to drug interference. *ECLIA,* Electrochemiluminescent assay; *ELISA,* enzyme-linked immunosorbent assay; *HMSA,* homogeneous mobility shift assay; *RGA,* reporter gene assay.

minimize drug interference, it is recommended by the American Gastroenterological Association to perform testing for drug and ADA at trough concentrations immediately before the administration of the next dose, when serum drug concentrations are the lowest.[68] Although several studies have shown that analytical methods used to detect TNF antagonist drug concentrations perform and compare well,[62,64,69–71] this is not necessarily true for ADA assays because of the reasons mentioned above. It is important to always interpret ADA results in the context of the assay used, and considering factors such as timing of blood samples (using trough concentrations when possible) and assay strategy and characteristics. Because of different units of measurement for quantification and lack of international standards, the agreement between ADA assays is qualitative at best, and quantitative correlations cannot be calculated, as ADA concentrations detected by different assays in different laboratories may vary.

In addition to TNF antagonists, other MAT targeted for assay development include natalizumab and interferon β used in multiple sclerosis. Laboratory monitoring of immunogenicity and detection of ADA have been shown to be associated with implementing more cost-effective individualized treatment strategy for patients with multiple sclerosis.[72] Testing for vedolizumab and ustekinumab drug concentrations and detecting ADA is also clinically available. These drugs, used for the treatment of IBD, are reported to be less immunogenic compared to TNF antagonists.[73] The clinical need for testing for MAT and associated ADA will likely increase in the future, as more and more of these protein-based drugs are introduced into clinical practice.

Enzyme-Linked Immunosorbent Assays

One of the most commonly used assays for TNF antagonist detection is capture ELISA. TNF antagonist drug concentrations are determined by adding patient serum to TNF-coated plates, followed by enzymatically labeled anti-human IgG reagent. Studies performed to compare several commercial ELISA kits indicated that although all of them were suitable for TDM, significant differences were observed in precision and assay agreement, the latter of which could be improved by assay standardization.[74]

Sandwich and bridging ELISA are the most common formats for detection of ADA. Sandwich ELISAs use plastic-immobilized Fab or F(ab')₂ fragments of the TNF antagonists for capture. Although this assay is affordable and easy to use, it can give false positive or aberrant results due to nonspecific binding of cross-reacting antibodies to the immobilized drug, or due to aggregation of drug molecules on the plastic surface, which can either create new epitopes or hide the existing epitopes.[24]

The bridging ELISA is an improved, modified ELISA method (Fig. 98.6A), which takes advantage of the bivalency or multivalency of the main antibody isotypes. It uses plastic-immobilized drugs as solid phase, which will bind and pull down the ADA from the patient's serum. Instead of using a detection antibody, enzyme-tagged drug is used for detection, with the ADA forming a bridge between the immobilized versus enzyme-tagged drug molecules due to the bivalency of IgG. This method is able to detect most types of IgGs and is easy to use, but there are several drawbacks that need to be recognized. False positive results can occur by the

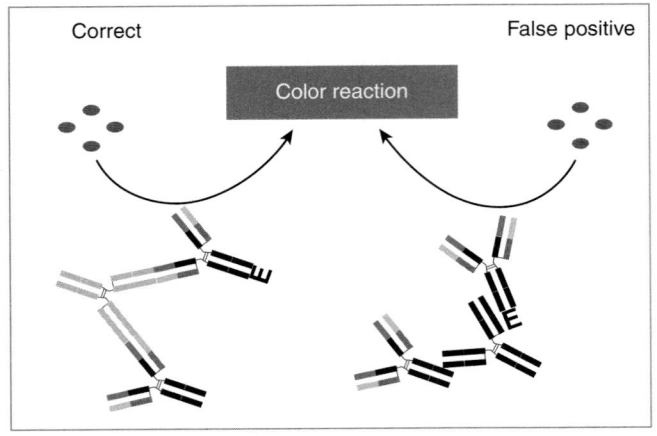
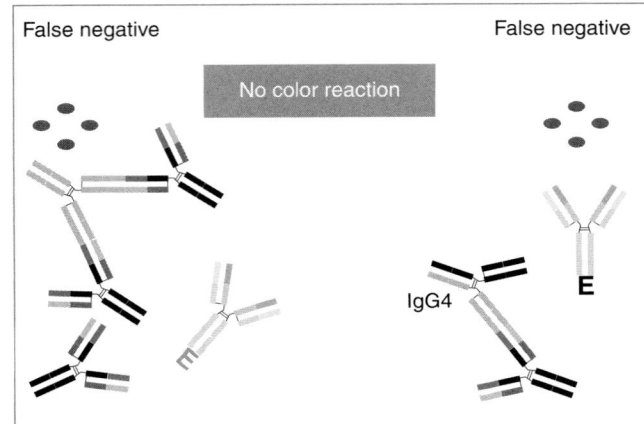

A Bridging elisa

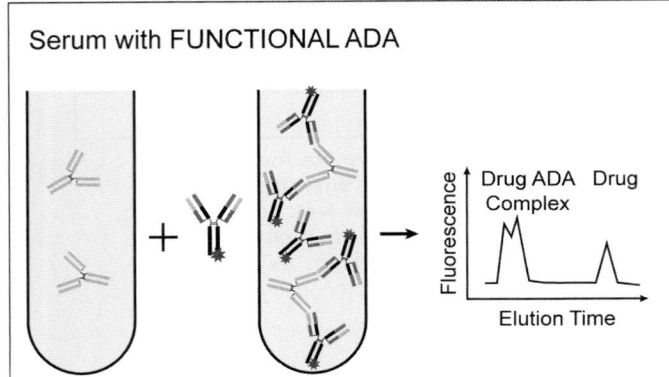
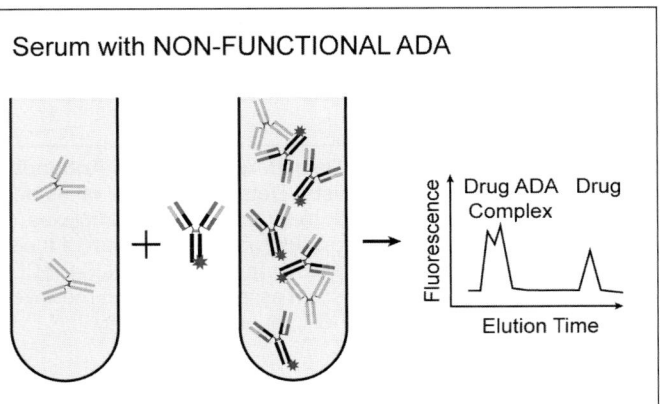

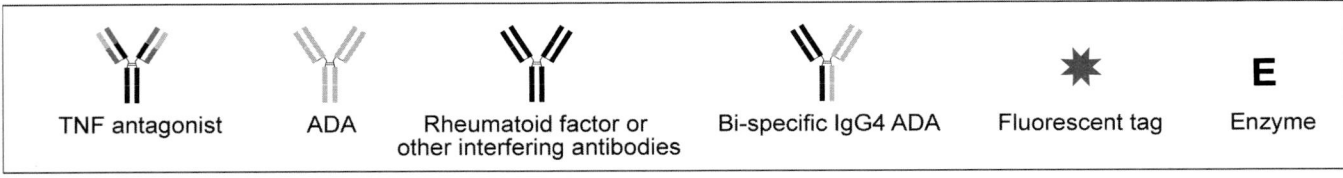

B Homogeneous mobility-shift assay (HMSA)

FIGURE 98.6 Binding-Based Assays Used for Detecting Antibodies to Tumor Necrosis Factor (TNF) Antagonists. (A) The solid phase bridging enzyme-linked immunosorbent assay is based on bivalency of IgG, which can bridge plate-bound unlabeled and soluble enzymatically labeled drug molecules. Nonspecific antibodies that can crosslink drug molecules will cause false-positive results. Excess drug or the presence of IgG4 type antidrug antibodies (ADA) will cause false-negative results. (B) The homogenous mobility shift assay detects ADA by complex formation with fluorescently labeled drug molecules added to the serum, followed by chromatographic (size-exclusion high-performance liquid chromatography) separation of ADA-bound versus free labeled drug. Binding-based methods detect any antibody that binds to the drug, including functional (neutralizing) and nonfunctional ADA.

presence of interfering antibodies that can crosslink the drug molecules added in the assay, such as rheumatoid factor that notoriously binds to the Fc part of IgG nonspecifically, or the presence of anti-idiotype antibodies (see Fig. 98.6A). False-negative results can occur due to drug interference, when the drug is present in high concentrations in the serum and forms complexes with the ADA, which will prevent its detection in the bridging ELISA (see Fig. 98.6A).[75] Furthermore, this method is unable to detect ADA that are IgG4 isotype since IgG4 is usually monovalent and bispecific, half

the molecule being exchanged after synthesis, which makes it invisible in bridging ELISA.[53]

While traditional ELISA methods can only measure free ADA in the serum, assay modifications have been implemented, which allow for measuring of total ADA. This is accomplished by adding acid to the serum sample in the preanalytical phase, which will disassociate drug-ADA complexes, followed by a neutralization step, before applying the sample on the ELISA well.[76] In this protocol, the time between neutralization and application of the sample on the plate is kept to less than 5 minutes to minimize re-association of dissociated residual infliximab to the ADA, thereby helping to ensure that ADA epitopes are available for binding in the ELISA. Several drug-tolerant ELISA assays have been developed but the percentage ADA positivity widely varies between the different assays.[66,77,78]

Electrochemiluminescence Immunoassay

ECLIA employ an electrical current to start the chemiluminescent reaction in the immunoassay system. The technology is commonly performed using streptavidin microparticles in a series of FDA-approved immunoassays. For MAT and ADA, the assays are still laboratory developed tests and employ platforms with streptavidin plates as a support system. The chemiluminescence principle is based on the use of a ruthenium (Ru) complex and tripropylamine. The use of voltage applied at a very specific time point allows for a precise and controlled start of the reaction. The principle is versatile and accommodates many types of immunoassay formats, already described in the ELISA section.

An example of ECLIA use for quantification of MAT is the test for adalimumab quantitation, which uses TNF labeled with biotin, and a second labeled TNF with the Ru complex.[79] The biotinylated TNF will act as capture molecule and bind to the streptavidin plate. In the presence of adalimumab, both labeled forms of TNF will bind to it, and once voltage is applied, the reporter labeled form of TNF with the Ru complex is reduced, causing light to be emitted. For detection of ADA, ECLIA is applied in the bridging immunoassay format. In the method used to detect and quantitate ADA against infliximab, this MAT is labeled either with biotin or Ru. In the presence of ADA against infliximab, a bridging large immunocomplex is formed. The bridging complex binds to the streptavidin plate and, after application of an electrical current, the Ru is reduced to an excited state, causing light to be emitted. When analyzed against a standard curve, the quantity of anti-infliximab antibodies is estimated.[80] Similarly to ELISA assays, ECLIA may be preceded by a step to improve the drug tolerance of the assays, using an acid dissociation strategy, although it is well known that no acid dissociation protocol is 100% effective. A small amount of ADA in the presence of a very high concentration of drug may not be detected, hence the general recommendation of having a blood draw at trough, immediately before the next infusion/injection.

Homogenous Mobility-Shift Assay

This method uses size exclusion HPLC for the measurement of both drug and ADA.[62] Drug concentrations are determined by incubation of fluorescently labeled TNF with patient serum. After equilibration, free TNF and TNF-drug complexes are resolved by HLPC and the peaks quantified by fluorescence using a standard curve of samples with known drug concentrations. ADA in patient serum is detected by adding fluorescently labeled drug, which will associate with the antibody present (fluid phase binding). This is followed by size exclusion HPLC-based separation of ADA-bound versus free labeled drug (Fig. 98.6B).

Since the antigen-antibody binding takes place in homogenous liquid-phase, the HMSA method is expected to show increased analytical specificity for ADA detection by overcoming potential artifacts related to solid-phase ELISAs, such as aggregation and nonspecific binding. Another advantage of the HMSA method compared to bridging ELISA is the ability to detect ADA of all isotypes and all subclasses, including IgG4. Due to the incorporation of an acid dissociation step during the ADA detection, the tolerance of HMSA for drug interference is dramatically improved, and allows for the detection of ADA in the presence of up to 60 μg/mL serum infliximab, although with over a 10-fold decrease in signal.[62]

Limitations include costly fluorescent labeling of TNF and drug, respectively. Another drawback of this test is its inability to distinguish between neutralizing and non-neutralizing antibodies, as their elution profiles are the same (see Fig. 98.6B). Method comparison studies have shown that the majority (68%) of HMSA-reported antibodies in infliximab-treated patients were not functionally active when tested in parallel with a functional test.[81] These antibodies may lack drug-neutralizing effect, or may be blocked from detection by functional assays due to being complexed with circulating drug in the serum, or they may just be nonfunctional antibodies, which may not result in treatment failure.

Functional Assays

Unlike binding assays that are not able to distinguish between functional neutralizing versus non-neutralizing ADA, functional assays allow for the detection of biologically active, drug-neutralizing antibodies, which interfere with the drug-mediated blocking of the TNF signaling pathway, and lead to therapeutic nonresponsiveness. It is important to note that regulatory authorities such as the FDA recommend that functional cell-based assays be used to measure neutralizing antibodies to therapeutic drugs, since bioassays are inherently more reflective of the in vivo situation.[82]

Initial attempts to develop cell-based assays were based on the ability of TNF to kill susceptible tumor cell lines.[83] However, these assays did not translate into clinical use since they were too cumbersome and difficult to standardize. Recently a cell-based RGA has become available,[84] which is currently the only method that allows for direct detection of functionally active drug and neutralizing antibodies, and is available for clinical use.[64] This method is based on the use of reporter cells carrying a TNF inducible, NF-κB regulated firefly luciferase reporter-gene construct. The reporter gene turns on when TNF is added to the cells and binds to TNF receptor, inducing firefly luciferase expression (Fig. 98.7). To control for serum matrix effects affecting viability and cell numbers, this signal is normalized to the constitutively expressed Renilla luciferase carried within the same reporter cell. To measure drug activity, the patient serum is mixed with a fixed amount of TNF and then added to the cells. If the drug is present, it will inhibit the activity of TNF and will prevent the expression of the reporter gene. Thus the amount of infliximab present in the serum will inversely correlate to the amount of luminescence produced by the cells (Fig. 98.7A).

For the detection of neutralizing ADA, the serum is pre-incubated first with a known concentration of drug and the assay is performed as described above. If the serum contains neutralizing antibodies, these antibodies will prevent the drug from interfering with the TNF induced induction of the reporter gene, resulting in a luminescent signal (Fig. 98.7B). The amount of neutralizing antibody in the serum directly correlates with the amount of luminescence produced by the cells. The antibody is currently quantified by testing serial

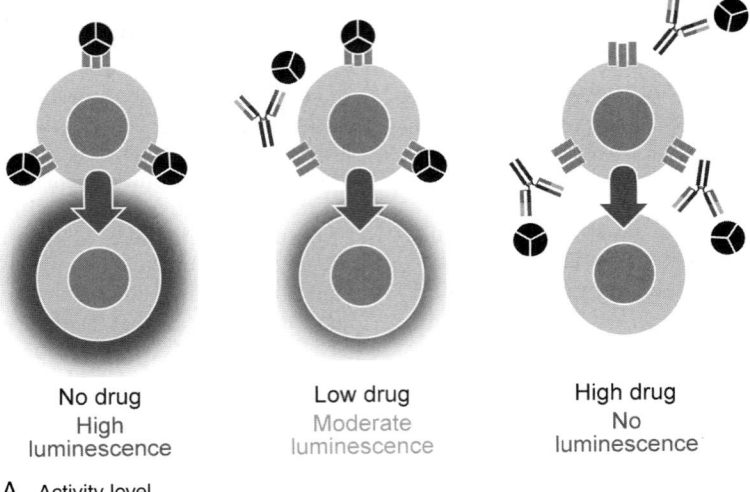

No drug
High
luminescence

Low drug
Moderate
luminescence

High drug
No
luminescence

A   Activity level

Patient serum with NO neutralizing antibodies

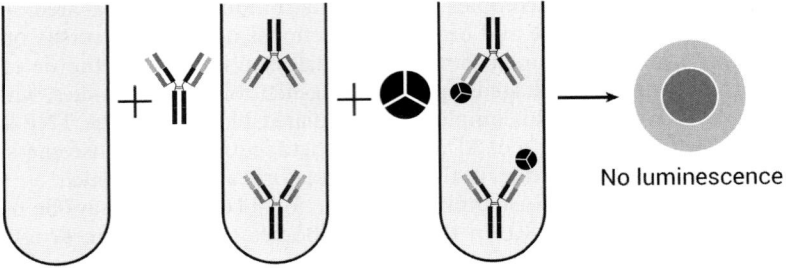

No luminescence

Patient serum WITH neutralizing antibodies

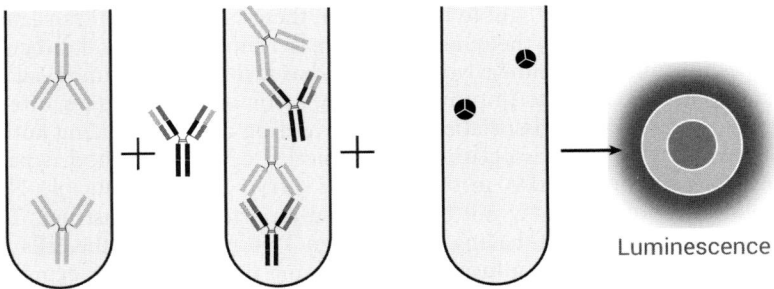

Luminescence

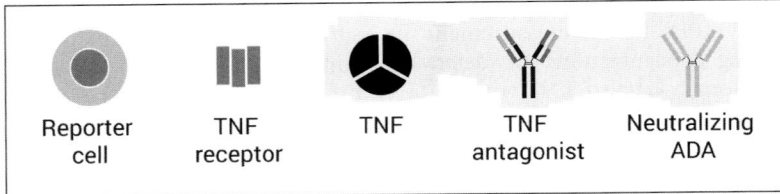

Reporter
cell

TNF
receptor

TNF

TNF
antagonist

Neutralizing
ADA

B   Neutralizing antibodies

FIGURE 98.7 Functional Cell-Based Reporter Gene Assay (RGA) for Detection of Antibodies to Tumor Necrosis Factor (TNF) Antagonists. RGA uses cells carrying a TNF-inducible luciferase reporter-gene construct, which is turned on by TNF receptor signaling, generating luminescence. (A) For drug activity assay, serum is mixed with TNF and incubated with the cells. The presence of drug in the serum blocks TNF activity, decreasing luminescence. (B) For measuring neutralizing antibodies, the same assay is used but the serum samples are preincubated with a fixed amount of drug. In the absence of neutralizing antibodies, the drug blocks TNF activity and there is no luminescence. When neutralizing antidrug antibodies (ADA) are present, the inhibition of TNF activity by the exogenous drug is released, the reporter gene is turned on, and luminescence is generated.

dilutions of the serum, and by identifying the highest dilution at which blocking of infliximab activity is no longer observed. The recently developed ADA standards to infliximab[76] and adalimumab[85] will allow for reporting absolute antibody concentrations, once these standards become widely available and appropriately validated and correlated against the existing methods.

In contrast to binding assays, RGA measures TNF bioactivity, providing a direct functional assessment of the biologically active drug and the neutralizing activity of ADA. Neutralizing ADA block the idiotype of the drug molecule directly or by steric hindrance, with sufficient strength to interfere with, or eliminate, the activity of the drug. Non-neutralizing ADA that do not directly interfere with the activity of the drug (e.g., bind to regions other than the idiotype, such as the Fc region) will not be detected. Because of this reason, RGA may be less sensitive for detection of ADA than binding assays (HMSA) or radioimmunoassays, but more specific, as it detects antibodies that truly neutralize and interfere with the biological activity, such as TNF signaling at the cellular level, thus better reflecting what happens in vivo.[81] Direct detection of functionally active, neutralizing antibodies provides a more direct understanding of why therapies fail in some individuals and not in others. Non-neutralizing antibodies may, however, still alter the pharmacokinetics of drugs by other mechanisms, such as formation of immune complexes and subsequent removal of the drug by the mononuclear phagocyte system.[28] The individual contributions of these different types of antibodies to therapeutic nonresponse are not well characterized, partly because the specific assays have not been widely available. Combined use of binding assays along with functional tests provides the necessary tools to clarify the role of both neutralizing and non-neutralizing antibodies in therapeutic response failure.

Due to the nature of the assay that it is measuring TNF activity, detection of ADA by RGA is sensitive to drug interference; increasing amounts of drug in the serum resulted in decreasing titers of ADA detected.[64] Therefore it is important to follow the recommended approach to test for ADA when drug concentrations are lowest (trough). Another cell-based method for measuring TNF inhibitors has been described for research use, which is based on measuring IL-6 released from a fibrosarcoma cell line upon TNF stimulation.[85] However, the longer turn-around time of this test will likely prevent its utility in clinical laboratories.

Applying Liquid Chromatography Tandem Mass Spectrometry for Measuring Tumor Necrosis Factor Antagonists

In addition to the binding and functional assays used to measure both drug and ADA, additional novel methodologies have been established for quantification of drug concentrations only, such as LC-MS/MS, which is available for clinical use.[63] The method is based on using clonotypic peptides obtained by trypsin digestion from the heavy and light chain variable regions of primarily chimeric Ig, which are then quantified using LC-MS/MS (Fig. 98.8). The principle of this method lies in being able to distinguish the tryptic peptides from the vast repertoire of endogenous Ig present in human serum, which is easier for chimeric antibodies such as infliximab, but can be more challenging for fully human antibodies such as adalimumab. In order to overcome this challenge,

a sample immunoenrichment would be necessary. While most assays for TNF antagonists are thought to measure predominantly free drugs (not complexed with ADA or TNF), the trypsin digestion step used in this method allows for the measurement of total infliximab, regardless of whether it is free or bound in immune complex. The difference in principle between methods, however, has not shown to impact measurement of infliximab obtained after trypsin digestion or using ECLIA[63] or RGA.[80] One explanation for these results is that infliximab is administered in excess of its target TNF, and ADA-infliximab complexes are rapidly cleared from circulation, so virtually all available infliximab is free. For MAT with different targets, the principle of measurement of free or total MAT could be of more significant difference.

Traditional tryptic peptide LC-MS/MS assays rely on a constant digestion of the protein mixture by trypsin. The use of stable isotopically labeled (SIL) peptide internal standards is important to correct for loss of analyte due to sample preparation and mass spectrometry analysis. Similar SIL internal standards are available only for a few MAT (e.g., infliximab, adalimumab, rituximab) where the original MAT patents have expired and allowed for production by other companies. Synthesizing an intact, full-length MAT incorporating SIL standards is a challenge since it is much larger than a peptide (>100-fold) and it must be expressed in a cell culture system, adding substantial cost. The lack of SIL standards has forced the field of proteomic to use alternative internal standards, including the use of other MAT with similar characteristics, winged peptides to be cleaved by trypsin or polyclonal animal Ig when commercial products do not fulfill the test prerequisites.[86]

Other Mass Spectrometry Methods for Monoclonal Antibody Therapeutics

While the trypsin digest method may be the mass spectrometry method of choice for several MAT, not every MAT will work with the digest method especially as newer MAT have only 5% murine sequences (e.g., eculizumab) or are considered fully human (e.g., adalimumab). Finding signature tryptic peptides may be challenging for these cases. For other MAT, sensitivity of the method will be the limiting factor. A time-of-flight mass spectrometer method referred to as monoclonal immunoglobulin Rapid Accurate Mass Measurement (miRAMM), originally developed for identifying endogenous monoclonal Ig in patients with multiple myeloma (MM),[87] has been adapted for the quantitation of rituximab in patients being treated for vasculitis.[88] While rituximab is a chimeric IgG1 MAT similar to infliximab, it was found that the tryptic method did not allow for the sensitivity needed for a clinical assay. The miRAMM method begins with an enrichment step to remove non-immunoglobulins followed by addition of dithiothreitol (DTT) to reduce the disulfide bonds that keep the heavy and light chains of Ig together. The reduced sample mixture is then analyzed by time-of-flight mass spectrometry. The light chains are smaller than heavy chains and ionize more efficiently and reproducibly. While full scan data is collected, the intact light chain mass of a particular MAT or one of the charge states can be monitored and used for quantitation against a standard curve of the pharmaceutical MAT spiked into pooled serum (Fig. 98.9).

The innovative aspect of the miRAMM methodology is that it does not rely on using the target antigen as part of the

LC-MS/MS

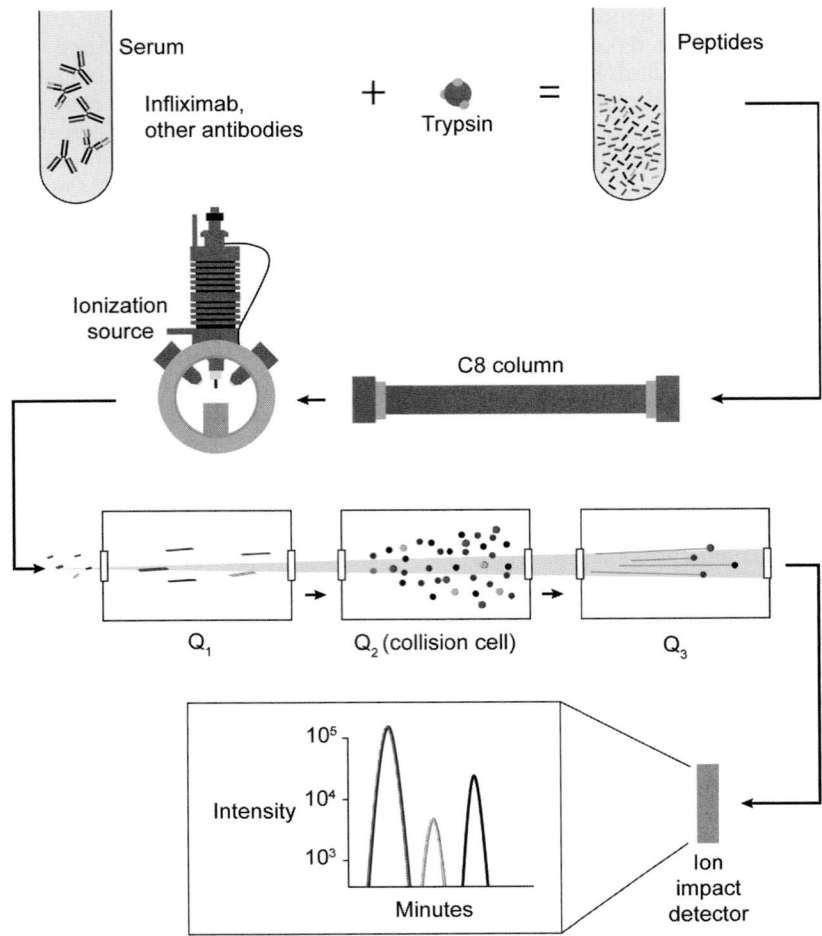

FIGURE 98.8 Liquid Chromatography Tandem Mass Spectrometry (LC-MS/MS) for the Quantitation of Infliximab. A trypsin digestion is performed and signature peptides unique to infliximab are measured by liquid-chromatography tandem mass spectrometry for quantitation of total infliximab. The parent (Q1) and fragment ions (Q3) mass-to-charge ratios from two different peptides, one from the light chain and one from the heavy chain are compared to known standards.

assay, and is capable of identifying and possibly quantitating multiple MAT at once by reviewing their specific mass. The instrumentation required for this assay, the time-of-flight mass spectrometer, is available in large toxicology laboratories performing drug screening testing. While this method has been found to work with MAT that are not ideal for the peptide method, there are still some limitations. For instance, the miRAMM method is not adequate for quantitation of adalimumab, as trough concentrations of adalimumab are below the limit of quantitation obtained for the assay, since adalimumab elutes on a spot with many other endogenous κ light chains. Furthermore, the enrichment step removes all non-immunoglobulins from the sample and it is possible that MAT/target bound complexes are depleted, resulting in under quantitation. These limitations have led to the exploration of new enrichment techniques for quantitation of other MAT. An example is eculizumab, a complement C5 component inhibitor with an IgG2/IgG4 hybrid structure. Using a matrix that selectively enriches for the IgG4 isotype, a 10-fold increase in sensitivity was gained for eculizumab quantitation compared to the original enrichment method.[89]

TEST GUIDED STRATEGY IN TUMOR NECROSIS FACTOR ANTAGONIST TREATMENT

Management of Therapeutic Failure

Until recently, therapeutic failure to TNF antagonists was usually managed by increasing the dose of the drug, or shortening the dose interval while continuing treatment with the same drug. If nonresponsiveness persisted, the patient was regularly switched to another type of TNF antagonist, anticipating the possible emergence of immunogenicity against the first drug. When treatment with the second drug failed, the patient was changed to a different class of biologicals since treatment history was suggestive of the involvement of non–TNF-mediated pathways. In this empiric strategy, no early attempt was made to identify the mechanism for loss of response to TNF antagonist.[90]

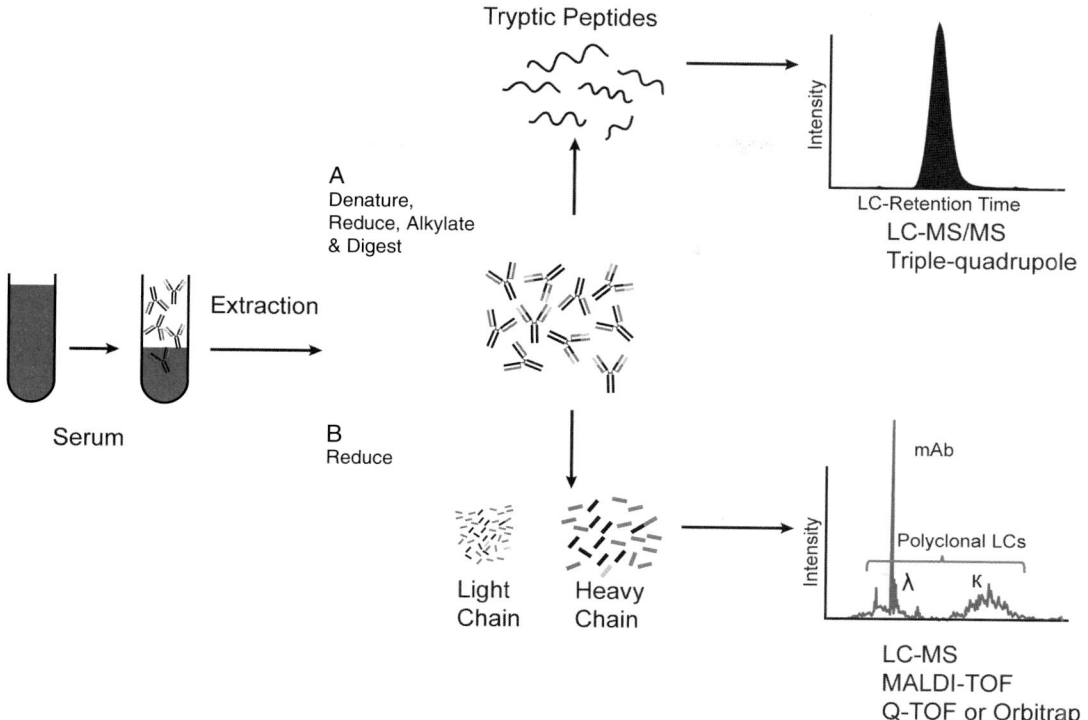

FIGURE 98.9 Mass Spectrometry Methods Applied to Monoclonal Antibody Therapeutics (MAT). Monoclonal antibodies can be quantitated by mass spectrometry. Immunoglobulin extraction or enrichment techniques (e.g., protein crash, Melon Gel IgG enrichment, or affinity matrix for specific IgG subclasses) will help reduce the amount of protein load in the sample and improve analytical sensitivity and specificity. (A) Liquid chromatography tandem mass spectrometry (LC-MS/MS) method. Extractions can promote denaturation (protein unfolded), reduction (cysteine reduction breaks disulfide bond connecting MAT light and heavy chains), alkylation steps (alkylation of cysteines prevents disulfide bonds from reforming), and digestion by trypsin into smaller peptides. The peptide mixture is separated by liquid chromatography before analysis by tandem mass spectrometry. The mass of the peptide of interest (parent ion) is recorded, the peptide is further cleaved inside the mass spectrometer (fragment ion), and the ion pair transition is utilized for quantitation. (B) LC-MS method. After immunoenrichment, sample mixtures are reduced with reducing agents such as dithiothreitol. The light and heavy chains are chromatographically separated, and the intact light chain mass is quantitated by mass spectrometry, a middle-up proteomics approach. The use of an appropriate internal standard is crucial for the success of this technique. *MALDI-TOF,* Matrix assisted laser desorption ionization time of flight; *O-TOF,* quadrupole time of flight mass spectrometer.

Given the risk of loss of response to TNF antagonists and their recognized immunogenic potential, a rational and mechanistic alternative to this empiric strategy has been adopted in clinical practice by employing laboratory testing to measure drug concentration, and detect ADA, in order to select the best treatment strategy based on the most likely mechanism responsible for loss of response. Support in favor of the test-guided strategy comes from recent studies showing significantly reduced average treatment costs per patient, compared to the empirical approach, without differences in clinical efficacy.[61,70,81,91] Testing-based strategies are not only cost-effective, but allow therapies to be tailored to the individual needs of patients, providing personalized rather than universal approach, reducing delays in effective treatment.[90]

The workup for therapeutic response failure includes measuring trough serum drug concentrations right before the patient is about to receive the next dose. Practices vary between laboratories; some laboratories measure both drug and ADA at the same time while others offer them as reflex tests, where if the drug is undetectable, or very low, then the sample is reflexed to an ADA test. Depending on the results of the two tests, and in the clinical context of therapeutic failure, four different scenarios may occur, which require different management strategies (Box 98.1). This algorithm has been proposed by several investigators,[24,27,81,90–92] and has been supported by clinical trials involving CD patients treated with infliximab.[93]

One scenario based on the test outcome is that both drug and ADA are below the level of detection at trough, despite the patient being compliant with therapy. In this group of patients the response failure is likely non–antibody mediated, but involving pharmacokinetic issues; therefore the recommendation is to intensify treatment using the same TNF antagonist by increasing the dose, or shortening the dose interval, followed by re-evaluation of clinical response.

The second scenario is when the drug is not detectable but ADA are present, ideally confirmed by serial measurements, providing laboratory evidence of the emergence of ADA, followed by declining drug concentrations. In the setting of persistent treatment failure, the recommendation is that these patients be switched to another TNF antagonist as there is evidence that they are receptive to the drug class, and antibodies are usually drug-specific.

The third scenario is when the patient has detectable trough drug concentrations and undetectable ADA. If trough concentration is low, compared to existing guidelines,[68] and no ADA are present, treatment escalation is recommended. If drug trough concentration is in the therapeutic range or higher but the patient is still not responding to treatment, this may indicate pharmacodynamic issue and the recommendation is to reassess the clinical condition, and to rule out other noninflammatory causes for treatment failure. Switching to another class of biologicals, targeting a different inflammatory mediator may be useful.[93]

Finally, the fourth and rarest scenario is when both drug and ADA are detected in the serum. In this case the recommendation is to repeat testing to rule out false positive results. This scenario is expected to occur predominantly when the ADA concentrations are tested using binding-based assays, which detect all antibodies, including those that are nonfunctional.[93] This group of patients would benefit from

cell-based testing to establish functionality of the drug and the antibodies. If the results of the repeat test are the same, and the response failure persists, switching to another type of therapy, as in the previous scenario, would be beneficial.

Therapeutic Drug Monitoring of Tumor Necrosis Factor Antagonists

Testing for serum concentrations of TNF antagonists and detecting ADA has been primarily recommended for the workup of treatment failure. However, therapeutic monitoring for these drugs is increasingly used in clinical practice. A guideline from the American Gastroenterological Association recommends TDM to guide changes in therapy in patients with active IBD. In addition, it also recommends target trough concentrations of at least 5 μg/mL for infliximab, and 7.5 μg/mL for adalimumab.[68] It is important to realize that specific TDM cut-off points need to be interpreted in the context of the assay used. While for many assay formats such as RGA, LC-MS/MS, and ECLIA the results obtained for the drug concentration correlate well, differences in analytical sensitivity and specificity between different assay platforms can lead to discrepancies in serum concentrations measured in different laboratories.[94] Although the guideline has its limitations since it is based on limited data, different methods used, and does not apply to all categories of patients, such as those with quiescent IBD, it is an important first step toward standardizing clinical practice for TDM of TNF antagonist drugs. Future studies are needed to characterize TDM of newly approved biological agents, and to establish appropriate testing intervals and clinical cut-off concentrations for TDM using different assays.

Another mode of TDM is the proactive monitoring of MAT drug concentrations. This approach of care has been suggested for TNF antagonists in the setting of IBD. The goal of proactive monitoring is to establish specific time-points in therapy with TNF antagonists associated with improved outcomes after long-term follow-up, where every patient with adequate response to therapy, in clinical response or remission, would be tested for serum drug concentration.[95,96] The evidence is particularly strong for TNF antagonists, but not so much for other classes of MAT, and suggests that proactive TDM may improve cost-effectiveness and safety of biologic therapy with implementation of potential de-escalation strategies in patients with supra-therapeutic concentrations by dose reduction, increased administration intervals, or suspending use of immunomodulators.[97–99] Several randomized clinical trials have compared patient outcomes with and without TDM during induction, postinduction, and maintenance phases. The results of these trials suggest that it is appropriate to perform TDM in responders at the end of the induction phase and at least once during maintenance phase for all TNF antagonists for IBD patients.[99] Proactive TDM of infliximab is associated with increased drug retention,[100] and the Trough Concentration Adapted Infliximab Treatment (TAXIT) randomized controlled trial showed that proactive TDM of infliximab was associated with lower frequency of sub-therapeutic drug concentrations and lower risk of relapse.[95] Infliximab concentrations greater than or equal to 5 μg/mL are associated with persistence on the drug, regardless of the use of monotherapy or combination therapy with immunomodulators.[101,102] Other assay thresholds associated with positive outcomes are not as well established. A group of

IBD specialists keeps an online tool regularly updated to assist in decision making based on TDM test results for several biologics, which includes the phase of therapeutic regimen. The tool is available at: www.bridgeibd.com.[99]

CLINICAL LABORATORY TESTING INTERFERENCE BY MONOCLONAL ANTIBODY THERAPEUTICS

The increased use of MAT for treatment of autoimmune diseases and malignancies has impacted several routine clinical testing methods, including detection and quantification of monoclonal proteins,[103–105] as well as methods performed in blood bank[106–108] or in histocompatibility laboratories.[109] The interference of certain MAT with clinical laboratory tests is an emerging concern that can trigger unnecessary additional testing and may delay important therapeutic decisions.[110]

Interference by Monoclonal Antibody Therapeutics in Histocompatibility Crossmatch Testing

Lymphocyte crossmatch is the final decisive test in histocompatibility testing for solid organ transplantation and allows for ruling out HLA antibodies in patients receiving a donor organ offer. Preformed HLA antibodies in patients following previous transplants, transfusions, or pregnancies are detrimental to the transplanted organ since they may trigger immunologic reactions leading to organ rejection. The lymphocyte crossmatch test evaluates binding between antibodies from the recipient's serum and donor lymphocytes, which can be detected by CDC or by flow cytometry assays. The use of crossmatch test greatly reduced the incidence of hyperacute rejection.[111] However, the presence of certain MAT such as rituximab in the recipient serum affects crossmatch results. Rituximab binds to CD20 on B cells and can produce false positive crossmatch, since complement used for CDC, or the anti-human IgG antibody used for flow cytometry detection are unable to differentiate between rituximab or HLA antibody bound to the B cells. Studies have shown that even residual rituximab concentrations in the serum many months after the last dose can interfere with CDC or flow cytometry crossmatch, resulting in false positive results.[112] Since measuring serum rituximab concentration is not part of the routine clinical practice, as it is the effect of the drug (decrease in B-cell counts) that is monitored, it is not known how much rituximab is present in the serum at any given time posttreatment; one study, however, found that serum rituximab concentrations as low as 0.2 μg/mL resulted in false-positive CDC crossmatch.[113] Rituximab interference may lead to denying transplant to a patient if previous medication history is not known at the time of the crossmatch result. In addition to requesting careful patient history including previous antibody-based medications, histocompatibility laboratories have developed methods to mitigate rituximab interference. One such approach employs pretreatment of the patient serum with an anti-idiotype antibody to rituximab, which will prevent rituximab from binding to CD20 on the B cells and thus giving a positive B-cell crossmatch result.[112,114,115] The success of this approach depends on the magnitude of serum rituximab concentration; although it works well with residual rituximab concentrations, it may not work when serum drug values are high, such as immediately after treatment. Other approaches include treatment of the donor lymphocytes with the proteolytic enzyme pronase, which cleaves off CD20 from

B cells, thus eliminating the target of rituximab binding.[116] However, as a nonspecific protease, pronase can also reduce the expression of HLA molecules on lymphocytes, decreasing the sensitivity of the crossmatch assay.[117] Other MAT shown to interfere with crossmatch testing include daclizumab (anti-CD25), alemtuzumab (anti-CD52), and anti-thymoglobulin, all of which are used to prevent and treat organ rejection.[118]

Interference by Monoclonal Antibody Therapeutics in Blood Bank Testing

MAT interference with transfusion medicine testing has been shown for daratumumab during Phase I and II trials. Daratumumab is a human monoclonal IgG1 κ antibody with high affinity for CD38 found on plasma cells, which effectively targets and kills malignant myeloma cells.[119,120] Patients treated with the drug showed panreactive positive antibody screens in red blood cell (RBC) panel testing, false positive agglutination, and positive direct antiglobulin test. This was consistent with a previously observed weak expression of CD38 on human RBCs.[121] Approaches to eliminate daratumumab interference include pretreatment of the plasma with a neutralizing anti-idiotype antibody to the drug at 5- to 10-tenfold excess, or with soluble CD38 at 10- to 20-fold excess.[106,108] Both methods work well, but disadvantages include higher cost and lack of widespread availability of these reagents. Another approach involves DTT treatment of the RBCs aimed to denature CD38.[106] The effect of DTT can be explained by the presence of six disulfide bonds in the extracellular domain of CD38, which are critical to the protein structure.[122] The advantage of this method is that DTT is inexpensive and it is already used by blood banks worldwide.[123] A potential drawback of DTT treatment is the disruption of blood group antigens such as those of the Kell blood group system, which may be missed on DTT-treated RBCs, and therefore group K negative units must be provided to patients unless they are known to be group K positive (more than 90% of donated RBCs are K negative). RBC antigen phenotyping is recommended before patients are started on daratumumab.[123]

Interference by Monoclonal Antibody Therapeutics in Detection and Quantitation of Monoclonal Proteins

MM is a malignant plasma cell dyscrasia associated with production of abnormal monoclonal Ig. Detection of monoclonal Ig, also known as monoclonal protein or M-protein, is performed by PEP and immunofixation electrophoresis (IFE) of serum and urine. The amount of M-protein measured by PEP and IFE in serum or urine correlates with tumor burden and disease progression.

MM is considered an incurable disease, with most patients showing good response to initial therapy but ultimately going into relapse regardless of the therapy used. Recently, two new MAT, daratumumab and elotuzumab, have been approved by the FDA for treatment of relapsed/refractory MM. Elotuzumab is a humanized IgGκ antibody that binds CS1/SLAMF7, a subunit of CD2 molecule predominantly expressed on plasma cells.[124] Both daratumumab and elotuzumab elicit plasma cell killing by a combination of actions including apoptosis, CDC, and ADCC.[125] Several additional MAT targeting plasma cells for the treatment of refractory MM are in early clinical trials, including isatuximab[126] and MOR202.[127]

Monitoring of patients with MM involves measuring of the M-protein by PEP and IFE in serum and urine at frequent intervals. The International Myeloma Working Group defines complete response in patients with MM as lack of evidence of initial M-protein isotype by IFE in the patient's serum and urine after the institution of any new therapy.[128] Misclassification of complete remission in patients with MM could occur during clinical trial evaluation of MAT therapy due to failure to differentiate between residual MAT and M-protein. The limit of detection of M-proteins by IFE is ~0.02 g/dL. However, patients with advanced MM often have hypogammaglobulinemia and the limit of detection of M-protein by IFE in these patients can be as low as 0.01 g/dL. Pharmacokinetic studies established that mean trough (predose) concentration of daratumumab is ~0.05 g/dL[129] and 0.01 g/dL for elotuzumab,[130] and experiments with spiked samples demonstrated that several other MAT can be detected by IFE down to 0.01 g/dL.[103] Thus it is possible that residual bands of MAT can be visible in IFE gels during patient monitoring depending on the time of testing.

Several studies have reported the detection of serum bands produced by MAT in patients with refractory MM by protein electrophoretic methods,[103,131,132] including ofatumumab, a MAT used for treatment of Waldenstrom macroglobulinemia.[133] Other MAT used to treat diseases other than MM (e.g., infliximab, eculizumab, natalizumab) do not produce IFE interference because these drugs are not administered at sufficiently high doses to achieve serum concentration that would be detectable by electrophoretic methods.[69,104]

Because of potential misclassification of patients receiving MAT for treatment of refractory MM, the International Myeloma Working Group recommends that laboratories involved

in clinical trials have a mechanism in place to differentiate between residual MAT and M-proteins on IFE reports.[134] One simple method is to establish the electrophoretic migration distance of commonly used MAT which then can be used to differentiate between residual MAT and M-proteins. For example, using electrophoresis it has been established that daratumumab runs at the cathodal end of the γ fraction, elotuzumab runs in the mid γ region, while isatuximab runs closer to the β γ region.[131] These patterns may assist laboratories in determining whether the band being visualized is due to one of these MAT. However, in practice, it is not always possible to use band migration mobility solely as a mean to distinguish whether the band is caused by residual MAT or M-protein. This is because M-proteins have unique electrophoretic migration patterns, some of which may run closely or completely overlapping with that of MAT on IFE (Fig. 98.10). This difficulty is even more pronounced given that the majority of MAT are of the IgG κ isotype. IgG κ M-proteins are the most common isotype found in patients with MM and therefore there is high potential for failure to differentiate between the two bands due to their close or overlapping electrophoretic migration pattern observed in IFE of these patients. Another complication is the use of combined methods for PEP and IFE by different laboratories. Some laboratories use capillary electrophoresis for PEP or IFE. Differences in the migration of MAT between capillary and agarose gel-based instruments due to corresponding differences in electrochemical properties of the buffer systems have been reported.[103] Furthermore, detection of MAT by serum IFE depends on their species of origin, since IFE typically uses anti-human reagent antibodies whereas detection of MAT by PEP (either agarose or capillary methods) does not

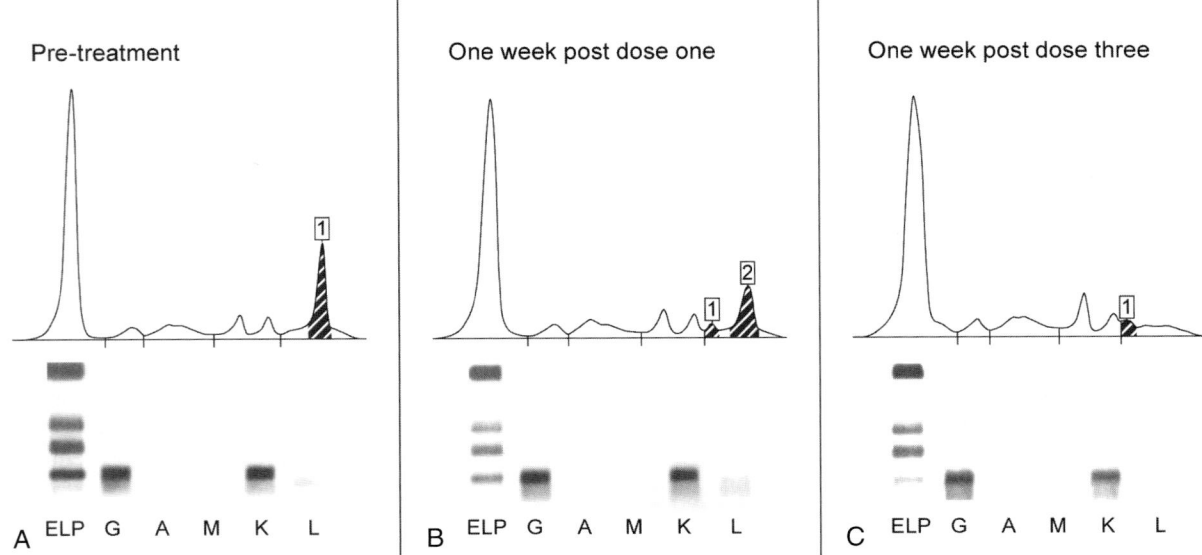

FIGURE 98.10 Interference of isatuximab with serum protein capillary electrophoresis and immunofixation results of a multiple myeloma patient. (A) Prior to treatment the patient had a single distinct M-protein of IgG κ isotype located in the mid-γ region. (B) One week after the first dose with isatuximab, the capillary electrophoresis result shows the presence of a second M-protein located in the β γ region. The two M-proteins observed by capillary testing overlap as a single IgG κ monoclonal band by immunofixation. (C) One week after the third dose with isatuximab, the capillary electrophoresis and immunofixation results show persistence of a small M-protein of IgG κ isotype.

depend on their species of origin. Therefore a mouse-derived MAT might be detectable by PEP but not IFE, which can further complicate the clinical assessment during patient monitoring.

There are other practical methods that clinical laboratories can use to mitigate the risk of reporting false-positive results due to MAT interference including making sure that sample collection is taken immediately before the next dose, ensuring close communication between laboratory staff and physicians to determine which patients are receiving MAT, review of electronic medical records by pathologists to confirm MAT use and time of doses, or including a disclaimer in the report stating that the appearance of a new M-protein could be suggestive of residual MAT. PEP and IFE results are typically reviewed by a pathologist or doctoral level laboratory director prior to reporting. However, there is substantial variation in result interpretation due to lack of standardization and many laboratories report all visible M-proteins without reference to patient medical history and interventions.[135] This is particularly true of PEP and IFE testing for clinical trial monitoring mainly performed at reference laboratories, which typically do not have access to patient medical records. Given the limitations of these approaches, new analytical methods and technologies are required to overcome these challenges.

Drug-specific Immunofixation Assays

Soon after the introduction of daratumumab for the treatment of refractory MM, it became clear that complete response could be misclassified in a subset of patients due to failure to differentiate between residual M-protein and drug. To help discriminate residual daratumumab from M-protein,

the daratumumab-specific immunofixation reflex assay (DIRA) was developed.[136] DIRA is based on the use of an anti-daratumumab antibody that binds to daratumumab, forming a complex that produces a change in the electrophoretic migration of the drug on serum IFE (Fig. 98.11). DIRA is currently indicated for disease monitoring of patients showing a single IgG κ M-protein on serum IFE. If the migration of the M-protein changes after addition of anti-daratumumab antibody (DIRA-negative result), the presence of residual drug can be confirmed and the presence of residual M-protein can be excluded. In contrast, samples showing no change of migration of the M-protein are considered DIRA positive likely due to presence of residual M-protein. DIRA has 100% analytical specificity and sensitivity at a concentration of 0.02 g/dL of daratumumab, which is below trough drug concentrations.[129]

Despite the great analytical sensitivity and specificity of DIRA to rule out daratumumab interference, this method has several limitations. DIRA is costly, not quantitative, and requires interpretation by a trained individual. DIRA result interpretation can be difficult in patients with high polyclonal Ig background and in patients with hypogammaglobulinemia, which decreases the limit of IFE detection of M-spike to as low as 0.01 g/dL. Additionally, serum IFE results from patients showing oligoclonal responses, commonly seen in patients treated with MAT, can also be difficult to interpret.[132] Finally, a drug-specific IFE assay such as DIRA is solely specific to daratumumab. Potential interference in patients receiving other MAT cannot be resolved using DIRA. A similar method is described for elotuzumab, although not yet available commercially.[137] Therefore additional methods that can address antibody interference in a more comprehensive manner are

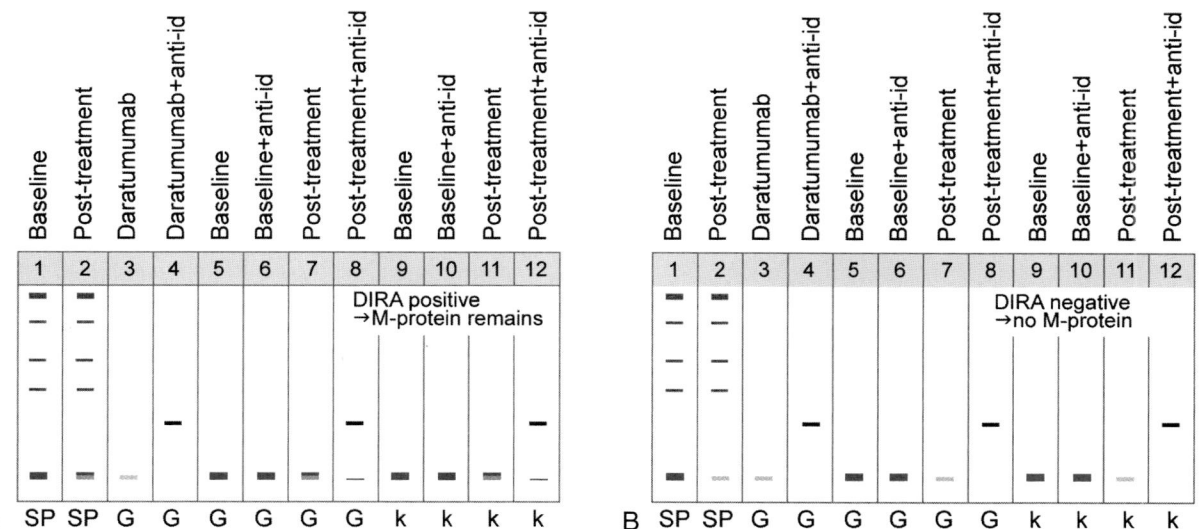

FIGURE 98.11 Diagram of Daratumumab-specific Immunofixation Reflex Assay (DIRA). The endogenous IgG κ M-protein (in red, baseline lane 1) comigrates with the daratumumab monoclonal band (in pink, control lane 3). The daratumumab specific anti-idiotype (anti-id) binds daratumumab and shifts its migration pattern (in gray, control lane 4). IgG (lanes 5–8) and κ (lanes 9 to 12) are separately analyzed by IFE. (A) In samples with residual IgG κ endogenous M-protein, a second band in the IFE gel remains visible (red lines in lanes 8 and 12), which corresponds to a positive DIRA test. (B) In samples where the endogenous M-protein is no longer visible, the only band visible is the shifted daratumumab complexes (gray lines in lanes 8 and 12), which indicates a negative DIRA test. G, Anti-IgG antisera; k, anti-κ antisera; SP, total serum protein fixation.

needed for patients receiving other MAT, or a combination of them, and in patients requiring quantitative testing.

Mass Spectrometry–based Approaches

Light chains confer antibody specificity due to unique amino acid sequences that provide each antibody with a distinct molecular mass. Differences in one amino acid, representing on average a 15-Da mass shift, can be accurately measured by high-resolution mass spectrometers. Following the improvement and refinement of preanalytical and postanalytical steps, a robust, analytically sensitive and specific mass spectrometry–based method was developed for the detection and monitoring of M-proteins in MM patients.[87] This method, known as miRAMM and referred to earlier in this chapter, is based on the identification of mass spectra of light chain portions of serum Ig, followed by the conversion of these mass spectra into molecular masses for each light chain variant. The identification of a peak above the polyclonal Ig background by miRAMM is consistent with the presence of an M-spike with the additional ability to accurately discern differences in molecular masses of M-proteins within 1 Da. This technique has shown high concordance and increased analytical sensitivity compared to electrophoretic methods for the identification and monitoring of M-proteins in MM patients.[138]

The practical use of miRAMM for evaluation of interference by MAT in electrophoresis testing was evaluated in samples from patients with MM spiked with different concentrations of MAT including infliximab and vedolizumab.[69] This method was able to differentiate M-spikes produced by these MAT from endogenous large M-proteins based on each antibody unique mass. Based on these preliminary results, miRAMM could be used to discern interference by MAT in patients with MM showing a previously undocumented IgG κ M-protein, undergoing treatment with MAT, regardless of the MAT used. This will require the development of a library containing the molecular masses of light chains from commonly used MAT. Daratumumab and a co-migrating IgG κ endogenous M-protein were tested in different ratios using miRAMM and the method was able to distinguish the two clones from each other.[139]

An interim approach to miRAMM is the use of matrix assisted laser desorption ionization time of flight (MALDI-TOF), a modification of the miRAMM method employed in the clinical laboratory as a replacement to immunofixation. In this qualitative method, the serum sample is immunoenriched using camelid-derived nanobodies against the constant domains of human heavy chains γ, α, and μ, and the light chains κ and λ in five separate vials. After the incubation period, the mixture is reduced to release the light chains from the heavy chains, followed by MALDI-TOF analysis. The spectra generated after this assay is overlaid for the five immunocapture agents: IgG, IgA, IgM, κ, and λ using a software. Similarly to miRAMM, the polyclonal light chains are distributed in multiple charge states (+2 and +1), which appear as overlapping Gaussian distributions corresponding to the λ and κ light chains. M-spikes show as distinct peaks above the polyclonal background, and the assay has been named MASS-FIX.[140,141] The mass accuracy of the MALDI-TOF is not as robust as the high-resolution mass spectrometers, and allows to accurately differentiate molecular masses within 10 Da. However, this is sufficient to identify the masses of daratumumab, elotuzumab, and isatuximab consistently as peaks and differentiating them from the mass of the endogenous M-protein, with similar limit of quantitation to what is observed on the immunofixation gels (Fig. 98.12). This method has potential to be quantitative when coupled to quantitation of total IgG, IgA, and IgM,[141] but that application is still not clinically available.

To date, these mass spectrometry–based methods are not used routinely in clinical laboratories. Due to initial instrumentation costs and analytical complexity for clinical validation of mass spectrometry-based techniques, it is likely that these methods will be initially offered by large regional or national reference laboratories. However, the increasing number of MAT currently introduced in clinical practice will require prompt validation and implementation of these methods for assessing interference by MAT in electrophoresis testing.

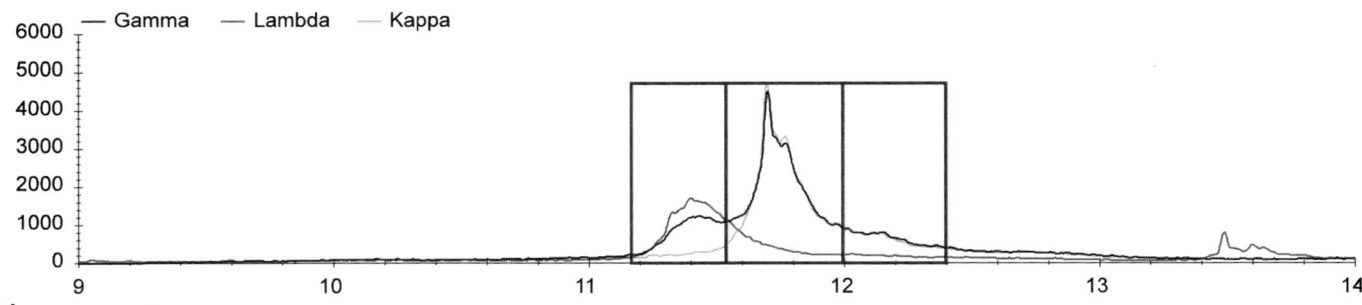

A Daratumumab

Figure 98.12 Mass spectrometric identification of the accurate mass of monoclonal antibody therapeutics (MAT) using matrix assisted laser desorption ionization time of flight. The images show the overlaid mass spectra of the +2 charge state of the lambda (first red box) and kappa polyclonal distributions (second and third red boxes), in the immunoenrichment vials for IgG, kappa and lambda. The three panels show distinct monoclonal IgG kappa peaks, with a mass-to-charge-ratio consistent with daratumumab (A), elotuzumab (B), and isatuximab (C), when compared to pharmaceutical preparation standards. In panel B, it is possible to note a residual amount of the endogenous M-protein, IgG lambda, indicating the absence of complete response to therapy for that sample, while other examples show only the presence of the MAT and no residual detectable M-protein.

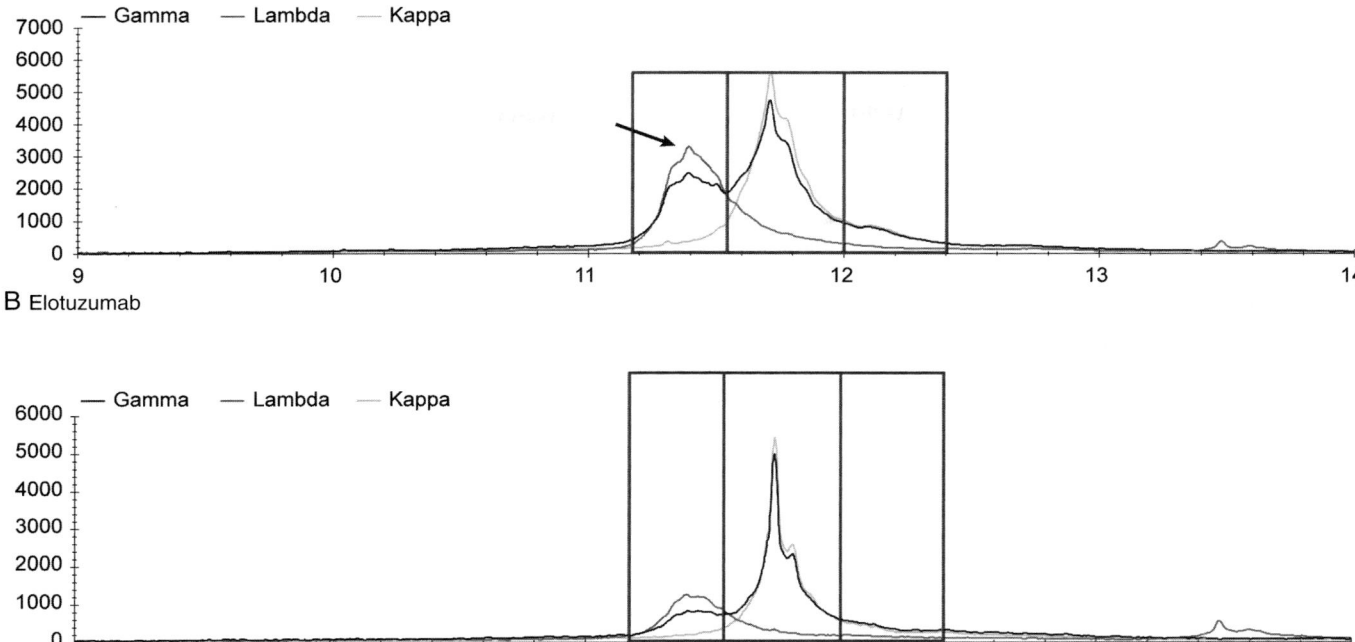

B Elotuzumab

C Isatuximab

FIGURE 98.12, cont'd

SELECTED REFERENCES

56. Bendtzen K, Geborek P, Svenson M, et al. Individualized monitoring of drug bioavailability and immunogenicity in rheumatoid arthritis patients treated with the tumor necrosis factor alpha inhibitor infliximab. Arthritis Rheum 2006;54: 3782–9.
57. Lazar-Molnar E, Delgado JC. Immunogenicity assessment of tumor necrosis factor antagonists in the clinical laboratory. Clin Chem 2016;62:1186–98.
61. Nanda KS, Cheifetz AS, Moss AC. Impact of antibodies to infliximab on clinical outcomes and serum infliximab levels in patients with inflammatory bowel disease (IBD): a meta-analysis. Am J Gastroenterol 2013;108:40–7.
62. Wang SL, Ohrmund L, Hauenstein S, et al. Development and validation of a homogeneous mobility shift assay for the measurement of infliximab and antibodies-to-infliximab levels in patient serum. J Immunol Methods 2012;382:177–88.
63. Willrich MA, Murray DL, Barnidge DR, Ladwig PM, Snyder MR. Quantitation of infliximab using clonotypic peptides and selective reaction monitoring by lc-ms/ms. Int Immunopharmacol 2015;28:513–20.
64. Pavlov IY, Carper J, Lazar-Molnar E, Delgado JC. Clinical laboratory application of a reporter-gene assay for measurement of functional activity and neutralizing antibody response to infliximab. Clin Chim Acta 2016;453:147–53.
68. Feuerstein JD, Nguyen GC, Kupfer SS, et al. American gastroenterological association institute guideline on therapeutic drug monitoring in inflammatory bowel disease. Gastroenterology 2017;153:827–34.
69. Willrich MAV, Ladwig PM, Andreguetto BD, et al. Monoclonal antibody therapeutics as potential interferences on protein electrophoresis and immunofixation. Clin Chem Lab Med 2016;54:1085–93.
80. Willrich MAV, Lazar-Molnar E, Snyder MR, Delgado JC. Comparison of clinical laboratory assays for measuring serum infliximab and antibodies to infliximab. J Appl Lab Med 2018;2:893–903.
81. Steenholdt C, Brynskov J, Thomsen OO, et al. Individualised therapy is more cost-effective than dose intensification in patients with crohn's disease who lose response to anti-TNF treatment: a randomised, controlled trial. Gut 2014;63:919–27.
84. Lallemand C, Kavrochorianou N, Steenholdt C, et al. Reporter gene assay for the quantification of the activity and neutralizing antibody response to TNFalpha antagonists. J Immunol Methods 2011;373:229–39.
85. Gils A, Vande Casteele N, Poppe R, et al. Development of a universal anti-adalimumab antibody standard for interlaboratory harmonization. Ther Drug Monit 2014;36:669–73.
86. Ladwig PM, Barnidge DR, Willrich MAV. Mass spectrometry approaches for identification and quantitation of therapeutic monoclonal antibodies in the clinical laboratory. Clin Vaccine Immunol 2017;24:e00545–16.
89. Ladwig PM, Barnidge DR, Willrich MA. Quantification of the Igg2/4 kappa monoclonal therapeutic eculizumab from serum using isotype specific affinity purification and micro-flow LC-ESI-Q-TOF mass spectrometry. J Am Soc Mass Spectrom 2017;28:811–7.
93. Steenholdt C, Bendtzen K, Brynskov J, Thomsen OO, Ainsworth MA. Clinical implications of measuring drug and anti-drug antibodies by different assays when optimizing infliximab treatment failure in Crohn's disease: post hoc analysis of a randomized controlled trial. Am J Gastroenterol 2014;109: 1055–64.
95. Vande Casteele N, Ferrante M, Van Assche G, et al. Trough concentrations of infliximab guide dosing for patients with inflammatory bowel disease. Gastroenterology 2015;148: 1320–9.e3.

103. McCudden CR, Voorhees PM, Hainsworth SA, et al. Interference of monoclonal antibody therapies with serum protein electrophoresis tests. Clin Chem 2010;56:1897–9.

110. Lazar-Molnar E, Delgado JC. Implications of monoclonal antibody therapeutics use for clinical laboratory testing. Clin Chem 2019;65:393–405.

132. van de Donk NWCJ, Otten HG, El Haddad O, et al. Interference of daratumumab in monitoring multiple myeloma patients using serum immunofixation electrophoresis can be abrogated using the daratumumab IFE reflex assay (DIRA). Clin Chem Lab Med 2016;54: 1105–9.

139. Mills JR, Kohlhagen MC, Willrich MAV, et al. A universal solution for eliminating false positives in myeloma due to therapeutic monoclonal antibody interference. Blood 2018;132:670–2.

Allergy Testing*

Lokinendi V. Rao

ABSTRACT

Background

Immunoglobulin E (IgE)-associated allergen conditions are increasing worldwide, affecting the quality of life of millions of individuals and are a burden on the health care system. The increasing availability of clinically relevant allergenic molecules has begun to change the way allergen-specific IgE antibody diagnostics are performed. Allergic diseases, respiratory infections, and autoimmune conditions have similar clinical presentations, and self-reported symptoms have low positive predictive value. Thus laboratory allergy and immunologic testing are useful in clarifying diagnosis and guiding treatment. They are also useful in identifying causative allergen in atopic dermatitis (eczema), contact dermatitis, urticaria, angioedema, and food or drug allergies. Testing helps provide clinically relevant information for avoidance and treatment.

Content

This chapter describes the basic concepts of allergy and hypersensitivity reactions of the immune system, cells involved in the allergy, and their functions. Fetal origins of allergy, including the route of exposure, and maternal and dietary influences, are discussed. Technological innovations are also changing the way allergies are diagnosed. Starting from skin testing to specific IgE measurements that are clinically relevant component tests, functional tests like basophil activation tests, microarrays, and nanosensor- and biosensor-based assays are evaluated. Details of various types of allergy including food, contact, inhalants, pollen, pets, fungal, trees, latex, animal epithelia, insect sting, ocular, occupational, and red meat allergy are outlined. Non-IgE and mixed IgE and non–IgE-mediated food allergies are discussed as they can be challenging due to the overall lack of noninvasive confirmatory tests. Various allergy-related disorders like asthma, COPD, hypersensitivity pneumonitis, rhinitis, urticaria, and angioedema are reviewed.

*The full version of this chapter is available electronically on ExpertConsult.com.

Primary Immunodeficiencies and Secondary Immunodeficiencies

Thomas F. Michniacki, Manisha Madkaikar, Kelly Walkovich, Maite de la Morena, and Roshini S. Abraham

ABSTRACT

Background

Over the last six decades, our understanding of human immunology, coupled with our ability to interrogate the immune system in detail, has gone through a period of rapid evolution. From the early pioneers of immunology, Sir Peter Medawar[1] and Sir MacFarlane Burnet,[2] who elucidated concepts such as tolerance in transplantation and cellular immunology, and the clonal selection theory of antibody diversity respectively, to Max Cooper and Jacques Miller, who discovered distinct classes of lymphocytes comprising the adaptive immune system—B and T cells, respectively—the field of immunology has been in "fast forward" mode. The understanding of the body's host defense mechanisms was paralleled by advances in technology, including flow cytometry and molecular biology, resulting in a powerful collision of knowledge derived from theoretical and experimental data.

Content

This chapter focuses on representative examples of inborn errors of immunity (primary immunodeficiencies [PIDs] and primary immune dysregulatory disorders [PIRDs]) and secondary immunodeficiencies, caused by extrinsic manipulation of the immune system, via either treatment, infections, or other causes. In the 2019 International Union of Immunological Societies (IUIS) classification of the inborn errors of immunity (IEIs),[3] 416 gene defects have been described associating with one or more distinct clinical phenotypes. In the current era, five or more new genetic defects are added to this list each year, making it impractical, if not impossible, to keep abreast of developments in the field. The goal of this chapter is to provide a high-level overview on illustrative examples of IEIs and an overview of diagnosis and treatment, as well as a discussion on and examples of secondary immunodeficiencies.

POINTS TO REMEMBER

1. Inborn errors of immunity refer to genetic disorders of any component of the immune system associated with susceptibility to infection or immune dysregulation (autoimmunity, lymphoproliferation, and malignancy).
2. There are now over 400 genetic disorders of the immune system.
3. Inborn errors of immunity are classified based on the main component of the immune system affected, although more than one component may often be involved in the phenotype.
4. Establishing genotype-phenotype correlations are important for diagnosis, prognosis, and management.
5. Not all inborn errors of immunity demonstrate Mendelian inheritance.
6. Diseases that phenotypically mimic inborn errors of immunity but are not caused by germline defects in genes associated with the immune system are considered phenocopies, and could be due to somatic variants or autoantibodies to biologically relevant molecules, such as cytokines.
7. Immune deficiencies may also be caused by nongenetic factors, such as medications, infections, and other diseases. These are considered secondary immunodeficiencies.

INTRODUCTION

The first primary immunodeficiency (PID) was reported in the 1950s by Colonel Ogden Bruton, who described a male patient without the gamma globulin fraction (immunoglobulin) in blood who was inherently susceptible to multiple and severe infections. It took approximately another four decades to identify the molecular basis of this X-linked recessive immune disorder, which is now called X-linked agammaglobulinemia (XLA) caused by pathogenic variants in the Bruton's tyrosine kinase (*BTK*) gene. Similarly, two physicians on two different continents approximately 15 years apart described male patients with a triad of bleeding diathesis, eczema, and diarrhea, which also appeared to be X-linked recessive in inheritance.[4,5] The disease was named Wiskott-Aldrich syndrome after the two physicians, and again it took almost four decades to identify the specific gene associated with this defect, now called Wiskott-Aldrich syndrome (*WAS*) gene.[6] Today in the 21st century we are aware of more than 400 single gene (monogenic) defects associated with various inborn errors of immunity, which includes primary immunodeficiencies (PIDs) and primary immune dysregulatory disorders (PIRDs).[3] We have come a long way in our understanding of human immunity, and our ability to diagnose, treat, and manage these conditions, but we still have a long way to go.

The cellular components of the immune system include both adaptive (T cells and B cells) and innate immune cells (natural killer [NK] cells, granulocytes, monocytes, dendritic cells). Additionally, there are other specialized cells including various types of innate lymphoid cells (ILCs) that along with a variety of cells and tissues play a key role in the modulation of the immune response. The immune system also produces and is regulated by several soluble biomarkers, including cytokines, chemokines, and other biologically active molecules that drive and modify the immune response. This chapter will not delve into the details of the development of the immune system or these cellular subsets, or the immune response and its regulation.

Key serum proteins of the immune system include antibodies or immunoglobulins produced by terminally differentiated B cells, plasma cells. A brief discussion of the role of antibodies is provided here. Antibodies are a critical component of the host defense mechanism able to neutralize toxins or viruses, or bind to bacteria or fungi and prepare them for killing by phagocytes and the complement system proteins. There are five major isotypes of immunoglobulin heavy chains—IgG, IgA, IgM, IgD, and IgE. Each of these has distinct functions within the humoral immune response, and pair with either kappa or lambda light chains. Within the IgG family of immunoglobulins, there are four subclasses (IgG1, G2, G3, and G4), while IgA has two subclasses (IgA1 and IgA2). The immunoglobulins either are secreted into plasma or present on the surface of B cells as membrane-bound immunoglobulin. Immunoglobulin allotypes are reflective of genetic differences in the constant region segments of antibody molecules and are either classified as Gm, Am, Em, or Km, depending on the alleles associated with each isotype. Idiotypes, on the other hand, are unique epitopes within the variable (V) regions of antibodies and allow discrimination of one antibody from another. IgG is the most abundant immunoglobulin in human serum and has a half-life of 23 days while IgM, IgA, IgD, and IgE have half-lives of 5, 7, 2.8, and 2.3 days, respectively. It is important to bear in mind that the half-life of IgG is not invariant but rather is related to the concentration of the immunoglobulin in circulation. Therefore for patients with low concentrations of IgG (hypogammaglobulinemia), the half-life may be as long as 35 days, while in patients with hypergammaglobulinemia, it can be as short as 10 days. The regulation of IgG half-life is mediated by the neonatal Fc receptor (FcRn) and permits recycling of the IgG molecule.[7] Deficiency of immunoglobulins is the most common of all inborn errors of immunity and falls into three broad categories, based on the degree of antibody deficiency, presence or absence of B cells, and whether there are other syndromic manifestations. Immunoglobulin is transferred through the placenta, especially IgG, while IgA is present in secretions, such as tears, breast milk, and saliva and is a critical component of mucosal immunity. Selective IgA deficiency is probably the most common immunodeficiency to be described, and most patients are clinically asymptomatic while some may have an increased incidence of infections. Maternal IgG is present in the first 6 months of life and gradually wanes allowing endogenous immunoglobulin production to take over. If the physiologic hypogammaglobulinemia of infancy persists beyond 6 months, it is often referred to as transient hypogammaglobulinemia of infancy (THI). Patients with THI may be either asymptomatic and normalize over time, or have

recurrent infections. Replacement with external immunoglobulin is commonly not recommended except if there is life-threatening infections. It may take several months to years to normalize immunoglobulin levels but typically most patients in this category would have normalized IgG levels by 4 years of age.

IgG subclass deficiencies, on the other hand, are conditions in which total IgG (and subclass IgG1, which is the most abundant subclass) is normal but one or more other subclasses are decreased due to reduction in production of one or more isotypes. As with THI, measurement of subclasses and treatment with replacement therapy is only recommended in the context of aberrant functional antibody responses and significant infections.

As previously alluded to in the abstract, inborn errors in immunity (IEIs), often referred to as primary immunodeficiencies (PIDs), are heterogeneous disorders affecting all components of the immune system, and occurring either as the dominant phenotype or in conjunction with other anomalies affecting one or more organ systems (syndromic immunodeficiencies). The spectrum of IEI can present with a clinical phenotype of susceptibility to infection, autoimmunity, predisposition to malignancy or atopy, lymphoproliferation, or combinations of these. While autoimmunity and immunodeficiency may appear mutually exclusive, studies of IEI reveal that monogenic defects can cause immune dysregulation, which not only predisposes to autoimmunity, but may also be associated with increased susceptibility to infections. With the advent of next generation sequencing (discussed later in this chapter), identification of molecular defects associated with aberrant immunity has become increasingly facile, and allowed for various permutations within the same gene associated with distinct phenotypes (e.g., gain-of-function [GOF] and loss-of-function [LOF] variants[8,9]) to be revealed. In addition, identification of specific molecular defects has opened the door to personalized therapies and targeted treatments.[10–13]

The IUIS classification of IEI[3,14] has grouped genetic defects associated with immunologic diseases into nine broad categories, based on the immune defect or predominant clinical phenotype (Fig. 100.1). A tenth category includes phenocopies of immunodeficiencies, which will be briefly described in this chapter. The nine categories include: (1) combined (T and B cell) immunodeficiencies, (2) combined immunodeficiencies (CIDs) with syndromic or associated features, (3) humoral or antibody deficiencies as the major phenotype, (4) defects of immune dysregulation, (5) congenital defects of phagocytes, (6) defects of innate/intrinsic immunity, (7) autoinflammatory conditions, (8) complement deficiencies, and (9) bone marrow failure syndromes. Representative examples of these monogenic disorders and phenocopies of PIDs are provided in this chapter along with an overview of treatment and management of IEI. The final section of this chapter is focused on secondary immunodeficiencies.

GROUP 1. COMBINED IMMUNODEFICIENCIES AFFECTING CELLULAR AND HUMORAL IMMUNITY

This category includes a variety of genetic defects associated with diverse clinical phenotypes but unified by a defect in both arms of adaptive immunity—T and B cells. Severe combined

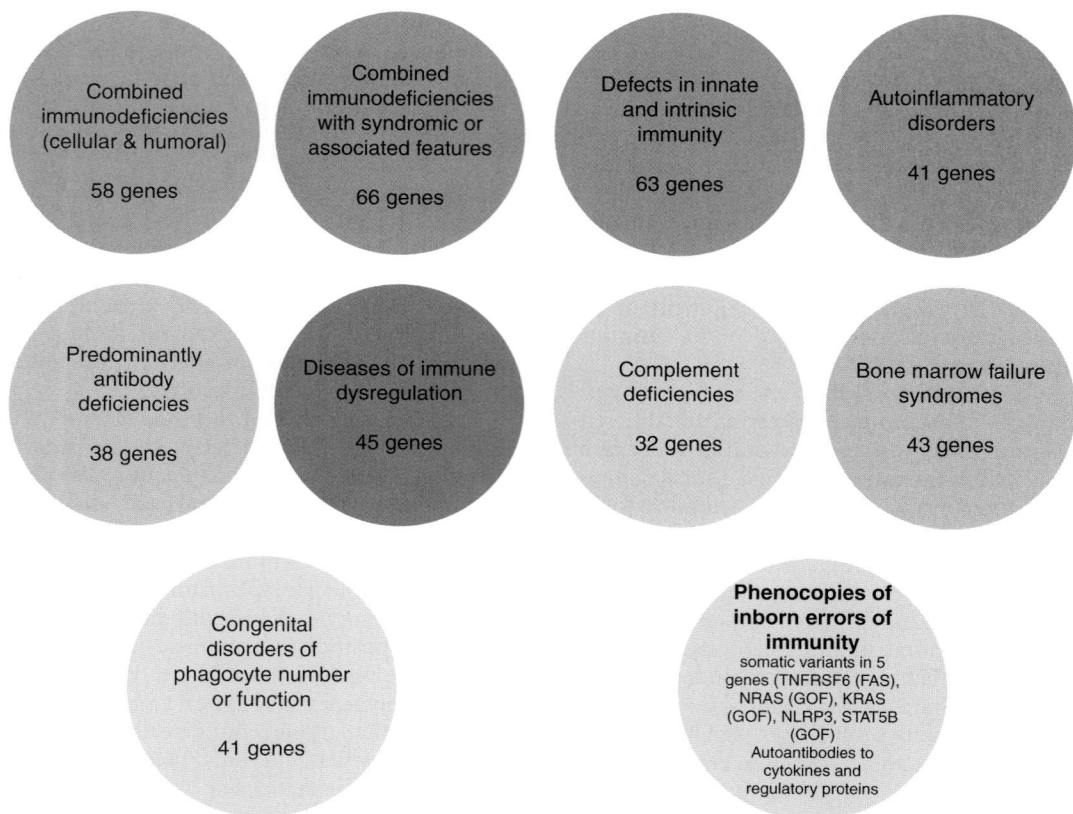

FIGURE 100.1 IUIS classification of inborn errors of immunity. The 10 categories of genetic disorders of the immune system (primary immunodeficiencies and immune dysregulatory disorders) are depicted here with the number of genes described in each category based on the 2019 classification.[3]

immunodeficiencies (SCIDs) are a prototype of this group of disorders.

Severe Combined Immunodeficiencies

SCID is characterized by defect in T-cell numbers and/or function. In addition, other components of the adaptive (B cells) and innate immune system (NK cells) may be affected. The disease manifests at a median of 4 to 6 months and most infants are asymptomatic at birth. Typical infections in these patients include recurrent viral, bacterial, and fungal opportunistic infections including pneumonias, diarrhea, and failure to thrive (FTT).[15–17] Due to compromised cellular immunity, live vaccines are contraindicated. The number of genetic defects associated with SCID has rapidly multiplied in recent years.[3,18] Most of the SCID defects present with an autosomal recessive inheritance except for a few, which demonstrate X-linked inheritance, including the prototypic SCID defect, X-linked SCID caused by pathogenic variants in the *IL2RG* gene, encoding the common gamma chain of the interleukin (IL)-2 receptor. SCID-associated conditions can be categorized based on whether B and NK cells are affected, in addition to T cells. The four main categories of SCID based on T-, B-, and NK-cell quantitation include T−B−NK−, T−B−NK+, T−B+NK−, and T−B+NK+ defects (Table 100.1). The clinical spectrum ranges from the classic or typical manifestations to leaky SCID, caused by partial loss-of-function (LOF) or hypomorphic gene defects in the same genes that cause the typical phenotype.[19] Also, if the leaky SCID presentation occurs in conjunction with

other features of erythroderma, elevated IgE, eosinophilia, organomegaly, or oligoclonal T cell expansion, then the phenotype is consistent with Omenn syndrome.[20,21] Most forms of SCID are associated with the absence of a thymic shadow on a chest X-ray, which ought to trigger suspicion for a primary immunodeficiency. However, there are certain forms of SCID, such as Coronin-1A and CD3 delta subunit deficiencies, which have a visible thymus.[22]

The diagnosis of SCID includes a combination of clinical features with laboratory testing. A simple complete blood count (CBC) can be informative as most patients with the classic forms of SCID have significantly decreased absolute lymphocyte counts (ALC < 2500 cells/μL; CD3+ T cells < 300 cells/μL). However, in some cases of leaky SCID or Omenn syndrome there may be either maternal engraftment or oligoclonal expansion of T cells, which can raise the ALC. Maternal engraftment (ME) can be ruled out by performing a karyotype analysis on peripheral blood of male infants, while for female infants, a short tandem repeat assay (STR) would be necessary to differentiate between maternal and infant T cells. The STR assay may also be used for ME in male infants and is likely less expensive than karyotyping. Flow cytometry for activated T cells expressing HLA DR and distribution of memory and naïve T cells can be informative, though these cannot discriminate between maternal engraftment and autologous oligoclonal expansion of T cells.

Most flow cytometry assays use a panel of basic markers for discriminating between naïve and memory T cells utilizing

TABLE 100.1 Examples of Classification of Severe Combined Immunodeficiencies Defects Based on Lymphocyte Subset Phenotyping

Category	Gene Defect
T−B+NK− SCID	
IL-2 receptor common gamma chain (X-linked)	*IL2RG*
Janus Kinase 3 (JAK3) deficiency	*JAK3*
T−B+NK+ SCID	
IL7 receptor chain α	*IL7RA*
CD45	*PTPRC*
CD3 δ	*CD3D*
CD3 ε	*CD3E*
CD3 ζ	*CD3Z*
Coronin 1A	*CORO1*
Winged helix deficiency	*FOXN1*
PAX1 deficiency	*PAX1*
T−B−NK+SCID	
Recombinase activating genes 1 and 2	*RAG1 and RAG2*
DNA crosslink repair enzymes 1C (Artemis)	*DCLRE1C*
DNA-dependent protein kinase catalytic subunit (DNA-PKcs)	*PRKDC*
DNA ligase IV deficiency	*LIG4*
CERNUNNOS/XLF deficiency	*NHEJ1*
T−B−NK− SCID	
Adenylate kinase 2 (reticular dysgenesis)	*AK2*
Adenosine deaminase 1 (ADA) deficiency	*ADA1/ADA*

NK, Natural killer; *SCID*, severe combined immunodeficiencies.

CD45RA and CD45RO, respectively, along with CD4 and CD8 to identify the main subsets in blood. However, additional markers such as CCR7 and CD62L are useful in ensuring the naïve T cells identified are truly naïve, and not antigen-experienced T cells that have re-expressed CD45RA (T-cell effector memory cells expressing CD45RA, TEMRA). More recently, a few studies have documented reference intervals for various lymphocyte and T-cell subsets in premature infants, neonates, healthy children, and adults.[23–28] It has also become common to assess recent thymic emigrants by flow cytometry using a combination of CD4, CD45RA, and CD31.[29,30] While immunophenotyping is the mainstay of the early laboratory diagnosis of SCID, functional assessment of T cells is also incorporated into most diagnostic algorithms. The most basic T-cell functional assay is measurement of T-cell proliferation after stimulation of whole blood or peripheral blood mononuclear cells with a polyclonal lectin stimulant, a mitogen such as phytohemagglutinin (PHA), or Pokeweed mitogen (PWM). The readout can utilize more traditional methods, such as radioactive thymidine (3H-t) or flow cytometry.[31] More complex T-cell proliferation assays can be performed depending on the specific clinical context (e.g., antigen-specific proliferation, stimulation with anti-CD3/anti-CD28 or anti-CD/IL-2),[31] the latter of which causes T-cell proliferation in response to CD3 receptor and other costimulatory molecule crosslinking. These assays are more

useful at an advanced diagnostic stage of evaluation rather than as a first-tier diagnostic test.

In addition to these laboratory criteria, the clinical phenotype and family history is very useful in identification of patients with asymptomatic SCID. Patients often have a failure to thrive and serious adverse reactions to live vaccines, such as the Bacillus Calmette Guerin (BCG) and rotavirus.[32]

Specific forms of SCID, which causes loss of enzyme function, such as adenosine deaminase (ADA) or recombinase activating gene (RAG) deficiencies, can also be confirmed by direct measurement of ADA enzyme activity and associated accumulation of toxic metabolites,[33] or measurement of recombinase activity in T cells, respectively,[34] in addition to the aforementioned laboratory tests. Hypomorphic (partial loss-of-function) forms of RAG1 and RAG2 deficiencies are often associated with a combined immunodeficiency along with autoimmunity and inflammatory manifestations, such as granulomatous disease[35,36] and can present at ages beyond infancy, including childhood and early adulthood.

Some forms of SCID are associated with defects in DNA repair and these tend to cluster within the T−B−NK+ grouping. These forms of SCID are frequently referred to as radiosensitive (rs)-SCID, and include genetic defects, such as DNA-PKcs (*PRKDC*), Artemis (*DCLRE1C*), Cernunnos (*NHEJ1*), and DNA Ligase IV (*LIG4*), among others. These radiosensitive forms of SCID along with other forms of syndromic combined immunodeficiency, such as ataxia telangiectasia (AT), can be rapidly diagnosed using a flow cytometry assay that measures the nonhomologous end-joining (NHEJ) pathway of DNA repair after induction of DNA double-strand breaks (DSBs) (Fig. 100.2).[37,38]

Newborn Screening for Severe Combined Immunodeficiencies

The early diagnosis of SCID has been revolutionized with the inclusion of this condition in the recommended uniform screening panel (RUSP) for newborn screening (NBS) in the United States 2010.[39–41] Several other countries also perform NBS for SCID though they may not have a RUSP.[42] SCID met all the criteria required for a public health initiative, such as NBS: (1) a lethal condition, which is asymptomatic in the newborn period, (2) availability of a biomarker, which can be used on dried blood spots (DBS), and (3) a curative treatment. The use of T-cell receptor excision circles (TREC), a by-product of T-cell receptor rearrangement, as a biomarker for T-cell production by the thymus revolutionized large-scale screening for SCID (Fig. 100.3), and though this condition was intended to be the primary target of NBS, it soon became apparent that other conditions associated with T-cell lymphopenia (TCL) could also be identified by NBS for SCID[40,43] as secondary targets. An early family-based study revealed that diagnosis by NBS SCID reduced the mortality associated with SCID,[44] by allowing life-saving interventions, such as hematopoietic cell transplantation (HCT), to be instituted early,[45,46] improving the long-term outcomes. Currently, all 50 states in the United States perform TREC-based NBS SCID, and several other countries or regions within countries have either implemented routine NBS SCID or are performing pilot studies.[42] While TREC-based screening facilitates detection of severe early-onset TCL, there are PIDs with late-onset TCL, which are not identified by NBS and are identified by other tests at ages beyond the neonatal period. The Clinical Laboratory Standards Institute (CLSI) produced a guidelines document on TREC-NBS-SCID (Clinical Laboratory Standards Institute, 2013, Newborn blood spot screening for Severe Combined Immunodeficiency by measurement of T-cell receptor excision circles; Approved Guideline) several years ago, and a current revision is underway, which will be published at the end of 2021.

NBS SCID has enabled assessment of the true population prevalence for SCID, and in an early study in the United States, it was estimated to be 1:58,000; more recently, from data in California, the incidence was estimated at 1:65,000 (95% confidence interval, 1:51,000 to 1:90,000).[43] However, certain ethnic groups have founder mutations for specific genes and thus have a higher incidence of those specific genetic forms of SCID, including the Navajo Nation (Artemis (*DCLRE1C*) SCID), Somali (ADA-SCID), and Amish and Mennonite (*RAG1, RAG2, IL7RA*).

Beyond the well-described genetic defects associated with the more classic SCID conditions, which are treated by HCT, NBS SCID has allowed for diagnosis of newer SCID defects, which are specific for thymic defects, and can only be treated with thymus transplantation (e.g., FOXN1 and PAX1 deficiencies).[47,48] Diagnosis of SCID caused by these defects can enable selection of the appropriate treatment reducing morbidity and mortality.

Measurement of TREC in blood can not only be used for population-based screening but also in the diagnostic laboratory for evaluation of TCL in various contexts and for monitoring recovery of thymic function post-HCT.[49–51] Since TREC is an extra-chromosomal product derived from VDJ gene rearrangement during production of the T-cell receptor, it is diluted by cell division in the periphery. Therefore infants have the highest levels of TREC, which steadily decreases with age, and this is particularly so after puberty and in adults (Fig. 100.4). Besides TREC measurements, diversity of the T-cell repertoire (TCR Vβ) can be analyzed by different methods including flow cytometry,[52] fragment length analysis (spectratyping), and next-generation sequencing. These assays can offer advanced diagnostic assessment of patients, especially with complicated phenotypes who have evidence of TCL or oligoclonal expansion of T cells.

As with any other clinical condition, there are several other immune defects that can present with overlapping phenotypes with SCID, and these may be either other primary immunodeficiencies or even secondary immunodeficiencies, including HIV or loss of T cells due to other conditions, such as chylothorax, gastroschisis, gestational diabetes, or prenatal exposure to maternal immunosuppression among many others. There are many genetic defects associated with CIDs, which can present with failure to thrive and opportunistic infections reminiscent of SCID, and while these cannot be addressed in detail in this chapter, beyond representative examples, they are described elsewhere in the literature.[3,14]

Molecular diagnosis of SCID, as with other PIDs and PIRDs is most frequently performed by next-generation sequencing (NGS) methods, which is discussed elsewhere in this chapter.

The definitive form of treatment for SCID and related conditions is hematopoietic cell transplantation (HCT) aimed at achieving immune reconstitution and correction of the underlying defect.[50,53–56] HCT has been shown to dramatically improve survival and outcomes in SCID patients.[57–59] For certain forms of SCID, such as ADA-SCID and X-linked SCID (*IL2RG*), gene therapy is available, either clinically or under a clinical trial, which has shown effective immune recovery.[60–64] For ADA-SCID, enzyme replacement therapy (ERT) with recombinant enzyme has proven effective at bridging therapies until a more definitive form of treatment is available.[65–67] In addition to these longer-term treatment options, supportive therapies, such as prophylactic antibiotics and replacement immunoglobulin, has proved efficacious in reducing infectious complications prior to transplant. If the patient has viral infections, such as cytomegalovirus (CMV), Epstein-Barr virus (EBV), adenovirus, or Varicella, virus-specific cellular therapies can be administered if antivirals have not proven effective.[68] Many of these supportive therapies are not restricted to SCID, and can be used for any of the PIDs and PIRDs, with significant complications and mortality.

GROUP 2. COMBINED IMMUNODEFICIENCIES WITH SYNDROMIC OR ASSOCIATED FEATURES—DIGEORGE SYNDROME

Angelo DiGeorge first recognized DiGeorge syndrome (DGS; OMIM #188400) in 1965 when he described a series of infants with hypoparathyroidism associated with thymic aplasia. Defective remodeling of the pharyngeal region during

Control

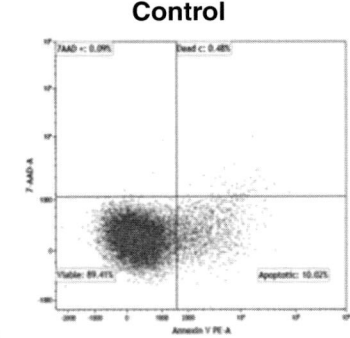

Patient

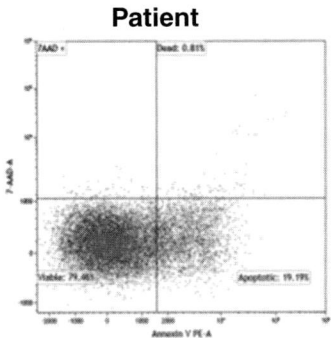

A

FIGURE 100.2 Assessment of cell viability and DNA repair defects by flow cytometry. (A) Cell viability of lymphocytes assessed based on exclusion of apoptotic cells, identified by Annexin V (*X*-axis), and dead cells, assessed by double-staining for 7-AAD (*Y*-axis) and Annexin V (upper right quadrant). Viable cells are present in the lower left quadrant and an example of a healthy control and a patient with ataxia telangiectasia (AT) is depicted. Panel (A) also shows the tabular data for the flow histograms in panel

Continued

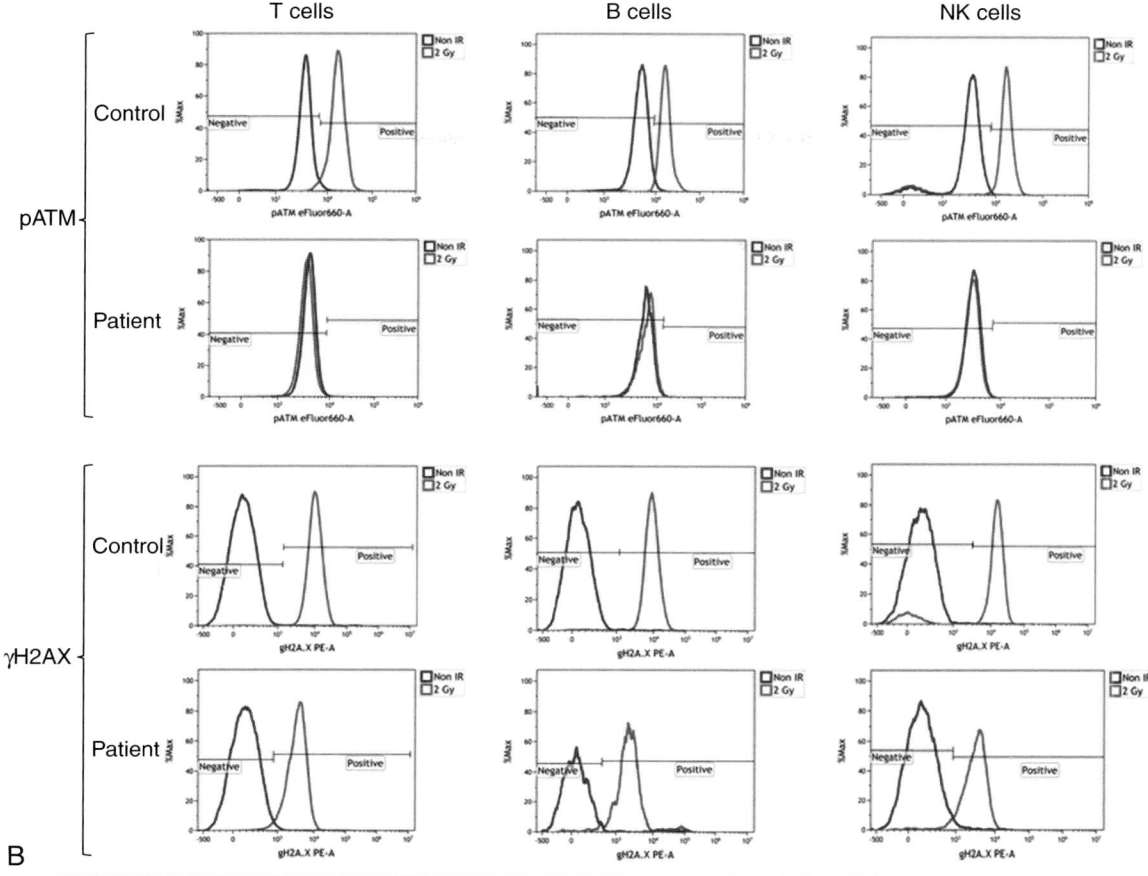

1h postIR	T cells		B cells		NK cells	
	Control	Patient	Control	Patient	Control	Patient
*Delta % pATM+	93.3	0	92.6	0	82.9	0
^Ratio MFI pATM	4.7	0.8	3.2	1.1	4.8	0.9
Delta % γH2AX+	98.1	95.4	96.4	91.4	83.9	90.9
Ratio MFI γH2AX	74	19	111	33.9	74.7	16.8

*Delta % = % 2 Gy irradiated – % nonirradiated (non-IR)
^Ratio median fluorescence intensity (MFI) = MFI 2 Gy IR / MFI non-IR
pATM= phosphorylated ATM
γH2AX = phosphorylated H2AX

FIGURE 100.2, cont'd (B). The nonhomologous end-joining (NHEJ) pathway of DNA repair is assessed in each lymphocyte subset (T, B, and natural killer [NK] cells), either without irradiation or exposure to low-dose irradiation (2 Gy). (B) Flow data for phosphorylated ATM (pATM) and gamma H2AX (γH2AX), key proteins involved in the DNA repair of double-stranded breaks, in a healthy control and patient with AT, at 1 hour postirradiation. The patient does not show any phosphorylation of ATM, and decreased γH2AX (also seen in the table in panel A), consistent with a diagnosis of AT. The table in panel (A) shows that the delta (irradiated value – unirradiated value) % (frequency of each cell subset expressing pATM or γH2AX) is essentially absent for pATM, while it is normal for γH2AX. However, the median fluorescence intensity (MFI) ratio (irradiated/unirradiated) is significantly decreased for γH2AX, due to the inability of ATM to phosphorylate H2AX, a histone involved in DNA repair.

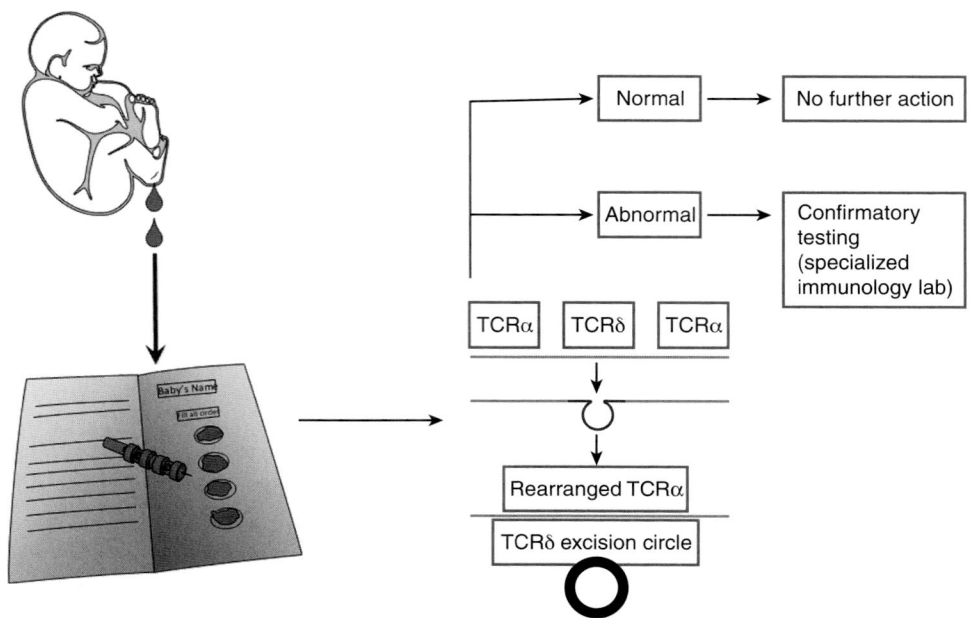

FIGURE 100.3 Newborn screening for severe combined immunodeficiencies (NBS SCID) using T-cell receptor excision circles *(TREC)* as a biomarker for T-cell production by the thymus. Blood is obtained by a heel-prick on a newborn on to a Guthrie card (filter paper), creating a dried blood spot (DBS), which is analyzed by a molecular method for TREC. A normal result is not pursued further, while an abnormal result is sent for additional follow-up diagnostic immunology evaluation. *TCR,* T-cell receptor.

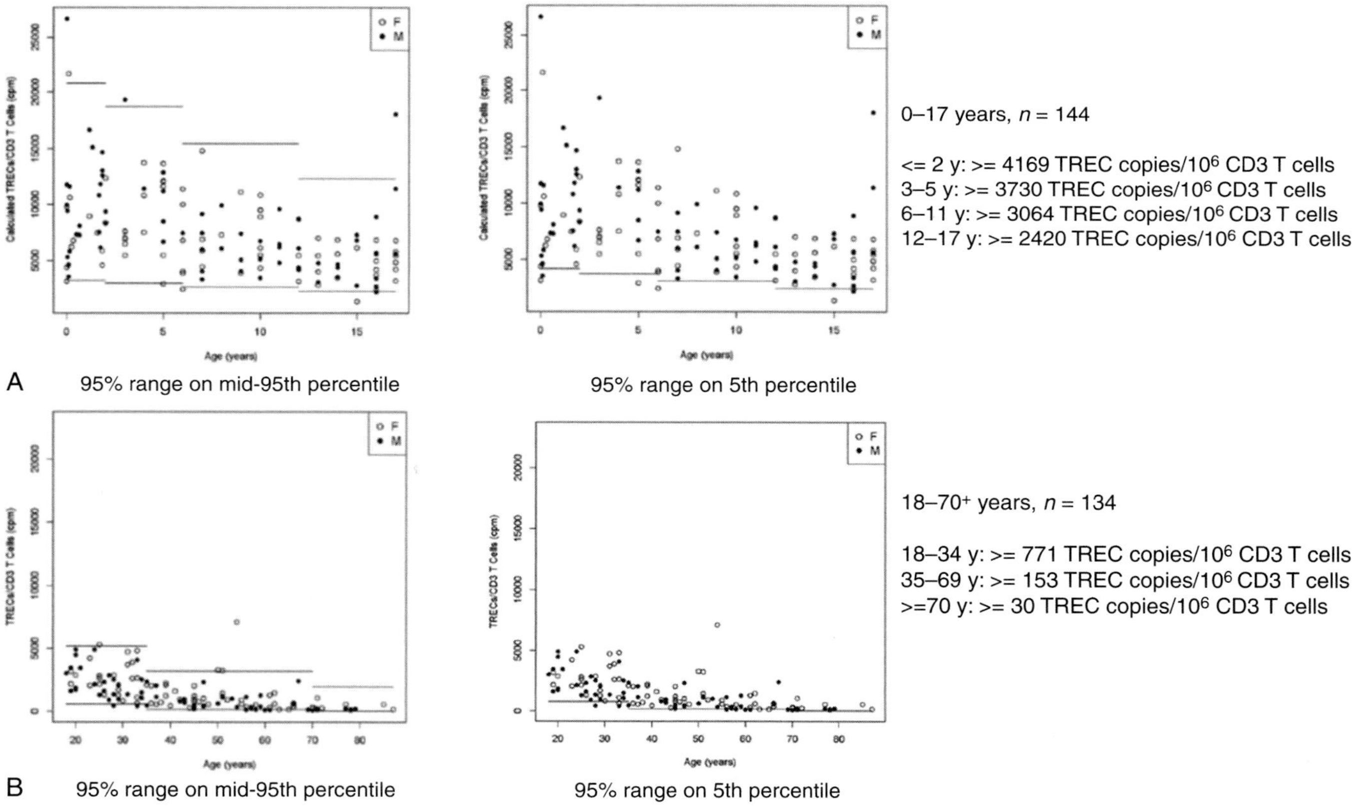

0–17 years, *n* = 144

<= 2 y: >= 4169 TREC copies/10⁶ CD3 T cells
3–5 y: >= 3730 TREC copies/10⁶ CD3 T cells
6–11 y: >= 3064 TREC copies/10⁶ CD3 T cells
12–17 y: >= 2420 TREC copies/10⁶ CD3 T cells

18–70⁺ years, *n* = 134

18–34 y: >= 771 TREC copies/10⁶ CD3 T cells
35–69 y: >= 153 TREC copies/10⁶ CD3 T cells
>=70 y: >= 30 TREC copies/10⁶ CD3 T cells

A   95% range on mid-95th percentile   95% range on 5th percentile

B   95% range on mid-95th percentile   95% range on 5th percentile

FIGURE 100.4 Reference values for T-cell receptor excision circles *(TREC)* in healthy pediatric and adult individuals. (A) Reference intervals obtained at either the 95th percentile or the 5th percentile on 144 healthy children of all ages. The final reference value is collected at the 5th percentile and the TREC copies are reported relative to the CD3+ T-cell counts, as copies per million CD3+ T cells. (B) Similar TREC reference interval data for healthy adults (*n* = 134) of all ages.

embryogenesis causes this syndrome. The classic triad of thymic hypoplasia/aplasia, congenital heart defects, and hypoparathyroidism with associated facial characteristics is recognized in most patients with DGS.[69,70] The majority (90%) of DGS patients have a microdeletion, either 3 or 1.5 Mb, on chromosome 22q11.2 (22q11.2del), which typically results in heterozygosity of 36 and 56 genes with the smaller and larger deletion, respectively.[71] Chromosome 22q11.2 deletion syndrome is the most common microdeletion syndrome reported in humans, reported in 1:4000 live births. This complex multiorgan disorder encompasses previously described overlapping genetic syndromes including velocardiofacial syndrome (VCFS; Shprintzen syndrome), the conotruncal anomaly face syndrome (CTAF; Takao syndrome), autosomal dominant Opitz G/BBB syndrome, Sedlackova syndrome, and Cayler cardiofacial syndrome.

In addition to 22q11.2del, the DiGeorge phenotype may be seen with other chromosomal abnormalities and genetic defects.[72–74] Congenital features overlapping with 22q11.2del/ DiGeorge phenotype are also observed in offspring of mothers with gestational diabetes or diabetic embryopathy, isotretinoin teratogenicity, and fetal alcohol syndromes.[75–77]

Thymic aplasia or hypoplasia results in absence or decreased levels of circulating T cells, especially naïve T cells in infants and children. Approximately 20% of DGS infants may be identified through NBS SCID due to decreased TREC copies. DGS infants with completely absent T cells are classified as complete DiGeorge syndrome (cDGS) and represent approximately 1% of DGS patients. These patients are phenotypically no different from classic forms of SCID and require immediate therapeutic intervention[40] for survival. Atypical forms of cDGS resembling Omenn syndrome have been reported.[78] The other DGS patients who do not have cDGS are classified as having partial DiGeorge syndrome (pDGS).

The clinical phenotype of 22q11.2del/DGS is extremely variable, differing from patient to patient, even within the same family. The congenital malformations frequently involve the heart (conotruncal malformations, tetralogy of Fallot, aortic arch abnormalities, truncus arteriosus, ventricular septal defects, and vascular rings), abnormalities of the palate (clefts and velopharyngeal incompetence), facial dysmorphism, renal and/or skeletal anomalies, hypoparathyroidism with hypocalcemia, and immunodeficiency. Developmental delay, autism and autism spectrum, attention deficit disorders, and psychiatric illnesses may become apparent with time.[79,80]

The clinical phenotype of DGS is extremely diverse.[81] Recurrent upper respiratory tract infections (URI) are a common feature and occur in 35 to 40% of children. These infections do not necessarily correlate with T-cell numbers, and may be related to a combination of factors including anatomic anomalies.[82] Opportunistic infections are rare and usually seen only in the cDGS phenotype. Autoimmunity has an overall frequency of 8 to 10% in DGS, with autoimmune cytopenias being the most common. DGS patients with autoimmune cytopenias have decreased naïve T cells and class-switched memory B cells.[83]

While cytogenetic analysis for the chr.22q11.2del by fluorescence in situ hybridization (FISH) was commonly used, more recently, use of single-nucleotide polymorphisms (SNP) or comparative genomic hybridization (CGH) arrays[84] and NGS for the *TBX1* gene have gained traction,[85] though

single gene haploinsufficiency is unlikely to account for all DGS phenotypes.[71] Other diagnostic immunology laboratory tests include a complete blood count (CBC), flow cytometry for lymphocyte subsets (T, B, and NK cells), and, if TCL is present, evaluation for naïve and memory T cells, and immunoglobulin levels, vaccine antibody responses, especially to inactivated vaccines. More complex immune studies, such as assessment of thymic function, B-cell differentiation subsets, T-cell receptor repertoire diversity, and T-cell proliferation to mitogens and antigens may also be performed but might require the use of a reference diagnostic immunology laboratory. Besides the immunologic studies, cardiac and renal evaluation, measurement of serum calcium and phosphorus, as well as a chest X-ray to assess for the presence of a thymic shadow should be obtained.

The degree of TCL in the majority of pDGS patients is variable, but patients with autoimmunity appear to have overall lower total T cells, CD4+ T cells, and naïve CD4+ T cells,[86] and there is an accelerated loss of naïve T cells and constrained T cell receptor repertoire diversity in older pDGS patients.[86] Defects in switched memory B cells have also been reported in DGS patients.[87] T-cell function, especially proliferation to mitogens and antigens, is also variable, and though most pDGS patients may respond to mitogens, such as PHA, the response to specific antigens, for example *Candida* and Tetanus toxoid, is less likely to be normal.[88]

Treatment of DGS patients requires a multidisciplinary approach to address the varied clinical needs unique to each patient.[89] Inactivated vaccines can be administered to all pDGS patients. However, the use of live vaccines demonstrates a lack of consistency in the immune parameters used to determine competence for these vaccines. Some criteria use a CD4+ T-cell count greater than 400 cells/μL with CD8+ T cells greater than 250 cells/μL and normal proliferation to mitogens; others do not use any T-cell proliferation criteria, and yet others do not perform any immunologic assessment.[90]

Patients with pDGS are typically managed conservatively with antibiotics, when needed, and use of immunoglobulin replacement if there is hypogammaglobulinemia and deficits in class-switched memory B cells. Complete DGS patients, on the other hand, typically require thymus transplantation, which is performed in very few centers, one in North America[91–96] and the United Kingdom.[97,98] While HCT has been attempted in cDGS and anecdotally reported as successful,[99] it is unlikely to serve the purpose for most patients as there is no appropriate environment for maturation of T-cell precursors differentiated from the hematopoietic stem cells. Therefore thymus transplantation would be the treatment of choice for these patients, though newer therapies with thymic organoids[100] may supplant or be used alongside thymus transplantation.

GROUP 2. COMBINED IMMUNODEFICIENCIES WITH SYNDROMIC OR ASSOCIATED FEATURES—WISKOTT-ALDRICH SYNDROME

Wiskott-Aldrich syndrome (WAS; OMIM #301000; gene *WAS*), caused by pathogenic variants in the *WAS* gene on chromosome Xp11.23, is a PID first described in 1937 by

Wiskott, and demonstrated as an inherited X-linked recessive disorder by Aldrich in 1954.[4,6,101] The estimated prevalence is reported between 1:100 to 250,000 live births. The protein encoded by *WAS*, WASp, is primarily expressed in the cytoplasm of hematopoietic cells and belongs to a family of proteins involved in the formation of actin filaments. Absence of WASp affects many immunologic processes including effective immunologic synapse formation, chemotaxis, migration and adhesion, NK cytotoxicity, peripheral regulatory T-cell (Treg) homeostasis, B-cell homeostasis, and Fas-mediated apoptosis.[101–103] A small amount of WASp has been found in the nucleus and a role in the prevention of DNA double strand breaks has been demonstrated in vitro.[104,105]

Clinical manifestations can be variable with all patients having microthrombocytopenia and risk for a bleeding diathesis. Beyond this, the spectrum of disease includes varying degrees of eczema, infections, diarrhea, autoimmunity (particularly autoimmune cytopenias), and cancer predisposition. Those patients with isolated thrombocytopenia with/without mild-to-moderate eczema and infrequent infections are classified as having X-linked thrombocytopenia (XLT), while those with the full spectrum of disease are classified as having "classic" WAS. The overall life expectancy of patients with XLT is reported similar to males in the general population, but many experience high morbidity related to disease-related complications. For "classic" WAS, long-term survival is limited if not treated with HCT, though gene therapy trials show promise.[106–108] The clinical phenotype can be highly variable and is related to the amount of WASp expressed, which in turn is dependent on the specific pathogenic variant.[109–111] *WAS* is a gene that shows several allelic variants, including the loss-of-function (LOF) phenotype associated with XLT, while a gain-of-function (GOF) phenotype is associated with X-linked myelodysplasia and X-linked neutropenia. WAS is also associated with a high degree of somatic reversion mosaicism[112] though this does not appear to influence the clinical phenotype.

WAS is diagnosed in the laboratory by platelet measurement—size and number. Small platelet size is a hallmark of the disease, but this requires laboratory expertise to ensure the measurements are accurate. A complete blood count (CBC) will provide a platelet count along with absolute lymphocyte count among other parameters. Serum IgG in WAS patients can be low or normal, but serum IgA is often increased, and IgA nephropathy can be seen as a complication in these patients. IgE levels are variable but can frequently be elevated, and this pattern of serum immunoglobulins may not always be apparent in the youngest patients. Other immunologic tests include measurement of T-cell and B-cell function, as well as immunophenotyping. These results can be variable, depending on the patient, and cannot be used independently for a diagnosis. Frequently, spontaneous NK-cell cytotoxicity is decreased resulting in increased viral infections in these patients. One of the most useful tests for the definitive diagnosis of WAS, besides gene sequencing, is intracellular flow cytometry in lymphocytes, monocytes, and granulocytes for WASp. Completely absent protein expression would support a more severe clinical phenotype while partially preserved protein expression is likely to reflect a milder clinical phenotype, though this may evolve over time. Carrier females can also be identified by flow cytometry due to the presence of two populations for

WASp, and occasionally somatic revertants can also be identified by this testing method.

The treatment for WAS is not unlike that for SCID with a variety of supportive therapies, including antibiotics and replacement immunoglobulin (and this is particularly essential if the patient has had a splenectomy for the management of autoimmune cytopenias). As with other combined immunodeficiencies on the more severe end of the spectrum, live vaccines should be avoided to prevent risk of vaccine-associated infection. Patients with autoimmune manifestations would require modulation with immunosuppression prior to HCT. For "classic" WAS patients and XLT patients at higher risk for developing malignancies, HCT remains a curative treatment.[106,113–116] Gene therapy trials for WAS show promise in early clinical trials.[117–119]

GROUP 3. ANTIBODY DEFICIENCIES—COMMON VARIABLE IMMUNODEFICIENCY

Common variable immunodeficiency (CVID), first described in 1954,[120,121] encompasses a heterogeneous group of antibody deficiency disorders defined by specific laboratory criteria[122–125] associated with a range of clinical manifestations, which encompass susceptibility to infection, autoimmunity, and lymphoproliferation. The term "CVID" appears a misnomer given the heterogeneity in clinical phenotypes and molecular defects, but nonetheless it persists, and the most recent IUIS classification[3] has redefined it as Common Variable Immunodeficiency Disorders. Not all the clinical phenotypes associated with this group of disorders appear to be monogenic and some may be oligogenic or polygenic.[126]

CVID is the most commonly diagnosed primary immunodeficiency in adults with an estimated prevalence of 1:25,000 to 1:50,000, affecting both genders equally. Most patients are diagnosed between the second and fourth decade of life though clinical manifestations may occur earlier, suggesting a bimodal distribution. Delay in diagnoses ranges between 4 and 7 years among adult patients.[127–129] While most cases of CVID occur sporadically, in 5 to 25% of patients a positive family history is encountered.[130]

The noninfectious clinical manifestations of CVID appear to be associated with the highest mortality.[127–129,131] Approximately 94% of CVID patients present with infections indicating that not all patients present with this manifestation, and in some patients, the presenting feature may be autoimmunity and/or lymphoproliferation.[128,129] As exemplified by humoral immunodeficiencies, sinopulmonary infections are the most common, along with gastrointestinal (GI) infections with norovirus, Giardia, etc. among the most pernicious.[132] Chronic lung disease due to infections and interstitial lung disease with or without noncaseating granulomas is not uncommon, though granulomas may be seen in other organs as well, including the central nervous system.[127,133–136] Other noninfectious complications are recognized in at least one-third of CVID patients, if not more, and include multiple target organs.[127–129] In particular, autoimmune cytopenias and GI complications have been recognized in this entity,[127–129,137] and may present before other clinical and laboratory features of the disease. Another significant complication is nodular regenerative hyperplasia of the liver, occurring in approximately 5% of these patients,[138] as well as lymphoid nodular hyperplasia, in other organs, including the gut. Malignancy in CVID is not rare, and largely tends to be hematopoietic neoplasias or adenocarcinomas of the gut or other organs.[127–129,131,132,139,140]

The laboratory diagnosis of CVID mandates primary hypogammaglobulinemia involving IgG and at least one or more of the other isotypes, along with abnormalities in functional antibody responses to vaccines (e.g., protein vaccines—Tetanus and Diphtheria toxoid, pneumococcal polysaccharide, Salmonella polysaccharide), B-cell differentiation (low switched memory B cells and other B-cell subset defects).[122–125,141,142] Most patients with CVID have normal numbers of circulating B cells, and 1% of patients may have decreased to absent B cells. This is relevant because some patients with X-linked agammaglobulinemia may be diagnosed in adulthood and incorrectly classified as "CVID."

Though not all diagnostic criteria recommend detailed B-cell subset immunophenotyping by flow cytometry, practical value in the evaluation of patients has been well established and is widely used.[142–146] The term "primary" hypogammaglobulinemia implies that other causes of hypogammaglobulinemia have been eliminated including infections, drugs, malignancies, and secondary losses due to lymphatic alterations. The challenges in interpretation of vaccine antibody responses in primary immunodeficiencies is a topic in itself, though several guidelines exist.[147,148]

Some patients diagnosed with CVID also appear to have defects in T cells—number and function. This has been referred to as late-onset combined immunodeficiency (LOCID)[149] and these patients may require different management strategies, therefore patients with a CVID diagnosis who have defects in total T cells or naïve T cells should be assessed more carefully for an underlying combined immunodeficiency.

While the current diagnostic criteria for CVID do not mandate genetic testing, it is part of accepted clinical practice to perform genetic testing by next-generation sequencing (NGS) methodologies,[150,151] as identifying the specific molecular defect has impact on prognosis and therapeutic management of disease. Even if only a small proportion of CVID patients (approximately 30%)[152,153] have monogenic defects identified by NGS, the value of knowing the specific molecular etiology has an immeasurable impact on clinical practice, patient care, and genetic counseling.

There are currently 14 different genetic defects with CVID phenotypes annotated in OMIM (Online Mendelian Inheritance in Man) (Table 100.2). The genetic defects in CVID may be inherited as autosomal dominant or autosomal recessive conditions, causing either LOF) GOF, or haploinsufficiency. There are other humoral immunodeficiencies with distinct clinical phenotypes, such as X-linked lymphoproliferative disease I (XLP1) caused by pathogenic variants in the *SH2D1A* gene, which may be mistakenly diagnosed as CVID, and therefore rare X-linked recessive conditions can also be included in the differential diagnosis of CVID. Other gene defects associated with antibody deficiencies described in the literature include *TNFSF12* (TWEAK deficiency), *IL21R* (IL-21 receptor deficiency), *PLCG2, PTEN, TRNT1, RAC2, VAV1, ATP6AP1* (X-linked), *ARHGEF1, SH3KBP1* (CIN85; X-linked), *SEC61A1, ITPKB* (haploinsufficiency due to microdeletion of chromosome 1q42.1–q42.3), and mannosyl-oligosaccharide glucosidase deficiency.[3,154]

TABLE 100.2 Common Variable Immunodeficiency Gene Defects Based on OMIM Classification

Gene Defect	OMIM Nomenclature	OMIM Number
ICOS	CVID1	604558
TNFRSF13B (TACI)	CVID2	604907/240500
CD19	CVID3	613493
TNFRSF13C (BAFF-R)	CVID4	613494
MS4A1 (CD20)	CVID5	613495
CD81	CVID6	613496
CR2 (CD21)	CVID7	614699
LRBA	CVID8	614700
PRKCD	CVID9	615559
NFKB2	CVID10	615577
IL21	CVID11	615767
NFKB1	CVID12	616576
IKZF1 (IKAROS)	CVID13	616873
IRF2BP2	CVID14	617765

CVID, Common variable immunodeficiency.

Several of the above noted gene defects have unique phenotypes, which has resulted in their reclassification from "classic CVID" diagnosis to distinct inborn errors of immunity classified by gene name. For example, patients with defects in *ICOS,* or dominant negative pathogenic variants in Ikaros (*IKZF1),* or *IL21/IL21R* gene defects, are now categorized among the combined immunodeficiency disorders. In addition, pathogenic variants within the same gene may cause either LOF or GOF consequences, further segregating them out as different diseases. For example, autosomal recessive deficiency of *PIK3CD* and *PIK3R1* causes a profound decrease or absence of B cells with agammaglobulinemia, while GOF mutations in *PIK3CD* causes an activation of p110δ and the resultant activated p110Delta syndrome (APDS1). An autosomal dominant defect in *PIK3R1* causes APDS2 (SHORT syndrome), and both these conditions are categorized under the CVID umbrella, in the genetics lexicon, while in immunology they are recognized and classified as distinct entities.[155–158] Other genetic defects grouped under "CVID" but with distinct immunologic and clinical phenotypes have also been re-classified based on the gene defect and its impact on immune function (e.g., LRBA, CTLA4 associated with LATAIE and CHAI disorders,[159–161] which affect Treg function) or CVID-like diseases associated with EBV driven lymphoproliferation (autosomal recessive defects in *TNFRSF7* causing CD27 deficiency).[162–164]

Treatment of CVID consists of passive replacement of immunoglobulin every 3 to 4 weeks by intravenous (IVIg) or subcutaneous (subcu Ig, SCIg) routes, antimicrobial therapy, and management of noninfectious manifestations with immunomodulatory therapies. A meta-analysis showed that a trough level of 1000 mg/dL of Ig replacement was effective in reducing pulmonary complications and demonstrated a significant inverse correlation between annual infection rate and serum IgG concentration.[165] Usually, higher doses result in higher IgG trough levels and are given to patients with end-organ damage including those with chronic lung disease, bronchiectasis, and enteropathy.[166] Hematopoietic cell transplantation (HCT) is typically not used for the management of "unspecified CVID" and is only considered in context of severe disease.[167] However, targeted therapies, such as abatacept for LRBA deficiency[11] or leniolisib for APDS1,[168] based on a molecular diagnosis has shown success along with other supportive therapies.

X-linked Agammaglobulinemia

X-linked agammaglobulinemia (XLA; OMIM #300755; gene *BTK*) is a rare humoral immunodeficiency affecting 1:100-379,000 live births and caused by pathogenic variants in the Bruton's tyrosine kinase gene (*BTK*).[169–171] The protein encoded by this gene, also called Btk, is essential for B-cell development and maturation. Consequently, patients with XLA lack or may have very few B cells in peripheral blood, have absent or hypoplastic secondary lymphoid organs, such as tonsils and adenoids, lymph nodes have a distorted architecture, plasma cells are not generated, serum concentrations of immunoglobulins are low or absent, and adaptive immunity is impaired. At least half of XLA patients are identified in the first year of life when maternal immunoglobulin starts to wane, and approximately 85% are identified in the first five years of life. Some patients with hypomorphic variants in *BTK* may have a progressive loss of B cells and hypogammaglobulinemia and may be started on treatment with replacement immunoglobulin without a diagnosis, or may be classified as CVID if a young adult. These patients have sinopulmonary infections, gastrointestinal infections, meningitis, and encephalitis, which could be either bacterial or viral in origin.[172–174] Noninfectious complications include inflammatory bowel disease, neutropenia, and arthritis, sometimes with rare pathogens, such as *Ureaplasma urealyticum*. Long-term outcome data suggest that despite IgG replacement therapy, patients with XLA continue to have sinopulmonary infections resulting in chronic lung disease, an important contributor to mortality.[175] From a large series of 783 XLA patients from 40 centers in 32 countries, it was shown that complications including enteroviral meningoencephalitis, inflammatory bowel disease, and arthritis contribute to morbidity.[176] While individually these complications may be uncommon, collectively these problems are seen in 20% of patients with XLA. Survival beyond 20 years depends on geographic location (lowest survival seen in Asia and Africa), with 62% of centers that followed adult patients reporting greater than 75% survival beyond 20 years of age.[176]

The laboratory diagnosis includes a complete blood count (CBC), serum immunoglobulins (IgG, IgA, and IgM), and flow cytometry for lymphocyte subsets (T, B, and NK cells). If B cells are absent or significantly decreased and serum immunoglobulins are low, intracellular flow cytometry for the Btk protein is performed in monocytes, as Btk is typically expressed in B cells, monocytes, and platelets. Since B cells are absent or very low in XLA, an alternative cell subset like monocytes is used for the specific protein analysis (Fig. 100.5). Depending on the detection antibody used in the flow cytometry assay, and the location of the variant in the *BTK* gene, protein may be present, decreased, or absent. Presence of protein does not negate a diagnosis of XLA, and in such cases, genetic testing of the *BTK* gene is required to confirm a diagnosis (Fig. 100.6). T-cell numbers and function are intact in patients with XLA.

Treatment of XLA consists of effective antimicrobial therapy for management of infections and therapeutic use of pooled human IgG immunoglobulin preparations (replacement immunoglobulin), similar to the treatment of CVID. Prophylactic antibiotics for those patients with chronic lung disease was found to be beneficial in a recent double blind, placebo-controlled, randomized trial of low-dose azithromycin prophylaxis.[177] Live vaccines should not be administered to XLA patients, particularly oral polio vaccine.[32] Given the selective advantage of functional Btk for normal B-lymphocyte lineage commitment, HCT can provide a cure.[178–180] Despite advancement in transplant practices, HCT is rarely offered to patients, especially in western countries, when medical management is readily available because the transplant-related morbidities, which include conditioning chemotherapy, graft versus host disease (GVHD), and infections while awaiting engraftment, may outweigh the potential benefit.[181]

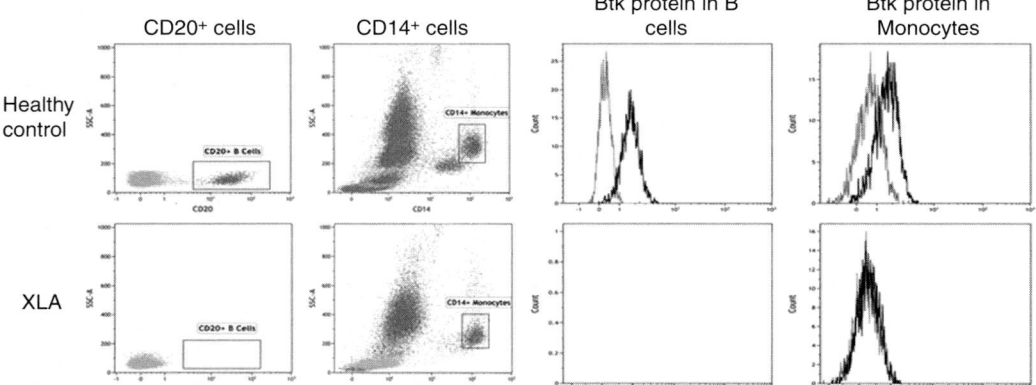

FIGURE 100.5 Flow cytometric analysis of Bruton's tyrosine kinase (Btk) protein. X-linked agammaglobulinemia *(XLA)* is caused by pathogenic variants in the *BTK* gene, encoding the Btk protein. Btk is an intracellular protein expressed in B cells, monocytes, and platelets. The flow histograms show data for a healthy control and a XLA patient. XLA patients do not have B cells (CD20+); therefore Btk protein is assessed in CD14+ monocytes. The patient has complete absence of Btk protein in monocytes as the antibody-specific histogram *(black)* overlaps with the isotype control *(gray)*, while there is separation of the two peaks in the healthy control, indicative of normal Btk protein expression.

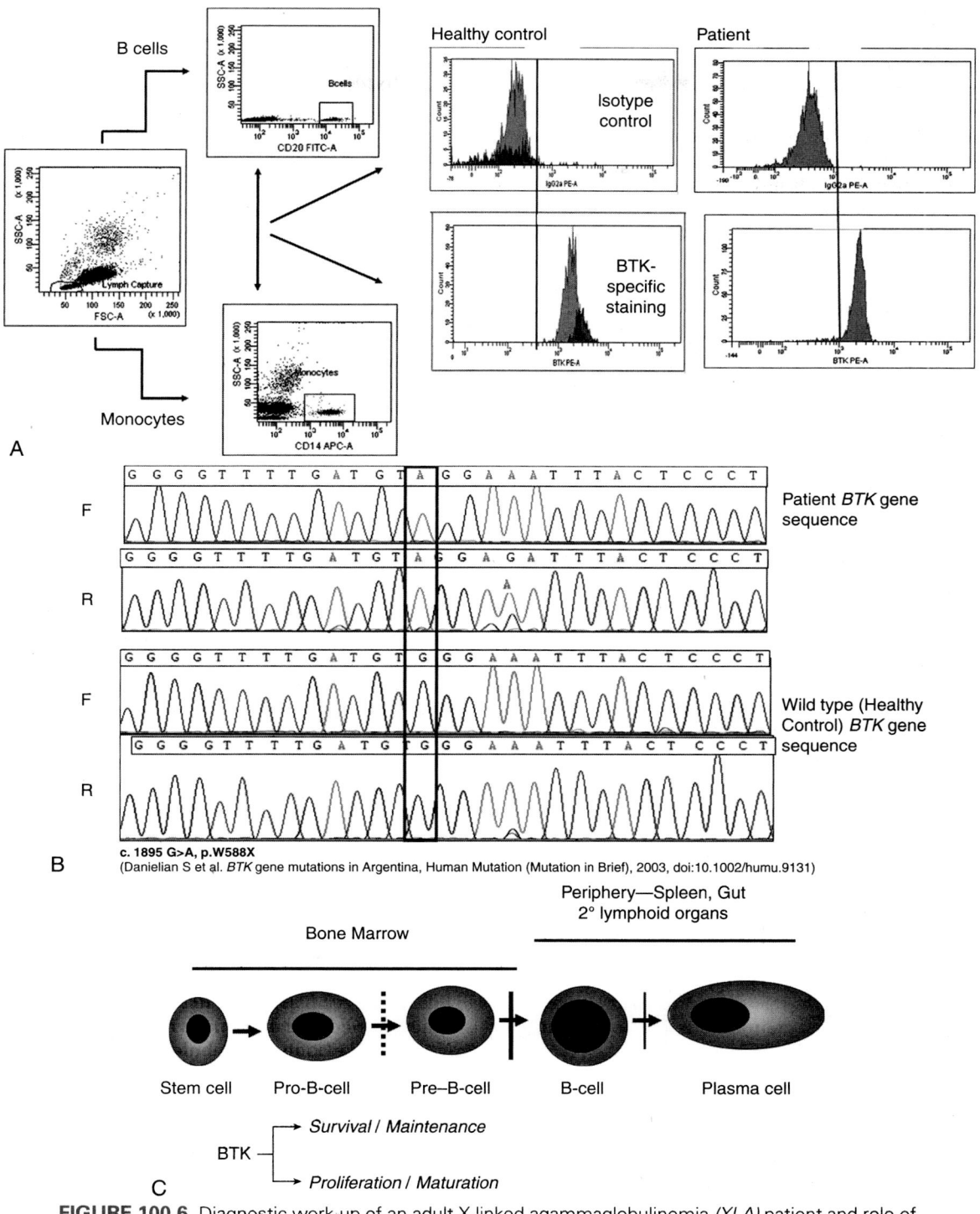

FIGURE 100.6 Diagnostic work-up of an adult X-linked agammaglobulinemia *(XLA)* patient and role of Btk protein in B-cell development and maturation. (A) Btk flow cytometry in B cells (only healthy control) and monocytes (both healthy control and patient) demonstrating that the patient has normal Btk protein expression. (B) The patient has a nonsense pathogenic variant in the *BTK* gene affecting the kinase domain of the protein. This result demonstrates that presence of protein does not preclude a diagnosis of an immunodeficiency, as depending on where in the gene the pathogenic variant is located, it may permit expression but affect function. Therefore genetic testing is required to confirm the diagnosis for this 51-year-old patient. Genetic confirmation is important to provide the right diagnosis and appropriate genetic counseling as the female offspring of a male patient with this X-linked recessive disorder will be obligate carriers of the variant. Each of their male offspring has a 50% chance of getting the disease, and each of the female offspring have a 50% chance of being a carrier for the disorder. (C) The role of Btk protein in B-cell development in the bone marrow, and blocks B-cell maturation beyond the pre–B-cell stage. Therefore patients with XLA have few to no B cells in blood. Btk is also important for survival of B cells in the periphery.

For the last two decades, knowledge of gene therapy strategies and genome editing methodologies has advanced such that *ex vivo* cellular engineering, utilizing viral vectors to treat monogenic disorders of immunity, and clinical trials are underway.[63,182–185] XLA is a unique disorder for gene correction because circulating levels of immunoglobulins have no effect on B-cell development or peripheral B-cell maturation, and human bone marrow provides an environment which permits B-cell reconstitution, independent of age. Preclinical work has demonstrated the rescue of Btk-dependent B-cell development, albeit incomplete, in the double knock-out mouse model for Btk- and Tec (Btk/Tec−/−) that phenocopies human XLA.[186,187] This provides proof-of-concept and a first step toward the development of gene-corrected autologous transplantation for XLA as an alternative therapeutic approach to conventional management and HCT.

GROUP 4. DISEASES OF IMMUNE DYSREGULATION—AUTOIMMUNE LYMPHOPROLIFERATIVE SYNDROME

Autoimmune lymphoproliferative syndrome (ALPS) (also known as Canale-Smith syndrome) encompasses a group of rare genetic disorders caused by defects in the extrinsic apoptotic pathway (FAS-mediated), resulting in dysregulated lymphocyte homeostasis.[188–191] The key characteristics include chronic nonmalignant, noninfectious proliferation with lymphadenopathy, hepatosplenomegaly, polyclonal hypergammaglobulinemia, and autoimmune cytopenias along with elevation of T cells lacking CD4 and CD8, "double-negative T cells" (DNT) (>1.5% of total lymphocytes or >2.5% of CD3+ lymphocytes).[189,192] Flow cytometry for DNT cells expressing the alpha-beta T-cell receptor (TCRαβ+) is one of the diagnostic laboratory tests (Fig. 100.7) and is used in conjunction with other immunophenotyping assays[193] along with evaluation of the B220 marker, which is aberrantly expressed on the above-described DNT cells.[194–196] Measurement of other biomarkers, including soluble Fas ligand (sFasL), vitamin B12, and IL-10 are useful in establishing the diagnosis of ALPS in patients who meet the Revised NIH diagnostic criteria.[189,197] Genetic testing is useful in confirming the diagnosis, and while most cases of ALPS are associated with germline variants, somatic variants in DNT cells can also cause a form of ALPS, which requires sorting of these specific cells and subsequent genetic analysis.[198] Assessment of apoptosis defects in vitro can also provide confirmation of a Fas-pathway defect. However, if patients have been previously treated, especially with steroids, the assay is nondiagnostic. A list of ALPS genetic defects and ALPS-like disorders is provided in Tables 100.3 and 100.4, respectively. Patients with an overlapping phenotype of ALPS and CVID have also been described[199] but these patients usually have hypogammaglobulinemia and not elevated levels of immunoglobulins.

The treatment of ALPS primarily focuses on reduction of lymphoproliferation and associated complications, as well as control of the autoimmune cytopenias. Steroids and sirolimus are frequently used for management with success.[192,200,201] HCT, though curative, is restricted to patients who are refractory to immunosuppression.[192] Patients with ALPS-like diseases are

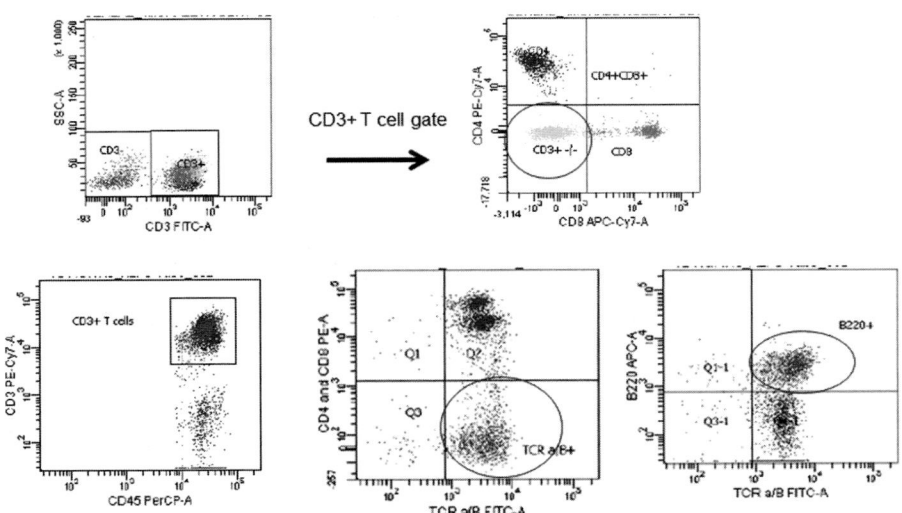

Total CD3 T cell count = 2198 cells/uL (ref range: 1000–2200 cells/uL)
Total CD3 T cell% of lymphs: 83% (ref range: 56–84%)
TCRαβ+ DNT cells; 36.1% of CD3 T cells; absolute count = 753 cells/uL
B220+ DNT cells; 3.3% of TCRαβ + DNT cells; absolute count = 69 cells/uL

Reference value for pediatric age for TCRαβ + DNT cells (2–18 y: <2% CD3 T cells; absolute count = <35 cells/uL)
B220 + DNT cells: <0.4% CD3 T cells; absolute count = <7 cells/uL

FIGURE 100.7 Flow cytometric evaluation of autoimmune lymphoproliferative syndrome (ALPS). One of the diagnostic criteria for ALPS includes expansion of a subset of CD3+ T cells that lack CD4 and CD8 receptors but express the T-cell receptor *(TCR)* (αβ+). The *upper right panel* demonstrates the presence of increased double-negative (CD3+CD4−CD8−) T cells *(DNTs)*. The *lower panels (middle and right)* demonstrate expansion of DNTs that express the TCRab. These cells also aberrantly express a CD45 isoform identified by the antibody, B220. This result is supportive of a diagnosis of ALPS, which, in the context of the clinical history and genetic analysis showing a heterozygous *FAS* gene variant, confirms the diagnosis.

TABLE 100.3 Autoimmune Lymphoproliferative Syndrome Diseases

Disease Name (Gene)	Inheritance	Clinical Features	Laboratory Parameters	Spectrum of Genetic Findings
ALPS-FAS (TNFRSF6)	AD/AR	Chronic nonmalignant lymphoproliferation with lymphocytosis, waxing and waning lymphadenopathy, splenomegaly, and hepatomegaly Late-onset autoimmunity- Coomb's positive hemolytic anemia, immune-mediated (AIHA) thrombocytopenia (ITP), glomerulonephritis and other autoimmune diseases Increased risk for Hodgkin and Non-Hodgkin lymphoma	Elevated DNTs (CD3+CD4−CD8− TCRαβ+) Defective apoptosis assay Elevated biomarkers: FASL, IL-10, IL-18, Vitamin B12 levels **Additional findings:** Coomb's positive hemolytic anemia Elevated IgG, IgA, and IgE Autoantibodies: ANA, RF, anti-neutrophil, anti-platelet, APLA Eosinophilia Lymph node biopsy-reactive lymphoid hyperplasia Expansion of γδ T cells, CD57+ senescent T cells	65–70% ALPS patients Pathogenic Variant spectrum: more than 70% variants affecting intracellular portion of FAS, usually in the death domain, 20% in extracellular domain and , 6–7% in transmembrane region (11) Most variants are heterozygous although homozygous variants have also been described **Somatic FAS** 15–20% ALPS patients Variants are identified in sorted DNT (TCR αβ+) cells
ALPS-FASLG (TNFSF6)	AD/AR	The clinical features are similar to ALPS-FAS	Elevated DNTs Low plasma sFasL levels Normal in vitro Fas-mediated apoptosis	<1% of ALPS patients Homozygous and heterozygous variants have been described
FADD deficiency (FADD)	AR	Recurrent bacterial and viral infections, encephalopathy, hepatic dysfunction, cardiovascular malformations, functional hyposplenism	Elevated DNTs Elevated plasma IL-10, sFasL levels	Rarely described
ALPS-CASPASE10 (CASP10)	AD	Cytopenias, autoimmunity, lymphoproliferation	Elevated DNTs may or may not be present Normal in vitro Fas-mediated apoptosis assay Elevated plasma IL-18 levels	3–6% of ALPS patients with heterozygous variants
ALPS-CASPASE8 (CEDS) (CASP8)	AR	Recurrent bacterial and viral infections, lymphadenopathy, splenomegaly	Marginally elevated DNT cells	Rarely described

AD, Autosomal dominant; ALPS, autoimmune lymphoproliferative syndrome; AR, autosomal recessive; DNT, double-negative T cells; Ig, immunoglobulin; IL, interleukin; TCR, T-cell receptor.

often treated with various immunomodulatory agents, depending on the underlying molecular defect, and aimed at reducing the morbidity associated with the various clinical features. ALPS patients require life-long surveillance due to the increased risk of developing lymphomas.

GROUP 5. PHAGOCYTIC DEFECTS—CHRONIC GRANULOMATOUS DISEASE

Chronic granulomatous disease (CGD) is a primary immunodeficiency largely affecting the innate immune system and caused by LOF variants in any of the five genes encoding the subunits of the phagocytic activity enzyme nicotinamide adenine dinucleotide phosphate (NADPH) oxidase, present mainly in phagocytes. The five subunits of the NADPH oxidase complex include the two membrane-bound proteins,

gp91phox (CYBB gene; X-linked) and p22phox (CYBA gene; autosomal recessive (AR)), and the three cytosolic components, p47phox (NCF1 gene; AR), p67phox (NCF2 gene; AR), and p40phox (NCF4 gene; AR) (Fig. 100.8). Very recently, a new gene defect associated with CGD has been described due to pathogenic variants in the CYBC1 gene encoding the EROS protein.[202,203] When phagocytes are stimulated, activated enzyme oxidase transfers electrons from the NADPH substrate to molecular oxygen resulting in the formation of reactive oxygen species (ROS), including superoxide (SO_2^-). NADPH oxidase deficiency results in defective production of ROS resulting in impaired microbial killing and excessive inflammation. CGD is characterized by severe recurrent bacterial and fungal infections and may be associated with hyperinflammatory complications, including inflammatory bowel disease.

TABLE 100.4   ALPS-like Diseases

Disease Name	Clinical Features	Laboratory Parameters	Gene Defect
RAS-associated autoimmune leukoproliferative disorder (RALD)	Splenomegaly, generalized lymphadenopathy, autoimmune manifestations like AIHA, ITP, and neutropenia (AIN)	Elevated granulocytes and monocytes Mild or no elevation of DNTs Expansion of B cells Autoantibodies: ANA, anti- phospholipid, anti-cardiolipin present In vitro Fas-induced apoptosis normal sFasL and vitamin B12 levels are normal Increase ERK phosphorylation (4)	Somatic GOF variants in *NRAS* and *KRAS*
Dianzani autoimmune lymphoproliferative disease (DALD)	Mimics ALPS clinically	DNTs not elevated Elevated serum OPN levels and IL-17 levels (15,16)	No molecular cause identified
Protein kinase C delta (PRKCD) deficiency	Lymphadenopathy, splenomegaly, Autoimmunity, recurrent infections, chronic EBV infection NK cell dysfunction	DNTs not elevated IL-10 overexpressed by B cells	Autosomal recessive variants in *PRKCD*
CTLA-4 haploinsufficiency with autoimmune infiltration (CHAI)	Lymphadenopathy, splenomegaly, organ-specific autoimmunity, autoimmune cytopenias	Hypogammaglobulinemia Normal in vitro apoptosis Elevated IL-18 levels Borderline elevated DNTs (17)	Heterozygous loss of function (LOF) variants in *CTLA4*
LRBA deficiency with autoantibodies, regulatory T-cell defects, autoimmune infiltration, and enteropathy (LATAIE)	Early-onset inflammatory bowel disease (IBD), lymphoproliferation, autoimmunity, interstitial lung disease	Low circulating B cells Hypogammaglobulinemia in most patients Defective autophagy	Heterozygous LOF variants in *LRBA*
A20 haploinsufficiency	Fever, hepatosplenomegaly, lymphadenopathy, skin rash with infiltration of T cells, Hepatitis with liver dysfunction	Thrombocytopenia polyclonal hypergammaglobulinemia Multiple autoantibodies (dsDNA, ssDNA) Increased IL-10, sFasL, IL-18	Heterozygous LOF variants in *TNFAIP3*
PASLI (p110δ-activating variant causing senescent T cells, lymphadenopathy and immunodeficiency) or APDS (Activated PI3Kδ syndrome)	Recurrent respiratory infections, bronchiectasis, sinus and ear damage, persistent infections with herpes viruses, lymphadenopathy, hepatosplenomegaly, increased risk of B cell lymphoma	Hypogammaglobulinemia with increased IgM levels decreased switched memory B cells increased transitional B cells impaired vaccine antibody responses reduced cytokine production and increased apoptosis on TCR-mediated restimulation increased effector memory T cells, senescent (CD57+) and exhausted T cells short telomeres	Heterozygous GOF variants in *PIK3CD* (p110δ) or *PIK3R1* (p85α) Homozygous LOF variants in these genes causes a completely different and rarer phenotype
STAT3-GOF	Recurrent infections, multi-organ autoimmunity, lymphoproliferation, autoimmune cytopenias, growth retardation	Hypogammaglobulinemia with increased IgM levels (some patients) increased DNT (some patients) decreased regulatory T cells (Tregs) increased naïve B cells expanded CD21dim B cells increased activated T cells elevated sFasL resistant to in vitro apoptosis	Heterozygous germline GOF variants in *STAT3* (somatic GOF variants have been reported in large granular leukemia (LGL) and hepatocellular adenoma

DNT, Double-negative T cells; *GOF,* Gain-of-function; *LOF,* loss-of-function; *OPN,* osteopontin.

The incidence of CGD varies based on population and the incidence in the West is approximately 1:200,000.[204,205] Infections in CGD patients are most frequently caused by catalase-positive microbes such as *Staphylococcus aureus*, *Burkholderia cepacia*, *Klebsiella*, *Serratia marcescens*, *Salmonella*, *Aspergillus*, and *Candida* species, though infections with catalase-negative organisms may also be seen.[206,207]

The laboratory diagnosis of CGD involves measurement of NADPH oxidase activity using the nonfluorescent dye, dihydrorhodamine (DHR) 123, which on stimulation of

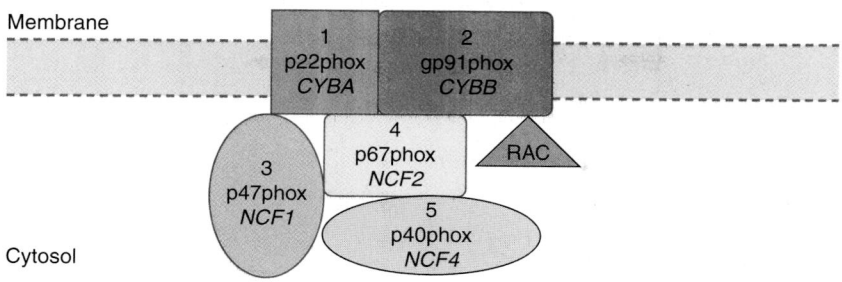

FIGURE 100.8 Schematic of the components of the nicotinamide adenine dinucleotide phosphate (NADPH) oxidase complex. The NADPH oxidase complex plays a key role in host defense in granulocytes. It is composed of five key subunits, two of which are on the membrane, and three in the cytosol. Pathogenic variants in any of the genes encoding these proteins can result in a diagnosis of chronic granulomatous disease (CGD).

neutrophils is oxidized to rhodamine 123, which is fluorescent and can be detected by flow cytometry. The Nitroblue tetrazolium (NBT) test[208] was widely used in the past but has largely been replaced by the flow cytometry-based DHR test, which is more sensitive and reliable and less subjective.[209] A variety of stimulants can be used to activate neutrophils; however, phorbol myristate acetate (PMA) is the most common in the clinical laboratory. Rac2 deficiency, which can partially overlap in phenotype with CGD,[210,211] shows a normal result in the DHR assay when stimulated with PMA but provides an abnormal result when stimulated with a synthetic bacterial peptide, N-formylmethionyl-leucyl-phenylalanine (fMLP). Rac2 deficiency has a mixed phenotype[212] and can overlap with CVID, but also has been identified by NBS SCID with TCL.[213,214] In the DHR test (Fig. 100.9), comparison is made to an unstimulated sample, and the median fluorescence intensity (MFI) data[215] is gathered for both the stimulated and unstimulated samples. The stimulation index (ratio of stimulated MFI to unstimulated MFI) is the most reliable measure of NADPH oxidase activity and can be used for serial measurement, both for diagnosis of disease and monitoring post-treatment. While the flow cytometry pattern can offer some correlation with the genotype, it is not always completely reliable, and therefore has to be confirmed independently, either by flow cytometric assessment of NADPH oxidase specific proteins[216] in neutrophils and monocytes, which can be useful in identification of atypical forms of CGD,[216] or genetic testing. Additionally, NADPH oxidase specific proteins can also be detected in B cells, while T cells can be used as a negative control. Confirmation of *NCF1* defects (p47phox deficiency) by genetic analysis is challenging due to the presence of two pseudogenes.[217–220] Therefore the p47phox flow assay is very useful for a rapid confirmation.[216] The phenotype of p40phox is somewhat different from the other CGD defects,[221,222] and has a different pattern by flow cytometry.[221] Complete myeloperoxidase deficiency (cMPO) can cause a false-positive (abnormal) result on the DHR flow assay, and therefore this has to be excluded before confirming a diagnosis of CGD, though this can often be triggered by a specific pattern on the DHR flow assay (see Fig. 100.9).[223] The DHR flow assay can also be used for identification of carrier females for X-linked CGD. Carrier females for *CYBB* variants (X-linked CGD) show skewed lyonization, and can develop clinical symptoms, especially with age (see Fig. 100.9).[224,225] The DHR flow assay can also be used

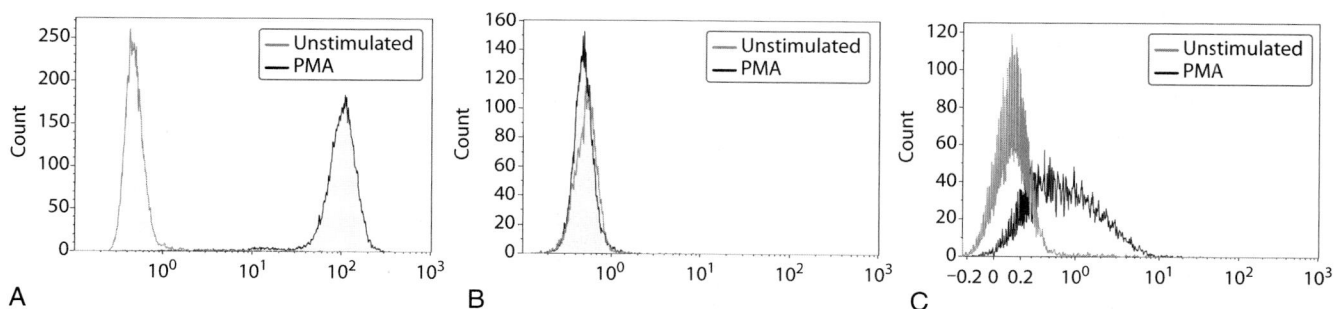

FIGURE 100.9 Examples of dihydrorhodamine (DHR) flow cytometry for the diagnosis of chronic granulomatous disease (CGD). Neutrophils when stimulated activate the nicotinamide adenine dinucleotide phosphate (NADPH) oxidase pathway, which can be measured by oxidation of the nonfluorescent dihydrorhodamine 123 to fluorescent rhodamine 123. (A) DHR flow data from a healthy control with the *green histogram* representing the baseline (unstimulated) NADPH oxidase activity, and the *red histogram* representing the activated NADPH oxidase, after phorbol myristate acetate *(PMA)* stimulation of neutrophils. (B) DHR flow data from a patient with classic X-linked CGD, where there is no NADPH oxidase activity and there is overlap of unstimulated and stimulated peaks. (C) and (D) The DHR flow data from patients with autosomal recessive CGD, due to NCF1 (C) and NCF2

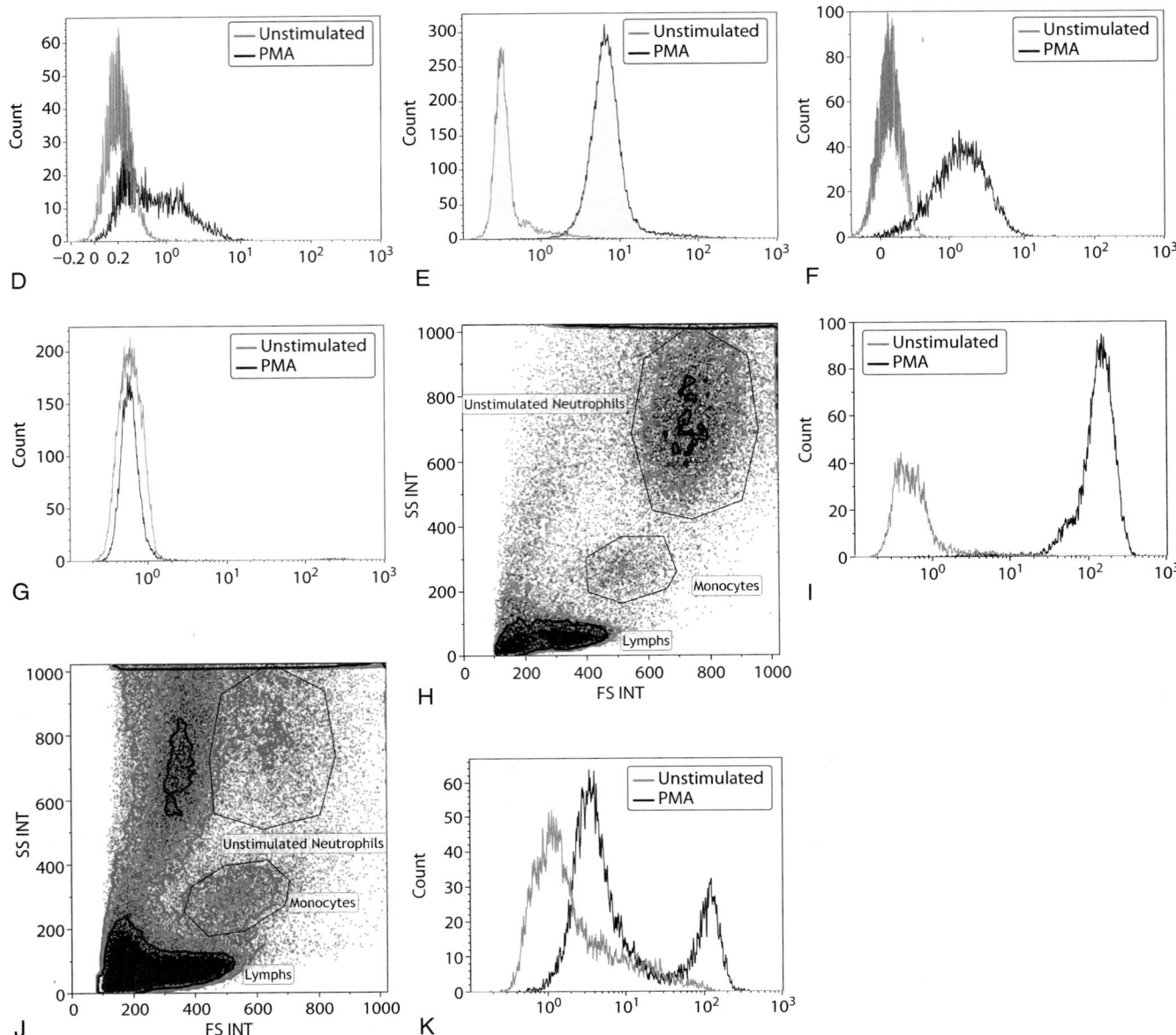

FIGURE 100.9, cont'd (D) pathogenic variants, respectively. (E) The DHR flow data from a patient with complete myeloperoxidase (cMPO) deficiency, which can provide a false-positive result for CGD on the DHR assay. (F) The DHR data from a boy with partial loss-of-function (hypomorphic) variants in the *CYBB* gene, encoding the gp91phox protein. (G) Completely skewed lyonization in a female carrier for X-linked CGD who presented with a *Burkholderia* pneumonia and a family history of CGD. (H)–(K) Importance of sample quality on the DHR flow result with panels (H) and (I) showing a good quality sample with normal DHR flow. (J) An aged sample from a healthy control with very few viable neutrophils and high background fluorescence in the unstimulated sample, and two populations of neutrophils with different fluorescent intensities suggestive of differing NADPH oxidase activity. Such poor-quality samples can affect the interpretation of patient results in this assay. *FS INT*, Forward scatter intensity; *SS INT*, side scatter intensity. (Reproduced from Abraham RS, Aubert G. Flow cytometry, a versatile tool for diagnosis and monitoring of primary immunodeficiencies. *Clin Vaccine Immunol* 2016;23:254–71.)

to monitor disease-specific chimerism post-hematopoietic cell transplant, and is useful for monitoring and prognosis.[215] The DHR assay is particularly sensitive to sample quality, and poor transport conditions can adversely affect the interpretation of the assay (see Fig. 100.9). Residual NADPH oxidase activity and production of ROS can be assessed by the ferricytochrome c assay, which is very specific and sensitive[215,226]; however, the assay requires fresh neutrophils, which makes it challenging for most clinical laboratories.

Treatment of CGD consists of life-long antifungal and antibacterial prophylaxis.[227,228] Recombinant IFN-gamma may be used along with antimicrobial drugs as an adjunctive therapy.[229–231] The only curative therapy that has gained widespread acceptance is HCT.[232,233] Pioglitazone, a drug used most commonly for the management of diabetes has been postulated to be useful in CGD as it can improve mitochondrial ROS formation and reduce inflammation by reversing impaired efferocytosis,[234] and is currently in a clinical trial. Gene therapy trials for X-linked CGD are available, and may be an alternative to HCT for some CGD patients.[235–239]

GROUP 6. DEFECTS OF INNATE IMMUNITY

The compartmentalization of the immune system, in an effort to simplify its complexity, has led to the binary organization of adaptive and innate immunity. The adaptive immune system, comprised mainly of T and B cells, requires generation of antigen-specific receptors, and thus can take a few days (~96 hours) to actively initiate participation in the immune response. Several of the preceding sections describe varied monogenic defects of the adaptive immune system. On the other hand, the innate immune system exists in the germline state and can immediately mount an immune response. They include not only cellular components, but also mucosal and epithelial barriers, naturally produced anti-microbial compounds, and receptors, called pathogen-recognition receptors, which recognize pathogen-associated molecular patterns (PAMPs) stimulating the secretion of bioactive substances, such as cytokines. The cells of the innate immune system include neutrophils, monocytes and macrophages, dendritic cells (DCs), NK cells, NKT cells, and other ILCs. There are several monogenic defects that affect either number or function of innate immune cells, or cytokines produced by these cells, which are critical for protection against infections with a variety of pathogens.[3,240,241] One example of an innate immune deficiency was described in the immediately preceding section, CGD. This section will briefly focus on Toll-like receptor (TLR) defects, as an example of innate immune defects.[242] TLRs are capable of recognizing specific microbial and host-derived molecules, and enabling rapid and early detection by the host of infection or other injurious signals. A variety of cells of the immune system express these TLRs, including T cells, B cells, DCs, macrophages, and epithelial cells among others. Signaling through the TLRs enables initiation of host defense mechanisms, which results in cytokine production or secretion of other bioactive moieties with

antimicrobial functions. Study of TLR defects enables our understanding of the critical role of the innate immune system and, in particular, these receptors in the host immune response. Human TLRs include both extracellular and intracellular receptors, and are ten in number. Each of these recognize different PAMPs, and danger-associated molecular patterns (DAMPs). A variety of ligands, microbial and endogenous (Table 100.5), stimulate these TLRs and mediate downstream signals and induce cellular functions. With few exceptions, TLRs utilize the MyD88 and IRAK (IL-1 receptor-associated kinase) complex to transduce intracellular signals. One of the most important effects of TLR signaling is the activation of the nuclear factor κB (NFκB) pathway. The NFκB family of proteins consist of five members, which in the inactive state are maintained in the cytosol, bound to inhibitory κB (IκB) proteins, or tethered by p100, in the canonical and noncanonical pathways respectively.[243] The five NFκB proteins include NFκB1 (p50), NFκB2 (p52), RelA (p65), RelB, and c-Rel, which are transcription factors that function as hetero- or homodimers.[244] While some of the gene defects affecting the NFκB pathway of signaling cause either a combined immunodeficiency (CID) or a humoral immunodeficiency, with a CVID-like phenotype, other defects affect individual TLRs, or MyD88, IRAK-4 or other components of the innate immune system, or cause an autoinflammatory phenotype.[3] As a prototype of innate immune defects, IRAK-4 (interleukin-1 receptor-associated kinase-4) deficiency causes recurrent infections, mainly by pyogenic, largely Gram-positive bacteria, like *Streptococcus pneumoniae*,[245] and results in a poor inflammatory response with low-grade fever. Another common infectious organism is *Staphylococcus aureus*. A few patients have had invasive infections caused by Gram-negative organisms. The most noteworthy feature of IRAK-4 deficiency is improvement in clinical phenotype with age, with most patients having infections in childhood prior to adolescence. This suggests an age-related compensation of immune function. Similar to phagocyte defects such as leukocyte adhesion deficiency (LAD) type 1, some patients with IRAK-4 deficiency can demonstrate delayed separation of the umbilical cord. Innate immune defects, such as IRAK-4 deficiency, are most often diagnosed in the laboratory by assessing cytokine production in response to TLR stimulation using a variety of

TABLE 100.5 Human Toll-Like Receptors and Their Ligands

TLR	Ligand	Extracellular (E) or Intracellular (I)	Adaptor
TLR1	Di-and tri-acylated lipoproteins	E	MyD88
TLR2	Lipoteichoic acid, lipoarabinomannan, zymosan and viral envelope antigens	E	MyD88
TLR3	dsRNA	I	TRIF
TLR4	Lipopolysaccharide (LPS)	E	MyD88/TRIF/TRAM/TICAM
TLR5	Flagellin	E	MyD88
TLR6	Di- and tri-acylated lipoproteins	E	MyD88
TLR7	ssRNA	I	MyD88
TLR8	ssRNA	I	MyD88
TLR9	Unmethylated DNA oligonucleotides	I	MyD88
TLR10	Unknown	E	MyD88

ds, Double-stranded; *MyD88*, myeloid differentiation factor 88; *ss*, single-stranded; *TRIF*, Toll/IL-1 receptor (TIR) domain-containing adaptor-inducing interferon β; *TRAM*, TRIF-related adaptor molecule; *TICAM*, TIR-containing adaptor molecule; *TLR*, Toll-like receptors.

ligands, and *IRAK4* gene sequencing. Flow cytometric detection of membrane-bound L-selectin on neutrophils has also been described as a rapid method for assessment of TLR defects.[246] Since this disease can be fatal in childhood, prophylactic antibiotics and replacement immunoglobulin therapy along with vaccination for encapsulated pathogens are mandatory. In general, though, the treatment of innate immune defects depends on the specific genetic defect and associated clinical phenotypes, and thus can be quite variable.

GROUP 7. AUTOINFLAMMATORY CONDITIONS

There is considerable overlap in the phenotypes and pathways affected by monogenic defects of the immune system, as evidenced by the IUIS categories[3] and the examples provided above. Nonetheless, single gene defects associated with an autoinflammatory phenotype are categorized as a distinct entity.[247–250] The concept of autoinflammation was proposed to explain the periodic fevers and systemic inflammation involving cells of the myeloid compartment but lacking features of classic autoimmune diseases, such as presence of autoantibodies or self-reactive T cells. Now it is recognized that autoinflammation involves aberrant activation and stimulation of the innate immune system. Inflammasomes, an integral part of the innate immune system, regulate the immune response to both extrinsic and intrinsic factors. Two groups of inflammasomes are recognized and include the NOD-like receptor (NLR) proteins—NLRP1, NLRP3, NLRP6, NLRP12, NLRC4 (IPAF), and the ALR-AIM2-like receptors, AIM2.[251,252] NLRP3, often regarded as the prototypic inflammasome, consists of a PRR (pathogen recognition receptor), a caspase-recruitment domain (ASC), which is an adaptor protein, and an enzyme, caspase 1, which promotes maturation of the pro-inflammatory cytokines, IL-1β and Il-18. The inflammasome is activated by triggering of the PRRs by PAMPs or DAMPs, and this in turn interacts with the ASC, leading to caspase 1 activation, which directs cleavage of the inactive precursors of IL-1β and IL-18 to their active forms. The periodic fever syndromes, a prototypic inflammasomopathy,[253] includes the cryopyrin-associated periodic syndrome (CAPS) due to GOF variants in the *NLRP3* gene, encoding the protein cryopyrin. The other most common form of periodic fevers is Familial Mediterranean Fever (FMF) due to pathogenic variants in the *MEFV* gene, encoding the pyrin protein, which is part of the inflammasome complex. Patients with FMF tend to have recurrent fever episodes, elevated acute phase reactants (APR) with inflammatory arthritis, and can also have inflammatory bowel disease. This condition is most typically seen in non-Ashkenazi Jews and other Eastern Mediterranean peoples. The list of autoinflammatory diseases continues to expand with identification of new monogenic defects,[3] and these are not exhaustively covered in this section. *NLRC4* GOF defects are associated with a severe form of infantile enterocolitis (AIFEC—autoinflammation with enterocolitis)[254] but can also be associated with a relatively milder phenotype, familial cold autoinflammatory syndrome type 4 (FCAS4). Besides germline GOF variants in *NLRC4*, somatic variants have been reported in one patient who presented with an AIFEC[255] phenotype, while another patient presented with a NLRP3-type phenotype of neonatal-onset multisystem disease (NOMID).[256] Treatment of most inflammasomopathies is with targeted therapies directed against IL-1β or IL-18.

Beyond the inflammasomopathies, genetic disorders associated with defective regulation of type I interferons, type I interferonopathies, are included under the umbrella of autoinflammatory conditions.[3,257] While the original designation of type I interferonopathies was confined to a few genetic disorders, such as Aicardi-Goutières syndrome (AGS), monogenic systemic lupus erythematosus (SLE), and spondyloenchondrodysplasia (SPENCD), now several others have been added to this group, including proteasome-associated autoinflammatory syndromes (PRAAS), Interferon (IFN)-stimulated gene 15 (ISG15) deficiency, Singleton-Merten syndrome and its atypical forms (SMS), and stimulator of IFN genes (STING)-associated vasculopathy with onset in infancy (SAVI).[258] Type 1 interferons are a key component of the host anti-viral and in some cases, anti-bacterial response. The viral and bacterial pathogens that stimulate a Type I IFN response are sensed by various PRRs, including the TLRs, RIG-I-like receptors (RLRs), NOD-like receptors (NLRs), and other sensors, including AIM2 (inflammasome) among others, in the cytoplasm or endosomes of infected cells. In addition to the family of type 1 IFNs, which includes 13 IFN-α and a single IFN-β, there are IFN regulatory factors (IRF), which translocate to the nucleus and induce transcription of the type I IFNs. Type I IFNs perform two key functions, antiviral activity and anti-proliferative activity. All type I IFNs can mediate antiviral activity at very low concentrations, in most cells, while the anti-proliferative function is very cell specific and depends on the expression of the type I IFN and its cellular receptors, and affinity of binding to the receptor. Genetic defects in many of these type I IFN-associated diseases results in susceptibility to severe viral infections, herpes, and influenza.[258]

Laboratory assessment of type I interferonopathies with enhanced type I IFN signaling is based on measuring increased expression of type I IFN. However, currently there is no such test available in a clinical laboratory. An assay has been developed and validated in the research setting, which measures expression of six interferon-stimulated genes (ISGs) as a surrogate for induction of type I IFN signaling.[259] These six ISGs include IFI27, IFI44L, IFIT1, ISG15, RSAD2, and SIGLEC1. While these have been shown to be of value in the diagnosis of specific interferonopathies, they have not been tested in all these disorders or indeed all autoinflammatory conditions.[259] In addition, increased expression of these six ISGs may be seen in other conditions with aberrant activation of innate immunity, but not classically considered as a type I interferonopathy (e.g., ADA2 deficiency, PRKDC defects among others). Increased Type I IFN signaling may also be seen in the context of cytokine blockade (IL-1β and tumor necrosis factor α [TNFα]) for other autoinflammatory diseases, which has clinical implications. An alternative scoring system was developed for IFN-response genes using 28 genes in the NanoString methodology, and used for the evaluation of a subset of patients with autoinflammatory diseases.[260] The value of such assays extends beyond diagnosis and could be used for monitoring disease activity, response to therapy, and long-term outcomes.

GROUP 8. COMPLEMENT DEFICIENCIES

Complement comprises several soluble and membrane-bound proteins and their associated receptors, which play a critical role in innate immunity and regulation of the

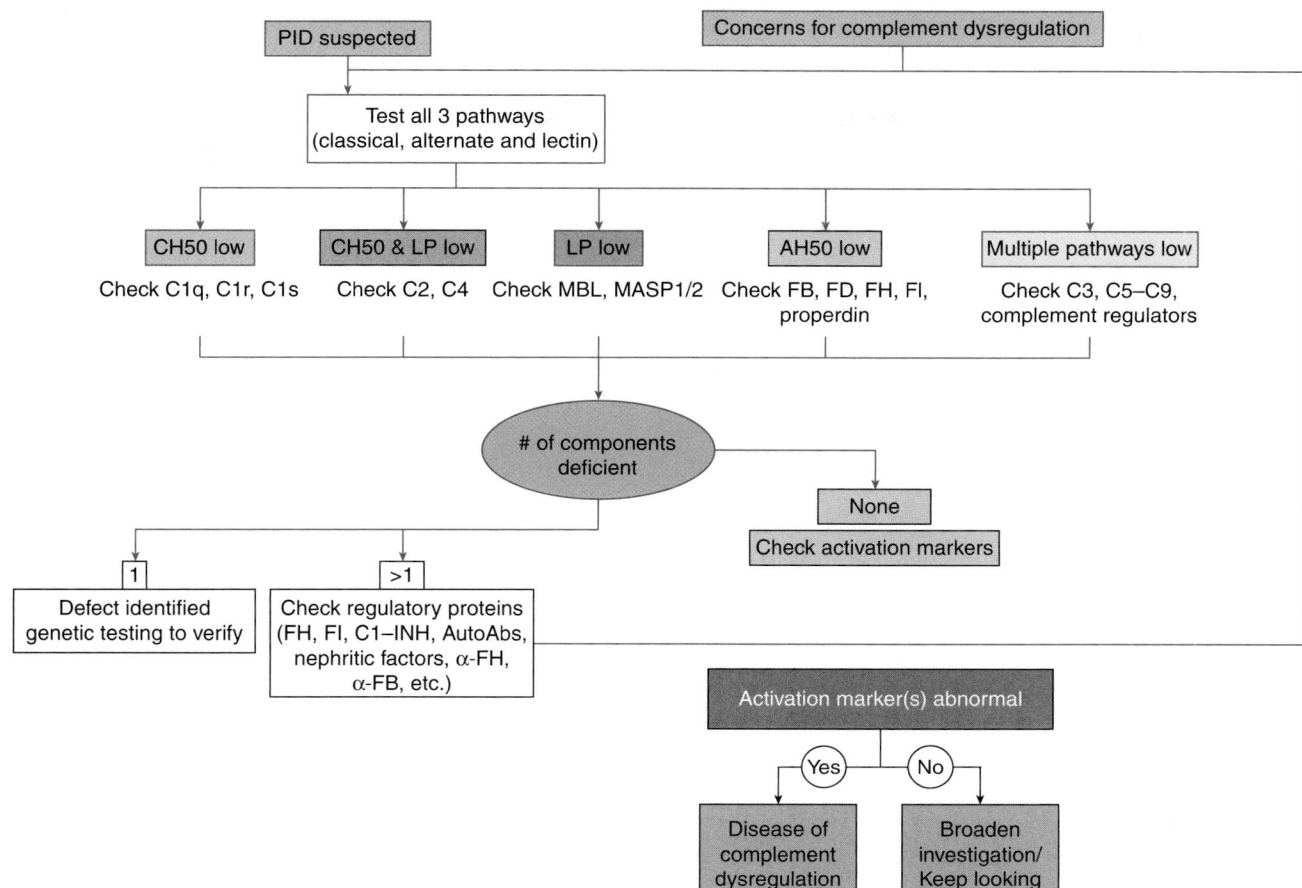

FIGURE 100.10 Diagnostic algorithm for complement deficiencies. Complement defects can affect all three pathways of complement—classical, mannose-binding lectin, and alternate. This is a schematic for diagnostic evaluation of a patient with suspected complement deficiency. *PID,* Primary immunodeficiencies. *AH50,* Alternate pathway; *AutoAbs,* autoantibodies; *C1-INH,* C1 inhibitor; *CH50,* classical pathway; *LP,* lectin pathway; *MASP,* mannan-binding lectin serine protease; *MBL,* mannose-binding lectin. (Adapted from Brodszki N, Frazer-Abel A, Grumach AS, et al. European Society for Immunodeficiencies [ESID] and European Reference Network on Rare Primary Immunodeficiency, Autoinflammatory and Autoimmune Diseases [ERN RITA] Complement Guideline: deficiencies, diagnosis, and management. *J Clin Immunol* 2020;40[4]:576–91.)

immune response. The prevalence of complement deficiencies has not been accurately ascertained in all populations, but several national or global registries consider it to account for 1 to 10% of all PIDs,[261] while another more recent review indicates an estimated prevalence of 0.03% in the general population.[262] This chapter will not discuss the complement system in detail, as it is covered elsewhere in this book. However, a very brief discussion on complement deficiencies will be provided here. Monogenic defects of the complement proteins can be organized into (1) susceptibility to infections, especially with encapsulated pathogens, (2) predisposition to autoimmunity, specifically SLE, (3) and dysregulation resulting in specific diseases, such as atypical hemolytic uremic syndrome (aHUS) and thrombotic microangiopathy (TMA). Fig. 100.10 provides an algorithm for the diagnostic evaluation, based on the European Society for Immunodeficiencies (ESID) review on complement defects,[262] and Table 100.6 is an overview of the known complement deficiencies, adapted from the European Society of Immunodeficiencies (ESID) review.[262]

GROUP 9. BONE MARROW FAILURE SYNDROMES—DYSKERATOSIS CONGENITA

The bone marrow failure syndromes (BMFSs) are a heterogeneous group of disorders, caused by either intrinsic (germline) or acquired defects resulting in ineffective hematopoiesis and cytopenias, affecting one or more lineages.[263,264] Inherited BMFS (iBMFS) are either autosomal recessive or X-linked conditions, many of them with high penetrance which usually, but not always, present in infancy. However, some of these have a broad clinical spectrum, and partial loss-of-function variants can result in a later onset. Other marrow-associated conditions, such as GATA2 deficiency or some of the short telomere syndromes (telomeropathies) have variable onset, are usually autosomal dominant, and manifest in adolescence or adulthood. Other iBMFS include dyskeratosis congenita, Hoyeraal-Hreidarsson syndrome, Fanconi anemia, Shwachman-Diamond syndrome, aplastic anemia, severe congenital neutropenia, and Diamond-Blackfan anemia, among others. Most of these conditions are identified by clinical phenotype and

TABLE 100.6 Complement Deficiencies

Complement Protein Defect	Clinical Phenotype	No. of Patients/Incidence/Inheritance
C1q, r, s	SLE, systemic infections with encapsulated pathogens	~80 patients
C2	Heterozygous deficiency is asymptomatic	1:20,000
Complete C4 deficiency	SLE, RA, systemic infections with encapsulated pathogens	~30 patients
C4A/ C4B deficiency	SLE, susceptibility to lymphoma, sarcoid, celiac disease, prolonged postinfection symptoms, intolerance to certain antibiotics	1:250
C3 GOF	Atypical HUS (aHUS)	2–8% of all aHUS
C3 LOF	Pyogenic infections, Neisserial infections, glomerulonephritis, age-related macular degeneration (AMD)	~40 patients
Factor H	Pyogenic infections, Neisserial infections, glomerulonephritis, AMD	~30 patients
Factor I	Pyogenic infections, Neisserial infections, glomerulonephritis, AMD	Rare
C5	Neisserial infections, recurrent meningitis	Rare
C6	Neisserial infections, recurrent meningitis	Rare in Caucasians; ~1:2000 in African Americans
C7	Neisserial infections, recurrent meningitis	Rare in Caucasians; ~1:10,000 in Moroccan Jews
C8	Neisserial infections, recurrent meningitis	
C9	Neisserial infections; mostly asymptomatic	Rare; 1:1000 in Japan
Factor B	Neisserial and pneumococcal infections; aHUS	aHUS (1 case)
Factor D	Bacterial infections	2 families
Mannose-binding lectin (MBL)	Controversial, possible susceptibility to bacterial infections and autoimmunity	5%
Ficolin 3	Various clinical phenotypes	<10 patients
MASP1	3MC	Rare
MASP2	Respiratory infections, mostly asymptomatic	0.03%
C1-INH	HAE	1:50,000
C4BP	Atypical Behçet, angioedema, protein S defect	1 patient
Properdin	Neisserial meningitis	Rare
CFHR1–3 gene deletion	aHUS, SLE	Variable
Thrombomodulin	aHUS	Rare
CD46/MCP	aHUS	Rare
CD55/DAF	PNH	1–2/million
CD55	CHAPLE	Rare
CD59	PNH	1–2/million
CD59	Chronic hemolysis, relapsing peripheral demyelinating disease, cerebral infarction	<20
CD21 (CR2)	Infections, CVID	Rare
CD18/CD11b (CR3)	LAD-I	1/million
CD18/CD11c (CR4)	LAD-I	1/million

3MC, Mingarelli, Malpeuch, Michels, Carnevale syndrome; *aHUS*, atypical hemolytic uremic syndrome; *CHAPLE*, complement hyperactivation, TMA, protein-losing enteropathy (PLE); *CVID*, Common Variable Immunodeficiency; *HAE*, hereditary angioedema; *LAD-I*, leukocyte adhesion deficiency type I; *MASP*, Mannan-binding lectin serine protease; *PNH*, paroxysmal nocturnal hemoglobinuria; *RA*, rheumatoid arthritis; *SLE*, systemic lupus erythematosus; *TMA*, thrombotic microangiopathy.
Adapted from Brodszki N, Frazer-Abel A, Grumach AS, et al. European Society for Immunodeficiencies (ESID) and European Reference Network on Rare Primary Immunodeficiency, Autoinflammatory and Autoimmune Diseases (ERN RITA) Complement Guideline: deficiencies, diagnosis, and management. *J Clin Immunol* 2020;40(4):576–91.

next-generation sequencing, though in some cases a molecular defect may not be clearly identified. As our understanding of the pathology of these disorders expands, other "classic" syndromic immunodeficiencies, such as Cartilage Hair Hypoplasia (CHH), may also be included in the overlap of iBMFS. Dyskeratosis congenita (DKC; Zinsser-Engman-Cole syndrome) is a prototypic iBMFS associated with a spectrum of immunodeficiency and telomere dysfunction.[265,266]

Hoyeraal-Hreidarsson syndrome is at the severe end of the spectrum of DKC and presents with a severe combined immunodeficiency phenotype along with other syndromic features (microcephaly, cerebellar hypoplasia) but milder forms may present with aplastic anemia. The clinical features of the classic form includes the triad of skin pigmentation anomalies, leucoplakia, and nail dystrophy. However, it is important to remember that not all DKC patients may present with this classic phenotype. In addition to these, there may be varying degrees of bone marrow failure, immunodeficiency, susceptibility to malignancy, and pulmonary fibrosis. DKC is also a prototype of telomere defects, as it is caused by pathogenic variants in the genes DKC1 (X-linked), TERC (autosomal recessive or dominant), and RTEL1 (autosomal recessive or dominant), all involved in maintenance of the telomere complex and its function. The autosomal recessive and dominant forms may present with different clinical features and age of onset. DKC is associated with a very high risk for developing malignancy and includes both hematopoietic and non-hematopoietic tumors.[267] Telomeres are "caps" on the end of chromosomes comprised of repetitive units of $(TTAGGG)_n$, and critical to cell survival and chromosome integrity.[268] They shorten with cell division, and several components of the telomere complex, including telomerase (includes TERT, the reverse transcriptase, and TERC, the RNA component) and dyskerin (encoded by *DKC1*) with others counteract this physiologic attrition. Short telomeres are associated with premature cellular senescence, and may result in abnormal organ function due to tissue ageing, even of a subset of cells within that tissue.[269] Patients with DKC who have bone marrow failure with associated immunodeficiency require HCT to rescue the hematopoietic/immunologic defect; however, outcomes are not very robust and require ongoing follow-up and improved approaches.[270] One of the key diagnostic tests to identify abnormally short telomeres in patients with relevant clinical phenotypes is to use a combination of flow cytometry and fluorescence in situ hybridization (FISH), called flow-FISH (Fig. 100.11), in various peripheral blood subsets.[271–273] This test is sensitive for measurement of telomere length, especially if less than the first percentile compared to healthy controls, though some patients may show evidence of short telomeres before the onset of clinical symptoms. While telomere length may be measured in many peripheral leukocyte subsets, the most meaningful information may be obtained

from analysis in lymphocyte and granulocyte subsets.[272] Telomere length measurement is available in the clinical diagnostic setting in only two laboratories in North America, and therefore it is a highly specialized test. It has proven utility in clinical management of at least a subset of patients with short telomeres[272] and associated clinical phenotypes, including selection of conditioning regimen for HCT.

GROUP 10. PHENOCOPIES OF PRIMARY IMMUNODEFICIENCIES

While inborn errors of immunity refers to genetic disorders of the immune system, within the IUIS classification, a category was included for disorders with no germline genetic defect, but rather caused by autoantibodies or somatic variants in genes associated with an immunodeficiency. These disease phenotypes mimicked those of germline immunodeficiencies and were thus called "phenocopies of inborn errors of immunity."[3] As would be expected with nongermline genetic defects, these diseases do not follow a Mendelian order of inheritance. This section focuses on autoantibody-associated phenocopies of errors of immunity, though somatic variants can result in phenocopies, and some examples have been provided in the Group 4 section (somatic FAS, NRAS, and KRAS defects associated with ALPS). Most phenocopies of PIDs are associated with anti-cytokine autoantibodies (Table 100.7), and these are usually high-titer, neutralizing IgG antibodies associated with a specific phenotype.[274–280] Diagnosis of autoantibody-mediated immunodeficiency requires measurement of the autoantibodies using immunoserology assays, either ELISA or multiplex bead-based assays, which detect ligand binding and offer assessment of the titer.[281] However, since not all autoantibodies which bind ligand mediate neutralizing function, it is useful to have alternate methods that assess biological impact and clinical significance. Flow cytometry has been used to detect the

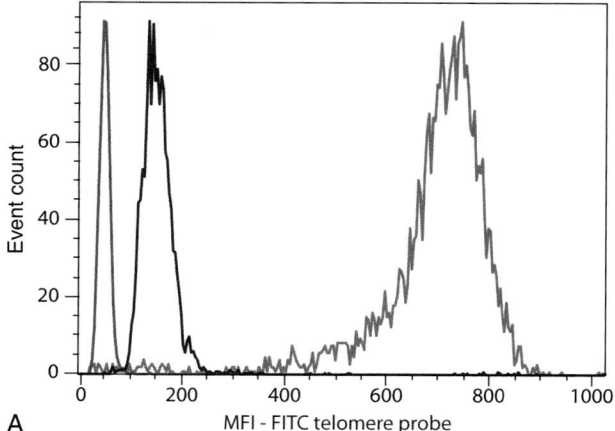

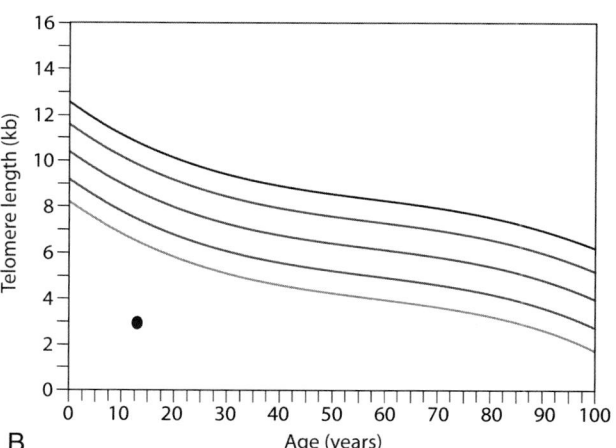

FIGURE 100.11 Flow-FISH for measurement of telomere length. Measurement of telomere length is diagnostically useful for patients with short telomere syndromes and certain bone marrow failure conditions. Flow-FISH is a sensitive method for assessment of telomere length in various leukocyte subsets, and the presence of short telomeres (less than first percentile) can be correlated with clinical phenotype and evidence of a short telomere syndrome or bone marrow failure and other clinical features. *FITC,* Fluorscein isothiocyanate; *MFI,* median fluorescence intensity. (Reproduced from Abraham RS, Aubert G. Flow cytometry, a versatile tool for diagnosis and monitoring of primary immunodeficiencies. *Clin Vaccine Immunol* 2016;23:254–71.)

TABLE 100.7 **Phenocopies of Immunodeficiencies Caused by Autoantibodies to Cytokines and Regulatory Proteins**

Autoantibody to Cytokine or Regulatory Proteins	Clinical Features
IFNγ	Nontuberculous mycobacterial infections (NTM), disseminated extrapulmonary, *Salmonella typhi* infections, reactivation of *Varicella zoster* (VZV) infection, cytomegalovirus (CMV), *Toxoplasma* infections
IL-17A and IL-17F	Autoimmune polyglandular syndrome 1(APS-1), chronic mucocutaneous candidiasis (CMC)
IL-22	APS-1 and CMC
IL-12	APS-1, thymoma-associated autoimmunity, Burkholderia lymphadenitis (single case)
IL-6	Recurrent staphylococcal infections with low C-reactive protein (CRP)
IFNα	SLE, APS-1, thymoma, hypomorphic RAG deficiencies, IPEX syndrome, NFκB2 deficiency (single case)
IL-1	Pemphigus, psoriasis, RA, Sjögren syndrome
IL-8	Acute respiratory distress syndrome (ARDS)
TNFα	SLE, MS, RA, psoriasis
GM-CSF	Pulmonary alveolar proteinosis (PAP)-autoimmune, infections with *Mycobacterium avium*, *Nocardia, Cryptococcus, Aspergillus*
G-CSF	Neutropenia, Felty syndrome
BAFF (B cell–activating factor)	SLE, CVID
Osteopontin (OPN)	RA, prostate cancer, hepatocellular carcinoma
Osteoprotegerin	Osteoporosis, celiac disease, enhanced bone resorption in RA
Erythropoietin (EPO)	Pure red cell aplasia (PRCA, autoimmune)
C1-INH	Acquired angioedema (aAE)
Complement factor H	Atypical hemolytic uremic syndrome (aHUS), thrombotic microangiopathy (TMA)

C1-INH, C1 Inhibitor; *CVID,* common variable immunodeficiency; *G-CSF,* granulocyte-colony-stimulating factor; *GM-CSF,* granulocyte-macrophage colony-stimulating factor; *IFN,* interferon; *MS,* multiple sclerosis; *RA,* rheumatoid arthritis; *SLE,* systemic lupus erythematosus; *TNF,* tumor necrosis factor.
Adapted from Merkel PA, Lebo T, Knight V. Functional analysis of anti-cytokine autoantibodies using flow cytometry. *Front Immunol* 2019;10:1517.

functional consequences of certain anti-cytokine autoantibodies, such as those to interferon-γ (IFNγ) and GM-CSF.[282] Consideration of a phenocopy of PID in the differential diagnosis depends on the clinical phenotype, age of the patient, and presence of negative genetic testing results (see Table 100.7).[274]

Treatment of anti-cytokine autoantibodies is focused on management of clinical symptoms, removal of the autoantibody or halting its production. Therefore removal of proteinaceous material from lungs of patients with pulmonary alveolar proteinosis (PAP) caused by autoantibodies to GM-CSF by therapeutic bronchoalveolar lavage (BAL) is one example. Others include plasmapheresis, use of B cell–depleting therapies such as anti-CD20 antibodies,[283] use of other immunomodulatory therapies, or treating the clinical consequences caused by autoantibodies.[284]

Genetic Testing for Primary Immunodeficiencies

In the preceding sections, various examples of inborn errors of immunity were discussed including some of the laboratory diagnostic tools widely used, such as flow cytometry. However, an equally important method for the evaluation of germline genetic disorders is genetic analysis for the identification of single gene defects associated with disease. A decade or two ago, most clinical laboratories performed single gene Sanger sequencing, however, in the last several years, the field of genetic testing has been revolutionized with the advent of high throughput, rapid, multi-gene analysis methods. Our understanding of PIDs has evolved over the years, from a linear, unidimensional concept of Mendelian disorders to a more multidimensional paradigm with complex single or multigene defects demonstrating variable expressivity and incomplete penetrance, and modulated by revertant or somatic mosaicism. Next-generation sequencing (NGS) methods are widely employed for diagnosis of inborn errors of immunity[285–288] and are essential for identification of the specific molecular defect, which would enable genotype-phenotype correlations, and use of personalized management strategies, including targeted therapies.[289] The NGS approaches for PIDs includes targeted analysis of genes known to be associated with inborn errors of immunity,[290,291] whole exome sequencing (WES) or whole genome sequencing (WGS).[292–294] However, exome analysis may not always be informative as coverage can be variable,[295] and with decreasing costs and turn-around-time (TAT) with improved bioinformatics WGS is becoming a more viable and attractive option.[296] Recently, the American Academy of Allergy, Asthma and Immunology (AAAAI) published guidelines for the interpretation of genetic results in PIDs,[297] which delineates the various genetic tools available to the clinician, and the pros and cons of each method. The accessibility of genetic analysis along with enhanced interpretive standards has significantly improved discovery of new PIDs, as well as expanded the genotypic and phenotypic spectrum of known PIDs.

In summary, the diagnostic armamentarium for PIDs[298] has revolutionized not only our understanding of human immunology by revealing the incredible and multifaceted complexity of the immune system, but also our ability to manage

TABLE 100.8 Secondary Causes of Immunodeficiencies

Hematologic Conditions Leading to Secondary Immunodeficiency	Infections
Aplastic anemia	HIV
Hematologic malignancies	Measles
Sickle cell disease	Epstein-Barr virus/cytomegalovirus
Non-hematologic conditions leading to secondary immunodeficiency	Parvovirus B19/adenovirus
Diabetes mellitus	Mycobacteria
Hepatic injury/cirrhosis	Parasites
Uremia/chronic kidney disease	Medications
Malnutrition/nutritional deficiencies	Cytotoxic chemotherapy
Ionizing radiation	Corticosteroids
Splenectomy/hyposplenism	Calcineurin inhibitors: Tacrolimus/cyclosporine
Trauma/significant stress	mTor inhibitors: sirolimus/everolimus
Thymoma	Purine synthesis inhibitors: azathioprine/mycophenolate
Recreational drug use	TNF inhibitors: infliximab/etanercept/adalimumab
Pregnancy	CD20 targeting antibody: rituximab
Extremes of age	CD30 targeting antibody: brentuximab
Disorders of immunoglobulin/lymphocyte loss	CD52 targeting antibody: alemtuzumab
Inflammatory bowel disease	C5 complement targeting antibody: eculizumab
Protein losing enteropathies	CTLA4 directed activity: abatacept
Intestinal lymphangiectasia	Interferon-gamma targeting antibody: emapalumab
Chylous effusions	JAK-STAT pathway inhibition: ruxolitinib
Severe dermatitis/burns	IL-1 targeting antibody: anakinra/canakinumab
Nephrotic syndrome	IL-2 targeting antibody: basiliximab
Congenital cardiac conditions	IL-6 targeting antibody: tocilizumab
Peritoneal dialysis	Lymphocyte destruction via immunoglobulins: antithymocyte globulin
Plasma exchange	Cancer immunotherapy: CAR-T, checkpoint inhibitors, bispecific T-cell engagers

CAR-T, Chimeric antigen receptor T cell; *CTLA,* cytotoxic T-lymphocyte-associated protein; *IL,* interleukin; *JAK,* Janus kinase; *mTOR,* mammalian target of rapamycin; *TNF,* tumor necrosis factor.

and treat these diseases through targeted therapies, based on the underlying molecular defect or specific etiology.

Secondary Immunodeficiencies

Infectious insults, pathologic medical conditions, various treatment modalities, and nonpathologic alterations in human physiology secondary to aging and pregnancy can all disrupt inherent immunity creating an elevated risk of infection, autoimmunity, and malignancy. Here we highlight the numerous intrinsic and extrinsic conditions and exposures that lead to secondary immunodeficiency in pediatric and adult patients (Table 100.8).

Selective Hematologic Conditions Leading to Secondary Immunodeficiency

Aplastic Anemia

Aplastic anemia as defined by peripheral cytopenias and concurrent bone marrow hypocellularity per the Camitta criteria leads to immunodeficiency primarily through reduced production of leukocytes, most prominently neutrophils.[299] Significant neutropenia greatly raises the risk of severe infection from fungal and bacterial organisms. In fact, a leading cause of death in aplastic anemia is invasive fungal infection, particularly *Aspergillus* species.[300] If lymphopenia is present, patients may additionally be susceptible to parasitic and viral (via primary infection or viral reactivation) illnesses. Various pathophysiologic mechanisms may lead to bone marrow failure, including infection, inherited genetic conditions that include

primary immunodeficiencies such as CTLA-4 haploinsufficiency, direct toxicity to hematopoietic stem cells via drugs/radiation/chemicals, and autoimmunity. In those with idiopathic aplastic anemia felt to be caused by immune-mediated destruction of bone marrow cells via cytotoxic T cells, further immunodeficiency is created via treatment modalities, such as calcineurin inhibitors and anti-lymphocyte globulin, which result in suppression of T lymphocytes.[301]

Hematologic Malignancies

Bone marrow infiltration by hematologic neoplasm results in abnormal proliferation of normal functioning lymphocytes, granulocytes, and monocytes. Altered lymphocyte function, hypogammaglobulinemia, decreased complement, and reduced plasma cell activity in individuals with multiple myeloma and chronic lymphocytic leukemia appear to further result in immune dysregulation.[302–305] Cellular immunodeficiency, resulting in an increased susceptibility to infections, is also a well-described phenomenon in those with classical Hodgkin lymphoma and is often present prior to a diagnosis of the condition.[306]

Sickle Cell Disease

Early splenic infarction secondary to misshaped red blood cells and oxidative stress in sickle cell patients results in significant impairment of splenic function and an elevated risk of infection with encapsulated organisms, including *Streptococcus pneumoniae, Haemophilus influenzae,* and *Salmonella* species. Susceptibility to infections prior to splenic dysfunction and microbes classically not considered encapsulated, such as *Mycoplasma pneumoniae* and *Escherichia coli*, raises the possibility of additional immunodeficiency factors in sickle cell. Complement activation defects, deficiencies in micronutrients causing immune impairment, and endothelial/osseous environment alterations may further lead to an increased predisposition to infections.[307] Prophylactic antimicrobial therapy, comprehensive vaccination administration, and aggressive management of suspected serious bacterial infections are imperative in those with sickle cell disease to prevent the potential for adverse outcomes as a result of immunodeficiency.

Nonhematologic Conditions Leading to Secondary Immunodeficiency

Diabetes Mellitus

Various disorders that cause biochemical homeostasis abnormalities bring about dysfunctional immunity through toxic metabolite production and nutrient imbalances. Diabetes mellitus is one such disorder, where both innate and adaptive immunity are weakened. Neutrophil chemotaxis, phagocytosis, and superoxide production all are impaired. The clinical presentation of diabetes mellitus can unmask previously clinically unrecognized myeloperoxidase deficiency, making patients more susceptible to *Candida* infections. Distorted cell-mediated immunity, particularly T-lymphocyte dysfunction, is the predominant adaptive immune abnormality observed in diabetics.[308] Humoral immunity overall seems to be less affected with an apparent adequate antibody response to vaccination in patients. Interestingly, immunodeficiency may be observed not only in the setting of hyperglycemia but additionally with hyperinsulinemia despite euglycemia. Those with diabetes mellitus not only have an increased risk of contracting common community-acquired microbes but also notably may be afflicted with rhinopulmonary mucormycosis, *Pseudomonas aeruginosa* otitis externa, and disseminated candidiasis.[308]

Hepatic Injury/Cirrhosis

Chronic hepatic injury can result in cirrhosis-associated immune dysfunction, a condition that manifests through alterations of various immuno-protective mechanisms provided by the liver. The liver plays an important role in immune surveillance and in the production of molecules crucial to effective immunity. Antimicrobial surveillance is achieved through various populations of lymphocytes and antigen presenting cells, notably Kupffer cells, within the hepatic architecture.[309] Significant hepatic fibrosis can also result in portal hypertension and altered splenic clearance of deleterious microbes. Reduced synthetic capabilities by the liver leads to decreased pattern-recognition receptors, such as lipopolysaccharide (LPS)-binding protein, and complement components. Elevated endogenous glucocorticoids from reduced hepatic metabolism and significant systemic inflammation in those with cirrhosis additionally damages circulating and intestinal immune cells leading to further immunodeficiency.[309]

Uremia/Chronic Kidney Disease

Significant renal injury leads to uremia, which causes poor antibody responses and ineffective neutrophil chemotaxis.[310]

Abnormalities in both innate and adaptive immunity along with chronic systemic inflammation and poor responses to bacterial infections that appear to underlie the complex immune dysfunction are also seen in chronic kidney disease patients.[311]

Malnutrition/Nutrient Deficiencies

Those with malnutrition suffer from chronic inflammation and recurrent infections; it is thought that the immune deficits in those undernourished are multifactorial.[312] Severe diarrhea may lead to stool losses of lymphocytes and immunoglobulins. Nutrient deficiencies lead to mucosal barrier abnormalities increasing the risk of invasion of infectious organisms. Those with kwashiorkor, a protein predominant malnutrition condition, are especially prone to hypocomplementemia and hypogammaglobulinemia. Significant nutrient inadequacies, including vitamin B12, zinc, and copper deficiencies, can also lead to bone marrow hypoproduction. Individuals with anorexia nervosa can manifest reduced immunity similarly as their undernourished bone marrow compartment is replaced with fat.[313] Improvement in nutritional status often resolves the immunologic deficits.[310]

Ionizing Radiation

Excessive exposure to irradiation may directly damage the bone marrow causing cytopenias. In addition to marrow toxicity, immunity is also reduced through modification of cytokine release and inhibition of antigen-presenting cells, particularly dendritic cells. Of note, it appears phagocytosis and humoral responses are relatively radioresistant.[310,314]

Splenectomy/Hyposplenism

Individuals with impaired splenic function or postsplenectomy are at risk for severe infections, especially with encapsulated organisms, given the importance of the spleen in maintaining adequate immunity. Total splenectomy should thus be deferred if possible until the age of 5 years in children, given their functionally more developed immune system at that time. Partial splenectomy should also be considered as it allows for some maintained immunologic splenic function.[315] Appropriate vaccinations (covering pneumococcal, *H. influenzae,* and meningococcal species) are imperative in these patients and antibiotic prophylaxis is also often administered, especially in children and those with a history of sepsis.[316,317]

Thymoma

Altered thymic architecture from a neoplastic thymoma can impact the normal development of T lymphocytes and diminish production of Tregs.[318] Thymoma may be associated with aplastic anemia and thus a quantitative decrease in immunity secondary to bone marrow suppression from autoreactive T cells. Patients with thymoma may also develop additional immune dysregulation and autoimmune conditions as a result of their malignancy.[319] Thymoma with B cell lymphopenia and hypogammaglobulinemia and an array of autoantibodies was described as Good syndrome more than half a century ago.[320,321]

Trauma/Significant Stress

Major trauma can result in immunodeficiency and an increased infection risk through the loss of epithelial barriers and elevated cortisol levels causing lymphocyte suppression.[310]

In the setting of severe trauma or burns, the body reacts initially with a systemic inflammatory response but then enters an immunosuppressed state known as the compensatory anti-inflammatory response syndrome (CARS), which further raises the possibility of infection acquisition.[322]

Conditions Associated With Protein/Lymphocyte Losses

Secondary hypogammaglobulinemia is much more common than primary antibody deficiency and can be caused by various disorders or treatments. Conditions that lead to excessive protein losses or alterations in lymphatic circulation may result in immunodeficiency through reduced antibody levels. Immunoglobulin losses may occur through the gastrointestinal tract in those with inflammatory bowel disease, protein losing enteropathies, or intestinal lymphangiectasias. Antibodies may also be quickly depleted with peritoneal dialysis, plasma exchange procedures, severe burns, significant dermatitis, and nephrotic syndrome.[304,323] Medications that negatively affect B cells will likely also result in secondary antibody deficiencies, which further increase their immunodeficient effects.[304] Lymphatic circulation abnormalities, such as chylothorax or intestinal lymphangiectasias, cause not only hypogammaglobulinemia, but also lymphopenia through direct loss of lymphocytes. There are also primary anomalies caused by germline or somatic variants in genes critical for lymphatic development.[324]

Particular attention must be paid to pediatric patients with a history of congenital cardiac anomalies as they are at risk for the development of quantitative lymphocyte and immunoglobulin abnormalities secondary to thoracic duct injury, surgical thymectomy, and protein-losing enteropathy from post-Fontan procedure hemodynamic changes. Interestingly, despite often impressive lymphopenia these patients do not appear at risk for significant opportunistic infections, although they may have difficulty with clearance of cutaneous viral lesions.[325]

Pregnancy

It is thought that reduced cellular immunity during pregnancy may develop to protect against immunologic rejection of the fetus, although some feel the unique immunity manifested during pregnancy should not be considered as a suppressed state but more so as merely modulated.[326] Changes in cellular immunity during pregnancy are not fully understood but may be related to suppressed T helper type 1 (Th1) responses, modified expression of MHC antigens, and altered cytokines release.[327]

Extremes of Age

Neonates, particularly those that are premature, have a poor ability to produce immunoglobulins given poor isotype class switching and plasma cell differentiation capabilities. Immaturity of antigen-presenting cells and a reduced differentiation of naïve CD4 T cells further renders neonates immunodeficient compared to older children or adults. Moreover, neonatal phagocytes have decreased chemotaxis and a reduced ability to phagocytose and destroy organisms as their NADPH-oxidase is not efficient at generating oxygen radicals.[328] Neonates also have a decreased storage pool of neutrophils and are not able to create effective neutrophil extracellular traps.[329] A relative immunodeficiency is further found in those of advanced age secondary to a limited ability to produce naïve

T cells, skewing of differentiated memory T cells, and decreased B-cell diversity. Bone marrow hypocellularity in the elderly further exacerbates immune dysfunction with an inability to often mount an appropriate phagocytic response to microbial infections.[310,330]

Recreational Drug Use

Various drugs and toxins used recreationally may lead to immunosuppression via direct impacts on immune cell function or via deleterious effects on the bone marrow. Those with a high intake of marijuana may experience reduced complement and immunoglobulin levels with additional decreased lymphocyte proliferation and NK-cell activity.[331,332] Levamisole-tainted heroin or cocaine can lead to neutropenia.[333] Cocaine and abusive opiate usage may additionally be associated with reduced cytokine production and altered phagocytosis, respectively.[331] Aplastic anemia with resultant neutropenia and bone marrow failure can occur with frequent inhalant or Ecstasy use.[334,335]

Infections Leading to Secondary Immunodeficiency

In addition to the immunosuppressive effects of the human immunodeficiency virus (HIV), which will not be discussed within this chapter but affects immunity primarily through devastation of CD4-positive T lymphocytes, many other microbes alter their host's immune system.

Measles

The measles virus results in significant immunosuppression secondary to dendritic cell dysfunction, suppressed macrophage activation, and reduced lymphocyte proliferation.[336,337]

Epstein-Barr Virus/Cytomegalovirus

The gamma-herpesvirus, EBV primarily infects dormant B lymphocytes, causing their dysfunction. The virus may then become latent and persist within B memory cells. Overall, cell-mediated immunity is often altered in those afflicted with the virus.[327] A similar virus, the CMV, can also modulate the host's immune system to cause chronic infection. NK-cell diversity and T-cell proliferation are modified by the virus.[338] Individuals with a genetic predisposition to inadequately control or monitor for the EBV following infection, such as those with SAP (XLP1) or XIAP (XLP2) deficiency, may manifest with fulminant infectious mononucleosis leading to significant morbidity and mortality.[339] The study of these conditions has led to a better appreciation of the role that natural killer, CD4+, and CD8+ lymphocytes play in the initial killing of and latent suppression of EBV, as patients with XLP1 and XLP2 appear to have broad lymphocyte dysfunction, rather than purely B-cell irregularities. Intracellular free magnesium, IL-2–inducible T-cell kinase, and PI(3)K have also now been found to play an important role in the prevention of EBV proliferation.[340–342]

Additional Viruses

In-addition to the prominent immunosuppressive effects of measles, EBV, and CMV, various other viruses can lead to immune dysfunction. The DNA virus parvovirus B19 replicates within erythroid progenitor cells resulting in possible reticulocytopenia and pure red cell aplasia. Those at particular risk for severe hematologic consequences of the virus include patients with underlying disorders with elevated red blood cell turnover, including sickle cell disease, thalassemia, and hereditary spherocytosis. Although anemia is the most common cytopenia observed in those infected with parvovirus B19, bone marrow suppression from the virus can lead to neutropenia and lymphopenia.[343] Patients' status post-hematopoietic stem cell transplantation (HSCT) may experience donor graft failure with parvovirus infection, resulting in a significant infectious risk.[344] Another DNA virus, adenovirus, can also have devastating effects on HSCT patients with de novo infection or viral reactivation leading to graft failure or severe immune dysregulation secondary to sepsis in the setting of viremia. In health individuals, the virus can also modify immunity and lead to latency via cytokine alterations, blockade of cellular apoptosis, and down-regulation of major histocompatibility complexes (MHC).[345]

Mycobacteria

Mycobacteria have the unique ability to avoid destruction by their host's immune system and reside within macrophages. Through chronic infection, the mycobacteria may alter normal immunity through modulation of cytokine production, inhibition of tumor necrosis factor-alpha release by macrophages, and possible alterations of toll-like receptor signaling.[346,347] These immunologic alterations are exacerbated in the immunodeficiency pathophysiology seen in patients with a diagnosis of Mendelian susceptibility to mycobacterial diseases (MSMD). MSMD occurs as a result of IFN-γ pathway defects, leading to reduced production of the cytokines IFN-γ or IL-12. The ability of mononuclear phagocytes to interact with T cells is thus hindered; intracellular organisms, such as mycobacteria, *Salmonella, Listeria monocytogenes,* and viruses (particularly cytomegalovirus and varicella), can subsequently flourish and become disseminated.[348]

Malaria and Other Parasites

It is thought that the elevated risk of EBV-associated Burkitt lymphoma in Africa is a result of malarial alterations in immunity against the Epstein-Barr virus. With *Plasmodium* spp. infection the ability of cytotoxic T cells to control EBV-infected B cells is hindered, thus allowing for excessive lymphoproliferation.[349] Infection by other parasitic organisms may additionally lead to immunosuppression by abnormal regulation of dendritic cells, suppression of antigen presentation, and inducing a T-regulatory cell response.[350,351]

Medications

Numerous medications act directly or indirectly to suppress immunity (Fig. 100.12). The recent propagation of biologic and targeted pharmaceutical therapies to treat autoimmune and malignant conditions has greatly added to the complexity observed regarding secondary immunodeficiency observed in clinical practice.

Cytotoxic Chemotherapy

Cytotoxic chemotherapy used for the treatment of malignancy or autoimmune conditions most commonly causes secondary immunosuppression through bone marrow suppression/toxicity leading to lymphopenia, monocytopenia, and neutropenia. Higher doses of the drugs can additionally

lead to mucosal breakdown with resultant ease of translocation of bacteria from mucosal surfaces to the immunodeficient patient's bloodstream.[310]

Corticosteroids

Corticosteroids are used broadly in clinical practice and result in the decreased production of cytokines crucial to immunity, including IL-6 and TNFα. Dendritic cells may have reduced maturation and function in the setting of glucocorticoids. Adverse effects on leukocyte chemotaxis and anergy are also observed with usage of corticosteroids. Proapoptotic leukocyte activity is increased and IL-2 levels are reduced leading to lymphopenia.[310,352] Deleterious immunosuppression appears to be dose and treatment chronicity dependent. Long-term high-dose use of corticosteroids significantly increases the risk of infections, including with opportunistic organisms such as *Pneumocystis jiroveci* and tuberculosis.[352]

Drugs classified as mammalian target of rapamycin (mTOR), inosine-5′-monophosphate dehydrogenase (IMPDH), and calcineurin inhibitors primarily cause acquired immunodeficiency through inhibitory actions on lymphocytes.

Calcineurin Inhibitors

The most commonly used calcineurin inhibitors in medical practice are tacrolimus and cyclosporine. Most often calcineurin inhibition is used in the setting of graft-versus-host disease prevention of post-hematopoietic stem cell transplantation or prevention of solid organ transplantation rejection. Through activation of the transcription factor nuclear factor of activated T cells (NFAT), calcineurin induces the expression of IL-2, resulting in the differentiation/proliferation of T cells and propagation of additional cytokines. Calcineurin inhibitors appear to predominantly affect lymphocyte-, primarily T cell–directed, immunity while mostly sparing neutrophil and macrophage functions.[310,353] Such drugs increase the risk of viral infections, including the EBV, which can lead to the malignant condition of post-transplant lymphoproliferative disease in patients taking the medications following hematopoietic stem cell or solid organ transplantation.

mTOR Inhibitors

Inhibition of the mTOR pathway, via drugs such as sirolimus or everolimus, has immunosuppressive effects through decreased cytokine production, most prominently IL-2, resulting in blockade of T- and B-cell activation and proliferation. Both agents are valuable agents in conditions necessitating immunomodulation, including post–solid organ transplantation, with sirolimus additionally having use in those with lymphangioleiomyomatosis.[354] Everolimus is currently used as a treatment modality against various neoplasms, including renal cell cancer, neuroendocrine tumors, and breast cancer.[355]

Purine Synthesis Inhibitors

IMPDH is a purine biosynthetic enzyme crucial to DNA/RNA synthesis, glycoprotein production, and signal transduction. Mycophenolate is a noncompetitive reversible inhibitor of the IMPDH enzyme that is particularly selective toward lymphocytes given their particular reliance on IMPDH for purine synthesis.[356] Azathioprine works similarly by reducing purine synthesis. The medication is a pro-drug and

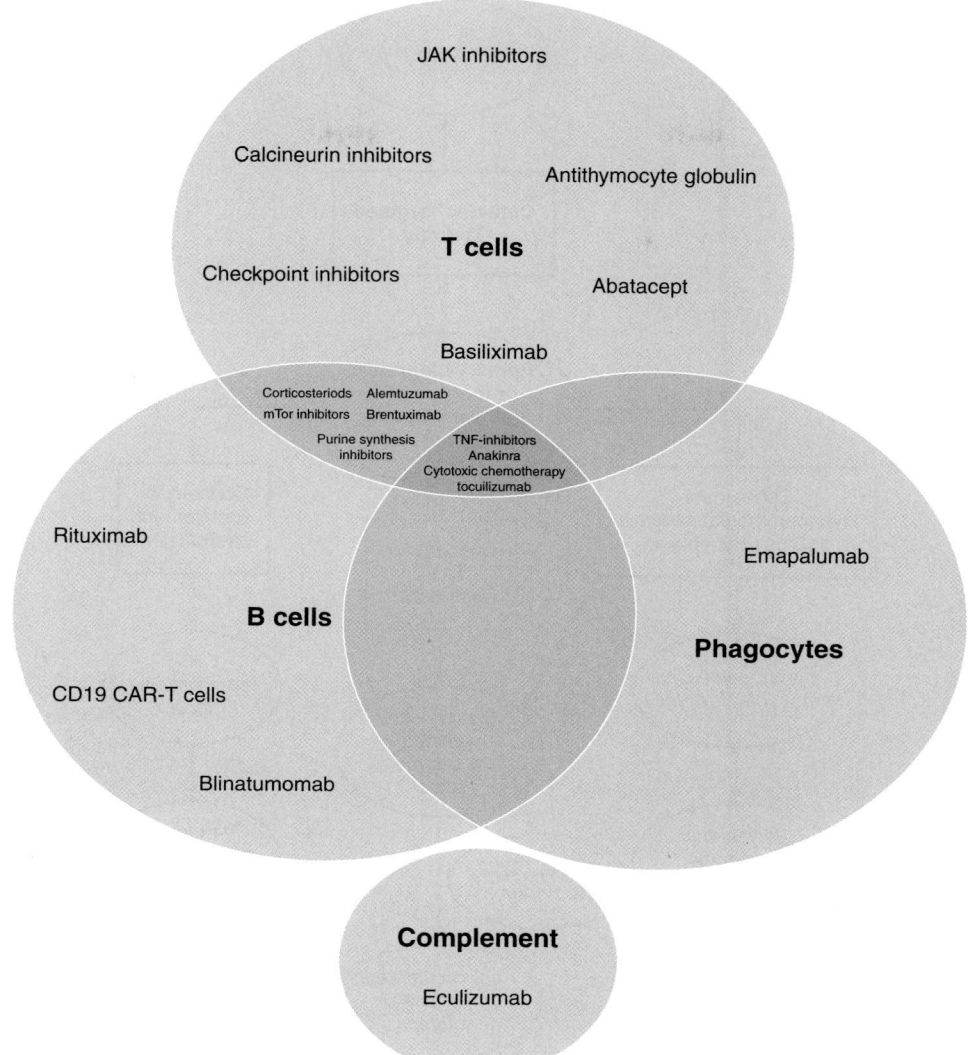

FIGURE 100.12 Target of immunomodulatory therapies. Pharmacologic interventions lead to immune dysregulation via targeting of various aspects of immunity, including T cells, B cells, phagocytes, and the complement system. *CAR-T*, Chimeric antigen receptor T cells; *JAK*, Janus kinase.

is converted to the active 6-mercaptopurine and 6-thioguanine molecules upon absorption. Further metabolism results in the formation of nonfunctional nucleotides that cause cessation of DNA replication and altered purine biosynthesis within lymphocytes.[357,358] Both medications are primarily used clinically in conditions with prominent autoimmunity or immune dysregulation.

Targeted Therapies/Biologics
The ever-growing list of medications that can be classified as biological disease-modifying therapies has not only greatly increased the available treatment options for oncology and rheumatology patients but has additionally expanded the scope of treatment modalities that may have a deleterious effect on immunity (Fig. 100.13). Patients on such therapies appear to be susceptible to a broad range of infectious organisms, including bacterial, parasitic, viral, and fungal, with risk

for each group of microbes somewhat dependent on drug class. Biologic or immune-modifying therapies also have the potential to unmask or exacerbate monogenic defects affecting similar pathways in those with a yet undiagnosed primary immunodeficiency. Furthermore, such drugs may lead to an elevated risk of malignancy or immune dysregulation that can further exacerbate immunodeficiency.[359]

Tumor necrosis factor (TNF) inhibitors, including infliximab, etanercept, and adalimumab, suppress the body's response to TNFα. These agents are used to treat various autoinflammatory conditions. TNFα is mostly produced by macrophages and functions as an acute phase reactant with the ability to upregulate leukocytes and cause systemic inflammation. TNFα inhibition may additionally adversely affect Tregs at times, leading to further immune dysregulation in patients.[360] There is a particular concern for a risk of fungal infection and tuberculosis reactivation in those receiving

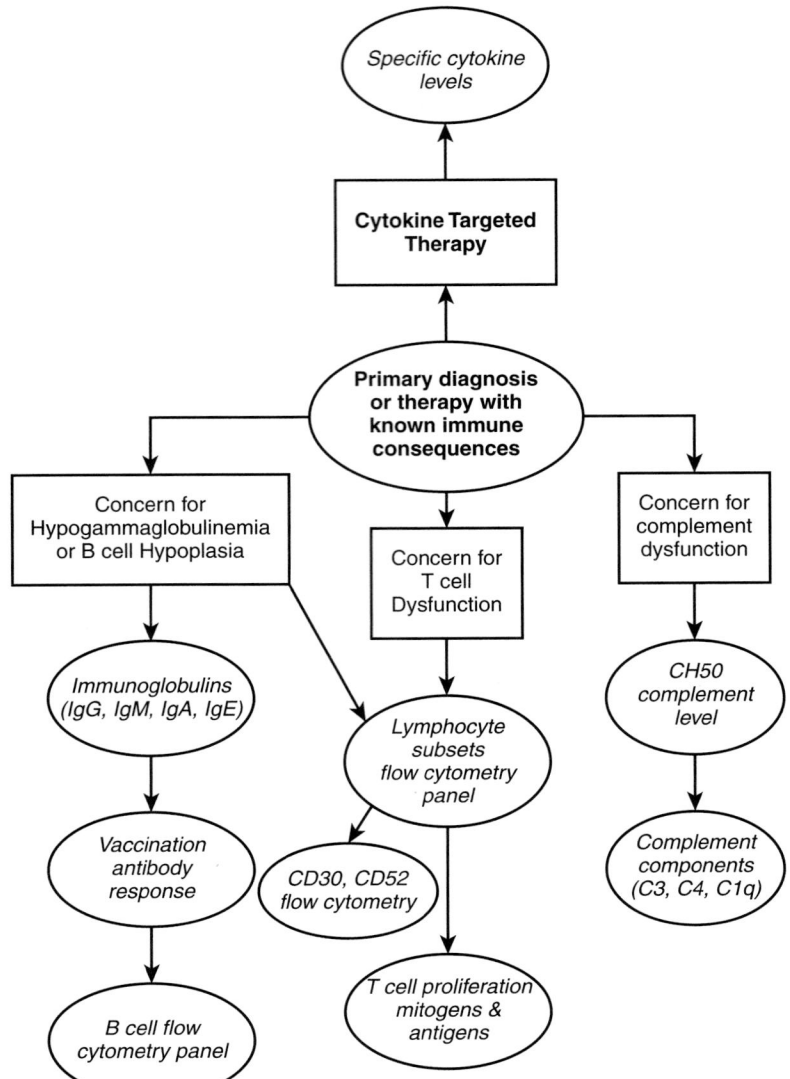

FIGURE 100.13 Diagnostic algorithm for secondary immunodeficiencies. When a suspected diagnosis that leads to secondary immunodeficiency is made or a therapy with known immune consequences is administered, quantitative and qualitative immune testing should be performed. Initial immunologic evaluations include serial immunoglobulin levels, T- and B-cell flow cytometry panels (including assessment of memory and naïve B cells, naïve, memory, activated, exhausted and senescent T cells), NK-cell subset quantitation, assessment of antibody production postvaccinations, lymphocyte proliferation to mitogens (PHA, anti-CD3 stimulants (including anti-CD28 and exogenous interleukin [IL]-2, and/or IL-7), and antigens (*Candida, Tetanus toxoid, Varicella*, Epstein-Barr virus, cytomegalovirus peptides), total complement activity via CH50 levels, and serum cytokine levels, when relevant.

TNF inhibition due to the importance of the protein in host control of these organisms.[361] Screening for tuberculosis should thus be completed prior to initiating therapy.[359]

Anakinra is an altered version of the IL-1 receptor antagonist used in autoimmune conditions and the excessive inflammatory condition of macrophage activating syndrome (MAS). Unlike other biologic agents, an elevated risk of opportunistic infections has not been apparent with Anakinra therapy, although the longer acting agent, Canakinumab, is associated with a higher rate of typical infections, such as urinary tract infections and nasopharyngitis.[361]

There are numerous biological agents targeting CD20,[362] of which rituximab has been the most widely used and studied.

CD20 is an attractive therapeutic target because it is expressed on the majority of peripheral B cells, and is thus useful in both B-cell malignancies and a variety of autoimmune diseases.[363] Hypogammaglobulinemia may occur transiently in patients treated with rituximab but additional reports have shown significant persistent B-cell lymphopenia in a subset of patients.[364] Those most at risk for impaired B-cell reconstitution and/or continued hypogammaglobulinemia include individuals with low IgG or B-cell lymphopenia pre-rituximab, and those receiving intensive combination therapy in addition to rituximab. Laboratory analyses assessing immunoglobulin levels (IgG, IgM, and IgA) and B-cell subset quantification via flow cytometry pre- and post-treatment may be beneficial in monitoring B-cell reconstitution.[364] Vaccination responses may be impaired as well post-rituximab. Granulocytopenia and lymphopenia has also been described.[363] Finally, black box warnings appear on the medication given concern for progressive multifocal leukoencephalopathy (PML) and hepatitis B reactivation, although these are rarely observed.[361] It is unclear to what extent these side effects are observed with other anti-CD20–depleting antibodies since there has been a paucity of immune monitoring data with these.

Similar to the anti-CD20–depleting drugs, there are several drugs that directly and indirectly target IL-6.[365] Of these, Tocilizumab is one of the most well known, and targets the IL-6 receptor. Both tocilizumab and sarilumab have been used with other cytokine-blocking drugs to treat the cytokine storm syndrome in SARS-CoV-2 infection.[366] Tocilizumab may also be used to treat autoimmune disorders or for cytokine release syndrome secondary to chimeric antigen receptor T-cell (CAR-T) therapy. Siltuximab, which directly blocks IL-6, is most often used in Castleman disease. IL-6 blockade negatively affects acute phase reactions and Th17 induction. In clinical trials, the drug was associated with a higher rate of cutaneous and respiratory tract infections. Drug-associated neutropenia and mycobacterium reactivation can occur with the medication but at a lower rate than other biologics.[361]

Emapalumab acts as an anti-interferon-γ antibody. Interferon-γ functions as an activator of macrophages, direct inhibitor of viruses, and assists in inducing MHC molecule expression. Aberrant production of the protein leads to excessive inflammation, which in the case of hemophagocytic lymphohistiocytosis (HLH) can be life-threatening. Those treated with the therapy for HLH do have an elevated risk of infections.[367]

Basiliximab functions as an antibody that competes with IL-2 binding and thus can prevent lymphocyte activation and replication. It is approved for use in renal transplant patients with concerns for organ rejection with further possible benefit in prevention of graft-versus-host disease in bone marrow transplant patients. Trials with the agent have shown an increased risk of infections but no clear pattern for infectious insults has yet been discovered.[361]

Eculizumab binds to the terminal complement component C5 causing its inactivation. The therapy seems to be most beneficial in those with atypical hemolytic uremic syndrome, generalized myasthenia gravis, paroxysmal nocturnal hemoglobinuria (PNH), and neuromyelitis optica spectrum disorder (NMOSD) in adults who are anti–aquaporin-4 (AQP4) antibody positive. Given its effects on complement, the drug causes a particular risk of meningococcal illness and thus immunization against all serotypes of meningococcus should be attempted before drug administration. Patients also appear to have an increased risk of encapsulated organism infection even with vaccination and strong consideration should be given to routine prophylaxis for encapsulated organisms while receiving eculizumab.[361]

Alemtuzumab is a monoclonal antibody that targets CD52-positive mature lymphocytes and thus causes significant prolonged lymphopenia and an elevated risk of fungal, bacterial, and viral infections. It is primarily used in the treatment of hematologic malignancies, multiple sclerosis, refractory HLH, and hematopoietic stem cell transplantation conditioning.[368]

Janus kinase (JAK) inhibitors work through downregulation of the JAK-STAT signaling pathway, which has numerous biologic functions but notably plays a significant role in the propagation of cytokine signaling through increased transcription of targeted genes necessary for inflammation and immunity. Alterations in the pathway inhibit dendritic cell and CD4+ T-cell function and result in additional NK-cell dysfunction.[369] Inhibition of JAK may cause serious and opportunistic infections with viral infections seeming to be most frequently observed.[370]

Abatacept, given its fusion to CTLA-4, prevents the costimulatory signal necessary for T cells to become fully activated. The medication is approved to treat rheumatoid arthritis and juvenile idiopathic arthritis with additional possible benefit of the medication in those with CTLA-4 haploinsufficiency and LRBA deficiency. Prior to beginning therapy, patients should be screened for latent tuberculosis and hepatitis given concern for reactivation with the medication. Infections have been noted in those receiving abatacept, but studies show no significant increase in overall infections.[361]

Antithymocyte globulin (ATG) compromises immunoglobulins derived from rabbits or horses exposed to human lymphoid cells. The therapy is used in induction regimens for hematopoietic cell and solid organ transplantation. It has also been found to be beneficial in the treatment of severe idiopathic aplastic anemia. The immunologic effects of ATG include inhibition of cutaneous delayed hypersensitivity and disruption of the interaction of antigen-presenting cells with T lymphocytes.[371] Such changes in immunity elevate susceptibility to most herpes viruses, especially cytomegalovirus. Serum sickness may also result from administration of the drug leading to a robust dysregulation in immune-mediated processes.[372]

Immunotherapy is increasingly becoming a treatment option for those suffering from refractory malignancies. Such therapies offer hope for a cure but additionally may alter the recipient's immunity. Chimeric antigen receptor T-cell (CAR-T) therapy involves modifying the patient's own T cells to improve recognition and cytotoxic immune destruction of their neoplastic cells. Most commonly used presently are CD19 CAR-T cells but T cells targeting CD20, CD30, CD38, and CD138 are also being assessed clinically in the treatment of hematologic cancers.[373] In particular such therapy has offered significant therapeutic benefit in patients with refractory/relapsed B-cell acute lymphoblastic leukemia, diffuse large B cell lymphoma, and chronic lymphocytic leukemia.[374] Clearance of healthy CD19 cells, in addition to malignant cells, often leads to B-cell aplasia necessitating regular immunoglobulin replacement. Prolonged cytopenias do occur with CAR-T administration even in the absence of lymphodepletion and can lead to an elevated infection risk. Indirect suppression of immunity may result after CAR-T delivery if an exuberant response to the therapy causes a condition known as cytokine release syndrome (CRS) that manifests as a severe systemic inflammatory response. The exact pathophysiology of CRS is not fully understood but appears to result from treatment-related activation of not only target neoplastic cells, but also bystander immune and nonimmune cells, including endothelial cells. This activation leads to a massive release of cytokines, most prominently interferon-gamma, IL-6, and IL-10.[374] CRS clinically presents with a range of symptoms, from a mild, flu-like illness to a life-threatening presentation characterized by multi–end-organ damage, massive vascular leakage with pulmonary edema, hypotension, and disseminated intravascular coagulation. Significant neurologic consequences may also occur following CAR-T therapy with aphasia, cranial nerve palsies, hemiparesis, seizures, and disorientation possible. CRS treatment involves administration of corticosteroids and the IL-6 receptor antagonist, tocilizumab, both of which function through immune depression.[373,375] Of note, CAR-T cell therapies are increasingly being used to treat solid neoplasms, but it has yet to be determined the immunologic consequences of such therapies that do not directly target lymphoid or myeloid cells.[376]

The bispecific T-cell engaging (BiTE) antibody, blinatumomab, consists of an anti-CD19 antibody linked to a CD3 specific antibody. Effector T cells can thus closely engage with malignant CD19+ cells resulting in their destruction. Just as in CD19 directed CAR-T cells, blinatumomab treatment can lead to B-cell aplasia and hypogammaglobulinemia.[369]

Brentuximab, an anti-CD30 antibody, is increasingly being used to treat various hematologic malignancies, including Hodgkin lymphoma, anaplastic large cell lymphoma, and CD30 expressing mycosis fungoides. The immunologic defects caused by Brentuximab are currently poorly defined but may include transient neutropenia and impaired memory cell creation.[369]

Checkpoint inhibitors function through altering the normal mechanisms employed by the body to dampen a response to an immunologic stimulus. Such therapies are now being used to block the inhibitory immune response to allow for increased clearance of cancerous cells. The most commonly used checkpoint inhibitors target CTLA4 (Ipilimumab), PD-1 (Nivolumab/Pembrolizumab), and PD-L1 (Atezolizumab/Avelumab). These therapies do not appear to have direct immunosuppressive effects but can lead to immune-related adverse events (irAEs). Patients most commonly experience dermatologic toxicities (pruritic rashes and vitiligo), asymptomatic transaminitis, arthritis, diarrhea secondary to colitis, and endocrinopathies (hypophysitis, adrenal insufficiency, and thyroid abnormalities). Serious and potentially fatal irAEs include pneumonitis, encephalitis/meningitis, immune-mediated cytopenias, severe hepatitis, and myocarditis/pericarditis.[377,378] The possibly significant secondary inflammatory consequences from checkpoint inhibitor usage may necessitate treatment with anti-inflammatory and immuno-modulatory agents, which may result in a risk of serious infections.[369,379] Finally, increasing usage of checkpoint inhibitors has led to the recognition of unforeseen consequences of the drugs, including at times promoting progression, rather than increasing destruction, of malignant cells.[380]

Interestingly, the irAEs observed following usage of checkpoint inhibitors mirror somewhat the signs and symptoms seen in individuals diagnosed with CTLA-4 haploinsufficiency and LRBA deficiency (these are caused by germline variants in either the *CTLA4* (cytotoxic T-lymphocyte protein-4) or *LRBA* (LPS-responsive beige-like anchor) genes. LRBA is crucial to the intracellular trafficking of CLTA4 by removing it from intracellular degradation and directing it to the cell surface,[11] although some differences are present. Dysregulated Tregs, hyperactivation of effector T cells, and organ infiltration by lymphocytes characterize the pathophysiology of the conditions.[10,381] Just as in those exposed to checkpoint inhibition, patients with LRBA deficiency or CTLA-4 haploinsufficiency may suffer from colitis, immune

dysregulation related rashes (eczema and psoriasis), endocrinopathies, and arthritis, although manifestations secondary to excessive lymphoproliferation (splenomegaly, lymphadenopathy, and lymphocytic brain infiltration) and immune-mediated cytopenias appear to be more prominent in those with primary defects in CTLA-4 or LRBA. Furthermore, immunodeficiency with elevated occurrence of infections resulting from lymphopenia (B and T cell) and hypogammaglobulinemia is also much more commonly observed in individuals with genetic alterations in the checkpoint pathway.[382] As noted above, re-establishing CTLA-4 activity through the usage of Abatacept appears to be beneficial in alleviating some of the disease manifestations of these disorders.[10,383]

Diagnosis of Secondary Immunodeficiency

The diagnosis of many of the causes of secondary immunodeficiencies involves specific laboratory and imaging studies in those with a high degree of clinical suspicion for a particular disorder. Bone marrow evaluation with pathologic assessment, flow cytometry, and cytogenetics is often necessary to make a diagnosis of a hematologic neoplasm or aplastic anemia. Imaging studies, including abdominal ultrasound, echocardiogram, chest x-ray, computed tomography with intravascular contrast, and magnetic resonance enterography may assist in the diagnosis of asplenia, congenital cardiac anomalies, thymoma, intestinal lymphangiectasia, and inflammatory bowel disease.

General laboratory studies, such as complete blood cell counts and comprehensive metabolic panels, can uncover a malignancy, renal disease, or significant hepatic dysfunction diagnosis. Blood polymerase chain reaction testing for CMV, EBV, parvovirus, and adenovirus is now becoming more common. Specific testing for HIV, measles, EBV, and CMV antibodies may also be beneficial. Direct visual inspection of stool and blood may locate parasitic organisms or their eggs (ova). Acid-fast bacilli (AFB) smear and culture testing assists in the diagnosis of mycobacterial infections. Testing via comprehensive genetic panels can discover a primary immunodeficiency/immune dysregulation condition only suspected once unmasked following treatment with an immunomodulatory agent.

Once a suspected primary diagnosis that leads to secondary immunodeficiency is made or a therapy with known deleterious immune consequences is administered, quantitative and qualitative immune testing can be completed. Serial immunoglobulin level testing and B cell flow cytometry panels (including ones that assess memory and naïve B cells) are useful in conditions/medications known to cause hypogammaglobulinemia or B cell hypoplasia. Assessment of antibody production postvaccination may also be helpful. If there is concern for T-cell abnormalities, flow cytometry of peripheral blood can yield absolute T-cell subclass numbers. Flow cytometry can be used to assess CD52 and CD30 status following Alemtuzumab and Brentuximab therapy, respectively. Lymphocyte proliferation to mitogens and antigens allows for further evaluation of T-cell dysfunction. Total complement activity may be measured via CH50 testing, with specific complement components, such as C3, C4, and C1, additionally capable of being assessed. For monitoring eculizumab therapy, it is most useful to measure CH50 with C5 function, as opposed to C5 levels, which will not be useful in patients being actively treated. Many commercial labs now offer the ability to monitor serum cytokine levels, which can be beneficial to monitor either the consequences or benefits of targeted immune therapies.

Treatment of Secondary Immunodeficiency

Treatment of secondary immunodeficiencies involves control of the underlying primary condition leading to immune dysregulation. Intravenous or subcutaneous immunoglobulin replacement may be beneficial in those with hypogammaglobulinemia.[384] Antimicrobial prophylaxis may be necessary if significant neutropenia or lymphopenia is present. Aggressive treatment with broad-spectrum antibiotics or antifungals may additionally be warranted in those with a high suspicion for fungemia or bacteremia. Supportive interventions may include use of irradiated blood products and avoidance of live vaccines.

SELECTED REFERENCES

3. Tangye SG, Al-Herz W, Bousfiha A, et al. Human inborn errors of immunity: 2019 update on the classification from the International Union of Immunological Societies Expert Committee. J Clin Immunol 2020;40:24–64.

14. Bousfiha A, Jeddane L, Picard C, et al. Human inborn errors of immunity: 2019 update of the IUIS phenotypical classification. J Clin Immunol 2020;40:66–81.

17. Rivers L, Gaspar HB. Severe combined immunodeficiency: recent developments and guidance on clinical management. Arch Dis Child 2015;100:667–72.

18. Tasher D, Dalal I. The genetic basis of severe combined immunodeficiency and its variants. Appl Clin Genet 2012;5:67–80.

19. Shearer WT, Dunn E, Notarangelo LD, et al. Establishing diagnostic criteria for severe combined immunodeficiency disease (SCID), leaky SCID, and Omenn syndrome: the primary immune deficiency treatment consortium experience. J Allergy Clin Immunol 2014;133:1092–8.

24. Amatuni GS, Sciortino S, Currier RJ, Naides SJ, Church JA, Puck JM. Reference intervals for lymphocyte subsets in preterm and term neonates without immune defects. J Allergy Clin Immunol 2019;144:1674–83.

27. Tate JR, Yen T, Jones GR. Transference and validation of reference intervals. Clin Chem 2015;61:1012–5.

30. Ravkov E, Slev P, Heikal N. Thymic output: assessment of CD4(+) recent thymic emigrants and T-Cell receptor excision circles in infants. Cytometry B Clin Cytom 2017;92:249–57.

31. Abraham RS. Assessment of functional immune responses in lymphocytes. In: Rich RR, Fleisher TA, Shearer WT, Schroeder HW, Frew AJ, Weyand CM, editors. Clinical immunology: principles and practice. 5th ed. Elsevier; 2018.

68. Keller MD, Bollard CM. Virus-specific T-cell therapies for patients with primary immune deficiency. Blood 2020;135:620–8.

80. Sullivan KE. Chromosome 22q11.2 deletion syndrome and DiGeorge syndrome. Immunol Rev 2019;287:186–201.

103. Candotti F. Clinical manifestations and pathophysiological mechanisms of the Wiskott-Aldrich syndrome. J Clin Immunol 2018;38:13–27.

125. Bonilla FA, Barlan I, Chapel H, et al. International Consensus Document (ICON): common variable immunodeficiency disorders. J Allergy Clin Immunol Pract 2016;4:38–59.

151. Chinn IK, Bostwick BL. The role of genomic approaches in diagnosis and management of primary immunodeficiency. Curr Opin Pediatr 2018;30:791–7.

208. Elloumi HZ, Holland SM. Diagnostic assays for chronic granulomatous disease and other neutrophil disorders. Methods Mol Biol 2007;412:505–23.

215. Kuhns DB, Alvord WG, Heller T, et al. Residual NADPH oxidase and survival in chronic granulomatous disease. N Engl J Med 2010;363:2600–10.

216. Sacco KA, Smith MJ, Bahna SL, et al. NAPDH oxidase-specific flow cytometry allows for rapid genetic triage and classification of novel variants in chronic granulomatous disease. J Clin Immunol 2020;40:191–202.

271. Abraham RS, Aubert G. Flow cytometry, a versatile tool for diagnosis and monitoring of primary immunodeficiencies. Clin Vaccine Immunol 2016;23:254–71.

298. Richardson AM, Moyer AM, Hasadsri L, Abraham RS. Diagnostic tools for inborn errors of human immunity (primary immunodeficiencies and immune dysregulatory diseases). Curr Allergy Asthma Rep 2018;18:19.

361. Henrickson SE, Ruffner MA, Kwan M. Unintended immunological consequences of biologic therapy. Curr Allergy Asthma Rep 2016;16:46.

Reference Information for the Clinical Laboratory*

Khosrow Adeli, Victoria Higgins, and Mary Kathryn Bohn[a]

ABSTRACT

Background

Accurate reference intervals established in healthy subjects are essential for appropriate interpretation of laboratory test results and to assist clinicians in diagnosis, monitoring, and treatment of disease. To facilitate interpretation of laboratory tests, reference intervals must be appropriately stratified based on key covariates, including age, sex, and ethnicity, which may alter "normal" analyte concentrations. When establishing or implementing reference intervals, it is important to consider the effect of these covariates as well as methodologic and regional variances. Notably, reference intervals may also be method and population dependent; thus reference intervals and clinical decision limits may vary across clinical laboratories. Reference intervals from one laboratory should not be adopted by another laboratory without first ensuring that proper transference and verification protocols have been completed.

Content

This chapter provides reference information for biochemical markers in serum, plasma, urine, and other body fluids, as well as for therapeutic drug monitoring and toxicology, hematologic parameters, and critical risk values. Where possible, method-, age-, and sex-specific partitions and values for both conventional and SI units are included. Reference publications are listed to support the values reported in this chapter. The reference information presented here has been updated using recently published studies where possible; however, some values were obtained from the previous edition. Most pediatric values were obtained from the Canadian Laboratory Initiative on Pediatric Reference Intervals (CALIPER) study.[2]

OVERVIEW

Reference intervals are defined as "limiting values within which a specified percentage (usually 95%) of apparently healthy individuals' results would fall"—usually the 2.5th and 97.5th centiles of the test result distribution in the reference (healthy) population (see Chapter 9).

Reference limits and intervals provide valuable information to medical practitioners in their interpretation of quantitative laboratory test results, serving as health-associated benchmarks to which individual test results can be compared. Although the concept of reference intervals and their utility appears straightforward, the process of establishing accurate and reliable reference intervals is considerably complex and involved, requiring recruitment of a large number of healthy individuals. This is particularly challenging for pediatric populations. Each clinical laboratory is responsible for ensuring the validity of reference intervals reported with their test results. Accrediting and licensing organizations and regulatory bodies governing medical laboratory best practices require that individual laboratories establish or verify reference intervals for all quantitative test methods, the exception being for tests that employ clinical decision limits (e.g., cholesterol, hemoglobin A_{1C}). It is important to note that values from apparently healthy and diseased populations may overlap significantly. Therefore reference intervals, although useful as a guide for clinicians, should not be used as absolute indicators of health and disease. Unfortunately, reference intervals are obtained with analytical procedures that produce results traceable only to the corresponding reference system and thus cannot be directly applied by any laboratory, because standardized methods, particularly for immunoassays, do not exist in most cases. As a result, the presented reference intervals are all, more or less, method-dependent. Moreover, it is not yet clear to what extent ethnicity and local environmental factors could influence the reference intervals for specific analytes. For these reasons, the reference intervals presented in the following tables are for general informational purposes only. Each individual laboratory should generate its own set of reference intervals or validate published reference intervals based on the CLSI C28-A3 guidelines (CLSI document C28-A3. Wayne PA Clinical and Laboratory Standards Institute 2008, p. 76).

*The full version of this chapter is available electronically on ExpertConsult.com.
[a]The chapter is based on Adeli K, Ceriotti F, Nieuwesteeg M. Reference information for the clinical laboratory. In: Rifai N, Horvath AR, Wittwer C, editors. Tietz textbook of clinical chemistry and molecular diagnostics. 6th ed. St. Louis: Elsevier; 2018. pp. 1745–818.

Reference Information Tables and Figures

CHAPTER OUTLINE

Tables A.1 to A.5 include up-to-date reference interval information obtained from recent initiatives to establish adult and pediatric reference intervals for a wide range of biochemical and hematologic markers. As much as possible, data from recent a priori reference interval studies have been used to update each table and provide robust reference information obtained from large studies based on healthy populations. Where no new data were available, original reference intervals were adopted from the previous (sixth edition) tables.[1]

Table A.1 combines biochemical marker reference interval information for both children and adults. Most pediatric reference intervals listed in this chapter are based on recent

data published by the Canadian Laboratory Initiative on Pediatric Reference Intervals (CALIPER), a national research project that has established age- and sex-specific reference intervals using data collected from thousands of healthy community children and adolescents.[3–26] The majority of CALIPER reference intervals included in this textbook were determined based on Abbott Architect assays. However, CALIPER transference data for common biochemical parameters and direct reference value data for immunochemical parameters are now available on other analytical chemistry systems, including the Beckman (AU, DxC & DxI),[12,21–23] Ortho (Vitros),[8,21,24] Roche (cobas & Modular),[21,25,26] and Siemens (ADVIA, EXL, Vista)[19,21] platforms. For some chemistry, hematology and special endocrine markers, both pediatric and adult reference values were obtained through the Canadian Health Measures Survey (CHMS) based on a study of approximately 12,000 children, adults, and elderly (3 to 79 years of age).[27–29] CHMS reference intervals were determined on a number of platforms (Ortho Clinical Diagnostics; Siemens and Beckman Coulter), as specified in the tables. Other reference intervals were adopted from reference tables in the sixth edition of this text[1] and other sources.[30–39]

Table A.2 lists reference intervals for routine tests performed on body fluids. Intervals were derived from the sixth edition of this text,[1] as well as from Zhang and associates.[40]

Table A.3 provides reference information for therapeutic drug monitoring, with toxicology tests shown in a separate table. Reference intervals were derived from the sixth edition of this text,[1] as well as from Hiemke and colleagues.[41]

Table A.4 depicts common hematologic markers based on the CHMS database (3 to 79 years),[29] the recent CALIPER hematology studies on the Beckman Coulter DxH 900 (birth to 19 years),[42] and on the Sysmex XN3000 analytical platform (birth to 19 years).[53]

Table A.5, in addition to reference intervals, provides a table of critical risk intervals. Notification of critical results to clinical staff is an important postanalytical process in all acute-care clinical laboratories. Data from a number of sources (references 1 and 44 to 48; CLSI, guideline GP47; Wayne PA: CLSI; 2015:100) have been used to generate a table of recommended intervals to assist laboratories when establishing and updating their critical risk result management policy.

Finally, biological variation is an important factor to consider when interpreting laboratory test results in a clinical setting. Biological variation represents the physiologic changes that occur within and between individuals for a specific analyte. Biological variation is important to consider for establishing the usual amounts of fluctuation for a given analyte when monitoring or following a patient, and for establishing quality specifications. Biological variation data have not been included in this chapter, but further information on biological variation in adults can be found from a number of sources.[49–51] Within-day pediatric biological variation information has also been published.[52] Chapter 8 provides detailed information about biological variation.

[b]CALIPER Cohort. *Canadian Laboratory Initiative on Pediatric Reference Intervals.* CALIPER Publications: Bailey et al. *Clin Chem* 2013;59(9):1393–405; Bevilacqua et al. *Clin Chem* 2014;60(12):1532–42; Bohn et al. *Clin Chem* 2019;65(4):589–91; Bohn et al. *Clin Biochem* 2020;76:31–4; Colantonio et al. *Clin Chem* 2012;58(5):854–68; Higgins et al. *Clin Chem Lab Med* 2018;56(2):327–40; Higgins et al. *Clin Chem Lab Med* 2018;56(6):964–72; Higgins et al. *Clin Chim Acta* 2018;486:129–34; Higgins et al. *EJIFCC* 2017;28(1):77; Karbasy et al. *Clin Chem Lab Med* 2016;54(4):643–57; Kavsak et al. *Clin Chem* 2014;60(12):1574–6; Kelly et al. *Clin Chim Acta* 2015;450:196–202; Konforte et al. *Clin Chem* 2013;59(8):1215–27; Kyriakopoulou et al. *Clin Biochem* 2013;46(7–8):642–51; Raizman et al. *Clin Chem Lab Med* 2015;53(10):e239–43; Raizman et al. *Clin Biochem* 2014;47:812–15; Tahmasebi et al. *Clin Chim Acta* 2019;490:88–97; Teodoro Morrison et al. *Clin Biochem* 2015;48(13–14):828–36
[c]Canadian Health Measures Survey. Adeli K et al. *Clin Chem* 2015; 61(8);1049–1062; Adeli K et al. *Clin Chem* 2015;61(8);1063–1074.
[d]Canadian Health Measures Survey. *Biochemical Markers.* Adeli K et al. *Clin Chem* 2015;61(8);1049–1062; Adeli K et al. *Clin Chem* 2015;61(8);1063–1074.

TABLE A.1 Pediatric and Adult Reference Intervals for Biochemical Markers (Serum, Plasma, and Urine)

Analyte	Specimen	Condition	REFERENCE INTERVALS			Reference Publication
			Conventional Units	Conversion Factor	SI Units	
Acetaldehyde	WB (F⁻/Ox)		mg/dL	22.7	µmol/L	
			<0.2		<4.5	1
		Occup exp	<0.5		<11.4	
		Toxic	1–2		22.7–45.4	
Acetylaspartic acid	U				mmol/mol creatinine	
					<14	1
α₁-Acid glycoprotein	S		mg/dL	0.01	g/L	
Pediatric values (0–19 y) based on Abbott Architect method		0–<6 mo	21–85		0.2–0.9	14
		6 mo–<5 y	48–201		0.5–2.0	
		5–<19 y	48–114		0.5–1.1	
		Adult (20–60 y)	50–120		0.5–1.2	
cis-Aconitic acid	U				mmol/mol creatinine	
		0–1 mo			5–31	1
		1–6 mo			10–97	
		6 mo–5 y			10–97	
		>5 y			3–44	
Adipic acid	U				mmol/mol creatinine	
		0–6 mo			9–37	1
		6 mo–5 y			<16	
		>5 y			<6	
Adipocarnitine	U				mmol/mol creatinine	
		0–7 d			0.04–0.40	1
		8 d–7 y			0.01–0.81	
		>7 y			0.00–0.13	
Adrenocorticotropic hormone (ACTH)	P, EDTA		pg/mL	0.22	pmol/L	
ACTH reference intervals may vary depending on immunoassay methods		Cord	50–570		11–125	1
		Newborn	10–185		2.2–41	
		Adult (0800–0900 h)	<120		<26	
		Adult (24 h, supine)	<85		<19	
Alanine	P		mg/dL	112.2	µmol/L	
		Premature, 1 d	2.44–4.24		274–476	1
		Newborn, 1 d	2.10–3.65		236–410	
		1–3 mo	1.19–3.71		134–416	
		2–6 mo	1.58–3.68		177–413	
		9 mo–2 y	0.88–2.79		99–313	
		3–10 y	1.22–2.71		137–305	
		6–18 y	1.72–4.85		193–545	
		Adult	1.87–5.88		210–661	
	S	0–<1 wk	1.56–3.81		175–427	20
		1 wk–<19 y	1.85–5.24		208–588	
	U, 24 h		mg/d	11.2	µmol/d	
		10 d–7 wk	4.1–9.3		46–104	
		3–12 y	9.1–39.2		102–439	
		Adult	7.9–48.3		88–541	
			µmol/g creatinine	0.113	µmol/mol creatinine	
		0–1 mo	554–2957		62.6–334.1	
		1–6 mo	613–2874		59.3–324.8	
		6 mo–1 y	428–2064		48.4–233.2	
		1–2 y	389–1497		44.0–169.2	
		2–3 y	255–1726		28.8–195.0	

TABLE A.1   Pediatric and Adult Reference Intervals for Biochemical Markers (Serum, Plasma, and Urine)—cont'd

Analyte	Specimen	Condition	REFERENCE INTERVALS Conventional Units	Conversion Factor	SI Units	Reference Publication
Alanine aminotransferase	S		U/L	0.017	µkat/L	
With pyridoxal phosphate		0–<1 y	5–51		0.08–0.85	7
Values (0–<3 y) based on Abbott Architect method		1–<3 y	11–30		0.18–0.50	
Values (3–79 y) based on OCD Vitros method		3–5 y	15–33		0.26–0.56	27
		6–8 y	16–37		0.27–0.63	
		9–11 y	18–39		0.31–0.66	
		12–17 y, M	17–50		0.29–0.85	
		12–49 y, F	14–41		0.24–0.70	
		18–49 y, M	18–78		0.31–1.33	
		50–79 y, M	20–62		0.34–1.05	
		50–79 y, F	16–44		0.27–0.75	
Without pyridoxal phosphate		0–<1 y	5–33		0.08–0.56	7
		1–<13 y	9–25		0.15–0.43	
		13–19 y	8–22		0.14–0.37	
Albumin (BCG)	S		g/dL	10	g/L	
Values (0–<3 y) based on Abbott Architect method	S	0–<15 d	3.3–4.5	10	33–45	7
		15 d–<1 y	2.8–4.7		28–47	
		1–<8 y	3.8–4.7		38–47	
		8–<15 y	4.1–4.8		41–48	
		15–<19 y F	4.0–4.9		40–49	
		15–<19 y M	4.1–5.1		41–51	
Values (3–79 y) based on OCD Vitros method		3–5 y	3.9–5.0		39–50	27
		6–15 y	4.1–5.1		41–51	
		16–29 y, M	4.6–5.3		46–53	
		16–54 y, F	3.9–5.0		39–50	
		30–54 y, M	4.4–5.1		44–51	
		55–79 y	4.2–5.0		42–50	
	CSF, lumbar	See Table A.2				1
		Adult				
		20–60 y	3.5–5.2		35–52	
		60–90 y	3.2–4.6		32–46	
		>90 y	2.9–4.5		29–45	
Values (3–79 y) based on OCD Vitros method	U		mg/L	1	mg/L	
		3–5 y	1.5–21.5		1.5–21.5	28
		6–8 y	1.5–37.8		1.5–37.8	
		9–19 y	1.5–169.6		1.5–169.6	
		20–29 y	1.5–74.6		1.5–74.6	
		30–39 y	1.5–36.8		1.5–36.8	
		40–79 y	1.5–47.2		1.5–47.2	
Albumin-creatinine ratio (NKDEP guidelines; see also Chapter 34)			mg/mmol		mg/g creatinine	
		M	<2.5		<22	
		F	<3.5		<30	
Aldolase	S		U/L	0.017	µkat/L	
		Child				1
		10–24 mo	10–40		0.17–0.68	
		25 mo–16 y	5–20		0.09–0.34	
		Adult	2.5–10.0		0.04–0.13	
Aldosterone	S		ng/dL	0.0277	nmol/L	
		Cord blood	40–200		1.11–5.54	1
		Premature infant	19–141		0.53–3.91	
		Full-term infant				
		3 d	7–184		0.19–5.10	
		1 wk	5–175		0.03–4.85	
		1–12 mo	5–90		0.14–2.49	

Continued

TABLE A.1 **Pediatric and Adult Reference Intervals for Biochemical Markers (Serum, Plasma, and Urine)—cont'd**

Analyte	Specimen	Condition	REFERENCE INTERVALS			Reference Publication
			Conventional Units	Conversion Factor	SI Units	
		1–2 y	7–54		0.19–1.50	
		2–10 y (supine)	3–35		0.08–0.97	
		2–10 y (upright)	5–80		0.14–2.22	
		10–15 y (supine)	2–22		0.06–0.61	
		10–15 y (upright)	4–48		0.11–1.33	
		Adult				
		Supine	3–16		0.08–0.44	
		Upright	7–30		0.19–0.83	
	U, 24 h		μg/d		nmol/d	
				2.77		
		Newborn (1–3 d)	0.5–5		1–14	1
		Prepubertal child				
		4–10 y	1–8		3–22	
		Adult	3–19		8–53	
Aluminum	S, P		μg/L	0.0371	μmol/L	
			<5.51		<0.2	1
		Patients on hemodialysis	20–550		0.74–20.4	
		Al medication	<30		<1.11	
	U		5–30		0.19–1.11	
Ammonia nitrogen	P (Hep)		μg N/dL	0.714	μmol N/L	
		Newborn	90–150		64–107	1
		0–2 wk	79–129		56–92	
		>1 mo	29–70		21–50	
		Adult	15–45		11–32	
	U, 24 h		mg N/d	0.0714	mmol N/d	
		Infant	560–2900		40–207	1
		Adult	140–1500		10–107	
Amylase	S		U/L	0.017	μkat/L	
Values (0–<19 y) based on Abbott Architect method		0–14 d	3–10		0.05–0.17	7
		15 d–<13 wk	2–22		0.03–0.37	
		13 wk–<1 y	3–50		0.05–0.83	
		1–<19 y	25–101		0.42–1.68	
IFCC, 37°C		Adult	31–107		0.52–1.78	30
Amylase (pancreatic)	S		U/L	0.017	μkat/L	
Values (0–<19 y) based on Abbott Architect method		0–<6 mo	<11.5		<0.20	14
		6 mo–<1 y	0.62–23.2		0.01–0.39	
		1–<2 y, F	2.63–27.8		0.04–0.47	
		1–<2 y, M	0.68–22.5		0.01–0.38	
		2–<19 y	4.10–31.3		0.07–0.53	
Androgen index, free (FAI)					%	
	S	0–<1 y, F			0.04–1.32	18
		1–<9 y, F			0.04–1.32	
		9–<14 y, F			0.12–2.63	
		14–19 y, F			0.59–6.50	
		0–<1 y, M			0.02–32.72	
		1–<9 y, M			0.03–0.60	
		9–<14 y, M			0.15–34.68	
		14–<19 y, M			3.58–83.30	
		Note: FAI should not be used in men if testosterone levels exceed SHBG binding capacity.				
3α-Androstanediol glucuronide	S	Levels may exceed SHBG binding capacity	ng/dL	0.0213	nmol/L	
		Child, prepubertal	10–60		0.2–1.3	1

TABLE A.1 Pediatric and Adult Reference Intervals for Biochemical Markers (Serum, Plasma, and Urine)—cont'd

Analyte	Specimen	Condition	REFERENCE INTERVALS Conventional Units	Conversion Factor	SI Units	Reference Publication
		Adult, M	260–1500		5.5–32	
		Adult, F	60–300		1.3–6.4	
Androstenedione (LC-MS/ MS)	S		ng/L			37
		6–24 mo	25–150			
		2–3 y	<110			
		4–5 y	23–170			
		6–7 y	10–290			
		7–9 y	30–300			
		10–11 y	70–390			
		12–13 y	100–640			
		14–15 y	180–940			
		16–17 y	300–1130			
		18–40 y	330–1340			
		40–67 y	280–890			
Vasopressin (Antidiuretic hormone [ADH])	P, EDTA	mOsm/kg	ng/L	0.926	pmol/L	
		270–280	<1.5		<1.4	1
		280–285	<2.5		<2.3	
		285–290	1–5		0.9–4.6	
		290–294	2–7		1.9–6.5	
		295–300	4–12		3.7–11.1	
Antimony	P (Hep)		μg/dL	82.1	nmol/L	
			0.014–0.090		1.15–7.39	1
	U		μg/L	8.21	nmol/L	
			<10		<82.1	
			mg/L		μmol/L	
		Toxic	>1		>8.21	
Antistreptolysin-O (ASO)	S		IU/mL	1	kIU/L	
Values (0–<19 y) based on Abbott Architect method		0–<6 mo	0–0		0–0	7
		6 mo–<1 y	0–30		0–30	
		1–<6 y	0–104		0–104	
		6–<19 y	0–331		0–331	
		Adult	<20–364		<20–364	32
Antithyroglobulin (Anti-Tg)	S		IU/mL	1	kIU/L	
Values based on Abbott Architect method		0–<19 y	0.4–17.7		0.4–17.7	4
α₁-Antitrypsin	S		mg/dL	0.01	g/L	
Values (0–<19 y) based on Abbott Architect method		0–<19 y	110–181		1.1–1.8	14
		Adult (20–60 y)	90–200		0.9–2.0	1
Apolipoprotein AI	S		mg/dL	0.01	g/L	
Values (0–<6 y) based on Abbott Architect method		0–14 d, F	71–97		0.7–1.0	7
		0–14 d, M	62–91		0.6–0.9	
		15 d–<1 y	53–175		0.5–1.8	
		1–<6 y	80–164		0.8–1.6	
Values (6–79 y) based on OCD Vitros method		6–15 y	100–180		1.0–1.8	28
		16–39 y, M	80–170		0.8–1.7	
		16–39 y, F	100–200		1.0–2.0	
		40–79 y, M	120–200		1.2–2.0	
		40–79 y, F	110–230		1.1–2.3	
Apolipoprotein B-100	S		mg/dL	0.01	g/L	
Values (0–<6 y) based on Abbott Architect method		0–14 d	9–67		0.1–0.7	7
		15 d–<1 y	19–123		0.2–1.2	
		1–<6 y	41–93		0.4–0.9	
Values (6–79 y) based on OCD Vitros method		6–13 y	50–100		0.5–1.0	28
		14–29 y	40–110		0.4–1.1	
		30–79 y	60–140		0.6–1.4	

Continued

TABLE A.1 Pediatric and Adult Reference Intervals for Biochemical Markers (Serum, Plasma, and Urine)—cont'd

Analyte	Specimen	Condition	REFERENCE INTERVALS Conventional Units	Conversion Factor	SI Units	Reference Publication
Arginine	P		mg/dL	57.4	μmol/L	
		Premature, 1 d	0.17–1.57		10–90	1
		Newborn, 1 d	0.38–1.53		22–88	
		1–3 mo	0.38–1.30		22–74	
		2–6 mo	0.98–2.47		56–142	
		9 mo–2 y	0.19–1.13		11–65	
		3–10 y	0.40–1.50		23–86	
		6–18 y	0.77–2.26		44–130	
		Adult	0.37–2.40		21–138	
	S	0–<1 mo	0.03–2.06		2–118	20
		1 mo–<1 y	0.82–2.40		47–138	
		1–<19 y	1.15–2.61		66–150	
	U, 24 h		mg/d	5.74	μmol/d	
		10 d–7 wk	<1.2		<7	1
		3–12 y	<5.1		<29	
		Adult	<50.2		<288	
			mg/g creatinine	0.65	mmol/mol creatinine	
		Adult	0–4		0–2.7	
Arsenic	WB (Hep)		μg/L	0.0113	μmol/L	
		Not exposed	2–23		0.03–0.31	1
		Chronic poisoning	100–500		1.33–6.65	
		Acute poisoning	600–9300		7.98–124	
		Not exposed	2–23		0.03–0.31	
Ascorbic acid (see vitamin C)						1
Asparagine	P		mg/dL	75.7	μmol/L	
		1–3 mo	0.08–0.44		6–33	1
		3 mo–6 y	0.95–1.90		72–144	
		6–18 y	0.42–0.82		32–62	
		Adult	0.40–0.91		30–69	
	S	0–<19 y	0.50–1.20		38–91	20
	U, 24 h		mg/d	7.57	μmol/d	
		Adult	4.5–13.2		34–100	1
			mg/g creatinine	0.86	mmol/mol creatinine	
		Adult	2–10		1.8–8.6	
Aspartate aminotransferase	S		U/L	0.017	μkat/L	
With pyridoxal phosphate		0–14 d	23–186		0.38–3.10	7
Values (0–<3 y) based on Abbott Architect method		15 d–<1 y	23–83		0.38–1.38	
		1–<3 y	26–55		0.43–0.92	
Values (3–79 y) based on OCD Vitros method		3–5 y	28–52		0.48–0.88	27
		6–11 y, M	25–47		0.43–0.80	
		F	23–44		0.39–0.75	
		12–17 y, M	18–36		0.31–0.61	
		12–19 y, F	15–34		0.26–0.58	
		18–54 y, M	18–54		0.31–0.92	
		20–54 y, F	18–34		0.31–0.58	
		55–79 y	18–39		0.31–0.66	
Without pyridoxal phosphate		0–14 d	32–162		0.54–2.75	7
Values (0–<19 y) based on Abbott Architect method		15 d–<1 y	20–67		0.34–1.14	
		1–<7 y	21–44		0.36–0.75	
		7–<12 y	18–36		0.31–0.61	
		12–19 y, M	14–35		0.24–0.60	
		F	13–26		0.22–0.44	

TABLE A.1   Pediatric and Adult Reference Intervals for Biochemical Markers (Serum, Plasma, and Urine)—cont'd

Analyte	Specimen	Condition	REFERENCE INTERVALS			Reference Publication
			Conventional Units	Conversion Factor	SI Units	
Aspartic acid	P		mg/dL	75.1	µmol/L	
		Premature, 1 d	0–0.39		0–30	1
		Newborn, 1 d	<0.2 1		<16	
		1–3 mo	0–0.15		0–8	
		9 mo–2 y	<0.12		<9	
		19 mo–10 y	<0.27		<20	
		6–18 y	<0.19		<14	
		Adult	<0.32		<24	
	S	0–< 2 wk	0.25–1.61		19–121	20
		2 wk–<19 y	0.27–0.56		20–42	
	U, 24 h		mg/d	7.51	µmol/d	
		3–12 y	<5.1		<38	1
		Adult	<26.2		<197	
			mg/g creatinine	0.85	mmol/mol creatinine	
		Adult	0–4		0.1–3.7	
Azelaic acid	U				mmol/mol creatinine	
					<1.1	1
Beryllium	U, 24 h		µg/L	0.111	µmol/L	
		Negative	None detected		None detected	1
		Toxic	>20		>2.22	
Bilirubin, direct (conjugated) Values (0–<19 y) based on Abbott Architect method	S		mg/dL	17.1	µmol/L	
		0–14 d	0.33–0.71		5.7–12.1	7
		15 d–<1 y	0.05–0.30		0.8–5.2	
		1–<9 y	0.05–0.20		0.8–3.4	
		9–<13 y	0.10–0.29		0.8–5.0	
		13–<19 y, F	0.10–0.39		1.7–6.7	
		13–<19 y, M	0.11–0.42		1.9–7.1	
Bilirubin, total Values (0–<3 y) based on Abbott Architect method	S		mg/dL	17.1	µmol/L	
		0–14 d	0.19–16.6		3.3–283.8	7
		15 d–<1 y	0.05–0.68		0.8–11.7	
		1–<3 y	0.05–0.40		0.8–6.8	
Values (3–79 y) based on OCD Vitros method		3–5 y	0.1–0.5		1.0–8.8	27
		6–15 y	0.1–0.9		1.0–15.6	
		16–48 y, M	0.2–1.1		3.0–18	
		F	0.1–0.9		1.0–16	
		49–79 y, M	0.1–1.2		2.0–19.9	
		F	0.1–1.0		1.0–16.6	
	U		Negative		Negative	1
	Amf	See Table A.2				
Conjugated	S		0.0–0.2		0.0–3.4	
Biotin	WB	Healthy			0.5–2.20 nmol/L	1
		Deficiency			<0.5 nmol/L	
BNP (see Chapter 48)	U					1
Cadmium	WB (Hep)		µg/L	8.897	nmol/L	
		Nonsmokers	0.3–1.2		2.7–10.7	1
		Smokers	0.6–3.9		5.3–34.7	
	U, 24 h		µg/L		µmol/L	
		Toxic range	100–3000		0.9–26.7	
Calcitonin	S, P		pg/mL	1	ng/L	
		Men	<8.8		<8.8	1
		Women	<5.8		<5.8	
		Athyroidal	<0.5		<0.5	
Calcium, ionized (free)	S, P (Hep)		mg/dL	0.25	mmol/L	
		Adult	4.6–5.3		1.15–1.33	1
Calcium, total	S, P (Hep)		mg/dL	0.25	mmol/L	

Continued

TABLE A.1 Pediatric and Adult Reference Intervals for Biochemical Markers (Serum, Plasma, and Urine)—cont'd

Analyte	Specimen	Condition	Conventional Units	Conversion Factor	SI Units	Reference Publication
Values (0–<3 y) based on Abbott Architect method		0–<1 y	8.5–11.0		2.13–2.74	7
		1–<3 y	9.2–10.5		2.29–2.63	
Values (3–79 y) based on OCD Vitros method		3–5 y	9.4–10.6		2.35–2.64	27
		6–15 y	9.3–10.5		2.33–2.62	
		16–19	9.2–10.4		2.3–2.60	
		20–39 y, M	9.1–10.4		2.28–2.60	
		20–39 y, F	9.0–10.1		2.24–2.53	
		40–79 y	9.0–10.2		2.24–2.56	
β-Carotene HPLC	S		μg/dL	0.0186	μmol/L	
			10–85		0.19–1.58	1
Cancer antigen 15–3	S		U/mL	1	kU/L	
Values (0–<19 y) based on Abbott Architect method		0–<1 wk	3.4–24		3.4–24	4
		1 wk–<1 y	4.9–33		4.9–33	
		1–<19 y	3.9–21		3.9–21	
		Adult	<30		<30	1
Cancer antigen 19–9	S		U/mL	1	kU/L	
Values (0–<19 y) based on Abbott Architect method		0–<1 y	<64		<64	4
		1–<19 y	<41		<41	
		Adult	<37		<37	1
Cancer antigen 27.29	S		U/mL	1	kU/L	
			<37.7		<37.7	1
Cancer antigen 50	S		U/mL	1	kU/L	
			<14–20		<14–20	1
Cancer antigen 72–4	S		U/mL	1	kU/L	
			<6		<6	1
Cancer antigen 125	S		U/mL	1	kU/L	
Values (0–<19 y) based on Abbott Architect method		0–<4 mo	2.4–22		2.4–22	4
		4 mo–<5 y	7.7–33		7.7–33	
		5–<11 y	4.7–30		4.7–30	
		11–<19 y, F	5.9–39		5.9–39	
		11–<19 y, M	5.4–28		5.4–28	
		Adult	<35		<35	1
Cancer antigen 242	S		U/mL	1	kU/L	
			<20		<20	1
Cancer antigen 549	S		U/mL	1	kU/L	
			<11		<11	1
Carbon dioxide, partial pressure (PCO_2)	WB, arterial (Hep)		mm Hg	0.133	kPa	
		Newborn	27–40		3.59–5.32	1
		Infant	27–41		3.59–5.45	
		Adult, M	35–48		4.66–6.38	
		Adult, F	32–45		4.26–5.99	
Carbon dioxide, total (tCO_2)	S		mEq/L	1	mmol/L	
Values (0–<6 y) based on Abbott Architect method		0–14 d	5–20		5–20	7
		15 d–<1 y	10–24		10–24	
		1–<5 y	14–24		14–24	
		5–<6 y	17–26		17–26	
Values (6–79 y) based on OCD Vitros method		6–79 y	19–26		19–26	27
	WB					1
	Arterial		19–24		19–24	
	Venous		22–26		22–26	
Carbon monoxide	WB (EDTA)		%HbCO	0.01	HbCO Fraction	
		Nonsmokers	0.5–1.5		0.005–0.015	1
		Smokers				

TABLE A.1   Pediatric and Adult Reference Intervals for Biochemical Markers (Serum, Plasma, and Urine)—cont'd

Analyte	Specimen	Condition	REFERENCE INTERVALS Conventional Units	Conversion Factor	SI Units	Reference Publication
		1–2 packs/d	4–5		0.04–0.05	
		>2 packs/d	8–9		0.08–0.09	
		Toxic	>20		>0.20	
		Lethal	>50		>0.5	
Carcinoembryonic antigen (CEA)	S		ng/mL	1	μg/L	
Values based on the Roche method		Nonsmokers	<3		<3	1
		Smokers	<5		<5	
Catecholamines						1
Epinephrine	P	Adult	pg/mL	5.46	pmol/L	
		Supine (30 min)	<50		<273	
		Sitting (15 min)	<60		<328	
		Standing (30 min)	<90		<491	
Norepinephrine	P	Adult	pg/mL	5.91	pmol/L	
		Supine (30 min)	110–410		650–2423	
		Sitting (15 min)	120–680		709–4019	
		Standing (30 min)	125–700		739–4137	
Dopamine	P	Adult	pg/mL	6.53	pmol/L	
		Supine (30 min)	<87		<475	
		Sitting (15 min)	<87		<475	
		Standing (30 min)	<87		<475	
Epinephrine *See Chapter 53, Table 53.1	U, 24 h					
Norepinephrine *See Chapter 53, Table 53.1	U, 24 h					
Dopamine *See Chapter 53, Table 53.1	U, 24 h					
Ceruloplasmin	P		mg/L	0.001	g/L	
		Cord (term)	50–330		0.05–0.33	
Pediatric values (0–19 y) based on Abbott Architect method		0–<2 mo	74–237		0.07–0.24	14
		2–<6 mo	135–330		0.13–0.33	
		6 mo–<1 y	137–389		0.14–0.39	
		1–<8 y	217–433		0.22–0.43	
		8–<14 y	205–402		0.21–0.40	
		14–<19 y, F	208–432		0.21–0.43	
		14–<19 y, M	170–348		0.17–0.35	
		Adult, M	220–400		0.22–0.40	1
		Adult, F with no contraceptive	250–600		0.25–0.60	
		Adult, F with contraceptives (estrogen)	270–660		0.27–0.66	

Continued

TABLE A.1 Pediatric and Adult Reference Intervals for Biochemical Markers (Serum, Plasma, and Urine)—cont'd

Analyte	Specimen	Condition	Conventional Units	Conversion Factor	SI Units	Reference Publication
		Adult, pregnant F	300–1200		0.3–1.20	
			mg/dL	0.01	g/L	
		Adult (20–60 y)	20–60		0.2–0.6	
Chloride (Cl)	S, P		mEq/L	1	mmol/L	
Values (0–2 y) based on Siemens EXL method		0–2 y	102–111		102–111	19
Values (3–79 y) based on OCD Vitros method		3–5 y	100–107		100–107	27
		6–11 y	101–107		101–107	
		12–29 y, M	101–106		101–106	
		F	100–107		100–107	
		30–79 y	102–108		102–108	
	U, 24 h		mEq/d	1	mmol/d	1
		Infant	2–10		2–10	
		Child <6 y	15–40		15–40	
		6–10 y, M	36–110		36–110	
		F	18–74		18–74	
		10–14 y, M	64–176		64–176	
		F	36–173		36–173	
		Adult	110–250		110–250	
		>60 y	95–195		95–195	
	Sweat (iontophoresis)	See Table A.2				
Cholesterol	S		mg/dL	0.0259	mmol/L	
Reference Limits						
Values (0–<3 y) based on Abbott Architect method		0–14 d, F	46–125		1.20–3.23	7
		0–14 d, M	42–109		1.09–2.82	
		15 d–<1 y	64–237		1.66–6.14	
		1–<3 y	112–208		2.90–5.39	
Values (3–79 y) based on OCD Vitros method		3–5 y	120–216		3.11–5.59	27
		6–15 y	116–205		3.00–5.31	
		16–19 y	100–182		2.59–4.71	
		20–29 y	116–228		3.00–5.91	
		30–39 y	147–266		3.81–6.89	
		40–79 y	139–274		3.60–7.10	
		Note: See more recent guidelines for recommendations on reducing the risk of atherosclerotic disease through cholesterol management (2018 AHA/ACC/AACVPR/AAPA/ABC/ACPM/ADA/AGS/APhA/ASPC/NLA/PCNA Guideline on the Management of Blood Cholesterol). See Chapter 36				1
Clinical Decision Limits		Coronary heart disease risk, Child				54
		Desirable	<170		<4.40	
		Borderline high	170–199		4.40–5.15	
		High	>200		>5.15	
		Coronary heart disease risk, Adult				55
		Desirable	<200		<5.18	
		Borderline high	200–239		5.18–6.19	
		High	>239		>6.19	
		Note: Cholesterol should not be used on its own for risk prediction. See Chapter 36.				
Cholinesterase	S		U/L	0.017	μkat/L	

TABLE A.1 Pediatric and Adult Reference Intervals for Biochemical Markers (Serum, Plasma, and Urine)—cont'd

Analyte	Specimen	Condition	REFERENCE INTERVALS Conventional Units	Conversion Factor	SI Units	Reference Publication
Pediatric values (0–<19 y) based on Abbott Architect method		0–14 d	4421–9722		75–165	7
		15 d–<1 y	5182–16027		88–272	
		1–<17 y	7769–15206		132–259	
		17–<19 y, F	7511–10904		128–185	
		17–<19 y, M	8186–12639		139–215	
(37°C)		Adult, M	40–78		0.68–1.33	1
		F	33–76		0.56–1.29	
Cholinesterase activity with dibucaine inhibitor (ChEDi)	S		U/L	0.017	µkat/L	
Pediatric values (0–<19 y) based on Abbott Architect method		0–<1 mo	797–2478		13–41	14
		1 mo–<19 y	1523–3280		25–55	
Chorionic gonadotropin intact molecule	S		mIU/mL	1	IU/L	
		Male and nonpregnant female	<5.0		<5.0	1
		Female, pregnancy (wk of gestation)				
		4 wk	5–100		5–100	
		5 wk	200–3000		200–3000	
		6 wk	10,000–80,000		10,000–80,000	
		7–14 wk	90,000–500,000		90,000–500,000	
		15–26 wk	5000–80,000		5000–80,000	
			*Values based on the Second International Standard for hCG.			
		Trophoblastic disease	>100,000		>100,000	
	U		Negative		Negative	
			Half of pregnancies are detected on the first day of the missed menstrual period.		Half of pregnancies are detected on the first day of the missed menstrual period.	
Chromium			µg/L	19.23	nmol/L	
	WB (Hep)		0.7–28.0		14–538	1
	S		0.1–0.2		2–3	
			µg/d	19.23	nmol/d	
	U, 24 h		0.1–2.0		1.9–38.4	
			µg/L	19.23	nmol/L	
	RBC		20–36		384–692	
Chymotrypsin (37°C)	F		U/g stool	1	U/g stool	1
			12		12	
trans-Cinnamoylglycine	U				mmol/mol creatinine	
					0.1–8.0	1
Citric acid	U				mmol/mol creatinine	
		0–1 mo			<1046	1
		1–6 mo			104–268	
		6 mo–5 y			0–656	
		>5 y			87–639	
Cobalt			µg/L	16.97	nmol/L	
	S		0.11–0.45		1.9–7.6	1
	U		1–2		17.0–34.0	
			µg/kg		nmol/kg	
	RBC		16–46		272–781	
Complement C3	S		mg/dL	0.01	g/L	

TABLE A.1 Pediatric and Adult Reference Intervals for Biochemical Markers (Serum, Plasma, and Urine)—cont'd

Analyte	Specimen	Condition	Conventional Units	Conversion Factor	SI Units	Reference Publication
					REFERENCE INTERVALS	
Values (0–<19 y) based on Abbott Architect method		0–14 d	50–121		0.5–1.2	7
		15 d–<1 y	51–160		0.5–1.6	
		1–<19 y	83–152		0.8–1.5	
		Adult (20–60 y)	90–180		0.9–1.8	1
Complement C4	S		mg/dL	0.01	g/L	
Values (0–<19 y) based on Abbott Architect method		0–<1 y	7–30		0.1–0.3	7
		1–<19 y	13–37		0.1–0.4	
		Adult (20–60 y)	10–40		0.1–0.4	1
Copper	S		μg/dL	0.157	μmol/L	
		Birth–6 mo	20–70		3.1–10.9	1
		Deficiency	<30		<5	
		6 y	90–190		14.1–29.8	
		12 y	80–160		12.5–25.1	
		Adult, M	70–140		10.9–21.9	
		F	80–155		12.5–24.3	
		Deficiency	50		8	
		Pregnancy, at term	118–302		18.5–47.4	
		Blacks	Blacks 8–12% higher		Blacks 8–12% higher	
	U, 24 h		μg/dL	0.157	μmol/L	
		Adult	<60 μg/24 h		1.0 μmol/24 h	
		Wilson disease	>200 μg/24 h		>3 μmol/24 h	
Corticosterone	S		μg/dL	28.84	nmol/L	
Pediatric values based on LC-MS/MS		0–<1 mo	0.00–0.69		0.14–20.0	16
		1 mo–<1 y	0.01–0.53		0.28–15.4	
		1–<4 y	0.02–0.13		0.62–3.72	
		4–<6 y	0.03–0.14		0.95–4.11	
		6–<15 y	0.02–0.32		0.44–9.19	
		15–<19 y	0.03–0.53		0.85–15.24	
Cortisol, free (see also Chapter 56)	S		μg/dL	27.6	nmol/L	
		0800 h	0.6–1.6		17–44	1
		1600 h	0.2–0.9		6–15	
	Sal	See Table A.2				
	U, 24 h	Child	μg/d	2.76	nmol/d	
		1–10 y	2–27		6–74	
		2–11 y	1–21		3–58	
		11–20 y	5–55		14–152	
		12–16 y	2–38		6–105	
		Adult	μg/d	2.76	nmol/d	
		Extracted	20–90		55–248	
		Unextracted (HPLC)	<50		<138 nmol/d	See Chapter 56
Cortisol, total	S		μg/dL	27.6	nmol/L	
		Cord blood	5–17		138–469	1
Pediatric values (2 d–<19 y) based on Abbott Architect method		2–<15 d	1–12		13–340	3
		15 d–<1 y	1–17		14–458	
		1–<9 y	2–11		48–297	
		9–<14 y	2–13		60–349	
		14–<17 y	3–16		77–453	
		17–<19 y	4–18		97–506	
		Adult	μg/dL	27.6	nmol/L	1
		0800 h	3–21		83–580	
		0800 h	5–23		138–635	
		1600 h	3–16		83–441	

TABLE A.1 Pediatric and Adult Reference Intervals for Biochemical Markers (Serum, Plasma, and Urine)—cont'd

Analyte	Specimen	Condition	REFERENCE INTERVALS			Reference Publication
			Conventional Units	Conversion Factor	SI Units	
		2000 h	<50% of 0800 h values		<50% of 0800 h values	
For LC-MSMS pediatric reference intervals please see: *Clinical Biochemistry* 2013;46:642–51						
Creatine kinase, myocardial bound (CKMB), mass* (see Chapter 48)						
C-reactive protein (CRP), high sensitivity	S		mg/L	1	mg/L	
Values (0–<3 y) based on Abbott Architect method		0–14 d	0.3–6.1		0.3–6.1	7
		15 d–<3 y	0.1–1.0		0.1–1.0	
Values (3–79 y) based on OCD Vitros method		3–5 y	0.1–2.4		0.1–2.4	28
		6–11 y	0.1–5.9		0.1–5.9	
		12–13 y	0.1–1.9		0.1–1.9	
		14–16 y	0.1–2.9		0.1–2.9	
		17–39 y, M	0.1–6.0		0.1–6.0	
		F	0.1–12.1		0.1–12.1	
		40–79 y	0.1–8.8		0.1–8.8	
		M				
		American	0.3–8.6		0.3–8.6	1
		White American	0.2–12.3		0.2–12.3	
		African American	0.1–8.2		0.1–8.2	
		Mexican American	0.2–6.3		0.2–6.3	
		European	0.3–8.6		0.3–8.6	
		Japanese	<7.8		<7.8	
		F				
		American	0.2–9.1		0.2–9.1	
		European	0.3–8.8		0.3–8.8	
Creatine kinase (CK)	S		U/L	0.017	μkat/L	
Pediatric reference values (0 to <19 years) based on Siemens ADVIA method		0–<13 y	68–293		1.16–4.98	19
		13–<19 y, F	48–200		0.82–3.40	
		13–<19 y, M	80–354		1.36–6.02	
IFCC, 37°C		M	46–171		0.78–2.90	1
		F	34–145		0.58–2.47	
CK isoenzymes	S	Fraction 2 (MB)	<5.0 μg/L	1	<5.0 μg/L	1
		Relative index MB/total	<3.9%	0.01	<0.039 fractional activity	
Creatinine			mg/dL	88.4	μmol/L	
Enzymatic	S	0–14 d	0.32–0.92		28–81	7
Values (0–<3 y) based on Abbott Architect method		15 d–<2 y	0.10–0.36		9–32	
		2–<3 y	0.20–0.43		18–38	
Values (3–79 y) based on OCD Vitros method		3–5 y	0.31–0.51		28–45	27
		6–7 y	0.36–0.56		32–49	
		8–9 y	0.37–0.63		32–56	
		10–11 y	0.43–0.68		38–60	
		12–15 y, M	0.47–0.91		42–81	
		12–16 y, F	0.48–0.84		42–74	
		16–79 y, M	0.71–1.16		63–102	
		17–79 y, F	0.56–0.96		49–85	

TABLE A.1 Pediatric and Adult Reference Intervals for Biochemical Markers (Serum, Plasma, and Urine)—cont'd

Analyte	Specimen	Condition	Conventional Units	Conversion Factor	SI Units	Reference Publication
	U		mg/dL	0.0884	mmol/L	
Values (3–79 y) based on OCD Vitros method		3–5 y	14.71–151.58		1–13	27
		6–11 y	13.57–195.70		1–17	
		12–13 y	21.49–214.93		2–19	
		14–29 y	19.23–305.43		2–27	
		30–79 y, M	14.71–294.12		1–26	
		F	12.44–229.64		1–20	
Jaffe			mg/dL	88.4	μmol/L	
	S	Cord	0.60–1.20		53–106	1
		0–14 d	0.42–1.05		37–93	7
		15 d–<1 y	0.31–0.53		28–47	
		1–<4 y	0.39–0.55		34–48	
		4–<7 y	0.44–0.65		39–57	
		7–<12 y	0.52–0.69		46–61	
		12–<15 y	0.57–0.80		50–71	
		15–<17 y, F	0.59–0.86		52–76	
		M	0.65–1.04		58–92	
		17–<19 y, F	0.60–0.88		53–78	
		M	0.69–1.10		61–97	
		18–60 y, M	0.90–1.30		80–115	1
		F	0.60–1.10		53–97	
		60–90 y, M	0.80–1.30		71–115	
		F	0.60–1.20		53–106	
		>90 y, M	1.00–1.70		88–150	
		F	0.60–1.30		53–115	
Jaffe, manual	U, 24 h		mg/kg/d	8.84	μmol/kg/d	
		Infant	8–20		71–177	1
		Child	8–22		71–194	
		Adolescent	8–30		71–265	
		Adult, M	14–26		124–230	
		F	11–20		97–177	
Creatinine clearance (see Glomerular filtration rate)						
C-Telopeptide	S		ng/L	1	ng/L	
		0–<1 y	210–4390		210–4390	14
Values (0–<19 y) based on Abbott Architect method		1–<6 y	350–4480		350–4480	
		6–<19 y	780–6790		780–6790	
		Men	<1009		<1009	1
		Premenopausal women	<574		<574	
	U, 24 h		mg/mol creatinine	1	mg/mol creatinine	
		Men	0–505		0–505	1
		Premenopausal women	0–476		0–476	
Cyanide	WB (Ox)		mg/L	38.5	μmol/L	
		Nonsmokers	<0.2		<7.7	1
		Smokers	<0.4		<15.4	
		Nitroprusside therapy	Up to 100 without toxicity		Up to 3850	
		Toxic	>1		38.5	
Cystatin C	S		mg/L	1	mg/L	
Pediatric values (0–<19 y) based on Abbott Architect method		0–<1 mo	1.49–2.85		1.49–2.85	14
		1–<5 mo	1.01–1.92		1.01–1.92	
		5 mo–<1 y	0.75–1.53		0.75–1.53	
		1–<2 y, F	0.60–1.20		0.60–1.20	

TABLE A.1   Pediatric and Adult Reference Intervals for Biochemical Markers (Serum, Plasma, and Urine)—cont'd

Analyte	Specimen	Condition	Conventional Units	Conversion Factor	SI Units	Reference Publication
		1–<2 y, M	0.77–1.85		0.77–1.85	
		2–<19 y	0.62–1.11		0.62–1.11	
		Adult, F	0.61–1.05		0.61–1.05	31
		M	0.71–1.21		0.71–1.21	
Cystine	S		mg/dL	83.3	μmol/L	
		Premature, 1 d	0.54–1.02		45–85	1
		Newborn, 1 d	0.43–1.01		36–84	
		0–<6 d, F	0.19–0.61		16–51	20
		0–<6 d, M	0.19–0.64		16–53	
		6 d–<2 wk	0.08–0.68		6.7–57	
		2 wk–<8 y	0.04–0.24		3.3–20	
		8–<19 y	0.05–0.34		4.2–28	
		Adult	0.40–1.40		33–117	1
	U, 24 h		mg/d	8.33	μmol/d	
		10 d–7 wk	2.16–3.37		18–28	
		3–12 y	4.9–30.9		41–257	
		Adult	<38.1		<317	
			mg/g creatinine	0.94	mmol/mol creatinine	
		Adult	2–14		1.9–13.1	
Dehydroepiandrosterone, unconjugated	S		ng/dL	0.0347	nmol/L	
		Children				1
		6–9 y, M	13–187		0.45–6.49	
		6–9 y, F	18–189		0.62–6.55	
		10–11 y, M	31–205		1.07–7.11	
		10–11 y, F	112–224		3.88–7.77	
		12–14 y, M	83–258		2.88–8.95	
		12–14 y, F	98–360		3.40–12.5	
		Adult				
		M	180–1250		6.25–43.4	
		F	130–980		4.51–34.0	
Dehydroepiandrosterone sulfate	S		μg/dL	0.027	μmol/L	
Pediatric values (0–<19 y) based on Abbott Architect method		Children				14
		0–<2 mo	1110–>1565		30.1–>42.5	
		2–<6 mo	25–599		0.7–16.3	
		6 mo–<1 y	6–184		0.2–5.0	
		1–<6 y	3–117		0.1–3.2	
		6–<9 y	5–159		0.2–4.3	
		9–<13 y	35–281		0.9–7.6	
		13–<16 y	58–479		1.6–13.0	
		16–<19 y, F	152–595		4.1–16.1	
		16–<19 y, M	129–700		3.5–19.0	
Tanner values based on Abbott Architect method		Pubertal levels, Tanner stage				1
		1, M	5–265		0.1–7.2	
		1, F	5–125		0.1–3.4	
		2, M	15–380		0.4–10.3	
		2, F	15–150		0.4–4.0	
		3, M	60–505		1.6–13.6	
		3, F	20–535		0.5–14.4	
		4, M	65–560		1.8–15.1	
		4, F	35–485		0.9–13.1	
		5, M	165–500		4.4–13.5	
		5, F	75–530		2.0–14.3	

Continued

TABLE A.1 Pediatric and Adult Reference Intervals for Biochemical Markers (Serum, Plasma, and Urine)—cont'd

Analyte	Specimen	Condition	Conventional Units	Conversion Factor	SI Units	Reference Publication
		Adult				
		18–30 y, M	125–619		3.4–16.7	
		18–30 y, F	45–380		1.2–10.3	
		31–50 y, M	5–532		1.6–12.2	
		31–50 y, F	12–379		0.8–10.2	
		51–60 y, M	20–413		0.5–11.1	
		61–83 y, M	10–285		0.3–7.7	
		F, Postmenopausal	30–260		0.8–7.0	
11-Deoxycortisol	S		ng/dL	0.0289	nmol/L	
		Cord blood	295–554		9–16	1
		Child and adult	20–158		0.6–4.6	
Pediatric values based on LCMS/MS		0–<1 y	0.00–183		0.00–5.30	16
		1–<2 y	3.46–30.4		0.10–0.88	
		2–<7 y	2.42–37.0		0.07–1.07	
		7–<12 y	3.11–78.5		0.09–2.27	
		12–<19 y	0.00–78.9		0.00–2.28	
Deoxypyridinoline	U		μmol/mol creatinine	1	μmol/mol creatinine	
		M	2.3–5.4		2.3–5.4	1
		F, Premenopausal	3.0–7.4		3.0–7.4	
Dihydrotestosterone	S		ng/dL	0.0334	nmol/L	
		Child, prepubertal	<3		<0.10	1
		Adult, M	30–85		1.03–2.92	
		Adult, F	4–22		0.14–0.76	
Dodecanedioic acid	U				μmol/mol creatinine	
					<0.06	1
Dopamines	P, S		pg/mL		nmol/L	
L-Dopa (1-dodecenoylcarnitine)		Adult, normotensive	1042–2366	0.0051	5.3–12.0	1
DOPAC (3,4-dihydroxyphenylacetic acid)			674–2636	0.0059	4.0–15.7	
DHPG (3,4-dihydroxyphenylglycol)			797–1208	0.0059	4.7–7.1	
DU-PAN-2			U/mL	1	kU/L	
			<401		<401	1
Estradiol	S		pg/mL	3.69	pmol/L	
Values (15 d–<19 y) based on Abbott Architect method		Child				15
		15 d–<1 y	<25		<92	
		1–<9 y, F	<10		<37	
		9–<11 y, F	<48		<176	
		11–<12 y, F	<94		<345	
		12–<14 y, F	11–172		39–631	
		14–19 y, F	<255		<936	
		1–<11 y, M	<13		<46	
		11–<13 y, M	<26		<95	
		13–<15 y, M	<28		<102	
		15–<19 y, M	<38		<141	
		Adult				1
		M	10–50		37–184	
		F				
		Early follicular phase	20–150		73–550	
		Late follicular phase	40–350		147–1285	

TABLE A.1 Pediatric and Adult Reference Intervals for Biochemical Markers (Serum, Plasma, and Urine)—cont'd

Analyte	Specimen	Condition	REFERENCE INTERVALS Conventional Units	Conversion Factor	SI Units	Reference Publication
		Midcycle	150–750		550–2753	
		Luteal phase	30–450		110–1652	
		Postmenopausal	<21		<74	
Tanner values based on Abbott Architect method		Pubertal levels Tanner stage				
		1, M	<19		<68	15
		1, F	<20		<74	
		2, M	<18		<67	
		2, F	<26		<96	
		3, M	<21		<76	
		3, F	<86		<317	
		4, M	<35		<128	
		4, F	13–141		49–517	
		5, M	17–34		64–126	
		5, F	19–208		69–762	
Estriol, free (unconjugated, uE3)	S		ng/mL	3.47	nmol/L	
		Males and non-pregnant females	<2.0		<6.9	1
		Pregnancy, wk of gestation				
		16 wk	0.30–1.05		1.04–3.64	
		18 wk	0.63–2.30		2.19–7.98	
		34 wk	5.3–18.3		18.4–63.5	
		35 wk	5.2–26.4		18.0–91.6	
		36 wk	8.2–28.1		28.4–97.5	
		37 wk	8.0–30.1		27.8–104.0	
		38 wk	8.6–38.0		29.8–131.9	
		39 wk	7.2–34.3		25.0–119.0	
		40 wk	9.6–28.9		33.3–100.3	
	Amf	See Table A.2				
For LC-MSMS reference intervals please see: *Clinical Biochemistry* 2013;46:642–51						
Estriol, total (E3)	S		ng/mL	3.47	nmol/L	
		Pregnancy, wk of gestation				1
		34 wk	38–140		132–486	
		35 wk	31–140		108–486	
		36 wk	35–330		121–1145	
		37 wk	45–260		156–902	
		38 wk	48–350		167–1215	
		39 wk	59–570		205–1978	
		40 wk	95–460		330–1596	
	U, 24 h		µg/d	3.47	nmol/d	
		M	1.0–11.0		3.5–38.2	
		F				
		Follicular phase	0–15.0		0–52.0	
		Ovulatory phase	13.0–54.0		45.1–187.4	
		Luteal phase	8.0–60.0		27.8–208.2	
		Postmenopausal	0–11.0		0–38.2	
		Pregnancy				

TABLE A.1 Pediatric and Adult Reference Intervals for Biochemical Markers (Serum, Plasma, and Urine)—cont'd

Analyte	Specimen	Condition	Conventional Units	Conversion Factor	SI Units	Reference Publication
		1st trimester	0–800		0–2776	
		2nd trimester	800–12,000		2776–41,640	
		3rd trimester	5000–50,000		17,350–173,500	
	Amf	See Table A.2				
Estrone	S		pg/mL	3.69	pmol/L	1
		M	15–65		55–240	
		F				
		Early follicular phase	15–150		55–555	
		Late follicular phase	100–250		370–925	
		Luteal phase	15–200		55–740	
Ethanol	WB (Ox)		mg/dL	0.217	mmol/L	
		Impairment	50–100		11–22	1
		Depression of CNS	>100		>21.7	
		Fatalities reported	>400		>86.8	
Ethylmalonic acid	U				mmol/mol creatinine 0.4–17	1
Ferritin	S		ng/mL	1	µg/L	
Values (4 d–<3 y) based on Abbott Architect method		4–<15 d	99.6–717.0		99.6–717.0	3
		15 d–<6 mo	14.0–647.2		14.0–647.2	
		6 mo–<1 y	8.4–181.9		8.4–181.9	
		1–<3 y	5.3–99.9		5.3–99.9	
Values (3–79 y) based on the Siemens Immulite method		3–5 y	10.7–85.2		10.7–85.2	28
		6–16 y, M	16.2–106.7		16.2–106.7	
		6–24 y, F	9.6–81.9		9.6–81.9	
		17–37 y, M	39.3–439.4		39.3–439.4	
		25–49 y, F	6.5–147.1		6.5–147.1	
		38–79 y, M	45.8–714.8		45.8–714.8	
		50–79 y, F	6.0–362.6		6.0–362.6	
α-Fetoprotein (AFP)	S		mg/dL	0.01	g/L	
		Fetal, 1st trimester	200–400		2.0–4.0	1
		Cord blood	<5		<0.05	
Pediatric values based on Abbott Architect method			ng/mL	1	µg/L	
		0–<1 mo	>2000		>2000	4
		1–<3 mo	9.80–1359.0		9.80–1359.0	
		3–<6 mo	4.15–274.70		4.15–274.70	3
		6 mo–<1 y	2.66–148.21		2.66–148.21	
		1–<3 y	2.88–20.94		2.88–20.94	
		3–<19 y	0.89–4.48		0.89–4.48	
		Adult (85% of population)	<8.5		<8.5	1
		Adult (100% of population)	<15		<15	
	Maternal serum		ng/mL (median)	1	µg/L (median)	
		Pregnancy, wk of gestation				
		14 wk	25.6		25.6	
		15 wk	29.9		29.9	
		16 wk	34.8		34.8	
		17 wk	40.6		40.6	

TABLE A.1   Pediatric and Adult Reference Intervals for Biochemical Markers (Serum, Plasma, and Urine)—cont'd

| Analyte | Specimen | Condition | REFERENCE INTERVALS | | | Reference Publication |
			Conventional Units	Conversion Factor	SI Units	
		18 wk	47.3		47.3	
		19 wk	55.1		55.1	
		20 wk	64.3		64.3	
		21 wk	74.9		74.9	
		Tumor marker	ng/mL	1	µg/L	
		Early marker	10–20		10–20	
		Cancer	>1000		>1000	
	Amf	See Table 82.2				
Fluoride	S		mg/L	52.6	µmol/L	
			0.2–3.2		10.5–168	1
Folate			ng/mL	2.265	nmol/L	
Values (5 d–<6 y) based on Abbott Architect method	S	5 d–<1 y	>10.6		>23.9	3
		1–<3 y	>3.9		>8.7	
		3–<6 y	>11.9		>27.0	
Values (6–79 y) based on Siemens Immulite method		6–18 y	8.2–30.6		18.6–69.3	28
		19–79 y	9.5–39.0		21.5–88.4	
	Erythrocyte	3–5 y	294.7–883.4		703.1–2012.9	1
		6–79 y	228.2–998.7		541.4–2110.6	
		Note: Reference limits for erythrocytes depend on the level of supplementation in the country.				
	S	Deficiency	<1.4		<3.2	
	Erythrocyte deficiency		<110		<252	
Follicle-stimulating hormone (FSH)	S		mIU/mL	1	IU/L	
Values (30 d–<19 y) based on Abbott Architect method		30 d–<1 y, F	0.4–10.4		0.4–10.4	15
		1–<9 y, F	0.4–5.5		0.4–5.5	
		9–<11 y, F	0.4–4.2		0.4–4.2	
		11–19 y, F	0.3–7.8		0.3–7.8	
		30 d–<1 y, M	0.1–2.4		0.1–2.4	
		1–<5 y, M	<0.9		<0.9	
		5–<10 y, M	<1.6		<1.6	
		10–<13 y, M	0.4–3.9		0.4–3.9	
		13–<19 y, M	0.8–5.1		0.8–5.1	
Tanner values based on Abbott Architect method		Pubertal levels, Tanner stage				
		1, M	<1.5		<1.5	
		1, F	0.6–4.1		0.6–4.1	
		2, M	<3.0		<3.0	
		2, F	0.3–5.8		0.3–5.8	
		3, M	0.4–6.2		0.4–6.2	
		3, F	0.1–7.2		0.1–7.2	
		4, M	0.6–5.1		0.6–5.1	
		4, F	0.3–7.0		0.3–7.0	
		5, M	0.8–7.2		0.8–7.2	
		5, F	0.4–8.6		0.4–8.6	
		23–70 y, M F	1.4–15.4		1.4–15.4	1
		Follicular phase	1.4–9.9		1.4–9.9	
		Midcycle peak	0.2–17.2		0.2–17.2	
		Luteal phase	1.1–9.2		1.1–9.2	
		Postmenopausal	19.3–100.6		19.3–100.6	

Continued

TABLE A.1 Pediatric and Adult Reference Intervals for Biochemical Markers (Serum, Plasma, and Urine)—cont'd

Analyte	Specimen	Condition	REFERENCE INTERVALS			Reference Publication
			Conventional Units	Conversion Factor	SI Units	
Fructosamine	S	Child	5% below adult levels			1
		Adult	μmol/L 205–285	1	μmol/L 205–285	
Fumaric acid	U				mmol/mol creatinine	1
		0–1 mo			10–45	
		1–6 mo			4–45	
		6 mo–5 y			1–27	
		>5 y			2–4	
Glomerular filtration rate (endogenous) based on KDIGO	Categories		mL/min/1.73 m²	0.00963	mL/s/m²	
	G1	Normal or high	≥90		≥0.87	34
	G2	Mildly decreased	60–89		0.58–0.86	
	G3a	Mildly to moderately decreased	45–59		0.43–0.57	
	G3b	Moderately to severely decreased	30–44		0.29–0.42	
	G4	Severely decreased	15–29		0.14–0.28	
	G5	Kidney failure	<15		<0.14	
Glucagon	P (Hep or EDTA)		ng/L		ng/L	
		Adult	70–180		70–180	1
	Amf	See Table A.2				
Glucose	S, fasting		mg/dL	0.0555	mmol/L	
		Cord	45–96		2.5–5.3	1
		Premature	20–60		1.1–3.3	
		Neonate	30–60		1.7–3.3	
		Newborn				
		1 d	40–60		2.2–3.3	
		>1 d	50–80		2.8–4.5	
		Child	60–100		3.3–5.6	
		Adult	74–100		4.1–5.6	
		>60 y	82–115		4.6–6.4	
		>90 y	75–121		4.2–6.7	
		Decision Limits				
		Normal glucose metabolism	≤100		≤5.55	
		Diabetes	≥126		≥7.00	
	CSF	See Table A.2				
	U		1–15		0.1–0.8	
	U, 24 h		g/d	5.55	mmol/d	
			<0.5		<2.8	
Glucose-6-phosphate dehydrogenase (G-6-PD) in erythrocytes, WHO and ICSH	WB (ACD, EDTA, or Hep)		U/g Hb	64.5	U/mmol Hb	1
			7.9–16.3		510–1050	
			U/10¹² RBC	10⁻³	nU/ RBC	
			230–470		0.23–0.47	
			2.69–5.53 U/mL RBC	1	2.69–5.53 U/mL RBC	
Glutamic acid	P		mg/dL	68	μmol/L	

TABLE A.1 Pediatric and Adult Reference Intervals for Biochemical Markers (Serum, Plasma, and Urine)—cont'd

Analyte	Specimen	Condition	REFERENCE INTERVALS			Reference Publication
			Conventional Units	Conversion Factor	SI Units	
		Premature, 1 d	0–1.98		0–135	1
		Newborn, 1 d	0.29–1.57		20–107	
		6 mo–3 y	0.28–1.47		19–100	
		3–10 y	0.34–3.68		23–250	
		6–18 y	0.10–0.96		7–65	
		Adult	0.21–2.82		14–192	
	S	0–<2 wk	1.34–5.90		91–401	20
		2 wk–<1 y	1.09–3.91		74–266	
		1<19 y	0.76–2.01		52–137	
	U, 24 h		mg/d	6.8	μmol/d	1
		10 d–7 wk	0.3–1.5		2–10	
		Adult	<33.8		<230	
			mg/g creatinine	0.77	mmol/mol creatinine	
		Adult	2–6		1.5–4.7	
Glutamine	P		mg/dL	68.5	μmol/L	
		3 mo–6 y	6.93–10.89		475–746	1
		6–18 y	5.26–10.80		360–740	
		Adult	5.78–10.38		396–711	
	S	0–<1 wk	6.58–16.2		451–1113	20
		1 wk–<1 y	4.85–11.5		332–789	
		1–<9 y	6.09–9.90		417–678	
		9–<19 y	6.82–11.0		467–755	
	U, 24 h		mg/d	6.85	μmol/d	
		10 d–7 wk	12.4–25.8		85–177	1
		3–12 y	20.4–113.7		140–779	
		Adult	43.8–151.8		300–1040	
			mg/g creatinine	0.77	mmol/mol creatinine	
		Adult	2–78		2–60	
γ-Glutamyltransferase	S		U/L	0.017	μkat/L	
Values (0–<3 y) based on Abbott Architect method		0–<14 d	23–219		0.38–3.65	7
		15 d–<1 y	8–127		0.13–2.12	
		1–<3 y	6–16		0.10–0.27	
Values (3–79 y) based on OCD Vitros method		3–5 y	11–20		0.19–0.34	27
		6–14 y, M	10–26		0.17–0.44	
		6–17 y, F	9–24		0.15–0.41	
		15–19 y, M	10–33		0.17–0.56	
		18–35 y, F	12–38		0.20–0.65	
		20–35 y, M	12–62		0.20–1.05	
		36–79 y, M	13–109		0.22–1.85	
		36–79 y, F	10–54		0.17–0.92	
Glutaric acid	U				mmol/mol creatinine	
					0.5–13	1
Glycated hemoglobin (HbA$_{1C}$)	WB (EDTA, Hep or Ox)		%		mmol/mol (IFCC)	
Values (6–79 y) based on OCD Vitros method		6–39 y	4.9–6.1		30–43	28
		40–79 y	5.0–6.3		31–45	
		Cutoff for diagnosis	≥6.5 (NGSP)		≥48	38
Glyceric acid	U				mmol/mol creatinine	
		0–1 mo			<40	1
		1–6 mo			<185	
		6 mo–5 y			<71	
		>5 y			<61	
Glycine	P		mg/dL	133.3	μmol/L	
		Premature 1 d	0–7.57		0–1010	1

Continued

TABLE A.1 Pediatric and Adult Reference Intervals for Biochemical Markers (Serum, Plasma, and Urine)—cont'd

Analyte	Specimen	Condition	REFERENCE INTERVALS Conventional Units	Conversion Factor	SI Units	Reference Publication
		Newborn 1 d	1.68–3.86		224–514	
		1–3 mo	0.79–1.67		106–222	
		2–6 mo	1.31–2.22		175–296	
		9 mo–2 y	0.42–2.31		56–308	
		3–10 y	0.88–1.67		117–223	
		6–18 y	1.18–2.27		158–302	
		Adult	0.90–4.16		120–554	
	S	0–<2 wk	2.24–5.87		299–782	20
		2 wk–<13 y	1.47–2.99		196–398	
		13–<19 y	1.64–3.05		218–407	
	U, 24 h		mg/d	13.3	μmol/d	
		10 d–7 wk	14.6–9.2		194–787	1
		3–12 y	12.4–106.8		165–1420	
		Adult	59.0–294.6		785–3918	
			mg/g creatinine	1.51	mmol/mol creatinine	
		Adult	12–108		18.2–163	
Glycolic acid	U				mmol/mol creatinine	
		0–1 mo			<63	1
		1–6 mo			<105	
		6 mo–5 y			2–121	
		>5 y			<167	
Glyoxylic acid	U				mmol/mol creatinine	
		0–1 mo			<14	1
		1–6 mo			<17	
		6 mo–5 y			<8	
		>5 y			<10	
Growth hormone	S		ng/mL	1	μg/L	
		Basal	2–5		2–5	1
		Insulin tolerance test	>10		>10	
		Arginine	>7.5		>7.5	
		L-Dopa	>7.5		>7.5	
Pediatric values (0–<19 y) based on Beckman DxI method	S	0–<3 mo	0.80–33.5		0.80–33.5	12
		3 mo–<2 y	0.14–6.27		0.14–6.27	
		2–<7 y	0.05–5.11		0.05–5.11	
		7–<12 y	0.02–4.76		0.02–4.76	
		12–<14 y	0.01–6.20		0.01–6.20	
		14–<19 y, F	0.03–5.22		0.03–5.22	
		14–<19 y, M	0.02–3.81		0.02–3.81	
Haptoglobin	S		mg/dL	0.01	g/L	
Values (0–<19 y) based on Abbott Architect method		0–14 d	0–10		0–0.1	7
		15 d–<1 y	7–221		0.1–2.2	
		1–<12 y	7–163		0.1–1.6	
		12–<19 y	7–179		0.1–1.8	
		Adult (20–60 y)	30–200		0.3–2.0	1
High-density lipoprotein cholesterol (HDL-C) *Reference Intervals*	S		mg/dL	0.0259	mmol/L	
Values (0–<3 y) based on Abbott Architect method		0–14 d	15–42		0.4–1.1	7
		15 d–<1 y	12–71		0.3–1.9	
		1–<3 y	32–63		0.8–1.6	
Values (3–79 y) based on OCD Vitros method		3–5 y	31–73		0.8–1.9	27
		6–14 y	35–81		0.9–2.1	
		15–79 y, M	31–70		0.8–1.8	
		F	35–89		0.9–2.3	

TABLE A.1   Pediatric and Adult Reference Intervals for Biochemical Markers (Serum, Plasma, and Urine)—cont'd

Analyte	Specimen	Condition	REFERENCE INTERVALS Conventional Units	Conversion Factor	SI Units	Reference Publication
Clinical Decision Limits		Pediatric	mg/dL	0.0259	mmol/L	
		Acceptable	>45		>1.2	54
		Borderline	40–45		1.0–1.2	
		Low	<40		<1.0	
		Adult				
		Low	<40		<1.0	55
		High	>59		>1.5	
Non-HDL cholesterol (calculated)	S		mg/dL	0.0259	mmol/L	
Calculated pediatric values based on Abbott Architect method		0–<1 y	27.8–202		0.72–5.22	10
		1–<10 y, F	79.9–165		2.07–4.28	
		1–<10 y, M	69.1–142		1.79–3.68	
		10–<19 y	64.9–156		1.68–4.04	
Histidine	P		mg/dL	64.5	µmol/L	
		Premature, 1 d	0.16–1.40		10–90	1
		Newborn, 1 d	0.76–1.77		49–114	
		1–3 mo	0.66–1.30		43–83	
		2–6 mo	1.49–2.12		96–137	
		9 mo–2 y	0.37–1.74		24–112	
		3–10 y	0.37–1.32		24–85	
		6–18 y	0.99–1.64		64–106	
		Adult	0.50–1.66		32–107	
	S	0–<2 wk	0.70–2.60		45–168	20
		2 wk–<19 y	1.01–1.75		65–113	
	U, 24 h		mg/d	6.45	µmol/d	
		10 d–7 wk	16.0–38.6		103–249	1
		3–12 y	47.4–199.2		306–1285	
		Adult	72.9–440.8		470–2843	
			mg/g creatinine	0.73	mmol/mol creatinine	
		Adult	1–141		1–103	
Homocysteine, total	S, P		µmol/L	1	µmol/L	
		Folate-supplemented diet				1
		<15 y	<8		<8	
		15–65 y	<12		<12	
		>65 y	<16		<16	
		No folate supplementation				
		<15 y	<10		<10	
		15–65 y	<15		<15	
		>65 y	<20		<20	
Values (5 d–<6 y) based on Abbott Architect method		5 d–<1 y	2.9–10.0		2.9–10.0	3
		1–<6 y	2.8–7.6		2.8–7.6	
Values (6–79 y) based on OCD Vitros method		6–12 y	1.7–6.9		1.7–6.9	28
		13–25 y, M	3.6–10.6		3.6–10.6	
		13–39 y, F	2.9–9.5		2.9–9.5	
		26–79 y, M	5.2–14.1		5.2–14.1	
		40–79 y, F	3.7–10.9		3.7–10.9	
Homogentisic acid	U				mmol/mol creatinine	
					<11	1
Homovanillic acid (HVA)	U, 24 h		mg/d	5.49	µmol/d	
		3–6 y	1.4–4.3		8–24	1
		6–10 y	2.1–4.7		12–26	

TABLE A.1 Pediatric and Adult Reference Intervals for Biochemical Markers (Serum, Plasma, and Urine)—cont'd

Analyte	Specimen	Condition	REFERENCE INTERVALS Conventional Units	Conversion Factor	SI Units	Reference Publication
		10–16 y	2.4–8.7		13–48	
		16–83 y	1.4–8.8		8–48	
	U	*See Chapter 53 Table 53.5				
						1
Human Epididymis Protein 4 (HE4)	S		pmol/L	1.0	pmol/L	
Values based on Abbott Architect method		0–<1 wk	159–618		159–618	4
		1 wk–<6 mo	55.7–178		55.7–178	
		6 mo–<2 y	30.9–98.6		30.9–98.6	
		2–<10 y	27.3–69.7		27.3–69.7	
		10–<19 y	22.5–61.8		22.5–61.8	
3-Hydroxybutyric acid	U				mmol/mol creatinine	
		0–5 y			<6	1
		>5 y			<11	
2-Hydroxyglutaric acid	U				mmol/mol creatinine	
					<16	1
5-Hydroxyindoleacetic acid		*See Chapter 53 Table 53.14				
4-Hydroxyphenyllactic acid	U				mmol/mol creatinine	
		0–1 mo			<51	1
		>1 mo			<11	
4-Hydroxyphenylpyruvic acid	U				mmol/mol creatinine	
		0–1 mo			<21	1
		>1 mo			<6	
17-Hydroxyprogesterone			ng/dL	0.03	nmol/L	
		Cord blood	900–5000		27.3–151.5	1
		Premature	26–568		0.8–17.0	
Values (4 d–<19 y) based on Abbott Architect method		4 d–<1 y	<130		<4.2	15
		1–<10 y	<35		<1.1	
		10–<15 y	13–90		0.4–2.7	
		15–<19 y, F	20–1030		0.6–32.6	
		15–<19 y, M	20–60		0.5–1.8	
Tanner values based on Abbott Architect method		Pubertal levels Tanner stage				
		1, M	<44		<1.4	
		1, F	<28		<0.9	
		2, M	<44		<1.4	
		2, F	13–41		0.4–1.3	
		3, M	<50		<1.6	
		3, F	16–47		0.5–1.5	
		4, M	<41		<1.3	
		4, F	19–72		0.6–2.3	
		5, M	13–50		0.4–1.6	
		5, F	<1028		<34.4	
		Adults				1
		M	27–199		0.8–6.0	
		F				
		Follicular phase	15–70		0.4–2.1	
		Luteal phase	35–290		1.0–8.7	
		Pregnancy	200–1200		6.0–36.0	

TABLE A.1 Pediatric and Adult Reference Intervals for Biochemical Markers (Serum, Plasma, and Urine)—cont'd

Analyte	Specimen	Condition	REFERENCE INTERVALS Conventional Units	Conversion Factor	SI Units	Reference Publication
For LC-MSMS reference intervals please see: *Clin Chem* 2006;52:1559–1567 & *Clinical Biochemistry* 2013;46:642–51		Post ACTH	<320		<9.6	
		Postmenopausal	<70		<2.1	
21-Hydroxyprogesterone Pediatric values based on LC-MS/MS method	S		nmol/L	1	nmol/L	
		0–<1 y	0.07–0.76		0.07–0.76	16
		1–<2 y	0.03–0.25		0.03–0.25	
		2–<12 y	0.00–0.15		0.00–0.15	
		12–<19 y	0.00–0.24		0.00–0.24	
Hydroxyproline	P		mg/dL	76.3	μmol/L	
		Premature, 1 d	0–1.56		0–120	1
		6–18 y, M	<0.66		<50	
		6–18 y, F	<0.58		<44	
		Adult, M	<0.55		<42	
		Adult, F	<0.45		<34	
	U, 24 h		mg/d	7.63	μmol/d	
		Adult	<1.4		<11	
			mg/g creatinine	0.863	mmol/mol creatinine	
		Adult	19–36		16–31	
Immunoglobulin A Values (0–<19 y) based on Abbott Architect method	S, P		mg/dL	0.01	g/L	
		0–<1 y	1–29		0.0–0.3	7
		1–<3 y	4–90		0.0–0.9	
		3–<6 y	26–147		0.3–1.5	
		6–<14 y	47–221		0.5–2.2	
		14–<19 y	53–287		0.5–2.9	
		Adult (20–60 y)	70–400		0.7–4.0	1
		Adult (>60 y)	90–4 10		0.9–4.1	
	Saliva	See Table A.2				
	CSF	See Table A.2				
Immunoglobulin D	S		IU/mL	1	kIU/L	
		Adult (20–60 y)	0–160		0–160	1
			ng/mL	1	μg/L	
			0–384		0–384	
Immunoglobulin E Values (0–<19 y) based on Abbott Architect method	S		kIU/L	2.4	μg/L	
		0–<7 y	<25–440		<60–1057	14
		7–<19 y	<25–450		<60–1079	
		Adult (20–60 y)	0–160		0–380	1
Immunoglobulin G Pediatric values (0–<19 y) based on Abbott Architect method	S		mg/dL	0.01	g/L	
		0–14 d	320–1407		3.2–14.1	7
		15 d–<1 y	108–702		1.1–7.0	
		1–<4 y	316–1148		3.2–11.5	
		4–<10 y	542–1358		5.4–13.6	
		10–<19 y	658–1534		6.6–15.3	
		Adult (20–60 y)	700–1600		7.0–16.0	1
		Adult (>60 y)	600–1560		6.0–15.6	
	CSF	See Table A.2				
Immunoglobulin M Values (0–<19 y) based on Abbott Architect method	S		mg/dL	0.01	g/L	
		0–14 d	5–35		0.1–0.4	7
		15 d–13 wk	12–71		0.1–0.7	
		13 wk–<1 y	16–86		0.2–0.9	
		1–<19 y, F	48–186		0.5–1.9	
		1–<19 y, M	39–151		0.4–1.5	

Continued

TABLE A.1 **Pediatric and Adult Reference Intervals for Biochemical Markers (Serum, Plasma, and Urine)—cont'd**

Analyte	Specimen	Condition	REFERENCE INTERVALS			Reference Publication
			Conventional Units	Conversion Factor	SI Units	
		Adult (20–60 y)	40–230		0.4–2.3	1
		Adult (>60 y)	30–360		0.3–3.6	
	CSF	See Table A.2				
Inhibin A	S		pg/mL	1	ng/L	
		M	1.0–3.6		1.0–3.6	1
		F (cycling; days of cycle)				
		Early follicular phase (−14 to −10 d)	5.5–28.2		5.5–28.2	
		Midfollicular phase (−9 to −4 d)	7.9–34.5		7.9–34.5	
		Late follicular phase (−3 to −1 d)	19.5–102.3		19.5–102 .3	
		Midcycle (d 0)	49.9–155.5		49.9–155.5	
		Early luteal (1–3 d)	35.9–132.7		35.9–132.7	
		Midluteal (4–11 d)	13.2–159.6		13.2–159.6	
		Late luteal (12–14 d)	7.3–89.9		7.3–89.9	
		IVF, peak levels	354–1690		354–1690	
		PCOS, ovulatory	5.7–16.0		5.7–16.0	
		Postmenopausal	1.0–3.9		1.0–3.9	
Insulin	S		µIU/mL	6	pmol/L	
Values (0–<6 y) based on Abbott Architect method		0–<1 y	1.0–23.4		7–163	14
		1–<6 y	1.3–40.2		9–279	
Values (6–79 y) based on Siemens Immulite and ADVIA Centaur methods		6–10 y	0.4–13.0		3–93	28
		11–19 y	2.1–19.5		15–140	
		20–79 y	2.4–21.8		17–157	
Insulin-like growth factor-I	S		ng/mL	1	µg/L	
		1–2 y				1
		M	31–160		31–160	
		F	11–206		11–206	
		3–6 y				
		M	16–288		16–288	
		F	70–316		70–316	
		7–10 y				
		M	136–385		136–385	
		F	123–396		123–396	
		11–12 y				
		M	136–440		136–440	
		F	191–462		191–462	
		13–14 y				
		M	165–616		165–616	
		F	286–660		286–660	
		15–18 y				
		M	134–836		134–836	
		F	152–660		152–660	
		19–25 y				

TABLE A.1 Pediatric and Adult Reference Intervals for Biochemical Markers (Serum, Plasma, and Urine)—cont'd

			REFERENCE INTERVALS			
Analyte	Specimen	Condition	Conventional Units	Conversion Factor	SI Units	Reference Publication
		M	202–433		202–433	
		F	231–550		231–550	
		Adult (25–85 y)				
		M	135–449		135–449	
		F	135–449		135–449	
Insulin-like growth factor II	S		ng/mL	1	μg/L	
		Child				1
		Prepubertal	334–642		334–642	
		Pubertal	245–737		245–737	
		Adult	288–736		288–736	
		GH deficiency	51–299		51–299	
Iodine	U		μg/dL	0.079	μmol/L	
Values based on manual microplate analysis		3–5 y	5–83		0.39–6.58	27
		6–79 y	1–49		0.09–3.88	
Iron			μg/dL	0.179	μmol/L	
Values based on Abbott Architect method		0–<14 y	16–128		2.8–22.9	7
		14–<19 y, F	20–162		3.5–29.0	
		14–<19 y, M	31–168		5.5–30.0	
Iron-binding capacity, total	S		μg/dL	0.179	μmol/L	
Values based on Siemens ADVIA method		0–<19 y	300–439		53.7–78.6	19
Isocitric acid	U				mmol/mol creatinine	
		0–1 mo			0–368	1
		1–6 mo			0–67	
		6 mo–5 y			0–77	
		>5 y			16–99	
Isoleucine	P		mg/dL	76.3	μmol/L	
		Premature, 1 d	0.26–0.78		20–60	1
		Newborn, 1 d	0.35–0.69		27–53	
		1–3 mo	0.59–0.95		45–73	
		2–6 mo	0.50–1.61		38–123	
		9 mo–2 y	0.34–1.23		26–94	
		3–10 y	0.37–1.10		28–84	
		6–18 y	0.50–1.24		38–95	
		Adult	0.48–1.28		37–98	
	S	0–<2 wk	0.33–1.69		25–129	20
		2 wk–<1 y	0.39–1.48		30–113	
		1<12 y	0.56–1.69		43–129	
		12–<19 y, F	0.42–0.89		32–68	
		12–<19 y, M	0.69–1.66		53–127	
	U		mg/d	7.62	μmol/d	1
		10 d–7 wk	Trace–0.4		Trace–3	
		3–12 y	2–7		15–53	
		Adult	5–24		38–183	
			mg/g creatinine	0.86	mmol/mol creatinine	
		Adult	1–5		0.8–4.4	1
L-Lactate	WB (Hep)		mg/dL	0.111	mmol/L	
		At bed rest	5–12		0.56–1.39	1
		Venous	<22		<2.5	
		Arterial	16–17		1.78–1.88	
	CSF	See Table A.2				
	U, 24 h	Adult				
					mmol/mol creatinine	
		0–1 mo			46–348	
		1–6 mo			57–346	

TABLE A.1 **Pediatric and Adult Reference Intervals for Biochemical Markers (Serum, Plasma, and Urine)—cont'd**

Analyte	Specimen	Condition	REFERENCE INTERVALS Conventional Units	Conversion Factor	SI Units	Reference Publication
		6 mo–5 y			21–38	
		>5 y			20–101	
	Gastric fluid	See Table A.2				
Lactate dehydrogenase (LD)	S		U/L	0.017	μkat/L	
Pediatric values based on Abbott Architect method		0–<15 d	309–1222		5.25–20.8	7
		15 d–<1 y	163–452		2.77–7.68	
		1–<10 y	192–321		3.26–5.46	
		10–<15 y, F	157–272		2.67–4.62	
		10–<15 y, M	170–283		2.89–4.81	
		15–<19 y	130–250		2.21–4.25	
		Adult	125–220		2.1–3.7	1
Lead	WB (Hep)		μg/dL	0.0483	μmol/L	
		Child	<25		<1.21	1
		Adult	<25		<1.21	
		Toxic	>99		>4.78	
	U, 24 h		μg/L		μmol/L	
			<80		<0.39	
Leucine	P		mg/dL	76.3	μmol/L	
		Premature, 1 d	0.26–1.58		20–120	1
		Newborn, 1 d	0.62–1.43		47–109	
		1–3 mo	10.58–2.14		44–164	
		9 mo–2 y	0.59–2.03		45–155	
		3–10 y	0.73–2.33		56–178	
		6–18 y	1.03–2.28		79–174	
		Adult	0.98–2.29		75–175	
	S	0–< 1 wk	0.60–2.16		46–165	20
		1 wk–<1 y	0.72–2.46		55–188	
		1–<11 y	1.11–2.96		85–226	
		11–<19 y, F	1.10–1.99		84–152	
		11–<19 y, M	1.35–2.98		103–227	
	U, 24 h		mg/d	7.624	μmol/d	1
		10 d–7 wk	0.9–2.0		7–15	
		3–12 y	3–11		23–84	
		Adult	2.6–8.1		20–62	
			mg/g creatinine	0.86	mmol/mol creatinine	
		Adult	0–8		0–6.8	
Lipase	S		U/L	0.017	μkat/L	
Values (0–<19 y) based on Abbott Architect method		0–<19 y	4–39		0.07–0.65	7
37°C		Adult	<38		<0.65	1
Low-density lipoprotein cholesterol (LDL-C) (calculated, Friedewald)			mg/dL	0.0259	mmol/L	
Calculated pediatric values based on Abbott Architect Method		0–<1 y	13.1–173		0.34–4.48	10
		1–<10 y, F	58.7–128		1.52–3.32	
		1–<10 y, M	47.1–121		1.22–3.14	
		10–<19 y	45.6–131		1.18–3.40	
Low-density lipoprotein cholesterol (LDL-C) (measured)	S		mg/dL	0.0259	mmol/L	
Reference Intervals		6–24 y, F	46–143		1.2–3.7	27

TABLE A.1　Pediatric and Adult Reference Intervals for Biochemical Markers (Serum, Plasma, and Urine)—cont'd

			REFERENCE INTERVALS			
Analyte	Specimen	Condition	Conventional Units	Conversion Factor	SI Units	Reference Publication
Values (6–79 y) based on OCD Vitros method		25–49 y, M	62–189		1.6–4.9	
		F	50–178		1.3–4.6	
		50–79 y	73–189		1.9–4.9	
		Note: See more recent guidelines for recommended LDL-C cut-offs for treatment initiation and LDL-C treatment targets to reduce risk of athero-sclerotic cardiovascular disease through cholesterol management (2018 AHA/ACC/AACVPR/AAPA/ABC/ACPM/ADA/AGS/APhA/ASPC/NLA/PCNA Guideline on the Management of Blood Cholesterol). See Chapter 36.				
Clinical Decision Limits			mg/dL	0.0259	mmol/L	
		Risk for coronary heart disease, Child				54
		Acceptable	<110		<2.8	
		Borderline	110–129		<3.3	
		High	>130		>3.4	
		Risk for coronary heart disease, Adults				55
		Optimal	<100		<2.59	
		Near/above optimal	100–129		2.59–3.34	
		Borderline high	130–159		3.37–4.12	
		High	160–189		4.15–4.90	
		Very high	>189		>4.90	
Lecithin-to-sphingomyelin ratio	Amf	See Table A.2				1
Luteinizing hormone (LH)			mIU/mL	1	IU/L	
Values (4 d–<19 y) based on Abbott Architect method		4 d–<3 mo F	<2.4		<2.4	15
		3 mo–<1 y F	<1.2		<1.2	
		1–<10 y, F	<0.3		<0.3	
		10–<13 y, F	<4.3		<4.3	
		13–<15 y, F	0.4–6.5		0.4–6.5	
		15–<17 y, F	<13.1		<13.1	
		17–<19 y, F	<8.4		<8.4	
Tanner values based on Abbott Architect method		Pubertal levels, Tanner stage				
		1, M	<1.2		<1.2	
		1, F	<0.1		<0.1	
		2, M	<1.2		<1.2	
		2, F	<2.3		<2.3	
		3, M	<2.3		<2.3	
		3, F	<7.4		<7.4	
		4, M	<4.9		<4.9	
		4, F	0.3–6.7		0.3–6.7	
		5, M	0.6–5.9		0.6–5.9	
		5, F	0.4–21.2		0.4–21.2	
		M (23–70 y)	1.2–7.8		1.2–7.8	1
		F				
		Follicular phase	1.7–15.0		1.7–15.0	
		Midcycle peak	21.9–56.6		21.9–56.6	

Continued

TABLE A.1 **Pediatric and Adult Reference Intervals for Biochemical Markers (Serum, Plasma, and Urine)—cont'd**

Analyte	Specimen	Condition	REFERENCE INTERVALS			Reference Publication
			Conventional Units	Conversion Factor	SI Units	
		Luteal phase	0.6–16.3		0.6–16.3	
		Postmenopausal	14.2–52.3		14.2–52.3	
Lysine	P		mg/dL	68.5	μmol/L	
		Premature, 1 d	1.01–4.53		70–310	1
		Newborn, 1 d	1.66–3.93		114–269	
		1–3 mo	0.54–2.46		37–169	
		9 mo–2 y	0.66–2.10		45–144	
		3–10 y	1.04–2.20		71–151	
		6–18 y	1.58–3.40		108–233	
		Adult	1.21–3.47		83–238	
	S	0–<2 wk	1.31–4.66		90–319	20
		2 wk–<19 y	1.49–3.78		102–259	
	U, 24 h		mg/d	6.85	μmol/d	1
		10 d–7 wk	5.7–10.9		39–75	
		3–12 y	9.3–93.7		64–642	
		Adult	3.1–153.0		21–1048	
			mg/g creatinine	0.77	mmol/mol creatinine	
		Adult	4–12		3.2–9.2	
α₂-Macroglobulin	S		mg/dL	0.01	g/L	
		Adult (20–60 y)	130–300		1.3–3.0	1
Magnesium AAS	S		mg/dL	0.4114	mmol/L	
		Newborn, 2–4 d	1.5–2.2		0.62–0.91	1
		5 mo–6 y	1.7–2.3		0.70–0.95	
		6–12 y	1.7–2.l		0.70–0.86	
		>12 y	1.6–2.6		0.66–1.07	
			mg/24 h	0.04114	mmol/24 h	
	U, 24 h		12–291		0.50–12.0	
Magnesium, free	S		mmol/L	1.0	mmol/L	
			0.45–0.60		0.45–0.60	1
Magnesium, total (enzymatic)	S		mg/dL	0.4114	mmol/L	
		0–14 d	1.99–3.94		0.82–1.62	7
		15 d–<1 y	1.97–3.09		0.81–1.27	
		1–<19 y	2.09–2.84		0.86–1.17	
Malic acid	U				mmol/mol creatinine	
		0–1 mo			0–52	1
		1–6 mo			8–73	
		6 mo–5 y			4–57	
		>5 y			17–47	
Manganese			μg/L	18.0	nmol/L	
	WB (Hep)		5–15		90–270	1
	S		0.5–1.3		9–24	
	U, collect in metal-free container		0.5–9.8		9.1–178	
		Toxic conc	>19		>342	
Mercury			μg/L	4.99	nmol/L	
	WB (EDTA)		0.6–59		3.0–294.4	1
	U, 24 h		<20		<99.8	
		Toxic conc	>150		>748.5	
		Lethal conc	>800		>3992	
Metanephrines (in serum, plasma)						1

TABLE A.1 Pediatric and Adult Reference Intervals for Biochemical Markers (Serum, Plasma, and Urine)—cont'd

Analyte	Specimen	Condition	Conventional Units	Conversion Factor	SI Units	Reference Publication
Normetanephrine (free)	S, P	*See Chapter 53				1
Metanephrine (free)	S, P	*See Chapter 53				1
Normetanephrine (total)	S, P	*See Chapter 53				1
Metanephrine (total)	S, P	*See Chapter 53				1
Metanephrines (total in urine)						
Metanephrine	U, 24 h	*See Chapter 53, Table 53.9				
Metanephrine	U	*See Chapter 53, Table 53.9				
Normetanephrine	U, 24 h	*See Chapter 53, Table 53.9				
Normetanephrine	U	*See Chapter 53, Table 53.9				
Methanol		See Tables A.3 and A.5				
Methemoglobin (MetHb)	WB (EDTA, Hep or ACD)		g/dL	155	μmol/L	
			0.06–0.24		9.3–37.2	1
			% of total Hb		Mass fraction of total Hb	
			0.04–1.52		0.0004–0.0152	
Methionine			mg/dL	67.7	μmol/L	
	P	Premature, 1 d	0.38–0.66		25–45	1
		Newborn, 1 d	0.13–0.61		9–41	
		1–3 mo	0.05–0.57		3–39	
		2–6 mo	0.24–0.73		16–49	
		9 mo–2 y	0.04–0.43		3–29	
		3–10 y	0.16–0.24		11–16	
		6–18 y	0.24–0.55		16–37	
		Adult	0.09–0.60		6–40	
	S	0–<19 y	0.19–0.65		13–44	20
	U		mg/d	6.7	μmol/d	1
		10 d–7 wk	0.1–1.9		0.7–13	
		3–12 y	3–14		20–95	
		Adult	<9.1		<63	
			mg/g creatinine	0.76	mmol/mol creatinine	
		Adult	0–9.5		0–7.2	
2-Methylbutyrylglycine	U				mmol/mol creatinine	
					0.2–5	1
Methylsuccinic acid	U				mmol/mol creatinine	
					0–12	1
β2-Microglobulin	S		mg/dL	10	mg/L	
Values (0–<19 y) based on Abbott Architect method		0–<3 mo, F	0.19–0.58		1.9–5.8	1
		0–<3 mo, M	0.19–0.47		1.9–4.7	
		3 mo–<2 y	0.13–0.45		1.3–4.5	
		2–<19 y	0.12–0.23		1.2–2.3	
			mg/dL (mean)	10	mg/L (mean)	
		0–59 y	0.19		1.9	
		60–69 y	0.21		2.1	
		>70 y	0.24		2.4	
Molybdenum			μg/L		nmol/L	
	S		0.1–3.0	10.42	1.0–31.3	1

Continued

TABLE A.1 Pediatric and Adult Reference Intervals for Biochemical Markers (Serum, Plasma, and Urine)—cont'd

Analyte	Specimen	Condition	REFERENCE INTERVALS Conventional Units	Conversion Factor	SI Units	Reference Publication
	U, 24 h		40–60 µg/d		416–625 nmol/d	
Myoglobin	S		ng/mL	1.0	µg/L	
Values based on OCD		0–<2 wk	13.9–234		13.9–234	8
Vitros method		2 wk–<1 y	7.29–60.9		7.29–60.9	
		1–<13 y	15.1–50.3		15.1–50.3	
		13–<19 y, F	11.7–47.3		11.7–47.3	
		13–<19 y, M	16.7–206		16.7–206	
Niacin	U, 24 h		mg/d	7.3	µmol/d	
			2.4–6.4		17.5–46.7	1
Nickel			µg/L	17	nmol/L	
	S or P (Hep)		0.14–1.0		2.4–17.0	1
	WB		1.0–28.0		17–476	
			µg/d		nmol/d	
	U, 24 h		0.1–10		2–170	
N-telopeptide (BCE = bone collagen equivalents)	S		nmol BCE/L	1.0	nmol BCE/L	
		Men	5.4–24.2		5.4–24.2	1
		Premenopausal women	6.2–19.0		6.2–19.0	
			nmol BCE/mmol creatinine	1.0	nmol BCE/ mmol creatinine	
		Men	3–63		3–63	
		Premenopausal women	5–65		5–65	
Nuclear matrix protein 22 (NMP-22)	S		U/mL	1.0	kU/L	
			<10		<10	1
Orotic acid					mmol/mol creatinine	
	U	0–1 mo			1.4–5.3	1
		1–6 mo			1.0–3.2	
		6 mo–5 y			0.5–3.3	
		>5 y			0.4–1.2	
Osteocalcin	S		ng/mL	1.0	µg/L	
		Adult, M	3.0–13.0		3.0–13.0	1
		Adult, F				
		Premenopausal	0.4–8.2		0.4–8.2	
		Postmenopausal	1.5–11.0		1.5–11.0	
Oxalic acid					mmol/mol creatinine	
	U	0–1 mo			51–931	1
		1–6 mo			7–567	
		6 mo–5 y			7–352	
		>5 y			<188	
2-Oxoglutaric acid	S				mmol/mol creatinine	
		0–1 mo			22–567	1
		1–6 mo			63–552	
		6 mo–5 y			36–103	
		>5 y			41–82	
Oxygen, partial pressure (PO_2)	Cord blood		mm Hg	0.133	kPa	
	Arterial		5.7–30.5		0.8–4.0	1
	Venous		17.4–41.0		2.3–5.5	
	WB, arterial	Birth	8–24		1.06–3.19	
		5–10 min	33–75		4.39–9.96	

TABLE A.1　Pediatric and Adult Reference Intervals for Biochemical Markers (Serum, Plasma, and Urine)—cont'd

Analyte	Specimen	Condition	Conventional Units	Conversion Factor	SI Units	Reference Publication
		30 min	31–85		4.12–11.31	
		1 h	55–80		7.32–10.64	
		1 d	54–95		7.18–12.64	
		2 d–60 y	83–108		11.04–14.36	
		>60 y	>80		>10.64	
		>70 y	>70		>9.31	
		>80 y	>60		>7.98	
		>90 y	>50		>6.65	
Oxygen, saturation (sO₂)	WB, arterial		Percent saturation	0.01	Fraction saturation	
		Newborn	40–90		0.40–0.90	1
		Thereafter	94–93		0.94–0.98	
Oxytocin	P, EDTA		μU/mL	1.0	mU/L	
		M	1.1–1.9		1.0–1.9	1
		F				
		Nonpregnant	1.0–1.8		1.0–1.8	
		Second stage of labor	3.2–5.3		3.2–5.3	
Pantothenic acid			μg/L	0.0046	μmol/L	
	WB		344–583		1.57–2.66	1
			mg/d	4.53	μmol/d	
	U, 24 h		1–15		5–68	
Parathyroid hormone, intact	S		pg/mL	0.106	pmol/L	
Values (6 d–<3 y) based on Abbott Architect method		6 d–<1 y	6–89		0.7–9.4	3
		1–<3 y	16–63		1.7–6.7	
Values (3–79 y) based on DiaSorin LIAISON method		3–5 y	7–29		0.7–3.1	28
		6–11 y	7–30		0.7–3.2	
		12–15 y	8–36		0.8–3.8	
		16–29 y	8–32		0.8–3.4	
		30–79 y	9–42		1.0–4.4	
Parathyroid hormone, (1–84)	S		pg/mL	1.0	ng/L	
			6–40		6–40	1
Parathyroid hormone-related peptide (PTHrP)	S		pmol/L	1.0	pmol/L	
			<1.4		<1.4	1
pH (37°C)	WB, arterial		pH	1.0	pH	
		Cord blood				1
		Arterial	7.18–7.38		7.18–7.38	
		Venous	7.25–7.45		7.25–7.45	
		Newborn				
		Premature, 48 h	7.35–7.50		7.35–7.50	
		Full term				
		Birth	7.11–7.36		7.11–7.36	
		5–10 min	7.09–7.30		7.09–7.30	
		30 min	7.21–7.38		7.21–7.38	
		1 h	7.26–7.49		7.26–7.49	
		1 d	7.29–7.45		7.29–7.45	
		Children, adults				
		Arterial	7.35–7.45		7.35–7.45	
		Venous	7.32–7.43		7.32–7.43	
		Adults				
		60–90 y	7.31–7.42		7.31–7.42	
		>90 y	7.26–7.43		7.26–7.43	

TABLE A.1 Pediatric and Adult Reference Intervals for Biochemical Markers (Serum, Plasma, and Urine)—cont'd

Analyte	Specimen	Condition	REFERENCE INTERVALS Conventional Units	Conversion Factor	SI Units	Reference Publication
Phenylalanine			mg/dL	60.5	μmol/L	
	Dry blood spot		<2.1		<122	1
	P	Premature	2.0–7.5		121–454	
		Newborn	1.2–3.4		73–205	
		Phenylketonuric 2–3 d	>4.5		>272	
		Phenylketonuric untreated	15–30		907–1815	
		Adult	0.8–1.8			
	S	0–<2 wk	0.81–1.77		49–107	20
		2 wk–<1 y	0.86–1.92		52–116	
		1–<19 y	0.91–1.67		55–101	
			mg/d	6.05	μmol/d	1
	U, 24 h	10 d DiaSorin LIAISON 7 wk	1.2–1.7		7–10	
		3–13 y	4.0–17.5		24–106	
		Adult	<16.5		<100	
			mg/g creatinine	0.68	mmol/mol creatinine	
		Adult	2–10		1.3–6.9	
3-Phenylpropionylglycine	U				mmol/mol creatinine	
					<0.7	1
Phosphate	S		mg/dL	0.323	mmol/L	
Values (0–<3 y) based on Abbott Architect method		0–14 d	5.6–10.5		1.80–3.40	7
		15 d–<1 y	4.8–8.4		1.54–2.72	
		1–<3 y	4.3–6.8		1.38–2.19	
Values (3–79 y) based on OCD Vitros method		3–5 y	4.4–6.0		1.41–1.94	27
		6–10 y	4.4–5.7		1.41–1.85	
		11–15 y, M	3.8–5.9		1.24–1.91	
		F	3.6–5.6		1.16–1.81	
		16–47 y	2.9–4.7		0.95–1.52	
		48–79 y, M	2.8–4.7		0.89–1.52	
		F	3.1–4.8		0.99–1.54	
	U, 24 h		g/d	32.3	mmol/d	
		Adults	0.4–1.3		12.9–42.0	
Phosphatase, acid tartrate resistant 37°C	S		U/L	0.017	μkat/L	
		Children	3.4–9.0		0.05–0.15	1
		Adult	1.5–4.5		0.03–0.08	
Phosphatase, alkaline IFCC, 37°C	S		U/L	0.017	μkat/L	
Values (0–<3 y) based on Abbott Architect method		0–14 d	90–273		1.50–4.55	7
		15 d–<1 y	134–518		2.23–8.63	
		1–<3 y	156–369		2.60–6.15	
Values (3–79 y) based on OCD Vitros method		3–5 y	144–327		2.45–5.56	27
		6–10 y	153–367		2.60–6.24	
		11–15 y, M	113–438		1.92–7.45	
		11–15 y, F	64–359		1.09–6.10	
		16–21 y, M	56–167		0.95–2.84	
		16–29 y, F	44–107		0.75–1.82	
		22–79 y, M	50–116		0.85–1.97	
		30–79 y, F	46–122		0.78–2.07	

TABLE A.1 Pediatric and Adult Reference Intervals for Biochemical Markers (Serum, Plasma, and Urine)—cont'd

Analyte	Specimen	Condition	REFERENCE INTERVALS Conventional Units	Conversion Factor	SI Units	Reference Publication
Phosphatase, alkaline (bone specific, by immunoabsorption)	S		U/L	1.0	U/L	
		Men	15.0–41.3		15.0–41.3	1
		Premenopausal women	11.6–29.6		11.6–29.6	
Phosphatase, alkaline isoenzymes						1
			Percentage of Total Activity	NA	*Fraction Activity*	
Biliary		<1 y	3–6		0.03–0.06	
		1–15 y	2–5		0.02–0.05	
		Adult	1–3		0.01–0.03	
		Pregnant women	1–3		0.01–0.03	
		Postmenopausal women	0–12		0.0–0.12	
Liver		<1 y	20–34		0.20–0.34	
		1–15 y	22–34		0.22–0.34	
		Adult	17–35		0.17–0.35	
		Pregnant women	5–17		0.05–0.17	
		Postmenopausal women	17–48		0.17–0.48	
Bone		<1 y	20–30		0.20–0.30	
		1–15 y	21–30		0.21–0.30	
		Adult	13–19		0.13–0.19	
		Pregnant women	8–14		0.08–0.14	
		Postmenopausal women	8–21		0.08–0.21	
Placental		<1 y	8–19		0.08–0.19	
		1–15 y	5–17		0.05–0.17	
		Adult	13–21		0.13–0.21	
		Pregnant women	53–69		0.53–0.69	
		Postmenopausal women	7–15		0.07–0.15	
Renal		<1 y	1–3		0.01–0.03	
		1–15 y	0–1		0.0–0.01	
		Adult	0–2		0.0–0.02	
		Pregnant women	3–6		0.03–0.06	
		Postmenopausal women	0–2		0.0–0.02	
Intestinal		<1 y	0–2		0.0–0.02	
		1–15 y	0–1		0.0–0.01	
		Adult	0–1		0.0–0.01	
		Pregnant women	0–1		0.0–0.01	
		Postmenopausal women	0–1		0.0–0.01	
Pimelic acid	U				mmol/mol creatinine	
					<1.1	1
Porphobilinogen	U, 24 h		mg/L	4.42	μmol/L	
			<2.26		<10	1
Porphyrins, total	U, 24 h				nmol/L	
					20–320	1
	Feces				nmol/L g dry wt	
					10–200	

Continued

TABLE A.1 **Pediatric and Adult Reference Intervals for Biochemical Markers (Serum, Plasma, and Urine)—cont'd**

Analyte	Specimen	Condition	REFERENCE INTERVALS Conventional Units	REFERENCE INTERVALS Conversion Factor	REFERENCE INTERVALS SI Units	Reference Publication
	Erythrocytes				μmol/L erythrocytes 0.4–1.7	
Potassium (K)			mEq/L	1.0	mmol/L	
	S	Premature cord	5.0–10.2		5.0–10.2	1
		Premature, 48 h	3.0–6.0		3.0–6.0	
		Newborn cord	5.6–12.0		5.6–12.0	
		Newborn	3.7–5.9		3.7–5.9	
		Infant	4.1–5.3		4.1–5.3	
Values (0–2 y) based on Siemens ADVIA method		0–<1 y, F	4.2–6.2		4.2–6.2	19
		0–<1 y, M	4.3–6.7		4.3–6.7	
		1–2 y	4.0–5.3		4.0–5.3	
Values (3–79 y) based on OCD Vitros method		3–5 y	3.9–4.6		3.9–4.6	27
		6–79 y	3.8–4.9		3.8–4.9	
			mEq/d	1.0	mmol/d	
	U, 24 h	6–10 y				
		M	17–54		17–54	1
		F	8–37		8–37	
		10–14 y				
		M	22–57		22–57	
		F	18–58		18–58	
		Adult	25–125		25–125	
Progastrin-Releasing Peptide (ProGRP)	S		pg/mL	1.0	ng/L	
Values based on Abbott Architect method		0–<1 wk	535–1889		535–1889	4
		1 wk–<6 mo	57–817		57–817	
		6 mo–<1 y	25–198		25–198	
		1–<12 y	22–129		22–129	
		12–<19 y	17–83		17–83	
Proinsulin	S		pmol/L	1.0	pmol/L	
			1.1–6.9		1.1–6.9	1
Prolactin	S		ng/mL	21.0	mIU/L	
		Cord blood	45–539		945–11319	1
Values (4 d–<19 y) based on Abbott Architect method		4–<30 d	13–213		273–4473	15
		30 d–<1 y	6–114		126–2394	
		1–<19 y	4–23		84–483	
Tanner values based on Abbott Architect method		Puberty, Tanner stage				
		1, M	3–20		63–420	
		1, F	2–20		42–420	
		2, M	4–19		84–399	
		2, F	4–23		84–483	
		3, M	4–23		84–483	
		3, F	4–23		84–483	
		4, M	6–20		126–420	
		4, F	6–23		126–483	
		5, M	7–32		147–672	
		5, F	5–23		105–483	
		Adult				1
		M	3.0–14.7		63.0–308.7	
		F	3.8–23.0		79.8–483.0	
		Pregnancy, 3rd trimester	95–473		1995–9933	

TABLE A.1   Pediatric and Adult Reference Intervals for Biochemical Markers (Serum, Plasma, and Urine)—cont'd

Analyte	Specimen	Condition	REFERENCE INTERVALS			Reference Publication
			Conventional Units	Conversion Factor	SI Units	
Proline			mg/dL	86.9	μmol/L	
	P	Premature, 1 d	0.92–4.36		80–380	1
		Newborn, 1 d	1.23–3.18		107–277	
		1–3 mo	0.89–3.73		77–325	
		9 mo–2 y	0.59–2.13		51–185	
		3–10 y	0.78–1.70		68–148	
		6–18 y	0.67–3.72		58–324	
	S	0–<1 y	1.46–3.36		127–292	20
		1–<13 y	1.36–4.28		118–372	
		13–<19 y	1.33–4.14		116–360	
	U, 24 h	Adult	1.17–3.86		102–336	1
			mg/d	8.69	μmol/d	
		10 d–7 wk	3.2–11.0		28–96	
		3–12 y	Trace		Trace	
		Adult	Trace		Trace	
			μmol/g creatinine	0.113	μmol/mol creatinine	
		0–1 mo	70–2300		7.91–259.9	
		1–6 mo	<600		<67.8	
		6 mo–1 y	<300		<33.9	
		1–2 y	<270		<30.5	
		2–3 y	<220		<24.9	
Propionylcarnitine					μmol/L	
	P	0–7 d			0.07–1.85	1
		8 d–7 y			0.17–1.27	
		>7 y			0.17–1.49	
	WB spots				0.55–8.01	
	Bile spots				0.36–8.10	
					mmol/mol creatinine	
	U	0–7 d			0.01–0.20	
		8 d–7 y			0.01–1.20	
		>7 y			0.00–0.06	
Prostate-specific antigen (PSA)	S		ng/mL	1.0	μg/L	
		M				1
		40–49 y	0–2.5		0–2.5	
		50–59 y	0–3.5		0–3.5	
		60–69 y	0–4.5		0–4.5	
		70–79 y	0–6.5		0–6.5	
Protein, total			g/dL	10	g/L	
	Cord		4.8–8.0		48–80	1
	S	Premature	3.6–6.0		36–60	
Values (0–<3 y) based on Abbott Architect method		0–14 d	5.3–8.3		53–83	7
		15 d–<1 y	4.4–7.1		44–71	
		1–<3 y	6.1–7.5		61–75	
Values (3–79 y) based on OCD Vitros method		3–5 y	6.3–8.1		63–81	27
		6–19 y	6.8–8.2		68–82	
		20–29 y	6.5–8.3		65–83	
		30–79 y	6.5–7.8		65–78	
	U, 24 h		mg/dL	10	mg/L	1
		Adult	1–14		10–140	
		Excretion	mg/d	0.001	g/d	
		Adult	<100		<0.1	
		Pregnancy	<150		<0.15	
	CSF	See Table A.2				

Continued

TABLE A.1 **Pediatric and Adult Reference Intervals for Biochemical Markers (Serum, Plasma, and Urine)—cont'd**

Analyte	Specimen	Condition	Conventional Units	Conversion Factor	SI Units	Reference Publication
Pyroglutamic acid	U				mmol/mol creatinine	
					<62	1
Pyruvic acid			mg/dL	0.114	μmol/L	
	WB, arterial	Adult	0.2–0.7		0.02–0.08	1
	WB, venous	Adult	0.3–0.9		0.03–0.10	
	CSF	See Table A.2				
	U, 24 h	Adult			<1.1 mmol/d	
					mmol/mol creatinine	
	U	0–1 mo			24–123	
		1–6 mo			8–90	
		6 mo–5 y			3–19	
		>5 y			6–9	
Remnant cholesterol (calculated)	S		mg/dL	0.0259	mmol/L	
Calculated pediatric values based on Abbott Architect method		0–<14 d	16.2–50.6		0.42–1.31	10
		14 d–<1 y	10.4–51.7		0.27–1.34	
		1–<19 y	8.88–39.0		0.23–1.01	
Retinol-binding protein (RBP)			mg/dL	10	mg/L	
	S	Birth	1.1–3.4		11–34	1
		6 mo	1.8–5.0		18–50	
		Adult	3.0–6.0		30–60	
Reverse triiodothyronine (rT$_3$)	S		ng/dL	0.0154	nmol/L	
		Cord (>37 wk)	130–300		2.00–4.62	1
		Children				
		1 d	83–194		1.28–2.99	
		2 d	107–209		1.65–3.22	
		3 d	102–166		1.57–2.56	
		1 mo–20 y	10–35		0.15–0.54	
		Adult	10–28		0.15–0.43	
		Maternal serum (15–40 wk)	11–33		0.17–0.51	
		Amniotic serum (17–22 wk)	163–599		2.51–9.22	
Rheumatoid factor (RF)	S		IU/mL	1	kIU/L	
Values (0–<19 y) based on Abbott Architect method		0–14 d	9.0–17.1		9.0–17.1	7
		15 d–<19 y	9.0–9.0		9.0–9.0	
		Adult	<7.5–14		<7.5–14	32
Riboflavin (vitamin B$_2$)			μg/dL	26.6	nmol/L	
	S		4–24		106–638	1
	Erythrocytes		10–50		266–1330	
			μg/g creatinine	0.3	μmol/mol creatinine	
	U		>80		>24	
			μg/d	2.66	nmol/d	
	U, 24 h		>100		>266	
Sebacic acid	U	0–1 mo			mmol/mol creatinine	1
		1–6 mo			3–16	
		>6 mo			3–26	
					<9	
Selenium	S		μg/L	0.0127	μmol/L	
		Neonates	<8.0 (deficiency)		<0.10 (deficiency)	1
		<2 y	16–71		0.2–0.9	

TABLE A.1   Pediatric and Adult Reference Intervals for Biochemical Markers (Serum, Plasma, and Urine)—cont'd

Analyte	Specimen	Condition	Conventional Units	Conversion Factor	SI Units	Reference Publication
		2–4 y	40–103		0.5–1.3	
		4–16 y	55–134		0.7–1.7	
		Adults	63–160		0.8–2.0	
	WB (Hep)		58–234		0.74–2.97	
	U, 24 h		7–160		0.09–2.03	
		Toxic conc	>400		>5.08	
Serotonin		*See Chapter 53, Table 53.15				
Sex hormone–binding globulin (SHBG)	S		nmol/L	1	nmol/L	
Values (4 d–<19 y) based on Abbott Architect method		4 d–<1 mo	14.4–120.2		14.4–120.2	15
		1 mo–<1 y	36.2–229.0		36.2–229.0	
		1–<8 y	41.8–188.7		41.8–188.7	
		8–<11 y	26.4–162.4		26.4–162.4	
		11–<13 y	14.9–107.8		14.9–107.8	
		13–<15 y	11.2–98.2		11.2–98.2	
		15–<17 y, F	9.8–84.1		9.8–84.1	
		17–<19 y, F	10.8–154.6		10.8–154.6	
Tanner values based on Abbott Architect method		Puberty, Tanner stage				
		1, M	23.4–156.8		23.4–156.8	
		1, F	21.1–210.1		21.1–210.1	
		2, M	27.5–133.4		27.5–133.4	
		2, F	29.6–140.7		29.6–140.7	
		3, M	17.4–160.1		17.4–160.1	
		3, F	23.7–101.7		23.7–101.7	
		4, M	12.2–79.4		12.2–79.4	
		4, F	12.1–125.6		12.1–125.6	
		5, M	7.7–49.4		7.7–49.4	
		5, F	15.3–92.5		15.3–92.5	
		Adult				33
		20 y	13.1–53.2		13.1–53.2	
		30 y	13.5–57.4		13.5–57.4	
		40 y	15.3–65.3		15.3–65.3	
		50 y	18.4–75.6		18.4–75.6	
		60 y	22.6–87.6		22.6–87.6	
		70 y	27.8–101.0		27.8–101.0	
		80 y	33.8–115.4		33.8–115.4	
Sodium (Na)			mEq/L	1.0	mmol/L	
		Premature cord	116–140		116–140	1
		Premature, 48 h	128–148		128–148	
		Newborn cord	126–166		126–166	
		Newborn	133–146		133–146	
		Infant	139–146		139–146	
Values (0–3 y) based on Siemens ADVIA method		0–3 y	139–146		139–146	19
Values (3–79 y) based on OCD Vitros method		3–5 y	135–142		135–142	27
		6–15 y	136–143		136–143	
		16–49 y, M	137–143		137–143	
		F	137–142		137–142	
		50–79 y	136–143		136–143	
	U, 24 h	6–10 y	mEq/d	1.0	mmol/d	1
		M	41–115		41–115	
		F	20–69		20–69	
		10–14 y				

Continued

TABLE A.1   Pediatric and Adult Reference Intervals for Biochemical Markers (Serum, Plasma, and Urine)—cont'd

Analyte	Specimen	Condition	Conventional Units	Conversion Factor	SI Units	Reference Publication
		M	63–177		63–177	
		F	48–168		48–168	
		Adult				
		M	40–220		40–220	
		F	27–287		27–287	
Suberic acid	U				mmol/mol creatinine	
		0–6 mo			4–20	1
		>6 mo			<9	
Succinic acid	U				mmol/mol creatinine	
		0–1 mo			35–547	1
		1–6 mo			34–156	
		6 mo–5 y			16–118	
		> 5 y			29–87	
Squamous Cell Carcinoma Antigen (SCC)	S		ng/mL	1.0	µg/L	
Values based on Abbott Architect method		0–<1 wk	>70		>70	4
		1 wk–<1 y	0.6–17		0.6–17	
		1–<19 y	0.4–1.6		0.4–1.6	
Testosterone, bioavailable (Vermeulen equation)	S		ng/dL	0.0347	nmol/L	
Values (0–<19 y) based on Abbott Architect method		0–<1 y, F	0.29–6.05		0.01–0.21	18
		1–<9 y, F	0.29–6.05		0.01–0.21	
		9–<14 y, F	0.58–10.95		0.02–0.38	
		14–<19 y, F	3.75–23.05		0.13–0.80	
		0–<1 y, M	0–121.9		0.01–4.23	
		1–<9 y, M	0.29–2.88		0.01–0.10	
		9–<14 y, M	0.58–161.69		0.02–5.62	
		14–<19 y, M	12.1–346.69		0.42–12.03	
		Adult				
		M	66–417		2.29–14.5	1
		F	0.6–5.0		0.02–0.17	
Testosterone, free (Vermeulen Equation)	S		pg/mL	3.47	pmol/L	
		Cord, M	5–22		17.4–76.3	1
		Cord, F	4–19		13.9–55.5	
Values (0–<19 y) based on Abbott Architect method		0–<1 y, F	0.1–2.6		0.4–9.0	18
		1–<9 y, F	0.1–2.6		0.4–9.0	
		9–<14 y, F	0.3–4.7		1.0–16.3	
		14–<19 y, F	1.4–9.9		4.9–34.4	
		0–<1 y, M	0.03–57.2		0.1–198.6	
		1–<9 y, M	0.1–1.2		0.4–4.2	
		9–<14 y, M	0.4–72.2		1.4–250.7	
		14–<19 y, M	5.0–142.3		17.4–494.1	
		Adult				
		M	50–210		174–729	
		F	1.0–8.5		3.5–29.5	
Testosterone, total	S		ng/dL	0.0347	nmol/L	
		Cord, M	13–55		0.45–1.91	1
		Cord, F	5–45		0.17–1.56	
		Premature				
		M	37–198		1.28–6.87	
		F	5–22		0.17–0.76	

TABLE A.1 Pediatric and Adult Reference Intervals for Biochemical Markers (Serum, Plasma, and Urine)—cont'd

Analyte	Specimen	Condition	Conventional Units	Conversion Factor	SI Units	Reference Publication
					REFERENCE INTERVALS	
Values (4 d–<19 y) based on Abbott Architect method		4 d–<9 y, F	1–62		0.0–2.15	15
		9–<13 y, F	<28		<0.98	
		13–<15 y, F	10–44		0.36–1.54	
		15–<19 y, F	14–49		0.49–1.70	
		4 d–<6 mo, M	9–299		0.3–10.37	
		6 mo–<9 y, M	<36		<1.24	
		9–<11 y, M	<23		<0.81	
		11–<14 y, M	<444		<15.42	
		14–<16 y, M	36–632		1.25–21.94	
		16–<19 y, M	148–794		5.13–27.55	
		Pubertal levels Tanner stage				
Tanner values based on Abbott Architect method		1, M	<18		<0.62	
		1, F	<19		<0.67	
		2, M	<25		<0.85	
		2, F	<20		<0.69	
		3, M	<543		<18.85	
		3, F	<42		<1.45	
		4, M	9–636		0.30–22.08	
		4, F	9–42		0.31–1.44	
		5, M	100–760		3.46–26.36	
		5, F	4–50		0.13–1.72	
		Adult				
		M	260–1000		9–34.72	1
		F	15–70		0.52–2.43	
For LC-MSMS pediatric reference intervals please see: *Clinical Biochemistry* 2013;46:642–51						
Tetradecanedioic acid	U				mmol/mol creatinine	
					<0.5	1
Thallium			µg/L	4.89	nmol/L	
	WB (Hep)		<5		<24 .5	1
			mg/L		µmol/L	
		Toxic	0.1–8.0		0.5–390	
			µg/L	4.89	Nmol/L	
	U, 24 h		<2.0		<9.8	
			mg/L		µmol/L	
		Toxic	1.0–20.0		4.9–97.8	
Thiocyanate	S		mg/dL	172.4	µmol/L	
		Nonsmokers	<0.4		<69	1
		Smokers	<1.2		<207	
		Nitroprusside therapy	0.6–2.9		103–500	
		Toxic	>5		>862	
Threonine	P		mg/dL	84	µmol/L	
		Premature, 1 d	1.14–3.98		95–335	1
		Newborn, 1 d	1.36–3.99		114–335	
		1–3 mo	0.75–2.67		64–224	
		2–6 mo	2.27–4.33		191–364	
		3–10 y	0.50–1.13		42–95	
		6–18 y	0.88–2.40		74–202	
		Adult	0.94–2.30		79–193	
	S	0–<1 y	0.96–3.73		81–313	20

TABLE A.1 Pediatric and Adult Reference Intervals for Biochemical Markers (Serum, Plasma, and Urine)—cont'd

Analyte	Specimen	Condition	REFERENCE INTERVALS			Reference Publication
			Conventional Units	Conversion Factor	SI Units	
	U, 24 h	1–<19 y	0.86–2.20 mg/d	8.40	72–185 μmol/d	
		10 d–7 wk	1.5–11.9		13–100	1
		3–12 y	10.1–29.6		85–249	
		Adult	14.3–46.7		120–392	
			mg/g creatinine	0.95	mmol/mol creatinine	
		Adult	0–28		0–27	
Thyroglobulin (TG)	S		ng/mL	1.0	μg/L	
Pediatric values (0–<19 years) based on Beckman DxI method		0–<2 y, F	7.82–79.5		7.82–79.5	12
		0–<2 y, M	2.99–56.0		2.99–56.0	
		2–<6 y	6.74–34.2		6.74–34.2	
		6–<9 y	5.01–28.5		5.01–28.5	
		9–<19 y	2.50–25.8		2.50–25.8	
		Adult euthyroid	3–42		3–42	1
		Athyroidic patient	<5		<5	
Thyroid uptake	S		%	1.0	%	
Pediatric values based on Beckman DxI method		0–<12 y	38.1–49.5		38.1–49.5	12
		12–<19 y, F	38.1–48.5		38.1–48.5	
		12–<19 y, M	39.6–48.8		39.6–48.8	
Thyrotropin (thyroid-stimulating hormone) (TSH)			μIU/mL	1.0	mIU/L	
	S	Premature, 28–36 wk	0.7–27.0		0.7–27.0	1
		Cord blood (>37 wk)	2.3–13.2		2.3–13.2	
Values (4 d–<19 y) based on Abbott Architect method		4 d–<6 mo	0.7–4.8		0.7–4.8	3
		6 mo–<14 y	0.7–4.2			
		14–<19 y	0.5–3.4		0.5–3.4	
		Adults				1
		21–54 y	0.4–4.2		0.4–4.2	
		55–87 y	0.5–8.9		0.5–8.9	
		Pregnancy	μU/mL	1.0	mU/L	
		1st trimester	0.1–2.5		0.1–2.5	36
		2nd trimester	0.2–3.0		0.2–3.0	
		3rd trimester	0.3–3.0		0.3–3.0	
	WB (heel puncture)	Newborn screen	<20		<20	
Thyroxine-binding globulin (TBG)			mg/dL	10	mg/L	
	S	Cord	3.6–9.6		36–96	1
		Children				
		4 mo–1 y	3.1–5.6		31–56	
		1–5 y	2.9–5.4		29–54	
		5–10 y	2.5–5.0		25–50	
		10–15 y	2.1–4.6		21–46	
		Adult				
		M	1.2–2.5		12–25	
		F	1.4–3.0		14–30	
		F (oral contraceptive)	1.5–5.5		15–55	

TABLE A.1   Pediatric and Adult Reference Intervals for Biochemical Markers (Serum, Plasma, and Urine)—cont'd

Analyte	Specimen	Condition	REFERENCE INTERVALS			Reference Publication
			Conventional Units	Conversion Factor	SI Units	
Thyroxine (T₄), total			μg/dL	12.9	nmol/L	
Values (7 d–<19 y) based on Abbott Architect method	S	7 d–<1 y	5.9–13.7		76–176	3
		1–<9 y	6.2–10.3		79–133	
		9–<12 y	5.5–9.3		71–120	
		12–<14 y, F	5.1–8.3		65–107	
		12–<14 y, M	5.0–8.3		65–107	
		14–<19 y, F	5.5–13.0		70–167	
		Adults (15–60 y)				1
		M	4.6–10.5		59–135	
		F	5.5–11.0		65–138	
		>60 y	5.0–10.7		65–138	
		Newborn screen				
		1–5 d	>7.5		>97	
		6 d	>6.5		>84	
Thyroxine, free (FT₄)	S		ng/dL	12.9	pmol/L	
		Newborns (1–4 d)	2.2–5.3		28.4–68.4	1
Values (5 d–<19 y) based on Abbott Architect method		5–15 d	1.1–3.2		13.5–41.3	3
		15–<30 d	0.7–2.5		8.7–32.5	
		30 d–<1 y	0.9–1.7		11.4–21.9	
		1–<19 y	0.9–1.4		11.4–17.6	
		Adults (21–87 y)	0.8–2.7		10.3–34.7	1
		Pregnancy				
		1st trimester	0.7–2.0		9.0–25.7	
		2nd and 3rd trimesters	0.5–1.6		6.4–20.6	
Thyroxine, free index (FT₄I)	S		μg/dL	12.9	nmol/L	
		Cord	6.0–13.2		77–170	1
		Infants				
		1–3 d	9.9–17.5		128–226	
		1 wk	7.5–15.1		97–195	
		1–12 mo	5.0–13.0		65–168	
		Children				
		1–10 y	5.4–12.8		70–165	
		Pubertal child and adult	4.2–13.0		54–168	
Transferrin	S		mg/dL	0.01	g/L	
Values (0–<19 y) based on Abbott Architect method		0–<9 wk	104–224		1.0–2.2	7
		9 wk–<1 y	107–324		1.1–3.2	
		1–<19 y	220–337		2.2–3.4	
		20–60 y	200–360		2.0–3.6	1
		>60 y	160–340		1.6–3.4	
Transferrin saturation Values based on Abbott Architect method	S		%	1.0	%	
		0–<1 y	4.1–59		4.1–59	11
		1–<14 y	6.5–39		6.5–39	
		14–<19 y, F	5.2–44		5.2–44	
		14–<19 y, M	9.6–58		9.6–58	
Soluble transferrin receptor (STfR)	S		mg/L		mg/L	

Continued

TABLE A.1   Pediatric and Adult Reference Intervals for Biochemical Markers (Serum, Plasma, and Urine)—cont'd

Analyte	Specimen	Condition	Conventional Units	Conversion Factor	SI Units	Reference Publication
Values based on Beckman DxI method		0–<1 y	0.98–1.99		0.98–1.99	
		1–<2.5 y	1.37–2.64		1.37–2.64	12
		2.5–<14 y	1.03–2.09		1.03–2.09	
		14–<19 y	0.79–1.68		0.79–1.68	
Transketolase, erythrocyte	Erythrocytes		U/g Hb	64.53	kU/mol Hb	
			0.75–1.30		48.4–83.9	1
Transthyretin (prealbumin)	S		mg/dL	10	mg/L	
Values (0–<19 y) based on Abbott Architect method		0–14 d	2–12		20–120	7
		15 d–<1 y	5–24		50–240	
		1–<5 y	12–23		120–230	
		5–<13 y	14–26		140–260	
		13–<16 y	18–31		180–310	
		16–<19 y, F	17–33		170–330	
		16–<19 y, M	20–35		200–350	
		Adult (20–60 y)	20–40		200–400	1
Triglycerides	S		mg/dL	0.0113	mmol/L	
Reference Intervals						
Values (0–<6 y) based on Abbott Architect method		0–14 d	82–259		0.9–2.9	7
		15 d–<1 y	53–258		0.6–2.9	
		1–<6 y	44–197		0.5–2.2	
Values (6–79 y) based on OCD Vitros method		6–29 y	35–186		0.4–2.1	27
		30–79 y M	44–301		0.5–3.4	
		30–79 F	35–212		0.4–2.4	
Clinical Decision Limits		Recommended cutoff points, Child 0–9 y	mg/dL	0.0113	mmol/L	54
		Acceptable	<75		<0.9	
		Borderline	75–99		0.9–1.1	
		High	≥100		>1.1	
		10–19 y				
		Acceptable	<90		<1.0	
		Borderline	90–129		1.0–1.5	
		High	≥130		>1.5	
		Recommended cutoff points, Adult	mg/dL	0.0113	mmol/L	55
		Normal	<150		<1.70	
		High	150–199		1.70–2.25	
		Hypertriglyceridemic	200–499		2.26–5.64	
		Very high	>499		>5.64	
Triiodothyronine (T₃), free			pg/dL	0.0154	pmol/L	
	S	Cord	15–391		0.2–6.0	1
Values (4 d–<19 y) based on Abbott Architect method		4 d–<1 y	234–487		3.6–7.5	3
		1–<12 y	279–442		4.3–6.8	
		12–<15 y, F	247–396		3.8–6.1	
		12–<15 y, M	286–435		4.4–6.7	
		15–<19 y, F	234–370		3.6–5.7	
		15–<19 y, M	227–383		3.5–5.9	
		Adult	210–440		3.2–6.8	1

TABLE A.1 Pediatric and Adult Reference Intervals for Biochemical Markers (Serum, Plasma, and Urine)—cont'd

Analyte	Specimen	Condition	REFERENCE INTERVALS			Reference Publication
			Conventional Units	Conversion Factor	SI Units	
Triiodothyronine (T$_3$), total	S	Pregnancy	200–380 ng/dL	0.0154	3.1–5.9 nmol/L	
		Cord (>37 wk)	5–141		0.08–2.17	1
Values (4 d–<19 y) based on Abbott Architect method		4 d–<1 y	85–234		1.33–3.60	3
		1–<12 y	113–189		1.74–2.91	
		12–<15 y	98–176		1.50–2.71	
		15–<17 y, F	92–142		1.42–2.18	
		15–<17 y, M	94–156		1.44–2.40	
		17–<19 y	90–168		1.38–2.58	
		Adults				1
		20–50 y	70–204		1.08–3.14	
		50–90 y	40–181		0.62–2.79	
		Pregnancy				
		1st trimester	81–190		1.25–2.93	
		2nd and 3rd trimesters	100–260		1.54–4.00	
Troponin I, high sensitivity	S		ng/L	1	ng/L	
Values based on Abbott Architect method, 99th percentile		0–<19 y	< 33.6		< 33.6	13
Troponin T, high sensitivity	S		ng/L	1	ng/L	
Values based on Roche cobas method, 99th percentile		0–<6 mo	<93		<93	5
		6 mo–<1 y	<21		<21	
		1–<19 y, F	<11		<11	
		1–<19 y, M	<14		<14	
Tryptophan			mg/dL	49	μmol/L	
	P	Premature, 1 d	0–1.23		0–60	1
		Newborn, 1 d	<1.37		<67	
		1–16 y	0.49–1.61		24–79	
		>16 y	0.41–1.94		20–95	
	U, 24 h		mg/d	4.9	μmol/d	
		Adult	5–39		25–191	
			mg/g		mmol/mol	
		Adult	<30		<16.5	
Tumor-associated trypsin inhibitor (TATI)			ng/mL	1.0	μg/L	
	S		3–21		3–21	1
	U		7–51		7–51	
Tyrosine	P		mg/dL	55.2	mmol/L	
		Premature, 1 d	0–5.79		0–320	1
		Newborn, 1 d	0.76–1.79		42–99	
		1–3 mo	0.54–2.42		30–134	
		2–6 mo	1.30–3.91		72–216	
		9 mo–2 y	0.20–2.21		1–122	
		3–10 y	0.56–1.29		31–71	
		6–18 y	0.78–1.59		43–88	
		Adult	0.40–1.58		22–87	
	S	0–<2 wk	0.49–3.39		27–187	20
		2 wk–<1 y	0.62–2.74		34–151	
		1–<13 y	0.82–2.28		45–126	
		13–<19 y	0.62–1.59		34–88	
	U, 24 h		mg/d	5.52	μmol/d	
		10 d–7 wk	4.0–7.2		22–40	1

Continued

TABLE A.1 **Pediatric and Adult Reference Intervals for Biochemical Markers (Serum, Plasma, and Urine)—cont'd**

Analyte	Specimen	Condition	Conventional Units	Conversion Factor	SI Units	Reference Publication
		3–12 y	7.2–30.4		40–168	
		Adult	12.0–55.1		66–304	
			mg/g creatinine	0.62	mmol/mol creatinine	
		Adult	0–23		0–14.2	
Uracil	U				mmol/mol creatinine	1
		0–6 mo			<33	
		6 mo–5 y			<22	
		>5 y			<18	
Urea	S		mg/dL	0.357	mmol/L	
Values (0–<3 y) based on Abbott Architect method		0–<14 d	3–23		1.0–8.2	7
		15 d–<1 y	3–17		1.2–6.0	
		1–<3 y	9–22		3.2–7.9	
Values (3–79) based on OCD Vitros method		3–5 y	9–19		3.1–6.9	27
		6–7 y	8–21		2.8–7.5	
		8–19 y, M	8–20		2.9–7.0	
		20–39 y, M	9–22		3.3–7.9	
		40–59 y, M	10–24		3.5–8.6	
		8–59 y, F	8–19		2.7–6.7	
		60–79 y	10–26		3.6–9.2	
	U, 24 h		g/d	0.0357	mol/d	
			10–20		0.43–0.71	1
Urea Creatinine Ratio (UCR)	S		mg/dL/mg/dL	4.04	μmol/L/ μmol/L	
Values based on Abbott Architect method, Enzymatic		0–<15 d	5–40		21–162	6
		15 d–<1 y	12–108		49–438	
		1–<3 y	31–104		127–419	
		3–<5 y	32–74		130–299	
		5–<8 y	22–61		87–246	
		8–<10 y, F	17–44		69–177	
		8–<10 y, M	21–47		83–189	
		10–<15 y	12–36		50–146	
		15–<19 y	11–26		44–107	
Values based on Abbott Architect method, Jaffe		0–<15 d	6–30		26–121	
		15 d–<1 y	9–39		35–156	
		1–<5 y	17–49		70–198	
		5–<8 y	17–40		69–160	
		8–<10 y, F	14–32		57–131	
		8–<10 y, M	16–39		66–156	
		10–<15 y, F	10–27		42–111	
		10–<15 y, M	12–33		50–134	
		15–<19 y	10–25		42–99	
Uric acid	S		mg/dL	59.48	μmol/L	
Values (0–<3 y) based on Abbott Architect method		0–14 d	2.8–12.7		167–755	7
		15 d–<1 y	1.6–6.3		95–375	
		1–<3 y	1.8–4.9		107–291	
Values (3–79 y) based on OCD Vitros method		3–<5 y	2.0–4.9		117–291	27
		5–8 y	1.9–5.0		116–295	
		9–10 y	2.4–5.5		142–326	
		11–12 y	2.6–5.8		156–345	
		13–79 y, M	3.7–7.7		218–459	
		F	2.5–6.2		147–366	
Valine	P		mg/dL	85.5	μmol/L	
		Premature, 1 d	0.34–2.70		30–230	1
		Newborn, 1 d	0.94–2.88		80–246	
		1–3 mo	1.13–3.4 1		96–292	

TABLE A.1   Pediatric and Adult Reference Intervals for Biochemical Markers (Serum, Plasma, and Urine)—cont'd

Analyte	Specimen	Condition	REFERENCE INTERVALS Conventional Units	Conversion Factor	SI Units	Reference Publication
		9 mo–2 y	0.67–3.07		57–262	
		3–10 y	1.50–3.31		128–283	
		6–18 y	1.83–3.37		156–288	
		Adult	1.65–3.71		141–317	
	S	0–<2 wk	1.02–3.81		87–326	20
		2 wk–<13 y	1.50–4.22		128–361	
		13–<19 y, F	1.81–3.03		155–259	
		13–<19 y, M	1.94–3.52		166–301	
	U, 24 h		mg/d	8.55	μmol/d	
		10 d–7 wk	1.4–3.2		12–27	1
		3–12 y	1.8–6.0		15–51	
		Adult	2.5–11.9		21–102	
Vanillylmandelic acid (VMA)	U, 24 h	*See Chapter 53, Table 53.5				
Vitamin A	S		μg/dL	0.0349	μmol/L	
Values (0–<19 y) based on Abbott Architect method		0–<1 y	8–54		0.3–1.9	17
		1–<11 y	28–44		1.0–1.6	
		11–<16 y	25–55		0.9–1.9	
		16–<19 y	29–75		1.0–2.6	
		Adult	30–80		1.05–2.8	1
Vitamin B$_1$ (thiamine diphosphate)	WB		90–140 nmol/L	1	90–140 nmol/L	
	Erythrocytes		280–590 ng/g Hb	0.146	40.3–85.0 μmol/mol Hb	1
Vitamin B$_2$ (see riboflavin)						
Vitamin B$_6$	P (EDTA)		ng/mL	4.046	nmol/L	
			5–30		20–121	1
		Deficiency	<5		<20.2	
Vitamin B$_{12}$			ng/L	0.733	pmol/L	
Reference Intervals						3
Values (5 d–< 3 y) based on Abbott Architect method		5 d–<1 y	259–1576		191–1163	
		1–<3 y	283–1613		209–1190	
Values (3–79 y) based on Siemens Immulite method		3–5 y	310–988		229–729	28
		6–8 y	321–985		237–727	
		9–11 y	276–969		204–715	
		12–79 y	188–908		139–670	
Clinical Decision Limits						
		Acceptable (WHO)	>201		>147	1
		Deficiency (WHO)	<150		<110	
Vitamin C (ascorbic acid)	S		mg/dL	56.78	μmol/L	
			0.4–1.5		23–85	1
		Deficiency	<0.2		<11	
	Leukocyte		20–53 μg/10^8 leukocytes	0.057	1.14–3.01 fmol/10^8 leukocytes	
		Deficiency	<10 μg/108 leuko- cytes		<0.57 fmol/108 leuko- cytes	
Vitamin D 25(OH)D	S		ng/mL	2.5	nmol/L	

Continued

TABLE A.1 **Pediatric and Adult Reference Intervals for Biochemical Markers (Serum, Plasma, and Urine)—cont'd**

Analyte	Specimen	Condition	REFERENCE INTERVALS Conventional Units	Conversion Factor	SI Units	Reference Publication
Values (5 d–<3 y) based on Abbott Architect method		5–<15 d	2–34		4–85	3
		15 d–<3 mo	6–41		15–101	
		3 mo–<1 y	7–47		17–118	
		1–<3 y	13–55		33–137	
Values (3–79 y) based on DiaSorin LIAISON method P		3–5 y	13–42		33–104	28
		6–79 y	8–46		21–116	
		Deficiency	<20		<50	39
Vitamin D (1,25(OH))	S		pg/mL	2.4	pmol/L	
Pediatric values based on DiaSorin LIAISON method		0–<1 y	32.1–196		77–471	9
		1–<3 y	47.1–151		113–363	
		3–<19 y	45.0–102		108–246	
		Adult	15–60		36–144	1
Vitamin E	S		mg/dL	23.2	µmol/L	
		Premature neonates	0.1–0.5		2.3–11.6	1
Values (0–<19 y) based on Abbott Architect method		0–<1 y	0.2–2.1		4.9–49.6	17
		1–<19 y	0.6–1.4		14.5–33.0	
		Adults	0.5–1.8		12–42	1
Vitamin E: Total cholesterol ratio		1–19 y			3.7–6.7	17
Vitamin E: Triglyceride ratio		1–19 y			8.5–44.5	
Vitamin K	S		ng/mL	2.22	nmol/L	
			0.13–1.19		0.29–2.64	1
Zinc	S		µg/dL	0.153	µmol/L	
			80–120		12–18	1
		Deficiency	<30		<5	
	U, 24 h		mg/24 h	15.3	µmol/24 h	
			0.2–1.3		3–21	

ACTH, Adrenocorticotropic hormone; *ADH*, antidiuretic hormone; *AGS*, American Geriatrics Society; *anti-Tg*, anti-thyroglobulin; *ASO*, antistreptolysin; *BCG*, bromocrescol green; *CEA*, carcinoembryonic antigen; *ChEDi*, cholesterase dibucaine number; *CK*, creatine kinase; *CK-MB*, creatine kinase myoglobin; *CRP*, C-reactive protein; *FSH*, follicle stimulating hormone; *IFCC*, international federation for clinical chemistry; *FAI*, free androgen index; *BNP*, brain natriuretic peptide; *OCD*, ortho clinical diagnostics; *PCO₂*, partial CO_2; *tCO₂*, total CO_2.

Reference Value Distributions: Age 3–80 years [CHMS]

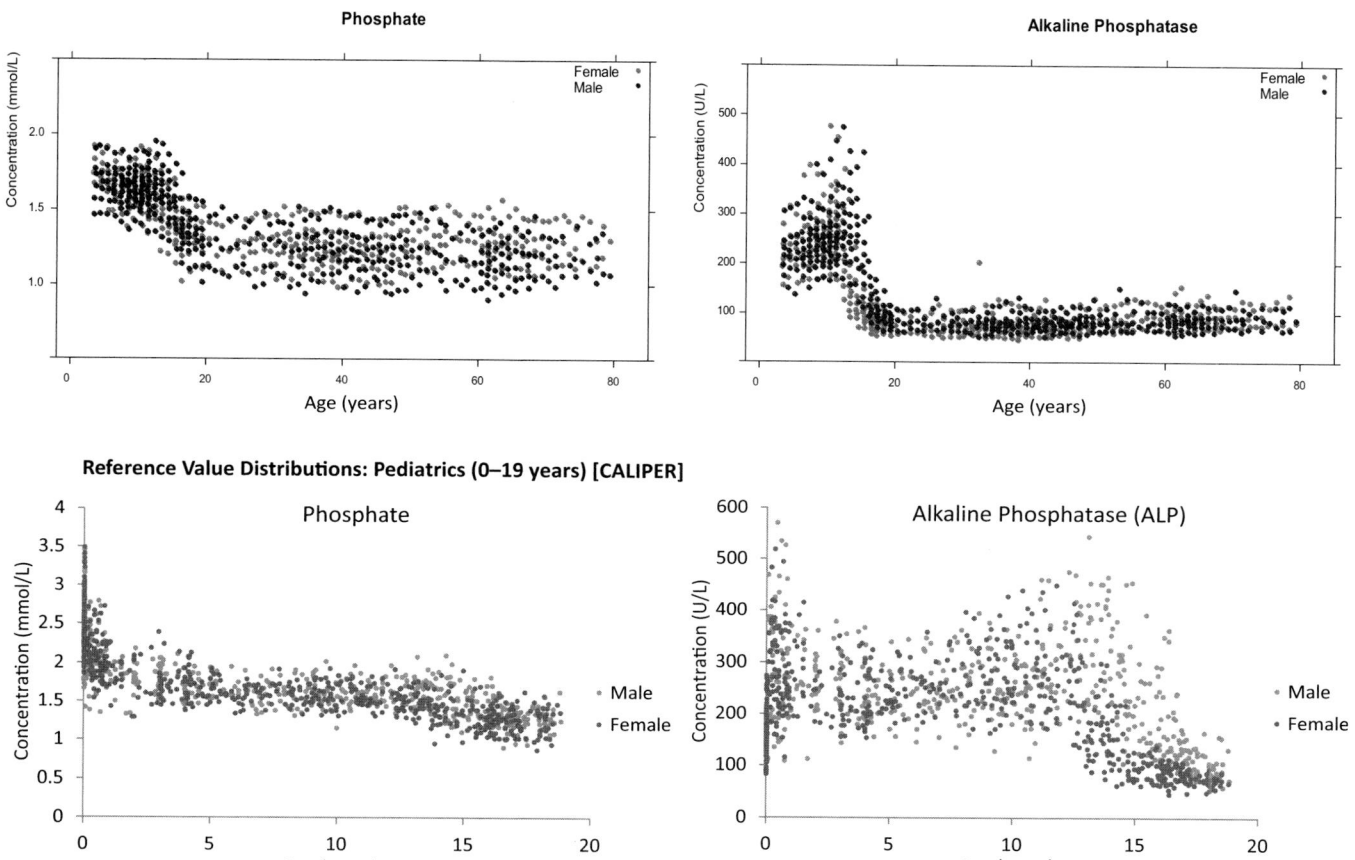

Reference Value Distributions: Pediatrics (0–19 years) [CALIPER]

FIGURE A.1 Reference value distributions for phosphate (mmol/L) and alkaline phosphatase (*ALP*; U/L) based on data from the Canadian Health Measures Survey *(CHMS)*[27] *(top panel)* or the CALIPER cohort of healthy community children and adolescents[7] *(bottom panel).*

Reference Value Distributions: Age 3–80 years [CHMS]

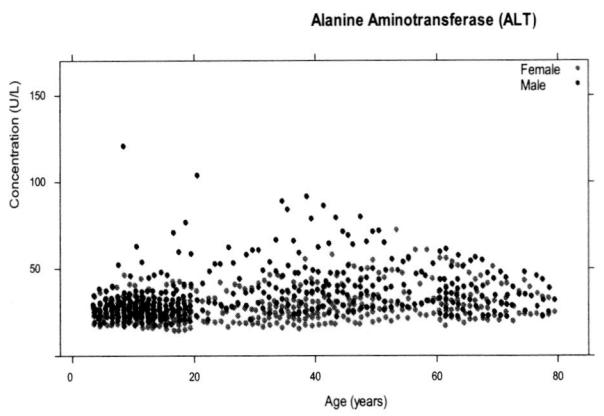

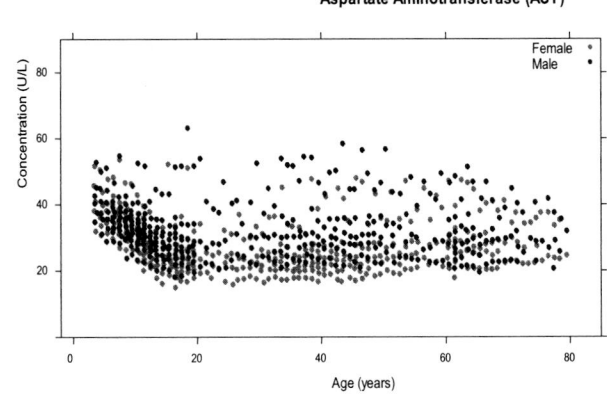

Reference Value Distributions: Pediatrics (0–19 years) [CALIPER]

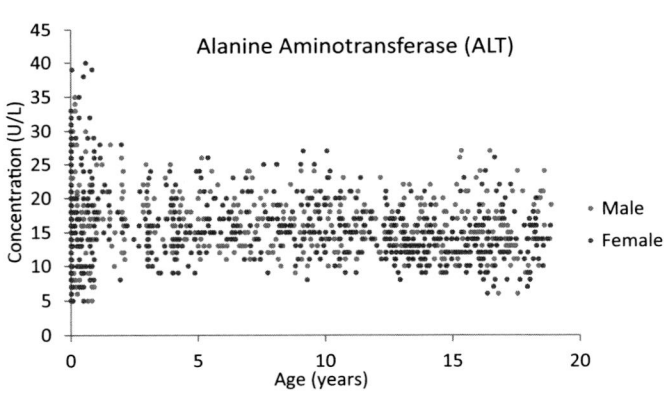

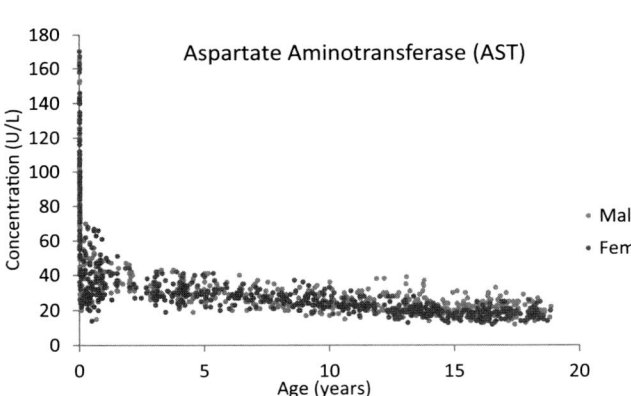

FIGURE A.2 Reference value distributions for alanine aminotransferase (*ALT;* U/L) and aspartate aminotransferase (*AST;* U/L) based on data from the Canadian Health Measures Survey *(CHMS)*[27] *(top panel)* or the CALIPER cohort of healthy community children and adolescents[7] *(bottom panel).*

Reference Value Distributions: Age 3–80 years [CHMS]

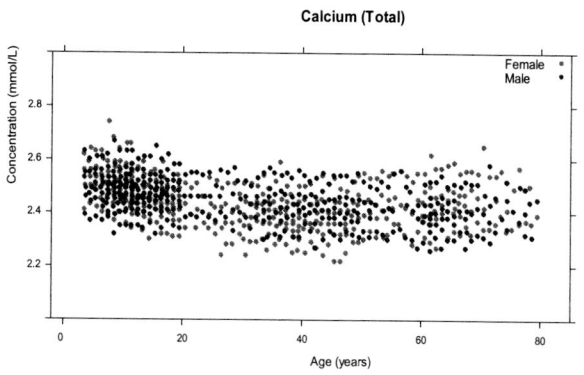

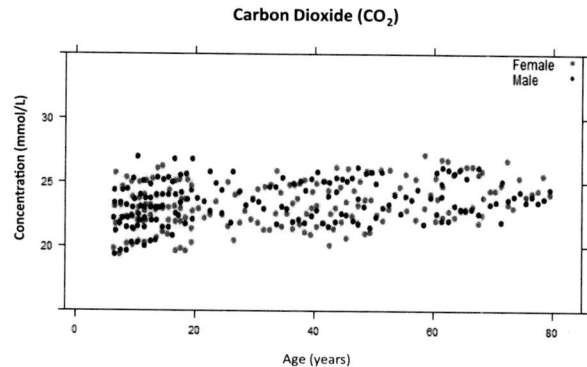

Reference Value Distributions: Pediatrics (0–19 years) [CALIPER]

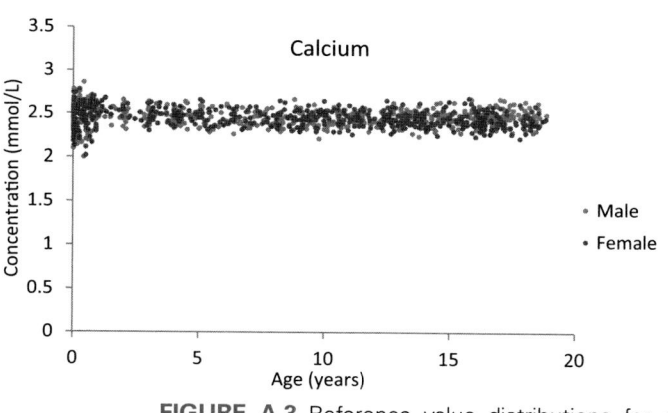

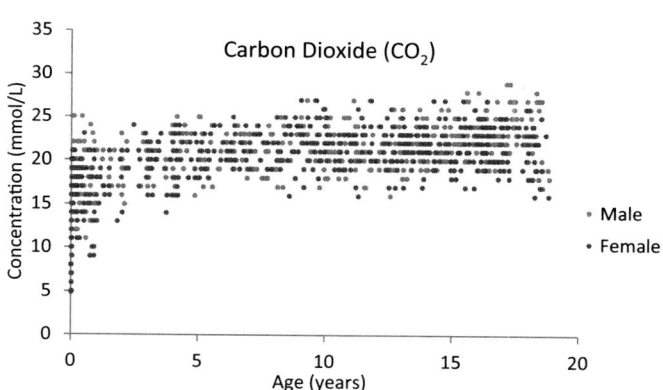

FIGURE A.3 Reference value distributions for calcium (total; mmol/L) and carbon dioxide (CO_2, mmol/L) based on data from the Canadian Health Measures Survey[27] *(top panel)* or the CALIPER cohort of healthy community children and adolescents[7] *(bottom panel)*.

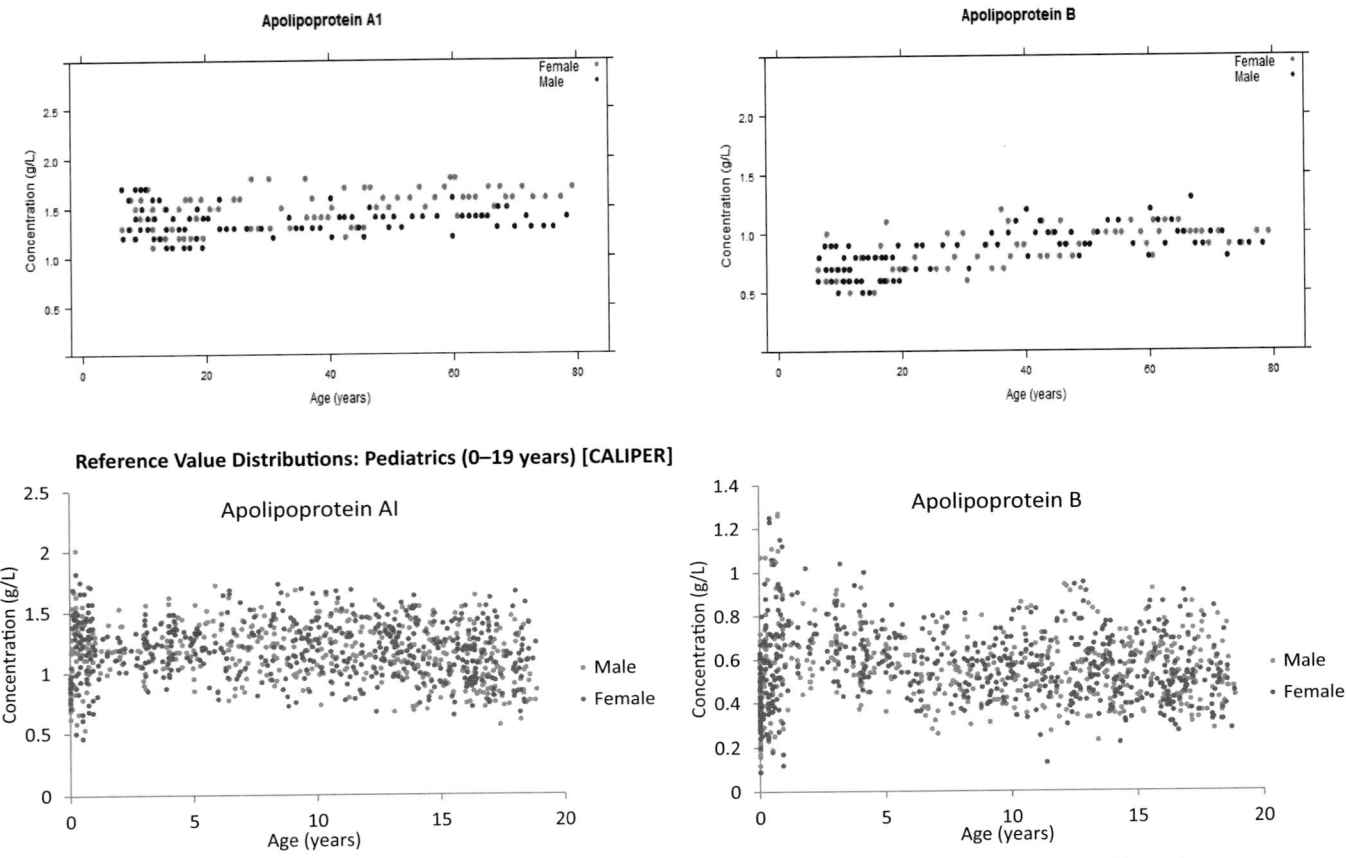

FIGURE A.4 Reference value distributions for apolipoprotein A1 (g/L) and apolipoprotein B (g/L) based on data from the Canadian Health Measures Survey[28] *(top panel)* or the CALIPER cohort of healthy community children and adolescents[7] *(bottom panel)*.

Reference Value Distributions: Age 3–80 years [CHMS]

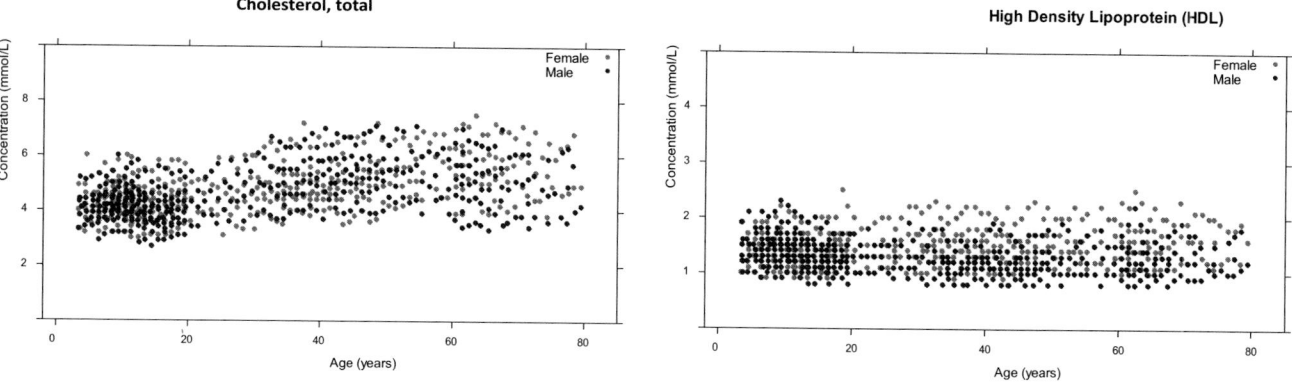

Reference Value Distributions: Pediatrics (0–19 years) [CALIPER]

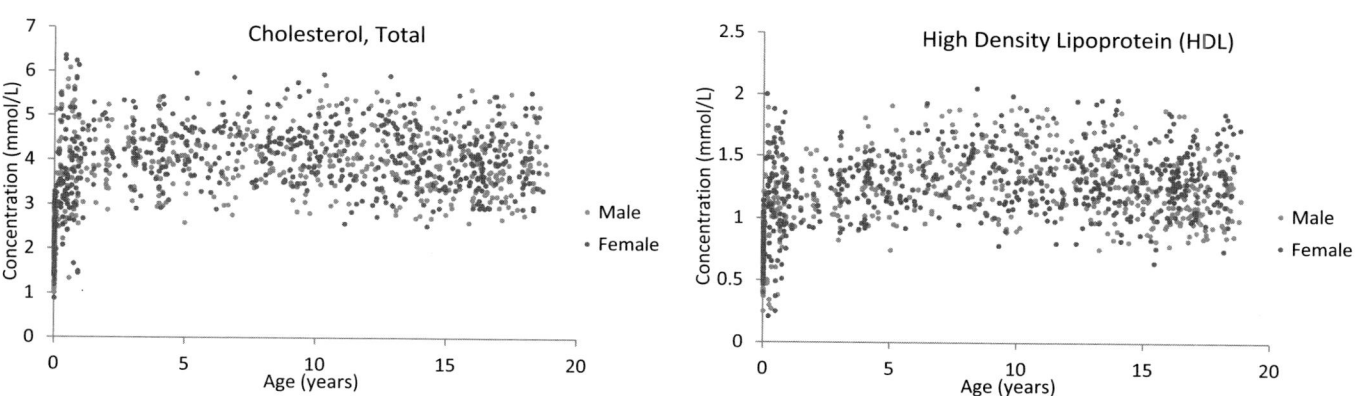

FIGURE A.5 Reference value distributions for cholesterol (total; mmol/L) and high-density lipoprotein cholesterol (*HDL;* mmol/L) based on data from the Canadian Health Measures Survey[28] *(top panel)* or the CALIPER cohort of healthy community children and adolescents[7] *(bottom panel).*

Reference Value Distributions: Age 3–80 years [CHMS]

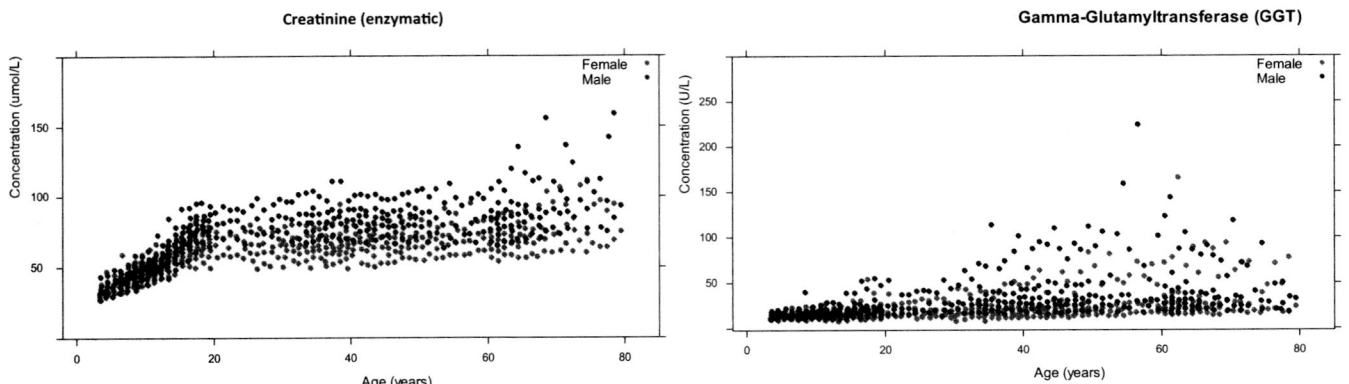

Reference Value Distributions: Pediatrics (0–19 years) [CALIPER]

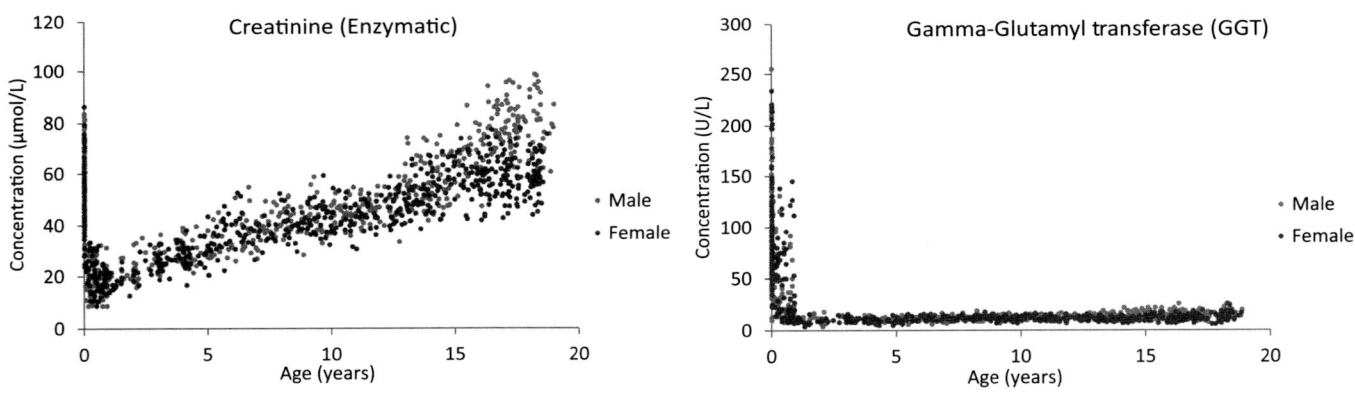

FIGURE A.6 Reference value distributions for creatinine (enzymatic; μmol/L) and γ-glutamyltransferase (*GGT*; U/L) based on data from the Canadian Health Measures Survey[27] *(top panel)* or the CALIPER cohort of healthy community children and adolescents[7] *(bottom panel).*

Reference Value Distributions: Age 3–80 years [CHMS]

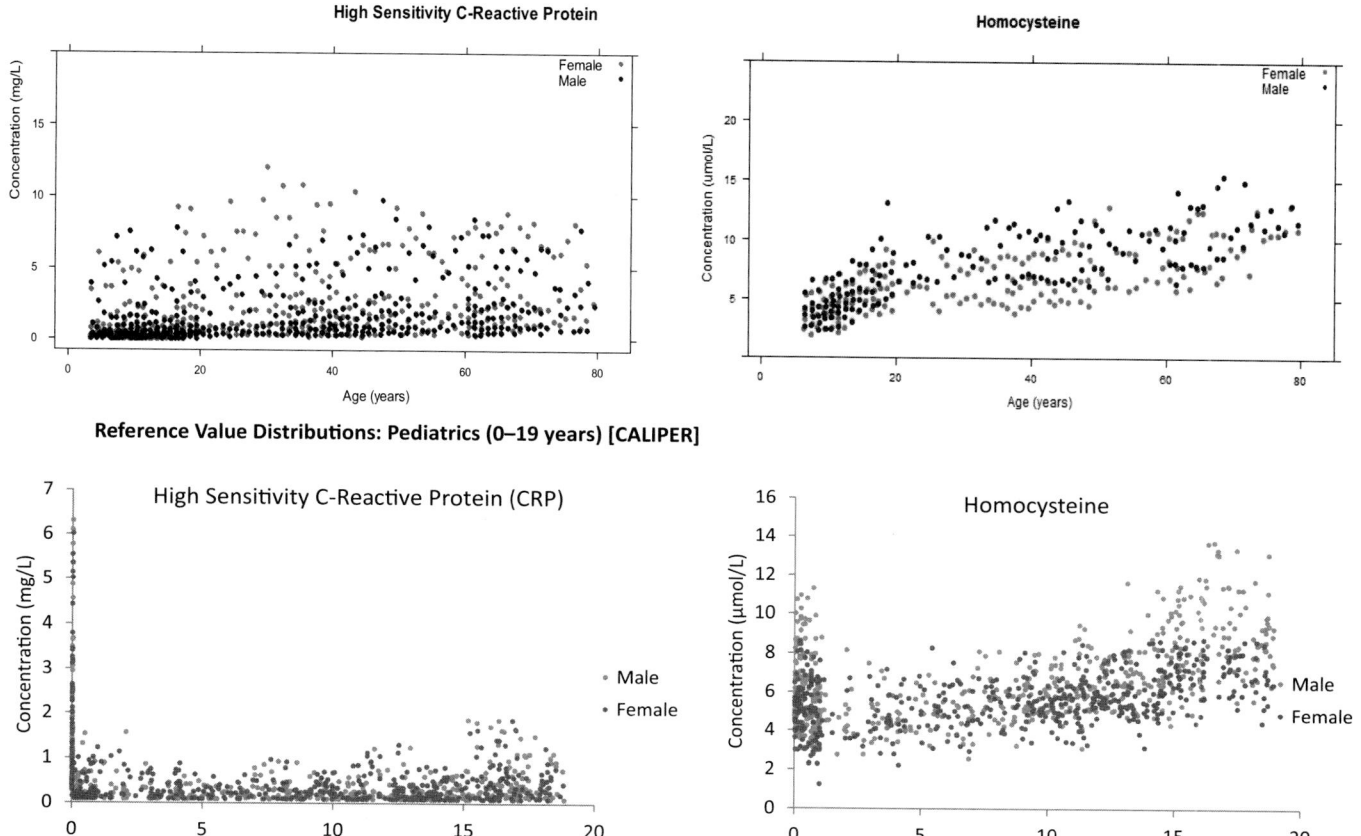

Reference Value Distributions: Pediatrics (0–19 years) [CALIPER]

FIGURE A.7 Reference value distributions for high-sensitivity C-reactive protein (*CRP*; mg/L) and homocysteine (μmol/L) based on data from the Canadian Health Measures Survey[28] *(top panel)* or the CALIPER cohort of healthy community children and adolescents[3,7] *(bottom panel)*.

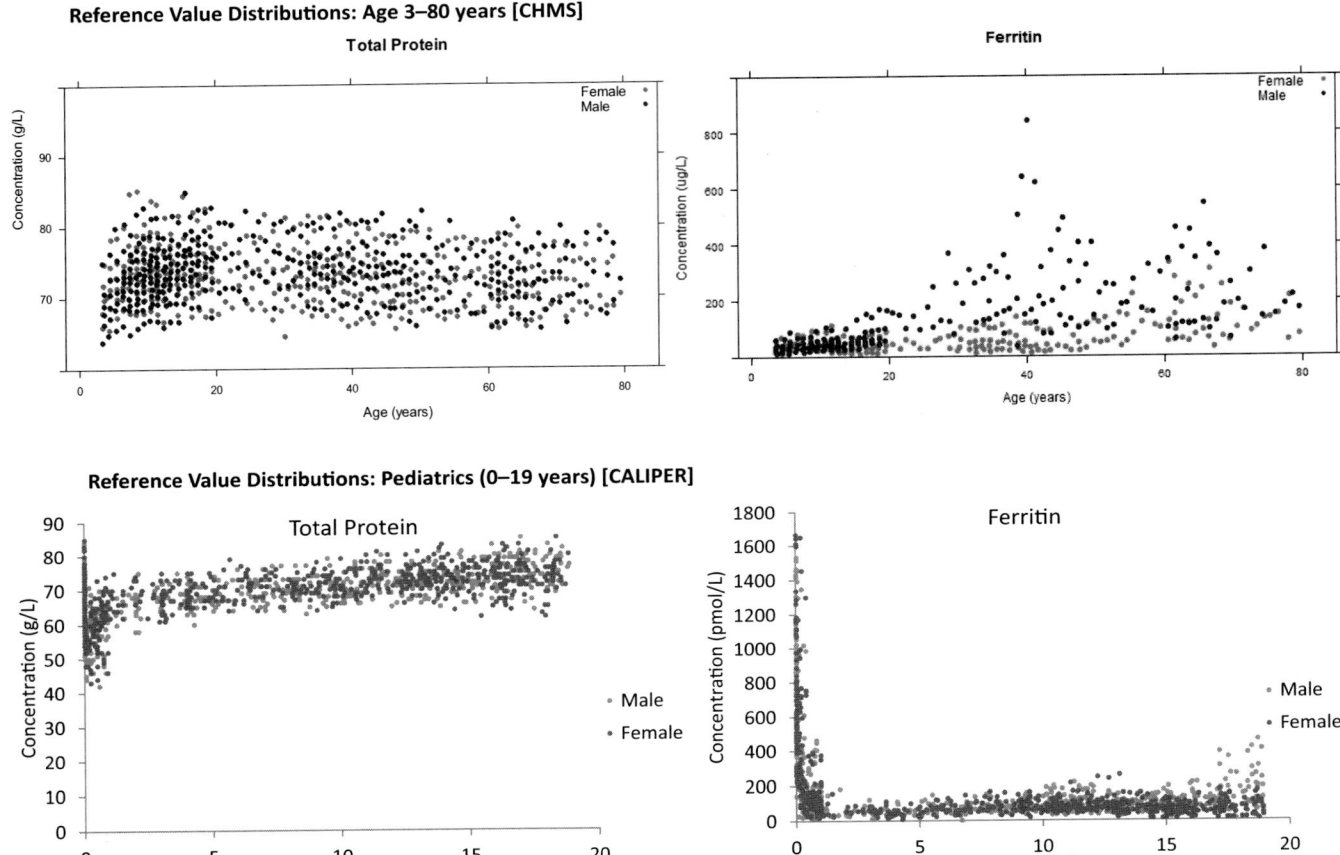

FIGURE A.8 Reference value distributions for total protein (g/L) and ferritin (μg/L) based on data from the Canadian Health Measures Survey *(CHMS)*[27,28] *(top panel)* or the CALIPER cohort of healthy community children and adolescents[2,7] *(bottom panel;* ferritin in pmol/L).

Reference Value Distributions: Age 3–80 years [CHMS]

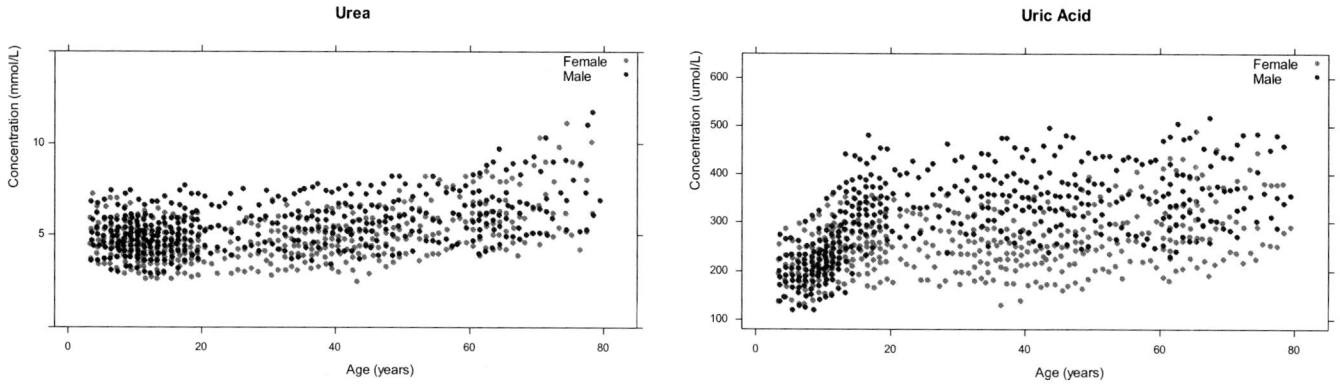

Reference Value Distributions: Pediatrics (0–19 years) [CALIPER]

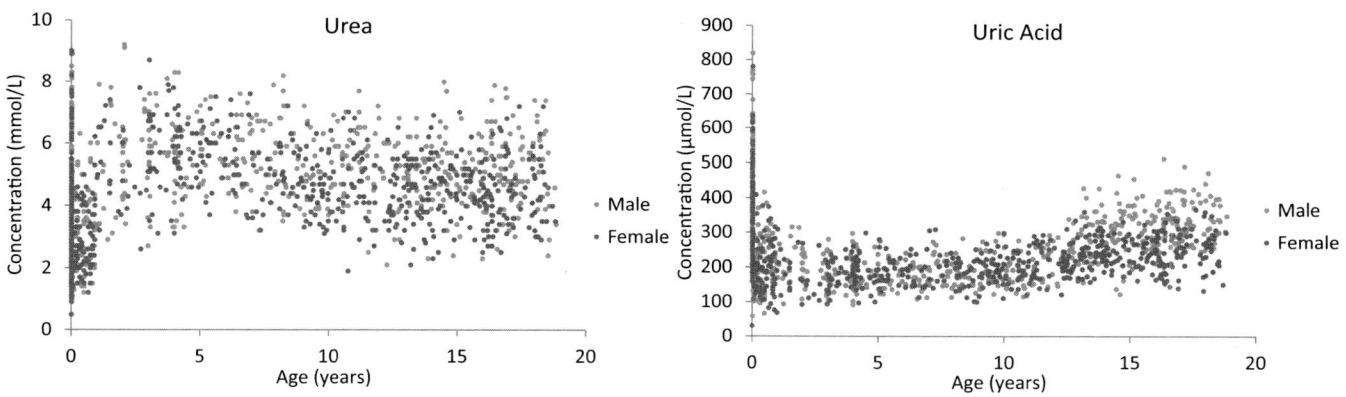

FIGURE A.9 Reference value distributions for urea (mmol/L) and uric acid (μmol/L) based on data from the Canadian Health Measures Survey[27] *(top panel)* or the CALIPER cohort of healthy community children and adolescents[7] *(bottom panel)*.

Reference Value Distributions: Age 3-80 yrs - [CHMS]

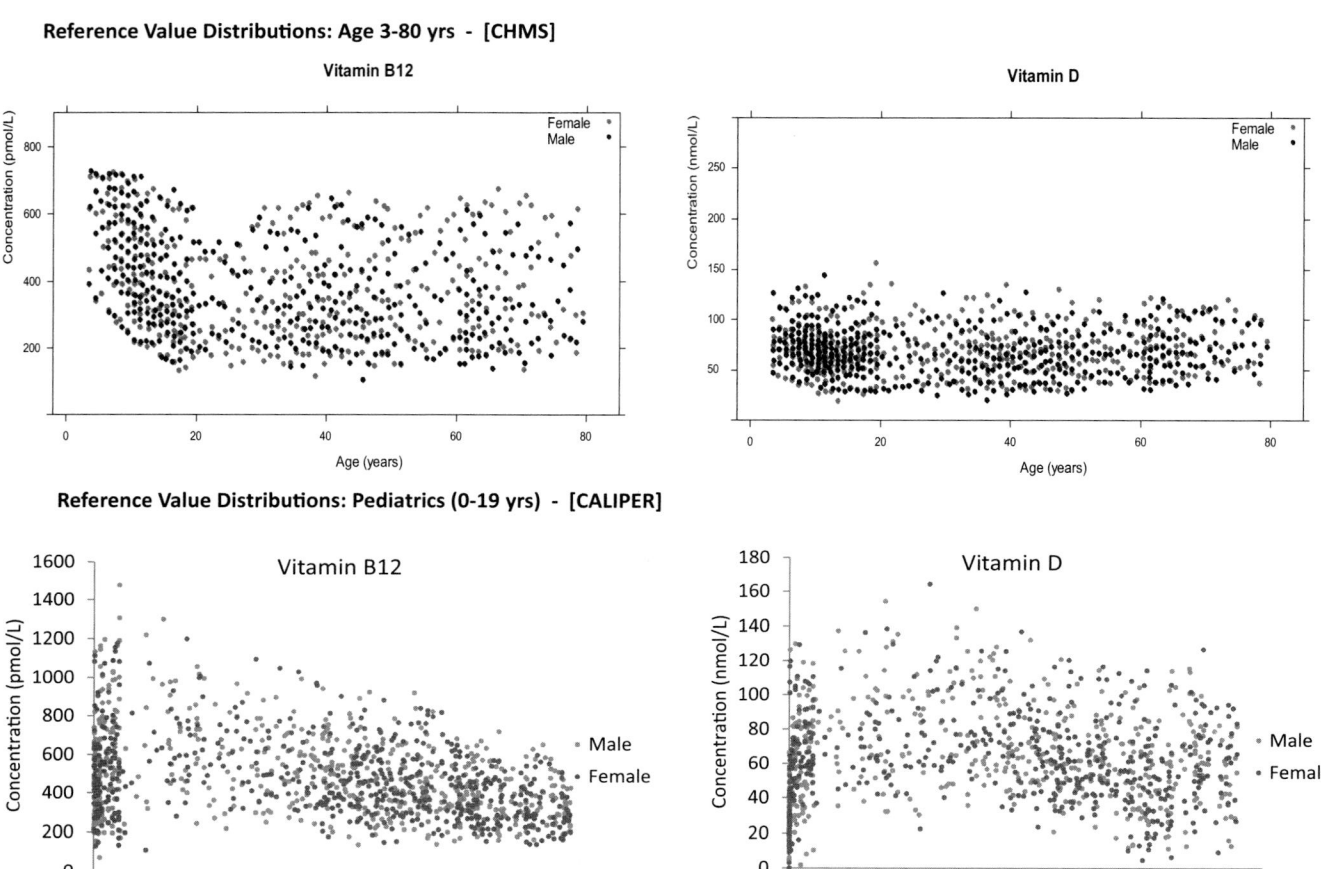

FIGURE A.10 Reference value distributions for vitamin B_{12} (pmol/L) and vitamin D (nmol/L) based on data from the Canadian Health Measures Survey[28] *(top panel)* or the CALIPER cohort of healthy community children and adolescents[2] *(bottom panel).*

TABLE A.2   Reference Intervals for Biochemical Markers in Other Body Fluids

Analyte	Specimen	Condition	REFERENCE INTERVALS Conventional Units	Conversion Factor	SI Units	Reference Publication
α-Fetoprotein (AFP)	Amf	Weeks of gestation	ng/mL	1	μg/L	1
		14	25.6		25.6	
		15	29.9		29.9	
		16	34.8		34.8	
		17	40.6		40.6	
		18	47.3		47.3	
		19	55.1		55.1	
		20	64.3		64.3	
		21	74.9		74.9	
Albumin	CSF, lumbar		mg/dL	10	mg/L	1
			17.7–25.1		177–251	
Bilirubin	Amf		mg/dL	17.1	μmol/L	1
		28 wk	<0.075		<1.28	
			ΔA_{450} <0.048			
		40 wk	<0.025		<0.43	
			ΔA_{450} <0.02			
Chloride	Sweat (iontophoresis)		mEq/L	1	mmol/L	1
		Normal	5–35		5–35	
		Marginal	30–70		30–70	
		Cystic fibrosis	60–200		60–200	
Cortisol, free	Sal		ng/mL	2.76	nmol/L	
		0700 h	1.4–10.1		4–30	1
		2200 h	0.7–2.2		2–6	
Estriol, free (unconjugated uE_3)	Amf	Weeks of Gestation	ng/mL	3.47	nmol/L	1
		16–20	1.0–3.2		3.5–11	
		20–24	2 .1–7.8		7.3–27	
		24–28	2.1–7.8		7.3–27	
		28–32	4.0–13.6		14–47	
		32–36	3.6–15.5		12–54	
		36–38	4.6–18.0		16–62	
		38–40	5.4–19.8		19–69	
Estriol, total (E_3)	Amf	Weeks of Gestation	ng/mL	3.47	nmol/L	1
		21–32	5–50		17–174	
		33–35	90–240		312–833	
		36–41	150–213		521–739	
Glucagon	Amf		ng/L	1	ng/L	1
		Midgestation	23–63		23–63	
		Term	41–193		41–193	
Glucose	CSF		mg/dL	0.0555	mmol/L	1
		Infant, child	60–80		3.3–4.5	
		Adult	40–70		2.2–3.9	
Immunoglobulin A	CSF		mg/dL	10	mg/L	1
			0.0–0.6		0.0–6.0	
	Sal		<11		<0.11	
Immunoglobulin G	CSF		mg/dL	10	mg/L	1
			0–5.5		0–55	
Immunoglobulin M	CSF		mg/dL	10	mg/L	1
			0.0–1.3		0–13	
L-Lactate	CSF	Child	mg/dL	0.0111	mmol/L	57
		Female	5.4–18.9		0.6–2.1	
		Male	8.1–19.8		0.9–2.2	
		Adult	mg/dL	0.111	mmol/L	40
			9.1–18.8		1.01–2.09	
	Gastric fluid		Negative		Negative	1

Continued

TABLE A.2 Reference Intervals for Biochemical Markers in Other Body Fluids—cont'd

Analyte	Specimen	Condition	REFERENCE INTERVALS			Reference Publication
			Conventional Units	Conversion Factor	SI Units	
L/S ratio	Amf	State of fetal maturity	Ratio	1	Ratio	1
		Immature	<1.5		<1.5	
		Transitional	1.6–2.4		1.6–2.4	
		Mature	>2.5		>2.5	
		Diabetic	>2.5		>2.5	
Protein, total	CSF		mg/dL	10	mg/L	1
		Premature	15–130		150–1300	
		Full-term newborn	40–120		400–1200	
		<1 mo	20 -80		200–800	
		>1 mo	15–40		150–400	
		Ventricular fluid	5–15		50–150	
		Cisternal fluid	15–25		150–250	
	Amf		g/dL	10	g/L	
		Early pregnancy	0.2–1.7		2.0–17.0	
		Late pregnancy	0.175–0.705		1.8–7.1	
Pyruvate	CSF		mg/dL	0.114	mmol/L	40
		Adult	0.3–1.3		0.03–0.15	
Serotonin	CSF		ng/mL	5.68	nmol/L	1
			1.0–2.1		5.7– 12.0	

Amf, Amniotic fluid; *CSF*, cerebrospinal fluid; *L/S*, lecithin-to-sphingomyelin ratio; *Sal*, saliva.

TABLE A.3 Reference Information for Toxicology and Therapeutic Drugs

Drug	Specimen	Status	REFERENCE VALUES			Reference Publication
			Conventional Units	Conversion Factor	SI Units	
Acetaminophen (Tylenol)	S or P		μg/mL	6.62	μmol/L	1
		Therap	10–30		66–199	
		Toxic				
		4 h after dose	>200		>1324	
		12 h after dose	>50		>331	
Amikacin (Amikin)	S or P		μg/mL	1.71	μmol/L	1
		Therap				
		Peak	25–35		43–60	
		Trough				
		Less severe infection	1–4		2–7	
		Severe infection	4–8		7–14	
		Toxic				
		Peak	>40		>68	
		Trough	>10		>17	
		Peak/MIC	>10		>17	
Aminocaproic acid (Amicar)	S or P		μg/mL	7.62	μmol/L	1
		Therap				
		Trough	100–400		762–3048	

TABLE A.3   Reference Information for Toxicology and Therapeutic Drugs—cont'd

Drug	Specimen	Status	REFERENCE VALUES			Reference Publication
			Conventional Units	Conversion Factor	SI Units	
Amiodarone (Cordarone)	S or P		μg/mL	1.47	μmol/L	1
		Therap	0.5–2.0		1–3	
		Toxic	>2.5		>4	
Amitriptyline (Elavil) + nortriptyline	S or P		ng/mL	3.61	nmol/L	1
		Therap	80–200		289–722	
		Toxic	>500 (sum)		>1805	
Amobarbital (Amytal)	S or P		μg/mL	4.42	μmol/L	1
		Therap	1–5		4–22	
		Toxic	>10		>44	
Amoxapine (Asendin) + 8-hydroxy amoxapine	S or P		ng/mL	3 .19	nmol/L	1
		Therap	200–600		638–1914	
		Toxic	>600		>1914	
Amphetamine (Adderall)	S or P		ng/mL	7.40	nmol/L	1
		Therap	20–30		148–222	
		Toxic	>200		>1480	
Bromide as bromine	S or P		μg/mL	0.0125	mmol/L	1
		Therap	750–1500		9–19	
		Toxic	>1250		>16	
Bupropion (Wellbutrin, Zyban)	S or P		ng/mL	3.62	nmol/L	1
		Therap	25–100		91–362	
		Toxic	>100		>362	
Caffeine	S or P		μg/mL	5.15	μmol/L	1
		Therap	8–20		41–103	
		Toxic	>20		>103	
Carbamazepine (Tegretol)	S or P		μg/mL	4.23	μmol/L	1
		Therap	4–12		17–51	
		Toxic	>15		>63	
Carbamazepine-10, 11-epoxide (carbamazepine metabolite)	S or P		μg/mL	3.97	μmol/L	1
		Therap	0.4–4		2–16	
		Toxic	>8		>32	
Carbenicillin (Geopen)	S or P		μg/mL	2.64	μmol/L	1
		Therap	Dependent on MIC of specific organism			
		Toxic	>250 (neurotoxicity)		>660	
Chloral hydrate (Noctec) as trichloroethanol	S or P		μg/mL	6.69	μmol/L	1
		Therap	2–12		13–80	
		Toxic	>20		>134	
Chloramphenicol (Chloromycetin)	S or P		μg/mL	3.09	μmol/L	1
		Therap	10–25		31–77	
		Toxic	>25		>77	

Continued

TABLE A.3   Reference Information for Toxicology and Therapeutic Drugs—cont'd

Drug	Specimen	Status	REFERENCE VALUES			Reference Publication
			Conventional Units	Conversion Factor	SI Units	
		Gray baby syndrome	>40		>124	1
Chlordiazepoxide (Librium) + nordiazepine	S or P		ng/mL	0.003	μmol/L	
		Therap	700–1000		2–3	
		Toxic	>5000		>17	
Chlorpromazine (Thorazine)	S or P		ng/mL	3.14	nmol/L	1
		Therap				
		Adult	30–300		94–942	
		Child	40–80		126–251	
		Toxic	>750		>2355	
Cimetidine (Tagamet)	S or P		μg/mL	3.96	μmol/L	1
		Therap				
		Trough	0.5–1.2		2–5	
		Toxic	>1.3		>5	
Ciprofloxacin (Cipro)	S or P		μg/mL	3.02	μmol/L	1
		Therap				
		Peak (oral dose)	0.5–1.5		2–5	
		Peak (IV dose)	<5.0		<15	
		Toxic	>5.0		>15	
		Gram positive AUC/MIC	>30			
		Gram negative AUC/MIC	>125			
Clomipramine (Anafranil) + norclomipramine	S or P		ng/mL	3.18	nmol/L	1
		Therap	175–450		556–1431	
		Toxic	>400 (sum)		>1272	
Clonazepam (Klonopin)	S or P		ng/mL	3.17	nmol/L	1
		Therap	20–70		63–222	
		Toxic	>80		>254	
Clonidine (Catapres)	S or P		ng/mL	4.35	nmol/L	
		Therap	1.0–2.0		4–9	1
		Toxic	>4.0		>17.4	56
Clorazepate (Tranxene) (see Nordiazepam)						
Clozapine (Clozaril)	S or P		ng/mL	3.06	nmol/L	1
		Therap	350–600		1071–1836	
		Toxic	>900		>2754	
Codeine	S or P		ng/mL	3.34	nmol/L	1
		Therap	10–100		33–334	
		Toxic	>1100		>3340	
Cyclosporin A (Sandimmune)	WB		ng/mL	0.83	nmol/L	1
		Therap				
		12 h after dose	50–350		42–291	
		Toxic	>350		>291	
Delavirdine (Rescriptor)	S or P		μg/mL	1.80	μmol/L	1
		Therap				
		Trough	3–8		5–14	
		Peak	14–16		25–29	
		Toxic	>16		>29	
Desipramine (Norpramin)	S or P		ng/mL	3.75	nmol/L	1

TABLE A.3 Reference Information for Toxicology and Therapeutic Drugs—cont'd

Drug	Specimen	Status	REFERENCE VALUES			Reference Publication
			Conventional Units	Conversion Factor	SI Units	
Diazepam (Valium) + nordiazepine	S or P	Therap	100–300		375–1126	
		Toxic	>400		>1502	
			ng/mL	3.51	nmol/L	1
Digitoxin	S or P	Therap	100–1000		351–3512	
		Toxic	>5000		>17,559	
			ng/mL	1.31	nmol/L	1
Digoxin (Lanoxin)	S or P ≥8 h after dose	Therap	10–30		13–39	
		Toxic	>45		>59	
			ng/mL	1.28	nmol/L	1
Disopyramide (Norpace)	S or P ≥12 h after dose	Therap	0.5–2.0		0.6–3.0	
		In heart failure	0.5–0.8		0.6–1.0	
		Toxic	>1.5		>2.0	
			μg/mL	2.95	μmol/L	1
Doxepin (Sinequan, Adapin) + nordoxepin	S or P	Therap	2.8–7.5		8–22	
		Toxic	>5		> 15	
			ng/mL	3.58	nmol/L	1
Efavirenz (Sustiva)	S or P	Therap	50–150		179–537	
		Toxic	>500		>1790	
			μg/mL	3.16	μmol/L	1
Ephedrine (Ectasule)	S or P	Therap	1–4		3–13	
		Toxic	>4		>13	
			μg/mL	6.05	μmol/L	1
Ethanol	WB (Ox)	Therap	0.05–0.10		0.3–0.6	
		Toxic	>2		>12	
			mg/dL	0.217	mmol/L	1
		Impairment	50–100		11–22	
		Depression of CNS	>100		>21.7	
		Fatalities reported	>400		>86.8	
Ethchlorvynol (Placidyl)	S or P		μg/mL	6.92	μmol/L	1
		Therap	2–8		14–55	
		Toxic	>20		>138	
Ethosuximide (Zarontin)	S or P		μg/mL	7.08	μmol/L	1
		Therap	40–100		283–708	
		Toxic	>150		>1062	
Everolimus (Zortress)	WB		ng/mL	1.04	nmol/L	1
		Therap	3–15		3–16	
		Toxic	>15		>16	
Felbamate (Felbatol)	S or P		μg/mL	4.2	μmol/L	1
		Therap	30–60		126–252	
		Toxic	>120		>504	
Fenoprofen (Nalfon)	S or P		μg/mL	4.12	μmol/L	1
		Therap	20–65		82–268	
Flecainide (Tambocor)	S or P		μg/mL	2.41	μmol/L	1
		Therap	0.2–1.0		0.5–2.0	
		Toxic	>1.0		>2.0	
5-Flucytosine (Ancobon)	S or P		μg/mL	7.75	μmol/L	1
		Peak	>25		>194	
		Toxic	>100		>775	
Fluoxetine (Prozac) + norfluoxetine	S or P		ng/mL	3.23	nmol/L	1
		Therap	120–300		388–969	
		Toxic	>1000		>3230	

TABLE A.3 Reference Information for Toxicology and Therapeutic Drugs—cont'd

Drug	Specimen	Status	REFERENCE VALUES Conventional Units	Conversion Factor	SI Units	Reference Publication
Fluphenazine (Modecate)	S or P		ng/mL	2.29	nmol/L	1
		Therap	0.5–2		1–5	
		Toxic	>100		>229	
Flurazepam (Dalmane)	S or P		μg/mL	2.58	μmol/L	
		Therap	>0.002		>0.005	56
		Toxic	>0.2		>0.5	1
Gabapentin (Neurontin)	S or P		μg/mL	5.84	μmol/L	1
		Therap	2–20		12–117	
		Toxic	>12		>70	
Gentamicin (Garamycin)	S or P		μg/mL	2.09	μmol/L	1
		Therap				
		Peak				
		Less severe infection	5–8		11–17	
		Severe infection	8–10		17–21	
		Trough				
		Less severe infection	<1		<2	
		Moderate infection	<2		<4	
		Severe infection	<4		<8	
		Toxic				
		Peak	>10		>21	
		Trough	>2		>4	
		Peak/MIC	>10		>21	
Glutethimide (Doriden)	S or P		μg/mL	4.60	μmol/L	1
		Therap	2–6		9–28	
		Toxic	>5		>23	
Haloperidol (Haldol)	S or P		ng/mL	2.66	nmol/L	1
		Therap	5–17		13–45	
		Toxic	>42		>112	
Hydromorphone (Dilaudid)	S or P		ng/mL	3.50	nmol/L	1
		Therap	1–3		4–11	
		Toxic	>100		>350	
Ibuprofen (Motrin)	S or P		μg/mL	4.85	μmol/L	1
		Therap	10–50		49–243	
		Toxic	>200		>970	
Imipramine (Tofranil) + desipramine	S or P		ng/mL	3.57	nmol/L	1
		Therap	150–300		536–1071	
		Toxic	>400 (sum)		>1428	
Indinavir (Crixivan)	S or P		μg/mL	1.41	μmol/L	1
		Therap				
		Trough	>0.1		>0.14	
		Peak	8–10		11–14	
		Toxic	>10		>14	
Isoniazid (Hyzyd, Nydrazid)	S or P		μg/mL	7.29	μmol/L	1
		Therap	1–7		7–15	
		Toxic	>20		>146	

TABLE A.3 Reference Information for Toxicology and Therapeutic Drugs—cont'd

Drug	Specimen	Status	REFERENCE VALUES Conventional Units	Conversion Factor	SI Units	Reference Publication
Itraconazole (Sporanox) + hydroxyitraconazole	S or P		μg/mL	1.42	μmol/L	1
		Therap	>1.5		>2	
Kanamycin (Kantrex)	S or P		μg/mL	2.06	μmol/L	1
		Therap				
		Peak	25–35		52–72	
		Trough				
		Less severe infection	1–4		2–8	
		Severe infection	4–8		8–17	
		Toxic				
		Peak	>35		>72	
		Trough	>10		>21	
		Peak/MIC	>10		>21	
Lamivudine (Epivir, 3TC)	S or P		μg/mL	4.36	μmol/L	1
		Therap	>0.4		>2	
Lamotrigine (Lamictal)	S or P		μg/mL	3.91	μmol/L	
		Therap	2.5–15		10–59	1
		Toxic	>20		>78	56
Levetiracetam (Keppra)	S or P		μg/mL	5.88	μmol/L	1
		Therap	12–46		71–270	
Lidocaine (Xylocaine)	S or P ≥45 min after bolus dose		μg/mL	4.27	μmol/L	1
		Therap	1.5–5		6–12	
		Toxic	>6		>26	
Lithium (Eskalith)	S or P		mEq/L	1.0	mmol/L	1
		Therap	0.5–1.2		0.5–1	
		Toxic	>2		>2	
Lorazepam (Ativan)	S or P		ng/mL	3.11	nmol/L	
		Therap	50–240		156–746	1
		Toxic	300–600		933–1866	56
Maprotiline (Ludiomil)	S or P		ng/mL	3.60	nmol/L	1
		Therap	125–200		450–720	
		Toxic	>300		>1080	
Meperidine (Demerol)	S or P		ng/mL	4.04	nmol/L	1
		Therap	70–500		283–2020	
		Toxic	>1000		>4004	
Mephobarbital (Mebaral)	S or P		μg/mL	4.06	μmol/L	1
		Therap	1–7		4–28	
		Toxic	>15		>61	
Meprobamate (Equanil)	S or P		μg/mL	4.58	μmol/L	1
		Therap	6–12		28–55	
		Toxic	>60		>275	
Methadone (Dolophine)	S or P		ng/mL	3.23	nmol/L	1
		Therap	100–400		320–1280	
		Toxic	>2000		>6460	
Methamphetamine (Desoxyn)	S or P		μg/mL	6.70	μmol/L	
		Therap	0.01–0.05		0.07–0.34	1
		Toxic	>0.5		>3	

Continued

TABLE A.3 Reference Information for Toxicology and Therapeutic Drugs—cont'd

Drug	Specimen	Status	Conventional Units	Conversion Factor	SI Units	Reference Publication
Methanol			mg/L	0.0312	mmol/L	1
	WB (F/Ox)		<1.5		<0.05	
		Toxic	>200		>6.24	
	U	Occup exp	<50		<1.56	
			ppm		mmol/L	
	Breath		0.8		0.03	
		Occup exp	2.5		0.08	
Methaqualone (Quaalude)	S or P		μg/mL	4.00	μmol/L	1
		Therap	2–3		8–12	
		Toxic	>10		>40	
Methotrexate (Trexall, Rheumatrex)	S or P		μg/mL	2.20	μmol/L	1
		Therap				
		24–72 h after high-dose therapy	0.05–0.45		0.1–1	56
		Toxic				
		24 h after high-dose therapy	≥10		≥22	
		48 h after high-dose therapy	≥1		≥2	
		72 h after high-dose therapy	≥0.1		≥0.2	
Methsuximide (Celontin) as normethsuximide	S or P		μg/mL	5.29	μmol/L	1
		Therap	10–40		53–212	
		Toxic	>40		>212	
Methyldopa (Aldomet)	S or P		μg/mL	4 .73	μmol/L	1
		Therap	1–5		5–24	
		Toxic	>7		>33	
Methyprylon (Noludar)	S or P		μg/mL	5.46	μmol/L	1
		Therap	8–10		43–55	
		Toxic	>50		273	
Mexiletine (Mexitil)	S or P		μg/mL	5.58	μmol/L	1
		Therap	0.5–2		3–11	
		Toxic	>2.0		>11	
Morphine	S or P		ng/mL	3.50	nmol/L	1
		Therap	10–80		35–280	
		Toxic	>200		>700	
Mycophenolate mofetil (CellCept) as mycophenolic acid	S or P		μg/mL	3.12	μmol/L	1
		Therap	1.3–3.5		4–11	
		Toxic	>12		>38	
Nefazodone (Serzone)	S or P		ng/mL	2.13	nmol/L	1
		Therap	25–2500		53–5325	
		Toxic	>2500		>5325	
Nelfinavir (Viracept)	S or P		μg/mL	1.76	μmol/L	1
		Therap	>1		>2	
		Toxic	>6		>11	
Netilmicin (Netromycin)	S or P		μg/mL	2.10	μmol/L	1
		Therap				
		Peak				
		Less severe infection	5–8		10–17	

TABLE A.3   Reference Information for Toxicology and Therapeutic Drugs—cont'd

Drug	Specimen	Status	Conventional Units	Conversion Factor	SI Units	Reference Publication
		Severe infection	8–10		17–21	
	Trough					
		Less severe infection	<1		<2	
		Moderate infection	<2		<4	
		Severe infection	<4		<8	
	Toxic					
		Peak	>10		>21	
		Trough	>2		>4	
Nevirapine (Viramune)	S or P		μg/mL	3.76	μmol/L	1
		Therap	>3.5		<13.2	
		Toxic	>12		>45.1	
Nordiazepine, active metabolite of several benzodiazepines	S or P		ng/mL	3.76	nmol/L	1
		Therap	100–500		376–1880	
		Toxic	>500		>1880	
Nortriptyline (Aventyl)	S or P		ng/mL	3.80	nmol/L	1
		Therap	70–170		266–646	
		Toxic	>500		>1900	
Olanzapine (Zyprexa)	S or P		ng/mL	3.20	nmol/L	1
		Therap	20–80		64–256	
		Toxic	>1000		>3200	
Oxazepam (Serax)	S or P		μg/mL	3.49	μmol/L	
		Therap	0.2–1.4		0.7–5	1
		Toxic	>2.0		>7	56
Oxcarbazepine (Trileptal) as monohydroxy oxcarbazepine (MHD)	S or P		μg/mL	3.97	μmol/L	1
		Therap	3–35		12–139	
		Toxic	>40		>159	
Oxycodone (Percodan)	S or P		ng/mL	3.17	nmol/L	1
		Therap	10–100		32–317	
		Toxic	>200		>634	
Paraldehyde (Paral)	S or P		μg/mL	7.57	μmol/L	1
		Therap				
		Sedation	10–100		76–757	
		Anesthesia	>200		>1514	
		Toxic	>200		>1514	
		Lethal	>500		>3785	
Paroxetine (Paxil)	S or P		ng/mL	3.04	nmol/L	1
		Therap	70–120		231–365	
Pentazocine (Talwin)	S or P		μg/mL	3.50	μmol/L	1
		Therap	0.05–0.2		0.2–0.7	
		Toxic	>1.0		>4	
Pentobarbital (Nembutal)	S or P		μg/mL	4.42	μmol/L	1
		Therap				
		Hypnotic	1–5		4–22	
		Therap coma	20–50		88–221	
		Toxic	>10		>44	

Continued

TABLE A.3 Reference Information for Toxicology and Therapeutic Drugs—cont'd

Drug	Specimen	Status	Conventional Units	Conversion Factor	SI Units	Reference Publication
			REFERENCE VALUES			
Perphenazine (Apo-Perphenazine)	S or P		μg/mL	2.48	μmol/L	1
		Therap	0.6–2.4		2–6	
		Toxic	>12		>30	
Phenacetin	S or P		μg/mL	5.58	μmol/L	1
		Therap	1–30		6–167	
		Toxic	50–250		279–1395	
Phenobarbital (Luminal)	S or P		μg/mL	4.31	μmol/L	1
		Therap	10–40		43–173	
		Toxic				
		Slowness, ataxia, nystagmus	35–80		151–345	
		Coma, with reflexes	65–117		280–504	
		Coma, without reflexes	>100		>431	
Phensuximide (Milontin) + norphensuximide	S or P		μg/mL	5.29	μmol/L	1
		Therap	40–60		212–317	
Phenylbutazone (Butazolidin)	S or P		μg/mL	3.24	μmol/L	1
		Therap	50–100		162–324	
		Toxic	>100		>324	
Phenytoin (Dilantin)	S or P		μg/mL	3.96	μmol/L	1
		Therap	10–20		40–79	
		Free	1.0–2.0		4–8	
		Toxic	>20		>79	
Posaconazole (Noxafil)	S or P		μg/mL	1.43	μmol/L	1
		Therap	>1.25		>2	
Primidone (Mysoline) + phenobarbital	S or P		μg/mL	4.58	μmol/L	1
		Therap	5–10		23–46	
		Toxic	>15		>69	
Procainamide (Pronestyl) + N-acetylprocainamide (NAPA)	S or P		μg/mL	4.25	μmol/L	1
		Therap	4–10		17–42	
			12–18 (NAPA)	3.61	43–65	
		Toxic	>12		>51	
			>40 (NAPA)		>144	
Propafenone (Rythmol)	S or P		μg/mL	2.93	μmol/L	1
		Therap	0.5–2.0		1.5–6	
		Toxic	>2		>6	
Propoxyphene (Darvon)	S or P		μg/mL	2.95	μmol/L	1
		Therap	0.1–0.4		0.3–1.0	
		Toxic	>0.5		>2	
Propranolol (Inderal)	S or P		ng/mL	3.86	nmol/L	1
		Therap	20–100		77–386	
		Toxic	>1000		>3860	56
		Fatal	>2000		>7720	
Protriptyline (Vivactil)	S or P		ng/mL	3.80	nmol/L	1
		Therap	70–260		266–988	
		Toxic	>500		>1900	

TABLE A.3 Reference Information for Toxicology and Therapeutic Drugs—cont'd

Drug	Specimen	Status	REFERENCE VALUES Conventional Units	Conversion Factor	SI Units	Reference Publication
Quetiapine (Seroquel)	S or P		ng/mL	0.00261	μmol/L	41
		Therap	100–500		0.26–1.3	
		Toxic	>1000		>2.6	
Quinidine (BioQuin)	S or P		μg/mL	3.08	μmol/L	1
		Therap	2–5		6–14	
		Toxic	>6		>19	
Risperidone + 9-hydroxyrisperidone (Risperdal)	S or P		ng/mL	2.44	nmol/L	1
		Therap	20–60		49–146	
Ritonavir (Norvir)	S or P		μg/mL	1.39	μmol/L	1
		Therap	>2		>3	
		Toxic	>22		>31	
Salicylates as salicylic acid or with chronic ingestion	S or P		μg/mL	0.00727	mmol/L	1
		Therap				
		Analgesia, antipyresis	<100		<0.7	
		Anti inflammatory	150–300		1–2	
		Toxic	>100		>0.7	
		Lethal, 24+ h after a dose	>500		>4	
Saquinavir (Fortovase, Invirase)	S or P		μg/mL	1.49	μmol/L	1
		Therap	>0.25		>0.4	
		Toxic	>6.0		>9	
Secobarbital (Seconal)	S or P		μg/mL	4.2	μmol/L	1
		Therap	1–2		4.2–8.4	
		Toxic	>5		>21.0	
Sertraline (Zoloft)	S or P		ng/mL	3.27	nmol/L	1
		Therap	10–50		33–164	
		Toxic	>300		>981	
Sirolimus (Rapamune, Rapamycin)	WB		ng/mL	1.10	nmol/L	1
		Therap	4–20		4–22	
		Toxic	>20		>22	
Sotalol (Betapace, Sorine)	S or P		μg/mL	3.67	μmol/L	1
		Therap	1–3		4–11	
Streptomycin	S or P		μg/ml	1.72	μmol/L	1
		Therap				
		Trough	<5		<9	
		Peak	20–30		34–52	
		Peak/MIC	>10		>17.2	
		Toxic	>50		>86	
Sulfonamides as sulfanilamide	S or P		mg/mL	5.81	mmol/L	1
		Therap	5–15		29–87	
		Toxic	>20		>116	
Tacrolimus (FK 506, Prodraf)	WB		ng/mL	1.24	nmol/L	1
		Therap	3–20		4–25	
		Toxic	>20		>25	
Teicoplanin (Targocid)	S or P		μg/mL	0.53	μmol/L	1
		Peak	>10		>5	

Continued

TABLE A.3 Reference Information for Toxicology and Therapeutic Drugs—cont'd

Drug	Specimen	Status	REFERENCE VALUES Conventional Units	Conversion Factor	SI Units	Reference Publication
Theophylline (Uniphyl)	S or P Therap		μg/mL	5.55	μmol/L	1
		Bronchodilator	8–20		44–111	
		Premature apnea	6–13		33–72	
		Toxic	>20		>111	
Thiopental (Pentothal)	S or P		μg/mL	4.13	μmol/L	1
		Hypnotic	1–5		4–21	
		Coma	30–100		124–413	
		Anesthesia	7–130		29–536	
		Toxic	>10		>41	
Thioridazine (Mellaril)	S or P		μg/mL	2.7	μmol/L	1
		Therap	0.2–2.0		0.5–5	
		Toxic	>10		>27	
Tiagabine (Gabitril)	S or P		ng/mL	2.66	nmol/L	1
		Therap	20–200		53–532	
		Toxic	>520		>1383	
Tobramycin (Nebcin)	S or P		μg/mL	2.14	μmol/L	1
		Therap				
		Peak				
		Less severe infection	5–8		11–17	
		Severe infection	8–10		17–21	
		Trough				
		Less severe infection	<1		<2	
		Moderate infection	<2		<4	
		Severe infection	<4		<9	
		Toxic				
		Peak	>10		>21	
		Trough	>2		>4	
		Peak/MIC	>10		>21	
Tocainide (Tonocard)	S or P		μg/mL	5.20	μmol/L	1
		Therap	6–15		31–78	
		Toxic	>15		>78	
Tolbutamide (Orinase)	S or P		μg/mL	3.70	μmol/L	1
		Therap	90–240		333–888	
		Toxic	>640		>2368	
Topiramate (Topamax)	S or P		μg/mL	2.95	μmol/L	1
		Therap	5–20		15–59	
		Toxic	>12		>36	
Trazodone (Desyrel)	S or P		ng/mL	2.68	nmol/L	1
		Therap	650–1500		1748–4020	
		Toxic	>4000		>10,720	
Trimipramine (Surmontil)	S or P		ng/mL	3.40	nmol/L	1
		Therap	150–350		510–1190	
		Toxic	>500		>1700	
Valproic acid (Depakene)	S or P		μg/mL	6.93	μmol/L	1
		Therap	50–100		346–693	
		Toxic	>100		>693	

TABLE A.3 Reference Information for Toxicology and Therapeutic Drugs—cont'd

Drug	Specimen	Status	Conventional Units	Conversion Factor	SI Units	Reference Publication
Vancomycin (Vancocin)	S or P		μg/mL	0.69	μmol/L	1
		Therap				
		Peak	20–40		14–28	
		Trough	>10		>7	
		Toxic	>80		>55	
Venlafaxine (Effexor) + desmethylvenlafaxine	S or P		ng/mL	3.61	nmol/L	1
		Therap	195–400		704–1444	
		Toxic	>1000 (sum)		>3610	
Vigabatrin (Sabril)	S or P		μg/mL	7.74	μmol/L	1
		Therap	0.8–36		6–279	
Voriconazole (Vfend)	S or P		μg/mL	2.86	μmol/L	1
		Therap	1–6		3–17	
		Toxic	>6		>17	
Warfarin (Coumadin)	S or P		μg/mL	3.24	μmol/L	1
		Therap	1–10		3–32	
		Toxic	>10		>32	
Zidovudine (AZT, Retrovir)	S or P		μg/mL	3.74	μmol/L	1
		Therap	>0.2		>0.8	
Zonisamide (Zonegran)	S or P		μg/mL	4.71	μmol/L	
		Therap	10–40		47–188	1
		Potential adverse effects	>80		>377	56

AUC, Area under the curve; *CNS,* central nervous system; *F,* fluoride ion; *MIC,* minimum inhibitory concentration; *Occup exp,* occupational exposure; *Ox,* oxalate; *P,* plasma; *S,* serum; *Therap,* therapeutic; *U,* urine; *WB,* whole blood.

TABLE A.4 Pediatric and Adult Reference Intervals for Hematologic Markers Based on the Canadian Health Measures Survey

Analyte	Age	Conventional Units	Conversion Factor	SI Units	Instrument/ Method	Reference Publication
Basophils		$10^3/\mu L$	1	$10^9/L$		29, 42, 53
	0–20 y	0.0–0.1		0.0–0.1	Sysmex XN-3000	
	0–20 y	0.0–0.1		0.0–0.1	Beckman Coulter DxH 900	
	3–5 y	0.0–0.1		0.0–0.1	Beckman Coulter HmX	
	6–79 y	0.0–0.9		0.0–0.9		
Eosinophils		$10^3/\mu L$	1	$10^9/L$		29, 42, 53
	0–3 y	0.0–0.8		0.0–0.8	Sysmex XN-3000	
	4–14 y	0.1–1.0		0.1–1.0		
	15–20 y	0.0–0.5		0.0–0.5		
	0–11 mo	0.1–0.9		0.1–0.9	Beckman Coulter DxH 900	
	1–12 y	0.1–0.5		0.1–0.5		
	13–20 y	0.1–0.5		0.1–0.5		
	3–5 y	0.0–0.5		0.0–0.5	Beckman Coulter HmX	
	6–11 y	0.0–0.5		0.0–0.5		
	12–79 y	0.1–0.2		0.1–0.2		

Continued

TABLE A.4 Pediatric and Adult Reference Intervals for Hematologic Markers Based on the Canadian Health Measures Survey—cont'd

Analyte	Age	REFERENCE INTERVALS Conventional Units	Conversion Factor	SI Units	Instrument/ Method	Reference Publication
Fibrinogen		mg/dL	0.01	g/L	Sysmex CA-500 SERIES analyzer	29
	12–13 y	180–350		1.8–3.5	Clauss method,	
	14–39 y, M	210–370		2.1–3.7	Photooptical clot	
	14–39 y, F	200–420		2.0–4.2	detection (turbidity	
	40–79 y	200–420		2.0–4.2	measurement)	
Hematocrit		%	0.01	L/L		29, 42, 53
	0–11 mo	28–39		0.28–0.39	Sysmex XN-3000	
	1–3 y	31–39		0.31–0.39		
	4–13 y	34–43		0.34–0.43		
	14–20 y, M	39–50		0.39–0.50		
	14–20 y, F	35–45		0.35–0.45		
	0–11 mo	27–40		0.27–0.40	Beckman Coulter DxH 900	
	1–3 y	30–40		0.30–0.40		
	4–13 y	34–42		0.34–0.42		
	14–20 y, M	39–48		0.39–0.48		
	14–20 y, F	34–44		0.34–0.44		
	3–5 y	34–42		0.34–0.42	Beckman Coulter HmX	
	6–7 y	34–42		0.34–0.42		
	8–11 y	35–43		0.35–0.43		
	12–15 y, M	38–47		0.38–0.47		
	16–79 y, M	40–50		0.40–0.50		
	12–79 y, F	35–43		0.35–0.43		
Hemoglobin		g/dL	10	g/L		29, 42, 53
	0–11 mo	9.3–12.9		93–129	Sysmex XN-3000	
	1–3 y	10.0–13.2		100–132		
	4–13 y	11.2–14.1		112–141		
	14–20 y, M	12.9–16.7		129–167		
	14–20 y, F	11.2–15.1		112–151		
	0–11 mo	9.3–13.4		93–134	Beckman Coulter DxH 900	
	1–3 y	9.9–13.4		99–134		
	4–13 y	11.4–14.1		114–141		
	14–20 y, M	12.9–16.5		129–165		
	14–20 y, F	11.3–14.9		113–149		
	3–5 y	11.4–14.3		113.5–143.1	Beckman Coulter HmX	
	6–8 y	11.5–14.3		114.7–143.0		
	9–10 y	11.8–14.7		118.4–146.9		
	11–14 y, M	12.4–15.7		124.2–156.5		
	15–19 y, M	13.3–16.9		132.5–169.0		
	20–79 y, M	13.6–16.9		136–168.9		
	11–79 y, F	11.9–14.8		119.3–148.4		
Lymphocytes		$10^3/\mu L$	1	$10^9/L$		29, 42, 53
	0–11 mo	1.96–8.94		1.96–8.94	Sysmex XN-3000	
	1–4 y	1.90–6.30		1.90–6.30		
	5–14 y	1.34–4.12		1.34–4.12		
	15–20 y	1.26–3.41		1.26–3.41		
	0–11 mo	3.3–8.8		3.3–8.8	Beckman Coulter DxH 900	
	1–4 y	1.8–7.1		1.8–7.1		
	5–14 y	1.4–4.1		1.4–4.1		
	15–20 y	1.1–3.6		1.1–3.6		
	3–5 y	1.6–5.3		1.6–5.3	Beckman Coulter HmX	
	6–11 y	1.4–3.9		1.4–3.9		
	12–79 y	1.0–3.2		1.0–3.2		

TABLE A.4 Pediatric and Adult Reference Intervals for Hematologic Markers Based on the Canadian Health Measures Survey—cont'd

Analyte	Age	REFERENCE INTERVALS			Instrument/ Method	Reference Publication
		Conventional Units	Conversion Factor	SI Units		
Mean corpuscular hemoglobin		Pg	1	pg		29, 42, 53
	0–11 mo	23.5–34.0		23.5–34.0	Sysmex XN-3000	
	1–3 y	23.5–28.2		23.5–28.2		
	4–13 y	25.1–30.3		25.1–30.3		
	14–20 y	25.6–32.0		25.6–32.0		
	0–11 mo	22.9–32.7		22.9–32.7	Beckman Coulter DxH 900	
	1–2 y	22.7–29.0		22.7–29.0		
	3–5 y	25.2–29.3		25.2–29.3		
	6–12 y	25.4–30.8		25.4–30.8		
	13–20 y	25.9–32.4		25.9–32.4		
	3–5 y	26.1–30.7		26.1–30.7	Beckman Coulter HmX	
	6–15 y	26.3–31.7		26.3–31.7		
	16–79 y	27.6–33.3		27.6–33.3		
Mean corpuscular hemoglobin concentration		g/dL	10	g/L		29, 42, 53
	0–11 mo	31.9–35.2		319–352	Sysmex XN-3000	
	1–20 y	31.0–34.5		310–345		
	0–20 y	32.3–35.0		323–350	Beckman Coulter DxH 900	
	3–5 y	32.4–34.9		324–348.8	Beckman Coulter HmX	
	6–79 y	32.5–35.2		324.5–352.3		
Mean corpuscular volume		fL	1	fL		29, 42, 53
	0–11 mo	72.0–98.6		72.0–98.6	Sysmex XN-3000	
	1–3 y	73.5–84.1		73.5–84.1		
	4–13 y, M	77.6–91.0		77.6–91.0		
	4–13 y, F	77.4–92.1		77.4–92.1		
	14–20 y	79.5–95.4		79.5–95.4		
	0–11 mo	70.5–94.9		70.5–94.9	Beckman Coulter DxH 900	
	1–3 y	72.8–85.2		72.8–85.2		
	4–13 y	77.4–89.9		77.4–89.9		
	14–20 y	77.6–95.7		77.6–95.7		
	3–5 y	77.2–89.5		77.2–89.5	Beckman Coulter HmX	
	6–11 y	77.8–91.1		77.8–91.1		
	12–14 y	79.9–93.0		79.9–93.0		
	15–79 y	82.5–98.0		82.5–98.0		
Mean platelet volume		fL	1	fL		29, 42, 53
	0–11 mo	8.6–11.3		8.6–11.3	Sysmex XN-3000	
	1–3 y	8.3–10.7		8.3–10.7		
	4–20 y	9.0–12.8		9.0–12.8		
	0–6 y	6.9–9.7		6.9–9.7	Beckman Coulter DxH 900	
	7–20 y	7.3–10.7		7.3–10.7		
	3–5 y	6.4–9.5		6.4–9.5	Beckman Coulter HmX	
	6–11 y	6.6–9.8		6.6–9.8		
	12–79 y	7.0–10.3		7.0–10.3		
Monocytes		$10^3/\mu L$	1	$10^9/L$		29, 42, 53
	0–4 y	0.37–1.45		0.37–1.45	Sysmex XN-3000	
	5–20 y	0.27–0.81		0.27–0.81		
	0–1 y	0.4–1.1		0.4–1.1	Beckman Coulter DxH 900	
	2–4 y	0.3–1.1		0.3–1.1		
	5–20 y	0.3–0.8		0.3–0.8		
	3–5 y	0.3–0.9		0.3–0.9	Beckman Coulter HmX	
	6–44 y	0.2–0.8		0.2–0.8		
	45–79 y, M	0.3–0.9		0.3–0.9		
	45–79 y, F	0.2–0.8		0.2–0.8		

Continued

TABLE A.4 **Pediatric and Adult Reference Intervals for Hematologic Markers Based on the Canadian Health Measures Survey—cont'd**

		REFERENCE INTERVALS				
Analyte	**Age**	**Conventional Units**	**Conversion Factor**	**SI Units**	**Instrument/ Method**	**Reference Publication**
Neutrophils		$10^3/\mu L$	1	$10^9/L$		29, 42, 53
	0–11 mo	0.7–5.8		0.7–5.8	Sysmex XN-3000	
	1–20 y	1.5–6.8		1.5–6.8		
	0–11 mo	0.9–4.6		0.9–4.6	Beckman Coulter DxH 900	
	1–20 y	1.5–6.4		1.5–6.4		
	3–5 y	1.6–7.8		1.6–7.8	Beckman Coulter HmX	
	6–16 y, M	1.4–6.1		1.4–6.1		
	6–14 y, F	1.5–6.5		1.5–6.5		
	15–50 y, F	2.0–7.4		2.0–7.4		
	17–50 y, M	1.8–7.2		1.8–7.2		
	51–79 y	2.0–6.4		2.0–6.4		
Platelet count		$10^3/\mu L$	1	$10^9/L$		29, 42, 53
	0–11 mo	253–552		253–552	Sysmex XN-3000	
	1–11 y	203–431		203–431		
	11–20 y	173–361		173–361		
	0–11 mo	287–589		287–589	Beckman Coulter DxH 900	
	1–11 y	212–480		212–480		
	12–20 y	170–380		170–380		
	3–5 y	187.4–444.6		187.4–444.6	Beckman Coulter HmX	
	6–9 y	186.7–400.4		186.7–400.4		
	10–13 y	176.9–381.3		176.9–381.3		
	14–26 y, M	138.7–319.6		138.7–319.6		
	F	158.1–361.6		158.1–361.6		
	27–50 y, M	152.6–322.4		152.6–322.4		
	F	141.7–362.1		141.7–362.1		
	60–79 y	142.6–347.7		142.6–347.7		
Red blood cell count		$10^6/\mu L$	1	$10^{12}/L$		29, 42, 53
	0–11 mo, M	3.00–5.18		3.00–5.18	Sysmex XN-3000	
	0–11 mo, F	3.05–4.85		3.05–4.85		
	1–3 y	3.90–4.96		3.90–4.96		
	4–13 y, M	4.14–5.14		4.14–5.14		
	4–13 y, F	3.95–5.00		3.95–5.00		
	14–20 y, M	4.26–5.74		4.26–5.74		
	14–20 y, F	3.98–5.40		3.98–5.40		
	0–11 mo	2.9–5.2		2.9–5.2	Beckman Coulter DxH 900	
	1–13 y, M	4.1–5.1		4.1–5.1		
	1–13 y, F	3.9–5.0		3.9–5.0		
	14–20, M	4.3–5.6		4.3–5.6		
	14–20, F	4.0–5.1		4.0–5.1		
	3–5 y	4.0–5.1		4.0–5.1	Beckman Coulter HmX	
	6–10 y	4.1–5.2		4.1–5.2		
	11–14 y	4.2–5.3		4.2–5.3		
	15–49 y, M	4.3–5.7		4.3–5.7		
	50–79 y, M	4.2–5.5		4.2–5.5		
	15–79 y, F	3.8–5.0		3.8–5.0		
Red cell distribution width		%	1	%		29, 42, 53
	0–11 mo	12.0–17.0		12.0–17.0	Sysmex XN-3000	
	1–13 y, M	11.9–15.3		11.9–15.3		
	1–13 y, F	11.5–14.5		11.5–14.5		
	14–21	11.5–15.6		11.5–15.6		
	0–1 y	12.2–17.7		12.2–17.7	Beckman Coulter DxH 900	
	2–20 y	12.2–15.2		12.2–15.2		
	3–5 y	11.3–13.4		11.3–13.4	Beckman Coulter HmX	
	6–80 y	11.4–13.5		11.4–13.5		

TABLE A.4 **Pediatric and Adult Reference Intervals for Hematologic Markers Based on the Canadian Health Measures Survey—cont'd**

Analyte	Age	REFERENCE INTERVALS Conventional Units	Conversion Factor	SI Units	Instrument/ Method	Reference Publication
White blood cell count		10³/µl	1	10⁹/L		29, 42, 53
	0–2 y	5.75–13.5		5.75–13.5	Sysmex XN-3000	
	3–4 y	4.92–11.8		4.92–11.8		
	5–20 y	4.23–9.99		4.23–9.99		
	0–2 y	5.3–13.2		5.3–13.2	Beckman Coulter DxH 900	
	3–4 y	4.8–11.5		4.8–11.5		
	5–20 y	4.2–10.2		4.2–10.2		
	3–5 y	4.4–12.9		4.4–12.9	Beckman Coulter HmX	
	6–79 y	3.8–10.4		3.8–10.4		

F, Female; *M,* male.

TABLE A.5 **Critical Values (Risk Thresholds) for Biochemical and Hematologic Markers**

Parameter	Conventional Units Lower Limit	Upper Limit	SI Units Lower Limit	Upper Limit	Reference Publication
Albumin (children)	g/dL		g/L		
	1.7	6.8	17	68	1
Aminotransferases	U/L		µkat/L		
	—	1000	—	16.7	43
Ammonia	µg/dL		µmol/L		
	—	187	—	110	1, 43, 44
Anion gap			mmol/L		
			—	20	43
Bilirubin (newborn)	mg/dL		mmol/L		
	—	15	—	257	1, 43
Calcium (total)	mg/dL		mmol/L		
	6.6	14	1.65	3.5	43, 44, 45
Calcium (children)	mg/dL		mmol/L		
	6.5	12.7	1.63	3.18	1
Calcium (free)	mg/dL		mmol/L		
	3.1	6.3	0.78	1.6	1, 43, 44, 45
Carbon dioxide, total			mmol/L		
			10	40	1
Chloride (adult)			mmol/L		
			80	120	1
Creatinine (adult)	mg/dL		mmol/L		
	—	5	—	442	1
Creatinine (children)	mg/dL		µmol/L		
	—	3.8	—	336	1
Creatine kinase	U/L		µkat/L		
	—	1000	—	16.7	43
Glucose	mg/dL		mmol/L		
	40	500	2.22	27.8	44
Glucose (children)	mg/dL		mmol/L		
	46	445	2.56	24.72	1
Glucose (newborn)	mg/dL		mmol/L		
	30	325	1.67	18.06	1,43
Glucose, CSF (adult)	mg/dL		mmol/L		
	40	200	2.22	11.11	1
Glucose, CSF (children)	mg/dL		mmol/L		

Continued

TABLE A.5 Critical Values (Risk Thresholds) for Biochemical and Hematologic Markers—cont'd

Parameter (units: conv; SI)	Conventional Units		SI Units		Reference Publication
	Lower Limit	**Upper Limit**	**Lower Limit**	**Upper Limit**	
(value continued from previous page)	31	—	1.72	—	1
Lactate CSF (mg/dL; mmol/L)	—	30.6	—	3.4	1
Lactate plasma (mg/dL; mmol/L)	—	45	—	5	43
Lactate plasma (children) (mg/dL; mmol/L)	—	36.9	—	4.1	1
Lactate dehydrogenase (U/L; µkat/L)	—	1000	—	16.7	43
Lipase (U/L; µkat/L)	—	700	—	11.7	43
Magnesium (mg/dL; mmol/L)	1	4.9	0.41	2	1, 43
Osmolality (mOsm/kg)	240	330			43
Osmolar gap (mOsm/Kg)	—	10			43
Phosphate (mg/dL; mmol/L)	1	9	0.32	2.9	1, 43
Potassium (mmol/L)	2.8	6.2			1, 43
Potassium (newborn) (mmol/L)	2.8	7.8			1
Protein (children) (g/dL; g/L)	3.4	9.5	34	95	1
Protein, CSF (children) (mg/dL; mg/L)	—	188	—	1880	1
Sodium (mmol/L)	120	160			1, 43, 44, 45
T_4 (free) (ng/dL; pmol/L)	—	3.5	—	45	43
Urea nitrogen (mg/dL; mmol/L)	—	100	—	35.6	43
Urea (mg/dL; mmol/L)	—	214	—	35.6	43
Urea nitrogen (children) (mg/dL; mmol/L)	—	55	—	19.6	1
Uric acid (mg/dL; mmol/L)	—	13	—	0.767	1, 43
Uric acid (children) (mg/dL; —)	—	12	—	0.708	1
pH	7.2	7.6	7.2	7.6	1, 43
PCO_2 (mm Hg; kPa)	20	70	2.7	9.45	1
PO_2 (mm Hg; kPa)	40	—	5.3	—	1
PO_2 children (mm Hg; kPa)	45	125	6.0	16.7	1
PO_2 newborn (mm Hg; kPa)	35	90	4.7	12.0	1
Hematocrit (adult) (%; L/L)	20	60	0.20	0.60	1
Hematocrit (newborn) (%; L/L)	33	71	0.33	0.71	1

TABLE A.5 Critical Values (Risk Thresholds) for Biochemical and Hematologic Markers—cont'd

| | REFERENCE INTERVALS | | | | |
| | Conventional Units | | SI Units | | |
Parameter	Lower Limit	Upper Limit	Lower Limit	Upper Limit	Reference Publication
Hemoglobin (adult)	g/dL		g/L		
	7.0	20	70	200	1
Hemoglobin (newborn)	g/dL		g/L		
	10.0	22	100	2204	1
Leukocytes (adult)	10^3/mL		10^9/L		
	2	30	2	30	1
Leukocytes (children)	10^3/mL		10^9/L		
	2	43	2	43	1
Neutrophil count	10^3/mL		10^9/L		
	0.5	—	0.5	—	44
Platelet count	10^3/mL		10^9/L		
	20	1000	20	1000	44, 47
Blasts	Any seen (first report only)				1
Drepanocytes	Presence of sickle cells or aplastic cells				1
Prothrombin time (INR)					
	—	5			44, 45, 47, 48
aPTT	Seconds		Seconds		
	—	110	—	110	47
Antithrombin	%				
	28	—	—		46
Factors II, V, VII, VIII, IX, X, and XI	IU/dL				48
(in emergency management [e.g. surgery])	—	5			
Factor XIII	IU/dL				48
(in emergency management [e.g., surgery])	—	3			
Fibrinogen	mg/dL		g/L		
	80	—	0.8	—	1, 47, 48
Digoxin	ng/mL		nmol/L		
	—	2.2	—	2.8	44
Digitoxin	mg/L		nmol/L		
	—	40	—	52	43
Ethanol	g/L		mmol/L		
CSF	—	3.5	—	66	43
CSF	Cells/µL				
WBC (0–1 y)	—	>30			1
WBC (1–4 y)	—	>20			
WBC (5–17 y)	—	>10			
WBC (>17 y)	—	>5			
Malignant cells, blasts, or microorganisms	Any				1
	Applies to other sterile body fluids				

aPTT, Activated partial thromboplastin time; *CSF*, cerebrospinal fluid; *INR*, international normalized ratio; T_4, thyroxine; *WBC*, white blood cell.

REFERENCES

1. Adeli K, Ceriotti F, Nieuwesteeg M. Reference information for the clinical laboratory. In: Rifai N, Horvath AR, Wittwer C, editors. Tietz textbook of clinical chemistry and molecular diagnostics. 6th ed. St. Louis: Elsevier; 2018. p. 1745–818.

2. Adeli K, Higgins V, Trajcevski K, et al. The Canadian laboratory initiative on pediatric reference intervals: a CALIPER white paper. Crit Rev Clin Lab Sci 2017;54(6):358–413.

3. Bailey D, Colantonio D, Kyriakopoulou L, et al. Marked biological variance in endocrine and biochemical markers in childhood: establishment of pediatric reference intervals using healthy community children from the CALIPER cohort. Clin Chem 2013;59:1393–405.

4. Bevilacqua V, Chan MK, Chen Y, et al. Pediatric population reference value distributions for cancer biomarkers and covariate–stratified reference intervals in the CALIPER cohort. Clin Chem 2014;60:1532–42.

5. Bohn MK, Higgins V, Kavsak P, et al. High-sensitivity generation 5 cardiac troponin T sex-and age-specific 99th percentiles in the CALIPER cohort of healthy children and adolescents. Clin Chem 2019;65:589–91.

6. Bohn MK, Higgins V, Adeli K. CALIPER paediatric reference intervals for the urea creatinine ratio in healthy children & adolescents. Clin Biochem 2020;76:31–4.

7. Colantonio DA, Kyriakopoulou L, Chan MK, et al. Closing the gaps in pediatric laboratory reference intervals: a CALIPER database of 40 biochemical markers in a healthy and multiethnic population of children. Clin Chem 2012;58:854–68.

8. Higgins V, Fung AW, Chan MK, et al. Pediatric reference intervals for 29 Ortho VITROS 5600 immunoassays using the CALIPER cohort of healthy children and adolescents. Clin Chem Lab Med 2018;56:327–40.

9. Higgins V, Truong D, White-Al Habeeb NM, et al. Pediatric reference intervals for 1, 25-dihydroxyvitamin D using the DiaSorin LIAISON XL assay in the healthy CALIPER cohort. Clin Chem Lab Med 2018;56:964–72.

10. Higgins V, Asgari S, Chan MK, et al. Pediatric reference intervals for calculated LDL cholesterol, non-HDL cholesterol, and remnant cholesterol in the healthy CALIPER cohort. Clin Chim Acta 2018;486:129–34.

11. Higgins V, Chan MK, Adeli K. Pediatric reference intervals for transferrin saturation in the CALIPER cohort of healthy children and adolescents. EJIFCC 2017;28:77.

12. Karbasy K, Lin DC, Stoianov A, et al. Pediatric reference value distributions and covariate-stratified reference intervals for 29 endocrine and special chemistry biomarkers on the Beckman Coulter Immunoassay Systems: a CALIPER study of healthy community children. Clin Chem Lab Med 2016;54:643–57.

13. Kavsak PA, Rezanpour A, Chen Y, et al. Assessment of the 99th or 97.5th percentile for cardiac troponin I in a healthy pediatric cohort. Clin Chem 2014;60:1574–6.

14. Kelly J, Raizman JE, Bevilacqua V, et al. Complex reference value distributions and partitioned reference intervals across the pediatric age range for 14 specialized biochemical markers in the CALIPER cohort of healthy community children and adolescents. Clin Chim Acta 2015;450:169–202.

15. Konforte D, Shea JL, Kyriakopoulou L, et al. Complex biological pattern of fertility hormones in children and adolescents: a study of healthy children from the CALIPER cohort and establishment of pediatric reference intervals. Clin Chem 2013;59:1215–27.

16. Kyriakopoulou L, Yazdanpanah M, Colantonio DA, et al. A sensitive and rapid mass spectrometric method for the simultaneous measurement of eight steroid hormones and CALIPER pediatric reference intervals. Clin Biochem 2013;46:642–51.

17. Raizman JE, Cohen AH, Teodoro-Morrison T, et al. Pediatric reference value distributions for vitamins A and E in the CALIPER cohort and establishment of age-stratified reference intervals. Clin Biochem 2014;47:812–15.

18. Raizman JE, Quinn F, Armbruster DA, et al. Pediatric reference intervals for calculated free testosterone, bioavailable testosterone and free androgen index in the CALIPER cohort. Clin Chem Lab Med 2015;53:e239–43.

19. Tahmasebi H, Higgins V, Woroch A, et al. Pediatric reference intervals for clinical chemistry assays on Siemens ADVIA XPT/1800 and Dimension EXL in the CALIPER cohort of healthy children and adolescents. Clin Chim Acta 2019;490: 88–97.

20. Teodoro-Morrison T, Kyriakopoulou L, Chen YK, et al. Dynamic biological changes in metabolic disease biomarkers in childhood and adolescence: a CALIPER study of healthy community children. Clin Biochem 2015;48(13-14):828–36.

21. Estey MP, Cohen AH, Colantonio DA, et al. CLSI-based transference of the CALIPER database of pediatric reference intervals from Abbott to Beckman, Ortho, Roche and Siemens Clinical Chemistry Assays: direct validation using reference samples from the CALIPER cohort. Clin Biochem 2013;46:1197–219.

22. El Hassan MA, Stoianov A, Araújo PA, et al. CLSI-based transference of CALIPER pediatric reference intervals to Beckman Coulter AU biochemical assays. Clin Biochem 2015;48:1151–9.

23. Araújo PA, Thomas D, Sadeghieh T, et al. CLSI-based transference of the CALIPER database of pediatric reference intervals to Beckman Coulter DxC biochemical assays. Clin Biochem 2015;48:870–80.

24. Higgins V, Truong D, Woroch A, et al. CLSI-based transference and verification of CALIPER pediatric reference intervals for 29 Ortho VITROS 5600 chemistry assays. Clin Biochem 2018;53:93–103.

25. Higgins V, Chan MK, Nieuwesteeg M, et al. Transference of CALIPER pediatric reference intervals to biochemical assays on the Roche cobas 6000 and the Roche Modular P. Clin Biochem 2016;49(1–2):139–49.

26. Bohn MK, Higgins V, Asgari S, et al. Paediatric reference intervals for 17 Roche cobas 8000 e602 immunoassays in the CALIPER cohort of healthy children and adolescents. Clin Chem Lab Med 2019;57(12):1968–79.

27. Adeli K, Higgins V, Nieuwesteeg M, et al. Biochemical marker reference values for pediatric, adult and geriatric age groups: establishment of robust pediatric and adult reference intervals based on the Canadian Health Measures Survey. Clin Chem 2015;61:1049–62.

28. Adeli K, Higgins V, Nieuwesteeg M, et al. Complex reference value distributions for endocrine and special chemistry biomarkers across pediatric, adult and geriatric age: establishment of robust pediatric and adult reference intervals based on the Canadian Health Measures Survey. Clin Chem 2015;61: 1063–74.

29. Adeli K, Raizman JE, Chen Y, et al. Complex biological profile of hematological markers across pediatric, adult, and geriatric ages: establishment of robust pediatric and adult reference

intervals based on the Canadian Health Measures Survey. Clin Chem 2015;61:1075–86.

30. Schumann G, Aoki R, Ferrero CA, et al. IFCC primary reference procedures for the measurement of catalytic activity concentrations of enzymes at 37 degrees C. Clin Chem Lab Med 2006;44:1146–55.

31. Ichihara K, Ceriotti F, Kazuo M, et al. The Asian project for collaborative derivation of reference intervals: (2) results of non-standardized analytes and transference of reference intervals to the participating laboratories on the basis of cross-comparison of test results. Clin Chem Lab Med 2013;51:1443–57.

32. Fuentes-Arderiu X, Ferré-Masferrer M, Gonzàlez-Alba JM, et al. Multicentric reference values for some quantities measured with Tina-Quant® reagents systems and RD/Hitachi analysers. Scand J Clin Lab Invest 2001;61:273–6.

33. Bjerner J, Biernat D, Fosså SD, et al. Reference intervals for serum testosterone, SHBG, LH and FSH in males from the NORIP project. Scand J Clin Lab Invest 2009;69:873–9.

34. KDIGO Clinical practice guideline for the evaluation and management of chronic kidney disease. Kidney Int Suppl 2013;3(1): Available from: http://www.kdigo.org/clinical_practice_guidelines/pdf/CKD/KDIGO_2012_CKD_GL.pdf.

35. National Heart, Lung and Blood Institute. Integrated guidelines for cardiovascular health and risk reduction in children and adolescents. Available from: http://www.nhlbi.nih.gov/health-pro/guidelines/current/cardiovascular-health-pediatric-guidelines. Accessed July 16, 2020.

36. Stagnaro-Green A, Abalovich M, Alexander E, et al. Guidelines of the American Thyroid Association for the diagnosis and management of thyroid disease during pregnancy and postpartum. Thyroid 2011;21:1081–125.

37. Kushnir MM, Blamires T, Rockwood AL, et al. Liquid chromatography: tandem mass spectrometry assay for androstenedione, dehydroepiandrosterone, and testosterone with pediatric and adult reference intervals. Clin Chem 2010;56:1138–47.

38. World Health Organization. Use of glycated hemoglobin A1c in the diagnosis of diabetes mellitus. WHO; 2011. p. 1–25.

39. Holick MF. Vitamin D deficiency. N Engl J Med 2007;357: 266–81.

40. Zhang WM, Natowicz MR. Cerebrospinal fluid lactate and pyruvate concentrations and their ratio. Clin Biochem 2013;46:694–7.

41. Hiemke C, Baumann P, Bergemann N, et al. AGNP Consensus guidelines for therapeutic drug monitoring in psychiatry: update 2011. Pharmacopsychiatry 2011;44:195–235.

42. Tahmasebi H, Higgins V, Bohn MK, Hall A, Adeli K. CALIPER hematology reference standards (I) improving laboratory test interpretation in children (Beckman Coulter DxH 900–Core Laboratory Hematology System). Am J Clin Pathol 2020.

43. Thomas L. Critical limits of laboratory results for urgent clinician notification. EJIFCC 2003;14(1):11–8. Available from: www.ifcc.org/ifccfiles/docs/140103200303.pdf.

44. Hashim IA, Cuthbert JA, Critical Values Working Group. Establishing, harmonizing and analyzing critical values in a large academic health center. Clin Chem Lab Med 2014;52: 1129–35.

45. Piva E, Pelloso M, Penello L, et al. Laboratory critical values: automated notification supports effective clinical decision making. Clin Biochem 2014;47:1163–8.

46. Pai M, Moffat KA, Plumhoff E, et al. Critical values in the coagulation laboratory: results of a survey of the North American Specialized Coagulation Laboratory Association. Am J Clin Pathol 2011;136:836–41.

47. Lippi G, Adcock D, Simundic AM, et al. Critical laboratory values in hemostasis: toward consensus. Ann Med 2017; 49:455–61.

48. Gosselin RC, Adcock D, Dorgalaleh A, et al. International Council for Standardization in Haematology recommendations for hemostasis critical values, tests, and reporting. In: Seminars in thrombosis and hemostasis.Thieme Medical Publishers; 2019.

49. Westgard J. Desirable biological variation database specifications. Available from: https://www.westgard.com/biodatabase1.htm. Accessed July 16, 2020.

50. Westgard J. Available from: https://www.westgard.com. Accessed July 16, 2020.

51. European Federation for Laboratory Medicine. Available from: https://biologicalvariation.eu/. Accessed July 16, 2020.

52. Bailey D, Bevilacqua V, Colantonio DA, et al. Pediatric within-day biological variation and quality specificaions for 38 biochemical markers in the CALIPER cohort. Clin Chem 2014;60:518–29.

53. Bohn MK, Higgins V, Tahmasebi H, et al. Complex biological patterns of hematology parameters in childhood necessitating age- and sex-specific reference intervals for evidence-based clinical interpretation. Int J Lab Hematol 2020;42(6):750–60.

54. Grundy SM, Stone NJ, Bailey AL, et al. 2018 AHA/ACC/AACVPR/AAPA/ABC/ACPM/ADA/AGS/APhA/ASPC/NLA/PCNA Guideline on the Management of Blood Cholesterol: A Report of the American College of Cardiology/American Heart Association Task Force on Clinical Practice Guidelines [published correction appears in J Am Coll Cardiol 2019 Jun 25;73(24):3237–41]. J Am Coll Cardiol 2019;73(24):e285–350. doi:10.1016/j.jacc.2018.11.003.

55. National Cholesterol Education Program (NCEP) Expert Panel on Detection, Evaluation, and Treatment of High Blood Cholesterol in Adults (Adult Treatment Panel III). Third Report of the National Cholesterol Education Program (NCEP) Expert Panel on Detection, Evaluation, and Treatment of High Blood Cholesterol in Adults (Adult Treatment Panel III) final report. Circulation 2002;106(25):3143–421.

56. Lexicomp Database. Available from: https://www.wolterskluwercdi.com/lexicomp-online/. Accessed September 2, 2020.

57. Benoist JF, Alberti C, Leclercq S, et al. Cerebrospinal fluid lactate and pyruvate concentrations and their ratio in children: age-related reference intervals. Clin Chem 2003;49:487–94.

ABBREVIATIONS

AACVPR:	American Association of Cardiovascular and Pulmonary Rehabilitation
AAPA:	American Association Academy of Physician Assistants
ABC:	Association of Black Cardiologists
ACC:	American College of Cardiology
ACD:	Anticoagulant Citrate Dextrose
ACPM:	American College of Preventive Medicine
ADA:	American Diabetes Association
AHA:	American Heart Association
Amf:	Amniotic fluid
APhA:	American Pharmacists Association
ASPC:	American Society for Preventive Cardiology
ATP:	Adult Treatment Panel
AUC:	Area under the curve
CALIPER:	Canadian Laboratory Initiative on Pediatric Reference Intervals
CHMS:	Canadian Health Measures Survey
CNS:	Central nervous system
CSF:	Cerebrospinal fluid
EDTA:	Ethylenediaminetetraacetic acid
F:	Female, fluoride ion
Hb:	Hemoglobin
HbCO:	Carboxyhemoglobin
hCG:	Human chorionic gonadotropin
Hep:	Heparin
HPLC:	High-performance liquid chromatography
ICSH:	International Council for Standardization in Haematology
IVF:	In vitro fertilization
KDIGO:	Kidney Disease Improving Global Outcomes
L/S:	Lecithin-to-sphingomyelin ratio
LC-MS/MS:	Liquid chromatography with dual mass spectrometry
M:	Male
NGSP:	National Glycohemoglobin Standardization Program
NKDEP:	National Kidney Disease Educational Program
NLA:	National Lipid Association
Occup exp:	Occupational exposure
Ox:	Oxalate
P:	Plasma
PCNA:	Preventive Cardiovascular Nurses Association
PCOS:	Polycystic ovary syndrome
RBC:	Red blood cell
S:	Serum
Sal:	Saliva
SHBG:	Sex hormone–binding hormone
U:	Urine
WB:	Whole blood
WHO:	World Health Organization

Answers to Multiple Choice Questions

CHAPTER 1

1. D	6. E
2. C	7. D
3. C	8. B
4. C	9. E
5. D	10. B

CHAPTER 2

1. D	6. B
2. D	7. D
3. E	8. D
4. E	9. A
5. E	10. A

CHAPTER 3

1. D	5. A
2. B	6. C
3. E	7. D
4. E	8. B

CHAPTER 4

1. D	6. B
2. D	7. C
3. A	8. A
4. C	9. C
5. A	10. C

CHAPTER 5

1. C	6. B
2. E	7. A
3. A	8. E
4. B	9. D
5. E	10. C

CHAPTER 6

1. C	6. A
2. C	7. D
3. D	8. E
4. C	9. D
5. B	10. B

CHAPTER 7

1. A	6. E
2. C	7. D
3. A	8. B
4. D	9. B
5. A	10. C

CHAPTER 8

1. D	6. D
2. C	7. C
3. B, E	8. D
4. E	9. A
5. B	10. A, D

CHAPTER 9

1. D	6. D
2. E	7. B
3. B	8. C
4. A	9. E
5. C	10. B

CHAPTER 10

1. C	6. D
2. B	7. B
3. E	8. D
4. C	9. A
5. E	10. D

CHAPTER 11

1. E	6. A
2. A	7. B
3. B	8. A
4. D	9. C
5. E	10. B

CHAPTER 12

1. B	6. D
2. D	7. B
3. D	8. B
4. B	9. A
5. C	10. B

CHAPTER 13

1. C	6. B
2. B	7. A
3. A	8. B
4. D	9. D
5. C	10. C

CHAPTER 14

1. C	8. A
2. D	9. C
3. D	10. A
4. A	11. C
5. E	12. A
6. A	13. E
7. B	

CHAPTER 15

1. E	6. B
2. A	7. D
3. D	8. E
4. A	9. A
5. A	10. E

CHAPTER 16

1. A	6. B
2. C	7. C
3. E	8. D
4. B	9. B
5. B	10. E

CHAPTER 17

1. C	6. D
2. A	7. E
3. B	8. A
4. B	9. D
5. D	10. C

CHAPTER 18

1. C	6. E
2. A	7. A
3. E	8. C
4. C	9. C
5. D	10. B

CHAPTER 19

1. D	6. B
2. B	7. B
3. C	8. C
4. C	9. A
5. D	10. D

CHAPTER 20

1. C	6. B
2. C	7. D
3. B	8. B
4. D	9. C
5. D	10. B

CHAPTER 21

1. C	6. D
2. C	7. B
3. E	8. B
4. D	9. E
5. A	10. C

CHAPTER 22

1. D	6. C
2. C	7. A
3. D	8. A
4. D	9. C
5. B	10. A

CHAPTER 23

1. B	7. E
2. A	8. D
3. A	9. C
4. C	10. D
5. B	11. D
6. D	

CHAPTER 24

1. A	6. C
2. C	7. A
3. E	8. D
4. D	9. D
5. B	10. B

CHAPTER 25

1. E	6. C
2. E	7. D
3. C	8. E
4. D	9. A
5. A	10. B

CHAPTER 26

1. C	6. B
2. A	7. E
3. C	8. B
4. E	9. E
5. A	10. D

CHAPTER 27

1. B	6. E
2. C	7. A
3. E	8. D
4. A	9. D
5. D	10. A

CHAPTER 28

1. B	6. D
2. C	7. C
3. D	8. B
4. B	9. D
5. B	10. C

CHAPTER 29

1. D	6. E
2. C	7. A
3. C	8. A
4. D	9. B
5. B	10. D

CHAPTER 30

1. D	6. C
2. C	7. E
3. C	8. A
4. A	9. B
5. C	10. C

CHAPTER 31

1. D	6. C
2. B	7. A, D
3. B	8. C
4. C	9. E
5. D	10. A, B

CHAPTER 32

1. A	6. A
2. A	7. D
3. C	8. A
4. A	9. B
5. D	10. E

CHAPTER 33

1. C	6. E
2. E	7. B
3. A	8. D
4. B	9. C
5. D	10. D

CHAPTER 34

1. A	6. E
2. B	7. D
3. B	8. C
4. C	9. E
5. C	10. A

CHAPTER 35

1. C	6. C
2. A	7. C
3. E	8. B
4. D	9. A
5. B	10. E

CHAPTER 36

1. D	8. B
2. C	9. C
3. D	10. D
4. A	11. A
5. B	12. B
6. C	13. C
7. A	

CHAPTER 37

1. D	6. D
2. A	7. D
3. A	8. E
4. A	9. C
5. B	10. A

CHAPTER 38

1. B	6. E
2. B	7. C
3. B	8. E
4. D	9. B
5. D	10. E

CHAPTER 39

1. C	6. D
2. A	7. E
3. C	8. C
4. E	9. E
5. C	10. D

CHAPTER 40

1. C	6. D
2. E	7. A
3. A	8. B
4. B	9. C
5. D	10. E

CHAPTER 41

1. D	6. D
2. B	7. A
3. C	8. C
4. D	9. B
5. E	10. C

CHAPTER 42

1. B	6. C
2. C	7. B
3. A	8. D
4. D	9. E
5. D	10. B

CHAPTER 43

1. A	3. C
2. D	4. E

CHAPTER 44

1. D	6. C
2. C	7. A
3. B	8. D
4. A	9. A
5. B	10. C

CHAPTER 45

1. E	9. E
2. A	10. D
3. D	11. B
4. B	12. A
5. C	13. C
6. C	14. C
7. B	15. A
8. D	16. C

CHAPTER 46

1. B	6. B
2. E	7. E
3. E	8. A
4. C	9. E
5. A	10. B

CHAPTER 47

1. A	4. B
2. C	5. D
3. D	

CHAPTER 48

1. B	6. C
2. A	7. D
3. C	8. C
4. C	9. D
5. D	10. A

CHAPTER 49

1. E	6. D
2. B	7. C
3. C	8. B
4. A	9. A
5. C	10. D

CHAPTER 50

1. C	6. E
2. B	7. D
3. D	8. B
4. E	9. C
5. A	10. A

CHAPTER 51

1. C	6. A
2. E	7. D
3. B	8. C
4. C	9. E
5. C	10. D

CHAPTER 52

1. C	6. D
2. A	7. C
3. A	8. A
4. D	9. C
5. B	10. D

CHAPTER 53

1. D	6. B
2. C	7. B
3. A	8. A
4. B	9. C
5. C	10. B

CHAPTER 54

1. C	6. A
2. B	7. A
3. B	8. A
4. A	9. B
5. C	10. A

CHAPTER 55

1. D	6. C
2. D	7. C
3. E	8. A
4. A	9. C
5. D	10. D

CHAPTER 56

1. A	6. A
2. E	7. D
3. B	8. A
4. B	9. D
5. E	10. C

CHAPTER 57

1. B	6. D
2. A	7. A
3. A	8. B
4. C	9. C
5. D	10. B

CHAPTER 58

1. A	6. E
2. C	7. A
3. D	8. A
4. B	9. B
5. C	10. B

CHAPTER 59

1. D	6. D
2. B	7. C
3. A	8. C
4. B	9. A
5. C	10. B

CHAPTER 60

1. D	6. D
2. C	7. D
3. D	8. E
4. A	9. C
5. D	10. E

CHAPTER 61

1. E	6. C
2. C	7. A
3. A	8. D
4. A	9. B
5. B	10. E

CHAPTER 62

1. D	7. A
2. A	8. E
3. B	9. A
4. E	10. C
5. D	11. B
6. C	

CHAPTER 63

1. D	6. B
2. B	7. D
3. A	8. C
4. B	9. A
5. A	10. C

CHAPTER 64

1. B	9. B
2. A	10. B
3. C	11. B
4. B	12. E
5. B	13. B
6. A	14. C
7. D	15. A
8. E	

CHAPTER 65

1. E	6. E
2. A	7. A
3. E	8. E
4. B	9. C
5. C	10. C

CHAPTER 66

1. C	6. D
2. B	7. B
3. E	8. C
4. A	9. D
5. C	10. C

CHAPTER 67

1. B	6. D
2. C	7. B
3. C	8. D
4. E	9. C
5. E	10. A

CHAPTER 68

1. E	6. B
2. D	7. B
3. A	8. B
4. B	9. C
5. A	10. A

CHAPTER 69

1. A	6. C
2. C	7. E
3. B	8. A
4. D	9. D
5. B	10. C

CHAPTER 70

1. B	6. D
2. D	7. E
3. A	8. C
4. C	9. D
5. C	10. A

CHAPTER 71

1. D	7. D
2. A	8. B
3. D	9. C
4. B	10. B
5. C	11. B
6. D	12. B

CHAPTER 72

1. E	6. B
2. B	7. A
3. A	8. D
4. D	9. E
5. C	10. B

CHAPTER 73

1. E	6. A
2. D	7. C
3. D	8. D
4. A	9. E
5. C	10. C

CHAPTER 74

1. D	6. D
2. A	7. D
3. C	8. D
4. D	9. A
5. A	10. A

CHAPTER 75

1. B	6. C
2. D	7. B
3. E	8. C
4. A	9. A
5. A	10. D

CHAPTER 76

1. D	6. E
2. B	7. B
3. E	8. C
4. B	9. C
5. A	10. E

CHAPTER 77

1. B	6. B
2. C	7. E
3. A	8. A
4. D	9. B
5. B	10. C

CHAPTER 78

1. B	6. B
2. A	7. A
3. B	8. B
4. C	9. D
5. D	10. A

CHAPTER 79

1. A	11. B
2. D	12. D
3. A	13. D
4. A	14. C
5. B	15. A
6. B	16. D
7. A	17. B
8. D	18. C
9. D	19. E
10. B	20. C

CHAPTER 80

1. E	12. B
2. A	13. C
3. C	14. E
4. D	15. C
5. B	16. A
6. A	17. B
7. A	18. E
8. D	19. C
9. A	20. B
10. B	21. A
11. E	22. C

CHAPTER 81

1. A	6. B
2. B	7. E
3. D	8. A
4. B	9. B
5. B	10. E

CHAPTER 82

1. A	6. A
2. B	7. B
3. C	8. C
4. D	9. D
5. E	10. E

CHAPTER 83

1. B	6. B
2. D	7. D
3. E	8. B
4. A	9. A
5. C	10. A

CHAPTER 84

1. C	6. D
2. A	7. D
3. D	8. C
4. C	9. B
5. B	10. D

CHAPTER 85

1. B	6. A
2. C	7. C
3. A	8. D
4. D	9. C
5. C	10. B

CHAPTER 86

1. B	6. C
2. C	7. B
3. D	8. C
4. C	9. B
5. E	10. C

CHAPTER 87

1. B	6. A
2. E	7. C
3. C	8. D
4. E	9. A
5. D	10. B

CHAPTER 88

1. B	6. E
2. E	7. A
3. A	8. B
4. C	9. C
5. D	10. E

CHAPTER 89

1. A	6. C
2. C	7. E
3. B	8. A
4. D	9. D
5. B	10. C

CHAPTER 90

1. A	6. C
2. C	7. D
3. E	8. A
4. B	9. B
5. D	10. E

CHAPTER 91

1. D	6. D
2. C	7. E
3. D	8. C
4. C	9. B
5. A	10. B

CHAPTER 92

1. D	6. A
2. B	7. D
3. E	8. C
4. A	9. E
5. C	10. B

CHAPTER 93

1. D	6. C
2. A	7. C
3. A	8. C
4. B	9. B
5. A	10. C

CHAPTER 94

1. C	9. D
2. B	10. D
3. E	11. B
4. D	12. E
5. D	13. B
6. B	14. A
7. C	15. E
8. C	

CHAPTER 95

1. C	6. A
2. B	7. A
3. B	8. A
4. B	9. B
5. D	10. A

CHAPTER 96

1. D	6. A
2. B	7. A
3. D	8. C
4. D	9. D
5. D	10. D

CHAPTER 97

1. C	6. B
2. E	7. D
3. E	8. C
4. B	9. B
5. A	10. C

CHAPTER 98

1. D	6. A
2. C	7. C
3. E	8. C
4. D	9. C
5. B	10. A

CHAPTER 99

1. D
2. A
3. A
4. A
5. A
6. B
7. B
8. A
9. A
10. B
11. C

CHAPTER 100

1. C
2. D
3. C
4. C
5. B
6. D
7. A
8. C
9. B
10. E

Page numbers followed by *f* indicate figures, *t* indicate tables, and *b* indicate boxes.